W9-BCO-178

MacBryde's
SIGNS and
SYMPTOMS

Applied Pathologic Physiology
and Clinical Interpretation

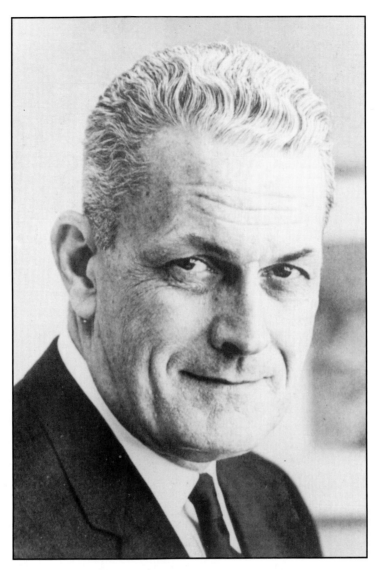

Cyril Mitchell MacBryde, M.D.
1906–1973

MacBryde's
SIGNS and
SYMPTOMS

Applied Pathologic Physiology and Clinical Interpretation

Sixth Edition
with 5 Color Plates

Robert S. Blacklow
A.B., M.D., F.A.C.P.

Professor of Medicine
Senior Associate Dean
Jefferson Medical College
    of Thomas Jefferson University
Attending Physician
Thomas Jefferson University Hospital
Philadelphia, Pennsylvania

with 50 Contributors

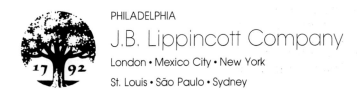

PHILADELPHIA
J.B. Lippincott Company
London • Mexico City • New York
St. Louis • São Paulo • Sydney

Acquisitions Editor: Micaela Palumbo
Sponsoring Editor: Darlene D. Pedersen
Manuscript Editor: June Eberharter
Indexer: Donald Smith
Art Director: Maria S. Karkucinski
Designer: Ron Dorfman
Production Supervisor: Tina Rebane
Production Coordinator: Charlene Catlett Squibb
Compositor: Waldman Graphics, Inc.
Printer/Binder: Halliday Lithograph

Sixth Edition

Copyright © 1983, by J. B. Lippincott Company.
Copyright © 1970, 1964, 1957, by J. B. Lippincott Company.
Copyright 1952, 1947, by J. B. Lippincott Company.
All rights reserved. No part of this book may be used or
reproduced in any manner whatsoever without written
permission except for brief quotations embodied in
critical articles and reviews. Printed in the United States
of America. For information write J. B. Lippincott
Company, East Washington Square, Philadelphia,
Pennsylvania 19105.

    5   6   4
Library of Congress Cataloging in Publication Data
Signs and Symptoms.
    MacBryde's Signs and symptoms.
    Rev. ed. of: Signs and symptoms.
    Includes bibliographies and index.
    1. Symptomatology. 2. Diagnosis. I. MacBryde,
Cyril Mitchell, DATE–   . II. Blacklow, Robert
Stanley, DATE–   . III. Title. [DNLM:
1. Diagnosis.   WB 141 M119s]
RC69.S53   1983   616.07′5   82-14843
ISBN 0-397-52094-8

The authors and publisher have exerted every effort to
ensure that drug selection and dosage set forth in this
text are in accord with current recommendations and
practice at the time of publication. However, in view of
ongoing research, changes in government regulations,
and the constant flow of information relating to drug
therapy and drug reactions, the reader is urged to
check the package insert for each drug for any change
in indications and dosage and for added warnings and
precautions. This is particularly important when the
recommended agent is a new or infrequently employed
drug.

With love
In memory of my Mother
and
To my Father,
still the compleat physician;
To my wife, Wini,
steadfast in all kinds of weather;
and
To Stephen, Kenneth, and David,
who represent our futures

Contributors

Richard D. Aach, MD

Physician-in-Chief
Department of Medicine
Sinai Hospital of Baltimore
Professor of Medicine
Johns Hopkins University School of Medicine
Baltimore, Maryland

Jack E. Ansell, MD

Associate Professor of Medicine and Pathology
University of Massachusetts Medical School
Worcester, Massachusetts

Elisha Atkins, MD

Professor of Medicine
Yale University School of Medicine
Attending Physician
Yale-New Haven Hospital
Attending Physician
West Haven V.A. Hospital
New Haven, Connecticut

Daniel B. Bauwens, MD

Instructor in Clinical Medicine
Washington University School of Medicine
Assistant Physician
Barnes Hospital
Staff Cardiologist
St. Luke's Hospital
St. Louis, Missouri

Robert S. Blacklow, AB, MD, FACP

Professor of Medicine
Senior Associate Dean
Jefferson Medical College
 of Thomas Jefferson University
Attending Physician
Thomas Jefferson University Hospital
Philadelphia, Pennsylvania

George F. Cahill, Jr., MD

Director of Research
Howard Hughes Medical Institute
Professor of Medicine
Harvard Medical School
Boston, Massachusetts

Francis I. Catlin, MD

Professor of Otorhinolaryngology
 and Communicative Sciences
Baylor College of Medicine
Houston, Texas

Sam L. Clark, Jr., MD

Departments of Anatomy and Medicine
Director, Center for Educational Resources
University of Massachusetts Medical Center
Worcester, Massachusetts

Cecil H. Coggins, MD

Associate Professor of Medicine
Harvard Medical School
Clinical Director
Renal Unit
Massachusetts General Hospital
Boston, Massachusetts

William F. Collins, MD

Harvey and Kate Cushing Professor of Surgery
Professor and Chief of Neurological Surgery
Yale University School of Medicine
Neurosurgeon-in-Chief
Yale-New Haven Hospital
Consultant
West Haven V.A. Hospital
New Haven, Connecticut

Richard A. Cooper, MD

Professor of Medicine
University of Pennsylvania School of Medicine
Chief, Hematology-Oncology Section
Hospital of the University of Pennsylvania
Philadelphia, Pennsylvania

William H. Daughaday, MD

Professor of Medicine
Director, Division of Endocrinology/Metabolism
* and Diabetes Research and Training Center*
Washington University School of Medicine
St. Louis, Missouri

Leon M. Edelstein, MD, FASCP, FACP

Clinical Associate Professor of Dermatology
Stanford Medical School
Palo Alto, California
Clinical Associate Professor of Dermatology and Pathology
University of California, Davis, Medical School
Director, California Age Research Institute
Director, American West Skin Pathology Laboratory
Yuba City, California

George L. Engel, MD

Professor of Psychiatry
Professor of Medicine
University of Rochester School of Medicine and Dentistry
Rochester, New York

Warren M. Gold, MD

Professor of Medicine
University of California, San Francisco
Senior Staff Member and Director
Adult Pulmonary Function Laboratories
Cardiovascular Research Institute
San Francisco, California

Arthur Hall, MD

Associate Clinical Professor of Medicine
Harvard Medical School
Department of Rheumatology and Immunology
Brigham and Women's Hospital
Boston, Massachusetts

Harley A. Haynes, MD

Associate Professor of Dermatology
Harvard Medical School
Chief, Dermatology Service
Department of Medicine
Brigham and Women's Hospital
Associate in Dermatology
Beth Israel Hospital
Chief, Dermatology Service, VAMC
Roxbury, Massachusetts
Consultant, Medical Oncology Division (Dermatology)
Sidney Farber Cancer Institute
Consultant in Dermatology
Massachusetts General Hospital
Boston, Massachusetts

Roger B. Hickler, MD

Lamar Soutter Distinguished University Professor
Director, Division of Geriatric Medicine
University of Massachusetts Medical School
Worcester, Massachusetts

John P. Howe, III, MD

Associate Professor of Medicine
Vice Chancellor/Academic Dean
University of Massachusetts Medical School
Worcester, Massachusetts

Harold Jeghers, MD, DSC (HON) FACP

Professor of Medical Education
The Northeastern Ohio Universities College of Medicine
Rootstown, Ohio
Consultant in Medical Education
Cleveland Health Sciences Library of Case Western Reserve
* University and The Cleveland Medical Library Association*
Cleveland, Ohio
Consultant in Medical Education
St. Elizabeth Hospital Medical Center
Youngstown, Ohio
Medical Director Emeritus and Consultant
* in Medical Education*
Saint Vincent Hospital
Worcester, Massachusetts
Professor of Medicine Emeritus
University of Medicine and Dentistry of New Jersey
New Jersey Medical School
Newark, New Jersey

Sylvia C. Johnson, MD

Group Health Medical Center
Assistant Professor of Medicine (Dermatology)
University of Washington School of Medicine
Seattle, Washington

Robert E. Kleiger, MD, FACC

Professor of Medicine
Washington University School of Medicine
Acting Chief, Cardiology Division
Jewish Hospital of St. Louis
St. Louis, Missouri

William M. Landau, MD

Andrew B. & Gretchen P. Jones Professor
* & Head of Neurology*
Washington University School of Medicine
Neurologist-in-Chief
Barnes Hospital
St. Louis, Missouri

Norman S. Lichtenstein, MD

Director of Medical Education
Waltham Hospital
Assistant Physician
Massachusetts General Hospital
Assistant Professor of Medicine
Harvard Medical School
Boston, Massachusetts

Bernard S. Lipman, MD, FACP, FACC

Clinical Professor of Medicine (Cardiology)
Emory University School of Medicine
Director Emeritus and Consultant to the Heart Station
St. Joseph's Hospital
Visiting Physician and Consultant in Cardiology
Grady Memorial Hospital
Area Consultant in Cardiology
*   to the Veterans Administration*
Consultant in Cardiology to the U.S. Department of Health
*   and Human Services*
Atlanta, Georgia

Robert J. McConnell, MD

Assistant Professor of Clinical Medicine
College of Physicians and
*   Surgeons of Columbia University*
New York, New York

James E. McGuigan, MD

Professor and Chairman
Department of Medicine
University of Florida College of Medicine
Gainesville, Florida

Edward Massie MD, FACC, FACP

Professor of Clinical Medicine
Washington University School of Medicine
Physician
Barnes Hospital and Jewish Hospital
Consultant to the Heart Station
Barnes Hospital
St. Louis, Missouri

Sarah L. Minden, MD

Clinical Fellow in Psychiatry
Harvard Medical School
Clinical Fellow in Medicine (Psychiatry)
Brigham and Women's Hospital
Boston, Massachusetts

James L. O'Leary, MD†

Professor Emeritus of Neurology
Washington University School of Medicine
St. Louis, Missouri

†Deceased

Martha Osnos, MA

Special Consultant
Memorial Sloan-Kettering Cancer Center
New York, New York

Robert Paine, MD

Professor of Clinical Medicine
Washington University School of Medicine
Assistant Physician
Barnes Hospital
Chief of Medical Service
St. Luke's Hospital
St. Louis, Missouri

Alan D. Perlmutter, MD

Professor of Urology
Wayne State University School of Medicine
Chief, Department of Pediatric Urology
Children's Hospital of Michigan
Detroit, Michigan

Malcolm L. Peterson, MD, PHD

Associate Professor of Medicine and Health Services
University of Washington School of Medicine
Seattle, Washington

John A. Pierce, MD

Professor of Medicine
Chief, Pulmonary Disease Division
Department of Internal Medicine
Washington University Medical Center
St. Louis, Missouri

Peter Reich, MD

Associate Professor of Psychiatry
Harvard Medical School
Senior Physician (Psychiatry)
Brigham and Women's Hospital
Boston, Massachusetts

Robert D. Reinecke, MD

Professor and Chairman
Department of Ophthalmology
Jefferson Medical College
Ophthalmologist-in-Chief
Wills Eye Hospital
Philadelphia, Pennsylvania

Richard S. Rivlin, MD

Chief, Nutrition Service
Memorial Sloan-Kettering Cancer Center
Professor of Medicine
Cornell University Medical College
Chief, Division of Nutrition
Department of Medicine
New York Hospital-Cornell Medical Center
New York, New York

Aldo A. Rossini, MD

Director, Division of Diabetes
Department of Internal Medicine
University of Massachusetts Medical School
Worcester, Massachusetts

Leon Schiff, MD, PHD, MACP

Emeritus Professor of Medicine
University of Cincinnati Medical School
Clinical Professor of Medicine
University of Miami Medical School
Miami, Florida

Sanford J. Shattil, MD

Associate Professor of Medicine and Pathology
University of Pennsylvania School of Medicine
Director, Coagulation and Thrombosis Laboratory
Hospital of the University of Pennsylvania
Philadelphia, Pennsylvania

John T. Stitt, PHD

Associate Professor of Epidemiology and Physiology
Associate Fellow, John B. Pierce Foundation Laboratory
Yale University School of Medicine
New Haven, Connecticut

Jay M. Sullivan, MD

Professor of Medicine
Chief, Division of Cardiovascular Diseases
University of Tennessee Center for the Health Sciences
Memphis, Tennessee

Alexander C. Templeton, MRCP, MRCPATH

Professor of Pathology
Rush Medical College
Senior Attending Physician
Rush-Presbyterian-St. Luke's Medical Center
Chicago, Illinois

Joan L. Venes, MD

Assistant Professor of Surgery
(Section of Neurosurgery)
University of Michigan School of Medicine
Ann Arbor, Michigan

N. Vijayan, MD

Sacramento Headache and Neurology Clinic
Sacramento, California
Associate Clinical Professor
Department of Neurology
University of California
Davis, California

Richard W. Vilter, MD, MACP

Gordon and Helen Hughes Taylor Professor of Medicine
  Emeritus
University of Cincinnati College of Medicine
Cincinnati, Ohio

Craig Watson, MD, PHD

Sacramento Headache and Neurology Clinic
Sacramento, California
Assistant Clinical Professor
Department of Neurology
University of California
Davis, California

Alfred D. Weiss, MD

Assistant Clinical Professor of Neurology
Harvard Medical School
Assistant Neurologist
Massachusetts General Hospital
Assistant in Otolaryngology (Otoneurology)
Massachusetts Eye and Ear Infirmary
Visiting Scientist
Man-Vehicle Laboratory
Department of Aeronautics and Astronautics
Massachusetts Institute of Technology
Boston, Massachusetts

M. Michael Wolfe, MD

Assistant Professor of Medicine
Division of Gastroenterology
Department of Medicine
University of Florida College of Medicine
Gainesville, Florida

Preface

It has been over 10 years since the last edition of *Signs and Symptoms* appeared. Preparations for a sixth edition coauthored by Blacklow and MacBryde were well under way when Cyril MacBryde died. MacBryde played a seminal role in integrating the teaching of clinical and basic science in American medical schools. A preliminary volume written by him in 1944 preceded the first (1947) edition of this book, whose purpose was, he wrote, ". . . to give the basis for analysis and interpretation of some of the commonest symptoms which bring patients to the physician, [emphasizing] the pathologic physiology of the symptom. . . ." Medical curricula and texts have adopted this approach over the last three decades. The sixth edition has been renamed *MacBryde's Signs and Symptoms* to honor his contributions.

There have been major changes in medical practice and education in the decade since the last edition. The revolutions in medical education begun in the 1960s continue into the 1980s. Although curricula have become more conservative, as resources diminish and educational costs increase, there are now available remarkable new ways for acquiring, storing, and analyzing data, which medicine is conscientiously attempting to make a part of its techniques for learning. The amount of factual detail relevant to medicine is constantly growing; medical educators must be more disciplined in identifying that which is most basic to it. The new biomedical and bioengineering technologies put continual strain on diagnosis and therapeutics; procedures learned today are often obsolete tomorrow. Novel ways of structuring choices, such as decision analysis, are now being applied to medicine at the levels of social policy and the individual patient. A more critical approach to the acquisition of the growing data base of medicine is needed and is the topic of much research.

Despite the impressive expansion of the scientific basis for clinical practice, ambiguity rather than certainty is prevalent in the clinical setting, where the crucial tasks include problem-solving, decision-making, and judgment. The development of the scientific basis for these intellectual skills has lagged far behind that of the factual underpinnings of clinical medicine. Recently, attempts have been made to fit observation of clinical practice into preexisting mathematical and psychological models of diagnostic problem-solving. Although our understanding of these strategies is, at the moment, quite fragmentary, certain fundamental principles have emerged as these models develop that elaborate on the process of eliciting the medical complaint and relating it to an abnormal or altered pathophysiologic state. Thus, the basic approach of *MacBryde's Signs and Symptoms* has been shown to be a rich and significant avenue of future knowledge.

Signs and symptoms are the basic parameters of medical diagnosis and are the final common pathways for the expression of disease. As our knowledge of the mechanism of disease processes unfolds, the significance of signs and symptoms becomes more clear. A book that approaches medicine in this fashion will need revision in order to remain up-to-date with changing interpretations of the mechanisms of disease and their relation to its clinical manifestations.

MacBryde's Signs and Symptoms is dedicated to the proposition that the physician with more insight into the processes of illness is better equipped to aid the patient. In each chapter, a major sign or symptom is analyzed, and the operations and interrelationships of the various factors in its causation are considered and wherever possible, clarified and logically related. The gap between the "preclinical" and "clinical" approaches that unfortunately exists in the

minds of many medical students, teachers, and practicing physicians is deplorable and artificial. The medical student studying human biology must be able to see the relationship between the normal and abnormal. The subject material needed for learning applied pathologic physiology and normal physiology, brought together and integrated in a fashion that recapitulates the steps in the process of thinking by which a physician reaches a diagnosis—by an analysis and an interpretation of symptoms and signs—often must be drawn from lectures, books, original articles, and other sources that often are fragmented and scattered. Since the major emphasis in the traditional introductory course, "Examination of the Patient," is, by necessity, on *techniques* of history-taking and physical examination, this course has failed to provide the needed synthesis of preclinical and clinical concepts. Likewise, the so-called integrated courses, such as "Pathophysiology" and "Mechanisms of Disease," often are a mere recitation of diseases and their protean manifestations without the necessary integration of preclinical and clinical.

This book attempts such a synthesis. It integrates available relevant information and makes it useful by explaining how and why certain signs and symptoms develop. An intelligent approach to a patient complaining of shortness of breath must involve a knowledge of the nature of dyspnea and the clinical setting in which it occurs, the workload imposed on the cardiopulmonary system needed to produce the sensation of dyspnea, the neuroanatomic pathways involved, and the pulmonary, cardiac, neurologic, and psychologic factors that might be responsible for its etiology. A discussion of pain, similarly, must integrate qualitative and quantitative descriptive aspects, such as location, intensity, and duration, with an understanding of the neural organization serving pain—receptors and afferent fibers, current ideas of neurotransmitters, a knowledge of the modulating effects of the higher centers on the perception of pain—and relate each of these to the psychological, social, and cultural background of the patient. Not only physicians, but medical students, now seeing patients at the beginning of the first year in many medical schools, should have anatomy, physiology, and biochemistry come alive! In this book the chief aim in the treatment of every subject discussed is the development of understanding and insight into disturbed mechanisms resulting in abnormal clinical findings. For these reasons, we believe that the need for *MacBryde's Signs and Symptoms* is even more pressing today than it was when the first edition appeared.

This volume has a multiple authorship, deriving breadth, depth, and vigor from the special talents and varied interests of 50 contributors who are teaching, doing research, and rendering patient care at medical centers throughout the country. Fresh insight into many fields is introduced by 29 authors who are welcome first-time contributors.

The sixth edition of *MacBryde's Signs and Symptoms* has combined dehydration and edema into one chapter for increased clarity of presentation and adds a separate chapter on acid-base regulation. Although not strictly a sign or a symptom, a thorough understanding of the principles of acid-base regulation will do much to help in the critical analysis of it.

Much effort has been devoted to interrelate the various parts of the book. The 40 chapters are parts of an interconnected whole, not an assemblage of unrelated monographs. An outline heads each chapter. Liberal use is made of illustrations, diagrams, and tables. Thorough reference lists follow each chapter. It is our hope that the newly available knowledge and concepts included in this sixth edition have been synthesized with older facts and hypotheses in a manner that will excite the interest of and be useful to medical students, graduate physicians, and other interested health professionals.

I am deeply grateful to the contributors who have patiently cooperated in revising their manuscripts, often more than once, so that this sixth edition of *MacBryde's Signs and Symptoms* could come to fruition.

Doris Bolef and the staff of the Rush University Library made the task of literature and citation search and verification easier by their willingness to provide rapid and accurate technical support even when pressed with the most unusual of requests.

To Micaela Palumbo, Darlene Pedersen, Maria Karkucinski, and June Eberharter of J. B. Lippincott Company go special thanks for guidance and constructive cooperation throughout the many phases of editing.

It is said that possession is nine points of the law. For many months, during the long process of rewriting and editing manuscripts and proofs for the sixth edition, I unilaterally took possession of as-

sorted tables, chairs, and areas in our house. My family has tolerated this state of siege and disorder goodnaturedly. I now have withdrawn my troops and return these areas, with thanks, to general family use.

Finally, on behalf of all who have contributed to this volume, I express the hope that our readers will find in this book a work that integrates the preclinical sciences with clinical medicine. We trust that this revised sixth edition will prove increasingly useful to practicing physicians, to teachers and students of medicine, and to all who labor to understand and relieve the diseases of man.

Robert S. Blacklow, M.D., F.A.C.P.

Preface to the First Edition

How convenient it would be for the physician if the new patient were able to announce: "I have a gastrointestinal disturbance," or, "My trouble is nephritis." A perusal of the usual textbooks of diagnosis or of medicine would lead one to believe this might be the case, for the chapters consider "infectious diseases," "intoxications," "deficiency diseases," "metabolic diseases," "respiratory diseases" and so on, in rigorous order, as though every sick person carried his presumptive diagnosis labeled on his chest. Where in such textbooks can the doctor seek help when the patient confronts him complaining, for example, of severe epigastric pain, or of headache, or of jaundice?

One must admit that monographic development of the complete picture of a disease is an important means of medical education, but there are serious defects in a system which encourages us to force the ailing person into a compartment, no matter how poorly it may fit him. It is widely recognized by experienced clinicians that a skillfully taken history, with a careful analysis of the chief complaints and of the course of the illness, will more frequently than not indicate the probable diagnosis, even before a physical examination is made or any laboratory tests are performed. A master diagnostician I know says: "Let me take the history and I will accept any good intern's word on the physical findings." In other words, even today the accomplished physician can learn more in the majority of cases from what his patient says, and the way he says it, than from any other avenue of inquiry. If one doubts this, let him remember that pain in one of its thousands of guises is by far the most common presenting symptom. How handicapped we would be if the patient could not tell us that he had pain, or where it was, or its nature, or duration, or radiation!

A useful aid in the interpretation of symptoms consists in grouping them together to form quickly recognizable complexes or syndromes. Every medical student learns that "dermatitis, diarrhea and dementia" means pellagra, and that "tremor, tumor and tachycardia" indicates hyperthyroidism. The veriest medical tyro knows that a chill, a pain in the chest and rusty sputum could hardly signify anything but pneumonia. Little medical rhymes, hallowed by word-of-mouth transmission to successive medical generations, honor *ileus,* "the symptom-complex known throughout the nation, characterized by pain, vomiting, tympanites and obstipation," and epilepsy, "the aura, the cry, the fall, the fits, the tonus, the clonus, the involuntary defecation." Indelibly stamped in many a physician's mind lies *"Charcot's triad"* of INSular (multiple or disseminated) sclerosis: Intention tremor, Nystagmus and Scanning speech. Frequently, however, in the commonly recognized syndromes very little is understood as to the actual origin or mechanism of production of the primary symptoms and signs. Thus these tricks, these aids to memory, lull us into a false complacency, based too often upon very little real knowledge.

The physician today has many techniques available to assist him in making accurate diagnoses. He

can peer into the recesses of the body: bronchoscopy, gastroscopy, thoracoscopy, peritoneoscopy, cystoscopy; he can study the shadows cast by the body's parts upon the x-ray film: simple x-ray, laminography, kymography, cholecystography, encephalography, gastroenterography, pyelography, bronchography; he can remove blood or lymph or abnormal fluid accumulations for physical and chemical analysis; he can remove bits of tissue from the surfaces or the cavities of the body and study them under the microscope and in the chemical and physiologic laboratory; the action potential, the very currents of life itself, he can record and analyze in the electroencephalogram and the electrocardiogram. However, without an understanding of the meaning of symptoms, how useless are these refined diagnostic techniques. They are but tools which are only as valuable as the mind which directs them. The informed mind will understand the meaning of the specific type of mucosal defect seen through the bronchoscope in relation to the patient's symptom of hemoptysis. The high icterus index observed in the laboratory study of a patient's serum has significance of one type if associated with recurrent attacks of right upper quadrant pain, but of another when found in association with a shrinking liver during pregnancy.

No mechanical measures can take the place of careful consideration of the patient's complaints. No device, be it ever so clever mechanically, electrically or chemically, can serve as a substitute in the art of medicine for the informed mind of the physician. The physician's ability as a diagnostician will determine the nature and the efficacy of the treatment he chooses to employ. His ability to diagnose will depend in only a minor degree upon his ability to use special technical measures. He must know when to use them, which tests to select, and how to interpret the physical findings, as well as the special laboratory tests. The physician's judgment in these matters will depend largely upon his ability to analyze and interpret symptoms.

This book attempts, so far as present knowledge permits, to give the basis for analysis and interpretation of some of the commonest symptoms which bring patients to the physician. Emphasis is placed upon the pathologic physiology of the symptom, while its correlation with other symptoms and with physical and laboratory evidence is considered as important, but secondary in the diagnostic method. Our knowledge concerning many of these symptoms is incomplete, but it is rapidly expanding. Although the final word often cannot be said, critical and analytical thinking in the manner followed in these chapters should prove productive for us all: patient, practitioner, professor and student.

Cyril Mitchell MacBryde, M.D., F.A.C.P.

Contents

LIST OF COLOR PLATES   xxiii

1 THE STUDY OF SYMPTOMS   1
Robert S. Blacklow

Patient and Physician—The Interview   1
Analyzing and Interpreting Symptoms   4
Environmental Hazards   10
Family History   12
Marital History   12
Social History   12
Occupational History   13
Interpreting Symptoms   13
Summary   15

2 GROWTH AND SEX DEVELOPMENT   17
William H. Daughaday

Body Size   17
Sex Development   33
Summary   40

3 PAIN   41
George L. Engel

Basic Characteristics of Pain   41
Neural Organization Serving Pain   43
Pain and Psychosocial Development   49
Clinical Interpretation of Pain   50
Summary   59

4 HEADACHE   61
N. Vijayan and Craig Watson

General Pathophysiology of
    Headaches   62
Mechanism of Pain   63
Pathophysiology of Pain   63
Classification of Headache   63
Migraine   64
Cluster Headache   69
Muscle Contraction Headache
    (MCHA)   72
Post-Traumatic Headache   74
Physical Causes of Headache   77

5 LOSS OF VISION—EYE PAIN   85
Robert D. Reinecke

Measurements of Visual Loss   85
Principal Locations of Pathologic
    Processes   86
Acute Visual Loss: Emergencies   86
Painless Loss of Vision with a Flashing
    Sensation: Retinal Detachment   88
Other Painless Acute Loss of Vision:
    Eye Hemorrhages   89
Acute Visual Loss with a Red, Painful
    Eye: Angle-Closure Glaucoma   92
Painless Chronic Visual Loss   95
Transient Visual Loss   97
Hemianopsias   97
Distorted Vision with Blurring   98
Sudden Traumatic Loss of Vision   98
Summary   100

6 PROBLEMS OF COMMUNICATION: SPEECH AND HEARING, EAR PAIN   101
Francis I. Catlin

How Human Beings Communicate   101
Normal Developmental Expectancies
    in Hearing and Speech   102
Possible Pathophysiologic
    Mechanisms   102
Hearing   102
Pain in the Ear   111
Speech   112
Summary   115

7 SORE TONGUE AND SORE MOUTH   117
Richard W. Vilter

Normal Morphology and Physiology
    of Tongue and Mouth   118
Medical History and Physical
    Examination   119

Systemic Diseases That May Cause
Sore Tongue and Sore Mouth   119
Other Systemic Diseases That May
Cause Sore Tongue and Sore Mouth   129
Local Oral Lesions   132
Summary   134

8 THORACIC PAIN   139
Daniel B. Bauwens and Robert Paine

Origin of Painful Stimuli   139
Pain Arising in the Chest Wall   141
Pain from the Trachea, Pleura, and
Diaphragm   144
Pain Arising from Mediastinal Organs 147
Cardiac Pain   151
Aortic Pain   160
Summary   161

9 ABDOMINAL PAIN   165
Richard D. Aach

History   165
Anatomy and Physiology   166
Pathways   166
Types of Deep Pain   167
Clinical Analysis   168
Etiologic Classification of Abdominal
Pain   173
Acute Abdomen   177
Summary   178

**10 URINARY TRACT PAIN,
HEMATURIA AND PYURIA   181**
Alan D. Perlmutter and Robert S. Blacklow

Urinary Tract Pain   181
Cells Normally in Urine   185
Hematuria   185
Pyuria   188
Summary   191

11 BACK PAIN   195
Arthur Hall

Anatomic and Physiologic
Considerations   195
Nerve Supply   196
Causes of Back Pain   198
Summary   207

**12 JOINT AND PERIARTICULAR
PAIN   211**
Arthur Hall

Anatomic Considerations   211
Physiologic Considerations   214
Pathogenesis of Articular Pain   215
Diagnostic Considerations   215
Monoarticular Pain   216
Single Joint Involvement   217
Polyarticular Pain   221
Nonarticular Rheumatism   224
Summary   225

13 PAIN IN THE EXTREMITIES   227
Joan L. Venes and William F. Collins

Pathophysiology   228
Regional Syndromes   240
Summary   244

**14 CLUBBED FINGERS AND
HYPERTROPHIC
OSTEOARTHROPATHY   245**
Bernard S. Lipman and Edward Massie

Relationship of Clubbing to
Hypertrophic Osteoarthropathy   245
Recognition   246
Association with Disease   252
Pathology   253
Pathogenesis   253
Summary   257

15 ARTERIAL HYPERTENSION   261
Jay M. Sullivan

The Circulatory Tree and the
Generation of Blood Pressure   261
Hemodynamics of Human
Hypertension   263
Consequences of Elevated Blood
Pressure   265
Rationale for Treatment   267
Labile or Borderline Versus Fixed
Hypertension   270
Systolic Versus Diastolic Hypertension 270
Therapeutic Goal   271
Evaluation of the Patient With
Hypertension   271
Essential Versus Secondary
Hypertension   277
Treatment of Hypertension   284
Therapeutic Implications of the
Renin–Angiotensin System   286
Hypertensive Emergencies   288

16 PALPITATION AND TACHYCARDIA   295
Edward Massie and Robert E. Kleiger

Palpitation   295
Tachycardia   299
Summary   314

17 COUGH   317
John A. Pierce

Mechanism of Cough   318
Stimuli That Produce Cough   320
Characteristic Types of Cough   321
Conditions in Which Cough Occurs   321
Complications of Cough   327
Sputum   328
Treatment of Cough   328
Summary   329

18 HEMOPTYSIS   331
John A. Pierce

Basic Pathophysiology   331
Localization of Bleeding Site   331
Study of Sputum   332
Causes of Hemoptysis   332
Summary   334

19 DYSPNEA   335
Warren M. Gold

Nature of Dyspnea   335
Setting in Which Dyspnea Occurs   336
Physical Tolerance in Occupational Activity   337
Physical Tolerance in Recreational Activity   338
Factors Determining the Load Imposed on the Cardiopulmonary System   338
Neuroanatomic Pathways   339
Theories of Dyspnea   340
Dyspnea in Chronic Pulmonary Disease   341
Psychogenic Dyspnea   342
Dyspnea in Cardiac Disease   342
Dyspnea in Anemia   344
Dyspnea in Neurologic Disease   344
Summary   346

20 CYANOSIS   349
Warren M. Gold

Definition   349
Oxygen Transport   349
Relationship of Cyanosis to CO_2 Exchange   357
Effects of Oxygen on Cyanosis   358

21 ANOREXIA, NAUSEA, AND VOMITING   361
James E. McGuigan and M. Michael Wolfe

Innervation of the Gastrointestinal Tract   361
Anorexia   363
Hunger   363
Nausea   365
Vomiting   365
Disturbances Associated with Anorexia, Nausea, and Vomiting   366
Summary   371

22 CONSTIPATION AND DIARRHEA   375
Malcolm L. Peterson

Normal Physiology of Propulsion of Intestinal Contents   376
Definitions   376
Causes of Constipation   378
Causes of Diarrhea   380
Diagnostic Assessment of Diarrhea   389
Summary   392

23 HEMATEMESIS AND MELENA   393
Leon Schiff

General Considerations   393
Etiology   397
History and Physical Examination   399
Radiographic Examination   400
Endoscopy and Selective Angiography   402
Bleeding Peptic Ulcer   405
Carcinoma of the Stomach   407
Bleeding Esophageal Varices   407
Gastritis and Esophagitis   409
Hiatal Hernia   410
Hematemesis and Melena From Miscellaneous Causes   410
Summary   417

24 JAUNDICE   423
Leon Schiff

Definitions and Classification   423
Clinical Approach   424
Radiologic Procedures   430
Needle Biopsy of the Liver   433
Conclusion   433

25 FEVER   441
Elisha Atkins and John T. Stitt

Definition   442
Regulation of Body Temperature   442
Body Temperature in Health   444
Limits of Body Temperature
  Compatible with Life   446
Fever   447
Summary   460

26 LYMPHADENOPATHY AND DISORDERS OF THE LYMPHATICS   467
Harold Jeghers, Sam L. Clark, Jr., and Alexander C. Templeton

Introduction   468
Functions of Lymphatics and Lymph
  Nodes   468
Lymph   469
Lymphatic Vessels   470
Lymphangitis   472
Dilatation of Lymphatic Capillaries
  and Vessels   473
Obstruction of Lymphatic Vessels   473
The Main Lymphatic Vessels   474
Lymph Nodes   476
Lymphoid Cells   478
Age Changes in Lymphoid Tissue   480
Modes of Lymph Node Involvement
  and Pathologic Changes   481
Diagnostic Methods   488
Regional Lymphadenopathy   493
Lymph Node Syndromes   517
Summary   522

27 PATHOLOGIC BLEEDING   535
Jack E. Ansell

Normal Hemostasis   535
Laboratory Approach to Hemostasis
  Evaluations   542
Approach to the Patient with
  Suspected Hemostatic Failure   543
Pathologic Bleeding Caused by
  Vascular Disorders   545
Pathologic Bleeding Caused by
  Platelet Disorders   547
Coagulation Disorders   551
Summary   558

28 ANEMIA, WEAKNESS, AND PALLOR   563
Sanford J. Shattil and Richard A. Cooper

Structure, Function, and Lifespan of
  Normal Human Red Blood Cells   564
The Signs and Symptoms of Anemia   566
Pathophysiology of the Anemias   571
Anemia Resulting from Decreased
  Red Cell Production   573
Hemolytic Anemias   578
Summary   585

29 NERVOUSNESS AND FATIGUE   591
Sarah L. Minden and Peter Reich

Introduction   591
Clinical Approach to Assessment of
  Nervousness and Fatigue   592
Theoretical Explanations of
  Nervousness and Fatigue   594
Differential Diagnosis   603
Summary   618

30 CONVERSION SYMPTOMS   623
George L. Engel

Definitions   624
Incidence, Prevalence, and Variety   625
Mechanisms of Conversion Symptoms
  and Conversion Complications   626
Clinical Diagnosis   630
Common Conversion Symptoms   635
Differentiation from Other
  Psychosomatic Symptoms   643

31 COMA AND CONVULSION   647
James L. O'Leary and William M. Landau

Historical Résumé   648
Neural Basis of Consciousness   649
Abnormal States of Consciousness
  and Their Etiologies   652
Convulsive Disorder   660
Narcolepsy   664
Summary   665

32 DISTURBANCES OF MOVEMENT   669
William M. Landau and James L. O'Leary

Impaired Movement   670
Distortions of Movement and Posture   678
Spontaneous Movement   681
Summary   686

33 FAINTING (SYNCOPE)   689
Roger B. Hickler and John P. Howe, III

Definition   689
Etiological Classification   689
Pathogenesis   690
Acute Reduction in Cerebral Blood
    Flow   691
Disturbance in Composition of Blood
    Flowing to the Brain   702
Neurophysiologic Factors   703
Summary   703

**34 VERTIGO AND DIZZINESS—
     DISORDERS OF STATIC AND
     DYNAMIC EQUILIBRIUM   707**
Alfred D. Weiss

Introduction   707
Functional Organization of the
    Systems   708
Principles of Neurologic Lesion
    Localization   713
Clinical Significance of Vertigo and
    Dizziness   715
Summary   723

35 DEHYDRATION AND EDEMA   725
Cecil H. Coggins

Anatomy and Definitions   726
Water Balance   726
Dehydration—Simple Water Loss   731
Water Excess   736
Salt Balance—The Regulation of
    Volume   737
Salt Lack—Extracellular Volume
    Depletion   740
Salt Excess—Edema   741
Summary   744

36 ACID BASE REGULATION   747
Norman S. Lichtenstein

Terminology   748
Acid Production   748
Body Buffers   749
Respiratory Regulation   750
Renal Regulation   751
Metabolic Acidosis   755
Metabolic Alkalosis   760
Respiratory Acidosis   762
Respiratory Alkalosis   763
Mixed Disorders   764
Summary   765

37 OBESITY   769
Aldo A. Rossini and George F. Cahill, Jr.

Definition   769
Methods for Estimating Obesity   770
Importance of Obesity   770
Differential Diagnosis   771
Physiology of Obesity   772
Multifactorial Etiologies and
    Complications of Obesity   773
Current Treatments of Obesity   778
Reasonable Approach to the Patient
    with Obesity   781

38 UNDERNUTRITION   787
Richard S. Rivlin, Robert J. McConnell,
and Martha Osnos

Introduction   787
Perspective of Nutrition Problems   788
Weight Loss or Subnormal Body
    Weight As Symptoms   788
Maternal Undernutrition and Child
    Development   788
Undernutrition Resulting from Drug
    Administration   792
Undernutrition in Cancer   795
Undernutrition and Aging   798
Undernutrition and Hormones   801
Summary   803

**39 SKIN COLOR IN HEALTH AND
     DISEASE   811**
Harold Jeghers and Leon M. Edelstein

Factors Involved in Normal Skin
    Pigmentation   811
Patterns of Normal Skin Color   818
Increased Pigmentation of the Skin   823
Decreased Skin Pigmentation   849
Value of Colored Illustrations in
    Medical Education   854
Summary   854

40 ITCHING (PRURITUS)   865
Harley A. Haynes and Sylvia Christine Johnson

Mechanisms of Itch   865
Pruritus Resulting from Systemic
    Disease   868
Pruritus Not Resulting from Systemic
    Disease   873
Pruritus Ani and Pruritus Vulvae   874
Approach to the Patient with Pruritus   875
Summary   876

INDEX   879

Color Plates

Plate 1. *(follows page 134)*
Sore tongue and sore mouth as manifestations of
systemic disorders: acute pellagrous glossitis,
magenta tongue of riboflavin deficiency, and
cheilosis of riboflavin deficiency.

Plate 2. *(follows page 134)*
Sore tongue and sore mouth as manifestations of
systemic disorders: geographiclike tongue of
diabetes mellitus, atrophic glossitis, and acute
scorbutic gingivitis.

Plates 3 and 4. *(follow page 406)*
Transilluminated ectasia.

Hemangioma of the cecum.

Plate 5. *(follows page 838)*
The mechanism of absorption, transmission, and
reflectance of incident white light by the skin.

MacBryde's
SIGNS and
SYMPTOMS

Applied Pathologic Physiology and Clinical Interpretation

The Study of Symptoms Robert S. Blacklow

Patient and Physician—The Interview
Analyzing and Interpreting Symptoms
  Importance of the History
  Patient Questionnaire
  Time with the Patient
  Technical Versus Clinical Methods
  Conduct of the Interview
  Considerations of Study
  Psyche and Soma
  Chief Complaints and Present Illness
  Association of Symptoms—Syndromes
  Patient's Attitude Toward His Symptoms
  Evolution of Symptoms
  Elaboration of the History
  Past History

Environmental Hazards
  Voluntary Use of Drugs and Chemicals
  Involuntary Exposure to Drugs and Chemicals
  Prescription Drugs
Family History
Marital History
Social History
  Sex Problems
  Drug Addiction
Occupational History
Interpreting Symptoms
  Guided Studies
  Basic Pathophysiology
Summary

Definitions. As broadly and generally employed, the word *symptom* is used to name any manifestation of disease. Strictly speaking, *symptoms* are subjective, apparent only to the affected person. *Signs* are detectable by another person and sometimes by the patient himself. Pain and itching are symptoms; jaundice, swollen joints, cardiac murmurs, and so forth are physical signs. Some phenomena, like fever, are both signs and symptoms. In this chapter the word symptom is often used to denote any evidence of disturbed physiology perceived by the patient or the physician.

PATIENT AND PHYSICIAN—THE INTERVIEW

The patient comes to the physician because he has a problem and wants help. The problem may be a simple one requiring only a health survey for school, employ-ment, insurance, or for personal information, and the patient may have no complaints. Nevertheless, the physician may discover in the course of such an examination one or more signs or symptoms of significance. The physician must respond to and alleviate these signs of ill health not yet apparent to the patient and maintain the patient in a state of well-being. Achieving these goals requires a broad orientation. Illness is rarely limited to one symptom, nor is it necessarily limited to a single disease, and whether the physician is a family practitioner, an internist who provides "primary care," a surgeon, or a subspecialist, the patient must be viewed not as an organ system but as a person. In this book we are concerned primarily with the study of the patient who presents himself with a disturbing sign or symptom. The aim of studying the patient's signs and symptoms must be kept in mind constantly: The purpose of analyzing the history care-

fully and of evaluating the physical findings thoughtfully is to determine the pathophysiologic processes involved. When these processes are understood, clinical interpretation may be attempted, and diagnosis may be possible. A sign or a symptom occurring in any person is not an isolated phenomenon; it may have multiple interrelationships including causes, associated phenomena, and effects. There may be interrelationships evidencing various types of disturbed physiology, and there is always a subjective, psychological component, sometimes of minor but often of major importance. The responses of the patient to his disorder, his reactions to it and understanding of it, are essential and often deeply revealing parts of the history.

Each illness has an emotional component, sometimes slight, sometimes amounting to an emotional crisis. The eventual health and well-being of the patient depend not only on his physical but also on his emotional recovery. From the very outset of the patient–physician relationship, at the beginning of the first interview, it is important to recognize that, no matter what the problem may be, every person has particular needs according to his individual personality. The patient should, by the physician's approach, be given reason to know at once that the doctor is interested in him as a person as well as in his disease. The patient has the right to expect kindness and humane consideration as well as professional competence.

The physician, as he starts to converse with his patient and to elicit the story of the illness, becomes engaged in the most intensely personal experience in medicine. With the account of complaints and medical problems may be yielded up embarrassing confidences and more or less pertinent information about past frustrations, present anxieties, and hopes for the future.

The young and inexperienced physician is often apt to neglect or to feel scorn for emotional and psychological manifestations unless they constitute well-defined and therefore "interesting" neuroses and psychoses. The physician who fails to use opportunities to consider and evaluate subjective aspects of the illness and confines his efforts unduly to objective data is not studying the patient as a whole and may be misled into inaccurate or incomplete conclusions and solutions.

To derive the fullest possible potential from the history, the physician must become skilled in eliciting the patient's story. Securing a meaningful history requires an interpersonal relationship involving cooperation between two strangers about one's intimate problems. This knowledge is gained by the physician listening to the patient and examining him. The relationship between physician and patient influences communications between them and the examinations conducted. It is the milieu in which interviews and examinations occur. A constructive physician–patient relationship cannot substitute for technical skill in history-taking and interviewing or medical knowledge. It is, however, a requirement of the best interviews and examinations.[1,2,3] With the patient distressed and distracted, the physician sometimes inexpert or inexperienced, and time pressing, it is small wonder that many histories are inadequate. Technical approaches are often overemphasized in the diagnostic work-up, since amassing laboratory data requires much less skill and experience than the ability to evaluate signs and symptoms.

The technical and the scientific aspects of medicine can be learned largely through reading and study; the arts and the skills required in the interpersonal parts of the patient–physician relationship cannot. The clinical ability to secure a good history is an art and a skill developed by imitation of accomplished preceptors and by practice and experience.

The accumulation, classification, and mathematical manipulation of great masses of technical data, with mechanical analysis of itemized information, can yield quickly, with the aid of computers, answers formerly obscure or requiring much time. Some have written that the computer will largely replace the mental processes heretofore required in diagnosis.[4] However, the role of the computer in clinical medicine is still in an evolutionary stage. Several medical centers have successfully developed computerized medical records for hospital and outpatient use.[5] The role of the computer in medical decision-making remains elusive but challenging. Considerable progress has been made in using the computer to facilitate differential diagnosis and to evaluate clinical decision-making.[6] Yet the nirvana of diagnosis and treatment by way of artificial intelligence remains illusory because of the misunderstanding of the meaning of diagnosis. True diagnosis means understanding thoroughly, and it necessarily involves human relationships: those of the person with his disease, with other persons, and so forth. These subtle and complex aspects of human problems cannot be programmed for computer analysis.[7] Machines can yield highly useful data based upon masses of other data fed into them.[8] Human understanding of human problems is possible only through human thought.

One must not confuse the accumulation and the interpretation of technical data (no matter how clever and helpful or even decisive) with the development of true insight into human problems.

Patient–physician relationships are changing. The

one-to-one relationship, which traditionally has been the goal of all physicians, is changing primarily because of the changing milieu in which medicine is being practiced. Individual patient management often requires the active participation of a variety of trained professionals—not only physicians but also nurses, physicians' assistants, social workers, dietitians, psychologists, and other health-care personnel. The patient can benefit greatly from this collaboration, but it is the responsibility of the physician to guide the patient through an illness. In order to carry out this task, the physician must have some familiarity with the techniques and skills of his colleagues in these fields allied to medicine. Their findings must not be interpreted as isolated phenomena but in terms of the whole clinical picture, and the physician must retain responsibility for the crucial decisions about diagnosis and treatment.

The patient's attitude toward the physician should be analyzed as the history is being obtained. It will depend on his background and on elements in the present situation, including responses to the appearance, the attitude, the actions, and the words of the physician. Excessive hopes or dependence must be forestalled. Insufficient trust in the doctor or anger or secretiveness may defeat the patient's objective in seeking medical help. The skillful physician guides the patient's attitude into desirable channels.

The physician's attitude toward the patient requires self-study. The examining physician is himself a human instrument, subject to reactions arising from his or her own background. This background will strongly influence the physician's responses to and understanding of the patient. His thought processes will be also influenced by those of the patient. His emotions will respond to those of the patient, and he must be aware of and evaluate his own emotional resonances. The physician must direct his own attitudes, words, and actions into a pattern most apt to promote the patient's welfare. Certain ingredients are taken for granted in a good physician: medical knowledge, self-confidence based upon competence, emotional self-control in the face of stress, dignity, kindness, graciousness, and good manners. The patient usually becomes aware of these quickly, even during a first interview.

In addition to these characteristics, other important qualities needed by the physician to be skillful in interviewing are interest, acceptance, warmth, and flexibility.

The physician's concern for his patient is conveyed by his actions, rather than by a statement. The confidence and cooperation of the patient are not secured by saying, "Trust me. I am trying to help you." It is best not to handicap oneself with such a bald, obvious, and superfluous remark, which may give the patient pause and make him distrustful. Proceed with the job at hand; the patient by his own observations will soon know whether the physician cares about him and his problem.

In the art of interviewing there is no substitute for genuine interest not only in the patient's problems but in the patient as a person. In trying to obtain a truly valuable history the physician will do well to keep these points in mind:

1. *Interest* springing from the desire to understand and to help is evident to the patient and encourages him to talk. It tells him he is talking to someone who wants to help. As a rule, the patient responds by answering questions and telling his story so as to assist the doctor as much as possible. Frequently, realization that the doctor really cares about him as a person, not just as "a case" of illness, will remind the patient of aspects of his problem and lead to illumination of facets of the situation of great diagnostic importance.

2. *Acceptance* of the patient is essential. The patient will reveal his inner feelings only to someone who, he feels, accepts him unconditionally. The physician must not reveal moral judgments he may have or his own emotional responses in regard to attitudes or behavior or statements of his patient. This does not necessarily imply approval, but the physician must be tolerant and understanding. The physician must be objective in evaluating the patient's story. In addition, he should convey to the patient his belief that the patient also is trying his best to be objective.

3. *Warmth and empathy.* No one can ever actually share the experiences of another person, but the effort to do so always brings one person closer to another. The physician who can combine sensitive insight and understanding (without oversympathizing or sentimentalizing) with a sensible, objective approach to the patient's problem usually will win the patient's friendship and confidence quickly.

4. *Flexibility.* The topics selected and the direction of the inquiry stem naturally (at least in the beginning) from the patient's presenting complaints. As the story is developed, the picture of the present illness will emerge. Then past history, family history, and other related subjects will be explored. This is the usual course along which the interviewer gently guides his patient in order to secure a coherent history, which may be recorded in some logical order. How-

ever, the physician often will find that adherence to a rigid pattern is a handicap and that the apparent wanderings of the patient's talk may be highly revealing. Frequently, what at first seems to be only a bypath will be found to be the main highway.

Sometimes the topics that the patient avoids are the most significant ones. If he shies away, changes the subject, becomes irritated, anxious, or confused, the interviewer may explore a more neutral area for a while, returning to the sensitive topic more productively later.

The expert interviewer must be flexible and prepared to allow the patient to vary the order in which topics are discussed. The interviewer may learn much by allowing the subject to run on freely with his story: He will observe what the patient wants to emphasize and thus may learn what seems to be important to the patient or what his motives are.

The responses of the physician must be flexible, natural, and appropriate. As a rule, the medical interview is serious business, but the physician tries to keep it on a constructive, optimistic level. He should respond with hopeful reassurance to the depressed patient, but not with excessive cheerfulness. To the patient who is anxious or fearful he should offer firm reassurance. If the patient is ill at ease, angry, or suspicious, the physician may establish more relaxed and friendly cooperative relations by discussing briefly a mutual interest or by inquiring into the possible causes for the patient's disquieting attitude before continuing the study of his medical problems.

The accomplished physician develops a technique in securing the history, and his technique must vary from patient to patient and according to circumstances. Knowledge of medicine and an understanding of human beings are limitless fields of endeavor; the physician's skill in obtaining the patient's story and interpreting it will grow in proportion to his progress in these very complex fields. Many believe that obtaining a good history requires practice of the greatest art in medicine.[17]

ANALYZING AND INTERPRETING SYMPTOMS

IMPORTANCE OF THE HISTORY

Symptoms are apt to appear some time before striking physical signs of disease are evident and before laboratory tests are useful in detecting disordered physiology. For this reason, and because a careful, detailed, properly analyzed, and properly interpreted history usually leads the physician more directly toward the correct conclusion than any other diagnostic method,

one should never neglect to elicit an accurate and sufficiently detailed history.

Persons vary greatly in their abilities to observe and describe their symptoms; intelligence, education, and verbal proficiency differ so much that eliciting a lucid and coherent account demands flexibility and adaptability. Routine or mechanical recording of data does not constitute a medical history. The emotional status of the patient colors his story; his background and environment always will condition his responses to stimuli as well as his efforts to describe such responses. Evaluation and perception of the patient as a person proceed simultaneously with the process of learning about his immediate symptoms.

Productive of insight, apparently simple yet truly complex, "taking the history" involves analysis and interpretation and requires the highest order of medical skill.

"Of all the technical aids which increase the doctor's power of observation, none comes even close in value to the skillful use of spoken words—the words of the doctor and the words of the patient. Throughout all of medicine, use of words is still the main diagnostic technique."[9]

PATIENT QUESTIONNAIRE

There is no doubt that a detailed printed history form or a computer-based questionnaire to be completed by the patient can be of great assistance under certain circumstances. When time permits and the patient is not acutely ill, and for use in screening for disease, in health surveys, and so forth, such a record of medical history may help to prevent omission of significant data and may save the physician much time.[8,10]

It might be suggested that such a multipaged questionnaire be presented to the patient after the initial history is obtained by the physician, if and when the intellectual, physical, and emotional status of the subject encourages such a method of assembling information. Such a detailed health record would then be very useful for later, more incisive, or pertinent inquiry by the physician.

However, when the patient's complaint is urgent or he is emotionally disturbed, as is usually the case in illness, he must not of course be confronted with a routine printed form or by a clerk or physician following any routine method of approach to his problem. The approach must vary appropriately with the problem and with the person affected.

No impersonal inquiry into the patient's complaints, no mechanical system, no tabular compilation with check marks or crosses or pressed buttons or electronic computer can substitute in diagnosis or care of the pa-

furnish important clues. "My headaches began about two years ago, a few weeks after my mother died." Follow the clue. Note that the patient is linking the symptom to psychic trauma. "My asthma came on in the summer, went away while we were in the mountains, but came back when we were on the desert ranch." An allergy to ragweed or to horse dander? "The dermatitis started on a Sunday; it gets better during the week but usually flares up on Sundays." An allergy to dyes in the ink of Sunday rotogravure or color sections?

"I've had this heart murmur since childhood. My heart never bothered me. My fever came on a few days after I had that tooth pulled three weeks ago." Look for petechiae. Get a blood culture. The diagnosis is very likely subacute bacterial endocarditis.

Take up each symptom or sign or complaint in order, following its course throughout the present illness. Even when the physician is unable to get the patient to give an orderly account, the written record should be ordered, consecutive, compact, and complete, but not verbose.

The evolution of one or several signs and symptoms constitutes the *clinical course* of the illness. Characteristics of the clinical course are apt to be highly significant in diagnosis.

ASSOCIATION OF SYMPTOMS—SYNDROMES

Certain disorders in physiology are characterized by the association of two or more related symptoms or signs. Investigation of either symptom will then lead to a further understanding of the related complaints and of the basic disease. For example, it is useful to know that a convulsion was preceded by carpopedal spasm, for that suggests hypocalcemia, whereas a convulsion preceded by hunger and perspiration suggests hypoglycemia. Likewise, vomiting accompanied by right lower abdominal pain and muscle spasm may indicate appendicitis, whereas vomiting with headache and failing vision leads one to suspect increased intracranial pressure.

Be alert to recognize characteristic groupings of certain signs and symptoms (syndromes). Often the anatomic location of the cause may be suggested (scalenus anticus syndrome, Horner's syndrome, Meniere's syndrome) or the organ or tissue or system involved (Banti's syndrome, Cushing's syndrome) or the etiology (Korsakoff's syndrome, Plummer–Vinson syndrome).

It is important, however, not merely to learn by rote, for instance, that sore tongue, pallor, digestive disorders, and numbness in the extremities suggest pernicious anemia but to try to understand as thoroughly as possible how these symptoms happen to be related and why the disease process results in these particular manifestations.

PATIENT'S ATTITUDE TOWARD HIS SYMPTOMS

An informative history is more than an orderly and complete listing of symptoms. Much can be learned from the manner and the method used by the patient in telling his story. In listening to the history, the physician discovers not only something about the disease but also something about the patient. If the patient is obviously oversensitive and apprehensive, the interpretation of his complaints usually differs from that of similar complaints of a calm and unemotional person. If he is exaggerating or minimizing his symptoms, evaluation must be correspondingly adjusted and motives must be sought. While the physician is taking the history he has an excellent chance to form preliminary impressions of the patient's personality.

Only rarely can a sick person present a relatively objective account of the illness. More often than not, the patient's presentation of his story to the physician is colored by emotional reaction or motivation. Among frequently encountered emotional states are fear, which sometimes leads to excessive emphasis and elaboration; embarrassment, usually leading to fragmentary or misleading statements; anger, resentment, or rebellion at being ill, which often causes the afflicted person to blame others in his family, his employer, his physician, or some element in his environment. Anger is often the expression of guilt feelings; sometimes anger is used as a cover for or defense reaction against anxiety or fear.

Among motives, one must consider first the usual one—the patient trying in his own way (which may be misguided) to assist the physician because he wants relief. One must consider the patient's self-diagnosis but beware of accepting it uncritically. For example, beware of the patient who has "just a little cough"; it may be tuberculosis. The patient who has "just a little constipation" may have rectal carcinoma. Second, consider motives that might lead to overemphasis or malingering, such as compensation neuroses. Third, remember motives leading to discounting of the importance of symptoms: ambition, religious faith wrongly employed, and so forth. A Christian Scientist, a man of 50, collapsed and died after having repeated tarry stools. Autopsy revealed a deep chronic duodenal ulcer. His sister said he had had epigastric pain relieved by food for years, but he would never admit it. We should teach everyone that it is admirable not to exaggerate symptoms, but it is foolish to be reticent or

to conceal clues. A symptom that may seem minor to the patient could prove important in the development of the diagnostic picture.

Symptoms as Buffers. Usually, diagnosis of an illness and removal of its cause is a welcome contribution to the patient's general health. One must realize, however, that in many chronic illnesses the handicap comes to play an essential part in the patient's life, so important a part sometimes that he may not gracefully part with it. For example, a man who for years had suffered with peptic ulcer was dramatically cured by gastrectomy and for the first time in years was free of pain. Surprisingly, instead of being happy he became depressed and attempted suicide. It became evident that his stomach symptoms had served as a crutch, buffer, or excuse to spare him from stress or unpleasant situations. His symptoms were gone and so was his protection.[9] Therefore, we must consider, What does this symptom mean to this patient?

EVOLUTION OF SYMPTOMS

Not only must the presenting symptom or symptoms be clearly understood, but they must be followed in their development from the onset to the date the history is obtained. Data should be sought indicating any alteration or change in the symptom. Has the pain changed its location? Has it changed in severity or nature? Is it now accompanied by any new phenomena? Was it first in the epigastrium and relieved by food or alkali but now not so relieved? Did the ankle edema at first disappear upon recumbency, but does it now persist all night?

The course or evolution of each sign or symptom forming the clinical picture of the present illness should be traced so that the significance of alterations may be considered in regard to possible changes in the pathologic physiology.

ELABORATION OF THE HISTORY

Every effort should be made to get a good history at the first interview. Later, further study of the patient's story may prove to be important. Often a useful procedure is repetition or elaboration or further cross-questioning concerning certain points in the history after some information is obtained from the physical examination or the laboratory tests. For example, a patient who has very dry or thickened skin will be questioned further about loss of energy, sensitivity to cold, drowsiness, and other symptoms that may be caused by hypothyroidism. If leukocytosis is revealed, further evidence of possible infection may be sought, or, if a cardiac murmur is discovered, inquiry should be made concerning previous episodes of joint soreness or febrile illness.

PAST HISTORY

The history of previous illnesses and health problems should be reviewed, and in some instances fully explored, particularly when information of help in understanding the present complaint is elicited. No listing of "measles, mumps, whooping cough, and chickenpox in childhood" is sufficient if, in the history of a man with edema, the information is omitted that he had scarlet fever and albuminuria as a child. Inquiry concerning trauma may be pursued, particularly if joint pain or back pain is the chief symptom. A careful analysis of the diet and inquiry concerning appetite, diarrhea, vomiting, or digestive disorders are indicated when weight loss is prominent.

ENVIRONMENTAL HAZARDS

Adverse reactions to natural elements in the environment formerly constituted a large part of medical histories: heat, cold, micro-organisms, and so forth. Today in our urban, industrialized society many illnesses are man-made, caused by machines, pollutants, chemicals, and drugs.

VOLUNTARY USE OF DRUGS AND CHEMICALS

Persons in the United States consume vast quantities of drugs, only a small fraction of which are prescribed by physicians. Among the substances most commonly used that cause druglike reactions but are not usually thought of as drugs are alcohol, tobacco, coffee, tea, and cola drinks. Alcohol and tobacco, both used chronically by a large percentage of our population, cause many disturbing symptoms and sometimes serious disease.

Aspirin is the drug most widely employed, and although generally considered safe, not infrequently has unpleasant or dangerous effects. Self-medication with easily-purchased over-the-counter pharmaceuticals is nearly universal, involving practically every man, woman, and child. Types of medications commonly ingested include preparations containing vitamins, iron, various "health foods," analgesics, soporifics, stimulants, and laxatives. In addition to those ingested are those applied externally, such as ointments, lotions, and douches, for eye irritation, dandruff, dermatitis, feminine hygiene and so forth.

A large proportion of our population is exposed to

chemicals contained in cosmetics: perfumes, powders, hair dyes, and bleaches, creams and lotions, rouges, nail applications, antiperspirants, deodorants, and so forth. The incidence of adverse reactions to these is high. Another class of chemicals to which everyone is exposed includes soaps, detergents, and other household cleaning agents.

INVOLUNTARY EXPOSURE TO CHEMICALS

We have discussed drugs and chemicals voluntarily employed that may or may not be beneficial and are often harmful. Practically everyone today is exposed to many chemicals involuntarily and usually without his knowledge. Even the experts are just beginning to realize the ubiquity of the contaminants of the environment, the high degrees of pollution often present, and the severity of the health hazards.

In many industries the worker is subjected to psychological, physical, or chemical hazards. The physician should be educated about these so that he can evaluate the part they play in many medical histories.

Man is also unwittingly and involuntarily "medicating" himself in many ways. We cannot discuss here in detail the various kinds of chemical threats to which human beings are increasingly subjecting themselves. However, we are concerned with the medical history, and it is highly important to emphasize that many signs and symptoms may be due to man-created environmental constituents of perilous significance.

In the health history of every person, in present illness or past, there may be pertinent data. Did the conjunctivitis occur after swimming in contaminated water? Did the bronchitis, asthma, or pneumonia begin during exposure to "smog"?

We are brought in contact with or ingest chemicals sprayed upon plants or put into soil. Exposure to organic phosphates constitutes a real danger. Fertilizers may be hazardous.

In the commercial processing of foods various chemical are often added as preservatives, or to affect taste, color, texture, and so forth. More studies are needed to determine which may be harmless and which are hazardous.

A widespread threat of which the public is becoming increasingly aware is the danger of exposure to radioactive material, not only from nuclear explosions and nuclear power plants but also from careless storage of dangerous radioactive waste products. Not only in Nagasaki or Hiroshima have human beings and animals absorbed appreciable quantities of such materials. Many of us now have radioactive iodine in our thyroid glands and radioactive strontium and phosphates in our bones and teeth.

Chemical pollutants of air and water and soil have already greatly damaged and increasingly threatened human and animal life. Sources of deleterious material include industrial wastes, human sewage, automobile exhausts, and so forth.

Man's technological skills have exceeded his judgment and wisdom. Man and his world are being despoiled by his own products. In a society largely controlled by technologists, the ability to accomplish a material, physical, mechanical, or chemical feat is considered a mandate: "We can do it; therefore we *must* do it." It should be obvious that such a philosophy is wrong. Knowledge and technologic skills should not alone control actions. Desirability or undesirability of consequences should be the paramount consideration. Judgment and wisdom should control and direct technology.

Our technologists today are usually mistakenly called "scientists." They are not, because science is a branch of knowledge and does not consist of materal manipulation and manufacture. Science does not consist of technology; it utilizes technology. Now, let us relate these considerations to the field of medicine.

Medical "scientists" (mostly technologists) have created a vast variety of drugs, too many drugs. Many have become highly useful; a few are truly essential. The great majority could be dispensed with without serious handicap to the physician or detriment to the health of our people. Reduction in the tremendous number of drugs would improve the practice of medicine, avoid the exposure of patients to many hazards, and save vast amounts of money and wasted effort. Physicians would not be compelled to learn the comparative merits and dangers of perhaps some 40 different antibiotics (or analgesics, or diuretics, and so forth), nor would pharmacies have to stock them. All drugs would be much less expensive if pharmaceutical companies were spared the astronomical expense involved in their promotion.

PRESCRIPTION DRUGS

Prescription drugs constitute only a small part of all the medications people are exposed to (and a tiny fraction of the combined exposure to all sorts of chemicals), but here physicians do exert limited control. Physicians write prescriptions, but there are many slips between lips and pen. Physicians can make mistakes unwittingly and innocently; it is inevitable also that every physician will sometimes advise medications to which certain persons will have unpredictable adverse responses. Also, many persons may be concerned with getting the drug from the pharmacy into the patient, and there is a possibility of error at every juncture.

Even when the correct drug arrives at the patient's bedside, he may take (or be given) an excessive amount, or he may get a wrong drug by mistake.

With the already tremendous and rapidly increasing therapeutic and diagnostic drug and chemical armamentarium at our disposal, no past history is complete without a history of present and past medications and a record of any bad effects from such agents. Even the most commonly used drugs, such as aspirin, propranolol, digitalis, the thiazides, and hormonal agents, such as thyroid, insulin, corticosteroids, and oral contraceptives, to name only a few, under certain conditions carry considerable risk to the patient. Drugs can be standardized, but patients cannot. Individual idiosyncrasy or hypersensitivity to many chemicals and drugs is quite common. The high frequency of untoward effects in private practice often has been reported.

Less well known are the chances of drug reaction during a closely supervised period of hospitalization in a university teaching situation. In one of the leading teaching hospitals, a record was kept of adverse responses attributed to widely accepted and well-intentioned diagnostic and therapeutic measures.[13] Every patient admitted to the medical service (1014 in all) over an eight-month period was included in the study. Twenty percent of patients had some untoward reaction. Forty-five percent of the adverse episodes were minor, twenty percent major, and the balance moderate. Overall, there was a five percent incidence of major (life-threatening) occurrences attributed to diagnostic or therapeutic procedures. One-half of all the untoward episodes were reactions to drugs used in treatment. Adverse responses observed were (in order of frequency) of the types indicated and due to the drugs specified: penicillin (allergic); antineoplastic agents (toxic); insulin (hypoglycemic); steroids and ACTH; sedatives; anticoagulants; and digitalis (toxic).

FAMILY HISTORY

The family history, a leading tool of clinical genetics, is all too often obtained in a routine, cursory fashion. It is not sufficient to ask if there are any known familial diseases. Such a vague and general question is usually answered in the negative. Information regarding symptoms like those of the patient that have occurred in blood relatives or "run in the family," along with knowledge of the ethnic origin of the parents and of consanguinity may be exceedingly helpful. The information must be obtained with tact, however, for patients may be embarrassed by such inquiries. If a patient has symptoms suggesting thyrotoxicosis, inquire specifically about the occurrence of goiter or nervous troubles in the family. Or if migraine is suspected, inquire particularly about headaches, epilepsy, and allergic or nervous disorders. When a growth or developmental problem is being studied, these characteristics of the close relatives are investigated. When an infectious disease, such as tuberculosis, is suspected, ask whether or not the patient could have been exposed to a relative suffering from it. If there is a question of allergic disease, ask about hay fever, hives, asthma, and other allergic manifestations in the family. In other words every effort should be made by specific inquiry to determine whether or not the family history will yield data helpful in understanding the patient's problems. Many disorders have genetic patterns, and the possibility of such conditions should be kept in mind and clues sought in the family history. When an hereditary trait is suspected, a diagram of the pedigree may clarify the nature of the disease. In such a case, the best family history may be obtained by actual examination of members of the family.

MARITAL HISTORY

Often much may be learned by inquiry concerning domestic and sexual happiness, compatibility, the emotional tone of the home, the health of the spouse, the number of children, pregnancies and miscarriages, housing conditions, diet, infections within the family, and family problems affecting husband, wife, or children.

SOCIAL HISTORY

In certain instances, especially of nervous or emotional disorders, the social history is of great importance. It may also bear an important relationship to the understanding of obviously organic disease. For example, it is important to know about the excessive use of tobacco by a patient with toxic loss of vision, or about alcoholism in a patient with vitamin deficiences or jaundice, or about what caused the poor food habits (possible food faddism or economic problems) when malnutrition or vitamin deficiency is suspected, or about the emotional factors that may precipitate attacks of angina pectoris or peptic ulcer symptoms.

Persons who are disadvantaged or frustrated economically, educationally, or socially are more subject to many types of disorders, both psychological and physical. Full information about the personal society history is of great importance in understanding illness. This should include information about the social habits and values of the family group and relations of members of the family with each other. These data have value chiefly insofar as they reveal to the physician the

influence of these people on the patient and on each other.

Information is obtained about the patient's education; home and family life; compatibility with siblings and parents; compatibility of parents; economic status; ambitions and interests; area (urban or rural), country, and climate of residence; business, work, and social life; recreations; sex experiences; personal habits; and any other factor that may assist the physician in understanding the patient more completely as an individual.

When sympathetically obtained and skillfully developed, such knowledge often is most important in revealing the origin and the nature of the patient's difficulties.

SEX PROBLEMS

Because of the openness that has overtaken discussion about sex, it seems only fitting that talking with patients about sex should move into the open, too. The sexual revolution and the new attitudes represent not only major quantitative shifts but also basic qualitative differences. The practice of medicine has been caught up in the sexual revolution. Patients today talk differently about sex to their physician, presenting the physician with new problems, asking new questions, and challenging the physician with them more directly. Patients may describe wife-swapping, perversions, homosexual marriages, transexualism, as well as accounts of oral sex, anal sex, and group sex, all told as if part of their regular sex habits. It seems likely that physicians who began to practice well before the sexual revolution may never become used to the new era, no matter how hard they try. The younger physicians, who come from the age of revolution, may turn out to be a different breed. To the doctor absorbed in caring for patients, neither side of this controversy is relevant, and taking sides is unnecessary. A confusing, ill-defined, hard-to-diagnose medical situation may mean the patient is in some kind of sexual trouble. Symptoms such as sleepiness, irritability, lack of pep, a sense of unfulfillment—regardless of what else they bring to the skilled clinician's mind—should not fail to register with him as a possible clue that the patient wants to talk about sex. Conversely, it should not be forgotten that sexual problems, themselves caused by neurotic problems, may lead to all sorts of other mental and physical symptoms.[1]

DRUG ADDICTION

There has been another revolution in the widespread, almost promiscuous, use of drugs in present-day western society. A good history will not neglect a tactful inquiry into their use as a possible cause of bizarre behavior, frequent accidents, attempted suicides, psychological disorders, and physical illnesses of certain kinds. Among the drugs commonly implicated are marijuana, LSD, amphetamines, barbiturates, phenothiazines, cocaine, and heroin. Alcohol, although not usually considered to be a drug, causes similar problems.

OCCUPATIONAL HISTORY

Certain occupations expose persons to particular hazards, such as physical injury, muscular or joint strain, nervous tension, viruses, bacteria, fungi, animal infections or animal products, dusts, gases, chemicals, noise, heat, cold, abnormal lighting conditions, unhygienic surroundings, and the possible presence of infected insects. It often is necessary to know what kind of work the patient does and under what conditions. Not only the physical conditions of the work itself, but relationships with employers and fellow workers may be important in determining, for example, whether irritability, headache, undue fatigue, tremor, or increasing inefficiency and inaccuracy may be a result of work problems.

The occupations of children likewise should be studied. School progress and conditions and play habits and environment may be related to the patient's symptoms.

INTERPRETING SYMPTOMS

The history largely consists of an analysis of the presenting symptom or symptoms and of the associated information that may be pertinent. The next step usually employed in the diagnostic method is the physical examination, and thereafter certain laboratory procedures may be used. The physician who pursues as far as possible the logical process of reasoning based upon and initiated by his analysis of the symptoms often finds that he can understand the pathologic physiology leading to the complaints with no data but the history. Thinking through as far as possible toward a diagnosis and writing down preliminary diagnostic impressions, arranged in order of probability or possibility at the end of the history, are useful clinical exercises.

Such a practice enables one to perform the physical examination with discrimination and curiosity, not as a routine requirement. If full advantage is to be gained from the physical examination, it must be performed systematically and thoroughly and extend to all parts of the body. Attention may be directed by the history

to certain offending systems or parts of the body. For example, if symptoms have suggested a blood dyscrasia, particular attention is paid to the skin color, to the mouth and the tongue, and to the lymph nodes and the spleen; or, if the patient has had arthritis or rheumatism, the heart, the extremities, the joints, the phalanges, and the tonsils are studied with special care.

GUIDED STUDIES

When certain diagnostic possibilities are under consideration, the choice of certain special studies, tests, and laboratory procedures is logical. Purpose, discrimination, and a guided curiosity depending upon the problem and the data yielded by the history and physical examination should direct the choice of special tests and laboratory studies. Other irrelevant studies may be omitted, and time, expense, discomfort, and possible untoward effects may be avoided. Thus, if epigastric distress relieved by food is present, gastroscopy, gastric analysis, and x-ray studies of the gastrointestinal tract may promptly yield the diagnosis. Or if pain that may originate in the ureter is present, a urinalysis and an x-ray at once give positive evidence of a kidney stone.

Interpretation of symptoms leads the clinician to choose valuable laboratory tests but to avoid compilation of useless data. He will secure blood sugar tests in diabetes, but not a glucose tolerance test. He will avoid bone-marrow puncture or liver-biopsy puncture if the hemotologic or hepatic diagnostic pictures are already clear. The wise doctor will protect his patient from even slight dangers or small pains or minimal expenses unless possible gains warrant them. He will not order a battery of tests in the hope that his shotgun diagnostic method will accidentally score a bull's-eye. Discrimination in the ordering of laboratory procedures and judgment in appraising their risk, expense, and possible benefit are important indicators of the effectiveness with which the art and science of medicine have been joined by the individual physician.

BASIC PATHOPHYSIOLOGY

As he attempts to interpret the signs and symptoms in each study of a patient, the physician will find his diagnostic impressions falling into one or more of four large groups on the basis of the chief types of pathophysiology involved. These groups are

Neuroses and psychoses
Psychosomatic diseases
Pathophysiologic diseases (functional disorders) without visible pathology
Organic diseases

There are many interrelationships and overlappings between these groups; each is not clearly distinct from the other. Also, any one person's problems may fit well into several of the categories, although his principal disorder may lie clearly in one group. Thus, the main problem may be pulmonary tuberculosis, but a neurosis also may cause serious symptoms; or an illness with early characteristics of a neurosis may be complicated by the development of a peptic ulcer.

It is highly useful to the physician engaged in the process of interpreting signs and symptoms to keep in mind these basic types of disease processes. Each is discussed briefly below.

Neuroses

Studies [14,15] have shown that from 30% to 50% of persons consulting internists and diagnosticians have psychoneuroses. These psychoneuroses may cause many of the symptoms discussed in the various chapters in this book: chest pain, backache, headache, malnutrition, obesity, nervousness, and fatigue, to name just a few.

Psychological problems may occur alone, may simulate organic disease, or be interrelated with true organic disease. Emotional illness can provoke symptoms duplicating those of somatic disorders; it can even produce definite somatic lesions. Physical illness can, of course, beget many emotional and psychological responses. This vast field is discussed in the chapter on conversion symptoms.

It is not possible, nor is it advisable, for the doctor to refer all such patients to psychiatrists. Often the mechanism of production of the symptom can be elucidated and the patient can be relieved through simple measures by the general physician. Careful history with proper interpretation of symptoms will reveal which patients are to be included in this large group with "functional" or "nervous" symptoms.

Psychosomatic Disease

In recent years there has been ample demonstration that not only functional or "nervous" symptoms may result from emotional or psychic disorders, but that organic disease may be so caused. Psychosomatic illness is common, and the more familiar the physician is with the two-way interplay of mental and emotional factors on body physiology and even on body structure, the better he will be able to interpret signs and symptoms.

Psychosomatic interrelationships are considered in all the chapters of this book because they are important in the study of every sign and every symptom, in every complaint of every patient. In the chapter on conversion symptoms, the pathophysiology involved is discussed.

Pathophysiologic Diseases (Functional Disorders) Without Visible Pathology

Many illnesses are attributed to *functional abnormalities,* which usually means that there is disturbed physiology but there is no known structural defect involved in the etiology. Physical or structural derangements as understood in the past were those visible through the microscope. Today we are aware that absence or excess of certain chemical entities, or abnormalities in the chemical configuration of many substances, can account for a number of diseases. Although not visible to the eye, these defects are detected and measured by other tests. They are, in a sense, therefore physical and structural.

Whether we should include such chemical abnormalities in the category of *organic* disease has been a problem, depending upon the meaning implied by the word "organic." If we mean by this word the old concept of a visible change in a tissue, these disorders are not organic. If, instead, we mean *structural,* including chemical composition of body constituents, chemical disorders are included as organic as contrasted with functional. We should adopt a different word; "organic" bears echoes of body organs. Structural seems a better term to carry the concept we intend.

Whether there is ultimately any disorder of function without a causative structural defect remains uncertain. As our knowledge increases, there is a steady dwindling in the number of disturbances still considered functional (without known material origin). Even various psychological illnesses are believed to have chemical etiologies.

Organic Disease

Possibly 60% of patients may be expected to have an organic basis for their symptoms. As one diagnostician has sagely pointed out,[15] clinical-pathologic conferences offer excellent training in the differential diagnosis of fatal diseases with an anatomic substratum, but there are many organic illnesses that are functional and nonfatal, and the clinician must be interested in these. He must be concerned not only in the diagnosis of anatomic disease, but in pathophysiologic disorders without visible causes and the personal and emotional problems of victims of disease. Study of differential diagnosis based upon autopsies[16] is recommended highly, but one must keep in mind that, fortunately, a large percentage of the clinician's practice will have similar symptoms with much less dire consequences.

It has been estimated that "about 55% of all internal diseases can be diagnosed from aspect and history alone, an additional 20% by physical examination, and another 20% by laboratory tests. The rest of the patients remain undiagnosed, regardless of whether they get well or die."[15]

SUMMARY

First the physician finds out what the signs and symptoms are (the patient's complaints) and traces their evolution through the clinical course of the presenting illness. He must determine their true character, not accept uncritically what the patient or someone else thinks they are. He must analyze the signs and symptoms to ascertain the pathophysiologic processes involved.

Interpretation of signs and symptoms involves aid secured from all parts of the history, from the physical examination, and from laboratory studies and special tests.

Interpretation may be faulty if based upon inaccurate or incomplete information. Therefore, analysis of the symptom or symptoms must precede interpretation. With a good history the physician, by virtue of his knowledge of the mechanisms of disease, of pathologic physiology, and of the causation of signs and symptoms, may arrive at a tentative conclusion concerning the malady present.

The physical examination can be done with curiosity and true interest when guided by a perceptive history. Examination so conducted is much more productive of significant information. There should be no such thing as a routine physical examination.

The choice of laboratory studies and special tests should be guided by the particular indications of each individual patient's history. Indiscriminate tests are wasteful and hazardous to the patient. Only studies that offer hope of giving pertinent data should be done. The diagnostic study must be guided throughout by consideration of the pathophysiologic processes believed to be likely causes of the patient's complaints. Unrelated physical findings or laboratory data of interesting or important nature may be discovered, but one's primary aim should be the detection of the cause of the symptoms. Thus may we progress in the understanding of disease and in the development of means to relieve or cure it.

REFERENCES

1. **Stevenson I:** The Diagnostic Interview, 2nd ed. New York, Harper & Row, 1971
2. **Enelow AJ, Swisher SN:** Interviewing and Patient Care, 2nd ed. New York, Oxford University Press, 1979
3. **Wittkower ED, White KL:** Bedside manners, Br Med J 1:1432, 1954
4. **Barnett GO:** Computers in patient care. N Engl J Med 279:1321, 1968
5. **Laska DM, Abbey SG:** Medical information systems. Annu Rev Biophys Bioeng 9:581, 1980

6. **Schoolman HM, Bernstein LM:** Computer use in diagnosis, prognosis and therapy. Science 200:926, 1978

7. **Jacquez J (ed):** The Diagnostic Process. Ann Arbor, Mallow Lithographing, 1964

8. **Wilson J, Jungner G:** Principles and Practice of Screening for Disease. New York, Columbia University Press, 1968

9. **Bird B:** Talking with Patients, 2nd ed. Philadelphia, JB Lippincott, 1973

10. **Forkner CE:** Record of medical history. Arch Intern Med 106:22, 1960

11. **Payson HE, Gaenslern EC, Stargardter FL:** Time study of an internship on a university medical service. N Engl J Med 264:439, 1961

12. **Cabot RC:** Differential Diagnosis. Philadelphia, WB Saunders, 1915

13. **Schimmel EM:** The hazards of hospitalization. Ann Intern Med 60:100, 1964

14. **Allan FN, Kaufman M:** Nervous factors in general practice. JAMA 138:1135, 1948

15. **Bauer J:** Differential Diagnosis of Internal Diseases, 3rd ed. New York, Grune & Stratton, 1967

16. **Harvey AM, Bordley J, Barondess JA:** Differential Diagnosis, 3rd ed. Philadelphia, WB Saunders, 1979

17. **Platt R:** Two essays on the practice of medicine. Lancet 2:305, 1947

2

Growth and Sex Development
William H. Daughaday

Body Size
  Genetic Endowment
  Prenatal Growth
  Postnatal Growth
  Body Proportions
  Skeletal Maturation
  Dental Development
  Body Weight
  Chemical Indication of Growth

Hormonal Regulation of Growth
Clinical Causes of Impaired Growth
Excessive Growth
Sex Development
  Endocrinology of Adolescence
  Body Changes During Adolescence
  Disturbances in the Pubertal Mechanism
  Premature Puberty
Summary

The human organism develops from a single cell to a sexually mature person of adult stature in a period of from 16 to 20 years. In view of the extraordinary complexity of the processes involved, derangement in normal growth and development provides one of the most sensitive manifestations of disease in childhood.

BODY SIZE

GENETIC ENDOWMENT

The fertilized ovum contains within it all the programmed information required for embryonic growth and postnatal development. Although it is legitimate to focus attention on the nucleus of the cell as the storehouse of genetic information, cytoplasmic influences should not be completely overlooked. It is known that mitochondria contain DNA, which participates in the regulation of protein synthesis independent of the nucleus. It is therefore possible that cytoplasmic changes may prove to be important in subsequent growth.

For the purpose of this discussion, the many detrimental mutations that impair normal growth by producing overt disease will be disregarded. There remain many other gene mutations that affect stature without impairing health or inducing deformity. Although the existence of these hereditary influences are widely accepted by the general public, the number of factors involved and the manner in which growth is determined remain very much a mystery. More is known of the participation of the sex chromosomes in the regulation of growth than of the autosomes because of the various effects of differences in number of the X and Y chromosomes that have been encountered.

In the early embryo, both X chromosomes of the female participate equally in cellular regulation, but after the 16th to the 18th day of fetal life, one of the two X chromosomes exists in a condensed form, which can be recognized in a heterochromatic bead (chromatin body) just inside the nuclear membrane. This sex chromosome plays a restricted role in determining ribonucleic acid synthesis and thereby influencing cellular processes. The X chromosome of the chromatin body

17

is also characterized by the fact that its DNA is replicated late in the process of cell division. If more than two X chromosomes are present, the maximum number of observed sex chromatin bodies is one less than the total number of X chromosomes. Once the choice has been made between one or the other X chromosome for full metabolic participation in any given cell line, this choice remains fixed for all subsequent cell divisions of that line. Although the choice between normal X chromosomes appears to be random, there is a beneficial bias for abnormal X chromosomes to be selected for formation of sex chromatin bodies.

Persons with a single X chromosome are phenotypically female but have only a streak representing the gonad. They present with the round facies, increased carrying angle of the arms, web neck, lymphedema, and other skeletal and visceral abnormalities that constitute Turner's syndrome (Fig. 2-1). The karyotype is 45 XO. Important for this discussion is the fact that persons with Turner's syndrome are usually short. We may conclude that the abnormalities of Turner's syndrome represent the consequence of deficiency of the functioning component of the X chromosome, which is present in the chromatin body. The clinical findings of the syndrome probably are due both to expression

of recessive genes of the unpaired X chromosome and to genic imbalance created by only a single dosage of a given locus. Studies of subjects with deletions or translocations of either the short or long arms of the X chromosomes suggest strongly that the genes important in skeletal growth that remain active in the X chromosome condensed in the chromatin body reside in the short arm of the chromosome.

In addition to the X chromosome, the Y chromosome has an important influence on growth, as well as on testicular and male sex duct differentiation. The difference in stature of patients with Turner's syndrome (monosomy X) compared with normal males (XY) can be attributed to growth-promoting genes within the Y chromosome. Some of these genes may be homologous to genes in the X chromosome. The greater stature of men compared with that of women can be explained by the greater positive influence of the Y chromosome than of the active short arm of the X chromosome in the chromatin body. If the dosage effect of Y chromosomes is increased, as in XYY persons, greater than normal stature is encountered. A similar but less evident increase in growth occurs in persons with XXY chromosome constitution. In this disorder, the subject has the positive growth influence of one X chromo-

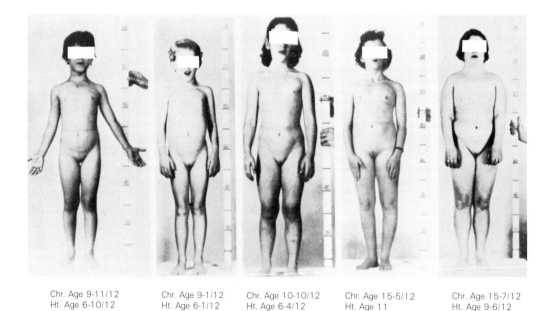

Chr. Age 9-11/12	Chr. Age 9-1/12	Chr. Age 10-10/12	Chr. Age 15-5/12	Chr. Age 15-7/12
Ht. Age 6-10/12	Ht. Age 6-1/12	Ht. Age 6-4/12	Ht. Age 11	Ht. Age 9-6/12
Sex Chrom. Neg.	Sex Chrom. Neg.	Sex Chrom. Neg.	Sex Chrom. Neg.	Sex Chrom. Neg.

Fig. 2-1. Variation in physical appearance in five patients with typical form of the syndrome of gonadal dysgenesis (Turner's syndrome). All of these patients had an XO karyotype, and all had differences between their height age and chronological age of three years or more. (From Van Wyk JJ, Grumbach MM: Disorders of sex differentiation. In Williams RJ (ed): Textbook of Endocrinology, 4th ed, p 170. Philadelphia, WB Saunders, 1968)

some and one Y chromosome and the partial effect of the X chromosome present in the chromatin body.

PRENATAL GROWTH

Growth in the intrauterine period is dependent on maternal health and nutrition and on the ability of the placenta to transport needed nutrients to the fetus and to remove waste products. Inadequacies or abnormalities in nutrients from the mother or in placental transport function may retard the rate of fetal growth so that the infant is born with decreased birth weight and size for the gestational age. More sophisticated measurements of muscle cell number in these newborn infants have demonstrated a significant decrease, indicating a critical loss of cell division *in utero.* Although these infants may show certain gross congenital abnormalities and a tendency toward hypoglycemia, more often decreased size is the only real manifestation of placental deprivation. In children who are undersized for gestational age, no make-up growth occurs after birth; they generally follow a subnormal growth pattern throughout life.

Fetal growth is affected by more specific extrinsic influences. Rubella, syphilis, and other infections may affect the fetus and produce general impairment of growth as well as abnormalities of the heart, central nervous system, eyes, and ears. Immunologic disorders resulting from incompatibility of maternal and fetal blood cells can adversely affect fetal growth when antibodies are transported from mother to fetus. The possibility that drugs taken by the mother may affect fetal growth has become an important consideration after the disaster with thalidomide. Even use of tobacco and excessive ingestion of alcohol by a pregnant female is suspected to have a detrimental effect on fetal growth. It is not surprising that the development of the fetus is sensitive to radiation damage. Infants born to mothers exposed to atomic bomb explosions in Japan have had a number of gross malformations of both somatic and sexual development and have shown a general tendency toward small stature.

Pituitary hormones in fetal life appear to exert relatively little effect on somatic growth. Growth hormone secretion becomes established during the latter weeks of the first trimester of gestation. Growth hormone concentrations of the fetal plasma are thereafter generally moderately to markedly higher than those encountered in normal children and adults. The significance of this relatively high level of plasma growth hormone is obscure because anencephalic fetuses and children with congenital growth hormone deficiency are generally of normal length and weight at birth.

Fetal growth is not appreciably impaired by failure of the fetal thyroid. This may be attributed to transfer of some thyroid hormone from the mother or the relative independence of fetal tissue from thyroid control. Evidence of thyroid hormone deficiency of the fetus can be recognized in certain tissues. A peculiar mottling of the epiphyseal ossification centers that dates back to intrauterine life has been described by Wilkins. It is also likely that the failure of prompt thyroid hormone treatment of cretins to restore normal intelligence indicates a disturbance in prenatal brain development.

POSTNATAL GROWTH

The physician is often asked to evaluate the growth of children to decide on the normality or abnormality of progress. Accurate measurement of children is required to answer these questions. It is surprising how frequently measurements are carelessly performed in the offices of otherwise careful and thorough physicians. Height may be determined simply by attaching a steel tape to a solid wall, ideally the steel frame of a door. The child is then positioned so that his heels are against the wall exactly on each side of the tape and close together. Gentle pressure is applied to the abdomen to assist the child in flattening his spine against the wall. With the head also against the wall in midposition, a right angle wooden or metal block with a width of at least 1½ inches is lowered until firm contact is made with the top of the child's head. Several independent measurements are desirable. With proper addition, measurements can be reproduced to within 0.3 cm.

To interpret the results of growth measurements, standard charts must be used. It is of utmost importance that the charts be appropriate for the environment and racial background of the subject. Most available growth charts were constructed from observations on Caucasians of predominantly northern European origin and are not appropriate for other population groups. It is also true that the information contained in certain growth charts was collected 20 or more years ago and does not reflect the secular trend for increased growth and earlier maturity that has been taking place for the past half century. The charts reproduced in Figure 2-2 can be considered representative. To help in interpretation, the lines indicating the first, 25th, 50th, 75th, and 99th percentiles have been indicated.

For many purposes, the height attainment type of chart is of little value to the physician in deciding the current rate of growth. For instance, one may want to evaluate the deceleration of growth of a child receiving

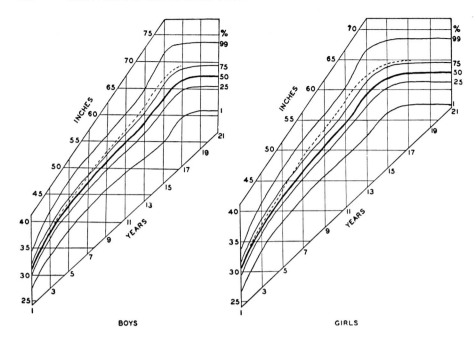

BOYS

GIRLS

Fig. 2-2. Charts adapted from Burgess show height of American boys and girls at various ages, the horizontal lines being inches and the vertical lines years. The diagonal curves represent percentile distributions in the population. The 50% curve represents the mean or average. The dotted curves show the way the growth of a particular child may be charted and illustrate the fact that a normal child frequently may pass from one channel to another. (From Wilkins L: The Diagnosis and Treatment of Endocrine Disorders in Childhood and Adolescence, 2nd ed. Springfield, Charles C Thomas, 1957)

corticosteroids or the degree of acceleration of growth that might follow the relief of a chronic ailment such as a congenital heart lesion. This is not easily seen by plotting data on the typical growth attainment chart. To serve this purpose, curves have been constructed by Tanner and associates for British children that depict the whole year increments in height expressed as a growth rate measured in centimeters per year (Figs. 2-3 and 2-4). As in the height attainment charts, the velocity standards give critical percentiles that permit a comparison of individual children with the larger experience.

A problem common to all tables and charts of growth is the variation in the age at onset of puberty. It is well known that any population of normal boys and girls will differ among themselves in the age at which puberty occurs by as much as 4 or 5 years. During the pubertal period, there is an acceleration of growth to about twice its preceding level. The growth rate progressively increases for about a year and a half and then just as precipitously decreases. The total period of significant growth is between 3 and 4 years from the onset of puberty. The pubertal growth spurt is greater in boys than in girls and it tends to be greater in early maturers compared with late maturers. Because of the difference in the age of onset of puberty, the magnitude and significance of the pubertal growth spurt are obscured in curves constructed from cross-sectional data obtained by measurements of populations of school children at different ages at only a single occasion. The characteristics of the pubertal changes

in growth become evident only when longitudinal studies are carried out by making repeated measurements on the same child. Replotting the data on the basis of years from the peak height velocity indicates the general uniformity of pattern of pubertal growth. The shaded areas in Figures 2-3 and 2-4 have been constructed from longitudinal data with normalization of the age of puberty.

BODY PROPORTIONS

In addition to measurement of height, it is frequently informative to make other simple measurements. These include (1) span (from finger tip to finger tip), (2) lower segment (top of symphysis pubis to the floor, (3) upper segment difference between total height and lower segment), (4) circumference of head, (5) circumference of chest, (6) circumference of abdomen. In Tables 2-1 and 2-2 the average normal measurements for females and males from birth to age 20 years are given, as compiled by Wilkins from data of Shelton and Engelbach for Caucasian Americans.

The most useful measurement of body proportions is the ratio of the upper to the lower segment of the body (U:L). At birth the trunk is relatively long, and therefore the ratio is approximately 1.7:1. Normally, this ratio falls with age so that after 10 or 11 years the two body segments are approximately equal. A number of characteristic changes in the ratio of body segments can be recognized in disease. In congenital hypothyroidism, the body proportions remain infan-

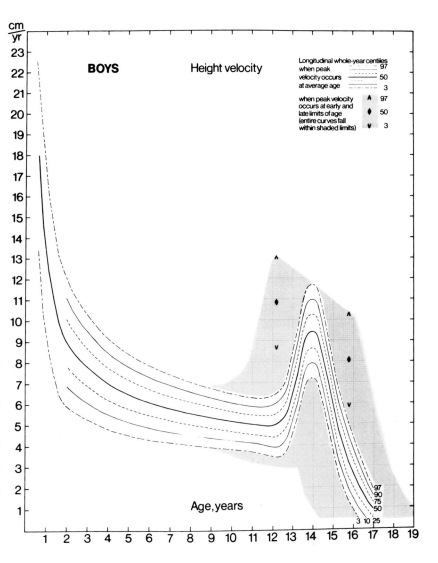

BOYS   Height velocity

Longitudinal whole-year centiles
when peak velocity occurs at average age — 97, 50, 3

when peak velocity occurs at early and late limits of age (entire curves fall within shaded limits) — ∧ 97, ◆ 50, ∨ 3

Age, years

Fig. 2-3. Whole year velocity standards for height of British boys. The percentile lines during the pubertal growth spurt give the range of velocities at the mean age of puberty. The shaded areas give the entire range of normal growth velocities at different ages of normal puberty. Also indicated are the mean plus 75% limits of growth velocities which occur at early and late limits of normal puberty. (Chart prepared by J.M. Tanner and R.J. Whitehouse, Institute of Child Health, London, Chart distributed by Creasey, Ltd., Hertford, England)

tile, with a failure of the U:L ratio to fall. In hypogonadism, the absence of sex hormones permits continued epiphyseal growth of extremities, so that U:L ratio is less than 1. A somewhat similar pattern in growth exists in Marfan's syndrome, despite the occurrence of puberty. It should be remembered that the norms for the U:L ratio have been obtained from Caucasians. A relatively greater lower segment length and span breadth are found normally in the black population.

Abnormalities in body proportions can be anticipated in congenital or acquired diseases that affect either the extremities or the spine. In achondroplasia, the predominant effect is shortening of the extremities, while in Morquio's disease the primary growth disturbance is in the spine.

SKELETAL MATURATION

Skeletal growth is the result of cartilage proliferation and the conversion of cartilage into bone. Growth ceases with the obliteration of the cartilage proliferation, which occurs at the epiphysial plates. Primary centers of ossification are established *in utero*; secondary centers of ossification develop after birth. The sequence in time of appearance of the secondary centers of ossification, as well as the order of the fusion of the epiphyseal and diaphyseal centers of calcification, is fairly predictable (Fig. 2-5).

Radiographs of the bones of growing children have long been used to estimate the relative maturity of any single subject compared with certain population norms. The most practical method in clinical practice is to ex-

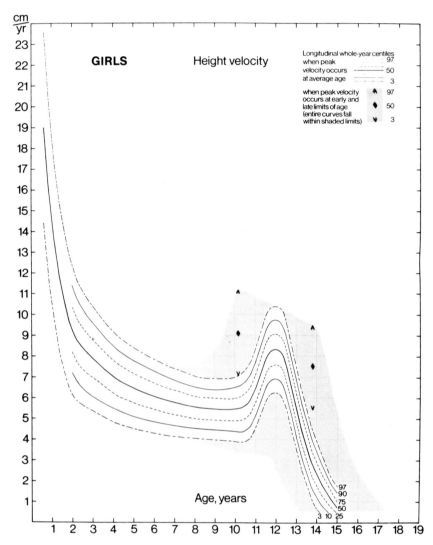

Fig. 2-4. Whole year velocity standards for height of British girls. The percentile lines during the pubertal growth spurt give the range of velocities at the mean age of puberty. The shaded areas give the entire range of normal growth velocities at different ages of normal puberty. Also indicated are the mean plus 95% limits of growth velocities which occur at early and late limits of normal puberty. (Chart prepared by J.M. Tanner and R.H. Whitehouse, Institute of Child Health, London. Chart is distributed by Creasey, Ltd., Hertford, England)

amine the hand and wrist by radiography. The films are then compared with an atlas of representative films accumulated from longitudinal studies of a relatively small group of normal children. The commonly used standards of Greulich and Pyle were derived from a study on California children who were primarily Caucasian. Their relevance to other populations and other social settings can be questioned.

The actual interpretation of the films is seldom uniform and may be influenced by subjective judgments, such as relative importance attached to carpal ossification centers compared with the characteristics of the phalangeal epiphyses. Radiography is of limited value in the early months of life when more reliable information can be obtained by examination of the knees.

A more elaborate system of interpretation of ra-

diographs has been recommended by Tanner and Whitehouse, based on a scoring system for each bone in the hand and wrist. Norms have been established for this grading system for a relatively large population of British children with varied social backgrounds. These norms would appear to be at least 1 year behind the Greulich and Pyle standards.

In 10% of cases, there may be asymmetry of skeletal maturation between the two sides of the body or maturation in the hands and wrist may not be representative of the maturation in epiphyseal centers in other parts of the body. Bilateral examination of all epiphyseal centers would lead to a greater reliability in estimating bone maturation, but the increased expense and greater radiation exposure negate the practicality of this approach.

Table 2-1. *Normal Measurements in Relation to Age (Male)**

Age	Height	Weight	Span	Upper Meas.	Lower Meas.	Ratio U/L	Head	Chest	Abdomen
Birth	20.2	7.4	19.1	12.7	7.5	1.69	13.9	13.8	13.4
1 Mo	21.9	10.4	21.1	13.7	8.2	1.67	15.2	14.3	13.8
2 Mo	23.1	12.0	22.0	14.4	8.7	1.65	16.0	15.6	15.2
3 "	24.1	13.6	23.0	15.0	9.1	1.65	16.6	16.4	16.0
4 "	25.0	15.0	24.0	15.5	9.5	1.63	17.0	16.9	16.5
5 "	25.7	15.8	24.4	15.9	9.8	1.62	17.4	17.2	16.8
6 "	26.4	17.3	25.4	16.3	10.1	1.61	17.7	17.5	17.1
7 "	27.1	18.0	25.9	16.6	10.4	1.61	17.9	17.7	17.3
8 "	27.6	18.7	26.4	16.9	10.7	1.58	18.1	17.9	17.5
9 "	28.1	19.4	26.9	17.2	10.9	1.58	18.2	18.0	17.6
10 "	28.6	20.0	27.3	17.4	11.2	1.55	18.4	18.2	17.7
11 "	29.1	20.7	27.8	17.6	11.5	1.53	18.5	18.3	17.8
12 "	29.5	21.4	28.3	17.9	11.6	1.54	18.6	18.5	17.9
15 "	30.7	22.7	29.3	18.5	12.2	1.52	18.9	18.8	18.2
18 "	31.9	24.6	30.8	19.2	12.7	1.51	19.1	19.1	18.5
21 "	32.9	25.9	31.8	19.6	13.3	1.47	19.3	19.4	18.7
24 "	33.9	27.2	32.7	20.0	13.9	1.44	19.4	19.7	18.9
30 "	35.7	29.2	34.2	20.8	14.9	1.40	19.6	20.2	19.2
36 "	37.3	32.0	36.2	21.3	16.0	1.33	19.8	20.6	19.5
42 "	38.8	34.0	37.7	22.0	16.8	1.31	20.0	21.0	19.8
48 "	40.2	35.5	38.8	22.5	17.7	1.27	20.1	21.4	20.0
54 "	41.5	37.7	40.3	22.9	18.6	1.23	20.3	21.7	20.2
60 "	42.7	39.3	41.4	23.4	19.3	1.21	20.4	22.1	20.4
5½ Yr	43.9	41.9	42.9	23.7	20.2	1.17	20.4	22.4	20.6
6 "	45.0	43.9	44.0	24.0	21.0	1.14	20.5	22.7	20.9
6½ "	46.1	45.9	45.1	24.3	21.8	1.11	20.5	23.0	21.1
7 "	47.2	48.1	46.2	24.7	22.5	1.10	20.6	23.3	21.3
7½ "	48.2	50.4	47.3	24.9	23.3	1.07	20.7	23.7	21.5
8 "	49.2	52.8	48.6	25.3	23.9	1.06	20.7	24.0	21.8
8½ "	50.2	55.3	49.8	25.7	24.5	1.05	20.8	24.3	22.0
9 "	51.2	58.0	51.0	26.0	25.2	1.03	20.9	24.6	22.3
9½ "	52.2	61.0	52.2	26.4	25.8	1.02	20.9	25.0	22.5
10 "	53.2	64.3	53.4	26.8	26.4	1.02	21.0	25.3	22.8
10½ "	54.2	67.7	54.5	27.1	27.1	1.00	21.0	25.7	23.0
11 "	55.2	71.2	55.6	27.5	27.7	0.99	21.1	26.1	23.3
11½ "	56.2	74.7	56.7	27.9	28.3	0.99	21.2	26.6	23.6
12 "	57.1	78.3	57.9	28.3	28.8	0.98	21.2	27.0	23.9
12½ "	58.0	82.0	59.1	28.7	29.3	0.98	21.3	27.5	24.2
13 "	58.9	85.8	60.2	29.1	29.8	0.98	21.4	28.0	24.6
13½ "	59.8	89.8	61.3	29.5	30.3	0.97	21.5	28.6	25.0
14 "	60.7	92.0	61.9	29.9	30.8	0.97	21.6	29.1	25.4
14½ "	61.6	96.5	63.0	30.3	31.3	0.97	21.7	29.7	25.9
15 "	62.4	101.4	64.1	30.7	31.7	0.97	21.8	30.3	26.4
15½ "	63.2	103.9	64.7	31.1	32.1	0.97	21.9	31.0	26.8
16 "	64.0	109.0	65.8	31.5	32.5	0.07	22.0	31.7	27.2
16½ "	64.7	111.7	66.4	31.9	32.8	0.97	22.1	32.3	27.5
17 "	65.4	117.7	67.5	32.2	33.2	0.97	22.2	32.9	27.8
17½ "	66.0	121.0	68.1	32.5	33.5	0.97	22.3	33.3	28.0
18 "	66.6	124.4	68.6	32.8	33.8	0.97	22.4	33.7	28.2
18½ "	67.1	127.8	69.2	33.2	33.9	0.98	22.4	34.1	28.4
19 "	67.5	131.4	69.8	33.4	34.1	0.98	22.5	34.4	28.5
19½ "	67.8	135.0	70.4	33.6	34.2	0.98	22.5	34.6	28.6
20 "	68.0	135.0	70.4	33.7	34.3	0.98	22.5	34.7	28.7

*Dimensions are in inches and weight in pounds (Williams, RH: Textbook of Endocrinology, 4th ed. Philadelphia, WB Saunders, 1968)

Table 2-2. *Normal Measurements in Relation to Age (Female)**

Age	Height	Weight	Span	Upper Meas.	Lower Meas.	Ratio U/L	Head	Chest	Abdomen
Birth	19.9	7.5	19.0	12.6	7.3	1.73	13.6	13.6	13.2
1 Mo	21.5	9.7	20.5	13.5	8.0	1.69	14.9	14.1	13.6
2 Mo	22.7	11.2	21.4	14.2	8.5	1.67	15.7	15.3	15.0
3 "	23.7	12.7	22.4	14.8	8.9	1.66	16.3	16.0	15.7
4 "	24.6	14.1	23.3	15.2	9.4	1.62	16.7	16.5	16.2
5 "	25.3	15.5	24.3	15.6	9.7	1.61	17.1	16.8	16.5
6 "	26.0	16.2	24.8	16.0	10.0	1.60	17.3	17.0	16.8
7 "	26.6	16.9	25.3	16.3	10.3	1.58	17.5	17.2	17.0
8 "	27.1	17.6	25.8	16.6	10.5	1.58	17.7	17.4	17.2
9 "	27.6	18.2	26.2	16.8	10.8	1.56	17.8	17.6	17.3
10 "	28.1	18.8	26.7	17.0	11.1	1.53	18.0	17.8	17.4
11 "	28.6	19.5	27.2	17.3	11.3	1.53	18.1	17.9	17.5
12 "	29.0	20.1	27.7	17.5	11.5	1.52	18.2	18.1	17.6
15 "	30.2	21.3	28.7	18.1	12.1	1.50	18.5	18.4	17.9
18 "	31.4	23.2	30.1	18.7	12.7	1.47	18.7	18.7	18.2
21 "	32.4	24.4	31.1	19.2	13.2	1.45	18.9	19.0	18.4
24 "	33.4	25.7	32.1	19.6	13.8	1.42	19.0	19.2	18.6
30 "	35.1	27.7	33.6	20.4	14.7	1.39	19.2	19.6	18.9
36 "	36.7	29.8	35.1	20.9	15.8	1.32	19.4	20.0	19.1
42 "	38.2	31.9	36.6	21.5	16.7	1.29	19.6	20.4	19.3
48 "	39.6	34.0	38.1	22.0	17.6	1.25	19.7	20.7	19.5
54 "	40.9	36.2	39.7	22.4	18.5	1.21	19.9	21.0	19.7
60 "	42.2	37.7	40.7	22.9	19.3	1.19	20.0	21.4	19.9
5½ Yr	43.4	40.2	42.3	23.2	20.2	1.15	20.1	21.7	20.0
6 "	44.6	42.0	43.3	23.7	20.9	1.13	20.1	22.0	20.2
6½ "	45.7	44.0	44.4	24.1	21.6	1.12	20.2	22.3	20.4
7 "	46.8	47.2	46.0	24.4	22.4	1.09	20.3	22.7	20.5
7½ "	47.9	49.5	47.1	24.7	23.2	1.06	20.3	23.0	20.7
8 "	48.9	52.0	48.2	25.0	23.9	1.05	20.4	23.4	20.8
8½ "	49.9	54.6	49.3	25.4	24.5	1.04	20.5	23.8	21.0
9 "	50.9	57.4	50.4	25.7	25.2	1.02	20.5	24.2	21.2
9½ "	51.9	60.7	51.5	26.1	25.8	1.01	20.6	24.6	21.5
10 "	53.0	63.6	52.6	26.7	26.3	1.01	20.7	25.0	21.8
10½ "	54.1	67.2	53.7	27.2	26.9	1.01	20.8	25.5	22.1
11 "	55.3	72.4	55.3	27.7	27.6	1.00	20.9	26.1	22.4
11½ "	56.5	76.2	56.3	28.2	28.3	1.00	20.9	26.6	22.8
12 "	57.6	80.6	57.5	28.7	28.9	0.99	21.0	27.1	23.2
12½ "	58.7	85.1	58.5	29.2	29.5	0.99	21.1	27.6	23.6
13 "	59.7	90.0	59.7	29.7	30.0	0.99	21.2	28.1	23.9
13½ "	60.6	95.4	60.8	30.3	30.3	1.00	21.3	28.5	24.2
14 "	61.4	101.4	61.3	30.6	30.8	0.99	21.4	28.9	24.5
14½ "	62.0	104.5	62.4	30.9	31.1	0.99	21.5	29.3	24.7
15 "	62.5	107.7	63.0	31.2	31.3	1.00	21.6	29.6	24.8
15½ "	62.9	110.9	63.6	31.4	31.5	1.00	21.7	29.9	25.0
16 "	63.2	110.9	63.6	31.6	31.6	1.00	21.7	30.1	25.1
16½ "	63.5	114.2	64.2	31.8	31.7	1.00	21.8	30.3	25.2
17 "	63.7	114.2	64.2	31.9	31.8	1.00	21.8	30.5	25.3
17½ "	63.9	117.5	64.8	32.0	31.9	1.00	21.8	30.7	25.4
18 "	64.0	117.5	64.8	32.1	31.9	1.01	21.9	30.8	25.5
18½ "	64.0	117.5	64.8	32.1	31.9	1.01	21.9	30.8	25.5
19 "	64.0	117.5	64.8	32.1	31.9	1.01	21.9	30.9	25.6
19½ "	64.0	117.5	64.8	32.1	31.9	1.01	21.9	30.9	25.6
20 "	64.0	117.5	64.8	32.1	31.9	1.01	21.9	31.0	25.7

*Dimensions are in inches and weight in pounds (Williams RH: Textbook of Endocrinology 4th ed. Philadelphia, WB Saunders, 1968)

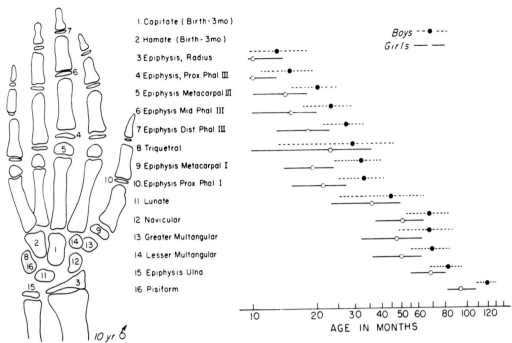

Fig. 2-5. Diagrammatic representation of hand and wrist of a 10-year-old boy. The circles on the accompanying chart represent the average at the time of ossification of the individual bones. The bars represent one standard deviation from the mean. (Data obtained from Greulich and Pyle, after Parker ML, Daughaday WH: The Pituitary in Disorders of Growth. Chicago, Year Book, 1962)

Bone maturation is expressed as "bone age" by matching the individual's radiographs with age standards. Wilkins has proposed a useful method of comparing bone age with height age and other developmental parameters. As shown in Figure 2-6, a plot is made of the developmental age versus the chronologic age of the subject. The developmental age is defined as the age at which the average child achieves the growth parameter in question, such as height, weight, bone maturity, mental development. In this way it is easy to detect whether specific alterations of one or more parameters is occurring. For instance, in hypothyroidism the bone age is more markedly retarded than height, while in hypopituitarism both height age and bone age are proportionately retarded.

The physician is frequently called upon to make a prediction concerning the future growth of a child. Some indication is provided by the percentile position on the height attainment charts. A better prediction is possible when the degree of bone maturation is also considered. The tables of Bayley and Pinneau were constructed from longitudinal studies of a relatively few children and indicate the percentage of mature stature reached at any given bone age. Separate tables are provided for boys and girls, and the tables are further subdivided for children whose bone age is retarded, parallel, or advanced as compared with chronologic age. In many cases, these tables are useful in reassuring concerned parents of short children with delayed maturation and parents of tall children with advanced skeletal maturity that final height will not be grossly abnormal.

DENTAL DEVELOPMENT

The development, eruption, and shedding of the deciduous teeth and the formation and eruption of permanent teeth follow a regular sequence, which is given in Table 2-3. Those disease processes that accelerate or retard bony development such as thyroid deficiency or pituitary deficiency often similarly affect dental development.

BODY WEIGHT

Measurement of body weight is a common procedure in any medical examination. The parameter is a less useful one than height in the assessment of growth

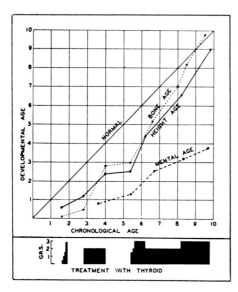

Fig. 2-6. Chart illustrates method of following and comparing growth and development. Chronologic age is plotted horizontally, and developmental age is plotted vertically. The patient's "height age" indicates that he has the height of an average child of the same sex of the age specified. Such a chart permits a comparison of the rate of growth with that of osseous and mental development.

The case shown is a cretin whose thyroid medication was omitted during two periods because of failure of the parents to cooperate. The resulting retardation in growth and development are shown. By this method of charting, inadequate treatment sometimes is detected by a lag in growth and development, even when other signs of deficiency are not obvious. (From Wilkins L: The Diagnosis and Treatment of Endocrine Disorders in Childhood and Adolescence, 2nd ed. Springfield, Charles C Thomas, 1957)

but it does provide an indication of the nutritional state of the subject. If the weight is greater than predicted for height and general build, it is usually assumed that the subject is obese, and when the weight is below the predicted value, reduced fat depots are assumed. The limitations of weight as an indication of body composition should be recognized from common experience. Many well-muscled athletes exceed the normal standards of weight and many older persons with atrophied muscles may have disproportionately large fatty depots, despite "normal" weight.

To provide more accurate measurements of the growth of individual constituents of the body, special methods are required that are not generally available clinically. Measurement of total body density can be performed by weighing in water or by displacement of gases. Knowing the density of fat and the density of "lean body mass," it is possible to calculate the relative contribution of each. An ingenious method for deter-

mining the metabolically active cellular mass is by measuring the body content of potassium 40. This isotope is naturally radioactive and emits gamma radiation with a characteristic spectrum that allows it to be distinguished from other radioactive atoms contained in the body. Because potassium is such an important and relatively uniformly distributed atom of intracellular water, its measurement in a total body counter provides an index of the cellular metabolic mass.

Although these methods require special, cumbersome, and expensive instrumentation and rarely are applicable to clinical problems, the results of such measurements have provided information of interest concerning human growth. The rise in lean body mass as a function of age is shown in Figure 2-7. The rise in lean body mass is progressive throughout the growing period of both males and females. The period of growth is essentially completed between age 14 and 16 in girls but persists beyond age 17 in boys.

The pattern of growth of fatty tissues is considerably different in males and females. This is most clearly shown when the percentage of fat is plotted as a function of age, as in Figure 2-8. In boys, relative fattiness increases during the prepubertal years and then falls after puberty. In females, there is no fall in proportion of body fat occurring with puberty; relative fattiness increases after puberty.

Because of the importance of measurements of body fat in health and nutrition surveys, simpler methods have been sought. Because about half the body fat is deposited under the skin, measuring the thickness of skin folds has been advanced as a technique to estimate adiposity or obesity. Special calipers have been devised that exert a defined pressure over a standard area. A number of studies have attempted to correlate skin fold thickness of different parts of the body with relative body fat content. Some have challenged the use of the triceps skin fold and have measured several skin areas.

For further discussion of body fat and body weight see Chapter 37.

CHEMICAL INDICATION OF GROWTH

A number of chemical measurements provide useful information concerning the growth of certain tissues. One such measurement is the determination of urinary hydroxyproline. The urine contains small amounts of free hydroxyproline and much larger quantities of hydroxyproline present as oligopeptides. Only very small amounts of larger hydroxyproline-containing peptides are present in the urine. All urinary hydroxyproline is derived from collagen catabolism. In the adult, the major site of collagen breakdown is in the skeleton and is

Table 2-3. *Chronology of Dentition*

	Tooth Name	Number	First Evidence of Calcification	Crown Completed	Eruption	Root Completed	Root Resorption Begins
Deciduous Teeth	Lower central incisors	L.I.	5th month in utero	4 mos.	6-8 mos.	1½-2 yrs.	5-6 yrs.
	Upper incisors	U.I. & II	5th month in utero	5 mos.	8-10 mos.	1½-2 yrs.	5-6 yrs.
	Lower lateral incisors	L.II	5th month in utero	5 mos.	10-14 mos.	1½-2 yrs.	5-6 yrs.
	Canines (cuspids)	III	6th month in utero	9 mos.	16-20 mos.	2½-3 yrs.	6-7 yrs.
	First molars	IV	5th month in utero	6 mos.	12-16 mos.	2-2½ yrs.	4-5 yrs.
	Second molars	V	6th month in utero	10-12 mos.	20-30 mos.	3 yrs.	4-5 yrs.
Permanent Teeth — Upper Jaw	Central incisor	1	3-4 mos.	4-5 yrs.	7-8 yrs.	10 yrs.	
	Lateral incisor	2	1 yr.	4-5 yrs.	8-9 yrs.	11 yrs.	
	Canine (cuspid)	3	4-5 mos.	6-7 yrs.	11-12 yrs.	13-15 yrs.	
	First bicuspid	4	1½-1¾ yrs.	5-6 yrs.	10-11 yrs.	12-13 yrs.	
	Second bicuspid	5	2-2¼ yrs.	6-7 yrs.	10-12 yrs.	12-14 yrs.	
	First molar	6	At birth	2½-3 yrs.	6-7 yrs.	0-10 yrs.	
	Second molar	7	2½-3 yrs.	7-8 yrs.	12-14 yrs.	14-16 yrs.	
	Third molar	8	7-9 yrs.	12-16 yrs.	17-30 yrs.	18-25 yrs.	
Permanent Teeth — Lower Jaw	Central incisor	1	3-4 mos.	4-5 yrs.	6-7 yrs.	9 yrs.	
	Lateral incisor	2	3-4 mos.	4-5 yrs.	7-8 yrs.	10 yrs.	
	Canine (cuspid)	3	4-5 mos.	6-7 yrs.	10-11 yrs.	12-14 yrs.	
	First bicuspid	4	1¾-2 yrs.	5-6 yrs.	10-12 yrs.	12-13 yrs.	
	Second bicuspid	5	2¼-2½ yrs.	6-7 yrs.	11-12 yrs.	13-14 yrs.	
	First molar	6	At birth	2½-3 yrs.	6-7 yrs.	9-10 yrs.	
	Second molar	7	2½-3 yrs.	7-8 yrs.	12-13 yrs.	14-15 yrs.	
	Third molar	8	8-10 yrs.	12-16 yrs.	17-30 yrs.	18-25 yrs.	

(Holt and McIntosh: Pediatrics, 12th ed. New York, Appleton-Century-Crofts)

related to the remodeling of bone. In growing children, a certain fraction of newly synthesized collagen is lost from the connective tissue before it can be incorporated into mature insoluble collagen. Some of the cleavage products of enzymatic action on collagen resist further peptidase digestion and appear in the urine as hydroxyproline-containing peptides.

Normally, total urinary hydroxyproline rises progressively during childhood, with peak excretion noted at the time of puberty (Fig. 2-9). Much lower values are found in adults. When growth is impaired, urinary hydroxyproline falls. When the cause of the growth failure is eliminated, the excretion of hydroxyproline returns to normal. This parameter has been of particular use in the study of the effects of growth hormone in treatment of dwarfism. The measurement cannot be directly equated with net growth of connective tissue, because some of the highest levels of urinary hydroxyproline are encountered in disease states associated with rapid bone turnover (*e.g.*, Paget's disease or hyperparathyroidism, in which no net accretion of collagen is occurring).

Another chemical parameter of body composition is the measurement of urinary creatinine. This constituent of urine is derived entirely from muscle creatine, or, more likely, its phosphorylated derivation. Nearly all body creatine is located within muscles, and the rate of conversion of creatine to creatinine is a relatively constant 2% per day. It is evident, therefore, that urinary creatinine provides a reasonable estimate of total muscle mass. By correlating urine creatinine with total calculated muscle mass, Cheek concluded that 1 g of urine creatinine was equivalent to about 20 kg of muscle mass. The measurement of urinary creatinine has two general applications that are based on these considerations. The constancy of urinary creatinine from day to day provides a reasonable indication of the completeness of urine collection. Comparison of the excretion of persons of different sizes may be achieved by expressing the urinary excretion of a given constituent per gram of creatinine. For instance, the excretion of urinary 17-hydroxycorticosteroids, when expressed per gram of creatinine, is relatively constant during the growing years.

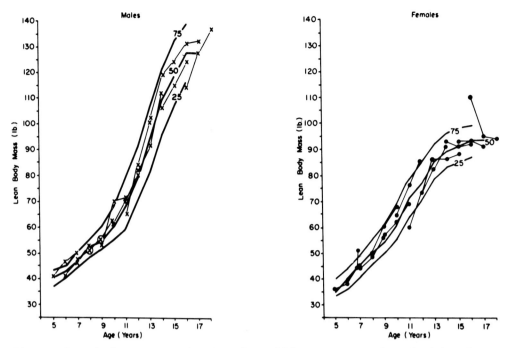

Fig. 2-7. Lean body mass as a function of age. Males are presented on the left and females on the right. The heavy lines described the 25th, 50th, and 75th percentiles from the 1963 sample. The thin lines plot a series of 3 annual values for individual children ranked as 50 percentile for their age from the 1965 sample. A circled point represents two children with the same value. Estimates were made on basis of multiple regression equations of Cheek by Rauh and Schumsky. (Reprinted by permission from Cheek DB: Human Growth, Energy and Intelligence, p 246. Philadelphia, Lea & Febiger, 1968)

HORMONAL REGULATION OF GROWTH

Normal growth is dependent on the secretion of several key hormones. The most important of these is the *pituitary growth hormone.* We now know that this hormone is a single-chain polypeptide of 191 amino acids. The somatotrophic cells of the pituitary synthesize the hormone and store it in large characteristic granules. The release of the hormone from the pituitary is regulated by hypothalamic hypophysiotropic hormones. There is much physiologic evidence of a growth hormone-releasing hormone, but only recently has evidence been obtained that it is a polypeptide of about 44 amino acids. The growth hormone release-inhibiting hormone or *somatostatin* has been isolated as a simple peptide of 14 amino acids and has been synthesized. In addition to inhibiting growth hormone secretion, this peptide can also inhibit the release of insulin, glucagon, and gastrin, as well as other hormones. It is still uncertain which of these actions occur physiologically.

Plasma growth hormone levels remain elevated in the newborn, but after several weeks plasma levels are about the same as in older children. The integrated mean level serum growth hormone (GH) is somewhat higher in children than in adults, and the level increases markedly at the time of puberty. After puberty the mean level of serum GH is higher in women than in men. A burst of GH secretion regularly occurs 60 to 90 minutes after the onset of deep sleep. Secondary peaks of GH secretion may occur during the night. During the day, GH is secreted in isolated bursts that occur about every three or four hours. Fasting, exercise, or other stresses may trigger bursts of GH secretion. During puberty the frequency and magnitude of these bursts are increased.

Growth hormone exerts multiple effects in the body other than augmenting growth, such as promoting lipolysis, and antagonizing the action of insulin. These effects are difficult to relate to the anabolic effect of the hormone. The promotion of protein synthesis is of obvious importance in consideration of human growth. The exact mechanism of this action on many tissues remains obscure because it has been extremely difficult to reproduce the effects observed *in vivo* by the direct addition of growth hormone *in vitro*. There is evidence

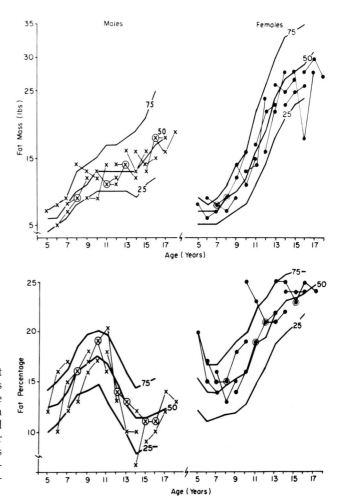

Fig. 2-8. Changes in body fat as a function of age. Fat mass is presented above and fat percentage below. Males are presented on the left and females on the right. The heavy lines described the 25, 50, and 75 percentiles from the 1963 sample. The thin lines plot a series of 3 annual values for individual children ranked as 50 percentile for their age from the 1965 sample. A circled point represents two children with the same value. (Reprinted by permission from Cheek DB: Human Growth, Energy and Intelligence, p 247. Philadelphia, Lea & Febiger, 1968)

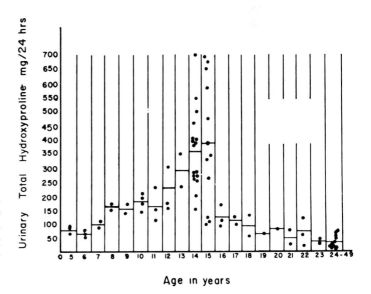

Fig. 2-9. Twenty-four hour urinary total hydroxyproline excretion by 80 normal subjects from 5 to 49 years of age on an *ad lib* diet. (Reprinted by permission from Jones RC, Bergman MW, Kittner PJ et al: Urinary hydroxyproline excretion in normal children and adolescents. Proc Soc Exp Biol Med 115:85, 1964)

that growth hormone acts on skeletal tissue by induction of secondary mediators, *the somatomedins*. Somatomedin C (also called IGF-I) can be measured in serum by radioimmunoassay. The concentration of this factor is low in pituitary dwarfism and is elevated in acromegaly.

Dependence on growth hormone for continued normal growth becomes evident within the first year of life. Thereafter through the years of childhood the role of growth hormone is vital. Although the cessation of skeletal growth can be attributed to closure of the epiphyses, it is also evident that soft tissues and viscera also cease to grow at maturity. Since we find that growth hormone persists in the plasma of adults, we can speculate that the tissues may lose their responsiveness. If so, such resistance is only relative, because visceral growth resumes with the elevated plasma growth hormone concentrations characteristics of active acromegaly.

CLINICAL CAUSES OF IMPAIRED GROWTH

Many classifications of growth failure that have been proposed have often been so inclusive that they are of relatively little practical use. The classification presented in Table 2-4 is an attempt to divide growth failure into four major physiologic types: (1) abnormal

Table 2-4. *A Functional Classification of Growth Impairment*

Abnormal Endocrine Regulation
  Decreased growth hormone activity
    Secondary (hypothalamic)
      hyposomatotropism
    Primary (pituitary) hyposomatotropism
      Genetic—monohormonal
      Sporadic mono- or polyhormonal
    Growth hormone receptor defect
  Hypothyroidism
  Hypoinsulinism
  Hyperadrenocorticism
Tissue Unresponsiveness—Genetic Factors
  Chromosomal imbalance
    Monosomy X and other X chromosome deficits
    Trisomy 21 (Down's syndrome)
  General tissue unresponsiveness
    Racial—pygmies
    Familial short stature
  Specific genetic disorders of bone and cartilage
Tissue Unresponsiveness—Nutritional Factors
  Major nutriments
    Vitamins
    Minerals
    Oxygen
Chronic Inflammation and Toxic States

endocrine regulation, (2) inherent defects of cellular responsiveness, (3) nutritional cause of cellular unresponsiveness, (4) cellular unresponsiveness due to inflammatory and toxic states.

Abnormal Endocrine Regulation

Deficiency of growth hormone production is the most important endocrine cause of growth failure. In some cases, this is the result of a hypothalamic disorder that presumably causes a decrease in the production of the growth hormone-releasing factor. It is likely that in many cases the hyposomatotropism occurring with suprasellar cysts is the result of hypothalamic insufficiency rather than direct destruction of the pituitary. Other tumors and inflammatory conditions may act similarly. Unfortunately, direct techniques for distinguishing secondary from primary hyposomatotropism have not yet been developed.

There is great interest in the possibility that emotional disturbances may act on the hypothalamus to produce secondary hyposomatotropism. Seriously disturbed children reared in an environment of deprivation of parental affection may exhibit impaired growth. In the more severe examples of this syndrome, a peculiar disturbance of appetite may develop in which these children eat all available food, even garbage. Absorption of food may be impaired by a functional malabsorption syndrome. It is difficult to attribute the growth failure to nutritional deficiency because of the absence of specific signs and the maintenance of fairly adequate adipose depots. Characteristically when these children are removed from a bad home environment and placed in more secure surroundings, they exhibit a characteristic make-up type of growth spurt. The suggestion has been made that the growth failure of the maternal deprivation syndrome is the result of functional hyposomatotropism. It has been difficult to establish this hypothesis because some of these children when tested in the hospital have normal plasma growth hormone responses to provocative stimuli. Unanswered is the question whether responsiveness might not be impaired if the test could be performed in the home environment.

Isolated growth hormone deficiency can be the result of a homozygous state for a specific gene. The pituitary dysfunction is limited to an inability to secrete growth hormone. All other pituitary hormones are secreted in near-normal concentrations. An autopsy of one case with this disorder demonstrated the presence of what appeared to be granulated somatotrophic cells. This suggests that the defect in this condition involved hypothalamic regulations of hormone release. The nonhereditary form of primary hyposomatotropism can also be monohormonal but more often

is polyhormonal. The pathologic lesion may be limited to an unexplained reduction of pituitary somatotropic cells, but in other cases a neoplastic, infiltrative, or infectious process can be recognized.

In congenital growth hormone deficiency, the growth rate slows within the first year of life (Fig. 2-10). Thereafter, it continues at about one-third to one-half the normal rate. Because of the common failure of puberty to occur, epiphyseal closure often does not occur, and slow growth persists through the third and fourth decades. Body proportions remain appropriate for height, and bone age is proportionately retarded compared with height age. Subcutaneous ''baby'' fat is retained in childhood. Underdevelopment of the face with small mandible and low nasal bridge suggests that the skull is inordinately large. Actually, however, head diameter is reduced. Secondary teeth appear late and may be crowded in the small jaw.

Pituitary deficiency may result from midline developmental abnormalities. There is an increased frequency of GH deficiency in children with cleft palate or cleft lip. In septoptic dysplasia, the optic disk is small, indicating failure of normal optic nerve development, and the septum pellucidum is absent when examined by computerized tomography. The sella turcica is abnormally small in 10% to 20% of cases of pituitary dwarfism.

Hypoplasia of laryngeal structures result in a high squeaky voice. Micropenis and cryptorchidism may be present in boys.

Dwarfism may result from the failure of growth hormone to induce the secondary mediator, somatomedin. Familial cases described by Laron with the physical features of hyposomatotropism have high growth hormone concentrations in plasma but a low plasma somatomedin, which does not rise following growth hormone treatment. The administration of growth hormone also fails to induce the expected acute changes of nitrogen retention and increased hydroxyproline excretion observed in true pituitary dwarfism. For this reason it seems most likely that dwarfism is due to an abnormality in growth hormone receptors in target tissues.

The thyroid gland is second in importance to the pituitary gland in the regulation of growth. In the rat, some of the growth failure of hypothyroidism is the result of depletion of pituitary somatotropin. Although some hypothyroid children fail to exhibit rises of plasma growth hormone following provocative stimuli, others have perfectly normal responses. It is likely that the direct cellular effects of thyroid hormone deficiency are paramount in many. In congenital hypothyroidism or cretinism, growth failure occurs in the early months of life. Bone maturation is retarded much more than height. Children with hypothyroidism are pale, dry-skinned,

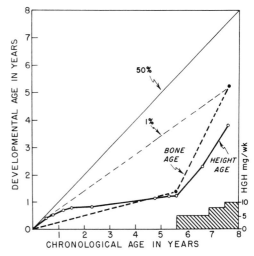

Fig. 2-10. Developmental chart for a boy with hypopituitary dwarfism. Before growth hormone treatment his height was below the first percentile curve. Note the excellent growth following human growth hormone administration. (From Daughaday WH, Parker ML: Pituitary in disorders of growth. Disease-a-Month, pp 1–47, August 1962)

and puffy. Umbilical hernias are common. The cry is hoarse. Feeding is poor and constipation is common. Prolongation of physiologic jaundice of the newborn is an important clue. The widespread introduction of neonatal screening for hypothyroidism should make cretinism a rare form of growth impairment.

When hypothyroidism occurs later in childhood, growth is also impaired but the clinical findings are less dramatic and may be overlooked. Intelligence is normal. Again, bone age is retarded out of proportion to height. Infrequently, premature puberty with inappropriate lactation occurs in girls with juvenile hypothyroidism.

It is likely that insulin is a true growth hormone that influences cellular growth directly. Moreover, the nutritional consequences of uncontrolled glycosuria and ketosis undoubtedly contribute to the short stature formerly common in poorly treated children with diabetes.

Recent investigations have established that somatomedin levels are reduced in patients with very poorly controlled diabetes. Inhibitors or somatomedin action may also be involved in the growth impairment.

Hyperadrenocorticism is a very important cause of growth failure. Fortunately, spontaneous Cushing's syndrome is rare in childhood but iatrogenic Cushing's syndrome occurs whenever corticosteroids are administered for long periods of time. In addition to the inhibition of growth, corticosteroids may lead to facial

and truncal obesity, atrophy of skin, muscle, and bone, and diabetes and lowered resistance to infection. Although large doses of corticosteroids block growth hormone release by the pituitary in response to provocative stimuli, this may not be a significant factor in children receiving typical therapeutic doses of corticosteroids. It has been shown that even when growth hormone is administered to children receiving corticosteroids, nitrogen retention is minimal and normal growth is not restored. In addition, plasma growth hormone responses to hypoglycemia are not consistently depressed in children receiving the usual doses of corticosteroids. From these observations it appears that the major factor responsible for growth impairment in children receiving corticosteroid therapy is not inhibition of the secretion of growth hormone but inhibition of somatomedin generation or action.

Genetic Tissue Unresponsiveness

Genetic factors are important in determining the responsiveness of tissues to circulating hormonal regulation. The polygenic control of growth has already been mentioned earlier in this chapter. Impairment in growth can be the result of imbalance of gene dosage due to chromosomal abnormalities or to gene substitutions in appropriate sites. *Monosomy X* (Turner's syndrome) with karyotype 45 XO is the most common type of chromosomal imbalance seen with short stature and can be easily recognized by the stigmata of the condition evident in Figure 2-1. Facial and body proportions often are less abnormal in cases of mosaicism, in which some of the cells contain the normal XX constitution and other cells contain only a single X chromosome or an abbreviated X chromosome. It is important to recognize that the presenting clinical findings of these children in the prepubertal years may be limited to short stature. A carefully performed cytologic examination of the buccal smear usually shows a decreased percentage of sex chromatin bodies, or the chromatin body may be abnormal in size. Definite diagnosis requires chromosomal analysis. It is usually sufficient to study the chromosomes derived from circulating lymphocytes, but in more difficult cases of mosaicism examination of fibroblasts and other cells may be required.

Abnormalities in the normal diploid number of other chromosomes generally produced impaired growth associated with gross maldevelopment of the brain and other organs. The only condition that is apt to be seen in the physician's office is *trisomy 21*. There are 47 chromosomes. The clinical condition is called Down's syndrome (mongolism). Again, the physical signs indicate disproportions in the growth process and should lead

one away from a consideration of endocrine deficiencies.

The general responsiveness of tissues to hormonal regulation of growth is determined by multiple genes. In the pygmies of Africa, selection has concentrated several of the specific genes that decrease the responsiveness to growth hormone. These people have normal amounts of circulating growth hormone and normal growth hormone responses to provocative stimuli. Somatomedin by bioassay is normal but one somatomedin peptide (IGF-I) is reported to be reduced when measured by radioimmunoassay. The finding of subnormal responses of plasma insulin to arginine and glucose administration is similar to that which occurs in growth hormone deficiency. Administered human growth hormone did not lower plasma urea nor increase insulin response to provocative stimuli. Although these studies were carried out under the most difficult field conditions, they do suggest subnormal responses to endogenous and exogenous hormones when compared with other racial groups.

It is likely that certain types of familial short stature may be attributed to a similar refractoriness to growth hormone, although studies of this problem are still fragmentary. Growth hormone treatment does not induce a sustained increase in growth velocity when administered in the same dosage that induces remarkable increments in patients with pituitary dwarfism. It is possible that when larger supplies of growth hormone become available, larger doses of hormone may successfully stimulate growth in such children.

Finally, consideration should be given briefly to the many genetic disorders of bone and cartilage that limit response to hormonal stimulation. Most familiar to physicians in this class are patients with achrondroplasia, with the characteristic short extremities and deformed skull. In the differential diagnosis of growth impairment, these cases seldom present problems because of their evident distortions of body proportions and the characteristic radiographic findings.

Defective Cellular Nutrition

In many cases, no primary abnormality in hormonal regulators or genetic defects in cellular responsiveness exists, but growth impairment is the result of a failure to provide the proper nutriments required for the synthesis of cellular constituents. Dietary deficiencies of calories, essential amino acids, vitamins, or essential minerals almost without exception produce growth impairment as one feature of the deficiency condition. Growth deficiency in these situations seldom presents specific characteristics. There have been a number of reports from the Middle East that zinc deficiency can

lead to growth deficiency and hypogonadism. The suggestion was made that pituitary deficiency was responsible for growth failure in zinc deficiency, but further studies indicate that the secretion of growth hormone is normal.

Growth deficiency is a common finding in patients with congenital heart disease. The disturbance is attributed to the failure of provision of oxygen to the tissues. Following correction of the cardiac defect by appropriate surgical operation, a period of accelerated "catch-up" growth often occurs.

Chronic Inflammation and Toxic States

A fall in growth velocity often provides an early indication of significant chronic disease. This is particularly evident in the collagen disease group such as juvenile rheumatoid arthritis or nonspecific inflammatory states such as regional enteritis and ulcerative colitis. Growth impairment is also a characteristic response to a number of chronic infections. This is particularly evident if predisposing factors such as cystic fibrosis or defective immune mechanisms are operative.

Growth failure is commonly observed in a number of chronic metabolic conditions such as the glycogenoses, defects in intermediary amino acid metabolism, and chronic renal disease. In renal tubular acidosis and azotemia, growth failure is usually associated with clinical or radiographic signs of osteitis fibrosa or osteomalacia.

EXCESSIVE GROWTH

When somatic growth exceeds the mean by two standard deviations, excessive growth can be considered to exist. Increased growth velocity can occur with overfeeding, an excess of anabolic hormones, or increased tissue responsiveness.

Forbes has pointed out that obese children are of two general types. The first is associated with increased height, increased lean body mass as well as total fat, and increased bone maturation. The second type of childhood obesity is unassociated with these changes in the nonfatty tissues. It is not known whether the increased growth of the first type is determined by nutritional factors, but its recognition is important for parental counseling.

Increased body growth as a result of excessive growth hormone secreted is seen infrequently. Pituitary gigantism resulting from a somatotrophic adenoma of the pituatary is a rare and dramatic condition that can be diagnosed with confidence using radioimmunoassay of plasma growth hormone. The diagnosis requires demonstration of elevated plasma GH under basal conditions, which remains elevated 1 to 2 hours after the administration of 75 g to 100 g of glucose by mouth. Serum somatomedin C by radioimmunoassay is elevated. It is possible that in the future a more detailed study of children with excessive growth will reveal additional cases of mild functional hypersomatotropism.

Sexual precocity leads to an acceleration of growth and a greater increase in bone maturation. Therefore, children with sexual precocity are taller than their peers during the early years of their precocity. Following epiphyseal closure they are overtaken in stature by their normal peers and are of short final stature.

Most cases of excessive stature are the result of increased tissue responsiveness to normal nutritional and hormonal factors. A family history of tall stature in one or both parents can usually be obtained. Parents bring tall girls to the physician hoping that growth can be curtailed. Unfortunately, after the pubertal growth spurt is underway, hormonal treatment is of little benefit. If the bone age is less than 11 years and the predicted height is in excess of 70 inches, there is a possibility of some control of eventual height with moderately high doses of estrogens. The author has employed the estrogen–progestin preparations such as those used for fertility control in these girls. The initial response to these hormone preparations is an acceleration of growth, but final height can be decreased by 1 inch to 3 inches. Following cessation of sex hormone administration, menses usually appear promptly. It is still unknown how frequently disturbed menstruation or other complications are associated with this therapy. The risks are not justified unless the projected height is likely to be a major psychologic and social barrier.

An unusual form of excessive growth has been reported in certain cases of mental deficiency and cerebral damage. It has not been possible to demonstrate excess growth hormone levels in these cases of cerebral gigantism. The mechanism of accelerated growth remains a mystery, and the validity of the syndrome remains open to question.

SEX DEVELOPMENT

ENDOCRINOLOGY OF ADOLESCENCE

At birth the gonads of both male and female infants show evidence of stimulation and secretory activity. Gonadal stimulation is the result of fetal pituitary secretion of follicle-stimulating hormone (FSH) and luteinizing hormone (LH) and the contribution of human chorionic gonadotropin (HCG) from the placenta. In the male fetus, HCG alone may not always provide

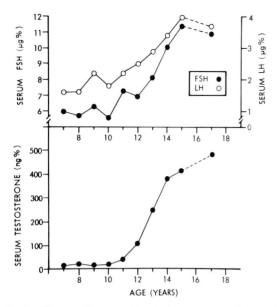

Fig. 2-11. Changes in mean level of serum FSH, LH, and testosterone during childhood and adolescence of boys. There is considerable individual variation at each age, partially because of the normal variation in the onset of puberty. (From Faiman C: Gonadotropin and sex hormone patterns in puberty. In Grumbach MM, Grave SD, Meyer FE (eds): Control of the Onset of Puberty. New York, John Wiley & Sons, 1974)

sufficient Leydig cell stimulation to ensure complete penile and scrotal development. A contributing role of growth hormone in the development of the penis is suggested by the occurrence of microphallus in a significant number of newborn infants with isolated growth hormone deficiency.

Gonadotropin levels fall during infancy to low levels during childhood and do not begin to rise again until just before puberty. During this period Leydig cells are inconspicuous in the testis, and the ovary contains only primary follicles. The increase in serum gonadotropin levels associated with changes in testosterone levels are shown in Figure 2-11. Similar changes in gonadotropin levels occur in girls, along with a dramatic rise in plasma estradiol (Fig. 2-12).

The basic change in the pubertal process must lie in the hypothalamus. For reasons that are still largely unknown, the hypothalamus begins to secrete increased amounts of the releasing factors for the gonadotropic hormones into the hypothalamic–pituitary portal system. It has been suggested that even in the prepubertal state there is a feedback system of regulatory control acting between pituitary and gonad. The event of puberty might result from a rise in the threshold of the hypothalamic centers that are sensing the concentra-

tion of gonadal steroids. With less feedback inhibition, the release of gonadotropins is promoted. Although this view has many attractive features, it does not explain the relatively low levels of gonadotropins in young children with gonadal agenesis.

Although measurements of gonadotropin levels in the basal state in the morning are revealing, these measurements give an incomplete picture of the secretory pattern throughout the day. It has been observed that in early puberty short bursts of gonadotropin secretion can occur in sleep. As puberty progresses, these bursts are replaced by a more sustained level of secretion.

The pubertal rise in gonadotropin titers stimulates the growth and secretion of the gonads. Not only do gonadal steroids promote the development of secondary sexual characteristics, but they induce character-

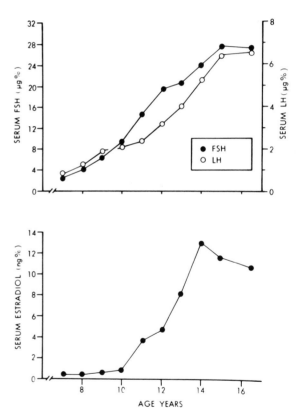

Fig. 2-12. Changes in mean level of serum FSH, LH, and estradiol during childhood and adolescence of girls. There is considerable individual variation at each age, partially because of the normal variation in the onset of puberty. (From Faiman C: Gonadotropin and sex hormone patterns in puberty. In Grumbach MM, Grave SD, Meyer FE (eds): Control of the Onset of Puberty. New York, John Wiley & Sons, 1974)

istic metabolic and psychic effects. Some of the effects of gonadal steroids on secondary sexual characteristics are indirectly mediated in the female. The development of axillary and pubic hair is not normally the result of ovarian hormones, but is a consequence of adrenal androgen secretion. In the prepubertal state, the adrenal glands secrete only small amounts of the potentially androgenic 17-ketosteroids. At puberty a change in adrenal enzyme composition occurs, possibly as a result of estrogen action, so that the secretion of 17-ketosteroids increases greatly. The androgenic activity derived from these steroids by extra-adrenal metabolism gives rise in normal girls to axillary and pubic hair, occasional acne, and slight lowering of the voice.

BODY CHANGES DURING ADOLESCENCE

The sequential stages of puberty in boys follow one another in a predictable pattern in the majority of cases. They are given in Table 2-5 and Figure 2-13. The first change detectable in boys is an increase in the size and firmness of the testis, due to gonadotropic stimulation. The accurate measurement of testicular size is important for physicians evaluating pubertal development. The author has found a series of testicular models of known volume to be the most satisfactory method of examination. Other physicians measure the length of the testicular axes. After the first increase in testicular size, penile development and scrotal development soon follow. Finally, the pubic hair becomes noticeable and scrotal skin becomes corrugated. It is important to recognize that pubic hair precedes the development of axillary hair by a year or two, and axillary hair precedes the development of beard growth by an equal period of time. The complete male escutcheon is not achieved until late in adolescence. During the most rapid phase of pubertal development there is normally limited proliferation of the male breast. Usually this escapes notice. Occasionally it is prominent enough to cause embarrassment and must be distinguished from pathologic gynecomastia resulting from Klinefelter's syndrome (a buccal smear will show sex chromatin bodies, and chromosomal studies will demonstrate an XXY pattern) or from adrenal or testicular tumors.

Associated with the changes in primary and secondary sexual characteristics, many other bodily changes occur. Linear growth velocity increases markedly (Figs. 2-3 and 2-4), and there is an acceleration of the process of epiphyseal closure. In boys there is a disproportionate increase in muscle mass and muscle strength. Body fat increases in absolute amounts during and immediately after puberty in adolescent boys, yet the percentage of body fat actually falls (Fig. 2-8).

Table 2-5. *Average Approximate Age and Sequence and Appearance of Sexual Characteristics in Both Sexes*

Age Years	Boys	Girls
9-10		Growth of bony pelvis, budding of nipples
10-11	First growth of testes and penis	Budding of breasts, pubic hair
11-12	Prostatic activity	Changes in vaginal epithelium and the smear Growth of external and internal genitalia
12-13	Pubic hair	Pigmentation of nipples, mammae filling in
13-14	Rapid growth of testes and penis Subareolar node of nipples	Axillary hair, menarche (average 13½ yr, range 9-17 yr) Menstruation may be anovulatory for first few years.
14-15	Axillary hair, down on upper lip, voice change	Earliest normal pregnancies
15-16	Mature spermatozoa (average 15 yr, range 11¼-17 yr)	Acne, deepening of voice
16-17	Facial and body hair, acne	Arrest of skeletal growth
21	Arrest of skeletal growth	

(Wilkins L: The Diagnosis and Treatment of Endocrine Disorders in Childhood and Adolescence, 3rd ed. Springfield, Ill, Charles C Thomas, 1965)

Pubertal changes in girls also follow a predictable sequence (Table 2-5). Mammary budding is followed by the appearances of the first wisps of pubic hair, which is followed by evident estrogenic effects on vaginal epithelium and uterine size. Menstruation usually develops about 1½ years after the first indication of puberty.

The changes in bodily composition at puberty in girls primarily involve the sudden disposition of body fat about the hips, in the breasts, and quite generally throughout the body. The pubertal growth spurt is less pronounced in girls than in boys, and the increase in lean body mass is much less accelerated during puberty.

Tanner and his colleagues have introduced a staging scale for characterizing the pubertal changes of the male

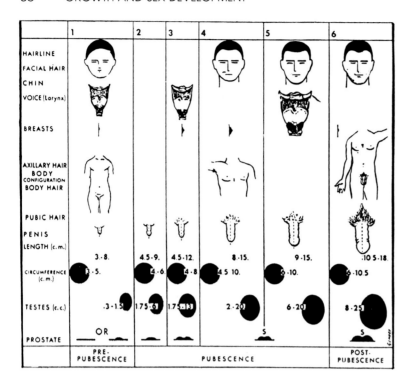

Fig. 2-13. Stages of sexual development and maturation. (From Schonfeld WA: Primary and secondary sexual characteristics. Am J Dis Child 65:535, 1943)

genitals, the female breast, and pubic hair in both sexes. Stage 1 in each scale is the prepubertal state and stage 5 is the full adult developmental state. The criteria used in staging are provided in Table 2-6. This staging scale has been widely accepted by endocrinologists and pediatricians.

Time of Occurrence of Puberty

The factors that determine the age of a child at puberty are still poorly understood. Nutritional, climatic, and racial influences have been recognized. Even in a single population under the same general environmental conditions, there may be great variability in the time of onset of pubertal changes. In some cases, distinct familial patterns of puberty development are recognized. Often the timing of puberty seems more closely correlated with other parameters of maturity than with calendar age. Children with advanced skeletal maturation and advanced height attainment tend to enter puberty at an earlier age, while poorly developed children with retarded bone maturation may be several years behind their peers at the onset of their puberty. The fact that many children with constitutionally delayed maturation have delayed pubertal growth spurt leads to exaggerated differences in height evident in peer groups from 12 to 15 years of age. These striking differences tend to decrease later in life.

Some indication of the variability of timing of normal puberty in boys is given in Figure 2-14. This chart shows

that normal puberty may commence any time between the ages of 10 and 14. In unusual cases, puberty may start quite early or quite late without being considered truly abnormal. Recognition of the important information set forth in this chart is of great assistance in counseling parents of children with minor disturbances of the timing of puberty.

The onset of puberty in girls precedes that of boys by about 2 years. The average age of peak velocity of growth occurs at about 12 years in girls and 14 years in boys (Figs. 2-3 and 2-4). The average age of menarche is a useful milestone for determining secular and geographic trends. In the United States, this is now about 12.7 years. The variability of the age of onset of puberty and the age of menarche in girls is equal to that in boys.

It has been observed in population studies of pubertal girls that the onset of menses correlates best with a weight of about 46 kg, suggesting that a critical body mass may be the important determinant of the timetable of puberty.

DISTURBANCE IN THE PUBERTAL MECHANISM

Delayed Puberty

Frequently physicians see children who have not shown pubertal changes by their 14th or 15th birthday. Fortunately, most of these children eventually enter a spontaneous puberty. A history of delayed puberty in

one or both parents with a comparable delay in height and skeletal maturation is reassuring. Malnutrition and chronic illness are important causes of delayed puberty. When none of these factors seems to be operative, serious consideration must be given to the possibility of endocrine disorders.

The physician should first determine whether the defect resides primarily in the gonads. Failure to find scrotal testes in boys suggests, but by no means establishes, primary hypogonadism as a cause of puberty failure. In the evaluation of delayed puberty in boys, the radioimmunoassay of FSH and LH in serum and urine has replaced the tedious and inaccurate bioassay of urinary gonadotropins. The presence of elevated concentrations of these hormones is indicative of gonadal failure. Decreased concentrations of these hormones does not necessarily mean that the gonads are capable of responding to tropic hormones because the pituitary phase of puberty may be delayed in some persons with gonadal causes of sexual infantilism.

When doubt exists concerning the adequacy of the gonads, the administration of chorionic gonadotropin (2000 IU, 2 to 3 times a week for 8 weeks), leads to unequivocal enlargement of the responsive testis and somatic evidence of testosterone production. In certain cases this procedure seems to be therapeutic as well as diagnostic, since the pubertal mechanism seems to follow shortly. It has been impossible to establish the validity of this clinical impression because some of these boys would have entered puberty spontaneously in the absence of gonadotropin administration. If there is little or no response to gonadotropin, gonadal inadequacy may be diagnosed.

In the presence of gonadal causes of sexual infantilism, the physician should consider developmental abnormalities of gonads related to sex chromosomal aberrations. A buccal smear may be sufficient to establish gonadal dysgenesis, but more elaborate chromosomal studies are required to define more complicated conditions. It is estimated that X chromosome abnormalities may account for as many as 40% to 50% of cases of sexual infantilism in girls.

Hypothalamicopituitary causes of failure of sexual development must be considered when levels of pituitary gonadotropins are low and the gonads are responsive to exogenous gonadotropins. The hypogonadotropism can be temporary (delayed puberty) or permanent (hypogonadotropic eunuchoidism). The deficiency of gonadotropic hormones need not be associated with deficiencies of other pituitary hormones. In the absence of recognizable gross pathology, it is often impossible to determine whether hypogonadotropism is due to a disturbance in pituitary or hypothalamic function. An increased gonadotropin

Table 2-6. *Tanner's Stages of Puberty*

Boys—genital development

Stage 1. Preadolescent. Testes, scrotum, and penis are of about the same size and proportion as in early childhood.
Stage 2. Enlargement of scrotum and testes. Skin of scrotum reddens and changes in texture. Little or no enlargement of penis at this stage.
Stage 3. Enlargement of penis, which occurs at first mainly in length. Further growth of testes and scrotum.
Stage 4. Increased size of penis with growth in breadth and development of glands. Testes and scrotum larger; scrotal skin darkened.
Stage 5. Genitalia adult in size and shape.

Girls—breast development

Stage 1. Preadolescent. Elevation of papilla only.
Stage 2. Breast bud stage. Elevation of breast and papilla as small mound. Enlargement of areola diameter.
Stage 3. Further enlargement and elevation of breast and areola with no separation of its contour.
Stage 4. Projection of areola and papilla to form a secondary mound above the level of the breast.
Stage 5. Mature stage. Projection of papilla only, owing to recession of the areola to the general contour of the breast.

Both sexes—pubic hair

Stage 1. Preadolescent. The vellus over the pubes is not developed further than that over the abdominal wall. No pubic hair
Stage 2. Sparse growth of long, slightly pigmented downy hair, straight or slightly curled, chiefly at the base of the penis or along labia.
Stage 3. Considerably darker, coarser, and more curled, the hair spreads sparsely over the junction of the pubes.
Stage 4. Hair now adult in type, but area covered is still considerably smaller than in the adult. No spread to the medial surface of thighs.
Stage 5. Hair adult in quantity and type with distribution of the horizontal (or classically feminine) pattern. Spread to medial surface of thighs but not up linea alba or elsewhere above the base of the inverse triangle. (Spread up linea alba occurs late and is rated stage 6.)

(Taken from the standard description in *Growth at Adolescence,* 2nd ed. Oxford, Blackwell Sci Publ, 1962. Used with permission)

concentration in the plasma following the administration of clomaphine or the gonadotropin-releasing hormone argues for a functional rather than an organic disease of the pituitary.

When the physician is considering the possibility of hypogonadotropic hypogonadism, the patient should be questioned concerning the acuteness of smell and tested with common odors such as coffee or crushed tobacco. If an abnormality is suspected, quantitative

and psychic factors frequently are involved in selective luteinizing hormone deficiency. Ovulation often follows clomaphine therapy.

Unresponsiveness of certain tissues to sex hormones may exist and distort pubertal development. In *testicular feminization,* partial or complete refractoriness to testosterone is present and the genotypic male develops into a phenotypic female lacking pubic and axillary hair and possessing labial testes. Inguinal hernias are often present. Vaginal examination discloses the absence of cervix and uterus. In less dramatic situations, the growth of facial, axillary, and pubic hair may not develop during puberty. Absence of facial hair is a racial characteristic of American Indians.

Increased sensitivity to mammogenic hormones may lead to mammary development long in advance of actual puberty and of the other physiologic and anatomic evidences of puberty. This condition has been called premature *thelarche.* Hormonal measurements have not clarified the nature of this disturbance. Plasma estrogens are at best only slightly elevated, and plasma prolactin levels are normal.

SUMMARY

Normal human growth is dependent on normal nutrition, normal endocrine function, and normal skeletal responsiveness. The fetus depends on the placenta for its nutrition; hormonal secretions of fetal endocrine glands are relatively unimportant in regulating fetal growth. While disorders of growth occur in abnormalities of X chromosome number, little is known of the autosomal genes that affect normal growth potential. Sequential accurate measurement of height, weight, and body proportions permit the early recognition of growth disorders. Growth hormone deficiency, thyroid hormone deficiency, and corticosteroid excess are important treatable endocrine causes of short stature. Accelerated growth velocity should alert the physician to the rare possibility of growth hormone excess or appropriate or inappropriate secretion of sex hormones.

Knowledge of the timing and sequence of normal pubertal development permits recognition of its abnormalities. Sexual precocity can result from the premature activation of the hypothalamic-pituitary-gonadal axis, or by sex steroid secretion by gonadal or adrenal neoplasms and by adrenal steroid dyshormonogenesis.

Failure of sexual development can be the result of hypothalamic, pituitary (gonadotropin), or gonadal disorders of hormone secretion.

BIBLIOGRAPHY

Bayley N, Pinneau, SR: Tables for predicting adult height from the skeletal age: Revised for use with the Greulich-Pyle hand standards. J Pediatr 40:423–441, 1952

Daughaday WH: Growth hormone and the somatomedins. In Avioli LV (ed): Endocrine Control of Growth. New York, Elsevier North-Holland, 1981

Falkner F, Tanner JM: Human Growth, Vol I, Principles and Prenatal Growth. Vol II, Postnatal Growth. Vol III, Neurobiology and Nutrition. New York, Plenum Press, 1978–1979

Greulich WW, Pyle SI: Radiographic Atlas of Skeletal Development of the Hand and Wrist, 2nd ed. Stanford, Stanford University Press, 1959

Powell GF, Brasel JA, Blizzard RM: Emotional deprivation and growth retardation simulating idiopathic hypopituitarism. I. Clinical evaluation of the syndrome. N Engl J Med 276:1271–1278, 1967

Rimoin DL, Horton WA: Medical progress, short stature. J Pediatr 92:523–528 and 697–704, 1978

Sizonenko PC: Endocrinology in preadolescents and adolescents. I. Hormonal changes during normal puberty. Am J Dis Child 132:704–712, 1978

Sizonenko PC: Preadolescent and adolescent endocrinology: Physiology and physiopathology. II. Hormonal changes during abnormal pubertal development. Am J Dis Child 132:797–805, 1978

Underwood LE, Van Wyk JJ: Hormones in normal and aberrant growth. In Williams RH (ed): Textbook of Endocrinology. Philadelphia, W B Saunders, 1981

3

Pain George L. Engel

Basic Characteristics of Pain
Neural Organization Serving Pain
  Receptors and Afferent Fibers
  Spinal Cord Modulating (Gate-Control) System
  Sensory-Discriminative System
  Motivational-Affective (Action) System
  Central Control (Cognitive) System
  Central Modulating Systems: Opioid and
    Nonopioid Mechanisms
  Summary
Pain and Psychosocial Development

Clinical Interpretation of Pain
  Clinical Implications of the Report of "Pain" or
    "No Pain"
  Profile of Pain
    Topographic Aspects (Location)
    Quantitative Aspects (Intensity)
    Temporal Aspects (Duration and Sequence)
    Qualitative Aspects (Descriptive Language)
    Associated Physiologic Aspects
    Behavioral and Psychosocial Aspects
Summary

BASIC CHARACTERISTICS OF PAIN

What is pain? At first glance the answer seems obvious enough. Every reader can at once refer to personal experience and be sure that he "knows" what pain is. Yet difficulties arise the moment one attempts to define pain in words. Perhaps before attempting to do so, it would be wise to consider the following facts about pain.[1–4] The reader will find it illuminating to be thinking about personal pain experiences while so doing:

1. *Pain is a private, subjective experience, information about which can come only from the sufferer.* Although one may sometimes be able to deduce from displayed behavior that a person is in pain, and even where the pain is located, details of the pain experience are contingent upon what the sufferer is able and willing to report. Consensual validation of the sensory experience is not possible. Hence the clinical diagnosis as well as the scientific investigation of pain must take into account the psychological processes governing how subjective experiences are communicated.

2. *Pain gives information primarily about the state of the body* and hence is more akin to thirst, hunger, and nausea than to seeing, hearing, tasting, smelling, or touching, which give information primarily about the environment.[5] Sensory experiences indicative of altered bodily states are not easily described, located, or quantified. Further, they tend to commit a person to a particular mode of behavior that serves specific bodily needs as well as survival in general. With pain this behavior is intimately related to avoidance of and recovery from injury.[5]

3. *What is experienced as pain commonly is combined with other bodily sensations such as pressure, stretching, pulling, heat, or cold.* To appreciate this the reader need only consider how one decides when a particular body sensation is, or is becoming, painful: the sensations experienced when sitting in an awkward position too long, when slowly pressing the point of a pencil into the palm of the hand, or when experiencing a strong intestinal contraction. Each of these involves a complex of sensations which, if intense enough, may ultimately be designated as

painful by some and merely as uncomfortable by others.

4. *Broadly speaking, the more intense a physical stimulation, the more likely is the ensuing sensation to be experienced as painful.* Further, this likelihood increases sharply as the stimulus approaches the threshold for tissue injury, (that is, as it becomes a noxious stimulus).[6] Yet it is also a fact that pain may be absent in the presence of injury and present in the absence of injury. *Thus, tissue injury is neither a necessary nor a sufficient condition for pain.*

5. *The experience of pain is inextricably linked with such disagreeable affective qualities* as suffering, discomfort, distress, misery, torture, and punishment. One suffers with pain, is afflicted with pain, is racked by pain, is tormented by pain. One is dominated by pain, is threatened by pain, is frightened by pain, is infuriated by pain, is exhausted by pain. Merely the prospect of pain characteristically evokes aversive responses. Yet paradoxically under some circumstances there can also be an element of pleasure or satisfaction in the suffering of pain, be it as pride in the ability ''to take it'' or as atonement and deserved punishment. Some persons knowingly or unknowingly even solicit pain. *Thus, pain, while basically unpleasant, may also be tinged with pleasure.*

6. *Only those parts of the body that have an afferent nerve supply belonging to the dorsal root system (or their analogues in the cranial nerves) can give rise to pain when physically stimulated.* Interrupting such nerve supply renders the part insensitive to direct stimulation and hence to pain. Yet a person may report pain in a limb that has been amputated (phantom pain), and psychological means (suggestion, hypnosis, conversion) may render what had been painful as painless and what had been painfree as painful. *Thus, neither physical stimulation of peripheral receptors nor an intact afferent nerve supply is necessary or sufficient for pain.* (See Chapter 30 for a more comprehensive discussion of conversion symptoms, malingering, and other psychological components of pain.)

7. *Both consciousness and attention are necessary to experience pain.* Pain may be ameliorated or eliminated by any influence that reduces consciousness or distracts attention. Conversely, pain may develop or intensify when attention is drawn to it. Yet, paradoxically, pain may be experienced during altered states of consciousness such as occur during dreaming and hypnosis.

8. *Psychological factors significantly influence how and when pain is experienced and reported.* An unpleasant body sensation is less likely to be experienced or reported as pain when it is familiar, understood, and known to be benign than when it is new, strange, and frightening. For some persons pain is a sign of weakness and must be hidden; for others it is a claim to special attention. For some it is an intolerable threat, which must be relieved at once; for others, it is a deserved punishment, which must be endured. For some, pain and suffering is a way of life; for others, it presents itself as an unwelcome intruder.

9. *Social and cultural influences also modify how different peoples react to and report pain.* In some cultures stoicism and self-control are virtues, whereas in others public expression of pain enjoys wide cultural approval. In some cultures pain has primarily health and medical implications, while in others it has magical and religious implications.

These nine characteristics identify pain as a complex psychological experience involving the concepts of injury and suffering but not contingent on actual physical injury. Simply the idea of injury, as well as the need to suffer, may lead to pain as readily as may an actual lesion or injury. Similarly, the wish not to suffer or not to accept the fact of injury may render an otherwise ''painful'' injury actually painless or at least cause it to be reported as ''painless.''

The clinician never deals directly with pain per se but only with what the patient is able to say about his pain. The reader need only try to put into words personal experiences of pain to appreciate the gap between what is experienced as pain and how it is reported. Pause for a moment and try it. The assessment of a particular sensory experience as ''pain'' rather than as some other sensation is clearly subject to the influences of the individual's current and past experience with pain. Thus, the same physical stimulus or psychological circumstance may be experienced and reported by different persons, or by the same person at different times, sometimes as pain, sometimes not. It also explains why actual injury is neither necessary nor sufficient for a sensation to be felt as pain, why pain may occur without input from peripheral afferents, and why pain and suffering may acquire pleasurable or satisfying qualities. In brief, pain does not exist as a felt experience and cannot be reported until and unless psychological processing of underlying physical events in the nervous system has already taken place.

Injury occupies a central position in the genesis of pain. Not only is physical injury the most reliable means of inducing pain, but aversive and protective responses are usual reactions to pain and serve to limit the effects of a noxious stimulus. Actually the stimulus threshold for pain is lower than that required to produce tissue damage.[6] Hence, pain may be felt *before*

actual injury takes place. Not only may pain mean that injury has taken place, it may also warn that injury *might* take place. In this way pain plays a critical role in learning which environmental circumstances may be injurious and how they are to be avoided. Psychologically speaking, the organism learns not what is injurious, but what is painful. This is the basis of aversive conditioning. Melzack showed that dogs raised in isolation from birth to maturity had markedly elevated thresholds for avoidance responses to electric shock, nose-burning, and pin pricks.[7] They behaved as if they did not know what was painful, what might be injurious, or how to avoid such stimuli. Evidently the development of the higher neural and psychic systems whereby the organism learns to appreciate and avoid what might be injurious requires experience with pain and injury early in life. Individuals born with congenital insensitivity to pain never seem to learn how to avoid injury; they suffer repeatedly from burns and fractures, and lose body parts.

By virtue of such superordinate systems to avoid injury, pain not only signals that the intensity of a stimulus is approaching the threshold for tissue damage, it also indicates that such a stimulus is currently present or that it *might* be present in the immediate future. *Thus, pain may signal that the threshold for injury is about to be or has already been exceeded, whereas absence of pain may convey the message "no injury," sometimes when injury is in fact present. Further, pain may come to symbolize injury, even in the absence of peripheral stimulation, if and when it serves the psychic need of the individual for it to do so.* In this way one may suffer pain when, for example, guilt imposes a need for punishment and atonement.

NEURAL ORGANIZATION SERVING PAIN

Despite great progress in the understanding of the neural organizations involved in pain, the clinical literature remains confusing because of the persistent use by many of the terminology and concepts of the outmoded 19th century specificity theory of pain. When pain is referred to as a specific sensation subserved by a straight-through "pain" transmission system from peripheral "pain" receptors to "pain" centers in the brain, a misleading concept of pain is generated and a logical category error is committed as well. To link the quality "pain" to receptors, fibers, or tracts, or to speak of "pain transmission," implies that their activation must always result in pain and only pain and that pain can originate only from direct stimulation of peripheral receptors or other components of the "pain" transmission system. Such a bias makes it difficult to understand how psychologic and social factors can contribute

to, and even at times be largely responsible for, pain as it occurs during dreams, hypnosis, suggestion, and conversion. Hence such mechanisms are generally omitted from discussions of the differential diagnosis of pain. This volume is no exception, and the reader will be well advised to regard as incomplete any discussion that limits pain mechanisms to those understandable only in terms of pain-sensitive structures. Every experienced clinician knows full well that many pain complaints simply cannot be explained on such a basis alone.

Another fault of traditional terminology is that anatomic, physiologic, and psychological frames of reference are confused, a category error. The neural system activity, which may ultimately result in the psychologic experience we call pain, serves many other functions as well, chiefly the general functions of warning against, escaping from, and recovering from tissue or bodily injury. Hence. it is more accurately designated the *nociceptive-nocifensive* system. Pain is not a form of stimulation; it is not something transmitted from one anatomic site to another. Rather, pain is a sensory and psychological function of the nociceptive-nocifensive system.

The gate-control theory of pain, developed since 1965 by Melzack and his coworkers, goes a long way to satisfy the requirements for a theory more capable of encompassing all the characteristics of pain.[8-10] It is also more consistent with the recent general systems approach to the understanding of biology and medicine (the biopsychosocial model).[11] Gate-control theory postulates a complex of feedback inhibitory and facilitory processes which operate at all levels of the neuraxis and which ultimately determine how and when activity of the nociceptive system is experienced, responded to, and reported as pain. Four levels of neural organization are involved:

1. *A modulating (gating) spinal cord system,* which controls the amount of input transmitted from receptors and peripheral fibers through the dorsal-horn transmission cells, which in turn project to the ascending fibers in the anterolateral cord

2. *A sensory discriminative system* whereby incoming stimuli are localized in space and time and along an intensity continuum

3. *A motivational-affective (action) system,* which serves as a central intensity monitor and which contributes to the quality of unpleasantness, mobilizes internal defenses, and drives the organism into behaviors aimed at avoiding or stopping the distress

4. *A central control (cognitive) system,* which evaluates and analyzes input in terms of past experience, probability of outcome, and symbolic meaning. It

regulates response and behavior through facilitating or inhibiting influences on the discriminative and action systems, as well as on input through the spinal gate-control system

Before elaborating on these four neural components, it is first necessary to describe the neural organization whereby potentially injurious physical stimuli are detected and fed into the central nervous system: receptors and afferent fibers.

RECEPTORS AND AFFERENT FIBERS

Two basic kinds of receptor organs serving body sensory function can be distinguished: bare nerve endings and specialized corpuscular receptors.[12–14] They differ in their capacity to transduce mechanical, thermal, and chemical energy into electrical impulses. The corpuscular endings are mainly responsive to various forms of deformation (mechanical energy), including vibration (Pacinian corpuscles). Free nerve endings, on the other hand, are sensitive to all the physical modalities, but different endings differ in their sensitivity as well as in their threshold to different stimuli. Particularly important are high-threshold, free nerve endings that respond only at levels of mechanical or heat stimulation where actual tissue injury is imminent. They are properly designated *nociceptors*. Such receptors characteristically show continued or delayed firing even after the initiating physical stimulus has been discontinued. They also show the property of sensitization after repeated or prolonged stimulation so that the threshold for their activation can diminish to levels of intensity that are ordinarily innocuous.[15] Chemical substances formed in tissues in response to injury may be responsible for this increased sensitivity, especially some of the humoral mediators released during acute inflammation.[16,17] The most promising candidates seem to be peptides of the bradykinin group, which have algesic effects in minute quantities, well within the range of naturally occurring biologic agents. Since kinin formation takes place after a latency period of 15 seconds to 30 seconds following tissue injury and does not reach a peak for another 10 seconds to 15 seconds, their effect on threshold could well contribute to the continued or delayed firing of high-threshold receptors. Important too are prostaglandins, which sensitize tissues to the pain-provoking and fever-inducing effects of other substances, especially the kinins.[18] All of these attributes of high-threshold receptors equip them to provide to higher neural levels information about high-intensity stimuli potentially or actually capable of inducing tissue damage.

The axons serving the receptors vary in size. The larger myelinated fibers (A-alpha and A-beta) serve low-threshold mechanoreceptors that provide information about innocuous mechanical stimuli. The higher threshold receptors are served by smaller fibers (A-delta and C). Fiber size also correlates with conduction velocity. The larger fibers are the most rapidly conducting. The smallest fibers are the slowest conducting. The larger fibers belong to the phylogenetically newer sensory systems, which ascend with few relays to posterior thalamus and project to the somesthetic cortex. The smaller fibers belong to the phylogenetically older sensory systems. They have shorter ascending pathways with multiple relays terminating variously in the reticular formation of the medulla and tegmentum, or in the intralaminar nuclei of the thalamus.[19]

The distribution of receptors and fibers is important for the understanding of the nature of sensory information derived from the body. The surface of the body, including orificial mucous membranes, is the most extensively innervated. The basic receptor supply of skin and mucous membrane is in the form of networks of free nerve endings, the so-called dermal-nerve networks, each of which is derived from several terminal fibers forming an interweaving arborization, although without fusion between axons of neighboring nerves.[20] Thus, stimulation at any point always invokes impulses flowing up several nerve fibers to the cells of the dorsal root ganglia. A wide spectrum of fiber sizes is involved in these networks, from the large A-beta to the small C fibers.

Except for the muscle spindle and the proprioceptors of joint capsules and tendons, all other innervated deep structures, visceral as well as somatic, are served by free nerve endings of fine fibers of the A-delta and C range. These are much more sparsely distributed than in skin. Most of the visceral receptors are mechanosensitive, but some may be sensitive to the chemical products of tissue damage. The latter are connected with small *paravascular* fibers (not to be confused with the *perivascular* plexus, which is sympathetic), which run parallel with small blood vessels down to the level of capillaries and which are peripheral axons of dorsal root ganglia.[21]

Afferent nerves have a definite segmental distribution, each dorsal root serving a particular segment. On the surface of the body they are topographically distributed as the cutaneous dermatomes, which overlap somewhat with each other and slightly cross the midline (Figs. 3-1, 3-2). For deeper somatic structures, such as muscles, tendons, and fascia, the distribution of afferents corresponds with the motor innervation. In

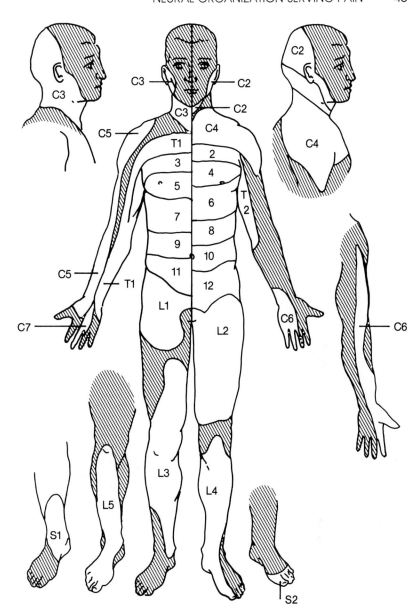

Fig. 3-1. Front view of dermatomal distribution. The right and left halves show the total distribution of alternating dermatomes, thereby illustrating the degree of overlap. In some regions, however, overlap is very great, and more than two dermatomes may be involved. Hence, additional figures (*insets*) are necessary to show the total distribution of certain dermatomes. (Adapted from Gardner E: Gross anatomy of the peripheral nervous system. In Dyck PJ, Thomas PK, Lambert EH (eds): Peripheral Neuropathy, Vol I. Philadelphia, WB Saunders, 1975)

contrast, the segmental innervation of the viscera derives from levels of embryologic origin rather than from the actual anatomic location. The visceral afferents run centripetally in the sympathetic and parasympathetic nerves, pass through the ganglia without synapse, and reach the posterior roots through the rami communicantes. Visceral and cutaneous afferents converge on some of the same sensory interneurons in the dorsal horn. The afferents from such structures as the heart, aorta, biliary ducts, and upper gastrointestinal tract pass through sympathetic ganglia, those from trachea and bronchi traverse the vagi, and those from the lower bowel, urinary bladder, uterine cervix, and prostate traverse the parasympathetic rami of the sacral nerves.[22]

SPINAL CORD MODULATING (GATE-CONTROL) SYSTEM

In the original formulation of their theory, Melzack and Wall postulated a mechanism whereby rostral flow of small-fiber activity through the dorsal horn could be modulated by large-fiber activity.[8-10] They designated this functionally as a "gating" mechanism regulating

on the dorsal horn transmission cells whose axons project to the brain. Large fibers were thought to excite the SG, thereby reducing presynaptic transmission (closing the gate), and small fibers to inhibit the SG, thereby reducing presynaptic inhibition (opening the gate). While this particular explanation has not been fully verified, the net effect is a mechanism controlling how much activity of small and large fibers, respectively, ultimately progresses rostrally. Evidence indicates that a relative preponderance of small-fiber activity favors the eventual interpretation of the stimulus as noxious, if not as pain, once some integrated form of the input is allowed to reach higher neural centers. As we shall discuss later, such rostral flow also may be inhibited or facilitated by downflowing activity originating from spinal cord, brain stem, limbic system, and even sensorimotor cortex before it is finally processed as "pain."

SENSORY-DISCRIMINATIVE SYSTEM

The sensory-discriminative system is composed of those medium to large-sized myelinated fibers that reach the ventral nucleus of the thalamus and project to the somesthetic area of the cortex.[8–10] It is served in part by two main tracts: the dorsal column-medial lemniscal and the neospinothalamic. The first, phylogenetically the most recently developed, arises from the large A-beta fibers, which ascend in the dorsal column to their first relay in the cuneate and gracile nuclei, from whence they pass upward in the medial lemniscus and terminate in the ventrobasal complex of the thalamus. The neospinothalamic tract, derived mainly from A gamma-delta fibers, originates in the ventral horn, crosses in the ventral white commissure of the cord, and ascends in the anterolateral column. Some fibers terminate in the posterior nuclear complex of the thalamus, while others join the medial lemniscus to terminate in the ventrobasal complex of the thalamus. The latter sends projections to the second sensory area of the cortex and probably makes the larger contribution to sensory-discriminative function.

The sensory-discriminative system is organized along precise topographic lines and shows high fidelity in following alterations in the spatial, temporal, and intensity properties of the stimulus constituting the input.[23] This is strikingly so with respect to the larger fiber input of the lemniscal system, less so with the input of the neospinothalamic tract, which terminates in the posterior thalamic nuclei. Various studies indicate exquisite preservation of specificity throughout the lemniscal system. As an impulse ascends from a single locus in the periphery, the receptive fields in the dorsal column nuclei, thalamus, and sensory cortex grow

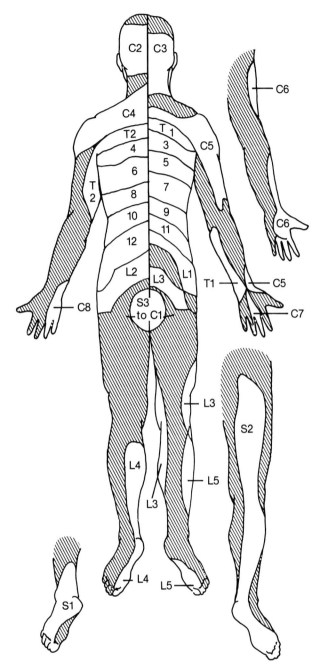

Fig. 3-2. Back view of dermatomes. (Adapted from Gardner E: Gross anatomy of the peripheral nervous sytem. In Dyck PJ, Thomas PK, Lambert EH (eds): Peripheral Neuropathy, Vol I. Philadelphia, WB Saunders, 1975)

inflow from the periphery and assigned it to substantia gelatinosa (SG) cells in the dorsal horn. It was suggested that SG cells exerted presynaptic inhibition on both large- and small-fiber terminals as they synapsed

progressively larger as one proceeds rostrally. Mount-castle proposes that information concerning spatial, temporal, and intensity relationships is extracted from the profile of activity in this large population of cells when activated from a discrete peripheral locus. Thus the lemniscal system provides discriminative information as to the origins of noxious stimuli. The very rapid transmission rates of these large fibers means that the lemniscal system receives information first and therefore can selectively modulate, through corticofugal impulses, slower messages along the smaller fibers before they get to the horn.[8]

The segment of the neospinothalamic tract that terminates in the posterior nuclear complex of the thalamus has much less specificity than does the lemniscal system. Thus, a given cell in the thalamus may be responsive to a variety of modalities of stimulation, and these unit cell responses may be evoked from distantly separated parts of the body. Since aversive functions may also be elicited from this region of the thalamus, it is possible that this part of the system contributes the quality of "hurting."[24,25] This view receives some support from the observation that surgical lesions in the ventrobasal nuclei of the thalamus of patients with intractable pain may produce profound deficit in sensory discrimination without relieving pain, whereas lesions in posterior nuclei may give pain relief without interfering with sensibility.[26,27]

MOTIVATIONAL-AFFECTIVE (ACTION) SYSTEM

The obvious role of pain in protecting the organism from injury warrants close attention to the neural system concerned with escape, avoidance, and defense.[8–10] The reticular system, particularly the bulbar reticular formation, is an important part of this neural complex. Cells in this region respond maximally to activation of A-delta and C fibers and to intense natural stimuli, which leads to escape behavior.[28,29] Involved is the phylogenetically older ascending tract (paleospino-thalamic), which originates in the small fibers (A gamma-delta, C range). This paramedial ascending system has numerous relays, and neither it nor the structures with which it connects are organized to provide discrete spatial or temporal information. A striking feature of the paramedial ascending system is its strategic relation to the limbic system and associated structures through reciprocal interconnections in the midbrain central gray area. It has been suggested that these systems may also function as a central intensity monitor. Cells in the medial brain stem that show summation and prolonged afterdischarge in relation to input from spatially separated and temporally dispersed units could transform discrete spatial and temporal information into intensity information.[30] Beyond a certain intensity level, it is suggested, the output of these monitoring cells would signal to the neural systems involved in protecting the organism against trauma that a noxious event is threatening or is already taking place. In this way are activated the affective and motivational behaviors that together constitute an integrated behavioral mode to deal with injury, of which pain is but one component.

CENTRAL CONTROL COGNITIVE SYSTEM

Pain thus far has been considered in terms of its sensory and affective components and the neural system serving each. Still to be accounted for are the central control factors determining how and whether the sensory input is perceived and/or the action system controlled. How do factors such as memory, attention, past experience, anticipation, and the symbolic meaning of pain determine when and how pain is experienced, responded to, and reported? These processes presumably are served by neocortical functions. It is now well established that forebrain structures, through corticofugal influences, can act on both the sensory-discriminative and the motivational-affective systems. As already discussed, descending inhibitory influences exerted at the dorsal horn cells can affect the gate-control system so that input is modulated before it even reaches either the discriminative or the motivational system. Extensive interconnection among sensory and associational cortical areas and reticular and limbic structures provides a means of mediating between cognitive activities and the motivational-affective features of pain. Such relationships may account for the effect of prefrontal lobotomy or certain drugs in reducing the suffering of pain without eliminating pain, for conversion pain, or for pain induced by suggestion or hypnosis, in which the idea of injury, but no actual injury, is implicated.

The central control system also serves to evaluate the input in terms of present and past experience and to modulate it before it activates the discriminative or motivational systems. In this way a "painful" injury may be rendered "painless" during the heat of battle or sport, or the "pain" of disease may be successfully denied; in brief, perception of "pain" does not take place. This is rendered possible by the rapid conduction properties of the pathways reaching the cortex, permitting information carried by them to undergo analysis, interact with other sensory input, and activate memory stores and preset response strategies so that the activation of central control processes can be begun *before* the pain response has developed (for example, the decision whether to drop a hot teacup or

to put it down gently). Subsequent pain behavior then undergoes integration and modification in terms of the continous monitoring of the central control system.

CENTRAL MODULATING SYSTEMS—OPIOID AND NONOPIOID MECHANISMS

A complex array of descending and ascending feedback loops provides a means of modulating the input and output of the nociceptive system. In this way are determined the ultimate patterns of response, including pain, to nociceptive information, whether it originates as small-fiber activity in the periphery or as psychological constructs in higher cortical areas. For example, the down-flowing corticospinal and corticoreticular tracts impinge on all levels of the reticular formation and spinal cord. The thalamic nuclei send tracts down to the reticular formation. They also receive messages from the cortex through motor, sensory, and association fibers, as well as from other structures. Stimulation of the periaqueductal gray (PAG) in midbrain and diencephalon, as well as (though less consistently) stimulation of the caudate nucleus, the septum, and posterior limb of the internal capsule results in relief of pain from various causes.[31] Similarly, distress vocalizations produced in guinea pigs by electrical stimulation of the dorsomedial thalamus or the ventral septum-preoptic area also are inhibited by PAG stimulation.[32] Such inhibition of nociceptive responses by PAG stimulation in man and animals demonstrates the modulating role of ascending pathways in response to nociceptive information. From the clinical perspective such observations underscore the misnomer "pain transmission." Pain is felt and expressed only after nociceptive information has undergone modulation at many levels of the neural system protecting the organism from injury. Pavlov's demonstration more than 50 years ago that hungry dogs could be conditioned to respond neutrally, even pleasurably, to burns or electric shocks as the stimuli for feeding is a case in point. Under such conditions they displayed not even the most subtle signs of pain, yet they continued to respond appropriately to other painful stimuli.[33]

Various mechanisms have been implicated in the central modulation of nociception. The discovery of opiate receptors and endogenous opioids in the brain quite naturally generated a veritable flood of interest in their role in endogenous pain control. Here again archaic language (e.g., "pain transmission") has tended to blur the distinction between pain as experience and the many other functions of the nociceptive system. Opioids (endorphins) and opiate receptors are in fact widely distributed in the nervous system, as well as elsewhere in the body, including areas not heretofore associated with pain or even nociception (e.g., globus pallidus).[34,35,36] Evidently opioid-mediated mechanisms are involved in a great variety of neural processes in addition to those specifically concerned with pain and nociception.

By the same token the modulation of nociception and of pain is not solely dependent on mechanism involving the opioids; other mechanisms are involved as well. Again, from the clinical point of view, it is well to remember that the action of opiates on humans is less a specific blunting of pain sensations than it is an emotional detachment from the state of suffering. Hence, while inhibition of aversive responses may be more dependent on descending controls "closing the gate" at spinal levels, the alleviation of pain as suffering may be more dependent on ascending influences on higher level feedback control systems.

Whatever else may be the functions of the opioid-mediated system, there is no question of its implication in the nociceptive apparatus.[31] Virtually all of the structures heretofore associated with the latter appear to be served by opioid-peptide sensitive neurons. An important relay is located in cells in the PAG and periventricular gray matter, which are activated by morphine and blocked by the morphine antagonist naloxone. Direct stimulation of PAG inhibits pain in humans and pain-associated behavior in animals. Well established in bringing about this effect is a descending efferent brainstem pathway that inhibits neuronal firing precisely in those cells that receive primary afferent input from small diameter somatic and visceral fibers and are maximally responsive to noxious stimuli. Little is as yet known about ascending connections with higher centers. The presence of such connections is suggested by the fact that pain relief brought about by electrical stimulation of the central gray matter in humans may exceed the period of stimulation by hours.[37] If actually experiencing pain is a precondition for activating the feedback loop, then descending connections from higher centers must also exist.

Other modulating systems not involving opioids also operate. Thus pain relief, sometimes prolonged, obtained by subcutaneous stimulation of peripheral nerves or of the dorsal column is not opioid-dependent.[38] These may depend on segmental mechanisms, perhaps involving antidromic activation of primary afferent collaterals that terminate in the dorsal horn.[31] The painful dysesthesias associated with deafferentation syndromes, which probably involve spontaneous firing of cells in the cord and brain, is relieved neither by opiates nor by PAG stimulation but is ameliorated by

chronic stimulation of the somatosensory system. Such stimulation is presumably mediated by an activation of the corticofugal fibers and does not involve opioids.[31] Inescapable foot shock yields profound analgesia in rats. When the shock is prolonged and intermittent, the opioid mechanism is involved; when brief and continous, a nonopioid system is activated.[39] With the prolonged shock schedule the animals appeared to become "behaviorally depressed." Analgesia induced in mice by defeat in a social confrontation is also opioid-dependent.[40] These observations suggest that the opioid mechanism may be more prone to be activated the more overwhelmed the animal is by the noxious circumstance. Even a threat of being overwhelmed may suffice. Thus, once an animal is conditioned to anticipate inescapable shock, a single shock is sufficient to activate the opioid system.[41,42] In addition, it has been found that hypnotic analgesia involves a nonopioid system unless the individual feels himself to be in a "no-solution" situation ("stress"), in which case opioids are involved.[43,44] It would appear that the opioid system is especially likely to be involved under circumstances where intolerable pain would threaten the organism's survival, as when it is necessary to continue to struggle despite injury or to be inactive and rest to recover from injury.[5] Under both of these circumstances alleviation of pain clearly would have survival value.

SUMMARY

Pain is the felt part of a nociceptive and nocifensive organization, the neural structures of which are widely represented throughout the neuraxis. For neural input or information to be experienced as pain, the higher neural processes involved in interpretation, evaluation, and feeling must be functionally intact. Inhibition of input may take place anywhere between the site of input and the cortex, where the highest level of psychological elaboration takes place. Pain may ultimately eventuate from stimulation of normal receptors (nociceptors) delivering their information into a normal nervous system; from stimulation of sensitized nociceptors firing into a normal nervous system; or from stimulation of nociceptors, normal or sensitized, firing into an abnormal nervous system. Pain may also eventuate from activity orginating within the central nervous system, as when peripheral or central lesions induce abnormal neuron states with spontaneous firing or interrupt control systems. Finally, pain may be experienced when psychological processes increase awareness of spontaneous firing from the periphery and/or reactivate memories of one's own or of witnessed pain experiences from the past ("psychogenic" pain). (See Chapter 30.)[3, 45]

PAIN AND PSYCHOSOCIAL DEVELOPMENT

Pain is not simply the expression of a biologic system concerned with protecting the body from injury.[3] As suffering it also contributes to moral and ethical values and plays a major role in the regulation of behavior and interpersonal relationships. It is a means whereby attributes of the environment are judged as safe or dangerous, as well as an instrument whereby power and control may be exercised. In the course of development, pain becomes complexly related in the mind to such polarities as good–bad, love–hate, innocent–guilty, reward–punishment, and victory–defeat. The learning processes involved in the development of such values for the most part take place in childhood and presumably are represented in the central control (cognitive) system, which provides the memory traces influencing whether and under what circumstances pain and suffering may be felt.

Among the earliest functions of pain in infancy is its contribution to the process of differentiation of the body from the environment and the formation of a body image. When the baby first bites too hard on his own finger, he is learning that what hurts is part of his own body. Szasz suggests that this early psychic equation may contribute to a later use of pain as a means of denying the loss of a body part (*e.g.*, phantom pain after amputation).[2]

Early pain experiences also form the basis for numerous conditioning experiences, which determine the readiness to feel pain or be relieved of pain under some circumstances and not under others. The familiar sequence of the pain of minor injuries disappearing as the child is comforted by the mother underlies the magical belief that mother's display of affection is what makes the pain go away. (Mother kisses the pain away.) This has its counterpart in the amelioration of pain often felt by patients as soon as the physician is seen as caring about their suffering and concerned with its relief (the placebo effect). The child also may find that by exhibiting pain and suffering one may influence others, as by gaining sympathy, earning love, or making others feel guilty.

The common association of pain with punishment provides the basis for a relationship between pain and feelings of guilt. For the child, pain is inflicted when one is bad. It is an easy step from this to the notion that pain signifies guilt, often expressed by patients as "What have I done to deserve such pain (suffering)"?

By the same token pain may also be used to expiate feelings of guilt. The development of such an association is especially likely to occur in children whose early relationships were marked by frequent painful punishments followed by contrite reconciliations. For such children suffering pain may come to represent a necessary condition for both the alleviation of guilt and the reconciliation with a loved one. In this way pain and suffering may anticipate pleasure, and some patients may suffer pain rather than feel guilt (the "pain-prone" patient).[3]

The child also is not long in discovering the association between pain and aggression and power. He soon realizes that he too can impose his will on others by inflicting or threatening to inflict pain, but he also learns that he may control his own aggression by threatening himself with pain. This provides an intrapsychic method of controlling aggression, since an aggressive act may be forestalled by experiencing pain instead.

When such psychic determinants are strong enough, the readiness to feel pain may be greatly enhanced and pain experienced with little or no afferent input from peripheral receptors. This may be an important consideration underlying some chronic pain syndromes, as will be discussed later.

CLINICAL INTERPRETATION OF PAIN

THE CLINICAL IMPLICATIONS OF THE REPORT OF "PAIN" OR "NO PAIN"

The compelling issue for the physician is to explain why a patient is complaining of pain. Equally important, paradoxically, he must also explain sometimes why a patient is *not* complaining of pain. Such an emphasis on whether the patient *reports* pain or no pain identifies operationally the data upon which the physician depends for evaluation of pain.

The complaint of "pain" may reflect any one, or combination, of the following:

1. *The presence of local tissue injury* or of a stimulus approaching the threshold of tissue injury in structures supplied with high-threshold afferents (nociceptors)
2. *A local afferent input that has become associated in the mind with the threat of injury or disease* so that a sensation not previously felt as painful is felt and reported as pain (*e.g.*, a vague abdominal sensation reported as pain by a patient fearful of cancer)
3. *Peripheral or central nervous system damage* that interferes with the normal modulation (*e.g.*, the neural-

gias, causalgia, deafferentation pain and "central" pain)
4. *A lowered threshold to fear or threat of injury*, as may occur with suggestion when under social or interpersonal pressure (*e.g.*, "sympathetic pain")[46]
5. *An unconscious psychological need to suffer or to be punished* or to assume the role of a sufferer, where a pain previously associated with physical trauma or the infliction of punishment is taken as the paradigm of suffering (*e.g.*, conversion, which is discussed in Chapter 30)
6. *A conscious and deliberate attempt to deceive others* for personal gain (malingering)

On the other hand, a report of "no pain" may indicate the following:

1. *No injury or tissue damage or no peripheral stimulation* approaching the threshold of tissue damage
2. *Destroyed receptors or blocked afferent nerves or pathways*, which are incapable of transmitting impulses centrally
3. *No afferent nerve supply capable of transmitting impulses into the dorsal root system* in the tissue or structure involved in a pathologic process (*e.g.*, lung parenchyma)
4. *The chemical or physical properties of a given pathologic process* are not such as to activate the receptors, fibers, or ascending connections of the dorsal root system (*e.g.*, acute lymphadenitis is painful; the lymphadenopathy of lymphoma is not)
5. *Insufficient level of patient consciousness or attention* to interpret the quality of the sensory experience as pain or to report it as pain
6. *Psychological factors* influencing the patient to reject notions of injury or suffering; hence, body sensations not experienced as pain
7. *Psychological or social factors* influencing the patient not to report that he is indeed suffering pain

THE PROFILE OF PAIN

The characteristics of pain as experienced and reported are the products of physiologic, psychological, and social determinants. The physiologic determinants include the nature of the physical stimuli impinging on receptors, the response characteristics of receptors and afferent fibers, the level of arousal (awareness), and the capability of the sensory-discriminative systems to analyze the input. Psychological and social determinants include the significance for the patient of the pain in terms of injury and of suffering; the role of the patient's past experiences, idiosyncratic as well as those determined by cultural influences; the life-setting and

psychological status of the patient at the time of the pain and its reporting; the patient's level of attention and his ability to communicate verbally the nature of what he is experiencing. The effects of such factors are by no means random. On the contrary, they endow pain experiences with a sufficient degree of predictability to enable the physician to reconstruct from the patient's verbal account the nature of the underlying physiologic and psychosocial processes responsible for the pain. It is precisely for this reason that a firm grasp of physiologic and psychosocial principles is essential for the diagnostic process.

For the purposes of diagnosis it is useful to classify pain according to the relative importance of the sources of input ("information") underlying each pain reported by the patient. Sources may be classified as peripheral, neurogenic, and psychogenic (Table 3-1).

Peripheral sources include all afferent input originating from receptors of the dorsal root system and its cranial nerve equivalents. These may be subdivided into *superficial somatic, deep somatic,* and *visceral.*

Neurogenic refers to input so modified by damage to the peripheral or central nervous system that it is experienced as pain. Such pain may result from abnormal processing of normal afferent activity or from paroxysmal activity generated within the nervous system itself.

Psychogenic sources include fantasies, memories, wishes, needs, conflicts, or impulses involving ideas of injury, aggression, sadism, punishment, atonement, masochism, or suffering, any of which may contribute to pain occurrence or pain intensification through such psychological mechanisms as suggestion, hypnosis, activation of memory traces of previous pains, and symbolization. "Sympathetic" pain, conversion pain, hypochondriacal pain, delusional pain, and malingered pain are important clinical examples.

The profile of pain includes six dimensions that reflect the respective roles of the underlying neurophysiologic and psychosocial processes implicated in pain and its reporting. The characterization of any pain experience requires exploration of all of these dimensions. They include

1. *Topographic aspects*—the bodily location
2. *Quantitative aspects*—intensity
3. *Temporal aspects*—duration and sequence
4. *Qualitative aspects*—descriptive language
5. *Associated physiologic aspects*—spontaneous physiologic processes that aggravate or alleviate the pain
6. *Behavioral and psychosocial aspects*—behavior induced by or associated with the pain and the psychologic and social meanings of pain

Topographic Aspects (Location)

As a source of information about bodily states, pain is always assigned a body location by one experiencing pain. Structures with the most extensive innervation are the most fully represented centrally in the body image and are the sites of the most precisely localized pain.

Superficial somatic structures, such as skin and subcutaneous tissue, fascia and fibrous tissue encasing the limbs and trunk (*e.g.,* intercostal fascia and parietal pleura), and periosteum, ligaments, and tendon sheaths situated subcutaneously, all are relatively richly supplied with receptors and fibers of widely ranging threshold and size. Hence, pain resulting from noxious stimulation of these regions is likely to be relatively well localized (see Figs. 8-5 and 8-6).

The more sparsely innervated, deeper somatic structures and viscera give rise to pain that is more diffuse and poorly localized. Further, pain from the deeper structure is not necessarily felt in its actual topographic location but is referred according to the spinal segmental distribution of its innervation. Such reference of pain to somatic areas of like dermatomal origin is thought to be due to the convergence of afferents from both deep and superficial structures on the same pool of cells in the posterior horn (see Fig. 8-1). Since the main contribution to the sensory-discriminative system arises from the larger fibers innervating more superficial structures, input from the viscera and other deep structures is thought to arise from these more familiar somatic segments. Occasionally, visceral disease may also be associated with segmental cutaneous hyperesthesia and hyperalgesia. This may be explained in terms of the facilitating effect of small-fiber activity from the affected viscus lowering the threshold of dorsal horn transmission cells to simultaneous small-fiber activity from the skin.

Since the afferent supply of individual viscera generally enters the cord through several adjacent roots, pain of visceral origin usually is felt somewhere within the segmental distribution of several roots. Sometimes it may be felt as well within the zone of immediately neighboring roots. For example, the sensory supply of the heart derives mainly from the first three thoracic roots (T1–T3), with the predominant input from the left (see Figs. 8-16 and 8-17). The most common sites of pain from myocardial ischemia include behind the sternum; the left pectoral region and shoulder; along the inner aspect of the left arm to the elbow; and occasionally in the back, usually in the midline or just to the left. All of these are within the distribution of T1 to T3. However, pain may also be felt on the right side,

Table 3-1. *Pain Profile in Relation to Source of Input*

	Location	Intensity	Temporal Aspects	Description	Associated Physiologic Aspects	Behavior
SUPERFICIAL SOMATIC	Surface; well localized	Basically correlated with intensity of stimulation	Correlates with tempo of input and extent of afterdischarge	In terms of familiar surface injuries; mainly determined by spatial-temporal intensity dimensions	Intensified by contact; alleviated by gentle stimulation in adjacent areas	Guarding of involved area; application of warmth, cold, soothing agent, counterirritation
DEEP SOMATIC	Segmental; deep; poorly localized; radiates; referred to surface	Basically correlated with intensity of stimulation	Correlates with tempo of input and extent of afterdischarge	Vague, aching, sharp, boring, pounding; mainly determined by spatial-temporal intensity dimensions	Intensified by movement, compression, pulsation (artery); alleviated by inactivity	Avoidance of movement, pressure; awkward movement owing to protective spasm
VISCERAL	Segmental; deep; poorly localized; radiates; referred to surface	Basically correlated with intensity of stimulation	Correlates with tempo of input and extent of afterdischarge	Gripping, cramping, aching, squeezing, crushing, stabbing, burning; mainly determined by spatial-temporal intensity dimensions	Intensified by motor activity or compression of involved viscus; correlates with secretory or motor rhythms of involved viscus	Trial and error behavior to relieve pain, based on physiologic concomitants, previous experience, psychic factors
NEUROGENIC	Within neural distribution; surface or deep; radiates	Excessive response to stimulation	No correlation with input; delayed	Indescribable; disagreeable; unlike any naturally occurring pain; unusual combination of painful sensations	Provoked by any peripheral stimulation in involved zone; trigger points "spontaneous" paroxysms	Vigilant guarding of involved part—apprehensive concern
PSYCHOGENIC	According to body image or appropriate to fantasy; surface or deep; well or poorly localized; may radiate	Variable; correlates with psychic needs for suffering, intensity of guilt, aggression, depression; inconsistent with severity of concurrent organic process	Variable; correlates with individual notions of injury, suffering, or disease	Vivid psychic imagery; correlates with notions of suffering, punishment, torture; variable; inconsistent; elaborated; spatial-temporal intensity dimensions vague or inconsistent with organic processes	Inconsistent or no correlation with physiologic processes	Emphasis on suffering; discrepancy between appearance and intensity of pain reported; distractible; background of violence or aggression; sadistic or masochistic attitudes. Importance of pain in past or current relationships; prominence of pain in family; pain seen as punishment or atonement; response to loss

behind the lower sternum, and even substernally (T4–T5), as well as down the inner side of the forearm to the fourth and fifth fingers (C8). Rarely it may be felt in the neck, throat, lower jaw, or ear, suggesting the spread to the lower and then upper cervical segments and to the sensory roots of the fifth and tenth cranial nerves.

Clinical experience also demonstrates that past or concurrent painful processes involving neighboring or overlapping segments may enhance the tendency to feel the pain in spinal segments shared by both distributions, sometimes resulting in an atypical location of the pain. Thus anginal pain may be referred to the right arm in a patient with a recent fracture of the humerus or to the epigastrium in a patient with a history of duodenal ulcer.[47]

Pain from deep structures, and especially from the viscera, is commonly reported as *radiating;* that is, it is felt to extend in some direction from some primary focus. Cardiac pain, for example, may be described as beginning retrosternally and radiating to the left shoulder and down the inner side of the left arm; gallbladder pain may be felt to originate in the right hypochondrium and to radiate to the angle of the scapula. Radiations are generally within the segmental innervation of the affected organ. They probably reflect the recruitment by the developing pathologic process of additional receptors so that more spinal segments become involved. Patterns of radiation with different disorders have a relatively high degree of consistency and hence are of diagnostic value. Occasionally pain may radiate toward the focus of the disease rather than away from it (*inverse radiation*). Thus, the pain of angina pectoris may sometimes begin the the hypogastrium and radiate upward; or it may radiate up to the sternum from the fingers, wrist, forearm, elbow, or arm on one or both sides.

When pain originates from actual involvement of a nerve root or trunk, its distribution typically follows quite exactly the afferent distribution of the root or nerve. Thus, a herniated intervertebral disc compressing the fifth lumbar root (L5) gives pain that extends down the posterior thigh and leg and is felt deeply as well as superficially (Fig. 11–6). Pain associated with thalamic damage has a contralateral hemiplegic distribution with a predilection for the extremities.

The locations of pain personally experienced or observed in someone else presumably are recorded centrally as part of the body image. Such pain memories provide the basis for conversion or for malingered pain, the location of which is determined by the meaning of the pain to the sufferer, not by the nature of the afferent innervation of the painful body region. Thus, conversion (or malingered) pain that the patient associates with his heart is more likely to be located in the region of the left nipple than retrosternally and down the left arm. However, when the symptom is modeled on a painful disorder previously experienced by the patient himself (*e.g.,* an injury or a myocardial infarction), its location may more closely approximate the usual distribution.

Quantitative Aspects (Intensity)

Patients report intensity of pain in such terms as slight, mild, bearable, severe, unbearable, or excruciating, but it is virtually impossible to know to what extent the report corresponds with the actual experience. While many factors influence how patients report the severity of pain, there is still often enough a sufficiently good correlation between the intensity of the noxious stimulation and the severity of the pain reported for it to have diagnostic value. This reflects the direct relationship between pain intensity and the amount or concentration of small-fiber activity transmitted through dorsal horn cells to activate the central intensity monitor of the action system. The important determinants of the reports of pain severity are as follows:

1. *Reduction in the level of consciousness at the time of the pain or in the interval before the pain is reported* may yield an understated account of its severity. Shock, prolonged syncope, or delirium may sometimes account for instances of coronary occlusion, dissecting aneurysm, or subarachnoid hemorrhage with little or no pain reported.

2. *Attention or distraction may significantly alter appreciation of pain severity.* Pain developing when the patient is alone often is reported as more intense than that developing when concerned persons are available. Relative isolation or sensory restriction, as when, for example, a patient is alone or immobilized in a body cast, may heighten awareness of pain, especially when chronic.[48] When pain is not too severe or too sudden in its development, even mild distraction, such as music or having the patient concentrate on something else, may ameliorate the pain.[49] Patients instructed preoperatively to take a deep breath from time to time with the explanation that it will relax tense abdominal muscles have been found to require less narcotic for pain relief postoperatively than do patients not so instructed.[50] Simply having ward personnel inquire at frequent intervals about the pain of postoperative patients may enhance the effects of placebo.[51] Here the reduction of feelings of anxiety and helplessness also plays a role. Endogenous pain-control mechanisms, both opioid and nonopioid, underlie such effects.

3. *Expectation, fear, and intolerance of suffering may influence the severity of the pain reported.* In their desperation not to suffer, certain patients may report almost any pain as unbearable, which is in effect a plea for help. Some patients show a progressive moderation in their report of pain severity as they gain confidence in the physician or are relieved of anxiety.

4. *A need to suffer or to assume the role of a sufferer,* sometimes determined by unconscious guilt and a wish for expiation and sometimes used as a means to influence or control others, may result in reports of pain of great severity. When the need to suffer is based on guilt, the patient may appear surprisingly composed despite the complaint of very severe pain.[3] Patients playing the role of sufferer, consciously or unconsciously, often exhibit more pain in the presence of persons important to them.

5. *A need to appear as strong, tough, and stoical, or a wish to overcome the fear of serious illness or death,* may lead some patients to minimize pain or deny it altogether. Some cultures foster such attitudes of stoicism and silent suffering, whereas others encourage a public display to bring family and professional support and sympathy.[52] The more pronounced the patient's need to be strong and in command, the more likely is he to block perception of pain successfully—a true psychic denial. Such patients may even fail to remember previous hospitalization or operations. Coronary patients with such personality features may not report pain or may attempt to deny serious implications by using terms other than pain or by ascribing their symptoms to "indigestion." Only after recovery may they acknowledge that the pain actually had been more intense than they had earlier described.[53]

6. *Apprehension about the doctor's intentions* may lead some patients, especially children, to claim pain to be inconsequential or absent. Concern about surgery or disagreeable diagnostic procedures, a wish to go home, or a hope to please the doctor may encourage such deceptive reports.

7. *Intrinsic variations in the neurobiologic system serving pain may be responsible for some individual differences in response to noxious stimuli.* Rare cases of congenital insensitivity (or indifference) to pain have been reported. In one case postmortem study revealed absence of small neurons in the dorsal ganglia, lack of small fibers in the dorsal roots, and absence of the shorter ascending pathway (dorsolateral fasciculus, Lissauer's tract).[54] Because an opioid antagonist (naloxone) lowered the threshold for withdrawal reflexes in such a patient, it has also been proposed that the syndrome may result from abnor-

mally high activity in the negative-feedback loop for pain.[55,56]

8. *Excessively severe pain in response to relatively minor stimulation is typical of peripheral or central nervous system lesions,* which may interfere with the modulating control mechanisms or induce abnormal neuron states with spontaneous firing. Neuralgia and causalgia are typical examples.[45]

9. *The severity of conversion pain bears no relationship to any concurrent afferent stimulus.* More important is the severity of suffering required to satisfy the need for punishment and atonement.

In the clinical evaluation of pain severity, it is helpful to have the patient compare the pain to pains experienced in the past, such as toothaches, injuries, or labor pains and to estimate its severity against the worst pain ever experienced. The degree to which a pain interferes with everyday activity provides another index whereby pain intensity can be gauged.

Temporal Aspects (Duration and Sequence)

Duration refers to how long any particular pain episode lasts, be it seconds or days, and to how long pain syndromes last, be they acute and short-lived or chronic and recurring.

The temporal sequence of a pain often accurately reflects the capability of the sensory-discriminative system to identify the spatiotemporal characteristics of the afferent input. For the most part the rate of rise and fall of a pain corresponds with the rate of stimulation and recruitment of receptors. A sudden prick or a blow will provoke a pain that reaches a peak within a fraction of a second and declines in a few seconds, only to resume in lesser intensity and persist for several minutes longer. This sequence reflects the sudden recruitment of receptors responding to mechanical energy (pressure, stretching, deformation), followed by the formation of chemical products of injury which stimulate chemoreceptors. The stretching of an inflamed pleura during inspiration evokes a volley of impulses felt as a sharp pain with each breath. The rhythmic peristaltic waves of a hollow viscus attempting to expel its contents against resistance, as with labor, renal colic, or intestinal obstruction, yields a characteristic sequence of pain that mounts in intensity over the course of 10 seconds to 20 seconds, is maintained for a minute or so, and then subsides, only to recur within a few minutes. Here one can readily visualize the recruitment of mechanical receptors responding as the region proximal to the obstruction is stretched with each successive peristaltic wave. Similarly, the throbbing character of the pain associated with arteritis or an abscess may be visualized. The

rhythmic stretch and relaxation with each systolic pulse of the sensitive arterial wall or of the tensely swollen inflammatory mass governs the pattern of afferent impulses.

The elaboration at the site of tissue injury of kinins and other chemical substances that lower receptor thresholds accounts for the steady pain and the exquisite tenderness typically associated with trauma and acute inflammation.[16] Such a mechanism probably also explains how structures ordinarily insensitive to pain, such as the mucosa of the gastrointestinal tract, may give rise to a steady pain with inflammation.[57]

Other irritating chemical substances, such as gastric juice, pancreatic enzymes, and bile, coming in contact with naked nerve terminals in the peritoneum or bed of the pancreas, are responsible for pain that mounts in intensity over a matter of minutes and is sustained for hours. The metabolic products of muscle ischemia act in a similar way to produce pain that is sustained as long as they are present and active, as in angina pectoris and intermittent claudication.

The time at which a pain begins to recede, whether minutes, hours, or days, may reflect the duration of activity of the responsible pathologic process, a change in its character, or damage to the receptors or afferent nerves involved. For example, the pain of angina pectoris, as induced by physical exertion in the patient with coronary insufficiency, disappears within a few minutes of cessation of exercise as reperfusion of the ischemic myocardium washes out the metabolic products of hypoxia. With coronary occlusion, on the other hand, pain persists until formation of the pain-inducing substances ceases or nerve endings in the ischemic myocardium are irretrievably damaged—a matter of hours.

Reduction in the level of attention or consciousness may also bring pain to an end, as with the use of drugs or with favorable psychological influences such as distraction or placebo effects.

When damage to a nerve involves chiefly the large fiber (nonnociceptive) system and disrupts the inhibitory balance with the small fiber (nociceptive) system, distinctive temporal characteristics are conferred upon the pain experienced. Thus, upon peripheral stimulation there may be a delay before onset of the pain, which may then be explosive, and once initiated, be sustained as an afterpain (hyperpathia) for some time after cessation of the provoking stimulus. This typically occurs in some forms of radiculitis, peripheral neuropathy, and neuralgia (e.g., trigeminal neuralgia).[4] The last may involve trigger zones. With injuries to the central nervous system involving central modulating mechanisms, pain may begin abruptly without evident peripheral stimulation. Such explosive and long-lasting bursts of pain are thought to result from spon-

taneous firing of spinal cord and brain cells no longer subject to ordinary inhibitory influences.[45]

The temporal characteristics of pain determined mainly by psychological factors, such as conversion and malingering, usually are not in keeping with temporal response patterns ordinarily associated with peripheral afferent activity. Rather, they correspond more with the patient's idiosyncratic notion of what the pain should be like. But when the conversion or malingered pain is based on a painful illness or injury previously experienced by the patient himself, then the patient's account of the time course of the pain may correspond closely with that of the original pain.

Qualitative Aspects (Descriptive Language)

In eliciting descriptions of pain it is important that the physician not bias the patient's account by proposing descriptive terms before the patient has been encouraged to use his own terms. Indeed, at times patients are describing sensations other than pain, such as "pressure," "tingling," or "fullness," and the clinical picture is only confused if the physician refers to these as "pain." Patients then say "pain" because that is the term used by the doctor when in fact it is not pain.

A limiting factor in pain description is the patient's verbal ability. One must accept the fact that some persons simply lack the vocabulary and fluency to report much beyond the fact that they are in pain. However, in evaluating the report of a patient who is unable to describe his pain, it is wise to inquire about other pain experiences, such as labor pain, toothache, or burn, for then one may discover that it is the pain that is "indescribable" rather than the patient who is incapable of describing the pain.

As a subjective experience, ultimately inaccessible to consensual validation, the available language for pain is limited. Some of the terms of widest currency reflect spatiotemporal characteristics such as "sharp," "dull," "throbbing," "aching," and "lightning." Often a pain is described in terms of some commonly familiar painful experience, such as "like a toothache," "a burn," "a sting," "a cramp," or "an electric shock." Such descriptions are usually also within the range of the personal experience of the physician and hence effectively convey a picture of the patient's pain. Or the description may be in terms of a pain previously experienced by the patient, such as labor pain, ulcer pain, or migraine—a very informative description when it is documented that the patient actually had the painful disorder referred to.

Very often patients make use of simile, often involving themes of violence.[1,58] They speak of a pain as "like a knife sticking in there," "like somebody hitting you," "like being burned with a red-hot poker," or "like hav-

ing the skin peeled off." Such similes demonstrate the intimate psychological association between pain and aggression. For some patients, such terms merely constitute the most lucid way for them to describe how the pain feels, in which case the complaint is reported in a quite matter-of-fact tone of voice. Other patients use such expressions in a dramatic way in order to impress upon the doctor the intensity of their suffering or the desperateness of their need for help. Often the more dramatic presentations also reflect powerful, underlying aggressive and self-punitive impulses. Their use is more prevalent among members of cultures that foster public display of suffering and dramatic appeals for help, as well as among patients with hysterical personality features. The latter are especially likely to exhibit conversion symptoms. Hence a dramatic pain presentation justifies looking for other evidence for conversion as the explanation of the pain.

Careful analysis of the similes used by patients to describe pain often reveal that they accurately convey the temporospatial characteristics of an underlying somatic process. For example, a patient with a herniated intervertebral disc said of his pain, "It was like a dog would bite you," and then, "As if somebody lit a match and went down the back of the leg with it." Upon further questioning he made it clear that he used the imagery of a dog biting into his thigh to describe how the pain would grab him and hang on—, its sudden onset and ensuing muscle spasm. The lighted match simile was intended to portray what must have been the radiation of burning pain along the root distribution. With conversion pain, the imagery offered in elaboration of these vivid terms would be more consistent with their symbolic meaning for the patient rather than being consistent with physiologic processes.

Some pains simply are not capable of being described in words because they do not correspond with any previous experience or fantasy. Pain that originates from injured nerves (*e.g.*, neuralgia, causalgia) or from lesions involving the central nervous mediating systems (*e.g.*, "central" pain) is especially likely to defy description.[59] Patients use terms such as "burning," "tingling," "knotting," "cramping," "boring," "gnawing," or "crushing," but above all they emphasize that the sensation is like nothing ever before experienced. This is understandable, for when an area innervated by a damaged nerve or central transmission pathway is stimulated, the characteristics of the resulting volley of impulses do not correspond with an input ever before experienced; it conveys information about the stimulus that is meaningless in terms of past experience. The patient, accustomed to reporting a skin sensation in terms of familiarity with the stimulus ("You're pricking me," "a pinch," "touch with cot-

ton"), now finds a familiar stimulus yielding unfamiliar sensations, often the only easily identifiable feature of which is that they are intensely unpleasant.[4]

Associated Physiologic Aspects

Body activities and physiologic processes serve to modify pain by increasing or decreasing afferent activity. Such relationships are helpful in identifying the site and nature of the pathologic process responsible for the pain.

1. *Skin.* Any modality of stimulation, including light contact of clothing, may intensify pain originating from the skin. On the other hand, gentle stimulation, such as stroking, warmth, or vibration, in adjacent uninvolved areas may reduce the pain, presumably through the inhibitory action of large-fiber activity on small-fiber transmission through the dorsal horn. Cooling may reduce pain of inflammatory origin, whereas dependency, which increases engorgement, may increase it. Cutaneous hyperesthesia and hyperalgesia may be referred from visceral disease or nerve lesions.

    Similar influences operate in pain originating in the sensitive mucous membranes of the nose and throat, conjunctiva, and anal and urogenital orifices.

2. *Subcutaneous structures.* Pressure or tension, and dependency in the case of inflammatory lesions, are the main influences increasing pain.

3. *Skeletal muscle pain* is intensified by use of the muscle as well as by mechanical forces, such as pressure. The sudden movements of coughing, sneezing, or laughing will increase pain coming from abdominal and trunk musculature. When pain is due to ischemia, as is characteristic of intermittent claudication, there is a direct relationship between the degree of circulatory insufficiency and muscle work. The interval between the beginning of muscle contraction and the onset of pain depends on how long it takes for hypoxic products of muscle metabolism to accumulate and exceed the threshold of receptor response. Hence, pain from an ischemic muscle builds up with the use of the muscle and subsides with rest.

4. *Movable skeletal parts,* including bones, joints, bursae, and tendons, give rise to pain when the structure is used and to relief when rested.

5. *Pain arising from arteries,* as with arteritis, migraine, and vascular headaches, increases with systolic impulse. Hence any process associated with increased systolic or pulse pressure, such as exercise, fever, alcohol, or bending over, may intensify the throbbing pain.[60]

6. *Pain from pleura*, as well as from trachea, correlates with respiratory movements.

7. *Heart pain*, a consequence of muscle ischemia, correlates with metabolic demand. Hence, with coronary insufficiency (angina pectoris), pain may develop when the work of the heart is increased, as with exertion, cold, or emotion, and subside with rest and composure.

8. *Pain from mediastinum* may be influenced by the activity of neighboring moving parts: esophagus (swallowing), musculoskeletal structures (movement), or aorta (increased systolic thrust).

9. *Pain from the gastrointestinal tract* tends to increase with peristaltic activity, particularly if there is any obstruction to forward progress. Hence it is increased with ingestion and may lessen with fasting or upon emptying the involved segment (vomiting or bowel movement). When hollow viscera are distended, body positions or movements that increase intra-abdominal pressure may intensify the pain, whereas positions that reduce pressure or support the structure may ease the pain. The patient with an acutely distended gallbladder may slightly flex his trunk and support his right hypochondrium with his hand. Pain secondary to the effect of gastric acid on esophagus, stomach, or duodenum correlates with *p*H; hence, it is relieved by the presence of food or other neutralizing material in the stomach and intensified when the stomach is empty and secreting acid.

10. *Viscera with capsules*, such as liver, kidneys, spleen, and pancreas, may give rise to pain when swollen; the pain increases with compression of the tense organ, as may occur with increased intra-abdominal pressure. Patients achieve some relief by assuming postures that decrease pressure on the organ. With pain arising from a tense, swollen kidney (or distended renal pelvis), the patient flexes his trunk and tilts toward the involved side; with pancreatic pain, he may sit up and lean forward or lie down with his knees drawn up to the chest.[61]

11. *Irritation of the parietal peritoneum*, local or generalized, yields pain that is intensified by any movement of the inflamed area. This may include movements of the trunk, respiratory movements, or movements of the underlying organ.

12. *Intracranial masses* that put pain-sensitive structures under tension are sensitive to processes that suddenly displace intracranial structures. Thus pain may be increased by jarring the head, jogging, or sudden alterations in intracranial pressure, as with coughing or sneezing.[60]

13. *Nerve and root pain* is intensified by any movement or posture that impinges on the involved nerve or root. Sudden increases in intraspinal pressure produced by coughing, sneezing, or straining typically exacerbate root pain. Pain may be intensified by stimulation of receptors within peripheral distribution of the damaged nerve. Any contact of the skin or pressure on deeper structures may be excruciating, although there may be a quite noticeable delay between the effective stimulus and the onset of the pain. Pain may also sometimes be induced by stimulation of receptor zones that feed impulses into the same spinal segment. Sometimes there are trigger points, the slightest contact with which will provoke an intense paroxysm of pain; this is characteristic of trigeminal and glossopharyngeal neuralgia.[4]

14. *Lesions of cord, bulb, pons, thalamus or the second sensory area of the cortex* may give rise to pain that often characteristically appears as unprovoked paroxysms but may also be steady and exacerbated by mild stimulation in the area of the body served by the damaged neural system (*e.g.*, the lightning pains of tabes dorsalis, the thalamic syndrome).[22]

15. *When pain is determined by psychological needs to any significant extent*, correlation with physiologic influences may be obscured or even absent altogether, as is typically the case with conversion pain or malingering. Indeed, such lack of correlation is criterion suggestive of conversion.

Behavioral and Psychosocial Aspects

Much behavior exhibited by the person in pain constitutes trial-and-error efforts at relief, and hence its elucidation has diagnostic value. Such behaviors include resting, physical activity, changing positions, altering eating patterns, efforts to induce regurgitation, eructation, urination, or defecation, and the use of heat, cold, message, compresses, pressure, or medications. For the most part, patients turn first to measures that they have found effective in the past with other pains. Some, they quickly discover, make matters worse; others have no effect. When nothing relieves the pain, the patient may persist in quite inappropriate and even dangerous activities; patients with acute myocardial infarction, for example, have been known to do pushups in a vain attempt to terminate the pain!

Some pain behavior is aimed at soliciting help. Here the setting and the individual's personal style, as well as cultural influences, affect the patterns of behavior manifested. The behavior of individuals for whom the pain is profoundly disturbing is primarily determined by their desperate need to be relieved of the pain. They may exaggerate the pain or be loudly insistent in their demand for relief. Others, those who take pride in their stoicism, may display little or no pain-related be-

havior. Patients for whom suffering serves important psychological ends behave as though they are more concerned with how others respond to them as sufferers than they are with the relief of pain. They include persons with deep underlying feelings of guilt and masochism or with intense aggressive impulses. Such persons are likely to invite injury or to suffer pain as a conversion symptom.[3,62]

Reported relationships between behavior and relief or exacerbation of pain must be interpreted with care. Patients are quick to ascribe significance to what may be merely coincidence. It is not uncommon, for example, for a patient to report that his pain was improved or made worse by a medication, when in fact the change reflected the natural progress of the underlying disorder, or perhaps the relief of anxiety or the intensification of anger or guilt.

Behavior and psychological reactions when pain is acute and relatively short-lived are likely to be different than when pain is chronic and recurring. For the most part, when the pain is new and acute, it is likely to be experienced as alien and threatening. It dominates attention, often frightens, and demands relief. On the other hand, when the pain is one with which the patient is already familiar, whether as a personal experience or from knowledge about the pain experience of others, the reaction is likely to be very much influenced by the outcome of the previous experience. Thus pains already known to be benign and to resolve spontaneously or with some specific measure are generally responded to with relative equanimity; when not, the physician must investigate why not. For example, careful inquiry may reveal that the pain is in fact a new one, the threat of which the patient is trying to deny by associating it with some more benign and familiar pain.

Recurrence of pains with ominous significance may also evoke paradoxical reactions, the patient sometimes minimizing or denying altogether the seriousness of the pain even to the extent of providing the doctor misleading information, if not avoiding or delaying medical attention altogether. Dangerous delay of hospitalization of patients with acute myocardial infarction often is based more on their reluctance to submit to the control of others than upon their failure to appreciate the significance of their symptoms or even the danger of death. Fear of cancer or other life-threatening diseases, however based, leads some patients to become preoccupied even with minor transient pains and others to try to ignore even severe pain. Appreciation of individual differences in patients' psychological and social backgrounds and circumstances helps to make such contrasting behaviors understandable.[63]

Once pain becomes chronic, whether unremitting or recurring, the behavior of the victim is likely to be quite different from that encountered with acute pain. Now the pain becomes part of the everyday life of the patient, a constant companion, so to speak. No longer is it experienced as a warning, a signal of impending injury or damage. Only with unexpected exacerbations or with changes in its character or location may the behaviors more typical of acute pain be noted. Chronic pain, of whatever origin, becomes a burden, something to be endured and somehow accomodated. It changes the course and goals of life, alters relationships. Attitudes of family and caretakers, including physicians, change. Frustrated by their inability to provide relief or meet demands, they readily become impatient, even angry with the patient, often disengaging or withdrawing altogether. A vicious cycle is readily engendered thereby: Some patients become more demanding and more frustrating, others seriously withdrawn and depressed.

Irrespective of the primary source of the pain, whether peripheral, neurogenic or psychogenic, the approach to the patient with chronic pain becomes increasingly determined by individual psychological and social factors. Chronic pain dominates the life of the sufferer. It intrudes into every facet of living, changing goals, attitudes, self-image, roles, and relationships, not only of the sufferer but also of all with whom he is involved. Pain experience and expression may be significantly influenced by how much expressions of suffering or disability are socially reinforced; by monetary compensation for pain through litigation and disability claims; by the relative availability of interpersonal and social support systems; by the degree to which the pain provides relief from unpleasant vocational and family responsibilities or justification for failure to live up to expectations, one's own or others'; as justification for dependence on alcohol or analgesics; and even by how good or how bad the prospects are for satisfying one's needs outside of the pain-patient role.[64]

A surprising number of patients do remarkably well even in the face of the severe unremitting pain often associated with cancer and other progressive or irremediable disorders. Pain may actually disappear when the patients come to terms with their fate. A woman in her 60s, convinced that her excruciating abdominal pain was due to cancer, required round-the-clock medication for relief. Careful diagnostic study, including exploratory laparotomy, failed to confirm the diagnosis of cancer. But after six months of suffering, during which her family drifted away, unmistakable evidence of metastatic cancer emerged. Informed of the diagnosis, her pain disappeared completely, never to recur again. Not only did she feel vindicated, but her family and the medical staff once again rallied around, and

she no longer felt isolated and abandoned. A young woman with metastatic breast cancer became tranquil and although not pain-free, she was at least detached from her pains once she resolved to live out the balance of her life in her own way.

For some pain may serve intrapsychic needs, be they to atone for intolerable feelings of guilt or as a means of controlling dangerous aggression. Such patients may display other sado-masochistic traits.[3,62] They may be designated "pain-prone," and efforts to provide relief to them may not be possible nor wise, since the pain may be playing a role in adjustment which the patient finds indispensable.[3,62,65,66] Paradoxically, some pain-prone patients become pain-free when they are being abused by others or by circumstances, only to relapse when conditions improve. They are accident-prone and surgery-prone. Pain relief, when it occurs, is likely to be transient; the same pain, or a new pain, soon again makes its appearance. Achieving better functioning despite the pain rather than relief of pain becomes the goal of treatment with such patients.

SUMMARY

Pain is a private, subjective experience, information about which can only come from the sufferer. It is the felt part of a nociceptive and nocifensive organization, the neural structures of which are widely represented throughout the neuraxis. For information to be experienced as pain, the higher neural processes must be functionally intact. The characteristics of pain as experienced and reported are the products of physiological, psychological, and social determinants. Any profile of pain must take into account the relative importance of the peripheral, neurogenic, and psychogenic sources of input underlying each pain and must consider the pain in terms of the six dimensions of location, intensity, duration, description, associated physiological factors, and behavioral and psychosocial factors. The compelling issue for the physician is to explain why a patient is complaining of pain or, paradoxically, why a patient is *not* complaining of pain.

REFERENCES

1. **Engel GL:** Primary atypical facial neuralgia. An hysterical conversion symptom. Psychosom Med 13:375–396, 1951
2. **Szasz T:** Pain and Pleasure. A Study of Bodily Feelings. New York, Basic Books, 1957
3. **Engel GL:** Psychogenic pain and the pain-prone patient. Am J Med 26:899–918, 1959
4. **Noordenbos W:** Pain. Amsterdam, Elsevier, 1959
5. **Wall PD:** On the relation of injury to pain. Pain 6:253–264, 1979
6. **Hardy HD, Wolff HG, Goodell H:** Pain Sensations and Reactions. Baltimore, Williams & Wilkins, 1952
7. **Melzack R, Scott TH:** The effects of early experience on the response to pain. J Comp Physiol Psychol 50:155–61, 1957
8. **Melzack R, Wall PD:** Pain mechanisms. A new theory. Science 150:071, 1965
9. **Casey KL, Melzack R:** Neural mechanisms of pain: A conceptual model. In Way EL(ed): Pain, New York, Academic Press, 1968
10. **Melzack R, Wall PD:** Gate control theory of pain. In Soulairac A, Cahn J, Charpentier J (eds): Pain. New York, Academic Press, 1968
11. **Engel GL:** The need for a new medical model. A challenge for biomedicine. Science 196:129–136, 1977
12. **Quillam TA:** Unit design and array patterns in receptor organs. In de Reuck AVS, Knight J (eds): Touch, Heat and Pain. Boston, Little, Brown & Co, 1966
13. **Cauna N:** Fine structures of the receptor organs and its probable functional significance. In de Reuck, AVS, Knight J (eds): Touch, Heat and Pain. Boston, Little, Brown & Co, 1966
14. **Iggo A:** Activation of cutaneous nocioceptors and their actions on dorsal horn neurons. In Bonica JJ (ed): International Symposium on Pain. Adv Neurol 4:1–9, 1974
15. **Bessou P, Perl ER:** Response of cutaneous sensory units with unmyelinated fibers to noxious stimuli. J Neurophysiol 32:1025–43, 1969
16. **Keele CA:** Chemical causes of pain and itch. Ann Rev Med 21:67–74, 1970
17. **Lim RKS:** Pharmacologic viewpoint of pain and analgesia. In Way EL (ed): New Concepts in Pain. Philadelphia, FA Davis, 1967
18. **Ferreira SH:** Prostaglandins, asprin-like drugs and analgesia, Nature 240:200, 1972
19. **Bishop GH:** The relation between nerve fiber size and sensory modality. Phylogenetic implications of the afferent innervation of the cortex. J Nerv Ment Dis 128:89, 1959
20. **Winkelman RK:** Similarities in cutaneous nerve endings. In Montagna W (ed): Advances in Biology of Skin, Vol 1, Cutaneous Innervations of the Skin, p 48. London, Pergamon Press, 1960
21. **Lim RKS, Liu CN, Guzman F, Braun C:** Visceral receptors concerned in visceral pain and the pseudoaffective response to intra-arterial injection of bradykinin and other algesic agents. J Comp Neurol 118:269, 1962
22. **White JC, Sweet WH:** Pain. Springfield, Charles C Thomas, 1955
23 **Mountcastle VB:** Duality of function in the somatic afferent systems. In Brazier MAB (ed): Brain and Behavior, Vol I, pp 67–93. Washington, American Institute for Biological Sciences, 1961

24. **Whitlock DG, Perl ER:** Thalamic projections of spinothalamic pathways in monkey. Exp Neurol 3:240, 1961

25. **Perl ER, and Whitlock DG:** Somatic stimuli exciting spinothalamic projections to thalamic neurons in cat and monkey. Exp Neurol 3:256, 1961

26. **Mark VH, Ervin FR, Yakovlev PL:** The treatment of pain by sterotaxic methods. Confin Neurol 22:238, 1962

27. **Sweet WH:** Pain, pp 287–303. New York, Raven Press, 1980

28. **Casey KL:** Somatosensory responses of bulbar-reticular units in awake cat: Relation to escape-producing stimuli. Science 173:77–80, 1971

29. **Casey KL:** Neural mechanisms of pain. In Caterette EC, Friedman MP (eds): Handbook of Perception, pp 183–230. New York, Academic Press, 1978

30. **Bell C, Sierra G, Buendia N, Segundo IP:** Sensory properties of neurons in the mesencephalic reticular formation. J Neurophysiol 27:961, 1964

3l. **Basbaum AI, Fields HL:** Endogenous pain control mechanisms: Review and hypothesis. Ann Neurol 4:451–462, 1978

32. **Herman BH, Pankseep J:** Ascending endorphin inhibition of distress vocalization. Science 211:1060–1062, 1980

33. **Pavlov IP:** Lectures on Conditioned Reflexes. New York, International Publishers, 1928

23. **Snyder SH:** The opiate receptor and morphine-like peptides in the brain. Am J Psychiatry 135:645–652, 1978

35. **Lewis ME, Mishkin M, Bragen E, et al:** Opiate receptor gradients in monkey cerebral cortex: Correspondence with sensory processing hierarchies. Science 211:1166–1169, 1981

36. **Cuello AC:** Endogenous opioid peptides in neurons of the human brain. Lancet 2:291–293, 1978

37. **Hosobuchi Y, Adams JE, Linchitz R:** Pain relief by electrical stimulation of the central gray matter in humans and its reversal by naloxone. Science 197:183–186, 1977

38. **Walker JB, Katz RL:** Non-opioid pathways suppress pain in humans. Pain 11:347–354, 1981

39. **Lewis JW, Cannon JT, Liebeskind JC:** Opioid and non-opioid mechanisms of stress analgesia. Science 208:623–625, 1980

40. **Miczek KA, Thompson ML, Shuster L:** Opioid-like analgesia in defeated mice. Science 215:1520–1522, 1982

41. **Fanselow MS:** Naloxone attenuates rats' preference for signaled shock. J Comp Physiol Psychol 7:30–74, 1979

42. **Grau JW, Hyson RL, Maier SF, et al:** Long-term stress-induced analgesia and activation of the opiate system. Science 213:1409–1411, 1981

43. **Goldstein A, Hilgard ER:** Failure of the opiate antagonist naloxone to modify hypnotic analgesia. Proc Natl Acad Sci USA 72:2041–2043, 1975

44. **Frid M, Singer G:** Hypnotic analgesia in conditions of stress is partially reversed by naloxone. Psychopharmacology (Berlin) 63:211–215, 1979

45. **Melzack R, Loeser JD:** Phantom body pain in parapleg-ics: Evidence for a central "pattern generating mechanism" for pain. Pain 4:195–210, 1978

46. **Schweiger A, Parducci A:** Nocebo: The psychologic induction of pain. Pavlov J Biol Sci 16:140–143, 1981

47. **Henry JA, Montuschi E:** Cardiac pain referred to the site of previously experienced somatic pain. Br Med J 520:1605–1606, 1978

48. **Blitz B, Lowenthal M:** The role of sensory restriction in problems with chronic pain. J. Chronic Dis 19:1119, 1966

49. **Melzack R, Weisz AZ, Sprague LT:** Strategems for controlling pain: Contributions of auditory stimulation and suggestion. Exp Neurol 8:239, 1963

50. **Egbert LD, Battit GE, Welch CE, Bartlett MK:** Reduction of post-operative pain by encouragement and instruction of patients. N Engl J Med 270:825, 1964

51. **Beecher HK:** Generalization from pain of various types and diverse origin. Science 130:267, 1959

52. **Zborowski M:** Cultural components in responses to pain. J. Social Issues 8:16, 1952

53. **Olin HS, hackett TP:** The denial of chest pain in 32 patients with acute myocardial infarction. JAMA 190:977, 1964

54. **Swanson AG, Buchan GC, Alvord EC:** Anatomical changes in congenital insensitivity to pain. Arch Neurol 12:12, 1965

55. **Buchsbaum MS, David GC, Bunney WE:** Naloxone alters pain perception and somatosensory evoked potentials in normal subjects. Nature 270:620–622, 1977

56. **Dehen H, Willer JC, Boureau F:** Congenital insensitivity to pain and endogenous morphine-like substances. Lancet 2:293–294, 1977

57. **Wolf S, Wolff HG:** Human Gastric Function. New York, Oxford University Press, 1943

58. **Klein RF, Brown W:** Pain descriptions in medical settings. J Psychosom Res 10:367, 1967

59. **Denny-Brown D:** The release of deep pain by nerve injury. Brain 88:725, 1965

60. **Wolff HG:** Headache. New York, Oxford University Press, 1963

61. **Macchia B:** Position relief of pain. Important clue to clinical diagnosis of carcinoma of the pancreas. JAMA 182:6, 1962

62. **Tinling DC, Klein RF:** Psychogenic pain and aggression. The syndrome of the solitary hunter. Psychosom Med 28:738, 1966

63. **Engel GL:** The clinical application of the biopsychosocial model. Am J Psychiatry 137:535–544, 1980

64. **Sternbach RA:** Pain Patients. Traits and Treatment. New York, Academic Press, 1974

65. **Delaney JF:** Atypical facial pain as a defense against psychoses. Am J Psychiatry 133:1151–1154, 1976

66. **Blumer D:** Psychiatric considerations in pain. In Rothran RH, Simeone FA (eds): The Spine, Vol II., pp. 871–906. Philadelphia, WB Saunders, 1975

4

Headache
N. Vijayan
Craig Watson

General Pathophysiology of Headaches
Mechanism of Pain
Pathophysiology of Pain
Classification of Headache
Migraine
　Definition
　Classification
　Epidemiology
　Diagnosis and Clinical Features
　　Duration
　　Frequency
　　Precipitating Factors
　　Premonitory Symptoms
　　Location and Type of Pain
　　Associated Features
　　Medication History
　Classic Migraine
　Common Migraine
　Hemiplegic Migraine
　Ophthalmoplegic Migraine
　Basilar Artery Migraine
　Migraine Equivalents
　Pathogenesis of Migraine
　　Neurovascular Abnormalities
　　Humoral Changes
Cluster Headache
　Definition
　Classification
　Clinical Features
　　Cluster Periods
　　Remission Periods
　　Cluster Attack
　Medical History
　Pathophysiology of Cluster Headache Pain
　　Vascular Aspects
　　Biochemical Aspects
　　Autonomic Nervous System Aspects
　　Hormonal Aspects
　Pathophysiology of Cluster Accompaniments
Muscle Contraction Headache (MCHA)
　Definition
　Incidence
　Classification
　Clinical Features
　Associated Features
　Combined Muscle Contraction and Vascular
　　Headache

　MCHA Due to Structural Disease
　Post-traumatic MCHA
　Conversion or Delusional Headache
　Mechanism of Pain in MCHA
Post-Traumatic Headache
　Clinical Features and Classification
　　Type 1: Muscle Contraction Headache
　　Type 2: Site of Injury Headache
　　Type 3: Vascular Headache
　　Type 4: Post-traumatic Dysautonomic
　　　Cephalalgia
　Post-traumatic Syndrome
　Natural History of Post-traumatic Syndrome
　Pathophysiology of Post-traumatic Headache
　　Muscle Contraction
　　Injury to Nerves
　　Scar Formation
　　Vascular Changes
　　Injury to Intracranial Structures
　　Psychological Factors
Physical Causes of Headache
　Nonmigrainous Vascular Headache
　　Nasal Vasomotor Headache
　　Fever Headache Due to Systemic Infection
　　Hypertension Headache and Hypertensive
　　　Encephalopathy
　　Hypoxic Headache
　　Post-seizure Headache
　　Headache Caused by Food and Chemicals
　Intracranial (Traction) Headache
　　Tumors
　　Arteriovenous Malformations
　　Aneurysms
　　Abscesses
　　Hematoma (Epidural, Subdural, Intracerebral)
　　Pseudotumor Cerebri (Benign Intracranial
　　　Hypertension)
　　Postlumbar Puncture Headache
　Headache Due to Overt Cranial Inflammation
　　Meningitis (Acute, Chronic, Chemical)
　　Subarachnoid Hemorrhage
　　Arteritis and Phlebitis
　Headache Due to Diseases of Cranial or Neck
　　Structures
　　Acute Nasal Sinusitis
　　Temporomandibular Joint Syndrome

Headache is a common malady. It can be the symptom of a systemic disease or it can result from physical or physiologic changes in the intra- or extracranial pain-sensitive structures. More often it is a disorder by itself. It is one of the most common complaints of the outpatient population. Despite this fact, it is very difficult to arrive at the exact incidence of headache in the general population because the severity of the symptom is so variable and often no medical attention is sought for its relief. For example, an epidemiologic study conducted by Waters and O'Connor found that only 23% of women with migraines had sought medical help.[1] It is estimated that approximately 80% of the population at one time in their life, experience headache as a symptom.[2] Of this population, 20% are thought to suffer from chronic headaches that require a physician's care.

A majority of headache surveys have been undertaken in Europe, and therefore there are only a few figures available for the incidence of headache in the United States.[3] The results of this study are very similar to those reported by European investigators. This means that at least 40 million people require the care of a physician for the treatment of their headaches on a regular basis. One can only estimate the loss of productivity engendered by absenteeism due to headaches, since no reliable figures are currently available.

GENERAL PATHOPHYSIOLOGY OF HEADACHES

Knowledge of the mechanism of production of pain from head and neck structures is essential for a clear understanding of the pathogenesis of headaches. This field has been greatly advanced by the contributions made by Wolff and his co-workers.[4] Their studies clearly defined the pain-sensitive and insensitive structures of the head and also the possible mechanisms by which these structures are affected to cause pain. These conclusions are the result of detailed human experimentation and clinical observations. The following is a list of the pain-sensitive and insensitive structures of the head:

Pain-Sensitive Structures
Scalp—all layers
Muscles
Periostium
Dura—mostly basal
Arteries
    Extracranial
    Dural
    Intracranial (proximal)
Veins
    Extracranial

Intracranial
Sinuses

Pain-Insensitive Structures
Cranial bone
Diploic veins
Pia-arachnoid
Brain parenchyma
Ependymal lining
Choroid plexus

One must also be knowledgeable about the anatomic pathways that carry pain from these structures so that headache pain mechanisms will be understood properly and any variations thereof can be accounted for. A brief description of the neural innervation of these structures follows.

Intracranial pain-sensitive structures, mainly the dura and the proximal portions of the large intracranial vessels, are supplied by the trigeminal nerve, the sensory fibers in the 9th and 10th cranial nerves, and the 2nd and 3rd cervical sensory nerve roots. The structures in the anterior and middle cranial fossa and the superior surface of the tentorium cerebelli are primarily innervated by the trigeminal nerve. Therefore, pain arising from these areas is referred to the anterior two-thirds of the head. It is worthwhile to remember that the superior surface of the tentorium is supplied by a recurrent branch of the ophthalmic division of the trigeminal nerve, and therefore pain from this location can actually be referred to the eye.

The posterior fossa structures are primarily innervated by the upper three cervical roots and to a very limited extent by the 9th and 10th cranial nerve sensory fibers. Therefore, pain from the posterior fossa is referred to the posterior portion of the head and neck. Another interesting clinical observation is the referral of pain arising from the neck to the frontal and orbital regions. It is believed that this results from the proximity or continuity of the pain pathways of the substantia gelatinosa, the spinal tract of the trigeminal nerve, and the central processes of the upper three cervical roots.

In general, pain originating from one side of the intracranial cavity is referred to the same side of the head. This holds true until the causative factors distort the intracranial anatomy across the midline or produce blockage of the cerebrospinal fluid pathways. The pain becomes bilateral when this happens. Therefore, at least in the initial stages, the location and lateralization of the headache give a good clue regarding the location of the causative factor. Generalization of the headache occurs very early in the course of a lesion in the posterior fossa because of the ease with which the cerebrospinal fluid pathways are obstructed by lesions in this location. Another important thing to remember

about posterior fossa lesions is that there could be sufficient referral of the pain to the neck causing reflex cervical muscle spasm. This clinical picture may be mistaken for a primary neck disorder or even a muscle contraction headache.

MECHANISM OF PAIN

An understanding of the mechanisms by which pain is produced from the pain-sensitive structures is essential because this will help explain how different pathologic processes lead to pain (which is perceived as headache) from these structures (see list).

Mechanism of Pain
Blood Vessels
   Traction
   Displacement
   Dilatation
Nerves
   Pressure
   Invasion
Ventricles
   Dilatation
   Collapse
Inflammation of all pain-sensitive structures

If these general principles are kept in mind, it will be easy to explain the genesis of headache pain under various circumstances. More details regarding the mechanism of production of pain from these structures will be provided when individual headache syndromes are discussed.

PATHOPHYSIOLOGY OF PAIN

There have been important advances in the understanding of central pain mechanisms during the last decade. One aspect of this development is the clarification of central pain pathways. No attempt will be made here to discuss this, since it has been dealt with independently in Chapter 3. Another aspect is the expansion of the knowledge of the chemical mediators involved in the genesis and control of pain. A number of these chemicals has been identified, including endorphins, encephalins, substance-P, serotonin, various types of kinins, dopamine and other catecholamines, and others. These advances have been applied to the study of headaches only in a very limited fashion so far. Some of the earliest studies were done by Chapman and associates in which they looked at the mechanism of localized changes in pain threshold in the region of the superficial temporal vessels in migraine patients.[5] They implicated the local release of certain

types of kinins for the focal changes in pain threshold. No follow-up observations have been undertaken in this field by anyone else so far.

Some of the preliminary studies involving endorphins are also interesting, but a lot more work in this area is required before any definite conclusions can be drawn regarding their role in the genesis of headache. It has been speculated that a deficiency of these inhibitory transmitters may be responsible for some of the spontaneous pain syndromes, including headache.

There are a number of other vasoactive amines specifically implicated in the genesis of migrainous vascular headaches. These will be discussed in detail in the section dealing with migraine.

CLASSIFICATION OF HEADACHE

Classification of any disease is necessary so that scientific communication in the field can be improved. This is especially true of headaches because the definition of various headache syndromes have always been vague. In the past, this has resulted in much confusion in scientific reports on evaluation of therapeutic modalities in headache because each investigator used his or her own criteria for diagnosis. As a result of this, no two studies could be adequately compared. This state of confusion still exists, but most of the publications now use the classification and the diagnostic criteria laid down by the *ad hoc* committee set up by the National Institute of Neurological Diseases and Blindness (NINDS).[6]

NINDS Classification of Headache
1. Vascular headache of migraine type
   a. "Classic" migraine
   b. "Common" migraine
   c. "Cluster" headache
   d. "Hemiplegic" and "ophthalmoplegic" migraine
   e. "Lower-half" headache
2. Muscle contraction headache
3. Combined headache: vascular and muscle contraction
4. Headache of nasal vasomotor reaction
5. Headache of delusional, conversion, or hypochondriacal states
6. Nonmigrainous vascular headache
7. Traction headache
8. Headache due to overt cranial inflammation
9–13. Headache due to disease of ocular, aural, nasal and sinusal, dental, or other cranial or neck structures
14. Cranial neuritides
15. Cranial neuralgias

Detailed definition of each category of headache can be found in the original publication and will not be repeated here. Most of the authors in the headache field use this classification. Since its publication in 1962, a lot more clinical and other basic information on headache has accumulated, which has already made this classification outmoded. Attempts are now underway to come up with a more comprehensive classification, but until such time, this classification is the one that is most extensively used.

A more compact clinical classification has been used by Dalessio in the last edition of Wolff's monograph.[7] The author identifies three major categories of headaches based on what structures are thought to be involved. He describes all headaches under *vascular, muscle contraction, and traction–inflammatory* categories. This is a very useful and practical approach even though the pathogenesis of pain in some of these categories of headaches is still uncertain. This will become more evident during subsequent discussions. There is one group of authors who believes that any such classification is worthless because most of the headache syndromes are associated with pain arising from multiple structures. Despite these problems, some type of generally agreed upon classification is essential for choosing appropriate drug therapy and scientific communication. Further subdivisions of each of the headache syndromes will be discussed in later sections.

MIGRAINE

DEFINITION

According to the *ad hoc* committee classification, "vascular headaches of the migraine type refers to recurrent attacks of headache widely varied in intensity, frequency and duration. The attacks are commonly unilateral in onset, are usually associated with anorexia, sometimes with nausea and vomiting and in some are preceded by or associated with conspicuous sensory, motor, and mood disturbances. They are often familial." The most important feature that is helpful in the diagnosis is the stereotyped pattern of occurrence of these attacks even if all the above criteria are not always present.

CLASSIFICATION

Migraine headaches have been subdivided based on the presence or absence of preceding or concomitant neurologic manifestations and the nature of these manifestations. Migraine headache without any neurologic manifestations is called *common migraine,* and

when such manifestations are present it is termed *classic migraine.* Typically, the neurologic manifestations precede the headache in classic migraine and the patient is free from these symptoms by the time the headache develops. However, in certain people these manifestations persist into the headache phase and may even outlast the headache. The term "complicated migraine" is used under these circumstances. Hemiplegic and ophthalmoplegic migraine are the typical examples of this variety of migraine. A summary of the varieties of migraine is listed below.

Classification of Migraine
1. Common migraine
2. Classic migraine
3. Complicated migraine
   a. Hemiplegic migraine
   b. Ophthalmoplegic migraine
   c. Basilar artery migraine
4. Migraine equivalents

A patient can suffer from a variety of these types of migraines at one time or other. It is very common to see a patient with frequent episodes of common migraine and infrequent classic migraine. Similarly, patients with ophthalmoplegic migraine often have a history of other varieties of migraine as well.

EPIDEMIOLOGY

The reported incidence of migraine varies remarkably from one study to the next. A survey in England revealed 19.44% of males and 25.72% of females suffered from migraine. Of these, 56.5% of the males and 61.6% of the females had a positive family history of migraine.[8] Another survey from the same country gave an incidence of 36.5% for males and 40% for females.[9] In general, women reported more severe headaches. This preponderance in women becomes obvious only after pubertal age. There is no clear-cut evidence that socioeconomic factors play a role in predisposition to migraine. Another question that is often posed is whether there is a "migraine personality." A majority of the studies so far do not support this concept, even though there is some evidence that migraine patients are somewhat more prone to anxiety and depression.[10,11]

DIAGNOSIS AND CLINICAL FEATURES

A majority of patients begin experiencing symptoms of migraine in their adolescence. However, it should be remembered that migraine can manifest at any age in a susceptible person. There are a number of patients in whom the typical manifestations occur as late as the

sixth decade. It is difficult to make a confident diagnosis of migraine at this age because the symptoms are very similar to transient ischemic attacks. Therefore, appropriate investigations to rule out underlying structural vascular diseases will have to be undertaken. There is only one well-documented published study in this category of patients.[12] On the other hand, very young children may also suffer from migraine. Manifestations are often atypical in children and diagnosis may be delayed or missed for a long time. Further details of these manifestations are provided in the discussion of migraine equivalents.

The female preponderance and family history are discussed under epidemiology. A positive family history is obtained in 60% to 70% of patients with classic migraine and in 30% to 40% of patients with common migraine.

Before discussing the specific clinical features, an outline for eliciting the history of migraine will be presented. This is very similar to the approach to any other medical problem. The only difference is that the history is the most important clue to the correct diagnosis because the physical examination is often normal. An adequate history should include the following minimum amount of information.

Duration

A long history of recurrent headaches spanning over a number of years is more indicative of migraine than of underlying structural diseases. Headaches associated with congenital arteriovenous malformations or benign lesions causing intermittent obstruction of spinal fluid pathways are the exceptions to this general rule.

Frequency

The frequency of headache occurrence gives an idea about the degree of disability caused by the headache and also forms a baseline for the assessment of therapeutic success. Fluctuations in frequency give an idea about the natural course and behavior of the headache. For example, clearly defined cycles of headaches are characteristic of episodic cluster headaches and are also seen in some patients with so-called cyclical migraine. Besides this, a sudden increase in the severity and frequency of the headaches may portend the development of some other underlying disorder like a tumor or vasculitis, which may have to be looked for.

Precipitating Factors

Identification of the precipitating factors of headaches, if any, and their avoidance may be of help in reducing the frequency of headaches. Besides, this information may specifically help in the differentiation of migraine from other headaches. For example, it is often reported by patients that muscle contraction headaches are improved by alcohol, whereas alcohol usually precipitates migraine in susceptible persons. See list for the most commonly reported precipitating factors reported by patients.

Precipitating Factors in Migraine

1. Alcohol, especially red wine
2. Emotional changes, especially "let-down" periods after stress
3. Hormonal changes, *e.g.*, menstruation, ovulation, birth control pills
4. Too little or excess sleep, exhaustion
5. Dietary, like chocolate, cheese, MSG, cured meats
6. Weather changes, *e.g.*, barometric pressure changes, exposure to sun

A majority of patients do not have any clearly identifiable precipitating factors. Lack of this history, therefore, does not go against the diagnosis of migraine. The role played by dietary factors in the genesis of migraine has been overemphasized in the literature. The mechanisms by which some of these agents cause migraine will be discussed in the section on pathogenesis.

Premonitory Symptoms

The presence or absence of premonitory symptoms help to categorize the headache. The duration, type, and time of occurrence of these manifestations may also help in evaluating the possible presence of other underlying neurologic diseases responsible for the headache. Typical manifestations will be discussed later.

Location and Type of Pain

Classically, the pain of migraine is described as unilateral, throbbing, or pounding in quality, which builds up gradually in severity (ingravescent). These features are not present in all patients. The typical features may be absent if the vasodilatation primarily involves the meningeal rather than the extracranial scalp vessels. Pain may often begin bilaterally. This is especially true of common migraine. In some patients, the neurologic symptoms predominate and headache may be very insignificant or even absent.

Associated Features

Symptoms like photophobia, phonophobia, nausea, vomiting, and localized or generalized dysautonomic features are helpful in the diagnosis of migraine but need not always be present.

Medication History

Medication history is an important part of the history and is often neglected. This information helps to identify any vasodilator agents that might precipitate mi-

graines. More important, it helps the physician in cataloging the pattern of response of the headaches to various medications in the past and their side-effects. Usually this information also uncovers the common fact that the most important causes of failure of drug treatment are the prescription of an inadequate amount of medication and inappropriate timing of medication doses. This also helps in choosing a drug that will be most effective in a particular patient.

A detailed review of the general physical health and the rest of the neurologic functions should be obtained so that symptomatic headaches can be differentiated from primary headache syndromes. Diagnostic and therapeutic measures will be inadequate or inappropriate unless full attention is paid to systemic causes that may be responsible for the genesis or perpetuation of headaches. After the physician acquires these historical details, he will be in a better position to categorize the headaches. A discussion of the specific clinical features of the different types of migraine follows.

CLASSIC MIGRAINE

Classic migraine, though best known and most easily recognized, constitutes only 10% of the total migraine population. Well-defined focal neurologic manifestations typically precede the onset of headaches. These manifestations are thought to be secondary to intracranial vasoconstriction. The clinical features vary depending on the location and extent of the area of maximum ischemia. The most common manifestations are visual and the most typical of these is the so-called "scintillating scotoma." This may proceed to a complete hemianopsia or occasionally even total blindness. Other types of visual symptoms, sensory, motor, or speech disturbances may also be experienced. Sometimes the aura consists of emotional changes or rarely symptoms suggestive of depersonalization or derealization, very similar to what is observed in patients with temporal lobe seizures. Most often these symptoms last for only a few minutes or up to or less than an hour. Once these symptoms subside the patient develops the typical unilateral, throbbing, ingravescent headache associated with nausea, vomiting, photophobia, and other symptoms. The headache may last anywhere from 1 to 12 hours. In some patients, episodes of neurologic manifestations may not be followed by a headache. Unless a diagnosis of migraine has already been made or headaches have been known to occur following some of these episodes in the past, a final diagnosis has to await other investigations to rule out the presence of underlying structural neurologic disorders.

COMMON MIGRAINE

As the name implies, this is the most common variety of migraine headache and constitutes about 80% of all migraines. The premonitory manifestations either are completely absent or may be very vague and ill-defined. These symptoms, if and when they occur, may consist of vague feelings of ill health, gastrointestinal upset, and, rarely, autonomic disturbances like chills, warmth, flushing, and pallor of the skin. Psychic or mood changes may also be experienced. Precipitation of headache in relation to stressful events is somewhat more commonly seen in common migraines. Headache itself is more often bilateral and diffuse even at the beginning and tends to last longer, sometimes for days. Other associated features, as described under classic migraine, occur with the same frequency in these patients also. Some features of muscle contraction headaches may be superimposed on this, and the term *combined headache* is often used to describe such a situation. It should be remembered that during exacerbations of chronic scalp muscle contractions, some symptoms suggestive of vasodilatory headaches may develop. The term, combined headache, is applied to this condition also. A detailed history will help in differentiating the initial process, and therapy should be directed toward that specifically.

HEMIPLEGIC MIGRAINE

In hemiplegic migraine, the neurologic manifestations appear as hemiplegia or hemiparesis that outlast the headache by hours to days. Eventually, full recovery occurs. This type of headache is very often familial and the manifestations are often "monotonously similar," as Wolff describes it. The whole family may have hemiplegia on the same side time and time again.

OPHTHALMOPLEGIC MIGRAINE

Another rare variety of migraine is one in which ophthalmoplegia accompanies the headache. Typically, the pain is located in the periorbital regions. Ophthalmoplegia develops 1 to 2 days after onset of headache, with the third nerve most commonly involved. The fourth, sixth, and the ophthalmic division of the fifth cranial nerve may also be affected. When the third nerve is paralyzed, the pupil is involved in only 30% of the patients. Cranial nerve paralysis is thought to be secondary to ischemia.[13] Ocular paralysis lasts for days to weeks but eventually makes a complete recovery in the majority of patients. Many of these patients have episodes of nonophthalmoplegic migraines also.

When neurologic manifestations outlast the head-aches, as in the above two examples, the term *complicated migraine* has been used in the literature. Besides this, some patients with classic migraine also develop permanent neurologic sequelae, thought to be secondary to prolonged cerebral vasospasm and ischemic infarction. These are also described under the term complicated migraine. CT scan studies have revealed unsuspected areas of cerebral lucencies in patients with repeated episodes of classic migraine. Most of these tend to disappear but some persist.[14]

BASILAR ARTERY MIGRAINE

Bickerstaff described a group of young females who had manifestations of brainstem ischemia characterized by loss of vision, ataxia, dysarthria, bilateral motor and sensory symptoms, and rarely loss of consciousness.[15] These symptoms are followed by biocciptal vasodilatory headaches. Though most frequently seen in young females, this has been well described in males and older patients.

MIGRAINE EQUIVALENTS

Migraine equivalents constitutes a conglomeration of ill-defined episodic bodily disturbances, most often seen in young children who later on develop typical migraines. A positive family history of migraine and the lack of other physical abnormalities help in arriving at this diagnosis. Typical manifestations included under this category are (1) abdominal migraine with episodic abdominal pain, nausea, vomiting, and diarrhea; (2) cyclical vomiting; (3) episodic confusional state and lethargy; and (4) benign paroxysmal vertigo of childhood. The relationship of some of these manifestations to migraine is conjectural.

PATHOGENESIS OF MIGRAINE

The exact pathogenesis of migraine remains elusive despite the accumulation of a large amount of clinical and experimental observations. The most relevant available information will be summarized. It can be stated, at the outset, that the cranial vasculature is the target organ for the major clinical manifestations of migraine. It is a well-known clinical observation that superficial temporal vessels are visibly dilated and local compression of these vessels or compression of the carotid artery in the neck relieve the pain temporarily. Graham and Wolff documented this by studying the amplitude of the pulsations of these vessels during the headache phase and also by correlating the reduction of the pulsation when the headaches are relieved with the administration of ergotamine.[16] However, other types of extracranial vasodilatation (*e.g.,* heat- or exercise-induced) are not associated with headaches. Obviously factors other than vasodilatation that make a person susceptible to migraine will have to be implicated in the genesis of pain. Despite the extracranial vasodilatation, patients appear pale during a headache. It has been suggested that this is due to constriction of small vessels in the skin. This is supported by the observation of lowered skin temperature on the side of the headache. This has been further confirmed by the tissue clearance studies of radioactive sodium.[17]

What happens to the intracranial vessels during migraine? The clinical manifestations of focal or diffuse cerebral or brainstem dysfunction have been attributed to intracranial vasoconstriction. On rare occasions patients develop permanent sequelae as a result of intracranial vasconstriction. All this fits very well with the concept of ischemia. This vasoconstriction has now been proven using the techniques of regional cerebral blood flow measurements. A majority of the measurements have revealed a reduction in the cerebral blood flow, sometimes to very low and critical levels, during the prodromal stage. This is followed by a stage of increased flow that can persist sometimes for more than 48 hours.[18-20] It is not known, however, whether these changes are primary or secondary to some other, probably metabolic, changes occurring in the brain.

Now that we have established that there are specific vascular changes that occur during migraines, the next obvious question concerns the mechanism of these changes and what makes a person susceptible to these changes. As discussed earlier, there is evidence for inheritance of migraine. What inherited factors make these persons go through the cycles of vasoconstriction and vasodilation is still mostly unknown. Another question to be raised is how the triggering factors set off these changes. At the present time, evidence points toward abnormalities in neural and humoral control of the blood vessels in these patients. Evidence for each of these is summarized in the following sections.

Neurovascular Abnormalities

It is believed that there is an inherited abnormality of vasomotor control in migraine patients. The evidence for this is not overwhelming but suggestive. Migraine patients suffer from orthostatic symptoms more often than normal people. It has been found that the pulsation of scalp arteries diminish when these patients stand up suddenly, unlike unaffected persons.[21] They seem to be abnormally sensitive to the vasodilatory effects of physical and chemical changes like exposure to sun,[22] alcohol, nitrites, and others. There is some evidence that the response of peripheral vessels to heat

and cold stimuli are inadequate in migraine patients.[23,24]

Humoral Changes

A number of chemical mediators have been implicated in the genesis of the vascular changes that occur in migraine. These can be divided generally into two groups. One group of investigators has studied the chemical changes responsible for the generalized vasomotor changes, and the other group has attempted to explain the focality of the headache often confined to certain vessels. Even though a number of chemicals has been studied, only a few of them has been found to have any reproducible and consistent influence.

One of the most extensively studied chemicals is the neurotransmitter, *serotonin*. It has been well established that there is a slight increase in the serotonin level just prior to a headache, followed by a sharp fall at the onset of a migraine headache.[25] A serotonin-releasing factor has also been found during the migraine attack.[26] The exact nature of this is not known, even though it is thought to be a free fatty acid or a related compound. In some patients there is an increased excretion of 5-HIAA, the breakdown product of serotonin, during migraine. Administration of reserpine is associated with a fall in serotonin levels, and this causes the development of headaches in migraine patients consistently. These headaches can be relieved by intravenous injection of serotonin.[25] Another interesting observation is the occurrence of serotonin-induced increased platelet aggregability in migraine patients. This, along with the hypercoagulable state observed in migraine, may be responsible for some of the permanent sequelae of migraine.[27] Decreased levels of serotonin are also known to lower the pain threshold. These observations suggest that serotonin does play a role in the genesis of migraine even though the exact mechanism remains unknown. It is possible that serotonin acts through the encephalin pathway. Serotonin is a known regulator of the inhibition of pain transmission by encephalins.

Other neurotransmitters like norepinephrine and acetylcholine have also been investigated in migraine. There is very little evidence so far that they are directly involved in the pathogenesis of migraine. Monoamine oxidase enzyme has been looked at, especially because some of the dietary factors that trigger migraine contain vasoactive amines like tyramine and phenylethylamine. These are known substrates for this enzyme. Sandler, Youdim, and Hannington have found diminished activity of this enzyme during migraine attacks.[28]

The exact significance of this is not clear, especially in view of the fact that migraines in some patients can be successfully treated with monoamine oxidase inhibitors.

The role of hormonal changes in the genesis of migraine has also been investigated in some detail. There are a number of women who develop migraines at the time of their menstrual periods or when they take birth control pills. Migraines may become less frequent during pregnancy. In menstrual migraines, Somerville has demonstrated that the withdrawal of estrogen initiates the development of headache.[29] The exact mechanism of this remains unknown. No difference has been found in the circulating levels of estrogens and progesterones during pregnancy in the women whose headaches get better compared with those who do not.

Prostaglandins have been studied in migraine and so far no alterations in the levels of these powerful chemicals have been found. However, infusion of very small doses of PGE1 intravenously can precipitate migraines.[30] Experimental studies have shown that intracarotid infusion of PGE1 in dogs causes constriction of intracranial vessels and dilatation of the extracranial vessels, a situation similar to that which happens during migraine. However, the exact role played by this chemical, if any, remains to be clarified.

So far, there is no good explanation for the selective involvement of certain blood vessels in migraine. Local humoral changes, in the vicinity of the affected vessels, have been considered. A polypeptide material has been found in the perivascular region on the side of the headache. This has been called "neurokinin."[5] Reduction in the number and degranulation of the mast cells in biopsy specimens of blood vessels taken during headaches have been reported by Sicuteri.[31] Increased amounts of basophils that were degranulated have been found in the blood taken from the earlobe on the side of headache.[32] It has been suggested from these studies that local perivascular changes in kinins, heparin, and histamine play a role in the localization of pain.

It is obvious from this discussion that so far there is no clear evidence of any single neural or humoral pathway being involved in the pathogenesis of migraine. In summary, it can be stated that persons with migraine inherit a neurohumoral abnormality that makes them susceptible for the development of migraines when exposed to the various triggering factors, whether internally modulated or externally introduced. This leads to intracranial vasoconstriction, in turn leading to the various neurologic manifestations and extracranial vasodilation causing the headache. Kinins, heparin, and histamine probably play a role in the localization of the headache to particular extracranial vessels.

CLUSTER HEADACHE

DEFINITION

Cluster headache is defined by the *ad hoc* Committee on Classification of Headache[6] as a "vascular headache, predominantly unilateral and usually associated with flushing, sweating, rhinorrhea, and increased lacrimation; brief in duration and usually occurring in closely packed groups separated by long remissions." It will become evident that this definition has many shortcomings. The chronic type of cluster headache is not included in the definition; nor are any of the so-called cluster variants. Furthermore, cluster headache is classified under vascular headaches of the migraine type; although most specialists in the field of cluster headache research consider this type of headache to be a separate and distinct entity from migraine. For a discussion of the evidence for and against the "common entity concept" of cluster and migraine the reader is referred to the excellent monographs by Kudrow[33] and Lance.[34]

CLASSIFICATION

The ***classification of cluster headache*** agreed upon by most authorities in the field is as follows:

1. Episodic
2. Chronic
   a. Primary
   b. Secondary
   c. Chronic paroxysmal hemicrania (CPH)
3. Cluster variants
   a. Cluster-migraine
   b. Cluster-tic
   c. Cluster-vertigo

Episodic cluster headache is the most common type of cluster headache, and the syndrome derives its name from the fact that headache attacks are grouped into well-defined "cluster periods." It was probably first described by Romberg in 1840.[35] Since that time there have been many published accounts of this or similar syndromes under a variety of names and eponyms (see Kudrow, 1980, for a list and discussion of these). Kunkle and associates first used the term "cluster headache" in describing the syndrome.[36] During a cluster period, headache attacks occur frequently and often with an amazing regularity, and there is an increased susceptibility to headache precipitating factors. The cluster periods are then followed by extended headache-free intervals termed *remission periods.*

Chronic cluster headache is defined as the presence of typical cluster headache without a remission period for at least one year. It was described by Rooke and associates[37] in 1962 and later emphasized by Ekbom and Olivarius.[38] Often headache attacks are more frequent in the chronic cluster than in the episodic type, and treatment is more difficult. Patients who have never experienced a remission period are termed *primary chronic cluster* patients. Those who evolve initially from the episodic type into a pattern without remissions are categorized as *secondary chronic cluster* patients. *Chronic paroxysmal hemicrania* (CPH) is a rare type of chronic cluster first described by Sjaastad and Dale.[39] It occurs more frequently in women, headache attacks are briefer and more frequent, and it responds dramatically to aspirin and indomethacin.

Cluster-migraine is a variant of cluster headache in which patients exhibit components of both types of headaches. Patients experience typical cluster symptoms during migraine attacks.[40]

Cluster-tic syndrome is a cluster variant characterized by the association of cluster headache and trigeminal neuralgia (tic douloureux) pain in the same patient in a cluster pattern.[34,41-43]

Cluster-vertigo was first described by Gilbert and consists of episodes of vertigo occurring during cluster periods but not during remission periods.[44,45]

CLINICAL FEATURES

The incidence of cluster headache in the general population is unknown. Even the comparative incidence of cluster to migraine in large series ranges all the way from 5.6:1 (migraine:cluster) to 47.1:1.[2] There is a strong male preponderance among cluster patients with most series reporting ratios of 4 to 6:1. The majority of patients with cluster headache experience the onset of headache between the ages of 10 and 40, with the mean age of onset in the 20s.[33,34,36,46,47,48,49]

Cluster Periods

Approximately 50% to 70% of cluster patients have one or two cluster periods per year.[47,50,51] The duration of cluster periods is from 2 to 8 weeks in about 50% of cases.[33,34,36,47,50,51] Factors that can precipitate a cluster period may include "stress" and infections.

Remission Periods

Remission periods generally last between 7 and 12 months with 80% lasting less than 2 years. The published range of remission period duration is from 6 weeks to 20 years.[33,50,51]

Cluster Attack

Within a cluster period, the frequency of headache attacks may range from 2 per week to 8 per day. The majority of patients experience between 1 to 3 attacks per day.[34,50] Patients with CPH, however, may have between 6 to 18 headaches per day.[39] Many patients note that the frequency of headaches is less in the beginning and at the end of the cluster period.

The average duration of a cluster attack is from 30 minutes to 2 hours with the range of 10 minutes to 9 hours.[33,34,47,50] Onset of the pain is rapid, and often the offset of the pain is the same.

The quality of the pain is described variously as severe, excruciating, bursting, boring, burning, or throbbing. The location of the pain is almost always unilateral. It can change sides from one cluster period to another, and, rarely, it may even change sides during a cluster period. Pain usually begins in the periorbital or deep retroorbital region and may then radiate to involve the ipsilateral supraorbital, frontal, and temporal areas[52] (Ekbom's "upper syndrome") or, alternatively, it may radiate to involve the ipsilateral maxilla, upper teeth and palate, nostril, and lower jaw[52] (Ekbom's "lower syndrome").

Fifty to sixty percent of cluster patients report that the headaches occur either entirely or more frequently at night while asleep.[34,36,47,50] Ekbom also reported that 47% of his patients experienced headache attacks with "clock-like regularity."[50]

A unique feature of the cluster attack is the wealth of "associated symptoms" that typically accompany the head pain. These are often termed "cluster accompaniments" and consist of a variety of local autonomic symptoms. The common accompaniments include ipsilateral tearing (82%–86% of cases), ipsilateral conjunctival injection (45%–82%), ipsilateral nasal stuffiness or rhinorrhea (55%–77%), and ipsilateral ptosis and miosis (33%–60%). Other symptoms such as facial flushing, alterations in facial sweating, and bradycardia are less common and less well established.[33,34,53] One other associated symptom that typically accompanies the cluster attack concerns the behavior of the patient. Kudrow has pointed out that during a cluster attack most patients are unable to sit or lie still.[33] They invariably pace the floor, rock back and forth, and may even bang their head against the wall or strike the wall with their fists.

Another feature of the cluster attack is that it is easily precipitated by vasodilator substances. This provocation of a typical attack occurs only while the patient is in the cluster period and is usually ineffective during a remission period. Ekbom was the first to describe that nitroglycerin, 1 mg, sublingually, would reliably provoke a typical cluster attack when administered to patients during the cluster period.[54] Many authors have commented on the fact that alcohol often brings on a cluster attack.[34,36,47,51,55] Horton and associates first described precipitation of cluster attacks by histamine injection[55] (0.3 mg–0.5 mg, subcutaneously). This finding led to the practice of using histamine desensitization as a treatment for cluster headache.

MEDICAL HISTORY

There is some indication that there is a relationship between cluster headache and coronary artery disease. Graham reported that one patient experienced relief of his intermittent claudication during cluster attacks.[56] Ekbom described a patient who had relief of angina pectoris during cluster periods.[50,57] Others have reported a higher incidence of coronary artery disease in patients with cluster headaches, although the differences have not reached statistical significance.[58,59]

Several authors have noted a relationship between cluster headache and peptic ulcer disease.[60-62] This relationship has now been well documented in several studies, and it appears that about 20% to 25% of cluster headeache patients have a current or past history of peptic ulcer disease.[33,50,52,58,59,63,64]

PATHOPHYSIOLOGY OF CLUSTER HEADACHE PAIN

Vascular Aspects

Neither the etiology nor the pathogenesis of cluster headache is known. However, most authorities agree that dilation of extracranial arteries is partly responsible for the pain of cluster headache. Support for this contention includes the facts that vasodilating substances are known to induce attacks, compression of the superficial temporal or carotid artery will reduce the pain, surface skin temperatures on the ipsilateral side of the head are 1° to 3° warmer than on the pain-free side, and vasoconstrictor agents are known to abort or prevent cluster attacks.[55,63,65-68] Facial thermography has also demonstrated a "cold spot" in the ipsilateral supraorbital area during the early part of a cluster attack (possibly indicating diminished arterial flow through the internal carotid artery), which is followed by increased skin temperature ipsilaterally as the attack continues.[69-71]

There is evidence that the pain arises in part from the internal carotid artery as well as from the external carotid branches. Lance makes the point that compression of the superficial temporal artery often relieves the pain in the temporal area, but some pain usually re-

mains in the deep retroorbital region.[34] Ekbom and Greitz demonstrated changes in the internal carotid artery by angiography during a cluster headache.[72] At the height of the attack, localized narrowing of the extradural part of the internal carotid artery was observed, just distal to its exit from the carotid canal. A few minutes later a repeat injection was performed and the narrowing of the artery had spread proximally into the carotid canal. The authors felt that this arterial narrowing represented edema of the vessel wall; although they could not rule out spasm of the artery. The ophthalmic artery was dilated during the cluster attack. Therefore, during a cluster headache, a segment of the internal carotid artery within the carotid canal narrows, becomes edematous, and expands, thereby compressing the artery and its perivascular sympathetic plexus against the bony confines of the carotid canal. This is felt by some to be a source of at least part of the pain of a cluster attack.[34,52]

Kudrow,[71] in a combined Doppler and thermographic study, found evidence of diminished arterial flow in the ipsilateral ophthalmic and supraorbital arteries during both the interim and attack states of cluster headache. He felt that this was compatible with decreased flow through a narrowed internal carotid artery. Sakai and Meyer found that during a cluster attack cerebral blood flow (CBF) increased more in the contralateral hemisphere than on the side ipsilateral to the pain.[73] This finding might also support the concept of ipsilateral internal carotid artery narrowing with subsequent diminished arterial flow.

Biochemical Aspects

It is possible that the vasodilation responsible for the pain in cluster headache is due to a locally liberated agent or chemical. This mechanism then would be similar to that proposed for migraine.[7] The locally liberated agent would then cause a circumscribed area of vasodilation and sterile inflammation.

Horton suggested that cluster headache was due to a sensitivity to histamine because he could reproduce all the features of a typical cluster attack by a subcutaneous injection of histamine.[74] However, others make the point that cluster patients may not be sensitive to histamine, but sensitive to many vasodilator agents.[7] Certainly, as previously mentioned, administration of nitroglycerin and ingestion of alcohol routinely provoke cluster attacks.[34,36,47,54] Anthony and Lance found that the level of serum histamine rose during a cluster attack, but did not change significantly during a migraine headache.[75] However, controlled studies using histamine H1 receptor antagonists alone and in combination with H2 antagonists have failed to show any benefit in the treatment of cluster headache when compared with studies using placebos.[33,76] Furthermore, other investigators have failed to demonstrate an alteration in histamine metabolism in cluster patients.[77]

Other biochemical agents that are felt to be instrumental in vascular headache syndromes have also been studied in cluster patients. Anthony and Lance found no significant changes in plasma serotonin levels during cluster attacks,[75] whereas there were significantly lower levels during migraine attacks. Kunkle found an acetylcholinelike substance in the CSF of 4 of 14 cluster patients.[78] None of the 7 migraine patients had this substance in their spinal fluid.

Autonomic Nervous System Aspects

Many authors have proposed that the greater (superficial) petrosal nerve, the nerve of the pterygoid canal (vidian nerve), and the sphenopalatine ganglion were the source of pain in cluster headache.[79-82] Although surgical procedures involving ablation of these structures often leads to pain relief initially, most patients undergoing such therapy have recurrence of pain at varying intervals postoperatively.[34,42]

Hormonal Aspects

Kudrow studied the relationship between plasma testosterone and LH levels in cluster patients during an active cluster period, in cluster patients during a remission period, and in normal controls.[83] He found that active cluster patients had significantly lower hormone levels than those in remission, and that cluster patients in remission had significantly lower levels of both hormones than normal controls. Since the LH level was also depressed, this indicated dysfunction in the hypothalamic–pituitary axis. Furthermore, other anterior pituitary hormone levels were normal, suggesting that the site of impairment was in the hypothalamus. In women, there appears to be no relationship between menstruation or pregnancy and cluster attacks or remission.[33]

PATHOPHYSIOLOGY OF CLUSTER ACCOMPANIMENTS

The pathogenesis of the common "cluster accompaniments" (tearing, conjunctival injection, nasal stuffiness and rhinorrhea, and ptosis and moisis) has not been clearly established. Many authors have attributed these symptoms to parasympathetic hyperactivity[78,79,82,84] or a combination of parasympathetic hyperactivity and sympathetic hypofunction.[85,86] However, most authorities now agree that the ipsilateral ptosis and miosis is due to a lesion in the postganglionic neurons somewhere between the superior cer-

vical ganglion and the effector organs. In view of the angiographic findings of Ekbom and Greitz,[72] the mechanism of this oculosympathetic paralysis is felt to be traction on and compression of the perivascular internal carotid sympathetic plexus against the bony confines of the carotid canal caused by the swelling and vasodilation of the internal carotid artery.[34,52,53,85-88] Recently, Vijayan and Watson documented that cluster patients have evidence of a lesion in the postganglionic neurons of their oculocephalic sympathetic pathways.[53] They suggested that all the common cluster accompaniments might be due to this sympathetic hypofunction, although certainly no studies have disproven the role of parasympathetic hyperactivity.

MUSCLE CONTRACTION HEADACHE

In the general population, muscle contraction or tension headache is the most common form of headache observed. The generally accepted term is *muscle contraction* headache (MCHA) because the message implied by the term tension headache is that this type of headache is always due to psychological tensions and anxieties. This is not entirely true because fairly typical symptoms of MCHA can occasionally be seen in patients with structural abnormalities. This will become more apparent later on when we discuss the clinical features of this particular variety of headache. Therefore, the term MCHA is accepted by most of the workers in the field. This terminology, however, implies that the headache is the direct result of excessive muscle contraction, which may or may not be really true as discussed in the section dealing with the mechanism of these headaches.

DEFINITION

The definition as proposed by the *ad hoc* committee for the classification of muscle contraction headache is as follows. "Ache or sensation of tightness, pressure or constriction, widely varied in intensity, frequency and duration, sometimes long lasting, and commonly suboccipital. They are associated with sustained contraction of skeletal muscles in the absence of permanent structural change, usually as part of the individual's reaction during life stress. The ambiguous and unsatisfactory terms 'tension,' 'psychogenic,' and 'nervous' headache refer largely to this group." Most of the scientific work published after this classification tends to follow this definition.

INCIDENCE

It is very difficult to obtain a correct estimate of the incidence of muscle contraction headache because many of the patients with mild to moderate or short-term episodes of MCHA do not often consult a physician. It is roughly estimated that approximately 80% of all headaches belong to this category. Most of the statistics from headache clinics indicate that migraine and MCHA occur with the same frequency. The patient population in a headache clinic obviously is a very selected group, and this does not clearly represent the true incidence in the general population.

CLASSIFICATION

Various clinical subdivisions of MCHA have been offered by different authors, depending on their clinical course and underlying causes. There is really no standardization so far. We like to divide the patients with MCHA into the following categories based on the clinical manifestations and the circumstances under which these symptoms occur:

Classification of Muscle Contraction Headache (MCHA)
1. Acute MCHA
2. Subacute MCHA
3. Chronic MCHA
4. Combined MC and vascular headaches
   a. as part of MCHA
   b. as part of migraine
5. MCHA due to structural disease
6. Post-traumatic MCHA
7. Conversion headache (very rare)

CLINICAL FEATURES

The major differences among acute, subacute, and chronic forms of MCHA are the constancy and duration of the pain. In the *acute* variety, the most common form of the so-called "tension headache," the pain is very often short-lived and associated with an acute stressful situation or fatigue. It usually lasts for a few hours and rarely requires any form of specific therapy except for an occasional mild analgesic like aspirin. Most often the pain is located in the back of the neck and the occipital regions or frontally. Sometimes it is generalized. The pain is usually aching in nature and is relieved by stretching or gentle massage. Most of the people who develop a headache toward the end of their working day find that getting home and relaxing relieves the headache.

In the *subacute* variety of MCHA, the headaches are more prolonged, sometimes lasting for days; often the pain is disabling. In patients with the chronic variety of MCHA, the physician is often told by the patient that initially the headaches were intermittent and that later they became chronic and continuous. The distribution of the pain again most often is generalized. Sometimes the pain is unilateral and may involve only one side of the head or may be confined to the back of the head and neck. The pain usually has an aching quality. Associated nausea and vomiting can occur if the pain is severe. Similar to the acute variety of MCHA, at least initially, specific precipitating factors may be identifiable in subacute MCHA. As the recurrences become more frequent, these factors become more and more difficult to identify. Gradually, the intervals between headaches become shorter and eventually merge into the chronic variety of MCHA.

As mentioned above, the *chronic* variety of MCHA may evolve from the subacute variety, but more often than not such a history is unavailable. Most patients start with the chronic variety *per se.* Patients with the chronic form of this headache have a very characteristic history. In some, onset may be related to a dramatic physical trauma like an injury or infection, and in others, it may follow a severe emotional trauma. In the majority, however, there is no specific initial precipitating factor that is identifiable. Characteristically, these headaches become gradually more and more severe. Pain is present continuously throughout the waking hours. It is also present at night if the patient happens to wake in the middle of the night, which is a common occurrence in chronic MCHA. Pain is noticed as soon as the patient wakes up; it tends to become progressively worse throughout the day and is still present at the time the patient goes to bed.

Active involvement in concentrated work and intake of alcohol often give some relief. The pain is most often generalized, involving the entire scalp, neck, and shoulder regions. It sometimes involves the upper part of the face, also. It is described as a dull aching or pressurelike sensation. It may also be described as a heavy weight on top of the head, a viselike feeling, a tight band around the head or a squeezing sensation. It is also described, rarely, as a feeling as if something is going to explode. Usually there is ever-present low-grade pain.

In the majority of patients, there are distinct exacerbations that are superimposed on top of this constant pain. These exacerbations are often associated with nausea and vomiting and may also develop some features of vasodilatory headaches with many of the usual symptoms described by patients with migraine headaches. These exacerbations may last for hours or days.

Frequently, these patients complain that they do not get any relief from the usual analgesic medications. Narcotic usage becomes a real problem because the headache persists for longer and longer periods of time.

ASSOCIATED FEATURES

A number of studies have indicated that a majority of patients with chronic MCHA have symptoms of depression. The incidence of depression has been variously estimated. According to one study, 30% of patients have significant depression[89]. The severity of the depressive symptoms varies from very mild to very severe. Besides the depressed emotional status, somatic symptoms of depression are very frequently reported by these patients. These include difficulty in falling asleep, frequent awakening, restless sleep, and waking up tired in the morning. Energy level is very low and vague descriptions of loss of memory and concentration are very common. Feelings of "fuzziness in the head" is also a common complaint.

Exacerbations of the headaches occur very frequently and cannot be correlated clearly with any added emotional stress. Patients often deny that headaches ever occur in relation to specific stressful stimuli. They may sometimes be related to the "let-down" periods. Mild degrees of photophobia and lightheadedness may be experienced by these patients, but none of them experience any of the neurologic manifestations seen in patients with migraine. Patients eventually become completely disabled physically and emotionally. They give up their jobs. Families have been known to break up because of these headaches. Chronic MCHA patients usually develop an existence of "living from pill to pill" during waking hours. These symptoms go on and on for years without relief.

COMBINED MUSCLE CONTRACTION AND VASCULAR HEADACHE

Features of muscle contraction and vascular headaches are often seen together. This phenomenon can occur in a patient with a severe exacerbation of MCHA. It has been reported by about 25% of patients. On the other hand, patients with prolonged migraine headaches develop muscle contraction components toward the later stages of the migraine attack. It is important to distinguish between MCHA and migraine because the primary therapy should be aimed at the original cause of the headache. About 10% of patients with muscle contraction headaches suffer from true migraine headaches also. These patients are usually able to differentiate one from the other.

MCHA DUE TO STRUCTURAL DISEASE

MCHA due to structural disease most commonly occurs in patients with cervical spine disease either in the form of spondylosis or as part of a traumatic disorder. Many of the other neurologic manifestations of spondylosis may be absent, and headache may be the only symptom in the beginning. Rarely, similar headaches can occur as a result of prolonged eyestrain due to close work, especially if there is uncorrected eyestrain. This is distinctly rare. Other diseases of the eyes like glaucoma may sometimes lead to similar symptoms. Temporomandibular joint disorders may also give rise to symptoms suggestive of scalp muscle contraction headaches. An adequate history, location of the pain, and a thorough clinical and, if necessary, radiologic examination of the joints will help in arriving at the correct diagnosis. On very rare occasions, a posterior fossa lesion may produce sufficient reflex muscle spasm, and the resultant pain may be mistaken for MCHA. A detailed history often reveals unusual features, and appropriate clinical and laboratory investigations often lead to the correct diagnosis.

POST-TRAUMATIC MCHA

Almost 90% of patients with post-traumatic headaches have all the characteristic features of chronic scalp muscle contraction headaches. They often have all the associated psychological features as described previously. Constant muscle spasm is considered to be one of the most important mechanisms in the genesis of post-traumatic headaches. An appropriate history of trauma and other associated features of the so-called "post-traumatic syndrome" should provide the correct diagnosis. The possibility of an associated structural lesion should always be considered under these circumstances and ruled out. (See Post-traumatic Headache for more details.)

CONVERSION OR DELUSIONAL HEADACHE

A conversion or delusional headache is a very rare psychiatric phenomenon. Patients with these types of headaches usually have evidence of very severe psychopathology. The headache itself may have all the features of a typical MCHA. However, very often the associated features of other bizzare psychiatric and behavioral patterns give the clue for the correct diagnosis.

MECHANISM OF PAIN IN MCHA

As implied by the name, most investigators believe that the pain of MCHA is due to chronic sustained contraction of scalp muscles. If one looks closely at the available information, the mechanism is certainly not all that clear. It has been reasonably well established that there is evidence of increased muscular activity in the scalp in patients with MCHA. Increased EMG activity has been demonstrated in the scalp muscles by a number of investigators.[90,91] Similarly, there is good correlation between the reduction of EMG activity and relief of headaches following biofeedback treatment.[90,92] But not all patients with increased muscular activity of scalp muscles develop headaches nor do all patients with MCHA have evidence of excessive muscle contraction.[93] There are other problems in attributing the entire pain mechanism to muscle contractions alone, such as (1) poor correlation between the degree of demonstrable muscle contraction and the severity of pain and (2) equally severe or sometimes more severe degrees of scalp muscle contraction in patients with migraine headaches. Therefore, other factors should be considered and studied.

Beginning with the original work of Harold Wolff, a number of investigators have demonstrated that vasoconstriction is a prominent accompaniment of MCHA.[94] They also reported that vasoconstrictor agents increased the severity of MCHA. The exact role played by vasoconstriction in the genesis of pain in MCHA is still not clearly established. It is possible that stress stimuli lead to neurohumoral changes that in turn lead to vasoconstriction, and subsequently to contraction of scalp muscles. Both these factors may be contributing to the pain. A lot more research needs to be done in this area to clear up these controversies.

There has been some suggestion that serotonin metabolism is abnormal in patients with chronic scalp muscle contraction headaches.[95] The authors found decreased levels of serotonin in the blood. Other theories about central abnormalities in pain sensitivity have been suggested. Further studies in these areas are required before any definite conclusions can be drawn. For the time being, one can conclude by saying that most of the evidence points toward constant muscle contraction as the primary cause for the development of pain in MCHA. Vasoconstriction may also play some adjunctive role in its pathogenesis.

POST-TRAUMATIC HEADACHE

Almost all persons who have had injury to their heads have local pain or tenderness at the site of impact for a few hours or even a few days following their injury, after which many become symptom-free.[7,96] A substantial number of these people complain of headache, vertigo, impairment of memory and concentration, and emotional instability for weeks, months, or even years after the injury. This syndrome, termed the *post-trau-*

matic or postconcussive syndrome, is not known to be associated with anatomic lesions of the central nervous system and may occur whether or not a person was rendered unconscious by the head trauma.[97] Certainly, headache is the most prominent and frequent symptom of the post-traumatic syndrome.

The actual incidence of post-traumatic headache is difficult to determine and varies in different series from 33% to 80%.[34,98-102] Post-traumatic headache may occur following major head trauma, but severe and prolonged headache may also follow seemingly trivial injury. The development of headache does not correlate with the duration of unconsciousness or post-traumatic amnesia, nor with EEG abnormalities, presence of skull fracture, or blood in the CSF.[102]

CLINICAL FEATURES AND CLASSIFICATION

Simons and Wolff classified post-traumatic headaches into three types, which they termed types 1, 2, and 3.[96]

Type 1: Muscle Contraction Headache

Type 1 headaches are the most common, being present in 100% of patients. The pain has a dull aching quality or steady pressurelike sensation. It is often described as a sensation of weight on the head, a "tightness like a cap" covering the whole head, or a sensation of a "tight band" around the head. It is diffusely distributed over the entire scalp. Patients tend to be anxious and depressed, and they often exhibit other vague symptoms of the post-traumatic syndrome. Therefore, they tend to share many characteristics with patients who have psychogenic muscle contraction headaches without a history of head trauma.

Type 2: Site of Injury Headache

Type 2 headaches occur in about 25% of patients. These patients characteristically have pain localized in the area of the actual scalp injury. There is usually a clearly defined and relatively superficial tender zone with or without scar formation. There is often a continuous pain in this location that is aggravated by any local stimulation such as wearing a hat or combing the hair. The pain is often described as burning, boring, aching, or stabbing in nature.

Type 3: Vascular Headache

Type 3 headaches occur in about 7% of patients. These patients have recurrent unilateral, throbbing headaches associated with anorexia, nausea, and vomiting. The headaches are usually episodic and of short duration, but most patients also have typical type 1 headaches between attacks of vascular headache.

Type 4: Post-traumatic Dysautonomic Cephalalgia

Recently, another type of post-traumatic headache has been described.[103,104] Patients with type 4 headaches have a history primarily of neck injury involving the anterior triangle of the neck. After recovery from the acute injury, they develop recurrent unilateral vasodilatory headaches. The headaches are associated with ipsilateral pupillary dilation, tearing, and sweating, and may be accompanied by nausea, vomiting, and photophobia. Following the headache, most patients develop an ipsilateral partial oculosympathetic paralysis that can be confirmed by appropriate autonomic testing. Unlike patients with typical forms of vascular headache, patients with type 4 headache do not respond to ergotamine preparations, but they are sensitive to propranolol.

POST-TRAUMATIC SYNDROME

Headache is the dominant symptom of the post-traumatic syndrome. It usually appears within 24 hours of the head injury, although about 6% of patients do not experience headache until some days or weeks afterward.[97]

Other common symptoms that occur as part of the post-traumatic syndrome include vertigo, lightheadedness, syncope, impaired concentration and memory, easy fatigability, irritability, lack of energy, depression, anxiety, phobia, and lowered tolerance for alcohol.[7,34,97,102]

NATURAL HISTORY OF POST-TRAUMATIC SYNDROME

Neither the severity nor the duration of post-traumatic symptoms correlates with the duration of unconsciousness. Approximately 10% of patients are symptom-free by one month after the accident. After one year, about 70% are recovered, and 85% are symptom-free within three years after their injury. Patients over 40 years old are more likely to develop persisting symptoms than those under 30.[105] Therefore, in general most patients with post-traumatic headache and post-traumatic syndrome note a gradual improvement in their symptoms over a period of one to three years.

PATHOPHYSIOLOGY OF POST-TRAUMATIC HEADACHE

There is no single identifiable factor responsible for the development of post-traumatic headache, and most often a multifactorial etiology is probably present. Most authors agree that an interplay of both physiologic and psychological factors are important in the genesis of post-traumatic headache and the post-traumatic syn-

drome. Injury to the pain-sensitive structures of the scalp, cervical spine, and intracranial contents leads to physiologic changes that ultimately result in headache. The initial insult may be to one or multiple structures, and the type of headache depends on the structure involved.

Muscle Contraction

The most common type of post-traumatic headache (type 1) is caused by sustained muscle contractions.[7,34,96] Electromyographic studies in patients with type 1 headache have revealed a fairly close correlation between the degree of muscular activity and the severity of the pain. Direct injury to muscle with increased irritability, scar formation, or increased reflex muscle spasm as a result of neural damage can lead to muscle contraction headache.[106] Psychological factors also undoubtedly play a role in this type of post-traumatic headache.

Injury to Nerves

Damage to either somatic or autonomic nerves can lead to the production of headache. Damage to the nerve supply of the scalp muscles can lead to irritability of the muscles and excess muscle spasm. In addition, entrapment of these nerves in the scar tissue of the scalp and the formation of neuromas in the scar tissue may be responsible for the development of type 2 post-traumatic headache.[107] Finally, dysfunction of the autonomic nerves may lead to vasomotor instability, which in turn causes vasodilatory headache (types 3 and 4).[104,105] This explanation is supported by the observation that injection of the perivascular plexus with local anesthetic may sometimes lead to relief of headache.[7,96]

Scar Formation

As already mentioned, scar formation in the scalp can lead to entrapment of nerves. This results in a painful scar at the site of injury, which is one cause of the type 2 post-traumatic headache. Other causes of this type of headache are thought to be traumatic myositis, fibrositis, and periostitis, which cause local tenderness and burning pain at the site of injury.[7,96]

Vascular Changes

Frequently, distended and excessively pulsatile scalp arteries can be observed or palpated during certain types of post-traumatic headache (types 3 and 4).[7,96,104,105] This vasodilation may result from local loss of vasomotor control, elaboration of vasodilatory chemicals, or lack of central vasomotor control. Studies have shown that cerebral circulation time is significantly slowed in patients with post-traumatic symptoms and that im-

provement of symptoms correlated with a return of the circulation time to normal.[108,109] These findings support the concept that vasomotor instability is an important mechanism in post-traumatic symptoms. This concept is further supported by the vascular quality of the headache in some types, "migrainous" phenomena in some patients, orthostatic and exertional aggravation of headache in many patients, responsiveness to ergotamine and other vasoactive drugs in some patients, reproduction of the headache by histamine injection, and relief of the headache by perivascular anesthetic infiltration.[7,96,97,101,102,106]

Injury to Intracranial Structures

Acute injury to various intracranial structures and subsequent scar formation have been considered to be other factors in the etiology of post-traumatic headache. Meningeal scarring leads to traction and distention of pain-sensitive structures. Some have attempted neurosurgical removal of these scarred areas with limited success.[98] Intracranial hemorrhage is most often responsible for the development of these scars. However, this mechanism probably plays only a minor role in most patients with post-traumatic headache.

Psychological Factors

The exact role of psychological factors in the genesis of post-traumatic headache and the post-traumatic syndrome is somewhat controversial. Many authorities believe that the premorbid personality is significant in the initiation and perpetuation of these symptoms. The fear that serious damage to the brain has occurred as a result of head trauma can lead to significant anxiety, especially if the patient is experiencing subtle difficulties in the realm of higher cortical functioning. The anxiety and depression, in turn, can result in muscle contraction headache, which may only exacerbate the patient's psychological symptoms.

Psychological testing has been abnormal in some studies and normal in others. Furthermore, the role played by monetary compensation and litigation, and even by malingering all seem to complicate the picture and must be considered when evaluating and treating the patient.

In any event, it is now clear that there is objective evidence of labyrinthine and CNS dysfunction in many patients with symptoms of the post-traumatic syndrome. Investigators have found abnormalities in visual-evoked potentials[110] (VEP), higher cortical functioning,[111] EEG,[112] vestibular functioning,[113,114] and the oculocephalic sympathetic pathways in the neck.[104,105]

It is obvious that post-traumatic headache and the post-traumatic syndrome are complex disorders with

multiple underlying mechanisms. Therapy should be directed toward these mechanisms and should include local measures, appropriate drug therapy, and psychological, social, and physical rehabilitation.

PHYSICAL CAUSES OF HEADACHE

Headache due to a recognizable lesion caused by a specific intracranial or extracranial disease process probably constitutes between 5% and 10% of serious headache problems. It is this small group of headache patients, however, that is a constant concern to the physician. To miss the diagnosis of this type of headache syndrome may not only prolong the patient's suffering, but also threaten his or her well-being.

NONMIGRAINOUS VASCULAR HEADACHE

A wide variety of medical diseases include headache associated with usually nonrecurrent dilation of cranial arteries as part of the overall symptomatic picture.[6] These headaches are not migrainous in character, but are usually bilateral and throbbing in nature. They rarely pose diagnostic difficulty, and treatment of the underlying condition usually relieves the pain.

Nasal Vasomotor Headache

Nasal vasomotor headache is predominantly anterior in location and associated with nasal discomfort resulting from congestion and edema of nasal and paranasal mucosae. This headache is often termed "'vasomotor rhinitis'' and is thought to represent a localized vascular reaction to stress.

Fever Headache Due to Systemic Infection

Fever headache is the most common type of nonmigrainous vascular headache, and may occur with any febrile illness.

Hypertension Headache and Hypertensive Encephalopathy

Headache is probably no more common in patients with hypertension than in normotensives.[34,115] In severe hypertension (diastolic pressure over 130mm Hg), headache may occur, especially if the blood pressure rises rapidly. The pain is frequently occipital in location, is present upon awakening, diminishes one to two hours after arising, and improves in those patients whose blood pressure responds to treatment.[116,117]

There are a number of conditions and situations in which the blood pressure rises dramatically, and these are typically accompanied by throbbing or bursting headache pain. Included in this category are headache associated with pheochromocytoma, autonomic hyperreflexia in high thoracic or cervical spinal cord injured patients, some cases of orgasmic cephalgia, exertional headache, and perhaps some cases of benign cough headache.[7,34,118-122] In hypertensive encephalopathy, headache is a common symptom, along with confusion, lethargy or obtundation, and occasionally focal neurologic signs.

Hypoxia Headache

Headache occurs in approximately 10% to 30% of patients with transient ischemic attacks and thrombotic or embolic cerebral infarcts.[123-125] Presumably, cerebral anoxia resulting in "postanoxic luxury perfusion" and/or "local factors," as well as in more generalized hypoxia, is responsible for the headache associated with these focal ischemic events.[7,34]

Post-Seizure Headache

Postictal headache is presumably due to widespread and marked cerebral vasodilation, and is present more often after a generalized convulsive seizure.[7,34]

Headache Caused by Food and Chemicals

Vascular headaches may be caused by a wide variety of chemicals and food. Many chemicals, drugs, and foods precipitate headache because of their vasodilator effect (nitroglycerin; nitrites, and nitrates in cured meats such as hot dogs, bacon, ham; monosodium glutamate; alcohol). Other substances cause headache by an acute rise in blood pressure, as in hypertensive crisis occurring in patients on MAO inhibitors after ingesting foods containing tyramine (e.g., cheddar cheese, red wine). Still other headaches result from withdrawal of vasoconstrictor substances (caffeine, sympathomimetic drugs, ergotamine).

INTRACRANIAL (TRACTION) HEADACHE

Headaches from intracranial sources are most often produced by traction on, displacement of, or inflammation in or about any of the intracranial pain-sensitive structures, or distention and dilation of intracranial arteries caused by an intracranial mass, infection, nonspecific brain edema, or lumbar puncture. Unless a tumor or other space-occupying lesion occurs in a strategic position along the CSF pathways or in the posterior fossa, it can grow to a considerable size before causing headache.

Tumors

Headache is an initial symptom in about 10% to 30% of patients with intracranial tumors. The pain of such lesions is usually a steady, nonthrobbing, deep, dull

ache that lasts from a few moments to several hours. It is usually most intense in the morning and may be increased by changes in head position, coughing, straining, or sneezing.

In the beginning, pain from tumor may be of some localizing value; when unilateral, the headache is usually on the side of the tumor. The pain is usually occipital when the tumor is in the posterior fossa, and more anterior when the mass is supratentorial. Later on, the headache tends to become generalized, since edema around the mass causes an increase in intracranial pressure.[7]

Posterior fossa tumors and those that develop within or adjacent to the ventricular system cause headache much earlier in their course than supratentorial masses. These may produce a "ball-valve action" within the ventricular system causing sudden attacks of severe headache when the head is moved to a specific position (e.g., 3rd and 4th ventricular tumors and tumors of the pineal region).

Tumors in the region of the sella turcica may exert pressure on the diaphragma sellae or pain-sensitive structures at the base of the brain, thus causing a headache often described as bursting.

Arteriovenous Malformations

Arteriovenous malformations can cause sudden headaches that recur in the same place. Often the headaches precede other symptoms, are on the same side as the AVM, and are confined to the area over the malformation. Occasionally, they produce neurologic symptoms associated with headache and thereby mimic classic migraine. Persistent focal neurologic findings, seizures, and a cranial bruit help make the diagnosis.

Aneurysms

Aneurysms of the internal carotid or posterior communicating arteries may cause a periorbital or frontal headache that, in some ways, mimics migraine. However, though the pain may be periodic, it is always in the same location. An exacerbation of pain may also be accompanied by a sudden or increasing paralysis of the oculomotor (III) or other parasellar cranial nerves, suggesting an enlargement of the aneurysm. An angiogram may be necessary to differentiate this entity from ophthalmoplegic migraine.[13]

Abscesses

Symptoms of an unruptured brain abscess are essentially the same as those of any expanding mass lesion in the brain. Brain scan, CT scan, angiography, and ultimately craniotomy may be required to differentiate this process from a tumor.

Hematoma (Epidural, Subdural, Intracerebral)

Although headache usually is a component of the initial symptoms of hematoma, it is rarely the only symptom, and the associated findings plus the history help in arriving at the correct diagnosis.

Pseudotumor Cerebri (Benign Intracranial Hypertension)

The term *pseudotumor cerebri* is applied to a condition in which CSF pressure is elevated without any demonstrable lesion (mass, CSF obstruction, and so on). The condition is usually self-limited, but there may be visual loss or recurrence of symptoms.

The etiology of pseudotumor is unknown, but a long list of "associated conditions" or "predisposing factors" exists. These include young obese women with menstrual dysfunction, obesity, menarche, steroid drugs or the discontinuance of steroids (including birth control pills), vitamin A toxicity, certain drugs (tetracycline, nalidixic acid, nitrofurantoin, phenothiazines), Addison's disease, hypoparathyroidism, systemic lupus erythematosus, and anemia (iron-deficient, vitamin B_{12}-deficient).

Diagnosis of pseudotumor is established by documenting an elevated CSF pressure with no other CSF abnormality, plus no other demonstrable CNS lesion (i.e., normal CT scan with normal or small ventricles).

The pathogenesis is somewhat controversial but may be (1) intracranial vascular engorgement, (2) decreased CSF resorption, and/or (3) increased CSF production.

Virtually all patients with pseudotumor present with headache, and it is the chief complaint in 90% of cases. It is described as generalized and intermittent and is generally worse in the morning. Its onset may be sudden or gradual. Other nonspecific complaints include dizziness, fatigue, and nausea. The most worrisome symptoms that occur in pseudotumor are visual and are present in about 35% of patients. These include transient obscurations or graying out of vision for 5 to 15 seconds, transient blurring of vision from minutes to hours, diplopia (usually due to VI nerve palsy), visual acuity changes usually preceded by blurring or obscurations, and visual field deficits. Papilledema is present in 100% of patients, is always bilateral, and occasionally asymmetric. The remainder of the neurologic examination is usually normal. Ninety percent of patients are obese.[126]

Laboratory studies are normal except for an elevated CSF pressure and occasional findings on skull x-ray film compatible with increased intracranial pressure. Specifically, no mass lesions or ventriculomegaly are present on CT scan, angiography, or pneumoencephalography.

Treatment for pseudotumor includes serial lumbar punctures, acetazolamide, and lumboperitoneal shunting if there is a deterioration in vision. The use of steroids in pseudotumor is still controversial; they should not be given for longer than two weeks in any case.[126–128]

Postlumbar Puncture Headache

Following lumbar puncture, headache occurs in from 15% to 41% of patients. The pathogenesis of this type of headache results from the continued leakage of CSF through the hole in the dura and arachnoid caused by the needle puncture.[129] This leakage of CSF from below causes the brain to "sag" and the bridging veins to dilate (due to pressure differences across their walls). The sagging brain places traction on pain-sensitive structures at the base of the brain, and that, plus the venous dilation, results in headache.[7,129–132]

The headache is usually a generalized dull, deep, nonthrobbing pain with a striking response to postural change. The headache is dramatically worsened by procedures that increase the traction on pain-sensitive structures, such as assuming an erect posture, bilateral jugular vein compression, or shaking the head. It generally begins 6 to 48 hours after lumbar puncture, commonly lasts for 24 to 48 hours, but may persist for weeks.

Through the years, many techniques have been suggested to prevent the development of postlumbar puncture headache. Procedures that probably do not affect the incidence of postlumbar puncture headache include: (1) forced recumbency in the supine position (for up to 24 hours after the tap); (2) the amount of CSF removed (unless more than 20 ml); and (3) administration of various drugs such as vasopressin or barbiturates.[130]

Procedures that do appear to decrease the incidence of postlumbar puncture headache include having the patient immediately assume a prone recumbent position for three hours and then become ambulatory.[131] This technique is probably the most effective preventive measure. It may work by (1) staggering the arachnoid and dural holes, (2) eliminating epidural negative pressure, (3) decreasing the tension on the dural and arachnoidal tears, (4) decreasing the epidural space, and (5) allowing gravity to help instead of hinder the situation. Use of a smaller needle probably is helpful, although this efficacy may be a result of tangential puncture of the dura rather than its size.[132] Adequate hydration also helps prevent postlumbar puncture headache.

Factors of questionable value include (1) abdominal binders, (2) skill of the physician, (3) configuration of the needle, and (4) needle insertion with the bevel parallel with dural fibers.

Treatment for postlumbar puncture headache is initiated with prone recumbency and increased fluid intake. If these measures fail and the headache persists, epidural blood patch is probably the most effective treatment.[129,130]

HEADACHE DUE TO OVERT CRANIAL INFLAMMATION

Headaches due to overt cranial inflammation are caused by readily recognized inflammation of cranial structures, either sterile or infectious. When the inflammatory process involves pain-sensitive structures or when inflammation causes an increase in intracranial pressure, headache results—the nature and location of which depend on the site of involvement. Treatment for this group of headaches should center around treating the underlying disorder.

Meningitis (Acute, Chronic, Chemical)

Acute meningitis causes a generalized severe headache associated with fever, photophobia, and a stiff and rigid neck (meningismus). Chronic meningitis produces a milder headache with less prominent meningeal signs. If communicating hydrocephalus occurs secondarily, mental status changes and other neurologic signs may develop.

Subarachnoid Hemorrhage

Headache associated with subarachnoid hemorrhage is typically rapid in onset, quite severe, and generalized in location. It is usually associated with photophobia, nuchal rigidity, and alterations in the level of consciousness. If vasospasm or intracerebral hematoma occurs, focal neurologic findings may be present. If the ruptured aneurysm is located in the internal carotid-posterior communicating artery area, an oculomotor (III) nerve palsy may result.

Arteritis and Phlebitis

Inflammation of the cranial arteries and veins causes headache, presumably due to inflammation of the vessel wall and surrounding perivascular regions. This inflammation may be secondary to an infectious process (viral, fungal, bacterial, tuberculous) or an autoimmune process (as in SLE, polyarteritis nodosa, rheumatoid arthritis, giant cell arteritis). Depending on which vessels are involved, the headache may be unilateral, bilateral, or generalized, and the pain may be described variously as throbbing, burning, or aching. If the involved vessels are extracranial, they may be

swollen, tender, nodular, erythematous, or eventually thrombosed and nonpulsatile.

The most discrete clinical arteritis is that of *giant cell (temporal) arteritis* (GCA). This disorder most often afflicts persons of both sexes over the age of 65, although women are affected more often than men.[7,34,133,134] Symptoms of a systemic disturbance such as malaise, weight loss, anorexia, low-grade fever, night sweats, arthralgias, myalgias, and weakness are commonly present, thus merging into the syndrome known as "polymyalgia rheumatica." Most patients complain of headache, and they usually have the symptoms listed previously. When present, jaw claudication, or pain in the masseter muscles on chewing, is almost pathognomonic for this disorder. Other arteries may also be involved, with large and medium-sized vessels being the principal sites of the inflammatory process. Scalp and temporal artery tenderness is often present.

The most dreaded complication of GCA is partial or complete loss of vision due to an ischemic optic neuropathy caused by occlusion of the central retinal artery or one of its branches. More than a third of patients with GCA are threatened by this manifestation. Other neurologic signs and symptoms such as diplopia, peripheral neuropathy, cerebral dysfunction, meningoencephalitis, stroke, lethargy, delirium, and coma have been reported.[7,133,134]

The cardinal laboratory finding in GCA is an elevated sedimentation rate, usually in the range of 45 mm–120 mm per hour.[34,134] Other common laboratory findings include moderate leukocytosis, mild anemia, elevated serum fibrinogen, elevated serum haptoglobin, and elevated liver function tests (SGOT, SGPT, alkaline phosphatase). The diagnosis is confirmed by a positive superficial temporal artery biopsy with multinucleated giant cells present. Treatment for this disorder, as in many of the arteritides, is with steroid preparations.

HEADACHE DUE TO DISEASES OF CRANIAL OR NECK STRUCTURES

Cranial and neck structure diseases are a broad group of diseases that cause headache due to the spread of effects of noxious stimulation of ocular, aural, nasal and paranasal, dental, and cervical structures (as by trauma, neoplasia, inflammation, and so on). For the sake of brevity, only two causes of headache from this group will be presented here.

Acute Nasal Sinusitis

Although many patients speak of severe chronic headache as being caused by "sinus problems," severe headache is rarely due to chronic sinusitis.[135,136] However, acute inflammation of one or more of the paranasal sinuses is frequently quite painful.

Conditions predisposing to acute sinusitis include severe upper respiratory infections, obstructions blocking the ostia of one or more sinuses (*e.g.,* septal and turbinate malformations, polyps, foreign bodies, enlarged adenoids), tooth abscess, and lowered host resistance.

The headache is usually referable to the site of infection, and the pain is usually dull and aching and described as a painful fullness. It is frequently periodic, depending on the drainage pattern of the involved sinus. In frontal and ethmoidal sinusitis, the intensity is greatest in the morning and diminishes toward the afternoon, because the upright posture facilitates drainage. In maxillary and sphenoidal sinusitis, drainage is better in the recumbent position. There may be tenderness over the affected sinus, and sinus x-rays frequently help confirm the diagnosis.

Treatment initially consists of antibiotics, analgesics, and mucosal vasoconstrictor agents. If these are ineffective, surgical drainage must be considered.

Temporomandibular Joint Syndrome

Patients with temporomandibular joint (TMJ) disorders fall into two groups: those with organic joint abnormalities (*e.g.,* ankylosis, neoplasm, trauma, arthritis) and those with facial pain, noise in the joint, and restricted movement without organic joint disease.[135,138] Those with organic disease make up only a small percentage of the total number.

The functional TMJ problem is a psychophysiologic condition that some prefer to call the "myofascial pain–dysfunction syndrome." The most common complaint is unilateral ear or preauricular pain, which may radiate to the temple or lateral neck. It is a dull constant ache that is worse in the morning, especially if the patient has bruxism at night. Limitation of jaw motion and pain with chewing may also be present. If pain and tenderness of the muscles of mastication, clicking in the joint, and limitation of jaw movement are present and there is no clinical or radiologic evidence of organic disease, the diagnosis of the myofascial pain–dysfunction syndrome may be made.

Treatment consists of counseling, local heat (or cold) therapy, ultrasound therapy, muscle relaxants and analgesics, elimination of gross occlusal discrepancies, and midline opening jaw exercises to restore normal muscle function. Many patients also benefit from antidepressant medications.[137,138] A small percentage of patients with TMJ syndrome develop secondary degenerative arthritis in the TMJ due to the constant trauma inflicted on the joint. A few of these patients may require high condylectomy for this problem.[137]

The organic TMJ problems consist of rheumatoid arthritis with ankylosis, chronic dislocation, ankylosis, hyperplasia, and neoplasia. These are best treated by a variety of surgical procedures.[137]

REFERENCES

1. **Waters WE, O'Connor PJ:** The clinical validation of a headache questionnaire. In Background to Migraine, Third British Migraine Symposium (April 24–25, 1969) London, Heinemann, 1970

2. **Newland CA, Illis LS, Robinson PK et al:** Epidemiological aspects of headache. Res Clin Stud Headache 5:1–20, 1978

3. **Ziegler DK, Hassanein RS, Couch JR:** Characteristics of life headache histories in a non-clinic population. Neurology 27:265–269, 1977

4. **Dalessio DJ:** Wolff's Headache and Other Head Pain, 3rd ed. New York, Oxford University Press, 1972

5. **Chapman LF, Ramos, AO, Goodell H, Silverman G, Wolff HG:** A humoral agent implicated in vascular headache of the migrainous type. Arch Neurol 3:223–229, 1960

6. Classification of headache. JAMA 179:717–718, 1962

7. **Dalessio DJ:** Wolff's Headache and Other Head Pain, 4th ed. Oxford University Press, New York, 1980

8. **Green JE:** A survey of migraine in England 1975–1976. Headache 17:67–68, 1977

9. **Turner DB, Stone AJ:** Headache and its treatment: A random sample survey. Headache 19:74–77, 1979

10. **Crisp AH, McGuinness B, Kalucy RS et al:** Some clinical, social and psychological characteristics of migraine subjects in the general population. Postgrad Med J 53:691–697, 1977

11. **Ziegler DK, Rhodes RJ, Hassanein RS:** Association of psychological measurements of anxiety and depression with headache history in a non-clinic population. Res Clin Stud Headache 6:123–135, 1978

12. **Fisher CM:** Late-life migraine accompaniments as a cause of unexplained transient ischemic attacks. Can J Neurol Sci 7:9–17, 1980

13. **Vijayan N:** Ophthalmoplegic migraine: Ischemic or compressive neuropathy? Headache 20:300–304, 1980

14. **Mathew NT, Meyer JS, Welch KMA et al:** Abnormal CT scans in migraine. Headache 16:272–279, 1977

15. **Bickerstaff ER:** Basilar artery migraine. Lancet 1:15–17, 1961

16. **Graham JR, Wolff HG:** Mechanism of migraine headache and action of ergotamine tartarate. Arch Neurol Psychiatr 39:737–763, 1938

17. **Elkind AH, Friedman AP, Grossman J:** Cutaneous blood flow in vascular headache of the migrainous type. Neurology 14: 24–30, 1964

18. **O'Brien MD:** Cerebral blood flow changes in migraine. Headache 10: 139–143, 1971

19. **Skinhoj E:** Hemodynamic studies within the brain during migraine. Arch Neurol 29:257–266, 1979

20. **Sakai F, Meyer JS:** Abnormal cerebral vascular reactivity in patients with migraine and cluster headache. Headache 19:257–266, 1979

21. **Wennerholm M:** Postural vascular reactions in cases of migraine and related vascular headaches. Acta Med Scand 169: 131–139, 1961

22. **Vijayan N, Gould S, Watson CE:** Exposure to sun and precipitation of migraine. Headache 20:42–43, 1980

23. **Appenzeller O, Davison K, Marshall J:** Reflex vasomotor abnormalities in the hands of migrainous subjects. J Neurol Neurosurg Psychiatry 26:447–450, 1963

24. **Downey JA, Frewin DB:** Vascular responses in the hands of patients suffering from migraine. J Neurol Neurosurg Psychiatry 35:258–263, 1972

25. **Anthony M, Hinterberger H, Lance JW:** Plasma serotonin in migraine and stress. Arch Neurol 16:544–552, 1967

26. **Anthony M, Hinterberger H, Lance JW:** The possible relationship of serotonin to the migraine syndrome. Res Clin Stud Headache 2:29–59, 1968

27. **Kalendowsky Z, Austin JH:** Complicated migraine: Its association with increased platelet aggregability and abnormal plasma coagulation factors. Headache 15:18–35, 1975

28. **Sandler M, Youdim MBH, Hannington E:** A phenylethylamine oxidizing defect in migraine. Nature 250:335–337, 1974

29. **Somerville BW:** The role of oestradiol withdrawal in the etiology of menstrual migraine. Neurology 22:355–365, 1972

30. **Carlson LA, Ekelund LG, Oro L:** Clinical and metabolic effects of different doses of prostaglandin-El in man. Acta Med Scand 183:423–430, 1968

31. **Sicuteri F:** Mast cells and their active substances: Their role in the pathogenesis of migraine. Headache 3:86–92, 1963

32. **Thonnard-Neumann E, Taylor WL:** The basophil leukocyte and migraine. Headache 8:98–107, 1968

33. **Kudrow L:** Cluster Headache: Mechanisms and Management. New York, Oxford University Press, 1980

34. **Lance JW:** Mechanism and Management of Headache, 3rd ed. London, Butterworth & Co, 1978

35. **Romberg MH:** A Manual of Nervous Diseases of Man Sieveking EH (trans). London, Syndenham Society, 1840

36. **Kunkle EC, Pfeiffer JB, Wilhoit WM et al:** Recurrent brief headache in "cluster" pattern. Trans Am Neurol Assoc 77: 240–243, 1952

37. **Rooke ED, Rushton JG, Peters GA:** Vasodilating headache: A suggested classification and results of prophylactic treatment with UML 491 (methysergide) Mayo Clinic Proc 37: 433–443, 1962

38. **Ekbom K, Olivarius B:** Chronic migrainous neuralgia—diagnostic and therapeutic aspects. Headache 11: 97–101, 1971

39. **Sjaastad O, Dale I:** Evidence for a new (?) treatable headache entity. Headache 14: 105–108, 1974

40. **Medina JL, Diamond S:** The chemical link between migraine and cluster headaches. Arch Neurol 34: 470–472, 1977

41. **Hornabrook RW:** Migrainous neuralgia. NZ Med J 63:774–779, 1964

42. **Sutherland JM, Eadie MJ:** Cluster headache. Res Clin Stud Headache 3:92–125, 1972

43. **Green MW, Apfelbaum RI:** Cluster-tic syndrome. Headache 18:112, 1978

44. **Gilbert GJ:** Meniere's syndrome and cluster headaches. JAMA 191:691–694, 1965

45. **Gilbert GJ:** Cluster headache and cluster vertigo. Headache 9:195–200, 1970

46. **Lance JW, Anthony M:** Some clinical aspects of migraine. Arch Neurol 15:356–361, 1966

47. **Friedman AP, Mikropoulos HE:** Cluster headaches. Neurology 8:653–663, 1958

48. **Ekbom K:** A clinical comparison of cluster headache and migraine. Acta Neurol Scand (Suppl 41) 46:1–48, 1970

49. **Ekbom K:** Clinical aspects of cluster headache. Headache 13:176–180, 1974

50. **Ekbom K:** Patterns of cluster headache with a note on the relations to angina pectoris and peptic ulcer. Acta Neurol Scand 46:225–237, 1970

51. **Symonds C:** A particular variety of headache. Brain 79:217–232, 1956

52. **Ekbom K, Kugelberg E:** Upper and lower cluster headache (Horton's syndrome). In Brain and Mind Problems, pp 482–489. Rome, Il Pensiero Scientifico Publishers, 1968

53. **Vijayan N, Watson C:** Evaluation of oculocephalic sympathetic function in vascular headache syndromes, Part II, Oculocephalic sympathetic function in cluster headache. Headache (in press)

54. **Ekbom K:** Nitroglycerin as a provocative agent in cluster headache. Arch Neurol 19:487–493, 1968

55. **Horton BT, MacLean AR, Craig WM:** A new syndrome of vascular headache: Results of treatment with histamine. Mayo Clin Proc 14:257–260, 1939

56. **Graham JR:** Proceedings of the conference on cluster headache. Headache Research Foundation, Faulkner Hospital, Massachusetts, 1968

57. **Ekbom K, Lindahl J:** Remission of angina pectoris during periods of cluster headache. Headache 11:57–62, 1971

58. **Graham JR:** Cluster headache. Headache 11:175–185, 1972

59. **Kudrow L:** Prevalence of migraine, peptic ulcer, coronary heart disease, and hypertension in cluster headache. Headache 16:66–69, 1976

60. **Horton BT:** Histaminic cephalgia resulting in production of acute duodenal ulcer. JAMA 122:59, 1943

61. **Alford RI, Whitehouse FR:** Histaminic cephalgia with duodenal ulcer. Ann Allergy 3:200–203, 1945

62. **Lovshin LL:** Clinical caprices of histaminic cephalgia. Headache l:7–10, 1961

63. **Ekbom KA:** Ergotamine tartrate orally in Horton's "histaminic cephalgia" (also called Harris's "ciliary neuralgia"). Acta Psychiatr Scand (Suppl) 46:106–113, 1947

64. **Graham JR:** Cluster headache. Headache 11:175–185, 1972

65. **Friedman AP, Elkind AH:** Appraisal of methysergide in treatment of vascular headaches of migraine type. JAMA 184:125–128, 1963

66. **Graham JR:** Methysergide for prevention of headache: Experience in five hundred patients over three years. N Engl J Med 270:67–72, 1964

67. **Ekbom K:** Prophylactic treatment of cluster headache with a new serotonin antagonist, BC 105. Acta Neurol Scand 45:601–610, 1969

68. **Kudrow L:** Comparative results of prednisone, methysergide, and lithium therapy in cluster headache. In Greene R: Current Concepts in Migraine Research. New York, Raven Press, 1978

69. **Lance JW, Anthony M:** Thermographic studies in vascular headache. Med J Aust 1:240–243, 1971

70. **Wood EH, Friedman AP:** Thermography in cluster headache. Res Clin Stud Headache 4:107–111, 1976

71. **Kudrow L:** Thermographic and doppler flow asymmetry in cluster headache. Headache 19:204–208, 1979

72. **Ekbom K, Greitz T:** Carotid angiography in cluster headache. Acta Radiol [Diagn] (Stockh) 10:177–186, 1970

73. **Sakai F, Meyer JS:** Regional cerebral hemodynamics during migraine and cluster headaches measured by the 133Xe inhalation method. Headache 18:122–132, 1978

74. **Horton BT:** Histaminic cephalgia: Differential diagnosis and treatment. Mayo Clin Proc 31:325–333, 1956

75. **Anthony M, Lance JW:** Histamine and serotonin in cluster headache. Arch Neurol 25:225–231, 1971

76. **Anthony M, Lord GDA, Lance JW:** Controlled trials of cimetidine in migraine and cluster headache. Headache 18:261–264, 1978

77. **Sjaastad O, Sjaastad OV:** Histamine metabolism in cluster headache and migraine. J Neurol 216:105–117, 1977

78. **Kunkle EC:** Acetylcholine in the mechanism of headaches of migraine type. Arch Neurol Psychiatr 84:135–141, 1959

79. **Gardner WJ, Stowell A, Dutlinger R:** Resection of the greater superficial petrosal nerve in the treatment of unilateral headache. J Neurosurg 4:105–114, 1947

80. **White J, Sweet W:** Pain. Its Mechanism and Neurosurgical Control. Springfield, IL, Charles C Thomas, 1955

81. **Robinson BW:** Histaminic cephalgia. Medicine 37:161–180, 1958

82. **Stowell A:** Physiologic mechanisms and treatment of histaminic or petrosal neuralgia. Headache 9:187–194, 1970

83. **Kudrow L:** Plasma testosterone levels in cluster headache: Preliminary results. Headache 16:28–31, 1976

84. **Graham JR:** Cluster headache. Postgrad Med 56:181–184, 1974

85. **Kunkle EC, Anderson WB:** Dual mechanisms of eye signs of headache in cluster pattern. Trans Am Neurol Assoc 85:75–79, 1960

86. **Kunkle EC, Anderson WB:** Significance of minor eye signs in headache of migraine type. Arch Ophthalmol 65:504–508, 1961

87. **Nieman EA, Hurwitz LJ:** Ocular sympathetic palsy in periodic migrainous neuralgia. J Neurol Neurosurg Psychiatry 24:369–373, 1961

88. **Riley FC, Moyer NJ:** Oculosympathetic paresis associated with cluster headaches. Am J Ophthalmol 72:763–768, 1971

89. **Lance JW, Curran DA:** Treatment of chronic tension headache. Lancet 1:1236–1239, 1964

90. **Budzynski TH, Stoyva JM, Adler CS et al:** EMG biofeedback and tension headache: A controlled outcome study. Psychosom Med 35:484–496, 1973

91. **Bakal DA, Kaganov SA:** Muscle contraction and migraine headache: Psychological comparison. Headache 17:208–214, 1977

92. **Peck CL, Kraft GH:** Electromyographic feedback for pain related to muscle tension. Arch Surg 112:889–895, 1977

93. **Martin PR, Mathews AM:** Tension headaches: Psychophysiological investigation and treatment. J Psychosom Res 22:389–399, 1978

94. **Tunis MM, Wolff HG:** Studies on headache: Cranial artery vasoconstriction and muscle contraction headache. Arch Neurol Psychiatr 7:425–434, 1954

95. **Rolf LH, Wiele G, Brune GG:** Serotonin in platelets of patients with migraine and muscle contraction headache. Excerpta Med 427:11–12, 1977

96. **Simons DJ, Wolff HG:** Studies on headache: Mechanisms of chronic post-traumatic headache. Psychosom Med 8:227–242, 1946

97. **Raskin NH, Appenzeller O:** Headache. In Smith LH: Major Problems in Internal Medicine, Vol 19. Philadelphia, WB Saunders, 1980

98. **Penfield W, Norcross NC:** Subdural traction and post-traumatic headache: Study of pathology and therapeusis. Arch Neurol Psychiatr 36:75–95, 1936

99. **Walker AE:** Chronic post-traumatic headache. Headache 5:67–72, 1965

100. **Rowbotham GF:** Complications and sequels of injuries to the head. Med Pr 205:379–384, 1941

101. **Merritt HH, Friedman AP, Brenner C:** Headache and the post-traumatic syndrome. Trans Am Neurol Assoc 70:56–60, 1944

102. **Brenner C, Friedman AP, Merritt HH et al:** Post-traumatic headache. J. Neurosurg l:379–391, 1944

103. **Vijayan N, Dreyfus PM:** Posttraumatic dysautonomic cephalalgia. Arch Neurol 32:649–652, 1975

104. **Vijayan N:** A new post-traumatic headache syndrome: Clinical and therapeutic observations. Headache 17:19–22, 1977

105. **Denker PG:** The post-concussion syndrome: Prognosis and evaluation of the organic factors. NY State J Med 44:379–384, 1944

106. **Friedman AP:** The so-called post-traumatic headache. In Walker AE, Caveness WF, Critchley M (eds): The Late Effects of Head Injury. Springfield, IL, Charles C Thomas, 1969

107. **Kredel FE:** Headache from lesions of scalp nerves. Ann Surg 122:1056–1059, 1945

108. **Taylor AR, Bell TK:** Slowing of cerebral circulation after concussional head injury. Lancet 2:178–180, 1966

109. **Oldendorf WH, Kitano M:** Radioisotope measurement of brain blood turnover time as a clinical index of brain circulation. J Nucl Med 8:570–587, 1967

110. **Ommaya AK, Gennarelli TA:** A physiopathologic basis for noninvasive diagnosis and prognosis of head injury severity. In McLaurin RL (ed): Head Injuries. New York, Grune & Stratton, 1976

111. **Gronwall D, Wrightson P:** Delayed recovery of intellectual function after minor head injury. Lancet 2:605–609, 1974

112. **Denker PG, Perry GF:** Postconcussion syndrome in compensation and litigation. Neurology 4:912–918, 1954

113. **Toglia JU, Rosenberg PE, Ronis ML:** Post-traumatic dizziness. Arch Otolaryngol 92:485–492, 1970

114. **Harrison MS:** Notes on the clinical features and pathology of post-concussional vertigo with especial reference to positional nystagmus. Brain 79:474–482, 1956

115. **Waters WE:** Headache and blood pressure in the community. Br Med J 1:142–143, 1971

116. **Bulpitt CJ, Dollery CT, Carne S:** Change in symptoms of hypertensive patients after referral to hospital clinic. Br Heart J 38:121–128,1976

117. **Badran RH, Weir RJ, McGuiness JB:** Hypertension and headache. Scott Med J 15:48–51, 1970

118. **Lance JW, Hinterberger H:** Symptoms of phenochromocytoma, with particular reference to headache, correlated with catecholamine production. Arch Neurol 33:281–288, 1976

119. **Lance JW:** Headaches related to sexual activity. J Neurol Neurosurg Psychiatry 39:1226–1230, 1976

120. **Paulson GW, Klawans HL:** Benign orgasmic cephalgia. Headache 13:181–187, 1974

121. **Rooke ED:** Benign exertional headache. Med Clin N Amer 52:801–808, 1968

122. **Diamond S:** Recurrent exertional headache. JAMA 237:580, 1977.

123. **Grindal AB, Toole JF:** Headache and transient ischemic attacks. Stroke 5:603–606, 1974

124. **Fisher CM:** Headache in cerebrovascular disease. In Vinken PJ, Bruyn GW (eds): Handbook of Clinical Neurology, Vol 5. Amsterdam, North Holland, 1968

125. **Mohr JP, Caplan LR, Melski JW et al:** The Harvard cooperative stroke registry: A prospective registry. Neurology 28:754–762, 1978

126. **Weisberg LA:** Benign intracranial hypertension. Medicine 54:197–207, 1975

127. **Gucer G, Viernstein L:** Long-term intracranial pressure recording in the management of pseudotumor cerebri. J Neurosurg 49:256–263, 1978

128. **Moffat FL:** Pseudotumor cerebri. Le Journal Canadien des Sciences Neurologiques 5:431–436, 1978

129. **Levine MC, White DW:** Chronic postmyelographic headache: A result of persistent epidural cerebrospinal fluid fistula. JAMA 229:684–686, 1974

130. **Jones RJ:** The role of recumbency in the prevention and treatment of postspinal headache. Anesth Analg (Cleve) 53:788–796, 1974

131. **Brocker, RJ:** Technique to avoid spinal-tap headache. JAMA 168:261–263, 1958

132. **Hatfalvi BI:** The dynamics of post-spinal headache. Headache 17:64–66, 1977

133. **Hamilton CR, Shelly WM, Tumulty PA:** Giant cell arteritis: Including temporal arteritis and polymyalgia rheumatica. Medicine 50:1–27, 1971

134. **Huston KA, Hunder GG, Lie JT et al:** Temporal arteritis: A 25-year epidemiologic, clinical, and pathologic study. Ann Intern Med 88:162–167, 1978

135. **Ryan Sr RE, Ryan Jr RE:** Acute nasal sinusitis. Postgrad Med 56:159–162, 1974

136. **Ryan Sr RE, Ryan Jr RE:** Headache of nasal origin. Headache 19:173–179, 1979

137. **Guralnick W, Kaban LB, Merrill RG:** Temporomandibular-joint afflictions. N Engl J Med 299:123–129, 1978

138. **Reik L, Hale M:** The temporomandibular joint pain-dysfunction syndrome: A frequent cause of headache. Headache 21:151–156, 1981

5

Loss of Vision—Eye Pain Robert D. Reinecke

Measurements of Visual Loss
Principal Locations of Pathologic Processes
Acute Visual Loss: Emergencies
   Without Pain or Flashes: Occlusion of Central
     Retinal Artery
Painless Loss of Vision with a Flashing
     Sensation: Retinal Detachment
Other Painless Acute Loss of Vision: Eye
     Hemorrhages
   Retinal Hemorrhages: Occlusion of Central
     Retinal Vein
   Painless Sudden Visual Loss with Diabetes
     Mellitus
Acute Visual Loss with a Red, Painful Eye:
     Angle-Closure Glaucoma
Acute Visual Loss and Painful Eye Movements:
     Retrobulbar Neuritis
Painless Chronic Visual Loss
   Macular Degeneration

Cataracts
Tunnel Vision
   Glaucoma
   Drug Toxicity
   Retinitis Pigmentosa
Transient Visual Loss
   Hemianopsias with Flashes
   Transient Monocular Visual Loss
Hemianopsias
Distorted Vision with Blurring
Sudden Traumatic Loss of Vision
   Head Trauma
   Electric Shock
   Direct Trauma to the Eye
     Physical Injury
     Chemical Contact
     Ultraviolet Exposure
Summary

MEASUREMENTS OF VISUAL LOSS

Visual loss may vary from slight and subtle to profound. In this chapter, most of the conditions discussed involve severe visual loss; that is, the loss is sufficient that the patient is well aware that the vision has changed dramatically, often from excellent vision to no light perception. Neither the more subtle visual losses nor the poor vision associated with amblyopia are discussed here; the latter can be considered a lack of development of vision rather than a loss of vision. In any instance of professed visual loss, careful evaluation and recording of central vision and of visual fields are of paramount importance.[1] Each eye is tested separately. By far the most satisfactory measurement of central acuity consists in determining the smallest line of a Snellen chart, which the patient can read accurately at 20 feet. Correction of refractive errors with lenses may be used, if helpful. Vision is usually considered to be within acceptable normal limits if it is 20/30 or better with or without glasses (correction by a lens). The second crucial measurement is that of the circumference of the visual field and detection within it of any areas of decreased or absent vision.

PRINCIPAL LOCATIONS OF PATHOLOGIC PROCESSES

Visual loss may be due to three principal types of pathologic processes. First, the optical properties of the eye may be impaired (cornea, aqueous, lens or vitreous). Second, the retina may be damaged so that no signal can be converted from light energy to neural impulses (as with retinal detachment or retinitis pigmentosa). Third, the neural pathway may be impaired at the optic disk (as in glaucoma), the optic nerve (as in ischemic optic atrophy), the chiasm (as in pituitary tumors), or in the brain. The first two principal causes usually can be seen with the ophthalmoscope, and the third can be studied with the visual field tests.

ACUTE VISUAL LOSS: EMERGENCIES

Sudden loss of vision requires emergency evaluation.[2] Of the several conditions that can cause acute loss of vision, occlusion of the central retinal artery and angle-closure glaucoma must be treated immediately. Even though there are only two disorders that require prompt treatment, all cases must be studied immediately to determine the diagnosis and thus to decide which merits emergency treatment. One of the conditions, occlusion of a central retinal artery, often produces irreversible blindness in the affected eye if the condition is not treated within 1½ hours; some observers believe the condition to be hopeless if the patient is not seen within ½ hour after the occlusion.

WITHOUT PAIN OR FLASHES: OCCLUSION OF CENTRAL RETINAL ARTERY

The central retinal artery is subject to the usual causes of occlusion—thrombosis, atherosclerosis, arteriolar sclerosis, and emboli.[3] Often, repeated showers of emboli are dramatic to watch but fortunately may spare the vision. There may be fat emboli after bone trauma, emboli from atheromatous plaques in the carotid (especially following arteriography), or off vegetations from diseased heart valves. Occasionally, emboli of lung carcinoma cells or tumors within the heart may be the cause. The site of occlusion in the artery usually shows fibrosis and intimal proliferation. If inflammation such as that sometimes associated with temporal arteritis is the cause, the site is usually in the nutrient arteries of the optic nerve; there, giant-cell proliferation can be seen in the wall of the artery.

After the retina has been permanently damaged by occlusion of the central retinal artery, the first pathologic change is edema of the entire retina with accentuated swelling of the internal layers. As the edema disappears, the inner layers show irreparable damage to the bipolar and ganglion cells. Often the rods and cones are surprisingly intact if the retina is sectioned within a few weeks of the occlusion. Later sectioning of the retina, years after the occlusion, shows complete gliosis of the retina with few recognizable structures.

Experimental studies with cats and rats have indicated that the retina cannot tolerate ischemia for more than 1½ hours.[4] If circulation is restored prior to that time, recovery from the ischemia seems complete, although histologic changes such as endothelial proliferation in the arterial wall can be identified. Case histories of recovered vision after occlusion of central retinal arteries in humans are common, although the exact etiology and extent of the occlusion typically are poorly if at all documented.

The patient with occlusion of a central retinal artery usually notes that vision is lost suddenly. He cannot distinguish light from dark. The symptom changes from blurring to complete loss of light perception in about 15 seconds, although in some patients there may be retention of light perception in the extreme temporal field. Others may report loss of the entire peripheral field and preservation of a small central field. In these patients, a cilioretinal artery provides a separate flow of blood to the macular area; hence, the central field is maintained. Unfortunately, the cilioretinal artery is present in only a small percentage of persons. On the other hand, occasionally the cilioretinal artery only is occluded. These patients report loss of central vision with preservation of the surrounding peripheral field. The rarity of the cilioretinal artery precludes this event from becoming common.

Examination of an eye after recent occlusion of the central retinal artery reveals a fundus that is whiter than usual, with a cherry-red spot in the macula. This change is due to the retinal edema, which occurs soon after the occlusion. The fovea is the thinnest portion of the retina; hence it is less swollen and shows the red choroid beneath it, giving the cherry-red spot. A more striking and dramatic feature is the visible stasis of blood in the retinal arterioles. The blood becomes separated into red clumps interspersed with areas of clear fluid. The degree of occlusion can be determined to some extent from this clumping; if the occlusion is complete, the blood clumps will not move. If, however, the occlusion is not complete, the blood will be seen moving slowly in the retinal arterioles. Even if the clumped blood is still moving to some extent, treatment should be employed because the retina will suffer irreparable damage if the condition is allowed to persist. Occasionally, the blood appears to be moving in the direction opposite to normal, and intermittently it may change direction of movement.

The diagnosis is relatively simple in the case of occlusion of a central retinal artery. The eye appears as in Figure 5-1. As soon as the diagnosis is firm, it is well to try to raise the patient's blood pressure. Vasodilators may bring about a sudden lowering of blood pressure, and thus have an untoward effect. The easiest means of temporarily raising the blood pressure is to have the patient exercise (*e.g.*, run in place for a few seconds). The fundus then can be checked intermittently to see whether the treatment has had any effect on the occlusion.

The principle behind this treatment is to raise the differential pressure of the artery proximal to the occlusion compared with the pressure in the artery distal to the occlusion. Raising the systemic blood pressure is an obvious means of accomplishing this. Another means is to lower the intraocular pressure. Intermittent massage of the eye is the quickest and easiest means of lowering intraocular pressure. Massage of the eye has the added advantage of causing sharp changes in the differential pressure, so that the embolus may be dislodged or broken up and can move to the periphery of the retina. Diamox (acetazolamide) also may be administered intravenously in a dose of 500 mg. This drug will lower the intraocular pressure several more millimeters of mercury.

Increasing the concentration of carbon dioxide in the blood causes a moderate dilatation of the central retinal artery and simultaneously raises the blood pressure. A 10% CO_2 in 90% O_2 mixture is used. If the CO_2 is to be effective, it must be inhaled in about this concentration. If the mask fits so loosely that room air leaks in or if the flow of gas is slower than the rate of inspiration, there is no appreciable effect. One can easily test the effect of the arrangement by breathing the mixture oneself and noting if (as expected) a slight giddiness accompanied by a moderate headache is produced with a few moments. An occasional patient benefits from this technique and reports some return of vision as he uses the gas mixture. One can judge results by looking into the eye and observing the blood flow.

With occlusion of the central retinal artery and the resultant blind retina, the direct pupillary reflex is extremely poor. Observation of the consensual reflex is valuable. It is elicited by shining a light into the fellow eye and observing that the reflex of the affected eye thus indirectly induced is normal. The poor direct pupillary reflex is of modest advantage to the doctor because it allows a good view of the fundus through a relatively large pupil.

From time to time during treatment, the intraocular pressure should be checked. If the preceding measures have failed to reduce the intraocular pressure substantially, one should lower the intraocular pressure by

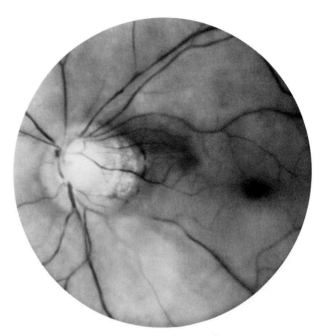

Fig. 5-1. The central retinal artery is occluded. Note the retinal edema. A small area has been spared temporal to the disc because a cilioretinal artery supplies the area. Note the dark (actually cherry-red) appearance of the macula.

removing a small amount of fluid from the eye. It is to be emphasized that this should be done only by an ophthalmologist because the potential complications of this maneuver can be severe and can result in as much damage to the eye as the occlusion of the central retinal artery. Until recently, the aqueous was removed with a small cataract knife. A tiny incision was made in the cornea to allow a drop of aqueous to escape. With the availability in most emergency rooms of the very small-caliber size-27 disposable needles, many ophthalmologists now prefer to use such a needle on a tuberculin syringe. The disposable needles are so sharp that they penetrate the cornea easily.

A question frequently asked is "Should anticoagulants be given at once and perhaps continued indefinitely?" There is no evidence that anticoagulants dissolve a thrombus or embolus, and if the occlusion is alleviated by the means just described, there seems to be relatively little danger that the same artery will occlude again.

Although the preceding treatment is continued in an effort to establish blood flow to the retina, blood should be drawn from the patient and an erythrocyte sedimentation rate measured. If the rate is elevated, temporal and retinal arteritis are immediately suspected until proven otherwise. When the sedimentation rate

report is available, approximately 2 hours will have elapsed, and the success or failure of the emergency treatment of the occluded retinal vessel is usually already apparent. An elevated sedimentation rate is an indication for biopsy of the temporal artery. When arteritis is suspected, corticosteroid therapy in large doses may be given immediately (before biopsy and microscopic confirmation) and continued until one is assured that the patient does not have temporal plus retinal arteritis.

Occasionally a patient may have all the symptoms of central retinal artery occlusion, yet on examination the blood flow may appear to be perfectly normal. There is nevertheless a sluggish pupillary reflex on direct stimulation and profound loss of vision. Upon comparison of the two disks, it is seen that the disk of the affected eye is ever so slightly boggy and slightly paler than the other disk. The only vision in the eye may be some light perception in the lower temporal field. The other eye is completely normal. This situation usually occurs in patients over 55 years old. The presumed diagnosis is occlusion of the nutrient artery of the optic nerve. The blood supply of the retina is intact, but the supply to the optic nerve has been interrupted just behind the eye. Although the etiology may be atherosclerosis, the most likely diagnosis is the syndrome of "temporal arteritis."

The sedimentation rate should be measured immediately and the patient should breathe the 10% CO_2 in 90% O_2 mixture. If the sedimentation rate is elevated, the diagnosis of temporal arteritis syndrome should be entertained. A biopsy of the temporal artery should be performed, but it will be several days before the pathology report is returned. This situation is an emergency, and prompt use of systemic steroids may save the sight of the involved eye and certainly may save the sight of the other eye. If steroids are not started quickly, the other eye may well become involved with the same condition, and the patient may end up with total blindness in both eyes. This unfortunate train of events may prevail even with steroid treatment.

The other possible serious effects of the temporal arteritis syndrome should be kept in mind when dealing with this disease. There may be a widespread polyarteritis. Coronary arteries may fatally occlude. General malaise and polymyalgia often occur, with daily spikes of fever to about 102°F.

PAINLESS LOSS OF VISION WITH A FLASHING SENSATION: RETINAL DETACHMENT

Detachment of the retina causes mechanical stimulation of the rods and cones as it tears away from the pigment epithelium and floats free. This produces a noticeable visual sensation of flash, which the patient usually remembers as the signal immediately or shortly preceding loss of vision.[5] He also may note that there appeared to be a "veil" over his eye either just before the flash or immediately after it. If the detachment involves only the peripheral portion of the retina, the patient will have only a partial visual field defect corresponding to the detachment. He often comments on this as a "veil" over a portion of his vision. If the macula is detached, the vision is poor in that eye and the emergency nature of the condition is reduced; the prognosis is much poorer once the macula is off, no matter how successful or immediate the surgery may be in mechanically reattaching the retina. If the macula is still attached, the prognosis for visual improvement following surgery is much better. When the symptoms of a flash and veil are reported, the patient should be referred to an ophthalmologist.

Two types of retinal detachment are by far the most common. Between the two, the rhegmatogenous is more common. *Rhegmatogenous* indicates that the cause of the detachment is a hole in the retina. For reasons that are not known, if a retina develops a hole in it, fluid may start to collect beneath the retina from the site of the hole. If this is allowed to continue, the entire retina becomes detached. The treatment consists of mechanically closing the hole with a tamponade and producing scar tissue, which permanently seals off the hole. Recent years have been fruitful in the development of new techniques, which cleverly accomplish that end.

The second most common form of retinal detachment occurs in the presence of an intact retina. In this condition, the fluid collects under the retina as a result of *transudation*, for example, when the blood is low in protein, as in advanced uremia. If the uremic condition is corrected, the retina reattaches itself. Tumors of the choroid, both primary and metastatic, also produce an exudation of fluid, which detaches the retina.

In retinal detachment, the fundus color is changed from bright red to dull pink. The blood vessels are not on one plane, but at various angles and at irregular distances; hence, they appear more tortuous than normal. If the detached retina has fluid under it, the raised blood vessels lie at various levels, and it is therefore hard to focus accurately; a high plus lens in the ophthalmoscope is required. Careful examination with a special ophthalmoscope usually reveals a hole in the retina. It is often difficult to determine whether the cause of the detachment is a hole or a tumor. Care is taken to be sure that no operation is undertaken on a retina that is detached by a tumor. Inflammatory conditions also may cause detachment of the retina, and these disorders must be considered in differential diagnosis.

When a retina becomes detached as a result of advanced renal failure, the retina repeatedly shifts position. The fluid that accumulates and causes the detachment is heavier than the surrounding fluid, and hence moves to the most inferior position possible in the eye. If the patient is sitting or standing, with the lower portion of the retina detached but the macula attached, the patient's vision is good. However, if the patient lies down for several hours, the fluid shifts to the most dependent part of the eye and the macula may detach. Such a patient complains of poor vision for several hours each morning and finds that his vision improves remarkably as the day progresses. If the renal problem can be corrected, the retinal detachment clears and the vision usually returns to normal. Occasionally a patient with no renal disorder or other known disease may have a retinal detachment that resembles the condition just described for the patient with renal failure. Such a serous detachment may continue for several years, resolve, or go on to blindness. Little is known of the etiology of these serous detachments.

OTHER PAINLESS ACUTE LOSS OF VISION: EYE HEMORRHAGES

Vitreous hemorrhages are common causes of sudden painless loss of vision. Typically, the patient's vision was normal until he noted that a series of floaters began to drift in front of his eye and that there appeared to be a red glow to everything. After a variable length of time, he notes that the vision gradually fades until all that remains is a vague awareness of light from darkness in that eye. Usually the history is noncontributory (see the exception noted under diabetes). The eye appears white, quiet, and painless. The pupillary reflex is good, although there may be a slight sluggishness on the affected side. Examination reveals only a black reflex. After dilatation of the pupil, the reflex may still be black, or one may glimpse a red reflex above. Somewhere within the eye a retinal blood vessel has ruptured and allowed blood to flow into the vitreous. There is no immediate treatment for this except bed rest to allow the blood to settle so that the retina can be examined carefully.

The most common cause of retinal vessel bleeding is a tear in the retina that includes a blood vessel. If the tear in the retina is across a fairly large blood vessel and can be seen to be under some tension from strands in the vitreous, surgical treatment is indicated. Research has led most authorities to implicate disturbances in the vitreous that cause traction bands, which in turn pull and tear the retina. The causes and mechanisms involved in vitreous traction bands are not known. Occasionally, blunt trauma causes retinal tears. If a tear is not found and treated successfully, it can lead to retinal detachment, which may in turn lead to loss of vision. A black reflex means an intraocular hemorrhage until proven otherwise.

While the patient is resting in bed, studies to detect possible pathologic bleeding from conditions such as hemophilia, sickle-cell anemia, and thalassemia should be undertaken. Hemophilia itself probably does not cause retinal hemorrhages, but rather allows an otherwise trivial damaged retinal vessel to continue to bleed. Sickle-cell anemia patients have tufts of new vessels growing out from the retina within the eye. These tufts may hemorrhage and can be treated with photocoagulation if found before severe hemorrhages occur. Thalassemia or cryoglobulinemia causes thrombosis of many veins, with resultant hemorrhages that can break out of the retina and produce vitreous hemorrhages.

Just as atherosclerosis may involve the arteries, so may it involve the central retinal vein and its branches. As the atherosclerosis proceeds, intimal proliferation continues until the stage is set for thrombosis at the exit of the vein from the eye. Some suggest that the continued normal pulsation, with complete collapse and dilation of the vein, predisposes the patient to thrombosis at this site. The immediate sequel to occlusion of either the central retinal vein or a branch is that the veins that feed the blocked vein become dilated and that any available collateral channels enlarge. If the central retinal vein is blocked, there are no effective collateral channels and the veins dilate to huge proportions with ensuing hemorrhages, which at first are in the nerve fiber layer, but may break through into the vitreous.

RETINAL HEMORRHAGES: OCCLUSION OF CENTRAL RETINAL VEIN

Localized hemorrhages within the retina may be extensive when there is occlusion of the central retinal vein.[6] The patient complains that vision in the eye has gradually blurred over the past few days. The amount of visual loss is variable and dependent upon whether or not the retinal hemorrhages are in the macula. The eye is normal in all external respects, including the pupillary reflex. The retinal picture, however, is striking, with marked tortuosity of the retinal veins. There are hemorrhages about the entire retina in a random fashion if the occlusion involves the central retinal vein, or only over the distribution of the occluded retinal vein if a branch is involved. Many of the hemorrhages are flame-shaped, indicating that they are in the nerve fiber layer of the retina, but some of the hemorrhages are also found in the deeper layers of the retina. The hemorrhages are everywhere and are especially prom-

inent about the disk. The tortuosity of the veins exceeds that seen in papilledema. The resultant fundus as shown in Figure 5-2 appearance is aptly termed "blood and thunder."

If the patient is under 40 years of age, there is a reasonably good chance that he will recover useful vision after occlusion of a central retinal vein. If he is well into his 60s, there is little likelihood that useful vision will be recovered. In fact, there is a fair chance in the older patient that within 3 months neovascularization of the iris may result in an intractable glaucoma, which may cause such pain that the eye must be removed. The etiology of the neovascularization of the iris that sometimes follows occlusion of the central retinal vein seems to be caused by a neovascular growth factor generated from the relatively ischemic retina. In these cases a delicate membrane of endothelial cells grows over the iris, and fine capillaries come with this membrane. The membrane covers the angle of the eye (the portion of the eye between the iris and cornea) where the aqueous normally drains. Because the outflow channels are blocked, an irreversible glaucoma develops. Few eyes survive this chain of events, even with the most radical surgery.

Even with early diagnosis of an occluded central retinal vein, there is little known effective therapy. Anticoagulants are ineffective. The main consideration is to detect possible causes that seem to favor the development of this condition. Raised intraocular pressure

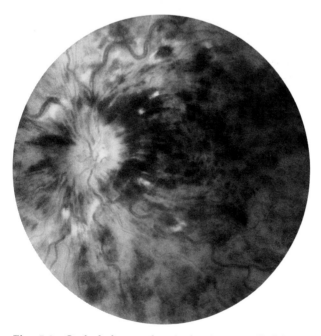

Fig. 5-2. Occluded central retinal vein—so-called blood and thunder.

(glaucoma), systemic hypertension, and diabetes seem to predispose patients to the development of occlusion of the central retinal vein, but their mechanism is not known. If early open-angle glaucoma is detected and treated, there is less probability that the central retinal vein will become occluded in the other eye. If diabetes is present, it should be controlled, since present evidence suggests prognosis for good vision to be related to the quality of diabetic control. Occasionally, especially in diabetes, the other eye becomes involved with the same dire outcome.

PAINLESS SUDDEN VISUAL LOSS WITH DIABETES MELLITUS

Young persons known to have diabetes for over 8 years are prone to serious eye involvement, apparently as a specific result of this metabolic disorder.[7] When visual loss is first reported, it is often the result of progression of diabetic retinopathy, the development of which has been observed as the diabetes has been treated, perhaps over a period of years. Occasionally, a diabetic develops edema of the central retina when no other ocular signs of diabetes are present. Over a few weeks the vision usually returns to normal. This maculopathy of diabetes may be the initial sign toward the diagnosis of diabetes mellitus.

Usually the first sign of diabetic retinopathy is slight engorgement of the retinal veins. At about this time, fine punctate hemorrhages can be observed. The fine-dot hemorrhages are from small aneurysms that are filled with blood. Serial photographs show that these small aneurysms are variable (Fig. 5-3). This variation is due to many of them scarring and becoming occluded and disappearing as the disease progresses. Concomitant with onset of aneurysms is enlargement of collateral fine venous channels. This is due to occlusion of other fine veins on the venous side of the capillary network. Many of these dilated collateral capillary channels can be seen ophthalmoscopically and are often termed neovascularization, although in fact they are just enlarged capillaries.

Kuwabara and Cogan have developed a technique that allows the retinal vessels to be studied on the flat after digesting away all other retinal tissue.[8] This technique reveals that there are two types of retinal vessel cells—mural cells and endothelial cells. Much of the damage in diabetic retinopathy seems to be due to damage to the mural cells. The reason for the susceptibility of the mural cells is not known. Although there are changes progressing in the vessel's wall, there are exudates being laid down in the deep layers of the retina. After a variable period of time, frank new vessel formation may begin and new vessels may break through the internal limiting membrane of the retina

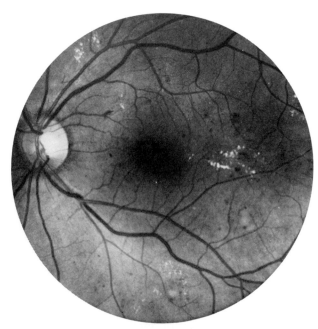

Fig. 5-3. Diabetic retinopathy. Note the scattered white "exudates" and the small dark spots, which are small hemorrhages and microaneurysms.

and appear as moving fronds, willowing in the vitreous. At any point the condition may suddenly become worse, often as a result of hemorrhage from the diseased vessels into the retina or into the vitreous.

Usually the sudden decrease in vision is due to a small hemorrhage in the macular area. This may be a small round hemorrhage similar to the many other small round hemorrhages that have been present elsewhere in varying degrees in the diabetic's eye (Fig. 5-4). Whether the hemorrhage hits the macular area seems to be a matter of chance. Macular involvement with consequent serious loss of vision may occur relatively early or late in the disease. If it is early, before there is a lot of scarring in the retina, the chances for absorption of the hemorrhage and the return of useful vision are much greater than if there is extensive scarring and if the region adjacent to the macula is already heavily involved with exudates, fibrous tissue, and other hemorrhages. The larger the hemorrhage, the poorer the prognosis for useful return of vision.

In a patient who has had the first decrease in vision due to diabetic retinopathy, the eye is white, quiet, and nonpainful. Upon examination of the fundus, the changes described previously probably will be seen with varying severity—the degree differing among patients. It is not unusual that the retina at the time of the first complaint of visual loss already has been seriously and extensively damaged, with new vessels growing out

of the disk into the vitreous, neovascularization of the retina and arteriovenous shunts in many places, exudates scattered about, many microaneurysms, and multiple hemorrhages. An eye in this condition has an extremely poor prognosis. Often a hemorrhage into the vitreous further decreases the chances for any useful vision. In such an eye, there may develop neovascularization of the iris with irreversible glaucoma. Occasionally there is bleeding from these new blood vessels, so that fresh blood can be seen in the anterior chamber. Once fresh blood is present in the anterior chamber, the outlook is poor for salvaging vision in that eye.

In recent years, retinopathy of some diabetic patients appeared to respond favorably to ablation of the pituitary gland, although the pathophysiology involved was not known. The results of a large controlled series were controversial, which, combined with the serious side-effects, caused the procedure to be deleted from the usual eye armamentarium. A recent large national study of the use of lasers in the treatment of the early stages of vascular lesions of diabetic retinopathy definitively proved the efficacy of this treatment. The treatment consists of placing about 1000 tiny burns in the retina. The side-effects of the laser ablative therapy include some reduction of the visual field and occasional hemorrhage.

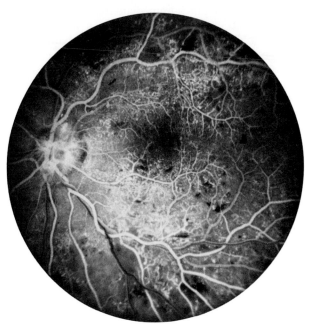

Fig. 5-4. Fluorangiogram of the retinal vessels of a diabetic patient. Note the many small leaks of dye from the vessels and the many fine dots, which represent aneurysms. Black areas represent retinal hemorrhages.

the hemianopsia usually leads to the correct localization of the lesion. Often the doctor is misled into discounting the likelihood of a hemianopsia simply because the field defect is not dense. Many times the only way in which a hemianopsia can be established is to have the patient describe the relative brightness of objects on either side of his visual fields. Basically, the hemianopsias are produced either by pressure on the optic nerve, tracts, radiations, or visual cortex or by ischemia of any part of the visual pathway.

The differential diagnosis of hemianopsias of all kinds appears elsewhere,[18] but it should be noted that most patients interpret hemianopsias as blurred vision rather than as field defects. When the patient has a left hemianopsia, he has difficulty in finding the starting letter of a line of print, consistently missing the first two or three letters on the vision chart of each line. The patient with a right hemianopsia is able to see each letter but often has difficulty in following the line and often skips the last letters of each line. Field defects may be severe, even if central visual acuity is still good. One patient who had most of her visual cortex ablated had a visual field of only 2 degrees to the left of fixation in each eye. Yet, with these 2 degrees, she was able to read slowly 20/15 letters.

DISTORTED VISION WITH BLURRING

Central serous retinopathy has been mentioned as a cause of sudden blurring of central vision.[19] However, vision is distorted more than blurred by this condition. The loss of vision typically is not permanent, occurs in males who smoke too much tobacco, and runs a course of several weeks, usually returning to normal after that time and often recurring about the same time in each of several consecutive years. The retina appears normal in all areas except the macula. A small amount of fluid collects under the macula, and the macula itself is slightly edematous. The changes are subtle and require careful examination to be seen. Only a relative field defect can be plotted with such a patient, and that done with difficulty.

The etiology of central serous retinopathy is not known, and little is known about the pathology. Fluorescein angiography of the retinal vessels shows tiny leaks in the vasculature in the affected area. This finding allows treatment of these cases with the laser if there are signs of advancement rather than the usual regression. Some authorities are skeptical of this treatment because it may offer a poorer long-term visual prognosis than the disease itself.

Occasionally, there is localized chorioretinitis of the macular area. The definitive causes of chorioretinitis are few and usually not found. However, toxoplasmosis may cause such a central lesion and should always be considered, particularly in the young. Occasionally a roundworm or other parasite may find its way into the eye and set up an inflammation about the macula. When some form of chorioretinopathy is discovered through the complaint of sudden visual loss, the eye specialist's opinion is valuable. Not uncommonly the patient may have had the condition for many years and discovers the loss of vision only when he accidentally covers one eye and finds that the vision in the other eye is poor. It is thus helpful to have an expert's opinion regarding the age and acuteness of the condition.

SUDDEN TRAUMATIC LOSS OF VISION[20]

HEAD TRAUMA

Severe head trauma with skull fractures, but without direct damage to the eyeball, occasionally is associated with loss of vision, either immediately at the time of the trauma or so shortly thereafter that it is hard to decide on the exact course of events that did take place. In such a case, one eye is normal, but the other may have varying amounts of vision—usually quite poor. The direct pupillary reflex of the involved eye is weak. The fundus is normal and the optic disk appears to be normal. Skull films or CT scans show that there is a fracture extending into the sphenoid bone and directly into the optic foramen.

The immediate question is "Should the optic foramen be unroofed so that the optic nerve can be spared the compression implied by the fracture line and possible hemorrhage?" This line of reasoning seems appropriate until one examines the results of unroofing the optic foramina in these patients. The statistics do not prove that this is a useful procedure. Often the general condition of the patient is sufficiently precarious that a major operation at that time seems unwise, especially since the chances of recovering vision are so poor. Most clinicians believe that the optic nerve is damaged at the time of the acute trauma, and the subsequent swelling does not add materially to the poor prognosis. Within 2 months, the patient with loss of vision due to trauma, with or without surgery, usually develops optic atrophy on the affected side. The only exception to the conservative conclusion not to operate is the patient who has documented good vision in the affected eye after the accident and subsequently loses vision. Such a case does merit surgical exploration, since

there may be severe retrobulbar hemorrhage. Care must be taken to see that such hemorrhage does not damage the eye from retrobulbar pressure on the eye and nerve. If progressive proptosis develops, a large needle can be inserted into the retrobulbar space to aspirate the hemorrhage. The needle must be placed carefully because the needle can damage the optic nerve. If proptosis develops without signs of hemorrhage in the lids or under the conjunctiva, there may be an arteriovenous communication in the cavernous sinus area. Arteriography is indicated in these cases.

ELECTRIC SHOCK

Severe electric shock to the head may result in sudden loss of vision from which it may take hours to recover. Typically, the patient receives a shock on his forehead of sufficient intensity to knock him down and cause a short period of unconsciousness. When he regains consciousness, he cannot see. Such a patient is often hysterical by the time the physician sees him. The eyes are white and quiet. The pupillary reflexes are absent or extremely sluggish. The fundi appear normal. The pupillary reflexes slowly come back to normal and objects begin to appear as gray forms; finally color perception and good vision return. The exact mechanism behind this series of events is not known, but some observers believe that the massive electric shock effectively depolarizes all cells in the retina and that time is needed for the resumption of normal electrical activity, and hence the return of vision.

DIRECT TRAUMA TO THE EYE

Physical Injury

After direct trauma, especially when it is severe enough to cause loss of vision, the eye should receive the gentlest treatment possible. Little is gained by forcing the lids open for a complete examination. The trauma attendant upon any manipulation may cause further severe damage to the eye. In such cases, it is best to examine the eyes as little as possible and to seek the consultation of an ophthalmologist. In all likelihood he will inspect the eye only briefly to determine whether an open wound is present. If such a wound is present, the complete examination is done after the patient is given general anesthesia. If the eye has no open wound, the patient is probably given bed rest to allow any blood that is present to clear, so that the ophthalmologist can see into the eye to determine the extent of damage. If he cannot be sure of the extent of damage, it may be necessary to explore the eye surgically to see whether there are any posterior ruptures. The prognosis for such eyes is poor.

Chemical Contact

A strong caustic agent such as lye splashed upon the eye causes severe damage.[21] The extent of injury depends on how quickly the harmful agent can be washed away. If prompt irrigation is done, eye and vision may be saved. If no irrigation is performed until the patient reaches the care of an ophthalmologist, the eye may be lost. In all cases in which a foreign substance is splashed upon the eye, the immediate treatment is generous irrigation with plain water. The eyelids should be forced open and a gentle but continuous stream of water directed into the eye for a minimum of 5 minutes. If there is reason to believe that the foreign substance was an acid or an alkali, it is important to test the pH of the eye from time to time with pH paper. The irrigation should be continued until the pH is 7. Then a period of 5 minutes may be allowed to pass, and the pH of the eye is again tested. If the pH has risen or fallen, further irrigation should be carried out until the pH remains normal after irrigation. Following irrigation, antibacterial eye drops may be put in the conjunctival *cul de sac*. If the cornea is chalky white, prognosis for vision is poor. However, if the eye looks reasonably good and the irrigation was thorough and carried out immediately after the accident, there is an excellent chance that vision will be saved without heroic measures such as corneal transplantation.

Ultraviolet Exposure

Loss of vision following exposure of the eyes to ultraviolet radiation is more imagined than real. What actually happens about 6 hours after exposure to rays from a sunlamp or welding arc without proper protection is onset of acute keratitis. The corneal epithelial cells are damaged and many of them die. The roughening of the corneas is extremely painful—so painful that the patient cannot voluntarily open his eyes, and hence maintains that he is blind. Application of 1 or 2 drops of ½% proparacaine hydrochloride relieves pain and allows examination. The patient can then open his eyes freely. The conjunctivae are moderately inflamed. The corneas are a bit hazy. A drop of fluorescein shows scattered staining of the cornea, indicating devitalization of many corneal epithelial cells. All other parts of the eye are normal. Within 24 hours, the eyes usually have recovered fully. One must not succumb to the pleas of the patient for proparacaine hydrochloride to apply for similar relief at home. Such local anesthetics have an inhibitory effect on healing of the cornea and should not be used more than a few times within 24 hours. Too frequent use may interfere with healing and cause chronic ulceration.

SUMMARY

Of the many possible causes of loss of vision, occlusion of the central retinal artery is the most urgent and requires immediate treatment aimed at increasing the pressure differential in the artery on the two sides of the occlusion. Breathing of a 10% CO_2 in 90% O_2 mixture may be helpful. Another condition requiring immediate medical attention is acute angle-closure glaucoma. A real possibility exists that the systemic effects of the high intraocular pressure may divert attention away from the eye to the gastrointestinal tract, resulting in unnecessary delay in the treatment of acute glaucoma. This delay may cause the sight of the patient to be irreparably damaged. In most conditions that cause a reduction of vision or pain in an eye, the symptoms are so characteristic and the signs are so prominent that the exact diagnosis can be made if an accurate history can be obtained and if the eye is examined carefully. Usually definitive diagnosis and treatment can be deferred to an ophthalmologist in serious or problem cases. However, the observations of the first physician to see the patient are invaluable in determining the probable diagnosis, in deciding whether emergency treatment is necessary, and in judging whether the attentions of an ophthalmologist are required.

REFERENCES

1. **Reinecke RD, Herm RJ:** Refraction, A Programmed Text. New York, Appleton-Century-Crofts, 1983

2. **Reinecke RD:** Ocular emergencies. In Eckert C (ed): Emergency Room Care, 4th ed, pp 347–358. Boston, Little, Brown & Co, 1981

3. **Henkind P, Chambers JK:** Arterial occlusive disease of the retina. In Duane TE (ed): Clinical Ophthalmology. Philadelphia, Harper & Row, 1981

4. **Reinecke RD, Kuwabara T, Cogan DG, Weis DR:** Retinal vascular patterns, Part V. Experimental ischemia of cat eyes. Arch Ophthalmol 67:470–475, 1962

5. **Straatsma BR, Foos RY, Krieger AF:** Rhegmatogenous retina detachment. In Duane TE (ed): Clinical Ophthalmology. Philadelphia, Harper & Row, 1981

6. **Jaeger EA:** Venous obstruction of the retina. In Duane TE (ed): Clinical Ophthalmology. Philadelphia, Harper & Row, 1981

7. **Benson WE, Tasman W, Duane TE:** Diabetic retinopathy. In Duane TE (ed): Clinical Ophthalmology. Philadelphia, Harper & Row, 1981

8. **Cogan DG, Kuwabara TK:** Capillary shunts in the pathogenesis of diabetic retinopathy. Diabetes 12:293, 1963

9. **Spaeth GL:** Glaucoma surgery. In Spaeth GL (ed): Ophthalmic Surgery, pp 215–359. Philadelphia, WB Saunders, 1982

10. **Dutton JJ, Burde RM, Klingele TG:** Autoimmune retrobulbar neuritis. Am J Ophthalmol 94:11–17, 1982

11. **Watske RC:** Laser photocoagulation of senile macular degeneration. Arch Ophthalmol 100:911, 1982

12. **Weinstein G:** Cataract surgery. In Spaeth GL (ed): Ophthalmic Surgery, pp 131–190. Philadelphia, WB Saunders, 1982

13. **Anderson DR:** Testing of The Visual Fields. St. Louis, CV Mosby, 1982

14. **Leopold IH:** Optic nerve. In Fraunfelder FT, Roy RH (eds): Current Ocular Therapy. Philadelphia, WB Saunders, 1980

15. **Berson E, Gouras P, Gunkel R, et al:** Dominant retinitis pigmentosa with reduced penetrance. Arch Ophthalmol 81(2):266, 1969

16. **Weinstein JM, Feman SS:** Ischemic optic neuropathy in migraine. Arch Ophthalmol 100:1099–1100, 1982

17. **Walsh FB, Hoyt WF:** Clinical Neuro-ophthalmology, 3rd ed, pp 1802–1832. Baltimore, Williams & Wilkins, 1969

18. **Newell FW:** Ophthalmology, Principles and Concepts, p 54. St. Louis, CV Mosby, 1982

19. **Watske RC:** Central serous retinopathy. In Fraunfelder FT, Roy FH, (eds): Current Therapy, pp 550–551. Philadelphia, WB Saunders, 1980

20. **Freeman HM:** Ocular Trauma. New York, Appleton-Century-Crofts, 1979

21. **Grant MW:** Toxicology of the Eye, pp 5–22. Springfield, IL, Charles C Thomas, 1974

6

Problems of Communication:
Speech and Hearing,
Ear Pain Francis I. Catlin

How Human Beings Communicate
**Normal Developmental Expectancies in Hearing
    and Speech**
Possible Pathophysiologic Mechanisms
Hearing
    Hearing Assessment in Children
        Auditory Responses
        Maternal High Risk Factors
        Infant High Risk Factors
    Otologic Evaluation
    Anatomy and Physiology of Auditory Apparatus
        Sound-Conduction Mechanism of the Ear
    Etiology of Conductive Hearing Impairment in
        the External Ear
    Etiology of Conductive Hearing Impairment in
        the Middle Ear
        Acute Otitis Media
        Serous Otitis Media

Tympanosclerosis and Otosclerosis
Tumor of the Middle Ear
Sensory-Neural Hearing Impairment
    Sudden Sensory–Neural Hearing Impairment
    Ménière's Syndrome
    Cerebello–Pontine–Angle Lesions
    Presbycusis
    Noise-Induced Hearing Impairment
    Acoustic Trauma
    Drugs
    Local Otitic Infection or Head Trauma
Pain in the Ear
Speech
    Basic Functions in Speech
    Disorders of Phonation
        Signs and Symptoms of Articulatory Disorders
    Language
Summary

HOW HUMAN BEINGS COMMUNICATE

Sound production by the voice and its reception through
hearing are the most common means employed for
interpersonal communication. Human beings transfer
messages between each other chiefly vocally, but regularly employ many other modalities. Beyond early
childhood the vocal expression is verbal; that is, the
child learns to form sounds with accepted meanings—
he employs language. Other sound transmission of
meaning can be conveyed by codes: through tapping
of a Morse key in telegraphy, by drumbeats, or gun-
shots, or music and so forth.

Language or code transmission can be sent by various means and perceived through sight, such as by
written or printed symbols, by colors, light flashes,
smoke signals, etc. Sight perception is regularly employed to receive messages conveyed by movements—
motion of another person's eyes, through facial expressions, through conscious or unconscious movements
of the head, hands, and body.

Meaning can be conveyed by touch—interpersonal
touch: a handshake, a caress, or a blow; or touch of
an object such as Braille.

We have mentioned the three senses most commonly acting as receivers in human communication:

101

hearing, sight, and touch. When a sense is impaired for reception, or a means of sending messages is incompetent, either temporarily or permanently, other techniques can be developed; the mute learn to speak with their hands, the blind learn to read by touch (Braille).

The other two senses regularly receive messages, sometimes purposefully intended, often involuntarily transmitted. Through smell we perceive numerous scents and odors, from delicate and pleasant to highly obnoxious. A perfume may say, "I want to be attractive to you." A detective entering a room may discover by sniffing the air that a shot has just been fired. Even *taste* can transmit information such as a certain spice in a food.

Problems of communication between human beings usually involve one or more of these four modalities:

1. *Voice production*—the ability to produce vocal sounds
2. *Word and sentence formation*—the ability to form accepted meaningful units or groups of sounds singly or in various interrelationships, that is, the use of language
3. *Hearing*—the ability to perceive sounds through the auditory apparatus
4. *The mental or intellectual ability to interpret the meaning of spoken sounds,* that is, to understand the language used. The language may range from the most primitive to the most sophisticated and complex; the intellectual equipment required may therefore vary widely.

In this chapter, our purpose is to discuss primarily the pathologic physiology concerned in disorders of speech and hearing.

NORMAL DEVELOPMENTAL EXPECTANCIES IN HEARING AND SPEECH

The signs and symptoms of disorders of human communication must be evaluated in terms of chronologic development of the patient. The general dictum: "a child talks as he hears, and in the manner in which he hears," presupposes a certain level of neurologic and intellectual development. The normal or abnormal child acquires language through certain patterns of learning procedure; the impaired adult, however, recovers impaired communicative skills through a learning mechanism that is often quite different, since relearning of acquired skills plus the development of secondary skills are involved. The diagnostician, therefore, must be acquainted with the normal developmental expectancies of communicative skills, which, for the child, are given in Tables 6-1, 6-2, and 6-3.[1]

Failure of any child to conform to these norms within a time lag of six months should lead to concern that a communicative problem may exist.

POSSIBLE PATHOPHYSIOLOGIC MECHANISMS

The child born with impairment of his ability to hear or to vocally or verbally communicate has defects which may be in his brain, in certain nerves, or in other organs; these defects may result: (1) from a genetic aberration, which may or may not be familial or hereditary; or (2) from a disorder affecting the maternal organism; or (3) from a disorder specifically affecting the individual fetus afflicted.

All infants are of course subject to genetic, maternal fetal, and postnatal influences and possible hazards. Such hazards may produce many other possible difficulties beside auditory and speech problems.

We are in this chapter first concerned with reminding ourselves of the primary elements in the pathophysiology of impairments of hearing and speech which may affect infants and young children, and are not attributable to postnatal factors.

Next we must consider all of the possible postnatal factors that may cause hearing or speech defects, the mechanisms through which they operate, and the types of derangements that result.

HEARING

HEARING ASSESSMENT IN CHILDREN

Auditory Responses

Hearing acuity in the very young child is judged by behavioral responses (Table 6-1), by tympanometric measurements of middle ear transmission of sound, and by electrophysiologic assessment of auditory neural responses to sound stimuli. Testing by pure tone audiometry becomes useful after the age of 3 years.

Current auditory screening procedures for the newborn and infant up to 8 months of age include a direct comparison of auditory performance with developmental expectancies plus a review of maternal and pediatric factors that might predispose the child to a communicative impairment, that is, the "high risk register." The use of such a register or questionnaire is highly recommended. The high risk factors are investigated and pursued as warranted by the information disclosed. (For details of the use of such checklists and questionnaires, see the system used by Utah.[2])

The following classification, which groups most of the types of factors, does go into detail, and is not exhaustive.

(Text continues on p. 106)

Table 6-1. Speech, Language, and Hearing Communication Chart (Newborn to Age Three Years)—Normal Developmental Expectancies; Responses to Acoustic Stimuli; the Learning of Language; Vocal, Verbal, and Speech Output

Age	Activities and Responses	Parental Observation	Office Procedures	Interpretations and Meaning
Newborn	1. Startle–reflex to sound; more often to sudden sounds of moderate-to-loud intensity 2. Arousal responses. Investigators have demonstrated that relatively loud sound will arouse the newborn infant from accustomed sleep state.	Not pertinent	Not pertinent	Not ideal time to test auditory responses. Lack of expected responses bears little relationship to later communication problems. Conditions that apparently lead to auditory or other communicative problems may not become operative until several days after birth. In neurologic terms, clinical motor responses in the early months are relatively simple (gross). At this stage, more complex "apparatus"—neurologic pathways (ultimately used for communicative purposes) may or may not be intact.
4 months	1. Typically turns eyes and head in direction of sound source. Awakens or quiets to mother's voice. May change facial expression or vocalize in response to sound. (During babbling, several speech sounds are used.) 2. May open eyes when sound is presented, or, when eyes are open, palpebral fissure size may increase. May frown, smile, or search for sound. May jerk head toward sound source.	What does he do when you talk to him? Does he react when he cannot see you? Do you see him turn toward sound of crib toys? How does he use his voice at home? After 4 to 6 months of age, if child actually has severely impaired hearing, previously noted babbling may cease or be diminished.	Tester should kneel or squat behind and to side of mother's chair. Baby is seated on mother's lap and held upright. Using quiet voice say baby's name; say s-s-s-s-s-s or k-k-k-k-k-k or use noisemaking toys. Keep sound source at ear level, but out of baby's peripheral vision. Be careful not to use a vowel (uh) after S or K.	With these procedures, one is not measuring baby's hearing, but indexing babies whose responses seem abnormal. Lack of expected response to sound does not necessarily mean impaired hearing, but that baby's status and development need to be studied carefully. Premature or mentally retarded infants may be slow in developing expected responses to sound.
8 months	1. Turns head and upper torso toward interesting sounds (at level of quiet conversational voice). 2. Vocalizes with variety of sounds and inflections. Done spontaneously when alone. Gives vocal responses when somebody talks to him; e.g., smiles, giggles, coos. 3. Usually responds to familiar sounds (his name, telephone bell, vacuum cleaner, barking dog), and quiets to mother's voice. 4. Usually awakens when mother talks to him.	1. Have you seen this? 2. What have you heard him say? What noises does he make? 3. What does he do if he hears father's footsteps, the vacuum cleaner, the telephone? 4. Does he respond to "no-no"? Does he jiggle to music? 5. Has babbling decreased?	Test at ear level. Baby should seek and find sound source. It is important to test from both sides out of baby's vision range. When baby does respond, reinforcement must be used to hold baby's attention. This is done by immediately repeating stimulus at a louder level while expressing approval of baby.	Response should be prompt. Delayed responses suggest possible hearing involvement. Persistent turning to one side or searching for sound, but not identifying appropriate direction of its source suggests hearing problem. Failure to turn quickly in presence of other evidence of hearing suggests developmental lag and need for careful follow-up. These responses indicate baby's developing ability to "understand" everyday sound around him (listening and discrimination).

(Continued)

Table 6-1. *Speech, Language, and Hearing Communication Chart (Newborn to Age Three Years)—Normal Developmental Expectancies; Responses to Acoustic Stimuli; the Learning of Language; Vocal, Verbal, and Speech Output (Continued)*

Age	Activities Responses	Parental Observation and Office Procedures		Interpretations and Meaning
12 months	1. Responds to a number of different sounds, often with different reactions, and seems to recognize them as different; *e.g.*, jabbers in response to human voice, may cry when there is thunder, quiets when hears mother nearby (vacuum cleaner), and may frown when scolded.	1. Direct query and observation. What kinds of sounds and noises does he make when you talk to him? What does he do when he hears a loud noise?		1. Average behavior is similar to 8-month period (Item 3), but responses should indicate more differentiation among speech sounds.
	2. Demonstrates understanding of some words by appropriate behavior, *e.g.*, points or looks at familiar objects on request.	2. Try to test with appropriate objects, by saying the word quietly without general conversation or instruction.		2. This behavior indicates early differentiation of speech sounds as symbolic meanings.
	3. Uses sounds. "Talks" to toys. This is an enjoyable experience for baby.	3. Direct query and observation. Does he "talk" to himself or make sounds as he plays with his toys?		3. One can look for changes in baby's "talking" as his attention and patterns of play change.
12 months (Cont'd)	4. Tries to imitate some simple words.	4. If possible, have mother demonstrate this; he is more used to her manner of speaking		4. This is evidence of developmental maturation. Many children use a few words at this age. However, babies may *not* imitate words at 12 months. Absence of verbal utterance indicates a need to inquire about verbal stimulation at home, parental attitudes, and expectancies; *e.g.*, "Do you have time to sit and talk with him and let him jabber back?" "Does his father?"
18 months	1. Expect some progressive increase in child's vocabulary (more definite words) from that observable at 12 months.	1. Query and demonstration. How many understandable words does he use? More or fewer than he used a few months ago?		1. Note any apparent loss of words that were previously used. With a child who has severely impaired hearing, one can expect cessation or regression of previously noted babbling.
	2. Begins to identify part of body, *e.g.*, may point to nose on request.	2. Demonstration, if possible. The baby should be able to show you his nose or eyes.		2. This is clear evidence of verbal symbolic understanding.
	3. Beginning to pay attention to, and identify, various sounds from considerable distance.	3. Note detail of parental anecdotes. It is important that auditory responses are identified without the use of visual cues. What does he do when refrigerator door opens in another room? When ice cream man's bell rings? When there is a fire siren? When you open a box of candy that he cannot see? Does he seem to react to music? with rhythm? Does he like to look at books with you, and turn the page?		3. Whereas at 8 to 12 months baby's auditory attention is limited to close environment, by 18 months he is responding to wider environment of sound *e.g.*, from another room, or from outside the house. If hearing loss has been acquired, he probably will not do this, and may show symptoms of regression in speech attempts previously made.

24 months

1. Can follow verbal commands with components without the aid of gestures, *e.g.*, "Pick up the block and give it to mother."
2. Can identify familiar objects when named.
3. Can spontaneously name familiar objects.
4. Initiates "sentences" of two or more "words," which are meaningful to listener.
5. Learns new (simple) word with only one presentation.

1 to 5. Screening requires demonstration as well as parental reporting. Often it is easier and more economic to let mother do the demonstrating. The responses should be observed and not simply accepted from parental statements. Mother can tell him to "Close the door and sit down," "Pick up the block and give it to me," "Get my purse and put it on that chair." Inquire whether he shows interest in musical introductions to regular television shows. Does he listen to music from a record player?

5. This is only one item in a battery of achievements for this age. If it can be demonstrated, this accomplishment represents a significant landmark. It is perhaps best to direct mother to undertake this. Failure to accomplish it on the part of a just 2-year-old may be related to various developmental states of affairs, any of which warrant careful investigation.

36 months

1. Can identify objects or activities with the use of pictures; *e.g.*, "Show me the one that is good to eat." "Show me the one that you wear."
2. Identifies his or her own sex.
3. Understands some verbs, adjectives, pronouns, and prepositions.
4. Repeats a 4-word sentence.
5. Uses some verbs, adjectives, pronouns, and prepositions.
6. May respond to pure tones from audiometer, as well as to speech.
7. Names familiar objects.

1. Should be readily demonstrated.
2. "Are you a boy or a girl?" Put correct reference first.
3. Preferably, this should be demonstrated with the use of toys in a doll house or other appropriate objects; up, down, in, on, under, big, little, you, me, I. "Put the baby in the big bed." "Make the dog jump." "Push the car."
4. Actually, he should be able to repeat and use 4 word sentences.
5. This requires observation, or acceptable reports, of the child's typical behavior.
6. To be determined in appropriate circumstances by qualified testers.
7. This should be readily demonstrated.

1 to 7. Child should be using speech socially. Deviations from normal development that may become apparent at this time, and that generally require extensive diagnostic evaluation, include "the retarded child," "delayed speech," "motor interference," "impaired hearing," and "emotional disturbance." If he does not quite readily demonstrate these verbal capacities, there is need for careful follow-up. If he uses jargon and gestures to try to control his environment, rather than words, hearing involvement may be suspected. There is always apt to be confusion between the dull child and the deaf child (frequently both conditions are present). Further definitive measurement of hearing is readily available for the child of this age. Various kinds of audiometry can be done. These require special equipment and experience. (Routine pure-tone audiometry can be carried out with confidence with about 50% of just 3-year olds.

(Adapted from unpublished report of Special Ad Hoc Committee of Children's Bureau; Chairman, William G. Hardy, Ph.D., 1965. Table constructed by Frances R. Tucker of the Maryland State Department of Health, in consultation with Francis I. Catlin, M.D., and William G. Hardy, Ph.D. of the Johns Hopkins Medical Institutions)

Table 6-2. *Vocabulary Growth**

Age		Number of Words
Years	*Months*	
0	10	1
1	0	3
1	6	22
2	0	272
2	6	446
3	0	896
3	6	1222
4	0	1540
4	6	1870
5	0	2072
5	6	2289
6	0	2562

Maternal High Risk Factors

1. *History of previous handicapped infant*
2. *History of prematurity, stillbirth,* and so on
3. *History of complications during pregnancy or at delivery*
4. *Illness* (endocrine, cardiovasculorenal, anemia, nutritional, Rh incompatibility, and so on.)
5. *Illness* (infections: rubella, syphilis, toxoplasmosis, influenza, cytomegalovirus, others)
6. *Other hazards* (drugs, alcohol, radiation)
7. *Age* (under 16 or over 36 primigravida; or over 40, multigravida)

Table 6-3. *Verbal Output**

Age		Average Length of "Sentences" (Number of Words)
Years	*Months*	
1	6	1.2
2	0	1.7 to 1.9
2	6	2.7 to 3.1
3	0	3.0 to 4.2
3	6	4.3 to 4.7
4	0	3.4 to 5.4
4	6	4.6 to 5.5
5	0	3.6 to 5.7
5	6	4.4 to 5.1
6	0	3.7 to 6.6
6	6	5.0 to 5.4
7	0	7.3
8	0	7.6

*These normative data can serve as a guide for checking status of vocabulary development and amount of expressive speech.

Infant High Risk Factors

1. *Gestational age* under 36 or over 42 weeks
2. *Birth weight* under 4 lbs† or over 11 lbs
3. *Trauma* at birth
4. *Apnea* at birth
5. *Neonatal shock, jaundice, bleeding or severe anemia, or severe hypoglycemia*
6. *Evidence of a genetic defect (e.g.,* phenylketonuria)
7. *Meningitis*

OTOLOGIC EVALUATION

A competent otologic examination to rule out disease of the ear is essential. When the otologic picture is normal, assessment of the neurologic and psychologic status of the child is most important.

Childhood auditory impairments may be genetic, congenital, or acquired. In small infants, this differentiation may be difficult because of the time lag between the causative event and the period during which impairment of performance is noticed. Some conditions may be recognized early: deformities of ear, lip, and palate are readily apparent. However, palatal incompetence and choanal atresia occasionally escape early diagnosis. Gross deformities of the inner ear structures fortunately are rare and usually are found in association with obvious external and middle ear malformations.

Hearing impairment may present in several ways. The age of onset, the character of the hearing impairment, and the nature of the underlying disease all exert a direct bearing upon the symptomatology. The 8-month-old infant may fail to turn toward the source of sound; the 2-year-old may be unable to identify familiar objects when named.

Mild hearing impairments may not be detected under average listening conditions. Under more difficult listening conditions, such as in the classroom, a child with a mild hearing impairment can be, and often is, classified mistakenly and unfairly as being uncooperative, unresponsive, erratic, or diffident, or as having a "behavior problem." The more severe hearing impairments create a recognizable communicative dysfunction unless the hearing loss is unilateral, although an alert parent or teacher may recognize the latter condition.

Hearing impairment in the pre-school (4- to 6-year-old) and school-age child is most commonly the result of upper respiratory infection and its sequelae. For the most part, such predisposing conditions are self-limiting, and the hearing impairment is therefore tran-

†Under 5.5 lbs if gestational age is less than 36 weeks.

sient. However, some of these conditions, though potentially reversible, can cause permanent damage to the auditory system unless the treatment is prompt and adequate. One must not forget that prolonged auditory impairment in the pre-school child may seriously delay and impair the normal acquisition of speech and language skills. Such delay may have long-term effects in many spheres upon the development of the person.

ANATOMY AND PHYSIOLOGY OF AUDITORY APPARATUS

Some knowledge of the normal mechanisms of the auditory system is essential for an understanding of the symptomatology of hearing impairment. Since the site of the underlying condition has a direct effect upon the symptomatology, these mechanisms will be described briefly (Fig. 6-1).

Sound-Conduction Mechanism of the Ear

The peripheral auditory system may be divided into three parts. Two of these, the external auditory canal, terminating in the tympanic membrane, and the middle ear, containing the sound-conducting ossicles (malleus, incus, and stapes) that transmit vibrations from the tympanic membrane to the inner ear by the stapes footplate, constitute the conductive mechanism by which airborne sound is effectively transmitted to the fluid-encased structures of the inner ear. Without the "transformer action" of the tympanic membrane and ossicles, airborne sound would be reflected from the inner ear, with a resultant loss of auditory sensitivity.

Impairment of the transmission mechanisms of the external and middle ear produces a *conductive hearing impairment.* The loss of auditory sensitivity tends to be fairly uniform over the useful frequency range of the ear: that is, low-pitched sounds are attenuated to the same extent as high-pitched sounds. Consequently, if

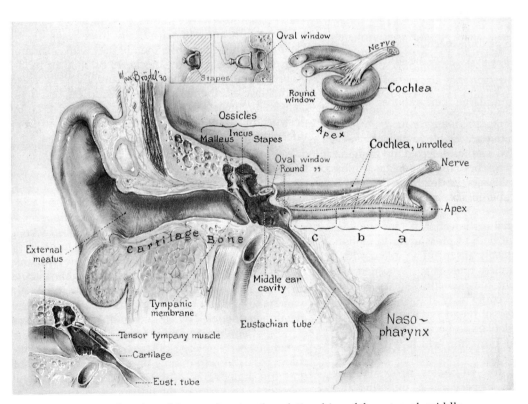

Fig. 6-1. Schematic drawing of the ear showing the relationships of the external, middle, and internal parts. The cochlea has been unrolled to show the relation of (*a*) the apical third, (*b*) the middle third, and (*c*) the basal third to the oval and round window niches of the middle ear space. (Department of Art as Applied to Medicine, Johns Hopkins University School of Medicine, an original drawing by Max Brödel)

SENSORY-NEURAL HEARING IMPAIRMENT

Disorders of the inner ear produce a sensory–neural hearing impairment if the sensory–neural elements of the organ of Corti are involved. The range of the hearing spectrum impaired follows certain general patterns. Thus, a hearing loss of sensory–neural type that affects the low-pitched frequencies is often encountered in those with early Meniere's disease, whereas a loss of hearing sensitivity in the higher frequencies is more characteristic of advanced Meniere's disease, noise-induced hearing loss, and the effects of aging.

Sudden Sensory–Neural Hearing Impairment

The loss of hearing may be abrupt in onset, as in acute idiopathic sensory–neural hearing impairment. The condition may be unilateral or bilateral, may be associated with vestibular dysfunction (or may not) and may improve spontaneously, although many unfortunately do not recover. Occasionally there is a history of a previous viral infection. The usual rapidity of onset suggests that impairment of the otic vascular supply may be at fault.

Meniere's Syndrome

When the sensory neural hearing impairment is accompanied by attacks of vertigo and tinnitus, (head noise), a diagnosis of Meniere's syndrome should be entertained. The vertigo should be of true rotatory or per-rotatory type, and usually persists during bedrest. The vertigo may even start while the patient is lying down. The initial episode of Meniere's syndrome tends to be incapacitating, with severe nausea, vertigo, and vomiting. The hearing impairment and tinnitus are confined to the affected ear; in late cases, however, about one-third of such patients show signs and symptoms of bilateral involvement. The frequency and severity of early attacks commonly subside within a week, often with simultaneous improvement of auditory acuity. Subsequent attacks may vary in intensity and frequency. Remission of symptoms may occur, at times for many years, and apparent recovery from a solitary attack has been reported. Although complete disappearance of hearing impairment may be found after early attacks, progression of hearing loss is typical among those who have subsequent attacks of vertigo.

Cerebello–Pontine–Angle Lesions

When the presenting symptom is unilateral hearing impairment with or without tinnitus and vertigo, dizziness or unsteadiness, one should suspect a cerebello-pontine-angle (c–p–a) tumor until proved otherwise. As Cushing[3] noted in his classic text on acoustic tumors, patients with these lesions usually exhibit early and steadily progressive signs and symptoms of impairment of hearing and vestibular function of the involved ear. The observer should examine the patient for stigmata of von Recklinghausen's disease and for other evidence of c–p–a tumor. Erickson[4] noted initial symptoms of hearing deficit with or without tinnitus (51%), headaches (16.5%), tinnitus without hearing deficit (12%), abnormality of gait (10%), dizziness and/or vertigo (9%), trigeminal symptoms (9%), symptoms of increased intracranial pressure (4%), visual impairment (3%), and facial weakness (2%) in his review of 126 unilateral cases. Approximately 2% to 3% of these tumors are bilateral, and most of these show evidence of von Recklinghausen's disease.

Presbycusis

Slowly progressive bilateral hearing impairment of the sensory–neural type (without vestibular signs, in the majority of persons) is a characteristic feature of aging in many countries, including the United States. Data by Spoor on normal persons show a gradual decrease in auditory sensitivity that is more pronounced for the higher audible frequencies.[5] This type of impairment starts in the teens or early 20s and becomes more severe with advancing age, especially in males. The degree of impairment for each decade of life shows wide variations; but for most this impairment, called *presbycusis*, does not produce any significant handicap until the fifth decade and above. Tinnitus is common, being more severe initially, but becoming less bothersome as age progresses and hearing acuity deteriorates. Distortions of hearing are common: "I can hear the voices, but I can't understand what they say," is the frequent complaint. Intolerance for any very loud sounds is occasionally noted.

Some familiar types of sensory–neural hearing impairment resemble the clinical picture of presbycusis, except that the age of onset is younger and the rate of deterioration of hearing tends to be more rapid over comparable periods of time.

The exact etiology of hearing loss in the aged is not definitely known. Presumably it is caused by arteriolosclerosis, with reduced blood supply to the inner ear (organ of Corti), the eighth cranial nerve itself, or the cortical and subcortical areas of the cerebrum involved in hearing.

Noise-Induced Hearing Impairment

Those who work in sufficiently noisy surroundings often notice three effects of such exposure: (1) difficulty in communicating with others while in the noisy environment (including use of the telephone), (2) tinnitus after leaving the noise, and (3) a muffled quality of sounds heard, including speech. This last effect is as-

sociated with a temporary loss of hearing, called a temporary threshold shift (TTS), and its existence suggests exposure to hazardous noise conditions. Recovery to previous hearing levels usually occurs within several hours. Pain is characteristically absent during and after the noise exposure unless the noise source is extremely loud (and extremely hazardous for the hearing mechanisms). Hazardous noise levels occur in many industrial settings, near jet aircraft engines and poorly muffled internal combustion engines, and possibly from contemporary amplified music.

When exposure to hazardous noise is prolonged or severe, the temporary threshold shift of auditory acuity may be replaced, in part, by a permanent threshold shift (PTS) which is called a noise-induced hearing impairment. Such impairment is almost always sensory–neural in nature; its development depends upon many factors; the loudness and composition of the noise, the duration of noise exposure, and the specific susceptibility of the individual to noise.

The signs and symptoms of noise-induced hearing impairment are indistinguishable from those of presbycusis. As yet, no test has been devised that distinguishes between these two conditions. Consequently, when the noise hazard is in doubt, or the individual is in an older age group, the clinician may find it difficult to determine the exact cause of the hearing impairment.

Acoustic Trauma

Exposure to very loud noise levels may produce a permanent sensory–neural hearing impairment within a short period of time, such as with a single episode of noise exposure. Such an impairment is called "acoustic trauma." In some instances, as from an explosion, the tympanic membrane may be ruptured, or disarticulation of the ossicular bones may occur, or both may occur. When this happens, the affected person suffers a mixed type of hearing impairment which is partly conductive and partly sensory–neural. At times, the degree of sensory–neural damage appears to be lessened when disruption of the ossicular conductive system takes place.

Drugs

Tinnitus and sensory–neural hearing loss may develop following the use of certain drugs, notably: systemic streptomycin, kanamycin, neomycin, and more recently, ethacrynic acid. The list of other chemical agents that may affect the eighth cranial nerve is legion: viomycin, quinine, ethyl alcohol, aspirin, lead, phosphorus, carbon monoxide, and oil of chenopodium, to name a few. With some of these agents, vestibular symptoms of dizziness and unsteadiness may occur, notably after streptomycin.[6]

Local Otitic Infection or Head Trauma

Local otitic infection or head trauma may be etiologic factors for sensory-neural hearing loss. Infection of the inner ear usually produces an associated ipsilateral labyrinthitis with spontaneous nystagmus, with the quick, or recovery, component to the side of involvement in the early or irritative phase, and toward the uninvolved ear in the late or paretic phase. Nausea, vomiting, and unsteadiness are common. Head trauma may evoke similar symptoms if a fracture through the otic capsule occurs. In some instances, there may be an associated cerebrospinal fluid otorrhea draining through the external auditory canal, if the tympanic membrane is torn, or through the eustachian tube, if the tympanic membrane is intact. Cerebrospinal otorrhea usually subsides spontaneously within a period of 2 to 3 weeks. Occasionally head trauma produces a "contre-coup" impairment of hearing in the ear opposite to the side on which the trauma occurs.

PAIN IN THE EAR

The differentiating characteristics between ear pain caused by otitis externa and by otitis media have previously been discussed. An outline of some of the common causes of pain in the ear with the localizing signs and symptoms follows:

Primary pain—arising from disorders of aural structures
  Auricular pain
    Frostbite
    Trauma
    Infection (soft tissue or perichondritis)
    (The foregoing conditions are usually self-evident, with an inflammatory reaction locally, hemorrhage or abrasions in the case of trauma, and swelling of the soft tissue.)
    Tumors
    Cysts (especially if infected)
  External auditory canal
    Abrasion or laceration (as with a foreign body)
    Furunculosis
    External otitis (swimmer's ear)
    Herpes oticus (with otic eruption, other signs of facial involvement; facial paralysis, sensory–neural hearing loss)
    Tumors
  Tympanic membrane
    Trauma

Laceration/perforation
Bullous myringitis
Middle ear
Aerotitis media (generally retraction of tympanic membrane and inflammation of middle ear mucosa)
Acute otitis media
Chronic otitis media with acute superinfection
Acute mastoiditis
Tumors
Referred pain—arising from adjacent structures
Nasopharynx
Acute nasopharyngitis
Tumors of the nasopharynx (usually invasive)
Dental origin
Pulpitis
Impaction
Sinusitis
Acute, usually sphenoid or maxillary
Pharynx, mouth
Infection (such as tonsils, pharyngeal spaces)
Tumors
Neck
Infection of the triangular spaces and their contents
Tumors (uncommon unless invasive)

SPEECH

BASIC FUNCTIONS IN SPEECH

Communicative oral expression involves a number of basic functions:[7]

1. *Respiration*—provision of the air flow for sound production
2. *Phonation*—the laryngeal aspect of sound production
3. *Resonance*—the selective modification of laryngeal-produced sound by the anatomic and physiologic characteristics of the speech mechanisms
4. *Articulation*—sound production and the selective modification of the voiced and unvoiced breath stream by the articulatory segments of the speech mechanisms (tongue, teeth, and lips); a function interrelated with resonance
5. *Pronunciation*—arrangement of speech sounds in prescribed sequences of syllables with the application of proper syllable stress
6. *Language comprehension and use*—the symbolization process involving the formulation and comprehension of language and other symbolic forms
7. *A communicative set*—enables the person to have a

willingness and readiness to speak, a confidence in his communicative ability, plus the urge to communicate

When an impairment of speech function is suspected, one must look for signs and symptoms of impairment of these basic functions, as well as of the speech-producing structures: the respiratory mechanism, larynx, tongue, teeth, hard and soft palate, lips, pharynx, and nasal cavities. In general, the respiratory or breathing mechanism is adequate if the speaker can provide adequate sublaryngeal pressures at appropriate times, accelerate or decelerate the volume of air flow at will, inspire and exhale at will, and otherwise regulate his breathing patterns. The respiratory mechanism is seldom a factor in major communicative problems unless there is paresis of the respiratory structures or a severely impaired pulmonary reserve.

DISORDERS OF PHONATION

Phonation is the auditory experience of laryngeal voice production that is culturally appropriate for human communication. Certain parameters, such as pitch, show normal variations with respect to age, sex and socio-economic status. Abnormalities of phonation (voice) cannot always be easily distinguished from impairments of articulation or of resonance.

Certain characteristics are commonly used to describe phonation:

1. *Pitch level*—the central tendency of fundamental frequency of vocal cord vibration about which intonation variations habitually occur
2. *Loudness level*—the average (characteristic) level of intensity of phonation
3. *Control*—the ability to initiate, maintain, and discontinue phonation at will
4. *Intonation*—the habitual variation of pitch, loudness, and control of phonation appropriate to speech meaning and the circumstances of the communicative situation
5. *Quality*—the overall characteristics of laryngeal-produced sounds that are not the results of articulatory or of resonance effects
6. *Loss or absence of the ability to phonate*

Voice disorders are frequently complex in nature. They are comparatively rare in incidence. Phonatory (voice) impairments may be classified as organic or nonorganic (functional). Every voice disorder should be studied for signs of organic impairment.

Hoarseness, a combination of the acoustical features of breathiness and harshness, is rare as a nonorganic disorder (as in ''false-cord'' phonation), but is rela-

tively common as a sign of laryngeal pathology. Painless hoarseness is one of the early symptoms of cancer of the larynx. Associated symptoms include voice fatigue, frequent need to clear the throat, and, on occasion, chronic dryness or rawness of the throat. One should question for a history of excessive smoking or voice misuse (as in singers and public speakers), as well as for signs and symptoms of hiatus hernia and esophageal regurgitation.

Hoarseness, breathiness, and weak voice intensity in the adult should lead to suspicion of a growth on the vocal cord, vocal cord paralysis, or myasthenia gravis. Vocal cord paralysis is most commonly the result of trauma (especially surgical trauma). Bilateral vocal cord paralysis with the cords approximated (bilateral abductor paralysis) can produce frightening symptoms in some patients: apprehension, dyspnea, and labored respiration and speech.

Hoarseness and its first cousin, *stridor* (harsh, high-pitched sound that is very audible), should lead the diagnostician to investigate the intrinsic as well as possible extralaryngeal causes. This study is especially urgent when these symptoms appear in small children. Intralaryngeal causes include inflammatory conditions, tumors, cysts, congenital anatomic abnormalities, neurologic problems, trauma and intralaryngeal foreign bodies. Among the extralaryngeal causes are: congenital anatomic abnormalities, tumors, cysts, inflammatory conditions of the neck and mediastinum, and foreign bodies in the esophagus.

Ventricular phonation is characterized by hoarseness, low pitch, a moderate-to-weak intensity, reduced inflection, and a raspy quality to the voice.

Diplophonia, the true production of two fundamental frequencies by the vocal cords, is rare.

Aphonia, or loss of voice, may result from organic causes, such as damage to the larynx, or from nonorganic conditions, such as psychogenic aphonia. With either organic or psychogenic aphonia, *whisper speech,* a sound produced by laryngeal air flow instead of by vocal cord vibration, may be employed.

Falsetto, a voice of higher pitch than appropriate for age and sex of the speaker, is most often the result of sociocultural conditions, although it has been reported following laryngitis, trauma or shock. Although use of falsetto may be appropriate for singing and under certain cultural conditions, it frequently dates from puberty and is more likely to occur if the true voice is bass. The falsetto voice does not necessarily have to be very high in pitch.

One should also consider other conditions that may affect phonation: hearing loss that impairs the person's self-monitoring mechanisms; reduced auditory memory span; poor or inconstant pitch placement; and faulty discrimination and use of intensity and quality. All these parameters of speech are affected by internal and external feedback systems. The functions of all these systems must be evaluated just as carefully as the physical apparatus for the production of speech sounds, if the interpretation of signs and symptoms is to be of value.

Signs and Symptoms of Articulatory Disorders

Learning to articulate the standard sounds of a language is an experience of all communicating persons. Since speech is a learned activity, the majority of speech disorders occur during the childhood or developmental period and, to a lesser degree, in the aging population in the form of aphasia and laryngeal disease.

Most childhood speech problems are articulatory disorders; that is, defective production of acceptable speech sounds. All physiologic measurements show ranges of variation. Speech sounds are no exception. As Van Riper and Irwin[8] have noted, however, certain criteria can be employed to describe abnormalities of articulation. These include:

1. *Intelligibility*—the degree to which intelligibility is impaired
2. *Frequency and consistency of error*—the number of errors heard by the listener and the consistency with which they occur
3. *Type of error*—some articulatory errors are more noticeable than others. Many errors are so close to the variations of normal utterance that they can scarcely be termed errors. Others deviate widely; for example, compare the effects of omissions, substitutions and distortions.
4. *Conditions of communication*—society uses different tolerance levels for variations in pronunciation in terms of the type of communication used. More variation is tolerated in casual conversation than in formal platform speech. Articulation errors tend to be overlooked by the listener during stressful or emotional environmental situations.
5. *Status within the culture*—judgment regarding the quality of articulation in speech is also based upon the listener's evaluation of the status of the speaker in his culture. Errors made by a child and accepted as normal would be considered abnormal for adult use. Two factors are apparent: the standards of language usage are frequently employed as signs of cultural status. Closely related to this factor of cultural status is the fact that the standards of acceptable pronunciation undergo continual change, just as do other cultural activities.
6. *Subjective criteria of abnormality*—the prior criteria have been defined primarily in terms of listener reaction.

In some instances, the speaker, because of anxiety, may attribute defects to his own speech that are nonexistent. Other persons may refuse to recognize articulatory errors that are real. A few refuse to believe that their speech is in any way defective. They are unable to isolate their errors sufficiently to perceive them.

Clearly, the identification and interpretation of articulatory disorders is not a task for the layman.

Other forms of defective speech include voice disorders that can mimic articulation disorders (and *vice-versa*). *Lalling* refers to slurred and defective articulation resulting from reduced tongue-tip activity. *Hyponasality,* as in muffling of the m, n, and ng sounds, occurs with nasal or nasopharyngeal obstruction (as in acute coryza). Although occasionally described as a voice disorder, Van Riper and Irwin consider hyponasality to be an articulation problem in which certain sounds are produced defectively.

Although cleft palate speakers are described as having characteristically hypernasal voices, their speech seems more nasal if it contains many consonant articulation errors than if it contains few. Apparently, hypernasality and misarticulation are closely related. Limitation of palatal closure by submucous cleft, palatal paralysis, or scarring should be considered in the presence of hypernasality. Indirect evaluation by cineradiographic studies or direct examination by the fiberoptic nasopharyngoscopy may be invaluable.

Misarticulations are also found in the speech of those with certain dental conditions, such as severe malocclusion. Misarticulation frequently occurs with cerebral palsy and as one of the speech defects of aphasia. Defective articulation, often accompanied by disorders of voice pitch and loudness, is frequently encountered in those whose learning mechanisms are hampered by severe hearing impairments, especially in young children.

Delayed speech is a common "wastebasket" diagnosis. Whereas the term properly refers to children with late onset of speech who nevertheless go through an orderly process of speech development, this diagnostic label is often applied to other conditions in which misarticulation and impairments of vocabulary, use of syntax, and general language awareness are intermixed in various proportions. Many of these children exhibit poor auditory memory (seldom better than the achievement of the normal 2-year-old) and impaired language comprehension. Many also have difficulty in reading. One should look for related emotional, intellectual (maturational), or socioeconomic factors.

Similarly, the person learning a new language needs to acquire new skills in articulation, vocabulary, syntax, intonation, and language comprehension. Traces of the characteristics of the first language learned in childhood are apt to remain to modify another language learned later in life.

Cluttered speech is described by Weiss[9] as "hurried in rate, yet hesitant," with repetition of syllables and short words, slurring with speed, and with syntactic deformation of longer sentences. Many of these speakers demonstrate poor auditory memory and omissions.

Stuttering, on the contrary, is not an articulatory problem but an interruption of the ongoing process of expressive speech that is characterized by part-word (syllable) repetitions, intermittent sound prolongations and irregularity in the rate of verbal expression. Stuttering becomes eminent when the performance of speech occurs under stress. Even speakers classified as "normal" may stutter if environmental conditions are sufficiently stressful. The debate over the behavioral versus organic etiology of stuttering remains unresolved.

LANGUAGE

Language comprehension and use implies the willingness and ability to formulate and use meaningful symbols for the comprehension of speech stimuli (*e.g.,* vision), and for the initiation of appropriate motor output (*e.g.,* speech output, gesture). A simplistic division of impairments of language comprehension into acquired versus developmental conditions is appealing but often unsatisfactory. Several reasons exist: too little is known about the relationship of language comprehension to the neurophysiology of the central nervous system; current tools for evaluation of the language function are, at best, gross; and the ability of the person to comprehend and use language changes continually.

Some authors have offered a diagrammatic outline in which the five stages of normal language development are compared with corresponding stages of aphasic disturbance found in impaired adults. (See Table 6-4.)

The average infant may be expected to reach stage III at a 12- to 18-month level, stage IV at about the 2-year level and stage V by 3 years of age. Failure to achieve these levels may be related to factors other than the ability to develop language. The diagnostician should consider the psychological stimulation provided (or not provided) by the child's environment, the presence and nature of associated hearing and speech defects, and the nonverbal mental age of the child, when compared with his peer group. A survey of the problems of classification may be found in: "Human Communication and Its Disorders," prepared by the National Institute of Neurological Diseases and Stroke.[10]

Table 6-4. *Language Development and Aphasia*

Stage	State of Development	Type of Aphasia
I	Prelanguage: characterized by speechlessness	Global
II	Prelanguage: characterized by meaningless autistic and echolalic phoneme use	Jargon
III	Progressive acquisition of comprehension. Oral expression of words and neologisms, largely unrelated to meaning or below level of comprehension.	Pragmatic
IV	The beginning use of substantive language, progressing through nominal, verbal, and adjectival words. Characterized by one- or two-word groups as complete expression.	Semantic
V	The use of syntax or grammar in oral expression	Syntactic

SUMMARY

Communication between human beings is a developmental process. The communicative act requires adequate hearing, the intellectual ability to interpret the meaning of spoken sounds, the ability to produce vocal sounds, and the ability to transmit meaning in the form of speech. An understanding of normal developmental expectancies for hearing, language, and speech is needed to assess the corresponding development of communication in the child. Impairments of ability to communicate may result from hearing, language, and speech disorders singly or in combination. Impairments of hearing, language, or speech function in the adult produce a slightly different symptomatology than when these impairments occur in the prelingual child. A review of the anatomy and physiology of the auditory apparatus and of the etiology of hearing loss is of benefit in understanding the signs and symptoms of hearing impairment. Pain is an important symptom that may or may not be associated with loss of hearing. Disorders of language are reviewed briefly, since the evaluation of language impairments requires specialized evaluative techniques beyond the scope of the chapter. A diagrammatic outline of the five stages of normal language development and the corresponding stages of aphasic disturbance in impaired adults is presented. In addition, language disorders frequently contribute to abnormal speech patterns. Disorders of phonation and articulation are reviewed in detail.

REFERENCES

1. **Tucker FR:** Speech and Hearing (adapted from unpublished report of Special Ad Hoc Committee of Children's Bureau, Chairman, William G Hardy, PhD, 1965). Maryland State Department of Health, 1969

2. **Utah State Division of Health, Maternal and Child Health Section:** Maternal and Infant High Risk Check Lists. Department of Health, Salt Lake City, 1967

3. **Cushing H:** Tumors of the Nervus Acusticus and the Syndrome of the Cerebellopontile Angle. Philadelphia, WB Saunders, 1917

4. **Erickson LS, Sorensen GD, McGavran MH:** A review of 140 acoustic neurinomas (neurilemmoma). Laryngoscope 75:601–627, April, 1965

5. **Spoor A:** Presbycusis values in relation to noise induced hearing loss. Int Audiology 6:48–57, 1967

6. **Worthington EL, Lunin LF, Heath M et al:** Index–Handbook of Ototoxic Agents 1966–1971. Baltimore, Johns Hopkins Press, 1973

7. **Johnson W, Darley FL, Spriestersbach DC:** Diagnostic Methods in Speech Pathology. New York, Harper & Row, 1963

8. **Van Riper C, Irwin JV:** Voice and Articulation. Englewood Cliffs, NJ, Prentice-Hall, 1958

9. **Weiss DA, Beebe HH:** The Chewing Approach in Speech and Voice Therapy. New York, S Karger, 1955

10. **National Institute of Neurological Diseases and Stroke, National Institutes of Health:** Human Communication and Its Disorders—An Overview. Bethesda, 1969

7

Sore Tongue and Sore Mouth Richard W. Vilter

Normal Morphology and Physiology of Tongue and Mouth
Medical History and Physical Examination
Systemic Diseases That May Cause Sore Tongue and Sore Mouth
  Nutritional Deficiency Diseases—Vitamin B Complex, Vitamin C, and Related Deficiency States
    Etiology
    Incidence of Nutritional Deficiency Diseases
    Pathology, Physiology and Chemistry
    Multiple Deficiency States
    Niacin Deficiency (Pellagrous Stomatitis and Glossitis)
    Riboflavin Deficiency (Ariboflavinosis)
    Other B Complex Deficiency States
    Atrophic Glossitis
    Vitamin C Deficiency
Other Systemic Diseases That May Cause Sore Tongue and Sore Mouth
  Cirrhosis—Alcoholic or Laennec's
  Leukemia, Hypoplastic Anemia, Idiopathic and Drug-Induced Neutropenia, and Thrombocytopenia

The Erythemas and "Collagen" Diseases
Lichen Planus
Psoriasis
Systemic Infections, Scarlet Fever, Syphilis
Exogenous Intoxication with Heavy Metals
Dilantin Gingivitis
Endogenous Intoxication, Uremia
Allergy
Antibiotics
Menopause
Neurologic Lesions
Psychoneuroses
Local Oral Lesions
  Vincent's Stomatitis
  Herpetic Gingivostomatitis
  Aphthous Stomatitis
  Isolated Simple Papillitis
  Enteritis
  Chronic Granulomas
  Hyperplasia and Dysplasia
  Leukoplakia
  Tumors
  Local Trauma
  Geographic Tongue
Summary

Since the earliest days of medicine, the tongue has been a barometer of health. Hippocrates correlated the dry, heavily coated, fissured tongue with fever and dehydration, and he associated a poor prognosis with the red, ulcerated tongue and mouth of the patient with protracted dysentery.[1]

With the medical renaissance of the 18th and 19th centuries, observations on the state of the tongue and mouth became as important as counting the pulse. Indeed, by 1844, glossology had become so important a part of the medical art that a physician named Dr. Benjamin Ridge proposed the fantastic theory that the viscera were represented by definite areas on the tongue and that an abnormality in a viscus was reflected in this predetermined area. The physician was not alone in holding the tongue in high regard. The patient and his family often considered it the only sure indicator of health or disease and held a physician in poor regard who did not greet his patient with the request, "Stick out your tongue, please." Such aphorisms as "raw red tongue—raw red gut" or "coated tongue—constipation" stem from this period.

During the first half of the 20th century, the science of medicine rapidly outstripped the art, and many reputable physicians, aware that the beliefs of previous centuries were frequently "old wives' tales," preferred to confine their observation to such newly developed instruments as the fluoroscope and the electrocardiograph. Observation of the tongue and mouth was so simple that it was frequently neglected and, in fact, often considered as the mark of the "old-timer."

In recent years, however, observations of the condition of tongue and mouth have assumed new diagnostic importance. Interpretations have been based upon controlled clinical observations rather than upon empiricism. The change began about 1900 with William Hunter's description of the glossitis of pernicious anemia.[2] Later, hematologists such as Minot and Murphy substantiated Hunter's observations and made use of them as diagnostic measures[3]; but the present emphasis on the significance of oral lesions primarily is due to the work of nutritionists such as Spies,[4,5] Jolliffe,[6] Sydenstricker,[7,8] Sebrell,[9] and Kruse,[10,11] who have stressed the importance of tongue and mouth lesions in the early diagnosis of nutritional deficiency diseases. The complicated mechanisms whereby the tongue and mouth mirror the abnormalities of the body as a whole have only begun to be unraveled, but knowledge of metabolic diseases is increasing rapidly. Already, the importance of questioning the patient concerning soreness or burning of the tongue have been reestablished.

This chapter is concerned with the description, interpretation, and differential diagnosis of *painful* abnormalities of the tongue and mouth that reflect metabolic disease. Wherever possible, the altered physiology responsible for the abnormalities provides the background for the discussion.

NORMAL MORPHOLOGY AND PHYSIOLOGY OF TONGUE AND MOUTH

Under normal conditions, the ventral surface of the tongue is covered with smooth pink, mucous membrane and lymphoid follicles. On its dorsal surface the filiform, fungiform, and circumvallate papillae, containing the end-organs of taste, produce a rough grayish red appearance. The 12 large mushroomlike circumvallate papillae are arranged in an inverted V shape at the base of the tongue. The hairlike filiform papillae, the most numerous type present, are fine projections of mucous membrane capped by tufts of squamous epithelial cells and usually arranged in rows parallel with the row of circumvallate papillae. These inverted V-shaped rows gradually merge into parallel straight lines on the anterior surface of the tongue, and finally at the tip this regular arrangement is lost. The fungiform papillae are conical or mushroom-shaped and covered by smooth, thin epithelium. They are larger than the filiform papillae among which they are scattered and usually occur in greatest abundance at the tip and sides of the tongue. The thick epithelial tufts of the filiform papillae give the tongue its characteristic gray white coating, whereas the globular, pale red fungiform papillae give the tongue a speckled pink appearance.

The tongue is usually not furrowed except for a midline groove. A common variant is the "scrotal" tongue, which appears more bulky than usual and many irregularly placed grooves and furrows transect it. However, the general arrangement and the appearance of the papillae are unaffected.

In health, the buccal mucous membrane has an even grayish red color and may be crossed by fine grayish ridges where it settles between the rows of teeth when the mouth is closed. On close inspection, particularly if a small magnifying glass is used, one can distinguish a meshwork of tiny blood vessels just under the epithelium from which this color is derived. The mucous membrane covering the gums has a somewhat lighter red color. The gingival margins and the interdental papillae (projections of gum between the teeth) have the same appearance as the rest of the gum.

The exposed portions of the lips are dry, vermilion in color, and usually marked by slight superficial vertical wrinkling. Inside "the line of closure," the lips are

moist and of the same even grayish red color as the rest of the oral mucous membrane. The hard palate is usually a pale pink and shades gradually into the deeper pink and red color of the soft palate and the uvula.

This highly vascularized mucous membrane, like the skin, is constantly shedding its outermost layers. Metabolic changes, particularly those affecting capillaries and the formation of new cells, may easily alter this process and thereby alter its appearance. Like the skin, the mucous membrane has many highly differentiated appendages (papillae of the tongue, interdental papillae, and teeth) that react in predictable fashions under abnormal conditions. The oral cavity is dark, moistened by saliva, and traumatized by the acts of chewing and smoking. Food, which collects in crevices and is attacked by bacterial saprophytes, ferments and forms the nidus for growth of pathogenic organisms. Such points of irritation have decreased tissue resistance and are frequently the first areas visibly affected by metabolic disturbances.

MEDICAL HISTORY AND PHYSICAL EXAMINATION

The physician may be approached by his patient primarily because of sore burning tongue and mouth "as though scalded by hot coffee," or this complaint may be uncovered only after careful history-taking in a patient who has some apparently unrelated difficulty, such as shortness of breath, weakness, or anxiety.

A careful investigation of the complaint of sore tongue and mouth is essential if the history is to be helpful. Such investigation should be directed toward establishing the onset, duration, and relationship of the sore tongue to seasons of the year, to types, quantity, and quality of food, to smoking, alcohol ingestion, therapy with drugs, and to emotional disturbances. The relationship to other symptoms, especially those of the gastrointestinal tract, is of great importance. Frequently an extremely accurate impression of the pathologic process responsible for the complaints can be gained by such a search. Even in the absence of a specific complaint referable to the oral cavity, this area deserves close scrutiny, because some patients with well-defined pathology either have no referable complaints or are so inured to them that they are ignored. Conversely, symptoms of sore tongue and mouth may be present and clinically significant even though no gross morphologic change is visible.

In most instances, a careful gross examination of the oral cavity gives the internist as much useful information as he could gain from biomicroscopic examination and the use of other technical refinements. Occasionally, a small hand lens is helpful in studying detail of very early lesions.

In considering the pathologic physiology or mechanisms that may lead to sore tongue or sore mouth, a division into (1) systemic and (2) local conditions may be made. The systemic disorders include those of nutritional origin and a large and varied miscellaneous group.

SYSTEMIC DISEASES THAT MAY CAUSE SORE TONGUE AND SORE MOUTH

NUTRITIONAL DEFICIENCY DISEASES— VITAMIN B COMPLEX, VITAMIN C, AND RELATED DEFICIENCY STATES

Etiology

Nutritional deficiency diseases usually occur for one of the following reasons: (1) deficient intake of essential nutrients because of poverty, ignorance, anorexia, food fads, or prescribed or self-imposed diets; or because alcohol or vitamin-free carbohydrate is substituted for foods rich in essential nutrients; (2) deficient absorption of essential nutrients because of gastroenteric tract diseases, such as regional ileitis and the malabsorption syndromes; (3) failure of utilization of essential nutrients as may happen when the liver is damaged; (4) requirements increased beyond the normal dietary intake as may occur in pregnancy, lactation, chronic febrile states, and hyperthyroidism; (5) increased elimination of essential nutrients in urine, feces, or vomitus as may occur in chronic diarrheal states; (6) decreased production of certain essential nutrients by colon organisms following prolonged oral administration of broad-spectrum antibiotic drugs; (7) blockade of chemical reactions by which essential nutrients are converted into biologically active compounds, competition of metabolically inactive analogues with their biologically active relatives for a locus on a protein apoenzyme, or destruction of the completed coenzyme. An example of blockade is the inhibiting effect of methotrexate (4-amino-N_{10}-methyl pteroylglutamic acid) on folic acid reductase, preventing the conversion of folic acid to its active form, tetrahydrofolic acid. An example of competition can be found in the inhibitory effect that 4–desoxypyridoxine (a vitamin B_6 antagonist) has on enzymatic reactions, such as transamination, in which pyridoxal phosphate serves as a prosthetic group.

Finally, irradiation may destroy coenzymes or apoenzyme-coenzyme complexes, or drugs like isonic-

otinic acid hydrazide may conjugate with pyridoxal to form an inactive isonicotinic acid hydrazone. If the history indicates that one of these situations may apply, a close search should be made for symptoms and signs of nutritional deficiency disease.

Incidence of Nutritional Deficiency Diseases

Nutritional deficiency diseases tend to occur in the spring and to a lesser degree in the autumn. This seasonal variation holds true whether the deficiency is due to inadequate diet or is secondary to one of the other etiologic factors listed in the preceding paragraph.[12]

Nutritional deficiency diseases are most common in women during the child-bearing period, in children and adolescents during the periods of rapid growth and development, and in men after their most productive years have passed. Bachelors and widowers who cook for themselves or eat in restaurants are prone to develop these diseases. Since wheat flour enriched with niacin, thiamin, riboflavin, and iron generally has been available throughout the United States, and with the improvement of the general standard of living of most American families, the incidence of full-blown nutritional deficiency disease has been reduced to nearly zero.

The diet may be inadequate in very low income families, food faddists, chronic alcohol and narcotic addicts, or in persons under the stresses of adolescence, pregnancy, lactation, chronic infections, hypermetabolic diseases, malabsorption, and old age. Between 5% and 10% of the robust people in the United States eat diets that are marginal in essential nutrients. Enough food is available, except in developing countries of the world, so that no one in the United States need eat a deficient diet. Only through continued elevation in the standard of living, improved food distribution, and repeated efforts at nutritional education for all people will nutritional deficiency disease be eliminated. Until this millenium is reached, the physician must be on the alert constantly for the symptoms and signs suggestive of the disordered metabolism resulting from insufficient essential nutrients.

Pathologic Physiology and Chemistry

A patient's sore tongue and mouth may be the only grossly visible signs that he has nutritional deficiency disease. Yet he is sick in every cell of his body and, indeed, has been biochemically sick for a variable period of time (prodromal period of the deficiency state) prior to the appearance of the first gross or microscopic lesion. The vascularity, constant moisture, bacterial flora, foci of infection, and recurring slight traumatization, which are characteristics of the oral cavity, account for the frequency with which the earliest morphologic changes occur here. The deficiency diseases do not induce changes in resting tissues as quickly as in tissues undergoing constant regeneration and repair.

The abnormalities that occur in the mouth and tongue as a result of two different deficiency states may be identical. Conditions unrelated to deficiency disease also may produce the same changes in these organs. Although these observations have always puzzled students of nutrition, it is probable that the explanation lies in the rather restricted spectrum of changes possible in the tongue and mouth. One possible change is vasodilation, causing hyperemia and redness. Atrophy or hypertrophy of the epithelium, capillary rupture with submucous hemorrage and infarction, ulceration, and necrosis are still others. When one considers these limits on the possibilities of reaction and the close chemical relationships of the nutritional deficiency diseases, it is not surprising that they frequently cause very similar changes in the tongue and mouth. These oral lesions are the readily visible manifestations of gross or microscopic cellular damage, tissue inflammation, and hyperemia occurring in the esophagus, stomach, and intestine,[13] of lesions of the skin that may at this time be visible only under the microscope,[14] and of chemical changes in muscle, liver, and other viscera[15] that may be detected with the aid of highly specialized biochemical and bacteriologic techniques.[16,17]

These chemical abnormalities of which we have some slight knowledge are the primary causes of the visible structural changes. Information gained from investigations in the respiration of yeast cells, bacteria, and various animal tissues indicates that many of the vitamins, particularly the vitamins of the B complex and probably vitamin C, are integral parts of complex respiratory enzymes or catalysts.[18-21] These vitamins, after undergoing certain changes in the body, enter into and implement oxidation–reduction reactions, which allow cells to breathe, perform work, and liberate energy. In the process, the catalyst is inactivated and then is regenerated, although the body is constantly incurring some loss of the catalyst or its progenitors through excretion. When these substances are absent, the cells lose their ability to use oxygen and they die. When there is a deficiency of these substances, the body uses whatever stores of these essential substances may be available for such emergencies. Alternate and possibly less efficient reactions, which do not require the deficient substance also may be called into play. Only after these protective mechanisms break down does the essential respiration of the cell suffer and illness occur. Thus, the process of depletion is usually a long one,

and all possible homeostatic mechanisms are used to protect vital cell functions.

Many of the B complex vitamins are essential for certain biochemical chain reactions, with each vitamin being responsible for the normal completion of one or more stages. The vitamins influence these processes after being chemically incorporated into coenzymes.

These coenzymes are organic compounds that, in the presence of specific protein enzymes, catalyze oxidation, reduction, transamination, decarboxylation, phosphorylation, and many other critical cellular reactions. Without either the coenzyme or the protein apoenzyme, the reaction stops. For instance, niacin, thiamine, riboflavin, and adenosine 5'-phosphate are essential for normal carbohydrate metabolism of yeast cells and probably of animal tissues also.

Figure 7-1 represents a simplification of the many reactions that may be involved in carbohydrate metabolism. It is included in this schematic form to facilitate visualization of the interrelated functions of many of the B complex vitamins.

Niacin is an essential part of nicotinamide adenine dinucleotide (NAD), formerly called diphosphopyridine nucleotide (DPN). It is also an essential component of nicotinamide adenine dinucleotide phosphate (NADP), formerly called triphosphopyridine nucleotide (TPN). Thiamine is a component of cocarboxylase (thiamine pyrophosphate, TPP) and transketolase. Riboflavin, also a precursor of several coenzymes, combines tightly with specific protein enzymes to form flavoproteins. It can fulfill its coenzyme role only when it is phosphorylated (riboflavin-5-phosphate) or when it is in the form of a nucleotide (flavin adenine dinucleotide). Adenosine 5'-phosphate may act as a means of carrying phosphate through reversible phosphorylation to adenosine diphosphate and adenosine triphosphate.

Nicotinamide adenine dinucleotide (NAD), in conjunction with its specific protein enzyme, catalyzes the conversion of a "triose phosphate" to phosphoglyceric acid (Fig. 7-1, step 1). In this oxidation reaction, it accepts a hydride ion (proton plus 2 electrons)—it acts as a dehydrogenase—and temporarily is reduced (to NADH), having oxidized the substrate, "triose phosphate." However, it may be regenerated by donating its excess hydride ion to flavin adenine dinucleotide,

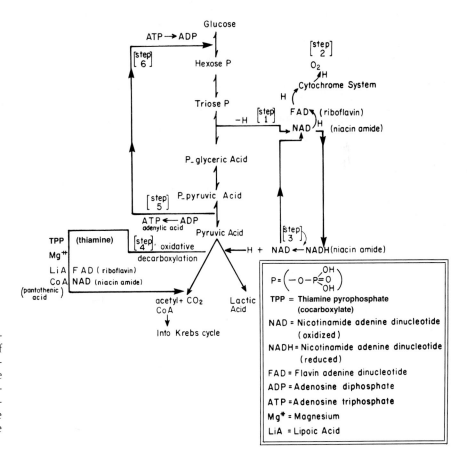

Fig. 7-1. A schematic representation of the Embden–Myerhof pathway of carbohydrate oxidation illustrating the probable mechanism through which B-complex vitamins control and implement these reactions and the chemical interrelationships of these vitamins.

and in this manner it regains its original oxidized form (NAD). The flavin adenine dinucleotide is reduced when it receives this hydride ion, but is reoxidized when it transfers the hydride ion through the cytochrome system to oxygen (step 2). On the other hand, NADH may donate its hydride ion to pyruvic acid, thus implementing the reduction of pyruvic acid to lactic acid (step 3). In either case, NAD is made available again for the primary dehydrogenating reaction. Energy released in this NAD⇋NADH reaction is utilized for the phosphorylation of adenosine diphosphate to form the triphosphate (ATP).

Cocarboxylase, in conjunction with its specific protein enzyme, catalyzes the decarboxylation and oxidation of pyruvic acid through intermediate metabolites to carbon dioxide and water. It is regenerated when lipoic acid accepts the carbon remnant of pyruvic acid (acetate) from it. The acetate finally is shifted to coenzyme A and thence into the Krebs tricarboxylic acid cycle, while lipoic acid is regenerated through the action of nicotinamide adenine dinucleotide and flavin adenine dinucleotide (step 4). Adenosine 5'-phosphate, after having been converted into adenosine diphosphate, acts as a phosphate carrier by accepting phosphate ion from phosphopyruvic acid. It becomes adenosine triphosphate (ATP), and in turn transfers its energy-rich phosphate to glucose (step 6). Through this reaction, hexose phosphate and adenosine diphosphate are formed.

The B complex vitamins are involved also in the direct oxidative pathway, which is frequently called the hexose monophosphate shunt (see Fig. 7-2). Glucose-6-phosphate is oxidized to 6-phosphogluconic acid by the enzyme glucose-6-phosphate dehydrogenase, for which NADP (nicotinamide adenine dinucleotide phosphate) is the coenzyme. Further NADP-dependent oxidation occurs when phosphogluconic acid is

converted to 3-keto-gluconic acid 6-phosphate. Carbon dioxide is lost from the first position, and ribulose-5-phosphate is formed. After some internal rearrangements, a 2-carbon ketone from xylulose-5-phosphate is transferred to ribose-5-phosphate to form sedoheptulose-7-phosphate. This transketolase reaction is catalyzed by thiamin diphosphate. Further rearrangements occur, leaving ultimately glyceraldehyde phosphate and fructose-6-phosphate.

It is probable that these and other vitamins of the B complex are essential for similar reactions in protein, fat, steroid, and nucleic acid metabolism. Pyridoxal phosphate, the coenzyme form of vitamin B_6 acts as a decarboxylase,[19] transaminase,[20] desulfurase,[21] and racemase[21] for certain amino acids. It is also essential for the conversion of tryptophane to nicotinamide derivatives (NAD),[22] and possibly for the interconversion of the essential fatty acids,[23] linoleic, and arachidonic acids. Pantothenic acid takes part in an enzyme system concerned with acetylation,[24] and folic acid and vitamin B_{12} are intimately connected with the formation of nucleotides and nucleic acid,[25,26] as well as phospholipid formation and the degradation of histidine through single carbon unit transfer.[27]

The relationship of the B complex vitamins to respiration and energy production has been stressed in the foregoing paragraphs. Emphasis also should be directed toward the role of these micronutrients in a much broader area of biochemistry. In many instances, the intermediates of these pathways as well as the level of reduction of the coenzymes exert a controlling influence on metabolic processes other than energy production. For instance, the level of NADH may be an important regulator for urate reabsorption by the renal tubule, for fat oxidation and mobilization, for the direction of carbohydrate metabolism. The hexose monophosphate shunt pathway links with the glucuronic acid pathway through which uridine diphosphoglucuronic acid is formed, an important mechanism for mucopolysaccharide formation. Many drugs and bilirubin are excreted as glucuronides,[28] and abnormal operation of the latter pathway may be important in producing the ground substance and basement membrane abnormalities found in patients with diabetes mellitus.[29]

A strong reducing agent, vitamin C, is probably essential to many oxidation-reduction systems and phosphatase activity, although its exact chemical function has not yet been defined. It is essential to the conversion of proline to hydroxyproline[30] in protocollagen, and to the normal metabolism of tyrosine and phenylalanine.[31] When vitamin C is deficient in animals, premature infants, or adult humans, intermediate phenolic products of the metabolism of these two amino

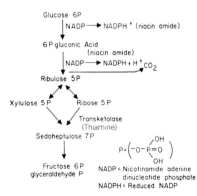

Fig. 7-2. Direct oxidative pathway for glucose or the hexose monophosphate shunt. The roles played by niacin and thiamine are indicated in this diagram.

acids appear in the urine in large amounts. A similar abnormality occurs when there is insufficient folic acid,[32] and it seems likely that a close biochemical relationship exists between ascorbic acid and folic acid. Ascorbic acid or other reducing agents are essential for the protection of the folic acid coenzymes (tetrahydrofolic acid and related compounds) from oxidative influences by protecting folic acid reductases. This is another example of vitamin interdependency.

The biochemical abnormalities attendant upon vitamin C depletion probably lead to the basic pathologic changes in the scorbutic state, the failure of normal formation of collagen and intercellular cement substance. These fundamental abnormalities result in increased fragility of capillaries and decreased strength of fibrous tissue and other tissues of mesenchymal origin—the basic abnormalities of clinical scurvy.[33]

A discussion of all of the possible chemical aspects of nutrition and nutritional deficiency diseases is beyond the scope of this chapter. Actually, biochemists have only scratched the surface of this very important subject. The chemical reactions cited, although they may be incomplete and possibly inaccurate in the light of future developments, illustrate most clearly the chemical relationships of the vitamins and in turn of the vitamin-deficiency diseases. These reactions show why nutrition must be adequate in all essential nutrients before health can be optimum.

Multiple Deficiency States

Deficiency diseases seldom occur as single clinical entities, although for didactic clarity they will be described as though they do. Under natural circumstances they almost always occur as multiple deficiency states. Deficient diets seldom if ever are lacking in only one essential nutrient. For instance, food deficient in one of the vitamins of the B complex is apt to be deficient in all of these vitamins and probably in minerals and protein also. In addition, many of the vitamins and minerals are essential for closely related biochemical reactions in the cells (Fig. 7-1), for the release of energy through the Krebs cycle and for the formation of the active coenzyme forms of other vitamins.

Niacin Deficiency (Pellagrous Stomatitis and Glossitis)

As the niacin concentration in the tissues decreases, the deficient person may become aware of burning sensations in the tongue following the intake of hot or spicy foods. The continuous burning resembles the sensation commonly experienced following the ingestion of extremely hot coffee. This complaint may come and go; it is usually most intense during spring and fall seasons and is associated with mild anorexia, fatigue, nervousness, irritability, alternating periods of constipation and diarrhea, and burning sensations in the epigastrium. As the deficiency becomes severe or a complicating disease develops that increases the body requirement for niacin, the mouth and tongue may become so sore that it is impossible for the patient to ingest or swallow anything but liquid food. Concomitantly, other symptoms and signs may develop such as severe watery diarrhea, burning erythematous skin eruptions, cheilosis, angular stomatitis, seborrhea or dyssebacea in the nasolabial folds, mental confusion, delirium, and occasionally spastic paraplegia.

While the deficiency is mild, there may be no gross abnormalities visible in the tongue and mouth, even though these structures may be hyperesthetic. If the deficiency continues or increases in severity, the fungiform papillae become increasingly vascular and prominent, imparting a distinctive redness to the tip and sides of the tongue, where these papillae are most numerous. At this stage, these papillae stand out as swollen red globules on a background of apparently normal filiform papillae. However, the filiform papillae may be affected later. Those at the tip and the lateral margins are affected first, and from these areas the process usually spreads backward toward the circumvallate papillae. The filiform papillae become swollen, denuded of epithelial tufts, hyperemic, and fused in certain areas, giving the tongue an edematous, slick, fissured, fiery scarlet-red appearance. All coating is absent, and the teeth leave indentations along the margins of the swollen organ. Minute ulcerations may appear that enlarge and become infected with staphylococci, hemolytic streptococci, Vincent's organisms, or fungi. These ulcers are frequently covered with a white or gray membrane. Occasionally only one portion of the tongue—usually an area located at the tip or the side—is involved. This involved area may move from place to place on the tongue, leaving atrophic spots behind. This type of localized painful excoriation of the tongue has been called "Moeller's glossitis" in older literature.

The same fiery redness observed on the dorsal surface of the tongue occurs on the ventral surface and in the smooth mucous membrane of the cheeks, gums, and soft palate. The mucous membranes of the stomach, rectum, vagina, and anterior urethra are affected similarly. The nasal mucous membrane frequently remains pallid in contrast to its boggy blue red appearance in virus diseases such as influenza. Often superficial ulcerations occur, particularly where the sharp edges of broken teeth irritate contiguous buccal mucous membrane. At this stage, the mouth and tongue are extremely painful, and saliva may drool from the mouth and over the pillow and the bedclothes. All

types of food are shunned by the patient because of pain.

Remissions and exacerbations in this clinical picture may be anticipated even though the patient receives no crystalline vitamin or diet therapy. Morphologic changes that tend to be permanent occur as the deficiency state continues over months or years. In point of time this may be called a chronic deficiency state. The hyperemic, swollen vascular papillae, both fungiform and filiform, become flattened and atrophic, and gradually disappear, leaving a ridged or furrowed "bald" tongue. During periods of remission this bald tongue may be quite pallid, but during periods of exacerbation may again become fiery red. Frequently, even at this stage, the hyperemic rudiments of the papillae can be seen with the naked eye as small pinpoint red dots, especially along the tip and sides of the tongue. The mucous membranes of the buccal cavity are affected by the same atrophic process, the interdental papillae of the gums recede, and secondary pyorrhea and other infections of the gums are common. Patients with chronic vitamin B complex deficiency diseases frequently lose their teeth at an early age because of these gum changes.[34]

The syndrome just described has been shown to be the result of lack of niacin and tryptophane. Such a deficiency state has been induced in human beings by corn diets deficient in these substances but fortified with other essential nutrients.[35] Glossitis occurred when the deficiency state was acute, whereas dermatitis was more likely when the deficiency state was induced more slowly. Whitish plaques and ulcerations developed under the tongue, and cheilosis and angular stomatitis were observed as were diarrhea, irritability, restlessness, and weakness. This clinical picture developed when the niacin and tryptophane daily intakes were 4 mg and 180 mg, respectively. Slightly more niacin and tryptophane provided by a "wheat diet" appeared to be protective.

With adequate therapy, acute pellagrous glossititis clears rapidly, frequently within 24 to 48 hours. In those patients with more chronic disease and glossal atrophy, regeneration of papillae may occur in time, usually after weeks of therapy. Much of the apparent regeneration observed early in the course of therapy is due to the disappearance of edema. The longer the period of deficiency, the slower and more incomplete the process of regeneration. Papillae may never regenerate on chronically scarred tongues, even after the most adequate therapy.

Riboflavin Deficiency (Ariboflavinosis)

Riboflavin deficiency once was the most common deficiency disease in the southern part of the United States.[36] Symptoms related to the tongue and mouth are usually mild. It is difficult to be sure that the usual burning sensations in the tongue experienced by the patient with riboflavin deficiency are caused by a lack of riboflavin or an associated deficiency of niacin. Tenderness and soreness at the corners of the mouth and along the lips usually are caused by cracking of the surface epithelium and secondary infection. In some patients, moderate or severe morphologic changes in the tongue and mouth due to riboflavin deficiency may produce no symptoms at all. The eyes, however, may burn, itch, or feel as if sand has found its way into them, and the patient is usually weak, irritable, and lacking in appetite.

As a rule, the first oral lesion is a painless grayish papule.[9] This lesion occurs at one or both angles of the mouth. The papule enlarges and gradually breaks down, resulting in a fissure, secondary infection, ulceration, and yellowish heaped-up crusts—angular stomatitis or perlèche (to lick).[37] The lips become red and fissured (cheilosis). Remissions are common, as in all deficiency diseases, but unless the diet is improved, relapse is almost certain. The process is extremely indolent, and remission or relapses may persist for months. After several relapses, the angles of the mouth may be scarred permanently.

The buccal mucosa of the cheeks is usually affected along with the angles of the mouth.[38] At first, the fine reticulated vascular pattern previously described as normal for this area is obliterated by engorgement, and the mucous membrane has a flat, dull red color. With progression, the mucous membrane becomes edematous, grayish, and pebbly. It tends to exfoliate in sheets, causing a distinctive mottled or moth-eaten appearance; some areas are gray pink and others, dull red. Because of the swelling, the occlusal line becomes prominent, and individual tooth imprints may be visible. The lips are involved in the same process. That part of the lips within the line of closure has the same pebbly, moth-eaten, dusk red appearance as the rest of the buccal mucous membranes. The vermilion borders of the lips exfoliate, dry, fissure, and crack (cheilosis). The line of closure is usually well demarcated and exhibits a striking dusky red color. The end-stage of this stomatitis is an atrophic moth-eaten mucous membrane.

The tongue is affected less frequently in riboflavin deficiency. The fungiform papillae enlarge and become hyperemic, followed by a similar process affecting the filiform papillae. However, they do not lose their shape or surface epithelium as in niacin deficiency. In contrast, the epithelium thickens and becomes edematous, which produces the rows of bulbous hyperemic papillae of the so-called "cobblestone tongue." (This term has been applied to syphilitic glossitis with leukoplakia in the older literature.) Since thickened

edematous mucous membrane covers the hyperemic vascular tuft of each papilla, the tongue is a diffuse dusky red or magenta color. This magenta tongue contrasts sharply with the brilliant scarlet red tongue of niacin deficiency.[7] The magenta color of the tongue may be deepened by the sluggish circulation in the dilated vessels of the papillae, essentially stagnation cyanosis.

Concomitantly, other grossly visible tissue changes due to riboflavin deficiency may occur. Conjunctival injection and diffuse superficial keratitis are common findings.[39] Erosions similar to cheilosis may occur at the ocular canthi, in the nasolabial folds, or at the mucocutaneous junction of the anus and of the vagina. Hypertrophy of the sebaceous glands over the bridge of the nose associated with plugging of the ducts of the glands may lead to a rough "sharkskin" effect. This process frequently affects the skin in the nasolabial fold as well as on the nose, and has been called dyssebacea. Seborrhealike dermatitis may occur in the nasolabial fold as well. Pure riboflavin deficiency induced in human beings by a diet containing 0.55 mg of riboflavin daily caused angular stomatitis and cheilosis, and seborrhealike lesions of the scrotum and the external genitalia, but the magenta tongue and the lesions of the oral mucosa and eyes were not reported.[40]

After repeated episodes of acute riboflavin deficiency, scars may be found at the angles of the mouth and less commonly in the corneae. The mucous membrane of the mouth is thin and mottled. The tongue and lips are fissured and dry. It is possible that some of the senile changes in conjunctivae, corneae, lenses, and skin, such as fatty and hyaline deposits, pinguecu lae, arcus senilis, cataracts, atrophy of the skin, senile hyperkeratoses, and so on, are in part the result of chronic riboflavin and other long-standing vitamin-deficiency states.

Other B Complex Deficiency States

No specific oral lesions in human beings can be related to a deficiency of thiamine or pantothenic acid. Rosenblum and Joliffe describe a lesion characterized by irregular desquamation of the mucous membranes of the tongue and buccal cavity leading to small whitish patches on a dull reddish purple background suggestive of riboflavin deficiency.[41] The lesion, however, responded to pyridoxine after niacin and riboflavin had failed to induce healing. Smith and Martin reported cheilosis typical of riboflavin deficiency that responded to pyridoxine after riboflavin had failed.[42] Angular stomatitis and glossitis of pregnancy have been reported to respond to both riboflavin and pyridoxine. In a crossover study, all 24 patients treated with pyridoxine responded, whereas 21 of 32 patients treated with riboflavin responded. Those that failed to respond to ribo-flavin responded to pyridoxine.[43] Vilter and his associates have described oral lesions in 50 patients with vitamin B_6 deficiency induced by desoxypyridoxine, a vitamin B_6 antagonist.[44]*

The B complex deficiency state could be induced most readily when the patient was on a diet poor in the vitamin B complex, but, with larger doses of the antagonist, it occurred in patients on a normal hospital diet. Erythema and atrophy of the tongue occurred in 14 patients, cheilosis and angular stomatitis in 3. The oral mucosa was involved also, in either a diffuse or spotty erythematous process. A much more common lesion was seborrheic dermatitis, beginning in the nasolabial folds and spreading over the cheeks, chin, eyebrows, and forehead, and down the neck and over the shoulders. Peripheral neuritis occurred also. Patients with this deficiency state excreted abnormally large amounts of xanthurenic acid in the urine after a test dose of tryptophane, suggesting that the conversion of tryptophane to nicotinamide coenzymes was impaired.[45] All these lesions failed to respond to niacin, thiamine, and riboflavin, but improved within 48 hours after the administration of any of the vitamin B_6 group (pyridoxine, pyridoxal, or pyridoxamine).

Patients studied by Sydenstricker, Singal, and Briggs developed manifestations of biotin deficiency on a diet poor in B complex vitamins but supplemented with the available crystalline members of this group, except biotin.[46] The absorption of biotin from the gastroenteric tract was limited sharply by including desiccated egg white, containing the protein avidin (which combines with biotin and prevents its absorption),in an amount equivalent to 30% of the total calories. The changes in the tongue varied from the geographic type to general atrophy of the lingual papillae or marginal atrophy. Cure resulted in 3 to 5 days after the administration of from 150 µg to 300 µg of biotin per day.

Acute folinic acid deficiency induced by amethopterin (methotrexate), an antagonist of the reaction that converts folic acid to folinic acid, may cause very severe soreness and ulceration of the mouth and tongue.[47] These lesions usually begin as erythematous patches on the buccal mucosa or gums; the superficial epithelium sloughs and ulcers appear. These spread and may involve the entire oral cavity. Since the drug mentioned above is among those used by persons with acute leukemia, the lesions frequently become purpuric, and infected with all varieties of organisms. If antibiotics and cortisone have been administered also,

---

*A vitamin antagonist is usually a chemical analogue of the essential nutrient, so similar in structure that the cell cannot differentiate between the two. The antagonist, or "antimetabolite," as it is sometimes called, is biologically inactive and induces deficiency of the active metabolite by replacing the active substance in biologic reactions, bringing the reaction to an end.[45]

fungal infections are frequent. The lesions cannot be differentiated with assurance on morphologic grounds from the purpuric secondarily infected ulcerating lesions of the acute leukemic process. However, lesions due to acute leukemia come and go regardless of the drug being administered and improve as clinical remission is induced, whereas the lesions due to methotrexate toxicity usually respond rapidly when folinic acid is given.[48]

These observations illustrate the morphologic counterparts of the biochemical interrelationships of the B complex vitamins that have already been stressed. The fact that deficiency of different vitamins should induce similar morphologic changes in the tongue and mouth is not surprising when one recalls these chemical interrelationships, and the probability that the tongue and mouth can respond only in a few ways to damage. These observations also illustrate the lack of specificity of a morphologic oral lesion for a deficiency of one member of the vitamin B complex. The lack of specificity of these lesions will be discussed in subsequent sections.

Atrophic Glossitis

Atrophic glossitis cannot be considered a disease entity. The acute glossal lesions of many systemic diseases (including those already described) may lead to atrophy of the glossal mucous membrane if adequate treatment is not given (see Fig. 7-3). We can only describe the lesion, catalogue the disorders that may be responsible, and speculate on their clinical similarities and probably metabolic interrelationships.[49-55]

The following are conditions with which atrophic glossitis is frequently associated;

1. *Vitamin B_{12} deficiencies*
   a. Addisonian pernicious anemia, due to a genetically and immunologically conditioned lack of the mucoprotein substance called "intrinsic factor," without which physiologic amounts of vitamin B_{12} cannot be absorbed from the intestinal tract [56-58]
   b. Postgastrectomy pernicious anemia, due to surgical removal of the stomach and elimination of intrinsic factor [58,59]
   c. Fish tapeworm infestation, which interferes with the activity of the intrinsic factor[60] by binding vitamin B_{12}
   d. Intestinal blind loop syndromes and other mechanical gastrointestinal abnormalities, which allow proliferation of microorganisms that bind vitamin B_{12}[61]
   e. The vegan syndrome, or pure vegetarianism, resulting in dietary deficiency of vitamin B_{12},[62] which is found primarily in foods from animal sources.
2. *Folic acid deficiencies*
   a. Megaloblastic anemia [63,64] of pregnancy, due to metabolic demands of the fetus for folic acid, maternal dietary inadequacy, and vomiting [65]
   b. Vitamin B_{12}-refractory megaloblastic anemia, due, it is thought, to failure of the metabolic processes responsible for the conversion of food folic acid to the coenzyme forms[66]
   c. Megaloblastic anemia of the alcoholic addict with cirrhosis, due to dietary lack of folic acid and to

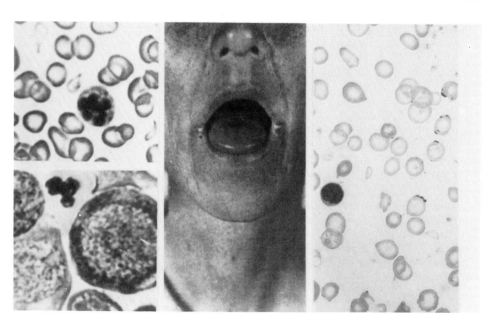

Fig. 7-3. (*Center*) Chronic atrophic glossitis and angular stomatitis in a patient with mixed vitamin B-complex deficiency disease. Similar lesions of tongue and mouth occur in patients with macrocytic megaloblastic anemia. (*Left, top*) Macrocytic erythrocytes and a hypersegmented neutrophil. (*Left, bottom*) Bone marrow megaloblast. Patients with microcytic hypochromic anemia of chronic blood loss and iron deficiency also develop this lesion of tongue and mouth. (*Right*) Microcytic hypochromic erythrocytes.

possible increased need for folic acid as a result of liver failure[67,68]

3. *Combined deficiencies of folic acid, vitamin B_{12}, and ascorbic acid*

   a. Nutritional macrocytic anemia[53]

   b. Megaloblastic anemia of malabsorption syndromes, particularly sprue, [69-71] a disease of obscure etiology, which results in deficiencies of all the hematopoietic vitamins, but especially folic acid. Diseases of the small bowel, such as gluten enteropathy, regional ileitis, intestinal lipodystrophy, lymphoma, and tuberculosis are other examples.[72]

   c. Megaloblastic anemia of infancy,[73] a combined dietary deficiency of folic acid and ascorbic acid due to an unsupplemented milk diet. (Ascorbic acid deficiency in the adult may result in megaloblastic anemia when the dietary supply of folic acid is marginal or when alcohol increases the requirements.)

4. *Iron deficiency (microcytic hypochromic) anemia* [74] due to chronic blood loss

5. *Idiopathic atrophic gastritis with achlorhydria*

6. *Chronic vitamin B complex deficiency disease*

7. *Glossal atrophy of unknown cause*

Symptomatically, the tongue and mouth feel dry, and there are exacerbations and remissions of burning and tingling sensations and paresthesias of taste. Atrophy is the most prominent morphologic feature. In a quiescent phase the tongue is small, slick, and glistening. All vestiges of papillae except the circumvallate are absent, and the mucous membrane is thin. It is usually ridged and furrowed where the atrophic process has involved muscle underlying mucous membrane. If the patient is very anemic, the color of the atrophic tongue is usually faint pink. If he is moderately anemic, the color is dull red.

With exacerbations of the pathologic process that may occur at any time before adequate therapy is administered, the mouth is extremely sore so that only liquid foods can be tolerated. Diffuse swelling may occur, and the color may become the raw, bluish red, shiny hue of rare beefsteak. Anemia must be severe (usually red blood cell count under 1.5 million or hemoglobin under 4 g) for the tongue to remain pallid.

If the tongue is examined closely during these periods of pathologic activity, multiple small pinpoint red dots corresponding with the hyperemic capillaries of the atrophied papillae are usually visible. Small superficial ulcerations, erosions, and hemorrhages may occur in the mucous membrane. The ulcerations may become secondarily infected with any of a number of pathogenic or saprophytic bacteria or molds. In periods of remission and exacerbation, the buccal mucous membranes have essentially the same appearance as the tongue. Erosions at the angles of the mouth similar to those seen in riboflavin deficiency occur frequently, especially in association with chronic iron deficiency.

Periods of exacerbation usually correspond with or immediately precede periods of activity in the causative disease, for example, a relapse in the anemia of pernicious anemia, although occasionally they occur while the anemia is under control or many years before anemia or other signs of the fundamental disease appear. Acute or atrophic glossitis also may appear as a manifestation of sprue before the appearance of steatorrhea.[75]

Each of these diseases with which atrophic glossitis is associated is usually characterized also by gastrointestinal disturbances, hypochlorhydria, achlorhydria or achylia gastrica, anemia that is macrocytic and megaloblastic (except in iron deficiency states), and multiple vitamin deficiencies. Among the macrocytic anemias with glossitis, separation can be made on the basis of historical or laboratory data including blood levels of vitamin B_{12} and folic acid or by demonstrating that a specific therapeutic agent will induce a remission of the glossal atrophy and anemia.

The use of vitamin B_{12} labeled with radioactive cobalt has improved the accuracy with which some of the conditions resulting in glossal atrophy and megaloblastic anemia can be differentiated. When labeled vitamin B_{12} is given orally to a patient with pernicious anemia, only a minute amount is absorbed. However, when the same dose is given with intrinsic factor, vitamin B_{12} is absorbed as effectively as in normal persons. Patients with sprue absorb vitamin B_{12} poorly whether or not intrinsic factor is given. Patients with dietary deficiencies of vitamin B_{12} or folic acid absorb vitamin B_{12} normally without added intrinsic factor. The physiologic defect of patients with intestinal lesions such as blind loops or pouches may be clarified by showing that tetracycline frequently improves vitamin B_{12} absorption under these conditions.[76,77]

Iron relieves the anemia, glossitis, and cheilosis of iron deficiency; niacin and riboflavin relieves the glossitis and cheilosis of pellagra. Idiopathic atrophic gastritis and glossitis sometimes are benefited by folic acid, vitamin B_{12}, or B complex vitamins. Only too often no effective therapeutic agent can be found.

There is no explanation that is entirely satisfactory for the morphologic similarity of the acute and chronic glossal changes that occur in these apparently different deficiency states.

Studies of the growth requirements of certain microorganisms and laboratory animals indicate that defi-

ciencies of the folic acid coenzymes and vitamin B_{12} interfere with the transfer of single carbon units, the former in a direct manner, the latter indirectly.[26,78,79] Vitamin B_{12} seems to be necessary for certain reduction reactions, also. Through these functions, both vitamins are involved in the formation of purine and pyrimidine nucleotides, particularly thymine deoxyribotide, as indicated in the following reactions:

$$uracil\ ribotide \xrightarrow[\substack{vitamin \\ B_{12} \\ coenzyme}]{reductase} uracil\ deoxyribotide \xrightarrow[\substack{folic\ acid \\ coenzyme \\ and \\ vitamin\ B_{12} \\ coenzyme}]{synthetase} thymine\ deoxyribotide$$

This reaction is essential for the formation of deoxyribonucleic acid, a major component of the nuclei of cells. Deficiencies of vitamin B_{12} or folic acid inhibit the completion of this essential reaction, and delay cell division. Since thymine,[80] uracil,[81] and orotic acid [82] (a precursor of pyrimidines) given in large doses induce remissions in patients with pernicious anemia, it is probably that the same relationships hold in human metabolism. Rapidly proliferating tissues, such as the bone marrow and mucosa of the digestive tract including the tongue, are most severely affected by such deficiencies. The megaloblast is a red blood cell precursor whose nuclear maturation is delayed by a deficiency of thymine deoxyribotide, whereas cytoplasmic maturation is less adversely affected, though the formation of all nucleotides must be delayed to some degree.

Cytologic changes similar to those of the megaloblast have been observed in the cells of the tongue, oral mucous membrane, and stomach, indicating the widespread involvement of tissues in these deficiency states.[83] Since ribonucleic acid (cytoplasmic and nucleolar type) controls the formation of protein, and deoxyribonucleic acid (the nuclear type) governs the process of cell division and is the template for the formation of messenger RNA, one can readily see that fundamental aspects of cellular growth and multiplication are involved when folic acid or vitamin B_{12} is lacking.

The B complex vitamins, niacin, riboflavin, vitamin B_6, and biotin (see preceding sections) have many different functions, most of which are concerned with the release of energy; iron is essential for the oxygen transport capacity of hemoglobin and for the activity of the respiratory enzymes, catalase, and the cytochromes. A deficiency of any of these substances adversely affects the metabolism of all the cells of the body, but certain areas, because of local conditions and demands, show the deficiency effects most strikingly. The tongue and mouth are such areas and react to all these deficiency states in essentially the same way—with vasodilatation, inflammation, and edema, followed eventually by atrophy of the papillae and the surface mucosa. It is true that there are few other ways in which these tissues can react to injury, and this may be the real explanation for the similarity of appearance. On the other hand, all these essential nutrients are chemically dependent upon each other and control fundamental reactions involved in the release of energy and the regeneration of cells. This, too, may be a common denominator.

Vitamin C Deficiency (Scurvy)

The principal complaints referable to the oral cavity in clinical scurvy are soreness, swelling, and bleeding of the gums. In advanced cases, the distress may be so great that the patient is unable to chew food. Lesions usually occur late in the development of the clinical disease. Pyorrhea and other diseases of the gums seem to be predisposing factors favoring earlier occurrence. Gross lesions seldom, if ever, occur in edentulous scorbutic patients.

The first oral lesions of scurvy usually occur in the interdental papillae,[11] and spread to the gingival margins and finally to the alveolar mucous membrane. They do not ordinarily extend beyond the alveolar–labial junction. Capillary dilatation and congestion are the earliest visible changes. The interdental papillae and then the gum itself become a deep blue red color as blood extravasates into these tissues. Swelling occurs, and the interdental papillae and the gingival margins may become so edematous that collars of swollen blue red friable mucous membrane surround the teeth, and in advanced cases may almost cover them. Debris and microorganisms collect or are already present in pockets along the gingival margins. Infection and ulceration may spread from these areas to involve and destroy much of the gum. Infarction and gangrene of the interdental papillae may occur. Only in the most severely affected cases does one observe spontaneous oozing of blood or frank hemorrhages. Usually trauma is necessary to induce bleeding. When bleeding does occur, it is seldom excessive or exsanguinating. The breath is fetid, and salivation is increased.

As the process subsides, atrophy of the interdental

papillae and retraction of the gums from around the teeth occur. With repeated exacerbations and remissions of the scorbutic process, there may be extreme recession of the gums from around the teeth. The net result may be the same as that following longstanding pyorrhea. The teeth loosen, rotate, or fall out in advanced cases because of rarefaction and reabsorption of alveolar bone. The gum becomes pale and scarred. If an acute deficiency of vitamin C supervenes, the gum may again become so blue red and swollen that the atrophic phase is completely masked.

Other characteristic lesions of scurvy are (1) follicular hyperkeratoses and perifollicular hemorrhages, especially on the extremities [84,85]; (2) larger confluent ecchymoses, especially around the joints and the popliteal spaces or at sites of slight trauma; (3) painful, tender, sometimes swollen joints (hermathroses); and (4) subperiosteal hemorrhages in children that may occur before the gum changes are visible. In adults, normocytic or moderately macrocytic anemia usually occurs after a prolonged period of severe vitamin C deficiency.[86,87] The bone marrow cytology may be normoblastic or megaloblastic. When it is normoblastic, the vitamin C deficiency may have had a direct inhibiting effect on the development of the erythroid marrow. When it is megaloblastic, the cause is probably a defect in the folic acid reductase reaction, one that is necessary for the formation of the folic acid coenzymes and that depends on the availability of reducing substances such as ascorbic acid to maintain the reductase in its reduced (i.e., active) form. Thus, ascorbic acid deficiency can convert a marginal intake of folic acid into a completely inadequate intake.

Scorbutic infants and young children may develop more severe anemia, sometimes quite rapidly because of loss of blood into tissues, particularly from subperiosteal hemorrhages.

OTHER SYSTEMIC DISEASES THAT MAY CAUSE SORE TONGUE AND SORE MOUTH

Many systemic diseases or local irritative processes may produce lesions that at some stage are morphologically similar to those that occur in the vitamin deficiency states. These various conditions must be recognized and understood in order to avoid mistakes in determining the mechanism producing the sore tongue or sore mouth.

Cirrhosis—Alcoholic or Laennec's

Vitamin deficiency diseases are common in patients with cirrhosis, particularly in those with the nutritional (alcoholic addict) type. Anorexia or vomiting may bring about deficiency states in persons with postnecrotic cirrhosis, too. When dietary deficiency disease is respsonsible, dietary improvement or supplementation of the diet with B complex vitamins overcomes the lesion. However, very frequently one finds a blue red tongue, sometimes with papillary atrophy, sometimes with papillary hypertrophy, but always with dilated, engorged capillaries in the papillae or their remnants. This has been called "liver tongue" and can be equated with palmar erythema and spider hemangiomas. Usually the oral mucosa is spotted with erythematous lesions also. These lesions usually do not cause pain, and they do not respond to any of the B complex vitamins. As the liver disease improves, these glossal and stomal lesions improve also. The reverse is true when liver failure ensues.

Leukemia, Hypoplastic Anemia, Idiopathic and Drug-Induced Neutropenia, and Thrombocytopenia

Sore, swollen gums from which blood constantly oozes may be found in patients with any type of acute or subacute leukemia, severe hypoplastic anemia, neutropenia, or thrombocytopenia. Thrombocytopenia and capillary damage are responsible for bleeding into the tissues, and the breakdown of the barriers against infection is responsible for the redness, ulceration, and swelling. Secondary infection and ulceration may make the mouth extremely sore and foul-smelling. Particularly in neutropenic states in which no polymorphonuclear neutrophils can be found in the blood, the mouth, pharynx, and tonsils may be severely inflamed, swollen, ulcerated, and necrotic (agranulocytic angina). So much tissue may be destroyed by the necrotic ulcers or noma that a sinus tract may form, and the lesion may present itself externally on the cheek. In acute monoblastic leukemia,[88] and occasionally in other types of acute leukemia, infiltration of the tissues of the gums with leukemic cells may account for some of the swelling and necrosis. Careful hematologic studies, with particular emphasis on the differential white blood cell count, platelet count, and bone marrow examination, establishes the diagnosis in these cases.

The Erythemas and "Collagen" Diseases

Certain diseases caused by altered immunologic reactivity, such as erythema multiforme, erythema nodosa, disseminated lupus erythematosus, and periarteritis nodosa may produce painful oral lesions.

Erythema multiforme, when severe, may affect the mouth as well as the skin, eyes, genitalia, lungs, and joints[89] (Stevens–Johnson syndrome). The lesions may be of any type. In severe cases, bullae or purpuric vesicles may form. Secondary infection usually is superimposed, and the mouth, gums, and tongue rapidly become extremely sore and foul-smelling. The oral le-

sions seldom occur in the absence of the skin eruption. These oral and dermal bullae must be differentiated from pemphigus and pemphigoid.

Disseminated lupus erythematosus may produce areas of purpura on the buccal mucosa that progress to infarction, secondary infection, and necrotic sloughs, and shaggy, grayish ulcer.[90] The diagnosis depends upon finding one or more of the other protean manifestations of the disease: (1) disseminated erythematous skin lesions, (2) serous pleural, pericardial, and peritoneal effusions, (3) arthralgia and arthritis, (4) nephritis, (5) myocarditis, (6) leukopenia, (7) the lupus cell phenomenon, and (8) antinuclear antibody.

A diffuse orange red discoloration of the tongue associated with burning sensations in the organ has been noted in persons with fulminating periarteritis nodosa. None of the vitamins of the B complex improves this glossitis. The etiology of the glossitis is obscure.

Lichen Planus

This dermatologic condition is frequently associated with oral lesions, plaques scattered irregularly over the tongue of a whitish cast, and pearly lacelike or spiderweblike threads on the oral mucous membrane. Occasionally, these occur without typical skin lesions. The etiology is unknown, but one usually finds strong psychogenic factors in affected patients.

Psoriasis

White elevated painless plaques occur occasionally on the tongue and buccal mucosa in persons with psoriasis. These lesions can be confused very early with leukoplakia.

Systemic Infections, Scarlet Fever, Syphilis

In the early stages of scarlet fever, the tongue is coated and dry. After 2 or 3 days, however, epithelial exfoliation begins. At first, only the swollen, red fungiform papillae can be seen which, on the gray background of the coated filiform papillae, give the tongue a "raspberry" appearance. The exfoliation continues until all papillae—filiform and fungiform alike—appear to be swollen red knobs. This is the so-called strawberry tongue. The oral mucous membranes and the lips may partake in the same process, and appear redder than normal. This enanthem is seldom painful; at least any soreness is obscured by the highly inflamed sore throat and cervical lymphadenitis so characteristic of the disease.

Secondary syphilis also produces oral lesions, the mucous patches that are painless unless secondarily infected. These lesions may appear anywhere in the oral cavity. They are usually circumscribed, flat, superficial white or gray patches, which bleed easily when scraped. They are teeming with spirochetes. If they are widespread over the tongue and if secondary infection occurs, the tongue may become fiery red, painful, and flecked with white patches. Under these conditions, secondary syphilitic glossitis may be easily confused with acute pellagrous glossitis. At times differentiation depends upon a careful history and search for other signs of primary and secondary syphilis or deficiency disease.

Tertiary syphilis usually does not produce painful lesions of the mouth. Solitary or multiple gummata may destroy large areas of tongue, palate, and gingiva without causing soreness or burning sensations. An obliterative endarteritis in the tongue during the secondary stage of syphilis may lead in the tertiary stage to atrophy of epithelium and muscle (glass tongue or sclerosing glossitis). This condition may be confused with atrophic glossitis, but in syphilitic glossal atrophy, the extensive replacement fibrosis can be determined by palpation. It is frequently the precursor of keratoses and leukoplakia. The rhagades or scars about the angles of the mouth and lips in congenital syphilitics must be differentiated from scars in the same areas due to chronic riboflavin and iron deficiencies.

Exogenous Intoxications with Heavy Metals

Subacute or chronic poisoning with mercury or one of its salts may cause severe swelling, redness, erosion, and ulceration of the mouth, tongue, and gums. Mercuric sulfide, formed in the mouth from mercuric salts excreted by the salivary glands, acts as the tissue irritant. Salivation is excessive and the salivary glands may be tender and swollen.

Bismuth and lead poisoning usually lead to the deposition of bismuth or lead sulfide in a black line along the gingival margins when teeth are present—the bismuth or lead line. The pigment may be deposited in any part of the mouth, pharynx, or gastroenteric tract, in which infection or putrefaction of food and debris liberated hydrogen sulfide. Stomatitis of varying degrees of severity may occur in either case, but more commonly with bismuth poisoning, since bismuth sulfide is a more potent tissue irritant than is lead sulfide.

Dilantin Gingivitis

Occasionally a patient who is taking Dilantin (diphenylhydantoin) for the control of epilepsy may develop hypertrophy of the gums, particularly when his oral hygiene is poor. The gums become sore and swollen, and bleed easily. As the condition progresses, the swollen gums may almost cover the teeth. Drug hypersensitivity is believed to be the cause. Dilantin may also precipitate folic acid deficiency by reducing folic acid absorption. This effect is significant, particularly in persons whose diets are of borderline adequacy. Glossitis and megaloblastic anemia may ensue.[27]

Endogenous Intoxication, Uremia

Ulcerated, bleeding, and necrotic lesions of the gums and oral mucous membranes may occur in the terminal stages of renal insufficiency, but are only rarely the presenting symptoms. Usually these lesions occur only when nitrogen retention is profound and when there is a high degree of metabolic acidosis. The lesion may be single and located at a point when a broken tooth has irritated the oral mucosa or the tongue or may be diffuse and involve large areas of the mouth. When the gums are principally involved and are swollen and oozing blood, a mistaken diagnosis of scurvy may be entertained. It is probable that these lesions are similar to the mucosal erosions that may occur throughout the gastroenteric tract in uremia, principally in the stomach, the duodenum, and the colon. The exact pathogenesis of these lesions is unknown, but it is probably related to capillary damage and tissue infarction.

Allergy

Local contact, inhalation, or ingestion of various allergens may cause localized or diffuse erythema, swelling and ulceration of the buccal mucosa, gums, and tongue with sensations of itching and burning.[91] It is reported that allergy to amalgam tooth fillings or minute galvanic currents induced between several types of metal fillings in the moist oral cavity may produce localized areas of irritation, erythema, and burning sensations. Local contact testing with the suspected allergen or the therapeutic test of elimination of the suspected allergen aids in differential diagnosis.

Antibiotics

Penicillin hypersensitivity has been implicated as a cause of the burning sensations of the tongue and the mouth that occur in many patients given this drug, particularly in the form of lozenges or troches.[92] Similar lesions occur in patients receiving tetracycline, chloramphenicol, and other antibiotics. Usually the tongue is swollen, the papillae are edematous and in some areas fused, producing a cobblestone, fissured appearance. The color most frequently seen is orange red, but occasionally the scarlet red of niacin deficiency or the magenta color of riboflavin deficiency is so closely mimicked that it is impossible to differentiate the lesions by appearance alone.

Diarrhea, itching and burning about the anus and vagina, and flatulence and intestinal discomfort occur even more frequently than the oral symptoms and have the same cause. There is no evidence that these lesions are due to interference by the antibiotics in the metabolism of the vitamins. A local allergic reaction is a more plausible explanation. More commonly, however, a different mechanism is responsible. Suppression of the normal bacterial flora of the oral cavity by the antibiotic allows uninhibited growth of other organisms, particularly fungi.[93] Moniliasis of the tongue, mouth, esophagus, and, in fact, any part of the gastroenteric, tracheobronchial, or genitourinary tracts has been found, particularly in debilated patients given broad-spectrum antibiotic or immunosuppresive drugs for extended periods of time. The tongue and mouth may become sore and inflamed, ulcers may form, and usually the physician can see small white or gray patches on the mucous membrane from which monilia can be obtained in smear or culture.

Persons taking penicillin, particularly by the oral route, occasionally have developed a painless, black hairy tongue.[94] The papillary tufts are much elongated, thickened, and fused, and pigment deposited on these unsloughed papillae gives the tongue a yellowish brown or black appearance. This type of tongue lesion may occur and remit spontaneously in persons who have not had contact with antibiotics. In either case, the cause is usually overgrowth with a fungus, such as Aspergillus niger.

The lesions do not respond to any of the vitamins, but disappear within a few days or several weeks after the antibiotiotic is discontinued.

Menopause

Burning sensations in the tongue and mild glossal atrophy may occur as manifestations of decreased production of estrogens after the menopause. These changes are probably similar to those that occur in the vagina—senile vaginitis. Improvement is prompt when estrogens are administered.

Prolonged use of oral contraceptive medications has been reported to cause hyperplastic erythematous painful gingivostomatitis. Remission follows elimination of the drug. A similar type of gingivostomatitis has been described during pregnancy.[95]

Neurologic Lesions

Hypoglossal nuclear lesions occurring in amyotrophic lateral sclerosis, syringomyelia, and related conditions may lead to glossal atrophy. The atrophy of the muscle is much more striking than the atrophy of mucous membrane. The tongue is smooth, deeply furrowed, and paretic. Fasciculations may be present, and inadvertent trauma from the teeth may lead to soreness and pain. Supranuclear lesions involving sensory and motor tracts may lead to contralateral paresthesias, numbness, and tingling sensations, as well as slight paresis. These lesions are seldom if ever the only cause for the patient's visit to the physician. Associated neurologic abnormalities suggest the correct diagnosis and interpretations.

Psychoneuroses

Sensations of burning, dryness, stinging, itching, soreness, or taste disturbance (metallic) in the tongue and mouth without any related objective evidence of inflammation or lack of salivation may occur as a manifestation of anxiety neurosis, which is said to be related to lack of sexual gratification and similar frustrations. Women in the postmenopausal period are affected most commonly. Men have this symptom only occasionally. Cancerophobia seems to be a commonly associated factor also.[96] Usually patients with neurotic glossodynia have had their symptoms for long periods of time with exacerbations and remissions related to emotional upsets rather than to seasons of the year, periods of dietary insufficiency, anemia, or local irritative factors. Frequently such patients date the onset of the symptom to the administration of an antibiotic. Occasionally tooth imprints may appear on the tongue of tense, anxious persons, who speak very infrequently and press the tongue forward against the teeth. This may occur in the absence of true glossal swelling. The underlying emotional factors must be clear before such a diagnosis is made.

It must be remembered that in the prodromal periods of niacin deficiency, burning of the tongue is common without change in gross morphology. During this prodromal period, the patient is usually emotionally unstable, irritable, and anxious. In the absence of a history suggestive of a psychoneurosis, a therapeutic test with niacin may be necessary. The physician also must be aware that a patient with a psychoneurosis manifesting itself by faulty function of the gastroenteric tract may not eat an adequate diet and therefore may develop niacin deficiency as a secondary disorder. Only through careful interpretation of all available historical data can the physician hope to understand the true sequence of events.

LOCAL ORAL LESIONS

The following types of local lesions of the oral cavity must be considered in differential diagnosis: acute and chronic oral sepsis, pyorrhea, granulomas, lesions due to local trauma and irritation, certain conditions thought to be developmental abnormalities, and lesions of unknown etiology.[95,97]

Vincent's Stomatitis

Of the acute infections, Vincent's stomatitis (trenchmouth) is probably the most common. This disease, caused by Vincent's spirochetes and fusiform bacilli, is highly contagious and may reach epidemic proportions. The acute inflammation may involve any or all structures of the oral cavity and throat. Painful ulcers form on the gingiva, the buccal mucosa, or the tongue. They are deep and may destroy a considerable amount of tissue. Fever and leukocytosis are common. There is considerable evidence that this disease usually attacks previously devitalized oral mucous membranes. The organisms are common secondary invaders of pellagrous lesions. Although the infection may be acquired by persons with no apparent underlying disease, the careful physician always searches for evidence of nutritional deficiency or other devitalizing processes when he is confronted by a patient with Vincent's stomatitis. Penicillin is effective therapy.

Herpetic Gingivostomatitis

Herpes simplex virus may attack the lips, tongue, and mouth and lead to very painful vesicular eruptions. In the nonimmune host, usually a child or in an immunosuppressed adult, primary gingivostomatitis occurs.[98] Vesicles, which collapse to form grayish white or yellow plaques and shallow ulcers surrounded by a zone of erythema, may occur anywhere in the mouth. The gingiva swell and may bleed easily. The ulcers are painful; new ones may appear for several days associated with local lymphadenopathy, but healing usually occurs in 1 or 2 weeks without scarring. Vesicles may also affect the skin, and rarely, the central nervous system may be involved in a very serious form of encephalitis.

Recurrent herpes simplex infection, the common fever blister or cold sore, begins with a sensation of burning on the lips, usually at the mucocutaneous junction. A papule or clusters of papules appear, evolve into vesicles surrounded by mild erythema, become purulent, and eventually rupture, forming shallow yellow ulcers covered with crusts. Healing occurs without scarring in 7 to 10 days. The appearance of herpetic lesions seems to be precipitated by febrile illnesses, emotional stress, trauma, or sunburn.

Herpes zoster may cause painful clusters of vesicles arranged in a linear pattern in the mouth, which may be followed by postherpetic neuralgia after they heal. The oral cavity may also be affected in chickenpox, but much less severely than the skin.

Herpangina, a disease primarily of infancy and childhood, is caused by the coxsackievirus A. It is characterized by fever, anorexia and dysphagia. The pharynx is inflamed and discrete vesicles may be seen, which eventually ulcerate. All parts of the oral cavity may be affected except the gingiva. Healing occurs in about 1 week without scarring. A variant, caused by coxsackievirus A$_5$, is called *hand, foot, and mouth disease*, since

maculopapular lesions may appear on the palms, soles, and heels, and the usual vesicles occur in the mouth.

Aphthous Stomatitis

Aphthous ulcers occur singly or in groups within the mouth, at the base of the tongue, or at the mucocutaneous junction of the lips. They are called the common canker sore and tend to recur in crops, much to the discomfort of the affected person. They usually heal without scar formation in 7 to 10 days.[95,99]

It is thought that Behçet's syndrome, a much rarer condition, characterized by similar ulcers affecting the vagina and anus as well as the mouth, is related to aphthous stomatitis. Behçet's syndrome, however, may cause dermatitis such as keratoderma blennorrhagica, iridocyclitis, arthritis, vasculitis, and encephalomyelitis. When arthritis is a major component and is associated with conjunctivitis and urethritis, the condition has been called Reiter's syndrome, which cultural and serologic studies relate to chlamydia and yersinia infections. The relationship of these various conditions is obscure.

There have been many unsuccessful attempts to culture etiologically relevant viruses and bacteria from aphthous ulcers. External allergens have been sought without success. An autoimmune mechanism seems to be a likely cause, perhaps initiated by cross-reactivity with a microbial antigen similar to that of oral mucosa. Histologic studies of aphthous and Behçet's ulcers demonstrate a lymphomononuclear infiltrate, and hemagglutination antibodies against oral mucosa, as well as lymphocyte transformation by oral mucosa, can be demonstrated in 70% to 80% of affected persons.[98,99]

Aphthous ulcers occur commonly in youths and in malnurished adults. They tend to occur also in persons with poor oral hygiene. Emotional stress may act as a precipitant, and there is frequently a strong family predisposition. Many therapeutic suggestions have been made, such as repeated vaccinations with vaccinia virus, hyposensitization to bacterial invaders, dusting with sodium chlorate micro-crystals, topical adrenocorticosteroid application, and improvement of nutrition, but efficacy has not been proved. If immune mechanisms are involved, early application of adrenocorticosteroid hormones has a reasonable rationale.[100]

Isolated Simple Papillitis

Isolated simple papillitis of the tongue is extremely common. It is the single swollen exquisitely tender papilla on the tip or sides of the tongue that appears suddenly, lasts a day or so, then disappears, leaving the tongue apparently normal. Occasionally under magnification, such an involved papilla appears as if it has burst and extruded a yellowish content. The cause of this phenomenon is unknown.

Enteritis

A virus type of enteritis in infants described by Buddingh and Dodd may cause painful vesicles on the tongue and in the mouth.[101] Coxsackie virus may cause minimally painful vesicles or a severe reaction such as herpangina, and it is probable that other related viruses may do likewise. Infections with yeasts and molds, such as thrush, ordinarily cause a dry sensation of the tongue, mouth, and throat with minimal burning.

Chronic Granulomas

Of the chronic granulomas, tuberculosis, histoplasmosis, actinomycosis, and blastomycosis may produce painful inflamed ulcerations of the tongue, lips, and mouth. Primary syphilitic chancre is usually nonpainful. Secondary syphilitic lesions, tertiary gummata, and sclerosing glossitis already have been described.

Hyperplasia and Dysplasia

Hyperplasia and dysplasia of the deep epithelial layers of the mouth and tongue frequently follow long-standing metabolic, infectious, or irritative glossitis. When these changes result in hyperkeratosis of the surface epithelium and the formation of white translucent plaques, we call the lesions *leukoplakia.*

Leukoplakia

Leukoplakia is usually asymptomatic. It frequently appears on a background of syphilitic or metabolic atrophic glossitis and commonly occurs in those who use tobacco and alcohol excessively. Its chief importance lies in the fact that it is a precarcinomatous lesion.

Tumors

Benign and malignant tumors of the tongue and oral mucosa are rare. They are usually nonpainful unless secondarily infected.

Local Trauma

Local trauma caused by poorly fitting dentures, sharp broken teeth, excessively hot coffee, or caustic and irritative medications may produce inflammatory changes and burning sensations lasting several days or as long as the trauma persists. Pipe smokers are acquainted with burning sensations in the tongue after excessive smoking.

An interesting lesion morphologically similar to the angular stomatitis of B complex deficiency diseases may occur in edentulous patients or those whose dentures no longer are satisfactory because of shrinking of the alveolar ridges.[102] Because of malocclusion, the closed

mouths of such patients often have deep crevices at the angles. Saliva and debris collect in these crevices, irritate and erode skin and the mucous membranes, and eventually cause deep, secondarily infected fissures. These perelèchelike lesions do not respond to vitamins of the B complex alone, but heal when the creases are eliminated by adequate dentures. It is probable that dietary deficiency in the beginning is often a contributory factor, but B complex vitamins do not induce healing until the local traumatic factors of stagnant saliva and secondary infection are removed by mechanically opening the "bite."

Pain or burning sensations in the tongue and mouth may occur in trigeminal neuralgia and xerostomia (particularly in mouth breathers), and has been described in *Costen's syndrome* (auriculotemporal nerve disturbance due to temporomandibular joint displacement). The appearance of the mucous membranes is not altered in these conditions.

Certain other conditions of the tongue of developmental or unknown etiology also must be considered in differential diagnosis. *Median rhomboid glossitis*, a congenital anomaly possibly arising from remnants of the tuberculum impar, appears as a plaque on the dorsum of the tongue just anterior to the circumvallate papillae. The surface is smooth and glistening and covered with stratified squamous epithelium. It is painless and harmless.

Geographic Tongue

Glossitis areata exfoliativa—wandering rash of the tongue—usually appears at an early age. The surface of the tongue is divided into irregular zones by zigzag white lines, which are formed from thickened hypertrophic filiform papillae. Within these lines, the filiform papillae have atrophied, and isolated fungiform papillae appear larger and redder than normal. These "hills and valleys" give the tongue the appearance of a relief map—the geographic tongue. The areas of atrophy and hypertrophy may migrate or remain stationary. Usually the condition is painless, although at times the patient may experience sensations of burning. The etiology is not established. In some cases, geographic tongue may be a manifestation of vitamin B complex deficiency disease. In others, it seems to be related to neurogenic disturbances; in still others, it seems to be congenital.

SUMMARY

A burning sensation or soreness in the tongue and mouth may be more commonly a manifestation of systemic disease than of local pathology. This chapter attempts to correlate these symptoms and the hyperemic, swollen, or atrophied mucous membrane of vitamin B complex deficiency diseases, scurvy, pernicious anemia, and related megaloblastic anemias, iron deficiency anemia, achlorhydria, and atrophic gastritis, and to explain these changes in light of deranged cellular biochemistry. Other systemic and local diseases are considered that may produce the same general complaints. A burning tongue and mouth, evaluated by careful history and physical examination, frequently provide the key leading to the solution of an otherwise obscure diagnostic problem.

REFERENCES

1. **Adams F:** The Genuine Works of Hippocrates, 2 vol. New York, William Wood & Co, 1886
2. **Hunter W:** Further observations on pernicious anemia (seven cases): A chronic infective disease. Lancet 1:331–224, 296–299, 371–377, 1900
3. **Minot GR, Murphy WP:** A diet rich in liver in the treatment of pernicious anemia: Study of 105 cases. JAMA 89:759, 1927
4. **Spies TD, Cooper C:** The diagnosis of pellagra. International Clinics 4:1, 1937
5. **Spies TD, Vilter RW, Ashe WF:** Pellagra, beriberi and riboflavin deficiency in human beings: diagnosis and treatment. JAMA 113:931, 1939
6. **Jolliffe N, Fein HD, Rosenblum LA:** Riboflavin deficiency in man. N Engl J Med 221:921, 1939
7. **Sydenstricker VP:** The clinical manifestations of nicotinic acid and riboflavin deficiency (pellagra). Ann Intern Med 14:1499, 1941
8. **Sydenstricker VP:** Clinical manifestations of ariboflavinosis. Am J Public Health 31:344, 1941
9. **Sebrell WH, Butler RE:** Riboflavin deficiency in man: Preliminary note. Public Health Rep 60:2282, 1938; 64:2121, 1939
10. **Kruse HD:** The lingual manifestations of aniacinosis with especial consideration of the detection of early changes by biomicroscopy. Milbank Mem Fund Q 20:262, 1942
11. **Kruse HD:** The gingival manifestations of avitaminosis C, with especial consideration of the detection of early changes by biomicroscopy. Milbank Mem Fund Q 20:290, 1942
12. **Bean WB, Spies TD, Blankenhorn MA:** Secondary pellagra. Medicine 23:1, 1944
13. **Spies TD, Bean WB, Ashe WF:** Recent advances in the treatment of pellagra and associated deficiencies. Ann Intern Med 12:1830, 1939
14. **Moore RA, Spies TD, Cooper ZK:** Histopathology of the skin in pellagra. Archives of Dermatology and Syphilology 46:100, 1942

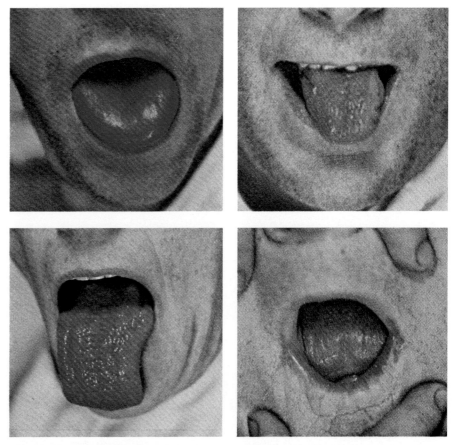

Plate 1.

(*Upper left*) Acute pellagrous glossitis in a patient with pancreatic insufficiency and steatorrhea. The tongue is scarlet red, swollen, and uncoated. Discrete hyperemic papillae are obscured by the swelling. Healing fissures are visible at the angles of the mouth.

(*Upper right*) Acute pellagrous glossitis superimposed on chronic pellagrous glossitis in a chronic alcoholic addict. The tongue is red, smooth, slick, and deeply furrowed. No papillae are visible.

(*Lower left*) Magenta tongue of riboflavin deficiency in a patient with long-standing congestive heart failure and anorexia. The blue-red color is distinctive. There is moderate papillary atrophy which is probably the result of an associated chronic niacin deficiency.

(*Lower right*) Cheilosis of riboflavin deficiency in a patient with hepatic cirrhosis. These are superficial fissures and erosions at the mucocutaneous junctions of the angles of the mouth. The tongue is magenta.

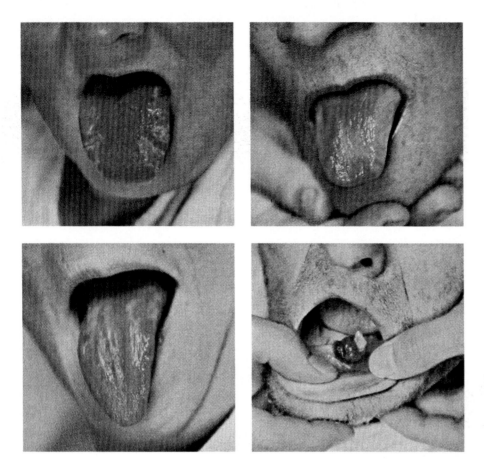

Plate 2.

(*Upper left*) Geographiclike tongue in a patient with uncontrolled diabetes mellitus and neurotic vomiting. The bulbous papillae at the tip are of the "cobblestone" variety. This lesion cleared when diabetes mellitus was controlled and an adequate diet was supplemented with niacin and riboflavin.

(*Upper right*) Atrophic glossitis in a black patient with microcytic hypochromic anemia. The tongue is extremely smooth, pale, and devoid of papillae.

(*Lower left*) Atrophic glossitis with leukoplakia. The posterior portion of the tongue is atrophic and streaked with thin, whitish, keratotic epithelium.

(*Lower right*) Acute scorbutic gingivitis. The gum surrounding the one remaining tooth snag is swollen and blue-red. The edentulous portion of the gum is normal.

15. **Axelrod AE, Spies TD, Elvehjem CA:** Effect of nicotinic acid deficiency upon coenzyme I content of human erythrocyte and muscle. J Biol Chem 138:667, 1941

16. **Evans EA Jr (ed):** The Biological Action of the Vitamins: A Symposium. Chicago, University of Chicago Press, 1942

17. **Baumann CA, Stare FJ:** Coenzymes. Physiol Rev 19:353, 1939

18. **Devlin TM:** The relation of diet to oxidative enzymes. In Wohl MG, Goodhart RS (eds): Modern Nutrition in Health and Disease, 4th ed, p 425. Philadelphia, Lea & Febiger, 1968

19. **Bellamy WD, Umbreit WW, Gunselus IC:** Function of pyriodoxine: Conversion of members of vitamin B_6 group into codecarboxylase. J Biol Chem 160:461, 1945

20. **Schlenk F, Snell EE:** Vitamin B_6 and transamination. J Biol Chem 157:425, 1945

21. **Snell EE:** Summary of known metabolic functions of nicotinic acid, riboflavin and vitamin B_6. Physiol Rev 33:509, 1953

22. **Ling CT, Hegsted DM, Stare FJ:** The effect of pyridoxine deficiency on the tryptophane-niacin transformation in rats. J Biol Chem 174:803, 1948

23. **Witten W, Holman RT:** Polyethenoid fatty acid metabolism. VI. Effect of pyridoxine on essential fatty acid conversion. Arch Biochem 41:266, 1952

24. **Lipman F, Kaplan NO, Novelli GD et al:** Coenzyme for acetylation, a pantothenic acid derivative. J Biol Chem 167:869, 1947

25. **Stokes JL:** Substitution of thymine for "folic acid" in the nutrition of the lactic acid bacteria. J Bacteriol 48:201, 1944

26. **Vilter RW, Will JJ, Wright T et al:** Interrelationships of vitamin B_{12} folic acid, and ascorbic acid in the megaloblastic anemias. Am J Clin Nutr 12:130, 1963

27. **Herbert V:** Folic acid and vitamin B_{12} In Goodhart RS, Shils ME (eds): Modern Nutrition in Health and Disease 5th ed, p 221. Philadelphia, Lea & Febiger, 1973

28. **Touster O:** Essential pentosuria and the glucuronate-xylulose pathway. Fed. Proc. 19:977, 1960

29. **Winegrad AI, Burden CL:** Hyperactivity of the glucuronic acid pathway in diabetes mellitus. Trans Assoc Am Physicians 78–158, 1965

30. **Peterkofsky B, Udenfriend SJ:** Enzymatic hydroxylation of proline in microsomal polypeptide leading to formation of collagen. Proc Nat Acad Sci USA 53:333, 1965

31. **Woodruff CW, Cherrington ME, Stockell AK et al:** The effect of pteroylglutamic acid and related compounds on tyrosine metabolism in the scorbutic guinea pig. J Biol Chem 178:861, 1949

32. **Govan CD, Gordon HH:** The effect of pterolyglutamic acid on the aromatic amino acid metabolism of premature infants. Science 109:332, 1949

33. **Wolbach SB, Bessey OA:** Tissue changes in vitamin deficiencies. Physiol Rev 22:233, 1942

34. **Mann AW:** Nutrition as it affects the teeth. Med Clin North Am 27:545, 1943

35. **Goldsmith GA, Sarett HP, Register VD, Gibbens J:** Studies of niacin requirements in man. I. Experimental pellagra in subjects on corn diets low in niacin and tryptophane. J Clin Invest 31:533, 1952

36. **Spies TD, Bean WB, Vilter RW et al:** Endemic riboflavin deficiency in infants and children. Am J Med Sci 200:697–701, 1940

37. **Stannus HS:** Problems in riboflavin and allied deficiencies. Br Med J 2:103–105, 140–144, 1944

38. **Sandstead HR:** Deficiency stomatitis. U.S. Public Health Reports (Suppl 169), 1943

39. **Cleckley HM, Kruse HD:** The ocular manifestations of ariboflavinosis: Progress note. JAMA 114:2437, 1940

40. **Horwitt MK, Hills OW, Harvey CC et al:** Effects of dietary depletion of riboflavin. J Nutr 39:357, 1949

41. **Rosenblum LA, Jolliffe N:** The oral manifestations of vitamin deficiencies. JAMA 117:2245, 1941

42. **Smith SG, Martin DW:** Cheilosis successfully treated with synthetic vitamin B_6. Proc Soc Exp Biol Med 43:660, 1940

43. **Iyengan L:** Oral lesions in pregnancy. Lancet 1:680, 1973

44. **Vilter RW, Mueller JF, Glazer HS et al:** The effect of vitamin B_6 deficiency induced by desoxypyridoxine in human beings. J Lab Clin Med 42:335, 1953

45. **Sauberlich EE et al:** Biochemical assessment of the nutritional status of vitamin B_6 in the human. Am J Clin Nutr 25:629, 1972

46. **Sydenstricker VP, Singal SA, Briggs AP et al:** Observations on "egg white injury" in man. JAMA 118:1199, 1942

47. **Rose JA:** Folic acid deficiency as a cause of angular cheilosis. Lancet 2:453, 1971

48. **Schoenbach EB, Greenspan EM, Colsky J:** Reversal of aminopterin and amethopterin toxicity by citrovorum factor. JAMA 144:1558, 1950

49. **Oatway WH Jr, Middleton WS:** Correlation of lingual changes with other clinical data. AMA Arch Intern Med 49:860, 1932

50. **Manson–Bahr P:** Glossitis and vitamin B_2 complex in pellagra, sprue and allied states. Lancet 2:317, 356, 1940

51. **Abels JC, Rekers PE, Martin HE et al:** Relationship between dietary deficiency and occurrence of papillary atrophy of tongue and oral leukoplakia. Cancer Res 2:381, 1942

52. **Harris S, Harris S Jr:** Pellagra, pernicious anemia, and sprue: Allied nutritional diseases. South Med J 36:739, 1943

53. **Moore CV, Vilter RW, Minnich VM et al:** Nutritional macrocytic anemia in patients with pellagra or deficiency of the vitamin B complex. J Lab Clin Med 29:1226, 1944

54. **Castle WB, Townsend WC:** Observations on etiological relationship of achylia gastrica to pernicious anemia: The

effect of the administration to patients with pernicious anemia of beef muscle after incubation with normal human gastric juice. Am J Med Sci 178:764–777, 1929

55. **Schieve JF, Rundles RW:** Response of lingual manifestations of pernicious anemia to pterolyglutamic acid and vitamin B_{12}. J Lab Clin Med 34:439, 1949

56. **West R, Reisner EH:** Treatment of pernicious anemia with crystalline vitamin B_{12}. Am J Med 6:643, 1949

57. **Herbert V, Castro Z, Wasserman LR:** Stoichiometric relation between liver receptor, intrinsic factor and vitamin B_{12}. Proc Soc Exp Biol Med 104:160, 1960

58. **Chanarin I et al:** Humoral and cell mediated intrinsic factor antibody in pernicious anemia. Lancet 1:1078, 1974

59. **Deller DJ, Witts LJ:** Changes in the blood after partial gastrectomy with special reference to vitamin B_{12}. I. Serum vitamin B_{12}. Q J Med 31:71, 1962

60. **Nyberg W:** The influence of Diphyllobothrium Latum on the vitamin B_{12} intrinsic factor complex. I. *In vivo* studies with Schilling test technique. Acta Med Scand 167:185, 1960

61. **Doscherholmen A, Hagen PS:** Absorption of CO^{60} labeled vitamin B_{12} in intestinal blind loop megaloblastic anemia. J Lab Clin Med 44:790, 1954

62. **Wokes F, Badenock J, Sinclair HM:** Human dietary deficiency of vitamin B_{12}, Am J Clin Nutr 3:375, 1955

63. **Eichner ER, Pierce HI, Hillman RS:** Folate balance in dietary induced megaloblastic anemia. N Engl J Med 284:938, 1971

64. **Jewett JF** Folic acid deficiency. N Engl J Med 287:252, 1972

65. **Gatenby PB, Lillie EW:** Clinical analysis of 100 cases of severe megaloblastic anemia of pregnancy. Br Med J 2:1111, 1960

66. **Mueller JF, Hawkins VR, Vilter RW:** Liver extract-refractory megaloblastic anemia. Blood 4:1117, 1949

67. **Jandl J, Lear AA:** The metabolism of folic acid in cirrhosis. Ann Intern Med 45:1027, 1956

68. **Sullivan LW, Herbert V:** Suppression of hematopoiesis by ethanol. J Clin Invest 43:2048, 1964

69. **Darby WJ, Jones E:** Treatment of sprue with synthetic *L. casei* factor (folic acid, vitamin M). Proc Soc Exp Biol Med 60:259, 1945

70. **Butterworth CE, Nadel H, Perez–Santiago E et al:** Folic acid absorption, excretion and leukocyte concentration in tropical sprue. J. Lab Clin Med 50:673, 1957

71. **Althausen TL, DeMelendez LC, Perez–Santiago E:** Role of nutritional deficiencies in tropical sprue. Am J Clin Nutr 10:3, 1962

72. **Vilter RW:** Treatment of macrocytic anemias. AMA Arch Intern Med 95:482, 1955

73. **May CD, Nelson EN, Lowe CV et al:** Pathogenesis of megaloblastic anemia in infancy: An interrelationship between pteroylglutamic acid and ascorbic acid. Am J Dis Child 80:191, 1950.

74. **Moore CV: Iron deficiency. In Goodhart RS, Shils ME**

(eds): Modern Nutrition in Health and Disease, 5th ed. Philadelphia, Lea & Febiger, 1973

75. **Jolliffe N, Fein HD:** Some observations on acute and chronic glossitis. Review Gastroenterology (USA) 15:132, 1948

76. **Schilling RF:** Intrinsic factor studies. II. The effect of gastric juice on the urinary excretion of radioactivity after the oral administration or radioactive vitamin B_{12}. J Lab Clin Med 42:860, 1953

77. **Jerzy–Glass GB:** Intestinal absorption and hepatic uptake of vitamin B_{12} in diseases of the gastrointestinal tract. Gastroenterology 30:37, 1956

78. **Chanarin I:** The biochemical lesion in vitamin B_{12} deficiency in man. Lancet 1:1251, 1974

79. **Herbert V:** Biochemical and hematological lesions in folic acid deficiency. Am J Clin Nutr 20:562, 1967

80. **Spies TD, Frommeyer WB Jr, Vilter CF et al:** Antianemic properties. Blood 1:185, 1946

81. **Vilter RW, Horrigan D, Mueller JF et al:** Studies on the relationships of vitamin B_{12}, folic acid, thymine, uracil and methyl-group donors in persons with pernicious anemia and related megaloblastic anemia. Blood 5:695, 1950

82. **Rundles RW, Brewer SS Jr:** Hematologic responses in pernicious anemia to orotic acid. Blood 13:99, 1958

83. **Klayman MI, Massey BW:** Further observations on gastric cytology of pernicious anemia. J Lab Clin Med 44:820, 1954

84. **Hodges RE, Baker EM, Hood J et al:** Experimental scurvy in man. Am J Clin Nutr 22:535, 1969

85. **King CG:** Present knowledge of ascorbic acid (vit. C). Nutr Rev 26:33, 1968

86. **Vilter RW:** Anemia related to nutritional deficiencies other than vitamin B_{12} and folic acid. In Williams WJ, Beutler E, Erslev A et al (eds): Hematology, pp 366–367. New York, McGraw–Hill, 1972

87. **Cox EV et al:** The anemia of scurvy. Am J Med 42:220, 1967

88. **Forkner CE:** Clinical and pathological differentiation of the acute leukemias. AMA Arch Intern Med 53:1, 1934

89. **Soll SN:** Eruptive fever with involvement of the respiratory tract, conjunctivitis, stomatitis, and balanitis, etc. Arch Intern Med 79:475, 1947

90. **Harvey AM:** Systemic lupus erythematosus. In Cecil Loeb (eds): Textbook of Medicine, 10th ed, p 641. Philadelphia, WB Saunders, 1959

91. **Goldman L, Goldman B:** Contact testing of buccal mucous membrane for stomatitis venenata. Archives of Dermatology and Syphilology 50:79, 1944

92. **Goldman L, Farrington J:** Contact testing of the buccal mucous membrane with special reference to penicillin. Ann Allergy 4:457, 1946

93. **Woods JW, Manning JH Jr, Patterson CN:** Monilial infections complicating the therapeutic use of antibiotics. JAMA 145:207, 1951

94. **Wolfron S:** Black hairy tongue associated with penicillin therapy. JAMA 140:1206, 1949

95. **Ship II et al:** Systemic significance of mouth ulcers. Postgrad Med 49:67, 1971

96. **Karshan M, Kutscher AH, Silvers HF et al:** Studies in the etiology of idiopathic orolingual paresthesias. Am J Dig Dis 19:341, 1952

97. **Thoma KH:** Oral Pathology: A Histological, Roentgenological, and Clinical Study of the Diseases of the Teeth, Jaws, and Mouth, 2nd ed. St Louis, CV Mosby, 1954

98. **Lennette EH, Magoffin RL:** Virological and immunological aspects of major oral ulcerations. J Am Dent Assoc 87:1055, 1973

99. **Editorial:** Recurrent oral ulcerations. Br Med J 3(5934):757, 1974

100. **Ship II, Merritt AD, Stanley HR:** Recurrent aphthous ulcers. Am J Med 32:32, 1962

101. **Buddingh CJ, Dodd K:** Stomatitis and diarrhea of infants caused by a hitherto unrecognized virus. J Pediatr 25:105, 1944

102. **Ellenberg M, Pollack H:** Pseudoariboflavinosis. JAMA 119:790, 1942

8

Thoracic Pain
Daniel B. Bauwens
Robert Paine

Origin of Painful Stimuli
  Tissue Tension
  Chemical Factors
  Pathways of Pain
Pain Arising in the Chest Wall
  Intercostal Nerve Pain
  Myalgia
  Ostalgia
  Dorsal Root Pain
  Breast Pain
Pain from the Trachea, Pleura, and Diaphragm
  Tracheobronchial Pain
  Pleural Pain
  Diaphragmatic Pain
Pain Arising from Mediastinal Organs
  Pericardial Pain

Esophageal Pain
Mediastinal Pain
Cardiac Pain
  Origin of Cardiac Pain
  Restriction of Coronary Flow
    Coronary Angiography
  Characteristics of Heart Pain
    Angina Pectoris
    Pain of Acute Myocardial Infarction
    Precordial Ache and Tenderness
  Tracts and Reference of Cardiac Pain
Aortic Pain
  Mechanisms of Aortic Pain
  Characteristics of Aortic Pain
Summary

Pain arising in the chest, in common with pain originating elsewhere, may occur in the presence of local lesions of no seriousness, or may indicate important somatic or visceral disease. Thoracic pain may be difficult to evaluate, particularly when it is the visceral type. Chest pain may be the only presenting indication of disease.

Information regarding many types and mechanisms of thoracic pain is fragmentary. Other forms of chest pain, such as that from the heart and the pleura, have been investigated more extensively. In the short space of this chapter, it is not possible to include detailed descriptions of all types of thoracic pain. The mechanisms of the common and important forms will be presented briefly.

ORIGIN OF PAINFUL STIMULI

There is now convincing evidence that there are nerve fibers specifically concerned with the transmission of pain impulses.[1,2] Further evidence indicates that tissue damage from trauma, bacterial invasion, or other disease stimulates pain nerve endings by tissue tension or by chemical factors present in the injured tissue, or by both these factors together.[1] It is clear that a wide variety of pathologic changes may lead to tension or chemical irritation to provoke pain; on the other hand, extensive tissue damage may be incurred, without pain, if these factors are absent.

TISSUE TENSION

That tissue tension can provoke pain is seen readily when a single hair is plucked. The pain is undoubtedly produced by direct tension exerted on the nerve endings.[3] Tension, applied to a wide area of normal skin, must be considerable before pain occurs; but tension (and chemical factors) in inflamed skin may produce exquisite pain. Inflammatory reactions are intensely painful when associated with much exudation[3] (as in the painful boil before pus issues from it) or with edema. Throbbing pain occurs with the rise of tension from each pulse wave into inflamed areas. Distention of the adventitia of blood vessels is said to be painful,[61,87] perhaps reaching a peak of severity in dissecting aneurysms of the aorta. Some workers have considered the pain of angina pectoris and myocardial infarction to arise from tension on the sheaths of the coronary arteries, although this explanation is now not widely accepted. Abnormal dilatation of hollow viscera has been shown to be painful.[5] The role of tissue tension in pain stimulation is therfore important. The preceding examples are only a few.

CHEMICAL FACTORS

The nature of the chemical excitants of pain in tissue injury is not known with certainty. It has been suggested that the liberation of potassium ions stimulates pain endings.[3] Moore and associates demonstrated that pain nerve endings are sensitive to potassium ions in certain concentrations.[4] Lewis spoke of a "pain producing substance" present in normal tissue that is liberated when injury to the tissue is sustained.[3] Possibly, Lewis's "substance" is a prostaglandin. These substances, found in virtually all tissue, produce marked hyperalgesia and pain when released in areas of damage. Drugs that inhibit prostaglandin release or synthesis (salicylates) are classic analgesics.[109] Acid accumulation (*i.e.,* ischemic muscle) may provoke pain.[4] It has been suggested that the pain of muscle ischemia results from accumulation of acid metabolites with irritation of pain nerve endings.[62] (See section on Cardiac Pain.) Lactic acid is likely to be one metabolite involved in ischemic pain. Others may accumulate in sufficient concentration to provoke pain in infections and other diseases. Whatever such chemical factors may be, they operate, often together with tension within the tissue, to cause discomfort.

With these fundamental pain stimuli in mind, many painful symptoms find reasonable explanations when considered in relation to the known or to the suspected pathology in a given clinical problem.

PATHWAYS OF PAIN

The impulses of all painful sensations below the level of the cranial nerves enter the spinal cord by fibers traversing the posterior ganglia and the dorsal roots and are transmitted to neurones in the posterior horns. The somatic and visceral pain fibers share these pathways. Therefore, impulses from visceral nerve endings arrive at the same reception point among the posterior horn cells as do impulses of somatic origin. An appreciation of this merger into a common path is essential to the understanding of the distributions of pain in visceral disease. Visceral pain will be noted in that somatic area with which it shares a final common path (see Fig. 8-1).

The precise localization of somatic pain differs from the wider distribution of visceral pain because, in general, visceral pain is transmitted to several segmental levels, whereas somatic pain is transmitted to a single level. However, it is important to realize that the intensity and duration of painful stimuli also influence the extent of spread of pain to adjoining segments, whether the reception is visceral or somatic. For instance, a traumatic injury to one digit may, after a time,

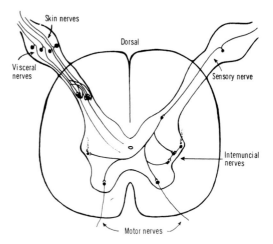

Fig. 8-1. Diagrammatic sketch of a cross section of the spinal cord illustrating certain nervous connections to explain the reference of pain. It is generally believed that visceral pain fibers may synapse in the spinal cord with certain neurones transmitting pain sensation from the skin. When these visceral pain fibers come under intense stimulation, the stimuli may affect the cutaneous neurones because of the crossed synapses, so that a sensation of cutaneous pain is simultaneously experienced. Referred pain may be due in part to reflex muscle spasm, also mediated through intraspinal nerve connections, as shown in the right of the diagram.

be followed by discomfort in the entire arm and shoulder.

Extension of pain to other levels demonstrates the existence of intermediate neurones connecting the posterior horn cells with other areas in the cord. These include the spinothalamic tract, the intermediolateral nuclei, and the anterior horn cells as well as internuncial cells connecting with the higher and lower segments of the cord. Impulses transmitted to the spinothalamic tract result in thalamic and cortical action in the awareness of pain. Impulses transmitted to the intermediolateral (sympathetic) nuclei may call forth motor responses (vasoconstriction and dilatation and sweating) and may be responsible for causalgic states, and impulses transmitted to the motor cells of the anterior horn produce the reflex muscular spasm associated with pain.

PAIN ARISING IN THE CHEST WALL

The integument and muscles of the chest wall are subject to essentially the same diseases as similar tissues elsewhere. The pain–sensory innervation of these tissues is conveyed to the dorsal roots through the cutaneous and intercostal nerves. Generally, pain arising from the thoracic integument and other superficial tissues is sharply localized. Furuncles and other infections, contusions, and abrasions of varying severity may produce superficial, well-localized pain. Because of the anatomic peculiarities of the thorax, pain of distinctive nature may arise from involvement of muscles, nerves, and bone. These will be considered separately.

INTERCOSTAL NERVE PAIN

Irritation of the intercostal nerves may arise from a neuritis of those nerves, resulting from trauma, systemic or upper respiratory infections or other toxic cause, or pressure upon the nerve.[7] The neuritis often is aggravated by exposure to cold. The onset of pain is usually sudden. The pain is localized in the intercostal space, the patient being readily able to identify the exact site of tenderness. The nature of the pain may be stabbing, lancinating, burning, and in severe cases, occurring in paroxysms when the patient breathes deeply, coughs, or moves suddenly. There has been interest in the frequency with which intercostal neuritis is localized about the precordium, leading the patient to believe that he has heart disease. However, in intercostal nerve irritation, localized tenderness may be found along the course of the inflamed nerve, and slight pressure elicits paroxysms of pain. Pressure points where tenderness is maximum may be located near the vertebrae, in the axillary lines, or near the parasternal lines.

Herpes zoster is a distinctive form of dorsal root irritation due to infection with varicellazoster virus in patients who previously have had chickenpox, usually in childhood.[8] It is assumed that zoster is a reactivation of latent varicella zoster infection of the dorsal root ganglia. Examination of these sensory ganglia reveal the virus particles in areas of hemorrhage and inflammation. The associated peripheral nerves may show degenerative and inflammatory changes. The pain is usually intense, often burning or knifelike, and may be punctuated by paroxysms of great severity. Pain usually precedes and often persists after the vesicular rash has subsided. Hypesthesia or, less commonly, hyperesthesia may occur. Frequency of zoster increases with age reaching a high of 16% in patients in the ninth decade of life.[9] Patients with malignancies, especially Hodgkin's disease, and patients receiving immunosuppressive therapy have been especially prone to becoming affected by zoster.[96] Indeed, zoster has appeared in the dermatomes subjected to irradiation for malignancy.[97]

Holmes has called attention to slipping rib cartilages as important causes of chest pain.[10] He notes that the costal cartilages of the eighth, ninth, or tenth ribs, on either side, may loosen from their fibrous attachments; this is followed by deformity—a curling upward of the end of the cartilage on the inner aspect of the rib, in close relation to the intercostal nerve. The condition is of traumatic origin. The manifestations of pain are varied. Usually the pain is a dull ache, often tolerated for years. Occasionally the pain is acute, stabbing, paroxysmal in type, incapacitating in severity. Localized tenderness to pressure over the lesion is present. The usual chronicity of the disease, together with the location of the pain and tenderness, ordinarily makes the diagnosis clear.

MYALGIA

Irritation of muscles is a common cause of somatic pain. Apparently muscle is a tissue from which only one sort of pain is produced; the discomfort is aching in nature.[6] The intense aching pain occurring during exercise of ischemic muscle is well known.[62] Muscle pain of the same nature was noted by Lewis when isotonic acids or hypertonic solutions were injected directly into the tissue. Firm squeezing of the muscle will likewise produce the pain. Muscle pain, if sufficiently intense, may be referred to other dermatomes common to the muscle itself, although often the pain is well localized at the site of muscle injury.

Inflammation of muscles and pain may occur in a variety of pathologic processes.[12,13] These processes may be local (*e.g.*, trauma, hematomas) or diffuse (*e.g.*, systemic infections, trichinosis, myositis ossificans). Perhaps the most common conditions provoking muscular pain about the chest result from exercise of "untrained" muscles of the shoulder girdle. Incessant or paroxysmal severe cough may render the intercostal muscles painful. Fibromyositis involving the shoulder muscles may occur; it presents no particular problem of identification because the shoulder and the arms may be tender on motion, and the muscles are readily palpated for tenderness. Myositis involving the intercostal muscles may give rise to marked discomfort and nodules and induration in the muscles may be present.[12] Elderly patients with polymyalgia rheumatica may experience severe pain in the neck, shoulders, upper arms, back, or thighs. In some patients the symptoms are widespread, and in others one particular area such as the shoulder girdle predominates. Polymyalgia rheumatica presents a paucity of physical findings, and responds dramatically to low-dose corticosteroid administration.[14]

OSTALGIA

The sources of pain from bone are the numerous sensory nerve endings in the periosteum and, to a lesser extent, in the endosteum. Therefore, bone disease may be present without pain until these structures are involved. Affections of the periosteum give rise to intense pain, usually well localized, whereas chronic disease, often affecting the bone marrow and endosteum, may result in poorly localized pain of varying degrees of severity. Reference of the pain to corresponding body segments may occur by the mechanism already described. Trauma (with or without fracture) and acute osteomyelitis may affect the bony thorax or the spine. Exquisite tenderness occurs over the affected point.[7] The pain is sharp and severe. In osteomyelitis, the pain may be continous for many hours.

Bone pain in syphilitic aortitis may be continuous and so severe that it is incapacitating. Aortitis with aneurysm may gradually erode the sternum or adjacent costal cartilages. In these cases there may be unremitting, well-localized pain, boring or burning in type.

Intense, aching, boring back pain may occur with malignant metastases to thoracic vertebrae; often the pain is referred to the corresponding dermatomes. The lesions may not be seen roentgenographically but may be recognized by nuclear bone scan. Mediastinal tumors, other than aortitis, may provoke chronic aching or dull chest pain (often substernal) by pressure against the spine or ribs. Hodgkin's disease and lymphosarcoma are common examples. Leukemia has long been known to produce costal pain in its advanced stages, particularly producing areas of point tenderness in the sternum.[16] Multiple myeloma, osteitis deformans, and sarcoma, involving the ribs or thoracic spine, may likewise cause ostalgia.

DORSAL ROOT PAIN

The clinical and the pathologic features of dorsal root pain and its differentiation from underlying visceral pain have been emphasized repeatedly.[98] Dorsal root pain refers to irritation—mechanical or otherwise—of the dorsal radicles in the proximity of the spinal cord. As with the other forms of somatic pain described before, root pain may be felt at the point of irritation, but is frequently referred to points along the peripheral course of a nerve. Root irritation of the thoracic spinal segments is often referred to the lateral and anterior chest wall.[18]

The lesions producing dorsal root pain may be toxic or infectious (*radiculitis*), but the pain is more frequently the result of mechanical irritation of the root due to spinal disease or deformity. Bony spurs about the intervertebral foramina in hypertrophic osteoarthritis may irritate the nerves upon motion of the spine.[19] Narrowing of the intervertebral spaces by compression of the intervertebral disks may bring pressure on the nerve trunks. Cervical ribs and apposition of the anterior scalene muscle to the brachial plexus have been noted to produce root pain referred to the chest wall.[19]

Dorsal root pain may be caused by thoracic deformity alone. In early osteoarthritis, swelling and thickening of the intervertebral disks straightens and lengthens the spine so that the spinal cord is drawn cephalad. This exerts tension on the spinal nerves in their exit through the intervertebral foramina, and they are irritated upon motion. As the spinal arthritis progresses, the vertebral bodies are thinned anteriorly with final anterior collapse to produce kyphosis (the characteristic hump). In this way, the spinal canal is even more lengthened, the spinal nerves are constantly taut, and irritation of nerves occurs upon motion of the column (Fig. 8-2).

The pain of dorsal root irritation often is a stabbing pain, or there may be twinges of sharp aching pain localized in the spinal region. The pain is accentuated upon motion, such as bending, use of the arms, or torsion of the trunk. Patients with spinal osteoarthritis commonly awaken at night in pain, presumably because relaxation in sleep allows the spine greater flexion and irritation of nerves by osteophytes or tension.

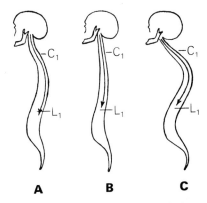

Fig. 8-2. Diagram showing position of the spinal cord with respect to abnormal degrees of vertebral flexion and extension. (*A*) Normal spinal curvature. The end of the cord lies at the level of L_1 or L_2, indicated by arrow point. (*B,C*) Abnormal dorsal straightening and kyphosis occurring in spinal osteoarthritis. In both instances the neural canal is lengthened and the cord is relatively displaced cephalad. Tension is exerted on the spinal nerves.

Reference of the pain to the lateral and anterior chest wall is common; it may be sharp; but is often dull and aching in nature. Occasionally the discomfort is projected to one or both arms through branches of the brachial plexus. Referred pain occurring about the sternum and shoulders, often paroxysmal, may closely resemble angina pectoris and sometimes is confused with it.[16,18] The confusion may be heightened by the partial relief obtained by the use of nitroglycerin.[18] Careful study of these patients reveals a history of back pain; the pain is more superficial than heart pain (See Cardiac Pain), is only indifferently relieved by nitrites, and usually is associated with exertion involving the upper part of the body.

Upper anterior and posterior chest pain can result not only from dorsal root irritation but also from cervical disorders, because the distribution of nerves originating as high as C3 and C4 may extend as far caudally as the nipple line. The pectoral, suprascapular, dorsal scapular, and long thoracic nerves originating in the lower cervical level can, upon irritation, cause pain in the chest, midscapular, and postscapular areas.

Although the anterior or ventral roots are motor in type, they can be productive of a dull, deep, boring type of discomfort when stimulated and can, therefore, produce a form of discomfort different from that attributed to posterior root disturbance. The anterior roots also play a role in the production of somatic motor echoes of visceral pain.

BREAST PAIN

With the accumulation of extensive data concerning disease of the mammary tissue, particularly carcinoma, increasing importance has been attached to the prompt investigation of the symptoms or signs of breast disease.

The sensory nerves of the breast are gathered into the second, third, fourth, fifth, and sixth intercostal nerves through the terminal brachial and medial antebrachial cutaneous twigs of the lower four of these nerves.[20] In addition, pain fibers in the second intercostal nerves have a common connection with the intercostobrachial nerve of the brachial plexus. A few pain fibers may ascend in the second and third cervical nerves from the region of the clavicles. Furthermore, sensory impulses from the medial brachial and medial antebrachial cutaneous nerves, as well as from the ulnar nerve, may enter the spinal cord in the same segments as sensory impulses from the breast tissue innervated by the upper intercostal nerves. Diffusion of pain from the breast passes around the chest and into the back, along the medial aspects of the arms and occasionally over the neck[21] (Fig. 8-3).

The integument of the breasts, including the nipples

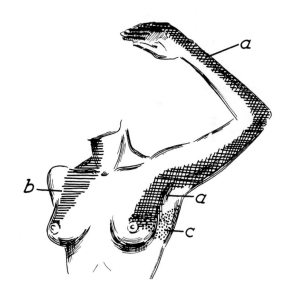

Fig. 8-3. Diagram illustrating diffusion of pain arising from the breasts. Cross-hatching (*a*) shows reference of mammary pain into axilla and along medial aspect of the arm. Pain (*b*) may be projected to supraclavicular level and into the neck. Breast pain may diffuse around the thorax (*c*) through the intercostal nerves (see text). Pain may be referred to the back and to the posterior aspects of the shoulder girdle (not shown).

and areolae, shows accurate localization of painful superficial stimuli in common with integumentary structures elsewhere. Pain from cutaneous incisions, furuncles, contusions of the surface, and similar lesions is superficial and is generally readily identified by the patient. Fissuring of the nipples and inflammation in the papillary ducts and areolae often produce intense, well-localized pain. The breast parenchyma seems to be peculiarly insensitive to painful stimuli, except when the stimulus occurs as the result of distention of the stroma.[20] Such stromal distention may be confined to a small segment of the parenchyma (e.g., in some cases of carcinoma), or may involve large portions of glandular tissue. Furthermore, it is possible that invading, malignant tumor tissue may involve pain nerve endings, so that pain may be severe and even constant. Inflammatory lesions, in addition to distending the stromal tissue, irritate sensory nerve endings and may produce severe pain.[22]

Inflammatory breast disease is a common cause of breast pain. The pain, often sharp, cutting and aching may refer to the axilla and along the medial aspect of the arms and the little and ring fingers. Veil studied a case of cellulitis of the breast displaying intermittent precordial pain and radiation of the discomfort to the left arm.[23] Angina pectoris was considered to be present; however, with a clearing of the cellulitis, all symptoms disappeared.

Benign and malignant tumors of the breasts are common cause of painful symptoms. It seems possible that a tumor that is situated to produce distention of the mammary parenchyma, or that involves pain nerve endings, may account for the pain.[20] However, large tumors may be present without necessarily provoking the symptom. The position and the nature of the neoplastic tissue would therefore appear to be primarily concerned in determining the presence of pain.

Mastodynia is one of the most common conditions producing mammary pain. It is almost always associated with ovulatory cycles and with chronic cystic mastitis. The discomfort is present particularly in the upper outer quadrant of the breast, which is firm, thick, and tender to palpation. The pain, at first, may be intermittent, occurring only at the premenstrual period, but later may be persistent. Jarring or movement of the breasts may accentuate the pain. It may radiate to the inner aspects of the arms as a dull (or intense) ache and is aggravated by motion of the arms. These breasts show imperfect lobular development with increased periductal stroma, epithelial proliferation, and changes tending toward cyst formation and adenosis.[21]

Other tumors and chronic inflammatory disease cause mammary pain that resembles mastodynia. Or, there may be an aching within the breast, a prickling sen-

sation, or lancinating pain projected along the side of the breast and into the axillae and arms.[22,24] Cheatle and Cutler state that the pain of carcinoma may be lancinating or stabbing, radiating to the characteristic places.[25] The breast may ache incessantly, and the patient attempts to support it to prevent jarring.

PAIN FROM THE TRACHEA, PLEURA, AND DIAPHRAGM

TRACHEOBRONCHIAL PAIN

The symptom of substernal pain from acute tracheitis is familiar to most persons. The discomfort is usually felt under the upper portion of the sternum and it is frequently described as a burning sensation. Coughing accentuates the discomfort. This pain is often accompanied by similar pain lateral to the sternum at points corresponding to the positions of the major bronchi. Sharp foreign bodies, such as fishbones, in the wall of the upper trachea may cause continuous pain in the anterior aspect of the neck.* Some patients with irritating foreign material, carcinoma,[28] or inflammatory lesions in the major bronchi can accurately identify the location of the pain in the right or left anterior chest, corresponding to the particular bronchus involved. Because of this, it is assumed generally that tracheobronchial pain is referred to sites in the neck or anterior chest at the same levels as the points of irritation in the air passages.

Although lower respiratory tract pain is common, the symptom has received scant attention. Investigation indicates that stimuli applied directly to the tracheal or bronchial mucosa, in patients under bronchoscopy, are construed as painful sensations in the anterior cervical or anterior thoracic area.[27] In addition, the pain is on the homolateral side of the neck or chest to the point of stimulation. The sites of pain are consistent and symmetric (Fig. 8-4). Morton and associates further showed that section of the vagus nerves (below the recurrent laryngeal branches but superior to the pulmonary plexus) abolished the pain on the side of the vagus section.[27] The cough reflex also was abolished. In a few instances, pain of tracheobronchial origin was referred to the contralateral side following vagotomy. These observations reaffirm the older suggestions that the pain–sensory innervation of the trachea and large bronchi is carried entirely in the vagus trunks. On the other hand, the finer bronchi and the lung parenchyma appear to be free of pain inner-

---

*Graham EA; Personal communication.

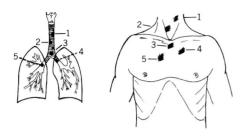

Fig. 8-4. When a bronchoscope is introduced into the tracheobronchial tree and when faradic stimulation is applied at points 1, 2, 3, 4, and 5, the patient may recall pain occurring at the corresponding points marked on the figure of the thorax. Note that the points of pain are homolateral to the areas of stimulation. (Diagram based on the observations of Morton DR, Klassen KP, Curtis GM: The effect of high vagus section upon the clinical physiology of the bronchi. Proceedings of the Central Society for Clinical Research (1949), J Lab Clin Med 34:1730, 1949)

vation.* Extensive disease may occur in the periphery of the lung without the occurrence of pain until the process extends to the parietal pleura. Pleural irritation then results in pain.

PLEURAL PAIN

It seems well established that the parietal pleura is amply supplied with pain endings, and that the visceral pleura is insensitive. These facts were brought out in the early experiments of Capps and Coleman.[29] They introduced a large trochar and cannula into the pleural space in patients with pleural effusion and stimulated various places on the pleural surfaces by means of a silver wire passed through the cannula. They found that the visceral pleura and the lung parenchyma were insensitive to these stimuli, but that stimulation of the parietal pleura gave rise to sharp pain. The location of the pain could be well identified by the subject (Fig. 8-5). It seemed clear, therefore, that pain arising from pleural irritation depends upon involvement of the parietal pleural membrane. Pain fibers, originating in the parietal pleura, are conveyed through the chest wall as fine twigs of the intercostal nerves. Irritation of these nerve fibers results in pain in the chest wall—usually construed as arising in the skin—which may be sharply localized, knifelike, and cutting in nature and accentuated on any respiratory movement. Arising in the most inferior portions of the pleura, the pain may be referred along the costal margins or into the

upper abdominal quadrants. The discomfort often is relieved dramatically by anesthetization of the skin.[30]

The mechanism by which painful stimuli are initiated in an inflamed parietal membrane has been the subject of some discussion. It has been held generally that friction between the two pleural surfaces, when the membranes are irritated and covered with fibrinous exudate, produces the sharp pain. Other theories suggest that intercostal muscle spasm due to pleurisy, or stretching of the parietal pleura, causes the characteristic pain. The latter theory is consistent with Bray's observation that during inspiration the superior excursion of the ribs widens the intercostal spaces appreciably.[31] The widening of the spaces, he reasoned, stretches the parietal pleural membrane; when the pleura is inflamed, such stretching irritates the pain fibrils, and sharp cutting inspiratory pain results. Although pleural stretching may be concerned in the production of pleural pain, other mechanisms have been suggested. There is evidence that pulling or tugging upon the membrane causes severe pain. Goldman observed that patients with artificial pneumothorax often develop pain when adhesions between the pleural surfaces are present.* He believed that if adhesions are present when a lung is forcibly collapsed in pneumothorax therapy, traction on the parietal pleura by the adhesions results in pain.

This suggestion affords an interesting explanation for the pain of acute fibrinous pleurisy (Fig. 8-6). The paroxysms of pain may be due to the many points of

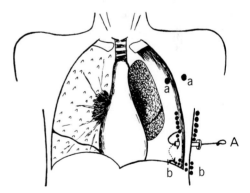

Fig. 8-5. Stimulation of the parietal pleural membrane by means of a silver wire (*A*) produces sharp pain. Such stimuli to the parietal pleura of the anterior, lateral, and posterior chest wall are referred to the superficial tissue at corresponding points in the wall (*a* and *b*) as shown in this sketch. Pain from pleural irritation is usually well localized.

*Graham EA: Personal communication.

*Goldman A: Personal communication.

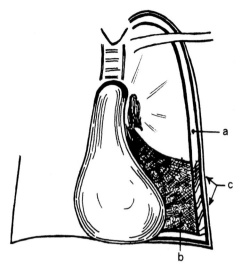

Fig. 8-6. Schematic diagram showing lobar consolidation and acute fibrinous pleurisy. The pleural space (*a*) is drawn in exaggeration, beneath which the consolidated lung lobe (*b*) is shown. Multiple fibrinous strands are represented by the small lines (*c*). Movement of the pleural surfaces in respiration exert tension upon the fibrinous strands, pulling upon the parietal pleural membrane. Such tension upon the parietal pleura probably produces the exquisite pain that characterizes the disease, in addition to tension caused by widening of the interspaces on movement and friction of the inflamed surfaces. Actually, the fibrinous deposit is dense so that individual strands are not visible, and the pleural membranes show acute inflammation.

traction upon the irritated parietal pleura by countless fibrinous strands, as well as by the stretching of the membrane upon costal movement. It also seems probable that irritation is further augmented by simple friction (clinically manifested by a friction rub) between the roughened surfaces of the pleural membranes.

Pleural pain is frequently encountered in acute fibrinous pleurisy complicating pulmonary inflammatory disease. Pneumonic processes reaching the extreme periphery of the lung cause a visceral pleuritis that quickly involves the contiguous parietal pleura. Pulmonary infarction may give rise to pleurisy if the infarcted tissue extends to the pleural surface. Krause and Chester found that pain was one of the most common symptoms in their series of cases of pulmonary infarction.[32] Tumor, especially bronchogenic carcinoma, may be attended by severe, continuous pain when the tumor tissue, extending to the pleurae through the lung, constantly irritates the pain nerve endings in the pleura.[33] The occurrence of spontaneous pneumothorax is often signaled by severe pain, usually in the upper and lateral thoracic wall, and is aggravated exquisitely by any movement and by the slight cough

and dyspnea that accompany it.[34] It is probable that adhesions, brought under tension by rapid recession of the lung, cause such pain (Fig. 8-7). Spontaneous pneumothorax may occur without pain.

As stated before, pleuritic pain is knifelike or "stabbing" in nature, and its position is usually easily defined by the patient. Laughing, coughing, or even normal respiratory movement produce paroxysms of exquisite pain. The notable exception is invasion of the parietal pleura by tumor, with which pain endings are constantly irritated.

DIAPHRAGMATIC PAIN

The diaphragmatic pleura receives a dual pain innervation through the phrenic and intercostal nerves. Capps and Coleman, using the technique described before, found that stimulation of the central portion of the diaphragmatic pleura with a wire resulted in sharp pain referred to the region of the superior ridge of the trapezius muscle[29] (the somatic segmental area innervated by nerves of common origin to the phrenic). The peripheral rim, anteriorly and laterally, and the posterior third of the diaphragmatic pleura have pain fibers reaching the fifth and sixth intercostal nerves.[35] Stimulation of the peripheral portions of the diaphragmatic pleura results in sharp pain felt along the costal margins. The latter pain may be projected to the epi-

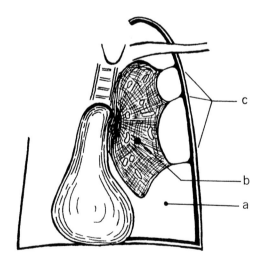

Fig. 8-7. Schematic diagram showing partial collapse of the left lung by air in the pleural cavity—pneumothorax (*a*). Complete collapse of the lung (*b*) is prevented by a number of "string" adhesions (*c*). It is readily understood how forcible collapse of the lung may produce tension upon the parietal pleural membrane when adhesions are present (as illustrated here); such tension explains the pain of pneumothorax when pleural adhesions are present.

gastrium, subchondral regions, or lumbar regions by the lower thoracic somatic nerves. The peritoneal surface of the diaphragm apparently is supplied by the same pain–sensory innervation, because stimulation of the central diaphragmatic peritoneum results in pain along the upper border of the trapezius.[29,36] Stimulation of the periphery of the diaphragmatic peritoneum causes pain reflected along the costal margins (Fig. 8-8).

It is easy to understand, therefore, how affections of the diaphragm may be localized clinically by the position of the referred pain. Diaphragmatic pleurisy, secondary to pneumonia or pericarditis, is common, and sharp pain occurs along the trapezius or costal margins, accentuated by the diaphragmatic motion in coughing or deep breathing. Subphrenic abscess may produce painful symptoms that are similar to diaphragmatic pleurisy. There may be tenderness to palpation about the costal margins with sharp pain occurring upon marked excursion of the diaphragm. Irritation of the central portion of the diaphragmatic peritoneum produces sharp pain in the shoulder on the affected side.

Herniation of abdominal viscera through a diaphragmatic hiatus may give rise to lower chest or upper abdominal pain.[37] It is often difficult to decide whether the pain originates in the diaphragm or from the anatomic distortion and disturbed function of the herniated viscus. Diaphragmatic hernias may provoke mild

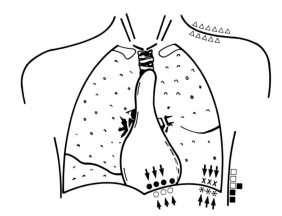

Fig. 8-8. Irritation of the pleural surface of the central area of the diaphragm (●●●) causes pain along the superior ridge of the trapezius muscle and supraclavicular fossa (△△△); stimulation of the marginal diaphragmatic pleura (*xxx*) provokes pain at corresponding points in the thoracic wall (□□□). Similarly, irritation of the central diaphragmatic peritoneal surface (○○○) produces pain in the shoulder and neck of the same side (△△△), and stimulation of the marginal peritoneal surface (***) results in pain referred to the abdominal wall (■■■).

epigastric distress or pain simulating that of peptic ulcer. Indeed, associated peptic esophagitis may be a major factor in the pain of hiatus hernia. Reference of discomfort to the lower sternal area may closely resemble seizures of cardiac pain.[38] The overlapping of symptoms appears to depend on pain reference mechanism of common distribution.

An interesting type of lower chest pain, attributed to the diaphragm, is a "stitch"—a sharp pain occurring about the costal margin upon exertion. It was attributed by Moor to interference with diaphragmatic motion.[39] Capps studied the sideache occurring on strenuous exertion at the right costal border in normal persons.[40] He reasoned that diaphragmatic anoxemia might precipitate the pain. It seems reasonable that pain originating in the muscle of the diaphragm may be referred to the level of the diaphragmatic attachment and the corresponding intercostal nerve.

PAIN ARISING FROM MEDIASTINAL ORGANS

Pain arising from the mediastinum or its contained organs is frequently difficult to evaluate. Regardless of its origin, pain arising from various mediastinal structurs has much in common and is frequently referred to identical peripheral sites. The subject is as difficult to present as such pain may be to interpret at the bedside. As an approach, it is good to recall that the mediastinum is a *space* bounded by structures that can in themselves give rise to pain (Fig. 8-9). Disease of the thoracic spine, affections of the esophagus, pericardium, pleurae, and other structures produce pain that may be referable to the mediastinum. On the other hand, inflammatory lesions and tumors within the mediastinum may provoke pain if extensive or critically located. A few of the more common forms of pain arising from the mediastinum and mediastinal organs will be considered briefly.

PERICARDIAL PAIN

The mechanism of pain arising in pericardial disease is puzzling. One might think of the acute pain of pericarditis as occurring from the movement of opposed, inflamed pericardial membranes, or one might consider that pain may be produced by marked distention of the sac by fluid. However, the experiments of Capps and Coleman indicate that there are very few pain fibers in the pericardium.[29] Using their cannula and silver-wire technique, they stimulated the endothelial surfaces of the pericardium in patients with pericardial effusion. No pain resulted from scratching the visceral surface. With the same stimulus, no pain occurred in

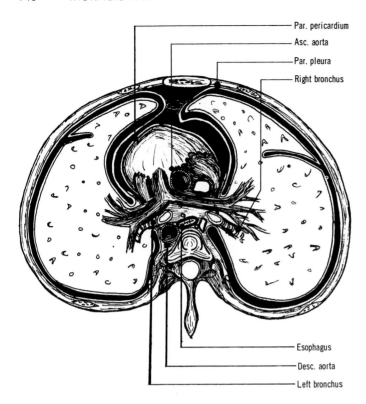

— Par. pericardium
— Asc. aorta
— Par. pleura
— Right bronchus

— Esophagus
— Desc. aorta
— Left bronchus

Fig. 8-9. Diagram of a transverse section through the thorax at a level immediately superior to the heart. The mediastinum and its contents are shown, together with the pleural and pericardial membranes. The pleuropericardial space is particularly exaggerated to accentuate its relationships clearly. (Based on an illustration in Gray's Anatomy of the Human Body, 29th ed. Philadelphia, Lea & Febiger, 1973)

the parietal layer except when the parietal membrane was stimulated opposite the fifth and sixth intercostal spaces. Such stimulation resulted in sharp pain about the superior border of the trapezius, as in central diaphragmatic stimulation (Fig. 8-10). From these findings, it seemed probable that a few pain fibers in the lower parietal pericardium, adjacent to the diaphragm, are carried in the phrenic nerves, but that elsewhere the pericardial membranes are devoid of pain sensation.

It remains to be explained why pain, usually substernal or immediately to the left of the sternum, occurs in some cases of acute pericarditis. Since the pericardium is largely insensible to pain, it seems probable that irritation of contiguous structures must occur to cause the pain of pericarditis. The parietal pleura and the pericardium are in close apposition (Fig. 8-9) in the mediastinal enclosure. Inflammation from an acute pericarditis then easily might spread to the neighboring pleura, producing pain, or even to other mediastinal tissues.[29] The situation of the pain (substernal or to the left of the sternum) is in keeping with the segment of pleura that may be involved. Barnes and Burchell, studying pain in apparently benign pericarditis, noted that difficulty in swallowing, deep breathing, or torsion of the trunk frequently accentuated the pain, suggesting that an associated inflam-

mation of the esophagus and other mediastinal structures was present.[41]

As noted, acute pericarditis may be accompanied by pain that is substernal, along the left sternal border, or occasionally, epigastric (Fig. 8-11). The pain is often

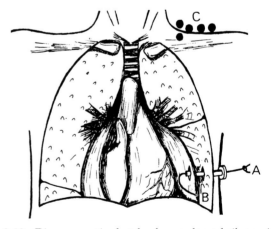

Fig. 8-10. Diagrammatic sketch of cannula and silver wire (*A*) in the pericardial sac. Most of the pericardial surface is insensitive to pain, but stimulation of the sac at the level of intercostal spaces 5 to 6 (*B*) produces pain referred to the superior border of the trapezius muscle and supraclavicular fossa (*C*).

sharp, lancinating, and paroxysmal; it may be continuous. The pain of pericarditis may be severe, closely resembling that of myocardial infarction[41] (see Cardiac Pain), although it is less agonizing and usually requires no narcosis for relief.

Pericardial effusion, often massive, is usually not accompanied by painful symptoms; however, in the series studied by Camp and White, pain occurred not infrequently.[42] Pericardial effusion may be manifested as a feeling of fullness within the chest, or as intermittent or continuous frank substernal pain, or ill-defined pain.[43] Distress of essentially the same nature may occur in tuberculous pericarditis.

ESOPHAGEAL PAIN

Esophageal pain, occurring as the only symptom, may be confusing because of its similarity to other visceral thoracic pain. Such pain presents itself as deep thoracic pain, or it is referred to corresponding somatic segments, conforming with visceral referred pain in general. However, other symptoms, such as progressive dysphagia, regurgitation of freshly eaten solid food, together with persistent pain or pain upon swallowing, suggest esophageal disease.

The esophageal mucosa, irritated by gastric acid, produces an unpleasant burning sensation in the upper thoracic, cervical and nasopharyngeal regions.[46] The installation of acid through a nasal tube into the esophagus has proven to be a useful method of diagnosis of esophageal pain. The induced pain, identical with the patient's symptom, is often a burning or tight substernal or cervical discomfort.[46]

Pain arising from the muscular portion of the tube is clearly demonstrated in the experiments of Paine and Poulton.[44] They introduced tubes, to the ends of which balloons were affixed, into the esophagus. When the balloons were inflated in the lower esophagus, a burning pain was induced, becoming "gripping" in character when the subject swallowed. Paine and Poulton reasoned that distention of the organ is painful, and that muscle contraction, attempting to overcome distention, results in paroxysmal cramping pain. These observers further noted that pain from the distended esophagus may be substernal or epigastric or may be referable to the back, but that the level of the referred pain corresponds closely to the level of the distended portion of the esophagus through successive spinal segments. Thus, the higher the pain in the esophagus, the higher the level of pain felt about the sternum and the back (Fig. 8-12).

Acute esophagitis may be caused by the swallowing of foreign bodies, such as bones or other sharp objects and spicy foods, or may be a complication of acute

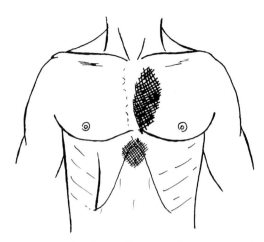

Fig. 8-11. Crosshatching illustrates the common sites of pain in pericardial disease. The pain may be substernal or to the left of the sternum and may be felt in the epigastrium. In some instances, pain may be more extensively referred (see text).

infectious disease. The mucosa as well as the muscle may be involved. Paroxysmal pain upon deglutition is one of the most constant symptoms, the pain being substernal and radiating to the back. There is often no discomfort when the esophagus is quiescent, although dull discomfort frequently persists. Chronic esophagitis, often seen in chronic alcoholics and heavy smokers, or seen following acute disease, may produce essentially the same symptoms. In phlegmonous esophagitis, painful symptoms are accentuated markedly, accompanied by fever, chills, nausea and vomiting and great fetor of the vomitus.[15] There may be constant substernal and back pain, so accentuated upon swallowing that taking food is nearly impossible. Carcinoma of the esophagus, in itself, provokes no pain, although pain occurs with the esophagitis that frequently complicates it.

Cardiospasm (spasticity of the cardia) may not be accompanied by distress.[45] However, pain upon deglutition often occurs, which is substernal, epigastric, or along the left border of the lower thoracic spine.

Esophageal pain, therefore, is referred to the sternum or back at the level of the lesion. Although the type and location of pain *per se* may be inconclusive, the occurrence of painful dysphagia and regurgitation of undigested food material, necessitating a liquid diet, and weight loss at once suggest esophageal disease.

MEDIASTINAL PAIN

Extensive mediastinal distortion from tumors or other disease may occur without producing painful symptoms. Indeed, enormous mediastinal tumors may be

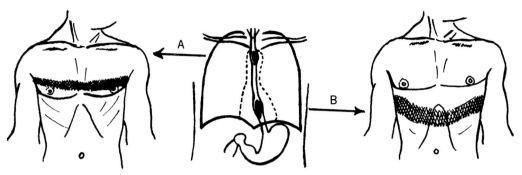

Fig. 8-12. Esophageal pain may be projected around the chest at the level of the spinal segment corresponding to the esophageal lesion. Schematically, pain from a lesion in the esophagus corresponding with the fourth thoracic spinal nerve (*represented by arrow A in the central figure*) may be referred as a band of pain about the thorax. An esophageal lesion at the level of the seventh or the eighth spinal nerve may manifest itself in pain about the chest following the course of those nerves (*arrow B*).

present with no discomfort to the patient other than cough, dyspnea, and moderate wheezing. Mediastinal lymph nodes involved by Hodgkin's disease,[52] neurofibromata, or other tumors may not give rise to pain unless nervous structures are involved. In explanation of such clinical phenomena, it seems possible that the mobility of the mediastinum, together with the resiliency of the tissues that bind it, may allow for considerable distortion without necessarily irritating pain-sensitive structures. However, many mediastinal tumors do provoke pain, usually in association with dyspnea and cough.[50] The pain first may be manifest by a sensation of substernal weight or "oppression" that is ill-defined. Over a period of weeks or months the pain may become severe. The discomfort usually remains substernal, but varies greatly in intensity. Involvement of the esophagus by tumor in the posterior mediastinum may produce pain upon swallowing. Certain tumors, such as carcinoma of the lung apex (Pancoast), may be accompanied by sharp axillary, shoulder, and subscapular pain radiating along the medial aspects of the arms.[53] Large aneurysms of the aorta may produce symptoms, particularly when they exert pressure upon the chest wall, although vague discomfort appears to arise from the aneurysms themselves in some instances[54] (see Aortic Pain).

Spontaneous mediastinal emphysema is frequently accompanied by agonizing pain. The syndrome has been vividly described by Hamman, who believes it to be more common than is generally thought.[49] From his observations, it appears that rupture of the lung may occur through an attenuated alveolus; the air then dissects along fascial planes to the mediastinum. Pneumothorax occasionally complicates mediastinal emphysema, and it has been suggested that some cases

of pneumothorax may result from unrecognized mediastinal emphysema. The condition often occurs when the person is making no effort and is sitting or lying quietly. The accident is generally heralded by intense agonizing substernal pain, radiating to the nape and to the shoulders. It seldom radiates to the arms. Such pain may persist for hours; indeed, a needle may have to be inserted into the mediastinum to permit the escape of air before relief is secured. In some instances the pain is milder, although it is "oppressive" and substernal in location. Frequently a distinctive crepitus is heard, synchronous with the heartbeat, indicating the presence of air about the heart.

Mediastinal pain may be caused by acute inflammatory disease or by traumatic rupture of the esophagus, or disintegration of the esophageal wall from carcinoma.[15,47] Occasionally, inflammation may be caused by the passage of infection through lymphatics or by burrowing along the fascial planes of the neck.[47,48] Under such conditions, the complaint of constant substernal pain is common, but the site of the pain is difficult to localize. The pain may seem to be present in the back, particularly if the vertebrae are involved, and percussion of the dorsal spine may elicit paroxysms of pain. Tenderness of the sternum occasionally has been noted. Pain may be accentuated upon swallowing if the esophagus is affected by the inflammatory process. Sudden motions of the trunk may be accompanied by severe discomfort. Painful symptoms of this nature should raise the question of mediastinitis, particularly if there are indications of infection in the neck, esophageal disease, or other lesions, such as retroperitoneal infection or pneumonia.

Chronic mediastinitis may arise as the result of tuberculosis, or following other chronic infections.[50] Oc-

casionally, mediastinitis occurs for which no cause can be elicited, as described by Pick.[51] Chronic mediastinal inflammation may give rise to pain (together with dyspnea). The discomfort may be a severe, unremitting substernal oppression, or a burning and aching sensation substernally or in the precordium. Some cases may run their course with little or no pain. Frequently, striking physical signs occur that point to the underlying disease.

CARDIAC PAIN

ORIGIN OF CARDIAC PAIN

In 1768, William Heberden accurately described the symptomatology of angina pectoris.[55] As Osler aptly put it, Heberden said little about the cause of the disease and had the "good fortune to get very close to the truth in what he did say." Herrick's classic description of acute coronary occlusion in 1912 gave impetus to the study of the recognition and cause of coronary insufficiency and cardiac pain.[56] One consideration was almost immediately apparent, namely, that cardiac pain results from diminution or cessation of blood flow to the myocardium.[57–59] Although early theories attributed the pain of angina pectoris and myocardial infarction to painful spasm or dilatation of the coronary arteries or of the aorta,[59–61] the conception of cardiac pain most widely held in explanation is that heart pain results from an accumulation of metabolites within an ischemic segment of the myocardium.

The theory had its inception in the work of Lewis, Pickering, and Rothschild.[62] They applied pressure to an arm by blood-pressure cuff and noted the occurrence of intolerable pain a short time (70 sec) after exercise of the arm was begun. Similar occlusion of the resting arm was not followed by pain despite the development of intense cyanosis. The conclusion was reached that during ischemic muscular contraction, a substance is produced that causes pain, but that anoxemia alone does not produce such discomfort. Katz and associates pursued this idea further and presented striking evidence that a substance, or substances, produced during muscular contraction, accumulates in the presence of ischemia and anoxia and provokes intolerable pain; angina pectoris and intermittent claudication were thought to be due to this mechanism.[63] Thus, it seems possible that ischemia of the myocardium, whether it is transient (causing angina pectoris) or prolonged (producing the pain of myocardial infarction), may set off pain impulses by causing rapid accumulation of metabolites within the heart muscle.

Although coronary angiography has provided precise information regarding the coronary arteries of the intact human, other catheterization techniques have extended the knowledge of myocardial functions from experimental animal preparations to the normal and diseased human heart.

These experimental and clinical investigations have demonstrated the predominantly aerobic nature of cardiac energy production. Oxidative processes within the heart muscle consume carbohydrate (glucose), fatty acids, lactate, and amino acids. The final combustion of each of these fuels is in the Krebs tricarboxylic acid cycle, which takes place within the mitochondria. Until the point of entry into this cycle, metabolic breakdown of glucose can proceed in the absence of oxygen and can produce small quantities of useful energy in the form of adenosine triphosphate. In the hypoxic state, pyruvate derived from glucose or amino acids is converted to lactate and is metabolized no further. The processes of the mitochondria are paralyzed in the absence of oxygen supply and the heart muscle, deprived of sufficient energy-rich ATP, rapidly loses the ability to contract.

In patients with coronary disease, areas of the myocardium deprived of normal arterial blood supply have been subjected to venous catheterization for analysis of the blood that drains the areas of ischemia. As anticipated, ischemic areas of myocardium have been distinguished by excessive quantities of lactate in their venous effluent. Other observations have demonstrated loss of contractility in these regions with reduction of stroke volume and ejection fraction during periods of coronary insufficiency.[106,107]

RESTRICTION OF CORONARY FLOW

From the foregoing discussion, it seems probable that the inception of cardiac pain results from myocardial ischemia. Furthermore, the evidence indicates that failure of myocardial nutrition occurs most frequently from insufficiency of the coronary circulation. The anatomic and physiologic factors governing the coronary blood flow have been investigated extensively and are of importance to the understanding of the genesis of ischemia of the heart muscle. These principles will be considered briefly.

The blood supply to the myocardium may be retarded or arrested by obstruction or constriction of the lumen of the arteries and by changes in dynamics of flow from valvular disease, heart failure, or other mechanical disturbances.

Obstructive lesions of the coronary vessels are encountered frequently by necropsy in the hearts of patients who have suffered attacks of cardiac pain.[64] The

lesions are atherosclerotic. Less commonly, the coronary ostia may be narrowed critically in syphilitic aortitis, or the arteries may be occluded by emboli from endocardial disease within the left cardiac chambers. Atherosclerotic narrowing of the lumina may be so marked that adequate coronary flow is maintained only at rest. Therefore, a rise in workload of the heart brought about by exertion or emotional stimulation may result in myocardial ischemia because of the failure of the vessels to provide the increased amounts of blood required. Under these conditions, the patient may suffer attacks of heart pain on effort. During rest, the coronary circulation again is adequate to meet the minimum requirements of the heart muscle; the attacks of pain cease.

Coronary Angiography

In recent years, coronary angiography has carried these studies from the postmortem table to the clinical radiology department, where, with minimal risk, the state of the major coronary vessels may be visualized in the living patient.[108]

By the insertion of an intra-arterial catheter in retrograde fashion through the aorta to the ostia of the coronary arteries, delineation of each coronary artery can be accomplished by injection of a radiopaque dye.

In patients afflicted with coronary disease, angiography may reveal a variety of lesions. There may be a single isolated segment of narrowing or occlusion. Of the three major coronary arteries (anterior descending, the left circumflex, and the right coronary arteries), the anterior descending is the most frequently diseased. It provides blood supply to the anterior and interventricular septal portions of the left ventricle and adjacent portions of the right ventricle. The right coronary artery is often the nutrient vessel for the conduction apparatus between the atria and ventricles and for the posterior, diaphragmatic portions of the ventricles. Because of their common blood supply, diaphragmatic or posterior myocardial lesions often are complicated by atrioventricular conduction defects, partial or complete heart block.

When isolated, lesions within the coronary tree most often lie within the proximal portions of the vessels near their ostia. Obstruction of the left main coronary artery is less common than significant disease of the anterior descending, left circumflex, and right coronary arteries and their major radicles, but the consequences may be catastrophic because of the large area of myocardium rendered ischemic by obstruction of the left main coronary artery.

Other patients present multiple lesions within the coronary tree, involving more than one of the three vessels with one or more points of narrowing or occlusion. In general, those patients in whom pain is most easily precipitated by exertion or for whom discomfort occurs during rest or upon the minimal stress of eating are found to have the more numerous angiography abnormalities. The specific referral of pain to arms, neck, or face does not appear to be related to the pattern of angiographic lesions.

Coronary angiography has documented the intermittent occurrence of spasm of major coronary arteries.[114] Episodes of spastic occlusion have usually appeared without provocation by emotion or exertion but have been provoked in experimental studies by alpha adrenergic and vasoconstrictive agents including ergonovine, an ergot alkaloid that is an alpha adrenergic agonist with a direct constrictive effect on vascular smooth muscle, and norepinephrine. Spasm of coronary arteries has been found in patients with and without evidence of arteriosclerotic coronary disease.

Patients found to have spastic coronary disease without atheromatous coronary disease have been found to be younger and more frequently female than those with atheromatous disease.

The mechanism whereby coronary spasm is precipitated is unknown. The demonstration of coronary narrowing after vagotonic and alpha adrenergic stimulation has suggested a neural process.

Although angiography may reveal discrete localized lesions in the coronary vessels, it should be emphasized that careful microscopic study of the coronary system of patients dying of coronary disease usually demonstrates diffuse involvement of the coronary apparatus with atherosclerotic lesions of varying stages.[110] In patients with diabetes mellitus, up to 70% of patients with coronary artery disease have small vessel narrowing or occlusion not visualized by angiography.[17] In diabetes mellitus and rarely in systemic small vessel inflammatory disease such as some collagen vascular diseases, the coronary disease may be limited to small vessels undetectable by coronary arteriography.[17,112]

The sudden restriction of flow in a major coronary vessel and the occurrence of frank myocardial infarction may be attended by violent pain. Fortunately, in many of these patients, the remainder of the coronary circulation is sufficiently intact to assure cardiac function until the infarct heals.

Extramural coronary arteries are diffusely involved by atherosclerotic plaques in fatal myocardial infarction. Coronary artery thrombi usually indicate the presence of shock or congestive heart failure or both during the development of myocardial necrosis. The infrequency of coronary thrombi in patients dying suddenly of cardiac disease and in those with transmural necrosis who never had shock or congestive heart fail-

ure suggests that thrombi are consequences of rather than causes of myocardial infarction.[26]

It is interesting that some patients may have extensive coronary artery disease without infarction and without having suffered pain or impairment of cardiac function. Blumgart and associates have pointed out that gradual occlusion of the principal coronary vessels may be accompanied by the development of extensive anastomoses between the branches of the right and left coronary arteries.[64] An effective collateral circulation then is established to enhance the circulation around points of obstruction (Fig. 8-13). Such enhancement of the circulation may sustain myocardial function for many years.

The devious networks of vessels that bridge the occlusions of large arteries have been shown in various ways.[64,65] Smith and Henry ligated major coronary vessels in the extirpated hearts of dogs.[65] Subsequent perfusion of the vessels with an opaque material indicated that the twigs included in the obstructed area were filled readily by the rich anastomoses derived from neighboring arteries (Figs. 8-14 and 8-15). Prinzmetal and co-workers were able to demonstrate that red blood cells labeled with radioactive phosphorus readily penetrated areas distal to the obstruction in the beating hearts of dogs and man, because of the rich collateral blood supply.[66] They suggested that blood flow through collateral channels operates to limit the size of infarcts, thereby lessening the danger of cardiac rupture as well as promoting the process of healing.

Levin studied the effect of collateral vessels on LV contractile function with coronary arteriography on pa-

tients with significant coronary artery disease. Collateral circulation was seen only when the degree of narrowing exceeded 90%. When adequate collateral circulation was present, there was a much smaller in-

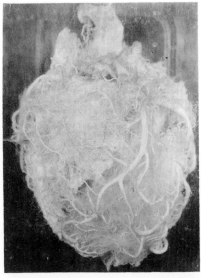

Fig. 8-14. Cast of the coronary arterial system of a dog heart filled with Neoprene latex. The heart muscle and blood vessels have been removed by digestion in concentrated hydrochloric acid. Delicate tracery of fine arteries and capillaries is preserved in the casting, which is suspended in water.

Fig. 8-13. (A) Diagrammatic sketch of a heart in which a theoretically *slow* occlusion has developed in the left circumflex coronary artery (*point K*), and a second partial occlusion has developed farther along the course of the vessel. Collateral channels from the left descending coronary artery (*LDC*) and from the right coronary artery (*RC*), shown in exaggeration, permit circulation about the point of occlusion. Establishment of such collateral blood supply may be important in sustaining anatomic and functional integrity of the myocardium following obstruction of major vessels. (B) Sketch of a heart in which the LDC is theoretically occluded *suddenly* (*point K*). Wide crosshatching indicates general area of ischemia distal to the obstruction. Although blood vessels near the point of occlusion may be filled, thorough irrigation of these vessels is lacking, and an infarct forms in the area indicated by dense shading.

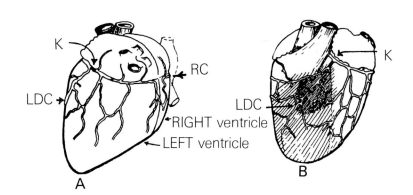

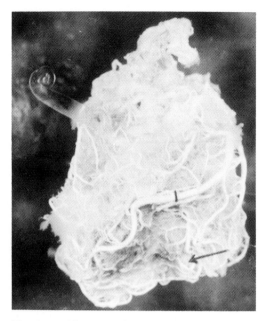

Fig. 8-15. Neoprene latex casting of the coronary arteries of a dog heart. The LDC is prominently displayed on the surface of the cast. Prior to injection of the arteries with Neoprene, the left descending coronary vessel was ligated at the point shown by the small black line. After injection with latex, the LDC distal to the ligation was filled from collateral vessels. The area below this artery (*arrow*) failed to fill with latex, leaving a depression in the casting. The specimen indicates that an abundance of anastomoses exists between the major coronary arteries and that the vessels that were not injected occupy a smaller area than would be expected from ligation of a large artery. (From Smith JR, Henry MJ: J Lab Clin Med 30:462, 1945)

cidence of regional left ventricular contraction abnormalities.[117] Excellent reviews on the functional importance of the collateral circulation have been published recently by Gregg and Patterson[118] and by Newman.[119] On the other hand, it is evident that further occlusions of arteries of the collateral system again may increase myocardial ischemia or result in infarction of the muscle, possibly with attacks of cardiac pain.

Convincing experimental evidence also has been evolved to show that other mechanisms may operate to increase the coronary flow. Gregg and associates observed marked increases in coronary arterial inflow when the right ventricle was placed under increased work by constriction of the pulmonary artery.[67] The increased flow was evident even when the aortic blood pressure diminished. They considered the augmented flow to be due to dilatation of the coronary arteries by metabolites present in the working cardiac muscle.

Similar observations were made by Smith and Jensen in experimental acute heart failure.[68] They demonstrated that, when the hearts of heart–lung preparations were made to fail by the administration of a toxic substance, there was a sharp increase in coronary inflow—even as the systemic blood pressure and cardiac output diminished. The phenomenon could be explained only by coronary dilatation. Therefore, it seems possible than an increase in work load for the heart muscle may result in greater blood flow from dilatation of the vessels. These experiments offer no clue as to the possible duration of coronary dilatation in hearts placed under chronic strain. Nevertheless, it is likely that the effects of coronary dilatation, and even of increased anastomotic circulation, may be neutralized largely by extensive narrowing and hardening of the vessel walls or by progressive occlusion of essential collateral channels. The flow may be insufficient to correct ischemia resulting from increased work, and exertional attacks of heart pain occur. Furthermore, it is observed often that drugs administered for the purpose of causing coronary dilatation appear to be ineffective, possibly because of previous continued dilatation of all of the vessels.

Interference with the dynamics of the coronary flow may be more difficult to understand. Passage of blood through the coronary vessels is dependent upon the head of pressure, the resistance to flow through the vascular bed, and the pressure existing at the venous end of the circuit. It must be assumed also that an optimum quantity of blood is available for irrigation of the system. The resistance of the vascular bed is modified further by the compression and relaxation of intramural vessels by myocardial motion; thus, an increase in intramyocardial tension as a result of hypertrophy or excess afterload may impair coronary flow. Certain alterations of any of these factors may be detrimental.

Aortic valvular disease (stenosis or insufficiency) may modify pressures at the aortic openings of the arteries, reducing the net flow into the system. In addition, it is possible that dilatation of the chamber, with stretch of the myocardium, impedes the flow. When the inflow of blood is measured into an atrial branch of the coronary system, dilatation of the atrial chamber inhibits the inflow into the artery even when a high perfusion pressure is maintained.[69] Other evidence indicates that most of the blood that passes through the coronary arteries is returned to the right cardiac chambers through the coronary sinus, the anterior cardiac veins, and the thebesian system of veins. Therefore, the elevation of right intraventricular pressure and right atrial tension (increased venous pressure) of sufficient degree may reduce the effective pressure gra-

dient between the pressure head (in the aorta) and the escaping venous blood, with consequent diminution of flow through the capillaries.[70] It is easy to visualize that in congestive heart failure, or in other conditions tending to raise tensions in the right cardiac chambers, the coronary flow may be impeded.

Clearly, coronary blood flow may be affected dramatically by variation in the tonus of the coronary arteries. As noted above, episodes of coronary spasm have been frequently observed in patients with and without atherosclerotic coronary disease. In a few instances spasm has been provoked by exposure to cold and by exercise,[115,116] providing one explanation for the adverse effects of chilling upon patients with angina pectoris.[71,72]

Demonstration of platelet aggregation upon the cracked and irregular surface of atheromatous plaques has led to the discovery of platelet emboli in the myocardial arterioles. Alterations in platelet function has been noted as platelets pass through atherosclerotic vessel beds. Platelets seem to be partially removed from the circulation after passing through atherosclerotic vessels as demonstrated by a gradient in platelet counts between the aorta and the coronary sinus.[120] Measured platelet functions were diminished implying the passage of biologically less active platelets. Inhibitors of platelet function (*e.g.*, aspirin, dipyridamole) tend to blunt platelet removal. Clumps of platelets, occluding the blood supply of small areas of cardiac muscle have been considered an important mechanism for random, atypical occurrences of chest pain.[111]

Occasionally, cardiac pain may be precipitated when the dynamics of the coronary circulation are normal. It is not uncommon for patients suffering from pernicious anemia to have attacks of angina upon exertion, presumably because of the primary lack of nutrition to the myocardium. Large doses of epinephrine may augment the work of the myocardium beyond the existing coronary flow, and cause pain.[73,105]

In some instances the administration of digitalis in cardiac failure has been noted to produce angina pectoris or to intensify the frequency and severity of attacks;[74] fortunately, this is not the usual occurrence with the use of digitalis.[75]

With reference to any of these mechanisms, it appears to be important that attacks of cardiac pain occur when critical myocardial ischemia is produced, either by an absolute diminution of the coronary blood or by increased demand on the heart out of proportion to the available blood supply. Clearly cardiac pain is most frequently the consequence of atheromatous disease of the coronary arteries, which renders inadequate flow of blood into the myocardium.

CHARACTERISTICS OF HEART PAIN

For convenience of discussion, cardiac pain will be considered as (1) paroxysmal (angina pectoris) and as (2) the pain of myocardial infarction.

Angina Pectoris

Typically, angina pectoris is characterized by the occurrence of substernal pain on exertion. Patients describe the pain as an "oppression," a tightness or crowding within the chest, or a heaviness substernally. Occasionally the sensation is said to be that of a vise-like gripping of the sternum and the lateral chest, and less commonly it is described as burning. The pain is rarely severe; more often it is of moderate intensity. It is never stabbing, never precipitated by coughing or respiratory movements. As the pain radiates to the upper extremities and elsewhere, the sensation is characterized as an ache, numbness, tingling, or other vague discomfort. The location of the pain is usually under the upper portion of the sternum, but it may be felt beneath the entire extent of the sternum. Anginal pain is usually, but not always, substernal. It may occur to the left of the sternum, in the precordium.[76] Under such conditions, the pain must be studied carefully, since pain in the precordium or in the region of the apical impulse is common to other disorders. Therefore, the occurrence of precordial pain must be interpreted with great care.[11]

The discomfort of angina pectoris commonly radiates from the substernal region. Frequently, the sensation is projected over the left pectoral region to the left shoulder and along the medial aspect of the left arm to the elbow.[76] The pain may be projected further through the forearm to the hand along the distribution of the ulnar nerve. Less commonly, the pain radiates to the right shoulder and arm with or without concomitant left-sided projection. Reference of the pain to the shoulders and to the inferior part of the neck has been described; these patients may have the sensation of a portmanteau clasped about the neck.[77] Occasionally, the pain is referred to the neck as a constriction, or as a pain in the left side of the neck and face. Radiation of the substernal discomfort to the epigastrium and the right costal margin also may occur, but such pain always has a thoracic component as well (Fig. 8-16).[76]

Attacks of angina pectoris often are precipitated by excitement or exertion. They may occur at night as in aortic valve disease, or after meals. The paroxysms usually last from a few minutes to one-half hour and usually disappear quickly when the patient rests;[76] frequently the subject is forcibly halted by the severity of

uncertain. Increased tension on papillary muscles or continuous myocardium as a result of the billowing mitral valve leaflet has been proposed as a mechanism of focal myocardial ischemia and pain in mitral valve prolapse.[121]

TRACTS AND REFERENCE OF CARDAIC PAIN

It seems well established that pain fibers from the heart pass from the cardiac plexus, enter the upper five or six thoracic sympathetic ganglia (through which they pass without interruption), and thence on through the rami communicantes to the corresponding spinal (or dorsal root) ganglia. The cell bodies of these fibers lie in the spinal ganglia.[107] Afferent pain neurones also pass through the inferior, middle, and superior cardiac nerves to the cervical sympathetic chains. They course downward to the inferior cervical and first dorsal (stellate) ganglion before passing across white rami into the dorsal roots. However, the majority of pain fibers from the heart course through the inferior cervical sympathetic and upper two or three thoracic ganglia. Elsewhere, they are much fewer in number. The pain neurones synapse with neurones of the second order in the posterior gray columns of the spinal cord (Fig. 8-17).

Consideration of the anatomic transmission of cardiac pain immediately suggests the mechanism of reference of heart pain. It seems probable that the greater part of pain impulses reaching the upper dorsal ganglia are projected as pain in one or both pectoral regions; pain occurring along the inner aspects of the arms may result from common connections through the brachial plexus.

Within the central nervous system, as in the sympathetic chain, considerable longitudinal dispersal of fiber occurs. Internuncial fibers extending from the cervical posterior horns may run cranially as far as the spinal nucleus of the trigeminal nerve in the medulla. These are neurones, which provide the passageway for pain impulses arising in the heart to a final common path with facial sensation. Whatever the site of origin, referral to visceral pain depends upon the merging of visceral and somatic afferents into a final common path. Although cardiac afferents in greatest numbers join with somatic sensory fibers in the upper thoracic and cervical area producing the commonplace pain referred to the arm, the sensory trigeminal nerve plays a comparable somatic role. Referral is less frequent, apparently because of the relative scarcity of interneural connections between the upper cervical cord and the medullary nucleus of the trigeminal nerve. The more frequent occurrence of pain in the angle of the jaw than in the upper portions of the face appears to reflect the proximity of that portion of the facial sensory supply to greater numbers of cardiac internuncials.

Potential merging of cardiac and cranial afferents also is seen in the parallel courses of the spinothalamic and trigeminal tracts ascending through the medulla, pons, and mesencephalon. Their termination in adjacent areas of the thalamus may afford a third point of overflow of cardiac sensory impulses into the facial stream.

Immediately following coronary occlusion, collateral coronary flow has been found to be doubled. Subsequently, the enlargement of anastomotic vessels provides significant supply to areas of myocardial ischemia so that the area of damage or necrosis may be much smaller than would be expected from occlusion of the vessel. That the establishment of "adequate" collateral flow following occlusion may require several weeks is a factor in the logic of gradual resumption of physical activity after infarction.

It has been suggested that the common anginal symptom of substernal oppression may be reflex muscular contraction of the anterior intercostal muscles. If the pain barrage is severe, mass excitation of visceromotor reflexes such as sweating, lowered blood pressure, ashy cyanosis and other evidence of vasomotor disturbance, and nausea and vomiting may become prominent.

The relationship between cardiac pain and pain in the upper abdominal region is less readily explained. Miller points out that difficulty in diagnosis arises when pain is referred to distant areas not directly related to the organ involved.[83] In most persons, visceral afferent fibers converge upon a limited number of dorsal roots that come into relation with a restricted number of afferent somatic fibers. Therefore, in diseases of the heart, gallbladder, stomach, and other viscera, pain usually is referred to characteristic localities.

With respect to the gallbladder, the visceral afferent pathways are numerous (extending from T1 to T12) and although the pain impulses are carried predominantly in the lower thoracic nerves, they may be included in many more segmental levels. In this way, gallbladder pain may be referred to segments commonly reserved for cardiac pain; acute heart pain may, in turn, be projected to the right upper quadrant and flank. Miller further notes that cardiac pain occasionally is transmitted over accessory afferent fibers. These are generally too few to carry impulses in any quantity, although in some persons they may be in sufficient concentration to refer pain to divergent sites. Possibly such a mechanism accounts for the radiation of pain to the upper abdomen in cardiac infarctions and for the pain that resembles heart pain in acute abdominal accidents. In this connection, it is interesting that Wertheimer and Leriche observed the occurrence of

Fig. 8-17. (*A*) Course of cardiac sensory fibers along sympathetic nerves through the white rami and into the posterior spinal root. (*B*) Pathways of the fibers in the cervical and dorsal region. (*C*) Intraspinal pain tracts transmitting pain impulses from the heart to corticosensory areas. The ascending internuncials pass from the posterior horn cranially as far as the spinal nucleus of the trigeminal and provide the pathways of referral of cardiac pain to the arm, neck, and face.

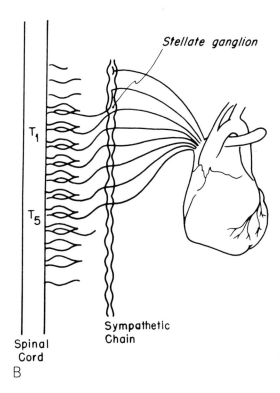

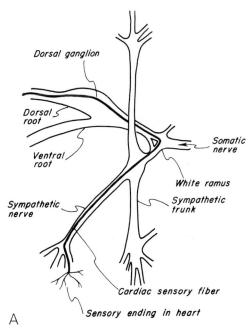

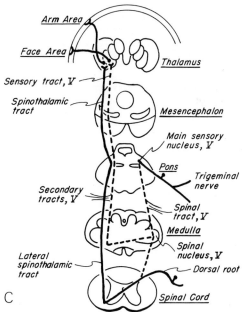

severe anginal symptoms upon stimulation of the central end of the severed greater splanchnic nerves in patients at operation.[84,85]

AORTIC PAIN

MECHANISM OF AORTIC PAIN

Clinical and experimental evidence indicates that the lesions of the aorta or of the smaller arteries in general may produce pain. The painful dilations of the cranial arteries in migraine and the pain produced by arterial punctures for clinical studies are common examples. It is generally held that the adventitia of large blood vessels contain pain fibers.[87] Spiegel and Wassermann found that acute stretching of the wall of the aortic arch produces pain.[88] They demonstrated also that coating the aorta with irritating substances had profoundly painful effects. These authors concluded that aortic pain results from stimulation of the adventitia.

Afferent aortic pain fibers appear to run in close relation to those from the heart. White has observed that the intractable pain of angina pectoris or aneurysm is abated by resection of the upper five thoracic ganglia, or the rami communicantes, or by interruption of the corresponding dorsal roots proximal to the root ganglia.[86] Aortic pain neurones pass to the sympathetic chain ganglia from the aortic plexus, traverse the rami communicantes, and reach their cell bodies in the dorsal root ganglia (Fig. 8-17).

It has been suggested that the pain of dissecting aneurysm of the aorta occurs because of marked distention of the adventitial coat.[86] On the other hand, syphilitic aortitis may lead to aneurysms of great size without discomfort to the patient. Syphilitic aortitis may give rise to attacks of angina pectoris by reducing the coronary flow through involvement of the mouths of the coronary arteries. Occasionally aoritis may provoke substernal discomfort that is dull, burning, and continuous. Mills and Horton have suggested that such pain in some cases of aortic aneurysm results from sudden distention of the aneurysmal sac.[54] They observed that the pain was frequently aggravated by recumbency, exercise, cough, or deep breathing. In our experience, aortitis and aneurysms due to syphilis have rarely been observed to produce painful symptoms, unless saccular dilatation had become so large as to impinge upon the chest wall or spine.

It is difficult to understand how the marked dilatation of syphilitic aortic aneurysm occurs with so little pain. Possibly in the slowly dilating aorta, adventitial distortion is gradual, and forceful stimuli to adventitial pain endings are not present. A further possibility is

that afferent nerve endings may be destroyed largely by extensive syphilitic involvement of the vasa vasorum and the adventitia.

Quite in contrast to syphilitic aneurysms are the sudden disruptions of the aortic coats termed aortic dissecting aneurysms that are frequently accompanied by agonizing pain. At present it is uncertain whether the primary pathologic event is rupture of a diseased intima with secondary dissection of the media or hemorrhage into a diseased media from a ruptured vasa vasorum with subsequent disruption of subjacent intima and propagation of the dissection through the intimal tear.[122] Blood enters the intimal tear under aortic pressure and splits apart the layers of the arterial wall. In the process of dissection, the muscle coats are torn apart and the adventitia in places may be lifted from the underlying media. Intense distention of the portions of the wall outside the burrowing column of blood occurs.

We have frequently observed dissecting aneurysms in open chest experimental dog preparations.* If the blood pressure is normal or high, and the aortic intima is then torn by a blunt instrument, blood burrows into the aortic wall so that the adventitia and a few strands of the medial coat are raised as a huge, bulbous purplish swelling, which creeps distally along the aorta. The aneurysmal sac becomes thin and tenuous in places where there is subadventitial dissection; elsewhere the sac may be firmer from support of underlying dissected layers of the media. Seepage from the thinner parts of the sac usually occurs, terminating in rupture. Pathologic evidence indicates that a similar mechanical rending of the vessel may occur in patients.[89] The basic lesion leading to aortic dissection appears to be medial cystic necrosis of the wall of the vessel.[90–92] The evidence offered by Bauersfeld indicates that cystic disease of the media causes a rupture of the vasa vasorum with the formation of medial hematomas;[94] the hematomas may split the aortic wall. Schlatmann believes there are continual processes of injury and repair within the aortic wall that are detected pathologically as cystic medial necrosis, elastin fragmentation, and fibrosis.[123,124] These processes may gradually lead to aortic dilatation, and, according to Laplace's law, a vicious cycle set up in which local circumstances determine whether a complete or incomplete dissection will occur. Most patients with dissecting aneurysms have had preexisting arterial hypertension. Marked elevation of blood pressure may facilitate rapid disruption and final rupture of the aortic wall when a small tear in the intima has occurred.

---

*Smith, JF, Paine R: Unpublished observations.

CHARACTERISTICS OF AORTIC PAIN

Clinically, aortic pain is recognized most clearly when dissecting aneurysms occur. Such pain may be dramatic; it is sudden in onset and quickly becomes severe and agonizing. When the aneurysm is confined to the aortic arch, the pain is substernal or diffuses over the upper anterior chest. It may be projected to the shoulders.[89,93] Projection into the arms is infrequent. As dissection proceeds over the arch and into the descending aorta, extreme pain may be felt at the base of the neck and along the back, particularly in the interscapular area. The agony is continuous and requires heavy narcotization. Although grayish cyanosis and other signs of visceromotor reflex disturbances appear, the blood pressure usually is sustained. In the grip of such pain, some patients may be distraught; they may climb in and out of bed, roll about, assume grotesque postures, or press their chests against chairs or walls in an effort to obtain relief.*

This behavior is in contrast to that of persons with myocardial infarction, who may lie quietly, and often exhibit signs of collapse. Dramatic relief from the pain of dissecting aneurysm may follow therapeutic reduction of blood pressure with hypotensive drugs. Specifically, those agents that reduce the abrupt systolic rise in aortic pressures appear to be effective in relief of pain and in prevention of further dissection. Cases of dissecting aneurysm are described in which symptoms have been transient or mild, suggesting angina pectoris.[89] In some cases (usually found unexpectedly at necropsy) no pain has occurred, although the aorta may be extensively damaged.

Perry has drawn attention to incomplete rupture of the aorta.[95] This lesion is produced by an intimal tear without dissection of the vessel wall. It may provoke severe substernal pain of a "stabbing" or "tearing" quality, but it is not as severe as that of dissecting aneurysm. This pain may be confused with that of coronary occlusion. Incomplete rupture of the aorta can give way to dissection of the aortic wall at any time.

SUMMARY

The essential clinical features of thoracic pain have been presented briefly, and the painful symptoms interpreted in light of the underlying, known pathologic physiology. Pain arising from the chest wall, thoracic respiratory system, mediastinum, esophagus, and cardiovascular system is discussed.

*Tillman C: Personal communication.

REFERENCES

1. **Heinbecker P:** Heart pain. J Thorac Surg 10:44, 1940
2. **Heinbecker P, Bishop GH, O'Leary J:** Pain and touch fibres in peripheral nerves. Arch Neurol Psychiatr 29:771, 1933
3. **Lewis T:** Pain. New York, Macmillan, 1942
4. **Moore RM:** Stimulation of peripheral nerve elements subserving pain-sensibility by intra-arterial injections of neutral solutions. Am J Physiol 110:191, 1934
5. **Hamilton JB:** The pathways and production of pain. Yale J Biol Med 9:215, 1936-1937
6. **Lewis T:** Suggestions relating to the study of somatic pain. Br Med J 1:321, 1938
7. **Behan RJ:** Pain. New York, Appleton-Century-Crofts, 1920
8. **Weller TH, Whitton HM, Bell JE:** The etiologic agents of varicella and herpes zoster: Isolation, propagation, and cultural characteristics in vitro. J Exp Med 108:843, 1958
9. **Hope-Simpson RE:** The nature of herpes zoster. A long term study and a new hypothesis. Proc R Soc Med 58:9, 1965
10. **Holmes JF:** Slipping rib cartilage, with report of cases. Am J Surg 54:326, 1941
11. **White PD:** Diseases of the Coronary Arteries and Cardiac Pain. New York, Macmillan, 1936
12. **Dixon RH:** Cure or relief of cases misdiagnosed "angina of effort." Br Med J 2:891, 1938
13. **Schmidt R:** Pain: Its Causation and Diagnostic Significance in Internal Diseases. Vogel KM, Zinsser H (trans): Philadelphia, JB Lippincott, 1911
14. **Healey LA:** Polymyalgia rheumatica, pp 681–684. In McCarty DJ (ed): Arthritis and Allied Conditions: A Textbook of Rheumatology, 9th ed. Philadelphia, Lea & Febiger, 1979
15. **Graham EA, Singer JJ, Ballon HC:** Surgical Diseases of the Chest. Philadelphia, Lea & Febiger, 1935
16. **Craver LF:** Tenderness of the sternum in leukemia. AM J Med Sci 174:799, 1927
17. **Zoneraich S:** Diabetes and the Heart. Springfield, Il, Charles C Thomas, 1978
18. **Davis D:** Spinal nerve root pain (radiculitis) simulating coronary occlusion: A common syndrome. Am Heart J 35:70, 1948
19. **Davis D:** Radicular syndromes with emphasis on chest pain simulating coronary disease. Chicago, Year Book Medical Publishers, 1957
20. **Fitzwilliams DCL:** On the Breast. St Louis, C V Mosby, 1924
21. **Geschickter CF:** Diseases of the Breast. Philadelphia, JB Lippincott, 1943
22. **Labbe L, Coyne P:** Traité des Tumeurs Bénignes du Sein. Paris, Masson, 1876

23. **Veil P:** Cellulite du sein et engine de poitrine. Arch Mal Coeur 25:703, 1932

24. **de Cholnoky T:** Benign tumors of the breast. AMA Arch Surg 38:79, 1939

25. **Cheatle G, Cutler M:** Tumors of the Breast. Philadelphia, JB Lippincott, 1931

26. **Roberts WC:** Coronary arteries in fatal acute myocardial infarction. Circulation 45:215, 1972

27. **Morton DR, Klassen KP, Curtis GM:** The effect of high vagus section upon the clinical physiology of the bronchi. Proceedings of the Central Society for Clinical Research, J Lab Clin Med 34:1730, 1949

28. **Bonner LM:** Primary lung tumor. JAMA 94:1044, 1930

29. **Capps JA, Coleman GH:** An Experimental and Clinical Study of Pain in the Pleura, Pericardium and Peritoneum. New York, Macmillan, 1932

30. **Dybdahl GL:** The control of pleuritic pain by the use of cutaneous anesthesia. Permanente Foundation Medical Bulletin 2:30, 1944

31. **Bray HA:** The tension theory of pleuritic pain. American Review of Tuberculosis 13:14, 1926

32. **Krause GR, Chester EM:** Infarction of the lung: Clinical and roentgenological study. AMA Arch Intern Med 67:1144, 1941

33. **Carlson HA, Ballon HC:** The operability of carcinoma of the lung. J Thorac Surg 2:323, 1933

34. **Ornstein GG, Ulmar D:** Clinical Tuberculosis, Vol II, G-21. Philadelphia, FA Davis, 1941

35. **Kiss F, Ballon HC:** Contribution of the nerve supply of the diaphragm. Anat Rec 41:285, 1928–1929

36. **Hinsey JC, Phillips RA:** Observations upon diaphragmatic sensation. J Neurophysiol 3:175, 1940

37. **Master AM, Dack S, Stone J et al:** Differential diagnosis of hiatus hernia and coronary artery disease. AMA Arch Surg 58:428, 1949

38. **Jones CM, Chapman WP:** Studies on the mechanism of the pain in angina pectoris with particular relation to hiatus hernia. Trans Assoc AM Physicians 57:139, 1942

39. **Moor F:** The cause of "stitch." Br Med J 2:282, 1923

40. **Capps R:** Cause of the so-called side ache that occurs in normal persons. AMA Arch Intern Med 68:94, 1941

41. **Barnes AR, Burchell HB:** Acute pericarditis simulating acute coronary occlusion. Am Heart J 23:247, 1942

42. **Camp PD, White PD:** Pericardial effusion: A clinical study. Am J Med Sci 184:728, 1932

43. **Harvey AM, Whitehill MR:** Tuberculous pericarditis. Medicine 16:45, 1937

44. **Paine WW, Poulton EP:** Experiments on visceral sensation. I. The relation of pain to activity in the human esophagus. J Physiol 63:217, 1927

45. **Hurst AF, Rake GW:** Achalasia of the cardia. Q J Med 23:491, 1929–1930

46. **Alvarez WC:** An Introduction to Gastroenterology. New York, Paul B Hoeber, 1941

47. **Neuhof H, Rabin CB:** Acute mediastinitis: Roentgenological, pathological and clinical features and principles of operative treatment. Am J Roentgenol 44:684, 1940

48. **Furstenburg AC:** Acute mediastinal suppuration. Transactions of the American Laryngological, Rhinological and Otological Society, p 210, 1929

49. **Hamman L:** Spontaneous mediastinal emphysema. Bulletin of the Johns Hopkins Hospital 64:1, 1939

50. **McLester JW:** Diseases of the mediastinum. In Christian HA (ed): Oxford Medicine. New York, Oxford University Press, 1949

51. **Pick F:** Über chronische unter dem Bilde der Lebercirrhose verlaufende Perikarditis (perikarditische Pseudolebercirrhose) nebst Bemerkungen über die Zuckergussleber (Curschmann). Zeitschrift Fur Klinische Medizin 29:385, 1896

52. **Middleton WS:** Some clinical caprices of Hodgkin's disease. Ann Intern Med 11:448, 1937

53. **Pancoast HK:** Superior pulmonary sulcus tumor. Tumor characterized by pain, Horner's syndrome, destruction of bone and atrophy of hand muscles. JAMA 99:1391, 1932

54. **Mills JH, Horton BT:** Clinical aspects of aneurysm. AMA Arch Intern Med 62:949, 1938

55. **Heberden W:** Pectoris dolor. In Major RH (ed): Classic Descriptions of Disease. Baltimore, Thomas, 1932

56. **Herrick JB:** Clinical features of sudden obstruction of the coronary arteries. JAMA 59:2015, 1912

57. **Sutton DC, Lueth HC:** Pain. AMA Arch Intern Med 45:827, 1930

58. **Pearcy JF, Priest WS, Van Allen CM:** Pain due to the temporary occlusion of the coronary arteries in dogs. Am Heart J 4:390, 1928–1929

59. **Keefer CS, Resnik WH:** Angina Pectoris: A syndrome caused by anoxemia of the myocardium. AMA Arch Intern Med 41:769, 1928

60. **Wenckebach KF:** Angina pectoris and the possibilities of its surgical relief. Br Med J 1:809, 1924

61. **Gorham LW, Martin SJ:** Coronary occlusion with and without pain. AMA Arch Intern Med 62:821, 1938

62. **Lewis T, Pickering GW, Rothschild P:** Observations upon muscular pain in intermittent claudication. Heart 15:359, 1931

63. **Katz LN, Linder E, Landt H:** On the nature of the substance(s) producing pain in contracting skeletal muscle: Its bearing on the problems of angina pectoris and intermittent claudication. J Clin Invest 14:807, 1935

64. **Blumgart HL, Schlesinger MJ, Davis D:** Studies on the relation of the clinical manifestations of angina pectoris, coronary thrombosis, and myocardial infarction to the pathological findings. Am Heart J 19:1, 1940

65. **Smith JR, Henry MJ:** Demonstration of the coronary arterial system with neoprene latex. J Lab Clin Med 30:462, 1945

66. **Prinzmetal M, Bergman HC, Kruger HE et al:** Studies on the coronary circulation. III. Collateral circulation of beating human and dog hearts with coronary occlusion. Am Heart J 35:689, 1948

67. **Gregg DE, Pritchard WH, Shipley RE et al:** Augmentation of blood flow in the coronary arteries with elevation of right ventricular pressure. Am J Physiol 139:726, 1943

68. **Smith JR, Jensen J:** Observations on the effect of theophylline amino-isobutanol in experimental heart failure. J Lab Clin Med 31:850, 1946

69. **Smith JR, Layton IC:** The flow of blood supplying the cardiac atria. Proc Soc Exp Biol Med 62:59, 1946

70. **Visscher MB:** The restriction of the coronary flow as a general factor in heart failure. JAMA 113:987, 1939

71. **Riseman JEF, Brown MG:** The duration of attacks of angina pectoris on exertion and the effect of nitroglycerine and amyl nitrite. N Engl J Med 217:470, 1937

72. **Freedberg AS, Spiegel ED, Riseman JEF:** Effect of external heat and cold on patients with angina pectoris: Evidences for the existence of a reflex factor. Am Heart J 27:611, 1944

73. **Herrick JB:** The coronary artery in health and disease. Am Heart J 6:589, 1930–1931

74. **Fenn GK, Gilbert NC:** Anginal pain as a result of digitalis administration. JAMA 98:99, 1932

75. **Gold H, Otto H, Kwit NT et al:** Does digitalis influence the course of cardiac pain? A study of 120 selected cases of angina pectoris. JAMA 110:895, 1938

76. **Harrison TR:** Clinical aspects of pain in the chest. I. Angina pectoris. Am J Med Sci 207:561, 1944

77. **Gallavardin L:** Syndromes angineux anormaux. Médecine 18:193, 1937

78. **Levine SA:** Coronary thrombosis, its various clinical features. Medicine 8:245, 1929

79. **Levine SA, Tranter CL:** Infarction of the heart simulating acute surgical abdominal conditions. Am J Med Sci 155:57, 1918

80. **Breyfogle HS:** The frequency of coexisting gallbladder and coronary artery disease. JAMA 114:1434, 1940

81. **Ernstene AC, Rinell J:** Pain in the shoulder as a sequel to myocardial infarction. AMA Arch Intern Med 66:800, 1940

82. **Askey JM:** The syndrome of painful disability of the shoulder and hand complicating coronary occlusion. Am Heart J 22:1, 1941

83. **Miller HR:** Interrelationship of disease of the coronary arteries and gallbladder. Am Heart J 24:579, 1942

84. **Wertheimer P:** A propos des doleurs provoquées par l'excitation des grands splanchniques. Presse Méd 45:1628, 1937

85. **Leriche R:** Des doleurs provoquées par l'excitation des grands splanchniques. Presse Méd 45:971, 1937

86. **White JC:** The neurological mechanism of cardio-aortic pain. J Nerv Ment Dis 15:181, 1935

87. **Singer R:** Experimentelle Studien über die Schmerzempfindlichkeit des Herzens und der grossen Gefässe und ihre Beziehung zur Angina Pectoris. Wiener Archiv Fur Innere Medizin 12:193, 1926

88. **Spiegel EA, Wassermann S:** Experimentelle Studien über die Entstehung des Aortenschmerzes und sein Leitung zum Zentralnervensystem. Zeitschrift Fur Die Gesamte Experimentelle Medizin 52:180, 1926

89. **Flaxman N:** Dissecting aneurysm of the aorta. Am Heart J 24:654, 1942

90. **Erdheim J:** Medionecrosis aortae idiopathica cystica. Virchow Archiv Fur Pathologische Anatomie 276:187, 1930

91. **Sailer S:** Dissecting aneurysm of the aorta. AMA Arch Pathol 33:704, 1942

92. **Niehaus FW, Wright WD:** Dissecting aneurysm of the aorta. J Lab Clin Med 26:1248, 1941

93. **Kountz WB, Hempelmann L:** Chromotropic degeneration and rupture of the aorta following thyroidectomy in cases of hypertension. Am Heart J 20:599, 1940

94. **Bauersfeld SR:** Dissecting aneurysm of the aorta: A presentation of fifteen cases and a review of the recent literature. Ann Intern Med 26:873, 1947

95. **Perry TM:** Incomplete rupture of the aorta: Heretofore unrecognized stage of dissecting aneurysm and cause of cardiac pain and cardiac murmurs. AMA Arch Intern Med 70:689, 1942

96. **Mazur MH, Dolin R:** Herpes zoster at the NIH: A twenty year experience. Am J Med 65:738, 1978

97. **Dolin R, Reichman RC, Mazur MH et al:** Herpes zoster–varicella infections in immunosuppressed patients. Ann Intern Med 89:375, 1978

98. **Davis D:** Radicular Syndromes with Emphasis on Chest Pain Simulating Coronary Disease. Chicago, Year Book Medical Publishers, 1957

99. **Steinbrocker O:** Shoulder–hand syndrome. Am J Med 3:402, 1947

100. **Edeiken J:** Shoulder–hand syndrome. Circulation 16:14, 1957

101. **Dressler W, Yurkoksky J, McStarr M:** Hemorrhagic pericarditis, pleurisy, and pneumonia complicating recent myocardial infarction. Am Heart J 54:42, 1957

102. **Dressler W:** A post-myocardial infarction syndrome. JAMA 160:1379, 1956

103. **Weiser NJ, Kantor M, Russell HK:** Posterior myocardial infarction syndrome. Circulation 20:371, 1959

104. **Gregg DE:** Physiology of the coronary circulation. Circulation 27:1128, 1963

105. **White JC:** Cardiac pain, anatomic pathways and physiologic mechanisms. Circulation 16:644, 1957

106. **Scheuer J, Brachfeld N:** Coronary insufficiency: Relations between hemodynamic, electrical, and biochemical parameters. Circ Res 18:178, 1966

107. **Herman MV, Eliot WC, Gorlin R:** An electrocardiographic, anatomic, metabolic study of zonal myocardial

ischemia in coronary heart disease. Circulation 35:834, 1967

108. **Proudfit WL, Shirey EK, Sones FM:** Selective cine coronary arteriography: Correlation with clinical findings in 1000 patients. Circulation 33:901, 1966

109. **Flower RJ:** Aspirin-like drugs and prostaglandins. Am Heart J 86:844, 1973

110. **Roberts WC:** Relationship between coronary thrombosis and myocardial infarction. Mod Concepts Cardiovasc Dis 41:7, 1972

111. **Mustard JF:** Platelets and thrombosis in acute myocardial infarction. Hosp pract 7:115, 1972

112. **Spencer IC:** Bypass grafting for pre-infarction angina. Circulation 45:1314, 1972

113. **Cosby RS, Giddings JA, See JR et al:** Variant angina. Am J Med 53:739, 1972

114. **Maseri A:** Coronary artery spasm, a cause of acute myocardial ischemia in man. Chest 68:5, 1975

115. **Hillis LD, Braunwald E:** Coronary-artery spasm. N Engl J Med 299(13):695, 1978

116. **Yasue H, Omote S, Takazawa A et al:** Circadian variations of exercise capacity in patients with Prinzmetal's variant angina: Role of exercise-induced coronary arterial spasm. Circulation 59:938, 1979

117. **Levin DC:** Pathways and functional significance of the coronary collateral circulation. Circulation 50:831, 1974

118. **Gregg DE, Patterson RE:** Functional importance of the coronary collaterals. N Engl J Med 303:1404, 1980

119. **Newman PE:** The coronary collateral circulation: Determinants and functional significance in ischemic heart disease. Am Heart J 102:433, 1981

120. **Mehta J, Mehta P:** Role of blood platelets and prostaglandins in coronary artery disease. Am J Cardiol 48:366, 1981

121. **Devereaux RB, Perloff JK, Reichek N et al:** Mitral valve prolapse. Circulation 54:3, 1976

122. **Slater EE, DeSanctis RW:** Diseases of the aorta. In Braunwald E (ed): Heart Disease. Philadelphia, W B Saunders, 1980

123. **Schlatmann TJ, Becker AE:** Pathogenesis of dissecting aneurysm of the aorta: Comparative study of significance of medial changes. Am J Cardiol 39:21, 1977

124. **Schlatmann TJ, Becker AE:** Histologic changes in the normal aging aorta: Implications for dissecting aortic aneurysm. Am J Cardiol 39:3, 1977

9

Abdominal Pain Richard D. Aach

History
Anatomy and Physiology
Pathways
Types of Deep Pain
  True Visceral Pain
  Deep Somatic Pain
  Referred Pain
Clinical Analysis
  History
    Location
    Quality Type of Onset
    Temporal Features
    Intensity
    Circumstances that Produce, Intensify, or
      Reduce Pain

  Associated Features
  Physical Examination
  Laboratory Tests and Diagnostic Procedures
Etiologic Classification of Abdominal Pain
  Intestinal Tract
    Esophagus
    Stomach
    Small and Large Intestines
  Pancreas, Liver, and Biliary Tract
  Peritonitis
  Genitourinary Tract
  Other Causes of Abdominal Pain
Acute Abdomen
Summary

Despite the many recent advances in diagnostic and laboratory procedures, a carefully taken detailed history still plays an invaluable role in the diagnosis of intra-abdominal diseases. Of paramount importance in the history is the evaluation of pain. It is the rare patient with an abdominal disorder who does not complain of pain. Often it is the only or the chief complaint. In contrast to pain in many other regions of the body, abdominal pain offers to the diagnostician a unique and at times frustrating challenge.

Intense pain in any portion of the abdomen may be the result of a variety of conditions, some benign, others demanding immediate attention. Pain can be experienced in an area that is far removed from the actual site of the disorder, and various disorders involving different organs can produce pain of similar character. Nevertheless, important patterns exist that can lead directly to the correct diagnosis. The assessment of ab-

dominal pain, therefore, demands critical judgment and a very careful search for all of its pertinent features.

HISTORY

Studies on the nature of abdominal pain date back more than 300 years. In 1760, the Swiss physiologist, von Haller, demonstrated that the visceral peritoneum, like the visceral pericardium and pleura, is insensible to mechanical stimuli, such as pinching and cutting. Despite the significance of these observations, little information was added until the turn of the last century. With the emergence of the fields of neuroanatomy and neurophysiology in the late 1800s, the problem of the sites of origin of abdominal pain became a subject of considerable interest. Soon there was controversy as

to the existence of true visceral pain, and heated debate continued well into the present century.

Essentially, there were two schools of thought on visceral pain. One school, with Ross as an early champion, held that there are two distinct types of visceral pain: splanchnic, or true visceral pain, experienced in the region of the stimulated organ; and somatic, or referred pain, experienced in somatic structures served by the same neural segment. The second school, with Mackenzie as the main protagonist, believed that all visceral pain is referred pain. According to this concept, abdominal viscera lack pain fibers; however, afferent pathways do exist that are capable of carrying nonpainful impulses from a visceral organ to the spinal cord by way of the sympathetics. These impulses could produce an "irritable focus" upon reaching the spinal cord, resulting in the stimulation of adjacent pathways, and thereby giving rise to the sensation of pain in somatic structures supplied by the same segment of the spinal cord. This view was supported by the studies of Lennander, who, like von Haller, demonstrated that abdominal viscera are insensible to the applications of heat and cold, clipping, cutting, and burning with caustics. On the other hand, pain was evoked when somatic nerves in the parietal peritoneum, mesentery, and subserous connective tissue were stimulated by torsion or traction.

The heat of this debate between the two schools has dissipated with time, and many of the hypotheses advanced during this early period of study have since been discarded. What remains, however, are many critical and careful observations. A notable example is the contribution of Head, who systematically mapped out the peripheral distribution of referred pain for each of the neural segments of the spinal cord. He also stressed that hyperalgesia was a common finding in an area of referred pain. To his credit, the term "Head zones of hyperalgesia" is still used to denote this important feature of referred pain.

It is now generally accepted that visceral structures do have a sensory apparatus that can give rise to the sensation of pain when properly stimulated. Although it is less well developed than the corresponding somatic sensory system with respect to size and number of nerve fibers, studies by Hertz, and later Ryle, demonstrate that pain can be elicited by stretching or distending visceral organs, or by contracting them if rapid and extreme in nature. The observations of René Leriche added further evidence that true visceral pain could be produced by vigorous contraction of the intestinal tract. However, under certain conditions, even ordinary mechanical stimuli can evoke pain. The very thorough studies of Wolff and Wolf convincingly demonstrated that pinching or faradic stimulation gives rise to visceral pain when the mucosal surface of a visceral organ is inflamed, congested, or edematous. Furthermore, ischemia due to vascular insufficiency also can lower the pain threshold so that ordinarily nonnoxious stimuli can give rise to the sensation of pain. Pain of intra-abdominal origin, therefore, may originate from the parietal peritoneum, mesentery, splanchnic vessels, and visceral organs themselves under the appropriate circumstances.

ANATOMY AND PHYSIOLOGY

Transmission of pain is carried in the peripheral nervous system by two types of nerve fibers. The first, A-delta fibers are myelinated, 2 $m\mu$ to 5 $m\mu$ in diameter, arising primarily from somatic structures, such as the integument, and are responsible for "bright" or "sharp" well-localized pain, which rapidly follows, for example, a blow to the finger. Impulses from these fibers are conducted at a rate of 12 m to 30 m per second. The second type of pain neurons are smaller unmyelinated C fibers, 0.4 μm–1.2 μm in diameter, which transmit impulses at a rate of 0.5 m to 2 m per second. These are the afferent neurons arising from the parietal peritoneum, abdominal and pelvic viscera, and the capsules of the liver, kidney, and spleen. Stimulation of C fibers produces pain of more gradual onset, "dull and aching" in character, usually poorly localized; it may be associated with nausea and automatic symptoms, such as sweating.

Intra-abdominal pain, as described in the previous section, can be elicited by (1) stretching of viscera, (2) distention, usually rapid, of a hollow structure, such as the intestine, ureter, or a biliary duct, (3) traction on the peritoneum or mesentery, and even mesenteric blood vessels that also contain afferent nerve fibers, (4) vigorous muscular contraction(s) of the intestine, (5) inflammation—whether infectious or chemical, (6) ischemia, and finally, (7) pain that may result from invasion of afferent neurons by neoplasm, such as carcinoma of the pancreas.

Crushing or cutting injuries to visceral structures do not ordinarily evoke pain unless the threshold for pain sensation has been lowered by other factors, such as inflammation or vascular insufficiency. There is some evidence that pain impulses are initiated by the release of a chemical agent, possibly a kinin, liberated at the site of injury or stimulation by proteolytic enzymes as a result of noxious stimuli.

PATHWAYS

The abdominal viscera and their supporting structures lack specific pain receptors. Rather, pain follows excitation of free nerve endings located in the viscera, mes-

entery, or parietal peritoneum. The number of visceral pain afferents are few in number in contrast to somatic structures; this in large part accounts for why visceral pain is poorly localized.

Pain felt in the abdomen is either transmitted through spinal roots T6 through T12 or referred to these segments through impulses traveling from neighboring structures in the chest, extremities, or pelvis. Some structures within the chest are innervated from segments as low as T9. Therefore, the location of the sensation of pain in the chest or abdomen does not necessarily establish the site of the disease with certainty.

Sensory impulses of somatic origin (integument and parietal peritoneum) travel by somatic afferent neurons to the dorsal root ganglia, and then into the region of the posterior horn of the spinal cord (Fig. 9-1). In the gray matter, the impulses are transmitted to a second neuron, which crosses to the opposite side of the cord and ascends to the thalamus through the lateral spinothalamic tract. In the thalamus, impulses pass to a third neuron, whose axon ends in the cerebral cortex in the region of the postcentral gyrus.

Sensory impulses from visceral structures within the abdomen are carried by visceral afferent nerve fibers, which accompany the sympathetics to the dorsal root ganglia by way of the rami communicantes. From the dorsal root ganglia, these fibers enter the posterior horn

of the spinal cord, along with somatic neurons. Once inside the central nervous system, sensory impulses of visceral origin travel along the same pathways as pain impulses arising in somatic structures. It is important to remember that on entering the spinal cord, these fibers may travel caudally or cranially for several segments in the posterior horn of the gray matter before synapsing with neurons in the dorsal horn, further contributing to the difficulty in precisely localizing the exact site of visceral pain. In addition, an extensive network of relays from other sensory neurons and from higher centers are also present within the dorsal horn. Impulses from these relays may substantially alter C fiber afferent sensations so as to intensify, diminish, or even abolish the sensation of visceral pain.

TYPES OF DEEP PAIN

There are three general categories of deep abdominal pain.

TRUE VISCERAL PAIN

True visceral pain is felt at the site of primary stimulation and may or may not be associated with referred pain. It is eliminated by infiltration of procaine into the site of noxious stimulation or by blocking of its afferent nerves. It is not altered by infiltration of procaine into other structures supplied by the same or adjacent neural segments. True visceral pain is characteristically dull and aching in character. It is diffuse and deep in location, often experienced in the midabdomen. The patient and physician may have a difficult time trying to localize the site of the pain, which roughly corresponds to the segmental location of the visceral structure producing the sensory impulses. Examples of true visceral pain are the initial midabdominal pain of acute appendicitis, and the discomfort experienced early in intestinal obstruction or cholecystitis.

DEEP SOMATIC PAIN

Deep somatic (parietal) pain arises from noxious stimulation of the parietal peritoneum and the root of the mesentery. Since pain impulses are transmitted by way of the cerebrospinal pathways, this form of pain is generally very intense and sharply circumscribed, and is appreciated in an area closely approximating that region being stimulated. Because the same central pathways subserve the more superficial areas of the same neural segment including the skin, deep somatic pain often is accompanied by referred pain. The sharply localized pain of acute appendicitis following the spread of inflammation to the parietal peritoneum or the in-

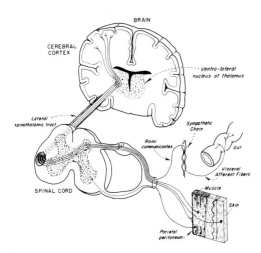

Fig. 9-1. Afferent pathways of abdominal pain. Afferent visceral fibers carried in the sympathetic chain pass through the rami communicantes to the spinal cord where their sensory impulses travel in the same pathways as do impulses of superficial and deep afferent somatic origins. After crossing to the opposite side, the afferent impulses ascend in the lateral spinothalamic tract to the ventrolateral nucleus of the thalamus and then to the postcentral gyrus of the cerebral cortex.

tense pain of peritonitis are examples of deep somatic pain.

REFERRED PAIN

Pain experienced at a site other than that stimulated, but in tissues supplied by the same or adjacent neural segments, is called "referred pain." Thus, painful stimulation of visceral or deep somatic structures gives rise to the sensation of pain in more superficial areas of the body (*e.g.*, skin) supplied by the same, and occasionally neighboring, segments of the spinal cord. Spread of excitation occurs because impulses from visceral organs, and both superficial and deep somatic structures, share common pathways inside the central nervous system. Referred pain may occur in addition to or in the virtual absence of true visceral and deep somatic pain. An entire dermatome or neural segment need not be involved. As a rule, however, referred pain usually is experienced only when the painful stimulus is sufficiently intense or when the pain threshold of a viscus or organ has been lowered by disease.

Characteristically, referred pain is sharp in character and relatively well localized, often to the lateral aspects of the abdomen or back. The right subscapular pain of acute cholecystitis or biliary colic is an example of referred pain. A heightened degree of discomfort to other painful stimuli applied to the area of referred pain (head zones of hyperalgesia) and local tenderness may frequently accompany and may rarely constitute the principal form to discomfort of an intra-abdominal disease. Alteration in effector or motor activity may also accompany referred pain. Skeletal muscle contraction, appreciated as "muscle guarding," often is demonstrable in the segment of referred pain. Muscular contraction, if prolonged, may itself be a new source of pain and local tenderness. In the same way, efferent impulses may stimulate other structures in the area of referred pain, including blood vessels and glands. This may be appreciated by observing a difference in the skin temperature and moisture in the region of referred pain. Hyperalgesia and muscle guarding are present to their fullest extent in association with the deep somatic pain of generalized peritonitis.

CLINICAL ANALYSIS

HISTORY

Because abdominal structures by and large have poorly developed sensory systems and because afferent impulses travel over a limited number of nerve pathways, determining the source of abdominal pain can be very difficult. All too often, the findings on physical examination are minimal or entirely absent. Therefore, the patient's history, past and present, is of extreme importance. Attention must be paid to details that are best obtained in a methodical fashion. If the patient is alert, the most accurate description is given when pain is being experienced or shortly thereafter. Questioning on more than one occasion may be required.

Patients vary widely in sensitivity to pain, in psychic and emotional reactions to pain, and in ability to describe their sensations of pain. Causes of variation among patients include such factors as age, education, and verbal ability. Patients may be able to describe even the most severe forms of abdominal pain in only very simple and general terms. Words such as "gas pains," "cramps," or "indigestion" are heard frequently by physician, and each may represent an entirely different pain experience to different persons. Therefore, the physician must not be content with only such vague descriptions, but must seek additional information by careful, systematic questioning. Abdominal pain should be characterized according to its (1) location, (2) quality, (3) type of onset, (4) temporal features, (5) intensity, (6) circumstances that produce or modify it, and (7) associated features.

Location

The site of pain can be a very valuable clue to its origin. Pain of the upper gastrointestinal tract is usually experienced low in the anterior chest or high in the abdomen, often in the midline. For example, esophagitis is felt as a burning sensation substernally or in the epigastrium, where the pain of a peptic ulcer also may be experienced. The pain of an active ulcer tends to be sharply localized; the patient may be able to point a finger to the exact site of pain. On the other hand, the abdominal pain experienced in gastroenteritis or in psychophysiologic gastrointestinal disease usually is diffuse and poorly localized.

Appendicitis and regional enteritis are examples of disorders that most often produce right lower quadrant pain, whereas diverticulitis usually gives rise to low abdominal pain, either in the midline or left lower quadrant. The pain of renal colic characteristically is felt in the flank, and radiates toward the groin, whereas the pain of cholecystitis usually is experienced in the right upper quadrant, where pain referred from basilar pneumonitis also may be felt.

Quality

Whether the pain sensation originates in the superficial or the deep structures often can be determined by the quality of the pain. Pricking or itching pains come

from superficial tissues such as the skin, whereas dull aching or colicky pain characteristically arises in deeper structures. The sensation of burning or "gnawing" is typical of peptic ulcer disease and peptic esophagitis.

Type of Onset

The type of onset, whether gradual or sudden, may provide very useful information. The pain of cholecystitis often begins gradually and builds in intensity, whereas the pain of renal colic, rupture of the viscus with resultant peritonitis, or mesenteric artery occlusion usually begins suddenly, and is maximal from the very onset.

Temporal Features

It is important to determine whether the pain is intermittent, continuous, pulsatile, or colicky in nature. The duration of a painful experience and its periodicity or frequency of occurrence in terms of minutes, days, or even season may provide valuable information. The colicky pain of biliary tract origin is likely to be intermittent, whereas the pain of acute pancreatitis and pancreatic carinoma often is persistent and unchanging; the pain of pancreatitis lasts hours to days, whereas the pain of a pancreatic neoplasm may be a constant feature for weeks to months. An abdominal aneurysm may produce pulsatile pain. Intestinal obstruction or gastroenteritis is characterized by intermittent cramping pain ("griping"), which comes and goes in a wave-like rhythm. In the female, intense but brief pain in the lower abdomen or back, known as "mittelschmerz," may occur at midmonth between menstrual periods, at the time of ovulation. Exacerbation of peptic ulcer disease are most common in the spring and fall of the year, whereas the pain of psychophysiologic gastrointestinal disease often is related to periods of emotional stress that the patient may or may not recognize.

Intensity

In general, the intensity of pain is related to the severity of the abdominal disorder, especially if acute. Thus, the pain of biliary and renal colic, the occlusion of a mesenteric vessel with intestinal infarction, acute pancreatitis, or a perforated ulcer with peritonitis usually is of high intensity, whereas the pain of psychophysiologic gastrointestinal disease and gastorenteritis is less severe. However, intensity is apt to be the most difficult feature of abdominal pain for the patient to describe accurately and for the physician to evaluate. This is because intensity of pain is largely a subjective quality and depends upon the patient's personality, his psychic and emotional state, as well as his previous pain experience and alertness. Furthermore, age and general health may also affect the degree to which a patient experiences pain; the pain of acute appendicitis may be much less intense in an elderly person, to the point that this diagnosis may be overlooked. To evaluate the intensity of pain, the patient can be asked to compare it with a previous painful experience. "Is the pain as severe as labor pains of childbirth, of a previous gallbladder attack, of appendicitis?" Also, the patient can be asked to grade the severity of the pain in terms of degree, from 1+ to 10+.

Circumstances That Produce, Intensify, or Reduce Pain

Most abdominal pain may be produced or intensified under certain specific circumstances, and this characteristic often is very helpful in making the correct diagnosis. In many instances, the onset, intensification, or reduction of abdominal pain can be related to a specific agent or event. Identification of such a pattern is frequently very helpful in making the correct diagnosis. For example, burning or gnawing pain that immediately follows the ingestion of alcohol is a tip-off that the patient may be suffering from peptic esophagitis or gastritis. The pain of vascular insufficiency of the small intestine ("abdominal angina") usually begins within an hour after eating (Bircher), whereas the pain of peptic ulcer disease is experienced later, 1 to 2 hours after a meal, when the stomach is empty of food. The intestinal cramping pain, bloating, and diarrhea associated with deficiency of the small intestinal disaccharidase enzyme lactase occurs 30 minutes to 2 hours after the ingestion of milk. Coughing, straining, or sneezing is likely to accentuate the pain from lesions involving spinal roots. Pleuritic pain, whether felt in the chest wall or referred to the abdomen, is associated with breathing. Sudden movement may intensify the pain of peritonitis or give rise to pain in patients with hepatic metastases.

Equally important are the factors that reduce abdominal pain. The pain of peptic ulcer characteristically is relieved by antacids or the ingestion of food. Right lower quadrant pain of regional enteritis frequently disappears after defecation, usually urgent in nature. Locally applied heat often reduces the intensity of pain from muscle tension. A particular posture may minimize abdominal pain. For example, pain from a hernia often is modified by changes in the position of the body. The pain of pancreatitis may be reduced by sitting up and leaning forward. Intestinal colic may also cause the patient to double up in a jack-knife position to seek relief. The patient with generalized peritonitis usually lies on his back absolutely motionless because any movement increases pain.

Associated Features

Other complaints that occur in relation to abdominal pain also represent invaluable information but an association may not be appreciated by the patient and must be carefully sought when taking the history. More obvious examples of related complaints include a history of nausea and vomiting of recently ingested food, indicative of obstruction due to peptic ulcer or a gastric neoplasm; or significant weight loss that attends a malignancy. Pancreatic carcinoma is strongly suspect when abdominal pain is associated with depression or the late appearance of jaundice. A change in the bowel habits or the character of the stool are also very important associated features of abdominal pain. A history of recurrent diarrhea associated with cramping abdominal pain, especially in the right lower quadrant, suggests Crohn's disease, particularly if accompanied by a history of fever, arthralgias, arthritis, rash, (e.g., erythema nodosum), ocular disturbances (uveitis), or perianal disease. Unformed or diarrheal stools mixed with blood and pus, lasting for several weeks, are typical of ulcerative colitis, and are usually more prominent features than abdominal pain in this condition. Patients with abdominal pain and diarrhea due to inflammatory bowel disease usually describe the need to defecate at night. In contrast, patients with psycho-physiological gastrointestinal disease (i.e., irritable bowel syndrome) rarely have nocturnal diarrhea or note blood in their stools (melena), unless they also have a bleeding hemorrhoid or anal fissure. Small amounts of fresh blood detected on the stool or in the toilet paper or observed only at the end of defecation are typical of rectal bleeding from a hemorrhoid or fissure and may be associated with rectal pain on defecation.

Finally, constipation or obstipation of recent origin, especially if accompanied by gradually increasing distention, should raise the possibility of low-grade obstruction due to colonic or rectal neoplasm.

PHYSICAL EXAMINATION

The same rules that apply to the general physical examination apply to examination of the abdomen. The examination must be systematic and thorough, beginning with inspection, then auscultation, and finally palpation and percussion. As the cardiac status is ascertained by evaluation of the patient in more than one position, so should the abdomen be examined. Abnormal masses may be felt only in certain positions, particularly if they are mobile. An enlarged spleen may be palpable only when the patient is lying on his right side. If at all possible, the patient should be examined during an attack of pain, because certain signs may be present only then. He should also be examined, if possible, when free from pain, when there is no muscle guarding masking other symptoms, and when other reactions to pain are absent.

General inspection should include careful attention to the position assumed by the patient when he is experiencing the pain. As mentioned earlier, strict immobility characterizes the patient with general peritonitis, whereas patients with biliary or renal colic writhe in agony. Lying with a flexed hip may indicate a psoas abscess, whether related to appendicitis or a perinephric abscess. An abnormally distended loop of bowel may be recognized simply by observing the anterior abdominal wall for visible peristalsis. Ascites can be suspected upon observing a protuberant abdomen, bulging flanks, or an umbilical hernia in an adult.

Although auscultation of the abdomen frequently does not yield meaningful information in a routine physical examination, it may be of extreme importance in the evaluation of abdominal pain. Complete absence of bowel sounds is found in advanced peritonitis or adynamic ileus of any cause. Pain coincidential with abnormally active, highly pitched bowel sounds is a feature of early mechanical bowel obstruction. The cessation of bowel sounds during an attack of pain of brief duration suggests biliary or renal colic with reflex ileus. Auscultation should not be limited to the characterization of bowel sounds. A systolic bruit or a friction rub heard over the liver may be an important clue in the diagnosis of a hepatoma or hepatic metastasis. Similarly, a friction rub heard over the spleen suggests pain due to a splenic infarct.

Palpation of the abdomen may be of value in discovering enlarged organs or masses not normally present, such as neoplasm. Muscular rigidity or "guarding" is one of the most important early signs of inflammation and must be carefully looked for in patients with acute abdominal pain. The examination is done by gently palpating both sides of the abdomen simultaneously with both hands, gradually moving toward the region in which the patient is complaining of pain. Muscular guarding is unilateral in the presence of a fairly localized inflammatory mass, such as a walled-off abscess, and is bilateral in generalized peritonitis. Palpation also elicits tenderness, which may be either superficial or deep. It is important to distinguish between superficial and deep tenderness, because deep tenderness implicates disease of visceral organs. However, it should be kept in mind that deep tenderness may be associated with overlying superficial tenderness through the mechanism of referred pain. An attempt should be made to elicit rebound tenderness, a sign of peritoneal irritation. The physician should be aware that the subjective reaction of the patient to the sudden release of pressure on the abdomen may limit the value of this maneuver. Palpation of the abdomen

is not completed until each of the sites of possible hernias (femoral and inguinal canals) have been examined.

Percussion of the abdomen usually does not play an important role in the assessment of abdominal pain. It may confirm the presence of an enlarged organ or abnormal mass found on palpation. Occasionally, the liver cannot be palpated but can be percussed. The percussion note over an abdominal mass (whether dull or tympanitic) distinguishes between a solid tissue mass or a distended bowel. Free fluid in the peritoneal cavity usually is best recognized by demonstrating shifting dullness.

It should be remembered that abdominal pain can be a feature of an extra-abdominal disease, not only of the chest or pelvis, but of the central or peripheral nervous system. For this reason, physical examination must not be limited to the abdomen. A carefully performed examination, including a neurologic evaluation, is mandatory.

The physical examination is not complete until a rectal and pelvic examination (in the female) have been performed. A rectal examination entails first inspecting the perineum for perianal disease (perirectal abscess, active or healed fistulae, fissures, hemorrhoids, and so on). After determining the competency of the rectal sphincter with a lubricated gloved finger, the prostate in the male should be palpated to note changes that indicate benign hypertrophy or prostatic cancer. The finger is then moved forward to determine whether a rectal carcinoma is present.

With the elderly and debilitated, a fecal impaction should also be sought that might account for signs and symptoms of intestinal obstruction attending abdominal pain. In addition, all quadrants of the lower pelvis should be palpated to search for evidence of a pelvic mass, either due to tumor or an abscess. A "rectal shelf" due to tumor infiltration in the area of the peritoneal reflection may be palpated in a patient with widespread metastatic adenocarcinoma. Tenderness and compression by a mass in the right pelvis represent an inflammatory process in the ileocecal region, due to either Crohn's disease or a walled-off appendiceal abscess. Tenderness in this region on rectal examination may be one of the only abnormal findings in a patient with an acutely inflamed appendix that is retrocecal in location. Finally, a specimen of stool should be obtained at the time of rectal examination and inspected for occult blood, if not grossly bloody. The stool should also be cultured for pathogens if acute bacterial gastroenteritis is suspected, and promptly examined microscopically for ova and parasites, if parasitic infestation, such as amebic dysentery, is a possible diagnosis.

A pelvic examination should also be part of the "routine" initial evaluation of all female patients. This examination is critical in determining whether abdominal pain is due to pelvic inflammatory disease, a twisted ovarian cyst, or an ectopic pregnancy.

A protoscopic examination with rectal biopsy should be performed early in the evaluation of patients in whom inflammatory bowel disease or a distal neoplasm is suspected as the cause of lower abdominal pain. Many physicians consider this to be a part of the initial evaluation to be done at the time of the physical examination unless the patient is desperately ill or the rectum is filled with feces. Approximately 60% of all adenocarcinoma arising in the large bowel can be seen with the proctoscope.

LABORATORY TESTS AND DIAGNOSTIC PROCEDURES

Especially in recent years, the diagnostician has had available a wide array of laboratory tests and procedures, which often play an essential role in establishing the cause of abdominal pain. The scope of this chapter does not permit a detailed discussion or even a list of all the useful tests, but mention should be made of some of the more recent diagnostic procedures now available in many medical centers and hospitals. These procedures do not supplant such time-tested studies as routine laboratory tests, barium examinations of the gastrointestinal tract, oral cholecystogram, and intravenous pyelograms. Rather, they are useful when the more conventional, easier to perform, less invasive tests have failed to establish a diagnosis.

Within the past few years, the flexible fiberoptic endoscope and colonoscope have come to play an increasingly important role in the evaluation of abdominal pain when radiographic procedures are not diagnostic (Morrissey). The newer panendoscopes enable excellent visualization of the esophagus, stomach, and duodenum, with a high yield of diagnosis in experienced hands when conditions such as esophagitis, peptic ulcer disease, or gastric neoplasm are possible sources of abdominal pain. Distinction between a benign gastric ulcer and gastric neoplasm is greatly facilitated by combining direct visualization with gastric washings, multiple biopsies, and brushing of the suspect lesion through the endoscope. Even more specialized techniques such as retrograde endoscopic pancreatic and biliary duct cannulation permit radiologic visualization of these structures in great detail by the installation of contrast media into the ampulla of Vater (Kasugai). This procedure has already shown considerable promise in detailing lesions in the biliary tree and pancreas, which were hitherto inaccessible except by surgical exploration, especially in the jaundiced patient. Percutaneous transhepatic cholangiography is another

nonsurgical procedure that can distinguish between jaundice due to intrahepatic disease (*e.g.,* drug-induced cholestasis) from extrahepatic obstruction produced by tumor or a common bile duct stone (Redeker). Fiberoptic colonoscopes are also available to directly view and biopsy either diffuse or localized lesions of the colon, which may be the source of abdominal pain.

Radioisotopic scanning is a diagnostic approach widely used in the work-up of patients with abdominal pain. Demonstration of a "cold area" in the liver that has failed to take up an isotopically labeled substance such as technetium-99 is suggestive of a hepatic neoplasm, abscess, or cyst (Drum).

Another new approach to the evaluation of abdominal pain of inflammatory or neoplastic origin is the use of the gallium-67 citrate scan. In contrast to other isotopic scanning techniques, gallium is taken up by hepatic neoplasms and areas of inflammation. A positive gallium scan therefore results in the demonstration of a "hot area" (Lomas). Unfortunately, none of the scanning procedures distinguishes between carcinomatous involvement of the liver and an abscess. However, the gallium scan may be useful in identifying a peripherally located hepatic lesion and has the added advantage of occasionally pinpointing an intraabdominal abscess not otherwise demonstrable (Littenberg).

Recently, radionuclide imaging of the gallbladder and distal biliary tract has been made possible by the introduction of technetium-99-labeled acetanilide iminodiacetic acid (99mTC-IDA) analogues (Rosenthall). Radionuclide imaging has proven quite useful in evaluation of patients with suspected cholecystitis; it can yield information even in the presence of jaundice. Following intravenous injection of any of the analogues, the gallbladder, common duct, and duodenum are normally visualized within one hour. In the typical patient with acute cholecystitis, the biliary tree but not the gallbladder is visualized owing to gallstone impaction in the cystic duct. Delayed filling beyond one hour suggests chronic cholecystitis, intrinsic liver disease, or partial extrahepatic obstruction.

Peroral and percutaneous biopsies of intra-abdominal structures have become commonplace in many medical centers. These techniques have the advantage of not requiring surgery or general anesthesia. The percutaneous needle liver biopsy, when performed by a physician experienced in the technique, is an established method for making definitive morphologic diagnosis of hepatic disease. Peroral biopsy of the small intestinal mucosa permits microscopic examination, which can reveal the changes of celiac sprue, Whipple's disease, or intestinal lymphangiectasia. Furthermore, analysis of the tissues for the activity of the

enzymes that split the disaccharide sugars can confirm the diagnosis of lactase deficiency, which causes milk intolerance with resultant abdominal cramping pain, flatulence, and diarrhea (Haemmerlie).

Another commonly used diagnostic approach is ultrasonography, which can demonstrate the presence of hepatobiliary and pancreatic disease (Ferrucci). This noninvasive procedure is highly effective in demonstrating gallstones and is an extremely valuable means of examining the common bile duct for dilatation in the jaundiced patient. It has become increasingly popular as the initial diagnostic procedure in patients thought to have acute cholecystitis. Ultrasound has also proven useful in identifying intrahepatic and intrarenal space-occupying lesions. By the echoes produced, it is possible to distinguish between cystic and solid-tissue masses. Ultrasound-guided liver biopsy has been used with increasing frequency in a number of medical centers when a single or small mass lesions are present within the substance of the liver.

The recent development and clinical application of computed tomography (CT) has greatly facilitated the work-up of selected patients with abdominal pain. This technique is also noninvasive and has much the same application as ultrasonography in the assessment of hepatobiliary and pancreatic disorders. It is also helpful in examining the patient for retroperitonal masses as a source of pain. A CT scan is more likely than ultrasonography to identify the site and etiology of obstructive jaundice. However, ultrasonography is usually the preferred first procedure because it is easier to schedule and generally less expensive to perform than a CT scan.

In selected cases arteriography may also be helpful in the work-up of a patient with abdominal pain. This radiographic procedure can be used to uncover a wide variety of intra-abdominal diseases, particularly vascular lesions and neoplasms. Neoplasm infiltrating the kidney, liver, or pancreas can be detected by the trained radiologist on the basis of alterations and the distribution and shape of blood vessels supplying these organs or by "tumor staining" or vise versa. The arteriogram is the only method except for surgery that can demonstrate narrowing of the celiac axis of the superior mesenteric artery and thus confirm the diagnosis of "abdominal angina."

Laparoscopy is a specialized procedure that can also be performed for evaluation of abdominal pain. Laparoscopy permits direct visualization of many intra-abdominal organs and some pelvic structures and permits the biopsy of lesions (*e.g.,* hepatic tumors) under direct view.

In the past when the cause of abdominal pain thought to be organic in nature could not be diagnosed after

extensive work-up, abdominal exploration (laparotomy) under general anesthesia was often recommended. Laparotomy is much less commonly performed today owing to the substantial improvement in the capability of the diagnostic procedures recently developed. In addition, it is now recognized that laparotomy infrequently provides diagnostic information when specific clues of involvement of a particular organ or structure are lacking.

Undoubtedly, present test and diagnostic procedures will be improved and supplemented by new and even better ones in the future.

ETIOLOGIC CLASSIFICATION OF ABDOMINAL PAIN

The common conditions and diseases that can cause abdominal pain can be divided into (1) those involving structures within the abdominal cavity and (2) those involving structures outside the abdominal cavity.

Etiologic Classification of Abdominal Pain
Pain originating within the abdomen
  Disease of hollow organs: bowel, gallbladder, ducts, and so on
  Peritonitis: chemical or bacterial
  Vascular disease: mesenteric thrombosis, "abdominal angina," dissecting aneurysm
  Tension on supporting structures: on mesenteries, distentions of capsules (liver, spleen, lymph nodes)
Pain originating outside the abdomen
  Referred pain: from thorax, genitourinary tract, spine, spinal cord, pelvis, and so on
  Metabolic pain
    Endogenous: Toxic—uremia, diabetic acidosis
    Allergic—food hypersensitivity
    Exogenous: Toxic—drugs, lead
    Biologic—bacterial toxins, insect and snake venoms, and so on
  Neurogenic pain: spinal cord or root pain; tabes, causalgia
  Psychogenic pain

Only those conditions seen most frequently will be discussed.

INTESTINAL TRACT

Esophagus

Pain impulses arising in the esophagus are carried by afferent nerve fibers, which course with the sympathetics and enter the spinal cord from the level of the lower cervical through the entire thoracic vertebrae. The fifth and sixth thoracic spinal segments are most heavily trafficked. In contrast to most of the other regions of the intestinal tract, esophageal pain corresponds relatively well to the site of the disease process. Thus, lesions of the upper esophagus give rise to pain in the suprasternal notch or beneath the manubrium; those in the midesophagus produce pain deep to the midsternum; and pain due to disease of the distal esophagus usually is experienced beneath the xiphoid process or in the epigastrium.

The most common pain from the esophagus is "heartburn," a burning pain felt substernally and fairly well localized over the site of stimulation. This pain has been shown by Jones to be due to spasm of the cardiac end of the esophagus. The spasm may be induced by mechanical, thermal, chemical, or electrical stimuli. The most common mechanism of heartburn in man is thought to include the regurgitation of highly acid gastric juice into the esophagus, which has already had its pain threshold lowered by the presence of engorgement or inflammation.

Stomach

The studies of Wolff and Wolf have shown convincingly that pain of considerable intensity is produced by either mechanical or chemical stimulation of the gastric mucosa, if it is inflamed, congested, or edematous. Deeper structures, either the muscular layer or serosa, can give rise to painful sensations when the stomach vigorously contracts, especially when the stomach wall is inflamed. Afferent impulses enter the cord at the level of the seventh to the ninth dorsal roots. Pain of gastric origin is most often felt in the epigastrium, usually in the midline or in the left upper quadrant.

Small and Large Intestines

Noxious impulses from the small intestine travel in splanchnic pathways, but enter the cord slightly lower than do those from the stomach from T9 to T11. The afferent innervation of the colon above the sigmoid is also carried in the sympathetic trunks. Below this level, it is probably supplied mainly by afferent fibers through its mesentery from the lower thoracic and upper lumbar segmental nerves, without involvement of sympathetic or parasympathetic pathways. The rectum, however, does receive afferent nerves through the parasympathetic rami from S2 to S4.

Like the pain of a gastric ulcer, that due to a peptic ulcer of the duodenum is most often experienced in the epigastrium, usually in the midline or close by. It may not be possible to distinguish between the pain of a gastric ulcer and that of a duodenal ulcer. Both may be sharply localized, burning in character, beginning approximately 1 to 2 hours after meals, and re-

lieved by eating or antacids. A change of any kind in this pattern of pain of ulcer disease should suggest penetration into neighboring structures, such as the pancreas. Such pain is apt to be deeper, boring, less localized, persistent rather than intermittent, and not relieved by food or antacids.

There is poor localization of pain in disease affecting other regions of the intestine. As a general rule, pain from the small intestine is periumbilical, with some tendency for jejunal lesions to be felt in the upper left quadrant and for ileal pain to be felt in the right lower quadrant. Pain arising from colonic disorders generally is experienced in the lower half of the abdomen, and is relatively diffuse. Cecal and ascending colon pain usually is felt in the right lower quadrant. Pain of transverse and descending colon origin is located typically in the left lower abdomen. Disease of the sigmoid colon often produces suprapubic pain, or pain posteriorly in the region of the sacrum.

As described earlier, intestinal pain is typically colicky in nature. Each wave of pain is brief, usually lasting less than a minute. In between attacks of pain, the patient may be entirely symptom-free. Audible bowel sounds can be heard at times synchronous with pain, and the patient may double up or feel the urge to defecate. Indeed, in gastroenteritis, "irritable colon syndrome," and regional enteritis, pain may abate following the passage of stool. Intestinal obstruction, whether due to adhesions, strangulated hernia, intussusception, volvulus, or a constricting neoplasm, generally is characterized by colicky pain. Partial obstruction may give rise to repeated attacks of colicky pain, eventually ending in complete obstruction. If the site of obstruction is high in the intestine, vomiting is a prominent feature, the vomitus at times appearing "fecal" in character. If the obstructive lesion is low in the intestinal tract, distention and obstipation are more prominent early features than vomiting. In patients with acute mesenteric artery occlusion, abdominal pain may be continuous rather than colicky. Persistent pain also characterizes peritonitis; muscular rigidity, hyperalgesia, and tenderness to palpation are frequent accompanying features.

Enzyme deficiency may cause colicky abdominal pain, bloating, and diarrhea. The lactase deficiency of infants with intolerance to the lactose of milk is an example of this. Lactase deficiency is also common in adults and is much more common among black than among white persons. Evidence suggests that the enzyme deficiency may be genetically transmitted (Bayless). The enzyme lacking in adults may not be the same one that is deficient in infants; adults with the disturbance have not commonly had milk intolerance as infants. Ingested lactose is not digested, and remains in the intestinal lumen. A great deal of fluid enters the lumen to dilute this hypertonic load. The excess fluid causes distention, abdominal cramps, and increased peristalsis. In addition, the undigested lactose is fermented to lactic acid, and this also acts as a cathartic. Carbon dioxide is also produced by this fermentation and contributes to the resultant bloating and frothy diarrhea.

Celiac disease of children or adults (nontropical sprue, idiopathic steatorrhea) is one of the malabsorption syndromes. Practically all patients suffering from this disease have abdominal discomfort; about 25% to 30% have, at times, quite severe cramping pain. Large, pale, fatty, bulky stools are characteristic, often with diarrhea. There is a typical histologic alteration of the jejunal mucosa (blunt or absent villi and lengthened crypts). Diagnosis may be made by peroral suction biopsy. Present concepts of the pathophysiology involved are that the mucosa lacks one or more peptide-hydrolyzing enzymes that normally complete the digestion of gluten; the remaining peptides (in the gliadin fraction of the cereal protein, gluten) damage the epithelial absorbing surface of the small intestine; multiple manifestations of malabsorption result. Gluten-free diets have resulted in remission of the symptoms and improvement in the appearance of the mucosa; resumption of gluten intake causes a relapse. Generalized disaccharidase deficiency due to epithelial cell damage occurs, affecting lactase particularly. Milk or lactose ingestion may cause cramping abdominal pain and diarrhea.

One of the most serious and yet most common causes of severe abdominal pain is acute appendicitis. It is a common illness, seen in both sexes and at all ages. Even laymen are familiar with it as often being the cause of right lower quadrant pain. However, in most instances, acute appendicitis begins not with right-sided pain, but with pain in the epigastrium or in the region of the umbilicus. Pain is soon followed by nausea and often by vomiting. Several hours after illness begins, pain classically shifts to the right lower quadrant, to an area frequently referred to as "McBurney's point," which is halfway between the umbilicus and the anterior superior spine of the ilium. In this region, deep tenderness, muscular rigidity, and cutaneous hyperalgesia usually can be demonstrated. Fever of 102° to 103°F and leukocytosis are characteristically present by this stage. If perforation of the appendix is to be avoided, surgery should not be delayed beyond this juncture.

In patients with a retrocecal or pelvic appendix, pain may begin in the right lower quadrant. In these patients and in elderly and debilitated persons, pain may be less intense, and deep tenderness and muscle guarding are correspondingly less evident. Rectal ex-

amination may be of considerable value because it may elicit pain in the region of the appendix and a tender inflammatory mass may be palpated.

Acute gastroenteritis may produce pain, sometimes similar to that of acute appendicitis. Distinguishing features usually are vomiting, more common at the onset in the former, soon followed by diarrhea, which is rare with appendicitis; muscle guarding and rebound tenderness and pain absent in the former, characteristic in the latter; often several associates or family members affected in the former.

Perforation of carcinoma of the colon may cause pain, tenderness, muscle spasm, vomiting, fever, and leukocytosis, and is difficult to distinguish from the clinical picture of acute appendicitis, especially in older persons.

Other conditions that may cause pain resembling that of acute appendicitis are discussed later in this chapter in the section of acute abdomen. Still other conditions causing pain resembling that of acute appendicitis may originate in the organs located in the pelvis of the female and are discussed in the section of the genitourinary tract.

Diverticulitis of the colon is yet another important cause of serious abdominal pain of intestinal origin. In contrast to appendicitis, this condition is limited to adults, almost always in middle age and beyond. Because the sigmoid colon is the most frequent site of diverticula, the pain of acute diverticulitis is located in the lower abdomen, either in the midline or the left hypogastrium. When experienced in the latter region, the clinical picture has been likened to "left-sided appendicitis." Diverticula also may occur in the cecum and ascending colon, and diverticulitis in these locations can be confused with acute appendicitis. A previous history of similar attacks, and of derangements in bowel habits, and the absence of early epigastric or periumbilical pain do not assure but favor the diagnosis of diverticulitis.

PANCREAS, LIVER, AND BILIARY TRACT

Afferent impulses from the pancreas, biliary tract, and liver appear to travel in the same pathways as do those from the stomach and duodenum. The common pathways explain, in part, the difficulty that can be encountered in the differential diagnosis of epigastric pain. The more common painful disorders involving these structures include cholecystitis, biliary colic, acute pancreatitis, pancreatic carcinoma, and rapid hepatic enlargement.

The pain of biliary tract origin is usually experienced along the distribution of T8 or T9. In acute cholecystitis, right upper quadrant or epigastric pain is most characteristic, but pain can be located anywhere in the abdomen, chest, or back. Pain referred posteriorly to the angle of the scapula suggests a stone impacted in the cystic duct, and may occur alone or in association with pain in the right hypochondrium. Occasionally, pain may be referred to the right shoulder through the phrenic nerve. In acute cholecystitis, it is common to obtain a history of the onset of pain several hours after the ingestion of a large meal. During an attack, severe pain may begin suddenly or gradually build in intensity over several hours. Although the pain may wax and wane, it does not entirely disappear until after the attack is over. Nausea and/or vomiting frequently accompanies biliary tract pain, and in some instances, vomiting may actually diminish the intensity of pain. In a prospective study of 107 patients with biliary tract pain, the mean duration of pain was 16 hours, with the most intense component lasting 2 to 3 hours (Gunn).

Tenderness and muscular rigidity in the right upper quadrant are common findings in patients with cholecystitis, and occasionally an inflammatory mass or distended gallbladder may be palpable. The patient with acute cholecystitis is febrile and appears toxic. It should be remembered that the pain of cholecystitis can be atypically located in the chest, and thus confused with pain of coronary insufficiency or acute myocardial infarction.

The passage of gallstones through extrahepatic bile ducts typically gives rise to biliary colic. The pain of biliary colic is sudden, intense, and paroxysmal. It is usually more localized than the pain of cholecystitis, but it can be felt either anteriorly in the right upper quadrant or posteriorly in the right subscapular area. Biliary colic is more frequently accompanied by vomiting and less often accompanied by muscular rigidity than is cholecystitis. In some instances, gallstones lodged in the common bile duct may be "silent," that is, they may not produce pain; rather, recurrent episodes of fever and chills (Charcot's fever) may be the principal abnormality. An elevated serum bilirubin and alkaline phosphatase, a nonvisualizing gallbladder or one containing stones, or a dilated common bile duct on radiographic studies of the biliary tract should lead to the correct diagnosis.

Diseases of the pancreas are among the most difficult intra-abdominal disorders to diagnose correctly. The pain of acute pancreatitis is usually sudden in onset, continuous in character, and epigastric in location; often it spreads to one or both flanks. It is almost always accompanied by vomiting. Shock may occur early in a severe attack. A history of alcoholism or gallstones, or the presence of mild jaundice and a very high level of amylase in the serum or urine, or peritoneal fluid (if present) should help establish the cor-

rect diagnosis. The pain of pancreatic carcinoma may be either continuous and unrelenting or intermittent. Although it is usually located in the upper left abdomen or epigastrium, the patient may complain only of back pain, poorly localized. Carcinoma of the pancreas is one of the most difficult causes of abdominal pain to diagnose. Anorexia, severe weight loss, or depression, in association with upper abdominal pain should suggest this diagnosis. Later signs of far advanced disease include biliary tract obstruction, steatorrhea, and diabetes. All too frequently, the correct diagnosis is made very late in the course of the disease, despite consultation with numerous physicians, including psychiatrists.

The hepatic parenchyma is insensitive to pain but the liver capsule, when rapidly distended, can evoke right upper quadrant pain. Acute fatty infiltration of the liver in the alcoholic, the swollen edematous liver of cardiac decompensation, the inflamed swollen liver of viral or toxic hepatitis, and the enlarged liver with tumor or hepatic abscess are examples.

PERITONITIS

Peritonitis is most commonly due to rupture of a diseased viscus. Appendicitis or perforated peptic ulcer are the most common causes of peritonitis. Other causes include rupture of the gallbladder, perforation of a diverticulum, and pancreatic disease. Gastric fluid, bile, or pancreatic juice in the abdominal cavity initiates a violent and severe peritonitis manifested by immediate and intense pain (chemical peritonitis), whereas perforation of a viscus lower in the intestinal tract produces a more slowly developing picture of peritonitis (bacterial peritonitis).

In the acute state, beginning as chemical peritonitis, the role of enzyme action and of secondary anaerobic infection is frequently of importance in causing a rapid and enormous accumulation of peritoneal fluid. The amount of fluid in the peritoneal cavity may reach as much as one-third of the total plasma volume. Very sudden intense pain may in itself cause shock as can massive fluid derangement. Together, they account for the high mortality rate of peritonitis.

Rupture of a liver abscess may be the cause of peritonitis (more frequently amebic, less often pyogenic). Perforation of an amebic ulcer of the colon provokes peritonitis.

Free blood in contact with the peritoneum causes peritonitis, and may result from trauma to a viscus (spleen, liver, gallbladder, intestinal tract) or from a ruptured graafian follicle, a ruptured tubal pregnancy, and so on.

Bacterial peritonitis, usually pneumococcal or due to enteric organisms, may occur from bacteremia or lymphatic spread of systemic infection. In adults, "spontaneous" peritonitis generally occurs in persons with cirrhosis who have preexisting ascites. Diagnosis is made by examination of peritoneal ascitic fluid that is characteristically an exudate containing more than 4 g of protein per 100 ml fluid, and more than 200 cells per mm^3 of fluid. Organisms may be seen on a Gram's stain of the ascitic fluid, and cultures should yield growth of the causative agent.

Streptococcal peritonitis is rare, but may occur from bacteremic spread from an upper respiratory infection, or scarlet fever or erysipelas, or as a complication of an operative procedure or puerperal infection.

Gonococcal peritonitis may spread from salpingitis. The onset may be severe and sudden, but systemic symptoms tend to subside in a few days and the signs usually become those of a localized pelvic infection.

Tuberculous peritonitis is a rare cause of abdominal pain. It may begin suddenly with severe abdominal pain, prostration, and high fever. Ascitic fluid may accumulate rapidly, causing distention and discomfort, and requiring tapping to afford relief. More characteristically, the onset is insidious, with moderate, poorly localized pain. The organism reaches the peritoneum by extension from lesions in the intestine, lymph nodes, or genital tract, or by hematogenous spread. The peritoneal infection may become chronic. Adhesions may form, matting the intestines and omentum together. The abdomen may be slightly or very tender and is usually distended.

Despite the classic description of the abdomen as "doughy," examination more often reveals findings typical of ascites of any cause, including "bulging flanks," and "shifting dullness." The fluid may have characteristics of a transudate rather than an exudate (Burack). The diagnosis of tuberculous peritonitis is established by the findings of a positive tuberculin skin test and demonstrating the causative organism. Although smear and culture of ascitic fluid may occasionally be positive, the highest diagnostic yield is derived by biopsy of the peritoneum, as with a Cope needle or by laparoscopy, demonstrating granuloma and acid-fast bacilli on stain and culture.

GENITOURINARY TRACT

Renal and urethral pain arise from afferent impulses that reach the spinal cord by way of the lower splanchnic trunks and the lower two thoracic and first lumbar segments. The pain of acute pyelonephritis is felt in the costovertebral angle posteriorly. Palpation or pressure over the area may elicit extreme discomfort. The passage of a renal stone or blood clot into the renal

pelvis or ureter gives rise to "renal colic." An unforgettable experience for those unfortunate enough to be afflicted, the pain of renal colic is excruciating. It comes and goes in waves and typically is located in the flanks, radiating to the lower abdomen, often ending in the groin. Extreme restlessness characterizes the patient with renal colic, and frequency of urination and hematuria also may be present. Bladder pain, as in cystitis, is experienced suprapubicly, although pain due to lesions of the bladder trigone and urethra is felt at the distal tip of the urethra. A more comprehensive discussion of the signs and symptoms of genitourinary tract pain can be found in Chapter 10.

Prostatic pain is experienced in the perineum or lower lumbar region, where it may be confused with skeletal, muscular, nerve, rectal, or even renal pain. Pain arising from the testes or spermatic cord is largely felt *in situ*, although occasionally it may be referred to the hypogastrium.

Although far less common than dysmenorrhea or the pain of labor, the more serious causes of acute abdominal pain arising in the female are those related to ectopic pregnancy, torsion of an ovarian cyst, and pelvic inflammatory disease, usually due to gonococcal infection. Ectopic pregnancy, with its ever-present danger of fallopian tube rupture, must be seriously considered in any female of reproductive age with lower abdominal pain of colicky type who has not menstruated for one for more months. The recent onset of "morning sickness," tender enlarging breasts, and scant uterine bleeding are helpful clues when present. Pain due to torsion of an ovarian cyst usually is experienced laterally low in the abdomen. If located on the right side, it may be confused with the pain of acute appendicitis. The pain of acute pelvic inflammatory disease generally is continuous and often is accompanied by signs of peritoneal irritation. An inflammatory mass that is exquisitely tender is found on pelvic examination, which may also reveal a purulent vaginal discharge containing intracellular gram-negative neisseria organisms.

OTHER CAUSES OF ABDOMINAL PAIN

Mention already has been made of the occurrence of abdominal pain due to thoracic disease. Thus, lower lobe pneumonia may produce severe upper quadrant abdominal pain, which may even be associated with muscular rigidity. However, the finding of pleuropulmonary abnormalities above the diaphragms in patients with abdominal pain does not ensure that the pain is thoracic in origin. Persons suffering from abdominal disorders frequently have pathologic changes above the diaphragm also. Pleural effusion may be seen

in patients with pancreatitis, and atelectasis is not an uncommon finding in cholecystitis and various forms of liver disease.

Since retroperitoneal and skeletomuscular structures share the same afferent pathways as visceral organs, lesions involving these structures also may give rise to abdominal pain. Spinal cord and vertebral lesions also can produce abdominal pain, usually in a segmental or radicular distribution. A history of trauma, the characteristics of the pain (particularly with respect to posture), and definitive findings in the physical examination should permit separation of visceral from somatic origin of pain in most instances.

Abdominal pain may be seen in a variety of systemic disorders. The abdominal pain of acute intermittent porphyria, uremia, or diabetic ketoacidosis may stimulate the pain of an "acute surgical abdomen." Finally, sickle cell crises, lead intoxication, and snake and insect bites are very rare causes of abdominal pain.

ACUTE ABDOMEN

Use of the term "acute abdomen" is usually reserved for a situation in which the patient is suddenly incapacitated by very intense abdominal pain, which may or may not be associated with fever, nausea, vomiting, and shock. The special feature on examination is finding spasm of the abdominal muscles, sometimes amounting to a boardlike rigidity. In such circumstances, a surgical consultation is imperative, although operative intervention may not necessarily be required. Many of the causes of acute abdomen have already been discussed. Appendicitis is the most common cause. Other causes include intestinal obstruction, perforation of a viscus with peritonitis, and vascular occlusion of mesenteric vessels with infarction of the bowel (Cope). The acute abdomen presents as an emergency problem, and yet more errors are made through failure to take time to question and examine the patient than from delay occasioned by a careful analysis of the problem. When the parietal peritoneum is an important source of the pain, an unusual or abnormal position of an organ such as a rotated sigmoid may cause confusion, as may the failure to take into account the complex peritoneal gutters through which pus may travel to a site distant from its origin. Thus, the corrosive fluid from a perforated ulcer may spread down the right pericolic gutter to produce intense pain and muscle spasm in the right lower quadrant. Conversely, fluid from a ruptured appendix may spread upward to the suprahepatic or infrahepatic spaces. The same principles apply to the diagnosis of the acute abdomen as to other less dramatic situations involving

abdominal pain. Again, intrathoracic conditions must be considered; careful examination of the chest is indispensable.

Among the laboratory tests that are particularly helpful in the differential diagnosis of the acute abdomen are the white blood cell count and the serum amylase determination. In acute appendicitis, the white blood cell count usually is elevated, but rarely above 25,000 per mm.[3] Pneumonia, however, which may produce a confusing picture of abdominal pain, is often associated with a very high white blood cell count. On the other hand, acidosis associated with diabetes or renal disease may be accompanied by abdominal pain and a normal white blood cell count, by the presence of ketonemia and ketonuria in the case of diabetes, or an elevated blood urea nitrogen level in the case of renal failure.

The serum amylase is most characteristically elevated in acute pancreatitis, and this diagnosis should be considered when serum levels of greater than 600 mg percent (or units) are found. However, the serum amylase may remain elevated for only a relatively short period of time and may return to normal levels in the first few days of an attack. An elevated serum lipase, increased rate of excretion of serum amylase, and elevated urine amylase-to-creatinine ratio may persist for a longer period of time, and therefore these tests are useful adjuncts when the initial serum amylase is not directly correlated with the severity of attack of acute pancreatitis. Furthermore, in an acute exacerbation of chronic pancreatitis, the serum amylase may never reach abnormal levels. Better correlates of severity include a serum calcium level of less than 7.5 mg % hyperglycemia, and hypotension. Perforation of a peptic ulcer near the pancreas may produce elevation of serum amylase reaching 400 mg %.

Other procedures that may be helpful in differential diagnosis include sickle cell preparations, examinations of the blood for hemoglobinopathies, and Ehrlich's test of urinary porphobilinogen. Radiographic examination of the abdomen is often helpful, particularly if there is free air in the abdominal cavity indicating an intestinal perforation, or air–fluid levels within the lumen of the gut indicating intestinal obstruction. Gallstones may, of course, be visualized, as may calcification of the pancreas or blood vessels occasionally be visualized. The introduction of barium into either end of the intestinal tract may help in diagnosis, but use of barium is to be avoided if perforation is suspected. Arteriography may demonstrate occlusion of a major mesenteric artery. Another procedure that may be of substantial help is the "peritoneal tap." Fluid so obtained should be examined by immediate inspection: Is it serous, hemorrhagic, purulent, or chylous?

It should be studied microscopically by proper cytologic and staining techniques for red blood cells, leukocytes, bacteria, and neoplastic cells. It should be cultured for possible infectious organisms and tested for pancreatic enzymes.

In conditions requiring prompt or possible surgical intervention, the diagnosis may be made quickly. An hour or two delay in surgery may increase the likelihood of a serious, and possibly fatal, outcome.

SUMMARY

The characterization of abdominal pain plays an essential role in the diagnosis of disorders of the abdomen, pelvis, and at times, the thorax. Abdominal pain may be of three types: true visceral pain, deep somatic pain, or referred pain. Clinical analysis should begin with a carefully taken detailed history. Abdominal pain should be defined as to its location; quality; type of onset; temporal features; intensity; the circumstances that produce, intensify, or reduce it; and its associated features. A thorough physical examination is mandatory. Like the cardiac examination, it should be systematic and include inspection, auscultation, palpation and percussion of the abdomen, as well as examination of surrounding regions of the body.

In recent years, an increasing number of diagnostically useful tests and procedures have become available. Studies should be ordered based upon the physician's clinical analysis and begin with the least invasive and least costly procedures.

The major causes of abdominal pain have been subdivided in this chapter by organ system, and the salient features of the more important disorders are reviewed. The chapter ends with consideration of the "acute abdomen."

BIBLIOGRAPHY

Bayless TM, Rosenweig NS: Incidence and implications of lactase deficiency and milk intolerance in white and Negro populations. Johns Hopkins Med J 121:54, 1967

Bircher J, Bartholomew LG, Cain JC et al: Syndrome of intestinal arterial insufficiency ("abdominal angina"). Arch Intern Med 117:632, 1966

Burack WR, Hollister RM: Tuberculous peritonitis: A study of forty-seven proved cases encountered by a general medical unit in twenty-five years. Am J Med 28:510, 1960

Cope Z: The Early Diagnosis of the Acute Abdomen, 13th ed. London, Oxford University Press, 1968

Drum DE, Christacopoulos JS: Hepatic scintigraphy in clinical decision making. J Nucl Med 13:908, 1972

Ferrucci JT: Body ultrasonagraphy. N Engl J Med 300:538–542, 590–602, 1979

Fredens M, Egeblad M, Holst-Nielsen F: The value of selective angiography in the diagnosis of tumors in the pancreas and liver. Radiology 93:765, 1969

Gunn A, Keddie N: Some clinical observations on patients with gallstones. Lancet 2:239, 1972

Haemmerli UP, Kisher H, Ammann R: Acquired milk intolerance in the adult caused by lactose malabsorption due to a selective deficiency of intestinal lactase activity. Am J Med 38:7, 1965

Head H: On disturbances of sensation with especial reference to the pain of visceral disease. Brain 16:1, 1893

Hertz AF: The Goulstonian lectures on the sensibility of the alimentary canal in health and disease. Lancet 1:1051, 1119, 1187, 1215; 1911

Jones CM: Digestive Tract Pain, Diagnosis and Treatment. Experimental Observations. New York, Macmillan, 1938

Kasugai T, Kuno N, Kizu M et al: Endoscopic pancreatocholangiography. II. The pathological endoscopic pancreatocholangiogram. Gastroenterology 63:227, 1972

Lennander KG: Uber die Sensibilitat der Bauchhohle und uber lokale und allgemeine Anasthesie bei Bruch und Bauchoperationen. Zentralbl Chir 28:209, 1901

Leriche R: The Surgery of Pain, p 434. Baltimore, Williams & Wilkins, 1939

Littenberg RL, Taketa, RM, Alazarki NP et al: Gallium-67 for localization of septic lesions. Ann Intern Med 79:403, 1973

Lomas F, Dibos PE, Wagner HN: Increased specificity of liver scanning with the use of [67]gallium citrate. N Engl J Med 286:1323, 1972

MacKenzie J: Some points bearing on the association of sensory disorders and visceral disease. Brain 16:321, 1893

Morrissey JF: Gastrointestinal endoscopy. Gastroenterology 62:1241, 1972

Redeker AG, Karvountzis GG, Richman RH et al: Percutaneous transhepatic cholangiography: An improved technique. JAMA 231:386, 1975

Rosenthall L: An update in radionuclide imaging in hepatobiliary diseases. JAMA 245:2065–2068, 1981

Ross J: On the segmental distribution of sensory disorders. Brain 10:333, 1888

Ryle JA: Visceral pain and referred pain. Lancet 1:895, 1926

von Haller A: Memoires sur la Nature Sensible et Irritable des Parties du corps Animal. Tome Quatrieme, contenant les Responses Faites a Differentes Objections, p 232. Lausanne, S D'Arnay, 1760

Wolff HG, Wolf SG: Pain. Springfield, IL, Charles C Thomas, 1948

10

Urinary Tract Pain, Hematuria, and Pyuria

Alan D. Perlmutter
Robert S. Blacklow

Urinary Tract Pain
  Anatomic and Physiologic Considerations
  Nerve Supply to the Urinary Tract
  Modes of Expression of Urinary Tract Pain
    Localizing Characteristics
Cells Normally in Urine
Hematuria
  Site of Origin
    Systemic Causes
    Nonrenal Parenchymal Pathology
    Renal Parenchymal Causes
    Trauma
    Undiagnosed Hematuria

Pyuria
  Bacterial Etiology
  Predisposing Factors
  Conditions Predisposing to Urinary Tract
    Infections
  Most Common Clinical Pictures of Pyuria
    Acute Pyelonephritis
    Chronic Pyelonephritis
    Cystitis
    Prostatitis
Summary

URINARY TRACT PAIN

ANATOMIC AND PHYSIOLOGIC CONDITIONS

The urinary tract consists of organs and structures serving varied functions. The kidneys are involved in the formation and excretion of urine by the filtration of plasma and by the secretion and reabsorption of small molecules and ions. The ureters conduct the urine, by peristalsis, to empty into the bladder. The bladder serves the dual functions of storage and evacuation. The urethra is the pathway to the exterior, and its voluntary sphincter helps provide urinary control.

The kidneys are paired organs in the upper retroperitoneum, below the diaphragm, usually opposite the T12 to L2 vertebral bodies. The ureters extend from the upper retroperitoneum into the true pelvis. The bladder in the adult is extraperitoneal and within the bony pelvis, except for the dome, which when distended can be palpated in the hypogastrium.

NERVE SUPPLY TO THE URINARY TRACT

The kidneys and ureters are innervated by both the sympathetic and the parasympathetic components of the autonomic nervous system (Figs. 10-1 and 10-2). Parasympathetic innervation to the kidney is derived from the vagus; the function is not known.[1] Vagal fibers terminate in synapses in the renal plexuses and do not directly reach the renal parenchyma.[2] Sympathetic fibers are derived from the thoracolumbar trunk, T6 to L3 inclusive, mainly T10 to L1. These fibers travel mainly in the superior, middle, and inferior splanchnic

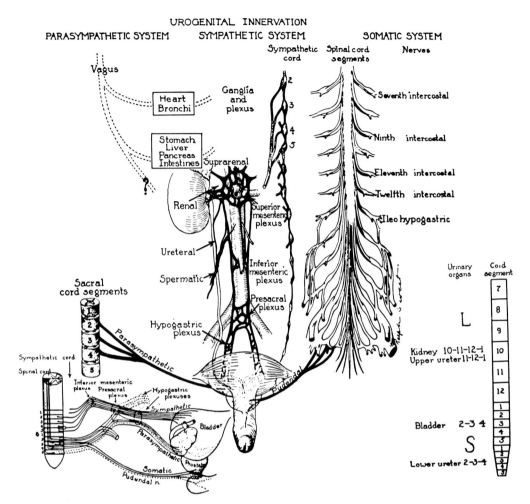

Fig. 10-1. Diagrammatic representation of urinary tract innervation. (From Campbell MF (ed): Urology, pp 1–46. Philadelphia, WB Saunders, 1963)

nerves, with some fibers from the lowermost lumbar segments by way of the pelvic plexus.[2,3] Preganglionic efferent fibers terminate in the semilunar (celiac) ganglion and for the inferior splanchnic nerve, in the aorticorenal ganglion. Postganglionic fibers enter the renal plexus, a network of nerves intimately associated with the renal vascular pedicle. From this plexus, fibers supply the intrarenal arterial system and calyces. Branches extend to the renal capsule, upper ureter, and adrenal. A few fibers connect to the opposite renal plexus.

The pathways of postganglionic nerves vary; the inferior splanchnic nerve is inconstant. Some nerve fibers pass directly to the renal plexus, together with branches of first and second ganglia of the lumbar sympathetic chain. Some of these direct connections may represent sensory (afferent) pathways traveling

with sympathetic afferent fibers.[1-4] Stimulation of efferent nerves to the kidney significantly reduces renal blood flow, with an acute decrease in urinary output. Despite some conflicting data, most investigators also note a redistribution of intrarenal blood flow.[5-9]

Afferent nerves from the kidney are both myelinated and unmyelinated. Some of these nerves monitor changes in renal venous pressure[10] and distention of the renal pelvis and capsule. The anatomy and neurophysiology of the renal sensory pathway are incompletely understood. Receptors have not been demonstrated in the human kidney, and sensory endings have not been identified in the renal pelvis or upper ureter, although myelinated fibers are present.[11,12] Despite a few autonomic nerve fibers crossing to the contralateral renal plexus, renal sensory innervation is

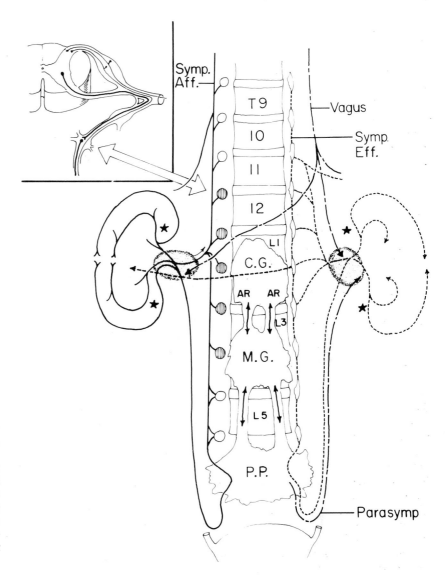

Fig. 10-2. Diagram of renal innervation (*C.G.* = celiac ganglion; A.R. = aorticorenal ganglion; M.G. = mesenteric ganglion; P.P. = pelvic plexus). Stippled area in each renal hilus represents renal plexus. Stars in kidneys represent intramural nerve cells. (Modified from Schvalev VN: Problems in the morphology and nature of renal innervation. Fed Proc 25:595–600, 1965)

generally unilateral. In human subjects undergoing a unilateral sympathectomy under procaine block, pain responses were elicited by stretching or compressing the ipsilateral renal pelvis, pedicle, or ureter near the ureteropelvic junction. Unilateral sympathectomy from T7 to L1, and division of the greater and lesser splanchnic nerves at the celiac ganglion eliminated these pain responses. No contralateral pain was sensed. During the same studies, upper ureteral pain was eliminated when the T12 and L1 ganglia were excised. Similarly, unilateral splanchnic block alone can eliminate ipsilateral renal pain.[13,14]

Innervation of the ureter is by multiple fibers extending from a meshwork of retroperitoneal plexuses. These include renal, spermatic, aortic, inferior mesenteric, hypogastric, and inferior vesical plexuses, and fibers from the celiac and aorticorenal ganglia. The distal ureter receives parasympathetic branches from S2, S3, and S4, which also supply the bladder.[2,3,15]

Ureteral afferents from the upper ureter are found in the 11th and 12th thoracic, the 1st, and possibly the 2nd lumbar nerves. Distal ureteral afferents enter the 2nd, 3rd, and 4th sacral segments. Although the proximal ureter has a sensory innervation, sensory terminations have been identified only for the lower ureter, where sensory fibers pass through the muscularis into the mucous membrane. Connections have been demonstrated among nerve fibers to the ureter and the

plexuses that supply the ovary, testis, and parietal peritoneum.[3,11,15,16]

The bladder has a triple innervation: sympathetic, parasympathetic, and somatic. The parasympathetic pathways of the bladder—S2, S3, and S4—provide motor function for coordinated voiding. Afferent parasympathetic fibers mediate the desire to void, proprioception, and pain. All these sensory and motor pathways run together in the pelvic nerves (nervi erigentes).

The sympathetic supply to the bladder is found in the hypogastric plexus, also referred to as the hypogastric or presacral nerve. In addition to supplying the internal genitalia, sympathetic motor pathways for both sexes provide alpha adrenergic innervation to the trigone and bladder neck. During seminal emission, closure of the vesical neck contributes to the process of ejaculation. In persons with normal bladder function, sectioning of these sympathetic fibers does not alter the voiding pattern, but in persons with neurogenic vesical dysfunction, these pathways may become important.[17] In some conditions, alpha adrenergic drugs are used to constrict the vesical neck and provide a secondary means of improving continence; in others, alpha adrenergic blocking agents are used to relax the vesical neck and enhance difficult voiding. Sympathetic afferents provide additional subjective awareness of bladder distention, pain, and less specific abdominal discomfort from vesical distention.[18,19] This sensory input reaches the cord at T9 or even higher. From studies in patients with traumatic paraplegia, it has been observed that awareness of distention is decreased as the cord lesion becomes more proximal and disappears completely between T6 and T4.[20]

Sensory receptors have been detected in the mucous membrane of the bladder, confirming that pain stimuli can originate in the mucous membrane. Since the sensory fibers run through the muscularis, contraction of the bladder wall may also cause pain. The sensory fibers are more concentrated near the ureterovesical junction, the bladder neck, and the trigone in decreasing density, and are less well developed in the remainder of the bladder.[11]

The urethra has a rich sensory innervation from S2, S3, and S4 through the pudendal nerve, a mixed somatic nerve which also contains motor fibers to the external urethral sphincter. Some sensory receptors within the urethra respond to flow, others to urethral distention.[21] Thermal sensation is also present in the urethra, and plays a role in awareness of urination. As contrasted with desire to void, imminence of voiding is from urethral sensation and from traction on the bladder neck and trigone by contracting bladder.[19]

MODES OF EXPRESSION OF URINARY TRACT PAIN

Because of the extensive and variable distribution of nerve fibers to the urinary tract, pain patterns are protean. The proximity of urinary organs to intraperitoneal structures and the extensive collateral nerve supply through the celiac and other plexuses are two reasons why localization of disease processes by site of pain may be difficult. As with other visceral pains, urinary tract pain is less well localized than corresponding somatic pain involving the same dermatomes; one reason for this is the decreased density of innervation of the involved viscus compared with that of skin. Visceral and skin afferents probably converge at different levels in the nervous system; impulses converge on the same secondary or tertiary neuron. Localization of visceral pain is also learned. Children do not localize urinary tract pathology as well as adults. Accuracy and body awareness tend to become greater with experience, growth, and development.[22,23]

Localizing Characteristics

Renal pain follows acute stretching of the renal vessels, peripelvic capsule or pelvis, or distention of the collecting system.[23] Pain of renal origin is classically felt in the posterior subcostal and costovertebral region, and is usually aching in nature, although severe, boring pain may be present. Hyperesthesia of associated dermatomes (usually T9–T10) may occur. Radiation forward around the flank into the lower abdominal quadrant (T11–T12), and ipsilateral or generalized abdominal pain, spasm of abdominal muscles, and even rebound tenderness occur with severe discomfort; often the latter symptoms exist alone or exceed the posterior pain. Nausea, vomiting, and paralytic ileus accompany severe acute pain. Pain referred to the contralateral abdomen has been described but is exceedingly rare.[23,24] A recent review classified renal pain into three types: visceral pain from stretching or other stimulation of renal hilar structures, renal colic from upper ureteral and pelvic distention with obstruction, and referred pain from common afferent pathways[23] (see Modes of Expression of Urinary Tract Pain).

Distention of the ureter is painful. The most common cause is an obstructing calculus which has descended from the kidney, with sudden dilatation of both kidney and ureter. Unusual pain patterns may result, but typically pain of ureteral origin starts in the costovertebral angle and radiates to the lower abdomen, upper thigh, testis, or labium on the same side. The pain is usually excruciating, and the patient writhes about, unable to obtain relief. In contrast, the patient

with peritonitis pain lies quietly because motion increases the discomfort.[25] If the calculus has reached the ureterovesical junction, urgency, frequency, and stinging referred to the urethra and glans of the phallus may be noted. Rectal tenesmus is sometimes another symptom of sudden low ureteral obstruction. As with renal pain, ileus with distention, nausea, and vomiting can occur. Acute urinary retention has also been noted.

Severe ureteral pain most often is felt as crescendo waves of colic. Once thought to be due to ureteral spasm or hyperperistalsis proximal to the acute obstruction, this pain has been shown to be caused by distention of and trauma to the ureter itself and includes the pain of renal pelvic distention. Experimentally, distention of the upper ureter and renal pelvis by a balloon catheter causes pain, but distention of the lower ureter above its terminal segment does not cause pain unless urinary flow is also blocked.[14] Amplitudes of contraction pressure higher than normal have not been recorded in acutely obstructed ureters; rather, the resting pressure rises and the amplitude of the contraction complexes falls as the ureter progressively dilates.[26] Upon physical examination, hyperesthesia of associated dermatomes (T12 and L1) and tenderness of palpation over the ureter and kidney with or without rebound, may be present.

Chronic renal and ureteral pain tend to be vague, poorly localized, and atypical, and easily confused with that from other visceral or somatic lesions.[27] Complete examination, including urinalysis and urographic study, is required for a differential diagnosis. Other possible causes of acute or chronic pain of a similar nature include a perforated viscus, intestinal obstruction, cholecystitis, retrocecal appendicitis, acute seminal vesiculitis, pelvic inflammatory disease, tubo-ovarian abscess, ruptured ectopic pregnancy, twisted ovarian cyst, and any other cause of peritonitis or peritonismus.

When inflammatory lesions of the upper urinary tract extend beyond the collecting system, adjacent structures become involved. Perinephritis or perinephric abscess may irritate the diaphragm, resulting in shoulder pain; with periureteral disease, pain may occur on movement of the adjacent iliopsoas muscle. Rebound tenderness results when the adjacent peritoneum becomes inflamed.

Bladder pain is suprapubic or low abdominal, usually associated with great urgency, tenesmus, and dysuria. Inflammation of the urethra and bladder neck may result in a "hot" or burning sensation because of stimulation of previously described thermal receptors in the urethra. Frequency and urgency result from stimulation of the proprioceptive and sensory receptors in the bladder wall and urethra. Upon examination, suprapubic and sometimes urethral tenderness may be observed, and if the infection arises in the prostate gland, a swollen, tender hot gland is palpable.

The foregoing review of urinary tract pain has considered the pertinent anatomic and physiologic factors. The modes of presentation and expression have been described. The reasons for the variability of symptoms that are encountered have been discussed.

Many of the disturbances resulting in urinary tract pain are inflammatory conditions of which hematuria or pyuria are important manifestations.

CELLS NORMALLY IN URINE

Both red blood cells and white blood cells (predominantly polymorphonuclear leukocytes) are found in normal urine in small numbers. Their route and mode of entry into the urinary tract are not clear. That the ratio of red blood cells to white blood cells in blood is 1000:1 and in urine is 1:30 suggests that these cells do not come from minute hemorrhages along the urinary tract.[28] In the presence of urinary tract disease, increased numbers of red cells and white cells are found in the urine; it is only when these blood elements are seen in casts that one may be certain that they derive from the kidney, unless red or white cells are collected by ureteral catheterization.[29,30]

HEMATURIA

Hematuria is the presence of red blood cells in the urine. Bleeding from the urinary tract, whether gross or microscopic, is a serious sign. It should be looked upon with the same gravity as abnormal bleeding elsewhere in the body. Gross hematuria is not always red. The color of bloody urine depends upon the amount of blood present and the pH of the urine. In an acid urine, the color is often brown or smoky; in an alkaline urine, the color is red. Not all red urine contains blood; cell-free hemoglobin or myoglobin stains the urine red. Drugs, food pigments, and metabolites may also color the urine red; azo dyes, phenolphthalein, indole alkaloids, beets, and porphyrins are among these substances.

Red blood cells may be found in the urine of healthy persons. The classic studies of Addis, Goldring, and others have established that the normal excretion of red blood cells per 12-hour period for healthy adults is up to 600,000.[31-34] The excretion of red blood cells in

the urine of infants during the first two weeks of life is greater than that in adults; in children aged 4 to 12 years, the normal range of red blood cell excretion is the same as that in adults.[35] An investigator from one insurance company diluted 600,000 red blood cells in 300 ml of clear urine and found about 2 red blood cells per high-power microscopic field after handling the specimen in the usual manner.[33] In 6000 consecutive male and female urine specimens examined by one observer, 78% had no red blood cells per high-power field, and 94% had one or less[36] (Fig. 10-3). These two studies suggest the normal limits of erythrocytes in urine as under 2 per high-power field.

Vigorous exercise, lordotic posture, acute febrile illness, dehydration, and unbalanced dietary intake may produce microscopic hematuria in the absence of serious disease of the urinary tract.[32,34,37]

SITE OF ORIGIN

Hematuria may be classified on an anatomic or an etiologic basis. Hematuria may also be classified into systemic causes, nonrenal parenchymal causes and renal parenchymal causes of glomerular or nonglomerular origin. Noting whether hematuria is initial, total, or terminal may help in the localization. *Initial hematuria* suggests the urethra as the source; *terminal hematuria* suggests the posterior urethra, trigone, or bladder base. *Total hematuria* means that red blood cells are dispersed throughout the urinary stream and suggests origins from the kidney, ureter, or bladder. Hematuria accompanied by red blood cell *casts* indicates a renal origin, such as acute or subacute inflammatory lesions of the glomeruli and renal parenchyma. In patients with unexplained hematuria, a careful urinalysis disclosing

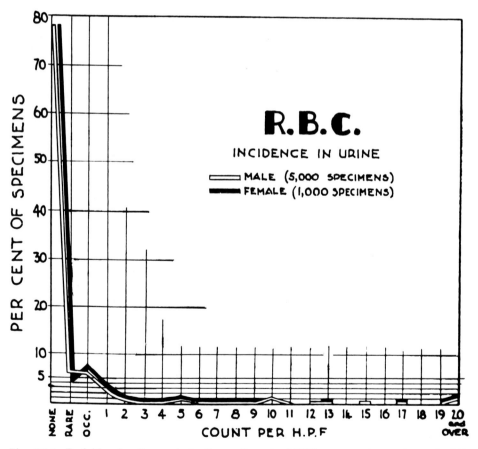

Fig. 10-3. Red blood cell counts in the sediment of 5000 consecutive male and 1000 consecutive female urine specimens received at the John Hancock Mutual Life Insurance Company. (Adapted from Wright WT: Cell counts in the urine. Arch Intern Med 103:76, 1959)

red blood cell casts localizes the lesion to the kidney and may save the patient from costly, uncomfortable, and potentially harmful urologic manipulations.

Systemic Causes

Systemic causes of bleeding may present with hematuria. A complete list is beyond the scope of this chapter, but some of the more common causes are the following: hemophilia, anticoagulant therapy with either heparin or vitamin K antagonists, thrombocytopenia, polycythemia vera, coagulation factor disturbances, hyperglobulinemic syndromes with generalized vascular bleeding, scurvy, and sickle-cell disease.

Nonrenal Parenchymal Pathology

Acute cystitis, urethritis or prostatitis, genitourinary tuberculosis, neoplasms of the kidney and urinary tract, ureteral and bladder calculi, and vascular malformations may cause hematuria. Extra-urinary tract pathology, such as endometrial, cervical, and rectal neoplasms, may invade the urinary tract and produce hematuria. Endometriosis involving the urinary tract produces cyclical bleeding with the menses.

Renal Parenchymal Causes

Renal parenchymal causes of hematuria of glomerular origin include those associated with primary renal disease, such as postinfectious acute glomerulonephritis, membranous and proliferative glomerulonephritis, chronic glomerulonephritis, and focal glomerulonephritis, as well as those associated with multisystem or heredity disease, such as systemic lupus erythematosus, polyarteritis, nodosa allergic purpura, malignant hyptertension, postradiation nephritis, the heredity nephritides, Wegener's granulomatosis, and Goodpasture's syndrome. Renal parenchymal causes of hematuria of nonglomerular origin include medullary sponge kidney, polycystic renal disease, leukemic infiltrates, interstitial nephritis, nephrocalcinosis, renal artery embolism, renal vein thrombosis, papillary or cortical necrosis, and acute tubular necrosis. If associated with a glomerulitis, red blood cell casts are also present. Proper history, physical examination, and laboratory studies, including (if necessary) renal biopsy and immunopathologic examination, help in the differential diagnosis.

Tumors, urinary tract obstruction, calculi, and infection account for over 60% of hematuria in adults. Painless total hematuria is suggestive of a tumor in the urinary tract, and at least 20% of people with this presenting symptom prove to have a urinary tract neoplasm. Tumors of the renal parenchyma produce hematuria when the kidney pelvis has been invaded. The bleeding may be intermittent and variable in volume and amount, often with clots.[38] Tumors of the upper collecting system and ureter (those parts of the urinary tract lined with transitional cell epithelium) also present with bleeding in over 74% of cases;[39] the bleeding is painless and has no distinctive characteristics as to amount and timing. Gross hematuria occurs in 60% to 90% of bladder tumors.[40]

Depending upon the anatomic location of a urinary tract neoplasm, the bleeding may be initial, terminal, or total. It is apparent that complete urologic visualization of both the upper and lower urinary tract is required to diagnose hematuria. Techniques used to localize the source of bleeding include intravenous urography, retrograde ureteropyelography, cystoscopy, ultrasonography, radionuclide imaging, and angiopathy with selective renal arteriography to outline the abnormal vascular supply of the tumor. Assays of certain enzymatic activities in the urine, while originally thought to constitute a potential screening method for genitourinary malignancies, have proved to be nonspecific.[41] Urinary cytologic examination including brushings, even when performed under proper supervision, awaits improvement in techniques and sensitivity and has not reached the sophistication of cervical cytopathology.[42]

Renal, ureteral, and bladder calculi, acute, chronic, and interstitial cystitis, vascular malformations of the bladder, prostatic venous congestion secondary to benign prostatic hyperplasia, and radiation cystitis are all common lower urinary tract causes of hematuria.

Hematuria may also occur in association with pyuria when there is urinary tract infection. In acute pyelonephritis, renal tuberculosis, and leptospirosis, the damaged blood vessels are probably in the kidney. Painless hematuria, "sterile" pyuria, and an acid urinary pH should suggest renal tuberculosis. The bladder is often the source of the hematuria in leishmaniasis and genitourinary schistosomiasis. Once again, history, physical examination, and appropriate laboratory studies aid in the diagnosis.

Trauma

Trauma must not be neglected as a significant cause of bleeding from the kidneys and bladder. Whether or not trauma is associated with pain depends upon the extent of renal capsule distention or tear and upon the extent of blood and urine extravasation into the retroperitoneum. A study on boxers by Kleiman demonstrated a correlation between injuries from boxing, hematuria, and morphologic and physiologic changes in the upper urinary tract.[43]

11

Back Pain Arthur Hall

Anatomic and Physiologic Considerations
Nerve Supply
Causes of Back Pain
  Disorders of the Spinal Column
  Lesions of the Joints and Intervertebral Disks
  Lesions of the Ligaments, Fascia, and Muscles

Lesions of the Spinal Cord and Meninges
Faulty Body Mechanics
Lesions of Thoracic, Abdominal and
    Pelvic Organs
Miscellaneous Causes
Summary

ANATOMIC AND PHYSIOLOGIC CONSIDERATIONS

Back pain is one of the most common complaints encounterd in the practice of medicine. The multiple causes of back pain are more easily understood if the anatomy and physiology of the back are clear in the mind of the practitioner.

The major structure of the back is the bony vertebral column with its stabilizing ligaments and muscles. These structures enclose and protect the spinal cord with its segmental spinal nerves and blood vessels. A column of vertebrae, each consisting of an anterior weight-bearing body and a posterior arch, surrounds the spinal canal. The bodies of the vertebrae are separated from each other by the intervertebral disks. The disks are not solid like poker chips but are semifluid substances like toothpaste, which can change in contour according to the pressure exerted on them. They therefore act as cushioning devices for the spine. Each disk is composed of a central expansile portion (nucleus pulposus) surrounded by a strong connective-tissue ring (annulus fibrosus) that holds the nucleus pulposus between the vertebral bodies. Each intervertebral disk tends to be spherical in shape, but in the erect position, the compression by the vertebrae between which the disk

is sandwiched, forces it into a flat, ovoid mass (Fig. 11-1).

Movement of the vertebral segments of the spine occurs through movement of the diarthrodial joints located in pairs between the posterior arches of the vertebrae. The strong ligaments that span the spinal column from vertebra to vertebra provide the stability of the spine. Some ligaments extend longitudinally throughout the length of the spinal column; others cross obliquely between two or three segments.

The spine articulates with the pelvis through the sacroiliac joints, composed of the cartilage-covered edges of the upper three sacral segments and the cartilage-covered surfaces of the iliac bones that oppose them. Strong fibrous tissue binds together the nonarticulating opposing surfaces of the spine and pelvis. Ribs, which enclose the thoracic organs, articulate with the dorsal spine.

An important part of the back is its musculature, composed of three layers of muscles. These help stabilize the trunk and produce many of the movements of the body (Fig.11-2). The muscles of the dorsal and lumbar back are surrounded by fascia. Some muscles attach directly into this strong fascia.

In the canal of the spinal column, the spinal cord extends from the brain distally and terminates in the

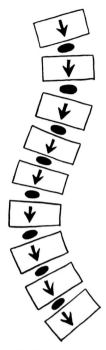

Fig. 11-1. This sketch illustrates the way in which the weight of the trunk of the body is balanced on the nuclei of the intervertebral disks.

lowermost nerves (cauda equina). From the spinal cord, pairs of nerves emerge at each intervertebral segment. These nerves innervate the trunk and extremities (described later).

The back serves several important functions. It provides the principal support and stability for the body as well as for motion of the trunk in all planes of motion. Many movements of the head and extremities in relation to the trunk are accomplished by the back muscles. All movements of locomotion, standing, and sitting are affected by the back muscles that produce movement at some joints and stabilize others.

The two important functions of the spinal muscles are to supply postural tone and to provide movement of the trunk and the structures attached to it. Postural tone, which is controlled by the autonomic nervous system, is normally maintained without effort or fatigue. In the erect position, the strong flexor and extensor muscles are kept in a balanced state of contraction by a static, postural, autonomic reflex system. If this function fails, voluntary contraction of the muscles is required to supplement the autonomic function. This quickly leads to fatigue, faulty posture, and backache. Maintenance of normal back function depends upon a physiologic integrity of bones, joints, tendons, muscles, and nerves.

Abdominal and pelvic organs are secured in their respective positions largely by suspending ligaments attached to the back. Sensory, motor, and autonomic nerves leading to supporting structures of the torso and the extremities and many nerves leading to viscera pass through the back.

NERVE SUPPLY

It is important to understand the innervation of the structures of the back. Pairs of nerves emerge from the spinal cord through foramina in the column at each vertebral segment (Fig. 11-3). These nerves derive from the cord through two roots: the anterior root is composed solely of motor fibers; the posterior root contains only sensory fibers. Just distal to the foramen, the two roots unite into one nerve, which divides near the spinal column into an anterior and posterior branch. Near the point of division, a recurrent branch is given off that innervates the meninges covering the cord. Motor and sensory fibers are supplied to most structures of the back through the posterior branch. The upper spinal nerves group themselves to form a plexus innervating the upper extremity; the lower spinal nerves form a plexus that supplies important nerves to the lower extremity.

Smaller branches of regional nerves follow closely along blood vessels to reach their termination. The vertebrae are innervated like other bones; the cortex and marrow cavity are poorly supplied, whereas the periosteum has rich sensory innervation. The numerous spinal ligaments also contain abundant pain fibers.[1] Muscles, fasciae, and tendons in the back are innervated as they are elsewhere. At their bony attachments, the regional periosteum shares the nerve distribution to the tendons. The posterior articulations of the spine have a nerve supply comparable to that of joints in the extremities (see Chap. 12, Joint and Periarticular Pain).

The parietal pleura, parietal peritoneum, and ligaments of the abdomen and pelvis that attach to the back are abundantly supplied with sensory fibers. In these structures the mechanism for initiating painful stimuli depends chiefly upon stretching, distending, tearing, or severing the membranes containing terminal nerve fibers and end-organs and upon chemical irritation (explained in Chap. 9, Abdominal Pain). Lesions affecting cartilage and bone without distorting the periosteal covering, or irritating the soft-tissue structures attached thereto, are relatively indolent; pain is produced chiefly when the periosteum, ligaments, fascia, and other richly innervated soft-tissue structures are affected.

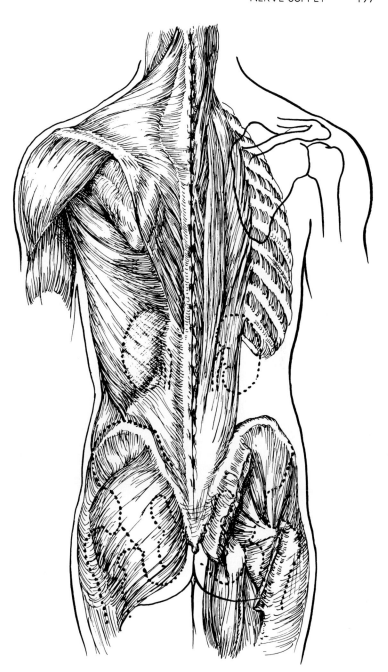

Fig. 11-2. The musculature of the back. On the left is shown the superficial layer of muscles; on the right the deeper paraspinous muscles are sketched. Note the strong attachments of the back muscles to the pelvic and shoulder girdles.

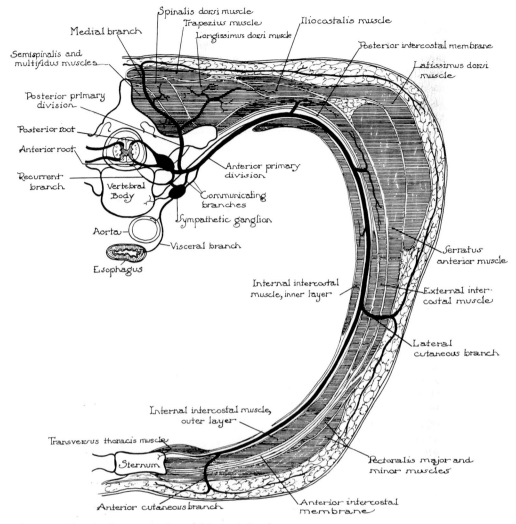

Fig. 11-3. A spinal nerve at the midthoracic level.

Within the spinal canal, painful stimuli may arise from irritation of sensory nerves, which are abundant in the meninges from stretching or pressure upon the sensory roots of spinal nerves or from stimulation of pain fibers in the spinal cord.

CAUSES OF BACK PAIN

It is clear that many different types of lesions affecting one tissue or other in the back may cause pain. Accurate knowledge of anatomic and biomechanical features of the back is required to understand its disorders. The analysis of backache depends on recognition of the nature and location of the underlying illness; this requires complete, systematic examination of the entire body and shrewd evaluation of all the findings in relation to the patient's complaints. No attempt will be made here to describe all the causes of back pain or the differential diagnosis. It is hoped that a discussion of the mechanisms of production of back pain by various causes will provide knowledge as a basis of accurate diagnosis and appropriate therapy.

DISORDERS OF THE SPINAL COLUMN

Most diseases of the spine cause pain. The spine is frequently injured. If trauma is sufficient to fracture the spine, the resulting irritation of the periosteum, the stretch of the ligaments, the pressure from edema and hemorrhage, and the spasm of muscles produce pain in the back. Spasm of the numerous large back muscles

may add greatly to the discomfort. Displacement of bone fragments may be sufficient to press on the meninges, on the pain tracts in the spinal cord, or on the spinal nerve roots, and so produce pain. Dislocation or fracture–dislocation of the spine causes pain in a manner similar to that of a simple fracture.

The most common traumatic lesion of the spine is a compression fracture of a vertebral body. This type of fracture usually occurs in older people with osteopenia as a result of aging or inactivity or because they have taken drugs such as corticosteroids that tend to remove calcium from bones.[2,3] Fracture may occur as the result of a relatively trivial trauma, such as stepping off a curb or bending over, and produces pain of sudden onset and marked severity. The pain is relieved by bedrest and gradually wanes over a period of one or two weeks. The pain is usually sharply localized but may be accompanied by considerable muscle spasm with its more diffuse pain. In some cases, the bone of the vertebral body may be so soft that the pressure of the intervertebral disk compresses the adjacent vertebral plate, causing a typical invagination seen on the radiograph known as a Schmorl's nodule. This is found most often in the lumbar or dorsal spine.

Osteopenia alone does not cause pain, and the degree of osteopenia observed on a radiograph does not correlate well with pain. When pain occurs without apparent change in the contours of the vertebral bodies, it suggests that microfractures have occurred without distortion of the vertebral bodies. Patients who have considerable kyphosis due to multiple compression fractures or ankylosing spondylitis or who have significant scoliosis often have muscular backache secondary to the chronic muscular effort necessary to maintain an erect posture. This pain is exaggerated by fatigue and is quickly relieved by lying down.

Spondylolisthesis (displacement of one portion of the spine on another) occurs most often in the lumbar spine. This lesion develops at the site of a congenital spine anomaly, at which point weakness or instability of the supporting structures allows displacement, usually at times of physical strain to the low back. The bony displacement causes strain on adjacent ligaments and articulations, protective muscle spasm develops, and all these changes contribute to the associated pain. Diagnosis is usually made accurately, based on the history of lumbar back strain, physical abnormalities including a palpable "shelf" at the site of the subluxation, painful flexion, and extension of the low back, with limitations of these motions and characteristic findings in the radiographs of the spine.

Infections may cause back pain. The most common infections are related to acute hematogenous osteomyelitis (due most often to *Staphylococcus, E. coli* or *Pseudomonas*) and tuberculosis of the spine (Pott's disease). Osteomyelitis in vertebrae has the characteristics of osteomyelitis elsewhere: suppuration, abscess formation, bone destruction, seqeuestration, involucrum formation, periosteal elevation, penetration and dissection along muscle or fascial planes, soft-tissue abscesses, and sinus formation. The type and intensity of the pain depend upon the degree of stretching of the periosteum, the amount of irritation from the products of inflammation, and the stimulation of nerve endings or compression of fibers caused by edema and muscle spasm.

Tuberculosis of the spine is always a metastatic process resulting from hematogenous dissemination of tubercle bacilli. It may begin in a vertebra or an intervertebral disk, from which it involves adjacent structures. In the early stages, pain and tenderness may be confined to a relatively small portion of the back in the region of the infection. As the tuberculous process advances, one or more vertebral bodies may collapse, causing an angular kyphosis (gibbus) that produces altered weight-bearing and strain of ligaments muscles and fascia. Muscle spasm may become extensive and cause more severe and widespread back pain. If a paraspinous tuberculous abscess develops, it may press upon nerve roots or fibers, causing pain in the distribution of the nerve. An abscess may dissect between fascial planes to produce pain quite remote from the original lesion, or it may point into the spinal canal and cause irritation of the meninges. Purulent meningitis may develop if infection is liberated within the spinal canal; cord compression may cause transverse myelitis. A diagnosis of Pott's disease usually is easily proved by characteristic radiographic changes and positive cultures.[4]

Malignant neoplasms may occur in the spine (primarily sarcoma, more often metastatic carcinoma or multiple myeloma). Whatever the nature of the neoplasm, if the tumor is small and does not irritate the periosteum, there may be no discomfort. When the tumor enlarges and erodes the cortex and tears or stretches the periosteum, or weakens the support in the back so that strain of ligaments or joint capsules and muscle spasm result, or when there is direct pressure on nerves, back pain may be agonizing. It is often described as "expansile" or "boring" pain. It is usually present constantly, but is intensified by weight-bearing or movement. In multiple myeloma, radiographic changes may not be found early in the disease. A serum protein electrophoresis, a search for Bence-Jones protein in the urine, and a bone marrow aspiration or biopsy are appropriate procedures in the evaluation of back pain in older patients. Radicular pain may accompany back pain or even predominate in these patients.

Spinal pain due to malignancy is characteristically not relieved by bed rest.

LESIONS OF THE JOINTS AND INTERVERTEBRAL DISKS

The apophyseal joints, which are true joints with articular cartilage, joint capsule, and synovial membrane, may become inflamed as do the joints of the extremities. The most common cause of joint inflammation to affect the apophyseal joints is ankylosing spondylitis (also known as rheumatoid spondylitis or Marie-Strümpell disease). Much doubt has arisen regarding this form of spinal arthritis.

Most investigators now do not believe ankylosing spondylitis to be a form of rheumatoid arthritis affecting the spine. First, the sex ration is different: males are predominantly affected by ankylosing spondylitis and females by rheumatoid arthritis. Patients suffering from the former are generally younger and lack rheumatoid factor in their sera. There are genetic differences as well. Most patients with ankylosing spondylitis exhibit the HLA-B27 histocompatability antigen in their sera, while this antigen occurs in a small minority of patients with peripheral rheumatoid arthritis. The histopathologic features of the disease in the spinal joints, however, are comparable to those of rheumatoid arthritis in the peripheral joints. The facts that some patients with classic ankylosing spondylitis also have peripheral joint involvement and that about 10% have rheumatoid factor may indicate a chance coincidence of both diseases. Spasm of the regional back muscles and paraspinous calcification under the spinal ligaments contribute to the stiffness, immobility, and pain. Irritation of the spinal nerve roots may produce radicular pain simulating that of a herniated disk. Consequently, this disease is usually characterized by severe back pain, stiffness, and loss of motion. In contrast to the spondylitis sometimes associated with psoriatic arthritis, which may start at any level in the spine, the spinous involvement in ankylosing spondylitis starts in the sacroiliac joints and the joints of the lumbar spine and ascends gradually with time.

Over the course of years, the sacroiliac joints usually become fused as do the affected posterior articulations and costovertebral joints. Often the symphysis pubis also becomes fused. Permanent stiffness and immobility of the spine result from intra-articular ankylosis or subligamentous calcification or from a combination of both of these pathologic processes.

In the preankylosing stages, pain is the major disabling problem. The mechanism of the production of pain in this type of spondylitis is the same as that in rheumatoid arthritis in the joints of the extremities. The pain that characteristically occurs in the early stages of this disease usually results from irritation of the fascia, the ligaments and the tendons that attach to the low back. The pain spreads upward as the inflammation ascends the spine, and the parts affected earlier become less painful as stiffness and ankylosis develop. The pain stops when motion stops. When spondylitis affects the dorsal spine, costovertebral joints are involved in the inflammatory process so that chest expansion becomes painful and restricted. In fact, loss of chest expansion is one of the earliest and most significant physical findings in the diagnosis of ankylosing spondylitis. Radicular pain resulting from nerve root irritation is common. Sneezing, coughing, or other movements that suddenly jar the back or increase the intraspinal pressure produce severe neuralgia in the back or along the thoracic or abdominal segmental nerves.

Whenever a teenage or young adult male complains of pain in the low back or thighs, ankylosing spondylitis should be suspected.[5] There may be an interval of months or years between the onset of pain and the appearance of radiographic changes, and therefore normal films do not exclude the diagnosis. In fact, radiographic changes in the sacroiliac joints may occur in Reiter's syndrome, psoriatic arthritis, or juvenile rheumatoid arthritis so that radiographic changes in the sacriliac joints are not specific for ankylosing spondylitis. Nevertheless, in the absence of skin abnormalities, urethritis, or conjuctivitis, radiographic changes in the sacroiliac joints almost always means ankylosing spondylitis.[6] Early diagnosis allows more effective treatment of this painful, crippling disease and is helpful in the maintenance of an erect posture.

Tuberculosis may affect one sacroiliac joint; it is very seldom bilateral. Disease of one sacroiliac joint causes unilateral, regional back pain, with or without muscle spasm. Tenderness is usually present only over the affected joint. Radiographs usually identify the lesion but a biopsy may be necessary to establish the diagnosis.

Low back pain that occurs after lifting or vigorous physical activity often is considered by the patient to be due to a "sacroiliac sprain." The concept that the sacroiliac joint can be sprained or "thrown out" is difficult to support with factual evidence.[7] Dislocation of the sacroiliac joint does not occur without fracture of the bones of the pelvis. Mechanical lesions of the sacroiliac joints, if they occur, are exceedingly rare.

The junctions between the vertebral bodies are not true articulations. Motion is not accomplished by gliding or hingelike movements at these junctions. Disk narrowing and reactive bone formation between the vertebral bodies in the cervical spine are therefore, not properly called osteoarthrits. The segmental bony

composition of the spine, however, with fibrocartilaginous disks between vertebrae, allows flexibility of the spine.

Because the spine shares so extensively in almost all physical activities, it commonly undergoes changes due to wear and tear. After a number of years, this results in degeneration of the intervertebral disks and hypertrophic lipping and spurring at the edges of the adjacent vertebrae. Complete bony bridging between vertebral bodies may result from osteophytic growths. These changes characterize oseoarthritis of the spine, more correctly labeled osteoarthrosis or degenerative disease of the spine.[8] These changes, so apparent on radiographs, are usually not the cause of back pain, with the exception of lumbar spinal stenosis, a condition that is discussed later in this section. In fact, a form of spinal osteoarthritis is commonly found in American Indians and yet they suffer back pain no more frequently than the general population.[9] Osteoarthritic changes discovered by radiographs should not be assumed to be the cause of back pain until proven. Osteophytic pressure on nerve roots may cause radicular pain, but more often the pressure results from herniation of the disk at the same level.

Intervertebral disk disease is the most common cause of sciatic pain.[10,11] Quite often, severe pain begins suddenly with a slipping or ''snapping,'' which the patient experiences in the act of stooping, lifting, or rising from a sitting or lying position. The pain is usually in the midline; the patient often cannot straighten his back because of pain and muscle spasm. Sneezing and coughing aggravate the pain. These attacks are believed by some investigators to represent the beginning of degenerative changes with softening and posterior displacement of the nucleus pulposus so that it produces pain by stretching the posterior spinous ligament (Fig. 11-4).[12] The symptoms of the disk lesion in this stage (with or without actual herniation) may be relieved by maneuvers that straighten the spine and readjust pressure so that the nucleus is returned to its

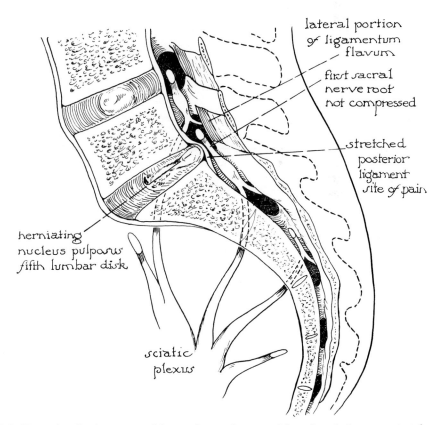

lateral portion
of ligamentum
flavum

first sacral
nerve root
not compressed

stretched
posterior
ligament
site of pain

herniating
nucleus pulposus
fifth lumbar disk

sciatic
plexus

Fig. 11-4. Posterior displacement of the nucleus pulposus without herniation may stretch the posterior spinous ligament, and it may not protrude sufficiently to compress nerve roots. (From Keegan, JJ: Diagnosis of herniation of lumbar intervertebral disks by neurologic signs. JAMA 126:868, 1944)

normal central position, thereby relieving pressure on adjacent ligaments and eliminating the irritation set up by the displacement.

True herniation of the nucleus pulposus occurs when there is a tear of the annulus and a sufficient amount of the nucleus escapes under the posterior longitudinal ligament. There is then a tumor within the spinal canal that causes pressure on a nerve root (Fig. 11-5). Such a rupture may be sudden or gradual. Symptoms indicating unilateral nerve root compression are the distinguishing characteristics. The patient usually complains of aching pain in the superior midgluteal region, with sharper, more variable pain radiating down the posterior thigh and lateral calf (sciatica).

Several factors are involved in the compression of a nerve root by herniation of an intervertebral disk. [13,14] Usually the herniation is located on one side of the midline directly beneath an emerging nerve root. If the spinal canal is large, the herniated fragment may displace the root and may not compress it. In such instances there may be several episodes of back pain without definite nerve root symptoms. In most persons, there is considerable flattening or narrowing of the spinal canal at the lumbosacral junction, so that herniation at this level usually compresses the nerve

root against the ligamentum flavum and lamina. The nerve root is fixed laterally, and the herniation of the disk occurs medial to it, so that the compression develops in the narrow lateral angle of the spinal canal beneath a portion of the ligamentum flavum.

The earliest and most common complaint of nerve root irritation from herniation of a disk in the lumbar region is superior midgluteal pain. This is best explained as resulting from compression of the posterior primary division of the nerve against the ligamentum flavum (Fig. 11-5). In this division are found the fibers that supply sensation to the central gluteal region. The central portion of the medial half of the root contain the sensory fibers that form the anterior primary division of the nerve to the leg. Greater compression may involve the anterior primary division of the root that joins with other roots to form the great sciatic nerve, which innervates most of the lower extremity below the knee.

Each of the roots forming the sciatic nerve has a segmental distribution, both motor and sensory (Fig. 11-6). The areas of the limb usually reported as sites of pain and paresthesia from disk lesions are the posterior thigh and the calf, the lateral portion of the ankle, and the foot. These segments are supplied by the

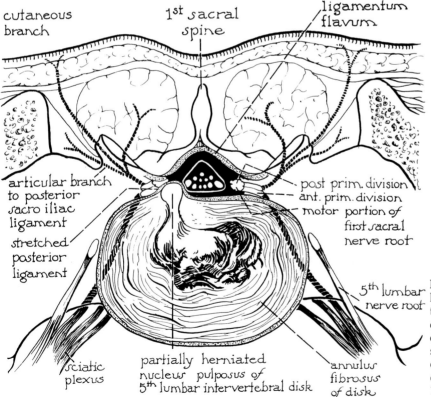

Fig. 11-5. Diagram showing how herniation of the nucleus pulposus through torn annular tissue may produce an intraspinal tumor that will compress a nerve root and cause sciatica. (From Keegan, JJ: Diagnosis of herniation of lumbar intervertebral disks by neurologic signs. JAMA 126:868, 1944)

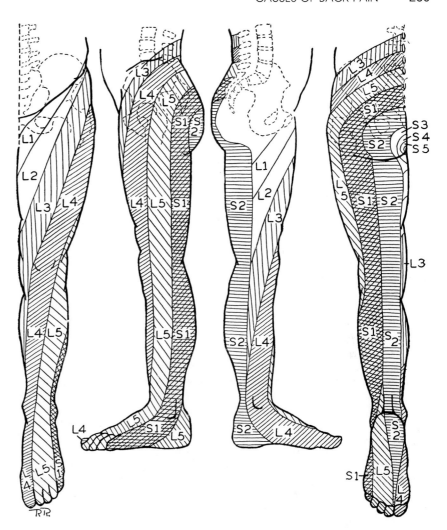

Fig. 11-6. Composite dermatome chart of the lower extremity determined by hypalgesia from single nerve root loss. (From Keegan JJ: Diagnosis of herniation of lumbar intervertebral disks by neurologic signs. JAMA 126:868, 1944)

first sacral root. The portion of the limb innervated by L5 is more lateral on the thigh and the leg, the front of the ankle, the top of the foot, and the second, third, and fourth toes. Since all the nerve roots have different dermatomes, determing the location of pain by careful history taking and demonstration of sensory changes in the limbs will indicate the nerve root involved and will locate the level of the disk lesion. If the roots supplying the heel or patellar areas are compressed, these deep tendon reflexes will be diminished or absent, contributing important diagnostic information.

The majority of disk lesions occur in the lumbar region at L4 or L5 accounting for the high incidence of low back pain and sciatica. The nerve root commonly compressed by protrusion of the L5 disk is S1; by disk L4 the compressed nerve is L5 and so forth. When unilateral nerve root pain, loss of reflex, and dermatone hypalgesia exist as the chief characteristics of a patient's illness, the pathologic conditions must be directly related to involvement of a nerve root on that side. The recognition of the first sacral root syndrome strongly suggests herniation or protrusion of the L5 disk and eliminates most other causes of back pain. If there is complete herniation of the nucleus pulposus through a tear in the annulus, tension on the annulus and longitudinal spinous ligament ceases and there is no longer pain in the back; there may be only nerve root irritation causing pain and sensory changes in the limb.[15]

Lesions of disks in the cervical portion of the spine produce the same type of pain in the back and pain and altered sensation from nerve root pressure as described for the lumbar disk syndrome. The only difference is the location of the back pain and involvement of the upper extremity instead of the lower. Movements of the head and neck aggravate the discomforts.

Lumbar spinal stenosis is a condition that is being recognized with increasing frequency. It is caused by narrowing of the spinal canal, nerve root canals and/or intervertebral foramina. As mentioned previously, the canal tends to be narrow at the lumbosacral junction and any combination of degenerative changes such as disk protrusion, osteophyte formation, or ligamentous thickening reduce the space needed for the spinal cord and its nerve roots. All diameters of the canal may be reduced, and the cross-sectional configuration assumes a triangular shape. A congenital form of spinal stenosis occurs in achondroplastic spines. The short, thick pedicles characteristic of this condition are due to the premature closure of the centers of ossification of the bodies with those of the lamina.

The more common acquired form has its peak incidence in the 7th decade.[16] It is primarily a male disorder characterized by pain in the back, buttocks, thighs, calves, and feet. There are often burning or numb sensations. All the symptoms are brought on by walking or standing and rapidly relieved by sitting or lying. Bodily positions that flex the lumbar spine tend to relieve the pain, while positions that extend the spine (and reduce the space within the canal) make the pain worse. Patients are more comfortable walking uphill, for example, than downhill. Unlike the situation in isolated disk protrusion, straight leg raising is usually not painful.

Because of the relationship of the pain to walking, the condition has been called "claudication of the cauda equina." Evidence that the pain may result from compression of the vessels supplying blood to the area has been provided by Evans who showed that breathing 12% oxygen reduced the pain on walking, while breathing pure oxygen allowed unrestricted walking.[17]

A variety of pathologic changes are found in these patients. There is usually disk protrusion into the anterior aspect of the canal with thickening of the lamina and ligamentum flavum. There is thickening of the nerve roots. Osteophytes are found along the margins of the vertebral bodies and around the posterior intervertebral joints. The ligaments are often thickened and buckled.[18]

Radiographically, the pedicles are often shortened and the posterior joints more medially placed. Plane films are usually inadequate for diagnostic purposes, however, and the diagnosis must be made by myelography or by computerized axial tomography.[19] Denervation may be revealed by electromyographic studies, but the changes are not specific. Since about 70% of patients with lumbar stenosis are relieved by extensive decompressive surgery, it is important to think of this diagnosis in older patients who have pain brought on

by walking, and to initiate the appropriate studies and therapy.

LESIONS OF THE LIGAMENTS, FASCIA, AND MUSCLES

Although involvement of the ligaments, fascia and muscles contribute much to the discomfort of disease primarily affecting the spinal column and its articulations, these structures are subject to relatively few primary pathologic processes causing backache. All or any of these soft tissues may be injured in performing heavy work, especially lifting, pushing, or pulling in a stooped position. In sports or accidental injuries, these structures may alone be traumatized. When there is no true joint dislocation, so-called back strain or sprain is the result of incomplete tears or stretching of the tendons at the site of their attachments or unusual use of muscles so that soreness and muscle spasm occur. The erector spinae, quadratus lumborum, latissimus dorsi, and trapezius are the muscles commonly injured in these ways. Diagnosis of such injuries depends chiefly upon knowledge of the circumstances of the injury and upon elimination of dislocation fractures, disk lesions, metastases, and so forth, by careful studies including radiographs.

Pain in the back frequently results from spasm of the muscles that occur as part of a protective mechanism for a lesion in the spinal column. Myalgia, muscle tenderness, is commonly experienced following unusual exercise or exposure to dampness and cold. Suppurative myositis in the back is very rare. Myositis usually exists as part of a generalized disease such as trichinosis. Muscle biopsy may be required to establish the diagnosis.

One of the diffuse systemic rheumatic diseases, polymyositis, may cause back pain, although usually associated with more widespread muscle pain.[20] It usually involves the muscles of the interscapular and shoulder girdle groups, and less often, the lower back muscles. Weakness of the inflamed muscles and atrophy commonly accompanies the pain. Tenderness varies considerably. Muscles biopsies showing inflammatory cell infiltration of muscle and muscle fiber degeneration is diagnostically characteristic. Polymyositis may be confused with polymyalgia rheumatica (see Chap. 12, Joint and Periarticular Pain) but in the latter condition muscle atrophy does not occur, the biopsy is normal, and there is no elevation of the serum muscle enzymes as is seen in active polymyositis.

Historically, a condition called fibrositis, myofibrositis, or muscular rheumatism has been described. The posterior neck, the shoulders, the interscapular region, and the lumbar region are tender and sore. Some of

these cases were undoubtedly cases of polymyalgia rheumatica. Since, in this form of nonarticular rheumatism, no histopathologic or other measurable changes have been found, there is considerable debate as to whether or not such a diagnosis is justifiable. In this condition, the onset may be abrupt so that it causes an acute painful stiff neck or a sore stiff lower back (lumbago). Severe muscle spasm prevents motion of the involved part and produces pain. The jarring of walking may produce so much pain that the patient prefers to remain in bed.

When fibrositis has a more insidious onset, the pain is usually a dull ache, worse after a night's rest or prolonged inactivity. With activity, pain and stiffness lessen; consequently through the middle of the day the patient is relatively comfortable, but toward evening with fatigue, stiffness and aching become worse. The affected tissues are usually tender to pressure and squeezing. Pressure over "trigger points" may produce more widespread discomfort.

LESIONS OF THE SPINAL CORD AND MENINGES

Trauma of sufficient violence to injure the spinal cord or the meninges almost invariably causes extensive injury to the supporting tissues of the back, which is the chief cause of the resultant back pain. Infection of the spinal cord and its coverings sometimes is the cause of back pain. Anterior poliomyelitis, for example, usually is characterized in the early stages by posterior headache and stiff neck. In the invasive stage of the disease, these symptoms appear to result from reflex phenomena caused by the inflammation, edema, and irritation of the invaded nervous tissue. If there is localization of the virus in motor cells supplying spinal muscles, pain and tenderness of the corresponding muscles result.

Diseases that irritate the meninges cause back pain by way of the recurrent branch of the spinal nerve, which carries sensory fibers from the meninges (Fig. 11-3). The discomfort results chiefly from reflex spasm of back muscles causing stiff neck (meningismus) and leg signs (Kernig's Lasègue's, and others) characteristic of meningitis. Back pain, however, is not a prominent symptom of meningitis. Culture of the spinal fluid establishes the diagnosis.

Neoplasms that originate in the spinal cord or its coverings may produce regional back pain by stretching of, or pressure on the meninges, or by invasion of supporting structures of the back. Pain from spinal cord tumors is referred to the sites of distribution of the peripheral nerves affected more often than it occurs in the back. When spinal cord tumors cause back pain or referred pain, there are usually characteristic sensory and motor changes as well. Clinical examination, study of the dynamics and characteristics of the spinal fluid, and radiographs of the spine usually indicate the nature of the trouble.

FAULTY BODY MECHANICS

Many people with dull back pain do not have a disease in any structure of the back; rather, they have a postural defect that strains the back as a whole. In order to understand backache that results from faulty body mechanics, it is only necessary to stand for several hours in an unnatural stooped position. Strain of the muscles, the tendon attachments, the fascia, the ligaments, and the joints causes aching that may persist for days. In like manner, defective posture may strain tissues that tend to compensate for a postural defect, and thus produce continuous and prolonged pain.[21]

Arthritis of the hip, scoliosis, and other lesions that cause imbalance of the paired structures of the back or alter the line of weight-bearing may cause back pain. The disturbance in the line of weight-bearing may be in the antero-posterior plane. Examples are dorsal kyphosis, increased lumbar lordosis, and "sway-back" from disproportionate abdominal obesity or gravidity. Any abnormal posture causes strain on some or the vertebral joint capsules, on the intervertebral ligaments, and the muscles of the back. Postural tone of the back muscles, normally maintained without effort or fatigue by the autonomic nervous system, is then partly maintained by voluntary contraction of the muscles in the back. This leads to fatigue and back pain. The discomfort is increased by the strain on the joint capsules and the ligaments in the spine at points where the increased curvature exists.[22]

The disturbed relationships of many parts of the body affected by the "slouch" position of the back (with increased dorsal kyphosis, increased lumbar lordosis, and a more horizontal position of the pelvis) are illustrated in Figure 11-7. Obesity with a protuberant abdomen produces added backache. Forward displacement and ptosis of the abdominal viscera cause strain on the suspensory ligaments that attach to the back, thus producing aching pain in the back.

Proper supports for pes planus, exercises to correct postural defects caused by weak torso muscles, restoration of good standing, sitting, and sleeping postures, and correction of accentuated spinal curvatures are beneficial remedial procedures. The relief obtained from proper correction attests to the importance of faulty mechanics as a cause of backache.[23]

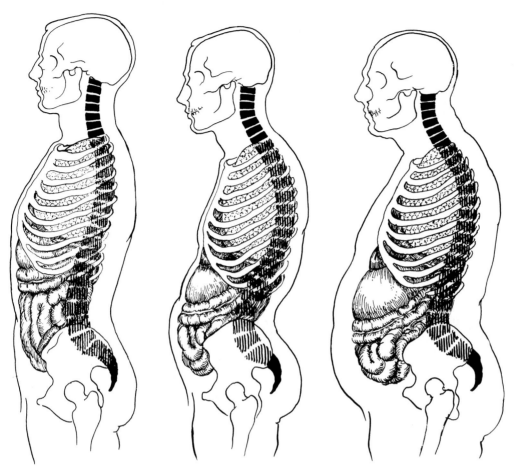

Fig. 11-7. The postural disorder of ''slouch back'' *(center)* and this abnormal posture combined with obesity *(right)* contrast sharply with normal posture *(left)*.

LESIONS OF THORACIC, ABDOMINAL, OR PELVIC ORGANS

In other chapters, the mechanism of reflex pain originating in somatic structures and referred to viscera is explained. The converse of this—viscerosomatic referred pain—is another cause of aching or severe pain in the back. Lesions in the peripheral portions of the lungs that may irritate the posterior parietal pleura may cause back pain in the thoracic region. With this type of back pain, there are usually important respiratory symptoms that do not accompany primary back pain. Mediastinal tumors (neoplasms and aortic aneurysms) may cause back pain. Saccular aneurysms may erode vertebrae and ribs causing severe boring pain or radicular pain from irritation of spinal nerve roots and distortion of the periosteum. Dissecting aortic aneurysms commonly cause agonizing pain in the back.

Pain in the back is more apt to result from visceral disease in the abdomen and pelvis than from intrathoracic disease. The mechanism by which gallbladder disease, liver abscess, or right subdiaphragmatic abscess cause pain referred to the right shoulder is well known. Backache or sharp pain in the back frequently results from lesions of the gastrointestinal tract. In most instances, visceral dysfunction causes prominent gastrointestinal symptoms, and backache is a lesser complaint, but many investigators have reported instances of duodenal ulcer in which back pain was the only symptom.[24-26] In most instances, back pain from peptic ulcer is a dull ache in the midline (or slightly to either side) between T5 and T10. Frequently these ulcer patients have been studied by an orthopedist, neurologist, neurosurgeon, gynecologist, or internist without finding the cause for the pain until hemorrhage or radiographs indicate the existence of the gastrointes-

tinal lesion. Examination of the stool for occult blood is a simple but valuable step in the workup of back pain.

Low back pain may be caused by disease of the colon or the rectum, especially if constipation exists. The classic balloon experiments by Jones indicate a mechanical basis for the backache due to disorders of the intestine.[24] A distended balloon in the duodenal cap sometimes caused pain in the back or pain that radiated from the xyphoid process through to the back. When a balloon was distended in the second portion of the duodenum, pain often occurred in the back or around the margin of the thoracic cage. Distention of the colon frequently caused low backache; sometimes this was the only symptom. These studies show that most, if not all, symptoms caused by these disturbances are fundamentally associated with local distention of the gut either above an area of spasm or above an area of organic disease that is constricting the bowel. The splanchnic nerves enter the cord from T5 to T12. Nerves to the stomach and the duodenum probably originate in the upper portion of this section of the cord. It has been shown that evulsion of the splanchnic nerves performed under local anesthesia causes severe pain. Often low back pain is caused by spasm or dilatation of the colon and promptly disappears when the bowel disorder is relieved. Lumbosacral pain due to distention of the sigmoid colon is promptly relieved by the enema, indicating that the pain is of a mechanical nature.

Perforation of a peptic ulcer may cause pain referred to the back. An ulcer in the posterior wall of the stomach or the duodenum and penetrating into the pancreas, or a carcinoma of the pancreas, sometimes causes low back pain. Agonizing lumbar back pain may be produced by acute pancreatitis or dissecting aneurysm of the abdominal aorta.[27]

There are records of a number of instances in which low back pain in the midline or slightly to the right was caused by an inflamed and distended retrocecal appendix. Sudden onset of pain in this region should make one suspicious of this lesion.

Painful disorders of the kidney parenchyma or capsule usually produce flank pain. The experimental studies of Ockerblad[28] indicate that obstructive uropathies which produce stretching of the capsule of the kidney, cause pain in the flank.[28] The average area of pain was small (8 cm–10 cm in diameter). If pain and tenderness exist in one or both costovertebral angles, the urinary tract should be investigated.

Inflammation in the prostate and the seminal vesicles may cause low lumbar or sacral pain. Many references have been made to the frequency with which chronic lower back pain is caused by infection or other diseases of the pelvic organs. Chronic lower back pain due to pelvic disease rarely occurs in patients who do not have other more prominent symptoms that would lead to consultation with a urologist or gynecologist.

It should be emphasized that low back pain in females is usually not due to pelvic disorders. Congestion at the time of menses, the mechanical burden of the late stages of pregnancy, and some pelvic tumors may cause backache for obvious reasons. Sometimes severe infection in the female pelvic organs may cause reflex pain in the low back. Uterine displacement however, and low-grade pelvic infection seldom cause backache.

MISCELLANEOUS CAUSES

In the prodromal stages of various febrile illnesses, backache may exist, along with generalized aching in the extremities. Sometimes septicemia may be ushered in by severe back pain, but soon malaise, fever, and other symptoms indicate the nature of the disease.

It is important to realize that some persons who complain of backache have no organic disease to cause it. Some of these persons are feigning pain that does not exist. Experiences in the armed forces have revealed a high incidence of "psychogenic rheumatism," occurring as a somatic manifestation of psychoneurosis.[29] Boland and Corr reported that the lower back is the most common site of this manifestation and that, in the group of soldiers studied, back pain was much more often due to psychoneurosis than to intrinsic disease of the spine or to organic rheumatic disease.[29] Psychogenic backache is very difficult to diagnose because there are few reliable characteristics. Careful study often reveals unusual localization of pain or bizarre radiation that does not conform to any anatomic pattern.[30] Usually it is uninfluenced by the factors that intensify or relieve the pain of organic disease. Other psychoneurotic manifestations are frequently present. Most difficult is the problem of proper evaluation of psychogenic back pain when it coexists with organic disease capable of producing back pain.[31, 32]

SUMMARY

Back pain may be caused by disease in any of the many structures in the back. Causes of back pain are explained on the basis of underlying pathologic physiology. The responsible disease is sometimes evident immediately; in the majority of cases, it can be determined through a thorough, systematic study. The complex structures of the back and the multiplicity of ailments to which the component tissues are subject

make it imperative to approach the problem in each patient with an unprejudiced viewpoint and to evaluate carefully all the evidence in an orderly fashion. Many mistaken diagnoses originate in the narrow viewpoint of specialists who fail to realize that the cause of the back pain may lie outside their specialty. The orthopedist must realize that back pain may not be due to structural disease of the back, the gynecologist cannot account for all cases of low back pain on the basis of pelvic disease, the neurologist can explain only some of the instances of back pain on lesions of the spinal cord or peripheral nerves, and the internist must realize that the different forms of arthritis or nonarticular rheumatism do not always account for pain in the back. Perhaps in no other medical problem is it so important to consider all the possibilities and to pursue a systematic study to a logical conclusion.

A carefully elicited and complete history of the manner of onset, the location, the radiation and nature of the pain, and the factors that aggravate or relieve it should be obtained. Thorough physical examination should include special back and leg maneuvers to allow recognition of disturbances of structure and function if they exist. Chest expansion should be measured. Examination of the thorax should be made whenever pain is located in the upper part of the back. When there is lower back pain, examination of the abdomen, pelvis, and rectum, including direct visualization of as many of these parts as can be seen, may be required. Radiographic examination of the spine and pelvis is an invaluable aid, including myelography, computerized axial tomography, and ultrasound examination. Studies of blood cytology, chemistry, erythrocyte sedimentation rate, and urinalysis are indicated. A systematic investigation supplemented by specialists' examinations should solve most problems of disease producing pain in the back. There are usually anatomic or physiologic disturbances that indicate a structural basis for back pain. Disturbances of posture usually can be recognized as a basis for faulty body mechanics. If back pain is referred from visceral disease, symptoms and signs of such a disease are usually found.

Pain in the back ranks among the most common problems of medical diagnosis. Knowledge of the structure and function of the back and the lesions that produce pain, together with intelligent interpretation of all findings, usually yield the solution.

REFERENCES

1. **Kellgren JH:** On distribution of pain arising from deep somatic structures with charts of segmental pain areas. Clin Sci 4:35–46, 1939

2. **Moldawer M:** Senile osteoporosis: The physiologic basis of treatment. Arch Intern Med 96:202, 1955

3. **Freyberg RH, Gascon J:** The problem of pathologic fractures in patients with rheumatoid arthritis receiving prolonged corticosteroid therapy. In Vol 1 pp 378–382. Proc X. Proc X International Congress on Rheumatic Diseases. Medica Turin, Minerva Medica 1961

4. **Berney S, Goldstein M, Bishke F:** Clinical and diagnostic features of tuberculous arthritis. Am J Med 53:56, 1972

5. **Polley HF:** Symposium on rheumatic diseases: diagnosis and treatment of rheumatoid spondylitis. Med Clin North Am 39:509, 1955

6. **Bluestone R:** Ankylosing spondylitis. In McCarty DJ (ed): Arthritis and Allied Conditions: A Textbook of Rheumatology, 9th ed, pp 610–631. Philadelphia, Lea & Febiger, 1979

7. **Cleveland M, Aldridge AH, Bosworth DM, Ray BS, Thomas SF:** Management of low back pain. Proc NY Acad Med 35:778–800, 1959

8. **Wilson JC Jr:** Degenerative arthritis of the lumbosacral joint, the end-space lesion. JAMA 169:1437, 1959

9. **Bennett PH, Henrard JC:** Hyperostosis of the spine in the Pima Indians. Arthritis Rheum 16:114, 1973

10. **Rose GK:** Backache and the disc. Lancet 1:1143, 1954

11. **Gill GG, White HL:** Mechanisms of nerve-root compression and irritation in backache. Clin Orthop 5:66, 1955

12. **Keegan JJ:** Diagnosis of herniation of lumbar intervertebral disks by neurologic signs. JAMA 126:868–873, 1944

13. **Jacobs JE:** Neuralgia and backache. Western Journal of Surgery 64:202, 1956

14. **Bradford FK:** Low back and sciatic pain. J Indiana State Med Assoc 50:559, 1957

15. **Morrell RM:** Herniated lumbar intervertebral disc: Cutaneous hyperalgesia as an early sign. Milit Med 124:257, 1959

16. **Blau JN, Logue V:** The natural history of intermittent claudication of the cauda equina: A long term followup study. Brain 101:211–222, 1978

17. **Evans JC:** Neurogenic intermittent claudication. Med J 2:985–987, 1964

18. **Hawkes CH, Roberts GM:** Lumbar canal stenosis. Br J Hosp Med 23:498–505, 1980

19. **Verbiest H:** The significance and principles of computerized axial tomography in the normal spine and in ideopathis developmental stenosis of the bony lumbar vertebral canal. Spine 4:379–390, 1979

20. **Pearson CM:** Polymyositis. Arthritis Rheum 2:127, 1959

21. **Denny–Brown D:** Clinical problems in neuromuscular physiology. Am J Med 15:368–390, 1953

22. **Gaston SR, Schlesinger EB:** Symposium on orthopedic surgery: Low back syndrome. Surg Clin North Am 31:329, 1951

23. **Levine DB:** The painful low back. In McCarty DJ (ed): Arthritis and Allied Conditions: A Textbook of Rheumatology, 9th ed, pp 1063–1064. Philadelphia, Lea & Febiger, 1979

24. **Jones CM:** Back pain in gastro-intestinal disease. Med Clin North Am 22:749–760, 1938

25. **Gilson SB:** Back pain in peptic ulcer. NY State J Med 61:625–627, 1961

26. **Compere EL:** Cymptom complex of visceral-spinal pain. Illinois State Med J 74:434–442, 1938

27. **Burt HA, Fletcher WD, Mattingly S:** Pitfalls in the diagnosis of backache. Ann Phys Med 2:1, 1954

28. **Ockerblad NF:** Urological backaches. Kansas City Med J 21:22–24, 1945

29. **Boland EW, Corr WD:** Psychogenic rheumatism. JAMA 123:805–809, 1943

30. **Levy RL:** Psychogenic musculoskeletal reactions. Medical Bulletin of the U.S. Army, Europe 13:175, 1955

31. **Wolff HG:** Stress and Disease. Springfield, Ill. Charles C. Thomas, 1953

32. **Sundt PE:** Psychogenic rheumatism. Proc R Soc Lond 48:66, 1955

12

Joint and Periarticular Pain Arthur Hall

Anatomic Considerations
Physiologic Considerations
Pathogenesis of Articular Pain
Diagnostic Considerations
Monoarticular Pain
Single Joint Involvement
    Finger
    Wrist
    Elbow
    Shoulder
    Hip
    Knee
    Ankle
    Foot

Polyarticular Pain
    Systemic Disorders
    Infectious Arthritis
    Rheumatic Fever
    Gouty Arthritis
    Rheumatoid Arthritis
    Degenerative Joint Changes
Nonarticular Rheumatism
    Fibrositis
    Polymyalgia Rheumatica
    Unexplained Arthralgias
Summary

Pain in and about the joints is one of the most common complaints with which the physician is confronted. Musculoskeletal pain, whether it arises from joints, tendons, muscles, bursae, or ligaments is usually described as joint pain. The patient who complains of hip pain may actually be describing pain along the iliac crest, pain in the trochanteric area (trochanteric bursitis), pain in the buttocks with the syndrome of sciatica, or true hip joint pain in the groin or in the corresponding posterior area in the buttock. Knowledge of the anatomic structures in which the inflammation may occur and of the mechanisms and patterns of articular and periarticular pain constitutes the basis for accurate diagnosis and proper treatment.

Not only is it important to identify the structures that are inflamed, but it is also helpful to divide musculoskeletal inflammatory conditions into those problems in which inflammation is part of a generalized disease process and those that reflect local problems.

Rheumatic fever is an example of a process that involves tissues and systems other than joints. Lateral epicondylitis (tennis elbow) is a local process.

ANATOMIC CONSIDERATIONS

Joints receive their nerve supply from nerves containing sensory fibers and autonomic fibers of various sizes. These nerves also innervate the muscles, bones, and skin of the surrounding area. There is usually an overlap of nerve innervation, with several nerves supplying a single joint area. Blocking a single nerve, therefore, does not solve the problem of pain in a particular joint. Following along the blood vessels to the joints, the articular nerve branches supply the joint capsule and adjacent ligaments. Terminal branches of unmyelinated and some finely myelinated fibers are distributed through the synovium and subsynovial tissue and

the regional periosteum. In the outer portion of the joint capsule, larger branches of the articular nerves divide to form a rich plexus from which finer branches course (usually along the arterioles into the subsynovial tissue, in which a secondary plexus may form close to the synovial surface). Some of the fine nerves terminate as individual fibers in synovial or subsynovial locations. Compared with the joint capsule, the synovium is relatively insensitive to pain, with most of the synovial nerves supplying blood vessels.

Nerves terminate to the joint capsule and synovium in one of three ways: (1) in a fine network, which often surrounds an arteriole close to the inner lining of the capsule (Fig. 12-1 A, B, E and Fig. 12-2 B), (2) as free nerve endings close to or actually in the surface of the synovial cells (Fig. 12-1 C, D and Fig. 12-2 A), (3) in a special end-organ that is an oval, laminated structure (Fig. 12-2 C, D) usually found deep in the fibrous portion of the capsule. This end-organ appears to be a form of pacinian corpuscle that is very sensitive to

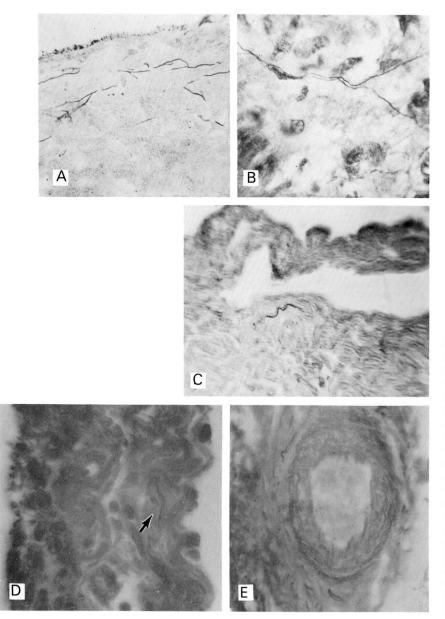

Fig. 12-1. Sections of human joint capsule, showing silver-impregnated nerve fibers. (A) Very near the synovial surfaces at the top of the section there is a rich plexus of small unmyelinated nerves. (B) A higher magnification of subsynovial tissue shows fine unmyelinated fibrils dividing, joining in a knotlike mesh, and separating again. (C) A single unmyelinated nerve very close to the synovial surface near the base of a villus. (D) High-power magnification of a villus (*arrow*) cut in longitudinal section, showing a single nerve fiber just beneath the surface. (E) High-power magnification of a synovial blood vessel, showing numerous unmyelinated nerve fibers in or near the adventitia.

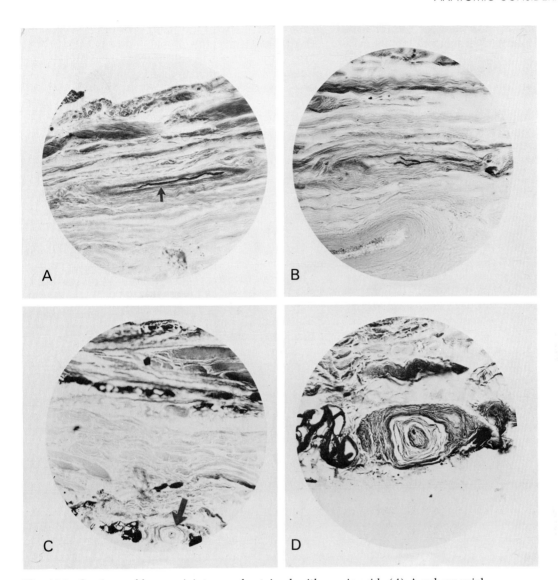

Fig. 12-2. Sections of human joint capsule stained with osmic acid. (*A*) A subsynovial nerve containing myelinated fibers. Note its proximity to the surface synovial cells at the top of the section. (*B*) Higher magnification of subsynovial tissue, showing a branching myelinated nerve alongside an arteriole. (*C*) Deep in a joint capsule (synovium at top) is a laminated nerve end-organ, a pacinian corpuscle. (*D*) Higher magnification of a pacinian corpuscle located deep in the fibrous tissue of the joint capsule.

changes in position or movement. The most painful stimuli are twisting, tearing, and stretching of the joint capsule or ligaments.

No nerves are found in articular cartilage or in the compact bone. Usually nerves travel to articular structures along blood vessels. Since joint cartilage is avascular, it is not surprising that cartilage should contain no nerves. This is important in understanding afflic-

tions primarily involving the articular cartilage, such as degenerative disease of joints (osteoarthritis).

Periarticular tissues are abundantly innervated, and in all these structures, the nerve endings are like those found in the joint capsule.[1,2] The smaller fibers from these various tissues form larger bundles that become parts of the dorsal spinal nerve root of the segment. The constituent parts of these nerves synapse in sim-

ilar spinal cord segments. It is clear, therefore, why stimuli originating in structures about the joints may give rise to a type of painful sensation considered by some patients as originating in the joint tissues.

PHYSIOLOGIC CONSIDERATIONS

Lennander found all the articular and periarticular structures (articular capsule, synovium, muscle, tendon, fascia, ligament, cancellous bone and periosteum) to be sensitive to pain: the articular cartilage and the cortical bone were insensitive.[3] These findings have been confirmed by others.[4-6] The only structures about which there is doubt concerning sensitivity to pain are the fibrocartilaginous menisci of the knee joints. It has been reported that direct stimulation of the menisci causes no pain, that displacement is painful, and that electrical stimulation causes pain. In these studies, the possibility that the pain might have originated in surrounding tissue to which the stimuli spread cannot be excluded.

The type, localization, and distribution of pain arising from structures in and about the joints have been studied extensively by Lewis and Kellgren.[7] Their fundamental research will be reviewed here in some detail. Kellgren injected muscles in various locations with hypertonic saline and observed that pain was always felt diffusely and was referred in a spinal segmental pattern. Ligaments irritated in a like manner gave rise to pain similar to that produced in muscle; a continuous ache was felt deep in the structures involved. The pain was associated with tenderness of the deep structures in a distribution corresponding to the localization of the pain; tenderness enabled the persons studied to localize the discomfort accurately to the areas stimulated.

Experiments repeated in the same subjects gave remarkably consistent results, even though weeks had elapsed between observations. Charts of the distribution of pain produced by the injection of intraspinous ligaments showed segmental areas of pain that did not correspond exactly with the dermatomes of skin tenderness. This variation suggests that distribution of deep pain and tenderness corresponds with the segmental innervation of the deep structures rather than that of the skin.

Pain that arose from the periosteum covering the tibia, the sternum, the vertebral spines, the acromion and the olecranon processes, or the phalanges (bony structures, all of which are close to the surface) was confined to the area of the point stimulated, whereas pain that arose from the deeply situated periosteum was felt more diffusely. Stimulation of nerve endings

in the deep fascia in the trunk and the limbs, in the subcutaneous ligaments in the tendon sheaths such as those in the wrists and ankles, and in the superficially placed tendons (patellar and Achilles tendon) also caused more localized pain like that from the superficial periosteum. Deeply situated intermuscular fascia and ligaments, when stimulated, gave rise to pain over a larger area, such as that arising from deeply located periosteum. Whether pain arising from a given structure is felt as localized or more diffuse pain depends upon the location of that structure (superficial or deep) more than upon the nature of the tissue (periosteum, ligament, tendon, or fascia).

Pain arising from muscles of the extremities usually is localized in the neighborhood of the joints that are moved by those muscles, if those joints are in the segmental pain area corresponding with the nerve supplying those muscles. Pain from smaller joints such as those in the hands and feet tends to be more localized, whereas pain arising in larger joints (hips and shoulders) usually is more segmental in distribution. Thus, pain arising from disease in the hip joint and the quadriceps femoris muscle often is felt in the knee, and pain arising from the tibialis anticus muscle may be localized in the ankle joint.

The extensive investigations of Gardner indicate that the joint capsule and the ligaments are sensitive to painful stimuli.[8-11] There is less clear evidence that the nerves shown in histologic specimens to terminate in the synovial lining of the joint capsules are pain receptors. Various methods used experimentally to stimulate nerve endings in the synovial lining may also have stimulated nerve receptors in the deeper layers of the joint capsule. The studies of Kellgren and Samuel, however, conducted in the human knee joint indicate that, although the synovial membrane is relatively insensitive, some areas of the synovia are definitely pain-sensitive.[6] The majority of the nerves in the synovial membrane are autonomic in origin and are contained in the blood vessel walls, whereas the fibrous joint capsule and articular ligaments are supplied with somatic nerves, with a variety of specialized and unspecialized nerve endings.[6,11]

Lewis and Kellgren studied referred somatic pain in relation to referred pain originating in a viscus.[12] It was found that, at its height, somatic pain experimentally produced in the trunk was accompanied by muscle rigidity and deep tenderness. With induced pain in the extremities, muscle spasm and tenderness were less evident. These features of somatic pain are similar to corresponding abnormalities associated with visceral pain. The nature of somatic pain was found to be exactly like that known to have visceral origin: it was constant and of unvarying intensity, and the quality

differed from the burning pain originating from the skin or mucous membranes. Induced somatic pain frequently was accompanied by paresthesias and subsequent hyperalgesia similar in type and location to such symptoms occurring with visceral pain. Lewis demonstrated that the pain of deep somatic origin cannot be distinguished from that of visceral origin and that deep somatic and visceral structures are supplied by a common set of afferent nerves, stimulation of which produces similar pain and reflex phenomena.[13] It is not surprising, therefore, that pains associated with various rheumatic disorders of the spine, thorax, shoulders, and arms may simulate the syndrome of angina pectoris caused by heart disease.[14]

Until recently it was thought that pain fibers were carried only in the somatic nerves entering the spinal cord through the posterior roots. The reports of Herfort indicate that at least a portion of the pain fibers from the lower extremities arrive at the cord centers through the autonomic pathways.[15,16] Herfort has reported substantial relief of pain due to arthritis in the hip and knee joints by performing "extended lumbar sympathectomy." Severing the lumbar sympathetic chain along the retroaortic plexus and sectioning the decussating fibers in the prevertebral plexus relieved joint pain in the lower extremities in the majority of arthritic patients in whom the operations were performed. Herfort believes that this surgical procedure accomplishes the benefit by "the ablation of afferent pain pathways running from the articular surfaces of the lower extremities and traversing the lumbar paravertebral sympathetic trunks and the retroaortic plexus."[15]

These observations appear to support the thesis that important sensory innervation of the articular structures of the hip, knee, and ankle joint is derived from the lumbar sympathetis ganglia. Support for this thesis is also provided by the report that transient diminution of pain resulted from the administration of tetraethylammonium bromide to patients with rheumatoid arthritis.[17] Furthermore, neuropathic joint changes did not occur in any of the sympathectomized patients. This indicates that the periarticular and extracapsular tissues are not denervated by section of the lumbar sympathetic trunks and that there is preservation of the extracapsular protopathic sensation providing the sense of joint position.

PATHOGENESIS OF ARTICULAR PAIN

The mechanism of excitation of pain-conducting nerve fibers in rheumatic disorders differs in the different diseases. The experiments of Lennander have shown that stimulation of tissues about joints by pinching, tearing, cauterizing with acid or heat, cutting, or sticking, or by the use electric currents produces the same type of pain.[3] Lewis confirmed these observations and also consistently initiated pain by injection of chemical irritants.[13] Knowing that pain can be induced by such different types of stimuli, one readily understands why most abnormalities of the joints and periarticular tissues are accompanied by pain.

The nature of the stimuli differs in various types of disease. Postural abnormalities and traumatic joint lesions produce pain by stretching, pinching, or tearing supportive tissues (ligaments, joint capsule, tendons, fascia, and periosteum). Neoplastic diseases, by reason of growth of the tumor and the resultant destructive changes, interrupt continuity, and stretch, pinch, or otherwise irritate pain nerve fibers and their endings. Inflammation, which characterizes so many rheumatic diseases (infectious arthritis, rheumatic fever, rheumatoid arthritis, gouty arthritis, bursitis, and tenosynovitis), excites pain by chemical irritation, stretching, tension, and, if there are any destructive changes of supporting tissues, by pressure on nerve endings that are normally protected. Swelling of the joint capsule and periaticular tissues by effusions in joints produces pain by stretching of the joint capsule. Typically, there is marked relief of pain when the fluid in the joint is aspirated. Absence of discomfort when joint tissues are loosely infiltrated by noninflammatory edema (as in the ankle edema of heart failure) indicates that pain accompanying inflammation of articular structure must result either from swelling within a closed space or from other stimuli. Chemical irritants formed by the inflammatory process appear to act as important excitants of pain in nerve endings. Current evidence indicates that the activation of the complement system and the kinin system is very important in the inflammatory and pain processes.[18]

Traumatic or inflammatory joint disease is often accompanied by spasm of adjacent muscles. Spasm contributes to the pain by adding the discomfort of muscle pain or by stimulating nerve endings in the periosteum at fascial and tendinous attachments. Faulty body mechanics may also add to the traction and strain.

DIAGNOSTIC CONSIDERATIONS

To understand the diagnostic implications of pain, it is necessary to know the nature of the pain, its localization and distribution, its constancy or variability, the features that accentuate or relieve it. Different patients may describe pain quite differently. Pain may be influenced by many things other than the nature of the

pain stimulus. Some people complain bitterly of pain that others may consider trivial. There are wide variations in the tolerance and threshold for pain. Common terms used to describe pain are dull, aching, sore, sharp, burning, and the like. One must try from the description of the pain to identify the structures that are involved and to decide which pathologic processes are most likely to have produced that involvement.

MONOARTICULAR PAIN

Pain in a single joint may result from a number of different disorders. Trauma, producing a significant injury to the joint, is usually of sufficient severity to make the diagnosis evident by history. Traumatic joint injuries commonly originate from the sports accidents, occupational injuries, violent or accidental injuries. Trauma usually results from strain, sprain, traumatic synovitis, fracture of the bone extending into the joint, tear of the ligaments, tendons or capsule, tear of the cartilage in the knee (which may thereafter cause recurrent episodes of joint pain), or joint dislocation. Since pain results from the fact that the architectural and mechanical integrity of the joint has been compromised, physical examination discloses mechanical problems. The joints tend to lock or give way on walking. One can feel crepitus or popping when the joint is moved, especially when the joint is moved against resistance. Asking the patient to step up on a low stool while the examiner's hand is on the knee may bring out these abnormalities. The patient may give a history of being able to take ten comfortable steps, with the next step resulting in knifelike pain in the joint. As opposed to inflammatory joint disease, monoarticular pain is often localized to one side of the joint or to the other. The usual description of hip pain is less informative. Since the hip is a deep structure, the pain is more visceral and diffuse. It is impossible to differentiate the pain resulting from rheumatoid arthritis from that caused by chronic obesity and osteoarthritis or from that found in a tuberculous hip. Pain from ankle or foot trauma is indistinguishable from the pain of osteoarthritis in these areas or from that of rheumatoid arthritis. Chronically pronated feet may produce the same type of pain.

Neoplastic disease afflicting only one joint is rare and usually is a primary tumor (fibroma, fibrosarcoma, or synovioma). A bone tumor adjacent to a joint may cause pain in the joint, or pain referred to it, especially during motion of the joint. Occasionally a tumor in the bone adjacent to a joint may cause a synovitis that cannot be distinguished from rheumatoid arthritis. Neoplasms are apt to cause severe pain described as "boring" or "expansile." The pain is not relieved by rest and nights are nearly sleepless. Radiographs usually reveal the lesion in the bone, but may be confused with subchondral cysts in patients with rheumatoid arthritis.

Degenerative joint disease is a common cause of joint pain in older adults. Although several joints are usually affected, a single joint may be painful. The hip and the knee are most commonly affected, but pain in the first carpometacarpal joint or one of the intercarpal joints is not uncommon. When degenerative changes occur in the first metatarsophalangeal joint, preventing extension of that joint, there may be pronounced pain, swelling, and redness in that joint. These cases are often misdiagnosed as gout. The fact that the toe cannot be dorsiflexed passively establishes the correct diagnosis (hallux rigidus).

Septic joints have become more common since our more permissive society has brought about an increase in gonorrhea, and the medical treatment of a number of diseases with immunosuppressive therapy has made these patients more susceptible to various infections. Staphylococcal infections are still common, especially in joints already afflicted with other problems such as rheumatoid arthritis. Joint sepsis should be suspected whenever a single joint is involved, or when, in a patient with preexisting polyarthritis, one joint becomes disproportionately painful and swollen compared with the other joints. In most cases the organism recovered from the joint is also recovered from the urinary tract or some other site representing the primary area of infection. Cultures should be taken, not only from the joint and blood, but from the urine, vagina, rectum, and any other site that might be infected. This disorder is usually characterized by severe, throbbing pain. The patient is unwilling to allow the affected joint to be palpated or moved. The pain increases as the joint capsule becomes distended with pus. The patient maintains the joint in the position of greatest comfort—that of flexion. Movement of the joint increases the pain because of increased stretching of and tension of the inflamed joint capsule.

Unless prompt and effective treatment for septic joints is instituted, there may be rapid and extensive destruction of articular cartilage and bone in a few days or weeks. It is vital that the joint be aspirated and the fluid cultured. Antibiotic treatment should be started even before the culture results are available. The antibiotic can be changed later if the sensitivity studies so indicate. By the time radiologic changes of septic arthritis are evident, marked joint destruction has already occurred.

Tuberculosis commonly affects a single joint. Tuberculosis infection may extend into a single joint from a

focus in an adjacent joint (*e.g.,* spinal tuberculosis extending into a disk space) or tuberculosis may be a metastatic lesion. Characteristically, the disease progresses slowly and the pain is initially mild. The pain is usually made worse by weight-bearing or movement. Destruction of cartilage and bone causes greater pain and dysfunction. After destructive changes occur, the radiographic appearance may be diagnostic.[19] The mild character of the inflammation accounts for the "cold" or "cool" joint. Since bone and joint tuberculosis is usually secondary to tuberculous infection elsewhere in the body, identification of the primary site is helpful in the diagnosis. Tuberculin tests should be carried out in suspected cases. Often, the true nature of the infection is not identified until the results of joint aspiration or biopsy are available. The possibility of tuberculous arthritis should be considered when a patient has painful monoarticular joint inflammation. This type of infectious arthritis is much less common since dependable treatment for tuberculosis has become available.

Neuropathic joint disease often is painless. Mild or moderate joint discomfort, however, occurring at a joint that exhibits much swelling and hypermobility should make one suspect neuropathic joint disease. Diabetes is a more common cause today than is syphilis, the traditional example of the cause of neuropathic joints. Special diagnostic studies such as a blood sugar or one of the serologic tests for syphilis usually clarify the diagnosis. From the functional point of view, the problem in these patients is one of a mechanically unsound joint. Loss of pain sensation has allowed fragmentation of the joint cartilage and bone producing loose bodies and irregular surfaces that produce grinding motion and loss of stability.

Rheumatoid arthritis commonly affects many joints, but in many instances, especially in children, may begin and persist for many months in only one or a few joints (pauciarticular juvenile arthritis). Brief attacks of joint pain accompanied by swelling lasting from 1 to 3 or 4 days are most likely due to rheumatoid arthritis. Attacks of gouty arthritis, if untreated, last from 10 days to 2 weeks. The distribution of the joints involved is especially useful in diagnosis. Pain and swelling in the second through fifth metacarpophalangeal joints, the wrists, or the elbows almost always indicates rheumatoid arthritis or one of its variants. Involvement of the shoulders and the weight-bearing joints is less helpful in diagnosis, since many conditions may cause pain in these joints. Prolonged morning stiffness, often lasting into the afternoon and at times more disconcerting than the pain, is very suggestive of rheumatoid arthritis. Early and impressive loss of grip strength is also very typical.

In nonarticular rheumatism, a bursa located near a joint may become inflamed as a result of trauma, infection, or in association with systemic rheumatic disease. The swelling and distention of the bursal sac as a result of the accumulation of fluid within it may stimulate the pain fibers that are numerous in and about all bursae. Bursal pain is elicited by those motions that disturb the relationships of the bursae. If the bursa overlies the joint, as in the shoulder, joint motion will exacerbate bursal pain. When bursae are removed some distance from the area of the joint, as with the trochanteric bursa, motion of the hip joint may not cause pain, yet palpation of the greater trochanter may be very painful. Trochanteric bursitis is especially common in those patients who sleep on their sides. Inflammation of the anserine bursa is common and is usually diagnosed as knee disease. The fact that motion of the knee is usually painless and that the area of tenderness is well below the joint line on the medial aspect of the knee establishes the fact that the problem is extra-articular. The tendons, tendon sheaths, and fascia near a joint may be stretched by joint motion and may give rise to "joint pain" in a similar manner. DeQuervain's syndrome, "tennis elbow" (lateral epicondylitis), and stenosing tenosynovitis in the palm are examples. Passive motion of the joint is usually painless, but attempts to move the joint against resistance that prevents motion is painful. In these cases, it is the stretching of the structures that indicates or prevents motion rather than the motion itself that causes pain.

SINGLE JOINT INVOLVEMENT

Finger

Pain in a single finger joint is usually due to trauma. Pain and a flexion deformity in a single distal interphalangeal joint are usually due to avulsion of the extensor tendon to the distal phalanx from an injury (baseball finger). Pain and enlargement of several distal or proximal interphalangeal joints usually suggest the form of osteoarthritis associated with Heberden's nodes. This inherited condition, more common in females (10:1), usually comes on within three years of menopause and is self-limited. It may involve the first metacarpophalangeal joint or the first carpometacarpal joint but not the other metacarpophalangeal joints. Pain and swelling in the second through the fifth metacarpophalangeal joints essentially always means systemic rheumatic disease.

Nodules in the flexor tendons of the fingers, usually proximal to the metacarpophalangeal joints, may cause pain and often "triggering" of the finger so that it is

caught in flexion. The pain is often felt in the meta-carpophalangeal joint or proximal interphalangeal joint and is described as joint pain.

Wrist

Sprains, strains, and fractures of the wrist are common. One lesion characteristically located at the wrist is the "ganglion." A ganglion is a herniation of the synovium of one of the carpal joints out into the soft tissue. It becomes closed off from the joint space forming a hard swelling, usually on the dorsum of the wrist. It is rarely tender. It is to be distinguished from swelling in the extensor tendon sheaths that represent true tenosynovitis, which provides evidence of rheumatoid arthritis or one of the other systemic rheumatic diseases. The fact that the swelling of a ganglion is clearly extra-articular and does not move with motion of the tendon suggest the true diagnosis.

Elbow

Swelling of the olecranon bursa, often accompanied by marked tenderness and a tense effusion may be due to trauma but more often is due to rheumatoid arthritis. Olecranon bursitis, when it occurs in gout, is often accompanied by one or more small tophi within the bursa and is rarely tender. By the time gout involves the olecranon bursa there have been a number of typical acute gouty attacks affecting weight-bearing joints.

Another cause of elbow pain is "tennis elbow," or epicondylitis, which results from repeated pulling of the forearm extensor muscles from their tendinous insertion into the lateral humeral epicondyle.[20] Pain, sharply localized to the lateral epicondyle, not accentuated by motion but markedly increased by attempting to extend the wrist against resistance is characteristic. Patients with this problem can pick up a weight comfortably with the palm facing up, but not with the palm down. The opposite is true with medical epicondylitis. In this case, the inflammation is at the tendinous insertion of the wrist and hand flexors at the medial epicondyle, a condition sometimes referred to as "golf elbow." Tenderness, sharply localized to one of the epicondyles, pain accentuated by forceful contraction of one of the muscles groups of the forearm, and the absence of pain on motion of the elbow are helpful signs in diagnosis.

Shoulder

Most shoulder pain is not due to arthritis, although shoulder pain in arthritis is common. Besides fractures and dislocations (concerning which there is usually no problem in diagnosis), there are several forms of periarthritis that cause pain about this joint. One or another form of periarticular soft-tissue inflammation commonly cause the painful stiff shoulder.[21,22] The most common cause of the painful shoulder is tendinitis,[23] with or without calcification. What is usually called "bursitis" of the shoulder has been shown to be, in fact, inflammation of one of the tendons inserting into the greater trochanter of the humerus, usually the tendon of the supraspinatus muscle.[24]

Tendinitis has an acute onset, characterized by severe tenderness in the subacromial area of the shoulder or in the bicipital groove anteriorly. In either case, the pain is usually referred to the upper arm at the site of the insertion of the deltoid muscle. The localization of pain by the patient is usually of little help in identifying the actual site of inflammation. Careful palpation is necessary for localization. Restricted motion in abduction and pain on abduction actively, and absence of pain on passive abduction are typical. Pain on rotation makes it difficult or impossible for the patient to get his hand behind his back at the level of the waist or neck.

In patients with chronic or recurrent tendon inflammation, calcium salts may be found deposited in the inflamed portion of the tendon; this condition is referred to as "'calcific tendinitis." If the calcium deposit ruptures through the peritendinous tissue, it may localize in the subacromial bursa that overlies the supraspinatus tendon. Then, the condition is complicated by calcific bursitis. Frequently tendinitis and bursitis coexist. From the character and localization of the pain, it is impossible to know whether the lesion is in the tendon, the bursa, or both. It should be emphasized that tendinitis and bursitis may be present whether or not calcification is visible on radiographs, and since calcification may have occurred months or years earlier, the fact that it appears on current radiographs does not guarantee that either tendinitis or bursitis is the cause of the patient's present discomfort.

Pain is produced, in part, by distention of the tendon, or the bursa, or both, and frequently is promptly relieved by puncturing the surface of the distended structure, or aspiration of the distended bursal sac.

When tendinitis or bursitis exists, there is pain upon abduction or rotation of the shoulder, movements that stretch the inflamed tendon or bursal walls. Flexion and extension of the shoulder usually do not cause as much pain. Arthritis of the shoulder produces pain in all planes of motion.

Tendinitis may develop insidiously. In such cases, pain and tenderness are similar in location to those of bursitis, but are less severe. Calcium salts may be deposited in the tendon; more often they are not. The character of the pain is the same unless a hard calcium deposit forms that may, in itself, mechanically cause or aggravate the pain started by tendinitis. Areas of

calcification seen on radiographs usually represent the natural healing of areas of inflammation. Like the calcified lung lesion of tuberculosis, calcification about the shoulder joint is the result of rather than the cause of inflammation.

Persistence of tendinitis and bursitis at the shoulder may cause irritation of other structures around the joint and cause the chronic condition of adhesive capsulitis. This is characterized by a dull aching pain and diffuse minor tenderness that causes progressive limitation of all motions of the shoulder until the motion is almost nil. This is the so-called "frozen shoulder," a poor but descriptive term for the almost motionless, painful, stiff shoulder.

If trauma causes a tear in the tendons attaching to the humeral trochanter or if there is a tear in the musculotendinous cuff, abduction of the shoulder cannot be initiated, a helpful diagnostic characteristic of this lesion. Tears of the musculotendinous cuff of the glenohumeral joint capsule account for a large percentage of cases of shoulder pain. In this case, pain is sharply localized to the site of the pathology. Tears are well demonstrated with shoulder arthrography. Fractures of the glenoid labrum require double-contrast arthrography for visualization.

Another form of periarthritis of the shoulder is bicipital tendinitis. This lesion is characterized by pain and tenderness over the bicipital groove and around the tendon of the long head of the biceps. The pain is initiated by movement of the arm requiring contraction of the biceps muscle, and there is persistent tenderness over the lesser tuberosity of the humerus. Holding the arm in abduction is painful even without motion, helping to differentiate bicipital tendinitis from arthritis of the shoulder.

Brachial neuritis characteristically causes a more severe and sharp pain that radiates through the distribution of the involved nerves, and in this way it can be differentiated from shoulder pain or periarticular disease. Associated abnormalities in these conditions also aid in diagnosis.[25]

A condition more recently recognized is that of the "impingement syndrome." In these cases, either due to an idiopathic laxity of the joint or to an anatomic variation, the humeral head rides high in the glenoid fossa and inpinges on the anterior, inferior edge of the acromion. This causes pain and a palpable bump on rotation of the shoulder in abduction. The solution is the surgical removal of this edge of the acromion.

Shoulder pain may rarely be the principal or only symptom of degenerative disk disease in the neck, commonly and erroneously called "osteoarthritis." Either disk protrusion or, less commonly, impingement on nerve roots by narrowed neural foramina at the C4-5 or C5-6 level may cause pressure on the spinal nerves that innervate the shoulder. Production or accentuation of the pain by movements of the head and neck are characteristic of this condition. Care must be taken in the interpretation of the radiographs, since most often the radiographic abnormalities clearly antedate the onset of the pain and remain after the pain is gone. The so-called "satisfaction of discovery" often leads the physician to assume that the changes so easily seen on the films are the cause of the pain and not to consider carefully alternative explanations. More often neck pain results from a shoulder that is painful or limited in motion. If the patient cannot abduct the shoulder well or comfortably, he raises his arm by hiking his shoulder with his lateral neck muscles. These muscles then become strained and sore.

Since the nature of pain from visceral disease has been found by Lewis and Kellgren to be indistinguishable from that caused by somatic disease, it is not surprising that the shoulder, innervated by nerves from the same segment that supplies the heart, should be the site of pain after myocardial infarction.[26,27] Absence of aggravation by shoulder motion of the signs and symptoms of cardiac or coronary artery disease help to establish the diagnosis.

Disease of the gallbladder, the liver, or the right basilar pleura may stimulate nerves in the right diaphragm and cause pain felt in the right shoulder. The pain may be sharp, stabbing, and severe and may be followed by a dull ache. It usually can be differentiated from the discomfort of shoulder disease by its characteristic location in the scapular region and the absence of shoulder joint abnormality.

Hip

Because of its deep location, this large, important weight-bearing joint cannot be examined as satisfactorily as most other joints. To learn the cause of hip pain, it is often necessary to conduct extensive studies. During childhood, osteochondritis of the femoral head, separation and displacement of the capital femoral ephiphysis, and tuberculosis frequently cause hip pain. Recalling the discussion concerning the reference of pain occurring in deep structures to more superficial areas supplied by nerves from the same spinal segment, it is understandable that persons with disease of the hip may complain of pain along the anterior aspect of the thigh or at the knee. Similarly, associated with hip pain from any cause, pain along the distribution of the femoral nerve is the rule. Such pain should suggest lesions in the hip rather than in the lower back, disorders of which are most frequently associated with leg pain of sciatic or obturator nerve distribution.

Sometimes hip pain and associated anterior thigh

INFECTIOUS ARTHRITIS

Gonococcal arthritis is a common form of specific infectious arthritis. Between 10 and 20 days after venereal exposure, the patient experiences marked malaise and generalized aching. A few days later the generalized aching and arthralgia, and often the fever and chills subside and the inflammation settles into a few extremely painful joints. Tenosynovitis may be a prominent finding and may be quite painful. These joints are septic joints, and irreparable damage may develop rapidly if the correct diagnosis is not made and adequate treatment begun.

Other infections, such as meningococcal and pneumococcal septicemia involving multiple joints, may be complicated by infectious arthritis, with clinical features similar to those described for gonococcal arthritis. Aspiration of the joint fluid with cell counts and cultures usually establishes the etiology of the joint pain.

RHEUMATIC FEVER

Rheumatic fever is a febrile disease occurring primarily in children and young adults. The joint pain of rheumatic fever is usually so characteristic that it is very helpful in diagnosis. Onset of the arthritis of rheumatic fever usually begins shortly after a hemolytic streptococcal infection in the tonsils or pharynx. Several joints, usually paired joints, become inflammed. The synovitis worsens rapidly, so that within 24 hours the joints are markedly swollen, red, hot, and extremely tender. The pain may be so severe that the slightest jarring of the bed or the weight of the bedclothes on the affected joints causes excruciating pain. After several days, inflammation subsides in the affected joints and moves to others. The disease is thus characterized by a "migratory" arthritis. No anatomic or functional residua remain after the joint inflammation subsides.

If one recognizes these typical features, the diagnosis usually can be made correctly. The presence of carditis, chorea, and a rising titer of antistreptococcal antibodies are helpful in the diagnosis. The joint pain is entirely due to the inflammation, is quantitatively related to its severity, and leaves as the synovitis subsides. Salicylates more quickly and completely relieve the pain and inflammation of acute rheumatic fever those of any other systemic rheumatic disease.

GOUTY ARTHRITIS

No discomfort produced by rheumatic disease is more characteristic than the pain of an acute attack of gouty arthritis. The disease occurs in a male-to-female ratio of 6:1. The sudden onset of severe pain of increasing intensity in one or more joints, often in the first metatarsophalangeal joint or in the arch of the foot, is typical. The pain usually reaches its maximum intensity within 12 hours of its onset. It is very unusual for a first attack to occur in a joint in the upper extremity. There is exquisite tenderness of the inflamed joint. Any pressure on the joint is intolerable. The patient axiomatically cannot stand the weight of the bedclothes on the affected joint, and the cut-out shoe has been considered a diagnostic sign. The untreated attack typically lasts from 10 days to 2 weeks if untreated. The brief attack of acute arthritis, lasting from 24 to 48 hours is almost always due to rheumatoid arthritis rather than gout. Between attacks of gouty arthritis the patient feels entirely well. Initially the attacks are usually separated by months or years. If the condition is untreated, the attacks tend to occur closer and closer together. In the late stages of the disease attacks are no longer separated by asymptomatic periods and there is continuing discomfort. This condition is referred to as "intercurrent gout" and is characteristically associated with the presence of tophi.

Gouty attacks may be precipitated by conditions that produce metabolic acidosis and a decrease in the excretion of uric acid in the urine.[28] Starvation, or even the relative starvation resulting from crash diets may produce attacks. Hyperuricemia induced by the use of thiazide diuretics is a common precipitating factor. It has been commonly observed that minor injury may produce an attack, presumably because the injury jars loose urate crystals from their position in the articular cartilage. Alcoholic excesses tend to produce attacks, also, through the production of acidosis and the resulting decrease in the excretion of uric acid. Joint destruction, with consequent pain, occurs when urate deposits replace the normal architecture of cartilage and bone.

Gout should be suspected when there is a history of typical acute attacks, especially in an adult male. The diagnosis can be proven only by the demonstration of urate crystals in the joint fluid or by the presence of tophi. The discomfort of acute gouty arthritis is entirely due to the synovitis produced by the crystals of sodium urate. Other similar crystals can produce a synovitis indistinguishable from that produced by urate crystals.[31,32] The most common example is the synovitis produced by calcium pyrophosphate crystals (pseudogout). In chronic tophaceous gout, structural changes in the joint add to the pain when joints are moved or support weight. The fact that the attacks of gout, in the early stages, is usually dramatically relieved by the use of colchicine makes this therapeutic application useful from the diagnostic point of view.[33]

Gouty arthritis is thus one of a number of micro-crystaline-induced arthritides. If the crystal is calcium prophosphate, one may be aided by the fact that the crystals may appear on radiographs as a fine line of density in the menisci or just below the surface of the articular cartilage (chondrocalcinosis).[34]

RHEUMATOID ARTHRITIS

A very common cause of polyarticular pain is rheumatoid arthritis. The joint abnormalities of this systemic disease begin with inflammation of the synovial lining of the joint and of the joint capsule. The pain is usually described as dull or aching in character but may be sharp and severe in particularly acute attacks, or if the joint capsule is markedly distended by fluid under pressure. Unlike gouty arthritis, the patient can usually walk on the joint in the early stages of the disease, although movement and weight-bearing increase the inflammation and discomfort.

As the disease progresses, the disease causes destruction of the cartilage, resulting in irregularities in the surface of the articular cartilage. A grating crepitus may be felt, and sometimes heard, on movement of the joint, accompanied by pain on motion. When the cartilage is destroyed, the grating assumes a harsher quality, as bone grinds on bone. Additional pain may be caused by muscles spasm, flexion contractures or joint effusion. It is the character of the disease, therefore, to destroy gradually the mechanical and architectural integrity of the joint. The joints become deformed, misaligned, and often unstable. Both muscles and ligaments are put under additional strain by the deformity and instability. The paresthesias and the neuralgic and myalgic pains that frequently occur in this disease are due, at least in part, to inflammatory infiltrations in the perineurium of peripheral nerves and of muscles.[35,36] When vasculitis complicates the picture, painful skin ulcers may occur.[37]

In the very early stages of rheumatoid arthritis, there may be little to differentiate it from other polyarticular nonpurulent inflammations. The distribution of joint involvement is often helpful. Involvement of the second through fifth metacarpophalangeal joints rarely occurs except in systemic rheumatic disease. An exception is found in hemochromatosis in which radiographs show what appears to be osteoarthritis in those joints where osteoarthritis otherwise does not occur. Involvement of elbows and wrists usually means systemic rheumatic disease in the absence of a history of trauma. The diagnosis usually turns out to be rheumatoid arthritis or one of its variants (e.g., psoriatic arthritis, Reiter's syndrome). As the disease progresses, with or without remissions and exacerbations,

its chronicity and the evidence of systemic involvement make the diagnosis clear. Fatigue is the single most common complaint, but there may be weight loss, low-grade fever, leukocytosis, elevation of the sedimentation rate, anemia, and various degrees of wasting and weakness. Demonstration of rheumatoid factor in the blood may be helpful, but in 15% to 20% of patients with rheumatoid arthritis, rheumatoid factor is never present. Juvenile rheumatoid arthritis (Still's disease) usually has characteristics similar to those in adults, although high fever and marked leukocytosis are much more common in children. Chronicity, joint deformities, the absence of a migratory pattern of joint involvement and the absence of carditis help to differentiate the disease from rheumatic fever, with which it may be confused.

Features clinically indistinguishable from classic rheumatoid arthritis frequently are seen in systemic lupus erythematosus. Sun sensitivity rashes, Reynaud's phenomenon, leukopenia, low serum complement levels and the demonstration of LE cells or antinuclear antibodies in the serum help to identify this syndrome.[38]

DEGENERATIVE JOINT CHANGES

Degenerative disease of joints is about as common a cause of joint pain as rheumatoid arthritis. This disorder begins as a degenerative change of articular cartilage that slowly progresses to cause thinning of the cartilage, irregular joint surfaces, and irritation of the periosteum covering the adjacent bone, with resultant spur formation at the joint margins and sclerosis of the subchondral bony plate. Since articular cartilage contains no nerves, as long as the disease is confined to that structure, the degeneration may progress subtly and indolently. After articular cartilage becomes eroded and osteophytes develop, movement of the joint and weight-bearing produce pain as the result of strain and tension on the sensitive supporting periarticular tissues. Joint pain in osteoarthritis is due largely to ligamentous or muscular strains of mild synovitis.[40] It is clear, however, that, when the cartilage is gone and bony crepitus is demonstrated, the grinding of bone on bone is in itself very painful. When the affected joints are not being subjected to weight-bearing or movement, the patient is usually comfortable.

The sharply contrasting pathology of these two forms of chronic arthritis—rheumatoid and osteoarthritis—fully explains the differences in the joint discomfort accompanying these disorders. Oteoarthritis is a disease of older adults who are usually constitutionally healthy. It is a local, mechanical disorder chiefly affecting the weight-bearing articulations. These char-

acteristics, together with the absence of physical or laboratory signs of inflammation, usually clarify the diagnosis.

Because degenerative changes occur in joints injured by any mechanism, it is not unusual for persons with rheumatoid arthritis to exhibit characteristics of osteoarthritis as well. Other causes of eventual degenerative disease include athletic injuries, prolonged periods of overweight, infectious arthritis, gout, or malalignment problems such as may be seen with valgus or varus deformities of the knee or with pronation of the foot.

There are two other conditions commonly referred to as "osteoarthritis" but they are unrelated to the osteoarthritis commonly seen in major weight-bearing joints. The first occurs in the hands and involves the distal interphalangeal joints with swelling, and often tenderness, on the medial and lateral aspects of the distal joints (Heberden's nodes). Some of these patients exhibit bony widening, and often, limitation of motion in the proximal interphalangeal joints as well. A smaller percentage have degenerative changes in the first metacarpophalangeal joints or in the first carpometacarpal joints. This is a familial, inherited condition. Females are afflicted more often than males in a ratio of 10:1. Fifty percent of the cases occur within three years of menopause. It is self-limited, always stopping in its progression eventually. The nodular enlargement does not go away, but the swelling stops increasing and the tenderness goes away. It is made worse by use of the hands, especially by strenuous use, such as typing and playing the piano. Patients should be advised that exercise of the affected joint makes the condition worse rather than better.

The term "osteoarthritis" is also commonly used to describe changes in the cervical or lumbar spine that are really due to degenerative disk disease. When the disk spaces have become narrowed, ostophytes develop at the margins of the vertebral bodies. These are secondary changes and rarely the cause of pain. More often than not the apophyseal joints are not involved.

NONARTICULAR RHEUMATISM

FIBROSITIS

Fibrosis is a term used to describe the painful symptoms in patients who have no measurable abnormality. The symptoms are predominantly muscular and the joints are clearly not involved. The aching, soreness, and stiffness are usually worse in the morning or after inactivity, and may also be increased with fatigue at the end of the day. There are no characteristic histo-

logic abnormalities in any of the periarticular tissues, so that the scientific basis for the diagnosis is in legitimate doubt. Many of the cases previously classified under the diagnosis of fibrositis have proven to be cases of polymyalgia rheumatica. It may be that, in the future, other conditions will explain the pain in the remaining patients. For the time being, the term "fibrositis" covers those patients with periarticular pain who have no demonstrable pathologic explanation for their pain.

POLYMYALGIA RHEUMATICA

During the recent years, a syndrome called polymyalgia rheumatica has been widely recognized, consisting of pain and stiffness in the shoulder girdle and hip girdle and medial thighs. The patients are usually female and over 50 years of age. There is usually no objective evidence of joint inflammation; raising the arms or trying to get out of a chair produces a great deal of muscular pain. Muscular tenderness may be present and the patients are often anemic. Fever may accompany the syndrome, and some patients present with fevers of unknown origin. A markedly elevated sedimentation rate is the rule, and the diagnosis of polymyalgia rheumatica cannot be made without this finding. In many patients, giant cell arteritis is found on biopsy of the temporal artery. The arteries may be nodular and tender to touch, and the patient may have recurrent headaches. Other cranial arteries may be involved as well, producing a variety of signs and symptoms. Gangrene of the tongue and trismus have been reported, for example. The most dreaded complication of cranial giant cell arteritis is blindness. The finding of giant cell arteritis on biopsy of the temporal artery proves the presence of cranial arteritis and alerts the physician to the threat of blindness and to the necessity for vigorous treatment. Symptoms usually respond dramatically to corticosteroid treatment, and the syndrome is usually self-limited, disappearing in a few months or years.[39,40]

UNEXPLAINED ARTHRALGIAS

Sometimes patients complain of intermittent or chronic pain involving their joints. Many young women complain of pain and stiffness in the proximal interphalangeal joints, worse in the morning and often making it difficult to get their rings on or off. On physical examination, it is difficult to see any swelling, there is no limitation of motion, and laboratory studies are normal. Many of these patients lose their symptoms after a period of time, and the cause of their discomfort never becomes apparent. Such complaints are partic-

ularly common after childbirth and may last from weeks to months. In other patients, the process gradually becomes more severe and becomes recognizable as a definite disease syndrome such as rheumatoid arthritis or systemic lupus erythematosus. It is important to observe these patients at intervals over the period of time that symptoms persist and not to write them off as hysterics or complainers.

SUMMARY

Joint pain and periarticular pain are very common symptoms resulting from a variety of disorders. To understand joint and periarticular pain, it is first necessary to identify the structure or structures from which the pain is arising. Once the anatomic location for the pain has been identified, it is necessary to analyze the pathologic basis for the pain and the mechanisms by which it is produced. This information, together with an understanding of the pathologic and clinical characteristics of the various diseases, leads to proper diagnosis.

The nature of the discomfort in some diseases of joints and periarticular structures is so characteristic that the correct diagnosis can be made from the history alone. In most cases, however, pain calls attention to the fact that a disorder exists. The nature of the pain suggests the cause, but a final diagnosis can only be made after correlating all the clinical, laboratory, and radiographic data with the symptoms and signs.

REFERENCES

1. **Stilwell DL Jr:** The innervation of tendons and aponeuroses. Am J Anat 100:289, 1957

2. **Stilwell DL Jr:** Regional variations in the innervation of deep fascia and aponeuroses. Anat Rec 127:635, 1957

3. **Lennander KG:** Mitt Grenzgeb Med Clin 15:465, 1906

4. **Lewis T:** Suggestions relating to study of somatic pain. Br Med J 1:321–325, 1938

5. **Kellgren JH:** On distribution of pain arising from deep somatic structures with charts of segmental pain areas. Clin Sci 435–46, 1939

6. **Kellgren JH, Samuel EP:** The sensitivity and innervation of the articular capsule. J Bone Joint Surg (Br) 32S:84, 1950

7. **Kellgren JH:** Observations of referred pain arising from muscles. Clin Sci 3:175–190, 1938

8. **Gardner E:** Nerve supply of muscles, joints and other deep structures. Bull Hosp Joint Dis 21:153, 1960

9. **Gardner E:** The innervation of the knee joint. Anat Rec 101:109–130, 1948

10. **Gardner E:** Physiology of movable joints. Physiol Rev 30:127–176, 1950

11. **Gardner E:** The nerve supply of diarthrodial joints. Stanford Med Bull 6:367–373, 1948

12. **Lewis T, Kellgren JH:** Observations relating to referred pain, viscero-motor reflexes and other associated phenomena. Clin Sci 4:47–71, 1939

13. **Lewis T:** Pain. New York, Macmillan, 1942

14. **Ernstene AC, Kinell J:** Pain in shoulder as sequel to myocardial infarction. Arch Intern Med 66:800–806, 1940

15. **Herfort RA:** Extended sympathectomy in treatment of chronic arthritis. J Am Geriatr Soc 5:904, 1957

16. **Herfort RA, Nickerson SH:** Relief of arthritic pain and rehabilitation of chronic arthritic patient by extended sympathetic denervation. Arch Phys Med Rehabil 40:133–140, 1959

17. **Howell TH:** Relief of pain in rheumatoid arthritis with Tetraethylammonium bromide. Lancet 1:204, 1950

18. **Fearon DT, Austen KF:** Acute inflammatory response. In McCarty DJ (ed): Arthritis and Allied Conditions: A Textbook of Rheumatology, 9th ed, pp 214–228. Philadelphia, Lea & Febiger, 1979

19. **Rose GK:** Tuberculosis of the knee joint. Br J Clin Pract 13:241, 1959

20. **Tegner WS:** Tennis elbow. Postgrad Med J 35:390, 1959

21. **Steinbrocker O, Neustadt D, Bosch SJ:** Painful shoulder syndromes their diagnosis and treatment. Med Clin North Am 39:563, 1955

22. **Albert SM, Rechtman AM:** The painful shoulder. American Practitioner 7:72, 1956

23. **Mosley HF:** Disorders of the shoulder. Clin Sympos 11:75, 1959

24. **Kozin F:** Painful shoulder and the reflex sympathetic dystrophy. In McCarty DJ (ed): Arthritis and Allied Conditions: A Textbook of Rheumatology, 9th ed, pp 1091–1111. Philadelphia, Lea & Febiger, 1979

25. **Bucy PC, Oberhill HR:** Pain in the shoulder and arm from neurological involvement. JAMA 169:798, 1959

26. **Morgan EH:** Pain in the shoulder and upper extremity: Visceral causes considered by the internist. JAMA 169:804, 1959

27. **Monnet JC:** Osteochondritis deformans. J Okla State Med Assoc 52:376, 1959

28. **Wyngaarden JB, Holmes EW:** Clinical gout and the pathogenesis of hyperuricemia. In McCarty DJ (ed): Arthritis and Allied Conditions: A Textbook of Rheumatology, 9th ed, pp 1193–1228. Philadelphia, Lea & Febiger, 1979

29. **Freyberg RH et al:** Rheumatic manifestations of systemic diseases. Clin Orthop 57:3–101, 1968

30. **Spilberg I, Meyer CJ:** The arthritis of leukemia. Arthritis Rheum 15:630, 1972

31. **McCarty DJ, Hollander JL:** Identification of urate crystals in gouty synovial fluid. Ann Intern Med 54:452, 1961

32. **Sigmiller JE, Howell RR, Malawista SE:** Inflammatory

reaction to sodium urate: Its possible relationship to genesis of acute gouty arthritis. JAMA 180:469, 1962

33. **Freyberg RH:** Gout. Arthritis Rheum 5:624, 1962

34. **McCarty DJ, Gatter RA, Brill JM:** Crystal deposition diseases: Sodium urate (gout) and calcium pyrophosphate (chondrocalcinosis, pseudo-gout). JAMA 193:129, 1965

35. **Freund HA, Steiner G, Leichtentritt B, Price AE:** Peripheral nerves in chronic atrophic arthritis. J Lab Clin Med 27:1256, 1942

36. **Freund HA, Steiner G, Leichtentritt B, Price AE:** Nodular polymyositis in rheumatoid arthritis. Science 101:202, 1945

37. **Johnson RL, Smyth CJ, Holt GW, Lubchenco A, Valentine E:** Steroid therapy and vascular lesions in rheumatoid arthritis. Arthritis Rheum 2:224, 1959

38. **Talbott JH, Ferrandis RM:** Collagen diseases. New York, Grune & Stratton, 1956

39. **Healey L:** Polymyalgia rheumatica. In McCarty DJ (ed): Arthritis and Allied Conditions: A Textbook of Rheumatology, 9th ed, pp 681–684. Philadelphia, Lea & Febiger, 1979

40. **Davison S, Spiera H:** Polymyalgia rheumatica. Clin Orthop 57:95, 1968

13

Pain in the Extremities
Joan L. Venes
William F. Collins

Pathophysiology
  Pain Originating in the Skin
  Pain Originating in Bone
  Pain Originating in Muscle
  Pain Originating in Joints
  Pain Originating in the Central Nervous System
  Radicular Pain
    Monoradicular Syndromes
    Polyradicular Syndromes
  Pain of Brachial and Lumbosacral Plexus Origin
  Pain Originating in Peripheral Nerve
    Mononeuropathy
    Trauma

    Entrapments
    Reflex Sympathetic Dystrophy
    Diabetic Mononeuropathy
    Polyneuropathy
Regional Syndromes
  Shoulder and Arm Pain
  Elbow Pain
  Forearm and Hand Pain
  Hip and Thigh Pain
  Knee and Calf Pain
  Foot Pain
  Multiple Extremity Involvement
Summary

Establishing the cause of pain in an extremity can be difficult because of the many elements that must be considered as possible pathophysiologic factors. Some of these are the numerous and various conditions that can affect the several different tissues of the extremity, the reactions of the tissues involved, and the secondary reactions that can occur in adjacent tissues. These include the possibility of pain radiating into the extremity from lesions of the spinal roots and peripheral nerve plexuses, referred pain from lesions of organs such as the heart or kidney, and pain from central nervous system lesions. They also include the problem of pain radiating to more proximal areas of the extremity from lesions of the foot or the hand, and into more distal portions of the extremity from lesions of the proximal joints or muscles. There is also the consideration of systemic disease that may appear first as pain in an extremity.

Probably the most difficult problem, however, is the differentiation between pain and suffering (which includes the emotional and psychological responses to the pain), or even more commonly, a determination of what portion of the complaint is actually pain caused by an organic lesion and what is the result of his suffering. The exposed position of the extremities and their constant use in the activities of daily living contribute not only to susceptibility to injury but also to the marked disability the patient suffers with the painful extremity. Disability appears to contribute frequently to conscious or subconscious fear that the pain signifies a more serious disease than is actually true. Suffering caused by this fear contributes to the complaints and to the physician's difficulty in determining the cause of pain.

In considering any complaint, the etiology is most easily determined from the history. If the information contained in the history is to be effectively used, the history must often contain not only the type, onset,

and duration of the complaint, as well as factors that alter the symptoms, but also the past history, the family history, and a review of systems. A history that is inaccurate or too brief is a common cause of error in discovery of the pathophysiology of pain in an extremity.

The physician must do a complete physical examination, as well as an examination of the extremity involved. Too often a complaint of pain in an extremity is investigated as if the extremity were isolated from the body, so that if the examination of the extremity reveals no positive findings, the physician concludes that the patient has no physical disease process as a basis for the complaint and diagnoses the cause as psychosomatic. The presence of possible contributory evidence such as contingent compensation for accident or injury may only strengthen the physician's confidence in his judgment instead of being simply another aspect of the history. Perhaps even worse than this is precipitous resort to unwarranted diagnostic tests or surgical approaches on finding an isolated positive physical sign such as a loss of reflex or change in muscle size in an extremity. This can be not only incorrect, but also dangerous for the patient.

PATHOPHYSIOLOGY

This chapter has been organized to provide both pathophysiologic and regional cross-reference. The well-known syndromes affecting an area are outlined, and the reader is referred to the appropriate section for a more detailed discussion of pathophysiology.

PAIN ORIGINATING IN THE SKIN

Lesions of the skin that can cause pain are numerous. They include trauma, tumors, allergic reactions, and infection, as well as many pathologic changes of unknown etiology and various reactions of the skin that reflect systemic disease. There are, however, characteristics of pain distinct from lesions of the skin. These distinctive attributes include accurate location and a special quality. The feeling is sharply localized and is described as similar to a previously experienced sensation from a burn, cut, or scrape of the skin. Typically there is alteration in the appearance of the skin or subcutaneous tissue in the area involved. If these criteria are not met, it is best to look elsewhere for the cause of the pain that the patient feels on the surface or in the subcutaneous tissue of an extremity.

The reason why the characteristics of pain are so constant in primary skin lesions is that the lesion involves sensory endings of the peripheral nerves. The deformation or injury of these primary endings conveys impulses that are similar to, if not the same as, impulses that are recognized through experience as coming from noxious stimuli on the surface of the body. The nervous system accurately localizes stimuli that arise on the surface of the body. The peripheral nerve ending must have an altered environment that through stretching, pressure, or alteration in metabolic function causes it to propagate impulses so that the subject feels pain. Changes in the skin detected by visual and tactile examination complete the reasons for these characteristics of painful skin lesions.

Pain that is perceived as being on the surface of the body but not well localized and not accompanied by an alteration in the skin, or pain that is described in an unusual fashion, should make the examiner consider alteration in the function of the nerves or blood supply to the area rather than a primary lesion of the skin. Disease affecting the blood vessels may cause cutaneous changes secondary to ischemia.

Raynaud's disease is an idiopathic bilateral paroxysmal contraction of the arteries and arterioles of the digits usually without local gangrene. It occurs secondary to peripheral stimuli such as cold or pain. The disease is much more common in women and although it may occur at any age, it most frequently appears in the second, third, and fourth decades. The attacks are precipitated by cold or emotion and may be relieved by warmth. In Raynaud's disease of many years' duration, one may occasionally see small superficial areas of gangrene, but in general the disease runs a benign course. Raynaud's phenomenon may be seen in scleroderma, sickle cell disease, leukemia, and myeloma. Prognosis in these disorders is that of the underlying disease process. Berger's disease, diabetes, periarteritis nodosa, and arteriosclerosis may cause changes in the skin with severe pain at rest from ulceration.

Failure of the deep venous system can cause chronic edema, petechial hemorrhages, poor drainage, and infection that may lead to chronic intractable ulcers of the lower leg; however, the pain is rarely as severe as that seen with the ischemic ulceration of the extremity secondary to arterial occlusion. It is the description of poorly localized discomfort and sensations that are difficult for the patient to describe in relation to previous experience that gives the clue that the pathology is not primarily in the skin. This group of afflictions in which peripheral nerve or blood vessel pathology is present causes the greatest difficulty in diagnosis of pain referred to the surface of an extremity. The distribution of the pain in the area of a dermatome, or a peripheral nerve, or over the specific area of the blood supply can be the clue that leads to the diagnosis of a systemic or proximal disease process.

PAIN ORIGINATING IN BONE

Pain from bone lesions is caused by irritation of or tension on the periosteum, alteration in the function of joints proximal or distal to the bone involved, or changes in the function of overlying tissues such as nerves, ligaments, tendons, or bursae. With the exception of mild discomfort from distention of the marrow cavity or compression of cancellous bone, bone itself appears to have little, if any, pain sensitivity. Pain caused by lesions of bone is less well localized than that from lesions of more superficial tissue and often is described as an ache or a deep pain in the general area of the diseased tissue. When a peripheral nerve is also involved, the pain radiates to the peripheral distribution of the nerve, thus sometimes causing difficulty in differentiating the lesion from a primary peripheral nerve lesion.

The pain from fractures comes from stretching, tearing, and irritation of the periosteum and surrounding tissue. The site of the fracture, besides showing anatomic deformity, also shows swelling and evidence of hemorrhage. There is tenderness locally and focal pain when stress is placed on the fracture site by proximal or distal manipulation of the bone. Pain of infections and tumors may resemble each other with aching discomfort, often made worse by dependency of the extremity. The severity of the pain reflects in general the rapidity with which the lesion is enlarging and the amount of irritation that the enlargement causes.

Infections such as syphilis (periostitis) or osteomyelitis from bacteria of low virulence may become very extensive before much discomfort is felt. Tumors that are slowly growing may act in the same fashion and, therefore, benign tumors are at times huge before any discomfort is felt. On the other hand, highly malignant, rapidly growing neoplasms or infections from highly virulent organisms may cause pain when the lesion is very small, even before it is detectable by x-ray examination. When either infection or tumor breaks through the periosteum, there is often a dramatic decrease in pain. These events illustrate and emphasize the part that the innervation of and stresses upon the periosteum have in the pain of these conditions.

Pain from metabolic disorders and from Paget's disease relate to a combination of factors including deformities of bone, irritation and stretching of periosteum, and stress on joints. The discomfort may vary markedly from patient to patient depending upon severity, location, and nature of the disease process.

Radiographs of bones and joints taken by proper techniques and studied by experts yield highly significant information concerning pathophysiologic processes causing bone pain.

When history and physical examination suggest possible bone involvement as a cause of pain, x-ray study is necessary. Because pain with bone disease is often poorly localized and since there is the possibility of soft-tissue and joint involvement at a distance from the lesion, radiographs should be made of the entire extremity. For comparison, radiographs of the opposite matching extremity are frequently of great help. Bone scans using radioactive substances can localize bone lesions often before other radiographic techniques. Technetium-99 attached to various organic phosphates is commonly used as the injectionable radiation source to localize bone tumors, while gallium-67 is more efficacious in demonstrating infections.

PAIN ORIGINATING IN MUSCLE

In contrast to bone, muscle is generously supplied with free nerve endings considered to be pain endings. Distribution of nerve endings is not as dense as in skin, therefore needle puncture or incision of muscle is much less painful than those of skin. Inflammation, compression, or alteration in the blood supply of muscle, however, results in severe agonizing pain partially localized to the area of the muscle involved, and also referred to overlying soft tissue and, at times, to the entire extremity. When a muscle is traumatized or involved in a painful disease process, it usually responds with increased tone, which may result in spastic contraction or cramping. Increased tone from injury or from spasticity of neurologic disease can in itself cause pain in muscle, related joints, fascia, or bursa by altering their normal function. Diffuse pain of an entire extremity arising from conditions affecting a single muscle or a group of muscles can, at times, be difficult to diagnose as being related to the muscle. Helpful findings in these conditions are tenderness of the muscle involved, increase in pain in the whole extremity when that muscle is compressed, and increase in the pain of the extremity when that muscle is used.

A traumatized muscle usually is painful, has increased tone, and is tender. The subject experiences increased pain when it is used and some relief of pain with rest. The mildest type of muscle trauma causing pain is that encountered after strenuous exercise by an unconditioned subject. The cause of the pain is not understood, but may relate to retained metabolic products. The pain usually begins at 4 to 6 hours after use and reaches its maximum intensity in 48 to 72 hours. Mild exercise, heat, and massage relieve the pain. The pain of muscle contusion is caused by hemorrhage within the muscle and begins within minutes after the injury; it may continue for days or weeks. Rupture of a muscle may consist of rupture of just a few fibers,

rupture of the fascial envelope of the muscle, rupture of the main muscle mass, or rupture of the tendon of the muscle. Examination reveals marked tenderness over the area of partial rupture. There is tenderness with rupture of the fascia, but the prominent finding is protrusion of the muscle mass through the fascia. With a major rupture of the body of the muscle or a rupture of the tendon, there is loss of function of the muscle, tenderness at the point of rupture, and contraction of the muscle mass proximal to the rupture. The pain of traumatic lesions of muscle may be localized or referred to the entire extremity. History of trauma and local findings clarify the diagnosis.

Polymyositis is a poorly understood condition in which inflammation of the muscles is associated with pain, tenderness, and weakness, which may be confused with a polyneuropathy. Onset may be acute, particularly in children, with severe inflammatory reaction in the muscle and subcutaneous and dermal tissue above the muscle. Myositis with involvement of the skin has been termed *dermatomyositis*. Inflammatory reaction is generally accompanied by fever, polymorphonuclear leukocytosis, and an elevated sedimentation rate. Chronic myositis in which an inflammatory reaction is lacking is more common in an older person. The fact that chronic polymyositis may accompany carcinomas of the stomach, breast, and lung has been known for many years. At times it is the first indication of the presence of a neoplasm, although in general it is seen only with dissemination of the tumor.

Less frequently, polymyositis may be seen after infection with Coxsackie virus or following a parasitic infection such as trichinosis. Polymyositis secondary to parasitic infection is rare and in general is a symptom of repeated infestation by the parasite. Inflammatory reaction is brief and not severe, usually lasting five to ten days. Viral infections of muscle also are usually relatively brief in duration, with a moderate inflammatory response.

Characteristically, the proximal muscles of the extremity are more commonly involved that the distal muscles, and they may become tender and weak. With weakness and tenderness of muscle, there may be alteration in joint function resulting in pain secondary to joint derangement. Examination may reveal fasciculations as well as tenderness and atrophy of the muscles. The diagnosis is best made by electromyographic studies and surgical biopsy.

The cause of diffuse myalgia of systemic infection with high fever or with viral infections with or without high fever is not known. The discomfort is usually a relatively mild pain that parallels the course of the fever or illness, and although it may involve proximal extremity muscles more than other muscle groups, it is generalized. A diagnostic problem is the occasional patient with residual focal areas of tenderness and pain in the area of the scapula or shoulder. This condition is usually diagnosed as focal myositis or fascitis and is particularly common after viral infections. These disorders seem to start with the illness but persist when the remainder of the muscle aches are gone. They frequently cause more difficulty and more pain with radiation into an extremity than when the entire myalgic syndrome was present.

One of the most severe pains known is that secondary to inadequate blood flow to a working muscle. A common cause of altered blood flow to an extremity is arteriosclerosis of either the major vessel of the limb or the more proximal arterial trunks. *Intermittent claudication,* cramping pain in the muscle with use, is a common presenting symptom of arterial insufficiency. Although most common in the lower extremities, it occurs in any extremity in which there is significant arterial insufficiency when the muscles are used. Diagnosis can be made from the history of recurrent pain with activity and confirmed by palpation of the peripheral pulses, comparison of blood pressure in the opposite limb, oscillometry in the extremity, and arteriography.

Acute venous thrombosis may also cause vascular insufficiency to a muscle in part by altered blood flow through the vessels secondary to increased venous pressure and in part from secondary arterial spasm. Venous obstruction causes some of the same complaints, but the discomfort is usually milder in degree and more frequently relates to dependency of the extremity and edema of the tissues as much as to activity of the muscle.

Primary tumors of the muscle such as rhabdomyosarcoma and desmoids are extremely rare and are usually diagnosed by the presence of tenderness, weakness, and a mass in the area of the pain and tenderness. The pain of such tumors is related to the rate of growth of the tumor and the alteration produced in the function of the muscle. Rhabdomyosarcomas are malignant, rapidly growing and often painful, and present an enlarging mass within the muscle. Tumors are rarely the cause of pain in an extremity.

PAIN ORIGINATING IN JOINTS

The causes and mechanisms that produce joint pain are discussed in Chapters 11 and 12. A few aspects of joint pain are, however, relevant to a discussion of pain in the extremities. Pain in joints is usually confined to the area of the joint involved, although more accurately in distal than in proximal joints. The pain is increased by movement of the joint and by pressure

on the joint. There is often tenderness of the tissues around the joint. Therefore, increased pain with movement of a joint and tenderness of the periarticular tissues are significant localizing signs. Pain from a joint, in addition, may be referred to the muscles acting on the joint, probably secondary to both altered tone in the muscle and altered mechanisms of action. Joint pain, as with other deep pain in an extremity, can be referred to the entire extremity or to a distal portion of the extremity (as in the *shoulder–hand syndrome*), or may be a basis for reflex sympathetic dystrophy. Such referred pain almost always contains elements of reflex sympathetic dystrophy and consists of an aching, burning stiffness with altered vasomotor tone in the hand distal to the painful shoulder.

When the reflex dystrophy in the extremity is the major part of the syndrome (most frequently in the upper extremity), sympathetic block with a local anesthetic is indicated. When the pain is primarily in the joint with mild referral to the distal part of the extremity, injection of tender areas around the joint with local anesthetic alone or in combination with corticosteroids often relieves both the joint and the extremity pain. Both sympathetic block and local injection have therapeutic as well as diagnostic merits, since their effects often long outlast the duration of action of the local anesthetic. Chronic conditions of joints that produce great limitation of joint function and severe alteration in anatomic configuration, particularly in rheumatoid conditions, do not respond to such injections unless local disease processes can be arrested and joint mobility restored. Therefore, injections for patients with chronic joint conditions have little diagnostic value.

PAIN ORIGINATING IN THE CENTRAL NERVOUS SYSTEM

Primary lesions of the central nervous system are seldom the cause of extremity pain other than pain that is secondary to the paralysis caused by these lesions. This secondary pain is almost always related to immobilization of a joint or spasticity. Lesions of the spinal cord, however, may be associated with paresthesias in the extremities variously described as numbness, tingling, or a feeling of coldness that may be interpreted by the patient as pain. The correct diagnosis is rarely made until there is definite evidence of loss of spinal cord function. The thalamic pain syndrome is a rare cause of painful dysesthesias (pain from usually nonpainful stimuli, such as light touch). This syndrome results from thrombosis of one of the thalamogeniculate branches of the posterior cerebral artery and causes transient paralysis, marked loss of position, vibratory and touch sensations on half of the body and moderate loss of pinprick perception.

RADICULAR PAIN

The upper extremity is innervated by the anterior rami of the fifth cervical through the first thoracic spinal nerves; the lower extremity is innervated by anterior rami of the second lumbar through the second sacral spinal nerves. The spinal nerves are formed in or just beyond the spinal foramina by the junction of the dorsal and ventral spinal roots peripheral to the dorsal root ganglia that lie outside the dura, usually in the spinal foramina. The central processes of the dorsal root ganglion cells enter the spinal cord in small bundles in an almost unbroken line along the dorsolateral sulcus. Similarly, the axons of the spinal motor neurons emerge from the ventrolateral sulcus as groups of small filaments that coalesce to form the ventral roots. The roots cross the spinal subarachnoid space and pierce the dura separately. The lower cervical and upper thoracic roots take a relatively short course obliquely downward through the subarachnoid space.

The lumbar and sacral roots, collectively called the cauda equina, have a long course in the spinal canal, since the end of the spinal cord, the conus medullaris, lies at the level of the first lumbar vertebra. This discrepancy between the vertebral level and the underlying spinal cord sements and nerve roots, is important in the anatomic localization of lesions of the spinal cord and nerve roots (Fig. 13-1). Soon after formation, the spinal nerves divide into a smaller posterior ramus and a larger anterior ramus. The posterior rami supply the paravertebral musculature and skin about the dorsal midline. The motor and sensory components of the anterior rami innervating the extremities undergo a somewhat complex rearrangement into the peripheral nerves within the brachial and lumbosacral plexuses.

The peripheral processes of a given dorsal root ganglion may be carried by more than one peripheral nerve, but the integrity of the area of skin supplied by that ganglion, the dermatome, is maintained (*i.e.,* unbroken). However, contrary to the impression that might be gained from dermatomal maps, a given area of skin is not solely supplied by fibers of one dorsal root ganglion. The dermatomes overlap in such a manner that the area of the skin supplied by one dorsal root ganglion is also usually supplied by adjacent ganglia. Thus, to surgically denervate a dermatome, at least three posterior roots—not one—must be sectioned. Overlapping of sensory innervation to the skin by adjacent peripheral nerves occurs as well, but not to such an extent since the peripheral nerves usually carry fibers from more than one dorsal root. Section of a major peripheral nerve almost invariably renders some area of skin anesthetic. The concept of the dermatome *versus* innervation by the peripheral nerves is important

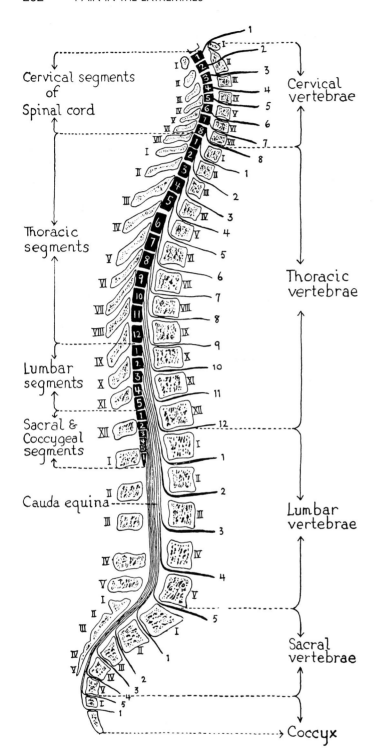

Fig. 13-1. Diagram of the position of the spinal cord segments with reference to the bodies and spinous processes of the vertebrae. Note also the place of origin of the nerve roots from the spinal cord and their emergence from the corresponding intervertebral foramina. (Modified from Tandler and Ranzi Strong and Elwyn: Human Neuroanatomy. Baltimore, Williams & Wilkins)

because it often aids in localization of a lesion and sometimes in the exclusion of disease in the malingerer or hysterical person.

Monoradicular Syndromes

A common cause of extremity pain is a lesion affecting one or more dorsal nerve roots. Because of their close proximity, the ventral as well as the dorsal roots are usually involved in the pathologic process with the consequence that weakness and reflex changes result as well as pain and sensory deficit. Exceptions to this rule may be found, for example, in herpes zoster infection, which may be confined to the dorsal root ganglion. The initial and usually the most prominent feature of the radicular syndrome is intermittent lancinating pain that radiates from one side of the midline of the body into the distribution of the involved root. Radicular pain is usually associated with actions that produce traction on the roots such as coughing or sneezing, movement of the adjacent spine or, in the case of lumbar root involvement, maneuvers such as straight leg raising that stretch the peripheral nerve trunks and, by contiguity, the nerve roots. By the same token, positions that reduce the tension on irritated nerve roots, such as holding the arm above the head when a lower cervical root is involved, may relieve the pain. Reflex spasm of the local paravertebral musculature is often present and may account for aching pain in the neck or back. With irritation of the lower cervical nerve roots, interscapular pain is often present, perhaps due to the distribution of the posterior primary rami.

The distribution of the radiating pain may be of some help in localizing the involved root, especially in the upper extremities, but of more aid is the distribution of associated paresthesias often described as a "pins and needles feeling" or "numbness," which often can be recognized as conforming to a dermatomal pattern. Examination of the patient with a radicular lesion usually reveals limitation of motion of the associated portion of the spine, tenderness over the spinous processes adjacent to the lesion or along the course of the peripheral nerves that convey the radicular fibers, and sensory loss conforming to a dermatomal pattern. Concomitant involvement of the corresponding anterior root produces a specific pattern of muscle weakness, while the combined lesion of both roots may produce loss of a specific stretch reflex. The patterns of sensory, motor, and reflex changes produced by lesions of the most commonly affected nerve roots innervating the extremities are illustrated in Table 13-1.

Table 13-1. *Common Monoradicular Syndromes*

Affected Nerve Root	Pain	Tenderness	Paresthesias and Sensory Deficit	Weakness, Fasciculation, and Atrophy	Reflex Changes
6th Cervical	Radiation from neck into lateral arm and forearm; interscapular pain	Lower cervical spine, brachial plexus, median nerve	Dorsal and lateral aspect of thumb	Biceps	Diminished biceps reflex
7th Cervical	Same as 6th cervical	Lower cervical spine, brachial plexus	Index finger and usually middle finger	Triceps	Depressed or absent triceps reflex
8th Cervical	Radiation from neck into medial arm and forearm; interscapular pain	Lower cervical spine, brachial plexus, ulnar nerve	5th and ulnar half of 4th finger ulnar side of hand	Intrinsic hand muscles	None
4th Lumbar	Bank pain radiation into anterior thigh	Midlumbar spine, femoral nerve	Anterior thigh just above knee	Quadriceps	Depressed or absent knee reflex
5th Lumbar	Bank pain radiating into buttocks and posterior aspect of thigh	Low lumbar spine, sciatic and occasionally superficial peroneal nerves	Dorsum of foot and great toe	Dorsiflexors of foot and great toe	None
1st Sacral	Same as 5th lumbar	Lumbosacral junction, sciatic nerve	Lateral aspect foot and small toe	Plantar flexors of foot (calf)	Depressed or absent ankle reflex

motor function in a peroneal nerve, evidence of peripheral neuropathy elsewhere in the body, and a familial incidence identify this condition. It rarely presents as pain in the back and thighs secondary to the muscle weakness of the lower extremities.

Inflammatory conditions involving multiple peripheral nerves (*i.e.,* polyneuritis) occur less commonly. Polyneuritis has been described following practically every acute infectious disease and although in some, particularly viral infections, there appears to be evidence of direct involvement of the nerves; usually the pathophysiologic process in the nerves appears to be a relatively nonspecific reaction to an infectious disease. The onset is usually signaled by paresthesia, with muscle and nerve tenderness followed by weakness and arreflexia. The sensory phenomena consisting of paresthesias, hyperesthesias, and dysesthesias in the hands and feet in a stocking and glove distribution may precede or be replaced by pain. The severity of the pain can be quite variable. Patients often complain that light touch, pressure, or movement of a joint increases the pain greatly. The resemblance between polyneuritis and polyradiculitis (Guillain-Barré syndrome) has been noted. Although in the former the sensory component is quite marked and the motor loss is distal, in the latter the sensory component is often minimal and mainly subjective, and there is striking weakness of the proximal musculature. The course of postinfectious polyneuritis may be acute or subacute, lasting days or weeks. It may progress so that the roots are involved and it is indistinguishable from the Guillain-Barré syndrome, or it may clear rapidly despite major loss of peripheral nerve function. Postinfectious polyradiculitis or Guillain-Barré syndrome is more common than postinfectious polyneuritis but rarely presents with complaint of pain in the extremities. At the onset, paresthesias that some patients describe as painful may occur, but the rapidly progressive areflexia, weakness, and paralysis are the main problems.

Syphilis must always be considered, and the shooting pains of tabes dorsalis should be easily recognized by the paroxysmal onset, the loss of deep tendon reflexes, impaired posterior column function and pupillary changes.

REGIONAL SYNDROMES

SHOULDER AND ARM PAIN

Most complaints in which pain is restricted to the shoulder region can be ascribed to affections of the joint and periarticular tissues (see Chapter 12). The orthopedic syndromes involving the shoulder joint are discussed in detail in that chapter. Differential diagnoses include fracture, dislocation, bursitis, tendinitis, and adhesive capsulitis. Shoulder pain is not uncommon complaint in patients with hemiplegia secondary to a cerebral vascular accident or other central nervous system lesions. In this condition, it is generally associated with a partial subluxation of the humeral head. Adhesive capsulitis ("frozen shoulder") is best managed by a combination of heat and exercise designed to increase range of motion.

Pain referred to the shoulder may occur in cervical spondylosis. The pain is generally secondary to spasm in the trapezius or rhomboid muscles and is unaffected by motion of the shoulder joint. Involved muscles may be tender to palpation, and the pain is often accompanied by restriction of neck motion. Pain in the rhomboid region, the neck, and occasionally the anterior chest is believed to be referred from the disk itself and is not diagnostic of the level of root involvement. Although radicular signs may often be absent in cervical spondylosis, the presence of long tract signs and pathologic reflexes such as the Babinski's and Hoffman's signs should be sought, since significant spinal cord compromise may exist without evidence of nerve root dysfunction.

Compression of the C5 cervical root by either a ruptured disk at the C4–C5 level or, less commonly, by a neoplasm causes pain in the shoulder with radiation down the lateral aspect of the arm to the elbow. Characteristically, pain does not radiate into the forearm. There may be marked weakness of muscles of the shoulder girdle and the biceps reflex may be depressed. Although shoulder and arm pain occur with disk diseases at lower levels, generally pain in the latter conditions radiates into the forearm and may even radiate into the fingers of the involved extremity. Posterolateral disk herniation in the cervical region impinges on the nerve roots exiting at the corresponding foramen, but because the first cervical nerve exists between the first cervical vertebra on the skull, the nerve roots involved likewise do not correspond to the interspace by number (*e.g.,* herniation at the C4–C5 interspace produces a radicular syndrome of the fifth cervical nerve). The differential diagnoses of monoradicular pain has been detailed previously.

Entrapment of the suprascapular nerve as it winds around the lateral edge of the spine of the scapula causes pain that is poorly localized to the area of the posterior and lateral aspects of the shoulder. It can usually be diagnosed by pain on palpation of the nerve at the scapular spine, weakness of the actions of the supraspinatus and infraspinatus muscles, and increase in pain with movement of the partially abducted arm to the opposite shoulder.

Spiller's neuritis (brachial plexus neuritis) is an inflammatory condition that presents with severe shoulder pain occurring several days to a week following a viral illness. The pain is initially quite severe and is followed by weakness and profound atrophy of the muscles of the shoulder girdle. The disease is usually self-limiting, and complete recovery is to be expected. A variant of this disorder is seen following the administration of tetanus and diphtheria antitoxins into the upper extremity. Paralysis of the proximal muscles of the arm with pain over the distribution of the upper brachial plexus is a common presentation, with onset two or three days after injection. Other syndromes that may involve the brachial plexus are discussed earlier in this chapter.

ELBOW PAIN

Pain in the elbow region is most commonly seen following trauma. The orthopedic conditions involving the elbow are discussed in Chapter 12.

FOREARM AND HAND PAIN

Diverse conditions may produce pain in the hand and forearm. Diseases associated with cutaneous manifestations are discussed earlier. Trauma, dislocation, fracture of the wrist and hand, as well as lesions involving the wrist joint primarily are common causes of pain in this area.

Radicular pain radiating into the forearm and hand is associated with the sensory, motor, and reflex changes outlined in Table 13-1. As was noted in the discussion of shoulder and arm pain, the nerve roots involved in posterior lateral disk herniation do not correspond to the interspace by number.

Entrapment of the median nerve at the wrist, or carpal tunnel syndrome, is the most common entrapment syndrome seen in the upper extremity. It occurs most often in persons with occupations necessitating considerable flexion, extension, and rotation of the wrist or in those who have marked alteration of the soft tissue around the wrist joints, as seen in rheumatoid arthritis, acromegaly, or wrist fractures. Loss of sensation in the palm over the distribution of the median nerve, atrophy of the thenar eminence, tenderness over the carpal ligament at the wrist, and Tinel's sign at the same area indicate the point of entrapment. Complaints of numbness, paresthesia, and weakness of the hand with the above findings and evidence of a decrease of nerve conduction across the wrist measured by electroneurography confirm the diagnosis. Resting of the wrist, particularly in a neutral or slightly flexed position is not only therapeutic, but often diagnostic.

Injection of steroids into the wrist to reduce inflammatory reaction in the area may be either temporarily or permanently curative. Surgical decompression, however, is often required. A less common entrapment of the median nerve may occur just below the antecubital fossa where the nerve is crossed by the pronator teres. The syndrome can be quite similar to entrapment at the wrist except that Tinel's sign is over the pronator teres and there is usually weakness of the flexors of the first four digits.

The second most common entrapment syndrome in the upper extremity is of the ulnar nerve at the elbow. This has often been termed "tardy ulnar paralysis," the description relating to the frequency with which it is seen following fractures at the elbow. It is more often seen as a result of recurrent minor injuries to the ulnar nerve as it passes below the medial epicondyle of the humerus where the nerve is covered only by fascia and skin. Such injury may occur from repetitive blows to the "funny bone" or by constant pressure exerted when leaning on the elbow while reading or writing. The presenting symptom is usually aching pain in the forearm, paresthesias in the ring and little finger, and progressive weakness of the ulnar musculature. Palpation of the ulnar nerve as it crosses the medial epicondyle may reveal tenderness and thickening compared with the opposite arm. Diagnosis is often confirmed by demonstrating loss of motor and sensory function within the distribution of the ulnar nerve and the slowing of conduction by electroneurography as it passes the epicondyle. The most effective therapy for ulnar entrapment is transplantation of the nerve to the antecubital fossa.

A less common entrapment is that of the radial nerve as it passes through the supinator muscle, causing weakness of extension of the fingers and pain in the midforearm.

Although most frequently affecting femoral and sciatic nerves, diabetic neuropathy may present as an isolated involvement of either the median or ulnar nerve. The absence of Tinel's sign and the presence of slowed conduction along the entire length of the nerve are aids in establishing the diagnosis. It is to be emphasized that a mild diabetic neuropathy that might otherwise to asymptomatic may make the involved nerve peculiarly sensitive to trauma caused by entrapment, and the two syndromes may coexist.

Pain in the forearm and hand is often the presenting symptom in a lesion of the brachial plexus variously called *scalenus anticus syndrome, cervical rib syndrome,* or *thoracic outlet syndrome.* This entity most often occurs in women of asthenic build, and it consists of pain in the medial arm and forearm often accompanied by a feeling of coldness in the affected hand and sometimes

associated with paresthesias involving the same distribution of the pain and in the fourth and fifth digits as well. The pain and dysesthesias may be made worse by turning the head to the opposite side and abducting the shoulder. On examination, the same maneuvers may reproduce the pain and at the same time cause obliteration of the peripheral pulse (Adson's test). However, pulse obliteration occurs in a large percentage of normal subjects under these conditions, and the presence of this sign, therefore, does not necessarily make the diagnosis. Radiographic demonstration of a cervical rib is of much more aid in the diagnosis, although its presence is not necessary for the syndrome to exist. The cause of this cervical rib syndrome is chronic pressure on the lower portion of the brachial plexus with or without associated compression of the subclavian artery. If a cervical rib, an unusually large transverse process of the seventh cervical vertebra, or a fibrous band from the transverse process to the first rib is present, the lower portion of the brachial plexus as well as the subclavian artery may be draped over it. Essentially the same anatomic abnormality may result from an unusually narrow thoracic outlet, with compression resulting from the abnormally narrow confines between the first rib and the scalenus anticus muscle and clavicle.

Syndromes associated with reflex sympathetic dystrophy constitute a group of devastatingly painful disorders in which involvement of either the median or the ulnar nerve is frequent. As noted earlier, the most characteristic complaint is that any stimulus, even a light touch or a cool breeze, causes an intense burning pain that spreads to the whole extremity.

HIP AND THIGH PAIN

Atherosclerotic disease of the aorta not infrequently presents with pain in the buttocks and thighs. Although generally bilateral early in the course of the disease, the pain may be limited to one extremity. The most common variety of this disorder is the Leriche syndrome, which may develop insidiously over a period of years. This disorder occurs most frequently in young and middle-aged males and is manifested by intermittent claudication in the buttocks and thighs, diminution in femoral pulses, muscular atrophy, and weakness of the legs, with occasional failure of penile erection. The legs are usually pale and cool, but unlike the situation in occlusive disease of the peripheral arteries, gangrene and trophic changes are rare except as a terminal complication. Since surgical reconstruction of the aorta often brings dramatic relief, it is imperative that the diagnosis be reached as early in the course of the disease as possible.

Lesions of the lumbosacral plexus may present with pain in the hip and thigh. It should be reemphasized that rectal and pelvic examinations are an important part of the diagnostic evaluation of the patient with low back and leg pain.

Radicular pain associated with herniation of an intravertebral disk usually occurs on a background of intermittent low back pain or is associated with trauma. Motion of the hip joint does not reproduce the pain, while flexion and extension of the low back, straight leg raising, and other motions designed to stretch nerve roots exacerbate the syndrome. Although local tenderness is not a prominent finding in radicular disease in this area, occasionally palpation of the sciatic nerve as it goes through the sciatic notch elicits a painful response.

Clinically significant, intravertebral disk herniation occurs most often at the last two lumbar interspaces, that is, between L4 and L5 or L5 and S1, with most of the remainder occurring at the L3–L4 interspace. Without objective evidence of nerve root compression, the diagnosis of a herniated intravertebral disk should rarely be made. In the lumbar region, the disposition of nerve roots is such that posterior lateral herniation does not compress the nerve exiting at the corresponding intravertebral foramen, but rather impinges on the set of anterior and posterior nerve roots that cross the disk in their course to the foramen immediately caudad. Thus, disk herniation at the interspace between the fourth and fifth lumbar vertebral bodies usually compresses the fifth lumbar nerve, and herniation at the lumbosacral junction produces signs and symptoms referable to the first sacral nerve. In addition to low back pain, the pain resembles that of the appropriate monoradicular syndrome listed in Table 13-1.

Fractures and dislocations of the hip and pelvis as well as disease of the hip joint such as aseptic necrosis and osteoarthritis may be excluded by appropriate radiographic findings. It should be noted that pain associated with hip disease may occasionally be referred to the medial knee, and the patient's primary complaint may be related to this area.

A common entrapment syndrome that presents as thigh pain is seen in obese patients who wear tight clothes or in whom sagging of the abdominal subcutaneous fat has become very prominent. The entrapment causes paresthesia and loss of sensation in the lateral aspect of the thigh. The syndrome is commonly known as *meralgia paresthetica* and relates to entrapment of the lateral femoral cutaneous nerve as it passes just anterior to the anterior superior iliac spine beneath Poupart's ligament. It is common in pregnant women, in obese persons, and in many persons who attempt to contain protuberant abdomens with firm undergar-

ments. It is usually best treated by making the diagnosis and reassuring the patient that it is not a serious condition. The pain is often self-limiting or can be decreased with exercises and strengthening of the abdominal muscles and loss of weight. A nerve entrapment of the lower extremity that can be quite confusing in relation to other causes of sciatica is the infrequent entrapment of the sciatic nerve at the sciatic notch (piriformis syndrome). This may produce symptoms indistinguishable from lumbar disk disease, but usually the patient has tenderness that is referred to the area of the sciatic notch with Tinel's sign at this point. Injection of the piriformis muscle and the administration of steroids to the area can be both diagnostic and therapeutic.

Involvement of the femoral nerve is the most common diabetic mononeuropathy. Mononeuropathy involving femoral or sciatic nerves can also appear as a mononeuropathy multiplex, or one affecting many peripheral nerves simultaneously. A common presentation in diabetic femoral neuropathy is the onset of acute or subacute pain in the proximal area of the extremity, particularly the hip, with asymmetric muscle wasting and weakness of the legs, but with very little sensory loss. As with other mononeuropathies, the process is usually self-limiting, but because of the extent of its involvement it can be quite disabling. There may be persistence of weakness and pain secondary to the altered function in the extremity after the neuropathy subsides.

KNEE AND CALF PAIN

Pain occurring at the knee secondary to primary involvement of the joint is discussed in Chapter 12. Lesions of the hip joint may on occasion refer pain to the medial aspect of the knee. Arterial insufficiency leading to ischemia of muscles of the calf is seen with occlusive disease of the aortic bifurcation and femoral artery.

Venous disease may or may not give rise to pain. Superficial venous thrombosis often presents as local painful swelling, and a tender thrombosed vein can usually be palpated. Thrombosis of the deeper vein should be suspected in patients whose complaint of lower extremity pain is associated with swelling of the calf or thigh. Examination for changes in girth of the calf, calf tenderness, and tenderness along the course of the major veins of the lower extremities should be part of the routine care of all postoperative and bedridden patients. Frequently, a positive Homan's sign is a diagnostic aid, but venous flow and impedance studies supplemented by venography are often required to confirm and localize the diagnosis. Pain and

pruritis secondary to the induration of chronic venous insufficiency may precede the development of skin ulcers and are not uncommon in these patients.

Ischemia secondary to prolonged exercise with consequent swelling and compromise of venous outflow may be seen in the anterior tibial compartment syndrome. Pain may be excruciating and is associated with muscle tenderness and weakness of the dorsiflexors of the foot. Since conservative therapy may be curative, early diagnosis is essential to avoid the need for fasciotomy.

Radicular pain associated with lumbar disk disease or other conditions affecting the nerve roots commonly radiates into the lower extremity and is usually associated with a history of back pain or discomfort. The associated sensory motor and reflex changes occurring in these disorders are outlined in Table 13-1.

FOOT PAIN

Diseases of the blood vessels causing cutaneous changes in the distal extremity have been discussed in the beginning of this chapter and are not dissimilar from those presenting in the hand. Foot pain relating to local conditions of the bones and joints of the foot has been discussed in Chapter 12.

Pain in the foot occurring with radicular lesions or with lesions of the lumbosacral plexus is usually associated with pain in the lower leg and back.

Entrapment neuropathies in the lower extremities are uncommon; however, there are several that may present with pain localized to the foot. The most common of these is entrapment of the digital nerve between the metacarpal heads with a production of a Morton's neuroma. The digital nerve most often involved is that between the third and fourth metacarpal heads. The pain radiates to the adjacent side of the toes with associated hypesthesia and hypalgesia. Increasing pain with pressure over the metacarpal heads or between the web of the toes can be diagnostic. The next most common peripheral nerve involved is the peroneal nerve. Loss of function is caused by repeated trauma or prolonged pressure on the nerve as it crosses the fibular head or from a severe blow to the same area. It is most commonly seen in patients with some mild peripheral neuropathy who have a habit of crossing their legs. Loss of motor function in the distribution of the nerve and mild hypesthesia with aching, usually referred to the dorsum of the foot or the arch of the foot, is a common complaint. Entrapment of the posterior tibial nerve as it enters the foot through the tarsal tunnel is an occasional cause of pain in the foot. The motor disturbance produced by this lesion is manifested by weakness in postural change in the foot,

with a pes cavus configuration and clawing of the toes. As with other peripheral nerve entrapment syndromes, conservative therapy may be sufficient to reverse the symptoms in these disorders, although occasionally surgical intervention becomes necessary.

MULTIPLE EXTREMITY INVOLVEMENT

The causes of pain affecting more than one extremity have been already reviewed in this chapter in a discussion of the polyneuropathies and polymyositis.

SUMMARY

Pain in the extremities may be a reflection of metabolic derangement involving the innervation or vascular supply of the limb (*e.g.*, diabetic neuropathy), or it may be related to a variety of causes acting locally (*e.g.*, tardy ulnar paralysis). A careful history is often the single most important diagnostic tool the physician has at his disposal, and tests indicating nerve or muscle function can only be interpreted in the context of a proper history. Careful analysis of the history is usually the only way in which the patient's suffering can be separated from the underlying physical pain, which requires diagnosis. Treatment that does not take into account both aspects of the problem is almost certain to fail in achieving a lasting positive result.

BIBLIOGRAPHY

Adair FD, McLean J: Tumors of peripheral nerve system with report of 2782 cases. Association for Research Nervous and Mental Disease Proceedings 16:440, 1937

Baile AA, Sayre GP, Clark EC: Neuritis associated with systemic lupus erythematosus: A report of five cases, with necropsy in two. Arch Neurol Psychiatry 75:251, 1956

Bennett AE: Horse serum neuritis with report of five cases. JAMA 112:590, 1939

Billig DM, Hallman GL, Cooley DA: Arterial embolism. Arch Surg 95:1, 1967

Brain R, Henson RA: Neurological syndromes associated with carcinoma: The carcinomatous neuromyopathies. Lancet 2:971, 1958

Chambers RA, Medd WE, Spencer H: Primary amyloidosis with special reference to involvement of the nervous system. Q J Med 27:207, 1958

Croft PB, Wadia NH: Familial hypertrophic polyneuritis: Review of a previously reported family. Neurology 7:356, 1957

Echlin F, Owens FM, Wells WL: Observations on major and minor causalgia. Arch Neurol Psychiatry 62:183, 1949

Fischer CM, Adams RD: Diphtheritic polyneuritis: A pathologic study. J Neuropathol Exp Neurol 15:243, 1956

Fleming R: Refsum's syndrome: An unusual hereditary neuropathy. Neurology 7:476, 1957

Gifford RW Jr, Hines EA Jr, Craig WM: Sympathectomy for Raynaud's phenomenon: Follow-up study of 70 women with Raynaud's disease and 54 women with secondary Raynaud's phenomenon. Circulation 17:5, 1958

Gilpin SF, Moersch FP, Kernohan JW: Polyneuritis: A clinical and pathologic study of a special group of cases frequently referred to as instances of neuronitis. Arch Neurol Psychiatry 35:937, 1936

Greenburg L: Diagnosis and treatment of occupational metal poisoning. JAMA 139:815, 1949

Gillain G, de Sèze S, Blondin–Walter M: Etude clinique et pathogénique de certaines paralysies professionelles du nerf sciatique poplite externe. Bull Acad Natl Med (Paris) 111:633, 1934

Keegan JJ, Garrett FD: The segmental distribution of the cutaneous nerves in the limbs of man. Anat Rec 102:409–438, 1948

Kirtley JA, Riddell DH, Stoney WS et al: Cervicothoracic sympathectomy in neurovascular abnormalities of the upper extremities: Experiences in 76 patients with 104 sympathectomies. Ann Surg 165:869, 1967

Kopell HP, Thomspon WAL: Peripheral Entrapment Neuropathies. Baltimore, Williams & Wilkins, 1963

Lewis T: Pain. New York, Macmillan, 1942

Love JA: The surgical management of the scalenus anticus syndrome with and without cervical rib. In Allen EV, Barker NW, Hines EA Jr (eds): Peripheral Vascular Diseases, 3rd ed. Philadelphia, WB Saunders, 1962

Martin MM: Diabetic neuropathy: A clinical study of 150 cases. Brain 76:594, 1953

Roos DB: Transaxillary approach for first rib resection to relieve thoracic outlet syndrome. Ann Surg 163:354, 1966

Semmes RD: Ruptures of the Lumbar Intervertebral Disc. Springfield, Ill, Charles C Thomas, 1964

Spencer FC: Peripheral arterial disease. In Schwartz SI (ed): Principles of Surgery. New York, McGraw–Hill, 1969

Spurling RG: Lesions of the Cervial Intervertebral Disc. Springfield, Ill, Charles C Thomas, 1956

Spurling RG: Lesions of the Lumbar Intervertebral Disc. Springfield, Ill, Charles C Thomas, 1953

Wechsler IS: Multiple peripheral neuropathy versus multiple neuritis. JAMA 110:1910, 1938

Woltman HW, Wilder RM: Diabetes mellitus: Pathologic changes in the spinal cord and peripheral nerves. Arch Intern Med 44:576, 1929

14

Clubbed Fingers and Hypertrophic Osteoarthropathy

Bernard S. Lipman
Edward Massie

Relationship of Clubbing to Hypertrophic Osteoarthropathy
Recognition
    Clinical Features
    Laboratory Tests

Radiographic Findings
Association with Disease
Pathology
Pathogenesis
Summary

Clubbing is a physical sign characterized by bulbous changes and diffuse enlargement of the terminal phalanges of the fingers and toes. No symptoms are present except for occasional burning or warmth of the terminal phalanges.

Hypertrophic osteoarthropathy generally is considered to be a further extension of the clubbing process. A chronic proliferative subperiosteal osteitis involves the distal ends of the extremities and is manifested by the digital clubbing and in addition by swelling, pain, and tenderness over the larger involved bones and over the accompanying joints. However, some authors still believe that real differences in clinical significance exist between clubbing and osteoarthropathy and that the etiology and the pathogenesis of these two conditions are different. It is important to define the terms separately.

Many different names have been proposed for what we now know as clubbing and hypertrophic osteoarthropathy. The phenomenon of clubbing has been called *Hippocratic fingers, drumstick fingers, parrot–beak nails, watch–glass nails,* and *serpent's head fingers.*

Hypertrophic osteoarthropathy has been called *pulmonary hypertrophic osteo-arthropathy* (originally by Marie[1]), *secondary hypertrophic osteo-arthropathy, hyperplastic osteo-arthropathy, toxigenic ossifying osteoperiostitis, Marie-Bamberger syndrome,* and numerous other names. As information accumulated, it became apparent that the bone lesions were characterized by the deposition of newly formed periosteal bone and that sometimes there were also joint manifestations; moreover, it became apparent that such changes were not limited strictly to an association with diseases of the lung.

The terms now generally accepted are hypertrophic osteoarthropathy for the changes in the larger bones and joints and clubbing for the distal extremity changes in toes and fingers.

RELATIONSHIP OF CLUBBING TO HYPERTROPHIC OSTEOARTHROPATHY

At first there was thought to be no relationship between clubbing and hypertrophic osteoarthropathy. They were described separately and considered to be

independent entities. Under the unified theory, they have been considered as variations of the same process—Hypertrophic osteoarthropathy being the more advanced stage, with manifestations not only in the fingers but also in the more proximal parts of the extremities. This relationship is supported by the following facts: (1) the two conditions, either separately or together, occur in association with the same diseases; (2) clubbing of the fingers is a constant characteristic finding in hypertrophic osteoarthropathy, although varying in degree; (3) the osseous changes in simple clubbing resemble those of hypertrophic osteoarthropathy.

As would be expected of the milder, earlier manifestation, clubbing is seen much more frequently than the more advanced state called hypertrophic osteoarthropathy.

As early as the 5th century B.C., Hippocrates described curving of the fingernails in a case of empyema.[2] In the latter part of the 19th century, von Bamberger and Marie drew attention to distinctive changes in the extremities associated with certain diseases of the lungs and heart[1,3] (Fig. 14-1). Since these early reports, numerous publications have appeared dealing with the intriguing physical evidences in the extremities of more serious internal disease and with the problem of how they are related. Mendlowitz in his review (1942) gave 337 references.[4] Howell in 1979 stated: "little more is known of the pathogenesis today than when recorded in 400 B.C. by Hippocrates."[103] Much remains obscure, particularly concerning the pathologic physiology. As Samuel West[5] stated in 1897, "clubbing is one of those phenomena with which we are so familiar that we appear to know more about it than we really do."

RECOGNITION

CLINICAL FEATURES

The symptoms of clubbing are almost entirely objective, particularly in cases that are developing slowly; usually the patient is not aware of the deformity until it is brought to his attention. Recognition is not difficult if one keeps the possibility in mind and observes the extremities carefully. Occasionally, especially in cases secondary to lung tumors, the more rapid onset of changes in the pulp and nail bed attract the attention of the patient manicurist and should alert the physician to the necessity of a chest radiograph. In cases of acute clubbing, a feeling of warmth, a burning sensation, sweating, and rarely pain in the fingertips may occur. It is important to detect early clubbing.

Because of its diagnostic implications the condition in its early stages may at times be confused with other abnormalities of the fingers. Early clubbing should be differentiated from (1) simple curving of the nail, which is seen normally, especially in the black population; (2) chronic paronychia, in which the soft tissues at the base of the nail are swollen and no change occurs in the nail bed itself; (3) Heberden's nodes, which lie more proximally and rarely cause diagnostic difficulty; (4) chronic infectious arthritis, in which the swelling is periarticular and no change is apparent in the nail bed; (5) epidermoid cysts of the bony phalanges; and (6) felons, where there is associated pain and absence of changes in the other fingers. Early in the process of clubbing, thickening of the fibroelastic tissue of the nail bed produces a definite firm transverse ridge at the root of the nail, best observed on the dorsal aspect of the finger. Lovibond[6] noted this "profile sign." When one views a normal finger from the side, one sees an obtuse angle of about 160° between the base of the nail and the adjacent dorsal surface of the terminal phalanx. This angle is referred to as the "base angle" and is clearly demonstrated in the normal thumb. In early clubbing, the base angle is obliterated and it becomes 180° or greater.[93] This "profile sign" is one of the best means of detecting the beginning stage of true clubbing.

Figure 14-2A illustrates the normal base angle of approximately 160°; Figure 14-2B shows curving, an alteration that may be present in many normal fingernails. Notice that the base angle is not interfered with, in spite of the fact that the distal nail is curved considerably downward. If the original nail is curved, clubbing is accordingly accompanied by curving. Figure 14-2C illustrates the characteristic base angle obliteration in early clubbing; Figure 14-2D shows advanced clubbing (base angle is greater than 180° and projects dorsally). In Figures 14-2E and F, illustrating chronic paronychia and Heberden's nodes, respectively, the base angle persists undisturbed.

Clubbing usually occurs first in the thumb and index

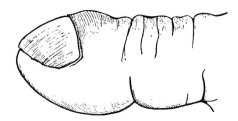

Fig. 14-1. Drawing of a clubbed finger from Marie's classic report. (Marie, P: De l'osteo-arthropatie hypertrophianate pneumique. Revue de Médicine 10:1, 1890)

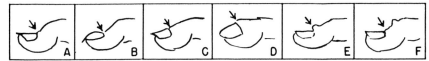

Fig. 14-2. Characteristic profile configurations of the finger. (*A*) Normal finger, illustrating the base angle of the nail (usually about 160°). (*B*) "Curving" of the nail, a variation of the normal. The base angle is undisturbed. (*C*) Early clubbing, with the base angle obliterated—positive "profile sign." (Club fingernails may also be curved.) (*D*) Advanced clubbing, with base angle greater than 180°. Base of nail projects upward, and overall area of nail is increased. (*E*) Chronic paronychia, with fundamental base angle unaltered. (*F*) Heberden's node, with normal base angle. (From Lovibond JL: The diagnosis of clubbed fingers. Lancet 1:363, 1938)

finger, and spreads to the other digits later. In the advanced stage, there is an increase in all tissues of the finger tips—soft tissues as well as nails—so that the ends of the fingers assume a bulbous appearance. In Figure 14-3, note the typical clubbed fingers in a girl with congenital heart disease. The overlying skin as well as the volar pads are smooth, shiny, and bright pink in color. The vascular bed gives a lilac or cyanotic hue to the nails. Witherspoon pointed out that the return of color following slight pressure on the fingernail is characteristically slower than normal.[7] The base of the nail may be elevated so that its outline is seen beneath the skin's surface. Furthermore, the nail can be rocked back and forth as if it were floating on a soft edematous pad.

Patients may complain of excessive sweating, a feeling of warmth, or a burning sensation in the fingertips; pain is rare but may occur in cases of very acute clubbing. Abnormally frequent filing or clipping of the fingernails is often necessary because of the accelerated rate of growth, and longitudinal striations in the nail may appear. Hangnails form readily, due to the rapid growth of the cuticle, resulting often in acute and chronic paronychia. In longstanding cases, particularly in congenital heart disease, dorsiflexion with hyperextensibility of the distal phalangeal joints may be present. Figure 14-4 illustrates the appearance of clubbed fingers in a man with carcinoma of the lung.

Various forms of clubbing (drumstick, watch-glass, parrot-beak, and serpent's head) have been described, and these variations now are known to be attributable to the duration and degree of the process as well as to differences in the initial anatomy of the digits. Clubbing of the toes nearly always develops in association with clubbing of the fingers but is more difficult to recognize because of the wide range in the shape of normal toes. The early stage may be recognized best in the large toe. Successive measurements of the nail surface are at times necessary to confirm the diagnosis. Several authors, Mendlowitz, Angel, and Buchman and

Hrowat, report the presence of clubbing (swelling, thickening, and furrowing of the skin) over the nose, the molar region, the eyelids, and the ears.[4,73,74]

Berry has divided clubbing into two general types, depending upon the difference in their appearances.[94] One type is associated with congenital, cyanotic heart

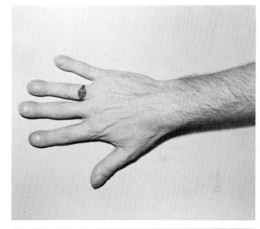

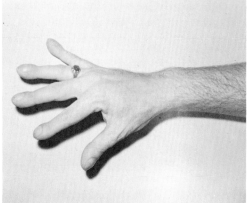

Fig. 14-3. Eleven-year-old girl with cyanosis from congenital heart disease (tetralogy of Fallot)

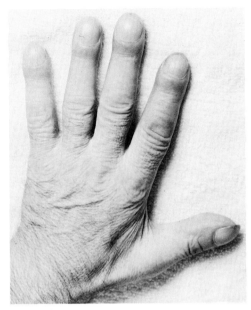

Fig. 14-4. Clubbed fingers in a 59-year-old man with carcinoma of the lung.

disease with terminal phalanges that are dusky, richly vascular, and frequently accompanied by a reddish brown pigmentation of the skin proximal to the lunula. This type of clubbing histologically is associated with increased vascularity, vasodilation, and increased flow of blood to the fingertips. There appears to be a relationship between the amount of clubbing and the degree of polycythemia. The other type of clubbing frequently is associated with chronic pulmonary disease, and the fingertips have a less engorged and more pallid and dry appearance. Histologically, the enlargement of the distal phalanx is composed mainly of connective-tissue overgrowth between the nail plate and the bone. Edema of the soft parts, thickening of the blood vessel walls, cellular infiltration, fibroblastic proliferation, and growth of new collagenous tissue account for the uniform enlargement of the terminal phalanges. Finger pulp mast cell counts have been found to be lower in clubbed finger than in controls.[109]

Hypertrophic osteoarthropathy should always be sought for in the presence of clubbing. Locke[8] stated that "every case of hypertrophic osteoarthropathy so far recorded has shown well-developed clubbing of the fingers and toes, and it is regarded as an absolutely constant sign of the disease." On the other hand, review of the literature reveals that clubbing occasionally may be absent in an otherwise typical case of pulmonary osteoarthropathy or that clubbing manifests itself later than the bone changes.[64,70,72] Locke reported 39

cases of "simple" clubbing in which 12 (30%) showed radiographic evidence of periosteal proliferation of the long bones indicative of hypertrophic osteoarthropathy. These findings illustrate the close association of these two conditions.

Hypertrophic osteoarthropathy in its early stages may be asymptomatic and detectable only on radiographs; on the other hand, the onset may be heralded by aching pains in the joints and tenderness along the shafts of the involved bones. The pain may be severe and aggravated by movement, and may precede detectable radiographic changes. It may vary in intensity from slight discomfort to deep, dull aching pain that is transient. The skin over the involved areas may be warm, reddened, and thickened by a brawny nonpitting edema. In some series, pain in the bones has been the only presenting complaint in as many as 40% of the cases—the underlying more serious disease having caused less evident symptoms or none at all. Such bone and joint symptoms warrant careful search for evidence of clubbing and osteoarthropathy and search for the underlying cause (chest radiographs, and so on).

Craig and others have implicated arthralgia as one of the earliest clinical manifestations of intrathoracic lesions, the hypertrophic osteoarthropathy in such cases being an early complication.[9,107] Symptoms of pulmonary osteoarthropathy may precede by 1 to 18 months the detection of localized lung lesions, particularly neoplastic disease of the chest, in contrast to suppurative lung processes in which the onset of symptoms of osteoarthropathy tends to lag behind respiratory and systemic manifestations.[65–67,71] Early diagnosis of cancer of the lung may be hastened by early detection of hypertrophic osteoarthropathy. The pains in the extremities are occasionally mistaken for rheumatoid arthritis or hypertrophic osteoarthritis. A moderate degree of joint effusion may be seen, along with some limitation of motion. Partial or complete ankylosis has been reported in advanced cases. Edema and hypertrophy of the subcutaneous tissue of the limbs are observed (Fig. 14-5).

The earliest histologic changes are round-cell infiltration and edema of the periosteum, articular capsule, synovial membrane,[111] and surrounding subcutaneous tissues. Lifting of the periosteum occurs with deposition of a bony matrix, eventually resulting in a sheath of new bone deposited over the cortex. Beneath the new bone, accelerated resorption of endosteal and haversian bone occurs, so that the new bony structure is weakened and pathologic fractures may occur. Synovial membranes adjacent to the involved bones are often edematous and infiltrated with plasma cells, lymphocytes, and polymorphonuclear leukocytes. Adjacent cartilage may also undergo degeneration. Electron

microscopic examination of the synovial membrane reveals alterations of the microcirculation, with dilatation of capillaries and venules, endothelial cells gaps, multilamination of basement membrane of the small vessels, and subendothelial electron dense deposits. These deposits that are present in patients with lung carcinoma and with circulatory tumor antigen–antibody complexes suggest that the synovities secondary to lung carcinoma might be immune complex-mediated.

Osteoarthropathy may occur at any age. Gottlieb and associates reported clubbing and osteoarthropathy in a 2-year-old infant with chronic pyopneumothorax.[75] Kennedy reported similar findings in a 7½-month-old infant with multiple lung abscesses since birth.

Hypertrophic osteoarthropathy was at one time confused with acromegaly, in which enlargement of the hands and feet is characteristic. There may be awkwardness of gait and clumsiness of movement in the hands and fingers due to the increased size and weight of the limbs in advanced stages of hypertrophic osteoarthropathy. The diagnosis also may be confused with thrombophlebitis, venous stasis, congestive heart failure, nutritional edema, and peripheral neuropathy. Several reports mention the presence of muscular weakness in association with osteoarthropathy; bone pain, which is deep-seated, burning in character, and

aggravated by lowering of the extremities; dusky discoloration of the fingertips; stiffness of the fingers; increased sweating; skin lesions, characterized by redness, glistening appearance, and warmth over the affected areas; increased hair growth; and broadened or cylindrical appearance of the distal thirds of the extremities produced by thickened skin and a firm, hard, pitting edema.[64,69] Spontaneous fractures may occur.

The changes associated with clubbing are usually gradual in onset, taking place over a period of many weeks, months, or years. However, they have been noted to appear within one week of onset of the underlying disease.* Similarly, hypertrophic osteoarthropathy may be evident in a few weeks, or it may not be evident for 20 years after onset of the associated malady. Clubbing and hypertrophic osteoarthropathy may disappear and reappear synchronously with remissions and exacerbations of the underlying disorder. Changes in the degree of clubbing have been used as a gauge of the activity of the concomitant disease as well as the effectiveness of treatment. Disappearance of the phenomena in the extremities has been reported following successful medical or surgical treatment of chronic pulmonary infections, subacute bacterial endocarditis, mediastinal and pulmonary tumors, cyanotic congenital heart disease, ulcerative colitis, regional ileitis, amebic dysentery, and sprue. Improvement, and even disappearance of symptoms of clubbing, have occurred also after therapy in pulmonary tuberculosis, following antiluetic therapy in syphilis of the lung, and, in subjects with chronic mountain sickness, after descent to sea level.[4,11] In fact, failure of improvement in the osteoarticular manifestations following successful management of chronic lung infections should arouse suspicion of an underlying malignant process.[68] Vogl and associates reported a case in which the general downhill course and the intractability of the pulmonary infection and of the symptoms of osteoarthropathy led to surgical exploration and detection of an underlying lung cancer.[64]

A remarkable occurrence confirmed by many observers is the very rapid disappearance of pain in the bone, which may occur following removal of a pulmonary tumor or other etiologic factor. Pain may disappear in 24 to 48 hours, thus suggesting the importance of circulatory or toxic (perhaps chemical) factors in the causation of the pain rather than the bone changes themselves being directly responsible. Flavell, believing that the manifestations of osteoarthropathy were caused by a neural reflex from the lung, reported five inoperable cases of carcinoma of the lung in which vagotomy on the affected side provided immediate re-

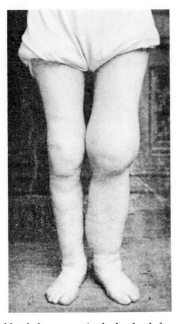

Fig. 14-5. Enlargement of both legs, particularly the left, in a case of hypertrophic osteoarthropathy. Note the large effusion in the left knee joint. (Norris GW, Landis HRM: Diseases of the Chest and Physical Diagnosis, 6th ed. Philadelphia, WB Saunders, 1938)

*Lipman B: Personal observations, 1978

lief of symptoms.[76] Steroid therapy and phlebotomies also have been suggested as therapy for symptomatic relief in inoperable cases[77]; the value of these measures is unproven.

LABORATORY TESTS

The most common abnormal laboratory finding in clubbing deformity is an elevated sedimentation rate. In addition, various other altered laboratory tests may occur as a result of the underlying disease processes. Since the concentrations of phosphorus and alkaline phosphatase in the blood may be elevated during destruction and repair of bone, these values also may be changed in hypertrophic osteoarthropathy. Examination of synovial fluid has been clear, of high viscosity, and generally "noninflammatory." White blood cell counts are usually below 2000 with less than 50% polymorphonuclear leukocytes. Serum and synovial fluid C3 and C4 levels have been within normal limits. The fluorescent antinuclear antibody and latex fixation tests have been negative.

RADIOGRAPHIC FINDINGS

The radiographic changes are variable and depend upon the intensity and duration of the pathologic process. In early clubbing, there is usually no radiologic evidence of alteration. Somewhat later, a burrlike proliferation of the tuft of one or more terminal phalanges may appear. In longstanding cases of clubbing, atrophic changes occur, ranging from simple osteoporosis to complete resorption (see terminal phalanx, 5th digit, Fig. 14-6). Erosion of the terminal tufts is rare; not infrequently, however, there is atrophy and spindling (narrowing of the shafts) of the terminal, and sometimes of the other phalanges and of the metacarpals and metatarsals (Fig. 14-6). The phalanges may show considerable elongation and prominent tufts when the clubbing occurs prior to cessation of growth. The development of newly formed periosteal bone in the terminal phalanges has been reported only rarely.

Fully developed hypertrophic osteoarthropathy produces distinct radiographic alterations.[106] These are generally extensive and involve earliest and most frequently the tibia, the fibula, the radius, the ulna, the femur, the humerus, the metacarpal, and the metatarsal bones. Later the phalanges, the clavicles, and the pelvis may be implicated and, very rarely, the tarsals, the carpals, the vertebrae, the ribs, the scapulae, and the skull.[4] Some authors state that the skull and mandible are never involved. Characteristically roughened, uneven, linear densities, which represent the newly

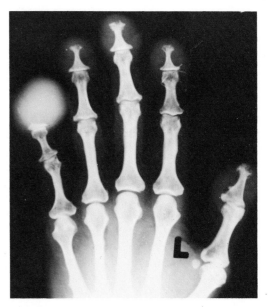

Fig. 14-6. Radiographic appearance of hand in patient also exhibiting changes in many other bones. Note the resorption of the terminal phalanx of the fifth digit and the narrowing of the shafts and osteoporosis of other phalanges of this digit. In some of the phalanges of the other fingers osteoporosis predominates; in others there is thickening of the cortical bone. (Courtesy of D.C. Weir, St. Louis)

formed periosteal calcium deposits, are observed along the shafts of the involved bones; the appearance suggests that the chronic periostitis (Fig. 14-7). The periosteal reaction is usually most evident along the distal half of the long bones. The densities are thickest in the region of the peripheral epiphyses and at the points of muscular insertions. With remissions and exacerbations of the underlying disease, the repeated layered calcification in the periosteum may give a laminated x-ray appearance. The periosteal new bone may vary from the simple, smooth, parallel type of normal new bone to the rough, irregular, lacelike appearance of abnormal periosteal proliferation.

In advanced cases, osteoporosis of the cancellous portion and thinning of the cortex of the original bone are found. Pathologic fractures may occur. Occasionally osteoporosis of the newly formed periosteal bone is seen. It should be pointed out that the radiographic diagnosis of hypertrophic osteoarthropathy is doubtful in the absence of definite periosteal proliferation. The new bone may be 1 mm–10 mm in thickness. Gall and associates noted that in the early stage of development, the periosteum showed signs of inflammation, thickening, and early division into two layers.[68] The outer layer showed an accumulation of inflammatory

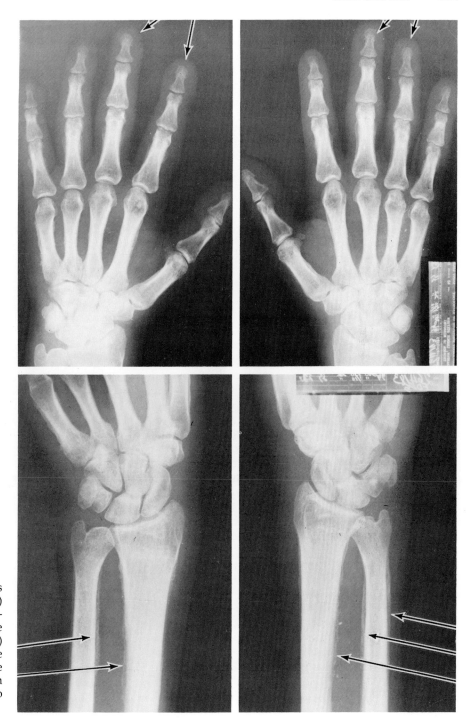

Fig. 14-7. Radiographs of hands (*top*) and distal forearms (*bottom*) in a case of clubbing and hypertrophic osteoarthropathy. Note the periosteal proliferation (*arrows*) along the shaft of the radius, the ulna, the metacarpals, and the phalanges. Burrlike proliferation of the distal phalanges is also present (*arrows*).

cells. The inner layer consisted of a fibrillary intercellular substance that was soon replaced by an osteoid matrix. The new subperiosteal bone layer fused with the original cortex, and numerous osteoclasts appeared and caused focal areas of bone resorption. A thickened spongy shaft with a rarefying osteitis of the older bone resulted.

The new subperiosteal bone is formed chiefly near the epiphyses and at the points of musculotendinous insertions. It tends to progress to the proximal ends of the bones, but these changes seldom are seen in areas covered by the articular capsule. If the new subperiosteal bone displaces the thickened periosteum rapidly, pain and tenderness may occur, but if the process progresses slowly there may be no discomfort. Various parts of the skeleton may show different stages of the disease, which may advance rapidly in one area while regressing another.[108]

ASSOCIATION WITH DISEASE

Clubbing and hypertrophic osteoarthropathy, though often relatively innocuous in themselves, owe their importance to the fact that they are usually associated with significant underlying diseases. However, these conditions may be absent even in the severe forms of the diseases with which they are often associated. Furthermore, clubbing may occur as an isolated condition, unassociated with any known systemic disorder, as in hereditary clubbing. The hereditary form, also known as the Touraine–Solente–Golé syndrome, is transmitted as a sex-limited autosomal dominant trait with low penetrance for females.[99,105]

The frequent association of these pathologic changes in bones with chronic pulmonary diseases is well recognized. Of the 144 cases of hypertrophic osteoarthropathy reported by Locke, 113 (78%) were associated with diseases of the respiratory tract.[8] Review of more recently published reports indicates that between 75% and 80% of cases with clubbing and hypertrophic osteoarthropathy are associated with diseases of the pulmonary system; 10% to 15% occur with diseases of the cardiovascular system; 5% to 10% are associated with lesions of the gastrointestinal tract, including the liver; and another 5% to 10% fall into a miscellaneous group. Of the associated pulmonary diseases reported by Locke, tuberculosis (20%), bronchiectasis (19%), malignancy (7%), and empyema (5%) occurred most frequently.[8] However, the great progress in the sophisticated procedures in the diagnosis of heart and lung diseases and in thoracic surgery has brought the realization that the percentage of persons who develop clubbing and hypertrophic osteoarthropathy secondary to bronchiectasis or pulmonary maligancy is higher than was

thought. Poppe reviewed 129 cases in which lobectomy was done at Barnes Hospital for bronchiectasis or chronic lung abscess.[12] Of these, 103 patients (79%) had clubbing in varying degrees. Of 276 tuberculous patients at Koch Hospital in St. Louis surveyed by Poppe, 71 (25%) revealed evidence of clubbing.[12]

Skorneck and Ginsburg emphasize a distinction between clubbing and osteoarthropathy.[78] In a 3-year radiographic study of 390 patients with pulmonary tuberculosis, they found no cases of osteoarthropathy; in three patients who were misdiagnosed as tuberculous and in whom osteoarthropathy was found, the final correct diagnoses were lung cancer in two and pyogenic abscess in one. The authors went so far as to state that the finding of osteoarthropathy without clubbing denies the presence of tuberculosis. In the presence of hypertrophic osteoarthropathy, intrathoracic neoplasm is the most important condition to be excluded.[110]

In the cardiovascular group of diseases, clubbed fingers were present in association with cyanotic congenital heart disease in 132 (13%) of Abbott's 1000 cases.[16] Friedberg noted clubbing in about 66% of fatal cases of subacute bacterial endocarditis, whereas Blumer reported the incidence of clubbed fingers in subacute bacterial endocarditis to be 18 of 48 cases (36%).[13,14] Trever described two cases of congenital cyanotic heart disease with longstanding clubbing and hypertrophic osteoarthropathy, emphasizing the distinction between simple osteoarthropathy and osteoarthropathy.[89] In congenital cyanotic heart disease, the literature shows a high incidence of clubbing but a low incidence of osteoarthropathy, and no case of osteoarthropathy occurred earlier than the age of 11 years. In the acyanotic child with clubbed fingers, a congenital heart malformation is unlikely, and an extracardiac cause should be sought. Moreover, when one congenital defect is discovered it is well to look for others, since multiple embryologic defects are the rule. Polydactyly, syndactyly, hypoplastic or absent thumb, simian creases, brachydactyly with index finger overlapping third finger and the fifth finger over the fourth with a tightly clenched fist, shortened fifth finger, arachnodactyly with lax joints, and telangiectasia of fingertips are some additional abnormalities of the hand, other than clubbed fingers, which are associated with congenital major cardiovascular defects.[93]

The various diseases that should be suspected in the presence of clubbing or hypertrophic osteoarthropathy are as follows:

Pulmonary Group. Bronchiectasis,[15] primary and secondary tumors of the lung,[16,17] bronchus,[9,18] mediastinum,[4] thymus,[19] and chest wall,[20] chronic empyema,[1,21,22] lung abscess,[23,24] fibroid pulmonary tuberculosis with excavation,[25,26] chronic pneumoni-

tis,[2,8] emphysema associated with chronic suppurative conditions,[27] pneumoconiosis,[2] neurogenic tumor of the diaphragm,[92] atelectasis,[10] cystic disease of the lung,[28] chest deformities,[21] syphilis of the lung,[29] actinomycosis,[30] Hodgkin's disease involving the lung or mediastinum,[31,32] pulmonary hemangioma,[33,34] and aortic aneurysm with compression of the lung.[35]

Levine has proposed another physical sign, the yellow rounded digit.[98] It combines tobacco-stained and clubbed fingers of cigarette smokers. The staining involves the terminal phalanges and nails of the index and middle fingers of either hand. Among 13 patients with the sign who were followed for one year, 10 patients or 77% proved to have bronchogenic carcinoma.

Cardiac Group. Cyanotic congenital heart disease with a venous-arterial shunt (right to left flow);[6,12,36–38] subacute bacterial endocarditis[4,13,14,43] (rare in the bacteria-free stage), chronic congestive heart failure,[39] and cardiac tumors.[4]

Hepatic Group. Cholangiolytic or Hannot's type of cirrhosis, obstructive biliary cirrhosis secondary to bile duct obstruction, cirrhosis associated with chronic malaria, hepatomegaly with amebic abscess, and, rarely, in portal cirrhosis.[40,104]

Gastrointestinal Group. Chronic ulcerative colitis, regional enteritis, intestinal tuberculosis, chronic bacillary and amebic dysentery, sprue, ascaris infestation, multiple polyposis of the colon and esophagus,[102] abdominal Hodgkin's disease, pyloric obstruction and gastrectasia associated with carcinoma of the pylorus or duodenal ulcer, and, rarely, in carcinoma of the colon.[4,41,43] Hollis reported a patient with severe hypertrophic osteoarthropathy secondary to a myxoma of the lower esophagus without local invasion or metastases and with regression of the osteoarthropathy following removal of the myxoma.[95]

Mixed Group. Idiopathic, hereditary, post-thyroidectomy, nasopharyngeal tumors, pituitary gland abnormality, myxedema due to ^{131}I, generalized lymphosarcomatosis, chronic mountain sickness (Monge's disease), chronic osteomyelitis with amyloidosis, and pseudohypertrophic muscular dystrophy.[4,10,44,45]

Miscellaneous Group. Unilateral clubbing may be present in aneurysm of the subclavian artery, the innominate artery, or the arch of the aorta, lymphangitis, brachial arteriovenous aneurysm, and superior sulcus tumor (Pancoast's tumor).[46–48]

PATHOLOGY

The pathology of clubbing and hypertrophic osteoarthropathy has received comparatively little consideration because of the difficulty in securing postmortem finger specimens for study, the inability to obtain suitable preparations for examination, and our inadequate knowledge of the normal histology of the fingertips. However, on the basis of various reports in the literature, the pathologic changes appear to consist chiefly of hypertrophy and hyperplasia.[2,8,11,49–53] There is increased proliferation of all tissues of the fingertip, especially in the fibrous elastic portion of the nail bed and in the fatty connective tissue of the ball of the finger. Corresponding with an increase in the underlying substance, there is an increase in the cross-sectional area of the nail. Newly formed capillaries have been observed, as well as dilation and increased thickness of the walls of the small blood vessels in the end of the finger. The terminal phalanx may show increased thickness of its periosteum and of the ungual process itself or, in advanced cases, complete resorption of the bone. Bigler stated that the shape of the clubbed digit is the result of the increased thickness of the nail bed.[79] He stated that the nail bed is loosely textured, with large fibroblasts in a reticular network. The glomera are increased, as are extravascular lymphocytes and eosinophils. In chronic clubbing, the increased thickness is due to increased collagen deposition in the nail bed with no evidence of edema.

In hypertrophic osteoarthropathy, there is calcification of the periosteum, and islands of newly formed periosteal bone may be found along the shaft of the long bones, thickest in the region of the peripheral epiphysis and at the points of musculotendinous insertions. There is thinning of the cortex of the original bone and osteoporosis of the cancellous portion. Bone resorption may extend to the new periosteal bone, leaving a thin trabeculated space between the cortex and the periosteum. In patients with exacerbations and remissions, there are multiple laminations suggestive of tree-trunk layers. Pathologic fractures may occur if thinning and osteoporosis exceed the capacities of the reparative processes. With joint involvement (which occurs in approximately one-third of the cases), the joint capsule and the synovial membrane occasionally are thickened, and there may be fluid collection within the joint capsule. Proliferation of the subsynovial granulation tissue associated with lymphocytosis and fibrinoid degeneration of the synovial membrane has been reported, resulting in pannus formation. Pressure from the pannus can produce degeneration of the cartilage with erosion; if this occurs, the process may terminate in ankylosis.

PATHOGENESIS

The pathogenesis of clubbing and hypertrophic osteoarthropathy has been in dispute since the time when these conditions were first recognized. Because of their

diagnostic significance, they have engaged the interest of many clinicians, and numerous theories have been proposed—none of which has been proved to this date. In the 18th century, it was thought that clubbing was due to emaciation, as described in the works of Laennec.[54] Pigeaux, in 1832, advanced the theory that circulatory alterations caused edema and increased cellularity of the connective tissue of the fingertip, resulting in clubbing.[54] In the latter part of the 19th century, following the classic papers of Marie and von Bamberger, the theory that chronic infection might by responsible was widely accepted.[1,3] The popularity of this theory soon was shared by the toxic hypothesis. (Circulating toxins were believed to act on susceptible peripherial capillaries and thus produce the characteristic changes.) However, the association of clubbing and hypertrophic osteoarthropathy with pulmonary neoplasms and congenital heart disorders provided evidence that these theories were inadequate. Verrusio and others later postulated the mechanical theory, which proposed that clubbing was due to capillary stasis resulting from back pressure.[55] The fact that clubbing was rarely seen in patients with heart failure and the fact that actual pressure measurements failed to substantiate the presence of stasis were cited as evidence against this hypothesis.[56] Numerous additional theories have been suggested, such as vitamin deficiency,[52] malfunction of the endocrine glands (pituitary,[57] thyroid,[55] parathyroid,[55] and gonads[55]), nerve injury,[27] lymph stasis,[58] change in blood volume,[59] increased intracranial pressure,[55] and reflex nerve impulses from peripheral pulmonic nerve fibers influencing the formation of arteriovenous anastomoses in the limbs.

Many attempts were made to study clubbing and hypertrophic osteoarthropathy in animals. A number of unsuccessful methods were tried to reproduce these conditions in rabbits, guinea pigs, dogs, cats, and monkeys.[2,23,60,61] It was not until 1940 that Mehdlowitz and Leslie successfully induced hypertrophic osteoarthropathy experimentally in one of three dogs by anastomosing the left and adjacent main pulmonary artery to the left auricle, resulting in a right-to-left heart shunt, simulating congenital heart disease with cyanosis.[62] By this method they were able to produce the gross and microscopic evidences of periosteal proliferation seen in hypertrophic osteoarthropathy (Figs. 14-8 and 14-9).

Careful studies revealed no change in the venous pressure, either circulation time, or oxygen comsumption. The main experimental finding was an increase in the cardiac output; the blood flow through the lungs remained relatively unchanged. Medlowitz also demonstrated the presence of increased peripheral blood flow in patients with acquired clubbed fingers by means of calorimetric and brachiodigital arterial blood pres-

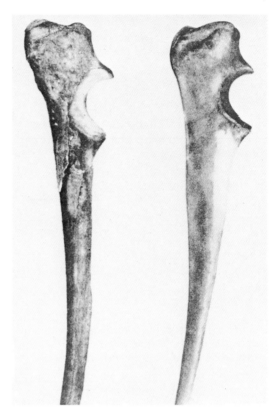

Fig. 14-8. Comparison of the ulna of a dog with experimentally induced hypertrophic osteoarthropathy (*left*) with ulna of a normal dog (*right*). Note the roughened, irregular, elevated areas of the newly formed periosteum on the left. (Mendlowitz M, Leslie A: The experimental simulation in the dog of the cyanosis in hypertrophic osteoarthropathy associated with congenital heart disease. American Heart Journal 24:141, 1942)

sure gradient methods.[56] Furthermore, he was able to show that the accelerated fingertip blood flow waxed and waned with exacerbations and remissions of clubbing and the underlying disease. In 1959, Wilson confirmed Mendlowitz's findings of increased blood flow in clubbed fingers. He concluded that the increased flow passed largely through numerous arteriovenous anastomoses and was in excess of physiologic requirements, resulting in accelerated growth due to "forced feeding." Wilson noted that clubbing on the left hand regressed after ligation of the left subclavian artery in patients with tetralogy of Fallot who underwent surgical correction by the Blalock technique.

Blood flow and temperature regulation of the distal phalanges are functions of the glomus, as observed by Wilkins, Grant and Bland, Popoff, and others.[80–82] The glomus is a highly specialized arteriovenous anasto-

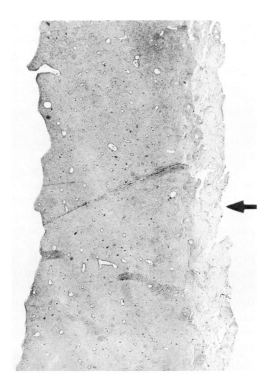

Fig. 14-9. Photomicrograph of transverse section of tibia of the dog with experimentally induced hypertrophic osteoarthropathy showing newly formed periosteum. (Mendlowitz M, Leslie A: The experimental simulation in the dog of the cyanosis in hypertrophic osteoarthropathy associated with congenital heart disease. American Heart Journal 24:141, 1942)

mosis present in the digital nail beds and pads. It consists of an afferent artery joining the so-called Sucquet–Hoyer canal, from which two to five arterioles arise; these subdivide into capillaries supplying the canal and related structures. The venous portion consists of a large receptacle forming a cape around the glomus and emptying into the subcapillary and deep veins of the digit. Reports concerning the influence of age on the number of glomera and the distribution of glomera vary according to the different counting techniques used. The fact that the glomus is a chief regulator of blood flow in the distal phalanx is established; its role therefore is inferred, but not proved, to be of major importance in the genesis of clubbing.[83]

Hall, in 1959, postulated that clubbing may be caused by a substance that is normally inactivated by the lungs and dilates the digital glomera.[84] He suggested that this substance might by ferritin. Shorr described a vasodepressor material (VDM) produced by ischemic skeletal muscle, spleen, and liver, which caused dilatation of the arteriovenous anastomoses in the mesentery and intestines of animals.[85] The VDM material produced by the liver was identified as ferritin. Ferritin, in its oxidized form, was inert against epinephrine; but in its reduced form blocked the vasoconstrictive action of epinephrine. Crismon reported that rutin, a flavonoid, blocked the vasodepressor effect of ferritin.[86] Using the reported findings on ferritin and rutin, Hall performed a study on subjects with and without clubbing.[84] The capillary blood flow through the fingertips was evaluated by a radiosodium ^{24}Na clearance technique before and after the intravenous injection of rutin. Hall concluded from his findings that one of the possible causes of clubbing was the long-term result of dilatation of the glomera in the nail beds by the reduced ferritin, which had evaded oxidation. In view of the fact that there is controversial evidence in the literature on rutin and its effect on vasodepressor materials (VDM) such as ferritin, Hall's concept is stimulating but needs confirmation, particularly in regard to determination of the amount of reduced ferritin as opposed to oxidized ferritin in subjects with clubbing.[87]

Mauer again raised the hypothesis that local tissue anoxia is the predisposing factor leading to clubbing.[63] His thesis is based upon the fact that in patients who have a disease associated with clubbing, the erythrocytes are altered physically, as evidenced by the elevated sedimentation rate. The delivery and uptake of oxygen by the tissues are thus hindered by the altered physical state of the red blood cells, and the local anoxia results. It is known, however, that tissue anoxia alone does not cause clubbing, since clubbing does not occur with the slow rate of flow and cold fingertips of Raynaud's syndrome. Mauer postulates that the increased blood flow present in clubbing is secondary to the anoxia, and that the rapid flow, the associated tissue warmth, and the rouleaux formation are all factors in the pathogenesis of clubbing.

On the other hand, it has been considered that the derangement of peripheral circulation may be dependent upon some pathologic intrathoracic reflex, which is promptly abolished by surgical removal of the primary lesion.[64] Flavell reported prompt relief of pain due to osteoarthropathy by vagotomy on the side of the affected lung cancer in five cases.[76] Trever reported a similar response of joint pains to atropinization.[89] Further evidence in favor of the neural reflex mechanism was furnished by Holling and associates, who observed eight canine and six human subjects with osteoarthropathy secondary to pulmonary neoplasm.[96] Division of the branches of the vagus in the hilus caused prompt regression of the osteodystrophy in all subjects. The validity of this neural concept could be investigated by preoperative and prompt postoperative capillary bed studies. Such studies may greatly con-

22. **Springthorpe JW:** Case of hypertrophic pulmonary osteoarthropathy. Br Med J 1:1257, 1895

23. **Phemister DB:** Chronic lung abscess with osteoarthropathy. Chicago Surgical Clinics 1:381, 1917

24. **Kerr J:** Pulmonary hypertrophic osteoarthropathy. Br Med J 2:1215, 1893

25. **Zesas DG:** An den Osteoarthropathien bein Lungentuberculose. Med Klin 5:1480, 1909

26. **Kaplan RH, Munson L:** Clubbed fingers in pulmonary tuberculosis. American Review of Tuberculosis 4:439, 1941

27. **Shaw HG, Cooper RH:** "Pulmonary hypertrophic osteoarthropathy" occurring in a case of congenital heart disease. Lancet 1:800, 1907

28. **Montuschi E:** Clubbing associated with congenital lung cyst. Br Med J 1:1310, 1938

29. **Munro WT:** Syphilis of the lung. Lancet 1:1376, 1922

30. **Wynn WH:** Case of actinomycosis (streptothrichosis) of lung and liver successfully treated with a vaccine. Br Med J 1:554, 1908

31. **Parkes Weber F, Ladinghaus JCG:** Uber einen Fall von Lamphadenoma (Hodgkinsche Krankeit) des Mediastinums verbunden mit einer hochgradigen hypertrophischen Pulmonalosteoarthropathie. Deutsche Archiv Klinishe Medicinische 96:217, 1909

32. **Shapiro RF, Zvaifler NJ:** Concurrent intrathoracic Hodgkin's disease and hypertrophic osteoarthropathy. Chest 63:912, 1972

33. **Rodes CB:** Cavernous hemangiomas of the lung with secondary polycythemia. JAMA 110:1915, 1938

34. **Plaut A:** Hemangioendothelioma of the lung. Arch Pathol 29:517, 1940

35. **Lang HB, Bower GC:** A report of a case of hypertrophic osteoarthropathy. Psychiatr Q 4:277, 1930

36. **Means MG, Brown NW:** Secondary osteoarthropathy in congenital heart disease. Am Heart J 34:262, 1947

37. **White PD, Sprague HB:** The tetralogy of Fallot. JAMA 92:787, 1929

38. **Wahl HR, Gard RL:** Aneurysm of the pulmonary artery. Surg Gynecol Obstet 52:1129, 1931

39. **Thorburn W:** Three cases of "hypertrophic pulmonary osteo-arthropathy" with remarks. Br Med J 1:115, 1893

40. **Rolleston HD, McNee JW:** Diseases of the Liver, Gallbladder, and Bileducts. London, Macmillan, 1929

41. **Schlicke CP, Bargen JA:** "Clubbed fingers" and ulcerative colitis. American Journal of Digestive Diseases 7:17, 1940

42. **Bennett I, Hunter D, Vaughan JM:** Idiopathic steatorrhoea (Gee's disease): Nutritional disturbance associated with tetany, osteomalatia, and anaemia. Q J Med 1:603, 1932

43. **Preble RB:** Gastrectasis with tetany and the so-called pulmonary hypertrophic osteoarthritis of Marie. Medicine 4:1, 1898

44. **Camp LJD, Scanlon RL:** Chronic idiopathic hypertrophic osteoarthropathy. Radiology 50:581, 1948

45. **Rynearson EH, Sacasa CF:** Hypertrophic pulmonary osteoarthropathy (acropachy) afflicting a patient who had postoperative myxedema and progressive exophthalmos. Mayo Clin Proc 16:353, 1941

46. **Smith T:** A case of aneurysm of the right axillary artery: Ligature of the subclavian; pyemia. Death on the twenty-second day. With remarks on clubbing of the fingers and toes. London, Transactions of the Pathology Society 23:74, 78, 1872

47. **Baur J:** De l'hippocratisme dans les affections cardiovasculaires. Revue de Médecine 30:993, 1910

48. **Poland A:** Statistics of subclavian aneurysm. Guy Hospital Report 15:47, 1870

49. **Campbell D:** The Hippocratic fingers. Br Med J 1:145, 1924

50. **Charr R, Swenson PC:** Clubbed fingers. Am J Roentgenology and Radium Therapy 55:325, 1946

51. **Parkes Weber P:** The histology of the new bone-formation in a case of pulmonary hypertrophic osteoarthropathy. Proc R Soc Med 2:187, 1908

52. **Crump C:** Histologie der allgemeinen Osteophytose (osteoarthropathie hypertrophiante pneumique). Virchows Arch [Pathol Anat] 271:467, 1929

53. **Thorburn W, Westamacott FH:** The pathology of hypertrophic pulmonary osteoarthropathy. London, Transactions of the Pathology Society 47:177, 1896

54. **Mendlowitz.** Clubbing and hypertrophic osteoarthropathy. Medicine 21:269, 1942

55. **Charr R, Swenson PC:** Am J Roentgenology and Radium Therapy 55:325, 1946

56. **Mendlowitz M:** Measurements of blood flow and blood pressure in clubbed fingers. J Clin Invest 20:113, 1941

57. **Fried BM:** Chronic pulmonary osteoarthropathy: Dyspituitarism as a probable cause. Arch Intern Med 72:565, 1943

58. **Bryan L:** Secondary hypertrophic osteoarthropathy following metastatic sarcoma of the lung. California and Western Medicine 23:449, 1925

59. **Pritchard E:** Familial clubbing of fingers and toes. Br Med J 1:752, 1938

60. **Compere EL, Adams WE, Compere CL:** Possible etiologic factors in the production of pulmonary osteoarthropathy. Proc Soc Exp Biol Med 28:1083, 1931

61. **van Hazel W:** Joint manifestations associated with intrathoracic tumors. J Thorac Surg 9:495, 1940

62. **Mendlowitz M, Leslie A:** The experimental simulation in the dog of the cyanosis in hypertrophic osteoarthropathy associated with congenital heart disease. Am Heart J 24:141, 1942

63. **Mauer EF:** Etiology of clubbed fingers. Am Heart J 34:852, 1947

64. **Vogl A, Blumenfeld S, Gutner LB:** Diagnostic signifi-

cance of pulmonary hypertrophic osteoarthropathy. Am J Med 18:51, 1955

65. **Berg R Jr:** Arthralgia as a first symptom of pulmonary lesions. Diseases of the Chest 16:483, 1949

66. **Deutschberger O, Maglione AA, Gill JJ:** An unusual case of intrathoracic fibroma associated with pulmonary hypertrophic osteoarthropathy. Am J Roentgenology and Radium Therapy 59:738, 1953

67. **Fischl JR:** Severe hypertrophic pulmonary osteoarthropathy: Report of a case due to carcinoma of the lung with operation and recovery. Am J Roentgenology and Radium Therapy 64:42, 1950

68. **Gall EA, Bennett GA, Bauer W:** Generalized hypertrophic osteoarthropathy. Am J Pathol 27:349, 1951

69. **Holmes HH, Bauman E, Ragan C:** Symptomatic arthritis due to hypertrophic osteoarthropathy in pulmonary neoplastic disease. Ann Rheum Dis 9:169, 1950

70. **Pattison JD, Beck E, Miller WB:** Hypertrophic osteoarthropathy in carcinoma of the lung. JAMA 146:783, 1951

71. **Robinson WD et al:** Rheumatism and arthritis: Review of American and English literature of recent years, part II. Ann Intern Med 39:498, 1953

72. **Shapiro L:** Ossifying periostitis of Bamberger–Marie. Bull Hosp Joint Dis 2:77, 1941

73. **Angel JH:** Pachydermo-periostosis (idiopathic osteoarthropathy). Br Med J 2:789, 1957

74. **Buchman D, Hrowat EA:** Idiopathic clubbing and hypertrophic osteoarthropathy. Arch Intern Med 97:355, 1956

75. **Gottlieb C, Sharlin HS, Feld H:** Hypertrophic pulmonary osteoarthropathy. J Pediatr 30:462, 1947

76. **Flavell G:** Reversal of pulmonary hypertrophic osteoarthropathy by vagotomy. Lancet 1:260, 1956

77. **Shapiro M:** Hypertrophic osteoarthropathy. AMA Arch Intern Med 98:700, 1956

78. **Skorneck AB, Ginsburg LB:** Pulmonary hypertrophic osteoarthropathy (periostitis): Its absence in pulmonary tuberculosis. N Engl J Med 258:1079, 1958

79. **Bigler FC:** The morphology of clubbing. Am J Pathol 34:237, 1958

80. **Wilkins RW, Doupe J, Newman HW:** The rate of blood flow in normal fingers. Clin Sci 3:403, 1938

81. **Grant RT, Bland EF:** Observations on arteriovenous anastomosis in human skin and in the bird's foot with special reference to reaction to cold. Heart 15:385, 1931

82. **Popoff NW:** Digital vascular system, with reference to the state of glomus in inflammation, arteriosclerotic gangrene, diabetic gangrene, thrombo-angiitis and supernumerary digits in man. Arch Path 18:295, 1934

83. **Ribot S:** Unilateral clubbing following traumatic obstruction of the axillary vein. AMA Arch Intern Med 98:482, 1956

84. **Hall GH:** The cause of digital clubbing. Lancet 1:750, 1959

85. **Shorr E:** Intermediary and biological activities of ferritin. Harvey Lect 50:112, 1954

86. **Crismon JM:** Rutin and other flavonoids as potentiators of terminal vascular responses to epinephrine and as antagonists of vasodepressor materials. Am J Physiol 164:391, 1951

87. **Williams J:** The etiology of digital clubbing. Am Heart J 63:139, 1962

88. **Barnes CG, Fatti L, Pryce DM:** Arteriovenous aneurysm of the lung. Thorax 3:148, 1948

89. **Trever RW:** Hypertrophic osteoarthropathy in association with congenital cyanotic heart disease. Ann Intern Med 48:660, 1958

90. **Cudkowicz L, Wraith DG:** A method of study of the pulmonary circulation of finger clubbing. Thorax 12:313, 1957

91. **Cudkowicz L, Armstrong JB:** Finger clubbing and changes in the bronchial circulation. Br J Tuberculosis and Diseases of the Chest 47:227, 1953

92. **Trivedi SA:** Neurilemmoma of the diaphragm causing severe hypertrophic pulmonary osteoarthropathy. Br J Tuberculosis and Diseases of the Chest 52:214, 1958

93. **Silverman ME, Hurst JW:** The hand and the heart. Am J Cardiol 21:116, 1968

94. **Berry TJ:** The Hand as a Mirror of Systemic Disease, p 104. Philadelphia, FA Davis, 1963

95. **Hollis WC:** Hypertrophic osteoarthropathy secondary to upper gastrointestinal-tract neoplasm. Ann Intern Med 66:125, 1967

96. **Holling HE, Danielson GK, Hamilton RW et al:** Hypertrophic pulmonary osteoarthropathy. J Thorac Cardiovasc Surg 46:310, 1963

97. **Gerbode F, Birnstingl M, Braimbridge M:** Experimental hypertrophic osteoarthropathy. Surgery 60:1030, 1966

98. **Levine H:** The yellow rounded digit. N Engl J Med 279:660, 1968

99. **Rodman PR:** Primer on rheumatic diseases. JAMA 224:785, 1973

100. **Nathanson L, Hall TC:** Paraneoplastic syndromes lung tumors: How they produce their syndromes. Ann NY Acad Sci 230:367, 1974

101. **Camiel MR, Benninghoff DL, Alexander LL:** Gynecomastia associated with lung cancer. Diseases of the Chest 52:445, 1967

102. **Melvin KEW:** Esophageal polyp with hypertrophic osteoarthropathy. Proc R Soc Med 1:576, 1965

103. **Howell DS:** Hypertrophic osteoarthropathy. In McCarty DJ (ed): Arthritis and Allied Conditions: A Textbook of Rheumatology, 9th ed, p. 977. Philadelphia, Lea & Febiger, 1979

104. **Epstein O, Ajdukifwicz AB, Dick R et al:** Hypertrophic hepatic osteoarthropathy. Am J Med 67:88, 1979

105. **Touraine A, Solente G, Golé L:** Un syndrome osteodermopathique: La pachydermie policaturée avec pachyperiostose des extremites. Presse Méd 43:1820, 1935

106. **Greenfield GB, Schorsch HA, Shkolnik A:** The various roentgen appearances of pulmonary hypertrophic osteoarthropathy. Am J Roentgenology, Radium Therapy and Nuclear Medicine 101:927, 1967

107. **Calabra JI:** Cancer and arthritis. Arthritis Rheum 10:553, 1967

108. **Freeman MH, Tonkin AK:** Manifestations of hypertrophic pulmonary osteoarthropathy in patients with carcinoma of the lung: Demonstration by ^{99m}Tc-pyrophosphate bone scans. Radiology 120:363, 1976

109. **Marshall R:** Observations of the pathology of clubbed fingers with special reference to mast cells. Am Rev Respir Dis 13:395, 1976

110. **Schumacker HR:** Articular manifestations of hypertrophic pulmonary osteoarthropathy in bronchogenic carcinoma. Arthritis Rheum 19:629, 1976

111. **Vidal AF, Altman RJ, Pardo V et al:** Structural and immunologic changes of synovium of hypertrophic osteoarthropathy (HPO). Arthritis Rheum 20:139, 1977

15

Arterial Hypertension Jay M. Sullivan

**The Circulatory Tree and the Generation
of Blood Pressure**
Hemodynamics of Human Hypertension
Consequences of Elevated Blood Pressure
Rationale for Treatment
Labile or Borderline Versus Fixed Hypertension
Systolic Versus Diastolic Hypertension
Therapeutic Goal
Evaluation of the Patient With Hypertension
  History and Physical Examination
    Examination of the Cardiovascular System
    Retinal Examination
  Laboratory Evaluation
    Cardiovascular Evaluation
    Renal Evaluation
Essential Versus Secondary Hypertension
  Oral Contraceptive Hypertension
  Renal Hypertension
    Renal Parenchymal Disease
    Renovascular Hypertension
  Adrenal Hypertension

Pheochromocytoma
Aldosteronism
Cushing's Syndrome
Adrenal Cortical Enzyme Deficiencies
Licorice Ingestion
Hyperparathyroidism
Coarctation of the Aorta
Treatment of Hypertension
Changes in Lifestyle
  Stress
  Exercise
  Obesity
  Tobacco
  Alcohol
  Salt
Pharmacologic Measures
**Therapeutic Implications of the Renin–Angiotensin
  System**
Hypertensive Emergencies
  Pathophysiology
  Differential Diagnosis
  Principles of Therapy

THE CIRCULATORY TREE
AND THE GENERATION OF BLOOD PRESSURE

Human beings face the problem of a multicellular organism trying to maintain life in a hostile environment. Unicellular organisms such as bacteria absorb nutrients from the surrounding environment and excrete waste products by simple diffusion across the cell membrane. Multicellular organisms must solve the problem of maintaining a suitable internal environment for cellular function, and they must transport nutrients over great distances to supply all cells and transport waste products over equally great distances to prevent accumulation of toxic levels. The way in which most animals have solved this problem has been through the evolution of a circulatory system that allows absorption of oxygen from the atmosphere and food products from the gut and arranges distribution of these compounds to cells throughout the body and transports water, carbon dioxide, and other waste products from the cells to lung, kidney, and skin for excretion. This function is served by the circulation of blood throughout the

261

body under the driving force of pressure generated by the heart.

In considering the problems of arterial hypertension, one should review the basic components of the circulatory system: the ventricle, a pressure generating pump; the aorta and other large elastic and muscular arteries, which serve as conduits; the resistance arterioles, which regulate flow of blood out of the arteries; the capillaries, which allow diffusion of materials into and out of cells; and the venules, veins, and atria, which serve as capacitance vessels, that is, chambers capable of storing a wide range of blood volumes without major changes in pressure.[1] The circulatory system is capable of intrinsic regulation due to the physical properties of its components and the autoregulation in each of the tissues it serves, and is under the overall control of the autonomic nervous system, which regulates function in response to changing physiologic circumstances (Fig. 15-1).

The hemodynamic expression of Ohm's law helps one to understand how the circulation is controlled. Ohm stated that electrical voltage equaled the product of current (amperage) and resistance (ohms). Poiseuille's equation for flow of homogeneous fluids states:

$$flow = \frac{(pressure\ gradient)(vessel\ radius)^4}{(vessel\ length)(viscosity)}\left(\frac{\pi}{8}\right)$$

Since vessel length and blood viscosity usually do not vary greatly in a given person, this equation can be simplified to state:

$$flow = \frac{(pressure)}{(resistance)},\ or$$

$$resistance = \frac{(arterial\ pressure)}{(cardiac\ output)}$$

Resistance is an approximation of the vasomotor tone of the vascular smooth muscle fibers in the resistance arterioles. The arteriole is influenced by both remote and local factors.[2] Inpulses traveling through the vasoconstrictor fibers of the sympathetic nervous system serve to increase resistance, while fibers in the parasympathetic nervous system have a weak vasodilator effect. The circulation also carries vasoactive compounds such as catecholamines, angiotensin II, vasopressin, serotonin, histamine, bradykinin, and the prostaglandins, which act directly to alter vasomotor tone.

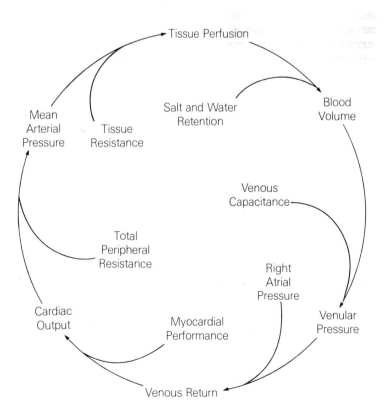

Fig. 15-1. Regulation of the circulation—interplay of factors to maintain arterial pressure and tissue perfusion.

A number of local factors have important effects on vascular smooth muscle. In metabolically active tissues, the release of adenosine, hydrogen, and potassium ion and the consumption of oxygen are associated with vasodilatation as the tissue autoregulates local blood flow. Vascular smooth muscle cells are myogenically active and display slow, rhythmic contraction due to spontaneous depolarization. The stretching effect of arterial blood pressure also stimulates contraction of vascular smooth muscles, the so-called Bayliss effect.[3] Finally, accumulation of sodium ion in vascular smooth muscle increases sensitivity to circulating angiotensin II and catecholamines[4] (Fig. 15-2).

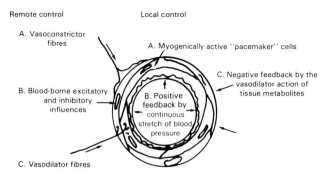

Fig. 15-2. Regulation of peripheral vascular resistance by remote and local factors. (Reproduced from Folkow B, Neil E: Circulation. New York, Oxford Press, 1971)

HEMODYNAMICS OF HUMAN HYPERTENSION

Several studies have shown that patients with mild to moderate fixed essential hypertension have a normal cardiac output.[5] Thus, the increase in blood pressure is accompanied by an increase in total peripheral resistance, the hemodynamic hallmark of established human essential hypertension.

Among the patients with the mildest hypertension are those who transiently show elevation of blood pressure to levels above 140/90 mm Hg but whose blood pressure is normal the rest of the time. This has been designated variously as labile or borderline hypertension. Several laboratories have studied the hemodynamic status of this group of hypertensive patients and have found that they differ from those with mild to moderate fixed essential hypertension.

The first studies in this area were reported by Widimsky and colleagues, who studied young patients and found that as a group, they had an elevated cardiac output at rest, a calculated total peripheral resistance that fell within the normal range, and an elevated blood pressure secondary to the increase in cardiac output.[6] Eich and his co-workers studied an older group of patients with labile hypertension and also found an elevated cardiac output with vascular resistance within the normal range.[7] Several other laboratories have confirmed the finding of an elevated cardiac output in this group and have also noted that these persons tend to have a higher left ventricular systolic ejection rate and a faster heart rate, leading several researchers to propose that a disorder of the autonomic nervous system might be involved in genesis of labile or borderline hypertension. Julius and his co-workers have studied this group of patients extensively.[8] One of their earlier findings was that a spectrum of hemodynamic changes was present in persons with labile hypertension, ranging from those with a very high cardiac output to those whose cardiac output was relatively reduced. It is now widely believed that labile or borderline hypertension is the initial phase of a disease process that eventually leads to sustained elevation of blood pressure and vascular resistance.

A number of studies have been carried out to find a reason for the elevation in cardiac output. Ulrych and coworkers found that those with labile hypertension did not have an increase in intravascular volume.[9] However, intravascular volume appeared to be redistributed toward the central circulation. Thus, an increased amount of blood was present in the cardiopulmonary circulation, increasing return to the right heart and stimulating an increase in cardiac output by the Starling mechanism. As the hypertensive process progressed and blood pressure inexorably became more and more elevated, the phenomenon of pressure diuresis was observed, resulting in a decrease in intravascular volume.

Another explanation for the increased cardiac output could be enhanced activity of the autonomic nervous system. The evidence in favor of this postulate is the fact that these persons have an increased heart rate and an increased left ventricular ejection rate. Julius and colleagues studied the effect of beta-adrenergic blockade and parasympathetic inhibition in young patients with hypertension secondary to an elevated cardiac output.[10] They found that this dual blockade resulted in a return of cardiac output to normal levels. They also studied the effect of various interventions such as sitting, mild exercise, and infusion of dextran upon the hemodynamic status of persons with borderline hypertension; they found that peripheral vascular resistance during any hemodynamic intervention was higher in the labile hypertensives than in the normotensive persons. Similarly, Sannerstedt and his coworkers have studied the degree to which cardiac output and vascular resistance change with exercise in patients with labile hypertension in comparison with normals, and have found that the slope of the line

relating output to resistance is shifted, indicating that peripheral vascular resistance is actually inappropriately elevated in persons with mild labile hypertension.[11]

Takeshita and Mark have studied the effect of stimuli causing maximum reactive hyperemia on forearm blood flow and resistance in normal subjects and subjects with borderline hypertension and have also demonstrated that forearm vascular resistance fails to fall as greatly during maximum reactive hyperemia in labile hypertensives.[12] It has also been observed that these patients have altered diastolic properties of the left ventricle and attenuation of the microvasculature.[13,14]

Thus, patients with labile, borderline hypertension are characterized by an increased cardiac output, a central redistribution of blood volume, and evidence of enhanced activity of the autonomic nervous system leading to an increased heart rate, an increase in left ventricular ejection rate, and an inability to drop forearm vascular resistance adequately in response to circumstances demanding an increase in blood flow.

Essential hypertension is further subdivided into categories of mild, moderate, and severe, depending upon the degree of elevation of diastolic pressure and the extent of involvement of target organs: brain, heart, kidneys, and peripheral vasculature. The hemodynamic pattern found in each of these subdivisions of patients appears to be determined by the interplay of three factors. The first relates to the degree of increase of peripheral vascular resistance and blood pressure. The second involves the degree of cardiac hypertrophy compensating for the elevated blood pressure and later the degree of cardiac impairment of function. The third factor relates to the degree to which pressure diuresis has taken place, resulting in a gradual contraction of intravascular volume and a redistribution of fluid volumes.

Meerson postulated that ventricular function undergoes three stages of change during the development of hypertension.[15] As afterload begins to increase, a stage of enhanced function of the ventricle occurs, during which time this pumping chamber can perform increased work. This can take place because of the hypertrophy that occurs in the left ventricle. During this phase, the heart has been affected by the increased blood pressure, but it can still function normally. Later, hypertrophy no longer suffices to compensate for the increased afterload, and the function of the left ventricle becomes impaired. Initially, this impaired function requires subtle techniques to detect. Later, the function worsens to the degree that the failure is clinically evident.

In early hypertension, there is no evidence of cardiac involvement by ECG or chest radiograph. Hemodynamic studies have shown that cardiac output remains normal. However, since vascular resistance and hence arterial pressure are higher, the ventricular workload is increased. Heart rate tends to be increased while stroke volume and left ventricular ejection rate, a reflection of ventricular contractility, are normal.

If the hypertensive process continues without treatment, the first evidence of cardiac involvement evolves with the appearance of a fourth heart sound on physical examination. The electrocardiogram may reveal evidence of left atrial enlargement. Measurement of systolic time intervals shows that the pre-ejection period is prolonged at this stage. Heart rate remains elevated and cardiac output remains normal although ventricular ejection rate begins to fall. At this point, although the chest radiograph may not reveal cardiac enlargement, careful echocardiographic techniques can demonstrate increased thickness of the left ventricle.

The progression of the hypertensive process leads to the development of cardiac enlargement on chest radiograph and the appearance of voltage and other criteria for left ventricular hypertrophy on the electrocardiogram. At this point, hemodynamic studies reveal further increases in total peripheral resistance and arterial pressure or cardiac output is reduced, even at rest, and systolic ejection rate falls further.

The third factor that has profound influence upon the hemodynamics of severe hypertension concerns the redistribution of fluid volumes. In human hypertension, studies have not revealed a change in either total body water or intracellular fluid volume. Thus, attention has focused on the distribution of extracellular fluid.

Over the years, a number of physiologic studies have pointed out that the kidney increases its output of urine as arterial pressure rises, thus reducing intravascular volume and lowering arterial pressure to the prior level.[16] Guyton and his colleagues have proposed that an impairment of the kidney's ability to respond appropriately to pressure is a major factor in the genesis of essential hypertension.[17] In the hypertensive patient, it is postulated that the kidney is set to begin pressure diuresis at a higher level. Thus, a patient with an expanded intravascular volume, secondary to a sodium load would initially increase cardiac output, thus stimulating total body autoregulation and leading to an increase in total peripheral resistance, blood pressure, and in volume of urinary excretion. This results in restoring cardiac output and intravascular volume to normal at the price of a higher vascular resistance and arterial blood pressure.

Changes in intravascular pressure also serve to redistribute intravascular volume. An increase in intravascular pressure tends to increase the amount of transport of water across the capillary walls into the

interstitial fluid, thus reducing intravascular volume. Similarly, a reduction of pressure is associated with an expansion of intravascular volume as tissue returns from the interstitial spaces.

Tarazi studied fluid volume in several forms of clinical hypertension, demonstrating that as blood pressure rises in the presence of normal renal function, intravascular volume falls on the basis of a decrease in plasma volume.[18] The higher the pressure, the smaller the intravascular volume, unless significant parenchymal renal disease is present, in which case the level of blood pressure elevation is directly proportional to the plasma volume. Thus, persons with severe hypertension presenting for urgent treatment might be anticipated to have a significantly contracted intravascular volume if they are free of renal failure; therefore, the excess of use of diuretic therapy in such persons is inappropriate.

Similarly, antihypertensive therapy based on the use of vasodilating agents might be anticipated to drop intravascular pressure allowing the return of fluid from the interstitium into the vascular tree, leading to a blunting of the antihypertensive effect or "pseudo-tolerance." Thus, careful use of diuretic agents to prevent this from occurring shortly after the initiation of antihypertensive therapy is most appropriate.

Measurements of interstitial fluid volumes in patients with essential hypertension has usually shown that the ratio of plasma volume to interstitial fluid volume is reduced, suggesting transcapillary passage of fluid into the interstitial spaces due to the high intravascular pressure.

Increasing degrees of severity of essential hypertension are marked by gradual increases in peripheral vascular resistance and blood pressure. The phase of increased cardiac output, characteristic of young labile borderline hypertensives, may sometimes persist into the phase of fixed mild essential hypertension. Alternatively, cardiac output may be normal in this group. These patients do not have clinically measurable damage to heart, kidneys, or brain. At times, persons in this group are found to have redistribution of blood volume to the cardiopulmonary circulation. They also have an increased heart rate and evidence of increased myocardial contractility with a normal stroke volume. The fact that the baroreceptor reflex does not act to slow the heart rate in an attempt to lower blood pressure at this point indicates that the baroreceptors have probably been reset. Intravascular volume may be reduced somewhat in these patients.

In patients with moderate essential hypertension, the first evidence of cardiac involvement might be detected. Careful renal function studies might reveal evidence of slight impairment. Total peripheral resistance

and arterial blood pressure is higher, cardiac output is ordinarily normal, and heart rate remains greater than normal. Plasma volume contracts in proportion to the increase in diastolic blood pressure in the absence of significant renal damage. As diastolic pressure exceeds 105 mm Hg, the decrease in intravascular volume becomes more apparent. The stroke volume remains normal or may, at this point, start to fall. Myocardial contractility is within normal range. In this phase, careful echocardiographic studies may reveal increased thickness of the left ventricular wall.

Severe essential hypertension develops as the diastolic pressure rises still farther, and evidence of target organ damage emerges clinically. The chest radiograph and electrocardiogram begin to reveal evidence of cardiac enlargement. Renal function studies reveal the first evidence of a decrease in creatinine clearance and perhaps a minor increase in blood urea nitrogen. The hemodynamic hallmark of this phase of hypertension is a still higher total peripheral resistance. Although left ventricular hypertrophy is present, cardiac output may begin to fall. Heart rate might remain elevated but stroke volume is less. Plasma volume decreases still further, and, as cardiac output and intravascular volume fall, plasma renin activity may rise. As arterial blood pressure is severely increased at this phase and cardiac enlargement has occurred, the left ventricular tension generated during each contraction is greatly increased.

CONSEQUENCES OF ELEVATED BLOOD PRESSURE

Since the vascular tree is designed to circulate fluids under pressure, why does elevated pressure ever cause a problem? The tough elastic aorta can withstand a pressure of around 500 mm Hg before rupture. Human beings cannot tolerate pressure this high. In order to evolve a rationale for treating patients with blood pressure elevation, one must examine the effects of hypertension on the cardiovascular system.

Since the development (around 1900) of methods for the indirect measurement of blood pressure, a vast amount of clinical data about blood pressure has emerged.[19] Within the next several decades, during which time patients were followed without effective antihypertensive therapy, it became apparent that severely elevated blood pressure was associated with an unfavorable prognosis. Patients with diastolic pressures of 130 and above tended to do poorly when the elevated pressure was associated with evidence of significant target organ damage, that is, papilledema, retinal hemorrhages or exudates, congestive heart failure,

and impaired renal function. The most frequently seen symptoms in these patients were visual impairment, acute headache, gross hematuria, dyspnea, edema, nausea, vomiting, epigastric pain, and malaise.[20] In one series of 105 cases, it was noted that most patients died within 4 months, and that very few patients survived longer than 16 months.[21]

The most frequently encountered underlying cause of malignant hypertension in these patients was either "essential" or parenchymal renal disease. In a series of 124 cases studied postmortem, chronic pyelonephritis was found in 21%, and chronic glomerulonephritis in 15%.[22]

With the development of effective treatment, it became apparent that prognosis was improved by the use of antihypertensive agents. The results of several studies suggested that antihypertensive therapy lengthened the half-time of survival of patients with malignant hypertension from approximately 6 months to about 2½ years.

Those patients with prior renal damage did not do as well as other patients when antihypertensive therapy was initiated because of the relentless progression of underlying renal disease.[23] The prognosis of this group has been changed by the availability of chronic hemodialysis and renal transplantation that allow the physician to support renal function while lowering blood pressure, thus preventing acute vascular complications.[24]

Hodge and Smirk noted that treated hypertensive patients ultimately died of different causes.[25] Prior to the era of antihypertensive therapy, 32% of hypertensive patients died with cerebral vascular accidents, 22% from congestive heart failure, 21% from coronary artery disease, 1.4% from uremia, and 24% from other causes. After the development of antihypertensive therapy, 42% of patients died from coronary disease, 23% from cerebral vascular accidents, 9.5% from uremia, 6% from congestive heart failure, and 20% from other causes.

Thus, although partial control of severe hypertension improved prognosis, those patients who still had some degree of blood pressure elevation continued to develop target organ damage. This called for further study of the adverse effects of lesser degrees of blood pressure elevation. The insurance companies were among the first to notice that minor elevation of blood pressure affected prognosis adversely. In 1959, the Build and Blood Pressure Study of the United States Society of Actuaries pointed out that blood pressure and longevity were inversely related, starting at levels of around 90/60 mm Hg.[26] Subsequent studies have clarified the details of this observation.

The Framingham study is one of the largest of these projects to study relationship of blood pressure and mortality.[27] In 1954, the residents of the town of Framingham, Massachusetts, were invited to participate in a long-term study of cardiovascular morbidity and mortality. This study was entirely observational, and no therapeutic interventions of any kind were initiated deliberately. The participants underwent a short physical examination and laboratory evaluation followed by re-evaluation at 2-year intervals. Of the 5127 men and women between 30 and 60 years of age who entered the study, 18% of the men and 16% of the women had systolic blood pressures greater than 160 or diastolic pressures greater than 95 mm Hg. Forty-one per cent of the men had blood pressure elevations above 140 mm Hg systolic and 90 mm Hg diastolic, while 48% of the women were in this range. For patients with moderate elevation of blood pressure, the risk of developing congestive heart failure was found to be six times greater than for subjects with a blood pressure less than 140/90. The risk of developing a stroke was three to five times greater and the risk of having a fatal heart attack was two to three times greater. The higher the blood pressure was, the shorter the life expectancy. The risk of developing cardiovascular disease was incremental, increasing with the level of blood pressure. These observations applied to men as well as women, were independent of age at the time of initial examination (at least between the ages of 30 and 62), and applied even when other risk factors such as gout, abnormal lipids, obesity, diabetes, and electrocardiographic abnormalities, were excluded. The risk included several forms of cardiovascular disease: atherothrombotic brain infarction, coronary heart disease, congestive heart failure, and intermittent claudication, and it applied to both hemorrhagic and nonhemorrhagic stroke. Cerebral vascular accidents were a greater cause of death and disability among women than among men with hypertension.[28]

Thus, the damage associated with blood pressure elevation is quite clear. In malignant hypertension, with very high pressures, retinopathy, and renal failure, death usually occurs from uremia and cerebral hemorrhage, with male and female patients sharing the risk equally. With moderate hypertension, morbidity, and mortality from coronary heart disease, hemorrhagic and thrombotic cerebrovascular accidents constitute a major risk. Women appear to tolerate mild hypertension better than men, perhaps because women have less coronary disease, before menopause, than men.

In 1962, data collected by the National Health Examination Survey of the Public Health Service on a random sample of the adult United States population between the ages of 18 and 79 years showed that 16%

of white adults and 30% of black adults had diastolic blood pressures higher than 90 mm Hg.[29] Using a diastolic pressure of 95 mm Hg as a cutoff point shows 9% of white adults and 22% of black adults above this level. This survey revealed that the prevalence of hypertension rose steadily with age. The frequency of hypertension was roughly two times higher in blacks than in whites. When hypertension was found in blacks, blood pressure levels tended to be higher than in whites. As a consequence, hypertensive heart disease was present from three to nine times more frequently in various subgroups of the black population than in comparable white subgroups.[30]

There is evidence suggesting that elevation of blood pressure itself causes vascular complications. In experimental animals, induced vasoconstriction is followed by sclerotic changes within the arterioles and necrosis of surrounding tissues.[31] In man, three conditions suggest that atherosclerotic changes are related to the level of blood pressure. In patients with coarctation of the aorta, atherosclerotic lesions are found in the high pressure area of the aorta but not in the low pressure area beyond the coarctation.[32] Patients with congenital heart disease and with longstanding pulmonary hypertension develop atherosclerotic lesions in the pulmonary arterial tree.[33] In patients with renal artery stenosis and associated hypertension, nephrosclerotic changes develop in the "healthy kidney," whereas the vascular tree distal to the stenosis in the ischemic kidney is usually protected from the development of nephrosclerosis.[34] Thus, hypertension is associated with serious cardiovascular morbidity and mortality. The complications are directly related to the level of the high blood pressure, but the risk imposed by a given level of arterial pressure is increased by the concomitant presence of additional risk factors—smoking, hypercholesterolemia, diabetes mellitus, and a family history of cardiovascular disease.

RATIONALE FOR TREATMENT

The goal of treating a patient with hypertension is to prevent the premature development of cardiovascular disease. The complications related to high blood pressure are further progression of hypertension, renal failure, hemorrhagic stroke, congestive heart failure, and dissecting aneurysm. Other complications are related to accelerated atherosclerosis associated with hypertension: acute myocardial infarction, atherothrombotic cerebral infarction, and intermittent claudication. Even patients with minimal blood pressure elevation are subject to these complications.

In the 1950s, it was found that antihypertensive medications prevented the development of necrotic and sclerotic changes in the arterioles of animals with experimental hypertension.[35] In clinical use, it became apparent that patients with accelerated or malignant hypertension could benefit from therapy.[36,37] Improved prognosis was limited by the presence of renal damage or underlying renal parenchymal disease. Patients with impaired renal function, that is, endogenous creatinine clearance less than 45 ml per minute, did not do as well with treatment. Only 4 out of 15 patients with less than this clearance were alive 1 year after the initiation of therapy, whereas 8 of 11 patients with more than this clearance were alive 1 year after beginning therapy.[38]

Thus, soon after effective antihypertensive drugs became available, it was apparent that patients with accelerated or malignant hypertension benefited from treatment, and since that time there has been little argument about treating these patients. It was not known whether patients with diastolic blood pressures between 90 and 129 mm Hg had anything to gain from the expense and inconvenience of chronic antihypertensive therapy. In 1964, Hamilton, Thompson, and Wisniewski reported that antihypertensive therapy prevented hypertensive complications in 10 men while complications in 8 of 12 untreated men followed concurrently.[39] In 1966, Wolff and Lindeman reported the results of a controlled 2-year study of 87 patients, which also showed only 33% as many cardiovascular complications in the treated group as in the group receiving placebo tablets.[40]

The next major study of this problem was the Veterans Administration Cooperative Study of Antihypertensive Agents.[41,42] In this project, male veterans were hospitalized for an evaluation, which excluded those with diastolic blood pressure above 129 mm Hg, those with secondary hypertension, and those whose blood pressure dropped beneath 90 mm Hg without therapy. Patients who already had evidence of cardiovascular complications were included in the trial. The patients were followed for 2 to 4 months, during which time they were placed on a placebo. During this period, the patients who were not taking their medications were eliminated, as well as those whose diastolic blood pressures accelerated to levels above 129 mm Hg. This left a cadre of patients, well characterized clinically, who could be relied upon to remain in the study long enough to yield meaningful information. At this point the patients were blindly divided into two random groups. One group received placebo tablets and the other group received hydrochlorothiazide 50 mg b.i.d., reserpine 0.1 mg b.i.d., and hydralazine 25 mg–50 mg t.i.d.

It soon became apparent that the patients who entered the study with the highest blood pressures were

developing complications rapidly. As a result, the subgroup of 143 patients who entered the study with diastolic blood pressures between 115 and 129 mm Hg were removed from the study after a period of about 20 months. This subgroup contained 70 patients in the control group and 73 in the treated group, roughly half of whom were white and half of whom were black. Analysis of events in the untreated group showed that 7 patients had developed grade 3 to 4 retinopathy; 3, accelerated hypertension; 3, renal failure; 3, dissecting aneurysm; 2, retinopathy with congestive heart failure; 2, strokes; 1, sudden death; 2, myocardial infarction; 2, congestive heart failure; and 2, minor strokes. In contrast, one patient in the treated group developed a drug reaction and one patient suffered a minor stroke. The difference between the two groups was highly significant, and it was proved that antihypertensive therapy benefited male patients with a diastolic blood pressure between 115 mm and 129 mm Hg.

This left a subgroup of 380 patients who had entered the study with average, resting diastolic pressures between 90 mm and 114 mm Hg on the fourth through sixth days of initial hospitalization. These patients were followed as long as 5 years, with an average follow-up of 3.3 years. Placebo tablets were given to 194 patients, while 186 received active therapy. There were 35 terminating morbid events in the control group, opposed to 9 in the treated group; 21 nonterminating cardiovascular events in the control group, opposed to 13 in the treated group; and 20 instances of accelerated hypertension in the control group opposed to none in the treated group. The fatalities consisted of 7 strokes in the control group, 3 myocardial infarctions in the control group, and 2 in the treated group; 8 instances of sudden death in the control group, opposed to 4 in the treated group, and 1 instance of ruptured arteriosclerotic aneurysm in the treated group. There were 12 strokes in the control group and only 1 in the treated group; 11 cases of coronary heart disease in the control group with 6 in the treated group; 5 cases of congestive failure in the control group and none in the treated group; 4 cases of accelerated hypertension in the control group and none in the treated group; and one instance of renal damage in the control group with none in the treated group.

Analyzing the data from the subgroup of patients with diastolic blood pressure between 90 mm and 114 mm Hg, it was found that the risk of developing a morbid cardiovascular event during a 5-year period was reduced from 55% in the group receiving a placebo to only 18% in the group on active treatment.[43] The difference between the treated and untreated group was statistically significant for patients with initial diastolic blood pressures of 105 mm Hg or more. For those pa-

tients who entered the trial with lower pressures, the risk of developing a cardiovascular event was not as great and the benefit from antihypertensive therapy was not as marked, although the patients in this subgroup also appeared to benefit from treatment. In no instance did it appear that antihypertensive therapy increased morbidity or mortality; indeed, this study suggests that long-term antihypertensive therapy is reasonably benign.

The Veterans Administration study established that treatment of male patients with diastolic blood pressure above 105 mm Hg conveys significant benefit to the patient. Women were not studied. Thus, there was no proof that they would benefit equally from therapy. Physicians remained cautious about applying the results of this trial for several reasons. First, the starting blood pressures were defined as the average of the resting diastolic pressures from the fourth through sixth days of hospitalization. When placed in the hospital, patients with significant levels of diastolic hypertension often become normotensive by the fourth day. Thus, those patients participating in the VA study probably had more sustained hypertension. Second, although patients with lesser degrees of blood pressure elevation are at risk of developing the cardiovascular damage, they have less risk than patients with higher levels of blood pressure. The VA study showed that patients with levels of diastolic blood pressure between 90 mm and 104 mm Hg benefited less from antihypertensive therapy than their counterparts with higher blood pressures. Thus, when treating patients with mild elevations of blood pressure, it was advisable to weigh the limited benefit of therapy against the greater inconvenience, greater expense, and greater risk of side-effects from antihypertensive therapy. Therefore, risk–benefit ratio in this group is not as favorable as it is in those with a persistent diastolic blood pressure above 105 mm Hg.

Considering the data from the Build and Blood Pressure Study, from the Framingham study, from the VA study, and from other sources, many authorities recommended that patients with sustained diastolic blood pressures of 90 mm to 104 mm Hg receive individualized treatment. A very important factor in reaching a decision to treat these patients was the presence or absence of additional cardiovascular risk factors. Since these factors appear to be cumulative, a patient with a slight risk imposed by a minor elevation of diastolic pressures has a much greater chance of developing cardiovascular disease if he also smokes, has diabetes mellitus, has elevated blood lipid levels, or has a family history of premature cardiovascular disease. In treating patients with additional risk factors, an attempt should be made to reduce as many risk factors as pos-

sible. The Inter-Society Commission for Heart Disease Resources recommends the approach shown in Figure 15-3.[44]

The results of the Veterans Administration study have been extended in an important way by the recent findings of the Hypertension Detection and Follow-up Program (HDFP), a 5-year, 14 center study involving 10,900 patients, which provided the first convincing evidence that mortality in patients with a diastolic blood pressure of 90 mm to 104 mm Hg was reduced by effective antihypertensive therapy.[45]

The participants in HDFP ranged in age from 30 to 69 years of age and included both males and females. Over 70% of the cohort had diastolic blood pressures between 90 mm and 104 mm Hg. The patients were stratified on the basis of age, sex, race, organ involvement, and prior treatment history, and separated randomly into one of two groups. One group received treatment from their usual source of medical care; the other received intensive antihypertensive therapy at special centers in which free medications were given, waiting time was short, extensive patient education measures used, and lost patients retrieved. Stepped-care therapy was used, consisting of thiazide diuretic, with the addition of reserpine, methyldopa, or, less frequently, propranolol, if needed. Hydralazine and then guanethidine were added in sequence if goal blood pressure had not been reached. The therapeutic goal of the centers was to lower diastolic blood pressure to levels beneath 90 mm or by 10 mm Hg, whichever figure was lowest. By the end of five years, goal had been achieved in 64.9% of the center-care patients and in 43.6% of the referred care group. Thus, both groups received antihypertensive treatment. The difference lay in the effectiveness. Although the average starting diastolic blood pressure was about 101 mm Hg, after five years blood pressure had fallen to 84.1 mm Hg in the center-care group, but to only 89.1 mm Hg in the referred-care patients.

Mortality from all causes was 17% lower in the center-care group and 20% lower in patients whose pretreatment diastolic pressure was 90 mm–104 mm Hg. The difference was highly significant ($p < 0.01$). Similarly, effective treatment lowered deaths from cerebrovascular disease by 45%, and death from acute myocardial infarction by 46%. Overall, there was a 15% reduction in the death rate from ischemic heart disease in the center-care group.

Similarly, an Australian trial of therapy in 3427 patients with mild hypertension has demonstrated a beneficial effect of treatment of patients whose diastolic blood pressure ranged between 95 mm and 110 mm Hg.[46] In this trial, mortality from cardiovascular disease was reduced by two-thirds over a 4-year-period.

Thus, there is now strong evidence to support the lowering of blood pressure in asymptomatic persons with diastolic blood pressure between 90 mm and 104 mm Hg, even if they are free of end-organ damage and are relatively old (some of the participants in HDFP were 74 at its conclusion). For those with deceptively "mild" hypertension, treatment might appropriately

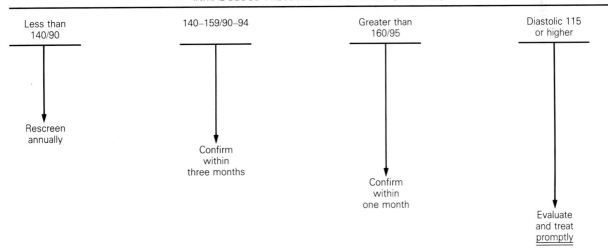

INITIAL BLOOD PRESSURE MEASUREMENT (ALL AGES)

Less than 140/90	140–159/90–94	Greater than 160/95	Diastolic 115 or higher
Rescreen annually	Confirm within three months	Confirm within one month	Evaluate and treat promptly

Fig. 15-3. Criteria for rescreening and referral of patients with elevated blood pressure. (Adapted from Report of Inter-Society Commission for Heart Disease Resources: Circulation 64:1079A–1089A, 1981)

begin with weight reduction, salt restriction, and regular exercise; pharmacologic agents may be added when these measures are unsuccessful.

LABILE OR BORDERLINE VERSUS FIXED HYPERTENSION

The criteria for entry into the Veterans Administration study and the Hypertension Detection and Follow-up Program required sustained diastolic hypertension. As a result, we have no firm data that proves that therapy of labile or borderline hypertension ultimately benefits the patient, although we do have information suggesting that labile hypertension places the patient at risk.

The World Health Organization defines labile hypertension as a stage at which blood pressure, determined casually, is found to be above 140 mm Hg (systolic) or 90 mm Hg (diastolic) on at least two occasions during a year of observation. At other times the blood pressure may be within what is arbitrarily considered the normal range.

A diagnosis of labile or borderline hypertension creates problems for the physician. A patient can have transient elevation of blood pressure to levels above 140/90 if he is in pain or discomfort or if he is anxious. It then becomes necessary to determine how often elevation of blood pressure occurs. Weekly determinations over a period of 3 weeks can help to resolve the question. Checking the pressure after rest, and having a nonphysician or family member check the pressure may give information about whether the patient's pressure has returned to normal or whether it is fluctuating around a mildly elevated average. Data from the Society of Actuaries suggests that mildly elevated casual blood pressure is associated with increased risk.[26]

The group with mild elevation of blood pressure had shortened longevity, and was composed of patients with both fixed and labile hypertension. The findings of the Framingham study were also based on casual blood pressure determinations and did not separate persons with mild fixed hypertension from those with mild labile hypertension. However, when the Framingham data were analyzed to assess the impact of lability, it was found that for any given average pressure, the degree of variability of the pressure did not affect the risk of cardiovascular events.[47] Thus, it is the average pressure around which repeated readings vary that determines risk.

Labile or borderline hypertension can follow several courses: some return to normal blood pressure levels; some continue to have labile blood pressure elevations, and others develop fixed hypertension.[48] The discovery of labile hypertension demands that the patient continue to be under medical surveillance so that the shortest possible time will elapse between the possible later development of fixed elevation of blood pressure and the initiation of effective antihypertensive therapy. Some authorities advocate the initiation of antihypertensive therapy for most patients with labile hypertension, since they are likely to develop fixed hypertension and early therapy might avoid years of target organ damage. However, there have been no controlled studies demonstrating that antihypertensive therapy of labile hypertension has any benefit.

Virtually any available antihypertensive agents serve to lower pressure in patients with mild, transient elevation. These patients respond to diuretic therapy. Because hemodynamic studies in these patients show a hyperkinetic circulation, they have been treated successfully with beta-adrenergic receptor blocking agents and can often respond to very low doses, for example, propranolol, 10 mg t.i.d.[49] Before deciding to treat, efforts must be made to evaluate the degree of risk faced by a patient with labile hypertension, that is, the degree, frequency, and duration of pressure elevation. Hypertensive damage is increased by the presence of other risk factors, and attention must be paid to use of cigarettes, family history, blood lipid levels, and diabetes mellitus. When several risk factors are present, therapeutic intervention appears to be reasonable.

SYSTOLIC VERSUS DIASTOLIC HYPERTENSION

Purely systolic hypertension (greater than 160 mm Hg) is often seen in older patients. Ejection of blood from the left ventricle into a rigid aorta causes a wide pulse pressure and an elevated systolic pressure. A few patients with elevated systolic pressure have disorders associated with high cardiac output, such as thyrotoxicosis, anemia, fever, and arteriovenous fistula. Because systolic hypertension is thought to reflect underlying atherosclerosis, systolic hypertension has not been an indication for antihypertensive treatment. However, in the Build and Blood Pressure Study, mortality increased with each increment of systolic pressure at any given level of diastolic pressure and applied to both men and women regardless of age.[26]

Multivariate analysis of the data from Framingham also shows that systolic blood pressure correlates with the risk of coronary heart disease better than diastolic or mean pressure. This observation applied equally to men and women over 45, but diastolic pressure seemed to be the strongest determinant of risk in younger men.[50]

In a study of older patients with isolated systolic hypertension, Colandera and associates found an increased incidence of coronary artery disease, strokes, and overall mortality during an 8-month period of ob-

servation.[51] However, patients with systolic pressure elevation also had diabetes mellitus, so the systolic hypertension might have been a reflection of increased susceptibility to vascular damage or of the presence of atherosclerosis in the elderly. The possibility exists that systolic hypertension, even though caused by atherosclerosis, may still act to further accelerate atherosclerosis, precipitate congestive heart failure, and thus contribute to morbidity and mortality. At present, one can conclude that such patients are at risk and reach decisions regarding antihypertensive therapy on an individual basis. However, when elderly patients are treated, antihypertensive agents should be started at a low dose and increased gradually with careful monitoring.

THERAPEUTIC GOAL

There is no clear dividing line between normal and elevated blood pressure. The lower the blood pressure, the lower the risk of cardiovascular disease. Since all must stand, we require sufficient pressure to maintain cerebral perfusion against gravity. There is no absolute goal in lowering blood pressure but rather one that must be individualized for each patient. Usually, attempts are made to lower blood pressure to levels less than 140/90 mm Hg or to levels approximately 120/80, if this can be accomplished without producing unacceptable side-effects.

When compared with a group treated to an average diastolic pressure of about 90 mm Hg, the results of the HDFP suggest that patients suffer fewer cardiovascular complications when diastolic pressures are lowered to 85 mm Hg or less. Thus, the HDFP has not only changed our indications for administering antihypertensive therapy, it has changed our therapeutic goals.

Reaching an ideal pressure must be weighed against side-effects. Persons can have blood pressure reduced to 140/90 on relatively moderate doses of medications and may be entirely free of side-effects. Yet, when medications are increased in an attempt to lower the pressure further, the patient may be unacceptably sleepy or fatigued, and may find that the medications are interfering with the quality of life. Here, the physician must use his skill to match medication with patient, and his judgment to assess how much risk the remaining minor elevation of blood pressure poses for his patient. If untoward effects occur that cannot be tolerated or avoided by changing antihypertensive agents, a compromise must be made. Data from the VA study suggests that even partial blood pressure control is beneficial.[52]

When arteriosclerosis narrows a blood vessel, flow across the stenosis depends on perfusion pressure. If arterial pressure falls, perfusion of the area distal to the lesion decreases. In the brain, this leads to symptoms of cerebrovascular insufficiency; in the heart, to angina pectoris; in the extremities, to claudication; and in the kidneys, to diminished renal function. In a patient with a history, physical findings, or laboratory tests that suggests the presence of underlying vascular disease, blood pressure must be lowered carefully, while looking for evidence of potentially adverse effects of the reduction. It is somewhat reassuring to note that the hypertensive survivors of strokes, when treated with antihypertensive agents, do not develop an increased rate of recurrence of stroke. In addition, antihypertensive therapy significantly decreases the development of congestive heart failure in such patients.[53]

EVALUATION OF THE PATIENT WITH HYPERTENSION

HISTORY AND PHYSICAL EXAMINATION

In the evaluation of patients with elevated blood pressure, the physician has three major goals. The first is to estimate the severity and rate of progression of the hypertensive process, the second is to assess target organ damage, and the third is to find curable forms of hypertension. A complete history and physical examination are essential steps in reaching these goals.

An attempt must be made to date the onset of hypertension. When was the elevation found? When was the last normal pressure recording? Can records be obtained for confirmation of blood pressure readings? Was the point of muffling or the point of disappearance of Korotkoff sounds used to determine the diastolic pressure? The point of muffling tends to overestimate the true diastolic intra-arterial pressure, while the point of disappearance tends to underestimate the true diastolic pressure and is influenced by arm thickness, length of stethoscope tubing, background noise, and acoustic activity.[54]

It is important to establish whether the patient has had frequent mild labile elevations when under periods of stress that have always returned to normal or whether evidence suggests a clear and relentless rise in blood pressure, which may not be greatly elevated, but has been climbing steadily for years and has now clearly reached a point requiring treatment.

The history should be evaluated for evidence of target organ damage. Ordinarily, moderate levels of blood pressure elevation are asymptomatic until an event occurs that reflects cardiovascular or renal disease. One study has suggested that symptoms of headache and dizziness most often develop after a patient has been

informed of his blood pressure elevation and now has reason to be concerned about hypertension. However, patients with diastolic levels above 130 noted headache and those above 110 noted dizziness before learning of their problem.[55,56]

Symptoms of hypertensive central nervous system damage reflect overlapping pathologic events. One includes the coma, convulsions, and mental obtundation associated with the encephalopathy of severe hypertension. Another reflects destruction of central nervous system tissue either from hemorrhage from a ruptured subarachnoid aneurysm or from a small Charcot-Bouchard aneurysm at the bifurcation of an intracerebral blood vessel. A third includes signs of ischemic damage that follows thrombotic occlusion of atherosclerotic lesions in the cerebral vessels. Finally, widespread atherosclerosis of cerebral vessels, which occurs prematurely in hypertensive patients, is reflected by symptoms such as memory loss and emotional instability.

The symptoms indicating impairment of the cardiovascular system are chest discomfort radiating to the neck, arms, shoulders, back, or upper abdomen related to exertion, meals, cold, or emotional excitement; discomfort at night; dyspnea on exertion; orthopnea, paroxysmal nocturnal dyspnea, ankle edema and palpitations.

Symptoms of renal impairment include loss of appetite, nausea, polyuria, ankle edema, hematuria, flank pain, proteinuria. A history of urinary tract infections is suggested by back pain, fever, urinary frequency, urgency, and dysuria.

Aching in the lower extremities after walking, which disappears with rest, suggests intermittent claudication secondary to atherosclerotic involvement of the vascular supply of the lower extremities.

Inquiry should be made about symptoms suggesting secondary hypertension. Renal parenchymal disease is the most common secondary cause of hypertension; it is suggested by a history of recurrent urinary tract infections or chronic pyelonephritis, or by episodes of edema, hematuria, and proteinuria in childhood, suggesting acute glomerulonephritis. The most common surgically curable form of secondary hypertension is renal vascular disease, which is suspected when the hypertension appears suddenly before the age of 35 or after the age of 55, or if the hypertension was preceded by flank pain or hematuria. Evidence of a source of emboli that might lodge in the renal artery also suggests a renal cause of hypertension and is suggested by a history of rheumatic fever, heart murmurs heard in the past (especially the murmur of mitral stenosis), cardiac arrhythmias, or cardiomyopathy.

To investigate adrenal causes of hypertension, one first looks for symptoms of pheochromocytoma. These chromaffin cell tumors usually release mixtures of epi-

nephrine and norepinephrine, and the symptoms depend on the relative amount of each catecholamine released. Patients who release norepinephrine show signs of intense alpha-adrenergic stimulation, which includes blanching of the skin, sweating, headache, and sometimes reflex slowing of the heart rate. Patients with tumors secreting epinephrine display the signs of beta-adrenergic receptor stimulation and present with flushing, tachycardia, and, at times, hypotension. Patients with pheochromocytoma frequently have postural hypotension. Because an undetected pheochromocytoma can have a fatal outcome, it is essential to keep this diagnostic possibility in mind.

Primary aldosteronism has less specific symptoms. The hallmark is hypokalemia, which is frequently asymptomatic. When symptoms are present, they consist of episodic muscle weakness, polyuria, polydipsia, nocturia, paresthesia, and tetany.

Cushing's syndrome is usually suspected from the physical examination. One should ask about the development of truncal obesity, bone pain, easy bruising, increasing hair growth, and development of a rounder, more florid face.

Patients with coarctation of the aorta are frequently asymptomatic. When the coarctation is severe, the patient may complain of intermittent claudication or he may have headaches because of the elevated blood pressure in the upper part of the body. This diagnosis should be considered in young patients with mild hypertension and a "functional" heart murmur.

Patients with hyperparathyroidism may also develop hypertension.[57] Points in the history that suggest this diagnosis are depression, constipation, peptic ulcer, and renal calculi.

Space-occupying intracerebral lesions can also present with blood pressure elevation. Most often this consists of systolic hypertension with a wide pulse pressure and a slow pulse rate. The examiner should direct appropriate questions about localizing neurologic symptoms to evaluate this possibility.

Patients with acute intermittent porphyria may display hypertension during an acute attack. One must look for a history of episodic hypertension, abdominal cramps, and precipitation by drugs such as the barbiturates.

It is now well established that the use of oral contraceptive agents can cause hypertension and that blood pressure elevation may take as long as 6 months to resolve.[58]

Inquiry should be made concerning the patient's habits relative to factors that complicate hypertension, such as caloric intake, salt intake, caffeine intake, chronic use of vasoconstricting agents for hay fever or asthma, or frequent use of licorice.

Knowledge of the patient's family history is impor-

tant. Although a strict genetic mode of inheritance of hypertension has not been found, blood pressure elevation tends to run in families. Patients often do not know whether their relatives have hypertension and should be questioned for evidence of premature death or vascular disease.

Examination of the Cardiovascular System

It is essential to measure blood pressure in both arms because atherosclerotic lesions or preductal coarctation of the aorta can result in asymmetric pressures. This might cause the physician to make a falsely low estimate of the central blood pressure or miss the fact that atherosclerotic lesions are present. A difference in arm readings of 20 mm strongly indicates obstruction. The next step is examination of the neck. The jugular venous pulse is inspected to determine whether it is elevated or whether the contour is abnormal. The carotid arteries must be examined. First, the neck is inspected visually for abnormal pulsations. Next, the arteries are palpated, and their relative contour assessed. In the hyperkinetic circulation of young patients with labile hypertension, the upstroke is brisk. Older patients who might have atherosclerotic lesions somewhere between the aortic valve and the jaw have a slow upstroke. The presence of carotid or subclavian bruits should be noted. On auscultation of the thorax and lungs, the examiner listens for basilar rales, indicative of congestive heart failure, and for extracardiac bruits, which might point to underlying coarctation of the aorta.

The complexities of cardiac examination will not receive detailed consideration in this chapter. In young hypertensive patients, cardiac examination can reveal vigorous precordial pulsations and a systolic ejection murmur, which together suggest a hyperkinetic circulation.

The examiner also looks for evidence of hypertensive cardiovascular disease. Inspection of the chest wall and palpation of the cardiac apex can disclose a palpable atrial gallop or S_4, a sign that the ventricle has begun to hypertrophy and that its compliance characteristics have changed; this results in the development of an audible sound as the left atrium forcefully ejects blood into the left ventricle.

Cardiac auscultation can reveal S_4 or S_3 gallops, systolic ejection murmurs suggesting calcification of the aortic valve, an apical holosystolic regurgitant murmur suggesting dilatation of the mitral valve anulus with valvular insufficiency, and in severe hypertension, the decrescendo diastolic murmur of aortic insufficiency suggesting dilatation of the aorta and aortic valve ring.

Examination of the cardiovascular system extends to the abdomen, where the presence of systolic bruits indicate underlying atherosclerosis of the aorta and bruits occupying both systole and diastole suggest renal ar-

tery stenosis. Physical examination should include palpation and auscultation of the femoral pulses for evidence of atherosclerosis or coarctation of the aorta. When significant coarctation of the aorta exists, the femoral pulse is diminished, the peak of the pulse is delayed relative to the pulse at the radial artery, and arterial pressure is lower in the legs than in the arms. The popliteal, posterior tibial and dorsalis pedis pulses are examined for evidence of peripheral atherosclerosis.

Neurologic examination should search for focal lesions, either as a cause of the hypertension or as a manifestation of previous intracerebral hemorrhage or infarction.

Retinal Examination

The changes that take place in the optic fundus can be divided into those due to arteriolosclerosis and those due to hypertension. Retinal exudates can result from other disorders, such as diabetes mellitus, emboli, malignancy, arteritis, hematologic malignancies, and primary renal disease.

The central artery of the retina is a muscular artery. After passing through the lamina cribosa of the sclera, the internal elastic lamina of the artery thins and usually disappears by the first bifurcation. The muscularis decreases in thickness as the vessels course away from the optic disk.[58] Thus, most of the vessels visualized are true arterioles, at least those beyond one or two disk diameters from the optic disk. The most characteristic change is vasoconstriction, but structural changes also may take place in the intimal and muscular layers.

Keith and associates described four grades of retinal changes in patients with hypertension—each associated with decreased survival.[59] Patients with grade 1 changes, generalized or segmental arteriolar narrowing, survived reasonably well. Prognosis was worse in grades 2, 3, and 4. Grade 2 changes refer to narrowing at the point at which the retinal vein crosses behind a thickened arteriole. Grade 3 changes also include retinal hemorrhages and exudates, and Grade 4 changes include papilledema.

Scheie has proposed a new classification that takes into account that certain retinal changes are arteriolosclerotic and that some are specifically due to hypertension.[60] In this system of nomenclature, grade 1 arteriolosclerotic changes consist of thickening of the vessel with slight depression of the veins at the arteriolar–venular crossing, while grade 1 hypertensive changes refer to arteriolar narrowing at the terminal branches. Grade 2 arteriolosclerotic changes consist of definite A–V crossing changes and moderate local sclerosis, while Grade 2 hypertensive changes refer to severe arteriolar narrowing with local constrictions. Grade 3 changes of arteriolosclerosis consist of loss of visibility of the vein beneath the arteriole and severe local

sclerosis with segmentation. The equivalent hypertensive changes include striate hemorrhages and soft exudates. Grade 4 arteriolosclerotic changes consist of the grade 1 through grade 3 changes, plus venous obstruction and arteriolar obliteration, while grade 4 hypertensive changes consist of the grade 1 through grade 3 changes, plus papilledema. The major difference between this classification and that of Keith and associates is the designation of A–V nicking as a nonhypertensive change.

Because hypertension is the most common predisposing factor for the development of arteriolosclerosis, the hypertensive patient might be expected to show the changes of both processes. Arteriolosclerosis can also develop in the absence of hypertension or in the presence of diabetes mellitus, old age, or hyperlipidema. In general, arteriolosclerotic changes correlate roughly with the duration of the blood pressure elevation, and the degree of the hypertensive changes corresponds with the severity of hypertension.[61]

Arteriolosclerosis is a diffuse process that involves thickening of the vessel walls.[62] This process begins with the deposition of hyaline material and lipid beneath the endothelium. The muscular layer is involved, and the adventitial layers are eventually involved. These changes are reflected by a wide arteriolar light reflex, a silver or copper-wire appearance, A–V crossing changes, and increased arteriolar tortuosity. Healthy young people can also show tortuous arterioles in the absence of underlying arteriolosclerotic disease. Arteriolovenous nicking begins with a mild depression of the vein, followed by obliteration for short distances on either side of the arteriole, and later by thickening of the vessel distal to the crossing.

The most striking hypertensive change is retinal hemorrhage, which is associated with severe hypertension and characteristically occurs near the optic disk. The lesions are usually flame-shaped because they occur in the nerve fiber layer and extend between the fibers.

Other forms of hemorrhage can occur in hypertension, but can be associated with other disease entities. When the hemorrhage is located in the periphery and is solitary and round in shape, it may be a sign of advanced arteriolosclerosis or of arteriolar or venous occlusion. Patients with anemia or leukemia can develop light-centered hemorrhages that can be flame-shaped. Patients with diabetes mellitus develop capillary aneurysms and may occlude small vessels leading to ischemic areas of hemorrhage. Patients with diabetes, stroke, trauma, leukemia, and normal subjects can develop hemorrhages in the deep layer of the retina. These hemorrhages are usually raised, bright red, and large with sharp borders.

Two types of retinal exudates can be seen on ophthalmoscopic examination. "Hard" exudates have a sharp margin and are thought to represent the residual of hemorrhages in layers deep to the retinal vessels. These exudates often appear after the initiation of antihypertensive therapy and can take as long as a year to resolve.[62]

The other common type of retinal exudate is the "cotton wool" or "soft" exudate, which appears suddenly and rapidly increases in size. With the initiation of antihypertensive treatment, the exudates become coarsely granular, develop small red microaneurysms and gradually disappear. Such exudates are usually located near the optic disk and are believed by some to represent ischemic infarcts.

The appearance of soft exudates with flame hemorrhages suggests that the hypertensive process is accelerating. These retinal changes can heal completely when the blood pressure is lowered, and the exudates often disappear after several days of successful antihypertensive therapy. Although soft exudates are ordinarily associated with severe hypertension, they can also be seen in lupus erythematosus and dermatomyositis, and after occlusion of the central retinal vein. The appearance of soft exudates and striate hemorrhages can also be associated with the development of retinal edema. One manifestation of retinal edema is the star figure that forms around the macula of hypertensive patients and resolves slowly with antihypertensive therapy.

When soft exudates and striate hemorrhages are accompanied by papilledema, malignant hypertension is present and the patient's prognosis is grave because the development of renal failure is imminent. The development of papilledema can be gradual. The patient may develop, in sequence, loss of physiologic cupping of the optic disk, blurring of the nasal margins of the disk, distention of the retinal veins, blurring of the temporal margins and, finally, elevation of the optic disk. With successful antihypertensive therapy, papilledema usually disappears in 2 to 3 months, although some irregularity around the edges of the optic disk may persist for a year. When papilledema appears, brain tumors, cerebral swelling secondary to trauma, intracerebral hemorrhage, pseudotumor cerebri, and lead poisoning should also be considered.

Controversy continues to exist over the role of vasospasm in producing the retinal changes of hypertension. There is agreement that acute forms of hypertension, such as eclampsia or acute glomerulonephritis, are accompanied by severe retinal arteriolar vasoconstriction. With chronic hypertension, it is difficult to distinguish sclerotic changes from acute vasoconstrictive changes if the vessels do not dilate and

constrict during the examination or change acutely in response to therapy. Irregularity of the vessel outline suggests chronic, sclerotic changes.

The development of hemorrhages or exudates signals a serious progression of hypertension. This progression from grade 2 to grade 3 retinal changes demands more aggressive management of the elevated blood pressure, often requiring prompt hospitalization.

LABORATORY EVALUATION

The findings of the HDFP indicate that persons with diastolic blood pressure higher than 90 mm Hg should be detected and treated.[45] Approximately 35 million Americans fit this description. Should they all have a costly work-up before being treated? In the 10,900 participants of the HDFP, the incidence of secondary hypertension was found to be less than 1%. Thus, an extensive laboratory evaluation to detect secondary causes of hypertension would not be cost-effective. Procedures such as the intravenous pyelogram, measurement of plasma or urinary catecholamines or their metabolites, and assay of the renin–angiotensin–aldosterone system should be ordered only when specific indications are uncovered by history or physical examination.

However, before the institution of antihypertensive therapy, every patient should undergo a limited number of baseline laboratory studies. The studies recommended by the Hypertension Study Group of the Intersociety Commission for Heart Disease Resources consist of an hematocrit, dipstick urinalysis for protein blood and glucose, serum potassium, blood glucose, BUN or creatinine, serum cholesterol, as well as uric acid, an ECG, and radiographic examination of the chest, if clinically indicated.[44] The Study Group has proposed this evaluation for patients regardless of age with a blood pressure over 140/90 on two or three successive determinations on different days. Children less than 15 years of age with blood pressure elevation above the norms for their particular age group should be evaluated. If the clinical history is suggestive, additional studies should be performed to rule out curable forms of hypertension.

Cardiovascular Evaluation

Electrocardiogram. The electrocardiogram can suggest the presence, and the severity, of left ventricular hypertrophy that alters the ECG in the following ways:[63] (1) increased voltage, duration, and direction of the main QRS vector; (2) prolonged onset of intrinsicoid deflection in the left precordial leads; (3) leftward and posterior change in direction of the initial (0.02 sec) QRS vector; (4) altered repolarization with more an-

terior and rightward direction of S–T segment and T wave vector; (5) left atrial abnormality or altered terminal P wave vector. It is postulated that some of these abnormalities are directly related to increased left ventricular muscle mass.

Increased left ventricular surface area and closer proximity of the enlarged heart to the chest wall account for increased voltage. As the left ventricle enlarges, a greater proportion of the total QRS voltage is composed of left ventricular potentials. Since the left ventricle occupies a posterior position, the mean QRS becomes more posteriorly directed. A greater period of time is required to depolarize the increased mass of left ventricular wall, resulting in increased duration of the QRS, increased duration of endocardial to epicardial activation, and prolongation of the onset of intrinsicoid deflection in the left precordial leads.

Other ECG changes do not appear to be related to the increase in left ventricular mass.

The initial 0.02 second of the QRS reflects septal depolarization. Alteration of these forces can be caused by septal fibrosis and subsequent block in the branches or fascicles of the left bundle. Such a block can also cause superior displacement of the mean QRS vector. Increasing amounts of septal fibrosis can be manifest as altered initial forces, superior and leftward displacement of the mean QRS vector, marked left axis deviation, widening of the QRS, or even complete left bundle branch block. The initial QRS vector can be displaced so far posteriorly that the initial R wave is lost in the right precordial leads, mimicking anterior myocardial infarction.

Left atrial abnormality may be present in any disorder of the left ventricle. This finding may be transient, due to altered conduction caused by elevated left atrial pressure, or permanent, as a result of left atrial dilatation and fibrosis.

The altered time course of repolarization in left ventricular hypertrophy causes nondiagnostic S–T and T wave abnormalities. Similar changes are caused by other factors, such as digitalis, electrolyte disturbance, and myocardial ischemia. S–T segment elevation and upright T waves in leads V_{1-2}, and S–T depression with inverted T waves in lead V_{5-6}, I and aVL, is referred to as a left ventricular "strain" pattern. The combination of altered depolarization and repolarization results in a wide QRS–T angle, normally less than 90° in any one plane. A QRS–T angle greater than 120° can be seen in left ventricular hypertrophy.

Despite characteristic electrocardiographic features, the ECG is a relatively insensitive means for detecting left ventricular hypertrophy. Romhilt and associates examined 33 ECG criteria in 360 prospective autopsy specimens.[64] Each criterion was compared for sensitiv-

ity in detecting left ventricular hypertrophy in 160 specimens and for presence in the absence of left ventricular hypertrophy in 200 (Table 15-1). It should be noted that the point-score system, which is more fully discussed below, is as sensitive and is more specific than any individual measure.

Combinations of increased precordial voltage were the most sensitive abnormality, but were present in less than 60% of patients with left ventricular hypertrophy and in about 10% of specimens without hypertrophy. Delayed onset of intrinsicoid deflection in leads V_{5-6} greater than 0.05, and increased voltage in the limb leads are more specific but are present less frequently.

Left axis deviation was present in 24% of specimens with left ventricular hypertrophy, but is frequently seen in the absence of hypertrophy.

Combining voltage, QRS duration, delayed intrinsicoid deflection, left axis deviation, ST–T wave abnormalities, and left atrial involvement, Romhilt and Estes have devised a weighted system for the detection of left ventricular hypertrophy with high sensitivity but without the high incidence of false–positives seen when voltage criteria were used alone[65] (Table 15-2). The vectorcardiogram has shown only slightly higher correlative values than the scalar ECG.

In a study by Dern as associates, 43 of 44 patients showed a reduction in precordial voltage during antihypertensive therapy.[66] The mean QRS vector in the frontal plane did not change significantly, suggesting

Table 15-1. *Sensitivity and Specificity of ECG Criteria for Left Ventricular Hypertrophy*

EKG Criterion	LVH Detected (%)	Present in Absence of LVH(%)
$S_{V1-2} + R_{V5} \geq 35$ mm	56.3	12.5
$S_{V1} + R_{V5-6} > 30$ mm	55.6	10.5
$S_{V1-2} + R_{V5-6} > 35$ mm	55.6	11.5
$S_{V2} + R_{V4-5} > 35$ mm	55.6	14.5
R + S > 40 mm	55	13.5
Point-score System	**54**	**3**
Delayed onset intrinsicoid $V_{5-6} \geq$ 0.05 sec	29	0.5
$R_{V5-6} > 26$ mm	25	1.5
Left axis—30° or greater	24.4	13
$R_{aVL} \geq 10$ mm	13.1	0.5
$R_I > 13$ mm	10.6	0
$R_I + S_{III} > 25$ mm	10.6	0

(From Romhilt DW, Bove, KE, Norris RJ et al: A critical appraisal of the electrocardiographic criteria for the diagnosis of left ventricular hypertrophy. Circulation 40:185–195, 1969)

Table 15-2. *Point-score System*

ECG Criteria	Score
Amplitude	3 points
Any of the following:	
Largest R or S wave in the limb leads $\geq$ 20 mm	
S wave in V_1 or $V_2 \geq$ 30 mm	
R wave in V_5 or $V_6 \geq$ 30 mm	
ST–T segment changes (pattern of left ventricular strain)	
Without digitalis	3 points
With digitalis	(1) point
Left atrial abnormality	3 points
Terminal negativity of the P wave in V_1 1 mm or more in depth and duration 0.04 sec or more	
Left axis deviation −30° or more	2 points
QRS duration $\geq$ 0.09 sec	1 point
Intrinsicoid deflection in $V_{5,6} \geq$ 0.05 sec	1 point
Left ventricular hypertrophy	5 points
Probable left ventricular hypertrophy	4 points

(From Romhilt DW, Estes EH: A point-score system for the ECG diagnosis of left ventricular hypertrophy. Am Heart J 75:752–758, 1968)

that QRS alterations in this plane are permanent and probably related to septal fibrosis. Leftward and superior mean QRS orientation was noted in patients with the highest systolic pressures, while more posterior QRS orientation was seen in patients with higher diastolic pressures. Repolarization changes showed early reversibility with therapy. Because of the nonspecific nature of these changes, the significance of their reversal is not clear.

Chest Radiograph. The routine posteroanterior and lateral chest radiograph are important in evaluating cardiac size, left ventricular and left atrial enlargement, pulmonary venous pattern, enlargement of the aortic root, tortuosity of the thoracic aorta, and signs of coarctation of the aorta.

Early left ventricular enlargement does not produce significant change in the cardiac silhouette or cardiothoracic ratio. With developing hypertrophy, there is increasing convexity to the left heart border due to enlargement of the left ventricular outflow tract. The lower left heart border enlarges leftward, and the apex points downward.

Dilatation, tortuosity, or elongation of the aortic root can result in a widened mediastinal shadow. Uncoiling or tortuosity of the aorta is present in fewer than 3% of persons under 40 years of age; therefore its presence suggests target organ involvement. In older patients, tortuosity is usually due to atherosclerosis.

In the lateral projection, a significant left ventricular

enlargement is suggested if its posterior border extends more than 2 cm beyond the shadow of the inferior vena cava. Slight left atrial enlargement is commonly seen in patients with hypertension and is apparent when the posterior left atrial wall indents the barium-filled esophagus.

The left anterior oblique view suggests left ventricular enlargement when posterior displacement of the cardiac border causes the spine to be overlapped.

The chest radiograph suggests coarctation of the aorta when the shadow of the dilated left subclavian artery on the upper mediastinal border, or rib-notching due to dilated intercostal arteries, is seen. Lateral views with barium swallow can demonstrate aortic dilatation proximal to the coarctation. The "reversed-three sign" or "E-sign" due to the aortic dilatation proximal to and distal to the coarctation is another characteristic radiographic finding.

Renal Evaluation

Routine Urinalysis. In the initial evaluation of a patient with newly discovered hypertension, one consideration to be kept in mind is the possibility of underlying renal disease, because chronic parenchymal renal disease is the most common secondary cause of hypertension. The intrarenal vasculature and glomerular capillaries are susceptible to hypertensive damage resulting in a loss of function.

The routine urinalysis is useful in assessing these possibilities. A clean-catch midstream specimen is less likely to give misleading results. The specific gravity screens for loss of concentrating ability. Urine should be collected when the patient is relatively dehydrated, as in the second voiding after rising. Severe proteinuria and glucosuria can cause elevated specific gravity. Attention must be paid to proteinuria. With the semiquantitative methods used in screening examination, trace amounts may reflect a normal amount of protein. A 1+ designation is abnormal in properly collected specimens and indicates protein concentrations of 10 mg to 30 mg/100 ml. These patients should have quantitative protein excretion measured.

Patients with glycosuria should be evaluated for diabetes mellitus, since glomerulosclerosis is associated with renal insufficiency and hypertension.

Microscopic examination of the urine sediment is essential. A normal urine sediment contains few formed elements, for example, one or two red blood cells, one to two white blood cells, occasional hyaline casts, and a few epithelial cells. Casts indicate parenchymal renal damage if present in an abnormal amount or type. Red blood cell or hemoglobin casts indicate active glomerular injury. Large amounts of white blood cells and bacteria indicate an infection in the urinary tract.

Renal Function Tests. Costly laboratory tests are not required in the evaluation of patients with hypertension. Serum creatinine is elevated when 50% of renal mass is not functioning. If an elevated value is obtained or there is other evidence of kidney disease, the endogenous creatinine clearance should be obtained to quantitate the degree of impairment of glomerular filtration rate.

There is little indication for the phenolsulfophthalein (PSP) test or measurement of insulin and para-aminohippuric acid (PAH) clearances in the evaluation of hypertensive patients.

ESSENTIAL VERSUS SECONDARY HYPERTENSION

Essential hypertension refers to patients who do not have a detectable cause for their blood pressure elevation. *Secondary hypertension* includes blood pressure elevation due to other disease processes. Discovery of an underlying cause can lead to surgical correction, thus eliminating the need of a lifetime of pharmacologic therapy. The timing of a work-up to detect secondary hypertension must be determined on an individual basis.

It is estimated that 80% of patients referred to a major medical center with hypertension that is severe or resistant to therapy, have essential hypertension, whereas 90% to 95% of patients in a community practice with blood pressure elevation usually have essential hypertension. In a group of patients with resistant hypertension, underlying renal disease is the cause of blood pressure elevation in approximately 14%. Of the total group, 5% of these patients will have renal artery stenosis; 2%, unilateral pyelonephritis; and 1%, a unilateral hypoplastic kidney. Thus, approximately one-half of the patients with hypertension due to renal disease are potential candidates for surgical cure of hypertension (Table 15-3).

About 4% of patients with resistant hypertension have adrenal causes of blood pressure elevation, and less than 1% of the patients have coarctation of the aorta, which is also curable by surgery. Thus, among patients with severe hypertension, the yield of surgically curable forms is relatively high—around 10% of the total. Therefore, patients with diastolic pressures above 115 mm Hg, or those who show evidence of target organ damage, probably should be evaluated for underlying causes of hypertension when they are first detected.

At present, efforts are being directed toward early detection and treatment of patients with mild blood pressure elevation to prevent cardiovascular morbidity. In these patients, the yield of surgically curable

Table 15-3. *Work-up of 500 Hypertensive Patients at Peter Bent Brigham Hospital, Boston, Massachusetts*

Type	Cause	Number of Patients	Subtotals (%)	Total (%)
Essential	Benign	386	77.2	
	Malignant	12	2.4	79.6
Renal	Unilateral pyelonephritis	10	2.0	
	Bilateral pyelonephritis	8	1.6	
	Renal artery stenosis	25	5.0	
	Chronic glomerulonephritis	11	2.2	
	Hypoplastic kidney	5	1.0	
	Polycystic kidney	7	1.4	
	Kimmelstiel–Wilson disease	2	0.4	
	Juxtaglomerular cell tumor	1	0.2	13.8
Adrenal	Cushing's	5	1.0	
	Primary aldosteronism	10	2.0	
	Pheochromocytoma	5	1.0	4.0
Miscellaneous	Hyperkinetic heart syndrome	4	0.8	
	Coarctation of the aorta	3	0.6	
	Others	3	0.2	
	Unclassified	5	1.0	2.6

(Sullivan JM: Unpublished data, 1974)

secondary forms of hypertension is much lower. Thus, it is reasonable to limit the initial evaluation of a patient with mild hypertension to these procedures listed here and pursue a more extensive evaluation of those patients who fail to respond to antihypertensive therapy. Also listed here is a reasonable initial work-up for patients suspected of having secondary hypertension.

Laboratory Evaluation of the Office Patient with Suspected Secondary Hypertension
1. Complete blood count, urinalysis
2. 2-hour postprandial blood sugar
3. Serum creatinine or BUN
4. Na, K (Repeat potassium × 2. If low, place patient on 10 mEq Na, 100 mEq K diet for 3 days, obtain peripheral venous renin levels after ambulating for 3 hours.)
5. Ca, PO_4
6. Urine culture and sensitivities
7. 24-hour urine for VMA (Metanephrines or Catecholamines), creatinine
8. ECG
9. Chest film for heart size and rib notching
10. Rapid-sequence IVP: If abnormal, renal arteriograms and renal vein renin; if suspicious, radioactive renogram and renal scan to confirm abnormality or go directly to renal arteriograms, according to clinical situation
11. If appearance suggests Cushing's syndrome, give decadron, 1 mg at midnight followed by measurement of plasma cortisol at 8:00 AM

ORAL CONTRACEPTIVE HYPERTENSION

In the late 1960s, investigators noted a fall in blood pressure when hypertensive women discontinued oral contraceptive agents, and that reinstitution of oral contraceptive therapy was followed by a reappearance of hypertension.[67,68] Later, prospective studies demonstrated that the administration of oral contraceptives causes a statistically significant rise in systolic blood pressure, which increased 7 mm Hg, while diastolic pressure tended to rise about 2 mm Hg.[69] The incidence of hypertension in users of oral contraceptive agents varies from 1% to 18% in various series.[70] An association has not been found between duration of treatment and incidence of hypertension. Blood pressure usually returns to pretreatment levels when contraceptives are discontinued, but the process may take as long as 6 months.

The pathophysiology of oral contraceptive hypertension is not yet fully understood. The estrogenic component stimulates increased hepatic synthesis of several proteins, including renin substrate. As substrate levels rise, plasma renin activity remains constant, and plasma renin concentration falls as enzyme release is

inhibited by increased angiotensin–II levels. These events occur in both normotensive and hypertensive women and therefore have not been firmly implicated as the cause of hypertension.

Patients who are found to develop hypertension must use other means of contraception. If blood pressure is significantly elevated, the patient should be treated with antihypertensive agents for about 6 months. The dosage should then be reduced or the drug discontinued to determine if it is still necessary. If blood pressure elevation is mild, the patient can be observed for a 6-month period before deciding to institute antihypertensive therapy or work-up for other secondary causes of hypertension.

Certain patients are at greater risk of developing hypertension on oral contraceptive agents: the elderly, the obese, those with a history of hypertensive pregnancies, and those with a family history of hypertension. Although these patients may cautiously start oral contraceptives, they must remain under careful medical observation, with blood pressure measured at least every 2 months for the first year, then two or three times a year. Malignant hypertension with irreversible renal failure has been reported due to oral contraceptive agents.[71] The problem is serious and deserves careful attention.

RENAL HYPERTENSION

Renal Parenchymal Disease

Renal parenchymal disease is the most common cause of secondary hypertension. The way in which this form of renal disease results in hypertension is not clear.[72] The possibilities include abnormal stimulation of the renin–angiotensin system with inadequate response to the negative feedback signals due to renal damage, inadequate control of sodium homeostasis, and impaired production of renal vasodepressor substances.[73]

Although the pathogenesis may differ, the approach to treatment of patients with renal parenchymal disease is the same as that of patients with essential hypertension, except for a few considerations.[74] Drugs that affect renal function adversely should be used with caution in patients with more than mild to moderate reduction of glomerular filtration, that is, those with a serum creatinine above 2.0 mg %. Thiazide diuretics, chlorthalidone, spironolactone, triamterene, metazozone, and guanethidine all increase nitrogen retention.

The second consideration regards adjustment of dosage. Furosemide and ethacrynic acid are useful in treating patients with moderate to severe renal insufficiency but a larger dose is required as function decreases. Failure to respond to antihypertensive therapy is often due to an inadequate dose of diuretic or to excessive sodium intake. The gastrointestinal side-effects seen with large doses of ethacrynic acid limits its usefulness in renal failure. Drugs that depend on renal excretion, such as methyldopa, must be given in lower doses as renal function deteriorates.

Renovascular Hypertension

In 1914, Volhard postulated that hypertension was caused by stenotic small arteries throughout the renal parenchyma with systemic arterial hypertension developing as the circulation attempted to drive blood through the kidneys' purification system.[75] In 1934, Goldblatt demonstrated that stenosis of the main renal artery caused systemic hypertension in the dog and that removal of the stenosis returned blood pressure to control levels.[76] Since this time, a number of studies have demonstrated that renal artery stenosis is a cause of hypertension in man and that correction of the stenosis frequently cures the hypertension. Renal artery stenosis is probably the most common surgically curable cause of hypertension in man.

There are two major forms of renal artery stenosis. The first is fibromuscular hyperplasia, a disorder with proliferation of vascular smooth muscle and collagen fibers within the wall of the artery. This condition affects females more often than males by a ratio of about 3 to 1 and often appears in younger patients. The lesions are usually present in the distal third of the renal artery, although they may also involve other sections (Table 15-4). On microscopic grounds, these lesions can be subdivided into four subgroups, based on which layer of the arterial wall is most involved.[77]

The second major type of renal artery stenosis is caused by atherosclerosis. This lesion occurs more often in males by a 2 to 1 ratio, characteristically occurs in older age groups, and usually involves the proximal third of the renal artery.

The clinical history is rarely of great help in diagnosing renovascular hypertension. Items that are consistent are hypertension with a diastolic pressure above 130 mm Hg; sudden onset of hypertension with a diastolic pressure above 110 mm Hg in patients less than 30 years old; accelerated hypertension with hemorrhages, exudates, or papilledema; prior history of flank pain, hematuria, or renal trauma; hypertension remaining resistant to pharmacologic therapy; and the presence of epigastric or flank bruits throughout systole and diastole. Systolic bruits are much less specific.

Rapid-sequence intravenous pyelograms are probably the best way to screen patients for renal artery stenosis.[78] The best indicator is late appearance of contrast material on the ischemic side. Another indication is a difference in renal size. As the left kidney is normally one-half centimeter longer than the right, a difference of 1.5 cm or greater when the left kidney is

Table 15-4. *Renal Arterial Lesions*

Lesion	Age	Sex	Angiographic Appearance	Pathology
Atherosclerosis	Older	——	Asymmetric narrowing Poststenotic dilation Occasional total occlusion	Atherosclerotic with plaques
Intimal fibroplasia	Young	——	Segmental circumferential narrowing, poststenotic dilation and aneurysm	Collagen deposit and elastic duplication
Medial fibroplasia with aneurysms	Middle age	Female predominance	String-of-beads	Destruction of media and intima with fibrosis
Fibromuscular hyperplasia	Young and middle age	Rare	Concentric narrowing with poststenotic dilation	Fibromuscular hyperplasia
Subadventitial fibroplasia	——	Female predominance	No aneurysm Severe stenosis often	Fibrosis of adventitia

(From Paine R, and Sherman W: Arterial hypertension. In MacBryde CM, and Blacklow RS (eds): Signs and Symptoms, 5th ed. Philadelphia, JB Lippincott, 1970)

larger, or 0.5 cm or more when the right kidney is larger, is significant. Because the ischemic kidney reabsorbs filtered water in excess of dye, delayed hyperconcentration is another sign of unilateral stenosis, as is scalloping along the course of the ureter, secondary to enlargement of collateral ureteric blood vessels.

The radioactive renogram and renal scan provide equally acceptable means for screening. The renogram is more expensive, has a higher incidence of false-positive results, and does not reveal the anatomic details yielded by intravenous pyelography, for example, hydronephrosis, pyelonephrotic scarring, and reduction in size secondary to glomerulonephritis. A multicenter cooperative study of renovascular hypertension shows that 10% of patients with essential hypertension have abnormal intravenous pyelograms, while 22% of patients with surgically correctable renal vascular hypertension have normal pyelograms.[79] Patients with hypertension and abnormal pyelograms have about a 50% chance of the presence of surgically curable renovascular hypertension. Computer-assisted intravenous angiography, a newly developed technique, offers the potential to improve detection of significant lesions without the risk of more invasive angiographic procedures.

Although average peripheral renin activity is higher in patients with renovascular hypertension than in patients with essential hypertension, there is so much overlap of values measured in those within the two groups that peripheral renin activity is not very useful in screening patients for renal vascular hypertension.[80]

However, the hypertension is related to increased activity of the renin–angiotensin system, and it has been shown that intravenous infusion of the angiotensin II receptor blocking agent saralasin reduces pressure to normal in patients with true renovascular hypertension, thus providing an additional way to screen for or assess the clinical significance of a renal artery stenosis.[81,82]

When an abnormal intravenous pyelogram or radioactive renogram have been obtained, the next diagnostic step is usually renal arteriography. This shows the anatomy of the lesion, if present. In postmortem studies, however, it has been found that about 50% of patients with renal artery stenosis were normotensive. Thus, functional assessment of a stenotic lesion is important. The most widely used method is measurement of renal vein renin activity in both renal veins. Elevated activity on the ischemic side and a renal vein renin ratio of ischemic to uninvolved side of 1.5 or greater allows correct prediction of the results of surgery in about 80% of cases.[83] When bilateral renal artery stenosis is present, this procedure is less valuable, although it might suggest which kidney contributes most to the elevation of blood pressure.

Studies by Strong and his colleagues have demonstrated that the sensitivity of renal vein renin measurement can be enhanced by sodium depletion.[84] Low sodium diet plus full doses of oral diuretics for 3 days prior to the measurement of renal vein renin activity improved the predictive value of the test from 35% to 90%. It is our impression that agents that act to reduce renin release tend to decrease the sensitivity of the test.

In experienced hands, bilateral ureteral catheterization and split renal function tests were of limited value in predicting the results of surgery, but the predictive value is not as great as that of renal vein renin ratios

and there is little reason at present to proceed with such a study.

An abnormal intravenous pyelogram, an arterial stenosis on arteriography, and a renal vein renin ratio of greater than 1:5 does not automatically indicate surgical correction. Many patients respond to pharmacologic therapy.

In a retrospective study of 24 patients who responded favorably to therapy, it was found that 7 patients with fibromuscular hyperplasia taking diuretics plus reserpine or methyldopa had an average fall in diastolic blood pressure of 20 mm Hg, while 17 of the other patients with arteriosclerotic lesions had a similar fall in blood pressure, but required additional vasodilator therapy.[85]

It has been found that corrective renovascular surgery in patients with significant extrarenal arteriosclerosis may improve blood pressure, but may not prolong life.[86] Thus, individual judgment must be applied to each case. It is reasonable to limit renal artery surgery to those patients who fail to respond to pharmacologic therapy. The recently developed technique, percutaneous transluminal angioplasty offers a less invasive way to relieve renal ischemia.[87] Unfortunately, many stenotic lesions cannot be dilated successfully with a balloon-tipped catheter.

ADRENAL HYPERTENSION

Pheochromocytoma

Pheochromocytomas are tumors of chromaffin cells of adrenal medulla or sympathetic ganglia. Neuroblastomas and ganglioneuromas arising from ganglion cells and chemodectomas arising from chemoreceptor cells are related tumors. Pheochromocytomas also occur in association with familial neurocutaneous disorders, with thyroid medullary carcinoma, and with hyperparathyroidism.

Pheochromocytomas contain the enzymes needed to metabolize tyrosine to catecholamine. After uptake, tyrosine is hydroxylated to dihydroxphenylalanine (dopa) by the rate-limiting tyrosine hydroxylase step. Dopa is decarboxylated to dihydroxphenethylamine (dopamine), which in turn is oxidized to norepinephrine in storage granules. In tissues containing phenethanolamine-N-methyl-transferase, norepinephrine is methylated to form epinephrine. This enzymatic step is usually confined to the adrenal medulla.[88]

Symptoms of pheochromocytoma occur as catecholamine mixtures are released into the circulation. The Valsalva maneuver, exercise, pregnancy, overeating, urination, and ingestion of tyramine-containing foods have all precipitated attacks. The most common symptoms are headache, sweating, palpitation, pallor, and nausea.[89] More than half of the patients with pheo-

chromocytoma have persistent hypertension with spikes; the remainder has intermittent hypertension. It is not unusual for such patients to go for several years before a diagnosis is reached. Postural hypotension is found in approximately two-thirds of patients. The cardiovascular effects of catecholamines cause most of the symptoms. Norepinephrine stimulates alpha-adrenergic receptors, causing systolic and diastolic hypertension, bradycardia, and cardiac arrhythmias. Epinephrine stimulates both alpha- and beta-receptors, causing tachycardia, elevated cardiac output, arrhythmias, and either hypotension or systolic hypertension. Both compounds decrease gastrointestinal motility, inhibit insulin release, and elevate blood sugar, free fatty acids, lactic acid, and basal metabolic rate. Norepinephrine is the major compound produced by most tumors, although predominant production of epinephrine has been reported.[90] Although the two types usually cannot be separated clinically, it is a sound assumption that attacks associated with bradycardia are norepinephrine-mediated, while attacks associated with hypotension are epinephrine-mediated.

The problems in management of patients with pheochromocytoma are to confirm the diagnosis by biochemical tests, and to locate the tumor and remove it with adequate monitoring after appropriate preparation of the patient.

Biochemical tests for urinary catecholamines or their metabolites form the mainstay of diagnosis.[91] Values twice normal or higher are usually found in the urine of affected patients. After release of catecholamines, relatively small amounts are excreted unchanged in the urine. Circulating catecholamines are converted to metanephrine and normetanephrine by hepatic catechol-o-methyl transferase (COMT). These products are excreted in the urine or metabolized throughout the body by monoamine oxidase to vanillylmandelic acid (VMA). Small amounts of norepinephrine are metabolized to dihydroxymandelic acid within the neuron, and converted to VMA by COMT.

Urinary (and plasma) catecholamines are present in small amounts and are difficult to measure. Elevated values are found in patients receiving methyldopa, levodopa or any catecholamine-containing medication. Measurement of urinary total metanephrine is a more reliable technique. Elevated values are found in patients receiving monoamine oxidase inhibitors. VMA can be measured by a colorimetric phenolic acid reaction, but results are elevated by ingestion of phenol-containing foods. A more specific spectrophotometric method is not influenced by diet, but is lowered by monoamine oxidase inhibitors or clofibrate, and falsely elevated by nalidixic acid.[92] If urinary levels of one product are elevated, a separate collection should be made and a different product found to be elevated be-

fore the patient is subjected to surgery. All urine collections should be made in an acid-containing bottle to prevent breakdown of catecholamine metabolites.

Bravo and his colleagues have compared the newer radioenzymatic assays of plasma catecholamines with 24-hour urinary VMA and metanephrine in 24 patients with pheochromocytoma and 40 without pheochromocytoma.[93] They found false-negative results in one patient using the radioimmunoassay, in 11 using VMA, and in 5 using metanephrine excretion. However, meticulous attention to patient preparation and specimen handling appeared to be essential.

The diagnosis of pheochromocytoma should never be made solely on the basis of pharmacologic testing. Provocative tests, that is, causing an elevation of blood pressure after administration of histamine, tyramine, or glucagon; or blocking tests, that is, causing a fall in pressure after administration of phentolamine, have a significant number of false-positive and false-negative results and also have an associated risk. However, pharmacologic testing is often useful in clarifying equivocal biochemical results.

When the diagnosis of pheochromocytoma has been confirmed, the surgeon is faced with the problem of locating the tumor. Approximately 80% of these tumors arise in the adrenals—most on the right. Another 10% to 15% arise from intra-abdominal sympathetic ganglia or from the organs of Zuckerkandl. Most extra-abdominal tumors arise from the thoracic sympathetic chain and can be seen on oblique chest films. Cervical tumors are usually palpable or cause local symptoms. Intravenous pyelograms or adrenal tomograms show displacement of the kidney by a suprarenal mass in 50% of cases.

Arteriography can localize tumors but can also precipitate acute attacks.[94] Patients should be treated with alpha-adrenergic blocking agents for 1 week before study. Finding one tumor on arteriography does not rule out the presence of multiple tumors, found in 15% to 20% of patients. Vena caval catheterization with catecholamine measurement at several sites has proved useful in localizing tumors. More recently, computerized axial tomography, echograms, and scintigraphy have been used successfully to locate pheochromocytomas.[95,96]

Because N-methyl transferase is usually limited to the adrenal medulla, it was hoped that the presence of significant amounts of epinephrine in the blood or urine placed the tumor in the adrenal glands.[97] Several case reports have now shown that epinephrine can be formed by extra-adrenal tumors.

Preoperative management of the patient with pheochromocytoma is based on pharmacologic stabilization for 1 or 2 weeks with alpha-adrenergic blockade.[98] Additional beta-adrenergic blockade is indicated when cardiac arrhythmia or serious tachycardia develops, but should not be used routinely because of the risk of inducing heart failure from catecholamine cardiomyopathy. Alpha-methylparatyrosine, an inhibitor of tyrosine hydroxylase, can eliminate symptoms by interfering with catecholamine synthesis. This may eventually prove to be the preoperative treatment of choice.

Aldosteronism

In 1953, Simpson and associates reported the isolation of a potent adrenal mineralocorticoid.[99] In 1955, Conn studied a patient with signs of mineralocorticoid excess, and reported the first case of an adrenal adenoma producing the syndrome of primary aldosteronism.[100]

Aldosterone causes resorption of sodium and secretion of potassium and hydrogen in the distal renal tubule. This leads to the two hallmarks of primary aldosteronism: hypertension and depletion of body potassium stores. Potassium depletion causes symptoms of muscle weakness and fatigue, and leads to the development of nephropathy with symptoms of polyuria and nocturia. The hypertension associated with primary hyperaldosteronism is ordinarily mild and well tolerated, although cases of more severe hypertension have been reported. Malignant hypertension secondary to primary aldosteronism is believed to be very rare.

At present, the best screening test for primary aldosteronism is measurement of serum potassium, which is usually less than 3.5 mEq per l. Since some patients with hyperaldosteronism have mild or borderline hypokalemia, it is advisable to repeat measurement of serum potassium in patients with borderline values. In order to rely on serum potassium for screening, it is necessary to be certain that the patient has not been taking potassium supplement nor restricting dietary sodium. When less sodium is presented to the distal renal tubules, less is exchanged for potassium, and thus serum potassium levels remain relatively normal.

Many circumstances other than primary aldosteronism result in hypokalemia. The most common is prior use of diuretic agents. Other causes are potassium-wasting renal disease, Cushing's syndrome, and aldosteronism secondary to renal vascular or renal parenchymal disease.

Plasma renin activity should be measured under well-defined conditions in patients with unexplained hypokalemia.[101] Patients with primary aldosteronism have retained sodium and water but "escape" before developing edema. Because of volume overexpansion,

plasma renin levels are usually suppressed. Our practice has been to place patients on a low sodium diet (10 mEq Na, 100 mEq K) for 4 days and to obtain a blood sample for measurement of renin at around noon on the morning of the fourth day, after the patient has been up and about all morning. The combination of upright posture and sodium depletion acts to stimulate renin release, but in patients with primary aldosteronism, because of the volume overexpansion, plasma renin activity remains suppressed.

A patient with suppressed renin activity has either aldosteronism or "low renin" hypertension. (See section on therapeutic implications of the renin-angiotensin system for a discussion of "low-renin" hypertension.) Definitive diagnosis of primary aldosteronism requires hospitalization for precise metabolic studies. The presence of a low plasma renin activity despite volume depletion must be confirmed, and elevated plasma or urinary aldosterone, which is not suppressed when the patient receives a salt load, must be demonstrated. Once the biochemical diagnosis of primary aldosteronism has been made, an attempt is made to locate the tumor by computerized axial tomography, which can detect bilateral enlargement or adenomas as small as 1 cm,[102] by bilateral adrenal venography and sampling of adrenal venous blood for assay of plasma aldosterone levels, or by surgical exploration of both adrenal glands.

Primary aldosteronism, though usually caused by a single adenoma, can also result from three other causes.[103] Surgical excision of an adrenal adenoma producing aldosterone ordinarily leads to correction of both hypertension and electrolyte abnormality. Some patients with biochemical evidence of aldosteronism have been found to have bilateral nodular hyperplasia of the adrenal cortex. Bilateral adrenalectomy results in correction of electrolyte abnormalities, but hypertension persists.[104] Although these two groups of patients show some differences in the way in which they respond to manipulations of salt and fluid balance, there is no certain way of separating the two groups prior to surgery, other than demonstration of a single adenoma by adrenal venography or demonstration of elevated levels of aldosterone in both adrenal veins.

A third group of patients has been described in whom signs and biochemical evidence of aldosteronism is present but who respond to the administration of deoxycorticosterone (DOCA) by suppressing urinary aldosterone secretion to normal levels.[105]

A fourth group of patients has glucocorticoid-remediable hyperaldosteronism. This rare disorder is found in children more often than in adults. The patients present signs, symptoms, and biochemical evidence of aldosteronism, but the administration of replacement doses of glucocorticoid results in correction of the blood pressure, suppression of urinary aldosterone secretion and correction of electrolyte levels.[106]

Cushing's Syndrome

Patients with syndromes of excessive cortisol secretion, either from adrenal cortical hyperplasia or adrenal cortical tumor, frequently develop hypertension. Ordinarily, Cushing's syndrome is apparent on physical examination, with the patient displaying truncal obesity, round face, buffalo hump, purple striae, multiple bruises over thin skin, and bone pain. To pursue the diagnosis, the next step is a rapid dexamethasone suppression test.[107] The patient receives 1 mg dexamethasone at midnight. This is perceived by the hypothalamus as an elevation of plasma corticosteroids, which leads to diminished pituitary ACTH release and diminished adrenal secretion of corticosteroids. In normal subjects, measurement of plasma cortisol at 8:00 A.M. the next morning should reveal marked suppression to less than 5μg/100 ml. Patients with the various forms of Cushing's syndrome fail to sustain cortisol suppression and require hospitalization for further evaluation.[108]

Adrenal Cortical Enzyme Deficiencies

Congenital disorders exist in which one of the hydroxylase enzymes necessary for the production of corticosteroids is absent, resulting in diminished serum levels of corticosteroids and elevated pituitary secretion of ACTH.[109] Because steroid synthesis cannot proceed through the normal pathways, the compensatory drive results in production of excess amounts of other steroid compounds, including some with salt-retaining properties. The syndrome more frequently seen in adults, involves deficiency of 17-hydroxylase, which catalyzes conversion of progesterone to 17-hydroxyprogesterone.[110] When this enzyme is missing, glucocorticoid, estrogen, and androgen production are impaired. The clinical syndrome consists of primary amenorrhea, hypertension, and defeminization. The diagnosis is suspected when urinary excretion of 17-ketosteroids and 17-hydroxysteroids is low or absent, despite hypertension. Dexamethasone, 1 mg daily for 7 to 14 days, should result in correction of the hypertension.

Licorice Ingestion

Licorice contains a salt-retaining compound, glycyrrhizic acid. Ingestion of large amounts of licorice on a daily basis results in sodium retention, potassium excretion, hypertension, and hypokalemia.[111] Because in-

travascular volume is expanded, plasma renin activity and plasma urinary levels of aldosterone are low.

Hyperparathyroidism

In a series of 40 patients with primary hyperthyroidism studied by Rosenthal and Roy, 13 were found to be hypertensive.[112] Nine patients initially presented with hypertension of whom 7 were discovered to have hyperparathyroidism through serum calcium determinations. In this series, the prevalence of primary hyperparathyroidism in hypertensive patients was 7.6%, whereas the frequency ranges between 0.1% and 0.2% in the general population. In a series of 80 patients reported by Madhavan, Frame, and Block, 17.5% were hypertensive, and one-half of these experienced significant improvement in their hypertension after parathyroidectomy.[113] This possibility should be considered in patients presenting with a history of depression, recurrent peptic ulcer, bone pain, renal calculus formation, and constipation. Increasing use of multiphasic screening procedures may bring more cases to medical attention.

Coarctation of the Aorta

Coarctation of the aorta causes hypertension in the upper extremities either by mechanical means or through an effect on renal blood flow. The diagnosis should be suspected in all patients with hypertension, particularly young men with "functional" heart murmurs. Patients with coarctation of the aorta are ordinarily asymptomatic. Certain symptoms, such as pain and coldness of the extremities on exercise, epistaxis, and headache, should suggest this diagnosis. On physical examination, there is a decrease, absence, or delayed peak of pulsation in the femoral arteries in comparison with the radial pulse. Measurement of blood pressure with a large cuff in the legs reveals a gradient. Radiographic examination of the chest may show the findings discussed earlier. Physical examination may reveal pulsations in the intercostal spaces, in the axilla, and in the interscapular space. A midsystolic murmur is frequently audible on the anterior chest, which radiates to the back. Murmurs may also be heard along the lateral chest wall over dilated collateral vessels.[114]

Coarctation of the aorta is often associated with other congenital cardiac abnormalities, most often bicuspid aortic valve, patent ductus arteriosus, ventricular septal defect or valvular aortic stenosis.

Unless contraindications exist, surgical correction is recommended to prevent complications of severe hypertension, rupture of cerebral aneurysm or of aorta, left ventricular failure, and bacterial endocarditis.[115]

TREATMENT OF HYPERTENSION

Mild blood pressure elevation gradually causes vascular damage in time. Successful long-term therapy demands that the patient fully understand the risk imposed by untreated hypertension and the need for lifelong therapy.

CHANGES IN LIFESTYLE

Contemporary therapy emphasizes early detection and treatment of mild hypertension. This approach gives rise to concern about the long-term effects of antihypertensive agents. Because the risk–benefit ratio cannot be calculated precisely, consideration should be given to nonpharmacologic therapy of mild hypertension before hypotensive drugs are prescribed.

Stress

Hypertension can be provoked in experimental animals subjected to recurrent stress. Emotional stress elevates blood pressure, even in persons whose blood pressure is ordinarily within normal limits. Constant monitoring of blood pressure shows elevation during periods of activity.

Unfortunately, it is difficult to do anything about stress. Major life changes, such as retirement from active professional life, can be followed by improved blood pressure, but most often this is not a realistic approach. Regular periods of rest during the day have not proved to be very effective in controlling blood pressure, nor has sedation.

It has been found that regular elicitation of the relaxation response for periods of 20 minutes, twice a day, results in lower blood pressure in some persons.[116] The therapeutic value of this approach requires further study.

Exercise

Strenuous exercise and isometric exercise tend to elevate blood pressure. It is unwise for hypertensive patients or patients in the coronary age group to attempt strenuous exercise without conditioning and isometric exercises, such as weight-lifting, should be avoided. Regular, moderate isotonic exercise is beneficial. Hypertensive patients on standard antihypertensive agents have been found to have better blood pressure control when following a program of regular exercise.[117] Boyer and Kasch observed an average fall in diastolic pressure of 11.8 mm Hg in a group of 24 hypertensive men participating in a walk–jog program.[118]

Obesity

Weight is positively correlated with blood pressure.[119] Although weight loss is not invariably followed by a great reduction in blood pressure, elimination of obesity is advisable for general medical reasons, such as control of hyperlipidemias.

Tobacco

Cigarette smoking increases blood pressure transiently. On the average, smokers tend to have lower blood pressure than nonsmokers. However, cigarette smoking is definitely a risk factor in the development of cardiovascular disease, which, when combined with hypertension, represents a potent combination. Moderate pipe or cigar smoking does not appear to have an adverse effect on cardiovascular mortality.

Alcohol

Moderate use of alcohol does not increase blood pressure. However, blood pressure rises as alcohol use increases.[120] Patients should also be aware of the caloric implications of alcohol, the adverse effect on the control of type 4 hyperlipidemia and the dangers of adding the sedative effects of alcohol to those of antihypertensive sympatholytic agents.

Salt

Populations with high average daily sodium intake contain a large number of hypertensive persons.[121] Kempner showed that improvement of severe hypertension required extreme salt restriction—less than 8 mEq sodium daily.[122] This is a very difficult diet to follow and requires special salt-free foods. More recent studies have shown that mild to moderate hypertension improves when sodium intake is lowered from 150 to 200 mEq to 50 to 90 mEq/day.[123,124,125] Although recent studies indicate that people vary considerably in their response to sodium,[126] until convenient and reliable methods are developed for the detection of salt-sensitive patients, it is prudent to advise the hypertensive patient to follow a no-added-salt diet.

PHARMACOLOGIC MEASURES

A wide variety of antihypertensive agents and combinations of agents have been placed on the market over the past two decades. As physicians have gained familiarity with these compounds and their side-effects, the number in general use has come to be reduced to a relatively small group: thiazide diuretics, agents that block the sympathetic nervous system, vasodilators, and the newly introduced agents that block

the renin–angiotensin system. It has become generally appreciated that the use of a large dose of a single antihypertensive agent tends to produce more side-effects for a given hypotensive effect than does the combined use of smaller doses of two antihypertensive agents with different mechanisms of action. As a result, the concept of "stepped-care" has emerged, which has been recommended by the Joint National Committee on Detection, Evaluation and Treatment of Hypertension.[127]

Unless contraindications exist, therapy is usually initiated with a thiazide or thiazidelike diuretic. Loop diuretics should be reserved for selected patients, such as those with renal failure. If the goal blood pressure has not been reached by 2 to 4 weeks of full-dose therapy, a sympatholytic agent, such as one listed here is added and gradually increased to a maximum tolerated dose. It is important to bear in mind that the step 2 agents are approximately the same in potency when given in the maximum recommended dose. However, all have side-effects and potentially adverse effects.

Stepped-Care Antihypertensive Therapy

STEP 1. Diuretic
STEP 2. Adrenergic inhibiting agent
        Beta-adrenergic receptor blocking agent
           Atenolol
           Metoprolol
           Nadolol
           Propranolol
           Timolol
        Central alpha-2 receptor agonist
           Clonidine
           Methyldopa
        Peripheral alpha-1 receptor blocking agent
           Prazosin
STEP 3. Vasodilator
        Hydralazine hydrochloride
        Prazosin (if not used in step 2)
STEP 4. Additional agents
        Captopril (angiotensin converting enzyme blocker)
        Guanethidine (adrenergic blocker—inhibits norepinephrine release)
        Minoxidil (vasodilator)

The art of successful antihypertensive therapy involves the careful matching of medication to patient, for example, selecting beta-blocking agents for patients with angina pectoris or with a history of recent acute myocardial infarction while avoiding them in the treatment of hypertensive patients with asthma, heart failure, or advanced degrees of heart block.[128] Similarly, methyldopa should be avoided in treating patients with

liver diseases; reserpine, in depressed patients; clonidine and methyldopa, in patients with chronic fatigue, and so on.

If a patient cannot tolerate the first step 2 agent selected, others should be tried before proceeding to step 3. If the combination of sympatholytic and diuretic therapy is not completely effective, hydralazine hydrochloride, a direct-acting vasodilator, is added to the antihypertensive program and gradually increased to a full dose. Prazosin hydrochloride may be used instead of hydralazine hydrochloride if it was not selected as the step 2 agent.

For some time, the potent adrenergic blocking agent guanethidine has been the mainstay of step 4 treatment of resistant hypertension. The recent introduction of minoxidil and captopril offers two additional options. Minoxidil is a potent vasodilator, which carries side effects of fluid retention, pericardial effusion, hirsutism, and headache.[129] Captopril, an angiotensin converting enzyme blocker, has possible side-effects of skin rash, proteinuria, granulocytopenia, and loss of taste.[130,131] Thus, none of the three agents is ideal, and a choice must be made based on individual considerations. Of the three, captopril clearly has the greatest patient acceptance.

In the majority of patients, control of blood pressure can be obtained with a simple program of antihypertensive agents with few side-effects. Around 50% of patients respond to diuretic therapy alone. Therefore, unless the hypertension is severe, therapy should be started with diuretics and additions made as needed. When diastolic pressure is greater than 115 mm Hg, a diuretic and a step 2 agent should be started simultaneously.

The pharmacologic properties of the most commonly used antihypertensive agents have been reviewed and are well described in the literature.[132]

THERAPEUTIC IMPLICATIONS OF THE RENIN–ANGIOTENSIN SYSTEM

In 1898, Tigerstedt and Bergman published a study of the hemodynamic effects of crude saline extracts of rabbit kidneys.[133] The extracts caused a rise in blood pressure that started within 10 seconds, peaked at 2 minutes, and disappeared in 20 minutes. The activity was heat-labile, nondializable and acetone-insoluble. In 1934, Goldblatt reported the production of hypertension by partial occlusion of the renal artery in the dog.[76] In 1939, Page noticed that renin, mixed with saline and injected into an ear vessel, did not cause vasoconstriction, but was vasoactive when mixed with blood.[134] He concluded that renin had to interact with

blood before a pressor substance was formed. In 1939, Braun-Menéndez found a pressor substance in renal vein blood, which did not have the physical properties of renin, and eventually proved to be angiotensin.[135] In 1953, Simpson and associates purified aldosterone.[99] In 1955, as a result of the work of several investigators, angiotensin I and II were isolated and angiotensin converting enzyme described. In 1960, Laragh and associates and Genest and his coworkers found elevated aldosterone excretion in patients with malignant hypertension and, in 1960, Laragh observed that infusion of angiotensin II caused increased urinary aldosterone.[136,137] Thus, all the components involved in the formation of a feedback loop were described[138] (Fig. 15-4).

The liver synthesizes renin substrate, a glycoprotein that is released into the circulation. Renin, a proteolytic enzyme, cleaves a decapeptide, angiotensin I, from the substrate molecule. During passage through the pulmonary circulation, angiotensin I is lysed by converting enzyme, leaving the octapeptide angiotensin II, a potent vasopressor, which is eventually destroyed by angiotensinases. Angiotensin II has several effects, among which are vasoconstriction and aldosterone release, which in turn causes sodium retention in the distal tubules of the kidney. The system works to maintain blood pressure in two ways, by increasing blood volume and by increasing peripheral vascular resistance. In addition, angiotensin II acts directly on the juxtaglomerular cells to inhibit renin release. Thus, any manipulation that tends to drop blood pressure, blood volume, or sodium concentration tends to activate the system. Hemorrhage, hypotension, sodium depletion, gastrointestinal fluid loss, upright posture, and renal artery stenosis all serve to stimulate renin release.

Stimulation of the autonomic nervous system also causes renin release. The control of renin release from the cells of the juxtaglomerular apparatus remains under study. There are stretch receptors in the afferent arterioles which, when subjected to increased pressure, reduce renin secretion. The cells of the macula densa respond to changes in sodium concentration or to the rate of sodium delivery and affect juxtaglomerular renin release. Potassium directly inhibits the release of renin, as does angiotensin II.

Potassium, as well as angiotensin II, stimulates aldosterone secretion. ACTH stimulates aldosterone secretion, and large increases in plasma sodium concentration inhibit aldosterone release.

The most valuable clinical use for measurement of components of the renin–angiotensin system is in the diagnosis of secondary hypertension. Patients with primary aldosteronism invariably have suppressed

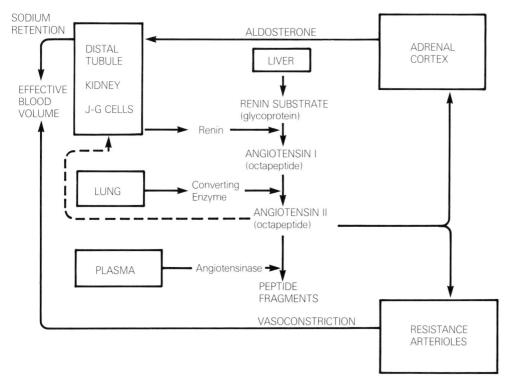

Fig. 15-4. The renin-angiotensin-aldosterone negative feedback loop for the regulation of effective blood volume.

plasma renin activity and measurement of differential renal vein renin activity in patients with renovascular lesions helps to predict the outcome of surgery.[83,101]

If plasma renin activity is measured in a group of normal subjects of comparable ages under standard conditions of posture, activity, diet, and time of day, values fall within a relatively narrow range.[104] If one measures renin activity prior to treatment under identical circumstances in patients with essential hypertension, the values for plasma renin activity spread over a much wider range. Roughly 20% to 30% of the patients have renin activity lower than normal, and around 10% to 15% have activity higher than normal. Thus, patients with essential hypertension can be subdivided on the basis of high, normal, or low plasma renin activity. The physiology of this system suggests that patients with low renin hypertension might be relatively volume overloaded, as in primary aldosteronism; while those with high renin activity might be volume-depleted and relatively vasoconstricted because of high circulating angiotensin II levels secondary to high renin activity. Thus, concepts of "volume-dependent" or low renin hypertension, and "vasoconstrictor dependent" or high renin hypertension, have evolved.[139]

The effects of various antihypertensive agents on pa-

tients with low renin hypertension have been studied to test the hypothesis that the patients are volume-dependent. Most workers now agree that such patients respond well to thiazide diuretics or to spironolactone, an aldosterone antagonist.[140,141]

Patients with high renin hypertension have been treated with propranolol, a beta-adrenergic blocking agent that blocks the release of renin. It has been reported that patients with high renin hypertension respond unusually well to this form of therapy.[142] Similarly, hypertensive patients with high plasma renin activity respond quite well to treatment with angiotensin-converting enzyme blocking agents.[130]

This type of characterization can be tried for patients who do not respond to the typical stepped-care antihypertensive therapy.[143] Roughly one-third of patients with essential hypertension have low renin, or volume-dependent hypertension, and another 60% have normal renin activity, which suggests that they too have a volume component to their blood pressure problem. Thus, 80% to 90% of patients with hypertension might be expected to respond in varying degrees to diuretic therapy. Those patients who fail to respond adequately to diuretics are ordinarily placed on sympatholytic drugs, which tend to decrease renin activity. Thus,

a stepped-care approach eventually covers the spectrum of high to low renin hypertension without adding the additional cost of renin profiling.

When faced with a patient who has had difficulty tolerating standard antihypertensive therapy, one could stop all drugs for 2 weeks, if possible, and measure plasma renin activity in a known state of sodium balance (or against locally established normograms based on urinary sodium excretion) to characterize the renin–angiotensin system. Once classified, the patient could be placed on either intensive diuretic or intensive converting enzyme or beta-blocking therapy. Despite the rational appeal of this approach, the results are often disappointing.[144]

Certain data suggest that renin is an additional risk factor for the development of cardiovascular disease.[145] Thus, for a given level of blood pressure elevation, a patient with low renin activity would have less tendency to develop the cardiovascular complications of hypertension than does a patient with the same level of blood pressure, but normal or high renin activity. This concept has not received widespread confirmation and should not form the basis for a decision exempting patients with low renin hypertension from adequate therapy.[146]

HYPERTENSIVE EMERGENCIES

In about 10% of patients, an accelerated or malignant phase occurs as a complication of almost all types of primary and secondary hypertension. Severe diastolic hypertension, grade 3 or grade 4 retinopathy, and progressive renal failure are the features that characterize this phase. Hypertensive encephalopathy, cerebral hemorrhage, left ventricular failure, and fluid retention are other common findings. Malignant hypertension is associated with a poor prognosis unless successfully treated before the vascular damage has taken place.[38]

PATHOPHYSIOLOGY

The control system for maintaining normal blood pressure involves several negative feedback loops. Normally, as blood pressure rises, a stimulus is created that decreases the output of one or more of the forces maintaining the pressure. Negative feedback loops are known to exist, which involve the renin–angiotensin–aldosterone system and the sympathetic nervous system among others.

Although the pathogenesis of the malignant phase is not completely understood, it has been proposed that conversion to a malignant phase occurs when increasing levels of blood pressure and an accelerating rate of vascular damage cause a normal negative feedback loop to become a positive loop. For example, plasma renin activity is usually elevated in patients with malignant hypertension, which is inappropriate because a rising pressure should be associated with a falling renin level as the body attempts to maintain pressure homeostasis. Because renin levels are high, angiotensin II and aldosterone levels rise and, as a result, sodium and water are retained, effective blood volume increases, and plasma renin levels should fall. However, high pressure injures the kidney, renin continues to be released despite the increased effective blood volume and blood pressure, and thus, a negative feedback loop becomes a positive factor in further elevating arterial pressure.

The malignant phase of hypertension can be reversed by aggressive antihypertensive therapy, which arrests progressive vascular damage. Therefore, during the malignant phase of hypertension, there is an urgent need for the reduction of blood pressure to normotensive levels.[147]

DIFFERENTIAL DIAGNOSIS

There are other hypertensive emergencies that require early, expert, and intensive treatment. These include subarachnoid hemorrhage, intracerebral hemorrhage, hypertensive encephalopathy, acute left ventricular failure due to hypertension, dissecting aneurysm, acute and advancing renal insufficiency due to hypertension, eclampsia, and pheochromocytoma.

Hypertensive Emergencies
1. Malignant hypertension
2. Hypertensive retinopathy with fundal hemorrhages and symptomatic reduction in visual acuity
3. Hypertensive encephalopathy
4. Acute left heart failure due to hypertension
5. Dissecting aneurysm with hypertension
6. Subarachnoid hemorrhage with hypertension
7. Intracerebral hemorrhage with severe hypertension
8. Acute or advancing renal insufficiency with severe hypertension
9. Hypertensive crisis in pheochromocytoma
10. Eclampsia

In addition to these hypertensive emergencies, there are less obvious situations that also require urgent therapy. Patients often experience a period of acceleration of hypertension in which the manifestations of vascular damage are not proportionate in all target organs; for example, patients may present with hypertensive encephalopathy in the absence of papilledema, hemorrhages, or exudates. Other patients may present

with blurred vision, retinal hemorrhages, and exudates, yet may have neither impairment of consciousness or renal function. It is important to realize that the urgency of blood pressure reduction varies with the hypertensive emergency and that the approach to treatment and the agent used vary.[149] Severely hypertensive patients with subarachnoid hemorrhage or patients with acute left ventricular failure and pulmonary edema secondary to hypertension require more immediate blood pressure reduction than an otherwise asymptomatic hypertensive patient with grade 3 hypertensive retinopathy and severely elevated diastolic pressure.

PRINCIPLES OF THERAPY

The primary aim in the management of hypertensive emergencies is the reduction of diastolic blood pressure to a normal range. This should be attempted with constant attention to maintaining perfusion of vital organs. Patients without pre-existing symptoms of vascular insufficiency rarely develop such complications when blood pressure is reduced, although a transient decrease in urine output with a slight rise in BUN is often noted. In the presence of significant coronary or cerebrovascular insufficiency, angina, electrocardiographic signs of ischemia, frank myocardial infarction, transient cerebral ischemia, convulsions, and cerebral infarction can occur, primarily as a result of a precipitous drop in the arterial pressure. This can usually be avoided if a more controlled reduction of pressure is achieved with close monitoring of vital organ functions. Persistence is often more important than speed of reduction.

Parenteral therapy falls into two categories. The first includes agents with a relatively long duration of action, which are given as a bolus followed by a blood pressure response of considerable variation in degree and duration. The second category comprises drugs with a short duration of action that require constant intravenous infusion and close supervision to effect a controlled and smooth fall of the blood pressure.[150] Gentle diuretic therapy should be employed in most cases to potentiate the effect of other agents and to prevent secondary retention of salt and water, but should not be given to the point of inducing intravascular volume depletion, reflex vasoconstriction, and additional renin release.[151] Oral antihypertensive therapy should be started as soon as possible, because it will be required eventually and the onset of action is relatively slow.

Hypertensive crises with concomitant renal failure present special management problems.[24] Not only do patients with malignant hypertension present with oliguria and renal failure, but also patients with dissecting aneurysms can develop oliguria due to obstruction of the renal arteries and patients with acute glomerulonephritis can develop acute renal failure. These patients retain salt and water, which makes them less sensitive to antihypertensive agents and can lead to problems with congestive heart failure. Effective hemodialysis can correct these problems and can sustain life while fibrinoid necrosis of renal arterioles resolves. Some patients recover enough renal function to be able to live without dialysis.

A few patients with end-stage renal failure become resistant to antihypertensive agents despite salt and water removal by dialysis. Such patients have extremely high levels of plasma renin activity and become normotensive when the kidneys are removed. It has become apparent that malignant hypertension does not prevent successful long-term dialysis and transplantation.[152] The results obtained in such patients are comparable to those obtained in patients with renal failure secondary to glomerulonephritis.

REFERENCES

1. **Rushmer RF:** Structure and Function of the Cardiovascular System. Philadelphia, WB Saunders, 1972

2. **Mellander S, Johansson B:** Control of resistance, exchange and capacitance function in the peripheral circulation. Pharmacol Res 20:117–196, 1968

3. **Bayliss WM:** On the local reaction of the arterial wall to changes of internal pressure. J Physiol (Lond) 28:220–231, 1902

4. **Folkow B, Neil E:** Circulation. New York, Oxford University Press, 1971

5. **Frohlich ED:** Hemodynamics of hypertension. In Genest J, Koiw E, Kuchel O (eds): *Hypertension.* New York, McGraw–Hill, 1977:15–49

6. **Widimsky J, Fejfarova MD, Fejfar Z:** Changes of cardiac output in hypertensive disease. Cardiologia 31:381, 1957

7. **Eich RJ, Peters RJ, Cuddy RP, Smulyan HI, Lyons RH:** Hemodynamics in labile hypertension. Am Heart J 63:188, 1962

8. **Julius S, Randall OS, Esler MD, Kashima T, Ellis C, Bennett J:** Altered cardiac responsiveness and regulation in the normal cardiac output type of borderline hypertension. Circ Res 36(Suppl 1):1994, 1975

9. **Ulrych M, Frohlich ED, Dustan HP, Page IH:** Cardiac output and distribution of blood volume in central and peripheral circulations in hypertensive and normotensive man. Br Heart J 31:570, 1969

10. **Julius S, Pascual AV, Sannerstedt R, Mitchell C:** Relationship between cardiac output and peripheral re-

sistance in borderline hypertension. Circulation 43:382, 1971

11. **Sannerstedt R:** Hemodynamic response to exercise in patients with arterial hypertension. Acta Med Scand 180(Suppl 458):1, 1966

12. **Takeshita A, Mark AL:** Decreased vasodilator capacity of forearm resistance vessels in borderline hypertension. Hypertension 2:610, 1980

13. **Al-Aouar ZR, Ratts TE, Cunningham BR, Sullivan JM:** Altered ventricular diastolic properties in borderline hypertension: Effect of sodium intake. Circulation 64(4):322, 1981

14. **Sullivan JM, Prewitt RL, Josephs JA:** Attenuation of the microcirculation in young patients with high output labile hypertension. Hypertension 5:844, 1983

15. **Meerson F:** The myocardium in hyperfunction, hypertrophy, and failure. Circ Res 25(Suppl 2):1, 1969

16. **Ledingham JM, Cohen RD:** The role of the heart in the pathogenesis of renal hypertension. Lancet 2:979, 1963

17. **Guyton AC, Granger HJ, Coleman TG:** Autoregulation of the total systemic circulation and its relation to control of cardiac output and arterial pressure. Circ Res 28(Suppl 1):93, 1971

18. **Tarazi RC:** Hemodynamic role of extracellular fluid in hypertension. Circ Res 38(Suppl II):73, 1976

19. **Riva–Rocci S:** Un nuovo sfigmonometro. Gazzetta Medica di Torino 47:981–1001, 1896

20. **Schottstaedt MF, Sokolow M:** The natural history and course of hypertension with papilledema (malignant hypertension). Am Heart J 45:331–362, 1953

21. **McMichael J, Murphy EA:** Methonium treatment of severe and malignant hypertension. J. Chronic Dis 1:527–535, 1955

22. **Kincaid–Smith P, McMichael J, Murphy EA:** The clinical course and pathology of hypertension with papilloedema (malignant hypertension). Q J Med 27:117–153, 1958

23. **Perry HM Jr, Schroeder HA, Catanzaro FJ et al:** Studies on the control of hypertension. VIII. Mortality, morbidity, and remission during twelve years of intensive therapy. Circulation 33:958–972, 1966

24. **Woods JW, Blythe WB:** Management of malignant hypertension complicated by renal insufficiency. N Engl J Med 277:57–61, 1967

25. **Hodge JV, Smirk FH:** The effect of drug treatment of hypertension on the distribution of deaths from various causes: A study of 173 deaths among hypertensive patients in the years 1959 to 1964 inclusive. Am Heart J 73:441–452, 1967

26. **Build and Blood Pressure Study.** Chicago Society of Actuaries, vol 2, 1979

27. **Kannel WB, Castelli WP, McNamara PM, Sorlie P:** The Framingham Study: Some factors affecting morbidity and mortality in hypertension, Part 2, Milbank Mem Fund Q 47(3):116–142, 1969

28. **Kannel WB, Schwartz MJ, McNamara PM:** Blood pressure and risk of coronary heart disease: The Framingham study. Dis Chest 56:43–52, 1969

29. **United States National Center for Health Statistics:** Vital and Health Statistics. Heart Disease in Adults: United States, 1960–1962 (PHS Publication No. 1000, Series 11, No. 6). Washington, D. C., Government Printing Office, 1964

30. **Stamler J, Kjelsberg M, Hall Y:** Epidemiologic studies on cardiovascualr–renal disease. I. Analysis of mortality by age–race–sex–occupation. J Chronic Dis 12:440–455, 1960

31. **Byrom FB:** Pathogenesis of hypertensive encephalopathy and relation to malignant phase of hypertension: Experimental evidence from hypertensive rat. Lancet 2:201, 1954

32. **Sako Y:** Effect of turbulent blood flow and hypertension on experimental atherosclerosis. JAMA 179:36, 1962

33. **Heath D, Wood EH, Dushane JW, Edwards JE:** The relation of age and blood pressure to atheroma in the pulmonary arteries and thoracic aorta in congenital heart disease. Lab Invest 9:259, 1960

34. **Brust AA, Ferris EB:** Diagnostic approach to hypertension due to unilateral kidney disease. Ann Intern Med 47:1049, 1957

35. **Gaunt R, Antonchak N, Miller GJ, Renzi AA:** Effect of reserpine (Serpasil) and hydralazine (Apresoline) on experimental steroid hypertension. Am J Physiol 182:63, 1958

36. **Perry HM Jr, Schroeder HA:** The effect of treatment on mortality rates in severe hypertension: A comparison of medical and surgical regimens. Arch Intern Med 102:418–428, 1958

37. **Dustan HP, Schneckloth RE, Corcoran AC et al:** The effectiveness of long-term treatment of malignant hypertension. Circulation 18:644–651, 1958

38. **Sokolow M, Perloff D:** Five year survival of consecutive patients with malignant hypertension treated with antihypertensive agents. Am J Cardiol 6:858–863, 1960

39. **Hamilton M, Thompson EN, Wisniewski TKM:** The role of blood pressure control in preventing complications of hypertension. Lancet 1:235–238, 1964

40. **Wolff FW, Lindeman RD:** Effects of treatment on hypertension: Results of a controlled study. J Chronic Dis 19:227, 1966

41. **Veterans Administration Cooperative Study Group on Antihypertensive Agents:** Effect of treatment on morbidity: Results in patients with diastolic blood pressures averaging 115 through 129 mm Hg. JAMA 202:1028–1034, 1967

42. **Veterans Administration Cooperative Study Group on Antihypertensive Agents:** Effect of treatment on morbidity: Results in patients with diastolic blood pressure averaging 90 through 114 mm Hg. JAMA 213:1143–1152, 1970

43. **Veterans Administration Cooperative Study Group on Antihypertensive Agents:** Effects of treatment on morbidity in hypertension III. Influence of age, diastolic pressure, and prior cardiovascular disease: further analysis of side effects. Circulation 45:991–1004, 1972

44. **Report of Inter-Society Commission for Heart Disease Resources:** Guidelines for the detection, diagnosis and management of hypertensive populations. Circulation 64:1079A–1089A, 1981

45. **Hypertension Detection and Follow-Up Program Cooperative Group.** Four Year Findings of the Hypertension Detection and Follow-Up Program. 1. Reduction in mortality of persons with high blood pressure, including mild hypertension. JAMA 242:2562–2571, 1979

46. **The Australian Therapeutic Trial in Mild Hypertension:** Report by the Management Committee. Lancet 1:1261–1267, 1980

47. **Kannell WB, Sorlie P, Gordon T:** Labile hypertension: A faulty concept. The Framingham Study. Circulation 61:1183–1187, 1980

48. **Harlan WR, Oberman A, Mitchell RE, Graybiel A:** A 30 year study of blood pressure in a white male cohort, In Gaddo Onesti (ed): Hypertension Mechanism and Management, pp 85–91. New York, Grune & Stratton, 1973

49. **Frohlich ED, Kozul VJ, Tarazi RC, Dustan HP:** Physiological comparison of labile and essential hypertension. Circ Res 27(Suppl I):55–69, 1970

50. **Kannel WB, Gorden T, Schwartz MJ:** Systolic versus diastolic blood pressure and risk of coronary heart disease: The Framingham study. Am J Cardiol 27:335–346, 1971

51. **Colandrea MA, Friedman GD, Nichaman MZ et al:** Systolic hypertension in the elderly: An epidemiologic assessment. Circulation 41:239–245, 1970

52. **Freis ED:** How far should blood pressure be lowered in treating hypertension? JAMA 232:1017–1018, 1975

53. **Hypertension–Stroke Cooperative Study Group:** Effect of antihypertensive treatment on stroke recurrence. JAMA 229:409–418, 1974

54. **Kirkendall WM, Burton AC, Epstein FH et al:** Recommendations for human blood pressure determination by sphygmomanometers. Central Committee for Medical and Community Responses. Dallas, American Heart Association, 1967

55. **Bandran RHA, Weir RJ, McGuiness JB:** Hypertension and headache. Scott Med J 15:48–51, 1970

56. **Weiss NS:** Relation of high blood pressure to headache, epistaxis and selected other symptoms: The United States health examination survey of adults. N Engl J Med 287:631–633, 1972

57. **Rosenthal FD, Roy S:** Hypertension and hyperparathyroidism. Br Med J, 4:396–397, 1972

58. **Friedenwald JS:** Retinal and choroidal arteriosclerosis. In Ridley F, Sorsby A (eds): Modern Trends in Ophthalmology, p 77, New York, Paul B Hoeber, 1940

59. **Keith NM, Wagener, HP, Barker NW:** Some different types of essential hypertension: Their course and prognosis. Am J Med Sci 197:332–343, 1939

60. **Scheie HG:** Evaluation of ophthalmoscopic changes of hypertension and arteriolar sclerosis. Arch Ophtholmol 49:117, 1953

61. **Kirkendall WM, Armstrong ML:** Vascular changes in the eye of the treated and untreated patient with essential hypertension. Am J Cardiol 9:663, 1962

62. Diseases of the ocular blood vessels. In **Friedenwald JS, Wilder HC, Maumenee AE, Sanders TE, Keys JEL, Hogan MJ, Owens WC, Owens EU (eds):** Ophthalmic Pathology, p 310. Philadelphia, WB Saunders, 1952

63. **Kossmann CE, Burchell HB, Pruitt RD, Scott RC:** The electrocardiogram in ventricular hypertrophy and bundle-branch block. Circulation 26:1336–1351, 1962

64. **Romhilt DW, Bove KE, Norris RJ, Conyers E, Conradi S, Rowlands DT, Scott RC:** A critical appraisal of the electrocardiographic criteria for the diagnosis of left ventricular hypertrophy. Circulation 40:185–195, 1969

65. **Romhilt DW, Estes EH:** A point-score system for the ECG diagnosis of left ventricular hypertrophy. Am Heart J 75:752–758, 1968

66. **Dern PL, Pryor R, Walker SH, Searls DT:** Serial electrocardiographic changes in treated hypertensive patients with reference to voltage criteria, mean QRS vectors, and the QRS-T angle. Circulation 36:823–829, 1967

67. **Laragh JH, Sealey JE, Ledingham JGC, Newton MA:** Oral contraceptives: Renin, aldosterone, and high blood pressure. JAMA 201:918, 1967

68. **Woods JW:** Oral contraceptives and hypertension. Lancet 2:653, 1967

69. **Fisch IR, Freedman SH, Myatt AV:** Oral contraceptives, pregnancy and blood pressure. JAMA 222:1507–1510, 1972

70. **Editorial: Blood pressure and the pill.** Br Med J 1:693, 1973

71. **Zacherle BJ, Richardson JA:** Irreversible renal failure secondary to hypertension induced by oral contraceptives. Ann Intern Med 77:83–85, 1972

72. **Tobian L:** A viewpoint concerning the enigma of hypertension. Am J Med 52:595–609, 1972

73. **Muirhead EE, Brooks B, Kosinski M, Daniels EG, Hinman JW:** Renomedullary antihypertensive principle in renal hypertension. J Lab Clin Med 67:778–791, 1966

74. **Hunt JC, Strong CG, Harrison EG Jr, Furlow WL, Leary FJ:** Management of hypertension of renal origin. Am J Cardiol 26:280–288, 1970

75. **Volhard F, Fahr T:** Die Brightsche Nierenkrankheit, Klinik, Pathologie und Attas. Berlin, Springer–Verlag, 1914

76. **Goldblatt H, Lynch J, Hanzal RF, Summerville WW:** Studies on experimental hypertension. I. The production of persistent elevation of systolic blood pressure by means of renal ischemia. J Exp Med 59:347, 1934

77. **Kincaid OW, Davis GD, Hallerman RJ et al:** Fibromuscular dysplagia of the renal arteries: Arteriographic features, classification and observations on the natural history of the disease. Am J. Roentgn., 104:271–282, 1968

78. **Hunt JC, Strong CG, Sheps SG et al:** Diagnosis and management of renovascular hypertension. Am J Cardiol 23:434–445, 1969

79. **Bookstein JJ, Abrams HL, Buenger RE et al:** Radiologic aspects of renovascular hypertension. 3. Appraisal of arteriography. JAMA 221:368–374, 1972

80. **Amsterdam EA, Couch NP, Christlieb AR et al:** Renal vein renin activity in the prognosis of surgery of renovascular hypertension. Am J Med 47:860–868, 1969

81. **Brunner, HR, Gavras H, Laragh JH et al:** Exposure of the renin and sodium components using angiotension II blockade. Circ Res 34–35 (Suppl I):35, 1974

82. **Streeten DHP, Anderson GH, Fiberg JM, et al:** Use of angiotensin II antagonist (Saralasin) in the recognition of angiotensinogenic hypertension. New Engl J Med 292:657, 1975

83. **Couch NP, Sullivan JM, Crane C:** The predictive accuracy of renal vein renin activity in the surgery of renovascular hypertension. Surgery 79:70–76, 1976

84. **Strong CG, Hunt JC, Sheps SG, Tucker RM, Bernatz PE:** Renal venous renin activity: Enhancement of sensitivity of lateralization by sodium depletion. Am J Cardiol 27:602–611, 1971

85. **Chassin MRG, Sullivan JM:** Pharmacologic management of renovascular hypertension. JAMA 227:421–423, 1974

86. **Kjellbo H et al:** Renal artery stenosis. III. Follow-up observations in operated and nonoperated patients. Scand J Urol Nephrol 4:49–57, 1970

87. **Grüntzig A, Vetter W, Meier B et al:** Treatment of renovascular hypertension with percutaneous transluminal dilatation of a renal artery stenosis. Lancet 1:801–802, 1978

88. **Wurtman RJ:** Catecholamines. N Engl J Med 273:637–646, 693–700, 746–753, 1965

89. **Thomas JE, Rooke ED, Krale WF:** The neurologists' experience with pheochromocytoma. JAMA 197:754–758, 1966

90. **Page LB, Raker JW, Berberich FR:** Pheochromocytoma with predominant epinephrine secretion. Am J Med 47:648–652, 1969

91. **Sjoerdsma A, Engleman K, Waldmann TA et al:** Pheochromocytoma: Current concepts of diagnosis and treatment. Ann Intern Med 65:1305–1326, 1966

92. **Rayfield EJ, Cain JP, Casey MP et al:** Influence of diet on urinary VMA excretion. JAMA 221:704–705, 1972

93. **Bravo EL, Tarazi RC, Gifford RW et al:** Circulating and urinary catecholamines in pheochromocytoma: Diagnostic and pathophysiologic implications. N Engl J Med 301:682–686, 1979

94. **Rossi P, Young IS, Panke WF:** Techniques, usefulness, and hazards of arteriography of pheochromocytoma. JAMA 205:547–553, 1968

95. **Epstein AJ, Patel SK, Petasnick JP:** Computerized tomography of the adrenal gland. JAMA 242:2791–2794, 1979

96. **Sisson JC, Frager MS, Valk TW et al:** Scintigraphic localization of pheochromocytoma. N Engl J Med 305:12–17, 1981

97. **Sullivan JM:** Editorial: Pheochromocytoma. Arch Surg 104:130–131, 1972

98. **Pertsemlidis D, Gitlow SE, Siegel WC, Kark AE:** Pheochromocytoma. 1. Specificity of laboratory diagnostic tests. 2. Safeguards during operative removal. Ann Surg 169:376–385, 1969

99. **Simpson SA, Tait JF, Wettstein A, Neher R, von Euw J, Reichstein T:** Isolierung eines neuen kristallisierten Hormons aus Nebennieren mit besonders hoher Wieksamkeit aus den Mineralstoffwechsel. Experientia (Basel) 9:33, 1953

100. **Conn JW:** Presidential address. II. Primary aldosteronism, a new clinical syndrome. J Lab Clin Med 45:6–17, 1955

101. **Conn JW, Cohen EL, Rovner DR:** Suppression of plasma renin activity in primary aldosteronism. JAMA 190:213–221, 1964

102. **Dunnick NR, Schaner EG, Doppman JF et al:** Computed tomography in adrenal tumors. Am J Roentgenol 132:43–46, 1979.

103. **Biglieri EG, Stockigt JR, Schambelan M:** Adrenal mineralocorticoids causing hypertension. Am J Med 52:623–632, 1972

104. **Laragh JH, Ledingham JGG, Sommers SC:** Secondary aldosteronism and reduced plasma renin in hypertensive disease. Trans Assoc Am Physicians 80:168–182, 1967

105. **Biglieri EG, Slaton PE, Kronfield SF, Schambelan M:** Diagnosis of an aldosterone-producing adenoma in primary aldosteronism: An evaluative maneuver. JAMA 201:510–514, 1967

106. **Sutherland DJA, Ruse JL, Laidlaw JC:** Hypertension, increased aldosteronism secretion, and low plasma renin activity relieved by dexamethasone. Can Med Assoc J 95:1109, 1966

107. **Tucci JR, Jagger PI, Lauler DP et al:** Rapid dexamethasone suppression test for Cushing's syndrome. JAMA 199:374–382, 1967

108. **Herrera MG et al:** Cushing's syndrome: Diagnosis and treatment. Am J Surg 107:144–152, 1964

109. **Bongiovanni AM, Root AW:** The adrenogenital syndrome. N Engl J Med 268:1283–1289, 1342–1351, 1391–1399, 1963

110. **Biglieri EG, Herron MA, Brust N:** 17-hydroxylation deficiency in man. J Clin Invest 45:1946–1954, 1966

111. **Koster M, David EK:** Reversible severe hypertension due to licorice. N Engl J Med 278:1381–1383, 1968

112. **Rosenthal FD, Roy S:** Hypertension and hyperparathyroidism. Br Med J 4:396–397, 1972

113. **Madhavan T, Frame B, Block MA:** Influence of surgical correction of primary hyperparathyroidism on associated hypertension. Arch Surg 100:212–214, 1970

114. **Campbell M:** Natural history of coarctation of the aorta. Br Heart J 32:633–640, 1970

115. **March HW, Hultgren HN, Gerbode F:** Immediate and remote effects of resection on the hypertension in coarctation of the aorta. Br Heart J 22:361–373, 1960

116. **Benson H, Marzetta BR, Rosner BA:** Decreased blood pressure associated with the regular elicitation of the relaxation response: A study of hypertensive subjects, In Eliot RS (ed): Contemporary Problems in Cardiology, vol 1: Stress and the Heart, p 293. New York, Futura, 1974

117. **Hanson JS, Nedde WH:** Preliminary observations on physical training for hypertensive males. Cir Res 27:I49–53, 1970

118. **Boyer JL, Kasch FW:** Exercise therapy in hypertensive men. JAMA 211:1668–1671, 1970

119. **Tyroler HA, Heyden S, Hames CG:** Weight and hypertension: Evans County studies of blacks and whites. In Paul O (ed): Epidemiology and Control of Hypertension, pp 177–201. New York, Stratton International Medical Book Conference, 1975

120. **Kannell WB, Sorlie P.:** Hypertension in Framingham. In Paul O (ed): Epidemiology and Control of Hypertension, p 553. New York, Stratton International Medical Book Conference, 1975

121. **Dahl LK:** Salt intake and salt need. N Engl J Med 258:1152–1157, 1205–1208, 1958

122. **Kempner W:** Treatment of hypertensive vascular disease with rice diet. Am J Med 4:545–577, 1948

123. **Parijs J, Joosens JV, Van der Linden L et al:** Moderate sodium restriction and diuretics in the treatment of hypertension. Am Heart J 85:22, 1973

124. **Carney S, Morgan T, Wilson MM et al:** Sodium restriction and thiazide diuretics in the treatment of hypertension. Med J Aust I:803, 1975

125. **Magnani B, Ambrosioni E, Agosta R et al:** Comparison of the effects of pharmacological therapy and a low sodium diet on mild hypertension. Clin Sci Mol Med 51:625s, 1976

126. **Sullivan, JM, Ratts TE, Taylor JC et al:** Hemodynamic effects of dietary sodium in man: A preliminary report. Hypertension 2:506–514, 1980

127. **Joint National Committee on Detection, Evaluation and Treatment of High Blood Pressure: 1980 Report.** Arch Intern Med 140:1280–1285, 1980

128. **Beta-blocker Heart Attack Study Group:** The beta-blocker heart attack trial. JAMA 246:2073, 1981

129. **Dormois JC, Young JL, Nies AS:** Minoxidil in severe hypertension: Value when conventional drugs have failed. Am Heart J 90:360, 1975

130. **Gavras H, Brunner HR, Turini GA et al:** Antihypertensive effect of the oral angiotensin coverting enzyme inhibitor SQ 14,225 in man. N Engl J Med 298:991, 1978

131. **Sullivan JM, Ginsburg BA, Ratts TE, Johnson JG, Barton BR, Kraus, DH, McKinstry DN, Muirhead EE:** Hemodynamic and antihypertensive effects of captopril, an orally active angiotensin converting enzyme inhibitor. Hypertension 1:397–401, 1979

132. **Page LB, Sidd J:** Medical management of primary hypertension. N Engl J Med 287:960–967, 1018–1023, 1074–1081, 1972

133. **Tigerstedt R, Bergman PG:** Niere und Kreishauf. Scand Arch Physiol 8:223–271, 1898

134. **Page IH:** On the nature of the pressor action of renin. J Exp Med 70:521–542, 1939

135. **Braun–Menéndez E, Fasciolo JC, Leloin LF, Muñoz JM:** La substancia hypertensova de la sangre del riñon isquemiado. Revta Soc Argent Biol 15:129, 1939

136. **Laragh JH, Ungers M, Kelly WG, Lieberman J:** Hypotensive agents and pressor substances: The effect of epinephrine, norepinephrine, angiotensin II and others on the secretory rate of aldosterone in man. JAMA 174:234–240, 1960

137. **Genest J, Nowaczynski W, Koiw E, Sandor T, Biron P:** Adrenocorticoid function in essential hypertension. In Boch KD, Cottier PT (eds): Essential Hypertension, pp 126–146. Berlin, Springer-Verlag 1960

138. **Peart WS:** Renin–angiotensin system. N Engl J Med 292:302–306, 1975

139. **Laragh JH, Baer L, Brunner HR, Buhler FR, Sealey JE, Vaughan ED Jr:** Renin, angiotensin and aldosterone system in pathogenesis and management of hypertensive vascular disease. Am J Med 52:633–652, 1972

140. **Laragh JH:** Vasoconstriction-volume analysis for understanding and treating hypertension: The use of renin and aldosterone profiles. Am J Med 55:261–274, 1973

141. **Carey RM, Douglas JG, Schweikert JR, Liddle GW:** The syndrome of essential hypertension and suppressed plasma renin activity: Normalization of blood pressure with spironolactone. Arch Intern Med 130:849–854, 1972

142. **Bühler FR, Laragh JH, Baer L, Vaughan ED Jr, Burnner HR:** Propranolol inhibition of renin secretion: A specific approach to diagnosis and treatment of renin-dependent hypertensive diseases. N Engl J Med 287:1209–1214, 1972

143. **Sullivan JM:** Physiological and biochemical profiles of hypertension for rational clinical management. Adv Intern Med 23:219, 1978

144. **Kaplan NM:** Renin profiles: The unfulfilled promises. JAMA 238:611, 1977

145. **Brunner HR, Sealy JE, Laragh JH:** Renin subgroups in essential hypertension: Further analysis of their pathophysiologic and epidemiologic characteristics. Circ Res 32(Suppl I):99–109, 1973

146. **Kaplan NM:** The prognostic implications of plasma renin in essential hypertension. JAMA 231:167, 1975

147. **Report of Inter-society Commission for Heart Disease Resources Hypertension Study Group, J. Edwin Wood, MD, Chairman.** Resources for the Management of Emergencies in Hypertension. Circulation 43 A:157–160, 1971

148. **Vaamonde CA, David NJ, Palmer RF:** Hypertensive emergencies. Med Clin North Am 55:325–334, 1971

149. **Finnerty FA:** Hypertensive encephalopathy. Am J Med 52:672–678, 1972

150. **Bhatia SK, Frohlich ED:** Hemodynamic comparison of agents useful in hypertensive emergencies. Am Heart J 85:367, 1973

151. **Sullivan JM, Schoeneberger AA, Ratts TE et al:** Short-term therapy of severe hypertension: Hemodynamic correlates of the antihypertensive response in man. Arch Intern Med 139:1233, 1979

152. **Woods JM, Blythe WR, Huffines WD:** Management of malignant complicated by renal insufficiency. N Engl J Med 291:10–14, 1974

16

Palpitation and Tachycardia

Edward Massie
Robert E. Kleiger

Palpitation
  Neurocirculatory Asthenia
  Mitral Valve Prolapse
  Relationship of Palpitation to Organic Heart
    Disease
  Relationship of Palpitation to Tachycardia
Tachycardia
  Chemical Control
  Nervous Control
  Types of Tachycardia
    Sinus Tachycardia

Paroxysmal Atrial Tachycardia
Paroxysmal Atrial Tachycardia with
  Atrioventricular Block
Atrial Flutter
Atrial Fibrillation
Paroxysmal Junctional Tachycardia
Multifocal Atrial Tachycardia
Bradycardia–Tachycardia Syndrome
Paroxysmal Ventricular Tachycardia
Ventricular Flutter and Fibrillation
Summary

PALPITATION

The word palpitation is a derivative of the Latin *palpitare,* which means to throb. Palpitation is usually a less dire heart symptom than pain and dyspnea and is extremely common. It consists of an unpleasant sensation of the heart's action, whether slow or fast, regular or irregular. It is more frequently the result of the less important disturbances of cardiac rhythm, namely, premature beats and atrial paroxysmal tachycardia, or of forceful regular heart action, either rapid or slow, resulting from effort, excitement, toxins (tobacco, caffeine, or alcohol), or infection. Minor degrees of disturbance more easily produce palpitation if the subject is a nervously sensitive person. Less frequently it may be caused by a more important disorder of heart rhythm such as atrial fibrillation, atrial flutter, or ventricular paroxysmal tachycardia.

It should be emphasized that palpitation and tachycardia often do not indicate a primary physical disorder but rather a psychic disturbance; they are the most important symptoms of cardiac neurosis. If these symptoms are analyzed critically, it is seen that subjectively they result in what is termed heart consciousness and that they may only be manifestations of enhanced normal function. Various associated symptoms sometimes occur that are largely the result of more appreciative sensibilities.

It is well known that when a person becomes nervously exhausted or hyperirritable his sense of values and judgment are often somewhat distorted, especially in matters concerned with his physical and psychic well-being. If at such a time the patient has occasion to lift some object or walk up an incline, he may instantly notice rapid and forceful beating of his heart. This symptom usually disappears rapidly, but if similar experiences are repeated, he may become con-

vinced that something serious has happened to his heart. The patient's nervous condition has brought about sufficient introspection, anxiety, and uncertainty to produce an increase in cardiac irritability and a decrease in the threshold at which palpitation, tachycardia, and the associated symptoms of cardiac neurosis become evident.

Often the threshold of consciousness of the heart's action is so lowered that palpitation may be complained of when the heart rate and rhythm are perfectly normal. The person who has done little in the way of physical activity for a prolonged period may, with relatively little exertion, experience untoward increase in heart rate with resultant feelings of palpitation.

Palpitation is one of the most characteristic symptoms of neurocirculatory asthenia. In this condition it probably results, along with other symptoms of the disease, from an imbalance of the autonomic nervous system. This imbalance may be more or less constant in certain nervously hypersensitive persons, but may also be precipitated in relatively normal persons by emotional or physical upsets acting reflexly on the autonomic nervous system.

The functional aspect of the symptom complex of palpitation was beautifully described in 1836 by John C. Williams* of Edinburgh who wrote a book on "Practical Observations on Nervous and Sympathetic Palpitation of the Heart, Particularly As Distinguished from Palpitation the Result of Organic Disease." He criticized the practice which was usually followed up to that time, of attributing functional derangement of the heart to true heart disease. He taught that palpitation was

> frequently, by a careless observer, regarded as symptomatic of some serious organic or structural change being established either in the covering of the heart, its muscular texture, or in some of its natural valvular appurtenances. A careful and deliberate inquiry, however, will, in the generality of cases, enable us to strip them of their apparent obscurity and danger and reduce them to their place in nosological arrangement. Latterly there has been too great a rage for tracing diseases almost exclusively to vascular derangement. I deprecate this, because I am convinced of the increasing influence of the nervous system, both in health and in disease. A deservedly popular writer on medicine of the present day says, "The longer we live, the more we see; and the deeper we study, so much the more we shall become convinced, that not only are the primary impressions of morbific causes sustained by the sentient system of the human fabric, but it is here the primary morbid movements first begin, and are thence

propagated to the vascular apparatus, which from that movement reacts upon, and is again influenced by the nervous system. No man, I am satisfied, can ever be a sound Pathologist, or a judicious practitioner, who devotes his attention to one of these systems in preference or to the exclusion of the other; through life they are perpetually acting, and inseparably linked together.

Williams went on to quote Dr. Baille as follows:

> There are in truth few phenomena which puzzle, perplex, and lead to error the inexperienced (and sometimes the experienced) practitioner, so much as inordinate action of the heart. He sees, or thinks he sees, some terrible cause for this tumult in the central organ of the circulation and frames his portentous diagnosis and prognosis accordingly. In the pride of his penetration he renders miserable for the time the friends and by his direful countenance damps the spirits of his patient. But ultimate recovery not seldom disappoints his fears and the Physician is mortified at his own success.

NEUROCIRCULATORY ASTHENIA

Palpitation is one of the most characteristic symptoms of neurocirculatory asthenia. This condition, first described during the Civil War, was very prevalent also in World War I and again in World War II; therefore, it certainly merits detailed discussion. Among the current synonyms for this disease are "effort syndrome," "cardiac neurosis," "disorderly action of the heart," "soldier's heart," and "Da Costa's syndrome." The last term is derived from Da Costa's classic article on the irritable heart, published in 1871 and based upon his experiences as surgeon in the Northern armies in the Civil War. The incidence of neurocirculatory asthenia has since been found to increase sharply in wartime and to vary greatly from only a few cases among soldiers in military training to a considerable number under the strain and the hardship of combat. Although this condition came into prominence in World War I, it appears to have been even more of a problem in World War II.

Neurocirculatory asthenia of a pronounced degree is not too common in civilian life, primarily because those likely to develop the condition are usually able to avoid the factors of effort and nervous strain that help precipitate the undesirable symptoms. There is, however, no way to determine its incidence, because in the slight and much more frequently unrecognized form, it is not likely to be recorded as a specific diagnosis. As a matter of fact, White and his associates were able to study a group of patients who had what was diagnosed in Army hospitals as neurocirculatory asthenia, and listed their various symptoms. Then, when a similar survey

*White PD: Heart Disease, 3rd ed. New York, Macmillan, 1944

was made of the symptoms of patients for whom the diagnosis of anxiety neurosis had been made in the psychiatric wards, the similarity in symptoms was striking. Thus, it seems that two patients with the same complaints and symptoms might have different diagnoses, depending entirely upon whether they were seen by a psychiatrist or an internist.

Clinically, neurocirculatory asthenia is characterized by such prominent symptoms as palpitation, chest pain, weakness, dyspnea, sighing respiration, sweating, tremulousness, dizziness, nervousness, headache, and faintness, all of which are aggravated by excitement or effort, and accompany or follow periods of anxiety, nervousness, or physical strain and infection. This symptom complex may occur as the only manifestation of illness, or it may be a complication of many diseases, including structural disease of the heart or other organ systems.

The disease appears to be a result of a fundamental imbalance of the autonomic nervous system. This imbalance may be more or less constant in certain nervously hypersensitive or constitutionally frail persons, but may also occur in relatively normal persons after psychic or physical upsets that act reflexly on the autonomic nervous system. The patient may be acutely aware of the most minor variations in the heart rhythm or rate. Palpitation may be so severe as a result of an occasional extrasystole or even mild exertion that the patient becomes more or less incapacitated.

In contrast to the characteristic symptoms listed above, there are no prominent physical signs in neurocirculatory asthenia. Tachycardia is often present, although the cardiac rate may be normal when mental and physical rest are established, only to increase again with slight exertion or with a disturbing thought. Such physical findings as cold, moist hands, excessive perspiration, tremor of the fingers, dermatographism, and variable and slightly elevated blood pressure are frequently encountered. The heart itself, in the majority of cases, is structurally normal and shows no significant murmurs. In addition, no characteristic laboratory findings have been identified in neurocirculatory asthenia. Many patients with these symptoms who previously would have been diagnosed as having neurocirculatory asthenia have been shown to have mitral valve prolapse that can produce identical symptomatology and may indeed be a cause of neurocirculatory asthenia.

MITRAL VALVE PROLAPSE

Mitral valve prolapse is quite a common condition and is found in approximately 10% of the population. From the clinical and symptomatic points of view, it occurs two to three times more frequently in women than in men. Although this condition may occur in association with ectodermal dysplasias, Marfan's syndrome, coronary artery disease, and ostium secundum defect among other conditions, it is usually idiopathic. These patients seem to have lax chordae tendeneae cordis, which allow the mitral valve to prolapse into the left atrium during systole. Many patients may also have tricuspid prolapse and some have abnormalities of the aortic valve as well. On physical examination, many of the patients have a murmur of mitral regurgitation that follows a midsystolic click. Others may be auscultatorily silent or have only a click. Various maneuvers such as standing using Valsalva technique and administration of amyl nitrate may accentuate or change the timing of either the click or the murmur.

The diagnosis of mitral valve prolapse is usually made by history and physical examination and then confirmed by echocardiogram. Since this condition is common, an argument can be made for obtaining an echocardiogram in a young patient with palpitation particularly if proved to be due to ventricular premature contractions. Almost half of these patients will at some time or another have complaints. These are often subjective palpitations, which on monitoring may not be associated with arrhythmias but often can be seen to correlate with diverse ventricular and atrial arrhythmias including ventricular premature contractions, ventircular tachycardia, supraventricular tachycardia, atrial fibrillation, atrial flutter, and sinus tachycardia. In many cases, the patient with mitral valve prolapse may exhibit a clinical picture closely resembling neurasthenia with complaints not only of palpitations but of fatigue, atypical chest pain, marked breathlessness, extreme anxiety, cold sweats, and so forth. Indeed, certain patients with mitral valve prolapse clearly meet all the diagnostic criteria for neurasthenia. Treatment of palpitations usually consists of reassurance, betablockers, and antiarrhythmic drug therapy if a specific arrhythmia is found warranting such therapy.

RELATIONSHIP OF PALPITATION TO ORGANIC HEART DISEASE

Persons with normal hearts may complain of palpitation whenever the force or the rate of the cardiac beat is increased to more than a moderate degree. On the other hand, patients with actual cardiac disorders as a rule are fortunately somewhat less sensitive than normal persons to the force and the rate of the cardiac beat. Perhaps this is a result in part of habituation, so that even in the presence of irregular rhythms or undue increase in rate, the abnormal stimuli do not penetrate the patient's consciousness and the reflex

phenomena at the basis of palpitation are not produced. Atrial fibrillation often is present when the patient has no sensation of any heart disorder. Occasionally these patients have palpitation temporarily after restoration to normal rhythm, although none was experienced when atrial fibrillation was present. In cardiac decompensation with profound disturbances of rate and rhythm, palpitation is not infrequently absent, even when dyspnea and orthopnea are severe.

Quite frequently extrasystoles are discovered of which the patient has no knowledge. Consciousness of an extrasystole is apt to be the awareness of a sudden premature forceful beat followed by a longer than usual pause, or, sometimes, there is chiefly perception of the hard postextrasystolic contraction. In contrast, patients with aortic valve disease including the lesions of stenosis or insufficiency, in which the cardiac beat may be extremely forceful and heaving, usually experience no palpitation. Sometimes the sensations that develop from benign extrasystoles can be very disturbing, as well as peculiar and distinctive, and it is well to be familiar with them since the description of the symptoms given by the patient may establish the diagnosis without further examination. The sensations are described in such varied ways as "a flop of the heart," "twisting or skipping of the heart," "sinking or fading away of the heart," "a sudden lump or choking feeling in the throat," "the heart turns a somersault," and "like the sensation of a fish turning in water." There may be fleeting lightheadedness or transient pain in the precordial or substernal area. These disturbances usually appear when the patient is relaxing or about ready to fall asleep, because at this time he is apt to become more conscious of any sensation occurring inside his body and because at rest the heart rate is slower and there is a greater opportunity during the longer diastolic pauses for premature beats to arise. The sensations are generally absent while the patient is active, walking, or busily engaged in his affairs.

Although it has been said repeatedly that extrasystoles are usually of no serious significance and that healthy people may have them, it was the animal experiments by Beattie and Brow that have made it possible to ascribe a definite neurogenic origin to them. They showed that if certain nerve tracts coming from the hypothalamic region were cut in animals with experimentally produced extrasystoles, the irregularity disappeared. They also found that if these tracts were cut beforehand, the extrasystoles could not be produced by the same technique that always produced them in animals not subjected to this treatment.

Thus it appears that there is a center in the brain that can initiate or is ultimately connected with the formation of premature heartbeats.

This demonstration points to a structural neurogenic basis for conditions that have long been regarded as functional. However, ventricular extrasystoles in the presence of organic heart involvement, and particularly coronary artery disease, are not benign. They may not only reflect the serious organic heart disease present but may predispose to fatal ventricular arrhythmias. The mechanism for these ventricular dysrhythmias may include increased automaticity of ischemic ventricular cells, conversion of some myocardial fibers into slow fibers with resultant delayed conduction, and increased temporal dispersion. Slow fibers also possess the characteristic of spontaneous fluctuations in resting potential, which may lead to the development of threshold potential and spontaneous activity. It has also been demonstrated in experimental myocardial infarction that some injured Purkinje cells may develop very prolonged durations of action potential. All these changes may give rise to ectopic ventricular activity, which may be potentially lethal.

RELATIONSHIP OF PALPITATION TO TACHYCARDIA

Palpitation, as previously stated, is a normal sensation when the force of the heartbeat and its rate are considerably elevated, and the subject may not only say he "feels his heart pounding" but that it is beating "too hard," "too fast," or both. Slight exertion in normal persons may cause only a little shortness of breath. When the activity is a little more strenuous, one is apt to become aware of the thumping of the heart against the chest wall. After rest the thumping sensation may persist for a while after the rate has returned to normal, showing that one may be aware of a "harder beat" (greater systolic contraction and cardiac output) when the rate is not increased. Persistence of tachycardia with greater cardiac activity beyond a normal or physiologic range of time suggests impaired cardiac reserve. Many of the physical fitness tests employed by the armed services are based upon accurate, graded observations of these phenomena in response to standard amounts of muscular effort.

Fortunately, persistent tachycardia is usually not accompanied by continual palpitation, or at least not to the degree that one might expect. Patients with cardiac decompensation whose pulse rates are over 100 per minute even at rest may have little or no palpitation. Although palpitation is a common symptom in thyrotoxicosis, there is often comparatively little consciousness of heart action. Persons with chronic infections resulting in longstanding fever and tachycardia often have no palpitation in spite of pulse rates that may be very rapid. It seems that in many of these instances physiologic readjustment takes place so that the subject becomes accustomed to the greater rate and

often the greater force of the cardiac contraction. A *sudden* alteration in rate or rhythm or in the force of the beat is apt to be perceived promptly whether the heart is normal or diseased. This is true whether the change is toward a slower, more orderly beat or toward rapid, irregular contraction. Static conditions, even though quite abnormal, may not be accompanied by palpitation.

TACHYCARDIA

The term *tachycardia* is derived from the Greek words *tachy* meaning quick and *cardia* meaning heart. Rapid action of the heart is the most common and obvious cardiac manifestation; accordingly, it is often the first to be discovered by the patient himself and by the physician. The rate of the heartbeat is the expression of the property of rhythmicity (automaticity) inherent in all parts of the heart muscle, but most highly developed in the specialized muscle cells that constitute the normal pacemaker. This pacemaker in the right atrium can keep the heart beating rhythmically independently of all extracardiac factors, as, for example, in the excised heart. However, in the body this inherent rhythm is always being modified. A great number of physiologic control mechanisms are capable of influencing the rate of the heartbeat. Practically all of these can be included under two headings, chemical control and nervous control.

CHEMICAL CONTROL

Chemical control of the heart is effected by certain ions and also by the more complex substances, hormones, which are secreted by the endocrine glands. The integrity of the living cell is dependent on a constant osmotic pressure of the surrounding extracellular fluid, which the body guards by various homeostatic mechanisms. The concentration of the sodium ion in extracellular fluid is responsible for almost all of the osmotic pressure due to cations, and its constancy may be regarded as a measure of the constancy of the osmotic pressure. When the concentration of sodium in the blood increases, the posterior pituitary gland is stimulated to secrete the antidiuretic hormone, water is retained by the kidney, and the normal concentration of sodium and the normal osmotic pressure are restored.

Potassium is the predominant intracellular electrolyte. A normal concentration of intracellular and extracellular potassium is essential for normal myocardial contraction. In the isolated heart, potassium antagonizes the tendency of calcium to cause systolic standstill (calcium rigor). When present in excess, potassium prolongs diastole and may cause complete inhibition with arrest of the heart. Various observations have suggested an intimate relationship between the action of the potassium ion and the action of acetylcholine, the humoral effector agent produced by vagal stimulation and muscular contraction by altering cell permeability. Changes in the concentration of potassium may produce clinical symptoms because of impairment of muscular activity or changes in the cardiac mechanism and the ECG.

Calcium ions (with sodium and potassium) are essential to proper cardiac contraction. The perfused isolated heart will stop in diastole if there is no calcium; an excess of calcium causes systolic arrest (calcium rigor). Like digitalis, calcium increases systolic contraction. Fear of a dangerous potentiating effect is a basis for the purported contraindication to the injection of calcium in digitalized patients.

Injected parathormone produces effects that are somewhat similar to those of calcium—an early increase in heart rate, followed by slowing and cardiac arrhythmia characterized by premature beats and shifting of the pacemaker.

The adrenal gland, when stimulated by its sympathetic nerve supply, secretes a mixture containing 80% *l*-epinephrine and 20% norepinephrine. The direct effect of *l*-epinephrine on strips of myocardium is to increase the speed, vigor, and power of myocardial contraction and to produce acceleration of the heart by acting on the pacemaker. In men, norepinephrine introduced into the bloodstream is reported to have a powerful vasoconstrictor effect on the peripheral vascular system but less effect on myocardial contraction. Increased contractile properties of the myocardium are noted, but the heart rate slows.

The circulatory response to hyperthyroidism resembles that of a normal person to strenuous exercise. The cardiac impulse is diffuse and forceful. The heart is accelerated. There is good evidence that the tachycardia from excess thyroid hormone (thyroxin) represents a direct effect on the pacemaker activity of the myocardium. Hyperthyroidism imposes a heavy load on the myocardium, which must put out more useful work to supply the augmented metabolic requirement of the body, while the efficiency of its contraction is diminished by tachycardia and by direct action of thyroid hormone on the myocardial fibers. When a patient with hyperthyroidism undertakes physical exertion, the circulatory reaction is exaggerated when compared with that of a normal person performing the same task. In young persons the heart may compensate for this excessive load, but in older persons cardiovascular reserves may become exhausted and heart failure supervenes. If coronary sclerosis is present, angina pectoris may become evident. Atrial fibrillation also is

likely to occur because of increased myocardial irritability.

Hypothyroidism, with its decrease in thyroxin, may result from spontaneous thyroid atrophy, surgical excision of thyroid tissue, or thyroid irradiation. One of its cardiac effects is the development of a slow heart rate. The thyroid hormones act primarily and directly upon the heart itself and may also affect it through the mediation of its autonomic nerve supply. The hormone control of the heart comes into play slowly, after a significant latent period following the original stimulus initiating the cardiac response. In contrast, cardiac responses evoked by nervous influences usually occur promptly, the latent period between the stimulus and the effect being short. Furthermore, the response by way of the nervous system is of relatively short duration, the effect disappearing promptly when the stimulus ceases, whereas effects produced by hormones tend to persist, outlasting the stimulus for some time.

NERVOUS CONTROL

Nervous control of the heart is effected through the vagus and the sympathetic nerves. Figure 16-1 is a diagrammatic representation of the cardiovascular reflex mechanisms. The vagus may be considered to be the more important of the two nerves. It is tonically active at all times and exerts a continuous restraining influence upon the heart, keeping it beating at a slower rate

than it would have if its intrinsic pacemaker, the sinoatrial node, were unchecked. This normal vagus tone is quite strong, and its removal leads to a marked and prompt increase in heart rate. Such removal or inhibition of the normal vagus tone is largely responsible for the tachycardia in nearly all the clinical conditions associated with acceleration of the heart.

Viewing the vagus nerve as the efferent limb of a reflex arc and the vagus center in the medulla as the center arc, the question arises as to what are the paths of the afferent impulses that reach the center and, by stimulating it, cause the heart to beat slower or, by inhibiting it, cause the heart to beat faster. Generally speaking, the potential afferent pathways capable of affecting the vagus center include all the afferent nerve fibers in the body. This concept means that all types of sensation from all parts of the body can affect the heart rate through the vagus center, although they may or may not do so according to circumstances. All afferent nerve impulses are conducted into some part of the central nervous system (spinal cord or brain), and, once within it, there is at least the possibility of a pathway to every center within the central nervous system. The actual flow of impulses from afferent to efferent paths is regulated by the very complex functional organization of the central nervous system. Thus, sudden distraction by a loud noise (8th cranial nerve) or immersion in hot water (cutaneous nerves) may precipitate a change in pulse rate (vagus nerve) by this

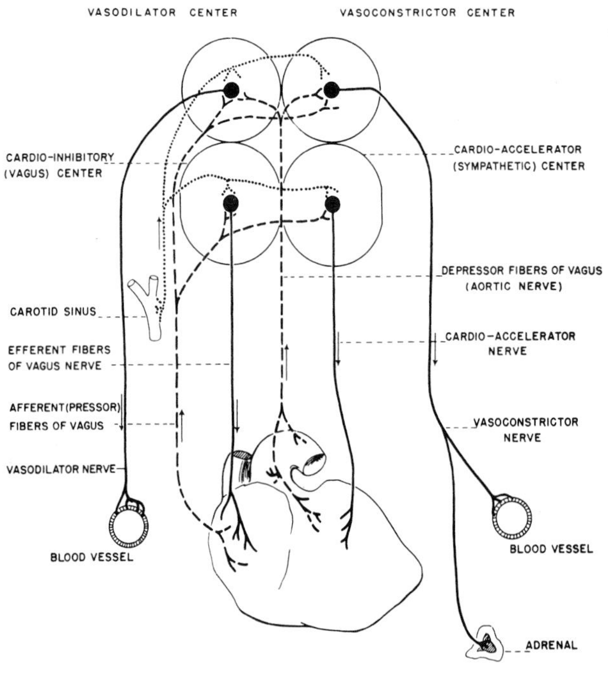

Fig. 16-1. Diagrammatic representation of the cardiovascular reflex mechanisms. Afferent vagal fibers are shown by broken lines; sinus nerve fibers, by a dotted line; efferent fibers to the heart and to the blood vessels, by a continuous line. The afferent fibers are represented as causing reciprocal effects upon the medullary centers. (From Best CH, Taylor NB: The Physiologic Basis of Medical Practice, 8th ed. Baltimore, Williams & Wilkins, 1968)

reflex mechanism. Obviously, not every type or intensity of sensation is uniformly potent in this respect, and the cardiac rate is not continuously interfered with by the usual sensations. Afferent impulses from certain regions are especially predominant in influencing the heart rate.

It is not surprising that the more important afferent impulses for controlling the heart arise in portions of the circulatory system itself, especially those regions from which the heart receives and into which it discharges the blood. On the venous or receiving end, the Bainbridge reflex causes acceleration of the heart when the venous return is so excessive that it overdistends the right atrium. The sensory endings of this reflex arc are in the right atrium and the adjacent portions of the venae cavae and are stimulated by increased tension. The resultant nerve impulses course along the afferent fibers in the vagus and inhibit the vagus center so that the heart beats faster, thus tending to raise the heart output to balance the inflow.

On the arterial side is the depressor reflex, whose afferent fibers arise from the root and arch of the aorta and run to the medulla within the vagus nerve. The initiating stimulus for these fibers is tension within the aorta; the higher the tension, the greater the stimulus. With elevation in the aortic pressure, afferent impulses ascend to and stimulate the vagus center so that the heart beats more slowly, and this action tends to reduce the blood pressure to its proper level. The reverse occurs also, since lowered aortic pressure gives rise to afferent nerve impulses that inhibit the vagus center and so accelerate the heart by diminishing the vagus tone. A similar depressor reflex, dependent primarily upon the pressure within the carotid artery for its activity, has its afferent nerve endings in the carotid sinus, which is a specially innervated part of the arteries and adjacent tissues located at the bifurcation of the common carotid artery. The afferent fibers from the carotid sinus reach the medulla by way of the glossopharyngeal and vagus nerves and the sympathetic trunk. The initiating stimulus is either increased or decreased intracarotid pressure, tending to slow or accelerate the heart by affecting the vagus center in a similar fashion to the aortic depressor fibers already described. The highly developed nerve endings located in the carotid body, which is situated at the bifurcation of the common carotid artery, are chemoreceptors and are sensitive to lack of oxygen and excess of carbon dioxide. When either of these conditions is present, impulses from the carotid body aid in accelerating the heart.

The higher centers of the brain itself also may be considered to be one of the special regions for initiating afferent impulses for cardiac control, since emotion may cause nerve impulses to descend to the medulla where they may affect the vagus center sufficiently to cause a change in heart rate. Increased intracranial pressure usually is associated with slowing of the heart, brought about by overstimulation of the vagus center. The stimulation may be due both to direct mechanical effect on the vagus center cells in the medulla and to ischemia of the center from the adverse effect of the pressure upon the blood supply. Furthermore, ischemia, when not too severe, stimulates practically all of the medullary centers including the vasomotor centers; therefore, increased intracranial pressure causes peripheral constriction and consequent elevation of blood pressure. The vascular hypertension thus produced in turn acts upon the aorta and the carotid sinus to stimulate the depressor reflexes already described and is therefore a secondary reason for cardiac slowing in increased intracranial tension.

The sympathetic and vagus centers in the medulla together from a functional unit referred to as the cardiac center. The quantity and quality of the blood reaching this center affect the heart rate. Slight hypoxia of the cardiac center causes increased cardiac rate, as does a small excess of carbon dioxide; a high degree of oxygen lack causes slowing of the heart, and a large excess of carbon dioxide may lead to heart block. These effects occur by means of efferent impulses coursing along the vagus, or the sympathetic nerves, or both. Increased temperature of the blood going to the center increases cardiac rate. Increased intracranial tension from any local cause tends to decrease the blood flow to the cardiac center and results in heart rate acceleration.

The sympathetic nerve control of the heart is subordinate to the vagus control, because under normal resting conditions it is quite inactive and upon stimulation the acceleration of the heart begins only after a definite latent period and then develops gradually. If the normal sympathetic acceleration influence is entirely removed, the resultant cardiac slowing is usually negligible. In addition, the latency of the response upon stimulation of the sympathetic trunk renders it relatively ineffective when there is need of prompt increase in the activity of the heart. However, since its effect manifests itself later than that wrought by the vagus, it persists longer and so maintains the responses initiated by the vagus. Usually increased sympathetic tone simultaneously induces secretion of adrenalin, which further prolongs the acceleration of the heart. The sympathetic efferent nerve center is in the medulla. The afferent paths by which impulses may reach and affect it are identical with those already mentioned in connection with the vagus cardiac center.

Similarly, the cardiovascular sensory areas of the right atrium, the root of the aorta, and the carotid sinus,

which are related to vagus control, have an analogously intimate relationship with sympathetic control. Consequently, cardiac acceleration from an overdistended atrium, though predominantly brought about by inhibition of the vagus center, is partially produced by sympathetic nerve stimulation, and slowing of the heart by the vagus in the depressor reflex is enhanced by concomitant decrease in sympathetic tone. In most instances, however, the chief portion of the total response is effected through the vagus, and to a much lesser extent through the sympathetic.

Stimulation of the right stellate ganglion shortens repolarization of the Q–T segment, whereas left stellate ganglion stimulation prolongs the Q–T interval and increases the duration of the action potential. Experimentally, stimulation of the latter is often accompanied by ventricular arrhythmias, since prolonged repolarization increases temporal dispersion and results in areas of the ventricle having markedly different potentials during repolarization, with potential excitation and response of ventricular tissues during the relative refractory period. Left stellate ablation has been used to treat the life-threatening ventricular arrhythmias associated with congenital prolongation of the Q–T interval.

TYPES OF TACHYCARDIA

The varieties and causes of tachycardia are so numerous that a classification is necessary. The most common type of tachycardia is that originating in the sinoatrial node. This is called sinoatrial tachycardia or simply sinus tachycardia. Next in frequency is paroxysmal atrial tachycardia, followed by rapid heart action associated with atrial fibrillation and atrial flutter. A relatively rare but more serious form of tachycardia is that arising from the ventricles called ventricular tachycardia; this may in turn predispose the heart to ventricular flutter and fibrillation. A less common form of paroxysmal tachycardia is that originating from the junctional tissue.

Sinus Tachycardia

Sinoatrial tachycardia, sinus tachycardia, or *simple tachycardia,* as it is otherwise known, is defined by Herrman as a "sustained increase in the heart rate beyond the normal limits of the individual." Usually a rate of 100 beats or more per minute in a person over the age of 18 years is evidence enough to justify a diagnosis of sinus tachycardia. Although there is a wide range of the normal pulse rate at rest, a rate of over 100 beats per minute in the heart of a normal resting adult is infrequent. In contrast, the upper range of normal in children is about 120, whereas in infants it is 150.

Etiology. Sinoatrial tachycardia occurs in persistent form in many healthy persons and is found normally as a trait in certain families. Transient sinus tachycardia is of daily occurrence in all persons as a physiologic response to physical exertion, ingestion of food, emotion, pain, and the application of heat to the body. It is particularly likely to appear when alcohol, tobacco, coffee, or the like are used to excess. Caffeine, for example, acts by direct stimulation of the myocardium. Rarely is a person found who can accelerate his pulse at will, and then usually because he has learned how to arouse an intense emotion. This ability has been used by malingerers to simulate heart disease. The effect is mediated through the sympathoadrenal system. Pathologic causes of sinoatrial tachycardia particularly include infections and fever; the pulse rate in general rises about 9 beats per minute for each degree Fahrenheit of temperature elevation. This increase probably is partly due to the direct effect the high temperature on the heart, because the beating of the excised heart has been shown to be accelerated by warming.

Another abnormal cause of tachycardia includes a group of noninfectious noxious disturbances, prominent among which is thyrotoxicosis. Thyroxin accelerates the heartbeat by direct action on the heart muscle fibers and also indirectly by increasing the metabolic rate.

Another pathologic cause of tachycardia is infarction of some part of the body in a sufficiently large area to give rise to reactions with fever and often leukocytosis. Shock and hemorrhage usually produce tachycardia as a compensatory reflex reaction to the lowered blood pressure.

Certain drugs, particularly epinephrine (by direct effect on the myocardium and conduction tissue), atropine (by blocking of vagal effects on the sinoatrial pacemaker), and the nitrites (through a carotid sinus reflex resulting in sympathoadrenal discharge), cause sinus tachycardia.

Episodes of neurocirculatory asthenia and mental shock often are associated with a rapid pulse. Sometimes the cause of tachycardia cannot be definitely discovered.

The heart in congestive failure accelerates to a greater or lesser degree in an effort to maintain the volume of blood flow. Acceleration of beat, however, is not an intrinsic adaptation of the heart to increased workload, since, in the heart–lung preparation, accommodation to increased arterial resistance or greater venous return is accomplished without any change in the rate of the heart. It is not that the heart in such a preparation is unable to accelerate, because elevation in temperature is followed promptly by increase in rate.

These observations on the isolated heart indicate that

extrinsic mechanisms—nervous or chemical—are involved in the production of compensatory tachycardia in heart failure. Among the mechanisms that appear to be concerned are the Bainbridge and carotid sinus and aortic reflexes, which have been discussed previously. It appears quite likely that, in the state of heart failure in which diminished cardiac output and elevated venous pressure are generally combined, these various reflexes are primarily responsible for the production of tachycardia.

Symptoms. The symptoms displayed by a person with sinoatrial tachycardia vary from little more than the objective sign of an increased pulse rate to a syndrome that may inhibit the normal activity of the patient. Palpitation is the most common of the symptoms encountered, although restlessness, agitation, apprehension, anxiety, and chest discomfort or pain also may be present, depending upon the symptom threshold and the nervous reactivity of the individual patient.

Diagnosis. As a rule, the diagnosis of sinoatrial tachycardia is obvious and clearly related to the exciting factor. The cardiac rhythm is usually regular, but shows fluctuations in rate in response to forced respiration and other physiologic stimuli, such as emotion and effort. In differentiating it from other forms of tachycardia, it should be remembered that sinus tachycardia has a gradual onset and a slight variation of the beat compared with the abruptness and marked regularity characterizing paroxysmal atrial or nodal tachycardia. Cases in which the increased pulse rate is due to psychogenic factors or an emotional imbalance generally exhibit a marked reduction in the pulse rate during sleep. Instances due to drug administration are easily singled out by a careful history. It is probable that many of the attacks called paroxysmal atrial tachycardia are really attacks of sinus tachycardia. This is especially true when the heart rate is not about 150 to 160. The electrocardiographic findings in sinus tachycardia are illustrated in Figure 16-2.

Prognosis. The prognosis of patients with sinoatrial tachycardia *per se* is good. In any given case, it depends primarily on the fundamental cause of the tachycardia. In those instances in which serious heart disease is already present, the myocardial or coronary reserve may be so limited that the tachycardia itself could precipitate heart failure.

Paroxysmal Atrial Tachycardia

Paroxysmal atrial tachycardia (PAT) is the most frequent of the abnormal or ectopic tachycardias. Its incidence is impossible to determine with any degree of accuracy because many persons may have short paroxysms of this type of tachycardia lasting seconds or minutes that are not interpreted as such, either because they are not sufficiently troublesome to excite concern on the part of the person affected or because there is no opportunity to obtain an ECG at the time of the paroxysms.

Mechanism. The mechanism of atrial tachycardia consists of a rapid and regular sequence of abnormal heartbeats originating in the atrium either from a given point outside the normal pacemaker or as a type of movement re-entering the atrial muscle, which in turn is recovering rapidly from its refractory stage. The site of origin of a paroxysm of atrial tachycardia may be in any part of the atrial musculature. The electrocardiographic picture resembles a series of premature atrial contractions occurring in quick succession. Electrocardiographically, the atrial complex differs from the normal P wave inasmuch as the origin of the impulse is abnormal and the course it takes through the atrium is likewise abnormal. The QRS complexes are similar in configuration to the QRS complexes of the basic mechanism unless aberration occurs. In such cases,

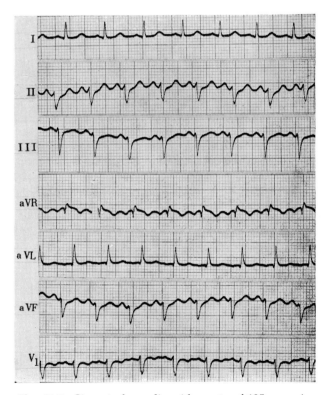

Fig. 16-2. Sinus tachycardia with a rate of 125 per min. (From Lipman B, Massie E: Clinical Scalar Electrocardiography, 5th ed. Chicago, Year Book, 1965)

slurring, notching, or widening of the QRS associated with defective conduction is present. There is now increasing evidence that paroxysmal atrial tachycardia is most often secondary to a re-entrant type of mechanism in which a circus type motion is produced by unidirectional block and slow conduction through junctional tissue. The area of block and slow conduction usually is in the atrioventricular node, but may also occur in the sinoatrial junction. Occasionally PAT or supraventricular tachycardia is secondary to increased automaticity in an ectopic atrial focus.

Atrial tachycardia may be confused with junctional tachycardia, particularly when the P waves are not identifiable. The two conditions, in this instance, are frequently grouped together under the term *supraventricular tachycardia*. At times difficulty may be encountered in differentiating slow paroxysmal atrial tachycardia from rapid sinus tachycardia. Paroxysmal atrial tachycardia has a rate that varies from 150 to 250 beats per minute.

Etiology. Paroxysmal atrial tachycardia may occur at any age, but it is rare in infancy. It is found more often in the absence of heart disease than in its presence; yet if we compare the relative incidence in normal persons and in cardiac patients, we find a higher incidence of paroxysmal atrial tachycardia in cardiac patients. It is frequently associated with indigestion, overexertion, fatigue, excess use of tobacco, alcohol, or coffee. It may be psychogenic in origin and may start with a specific emotional reaction. It may be associated with various infections. Thyrotoxicosis should be suspected in every case until eliminated. Among the various forms of organic heart disease accompanied by paroxysmal atrial tachycardia, mitral stenosis probably has the highest incidence.

Paroxysmal atrial tachycardia also occurs frequently in the Wolff–Parkinson–White syndrome or pre-excitation syndrome. In this condition, there is an anomalous pathway between the atrium and ventricle that bypasses the normal conducting pathway; thus conduction along this anomalous path produces a shortened PR interval and an abnormal QRS, since the ventricle is excited away from the usual site. Because of the dual pathways, re-entrant tachycardias are likely to occur. Usually the re-entrant pathway is such that antegrade conduction is through the A–V node and retrogade through the accessory pathway.

Symptoms. In most cases of PAT the patient is conscious of the disturbance of heart rhythm. The attack itself is instantaneous in onset and offset, and the patient is usually aware of this, describing it as coming on suddenly and stopping with a "thump." The patient complains of palpitation or fluttering of the heart, pounding in the chest, fullness in the neck; he becomes uneasy, nervous, dizzy, and apprehensive, and desires to lie down. Occasionally there is pain over the heart, and there may be typical anginal distress even with radiation to the arms. Sometimes nausea and vomiting occur, and then attacks often cease. This experience suggests to the patient that it is all produced by indigestion or some recently eaten food. After a length of time, varying from minutes to hours or even days, the attack ends and the patient quickly recovers either in good condition or in a sufficiently weakened state to remain inactive for a day or two. The distress experienced depends primarily on the duration of the attack, the cardiac rate, and the condition of the heart before the attack occurred.

Diagnosis. The diagnosis of paroxysmal atrial tachycardia is simple in most cases. It is important to elicit evidence of an abrupt change in rhythm with an approximate doubling of heart rate. Usually the cardiac beat ranges from about 150 to 250 per minute. Although usually sudden cessation of the episode occurs, sometimes the attack does not appear to stop abruptly. This is because, in spite of the considerable drop in rate at the end of the paroxysm, the sinoatrial rate when the heart resumes normal rhythm is elevated by excitement or other causes, preventing the obvious sensation of marked change in the cardiac rhythm that occurred at the onset of the attack. Not only is the heart rapid and regular but its rate is very fixed for long intervals of time and cannot be altered by simple procedures like breathing or exercise, which affect the rate of the normal heart. If repeated counts of the heartbeat taken at the bedside several minutes apart show a significant difference in rates, it speaks against the diagnosis of paroxysmal atrial tachycardia.

The various methods that are used to stop an attack also serve as diagnostic procedures, because there is no other type of rapid heart action that can be made to return to a normal rate by such simple means and so quickly. If vagus stimulation is produced by pressure over the carotid sinus in this type of arrhythmia, the rate either remains unaltered or abruptly falls to the normal sinus range. With normal tachycardia or atrial flutter, there is apt to be temporary slowing with gradual return to the previous rate, and when ventricular tachycardia is present vagus stimulation produces no effect. The ECG is almost invariably diagnostic (see Fig. 16-3), but there are a few puzzling records in which the tracing, unless it is taken at the beginning of the paroxysm, is not adequate to eliminate definitely a rare case of sinus tachycardia or atrial flutter. Another both diagnostic and therapeutic measure helpful in paroxysmal atrial or supraventricular tachycardia (SVT) is

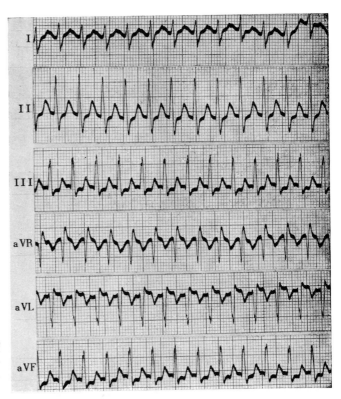

Fig. 16-3. Paroxysmal atrial tachycardia with a rate of 190 per min. The P and T waves are superimposed. (Lipman B, Massie E: Clinical Scalar Electrocardiography, 5th ed. Chicago, Year Book, 1965)

the infusion of 5 mg or 10 mg of verapamil over two minutes. Over 90% of PAT or SVT reverts to normal sinus rhythm with this procedure.

Prognosis. The prognosis of paroxysmal atrial tachycardia is usually excellent as to life expectancy, but there are rare instances in which the tachycardia is so excessive that cardiac failure results even in a normal person. It is always a more important disturbance, however, in the presence of serious heart disease. The cardiac conditions that are likely to be overburdened by this type of tachycardia include mitral stenosis, coronary insufficiency, and enlargement of the left ventricle. The tendency to recurrence of attacks varies greatly from only a few attacks in a lifetime to almost daily paroxysms.

PAROXYSMAL ATRIAL TACHYCARDIA WITH ATRIOVENTRICULAR BLOCK

There is another form of atrial tachycardia that is associated with varying degrees of atrioventricular block. The rising incidence of this arrhythmia and its significance with reference to digitalis intoxication have been gaining attention in recent years. Levine and Lown observed a number of patients with paroxysmal atrial

tachycardia with atrioventricular block (PAT with block). In their series, originally it was considered that only a comparative few of these patients had attacks in which digitalis intoxication could not be implicated as a causative factor; however, as time has gone on, it now appears that, in a certain number of instances (perhaps as many as half), digitalis is not involved. Many of the patients who have developed paroxysmal atrial tachycardia with block have this rhythm precipitated by potassium loss during excessive diuresis.

The electrocardiographic features of PAT with block are as follows:

1. *The onset is more gradual than that of supraventricular tachycardia without A–V block.* The normal P waves become progressively altered in appearance as the ectopic forces stimulate the atrium. Then the rate of this pacemaker speeds up with a 1:1 atrioventricular response initially, followed by the onset of variable atrioventricular block.

2. *The differentiation of the atrial flutter pattern from PAT with block may be difficult at times,* especially if the atrial rate is approximately 200 beats per minute. The atrial rate in the latter rhythm is usually between 150 and 190 beats per minute, and seldom exceeds 200 beats per minute.

3. *The A–V block is a constant 2:1 in only 30% of the pa-*

tients, the remainder showing variable and often inconstant degrees of block. The degree of A–V block can be increased by vagal stimulation and decreased by atropine or exercise.

4. *Unlike the common form of supraventricular tachycardia, the atrial mechanism in PAT with block, with rare exceptions, cannot be converted to sinus rhythm by carotid sinus stimulation or other simple measures that increase the vagal tone.* Generally, its response to various therapeutic agents more closely resembles that of atrial flutter than that of atrial tachycardia. When the P wave is superimposed on the QRS and T deflections, as is often the case, the diagnosis may be overlooked easily. Recognition of the mechanism often depends on a high degree of suspicion, as well as on vagal maneuvers that increase the degree of A–V block and uncover the concealed P wave. Suspicion may be aroused by a knowledge of the clinical picture or by the appearance of a newly developed, unexplained, persistent deformity of the QRS complex, the ST segment, or the T wave. Figure 16-4 shows an example of paroxysmal atrial tachycardia with 2:1 atrioventricular block.

5. *The interatrial intervals in paroxysmal atrial tachycardia with block are isoelectric,* and the P waves are upright in leads II, III, and AVF. The reverse is usually the case, with atrial flutter.

6. *Digitalis-induced paroxysmal atrial tachycardia with block has a characteristic response to potassium or Dilantin administration.* The atrial rate slows and the atrioventricular conduction improves with eventual 1:1 conduction. At this point, the ventricular rate may actually accelerate. Further administration of potassium or Dilantin then results in conversion to normal sinus rhythm.

Atrial Flutter

A still higher degree of atrial disturbance is atrial flutter. It is relatively uncommon, its incidence being less than one-twelfth that of atrial fibrillation.

Mechanism. The mechanism producing atrial flutter (and also that causing atrial fibrillation) has been the subject of lively controversy for much of the last decade, and the divergence of opinion is just as marked now as ever. Although investigations in recent years

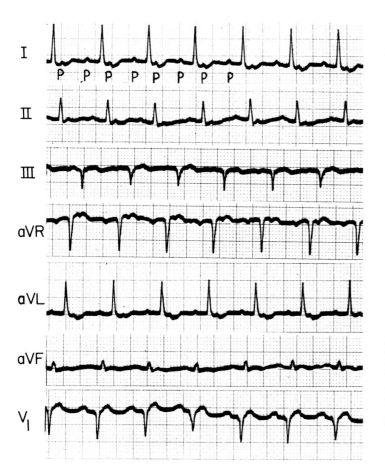

Fig. 16-4. Paroxysmal atrial tachycardia with 2:1 atrioventricular block associated with digitalis intoxication in a man 55 years of age. The rate of the paroxysmal atrial tachycardia is 200 beats per min, while the ventricular rate is exactly one-half as fast. The symbol *P* indicates the ectopic atrial beats in Lead I. (Massie E, Walsh T: Clinical Vectorcardiography and Electrocardiography. Chicago, Year Book, 1960)

have provided new and important information concerning the genesis of these two rhythms, none of these data incontestably prove or refute any of the theories currently favored. These theories are three in number: the concept of circus movement, the theory of multiple re-entry, and the theory of focal or multifocal impulse formation.

Atrial flutter is a very rapid regular atrial beat that replaces the normal atrial contraction. A rapid series of impulses is initiated in an ectopic area in either atrium. The atrial rate varies between 200 and 400 beats per minute, but following quinidine administration it may slow to less than 150. Usually the ventricular rate is only a fraction of that of the atria, since junctional tissue cannot conduct impulses so rapidly and a certain degree of atrioventricular block results. In exceptional cases, all atrial beats come through the ventricles; then the heart rate is extremely rapid. Commonly the ratio of atrial to ventricular beats is 2:1 and less often 4:1, or even 5:1 or 6:1. Not infrequently the ventricular response is irregular as a result of a changing atrioventricular block.

Etiology. Unlike paroxysmal atrial tachycardia, which usually occurs in otherwise normal hearts, atrial flutter is apt to be associated with organic heart disease, either valvular or myocardial, although it can occur as a purely functional disturbance. Its incidence is probably highest in cases of mitral stenosis, hypertension, and coronary heart disease. Occasionally one encounters it in patients with severe thyrotoxicosis. It can also occur in pericarditis. Atrial flutter occurs chiefly in adults, and the exciting factors are the same as those for paroxysmal atrial tachycardia.

Symptoms. Symptoms of atrial flutter are produced when the rate of the ventricle is rapid, but are more common in the paroxysmal form of atrial flutter or if heart disease is advanced. The typical symptom is rapid, regular, forceful palpitation subjectively indistinguishable from paroxysmal tachycardia. Symptoms of congestive heart failure may be coincidental or may result from the rapid ventricular action. Pain is rare, although precordial aching may occur. The patient may be made nervous and apprehensive from the alarm occasioned by the attack. If the ventricular rate is very rapid, as in 1:1 rhythm, and the heart rate approaches 300 per minute, dizziness, weakness, and partial or complete syncope may result as a consequence of cerebral anemia and other effects of greatly reduced cardiac output.

Diagnosis. The diagnosis of atrial flutter is easily made with ECG but with difficulty any other way. Atrial flutter is characterized at the bedside by long-continued rapid beating at a precise rate. Temporary halving of the heart rate spontaneously, by exercise, or by carotid sinus pressure is suggestive of this arrhythmia. Carotid sinus pressure slows the ventricle in "jumps" because it does not, as a rule, alter the atrial rate but only the ratio of atrial impulses conducted to the ventricle. Upon removal of the carotid sinus pressure, the ventricular rate returns to its previous level, but often the return occurs in an irregular though rapid fashion. Strenuous exercise, on occasion, also causes a sudden change in the ventricular rate that reverts to its original level when the exertion is over. The neck veins always should be inspected for the presence of the rapid regular atrial waves. For this type of examination, the patient should be placed in such a position that the neck veins are only partially filled.

The ECGs of atrial flutter are very peculiar and characteristic. In lead I, the atrial waves are represented by small notches. In leads II and III, the waves have a triangular form. The upstroke is sharp and smooth and the downstroke more prolonged and notched at its midpoint. The flutter waves are continuous, and as one cycle ends the next begins. They often resemble a tuning–fork record and at other times a picket fence. The rhythm of the atria is strikingly regular. The ventricular rate and rhythm depend on the degree of heart block. With experience, one learns to detect flutter from the appearance of the ECGs, but if there is any doubt as to the underlying mechanism, slowing of the ventricular rate by vagal stimulation may allow the flutter waves to be more evident. Lead V_1 may be helpful in differentiating questionable cases, since it often shows most clearly evidences of atrial activity if carefully examined. Figure 16-5 shows the ECG of a patient with atrial flutter and 2:1 atrioventricular block.

Prognosis. The prognosis is less favorable for the atrial flutter than for paroxysmal atrial tachycardia because of the higher incidence of heart disease in association with flutter and because of the longer paroxysms. Sometimes the flutter continues in more chronic form lasting for years.

Atrial Fibrillation

Atrial fibrillation is closely allied with atrial flutter and has about 12 to 15 times the clinical incidence. It is one of the most common and most important disorders of cardiac rhythm. It is probably fourth in frequency as a disturbance of rhythm; sinoatrial tachycardia, premature beats, and paroxysmal atrial tachycardia rank first, second, and third, respectively. Atrial fibrillation, even the paroxysmal type, rarely escapes notice and with rare exceptions comes eventually under the scrutiny of a physician.

Mechanism. Atrial fibrillation represents the highest degree of atrial disturbance. In this condition, the

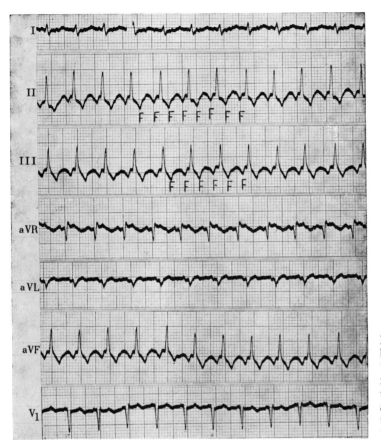

Fig. 16-5. Atrial flutter with 2:1 atrioventricular block. The atrial rate is 300 and ventricular rate 150 per min. Note that the atrial waves (*F*) are represented by small notches in Lead I and by triangular form of *P* waves in Leads II, III, and aVF. (Lipman B, Massie E: Clinical Scalar Electrocardiography, 5th ed. Chicago, Year Book, 1965)

number of atrial impulses per minute is very great, varying between 350 and 500. The impulses travel in a circus pattern in which the path is impure and irregular. The atria do not actually contract but rather remain distended in diastole and show fibrillary twitching. The speed of the atrial impulses is so great that areas of block or refractory points develop in the circuit, accounting for the irregularity of rate seen in the ECG. There is no constant pathologic finding in the atria to account for atrial fibrillation; accordingly, it is regarded as a functional derangement accompanying a number of conditions. This arrhythmia can be reproduced in a dog's atrium by a rapid series of faradic stimulations. The number of atrial impulses is so great that only a portion of them can be conducted through the junctional tissue. Consequently, there is always some degree of atrioventricular block associated with this arrhythmia. The ventricular response occurs in a grossly irregular fashion. The peripheral pulse is necessarily irregular both in time and in force. The ventricles respond irregularly, with an average rate of 100 to 140 per minute in untreated cases, but rates above 200 sometimes occur.

Etiology. Atrial fibrillation occurs chiefly in adults of both sexes and is very rare in early childhood. The incidence of atrial fibrillation increases with increasing years; it is common in old age. The most common conditions with which this arrhythmia is associated are rheumatic valvular disease with mitral stenosis, hypertensive heart disease, coronary artery disease, hyperthyroidism, various myopathies, and atrial septal defects, and it is associated with surgical procedures. It may develop precipitously during acute infections such as pneumonia and rheumatic fever. It is seen not infrequently during the early stages of an acute coronary thrombosis. Very rarely, it develops as a result of excessive digitalis therapy. In addition, there is the important group in which it is present either paroxysmally or permanently in otherwise healthy persons and without any apparent cause such as organic heart disease or even excesses of tobacco or alcohol. It may follow excitement, trauma, operations, or intoxications, particularly in nervously high-strung people or those with pericarditis.

Symptoms. Symptoms vary with the ventricular rate,

the underlying functional state of the heart, and the duration of the atrial fibrillation. In the chronic form, atrial fibrillation may exist without symptoms. Usually, however, the patient is aware of the irregular heart action and has such sensations as fluttering, skipping, irregular beating or a pounding, and heaving action. Palpitation is usually present and may be considered as the characteristic symptom of atrial fibrillation. Dyspnea and pain are much less common, but they may develop as a part of neurocirculatory asthenia if there is an associated marked psychic element. Although angina pectoris may appear, due to the extra work imposed by rapid heart action on a damaged myocardium, it is comparatively rare in atrial fibrillation, a fact that is best explained by the limitation of activity imposed by the arrhythmia itself and by medical advice. The entire symptomatic picture is particularly striking in the paroxysmal form, and there may also be the more general symptoms of anxiety, nervousness, pallor, cyanosis, and collapse. The patient may even harbor feelings of impending death. Successive attacks are apt to cause sufficient psychic trauma that chronic invalidism results even in the absence of signs of heart failure. Congestive failure may be coincidential with, precipitated by, or entirely caused by the rapid irregular ventricular action.

Diagnosis. The bedside recognition of atrial fibrillation is generally simple. A rapid, apparently grossly irregular heartbeat with an appreciable pulse deficit of 10 or more is due to atrial fibrillation in the majority of cases. In addition, any tachycardia at a rate of over 120 that is grossly irregular is most likely the result of this arrhythmia. When the patient has a history of rheumatic fever and the signs of mitral stenosis, atrial fibrillation occurs frequently and should be suspected if an arrhythmia is found.

The ECG gives immediate evidence of the condition and is of great diagnostic aid when there is a question of clinical interpretation. The normal P waves in the tracing are absent, and instead there are found irregular, rapid undulations (F waves) of varying amplitude, contour, and spacing. These F waves vary in form all the way from being clearly visible in most leads in coarse atrial fibrillation and impure flutter to being imperceptible in fine atrial fibrillation. There is a totally irregular ventricular spacing except in complete atrioventricular block, but, inasmuch as the course of impulses that succeed in reaching the ventricles travel down the normal atrioventricular conduction path, the ventricular complexes are normal in form. Figure 16-6 shows an example of the electrocardiograph finding in atrial fibrillation.

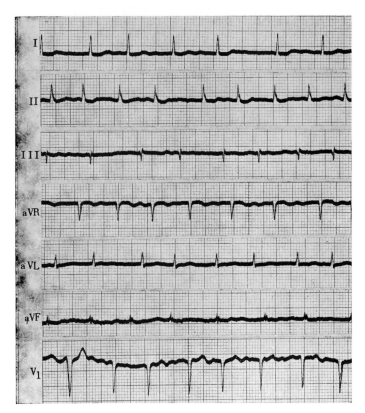

Fig. 16-6. Atrial fibrillation with an irregular ventricular rate of 75 to 110 per min. (Lipman B, Massie E: Clinical Scalar Electrocardiography, 5th ed. Chicago, Year Book, 1965)

Prognosis. The prognosis for patients with atrial fibrillation depends on the underlying heart condition and the treatment. In the absence of cardiac muscle or valve involvement, the prognosis is excellent. The attack, even though subsiding spontaneously, may in some instances recur. In the presence of heart disease, the result depends on the severity of the cardiac lesion and the ease of controlling the ventricular rate. It is possible to have recurrent episodes of atrial fibrillation over periods of many years in some patients, yet in those cases in which the heart is seriously involved, an attack may cause death in a matter of hours.

Paroxysmal Junctional Tachycardia

Paroxysmal junctional tachycardia is a relatively uncommon variety of paroxysmal tachycardia. It may be diagnosed only by electrocardiographic means, and even then the diagnosis is sometimes difficult. Because of the difficulty of distinguishing between paroxysmal junctional tachycardia and paroxysmal atrial tachycardia, these arrhythmias are frequently grouped together under the term *supraventricular tachycardia.* Paroxysmal junctional tachycardia is due to rapid impulse formation in the junctional tissue, both ventricles and atria being controlled from that center. The P waves of the ECG are inverted and just follow, precede, or occur simultaneously with the QRS complexes. An example is shown in Figure 16-7.

The etiology, symptomatology, and prognosis of this arrhythmia are similar to those of paroxysmal atrial tachycardia.

Multifocal Atrial Tachycardia

Multifocal atrial tachycardia is a rhythm characterized by a rapid, grossly irregular rate. Clinically, it is usually indistinguishable from atrial fibrillation since it is rapid, very irregular, and often associated with a pulse deficit. Electrocardiographically, however, there are P waves, but in any given lead there are three or more P wave morphologies. Frequently there are blocked atrial premature contractions, and also junctional premature beats. The ventricular rate is generally greater than 120 and on occasion may exceed 200 beats per minute. An example is shown in Figure 16-8. It is most often seen in the context of severe pulmonary disease, respiratory failure, with or without marked cardiac disease. Its presence often presages atrial fibrillation or flutter. Generally the therapy is that for the underlying disorder. It has an unfavorable prognosis and responds poorly to drug therapy. Occasionally it may be

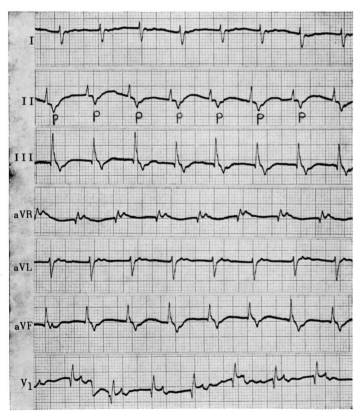

Fig. 16-7. Junctional rhythm with a rate of 108 per min. The atrial complexes (labeled *P* in Lead II) are retrograde in nature and may be seen in all the leads. (Lipman B, Massie E: Clinical Scalar Electrocardiography, 5th ed. Chicago, Year Book, 1965)

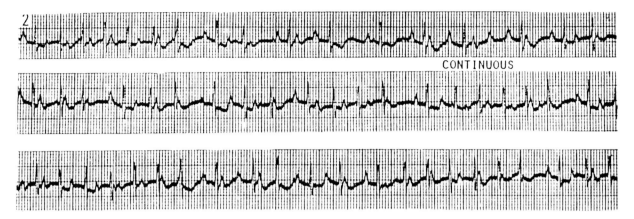

CONTINUOUS

Fig. 16-8. Multifocal atrial tachycardia with variable *P*-wave contour, rapid atrial rate, and fast and irregular ventricular response. (Courtesy of Marvin Dunn, MD, Director of the Division of Cardiovascular Diseases, University of Kansas School of Medicine)

made worse by theophylline or digitalis administration.

Bradycardia–Tachycardia Syndrome

Bradycardia–tachycardia syndrome is a type of so-called "sick sinus syndrome." There is marked dysfunction of sinoatrial activity so that patients may have periods of bradycardia due to a variety of mechanisms such as sinus bradycardia, sinoatrial block, junctional escape rhythm, ventricular and atrial standstill, alternating with periods of rapid rhythm, usually atrial fibrillation, atrial flutter, or paroxysmal atrial tachycardia, and sometimes even ventricular tachycardia. Following the bursts of tachycardia, the patient may have episodes of standstill, producing syncope of transient cerebral ischemic attacks. An example is shown in Figure 16-9. The tachycardia episodes often produce the complaints of palpitation, breathlessness, and chest pain. Therapy consists of implantation of a permanent pacemaker for the bradycardia and treatment with drugs such as digitalis, propranolol and quinidine for the tachyarrhythmias.

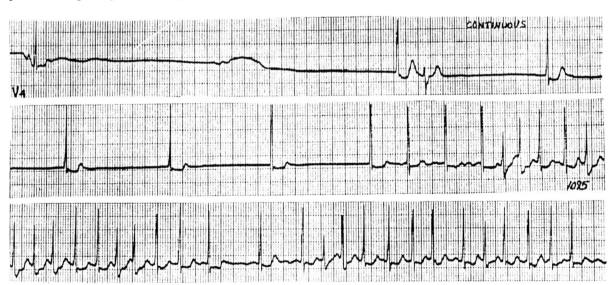

Fig. 16-9. Bradycardia–tachycardia syndrome in an elderly patient. Note periods of sinus bradycardia, sinoatrial block, junctional escape rhythms, and atrial and ventricular standstill alternating with periods of rapid rhythm, mostly atrial fibrillation. (Courtesy of Marvin Dunn, MD, Director of the Division of Cardiovascular Diseases, University of Kansas School of Medicine)

Paroxysmal Ventricular Tachycardia

Paroxysmal ventricular tachycardia is a comparatively rare arrhythmia and occurs approximately in the ratio of 1:8 compared with paroxysmal atrial tachycardia.

Mechanism. Paroxysmal ventricular tachycardia may be regarded as a consecutive series of ventricular extrasystoles arising from an ectopic focus in the ventricle. There is much in the nature of this mechanism that resembles a circus motion. Since it starts from an abnormal focus in the ventricle and the impulse travels an abnormal course, the resultant complex is necessarily unlike the normal configuration. Each complex resembles a ventricular extrasystole. The impulses may travel in a retrograde fashion up the junctional tissue and produce atrial contractions. Because the rate is rapid there may be a retrograde block, so that only every other ventricular impulse produces an atrial contraction. At other times the atria contract independently and follow their own pacemaker in the sinoatrial node.

Etiology. Paroxysmal ventricular tachycardia occurs in both sexes and, unlike paroxysmal atrial tachycardia, is much more common in older persons. It appears rarely in youth. It is a serious condition because of its much higher incidence among patients with important cardiac involvement or toxic states. Precipitating factors include acute myocardial infarction, toxic doses of digitalis, manipulation during cardiac catheterizations, coronary arteriography, and surgical procedures, particularly those involving manipulation of the heart and great vessels. The authors have recently encountered a 44-year-old male patient, who has had recurrent bouts of this arrhythmia associated with subacute lupus erythematosus. It very rarely occurs transiently in normal people.

Paroxysmal ventricular tachycardia is also rarely seen with mitral valve prolapse. A very special type of ventricular tachycardia called polymorphous ventricular tachycardia or *torsades de pointes* is seen in patients with prolonged QT intervals on their ECG. The prolonged QT may occur as a result of drugs such as quinidine, tricyclic antidepressants, or phenothiazines, as a result of a cerebral vascular accident, congenitally with or without deafness, or occasionally with ischemic heart disease. The rate of ventricular tachycardia is usually rapid, is between 160 and 280, has variable morphology often with twisting around the baseline, and may also be accompanied by isolated ectopic beats and short runs of three or four consecutive ventricular ectopic beats. This rhythm disturbance often progresses to ventricular fibrillation. Most patients with torsades have as their chief complaint, syncope but suggestive palpitations are also frequent.

Symptoms. The symptomatology of paroxysmal ventricular tachycardia resembles that of paroxysmal atrial tachycardia with the exception that these patients are usually seriously ill with some underlying disease; consequently, the tachycardia produces symptoms that are much more accentuated.

Diagnosis. Diagnosis can be made with certainty only by examining the ECG, which reveals abnormal-shaped QRS waves resembling repeated ventricular premature beats; the heart rate usually is about 160 to 180 per minute, and very rarely reaches the high levels of 220 or more that occur in atrial tachycardia. The atria beat independently, and the P waves sometimes may be seen clearly superimposed on the QRS and T waves. Paroxysmal ventricular tachycardia is sometimes difficult to differentiate from paroxysmal atrial tachycardia with bundle branch block when the P waves are hard to identify. A typical electrocardiogram is shown in Figure 16-10.

There are some bedside methods that enable one to elicit the presence of paroxysmal ventricular tachycardia. When paroxysmal, the attacks begin and end suddenly. The rate is rapid, but occasionally slight irregularities can be detected by auscultation, in contrast to that found with atrial tachycardia. The condition may be suspected if the heart rate rises abruptly to a level between 140 to 160 per minute or if the rate is above 160 and the rhythm is slightly irregular. In addition, upon careful examination, slight but suggestive differences in the intensity and quality of the first sound are heard in some cases as a result of the different relationship between the ventricular and atrial systoles in various cycles. Atrial pulsations as seen in the jugular vein are fewer in number than the ventricular rate, but this observation is especially difficult to make. However, in most cases of ventricular tachycardia there is independent beating of atria and ventricles (A–V dissociaton). As a result, periodically the atria and ventricles beat simultaneously, and thus the atrial contractions occur against a closed A–V valve. This produces a prominent jugular wave pulsation (cannon A wave) that occurs intermittently and establishes A–V dissociation. Because of the abnormal duration of ventricular excitation in this rhythm, both the first and second heart sounds may be abnormally widely split, and because of poor ventricular performance there is often a prominent diastolic gallop. Because of the A–V dissociation and changing P–R intervals, beats that by coincidence have normal P–R intervals have had better ventricular filling, since there is normal atrial contribution during diastole. These beats then have a higher stroke volume and thus engender a higher systolic blood pressure. Hence, ventricular tachycardia with

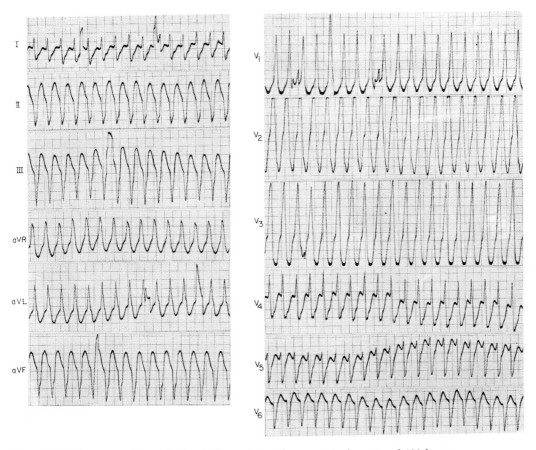

Fig. 16-10. Paroxysmal ventricular tachycardia with a ventricular rate of 188 beats per min. The ventricular complexes are bizarre in appearance and prolonged in duration. (Massie E, Walsh T: Clinical Vectorcardiography and Electrocardiography. Chicago, Year Book, 1960)

A–V dissociation is characterized by a phasic change in blood pressure that is not induced by respiration.

In some cases, the differentiation of ventricular tachycardia from supraventricular tachycardia with aberration requires invasive electrophysiologic cardiac studies. In these studies, surface recordings can be correlated with recordings from the high and low atrium, the His bundle, and from either right or left, or both ventricles, and atrial and ventricular pacing can be used to induce the arrhythmia under study. These studies are also useful in establishing appropriate therapeutic regimens. Finally, this type of rapid heart action is not influenced by any of the methods that stimulate the vagus nerve. The duration of the attacks is somewhat like that of paroxysmal atrial tachycardia (*i.e.,* minutes or hours, and rarely days).

Prognosis. The prognosis for patients with paroxysmal ventricular tachycardia is unfavorable because of the severe underlying heart disease or toxic condition. The occurrence of paroxysmal ventricular tachycardia usually indicates a short life, sometimes only a few hours and infrequently more than a few months or years.

Ventricular Flutter and Fibrillation

Ventricular flutter and fibrillation are related in the same way as are their analogous rhythms in the atria. Ventricular flutter is extremely rare. Ventricular fibrillation is, with few exceptions, an irreversible condition found in moribund patients and is one of the causes of sudden death. As in atrial fibrillation, the synergic contractions of the heart are replaced by an incoordinate quivering, each part of the ventricle beating independently. This incoordination directly suspends the pumping action of the heart, and fainting, coma, convulsions, and death occur unless the attack quickly

subsides. The pulse is absent, and the attack may resemble Adams–Stokes syndrome.

Diagnosis can be made only by electrocardiographic means. Ventricular flutter can be diagnosed in the ECG when regular continuous waves of large amplitude occur at a rate of over 250 per minute. In these deflections no distinction can be made between the QRS complex and the T wave. Ventricular fibrillation is diagnosed in the tracing by the absence of QRST complexes and the presence of irregular undulations of varying amplitude, contour, and spacing. The rate of these may vary from 250 to 500 per minute. The waves are larger than in atrial fibrillation, and no ordinary QRST complexes are seen. Transient ventricular fibrillation and/or torsades de pointes (see above) may be seen with quinidine syncope, in complete heart block, and with acute coronary vasospasm (Printzmetal's angina).

SUMMARY

Palpitation and tachycardia are among the most common complaints that cause patients to seek medical aid. Often, however, the complaint is the most grievous in the presence of the least serious organic disturbance. On the contrary, mild or moderate symptoms may indicate serious underlying disease. Palpitation often results from emotional or psychic disturbance and does not necessarily imply an organic cardiac condition. Increase in the force or rate of the heartbeat and the various cardiac arrhythmias may cause palpitation. Tachycardia, strictly speaking, is a physical sign, but it is often a symptom, with the subject complaining not so much of an awareness of the heartbeat (palpitation) as of a consciousness that the rate is excessive. Frequent or persistent tachycardia may result from metabolic or hormonal disorders, emotional disturbances, psychic or nervous system disease, infections and other conditions affecting the total organism, as well as cardiac disease. Every such complaint, therefore, deserves careful study until the mechanism is adequately understood. In this way the proper and logical therapeutic approach should become evident.

Particularly useful laboratory procedures in evaluating a complaint of palpitation may include the resting electrocardiogram, the stress ECG, extended ECG monitoring by either fixed wire, telemetry, or Holter systems, or event recorders activated by the patient that record on magnetic tape the ECG while the patient is symptomatic and allow phone transmission of the ECG. Often these tests establish that the subjective feeling of palpitations has no electrocardiographic basis or is solely due to relatively benign sinus tachycardia. On the other hand specific arrhythmias requiring appropriate therapy may be uncovered. Also useful are M mode and 2-dimensional echocardiography. These often reveal subtle structural abnormalities such as mitral valve prolapse or hypertrophic myopathy responsible for arrhythmias but not readily apparent.

BIBLIOGRAPHY

Barker PS, Wilson FN, Johnston FD: Mechanism of auricular paroxysmal tachycardia. Am Heart J 26:435–445, 1943

Barlow JB, Pocock WA: The problem of nonejection systolic clicks and associated mitral systolic murmurs: Emphasis on the billowing mitral leaflet syndrome. Am Heart J 90:636, 1975

Beattie J, Brow GR, Long CNH: Physiological and anatomical evidence for existence of nerve tracts connecting the hypothalamus with spinal sympathetic centres. Proc Roy Soc [Biol] 106:253–275, 1930

Bellet S: Current concepts in therapy: Drug therapy in cardiac arrhythmias, II. N Engl J Med 262:979–981, 1960

Bellet S: Clinical Disorders of the Heart Beat, 2nd ed. Philadelphia, Lea & Febiger, 1963

Best CH, Taylor NB: The Physiological Basis of Medical Practice, 8th ed. Baltimore, Williams & Wilkins, 1966

Bristowe JS: On recurrent palpitation of extreme rapidity in persons otherwise apparently healthy. Brain 10:164–198, 1887

Burchell HB: Cardiac manifestations of anxiety. Proc Staff Meet Mayo Clin 22:433–440, 1947

Campbell M, Elliott GA: Paroxysmal auricular tachycardia. Br Med J 1:123–160, 1939

Cooksey JD, Dunn M, Massie E: Clinical Vectorcardiography and Electrocardiography. Chicago, Year Book Medical Publishers, 1966

Cookson H: Aetiology and prognosis of auricular fibrillation. Q J Med 23:309–325, 1930

Criteria Committee of the New York Heart Association: Nomenclature and Criteria for Diagnosis of Diseases of the Heart and Blood Vessels, 6th ed. Boston, Little Brown & Co, 1964

Devereux RB, Perloff JK, Reichek N, Josephson ME: Mitral valve prolapse. Circulation 54:3, 1976

Ernstene AC: Diagnosis and treatment of the cardiac arrhythmias. Cleve Clin Q 16:185–195, 1949

Friedberg CK: Diseases of the Heart, 3rd ed. Philadelphia, WB Saunders, 1966

Goodman L, Gilman A: The Pharmacological Basis of Therapeutics, 3rd ed. New York, Macmillan, 1965

Hoffman BF, Cranefield PF: Electrophysiology of the Heart. New York, McGraw–Hill, 1967

Katz LN, Pick A: Clinical Electrocardiography, Part I: The Arrhythmias. Philadelphia, Lea & Febiger, 1956

Korth C: Production of extrasystoles by means of the central nervous system. Ann Intern Med 11:492–498, 1937

Levine SA: Clinical Heart Disease, 5th ed. Philadelphia, WB Saunders, 1958

Levine SA, Harvey WP: Clinical Auscultation of the Heart, 2nd ed. Philadelphia, WB Saunders, 1959

Lewis T: The Soldier's Heart and the Effort Syndrome, 2nd ed. London, Shaw & Sons Ltd, 1940

Lewis T: The Mechanism and Graphic Registration of the Heart Beat, 3rd ed. London, Shaw & Sons Ltd, 1925

Lewis T, Feil HS, Stroud WD: The nature of auricular flutter. Heart 7:191–243, 1920

Lipman BS, Massie E, Kleiger RE: Clinical Scalar Electrocardiography, 6th ed. Chicago, Year Book Medical Publishers, 1972

Luten D: The Clinical Use of Digitalis. Springfield, Ill, Charles C Thomas, 1936

Massie E, Walsh TJ: Clinical Vectorcardiography and Electrocardiography. Chicago, Year Book Medical Publishers, 1960

Mills P, Rose J, Hollingsworth J, Amara I, Craige E: Longterm prognosis of mitral-valve prolapse. N Engl J Med 297:13, 1977

Nash J: Surgical Physiology. Springfield, Ill, Charles C Thomas, 1942

Oppenheimer BS: Neurocirculatory asthenia and related problems in military medicine. Bull NY Acad Med 18:367–382, 1942

Prinzmetal M, Corday E, Brill IC, Oblath RW, Kruger HE: The Auricular Arrhythmias. Springfield, Ill, Charles C Thomas, 1952

Prinzmetal M, Corday E, Brill IC, Sellers AL, Oblath RW, Flieg WA, Kruger HE: Mechanism of the auricular arrhythmias. Circulation 1:241–245, 1950

Ravin A: Auscultation of the Heart, 2nd ed. Chicago, Year Book Medical Publishers, 1967

Rushmer RF: Cardiovascular Dynamics, 3rd ed. Philadelphia, WB Saunders, 1970

Sodi–Pallares D, Calder RM: New Bases of Electrocardiography. St Louis, CV Mosby, 1956

Stroud WD: Diagnosis and Treatment of Cardiovascular Disease, 3rd ed, vols 1 and 2. Philadelphia, FA Davis, 1945

Waldman S, Moskowitz SN: Treatment of attacks of sinus tachycardia with prostigmin. Ann Intern Med 20:793–805, 1944

Weiss E, English OS: Psychosomatic Medicine, 3rd ed. Philadelphia, WB Saunders, 1957

White PD: Tachycardia and its treatment: Mod Concepts Cardiovasc Dis 9:8, 1940

White PD: Neurocirculatory asthenia (Da Costa's syndrome, effort syndrome, irritable heart of soldiers). Mod Concepts Cardiovasc Dis 11:8, 1942

White PD: Heart Disease, 4th ed. New York, Macmillan, 1951

Wiggers CJ: Mechanism and nature of ventricular fibrillation. Am Heart J 20:399–412, 1944

Willius FA: Cardiac Clinics. St Louis, CV Mosby, 1941

Winkle RA, Harrison D: Propranolol for patients with mitral valve prolapse. Am Heart J 93:422, 1977

17

Cough John A. Pierce

Mechanism of Cough
Stimuli That Produce Cough
  Mechanical Stimuli
  Inflammatory Stimuli
  Chemical Stimuli
  Thermal Stimuli
  Psychogenic Stimuli
Characteristic Types of Cough
Conditions in Which Cough Occurs
  Inflammations
    Acute Pharyngitis
    Acute Laryngitis
    Acute Tracheobronchitis
    Pertussis
    Chronic Bronchitis
    Bronchiectasis
    Lobar Pneumonia
    Bronchopneumonia
    Lung Abscess
    Pulmonary Tuberculosis
    Deep Fungal Infections
    Parasitic Lung Diseases
    Opportunistic Lung Infections
  Cardiovascular Disorders
    Acute Pulmonary Edema
    Pulmonary Infarction
    Aortic Aneurysm

Trauma and Physical Agents
  Irritant Gases
  Pneumonoconioses
Neoplasms
  Primary Bronchogenic Carcinoma
  Metastatic Lung Tumor
  Bronchioalveolar Cell Carcinoma
  Mediastinal Tumors
  Bronchial Adenomas
Allergic Disorders
  Bronchial Asthma
  Hay Fever and Vasomotor Rhinitis
Other Causes of Cough
  Eosinophilic Granuloma
  Wegener's Granuloma
  Sarcoidosis
  Diffuse Fibrosing Alveolitis
  Alveolar Proteinosis
  Right Middle Lobe Syndrome
  Transvenous Endocardial Pacemakers
Complications of Cough
  Cough Fractures
  Cough Syncope
Sputum
Treatment of Cough
Summary

Respiratory gas exchange requires such large volumes with ventilation that particulate matter inevitably enters the airways with the inspired air. The tracheobronchial tree branches in a manner that effectively filters out particulate matter by impaction. Particles larger than 20 μ usually deposit in the nose, mouth, or nasopharynx. Particles 10 to 20 μ in diameter may reach the trachea. Smaller particles deposit in the bronchi so that the only particles that reach the respiratory bronchioles and more distal lung parenchyma are less than 2 μ in diameter. The ideal size for particle deposition in the lung parenchyma is 1 μ, and particles 0.1 μ or smaller that enter the parenchyma generally are not deposited but return suspended in the expired air.

Two specific mechanisms exist for clearance of such particles from the parenchyma of the lung. (1) A thin layer of mucus is propelled by continuous ciliary motion from the level of the terminal bronchioles toward the trachea. Particles that land on this surface may move toward the larynx at a rate of 1 mm–15 mm per minute. (2) The second protective clearance mechanism is cough. Cough may effectively empty the tracheobronchial tree of secretions proximal to the level of the segmental bronchi. If the mucous blanket is considered the escalator to the lungs, cough is the high speed elevator. Cough has been referred to as a backup defense mechanism that is called into play whenever mucociliary clearance is ineffective or overloaded. Few words are more precisely onomatopoetic than cough. The act is under voluntary control, but occurs involuntarily when stimulated through a reflex arc. A cough that is not followed by expectoration is termed nonproductive or dry. Cough that is followed by expectoration is termed productive and qualified as loose or wet. The sound of wet cough is rather characteristically a wheeze interrupted by sharp rasping noises that are produced as secretions move from the distal to the more proximal bronchi.

MECHANISM OF COUGH

Cough occurs in three distinct phases. Air drawn into the lungs immediately before cough constitutes the inspiratory phase. Closure of the glottis and contraction of the thoracic and abdominal muscles comprise the compressive phase. Abrupt decompression occurs with sudden opening of the glottis and acceleration of the intrathoracic gas during the expulsive phase of the cough. The vigor of the cough is determined by the volume of the precough inspiration, the intensity of the compressive effort, and the rapidity of onset of the expulsive phase of the cough. Although the precough activity of inspiration and compression are essential components, the useful effect of cough occurs only during the expulsive phase.

Understanding the mechanics of cough requires an understanding of the forces involved. Figure 17-1 presents a diagram of maximal pressure–volume of the lungs–thorax system. Pressure from the contraction of the thoracic muscles has been measured at the nose, but with the glottis open. It is apparent that muscular contraction produces maximal positive intrathoracic pressure (relative to atmospheric pressure) when the lungs are fully inflated. Conversely, maximal negative intrathoracic pressure is achieved at levels near full expiration, or residual volume level of lung inflation. At moderate levels of lung inflation, the maximal deviations (from atmospheric pressure) of which the thoracic muscles are capable approximates −60 to +70 Torr (mm Hg).

It should be mentioned that all deviations of intrathoracic pressure from atmospheric pressure are imposed on the heart and great vessels. This, naturally, has no relevance to the relationships between thoracic intravascular pressures as, for example, between aortic and left atrial pressure. However, these pressures are important in altering the relationships between intra- and extrathoracic pressures within the vessels. A high positive intrathoracic pressure, for example, precludes the entry of blood into the right atrium and during intense cough compression may result in an intense facial cyanosis due to the regurgitation of blood from the superior vena cava into the facial veins.

It is pertinent that free venous communication exists between intrathoracic and intracranial veins. Cerebrospinal fluid pressure thus parallels intrathoracic pressure.

Reflexes from the respiratory tract, as with all reflexes, require five components. These include peripheral receptors, afferent pathways, centers, efferent pathways, and effector mechanisms. From the lungs the afferent pathways are mainly through the vagal and superior laryngeal nerves. The cough center lies in the medulla near the midline. The efferent pathways are mainly through the phrenic and intercostal nerves, and the principal effector organs are the diaphragmatic and intercostal muscles. Histologically, there are no differences in the appearance of the epithelial nerve endings in the different parts of the respiratory tract. Cough receptors are localized mainly in the trachea, especially in the posterior wall, and in the large bronchi. The bronchial nerve endings are localized at bifurcations. These receptors are sensitive to touch or pressure. The afferent pathway is through myelinated fibers in the vagus nerve.

The smaller airways contain irritant receptors sensitive to chemicals such as ethyl ether and ammonia

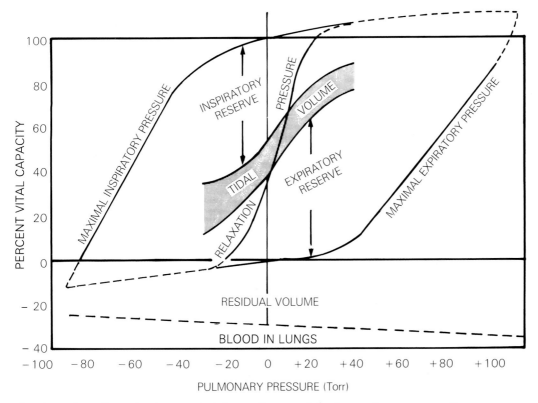

Fig. 17-1. Overall maximal pressure-volume diagram of the lungs–thorax system. Pressure attained by contraction of thoracic muscles was measured at the nose with glottis open. Note the maximal positive intrathoracic pressure is produced when the lungs are fully inflated; conversely, maximal negative intrathoracic pressure is achieved at levels near full expiration, or residual volume level of lung inflation.

vapor, smoke, and inert dust. These receptors may also be activated by smooth muscle contraction, or distortion of the airway walls as produced by pneumothorax and atelectasis. Both types of receptors can be blocked with topical Xylocaine or by cooling the vagus nerve to 7° to 15° C.

The larynx is strategically located and effectively structured to prevent the entry of fluid and food from the mouth into the lungs. This watchdog function of the larynx is enhanced by the presence of at least three different types of neural receptors that can provoke at least seven types of reflex effects. These reflexes include laryngeal constriction, bronchial constriction, cough, swallowing, apnea, increased systemic blood pressure, and cardiac arrhythmias. Virtually everyone has experienced the unpleasant mishap in which liquid or food has entered the larynx. This usually triggers a series of violent coughs accompanied by an uncomfortable choking sensation. Laryngospasm may occur as indicated by audible inspiratory stridor and one may even retch and vomit. The *Heimlich maneuver* (forceful

compression of the abdomen while standing behind the subject) can be successful for the removal of solid food particles (frequently beef steak) from the larynx. This kind of accident commonly occurs in the setting of a formal cocktail supper due to haste or carelessness in eating.

Knowledge of the mechanical efficiency of a cough is fundamental. Measurements of peak intrathoracic pressures during cough are reproducible in the same subject, but range from about 110 Torr to 250 Torr from subject to subject. The resistance to expiratory air flow tends to be much higher than normal at the time of peak flow and higher still at the time of peak pressure. Material is removed from the walls of the larger airways by the scrubbing action of air flow. This action is equal in magnitude to the resistance encountered by the air flow, which depends upon the linear velocity of the air column and the size of the airway. Peak flow occurs during the initial part of the cough, before maximum tracheal narrowing has occurred, so that maximal linear air velocity does not coincide with peak flow.

Maximum tracheal narrowing occurs at the time of peak pressure and a more sustained but lower flow rate. The time interval between peak flow and peak pressure in healthy subject averages around 72 msec, and is approximately twice that in subjects with obstructive pulmonary disease. It has been estimated that only about one-fourth of the scrubbing action occurs during the phase of peak flow.

Cineradiographic studies have shown that tracheal narrowing occurs during only about 50% of the period of air flow. Since linear velocity is greatest at the time of the maximal narrowing of the large airways, the period of sustained air flow during coughing has the most significance relative to the effectiveness of the cough. There is evidence of differential behavior of the airway at different levels in the tracheobronchial tree. Airways peripheral to the trachea may collapse more rapidly than the trachea, and thus offer more airway resistance. As the level of lung inflation diminishes, narrowing occurs more readily in the peripheral bronchi.

These events may be considered in the context of equal pressure points. At the end of inspiration with the glottis open, alveolar pressure is atmospheric. During expiration, alveolar pressure exceeds intrathoracic (pleural) pressure by an amount that may equal the retractive force of the lungs (static recoil pressure). When expiration is forced, and alveolar pressure becomes positive relative to the atmosphere, there is a point in the airways in which extraluminal (intrathoracic) pressure equals intraluminal (airway) pressure. From this equal pressure point toward the glottis, the intrathoracic pressure exerts a compressive effect on the airway wall. In healthy young people at moderate volumes of lung inflation, this equal pressure point is located in the lobar bronchi. In those with disease and with lower levels of lung inflation during health, the equal pressure point moves toward the alveoli. Thus, a cough from a high level of lung inflation tends to clear the large airways. The smaller bronchi may be cleared more effectively with a series of coughs that occurs at lower levels of lung inflation. Patients with obstructive airways disease often initiate a series of coughs without much antecedent inspiration. This mechanism probably serves to clear secretions from the more distal bronchi.

Maximal expiratory flow over the lower 80% of the vital capacity is independent of effort. With the glottis open, it is a unique function of the relationship between the static retractive force of the lungs and the resistance to air flow. Since these factors are volume-dependent, maximal expiratory flow ($\dot{V}max$) is determined by lung volume. But there is a mechanism during cough that permits air flow to exceed $\dot{V}max$ over a wide range of lung volumes.

With rapid opening of the glottis, the bulk air flow occurs from the distal lung parenchyma but air also is expired from compression of the larger airways (from the equal pressure point mouthward). This extra volume of air (50 ml–150 ml in normal subjects) results in the achievement of "supramaximal" flow. The time constants for displacement were between 3 msec and 8 msec in normals and between 20 msec and 60 msec in patients with obstructive airways disease.

STIMULI THAT PRODUCE COUGH

Stimuli that provoke an activation of the cough or irritant receptors in the conducting airways may be mechanical, inflammatory, chemical, thermal, or psychogenic.

MECHANICAL STIMULI

The inhalation of dust, smoke, or small foreign bodies is one of the commonest causes of cough. Cigarette smokers often have a chronic cough, produced sometimes by the foreign body activity (inhaled smoke) present during the period of active smoking, but more often due to the excessive mucus production associated with smoker's bronchitis. Small particles of any nature in the inspired air may result in cough.

Miners and other industrial workers exposed to dusty environments commonly are afflicted with chronic cough.

The involuntary aspiration of oral or nasal secretions, or of food particles, or the presence of inflammatory exudates on the mucosal surface of the nasal passages, pharynx, larynx, trachea, or bronchi may thus act as mechanical stimulants to coughing. The pressure or tension upon structures in the air passages that may result from mediastinal or bronchogenic tumors, aortic aneurysms, the enlarged peribronchial and mediastinal nodes in Hodgkin's disease, tuberculosis, or neoplasms constitute other types of mechanical stimulation. Tension or pressure produced by distortion of the respiratory tract due to pulmonary fibrosis, atelectasis, or pleural effusion may likewise be capable of initiating the stimulus for cough.

INFLAMMATORY STIMULI

Inflammation may activate cough receptors through hyperemia or edema of the mucous membrane, or mechanically from the presence of exudate on the membrane surface. Acute laryngitis is usually accompanied by hoarseness and sore throat as well as cough. Tuberculous laryngitis is associated with a cough notorious for the aerosolization of infective particles.

CHEMICAL STIMULI

A variety of irritant gases may result in cough. These tend to be strongly acidic or basic vapors as well as many organic compounds. The more commonly encountered gases probably are ammonia, chlorine, and nitric and sulfuric acid vapors, and nitrogen dioxide. A particular hazard for firefighters is the production of phosgene when carbon tetrachloride is incompletely combusted. Many other irritant compounds may result from the combustion of plastic materials.

THERMAL STIMULI

Thermal stimuli include the inhalation of very hot or very cold air. However, it is rare for sudden change in the temperature of the inspired air to be the sole cause of cough. Usually pathology in the respiratory tract initiates the stimulus for coughing, which is merely accentuated by the temperature change.

PSYCHOGENIC COUGH

Psychogenic cough is not uncommon. It is found (1) in persons who have some organic basis for cough, but either consciously or unconsciously cough excessively. The cough may serve to gain attention and sympathy or to express hostility. It is also found (2) in persons with little or no organic basis for cough in whom it may serve as release of nervous tension during embarrassment. When chronic, psychogenic cough may assume the clinical characteristics of a tic, becoming an involuntary reflex.

CHARACTERISTIC TYPES OF COUGH

As with many other symptoms, cough is more troublesome at night because of few distractions and because secretions accumulate and provoke cough, thus disturbing sleep. Bronchiolitis, or croup, is accompanied by short, rapid, bursts of coughing. Cough occurs upon awakening, and often is productive. Smoker's cough characteristically results in the morning production of brownish mucoid sputum. Patients with bronchial asthma usually cough during attacks. Occasionally, coughing occurs as the initial and sometimes the only symptom of an asthmatic attack. Usually the cough during asthma is dry, but it may be productive of much thin watery sputum. Typically, wheezing is prominent during the cough. Rarely, a special syndrome occurs in patients with asthma during the formation of bronchial casts. This is accompanied by a vigorous, intractable, cough and has been called "plastic" bronchitis. It occurs together with exacerbation of the asthmatic

symptoms, usually following respiratory tract infection. The sputum always contains bronchial casts, and sometimes *Aspergillus fumigatus* is identified upon culture of the sputum. Acute episodes of pulmonary insufficiency may cause death in some of these patients.

Patients with obstructive pulmonary disease have a characteristic loose cough with a prolonged expulsive phase. This long, slow cough frequently is accompanied by expiratory wheezing. Such patients commonly laugh in a manner typical for its wheezing character.

Cough often is troublesome during acute respiratory infections, but in this case has no characteristic features. Pneumonia occasionally produces intractable coughing, presumably through stimulation of the peripheral, chemical sensitive receptors. Bronchiectasis is remarkable for the frequent ease with which secretions are produced. Cough in pulmonary infarction secondary to thromboembolism is not often troublesome except for aggravation of pleuritic pain. Pleural friction rubs may persist for several weeks in pulmonary infarction, but usually are more transient when due to other causes.

The most distinctive of all coughs is that encountered in pertussis, because of the characteristic sound of the whoop. The inspiratory whoop is a function of the intensity of the effort of cough and the spasm of laryngeal muscles. The whoop lacks specificity for diagnosis, but it should point out the need for bacteriologic methods. In areas in which pertussis continues to be a common infection, the presumptive diagnosis of whooping cough can be made from the whoop.

Observations on healthy medical students during class indicate a mean cough frequency of 2.5 coughs per minute per 100 students. Cough frequency was found to increase during the colder winter months. Men coughed about twice as often as women. Defined simply as persons who were observed to smoke cigarettes during the periods of observation, smokers coughed about twice as often as nonsmokers. The number of coughs was not, however, increased acutely, that is, within 15 minutes after smoking.

CONDITIONS IN WHICH COUGH OCCURS

The conditions in which cough may be an important symptom can be classified as follows:

Inflammations
Cardiovascular disorders
Trauma and physical agents
Neoplasms
Allergic disorders
Other causes

INFLAMMATIONS

The most common cause of cough in otherwise healthy young people is the common cold. Characteristically, the onset is rhinitis, sneezing, and nasal discharge. The cause is viral and the incubation period is short (1–3 days). The infection may progress rapidly (within 24 hours) or gradually (over several days) to involve the lower respiratory tract. Conjunctivitis may be apparent, with burning, itching, and running eyes.

Acute Pharyngitis

Acute pharyngitis frequently occurs in this setting with sore throat and a diffuse redness of the oropharyngeal mucosa. The tonsils are often enlarged. Patchy areas of exudate may be present, or the oropharynx may be covered with an extensive grayish membrane composed of pus cells, bacteria, fibrin, and tissue debris. Since viral pharyngitis is indistinguishable on clinical grounds from bacterial pharyngitis, it is necessary to examine material obtained with a sterile cotton swab. Gram staining of the pharyngeal smear may permit a presumptive diagnosis of streptococcal, corynebacterial (diphtheria), or fusospirochetal infection. Throat cultures for streptococcal involvement are essential if one is to prevent rheumatic fever. Diphtheria must be confirmed by culture as well. An acute necrotizing pharyngitis may appear during the course of agranulocytosis from any cause.

Acute Laryngitis

Acute laryngitis may occur separately or as a part of a viral or bacterial inflammation of the upper or lower respiratory tract. In addition to hoarseness and cough, these patients often have a sore throat, and with tuberculous laryngitis, patients are also apt to suffer from very painful swallowing. Tuberculous laryngitis seldom occurs in the absence of active, infectious pulmonary or endobronchial tuberculosis. The diagnosis is best made by biopsy and culture.

Acute Tracheobronchitis

Acute tracheobronchitis, due to viral or bacterial agents, may occur as a separate illness or as a part or complication of an acute upper respiratory infection. This syndrome also occurs as part of a number of specific infections, including influenza, measles, pertussis, and occasionally typhoid fever. Symptoms include fever, dyspnea, substernal pain, and a severe, irritative, often productive cough.

Influenza is a viral infection characterized by sudden onset of fever, headache, myalgia, prostration, and weakness. The acute symptoms usually subside in 3 or 4 days. Severe dry cough occurs in most cases. The cough may become more prominent as the earlier systemic symptoms diminish. The cough, usually nonproductive, may be productive of small amounts of tenacious mucoid sputum.

Influenza is often complicated by a viral or bacterial pneumonia. If the causative virus belongs to one of the A strains, the disease is apt to be severe, to have a high incidence of complications, and to occur in epidemic or pandemic waves.

Primary influenza virus pneumonia is often fatal. Within hours of the onset of influenza symptoms, the patient may experience high fever and a cough productive of bloody sputum. Intense dyspnea and cyanosis usually appear with progressive diffuse pulmonary infiltrates on the chest radiograph. Death usually occurs within a week.

Pertussis

Pertussis is an acute respiratory infection that mainly affects infants and small children. The etiologic agent is usually *Bordetella pertussis*. The course of the illness may be divided into three phases of roughly two weeks each. After an incubation period of one to two weeks, the patient experiences symptoms similar to those of any viral upper respiratory infection. But the symptoms persist and low-grade fever occurs (catarrhal stage). Within one to two weeks, the patient develops typical paroxysms of coughing. These consist of a burst of 15–20 short coughs followed by a sudden, forceful, "whooping" inspiration; hence, the name. Cough is a predominant feature of pertussis because the organisms selectively attack the respiratory mucous membranes, in which they cause an intense catarrhal inflammation and interference with ciliary action. The disease is also characterized by inflammatory swelling of the tracheobronchial lymph nodes, a fact that also may play a part in the genesis of the severe cough. Pertussis is frequently complicated by interstitial pneumonia or bronchopneumonia; if these complications are slow in resolving, patchy necrosis of the bronchi and adjacent tissues may lead to the late complication of bronchiectasis.

Chronic Bronchitis

Chronic bronchitis is defined clinically as a chronic productive cough for at least 3 months of each year for at least 2 consecutive years. It is characterized pathologically by hypertrophy of the tracheobronchial mucous glands and increased numbers of goblet cells in the small bronchi and bronchioles. The hallmark of this disorder is the overproduction of mucus. The disease is associated closely with cigarette smoking, heavy in-

dustrial air pollution, cold damp climate, and repeated deep viral and bacterial respiratory infections. Patients with chronic bronchitis tend to start their days with an episode of severe dry coughing, culminating in the production of sputum. Most often the sputum is mucoid, and frequently contains brownish pigment. At times of acute infection, the sputum is usually purulent and opaque with a yellow or green color. Lower respiratory tract infections tend to be more severe and prolonged in patients with chronic bronchitis than in healthy subjects. While bronchitis does not eventuate in development of emphysema, the inflammatory response to tobacco tars in the lung parenchyma can provoke a remodeling of the lung structure from normal to an emphysematous form. It seems certain that patients with severe obstructive airways disease, have impaired tracheobronchial clearance, whether the major disease is bronchitis or emphysema. Double jeopardy occurs in the bronchitic smoker who has hypersecretion of mucus, since each cigarette smoked acutely impairs the ciliary function in his respiratory tract.

The mean frequency of night cough in patients with chronic obstructive pulmonary disease is about equal to that found in acute pneumonia. The cough mechanism differs from the normal in subjects with obstructive pulmonary disease because peak flow tends to be slightly higher during the cough than during forced expiration in the patient with obstructive disease. More important, the resistance to air flow during cough exhibits a striking increase, which reflects a greater than normal narrowing of the bronchi during the fast expulsive phase. It should be recalled that the lag between peak flow and peak pressure is twice normal, and, of course, the peak flow rates are much lower in the patients with obstructive diseases than in normal subjects. Since the effectiveness of cough depends on linear velocity as well as volume of flow, the patient with obstructive disease may gain some mechanical advantage from the unusual narrowing of the airways, since this will result in an increased linear velocity during the period around peak pressure. If the bronchi were less compressible, the patient with obstructive disease, with his sharply limited flow rate, would have a much less effective cough.

Bronchiectasis

Bronchiectasis is, by definition, an irreversible destruction of the bronchial walls. It may result from severe pneumonia during childhood, especially when due to necrotizing microorganisms. Bronchiectasis may also occur following the inhalation of a foreign body and following pertussis. A congenital or developmental form is recognized in which multiple epithelium-lined spaces, reminiscent of bronchogenic cysts, become acutely and then chronically infected. The cough in bronchiectasis is usually chronic and is typically worse in the morning. It is characteristically "loose" and relatively productive of large quantities of purulent, often foul, sputum. The sputum tends to settle into 2 or 3 layers upon standing. The diagnosis of bronchiectasis is confirmed by a bronchogram showing localized or widespread dilatation of bronchi and pooling of contrast medium. The dilations are usually irregular or saccular and often interspersed with areas of narrowing. The number of patients developing bronchiectasis has decreased sharply following the introduction of effective antibiotic therapy for pneumonia.

Lobar Pneumonia

Lobar pneumonia is usually caused by *Streptococcus pneumoniae*, less commonly by other streptococci, staphylococci, and pus-forming bacteria. This disease occurs after exposure to cold, after an upper respiratory infection, after an alcoholic debauch, or without any predisposing cause. Its onset is characteristically sudden, with severe prostration, a tooth-chattering chill, localized severe pleurisy, high fever, and a slight but irritative cough. Within 1 to 2 days, the cough tends to become productive of "rusty," frankly bloody or purulent sputum. The cough gradually becomes more severe and finally productive of copious amounts of purulent sputum as the process begins to resolve.

Bronchopneumonia

Bronchopneumonia may be caused by pneumococci, staphylococci, streptococci, Klebsiella and various other bacteria, or by various viral agents. Bronchopneumonia is apt to occur in the aged and infirm, or in the very young following an alcoholic debauch. It is often a complication of influenza or some other severe infection involving the respiratory tract; it may follow the inhalation of food or other foreign material or various irritant gasses. When due to one of several different viral agents, it is labeled *viral pneumonia*. Primary atypical pneumonia, often with positive cold hemagglutinins that appear during the second or third week, is caused by *Mycoplasma pneumoniae*. Cough in these pneumonias tends to be relatively dry and irritative at the outset, and only becomes severe and frankly productive as the process begins slowly to resolve.

Lung Abscess

Lung abscess most commonly is caused by the aspiration of material from the upper airway into the lung. The illness often follows dental work or a period of

unconsciousness due to alcoholism or a convulsive seizure. Putrid lung abscess typically is associated with anaerobic organisms. These organisms are present in large numbers in patients with poor dental hygiene. At first the patient may develop a dry, nonproductive cough, but when the fluid contents of the abscess gain access to the bronchus, the cough becomes productive of large amounts of sputum. Often this is purulent, blood-tinged, and at times, putrid.

Pulmonary Tuberculosis

Pulmonary tuberculosis occurs typically in two forms. The childhood form, called primary tuberculosis, is an acute pneumonic consolidation that occurs following the deposition of the tubercle bacillus in the peripheral air space. Associated regional lymph node enlargement is characteristic, and the pneumonia usually subsides without therapy. The adult forms of tuberculosis include reactivation and reinfection types, of which reactivation is most common. Frequently the disease is located in the posterior portion of the upper lobe. Without treatment, cavitation usually occurs and lung tissue is destroyed. The factors most important in determining how a tuberculous process will behave are host resistance, the virulence of the individual infecting microorganisms, the presence of other diseases and conditions such as diabetes, silicosis, and pregnancy, and the effectiveness of any chemotherapy that may be given.

Cough in pulmonary tuberculosis may be due to the presence of exudate in the bronchi, to actual inflammation of the bronchi, usually near an area of parenchymal involvement, to complicating bronchial damage or bronchiectasis, to pleural irritation, or to pressure upon bronchi caused by distortion, which is in turn caused by fibrous tissue contraction or atelectasis. Cough may be dry, but with cavitary disease is most often productive of purulent sputum before chemotherapy. Cough frequency varies directly with the extent of disease as seen on the chest radiograph. Other symptoms commonly seen in tuberculosis are hemoptysis, pleurisy, weakness, easy fatigability, fever, and weight loss.

Deep Fungal Infections

Deep fungal infections that are apt to occur in the lungs include especially histoplasmosis and coccidioidomycosis; others are actinomycosis, nocardiosis, blastomycosis, cryptococcosis (torulosis), aspergillosis, and mucormycosis. Pathologically, these diseases attack the lung in much the same way as does tuberculosis. Cough is frequently present. It is either dry or productive, depending on whether a necrotic area has begun to slough into an open bronchus.

Chest radiographs in the pulmonary fungal diseases are not diagnostic and often are similar to or indistinguishable from those of pulmonary tuberculosis. Definitive diagnosis of fungal diseases of the chest rests with isolation and culture of the agent.

Histoplasmosis. Histoplasmosis is endemic in the valleys of the Mississippi, and Ohio rivers and tributaries. The acute form of the disease is commonly acquired by inhaling dried bat, pigeon, or chicken dung (in caves, old buildings, or especially in abandoned chicken yards). Despite the fact that 50% to 75% of adults in the endemic area have been infected (positive histoplasmin skin test), the primary infection in most cases is unapparent, and both the acute and chronic active forms of the disease remain quite uncommon.

Coccidioidomycosis. Coccidioidomycosis is endemic in various hot arid parts of the world; southern California, New Mexico, and Arizona and western Texas are the endemic areas in the United States. As is true of histoplasmosis, far more persons have the infection than the disease. In the acute nondisseminated form, the disease is often manifested by a pulmonary nodule or a thin-walled cavity.

Actinomycosis. Actinomycosis (caused by *Actinomyces bovis*) is apt to spread through natural tissue barriers and thus lead to chronic draining sinuses. Tissue sections and cultures reveal the characteristic ''sulfur granules.''

Nocardiosis. Nocardiosis (due to *Nocardia asteroides*) usually attacks debilitated persons and those with other serious pulmonary diseases, and is often fatal. The mycelia are faintly acid-fast and may break up into rodlike forms, which may be mistaken for tubercle bacilli.

North American Blastomycosis. North American blastomycosis behaves much like actinomycosis. About one-third of cases have pulmonary involvement, usually with patchy pneumonia, cavitation, and fibrosis. The skin and lymph nodes are commonly involved.

Pulmonary Cryptococcosis. Pulmonary cryptococcosis commonly presents a solitary pulmonary nodule or cavity. A chronic low-grade meningitis, which often ultimately proves fatal, is a common complication.

Aspergillosis. Aspergillosis occurs most commonly as a saprophytic ''fungus ball'' or mycetoma in an old inert pulmonary cavity caused by previous tuberculosis, fungus disease, or lung abscess. A severe bronchitis often lasting for two or three months is occasionally seen.

Mucormycosis. Mucormycosis is a rare, terminal

complication seen especially in older persons with severe uncontrolled diabetes.

Parasitic Lung Diseases

Parasitic lung diseases may also cause cough due to bronchial irritation; these include paragonamiasis, schistosomiasis, and ecchinococcal disease, in particular.

Opportunistic Lung Infections. The modern use of chemotherapeutic agents for the treatment of malignant disease, together with the requirement for prolonged immunosuppression in patients who receive organ transplants, has resulted in a segment of the population with high susceptibility to infection. Infection in such patients may be caused by a variety of organisms, including many agents of low virulence. Cough may be a prominent symptom in the presentation of any patient with diffuse lung involvement by these organisms. Occasionally the process is extensive enough to produce respiratory insufficiency. Herpes strains, cytomegalovirus, anonymous mycobacteria, *Pneumocystis carinii, Candida albicans, Aspergillus fumigatus* and *Cryptococcus neoformans* are common opportunistic agents. A definitive diagnosis can frequently be established with transbronchial lung biopsy.

CARDIOVASCULAR DISORDERS

Acute Pulmonary Edema

Acute pulmonary edema is usually due to acute left ventricular failure. It may also follow the inhalation of smoke or noxious gases such as NO_2. It is characterized by intense vascular engorgement and by transudation of fluid from congested capillaries into both the air spaces and interstitial tissues of the lungs. Cough in pulmonary edema is typically frequent, loose, and productive of frothy, often pink, sputum. There is also severe dyspnea and orthopnea. An attack is often ushered in by an attack of paroxysmal nocturnal dyspnea (cardiac asthma). Fine crepitant rales can be heard throughout the lungs. The most common causes of acute left ventricular failure are hypertensive and arteriosclerotic heart disease and aortic regurgitation. A somewhat special form of pulmonary edema is seen in severe mitral stenosis. This form is more chronic and often less severe than others. It may be accompanied by frequent small hemoptyses, and in some cases, by gross hemoptysis following vigorous exercise. Other special forms of pulmonary edema are sometimes seen in uremia, in acute rheumatic fever with carditis, and rarely in persons exposed to high altitude. The radiographic picture of pulmonary edema is diagnostic, characterized by small to large symmetric or assymmetric patches of cloudy infiltration around the region of the lung roots.

Pulmonary Infarction

Pulmonary infarction may cause mild to moderate cough, which is usually dry, but sometimes productive of blood or blood-tinged sputum. The patient may or may not also have pleurisy with or without effusion and may or may not have some obvious source of pulmonary emboli.

Aortic Aneurysm

Aortic aneurysm may cause severe cough by pressure on the trachea, bronchi, or lung parenchyma, or by interference with one of the recurrent laryngeal nerves. When an aneurysm presses on the trachea, the cough is apt to have the brassy quality of major airway obstruction.

TRAUMA AND PHYSICAL AGENTS

Foreign bodies of many kinds may be aspirated in the airways. The resulting cough depends on the nature and location of the foreign material. Obstruction farther down the bronchial tree is apt to cause severe paroxysmal cough, often followed by pneumonitis, atelectasis, or both. Atelectasis and pneumonia are particularly likely to occur when the inhaled object consists of vegetable matter, such as a peanut, which tends to incite an intense inflammatory reaction in the lung. Bacterial infection occurs secondarily and may result in lung abscess.

Irritant Gases

Irritant gases such as phosgene, chlorine, NO_2, SO_2, ozone, dichlorethyl sulfide, dichlormethylether, and other organic solvents can cause intense inflammation of the respiratory mucosa and a severe irritative cough, and ultimately, acute pulmonary edema. Patchy pneumonia is a common complication. Later changes that can prove fatal may occur, such as bronchiolitis obliterans, especially following NO_2 inhalation. Intensely cold air may also act as a mild cough-inducing irritant, especially in persons with some underlying chronic pulmonary pathology. Furthermore, any noxious or irritating gas is considerably more irritating when inhaled through the mouth than when inhaled through the nose, since the nose filters, warms, and moistens inhaled gases to a remarkable degree.

Pneumoconioses

The pneumoconioses seldom cause cough unless complicated by extensive fibrosis, chronic bronchitis, or

pulmonary infection. *Beryllium granulomatosis* is a rather special exception in that intense paroxysmal dry cough, marked weight loss, and respiratory failure may occur without much impairment of ventilation. The radiographic appearance is like miliary tuberculosis or miliary sarcoidosis.

NEOPLASMS

Primary Bronchogenic Carcinoma

Primary bronchogenic carcinoma is a common cause of cough, especially a severe or changing cough. The cough in bronchogenic carcinoma may be caused by partial airway obstruction or by bronchial mucosal irritation either directly or secondary to infection distal to an obstructed bronchus. Cough, chest pain, and hemoptysis form a triad of symptoms characteristic of this disease. Affected persons usually have been cigarette smokers for many years and often have been accustomed to a chronic cough, especially in the mornings. The associated chest pain is a poor prognostic sign that may be pleuritic with or without a clear or bloody effusion.

Various other manifestations that should arouse suspicion of bronchogenic cancer in a person with a chronic or changing cough include personality change or seizures suggesting a metastatic brain lesion; evidence of involvement of the brachial plexus or of a recurrent laryngeal, phrenic, or cervical sympathetic nerve; recurrent pneumonitis, especially if in the same segment or lobe; or a wheeze, which is either made worse or relieved by one or the other lateral recumbent positions.

The diagnosis may be confirmed by radiographic examination of the chest (including fluoroscopy and tomography), bronchoscopy, and sputum cytology. A blind scalene node biopsy is only occasionally helpful, but biopsy of a palpable cervical node, especially when hard and located just behind the medial end of either clavicle, is apt to be diagnostic. Computerized tomography has proved useful for delineating the extent of the tumor and for the detection of mediastinal lymph node involvement that may not be apparent on the chest radiograph. Sometimes the diagnosis can be established only by thoracotomy.

Metastatic Lung Tumors

Metastatic lung tumors are not likely to cause cough except in two circumstances: when the metastasis occurs in a bronchus or when pulmonary metastases are lymphangitic. In these forms, cough may be severe, is usually dry, and is often associated with hypoxic respiratory failure.

Bronchial Adenomas

Bronchial adenomas may compress or invade a bronchial wall and cause severe cough, often with severe hemoptysis.

Bronchioalveolar Cell Carcinoma

Bronchioalveolar cell carcinoma usually causes chronic cough. Occasionally, this tumor secretes mucus causing the patient to produce large quantities of clear watery mucoid sputum. The radiographic picture is that of an infiltrative alveolar process.

Mediastinal Tumors

Tumors of the thyroid or thymus; teratomas, nerve tissue tumors, lymphomas, aneurysms, or inflammatory enlargement of hilar or paratracheal lymph nodes may cause cough by pressure or invasion of the trachea or bronchi.

ALLERGIC DISORDERS

Bronchial Asthma

Bronchial asthma may be defined as hyperreactivity of the bronchial smooth muscle. Patients have episodes of dyspnea associated with wheezing. These may be induced by contact with a specific substance (allergen). A family history of allergy is common, and blood and sputum eosinophilia may be present. Such patients are apt to show temporary relief after the administration of epinephrine or some other bronchodilator. Although one may thus describe the so-called extrinsic type of asthma, the intrinsic variety may not exhibit these features, but is often related to recurrent deep bronchial infections. The cough in asthma is dry, tight, and wheezy, and usually occurs in paroxysms. A chest examination during an attack characteristically reveals a prolonged expiratory phase with diffuse musical rales. Status asthmaticus is a protracted attack and a critical phase of asthma, in which response is no longer obtained with standard treatment. Death may occur in such an attack. Postmortem examination reveals extensive blocking of the finer airways with inspissated mucus plugs.

Hay Fever and Vasomotor Rhinitis

Hay fever and vasomotor rhinitis both may cause a mild, usually dry cough because of the postnasal drip so frequently accompanying these conditions.

OTHER CAUSES OF COUGH

Other causes of cough include a wide range of conditions involving the lungs and tracheobronchial tree.

Calcified parenchymal foci or lymph nodes may ulcerate into a bronchus (broncholithiasis) and cause an intense irritative cough. Occasionally patients expectorate calcified material.

Eosinophilic Granuloma

Eosinophilic granuloma is characterized by diffuse radiographic involvement out of proportion to the mildness of symptoms, which may include cough, episodes of spontaneous pneumothorax, and occasionally diabetes insipidus.

Wegener's Granulomatosis

Wegener's granulomatosis is a rare disease characterized by asymmetric pulmonary infiltrates, often with large nodules that may cavitate, granulomatous involvement of the nasal septum and sinuses causing severe catarrh, widespread necrotizing angiitis, and a focal glomerulonephritis that causes terminal renal insufficiency.

Sarcoidosis

Sarcoidosis is a relatively common cause of hilar and paratracheal lymph node or lung parenchymal involvement that may result in dry cough and dyspnea.

Diffuse Fibrosing Alveolitis

Diffuse fibrosing alveolitis is an uncommon disease of unknown cause, usually presenting with evidence of diffuse bilateral pulmonary fibrosis and arterial hypoxemia due to impaired gas transfer, with relatively little ventilatory impairment.

Alveolar Proteinosis

Alveolar proteinosis is a disease of unknown cause in which the radiographic picture is a bilateral homogeneous increase in density due to accumulation of proteinaceous material within the alveolar spaces. The specific defect seems to be failure of the clearance mechanisms for pulmonary surfactant and proteins released into the alveolar spaces. The principal symptom is dyspnea, and cough is not usually prominent. The disease may be fatal if not diagnosed.

Right Middle Lobe Syndrome

Right middle lobe syndrome also may cause cough because of narrowing of the right middle lobe bronchus with associated atelectasis and pneumonitis. The right middle lobe bronchus is particularly vulnerable to compression by one or more enlarged lymph nodes situated at its origin from the right bronchus. Enlargement of the peribronchial lymph nodes at the site is most often caused by tuberculosis, but histoplasmosis and other infections and bronchogenic carcinoma also may cause this syndrome.

Transvenous Endocardial Pacemakers

On rare occasions transvenous endocardial pacemakers may cause paroxysmal cough, presumably due to the electrical stimulation of afferent nerve endings in the diaphragm or pericardium; this complication has required an interruption of the pacing.

COMPLICATIONS OF COUGH

Cough interferes with normal activity in a number of inconvenient ways. Most of these effects are minor and inconsequential, for example, embarrassment, hoarseness produced by laryngeal irritation, loss of sleep, or thoracic muscular soreness. However, two rare complications deserve special consideration.

COUGH FRACTURES

Cough fractures of the ribs occur laterally, at the point of maximal mechanical stress, usually in the middle third of the rib. They occur more commonly in patients with diseases of the bones, such as multiple myeloma, metastatic carcinoma, hyperparathyroidism, or senile osteoporosis. However, they occur also in patients who do not have pre-existing intrinsic disease of the bones. In such instances, the usual history is that an uncommonly vigorous cough effort was accompanied by a sensation of a break, or rupture. Some patients hear the rib break. Pain and soreness follow. Chronic bronchitis is the disease most often associated with "benign" cough fracture of the ribs. The bronchitis should be treated but the fracture usually requires no therapy.

COUGH SYNCOPE

Cough syncope is another rare but important complication of cough. Chronic bronchitis is, again, the most common associated pulmonary disease. The cause of cough syncope is cerebral ischemia. Usually it occurs in obese men past middle life who are heavy cigarette smokers. A typical history is of a coughing fit with syncope during cough. The patient is unconscious only a few seconds, but may fall. The potential for accidents is obvious. A convenient aid in establishing the diagnosis of cough syncope is measurement of the intrathoracic pressure. This can be done simply with a blood pressure manometer fitted with a mouthpiece, with the nose occluded.

Cerebral ischemia may result from severe cough

through two mechanisms. (1) As intrathoracic pressure exceeds arterial pressure, blood is prevented from entering the cranial vault because cerebrospinal fluid, and hence intracerebral pressure, parallels intrathoracic pressure. (2) Because cough causes high intrathoracic pressure, blood also is prevented from entering the right atrium, and cardiac output falls. Because cerebral ischemia can be sustained in this manner for several seconds, syncope occurs. Therapy is simple and is directed against the bronchitis. In order to avoid the syncope, the patient need only understand that he must not take a deep breath prior to cough. By avoiding precough inspiration, he limits the amount of pressure developed within the thorax and avoids syncope.

Pneumomediastinum complicates severe and prolonged paroxysms of coughing. It is seen especially in children with pertussis and may be encountered in patients with asthma. A xiphisternal crunch is a peculiar noise that occurs in the rhythm of the heartbeat as the air shifts about in the mediastinum. Subcutaneous emphysema is a benign complication that may appear at the base of the neck anteriorly. Blood vessels may rupture in the conjunctivae or nose as a result of the increased systemic venous pressure during cough. Reflex vagal stimulation during cough may provoke bradycardia or even heart block.

SPUTUM

A discussion of cough is incomplete without consideration of secretions. The study of sputum has primary importance in the evaluation of pulmonary disease. Except for microbiologic examination in pneumonia, fungus disease, and tuberculosis, the study of sputum often is neglected. Patients dislike sputum and dispose of it as promptly as possible since they find it unpleasant esthetically. Its production frequently is denied or minimized by the patient. The physician must not rely entirely on the results of interview for determination of the volume and appearance of sputum.

The exact quantity of tracheobronchial mucus produced daily in healthy people is somewhat uncertain, but may be as much as 100 ml per day. In the normal subject, mucus is moved rapidly toward the glottis by ciliary action. Only 30 to 60 minutes are required for transit from the level of the respiratory bronchiole to the glottis, at which point its removal from the respiratory tract occurs without notice. This rapid and efficient transit of mucus is a principal factor in maintaining the lower respiratory tract free of microorganisms. Since the ciliated epithelium does not extend beyond the level of the terminal bronchioles, other mechanisms operate to remove organisms deposited in the peripheral lung parenchyma.

Just as a cough is always abnormal, so the production of sputum is always a sign of disease. Smokers accept the production of a few milliliters per day of mucoid sputum as part of their daily lives. The pathology of smoker's bronchitis, a common form of chronic bronchitis, is hyperplasia of the mucus-secreting cells in the respiratory tract. Most parenchymal diseases of the lung lead to sputum production. Persistent daily sputum in a volume exceeding 100 ml suggests bronchiectasis.

Patients cooperate well in the submission of sputum samples when they learn that the physician is interested. Medication vials of clear plastic with a snap-on cap are convenient for the collection of sputum samples. Ambulatory patients are instructed to collect all sputum from time of awakening until they report. Hospital patients may desire to avoid the sight of sputum samples on the bedside table and find it convenient to place a paper cup upside down over the sample. Some of the more useful studies to be performed on sputum are listed below:

Sputum Examination
Collection period   6–24 hours
Volume   2–120 milliliters
Appearance   Clear, buff, yellow, green, red
Layers   Single gel, single watery, double, triple
pH   4–8
Purulence   1+ a few particles of pus in a mucoid gel; 4+ pure pus gel
Viscosity   1+ watery; 4+ solid gel
Peroxidase reaction
Microscopic examination
    Unstained: worms, pigmented macrophages, respiratory epithelial cells, polymorphonuclear leukocytes, and eosinophils
    Wright's stain (or modified Giemsa) for eosinophils, and other cells
    Papanicolaou for malignant cells
    Gram stain for bacteria
    NaOH wet preparation for fungi
    PAS stain for fungi, alveolar proteinosis
    Ziehl-Neelsen, or auramine-rhodamine stain for mycobacteria
Microbiologic examination
    Routine culture
    Anaerobic culture
    Mycobacterial culture
    Fungal culture

TREATMENT OF COUGH

Treatment of cough is most effective when one can identify a specific cause. For example, a foreign body

(usually a hair) in the external auditory meatus may stimulate vagal afferent fibers and provoke a troublesome dry cough. Removal of the hair is curative. If one can eliminate exposure to toxic (cigarette smoke) or allergenic inhalants, the result is usually definitive and rewarding.

Cough from whatever cause that is persistent enough to interfere with sleep may be modified with one of the centrally acting cough suppressants, such as codeine phosphate (20 mg–60 mg) given as a single oral dose. Other narcotics are also effective. Several nonnarcotic antitussives are available. Among these, dextromethorphan hydrobromide (given in a single oral dose of 15 mg–50 mg) has been estimated to account for three-fourths of all over-the-counter sales of antitussives in this country. The product is available only in mixtures with other compounds, but it has no central effects other than cough suppression. Both codeine and dextromethorphan have the potential to release histamine in the tissues, and thus the ability to provoke or aggravate bronchospasm.

Topical anesthetic agents effectively block the pressure-sensitive cough receptors in the large airways. Many commercially available cough preparations contain sympathomimetics and/or antihistamines. If the cough is associated with or due to bronchospasm, the sympathomimetic drugs may be indicated. Antihistaminic agents tend to produce dryness in the respiratory tract that may be undesirable.

Expectorant agents are intended to increase the volume of sputum, in the hope that this will facilitate its removal. The oral intake of large amounts of water has been suggested. Steam vapor or ultrasonic nebulizer mists may be inhaled. Drugs that affect the viscosity of mucus tend to have untoward side reactions. For example, inorganic iodides provoke the formation of thin watery mucus but only in toxic doses. Glyceryl guaiacolate is a commonly used expectorant of doubtful value. Acetylcysteine is an effective mucolytic agent that can be administered as a liquid aerosol or by direct instillation into the airways.

SUMMARY

Cough is an important protective clearance mechanism for the lung. Essentially an explosive expiration, cough may be voluntary or involuntary. When involuntary, the reflex arc from the respiratory tree responsible for cough consists of afferent impulses arising from irritation or pressure to the trachea and large bronchi or chemical and mechanical irritation to the smaller airways. These impulses are transmitted by the vagal and superior laryngeal nerves to an area in the medulla near the midline. The efferent impulses then descend to the various muscles of expiration, principally the diaphragm and intercostal muscles, and to the glottis.

The stimuli that can give rise to cough may be inflammatory, mechanical, chemical, thermal, or psychogenic.

The specific diseases that may cause cough were discussed under the following headings: Inflammations, Cardiovascular Disorders, Trauma and Physical Agents, Neoplasms, Allergic Disorders, Other Causes.

Complications of cough, especially cough fractures of ribs and cough syncope, are discussed.

Sputum production and characteristics are described; their study is an important adjunct to the study of cough.

Treatment of cough should be directed at thinning bronchial secretions, at avoiding or removing abnormal irritation, or at suppressing the sensitivity of the sites of origin of afferent cough impulses. An intelligent attack upon cough thus requires an accurate knowledge of its etiology.

BIBLIOGRAPHY

Bickerman HA, Barach AL: The experimental production of cough in human subjects induced by citric acid aerosols. Am J Med Sci 228:156–163, 1954

Bucher K: Pathophysiology and pharmacology of cough. Pharmacol Rev 10:43–58, 1958

Cohen BM, Elizabeth NJ: Respiratory and cough mechanics in antitussive trials: Responsivity of objective indices to the treatment of acute upper respiratory tract infections. Respiration 32:32–45, 1975

Currens JH, White PD: Cough as a symptom of cardiovascular disease. Ann Intern Med 30:528–543, 1949

Dawes GS, Comroe JH: Chemoreflexes from the heart and lungs. Physiol Rev 34:167–201, 1954

Fenn WO: Mechanics of respiration. Am J Med 10:77, 1951

Harris RS, Lawson TV: The relative mechanical effectiveness and efficiency of successive voluntary coughs in healthy young adults. Clin Sci 34:569–577, 1968

Irwin RS, Rosen, MJ, Braman SS: Cough. A comprehensive review. Arch Intern Med 37:1186–1191, 1977

Kang J, Gupta M, Catangay P, Raia F: Paroxysmal cough induced by transvenous pacemaker. Am Heart J 81:719–720, 1971

Korpas J, Tomori Z: Cough and other respiratory reflexes. Progress in Respiration Research 12:1–281, 1979

Knudson RJ, Mead J, Knudson DE: Contribution of airway collapse to supramaximal expiratory flows. J Appl Physiol 36:653–667, 1974

Lawson TV, Harris RS: Assessment of the mechanical efficiency of coughing in healthy young adults. Clin Sci 33:209–224, 1967

Leith DE: Cough. In Brain JD, Proctor DF, Reid LM (eds): Lung Biology in Health and Disease, vol 5, Part II, Respiratory Defense Mechanisms. New York, Marcel Dekker, 1977

Loudon RG: Cough: A symptom and a sign. Basics of Respiratory Disease, American Thoracic Society, New York, 9:4, 1981

Loudon RG, Shaw GB: Mechanics of cough in normal subjects and in patients with obstructive respiratory disease. Am Rev Respir Dis 96:666–667, 1967

Ross BB, Gramiak R, Rahn H: Physical dynamics of the cough mechanism. J Appl Physiol 8:264–268, 1955

Sanzari NP, Fainman FB, Emele JF: Cough induced by 1, 1-dimethyl-4-phenylpiperazinium iodide: A new antitussive method. J Pharmacol Exp Ther 162:190–194, 1968

Sharpey–Schafer EP: Effects of coughing on intrathoracic pressure, arterial pressure and peripheral blood flow. J Physiol 122:351–357, 1953

Sharpey–Schafer EP: The mechanism of syncope after coughing. Br Med J 2:860–863, 1953

Whipple HE: Mucous secretions. Ann NY Acad Sci 106:157–809, 1963

Widdicombe JG: Respiratory reflexes. In Fenn WO, Rahn H (eds): Handbook of Physiology, section 3: Respiration, vol 1, Washington, D.C., American Physiological Society, 1963

Williams DM, Krick JA, Remington JS: Pulmonary infection in the compromised host. Am Rev Respir Dis 114:359–394, 593–627, 1976

18

Hemoptysis John A. Pierce

Basic Pathophysiology
Localization of Bleeding Site
Study of Sputum
Causes of Hemoptysis
  Trauma
  Foreign Bodies
  Inflammation
    Tuberculosis
    Pneumococcal Pneumonia

Necrotizing Pneumonias
Fungus Infections
Parasitic Diseases
Saccular Bronchiectasis
Bronchitis
Neoplasms
Vascular and Circulatory Conditions
Miscellaneous Causes
Summary

Hemoptysis is one of the most alarming and startling of all symptoms. It occurs typically after cough, and frequently recurs over several hours or days. Some patients have hemoptysis daily for many years, whereas others may become exsanguinated in a few seconds. True hemoptysis is defined as the spitting of some quantity of blood, usually more than 2 ml. It is remarkable that hemoptysis is not often fatal. Massive hemoptysis (bleeding that exceeds 600 ml loss within 48 hours) often is fatal.

BASIC PATHOPHYSIOLOGY

The basic pathophysiologic mechanisms involved in bleeding into the respiratory tract are (as with bleeding anywhere) (1) disturbances in the integrity of vascular walls (from trauma, inflammation, neoplastic destruction, pressure disruption, vitamin C deficiency, and so on); and (2) disorders in blood clotting mechanisms (platelet deficiency, prothrombin deficiency, lack of antihemophilic factor). Two or more of the basic mechanisms often operate together to cause "hemorrhage." (See Chapter 27, Pathologic Bleeding.)

LOCALIZATION OF BLEEDING SITE

It is always important to locate the site of origin of pulmonary hemorrhage. Examination of the nose and throat must be done in all patients to determine whether the expectorated blood may have come from the nasal passages or pharynx. Many patients experience a pulling or drawing sensation in the chest with hemorrhage, often localized to the general area of the bleeding. Rales or rhonchi may be localized to one area of the lungs and may aid in establishing the site of hemorrhage. Bronchoscopy during hemorrhage is useful to determine the origin of hemorrhage. However, during active bleeding, it may be difficult to localize the origin at bronchoscopy. Smiddy has reported successful use of the fiberoptic bronchoscope for the localization of bleeding, pointing out that its flexibility has reduced discomfort to the patient. Other workers (Ores and Baker) have employed an intravenous injection of fluorescein and an ultraviolet light through the fiberscope to detect the appearance of fluorescence in the pulmonary hemorrhage. Selective bronchial arteriography has also been used successfully to determine the bleed-

ing site. Brisk hemorrhage calls for emergency measures in diagnosis and therapy.

STUDY OF SPUTUM

Years ago, the most common cause of hemoptysis in the United States was tuberculosis. Today, hemoptysis is most often caused by chronic bronchitis. Bronchogenic carcinoma, pulmonary infarction, and lung abscess each account for more episodes of hemoptysis than does tuberculosis. The underlying cause of hemoptysis must be carefully sought in each instance. The history, physical examination, and radiographic studies frequently permit a presumptive diagnosis to guide the laboratory investigation. Examination of sputum should be pursued exhaustively whenever the cause of hemoptysis is obscure. In addition to culture studies for common pathogens, microbiologic examination should include special cultures for tubercle bacilli and fungi. Anaerobic cultures are likely to be helpful whenever the sputum is foul or putrid.

The importance of sputum cytology cannot be overemphasized. This examination, carefully performed, often is positive in patients with bronchogenic carcinoma. When bleeding is brisk, the sputum hematocrit should be recorded to aid the assessment of blood loss. We recommend bronchoscopy to localize the site of bleeding and to obtain washings for culture, and especially for cytologic examination.

It is important to determine the amount of hemoptysis. Thus, the patient should be instructed to collect all of his sputum so that the volume and appearance can be recorded. Careful examination of the sputum occasionally reveals bits of tumor tissue or calcified particles. The coughing of blood should be observed directly by the physician whenever possible.

CAUSES OF HEMOPTYSIS

The causes of hemoptysis may be classified as follows: (1) trauma, (2) foreign bodies, (3) inflammation, (4) neoplasms, (5) vascular and circulatory conditions, and (6) miscellaneous causes.

TRAUMA

Hemoptysis may result when the lungs are punctured by a fractured rib or lacerated with a stab or gunshot wound. The inhalation of noxious fumes or smoke gives rise to tracheobronchitis; the area bleeds when ulcerated. The tracheobronchial tree may be lacerated or fractured by blunt trauma, such as that from a steering wheel in an automobile collision. Severe protracted coughing may also lead to mucosal lacerations, and thus to hemoptysis.

FOREIGN BODIES

Foreign bodies cause bleeding by direct trauma, producing laceration or ulceration of the mucosa of the airways. Marks has pointed out that whenever hemoptysis recurs in a child with allergic asthma, presence of a foreign body in the lung must be ruled out.

INFLAMMATION

Bleeding from infectious lesions may arise in the pharynx, larynx, trachea, bronchi, or lungs. It is particularly apt to occur with necrotizing infections such as tuberculosis, fungal infections, and pneumonias due to staphylococci and gram-negative organisms.

Tuberculosis

Hemorrhage early in tuberculosis occurs because necrosis involves the walls of vessels, but it is not uncommon to encounter hemoptysis in patients whose tuberculosis is inactive. Presumably, this occurs because of aneurysmal deformity of vessels, because of bronchiectasis, or because of the erosion of calcific particles through the bronchial mucosa.

Pneumococcal Pneumonia

Pneumococcal pneumonia often can be diagnosed clinically from the abrupt onset of a shaking chill followed by fever, pleuritic pain, and cough with hemoptysis. Characteristically, the sputum is pink or rust-colored, but hemorrhage at times may be brisk. Viral pneumonias may be associated with blood-streaked sputum, but rarely cause significant hemoptysis.

Necrotizing Pneumonias

Necrotizing pneumonias often cause hemoptysis. This is apt to occur several days after onset of the illness and may be abrupt and brisk. Gram-negative organisms are the most common causes, but staphylococci also may be responsible. Anaerobic organisms frequently are present in patients with putrid lung abscess. These patients often have advanced periodontoclasia and frequently give a history of dental manipulation just prior to the onset of symptoms. Many are alcoholic or epileptic and have inspired regurgitated or vomited material.

Fungus Infections

Fungus infections of the respiratory tract cause bleeding because of tissue necrosis or cavitation. Hemop-

tysis may occur after the healing of fungal infections, presumably from erosion of calcium deposits, or because of secondary bacterial infection in deformed bronchi.

Parasitic Diseases

Parasitic diseases of the lung occasionally cause hemoptysis. An amebic abscess of the liver may erode into the lung through the right hemidiaphragm; the patient may cough up a large volume of thin chocolate-colored fluid, which has been likened to anchovy sauce.

Saccular Bronchiectasis

Hemoptysis frequently occurs in patients with saccular bronchiectasis. The deformity of the bronchi renders these patients susceptible to persistent bacterial infections, which may from time to time lead to mucosal ulcerations and hemoptysis. The bronchial arteries enlarge considerably with severe bronchiectatic deformity, and hemorrhage from this systemic arterial source may be brisk.

Bronchitis

Hemoptysis occurs in patients with bronchitis and it is often difficult or impossible to identify the site of bleeding. The radiograph of the chest often is not helpful, but occasionally shows aspirated blood. The radiographic change almost invariably appears abruptly, during a time of active hemoptysis, and may occur with hemoptysis due to any cause. Considerable blood may be aspirated without the production of symptoms. The shadows on the radiograph usually disappear within a few days after bleeding stops.

NEOPLASMS

The most common cause of chronic hemoptysis in persons past the age of 45 is primary bronchogenic carcinoma. Hemoptysis, together with severe and changing cough, and nondescript chest pain form the characteristic triad of symptoms of this neoplasm. Unfortunately, all these symptoms appear very late in the course of this disease. Bleeding in primary bronchogenic cancer may occur because of mucosal ulceration, because of necrosis within the center of a tumor, or secondary to a pneumonic or bronchitic process distal to an obstructing bronchial tumor.

Hemoptysis caused by metastatic cancer in the lung is rare. Although primary bronchial adenoma is not common, when this lesion is present, bleeding is common and apt to be severe. If a bronchoscopist sees what he believes may be a bronchial adenoma, he should not attempt to biopsy it, since the danger of starting an uncontrollable hemorrhage is great.

Hemangioma is a rare tumor of the lung or tracheobronchial tree which may cause severe pulmonary hemorrhage. It may be benign or malignant.

VASCULAR AND CIRCULATORY CONDITIONS

Patients with acute pulmonary edema due to left ventricular failure may cough up large quantities of pink frothy sputum. Pulmonary edema due to severe mitral stenosis is more often associated with brisk frank hemoptysis. This is an expression of the severe degree of pulmonary hypertension that occurs with mitral stenosis.

Pulmonary embolism and thrombosis are extremely common causes of hemoptysis, when complicated by true infarction. It should be stressed that many pulmonary emboli occur without hemoptysis or pleurisy and without any obvious source of an embolus. Pulmonary infarction occurs more often in patients with cardiac disease and in hospitalized patients following acute illness and surgery than in healthy people. Whenever frank hemoptysis occurs in a patient with left ventricular failure, a presumptive diagnosis of pulmonary infarction is warranted.

Occasionally, an aortic aneurysm erodes into the tracheobronchial tree and causes an exsanguinating hemorrhage.

Patients with hereditary hemorrhagic telangiectasia may have hemoptysis from pulmonary arteriovenous fistulae. Typical angiomata often are present on the lips, face, tongue, ears, and fingers. When pulmonary fistulae are present, the patients also have cyanosis, clubbing of the fingers, and a bruit over the fistula. Bleeding may be severe.

MISCELLANEOUS CAUSES

Hemoptysis may occur with any type of hemorrhagic diathesis. It occurs with thrombocytopenia, hemophilia, hypoplastic anemia, and leukemia. It may occur with uremia, or in scurvy. The mechanisms involved in these and other clinical disorders are discussed in the chapter on pathologic bleeding.

Pulmonary hemosiderosis is a rare disease without known cause that usually occurs in young adult males. It is characterized by recurrent episodes of hemoptysis, by dyspnea on exertion, and by the appearance of a diffuse, almost miliary, infiltrate on the chest radiograph. Anemia is a constant feature in these patients.

The *right middle lobe syndrome* is due to a partial or complete obstruction of the long and narrow right middle lobe bronchus. This causes right middle lobe atelectasis, pneumonitis, or both. The obstruction often

is due to scar tissue formation and inflammation, but may result from physical compression of the lumen of the bronchus by an enlarged lymph node. Hemoptysis occasionally accompanies this syndrome.

Lung purpura with nephritis (Goodpasture's syndrome), *Wegener's granulomatosis,* and *polyarteritis nodosa* are all disorders of obscure etiology that may give rise to hemoptysis.

Patients with *cystic fibrosis* are subject to episodes of hemoptysis during acute exacerbations of chronic infection. Improved medical management with modern antibiotic therapy has permitted many of these patients to reach the third and fourth decades. Chronic inflammation during growth and development of the lung frequently leads to the formation of bronchopulmonary anastomoses. These anomalous vessels may be subjected to the same high pressures found in the dilated bronchial arteries. Death due to hemoptysis is being reported with increasing frequency in these patients. As with the other causes of hemoptysis, the mode of death is more often asphyxiation than exsanguination.

Pulmonary microlithiasis, pulmonary amyloidosis, chronic lipoid pneumonia, and endometriosis of the lung also are reported causes of hemoptysis.

One should not overlook the fact that certain drugs are capable of inducing hemorrhage, such as anticoagulants. These may cause bleeding anywhere, especially if there is an added factor, such as blood vessel fragility or trauma, or infection damaging blood vessels. Therefore, persons receiving anticoagulant drugs who have congestive heart failure, bronchitis, or severe cough or high blood pressure are particularly prone to hemoptysis.

Severe hypertension, which is so often associated with degenerative changes in small arteries and arterioles, often leads to rupture of these fragile vessels. Bleeding may occur in the brain, heart, kidney, eye, or other areas. If bleeding occurs in the respiratory tract, hemoptysis may result.

SUMMARY

Recent years have witnessed an increased number of emergency lobectomies for massive hemoptysis. The more conservative and time-honored methods of rest, reassurance, sedation, and blood replacement are inappropriate if bleeding is massive and the patient has adequate pulmonary reserve to permit resectional surgery. If excisional surgery is to be undertaken, there is great urgency for accuracy in localization of the bleeding. Some workers have successfully used tamponade to control bleeding during preparation for surgery.

BIBLIOGRAPHY

Abbott OA: The clinical significance of pulmonary hemorrhage: Study of 1316 patients with chest disease. Diseases of the Chest 14:824, 1948

Crocco JA, Rooney JJ, Fankushen DS, Dibenedetto RJ, Lyons HA: Massive hemoptysis. Arch Intern Med 121:495, 1968

Fellows KE, Stigol L, Shuster S, Khaw KT, Schwachman H: Selective bronchial arteriography in patients with cystic fibrosis and massive hemoptysis. Radiology 114:551, 1975

Gourin A, Garzon AA: Control of hemorrhage in emergency pulmonary resection for massive hemoptysis. Chest 68:120, 1975

Johnston RN, Lockhart W, Richie RT, Smith DH: Hemoptysis. Br Med J 1:592, 1960

Marks MB: Significance of recurrent hemoptysis in allergic asthma: Always think of a foreign body in the lung. Clin Pediatr 10:479, 1971

Ores CN, Baker DC: Localization of hemoptysis in patients with cystic fibrosis. Am Rev Respir Dis 99:790, 1969

Smiddy JF, Elliott RC: The evaluation of hemoptysis with fiberoptic bronchoscopy. Chest 64:158, 1973

Sonders CR, Smith AT: The clinical significance of hemoptysis. N Engl J Med 247:791, 1952

Yeoh CB, Hubaytar RT, Ford JM, Wylie RH: Treatment of massive hemorrhage in pulmonary tuberculosis. J Thorac Cardiovasc Surg 54:503, 1967

19

Dyspnea Warren M. Gold

Nature of Dyspnea
Setting in Which Dyspnea Occurs
Physical Tolerance in Occupational Activity
Physical Tolerance in Recreational Activity
**Factors Determining the Load Imposed on the
    Cardiopulmonary System**
Neuroanatomic Pathways
Theories of Dyspnea
Dyspnea in Chronic Pulmonary Disease
Psychogenic Dyspnea
Dyspnea in Cardiac Disease

Cardiac Asthma
Dyspnea Without Pulmonary Congestion
Dyspnea in Anemia
Dyspnea in Neurologic Disease
    Midbrain Lesions
    Spinal Cord, Peripheral Nerve, and Respiratory
     Muscles
    Pontine Lesions
    Medullary Lesions
Summary

Dyspnea is difficult, uncomfortable, unpleasant breathing, but it is not painful. Dyspnea is often confused with abnormalities in the pattern of breathing; however, it is not rapid breathing (*tachypnea*), increased ventilation in proportion to increased metabolism (*hyperpnea*), or ventilation in excess of metabolic needs (*hyperventilation*). Although physicians tend to call all kinds of unpleasant breathing "dyspnea," there appear to be many different sensations.

More specific descriptions of dyspnea in the words used by the patient might lead to better correlations with the responsible mechanisms. Not only is a more precise description of the quality of dyspnea important, but also a description of the setting in which it occurs is important. Does it occur at rest, or only during exercise? Quantitation of the degree of limitation of activity is valuable to determine how far to pursue diagnostic studies, to determine the natural history of the disease that causes the dyspnea, and to evaluate the effect of treatment on the disease. The critical criterion is to determine whether the symptom has forced the patient to significantly alter his or her lifestyle. If dyspnea is so severe that the patient has changed his (or her) way of life, the symptom requires a specific diagnosis and appropriate therapy.

NATURE OF DYSPNEA

Is there a difference between the breathlessness of healthy subjects and that of those with disease? In evaluating the patient with dyspnea, it is useful to compare the patient with persons of the same age, sex, and degree of physical conditioning. However, it is unclear whether the dyspnea experienced by the patient with cardiac asthma or bronchial asthma is ever similar to the feelings of a healthy person after running to catch a bus, or during recovery after running a mile in 5 minutes. Indeed, one of the difficulties that has resulted from the tendency of physicians to lump together all forms of dyspnea is that clear distinctions and associations have not been made.

Careful observers suggest that some distinctions can be made. The distress experienced during experimen-

Table 19-1. *Relationship between Various Activities and Maximal Available Work Rate in Children*

Activity	Girls	Boys
Walk ½ mile	27† (21–43)*	25† (15–32)*
Stairs	40 (25–51)	43 (26–57)
Calisthenics	64 (50–81)	54 (47–68)
Bicycle	86 (74–100)	89 (81–100)
Run	95 (89–100)	94 (96–100)

n = 21, ages 11–15 years old;
† mean
* range of percentage of maximal available working capacity
(Goldberg SJ, Weiss R, Kaplan E, Adams FH: Comparison of work required by normal children and those with congenital heart disease to participate in childhood activities. J Pediatrics 69:56, 1966)

egory when it requires walking or standing to a significant degree, or when it involves sitting most of the time with a degree of pushing and pulling of arm and or leg controls.''

Medium work includes ''lifting 50 pounds maximum with frequent lifting and/or carrying of objects weighing up to 25 pounds.''

Heavy work is defined as ''lifting 100 pounds maximum with frequent lifting and/or carrying of objects weighing up to 50 pounds.''

Very heavy work involves ''lifting objects in excess of 100 pounds with frequent lifting and/or carrying of objects weighing 50 pounds or more.''

Levels of energy expenditure for peak loads mostly correspond to those given in Table 19-2, and the levels for tasks frequently carried out are approximately equal to one-half the peak load. However, these job classifications are based on a limited number of studies of each job situation, and variations may occur from one situation to another.

The peak expenditure of energy for most professional activities, domestic work, and most tasks in light industry, laboratory, and hospital work, retail and distribution trades is less than 5 Cal/min. Some jobs in building and construction, agriculture, the steel indus-

try, and the armed forces require peak energy expenditures up to 7.5 Cal/min. The highest levels of energy expenditure are found in commercial fishing, forestry, mining, and dock labor, and occasionally exceed 10 Cal/min.

PHYSICAL TOLERANCE IN RECREATIONAL ACTIVITY

It is almost impossible to classify recreational activities with respect to energy demands and estimates of the load on the cardiopulmonary system without introducing a very elaborate set of qualifications. Different people pursue recreational activities with different degrees of vigor. Swimming may require less than 5 Cal/min during a quiet breaststroke or more than 20 cal/min during freestyle competition. The energy demand of activities such as walking, running, or bicycle riding show a similar range of energy expenditure, depending on the speed and the terrain. The skills of the individual person may set an upper limit of energy expenditure in some sports such as tennis, while the intensity of participation is frequently as important as the type of activity in determining the energy demands on the body.

FACTORS DETERMINING THE LOAD IMPOSED ON THE CARDIOPULMONARY SYSTEM

Estimates of the demands imposed on the circulatory system during various activities and classification of jobs as light or heavy primarily reflect levels of energy expenditure. The factor that limits physical work capacity in many patients with heart disease is a restricted systemic cardiac output. Maximal oxygen uptake and maximal rate of energy expenditure are largely determined by the magnitude of the patient's maximal cardiac output. Energy requirement is, therefore, a highly relevant variable in determining whether a car-

Table 19-2. *Relationship between Exercise Intolerance, Energy Expenditure, and Work Intensity*

Category	Maximum Allowed	Peak Load Cal./Min.	Example
1. No restriction	Very heavy and heavy	7.6 and above	Lifting objects 100 lbs or more
2. Mild restriction	Medium	5.0–7.5	Lifting objects of 50 lbs maximum
3. Moderate restriction	Light	2.6–4.9	Lifting objects of 20 lbs maximum
4. Severe restriction	Sedentary	2.5 and below	Mostly sitting with some walking. Lifting objects of 10 lbs maximum

(Dictionary of Occupational Titles, Suppl 2, 3rd ed. Washington: U.S. Department of Labor, 1968)

ness, leading to dyspn
is negligible in man b
Moreover, dyspnea car
breaths, or during rh
bly, collapse of air spa
mitted directly to co
perceived as dyspnea.

Campbell and Howe
when there is a state of
pathways involved in
ical demand is inappro
altitude), when neurc
to the ventilation achie
effort is inappropriate
(e.g., muscle paralysi
sensed unconsciously
logic mechanism; wh
priateness is reached,
and is perceived as
ness" is detected is u

Any theory of dys
the usual conditions
exercise or with asthn
types of dyspnea rep
sistance and compliar
cular obstruction, hea
neuromuscular paral
ralysis of their muscle
specific brain or spin

DYSPNEA IN CHRC

Acute and chronic d
the most common ca

When patients wit
describe their sympto
difficulty in doing so
is involved. The only
one in which dyspne
exertion. Therefore,
tween symptoms that
that do not. Effort d
is inappropriate to
other type of respirat
less of the circumsta

Respiratory symp
usually develop wh
monary function. Th
orders are of two typ
with fibrosing alveo
disorders associated
sema or intermittent
asthma. By history,

---

diac patient will be limited during exercise. However, the type of cardiac defect, the characteristics of the task to be performed, various environmental factors, and intrinsic individual differences (physical conditioning, motivation) may greatly modify the circulatory response to a given level of energy expenditure.

The duration of work is also important. Energy demands during maximal effort lasting less than 2 minutes are usually met by anaerobic metabolism, and performance capacity is, therefore, not related directly to oxygen uptake or cardiac output.[2] A person with restricted aerobic capacity can frequently tolerate heavy workloads, provided that the work is of short duration and followed by adequate periods of rest or work at low intensity.

The nature of the work in terms of static or isometric effort versus dynamic or isotonic effort significantly affects the response of the circulation. It has been well established that isometric work and work with an isometric component (e.g., lifting, holding, or carrying of objects of all kinds, pushing heavy objects, or working with the arms overhead) is associated with a much larger increase in systemic blood pressure, and therefore left ventricular load, than work at a similar level of oxygen uptake without an isometric component. Work at high altitude obviously imposes an extra pressure load on the right ventricle. High altitude and environmental temperatures also require an increased systemic cardiac output to compensate for lowered arterial oxygen saturation and increased blood flow to the skin, respectively. The load on the circulatory system during prolonged work may also be increased by the resulting increase in body temperature, as well as by dehydration. Emotional stress may produce profound circulatory changes and add significantly to the load on the heart during physical work without affecting the level of energy expenditure.

Thus, the level of energy expenditure is a useful index to assess demands imposed on the cardiovascular system, but is of limited accuracy. The magnitude of the load is likely to be overestimated for tasks of short duration; a variety of factors may disproportionately increase the load above that predicted by the task.

Data on energy demands are usually given in terms of kilocalories per minute (kcal/min, or Cal/min). The caloric equivalent of oxygen is approximately 5, and depends largely on the relative rates of carbohydrate and fat metabolism. Values given in Cal/min may be converted to oxygen uptake in l/min without any significant error, simply by dividing by 5. An energy expenditure of 5 Cal/min corresponds to an oxygen uptake of 1 l/min which, in turn, corresponds to a work rate of approximately 400 kg-m/min, or a power output of approximately 45 watts. Data on energy expenditures

---

in Cal/min usually refer to a standard body weight of 70 kg or 150 lb. Some investigators report their results in net calories after deducting a value for estimated basal metabolism, but gross calories provide a more meaningful index of the total demand on the circulatory system.

Body size has to be taken into consideration in any discussion of energy demands. In general, a smaller person is not at a disadvantage so long as the task consists primarily of locomotion. The energy cost of walking and running is proportional to body weight. On the other hand, the energy cost of moving objects is largely independent of body size. A small person is therefore at a distinct disadvantage, since physical work capacity is proportional to body weight.

There appears to be a distinct difference between sexes in work capacity, not related to body size. Gold and associates, for example, found that in young adults, males were capable of approximately 33% more maximal work when corrected for body weight than young women.[6]

The mechanical efficiency of working muscles (calories of external work divided by energy expenditure) is approximately 21% and does not vary among individuals, even considering age, physical conditioning, or disease.[2] The energy expended to accomplish a given task tends to be higher in children and elderly subjects, although probably reflecting variations in the amount of surplus muscular activity (e.g., children tend to be unnecessarily vigorous in their movements).

NEUROANATOMIC PATHWAYS

What are the sensory receptors that cause dyspnea? Are there different mechanisms for each sensation, or is there a common mechanism for all the sensations of dyspnea? Is dyspnea caused by activation of special receptors that send impulses directly to areas of consciousness? Is the dyspnea caused when those impulses directed to the same receptors that regulate rate and depth of breathing in the medullary respiratory center are in excess and spill over into areas of consciousness? Or, does dyspnea result from changes in patterns of impulses? What is the anatomic location of the receptors? What sensory modality activates them? Do they send impulses to the brain in somatic nerves, sympathetic nerves, phrenic nerves, or in the vagus nerves? The answers to most of these questions are unknown.

An increasing number of experiments have been carried out on conscious subjects in an attempt to abolish dyspnea by blocking one or more of these nervous pathways. Guz and associates observed that bilateral

blockade of vagus
of breath-holding
ated with it.[7] One c
the breaking-point
not acute in inten
assessment of time

The sensation th
associated with in
mixtures was also
other hand, the p
decreased compliɑ

In patients witl
cardiac and pulmɑ
ade decreased res
(those with pulmc
pulmonary vascul
effect on others (tl
physema, and a ri
transient relief of
vagal blockade, s
caused similar rel
dyspnea from ur
elimination of spɑ
or elimination of
ilar relief of dyspι
ers in treating as
been confirmed b
dyspnea can be ι
pulses in some ε
but that the affe
contribute to this

Investigators h
afferent impulses
to the sensation
blocked by spinal
fering from trar
workers have exa
piration are para
unteers receiving
curare). Investigɑ
nerve blockade (
fecting movemei
blockade of inter

The results of
involved in the
compliance are i
blocks and, ther
arising in the up
sociated with bι
ade of the respi
must arise in p
Dyspnea associɑ
dioxide mixtures
(not by sensory

sure to dust in cotton mill workers induces a condition characterized by chest tightness that is worse on the first day of the week and may not recur on subsequent days. In many patients airway obstruction and other pulmonary function abnormalities were the same at the end of the day as they were before the patients started work in the morning. This finding suggests that the symptom is not due to the abnormal mechanical properties of the lungs, but might be due to nervous impulses arising in the bronchi. Furthermore, none of the patients with pure byssinosis felt that elastic loading caused a sensation similar to that caused by cotton dust; whereas, patients with byssinosis complicated by chronic bronchitis felt that elastic loading and cotton dust caused similar sensations.[20]

The fact that stimulation of sensory nerve endings in the airways by inhaled irritants may cause respiratory symptoms should surprise no one living in an urban industrial center during conditions producing heavy concentrations of air pollution. Although several possible nervous pathways might be responsible, several arguments suggest that these sensations are mediated by the vagus nerves: (1) in patients with transsection of the spinal cord at C3, added expiratory loads or suction applied to the trachea caused chest tightness. The only sensory connection in these patients between the thorax and the central nervous system was by way of the vagus nerves. (2) Petit reported that dyspnea induced by histamine in an asthmatic subject was inhibited by vagal block.[9] Similar findings have been reported by Eisele, Guz, and Dimitrov.[7,8,10]

Studies in a small number of patients by Culver and Rahn, and Guz suggest that right vagal block in patients with asthma decreased tachypnea and produced marked relief of dyspnea, whereas left vagal block did not.[7,11] No significant changes in arterial blood gases or spirometry occurred despite the subjective improvement. These reports suggest that "tightness" is not a single symptom and that one type may arise from sensory receptors in the bronchi and be carried centrally in the vagi. The other component of this symptom appears to be related to changes in mechanical properties of the lungs and may be detected by somatic mechanisms.

PSYCHOGENIC DYSPNEA

Many patients complain of dyspnea, but have no objective changes to account for their disability. Moreover, patients with obscure causes of dyspnea (such as pulmonary vascular obstruction) may become emotionally disturbed by the inability of the physician to make a diagnosis, let alone relieve the symptom. These patients tend to have a grossly irregular pattern of

breathing with frequent sighs, if not at rest, definitely during exercise; attacks of dyspnea associated with progressive increases in end–expiratory level; acute hyperventilation at rest, but ventilation appropriate for metabolic needs during exercise; and disability during exertion that tends to be independent of the work rates. The patient may complain of "smothering," or of being "unable to get a deep breath." The patient may have a hyperventilation syndrome manifested by lightheadedness, dizziness, and "numbness" of the hands, feet, and skin around the mouth.

However, patients with chronic psychogenic breathlessness are not a homogeneous group.[24] Many patients are depressed. Of these, some have reactive depression to stress, including primary pulmonary disease. Others have depressive psychosis with anorexia, weight loss, early morning awakening, psychomotor retardation, and diurnal variation in moods. Many other patients have prolonged anxiety or tension states in which general muscular relaxation is not attained and the chest cage is held in the inspiratory position, not surprisingly resulting in the patient's feeling unable to inhale enough air. These patients are perfectionists with a constant doubt pervading everything they do, which leads to a feeling of continual insecurity. In a small group of subjects, breathlessness may be linked to the desire for financial compensation; these patients vary from genuine to malingering. In all groups, psychogenic factors are critical, especially iatrogenic factors. Many of these patients have heard specialists label them with a particular diagnosis that may have altered their entire life style and life outlook.[24]

DYSPNEA IN CARDIAC DISEASE

Although dyspnea may occur in any of the various diseases of the heart, it is most prominent and most disabling in those associated with pulmonary congestion. Left ventricular failure from any cause and mitral stenosis are excellent examples. Hemodynamic studies in these conditions have revealed elevation of pressures in all segments of the pulmonary vascular bed consequent to increase in left atrial pressure.[25,26] The high pressures in the pulmonary veins and the capillaries are particularly noteworthy, since they are responsible for the increased rate of transudation of fluid into the interstitial tissues and the alveoli and for the consequent expansion of the interstitial fluid volume of the lungs.[27–30] In tight mitral stenosis, the pressure at rest in the pulmonary capillaries is usually in the range of the plasma protein osmotic pressure.[31] This indicates that such patients live under the constant threat of pulmonary edema.

Because of the gravitational effects, the increase in

interstitial fluid volume within the lungs is greater in the lower lobes. The accumulation of edema fluid about the capillaries and small vessels produces an increase in resistance to blood flow in these lobes and a preferential distribution of flow to the upper lobes.[32–34] When pulmonary venous hypertension is more pronounced, perivascular edema and increased vascular resistance are more widespread, and the distribution of pulmonary blood flow tends to revert to the normal pattern.[34]

With longstanding pulmonary venous hypertension, anatomic alterations develop, characterized by fibrosis of the alveolar walls and medial hypertrophy and intimal proliferation of the small pulmonary arteries.[35-37] These vascular lesions result in an increase in pulmonary arterial pressure that is greatly disproportionate to the elevation of pulmonary venous pressure.[25,26,31]

The secondary effects on the pulmonary parenchyma of these abnormalities in pulmonary circulation increase the stiffness of the lungs as much as three times the normal resistance.[38] This alteration in the viscoelastic properties of the lungs is mainly responsible for large swings in intrapleural pressure, increase in the work of breathing, and the large oxygen requirement for each liter of ventilation.[38]

In a number of patients, the resistance to air flow in the intrapulmonary airways is also greater than normal and is responsible for a further increment in breathing work.[38] Although in the past it has been questioned whether such changes in the mechanical properties of the lungs can occur without the anatomic lesions of pulmonary venous congestion, recent observations leave no doubt that pulmonary congestion alone results in decreased compliance and increased resistance to airflow of the lungs and that these abnormalities are accentuated by expansion of pulmonary interstitial fluid volume.[33]

During exercise, the pulmonary vascular pressures of patients with left ventricular disease, and particularly of those with mitral stenosis, rise considerably above the resting level.[25,26,31] With the resultant extravasation of fluid, the compliance of the lungs is less than that in the resting state. This change in the elastic properties of the lungs is distinctly abnormal, since normally pulmonary vascular pressures do not rise, and the dynamic compliance of the lungs increases with exercise.

Hyperventilation of variable degree during both rest and exercise is usually present in patients with pulmonary congestion and serves to increase the burden imposed on the ventilatory apparatus. The degree of hyperventilation is not great and therefore of itself is not responsible for the dyspnea. The hyperpnea is out of proportion to metabolic demands, since the arterial carbon dioxide tension is usually low or normal.[39] Hypoxemia also may contribute to hyperventilation, although it is usually mild in the absence of significant pulmonary edema.

Reduction of cardiac output and inability to increase output appropriately with exercise bear only a general relationship to the severity of dyspnea in patients with pulmonary congestion. In mitral stenosis the symptom may be quite disabling, even though the cardiac output is normal. Early fatigue of exercising muscles is perhaps the most common symptom of an inadequate cardiac output. Since the respiratory muscles are performing two to three times as much work as normal in achieving a particular level of ventilation, their early fatigue when blood flow is deficient may be an important contributing factor in respiratory distress.

Orthopnea is a common symptom of pulmonary congestion. It is the term applied to the phenomenon of dyspnea that occurs at rest in the recumbent, but not the upright or semivertical position. It is usually relieved by two or three pillows under the head and the back. Marshall and associates have observed in patients with mitral stenosis considerable decrease in pulmonary compliance in the supine compared with the upright position.[15] The swings in intrapleural pressure during the respiratory cycle were consequently greater (over 40 cm of water) and the work of breathing was two to three times greater in recumbency than in the upright position. The respiratory rate also increased to a frequency that corresponded strikingly to the frequency at which the work of ventilating the more rigid lungs was at a minimum.

The decrease in compliance upon lying flat probably is related to the fact that more of the lung lies at or below the level of the heart. Thus, the increased vascular pressures are distributed throughout a greater portion of the lungs and are augmented in the most dependent regions by the overlying column of blood. In the upright position a greater portion of the lungs lies above the heart. In these regions pulmonary venous and capillary pressures are lowered by hydrostatic effects.

Vigorous movements of the chest bellows are achieved more readily in the upright position. This probably explains why some patients with chronic lung disease or bronchial asthma are also intolerant of the recumbent position.

Paroxysmal nocturnal dyspnea may occur in the presence of mitral stenosis or in any condition that taxes the left ventricle sufficiently to cause it to fail, such as hypertension or aortic insufficiency. The attack may be severe, dramatic, and terrifying. The patient is aroused from his sleep gasping for air, and must sit up or stand to catch his breath. He may sweat profusely. Sometimes he throws open a window widely in an attempt to relieve the oppressive sensation of

suffocation. The chest tends to become fixed in the position of forced inspiration. Both inspiratory and expiratory wheezes, often simulating typical asthma, are heard. In some cases overt pulmonary edema occurs, with many moist rales. The acute pulmonary edema rarely terminates fatally. Occasionally the attacks may recur several times a night, necessitating sleeping upright in a chair.

The mechanism of these attacks includes those factors that produce orthopnea, as well as the hypervolemia that occurs during the redistribution of peripheral edema fluid when body position is changed from vertical to horizontal upon retiring.[40] The hypervolemia constitutes an additional burden to the heart and of itself increases pulmonary venous and capillary pressures.[41] The actual attack may be "triggered" by coughing, abdominal distention, the hyperpneic phase of Cheyne–Stokes respiration, a startling noise or anything causing a sudden increase in heart rate and further acute elevation of pulmonary venous and capillary pressures. Usually the attack is terminated by assumption of the erect position and a few deep breaths of air. Cough, an important manifestation of pulmonary congestion, frequently occurs during the attack.

Cardiac Asthma

The asthmatic wheezes often heard in patients with pulmonary congestion have given rise to the term, cardiac asthma. The wheezes are a manifestation of pulmonary edema, and often are accompanied by other signs of this condition. Reduction in lumen of the small intrapulmonary airways by edema fluid and thickening of bronchiolar walls by edema is responsible for the wheezes. In addition, the high intrathoracic pressure required to overcome the obstruction during expiration tends to narrow the small bronchioles further and even collapse them.[38] Mills and associates have demonstrated that pulmonary congestion is associated with increased discharge from rapidly adapting vagal sensory receptors in the airways, perhaps due to deformation of the receptors by edema, resulting in reflex bronchoconstriction.[42] Increased resistance to air flow during both inspiration and expiration has been measured in pulmonary congestion and has been found to be especially high (4 times normal) in frank pulmonary edema.[33,38] The compliance of the lungs is reduced greatly in pulmonary edema, with values as low as 1/10 normal having been recorded. With recovery from edema, very significant reductions in airway resistance and increases in pulmonary compliance occur.[43,44]

Dyspnea Without Pulmonary Congestion

Dypsnea occurs in many forms of heart disease that are not associated with congestion of the lungs. Uncomplicated pulmonic stenosis is an excellent example.

Probably the symptom is related to an inadequate cardiac output during exercise. In tetralogy of Fallot, dyspnea may be severe and often is relieved by assuming a squatting position. In this and other forms of cyanotic heart disease, preexisting hypoxemia is aggravated by exercise. It is of note that both dyspnea and fatigue appear during exertion when the arterial oxyhemoglobin saturation has fallen significantly below the resting level.

DYSPNEA IN ANEMIA

Exertional dyspnea is a common symptom of anemia, and is particularly marked in the more acute and severe forms. Its pathogenesis is also not completely understood.

The supply of oxygen to the tissues is dependent upon transport by hemoglobin. If the hemoglobin concentration and arterial oxyhemoglobin saturation are normal, the mixed venous blood in the resting state is about 75% saturated with oxygen, since the mean extraction of oxygen by the tissues from each 100 ml of blood is 4 ml. With reduction in hemoglobin concentration and hence in the amount of oxygen in the arterial blood (normally 19.4 ml per 100 ml), the mixed venous blood saturation decreases if extraction of oxygen from each 100 ml of blood continues as usual, so that tissue oxygen pressure falls. This hypoxic effect is greatest in those tissues, such as contracting muscle, in which the extraction rate of oxygen is high.

The hypoxia is prevented partially by an increase in the cardiac output, which permits tissue oxygen needs to be met at a lower extraction rate of oxygen from the blood.[45] In severe anemia, the adjustment in output may fall short of the mark. If the hemoglobin concentration is 4 gm/100 ml of blood, the cardiac output would have to be tripled to merely maintain tissue oxygen exchange at a normal level in the basal state.

The heart under these circumstances does not respond normally to stress and may fail.[46] In the production of dyspnea, the roles played by the augmented blood flow through the lungs and by pulmonary congestion resulting form left ventricular failure or strain during exercise may only be speculated upon.[47]

Although the arterial oxyhemoglobin saturation is within normal limits, the oxygen pressure has been demonstrated to be decreased.[48] This may be responsible in part for the hyperventilation that is characteristic of anemia.

DYSPNEA IN NEUROLOGIC DISEASE

According to Plum, the effect of neurologic disease on respiration and sensations of breathing depends on the anatomic distribution of the lesion, rather than on a

specific disease.[49] Figure 19-2 summarizes the changes in respiratory pattern following brain injury at various levels in the central nervous system. The figure illustrates Cheyne–Stokes respiration associated with lesions of the forebrain, neurogenic hyperventilation associated with a midbrain lesion in the upper pons, apneustic breathing associated with lesions of the lower pontine tegmentum, cluster breathing associated with lesions in a similar location, and irregularly irregular, ataxic breathing associated with lesions in the medullary respiratory center.

The net effect of cerebral disease is to increase instability of respiration. Cerebral lesions (1) impair voluntary and involuntary control of the behavioral component of breathing, resulting in apraxia or pseudobulbar palsy; (2) destroy cortical influences on rhythmic breathing when chemical stimuli are removed, resulting in posthyperventilation apnea; and (3) remove normal cortical influences on subcortical structures, resulting in hyperactive ventilatory responses to inhaled carbon dioxide. Cheyne–Stokes respiration results in dyspnea, but not out of proportion to the chemical stimulus.

Midbrain Lesions

These patients have central hyperventilation associated with coma. It has been suggested that this probably represents a respiratory reflex response to pulmonary congestion.

Spinal Cord, Peripheral Nerve, and Respiratory Muscles

Most illnesses involving these structures produce respiratory insufficiency and dyspnea. Paralysis of the muscles of the chest is usually associated with the need for hyperventilation to prevent dyspnea. In many cases,

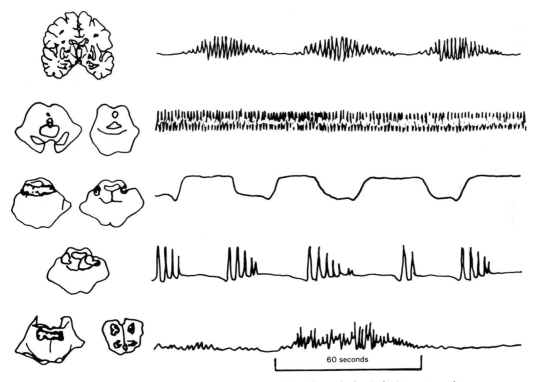

60 seconds

Fig. 19-2. Abnormal respiratory patterns associated with pathologic lesions at various levels of the brain. Tracings obtained with a chest–abdomen pneumograph, inspiration up. Cheyne–Stokes respiration (*top tracing*) is associated chiefly with forebrain dysfunction; neurogenic hyperventilation (*second tracing*) arises when dysfunction affects the midbrain or upper pons; apneustic (*third tracing*) or cluster breathing (*fourth tracing*) results from lesions of the lower pontine tegmentum; and patients with lesions of the medullary respiratory centers (*bottom*) tend to develop an irregularly irregular ataxia. (From Plum F: Breathlessness in neurological disease: The effects of neurological disease on the act of breathing. In Howell JBL, Campbell EJM (eds): Breathlessness. Philadelphia, FA Davis, 1966)

the degree of breathlessness is related to the muscles involved rather than the absolute level of ventilation. Patients dependent on high intercostal muscles are dyspneic, while patients dependent on their diaphragms are not. This may be due to increased energy expenditure and ease of fatiguability of the intercostal muscles. Alternatively, activity of central structures may be conditioned to recruit intercostal and accessory muscles late, after first activating the diaphragm and lower intercostal muscles. These clinical observations imply that the respiratory center must discharge to its limit in order to activate the accessory muscles of respiration, and this fully excited state spills over to areas of consciousness and is perceived as dyspnea. The finding correlates with the fact that normal subjects experience dyspnea when they approach 30% to 35% of their maximal voluntary ventilation. The sensation of breathlessness in these patients may be due either to massive output from central respiratory centers or to a mismatch between maximal central demand and minimal peripheral proprioceptor feedback.

Pontine Lesions

In addition to causing respiratory ataxia and other problems with control of respiration, pontine lesions abolish alert wakefulness so that dyspnea cannot be accurately evaluated.

Medullary Lesions

Medullary lesions destroy the automatic control of breathing without any accompanying sensation of breathlessness. This fact suggests that dyspnea is in some way related to the output from the medullary respiratory area.

It is known in a general way that dyspnea reflects an increased activity in the respiratory system and that the symptom disappears when many respiratory stimuli are inhibited. Since neurologic disease of the lower brainstem not only abolishes the act of breathing but also the sensation of dyspnea, this clinical association suggests that dyspnea is somehow related to the output of the medullary center.

When neurologic disease paralyzes the chest muscles, the intensity of dyspnea depends on which muscles are involved and not just the degree of ventilatory dysfunction. This association also suggests a possible central origin of the sensation if the pattern of automatic supraspinal respiratory discharge is fixed, requiring increased central excitation to drive intercostal and accessory muscles, regardless of whether the diaphragm can be activated initially in the respiratory act. Paralysis of chest muscles may also affect breathlessness by the failure to inflate the lungs, and may reflexly stimulate central structures or fail to inhibit them.

Finally, studies of patients with poliomyelitis suggest that contraction of the chest muscles may lead to a satisfying sensation during breathing, since the voluntary demand increases in excess of metabolic needs when these muscles are rested during passive ventilation with a respirator.

The role of wakefulness and higher cerebral function on the respiratory act is unclear; however, voluntary control can override the automatic mechanism to stimulate or inhibit automatic drive, both during rest and during exercise.

SUMMARY

Dyspnea is a subjective symptom related to the effort of breathing, and as such must be regarded as originating in the ventilatory apparatus, although the stimuli, sensory receptors, and nerve pathways that participate in its appreciation are unknown.

Numerous acute and chronic diseases may affect the various components of the ventilatory apparatus—ribs, spine, respiratory muscles, their peripheral and central nervous control, the extrapulmonary and intrapulmonary airways, alveolar tissue, pleura, and pulmonary vessels. These disturbances, if sufficiently severe, decrease the capacity of the apparatus to ventilate and exaggerate the effort necessarily expended to make it function. Alterations in the parenchyma and the airways of the lung produced either by primary lung disease, or secondarily by heart disease, are the most common clinical causes of ventilatory dysfunction and dyspnea.

In many conditions the levels of ventilation required at rest, and especially during exercise, are greater than normal and serve to overtax a disabled ventilatory apparatus. Severe grades of hyperventilation, such as may occur during vigorous exertion, can provoke dyspnea even in a normal person.

The rate of alveolar ventilation is adjusted to meet the wide fluctuations in metabolic needs for exchange of oxygen and carbon dioxide that occur in the course of human activity. These adjustments are initiated primarily by alterations in the gas composition and pH of the arterial blood and are designed to minimize such changes. Many additional reflex and emotional factors, which may assume importance in disease, are capable of modifying ventilation.

In order to appraise dyspnea adequately, it is necessary to ascertain the severity of the symptom and the conditions under which it occurs. Through the history and physical examination, all evidence of disability of the ventilatory apparatus and factors that increase the demands for ventilation must be sought. Detailed

studies of pulmonary and cardiac function may be necessary, particularly in those persons in whom adequate cause for dyspnea cannot be found, or in whom the symptom appears out of proportion to the evidence of disease. In most instances, simple studies such as observation of the patient during exercise, radiographic examination of the heart and lungs, determination of blood carbon dioxide pressure and hematocrit, spirometry and electrocardiogram suffice to determine the organ system responsible for this important symptom, although the mechanism that causes dyspnea is still unknown.

REFERENCES

1. **Wasserman K, Whipp BJ, Koyal SN, Beaver WL:** Anaerobic threshold and respiratory gas exchange during exercise. J Appl Physiol 35:236–243, 1973

2. **Wasserman K, Van Kessel AI, Burton GG:** Interaction of physiological mechanisms during exercise. J Appl Physiol 22:71–85, 1967

3. **Goldberg SJ, Weiss R, Kaplan E, Adams FH:** Comparison of work required by normal children and those with congenital heart disease to participate in childhood activities. J Pediatr 69:56–60, 1966

4. **American Heart Association Council on Rheumatic Fever and Congenital Heart Disease, Ad Hoc Committee on Habilitation of the Young Cardiac:** Recreational activity and career choice recommendations for use by physicians counseling physical education directors, vocational counselors, and young patients with heart disease. 1970

5. Selected Characteristics of Occupations by Worker Traits and Physical Strength. Suppl. 2, Dictionary of Occupational Titles, 3rd ed. Washington, D.C., U.S. Department of Labor, 1968

6. **Gold WM, Mattioli LF, Price AC:** Response to exercise in tetrology of Fallot. Pediatrics 43:781, 1969

7. **Guz A, Noble MIM, Eisele JH, Trenchard D:** Experimental results of vagal block in cardiopulmonary disease. In Porter R (ed): Breathing: Hering–Breuer Centenary Symposium, pp 315–354. London, J & A Churchill, 1970

8. **Dimitrov–Szokodi D, Husveti A, Balogh G:** Lung denervation in the therapy of intractible bronchial asthma. J Thorac Surg 33:166, 1957

9. **Petit JM:** Dyspnea in bronchial asthma. in Howell JBL, Campbell EJM (eds) Breathlessness, pp 178–181. Philadelphia, FA Davis, 1966

10. **Eisele JH, Jain SK:** Circulatory and respiratory changes during unilateral and bilateral cranial nerve ix and x block in two asthmatics. Clin Sci 40:117, 1971

11. **Culver GA, Rahn H:** Reflex respiratory stimulation by chest compression in the dog. Am J Physiol 168:686–693, 1952

12. **Phillips EW, Scott WJM:** The surgical treatment of bronchial asthma. Arch Surg 19:1425, 1925

13. **Gold WM, Nadel JA:** Dyspnea and hyperventilation associated with unilateral disease of the chest wall relieved by blocking the intercostal nerves. In Howell JBL, Campbell EJM (eds): Breathlessness, pp 203–222. Philadelphia, FA Davis, 1966

14. **Gad J:** In Luciani L: Human Physiology, vol 1, pp 458–459. London, MacMillan, 1911

15. **Marshall R, Stone RW, Christie RV:** The relationship of dyspnea to respiratory effort in normal subjects, mitral stenosis and emphysema. Clin Sci 13:625, 1954

16. **Harrison TR:** Principles of Internal Medicine, pp 111. Philadelphia, P Blakiston & Son Co, 1950

17. **Wright GW, Branscomb BV:** Origin of the sensation of dyspnea. Trans Am Clin Climatol Assoc. 66:116, 1954

18. **Comroe JH Jr:** Some theories of the mechanism of dyspnea. In Howell JBL, Campbell EJH (eds): Breathlessness, pp 1–7, Philadelphia, FA Davis, 1966

19. **Campbell EJM, Howell JBL:** The sensation of breathlessness. Br Med Bull 19:36–40, 1963

20. **Howell JBL:** Respiratory sensation in pulmonary disease. In Porter R (ed): Breathing: Hering–Breuer Centenary Symposium, pp 287–295. London, J & A Churchill, 1970

21. **Simonsson BG, Jacobs FM, Nadel JA:** Role of autonomic nervous system and the cough reflex in the increased responsiveness of airways in patients with obstructive airway disease. J Clin Invest 46:1812, 1967

22. **Empey DW, Laitinen LA, Jacobs L, Gold WM, Nadel JA:** Mechanisms of bronchial hyperreactivity in normal subjects after upper respiratory tract infection. Am Rev Respir Dis 113:131, 1976.

23. **Howell JBL:** Breathlessness in pulmonary disease. In well JBL, Campbell EJM (eds): Breathlessness, pp 5–177. Philadelphia, FA Davis, 1966

24. **Burns BH:** Discussion of breathlessness in pulmonary disease. In Howell JBL, Campbell EJM (eds): Breathlessness, pp 183–184. Philadelphia, FA Davis, 1966

25. **Lewis BM, Houssay HE, Haynes FW, Dexter L:** The dynamics of both right and left ventricles at rest and during exercise in patients with heart failure. Circ Res 1:312, 1953

26. **Lukas DS, Dotter CT:** Modifications of the pulmonary circulation in mitral stenosis. Am J Med 12:639, 1952

27. **Guyton AC, Lindsey AW:** Effect of elevated left atrial pressure and decreased plasma protein concentration on the development of pulmonary edema. Circ Res 7:649, 1959

28. **Levine OR, Mellins RB, Fishman AP:** Quantitative assessment of pulmonary edema. Circ Res 17:414, 1965

29. **Levine OR, Mellins RB, Senior RM, Fishman AP:** The application of Starling's law of capillary exchange to the lungs. J Clin Invest 46:934, 1967

30. **De Martino AG, Kozam RL, Lukas DS:** The control of rapidly exchanging water volume of the lung by left atrial pressure. Clin Res 12:293, 1964

31. **Araujo J, Lukas DS:** Interrelationships among pulmonary "capillary" pressure, blood flow and valve size in

mitral stenosis: The limited regulatory effects of the pulmonary vascular resistance. J Clin Invest 31:1082, 1952

32. **Dollery CT, West JB:** Regional uptake of radioactive oxygen, carbon monoxide and carbon dioxide in the lungs of patients with mitral stenosis. Circ Res 8:765, 1960

33. **West JB, Dollery CT, Heard BE:** Increased vascular resistance in the lower zone of the lung caused by perivascular edema. Lancet 2:181, 1964

34. **Dawson A, Kaneko K, McGregor M:** Regional lung function in patients with mitral stenosis studied with xenon[133] during air and oxygen breathing. J Clin Invest 44:999, 1965

35. **Parker F Jr, Weiss S:** Nature and significance of structural changes in lungs in mitral stenosis. Am J Pathol 12:573, 1936

36. **Larrabe WF, Parker RL, Edwards JE:** Pathology of intrapulmonary arteries and arterioles in mitral stenosis. Proc Mayo Clin 24:316, 1949

37. **Harris P, Heath D:** The Human Pulmonary Circulation: Its Form and Function in Health and Disease. Baltimore, Williams & Wilkins, 1962

38. **Brown CC Jr, Fry DL, Ebert RV:** The mechanics of pulmonary ventilation in patients with heart disease. Am J Med 17:438, 1954

39. **West JR, Bliss HA, Wood JA, Richards DW Jr:** Pulmonary function in rheumatic heart disease and its relation to exertional dyspnea in ambulatory patients. Circulation 8:178, 1953

40. **Perera GA, Berliner RW:** The relation of postural hemodilution to paroxysmal dyspnea. J Clin Invest 22:25, 1943

41. **Doyle JT, Wilson JS, Estes EH, Warren JV:** The effect of intravenous infusions of physiologic saline solution on the pulmonary arterial and pulmonary capillary pressure in man. J Clin Invest 30:345, 1951

42. **Mills JE, Sellick H, Widdicombe JG:** Activity of lung irritant receptors in pulmonary microembolism, anaphylaxis, and drug-induced bronchoconstrictions. J Physiol [London] 203:337, 1969

43. **Sharp JT, Griffith GT, Bunnell IL, Greene DG:** Ventilatory mechanics in pulmonary edema in man. J Clin Invest 37:111, 1958

44. **Sharp JT, Bunnell IL, Griffith GT, Greene DG:** The effects of therapy on pulmonary mechanics in human pulmonary edema. J Clin Invest 40:665, 1961

45. **Brannon ES, Merrill AJ, Warren JV, Stead EA:** The cardiac output in patients with chronic anemia as measured by the technique of right atrial catheterization. J Clin Invest 24:332, 1945

46. **Sharpey–Shafer EP:** Transfusion and the anemic heart. Lancet 2:296, 1945

47. **Leight L, Snider TH, Clifford GO, Hellems HK:** Hemodynamic studies in sickle cell anemia. Circulation 10:653, 1954

48. **Ryan JM, Hickam JB:** The alveolar–arterial oxygen pressure gradient in anemia. J Clin Invest 31:188, 1952

49. **Plum F:** Breathlessness in neurological disease: The effects of neurological disease on the act of breathing. In Howell JBL, Campbell EJH (eds): Breathlessness, pp 203–222, Philadelphia, FA Davis, 1966

20

Cyanosis Warren M. Gold

Definition
Oxygen Transport
  Cutaneous Circulation
  Peripheral Cyanosis
  Central Cyanosis

Pulmonary Abnormalities
Cardiac Abnormalities
Abnormalities of Hemoglobin
Relationship of Cyanosis to CO_2 Exchange
Effects of Oxygen on Cyanosis

DEFINITION

Cyanosis is a blue color that is due to increased amounts of deoxygenated hemoglobin in the subpapillary venous plexus of the skin. It may be confused with the leaden-gray color caused by methemoglobin or sulfhemoglobin in the blood, or with the bluish, slate-colored generalized pigmentation of the skin that results from the use of silver compounds (argyria). Cyanosis is not synonymous with hypoxemia (a decreased amount of O_2 in arterial blood), or hypoxia (a decreased amount of O_2 in any part of the body). A decrease in functioning hemoglobin owing to either a decrease in total hemoglobin (anemia) or a decrease in active O_2-binding hemoglobin (carbon monoxide poisoning or methemoglobinemia) causes hypoxemia without decreased arterial pO_2, unsaturation of active hemoglobin, or cyanosis. Profound tissue hypoxia and death can occur in cyanide poisoning without hypoxemia or cyanosis. Thus, the presence of cyanosis implies hypoxemia (local or generalized), but the absence of cyanosis does not preclude severe hypoxia or hypoxemia.

Skin pigmentation and thickness may modify the appearance of cyanosis or may mask it completely. The presence of other pigments in the blood, such as methemoglobin or bilirubin, may impair recognition, whereas dilatation of superficial vessels makes the color more obvious. Cyanosis can best be seen and recognized in regions where the skin is thick, unpigmented, and flushed, such as the ear lobes, cutaneous surfaces of the lips, and the fingernail beds.

Cyanosis is less apparent in the mucous membranes and in the retina, but these sites may be useful to examine in patients with dark skin. The nature of the light under which the subject is examined is important in detecting cyanosis: natural, bright daylight is best, whereas certain fluorescent lights cause even normal subjects to appear cyanotic. The visual perception of "blueness" varies greatly among physicians; the average physician does not perceive cyanosis with certainty until the O_2 saturation falls to 85%, and some not until 75%. The contribution of the vascular contents to the color of the skin can be assessed by applying sufficient pressure to the skin to empty its vessels.

OXYGEN TRANSPORT

Total O_2 transport depends on (1) pulmonary ventilation and diffusion to provide a proper alveolar and arterial pO_2 and pCO_2 for loading O_2 into mixed venous blood in the pulmonary capillaries; (2) the proper type and quantity of hemoglobin for optimal loading and unloading of O_2; and (3) the heart and blood vessels to deliver the proper amount of oxygenated blood to

the tissues according to their needs. At rest, the total O_2 delivered to body tissues is 1000 ml per minute (cardiac output in liters per min $\times$ ml of O_2 contained in 1 liter of arterial blood = 5 $\times$ 200), but only one fourth of the O_2 is used by the tissues, while three fourths is returned in mixed venous blood. During maximal exercise, the total O_2 delivered to the tissues is markedly increased to about 5000 ml per minute. This results from a marked increase in cardiac output despite a constant O_2 content (25 liters per min $\times$ 200 ml O_2 per liter of blood); but under these conditions, the tissues consume three fourths of the O_2 delivered and return only one fourth to the heart in mixed venous blood. This change in the fraction of O_2 used means that the O_2 unloading and loading systems work more efficiently:

By changing temperature, acidity, pO_2, and pCO_2, the tissues extract three times as much O_2 from each liter of blood as they did during rest

By increasing frequency and tidal volume and by markedly improving the matching of alveolar ventilation and blood flow, the lungs add three times as much O_2 to each liter and almost 15 times as much O_2 to blood per minute as they did at rest

By increasing rate and stroke volume, the heart pumps almost five times as much O_2 to the tissues per minute

By perfusing the exercising muscles and vital organs while decreasing unnecessary blood flow, the oxygenated blood is distributed more efficiently, and energy demands can be met without resorting to glycolytic metabolic sources.

In this transport process, hemoglobin plays a key role because the concentration of O_2 in plasma under normal conditions is small. One ml of plasma at 37° C takes up 0.00003 ml of O_2 for each 1 torr increase in pO_2. Since the tissues use 250 ml O_2 per minute in an adult at rest, if blood were plasma and the subject breathed air, the cardiac output would have to be over 80 liters per minute, assuming every molecule of O_2 was removed from plasma in the tissue capillaries. If such a person merely doubled the amount of O_2 needed during exercise, the cardiac output would have to be increased to more than 160 liters per minute.

However, blood contains hemoglobin as well as plasma, which permits whole blood to load 65 times as much O_2 as plasma at a pO_2 of 100 torr. When fully saturated with oxygen, each gram of hemoglobin binds 1.34 ml of O_2; thus, at a normal hemoglobin concentration of 15 g per 100 ml of blood, 20.1 ml O_2 per 100 ml can be carried by hemoglobin, while 0.3 ml O_2 per 100 ml can be carried in physical solution in the plasma. The binding of O_2 to hemoglobin is determined by in-

teraction of the four chains in the globin molecule, which create an S-shaped curve of O_2 uptake that is uniquely suited for loading O_2 in the lungs and unloading O_2 in the tissues. When blood passes through the pulmonary capillaries, exposed to an alveolar pO_2 of 100 torr, the hemoglobin in 100 ml of blood combines with almost 20 ml O_2 and is 97.4% saturated. No matter how high the alveolar pO_2 is raised, the saturation of hemoglobin can increase only 2.6%, and the O_2 bound to hemoglobin can increase only 0.5 ml per 100 ml of blood. Since maximal hyperventilation with air rarely raises alveolar and arterial pO_2 greater than 130 torr, it can add only 0.3 ml of O_2 (dissolved plus combined) to each 100 ml of blood in a healthy subject. This is not true for removal of CO_2: Doubling alveolar ventilation halves alveolar pCO_2 (from 40 torr to 20 torr) and decreases the CO_2 content from 48.4 ml per 100 ml to 36.3 ml per 100 ml. This means that hyperventilation of some regions of lung can compensate for hypoventilation of others in removing CO_2 but not in loading O_2 (unless the patient is hypoxemic and the percent saturation of hemoglobin by O_2 is on the steep part of the curve).

Because the O_2 curve is relatively flat between pO_2 of 100 and 70 torr, the saturation decreases from 97.4% to only 94%. This means that it is possible to live at high altitude, where inspired pO_2 is much lower than at sea level, without much difficulty in loading O_2. It also means that a patient can have significant respiratory disease resulting in an arterial pO_2 of 70 torr with an arterial saturation only 3.3% below normal.

Although the O_2 curve is not fixed and varies with temperature and pH, the amount of O_2 loaded is relatively unaffected compared to the effect on dissociation, or unloading O_2 in the tissues.

As blood passes through the systemic capillaries, O_2 is removed to meet the metabolic demands of the tissues. At low pO_2, the O_2 curve is very steep and hemoglobin releases O_2; thus, the steep middle and lower parts of the curve protect the tissues by enabling them to withdraw large quantities of O_2 from the blood for relatively small decreases in pO_2. Furthermore, the increased temperature and decreased pH of active tissues shifts the curve to the right, far more in the dissociation part than in the association part, ensuring that blood unloads more O_2.

Recently, an important chemical mechanism controlling hemoglobin affinity for O_2 has been elucidated. A specific chemical, 2,3-diphosphoglycerate (DPG), formed during anaerobic glycolysis in red cells, regulates release of O_2 from oxyhemoglobin. The effect of DPG is usually reported in terms of the pO_2 required to produce 50% saturation of hemoglobin. The oxygen

tension at which hemoglobin is half-saturated with oxygen (P_{50}), determined at 37°C and pH 7.4, is approximately 26 torr with DPG of 15 moles per gram of hemoglobin. P_{50} is increased, favoring release of O_2 in many conditions: high altitude, anemia, hypoxia, sickle cell anemia, exercise, and deficiency of pyruvate kinase in red cells; and in the presence of certain hormones, including thyroid, testosterone, and growth hormone. P_{50} is decreased and O_2 release is hindered in many conditions: storage of red cells in blood banks, deficiency of hexokinase in red cells, high-affinity variants of hemoglobin, and carbon monoxide poisoning.

Although it is clear that free DPG influences O_2 release, the factors regulating DPG formation are still uncertain; active tissues generate heat which may stimulate glycolysis. Increased deoxygenated hemoglobin may bind more DPG, stimulating glycolysis by producing low levels of unbound DPG in cells or increase pH of red cells, increasing glycolysis. Hormones (*e.g.*, thyroid, testosterone, or growth hormone) may also increase glycolysis, or catecholamines may decrease DPG-binding.

The arteriovenous blood oxygen difference for the whole body at rest is 4.07 ± 0.66 ml per 100 ml (mean $\pm$ standard deviation). The mixed venous blood in the pulmonary artery contains slightly more than 15 ml O_2 per 100 ml, which represents an oxyhemoglobin saturation of 75% and an arterial pO_2 of 40 torr.

The actual O_2 pressure of blood leaving the capillaries in the tissues is uncertain, but the measured values are well below those of simultaneously measured venous O_2, indicating that marked O_2 differences exist in the tissues. Indirect estimates of O_2 pressure within the mitochondria are less than 1 torr. However, oxidative metabolism appears to proceed unimpeded at even lower O_2 pressures, and electrical activity in the brain ceases only when mitochrondrial O_2 pressure decreases to well below 1 torr.

CUTANEOUS CIRCULATION

The most superficial cutaneous capillaries contribute relatively little to skin color in most areas of the body. These capillaries originate from subpapillary arterioles, course perpendicularly to the surface, and form tight hairpin loops in the papillae. Thus, only the small apical segment of each loop is visible from the surface of the skin. These capillaries drain into venules, which form an extensive vascular plexus lying immediately below the papillae, parallel to the surface of the skin. The vessels of this plexus are thin-walled and make the largest vascular contribution to skin color.

In nail folds, the capillary loops are profuse and lie parallel to the surface; their contents contribute to the color in these regions. In nail beds, the capillary loops in each papilla are numerous and tortuous, and their density is sufficient to contribute substantially to the color of these regions.

Brachial venous blood does not drain the capillaries of the skin alone and cannot be used to estimate O_2 saturation of cutaneous capillary blood. Indirect estimates of cutaneous venous oxyhemoglobin saturation, based on measurements of skin blood flow and cutaneous oxygen consumption, suggest that the skin is relatively overperfused and that its venous O_2 saturation is high relative to the body as a whole. These findings are consistent with the fact that cutaneous blood flow is of critical importance to heat exchange and temperature control and not simply to subserve the metabolic needs of skin alone.

When ambient temperature increases, cutaneous blood flow increases in excess of the associated increase in cutaneous metabolic rate. Roddie and associates found that the oxyhemoglobin saturation in blood taken from a superficial vein of the forearm was 40% to 72% in normal subjects in a cool room (17°C–19°C) and with heating the saturation increased to 85% to 95%.[1] This well-known effect is why samples of capillary blood are obtained from heated ear lobes or fingertips, which approximate arterial blood values for oxygen saturation and pressure. This increased cutaneous blood flow caused by heating probably results from reflex vasodilation as well as from the opening of multiple, arteriovenous communications.

Despite the complexity of the anatomy and physiology of the cutaneous circulation and the technical difficulty of estimating accurately oxygen saturation and oxyhemoglobin concentration in skin capillaries by measuring arterial and brachial venous blood oxygen values, the results of the classical studies of cyanosis by Lundsgaard and Van Slyke[2] are still clinically relevant: An increased concentration of deoxyhemoglobin in cutaneous vessels is responsible for cyanosis. The intensity of the cyanosis depends on the absolute concentration of deoxyhemoglobin and not on the ratio of oxyhemoglobin and deoxyhemoglobin. On the basis of results obtained in a variety of diseases and physiologic conditions, skin becomes cyanotic when the numerical average of the oxygen deficits in the arterial and venous blood in the arm exceeds 6 ml to 7 ml per 100 ml of whole blood. In anemia, the concentration of hemoglobin may be too low for cyanosis to develop. In polycythemia, cyanosis may occur with less unsaturation. When oxyhemoglobin is 75% saturated, blood with a hemoglobin concentration of 20 g per 100 ml contains 5 g deoxyhemoglobin, whereas at the same

O_2 saturation, blood with a hemoglobin of 5 g per 100 ml contains 1.25 g deoxyhemoglobin only.

PERIPHERAL CYANOSIS

Peripheral cyanosis is caused by increased extraction of O_2 from the systemic capillaries by the tissues. It results either from increased utilization (*e.g.*, muscular exercise) or decreased blood flow (*e.g.*, polycythemia). The Fick principle relates the O_2 consumption of an organ, the blood flow to it, and the arteriovenous O_2 concentration difference across it:

Blood flow to the organ =
$$\frac{O_2 \text{ consumption by the organ}}{\substack{O_2 \text{ content} \\ \text{(arterial blood minus venous blood} \\ \text{from the organ)}}}$$

The most common type of peripheral cyanosis is caused by decreased blood flow to the peripheral capillaries, resulting in increased O_2 extraction from the blood during its passage through the capillary bed. In normal subjects this condition may result from chilling, cold applications, or exposure to low environmental temperature. Cyanosis is particularly apparent in the nail beds of the extremities under these circumstances. At very low temperatures, however, cutaneous metabolism is reduced, O_2 extraction decreases, and the oxyhemoglobin dissociation curve shifts to the left, so that less O_2 is lost to tissues. Then, despite almost complete cessation of cutaneous blood flow, the skin of the ears and nose may appear bright red.

During anxiety, normal subjects may also have cyanosis of the nail beds (usually associated with pale, cold skin), owing to the constriction of superficial cutaneous blood vessels.

Peripheral cyanosis may result from decreased cutaneous blood flow in polycythemia (owing to increased blood viscosity); in Raynaud's disease (owing to spasmodic contraction of arteries, especially in the fingers); in thromboangiitis; or in phlebitis, venous thrombosis, or even venous varicosities (owing to venous obstruction of capillary flow).

Cardiac diseases are commonly associated with peripheral cyanosis. In congestive cardiac failure with low cardiac output, although the arteriovenous O_2 difference is seldom greater than 9 ml per 100 ml at rest for the body as a whole, blood flow to the extremities is often reduced disproportionately, leading to increased O_2 extraction and peripheral cyanosis. Cyanosis becomes even more apparent during exercise, because O_2 extraction increases as cardiac output fails to increase appropriately for the increased O_2 demands of the tissues. This situation may be aggravated by pulmonary congestion or edema, causing hypoxemia and worsening cyanosis on a central basis. Cyanosis is also found in other conditions associated with reduced cardiac output such as shock; moreover, in severe hypotensive states, mismatching of ventilation and perfusion in the lungs may cause hypoxemia and worsening cyanosis on a central basis.

In cardiac conditions associated with increased venous pressure, such as tricuspid disease, the subpapillary venous plexus becomes congested, and skin color is affected by these dilated, prominent venules. In advanced tricuspid valvular disease, jaundice may be associated with cyanosis, resulting in a skin color called *icterocyanosis*.

The peripheral cyanosis of cardiac failure is characteristically most marked in distal regions such as the hands, the feet, and the tip of the nose. Peripheral cyanosis may be differentiated from central cyanosis resulting from hypoxemia, as Sir Thomas Lewis suggested, by massaging the cyanotic part or applying heat to it. The resultant increased blood flow will abolish peripheral but not central cyanosis.

CENTRAL CYANOSIS

Hypoxia may present as cyanosis; however, cyanosis is an unreliable indicator of the state of arterial oxygenation (Table 20-1). Severe arterial hypoxemia may occur without cyanosis; unless cardiac output increases, tissue hypoxia is inevitable. This may be manifested by abnormal brain function (poor judgment, irritability, dizziness, paranoia, confusion, coma) and by abnormal cardiac function (hypotension and cardiac arrhythmias, particularly atrial flutter).

Hypoxia evokes a series of compensatory responses, including (1) hyperventilation secondary to stimulation of chemoreceptors, and (2) increased sympathetic activity secondary to both chemoreceptor and vasomotor center discharge. The increased sympathetic activity leads to increased heart rate, which causes increased cardiac output. Selective peripheral vasoconstriction preferentially directs blood flow to vital organs. The combination of increased cardiac output and peripheral resistance results in systolic hypertension. In the absence of this sympathetic activation of the circulation, bradycardia, hypotension, and circulatory arrest ensue.

Hypoxia may be promoted by many patient factors, such as old age, obesity, or cardiopulmonary disease; restrictive factors, such as pain or abnormal posture; and depressive factors, such as narcotics or sedatives which depress central nervous system (CNS) function. Circulatory compensation may be compromised by coronary artery disease, obesity, anemia, and other pa-

Table 20-1. *Causes of Hypoxia*

	Effect on Arterial Blood			
Cause of Hypoxia	O_2 Pressure	O_2 Content	O_2 Saturation	CO_2 Pressure
Normal lungs, inadequate oxygenation				
Deficiency of O_2 in atmosphere	↓	↓	↓	↓
Hypoventilation (CNS or neuromuscular disease)	↓	↓	↓	↑
Venous-to-arterial shunts				
Intracardiac	↓	↓	↓	↓,↔, or ↑
Intrapulmonary	↓	↓	↓	↓,↔, or ↑
Pulmonary disease				
Hypoventilation	↓	↓	↓	↑
Uneven distribution of ventilation/perfusion	↓*	↓*	↓*	↓,↔, or ↑
Diffusion defect	↓*	↓*	↓*	↓
Inadequate transport/delivery of O_2				
Anemia; abnormal hemoglobin	↔	↓	↔‡	↔
General circulatory deficiency	↔	↔	↔	↔
Localized circulatory deficiency	↔	↔	↔	↔
Inadequate tissue oxygenation				
Tissue edema	↔	↔	↔	↔
Abnormal tissue demand	↔	↔	↔	↔
Poisoning of cellular enzymes	↔	↔	↔	↔

*Unless hyperventilation present
‡Saturation of active hemoglobin normal, ↑ = increased, ↔ = no change, ↓ = decreased.
(After Comroe, JH, Forster II, RE, Dubois, AB: The Lung, p 149. Chicago, Year Book, 1962)

tient factors, as well as by drugs, such as narcotics and anesthetics.

In any event, cyanosis is a late sign, since in a normal subject with 15.6 g of hemoglobin per 100 ml of blood, cyanosis does not occur until arterial oxygen saturation decreases to 80%. If the patient is anemic, (hemoglobin of 10 g per 100 ml), cyanosis does not occur until there is a decrease to 70% to 75% saturation, corresponding to an arterial pO_2 of 35 torr or an altitude of 20,000 feet. If blood flow is doubled to a tissue, the threshold for cyanosis would be 60% arterial O_2 saturation for a patient with 10 g of hemoglobin, and 70% saturation for a patient with normal hemoglobin. Thus, cyanosis appears even later in patients capable of increasing their blood flow in response to hypoxia. If anemic, such a patient might suffer irreversible tissue injury without even becoming cyanotic (Fig. 20-1).

PULMONARY ABNORMALITIES

Hypoxia may result from decreased arterial pO_2 if the airway is obstructed. It may also occur with alveolar hypoventilation from any cause (Table 20-2): increased work of breathing related to an abnormally stiff chest wall (obesity, kyphoscoliosis), impaired respiratory muscle function (poliomyelitis, myasthenia); CNS depression (drug overdose, idiopathic); or certain pul-

monary diseases, especially of the obstructive type (asthma, bronchitis, or bronchiolitis). In the last situation, McNicol and Campbell have emphasized that most patients with chronic respiratory failure enter the hospital with severe hypoxemia, modest hypercapnea, and mild acidemia; they are usually conscious, without shock, and have an effective cough.[3] The explanation of the modest hypercapnea and acidemia is in the reciprocal relationship between alveolar pO_2 and pCO_2. The higher the alveolar pCO_2, the lower the alveolar pO_2. When the patient is breathing air, the highest tolerable pCO_2 is 80 to 90 torr with a severely decreased pO_2 of 20 to 30 torr (Fig. 20-2).

Hypoxemia may result from decreased O_2 in inspired air. This can occur at high altitude: At 17,600 feet, arterial O_2 saturation is 68%, comparable to an arterial pO_2 caused by breathing 10% O_2 at sea level. Hypoxemia may also result from breathing a subnormal concentration of O_2 in air at sea level, such as might occur in respiratory failure, after an error in O_2 therapy, or in an anesthesia accident or error.

Decreased oxygen pressure may also result from anatomic shunts or shuntlike effects within the lungs. Shuntlike effects within the lungs occur with atelectasis, pneumothorax, or pneumonia when regions of lung are perfused but not ventilated.

Diffusion defects, as seen in restrictive disorders such as pulmonary fibrosis or vascular disorders such as

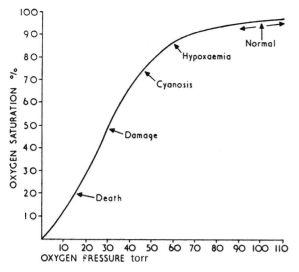

Fig. 20-1. Oxygen dissociation curve. The O_2 dissociation curve relates the saturation of the hemoglobin to the partial pressure of oxygen (pO_2) in the blood. In a normal subject at sea level, the arterial pO_2 is 90 to 110 torr and saturation is 95% to 98%. The threshold of hypoxemia occurs at the shoulder of this curve ($pO_2 = 60$ torr and saturation = 90%). Cyanosis cannot be detected reliably until the saturation falls to almost 70%. Although hypoxia even of slight degree has effects on the respiration, circulation, and bone marrow, they are essentially adaptive; unless there is some complicating factor, damage occurs only at a pO_2 of 0 torr to 40 torr (saturation about 50%). An arterial pO_2 below 20 torr seems insupportable. Note that a fall of pO_2 over 40 torr is required to produce cyanosis that can be detected reliably; a further fall of only 20 torr may be fatal. The oxygen dissociation curve has been shifted to the right in the lower portion because of the usual acidemia present in respiratory failure. (After Campbell, EJM: Respiratory failure. Br Med J 1:1451, 1965)

systemic lupus erythematosus, seldom cause decreased arterial pO_2 at rest but may contribute to hypoxia during exercise. Recent studies indicate that O_2 diffusion is not impaired significantly by increased thickness of the alveolar capillary membrane but can be impaired when the capillary bed is reduced, resulting in insufficient time for O_2 to equilibrate with the red cell in the pulmonary capillary. As cardiac output increases with exercise, velocity of blood flow increases through the restricted capillary bed, leading to hypoxemia.

The most common cause of hypoxia and decreased arterial pO_2 associated with pulmonary disorders is regional hypoventilation relative to perfusion. This abnormality can occur with any pulmonary disorder but most commonly occurs with chronic airway obstruction.

Table 20-2. *Causes of Hypoventilation*

Diseases of	Examples
Brain	Sedative overdose, CVA, head trauma
Spinal cord	Poliomyelitis, Guillain–Barré syndrome Spinal cord trauma
Chest wall	Flail chest, rheumatoid spondylitis
Upper airways	Tumor of cords Laryngospasm
Lower airways/lungs	Bronchitis, asthma, emphysema Severe pneumonias
Heart	Congestive heart failure

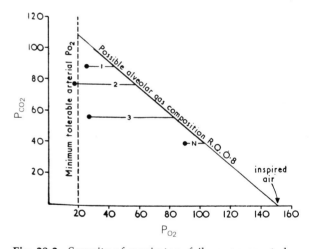

Fig. 20-2. Severity of respiratory failure represented on a carbon dioxide–oxygen diagram. This CO_2:O_2 diagram is based on a barometric pressure of 760 torr. The value of 20 torr (equivalent to a saturation of 30% to 40%) chosen for the minimal tolerable arterial pO_2 is based on general experience. The horizontal lines are observed values; the height of the line is the arterial pCO_2. At the right is the alveolar pO_2; at the left is the arterial pO_2. The horizontal length is the alveolar-arterial pO_2 difference. The line N gives average normal values. The other lines are taken from a series of 81 patients with hypercapnia whose arterial blood was examined soon after admission to hospital and before administration of O_2: No. 1 is patient with highest pCO_2 (88 torr); No. 2 is patient with lowest pO_2 (19 torr); and No. 3 is patient with greatest alveolar-arterial pO_2 difference (57 torr). The data are based on studies of McNicol and E.J.M. Campbell. (From Campbell EJM: Respiratory failure. Br Med J 1:1457, 1965)

CARDIAC ABNORMALITIES

Cyanosis in congenital heart disease is mainly attributable to contamination of the arterial stream by venous blood. Such a right–left shunt may occur through any of the various abnormal communications that may exist between the right and left cardiac chambers or great vessels. Whether a shunt exists depends on the size of the communication and the relationship between the pressures on either side of the communication. Normally both the systolic and the diastolic pressures in the left cardiac chambers and great vessels exceed those in the corresponding right chambers and vessels. In atrial and ventricular septal defects and patent ductus arteriosus, the shunt is from left to right, and cyanosis is absent. If the pressures in the pulmonary artery, right ventricle, and right atrium are increased greatly, as they often are when pulmonary vascular lesions develop or cardiac failure supervenes, the shunt may become bidirectional or may be reversed completely. In pulmonic stenosis, pressures in the right ventricle, and also secondarily in the right atrium, are increased and may give rise to a right–left shunt through a ventricular septal defect, a patent foramen ovale, or an atrial septal defect. Pressure relationships between the atria may be altered by vigorous crying, the Valsalva maneuver, or heavy exertion, which can cause transient reversal of a left–right interatrial shunt.

Several factors determine the presence or absence and degree of cyanosis in congenital heart disease. Most important is the size of the shunt relative to the systemic blood flow. If the systemic blood flow is normal, it is possible for one third of it to be composed of venous blood without the appearance of cyanosis, since the arterial oxyhemoglobin saturation would be greater than 85%. This is demonstrated in Table 20-1.

Another factor is the oxyhemoglobin saturation of the venous blood. If the systemic blood flow is less than normal in a patient with cyanotic congenital heart disease, the arteriovenous oxygen difference is increased, and the mixed venous blood that is shunted into the arterial circulation is less saturated with oxygen. Under these circumstances, a small shunt may produce a significant degree of hypoxemia. During exercise, the oxyhemoglobin saturation of mixed venous blood normally falls. This change may be exaggerated in cyanotic congenital heart disease because of an inability to increase cardiac output appropriately. This factor, as well as an increase in the size of the shunt, accounts for the exaggerated hypoxemia and cyanosis that develop during exertion. In some patients, cyanosis may not be evident except with exertion. Therefore, observation of the patient during some simple form of exercise constitutes an important part of the examination. In extensive bidirectional shunting through a defect, the saturation of the blood shunted from right to left depends on the ratio of pulmonary and systemic blood flows. If the ratio is high, a large right–left shunt may not produce much arterial desaturation.

Secondary polycythemia occurs frequently and is another factor that is responsible for the very profound degree of cyanosis that is observed in these disorders.

Pulmonary factors ordinarily do not play a role in producing the hypoxemia unless cardiac failure with pulmonary congestion develops. The arterial lesions responsible for the production of marked pulmonary arterial hypertension in some cases of congenital heart disease do not interfere greatly with pulmonary gas exchange, and pulmonary venous saturation in such patients is usually within the normal range. Pulmonary arteriovenous fistula, a congenital vascular lesion, may give rise to cyanosis and polycythemia without disturbing cardiac function. In some cases multiple fistulae occur, and the cyanosis may be pronounced.

The anatomic distribution of cyanosis in the various congenital cardiovascular disorders is like that in arterial hypoxemia of any cause. However, there are instances in which the distribution is not uniform. Cyanosis of the lower extremities, with absence or a lesser degree of cyanosis in the upper extremities, occurs in patent ductus arteriosus when the usual direction of blood flow through the ductus is reversed as a result of severe pulmonary arterial hypertension.[4] Since the ductus is inserted into the aorta distal to the bronchiocephalic arteries, the venous blood is directed mainly into the descending aorta. Occasionally the left hand is more cyanotic than the right because the left subclavian artery, which arises almost opposite the ductus, receives some of the shunt. The differential cyanosis between the upper and lower extremities often is associated with differential clubbing and is of diagnostic importance. The "machinery" murmur typical of a patent ductus is absent under these circumstances (reversed flow).[4] Reversal of ductus flow also occurs in coarctation of the aorta when a coexisting ductus inserts into the aorta beyond the coarctation.

Normally, a very small quantity of venous blood is shunted into the systemic arterial stream through anastomotic connections between the bronchial and the pulmonary veins, and by drainage of the thebesian and the anterior cardiac veins into the left heart. This venous admixture does not exceed 1% of the pulmonary blood flow.[5] In some patients with cirrhosis of the liver, venous admixture is increased by the development of anastomoses between the portal, the mediastinal, and the pulmonary veins.[6] This venous admixture, although apparently not large, may contribute to the

decreased arterial oxyhemoglobin saturation and the consequent cyanosis that occur in some patients with alcoholic cirrhosis.

ABNORMALITIES OF HEMOGLOBIN

Hemoglobin, a metalloprotein of molecular weight 64,500, contains four ferroprotoporphyrin or heme units, each of which is capable of binding a single molecule of oxygen. (Truly phenomenal advances in peptide chemistry have resulted in identification of the amino acids and their sequence in the peptic chains that constitute the protein moiety of hemoglobin, and x-ray diffraction studies have revealed the conformation of the entire molecule.)[7,8,9] Normal adult human hemoglobin is composed of four polypeptide chains. The sequence of the 141 amino acid residues in each of two of these chains, designated α, is identical and differs from that of the 146 residues in the other two identical β chains. These chains appear to be crumpled together, and the heme units, which are bonded by their iron atoms to the imidazole nitrogen of histidines at position 87 in the α chains and position 92 in the β chains, are imbedded in them.

It has been known for some time that binding of an oxygen molecule by one of the heme units successively facilitates binding of the gas by the other heme groups in the molecule. This phenomenon, known as the heme–heme interaction, accounts for the distinctive configuration of the oxyhemoglobin dissociation curve and has been the subject of extensive theoretical analyses.[8] A complete explanation of the phenomenon is still not at hand, but an essential component of the mechanism is a conformational change in the hemoglobin molecule that occurs when it binds oxygen.[9] Hemoglobin is capable of dissociating into two symmetrical dimers, each containing an α and a β chain, and by current theory the dimer is the primary functional unit. Oxygenation enhances the tendency of hemoglobin to dissociate. Heme–heme interaction is regarded as the result of the effect of oxygen-binding on the dissociation of the hemoglobin molecule to dimers and of the rapid exchange of oxygen among dimeric units.[10,11]

Decreased O_2 content of arterial blood occurs when the arterial pO_2 is decreased, but also in association with anemia (discussed earlier), carbon monoxide poisoning, and abnormal hemoglobins. Carbon monoxide has an affinity for hemoglobin 210 times that of O_2. Thus, blood equilibrated with air plus 0.1% CO (210:1 ratio) will contain 50% oxyhemoglobin and 50% carbon monoxyhemoglobin. This saturation would not result instantaneously; in fact, with a normal level of cardiac output and ventilation in an average adult, it might take almost 2 hours to reach such a concentration of carbon monoxyhemoglobin. Since CO is colorless, odorless, tasteless, nonirritant, and causes no change in ventilation or respiratory symptoms, it is a particularly dangerous gas and may be inhaled long enough to cause severe hypoxia and death. The effect of CO on O_2 transport is not only to exclude O_2 from hemoglobin (an effect like several anemia), but also to shift the O_2 dissociation curve to the left so that less O_2 is released to the tissues or is available only at very low pO_2. This is particularly dangerous in heart muscle where 60% to 70% of O_2 in the arterial blood is extracted and a significant amount of carbon monoxyhemoglobin might prevent unloading of O_2 needed by the heart. Small amounts of CO (as found in heavy smokers) may impair O_2 delivery to tissues more than a loss of 5% to 8% of hemoglobin, by bleeding or marrow failure. But the reduction of tissue O_2 from 40 to 35 torr would probably be significant only in patients with ischemic disease and already borderline O_2 supply.

There are now over 120 variants of normal adult hemoglobin. Abnormal hemoglobins may affect O_2 transport, usually by altering the unloading of O_2 from hemoglobin. In only one, hemoglobin M, is the abnormality in the heme group. In another, hemoglobin Kansas, there is a marked change in association: Only 70% to 75% saturation occurs at normal arterial pO_2.

Several genetic variants of hemoglobin have been discovered that differ chemically from hemoglobin A only by a substitution of a single amino acid residue in either the α or β peptide chains. The physical properties of these hemoglobins, as in the case of sickle cell hemoglobin (S) or hemoglobin C, differ from those of hemoglobin.

One such hemoglobin was obtained from a 14-year-old boy who was completely normal except for cyanosis, which had been present since birth.[12] His hemoglobin showed a striking reduction in its affinity for oxygen; although the arterial blood oxygen tension was normal (100 torr), the hemoglobin was only 60% saturated with oxygen. Saturation attained a level of 94% during oxygen breathing. Hemoglobin from the patient's mother showed a quantitatively similar decrease in ability to bind oxygen.

This hemoglobin, now designated as *Kansas hemoglobin,* has a threonine residue instead of the normal asparagine residue in position 102 of the β chain, but its primary structure is otherwise identical to that of hemoglobin A.[13] The striking decrease in its affinity for oxygen has been attributed to its increased tendency to dissociate into dimeric units when oxygenated.[13,14] This dissociation constant of the oxygenated tetramer is almost 200 times that of hemoglobin A.[13] P_{50} is 3.3

times greater than that of normal hemoglobin. The ease with which this hemoglobin unloads its oxygen in the systemic capillaries prevents the development of hypoxia.

Hemoglobin variants with a single amino acid substitution that have been characterized as having increased affinity for oxygen are called Chesapeake, Yakima, Kempsey, Rainier, Hiroshima, and J-Cape Town. All, with the exception of J-Cape Town, are associated with erythrocytosis in members of families who are homozygous for these hemoglobins.[14] The high affinity of hemoglobin Chesapeake for oxygen has been attributed to decreased dissociation of the oxygenated hemoglobin tetramer.[14]

Fetal hemoglobin (F) differs from adult hemoglobin in that it contains two γ peptide chains instead of the two β chains. This hemoglobin constitutes 60% to 90% of circulating hemoglobin at birth and is gradually replaced by hemoglobin A; by age 4 months, only traces of hemoglobin F persist.[7] Although the oxygen affinity of umbilical cord blood is greater than that of adult blood, this is not an intrinsic property of hemoglobin F but is related to some factor in the intracellular environment, since the difference disappears after dialysis of the protein.[7]

Two hemoglobins associated with a thalassemialike clinical picture are hemoglobin H and hemoglobin Bart's. All the polypeptide chains in H are β, and in Bart's they are all γ.[7] Both hemoglobins have an abnormally large affinity for oxygen; that of H is 10 times normal.[15]

It has been shown recently that certain organic phosphates, especially adenosine triphosphate and DPG affect the affinity of hemoglobin for oxygen.[16] This compound is an intermediary product of red cell glycolytic metabolism and is present in relatively high concentration. It binds specifically with deoxyhemoglobin, consequently reducing affinity of hemoglobin for oxygen. It is believed that the reduction of intracellular concentration of unbound DPG that occurs with an increase in deoxyhemoglobin stimulates glycolytic production of the compound and raises its total concentration in the cell. Thus, DPG might be a cardinal component of a feedback system that relates red cell metabolism to the functional properties of the hemoglobin and thereby regulates the interaction of hemoglobin and oxygen to a level appropriate for the existing physiologic state.

One of the adaptations to high altitude is a decreased affinity of hemoglobin for oxygen (increased P_{50}), which acts to make hemoglobin-bound oxygen more available to the tissues. Studies have shown that the increased P_{50} that occurred in the hemoglobin of intact red cells within 24 hours after ascent to 4350

meters was accompanied by an increase of more than 50% in the concentration of DPG, and that these changes were reversed by descent to sea level.[17] The marked increase in oxygen affinity of red cells during storage has been correlated with a drastic fall in red cell DPG concentration; this defect can be partially corrected by partial metabolic repletion of erythrocyte DPG.[18] Young red cells have a much lower oxygen affinity than do old red cells, and this has been attributed to the fact that DPG concentration in young cells is 40% greater than that in old cells.[18,19] Increased P_{50} of erythrocytes has been observed in patients with chronic hypoxemia secondary to either pulmonary disease or congenital heart disease and in patients with chronic low cardiac output;[20,21] it has been suggested that this change may be related to higher intracellular concentrations of DPG.

Hemoglobin M is of interest because of its tendency to form methemoglobin. In the several variants of this protein that have been characterized, a single amino acid substitution has been found in the α or β chains, usually at or in proximity to the point of attachment of the heme group.[22] The oxidized or ferric form of the heme units in the abnormal chains resists the action of intracellular enzyme systems that maintain heme iron in the ferrous form, and consequently concentrations of circulating methemoglobin rise to values well above the normal of 2%.[22] Not only is methemoglobin not capable of binding oxygen, but it shifts the dissociation curve of coexisting normal hemoglobin to the left. Patients with methemoglobinemia may experience fatigue, dyspnea, and palpitation, and polycythemia may develop. The skin has a peculiar leaden, blue-gray color, and the blood has a chocolate hue.

Hemoglobin-M disease should not be confused with another form of congenital methemoglobinemia in which the hemoglobin protein is normal but methemoglobin reductase in the red cell is deficient. Reduced nicotinamide adenine dinucleotide diaphorase is the most active enzyme performing this function and is specifically deficient in this disorder.[22]

RELATIONSHIP OF CYANOSIS TO CO_2 EXCHANGE

When hypoxemia is due to an overall diminution of alveolar ventilation, the tension of CO_2 in alveolar air and arterial blood also is increased (see chapter 19, Dyspnea). Characteristically, in instances of uneven distribution of air and blood among the alveoli (such as may be caused by obstruction of the intrapulmonary airways in emphysema, asthma, or pulmonary edema), there is an increase in CO_2 tension and consequent

respiratory acidosis only when many alveolar areas are underventilated and there is already advanced anoxemia. This phenomenon is explained by the fact that other areas of the lung are hyperventilated. CO_2 output from the overventilated alveoli can balance or even overcompensate for the retention of this gas in the blood of poorly ventilated alveoli because of the steepness of the blood CO_2 dissociation curve. On the other hand, the oxyhemoglobin dissociation curve is relatively flat in the usual physiologic range. The additional amount of O_2 that can be bound by the blood in the overventilated alveoli is not sufficient to compensate for the inadequate oxygenation of the blood in the underventilated regions.

If the alveolar-capillary membrane is abnormal, hypoxemia may be severe, but because of the much greater diffusibility of CO_2 as compared to O_2, exchange of CO_2 is relatively undisturbed unless inadequacy of alveolar ventilation and ventilation/perfusion defects are superimposed.

Until recent years, the clinical importance of CO_2 has been poorly appreciated. In high concentrations this gas produces unconsciousness. In lesser concentration, delirium, stupor, and somnolence are common effects. In very high concentrations it can produce death. The exact concentrations at which these phenomena occur is not known. Stupor has been observed in young men breathing 10.4% CO_2 for 3 minutes to 4 minutes.[23,24,25] Patients with pulmonary disease whose arterial CO_2 tension rises to the range of 100 torr frequently become comatose. Normal subjects lose consciousness in 20 seconds to 30 seconds upon breathing a mixture of 30% CO_2 and 70% O_2.[26]

CO_2 is a powerful dilator of the cerebral vessels.[27] The sudden dilatation of these vessels that occurs with increments in arterial CO_2 tension causes an abrupt increase in cerebrospinal fluid pressure.[28] This change may be of sufficient degree to produce papilledema.[29] CO_2 directly constricts other systemic vessels and may produce a rise in blood pressure. In high concentrations it may cause cardiac arrhythmias, both auricular and ventricular.[26]

EFFECTS OF OXYGEN ON CYANOSIS

When pure O_2 is breathed, the pressure of O_2 in the alveolar air and arterial blood is increased sixfold. The concentration of O_2 carried in solution consequently rises to 1.8 ml per 100 ml; an additional 0.6 ml per 100 ml is bound by the hemoglobin, since it becomes fully saturated. The net increase in arterial O_2 content is,

therefore, 2.4 ml per 100 ml. The additional increase in dissolved O_2 that can be achieved by breathing O_2 under increased pressure in a hyperbaric chamber is directly related to the ambient pressure.

Amelioration of any type of cyanosis will occur on breathing pure O_2. For example, in peripheral cyanosis with normal hemoglobin concentration, if the arterial blood O_2 content is raised from 19.8 ml to 22.2 ml per 100 ml, and the amount of O_2 extracted by the tissues continues at 12 ml per 100 ml, the venous blood will be only 9.9 ml per 100 ml unsaturated. The average deficit of O_2 in the capillary blood will be 4.4 ml per 100 ml (equivalent to 3.3 g per 100 ml of deoxyhemoglobin) instead of 6.5 ml per 100 ml, and cyanosis will disappear. However, O_2 will not abolish cyanosis when the peripheral blood flow is more restricted and the arteriovenous O_2 difference in the tissue being examined is consequently greater than that in this example.

In the case of a right–left shunt, breathing of O_2 will also lessen the hypoxemia and relieve cyanosis by increasing the amount of O_2 in both the pulmonary venous blood and in the systemic venous blood that is being shunted. In the mixture calculation described in the section on congenital heart disease, the pulmonary venous O_2 content will increase to 22.2 ml per 100 ml, the right–left shunt content to 15.8 ml per 100 ml, and the arterial content to 20.07 ml per 100 ml, which corresponds to an oxyhemoglobin saturation of 98%. Although arterial saturation may reach the normal range, O_2 tension will fall far short of 650 torr, the value normally found during O_2 breathing. Measurement of arterial blood O_2 tension while the subject is breathing O_2 is a simple procedure, and the value can be used in a simple shunt formula interrelating calculated concentrations of dissolved O_2 in pulmonary venous, mixed venous, and arterial blood to estimate the relative magnitude of the shunt. Complete saturation of the arterial blood with O_2, however, will not occur if the shunt is greater than 40% of the systemic blood flow or if the arteriovenous O_2 difference is greater than normal.

Measurement of alveolar-arterial O_2 pressure differences during administration of pure O_2 is useful to detect abnormalities in gas exchange and clinical problems such as atelectasis, pneumonia, or pneumothorax even before the radiograph is abnormal. The most dramatic relief of hypoxemia and cyanosis that is achieved by administration of O_2 occurs when gas exchange is impaired by disturbances in pulmonary function. Regardless of whether these disturbances consist of marked generalized alveolar hypoventilation, maldistribution of air and blood among the alveoli, decrease in the pulmonary O_2 diffusing capacity, or a combination of these factors (as is so often the case), administration

of O_2 will almost always increase the arterial blood oxyhemoglobin saturation to or near normal. O_2 therapy is therefore of considerable value, especially in acute conditions such as pulmonary edema, pneumonia, chronic pulmonary disease complicated by a respiratory infection, and severe asthma. Frequently it is life-saving (Fig. 20-1).

Some reservations about the use of O_2 should be noted. When alveolar ventilation is decreased seriously by respiratory paralysis resulting from poliomyelitis or depression of the respiratory center, O_2 will promptly abolish hypoxemia and cyanosis, but it will not correct the coexisting hypercapnia. The patient may be spared the danger of anoxia while receiving O_2 but may develop all the serious mental and neurologic consequences of a markedly increased blood CO_2 tension and respiratory acidosis. Mechanical ventilation is the essential therapy in these conditions and is the only way to control the concentration of CO_2 in the alveolar air and the arterial blood.

In chronic pulmonary disease complicated by chronic hypoxemia and respiratory acidosis, as is often the case in emphysema, O_2 may produce undesirable sequelae, especially if it is administered in concentrations approaching 100%. The respiratory centers of such patients are relatively insensitive to CO_2 and increase in blood hydrogen ion concentration. A greater than normal portion of central neurogenic drive to respiration arises from hypoxic reflexes originating in the O_2-sensitive aortic and carotid bodies, although recent evidence suggests that, in part, the increased drive is the result of hypoxia-induced lactic acidosis, causing central hydrogen ion drive to ventilation. In either case, elevation of the arterial O_2 tension to normal or above on breathing O_2 abolishes the hypoxia-induced impulses, and ventilation may drop precipitously. Preexisting inadequacy of alveolar ventilation is aggravated thereby. Alveolar and arterial CO_2 tensions rise sharply, and the various manifestations of CO_2 narcosis syndrome may appear.

If O_2 therapy is required, as it often is when the chronic pulmonary insufficiency is acutely aggravated, it is best given in concentrations of 24% to 28%. Such concentrations will improve arterial oxyhemoglobin saturation substantially without producing intolerable depression of respiratory drive. In the range of arterial pO_2 25 to 40 torr, arterial oxygenation and tissue O_2 supply are very sensitive to a small change in inspired O_2 concentration. The worse the hypoxemia, the steeper the portion of the O_2 dissociation curve on which O_2 uptake occurs: For a given increase in pO_2, the greater the increase in arterial O_2 content and the greater the relative increase in O_2 supply. Therefore, the aim of

O_2 therapy is to increase inspired O_2 a small amount to greatly improve oxygenation or greatly reduce the threat of hypoxia. If the increased O_2 causes a decrease in ventilation, the reciprocal relationship between pO_2 and pCO_2 implies that pCO_2 cannot rise by as much as the increase in pO_2. Breathing 25% O_2 is unlikely to cause arterial pCO_2 to increase more than 10 torr (Fig. 20-3). With judicious use of O_2 enriched air, guided by careful monitoring of the patient and his arterial blood gas concentrations and supplemented by a vigorous therapeutic attack on underlying bronchial obstruction, pulmonary infection, and cardiac failure, the clinician can maintain ventilation without resorting to mechanical respirators.[30,31] The treatment of pulmonary insufficiency and the use of O_2 and mechanical ventilators and their potential dangers are beyond the scope of this chapter; the interested reader is referred to the extensive and growing literature on these subjects.[32]

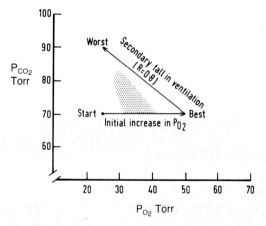

Fig. 20-3. Effects on arterial blood gases of increasing inspired pO_2 from 150 torr (21% O_2, air at sea level) to 175 torr (24.5% O_2). Assumed conditions breathing air (*start*): arterial pCO_2 70 torr, pO_2 25 torr, respiratory gas exchange ratio (R) 0.8. When the inspired pO_2 is increased by 25 torr, the initial increase in arterial pO_2 is difficult to predict but is unlikely to be greater than 25; so the "best" result that might occur would be an increase in pO_2 to 50 torr and no change in pCO_2. If a secondary fall in ventilation occurred before the original pO_2 was restored, the "worst" result might be an increase in pCO_2 of 20 torr (*i.e.,* the increase in inspired $pO_2 \times R$). In clinical practice, the initial rise in arterial pO_2 is not more than 15 torr (nor less than 7 torr) and pCO_2 rarely increases more than 12 torr, so the net result is that the blood gas changes are limited to the shaded area. (From Campbell EJM: The management of acute respiratory failure in chronic bronchitis and emphysema. The J. Burns Amberson Lecture. Am Rev Respir Dis 96:626, 1967)

REFERENCES

1. **Roddie IC, Shepherd JT, Whelan RF:** Evidence from venous saturation measurements that the increase in forearm blood during body heating is confined to the skin. J Physiol 134:444, 1956

2. **Lundsgaard C, Van Slyke DD:** Cyanosis. Medicine 2:1, 1923

3. **McNicol MW, Campbell EJM:** Severity of respiratory failure: Arterial blood-gases in untreated patients. Lancet 1:336, 1965

4. **Lukas DS, Araujo J, Steinberg I:** The syndrome of patent ductus arteriosus with reversal of flow. Am J Med 17:298, 1954

5. **Fritts HW Jr, Hardewig A, Rochester DF, Durand J, Cournand A:** Estimation of pulmonary arteriovenous shunt-flow using intravenous injections of T-1824 dye Kr[85] J Clin Invest 39:1841, 1960

6. **Calabresi P, Abelmann WH:** Porto-caval and porto-pulmonary anastomoses in Laennec's cirrhosis and in heart failure. J Clin Invest 36:1257, 1957

7. **Lehmann H, Huntsman RC, Ager JAM:** The Hemoglobinopathies and thalassemia. In Stanbury JB, Wyngaarden JB, Frederickson DS (eds): The Metabolic Basis of Inherited Disease, p 1100. New York, McGraw–Hill, 1966

8. **Roughton FJW:** Transport of oxygen and carbon dioxide. In Fenn W, Rahn H (eds): Handbook of Physiology. Respiration, vol I, sec 3, p 767. Washington, D.C., American Physiological Society, 1964

9. **Muirhead H, Perutz MF:** A three-dimensional Fourier synthesis of reduced human hemoglobin at 5.5 A resolution. Nature 199:633, 1963

10. **Benesch RE, Benesch R, Macduff G:** Subunit exchange and ligand binding: A new hypothesis for the mechanism of oxygenation of hemoglobin. Proc Nat Acad Sci USA 54:535, 1965

11. **Guidotti G:** Studies on the chemistry of hemoglobin. IV. The mechanism of reaction with ligands. J Biol Chem 242:3704, 1967

12. **Reissmann KR, Ruth WE, Nomura T:** A human hemoglobin with lowered oxygen affinity and impaired heme–heme interactions. J Clin Invest 40:1826, 1961

13. **Bonaventure J, Riggs A:** Hemoglobin Kansas: A human hemoglobin with a neutral amino acid substitution and an abnormal oxygen equilibrium. J Biol Chem 243:980, 1968

14. **Bunn HF:** Subunit dissociation of certain abnormal hemoglobins. J Clin Invest 48:126, 1969

15. **Benesch R, Ranney HM, Benesch RE:** Some properties of hemoglobin H. Fed Proc 20:70, 1961

16. **Benesch R, Benesch RE, Yu CI:** Reciprocal binding of oxygen and diphosphoglycerate by human hemoglobin. Proc Nat Acad Sci USA 59:526, 1968

17. **Lenfant C, Torrance J, English E, Finch CA, Reyafarje C et al:** Effect of altitude on oxygen binding by hemoglobin and on organic phosphate levels. J Clin Invest 47:2652, 1968

18. **Bunn HF, May MH, Kocholaty WF, Shields SE:** Hemoglobin function and stored blood. J Clin Invest 48:311, 1969

19. **Edwards MJ, Rigas DA:** Electrolyte labile increase of oxygen affinity during in vivo aging of hemoglobin. J Clin Invest 46:1597, 1967

20. **Edwards MJ, Novy MJ, Walters C, Metcalfe J:** Improved oxygen release: An adaptation of mature red cells to hypoxia. J Clin Invest 47:1851, 1968

21. **Metcalfe J, Dhindsa DS, Edwards MJ, Mourdjinis A:** The oxygen dissociation curve of blood from patients with low rates of peripheral blood flow. Clin Res 16:240, 1968

22. **Gerald PS, Scott EM:** The hereditary methemoglobinemias. In Stanbury JB, Wyngaarden JB, Frederickson DS (eds): The Metabolic Basis of Inherited Disease, p 1100. New York, McGraw–Hill, 1966

23. **McNicol MW:** The management of respiratory failure. Hosp Med 1:601, 1967

24. **Haldane JS:** Respiration. New Haven, Yale University Press, 1922

25. **Dripps RD, Comroe JH Jr:** The respiratory and circulatory response of normal men to inhalation of 7.6 and 10.4 per cent O_2 with a comparison of the maximal ventilation produced by severe muscular exercise, inhalation of CO_2 and maximal voluntary hyperventilation. Am J Physiol 149:43, 1947

26. **MacDonald FM, Simonson E:** Human electrocardiogram during and after inhalation of 30 per cent carbon dioxide. J Appl Physiol 6:304, 1953

27. **Schieve JF, Wilson WP:** The changes in cerebral vascular resistance of man in experimental alkalosis and acidosis. J Clin Invest 32:33, 1953

28. **Davies CE, Mackinnon J:** Neurological effects of oxygen in chronic cor pulmonale. Lancet 2:883, 1949

29. **Simpson T:** Papilloedema in emphysema. Br Med J 2:639, 1948

30. **Smith JP, Stone RW, Muschenheim C:** Acute respiratory failure in chronic lung disease: Observations on controlled oxygen therapy. Am Rev Resp Dis 97:791, 1968

31. **Campbell EJM:** Respiratory failure. Br Med J 1:1451, 1965

32. **Campbell EJM:** The J Burns Amberson Lecture: The management of acute respiratory failure in chronic bronchitis and emphysema. Am Rev Resp Dis 96:626, 1967

21

Anorexia, Nausea, and Vomiting

James E. McGuigan
M. Michael Wolfe

Innervation of the Gastrointestinal Tract
Anorexia
Hunger
  Appetite
Nausea
Vomiting
  The Physiology of Vomiting
  The Act of Vomiting
Disturbances Associated with Anorexia, Nausea, and Vomiting
  Psychic and Neurologic Factors
  Drugs and Toxic Agents

Intra-abdominal Disorders
  Mechanical Obstruction of the Gastrointestinal Tract
  Intra-abdominal Inflammatory Disorders
Nausea and Vomiting of Pregnancy
Other Factors
  Endocrine Disorders
  Cardiac Disease
  Malnutrition
  Motion Sickness
  Meniere's Disease
Summary

Anorexia, nausea, and vomiting are among the most common and distressing symptoms that afflict man. So widespread and significant are these symptoms that very commonly patients equate being "sick" with the presence of these symptoms. Anorexia, nausea, and vomiting are associated with a wide variety of clinical disorders, some of which are relatively trivial, others of which may reflect diseases of a most severe and disabling nature. Anorexia, nausea, and vomiting may be evoked by disorders of the gastrointestinal tract but also may reflect psychic, neurologic, or metabolic conditions, or other visceral abnormalities.

INNERVATION OF THE GASTROINTESTINAL TRACT

In order to understand the mechanisms by which nausea and vomiting are provoked, it is necessary to discuss the portion of the peripheral and central nervous system that innervates the gastrointestinal tract, regulating and modifying its function.

The gastrointestinal tract receives it extrinsic nerve supply from components of the autonomic nervous system.[1] In purely anatomic terms, autonomic outflow is limited to craniosacral and thoracolumbar spinal seg-

ments, craniosacral outflow designated as parasympathetic and thoracolumbar as sympathetic. Adrenergic nerves act by liberation of norepinephrine or epinephrine; cholinergic nerves liberate acetylcholine. Most sympathetic nerves are adrenergic, whereas most, but perhaps not all, parasympathetic nerves are cholinergic.

Thoracolumbar sympathetic preganglionic fibers synapse with cells in paravertebral ganglia. Postganglionic efferent fibers arising in these ganglia supply most of the gut through the splanchnic nerves. Efferent fibers from the celiac plexus supply the stomach. In addition, the gut is partially supplied through the aortic plexi, the para-aortic nerves, branches from the lumbar portions of the sympathetic trunks, and from fibers carried in the vagus nerves.

In addition to classic cholingeric and adrenergic nerve pathways, much of the function of the gastrointestinal tract is mediated through noncholinergic–nonadrenergic pathways. Elucidation of the precise neurotransmitters involved in these pathways is presently an area of intense research. One amine that probably plays a role is dopamine, which is stored in very large quantities in the mucosa of the gastrointestinal tract.[2] Dopamine is synthesized by enteric neurons. It is released by a calcium-dependent mechanism upon nerve stimulation. It mimics a variety of effects of enteric nerve stimulation, and there is an efficient and specific inactivating mechanism for dopamine. Other candidates for the role of enteric neurotransmitter include adenosine triphosphate (ATP), vasoactive intestinal peptide (VIP), substance P, somatostatin, enkephalins, pancreatic polypeptide, gastrin or cholecystokinin (CCK), neurotensin, and gastrin releasing peptide.[2]

Neural plexi extend throughout the alimentary tract. These plexi lie on the surfaces of the pharynx and uppermost esophagus, but in the remainder of the gastrointestinal tract they comprise collections and networks of interconnected ganglion cells located in the submucosa and interspersed between longitudinal and circular smooth-muscle layers. In the gut, many adrenergic nerves connect with intramural ganglion cells,[3,4] most of which are cholinergic. Thus, most adrenergic effects on gastrointestinal motility are caused principally by postganglionic cholinergic cells.

With certain exceptions, sympathetic innervation of the gastrointestinal tract is generally inhibitory. Adrenergic receptors have been classified as α and β,[5] α receptors being those that are excited by sympathetic stimulation or sympathomimetic agents, and β receptors being those that are inhibited by these same factors. The ergot alkaloids and haloalkylamines antagonize α receptor responses, whereas β receptor responses are inhibited by propranolol, nethalide, and dichloro-

isoproterenol. Stimulation of either α or β receptors results in inhibition of intestinal smooth-muscle activity.[6] In certain areas of the guinea pig gastrointestinal tract, α receptors are excitatory: these include the esophagus,[7] bile duct,[8] and terminal ileum.[9] In spite of our knowledge of neural circuitry and receptor function, the role of sympathetic activity in the control of gastrointestinal motility is largely unknown.

Parasympathetic activity usually produces increased tone and motility of the gastrointestinal tract, with reinforcement of activity mediated through local nerve plexi.

Efferent parasympathetic innervation of the stomach and most of the intestinal tract (except for its lowermost portions) is supplied by vagal fibers, which follow blood vessels to synapse with cell bodies located in the myenteric and submucosal plexi. The smooth muscle of the gastrointestinal tract is supplied by postganglionic efferent fibers arising in these plexi.

Visceral afferent fibers, with sensory endings in the gut, synapse in gastrointestinal ganglia, muscle layers, or mucosal epithelium. These postganglionic fibers accompany vagal and sympathetic rami to the dorsal roots of the spinal cord. Some afferent fibers pass centrally with the sympathetics through celiac and other ganglia without synapsing. Other afferent fibers synapse in the celiac plexus ganglia, with postganglionic sympathetic fibers constituting the afferent limbs of visceral reflex arcs.

Many gastrointestinal visceral reflexes are conducted without participation of higher central connections. Other reflexes appear to be modified or controlled by medullary and hypothalamic activity. Simultaneous visceral and somatic expression appear to be coordinated by the hypothalamus.[10] Sensory and motor autonomic and somatic functions are connected principally with the cerebral cortex and the cerebellum. It is through these connections that psychic influences modify activity of the gastrointestinal tract.

Currently much investigation is being conducted relating to motor activity and neural control of gastrointestinal functions. Our present level of understanding does not permit us to interrelate these investigations, such as observations of electrical activity and changes in intraluminal pressure with human symptoms in disease states associated with anorexia, nausea, and vomiting. Widespread interest has evolved in the polypeptide hormone gastrin,[11] which has as its principal activity the capacity to powerfully evoke gastric secretion of hydrochloric acid. However, gastrin also exerts effects on motor activity of the stomach and of the small intestine. Similarly, other gastrointestinal peptides, including secretin, motilin, CCK, VIP, glucagon, and gastric inhibitory peptide (GIP), influence

gastrointestinal motility.[12,13] It remains to be determined whether these peptides play a significant role in disturbances of motor activity related to anorexia, nausea, and vomiting.

ANOREXIA

Anorexia may be defined as lack or loss of appetite for food, or as disinterest in the ingestion of food. The concept of *appetite* is somewhat more elusive but may be regarded as a favorable disposition toward or simply a desire for food. Lack of interest in consumption of a particular variety of food or foods may reflect individual and personal preferences and does not have the same connotation as the somewhat more generalized and at times active disinterest in consumption of all foods, which is termed anorexia. When a man consumes sufficient food, interpreted by complex physiologic signals as adequate for his present requirements, a state of satiety is achieved. No further food is then desired, but the subjective sensation is somewhat different from that actively disinterested state that we define as anorexia. Anorexia is frequently associated with a disinterest in consumption of even those foods toward which the individual may habitually manifest his greatest gustatory interest. Sensations of appetite, hunger, and satiety may be looked upon as normal psychophysiologic mechanisms of control of food ingestion. However, in certain states, individuals may consume or reject food independent of sensations of appetite, hunger, or satiety.

HUNGER

Hunger has been defined as a craving for food, the driving sensation or urge to eat that follows a period of fasting. Hunger concerns itself with the satisfaction or fulfillment of the requirement for food. Undoubtedly, many cultural, physiologic, and psychological factors influence the subjective appreciation of hunger. It is well known that the sensation of hunger often is associated temporally with rhythmic contractions of the stomach,[14] but the speculation that the hunger sensations are the results of these contractions has been largely discarded. Data to the contrary include the following:

Humans and experimental animals without stomachs experience hunger
Vagally transmitted hunger "pangs" are not correlated in time with gastric contractions
Gastric contractions even greater than those observed in the fasting state are observed following ingesting of food
Gastrectomized animals are able to regulate their caloric intake

However, hunger probably does cause motor activity of the stomach. Many of the drugs that suppress the intake of food decrease gastric motor activity.

The precise mechanisms by which hunger is produced are not known. Evidence from investigations in experimental animals and correlative clinical states supports the existence of two hypothalamic centers whose function relates to hunger and food ingestion. The first of these, the "feeding center," is located in the ventrolateral portion of the hypothalamus caudolateral to the mamillary bodies. Electrical stimulation of the feeding center results in hyperphagia, whereas ablation of it is associated with reduced food intake, emaciation, and death. The second center, the "satiety center," is located in the ventromedial region of the hypothalamus. Stimulation of this center causes inhibition of food intake, and destruction of its results in excessive food ingestion. There is evidence that the activities of these centers are influenced by blood glucose levels and arteriovenous glucose differences.[15] The satiety center can be inactivated experimentally by administration of goldthioglucose but not by a number of other organic gold compounds. Inactivation of the satiety center, associated with cytotoxicity owing to gold, is accompanied by the deposition of gold in cells of the ventromedial hypothalamic area.

It has been proposed that the mechanism determining the expression of hunger or satiety is related to the rate of utilization of glucose and that this is sensed by glucoreceptors located in the hypothalamus. This hypothesis proposes that large arteriovenous glucose differences stimulate the satiety center and inhibit the feeding center. Low arteriovenous differences in glucose levels, such as those produced by insulin administration, are proposed to produce converse effects. In certain persons, hypoglycemia may provoke hunger, as is seen in states of hyperinsulinism induced in experimental animals, in functional hypoglycemia, and in association with excessive circulating insulin, as from β-cell islet tumors. Hunger is also provoked following injection of exogenous insulin in diabetic and nondiabetic patients, in Addison's disease, and in hypoglycemia associated with certain tumors, particularly certain sarcomas. Relief of hunger of this variety promptly follows administration of intravenous glucose. The central nature of stimulation of hunger of this variety was amply demonstrated by its occurrence following insulin injection even after complete denervation of the gastrointestinal tract.[16] Glucagon administered intra-

venously reduces hunger, elevates the venous glucose levels, and according to some investigators increases arteriovenous glucose differences.[17] There are several objections to acceptance of the hypothesis that blood glucose levels serve as the sole determinants for hunger. Intravenous glucose does not relieve hunger in normal individuals in the absence of insulin administration. To date, there have not been good correlations between venous glucose levels or arteriovenous glucose differences and hunger in normal individuals. Hunger sensations may follow insulin administration in the absence of substantial differences in arteriovenous glucose levels.

The peptide hormone CCK has recently evoked great interest regarding its potential role in the control of appetite. Several investigators have shown that injections of either CCK33 or CCK8 can induce not only cessation of eating but the full sequence of satiety behavior in rats.[18,19,20] In addition, it has been shown that CCK injected directly into cerebral ventricles can diminish the hunger drive in rats.[21] These observations combined with the discovery of large concentrations of CCK within the central nervous system and the demonstration of reduced CCK concentrations in the brains of a strain of genetically obese mice, have suggested a potential function of CCK as a mediator of satiety within the central nervous system and periphery.[20]

Although blood glucose levels and differences in arteriovenous glucose levels may participate in certain situations in the production of hunger, it is apparent that gastric distention also serves as an important satiety signal. Insertion of nonfood bulk [22,23] (or of food) into the stomach produces short-termed inhibition of eating. Distention of the stomach produces afferent impulses carried through cervical vagal fibers.[24] Certain of these units respond to as little increase in intragastric pressure as 2 mm of water. It has been suggested that there are distention-sensitive gastric receptors in the outer layers of the stomach wall, that these units are "in series"[25] with smooth-muscle fibers, and that these receptors initiate signals resulting from increases in gastric-wall tension as well as from gastric distention or contractions. These mechanoreceptors are present in the walls of the stomach and of the small and large intestines.[25,26] In experimental animals, increasing gastric distention produces an increase in electrical activity in the hypothalamic satiety center,[27] accompanied by a lack of activity in the region of the hypothalamic feeding center. Intestinal distention produces similar results. In rats, inflation of small intragastric balloons results in decreased food-investigative activity.[28] This decrease of food investigation and consumption with gastric distention is eliminated by subtotal vagotomy. Food intake of rats has been demonstrated to be decreased in association with distention of exteriorized small intestinal segments.[29] When these intestinal loops were denervated, decrease in food consumption was inhibited. In addition to the mechanoreceptors, there are also apparently chemoreceptors[30,31] in the wall of the gastrointestinal tract. Glucose perfusion of the stomach and the small intestine of humans and experimental animals produces increased afferent electrical activity in small fiber groups transmitted through fibers contained in mesenteric and splanchnic nerves.

It has been proposed that "long-term" regulation of food intake, as opposed to "short-term" regulation described previously, may be influenced by the magnitude of the adipose tissue reservoir in the organism.[32] This hypothesis is based on observations that rats made hypophagic from hypothalamic lesions reach a plateau of obesity at which food intake falls. If one member of a pair of parabiotic rats is made hyperphagic, the other member progressively loses weight, presumably on the basis of stimulation of its satiety center by the adiposity of its parabiotic mate.

It is apparent from the foregoing discussions that we do not understand completely the mechanisms involved in the production and regulation of hunger. The psychophysiologic phenomenon of hunger appears to be influenced by a variety of mechanisms: central regulation mediated through the hypothalamic centers, biochemical alterations in blood and tissue components, and afferent nervous stimuli resulting from mechanical and chemical events occurring in the gastrointestinal tract. The way, or ways, in which these factors are interrelated in their influence upon hunger in the short and long-term regulation of food intake remain to be defined.

APPETITE

Appetite may be regarded as an agreeable attitude toward ingesting food, often toward a particular variety or varieties of food. The central nature of appetite is reaffirmed by observations that appetite remains unaffected following autonomic denervation of the stomach, small bowel, and proximal colon. Not only does hunger remain following a gastrectomy, but selective desires for individual food remain. The parietal and frontal regions of the brain have been known to be associated with appetite. Desire for food is associated with increased rates of gastric hydrochloric acid secretion, with gastric hyperemia, and hypermotility.[33] *Anorexia*, the absence of hunger or appetite, has been associated with the opposite: decreased gastric hydrochloric acid secretion with hypomotility of the stomach and pallor of the gastric mucosa. Anorexia may be induced by unpleasant or revolting experiences. Appre-

hension, fear, or anxiety may result in the sensation of anorexia. However, excitement of pleasurable and desirable types also may be associated with anorexia.

NAUSEA

Nausea is an ill-defined but distinctly unpleasant sensation usually associated with a profound revulsion toward the ingestion of food. Most states proceeding to vomiting are accompanied by anorexia and nausea. Anorexia is commonly followed by nausea, which in turn is followed by vomiting. It must be recognized, however, that any of these three symptoms may be experienced by the patient in the absence of either or both of the other two. Nausea is often but not invariably preceded by anorexia. Nausea without some degree of anorexia is very unusual. Stimuli that evoke anorexia in susceptible persons, when amplified, will often cause the subjects to become nauseated. Chemical agents, food, drugs, and other stimuli that in small doses produce anorexia often produce nausea when given in greater doses. The anorectic individual often becomes frankly nauseated when confronted with food; his revulsion toward food has been thrust into his consciousness. Both nausea and anorexia are associated with decreased motor activity of the stomach and pallor of the gastric mucosa; the changes are more conspicuous with nausea than with anorexia. In contrast to the hypotonicity of the stomach, there is contraction of the proximal duodenum. It is possible to induce nausea by distention of an air-filled balloon located in the distal esophagus, stomach, or most especially, in the duodenum. Nausea or vomiting is frequently associated with evidence of diffuse autonomic discharge, including profuse watery salivation; often sudden, drenching sweating; and tachycardia. Bradycardia is often experienced concurrently with the act of vomiting.

Patients often have great difficulty in describing the nature of the extremely unpleasant phenomenon that they experience as nausea. The sensation of nausea is commonly described by the patient as a vague unpleasantness located in the epigastrium or diffusely in the abdomen. When nauseated, some patients experience distressing sensations in the region of the throat. The unpleasant abdominal sensations experienced as nausea often have to be distinguished from visceral abdominal pain of mild degree, which is also frequently poorly localized in the abdomen.

The mechanism by which acid secretion is reduced while nausea is experienced has not been defined. The fact that denervation of the stomach does not abolish nausea suggests that the phenomenon is not solely under neural regulation and that other factors (*e.g.,* vascular or hormonal mechanisms) may be involved.[34] The mucosal pallor associated with nausea makes it tempting to speculate that vascular changes within the gastric mucosa are responsible for both reduction in acid secretion and gastric mucosal pallor.

VOMITING

Vomiting may be defined as the sudden forceful peroral expulsion of the contents of the stomach. It often, but not invariably, is preceded by nausea, which may become acutely more severe immediately prior to the act of vomiting.

THE PHYSIOLOGY OF VOMITING

The vomiting center is believed to be located in the dorsal portion of the lateral reticular formation in the medulla. Destruction of the vomiting center in dogs and cats has been shown to ablate the vomiting response to the usual methods of provocation of vomiting. Apormorphine, an agent capable of inducing vomiting when administered orally or intravenously, produces vomiting when applied to this region of the medulla. A "chemoreceptor trigger zone"[35] has been described adjacent to the vomiting center. They appear to be connected to each other by the fasciculus solitarius, which has recently been shown to be rich in enkephalins.[36] From investigations in experimental animals, it has been proposed that this chemoreceptor trigger zone may be stimulated by humoral agents, including certain toxic chemicals, and that stimulation of this chemoreceptor center results in transmission of neural impulses to the vomiting center, with resultant vomiting. Input originating from three other sources—the vestibular apparatus, the periphery, and higher cortical and brain stem structures—can induce vomiting through the vomiting center without necessary mediation through the chemoreceptor trigger zone.[35] Peripheral input originates primarily from the pharynx and gastrointestinal tract, with afferent nerve fibers carried principally by the vagus nerve and, to a lesser extent, by other cranial and sympathetic nerves. Gastric dopamine[37] and opiate[38] receptors may play important roles in mediating either afferent or efferent limbs of the vomiting pathway.

THE ACT OF VOMITING

Exaggerated and frequently extreme vasomotor phenomena often immediately precede and accompany the act of vomiting. These include abundant watery salivation and sweating, vasoconstriction with pallor, and changes in pulse rate. The hypersalivation is probably

due to the proximity of the medullary salivary and vomiting centers. The patient often may become tremulous, weak, lightheaded, and "dizzy" but seldom experiences true vertigo. A gradually accelerating rate of respiration with some irregularity of breathing may occur immediately prior to the act of vomiting. Retching commonly but not invariably precedes vomiting. During retching, which is characterized by spasmodic respirator movements of the chest wall and diaphragms, which are opposed by expiratory contractions of the abdominal muscles, the mouth and glottis are closed. The blood pressure may fall just prior to vomiting and often fluctuates during the act of vomiting. This phenomenon may reflect in part modification of cardiac output resulting from abrupt changes in intrathoracic pressure. The heart rate, which is often rapid prior to vomiting, slows to the point of bradycardia during the act of vomiting. Cardiac arrhythmias, sometimes induced in animals made to vomit, may be inhibited by atropine. Respirations cease during the act of vomiting.

The sequence of events during the act of vomiting is as follows: The upper half of the stomach and the region of the gastroesophageal sphincter relax. Peristaltic contractions from the midportion of the stomach proceed to the angulus of the stomach, where a violent contraction occurs. With the pylorus contracted, the diaphragm undergoes violent descent, with simultaneous contractions of the abdominal muscles expelling gastric contents up, into, and through the esophagus. Descent of the diaphragm and acute contraction of the abdominal muscles operate in concert to elevate acutely the intra-abdominal pressure. During the forceful expulsion of food up and out through the esophagus, the glottis is closed, respirations cease, and the soft palate is thrust upward against the nasopharynx.

There is no evidence that reverse (cephalad-directed) peristalsis occurs in the stomach or plays any part; nor has it been shown that reverse peristalsis in the small intestine plays a significant role in the act of vomiting.[39]

DISTURBANCES ASSOCIATED WITH ANOREXIA, NAUSEA, AND VOMITING

Anorexia, nausea, and vomiting may be observed in a variety of psychophysiologic and organic disorders. For purposes of description and discussion causes of vomiting will be classified as associated with psychic and neurologic factors, drugs and intoxications, intra-abdominal disorders, and other assorted factors. No classification is satisfactory for these purposes, since one or more of these symptoms may be associated with disturbances of well-being in virtually every disease to which man is prone.

PSYCHIC AND NEUROLOGIC FACTORS

In many patients, emotional factors may play an important role in the production of anorexia, nausea, or vomiting. Life situations that evoke subjective responses of fear, depression, frustration, apprehension, and anxiety may commonly be associated with these symptoms. In not all instances are the predisposing or conditioning emotional responses unpleasant ones. We are all familiar with the loss of appetite associated with apprehension regarding a forthcoming event, even one which may be anticipated with the greatest pleasure. More commonly, however, unpleasant experiences (which may not necessarily be recognized as unpleasant) are associated with these symptoms. However, hyperphagia is a more common symptom of chronic anxiety than loss of appetite. Anorexia is commonly a manifestation of depressed states and may be an early warning signal in the depressed patient. Unpleasant prior life experiences may have conditioned the patient in such a way that he experiences revulsion toward a life situation over which he feels he can exert no control. His response may be to be "sick"—to vomit. Vomiting that is principally on a psychic basis frequently occurs during or shortly after meals. Often it may be unaccompanied by nausea and retching. Vomiting of this variety frequently does not empty the stomach. Following vomiting, the patient may wish to continue to eat and often can do so without immediate recurrence of vomiting.

The ingestion of food for maintenance of adequate nutrition relates to basic needs and requirements for survival. Therefore, it is not surprising that abnormalities in these primitive attitudes toward food intake and rejection are observed with subtle or profound psychological disturbances.

Although some patients with severe psychoses may have disturbances of food intake, most such patients do not. The most profound disturbance of impairment of food intake of neuropsychiatric origin has been termed *anorexia nervosa*. This is a state in which there is anorexia and rejection of food to an extraordinary degree.[40] The patient is usually a young woman. The age of onset is usually between menarche and age 18 years, with symptoms rarely, if ever, beginning after age 25 years. The subject may become extremely emaciated. It is not unusual to have patients with anorexia nervosa die of malnutrition. Vomiting, which may be self-induced, may be a prominent or dominant symptom in young women with anorexia nervosa. In general, vomiting is a bad prognostic sign.[41] The patient with anorexia nervosa may develop a picture of sec-

ondary panhypopituitarism, which has to be distinguished from primary pituitary disease. Amenorrhea is almost invariably present in these patients. The secondary hypopituitarism found in these patients may result from nutritional deficiency of amino acid building blocks required for assembly of proteins and polypeptide hormones. Onset of symptoms of anorexia nervosa frequently follow a weight-reduction diet program. Patients with anorexia nervosa usually deny their illness, appear to enjoy losing weight, and appear to take pleasure in refusal of food, which they may handle excessively or hoard. Although depressive and obsessive-compulsive manifestations may be present in these patients, the precise basis of the primary psychological disorder associated with the starving state of anorexia nervosa has not been defined. Repeated vomiting of food ingested more than 12 hours earlier rarely, if ever, is due to psychogenic vomiting.

Vomiting can be induced by the experimental production of hypoxemia of the vomiting center. This fact has been demonstrated in experimental animals in which the carotid arteries have been ligated. Vomiting, which probably reflects oxygen deprivation of the vomiting center, may be seen in association with severe anemia of a variety of causes; local or regional vascular occlusion; inadequate perfusion of the brain stem, as may be observed acutely following excessive blood loss; or in states with diminished cardiac output. It has been postulated that the enhanced sensitivity of the vomiting center with the production of vomiting that accompanies increased intracranial pressure is a result of impedance of blood flow to the vomiting center, with resultant hypoxia. Inadequate perfusion and oxygenation of the vomiting center with resultant irritability supplies the most likely explanation for the vomiting that often is observed in association with vascular shock. Vomiting also may be seen in association with reductions in environmental oxygen, as in high-altitude activities such as mountain climbing or riding in incompletely pressurized aircraft. It is presumed that vomiting observed with exposure to high altitude, particularly when associated with vigorous, oxygen-requiring activity, occurs as a result of relative hypoxemia of the vomiting center.

Increased intracranial pressure may be associated with a "projectile" variety of vomiting. Projectile vomiting associated with increased intracranial pressure commonly is not preceded by nausea. Expulsion of the gastric contents is more forceful with projectile vomiting than with other types of vomiting and may result in gastric contents being hurled across the room. Projectile vomiting with increased intracranial pressure may occur with lateral sinus thrombosis, meningitis of any etiology, internal hydrocephalus, and various space-occupying intracranial lesions including tumor, hemorrhage, and abscess. One must be cautioned, however, that vomiting in association with increased intracranial pressure is not invariably projectile in nature and often may be preceded by nausea and retching. In addition, forceful vomiting of a projectile nature may occur in a variety of conditions other than those associated with abnormalities of the central nervous system. It should be emphasized that in addition to the production of vomiting secondary to increased intracranial pressure, certain intracranial tumors may result in a clinical state similar to anorexia nervosa. Tumors involving the hypothalamus, presumably influencing the function of the hypothalamic center(s) participating in the regulation of food intake, have been observed to be associated with anorexia of the severity seen in anorexia nervosa. The clinical syndrome of severe anorexia nervosa has been noted in a child with a tumor in the region of the fourth ventricle.[42] Vomiting is often seen with cerebellar lesions. Some degree of nausea or vomiting is a frequent accompaniment of migraine headaches. The mechanism by which vomiting occurs in migraine disorders has not been defined; however, hypoxemia of the vomiting center secondary to vascular changes recognized to occur with migraine has been suggested as the possible mechanism. Nausea and vomiting of this migraine variety may be seen in the absence of headache and with or without abdominal pain. Often the associated visual disturbances afford a clue as to the nature of the vomiting.

Cyclic vomiting consists of a syndrome of recurrent episodes of vomiting, often of a severe degree and usually without apparent cause, which occurs in children. The onset is sudden and the episode of vomiting may last several days, with spontaneous recovery. Since the vomiting may be severe, it may produce severe alkalosis and dehydration. The frequency of episodes may vary from more than once a month to three times per year.[43] The onset is in childhood with disappearance of symptoms usually by the time of menarche. The cause, or causes, of cyclic vomiting has not been established. Many of these children have headaches associated with the vomiting, often with a family history of migraine headaches, and frequently these children have abnormal EEG patterns. Many investigators propose psychogenic factors to explain cyclic vomiting, whereas others attribute the syndrome to perinatal and postnatal brain injury.

DRUGS AND TOXIC AGENTS

Many chemicals, drugs, and toxic agents possess the capacity to induce nausea and vomiting. Some agents appear to act centrally by stimulation of the medullary chemoreceptor trigger zone, which conveys neural

stimulatory impulses to the adjacent vomiting center with the subsequent production of vomiting. Other agents appear to have direct effects on the gastrointestinal organs whereby they induce vomiting. The vomiting center may be stimulated by afferent impulses from the stomach and the small bowel which accompany stimulation of the vagal nerves.

Mucosal damage of the upper gastrointestinal tract follows ingestion of mercury bichloride, ammonium chloride, copper sulfate, or aminophylline.[35,44] Ingestion of these compounds commonly is associated with the production of vomiting, which probably results from local stimulation of the damaged gastrointestinal organs. It has been concluded that the receptor site for the provocation of emesis observed following oral administration of sodium salicylate is in the upper gut. When copper sulfate is applied to the region of the medullary chemoreceptor trigger zone, vomiting can be evoked. Bilateral vagotomy will inhibit the usually observed immediate vomiting seen in dogs in whose stomachs copper sulfate has been placed. Vomiting in these vagotomized dogs occurs but is delayed. The delay in vomiting is interpreted as reflecting the time required for absorption and circulation of copper sulfate until adequate concentration is reached in the medullary chemoreceptor trigger zone to induce nausea of central origin.

Nausea and vomiting are common accompaniments of a variety of febrile infectious disease. It has been shown experimentally that administration of microgram quantities of staphylococcal enterotoxin and enterobacteriaceal endotoxin induces emesis in cats.[45] The site of action of the staphylococcal enterotoxin in inducing vomiting in the rhesus monkey appears to be located in the abdominal viscera.[46] Sensory responses provoked by stimulation from the staphylococcal toxin in the gastrointestinal tract appear to be transmitted through afferent fibers traveling with the vagus and sympathetic nerves. In rhesus monkeys, following vagotomy and abdominal splanchnicectomy, vomiting is not induced after administration of enterotoxin, even in amounts proving lethal to intact animals. The vomiting reflexes in these autonomically denervated monkeys is not suppressed because of a lack of capacity to perform the act of vomiting, since vomiting in response to the emetic agent Veriloid is maintained in these animals.

Vomiting is frequently observed following ingestion of large quantities of alcohol. Gastroscopic examination of such patients frequently shows gastric mucosal hyperemia, and in some instances, erosive gastritis. However, in many patients who vomit following the ingestion of alcohol no abnormalities of the gastric mucosa can be visualized. In most instances vomiting following ingestion of alcohol is probably of central origin,

since the action of alcohol is similar to that of other pharmacologically active anesthetic agents: stimulation of hypothalamic nuclei. A variety of chemical agents including apomorphine, morphine, emetine, histamine, and epinephrine are capable of inducing vomiting when directly applied to the chemoreceptor trigger zone of the hypothalamus.

Certain amphetamines and amphetamine derivatives have been used widely to induce anorexia for purposes of weight reduction. These drugs behave as central nervous system stimulants. The mechanisms by which amphetamines reduce appetite is not known. Complete extrinsic denervation of the stomach and intestinal tract does not diminish the effect of amphetamines in reducing appetite.[47]

Nausea and vomiting are commonly observed in patients receiving cancer chemotherapy and are sometimes the most unpleasant symptoms they must endure. Drugs with high emetic activity include cisplatin, dacarbazine, actinomycin-D, doxorubicin, streptozocin, and mechlorethamine.[48] Surprisingly little research has been aimed at elucidation of the site of emetic action of these chemotherapeutic agents. The best studied drug, mechlorethamine, appears to initiate vomiting at the chemoreceptor trigger zone in dogs, but in cats its emetic actions are primarily peripheral.[48] Cisplatin, which poorly penetrates the blood-brain barrier and which has delayed emetic action, is felt to induce vomiting through peripheral pathways.[49]

To date there is no evidence that the vomiting that is seen in association with digitalis glycoside administration is caused by a direct effect on the gastrointestinal tract. In experimental animals digitalis does induce vomiting when applied to the medullary chemoreceptor trigger zone.

INTRA-ABDOMINAL DISORDERS

A wide spectrum of intra-abdominal disorders, a generous portion of which reflect abnormalities of the gastrointestinal tract, may cause anorexia, nausea, and vomiting. The varieties of intra-abdominal abnormalities that may be associated with nausea and vomiting are so numerous that they defy meaningful and worthwhile tabulation and categorization. However, certain intra-abdominal conditions that produce vomiting, as well as certain generalizations regarding abdominal causes of vomiting, merit discussion.

Mechanical Obstruction of the Gastrointestinal Tract

Nausea and vomiting brought to the attention of the physician frequently and appropriately provoke the immediate suspicion that these symptoms may reflect mechanical obstruction of the normal passage of the

contents of the gastrointestinal tract. Mechanical obstruction is a relatively uncommon cause of vomiting; however, anorexia, nausea, and vomiting are prominent symptoms of gastrointestinal tract obstruction and may be seen with obstruction at virtually any level. Vomiting found with mechanical obstruction of the gastrointestinal tract is the result of distention of the lumen.[50] This distention activates mechanoreceptors in the gastric and bowel walls, which evoke vomiting through visceroviseral reflexes or activation of the medullary vomiting center through the neural pathways already outlined. Vomiting in association with gastrointestinal visceral distention that is not the result of mechanical obstruction (e.g., paralytic ileus) is believed to be produced by these same mechanisms.

Vomiting with gastrointestinal tract obstruction is seen most commonly when the obstruction is high. Pyloric obstruction, whether associated with congenital hypertrophic pyloric stenosis, pyloric stenosis in the adult, peptic ulcer disease, or tumor, constitutes the major gastric site of obstruction resulting in nausea and vomiting. The nausea and vomiting owing to obstruction at the level of the pylorus commonly are observed shortly following eating, and the severity of vomiting often correlates with the acuteness of development and degree of obstruction. With pyloric obstruction, the vomited material often contains undigested food. Bile may be present in the vomitus of patients with pyloric obstruction, even though the ampulla of Vater is distal to the obstructive site. The presence of bile in vomited material from patients with pyloric obstruction reflects incompleteness of the obstruction with regurgitation of intestinal contents. For example, both peptic ulcer disease and tumor may involve the region of the pylorus, producing both relative obstruction and incompetency of the pyloric sphincter mechanism.

With long-standing pyloric obstruction dilation of the stomach may develop, gradually creating an enormous fluid reservoir; when vomiting occurs it may be of extraordinarily large volumes of material. These patients often have a succussion splash and often visible gastric peristaltic waves. Associated or preceding symptoms often may supply clues as to the disease responsible for the pyloric obstruction. Examples would be the history of relief of epigastric pain with eating in patients with peptic ulcer disease, or excessive fullness following ingestion of meals of a size previously readily accommodated by the patient who has carcinoma of the stomach.

Early morning vomiting before breakfast may occur not only in pregnancy but also after gastric surgery and with metabolic abnormalities including uremia and alcoholism. The pain of peptic ulcer is often relieved by vomiting; however, no relief of pain from pancreatic or biliary disease is provided by vomiting.

Intestinal obstruction at virtually all levels, particularly in the upper small intestine, may be associated with vomiting. Fecal vomiting, especially when protracted, is particularly characteristic of obstruction at the intestinal level. Intestinal obstruction may be caused by a large number of abnormalities, including among others tumor, volvulus, intussusception, adhesion, foreign bodies, inflammatory disease, and vascular insufficiency. As in pyloric obstruction, severity of the vomiting owing to intestinal obstruction often correlates with the degree of completeness of the obstruction. Acute obstruction more commonly results in vomiting than does chronic incomplete obstruction. Anorexia, nausea, and vomiting are extremely common symptoms with paralytic ileus in which there are dilated nonmotile regions of bowel in the absence of mechanical impedance of the flow of gut contents. Thus, these symptoms do not assist in the differentiation of dilated loops of bowel in either paralytic ileus or mechanical intestinal obstruction. Splanchnic sympathectomy or spinal cord transection (C_7 to T_1) will eliminate vomiting owing to intestinal obstruction in experimental animals; however, transthoracic subdiaphragmatic vagotomy was unsuccessful in blocking vomiting under those circumstances.[52]

Intra-abdominal Inflammatory Disorders

Inflammatory involvement of virtually any abdominal or pelvic organ may be associated with production of anorexia, nausea, and vomiting. Vomiting in these instances is a result of stimulation of visceral afferent pathways. Stimuli are conducted from the involved organ through the vagi and splanchnic afferent trunks to the vomiting center in the medulla. Their synaptic connections are made with efferent vagal splanchnic and spinal nerves to the pharynx, the esophagus, the cardioesophageal junction, the stomach, muscles of the abdominal wall, and the diaphragm. Inflammation with irritation of the visceral peritoneum[51] results in vomiting in the same manner.

Anorexia, nausea, and vomiting are particularly common accompaniments of acute appendicitis. Anorexia is usually the initial symptom experienced by patients with acute appendicitis and occurs almost invariably. In acute appendicitis anorexia may be overshadowed later in the course of the attack by acute and sometimes severe abdominal pain.

Vomiting is seen in some patients with viral hepatitis, but this is not the rule. On the other hand, a profound degree of anorexia, which usually precedes more overt clinical manifestations, is almost invariably found in patients with viral hepatitis. Disappearance of anorexia in patients with viral hepatitis may correlate with morphologic and biochemical evidence of hepatic improvement.

Nausea and vomiting are often found with urinary tract infections, especially when associated with urinary tract obstruction such as is seen with ureteral colic owing to impaction of a stone. Obstruction of the ureter may be heralded by severe nausea and vomiting, even in the absence of the colicky pain usually associated with obstruction of the ureter.

Vomiting is frequent in patients with acute pancreatitis. Vomiting with pancreatitis often may occur in the absence of severe abdominal pain. One must be alert to the possibility that the vomiting in pancreatitis reflects a condition associated with the pancreatitis, and in certain instances may not necessarily be due to the pancreatitis itself. The following are given as examples:

The vomiting may reflect biliary tract disease, which so frequently accompanies pancreatitis.

Hyperparathyroidism with hypercalcemia may be the principal cause of vomiting in certain patients with pancreatitis.

Peptic-ulcer disease, sometimes with penetration of the pancreas and resultant pancreatitis, may result in vomiting.

It must be borne in mind that vascular insufficiency and occlusion of the arterial and venous splanchnic and mesenteric circulation, as well as inferior vena caval obstruction, may produce anorexia, nausea, and vomiting. In addition, cicatricial stenosis of limited regions of the intestines following episodes of acute vascular insufficiency may produce intestinal obstruction, accompanied by these symptoms.

NAUSEA AND VOMITING OF PREGNANCY

Nausea and vomiting of pregnancy is a designation intended to describe a frequent set of symptoms that are usually mild and, in general, limited to the first four months of pregnancy.[55] The symptoms, which occur predominantly in the morning, usually are not severe nor persistent, nor are they associated with significant fluid and electrolyte depletion. *Hyperemesis gravidarum* refers to severe, usually persistent vomiting in early pregnancy, which may result in profound nutritional and metabolic abnormalities, including sodium, water, and potassium depletion. The mechanism producing nausea and vomiting in pregnant women in the absence of other demonstrable disease associated with these symptoms is not known. A variety of chemical alterations found in pregnancy has been suspected, but none has been demonstrated to be of importance in the pathophysiology of vomiting. Psychic influences appear to play a part in producing nausea and vomiting in some pregnant women, but whether psychologic factors constitute the entire explanation for

this variety of vomiting is not known. Nausea and vomiting are produced in about 10% of women receiving certain oral contraceptives containing norethynodrel.[54] These agents, by their metabolic effects, simulate pregnancy. The intensity, the incidence, and the variability of symptoms among nonpregnant women receiving these agents are similar to those observed in women who are actually pregnant. It is conceivable that steroid hormones elaborated and released during pregnancy may be responsible for the observed nausea and vomiting in a similar manner.

OTHER FACTORS

Nausea and vomiting are common accompaniments of a variety of generalized and systemic disorders. They are particularly common symptoms in children, especially during the course of febrile illnesses. There is not a good temporal correlation between the occurrence of fever and vomiting, nor can nausea and vomiting be induced experimentally by production of levels of pyrexia comparable to those observed in certain febrile illnesses. It is conceivable that chemical agents are elaborated and released into the peripheral circulation in association with certain illnesses in which fever is observed, and that these toxic substances, as yet undefined, may induce vomiting by stimulation of the medullary chemoreceptor trigger zone or by action at peripheral sites. Nausea and vomiting commonly occur in patients with uremia, as well as in patients with diabetic ketoacidosis. The agent or agents responsible for the production of nausea and vomiting in patients with uremia have not been defined, but it appears that it is not urea. However, in uremic patients, anorexia, nausea, and vomiting commonly disappear when effective hemodialysis corrects the grossly disordered biochemical state. Nausea and vomiting associated with diabetic ketoacidosis usually are relieved after the correction of ketoacidosis.

Endocrine Disorders

Anorexia, nausea, and vomiting are common afflictions with patients suffering from Addison's disease. When anorexia, nausea, and vomiting occur in Addison's disease, there are often profound changes in electrolyte levels, with evidence of metabolic alkalosis, hyperkalemia, and elevation of blood urea nitrogen levels. Nausea and vomiting in patients with Addison's disease usually disappear after replacement therapy with required adrenocorticoids.

Hyperparathyroidism may be signaled by profound anorexia, nausea, and vomiting. In many such patients, vomiting is accompanied by abdominal pain, which is often cramping in nature but may be constant.

In some patients whose hyperparathyroidism is manifested by anorexia, nausea, and vomiting, abdominal pain is absent. The abdominal distress in certain patients with hyperparathyroidism may be vague and difficult to distinguish from the nausea that commonly accompanies it. Vomiting is frequently seen in association with hyperthyroidism, particularly in patients in hyperthyroid crisis. It has been postulated that the vomiting is a manifestation of the central nervous system irritability that characterizes hyperthyroidism and that it reflects reduction of the threshold of excitation of the medullary vomiting center.

Cardiac Disease

Vomiting with or without abdominal pain is not unusual with acute myocardial infarction. It may occur in association with or distinct from chest and arm pain characteristic of myocardial infarction. Vomiting that is presumed to be secondary to congestion of abdominal viscera may accompany severe congestive heart failure, particularly when it is relatively acute in its development. Other factors may contribute to or be responsible for the vomiting seen in patients with heart disease. These include the administration of drugs that are known to be capable of inducing vomiting, such as digitalis or aminophylline. Severe fluid and electrolyte disturbances, such as may result from too vigorous use of diuretic agents in patients with heart disease, also may provoke anorexia, nausea, and vomiting.

Malnutrition

Extended periods of fasting or starvation result in anorexia. In certain patients, this effect may be due to the anorexigenic effects of the ketosis that develops secondary to utilization of lipid stores as caloric sources. Protracted periods of malnutrition are associated with multiple deficiencies of nutrients including vitamins, minerals, and sources of calories. It has been shown clearly that anorexia may be produced by administration of a diet deficient in thiamine.[55] It is probable that additional factors in individuals with severe general malnutrition also contribute to the anorexia so commonly observed.

Motion Sickness

Anorexia, nausea, and vomiting may be the most prominent manifestations of the clinical entity referred to as motion sickness. This distressing constellation of symptoms occurs in susceptible persons during or following transportation by a variety of moving vehicles including trains, planes, ships, and cars. As the symptoms develop, the affected individuals become initially anorectic and then experience profound apathy, salivation, and sweating. These symptoms proceed to their culmination in nausea and vomiting. Similar symptoms can be produced by caloric stimulation of the otic labyrinth. Other factors in addition to labyrinthine stimulation appear to play a part in the production of motion sickness including psychic, tactile, visual, and proprioceptive impulses.

Meniere's Disease

Meniere's disease is a disorder in which there is distention of the membranous labyrinth with degeneration of the organ of Corti. These patients experience genuine vertigo, accompanied by tinnitus and deafness. During or following these acute episodes, nausea and vomiting may be prominent symptoms. Meniere's disease, or syndrome, has its onset most commonly in the fifth decade; however, it may occur in younger adults and the aged. It is not common in children. Identification of Meniere's disease as the cause of vomiting in such patients usually can be obtained by recognition of the associated symptoms reflecting labyrinthine stimulation, as well as by the acute recurrent nature of the symptoms.

SUMMARY

Anorexia, nausea, and vomiting are common manifestations of various disease entities that affect man. Anorexia is a prominent symptom in a variety of gastrointestinal and extragastrointestinal disorders. Normally, food intake is regulated by two hypothalamic centers, the ventrolateral or "feeding center" and the ventromedial or "satiety center." The mechanisms by which hunger and appetite are regulated under normal conditions and modified in various disease states are not completely understood. It does appear, however, that blood glucose levels and various peptide hormones, such as insulin, glucagon, and cholecystokinin, are involved. Anorexia is commonly present in diseases of the liver, such as hepatitis, and of the gastrointestinal tract, as in mechanical obstruction. It may also be a prominent manifestation of extraintestinal disease, including metabolic, cardiorespiratory, renal, neurologic, and psychiatric disorders.

Nausea, an ill-defined but distinctly unpleasant sensation associated with a profound revulsion toward the ingestion of food, is commonly associated with both anorexia and vomiting. When amplified, stimuli that evoke anorexia will often precipitate nausea and vomiting. These stimuli include chemical agents, food, drugs, and several disease entities, such as those associated with increased intracranial pressure, which may produce projectile vomiting. The vomiting center is located in the dorsal portion of the lateral reticular for-

mation in the medulla. Impulses are transmitted to this center by humoral and chemical stimulation of an adjacent "chemoreceptor trigger zone," from higher cortical and brain centers, from the vestibular apparatus, and peripherally from the pharynx and gastrointestinal tract, principally by the vagus nerve.

Nausea and vomiting are prominent manifestations of diseases of the gastrointestinal tract, such as mechanical obstruction and various intra-abdominal inflammatory disorders, including hepatitis, pancreatitis, and ureteral colic. Nausea and vomiting are also common accompaniments of pregnancy, especially in the first trimester, and of various metabolic and endocrine disorders.

REFERENCES

1. **Mitchell GAG:** Anatomy of the Autonomic Nervous System. Edinburgh, E & S Livingston, 1953
2. **Gershon MD, and Erde SM:** The nervous system of the gut. Gastroenterology 80:1571–1594, 1981
3. **Norberg KA:** Adrenergic innervation of the intestinal wall studied by fluorescence microscopy. Int J Neuropharmacol 3:379–382, 1964
4. **Jacobowitz D:** Histochemical studies of the autonomic innervention of the gut. J Pharmacol Exp Ther 149:358–364, 1965
5. **Ahlquist RP:** A study of the adrenotropic receptors. Am J Physiol 153:586–600, 1948
6. **Levy B, Ahlquist RP:** An analysis of adrenergic blocking activity. J Pharmacol Exp Ther 133:202–210, 1961
7. **Bailey DM:** The action of sympathomimetic amines on circular and longitudinal smooth muscle from the isolated esophagus of the guinea-pig. J Pharm Pharmacol 17:782–787, 1965
8. **Crema A, Benzi G, Frigi GM, Berte F:** Occurrence of alpha and beta receptors in the bile duct. Proc Soc Exp Biol Med 120:158–160, 1965
9. **Reynolds DG, Demaree GE, Heiffer MH:** An excitatory adrenergic alpha-receptor mechanism of the terminal guinea pig ileum. Proc Soc Exp Biol Med 125:73–78, 1967
10. **Thomas JE:** Recent advances in gastrointestinal physiology. Gastroenterology 12:545–560, 1949
11. **Gregory RA, Tracy HJ:** The constitution and properties of two gastrins extracted from hog antral mucosa. I. The isolation of two gastrins from hog antral mucosa. II. The properties of two gastrins isolated from hog antral mucosa. Gut 5:103–114, 1964
12. **Debas HT, Yamagishi T, Dryburgh JR:** Motilin enhances gastric emptying of liquids in dogs. Gastroenterology 73:777–780, 1977
13. **Thomas PA, Akwari OE, Kelly KA:** Hormonal control of gastrointestinal motility. World J Surg. 3:545–552, 1979
14. **Cannon WB, Washburn AL:** An explanation of hunger. Am J Physiol 29:441–454, 1912
15. **Mayer J:** Genetic traumatic and environmental factors in the etiology of obesity. Physiol Rev 33:472–508, 1953
16. **Grossman MI, Cummins GM, Ivy AC:** The effect of insulin on food intake after vagotomy and sympathectomy. Am J Physiol 149:100–106, 1947
17. **Magee DF:** Gastro-intestinal Physiology, p 194. Springfield, Ill, Charles C Thomas, 1962
18. **Gibbs J, Young RC, Smith GP:** Cholecystokinin elicits satiety in rats with open gastric fistulas. Nature 245:323–325, 1973
19. **Gibbs J, Smith GP:** Cholecystokinin and satiety in rats and rhesus monkeys. Am J Clin Nutr 30:758–761, 1977
20. **Schneider BS, Monahan JW, Hirsch J:** Brain cholecystokinin and nutritional status in rats and mice. J Clin Invest 64:1348–1356, 1979
21. **Maddison S:** Intraperitoneal and intracranial cholecystokinin depress operant responding for food. Physiol Behav 19:819–824, 1977
22. **Janowitz HD, Grossman MI:** Some factors affecting the food intake of normal dogs and dogs with esophagostomy and gastric fistula. Am J Physiol 159:143–148, 1949
23. **Janowitz HD, Grossman MI:** Effect of prefeeding, alcohol and bitters on food intake of dogs. Am J Physiol 164:182–186, 1951
24. **Iggo A:** Gastrointestinal tension receptors with unmyelinated afferent fibers in the vague of the cat. Q J Exp Physiol 42:130–143, 1957
25. **Iggo A:** Tension receptors in the stomach and the urinary bladder. J Physiol 128:593–607, 1955
26. **Paintal AS:** Responses from mucosal mechanoreceptors in the small intestine of the cat. J Physiol 139:353, 368, 1957
27. **Paintal AS:** A study of gastric stretch receptors: Their role in the peripheral mechanism of satiation of hunger and thirst. J Physiol 126:255–270, 1954
28. **Chernigovsky VN:** The significance of interoceptive signals in the food behavior of animals. In Second Conference on Brain and Behavior, Los Angeles, 1962. Brain and Behavior. II. The Internal Environment and Alimentary Behavior, pp 319–348. Washington, D.C., American Institute of Biological Sciences, 1962
29. **Sharma KN:** Alimentary receptors and food intake regulation, In Kare MR, Maller O (eds): The Chemical Senses and Nutrition, p 286. Baltimore, John Hopkins University Press, 1967
30. **Iggo A:** Gastric mucosal chemoreceptors with vagal afferent fibers in the cat. Q J Exp Physiol 42:398–409, 1957
31. **Sharma KN, Nasset ES:** Electrical activity in mesenteric nerves after perfusion of gut lumen. Am J Physiol 202:725–730, 1962
32. **Magee DF:** Gastro-intestinal Physiology, p 195. Springfield, Ill, Charles C Thomas, 1962

33. **Wolf S, Wolff HG:** Human Gastric Function, p 111. London, Oxford, 1947

34. **Grossman MI, Woolley JR, Dutton DF, Ivy AC:** The effect of nausea on gastric secretion and a study of the mechanism concerned. Gastroenterology 4:347–351, 1945

35. **Borison HL, Wang SC:** Physiology and pharmacology of vomiting. Pharmacol Rev 5:193–230, 1953

36. **Atweh SF, Kuhar MJ:** Autoradiographic localization of opiate receptor in rat brain, II. The Brain Stem. Brain Res 129:1–12, 1977

37. **Valenzuela JE:** Dopamine as a possible neurotransmitter in gastric relaxation. Gastroenterology 71:1019–1022, 1976

38. **Ambinder RF, Schuster MM:** Endorphins: New gut peptides with a familiar face. Gastroenterology 77:1132–1140, 1979

39. **Gregory RA:** Changes in intestinal tone and motility associated with nausea and vomiting. J Physiol 105:58–65, 1946

40. **Bruch H:** Anorexia nervosa and its differential diagnosis. J Nerv Ment Dis 141:555–566, 1965

41. **Halmi K, Brodland G, Loney J:** Prognosis in anorexia nervosa. Ann Intern Med 78:907–909, 1973

42. **Udvarhelyi GB, Adamkiewicz JJ Jr, Cooke RE:** "Anorexia nervosa" caused by a fourth ventricle tumor. Neurology 16:565–568, 1966

43. **Hoyt CS, Stickler GB:** A study of 44 children with the syndrome of recurrent (cyclic) vomiting. Pediatrics 25:775–780, 1960

44. **Wolf S:** Studies on nausea: Effects of ipecac and other emetics on the human stomach and duodenum. Gastroenterology 12:212–218, 1949

45. **Martin WJ, Marcus S:** Relation of pyrogenic and emetic properties of enterobacteriaceal endotoxin and of staphylococcal enterotoxin. J Bacteriol 87:1019–1026, 1964

46. **Sugiyama H, Hayama T:** Abdominal viscera as site of emetic action for staphylococcal enterotoxin in the monkey. J Infect Dis 115:330–336, 1965

47. **Harris SC, Ivy AC, Searle LM:** The mechanism of amphetamine-induced loss of weight. JAMA 134:1468–1475, 1947

48. **Siegel LJ, Longo DL:** The control of chemotherapy-induced emesis. Ann Intern Med 95:352–359, 1981

49. **Gylys JA, Doran KM, Buyniski JP:** Antagonism of cisplatin-induced emesis in the dog. Res Commun Chem Pathol Pharmacol 23:61–68, 1979

50. **Herrin RC, Meek WJ:** Afferent nerves excited by intestinal distension. Am J Physiol 144:720–723, 1945

51. **Walton FE, Moore RM, Graham EA:** The nerve pathways in the vomiting of peritonitis. Arch Surg 22:829–837, 1931

52. **Sharma RN, Dubey PC, Dixit KS, Bhargaua KP:** Neural pathways of emesis associated with experimental intestinal obstruction in dogs. Ind J Med Res 60:291–295, 1972

53. **Fairweather DVI:** Nausea and vomiting in pregnancy. Am J Obstet Gynecol 102:135–175, 1968

54. **Bakker CB, Dightman CR:** Side effects of oral contraceptives. Obstet Gynecol 28:373–379, 1966

55. **Williams RD, Mason HL, Wilder RM, Smith BF:** Observations on induced thiamin deficiency in man. Arch Intern Med 66:785–789, 1940

22

Constipation and Diarrhea Malcolm L. Peterson

Normal Physiology of Propulsion of Intestinal Contents
Definitions
Causes of Constipation
  Neurogenic Basis
    Psychological Factors
    Spinal Cord Lesions
    Postganglionic Disorders
  Muscular Basis
    Muscular Atony from Laxative Abuse
    Weakness of the Voluntary Muscles
  Mechanical Basis

Causes of Diarrhea
  Malabsorption
    Basic Pathophysiology
    Malabsorption of Fat
    Bile Salt Disorders
    Malabsorption of Carbohydrates
    Malabsorption of Water
    Secondary Malabsorption Syndromes
  Neuromuscular Origin of Diarrhea
  Mechanical Basis of Diarrhea
  Inflammatory Basis of Diarrhea
Diagnostic Assessment of Diarrhea
Summary

When a patient describes a change in bowel habit the clinician must try to determine the specific pathophysiology involved in the disturbance of intestinal absorption and motility. Diagnosis is facilitated by the development of such information. Rational therapy is possible only if there is a sound understanding of the factors that regulate intestinal transit.

In most American and European populations, the usual bowel habit is passage once daily of a plastic, intact fecal mass measuring 150 g to 300 g (about the shape of a thin, medium-sized potato or often in the form of one to several segments shaped like small bananas). Normally the stool, although appearing to be a soft solid, contains about 70% water. Form, color, odor, and consistency are subject to some variation resulting from dietary and bacterial influences, but the familiar, olive-drab stool is usually only slightly odoriferous and remains intact in the toilet bowl. Significant and sustained variation from this pattern is worthy of clinical attention. To avoid a pitfall of history-taking, the clinician should ask for a specific description of bowel habit and fecal characteristics rather than phrase the question in terms of "normal."

It is important to define in what sense the terms "constipation" and "diarrhea" are used, since the patient's meanings of these complaints are often not consonant with medical definitions. This is particularly true with regard to constipation, because individuals vary widely in their concepts of what constitutes normal bowel action. Does the patient mean that he does not have a bowel action every day, that the stool is too hard or too small, or that he never has a feeling of complete evacuation? The details may reveal that he needs reassurance rather than a laxative. Before at-

tempting a precise definition, therefore, it is necessary to discuss the normal physiology concerned with the formation of feces.

NORMAL PHYSIOLOGY OF PROPULSION OF INTESTINAL CONTENTS

Within a few minutes after food enters the stomach, some of it passes into the duodenum. The rate of gastric-emptying depends upon a number of factors, among them the quantity and the quality of the food, the emotional state of the individual, his nutritional status, and the time interval since the previous food intake. On the average, after an ordinary mixed meal, the stomach is empty of the ingested food in three hours to four hours.

As judged by the rate of movement of a barium meal, the rate of passage of chyme is relatively rapid in the duodenum and jejunum, slowing considerably in the ileum, particularly in the distal 25 cm to 30 cm. The residue of a mixed meal will begin to pass through the ileocecal valve in from two hours to 3 hours after it is consumed and will have completed its passage into the cecum in from six hours to nine hours.[1] A great deal of the water content is absorbed, including the fluid derived from mucus, but the consistency of the contents of the distal small gut is still semiliquid.

Transit time in the colon is more variable. From cecum to sigmoid, the transit time is normally several hours to one to two days. In persons with chronic diarrhea the colonic transit time has been shown to be 17 hours ± 4 hours; in persons with chronic constipation this same transit time has been shown to be 118 ± 4 hours.[2]

Even when there is little or no fluid ingested, there is a large volume of fluid secreted into the gastrointestinal tract. The various types of secretion are essential to normal distal propulsion of gastrointestinal contents and to physiologic digestion and absorption. The sources and approximate 24-hour volumes in an average adult are listed below:

Saliva	1 liter
Gastric secretions	2 liters
Bile	1 liter
Pancreatic juice	2 liters
Small intestine	1 liter
Total digestive secretions	7 liters

Absorption of all but about one liter of fluid, plus ingested water, is complete in the small bowel. Another 0.8 liter to 0.9 liter of water is absorbed in the colon.[3]

The assimilation or excretion of ingested material by the gut is regulated by the combined secretory and motor phenomena of the alimentary tract;[4] these, in turn, are regulated by the interplay of both nervous and hormonal factors. Cholinergic and adrenergic mediation of the pathways of the autonomic nervous system maintain the base of muscular function on which modulations are superimposed by gastrin, cholecystokinin (pancreozymin), secretin, glucagon, and the prostaglandins.[5] In the normal circumstance of this interplay, the major force that tends to accentuate gastrointestinal transit is parasympathetic activity, stimulated or enhanced by gastrin, cholecystokinin, serotonin, and the prostaglandins, and that which reduces it is sympathetic activity stimulated or enhanced by secretin and glucagon (Table 22-1).[6]

Motion of the intestinal wall achieves mixing, which facilitates both digestion and the flux of water and solutes across the mucosa, and propulsion of the contents. Movement of the villi are particularly important in achieving transepithelial absorption and secretion. Seemingly random contraction and relaxation of narrow rings of the small intestinal wall (segmentation) churn and displace the chyme to and fro, but longitudinal muscular contractions and relaxations do not appear to move the contents. Peristalsis, perhaps coordinated by slow waves (action potentials that progress aborally, depolarizing the longitudinal smooth muscles), is of questionable importance in moving chyme.[4] Since stretch receptors can initiate peristalsis, volume of chyme in segments undergoing segmentation may be the major influence in origination of propulsive movements.[7]

The normal stimuli for the evacuation of material from the colon (Table 22-2) are moderated by psychological control imposed over afferent signals from pudendal and pelvic splanchnic nerves, which arc in the same segments back through the splanchnic nerves to stimulate colonic contractions and internal anal sphincter relaxation.[8]

Obviously, these neurohumoromuscular systems depend upon the integrity of cell membranes and the subcellular biochemical mechanisms that form the intricate networks of biophysical controls. Aberrations in these, whether induced by exogenous pharmacologic agents, endogenous hormonal imbalances, or imbalances in impulses in the nervous pathways, may alter the normal circumstances to create abnormal patterns of defecation—constipation or diarrhea.

DEFINITIONS

Constipation may be considered as simply undue delay in the evacuation of feces. This does not imply that there need normally be a bowel movement every 24 hours; there are healthy persons who pass a well-formed

Table 22-1. *Factors That Alter Motor Activity of the Alimentary Canal*

	Increased Motor Activity	Decreased Motor Activity	Region Affected
Physiologic			
Parasympathetic activity	+		Stomach
Gastrin	+		Small intestine
Cholecystokinin	+		Small intestine
Serotonin	+		Small intestine
Prostaglandins	+		?Colon
Sympathetic activity		+	Colon (small intestine*)
Secretin		+	Small intestine
Glucagon		+	Small intestine
Pharmacologic			
α-adrenergic blockade	+		Small intestine
β-adrenergic blockade	+		Colon
α-adrenergic stimulation		+	Small intestine
β-adrenergic stimulation		+	Colon

*Minor effect

stool of normal consistency once every two or even three or more days. They are not constipated. Persons who are constipated usually pass hard, dry stools or no stool at all for an inordinate number of days. The evacuation of hard stools is usually accomplished only with some difficulty involving excessive use of the voluntary muscles. Constipation does not mean that the stool must be small, although it often contains very little water. Neither does it imply that there need be a feeling of complete evacuation after defecation, although this normally occurs. A feeling of incomplete evacuation may be due to local conditions in the rectum, or, more frequently, to psychic factors.

Diarrhea, as the opposite of constipation, means discharge of watery or semisolid stools. It may, or may not, be accompanied by abdominal cramping or tenesmus. The number of stools need not enter into the definition of diarrhea, although usually the frequency of the bowel movements is increased to three or more per day. *Dysentery* is a term misused by many persons to describe any severe diarrhea. The term should be restricted to inflammations of the intestine characterized by severe diarrhea with frequent passage of mucus and blood and accompanied by systemic disturbances, such as fever. The most common forms are bacillary dysentery and amebic dysentery.

Useful guidelines for definitions of diarrhea and constipation emerge from consideration of the distribution of persons with different "normal" patterns of bowel habit. Ninety-four percent of adults describe their stool habits to be within the range of two or fewer stools per day to five to seven stools per week. Ninety-nine percent report a stool frequency from three per day to three per week.[9] Thus, *diarrhea* is an intermittent or continuous increase in bowel frequency to three or more stools daily, the stool usually being watery or semisolid. *Constipation* is characterized by decrease in frequency of bowel movements to passage less than three times per week of stools that are usually hard and often covered with mucus.

Table 22-2. *Dominant Neurophysiologic Pathways of Control of Release of Gastrointestinal Contents*

Region	Pathways	Mechanisms Affected
Stomach	Parasympathetic	Pyloric relaxation and gastric peristalsis
Small intestine	Sympathetic	Segmentation
Colon	Sympathetic	Peristalsis
Rectum	Parasympathetic	Mass contraction with defecation
Anus	Parasympathetic	Anal relaxation

CAUSES OF CONSTIPATION

The volume of laxatives and "natural regulators" sold in the United States would suggest that constipation tends to be a national preoccupation. The reported symptom, undue delay in fecal evacuation, demands careful individual study by the clinician before the complaint can be considered symptomatic of underlying disease. Many persons without disease have only one stool every two to three days, but in others a sustained change from a bowel habit of one stool daily to such a schedule can be a very important clue to disease. The normal stimuli to evacuate the sigmoid colon initiate such basic reflexes that relatively few factors can appreciably postpone fecal elimination.

Causes of constipation can be neurogenic, muscular, or mechanical. As with any classification based on our incomplete knowledge of gastrointestinal physiology, some overlap will occur, and an etiologic factor, if completely elucidated, might account for disturbances under several of these functional headings. In Table 22-3, etiologies are classified under the pathophysiologic processes believed to be primarily operative.

Table 22-3. *Causes of Constipation*

Neurogenic
  Cortical, voluntary, or involuntary delay of evacuation
  Central nervous system lesions
    Multiple sclerosis
    Cord tumors
    Tabes dorsalis
    Traumatic spinal cord lesions
  Postganglionic disorders
    Hirschsprung's disease (congenital megacolon)
    Chagas' disease

Muscular
  Atony
  Laxative abuse
  Severe malnutrition
  Metabolic defects
  Hypothyroidism
  Hypercalcemia
  Potassium depletion
  Porphyria
  Hyperparathyroidism

Mechanical
  Bowel obstruction
    Neoplasm
    Volvulus
    Diverticulitis
  Extra-alimentary tumors (including pregnancy)
  Rectal lesions
    Lymphogranuloma venereum
    Thrombosed hemorrhoids
    Fissure-in-ano
    Perirectal abscess

NEUROGENIC BASIS

Psychological Factors

Certainly the most common cause of delayed evacuation is voluntary restriction of defecation. When stool enters the rectum in sufficient quantity to stimulate the pressure receptors, one is aware of the urge to defecate, but by voluntarily contracting the external sphincter and associated muscles, he can postpone the need to defecate signaled by the mass contraction, reflex relaxation of the internal and sphincter, and propulsion of the fecal mass.[10] The rectum then adjusts itself to the increased tension and ceases transmission of afferent impulses, or the rectum may actually return stool into the sigmoid. If such voluntary delay is habitual, the reflex ceases to function.

The signal in most normal persons occurs shortly after the first meal of the day and is initiated by the gastrocolic reflex. Students, office employees, factory workers, and others who must leave home soon after breakfast often learn to disregard signals to move the bowels. The signal may be repeated, perhaps after a midmorning coffee break, and again perhaps after lunch. If repeatedly, consciously disregarded, the impulse to evacuate may become unconsciously blocked. The affected person, not understanding the origin of his problem, often considers himself to be constipated and becomes involved in the laxative habit, which leads to further constipation.

Remarkable conscious and unconscious disregard of the impulse to defecate is possible. Occasional voluntary inhibition of the impulse is not harmful; everyone uses this control occasionally. Combat troops and travelers find control of the urge essential. Facility for conditioning of the reflex was built into the training of some of the first Soviet cosmonauts. Children may develop constipation in deliberate efforts to manipulate their parents.[11]

A large group of chronically constipated persons has been shown to have excessive tone of the circular muscle of the distal colon, mediated by signals through the autonomic nervous system. Experimentally, markedly increased contraction of the colon has been observed with a wide variety of stressful situations, such as exposure to cold, pain, compression of the head, and discussion of troublesome life situations.[12]

Since it is believed that excessive tone interferes with the propulsive motility, the constipation of patients with chronic anxiety is usually attributed to this mechanism. Constipation may be associated with certain types of acute emotional disturbances (grief, anger, abject fear) shown to be associated with inhibition of intestinal muscular activity (Table 22-2).[13] Psychotic states can be accompanied by constipation.

Spinal Cord Lesions

Traumatic lesions and organic diseases of the nervous system, such as tabes dorsalis, multiple sclerosis, brain and cord tumors, meningitis, and the like, may produce constipation. Stimuli from the higher nerve centers may influence bowel activity directly. Such influences are evident from both clinical and experimental studies. However, cord involvement is more likely to alter gastrointestinal motility than are diseases of the brain, possibly because the effect may be on only the parasympathetic or sympathetic nerves, leaving the "opposing" set in control. For example, various lesions may destroy efferent nerves concerned with the defecation reflex. When the spinal cord is unable to recognize the presence of stool in the rectum, there is no stimulus to start the reflex. Many patients with strokes are unable to recognize the pressure produced by accumulation of stool in the rectum. These patients may be constipated at first, but they are likely to have involuntary liquid stools when reflex is at the spinal level.

Postganglionic Disorders

Megacolon. In Hirschsprung's disease, regions of the bowel, usually in the colon, are congenitally without myenteric or submucosal plexuses.[14] Blockage occurs because peristalsis cannot pass through this section. Further, this segment is narrowed because the smooth muscle contracts when separated from the nearest ganglion cell.

The functional blockade is overcome only by forceful propulsion from above the affected segment, and there may be long intervals between defecations. Evacuation often requires enemas. Diagnosis demands careful assessment of history, proctoscopic findings, barium enemas, and bowel wall biopsy.

The aganglionic segment may be located just inside the anal margin only or may extend upward into the rectum or even into the sigmoid. The narrow, usually empty rectum connects by a short conical portion with a greatly dilated descending colon. Rarely, the transverse colon also is dilated. The distended bowel segments have normal myenteric ganglia, normal propulsive activity, and hypertrophic muscular coats; they usually are filled with puttylike feces. Typically, the condition involves the rectum and is observed in infants with severe constipation. They may develop huge protruberant abdomens. Removal of the congenitally aganglionic segment is curative.

Acquired megacolon sometimes occurs as a late complication of Chagas' disease (South American trypanosomiasis). Tissue reaction to the parasite destroys the ganglia.

Drugs. Some drugs, given orally or parenterally, delay the passage of intestinal contents. Opiates and meperidine compounds are notorious as constipating agents. Addicts usually are constipated while using these drugs.

Morphine and, to a lesser extent codeine, increase the tone of the small intestine and the colon. Efforts to block the effect of morphine by various means have shown that its spasmogenic action is mediated through postganglionic fibers of the extrinsic intestinal nerves, but whether this results from stimulation of the cholinergic fibers or from blocking the adrenergic inhibitory supply is not known. The latter is suggested by *in vitro* experiments.[15]

Anticholinergic drugs, usually only in doses that already have produced other atropinelike effects, can produce constipation. Atropine decreases motility by functionally paralyzing parasympathetic nerves, as do the synthetic parasympathetic drugs, such as tricyclamol and propantheline. Tetraethylammonium chloride, which blocks both parasympathetic and sympathetic nerves, produces almost complete inertness of the bowel, as does dibutoline; like atropine, dibutoline is parasympatholytic but also has a direct inhibitory action on smooth muscle. In peptic ulcer patients, constipation may result from side-effects of intensive therapy with anticholinergic drugs plus aluminum-containing antacids. The constipating action of these latter drugs occurs by an unknown mechanism.

MUSCULAR BASIS

The bowel may be unable to move the stool distally in the usual length of time because of weakness of the bowel muscles or weakness of the voluntary muscles of defecation. In these situations, there may be no abnormal reflex activity nor any disturbing impulses directly from the central nervous system.

Muscular Atony From Laxative Abuse

Perhaps the most vexing type of constipation to manage is the end-stage of laxative abuse. This problem results from muscular atony. Patients, many of whom are started on this road by well-intentioned clinicians, family members, friends, or nonallopathic practitioners, take increasing amounts of varied types of laxatives until even various potent plant extracts become less and less effective. The patient may be sent to a specialist, sometimes referred with the diagnosis of Hirschsprung's disease. Patient and physician are frustrated by the necessarily protracted therapeutic program to solve a problem that was years in development. Success is usually possible by making clear to the patient the cause of the trouble and by use of stepwise reductions of senna alkaloids over many weeks or months.

Weakness of the Voluntary Muscles

Because of the important role of the abdominal, pelvic, and diaphragmatic muscles in initiating and completing defecation, diseases affecting the strength of these muscles obviously make evacuation difficult. Weakness of the voluntary muscles occurs with obesity, pregnancy, ascites, emphysema, and cachexia. Some patients with large ventral hernias or severe diastasis recti are constipated. The stretching and thinning of muscle tissue associated with severe rectocele is often associated with constipation; an additional mechanical factor is the angulation of the ampulla, causing the propulsive force to be directed against the perineum rather than toward the anus.

MECHANICAL BASIS

An abnormal physical state of the bowel content or actual physical obstruction of various degrees may retard propulsion. Narrowing of the lumen of the colon which develops slowly may cause *obstipation* (severe refractory constipation). This may result from constricting neoplasms or inflammatory lesions, especially lymphogranuloma venereum. Two types of pathophysiologic process are involved: (1) actual physical blockade, and (2) reflex inhibition of the gut above the lesion.

Occasionally, painful rectal conditions (inflamed hemorrhoids, fissures, abscesses, and so forth) can cause excessive sphincter tone, resultant failure to evacuate, and consequent constipation. A patient may postpone defecation in order to avoid *dyschezia*, so *tenesmus* is a common consequence of these inflammations.

Mechanical obstruction of such a degree that even strong intestinal and abdominal muscles cannot force the intestinal content through it usually is acute. Common causes of acute obstruction are strangulated hernia, intussusception, and volvulus. A gradually developing stenosis is more likely to produce constipation through inhibition of reflexes.

Large extra-alimentary tumors (*e.g.* fibroids, ovarian cysts, or pregnancy) are associated with constipation, but this effect may be more a consequence of loss of mechanical advantage of voluntary muscles than any direct influence on the gut itself.

CAUSES OF DIARRHEA

By definition, any factor that hastens evacuation of the feces may be a cause of diarrhea. However, hypermotility in the small bowel and the proximal colon can be compensated for by slightly longer retention and dehydration in the distal colon. Furthermore, hypermotility in the distal colon may result in little abnormality if the stool is already of normal consistency.[16] It is helpful to recall in this regard that a liquid stool contains only about 10% more water than the hardest scybalum, so that addition or removal of relatively small amounts of fluid can alter physical characteristics of excreta enormously.

Austin Flint's definition in 1880 of the term *diarrhea,* "to denote morbid frequency of intestinal dejections which are also liquid or morbidly soft, and often otherwise altered in character," is still useful, because diarrhea (Gr. διαρροια, a flowing through) means many different things in lay *and* medical argot. Some patients emphasize stool frequency and others note stool consistency; clinicians may translate the term through their personal as well as medical experience.

From the patient's description of alterations in his stools, useful clues can be selected in directing the clinician's attention to one or the other of the possible causes of diarrhea.[17] Age, sex, race, exposure (travel, epidemic, and so forth), dietary relationships, associated symptoms, presence of other diseases, and use of specific drugs are aspects of the history that may be key in establishing the cause of diarrhea. Table 22-4 lists the categories and some of the specific conditions that can result in diarrhea.

As with constipation, many classifications of diarrhea have been suggested. None is completely satisfactory because it is impossible to include all of the many factors involved, such as the etiology, pathology, chemistry, clinical picture, and characteristics of the excreta.

MALABSORPTION

Anything that can influence the complex processes involved in water, solute, or fat absorption can initiate a series of malabsorptive events that results in diarrhea.[3] In the normal person 9 liters to 10 liters of fluid pass the ligament of Treitz (at the duodenojejunal junction) every day. Anything that interferes with the absorption of that fluid or its contents can lead to excessive stool production. Malabsorption may involve primarily water, fat, protein, or carbohydrate, or various combinations of these. With these absorptive deficiencies there also may be significant associated failure in uptake resulting in excretory losses of certain vitamins and other trace elements of vital nutritional importance.

Basic Pathophysiology

There are a number of possible basic causes of malabsorption, especially the following:

Table 22-4. *Causes of Diarrhea*

Malabsorption
  Malabsorption of fats
    Maldigestion secondary to lipase insufficiency
      Pancreatitis
      Carcinoma of the pancreas
      Mucoviscidosis
      Kwashiorkor
    Maldigestion secondary to bile salt deficiency
      Resection or disease of distal ileum
      Regional enteritis
      Ileectomy for tumors or inflammatory disease
      Bacterial growth
        Postgastrectomy afferent loop syndrome
        Jejunal diverticulosis
    Malassimilation secondary to defective paths of
      absorption
      Acanthocytosis
      Intestinal lymphangiectasia
      Whipple's disease*
  Malabsorption of carbohydrates
    Primary lactase deficiency
    Primary sucrase deficiency
    Secondary disaccharidase deficiencies
    Defective glucose transport system
  Malabsorption of water
    Interference with absorption
      Mucosal cell damage
        X-ray
        Metallic poisons
        Gluten
        Colchicine*
        Mesenteric vascular occlusion*
      Osmotic effects of nonabsorbable solutes and ions
        (mannitol, $Mg++$, and so forth)
    Excessive secretion
      Villous adenoma
      Bile acid toxicity in colon

Neuromuscular
  Autonomic system imbalance
    Postvagotomy
    Diabetic enteropathy
    Irritable bowel syndrome*
    Narcotic withdrawal*
  Hormonal and pharmacologic influence
    Serotonin (chromaffin tumors)
    Thyroxin (thyrotoxicosis)
    Gastrin (Zollinger-Ellison tumor)
    Histamine (mastocytosis)
    Phospholine iodide

Mechanical
  Incomplete obstruction
    Neoplasm
    Adhesions
    Stenosis
  Fecal impaction
  Muscular incompetency
    Scleroderma
  Postsurgical effects
    Short bowel syndrome
    Ileal bypass

Inflammatory basis and direct toxins
  Infections
    Parasites
      Giardia lamblia
      Endameba histolytica
      Helminths
    Bacterial
      Cholera and other *Vibrios*
      Campylobacter
      Escherichia coli (toxigenic)
      Clostridium difficile
      Yersinia
      Salmonella
      Shigella
      Staphylococcus
      Tuberculosis
    Viral
      Reovirus
      Adenovirus
      Rotavirus
      Parvovirus
  Nonspecific
    Jejunitis (tropical sprue)
    Regional enteritis
    Ulcerative colitis
    Postantibiotic proctitis*
    "Turista"*
    Amyloidosis
    Diverticulitis
  Cathartics—cascara, senna, and so forth
  Poisons—mercury, arsenic, and so forth

*Assignment of this diagnosis to the indicated category is based upon incomplete evidence or speculation.

1. *A defect in the mucosal cells of the small intestinal cells that may be of genetic origin (e.g., acanthocytosis) or acquired (e.g., Whipple's Disease)*
2. *Temporary inflammatory changes in the intestinal mucosa (from toxins, chemicals, viruses, bacteria, parasites, and so forth, which limit absorption*
3. *Factors that cause excess secretion by the mucosa (cholera, villous adenoma, bile acid toxicity)*
4. *Derangement of bile salt metabolism*
5. *Lack of certain digestive enzymes from pancreas or intestinal mucosa*
6. *Osmotic effects (mannitol, magnesium ion, and so forth)*

Malabsorption of Fat

Obviously, whenever the ingested or secreted contents of the gut cannot be absorbed, changes in bowel habit ensue. Failure to absorb fat results in a pasty stool, which has a relatively high water content. It is often malodorous, light-colored, and floats, making it difficult to flush the stool down the toilet.

Pancreatic lipase hydrolyzes digested triglycerides (Fig. 22-1) into free fatty acids and β-monoglycerides. These relatively more polar lipids can form macromolecular aggregates with bile salts, and they are dispersed as mixed micelles in a fashion that permits the products of enzymatic lipolysis to approach and, presumably, dissolve in the lipid membrane of the microvilli (Fig. 22-2). Triglyceride cannot be so readily dispersed and is, therefore, not available for absorption in the absence of lipase. Lipase acts by cleaving off first the α- and then the α^1-acyl groups, leaving a β-monoglyceride, which can be absorbed. This lipolytic action is optimum at slightly basic *pH*, and diminished lipase activity will result if the duodenal *pH* is lowered. Thus, gastrin-producing tumors provoke such profound gastric acid secretion that the bicarbonate-rich pancreatic secretions fail to neutralize the duodenal contents, and the reduction in lipase activity in this acidified milieu interferes with fat digestion.

Hydroxylation of free fatty acids by organisms in the lumen of the gut has been shown to produce hydroxy compounds similar to the active agent in castor oil (ricinoleic acid). Hence, malabsorption of fat may be a cause of diarrhea because it produces a circumstance of pharmacologically-induced diarrhea as well.[17]

Pancreatic destruction must be relatively extensive to result in enzyme deficiency sufficient to cause steatorrhea. This does not usually occur in acute pancreatitis but may be a permanent dysfunction after prolonged and recurrent attacks of pancreatitis. Blockade of the ducts or replacement of the pancreas by

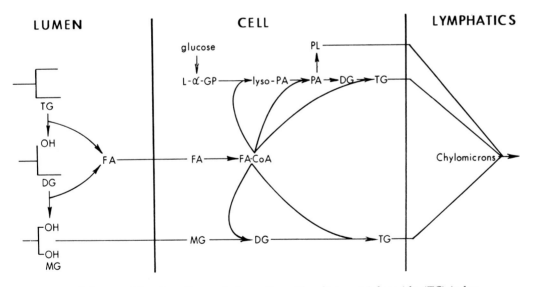

Fig. 22-1. Scheme of fat digestion and absorption. The dietary triglyceride (*TG*) is hydrolyzed in the lumen into α, β-diglyceride (*DG*) and then β-monoglyceride (*MG*) and fatty acids (*FA*) by pancreatic lipase. These lipolytic products enter the cell where the coenzyme A-activated fatty acids (*FA-CoA*) are reassembled into *TG* through intermediate steps involving synthesis of phospholipid (*PL*), glycerophosphate (L-α-GP), lysophosphatidic acid (lyso-*PA*), and phosphatidic acid (*PA*) or addition to partial glycerides. Then the dietary fat is circulated as chylomicrons through the lacteal and thoracic duct.

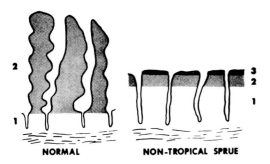

Fig. 22-5. Epithelial zonation in the human jejunum. The zonation of the normal and abnormal intestinal epithelia is derived from histochemical characteristics. Zone I comprises the crypts, and this germinal region is more extensive in nontropical sprue. Zone 2 represents the villous epithelium; in sprue this area is considerably smaller. Zones 1 and 2 in sprue are identical histochemically to Zones 1 and 2, respectively, of the normal intestine. Zone 3 is the location of the peculiar surface epithelium of sprue, and it shows striking deviations from the normal absorptive epithelium. (From Padykula HA, Strauss EW, Ladman AV et al: A morphologic and histochemical analysis of the human jejunal epithelium in non-tropical sprue. Gastroenterology 40:738, 1961)

basis, the result is defective absorption of electrolytes, water, protein, lipids, and vitamins, not only because of decreased mucosal surface, but also because of deficiency in the chemical organization of absorptive cells, especially in relation to active transport.

NEUROMUSCULAR ORIGINS OF DIARRHEA

Dysfunction of the autonomic nervous system or the intestinal musculature it innervates can result in altered absorption and transit time. Generally there is a direct relationship between intestinal motility and absorption; that is, agents or circumstances that produce atony usually impair water absorption, whereas increased motility may be associated with greater absorption of water and prolonged transit time. Since motility is under both neural and endocrine control, it is not surprising that a variety of disease states and medications can influence bowel habit.

After complete vagotomy, gastric motility is severely diminished, but intestinal motility is not markedly affected. Nevertheless, a certain number of patients have transient diarrhea after vagotomy. Whether this is only a reflection of interrupted parasympathetic innervations or some other direct consequence of the operation is not clear. Parallel observations in other states of neuropathy (*e.g.*, diabetic enteropathy) have led to the speculation that surgical or neuropathic parasympathetic denervation results in diminished motility with corresponding reduction in absorption.

Irritable bowel syndrome has shown manifestations of autonomic dysfunction when pharmacologic studies of intestinal motility have been carried out.[23] The common history is one of episodes of watery diarrhea occurring during or just after periods of stress. Often the pressure of unusual situations at home or at work will be associated with the symptoms. With the diarrhea the patient experiences abdominal discomfort, often located in the left upper quadrant, giving rise to the term *splenic flexure syndrome.* The stool volume usually is not very great, but the patient experiences urgency and frequency of defecation. Often the stools are more watery or numerous after midday, but patients with this disorder rarely are awakened by an urge to move their bowels. In the absence of blood in the stools, constitutional symptoms, and dietary relationship of the diarrhea, the diagnosis of irritable bowel syndrome is very likely. Confirmation is afforded by finding normal mucosa upon sigmoidoscopy and by obtaining relief of symptoms with administration of diphenoxylate. Sometimes the distinction between lactase deficiency and irritable bowel syndrome can be difficult.

Narcotic addiction usually is associated with constipation attributed to neuromuscular effects of the drug. Conversely, diarrhea is associated with the withdrawal syndrome, but whether this represents compensatory rebound phenomena in the nervous or muscular tissues has not been established.

Many hormones affect the gut, but their mechanisms of action are not well understood. In overproduction of serotonin by chromaffin tumors, diarrhea can be a prominent symptom. Hyperthyroidism is often accompanied by increased frequency of defecation without marked change in the characteristics of the stool. Although there are multiple reasons for the diarrhea associated with Zollinger–Ellison syndrome, this altered bowel habit results in some measure from the stimulatory effect of gastrin on smooth muscle. Histamine has a profound effect on smooth muscle, and in patients with mastocytosis this substance may effect colonic contractions in such a fashion that diarrhea results.

Diarrhea can be an undesirable side-effect of numerous drugs. Excessive doses of colchicine, quinidine, and various cytotoxic agents often is signaled by appearance of diarrhea. Even therapeutic doses of certain medications can produce diarrhea. For example, the organophosphorus compound echothiophate (phospholine iodide) is used as eye drops by some patients with glaucoma. This potent cholinesterase inhibitor can produce diarrhea resulting from the accumulation of acetylcholine in the neuromotor end-plates of the intestinal muscles, especially the colon.

Cathartic abuse can create severe diarrhea. Such drugs are variously classified as saline, emollient, bulk, or irritant types. In fact, most mechanisms of action are

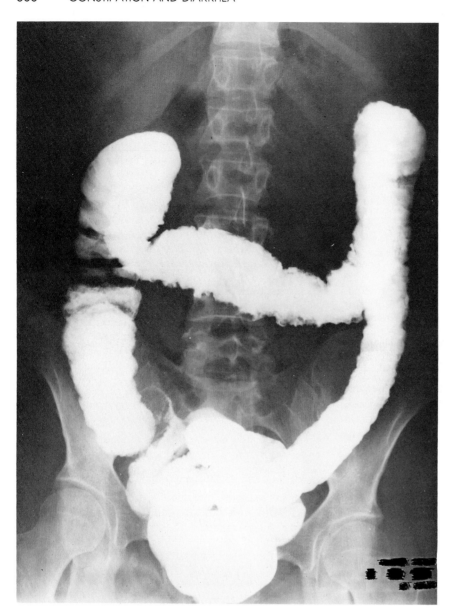

Fig. 22-6. The colon in acute ulcerative colitis with barium clearly outlining many of the ulcers. Admixture of mucus, pus, and blood to the mushy fecal content results in a characteristic type of diarrhea.

poorly understood. The saline cathartics, such as magnesium sulfate and magnesium citrate, exert osmotic effects. Because the cations are not absorbed well, they cause retention of water within the bowel. Presumably mineral oil, certain surfactants, and even cellulose laxatives exert their actions by entrapping bile salts and other amphipathic materials, thereby increasing stool volume with water.

MECHANICAL BASIS OF DIARRHEA

For reasons that may be more complicated than we now appreciate, incomplete obstruction of the bowel may be associated with diarrhea. Stenosis of the large bowel caused by inflammatory changes, extraluminal constriction from adhesions, or invasion of cancer can produce diarrhea. Whether these conditions create circumstances that enhance bacterial overgrowth, resulting in bile salt deconjugation and choleretic diarrhea, has not been clarified. Clearly, the evaluation of any patient with diarrhea demands a rectal examination, which may disclose fecal impaction, a frequent cause of diarrhea in elderly, bedridden, postoperative, or malnourished patients.

Scleroderma can be associated with diarrhea. In such instances histologic study of the intestinal muscle shows

that there is considerable atrophy and replacement by collagen. Resulting atony probably causes impairment of water absorption and diarrhea.

INFLAMMATORY BASIS OF DIARRHEA

Mucosal damage from organisms or their toxins can produce diarrhea that may be brief and self-limited but can be so profuse that dehydration and death ensue.[24] In the usual instance, pathogenic bacteria are not cultured from the stool, although *Shigella* and *Salmonella* are frequently found.

Salmonellosis is a ubiquitous public health problem. Clusters of patients with acute diarrhea in families, schools, or institutions can lead one to suspect this cause, but certainly many of the infectious agents in Table 22-4 can give a similar epidemiologic pattern.

The cause of *traveler's diarrhea* (turista, "Montezuma's revenge," and so forth), an explosive diarrhea which affects a large proportion of international travelers, has long been the subject of speculation. It is not restricted to tropical climes. While only dietary changes (or indiscretions) are commonly indicted, especially by those afflicted briefly after a gastronomic overindulgence, the best evidence shows that unusual bacterial and viral infection of the gut is associated with this scourge of the holiday or business traveler.[25] Controlled studies have failed to give convincing evidence that prophylaxis with various antibiotics is feasible.

"Intestinal flu" is a very common epidemic dysentery. Many types of enteroviruses, including ECHO and Coxsackie viruses, have been established as capable of causing this sudden, usually brief illness.[24]

Regional enteritis commonly produces diarrhea, particularly if it involves the distal ileum, blocking the enterohepatic recirculation of bile salts. Other factors may be responsible for the diarrhea if the inflammation has resulted in a secondary disaccharidase deficiency or in rectal irritability. The stools are usually watery and contain blood; sometimes steatorrhea is a prominent feature if bile salt deficiency is severe.

The diarrhea that characterizes ulcerative colitis is bloody, watery, and associated with urgency and tenesmus. Since not every patient with ulcerative colitis has blood in the stool (or even diarrhea), this diagnosis is worthy of consideration in dealing with a variety of gastrointestinal, hepatic, or dermatologic complaints. Occasionally patients given certain *broad-spectrum antibiotics* develop a pattern of diarrhea resembling that seen in mild ulcerative colitis.[26] Even upon proctoscopic examination, the distinction may be impossible to make, and reliance on history plus the self-limited course of the antibiotic effect may be the only basis of

differentiation. (For radiographic characteristics of acute and chronic ulcerative colitis, see Figs. 22-6 and 22-7.)

Although colonic amebiasis is a relatively uncommon problem, it is endemic in the United States. In addition, world travelers add to this constant background level of amebic infestation. Giardiasis is recognized as a cause of a malabsorptive pattern of diarrhea. Reports of outbreaks should lead to a search for *Giardia lamblia* (a flagellate protozoon) in the jejunal aspirates of the diarrhea victim who has been exposed. Tropical sprue remains an enigma today, but there is little question that it is the cause of diarrhea in many native and foreign residents of certain tropical areas. The frequency of jejunitis in Americans assigned to work in Pakistan or Southeast Asia has approached 40%, but ascribing diarrhea to this cause is untenable in the absence of jejunal biopsy and proper exclusion of other causes.

DIAGNOSTIC ASSESSMENT OF DIARRHEA

A diagnostic approach to the evaluation of diarrhea can be summarized as follows:

History
Physical examination (including rectal examination and sigmoidoscopy)
Examination of stool
    Inspection
    Microscopic examination for ova and parasites or leukocytes
Chemical analyses
    Fecal fat measurements (3-day on known fat intake)
    Guaiac
    Alkalinization
    Osmolarity
    Clostridium difficile exotoxin
Radiographic examination of alimentary tract
Examination of duodenal or jejunal contents
    Microscopic examination
    Culture
    Secretin test
Examination of tissue
    Jejunal biopsy
        Disaccharidase assay
    Rectal biopsy
        Light microscopy
        Electron microscopy
Urine tests
    5-hydroxyindolacetic acid
    Histamine
    Xylose absorption test
Blood tests

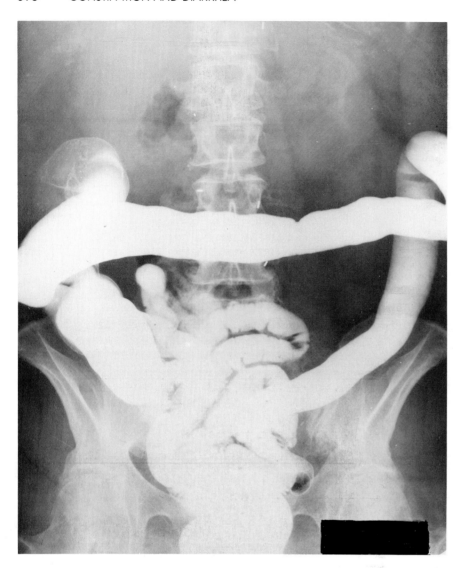

Fig. 22-7. In the patient with chronic ulcerative colitis, the tubular shortened colon discharges the fecal content in the same mushy state in which it is received from the ileum. Because of extensive damage to the mucosal cells, very little water can be absorbed.

Disaccharide tolerance test
Serological test for amebiasis
Serum gastrin assay
Serum carotene
Breath tests

If one uses the insights afforded by understanding the pathophysiology of diarrheal states, the history can provide the information necessary to establish the correct diagnosis in most instances. Asking about characteristics of the stool, duration of diarrhea, drugs, recent travel, exposure to others with diarrhea, sexual preference, dietary patterns, occupation, and other relevant historical data can enable the clinician to distin-

guish among the likely and unlikely causes of the symptom. The physical examination can uncover important diagnostic leads, such as indolent perianal fistula associated with regional enteritis; erythema nodosum, pyoderma, or uveitis associated with ulcerative colitis; dermographia of mastocytosis (urticaria pigmentosa); dermatitis herpetiformis in celiac disease; various cutaneous expressions of nutritional deficiencies; and many others. Patients with irritable colon syndrome may show persistent spasms of the rectosigmoid, causing considerable difficulty in passing the sigmoidoscope.

Inspection of the stool is mandatory in the assessment of the basis of the diarrhea. These observations

and tests usually should be done before the radiologist has given the patient barium sulfate. Odor, color, consistency, presence of absence of mucus, pus, or blood, and the recognition of parasites or undigested food can be reliably determined only by first-hand observation. Microscopic examination for ova and parasites should be done on very fresh warm specimens or those preserved in polyvinyl alcohol. Examination of wet specimens stained with methylene blue to detect leukocytes is useful in recognizing infectious causes of diarrhea.

If a sample of liquid stool should turn pink on the addition of a few drops of sodium or potassium hydroxide solutions, a factitious diarrhea caused by ingestion of phenolphthalein cathartics is likely. Another type of factitious diarrhea can be suspected if liquid stool osmolarity is high, suggesting ingestions of saline cathartics.

Culture of fresh stools on selective media and appropriate subcultures or fermentative classification tests should be done as early as possible in the evaluation. Incubation of the cultures must be done at various temperatures and with special media to detect unusual organisms.

Analysis of fecal fat levels is valid only when the patient is fed a diet of known fat content (usually 60 g–100 g/day), and a 72-hour stool collection is carefully done. Less than 7% of fat (van de Kamer method) is normally excreted in a three-day period under these conditions. Substitutes for this rather tedious determination are not reliable; use of radioiodinated fat absorption studies or spot checks for visible or chemical fat is of little diagnostic benefit.

Radiologic examination of the gut with contrast media can reveal stenosis, diverticula, postsurgical deformities, fistulae, and various neoplastic or inflammatory deformities. A pattern of flocculation of barium in the small bowel is nonspecific in states of malabsorption from various causes. Plain films of the abdomen can reveal perforation (with appropriate position of the patient), pancreatic calcification, and unusual distribution of intraluminal gas. Barium enema can usually facilitate the distinction between regional enteritis of the colon (granulomatous colitis) and ulcerative colitis.

In some instances, examination of duodenal or jejunal contents may be useful, especially for G. lamblia or for overgrowth of bacteria in postgastrectomy diarrheal states. Chemical or cytologic examination of duodenal fluid after intravenous secretin may provide evidence for pancreatic dysfunction or neoplasm.

One of the most useful studies for differentiation of causes of the malabsorptive state is the jejunal biopsy; however, without proper care of the tissue in mounting, sectioning, and staining, little reliable assistance can be expected. The characteristic appearance of celiac disease, intestinal lymphangiectasia, Whipple's disease (especially on PAS stain and under electron microscopy), and acanthocytosis can provide diagnostic certainty. Assay of a small portion of the tissue for lactase, sucrase, and maltase provides the most useful evidence for primary or secondary disaccharidase deficiencies.

Rectal biopsy can reveal granulomata (regional enteritis), schistosomiasis, amyloidosis, or the mucosal ulcers seen in ulcerative colitis (which unfortunately are not specifically characteristic).

Urinary levels of 5-hydroxyindolacetic acid can be of use in establishing the diagnosis of a serotonin-producing neoplasm. Histamine levels in urine have been grossly elevated in patients with diarrhea associated with mastocytosis.

Biopsy of the gut or direct observation of luminal or fecal material usually provides the best diagnostic approach. Most indirect tests are inferior and entail much higher cost: benefit ratios in their use.

The observation that blood levels of glucose do not change significantly following ingestion of disaccharides is less useful than the direct enzyme assay in establishing the diagnosis of disaccharidase deficiency. Nevertheless, disaccharide tolerance tests, done with great care, can be informative, especially if the diarrhea and other symptoms are provoked by the carbohydrate test meal. Serum levels of carotene are sometimes low in certain malabsorptive states, but this test is of much less use than fecal fat measurement and is no more specific as to the cause of lipid malabsorption.

Urinary levels of xylose following ingestion of 25 g of this pentose may be low (less than 5 g in 5 hr) if there is impaired mucosal absorption reflecting intestinal epithelial disease. Unfortunately, this test can be falsely positive if gastric-emptying is delayed and falsely negative if there is renal disease or only limited bowel involvement.

Analysis of a patient's breath after ingestion of a substance that is poorly absorbed because of a disease state can yield useful diagnostic information.[27] A carbohydrate that is not hydrolyzed or assimilated will be the source of excessive hydrogen in the breath after intestinal organisms have metabolized the substrate that is fed as a test substance. Similarly, isotopically-labeled test materials can yield valuable diagnostic data through breath tests when bile acids or carbohydrates produce labeled carbon dioxide after bacterial action in the gut.

In the interest of patient comfort and risk, cost control, appropriate use of resources, and precision, the dictum of Sutton's Law ("Go where the money is") should be kept in mind whenever the diagnostic approach to diarrhea is planned.

SUMMARY

Abnormal motility or deranged absorptive functions of the gut can be manifested by constipation or diarrhea. Appreciation of the normal physiology of propulsion, secretion, and absorption of intestinal contents is the basis of differentiating among neuromuscular, metabolic and hormonal, pharmacologic, and mechanical causes of these symptoms.

Constipation is most commonly induced by laxative abuse that affects intestinal musculature. Obesity, pregnancy, and other causes of abdominal distention leading to attenuation of the strength of the voluntary muscles used in defecation are also frequent causes.

Diarrhea most commonly results from psychological factors, but any of a host of infectious agents can cause watery stools through interference with electrolyte or water absorption. Maldigestion of dietary components leading to diarrhea can be caused by genetic, infectious, metabolic, or mechanical factors that interfere with enzymatic or transport processes. Definition of the precise cause of diarrhea can be achieved by careful selection from among myriad diagnostic techniques, by formulating a logical sequence deduced from the clinical picture, and by reasoning based on basic physiologic principles. The characteristics of the bowel pattern and the stool itself, the temporal features, and the physical findings can permit judicious use of diagnostic and therapeutic modalities in a cost-effective manner.

REFERENCES

1. **Waller SL:** Differential measurement of small and large bowel transit times in constipation and diarrhea: A new approach. Gut 16:372–378, 1975
2. **Waller SL, Misiewicz JJ, Kiley N:** Effect of eating on motility of the pelvic colon in constipation or diarrhea. Gut 13:805–811, 1972
3. **Phillips SF:** Diarrhea: A current view of the pathophysiology. Gastroenterology 63:495–518, 1972
4. **Bartoff A:** Digestion: Mobility. Annu Rev Physiol 34:261–290, 1972
5. **Grossman MI:** Gastrin, cholecystolkinin and secretin act on one receptor. Lancet 1:1088–1089, 1970
6. **Hubel KA:** Secretin: A long progress note. Gastroenterology 62:318–341, 1972
7. **Christensen J:** The controls of gastrointestinal movements: Some old and new views. N Engl J Med 285:85–98, 1971
8. **Christensen J:** Colonic motility. Viewpoints on Digestive Disease 13(3):9–12, 1981
9. **Connell AM, Hilton C, Irvine G et al:** Variation of bowel habit in two population samples. Br Med J 2:1095–1099, 1965
10. **Duthie HL:** Anal continence. Gut 12:844–852, 1971
11. **Bently JFR:** Constipation in infants and children. Gut 12:85–90, 1971
12. **Almy TP, Hinkle LE Jr, Berle B et al:** Alteration in colonic function in man under stress. Gastroenterology 12:437–444, 1949
13. **Grace WJ, Wolf S, Wolff HG:** Life situations, emotions, and colonic function. Gastroenterology 14:93–108, 1950
14. **Fisher JH, Swenson O:** Aganglionic lesions of the colon. Am J Surg 99:134–136, 1960
15. **Daniel EE, Sutherland WH, Bogoch A:** Effects of morphine and other drugs on motility of the terminal ileum. Gastroenterology 36:510–523, 1959
16. **Connell AM:** The motility of the pelvic colon. Part II. Paradoxical motility in diarrhea and constipation. Gut 3:342–348, 1962
17. **Low-Beer TS, Read AE:** Diarrhea: Mechanisms and treatment. Gut 13:1021–1036, 1971
18. **Hofmann AF:** A physiochemical approach to the intraluminal phase of fat absorption. Gastroenterology 50:56, 1966
19. **Gray GM:** Assimilation of dietary carbohydrate. Viewpoints on Digestive Disease. 12(3):9–12, 1980
20. **Peterson ML, Herber R:** Intestinal sucrase deficiency in adults. Trans Assoc Am Physicians 80:275, 1967
21. **Binder HJ:** Net fluid and electrolyte secretion: The pathophysiological basis of diarrhea. Viewpoints on Digestive Disease. 12(2):5–8, 1980
22. **Banwell J, Sherr H:** Effect of bacterial entertoxin in the gastrointestinal tract. Gastroenterology 65:467–497, 1973
23. **Thompson WG, Heston KW:** Functional bowel disease in apparently healthy people. Gastroenterology. 79:283–288, 1980
24. **Ericcson CD, DuPont HL:** Infectious diarrheas: Newer knowledge and current concepts. In Berk JE (ed): Developments in Digestive Diseases, Chap. 5. Philadelphia, Lea & Febiger, 1980
25. **Merson MH, Mouns GK, Sack DA et al:** Travelers' diarrhea in Mexico: A prospective study on physicians and family members attending a congress. N Engl J Med 294:1299–1305, 1976
26. **Bartlett JG:** Antibiotic associated Pseudomonadaceae colitis. Rev Infect Dis 1:530–539, 1979
27. **Toskes PP:** Breath tests: Concept and role in digestive disorders. In Berk JE (ed): Developments in Digestive Disease, Chap 3. Philadelphia, Lea & Febiger, 1980

23

Hematemesis and Melena Leon Schiff

General Considerations
  Source of Hemorrhage
    Melena Without Hematemesis
    Color of Stools
  Characteristics of Melena
  Severity of Hemorrhage
  Azotemia
  Fever
Etiology
History and Physical Examination

Radiographic Examination
Endoscopy and Selective Angiography
Bleeding Peptic Ulcer
Carcinoma of the Stomach
Bleeding Esophageal Varices
Gastritis and Esophagitis
Hiatal Hernia
Hematemesis and Melena from Miscellaneous
    Causes
Summary

GENERAL CONSIDERATIONS

Hematemesis is the vomiting of blood, whether fresh and red or digested and black. *Melena,* by derivation, means black and usually describes the passage of stools with the coal-black, clotted, gummy appearance of tar. However, melena is used clinically in a wider sense to describe the passage of blood in the stools whether the color is visibly altered or not and whether the color is light, reddish, or (as is more common) dark brown or blackish. In general, rapid bleeding tends to cause hematemesis while slower bleeding causes melena.

SOURCE OF HEMORRHAGE

The vomiting of large amounts of blood or the passage of tarry stools are symptoms that usually appear with dramatic suddenness. They may supervene in patients with preexisting digestive disturbances or may of themselves prove the harbingers of disease. Their occurrence may clarify the significance of existing symp-

toms or may constitute the sole evidence of disease. It is well known that they occur most commonly in a number of disorders, which will be considered separately. The occurrence of hematemesis indicates a bleeding point proximal to the ligament of Treitz. The appearance of the vomitus, whether resembling coffee grounds or bright red and obviously bloody, has proved of little diagnostic value.

Melena Without Hematemesis

Although it is generally true that the occurrence of tarry stools without hematemesis indicates a lesion distal to the pylorus (usually a duodenal ulcer), this is not invariably so. We have seen melena without hematemesis in cases of ruptured esophageal varix associated with hepatic cirrhosis and in cases of gastric cancer. Ratnoff and Patek noted 9 instances of melena without hematemesis in 386 cases of hepatic cirrhosis.[1] Benedict reported melena alone in 5 of 20 cases of hemorrhage from gastritis.[2] Jones observed melena only in 6 fatal cases of bleeding gastric ulcer.[3] A common fea-

ture of these 6 patients was their extremely poor general condition, and it was suggested that they may have been too weak to vomit.

Color of Stools

While the presence of bright blood in the stools usually indicates a bleeding point low in the intestine, this is not an infallible sign. In the presence of hypermotility, the blood may be swept through the intestinal tract so rapidly as to appear unaltered in the feces. The presence of bright blood in the stools has been noted in three patients 4 hours to 17 hours after they were given 1000 ml of citrated human blood intragastrically; none of them passed a tarry stool.[4] Truly tarry stools almost always indicate a bleeding site proximal to the transverse colon and hepatic flexure. As a rare exception, they have been reported in bleeding from diverticula in the descending colon. Blood on the surface of the stool almost certainly originates in the distal part of the rectum or anal canal. Patients who have had small polyps of the rectum snared through a proctoscope and who then have bled profusely, retaining a liter or two of blood in the rectosigmoid colon for approximately 24 hours, evacuate red, rarely black blood.[5] Tarry stools are said to occur when blood is introduced in the cecum, particularly in the presence of delayed colonic motility.[5] The author has seen truly tarry stools in the hemorrhage arising just distal to the ileocecal valve, but not when bleeding took place beyond this area. According to Hilsman, the color of the stools (whether bright red, dark red, brown, or tarry) depends more on the time the blood remains in the intestine than on the level at which the bleeding occurs.[5]

CHARACTERISTICS OF MELENA

Amount of Blood Necessary. Daniel and Egan reported the occurrence of tarry stools after the oral administration of 50 ml to 80 ml of fresh human blood.[6] The writer and his associates have reported the occurrence of tarry stools after the oral administration of 100 ml of citrated human "bank" blood. These observations indicate that the passage of a tarry stool does not necessarily indicate severe blood loss.

Duration of Tarry Stools. Tarry stools may be passed for from three days to five days following the intragastric administration of 1000 ml to 2000 ml of citrated human blood to human subjects.[4] This indicates that the passage of a tarry stool is no proof that hemorrhage is continuing. The number of tarry or bloody stools that follow the intragastric administration of blood is not necessarily related to the quantity of blood introduced.

Duration of Occult Blood. Hesser has pointed out that occult blood is usually present in the stools for about two weeks to three weeks following hematemesis or melena in patients with bleeding peptic ulcer.[7] We have been able to confirm this experimentally upon oral or intragastric administration of citrated human blood. The persistence of a positive test for occult blood is, therefore, not necessarily an indication that hemorrhage is continuing.

SEVERITY OF HEMORRHAGE

It is difficult to estimate the quantity of blood lost by judging from the amount apparently present in the vomitus because of the admixture of gastric contents and because only part of the effused blood is vomited. One not infrequently hears a patient proclaim that he has vomited a gallon or two of blood! Cullinan and Price have put it well: The amount of blood vomited varies with the patient's imagination.[8]

It may be difficult to estimate the severity of the bleeding with the patient is first seen clinically, for, as Black has stated, the rate of blood loss may influence the patient's appearance. Thus, "the rapid loss of a small amount of blood may produce as much appearance of circulatory failure" as the gradual loss of a larger quantity.[9] The pulse rate may be misleading, as Wallace and Sharpey–Schafer have shown, because the heart rate may be slowed, increased, or unchanged after the rapid removal of up to 1150 ml of blood in control subjects.[10] We have been impressed with the frequency of a normal pulse rate in the presence of a rather marked fall in blood pressure soon after massive hematemesis or melena. The hematocrit may prove unreliable shortly after hemorrhage, since the lowest values are usually obtained 6 hours to 48 hours later as a result of dilution of the blood by tissue fluids.[9] Wallace and Sharpey–Schafer obtained maximum blood dilution (and lowest hemoglobin percentage) 3 hours to 90 hours after the rapid removal of as much as 1150 ml of blood in control subjects. They found the time of maximal dilution to vary in the same individual on different occasions.[10]

Ebert, Stead, and Gibson removed amounts ranging from 760 ml to 1220 ml of blood from six normal subjects in 6 minutes to 13 minutes. They found a sharp drop in plasma volume immediately after hemorrhage; thereafter the plasma volume gradually increased, until, at the end of three to four days, it was greater than the original plasma volume by an amount approximately equal to the volume of red cells removed. After the first two hours, the change in plasma volume was much more accurately reflected by the hematocrit value than by the protein concentration. "If the difference

between the original hematocrit reading and that made 72 hours after venesection is taken as 100%, it is found that 14% to 36% of this drop occurred in 2 hours, 36% to 50% in 8 hours, and 63% to 77% in 24 hours."[11]

Howarth and Sharpey–Schafer describe three low-blood-pressure phases after hemorrhage. The first phase is that of sudden vasovagal reaction, with bradycardia and muscle vasodilatation, which develops suddenly during or after bleeding. The second phase is associated with increased heart rate, low right atrial pressure, and low cardiac output. Large transfusions raise right atrial pressure, cardiac output, and blood pressure. The third phase "takes time to develop and persists over long periods. Severe anemia may be a causal factor in this phase. Right atrial pressure and cardiac output are increased. Large transfusions may be dangerous from overloading."[12] I have seen instances of pulmonary edema following blood transfusions in patients with severe gastroduodenal hemorrhage who were probably in phase three of Howarth and Sharpey–Schafer and in whom the cardiac output probably fell as the result of the transfusion instead of increasing as it would normally, according to Sharpey–Schafer.[13]

AZOTEMIA

The frequent occurrence of azotemia following hematemesis and melena has been confirmed by numerous observers since it was first pointed out by Sanguinetti in 1933 in cases of bleeding gastric and duodenal ulcer.[14] The writer and his associates reported an elevation of the blood urea nitrogen to 30 mg/dl or more in about two-thirds, and elevation of 50 mg/dl or more in one-fifth of 135 cases of hematemesis or melena owing to various causes.[15] Following a single nonfatal hemorrhage, the blood urea nitrogen may increase within a few hours and usually reaches a maximum within 24 hours, dropping sharply to normal by the third day (Fig. 23-1).[16]

The rate of subsidence of the azotemia can be increased by slow drip blood transfusion but not by infusion of plasma in a comparable amount.[17] In cases in which there is a second (nonfatal) hemorrhage, there is a secondary increase within 24 hours, with a drop to normal by the third day. In cases in which repeated hemorrhages occur and ultimately prove fatal, there is an increasingly or persistently high level of the urea nitrogen in the blood. The kidneys have generally been found normal at autopsy.

The mechanism of the azotemia is not the same as that associated with high intestinal obstruction because it occurs in the absence of any vomiting (that is, in the presence of melena alone) and is associated with a normal or increased blood chloride concentration and a normal carbon dioxide combining power of the blood.

Other things being equal, the degree of azotemia is determined by the amount of blood entering the intestinal tract in a given period of time. The time factor is important, since it has been shown that, if a given quantity of blood is introduced into the gastrointestinal

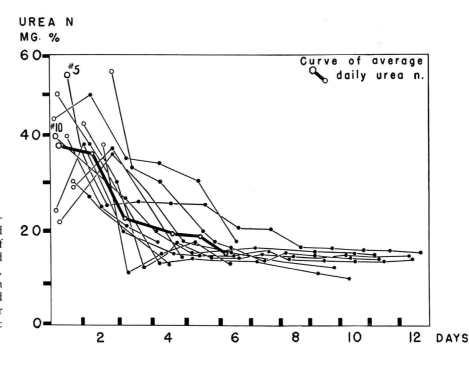

Fig. 23-1. Repeated determinations of the value for blood urea nitrogen in 12 cases of single hemorrhage followed by recovery. (From Schiff L, Stevens RJ: Elevation of urea nitrogen content of the blood following hematemesis or melena. Arch Intern Med 64: 1239, 1939)

tract over a period of days, the maximum elevation of the blood urea nitrogen obtained on any single day may be much less than if a fraction of the blood is given quickly. (Thus, the administration of 250 ml of citrated human blood daily to a control subject for eight days yielded a maximum blood urea nitrogen value of 26 mg/dl; whereas giving 1000 ml of blood intragastrically during a half-hour period yielded a maximum elevation of 47 mg/dl (Fig. 23-2).[18] The time element may explain the disparity between the degree of anemia and the level of the blood urea nitrogen in some patients with hematemesis. Thus, if a patient loses 2000 ml of blood over a period of eight days, one might not expect the same degree of elevation of the blood urea nitrogen that would follow the sudden loss of this quantity of blood, although comparable degrees of anemia might develop.

The azotemia occurs regardless of the cause of hemorrhage into the upper digestive tract. It does not appear in hemorrhage from the colon, a fact that may prove of value in differential diagnosis. It does not follow the sudden withdrawal of as much as 1150 ml of blood in control subjects except in the presence of renal impairment.[10]

The factors that may influence the azotemia include dehydration, shock, impairment of renal function, increased catabolism of tissue protein, and absorption of products of decomposition of the blood liberated into the intestinal tract. Observations on both man and an-

imals indicate the importance of the digestion and the absorption of the blood liberated into the intestinal tract in the production of the azotemia.[18,19,20,21,22] Black, although admitting the role of the blood in the intestinal tract, nevertheless believes that functional renal failure, resulting from a fall in the pressure and in the amount of the blood supplied to the kidneys, plays an important role at the time of the blood urea nitrogen is rising. He finds that the rise of the blood urea that follows the giving of large amounts of blood by mouth is smaller and slower in onset than the azotemia of severe hematemesis.[9] The observations of Gregory and associates in experimental animals indicate that the azotemia may be due to decreased renal function caused by low blood pressure and dehydration or to absorption of digested blood protein. They found the rise in the blood urea nitrogen that followed maintenance of a low blood pressure through bleeding to be slower and more sustained than that which followed the administration of blood by stomach tube.[22]

Although functional renal failure may occur in the presence of shock, it is not essential to the genesis of the azotemia. This is substantiated by the production of azotemia through the intragastric administration of blood to individuals without obvious renal disease (producing in some instances a curve almost exactly the same as that which followed hematemesis in the same subject), by the demonstration that the introduction of such blood does not cause impairment of renal

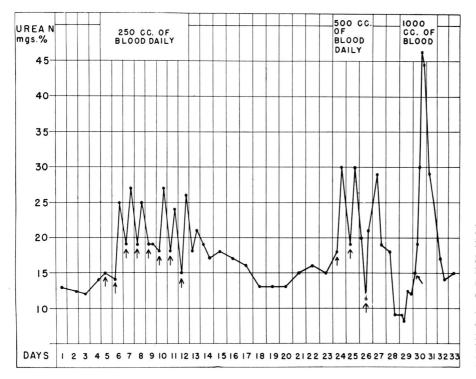

Fig. 23-2. Blood urea nitrogen in one patient following intragastric administration of varying quantities of citrated blood. (From Schiff L, Stevens RJ, Goodman S, Garber E, Lublin A: Observations on the oral administration of citrated blood in man I. The effects on the blood urea nitrogen. Am J Dig Dis 6:597, 1939)

function, and by the demonstration of normal renal function in the presence of azotemia.[23]

We thoroughly endorse Black's statement that "the level to which the blood urea nitrogen rises is of value in judging the severity of gastroduodenal hemorrhage and repeated estimation a good measure of progress."[9] In a series of 135 cases, the writer and his associates reported a maximum blood urea nitrogen of less than 30 mg/dl to be a favorable prognostic sign in patients with hematemesis owing to peptic ulcer, hepatic cirrhosis, or undetermined cause.[15] Exceptions noted were two cases of ruptured aortic aneurysm and one of perforated peptic ulcer. (Subsequent observations include a fatal case of bleeding peptic ulcer without significant elevation of the blood urea nitrogen, in which death was due to pneumonia.) The presence of a maximum blood urea nitrogen content of 50 mg/dl or more was followed by a fatal outcome in one-third of the cases, whereas an elevation of 70 mg/dl or more was accompanied by a fatal outcome in about two-thirds of the cases. In interpreting azotemia in a given case, one should keep in mind that the blood urea nitrogen level may be affected by such complicating factors as starvation, dehydration, alkalosis, or preexisting renal disease. In our experience, a blood urea nitrogen content of over 100 mg/dl has been found to indicate preexisting kidney disease. Evidently the functional renal failure and the amount of blood entering the intestinal tract are, clinically, not sufficient to produce a degree of azotemia above this level.

FEVER

Fever occurs in the majority of patients with hematemesis and melena, regardless of the cause of hemorrhage (Figs. 23-3 to 23-6). It usually appears within 24 hours, lasts from a few days to a week or slightly longer, and may reach a maximum of 103°. It more frequently follows massive or moderately severe than mild hemorrhage. To the unwary clinician, it may initiate an unnecessary search for a complicating infection.

The cause of the fever is not known. According to Dill and Isenhour, numerous factors have been invoked, including absorption of blood decomposition products, reduction in blood volume, anemia, associated gastritis, or increased lability of the heat-regulating center as a result of asthenia or shock.[24] The absorption of blood decomposition products has been considered the most likely cause by a number of European observers. Black suggests that the fever may be related to the endogenous breakdown of the body protein that may occur after hemorrhage.[9] However, the experimental observations of Dill and Isenhour in man and in animals, and our own observations in man[25] indicate that the intragastric administration of large quantities of citrated blood is not followed by any significant elevation in temperature. Incidentally, no change in the white-blood-cell count followed the administration of such blood.

ETIOLOGY

Vomiting of blood or the passage of tarry stools may be due to a variety of disorders. The most common of these is bleeding peptic ulcer.

In our own experience with 640 cases of hematemesis and melena admitted to the Cincinnati General Hospital over a 10-year period (1937–1947), peptic ulcer constituted 339, or 52.9% of the causes; the cause was undetermined in 132, or 20.6%; hepatic cirrhosis was

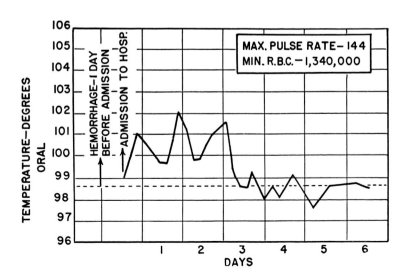

Fig. 23-3. Temperature curve following hemorrhage in patient J. P. (bleeding gastric ulcer).

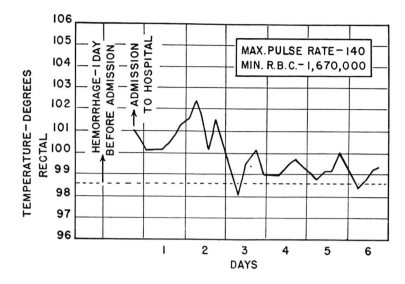

Fig 23-4. Temperature curve following hemorrhage in patient J. W. (bleeding duodenal ulcer).

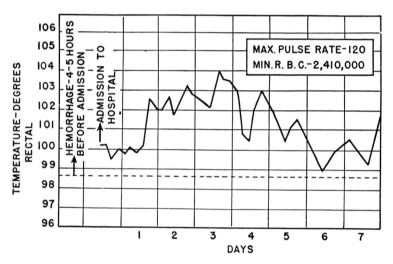

Fig. 23-5. Temperature curve following hemorrhage in patient L. G. (gastric carcinoma).

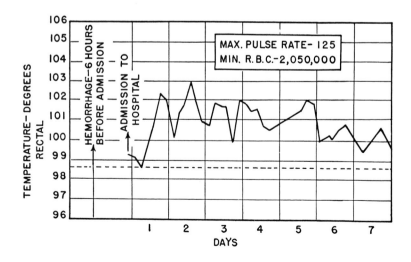

Fig. 23-6. Temperature curve following hemorrhage in patient F. W. (hepatic cirrhosis with ruptured esophageal varix).

present in 80, or 12.5%; gastric carcinoma in 15, or 2.3%; hiatal hernia in 14, or 2.1%; gastritis with mucosal erosions in 7, or 1.1%; aortic aneurysm rupturing into the esophagus in 5, or 0.8%; and miscellaneous causes were found in 48, or 7.5%.

The etiologic factors in other groups of cases are listed in Tables 23-1 and 23-2. In Palmer's series, the diagnoses were based on the author's "vigorous diagnostic approach," which consists of ice-water lavage of the stomach as soon as the history and physical examination have been completed, followed by immediate esophagogastroscopic and contrast radiographic examinations.[26] Using this type of approach, Palmer reports a diagnostic accuracy of 87.1% in 650 patients, as compared with an accuracy of 34.9% obtained in 212

Table 23-2. *Causes of Lower Gastrointestinal Bleeding When Extravasation Is Noted at Angiography*

Cause	Percentage of Patients
Diverticulosis	70%
Angiodysplasia	10%
Peptic ulcer	5%
Meckel's diverticulum	3%
Neoplasms	3%
Vascular-enteric fistula	2%
Jejunal diverticulum	2%
Other	5%

(Courtesy of Walter Pederson, MD, Medical Grand Rounds, Southwestern Medical School, September 17, 1981)

Table 23-1. *Bleeding Sources Among 1500 Patients with Active Bleeding Studied by the Vigorous Diagnostic Approach*

Source	Number of Patients
Duodenal ulcer	406
Esophagogastric varices	295
Erosive gastritis	193
Gastric ulcer	186
Erosive esophagitis	109
Mallory–Weiss syndrome	77
Stomal (anastomotic) ulcer	47
Gastric carcinoma	21
Esophageal ulcer	10
Rendu–Osler–Weber disease	8
Gastric sarcoma	7
Esophageal carcinoma	5
Gastric leiomyoma	5
"Cirsoid" aneurysm into stomach	3
Gastric leukemia	2
Gastric and duodenal ulcer	2
Mucosal prolapse into esophagus	2
Duodenal leiomyoma	2
Liver, posttraumatic	2
Aortoesophageal fistula	2
Gastric biopsy site	2
Adenoma at gastroenteric stoma	2
Ulcer in duodenal diverticulum	1
Metastasis to stomach	1
Duodenal ulcer to varices	1
Gastric sarcoidosis	1
Aortic aneurysm into duodenum	1
Splenic artery aneurysm into gastric stump	1
Splenic artery aneurysm into duodenum	1
Pancreatic pseudocyst into stomach	1
Undetermined or wrong	104

(From Palmer ED: Upper Gastrointestinal Hemorrhage. Springfield, Charles C Thomas, 1970)

patients using the classical approach. The advantage of Palmer's method lies in the greater frequency with which bleeding can be traced, as contrasted with the mere radiologic demonstration of a lesion capable of explaining bleeding.

HISTORY AND PHYSICAL EXAMINATION

Inquiry should be made regarding bleeding tendencies during childhood and early adulthood which, if present, should suggest a blood dyscrasia. A family history of gastrointestinal bleeding is suggestive of hemophilia or Osler-Rendu-Weber disease. Questioning should be directed toward eliciting a history of ingestion of drugs capable of inducing gastrointestinal bleeding, such as steroids, aspirin, butazolidin, and rauwolfia alkaloids. A history of alcoholism should favor erosive gastritis or bleeding esophageal varices. The passage of tarry stools should be checked by inquiry regarding concomitant faintness or weakness, ingestion of iron and bismuth compounds, and the eating of licorice candy. The typical peptic-ulcer syndrome may frequently be absent prior to ulcer bleeding. Prominent heartburn and belching and epigastric or low substernal discomfort or pain, particularly in the recumbent position, which are brought on by large meals, by stooping over as in lacing one's shoes, or ingestion of citrus juices should suggest the presence of erosive esophagitis, which is frequently associated with hiatal hernia. These symptoms most often occur about an hour after meals and are promptly relieved by antacids. An unequivocal symptom of esophageal reflux is the regurgitation of fluid into the mouth, usually at night, or upon bending over. The patient may state that he wakes up coughing and strangling or that he wakes up with a mouth full of fluid. Mucus, bile, or gastric acid may be found on

the pillow. Regurgitation reflects rather severe reflux.[28] It may be accompanied by pulmonary symptoms.

Although the patient may give a history of other symptoms of reflux esophagitis, it is not uncommon for bleeding to be the first clinical manifestation of this disorder. It would seem that patients without the early warning system of heartburn are those in whom bleeding is a manifestation of this particular illness.[28]

The examination of a patient with massive hematemesis or melena must of necessity be cursory. Attention should be concentrated on pulse rate, blood pressure, and general appearance. Icterus, if present, should direct attention to disease of the liver, as should the presence of vascular spiders on the face, neck, upper trunk, or upper limbs. Search should be made on the skin of the face, the lips, the mucocutaneous junction, and the mucous surfaces of the mouth for the brownish, freckle-like melanin spots of the Peutz–Jeghers syndrome. The telangiectasia of the Osler–Rendu–Weber syndrome are usually reddish (occasionally purplish) and are most commonly found on the lips, the tongue, the ears, the fingers, and the toes; frequently, they can be demonstrated to pulsate (Fig. 23-7). Also to be looked for are the skin changes characteristic of pseudoxanthoma elasticum: the yellowish discoloration and the lax, redundant, and relatively inelastic quality with thickening and a grooved appearance of "coarse Moroccan leather."[29,30] According to McKusick, the regions prone to be involved are the face, the neck, the axillary folds, the cubital areas, the inguinal folds, and the periumbilical area (Fig. 23-8).[30] Examination of the ocular fundi may reveal the angioid streaks of pseudoxanthoma elasticum.[31] These streaks are brownish or gray, are four or five times wider than veins, and resemble vessels (Fig. 23-9). The left supraclavicular space should be felt for the presence of "sentinel glands." The time-honored practice of palpating the abdomen gently and briefly in cases of upper digestive tract hemorrhage for fear of reinducing bleeding by the usual form of palpation is no longer tenable. It is indeed difficult to picture dislodgement of a clot from an esophageal varix by pressing on the abdomen. Hemostasis in the capillary bleeding of erosive gastritis and esophagitis is said to be accomplished by the prevention of filling of the injured capillaries through the opening of arteriovenous shunts of the mucosal vascular system, rather than by clot formation. Furthermore, the importance of surface clotting in the hemostasis of bleeding peptic ulcer has been seriously questioned.[27]

A palpable liver of increased consistency should strongly suggest the presence of hepatic cirrhosis, as should the presence of splenomegaly, ascites, vascular spiders, or distended veins over the chest and the abdomen. It should be remembered that the spleen contracts after hemorrhage and thus, for a time, may not be palpable. It is needless to add that the presence of an abdominal tumor should suggest carcinoma. A search for the characteristic continuous murmur of splenic arteriovenous fistula should be made over the lower left posterolateral ribs in young patients with suspected portal hypertension and hypersplenism in the absence of hepatomegaly and abnormal liver function tests.[32]

RADIOGRAPHIC EXAMINATION

Gastric and duodenal ulcer and gastric cancer may be readily diagnosed radiographically. A gastric leiomyoma—though a rare cause of hematemesis—characteristically presents as a smooth, rounded filling defect, often with a pit or crater in its center (see Fig. 23-12). In the presence of active bleeding it is sometimes difficult to differentiate filling defects owing to tumor from those owing to blood clots. Unfortunately, the radiograph has proved to be of little value in the diagnosis of gastritis.[32] Gastric erosions are rarely demonstrated radiographically. Radiographic examination may prove of particular value in the diagnosis of esophageal varices, although it does not indicate whether the varices are the source of bleeding (Fig. 23-10).

In an excellent discussion of the subject, Schatzki points out that the principle of radiographic visualization of esophageal varices rests on the fact that the dilated veins bulge into the lumen of the esophagus and produce an "uneven wormlike surface."[23] Large varices may be detected fluoroscopically, whereas small ones may be visible only on a radiograph. Occasionally, varices may be seen in the cardiac end of the stomach and be mistaken for the enlarged folds of a localized hypertrophic gastritis, or even for a tumor (Fig. 23-11).[34] Schatzki advises that the examination be made with the patient in the horizontal position, as varices become smaller in the erect position. He uses a suspension of equal parts of barium and water and advises coating the inner surface of the esophagus with only a thin layer of barium, because filling the organ with a large amount of the opaque medium will obliterate the protruding vessels. Films should be taken in several projections after slight inspiration, since during this phase the lower end of the esophagus is stretched slightly; the radiologist thus avoids misinterpreting tortuous folds in a slack esophagus.[33] Nelson recommends the admixture of carboxymethylcellulose (0.25% to 0.75%) to increase the adherence of the barium to the esophageal and gastric mucosa, or the administration of atropine (0.5 mg to 1.0 mg) subcutaneously 30 minutes before the examination. He stresses the value

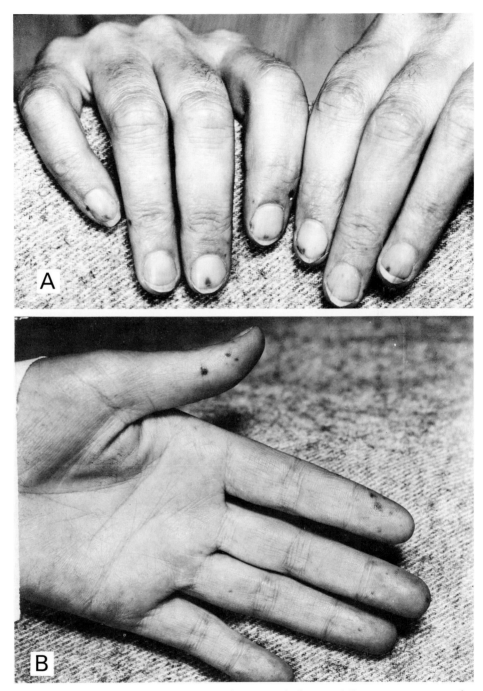

Fig. 23-7. Osler's disease. Telangiectatic lesions with characteristic punctate areas on the palmar surface of the fingers and the typical diffuse, sometimes linear spots under the nails. These ordinarily do not have very sharply defined margins. (Bean WB: Vascular Spiders and Related Lesions of the Skin. Springfield, IL, Charles C Thomas, 1970)

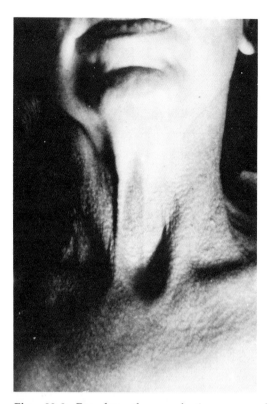

Fig. 23-8. Pseudoxanthoma elasticum, revealing the leathery, ridged, yellowish skin of the anterior portion of the neck. (Bean WB: Vascular Spiders and Related Lesions of the Skin. Springfield, IL, Charles C Thomas, 1970)

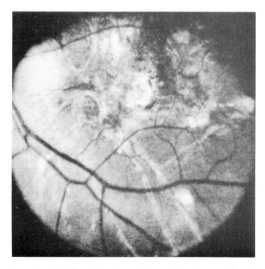

Fig. 23-9. Angioid streaks and proliferative changes in fundus oculi. (McKusick VA: Heritable Disorders of Connective Tissue, 2nd ed. St. Louis, CV Mosby, 1960)

of the Valsalva maneuver in demonstrating varices and states that the Müller maneuver may occasionally show varices when all other methods have failed.[35] Barium studies of the esophagus are much less reliable than either esophagoscopy or splenoportography for the demonstration of esophageal varices.[36] It has been estimated that the radiologist is able to visualize varices in only about 30% to 50% of the cases.[35] Even when special techniques are employed, only 70% are said to be demonstrated.

It was formerly customary to defer x-ray examination of the upper digestive tract in patients with hematemesis or melena until two or three weeks after the hemorrhage. The reason for this delay was the fear of reinducing hemorrhage through the manipulation of the abdomen. The disadvantage of deferring the examination has been twofold: (1) an ulcer may heal within one to three weeks after hemorrhage and thus escape detection;[2,3,37] and (2) it withholds the means of establishing promptly the diagnosis of peptic ulcer in patients past 50 years of age with massive hemorrhage, in whom emergency surgery may be contemplated.

Hampton devised a technique for the radiographic demonstration of bleeding duodenal ulcers in which neither abdominal palpation nor compression is used in order to obviate the danger of reinducing hemorrhage if such existed.[37] At the Cincinnati General Hospital, the Hampton technique was carried out in many patients with severe hematemesis and melena, often within a few hours after admission to the hospital. The procedure proved to be quite safe and of great value in establishing an early diagnosis in cases of severe gastroduodenal hemorrhage.[38]

The Hampton technique has been virtually replaced by endoscopy and selective angiography. In hospitals not staffed for these procedures, prompt barium radiographic study should be employed in cases of bleeding gastric and duodenal ulcer and gastric cancer. A leiomyoma of the stomach—an uncommon cause of upper gastrointestinal bleeding—presents a characteristic change on x-ray film (Fig. 23-12).

ENDOSCOPY AND SELECTIVE ANGIOGRAPHY

Gastrointestinal endoscopy has developed rapidly in the past two decades because of advances in fiberoptic equipment, which have enabled visualization (with target biopsy and photography) of portions of the upper digestive tract not attainable with the older types of separate instruments (esophagoscope and gastroscope) and with less discomfort and greater safety. Present fiberoptic instruments permit inspection of the esophagus, stomach, and duodenum (up to the third

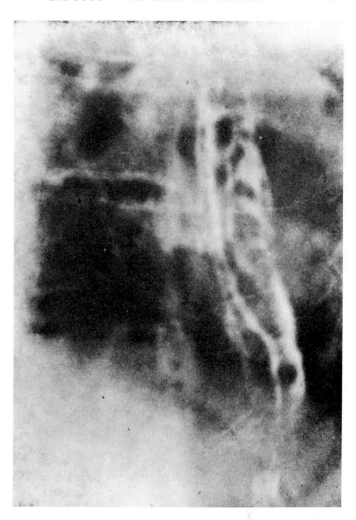

Fig. 23-10. Radiograph showing esophageal varices in patient R.R. (hepatic cirrhosis).

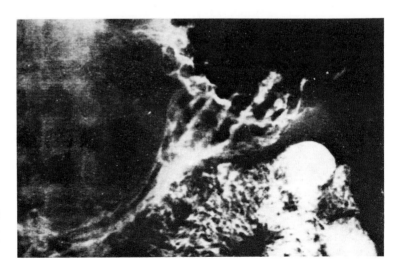

Fig. 23-11. Film showing a lobulated mass at the esophagogastric junction. (From Karr S, Wohl GT: Clinical Importance of Gastric Varices. N Engl J Med 263:667, 1960)

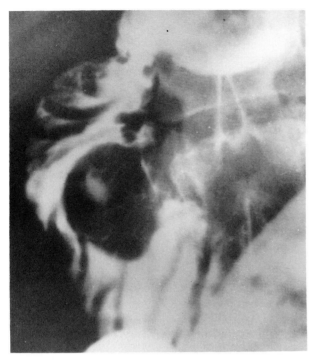

Fig. 23-12. Leiomyoma of duodenum. Radiograph of descending portion of duodenum showing large circular filling defect owing to the tumor with a collection of barium slightly above the center. (From Balint JA, Sarfeh IJ, Fried MB: Gastrointestinal Bleeding: Diagnosis and Management. New York, John Wiley & Sons, 1977)

portion) at one sitting. Because of the frequent association of several lesions capable of producing hemorrhage in the upper three segments of the gut, it is important to examine the esophagus, stomach, and duodenum simultaneously.

Gastrointestinal endoscopy has proved of greatest value when promptly employed in upper gastrointestinal bleeding, as originally stressed by Palmer.[27] It has been stated that if esophagogastroduodenoscopy is performed during the bleeding or within 4 to 12 hours after apparent cessation of bleeding, the correct diagnosis of the cause can be made in 90% of actively bleeding upper gastrointestinal lesions.[39]

In about one fourth to one half the patients with known esophageal varices, the source of the bleeding may prove to be erosive gastritis or peptic ulcer. The failure to demonstrate an actively bleeding site in the esophagus, stomach, or duodenum would indicate prompt recourse to other diagnostic procedures, such as a barium swallow or selective celiac and mesenteric arteriography. If endoscopy is postponed for more than 48 hours, normal mucosa may be found in patients with suspected erosive gastritis, or potential bleeding

lesions may be found without proof of their having bled. The diagnostic accuracy falls from 93% to less than 50% in these 48 hours.

Since its introduction in 1963, selective celiac angiography has become established as a safe and important means of evaluating patients with unexplained gastrointestinal hemorrhage. Emergency angiography is employed for both localization and therapy in the management of patients with acute gastrointestinal bleeding.[40] Bleeding sites may be demonstrated and the hemorrhage may be stopped with infusions of vasoconstricting agents or transcatheter vessel occlusions.

Selective celiac angiography is particularly valuable in the localization of bleeding lesions of the lower digestive tract. Its use depends on continuation of blood loss at the rate of 0.5 ml/minute to 0.6 ml/minute for the extravasated dye to be seen on x-ray film. As Baum has stressed, any discussion of the relative priorities of barium studies versus angiography is without meaning unless the institution has available the services of a skilled angiographer capable of performing the examination quickly and safely.[41]

In addition to being prerequisite in the clinical diagnosis of gastritis, endoscopy is particularly valuable in revealing erosions or small superficial or acute ulcers that usually are not demonstrable on radiographic examination (Figs. 23-13 and 23-14). In some cases of gastritis, there may be oozing from the mucosa without definite erosion. Schindler believed that hemor-

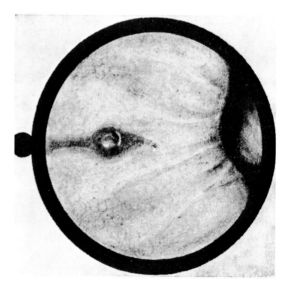

Fig. 23-13. Photograph of a drawing of a bleeding mucosal erosion seen at gastroscopy. There was associated hypertrophic gastritis as evidenced by the polygonal pattern of the nearby mucosa.

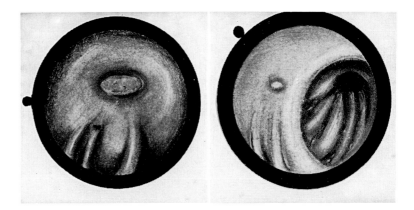

Fig. 23-14. (*Left*) Photograph of a drawing of a superficial gastric ulcer made at gastroscopy, 3 days after massive hematemesis. (*Right*) Gastroscopic findings after 15 days on Meulengracht diet. Note marked reduction in size of the ulcer.

rhagic erosions may occur in the absence of demonstrable gastritis, and our experience would confirm this view.[42] The erosions are small, usually less than 5 mm in diameter, and deep. They may be reddish, grayish-red, or brownish-red in color, and they usually heal within two or three days. Occasionally a gastric ulcer containing clots may be seen without an antecedent or subsequent history of hemorrhage (Fig. 23-15).

Mucosal hemorrhages may not be necessarily significant, since they may be present in the normal stomach. Ruffin and Brown believe that they may result when suction is employed prior to introduction of the gastroscope.[43] In this connection, the important observations that Wolf and Wolff made in their experimental subject must be kept in mind, namely, that acceleration of acid production and motor activity were always accompanied by hyperemia and engorgement of the mucosa.[44] When vascular engorgement was prolonged, the rugae became intensely red, thick, and turgid, presenting the picture of what has been called hypertrophic gastritis. In this state, the mucosa was unusually fragile, hemorrhages and small erosions resulting from the most minor traumata.

BLEEDING PEPTIC ULCER

According to Crohn and Hurst, the frequency of hemorrhage in peptic ulcer is probably about 10% if patients who are not admitted to the hospital as well as hospital patients are included.[45,46] Hemorrhage in patients with peptic ulcer is generally due to erosion of an artery lying at the base of the ulcer. Ulcers on the posterior wall of the superior portion of the duodenum are unusually prone to bleed. In some cases, the stomach itself may be eroded as the result of an associated gastritis.[2] Chronic gastric ulcers are apt to bleed more severely than duodenal ulcers, probably because of

erosion of the larger-sized arteries—the main trunks of the right or the left gastric arteries—as compared with branches of the gastroduodenal or pancreatioduodenal arteries.[47]

In discussing cases of bleeding peptic ulcer, Jones states the following:[3]

At necropsy it was usual to find one large open vessel in the floor of the ulcer, and it was remarkable that death had occurred usually not quickly but after several recurrent bleedings in the course of as many days. Bleeding with acute collapse must have occurred from the large exposed vessel, not once but perhaps six times. It would seem probable that in most cases bleeding

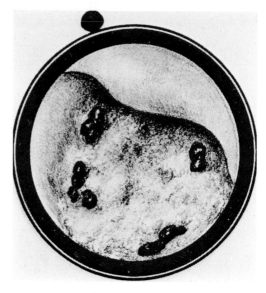

Fig. 23-15. Photograph of a drawing made at gastroscopy of a large benign gastric ulcer containing several large clots (patient C. F.). There was no antecedent history of hematemesis or melena. The lesion disappeared following medical therapy.

from such a large vessel could have occurred for only a short period, perhaps 10 to 15 minutes, and then ceased. At operation the vessel usually did not begin to spurt until it was manipulated.

If the loss of blood is severe, there is a prompt fall in blood pressure, which in itself, if not too great, is advantageous, since it helps curtail further bleeding. Clotting of the blood serves to close the opening of the blood vessel. Effectual sealing of the vascular wall is furthered by the retraction of the open end of the artery. Only after a few days does the clot begin to harden. It is apparent that if the eroded artery is sclerotic it may not be able to retract sufficiently to prevent further bleeding, which may prove fatal.

It is generally agreed that during hunger the stomach exhibits active contractions, and it is conceivable that such contractions may dislodge the clot. The administration of food has a quieting effect on these hunger contractions.[48] This fact, among others, led Meulengracht to begin the immediate feeding of patients suffering from bleeding peptic ulcers.[49]

The relative frequency of hematemesis versus melena varies in different statistics. In hospital cases, hematemesis accompanied by melena occurs more frequently than melena alone. This may be explained by the fact that melena may be unnoticed or disregarded by the ambulatory patient, whereas hematemesis is more apt to cause him to seek hospital care.

Hemorrhage is an indication of activity of the ulcerative process. It is said to occur rarely in patients under strict treatment. In most cases, ulcerlike symptoms precede hemorrhage for varying periods of time, usually for many years. In some cases, however, there are no antecedent symptoms, or symptoms have been present for only a few days or weeks.

Disappearance of pain for weeks or longer following hemorrhage has been pointed out by Hurst and has been quite striking in our experience.[46] The cause of this phenomenon is not clear. In some instances it has been found to be associated with actual healing of the ulcer. It is possible that the lack of gastric tone occurring as a result of the anemia may play a role.* Bonney and Pickering suggest that the blood in the crater may increase the thickness of the protective layer of slough, which may cover the pain nerve endings and hinder their excitation by the hydrochloric acid.[50] Another explanation of the initial loss of pain may be the neutralizing effect of the blood in the stomach on the gastric acidity.

The symptoms of bleeding peptic ulcer depend upon the severity of the hemorrhage. In mild cases there may be little more than hematemesis or melena. In more severe hemorrhage there may be weakness, dizziness, faintness, excessive perspiration, thirst, or actual syncope and shock. Headache may be quite severe; in several of our patients, this was relieved by inhalation of oxygen or by a blood transfusion. Hematemesis may precede or follow the passage of loose, tarry stools. Syncope, not infrequently, takes place in the bathroom and may be due to a fall in blood pressure upon assumption of the erect position. In this connection, Wallace and Sharpey-Schafer reported syncope following assumption of the erect position as long as five or six hours after venesection in some of their control subjects. They found that the rapid removal of from 900 ml to 1150 ml of blood resulted in an exaggerated "postural response" in every instance immediately following the removal.[10]

In one patient with duodenal ulcer and a rather severe hemorrhage manifesting itself by melena, the first complaint was marked shortness of breath, which she experienced after climbing two flights of stairs on her way to dinner. Earlier in the day she had fainted at the hairdresser's, and she had felt faint on two other occasions. She had passed a tarry stool the day before the attack of dyspnea but recalled this only after passing several more tarry stools the following day. Another patient felt a little weak and sweated a little after a round of golf on a cool October day. He was driven home by a friend. Before entering his home, he sat on the porch, but he grew weaker and became frightened. He called his family physician, who advised a suppository. He noticed that his stool was black, but he went to bed without notifying anyone. He passed three black stools during the night and the following morning fainted in the bathroom. Another patient, not included in this study, became a little faint and sweated as he was dictating a letter to his stenographer. That night he passed a tarry stool and was brought to a hospital.

Although coronary thrombosis has been precipitated by gastroduodenal hemorrhage, electrocardiographic changes may occur after acute gastrointestinal hemorrhage without subsequent evidence of coronary artery disease.[3,51,52,53,54] Rasmussen and Foss reported flattening, isoelectric, or negative T-waves, and lowering of the S–T interval in about half of the cases.[55] They were unable to correlate the changes with anemia or fall in blood pressure but did find some relationship to azotemia. Like Scherf and his associates, they attribute the changes to myocardial anoxemia secondary to coronary spasm associated with the generalized vasoconstriction following hemorrhage.[56] On the other hand, Master and his associates stress the degree of shock, drop in blood pressure, tachycardia, and decrease in hemoglobin level as factors responsible for precipitating these changes, which they interpret as evidence of acute coronary insufficiency.[57] They regard

*Carlson AJ: Personal communication.

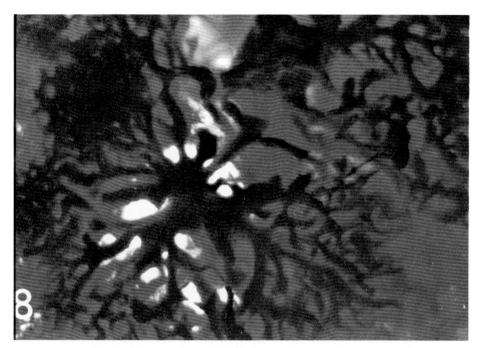

Plate 3. Transilluminated ectasia showing the pronounced distortion of the deeper veins and venules of the mucosa and submucosa. (From Boley SJ et al: On the nature and etiology of vascular ectasias of the colon: Degeneration lesions of aging. Gastroenterol 72:650, 1977)

Plate 4. Bright red, flat, irregular hemangioma of the cecum.
(After Rogers BHG, Adler F: Hemangiomas of the cecum.
Gastroenterol 71:1079, 1976)

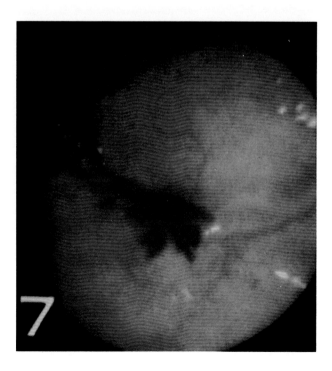

the decreased blood volume resulting from hemorrhage as the major mechanism.

Association of acute emotional distress with gastroduodenal hemorrhage is frequent.[3,58,59] The engorging effect on the gastric mucosa of sustained resentment, frustration, and anxiety may play an important role in the genesis of the ulceration. The additional factors of missed meals, extra smoking, and drinking have been suggested as possibly causing sudden extension of the ulceration.[3]

The diagnosis of a bleeding anastomotic ulcer is frequently difficult to make by any technique. Barium studies and even endoscopy may be unsuccessful in diagnosing these lesions, since thay may be very shallow and hidden behind edematous gastric or jejunal folds. In the face of active bleeding from an anastomotic ulcer, selective arteriography demonstrates the site of extravasation, which is usually from a jejunal branch of the superior mesenteric artery (Fig. 23-16). Infusion of pituitrin will frequently stop the bleeding.

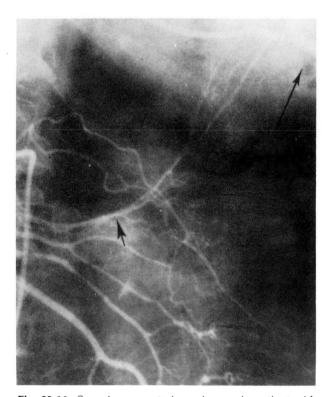

Fig. 23-16. Superior mesenteric angiogram in patient with marginal ulcer demonstrating extravasation of contrast medium (*long arrow*) from the first jejunal artery (*short arrow*). (From Cho KJ, Adams DF: Diagnostic angiography in gastrointestinal hemorrhage. In Fiddian–Green RG, Turcotte JG (eds): Gastrointestinal Hemorrhage, p 57. New York, Grune & Stratton, 1980)

CARCINOMA OF THE STOMACH

Bleeding in cases of gastric carcinoma is usually due to ulceration of the stomach or necrosis and sloughing of papillary growths. "Because of the small vessels involved, the bleeding is usually in the form of oozing or seepage."[60] However, if there is erosion of a medium-sized or large vessel, massive hemorrhage may result, as occurred in the case shown in Figure 23-17. In one patient with a large carcinomatous ulcer 15 small vessels were seen projecting from the base of the lesion at autopsy, 3 of which were capped with thrombi.

Massive hemorrhage may be the initial symptom in patients with gastric carcinoma and is probably not as rare as is generally supposed. It was the presenting symptom in 10 such patients seen at the Cincinnati General Hospital, taking the guise of hematemesis followed by melena in eight and of melena alone in two. Massive hemorrhage in gastric carcinoma may occur in the absence of any demonstrable lesion either by physical or radiographic examination.*[61] Temporary improvement may occur in patients with gastric cancer and may suggest the presence of a benign rather than a malignant ulcer. If the disease is sufficiently advanced, physical examination may reveal the presence of enlarged supraclavicular glands on the left, an abdominal mass, an enlarged nodular liver, or a "Blumer's shelf."

X-ray and gastroscopic examinations are of recognized value in the diagnosis of gastric carcinoma. The presence of a persistent posthistamine achlorhydria in a patient with hematemesis and melena should exclude the possibility of peptic ulcer and should lead to a suspicion of gastric cancer. It is now well recognized that gastric cancer is becoming much less frequent in this country.

Exfoliative cytology as applied to gastric aspirates has proved of diagnostic value in areas where it is properly performed. Determination of the lactic dehydrogenase activity of gastric juice may also prove helpful in diagnosis.[62]

BLEEDING ESOPHAGEAL VARICES

Hematemesis in patients with hepatic cirrhosis is usually due to a ruptured varix in the lower end of the esophagus. Rupture may occur spontaneously or may follow excessive physical activity, uncontrolled vomiting, or coughing. Esophageal varices develop because of obstruction to the return of the portal blood to the systemic venous system. The site of the portal block may be either in the liver (the intrahepatic type

*Schiff L: Unpublished observation.

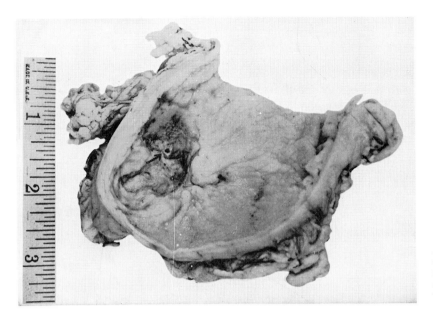

Fig. 23-17. Photograph of a specimen of stomach showing malignant gastric ulcer with a gaping sclerotic artery in its base (patient J. S.).

secondary to portal cirrhosis), or in the portal vein itself (the extrahepatic type as seen in Banti's syndrome).[63]

Bleeding varices may occur in the absence of either intrahepatic or extrahepatic obstruction of the portal vein.[65] To explain this occurrence, Tisdale postulates functional or structural alterations of the vessels of the gastrointestinal tract, the spleen, and the liver as permitting increased flow of blood into the portal vein, with a resultant rise in pressure.[66] On the basis of a similar mechanism, portal hypertension may result from splenic arteriovenous fistulas. Aneurysm of the hepatic artery may produce portal hypertension and bleeding esophageal varices by compression of the portal vein or by direct communication with the portal vein in the nature of an arteriovenous shunt.[67] Bleeding varices also have been noted in obstruction of the superior vena cava from idiopathic mediastinal fibrosis.[68] They have also been described as arising from previous thyroid surgery.[69] Their occurrence in young people without demonstrable liver disease or abnormalities of liver function tests should suggest the possibility of polycystic liver.[70,71] Opinion differs as to the relative importance of the increase in portal venous pressure and the presence of peptic esophagitis in the causation of variceal rupture.[72] Whipple believed that the esophageal veins are prone to thinning, dilation, and varix formation because of a combination of portal hypertension and meager support by the tissues and organs in the mediastinum. He also pointed out that the varices are subject to trauma because of the frequent contractions of the esophagus and the pressure and passage of boluses of ingested food. Wangensteen suggested that rupture of esophageal varices may be due to peptic ulceration of the esophageal mucosa over them because of the reflux of acid contents into the esophagus.[73] Orloff and Thomas found esophagitis by biopsy in the course of transesophageal varix ligations in only one of 20 patients bleeding from varices.[74] "Varices don't bleed because of reflux esophagitis; they bleed because they blow out as a result of increased hydrostatic pressure."[75] Another possible cause of esophageal bleeding that has been postulated is based on the assumption that intravariceal pressure is sufficient to cause necrosis of the thin-walled vessel and overlying attenuated mucosa. In some instances, the source of the blood may be an erosive gastritis, a gastric varix, or a coexisting peptic ulcer.

Esophagoscopy correctly distinguished bleeding esophageal varices from other lesions in 91% of the bleeding episodes in which it was successfully carried out. It almost always correctly identified bleeding esophageal varices or a completely normal esophagus.[76] In a group of 13 patients in whom varices were seen but were not thought to be the cause of bleeding, the implied diagnosis of nonvariceal bleeding was correct in only 5.[77] This stresses an important factor: Failure to demonstrate active bleeding at a given time does not *per se* exclude varices as the source of hemorrhage. They may bleed intermittently, as is true of gastrointestinal bleeding in general.

Ratnoff and Patek[1] reported 9 instances of melena without hematemesis in a series of 386 cases of Laennec's cirrhosis. They also pointed out the frequency of

other hemorrhagic phenomena, such as epistaxis, purpura, and bleeding from the gums. Morlock and Hall have emphasized the occurrence of thrombopenia, which they believe may increase the bleeding hazard.[78]

Hematemesis occurs in about one fourth of patients with hepatic cirrhosis, the initial bout being fatal in about one third of the cases in which it occurs.[1] It may be the first manifestation of disease in about 10% of cases. Although frequently fatal, hematemesis sometimes recurs over long periods of time. In one of our patients who subsequently came to autopsy, it recurred during a 10-year period. In some instances it may be followed by a decline in serum protein and development of ascites.[1] Hematemesis is frequently a forerunner of hepatic coma. The presence of blood in the intestinal tract may produce an elevation of the blood ammonia concentration.[79]

Gastrointestinal symptoms, such as anorexia, morning nausea, vomiting, flatulence, and not infrequently, diarrhea, may precede the attacks of hematemesis. Of value in establishing a diagnosis of hepatic cirrhosis are a history of chronic alcoholism; the presence of icterus; ascites; vascular spiders on the skin of the face, the neck, the upper chest, and the upper extremities; distended veins on the abdomen and the chest; a firm palpable liver; and a palpable spleen. Laboratory tests suggesting cirrhosis include retention of bromsulphalein, reduction of serum albumin content and elevation of gamma globulin, and elevation of the serum transaminases, especially the serum glutamic-oxaloacetic transaminase (SGOT). Needle biopsy of the liver is extremely helpful in diagnosis but is best carried out following recovery from hemorrhage. The demonstration of esophageal varices by radiographic examination, esophagoscopy, or portal venography may clinch the diagnosis if congestive splenomegaly owing to extrahepatic portal block or hepatoma can be excluded.

Merigan and his associates found that patients with cirrhosis who underwent acute hepatic decompensation were more apt to be bleeding from esophageal varices and less apt to be bleeding from sites other than varices than those who bled without hepatic decompensation.[80] Bleeding in patients who have had a recent portacaval shunt may not necessarily indicate recurrence of esophageal varices but rather prove to be due to a peptic ulcer developing following the shunt.[81,82] In dogs, the secretion of hydrochloric acid from a Heidenhain pouch has been shown to increase greatly after portacaval transposition. This may be due to the increased effect of a humoral secretagogue that originates in the abdominal viscera and is normally inactivated by the liver.

Panke and his associates have stressed the value of determining the intrasplenic pulp pressure (a measure of the portal venous pressure) in patients with upper digestive tract hemorrhage.[83] In a series of 130 patients, they found that bleeding esophagogastric varices were never associated with a splenic pulp pressure below 250 mm of water. Contrariwise, bleeding from other lesions were never associated with pressures above 290 mm of water. Variceal bleeding was associated with high splenic pulp pressures regardless of the presence of shock. They reported a 90% accuracy in determining the presence or absence of varices. Nowadays, hepatic vein free and wedged pressure determination have virtually replaced estimation of splenic pulp pressure largely because of greater safety.

The angiographer welcomes prior endoscopy because the preangiographic knowledge of the location of the bleeding site makes catheterization of the appropriate vessel much less difficult. Endoscopic confirmation of the presence of a bleeding varix means that the angiographer need only catheterize and infuse the superior mesenteric artery. Without this endoscopic confirmation, angiograms of the left gastric artery must be performed to exclude bleeding gastritis, and of the gastroduodenal artery to exclude a bleeding duodenal ulcer.[41]

GASTRITIS AND ESOPHAGITIS

Gastritis has long been recognized as a cause of varying degrees of hemorrhage, particularly by European observers. This relationship has been stressed by Faber,[84] Moutier,[85] Henning,[86] and Benedict,[2] among others. In a series of 42 cases of hemorrhage from gastritis, Benedict reported a mild degree of hemorrhage in 7, a moderate degree in 14, and a severe degree in 21. The bleeding occurring in chronic gastritis usually takes place from erosions in the mucous membrane (Fig. 23-18), which most commonly occur on the crests of the folds. In some cases there may be oozing from the mucosa without definite erosion.[2,55] Benedict stresses excessive use of alcohol as the most important etiologic factor in massive bleeding from gastritis. Dagradi and colleagues found that 27 of 40 patients bleeding from erosive gastritis had ingested either alcohol or aspirin or both shortly prior to the onset of bleeding.[87] According to Palmer, ingestion of large amounts of alcohol during a brief period produces an acute gastritis with frequently demonstrable erosions and with return of the gastroscopic appearance to normal soon after avoidance of alcohol.

The relatively high incidence of subacute erosive esophagitis and acute erosive gastritis as a cause of upper digestive tract hemorrhage in Palmer's series of cases is testimony to the diagnostic value of early en-

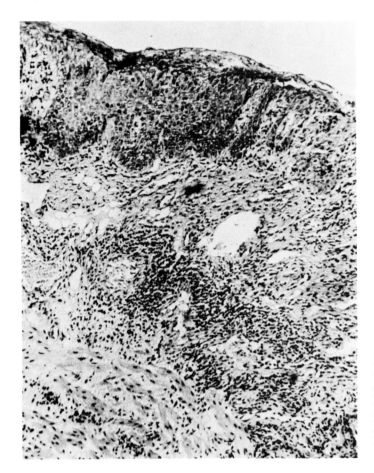

Fig. 23-18. Biopsy at the edge of erosion in a case of erosive esophagitis. The hemorrhage stopped about half an hour before the specimen was taken. No clot has formed on the erosion's surface, in the mucosa's capillaries, or in the other vessels. (From Palmer ED: Diagnosis of Upper Gastrointestinal Hemorrhage. Springfield, IL, Charles C Thomas, 1970)

doscopy, particularly in cases where radiographic examination is apt to prove negative. Palmer recommends a swallow of 10% fluorescin several minutes before the procedure to improve the visualization of both esophageal and gastric erosions, particularly following ice-water lavage.

HIATAL HERNIA

Bleeding in cases of hiatal hernia may be due to congestion of the blood vessels in the herniated portion of the stomach, gastritis, or ulceration.[88] There may be ulceration of the esophagogastric junction, or there may be a gastric ulcer adjacent to the neck of the sac where it passes through the diaphragm. The symptoms of hiatal hernia have been well described.[89–91] At the time of admission it may be difficult to prove the hiatal hernia as the cause of the bleeding. Endoscopy may prove helpful. In some instances presumptive proof

may be based on the lack of recurrence of bleeding following repair of the hernia.

HEMATEMESIS AND MELENA FROM MISCELLANEOUS CAUSES

Miscellaneous causes of hematemesis and melena found in 43 patients (48 cases) from a series of 640 cases seen at the Cincinnati General Hospital are listed in Table 23-3. Other causes include hemorrhage from localized arteriosclerosis of gastric vessels,[92] hereditary telangiectasia,[93–95] tumors of the small intestine,[96] rupture of aneurysm of the hepatic artery[97] or splenic artery,[98] pseudoxanthoma elasticum,[30,31] ruptured aortic aneurysm, periarteritis nodosa,[99] jejunal diverticulosis,[100] multiple hemangiomas of the jejunum,[101] and gastric carcinoid.[102] Bleeding may also arise from Meckel's diverticulum or diverticula of the colon. Potential causes of bleeding of obscure origin are listed in Table 23-4.

Hematemesis and melena have been ascribed to as-

Table 23-3. *Causes of Hematemesis and Melena in Miscellaneous Group of 43 Patients Over a 10-Year Period*

Causes of Hemorrhage	Number of Patients
Acute esophagitis with pancreatic necrosis	1
Banti's syndrome (extrahepatic block)	2
Benign tumor of the stomach	1
Blood dyscrasia	8
Carcinoma of the esophagus	3
Chronic relapsing pancreatitis	1
Cirrhosis with esophageal diverticulum	1
Cholecystoduodenal fistula	1
Curling's ulcer	1
Erosive esophagitis or erosive gastritis associated with liver disease	8
Erosion of the aorta owing to periaortitis	1
Gastric varices	1
Lymphosarcoma of the stomach	1
Malignancy eroding the gastrointestinal tract	3
Mesenteric thrombosis	5
Prolapsed gastric mucosa	1
Ulcerative esophagitis	3
Ulcerated heterotopic gastric tissue	1

pirin ingestion. Muir and Cossar[103,104] found that 72 out of 157 patients admitted with upper gastrointestinal hemorrhage had taken aspirin within 24 hours of the onset of bleeding. Overt bleeding, on the other hand, may follow the ingestion of a single tablet of aspirin. Slight to intense hyperemia, and even a submucous hemorrhage, have been reported at gastroscopic examinations made upon patients following the ingestion of three crushed aspirin tablets. Acute gastric erosions attributed to salicylates have been described at gastroscopy[105] and laparotomy. Gastrointestinal bleeding is more apt to occur following aspirin ingestion, especially with concomitant alcohol ingestion.

Muir and Cossar gave aspirin shortly before partial gastrectomy and found less reaction in the resected specimens when soluble aspirin was given as contrasted with ordinary aspirin. In one case, half of an aspirin tablet was found imbedded in the mucosa of the greater curvature, lying beneath overlapping edematous and congested rugae.[106] According to Winkelman and Summerskill, factors involved in mucosal damage and resistance seem more important than hydrochloric acid secretion in relation to gastrointestinal bleeding following the consumption of aspirin.[106] Aspirin is reported either to have no effects on gastric secretion of humans or animals, or, if anything, to lower gastric secretory activity.[107]

In experiments conducted on both dogs and rats, Menguy found that aspirin administered so as to avoid contact with the gastric mucosa profoundly decreased the rate of mucus secretion.[108] It also altered the composition of mucus in such a way as to render it theoretically less efficient as a protective barrier. "It is entirely possible then that the altered mucus production represents simply the result of aspirin-induced cellular injury which in turn might render the cells more friable, with ensuing appearance of superficial erosions." The mechanism of aspirin-produced gastric injury still requires further elucidation. It is quite possible that its well-known ability to inhibit synthesis of endogenous prostaglandins may play an important role.

Hemorrhage from gastroesophageal lacerations at the cardiac orifice of the stomach—the so-called Mallory–Weiss syndrome,[109–111] which was formerly considered an uncommon cause of upper gastrointestinal hemorrhage—has recently been reported to have reached an incidence of approximately 10% to 15% as the cause of massive bleeding (Figs. 23–19, 23–20). The importance of a history of alcoholism and violent or protracted retching preceding the bleeding from the lacerations has been de-emphasized. A history of alcoholism may be absent, as in the vomiting of pregnancy and obstructing ulcer; hematemesis *per se* may be the first manifestation of the syndrome. There may be one laceration[28] or two to four, as originally described. Mallory and Weiss reported the lesions to be arranged characteristically around the circumference of the cardiac opening, along the longitudinal axis of the esophagus.[109] In their report, the size of the lesions varied from 3 mm to 20 mm in length and from 2 mm to 3 mm in width. According to Palmer, the laceration is found at gastroscopy to be a straight cleft running roughly parallel to the esophageal axis. The cleft is usually estimated to be a centimeter in length and rarely, may extend up to 4 cm. A characteristic feature of the laceration is rather steep elevation of its edges, with fairly wide gaping. The cleft is always filled with clot, and it is presumed that the ridgelike elevation is due to bleeding beneath the laceration's edges. Mallory and Weiss considered the pressure changes in the stomach during the disturbed mechanism of vomiting, together with regurgitation of the gastric juice and the corrosive effect of alcohol, to be responsible for the lesions described in their cases. Axon and Clarke reported three patients with symptoms suggesting a Mallory–Weiss syndrome but who on endoscopy showed a localized demarcated area of bright red mucosa (with an appearance of acute gastritis with severe inflammation) near the gastroesophageal junction with an area of normal gastric mucosa interposed between the lesion and

Table 23-4. *Potential Causes of Gastrointestinal Bleeding of Obscure Source*

Disease	Cardinal Features	Diagnosis
Meckel's diverticulum	Usually reddish blood with pain; < 25 years old	Pertechnitate scan Angiography during bleed
Small-bowel tumors	Recurrent anemia; melena or red blood; > 25 years old	Repeated SBFT* Angiography; string test
Vascular lesions Arteriovenous aneurysm Telangiectasia Angiodysplasia	Recurrent, painless bleeds; may have mucocutaneous lesions	Angiography Telangiectasia by PE or endoscopy
Cardiovascular Aortic stenosis‡	Recurrent hemorrhage with aortic stenosis	Angiography
ASHD†	Recurrent hemorrhage	Angiography
Hematologic disorders Lymphoma	Usually asymptomatic bleeding; may have pain	Radiology, endoscopy
Clotting disorders	Bleeding tendency	Clotting tests
Hereditary disorders Pseudoxanthoma elasticum Ehlers–Danlos	Family history; cutaneous lesions Abnormal skin elasticity; hyperextensible joints	Clinical Clinical
Peutz–Jeghers	Perioral pigmentation	Clinical and radiology

*Small-bowel follow-through examination
†Arteriosclerotic heart disease
‡Most commonly found to have angiodysplasia
(From Balint JA, Sarfeh IJ, Fried MB: Gastrointestinal Bleeding: Diagnosis and Management, p 92. New York, John Wiley & Sons, 1977)

the cardioesophageal junction tears.[112] The authors postulate the lesion to have arisen by retrograde intussusception of the stomach during vomiting or retching.

Heuer reported a case in which the pathologist failed to find any erosion of the mucosa of the stomach or duodenum.[113] Upon injecting the gastric artery with saline from a pressure bottle, however, he was able to observe a jet of fluid from the mucosal lining. Serial sections of the area showed a small ruptured aneurysm concealed by overlying, mucosal folds. It appears quite plausible that this type of lesion may be the underlying cause of hemorrhage in some otherwise unexplained cases.

Retrograde jejunogastric intussusception occurs more often in women than in men, is much more frequent after gastroenterostomy than after gastric resection, and may occur as long as 18 years after the operation, with an average interval of 6 years (Fig. 23–21).[114] In the majority of cases, vomiting of food and bile precedes hematemesis. A mass may be palapable above and to the left of the umbilicus in more than half of the cases. The x-ray finding within the lumen of the stomach of a partially moving filling defect simulating the normal pattern of small intestinal folds (Kerckring folds or valvulae conniventes) is characteristic.

Fistulization between the intestinal tract and an abdominal aortic prosthesis is a common cause of late graft failure and usually occurs at suture lines that are contiguous with bowel loops. "Any massive gastrointestinal hemorrhage after an abdominal aortic operation should be considered of aortic origin until proved otherwise."[115]

Massive gastrointestinal bleeding may result from hemorrhage into the bile duct. *Hemobilia*, as this condition has been designated, occurs when disease or

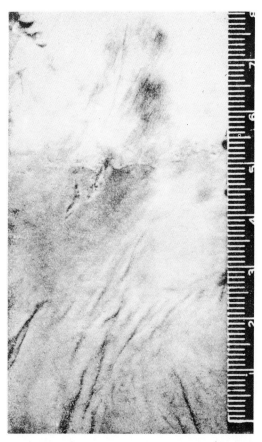

Fig. 23-19. Specimen showing two small (1-cm) lacerations just inferior to the gastroesophageal junction. (From Decker JP, Zamcheck N, Mallory GK: Mallory–Weiss syndrome: Hemorrhage from gastroesophageal lacerations at the cardiac orifice of the stomach. N Engl J Med 249:957, 1953)

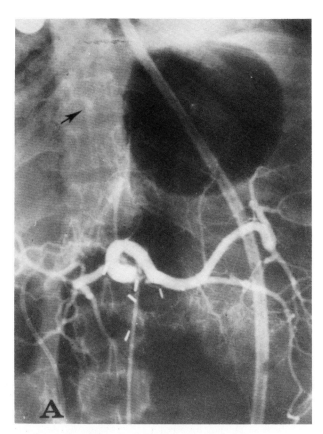

Fig. 23-20. Celiac angiogram in 37-year-old man with bleeding Mallory–Weiss tears shows extravasation of contrast medium (*arrow*) near cardioesophageal junction. (From Cho KJ, Adams DF: Diagnostic angiography in gastrointestinal hemorrhage. In Fiddian–Green RG, Turcotte JG (eds.): Gastrointestinal Hemorrhage, p 55. New York, Grune & Stratton, 1980)

trauma produces an abnormal communication between blood vessels and bile ducts. In instances of minor bleeding, the blood mixes with bile and enters the intestine in a liquid state, but when the proportion of blood exceeds 70%, it coagulates. A blood clot may lodge in the common bile duct and simulate a common duct stone (Fig. 23–22). The pathognomonic symptom triad consists of gastrointestinal bleeding in almost 100% of cases, biliary colic in 70%, and jaundice in 60%. The patient having previously experienced such pain before bleeding may rightly warn the physician that he is about to bleed again.[116–118]

The most common cause of hemobilia in the western world is said to be accidental or iatrogenic, operative trauma being as frequent a cause as traffic accidents. During biliary tract surgery, the hepatic artery may be damaged by a suture or by the dissection, which can result in an arteriobiliary fistula or in a false aneurysm leading or eroding into the extrahepatic bile ducts. Intrahepatic lesions are caused more commonly by instrumentation of the biliary tree. Selective celiac arteriography affords the best means of establishing the diagnosis and may prove of particular value in revealing central liver lesions, which may be difficult or impossible to localize, even at exploratory laparotomy (Fig. 23–23).

Pseudoxanthoma elasticum should be recognized by the characteristic skin changes and the angioid streaks in the retina. Superficial ulceration has been observed at gastroscopy and in the resected stomach. In some cases, gastroscopy soon after hematemesis has been negative.[119] The bleeding point may be in the duo-

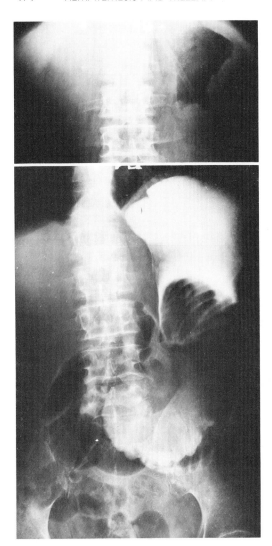

Fig. 23-21. (*Top*) A lobulated mass is shown projecting into the lumen of the distal stomach. (*Bottom*) Following a barium swallow, the mass in the stomach shows valvulae conniventes on its surface. There is obstruction of the duodenum and proximal jejunum secondary to the intussusception.

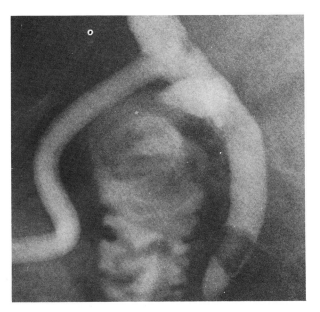

Fig. 23-22. A blood clot in the common duct caused by postoperative hemobilia. Three weeks after the difficult removal of a common duct stone, a cholangiogram showed this defect in the contrast. It was interpreted as owing to a retained calculus. (Sandblom P: Hemobilia. In Schiff L (ed): Diseases of the Liver, 5th ed. Philadelphia, JB Lippincott, 1982)

denum, or there may be multiple bleeding points in other parts of the intestine.

Colonic diverticular disease is the most common cause of massive acute lower gastrointestinal hemorrhage.[120,121,122] The patients involved, as in vascular ectasia, are usually elderly with coexisting diseases that make them poor operative risks, and thus it is fortunate that bleeding usually stops with conservative therapy and blood replacement. Massive bleeding from diverticulosis is most likely to occur in patients with diverticula involving the entire colon; but despite the great number of diverticula present, the source of the hemorrhage is most frequently a single diverticulum in the right colon[122] as confirmed by angiography (Figs. 23–24, 23–25).

Casarella and associates[123] stress the close relation of perforating arterioles to the base of colonic diverticula; these arterioles are the source of massive bleeding. Apparently there is erosion by a fecalith in the base of a single diverticulum. In most patients with significant bleeding, there is no history of a previous bout of diverticulitis. The stool color is usually bright red or maroon, but it may be black if the rate of bleeding is slow. Selective visceral angiography is the diagnostic procedure of choice.

Vascular ectasias (angiodysplasia), a common cause of episodic colonic bleeding in elderly patients, has been identified as a collection of ectatic thin-walled mucosal vessels invariably associated with severely dilated, tortuous submucosal veins (Figs. 23–26, 23–27). It has been suggested that the ectasias are secondary to chronic obstruction of the submucosal veins by tension in the muscularis propria. The abnormal intra-

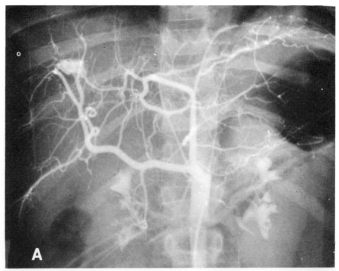

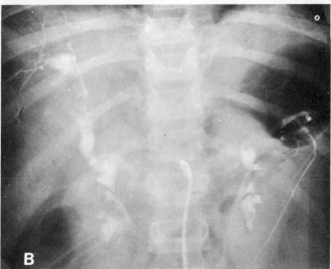

Fig. 23-23. Celiac arteriogram in a case of central liver rupture. (*A*) Arterial phase. Pooling of contrast medium in the center of the right lobe. (*B*) Early parenchymatous phase. Note filling of dilated right hepatic duct with contrast medium directly from the lesion. With skill and a measure of good luck, the radiologist has managed to catch the passage of blood and contrast medium from the central lesion down into the common duct. (From Enge I, Knutrud O, Normann T: Central rupture of the liver with traumatic haemobilia. A pre- and post-operative angiographic study. Br J Radiol 41:789, 1968)

mural vasculature in the right colon has been variously designated as arteriovenous malformation, hemangioma, angiodysplasia, vascular dysplasia, and most recently, vascular ectasia[40,124–132] (Fig. 23–28, Col. plates 3,4).

Associated heart disease has been noted in more than 50% of patients with vascular ectasias; the most common is aortic stenosis. The bleeding is characteristically recurrent and usually stops spontaneously; exsanguination is exceptional and more likely attributable to diverticulosis. Colonoscopy and selective visceral angiography offer the most valuable diagnostic procedures, as the lesions are apt to be missed on radio-

logic examination and even exploratory laparotomy (Figs. 23–28, Col. plate 4)

Coagulation biopsy appearances permit confirmation of the diagnosis at the time of therapeutic electrocoagulation. Endoscopic photography of the lesion is said to provide an essential confirmation for the pathologist and endoscopist.[124] The introduction of specimen angiography using a colloid barium sulfate solution has facilitated gross dissection of the resected colon and identification of the abnormal vessels.[125]

Czaja and associates[133] reported the occurrence of gastric erosions in 25 of 29 patients with large burns

Text continues on p. 417

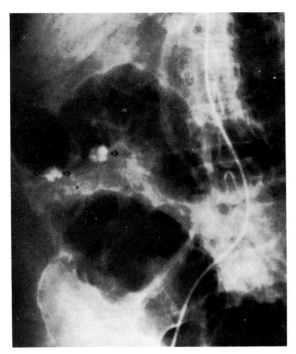

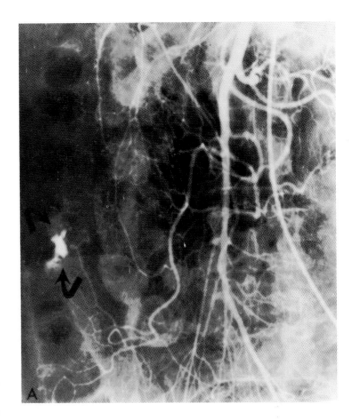

Fig. 23-24. Venous phase of a superior mesenteric arteriogram in a 63-year-old woman. Extravasation of contrast material onto the lumen of two diverticula in the hepatic flexure is clearly seen. The contrast persists throughout the venous phase of the study and is apparently pooled in the confines of the diverticular sacs (*arrows*). (From Casarella WJ, Kanter IE, Seaman WB: Right-sided colonic diverticula as a cause of acute rectal hemorrhage. N Engl J Med 286:450–453, 1972)

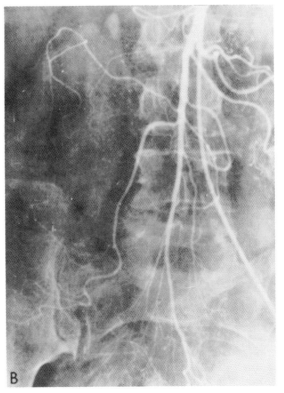

Fig. 23-25. (*A*) Massive bleeding from diverticulum of right colon showing extravasation in the ascending colon (*arrows*) from a branch of the ileocolic artery. (*B*) Repeat arteriogram after 20 min of vasopressin infusion showing constriction of the mesenteric arterial branches and no extravasation. (From Athanasoulis CA, Waltman AC, Ring EJ et al: Angiography, its contribution to the emergency management of gastrointestinal hemorrhage. Radiol Clin North Am 14:265, 1976)

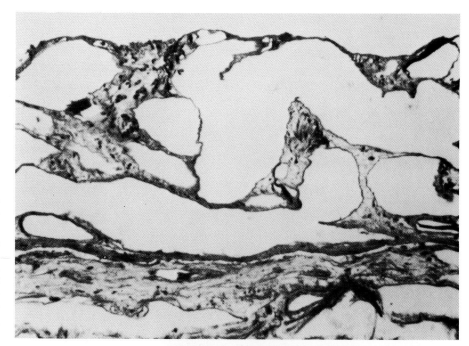

Fig. 23-26. End stage demonstrating loss of mucosal supporting structures and glands. Only the thin wall of the vessel separates the vascular lumen from the bowel lumen. (From Mitsudo SM, Boley SJ, Brandt LJ et al: Vascular ectasias of the right colon in the elderly; a distinct pathologic entity. Hum Path 10:585, 1979)

(involving more than 35% of body surface), 17 of 23 having lesions within 72 hours after the burn. A gastric ulcer developed in 7 of 32 patients, while 9 of 32 had duodenal ulceration. Life-threatening hemorrhage or perforation occurred mainly in patients with ulcers (8 of 9 cases). Over 40% of patients with thermal injury are said to have occult blood in their stools, whereas less than 5% are said to have life-threatening hemorrhage.

Polyarteritis[134] is one of the rarer causes of intestinal hemorrhage. Celiac arteriography may demonstrate multiple aneurysms in the small and medium-sized visceral arteries; extravasated contrast medium may mark the site of bleeding.

SUMMARY

Bleeding into the gastrointestinal tract may be brought to the attention of the patient and the physician through vomiting of blood (hematemesis) or through the passage of blood in the stools. One should be comforted, however, by the thought that gastrointestinal hemorrhage is usually intermittent and stops in most cases when the patient is put to bed and given supportive therapy. If bleeding continues and fresh blood is aspirated from the stomach upon lavage with ice water, endoscopy is the diagnostic procedure of choice. If this is unrevealing and the patient is still bleeding (with blood loss greater than ½ ml per min), selective celiac and mesenteric arteriography should be carried out in

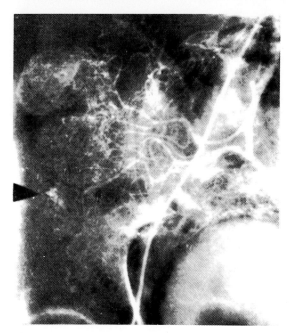

Fig. 23-27. Superior mesenteric angiogram showing a single area of angiodysplasia in the right colon (*arrow*). At colonoscopy, seven vascular lesions were found scattered from the cecum to the distal transverse segment. (From Rogers BHG: Endoscopic diagnosis and therapy of mucosal vascular abnormalities of the gastrointestinal tract occurring in elderly patients and associated with cardiac, vascular, and pulmonary disease. Gastrointestinal Endoscopy 26:134, 1980)

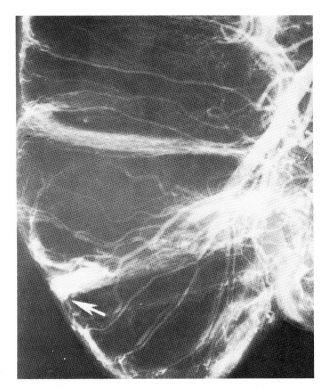

Fig. 23-28. Vascular ectasia. Specimen angiogram of resected colon showing vascular ectasia (*arrow*) at the antimesenteric border of the cecum. (From Cho KJ, Adams DF: Diagnostic angiography in gastrointestinal hemorrhage. In Fiddian–Green RG, Turcotte JG (eds): Gastrointestinal Hemorrhage, p 71. New York, Grune & Stratton, 1980)

properly equipped clinics staffed with a skilled and experienced team of workers. Should this approach prove nonproductive, x-ray examination with barium should be undertaken. In selected instances clinical judgment is required to determine the order in which these procedures should be used, as, for example, in some cases of severely bleeding peptic ulcers in which x-ray confirmation is desirable prior to emergency surgery. In certain instances it may be most helpful to employ all three diagnostic procedures. When bleeding stops and does not recur, elective barium studies on the third hospital day have been recommended.[49] Discovery of the cause should be as prompt as possible so that proper therapy can be used to prevent death, various complications, or chronic disability.

REFERENCES

1. **Ratnoff OD, Patek AJ Jr:** The natural history of Laennec's cirrhosis of the liver: An analysis of 386 cases. Medicine 21:207, 1942

2. **Benedict EB:** Hemorrhage from gastritis: A report based on pathological, clinical, roentgenological and gastroscopic findings. Am J Roentgenol 47:254, 1942

3. **Jones FA:** Haematemesis and melaena with special reference to bleeding peptic ulcer. Br Med J 2:441; 477, 1947

4. **Schiff L, Stevens RJ, Shapiro N, Goodman S:** Observations on the oral administration of citrated blood in man. II. The effect on the stools. Am J Med Sci 203:409, 1942

5. **Hilsman JH:** The color of blood-containing feces following instillation of citrated blood at various levels of the small intestine. Gastroenterology 15:131, 1950

6. **Daniel WA Jr, Egan S:** Quantity of blood required to produce a tarry stool. JAMA 113:2232, 1939

7. **Hesser S:** Uber die Dauer von Magengeschwürblutungen. Acta Med Scand (Suppl 59): 367, 1934

8. **Cullinan ER, Price RK:** Haematemesis following peptic ulceration: Prognosis and treatment. St. Bartholomew Hospital Reports 65:185, 1932

9. **Black DAK:** Critical review: Azotaemia in gastroduodenal haemorrhage. Q J Med 11:77, 1942

10. **Wallace J, Sharpey–Schafer EP:** Blood changes following controlled haemorrhage in man. Lancet 2:393, 1941

11. **Ebert RV, Stead EA Jr, Gibson JG II:** Response of normal subjects to acute blood loss, with special reference to the mechanism of restoration of blood volume. Arch Intern Med 68:578, 1941

12. **Howarth S, Sharpey–Schafer EP:** Low blood-pressure phases following haemorrhage. Lancet 1:18, 1947

13. **Sharpey–Schafer EP:** Transfusion and the anaemic heart. Lancet 2:296, 1945

14. **Sanguinetti LV:** Curvas azohemicas en las hemorragias retenidas del tubs digestiva. Arch Argent Enferm Apar Dig y Nutr 9:68, 1933

15. **Schiff L, Stevens RJ, Moss HK:** The prognostic significance of the blood urea nitrogen following hematemesis or melena. Am J Dig Dis 9:110, 1942

16. **Schiff L, Stevens RJ:** Elevation of urea nitrogen content of the blood following hematemesis or melena. Arch Intern Med 64:1239, 1939

17. **Black DAK, Smith AF:** Blood and plasma transfusion in alimentary haemorrhage. Br Med J 1:187, 1941

18. **Schiff L, Stevens RJ, Goodman S, Garber E, Lublin A:** Observations on the oral administration of citrated blood in man. I. The effects on the blood urea nitrogen. Am J Dig Dis 6:597, 1939

19. **Kaump DH, Parsons JC:** Extrarenal azotemia in gastrointestinal hemorrhage. II. Experimental observations. Am J Dig Dis 7:191, 1940

20. **Chunn CF, Harkins HN:** Experimental studies on alimentary azotemia. I. Role of blood absorption from the gastrointestinal tract. Surgery 9:695, 1941

21. **Chunn CF, Harkins HN:** Alimentary azotemia due to whole blood absorption from the gastrointestinal tract. Proc Soc Exp Biol Med 45:569, 1940

22. **Gregory R, Ewing PL, Levine H:** Azotemia associated with gastrointestinal hemorrhage: An experimental etiologic study. Arch Intern Med 75:381, 1945

23. **Stevens RJ, Schiff L, Lubin A, Garber ES:** Renal function and the azotemia following hematemesis. J Clin Invest 19:233, 1940

24. **Dill LV, Isenhour CE:** Observations on the incidence and cause of fever in patients with bleeding peptic ulcers. Am J Dig Dis 5:779, 1939

25. **Schiff L, Shapiro N, Stevens RJ:** Observations on oral administration of citrated blood in man. III. The effect on temperature and the white blood cell count. Am J Med Sci 207:465, 1944

26. **Palmer ED:** Diagnosis of Upper Gastrointestinal Hemorrhage, Publ 443, American Lecture Series. Springfield, Ill, Charles C Thomas, 1961

27. **Palmer ED:** Upper Gastrointestinal Hemorrhage. Springfield, Ill, Charles C Thomas, 1970

28. **Pope CE II: Sleisenger MH, Fortdran JS:** Gastrointestinal Disease. Philadelphia, WB Saunders, 1973

29. **Strandberg J:** Pseudoxanthoma elasticum. Zentralblatt für Haut-u.-Geschlechtskrankheiten 31:689, 1929

30. **McKusick VA:** Heritable Disorders of Connective Tissue, 2nd ed. St Louis, CV Mosby, 1960

31. **Grönblad E:** Angioid streks–pseudoxanthoma elasticum: Verlaüfige mitheilung. Acta Ophthalmol 7:329, 1929

32. **Murray MJ, Thal AP, Greenspan R:** Splenic arteriovenous fistulas as a cause of portal hypertension. Am J Med 29:849, 1960

33. **Schatzki R:** Roentgen demonstration of esophageal varices: Its clinical importance. Arch Surg 41:1084, 1940

34. **Karr S, Wohl GT:** Clinical importance of gastric varices. N Engl J Med 263:665, 1960

35. **Nelson SW:** The roentgenologic diagnosis of esophageal varices. Am J Roentgenol 77:599, 1957

36. **Leevy CM, Cherrick GR, Davidson CS:** Medical progress. Portal hypertension. N Engl J Med 262:397–403, 451–456, 1960

37. **Hampton AO:** A safe method for the roentgen demonstration of bleeding duodenal ulcers. Am J Roentgenol 38:565, 1937

38. **Knowles HC, Felson B, Shapiro N, Schiff L:** Emergency diagnosis of upper digestive tract bleeding by roentgen examination without palpation ("Hampton technic"). Radiology 58:536, 1952

39. **Dent TL:** Diagnostic Endoscopy. In Fiddian–Green RG, Turcotte JG (eds): Gastrointestinal Hemorrhage, p 39. New York, Grune & Stratton, 1980

40. **Athanasoulis CA, Waltman AC, Ring EJ et al:** Angiography: Its contribution to the emergency management of gastrointestinal hemorrhage. Radiol Clin North Am 14:265, 1976

41. **Baum S, Athanasoulis CA, Waltman AC, Ring EJ:** Angiographic diagnosis and control. Adv Surg 7:149, 1973

42. **Schindler R:** Discussion: Hemorrhage from gastritis: A gastroscopic study. Am J Dig Dis 4:657, 1937

43. **Ruffin JM, Brown IW Jr:** The significance of hemorrhagic or pigment spots as observed by gastroscopy. Am J Dig Dis 10:60, 1943

44. **Wolf S, Wolff HG:** Human Gastric Function, 2nd ed p 149. New York, Oxford, 1947

45. **Crohn BB:** Affections of the Stomach. Philadelphia, WB Saunders, 1927

46. **Hurst AF, Stewart MJ:** Gastric and Duodenal Ulcer. London, Oxford University Press, 1929

47. **Shapiro N, Schiff L:** Ten years' experience with bleeding peptic ulcer with emphasis on 45 fetal cases. Surgery 31:327, 1952

48. **Meulengracht E:** Behandlung von Hämatemesis und Meläna mit uneingeschränkter Kos. Wien Klin Wochenschr 49:1481, 1936

49. **Meulengracht E:** Treatment of haematemesis and melaena with food: The mortality. Lancet 2:1220, 1935

50. **Bonney GLW, Pickering GW:** Observations on mechanism of pain in ulcer of stomach and duodenum; nature of the sttimulus. Clin Sci 6:63, 1946

51. **McLaughlin CW, Baker CP, Sharpe JC:** Bleeding duodenal ulcer complicated by myocardial infarction. Nebr Med J 25:266, 1940

52. **Blumgart HL, Schlesinger MJ, Zoll PN:** Multiple fresh coronary occlusions in patients with antecedent shock. Arch Intern Med 68:181, 1941

53. **McKinlay CA:** Coronary insufficiency precipitated by hemorrhage from duodenal ulcer. Lancet 63:31, 1943

54. **Kinney TD, Mallory GK:** Cardiac failure associated with acute anemia. N Engl J Med 232:215, 1945

55. **Rasmussen H, Foss M:** The electrocardiogram of acute hemorrhage from stomach and intestines. Acta Med Scand 111:420, 1942

56. **Scherf D, Reinstein H, Klotz SD:** Electrocardiographic changes following hematemesis in peptic ulcer. Rev Gastroenterol 8:343, 1941

57. **Master AM, Dack S, Grishman A, Field LE, Horn H:** Acute coronary insufficiency: An entity: Shock, hemorrhage and pulmonary embolism as factors in its production. J Mt Sinai Hosp (NY) 14:8, 1947

58. **Davies DT, Wilson ATM:** Personal and clinical history in haematemesis and perforation. Lancet 2:723, 1939

59. **Gainsborough H, Slater E:** A study of peptic ulcer. Br Med J 2:253, 1946

60. **Rivers AB:** Hemorrhage from the stomach and duodenum. In Eusterman GB, Balfour DC (eds): The Stomach and Duodenum, p 759. Philadelphia, WB Saunders, 1935

61. **Palmer WL:** Peptic ulcer. In Portis SA (ed): Diseases of the Digestive System, 2nd ed, p 208. Philadelphia, Lea & Febiger, 1944

62. **Smyrniotis F, Schenker S, O'Donnell J, Schiff L:** Lactic dehydrogenase activity in gastric juice for the diagnosis of gastric cancer. Am J Dig Dis 7:712, 1962

63. **Linton RR:** The surgical treatment of bleeding esophageal varices by portal systemic venous shunts, with a report of 34 cases. Ann Intern Med 31:794, 1949

64. **Whipple AO:** Portal Bed Block and Portal Hypertension, In Advances in Surgery, vol 2, p 155. New York, Interscience, 1949

65. **Garrett N Jr, Gall EA:** Esophageal varices without hepatic cirrhosis. Arch Pathol 55:196, 1953

66. **Tisdale WA, Klatskin G, Glenn WWL:** Portal hypertension and bleeding esophageal varices: Their occurrence in the absence of both intrahepatic and extrahepatic obstruction of the portal vein. N Engl J Med 261:209, 1959

67. **Liebowitz HR:** Bleeding Esophageal Varices, Portal Hypertension. Springfield, Ill, Charles C Thomas, 1959

68. **Snodgrass RW, Mellinkoff SM:** Bleeding varices in the upper esophagus due to obstruction of the superior vena cava. Gastroenterology 41:505, 1961

69. **Fleig WE et al:** Upper gastrointestinal hemorrhage from downhill esophageal varices. Digestive Diseases & Sciences 27:23, 1982

70. **Campbell GS, Bick HD, Paulsen EP, Lober PH, Watson CJ, Varco RL:** Bleeding esophgeal varices with polycystic liver. N Engl J Med 259:904, 1958

71. **Sedacca CM, Perrin E, Martin L, Schiff L:** Polycystic liver: An unusual cause of bleeding esophageal varices. Gastroenterology 40:128, 1961

72. **Liebowitz HR:** Pathogenesis of esophageal varix rupture. JAMA 175:874, 1961

73. **Wangensteen OH:** The ulcer problem (Listerian oration). Can Med Assoc J 53:309, 1945

74. **Orloff MJ, Thomas HS:** Pathogenesis of esophageal varix rupture. Arch Surg 87:301, 1963

75. **Orloff MJ:** Emergency treatment for bleeding esophageal varices. Hosp Pract 10, No. 5:28, April 1975

76. **Conn HO, Brodoff M:** Emergency esophagoscopy in the diagnosis of upper gastrointestinal hemorrhage. Gastroenterology 47:505, 1964

77. **Conn HL, Simpson JA:** A rational program for the diagnosis and treatment of bleeding esophageal varices. Med Clin North Am 52:1457, 1968

78. **Morlock CG, Hall BE:** Association of cirrhosis, thrombopenia and hemorrhagic tendency. Arch Intern Med 72:69, 1943

79. **Young PC, Burnside CR, Knowles HC Jr, Schiff L:** The effect of the intragastric administration of whole blood on the blood ammonia, blood urea nitrogen and nonprotein nitrogen in patients with liver disease. J Clin Invest 35:747, 1956

80. **Merigan TC Jr, Hollister RM, Gryska PF, Starkey GWB, Davidson CS:** Gastrointestinal bleeding with cirrhosis. N Engl J Med 263:579, 1960

81. **Clarke JS, Ozeran RS, Hart JC, Cruze K, Crevling V:** Peptic ulcer following portacaval shunt. Ann Surg 148:551, 1958

82. **Dubuque TJ Jr, Mulligan LV, Neville EC:** Gastric secretion and peptic ulceration in the dog with portal obstruction and portacaval anastomosis. Surg Forum 8:208, 1958

83. **Panke WF, Moreno AH, Rousselot LM:** The diagnostic study of the portal venous system. Med Clin North Am 44:727, 1960

84. **Faber K:** Gastritis and Its Consequences. London, Oxford, University Press, 1935

85. **Moutier F:** Traité de gastroscopie et de pathologie endoscopique de l'estomac. Paris, Masson, 1935

86. **Henning N:** Die Entzündung des Magens. Leipzig, Barth, 1934

87. **Dagradi AE, Stempien SJ, Lee ER, Juler G:** Hemorrhagic–erosive gastritis. Gastrointest Endosc, 14:147, February, 1968

88. **Sahler OD, Hamptom AO:** Bleeding in hiatus hernia. Am J Roentgenol 49:433, 1943

89. **Jones CM:** Hiatus esophageal hernia, with special reference to a comparison of its symptoms with those of angina pectoris. N Engl J Med 225:963, 1941

90. **Harrington SW:** Diagnosis and treatment of various types of diaphragmatic hernia. Am J Surg 50:377, 1940

91. **Olsen AM, Harrington SW:** Esophageal hiatal hernias of the short esophagus type: Etiologic and therapeutic considerations. J Thorac Surg 17:189, 1948

92. **Frank W:** Hematemesis associated with gastric arteriosclerosis: Review of literature with case report. Gastroenterology 7:231, 1946

93. **Griggs DE, Baker MQ:** Hereditary hemorrhagic teleangiectasia with gastrointestinal bleeding. Am J Dig Dis 8:344, 1941

94. **Kushlan SD:** Gastro-intestinal bleeding in hereditary hemorrhagic telangiectasia: Historical review and case report with gastroscopic findings and rutin therapy. Gastroenterology 7:199, 1946

95. **Bean WB:** Enteric bleeding in rare conditions with diagnostic lesions of the skin and mucous membrane. Trans Am Clin Climatol Assoc 69:72, 1957

96. **Segal HL, Scott WJM, Watson JS:** Lesions of small intestine producing massive hemorrhage, with symptoms simulating peptic ulcer. JAMA 129:116, 1945

97. **Gordon–Taylor G:** Rare causes of severe gastro-intestinal haemorrhage, with note on aneurysm of hepatic artery. Br Med J 1:504, 1943

98. **Murphy B:** Aneurysm of splenic artery: death from haematemesis. Lancet 1:704, 1942

99. **Lee HC, Kay S:** Primary polyarteritis nodosa of the stomach and small intestine as a cause of gastrointestinal hemorrhage. Ann Surg 147:714, 1958

100. **Denkewalter FR, Molnar W, Horava AP:** Massive gastrointestinal hemorrhage in jejunal diverticulosos. Ann Surg 148:862, 1958

101. **Evans AL, Cofer OS, Gregory HH:** Multiple hemangiomas of the jejunum as a cause of massive gastrointestinal bleeding. J Med Assoc Ga 47:600, 1958

102. **Schoenfeld R, Cahan J, Dyer R:** Gastric carcinoid tumor: An unusual cause of hematemesis. Arch Intern Med 104:649, 1959

103. **Muir A, Cossar IA:** Aspirin and gastric haemorrhage. Lancet 1:539, 1959

104. **Muir A, Cossar IA:** Aspirin and ulcer. Br Med J 2:7, 1955

105. **Douthwaite AH, Lintott GAM:** Gastroscopic observation of the effect of aspirin and certain other substances on the stomach. Lancet 2:1222, 1938

106. **Winkelman EI, Summerskill WHJ:** Gastric secretion in relation to gastrointestinal bleeding from salicylate compounds. Gastroenterology 40:56, 1961

107. **Lynch A, Shaw H, Milton GW:** Effect of aspirin on gastric secretion. Gut 5:230, 1964

108. **Menguy R:** Gastric mucosal injury by aspirin. Gastroenterology 51:430, 1966

109. **Mallory GK, Weiss S:** Hemorrhages from lacerations of the cardiac orifice of the stomach due to vomiting. Am J Med Sci 178:506, 1929

110. **Decker JP, Zamcheck N, Mallory GK:** Mallory–Weiss syndrome: Hemorrhage from gastroesophageal lacerations at the cardiac orifice of the stomach. N Engl J Med 249:957, 1953

111. **Saylor JL, Tedesco FJ:** Mallory–Weiss syndrome in perspective. Digestive Diseases & Sciences 20:1131, 1975

112. **Axon ATR, Clarke A:** Haemetemesis: A new syndrome? Br Med J 1:491, 1975

113. **Heuer GJ:** The surgical aspects of hemorrhage from peptic ulcer. N Engl J Med 235:777, 1946

114. **Foster DG:** Retrograde jejunogastric intussusception: A rare cause of hematemesis. Review of the literature and report of two cases. Arch Surg 73:1009, 1956

115. **Cordell AR, Wright RH, Johnston FR:** Gastrointestinal hemorrhage after abdominal aortic operations. Surgery 48:997, 1960

116. **Sandblom P:** Hemorrhage into the biliary tract following trauma: "Traumatic hemobilia." Surgery 24:571, 1948

117. **Sandblom P:** Hemobilia. Springfield, Ill, Charles C Thomas, 1972

118. **Sandblom P:** Hemobilia. In Schiff L (ed): Diseases of the Liver, 4th ed. Philadelphia, JB Lippincott, 1975

119. **Stokes JF, Jones FA:** Haematemesis due to pseudoxanthoma elasticum. Gastroenterologia 89:345, 1958

120. **Knight CD:** Massive hemorrhage from diverticular disease of the colon. Surgery 42:853, 1957

121. **Nusbaum M, Baum S:** Radiographic demonstration of unknown sites of gastrointestinal bleeding. Surg Forum 13:374, 1963

122. **Thompson NW:** Vascular ectasias and colonic diverticula. In RG, Fiddian–Green, Turcotte JG (eds): Gastrointestinal Hemorrhage. New York, Grune & Stratton, 1980

123. **Casarella WJ, Kanter IE, Seaman WF:** Rightsided colonic diverticula as a cause of acute rectal hemorrhage. N Engl J Med 286:453, 1972

124. **Buchanan JD, Hunt RH:** Photography and coagulation biopsy confirms the diagnosis of angiodysplasia. Gut 21:A927, 1980

125. **Baum S, Athanasoulis CA, Waltman AC et al:** Angiodysplasia of the right colon: A cause of gastrointestinal bleeding. Am J Roentgenol 129:789, 1977

126. **Hunt R:** Massive bleeding from the large bowel. Br Med J 280:320, 1980

127. **Howard OM et al:** Angiodysplasia. Lancet II: 1340, 1981

128. **Rogers BHG:** Endoscopic diagnosis and therapy of mucosal vascular abnormalities of the G.I. tract occurring in elderly patients and associated with cardiovascular and pulmonary disease. Gastroint Endosc 26:134, 1980.

129. **Hunt RH, Buchanan JD:** The diagnosis and management of angiodysplasia. Gastroint Endosc 27:123, 1981

130. **Mitsudo SM, Boley SJ, Brandt LJ et al:** Vascular ectasias of the right colon in the elderly: A distinct pathological entity. Human Pathol 10:585, 1979

131. **Boley SJ, Sammartano R, Adams A et al:** On the nature and etiology of vascular ectasias of the colon: Degenerative lesions of aging. Gastroenterology 72:650, 1977

132. **Rogers BHG, Adler F:** Hemangioma of the cecum: Colonoscopic diagnosis and therapy. Gastroenterology 71:1079, 1976

133. **Czaja AJ, McAlhany JC, Pruitt BA Jr:** Acute gastrointestinal disease after thermal injury. N Engl J Med 291:925, 1974

134. **Cabal E, Holtz S:** Polyarteritis as a cause of intestinal hemorrhage. Gastroenterology 61:99, 1971

24

Jaundice Leon Schiff

Definitions and Classification
Clinical Approach
  History
  Physical Examination
  Routine Tests
  Liver Profile

Prothrombin Response to Vitamin K
Duodenal Drainage
Minilaparotomy
Radiologic Procedures
Needle Biopsy of the Liver
Conclusion

DEFINITIONS AND CLASSIFICATION

Jaundice, or icterus, is the condition recognized clinically by a yellowish discoloration of the plasma, the skin, and the mucous membranes, which is caused by staining by bile pigment. It may be the first, and sometimes the sole, manifestation of disease. It is detected best in the peripheral portions of the ocular conjunctivae and can be observed also in the mucous membrane of the hard palate or in the lips when compressed with a glass slide. It may be overlooked in poor or artificial light. Attention may be first directed to it by a laboratory report of "serum icteric." It may be preceded for a day or more by the passage of dark urine or light-colored stools. As Osler so well stated, "Jaundice is the disease your friends diagnose."[1] Icterus may be detected when the concentration of serum bilirubin exceeds 2 mg/100 ml.

As a rule, the clinician has little difficulty in distinguishing hemolytic from hepatocellular and obstructive jaundice. His usual task is to distinguish jaundice owing to primary liver disease or dysfunction from that owing to obstruction of the extrahepatic bile ducts, or in other words, to distinguish "medical" from "surgical" jaundice.

The physician should first rule out such hereditary forms of icterus as Gilbert's,[2] Dubin–Johnson,[3] or Ro-

tor's syndrome,[4,5] in which no treatment is indicated. When considering the more common forms of liver disease that produce jaundice, he usually has to decide between an acute viral, drug-induced, or alcoholic hepatitis; subacute or chronic hepatitis; or cirrhosis. In the case of biliary tract obstruction, he must consider common duct stone, intraductal or extraductal neoplasm, sclerosing cholangitis, and in patients with previous gallbladder surgery, common duct stricture, or residual stone.

In the differentiation of the various causes of jaundice, he should stress the clinical examination and laboratory tests and if necessary, select one or more of the newer diagnostic maneuvers, which include abdominal ultrasonography,[6,7,8,9,10] computerized axial tomography,[11,12,13] HIDA scan,[14,15] percutaneous transhepatic cholangiography (PTC),[16–18] and endoscopic retrograde cholangiopancreatography (ERCP).[19] In cases in which a definitive diagnosis is not reached, he has recourse to needle biopsy of the liver with or without guidance by ultrasonography or computerized tomography, and in selected instances, exploratory laparotomy. Less and less used because of overlapping results but of occasional help are the response of the serum bilirubin concentration to steroid administration[20,21] and the use of transduodenal biliary drainage.[22] Minilaparotomy[23] has been employed by

some observers in especially puzzling cases, particularly in the presence of coagulation disorders, ascites, or obstructive jaundice.

CLINICAL APPROACH

About 20 years ago Steven Schenker, John Balint and the author[24] reported that a careful history, physical examination, and review of the standard liver chemistries in a group of jaundiced patients yielded a diagnostic accuracy of approximately 85%. A recent report by Lumeng and colleagues[25] not only confirmed these observations but also pointed out that the clinical examination was an efficient as individual diagnostic procedures in current use. Because of technical advances, the clinical examination is being relegated regrettably to a secondary role.

HISTORY

The familial occurrence of icterus should suggest the possibilities of congenital hemolytic jaundice, Gilbert's syndrome,[2] the Dubin–Johnson syndrome,[3] Rotor's syndrome,[4,5] or benign recurrent intrahepatic cholestasis.[26,27] A history of consanguinity of parents should arouse suspicion of Wilson's disease. A history of allergic disorders may predispose to drug-induced liver injury.

Recent foreign travel with particular reference to areas of endemic hepatitis and to contact with jaundiced persons should arouse suspicion of viral hepatitis. A high index of suspicion of hepatitis should be held in homosexuals, drug addicts, patients undergoing hemodialysis and attendants in such units, and in clinical laboratory personnel. Inquiry should be made regarding the recent ingestion of raw oysters or raw or steamed clams.[28,29] All medications the patient has been taking should be brought in and listed, particularly anabolic steroids, oral contraceptives, thorazine, isoniazid, methyldopa, acetaminophen in doses of 4 g per day, and aspirin in doses sufficient to produce blood salicylate levels of > 15 mg/dl in patients with rheumatic fever, systemic lupus erythematosis, and juvenile rheumatoid arthritis.[30] Liver injury owing to drugs may be indistinguishable from viral hepatitis, especially when caused by isoniazid[31] or methyldopa,[32] or it may present as cholestasis, especially following use of anabolic steroids, thorazine, or oral contraceptives. The clinician must guard against mistaking drug-induced cholestasis for extrahepatic obstructive jaundice.

Blood transfusions administered two weeks to six months prior to the onset of jaundice should lead to suspicion of posttransfusion hepatitis, the more blood used the stronger the suspicion. The incidence is said to be six or seven times higher in recipients of commercial blood than volunteer blood.[33] Hepatitis A is rarely, if ever, transmitted by transfusion.[34] Up to about 90% of cases of posttransfusion hepatitis are of the non-A, non-B types, outbreaks of which have been reported after the administration of blood clotting factors VIII and IX.

A history of alcoholism should always be sought and in doubtful situations an interview arranged with spouse, minister, golfing partner, or bartender. The importance of determining the alcoholic content of the urine has recently been stressed in assessing the patient's estimate of the quantity of alcohol consumption.[35] In young people, a history of alcoholism may detract from consideration of viral hepatitis. In older patients, the symptoms of anorexia, weakness, and weight loss (and the presence of hepatomegaly) may wrongly suggest a malignant tumor of the liver. On the other hand, a bout of alcoholic hepatitis with its acute abdominal pain, nausea and vomiting, fever, right upper abdominal tenderness, and leukocytosis may be mistaken for an acute surgical abdominal disorder.

The physician should adopt a conservative attitude in cases of postoperative jaundice.[36–38] If much blood accumulated in the peritoneal or pleural cavities and resulted in shock, anoxia, and liver damage, and if much blood was transfused, the damaged liver is unable to excrete the increased bilirubin load, although it is able to conjugate it. The resulting cholestasis is not harmful *per se* and does not require specific therapy. In case of a cholecystectomy, accidental injury to the common bile duct should be suspected. If the duct has been ligated, jaundice will appear early; if it has been severed or incised, prolonged drainage of bile from the operative area will ensue, to be followed later by icterus and evidences of associated cholangitis. On the other hand, the resulting stricture may not become manifest for a year or more—seldom longer than two years—after the bile duct injury.[39]

If halothane was the anesthetic employed, and more particularly if it had been administered in the past and followed by an unexplained fever, toxic hepatitis owing to halothane must be strongly considered. The first exposure is apt to trigger symptoms after seven days, while following multiple exposures, symptoms tend to appear in three days. It is well to remember that children are relatively resistant to halothane hepatotoxicity.

Careful inquiry should be made regarding abdominal pain. It is usually improminent—more of a heavy or dragging sensation—in viral hepatitis, although oc-

casionally it is severe enough to simulate gallstone colic.*†‡[40] Perhaps as Watson has suggested the basis in such cases may be a true catarrhal choledochitis, as originally postulated by Virchow. In about 10% of elderly patients, common duct stone may be painless[41] and may manifest itself many years after cholecystectomy for calculous cholecystitis, a fact not generally appreciated by the medical profession. The stone may be residual or may have formed *de novo* in the bile duct. Glenn believes that "any calculus recognized within the biliary ductal system during a period of one year or less following surgery for calculous biliary tract disease is indeed a retained stone." The longer the stones have been present in the gallbladder the more likely they are to migrate into the common bile duct.[41] A case of common duct stone has been reported with neither pain nor icterus, presenting itself as a fever of undetermined origin.[42]

The pain caused by pancreatic cancer is quite characteristic, as originally pointed out by Chauffard.[43] It is usually located in the upper abdomen or right upper quadrant and radiates to the back. It is worse in the recumbent position and is lessened by turning on either side, by assuming the prone position, or by sitting up and flexing the spine. It is usually severe and often requires an opiate, though aspirin at frequent intervals may provide relief also. The pain, when accompanied by weakness, weight loss, pruritus, jaundice, and frequently hyperglycemia, warrants the strongest suspicion of pancreatic cancer and may provide the sole basis for diagnosis.

Tumors of the liver, both primary and metastatic, may present with abdominal pain, which may be dull or boring or sharp and usually localized to the right hypochondrium. The pain may radiate to the back, right infrascapular area, or right flank, and it may be increased by deep breathing, cough, exertion, or changes in posture.[44] The pain is presumably due to invasion or stretching of the liver capsule by the neoplasm. Hemorrhage into a tumor may result in sudden severe pain. Rupture of the tumor may produce an acute catastrophic hemoperitoneum.

Although a history of chronic jaundice—recurrent or continuous—with chills, fever, and usually, abdominal pain is generally indicative of common duct stones, it nevertheless warrants a search for sclerosing carcinoma of the bile ducts;[45,46] sclerosing cholangitis, especially in the presence of ulcerative colitis;[47–49] and much less commonly, congenital malformation of bile ducts,

*Schiff L: Unpublished observation

†Redeker A: Personal communication.

‡Watson CJ: Personal communication.

especially choledochal cyst and Caroli's disease. In patients with previous biliary tract surgery, iatrogenic stenosis (stricture) or a residual stone should be suspected.

Chills and fever do not occur in extrahepatic obstruction owing to pancreatic tumor because the bile is not infected, in contrast with common duct stones. Chills and fever may be present during the preicteric phase of viral hepatitis and may occur in thorazine or other drug-induced liver injury, leptospirosis, and chronic active hepatitis. In the experience of the author, their appearance after the onset of jaundice would be unusual in uncomplicated acute viral hepatitis.

Over one hundred years ago, Budd pointed out that pruritus is most pronounced in cases of occlusion of the common bile duct, particularly by tumor.[50] According to Schoenfield, pruritus occurs with extrahepatic obstruction in 75% of patients with malignant lesions and in 50% of those with benign conditions.[51] He believes that the itching that occurs in 20% of patients with hepatitis and 10% of those with cirrhosis is often associated with clinical and laboratory evidence of intrahepatic cholestasis, and he finds that about 75% of patients with bile duct stricture or primary biliary cirrhosis have pruritus. Itching is prominent in recurrent intrahepatic cholestasis and in the recurrent jaundice of pregnancy.[52]

While an increase in serum bile acids has long been suspected as the cause of the pruritus, clinicians have been aware that itching of the skin not infrequently precedes or follows the appearance or disappearance of icterus. It is not surprising, therefore, that pruritus may occur with low serum bile acid concentrations or may not occur with very high serum bile acid values, and relief of itching may follow the use of norethandrolone without concomitant decrease in serum bile acids.[53]

According to Javitt, the pruritus occurring in cholestatic syndromes can be distinguished from that occurring in other diseases by its diurnal variation: it is worst at bedtime and gone by morning. He points out that serum bile acids are highest in the evening after dinner and can become normal by morning. He feels that the lack of pruritus in some individuals regardless of the height of the serum bile acid concentration implies "some variation in the perception of pruritus as a sensory phenomenon, or variation in the type of bile acid and the moderating effects of bilirubin and other components that are also retained in the skin and other tissues."[54,55]

The appearance of dark urine—"looking like tea or Coca Cola"—is the most reliable criterion of the onset of jaundice and is apt to precede the yellowish discol-

oration of the skin or sclerae by days. In cases of viral hepatitis the stools may be clay-colored for a few days or more, while in common duct stone they may alternate between acholic and cholic. Occasionally, a seemingly acholic stool may be due to admixture of barium ingested during an upper gastrointestinal x-ray study. The occurrence of brown stools in the presence of deep jaundice is usually indicative of hepatocellular disease but may occur rarely in carcinoma of the head of the pancreas.[56] Although it may prove to be caused by a bleeding peptic ulcer or ruptured esophageal varices, the passage of tarry stools by an icteric patient should arouse suspicion of carcinoma of the ampulla of Vater or pancreas eroding the duodenum or stomach, or hemobilia.[57]

PHYSICAL EXAMINATION

Age and Sex. The age and the sex of the patient may prove of diagnostic help. Viral hepatitis type A is seen most commonly in children of school age, whereas common duct stone and neoplastic jaundice usually occur in middle-aged or older patients. Leptospirosis is primarily a disease of children and young adults and occurs predominantly in males.[58] Portal cirrhosis, chronic Type B hepatitis, hepatoma, pancreatic cancer, sclerosing cholangitis, and primary hemochromatosis predominate in the male, while common duct stone, primary biliary cirrhosis, and carcinoma of the gallbladder are more prevalent in the female.

Eyes. Mild degrees of icterus may be detectable only in the scleral periphery and may be overlooked in artificial light. Kayser-Fleischer rings should be looked for in all patients under 30 years of age with chronic active hepatitis, since Wilson's disease may present in this form.[59] Pigmented corneal rings have also been described in non-Wilsonian liver disease, notably primary biliary cirrhosis.[60] Conjunctival suffusion, occasionally accompanied by conjunctival hemorrhage, should suggest leptospirosis.[61]

Vascular Spiders. These structures should be looked for carefully with the aid of a good light. They usually occur on the face, neck, arms, fingers, and upper trunk, and exceptionally, on the lower trunk and lower extremities. Inspection with a hand lens may be necessary to distinguish them from small papular lesions. They may pulsate and can be obliterated by pressing on their center point with the point of a pencil.[62,63] They usually indicate the existence of hepatic cirrhosis and have been linked with esophageal varices.[64] They seldom occur in patients with jaundice resulting from neoplasm or common duct stone. They may be seen in acute hepatitis, chronic active hepatitis, pregnancy, and occasionally in normal persons, in whom they are more apt to be solitary.

Breath. A peculiar, sickly sweetish breath (hepatic foetor) is characteristic of severe hepatic disease with necrosis,[65] but it may be encountered in cases of extensive collateral circulation.[66] The foetor is probably due to a mixture of the three related volatile compounds: metanethiol, dimethyl sulfide, and dimethyl disulfide.[67] Detection of the peculiar foetor in a patient in coma should arouse suspicion of hepatic encephalopathy.

Skin. Brownish pigmentation of the skin owing to deposition of melanin should suggest primary biliary cirrhosis or hemochromatosis, in which the skin may also assume a blue-gray color owing to deposition of hemosiderin. Reynolds has noted the frequent development of a butterfly-shaped area of lesser pigmentation over the back where the patient cannot easily reach to scratch.[68] In primary biliary cirrhosis, *xanthomata*—the yellowish infiltrations of the skin—are generally first observed in the eyelids, usually at the inner canthi. The flat type similar to those around the eyes may involve the palms, the neck, and the chest or back. The tuberous variety are usually found over the knuckles, wrists, elbows, ankles, and Achilles tendons and also may involve the buttocks.

Abdominal Examination. I cannot overemphasize the importance of Osler's advice: ''Do not touch the patient. State first what you see—cultivate your powers of observation.''

Prominent superficial abdominal veins are observed most often in patients with hepatic cirrhosis but may occur in the presence of peritoneal tumor implants, obstruction of the portal vein by tumor, or in cases of inferior caval obstruction. In portal hypertension the blood flow in the abdominal veins is radially away from the umbilicus, whereas in inferior caval obstruction, it is upward over the abdominal wall.[69] Normal veins may be made more prominent by the stretching and thinning of the overlying skin resulting from abdominal distention in the absence of portal hypertension.

It is good practice to examine the abdomen on more than one visit, since variations in the degree of abdominal relaxation, in the examiner's own perceptivity, and in the time he devotes to the examination will explain the ability to palpate the liver, gallbladder, or spleen on one day and failure to do so on another. Having the patient think of something pleasant may help promote abdominal relaxation.

I recall a patient with portal systemic encephalop-

athy who had had a portacaval shunt three years before. His liver was not palpable on the initial examination; however, repeated abdominal palpation during a two-week period revealed a steady increase in liver size with appearance of surface nodules, which led to a diagnosis of hepatoma.

Hanger has noted, "One good feel of the liver is worth any two liver function tests."[70] Through the years I have been so impressed with the truth of this dictum that I cannot sufficiently emphasize the importance of a careful examination of the liver. To obtain a good "feel" of the liver, the examiner's hand should be warm. The patient should lie on his back, with head slightly raised, arms at his sides, and knees flexed. It is best to begin palpation over the lower right abdomen, to avoid pressing too heavily, and to proceed upward, while asking the patient to breathe deeply. This is a more productive procedure than commencing just below the right costal margin and proceeding downward. The first "feel" is often the best, because flipping the liver edge at the end of inspiration may be painful and cause the patient to restrict subsequent inspirations. Yet two feels may prove better than one!

The normal liver is soft, has a thin edge, and may be tender. It may extend below the costal margin and yet remain impalpable. Percussion is more accurate in estimating the lower border but less accurate in determining the upper border. It is safe to assume that a liver that extends three fingerbreadths or more below the right costal margin is probably enlarged, provided that one may exclude a hyposthenic body habitus or downward displacement by right pleural effusion or pulmonary emphysema. Variations in the shape and position of the liver appear to be related to body type.[71] In a stocky person, the liver often extends to the left lateral abdominal wall with its lower edge lying relatively high; it may not be palpable beneath the costal margin. In a lanky individual, the normal liver, including the left lobe, may lie entirely in the right abdomen and may extend five fingerbreadths below the costal margin.

A liver that is unduly firm is apt to be diseased, as is one with a blunted edge or irregular contour. A nodular liver is most commonly indicative of intrahepatic malignant neoplasm. However, the large regenerating nodules of postnecrotic cirrhosis or multiple cysts may produce changes that closely simulate those produced by tumor.

The liver usually extends one to two (or two to three) fingerbreadths below the right costal margin in viral hepatitis and is frequently tender. A very large liver (one extending four to five fingerbreadths or more below the right costal margin) is usually indicative of fatty vacuolization, cirrhosis, tumor, amyloidosis, cystic disease, or congestive failure (Fig. 24-1).

A friction rub over the liver is usually due to a ma-

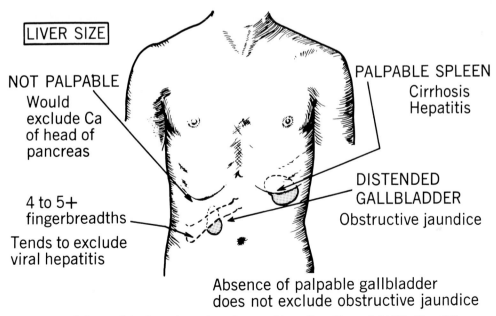

Fig. 24-1. Abdominal findings in various forms of jaundice. (From Schiff L: The differential diagnosis of jaundice. Postgrad. Med. 41:39, 1967)

lignant tumor[72] invading or breaking through the liver capsule; but it may be encountered in acute gonococcal perihepatitis or hepatic syphilis, or it may follow percutaneous liver biopsy. It has been described in acute cholecystitis, presumably caused by fibrinous exudate on the serosal surface of the gallbladder.[73]

A harsh (arterial) murmur over the liver has been reported in hepatoma, alcoholic hepatitis,[74] and anemia.[75] It should be contrasted with the low-pitched venous hum arising in collateral venous channels, which unlike the arterial murmur, is altered by posture, respiration, or firm pressure with the stethoscope.[74]

The absence of a palpable liver in a patient who has been jaundiced for two to three weeks or more would tend to exclude neoplastic obstruction of the common bile duct by carcinoma of the head of the pancreas, because enlargement usually results from the intrahepatic bile stasis that is secondary to complete biliary tract obstruction.[76]

The presence of a smooth, nontender, distended gallbladder in a patient with jaundice, once considered to be pathognomonic of neoplastic obstruction of the common bile duct in accordance with Courvoisier's law, was reported in 25% of cases of common duct stone by Flood and associates.[77] It is such a reliable indicator of obstructive jaundice as to warrant limiting the choice of diagnostic maneuvers used to establish biliary tract obstruction.

A distended gallbladder may be more visible than palpable, particularly when the abdominal wall is tense and the patient apprehensive. It may be found in the lower right abdominal quadrant, may attain the size of a grapefruit, and may be mimicked by a tumor of the colonic flexure or of the right kidney. Lateral mobility, descent on inspiration, and lack of forward displacement by pressure over the right lumbar region may prove helpful in identifying it. The author has on occasion followed Watson's practice of beginning palpation of the abdomen in the left lower quadrant, at the same time observing the right upper quadrant for movement during inspiration.[65] It has been the author's experience that when there is some doubt at the bedside as to whether the gallbladder is palpable, it will usually prove to be so.

Palpation of the spleen should be gentle, as Galambos has emphasized, since the organ is quite superficial and may be missed with very deep palpation.[78] It may occasionally be more readily palpable with the patient in the supine position than in the preferred right lateral decubitus with the left arm extended over the head. As in the case of the liver, palpation should proceed upward from well below the costal margin. The spleen is palpable in about one-half of patients

with hepatic cirrhosis, in about 10% to 15% of patients with viral hepatitis, and in about 20% of patients with hepatic neoplasm.[44] In obstructive jaundice of long standing, splenomegaly may be a manifestation of secondary biliary cirrhosis. In cancer of the body and tail of the pancreas, splenic enlargement may result from encroachment of the tumor on the splenic vein.[79]

The presence of ascites in a jaundiced patient is usually indicative of hepatic cirrhosis but may also be observed in massive or submassive hepatic necrosis, in the presence of peritoneal tumor implants, or in invasion of the portal vein by tumor. Because of its occurrence in alcoholics, pancreatic ascites may at times be mistaken for cirrhotic ascites.[80] Marked elevation of amylase and higher protein values characterize pancreatic ascites. A high protein content (over 3 gm/ml) and a lactic dehydrogenase level of over 400 sigma units are strongly suggestive of peritoneal carcinoma.[81] Relatively small quantities of ascitic fluid may escape clinical detection but may be revealed by abdominal ultrasonography in amounts as little as 300 ml.[82] An enlarged spleen may obscure shifting dullness when the patient turns on his right side.[78]

A cell count of more than 500 per cu mm of ascitic fluid with more than 50% polymorphonuclear leukocytes is very much in keeping with spontaneous bacterial peritonitis[83] but may also occur in peritonitis secondary to perforated peptic ulcer or gallbladder, as may a positive culture for enteric organisms. When the ascitic fluid white cell count is greater than 500/cu mm and monomuclear cells are predominant, tuberculosis, malignant neoplasm, and pancreatic ascites should be considered.[81] Hoefs has recently pointed out that ascitic fluid protein and cell counts may rise during diuresis.[84]

Ascitic fluid may conceal an enlarged liver even on palpation by dipping or ballotting. The author recalls instances in which he could no longer palpate an enlarged tumorous liver following development of ascites, only to readily feel it again after abdominal paracentesis. Hemorrhagic ascitic fluid should suggest hepatoma, peritoneal tumor implants, or tuberculous peritonitis. Palpation of the umbilicus, especially in patients with ascites, may at times reveal small metastatic nodules.

Miscellaneous findings include the presence of an abdominal mass, usually indicative of intra-abdominal tumor. Absence of axillary or pectoral hair is suggestive of cirrhosis of the liver, as are testicular atrophy and gynecomastia, although the last two have been reported in hepatitis. Parotid enlargement, Dupuytren's contracture, and palmar erythema may also be noted in cases of cirrhosis. The presence of multiple

venous thrombi in a jaundiced patient should suggest cancer of the body or the tail of the pancreas,[85] and calf tenderness, leptospirosis.

ROUTINE TESTS

Blood Count. The white cell count is usually reduced during the preicteric and normal during the icteric phase of viral hepatitis, but it rises in fulminant hepatitis. The leukocyte count may help differentiate uncomplicated viral hepatitis from disorders accompanied by leukocytosis, such as toxic hepatitis, amebic abscess, metastatic hepatic neoplasm, common duct stone (with cholangitis), and leptospirosis. Eosinophilia should suggest toxic hepatitis.

Blood Urea Nitrogen (BUN). In addition to complicating renal failure, azotemia in a patient with jaundice should suggest the possibility of leptospirosis or exposure to an hepatotoxic agent simultaneous injurious to the kidney, such as carbon tetrachloride. According to Galambos, depression of the BUN below 5 mg/dl is characteristic of alcoholic cirrhosis and is uncommon in other forms of cirrhosis.[78]

Urine Analysis. The presence of albuminuria should suggest the possibility of leptospirosis, although it may occur in the preicteric and the early icteric phases of viral hepatitis. Since jaundice may occur in amyloidosis, the simultaneous occurrence of marked albuminuria should also arouse suspicion of this disorder.

Stool Examination. Strongly positive tests for occult blood in the stools should lead to suspicion of an ulcerating periampullary lesion or a pancreatic cancer eroding the stomach or duodenum, as well as to consideration of bleeding esophageal varices or peptic ulcer.

Serum Lipids. Increase in serum lipids should suggest biliary cirrhosis, fatty liver, or Zieve's syndrome.[86]

LIVER PROFILE

Among the laboratory tests constituting the so-called liver function tests, the serum bilirubin determination possesses diagnostic value that is not fully appreciated. Watson has emphasized the value of the ratio of conjugated to total serum bilirubin in subdividing cases of jaundice.[65] A ratio of less than 15% would indicate unconjugated hyperbilirubinemia comprising hemolytic disease, Gilbert's syndrome, and the Crigler–Najjar syndrome, while a value between 15% and 40%, which he designates as semiconjugated, charac-

terizes liver disease with a hemolytic component or hypersplenism and hemolytic disease with liver injury. Ratios exceeding 40% are to be found in cholestasis owing to biliary obstruction or liver disease.

A total serum bilirubin value of less than 10 mg/dl is usually encountered in common duct stone, largely because of intermittent obstruction, while greater concentrations favor the persistent and often complete obstruction owing to neoplasm. The peak concentration of total serum bilirubin in acute viral hepatitis is usually 15 mg/dl but may reach higher levels. A peak concentration above 25 mg/dl is unusual in extrahepatic obstruction unless complicated by oliguria or hemolysis. A total serum bilirubin concentration of less than 5 mg/dl is characteristic of uncomplicated primary biliary cirrhosis, particularly in its relatively earlier stages.

A daily increase of 1.5 mg/dl 2 mg/dl in the total serum bilirubin is characteristic of extrahepatic biliary obstruction;[36] more dramatic rises point to hepatitic or hemolytic states. The author recalls a consultation in which he rightfully suspected extrahepatic obstruction (which was proved to be due to a pancreatic tumor) because of a reported daily increase in the serum bilirubin of approximately 1.5 mg/dl. A diagnosis of viral hepatitis had been based on serum transaminase values exceeding 1000 units.

Although obstructive jaundice is accompanied almost always by an increase in the serum alkaline phosphatase, this increase may be of moderate degree, even in cases of biliary obstruction owing to neoplasm.[24] A steadily rising concentration of both serum alkaline phosphatase and serum bilirubin in the absence of corresponding increases in the serum transaminases constitute a most reliable index of obstructive jaundice. One may exclude increases in the enzyme concentration attributable to bone disease by determining the level of serum 5-nucleotidase, or gamma glutamyl transpeptidase, which are not influenced by osseous factors.[87] It is being increasingly realized that elevation of the serum alkaline phosphatase may prove to be the forerunner of pruritus and jaundice by years in primary biliary cirrhosis.[88–92]

Determination of the serum glutamic oxaloacetic transaminase (SGOT) and serum glutamic pyruvic (SGPT) transaminase levels has proved of great value in the distinction between hepatocellular and obstructive jaundice. In obstructive jaundice the concentration of these enzymes is usually not greater than 300 to 400 units, whereas in the very early stages of hepatitis, an increase of 1000 or more units is frequent. The diagnostic value of these enzyme determinations varies with the duration of jaundice, since the most marked increases occur in the very early stages of hepatitis. Thus,

in patients first seen two or three weeks after the onset of hepatitis, the enzyme level may have fallen to that ordinarily observed in obstructive jaundice.[24] In cirrhosis the SGOT is usually greater than the SGPT, which may even be normal, while the reverse is usually true in viral hepatitis.

While serum transaminases exceeding 500 Karmen units are unusual in extrahepatic obstructive jaundice, exceptions do occur, which may lead to erroneous diagnosis of viral hepatitis.[93,94] Such elevations are apt to be more transient than those occurring in viral hepatitis, and there is evidence to suggest that they may follow a hypodermic injection of morphine with resultant spasm of the sphincter of Oddi.[95]

Tests should be made for HB_sAg in all cases of jaundice that appear to be of hepatocellular origin, and if indicated, determinations should be made of HB_s antibody, HB_c antibody, E antigen and antibody, and IgM-A antibody. The mitochondrial antibody test, while not specific for primary biliary cirrhosis, has proved of inestimable value in differentiating this disorder from extrahepatic obstructive jaundice,[96] thus virtually eliminating the need for laparotomy to rule out obstructive jaundice.

PROTHROMBIN RESPONSE TO VITAMIN K

Four of the clotting factors in plasma appear to be synthesized exclusively in the liver: prothrombin, Factor VII (pro-SPCA or proconvertin), Factor X (Stuart–Power factor), and Christmas factor (plasma thromboplastin component). Their formation depends on the normal absorption of vitamin K from the intestine and the functional integrity of the liver cells. Three of these factors (prothrombin, Factor VII, and Factor X) influence the one-stage prothrombin time. Thus, a long prothrombin time may be due to the exclusion of bile from the intestine or severe liver injury. If the prothrombin time of the blood of an icteric patient is markedly prolonged (that is, if the prothrombic activity is under 40% of normal) and becomes normal within 24 hours after parenteral administration of vitamin K, it is probable that liver cell function is reasonably good and that the jaundice is due to extrahepatic obstruction. The failure of the prothrombin time to shorten under these circumstances would indicate the presence of parenchymal liver disease. An adequate amount of vitamin K is provided by 10 mg of menadione sodium bisulphite (Hykinone) given subcutaneously. In order to exclude intrinsic errors in the test itself, it is best to determine the blood prothrombin time on two separate days, both before and after the administration of the vitamin K.

DUODENAL DRAINAGE

Although infrequently employed nowadays, duodenal drainage may be of value in the differential diagnosis of jaundice by furnishing bile for microscopic examination. The finding of calcium bilirubinate and cholesterol crystals would be suggestive of cholelithiasis. Cytologic examination of the sediments of duodenal aspiration may prove of value in the diagnosis of tumors of the gallbladder, the extrahepatitic bile ducts, ampulla or Vater, or pancreas.[22]

MINILAPAROTOMY

Minilaparotomy has been best performed by a selected team using a 5-cm midline subxyphoid incision, expediting the performance of transhepatic cholangiography, liver biopsy, and omentoportography with a high degree of success in diagnosis and a low complication rate. The procedure, among other things, has the advantage of permitting guided needle biopsy of the liver in the presence of abnormal blood coagulation, ascites, or extrahepatic obstructive jaundice.[23]

RADIOLOGIC PROCEDURES

A plain film of the abdomen may reveal enlargement of the liver and spleen, pancreatic calcification, gallstones, a ground-glass appearance suggestive of ascites, or an elevated right diaphragm indicative of hepatic tumor or abscess. The mere demonstration of gallstones does not necessarily implicate them as the cause of the jaundice. The use of the conventional gastrointestinal x-ray examination in patients with suspected extrahepatic biliary obstruction has dwindled considerably in view of the advances in biliary tree imagery, but it nevertheless still possesses value. It may furnish evidence of an enlarged liver by demonstrating displacement of the stomach posteriorly or to the left, or displacement of the hepatic flexure of the colon downward. A pancreatic tumor may produce anterior displacement of the duodenal loop, downward displacement of the duodenal-jejunal juncture, compression or invasion of the duodenum or the stomach, or widening of the duodenal loop. Periampullary tumor may produce a filling defect in the descending duodenum or Frostberg's reversed-3 sign (Fig. 24-2). The radiologic examination may help to confirm the diagnosis of metastatic hepatic tumor by revealing a primary site.

Cholecystography is virtually valueless in cases of

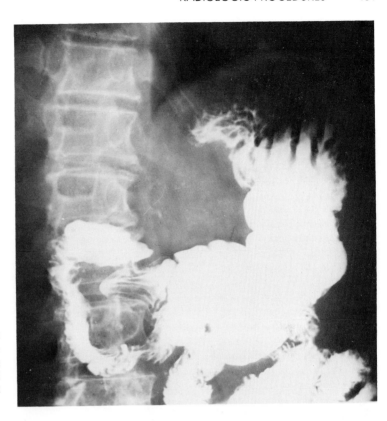

Fig. 24-2. (W.B. 539). Reversed-3 sign in the descending portion of the duodenum with clinical evidence suggestive of carcinoma of the ampulla of Vater. (From Schiff L: Differential Diagnosis of Jaundice. Chicago, Year Book Publishers, 1946)

jaundice, since the liver's impaired ability to excrete the dye interferes with gallbladder filling. In the presence of jaundice the HIDA scan has been found most useful in the diagnosis of acute cholecystitis.[14,15] Intravenous cholangiography is being replaced largely by superior and less hazardous percutaneous and retrograde cholangiography.

PTC (Figs. 24-3 to 24-5) and endoscopic retrograde cholangiopancreatography (ERCP) (Figs. 24-6, 24-7) have proved quite safe and of great value not only in delineating the bile ducts but also in depicting the site and frequently, the presumed cause of bile duct obstruction, especially by common duct stone or tumor of the head of the pancreas.[16–19] On the other hand, demonstration of a normal biliary tree would exclude common duct stones with rare exceptions.[97] ERCP is preferred in some clinics but requires more experience and skill. It has the advantage of outlining the pancreatic duct in addition to the bile ducts and visualizing ampullary tumors and the constricted ducts of a sclerosing cholangitis more readily than PTC. It is not contraindicated by blood coagulation defects. On the other hand, when ERCP demonstrates a defect in the distal duct with failure of visualization of the proximal duct system, a supplementary transhepatic approach would

be indicated. A defect owing to iatrogenic stenosis may be indistinguishable from one owing to a tumor at the bifurcation of the common hepatic duct (Figs. 24-8, 24-9), both being best visualized by PTC. Bile aspirated at the time of the percutaneous cholangiography may yield organisms not recovered on repeated blood cultures. Endoscopic cholangiographic diagnosis of ascaris in the common bile duct has been reported.[98]

Abdominal ultrasonography (Figs. 24-10, 24-11) and computed tomography (CT—Figs. 24-12, 24-13) are being used increasingly in cases of jaundice and have the advantage of noninvasiveness. The former may prove fruitless in the obese and gaseously distended, while the latter is least helpful in the very thin. They are most valuable in visualizing distended bile ducts, especially intrahepatic, and in the case of the CT scan, tumors of the pancreas. The ultrasonogram is very efficient in revealing stones in the gallbladder but of little help in depicting ductal calculi.

Our own practice is to employ abdominal ultrasonography as a screening procedure when obstructive jaundice is suspected. If the ducts are dilated (Fig. 24-10, we proceed with PTC prior to surgery. Otherwise we may employ ERCP, and if this proves normal, needle

Text continues on p. 433

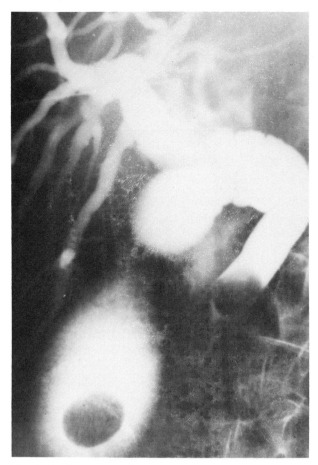

Fig. 24-3. Stone in gallbladder and common bile duct delineated by PTC. (Courtesy of Raul Pereiras)

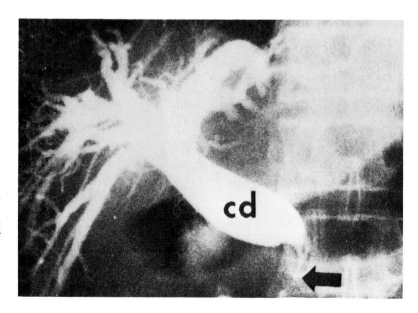

Fig. 24-4. Carcinoma of the pancreas delineated by PTC. Arrow shows the stricture of the common duct (*cd*) by the pancreatic carcinoma. (From Pereiras R et al: Relief of malignant destructive jaundice by percutaneous insertion of a permanent prosthesis in the biliary tree. Ann Int Med 89:589, 1978)

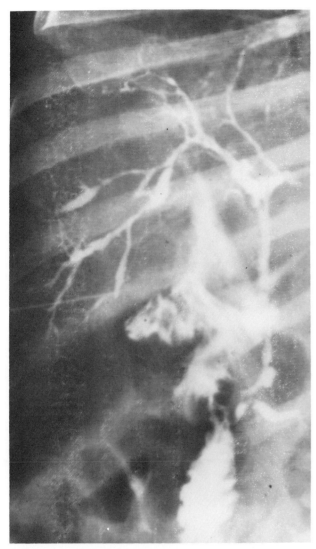

Fig. 24-5. Sclerosing cholangitis delineated by PTC. (From Pereiras R: Special radiologic procedures in liver diseases. In Schiff L, Schiff ER (eds): Diseases of the Liver, 5th ed. Philadelphia, JB Lippincott, 1982)

biopsy of the liver. If a definitive diagnosis is still lacking, and especially if the clinical features favor obstructive jaundice, the author recommends exploratory laparotomy.

NEEDLE BIOPSY OF THE LIVER

Needle biopsy of the liver is being used more sparingly than formerly in the differential diagnosis of jaundice owing largely to the contributions of biliary tract im-

agery. Though its hazard in obstructive jaundice has been exaggerated, it should not be used in the presence of a Courvoisier gallbladder because of the reliability of this finding as a sign of extrahepatic obstructive jaundice; the great increase in intrabiliary pressure it reflects would predispose to bile peritonitis on liver puncture. Another reason for the decline in the use of liver biopsy in the jaundiced patient is the frequent difficulty in distinguishing intrahepatic from extrahepatic cholestasis. Nevertheless, the procedure retains its value in the diagnosis of alcoholic and chronic hepatitis and primary biliary cirrhosis. The changes in alcoholic hepatitis, once considered pathognomonic, have been described following jejuno-ileal bypass and in nonalcoholics.[99–101]

Sampling errors in needle specimens of the liver are most likely to occur in cases of cirrhosis, chronic hepatitis, and in a third or more cases of neoplastic invasion. A sample obtained from one area may be interpreted as normal, from another as questionable cirrhosis, and from a third as micronodular cirrhosis.[102] Soloway and associates have observed five instances in which a biopsy specimen did not show cirrhosis but was preceded and followed by specimens that did,[103] and Edmondson has had a somewhat similar experience.*

CONCLUSION

Clinical examination of the jaundiced patient retains its importance in providing valuable clues to accurate diagnosis and to selection of the more helpful laboratory procedures to the exclusion of the unnecessary or least helpful. Not only is appropriate therapy thus expedited, but the cost and hazards of medical care are reduced concomitantly.

Repeated abdominal examination may detect abnormalities overlooked because of a hurried and less perceptive examination or poor abdominal relaxation.

The advances in the radiologic imaging of the liver and biliary tract have been great and will in all likelihood continue to expand, but they should neither replace nor lessen the importance of the clinical examination. After all, there is, as yet, no substitute for the patient!

Finally, keep in mind the words of Nellis B. Foster: "... The most brilliant discoveries in therapeutics or the most skillful surgery avail nothing if the patient's disease is not correctly diagnosed."[104]

*Edmondson H: Personal communication.

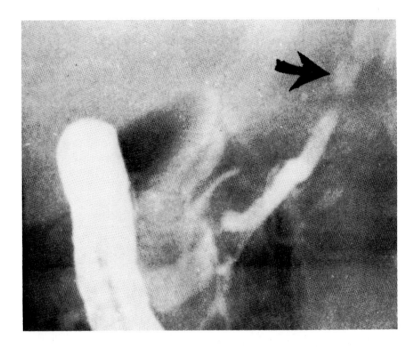

Fig. 24-6. Carcinoma of pancreas delineated by ERCP. There is abrupt and irregular termination of the pancreatic duct in the head of the pancreas; contrast fills a small cavity (*arrow*). (From Epstein RJ, Protell RL, Silverstein FE et al: The role of ERCP in the diagnosis of pancreatic malignancy presenting as steatorrhea. Gastrointest Endosc 26:98–101, 1980)

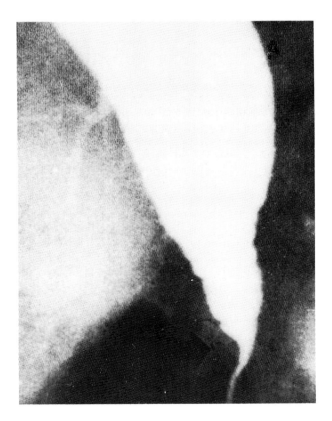

Fig. 24-7. Chronic pancreatitis delineated by ERCP shows the characteristic smooth, symmetrical narrowing of the intrahepatic portion of the common bile duct. (From Gremillion DF Jr, Johnson LF, Commarer RC et al: Biliary obstruction: A complication of chronic pancreatitis diagnosed by endoscopic retrograde cholangiopancreatography (ERCP). Dig Dis Sci 24:145, 1979)

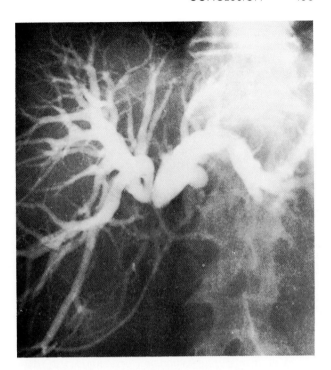

Fig. 24-8. Cholangiogram of patient with carcinoma of bile duct arising at confluence of right and left hepatic ducts. (From Longmire WP: When is cholangitis sclerosing? Am J Surg 135:312–320, 1978)

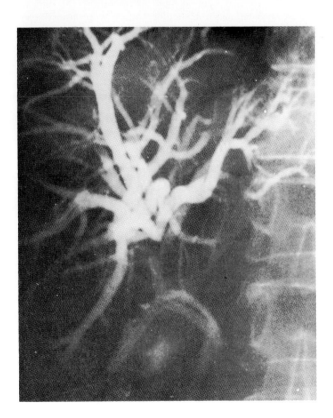

Fig. 24-9. Cholangiogram of iatrogenic stenosis of hepatic ducts at hilus of liver. (From Longmire WP: When is cholangitis sclerosing? Am J Surg 135:312–320, 1978)

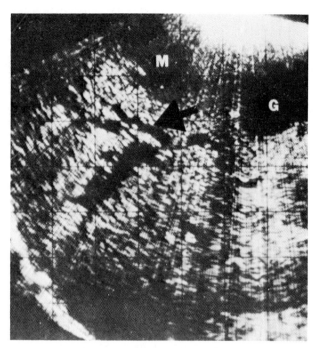

Fig. 24-10. Parasagittal section of liver demonstrating distended biliary canaliculi (*arrow*). At operation, the lymph nodes involved with testicular tumor were found obstructing the common bile duct. Superior to the gallbladder (*G*) is a liver metastasis (*M*). (From Taylor KJW, Rosenfeld AT: Grey-scale ultrasonography in the differential diagnosis of jaundice. Arch Surg 112:822, 1977)

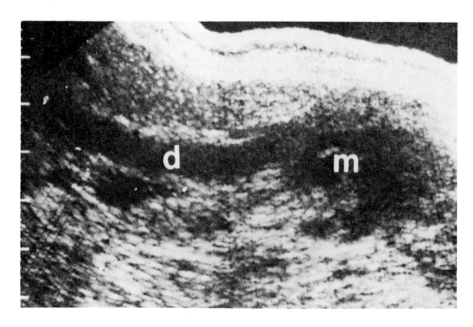

Fig. 24-11. Dilated common bile duct (*d*) ending in solid mass (*m*). (From Zeman R et al: Ultrasound demonstration of anicteric dilatation of the biliary tree. Radiol 134:689, 1980)

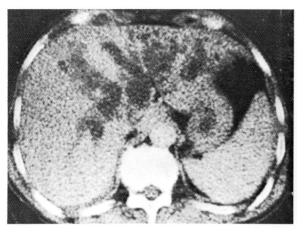
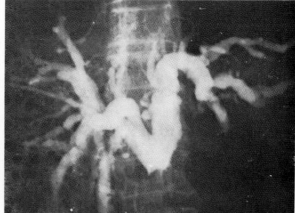

Fig. 24-12. Severe dilatation of the intrahepatic bile ducts in carcinoma of common hepatic duct. (From Shimizu H, Masohiro I et al: The diagnostic accuracy of computed tomography in obstructive biliary disease: A comparative evaluation with direct cholangiography. Radiol 138:411–16, 1981)

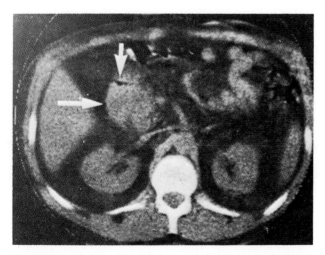

Fig. 24-13. Carcinoma of the pancreas. Mass of soft-tissue density in head of pancreas (*arrows*). (From Morris AI, Fawcett RA, Wood R et al: Computed tomography, ultrasound and cholestatic jaundice. Gut 19:685–688, 1978)

REFERENCES

1. **Bean NB:** Osler Aphorisms. New York, Henry Schuman, 1950

2. **Billing BH:** Bilirubin Metabolism. In Schiff L, Schiff ER: (eds): Diseases of the Liver, 5th ed. Philadelphia, JB Lippincott, 1982

3. **Dubin IN:** Chronic idiopathic jaundice: A review of 50 cases. Am J Med 24:268, 1958

4. **Rotor HB et al:** Familial non-hemolytic jaundice: With direct Van den Bergh reaction. Acta Med Phillip 5:37, 1948

5. **Schiff L et al:** Familial non-hemolytic jaundice with conjugated bilirubin in the serum: A case study. N Engl J med 260:1315, 1959

6. **Taylor KJW et al:** Diagnostic accuracy of gray-scale ultrasonography for the jaundiced patient: A report of 275 cases. Arch Intern Med 139:60, 1979

7. **Taylor KJW et al:** Ultrasonography, scintigraphy and computerized axial tomography of the liver. In Schiff L Schiff ER (eds): Diseases of the Liver, 5th ed. Philadelphia, JB Lippincott, 1982

8. **Wild SR et al:** Grey-scale ultrasonography and percutaneous transhepatic cholangiography in biliary tract disease. Br Med J 281:1524, 1980

9. **Cooperberg PL, Burhenne HS:** Real-time ultrasonography: Diagnostic technique of choice in calculous gall bladder disease: N Engl J Med 302:1277, 1980

10. **Ferruci JT Jr:** Body ultrasonography. N Engl J Med 300:590, 1979

11. **Morris AI et al:** Computerized tomography, ultrasound and cholestatic jaundice. Gut 19:685–688, 1978

12. **Shimizu H et al:** The diagnostic accuracy of computed tomography in obstructive biliary disease: A comparative evaluation with direct cholangiography. Radiology 138:411–416, 1981

13. **Haaga JR et al:** CT guided biopsy. Cleve Clin 44:27, 1977

14. **Harvey E et al:** Tc 99m HIDA: A new radio-pharmaceutical for hepatobiliary imaging. J Nucl Med 16:533, 1975

15. **Weisman HS et al:** Cholescintigraphy, ultrasonography and computerized tomography in the evaluation of biliary tract disorders. Semin Nucl Med 9:22–35, 1979

16. **Okuda K et al:** Non-surgical, percutaneous transhepatic cholangiography: Diagnostic significance in medical problems of the liver. American Journal of Digestive Diseases 19:21, 1974

17. **Pereiras R Jr et al:** Percutaneous transhepatic cholangiography with the "Skinny" needle: A rapid, simple and accurate method in the diagnosis of cholestasis. Ann Int Med 86:562, 1977

18. **Harbin WP et al:** Transhepatic cholangiography: complications and use patterns of the fine needle technique. Radiology 135:15, 1980

19. **Zimmon DR:** ERCP for the diagnosis and management of liver disease. In Schiff L, Schiff ER (eds): Diseases of the Liver, 5th ed. Philadelphia, JB Lippincott, 1982

20. **Chalmers TC et al:** Evaluation of a four day ACTH test in the differential diagnosis of jaundice. Gastroenterology 30:894, 1956

21. **Williams R, Billing BH:** Action of steroid therapy in jaundice. Lancet 2:392, 1961

22. **Raskin HF et al:** Gastrointestinal cancer definitive diagnoses by exfoliative cytology. Arch Surg 76:507, 1958

23. **Strack RP et al:** An integrated procedure for the rapid diagnosis of biliary obstruction, portal hypertension, and liver disease of uncertain etiology. N Engl J Med 285:1225, 1971

24. **Schenker S et al:** Differential diagnosis of jaundice: A report of a prospective study of 61 proved cases. American Journal of Digestive Diseases 7:449, 1962

25. **Lumeng L et al:** Final report of a blended prospective study comparing current non-invasive approaches in the differential diagnosis of jaundice (Abstr). Gastroenterology 78:1312, 1980

26. **Summerskill WHJ, Walshe JM:** Benign recurrent intrahepatic "obstructive jaundice." Lancet 2:686, 1959

27. **Spiegel EL et al:** Benign recurrent intrahepatic cholestasis, with response to cholestyramine. Am J Med 39:682, 1965

28. **Koff RS et al:** Viral hepatitis in a group of Boston hospitals. III. Importance of exposure to shell fish in a non-epidemic area. N Engl J Med 276:703, 1967

29. **Koff RS, Sear HS:** Internal temperature of steamed clams. N Engl J Med 276:137, 1967

30. **Zimmerman HJ:** Effects of aspirin and acetaminophen on the liver. Arch Intern Med 141:333, 1981

31. **Black M et al:** Isoniazid-associated hepatitis in 114 patients. Gastroenterology 69:289, 1975

32. **Maddrey WC, Boitnott JK:** Severe hepatitis from methyldopa. Gastroenterology 68:351, 1975

33. **Editorial:** Post-transfusion hepatitis. Br Med J 283:1, 1981

34. **Zuckerman AJ:** Acute viral hepatitis. J R Coll Physicians Lond 15(2):88, 1981

35. **Orrego H et al:** Reliability of assessment of alcohol intake based on personal interview in a liver clinic. Lancet 22(29):1354, 1979

36. **Morgenstern L:** Post-operative jaundice. In L Schiff (ed): Diseases of the Liver, 4th ed. JB Lippincott, Philadelphia, 1975

37. **Schmid M et al:** Benign post-operative intrahepatic cholestasis. N Engl J Med 272:545, 1965

38. **Kantrowitz PA et al:** Severe post-operative hyperbilirubinemia simulating obstructive jaundice. N Engl J Med 276:591, 1967

39. **Way LW:** Biliary stricture (Abstr). In Hepatobiliary Disease in Clinical Practice, University of Miami, March 2–4, 1978

40. **Pickles WN:** Epidemiology in Country Practice. Baltimore, Williams & Wilkins, 1939

41. **Glenn F:** Common Duct Stones. Springfield, Ill, Charles C Thomas, 1975

42. **Taub S, Schiff L:** Common duct stone and cholangitis simulating fever of unknown origin. South Med J 74:230, 1981

43. **Chauffard MA:** Le cancer de corps de pancreas. Bull Acad Nat Med 60:242, 1908

44. **Fenster F Klatskin G:** Manifestations of metastatic tumors of the liver: A study of eighty-one patients subjected to needle biopsy. Am J Med 31:238, 1961

45. **Altemeier WA et al:** Sclerosing carcinoma of the major intrahepatic bile ducts. Arch Surg 75:450–461, 1957

46. **Altemeier WA, Culbertson WR:** Sclerosing carcinoma of the hepatic bile ducts. Surg Clin North Am 53:1229, 1973

47. **Holubitzky IB, McKenzie AD:** Primary sclerosing cholangitis of the extrahepatic bile ducts. Can J Surg 7:277, 1964

48. **Longmire WP:** When is cholangitis sclerosing? Am J Surg 135:312, 1978

49. **Warren K, Tan E:** Diseases of the gall bladder and bile ducts. In Schiff L, Schiff ER (ed): Diseases of the Liver, 5th ed. Philadelphia, JB Lippincott, 1982

50. **Budd G:** On Diseases of the Liver, Philadelphia, Lea & Blanchard, 1846

51. **Schoenfield LJ:** The relationship of bile acids to pruritus in hepatobiliary disease. In Schiff et al (eds) Bile Salt Metabolism. Springfield, Ill, Charles C Thomas, 1969

52. **Krejs GJ, Haemmerle WP:** Jaundice during pregnancy. In Schiff L, Schiff ER (eds): Diseases of the Liver, 5th ed. Philadelphia, JB Lippincott, 1982

53. **Osborn EC et al:** Serum bile acid levels in liver disease. Lancet 2:1049, 1959

54. **Javitt NB:** Cholestatic liver disease: Mechanisms, diagnosis and therapy. Adv Intern Med 25:147, 1980

55. **Javitt NR:** Bile acids and hepatobiliary disease. In Schiff L, Schiff ER (eds): Diseases of the Liver, 5th ed. Philadelphia, JB Lippincott, 1982

56. **Schiff L:** The differential diagnosis of jaundice. Postgrad Med 41:39, 1967

57. **Sandblom P:** Hemobilia (Biliary Tract Hemorrhage):

History, Pathology, Diagnosis, Treatment. Springfield, Ill, Charles C Thomas 1972

58. **Sanford JB:** Leptospirosis. In Schiff L, Schiff ER (eds): Diseases of the Liver, 5th ed. Philadelphia, JB Lippincott, 1982

59. **Sternlieb I, Scheinberg IH:** Chronic hepatitis as a first manifestation of Wilson's disease. Ann Int Med 76:59, 1972

60. **Fleming CR et al:** Pigmented corneal rings in non-Wilsonian liver disease. Ann Int Med 86:285, 1977

61. **Heath CW et al:** Leptospirosis in the United States. N Engl J Med 273:857, 1965

62. **Bean WB:** The cutaneous arterial spider: Survey Medicine 24:243, 1945

63. **Bean WB:** Vascular Spiders and Related Lesions of the Skin. Springfield, Ill, Charles C Thomas, 1958

64. **Brick IB, Palmer ED:** Esophageal varices and vascular spiders (nevi araneosi) in cirrhosis of the liver JAMA 155:8, 1954

65. **Watson CJ:** Jaundice: Compelling clinical signs and some differential laboratory aids. In Najarian JS, Delaney JP: Surgery of the Liver, Pancreas and Biliary Tract. New York, Stratton Intercontinental, 1975

66. **Sherlock S:** Diseases of the Liver and Biliary System, 5th ed. Blackwell Scientific Publications, 1975

67. **Zieve L:** Hepatic encephalopathy. In Schiff L, Schiff ER (ed): Diseases of the Liver, 5th ed. Philadelphia, JB Lippincott, 1982

68. **Reynolds TB:** The "butterfly" sign in patients with chronic jaundice and pruritus. Ann Int Med 78:545, 1973

69. **Sherlock S:** Cirrhosis of the liver. Postgrad Med 26:472, 1950

70. **Schiff L:** One feel of the liver. Gastroenterology 26:506, 1954

71. **Fleischner FG, Sayegh V:** Assessment of the size of the liver: Roentgenologic considerations. N Engl J Med 259:271, 1958

72. **Fred HL, Brown GR:** The hepatic friction rub N Engl J Med 266:554, 1962

73. **Nicholas GG, Williams R:** Friction rub in acute cholecystitis: An unusual finding. JAMA 218:13, 1971

74. **Clair H et al:** Abdominal arterial murmurs in liver disease. Lancet 2:516, 1966

75. **Konar NR et al:** Murmurs over liver in cases of severe anemia. Br Med J 4:154, 1967

76. **Schiff L:** Absence of a palpable liver: A sign of value in excluding obstructive jaundice due to pancreatic cancer. Gastroenterology 32:1143, 1957

77. **Flood CA et al:** The differential diagnosis of jaundice: A study of 235 cases of nonhemolytic jaundice due to carcinoma, calculus in the common bile duct and liver degeneration. Am J Med Sci 185:358, 1953

78. **Galambos J:** Cirrhosis. Philadelphia, WB Saunders, 1979

79. **Duff GL:** The clinical and pathological features of carcinoma of the body and tail of the pancreas. Bull Johns Hopkins Hosp 65:69, 1939

80. **Cameron JL et al:** Pancreatic ascites. Surg Gynec Obstet 125:328, 1967

81. **Boyer TD et al:** Diagnostic value of ascitic fluid, lactic dehydrogenase, protein and WBC levels. Arch Intern Med 138:1103, 1978

82. **Goldberg BB:** Ultrasonic evaluation of intraperitoneal fluid. JAMA 235:2427, 1976

83. **Conn H, Fessel JM:** Spontaneous bacterial peritonitis in cirrhosis: Variations on a theme. Medicine 50:161, 1971

84. **Hoefs JC:** Increase in ascites white blood cell and protein concentrations during diuresis in patients with chronic liver disease. Hepatology 1:249, 1981

85. **Kenney WE:** The association of carcinoma of the body and tail of the pancreas with multiple venous thrombi. Surgery 14:600, 1943

86. **Zieve L:** Jaundice, hyperlipemia and hemolytic anemia: A heretofore unrecognized syndrome associated with alcoholic fatty liver and cirrhosis. Ann Intern Med 48:471, 1958

87. **Young II:** Serum 5-nucleotidase: Characterization and evaluation in disease states. Ann NY Acad Sci 73:357, 1958

88. **Sherlock S, Scheuer PJ:** The presentation and diagnosis of 100 patients with primary biliary cirrhosis. N Engl J Med 289:674, 1973

89. **Fleming LC et al:** Asymptomatic primary biliary cirrhosis. Mayo Clin Proc 53:587, 1978

90. **Christensen E et al:** Clinical pattern and course of asymptomatic and course of disease in primary biliary cirrhosis based on an analysis of 236 patients. Gastroenterology 78:236, 1980

91. **Roll J et al:** Long term survival of asymptomatic and symptomatic patients with primary biliary cirrhosis. Gastroenterology 79:1050, 1980

92. **James O et al:** Primary biliary cirrhosis: A revised clinical spectrum. Lancet 1:1278, 1981

93. **Schiff L:** Clinical Pearls and Perils. J Fla Med Assoc 69:959, 1978

94. **Abbruzzese A, Jeffrey RL:** Marked elevation of serum glutamic oxaloacetic transaminase and lactic dehydrogenase activity in chronic extrahepatic biliary disease. Am J Dig Dis 14:332, 1969

95. **Burckhardt D, Ladue JS:** Provocation of serum enzyme activity in cholecystectomized patients given opiates. Am J Gastroenterol 46:43, 1966

96. **Doniach D, Walker G:** Progress report mitochondrial antibodies (AMA) Gut 15:664, 1974

97. **Greenwald RA et al:** Jaundice, choledocholithiasis, and a non-dilated common duct. JAMA 240:1983, 1978

98. **Kaplowitz N:** Cholestatic liver disease. Hosp Pract 13(8):83, 1978

99. **Peters R et al:** Post-jejunoileal by-pass hepatic disease. Am J Clin Pathol 63:318, 1975

100. **Miller DJ et al:** Non-alcoholic liver disease mimicking alcoholic hepatitis and cirrhosis. Gastroenterology 77:A27, 1979

101. **Adler M, Schaffner F:** Fatty liver, hepatitis and cirrhosis in obese patients. Am J Med 67:811, 1979

102. **Thaler H:** Leberbiopsie. Berlin, Springer–Verlag, 1969

103. **Soloway et al:** Observer error and sampling variability tested in evaluation of hepatitis and cirrhosis by liver biopsy. American Journal of Digestive Diseases 17:1082, 1971

104. **Foster NB:** The Examination of Patients. Philadelphia, WB Saunders, 1923

perature. Furthermore, it is apparent that body temperature varies within different regions of the body, the inner core being the warmest and the skin of the extremities the coolest. Consequently, any discussion of the normality of body temperature is meaningless unless one specifies the site at which temperature is taken. Clinically, for convenience, body temperature is measured either orally or rectally.

ORAL TEMPERATURE

Although oral temperature in man is widely regarded as being a constant at the proverbial 98.6°F (37°C), many studies have shown that this is not so and that in any population of healthy individuals considerable variations exist. While both the findings and conditions of these studies varied somewhat, and in some instances morning temperatures were taken before arising whereas in others temperatures were taken after breakfast and activity, it is clear that normal oral temperature differs among individuals. The mean value for oral temperature in several of these studies was 98.34°F ± 0.47°F SD.[23] It can be assumed, then, that in a normal distribution for a population of people (with the conventional mean of 98.6°F), the range of oral temperatures in normal, healthy adults extends from 97°F to 100.2°F.[24]

RECTAL TEMPERATURE

Rectal temperature is usually somewhat higher than oral, the average difference being about 0.7°F. However, there are comparatively wide variations from person to person, and it is not unusual to find a healthy person who has a higher oral than rectal temperature. Rectal temperature is somewhat less variable and has been generally assumed to be a more accurate and reliable index of internal body or "blood" temperature. From a clinical standpoint rectal temperatures are certainly preferable with children or others who cannot keep their mouths closed while temperatures are being taken. Furthermore, oral temperatures may be grossly disturbed immediately after drinking hot or cold liquids.

TYMPANIC MEMBRANE AND ESOPHAGEAL TEMPERATURES

In experimental studies on thermoregulation, tympanic membrane or esophageal temperature is generally used as a measure of core temperature. It has been claimed that these temperatures reflect alterations in body heat balance more accurately and rapidly than do oral or rectal temperatures, presumably because they closely approximate the temperature of blood perfus-

ing the hypothalamus. Benzinger developed a thermocouple that fits within the ear and rests next to the tympanic membrane, anatomically quite close to the hypothalamus.[4] Esophageal temperature is generally measured by a thermocouple inserted through the nasopharynx to the level of the heart.[25] By this means, core temperature can be measured at the aortic arch, which, in turn, closely reflects the temperature of the arterial blood perfusing the brain and hypothalamus. Although uncomfortable to insert, esophageal thermocouples are more readily tolerated than those on the tympanic membrane.

DIURNAL VARIATION

There is a daily rhythmic change in body temperature, amounting to as much as 2°F or 3°F. The highest point is usually reached between 8 PM and 11 PM and the lowest during sleep between 4 AM and 6 AM.[26] This variation does not depend upon the environmental temperature and is not abolished by confinement to bed or by fasting. However, it is likely that the effects of muscular activity and digestion of food do contribute to higher temperatures during waking hours and that lower temperatures occur during sleep when activity is at a minimum. It has been found that the pattern of diurnal variation may be inverted in persons who work at night (nurses, watchmen, and so forth).[27] This alteration in the temperature rhythm is not uniform in all people; some readily adapt to a new cycle, whereas others retain their former cycle for weeks.

Finally, we should note that occasional normal individuals have higher morning than evening temperatures, while others show a rapid morning rise, then a plateau until after going to sleep at night.

BODY TEMPERATURE IN CHILDREN

In infancy the regulation of body temperature is imperfect, and marked variations occur, depending on changes in environment. Because of this, babies must be protected against excessive cold or heat. The normal diurnal temperature rhythm becomes established some time during the second year of life, usually about the time the child begins to walk. Some lability of temperature regulation persists until about the time of puberty. Van der Bogert and Moravec studied the temperatures in more than 700 healthy children and noted oral temperatures higher than 98.6°F at some time in 43% of the children aged 7 and 8, but in the group between 13 and 15 years of age only 8% ever had temperatures higher than 98.6°F.[28] The effect of exercise on body temperature is particularly marked in children; it is not uncommon for them to have temperatures of 100°F after ordinary play, such as baseball.

This fact should be kept in mind in estimating the significance of fever in children.

BODY TEMPERATURE IN THE ELDERLY

The average body temperature is somewhat lower in the aged and is more likely to be low in cold weather. It has been recognized only recently that a proportion of the elderly population runs a significant health risk in the cold because of a condition called accidental hypothermia.[29] This can occur even in moderately cool environments (<65°F) when body temperature is not maintained and falls below 95°F. The cause of this condition and why only a small portion of the over-65 population (~1%) is susceptible are unknown. However, it has been postulated that with increasing age thermoregulatory abilities are progressively blunted so that vasoconstriction and shivering are insufficient to sustain body temperature, even in moderately cold, stressed, elderly individuals. In the current era of high energy prices and an emphasis on energy conservation, physicians should be on the lookout for cases of accidental hypothermia among the elderly, especially during cold weather.

BODY TEMPERATURE DURING THE MENSTRUAL CYCLE

There is a rhythmic variation in body temperature associated with the menstrual cycle. Immediately before the onset of menstruation the temperature falls 0.5° to 0.75°F below its previous level. This relatively low temperature is maintained until the time of ovulation, which is usually about the 13th or 14th day of the cycle. Then there is a rise of 0.5° to 0.75°F, which is maintained until just before the next menstrual period. Such variations may be exaggerated in women who have a fever from another cause, such as pulmonary tuberculosis. Anovulatory women have no cyclic temperature change and in them it has been reported that estrogen therapy depresses body temperature whereas progesterone provokes a rise. Therefore, it has been assumed that endogenous estrogens and progesterone are responsible for the biphasic basal temperature of the menstrual cycle. However, certain clinical observations indicate that body temperature change does not always coincide with these phases of the ovarian follicle cycle.[30]

BODY TEMPERATURE DURING PREGNANCY

Early in pregnancy there is a slight rise in average temperature. About the fourth month of gestation a gradual fall begins, and this continues until parturition, when there is a quick return to the normal level.[31]

LIMITS OF BODY TEMPERATURE COMPATIBLE WITH LIFE

LOW TEMPERATURES

Formerly it was believed that life would cease if the body temperature fell below about 90°F. Smith and Fay have shown, however, that by administering sedatives and then applying cold, the body temperature can be reduced to from 75°F to 80°F and maintained there for days without evident harm.[32] An extreme example of hypothermia is reported by Laufman.[33] The subject, under influence of alcohol, lay unconscious for many hours out of doors in cold weather. When brought to a hospital the rectal temperature, obtained 90 minutes after warming had begun, was 64.4°F. It was calculated that on admission the rectal temperature must have been in the vicinity of 61°F. This is the lowest recorded internal body temperature in a patient who survived.

Profound hypothermia with a fall in rectal temperature to 87.8°F has been reported in a patient with systemic lupus erythematosus treated with cortisone.[34] There were signs of active heat loss with sweating and vasodilatation despite the low temperature, which was felt to be caused by the action of steroid on the thermoregulatory center. ACTH and cortisone also have a marked antipyretic effect in many febrile states, presumably because, like other antipyretics, they have a direct action on the hypothalamus. Certain drugs affect normal body temperature as well, as several (such as chlorpromazine) have been used in conjunction with cooling to induce hypothermia in surgery.[35]

HIGH TEMPERATURES

In the medical literature there are reports of fantastic fevers, 130°F or even 150°F. These are undoubtedly the results of fraud or error on the part of either the patient or the physician. Experiments in animals and acceptable observations in human beings indicate that living tissues are irreversibly damaged at temperatures above the region of 115°F. Richet placed the upper possible limit at 114.8°F (46°C), and this has been endorsed by MacNeal after a careful study of the evidence.[36] There are a number of acceptable reports of temperatures as high as 112°F or 113°F with recovery. In a case of staphylococcal septicemia the fever ranged between 104°F and 112°F continuously for three months.[37] More recently, Simon has reviewed the histories of 28 patients with temperatures ranging from 106°F to 108°F admitted over a five-year period to a single hospital. Infection alone or in conjunction with thermoregulatory defects accounted for two thirds of these fevers, with gram-negative bacteremia the most common cause. Fe-

ver in most patients responded well to simple measures of antipyretics and cooling by various routes. There was little evidence of direct tissue damage caused by fever itself.[38]

As has been pointed out by DuBois, there is a sort of temperature "ceiling" in most febrile disease at about 105°F or 106°F.[39] It would appear that the body's thermostat can rarely be disturbed sufficiently to permit an elevation much beyond this level.

FEVER

TYPES AND TERMINOLOGY

Fever is an elevation of the body temperature due to disease. As was pointed out earlier, thermoregulation is still functional during fever, but both the heat-producing and heat-dissipating mechanisms appear to be activated at body temperature thresholds that are higher than normal. This causes body temperature to be maintained and regulated at a higher level than is normal.

Pyrexia is a term that is now largely confined to the British literature. Though usually considered synonymous with fever, some writers have used it to indicate elevations in body temperature not resulting from infection.

Hyperthermia is a generalized term that physiologists have applied to all situations in which body temperature is elevated above its normal range.[1] Hyperthermia may be mild to moderate during physical exercise or severe during work in hot and humid environments, in fever, or when heat-dissipative mechanisms are impaired due to disease or damage to the CNS. In clinical medicine the term "hyperthermia" is usually restricted to those situations in which body temperature exceeds limits ordinarily attained in fever (105°F–106°F).

An *intermittent* or *quotidian fever* is one in which the temperature falls to normal and rises again each day.

In a *remittent fever* there is a marked variation in the temperature level each day, but the low point is still above the normal line.

A *relapsing fever* is one in which short, febrile periods are interspersed by periods of one or more days of normal temperature. Figure 25-2 illustrates this in a case of rat-bite fever.

A *hectic* or *septic fever* is an intermittent fever in which the daily oscillations are very large; it often is associated with chills and sweating.

THERMOREGULATION DURING FEVER

As early as 1875, von Liebermeister observed that the internal body temperature appeared to be regulated at a new, higher level during fever.[40] Despite the periodically recurring contention that fever is produced by a decrease or loss of central thermosensitivity, both clinical and experimental evidence support von Liebermeister's view.[41,42] It has been shown that man can still thermoregulate effectively, albeit at a higher body temperature, both during exposure to high ambient temperatures[43] and during exercise.[42] Thus, pyrogens appear to raise the thermoregulatory set point in the hypothalamus so that body temperature is maintained at a higher than normal level during fever. Such a phenomenon may be likened to the response of a house heating system when its thermostat setting is increased. After the setting is raised, the furnace will increase its heat production until the room temperature attains the new, higher level "called for" by the thermostat. Thereafter, it will cycle on and off as before, except that it will maintain the room at a higher temperature than before.

Direct heating of the hypothalamus can suppress or modify the febrile response to bacterial pyrogens, presumably by supplying locally the increase in temperature "called for" by the action of the pyrogen.[44] Experiments that have compared hypothalamic thermosensitivity in animals in both afebrile and febrile conditions indicate that thermosensitivity remains unaltered but that the threshold temperatures for the

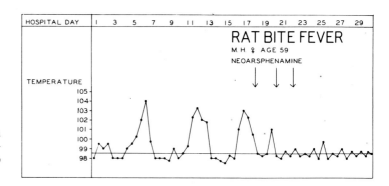

Fig. 25-2. Rat bite fever, due to infection with *Spirillum minus,* is an example of a relapsing fever. Short febrile periods are separated by two or three days of normal temperature.

thermoregulatory responses (*i.e.*, shivering, sweating, or vasodilatation) are elevated.[45] The mechanisms that raise body temperature after an injection of pyrogen depend on the thermal environment. In the cold, the extra heat in man is produced by vigorous shivering; in neutral to warm environments it is produced by vasoconstriction and a chill, while in the heat, body temperature is increased by cessation of sweating and by the onset of vasoconstriction and a mild chill only.[43]

For these reasons, then, it is important to differentiate between fever and a malignant, unregulated hyperthermia. It is evident that attempts to reduce body temperature in fever by physical cooling will be resisted by the thermoregulatory system. On the other hand, antipyretics appear to act on the hypothalamus to "reset" downward the regulated level of body temperature and reduce fever.[46] In the case of malignant hyperthemias, however, this central regulation is absent, and body temperature can rise to fatal levels. In these circumstances, rapid and vigorous body cooling is essential in preventing fatal hyperpyrexia, while antipyretics, of course, are ineffective in lowering body temperature.[1]

PATHOGENESIS

A satisfactory explanation of the genesis of fever must encompass two facts: (1) Fever is a manifestation of many kinds of disease processes, not only infectious diseases but also injuries, neoplastic diseases, vascular accidents, hypersensitivity reactions, certain metabolic disorders, and so forth. The most obvious common factors in them are tissue injury and associated inflammation. (2) Fever may occur in disease of practically any tissue of the body.[47]

Several older theories of the mechanism of the production of fever, including abnormal shifts in body water that interfere with heat dissipation or increased activity of the thyroid and adrenals, have been discarded. It is now clear that in fever, the regulation of body temperature by the CNS is changed in such a way that the normal "thermostatic set point" (usually 37°C or 98.6°F) is shifted upward to a new level around which body temperature is now regulated, as in health.

A great deal of work has been carried out in the past 30 years to elucidate the nature of the stimulus to the hypothalamic thermoregulatory center (TRC) that initiates these changes.[48-50]

The data accumulated from experimental studies in both animals and humans indicate that the interaction of a number of stimuli of microbial and nonmicrobial origin (so-called exogenous pyrogens) with various cells of the host results in the production of an endogenous pyrogen (EP). This group of molecules has been detected in the circulation of animals during experimentally induced fevers and collectively appear to be the agents that act on the TRC to cause the rise in body temperature.[51,51a]

The action of most fever-inducing agents ("pyrogens") on the thermoregulatory system appears, therefore, to occur either directly or indirectly within the CNS rather than in the periphery. It has been demonstrated that intracarotid arterial infusions of an EP derived from leukocytes produce fever more rapidly and at lower dose levels than do intravenous injections.[52] When injected into the cerebroventricular system, 1/500th of the normally required intravenous dose of bacterial pyrogen produces prompt and high fevers.[53] Finally, several studies in which minute amounts of EP have been injected into various areas in the brain indicate that the major and perhaps sole site of pyrogen action lies within the anterior hypothalamus.[54-56] It has also been shown in studies of animals with serial truncations of the brain stem that the ability to develop pyrogen-induced fever requires the functional integrity of the hypothalamic thermoregulatory mechanisms.[57]

Recent studies on the pathogenesis of fever originated with the independent observations by Menkin, Bennett, and Beeson that a pyrogenic material could be extracted from sterile inflammatory exudates. Although it seems likely that Menkin's material was contaminated with extraneous bacterial pyrogens, it was clearly established in a subsequent study in rabbits by Bennett and Beeson that leukocytes derived from exudates, blood, or various inflammatory lesions were sources of EP.[58]

Initially, EP was thought to be derived only from granulocytes; later, monocytes or macrophages from various sites (blood, lung, liver, or peritoneal exudates) were shown to be potent sources of EP. Using phagocytosis of staphylococci as a stimulus, Murphy and his associates have shown recently that EP production in mixed populations of blood cells can be entirely attributed to their monocyte content. When sufficiently purified, granulocytes, though functioning normally in other ways, do not generate detectable amounts of EP *in vitro*.[59]

Among the microbial agents that have been shown to evoke release of EP both *in vivo* and *in vitro* are the lipopolysaccharides that form part of the cell wall of the gram-negative bacteria (so called endotoxins), as well as various gram-positive bacteria, pathogenic fungi, and viruses.[60] The mechanisms by which these agents activate cells to release pyrogen are multiple.[61,62] They probably include certain particulate stimuli (including phagocytosis), as well as chemical stimulation, probably of the cell membrane. In studies of rabbits with

fever accompanying peritoneal infections with pneumococci, it has been shown that pyrogen is rapidly liberated by cells in the inflammatory exudate and subsequently reaches the blood by way of the thoracic duct lymph. Experimentally induced fevers resulting from the injection of both microbial and nonmicrobial antigens into specifically sensitized animals appear to be caused by a circulating EP, although its cellular source has not been conclusively demonstrated. In mixed lymphocyte reactions with human cells[63] or in experimental states of delayed hypersensitivity,[64] lymphocytes activated by specific antigen(s) produce a lymphokine that stimulates blood or exudate monocytes to produce EP. Lymphocytes themselves, however, do not appear capable of producing EP directly.

In man, buffy coat incompatibilities and certain immune hemolytic reactions are associated with marked leukopenias and fevers. Presumably, these are examples of hypersensitivity phenomena leading to EP release, but the site of pyrogen release and the exact immune mechanisms involved are unknown.

In all these experimental situations it seems clear that an intermediary pyrogen, liberated from tissues of the host, plays a major role in producing the febrile response. Recent evidence suggests that EP itself may initiate synthesis of another mediator protein, although the nature and location (blood or brain) of this substance remain to be defined.[65]

EP derived from rabbit leukocytes has now been purified to a considerable extent and appears to consist of several molecular species of proteins with a molecular weight of 13,000 to 15,000,[66,67] although a presumable trimer with a molecular weight of 38,000 has been described.[68] Collectively, EP is clearly different from all known exogenous pyrogens including endotoxins, which are lipopolysaccharides with much larger molecular weights in their natural aggregated state.[69]

Studies by several investigators on the mechanism of EP production in vitro have shown that it is an active metabolic process, which is dependent upon temperature and intact cellular structure and which may be blocked by certain enzyme inhibitors during an early critical period after addition of the activator.[70,71] After this initial period, production of EP continues despite addition of various inhibitors of DNA synthesis or of aerobic or anaerobic metabolism. Production of pyrogen is suppressed, however, by inhibitors of protein synthesis long after the initial period required for activation of the cell, suggesting that it is an active synthetic process.[72]

More recent studies in a number of different animals have implicated two additional classes of agents in the brain that may be important, both in normal thermoregulation and in the pathogenesis of fever. Feldberg, Myers, and their associates have shown that intracerebral injection of several monoamines—including catecholamines and serotonin, both of which occur normally in high concentration in the region of the third ventricle—produces profound effects on the body temperature of various conscious animals.[73,74] The change in temperature (whether rise or fall) varies with different species, but clearly, marked elevations in body temperature may be produced in this manner.[75]

Similarly, certain prostaglandins (especially PGE$_1$), long-chain fatty acids of endogenous origin, produce immediate high fevers when injected in minute amounts directly into the TRC of a number of animals.[76] Unlike the effects of EP when given intracerebrally, the pyrogenic action of PGE$_1$ is not suppressed by aspirin. Since aspirin is known to block the synthesis of prostaglandins, this finding suggests that other pyrogenic agents may indeed activate the cells in the TRC by synthesizing prostaglandins or other derivatives of arachidonic acid metabolism which, in turn, would function as the final common pathway in the pathogenesis of fever.[77] In conformity with this hypothesis, human EP stimulates prostaglandin synthesis in vitro when incubated with rat brain slices.[78] Rosendorff has postulated a more complex scheme involving, sequentially, prostaglandins, catecholamines, and, ultimately, cAMP as the final stimulus to the specialized temperature-sensitive neurons in the hypothalamus that presumably control thermoregulation in health and fever.[79]

At present, the actual sequence of events in the brain that mediates fever is uncertain. After intravenous injection of various pyrogens, prostaglandin levels increase in the cerebrospinal fluid (CSF)[80] and, more conclusively, near the hypothalamus of rabbits.[81] However, fever and CSF prostaglandin levels can be dissociated under certain experimental conditions.[82]

Unsolved Questions

It is apparent from this discussion that many questions concerning the pathogenesis of fever remain unanswered. Are there other as yet undiscovered types of EP? Are monocytes and tissue macrophages the only souce of EP? Although EP seems to be the chief factor in producing fever of microbial origin, little is known about the cause of fever in patients with malignant tumors, lymphomas, collagen diseases, or certain metabolic diseases, such as acute gout and porphyria. In some of these conditions, factors known to contribute to fever in various infectious diseases, such as inflammation and hypersensitivity, may play a role. As yet, there is no known endogenous agent or component of the inflammatory response that is, by itself, capable of activating cells to produce EP, although the pyrogenicity of synthetic, double-stranded RNA, Poly I:C,[83]

suggests an intriguing analogy with endogenous RNA or DNA. The discovery of such an agent would provide an explanation for fevers in diseases where tissue damage and inflammation are unaccompanied by infection or hypersensitivity (*e.g.,* acute myocardial or pulmonary infarction or thrombophlebitis).

Also, little is known of the location or precursors of EP in the cell or of the specific mechanisms by which EP is activated or disposed of in the body, although a metabolite of radioactively labeled EP has been found in the urine.[84]

An exciting new development has been the discovery that EP is, in all probability, identical to lymphocyte-activating factor (LAF), a monokine now known as interleukin-1 (IL-1) that potentiates the mitogenic effect of antigen and mitogens (*e.g.,* concanavalin A) on thymus-derived lymphocytes.[85,86] Since the mitogenic assay for LAF is about 1000-fold more sensitive than is the pyrogenic assay for EP in rabbits, it is likely that other new functions of this substance will be discovered in the near future. A partial radioimmunoassay for human EP has been recently described that should also facilitate study of the intracellular synthesis of EP as well as detect its presence in various tissues during clinical fever.[87] EP derived from clinical exudates or human blood leukocytes activated *in vitro* can be readily detected by pyrogenic assay in humans, in rabbits, and in much smaller amounts, in mice. However, it is much more difficult to measure EP in the circulation of humans with fever than in most experimental models in animals.[88]

CLINICAL FEATURES OF FEVER

The basal metabolism is elevated in fever in proportion to the height of the temperature—roughly 7% for each degree Fahrenheit. In other words, the effect of fever on the metabolic rate follows the principle of van't Hoff that the velocity of chemical reactions is proportional to the temperature at which they occur. At a temperature of 105°F the basal metabolism is approximately 50% above normal.

The biochemical disturbances that have been noted in fever are not very distinctive. During the first week or two of a febrile disease, there is always some destruction of body protein, evidenced by negative nitrogen balance. Fever often is accompanied by mild to severe dehydration. The biochemical disturbances characteristic of dehydration may become evident: passage of Na and Cl into cells; loss of K, P, and N from cells; and loss of cell water as well as of extracellular (plasma and interstitial) water (Chap. 35). Achlorhydria is usually present in persons with high fever, but gastric secretion of acid is resumed when the temperature falls. Mild acidosis is common during infectious fevers.

As stated, the endocrine, metabolic, and biochemical evidences of fever are not distinctive but appear to be shared by many conditions associated with stress. In general, fever and the disorders that cause fever also stimulate the hypothalamic-pituitary-adrenocortical system. Thus, adrenocortical hyperactivity is not part of the mechanism that produces fever; it is an important part of the *response* to fever.

A febrile episode can normally be divided into three components that correlate with the physiologic processes underlying thermoregulation during fever. The prominence and duration of these phases depend on the thermal environment and on the nature of the disease process producing the fever. The three phases are (1) chill, (2) plateau, and (3) defervescence.

The chill phase is caused by the action of the pyrogen in the circulation on the thermoregulatory center, and it produces the initial rise in body temperature. It is characterized by the onset of vigorous shivering, an intense vasoconstriction that causes the skin to blanch or even to become cyanotic in the extremities, and by the appearance of "gooseflesh."[89] The muscular activity producing shivering appears to be controlled through the extrapyramidal motor system, while vasoconstriction is mediated by the sympathetic division of the autonomic nervous system.[90] Other observations of the circulatory changes during fever have been reviewed by Altschule and Freedberg.[91] The patient feels intensely cold and seeks warmth and extra clothing. During the chill most of the extra heat produced is retained within the body and consequently there is a very rapid rise in body temperature of from 2° to 7°F. Chills appear to be most intense in septicemias and malaria, although severe chills may be experienced by patients with lymphomas or hypernephromas.

When body temperature has attained the new higher level "dictated" by the fever, it then levels off. This plateau marks the end of the chill phase. Heat production returns to a normal level, the vasoconstriction passes, and the feeling of coldness disappears. Outwardly the patient may appear normal, but body temperature remains elevated and he may feel somewhat restless. Some fevers, such as the enteric fevers and those of pneumococcal pneumonia, are characterized by sustained plateaus that can last from a few days up to several weeks if untreated. On the other hand, the fevers of malaria or brucellosis are marked by a short plateau with a rapid return of body temperature to normal. This return to normal, formerly called "crisis," constitutes the third phase of fever and is termed "defervescence." During this phase heat loss is intense and is characterized by a pronounced vasodilation and

profuse sweating. The patient feels excessively warm, seeks a cold environment, or removes clothing and coverings. The stage of defervescence is often brief, and the body temperature falls rapidly. Sweating is particularly common in diseases associated with intermittent fever, such as miliary tuberculosis, acute brucellosis, or rheumatic fever. In these diseases it is common to have a series of chills and sweats with brief plateaus. Other examples of intermittent fever are malaria; many acute viral diseases, such as influenza; and such pyogenic infections as pylonephritis, acute osteomyelitis, and postpartum infections. When fevers are treated with an antipyretic drug, the fall in body temperature is usually accompanied by marked sweating and vasodilatation.[92]

COMPLICATIONS OF FEVER

Herpes Simplex. Herpetic lesions about the mouth occur so frequently in certain febrile diseases that they are described in textbooks as manifestations of those diseases. Meningococcal meningitis and pneumococcal pneumonia are particularly likely to be so complicated, whereas, peculiarly, typhoid fever, typhus fever, and primary atypical pneumonia are accompanied only rarely by herpes. Actually, "fever blisters" are due to a separate infection by the virus of herpes simplex, which apparently is activated by the rise in body temperature. The purest example of the association with fever is found in persons who are given artificial fever therapy; in them the incidence of labial herpes may be as high as 46%.[93] The lesions appear 30 hours to 48 hours after a treatment.

Albuminuria. Albumin is frequently present in the urine of patients with fever. In many cases this is certainly due to a direct effect of the disease on the kidneys; consequently, there has been some controversy as to whether fever alone may cause albuminuria. Welty, however, by studying a group of patients being treated with fever in the Kettering Hypertherm, found that albuminuria occurred solely from the artificially induced rise in body temperature. He reported "true febrile albuminuria" in more than 75% of his patients.[94]

Convulsions. Convulsions may occur at the onset of infectious diseases. This phenomenon is limited to children, and in them it appears to be dependent largely on the rapidity with which the temperature rises. Wegman experimented with kittens and noted that they frequently had convulsions if subjected to rapid rise in body temperature; adult cats under the same conditions seldom had convulsions.[95]

The question that is not yet settled is whether febrile convulsions are essentially benign or whether they indicate some abnormality in the CNS. Some follow-up studies have provided evidence that children who have suffered febrile convulsions are liable to nonfebrile seizures later or to exhibit signs of cerebral damage suggestive of conditions such as birth trauma or encephalitis.[96,97]

Delirium. Fever and delirium are often associated. In general, it may be said that delirium seldom is present when the fever is less than 104°F, although in exceptional instances and in elderly patients it may accompany only a moderate elevation of the temperature. The reason is that delirium depends on several factors: the degree of the fever, the temperament of the patient, previous health, medications, and the nature of the underlying disease.

FACTITIOUS FEVER

MacNeal has described some of the ways in which high temperature has been faked by patients.[36] The most common method is to heat the thermometer with a hot water bottle or other source of heat. This is especially easy if the patient has previously obtained a spare thermometer to substitute for the one given him. Another trick is to hold the bulb of the thermometer tightly between the fingers and rub it against the bedclothes. Skilled malingerers can raise the reading by tapping the bulb end of the thermometer, jarring the mercury upward. Vigorous chewing motion can raise the mouth temperature by as much as 1°F. To detect trickery, it is recommended that simultaneous temperatures be taken in the axilla, the rectum, and the mouth, with a different observer holding each thermometer in place. The temperature of a freshly voided sample of urine is also a useful means of corroborating fever in patients.[98] The use of disposable thermometers with instant digital readout will probably reduce the number of factitious fevers in the future.

Useful clues from the patient's chart for detecting this state include failure of the temperature curve to follow normal diurnal variation and the absence of correlation of the fever pattern with pulse rate or sweats.[99] There is a recent review of this problem.[100]

EFFECTS OF FEVER

It is often said that fever assists the host in combating infection. There is no question of the value of fever therapy that was once used in the treatment of neurosyphilis. It has also been observed that failure to develop fever in the presence of severe infection signifies a grave prognosis. However, in most of these instances the absence of fever is probably related to circulatory

failure, and death is due to this complication rather than to the lack of benefit conferred by a febrile response *per se* to the infected host.

Under natural circumstances of infection, it seems unlikely that the increase in body temperature itself directly affects the invading microorganism.[101] Thermolabile microbes, like treponemes, rarely induce in the host high temperatures that would destroy themselves. On the other hand, those microbes that do evoke high fevers, such as the malaria parasite, are clearly unaffected by these temperatures. However, it has long seemed probable from the evolutionary standpoint that fever is somehow beneficial to the host and might indirectly modify the virulence of the invading microorganism by accelerating or enhancing some aspect of host resistance to infection, such as the inflammatory or immune responses. A study in lizards was the first to show conclusively that the ability to develop fever in infection is clearly correlated with survival.[102] Reptiles, being poikilotherms, regulate their body temperature by behavioral means and were found to develop a 2°C fever (to 40°C) by selection of an appropriately warm environment when infected with a gram-negative bacterium. Lizards kept at this febrile temperature after infection had a significantly enhanced survival as compared with others maintained at low or neutral temperatures (34°C or 38°C, respectively). In a later study with the same species of lizard, Bernheim and colleagues showed that the febrile temperature was correlated with the development of an early inflammatory response at the site of infection and a dramatic reduction in the number of bacteria in various organs.[103] More recent studies in rabbits given antipyretics have confirmed that moderate (but not extreme) fevers are associated with decreased mortality in experimental infection.[104]

The previously mentioned finding that EP and LAF are presumably identical and that inflammation as well as lymphocyte proliferation and function are increased at febrile temperatures[105] provide powerful evolutionary arguments for the usefulness of fever.[48,62,105a] Furthermore, it appears likely that EP is also the same as a substance known as leukocyte endogenous mediator (LEM), which produces a number of bodily defense reactions[106] including lowering serum iron (necessary for bacterial metabolism); promoting synthesis of acute-phase proteins;[107] and increasing the number of circulating granulocytes and, under the guise of "purified EP," activating certain of their bactericidal mechanisms.[108,109] Thus, this single mononuclear cell product seems to be one of the main modulators of the inflammatory response with an array of functions that are astonishingly well integrated to protect the host against infection.

The fever that accompanies noninfectious conditions, however, does not appear to serve any useful purpose and may at times be harmful. In malignant disease, for example, high temperature accelerates weight loss and causes malaise, though it may also be cytostatic for neoplastic cells. Likewise, fever that follows myocardial infarction increases the metabolic rate, thereby placing an extra load on the weakened myocardium, but may promote scar formation. Much remains to be learned in these important areas about the possible usefulness of fever.

CLINICAL CAUSES OF FEVER AND HYPERTHERMIA

Infections

Infections are certainly the most frequent causes of fever. In general it may be said that any known infection may cause fever; to list a large number of infectious diseases would serve no purpose here. Instead, a few instances will be cited wherein certain infections cause fevers that are particularly characteristic. These are less commonly observed now than formerly, because effective chemotherapy alters their natural courses.

In typhoid and parathyroid fevers there is a classical temperature course; it consists of a "staircase" rise for several days, a plateau of remittent fever for 1 to 3 weeks, then a steplike return to normal temperature. Dissociation of temperature and pulse is often prominent in these fevers, as in some viral illnesses.

Typhus fever produces a fairly uniform temperature curve. After a sudden elevation there is a sustained high fever for 9 or 10 days, then a fall by lysis, returning to normal about the 14th to the 18th day of disease. An example of this is shown in Figure 25-3.

Gonococcal endocarditis may have a unique fever: two steeplelike rises and falls in each 24-hour period—

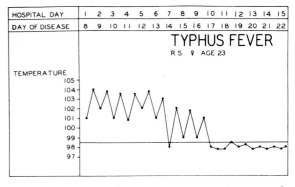

Fig. 25-3. The typical temperature course in a case of murine typhus fever. There is a remittent fever for about 10 days, then a fall by lysis, usually reaching normal between the 14th and 18th days of illness.

double quotidian.[110] This also is described as a feature of kala-azar. It may be present occasionally in other severe infections. We have seen a double quotidian fever in miliary tuberculosis.

In dengue a "saddle-back" temperature curve is typical. By this is meant a fever that rises rapidly, declines somewhat during the succeeding 2 or 3 days, then rises again to a peak on about the 6th day, after which it subsides quickly.

Localized collections of pus, as in subdiaphragmatic abscess or osteomyelitis, frequently lead to a hectic type of fever, associated with chills and sweating. This may also be seen in patients with pyelonephritis, ascending cholangitis (Charcot's biliary fever), and thrombophlebitis.

Diseases that cause relapsing fevers are not very frequent in the United States. The following diagnostic possibilities should receive special consideration: (1) malaria; (2) rat-bite fever, caused by either *Spirillum minus* or *Streptobacillus moniliformis* (see Fig. 25-2); (3) relapsing fever, caused by *Spirillum recurrentis;* and (4) chronic meningococcemia.

It should be stressed, however, that despite some of the distinctive characteristics described above, fever patterns generally have little clinical significance.[111] Certain tumors or collagen vascular diseases, for instance, may produce spiking intermittent fevers often seen in patients with septicemia.

Most infectious diseases associated with the toxins of gram-positive bacteria (*e.g.* botulism, gas gangrene, tetanus, and diphtheria) are not usually characterized by significant fever. Exceptions to this rule are scarlet fever and a newly described entity, toxic shock syndrome,[112] both diseases in which fever and rash are conspicuous features, presumably because of toxins associated with certain strains of Group A streptococci and staphylococci, respectively.[113]

Diseases of the Central Nervous System

Head Injury. Fever is nearly always present after head injury, and the height of the temperature may be of some value in estimating prognosis. In slight concussions there is a rise to 101°F or less, whereas in more serious cases the fever is often higher, and in the most severe injuries there may be a rapid ascent to a hyperthermic level before death. Erickson states that following middle meningeal hemorrhage, a person may be more or less poikilothermic, his body temperature fluctuating markedly with changes in the environmental temperature.[114]

Cerebrovascular Accident. Hemorrhage or thrombosis in the vessels of the brain is often attended by a moderate fever—100°F to 102°F. In large hemorrhages very high fever may develop just before death. Recent work suggests that release of prostaglandins from the affected tissue may be responsible for some of these fevers.[115]

Neurogenic Hyperthermia. Following surgical operations in the region of the pituitary fossa and the third ventricle, a serious hyperthermia sometimes occurs. The rectal temperature rises steadily during the first few hours after operation. The skin of the extremities is cold, while that of the trunk is relatively warm. There is complete absence of sweating. Energetic cooling is indicated: application of ice bags, alcohol rubs, cold air fan, and so forth.[114]

Brain Damage Following Infection or Trauma. Disturbances in temperature regulation are occasionally noted after recovery from encephalitis. Children who have sustained cerebral trauma in a birth injury often have impaired temperature regulation.

Spinal Cord Injury. Holmes made a study of the effects of spinal cord injuries and observed that injury to the cervical cord was frequently followed by severe disturbance of temperature regulation. Injury to the lower cervical cord usually resulted in very low body temperature, whereas patients with upper cervical cord injury often had high, irregular temperatures.[116] The cause of this temperature disturbance probably is the interruption of the tracts leading to and from the hypothalamus.

Neoplasms

Malignant growths frequently cause fever.[117,118] Sometimes, for example, in bronchogenic carcinoma, this fever may be the result of an associated infection; but often the tumor alone appears to be responsible. Hypernephroma is notorious in this respect; it may even cause a hectic fever with chills and sweats. Primary or metastatic carcinoma in the liver is also frequently attended by fever.[119] Figure 25-4 shows the temperature chart of a patient with primary carcinoma of the pancreas, with metastasis to the liver. Harsha has reviewed the literature on fever in malignant disease and reports a case in which there was dramatic cessation of a hectic fever after removal of a retroperitoneal malignant tumor.[120] Similar defervescence has followed extirpation of mesotheliomata of the pleura.[121] Infection with or without obstruction is a more frequent cause of fever in malignancy than is the disease itself.[122] The fever of malignancy presents no characteristic features, although low-grade or regularly recurrent fevers seem more common in tumors not associated with infection.[123] Several studies have shown that fe-

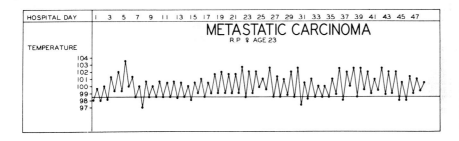

Fig. 25-4 Temperature chart of a young woman with fever due to carcinoma of the pancreas with metastasis to the liver.

vers associated with tumors are responsive to the antipyretic action of indomethacin.[124]

Lymphoma. Fever frequently accompanies this group of neoplastic diseases and is often the first sign. Consequently, such conditions as Hodgkin's disease, lymphosarcoma, and leukemia always must be considered in investigating cases of obscure fever. A few persons with Hodgkin's disease exhibit a peculiar relapsing fever in which periods of about 7 to 10 days of normal temperature alternate with equal periods of fever. This is called the Pel-Ebstein fever. An example is shown in Figure 25-5.

Bodel has shown that certain tissues, including hypernephromas, as well as spleens and lymph nodes from some patients with Hodgkin's disease, release EP spontaneously *in vitro*, unlike those obtained from patients with nonmalignant diseases.[125] Although pyrogen release from tissue cells *in vitro* did not correlate well with the febrile status of the patient or with microscopic evidence of tumor, this clearly abnormal finding suggests that such cells may be a source of the pyrogen that produces fever in these diseases. The cause of this "spontaneous" pyrogen release is obscure, although activation of the cells by oncogenic factors or by an immunologic reaction to tumor antigens are clearly possibilities to be considered.

Diseases of Blood

Acute leukemia is usually a febrile disease, even in the absence of discernible infection.[126,127] Certain acute hemolytic anemias also are associated with fever, especially those due to an immunologic process or sickle-cell anemia in crisis.[128] Hemorrhagic disorders, such as thrombocytopenic purpura, hemophilia, and scurvy, may cause fever if there is hemorrhage into the tissues. Severe anemia from chronic blood loss is not a cause of fever. Chronic aplastic anemia, chronic lymphocytic leukemia (in the absence of infection), multiple myeloma, and myelofibrosis are rarely febrile diseases, but high fevers often are present in acute agranulocytosis and cyclic neutropenias. When infection is not a cause, the fevers may be due to absorption of endotoxins from the gut, as serum samples from such patients are often positive in the sensitive limulus test for endotoxin.[129]

Embolism and Thrombosis

Embolism or aseptic thrombosis in a large artery or vein often is associated with fever.[130] This probably depends on the occurrence of tissue necrosis (and attendant inflammation) due to interference with the nutrition of the part supplied by the vessel. In myocardial infarction, for example, low fever is expected during the first few days, but elevations as high as 103°F to 104°F may be seen occasionally.

Septic thrombophlebitis in postpartum patients occasionally may give rise to persistent spiking fevers with either positive or negative blood cultures but without local signs of infection. The fever often responds dramatically to anticoagulants after trials with various antibiotics have been unsuccessful.[131]

Heat Stroke

Heat stroke is a serious condition characterized by high temperatures, coma, and absence of sweating. It should not be confused with heat cramp or heat exhaustion, neither of which causes a change in body temperature. Heat stroke is induced by prolonged high environmental temperature; it occurs most commonly in old people, in those who have been consuming alcohol, and especially in those who have been exercising. Apparently the fault here is failure of the cerebral centers of heat regulation. The onset of symptoms is usually sudden, with loss of consciousness. The affected person ceases to sweat just prior to his collapse. Ferris and his associates carried out an excellent study on 44 patients with heat stroke during a single period of hot weather.[132] The body temperatures of their patients ranged from 104°F to 112°F. Absence of sweating was noted in all of them. Biochemical studies revealed normal blood chlorides, but there was some acidosis and hemoconcentration. The reason for the sudden cessation of sweating could not be ascertained. Of the 44 patients, 17 died. It was concluded that energetic measures must be employed in an effort to reduce the body temperature quickly; the procedures recommended were ice-water tubbing combined with massage and IV fluids. Since this is not a true fever with a regulated elevation of body temperature, antipyretics, of course, have no place in therapy.

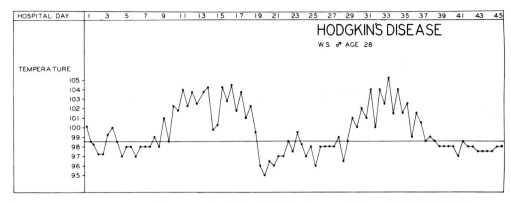

Fig. 25-5. An example of the Pel-Ebstein type of fever in Hodgkin's disease.

Patients with heat stroke may present with numerous other complications, including jaundice, acute renal failure, myocardial infarction, and hematologic complications.[133-135]

Disturbances in Fluid Balance

Dehydration is commonly held to be responsible for fever. However, there is little evidence that this is true in adults, and the best clinical practice is to search for some other cause.

There can be little doubt that infants during the first few days of life can have temperature elevation due to lack of fluids—the so-called dehydration or inanition fever. Administration of adequate fluid is followed by prompt cessation of the elevated temperature. The mechanism of this is obscure.

Fever may be observed in severe diabetic acidosis, and some persons have ascribed this to dehydration. Himwich produced acidosis and high fever in depancreatized dogs by withholding water and insulin; then by giving fluids he found that the temperature returned to normal. Insulin alone did not have this effect.[136] However, the temperature is frequently normal or subnormal in diabetic acidosis; consequently the presence of fever should stimulate a search for some other disease.

Thyroid Disease

It is common to find a slight temperature elevation—99.5°F to 100.5°F—in persons who have thyrotoxicosis.[137] This is probably due to the excessive heat production that accompanies the increased metabolism. In a thyroid crisis, which may appear spontaneously or may occur immediately after surgery on the thyroid (occasionally also after other surgical procedures) there is a rapid rise in body temperature to 104°F or higher accompanied by tachycardia, thready pulse, restlessness, sometimes mania, and eventually stupor.

Many of the clinical manifestations of so-called thyroid storm, including elevated temperature, have been attributed recently to exaggerated responses of the thyrotoxic patient to catecholamines. In support of this hypothesis, such patients have responded well to reserpine, guanethidine, or propranolol—agents that deplete or impair release of catecholamines or block β-adrenergic receptors, respectively.[138] Several other, more unusual endocrine disorders associated with fever have been reviewed recently.[139]

Steroid Fever

There is a poorly defined group of diseases in which fever occurs either at regular or irregular intervals (so-called cyclic or periodic fever, respectively).[140] The febrile episodes often are associated with bouts of aseptic arthritis or peritonitis. Although symptoms may recur for years, patients generally remain healthy, and the prognosis is benign in most instances. Recently, evidence has accumulated that "periodic disease" may include several distinct diseases of varying etiology.

In familial Mediterranean fever, a form of periodic febrile disease that is associated with amyloidosis and appears to be almost entirely restricted to Jews and Armenians,[140a] the cause of fever is still unknown, although the febrile bouts are associated with recurrent serositis and can be suppressed by colchicine.[141]

A number of steroid metabolites of the pregnane and etiocholane type, when given by either intravenous or intramuscular routes, produce marked pyrogenic responses in man, associated with leukocytosis, headache, myalgia, and arthralgia.[142] At present, the mechanism by which these agents cause fever is unknown, but since there is a prolonged delay before onset of fever, it seems doubtful that they act directly on the thermoregulatory center. Human leukocytes can be stimulated by etiocholanolone *in vitro* to release EP.[143] This action appears to be highly specific, since minor structural modifications of the molecule abolish its pyrogenic properties both *in vivo* and *in vitro*. These sim-

ilarities between *in vitro* and *in vivo* activity suggest that pyrogenic steroids may act like other fever-inducing agents by releasing an intermediate pyrogen from leukocytes. These steroids appear to produce fever only in man and hence may be distinguished clearly from various pyrogens of microbial origin which, as noted previously, are effective in a number of animals.

At present, none of these compounds has been conclusively shown to play a role in clinical fevers, although the urinary ketosteroid, etiocholanolone, was initially thought to be a cause of some benign recurrent fevers.[144] However, since many transformation products of endogenous adrenocortical and gonadal hormones, as well as some bile acids, are pyrogenic, these agents may well be implicated in certain hitherto unexplained fevers associated with various hepatic and endocrine disorders. In this regard, estrogens, which reduce pyrogen release from blood leukocytes simultaneously activated *in vitro* by other means, were found to be effective in suppressing fever when given intermittently to several patients with long-standing "benign" recurrent episodes of fever.[145]

Liver Diseases

Various diseases of the liver are prone to produce fever. Liver abscess, amebic or bacterial, may cause a hectic type of fever. The frequency of temperature elevation in neoplastic disease of the liver already has been mentioned. About one half of all patients with cirrhosis of the liver have temperature elevations, which are typically moderate and prolonged in uncomplicated cases.[146]

Diseases Affecting the Heart

Some degree of fever is often present in patients with congestive heart failure, but there is usually some associated complication that could cause it, such as bronchopneumonia, pulmonary infarction, myocardial infarction, thrombophlebitis, or rheumatic fever. Nevertheless, there are occasional instances in which no such complication is obvious and where fever appears with failure and disappears when compensation is regained. Decompensation alone, however, is unlikely to cause a temperature elevation of more than 1°F.[147]

Patients occasionally have fever during paroxysms of tachycardia, in the absence of any other disease.[148] This may be due to the combined effect of impaired circulation and extra heat production resulting from the muscular activity of the heart. Fever almost invariably accompanies either acute or subacute endocarditis.[149] Certain clinical features of this disease, including fever, anemia, petechiae, peripheral embolic phenomena, and changing cardiac murmurs may be mimicked

closely by myxomas of the left atrium.[150] A febrile illness associated with a pleuropericardial inflammatory reaction may follow shortly after extensive closed heart surgery involving either mitral valvulotomy or pericardiotomy.[151] Originally this syndrome was attributed to reactivation of rheumatic fever, but as it may occur in patients undergoing cardiac surgery without other evidence of this disease, as well as in other patients after nonpenetrating chest injuries[152] or myocardial infarction,[153] it has been suggested that the symptoms are due to an autoimmune reaction.[154,155]

Another febrile syndrome due to infection with cytomegalovirus[156] has been described in a small number of patients undergoing open heart surgery with cardiopulmonary bypass through a pump oxygenator. These patients develop a viral-like illness that resembles infectious mononucleosis, with fever, splenomegaly, and atypical lymphocytes.[157] The fever, which usually begins several weeks after operation, follows an intermittent daily course and gradually subsides after a month or so.

Patients undergoing rejection of transplanted organs may respond with fever one or two weeks after operation, presumably because of a hypersensitivity reaction of the delayed type to homologous tissue. Since the immune mechanisms of such patients have been suppressed by various agents, infection remains an important possible cause of fever in these instances.[158]

The many possibilities to be considered in the febrile patient with heart disease have been summarized by Silber and Katz.[159]

Sarcoid

Nearly half the patients with sarcoid, a granulomatous disease of unknown etiology involving the lymph nodes, liver, spleen, eyes, and skin, present with a significant degree of fever. The cause of fever in such patients is obscure, and since it follows no characteristic pattern, fever is unfortunately of little help in diagnosis.[160]

Tissue Trauma and Postoperative Fevers

Crushing injuries and fractures of large bones are followed by some rise in body temperature. Mild elevations in body temperature are regularly present for a day or two after major surgery and are believed to be due to inflammation associated with tissue injury and repair. Atelectasis is another frequent cause of postoperative fever resulting from pulmonary obstruction and incipient pulmonary infection; it may be aborted by vigorous measures to clear the patient's airways. Roe has called attention to an entity he has called "benign postoperative fever."[161] Typically, patients presenting with this condition have undergone abdominal operations with wide exposure of peritoneal contents

and have received a number of cold intravenous infusions. Upon recovery from anesthesia, the thermoregulatory center responds to the lowered core temperature by instituting mechanisms for heat conservation and production, and there is a transient "overshoot" in body temperature, which may be misdiagnosed as a fever due to other causes. Such "fevers" may be prevented by measures aimed at maintaining body temperatures near the normal range during the operation.

Other more serious causes of postoperative fever include infections, especially of the lungs and urinary tract, resulting from intubation and indwelling catheters, respectively; suppurative complications of the operative site; and pulmonary embolism, thrombophlebitis, pancreatitis, and so on.

The time of onset of fever after surgery may be helpful in suggesting the cause. Fever developing during or immediately after operation can be often attributed to an idiosyncratic reaction to the anesthesia (which is discussed later in this chapter), to pyrogen-contaminated intravenous infusions, or to sepsis, especially in the case of cardiac surgery. Atelectasis as a cause of fever usually appears within the first 24 hours, whereas the fevers resulting from wound infections generally make their appearance several days after operation. Similarly, fever associated with allergic reactions to the anesthetic (particularly halothane, which may induce a hepatitis)[162] or to medications appears between the first and second week after initial exposure but may appear earlier (within hours or several days) upon subsequent exposure. Surgical aspects of fever and their management are comprehensively discussed in Roe's monograph.[161]

Peptic Ulcer

European physicians have reported fever in 8% to 25% of patients with uncomplicated peptic ulcer.[163] The elevation seldom exceeds 100.5°F. Dill and Isenhour in this country found fever in 46% of a group of patients with uncomplicated peptic ulcer, but the significance of the finding was somewhat clouded by the fact that the same criteria for fever were satisfied in 37% of their control group—persons with digestive symptoms but without demonstrable organic lesions.[164] Upon the basis of the available evidence, the statement that uncomplicated peptic ulcer is a cause of fever is still open to question.

Massive hemorrhage from a peptic ulcer results in fever in at least 80% of cases. However, attempts to produce this type of fever in normal subjects by the introduction of large quantities of blood into the intestinal tract were unsuccessful.[165] One factor, which perhaps is not appreciated sufficiently in evaluating fever

after gastrointestinal hemorrhage, is the effect of blood transfusions that these patients receive. The findings of Selesnick and White indicate that the fever of gastrointestinal hemorrhage rarely exceeds 100°F except after transfusion.[166]

Abnormalities of the Skin

Persons who have congenital absence of the sweat glands or other generalized skin disease may be handicapped seriously in hot weather, when vaporization is the principal means of heat loss. Under such conditions they may develop fever.[167] Woodyatt reported this in the case of a woman with extensive ichthyosis. In the winter she was able to work normally, but in summer she would develop fever and symptoms resembling those of effort syndrome.[168]

Serum Sickness and Allergy

Serum sickness, with fever, arthralgia, and urticaria, may occur from 5 to 10 days after administration of an animal serum to a human being and apparently results from a vigorous immune reaction to the foreign protein. The temperature elevation may be considerable—103°F to 105°F. Presumably the syndrome is due to EP released by the patient's tissues following an antigen-antibody reaction. Circulating EP has been detected in sensitized rabbits that develop fever after intravenous injection of antigen. It seems likely that a similar mechanism is responsible for the fevers that are frequently seen in patients with many collagen–vascular diseases of so-called autoimmunity (acute rheumatic fever, lupus erythematosus, juvenile rheumatoid arthritis, polyarteritis, and so forth).[169–171]

It has been suggested that allergy may cause certain obscure fevers, but there is not a great deal of evidence to support the idea. Rowe, however, has reported a case in which the evidence was strong that a prolonged obscure fever was due to food allergy.[172]

Anesthesia

Dangerous hyperthermia is an occasional complication of anesthesia. This is a special hazard in the case of young children, and the danger is increased in operations about the face, such as those for cleft palate.[173,174] This syndrome closely resembles neurogenic hyperthermia, including the absence of sweating and the coldness of the skin of the extremities. Death may ensue. Mangiardi reported on three such cases in adults and advocated therapy with oxygen inhalation, alcohol sponging, and continuous intravenous administration of 50% dextrose solution.[175]

A rare disorder known as malignant hyperthermia (inherited in some, but not in all instances) has been recognized recently following the use of a number of

inhalation anesthetics as well as muscle relaxants.[176] The syndrome is characterized by a rapid, progressive rise in body temperature often to fatal levels, accompanied by muscular rigidity, tachycardia, tachypnea, and a severe metabolic acidosis. The hyperthermia (usually a late sign) appears to be due to a disorder of muscle metabolism leading to increased heat production, triggered by release of calcium from the sarcoplasmic reticulum of skeletal muscle. Many potentially susceptible subjects may be identified by elevated levels of serum creatinine phosphokinase. Perhaps because of anesthesia, the thermoregulatory center fails to activate heat loss mechanisms when the body temperature exceeds the ceiling reached in febrile disease (see previous discussion). This, then, clearly separates the syndrome from most cases of clinical fever and, as in the case of heat stroke, necessitates emergency measures to lower body temperature. Treatment is controversial, though various agents (intravenous dantrolene, procaine, or procainamide) as well as physical cooling methods have been used successfully.

DRUG FEVERS AND HYPERTHERMIAS

A number of drugs may cause elevated body temperature after prolonged administration. Some of the important ones are antihistamines, antitumor agents (*e.g.* chlorambucil and bleomycin) atropine, barbiturates, bromides, iodides, isoniazid, mercurials, methyldopa, morphine, penicillin, phenylbutazone, phenytoin, quinidine, salicylates, streptomycin and other aminoglycosides, sulfonamides, and thiouracil. Drug fevers caused by antibacterial agents may be difficult to identify because they occur in persons who may already have fever due to infection. In many cases, drug fevers are due to hypersensitivity, and since they are often associated with skin eruptions, the simultaneous appearance of rash and fever may make the diagnosis easy.

A helpful clinical point is that most drug fevers subside within 48 hours after the medication is discontinued. Several commonly used medications that rarely if ever produce fever are digitalis and most hormones and diuretics (except mercurials), as well as the tetracyclines and chloramphenicol among the antibiotics. The various causes and manifestations of drug fevers have been reviewed comprehensively by Cluff and Johnson.[177] There are two recent summaries.[178,178a]

Temperature elevations of as much as 2°F may occur when morphine is withheld from an addict.[179]

Another type of febrile reaction, which occurs in the therapy of syphilis and other spirochetal illnesses, is known as the Jarisch–Herxheimer reaction. It may result from treatment either with an arsenical or with penicillin and is undoubtedly related to the effect on the syphilitic infection. Within a few hours after the first injection, the patient develops fever and malaise; these may be associated with an intensification of a skin eruption or severe pain in a syphilitic lesion of bone. The symptoms seldom last more than 24 hours to 48 hours. Endotoxins (possibly absorbed from the gut) may play a role in such reactions, as they have been found in the circulation during the Jarisch–Herxheimer-like reactions associated with antibiotic treatment of patients with *Borrelia recurrentis* infection.[180]

Other drugs that may elevate body temperature under certain conditions are epinephrine, dinitrophenol (DNP) and lysergic acid diethylamide (LSD), an inhibitor of serotonin.[181] As previously mentioned, both serotonin and norepinephrine are normally present in high concentration in the region of the hypothalamus and are capable of modifying thermoregulation when injected directly into the cerebral ventricles of various animals.[73,74] Fatal hyperpyrexias occasionally follow the concurrent administration of tricyclic antidepressants (imipramine, amitriptyline and others) and MAO inhibitors. Presumably, these agents modify the local metabolism of serotonin or catecholamines in the region of the thermoregulatory center and in some fashion prevent the normal activation of heat loss mechanisms (as occurs in most clinical fevers) when body temperature reaches levels of about 106°F.

Patients with pheochromocytoma characteristically have a moderate elevation in temperature during an attack and may occasionally have signs that simulate overwhelming infection.[182]

Little is known about the mechanisms by which all these agents raise body temperature, and it seems probable that some are direct stimulants to the CNS, whereas others, such as DNP, the anticholinergics and phenothiazines (which may modify heat production or heat elimination directly), act peripherally rather than on the thermoregulatory center itself.

Clearly, in some of these instances these temperature elevations are hyperthermias rather than true fevers and therefore will not respond to antipyretics.

Fever Due to Heavy Sedation

It is not unusual for fever to occur in persons who have received heavy sedation (amytal narcosis for psychiatric therapy, barbiturate intoxication in suicide attempt, patients being treated for delirium tremens or tetanus). This temperature elevation suggests a pulmonary complication, such as atelectasis or pneumonia.[183]

"Pyrogens"

Chill and high fever occasionally follow the intravenous administration of saline solutions, serums, and other biologic preparations because of the presence of

bacterial pyrogens, a term usually applied to lipopoly-saccharide endotoxin (see above). These agents gain access through contamination of the material at some stage of preparation. Special precautions must be taken to avoid pyrogen contamination of any material that is to be given intravenously. Pyrogens are exceedingly difficult to remove from biologic preparations, because they can pass through bacterial filters and can withstand autoclaving as well as certain other methods of sterilization. Serious reactions caused by equipment or solutions inadvertently contaminated with bacterial pyrogens continue to present a problem in medicine. One such epidemic occurring in a cardiac catheterization laboratory where materials were sterilized by ethylene oxide has been reported.[184]

MISCELLANEOUS CAUSES OF FEVER

Cotton Dust Fever. Persons who handle raw cotton, in mills or in making mattresses, are subject to a febrile disorder. Toward the end of the day there is malaise, chilliness, and fever of 100°F to 102°F. The symptoms subside during the night, and the person usually feels well enough to return to work the next day. A tolerance develops within a few days so that there are no symptoms as long as employment is continued. However, tolerance is lost when the worker takes a short vacation. Studies have indicated that the febrile reaction is related to the presence of a species of *Aerobacter cloacae* in the cotton fibers. This organism has been shown to be a potent pyrogen producer, and the presumption is that the symptoms are caused by absorption of the pyrogen from the respiratory mucosa.[185]

Metal Fume Fever. Workers in certain metal industries are subject to illness of the type just described for cotton workers, including the development of tolerance. The workers particularly susceptible are those exposed to fumes containing zinc oxide.[186] It has been impossible to produce fever in animals exposed to the same fumes. The suggestion has been offered that in man the metal fumes cause increased absorption of bacterial products from the respiratory mucosa. However, the fever (which also occurs after inhalation of certain polymer fumes)[187] may be due to an immunologic response[188] or to absorption of finely divided particles *per se,* as in some experimental fevers.

"Catheter Fever." Occasionally the passage of a catheter or other instrument through an infected urethral tract is followed in an hour or two by the development of fever, sometimes with a chill. It has been shown that this fever is caused by a bacteremia, which is usually transient. A similar fever may follow digital dilation of rectal stricture.

Teething. Lay people regard teething as a frequent cause of fever in children, whereas physicians are somewhat reluctant to take this view. However, most pediatricians believe that now and then, especially when there is swelling and inflammation of the gum over the erupting tooth, teething may cause a rise in temperature.

"Milk Fever." In the last century, when puerperal infection was more frequent than it is today, physicians were so accustomed to the appearance of fever about the third day after delivery that they came to regard engorgement of the mother's breasts as a process that could cause fever. However, modern obstetricians now believe that fever that occurs coincidentally with the onset of lactation is probably due to some undetected infection.

Habitual Hyperthermia. Reimann was interested in the problem of persons whose temperatures are set at a level slightly above the average normal (habitual hyperthermia) and reported on a group of 16 such cases.[189] Each one was subjected to thorough examination and was observed over a period of years without finding evidence of organic disease. Reimann believed that such people are not rare and often are improperly managed because of the assumption that even a slight fever means disease. He thought that certain persons, particularly those with neurotic dispositions, maintain a body temperature that is always slightly above normal and that long-continued low-grade fever in them should not be interpreted as an indication of infection or other febrile disease. All physicians are familiar with this clinical problem,[190] and after a thorough work-up to eliminate the possibility of organic disease, it seems advisable at times to make a positive diagnosis of habitual hyperthermia in order to spare these patients the anxiety and expense of repeated examinations and treatment.

Psychogenic Fever. Most physicians are convinced that under certain conditions an emotional stimulus may induce an elevation of temperature. Dunbar has reviewed the evidence on the subject.[191] The slight rise so often observed at the time of admission to a hospital appears to be an example of psychogenic fever. We have all noticed that occasionally a patient who has no apparent cause for fever will show a slight elevation on the day of admission but a normal temperature thereafter. Similarly, it is not unusual to find a number of slight elevations immediately after visiting hours in pediatric wards.

Wynn took the temperatures of 40 nurses immediately before and immediately after the writing of a state board examination and found that the average was

98.9°F before and 98.3°F after the examination. Similarly, he found that among 324 draftees who were awaiting physical examination for the Army, the average temperature was 99.3°F. Indeed, 17% of the men had temperatures above 100°F. He attributed these elevations to anxiety and excitement.[192]

Wolf and Wolff[193] reported another interesting example of psychogenic fever. Their patient, a man, had had periodic bouts of fever for 13 years. He had suffered from migraine previously, and with the appearance of the fever, his migraine ceased. After extensive negative studies for other causes of fever, therapy directed toward certain personality disorders seemed to relieve him of both the fever and the headaches. It is evident from the previous discussion that in most of these instances the elevation of temperature represents nonspecific hyperthermia and not a true fever.[1]

FEVER OF UNKNOWN ORIGIN

One of the most intriguing and difficult problems of diagnosis in medicine is the fever of unknown origin (FUO). The causes of most such fevers of short duration are probably infectious diseases, especially viral. Other pyrexic states, which follow a more prolonged course (two or three weeks or longer), are due to a variety of causes, as is evident by the number of diseases that may present at some time or other with fever. A point stressed in one large series is that most patients with FUO are not suffering from rare diseases but have unusual manifestations of common illnesses.[194] In over one third of the patients in this series the fevers were found after careful study to be of infectious origin, and nearly two thirds of these patients recovered or benefited from specific treatment. One clearly must make every effort to arrive at a correct diagnosis before blindly subjecting such patients to various therapeutic trials.

There appears to be little difference in the relative contribution of various disease categories in the several series of FUO reported over the past 30 years, with infections responsible for 25% to 50% of the cases, neoplasms (including blood dyscrasias) about 20%, and collagen diseases 10% to 15%. However, within the fevers of obscure origin due to infectious diseases, there has been a diminution of those caused by gram-positive cocci and a corresponding increase in gram-negative enteric infections. Tuberculosis continues to cause many a chronic obscure fever. Discussions of the problems of diagnosis and treatment of patients with FUO are presented in a number of recent reviews of this subject.[194-203] It seems likely that with our many new diagnostic techniques we shall remove a higher percentage of cases from the unknown category.

SUMMARY

Body temperature is maintained relatively constant by centers in the hypothalamus that regulate heat production and loss through the nervous system. Body heat is derived principally from combustion of food in the liver and voluntary muscles. Heat is lost by radiation, convection, and evaporation. Under normal conditions, the nervous system is able to keep body temperature stable simply by varying the caliber of peripheral blood vessels and hence regulating the loss of heat from the surface of the body.

There is no set "normal" body temperature. The temperature varies considerably in different parts of the body; furthermore, there are small differences in rectal temperatures among healthy individuals. In all persons there is a diurnal variation, amounting to as much as 3°F, the peak usually being attained in the evening, the low point during sleep in the early morning hours.

Certain physiologic conditions influence the body temperature; among these are exercise, digestion of food, ovulation, and pregnancy. Knowledge of the possible effect of exercise may be of particular importance to clinicians in evaluating "fever" in children.

Experimental studies on the pathogenesis of fever in animals and man indicate that most fever-inducing agents—both microbial and nonmicrobial—(so-called exogenous pyrogens) mobilize one or more endogenous pyrogens (EP) from certain tissues of the host, presumably those containing mononuclear phagocytes, including the blood and reticuloendothelial system. EP is a collective term for several immunologically distinct proteins of relatively small molecular weight (about 14,000) that enter the circulation and appear to act on the hypothalamic thermoregulatory center to cause the increase in body temperature (by a combination of reduced heat loss and increased heat production).

The local effect of EP on the brain appears to be mediated by one or more derivatives of arachidonic acid (including prostaglandins). Whether these agents act directly on the hypothalamic neurons that control heat loss and production or through other local chemical changes in this region is unknown. It seems likely that fever in most clinical diseases is due to the same sequence of events, although this remains to be proven.

Many different types of disease cause fever. Among the most important are infections, diseases of the CNS, neoplasms, collagen–vascular diseases, and vascular accidents. An understanding of the characteristics and mechanisms of fever is of great value in the study of disease, especially as recent evidence suggests that fever itself, as well as other activities of the endogenous

agent that induces fever, play important evolutionary roles in modulating the immune and inflammatory responses and, hence, in mobilizing bodily defenses against infection.[204]

The authors are grateful to Dr. P. B. Beeson, who generously has allowed the incorporation of major sections of his text from the third edition of this chapter; we also wish to acknowledge our deceased colleague, Dr. Phyllis Bodel, for her keen editorial help throughout, and Dr. Gordon Duff, who read the entire manuscript and made a number of helpful suggestions.

REFERENCES

1. **Stitt JT:** Fever versus hyperthermia. Fed Proc 38:39, 1979
2. **Bazett HC:** The regulation of body temperature. In Newburgh LH (ed): Physiology of Heat Regulation and the Science of Clothing, p 109. Philadelphia, WB Saunders, 1949
3. **DuBois EF:** Basal Metabolism in Health and Disease. Philadelphia, Lea & Febiger, 1927
4. **Benzinger TH, Pratt AW, Kitzinger C:** The thermostatic control of human metabolic heat production. Proc Nat Acad Sci 47:730, 1961
5. **Spealman CR:** A characteristic of human temperature regulation. Proc Soc Exp Biol Med 60:11, 1945
6. **Robinson S:** Physiological adjustments to heat. In Newburgh LH (ed): Physiology of Heat Regulation and the Science of Clothing, p 193. Philadelphia, WB Saunders, 1949
7. **Hardy JD, Opel TW:** Studies in temperature sensation. III. The sensitivity of the body to heat and the spatial summation of the end organ responses. J Clin Invest 16:533, 1937
8. **Ranson SW:** Hypothalamus and central levels of autonomic function. Nerv Ment Dis Monog 20:342, 1940
9. **Hammel HT, Hardy JD, Fusco MM:** Thermoregulatory responses to hypothalamic cooling in unanesthetized dogs. Am J Physiol 198:481, 1960
10. **Simon E, Rautenberg W, Thauer R et al:** Die Auslösung von Kältezittern durch lokale Kühlung im Wirblelkanal. Pflügers Arch 281:309, 1964
11. **Rawson RO, Quick KP:** Evidence of deep-body thermoreceptor response to intra-abdominal heating of the ewe. J Appl Physiol 28:813, 1970
12. **Bligh J:** Possible temperature-sensitive elements in or near the vena cava of sheep. J Physiol 159:85, 1961
13. **Meyer FR, Robinson S, Newton JL et al:** The regulation of the sweating response to work in man. Physiologist 5:182, 1962
14. **Hardy, JD:** Physiology of temperature regulation. Physiol Rev 41:521, 1961
15. **Barbour HG:** Die Wirkung unmittelbarer. Erwärmung und Abkühlung der Wärmezentra auf die Körpertemperatur. Arch Exp Pathol Pharmakol 70:1, 1912
16. **Isenschmid R, and Krehl L:** Uber den Einfluss des Gehirns auf die Wärmeregulation. Arch Exp Pathol Pharmakol 70:109, 1912
17. **Ström G:** Central nervous regulation of body temperature. In Field J, Magoun HW, Hall VE (eds): Handbook of Physiology. Sec. 1. Neurophysiology, Vol 2, p 1173. Washington, American Physiological Society, 1960
18. **Keller AD:** Temperature regulation disturbances in dogs following hypothalamic ablations. In Herzfeld CM (ed): Temperature: Its Measurements and Control in Science and Industry, Vol 3, p 571. New York, Reinhold, 1963
19. **Meyer HH:** Theorie des Fiebers und seiner Behandlung. Zentbl ges inn Med 6:385, 1913
20. **Nakayama T, Hammel HT, Hardy JD et al:** Thermal stimulation of electrical activity of single units of preoptic region. Am J Physiol 204:1122, 1963
21. **Hellon RF:** Thermal stimulation of hypothalamic neurones in unanaesthetized rabbits. J Physiol 193:381, 1967
22. **Nadel ER, Bullard RW, Stolwijk JAJ:** Importance of skin temperature in the regulation of sweating. J Appl Physiol 31:80, 1971
23. **Horvath SM, Menduke H, Piersol GM:** Oral and rectal temperatures of man. JAMA 144:1562, 1950
24. **Reimann HA:** Habitual hyperthermia: A clinical study of four cases with long-continued lowgrade fever. Arch Intern Med 55:792, 1935
25. **Gerbrandy J, Snell ES, Cranston WI:** Oral, rectal, and esophageal temperatures in relation to central temperature control in man. Clin Sci 13:615, 1954
26. **Mellette HC, Hutt BK, Askovitz SI et al:** Diurnal variations in body temperatures, J Appl Physiol 3:665, 1951
27. **Kleitman N:** Biological rhythms and cycles. Physiol Rev 29:1, 1949
28. **Van der Bogert F, Moravec CL:** Body temperature variations in apparently healthy children. J Pediatr 10:466, 1937
29. **Exton–Smith AN:** Accidental hypothermia. Br Med J 4:727, 1973
30. **Whitelaw MJ:** Hormonal control of the basal body temperature pattern. Fertil Steril 3:230, 1952
31. **Seward GH, Seward JP Jr:** Changes in systolic blood pressure, heart rate, and temperature before, during, and after pregnancy in healthy women. Hum Biol 8:232, 1936
32. **Smith LW, Fay T:** Observations on human beings with cancer, maintained at reduced temperatures of 75°–90° Fahrenheit. Am J Clin Pathol 10:1, 1940
33. **Laufman H:** Profound accidental hypothermia, JAMA 147:1201, 1951
34. **Kass GH:** Hypothermia following cortisone administration. Am J Med 18:146, 1955
35. **Dripps RD (ed):** The physiology of induced hypothermia. Proceedings of a Symposium, Pub 451. Washing-

ton, National Academy of Sciences–National Research Council, 1956

36. **MacNeal WJ:** Hyperthermia, genuine and spurious. Arch Intern Med 64:800, 1939

37. **MacNeal, WJ, Ritter HH, and Rabson, SM:** Prolonged hyperthermia; report of a case with necropsy. Arch Intern Med 64:809, 1939

38. **Simon HB:** Extreme pyrexia. JAMA 236:2419, 1976

39. **DuBois EF:** Why are fever temperatures over 106°F rare? Am J Med Sci 217:361, 1949

40. **von Liebermeister C:** Handbüch der Pathologie und Therapie des Fiebers. Leipzig, Vogel, 1875

41. **Cooper KE, Cranston WI, Snell ES:** Temperature regulation during fever in man. Clin Sci 27:345, 1964

42. **Macpherson RK:** The effect of fever on body temperature regulation in man. Clin Sci 18:281, 1959

43. **Palmes ED, Park CR:** The regulation of body temperature during fever. Arch Environ Health 11:749, 1965

44. **Andersen HT, Hammel HT, Hardy JD:** Modifications of the febrile response to pyrogen by hypothalamic heating and cooling in the unanesthetized dog. Acta Physiol Scand 53:247, 1961

45. **Stitt JT, Hardy JD, Stolwijk JAJ:** PGE_1 fever, its effect on thermoregulation at different low ambient temperatures. Am J Physiol 227:622, 1974

46. **Clark WG:** Mechanisms of antipyretic action. Gen Pharmacol 10:71, 1979

47. **Atkins E, Bodel P:** Clinical fever: Its history, manifestations and pathogenesis. Fed Proc 38:57, 1979

48. **Kluger MJ:** Fever: Its Biology, Evolution and Function. Princeton, Princeton University Press, 1979

49. **Lipton JM (ed):** Fever. New York, Raven Press, 1980

50. **Cox B, Lomax P, Milton AS, et al (eds):** Thermoregulatory Mechanisms and Their Therapeutic Implications. Basel, Karger, 1980

51. **Atkins E, Bodel P:** Fever. In Zweifach BW, Grant L, McCluskey RT (eds): The Inflammatory Process, 2nd ed, p 467. New York, Academic Press, 1974

51a.**Dinarello CA, Wolff SM:** Molecular basis of fever in humans. Am J Med 72:799, 1982

52. **King MK, Wood WB, Jr:** Studies on the pathogenesis of fever. IV. The site of action of leucocytic and circulating endogenous pyrogen. J Exp Med 107:291, 1958

53. **Sheth UK, Borison HL:** Central pyrogenic action of *Salmonella typhosa* lipopolysaccharide injected into the lateral cerebral ventricle in cats. J Pharmacol Exp Ther 130:411, 1960

54. **Cooper KE, Cranston WI, Honour AJ:** Observations on the site and mode of action of pyrogens in the rabbit brain. J Physiol 191:325, 1967

55. **Jackson DL:** A hypothalamic region responsive to localized injection of pyrogens. J Neurophysiol 30:586, 1967

56. **Rosendorff C, Mooney JJ:** Central nervous system sites of action of a purified leucocyte pyrogen. Am J Physiol 220:597, 1971

57. **Bard P, Woods JW:** Central nervous region essential for endotoxin fever. Trans Am Neurol Assoc 87:37, 1962

58. **Bennett IL, Jr, Beeson PB:** Studies on the pathogenesis of fever. I. The effect of injection of extracts and suspensions of uninfected rabbit tissues upon the body temperature of normal rabbits. J Exp Med 98:477, 1953

59. **Hanson DF, Murphy PA, Windle BE:** Failure of rabbit neutrophils to secrete endogenous pyrogen when stimulated with staphylococci. J Exp Med 151:1360, 1980

60. **Dinarello CA, Wolff SM:** Exogenous pyrogens. In Milton AS (ed): Handbook of Experimental Pharmacology, Vol 60, p 73. New York, Springer-Verlag 1982

61. **Dinarello CA, Wolff SM:** Pathogenesis of fever in man. N Engl J Med 298:607, 1978

62. **Bernheim HA, Block LH, Atkins E:** Fever: Pathogenesis, pathophysiology, and purpose. Ann Intern Med 91:261, 1979

63. **Dinarello CA:** Demonstration of a human pyrogen-inducing factor during mixed leukocyte reactions. J Exp Med 153:1215, 1981

64. **Atkins E, Francis L, Bernheim HA:** Pathogenesis of fever in delayed hypersensitivity: Role of monocytes. Infect Immun 21:813, 1978

65. **Cranston WI, Hellon RF, Townsend Y:** Suppression of fever in rabbits by a protein synthesis inhibitor, anisomycin. J Physiol 305:337, 1980

66. **Murphy, PA, Cebula TA, Windle BE:** Heterogeneity of rabbit endogenous pyrogens is not attributable to glycosylated variants of a single polypeptide chain. Infect Immun 34:184, 1981

67. **Murphy PA, Cebula TA, Levin J et al:** Rabbit macrophages secrete two biochemically and immunologically distinct endogenous pyrogens. Infect Immun 34:177, 1981

68. **Dinarello CA, Goldin NP, Wolff SM:** Demonstration and characterization of two distinct human leukocytic pyrogens. J Exp Med 139:1369, 1974

69. **Morrison DC, Ryan JL:** Bacterial endotoxins and host immune responses. Adv Immunol 28:293, 1979

70. **Nordlund JJ, Root RK, Wolff SM:** Studies on the origin of human leukocytic pyrogen. J Exp Med 131:727, 1970

71. **Bodel P:** Studies on the mechanism of endogenous pyrogen production. I. Investigation of new protein synthesis in stimulated human blood leucocytes. Yale J Biol Med 43:145, 1970

72. **Bodel P:** Studies on the mechanism of endogenous pyrogen production. III. Human blood monocytes. J Exp Med 140:954, 1974

73. **Feldberg W, Myers RD:** Effects on temperature of amines injected into the cerebral ventricles. A new concept of temperature regulation. J Physiol 173:226, 1964

74. **Myers RD, Yaksh TL:** Control of body temperature in the unanaesthetized monkey by cholinergic and aminergic systems in the hypothalamus. J Physiol 202:483, 1969

75. **Hellon RF:** Monoamines, pyrogens and cations: Their

actions on central control of body temperature. Pharmacol Rev 26:289, 1975

76. **Milton AS, Wendlandt S:** Effects on body temperature of prostaglandins of the A, E and F series on injection into the third ventricle of unanaesthetized cats and rabbits. J Physiol 218:325, 1971

77. **Stitt JT, Hardy JD:** Microelectrophoresis of PGE₁ onto single units in the rabbit hypothalamus. Am J Physiol 229:240, 1975

78. **Dinarello CA, Bernheim HA:** Ability of human leukocytic pyrogen to stimulate brain prostaglandin synthesis in vitro. J Neurochem 37:702, 1981

79. **Rosendorff C:** Neurochemistry of fever. S Afr J Med Sci 41:23, 1976

80. **Philipp–Dormston WK, Siegert R:** Prostaglandins of the E and F series in rabbit cerebrospinal fluid during fever induced by Newcastle Disease Virus, *E. coli*-endotoxin and endogenous pyrogen. Med Microbiol Immunol 59:279, 1974

81. **Bernheim HA, Gilbert TM, Stitt JT:** Prostaglandin E levels in third ventricular cerebrospinal fluid of rabbits during fever and changes in body temperature. J Physiol 301:69, 1980

82. **Cranston WI, Duff GW, Hellon RF et al:** Evidence that brain prostaglandin synthesis is not essential in fever. J Physiol 259:239, 1976

83. **Nordlund JJ, Wolff SM, Levy HB:** Inhibition of biologic activity of poly I poly C by human plasma. Proc Soc Exp Biol Med 133:439, 1970

84. **Dinarello CA, Weiner P, Wolff SM:** Radiolabeling and disposition in rabbits of purified human leukocytic pyrogen. Clin Res 26:522A, 1978

85. **Rosenwasser LJ, Dinarello CA, Rosenthal AS:** Adherent cell function in murine T-lymphocyte antigen recognition. IV. Enhancement of murine T-cell antigen recognition by human leukocytic pyrogen. J Exp Med 150:709, 1979

86. **Murphy PA, Simon PL, Willoughby WF:** Endogenous pyrogens made by rabbit peritoneal exudate cells are identical with lymphocyte-activating factors made by rabbit alveolar macrophages. J Immunol 124:2498, 1980

87. **Dinarello CA, Renfer L, Wolff SM:** Human leukocytic pyrogen: Purification and development of a radioimmunoassay. Proc Natl Acad Sci 74:4624, 1977

88. **Greisman SE, Hornick RB:** On the demonstration of circulating human endogenous pyrogen. Proc Soc Exp Biol Med 139:690, 1972

89. **Fremont–Smith F, Morrison LR, Makepeace AW:** Capillary blood flow in man during fever. J Clin Invest 7:489, 1929

90. **Perera GA:** Clinical and physiologic characteristics of chill. Arch Intern Med 68:241, 1941

91. **Altschule MD, Freedberg AS:** Circulation and respiration in fever. Medicine 24:403, 1945

92. **Adler RD, Rawlins M, Rosendorff C, et al:** The effect of salicylate on pyrogen-induced fever in man. Clin Sci 37:91, 1969

93. **Warren SL, Carpenter CN, Boak RA:** Symptomatic herpes; a sequela of artificially induced fever; incidence and clinical aspects; recovery of a virus from herpetic vesicles, and comparison with a known strain of herpes virus. J Exp Med 71:155, 1940

94. **Welty JW:** Febrile albuminuria. Am J Med Sci 194:70, 1937

95. **Wegman ME:** Factors influencing the relation of convulsions and hyperthermia. J Pediat. 14:190, 1939

96. **Lennox WG:** Significance of febrile convulsions. Pediatrics 11:341, 1953

97. **Ouellette EM:** The child who convulses with fever. Pediatr Clin North Am 21:467, 1974

98. **Murray H, Tuazon CU, Guerrero IC et al:** Urinary temperature. N Engl J Med 296:23, 1977

99. **Petersdorf RG, Bennett IL, Jr:** Factitious fever. Ann Intern Med 46:1039, 1957

100. **Aduan RP, Fauci AS, Dale DC et al:** Factitious fever and self-induced infection: A report of 32 cases and review of the literature. Ann Intern Med 90:230, 1979

101. **Bennett IL, Jr, Nicastri A:** Fever as a mechanism of resistance. Bact Rev 24:16, 1960

102. **Kluger MJ, Ringler DH, Anver MR:** Fever and survival. Science 188:166, 1975

103. **Bernheim HA, Bodel PT, Askenase PW et al:** Effects of fever on host defence mechanisms after infection in the lizard *Dipsosaurus dorsalis*. Br J Exp Path 59:76, 1978

104. **Kluger MJ, Vaughn LK:** Fever and survival in rabbits infected with *Pasteurella multocida*. J Physiol 282:243, 1978

105. **Roberts NJ, Jr:** Temperature and host defense. Microbiol Rev 43:241, 1979

105a. **Dinarello CA:** Human pyrogen: A monocyte product mediating host defenses. In Gallin JI, Fauci AS (eds): Advances in Host Defense Mechanisms, Vol 1, pp 57–74. New York, Raven Press, 1982

106. **Kampschmidt RF:** Leukocytic endogenous mediator/endogenous pyrogen. In Powanda MC, Canonico PG (eds): Infection: The Physiologic and Metabolic Responses of the Host, p 55. New York, Elsevier/North-Holland Biomedical Press, 1981

107. **Bornstein DL, Walsh EC:** Endogenous mediators of the acute-phase reaction. I. Rabbit granulocytic pyrogen and its chromatographic subfractions. J Lab Clin Med 91:236, 1978

108. **Klempner MS, Dinarello CA, Gallin JI:** Human leukocytic pyrogen induces release of specific granule contents from human neutrophils. J Clin Invest 61:1330, 1978

109. **Klempner, MS, Dinarello CA, Henderson WR, and Gallin JI:** Stimulation of neutrophil oxygen-dependent metabolism by human leukocytic pyrogen. J Clin Invest 64:996, 1979

110. **Futcher PH:** The double quotidian temperature curve of

gonococcal endocarditis; a diagnostic aid. Am J Med Sci 199:23, 1940

111. **Musher DM, Fainstein V, Young EJ, et al:** Fever patterns: Their lack of clinical significance. Arch Intern Med 139:1225, 1979

112. **Todd J, Fishaut M, Kapral F et al:** Toxic-shock syndrome associated with phage group-1 staphylococci. Lancet 2:1116, 1978

113. **Schlievert PM, Schoettle DJ, Watson DW:** Purification and physicochemical and biological characterization of a staphylococcal pyrogenic exotoxin. Infect Immun 23:609, 1979

114. **Erickson TC:** Neurogenic hyperthermia (a clinical syndrome and its treatment) Brain 62:172, 1939

115. **Ackerman D, Rudy TA:** Thermoregulatory characteristics of neurogenic hyperthermia in the rat. J Physiol 307:59, 1980

116. **Holmes G:** Goulstonian lectures on spinal injurnies of warfare. II. The clinical symptoms of gunshot injuries of the spine. Br Med J 2:815, 1915

117. **Lobell M, Boggs DR, Wintrobe MM:** The clinical significance of fever in Hodgkin's disease. Arch Intern Med 117:335, 1966

118. **Klastersky J, Weerts D, Hensgens C et al:** Fever of unexplained origin in patients with cancer. Eur J Cancer 9:649, 1973

119. **Fenster LF, Klatskin G:** Manifestations of metastatic tumors of the liver. Am J Med 31:238, 1961

120. **Harsha WN:** Fever in malignant disease. Am Surg 18:229, 1952

121. **Clagett OT, McDonald JR, Schmidt HW:** Localized fibrous mesothelioma of the pleura J Thorac Surg 24:213, 1952

122. **Browder AA, Huff JW, Petersdorf RG:** The significance of fever in neoplastic disease. Ann Intern Med 55:932, 1961

123. **Boggs DR, Frei E, III:** Clinical studies of fever and infections in cancer. Cancer 13:1240, 1960

124. **Warshaw AL, Carey RW, Robinson DR:** Control of fever associated with visceral cancers by indomethacin. Surgery 89:414, 1981

125. **Bodel P:** Tumors and fever. Ann NY. Acad Sci. 230:6, 1974

126. **Silver RT, Utz JP, Frei E, III et al:** Fever, infection and host resistance in acute leukemia. Am J Med 24:25, 1958

127. **Raab SO, Hoeprich PD, Wintrobe MM et al:** The clinical significance of fever in acute leukemia. Blood 16:1609, 1960

128. **Margolies MP:** Sickle-cell anemia. A composite study and survey. Medicine 30:357, 1951

129. **Greenberg PL, Bax I, Levin J et al:** Alteration of colony-stimulating factor output, endotoxemia and granulopoiesis in cyclic neutropenia. Am J Hematol 1:375, 1976

130. **Murray HW, Ellis GC, Blumenthal DS et al:** Fever and pulmonary thromboembolism. Am J Med 67:232, 1979

131. **Dunn LJ, Van Voorhis LW:** Enigmatic fever and pelvic thrombophlebitis. Response to anticoagulants. N Eng J Med 276:265, 1967

132. **Ferris EB, Jr, Blankenhorn MA, Robinson HW et al:** Heat stroke; clinical and chemical observations on 44 cases. J Clin Invest 17:249, 1938

133. **Knochel JP, Beisel WR, Herndon EG, Jr et al:** The renal, cardiovascular, hematologic and serum electrolyte abnormalities of heat stroke. Am J Med 30:299, 1961

134. **Shibolet S, Lancaster MC, Danon Y:** Heatstroke: A review. Aviat Space Environ Med 47:280, 1976

135. **Clowes GHA, Jr, O'Donnell TF, Jr:** Current concepts: Heat stroke. N Engl J Med 291:564, 1974

136. **Himwich HE:** The metabolism of fever, with special reference to diabetic hyperpyrexia. Bull NY Acad Med 10:16, 1934

137. **Edelman IS:** Thyroid thermogenesis. N Engl J Med 209:1303, 1974

138. **Rosenberg IN:** Thyroid storm. N Engl J Med 283:1052, 1970

139. **Simon HB, Daniels GH:** Hormonal hyperthermia: Endocrine causes of fever. Am J Med 66:257, 1979

140. **Reimann HA:** Periodic Diseases, pp 41–69. Oxford, Blackwell, 1963

140a.**Meyerhoff J:** Familial Mediterranean fever: Report of a large family, review of the literature, and discussion of the frequency of amyloidosis. Medicine 59:66, 1980

141. **Dinarello CA, Wolff SM, Goldfinger SE et al:** Colchicine therapy for familial Mediterranean fever. A doubleblind trial. N Engl J Med 281:934, 1974

142. **Kappas A, Palmer RH:** Selected aspects of steroid pharmacology. Pharmacol Rev 15:123, 1963

143. **Bodel P., and Dillard M:** Studies on steroid fever. I. Production of leukocyte pyrogen in vitro by etiocholanolone, J Clin Invest 47:107, 1968

144. **George JM, Wolff SM, Diller E, and Bartter, FC:** Recurrent fever of unknown etiology: Failure to demonstrate association between fever and plasma unconjugated etiocholanolone. J Clin Invest 48:558, 1969

145. **Bodel P, Dillard GM:** Suppression of periodic fever with estrogen. Arch Intern Med 131:189,1973

146. **Tisdale WA, Klatskin G:** The fever of Laennec's cirrhosis. Yale J Biol Med 33:94, 1960

147. **Kinsey D, White PD:** Fever in congestive heart failure. Arch Intern. Med 65:163, 1940

148. **Lian C, Facquet J, Brawerman:** Fièvre et tacycardies paroxystiques. Arch Mal Coeur 32:566, 1939

149. **Kerr A, Jr:** Subacute Bacterial Endocarditis. Springfield, Il, Charles C Thomas, 1955

150. **Goodwin JF, Stanfield CA, Steiner RE et al:** Clinical features of left atrial myxoma. Thorax 17:91, 1962

151. **Goodyer AVN, Glenn WWL:** Management of the circulatory, inflammatory and metabolic complications of mitral valvulotomy. N Engl J Med 257:735, 1957

152. **Goodkind MJ, Bloomer WE, Goodyer AVN:** Recurrent pericardial effusion after nonpenetrating chest trauma. Report of two cases treated with adrenocortical steroids. N Engl J Med 263:874, 1960

153. **Dressler W:** Post-myocardial-infarction syndrome: Report on forty-four cases. Arch Intern Med 103:28, 1959

154. **Engle MA, Ito T:** Postpericardiotomy syndrome. Am J Cardiol 7:73, 1961

155. **Drusin LM, Engle MA, Hagstron JWC et al:** The postpericardiotomy syndrome. A six-year epidemiologic study. N Engl J Med. 272:597, 1965

156. **Lang DJ, Scolnick EM, Willerson JT:** Association of cytomegalovirus infection with the post-perfusion syndrome. N Engl J Med. 278:1147, 1968

157. **Wheeler EO, Turner JD, Scannell, JG:** Fever, splenomegaly and atypical lymphocytes. A syndrome observed after cardiac surgery utilizing a pump oxygenator. N Engl J Med 266:454, 1962

158. **Rifkind D, Marchioro TL, Waddell WR et al:** Infectious diseases associated with renal homotransplantation. I. Incidence, types and predisposing factors. JAMA 189:397, 1964

159. **Silber EN, Katz LN:** Fever in patients with heart disease. Med Clin North Am 50:211, 1966

160. **Nolan JP, Klatskin G:** The fever of sarcoidosis. Ann Intern Med 61:455, 1964

161. **Roe CF:** Surgical aspects of fever. Curr Probl Surg, November 1968

162. **Klatskin G:** Mechanisms of toxic and drug induced hepatic injury. In Fink RB (ed): Toxicity of Anesthetics, p 159. Baltimore, Williams & Wilkins, 1968

163. **Bang S:** Fever in gastric and in duodenal ulcer. Arch Intern Med 41:808, 1928

164. **Dill LV, Isenhour CE:** Observations on the incidence and cause of fever in patients with bleeding peptic ulcers. Am J Dig Dis 5:779, 1939

165. **Schiff L, Shapiro N, Stevens RF:** Observations on the oral administration of citrated blood in man. III. The effect on temperature and the white blood cell count. Am J Med Sci 207:465, 1944

166. **Selesnick S, White BV:** Body temperature in persons with bleeding peptic ulcer. Gastroenterology 20:282, 1952

167. **Stiles FC, Weir JR:** Ectodermal dysplasia presenting as fever of unknown origin. JAMA 158:1432, 1955

168. **Woodyatt RT:** Ichthyosis, fever and effort syndrome. Trans Assoc Am Physicians 50:105, 1935.

169. **Harvey AMcG, Shulman LE, Tumulty PA et al:** Systemic lupus erythematosus: Review of the literature and clinical analysis of 138 cases. Medicine 33:291, 1954

170. **Calabro JJ, Marchesano, JM:** Fever associated with juvenile rheumatoid arthritis. N Engl J Med 276:11, 1967

171. **Bujak JS, Aptekar RG, Decker JL et al:** Juvenile rheumatoid arthritis presenting in the adult as fever of unknown origin. Medicine 52:431, 1973

172. **Rowe AH:** Fever due to food allergy. Ann Allergy 6:252, 1948

173. **Bigler JA, McQuiston WO:** Body temperatures during anesthesia in infants and children. JAMA 146:551, 1951

174. **Pickrell HP:** Hyperpyrexia pallida and its prevention. Aust NZ J Surg 21:261, 1952

175. **Mangiardi JL:** Experiences with post-operative temperatures above 108°F. Am J Surg 81:189, 1951

176. **Henschel EO (ed):** Malignant Hyperthermia: Current Concepts. New York, Appleton Century-Crofts, 1977

177. **Cluff LE, Johnson JE, III:** Drug fever. Prog Allergy 8:149, 1964

178. **Lipsky BA, Hirschmann JV:** Drug fever. JAMA 245:851, 1981

178a. **Young EJ, Fainstein V, Musher DM:** Drug-induced fever: Cases seen in the evaluation of unexplained fever in a general hospital population. Rev Infect Dis 4:69, 1982

179. **Vogel VH, Isbell H, Chapman KW:** Present status of narcotic addiction; with particular reference to medical indications and comparative addiction liability of the newer and older analgesic drugs. JAMA 138:1019, 1948

180. **Galloway RE, Levin J, Butler T et al:** Activation of protein mediators of inflammation and evidence for endotoxemia in *Borrelia recurrentis* infection. Am J Med 63:933, 1977

181. **von Euler C:** Physiology and pharmacology of temperature regulation. Pharmacol Rev 13:361, 1961

182. **Fred HL, Allred DP, Garber HE et al:** Pheochromocytoma masquerading as overwhelming infection. Am Heart J 73:149, 1967

183. **Swank RL, Smedal MI:** Pulmonary atelectasis in stuporous states; a study of its incidence and mechanism in sodium amytal narcosis. Am J Med 5:210, 1948

184. **Lee RV, Drabinsky M, Wolfson S et al:** Pyrogen reactions from cardiac catheterization. Chest 63:757, 1973

185. **Ritter WL, Nussbaum MA:** Occupational illnesses in cotton industries: "Cotton fever." Miss. Doctor, p 96, September 1944

186. **Sayers RR:** Metal fume fever and its prevention. Public Health Rep 53:1080, 1938

187. **Harris DK:** Polymer-fume fever. Lancet 2:1008, 1951

188. **McCord CP:** Metal fume fever as an immunological disease. Industr Med Surg 29:101, 1960

189. **Reimann HA:** The problem of long-continued, low-grade fever. JAMA 107:1089, 1936

190. **Richardson JS:** Pyrexia of uncertain origin and psychogenic fever. Practitioner 170:61, 1953

191. **Dunbar HF:** Emotions and Bodily Changes, 2nd ed. New York, Columbia, 1938

192. **Wynn FB:** The psychic factor as an element in temperature disturbance; shown by some observations in the selective draft. JAMA 73:31, 1919

193. **Wolf S, Wolff HG:** Intermittent fever of unknown origin; recurrent high fever with benign outcome in a pa-

tient with migraine and notes on "neurogenic" fever. Arch Intern Med 70:293, 1942

194. **Petersdorf RG, Beeson PB:** Fever of unexplained origin: Report on 100 cases. Medicine 40:1, 1961

195. **Tumulty PA:** The patient with fever of undetermined origin: A diagnostic challenge. Bull Johns Hopkins Hosp 120:95, 1967

196. **Baker RR, Tumulty PA, Shelley WM:** The value of exploratory laparotomy in fever of undetermined etiology. Johns Hopkins Med J 125:159, 1969

197. **Molavi A, Weinstein L:** Persistent perplexing pyrexia: Some comments on etiology and diagnosis. Med Clin North Am 54:379, 1970

198. **Jacoby GA, Swartz MN:** Fever of undetermined origin. N Engl J Med 289:1407, 1973

199. **Wolff SM, Fauci AS, Dale DC:** Unusual etiologies of fever and their evaluation. Annu Rev Med 26:277, 1975

200. **Pizzo P, Lovejoy F, Smith D:** Prolonged fever in children: Review of 100 cases. Pediatrics 55:468, 1975

201. **Esposito A, Gleckman R:** A diagnostic approach to the adult with fever of unknown origin. Arch Intern Med 139:575, 1979

202. **Weinstein L, Fields BN:** Fever of obscure origin. Semin Infect Dis 1:1, 1978

203. **Larson EB, Featherstone HJ, Petersdorf RG:** Fever of undetermined origin: Diagnosis and follow-up of 105 cases, 1970–1980. Medicine 61:269, 1982

204. **Dinavello C:** Interleukin-I. Rev. Infect Dis 6:51, 1984

26

Lymphadenopathy and Disorders of the Lymphatics

Harold Jeghers,
Sam L. Clark, Jr.,
Alexander C. Templeton

Introduction
Functions of Lymphatics and Lymph Nodes
Lymph
Formation of Lymph
Composition of Lymph
Lymphatic Vessels
Transport of Lymph
Volume of Lymph
Uncommon Pathways of Lymph Flow
Areas Lacking Lymphatic Drainage
Lymphangitis
Dilatation of Lymphatic Capillaries and Vessels
Obstruction of Lymphatic Vessels
The Main Lymphatic Vessels
Anatomy
Chylous Effusions
Lymph Nodes
Stroma
Architecture of Lymph Nodes
Filtration of Lymph
Cellular Populations in Lymph Nodes
Lymphoid Cells
Age Changes in Lymphoid Tissue
**Modes of Lymph Node Involvement and
         Pathologic Changes**
Hereditary Causes
Immunodeficiency Diseases
Lysosomal Storage Diseases
Acquired Diseases
Inflammatory Reactions in Lymph Nodes
Neoplastic Diseases in Lymph Nodes
Diagnostic Methods
Lymphography
The Normal Lymphogram

The Abnormal Lymphogram
Advantages of Lymphogram
Xeroradiography
Diagnostic Ultrasound
Computed Tomographic Scanning
Scintigraphy
Regional Lymphadenopathy
Lymph Nodes of Head and Neck
Group I—Clinically Important and Readily
Palpable Lymph Nodes
Group II—Less Clinically Important and Not
Readily Palpable Lymph Nodes
The Axillary Nodes
The Epitrochlear (Superficial Cubital or
Supratrochlear) Nodes
The Inguinal Lymph Nodes
The Popliteal Nodes
The Mediastinal Lymph Nodes
Abdominal Lymph Nodes
Clinical Syndromes of the Intra-abdominal
Nodes
Lymph Node Syndromes
Extremity Lesion and Regional
Lymphadenopathy Syndrome
Oropharynx Lesion with Cervical Satellite
Lymphadenopathy Syndrome
Genital Lesion and Groin Lymphadenopathy
Syndrome
Lymphatic Metastases from Breast Cancer
Syndromes
Suppuration of Lymph Nodes
Generalized Lymphadenopathy
Summary

INTRODUCTION

Lymphatic vessels and lymph nodes constitute only a part of the lymphoid system, which also includes the thymus, spleen, tonsils, appendix, Peyer's patches, and other lymphoid aggregations of the intestine, as well as other less well organized accumulations of lymphoid cells scattered through the connective tissues of the body. Thus, lymphatics and lymph nodes function interdependently with the rest of the lymphoid system, participating in its constant traffic of wandering lymphocytes, in the immune reactions, and in the diseases that affect the rest of the system. Therefore, the diseases to be considered here cannot be viewed in isolation from the lymphoid system and generalized immune reactions. The term *lymphatic system* has been used to encompass the lymphatics and lymph nodes, but for the reasons stated, it does not define a distinct and independent organ system. Its use has been confused by those who make it ambiguously synonymous with the more comprehensive term *lymphoid system*. Therefore, *lymphatic system* will not be used in this discussion. The even more ambiguous term *reticuloendothelial system* will also be avoided, because in the light of newer knowledge the term appears to be more misleading than helpful in understanding the distribution and lineages of phagocytic cells.

Although lymphatics and lymph nodes are part of a larger system and are dispersed widely throughout the body, lymph is drained and filtered locally through lymph nodes before combining with lymph from other regions of the body to rejoin the blood stream. Thus, lymph nodes serve to isolate disease, preventing its spread to other parts of the body. Many lymph nodes are subcutaneous, palpable when enlarged, and amenable to biopsy; histologic examination gives clues to both the nature and geographic extent of disease processes. For these reasons, a knowledge of the regional anatomy and histology of lymphatics and lymph nodes is critical to proper diagnosis and treatment of many diseases.

The major categories of disease involving lymphatics and lymph nodes include (1) disorders of immune function, (2) primary hematopoietic diseases, (3) infectious lymphadenopathy, (4) lymphadenopathy caused by the sequestration of irritating foreign materials, (5) storage of the accumulated products of a genetically disordered metabolism, and (6) carcinomatous invasion.

The following discussion of normal structure and function of the lymphatics and lymph nodes may be documented and extended by reference to the comprehensive monograph of Yoffey and Courtice[1] and the more specialized monographs by Battezzoti and Donini;[2] Greaves, Owen, and Raff;[3] Weiss;[4] Barrowman;[5] and Clouse.[6] The appropriate chapters in the tenth edition of Bloom and Fawcett's *Textbook of Histology* provide a concise yet scholarly and provocative synthesis of our rapidly growing knowledge concerning the relationships between the structure of lymphoid tissues and the functions of immunity.[7]

Lymphatics form a converging system of vessels which begins blindly with plexuses of lymphatic capillaries deployed throughout the loose connective tissues of the body; it continues through progressively larger lymphatics, interrupted by lymph nodes; and it terminates at several points where major lymphatic ducts join major veins. Lymphatics develop in the embryo as endothelial outgrowths of veins in the neck and trunk. They follow the major blood vessels, and lymph nodes develop in groups, particularly at the junctions of lymphatics. The original outgrowths of lymphatics in the neck—the jugular lymph sacs—become the terminal portions of the thoracic and right lymphatic ducts. Sites of lymphatic outgrowth from veins in the trunk remain, at least potentially, as alternative pathways for the return of lymph to the blood stream.

FUNCTIONS OF LYMPHATICS AND LYMPH NODES

Lymphatics conduct lymph from its site of formation in loose connective tissue to its destination in the blood stream. Lymph formed in the lamina propria of the small intestine is rich in absorbed nutrients, particularly lipids and lipid-soluble vitamins; thus the intestinal lymphatics participate in intestinal absorption, particularly of neutral fats, providing a pathway to the blood stream that bypasses the liver. Microorganisms that gain access to the connective tissues may also enter lymphatics, with the potentiality of causing infection of the lymphatics (tubular lymphangitis) or of lymph nodes (lymphadenitis). If lymph nodes fail to confine an infection, microorganisms may enter the blood stream (bacteremia) and cause septicemia.

Lymph nodes are very effective filters of lymph. Phagocytic cells lining sinuses ingest microorganisms and other particulate or antigenic material as it percolates slowly through the lymph node; nearly all such material is removed by passage through a single node. The phagocytosis of antigenic material, potentiated by its combination with specific antibody, plays a role in the induction of immune responses.

Lymph nodes, like other lymphoid tissues, produce lymphocytes and plasma cells in response to antigenic

stimulation. These, in turn, carry out cell-mediated immune responses, are the repositories of immunologic memory, and secrete antibody. Under pathologic conditions, lymph nodes may also become sites of extramedullary hemopoiesis, but this activity is not necessarily the work of cells indigenous to lymph nodes; the relationships between lymphoid cells and other hematopoietic cells remain incompletely understood.

LYMPH

FORMATION OF LYMPH

Lymph is, indirectly, an ultrafiltrate of blood plasma somewhat analogous in formation and composition to glomerular filtrate. It represents the excess of fluid that leaves the blood capillaries over that which is reabsorbed farther down the blood stream. However, lymph is the direct product of the extracellular fluid of connective tissue, altered from the original ultrafiltrate by the actions of neighboring cells, which remove nutrients and discharge waste, as well as by the incursion of invading microorganisms and wandering cells.

Blood capillaries are freely permeable to water and small molecules but relatively impermeable to proteins. The diffusion of water and small molecules between the blood stream and surrounding connective tissue is modulated by (1) a variable difference in hydrostatic pressure between the two compartments and (2) a difference in colloid osmotic pressure owing to the high concentration of proteins in blood plasma and the low concentration of dissolved proteins in extravascular extracellular fluid. The relatively constant difference in colloid osmotic pressure promotes movement of water from an extravascular to an intravascular position. In capillaries fed by open arterioles, the hydrostatic pressure of the blood exceeds both tissue pressure and colloid osmotic pressure sufficiently to cause movement of fluids out of the vessel into the extracellular perivascular spaces. In venules, or in capillaries supplied by temporarily constricted arterioles, the sum of colloid osmotic pressure and tissue pressure exceeds blood pressure, and fluid is reabsorbed from the connective tissue into the blood stream. In nondistensible tissues such as bone, there is no room for fluid to accumulate, and reabsorption is in equilibrium with transudation. In loose connective tissue, where extracellular fluid can accumulate without causing a commensurate increase in tissue pressure, more fluid inevitably leaves the blood stream than can return to it. If this excess is not removed as lymph, it continues to accumulate as edema fluid.

Any physiologic or pathologic process that alters the parameters of transudation and reabsorption just described will alter the rate of accumulation of extracellular fluid, which is the rate of production of lymph. Such processes include

Decreased arterial blood pressure, as in traumatic shock
Reduction in the colloid osmotic pressure of plasma, as in the hemodilution produced by parenteral administration of fluid, the hypoproteinemia of starvation, or the nephrotic syndrome
Changes in capillary blood pressure produced by arterial dilation or constriction, either locally, as in the regulation of body temperature, or generally, as in the maintenance of arterial blood pressure
Increased capillary permeability to proteins produced by physical injuries, such as burns; by hypoxia; by the release of mediators of acute inflammation, such as histamine or serotonin; or by the administration of similar substances, such as drugs
Increased venous pressure owing to the effects of gravity, venous obstruction, or cardiac failure.

COMPOSITION OF LYMPH

The composition of lymph is altered from that of the original ultrafiltrate of blood plasma by the actions of neighboring cells and tissues. Hence it varies from time to time and in different regions of the body. In its content of nutrients, waste products, and respiratory gases, it is generally in equilibrium with venous blood leaving the region. Because of its content of waste products, removal of lymph from the thoracic duct has been reported to reduce blood urea nitrogen in uremic patients.

Although blood capillaries are relatively impermeable to protein, all the plasma proteins diffuse into connective tissue to some extent; the increased capillary permeability at sites of acute inflammation offers almost no barrier to diffusion of plasma proteins. As a result, lymph from peripheral regions of the body contains most plasma proteins at approximately one third their concentration in the blood; such lymph clots slowly. Capillary endothelium is more permeable to albumin than to other plasma proteins; it may reach levels in peripheral lymph 50% of those in plasma. Immunoglobulins, produced by plasma cells in lymph nodes, enter the lymph as it traverses lymph nodes, constituting a major source of immunoglobulin for the blood. Hepatic lymph is rich in the other plasma proteins, which are synthesized by the liver. Apparently, the space of Disse, lying between hepatic parenchymal cells and sinusoidal endothelium, is in functional continuity with lymphatic capillaries surrounding branches

of the portal vein. In sum, thoracic duct lymph is rich in protein and supplies the blood plasma with a major proportion of its proteins.

Intestinal lymph contributes much neutral lipid and other absorbed nutrients to thoracic duct lymph.

In addition to soluble materials, lymph also carries lymphocytes from three major sources:

1. *The loose connective tissues,* where lymph is formed, constitute a minor source. Lymphocytes leave the blood stream by diapedesis, especially at sites of inflammation or where antigens enter the body through epithelial surfaces. Diapedesis of lymphocytes is particularly marked at sites of cell-mediated immune responses, such as delayed hypersensitivity. Lymphocytes that enter connective tissue may penetrate the walls of lymphocytic capillaries to join the lymph stream.

2. *The intestinal lymphoid aggregations,* including tonsils, Peyer's patches, and appendix, are a major source. Lymphocytes accumulate in these structures by two mechanisms: cellular proliferation and diapedesis of lymphocytes from the blood through the walls of specialized venules with high endothelium. Large numbers of lymphocytes from these sources enter intestinal and pharyngeal lymphatics.

3. *Lymph nodes* constitute another major source of lymphocytes in lymph. Lymphocytes enter lymph nodes not only through afferent lymph, but also by diapedesis through high-endothelial venules similar to those in intestinal aggregations. Lymphocytes are also produced by cellular proliferation in germinal centers and in the diffuse thymus-dependent inner cortex. Many of these lymphocytes enter lymphatic sinuses and leave the node through efferent lymph in far greater numbers than entered the node with the afferent lymph.

From these sources, very large numbers of lymphocytes enter the blood stream by way of the thoracic and right lymphatic ducts—enough to replace the population of lymphocytes in the blood several times daily. Contrary to former beliefs, this rapid turnover does not represent the rate of death and production of lymphocytes but represents instead a massive continuous recirculation of lymphocytes from lymphoid tissues to the blood stream and back to lymphoid tissues to begin the cycle again. Many lymphocytes survive for months or years, wandering through the connective tissues of the body, entering the intercellular spaces of epithelia, reaching lymphoid tissues through the lymph or by diapedesis through the walls of high-endothelial venules, and recirculating back to the blood stream through the lymphatics. Most of these recirculating lymphocytes are derived from the thymus (T-cells). The con-

tinual movement of these cells through connective tissue and epithelia probably represents a mechanism for surveillance of the body, providing immunologic protection against invading microorganisms or the advent of antigenically recognizable malignant cells.

Other wandering cells of the blood and connective tissues also enter the lymph in small numbers, potentiated by local inflammatory and allergic reactions, but most of these are removed in lymph nodes and do not reach the thoracic duct.

Lymph also carries invading microorganisms and foreign particulate material from the connective tissues to be removed by phagocytosis in lymph nodes. Cells of malignant tumors may invade lymphatic vessels to settle down and grow locally or produce emboli of tumor cells that travel with the lymph stream to regional lymph nodes.

LYMPHATIC VESSELS

Lymphatic capillaries, forming ubiquitous plexuses in loose connective tissue, are particularly concentrated adjacent to epithelia. Such plexuses are found in glands; in serous membranes lining the pleural, peritoneal, and pericardial cavities; in synovial membranes of joints and bursae; and underlying body surfaces in the skin and in the mucous membranes of the respiratory, gastrointestinal, and urinary systems. In the skin and mucous membranes, the plexuses are usually arranged as a superficial and a deep set. The superficial plexus beneath the epidermis may be a site for *localized infectious lymphangitis* (erysipelas).

Lymphatic capillaries have no afferent vascular supply except other anastomosing capillaries; some, such as the lacteal in each intestinal villus, begin blindly. Capillary plexuses are drained by larger lymphatics, which usually accompany veins, often as a freely anastomosing network of vessels. Groups of lymph nodes lie at junctions where lymphatics converge to form larger lymphatics.

Lymphatic capillaries are larger in diameter and more irregular in shape than blood capillaries. Their walls comprise only a thin and very permeable endothelium surrounded by an incomplete basal lamina. The thin and sometimes fenestrated endothelial cells are joined at intervals by junctional complexes, leaving at least potential gaps between the endothelial cells, large enough for erythrocytes and leukocytes to squeeze through.

Overlapping flaps of endothelial cytoplasm may serve a valvelike function at these gaps, allowing penetration into, but not out of, the lymphatic capillary. The great permeability of lymphatic capillaries would not, by it-

self, ensure escape of excess extracellular fluid and particulate material from connective tissue; a pressure gradient is needed to force interstitial fluid from connective tissue spaces into lymphatic capillary lumens.

Until recently it was believed that the increased tissue pressure produced by passive movements and contractions of skeletal muscle provided the motive power, milking lymph centrally, where it is retained by valves, and forcing interstitial fluid down a pressure gradient into capillary lymphatics held open by fine, collagenous guy-wires extending from the lymphatic endothelium into surrounding tissues.

However, direct measurements of interstitial and lymphatic capillary pressures have failed to demonstrate such a hydrostatic pressure gradient; if anything, hydrostatic pressures tend to be higher in the lymphatics than in the surrounding tissues. The best current explanation—not yet completely established as fact—identifies the needed pressure gradient as a gradient in colloid osmotic pressure, created by mechanisms that concentrate proteins in lymphatic capillaries.[8] Once this gradient has pulled interstitial fluid into lymphatic lumens through intercellular slits in the endothelium, passive movement and contractions of skeletal muscle serve to squeeze lymph from lymphatic capillaries into valved lymphatics draining the area. Lymphatic capillaries have also been observed to contract actively and to develop pulsatile increases in intraluminal pressure, although the mechanism for these contractions has not been identified.

Larger lymphatics have walls reinforced by connective tissue and a few smooth muscle cells. The thickness and degree of organization of the vascular walls increase with increasing size of vessel, but the wall is never as thick or as well organized as that of veins of corresponding size. Lymphatics are plentifully supplied with valves which, by preventing backflow, ensure that any net flow of lymph will be toward the blood stream. There is an enlargement of the vessel at the site of each valve, which gives lymphatics a beaded appearance.

Usually, lymphatic vessels are disposed in two sets: superficial and deep. This is particularly true of the lymphatic vessels of the extremities. The superficial set lies in the dermis and the superficial fascia. The lymphatic vessels of this set accompany the superficial veins (cephalic and basilic in the upper extremity, long and short saphenous in the lower). The deep set lies beneath the deep fascia and runs with the deep arteries and their accompanying veins in the intermuscular planes. Usually there is little communication between the superficial and deep lymphatic vessels, except where superficial vessels pierce the deep fascia to empty into deep lymph nodes. Since lymphatic vessels accom-

pany both superficial and deep veins and the deep arteries, lymphatic and venous drainages coincide closely. This is of practical value from the surgical point of view, because veins and arteries can be seen easily, whereas lymphatic vessels cannot.

TRANSPORT OF LYMPH

Slow pulsations (frequency of 1–30 contractions/min) of larger lymphatics have been recorded in man and in other mammals. It has been proposed that smooth muscle in the wall of lymphatic vessels contracts in response to an increase in intraluminal pressure.[10] Because lymphatic vessels are subdivided into short segments by valves, contraction in one segment could propel lymph into the next proximal segment, where the resultant increase in intraluminal pressure would stimulate contraction in that segment to propel the lymph still further proximally. There is growing evidence that such intrinsic pumping may be important in the transport of lymph, particularly in the mesenteric lymphatics, which are not so subject to intermittent external pressures as are lymphatics in the limbs.

The major factors promoting transport of lymph are extrinsic to the lymphatics. Anything that increases tissue pressure locally will move lymph into more proximal lymphatics. Such pressures are produced by contraction of skeletal muscles; by passive movement and pressures from the external environment; by pulsation of arteries along which lymphatics run; and by contraction of smooth muscle in viscera, such as intestinal peristalsis. During respiration, intermittent increases in intra-abdominal pressure and decreases in the intrathoracic pressure propel lymph into the thoracic duct. A pathologic increase in venous pressure in the neck and the force of gravity on dependent portions of the body both interfere with the flow of lymph. When a person stands at attention, the contribution of active and passive motion to the flow of lymph is eliminated, and the force of gravity retards lymphatic drainage. In addition, a coincident increase in venous pressure from the same causes reduces reabsorption of fluid from the connective tissues. The edema that results is a graphic demonstration of the influence of extrinsic factors on the flow of lymph.

VOLUME OF LYMPH

It has been estimated that in a resting human adult the average flow of lymph from the thoracic duct amounts to 0.9 ml per min or 1.4 ml per kg of body weight per hr. The maximum rate of flow induced by a heavy meal was 3.9 ml per min, whereas the minimum was 0.4 ml per min. The rate of flow can be increased by the inges-

tion of food or water or by abdominal massage. In a report of a thoracic duct fistula in a carefully studied patient, the lymph flow varied from 1.06 ml to 1.86 ml per kg per hr.[11]

UNCOMMON PATHWAYS OF LYMPH FLOW

Although as a rule lymph must traverse at least one group of lymph nodes before reaching the thoracic duct and the blood stream, there are cases of the spread of infection or cancer that appear to belie this rule in one of three ways: (1) disease rapidly spreads to distant sites or reaches the blood stream, as if it had bypassed one or more groups of lymph nodes; (2) disease spreads in a retrograde direction, against the flow of lymph; (3) disease spreads rapidly to the opposite side of the body.

Lymphatic spread of disease that bypasses one or more groups of lymph nodes may be real or only apparent. Some lymph nodes do not completely interrupt the flow of lymph but are bypassed by one or more lymphatic vessels connecting afferent and efferent lymphatics. This may be the result of normal development or the regeneration of damaged or obstructed lymphatics. However, lymph nodes also may lose their filtering function and become mere conduits for lymph as a result of replacement of the lymphoid tissue by tumor or scar tissue. The lymphaticovenous communications with veins in the trunk, which develop embryologically, may allow tumor cells or microorganisms to reach the blood stream without traversing a lymph node. Apparently these communications are not functionally patent under normal conditions but may open if the normal drainage of lymph is obstructed. In other cases, anomalous spread of disease may not be lymphatic at all but may involve the vertebral system of veins, which communicates freely, without valves, throughout the length of the vertebral column.[12]

Retrograde lymphatic spread probably occurs only in cases of lymphatic obstruction, when valves apparently become incompetent. In addition, collateral lymphatic pathways may open up and drain lymph to more distal lymph nodes.

Lymphatic spread of disease to the opposite side of the body may occur in one of the following ways:

1. *Lymphatic efferents* from an organ may terminate in the regional lymph nodes of both sides. This is characteristic of the spread of cancer of the tongue and lip.
2. *Cutaneous lymphatics* anastomose across the midline. This is particularly significant for the spread of cancer of the mammary gland and perineum.
3. *Regional lymph nodes* near the midline are connected anastomotically with those of the opposite side. This is characteristic of para-aortic lymph nodes and accounts for contralateral spread of cancers of the ovary, testis, kidney, bladder, and adrenal gland.
4. *The thoracic duct* may terminate anomalously on the right or on both sides, accounting for the spread of distant tumors to the right subclavian region.

AREAS LACKING LYMPHATIC DRAINAGE

Just as lymph is formed from extracellular fluid of connective tissues, so lymphatics are confined to the loose connective tissues of the body. Nondistensible connective tissues, such as cartilage, bone, and bone marrow, cannot accumulate excess extracellular fluid and are not supplied with lymphatics. Epithelia lack lymphatics but generally are in close relationship to a lamina propria of loose vascular connective tissue rich in lymphatics. The central nervous system (CNS), a solid epithelial organ almost devoid of connective tissue, lacks lymphatics. Vascular endothelium in the CNS appears to be less permeable than other endothelia, thus limiting the leakage of extracellular fluid. Apparently, excess fluid that accumulates in the brain reaches the ventricular or subarachnoid spaces to join the cerebrospinal fluid and eventually reenter the blood stream. The eye lacks lymphatics, intraocular fluid being produced and reabsorbed by mechanisms analogous to those pertaining to cerebrospinal fluid. The thymus and spleen, encapsulated lymphoid organs intimately associated with the blood vascular system but almost totally lacking in loose connective tissue, have lymphatics only in the trabeculae and connective tissue accompanying the larger blood vessels at the hilum. The placenta lacks lymphatics.

Areas without lymphatic drainage do not contribute directly to the antigenic content of lymph. With the exception of the spleen, such tissues occupy an immunologically sequestered position. Antigens from these tissues are less likely to reach the lymphoid system and induce an immune response. As a result, these are protected sites for infections, cancer, and grafted tissues. Because the indigenous antigens of these tissues are less likely to reach the lymphoid system in early life, the body is less likely to develop tolerance for these organs, and they are susceptible to the development of autoimmune disease in later life.

LYMPHANGITIS

Lymph vessels may be affected by acute, subacute, or chronic inflammatory processes. Lymphangitis usually arises from superficial wounds, such as punctures, small

abrasions, cuts, and scratches. Consequently, it affects primarily the superficial lymphatic vessels.

Lymphangitis involving the lymphatic capillar plexuses of the skin is called capillary or reticular lymphangitis. Streptococci and pyogenic staphylococci are the most common causative organisms in lymphangitis.

Capillary (reticular) lymphangitis may occur in any part of the body. It is seen most characteristically in erysipelas. Capillary lymphangitis is marked by an intense hyperemia, with exudation about the rich cutaneous lymphatic capillary plexuses. The lymphatic capillaries themselves may become plugged by clotting of the lymph within them. There is accompanying intense heat, moderate swelling, and redness of the skin. Pain may be present or absent. The face is the area most commonly involved. If the infection occurs in the extremities, the capillary lymphangitis may be the starting point of a tubular lymphangitis. As a rule, the condition is self-limited, ending after a few days without suppuration or necrosis. Occasionally it may be very virulent and rapidly fatal.

Tubular lymphangitis occurs almost exclusively in the extremities[13,14] but rarely, it may involve the trunk.[15] It is due to infection of lymphatic vessels that drain a wounded, infected area. The wound may be very slight and often is not noticed or is forgotten. It is characterized by the appearance, some time after the infliction of the wound, of subcutaneous red streaks coursing up an extremity from the area of the wound to the nearest regional lymph nodes. If the involved lymph vessels are large, they may be felt as tender cords upon palpation. The lymph nodes into which the inflamed vessels drain also react and become enlarged, tender, and painful. Toxemia is often severe in such cases. The lymph node reaction may not occur until the acute tubular lymphangitis has subsided, so that errors in diagnosis may arise, particularly if the initial wound has healed.

The involved lymph vessels are surrounded by a zone of hyperemia and exudate. The vessels may become obstructed by an accumulation of desquamated endothelial cells, leukocytes, and coagulated lymph. Local abscesses may develop. A diffuse cellulitis may complicate the lymphangitis. Usually, prompt resolution follows the early and adequate treatment of the initial wound. On the other hand, with injudicious treatment or inability of the regional lymph nodes to cope with a particularly virulent organism (usually the streptococcus), the infection may rapidly progress within 48 hours to a serious, often fatal, systemic involvement which results from the entrance into the blood stream of the infecting organism and its toxins. This condition is known as *septicemia.*

Chronic tubular lymphangitis may follow acute lymphangitis, but more often it is the result of repeated subacute attacks of infection.

DILATATION OF LYMPHATIC CAPILLARIES AND VESSELS

Dilation of lymphatic vessels is found as lymphangiectasis, capillary lymphangioma, cavernous lymphangioma, and solitary lymph cyst.

Acquired dilation of lymphatic vessels is due to obstruction of the main collecting lymphatics.

Lymphoceles (accumulation of lymphatic fluid) may occur as an infrequent complication of renal transplantation[16] or certain gynecologic operations.[17]

Lymphangiectasis may involve various parts of the body and lead to enlargement of the affected part. It is most commonly seen in the tongue (macroglossia)[18] and lip (macrocheilia).[19] It may occasionally involve the subcutaneous lymphatics of an extremity (Milroy's disease).[20]

Capillary lymphangioma occurring in the skin is known as *lymphatic nevus.* This consists of brownish papules covered with small vesicles containing lymph.

Cavernous lymphangioma consists of an aggregation of lymphatic cysts. This condition is found most often in the neck and in the axilla. In the neck it is usually known as *cystic hygroma* and should be differentiated from lymphadenopathy.[21] Here it appears during early infancy or may be present at birth. Typically, the cystic hygroma occupies the lower part of the neck and may extend upward to the ear or downward behind the clavicle, where it comes into relation with the cervical pleura. Cavernous lymphangioma is due to lack of communication during development between the primitive lymphatic system and the collecting lymphatic vessels or the venous system.

OBSTRUCTION OF LYMPHATIC VESSELS

Lymphatic vessels may undergo obstruction from various causes. The end result is lymphatic edema, which involves the region drained by the obstructed vessels. Lymphatic edema is characterized by little tendency to pit upon pressure (so characteristic of venous obstruction) and by brawny induration of the subcutaneous tissues. Eventually, the skin becomes coarse and rough, and the part involved often undergoes tremendous swelling (elephantiasis). Sometimes, lymphatic vesicles develop in the affected area, which may rupture and lead to ulceration and recurrent infection. Leakage of lymph is known as *lymphorrhea.*[22]

Primary lymphedema may result from lymphagiectasis, as already described, or it may be due to other congenital changes.[23] Acquired obstruction[24] may result from the following:

1. *Surgical procedures,* such as radical mastectomy, extensive removal of the axillary lymph nodes, and the division of lymphatic vessels, may result in massive lymphatic edema of the upper extremity. Similar effects may follow radiation therapy. Factitial proctitis is an example of a localized disorder by which radium therapy of malignancy of the cervix uteri may occasionally, as a complication, destroy the lymphatics of the rectum, producing lymphatic block, lymphedema, and an annular type of rectal constriction.[25]

2. *Inflammation, followed by fibrosis of the lymphatic vessels,* may occur following an attack of acute lymphangitis, recurring erysipelas, or certain persistent chronic infections, such as tropical ulcers.

3. *Neoplastic invasion of lymphatic vessels* may occur. Thus, in the case of breast cancer, obstruction of the subcutaneous lymphatics through their permeation by cancer cells leads to the formation of discrete nodules in the skin (orange peel or *peau d'orange*). Likewise, the brawny arm, which develops some months or years after radical mastectomy for cancer, may occur from lymphatic permeation by malignant cells. Invasion of the lymphatics of the ligaments of Cooper of the breast eventually results in gross retraction of the skin.

   It is well to remember that rarely, unilateral lymphedema may be the presenting manifestation of neoplasm, especially in older adults. The most frequent example of this is swelling of one lower extremity as a result of a lymphoma, carcinoma of the prostate,[26] or other malignant tumor.[27,28]

4. *Parasitic infections.* The most dramatic form of elephantiasis occurs in connection with infections of *Filaria sanguinis hominis.* The resulting lymphatic edema affects particularly the scrotum or the vulva and the lower extremity, and there is enormous thickening of the subcutaneous tissues.

THE MAIN LYMPHATIC VESSELS

ANATOMY

The main lymphatic vessels include the following: (1) the right and left jugular trunks, (2) the right and the left subclavian trunks, (3) the right and the left bronchomediastinal trunks, (4) the right lymphatic duct, (5) the intestinal trunk, (6) the right and the left lumbar trunks, and (7) the thoracic duct.[29,30] (See Figs. 26-11, 26-12.)

The *jugular trunk* is formed on each side of the union of the efferents from the inferior deep cervical lymph nodes. It terminates at the junction of the subclavian and the internal jugular veins. Instead of emptying independently into the systemic venous circulation, it may join with the subclavian trunk to form the right lymphatic duct; on the left side, it may join the thoracic duct. The jugular trunk receives lymph from the inferior and the superior deep cervical nodes, the axillary nodes, the back of the scalp, the skin of the arm, and the pectoral region. The jugular trunk thus is concerned with the lymphatic drainage of the head, the neck, the arm, and part of the thorax.

The *subclavian trunk* is formed on each side by the union of the efferents from the apical axillary (infraclavicular) lymph nodes. It terminates on the right side in the subclavian vein or joins the right jugular trunk to form the right lymphatic duct; on the left side, it either joins the thoracic duct or empties independently into the left subclavian vein. The subclavian trunk receives lymph by way of the axillary nodes from the upper extremity, the posterior surface of the thorax, the mammary gland, the front of the chest, and the lateral wall of the chest.

The *bronchomediastinal trunk* is formed on each side by the union of the efferents from the tracheobronchial and the superior mediastinal nodes. Although it usually terminates in the subclavian vein, it may join the right lymphatic or the thoracic duct. The bronchomediastinal trunk receives lymph from the lungs, the bronchi, the trachea, the esophagus, and the heart.

The *right lymphatic duct* is formed on the right side at the root of the neck by the junction of the right jugular, the right subclavian, and the right bronchomediastinal ducts. It may be absent if one or more of these open independently into the right internal jugular, the right subclavian, or the left innominate veins, respectively.

The right lymphatic duct is concerned with the lymphatic drainage of the right half of the head and neck, the right upper extremity and mammary gland, and the right half of the thorax. When present, it is about ½-in long. Its tributaries normally communicate with the thoracic duct. Its importance thus lies in the fact that it provides an alternate route for passage of lymph into the systemic venous circulation in cases of obstruction of the thoracic duct.

The *intestinal trunk* is a single short trunk extending from the celiac preaortic nodes to the cisterna chyli. It may enter the latter independently but often joins the right or the left lumbar trunk. It receives lymph from the preaortic nodes (celiac, superior, and inferior mes-

enteric) and hence is concerned with the lymphatic drainage of the lower part of the esophagus, the stomach, the liver, the gallbladder, the pancreas, and the small and large intestines, exclusive of the anal canal.

The *lumbar trunks,* right and left, are two short lymphatic vessels extending from the uper para-aortic nodes on each side of the abdominal aorta to the cisterna chyli. The left lumbar trunk passes behind the abdominal aorta. They are concerned with the lymphatic drainage of the lower extremities, the perineum, the pelvis and the pelvic organs, the kidneys, the suprarenals, and the deep structures of the abdominal walls.

The *thoracic duct* is the main collecting duct of the lymphatic system.[31] It transports lymph to the systemic venous system from both lower extremities, the perineum, the pelvic and the abdominal organs, the abdominal walls, and the left half of the body above the xiphisternal junction.

The thoracic duct extends from the cisterna chyli to the root of the neck. The *cisterna chyli* is a lymph sac about 2-in long, lying in front of the first and the second lumbar vertebrae, beneath the diaphragm. It is formed mainly by the confluence of the intestinal and the two lumbar lymphatic ducts.

The thoracic duct measures 16 in to 18 in (40 cm–45 cm) in length and approximately ⅛-in (0.3 cm) in width. However, its caliber is not uniform.

Structurally, the thoracic duct resembles a vein, differing from the latter by a lesser content of smooth muscle and a greater number of bicuspid valves.

In its ascending course from the cisterna chyli, the thoracic duct is in close proximity to larger arteries, whose pulsations aid considerably in propelling the flow of lymph toward the root of the neck. Thus, the thoracic duct enters the posterior mediastinum by passing through the aortic hiatus of the diaphragm. Here it lies between the azygos vein and the aorta, the right border of which overlaps it. In the posterior mediastinum, it ascends in or near the midline, lying here on the thoracic vertebrae behind the esophagus and close to the right border of the descending thoracic aorta.

At about the level of the fourth or the fifth thoracic vertebra, it turns to the left and enters the superior mediastinum to ascend along the left border of the esophagus and behind the left subclavian artery. Upon reaching the root of the neck, it curves to the left behind the left common carotid artery, the vagus, and the internal jugular vein. After a short downward course, it joins the beginning of the left innominate vein. Near its termination, the thoracic duct is joined by the left bronchomediastinal, the left subclavian, and the left jugular lymphatic trunks. The mouth of the thoracic duct is guarded by a sentinel valve, which

prevents the entrance of blood into it during life. After death, this valve no longer functions, so that at autopsy the terminal part of the thoracic duct may contain a variable amount of blood.

The tributaries of the thoracic duct are as follows:

In the abdomen it receives the intestinal and the right and the left lumbar trunks and efferents from the intercostal lymph nodes of the lower six intercostal spaces.

In the thorax, it receives (1) afferents from the right and the left para-aortic and the retroperitoneal lymph nodes, which enter it after passing through the crura of the diaphragm; (2) efferents from the posterior mediastinal nodes; and (3) efferents from the intercostal lymph nodes of the upper five or six intercostal spaces.

On the other hand, the thoracic duct sends afferents to the superior mediastinal nodes and has communications with the azygos system of veins. Both of these types of anastomoses are found chiefly above the level of the eighth thoracic vertebra. Below this level, the thoracic duct is a single tube. Therefore, traumatic injuries of the thoracic duct below the level of the eighth thoracic vertebra are prognostically far more serious and may prove fatal unless the torn duct is ligated.

The thoracic duct may show important anomalies: It may veer to the right and open into the right innominate vein, or it may bifurcate, one branch opening into the left and the other into the right innominate vein.[32]

CHYOUS EFFUSIONS

Since the thoracic duct drains lymph from the greater part of the body, its severance entails a considerable loss of fluid, fat and protein, and lymphocytes.[33] Hence such injuries are followed by

Dehydration, producing excessive thirst, decreasing urinary output, and dry skin

Loss of weight because of rapid depletion of body fat depots

Marked weakness

Loss of fat-soluble vitamins A and D absorbed from the gastrointestinal tract

Striking drop in number, or complete disappearance of, lymphocytes in the circulating blood. This marked drop in the lymphocyte count can be of great diagnostic value, especially in accident cases with chest injury but no evidence of injury to the thoracic duct

Loss of protein

To these would be added the effects of compression by the accumulation of the extravasated lymph or chyle. Extravasated lymph or chyle usually does not clot like

blood; hence the wound may not heal. Consequently, life may be endangered unless operative repair or ligation of the duct is carried out. Because of the bacteriostatic action of lymph, severance of the thoracic duct is not accompanied by infection unless this is introduced by the traumatic agent.

Rupture of the thoracic duct may result from trauma, operative procedures, or obstruction. It may occur in the cervical, the thoracic, or the abdominal segments of the thoracic duct.

Chylous effusions into the root of the neck may result from trauma and embolism, as well as from operations on the neck by the anterior approach. The extravasated lymph or chyle accumulates in the lower part of the neck, and since it does not clot, it forms a doughy swelling. Cervical chylous effusions rarely are associated with the thrombosis of the neck veins.

Rupture of the duct in its thoracic course may be due to trauma or certain operations, such as thoracic sympathectomy, pneumonectomy, rib resection, or thoracolysis. In such cases, the chylous effusion first involves the mediastinum and finally one or both pleural cavities, with resulting *chylothorax*.[33] The chylous effusion usually assumes such proportions that compression of one or both lungs leads to serious embarrassment of respiration. Compression of the thoracic vessels may lead to vascular collapse, resembling shock from hemorrhage. Chyle extravasated into the pleural cavity causes an inflammatory reaction, resulting in thickening of the pleura, with loss of its elasticity and deposition on its surface of heavy exudate.

In the abdominal cavity, chylous effusions usually are due to obstruction, with consequent increase in the intraductal pressure, dilatation, and rupture of the distal afferents of the thoracic duct. The chylous effusion may enter the peritoneal cavity, with resulting chylous ascites (*chyloperitoneum*), or it may enter the urinary passages, with the occurrence of *chyluria*.[34]

Chylous fluid obtained by aspiration in cases of chylous effusions has the following characteristics:

It is a milklike fluid, which forms three layers upon standing: an upper "cream" layer, a middle "milk" layer, and a lower sediment layer, consisting chiefly of cellular elements.
Upon standing for a long time, a small coagulum forms.
The specific gravity varies from 1.016 to 1.025.
The protein content varies from 3 g to 6 g per 100 ml[33]

LYMPH NODES

Lymph nodes, usually flattened and ovoid or kidney-shaped, vary greatly in size, from 1 mm to 25 mm in greatest diameter and even larger when hypertro-

phied. They are disposed for the most part in groups along the great vessels of the neck, thorax and abdomen, in the mesentery, and in adipose tissue near joints. Although their apparent number may increase in an area of infection or cancerous invasion, it is not yet clear whether this represents formation of new lymph nodes or merely hypertrophy of previously undetectable ones.

Lymph nodes consist of a stromal framework of connective tissue traversed by lymphatic sinuses and populated with lymphoid cells.

STROMA

A thin capsule of dense collagenous connective tissue surrounds each lymph node and extends into the interior as slender trabeculae. The capsule is particularly well developed at the hilum where it reinforces arteries, veins, and efferent lymphatics. The remainder of the stroma, which pervades the entire lymph node, consists of reticular connective tissue, a specialized tissue characteristic of hemopoietic and lymphoid organs.

Reticular connective tissue has an extracellular framework of very thin bundles of collagenous filaments called *reticular fibers*. These fibers form a delicate three-dimensional meshwork in which the intervening spaces are not filled with ground substance as in most connective tissue. Instead, each reticular fiber is wrapped closely about by the extended processes of fibroblastlike cells called *reticular cells*. The spaces between the fibers form an extracellular labyrinthine space, free of both fibers and ground substance and lined by reticular cells. It is the quasivascular nature of this space that makes reticular connective tissue unique among connective tissues; this is the space where lymphoid cells reside.

Reticular cells resemble fibroblasts in many respects. They have the same slender, branched processes, but in the case of reticular cells, these processes are extended along reticular fibers and joined by junctional complexes to those of neighboring reticular cells, enclosing the reticular fibers in a cellular sheath. Reticular cells have the same, well-developed protein-secretory apparatus as fibroblasts—large pale nucleus, prominent nucleolus, rough endoplasmic reticulum, and Golgi complex; presumably they also produce collagen—the collagen of reticular fibers. Reticular cells differ from fibroblasts in that some are phagocytic. These are the so-called fixed or reticular macrophages of lymphoid tissue. It is not yet certain whether phagocytic reticular cells represent only a functional state in the life of all reticular cells or an independent population with a different origin from other reticular cells.

Reticular cells, at least nonphagocytic ones, form a population distinct from and apparently unrelated to

lymphoid cells. When irradiation has destroyed most of the lymphoid cells of the body, reticular cells survive but proliferate little and do not appear to participate in regeneration of the lymphoid system. Therefore, they are not the primitive hemopoietic stem cells they were long thought to be; this misconception is still reflected in a confusing pathologic nomenclature.

Reticular connective tissue in lymph nodes assumes two forms: lymph sinuses and dense lymphoid tissue.

Lymph sinuses are irregular tubular vessels bordered by reticular cells that form a continuous lining in most places. This lining is reinforced by reticular fibers that surround the sinus and also cross its lumen, ensheathed in reticular cells. A tortuous, extended surface is thus created, slowing the flow of lymph and providing an opportunity for its contents to make contact with phagocytic reticular cells that carry out the filtering functions of the lymph node.

In *dense lymphoid tissue,* the space between reticular cells is labyrinthine rather than tubular so that lymphoid cells can move through this tissue in any direction without leaving its quasivascular intercellular space. Lymphocytes apparently also can migrate between dense lymphoid tissue and sinuses by penetrating potential gaps in the wall of the sinus. Some of the reticular cells in dense lymphoid tissue are also phagocytic.

ARCHITECTURE OF LYMPH NODES

On the basis of stromal architecture and cellular populations, lymph nodes may be divided into cortex and medulla. The cortex may be subdivided further into a nodular outer cortex and diffuse inner cortex (Fig. 26-1).

Afferent lymphatics pierce the capsule at sites opposite cortical tissue to empty into the peripheral or subcapsular sinus. This is a flattened cleft immediately subjacent to the capsule that surrounds almost the entire lymph node. Sinuses running along the trabeculae—trabecular sinuses—drain the subcapsular sinus and deliver lymph to the dense network of sinuses in the medulla. Most of the cortex appears to be free of lymph sinuses, although there may be additional cortical sinuses that are relatively invisible in histologic sections because they are filled with densely packed lymphocytes. The medullary sinuses drain into one or more efferent lymphatics, which leave the lymph node at the hilum, completing the circulation of lymph through the lymph node.

The outer cortex consists of lymphoid nodules, which are spheres of densely packed, small lymphocytes. Most lymphoid nodules contain a germinal center—a central, less dense region filled with proliferating lymphoblasts and macrophages ingesting dying lymphocytes. These lymphoid nodules lie closely adjacent to the subcapsular sinus, the inner wall of which forms a border crossed by heavy traffic between sinus and outer cortex. Numerous small lymphocytes may be seen, in section, breaching the inner wall of the subcapsular sinus, although in such preparations it is not possible to determine the direction of migration. Presumably, small lymphocytes produced in the germinal centers enter the subcapsular sinus to leave the lymph node with the efferent lymph. Antigens and particulate materials that reach the lymph node through afferent lymph also cross the inner wall of the subcapsular sinus to enter the outer cortex.

The diffuse cortex extends from medulla to cortical nodes and between cortical nodes as far as the subcapsular sinus. It is diffusely but tightly packed with cells, mostly small lymphocytes. The diffuse cortex is also the location of high-endothelial venules, through the walls of which lymphocytes leave the blood stream to enter lymphoid tissue; the diffuse cortex thus lies on a major route for recirculation of lymphocytes.

The medulla contains a rich network of most of the sinuses of the lymph node, interspersed with cords of dense lymphoid tissue. These sinuses, with phagocytic

Fig. 26-1. Structure of a lymph node.

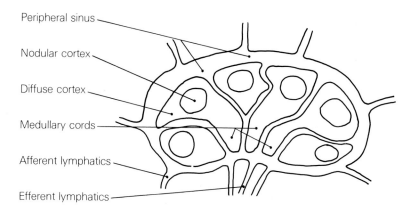

Peripheral sinus

Nodular cortex

Diffuse cortex

Medullary cords

Afferent lymphatics

Efferent lymphatics

reticular lining cells and free macrophages in the lumen, are the major sites of phagocytosis of antigenic and particulate materials carried in the lymph. The medullary cords are occupied chiefly by plasma cells in various stages of differentiation, the cells responsible for secretion of immunoglobulin.

Although lymph nodes are considered as organs associated with the lymph stream, they also have an important blood supply. One or more small arteries enter at the hilum, give branches to a capillary plexus in the medullary cords, and send relatively straight arteriolar branches through the diffuse cortex to the outer cortex. There terminal arterioles supply a capillary plexus, which is particularly well developed in each germinal center. This outer cortical capillary plexus drains into the characteristic, high-endothelial postcapillary venules of the diffuse cortex, through which blood reaches the medulla to leave the lymph node by veins at the hilum. Thus, medullary cords and cortical nodules have the most immediate and richest blood supply. Much remains to be learned concerning the relationships of blood supply to movements of antigens and lymph cells.

Small nerves enter at the hilum. Some are vasomotor to the blood vessels and some end in the capsule where, presumably, they are sensory, mediating the pain and tenderness that emanate from the stretched capsule of an engorged, inflamed lymph node.

FILTRATION OF LYMPH

The process begins where afferent lymphatics deliver lymph to the subcapsular sinus. Its irregular shape, large extended surface, and bridging reticular fibers serve to slow the flow of lymph and offer maximum opportunity for antigens and particulate materials to contact phagocytic reticular lining cells and free macrophages in the lumen of the sinus. The phagocytosis of antigen is potentiated by specific humoral antibody which, by combining with antigen, renders it more attractive to phagocytic cells, which recognize and are stimulated by immunoglobulin. Antigens and particulate materials are also filtered from the lymph by penetrating the inner walls of the subcapsular sinus to reach phagocytic reticular cells and macrophages in the outer cortex. Presumably, antigen ingested by phagocytic cells in the outer cortex plays a direct role in stimulating proliferation of lymphoid cells to form germinal centers and cortical nodules.

Practically all particulate material in lymph is removed by passage through a single lymph node. Indigestible materials, such as inhaled carbon particles in lymph nodes at the hilum of the lung, or the products of disordered metabolism in storage diseases, may be stored in large quantities by phagocytic cells. Cancer cells reaching a lymph node in the lymph apparently settle down in the sluggish stream of the sinuses to grow and fill the node unless they are destroyed by immune mechanisms.

CELLULAR POPULATIONS IN LYMPH NODES

The major populations of free cells inhabiting lymph nodes are lymphoid cells and macrophages. Granular leukocytes and mast cells may be found in small numbers under normal conditions, or in increased quantities under pathologic conditions. Little is known concerning the function of granular leukocytes or mast cells in lymph nodes.

The free macrophages of lymph nodes may be found in sinuses and in dense lymphoid tissue, particularly in germinal centers. They participate, as already stated, in the phagocytosis of antigenic and particulate materials. In germinal centers they are also involved in removing the large number of lymphocytes that die there. The free macrophages appear to be derived from monocytes of the blood stream, which are produced in bone marrow. The traffic of monocytes into lymph nodes is poorly understood. The relationship between free macrophages and phagocytic reticular cells remain unknown.

LYMPHOID CELLS

These cells form a large, interrelated family, including lymphocytes of all sizes, plasma cells, and lymphoblasts. The latter form the proliferating, relatively undifferentiated links between the branches of the lymphoid cell family. It has been known for a long time that plasma cells secrete antibody, but until recently, our ignorance concerning the small lymphocyte—one of the most numerous cells in the body—amounted to a scandal in biology. The only things small lymphocytes had been observed to do were to circulate in the blood to accumulate at sites of chronic inflammation in connective tissues and to die in large numbers in germinal centers and elsewhere. In some species small lymphocytes are killed by adrenal glucocorticoids, which thus produce involution of lymphoid tissues under conditions of stress. Accordingly, leading theories concerning small lymphocytes have included the proposition that their major function was to die and release their contained nutrients for other, more deserving tissues to use. During the last two decades, there has been an explosive increase in our understanding of lymphocytes, which can now be identified unequivocally as serving major immunologic functions. How-

ever, our growing knowledge is incomplete; it still serves to define ever larger areas of ignorance and complexity. Therefore, what follows is based upon reasonable inference as well as established fact.

The entire family of lymphoid cells is derived embryologically, and to some extent throughout life, from lymphocytes produced in the bone marrow. It has been proposed that such lymphocytes also may serve as stem cells for erythropoiesis and granulopoiesis, but this remains unproven; under most circumstances, lymphoid cells remain uninvolved with other lines of hemopoiesis. There are two major categories of immune response: humoral immunity, expressed in the secretion of soluble immunoglobulin by plasma cells, and cell-mediated immunity, expressed by development of delayed hypersensitivity, contact sensitivity, the rejection of grafted tissues, and perhaps, immunologic resistance to cancer. Likewise, there are two major branches of the family of lymphoid cells: T-cells and B-cells. *B-cells* are derived directly from the lymphocytes of bone marrow, which migrate to lymph nodes and other peripheral lymphoid tissues to carry out the functions of humoral immunity. Thus, they are the progenitors of plasma cells in the medullary cords and the B-lymphocytes, which produce germinal centers and cortical nodules. *T-cells* are derived indirectly from bone marrow lymphocytes, which migrate to the thymus and proliferate there to produce large numbers of small thymic lymphocytes. These cells acquire unique characteristics in the thymus and migrate to peripheral lymphoid tissues as T-lymphocytes, populating the diffuse cortex of lymph nodes and carrying out the functions of cell-mediated immunity. The diffuse cortex, therefore, depends upon the thymus for the major portion of its lymphocytes.

Nearly all lymphocytes are small: 5 μm to 10 μm in diameter. They have a small, highly condensed nucleus and very little cytoplasm, containing few organelles. These cells are as inactive as they look; they do not synthesize DNA or proliferate. They synthesize little RNA, but the ribosomes in the cytoplasm make some protein, at least part of which is immunoglobulin destined to be incorporated into the plasma membrane of the lymphocyte. Growing evidence indicates that this immunoglobulin serves for the recognition of antigens by lymphocytes, the event that initiates an immune response. B-lymphocytes are rich in surface immunoglobulin, whereas T-lymphocytes have only a little. Lymphocytes do not engage in phagocytosis, and the evidence that they can transform into macrophages is equivocal. When outside the blood stream, they can progress slowly by ameboid motion.

Although small lymphocytes are so inactive, and despite earlier theories that they were short-lived, there is now a large body of evidence to indicate that many small lymphocytes live for months or years. When properly stimulated, they grow into large lymphoblasts that proliferate and differentiate to produce other lymphocytes and, in the case of B-lymphocytes, plasma cells. Small lymphocytes represent only one stage in the life cycle of a protean cell; one must think dynamically to understand the lymphoid system.

The medium-sized and large lymphocytes seen in the blood are not much different in structure from small lymphocytes but form a continuum in cellular size and cytologic characteristics between lymphocytes and lymphoblasts, as would be expected of cells that lie along a reversible developmental pathway between these two extremes. Thus, medium-sized and large lymphocytes are cells in transition, either proliferating to produce small lymphocytes or being produced by growth of small lymphocytes.

The result of activation and growth of a small lymphocyte is a blast cell, called interchangeably a lymphoblast or immunoblast. Lymphoblasts are pivotal in the lymphoid cell family. T-lymphoblasts proliferate to produce eventually more small T-lymphocytes. B-lymphoblasts proliferate and differentiate to produce eventually more small B-lymphocytes or plasma cells. Lymphoblasts are larger and more active synthetically than even the largest lymphocytes to be found in the blood. Nuclear chromatin is in the highly dispersed state necessary for synthesis of DNA and RNA. Prominent nucleoli give evidence of the assembly of ribosomes, which pack the voluminous cytoplasm and confer upon it an intense basophilia.

Plasmablasts, derived from lymphoblasts, may be distinguished from their progenitors by the gradual accumulation of rough-surfaced endoplasmic reticulum and prominent Golgi complex (the apparatus for synthesis and secretion of immunoglobulin) in the cytoplasm. Eventually, cytoplasmic differentiation reaches full development, proliferation and synthesis of RNA cease, the nucleus becomes condensed into a characteristic clumped pattern, and a mature plasma cell has been produced. Mature plasma cells are truly effete; no longer capable of proliferation or synthesis of RNA, they secrete immunoglobulins for several days and then die. Thus, the secretion of antibody in response to a brief exposure to antigen is a self-limiting process.

On the basis of this knowledge concerning lymphoid cells, it is now possible to provide what is still a partly hypothetical reconstruction of the sequence of events induced by antigenic stimulation. Antigen reaching a lymph node with afferent lymph is sequestered by macrophages and phagocytic reticular cells in the subcapsular sinus, medullary sinuses, and dense lymphoid tissues of the cortex. A lymphocyte recognizes

antigen when immunoglobulin in the surface of the lymphocyte has the structure to combine with that antigen as a specific antibody. This leads to an unknown sequence of events that causes the lymphocyte to grow into a lymphoblast. In the case of T-cells, lymphoblasts develop in the diffuse cortex, proliferate there, and produce a large number of small T-lymphocytes, all capable of recognizing that antigen. These recirculate through the body to produce cell-mediated immune responses such as tuberculin hypersensitivity and contact allergy. They also serve as a reservoir of cells able to recognize the particular antigen and produce an even greater immune response if the body is exposed to that antigen subsequently. In the case of B-cells, lymphoblasts produced in the outer cortex form germinal centers. It has been proposed that each germinal center represents the clonal product of a single, stimulated B-lymphocyte. Germinal centers produce the large number of B-lymphocytes in the surrounding lymphoid nodules, which serve as memory cells for humoral immunity. Immunoblasts produced in the medulla form large numbers of plasma cells, which secrete antibody against that antigen for a few days or a week. Because of this segregation of the various facets of immunologic function in lymph nodes, one can judge the type of immunologic response going on by the microscopic appearance of a lymph node.

Activation of small lymphocytes and the production of proliferating lymphoblasts also may be induced nonspecifically. In other words, there are substances that stimulate proliferation of lymphocytes, regardless of their antigenic specificity. These include plant lectins, which are unlikely to be found in man but have been very useful in studying lymphoid cells in the laboratory. They also include the lipid coat of the tubercle bacillus and bacterial lipopolysaccharides, endotoxins produced by bacteria of the intestinal flora. These bacterial products may cause hyperplasia of lymphoid tissues in man.

Research continually reveals more and more diversity and interactions among lymphocytes and macrophages in the induction of immune responses. In addition to receptors for specific antigens, lymphocytes express a great variety of surface antigens and receptors for immunologically important molecules, such as complement. Through the agency of these substances, lymphocytes and macrophages communicate, macrophages presenting antigens to lymphocytes and T-cells helping or suppressing B-cell responses to antigens in a bewildering variety of interrelationships. Growing knowledge of these interrelationships will become increasingly important in understanding cancer and a host of so-called auto-immune diseases, such as arthritis and juvenile-onset diabetes. There is growing evidence that susceptibility to such diseases has a genetic component.

AGE CHANGES IN LYMPHOID TISSUE

The amount of lymphoid tissue and general distribution of lymph nodes bear a definite relation to age.[35] The rate of growth of lymphoid tissue is highest in infancy and continues at a high level throughout childhood. It reaches its peak at about puberty and declines thereafter. At 2 years of age, the child has 50% of the lymphoid tissue of a 20-year-old person; at 4 years, 80%; at 8 years, 120%; at 12 years, 190%; at 16 years, 120%. The maximal development of lymphoid tissue occurs during the time when acute infections of the respiratory and the alimentary tracts are most common and during the period of greatest increase in weight and height. This suggests that it is part of a natural defense mechanism. During infancy and childhood, moreover, lymphoid tissue responds characteristically to infection by prompt and excessive swelling and hyperplasia. With advancing age, such dramatic changes become less frequent.

Lymph nodes are more numerous and larger in children than in adults. There is marked hypertrophy during childhood and involution during adult life. However, there is no real atrophy, as a rule, since at any age local or generalized infections may induce hypertrophy. Involutional changes in the lymph nodes consist of reduction in the size of the nodes and of the germinal centers, accompanied by infiltration with fat.

The fact that certain groups of lymph nodes disappear in adult life and that certain areas of lymphoid tissue, although they do not disappear, undergo involution, is of practical significance, since it serves to explain the relative incidence of certain pathologic conditions with reference to age. Perhaps the most significant diseases from this point of view are adenoiditis, tonsilitis, retropharyngeal abscess, appendicitis, and mesenteric adenitis.

Adenoid tissue is present in the nasopharynx at birth. It increases in size and reaches its maximum at 3 years to 5 years of age. Hypertrophy during infancy is a normal physiologic process and must not be interpreted as pathologic unless there is evidence of infection (adenoiditis). A regressive process eliminates the adenoid tissue of the nasopharynx (pharyngeal tonsil) as a source of obstruction in older children.

The palatine tonsils are present in the newborn. They gradually increase in size during the second and the third years, and become relatively smaller after the age

of 5 years. This corresponds with the marked reduction in the incidence of tonsillitis after this age.

Retropharyngeal abscess occurs most commonly in infants up to the age of 2½ or 3 years and more rarely in older children. Such abscesses are due to pyogenic infections of the small retropharyngeal lymph nodes, which lie on either side of the midline between the posterior wall of the pharynx and the prevertebral fascia. These nodes undergo involution early in life.

Appendicitis occurs most commonly in childhood, adolescence, and early adulthood. In childhood, it is an important pathologic condition, being the most common lesion requiring intra-abdominal surgery. It is rare during infancy but becomes more common after the age of 2 years. This relation between the incidence of appendicitis and age definitely is correlated with the fact that in early life the appendix contains much lymphoid tissue, disposed in the form of a circumferential aggregation of lymph follicles, which is especially prone to infection. The subsequent atrophy of this tissue accounts to a high degree for the markedly reduced frequency of appendicitis in later years.

The mesenteric nodes are more hyperplastic in childhood and adolescence than in adult life. Correspondingly, mesenteric adenitis, both acute and chronic, usually occurs between the ages of 3 years and 13 years.

MODES OF LYMPH NODE INVOLVEMENT AND PATHOLOGIC CHANGES

Pathologic abnormalities of the lymph nodes may be broadly classified into *hereditary* and *acquired* (Table 26-1). Changes found in the different diseases are most easily understood if one remembers the internal architecture of the node and the location of different types of cells. These were outlined previously in the section describing the histology of the lymph node, schematized in Figure 26-1.

Histologic diagnosis requires the examination of good material that has been well handled. A number of rules of biopsy technique need to be observed. Lymphocytes and especially neoplastic cells are extremely sensitive to trauma. This predicates that the node be handled as little as possible before, during, and after the biopsy procedure. When there is a mass of neoplastic nodes, the smaller ones around the edge, which are the easiest to biopsy, may show only reactive changes. The largest node in a group may show extensive necrosis. Biopsy should, therefore, select a node from the main mass of moderately large size. Histologic interpretation is difficult in nodes that have been involved in previous episodes of infection. For this reason, in-

Table 26-1. *A Classification of the Causes of Lymphadenopathy*

Hereditary
Immunodeficiency diseases
    All systems—Swiss-type combined deficiency
    T-cell defects—DiGeorge's syndrome
    B-cell defects—Bruton-type agammaglobulinemia; selective deficiencies
Lysosomal storage diseases
    Mucopolysaccharidoses
    Lipoidoses
    Carbohydrate abnormalities

Acquired
Inflammatory
    Acute lymphadenitis
    Follicular hyperplasia
    Paracortical hyperplasia
    Histiocytic patterns
    Granulomatous patterns
    Miscellaneous reactions
Neoplastic
    Malignant lymphoma/leukemia
        Hodgkin's disease
        Non-Hodgkin's lymphoma
            Nodular lymphomas
            Diffuse lymphomas
            Other patterns of lymphoma
    Metastatic neoplasms

guinal node biopsy should be avoided. Lymph nodes in the porta hepatis almost invariably show lipid granulomata, which also obscures early pathologic changes. When there is a choice, therefore, biopsy should be taken from other sites. Fixation is critical to diagnosis, and this is best achieved if the node is bisected along its long axis before immersion in adequate volumes of fixative. The histologic preparation should be done carefully and slowly. Frozen sections and attempts at rapid diagnosis may lead to errors that may prove disastrous for the patient. Touch preparations stained by one of the Romanovsky methods are often invaluable in diagnosis.[36] Consideration should always be given to culturing nodal tissue, since microscopic diagnosis of infective disease is usually much less sensitive.[37] Errors in lymph node diagnosis are made more often than with any other tissue. In one series, for example, the author disagreed with the diagnosis of Hodgkin's disease suggested by a pathologist colleague in 47% of cases.[38]

HEREDITARY CAUSES

Immunodeficiency Diseases

Only representative examples of these diseases will be considered here; fuller treatment is available else-

Table 26-2. *Hereditary Immunodeficiency Diseases and Their Relationship to Normal Maturation*

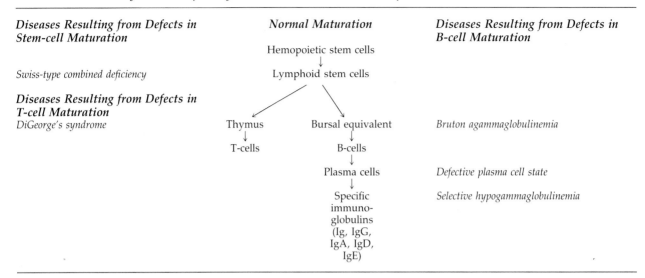

Diseases Resulting from Defects in Stem-cell Maturation	*Normal Maturation*	*Diseases Resulting from Defects in B-cell Maturation*
	Hemopoietic stem cells ↓	
Swiss-type combined deficiency	Lymphoid stem cells	
Diseases Resulting from Defects in T-cell Maturation		
DiGeorge's syndrome Thymus	Bursal equivalent	*Bruton agammaglobulinemia*
↓	↓	
T-cells	B-cells	
	↓	
	Plasma cells	*Defective plasma cell state*
	↓	
	Specific immuno-globulins (Ig, IgG, IgA, IgD, IgE)	*Selective hypogammaglobulinemia*

where.[39,40,41] Hereditary immunodeficiency is a result of failure in cell maturation at different stages (Table 26-2). In the case of stem cell arrest or failure of helper T-cell differentiation, there will be a profound abnormality of both T- and B-cell systems (Swiss-type combined deficiency). This condition is almost universally fatal unless bone marrow transplant can be successfully undertaken. Pure B-cell agenesis is seen in Bruton-type agammaglobulinemia and pure T-cell deficiency in DiGeorge's syndrome. In Bruton's disease the patient has no circulating antibody, and no plasma cells are seen in the tissues. The T-cell system is intact, and the patient is able to live an essentially normal existence except for recurrent infections with gram-positive cocci. By contrast, in DiGeorge's syndrome there is a failure to development of the third brachial arch and therefore of the thymus. As a consequence, there are no mature T-cells present, and the patient is unable to handle viruses, mycobacterial fungi, or gram-negative bacteria. The nodes are initially small in all of these patients. A profound failure of cellular proliferation affecting the entire node is seen in the Swiss-type disease. In Bruton's agammaglobulinemia the follicles are absent, and no plasma cells are seen in the cords. Reciprocally, in DiGeorge's syndrome the follicles and medulla may be normal or even hyperplastic, but the paracortex is depopulated. In other forms of immunodeficiency, such as selective IgA deficiency, a marked proliferation of cells may be seen, particularly around the small intestine. Only very seldom does this involve the nodes.

Lysosomal Storage Diseases

There are over 25 diseases of this type described.[42] Each is a result of a hereditary deficiency of a specific lysosomal enzyme involved in the handling of mucopolysaccharides, lipids, or carbohydrates. This causes an accumulation of the substrate or its precursors and a deficiency of the product of enzyme action. The type and distribution of accumulated material depends upon the enzyme that is absent. The better known diseases of the group included Pompe's disease, Fabry's disease, Niemann–Pick's disease, and Gaucher's disease. Only rarely is lymph node enlargement clinically significant. However, since the inherited defect involves all lysosomes that normally contain enzyme, macrophages are also affected. Histologically, one may see cells distended by phagocytosed material lying within the sinuses of the node. This histologic appearance causes difficulty in differential diagnosis from some inflammatory reactions.

ACQUIRED DISEASES

Inflammatory Reactions in Lymph Nodes

Macrophages, B-cells, T-cells, blood vessels, and granulocytes may each proliferate in response to suitable antigenic stimuli within a lymph node. Acute changes result in pain caused by tension in the nodal capsule. More chronic reactions with less rapid changes in volume are seldom painful. In many instances, the histologic picture is that of nonspecific hyperplasia; sometimes a specific pattern may be seen that enables

the pathologist to predict the nature of the antigen. Histologically the reactions are broadly classifiable into one of six groups (see Table 26-1). It should be remembered that only rarely is one histologic pattern present in a given node, and diagnosis is made on the dominant picture. The following account will mention only representative examples of diseases producing the various nodal patterns.

Acute Lymphadenitis. This pattern most frequently occurs when bacteria, concentrated by the filtering action of the sinuses, are living and replicating in the node itself. The node is edematous, containing varying numbers of granulocytes. In extreme examples, it may become converted into an abscess cavity. Such lesions may progress to septicemia if the immune defense of the node is overwhelmed. Alternatively, superficial nodes may ulcerate to the skin surface and suppurate. More commonly there is complete resolution, but extensive scar formation may cause lymphedema if repeated episodes of infection occur. Acute painful lymphadenitis with microabscess formation may also be seen with viral diseases such as, cat-scratch disease[43] and lymphopathia venereum.[44]

Follicular Hyperplasia. Germinal center formation indicating intense B-cell activity is seldom seen in pure form, since macrophage and T-cell proliferation often accompanies it. Typically, such a reaction may be seen in nodes draining an area of infection by gram-positive bacteria when the node itself is not infected. In this case the nodes are moderately enlarged but seldom painful.

Paracortical Hyperplasia. T-cell replication also is seldom seen in pure form except in such artificial circumstances as challenge by dinitrochlorobenzene. Combined paracortical and follicular hyperplasia is seen in a variety of infections, particularly with many viruses. In infectious mononucleosis, caused by Epstein–Barr virus, the reaction is particularly intense. The nodes are swollen and tender and, on biopsy, they appear firm and pale. Microscopic examination shows a vigorous replication of lymphocytes in all areas of the node with large active follicles and gross paracortical proliferation. In some instances the differentiation of paracortical proliferation of infectious origin from a follicular lymphoma may be extremely difficult.[45]

Cytomegalovirus (CMV) may induce a disease that is clinically very similar to mild cases of infectious mononucleosis. The histologic picture is very similar, except that careful search usually reveals CMV inclusion bodies. In addition, heterophil antibody is not present, and lymph nodes are not markedly enlarged.[46] Reactions to smallpox vaccination may be similarly brisk and closely mimic neoplasia.[47]

Histiocytic Patterns. Proliferation of macrophages, particularly in and around the sinuses, is seen in any node clearing particulate matter from the afferent lymph. Thus, axillary lymph nodes draining a breast that contains cancer may show hyperplasia of the sinuses. Macrophages in the sinuses of nodes at the pulmonary hilum usually contain carbon and other inhaled foreign material. Skin rashes may induce proliferation in draining nodes, and these nodes may become markedly enlarged if the condition is chronic. In this case, the nodal changes are referred to as *dermatopathic lymphadenopathy* or *lipomelanic reticulosis*. The first term explains the etiology of the reaction, whereas the second refers to its histologic appearance. Thus macrophages containing large quantities of lipid or melanin, presumably derived from the disturbed skin, accumulate in the nodal sinuses. Reactive changes in the T- or B-cell areas are frequently superadded. Typhoid fever induces an accumulation of macrophages in all parts of the lymphoid system that appears as sinusoidal hyperplasia in a lymph node. Giant nodal hypertrophy with sinusoidal histiocytosis affects the cervical nodes of young children and is a benign, self-limiting disorder of unknown etiology. Both clinically and histologically it may be difficult to distinguish this condition from Hodgkin's disease.[48] Marked histiocytic proliferation often arranged in clumps may be seen in leprosy of the lepromatous type[49] and also in toxoplasmosis.[50]

Granulomatous Patterns. Granulomas are accumulations of large pale cells that have the appearance of histiocytes surrounded by a rim of lymphocytes that are mainly T-cells. There may or may not be a rim of fibroblasts around this reaction, with giant cell formation or necrosis in the center. Such a reaction is seen not only in tuberculosis, but is indicative of exposure to any antigen that cannot be disposed of by the ordinary process of inflammation. Granulomas will be formed in normal people when exposed to a relatively small number of antigens. Some individuals, such as patients with chronic granulomatous disease of childhood, produce granulomas in response to many bacterial antigens. This is because a defect in lysosomal peroxide production prevents normal disposal of many organisms. Distinction of one cause of granulomatous diseases from another is made by searching for the causative agent, by morphology, by culture, and by chemical and physical analyses. Diseases that should be considered in the differential diagnosis of granulomatous lymphadenopathy include tuberculosis,

atypical mycobacterial infections, tularemia, *Yersinia* infections, leprosy, fungal diseases (particularly histoplasmosis), syphilis, brucellosis, berylliosis, sarcoidosis, Crohn's disease, reactions to zirconium, various foreign body reactions (particularly following lymphangiography), and response to necrotic neoplasms.

Miscellaneous Reactions. Reactive lymphadenopathy with a mixed histologic picture is seen in rheumatoid arthritis[51] and other collagen diseases. Measles or measles vaccination may cause lymphadenopathy.[52] Characteristically, Warthin–Finkeldy giant cells are seen in the node but may be absent in early cases. Anticonvulsant therapy may produce generalized nodal enlargement.[53]

Lymph node enlargement of massive degree may occur in the mediastinum or more rarely in the mesentery owing to a condition variously called angiofollicular lymph node hyperplasia, giant mediastinal node hyperplasia, lymph node hamartoma, or Castleman's disease.[54] The nature of the lesion and its cause are unknown. It is a benign disorder, but surgical extirpation is required to make the diagnosis and to relieve pressure symptoms. Another condition in which generalized lymphadenopathy occurs, characterized by a mixed lymphoid and vascular proliferation of unknown cause, is angioimmunoblastic lymphadenopathy.[55] The disease may be associated with a dysproteinemia and carries a considerable risk of subsequent development of lymphoma. The nature of the disease is unknown.[56]

Neoplastic Diseases in Lymph Nodes

Neoplastic involvement of nodes may occur in primary tumors of the lymphoid system or as a result of lymphatic metastases. Most metastatic tumors are carcinomas derived from tissues within the lymphatic drainage territory of the involved gland. Clinically, it is usually fairly easy to discern the primary tumor provided the anatomy of lymph flow is recalled. Difficulties are experienced in certain sites where primary neoplasm is small and inaccessible. Nasopharyngeal carcinomas, for example, are notorious for producing cervical node enlargement without local symptoms.[57,58] Inguinal node enlargement may be caused by lesions in the anus, as well as in the more obvious primary sites such as the limbs or genitalia.

Lymphoreticular neoplasms may present with local or generalized nodal involvement. Generalized involvement, particularly when associated with splenomegaly, is characteristic of lymphomas, and the differential diagnosis is usually straightforward. Localized enlargement often poses more problems, and the exclusion of infective or metastatic disease requires biopsy with culture and careful histologic examination.

Malignant Lymphomas. These neoplasms may arise from lymphoid cells where ever they are located in the skin, bowel, nodes, brain, spleen, liver, or bone marrow. Widespread involvement of many parts of the body is characteristically seen in these diseases. This pattern is predictable when it is recalled that lymphocytes wander around most tissues. Studies of genetic markers of lymphoma cells have shown that all the tumor cells from a given patient are identical and therefore almost certainly monoclonal in origin.

The classification of malignant lymphomas[59–61] is complicated by the fact that the nomenclature has changed at frequent intervals as the understanding of immune function has evolved (Fig. 26–2). Most of the classifications have been based on morphology as seen by light microscopy. Unfortunately, fixation and processing artifacts influence morphology drastically. Also, it is intrinsic to the nature of the immune system that different cell lines may share a similar appearance and conversely, that a single cell may change its appearance in size and shape in response to various stimuli. It is not surprising, therefore, that morphologic classification would be supplemented by other means of identifying cells when these become available.[62] Gradually, information derived from electronmicroscopy, immunofluorescence, and various dynamic tests of membrane receptor function[63] are being incorporated into our knowledge of lymphomas. In the present state of the art, however, most authorities agree that the tried and trusted morphologic criteria should continue to be used.

Hodgkin's Disease. The histologic and diagnostic criteria of Hodgkin's disease have been well defined and are relatively easily applied. Therefore, the separation of this group of diseases from other lymphomas constitutes the primary axis of classification (Fig. 26-2).

First described by Thomas Hodgkin in 1832,[64] the precise taxonomic position of this disease is still uncertain. It is identified by the concomitant proliferation of large histiocytic cells, lymphocytes, and specific giant cells with or without eosinophils and fibroblasts. The precise nature of Hodgkin's disease has remained obscure, partly because many cell lines are present. It is currently believed that Hodgkin's disease is a viral-induced tumor of T-cells with a prominent B-cell reaction.[65] The tumor is almost certainly induced initially in one node and spreads to neighboring contiguous nodes. This produces the classic appearance of Hodgkin's disease: a mass of matted but separable nodes that are firm but seldom as hard as epithelial neo-

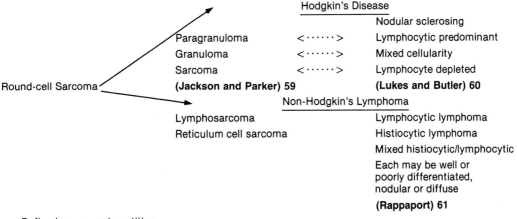

Fig. 26-2. The evolution of classifications of malignant lymphomas.

plasms. Spread occurs by involvement of contiguous groups of nodes through lymphatic channels. Deposits in parenchymal organs occur but are relatively unusual. Splenic involvment probably takes place through the blood stream.

Histologically, Hodgkin's disease is divided into four main types (Fig. 26-2). Nodular sclerosing disease is recognized by the presence of fibrous tissue within the node, which may eventually scarify completely. The cellular component is comprised of malignant histiocytic cells with a variable admixture of lymphocytes, plasma cells, and eosinophils. The giant cells present are characteristically shrunken in paraffin sections and appear to be surrounded by a clear zone (lacunar cells). The other patterns of Hodgkin's disease are diffuse in their arrangement. The giant cells present are of the classic Sternberg–Reed type. The names applied to the different subtypes are indicative of the means of making the diagnosis. Thus tumors composed mainly of lymphocytes with few histiocytic or giant cells are diagnosed as lymphocyte predominant, whereas lym-

phocyte-depleted tumors are composed mainly of large histiocytic cells with few lymphocytes.

The presentation, epidemiology, and prognosis of each type of tumor is different.[66] Some authorities argue that they should be regarded as different diseases. Thus, nodular sclerosing disease, usually with a mediastinal mass, occurs predominantly in young adult Caucasian females. The prognosis is intermediate between that for lymphocyte-predominant tumors and those of mixed cellularity. Lymphocyte-depleted disease is found in elderly Caucasian patients or in younger patients resident in developing countries. In both instances, the tumor frequently involves the liver, spleen, abdominal lymph nodes, and sometimes the wall of the bowel. The prognosis of these patients has been poor until recently, when some long-term remissions have been obtained using combination chemotherapy. Lymphocyte-predominant disease is a slowly progressive form, often presenting as localized cervical nodal enlargement and having an excellent prognosis. Mixed cellularity disease also usually presents with enlarged

cervical nodes, but in this case there is a greater chance of involvement of the spleen, bone marrow, and other nodes found at staging procedures. The prognosis for this group lies between that of lymphocyte-depleted and nodular-sclerosing types.

Some patients who eventually develop Hodgkin's disease present with enlarged lymph nodes that show only reactive changes with or without granulomata. These histologic features may precede the onset of diagnosable Hodgkin's disease by up to several years. It is possible that this represents a prodromal phase of the disease or perhaps a reaction to a virus.

Non-Hodgkin's Lymphoma. The major axis of classification of these lymphomas is morphologic. Tumors composed of cells with small, dark, round nuclei with little cytoplasm, closely resembling lymphocytes, are called lymphocytic lymphomas. Cells with larger, paler, folded nuclei surrounded by abundant cytoplasm closely resemble macrophages, and such tumors are called histiocytic lymphomas. In some cases, the tumor cells are arranged in spheres resembling lymphoid follicles, and sometimes there is no discernible structure or organization. These two types of lymphomas are referred to as nodular (follicular) and diffuse, respectively.[61] Tumor cells, which show prominent nucleoli, marked nuclear pleomorphism, and a high mitotic rate, are said to be poorly differentiated. Application of these three criteria to each lymphoma results in a classification of eight theoretically possible entities. Thus there are four possible lymphocytic tumors: well-differentiated nodular, well-differentiated diffuse, poorly differentiated nodular, and poorly differentiated diffuse. Similarly, there are four possible histiocytic lesions. In some tumors both lymphocytes and histiocytes appear to be proliferating together, and this is referred to as a mixed lymphocytic-histiocytic tumor. These tumors may also be theoretically subdivided into four subtypes, as with the pure cell proliferations.

To a considerable degree the histologic pattern of lymphoma predicts the clinical pattern and the response to therapy. In general, non-Hodgkin's lymphoma shows evidence of spread throughout the body with involvement of the spleen and bone marrow being particularly frequent in a much higher proportion of cases than Hodgkin's disease.

Nodular Lymphomas. Nodular lymphomas[67] are seen most commonly in older people. They produce few symptoms beyond painless enlargement of the nodes. Involvement of the spleen and bone marrow at the time of presentation is seen in most patients.[68] Histologically, three subtypes are distinguished: lymphocytic, mixed lymphocytic-histiocytic, and histiocytic. Prognosis is best in the lymphocytic type; it is poorer in the histiocytic types. Well-differentiated nodular lymphomas do not occur.

Diffuse Lymphomas. Diffuse lymphomas in general carry a poorer prognosis than the nodular varieties. Well-differentiated, diffuse lymphocytic lymphoma is the exception. Patients with this pattern pursue a very indolent course and may be associated with chronic lymphatic leukemia. Prolonged survival is usually seen, even when disease is widespread at presentation.[69] Poorly differentiated diffuse lymphocytic lymphoma probably includes a number of entities with a similar morphology. The cells in some tumors of adults show many of the morphologic features of follicular center cells (large dendritic cells of lymphoid follicles) and may represent follicular tumors that have spread diffusely prior to biopsy. Children and young adults with this disease may present with mediastinal masses, and such patients have a particularly poor prognosis and often progress to leukemia. Another group of young patients with similar light microscopic histologic appearances show widespread nodal involvement, frequently with parenchymal organ involvement. Diffuse mixed histiocytic-lymphocytic lymphoma may derive from the nodular variety or sometimes may arise *de novo*. Diffuse histiocytic lymphoma probably also comprises a number of different diseases with similar morphology. All show a rapidly progressive clinical course, and response to therapy is disappointing. However, this type of tumor shows less tendency to be widespread at presentation, and aggressive local therapy using surgery or radiotherapy may on occasion be curative. Morphologically, these tumors show a variable degree of pleomorphism. Some are relatively regular and homogeneous, and others show gross variation in the nuclear size. The significance of these differences is not yet fully clear.[70]

Other Patterns of Lymphoma. *Histiocytic medullary reticulosis*,[71] also called malignant histiocytosis, shows a characteristic clinical picture of a fulminating, rapidly fatal disease occurring in young people. The patient presents with fever and a hemolytic anemia. Hepatosplenomegaly is prominent, and nodes may show modest generalized enlargement. Histologically the sinuses are lined by prominent histiocytic cells, many of which are extremely bizarre and may show erythrophagocytosis. An apparently closely related disease is *malignant histiocytosis*, characterized by a skin rash and peripheral eosinophilia.[72]

Burkitt's lymphoma was first described in African children and typically involves the jaws in males and the ovaries in females.[73] It has now been diagnosed in most countries of the world but is rare in those areas where the temperature falls below 63°F or where the annual

rainfall is less than 20 in.[74,75] The pattern of lymph node involvement is different from that seen in other lymphomas. The cervical, axillary, and medistinal nodes are virtually never enlarged and inguinal nodes only rarely; retroperitoneal nodes are frequently involved. The reason for this marked anatomic variation is unknown.

Mycosis fungoides and *Sézary's syndrome,* which are probably cytogenetically identical,[76] present with cutaneous infiltration by lymphoid cells. In mycosis, nodal involvement takes place late in the course of the disease and is characterized by a pleomorphic infiltrate, including a large cell with a much-folded nucleus (mycosis cell) mainly in the nodal sinuses.[77]

Hairy cell leukemia (leukemic reticuloendotheliosis) presents as a diffuse infiltration of the marrow, spleen, and to a lesser extent, lymph nodes with cells that are remarkably cohesive—probably a result of numerous microscopic projections from the cell surface.[78] The number of tumor cells in the peripheral blood is usually small. Hypersplenism is present and contributes to the anemia and thrombocytopenia. Treatment consists of splenectomy if indicated, but cytotoxic chemotherapy has been found to worsen the prognosis. The cytogenesis is unknown, and the cell appears to be midway between a lymphocyte and a macrophage.[79]

Histiocytosis X comprises a group of related diseases with a marked variation in clinical appearance.[80] They are considered together because there are cases that lie midway between the classic entities, and electronmicroscopic studies have shown rather distinctive, tennis-racquet-shaped inclusions in the cytoplasm of the histiocytes. Similar inclusions are seen also in the Langerhans' cells in the epidermis. The connection between these two cell lines is obscure.

Waldenström's macroglobulinemia is a variant of B-cell lymphoma in which the cells secrete large quantities of IgM.[81] Diffuse enlargement of the lymph nodes is seen as a result of infiltration by cells with characteristics midway between lymphocytes and plasma cells. This condition is seen almost exclusively among elderly people and has a long, relatively benign course. Interestingly, Burkitt's lymphoma is also a tumor of IgM secreting cells, and the clinical picture could hardly be more different.

The classification of lymphomas just outlined has been found to have considerable clinical usefulness. It predicts the probable distribution of disease within the body and the response to therapy fairly accurately. It is relatively easily reproducible throughout the world, is widely understood by pathologists and clinicians, and requires a minimum of sophisticated equipment to diagnose. Everyone is therefore unwilling to give it up without good reason. Unfortunately, there are sev-

eral good reasons to believe that it is based on fallacious assumptions.[82] Most so-called histiocytes have been shown to possess surface markers of lymphocytes, and only a few tumor cells have a demonstrable phagocytic ability. Thus, most so-called histiocytic tumors are indeed lymphocytic, and mixed cell tumors are better regarded as pure lymphocytic tumors with variable degrees of differentiation. The tests needed to differentiate T-cells from B-cells from monocytic cell lines are complex and time-consuming. They require that tissue be studied fresh and in culture, and the facilities to do these tests are not universally available.

Other morphologic classifications using electron microscopic and immunofluoescence data have been proposed.[83,84,85] Most of these are based essentially on the characteristics of the nuclear membrane in terms of folds, clefts, and indentations. These may become valuable in the future, but at present they have not been proven to be superior for clinical purposes to the Rappaport classification, even though they may be more correct cytogenetically. Probably in the near future a classification based on information from histochemistry, immunology, receptor sites, cellular ultrastructure, anatomic location, geography, and etiology will become acceptable.

Metastatic Neoplasms. Lymphatic metastases occur most commonly from carcinomas, whereas sarcomas are more often spread by the blood stream. Permeation of lymph vessels by tumor is frequently seen in the region of the primary tumor, and a solid column of cells may grow for considerable distances along the lumen. This involvement may give rise to local lymphedema (*peau d'orange*) overlying a tumor. Tumor involvement of lymph channels in the lung produces a fibrotic contraction and loss of compliance (*lymphangitis carcinomatosum*).[86] Most commonly, nodes are involved by embolic deposits rather than by direct extension. Tumor emboli lodge in the peripheral sinus of the node and if they grow successfully, may then gradually encroach upon the remainder of the node, eventually destroying it completely. The node may also show evidence of reaction to the tumor, either in the form of follicular hyperplasia, paracortical proliferation, granuloma formation, or sinusoidal hyperplasia. The presence of reactive changes in draining lymph nodes correlates with a better prognosis than when the node appears depleted.

Palpation of superficial nodes to determine the presence of metastasis is part of the examination in all cancer patients. Involved nodes are usually much harder than uninvolved, and nodes greater than 5 cm in any dimension are usually the seat of tumor. Unfortunately, clinical examination alone is not very accurate. For example,

palpation of axillary nodes in carcinoma of the breast leads to an incorrect diagnosis in about 40% of cases when compared with histologic examination. This is because not all involved nodes are enlarged, and not all enlarged nodes are involved by tumor. The frequency with which nodes are found to be involved also depends upon the patience of the histologist. Thus, clearing the axillary contents with xylene increases the average number of nodes found in a radical mastectomy specimen from 5 to 36. Serial section increases the number of patients found to have metastases by about 25%.[87]

The site of involvement is usually easily explicable in terms of lymph flow in the area. However, once a node or lymphatic channel is involved by tumor the flow of lymph may be obstructed. Under these circumstances, retrograde flow of lymph fluid and contained tumor emboli may occur. Thus, metastatic tumor from the lung may involve mediastinal nodes and then spread inferiorly to the pericardium or the abdominal nodes. Tumor emboli in lymph channels may involve the blood stream through lymphaticovenous shunts.[88]

DIAGNOSTIC METHODS

LYMPHOGRAPHY

The lymphatic system plays a major role in various diseases, such as infection, metastatic cancer, and lymphomas. Its opacification by radiopaque media, *lymphography*, has long been an important and useful diagnostic tool, but two newer imaging procedures, ultrasonography and computed tomography (CT), are competing successfully with it.[89–91] In addition to being noninvasive, these newer techniques visualize several abdominal and pelvic lymph node groups not opacified routinely on bipedial lymphography. Not withstanding, only lymphography has the resolution to allow architectural abnormalities to be detected in normal-sized nodes, and it continues to have an important role in the management of patients with lymphomas and certain other tumors, particularly those of the urogenital system.[92–97]

The term *lymphography* refers to the visualization of both lymphatic vessels and lymph nodes. Visualization of the lymphatic vessels alone is properly called *lymphangiography*, whereas visualization of the lymph nodes is termed *lymphadenography*. Since the modern method of radiographic visualization of the lymphatic system simultaneously demonstrates both lymphatic vessels and nodes, the term *lymphography* is preferred. This term is less cumbersone than the term *lymphangioadenography*.

In the past, lymphography has been practiced by direct and indirect approaches. The indirect method consisted of the introduction of vital dyes or radiopaque media into the subcutaneous tissue or peritoneal cavity. Although this method was used experimentally, it is of no value in human medical and surgical practice.

The presently used method of direct lymphography consists of the subcutaneous injection of a vital dye, which renders the subcutaneous lymphatics visible, aiding in their subsequent surgical exposure and cannulation. Following cannulation, radiopaque contrast material is injected. Radiographs are obtained immediately following the injection of contrast (filling phase) and at 24 hr (storage or nodal phase). This method was first made practical by Kinmonth, Taylor, and Harper.[98] It has been modified in various ways by Wallace and associates[99] and others. Review articles or monographs can be consulted for more detail.[100–102]

The Normal Lymphogram

Normally peripheral lymph vessels are fine in caliber (usually less than 1 mm in diameter), run parallel to the superficial veins (demonstrable by phlebography), and present a characteristic beaded appearance because of the presence of valves (Fig. 26-3).[97,98,102,103] The lymphatic vessels bifurcate and anastomose with each other. They are in uniform diameter until they reach the pelvis, at which point they increase slightly in diameter. Ordinarily, when the injection is made unilaterally, lymphatics crossing over to the opposite side are demonstrable in the upper sacral and in the lumbar regions, in the case of the lower extremity. This feature is highly significant in the planning and follow-up of radical surgery and therapy in the retroperitoneal region.

Normal lymph nodes, although usually present singly or in groups at certain locations, do not show a constant pattern. They vary both in number and size from patient to patient. There is also a dissimilarity between the two sides in the same patient. In size, nodes may measure up to 2 cm to 3 cm in maximum diameter. The peripheral contour is regular, and there is usually a slight indentation in the region of the hilus. In shape, normal nodes appear as globular or reniform. Usually, 8 to 12 afferent vessels enter the node, the efferent vessels being fewer in number. The opacification of the normal node by the contrast medium is homogeneous, giving the node a fine reticular pattern in the radiograph.

Irregularities of nodal architecture, simulating neoplastic disease, may be observed in nodes in the absence of neoplasia. Such irregularities consist primarily of filling defects produced by fatty infiltration or fi-

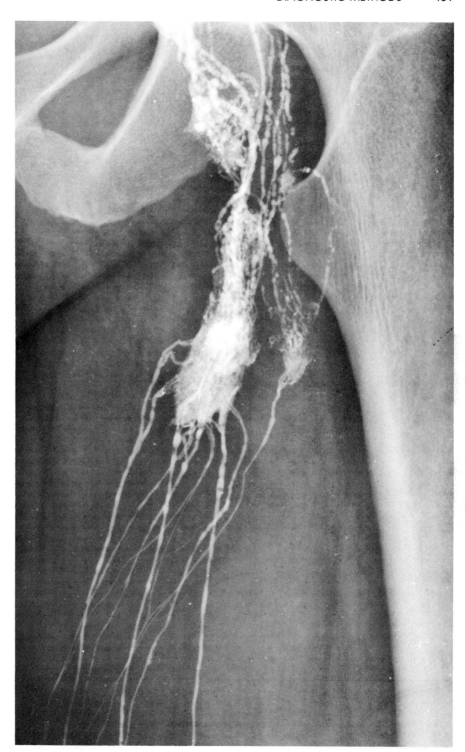

Fig. 26-3. Magnification radiograph of normal left superficial sublinguinal lymph node with afferent and efferent lymphatic channels in a 40-year-old woman. (From Isard HJ, Ostrum BJ, Cullinan JE: Magnification roentgenography: A "spot-film" technic. Med Radiogr Photogr 38:92–109, 1962)

brous replacement consequent to previous infections (fibrolipomatosis). Such defects are seen most frequently in the femoral and the inguinal lymph nodes, which represent the primary drainage from the lower extremity. However, they may also occur in the iliac and para-aortic nodes. Small defects may be caused by hilar vessels, by superimposition of separate nodes, or by wrapping of the node around a blood vessel. Oblique and stereoscopic radiographs as well as CT can often clarify the situation under such circumstances.

The Abnormal Lymphogram

Abnormalities of the lymphatic channels are observed in primary and secondary lymphedema and in lymphatic obstruction. Kinmonth and associates[104] describe four types of lymph vessel abnormality in idiopathic lymphedema—hypoplasia, aplasia, dilatation, and varicosity of lymphatic vessels.

Various radiographic abnormalities are produced by disease of the lymph nodes. Briefly, these consist of enlargement, focal or diffuse filling defects, irregularities of the marginal outline, displacement and obstruction of adjacent lymphatic vessels, and reflux opacification of collateral vessels. Although the specific pattern of abnormality may permit the determination of the type of disease (inflammation, metastasis, neoplasms of epithelial origin, or lymphoma) considerable overlap in lymphographic patterns is found, making it impossible to render a specific diagnosis in many cases. Because of this, lymphography is more often performed to delineate the extent of known disease than to make a primary diagnosis.

Inflammatory Nodes. In nodes involved only by inflammatory processes, the usual radiographic findings are (1) enlargement, the nodes usually measuring 2 cm to 4 cm in diameter; (2) preservation of peripheral contours; and (3) diffuse reticular alteration of internal architecture that may be difficult to distinguish from the normal homogeneous granular pattern (reactive hyperplasia). However, granulomatous and necrotizing inflammations may be present with focal and diffuse filling defects mimicking the metastatic and lymphomatous patterns described below.

Metastatic Nodes. Early metastatic lesions may not cause any abnormality. As a rule, a metastatic lesion, to be visible on the radiographs, must attain a diameter of at least 4 mm. If the node is completely filled with metastases, it is not visualized on the lymphangiogram. However, its presence may be revealed by deviation and obstruction of adjacent afferent lymphatic vessels. Nodes that are partially occupied by metastases of sufficient size are characterized by (1) filling defects along the margin of the node so that the normal

regular peripheral contour is altered, and (2) dilation of the afferent lymph vessels secondary to obstruction. Metastatic nodes may be normal in size or only slightly enlarged (Fig. 26-4). When a whole group of nodes is completely replaced by metastatic disease, this may be recognized because of discontinuity of lymph node chains.

Lymphomatous Nodes. In general, lymphomatous nodes are characterized by a more diffuse alteration of nodal architecture than is seen in metastatic nodes. The degree of node enlargement is variable and is somewhat related to the type of lymphoma, as is the pattern of architectural change. Thus, large lymph nodes with a foamy or lacy pattern are typical of lymphocytic or histiocytic lymphomas but may be seen in Hodgkin's disease. The latter often presents with multiple discrete filling defects in nodes that are only slightly enlarged.

There is now an extensive literature on lymphography that can be consulted for more detail.[101,102]

Complications. As a rule, the use of lymphography is not attended by significant complications. It has been shown repeatedly that lymphography is not associated with any functional or anatomic changes in the lymphatic vessels and lymph nodes. Some of the injected oily contrast material does not enter nodes, but it does reach the thoracic duct and subsequently, the venous system. Thus, minute oil emboli occur in the lungs in 100% of patients undergoing lymphography. This does not impair ventilation but does decrease the diffusing capacity for up to several days. For this reason, lymphography should be performed with caution, if at all, in patients with pulmonary insufficiency. Such patients should be evaluated with pulmonary function tests prior to the examination.

Other minor complications that may occur include (1) transient fever, (2) transient lymphangitis, (3) local wound infection, and (4) occasional sensitivity reaction to the vital dye or to iodine.

More serious complications, fortunately rare, include bronchopneumonia, pulmonary infarction, pulmonary edema, hemoptysis, and systemic embolization.

A theoretical complication is the spread of tumor emboli by the lymphographic procedure itself. Its occurrence would be difficult to substantiate. The literature should be consulted for detail on these and other rarer complications.[101,102,105–108]

Advantages of Lymphography

Lymphography has these distinct advantages:

It makes possible a more exact location of involved lymph nodes and indicates the status of such nodes.

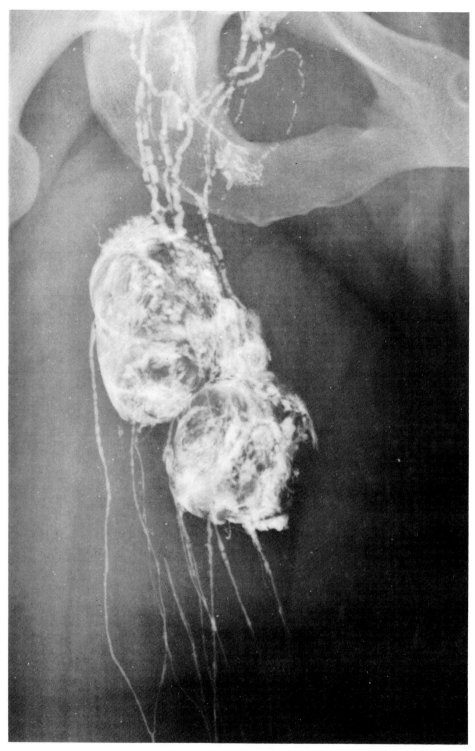

Fig. 26-4. Magnification radiograph of enlarged right superficial subinguinal lymph node with malignant infiltration secondary to primary melanoma of skin of heel (same patient as Fig. 26-3). (Isard HJ, Ostrum BJ, Cullinan, JE: Magnification roentgenography: A "spot-film" technic. Med Radiogr Photogr 38:92–109, 1962)

It helps to demonstrate involved nodes in case of unsuspected disease.

It demonstrates unsuspected extension of malignancy.

It determines the feasibility of radical surgery.

It helps assess the degree of thoroughness of radical surgery.

It is helpful in the followup of malignant nodal disease after radiotherapy or chemotherapy, since opacification of abnormal nodes persists for many months.

It aids in the detection of metastatic lesions in the absence of palpable nodes.

It may demonstrate the cause of displacement of the kidney and the ureters.[109]

It aids in the study of abnormalities of the thoracic duct.

It aids in differentiating between primary and secondary lymphedema.

XERORADIOGRAPHY

Xeroradiography, as a method of recording x-ray images of soft-tissue masses, has gained wide application in medical practice, particularly in examination of the breast. Striking images can also be obtained of soft-tissue parts, such as the extremities of axilla where enlarged lymph nodes can be readily detected. The cause of the enlargement is sometimes evident; for example, an enlarged node consisting primarily of fatty tissue might be expected following an inflammatory condition. Correspondingly, a node with irregular, indistinct margins might be seen secondary to malignant infiltration. Unfortunately, the xeroradiographic appearance is so often nonspecific that an etiology for the nodal enlargement cannot be stated. At present, this technique seems to have limited usefulness for the study of adenopathy. Recent reports discuss xeroradiography of axillary lymph node disease.[110,111]

DIAGNOSTIC ULTRASOUND

Ultrasonography is a noninvasive imaging procedure without known harmful effect. It can be used safely in those patients who are allergic to lymphographic contrast material. Cross-sectional body images are produced by detecting the reflected portions of the nonaudible, high-frequency sound waves directed into the body by a transducer, usually in direct contact with the patient's skin. The transducer is simultaneously the transmitter and receiver of the ultrasonic signals.

Diagnostic ultrasound is of great value in identifying enlarged lymph nodes in the retroperitoneum, abdomen, and to a lesser extent, the pelvis.[89,112] It is not capable of determining the etiology of lymph node masses. Lymph nodes in the 2 cm to 3 cm range may be visualized.[113] Body computed tomography (BCT) appears to be superior to ultrasonography in detecting slight lymph node enlargement because of its better spatial resolution.[89,91] Nonetheless, BCT has the disadvantages of employing ionizing radiation and of being a generally less available and more expensive procedure.

Ultrasonography can be repeated with impunity and is of particular value in the serial followup of masses undergoing chemotherapy or radiation therapy. In many cases, it gives a better picture of the extent of nodal involvement than does the lymphangiogram. The latter is limited to imaging the pelvic and retroperitoneal lymph node chains paralleling the abdominal aorta and the iliac arteries, whereas ultrasonography can evaluate not only these nodes but also those present in the porta hepatis, renal hila, mesentery, and upper para-aortic region. In addition, if lymph nodes are totally replaced by tumor, they will not be opacified by lymphography but are readily detected by ultrasonography (or BCT).

The characteristic sonographic appearance of a lymph node mass is a sonolucent (echo free) area, not unlike that seen in retroperitoneal sarcomas.[113,114] Loculated collections of fluid, aneurysms, and cysts may mimic lymphadenopathy, but in most instances it is possible to make the differentiation. Recent literature can be consulted for more details.[89,112–115]

COMPUTED TOMOGRAPHIC SCANNING

Computed tomography (CT) presents cross-sectional images. Scans of both thorax and abdomen may identify abnormal lymph nodes in the mediastinum, hila, and around the descending aorta in the chest and in the retroperitoneum, mesentery, and iliofemoral regions of the abdomen and pelvis. Abnormal nodes present as discrete nodules or as bulky amorphous masses of tissue density obliterating normal structures. However, the presence of such findings does not, of itself, establish the presence of lymphadenopathy. Cellulitis, hemorrhage, and nonlymphatic tumors arising in the usual node-bearing areas can be mistaken for lymph node abnormality. Nevertheless, the presence of abnormal tissue masses in the appropriate locations is very strong evidence of nodal involvement in the appropriate clinical context. If needed, fine-needle aspiration biopsy, under CT control, with cytological evaluation almost uniformly establishes the tissue type without morbidity.[116] Widespread adoption of the noninvasive CT scanning for detection of visceral lymphadenopathy inevitably followed demonstration of its reasonable accuracy.[90,91,117]

In addition, CT enables patients with known lymphoma to be staged for distant disease quite accurately.[118,119] Similarly, patients with proven pelvic

malignancy can be evaluated preoperatively to determine not only local tissue extension but spread to local and distant lymph nodes.[91,117] The effects of radiation or chemotherapy can be assessed by sequential CT scans.

Despite the quite high sensitivity of CT, negative scans do not exclude lymph nodal involvement by either lymphoma or metastatic disease. The ability of contrast lymphography to identify even single diseased lymph nodes of normal size retains an important place for this study in the evaluation of patients with suspected visceral nodal disease.

SCINTIGRAPHY

Introduction of radiocolloids interstitially allows imaging by scintillation cameras or scanners of the regional lymph nodes that drain a particular area.[120,121] Early experience with lymphatic scintigraphy offered promise that this technique might be useful in detecting malignant involvement of regional nodes. However, the lesser sensitivity of the technique compared to contrast lymphography was also noted quite early.[121] The advent of modern ultrasonography and CT has rendered this technique almost useless for identifying tumor-bearing nodes noninvasively.

Scintigraphy has been useful in planning radiation therapy portals. The location of the regional lymph nodes must be known in order to include them in the radiation field, and they can be demonstrated by the radioisotope procedure. Internal mammary nodes can be located to within 3 mm of actual location by scintigraphy following injection of radiocolloid into the posterior sheath of the rectus abdominus below the xiphoid.[123] The technique may also be applied to other anatomic sites.

Several radionuclides concentrate in abnormal lymph nodes following intravenous administration. The only widely used such method uses [67]gallium citrate. Localization of the radiogallium occurs in both inflammatory nodes and in a variety of malignant epithelial and lymphomatous neoplasms. The mechanism of localization is uncertain, but the best evidence indicates that physicochemical binding to a lactoglobulin elaborated by the neoplasm or inflammation is the primary determinant.[122] The technique has a rather low sensitivity (approximately 60%–75%) but occasionally demonstrates involved nodes not otherwise detected. Technical problems include high liver and spleen and frequently, large bowel concentration that obscures abdominal lymph nodes.

The appropriate tactic to detect nodal disease, at least cost and morbidity, is not as yet universally agreed upon. Many accept CT or ultrasound evidence of nodal involvement as diagnostic. Some also accept normal studies as sufficient indication of absent nodal disease, while others follow a normal noninvasive study (CT scan or ultrasonogram) with contrast lymphography to increase the detection rate of nodal involvement.

In the chest, CT scanning is the most accurate means of demonstrating abnormal mediastinal and para-aortic nodes. Oblique standard tomography may better evaluate the hila for lymphadenopathy.

REGIONAL LYMPHADENOPATHY

In the following sections, lymphadenopathy involving various regions will be described, its pathologic physiology analyzed, and its clinical significance discussed.

Any regional group of nodes may, of course, be involved in a disease producing a generalized lymphadenopathy, which fact will not be mentioned under each region unless of special importance. Generalized lymphadenopathy will be discussed separately later. The sections under head and neck nodes will stress instead the clinical significance of enlargement of nodes in each area or certain combination of areas. Reference to Figure 26-5 while reading this section will help in visualizing the anatomic locations of nodes and their drainage areas.

The importance of proper preparation of lymph nodes obtained by biopsy for appropriate histologic examination has been commented upon previously in this chapter. The value of this procedure, the indications for doing biopsies, and their interpretations will not be commented upon in the following sections concerned with regional and generalized lymphadenopathy because of a lack of space. This information is covered appropriately and in detail in various articles quoted.

Particular attention should be paid to patients with suspected systemic disease if the original biopsy diagnosis of a superficial lymph node is reported as *hyperplasia*. One should carefully follow the clinical course of this type of patient, whether the nodes are regional or generalized, for possible development of a recognizable serious illness, particularly a disease of collagen tissue or malignancy. There is much helpful literature concerned with such studies,[124,125,128–132] as well as discussion of nonneoplastic lesions of lymph nodes, which histologically resemble the appearance of a malignant lymphoma.[126,127]

LYMPH NODES OF HEAD AND NECK
Group I—Clinically Important and Readily Palpable Lymph Nodes

Of the numerous lymph nodes of the head and the neck, only the following are easily palpable when enlarged: (1) occipital; (2) posterior auricular; (3) anterior

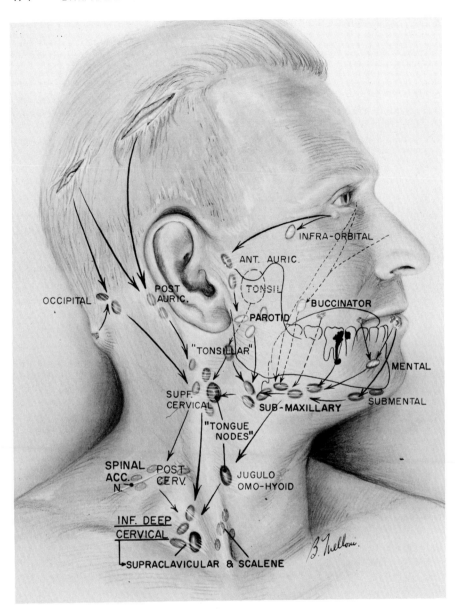

INFRA-ORBITAL

ANT. AURIC.

TONSIL

POST
AURIC.

BUCCINATOR

OCCIPITAL

PAROTID

"TONSILLAR"

MENTAL

SUPF.
CERVICAL

SUB-MAXILLARY

SUBMENTAL

"TONGUE
NODES"

SPINAL
ACC.
N.

POST.
CERV.

JUGULO
OMO-HYOID

INF. DEEP
CERVICAL

SUPRACLAVICULAR & SCALENE

B. Mellow.

Fig. 26-5. Diagrammatic view of the lymph nodes of the head and the neck with directions and channels of lymph flow. Nodes drawn darker are those generally palpable clinically, while nodes drawn lighter (infraorbital, parotid, buccinator, and mental) are either less constant or deeper and generally not detectable clinically.

auricular; (4) "tonsillar" and other superior deep cervicals; (5) superficial cervicals; (6) submaxillary; (7) submental; (8) posterior cervical; (9) inferior deep cervicals, including the supraclavicular nodes, jugulo-omohyoid (tongue node), and so forth. The scalene nodes, although not palpable, belong in this group.

The Occipital Nodes. *Anatomy.* The occipital nodes, one to three in number, lie midway between the external occipital protuberance and the mastoid process, in close relation to the great occipital nerve, near the occipital insertion of the semispinalis capitis muscle.

Enlarged occipital nodes may cause pressure on this nerve and neuralgia in its distribution. These nodes receive afferents from the back of the scalp and the back of the head and drain into the deep cervical nodes.

Clinical Significance. Any infectious lesion in the scalp of this drainage area, whether localized or diffuse, may produce isolated occipital lymphadenopathy which, depending upon the nature and the extent of the primary infection, may be unilateral or bilateral. A small primary lesion may be easily overlooked when the hair is heavy. Pediculosis capitis, which may be suspected from the presence of nits in the hair, and ringworm of

the scalp are particularly common initiating conditions in children. Hair style (*e.g.,* tightly braided in rows against the scalp) may lead to lymphadenopthy in the scalp drainage areas, probably by causing acute recurrent folliculitis.[133]

Being so readily detectable, occipital lymphadenopathy may be a conspicuous part of a generalized lymphadenopathy, and for this reason it is often the first node enlargement to be detected. At one time, painless occipital nodes, and also epitrochlear nodes without local reason, were considered suggestive of systemic syphilis. This is now a rare cause. Cancer with primary site in this drainage area is quite rare.

The Posterior Auricular Nodes.
Anatomy. The posterior auricular nodes, usually two in number, lie on the mastoid process behind the pinna of the external ear, on the insertion of the sternocleidomastoid muscle. They receive afferents from the external auditory meatus and the skin of the back of the pinna and of the temporal region of the scalp. They drain into the upper part of the superficial cervical nodes.

Clinical Significance. Comments made about the occipital nodes with relation to scalp infections apply also to posterior auricular lymphadenopathy. If the primary scalp lesion of the drainage area is overlooked, pain, fever, and local tenderness behind the ear may stimulate mastoiditis, especially if the middle ear is acutely or chronically infected. The auditory meatus as a site for an infectious process (or rarely, a neoplasm) should not be overlooked. The Ramsay–Hunt syndrome of herpes zoster may involve the auditory meatus with lymphadenopathy.

Enlargement of posterior auricular lymph nodes generally has been considered a characteristic and often diagnostically suggestive finding in rubella (German measles), accompanied at times by suboccipital and posterior cervical lymphadenopathy, and less commonly by axillary and inguinal adenopathy. This may not always be true, as shown by the study of Kalmansohn, who found posterior cervical lymphadenopathy to be more common and often more marked in 100 adults with this disorder.[134] At any rate, the frequent presence of marked posterior auricular lymphadenopathy in rubella and the rarity of this sign in regular measles is a finding of considerable diagnostic value.

Anterior Auricular Nodes.
Anatomy. The anterior auricular nodes lie immediately in front of the tragus, superficial to the parotidomasseteric fascia. They receive afferents from the lateral portion of the eyelids and its palpebral conjunctivae, from the skin of the temporal region, the external auditory meatus, and the anterior surface of the pinna of the external ear.

Clinical Significance. The skin drainage area of this node is limited and conspicuously apparent, so that any infections or neoplastic process is readily detected early. Particularly significant as primary lesions in this area are squamous cell carcinoma, primary syphilitic chancre, or any infectious skin disorder of the face. While basal cell carcinoma occurs in this region, metastases are late and rare. Erysipelas may at times produce significant lymphadenopathy because of its common initiation about the upper cheek and the eyelids.

Herpes zoster ophthalmicus commonly produces unilateral enlargement of the anterior auricular nodes, which, in fact, is considered part of the clinical picture.[135] It has been noted at times before the appearance of the skin eruption and results from the primary viral infection, although subject to exacerbation when the skin vesicles become infected secondarily.

Kalmansohn noted anterior auricular lymphadenopathy in 52% of adults in a large outbreak of German measles, coupled at times with ocular complaints and palpebral conjunctivitis.[134] Rice reported a 27% incidence of anterior auricular lymphadenopathy in a large series of 112 cases of trachoma with lid activity.[136]

The intact conjunctiva may serve as the portal of entrance for a variety of etiologic infectious agents carried to the area by finger contact, fomites, kissing, spray droplets, contact with cats, and so forth, producing conjunctivitis and regional anterior auricular lymphadenopathy, with spread at times to cervical nodes and with varying systemic features. The submaxillary nodes, draining as they do the inner aspect of the eyelids, often are involved coincidently when the anterior auricular nodes are involved and should be searched for, since they are less conspicuous clinically. The nature of the primary inoculation makes unilateral involvement much more common than bilateral.

Acute suppurative conjunctivitis, such as is produced by the gonococcus, seldom produces significant lymph node enlargement.

Oculoglandular Syndrome.
Of particular interest is the ability of the intact conjunctiva to be the site of entrance of a number of infectious agents, which may produce a more chronic disorder characterized by involvement of the conjunctiva and significant lymphadenopathy of the anterior auricular nodes. Sometimes these disorders are characterized under the name *oculoglandular syndrome* or *Parinaud's syndrome* (not to be confused with the neurologic Parinaud's syndrome). The early description of a disorder in this group was that of a glandular type of conjunctivitis associated with painful and enlarged anterior auricular nodes with minimal systemic symptoms. A leptothrix organism was demonstrated in some cases by Verhoeff in 1933.[137]

There may be a mild irregular fever and the minimal systemic symptoms associated at times with mild blood eosinophilia. Lymphadenopathy commonly is limited to the anterior auricular group, which becomes painfully enlarged, and rarely, as is true for all disorders in this group, involves nodes in the neck area, particularly in the submaxillary nodes, which drain the inner aspect of the eyelids. Rarely, the facial nodes and the infraorbital nodes may become involved also.

The virus of lymphopathia venereum may rarely be a cause of this syndrome.[138] Specific diagnosis by use of the Frei test is possible. Tularemia may occur as a pure oculoglandular syndrome when the *Bacillus tularensis* enters the body through an intact conjunctiva.[139,140] Nodular conjunctivitis ensues, often ulcerative and followed by marked anterior auricular lymphadenopathy, extending at times to include the cervical nodes. The systemic response and the ocular disability may last for weeks to months. Diagnosis by bacterial culture and agglutination tests usually firmly establishes the etiology. As a rule, the systemic response of this form of tularemia is less marked than the usual type, with a consequent lower mortality.

A significant advance in explaining obscure instances of the oculoglandular syndrome has been the demonstration that cat-scratch disease may be manifested by conjunctivitis, with granulation, followed by anterior auricular lymphadenopathy and the usual systemic features of this disorder.[141,142,143] A history of contact with cats is common. Diagnosis is possible by a specific skin test. The propensity of this type of lymphadenopathy to suppuration is well known but rare in this syndrome.

Not to be overlooked is the possibility of tuberculosis, syphilis, or sporotrichosis, which occasionally produce this syndrome, nor, more rarely still, other unusual infections, such as glanders, chancroid, and so forth.[144–147] Neoplasm of the eyelid with regional anterior auricular metastasis can closely simulate the oculoglandular syndrome, particularly if the primary lesion on the eyelid is infected.

The viral disorder epidemic keratoconjunctivitis produces an oculoglandular syndrome, commonly unilateral.[148,149] The more acute form is of about two weeks' duration accompanied by conjunctivitis with a watery discharge containing demonstrable lymphocytes. Diagnostic criteria include the absence of purulent discharge in the presence of acute bulbar and palpebral conjunctival inflammation, occasionally with a pseudomembrane; multiple cases occurring in an epidemic; and the absence of a detectable organism in the eye by the usual bacteriologic techniques. A definitive diagnosis depends on special laboratory studies. The edematous erythema of the skin about the eye suggests infection of the reticular lymphatics and resembles erysipelas. In some cases, corneal involvement damages sight. Anterior auricular nodes are large and tender in over 90% of cases; such changes are occasionally followed by submaxillary and cervical lymphadenopathy. If present, systemic features are mild but rarely may be marked.

Pharyngoconjunctival fever of adenoidal-pharyngeal-conjunctival (APC) viral etiology is characterized by fever, various systemic complaints, nasopharyngitis, and lymphadenopathy of cervical or submaxillary and occasionally anterior auricular groups of nodes.[150] It can be added to the already large group of disorders manifesting the oculoglandular syndrome.

Eyelid edema, occasional enlargement of lacrimal gland, slight conjunctival reaction, anterior auricular and occasionally submaxillary lymphadenopathy, all unilateral, is known as the oculonodal complex (sign of Chagas–Romaña),[151] an early phase of Chagas' disease of South America. In this syndrome, the eye is apparently the inoculation site for the etiologic agent contained in the excreta of the reduviid bug vector.[152]

The Superior Deep Cervical Nodes, Including the Tonsillar and the Tongue (Jugulodigastric) Nodes.

Anatomy. The tonsillar node, the main node of the tonsil, belongs to the superior deep cervical nodes. This node lies below the angle of the mandible, between the internal jugular and the common facial veins, at the posterior side of the posterior belly of the digastricus.

The jugulodigastric node is an important node in the lymphatic drainage of the tongue, receiving afferents from the greater part of the tongue, with the exception of the apex. It lies just below the great cornu of the hyoid bone, close to the bifurcation of the common carotid artery.

Clinical Significance. The tonsillar node undergoes enlargement with infections of the palatine tonsil and, to some degree, of the pharynx. The jugulodigastric node undergoes enlargement because of neoplastic invasion by cancer of the tongue, faucial arch, tonsil, larynx, or pharynx, or because of lymphomas of the tonsil or base of the tongue, such as Waldeyer's ring.

Superficial Cervical Nodes.

Anatomy. The superficial cervical nodes lie on the external surface of the sternomastoid muscle, in close relationship to the external jugular vein as it emerges from the parotid gland. They receive afferents from the pinna of the external ear and the parotid region and send efferents around the anterior border of the sternomastoid muscle to the superior deep cervical nodes.

Clinical Significance. These are the most important and obvious nodes involved with cervical lymphoma, both the Hodgkin's and non-Hodgkin's types. They are distinguished from the cervical lymph node metastases of

squamous cell carcinoma by being more rubbery and mobile and anatomically more superficial.

Submaxillary Nodes. Anatomy. The submaxillary nodes lie within the submaxillary fascial compartment surrounded by deep cervical fascia. Some of the nodes are imbedded within, and others lie on, the submaxillary gland. In cancer, removal of submaxillary nodes necessitates removal of the submaxillary salivary gland. One of the nodes, the node of Stöhr, lying in relation to the external maxillary artery, is concerned particularly in lymphatic drainage of the tongue. These nodes receive efferents from the submental nodes. The submaxillary nodes receive afferents from the sides of the tongue, the gums, the lateral part of the lower lip, the entire upper lip, the angle of the mouth and the cheek, and the medial angle of the eye. Since the submaxillary nodes drain not only cutaneous areas but also parts of the mucous membrane of the lips and the mouth, their efferents drain not only into the superficial but also into the deep cervical lymph nodes.

Clinical Significance. Enlargement follows infection or neoplasm primarily in the drainage area. The initial lesion in the mouth may not always be readily detectable upon clinical inspection and may require palpation of the mouth with the gloved hand. Infections of dental origin are very common as a cause of submaxillary lymphadenopathy and may require dental and radiographic examination for evaluation. The lip, the tongue, or the inside of the mouth are common locations for primary syphilitic chancre or for neoplasm. Rarely, the inside of the mouth is the site of primary oral tuberculosis.[153]

Submaxillary salivary glands, if enlarged because of mumps, sarcoidosis, or reaction to iodine-containing medications, may be confused with lymph node enlargement, especially when the parotids are not involved.[154]

One should not overlook the fact that the area of the medial aspects of the conjunctiva and the eyelids drain to the submaxillary lymph nodes, which may be enlarged along with the anterior auricular nodes as part of the oculoglandular syndrome.

The Submental Nodes. Anatomy. The submental nodes lie in the submental triangle, bounded by the inferior border of the mandible, the anterior bellies of the two digastric muscles, and the hyoid bone. They usually lie near the midline. They drain the central part of the lower lip, the floor of the mouth, the tip of the tongue, and the skin of the chin; their efferents pass either to the submaxillary nodes or to the deep cervical nodes.

Clinical Significance. Enlargement follows infection or neoplasm that is primary in the drainage area. The initial lesion in this area is easily seen, or at least detectable, by palpation of the mouth with the gloved hand. Infections of dental origin are very common as a cause of the submental lymphadenopathy.

Submental lymphadenopathy should not be confused with sublingual mumps. In all instances in which the submental and the submaxillary nodes are enlarged, the physician should palpate the drainage areas within the mouth with his gloved hand to detect a primary infection or a neoplastic lesion not clinically observable.

Posterior Cervicals. Anatomy. The posterior cervical nodes belong to the deep cervical nodes but often are palpable as a separate group. They are located in the occipital triangle, above the level of the inferior belly of the omohyoid. They are related intimately to the spinal accessory nerve, which crosses this triangle.

Clinical Significance. The posterior cervical nodes are commonly involved in scalp infections, pediculosis, and tuberculosis. Rarely, other infections and neoplasms are the cause. This site of neoplastic lymph node involvement is characteristic of carcinoma of the nasopharynx. Because of their close relationship to the spinal accessory nerve, removal of these nodes in the surgical treatment of tuberculous cervical adenitis or biopsy of these nodes in suspected primary or secondary neoplasms may produce damage to this nerve with consequent spinal accessory nerve paralysis.[155]

Although generalized lymphadenopathy is common in African trypanosomiasis, bilateral enlargement of the posterior cervical nodes is especially prominent and constitutes a diagnostic feature of this disease known as *Winterbottom's sign.*[156] A recent report commenting on imported cases diagnosed and treated in the United States stresses the value of this clinical sign.[157]

The Inferior Deep Cervicals. Anatomy. The inferior deep cervical nodes lie in the lower part of the neck below the level of the inferior belly of the omohyoid muscle. Some of these nodes lie behind the sternomastoid muscle in the fat covering the anterior scalene muscle; these are known as the scalene nodes. Others lie beyond the posterior border of the sternomastoid muscle in the supraclavicular triangle (the supraclavicular nodes; Virchow's node).

The inferior deep cervical nodes receive afferents from the back of the scalp and neck, from many of the superior deep cervical nodes, from some of the axillary nodes, and even from lymph vessels directly from the skin of the arm and from the pectoral region. Altogether, therefore, the inferior cervical nodes receive a great deal of the lymphatic drainage of the entire head and neck, as well as some drainage from the arm and the superficial aspects of the thorax.

Clinical Significance. Because of their wide connections, the inferior deep cervical nodes may be involved in carcinoma originating anywhere in the head or the

neck; in addition, the supraclavicular nodes may be involved by carcinoma originating within the abdomen or the thorax. The nodes on the left are involved more frequently, probably because of their relationship to the thoracic duct, whereas the nodes on the right usually are involved only when there are tumors in the thorax. The supraclavicular and the scalene nodes will be discussed separately.

A number of papers present excellent general information on the problem of cervical lymphadenopathy.[154,158–162,413] Persistent jugular lymph sac must be differentiated from cervical lymphadenopathy.[163]

Special comment about several newer diseases in which cervical lymphadenopathy is prominent will be helpful. Mucocutaneous lymph node syndrome (*Kawasaki's disease*), described in Japan in 1967 and now being reported with increasing frequency in the United States, is an example.[164] This disorder occurs in infants and small children and is characterized by an acute febrile course, a focal nonsuppurative (predominantly unilateral) cervical lymphadenopathy, conjunctivitis, lingual and oral mucosal involvement, skin rash, and indurative edema of hands and feet. There may be various types of other systemic manifestations. Death occurs rarely, with autopsies showing coronary arteries involved with arteritis, aneurysmal dilatation, and extensive thrombosis.[164]

There is a growing literature on another unique disorder named *sinus histiocytosis with massive lymphadenopathy* (SHML),[165] which has proved to have worldwide distribution. It is most frequent in the first decade of life, rare in adults, common in blacks, and characterized clinically by bilateral, painless, often massive but predominantly cervical lymphadenopathy, running a febrile, prolonged, progressive course, with eventual recovery in most cases.[166]

Enlargement of cervical lymph nodes in Graves' disease may occur, but it is not diagnostic. However, there has been recent re-emphasis of older observations that in this disorder the painful enlargement of the lymph nodes of the left subtrapezoid or pretrapezoid chain may constitute a useful diagnostic sign.[167]

The Jugulo-omohyoid (Tongue) Node.

Anatomy. The jugulo-omohyoid node belongs to the inferior deep cervical group. It is situated in relation to the internal jugular vein and the common carotid artery, just above the point at which these vessels are crossed by the superior belly of the omohyoid muscle. It receives lymph from apex of the tongue by lymphatics that bypass the submental nodes.

Clinical Significance. Cancer originating in the apex of the tongue may spread by lymphatics to the submental nodes but also by a direct route to the jugulo-omohyoid node (tongue node).[168] This node should not be confused with the large node of the superior deep cervical group, often called the *main tongue node* (*jugulodigastric*). The latter is located at the level of the bifurcation of the common artery, just below the great cornu of the hyoid bone, and becomes involved from cancer of the margin and the posterior part of the tongue. (See reference to these two tongue nodes on Fig. 26-5.)

Supraclavicular Nodes.

Anatomy. The supraclavicular nodes on each side are essentially part of the homolateral deep cervical node group and when enlarged are usually palpable behind the clavicular insertion of the sternomastoid muscle. The Valsalva maneuver may aid in detecting a supraclavicular lymphadenopathy not readily palpable.[169] Being intercalated in the drainage system from the head, the arm, the chest wall, and the breast, supraclavicular nodes are involved frequently in infectious and neoplastic processes developing in these drainage areas.

Clinical Significance. The particular interest of the supraclavicular nodes, especially those on the left, centers in their occasional and peculiar metastatic involvement from neoplasms originating with the abdominal cavity and rarely from lesions located anywhere in the drainage area of the thoracic lymphatic duct. Because its lymphatic drainage is from the lungs and the mediastinum, the right supraclavicular node is enlarged primarily from metastases from the lung and the esophagus. It has been reported to be involved from cancer of the pancreas[170] and rarely from other intraabdominal tumors, probably as a result of lymphatic crossover in the mediastinum.

After exclusion of a nonvisceral site for a malignancy, metastatic involvement of the supraclavicular nodes has been accepted as diagnostic of distant intrathoracic or intra-abdominal neoplasm and is known by various special names, such as sentinel node, signal node, and the eponyms, *Virchow's node* and *Troisier's node*.[170] Although this sign was introduced in 1848 by Virchow as associated with cancer of the stomach,[171] its present meaning is much broader. In an extensive study of supraclavicular metastases, Viacava and Pack noted it in 28% of 4365 cases of cancer.[170] The order of the primary site was 13.27% from the lung, 8.1% pancreas, 7.1% esophagus, 6.9% kidney, 6.1% ovary, 4.8% testicle, and 2.6% stomach.[170] These figures indicate that this diagnostic sign is not particularly common and when present is of ominous prognostic interest rather than of helpful early diagnostic value. Recent reports stress that carcinoma of the prostate may metastasize to the supraclavicular lymph node.[172] Its occurrence with testicular tumors has received special attention.[173] Biopsy of this node has been used for staging, therapy, and determining prognosis. It is actually infrequent in cancer of the stomach, the neoplasm with

which it is usually thought to be commonly associated. McKusick, in an interesting report, stresses that the *Virchow–Troisier* node may be a noticeable metastatic lesion with cancer of the gallbladder.[171]

In general, a right-sided or bilateral supraclavicular node is suggestive of a lung or an esophageal lesion, whereas an isolated left supraclavicular metastasis suggests a primary site in the kidney, the ovary, the testes, the gallbladder, or the stomach.[170,171]

Controversy has centered on whether tumor spreads to the supraclavicular nodes by lymphatic permeation or by embolization. To support the former view are reports of lymphatic ducts completely filled with tumor cells.[174] Some interesting experimental studies by Zeidman support the tumor emboli theory and indicate strongly that tumor emboli can reach the supraclavicular node from the thoracic duct through afferent branches and need not be explained by retrograde passage through efferent channels.[175] In one study, there was a positive correlation between supraclavicular metastasis and the presence of neoplastic cells in the thoracic duct lymph.[176]

One should not overlook the fact that any intra-abdominal infection, especially if of chronic nature such as tuberculous peritonitis, may produce a left supraclavicular infectious lymphadenopathy.[171] Patients vaccinated against smallpox in the left deltoid region may develop a noticeable postvaccinal lymphadenitis of the left supraclavicular lymph node.[177] If its cause is overlooked, the enlarged supraclavicular node may be confused with lymphoma.[47,177]

Scalene Nodes and Scalene Node Biopsy. *Anatomy.* Extensive studies[178,181,182] have reported on the value of the scalene node biopsy, a procedure introduced by Daniels in 1949 for the diagnosis of intrathoracic disease.[183] This operation can be performed under local anesthesia and is neither complicated, dangerous, nor prolonged. Figure 26-6 indicates in diagrammatic fashion the anatomic relations of the scalene nodes. This operation permits entrance to a fat-filled space bound medially by the internal jugular vein, laterally by the omohyoid muscle, below by the subclavian vein and overlying the scalenus anticus muscle. The fat pad in this space constantly contains several lymph nodes, even if they are not enlarged enough to detect upon physical examination.

Clinical Significance. Shefts, Terrill, and Swindell, in a report of 314 biopsies in 293 patients, secured a positive histologic diagnosis in 102 patients (35%). In-

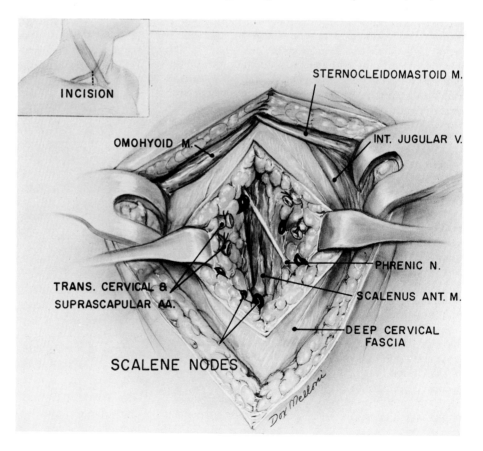

Fig. 26-6. Diagram to illustrate anatomic location and relations of scalene nodes.

cluded in their series of cases were 60 patients with Boeck's sarcoid, 20 with bronchogenic carcinoma, 9 with tuberculosis, 7 with primary lymphoma, and 4 with metastases to lung.[181] Skinner[182] and others[184–187] have reviewed this subject, and the reader is referred to these sources for a critical discussion. In a large series of proven lung carcinomas, the scalene node biopsy was positive in 93% of patients with palpable nodes and in 23.8% with nonpalpable nodes.[188] An extensive literature exists on this procedure. Aside from malignancy, the procedure has proved particularly valuable by frequently proving Boeck's sarcoid to be the cause of obscure lung and hilar node pathology. It has also shown that silicosis can involve the scalene node.

The report of Harken and associates in 1954 added much data supporting the diagnostic importance of this procedure and emphasized extending the scope of the operation, especially to exploration of the upper mediastinum, since approximately half of their positive results came from tissue removed from the mediastinum when the scalene node biopsy was negative. The authors reported a positive histologic diagnosis of 45 of 142 cases (31.7%) with the use of this complete technic.[178]

Anatomic peculiarities of the lymph drainage of the right and the left lung into the hilar area and to the scalene nodes must be understood to secure the best results (see Fig. 26–11). Homolateral biopsy can be used in all cases with the exception of lesions in the left lower lobe, a point emphasized by Harken and associates.[178] Figure 26–11 shows clearly that the left lower lobe has lymphatic drainage through the intertracheal-bronchial nodes to both lateral chains. Bilateral scalene node and upper mediastinal node biopsies are indicated when a primary site is suspected to be in the left lower lobe. Radner in 1955 also used exploration of the superior mediastinum to biopsy nodes.[179]

Mediastinoscopy was introduced in 1959 by Carlens who developed the technic and special instruments suitable for exploration of the mediastinum.[180] It is essentially a surgical-endoscopic technic, making use of a suprasternal incision and a specially designed endoscopic instrument called a mediastinoscope. The procedure provides for biopsy of certain lymph nodes and other lesions in the mediastinum under visual guidance.

The technic is well documented in many publications.[189,190] Mast and Jafek have provided an excellent account of the mediastinal anatomy involved.[191] The procedure has received wide acceptance in Europe and in the United States. Several excellent reviews provide access to an extensive literature.[189,190,192] Study of published data indicates that in the absence of palpable supraclavicular nodes, mediastinoscopy is superior to scalene node biopsy in accuracy of diagnosis and prognosis.[189]

Mediastinoscopy was a logical diagnostic extension to the scalene node biopsy, which it has replaced to a considerable degree. Recent reports comment on an appropriate current role for scalene node biopsy.[199,200]

Several recent publications described the use of percutaneous fine needle aspiration biopsy of hilar and mediastinal masses as another method of diagnosis.[201,202]

Group II—Less Clinically Important and Not Readily Palpable Lymph Nodes

In the anterior part of the face are several groups of nodes not ordinarily searched for or detectable routinely but which may occasionally become clinically significant and produce signs or symptoms. These include the infraorbital, the facial, the parotid, and the mental. (See Fig. 26-5.)

Here we shall not discuss other nodes of the head and the neck, such as the anterior cervicals, the retropharyngeal, and the many deep neck nodes likely to be encountered only in surgical procedures, especially radical dissections, since such nodes are detectable only indirectly through clinical manifestations or biopsies.

Infraorbital Nodes. Anatomy. The infraorbital nodes lie just below the orbit; they help drain the outer aspect of the eyelids and the conjunctiva. Their efferents join the anterior auricular as well as the submaxillary nodes.

Clinical Significance. This node sometimes becomes enlarged and tender from infections of the conjunctiva and the eyelid and therefore may constitute part of the oculoglandular syndrome.

The Facial Lymph Nodes. Anatomy. The superficial facial lymph nodes (buccinator nodes) lie on the buccinator muscle and are inconstant. They drain the medial aspect of the eyelids, the conjunctiva, the nose, and the cheek, and they send efferents to the submaxillary nodes.

Clinical Significance. These nodes are rarely detectable since they are inconstant and lie in the deep and not readily palpable areas.[193] They may occasionally be involved as the only manifestation of metastasis from facial malignancy.[194] If enlarged, they may be detected by bimanual palpation of the cheek with one hand gloved for examination within the mouth. More rarely, they present as a detectable lump in the cheek which, according to Bailey,[195] must be differentiated from a lipoma of the sucking pad and tumor or cyst of a molar gland.[196] A suppurating gland can leave a scar on the cheek.

The Parotid Group. Anatomy. The parotid group is fairly large, usually containing from 10 to 16 nodes.

They lie within the parotid fascial compartment, enclosed by the superficial layer of the deep cervical fascia. Some of the nodes are imbedded within the substance of the parotid, and others are outside of the parotid but within the parotid fascial compartment. The intraparotid nodes receive afferents from the eyelids, the external auditory meatus, the skin of the temporal and the frontal regions, and the tympanic cavity. The deep parotid nodes drain the back of the nose and the nasopharynx, as well as the parotid gland.

Clinical Significance. These nodes are not commonly palpable. Occasionally pain or enlargement in the parotid area may be explained by some infection or tumor in the drainage area, which includes locations not readily accessible to clinical inspection, such as the back of the nose and the nasopharynx. These nodes are best studies by endoscopic or mirror examination.

Late formation of the parotid salivary gland capsule may result in parotid lymph nodes being incorporated within this gland. As a result, it is clinically difficult to distinguish enlargement of those lymph nodes from swelling of the parotid gland itself.[197] Most cases of malignant lymphoma of the parotid region are in reality located in these nodes. Similarly, adenolymphoma (*Warthin's tumor*) also may arise within lymph nodes rather than in the parotid itself.

Mental Node. Anatomy. This node lies in relation to the mental foramen of the mandible. It helps to drain the lower lip, the tip of the tongue, and the floor of the mouth. Although its efferents drain chiefly into the submaxillary nodes, some of these efferent lymphatic channels enter the mandibular foramen.

Clinical Significance. This node permits cancer emboli to involve the mandible in metastatic cancer from the lip or the tip of the tongue. This is the reason for *combining hemimandibulectomy with radical neck dissection in treatment of cancer of the lip and the tongue.*[198]

Cancerous Metastasis to Head and Neck Nodes. Any of the head and neck nodes may be involved with metastatic cancer, the primary site of which lies externally on the scalp or face or more commonly, in the upper food and air passage epithelium, such as the oral cavity, including tongue, floor of mouth, or buccal mucosa; oropharynx, including tonsil, tonsillar fossa, or posterior pharyngeal wall; larynx, including vocal cords, laryngeal ventricle, false cord, epiglottis, or aryepiglottic fold; hypopharynx, including pyriform sinus and postcricoid area; or finally, nasopharynx or paranasal sinuses. Martin and Morfit have emphasized the importance of always considering this etiology when any of these nodes manifest a chronic enlargement characterized by unilateral location and firmness to touch with absence of pain.[203] Hendrick notes that 50%

of patients with supraglottic and hypopharyngeal carcinomas present with painless neck nodes.[204] Figure 26-7 shows the more common sites for such metastatic lesions. If an infectious focus can be excluded, the drainage area of the involved node should be searched for a primary site of a neoplasm. The reader is referred to the excellent coverage of this subject by Feind for more detail.[205]

Cancerous lymphadenopathy in the neck may present a difficult diagnostic problem, since it must be differentiated from such benign masses as chronic infectious lymphadenopathy, sebaceous cyst, lipoma, thyroglossal cyst, bronchogenic cyst, and so forth.[206] The diagnosis of malignancy should be suspected in adults, especially in cigarette-smoking males, and a thorough head and neck examination, including direct laryngoscopy and nasopharyngoscopy with biopsies performed to reveal the source of the tumor. In approximately 10% of patients, the most complete investigations fail to uncover such primary cancer. Such patients should then undergo cervical lymph node biopsy to confirm the malignant diagnosis and receive definitive treatment.[207,208] Frequent follow-up examinations eventually reveal the occult primary site, usually in the structures of *Waldeyer's ring* (nasopharynx, base of tongue, or tonsil) or the pyriform sinus. These sites are generally inaccessible to routine inspection and have irregular surfaces and sparse sensory nerve supplies, causing symptoms late in their course but sharing the propensity for early cervical lymph node metastases.

THE AXILLARY NODES

Anatomy. The axillary nodes are subdivided into five groups: lateral, posterior, central, anterior, and apical.

The lateral axillary nodes lie near the junction of the axillary and the brachial veins on the medial aspect of the humerus and constitute the main termination of afferent channels of the superficial and the deep lymphatics of the upper extremity. Although their efferents drain mostly into the central and the apical nodes, some channels pass directly to the supraclavicular group. The posterior axillary nodes lie along the axillary border of the scapula, in relation to the subscapular vein, and receive afferent lymph channels from the upper extremity and the posterior thoracic wall, draining efferently into both the lateral and the central axillary nodes. The central axillary nodes lie in the deep fat of the axilla or between layers of the axillary fascia at its base, receiving afferents from the lateral, the posterior, and the anterior axillary nodes and terminating their efferents in the apical axillary nodes. The anterior axillary nodes, situated along the lower border of the

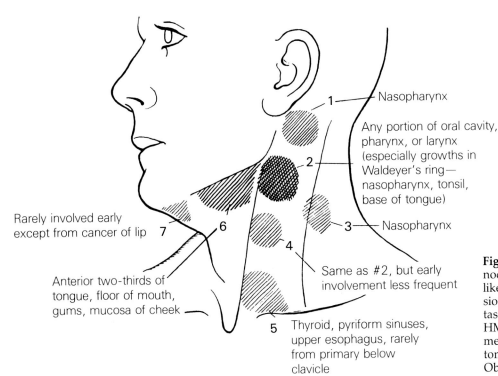

1 — Nasopharynx

2 — Any portion of oral cavity, pharynx, or larynx (especially growths in Waldeyer's ring — nasopharynx, tonsil, base of tongue)

3 — Nasopharynx

4 — Same as #2, but early involvement less frequent

5 — Thyroid, pyriform sinuses, upper esophagus, rarely from primary below clavicle

6 — Anterior two-thirds of tongue, floor of mouth, gums, mucosa of cheek

7 — Rarely involved early except from cancer of lip

Fig. 26-7. Various lymph node groups with the most likely sites of the primary lesion that may cause the metastases. (Martin H, Morfit HM: Cervical lymph node metastasis as the first symptom of cancer. Surg Gynecol Obstet 78:133–159, 1944)

pectoralis major, in relation to the lateral thoracic vein, drain the greater part of the lymph from the mammary gland and also receive efferents from the anterior chest wall. The efferents end in the central and the apical axillary nodes. The apical axillary or the intraclavicular nodes lie along the upper part of the axillary vein in the interval between the costocoracoid membrane anteriorly, the axillary vein posteriorly, and the first intercostal space inferiorly. These nodes receive afferents from the other axillary nodes, as well as direct afferents from the superior part of the subclavian trunk (Fig. 26–8).

Clinical Significance. Axillary lymphadenopathy is a common clinical problem and suggests mainly an infectious process or neoplasm in the drainage area, which includes part of the hand and the arm, chest wall, upper and lateral abdominal wall, and part of the breast (Fig. 26-8). It may follow lesions in the drainage area of the epitrochlear nodes if the pathologic condition spreads beyond this lymph node barrier. Evaluation is made more difficult in that nodes may be palpated at times in supposedly "normal" persons.[209] There are many reports on the value of careful study of axillary lymphadenopathy.[210,211] A recent study of axillary lymph nodes from 487 random autopsies provides valuable data on correlation of histology with age of the deceased and cause of death.[212]

In most instances, infectious lymphadenopathy is responsible for axillary node involvement, since the fingers and the arm are subject to so many potentially infectious traumatic episodes. The finding of a unilateral axillary lymphadenopathy suggests the need to consider use of injectable addicting drugs in the arm on the same side.[213] Likewise, many infectious systemic diseases commence by inoculation in this drainage area, producing axillary lymphadenopathy with one or more satellite nodes prior to systemic invasion. Representative examples include extragenital chancre of syphilis, brucellosis in veterinarians, inoculation tuberculosis, tularemia, cat-scratch disease, sporotrichosis, and so forth. The axillary nodes are especially likely to be involved in streptococcal infections of the hand with tubular lymphangitis. Axillary nodes commonly suppurate in certain types of infections. They may enlarge in rheumatoid arthritis of the arm.[214,215]

Although any skin neoplasm primary in the drainage area, particularly malignant melanoma and epidermoid carcinoma, may metastasize to the axillary nodes, special attention in these nodes centers about the frequency with which they are involved with carcinoma primary in the female breast. The number of axillary nodes involved markedly influences the prognosis and the management of this disease. It is well to note that metastasis to the supraclavicular lymph nodes from carcinoma of the breast is unusual unless the ax-

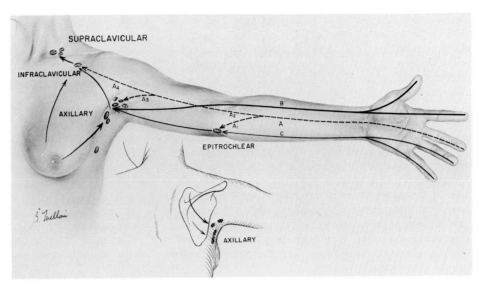

Fig. 26-8. Lymphatic drainage of the upper extremity. The lymphatic vessels draining the fingers and the hand converge on the dorsum of the hand. From here the lymphatic drainage pursues three courses: (1) The lymph vessels draining the ulnar aspect (little finger and ring finger) accompany (C) the basilic vein and drain into the epitrochlear nodes and thence into the axillary nodes, (2) the lymph vessels draining the thumb and the index fingers (B) bypass the epitrochlear nodes and go directly to the axillary nodes, and (3) the lymph vessels draining the middle fingers (A) may drain into the epitrochlear (A_1), the axillary (A_2, A_3), or may bypass both of these groups of nodes to drain directly into the infraclavicular (A_4), and thence into the supraclavicular, and finally into the bloodstream. The axillary nodes also receive lymph from the posterior scapular region (*inset*).

illary nodes are also invaded.[216] Occasionally, axillary metastasis from breast cancer is striking when the primary lesion is small and readily overlooked.[217,218] Rarely, lymph node enlargement of infectious nature, if located very anteriorly in the axilla, may simulate a cancer of the breast.

Lesions in the axillary tail of the breast[219] may be confused readily with axillary lymphadenopathy, especially when such breast tissue is the site of painful enlargement during or after pregnancy. This location also may be the site of a malignancy. Likewise, necrosis of fat in the axillae may simulate lymphadenopathy as may fatty infiltration of axillary nodes.[220,221]

Other rare causes of axillary lymphadenopathy include epithelial inclusion cysts,[222] metastases from unknown primary sites,[223] and silicone lymphadenopathy as a complication from silicone elastomer finger joint prostheses[224] or silicone gel prosthetic mammoplasty.[225]

Prophylactic vaccines, BCG vaccine, and serum are often injected in the shoulder area and may occasionally initiate axillary lymphadenopthy of marked degree on the same side,[226,227] followed rarely by suppuration. BCG vaccine used in infancy may lead to calcification

of the axillary nodes, a finding readily detected on the radiograph of the chest area.[228] An infectious process of the umbilicus may result in lymphadenitis of both axillae and both groins.[229]

Also worth noting is the rare presence of *Irish nodes*, lymph nodes beneath the lateral edge or deeper in the left axilla in the absence of similar nodes on the right side.[230] They have a diagnostic significance for cancer of the stomach similar to the Virchow node.

Rarely, an anomalous axillary pectoral muscle (*Langer's arch*) may present as an axillary mass and may cause a diagnostic problem.[231]

Subpectoral Abscess (Suppurative Infraclavicular Lymphadenitis). Acute subpectoral abscess is an unusual and relatively uncommon clinical entity produced by suppuration of the infraclavicular apical axillary nodes on one side of the body, a result usually of infection with a hemolytic streptococcus. When infected, these nodes become enlarged and may suppurate to involve the surrounding fat in a suppurative, necrotic process. Because it is enclosed in tight, fascialined pockets, the infectious process produces a severe disability characterized by high fever, a toxic state, ten-

derness to palpation over the affected area, and much pain in the region of the shoulder, especially upon abduction of the arm.[232,233] If not treated, the pus dissects extensively along the fascial planes and may reach the axilla with spontaneous drainage, or it may cause septicemia.

The infraclavicular nodes are most likely to become involved in those persons with an infection of the middle finger in whom the lymphatic drainage is directly to the infraclavicular nodes without passage through the epitrochlear or axillary nodes (see A_4 in Fig. 26-8). It may also follow failure of inadequate defense reaction of the latter nodes in cases in which they are intercalated in the lymphatic pathway to the infraclavicular nodes. The initial infection may originate elsewhere on the hands, the arms, or the shoulder. There is a close analogy between acute infraclavicular adenitis and deep inguinal adentitis.

THE EPITROCHLEAR (SUPERFICIAL CUBITAL OR SUPRATROCHLEAR) NODES

Anatomy. The epitrochlear nodes lie on the back of the elbow in the superficial fascia above the medial epicondyle of the humerus and in relation to the basilic vein. Their afferents drain lymph from the little, the ring, and the ulnar half of the middle finger (but not from the thumb and the index fingers), and also from the ulnar part of the palm of the hand and the forearm. Their efferents terminate in the axillary nodes.

Clinical Significance. Acute enlargement of the epitrochlear nodes in one arm, as a result of local infection or of neoplasm primary in the drainage area, is common and well understood.[234] More difficulty may be encountered when the drainage area in one arm is the inoculation site for an infectious agent capable of producing a systemic disease, and enlargement of the epitrochlear lymph node is only a satellite response in a more complex picture. Representative examples would include lesions such as extragenital chancre of syphilis, tularemia, cat-scratch disease, inoculation tuberculosis, and other examples noted in the section on extremity lesion and regional lymphadenopathy syndrome.

Being intercalated in the drainage to the axillary nodes, enlargement of the latter nodes may follow epitrochlear adenopathy if the defense mechanism at this level fails.

Of course, epitrochlear nodes may be involved in any disease capable of producing a generalized lymphadenopathy. Being easily palpated, enlargement of these nodes is readily detected clinically. In the older literature, much interest has centered on the frequency and the diagnostic significance of bilateral, painless epitrochlear lymphadenopathy with regard to the systemic phase of syphilis.[235,236,237] However, any diagnostic value assigned to this finding must be conditioned by the fact that lymph node enlargement in this region is often a chronic, nonspecific lymphadenitis resulting from repeated minor trauma and infections in the drainage area; it is more common in men than women and more frequent and striking in those doing manual labor.[236,237] It has been noted with rheumatoid arthritis.[214] Comment has been made of the consistent involvement of this node with tuberculous elbow.[238] Epitrochlear involvement is said to be minimal or absent with generalized tuberculous lymphadenopathy[239] and has been noted more commonly in patients with nodular lymphocytic lymphoma (11%) as compared with those with the diffuse lymphocytic types (2%).[240] It is less common in Hodgkin's disease and "extremely rare" as the first and only manifestation.[241]

THE INGUINAL LYMPH NODES

Anatomy. The inguinal lymph nodes are arranged in two groups: superficial and deep (Fig. 26-9). The superficial inguinal nodes lie in the superficial fascia and are disposed in an upper horizontal and a lower vertical group. The horizontal group lies parallel to the inguinal ligament, below the attachment of the fascia of Scarpa to the fascia lata. These nodes drain lymph from the skin of the anterior abdominal wall below the umbilicus, the skin of the penis and the scrotum in the male, the skin of the vulva and the mucosa of the vagina in the female, the skin of the perineum and the gluteal region (Fig. 26-10), and the lower part of the anal canal. They receive no lymph from the testis or the ovary. The vertical group lie on either side of the upper part of the greater saphenous vein. They receive all of the superficial lymphatic vessels of the lower extremity that accompany the greater saphenous vein. They do not receive the lymphatic vessels accompanying the shorter saphenous vein; these end in the popliteal nodes. In addition, the vertical group also receives lymph from the penis, the scrotum, and the gluteal region. The superficial inguinal nodes drain into the deep inguinal nodes (see Figs. 26-9 and 26-12).

The deep inguinal nodes, one to three in number, lie beneath the fascia lata, on the medial side of the femoral vein and below the femoral canal. One node (*node of Cloquet*) lies within the fat of the femoral canal. The deep inguinal nodes receive the deep lymphatic vessels accompanying the femoral vein, including those draining the popliteal nodes. They also receive lymph from the glans penis or the glans clitoris and from the superficial inguinal nodes. They drain into the external iliac nodes by efferents that partly traverse the femoral canal and partly course in front of and lateral to the femoral sheath.

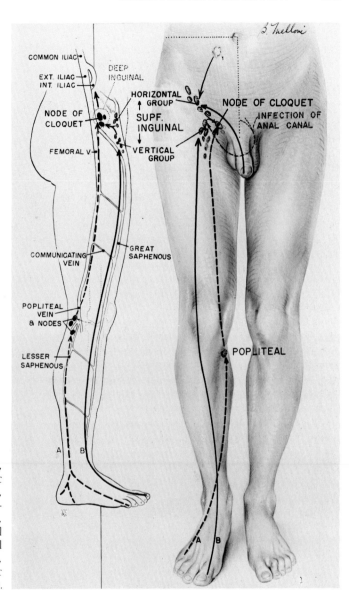

Fig. 26-9. Lymphatic drainage of lower extremity, genitalia, and lower abdomen. (*Right*) Lymphatic drainage of medial and middle aspects of foot (*B*), heel, and outer aspects of foot (*A*). Channel B shows superficial drainage of inner and middle aspects of foot, leg, genitalia, perineum, and lower abdomen to superficial inguinal nodes. (*Left*) Channel A shows superficial drainage of small toe and outer aspect of foot, heel, and knee to the popliteal nodes with major lymphatic channel deep along femoral vein in deep inguinal nodes.

Clinical Significance. Persistent enlargement of the superficial inguinal nodes of minimal degree is a common clinical finding. It represents the effect of chronic hyperplasia of these nodes from constant and often unnoticed or forgotten minor infections and irritations in the drainage areas to which most people are subjected at various times. These are more likely in those who go barefoot. For this reason, a minimal degree of superficial inguinal lymphadenopathy is difficult to evaluate. Physicians learn to accept a so-called unusual life baseline degree of groin lymphadenopathy. Diagnostic interest should be aroused when the nodes are

(1) increasing in size under observation, (2) larger than expected, (3) painful, or (4) suppurating.

Significant lymphadenopathy of the superficial inguinal nodes is related most commonly to (1) local infectious process of the drainage area, (2) systemic infection in which the infectious agent enters the body in the drainage region, or (3) primary neoplasm in this area, chiefly a malignant melanoma or squamous cell carcinoma. Inguinal node metastases must also be considered.[242,243] The number of disorders possible in the large and anatomically complicated drainage area is infinitely greater than in the axillary node drainage area.

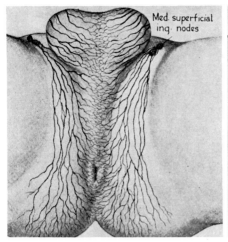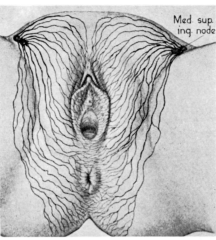

Fig. 26-10. Diagram of the cutaneous lymphatics of the perineum showing their communication across the midline and drainage into the superficial inguinal nodes (*left* = male, *right* = female). (From Pack, GT, Rekers P: The management of malignant tumors in the groin: A report of 122 groin dissections. Am J Surg 56:545–565, 1942)

Rarely, regional lymphadenopathy may be the initial manifestation of scleroderma.[244]

The ease with which a local infection or small primary neoplasm can be overlooked if located on the scrotum, between the buttocks, on the labia, under the prepuce, in the umbilicus, in the cutaneous zone of the anus, or between the toes is well known *since these areas are not examined as frequently and thoroughly as the upper extremities or head and neck.*

Lesions of the penis that are especially important include syphilitic chancre, gonorrhea, herpes genitalis, lymphopathia venereum, chancroid, and malignancy. Granuloma inguinale is not a lymph node disease but may predispose to secondary infectious lymphadenitis.

Minor but often overlooked causes include pediculosis pubis, tinea crurum of the inguinal area, ringworm between the toes, and the irritation incident to wearing a truss to restrain a hernia.

An infectious or neoplastic lesion is not easily overlooked on the legs, the lower abdomen, the buttocks, or the lower back, but it may be missed readily if present on the scrotum, the perineum, the anus, or the labia. Tumors of the testis metastasize directly to the upper para-aortic nodes (see Fig. 26-12) and involve the superficial inguinal nodes only when the tumor breaks through the tunica vaginalis to invade the scrotum (see Figs. 26-9 and 26-10).

All infections or neoplastic lesions primary in these skin areas do not necessarily involve the superficial inguinal nodes. The skin of the heel and the posterior half of the outer aspects of the foot drain into the popliteal nodes and from these directly to deep inguinal nodes (see Fig. 26-9 and discussion in the following section on popliteal nodes). In an occasional anomaly, lymphatics from upper posterior thigh and lower buttocks penetrate the fascia and reach the common iliac nodes along the sciatic nerve sheath, thus permitting lesions in this drainage area to bypass the superficial inguinal nodes. Lesions of the glans penis or the glans clitoris may drain not only to the superficial inguinals, but also directly into the deep inguinal and the other deep nodes. There is also the possibility of drainage of the penis to the prepubic lymph nodes and thence to the external iliac lymph nodes without passage to the superficial inguinals. Therefore, absence of palpable superficial inguinal nodes does not rule out infections or tumor metastases from these areas. See the excellent paper by Pack and Rekers for a detailed discussion of this subject.[245]

Several infectious systemic diseases in which the etiologic agent enters the drainage area of the superficial inguinal nodes may produce a satellite enlargement in these nodes or, if lymphadenopathy is general, exaggeration of the nodes in this location. This is particularly likely to occur with bubonic plague, scrub typhus, rat-bite fever, and filariasis. Superficial inguinal adenitis has been noted in swamp fever (owing to leptospirae).[246] This suggests the possibility that the infection was acquired through the skin of the leg. Atypical mycobacterial infection of the genital region in a female child was reported as a cause of bilateral inguinal adenitis.[247]

Superficial inguinal adenitis may be noted in infants and small children when the thigh is used as a site for subcutaneous prophylactic inoculation with vaccines against the various diseases of childhood, smallpox vaccination, or BCG vaccine.[226,227,248] In infants suppuration of the superficial inguinal nodes with thigh injections was much more frequent than suppuration of the axillary nodes when comparable injections of BCG vaccine were given in the shoulder area.[248] A pos-

sible explanation is that in infants the superficial inguinal nodes are already under continuous phagocytic stress because of constant irritation and soilage from urine and feces in the diaper area and are unable to accept the added phagocytic load resulting from the vaccination. Inguinal lymphadenopathy has been reported following the administration of live attenuated measles virus vaccine injected in the buttock.[249]

In contrast with the paucity of subcutaneous masses in the axillary area capable of simulating lymphadenopathy are the variety of conditions present in the groin. Tumefactions in the groin that must be distinguished from lymphadenopathy include hernia, varix, lipoma, aneurysm, tuberculosis of bursa of short head of rectus femoris muscle, psoas abscess, ectopic testis, ectopic spleen, inguinal endometriosis, and so forth.[245,250–252] For this reason, the differential diagnosis of masses in the groin is not always easy and must be considered carefully before a palpable ''lump'' is called an enlarged node. Rarely, painful swelling in superficial lymph nodes may be caused by spontaneous infarction.[253]

In females, a primary lesion of lymphopathia venereum deep in the vagina or the fornix does not produce superficial lymphadenopathy. Instead, the lymph drainage is to the lymphatics about the rectum, with production of a periproctitis, which may eventuate in a rectal stricture.[138]

Acute Iliac Lymphadenitis. Although the nodes are classified as in the retroperitoneal group, suppuration of the external iliacs bears a closer relationship to infections of the extremities and will be better understood if viewed in this light.

Suppuration of the external iliac nodes, most commonly unilateral, may manifest a striking analogy to subpectoral abscess (suppurative infraclavicular lymphadenitis).[254–256] These nodes, located retroperitoneally deep in the iliac fossa, adjacent to the external and the common iliac vessels and anterior to the psoas muscle, receive drainage from the superficial and the deep inguinals, the penis, the urethra, the prostate, the bladder, the uterus, the deep lymphatics of the abdominal wall, and the upper thigh. The nodes enlarge to a clinically significant degree two or three weeks after onset of an infection primary in one of the drainage sites usually resulting from coagulase-positive staphylococcus or hemolytic streptococcus. Such lymphadenitis is most common in children and young adults and may occur without obvious involvement of the superficial inguinal nodes. The clinical picture is one of high fever, leukocytosis, occasionally bacteremia, lower abdominal pain but without sign of peritoneal irritation, psoas muscle spasm limiting extension of the leg on the involved side, and abdominal tenderness with rectus muscle spasm. At times, the greatly enlarged nodes are detectable as a palpable tender mass just above Poupart's ligament. Often the nodes suppurate to form an extraperitoneal abscess requiring surgical drainage.

At times, suppurative iliac lymphadenitis may localize to the retroperitoneal iliac fossa and present as a distinct clinical picture.[257]

THE POPLITEAL NODES

Anatomy. The popliteal nodes, five or six in number, lie under the deep fascia in the fat around the popliteal vessels in the popliteal fossa. They receive lymph vessels from the knee joint and skin of the lateral side of the lower part of the leg, foot, and heel. They receive lymph from the deep structures of the leg and foot by lymphatic vessels coursing along the anterior and posterior tibial arteries and veins. Their efferents drain into the deep inguinal nodes by lymphatic vessels that accompany the popliteal and femoral veins. An inconstant anterior tibial node may be intercalated between the heel area and the popliteal node, but this is only rarely clinically important.

Clinical Significance. Except for the previously described drainage area, infections and neoplasms of the foot and the lower leg spread lymphatically directly to the superficial inguinal lymph nodes without filtering through the popliteal nodes. Infections of the knee joint and lesions on the heel and the outer side of the posterior half of the foot drain into the popliteal nodes (see Channel A, Fig. 26-9). Popliteal nodes are not easy to palpate unless greatly enlarged because of· their subfascial location. Study of the popliteal nodes by use of lymphangiograms can often be helpful in evaluating these lymph nodes.[258] It is well to remember that the afferent lymphatic channels from the popliteal nodes course along with the femoral artery to drain directly into the deep femoral and the external iliac nodes, bypassing completely the superficial inguinal nodes.[245] It is a practical clinical point that the abscess of enlarged superficial inguinal nodes does not rule out spread beyond the popliteal nodes of a tumor of heel and outer foot. This is particularly important in the management of malignant melanoma.

THE MEDIASTINAL LYMPH NODES

Anatomy. The mediastinum contains a large number of nodes, the most important of which may be divided into two groups: (1) the superior mediastinal and (2) the tracheobronchial (Fig. 26-11).

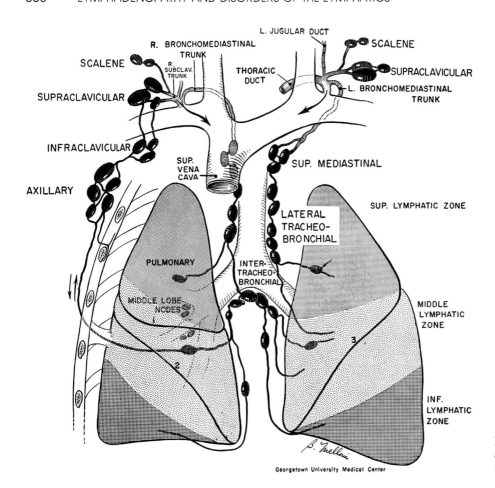

Fig. 26-11. Lymphatic drainage of the lungs and mediastinum.

The superior mediastinal nodes lie in front of the aortic arch, in relation to the large arterial trunks arising from the aortic arch and also to the innominate veins. They receive afferents from the thymus, the pericardium, the heart, the esophagus, and the trachea, as well as from the parasternal nodes. Their efferents join with those from the tracheobronchial on each side to form the corresponding bronchomediastinal trunk.

The tracheobronchial nodes include some of the largest nodes in the body. They may be subdivided into (1) the lateral tracheobronchial, (2) the intertracheobronchial, and (3) the pulmonary.

The lateral tracheobronchial nodes lie in relation to the trachea and lateral to the primary bronchi.

The intertracheobronchial nodes lie at bifurcation of the trachea, between the primary bronchi.

The pulmonary nodes are both extrapulmonary and intrapulmonary in location. The extrapulmonary nodes lie in the hilum of each lung; these are the so-called hilar nodes. The intrapulmonary nodes lie along the secondary branches of the primary bronchi and are related to the lobes of the lungs. Of these, the nodes related to the right middle lobe are of special importance since they drain not only the middle but also the lower lobe of the right lung and almost completely surround the secondary middle lobe bronchus. Compression or obstruction of this bronchus is particularly likely to occur when they enlarge. This interferes with normal function of the middle and lower lobes. The tracheobronchial nodes drain lymph from lungs, bronchi, and thoracic portion of the trachea, heart, esophagus, and liver; their efferents join the bronchomediastinal lymphatic trunk.

It is to be noted that the lymphatic drainage of the lung does not conform to the anatomic division of the lobes. Hence, in the surgical treatment of cancer of the lung, pneumonectomy and not lobectomy is indicated. The pulmonary nodes drain into the intertracheobronchial and the lateral tracheobronchial nodes, which in turn drain into the superior mediastinal nodes. From the mediastinal nodes of each side, the lymph passes through the corresponding bronchomediastinal trunk into the venous system. Blockage of the mediastinal

nodes leads to retrograde flow, and, in the presence of pleural adhesions, cancer may spread to the axillary nodes. Similarly, with blockage of the axillary nodes, retrograde flow will carry cancer emboli across the chest wall to the mediastinal nodes.

Clinical Significance—Mediastinal Lymphadenopathy. Only rarely does a clinically significant degree of hilar lymphadenopathy follow bacterial infections of the lung, such as pneumonia. Diffuse staphylococcal or streptococcal bronchopneumonias, multiple lobe bronchiectasis, or abscess formation rarely may produce a bilateral form, whereas unilateral hilar lymphadenopathy may occasionally follow bronchiectasis, lung abscess, or viral infection. Tuberculosis, in sharp contrast, whether as a primary complex or in hematogenous form, often involves the hilar lymph nodes on one or both sides. Enlargement may persist for long periods and terminates by healing and constriction, calcification, or rarely, caseation. A lung infection that has cleared may leave a hilar adenitis, which persists for a time. Coccidioidomycosis, histoplasmosis, and especially sarcoidosis may produce bilateral, symmetrical mediastinal lymph node enlargement, the latter being a particularly common benign type.[259–261]

In sarcoidosis the enlarged hilar lymph nodes are bilateral, rarely calcify, occur early in the course, are harmless as such, and generally regress.[262]

Silicosis and other pneumoconioses, asbestosis, and beryllium intoxication may all manifest by chest radiography evidence of both bilateral lymphadenopathy and pulmonary (lung field) involvement.[260] The pathology of the nodes in these conditions is one of an infiltrative nature.

Bilateral mediastinal lymphadenopathy, often without pulmonary involvement and occasionally with arthralgia, is commonly associated with erythema nodosum.[259,263,264] Although various etiologies for this syndrome have been proposed, much attention centers on sarcoidosis as one of the interesting causes.[265–267] Rare causes of bilateral mediastinal lymphadenopathy without lung changes are infectious mononucleosis[268] and collagen diseases.

Metastasis to hilar nodes, irregularly unilateral, especially from the lungs and more rarely from distant organs such as the kidney and the testis, may occur.

Lymphoid neoplasms may involve mediastinal nodes. This is seen particularly frequently with nodular sclerosing Hodgkin's disease and diffuse lymphocytic lymphomas.

Rarely, cardiophrenic lymphadenopathy[269,270] may radiologically simulate pericardial fat pad, while intrapulmonary lymphadenopathy, situated distally from the hilum, may simulate a pulmonary solitary nodule or coin-type lesion.[271,272] Because of the limitation of the physical examination in this area, radiographs and other specialized studies should always be used. They give much helpful information in evaluating mediastinal lymphadenopathy.

A considerable literature documents the details about angiofollicular lymph node hyperplasia, first described by Castleman.[273] Of interest is its propensity to characteristically but not always involve the mediastinal and hilar lymph nodes and occasionally the cervical or retroperitoneal ones. The course is usually symptomless. Occasionally there are local pressure symptoms. More rarely, it manifests systemic symptoms. These are all relieved by surgical removal. The course has been benign in cases recorded to date.[274]

Lymphangiomyoma is a disorder of smooth muscle and lymphatic channels, occurring exclusively in females, which may involve the thoracic duct or the mediastinal and hilar nodes and the lymphatics of the lungs and produce such clinical features as dyspnea, chylothorax, and pneumothorax.[299]

Mediastinal lymph node enlargement may or may not cause symptoms. The use of routine chest radiographs in miniature or standard size in mass population surveys for chest disease, pre-employment examination, induction station surveys, preadmission to many hospitals, and so forth, has resulted in detection of many instances of hilar adenopathy that are apparently asymptomatic. Perhaps the majority fall in the asymptomatic group. However, an extensive literature based on the study of certain patients admitted to hospitals indicates that a variety of signs and symptoms may be produced by various forms of hilar lymphadenopathy. A study of these clinical observations is important in understanding the mechanism of their production and the basic pathology responsible.

Symptoms of mediastinal lymph node enlargement include the following:

Cough. Regional nodes about the trachea and the bronchi, when sufficiently enlarged, are said to produce a cough by an irritative process or by pressure; often it is of a type commonly called "brassy." The exact mechanism in any instance is difficult to evaluate, since many patients also have intrinsic lung and bronchial disease. Pulmonary or bronchial infection, granulation tissue, neoplasm, and bronchial lithiasis are other possible mechanisms for the production of the cough.

Obstructive phenomena. Early partial bronchial obstruction by lymph nodes may cause obstructive emphysema because the bronchial lumen is greater upon inspiration than expiration, and the inspiratory phase is more forceful. Ingress is thus easier than egress.

This condition is more common in children because their bronchial structure is compressed more easily, and the lymph node enlargement is proportionately greater in that age group. The resulting physical signs are usually lobar in distribution rather than generalized because of the nature of the process initiating the lymph node enlargement.

Prolonged or repeated partial obstruction may lead to bronchiectasis by preventing normal movement of secretions and thus predisposing to low-grade, persistent infection. Chronicity leads to slow progression of the infectious process, which as in emphysema usually is localized and segmental. More rarely, lung abscess may follow partial bronchial obstruction.

Complete bronchial obstruction may lead to atelectasis, productive of characteristic physical and radiographic findings. At times, atelectasis may result from intraluminal rupture of suppurated mediastinal nodes or extrusion of a broncholith into the lumen. Some feel that atelectasis on this basis may be the explanation for most cases of epituberculosis among infants and children. At this age tuberculosis is especially likely to involve bronchial and hilar nodes primarily with the lung involvement being atelectatic from mechanical compression of the lumen and not parenchymal.

However, it should be pointed out that edema and inflammation of the bronchial wall alone may lead to bronchial obstruction and that extrinsic pressure is not necessary.[266]

Although such obstruction from lymph node pressure may occur in any lobe of the lung, the bronchus of the right middle lobe is peculiarly susceptible to compression because it is surrounded by a group of lymph nodes draining both the adjacent lower lobe and the middle lobe, an anatomic situation first stressed by Brock and associates.[275,276] Therefore, infection in either of these two lobes can predispose to lymph node changes in this particular anatomic group. The small lumen size of the middle lobe bronchus and its almost right-angle drainage into intermediate bronchi constitute further peculiar hazards to drainage of this lobe.[277] The clinical features produced by obstruction of the right middle lobe bronchus have become popularly known as *middle lobe syndrome* as the result of the description by Graham, Burford, and Mayer.[278] Clinical features are often chronic and most characteristically include obstructive phenomena of the right middle lobe with wheezing, pneumonitis or bronchiectasis, chest pain, periodic hemoptysis, and demonstrable radiographic findings.[277,278] This syndrome of extrinsic bronchial obstruction of the right middle lobe should not be confused with obstruction of intraluminal origin, such as that produced by a bronchial tumor, granulomatous lesion of the bronchus, and so forth.

Hemoptysis. Next to cough, this is probably the most common indirect manifestation of hilar and bronchial lymphadenopathy. Mechanisms include friability of granulation tissue, mechanical erosive process, chronic obstruction with bleeding produced by associated infections (bronchiectasis, lung abscess, and so forth), and the irritating and cutting effects of broncholithiasis with rupture of bronchial pulmonary vessels. Periodic hemoptysis is especially characteristic of the middle lobe syndrome.[277,278]

Calcification of lymph nodes. A variety of mechanisms may predispose to calcification of intrathoracic lymph nodes. Calcification of lymph nodes is commonly due to tuberculosis or histoplasmosis but may be caused by fungus infection, coccidioidomycosis, and so forth. Its rarity in Hodgkin's disease has been stressed.[280,281] Large calcified lymph nodes in the hilar area can produce any of the features discussed in this section. However, there are certain clinical features peculiar to calcified nodes.[282–285] They show a propensity to penetrate the bronchial wall, possibly by erosive action of the calcified node against a bronchial wall in constant motion.[283] Extrusion of the calcified node into the lumen of a bronchus may produce bronchial obstructive symptoms of various types: occasionally an intractable localized wheeze, paroxysms of coughing productive of gritty particles and even of the broncholith itself, hemoptysis, and other features. Calcified nodes may compress a bronchus and cause atelectasis, produce a traction diverticulum of the esophagus, cause dysphagia, or rarely, even compress the superior vena cava.[286] Bronchoscopic examination and radiographic studies are helpful. Reports of 41 cases by Schmidt, Clagett, and McDonald indicate that broncholithiasis is by no means rare.[287] Storer and Smith have reviewed this intriguing subject.[286]

Calcification of an entire lymph node should not be confused with peripheral calcification, the so-called eggshell calcification considered diagnostic of silicosis of mediastinal lymph nodes but seen very rarely in other conditions, such as sarcoidosis.[259,288]

Caseation. Caseation of hilar nodes may lead to traction diverticulum of the esophagus, with its attendant disturbance of swallowing, and of the morphology of this organ.[289]

Mediastinitis. Infectious lymphadenopathy of the hilar area may lead to mediastinitis. However, considering the great frequency of infections of hilar nodes from various pulmonary infections, mediastinitis owing to this cause is a rare complication. A posterior mediastinal mass may represent an infectious lymphadenitis as a result of an esophagitis.[279]

Superior vena caval obstruction. Hilar lymphadenopathy rarely may produce superior vena caval obstruction. This may be a late feature resulting from cicatrization of tissue about the superior vena cava from mediastinal infection of lymph node origin, or obstruction may result from compression. Compression occurs particularly from lymph node enlargement as a result of metastasis from a bronchial carcinoma, commonly on the right, because of the peculiar anatomic relationships in that area.

Hoarseness. This is an uncommon manifestation that may occur with lymph node metastasis from cancer, particularly of the breast, compressing the recurrent laryngeal nerve, or it may possibly result from venous obstruction of the superior vena cava, producing edema of the larynx.

Bronchoesophageal fistula. This is an unusual complication that may result from an infectious erosive process originating in tuberculous lymph nodes and resulting in the formation of a fistulous tract between a bronchus and the esophagus. A coughing spell that *comes on a short interval after swallowing* is diagnostically suggestive. A coughing paroxysm from aspirating food or fluid into the larynx owing to an upper esophageal difficulty in swallowing *comes on at once without the latent interval* necessary for esophageal peristalsis to carry food or fluid to the fistulous opening into the bronchus.

Dysphagia is likewise an unusual feature, sometimes caused by bronchoesophageal fistula,[290] traction diverticula of the esophagus, or enlarged mediastinal nodes.

Chest pain has been neither severe nor common with mediastinal lymphadenopathy. It may result from broncholithiasis, traction diverticula of the esophagus, or bronchoesophageal fistula.

Radiographic studies give much helpful information in evaluating mediastinal lymphadenopathy.[291,292]

A palpable swelling of the chest wall in the region of the second and the third intercostal spaces near the sternum may occur rarely when a lymphoma involves the sternal nodes.[293,294]

Occasionally, in neoplasm of the breast and very rarely from primary tumors elsewhere, there may be metastases to the parasternal nodes.[295] It is well to carefully palpate each of the upper five intercostal areas on both sides close to the sternum as part of a search for nodal metastases. This is an area easily overlooked in the physical examination.

ABDOMINAL LYMPH NODES

Anatomy. The lymph nodes of the abdominal cavity are divided into two large groups: (1) the intra-abdominal or visceral, and (2) the retroperitoneal or parietal.[30] (Fig. 26-12). A more detailed description can be obtained from standard sources.[29]

The intra-abdominal nodes or visceral nodes consist of a large number of nodes that are located in the various peritoneal ligaments (lesser and greater omentum, gastrosplenic ligament, mesentery, and mesocolon) and at the root of the large visceral branches of the aorta. The latter are called preaortic nodes and are subdivided into the celiac, the superior mesenteric, and the inferior mesenteric.

The celiac preaortic nodes are disposed about the origin of the celiac artery. They receive lymph from the organs supplied by the branches of the celiac artery: the lower part of the esophagus, the liver, the gallbladder, the stomach, the spleen, the pancreas, and the duodenum. Lymph from these organs first passes through nodes that are located close to these organs within the peritoneal ligaments traversed by the nutritive branches of the celiac artery. Such nodes include the gastric nodes (in the lesser and the greater omenta), the hepatic and the cystic nodes (in the lesser omentum), and the pancreaticolienal nodes (in the gastrosplenic ligament).

The superior mesenteric preaortic nodes lie about the origin of the superior mesenteric artery. The inferior mesenteric preaortic nodes surround the origin of the inferior mesenteric artery. These two groups of nodes receive lymph from the small and the large intestines, not directly but indirectly, after its passage through a series of nodes located within the mesentery and the mesocolon. The latter nodes are collectively known as the mesenteric nodes. They are arranged in two groups: (1) the proximal, lying about the arterial arcades formed by the branches of the superior and the inferior mesenteric arteries; and (2) the distal, located along the wall of the gut beside the vasa recta, branches of the arterial arcades.

The efferents of the preaortic nodes unite to form a single trunk, the intestinal trunk, which joins the cisterna chyli.

The retroperitoneal or parietal nodes are composed of (1) the sacral, (2) the internal iliac, (3) the external iliac, (4) the common iliac, and (5) the para-aortic.

The sacral nodes lie in the hollow of the sacrum, in relation to the middle and the lateral sacral arteries. They receive lymph from the rectum, the posterior wall of the pelvis, the prostate, and the cervix of the uterus. Their efferents join the internal iliac and the para-aortic nodes.

The internal iliac nodes are disposed about the internal iliac vessels and their branches. A special group is located about the obturator canal and constitutes the obturator nodes. They receive a large part of the lymph from the rectum, the bladder, the urethra, the pros-

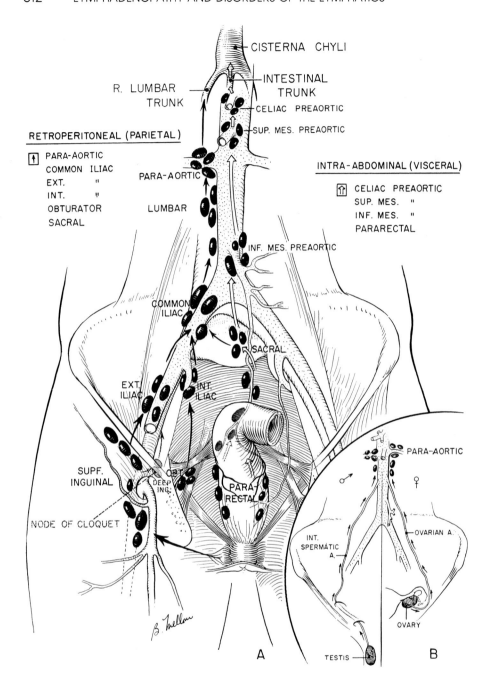

Fig. 26-12. Lymph nodes of the abdominal cavity. (*A*) Retroperitoneal (parietal) and intra-abdominal (visceral) nodes. (*B*) Lymphatic drainage of ovary or testis directly to upper para-aortic nodes without passage through the lower retroperitoneal nodes.

tate, the uterus, and the buttocks. Their efferents drain into the common iliac nodes.

The external iliac nodes are located about the external iliac vessels, just behind the inguinal ligament and in relation to the genitofemoral nerve. They receive lymph from superficial and deep inguinal nodes, internal iliac nodes, deep structures of the anterior abdominal wall below the level of the umbilicus, glans

penis or glans clitoris, bladder, cervix and body of the uterus, upper part of the vagina, prostate, and membranous urethra. Their efferents join the common iliac nodes.

The common iliac nodes are disposed about the common iliac vessels. They receive afferents from the external iliac, the internal iliac, and the sacral nodes. In addition they also receive lymph directly from the rec-

tum, the vagina, the uterus, and the prostate. Their efferents empty into the right and the left para-aortic nodes.

The para-aortic nodes form an almost continuous chain on each side of the abdominal aorta. They rest on the psoas major muscle. Those on the right side are related also to the inferior vena cava. They receive the efferents of the common iliac nodes (hence the lymph from the lower extremities, the external genitalia, and most of the lymph from the pelvis). In addition, they receive lymph from the lateral abdominal wall by lymphatics accompanying the lumbar arteries, the kidneys, the suprarenals, the testes, the ovaries, the fallopian tubes, and the body of the uterus. Their efferents unite on each side to form the right and the left lumbar lymphatic trunks, which unite to form the cisterna chyli. Some of the efferents join the preaortic nodes, as well as some relatively unimportant nodes, behind the abdominal aorta (retroaortic nodes). Still other efferents, instead of joining the lumbar trunks, pass through the crura of the diaphragm to join the thoracic duct directly. Lymphography, CT, and echographic techniques are of great use in investigating retroperitoneal lymph node enlargement.[117,296]

Clinical Significance. The lymph nodes of the abdomen and the pelvis constitute the largest group of nodes of the body. These nodes drain lymph not only from the lower extremities, but also from all of the pelvic and the abdominal organs. Because of their anatomic proximity to blood vessels and nerve plexuses of the abdominal cavity and to the various segments of the gastrointestinal tract, their enlargement from neoplastic or infectious involvement produces a rich symptomatology, the analysis of which is of great value in diagnosis.[297,298,300,301]

Of interest is the frequent involvement of major lymphatic trunks and nodes in the retroperitoneum by Burkitt's lymphoma[74] and its occasional localization here by angiofollicular lymph node hyperplasia[274] and lymphangiomyoma.[299]

Clinically, the most important symptoms are abdominal discomfort, digestive disturbances, abdominal pain, backache, and fever. Less frequent in occurrence but nevertheless significant are the following: constipation, ascites, edema, chyloperitoneum, urinary disturbances, jaundice, and intestinal obstruction. Although the clinical picture is characterized by a variety of symptoms, the physical signs of neoplastic involvement of the abdominal nodes are few and consist of demonstration of palpable nodes, of localized tenderness, and occasionally, of abnormal bruits.[297,298] A fuller discussion of the more important signs and symptoms follows.

Abdominal Discomfort. Abdominal discomfort occurs as soreness, sense of heaviness or fullness in the epigastric region after meals, and inability to eat a full meal. It is caused by the crowding of the stomach and the intestine by enlarging para-aortic and intra-abdominal nodes. The stomach and intestines are unable to expand as their contents increase with the ingestion of meals. There is also delay in emptying of the stomach and passage of food down the intestine because of impaired peristaltic activity.[298]

Digestive Disturbances. Bloating and belching may be the only symptoms of digestive disturbances and may be misinterpreted as resulting from cholecystitis, peptic ulcer, neurasthenia, or even malingering. Nausea and vomiting are less frequent and may occur irregularly or become constant and progressive with rapid loss of weight. Diarrhea is not common. When it occurs, it may be irregular or may continue indefinitely. It has a tendency to increase progressively in severity. It is associated with loss of weight and strength in spite of a normal or ravenous appetite. Usual therapeutic measures are unavailing, and whatever improvement may be obtained proves to be only temporary. Diarrhea may be associated with melena; it usually sets in when the intramural lymphoid tissue of the bowel (solitary lymph follicles, patches of Peyer, and annular follicles of the appendix) become involved by the neoplastic process.[297,298]

Abdominal Pain. The para-aortic and the pelvic retroperitoneal, as well as the preaortic intra-abdominal lymph nodes, are associated intimately with the abdominal autonomic nervous system, which contains parasympathetic, sympathetic, and pain fibers. The parasympathetic fibers regulate the motility and the secretory activity of the gastrointestinal tract. The sympathetic fibers are concerned especially with regulation of vasomotor tone of the blood vessels of the gut. The pain fibers relay pain impulses from all of the abdominal and the pelvic organs. After passing through the abdominal autonomic nervous system, which is intimately related to the whole length of the abdominal aorta and its branches, the pain impulses are finally transmitted to the spinal cord by the lumbar and the thoracic splanchnic nerves.

The intra-abdominal lymph nodes, located within the lesser and the greater omenta, the mesentery, and the mesocolon, also are related intimately to the branches of the celiac, the superior, and the inferior mesenteric arteries, which are accompanied throughout their course by the peripheral fibers of the parasympathetic and sympathetic nerves and by pain fibers.

Enlarged retroperitoneal as well as intra-abdominal

lymph nodes may irritate both autonomic and pain fibers and thus lead not only to impairment of the secretory and motor activity of the gastrointestinal tract, but also to pain. Pain may be caused in another way by the effects of direct neoplastic infiltration of the wall of the digestive tube, gaseous distention, and excessive motor activity ("spastic" pain).

Pain owing to compression by enlarged lymph nodes is at first characteristically dull in character and felt as soreness. Its distribution depends entirely upon the nerves involved by the pressure. Thus, enlarged para-aortic or preaortic nodes compressing the pain fibers coursing through the abdominal autonomic nerves related to the aorta may produce pain suggestive of disease of various organs such as the gallbladder, the pancreas, or the appendix. If the pain is severe, the clinical picture may suggest an acute abdominal emergency. Surgery in such cases may bring temporary relief. However, the underlying neoplastic process is relentless in its progress, and the pain may recur with even greater intensity. With progressive enlargement of the nodes, the pain may be so severe as to simulate the intractable pain of interstitial pancreatitis. The distribution of the pain will become more extensive as more and more of the para-aortic and the preaortic nodes become enlarged.

Spastic pain is cramplike or colicky and occurs in waves. Pressure on the ureter may lead to ureteral spastic pain, simulating pain from ureteral stone.[302] In mesenteric adenitis, the spastic pain occasionally may be due to ileocecal intussusception.[301]

Backache. This type of pain is especially characteristic of pressure by enlarged para-aortic and mesenteric nodes on branches of the lumbar and the sacral plexuses and may be felt at various levels of the trunk or in the lower extremities. Depending on the particular nerve irritated, it may be localized in the hip, the thigh, the knee, the ankle, or the feet. It may first be felt in the hip and then extend to the foot, simulating sciatic neuritis. It may be unilateral or bilateral. At first, the pain is dull in character. Later, when the nerves become infiltrated with cancer metastases, or when metastases to the pubic bones or to the bones of the lower extremities have occurred, the pain becomes boring and severe.[298]

Fever. Often enlargement of the para-aortic and intra-abdominal nodes in Hodgkin's disease and lymphocytic lymphoma is characterized by fever, which is conspicuously absent if the lymphadenopathy in these diseases is confined to the cervical nodes. Fever also develops with involvement of mediastinal nodes. Usually the fever is continuous, but occasionally it may be of the relapsing or intermittent *Pel-Ebstein* type. Periodic nodal enlargement, synchronous with this type of fever, has been demonstrated.[303]

Constipation. Enlargement of both para-aortic and intra-abdominal (mesenteric) nodes may lead to mechanical interference with the motor activity of the gut and thus cause constipation, which is proportional to other preceding or concomitant symptoms, such as abdominal pain, backache, bloating, and belching. It is characteristic of this type of constipation that it often diminishes or disappears with retrogression of the enlarged nodes following irradiation to reappear when the nodes enlarge again with advance of the neoplastic process.

Ascites. Ascites may be caused by portal vessel compression from lymph nodes or by metastases to peritoneal surfaces, the latter being more common.

Edema. Enlargement of the iliac and the pelvic retroperitoneal nodes may compress the iliac veins, especially the external iliac, with resulting edema of the lower extremities. However, this is rarely of a degree to involve an entire lower extremity. Usually, the edema first appears in the feet and ankles. Compression of the common iliac vein by enlarged common iliac nodes results in edema not only of the lower extremity, but also of the scrotum, penis, pubic region, and lower abdomen. Deep palpation of the iliac region may reveal a nodular mass of enlarged nodes or a matted mass, tender to pressure.

Chyloperitoneum. Marked enlargement of the celiac preaortic or of the para-aortic nodes in the immediate vicinity of the celiac artery may block the cisterna chyli, with the production of chyloperitoneum. At the same time, such blockage, because of retrograde flow, may result in cancerous infiltration of the stomach and the duodenum, causing gastrointestinal bleeding.

Urinary Disturbances. Such disturbances, when present, usually take the form of increased frequency of urination and hematuria. Urinary disturbances are not a common complication. They may be due to compression of the ureter by enlarged iliac nodes, resulting in hydronephrosis or pyonephrosis. However, urinary disturbances may also result from cancerous infiltration of the ureter by the lymphatic spread from the primary cancer or by direct extension from involved adjacent para-aortic nodes.

Jaundice. Jaundice, occurring with intra-abdominal lymphoid tumors or lymph node metastases, usually

indicates liver metastases and only rarely results from lymph node obstruction of extrahepatic biliary passages, as indicated by an earlier paucity of even isolated case reports in the literature.[304,305] More recently Warshaw and Welch, in a most informative and helpful paper, present their experience with extrahepatic biliary obstruction owing to cancer metastasis from the colon to lymph nodes compressing bile ducts.[306]

Intestinal Obstruction. Such obstruction may involve the duodenum, the cecum, or the other parts of the intestine and is due either to compression by enlarged nodes adjacent to these structures or to actual infiltration of the bowel by the neoplastic process affecting the nodes. The intestinal obstruction is accompanied by pain of increasing severity, nausea, and vomiting.

Physical Signs. The physical signs associated with enlarged retroperitoneal and intra-abdominal nodes are minimal and usually consist of the demonstration of the enlarged nodes by palpation and the elicitation of tenderness upon pressure over the nodes. Occasionally, abnormal bruits may be heard.

Physical signs are conspicuously absent in the early stages and may also be absent in cases in which the clinical symptoms are marked. Evidence of nodes may be obscured by cancerous involvement of the gastrointestinal tract, the liver, and the spleen, as well as by peritoneal carcinomatosis.

As a rule, the physical signs do not become apparent until the involved nodes have reached a certain size. Under such conditions, by careful palpation through relaxed abdominal walls over the iliac region or over the course of the abdominal aorta, the enlarged nodes can be felt as nodular masses of irregular size. Should the nodes be matted together, only a deep resistance may be felt upon deep palpation. This must not be mistaken for muscular rigidity. The palpable nodes or resistance may be confined to one side. This is particularly true with lymphadenopathy associated with cancer of the testis. In such cases, the palpable nodes are always confined to one side or the other, depending upon the site of the primary cancer, since, with cancer of these organs, the spread is always to the homolateral nodes at first. The enlarged nodes are situated high in the abdomen at the level of the renal vessels, because the lymphatics drain directly into the upper para-aortic nodes (See Fig. 26-12). Later, with retrograde involvement of the iliac para-aortic nodes, the palpable nodular mass extends vertically toward the iliac region.

Palpable, enlarged para-aortic nodes are fixed characteristically and show practically no mobility, not even with respiration. By contrast, enlarged intra-abdominal nodes, particularly the mesenteric or the mesocolic, display a noticeable degree of mobility and shifting and may give the impression of a pedicled mass. At the same time, the mass gives a sensation of solidity and lack of resilience. If these physical aspects of enlarged para-aortic and intra-abdominal nodes are kept in mind, their confusion with enlarged liver, spleen, or kidney can be avoided. The liver and the spleen may be displaced forward and downward by greatly enlarged para-aortic nodes.

The palpable enlarged nodes may vary in size at intervals. This is particularly true in cases of abdominal lymphadenopathy owing to Hodgkin's disease or lymphocytic lymphoma. In these diseases, there is an abnormal predisposition to respiratory infections. With each infection there occurs a rapid enlargement of the nodes. With subsidence of the infection, the nodes may regress in size, but the enlargement seldom disappears. Eventually, there is progressive enlargement, although there are cases in which the nodes remain small throughout the disease.

In nodular lymphatic lymphomas, there may be enlargement of all retroperitoneal and intra-abdominal nodes, but in addition all aggregations of lymphoid tissue of the small and large bowel may become infiltrated with neoplastic cells. Also, there is a marked tendency for retroperitoneal nodes of the two sides to become matted together along the whole length of the abdominal aorta.

Enlarged nodes may be demonstrated not only by abdominal palpation, but also by rectal or vaginal examination. In women, enlarged pelvic nodes must be differentiated from uterine fibroids, ovarian cysts, or pyosalpinx. At the same time it must be remembered that these conditions may be coincidental.

In palpating for enlarged retroperitoneal and intra-abdominal nodes, careful attention must be paid to certain procedural details. The patient must be placed in the recumbent position; the head should be flexed on the chest; and the arms should be relaxed and placed by the side of the body. In order to relax the anterior wall as completely as possible, the patient should be encouraged to breathe through the mouth. Further relaxation may be achieved by placing a pillow under the small of the back.

The second significant physical sign of enlarged nodes is tenderness elicited by pressure. Such tenderness is usually slight or moderate.

Abnormal Bruits. Enlarged para-aortic nodes may interfere with normal expansion of the aorta and thus produce abnormal bruits. Constriction of the abdominal aorta may also result from either bilateral or unilateral enlargement of the para-aortic nodes.

Clinical Syndromes of the Intra-abdominal Nodes

Malabsorption. That lymphomatous involvement of the small intestine and mesenteric nodes may lead to the syndrome of malabsorption is well documented in the literature.[307–309] The Mediterranean type of abdominal lymphoma—a disorder affecting primarily young people of Mediterranean origin—may do this as well.[310,311] In some of these cases, alpha heavy chain disease is present.[310,311] This may be a variant of Mediterranean lymphoma.[310] Another form of lymphoma occurs as a late complication of idiopathic steatorrhea or adult celiac disease.[309]

Infiltration of the wall of the gastrointestinal tract may block the intestinal lacteals and result in malabsorption. Enlarged lymphomatous nodes, through pressure on the gut or the pain fibers, may produce pain related to eating. There may also be interference with motor functions of the gut, leading to diarrhea. If this is marked, there is loss of fluid, electrolytes, and nutritive elements.

Syndrome of Calcified Intra-abdominal Lymph Nodes. Calcified intra-abdominal nodes may produce no symptoms and may be discovered upon routine x-ray examination or as an incidental finding in x-ray studies of the urinary or the genital tracts. Such asymptomatic calcified nodes may cause confusion in the presence of renal, ureteral, and vesical calculi.

However, calcified intra-abdominal nodes in the mesentery may cause symptoms that suggest the advisability of x-ray studies of the gastrointestinal tract, particularly the mesenteric nodes near the ileocecal junction. Almost invariably, such symptomatic calcified nodes are due to tuberculosis. In addition to the calcified nodes, the patient may show evidences of a tuberculous process involving the wall of the gut itself. The calcified nodes are tender upon pressure, usually slightly movable. Since they are associated intimately with blood vessels and nerves coursing through the mesentery, there is usually distortion of the affected segments of the blood vessels. The mesentery itself often shows scarring and puckering, interfering with normal motor function of the intestine.[312,317]

Clinically, the syndrome of calcified mesenteric nodes is characterized by repeated attacks of abdominal pain in the right lower quadrant accompanied by nausea, vomiting, and weakness. There is no elevation of temperature and no leukocytosis during the attack. There is usually a history of underweight and lack of endurance in spite of good appetite, of repeated visits to a physician, and of slow convalescence following various attacks of infections.

Radiographic studies show not only the calcified nodes, but barium studies demonstrate spasm of the loop of the intestine at the site of the calcified nodes, delay in emptying of the ileum, and reversed peristalsis.[313]

Syndrome of Tuberculous Mesenteric Lymphadenitis. This condition is usually secondary to tuberculosis elsewhere. The process begins in the patches of Peyer and the solitary lymph follicles of the ileum. These lymphoid structures enlarge, fuse, caseate, and ulcerate. The ulcers enlarge laterally since the tuberculous process follows the intestinal lymphatics, which course at right angles to the longitudinal axis of the bowel. Accompanying this process there is massive involvement of the mesenteric lymph nodes.[314,315] As a rule, tuberculous mesenteric lymphadenitis is confined to the ileum. However, in some cases, it may also involve the jejunum and the duodenum as well as the cecum and the colon.[316] The nodes may remain discrete or become matted together to form large masses. Eventually, gradual calcification of the involved nodes takes place.

Some cases are asymptomatic. Calcified nodes may be seen on routine radiographs of the gastrointestinal or urinary tracts. When the infection is active, there is fever, malaise, loss of weight, and abdominal pain. Since the mesenteric nodes near the ileocecal junction are involved most often, the pain and associated tenderness in the right iliac fossa may simulate that of appendicitis. The nodes are usually not palpable unless they are enlarged considerably.

The tuberculous nodes may break down and discharge their contents into the peritoneal cavity, with resulting localized peritonitis (cold abscess) or generalized tuberculous peritonitis. Fistulas may develop between different segments of the small intestine. The enlarged, fused nodes may also produce multiple obstructions of the bowel.[316,317]

Syndrome of Acute Mesenteric Lymphadenitis. This syndrome is characterized by acute abdominal pain and tenderness in the right iliac fossa, a febrile course, leukocytosis, and enlarged mesenteric (intra-abdominal) nodes. It is seen most commonly in childhood but rarely beyond puberty. Its ability to closely simulate acute appendicitis often leads to a laparotomy. The mesenteric adenitis is then evident.[318–321] Earlier studies were often unrewarding in detecting an etiologic cause, leading to this disorder being designated as acute, nonspecific mesenteric adenitis.

In recent years, in some of the cases, etiologic agents are being shown to be or suspected of being a common bacteria, adenovirus, or other miscellaneous causes.[321,322] Of particular interest is the demonstration with increasing frequency and effective documentation in some cases that either *Yersinia pseudotuberculosis* or *Yersinia*

enterocolitica are present.[323,324] Laparotomy enables observation of the characteristic mesenteric adenitis with enlargement of the ileocecal lymph nodes with, as a rule, a normal appendix.[323] While the course is usually benign and brief, serious complications may occur rarely, such as terminal ileitis—a recurrent or chronic course,[325] septicemia,[324] initiation of an intussusception,[341] or suppuration of the involved nodes.[326] Therapy depends on the nature of the responsible organism, if this can be determined.

Syndrome of Peritonitis from Lymph Node Suppuration. Very rarely, peritonitis may follow suppuration of an intra-abdominal lymph node.[326,340]

LYMPH NODE SYNDROMES

A considerable literature attests to the wide interest in lymph node disease. In the section to follow, a number of characteristic lymph node syndromes are briefly described. The reader is also referred elsewhere to representative articles that discuss various classifications and clinical features of, and give fuller details about, various types of lymphadenopathy.[327–334]

In addition to the regional types of lymphadenopathy, which are related mostly to local area disease as already described, there are other clinical states not so easily classified. The following groupings of syndromes have been found to be a helpful method of presenting certain of the lymphadenopathies.

EXTREMITY LESION AND REGIONAL LYMPHADENOPATHY SYNDROME

A number of diseases, mostly infections, fit into a clinical pattern or syndrome characterized by a primary sore or entrance lesion on an extremity, regional (satellite) lymphadenopathy, fever, and systemic symptoms with or without a rash. The initial inoculation of the infectious agent, although much more common on the more exposed limb, may occur occasionally on the chest or the abdomen, with axillary or superficial inguinal lymphadenopathy, respectively, with a similar clinical picture.

The best-known syndrome consists of a wound or abrasion at site of entry with tubular lymphangitis and septicemia owing to *Streptococcus hemolyticus*,[335] referred to in the past by the old-fashioned term *blood poisoning*. It is now rare since the advent of sulfa and antibiotic therapy. The unusual occurrence of a primary syphilitic chancre and regional lymphadenopathy, not yet subsided, simultaneously with the presence of the systemic features of the secondary stage of syphilis, fits into this category. The nonvenereal site of ex-

tragenital chancre (*e.g.*, the finger of a dentist or a physician) often makes the diagnosis confusing.[336] Primary extragenital cutaneous gonorrhea with a local pustule, lymphangitis, and regional lymphadenopathy may occur rarely.[337] Rarely, primary inoculation of tuberculosis in the skin of an extremity in a person who is tuberculin-negative may produce an indolent ulcer at the inoculation site, lymphangitis, and satellite lymphadenopathy. There is usually only minimal systemic reaction and fever, but there is transition of the tuberculin test to positive as healing occurs.[338,339] In a sense, this constitutes, by analogy with the primary lung infection, a dermatologic, primary Ghon tubercle, with a primary skin lesion and its satellite adenopathy forming a complex like the Ghon pulmonary complex.[339]

Sporotrichosis of the lymphangitic type may commence as indolent ulcers at the inoculation site with chronic nodular and often painless lymph channel involvement but without marked regional lymphadenopathy or systemic symptoms.[342]

Anthrax usually commences as a firm red papule, progressing through vesicular formation to a painless ulcer surrounded by a zone of erythema and edema, and followed by tender regional lymphadenopathy with severe systemic symptoms, often with bacteremia.[344,345]

Inoculation of the skin by the *Erysipelothrix rhusiopathia*, commonly from handling fish or dead animal matter, may produce a local lesion, lymphangitis, and regional adenitis, with variable systemic symptoms. This constitutes the clinical picture of the occupational disease known as erysipeloid of Rosenbach.[346]

A classic picture of the ulceroglandular type of *tularemia* comprises a sensitive ulcer on a finger, regional lymphadenopathy, fever, and systemic symptoms with or without a rash, often with bacteremia, in a person who has handled rabbits.[347,348]

Bubonic plague is another classic example of this syndrome. A vesicle forms at the site of bite of an infected flea, followed by a very large painful regional adenitis, often suppurative or hemorrhagic, with severe systemic symptoms.[349]

Several rickettsial diseases fit into this pattern. Best known, as a result of World War II experiences, is *scrub typhus* owing to *Rickettsia orientalis*.[350] A black eschar forms at the site of a mite bite, followed by regional adenopathy (usually without lymphangitis), systemic spread, fever, and rash. At times, the eschar, regional lymphadenopathy, and rash may be absent. It may present without these, in the form of illness with generalized lymphadenopathy and lymphocytosis; it is often mistakenly diagnosed as infectious mononucleosis.[351] *Boutonneuse fever* (owing to *Rickettsial conorii* and carried

by a dog tick), *South African tick bite fever*, and possibly *Kenya typhus* have a systemic picture similar to scrub typhus.

Rickettsialpox (owing to *Rickettsia akari*), a relatively new American rickettsial disease, is somewhat similar, manifesting an initial painless lesion at the site of the infecting mite bite, painful regional adenitis, systemic spread, fever, and a characteristic rash.[352]

Filariasis does not entirely fit this syndrome. Usually the legs are involved, but they fail to show a primary entrance lesion. However, lymphangitis, regional lymphadenopathy, and various systemic symptoms may occur.

Rat-bite fever is characterized by a late local lesion at the rat-bite site, followed by lymphangitis, regional lymphadenopathy, systemic symptoms, rash, and fever, all of which may show remissions and relapses. The *Spirillum minus* organism does this more strikingly than the *Streptobacillus moniliformis*.[353,354]

Cat-scratch disease (inoculation lymphoreticulosis) is now known to be a frequent cause of this syndrome. It is probably a viral infection and usually follows a cat scratch. It may follow trauma from other animals. This is followed by regional or single lymph node enlargement, which only rarely suppurates. Systemic symptoms and a transitory rash are unusual but are more commonly seen in hospitalized cases.[355] Diagnosis is established by a positive skin test, absence of bacteria in the node, and histologic features of node biopsy.[355] Carithers and associates reviewed their experience with 152 cases during 13 years of pediatric practice. All had nodal enlargement, which was usually the chief complaint. The axilla was most commonly involved, and often only a single node was enlarged. Suppuration occurred in 10% of cases.[356]

The virus of *orf*, a poxvirus disease of sheep, may rarely infect humans, producing a characteristic local lesion at site of inoculation. Lymphangitis, lymphadenitis, fever, and rash may occasionally occur but are seldom marked.[357]

Erythema chronicum migrans (as the early phase of Lyme arthritis) may present with a vector bite, skin lesion, and regional lymphadenopathy, followed by systemic symptoms, including arthritis.[358,409]

Although all of these syndromes are infectious, one never should overlook the fact that a primary neoplasm may occur on an extremity, cause regional metastasis, and manifest systemic symptoms and fever as a result of visceral metastases.

Lymphomas may commence at times in a local form before becoming more generalized.[343] If at the same time there is exposure to one of the infectious diseases involving skin inoculation mentioned in this section, the entire clinical picture could be attributed to the infectious cause.

OROPHARYNX LESION WITH CERVICAL SATELLITE LYMPHADENOPATHY SYNDROME

Infection by many different bacteria, such as streptococcal sore throat, scarlet fever, diphtheria, and so forth, may produce this constellation. Lymphadenopathy in throat infections of viral etiology is usually less striking than it is for bacterial infections. Most characteristic of diseases illustrating this syndrome is infectious mononucleosis, when associated with a severe sore throat, as well as cytomegalic inclusion disease. Likewise, cervical lymphadenopathy may occur as a manifestation of toxoplasmosis.[359] Weil's disease occasionally produces cervical adenopathy as part of the total clinical picture.

Cat-scratch disease occasionally may have an oropharyngeal site of origin, with striking lymph node enlargement of the neck, progressing at times to suppuration.[355] Rarely, this disease may be responsible for a persistent cervical lymphadenopathy.[360] An oral cavity syphilitic chancre with regional neck lymphadenopathy, followed by the secondary systemic phase, is an especially classic manifestation of this syndrome. An edematous reaction in the primary lesion and an increase in the degree of satellite adenopathy may occur if a Herxheimer reaction follows the initiation of therapy.[361] Another classic manifestation is cervical node tuberculosis, which rarely may spread systemically.

GENITAL LESION AND GROIN LYMPHADENOPATHY SYNDROME

Most of the diseases described for an extremity site of origin could occur if the inoculation site of the infectious agent is on the genitalia instead of an extremity. In general, however, infectious disorders with a primary genital site are of venereal origin and include primarily syphilis,[364,365] gonorrhea, chancroid, and lymphopathia venereum. Gonococcus rarely may cause inguinal adenitis even in the absence of urethritis.[362] Inguinal nodes secondary to gonococcal urethritis may be tender.[363] Rarely, a tuberculous infection may be responsible. Infection with other organisms is distinctly unusual. Cancer of the penis with regional groin metastases and systemic metastatic spread fits into this pattern quite readily.

LYMPHATIC METASTASES FROM BREAST CANCER SYNDROMES

Cancer of the mammary gland may metastasize by several lymphatic pathways (Fig. 26-13). Cancer arising in the upper outer quadrant of the gland metastasizes to the axillary nodes (A_1), the infraclavicular, and the supraclavicular nodes. Supraclavicular lymph node in-

volvement is unusual if there is no spread to the axillary nodes. From here, cancer emboli can reach the venous system through the jugular trunk. Cancer metastasizing in this manner has the most favorable prognosis. Supraclavicular lymph node metastases may develop after radical mastectomy as the first clinical evidence of recurrence. This circumstance is often a sign of widespread dissemination.[366]

In the upper inner quadrant it may metastasize first to the intercostal, then to the parasternal nodes (A_2), or it may reach the parasternal nodes directly (A_3). The parasternal nodes drain into the mediastinal nodes, from which cancer emboli can reach the venous system by way of the bronchomediastinal trunk. Because of the involvement of the mediastinal nodes, cancer spreading by this route has a dangerous prognosis. Internal mammary lymph nodes (parasternal lymph nodes A_3) should be searched for by careful palpation in the upper five intercostal spaces, on both sides, close to the sternum;[295] they can also be identified by scintographic scan,[367] as well as by transsternal phlebography.[368] Their enlargement may be the first sign of recurrence after surgery for cancer of the inner side of the breast, most commonly located in the second and third intercostal spaces. Marked involvement of these nodes is uncommon in lymphoma.[295]

The lymphatics of the skin of one mammary gland communicate directly across the midline (A_4) with those of the opposite side. Hence, unilateral cancer may become bilateral by this lymphatic route. Contralateral axillary metastases indicate a poor prognosis.[369]

Cancer developing in the lower quadrants, particularly the lower inner, may spread by lymphatics that traverse the pectoralis major, the external oblique, and the upper thin part of the linea alba and communicate with the subperitoneal lymphatic plexus (A_5). Thus, cancer emboli may reach the peritoneal cavity and set up secondary foci on any of the abdominal organs. Cancer cells may also drop by gravity from the peritoneal cavity into the pelvic cavity and thus give rise to secondary pelvic metastases. Because of the possibility of invasion of the peritoneal cavity, this type of spread has the more dangerous prognosis. Furthermore, because of this possible mode of metastasis, every patient with breast nodules should have careful rectal and vaginal examination.

The mammary gland and its overlying skin is anchored to pectoral fascia covering the pectoralis major by bands of fibrous tissue called the *ligaments of Cooper.* When these ligaments become invaded by cancer emboli, contraction occurs along them. As a result, the skin of the breast may become attached to the subjacent neoplastic growth so that the skin cannot be pinched up from the tumor. With further extension of the cancer, the entire breast may be bound to a pectoral

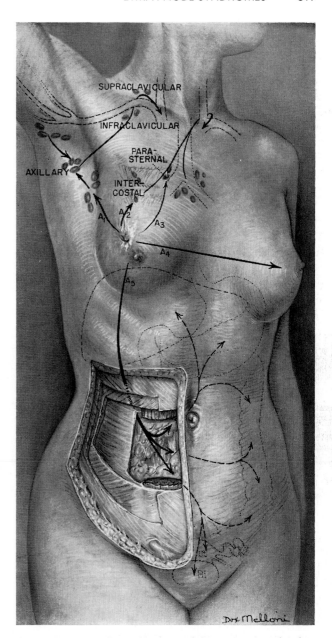

Fig. 26-13. Lymphatic drainage of the mammary gland. Metastases from cancer of the mammary gland may follow several lymphatic pathways: (A_1) Upper outer quadrant to axillary, infraclavicular, supraclavicular nodes, and so forth. (A_2) Upper inner quadrant to intercostal and parasternal nodes. (A_3) Upper inner quadrant directly to parasternal nodes. (A_4) Directly across midline to opposite breast. (A_5) Lower quadrants, particularly inner aspect, through pectoralis major, external oblique, and linea alba to subperitoneal lymphatic plexus, followed by abdominal and pelvic spread.

fascia so that it can no longer move in the long axis of the pectoralis major. Finally, with continued contraction of the involved ligaments of Cooper, there is dimpling of the skin or the nipple of the mammary gland (Fig. 26-14A).

The lymphatic vessels draining the skin over the mammary gland may become blocked with consequent stagnation of lymph and edema of the skin. Since the hair follicles are attached more firmly to the underlying superficial fascia, the edematous skin projects in between the hair follicles. This skin thus presents pitting. This condition is called *peau d'orange* (Fig. 26-14B). Extensive infiltration by tumor throughout the dermal lymphatics may excite a considerable fibrotic response.

This causes an almost armor-plated appearance to the skin (cancer *en cuirasse*). *Peau d'orange* may occur in other parts of the body in which blockage of the skin lymphatics occurs (*e.g.,* ischiorectal abscess).

SUPPURATION OF LYMPH NODES

A distinctive phenomenon that occasionally follows infectious lymphadenopathy occurs when the infecting organism overwhelms the local defensive mechanism within the node to produce excess cellular reaction and collection of pus. Suppuration may subside spontaneously, it may require incision and drainage, or it may lead to destruction of the node with spontaneous

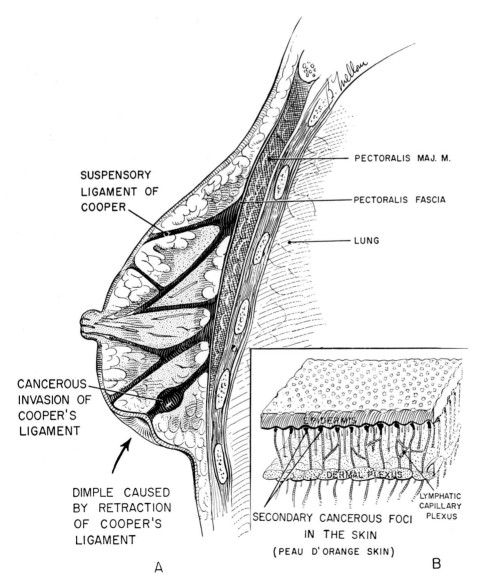

SUSPENSORY LIGAMENT OF COOPER

PECTORALIS MAJ. M.

PECTORALIS FASCIA

LUNG

CANCEROUS INVASION OF COOPER'S LIGAMENT

DIMPLE CAUSED BY RETRACTION OF COOPER'S LIGAMENT

A

EPIDERMIS

DERMAL PLEXUS

SECONDARY CANCEROUS FOCI IN THE SKIN
(PEAU D'ORANGE SKIN)

LYMPHATIC CAPILLARY PLEXUS

B

Fig. 26-14. (*A*) Retraction of the skin in cancer of the breast when ligaments of Cooper contract following cancer invasion. (*B*) Secondary cancerous foci in skin producing *peau d'orange* skin.

rupture and drainage. This may occur in a single node or lead to coalescence of multiple nodes with suppuration, at times from several sites.

The nodes most likely to suppurate are the cervical and superficial inguinal, occasionally the axillary, and much less often the epitrochlear or popliteal. The rarity of suppuration of the intrathoracic and the intra-abdominal nodes deserves comment, considering the frequency of involvement of these nodes.

Of the many regional and systemic infections leading to adenopathy, relatively few produce lymph node suppuration with any regularity. Those most commonly responsible are listed below:

Streptococcal pharyngitis
Streptococcal wound infection
Tuberculous lymphadenitis
Staphylococcal lymphadenitis
Lymphopathia venereum
Coccidioidomycosis
Anthrax
Cat-scratch disease
Chancroid
Sporotrichosis
Plague
Tularemia

Hemolytic streptococcus infections of the pharynx and tonsils, producing cervical and more rarely retropharyngeal suppuration (most commonly in children under age 5 years), were the most common causes of lymph node suppuration prior to the sulfonamide era. There is some question whether the occasional peritonsillar abscess or cellulitis of the neck complicating tonsillitis is due to another superimposed bacterial infection. Streptococcus infections in extremity wounds often produce tubular lymphangitis (characterized by painful red streaks) and suppurative regional lymphadenitis. The pus is often thin, possibly because of the presence of the enzymes streptokinase and streptodornase. *Staphylococcus infection* is manifested by a thick, yellow-white type of pus. *Lymphopathia venereum* (of viral origin), especially in the male, and *chancroid* (owing to *Bacillus ducreyi*) are common genital infections predisposing to suppurative superficial inguinal adenitis. *Cervical tuberculous lymphadenitis with suppurative scrofula*, now rare in Europe and America, was in the past years a classic and common form of cervical node suppuration with localization at a lower level in the neck than that of streptococcus adenitis. Cervical lymphadenitis caused by atypical mycobacteria has recently been shown to be a common cause of suppuration in young children.[412] Pediculosis of the scalp, probably by permitting secondary infection, occasionally may produce suppuration of occipital and posterior neck nodes.

Anthrax and *plague* represent serious systemic disorders, with regional nodes draining the entrance area manifesting marked suppuration, which occasionally may be hemorrhagic or manifest necrotic liquefaction. Fungus infections, especially *sporotrichosis* (usually on an extremity) and *coccidioidomycosis* (cervical area), occasionally may produce suppuration. Cat-scratch disease (inoculation lymphoreticulosis), of probable viral etiology, has been found to be a common cause of lymph node suppuration that most commonly appears in the groin or the axilla, occasionally in the epitrochlear, and rarely in the cervical nodes.[355] Early, the enlarged nodes may simulate a lymphoma. Following suppuration they simulate tularemia. Bacteriologically negative pus, history of contact with cats, and use of the cat-scratch antigen skin test assist in diagnosis.

Chronic granulomatous disease of childhood is a hereditary disease resulting from inadequate peroxidase function in leucocyte lysosomes.[370–373] A review of published cases notes suppuration of lymph nodes in 104 of 137 cases.[414] Other signs include hepatosplenomegaly, pulmonary infiltration, lymphoreticulosis, and eczemoid dermatitis.

BCG vaccination in infants may lead to suppuration of the axillary nodes when the shoulder is the site of injection and suppuration of the superficial inguinal nodes when the thigh is the injection site. Suppuration may not take place until months following the injection and appears to be related to the dose. Groin suppuration is much more common than axillary suppuration for reasons explained in the section on inguinal adenitis.

The enlarged lymph nodes of advanced lepromatous leprosy during an exacerbated phase may become necrotic and break down, producing a clinical picture somewhat similar to those just discussed.[374]

GENERALIZED LYMPHADENOPATHY

By common understanding, the term *generalized lymphadenopathy* has come to mean involvement of two, and preferably three, regionally separated lymph node groups in which enlargement results from a systemic disorder acting on lymphoid tissue. Inflammatory reactions and lymphoid neoplasms account for the majority of cases. Many miscellaneous etiologies account for the balance. Although the basic stress is generalized, enlargement of nodes often occurs in irregular fashion and need not appear simultaneously and to an equal degree in all body areas. At times, the pattern is clinically helpful.

Generalized lymph node enlargement obviously can occur as a result of various diffuse skin disorders, which permit infectious and toxic multiple regional lymph node involvement of a chronic reactive type.[375] A specific

syndrome can be identified in this general category: lipomelanotic reticular hyperplasia of lymph nodes, usually related to erythematous and exfoliative types of pruritic dermatosis in which the lymphadenopathy is characterized by lipid and melanin infiltration and reticulum cell reaction (at times suggesting a lymphoma).[376,377] The diagnostic problem is compounded when the generalized cutaneous condition is itself due to neoplasms, such as Sézary's syndrome[378] and the related disease of mycosis fungoides.[379] The latter condition almost always develops as a chronic benign dermatitis followed in the majority of cases by clinically detectable lymphadenopathy.[379] Generalized lymphadenopathy is fairly common in the exacerbated phase of advanced lepromatous leprosy, as is hepatosplenomegaly.[374]

Generalized involvement of systemic infectious origin may occur, in addition to a more prominent regional adenopathy of the drainage area of the inoculation site, in a number of the disorders described in the preceding sections, such as cat-scratch disease,[355] infectious mononucleosis, tularemia,[348] plague,[349] secondary syphilis,[380] postvaccinal lymphadenitis,[47] and so forth. Although some of the infectious diseases that produce a generalized type of lymphadenopathy are well known, others are less commonly appreciated. The latter include brucellosis,[381,382] generalized peripheral lymphadenopathy of tuberculous origin,[383] certain tropical diseases,[384,385] and others.[386]

Children often manifest a greater degree of generalized lymph node response to a particular infection than do adults for reasons commented upon previously (*e.g.,* in measles, rubella, and scarlet fever).[387]

Virtually all metastatic neoplasms and most malignant lymphomas produce regional lymphadenopathy. Generalized involvement is seen most frequently with histiocytic medullary reticulosis,[388,389] diffuse or nodular lymphocytic lymphoma, lymphatic leukemia, and hairy cell leukemia. The patient with histiocytic medullary reticulosis also has a marked fever and signs of a hemolytic anemia. Patients with lymphocytic lymphoma usually show marrow involvement, and leukemia may also be present; hairy cell leukemia is usually accompanied by pancytopenia and splenomegaly.

Rarely, Kaposi's sarcoma may produce generalized nodal enlargement in children with minimal cutaneous involvement;[390] recently, an epidemic of nodal Kaposi's sarcoma has been noted in homosexual men.[391]

General lymph node enlargement may be of metabolic origin, as in Neimann-Pick's disease, Gaucher's disease, hyperthyroidism, primary amyloidosis, Addison's disease, and primary macroglobulinemia. Generalized lymphadenopathy commonly occurs in the γ-chain form of heavy-chain disease, characterized by the unusual findings in about one fourth of cases of

waxing and waning in the size of the nodes and in about one third by erythema and edema of the palate, which is probably related to nodal involvement of this drainage area.[392]

Such immunologically mediated diseases as serum sickness, generalized drug reactions (especially if accompanied by a rash), autoimmune hemolytic anemia,[393] and so forth may produce a generalized lymphadenopathy. A generalized lymphadenopathy may occur in heroin addiction, perhaps as a result of altered circulating lymphocytes and changes in the immunoglobulin system.[213]

Reactive proliferation of lymph nodes of unknown cause is seen in sarcoidosis.

Generalized lymphadenopathy may occur in some of the disorders of the collagen tissues. It is particularly well documented in rheumatoid arthritis (nodes are rare above the clavicle),[394] Still's disease,[395] dermatomyositis, and disseminated lupus erythematosus.[396,397]

Lymphadenopathy of generalized distribution may occur occasionally in the adult-acquired form of toxoplasmosis, and the entire syndrome may resemble, to a remarkable degree, acute infectious mononucleosis. One should especially suspect toxoplasmosis if this picture occurs in a person ingesting uncooked meat or one exposed to fecal litter from cats. The diagnosis can be confirmed by various laboratory tests.[398] At times, the lymphadenitis may be relapsing.[399] Rarely, leishmaniasis may be localized to lymph nodes and may cause enlargement at multiple sites.[400] Prominent in the literature are reports of hydantointype anticonvulsant drugs producing a lymphadenopathy mimicking a lymphoma clinically and even pathologically, but this is reversible upon cessation of their use.[401,402]

Gantz and Gleckman and others have provided excellent discussions of the causes of generalized lymphadenopathy and persistent fever.[407,408]

A growing literature documents more recently described disorders in which generalized adenopathy is present. Included are Rademacher's disease,[403] immunoblastic lymphadenopathy,[404] and others.[405,406,410,411]

It is well to remember that generalized lymph node enlargement may occur rarely or occasionally in some disorders or consistently or characteristically in others. It is impossible to document in this chapter all the possible causes mentioned in the literature.

SUMMARY

Lymph nodes, lymphatic vessels, and other lymphoid aggregates function interdependently with the rest of the lymphoid system and participate in the motion of wandering lymphocytes, in the immune reactions, and

27

Pathologic Bleeding Jack E. Ansell

Normal Hemostasis
Laboratory Approach to Hemostasis Evaluations
Approach to the Patient with Suspected Hemostatic
  Failure
Pathologic Bleeding Caused by Vascular Disorders
  Direct Vascular Injury
  Decreased Mechanical Strength of the
    Microcirculation
Pathologic Bleeding Caused by Platelet Disorders
  Quantitative Disorders: Thrombocytopenia
    Deficient Thrombopoiesis

Accelerated Destruction, Utilization, or Loss of
  Platelets
Qualitative Disorders: Congenital and Acquired
  Platelet Dysfunction
Coagulation Disorders
  Factor Deficiency: Production Defect
  Factor Deficiency: Accelerated Factor Destruction
    or Loss
  Inhibitors (Anticoagulants)
Summary

Hemorrhage does not always imply defective hemostasis because bleeding can be initiated by severe trauma placing excessive stress upon a normal hemostatic system. Hemorrhage that is inappropriate to the inciting event is evidence of hemostatic failure. This phenomenon is the focus of this chapter.

Three major components of the hemostatic system must be intact for normal hemostasis and the prevention of pathologic bleeding. These include the vascular, cellular (platelet), and plasmatic (coagulation) components of hemostasis (Fig. 27-1). The physiology and pathophysiology of these components are reviewed and an approach to the evaluation of hemostatic failure is discussed. Because this evaluation relies heavily upon the hemostasis laboratory, the laboratory diagnosis of hemostatic failure is an essential component of this review as well.

NORMAL HEMOSTASIS

Vascular Component. The vascular contribution to the maintenance of normal hemostasis is commonly underemphasized, perhaps because of our inability to easily assess its function. The vascular component can be functionally and anatomically divided into three divisions: the vascular supporting tissue, the blood vessel wall, and the vascular endothelium and subendothelium.[1,2] The composition of supporting and surrounding tissue adjacent to sites of vascular injury influences the amount of blood loss by the ability of this tissue to impede blood accumulation and create external compression, which tamponades further bleeding. Thus, hemorrhage from vessels in soft-tissue spaces is likely to be much greater than hemorrhage that occurs in small, tightly bound, fascial compartments. The type and size of injured vessels also influence the amount of hemorrhage. Vascular contraction is a normal physiologic response to injury and plays an important role in the initial control of bleeding, especially in the arterial system where larger arterioles and arteries are supplied with abundant muscular and elastic tissue. Vascular contraction is initiated and controlled by reflex neurogenic stimuli, humoral vasospastic stimuli, and precapillary sphincter constriction.[2] Arterial injury induces circumferential and longitudinal contraction at the site of injury and vasospasm proximal to the injury. These reactions may completely

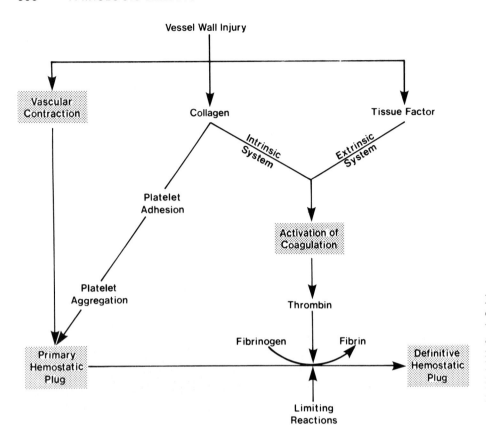

Fig. 27-1. The three major components of hemostasis—vascular, cellular (platelet), and plasmatic (coagulation)—interact to form a definitive hemostatic plug. (Adapted from Deykin D: Hemostasis. In Reich PR: Hematology. Boston, Little, Brown & Co, 1978)

control initial bleeding, but without concomitant platelet aggregation and fibrin deposition, hemorrhage quickly resumes.

The vascular endothelium and subendothelium have received much scientific scrutiny as a hemostatic barrier.[3] Attention has been focused on the low thrombogenicity of intact endothelium. Endothelial cells produce a number of substances important in initiating, as well as retarding, thrombosis. These include prostacyclin, a potent vasodilator and inhibitor of platelet aggregation, plasminogen activator, and von Willebrand factor. The importance of these substances is discussed below. Subendothelial constituents in the vessel wall also play an important role because they serve as the site of platelet adherence and the stimulus for platelet aggregation.

Cellular Component (Platelets). Knowledge of platelet production, development, and structure are important prerequisites for an understanding of platelet physiology.[4] Platelets originate in megakaryocytes, the large multinucleated cells of the bone marrow, as cytoplasmic fragments that break off and enter the circulation. They survive an average of 9 to 12 days in the circulation. In normal individuals, approximately 30% of circulating platelets are pooled in the spleen. Platelets are removed in the spleen according to their senescence, although random platelet loss also occurs.

Platelets circulate as disc-like elements in an inactive state (Fig. 27-2). Morphologically, the platelet can be divided into three zones: the outer or peripheral zone, the sol-gel zone, and the organelle zone.[5] The outer or peripheral zone is made up of an exterior coat, a trilaminar membrane, submembranous filaments, and an open canalicular system. The exterior coat contains the antigenic characteristics, the receptor sites, and the properties responsible for platelet adhesiveness. The platelet membrane is similar to other cell membranes and contains the phospholipid substance that accelerates blood coagulation known as *platelet factor 3* (PF_3). The submembrane filaments resemble microfilaments and probably serve as a form of stress fiber that produces tension at the cell surface to maintain the discoid shape.[6] The open canalicular system is a specialized system of cell-membrane invaginations that increases the surface area of the platelet and serves as a conduit for the uptake and the discharge of substances that participate in platelet reactions.

The sol-gel zone is made up of microtubules, microfilaments, submembrane filaments, and glycogen. The

microtubules support and regulate the discoid shape of the platelet and play a role in platelet-shape change during the release reaction. Microfilaments are composed of thrombosthenin (actin-myosin elements) and function in the contractile process during platelet release as well as in the maintenance of the cytoskeleton.

The organelle zone contains granules of various electron densities, mitochondria, and a dense tubular system. The delta granules, or dense bodies, function as storage granules for adenosine diphosphate (ADP), adenosine triphosphate (ATP), serotonin, and small amounts of calcium, substances that are important for normal platelet function. Alpha granules contain a number of platelet-specific proteins, including platelet factor 4 (PF_4), beta thromboglobulin (BTG), platelet-derived growth factor (PDGR), fibrinogen, and others.[7] Although much is known about many of these proteins, their true physiologic role is not entirely clear. A third type of granule is the lysosomal granule. The dense tubular system is derived from the endoplasmic reticulum. It is located close to the open canalicular system and serves as a major site of calcium storage.[8]

Platelet reactions can be divided into three distinguishable events: adhesion, release, and aggregation. Adhesion is the property of adhesiveness whereby platelets interact with certain surfaces. Subendothelial collagen of a specific type with certain structural requirements appears to provide the physiologic surface to which platelets adhere *in vivo*.[9] To a lesser extent, basement membrane and other amorphous subendothelial supporting elements may be similarly effective. Platelets also require a specific structural property of coagulation factor VIII known as *von Willebrand factor* (vWF) for normal adherence.[10] The platelet membrane has a variety of glycoproteins exposed on its surface.[11] A specific glycoprotein identified as *glycoprotein I_b* appears to be a receptor for vWF on the surface of platelets. Although the exact mechanism is unknown, both of these elements are essential for adherence of platelets to collagen. In the absence of vWF (*i.e.*, von Willebrand's disease), or the absence of glycoprotein I_b, (*i.e.*, Bernard Soulier syndrome), platelet adhesion is abnormal, whereas other platelet functions are generally maintained. Following adherence of platelets to collagen, a series of reactions are triggered that eventually lead to platelet aggregation and formation of a primary hemostatic plug. During this process, platelets release a number of vasoactive substances such as serotonin and prostaglandin intermediates that contribute to the humoral stimulus for vascular contraction.

The precise order of events that occur following platelet adherence to collagen is not entirely clear.[12] It is generally believed that, as a result of adherence,

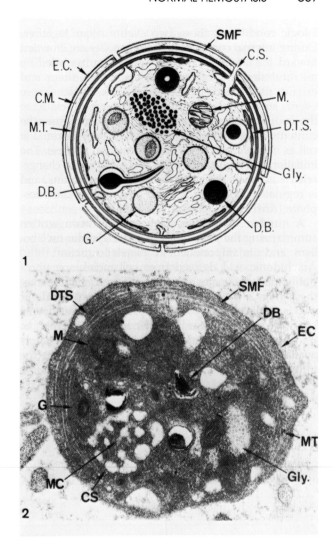

Fig. 27-2. Ultrastructural platelet morphology. (*EC* = exterior coat; *CM* = trilaminar unit membrane; *SMF* = submembrane filaments; *CS* = canalicular system; *MT* = microtubules; *Gly* = glycogen; *M* = mitochondria; *G* = granules; *DB* = dense bodies; *DTS* = dense tubular system; *MC* = membrane complex. Reprinted from White JG, Gerrard JM: Platelet morphology and the ultrastructure of regulatory mechanisms involved in platelet activation. In de Gaetano G, Garattini S (eds): Platelets: A Multidisciplinary Approach, p 18. New York, Raven Press, 1978)

platelets are stimulated to release a number of endogenous substances (*i.e.*, release reaction) that then stimulate other platelets in the surrounding medium to release and to clump together (*i.e.*, aggregation). Immediately prior to the release reaction, platelets undergo a shape change from a discoid structure to a sphere.[13] This process of shape change involves pseudopod extension and internal contraction. Under certain phys-

of neoplasia cause a predictable decrease in thrombopoiesis as well as general hematopoiesis by well-defined mechanisms.[52] These agents interfere with DNA synthesis and cell replication, leading to marrow hypoplasia. Ionizing radiation is also included in this group of marrow-toxic substances. Some drugs selectively suppress thrombopoiesis by unknown mechanisms. The thiazide diuretics and alcohol have also been reported to produce megakaryocytic hypoplasia.[53]

Bone marrow infiltration (myelophthisis) by malignant or granulomatous disease can lead to thrombocytopenia by interfering with thrombopoiesis. Whether the mechanism is simply a "crowding out" phenomenon or whether a humoral factor is involved is unclear.[54] Cancer can cause thrombocytopenia by mechanisms other than suppression of thrombopoiesis.

Ineffective Thrombopoiesis. In the presence of vitamin B_{12} or folate deficiency, thrombocytopenia can result from ineffective production of platelets, presumably due to defective DNA synthesis.[55] Megaloblastic changes occur in megakaryocytes just as in red cells. This is rarely severe, although severe bleeding can occur in some cases. Ineffective thrombopoiesis is also seen in some of the preleukemic disorders and certain myeloproliferative diseases, such as paroxysmal nocturnal hemoglobinuria, presumably because of a stem cell abnormality.

Thrombocytopenia is commonly found in a number of hereditary disorders such as the Wiskott–Aldrich syndrome, Chediak–Higashi anomaly, May–Hegglin anomaly, and others, in which the thrombocytopenia is only one of a number of associated clinical or laboratory abnormalities.

Accelerated Destruction, Utilization, or Loss of Platelets

Peripheral destruction of platelets is a common cause of thrombocytopenia. In this situation, megakaryocytes are increased, as is platelet production, and platelet survival is shortened. Circulating platelets are larger and younger in age. Studies suggest that young platelets are more hemostatically effective and clinical studies support this.[56] The correlation between a rising bleeding time and a falling platelet count breaks down and patients in whom this occurs occasionally have bleeding times shorter than expected.

Immunologic Destruction of Platelets. Antibodies to platelets alter the platelet membrane such that they are recognized as abnormal and destroyed by macrophages in the reticuloendothelial system (RES). As a result, their survival is shortened and platelet production in the bone marrow is increased. Platelet antibodies are either autoantibodies, as occur in some autoimmune diseases such as lupus erythematosus, or isoantibodies, as occur in sensitization to foreign antigens following blood- or platelet-transfusion. Drug-induced platelet antibodies are not primarily directed against the platelet membrane. Studies suggest that the platelet behaves as an innocent bystander and is sensitized by attachment of the drug-carrier protein that stimulates antibody production.[57] Immune complexes can also lead to thrombocytopenia by attaching to platelets, leading to their removal in the RES.[58]

Idiopathic thrombocytopenic purpura (ITP) is the most common form of immune thrombocytopenia. With the development of more sensitive techniques to detect immunoglobulin on the platelet membrane, it appears that most incidences are caused by platelet antibody.[59] These sensitized platelets are removed by macrophages in the reticuloendothelial system, primarily in the spleen.[60] The spleen is also the major source of antibody-producing cells. Thus, therapeutic splenectomy not only removes the site of platelet destruction, but also a major site of antibody production. Almost all patients with ITP have increased megakaryocytes in the bone marrow, although there are rare cases associated with decreased megakaryocytes. This suppression of megakaryopoiesis has been attributed to a humoral factor elaborated by the spleen. Whether this humoral factor exists is unclear, but it certainly is a rare situation in ITP.

ITP occurs in a *chronic* or *acute* form.[61] ITP in children is of the acute form in 90% or more of cases. There is a peak incidence between 2 to 6 years of age and boys and girls are equally affected. The problem is usually brought to the attention of a physician because of the sudden appearance of petechiae on the lower extremities. A history of an antecedent infection, usually a viral-like upper respiratory infection, is found in more than 80% of children suffering acute ITP. Symptoms other than petechiae or minor bleeding are usually lacking, and physical examination is unremarkable. Splenomegaly rarely occurs and, if it is found, the possibility of another cause of thrombocytopenia should be entertained. Severe bleeding almost never occurs, especially the dreaded complication of CNS hemorrhage, in spite of the rather severe thrombocytopenia that is usually present. Treatment is supportive and the illness is self-limited, with 90% or more of cases involving children resolving over a few months. Glucocorticosteroids may elevate the platelet count when administered, but they are not thought to alter the natural course of the disease.

Chronic ITP occurs predominantly in adults and in about 10% of children with ITP. The onset is more insidious in patients with a history of easy bruising or

minor bleeding dating back several months. Women are more commonly affected with chronic ITP than men. Bleeding manifestations include petechiae and ecchymoses, menorrhagia, hematuria, melena, epistaxis, and gingival bleeding. The onset is not associated with an antecedent infection. The physical examination is unremarkable and splenomegaly is rarely found. Treatment is considerably more complex than in cases of acute ITP. Glucocorticosteroids are indicated initially, but a maintained good response is uncommon. Splenectomy is generally indicated next in a healthy subject who is a low surgical risk. Other forms of treatment include immunosuppressive agents and plasmapheresis. After all modalities of therapy have been exhausted, there is generally a small group of 10% to 25% of patients who remain refractory to treatment.[62] Some of these patients may remit spontaneously after several years. Others may succumb to the illness from bleeding complications.

Autoimmune thrombocytopenia similar to ITP may occur in the presence of, or as the presenting sign of, various autoimmune diseases such as systemic lupus erythematosus. The treatment is similar to that of ITP, but, with active underlying disease, treatment of the primary disease is essential.

Thrombocytopenia due to isoantibodies occurs following multiple platelet transfusions or, classically, in a syndrome called *posttransfusion purpura*.[63] This disorder is due to antibodies directed against a common platelet-associated antigen called PL^{A1}. All patients with the syndrome have been PL^{A1}-negative, and have usually been sensitized by receiving blood containing PL^{A1}-positive platelets. The exact reason why these patients who lack PL^{A1} should develop thrombocytopenia is unclear.

Thrombocytopenia is occasionally seen in certain types of systemic infections. The pathophysiology is multifactorial and includes direct effects of bacteria upon platelets and indirect effects by means of immune reactions and vascular damage.[3,64,65]

Nonimmunologic Thrombocytopenia. Activation and consumption of platelets in the syndrome of disseminated intravascular coagulation (DIC) is secondary to the activation of coagulation and the formation of thrombin and intravascular fibrin thrombi upon which platelets are consumed. In a similar syndrome, thrombotic thrombocytopenic purpura (TTP), platelets are aggregated and consumed directly by an unknown stimulus resulting in intravascular platelet thrombi that then behave much like intravascular fibrin thrombi and predispose to further thrombocytopenia.[66] TTP is a complex and controversial syndrome. Evidence suggests that there is either a platelet-aggregating factor in the blood that can be effectively removed by plasmapheresis, or a missing factor that normally inhibits platelet activation that can be replaced by plasma infusion.[67,68] Some investigators have found a deficiency of prostacyclin production in vascular tissue of patients with TTP.[69] The clinical hallmarks of TTP include thrombocytopenia, hemolytic anemia, transient neurologic abnormalities, fever, and renal failure. Hemolytic-uremic syndrome, the counterpart of TTP that occurs in children, probably has a similar pathophysiology, but, for unknown reasons, primarily affects the kidneys and has a considerably better prognosis than TTP.

Dilutional thrombocytopenia may occur in patients who have been transfused with large volumes of blood over a short interval of time. This is because platelet viability in banked blood is very poor. This can typically be seen in the patient who has sustained severe injury and bleeding, and who receives 10 to 20 units of blood over a 24-hr period or less.

Under normal circumstances, the spleen contains approximately one third of the total platelet mass. In the presence of splenomegaly, a larger percentage of platelets can be sequestered in the spleen, leading to a condition called *hypersplenism*. This occurs in disease states such as cirrhosis, lymphoma, Felty's syndrome, and Gaucher's disease. Platelets are not only sequestered in these conditions, but, according to platelet kinetic studies, also show a reduction in survival. Not uncommonly, hypersplenism involves all three cell lines and, occasionally, splenectomy is necessary to reverse the drop in blood counts.

QUALITATIVE DISORDERS: CONGENITAL AND ACQUIRED PLATELET DYSFUNCTION

A reduction in the number of platelets is not the only cause of a defective platelet phase of hemostasis. Poorly functioning platelets can also be responsible for bleeding (see Table 27-2).[70,71] The most common cause of bleeding due to a platelet disorder is a drug-induced (*e.g.,* aspirin) qualitative platelet defect. The basic test in functional platelet disorders to identify platelet dysfunction is a bleeding time that is usually prolonged. However, for purposes of classification, platelet aggregation studies are more useful (Table 27-3).

Adhesion Defect. There are two congenital disorders characterized by an inability of platelets to adhere to certain surfaces such as collagen. Von Willebrand's disease is a defect extrinsic to the platelet that is due to a plasma-factor deficiency normally expressed as a property of factor VIII (see von Willebrand's disease below). This factor interacts with a glycoprotein in the

Table 27-3. *Congenital Disorders of Platelet Function (Based Upon Platelet Aggregation)*

	Bleeding Time	Clot Retraction	Adhesion	Platelet Factor 3	Storage Pool	Release	Electron Microscopy	Aggregation 1°	2°	Ristocetin
Absent 1° & 2° Aggregation → Thrombobasthemia	↑	↓	↓	↓	N	N	↓	↓	↓	N
Absent 2° Aggregation ↗ Storage pool disease	↑	N	↓	↓	↓	N	A	N	↓	N
↘ Release defect	↑	N	↓	↓	N	↓	N	N	↓	N
Absent ristocetin Aggregation ↗ von Willebrand syndrome*	↑	N	↓	N	N	N	N	N	N	↓
↘ Giant platelet syndrome†	↑	N	↓	↓	N	N	A	N	N	↓

↑ (Increased); ↓ (Decreased); N (Normal); A (Abnormal)
*Long PTT; ↓ VIII$_C$; ↓ VIII$_{Ag}$; ↓ VIII$_{VWF}$
†(May have thrombocytopenia)

platelet membrane important for adherence. Platelet aggregation induced by collagen, ADP, and epinephrine are normal in von Willebrand's disease. Platelets from patients with Bernard Soulier syndrome also have abnormal adherence with normal aggregation to collagen, ADP, and epinephrine.[72] The defect, however, is in the platelet membrane, which lacks glycoprotein I$_b$.[73] Platelets from Bernard Soulier syndrome and von Willebrand's disease fail to aggregate in response to ristocetin, an antibiotic no longer in clinical use that requires glycoprotein I$_b$ and von Willebrand factor to induce aggregation. Bernard Soulier syndrome is inherited as an autosomal recessive trait. It is associated occasionally with mild thrombocytopenia and morphologically giant platelets. Bleeding may be severe and is usually of the purpuric type. Von Willebrand's disease is described in greater detail below. Uremia, as well as some drugs, may also lead to an acquired adhesion defect. Von Willebrand's disease can rarely develop as an acquired disorder.

Release Defect. A release, or secretion, defect can be due to a primary abnormality in the release mechanism or to a deficiency in the granular elements within the platelet such that, upon release, there is nothing to be secreted (storage pool disease). Delta- and alpha-granule deficiencies are seen in storage pool disease, and can occur singly or in combination. Patients with the

Hermansky-Pudlak syndrome, a disorder characterized by oculo-cutaneous albinism, have a bleeding tendency owing to a deficiency of platelet delta granules.[74] They have a prolonged bleeding time, no secondary platelet aggregation in response to ADP or epinephrine, and no platelet-dense granules by electron microscopy. Similarly, a condition called the *gray platelet syndrome* is due to a deficiency of alpha granules and patients suffering from this syndrome fail to secrete PF$_4$, beta thromboglobulin, and PDGR, all proteins found in alpha granules.[75]

Platelets of some patients with immune thrombocytopenia, or patients with normal platelet counts but with increased platelet associated IgG, have also been shown to have deficient granular contents and a storage-pool-like platelet defect.[76] This may be due to subclinical platelet activation and release without aggregation, causing these platelets to exhaust their storage pool. Storage-pool deficiency can also be seen during the use of certain drugs, such as serotonin antagonists, that inhibit the uptake and storage of certain granular elements.

Patients with a primary release defect show no secondary wave of platelet aggregation, but the granular content of the platelet is normal (by electron microscopy and biochemical measurement) and the fault lies with a defect in the release mechanism.[70] Congenital release defects are very uncommon; a release defect is

most often seen as an acquired defect in thromboxane production due to inhibition of prostaglandin cyclo-oxygenase by drugs such as aspirin or other nonsteroidal, anti-inflammatory agents. Acetylsalicylic acid irreversibly acetylates cyclo-oxygenase and impairs the platelet for the remainder of its lifespan.[77] Other nonsteroidal, anti-inflammatory agents reversibly inhibit cyclo-oxygenase only while the drug is present in the blood. Only recently have patients with a congenital cyclo-oxygenase deficiency been described.[78] Myeloproliferative disorders such as myelofibrosis, chronic myelogenous leukemia, essential thrombocythemia, and others are also associated with platelet dysfunction most often characterized as a release defect.[79] The defect in these disorders is attributed to an abnormal stem cell that gives rise to the myeloproliferative disease. However, the precise defect is unknown.

Aggregation Defect. Glanzmann's thrombasthenia is a rare autosomal condition in which platelets are unable to aggregate and clot retraction is abnormal.[80] Although the bleeding time is prolonged, adherence, measured more specifically by other techniques, is normal. These platelets undergo shape change and release and their granular contents are normal. Analysis of thrombasthenic platelet membranes reveal a deficiency of two glycoproteins, II_b and III_a.[73] It is believed that these glycoproteins are required for fibrinogen binding, which is necessary for platelet aggregation.

Platelet Coagulant Activity Deficiency. Most qualitative platelet disorders are associated with a deficiency of platelet coagulant activity or PF_3. However, in these disorders, the PF_3 defect is secondary to other abnormalities of the platelet. To date, only one patient with a well-documented isolated PF_3 defect has been described.[81] The defect was associated with decreased binding of factor X_a and V_a to its surface. This patient had a moderately severe hemorrhagic diathesis.

COAGULATION DISORDERS

Hemorrhagic coagulation disorders can be due to absolute or functional factor deficiencies or to the presence of an inhibitor or anticoagulant (see Table 27-2). Deficiencies can be caused by a congenital or acquired defect in production or by increased consumption, dilution, or loss of a factor. Inhibitors occur endogenously or result from the administration of an exogenous anticoagulant. Table 27-4 summarizes the results of the routine screening tests in these various conditions.

Table 27-4. *Presumptive Diagnosis of Common Bleeding Disorders Based Upon Routine Screening Tests*

Platelet Count	Bleeding Time	Pro-thrombin Time (PT)	Partial Thrombo-plastin Time (PTT)	Thrombin Time (TT)	Miscellaneous	Presumptive Problem
↓	N, ↑	N	N	N		Thrombocytopenia
N	↑	N	N	N		Platelet-function defect or vascular defect
N	↑	N	↑	N	↓ VIII_c, ↓ VIII_{ag}, ↓ VIII_{vwf}	Von Willebrand's disease
N	N	↑	N	N		Extrinsic pathway defect (VII)
N	N	N	↑	N		Intrinsic pathway defect (VIII, IX, XI, XII, prekallikrein, high-molecular-weight kininogen, inhibitor)
N	N	↑	↑	N		Common pathway or multiple pathway defects excluding fibrinogen
N	N	↑	↑	↑	High levels of fibrin(ogen) degradation products (FDP)	Fibrinogen deficiency or dysfunction, vitamin-K deficiency, liver disease, primary fibrinolysis
↓	N, ↑	↑	↑	↑	High levels of FDP	Disseminated intravascular coagulation
N	N	N	N	N	Positive clot solubility	XIII deficiency

N = normal; ↓ = decreased; ↑ = increased

FACTOR DEFICIENCY: PRODUCTION DEFECT

Congenital Deficiency of Factors VIII and IX. The most common inherited deficiencies are those of factor VIII (classical hemophilia A) and factor IX (hemophilia B, Christmas disease). Because deficiencies of either factor VIII or factor IX lead to identical clinical syndromes, they are discussed together. Factor VIII is a glycoprotein with a molecular weight of at least 1.2 million daltons. It is composed of subunits of approximately 230,000 molecular weight held together by disulfide bonds.[82] Factor-VIII complex has three properties: procoagulant activity (VIII_c—the ability of normal factor VIII to correct the abnormal coagulation time of hemophilic plasma); antigenic activity (VIII_{ag}—the ability of normal factor VIII to precipitate in reaction with a heterologous antisera); and vWF activity (VIII_{vwf}—the ability of normal factor VIII to correct the prolonged bleeding time *in vivo* in a patient with von Willebrand's disease, or to correct *in vitro* ristocetin-induced platelet aggregation of platelets from a patient with von Willebrand's disease). Thus, factor VIII participates in the intrinsic coagulation pathway (VIII_c) and is necessary for normal platelet adhesion (VIII_{vwf}), which is important in determining the bleeding time. Whether these properties are all part of one large molecular complex or are properties of separate molecules that are closely associated *in vivo* is still debated.[83] Most recent evidence suggests that VIII_{ag} and VIII_{vwf} are components of one protein and that VIII_{vwf} activity is dependent upon the degree of polymerization of the molecular subunits.[84] The more highly polymerized the protein is, the greater the vWF activity. The VIII_{ag-vwf} protein is synthesized in endothelial cells and is under autosomal genetic control.[23] Factor VIII_c may be a separate molecule produced elsewhere in the body under X-chromosome control that then becomes associated with factor VIII_{ag-vwf} in the blood.

Factor IX is a vitamin-K-dependent coagulation factor synthesized under X-chromosome control and is produced in the liver (see earlier discussion of factor IX physiology).

The inherited clinical bleeding disorders due to deficiencies of factor VIII or factor IX have been recognized for centuries, but it was not until the 1930s that a factor present in normal plasma was shown to correct the prolonged coagulation time of hemophilic plasma *in vitro*.[85] Antihemophilic globulin, as it was known, later became designated as factor VIII. It was subsequently shown that a similar disorder was caused by a deficiency of another factor, later designated factor IX.[86] In classical hemophilia A, patients suffer from a deficiency of factor-VIII procoagulant activity while levels of VIII_{ag} and VIII_{vwf} are normal. Two thirds of cases of factor-IX deficiency have an absolute reduction of factor-IX procoagulant activity and antigen, whereas approximately one third are discordant with normal or higher levels of factor-IX antigen, but with reduced functional activity, suggesting the presence of a dysfunctional protein.[87]

Severe hemophilia occurs in approximately 1 per 25,000 of the population. As for mild hemophilia, the incidence may be 1 per 3,000 to 4,000 live births. Both disorders are X-linked recessive diseases: a male inherits the normal or affected X chromosome from his carrier mother and a female inherits one affected X chromosome from her carrier mother or affected father. The female offspring thus become carriers of the disease.[88] Not uncommonly, an affected child has no family history of hemophilia and the genetic defect is presumed to arise as a spontaneous mutation.

Severity of clinical bleeding depends upon the concentration of factor-VIII or factor-IX activity. Patients with factor-activity levels above 5% to 10% are considered mild hemophiliacs and have fewer episodes of spontaneous hemorrhage. Spontaneous bleeding into muscles or joints is the most common and damaging problem in hemophilia. Excluding circumcision, it does not generally become a problem until an affected child begins to crawl or walk (6 to 18 months), at which time the knees and ankles are mainly affected. Upper extremity joints, however, are by no means spared as time goes on. Bleeding into muscles and joints causes pain, stiffness, and swelling. The onset of bleeding may be preceded by an "aura" or a feeling that hemorrhage has begun. There may be little, if any, bluish discoloration around the joint to signify bleeding. Bleeding stops as a result of blood accumulation and tamponade, and the blood is slowly resorbed. Joint damage occurs as the result of repeated bleeding, high intra-articular pressure, inflammation, and necrosis of the synovium. Recurrent hemarthroses predispose to future episodes because of the vascular synovial proliferation and joint instability that develop. Vascular and nervous supply to the joint and extremity can also be compromised by hematoma formation. Repeated hemorrhages can lead to joint destruction and ankylosis, causing contractures and crippling deformities. In children, epiphyseal areas may become involved, leading to premature closure and subsequent shortening of the bone.

The usual signs of acute joint or muscle hemorrhage diminish as scarring develops. Diagnosis is commonly based upon the onset of pain. A noticeable drop in hemoglobin is only likely to occur during major hemorrhage such as can occur in the iliac or psoas muscles when a patient presents with acute abdominal pain that can be confused with acute appendicitis. The diag-

nosis of intra-abdominal bleeding has been aided by the development of CT scanning capabilities. With the advent of home therapy and the improved care of hemophiliacs, the frequency of hemarthroses has diminished as have the frequency and severity of disabling contractures.[89]

Mucous-membrane bleeding is another major problem in hemophiliacs. Excessive and life-threatening hemorrhage can result from simple tooth extractions, and epistaxis and bleeding from erupting teeth is a common childhood problem. Bleeding into the soft tissues around the trachea or esophagus can be life-threatening. Hematuria occurs in approximately 30% of hemophiliacs and may be quite persistent, leading to obstruction of the ureters by clot and permanent renal damage. CNS bleeding is relatively rare and is usually initiated by trauma or severe hypertension. Intracranial hemorrhage, however, is often serious and requires immediate treatment. Signs and symptoms depend upon the location of bleeding.

Approximately 10% to 20% of patients with hemophilia A develop antibodies to factor VIII, usually in childhood and after exposure to transfused plasma products.[90] These antibodies can quickly and effectively neutralize any transfused factor VIII and make the treatment of bleeding in a hemophiliac extremely difficult. Not all patients who develop such antibodies necessarily have high titers, and the antibody titers are known to fluctuate widely from patient to patient or even within the same patient from time to time. Treatment of such patients with massive quantities of factor-VIII concentrate in an effort to overcome the inhibitor, or with immunosuppressive agents trying to suppress antibody production, are not uniformly successful. Newer modes of therapy with preparations containing activated factor X, which bypasses the factor-VIII stage, are promising.[91]

Hemophilia is not difficult to diagnose. The patient's history should support the presence of a congenital disorder, although mild hemophiliacs may not experience hemorrhagic problems until an older age. The family history might suggest an X-linked recessive disorder although spontaneous mutations do occur. Bleeding into joints or muscles, mucous-membrane bleeding, delayed-onset bleeding, or ecchymoses indicate a coagulation-factor deficiency. The laboratory provides definitive evidence of a coagulation disorder by means of an abnormal PTT, normal PT, and TT. A normal bleeding time suggests that platelet function is intact. Distinguishing between a deficiency of factor VIII or factor IX requires specific assays for each factor. A factor-XI deficiency is rarely severe enough to be confused with a factor-VIII or a factor-IX deficiency. A factor-XI deficiency is most often manifested by a mild hemorrhagic tendency or by no hemorrhagic tendency at all.

Von Willebrand's disease is another form of factor-VIII deficiency in which all three properties of factor VIII (coagulant, antigen, vWF) are usually reduced concordantly. Thus, von Willebrand's disease is often a true deficiency of factor-VIII production whereas hemophilia A is consistent with a partial defect of factor VIII with loss of coagulant activity but retention of antigen and vWF properties. Von Willebrand's disease is an autosomal disorder first described by von Willebrand in 1926 in inhabitants of the Aland Islands off the coast of Finland.[92] Initially called pseudohemophilia, von Willebrand's disease was characterized by hemophilic-like bleeding, but of much less severity without hemarthroses and joint deformities. It was originally thought to be a platelet disorder and vascular defect, but was subsequently shown to be associated with factor-VIII deficiency.[93] Current studies now confirm that most cases of von Willebrand's disease are predominantly caused by an overall decrease in the properties that make up the factor-VIII complex. The reduction in VIII_c predisposes to a coagulation defect characterized by a prolonged PTT. The reduction in VIII_{vwf} predisposes to a defect in platelet adhesion (not aggregation, except in response to ristocetin) and is characterized by a prolonged bleeding time, reduced platelet retention in a glass bead column, and reduced platelet aggregation in response to ristocetin. However, another form of von Willebrand's disease has been described that appears to be both a qualitative and quantitative abnormality.[94] This is shown by the immunoelectrophoretic pattern of VIII_{ag} on crossed immunoelectrophoresis where there is a relative decrease in the larger-molecular-weight forms of factor VIII. This type is characterized by a marked heterogeneity in the patterns of reduction of the components of the factor VIII complex.[95] Thus, type I disease is the classical pattern with equivalent reduction of VIII_c, VIII_{ag}, and VIII_{vwf} and a normal electrophoretic profile. Type II disease includes those individuals with an abnormal electrophoretic pattern but with variable levels of VIII_c, VIII_{ag}, and VIII_{vwf}. In type IIa, VIII_{vwf} is reduced but VIII_{ag} may be normal or only slightly reduced. In type IIb, VIII_{vwf} is enhanced (more than normal) with normal or slightly reduced VIII_{ag}.[95] Factor VIII_c in type IIa and type IIb is variable. Interestingly, the bleeding time in type IIb (enhanced vWF activity) is still prolonged, suggesting that ristocetin-cofactor activity (used to measure vWF activity) cannot always predict the bleeding time abnormality.

Clinically, von Willebrand's disease is not associated with the high incidence of spontaneous hemorrhage seen in hemophilia, except in severe cases. Bleeding

more typical of a platelet disorder is commonly seen, such as prolonged bleeding from superficial abrasions and from the oral and nasal mucosa, gastrointestinal tract, or uterus. Von Willebrand's disease is occasionally associated with abnormal superficial vessels in the gastrointestinal tract or oral mucosa. A syndrome of angiodysplasia has also been associated with von Willebrand's disease.[96]

The diagnosis of von Willebrand's disease is based upon the clinical history of a variable hemorrhagic diathesis, autosomal inheritance, and laboratory studies of the factor-VIII complex and of platelet function. Screening tests such as the PTT and bleeding time are usually abnormal with a normal PT, normal TT, and normal platelet count. More detailed studies of platelet function are all normal except for platelet aggregation in response to ristocetin when the patient's plasma is used as the source of vWF. Measurement of VIII_c and VIII_{ag} are generally reduced but may vary considerably from patient to patient as discussed above.

A peculiar phenomena in von Willebrand's disease is the response to infusion of products containing factor VIII. Patients initially demonstrate the expected rise in VIII_c, VIII_{ag}, and VIII_{vwf} based upon the amount of factor VIII infused. The level of VIII_{ag} and VIII_{vwf} subsequently decrease in accordance with the normal half-life of factor VIII. However, VIII_c shows a paradoxical additional rise thereafter, until it begins a gradual decrease over the following 24 to 48 hours as if new VIII_c were being synthesized. The reason for this response following factor-VIII infusions remains unexplained.

Other Congenital Deficiencies. Deficiencies of all other coagulation factors have been described. Detailed descriptions of these syndromes are beyond the scope of this text, but can be obtained from several other sources.[36,97,98] Factor-I deficiency (congenital afibrinogenemia) is a rare autosomal recessive disorder that is clinically milder than severe hemophilia, even in its severe forms. Because fibrinogen is markedly reduced in the homozygous state, the characteristic laboratory findings are an infinitely prolonged PT, PTT, TT, and whole blood-clotting time. Inherited abnormal fibrinogens (dysfibrinogenemias) have also been described. These are characterized by a prolonged TT with normal levels of fibrinogen according to immunologic assays. Factor-II deficiency is also an extremely rare disorder that affects both sexes. Manifestations are generally mild and, surprisingly, the one-stage PT is abnormal in only the most severe deficiency states. Other coagulation tests are quite variable. Factor-V deficiency is an autosomal recessive condition that is more common than factor-I or factor-II deficiency. Epistaxis bruising and hemorrhagia are the usual clinical problems. The PT is characteristically prolonged and in some cases a

prolonged bleeding time has been found. Factor-VII and factor-X deficiencies are rare autosomal recessive disorders characterized by a mild hemorrhagic tendency. Factor-VII deficiency is characterized only by a prolonged PT. Because factor X functions in the common pathway relative to both the intrinsic and extrinsic systems, the PT and PTT are abnormal. Factor-XI deficiency is probably the third most common congenital deficiency after factor-VIII and factor-IX deficiencies and von Willebrand's disease. It is inherited as an autosomal recessive trait and is more common in patients of Jewish ancestry. The bleeding manifestations are usually mild even with very low levels of factor XI. Post-operative or post-traumatic bleeding is the most troublesome feature. The characteristic laboratory abnormality is a prolonged PTT. Factor-XII deficiency (Hageman trait) is a rare autosomal recessive disorder that is not associated with a hemorrhagic tendency in spite of a prolonged PTT and whole blood-clotting time. Deficiencies of prekallikrein, also known as *Fletcher-factor deficiency*, and HMWK deficiency, or *Fitzgerald-factor deficiency*, have also been described. HMWK deficiency may predispose to a slightly greater hemorrhagic tendency than Fletcher-factor deficiency, but both are clinically mild, and prekallikrein deficiency may well be asymptomatic. Both disorders are characterized by a prolonged PTT, but in prekallikrein deficiency, the PTT can be corrected by incubating the reaction mixture (plasma, activator, and phospholipid) for a longer period of time because the defect is one of delayed activation of factor XII. Both deficiencies can be diagnosed by assays for the specific factors. Factor-XIII deficiency is an uncommon autosomal recessive defect that leads to abnormal clot formation. Bleeding manifestations are delayed 24 hours or more after injury and defective wound healing and scar formation may occur. Routine screening coagulation tests are normal because the fibrin-clot end point of most assays is not dependent upon factor XIII for initial clot formation. Clot stability is poor, however, and such fibrin clots are soluble in solutions of high ionic strength such as 5 molar urea or 1% monochloracetic acid. Specific quantitative assays for factor XIII are also available.

In addition to inherited single factor deficiencies, the reader is referred to an excellent review and classification of familial multiple factor deficiencies.[99]

Acquired Deficiencies. Acquired factor deficiencies due to inadequate factor synthesis almost always involve multiple factors and can be attributed primarily to vitamin-K antagonists, vitamin-K deficiency, or liver disease. The coumarin or indanedione anticoagulant drugs interfere with vitamin-K metabolism and produce a deficiency of the vitamin-K-dependent coagulation factors, thus producing a clinical state of apparent vitamin-

K deficiency. Vitamin K is necessary for the normal synthesis of factor II, factor VII, factor IX, and factor X. It participates in an unknown way in the gamma carboxylation of several glutamic acid residues in the precursors of these factors in hepatocytes.[24,100] These gamma-carboxyglutamic-acid moieties enable the zymogens to bind calcium, which is required for binding to phospholipid. In the absence of vitamin K, the precursor proteins circulate as nonfunctional coagulation factors because they cannot bind to phospholipid. As a result, measurement of the factors by functional assays such as the PT or PTT reveal very low levels, whereas immunologic assays using a precipitation reaction with heterologous antibodies reveal normal levels. This is because the nonfunctional proteins retain their antigenic characteristics.

Vitamin K is obtained from the diet (leafy colored vegetable, fish, alfalfa) as well as a by-product of metabolism of endogenous intestinal gram-positive bacteria. It is a fat-soluble vitamin and requires bile salts for normal absorption. It is very unusual for a patient to become vitamin-K deficient on the basis of poor intake alone because the bacterial production of vitamin K is enough to maintain adequate factor production. Clinical states of vitamin-K deficiency most commonly occur as a result of malabsorption due to biliary disease, which leads to fat malabsorption. Patients who are severely malnourished and are receiving antibiotics that suppress the gram-positive flora of the gut may also develop vitamin-K deficiency.[101] This can be seen in the post-operative patient on antibiotics who is also unable to eat for some time. Hematuria, melena, epistaxis, and ecchymoses are common manifestations of vitamin-K deficiency. Severe gastrointestinal bleeding can occur if the deficiency persists, and CNS bleeding can be fatal. The characteristic laboratory findings in vitamin-K deficiency include an initial prolongation of the PT owing to the rapid decline of factor VII, which has the shortest half-life of the vitamin-K dependent coagulation factors (approximately 6 hours). A gradual prolongation of the PTT follows, owing to depression of factor IX. A common clinical problem is the differentiation between liver impairment and vitamin-K deficiency when both conditions may exist in a patient with a prolonged PT and PTT. The diagnosis can be established by assaying the activity of two coagulation factors, both of which are synthesized in the liver but only one of which is vitamin-K-dependent (*e.g.*, factor VII and factor V). Another means of establishing the diagnosis is a therapeutic trial of parenteral vitamin K. Full correction of the coagulopathy should occur within 24 to 48 hours if the abnormality is due to vitamin-K deficiency.

Hemorrhagic disease of the newborn, once a common syndrome due to vitamin-K deficiency in the neonate, is now encountered less often because of routine administration of vitamin K.[102] Hemorrhage occurs at, or a few days following, birth and manifests itself as umbilical-stump oozing or ecchymoses. Serious gastrointestinal or CNS bleeding can occur as well. The vitamin-K-dependent coagulation factors are usually lower than normal at birth, and vitamin-K deficiency exaggerates this depression.

Advanced liver disease is commonly associated with pathological bleeding as a result of an accompanying coagulopathy.[103] Altered coagulation occurs as a result of decreased factor synthesis, production of an abnormal factor, increased factor consumption, or primary fibrinolysis. Because most of the coagulation factors are produced in the liver, the most common coagulopathy is due to impaired factor synthesis and results in multiple factor deficiencies. The vitamin-K-dependent factors are particularly sensitive to liver impairment, especially factor VII. The contact activation factors (XII, XI, prekallikrein, HMWK) are less severely affected. The liver has great potential to produce fibrinogen and thus its concentration is not depressed until late stage liver failure occurs. In certain states, dysfunctional fibrinogens may also be produced.[104] This can be seen with hepatomas, cirrhosis, chronic active liver disease, and acute hepatic failure. Extensive studies have failed to reveal a consistent abnormality in fibrinogen structure responsible for its inactivity. Many investigators have shown that the coagulation mechanism can also be activated in liver disease and result in DIC.[105] Activation is postulated to result from necrosis of hepatocytes and release of tissue thromboplastin, inadequate clearance of already activated factors, and depressed levels of naturally occurring inhibitors produced in the liver such as antithrombin III. Intravascular coagulation results primarily in the consumption of factor II, factor V, factor VIII, factor XIII, and fibrinogen, as well as in the secondary activation of fibrinolysis and the generation of fibrin-split products that further inhibit the polymerization of fibrin, thus impairing clotting.

The occurrence of primary fibrinolysis in liver disease is controversial. Regardless of whether primary fibrinolysis occurs, fibrinolysis would lead to hypofibrinogenemia and high titers of fibrin-split products, both of which lead to impaired coagulation. Proposed mechanisms of primary fibrinolysis include reduced synthesis of antiplasmins and reduced clearance of plasminogen activators.

FACTOR DEFICIENCY: ACCELERATED FACTOR DESTRUCTION OR LOSS

Consumption. DIC is a syndrome of accelerated destruction or consumption of certain coagulation factors.[106] It involves the pathologic activation of

coagulation by an underlying disease process leading to fibrin-clot formation and secondary fibrinolysis and producing consumption of coagulation factors, platelets, and red cells. It may be clinically inapparent or it may be manifested by thrombosis, hemorrhage, or both, depending upon the degree of activation and compensatory efforts of the body. The fulminant syndrome is most often a life-threatening bleeding disorder. Bleeding results from the developing factor deficiency (primarily factor I, factor II, factor V, factor VIII, and factor XIII), thrombocytopenia, excessive fibrinolysis, and high levels of fibrin-split products superimposed upon a vascular system damaged by diffuse microvascular thrombi. Bleeding is typically manifested by diffuse, superficial hemorrhage in the form of ecchymoses and petechiae, as well as oozing from the gingiva and other areas of the oral mucosa, the gastrointestinal tract, and the urinary tract. Hemorrhage is classically from the microvasculature, but major vascular hemorrhage can occur as well. CNS bleeding, which is not unusual, can be fatal. The most common causes of DIC include gram-negative septicemias, certain malignancies, surgery, trauma, and obstetrical complications. Table 27-5 lists several other potential causes of DIC. The pathophysiology of DIC depends upon the underlying disease process or initiating event. The common underlying mechanism is activation of the extrinsic, intrinsic, or common pathway of coagulation (Fig. 27-7). In infections with gram-negative organisms, the lipopolysaccharide component of endotoxin can directly activate factor XII and the intrinsic pathway. More importantly, endotoxemia causes lysis and degranulation of granulocytes. Granulocytes release a substance with thromboplastic activity, initiating the extrinsic system of coagulation. This is the major pathway of intravascular coagulation in these infections.[107] Acute promyelocytic leukemia is the neoplasm most commonly associated with DIC. Lysis and release of a thromboplastic activity from promyelocytes is the cause of the intravascular coagulation.[108] Mucin-producing adenocarcinomas similarly release a thromboplastic substance (mucin) with a potential for activating the extrinsic system.[109] The pathophysiology of DIC in obstetrical complications is variable. Puerperal sepsis with a gram-negative organism initiates coagulation through endotoxin. Abnormalities of, or complications affecting, the placenta generally affect coagulation by releasing thromboplastic activity into the maternal circulation.

The diagnosis of DIC is complicated by the fact that the clinical manifestations range from none to an extensive thrombotic disease to a severe hemorrhagic disorder. Unless there are large vascular defects, bleeding is usually from the microvascular system and is generalized. The patient usually shows evidence of

Table 27-5. *Disorders Associated with Disseminated Intravascular Coagulation (DIC)*

Infection
  Gram-negative endotoxemia with hypotension or shock
  Severe gram-positive septicemia
  Rocky Mountain spotted fever
  Viral infections (herpes)
  Malaria (*Plasmodium falciparum*)
Complications of Pregnancy and Delivery
  Gram-negative sepsis
  Abruptio placentae
  Amniotic fluid embolism
  Retained dead fetus
  Toxemia
Pediatric Disorders (especially in newborn)
Malignant Diseases
  Metastatic carcinoma (prostate, pancreas, lung, stomach, colon, breast)
  Leukemia (especially acute promyelocytic leukemia)
Liver Diseases (cirrhosis)
Complications of Surgery
  Extracorporeal circulation
Critical Tissue Damage
  Brain tissue destruction
  Massive trauma
  Heat stroke
  Extensive burns
Miscellaneous
  Hemolytic transfusion reactions
  Vasculitis
  Aneurysms
  Giant hemangioma
  Snake bites

an underlying disorder known to predispose to DIC. The definitive diagnosis is established in the laboratory.

Factor consumption and high titers of fibrin(ogen) degradation products (FDP) that inhibit fibrin monomer polymerization produce prolongations of the PT, PTT, and TT, as well as measurably high FDP. Thrombocytopenia occurs as a result of platelet consumption on microvascular clots. Red blood cells are fragmented and lysed as a result of impact with intravascular fibrin strands, producing a microangiopathic hemolytic anemia with a low hemoglobin, high reticulocyte count, and signs of intravascular hemolysis. More sophisticated tests can be performed looking specifically for fibrin-monomer formation or activation of fibrinolysis, but are seldom necessary to confirm the diagnosis in clinically significant cases of DIC.

Fibrinolysis is often the result of the activation of the coagulation cascade and so can usually be considered a secondary phenomenon. Whether conditions exist that initiate fibrinolysis primarily is unclear, but there are conditions in which fibrinolysis is the major physiologic response.[110] In this situation, plasminogen is

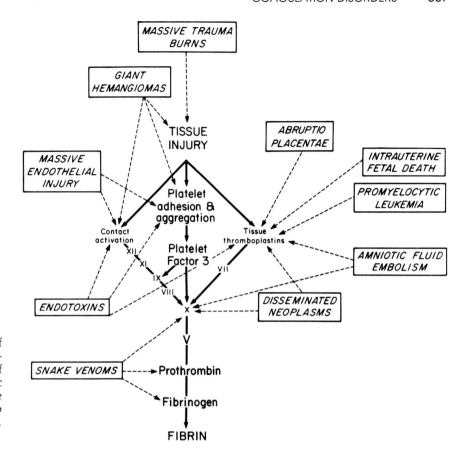

Fig. 27-7. The pathophysiology of DIC and points of initiation of coagulation or other mechanisms of hemostasis by multiple etiologic factors. (Reprinted from Wintrobe MM: *Clinical Hematology*, 8th ed, p 1216. Philadelphia, Lea & Febiger, 1981)

activated by plasminogen activators and plasmin enzymatically attacks fibrinogen, producing high levels of FDP. Low levels of fibrinogen and high titers of FDP cause a prolongation of the TT, PT, and PTT. Plasmin also destroys factor V and factor VIII, but other factors would be normal and fibrin monomer would not be detectable. Conditions under which primary fibrinolysis is said to occur include the existence of certain tumors such as carcinoma of the prostate, and extracorporeal open-heart surgery.[111,112]

Amyloidosis is occasionally associated with a coagulopathy due to factor-X deficiency. Investigators have shown by means of ^{131}I-labeled factor X that this factor is absorbed onto amyloid fibrils distributed throughout the vascular system.[48] Vascular fragility is also a potential cause for bleeding in amyloidosis.

Factor Loss. Isolated, acquired single-factor deficiencies have been described in patients with the nephrotic syndrome. Deficiency of factor IX or factor XII has been attributed to loss of the proenzyme in the urine along with the massive proteinuria that occurs with this disease.[113,114] More commonly, the nephrotic syndrome is associated with the loss of antithrombin III resulting

in reduced plasma levels.[115] It is presumed that this deficiency accounts for the high incidence of thrombosis in patients with nephrotic syndrome.

Dilutional Factor Loss. A mild bleeding tendency may be associated with massive blood transfusions, particularly when the amount of blood received is given over a short interval and approximates the patient's normal blood volume. Labile coagulation factors (V and VIII) and platelets do not survive long in stored blood and dilutional deficiencies of platelets and these labile coagulation factors may account for the hemorrhagic tendency.[116] However, patients receiving such large amounts of blood are often very ill and it is difficult to attribute bleeding to one etiology.

INHIBITORS (ANTICOAGULANTS)

Endogenous or spontaneously occurring pathologic inhibitors of coagulation may either be antibodies or soluble fragments of fibrinogen or fibrin that interfere with the coagulation of blood and can lead to a hemorrhagic disorder. Inhibitor antibodies function by direct neutralization of a specific coagulation factor or by reacting

with phospholipid and interfering with coagulation factor interaction. FDP interfere with the polymerization of fibrin monomer.

Antibodies to Specific Factors. Antibodies directed toward factor VIII are the most common neutralizing factor-specific antibodies. They occur in 10% to 20% of patients with hemophilia but may be found in nonhemophilic individuals with autoimmune disorders such as systemic lupus erythematosus and rheumatoid arthritis. These antibodies also occur in postpartum women and even in some elderly patients who lack a demonstrable underlying disease.[117] Factor VIII antibodies generally occur initially in hemophiliacs under 10 years of age, usually with severe disease, who have received multiple transfusions of factor-VIII-containing products. Why only some patients develop antibodies is unknown. It seems to occur as a random event and is not restricted to specific kindreds nor limited to only those few hemophiliacs who lack immunoreactive factor VIII (VIII_{ag}). The antibody is directed toward the coagulant moiety of the factor-VIII complex and its interaction is time- and temperature-dependent. The antibody is usually an IgG immunoglobulin and its heterogeneity is often more restricted in hemophiliacs than in nonhemophiliacs.

Factor-VIII antibodies most often have a strong affinity or neutralizing capacity, producing a hemorrhagic state equivalent to severe hemophilia. Weak antibodies are occasionally seen in hemophiliacs. Hemophiliacs with inhibitors typically respond to an infusion of factor VIII with a dramatic rise in inhibitor titer that effectively neutralizes any transfused factor VIII. These patients are notoriously difficult to treat when bleeding occurs because replacement therapy with factor VIII is ineffective. The diagnosis of factor-VIII antibody can be made on the basis of failure to respond to factor-VIII infusions or by various mixing experiments. More specific quantitative assays are also available.[118]

Factor-IX inhibitors are relatively less common compared to factor-VIII inhibitors, and occur in approximately 5% of patients with factor-IX deficiency. They have not been described in diseases other than hemophilia B. Inhibitors of fibrinogen, factor V, factor VII, factor XI, factor XII, and factor XIII, as well as vWF have been described much less frequently.[117] Streptomycin and isoniazid have been implicated in the etiology of inhibitors to factor V and factor XIII respectively.

Antibodies to Phospholipid. The other major variety of endogenous inhibitor is referred to as the *lupus inhibitor* and is present in as many as 10% of patients with systemic lupus erythematosus.[117,119] However, a similar inhibitor has now been demonstrated to occur in a number of other disease states, including other autoimmune disorders, various malignancies, and with certain drugs, particularly those known to produce a lupuslike syndrome (*e.g.,* procainamide, hydralazine, chlorpromazine). The inhibitor is an immunoglobulin, most often of the IgG class but occasionally of the IgM class. Its interference with coagulation is instantaneous and is not time-dependent as are factor-VIII antibodies. Investigations have shown it to inhibit various factors in the coagulation cascade, especially in the intrinsic and common pathways. However, most consistent findings favor the evidence that the antibody interacts with phospholipid and exerts its major influence on the interaction between activated factor X and factor II by interfering with their interaction with phospholipid.[120]

Interestingly, the *in vivo* significance of this inhibitor is minimal because patients generally do not manifest a bleeding tendency unless coexistent defects such as thrombocytopenia or other factor deficiencies are also present.

Dysproteinemias and FDP. Patients with multiple myeloma and other paraproteinemias have been found to have inhibitors attributable to the paraprotein.[117] They may act by absorption to fibrin monomer and interference with fibrin-monomer polymerization.[121] High concentrations of FDP as a result of plasmin digestion act as inhibitors of fibrin-monomer polymerization by binding to fibrin monomers and keeping them in solution.[122] They are a contributing factor to the hemorrhagic tendency in DIC.

SUMMARY

Faulty hemostatic mechanisms leading to pathologic bleeding usually imply a defect in the vascular, platelet, or coagulation phases of hemostasis. Vascular defects commonly result from deficient or abnormal vascular supporting structures. Platelet defects result from quantitative or qualitative abnormalities of platelets. Coagulation deficits occur when clotting factors are deficient or their activity is neutralized.

Specific laboratory tests can assess each phase of hemostasis as well as specific interactions within each system. Tests of vascular function are few and of limited value. The bleeding time assesses vascular competency but also reflects adequacy of platelet number and function. The platelet count directly measures quantitative abnormalities of platelets, and platelet aggregation studies distinguish various types of func-

tional defects. The prothrombin time, partial thromboplastin time, and thrombin time are general screening tests of the coagulation cascade.

Disorders of the vascular and platelet phase of hemostasis commonly result in subcutaneous hemorrhage characterized as petechiae and purpura, as well as bleeding from mucosal surfaces. Coagulation disorders also give rise to subcutaneous bleeding manifested as ecchymoses. Hemarthroses and mucosal bleeding may occur with coagulation defects as well.

Congenital or acquired hemorrhagic vascular disorders are generally uncommon and infrequently result in serious bleeding. Inherited platelet disorders are also uncommon, but acquired defects are seen quite often. Immune thrombocytopenias (*e.g.*, idiopathic or drug induced) or drug-induced megakaryocyte hypoplasia (*e.g.*, chemotherapy induced) are frequently responsible for major hemorrhagic problems. Drug-induced platelet dysfunction (*e.g.*, as a result of aspirin ingestion) is widespread and may result in bleeding, particularly after invasive procedures. Acquired coagulation disorders occur with great frequency in patients with other diseases (*e.g.*, disseminated intravascular coagulation, liver disease) and are frequently responsible for major hemorrhagic sequelae. Inherited coagulation disorders are less common, factor VIII deficiency (hemophilia) and von Willebrand's disease being the most frequent disorders encountered.

When confronted with a patient who is bleeding, one must determine whether or not there is an underlying hemostatic defect and, if so, what aspect of hemostasis is at fault. This knowledge will directly aid in making the correct therapeutic intervention. The clinical and laboratory assessment of the patient is essential in making this determination.

REFERENCES

1. **Tocantins LM:** The mechanism of hemostatis. Ann Surg 125:292–310, 1947

2. **Mason RG, Saba HI:** Normal and abnormal hemostasis. An integrated view. Am J Pathol 92:775–811, 1978

3. **Barnhart MI, Baechler CA:** Endothelial cell physiology, perturbations and responses. Semin Thromb Hemostas 5:50–86, 1978

4. **Pennington DG:** Thrombopoiesis. In Bloom AL, Thomas DP (eds): Haemostasis and Thrombosis, pp 1–21. New York, Churchill Livingstone, 1981

5. **White J:** Platelet morphology. In Johnson SA (ed): The Circulating Platelet, pp 45–121. New York, Academic Press, 1971

6. **White J:** Platelets and their role in hemostasis. Ann NY Acad Sci 201:205–233, 1972

7. **Niewiorowski S:** Platelet release reaction and secreted platelet proteins. In Blood AL, Thomas DP (eds): Haemostasis and Thrombosis, pp 73–83. New York, Churchill Livingstone, 1981

8. **White JG:** Interaction of membrane systems in blood platelets. Am J Pathol 66:295–312, 1972

9. **Michaeli D, Orloff KG:** Molecular considerations of platelet adhesion. Prog Hemost Thromb 3:29–59, 1976

10. **Tschopp TB, Weiss HJ, Baumgartner HR:** Decreased adhesion of platelets to subendothelium in von Willebrand's disease. J Lab Clin Med 83:296–300, 1971

11. **Shattil SJ, Bennett JS:** Platelets and their membranes in hemostasis: Physiology and pathophysiology. Ann Intern Med 94:108–118, 1980

12. **Holmsen H:** Are platelet shape change, aggregation and release tangible manifestations of one basic platelet function? In Baldini MG, Ebbe S (eds): Platelets, Production, Function, Transfusion and Storage, pp 207–220, New York, Grune & Stratton, 1974

13. **Hovig T:** The ultrastructural basis of platelet function. In Baldini MG, Ebbe S (eds): Platelets, Production, Function, Transfusion and Storage, pp 221–233. New York, Grune & Stratton, 1974

14. **Gerrard JM, White JG:** Prostaglandins and thromboxanes: "Middlemen" modulating platelet function in hemostasis and thrombosis. Prog Hemost Thromb 4:87–125, 1978

15. **Smith JB:** Involvement of prostaglandins in platelet aggregation and haemostasis. In Bloom AL, Thomas DP (eds): Haemostasis and Thrombosis, pp 61–72. New York, Churchill Livingstone, 1981

16. **Nalbandian RM, Henry RL:** Platelet-endothelial cell interactions: Metabolic maps of structure and actions of prostaglandins, prostacyclin, thromboxane and cyclic AMP. Semin Thromb Hemostas 5:87–111, 1978

17. **Moncada S, Gryglewski R, Bunting S et al:** An enzyme isolated from arteries transforms prostaglandin endoperoxides to an unstable substance that inhibits platelet aggregation. Nature 263:663–665, 1976

18. **Gorman RR, Bunting S, Miller OV:** Modulation of human platelet adenylate cyclase by prostacyclin (PGX). Prostaglandins 13:377–388, 1977

19. **Sutherland EW:** Studies on the mechanism of hormone action. Science 177:401–408, 1972

20. **Phillips DR:** An evaluation of membrane glycoproteins in platelet adhesion and aggregation. Prog Thromb Hemost 5:81–109, 1980

21. **Rosenberg RD:** Hypercoagulability and methods for monitoring anticoagulant therapy. In Fratantoni J, Wessler S (eds): Prophylactic Therapy of Deep Venous Thrombosis and Pulmonary Embolism, pp 28–42. Washington DC, USGPO, 1975 (DHEW Pub # (NIH) 76-866).

22. **Wintrobe MM:** Clinical Hematology, 8th ed, pp 405–452. Philadelphia, Lea & Febiger, 1981

23. **Jaffe EA, Hoyer LW, Nachman RL:** Synthesis of anti-

hemophilic factor by cultured human endothelial cells. J Clin Invest 52:2757–2764, 1973

24. **Suttie JW:** Oral anticoagulant therapy: The biosynthetic basis. Semin Hematol 14:365–374, 1977

25. **Munrano G:** A basic outline of blood coagulation. Semin Thromb Hemostas 6:140–162, 1980

26. **Osterud B, Rapaport SI:** Activation of ^{125}I-factor IX and ^{125}I-factor X: Effect of tissue factor and factor VII, factor X_a and thrombin. Scand J Haematol 24:213–226, 1980

27. **Griffin JH, Cochrane CG:** Recent advances in the understanding of contact activation reactions. Semin Thromb Hemostas 5:254–273, 1979

28. **Wintrobe MM:** Clinical Hematology, 8th ed, pp 405–452. Philadelphia, Lea & Febiger, 1981

29. **Rosenberg RD:** Actions and interactions of antithrombin and heparin. N Engl J Med 292:146–151, 1975

30. **Stenflo J:** A new vitamin K-dependent protein. J Biol Chem 251:355–363, 1976

31. **Esmon NL, Harris KW, Esmon CT:** The effect of thrombomodulin (Protein C activation cofactor) on the catalytic properties of thrombin. Blood (Suppl 1) 58:215a, 1981

32. **Marlar RA, Griffin JH:** Deficiency of protein C inhibitor in combined factor V/VIII deficiency disease. J Clin Invest 66:1186–1189, 1980

33. **Wintrobe MM:** Clinical Hematology, 8th ed, pp 432–434. Philadelphia, Lea & Febiger, 1981

34. **Deykin D:** The role of the liver in serum-induced hypercoagulability. J Clin Invest 45:256–263, 1966

35. **Wintrobe MM:** Clinical Hematology, 8th ed, pp 1050–1051. Philadelphia, Lea & Febiger, 1981

36. **Biggs R:** Human Blood Coagulation, Haemostasis and Thrombosis, 2nd ed. Oxford, Blackwell Scientific Publications, 1976

37. **Bloom AL, Thomas AL:** Haemostasis and Thrombosis. New York, Churchill Livingstone, 1981

38. **Kitchens CS:** The anatomical basis of purpura. Prog Hemost Thromb 5:211–244, 1980

39. **Burke M, Marks J:** Purpura associated with vomiting in pregnancy. Br Med J 1:488, 1973

40. **Pitt PW:** Purpura associated with vomiting. Br Med J 1:667, 1973

41. **Ackroyd JF:** Allergic purpura including purpura due to foods, drugs and infections. Am J Med 14:605–632, 1953

42. **Gaynor E, Bouvier C, Spaet TH:** Vascular lesions: Possible pathogenetic basis of the generalized Shwartzman reaction. Science 170:986–988, 1970

43. **Braverman IM, Yen A:** Demonstration of immune complexes in spontaneous and histamine-induced lesions and in normal skin of patients with leukocytoclastic angiitis. J Invest Dermatol 64:105–112, 1975

44. **Wintrobe MM:** Clinical Hematology, 8th ed, pp 1072–1077. Philadelphia, Lea & Febiger, 1981

45. **Bick RL:** Vascular disorders associated with thrombohemorrhagic phenomena. Semin Thromb Hemostas 5:167–183, 1979

46. **Wallerstein RO, Wallerstein RO, Jr:** Scurvy. Semin Hematol 13:211–218, 1976

47. **Feinstein RJ, Halprin KM, Penneys NS et al:** Senile purpura. Arch Dermatol 108:229–232, 1973

48. **Furie B, Green E, Furie BC:** Syndrome of acquired factor X deficiency and systemic amyloidosis. N Engl J Med 297:81–85, 1977

49. **Goodman TF, Abele DC, West CS:** Electron microscopy in the diagnosis of amyloidosis. Arch Dermatol 106:393–397, 1972

50. **Wintrobe MM:** Clinical Hematology, 8th ed, pp 1110–1111. Philadelphia, Lea & Febiger, 1981

51. **Hall JG, Levin J, Kuhn JP et al:** Thrombocytopenia with absent radius. Medicine 48:411–439, 1969

52. **Wintrobe MM:** Clinical Hematology, 8th ed, pp 1855–1882. Philadelphia, Lea & Febiger, 1981

53. **Post RM, Desforges JF:** Thrombocytopenia and alcoholism. Ann Intern Med 68:1230–1236, 1968

54. **Brodie GN, Bliss D, Firkin BG:** Thrombocytopenia and carcinoma. Br Med J 1:540–541, 1970

55. **Harker LA, Finch CA:** Thrombokinetics in man. J Clin Invest 48:963–974, 1969

56. **Karpatkin S:** Heterogeneity of human platelets. II. Functional evidence suggestive of young and old platelets. J Clin Invest 48:1083–1087, 1969

57. **Shulman NR:** A mechanism of cell destruction in individuals sensitized to foreign antigens and its implications in autoimmunity. Ann Intern Med 60:506–521, 1964

58. **Storck H, Hoigne R, Koller F:** Thrombocytes in allergic reactions. Int Arch Allergy Appl Immunol 6:372–384, 1955

59. **Dixon RH, Rosse WF:** Platelet antibody in autoimmune thrombocytopenia. Br J Haematol 31:129–134, 1975

60. **Gugliotta L, Isacchi G, Motta MR et al:** Chronic idiopathic thrombocytopenic purpura: ^{51}Cr platelet kinetics and splenectomy in 197 patients. Thromb Haemost 42:47, 1979

61. **Mueller–Eckhardt C:** Idiopathic thrombocytopenic purpura: Clinical and immunologic considerations. Semin Thromb Hemostas 3:125–159, 1977

62. **Difino SM, Lachant NA, Kirshner JJ et al:** Adult ITP: Clinical findings and response to therapy. Am J Med 69:430–442, 1980

63. **Mueller–Eckhardt C, Lechner K, Heinrich D et al:** Post-transfusion thrombocytopenic purpura: Immunological and clinical studies in two cases and review of the literature. Blut 40:249–257, 1980

64. **Clawson CC:** Platelet interaction with bacteria. Am J Pathol 70:449–462, 1973

65. **Kelton JG, Neame PB, Gauldie J et al:** Elevated platelet-associated IgG in the thrombocytopenia of septicemia. N Engl J Med 300:760–764, 1979

66. **Neame PB, Hirsh J, Browman G et al:** Thrombotic thrombocytopenic purpura: A syndrome of intravascular platelet consumption. Can Med Assoc J 114:1108–1112, 1976

67. **Ansell J, Beaser R, Pechet L:** Thrombotic thrombocytopenic purpura fails to respond to FFP infusion. Ann Intern Med 89:647–648, 1978

68. **Byrnes JJ, Khurana M:** Treatment of thrombotic thrombocytopenic purpura with plasma infusion. N Engl J Med 297:1386–1389, 1977

69. **Remuzzi G, Misiani R, Marchesi D et al:** Hemolytic-uremic syndrome: Deficiency of plasma factors regulating prostacyclin activity? Lancet 2:871–872, 1978

70. **Weiss H:** Congenital disorders of platelet function. Semin Hematol 17:228–241, 1980

71. **Malpass TW, Harker LA:** Acquired disorders of platelet function. Semin Hematol 17:242–258, 1980

72. **Weiss HJ, Tschopp TB, Baumgartner HR et al:** Decreased adhesion of giant (Bernard–Soulier) platelets to subendothelium: Further implications on the role of the von Willebrand factor in hemostasis. Am J Med 57:920–925, 1974

73. **Nurden AT, Caen JP:** The different glycoprotein abnormalities in thrombasthenic and Bernard–Soulier platelets. Semin Hematol 16:234–250, 1979

74. **Hardisty RM, Mills DCB, Ketsa–Ard K:** The platelet defect associated with albinism. Br J Haematol 23:679–692, 1972

75. **White JG:** Ultrastructural studies of the gray platelet syndrome. Am J Pathol 95:445–453, 1979

76. **Zahavi J, Marder VJ:** Acquired "storage pool disease" of platelets associated with circulating antiplatelet antibody. Am J Med 56:883–890, 1974

77. **Roth GJ, Stanford N, Majerus P:** Acetylation of prostaglandin synthetase by aspirin. Proc Natl Acad Sci USA 72:3073–3076, 1975

78. **Malmsten C, Hamberg M, Svensson J et al:** Physiological role of an endoperoxide in human platelets: Hemostatic defect due to platelet cyclo-oxygenase deficiency. Proc Natl Acad Sci USA 72:1446–1450, 1975

79. **Cardamone JM, Edson JR, McArthur JR et al:** Abnormalities of platelet function in the myeloproliferative disorders. JAMA 221:270–273, 1972

80. **Hardisty RM, Dormandy KM, Hutton RA:** Thrombasthenia. Br J Haematol 10:371–378, 1964

81. **Weiss HJ, Vicic WJ, Lages BA et al:** Isolated deficiency of platelet coagulant activity. Am J Med 67:206–213, 1979

82. **Hoyer LW:** The factor VIII complex. Structure and function. Blood 58:1–13, 1981

83. **Bloom AL, Peake IR:** Factor VIII and its inherited disorders. Br Med Bull 33:219–224, 1977

84. **Meyer D, Obert B, Pietu G et al:** Multimeric structure of factor VIII/von Willebrand factor in von Willebrand's disease. J Lab Clin Med 95:590–602, 1980

85. **Patek AJ, Taylor FHC:** Hemophilia II: Some properties of a substance obtained from normal human plasma effective in accelerating the coagulation of hemophilic blood. J Clin Invest 16:113–124, 1937

86. **Biggs R, Douglas AS, MacFarlane RG et al:** Christmas disease: A condition previously mistaken for hemophilia. Br Med J 2:1378–1382, 1952

87. **Pechet L, Tiarks CY, Stevens J et al:** Relationship of factor IX antigen and coagulant in hemophilia B patients and carriers. Thromb Hemost 40:465–477, 1978

88. **Green D:** Hemophilia and von Willebrand's disease: Genetic considerations. Ann Clin Lab Sci 10:123–127, 1980

89. **Levine PH, Britten AFH:** Supervised patient-management of hemophilia. Ann Intern Med 78:195–201, 1973

90. **Penner JA, Kelly PE:** Management of patients with factor VIII or IX inhibitors. Semin Thromb Hemostas 1:386–399, 1975

91. **Sjamsoedin LJM, Heijnen L, Mauser–Bunschoten EP et al:** The effect of activated prothrombin complex concentrates (FEIBA) on joint and muscle bleeding in patients with hemophilia A and antibodies to factor VIII. N Engl J Med 305:717–721, 1981

92. **Willebrand EA, von:** Hereditare pseudohemofili. Finska Lakaresallsabits Handlingar 67:7–12, 1926

93. **Alexander B, Goldstein R:** Dual hemostatic defect in pseudohemophilia. J Clin Invest 32:551, 1953

94. **Gralnick HR, Coller BS, Sultan Y:** Studies of the human factor VIII/von Willebrand factor protein: III Qualitative defect in von Willebrand's disease. J Clin Invest 56:814–827, 1975

95. **Ruggeri ZM, Pareti FI, Mannucci PM et al:** Heightened interaction between platelets and factor VIII/von Willebrand factor in a new subtype of von Willebrand's disease. N Engl J Med 302:1047–1051, 1980

96. **Ahr D, Rickles FR, Hoyer LW et al:** von Willebrand's disease and hemorrhagic telangiectasia: Association of two complex disorders of hemostasis resulting in life threatening hemorrhage. Am J Med 62:452–458, 1977

97. **Bloom AL:** Inherited disorders of blood coagulation. In Bloom AL, Thomas DS (eds): Haemostasis and Thrombosis, pp 321–370. New York, Churchill Livingstone, 1981

98. **Wintrobe MM:** Clinical Hematology, 8th ed, pp 1158–1205. Philadelphia, Lea & Febiger, 1981

99. **Soff GA, Levin J:** Familial multiple coagulation factor deficiencies. Semin Thromb Hemostas 7:112–148, 1981

100. **Esmon CT, Sadowski JA, Suttie JW:** A new carboxylation reaction. The vitamin K-dependent incorporation of $H^{14}Co_3^-$ into prothrombin. J Biol Chem 250:4744–4748, 1975

101. **Ansell JE, Kumar R, Deykin D:** The spectrum of vitamin K deficiency. JAMA 238:40–42, 1977

102. **Sutherland JM, Glueck HI, Gleser G:** Hemorrhagic disease of the newborn. Am J Dis Child 113:524–533, 1967

103. **Lechner K, Niessner H, Thaler E:** Coagulation abnormalities in liver disease. Semin Thromb Hemostas 4:40–56, 1977

104. **Palascak JE, Martinez J:** Dysfibrinogenemia associated with liver disease. J Clin Invest 60:89–95, 1977

105. **Straub PW:** Diffuse intravascular coagulation in liver disease. Semin Thromb Hemostas 4:29–39, 1977

106. **Muller–Berghaus G:** Pathophysiology of generalized intravascular coagulation. Semin Thromb Hemostas 4:209–246, 1977

107. **Horn RG, Collins RD:** Studies on the pathogenesis of the generalized Shwartzman reaction: The role of granulocytes. Lab Invest 18:101–107, 1968

108. **Gralnick HR, Abrell E:** Studies of the procoagulant and fibrinolytic activity of promyelocytes in acute promyelocytic leukemia. Br J Haematol 24:89–99, 1973

109. **Pineo GF, Regorczi F, Hatton MWC et al:** The activation of coagulation by extracts of mucin: A possible pathway of intravascular coagulation accompanying adenocarcinomas. J Lab Clin Med 82:255–266, 1973

110. **Kwaan HC:** Disorders of fibrinolysis. Med Clin North Am 56:163–176, 1972

111. **Bick RL:** Alterations of hemostasis associated with cardiopulmonary bypass: Pathophysiology, prevention, diagnosis and management. Semin Thromb Hemostas 3:59–82, 1976

112. **Tagnon HJ, Schulman P, Whitmore WF et al:** Prostatic fibrinolysin. Am J Med 15:875–884, 1953

113. **Natelson EA, Lynch EC, Hettig RA et al:** Acquired factor IX deficiency in the nephrotic syndrome. Ann Intern Med 73:373–378, 1970

114. **Honig GR, Lindley A:** Deficiency of Hageman factor (factor XII) in patients with the nephrotic syndrome. J Pediatr 78:633–637, 1971

115. **Kauffmann RH, Veltkamp JJ, van Tilburg NH et al:** Acquired antithrombin III deficiency and thrombosis in the nephrotic syndrome. Am J Med 65:607–613, 1978

116. **Ingram GIC:** The bleeding complications of blood transfusion. Transfusion 5:1–5, 1965

117. **Shapiro SS, Hultin M:** Acquired inhibitors to the blood coagulation factors. Semin Thromb Hemostas 1:336–385, 1975

118. **Kasper C:** A more uniform measurement of factor VIII inhibitors. Thrombosis et Diathesis Haemorrhagica 34:869–872, 1975

119. **Schleider MA, Nachman RL, Jaffe EA et al:** A clinical study of the lupus anticoagulant. Blood 48:499–509, 1976

120. **Thiagarajan P, Shapiro SS, DeMarco L:** Monoclonal immunoglobulin M lambda coagulation inhibitor with phospholipid specificity. J Clin Invest 66:397–405, 1980

121. **Coleman M, Vigliano EM, Weksler ME et al:** Inhibition of fibrin monomer polymerization by lambda myeloma globulins. Blood 39:210–223, 1972

122. **Fletcher AP, Alkjaersig N, Sherry S:** Pathogenesis of the coagulation defect developing during pathological plasma proteolytic ("fibrinolytic") states. I. The significance of fibrinogen proteolysis and circulating fibrinogen breakdown products. J Clin Invest 41:896–913, 1962

28

Anemia, Weakness, and Pallor

Sanford J. Shattil
Richard A. Cooper

Structure, Function, and Life Span of Normal
    Human Red Blood Cells
The Signs and Symptoms of Anemia
  General Considerations
  Constitutional Symptoms
  Cardiovascular System
  Gastrointestinal System
  Genitourinary System
  Neurologic System
  Constitutional Signs
Pathophysiology of the Anemias
  Classification of Anemias
Anemias Resulting from Decreased Red Cell
    Production
  Anemias Resulting from Defective Proliferation of
    Red Cells
    Erythropoietin Lack
    The Anemia of Chronic Inflammatory Disease
      and Malignancy
    Marrow Disease

    Myelophthisic Anemias
    Iron-Deficiency Anemia
  Anemias Resulting from Defective Maturation of
    Red Cells
    Megaloblastic Anemias
    Sideroblastic Anemias
    Thalassemia Syndromes
Hemolytic Anemias
  General Considerations
  Extrinsic Causes of Hemolysis
    Splenomegaly
    Red Cell Antibodies
    Microangiopathic Hemolysis
    Toxins
  Membrane Defects (Acquired)
  Membrane Defects (Hereditary)
  Intrinsic Causes of Hemolysis
    Enzyme Defects
    Hemoglobinopathies
Summary

Anemia is a reduction in the oxygen-carrying capacity of the blood due to an abnormality in the quantity or quality of the red blood cells. In the great majority of cases, anemia involves a reduction in the quantity of hemoglobin and the volume of packed erythrocytes in a given volume of whole blood. This is usually due to a reduction in the total circulating hemoglobin mass, but may also result from an expansion of plasma volume (dilutional anemia). In certain conditions, such as methemoglobinemia and carboxyhemoglobinemia, the concentration of hemoglobin in the blood is normal but it is in a chemical form that will not transport oxygen (O_2).

It is important to emphasize that the normal ranges of red-cell count, hemoglobin concentration, and hematocrit are considerably greater than is generally appreciated. Normal values vary with age and sex (Fig. 28-1). In adults, the normal range of hemoglobin is approximately 14 g/dl to 18 g/dl for men and 12 g/dl to 16 g/dl for women. When a patient's hemoglobin con-

563

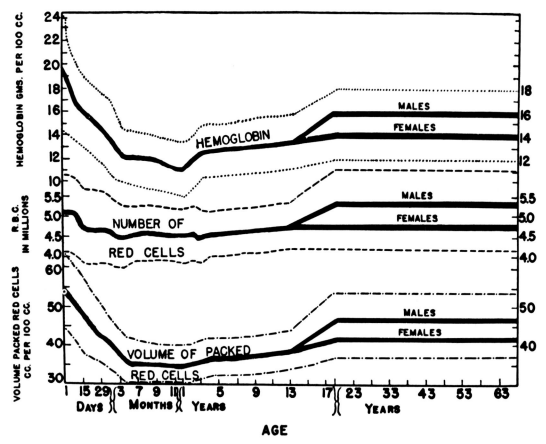

Fig. 28-1. Normal curve for hemoglobin concentration, red blood cell count, and volume of packed red cells from birth to old age. The mean values are heavily outlined, and the range of variation is indicated by dotted lines for hemoglobin, interrupted lines for red blood cell count, and dotted interrupted lines for volume of packed red cells. The scales for hemoglobin, red blood cell count, and volume of packed red cells are similar, and therefore the relative changes in these three values are apparent on inspection. The scale for age, however, is progressively altered. (From Wintrobe M: The Erythrocyte. In Wintrobe M (ed): Clinical Hematology, 6th ed, p. 91. Philadelphia, Lea and Febiger, 1967)

centration is in the uncertain area between normal and abnormal, it is helpful to secure previous values obtained over a period of years to determine whether a specific value is normal for a given patient.

STRUCTURE, FUNCTION, AND LIFE SPAN OF NORMAL HUMAN RED BLOOD CELLS

Red-Cell Membrane. The mature red cell is nonnucleated and made up of a plasma membrane and cytoplasm. The red-cell membrane contains approximately 50% protein, 40% lipid, and 10% carbohydrate.[1] The predominant membrane lipids are phospholipid and cholesterol, which appear to exist primarily in a bilayer structure. Membrane proteins are associated with the lipid bilayer to various degrees. Some are located only on the inside surface of the membrane, while others traverse the bilayer partially or completely.[2] The fluidity of the lipid bilayer and the mobility of membrane proteins appear important for normal membrane function.[3,4]

Normal red cells are approximately 7.5 μ in diameter and have the shape of biconcave discs. It is an excess of membrane relative to cytoplasmic volume and the viscoelastic properties of the membrane itself that allow the red cell to deform markedly during its sojourn in the circulation.[5] In fact, in order for red cells to enter the venous sinuses of the spleen, they are required to deform to less than one third of their normal diame-

ter.[6] Other functions of the red-cell membrane include glucose and ion transport; the regulation of intracellular ion content in turn maintains the constancy of intracellular water.[7] In addition, glycoproteins carry the A, B, M, N, and other surface antigens.[8]

Red-Cell Cytoplasm. The cytoplasm contains water and electrolytes in appropriate proportions to support the functions of intracellular enzymes and hemoglobin. Most cytoplasmic enzymes are part of either the Embden-Meyerhof (glycolytic) pathway, which produces adenosine triphosphate (ATP), or the hexose-monophosphate shunt, which generates NADPH, which is necessary for the maintenance of globin in the reduced state. Glutathione (GSH) serves as a reservoir of reducing substance capable of buffering transient oxidant threats, thereby affording further protection to globin.

The primary function of the red cell is delegated to the hemoglobin molecule and involves the transport of O_2 from the lungs to its sites of utilization in the tissues. In addition, much of the carbon dioxide (CO_2) formed during metabolism in tissues is carried by the red cell to its site of excretion in the lungs.[9] Normal adult hemoglobin consists of 4 polypeptide globin chains, 2 α-chains, and 2 β-chains. Each is associated with a heme group. Each polypeptide chain is arranged in a precise three-dimensional relationship to the other polypeptide chains, and each is capable of binding 1 molecule of O_2.[10] Therefore, 1 hemoglobin tetramer is capable of binding 4 molecules of O_2. The ability of a single hemoglobin monomer that has already bound an O_2 molecule to influence the molecular configuration and O_2-binding properties of the remaining heme groups (heme–heme interaction) accounts for the sigmoidal shape of the hemoglobin O_2 dissociation curve.[11] At the high partial-pressure of O_2 (pO_2) in the pulmonary capillaries (about 100 torr), oxyhemoglobin

predominates and the uptake of O_2 by the red cell is facilitated. In contrast, at the lower pO_2 on the venous side of capillaries (about 40 torr), deoxyhemoglobin predominates and O_2 release to the tissues is facilitated. The O_2 affinity of hemoglobin at any given pO_2 is further modulated by both pH and the red-cell content of 2,3-diphosphoglyceric acid (2,3-DPG) and the partial pressure of CO_2 (Fig. 28-2).[12,13]

Red-Cell Life Span. The earliest recognizable red-blood-cell precursor in the bone marrow undergoes approximately 3 mitotic divisions over a period of 3 or 4 days in the process of developing into a reticulocyte. The bulk of hemoglobin is synthesized during this time. Red-cell production is stimulated by the hormone erythropoietin, a glycoprotein that is derived from the action of humoral *renal-erythropoietic factor* on an $\alpha2$-globulin-plasma substrate.[14] Elevated blood levels of erythropoietin are detectable in most anemias, except those secondary to renal, inflammatory, and malignant diseases.

It is thought that 10% to 15% of the developing red blood cells in the bone marrow of normal healthy persons disintegrate without ever reaching maturity (ineffective erythropoiesis). In pernicious anemia, thalassemia, and certain other anemias, the degree of ineffective erythropoiesis is much greater, leading to hyperbilirubinemia. The serum level of the enzyme lactic dehydrogenase (LDH) correlates well with the severity of ineffective erythropoiesis.[15] When released from the marrow, many red blood cells are at the reticulocyte stage of development, but some of the cells lose their reticular substance prior to release. The reticular substance stains with supravital dyes and serves to identify reticulocytes on peripheral blood smears. Under conditions of greatly increased erythropoiesis, the release of reticulocytes is accelerated, and the percentage of reticulocytes in the peripheral blood roughly paral-

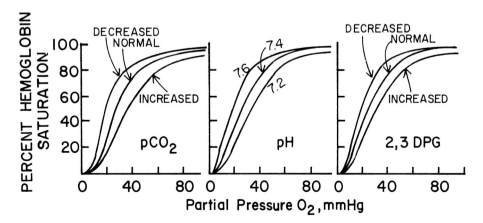

Fig. 28-2. The relationship between percent hemoglobin saturation and the partial pressure of oxygen as influenced by changes in the partial pressure of carbon dioxide (*left*), pH (*middle*) and red cell content of 2,3 DPG (*right*).

lels the rate of red-blood-cell production.[16] Some reticulocytes stain basophilic with Wright's stain as a result of retained RNA (polychromatophilia).

The life span of normal red cells in the circulation is approximately 120 days. Therefore 1/120, or 0.8%, of the total red-blood-cell mass is broken down and must be replaced each day. As erythrocytes age, the concentration of certain vital enzymes decreases and other changes occur, such as the loss of membrane lipids and sialic acid.[17,18] However, the sequence of events whereby senescent red cells are removed from the circulation is unclear.

THE SIGNS AND SYMPTOMS OF ANEMIA

GENERAL CONSIDERATIONS

Deficiency in the O_2-carrying capacity of blood may result in disturbances in the function of many organs and tissues. These disturbances may lead to a variety of symptoms. The complaints vary from patient to patient, as do the rapidity of development of the anemia and its severity. In general, an anemia of slow and insidious onset is surprisingly well tolerated by young, otherwise healthy persons, and there may be no symptoms whatever until the hemoglobin concentration and the hematocrit fall to levels below 50% of normal. The anemic person may first seek medical attention, not because he has any complaints, but because friends have commented upon his pale appearance. In contrast, when anemia is of rapid onset, dyspnea and palpitations may occur when the hemoglobin and hematocrit values are considerably above 50% of normal. When blood loss from the intravascular space is sudden or very severe, shock may ensue as a result of a decrease in O_2-carrying capacity and a decrease in intravascular volume.

Anemia itself may cause certain signs and symptoms, but other unrelated diseases often play an important part in determining the degree of anemia required to precipitate symptoms. For example, a patient with asymptomatic coronary atherosclerosis may first have chest pain when anemia further decreases O_2 delivery and produces myocardial ischemia.

A second group of signs and symptoms is caused by the effect of anemia on the various organs. This is discussed in the next section. Reference has already been made to the fact that anemia may precipitate angina. In certain circumstances, the sudden onset of a severe anemia may be the immediate precipitating cause of infarction of the myocardium, brain, or bowel.

A third group of signs and symptoms is not caused by the anemia itself, but rather is related to the etiology of the anemia. In pernicious anemia, vitamin-B_{12} deficiency results in anemia, but also gives rise to soreness of the tongue, numbness and tingling of the extremities, and diarrhea. Hypothyroidism is often associated with a mild to moderate reduction in hemoglobin concentration, but symptoms such as hoarseness, constipation, cold intolerance, and hypermenorrhea are due solely to the lack of thyroid hormone.

The pathophysiology of the symptoms and signs occurring in association with various types of anemia are discussed below. Under each symptom or sign, emphasis is placed on whether the clinical manifestation is due to the anemia itself, to the underlying deficiency or disease responsible for the anemia, or to aggravation by the anemia of some unrelated disorder.

CONSTITUTIONAL SYMPTOMS

Weakness and Fatigue. There is a widely held misconception that anemia is the most common cause of weakness and fatigue. Many patients have moderately severe anemia without any weakness or fatigue and, conversely, weakness and fatigue may be due to a variety of causes, prominent among which are boredom, depression, and anxiety (see Chap. 29 on nervousness and fatigue). Although an adult with moderately severe anemia may not complain of weakness or fatigue at rest, exercise intolerance is often present. In children, however, even severe anemia may be associated with very little decrease in exercise tolerance.[19]

Apathy and Lassitude. The anemic patient sometimes shows a lack of interest in his surroundings and a diminished enthusiasm for work. Although anemia is not the most common cause of apathy and lassitude, these symptoms do occur in association with moderate to severe anemia. Their pathogenesis is not clear. However, no close correlation exists between these symptoms and the degree of anemia, and it would seem that psychologic mechanisms contribute to the development of these complaints in some cases.

Pallor and Skin Changes. *Pallor* refers to an abnormally pale appearance of the patient. Although pallor may be manifest on examining the skin, it can be misleading because there is a wide normal variability in skin color because of individual differences in the size and depth below the skin surface of the small skin blood vessels. Thus, some individuals with normal blood counts may appear pale, whereas others with similar blood values may appear plethoric. Hence, a change in skin color may be more important than the absolute shade. There is less normal variation in the color of mucous membranes, and the physician can estimate the degree of anemia more accurately by examining the

conjunctivae, buccal mucosa, pharynx, and lips. The color of the fingernail bed is also more reliable than skin color in diagnosing anemia. It is common practice to inspect the hands for pallor. As the hemoglobin level drops, the palms become pale first, but the creases of the palms become pale only with severe anemia. Inspection of the palms, although a more reliable index of anemia than examination of other parts of the skin, is valid only if the hands are warm and held at the level of heart. Cold hands may appear pale because of vasoconstriction.

A light, lemon-yellow tint to the skin is characteristic of severe, untreated pernicious anemia and is due to mild hyperbilirubinemia plus pallor. The severe anemia resulting from acute hemorrhage gives rise to a very white, waxy appearance of the skin. With more chronic blood loss, the skin color is sallow. Pallor is often severe in leukemia and it has been stated that the skin may have a greyish tint.

Nails become brittle in severe, long-standing iron-deficiency anemia, and koilonychia (concave rather than convex nails) may occur.[20] Thinning and premature greying of the hair may occur in pernicious anemia.

Chronic ulcers around the ankles occur in association with various blood dyscrasias, but particularly in sickle-cell anemia and other chronic hemolytic anemias.[21,22] The leg ulcers in sickle-cell anemia are probably due to a combination of factors. Occlusion of small vessels and the anemia itself lower the O_2 tension in the areas where the circulation is normally sluggish. The lowered O_2 tension then further aggravates the situation by causing an increase in the viscosity of the sickle-cell blood.

CARDIOVASCULAR SYSTEM

Cardiovascular Adaptations to Anemia. Cardiovascular symptoms and signs in anemic patients may be considered either secondary to the adaptive physiological responses of the cardiovascular system to anemia or secondary to aggravation of pre-existing cardiovascular disease. Whatever their cause, the presence of symptoms and signs in a given person is determined by several factors including the severity of the anemia, the speed with which it has occurred, the patient's age, and the functional status of the heart and peripheral vessels.

Anemia evokes compensatory changes within the red blood cell, the heart, and the peripheral vasculature. A relationship exists between the degree of anemia and a decrease in the affinity of hemoglobin for O_2.[23] The decrease in O_2 affinity is mediated by intracellular organic phosphates, the most prevalent being 2,3-DPG. The 2,3-DPG levels in red cells appear to be regulated by many factors, but *pH* may be the most important.[24] There is a cavity in the center of the hemoglobin molecule into which 2,3-DPG fits, where it stabilizes the molecule in the deoxy form. This decreases the affinity of hemoglobin for O_2 and results in a shift of the hemoglobin-O_2 dissociation curve to the right (see Fig. 28-2). Thus, at any given pO_2, the hemoglobin in a given volume of blood is less saturated with O_2. This facilitates the release of O_2 at the tissue level, where O_2 tension is low. This intraerythrocytic response to anemia occurs within hours and is also observed in acute or chronic hypoxemia.[25,26] Quantitatively, it appears to be a major mechanism for increasing O_2 supply to tissues in anemia and may therefore lessen the magnitude of the cardiovascular adaptation that must occur.

Blood volume in anemia is not significantly different from normal blood volume; however, it is increased if congestive failure supervenes and decreased if acute blood loss occurs.[27] There is a redistribution of blood in anemia, resulting from variations in the degree of constriction of small blood vessels. This brings about a proportionately greater distribution of blood to the organs that are most sensitive to O_2 deprivation, with less blood going to organs that can better tolerate decreased blood flow. For example, in severe anemia, the blood flow to the hands and kidneys may decrease, whereas blood flow to the heart, muscles, and brain are increased.[28,29] Systolic blood pressure may be unaffected, but diastolic pressure may be lower than normal and pulse pressure may therefore be increased.[30]

Resting cardiac output is usually normal in patients with mild anemia, but cardiac output increases with exercise more than in nonanemic persons.[31] As the anemia becomes more severe, resting cardiac output increases. This is brought about by increases in stroke volume and heart rate and may be related to decreased blood viscosity in anemia and to decreased peripheral resistance.[32] The adrenal glands, sympathetic nervous system, or increased cardiac-filling pressure appear to be unnecessary, and the precise explanation for increased cardiac output in anemia is unknown.[33] Nonetheless, the net effect of cardiac-adaptive efforts is an increased blood flow to tissues, resulting in a decreased extraction of O_2 from a given volume of blood and a decreased arteriovenous O_2 difference.[34]

That cardiac output must increase in anemia is evident from a consideration of the relationship of cardiac output to O_2 consumption and to the arteriovenous-O_2 difference. Cardiac output is directly related to O_2 consumption and inversely related to arteriovenous O_2 difference.[35] The O_2-carrying capacity of blood is determined by the hemoglobin content because 1 g of hemoglobin will combine with 1.34 ml of O_2. Thus, the O_2 content of normal arterial blood is about 20% of the

blood volume. At venous pO_2, the hemoglobin is less saturated with O_2, and the venous O_2 content is about 15% of blood volume. Thus, the normal arteriovenous-O_2 difference is about 5% blood volume. However, in anemia, the total O_2 content of arterial blood is reduced due to the reduction in hemoglobin content, and the arteriovenous-O_2 difference is decreased. In order for O_2 consumption to remain normal in the face of a reduced arteriovenous-O_2 difference, cardiac output must increase.

Cardiovascular Symptoms and Signs. Most otherwise healthy patients who have mild or moderate anemia have no cardiorespiratory symptoms at rest, although they may have diminished exercise tolerance. As anemia becomes more severe, exercise tolerance progressively decreases until finally dyspnea, tachycardia, and palpitations are present even at rest and without superimposed congestive heart failure.[28] Dyspnea correlates with a decrease in vital capacity, and minute ventilation is increased.[36,37] Palpitations are evidently the subjective counterparts of increased stroke volume and heart rate. When anemia is due to acute blood loss, additional symptoms of postural dizziness and syncope are indicative of intravascular volume depletion.

Most cardiovascular signs in anemia can be accounted for by the increased velocity of blood in various areas of the circulation brought about by increased cardiac output and decreased peripheral resistance. Tachycardia, increased pulse pressure, bounding peripheral pulses, and an increased cardiac impulse all indicate a high-cardiac-output state. *Bruits* are sometimes heard bilaterally over the carotid arteries in association with severe anemia when there are no diseases of the arteries.[38] The continuous sound of a venous hum may be heard on auscultation over the jugular vein, particularly on the right side with the patient sitting.[39] This may be a normal finding in children, and is seen in other high-cardiac-output states as well.

Heart murmurs are common in association with severe anemia and those caused by blood abnormalities are called *hemic murmurs.* They occur most commonly at the apex, but almost as frequently at the pulmonic area; occasionally, the murmur may be audible over the whole precordium, but in this circumstance it tends to be loudest in the apical or pulmonic areas.[40] The functional murmur of anemia is almost always early to mid-systolic in time and the aortic second sound is normal. However, diastolic murmurs are rarely heard in patients with severe chronic anemia without organic heart disease.[41] The diastolic murmur may be mid-diastolic or pre-systolic and may be best heard at the apex, thus simulating the murmur of mitral stenosis.

The classical systolic murmur heard in association with moderate to severe anemia has been attributed to the increased velocity and turbulence of blood of low viscosity passing through a normal pulmonic valve. This has been referred to as a *systolic flow murmur.* Another mechanism of production of systolic murmurs in severely anemic patients is ventricular dilatation resulting in insufficiency of the mitral or tricuspid valve apparatus.[42] The rare diastolic murmurs heard in association with very severe anemia have been attributed to greatly increased blood flow across the mitral or tricuspid valves. Both the systolic and diastolic murmurs tend to disappear when the anemia is relieved.

Electrocardiographic Changes. Mild anemia does not produce any electrocardiographic abnormalities. When electrocardiographic changes do occur, they usually signify underlying heart disease. However, in one study, 11 of 100 patients with severe anemia due to various causes had electrocardiographic changes that did not appear to be due to associated cardiac disease or hypokalemia. The most common abnormalities are S–T segment depression, and flattening or depression of the T waves.[40,43] These changes are presumably attributable to myocardial hypoxia. Similar changes have been observed in anemia resulting from acute blood loss.[44] Other changes including low voltage of the QRS complexes and prolongation of the P–R interval have been noted occasionally. The electrocardiographic findings usually return to normal when the anemia is corrected.[45]

Sickle-Cell Anemia. The cardiovascular disturbances that are observed in association with the sickle-cell anemia deserve special mention. Homozygous sickle-cell disease is one of the few disorders in which the anemia is consistently severe enough that in nearly every case cardiac symptoms eventually develop. Furthermore, sickle-cell anemia is often accompanied by loud cardiac murmurs and signs and symptoms such as aching pains in the joints and elsewhere, which may lead to an incorrect diagnosis of acute rheumatic fever or subacute bacterial endocarditis. Multiple occlusions of small pulmonary arteries may be so extensive that pulmonary hypertension develops, leading eventually to cor pulmonale.[46,47]

Congestive Heart Failure. Congestive heart failure, angina pectoris, and myocardial infarction are cardiovascular events that are almost always related to underlying cardiac disease and are only aggravated or precipitated by anemia. Dyspnea on exertion, palpitations, tachycardia, cardiomegaly, and edema may all occur in anemia without concomitant congestive heart failure.[28,48] The diagnosis of cardiac decompensation is justified clinically only if the patient also has orthopnea, pulmonary rales, third heart sounds, or distended

neck veins signifying increased right-sided venous pressure.

When frank congestive heart failure does develop in an anemic individual, the possibility of underlying organic heart disease should be considered. There may be unsuspected coronary artery disease; or a murmur, considered to be hemic in origin, may actually be due to rheumatic heart disease. With increasingly severe anemia, however, compensatory physiologic adjustments may fail to maintain the circulation, and congestive failure may occasionally occur in the absence of organic heart disease.[49] High-output congestive failure may also be seen in thyrotoxicosis, beri–beri heart disease, and with systemic arteriovenous fistulas.

Myocardial Infarction. A patient with fairly marked atherosclerosis of the coronary arteries may be able to maintain reasonably normal circulatory dynamics for a considerable period of time. However, the sudden development of acute blood-loss anemia, or even acute hemolytic anemia, may lower the O_2 tension in the myocardium below a critical level with resultant myocardial infarction. In this situation, the sudden development of anemia is an important contributory cause of myocardial infarction. Anemia alone probably never causes myocardial infarction in patients with an otherwise normal heart.

GASTROINTESTINAL SYSTEM

A great variety of gastrointestinal symptoms commonly occur in conditions characterized by anemia. These symptoms may be due directly to the anemia, or may be the result of a deficiency state that simultaneously affects the hematopoietic organs and the gastrointestinal tract. They may potentiate the anemia by interfering with proper nutrition. The symptoms include sore mouth, a sore tongue, dysphagia, anorexia, abdominal distention and flatulence, nausea, vomiting, diarrhea or constipation.

Almost any part of the digestive system may be involved. Recurrent episodes of sore tongue (glossitis) are common in cases of untreated pernicious anemia. During these episodes, the patient may complain of marked soreness or actual pain in the tongue. The tongue appears beefy red either over its whole dorsum or in a patchy distribution. Occasionally, vesicles or small white ulcers simulating aphthous stomatitis may appear. Rarely, the patient may complain of burning of the entire mouth and pharynx and even pain on swallowing. The glossitis tends to subside spontaneously in the absence of treatment, only to recur again. With the passage of time, the epithelium of the tongue becomes smooth and, upon examination with a magnifying glass, it is seen to be devoid of papillae. These atrophic changes develop even in patients who have never had any soreness of the tongue. Adequate therapy usually results in partial restoration of the papillae.[50]

The primary defect of pernicious anemia is lack of secretion of intrinsic factor by the gastric mucosa, associated with atrophy of the gastric mucosa. Although the prominence of some of the gastrointestinal symptoms in pernicious anemia may be the result of gastric atrophy, most of the symptoms are due to the effects of vitamin-B_{12} deficiency.

Cheilosis and glossitis are common in association with chronic iron-deficiency anemia and can be relieved by iron therapy.[51] Dysphagia, which is the outstanding symptom in the Plummer–Vinson's syndrome, has also been attributed to iron deficiency.[52] However, cheilosis, glossitis, and dysphagia are rare in East Africans with severe iron deficiency.[53]

Ulcerated and necrotic lesions may be seen in the mouth, the pharynx, the rectum, and the vagina in association with severe granulocytopenia such as that seen in aplastic anemia, acute leukemia, or drug-induced agranulocytosis. Although their etiology is unclear, examination of such lesions at necropsy usually shows acute and chronic inflammation, necrosis, and, in leukemia, infiltration with leukemic cells.

GENITOURINARY SYSTEM

Menstrual disturbances are common in association with anemia. The most common disturbance is amenorrhea, but menorrhagia also occurs and may be severe. Anemia in a man may lead to loss of libido. The pathogenesis of these symptoms has not been defined.

Sickle-cell trait may be associated with microscopic or gross hematuria, in part due to necrosis of the renal papillae.[54] In addition, isosthenuria is a constant feature of both sickle-cell trait and sickle-cell disease and is probably due to damage resulting from sickling within the renal medulla.

It has been shown that effective renal blood flow is markedly reduced in chronic anemia, presumably as a result of constriction of afferent glomerular arterioles.[55] Tubular excretion may also be significantly reduced in chronic anemia. Nonetheless, when overt renal insufficiency and azotemia occur in the anemic patient, the physician must consider either a disease that causes both anemia and azotemia (*i.e.,* multiple myeloma) or an intrinsic renal disease unrelated to the anemia.

NEUROLOGIC SYSTEM

Headache (often pounding in character), fainting, dimness of vision, tinnitus, vertigo, irritability, restlessness, inability to concentrate, and drowsiness are all

common in association with severe anemia. Presumably, these symptoms are due to hypoxia of the nervous system, and thus are attributable to the anemia itself.

Papilledema in association with severe, chronic blood-loss anemia has been reported.[56] Retinal hemorrhages are seen frequently in severely anemic patients with leukemia, aplastic anemia, and pernicious anemia. Thrombocytopenia and hemorrhagic diathesis occur in many of these conditions and these, plus a direct effect of anemia on capillary permeability, account for the hemorrhages.[57] The retinal hemorrhages may be of almost any type.[58]

The neurologic manifestations of pernicious anemia are not due solely to the anemia; they may appear in the absence of significant anemia. Indeed, paresthesias may be the first clinical manifestation of pernicious anemia. Vitamin B_{12} is apparently essential to the maintenance of normal nervous tissue metabolism, and vitamin-B_{12} deficiency due to any cause may lead to degeneration of the dorsal and lateral columns of the spinal cord, and even to degenerative changes in the peripheral nerves and in the brain itself. However, the pathogenesis of these pathologic changes is not clear.

Symptoms referable to the nervous system occurred in from 70% to 95% of cases of pernicious anemia, according to reports published prior to 1935.[59,60,61] In 25% of cases, the neurologic manifestations occurred prior to the development of recognized anemia. Because effective therapy and much better diagnostic tests for pernicious anemia have come into general use, the frequency of severe neurologic manifestations has markedly decreased.[62] The earliest neurologic symptoms of pernicious anemia are paresthesias in the extremities and difficulty in walking. The earliest physical signs are first, loss of vibratory sense, and next, loss of position sense in the distal portions of the extremities. There may be impaired touch sensation, but pain and temperature sensation usually remain intact. Ataxia, Romberg's sign, decreased or increased deep tendon reflexes, Babinski's sign, muscle flaccidity or spasticity, and sphincteric disturbances may occur as the degenerative process in the spinal cord progresses. Visual disturbances and optic atrophy occasionally occur. Peripheral nerve degeneration occurs and may be responsible in part for the numbness as well as the rare instances of stocking hypoesthesia and hyperesthesia of the soles of the feet.

Numerous neurologic manifestations occur in association with sickle-cell anemia, including headache, convulsions, drowsiness, stupor, coma, aphasia, hemiplegia, stiff neck, nystagmus, pupillary changes, blindness, cranial nerve palsies, and paresthesias.[63] It is likely that these manifestations are due to impairment of circulation to the nervous system resulting from sickling of red blood cells.

CONSTITUTIONAL SIGNS

Fever. Fever in hematologic disease is almost always secondary to infection. However, it may be seen in the absence of infection in chronic myelogenous leukemia and severe pernicious anemia.[64,65] Acute hemolytic anemia, such as that seen with the transfusion of incompatible blood, may be accompanied by symptoms suggesting an acute infection, such as malaise, headache, severe aching pain in the back, extremities, or abdomen, and chills and fever. In extreme cases, prostration and shock may develop.

Splenomegaly, Hepatomegaly and Lymph Node Enlargement. These physical signs are not due solely to anemia, but are often encountered in disorders characterized by anemia. The spleen, the liver, and the lymph nodes are commonly enlarged, firm, and non-tender in the leukemias and malignant lymphomas. The enlargement is usually due to direct involvement of these organs by the neoplastic cells. Splenomegaly is an essential feature of chronic congestive splenomegaly (Banti's syndrome). In this syndrome, the liver may or may not be enlarged, and there is usually an associated leukopenia and thrombocytopenia. Splenomegaly commonly occurs in chronic hemolytic states due to the "work hypertrophy" related to the processing of dying red cells.[66] Minimal enlargement of the spleen also occurs in severe pernicious anemia and iron-deficiency anemia, possibly because, in their most severe forms, both are associated with a hemolytic component. Splenomegaly is more common in children with iron deficiency than in adults, and it appears that the incidence in adults is far more rare than suggested by an early, often quoted report.[67] In sickle-cell anemia, the spleen is enlarged early in life, but later undergoes multiple infarctions, fibrosis, and shrinkage so that at autopsy it often weighs less than 50 g.[68] Splenomegaly persisting into adult life is common in many other hemoglobinopathies, and also in the thalassemias. If an adult patient has significant splenomegaly and sickle cells are seen in the blood smear, the most likely diagnosis is that the patient is doubly heterozygous for hemoglobin S (HgS) and another abnormal hemoglobin (often HgC), or thalassemia.

Localized bone tenderness unrelated to trauma and not accompanied by spontaneous bone pain, is an important physical sign that often indicates acute leukemia. This sign is most readily elicited by moderate pressure over the sternum. It is present less commonly in patients with myelophthisic anemia due to metastatic cancer invading the bone marrow.

Jaundice. When jaundice occurs in association with anemia, it may be due either to a hemolytic process, in which case there is increased production of biliru-

bin, or to a disease in the hepatobiliary system, in which case there is either decreased hepatic conjugation or hepatobiliary excretion of bilirubin.

Most hemolytic anemias are characterized by red-blood-cell destruction in the spleen and other reticuloendothelial organs. The reticuloendothelial cells in which red cells are destroyed are the same cells in which hemoglobin pigment is converted to bilirubin. However, in hemolytic anemias in which red cells are primarily destroyed in the circulation (such as paroxysmal nocturnal hemoglobinuria) free hemoglobin is released into the plasma, where its fate depends on the rate of hemolysis.[17]

In mild intravascular hemolysis, plasma hemoglobin becomes bound to an α2 globulin, haptoglobin, and this complex is cleared from the circulation rapidly (in minutes) by reticuloendothelial cells. This also results in depletion of serum haptoglobin. In addition, free hemoglobin in the plasma may be oxidized irreversibly to methemoglobin. The oxidized heme (ferriheme) moiety of methemoglobin transfers from globin to albumin or to *hemopexin*, a heme-binding protein found normally in plasma.[69] The ferriheme–hemopexin complex is cleared from the circulation by hepatocytes with a half-time (T½) of 7 to 8 hours, whereas methemalbumin is cleared more slowly (T½ of 20 hours). The end result of all these processes is clearance of free hemoglobin from plasma and its subsequent conversion to bilirubin. If hemolysis is chronic, the pigment-binding proteins of plasma become depleted and hemoglobin αβ dimers, which are more stable in solution than tetramers, enter the glomerular filtrate.[70] Hemoglobin is reabsorbed by renal tubular cells in which globin and porphyrin are rapidly catabolized and the heme iron enters a storage form, hemosiderin. Tubular cells are eventually shed into the urine and the presence of hemosiderin in the urinary sediment serves as a sensitive diagnostic test for chronic intravascular hemolysis. If the capacity of the tubular cells for hemoglobin is exceeded, as in severe or acute hemolysis, hemoglobinuria may ensue. This results in a positive "dipstick" for blood in the urine. Free hemoglobin in the urine must be differentiated from hematuria (red blood cells in the urine) and from myoglobinuria.[71]

In hemolytic anemias, bilirubin is present in the serum primarily in the form of unconjugated, or indirect-reacting, bilirubin, a form that is not excreted by the kidney. In the absence of liver disease, icterus is mild (bilirubin <5 mg/dl) owing to the great capacity of the normal liver to handle an increased bilirubin load.[72] Unconjugated bilirubin enters hepatocytes where it is conjugated with glucuronic acid and excreted in the bile. Intestinal bacteria convert bilirubin to urobilinogen, some of which is reabsorbed from the intestine and excreted into the urine. Thus, fecal- and urine-urobilinogen content are increased, but bile in the urine (*choluria*) is not usually observed in hemolysis.

PATHOPHYSIOLOGY OF THE ANEMIAS

CLASSIFICATION OF ANEMIAS

Anemias may be classified in several ways. For example, they may be categorized by their morphology on peripheral blood smears on the basis of red-cell size (normal size termed *normocytic*; large size termed *macrocytic*; small size termed *microcytic*), by their degree of hemoglobinization (normal is termed *normochromic*; decreased is termed *hypochromic*), or by their shape (target cell, sickle cell, fragmented red cell, and so on). An ideal classification would be based upon specific etiology; however, the precise cause of many anemias is unknown. The classification of anemias suggested by Hillman and Finch and based on data derived from ferrokinetics and erythrokinetics is particularly useful as a diagnostic approach to the anemic patient.[73] Such a classification appears in Table 28-1, which also lists etiologic examples and a description of typical red-cell morphology associated with the various disease entities. Anemias are classified broadly into those due to decreased red-cell production or those due to increased destruction (hemolysis) or loss (hemorrhage) of red cells. In most clinical situations, all that is required in order to classify an anemia pathogenetically is a knowledge of the reticulocyte count, an analysis of the degree of marrow erythroid cellularity, and a stool guiac or other test for gastrointestinal blood loss. Thus, anemia associated with a decreased reticulocyte count must be due to decreased production of red cells. Furthermore, if the erythroid marrow is hypocellular, there is a defective proliferation (or division) of red-cell precursors. On the other hand, if the reticulocyte count is decreased but the erythroid marrow is hypercellular, then there is defective maturation of red-cell precursors such that they proliferate normally but do not mature normally. As a result, these red cells die in the marrow before entering the peripheral circulation. This is also known as ineffective erythropoiesis. If the reticulocyte count is increased and the anemia does not improve with time, then the problem is either increased destruction (hemolysis) of red cells or loss of red cells from the circulation (acute blood loss). In either case, the erythroid marrow is hypercellular, reflecting increased effective erythropoiesis. Serial stool tests for occult blood will confirm or exclude gastrointestinal blood loss in this situation. Once a patient's anemia is classified, a specific etiologic diagnosis can usually be made with the aid of data from the patient's history, physical examination, and peripheral blood smear. If

Table 28-1. *Pathophysiologic Classification of Anemias*

Classification	Examples	Red Cell Morphology
I. Decreased Red Cell Production		
A. Defects of Proliferation		
1. Erythropoietin lack	Renal failure	Normochromic, normocytic, burr cell
2. Erythropoietin lack or diminished marrow responsiveness	Starvation, hypothyroidism, anemia of chronic inflammatory disease and malignancy	Normochromic, normocytic or slightly hypochromic
3. Marrow disease	Aplastic anemia, myelophthisic (neoplasia, granulomas)	Normochromic, normocytic, tear-drop red cells, leukoerythroblastic
4. Iron deficiency	Iron-deficiency anemia	Hypochromic, microcytic
B. Defects of Maturation		
1. Defective nuclear maturation		Macrocytic (oval)
a) B_{12} deficiency	Pernicious anemia	
b) Folate deficiency	Poor dietary intake	
c) Other	Cytotoxic drugs, preleukemia	
2. Defective cytoplasmic maturation		
a) Thalassemia syndromes	α-thalassemia, β-thalassemia	Hypochromic, microcytic, target-shaped cells, bizarre shapes
b) Sideroblastic anemias	Congenital	Hypochromic, microcytic
	Acquired: idiopathic, secondary (alcohol, lead, leukemias, etc.)	Hypochromic, microcytic, or macrocytic
II. Increased Red Cell Destruction (Hemolysis)		Polychromatophilia
A. Extrinsic Causes		
1. Splenomegaly	Congestive splenomegaly	Normal or rare spherocytes
2. Antibody mediated		
a) Alloantibodies	Hemolytic transfusion reactions	Spherocytes
b) Warm antibody type	Idiopathic,	Spherocytes
	lymphoma,	Spherocytes
	systemic lupus erythematosus	Spherocytes
c) Drug related		
Autoimmune	Aldomet	Spherocytes
Haptenic	Penicillin	Spherocytes
Immune complex	Quinine	Normal (some with spherocytes)
d) Cold antibody type		
Cold agglutinins	Idiopathic, lymphoma, mycoplasma pneumonia	Normal, occasional spherocytes
Paroxysmal cold hemoglobinuria	Syphilis, infectious mononucleosis	Normal
3. Trauma		
a) External impact	March hemoglobinuria	Normal
b) Cardiac hemolysis	Aortic valve prosthesis	Fragments (schistocytes)
c) Fibrin deposition	Disseminated intravascular coagulation	Fragments (schistocytes)
4. Toxins	Clostridial sepsis,	Spherocytes
	burns	Fragments, budding
B. Membrane Abnormalities	Spur-cell anemia	Spur cells (Acanthocytes)
	Paroxysmal nocturnal hemoglobinuria	Normal
	Hereditary spherocytosis	Spherocytes
	Elliptocytosis	Elliptocytes
	Abetalipoproteinemia	Acanthocytes
	Stomatocytosis	Stomatocytes
C. Intrinsic Causes		
1. Enzyme defects		
a) Glycolytic	Pyruvate kinase deficiency	Rare crenated cells
b) HMP Shunt	G6PD deficiency	"Bite" cells
2. Hemoglobinopathies	Sickle-cell anemia,	Sickle cells
	unstable hemoglobins	Heinz bodies
III. Red Cell Loss	Acute blood loss anemia	Polychromatophilia

572

the etiology is still obscure, special tests chosen on the basis of the existing data base can be ordered.

ANEMIAS RESULTING FROM DECREASED RED CELL PRODUCTION

ANEMIAS RESULTING FROM DEFECTIVE PROLIFERATION OF RED CELLS

The entry of stem cells into the committed erythroid marrow pool and the subsequent proliferation (cell division) of erythroid precursors is dependent upon (1) a normal level of erythropoietin, (2) a normal marrow environment capable of supporting erythropoiesis, and (3) an adequate supply of iron.[74] Abnormalities of any of these results in defective red-cell proliferation.

Erythropoietin Lack

This is a major cause of anemia in patients with chronic renal failure. It is usually irreversible and is presumably caused by damage to those parts of the kidney that normally sense tissue hypoxia or that produce the renal erythropoietic factor.[14] The degree of azotemia correlates poorly with the degree of anemia, although most individuals with a blood-urea nitrogen over 100 mg/dl have a hematocrit of less than 30%.[75] Although quantitatively less important, other etiologic types of anemia commonly occur in the patient with chronic renal disease. Iron deficiency, folic-acid deficiency, and a relative marrow unresponsiveness to erythropoietin may each contribute to the degree of anemia and are important to diagnose because iron and folate deficiency respond to replacement therapy and marrow unresponsiveness may improve with chronic hemodialysis.[76,77] The anemia of chronic disease may be operative in chronic pyelonephritis. Hemolysis due to red-cell fragmentation may occur with renal vasculitides or with thrombotic thrombocytopenic purpura or disseminated intravascular coagulation. Mild hemolysis without red-cell fragmentation is frequent in chronic renal failure and its etiology is unclear. Hemolysis is more prominent in acute renal failure and in general the anemia improves if other renal functions improve.[78] Crenated red cells (burr cells) as commonly seen in acute or chronic renal failure are caused by a nondialyzeable substance in uremic plasma.[79] Their relation to hemolysis is unclear. The kidney is not the only source of erythropoietic factor; erythropoietin production continues in nephrectomized patients, albeit at markedly reduced levels, and is responsive to hypoxic stimulae.[80] Erythropoietin lack or diminished marrow re-

sponsiveness to erythropoietin are believed to be operative in the anemias associated with endocrinopathies (such as hypothyroidism, hyperthyroidism, Addison's disease), and starvation and protein malnutrition.

The Anemia of Chronic Inflammatory Disease and Malignancy

Persons with chronic infections, chronic inflammatory diseases (such as rheumatoid arthritis), and malignancy often demonstrate a mild to moderate anemia with a depressed reticulocyte count.[81] This is seen in patients with malignancy even when other obvious causes of anemia, such as neoplastic invasion of the bone marrow or gastrointestinal blood loss, are excluded. Red-cell production is decreased and red-cell life span is mildly reduced. The pathogenesis of this type of anemia is unclear but in many cases is associated with reduced plasma levels of erythropoietin, or defective release of iron from reticuloendothelial stores.[82,83,84]

Marrow Disease

Aplasia rarely involves only marrow erythroid elements (pure red-cell aplasia). In some patients this is associated with thymoma, lymphomas, or certain drugs, but in most it is idiopathic.[85] Serum antibodies against erythroblast nuclei have been demonstrated in some patients.[86] More commonly, aplastic anemia involves all blood elements, resulting in pancytopenia in the peripheral blood associated with marrow aplasia on bone marrow aspiration and biopsy. Aplastic anemia may be idiopathic, or may be associated with drugs such as the antibiotic, chloramphenicol, the anti-inflammatory agent, phenylbutazone, or with chemicals such as benzene.[87] The pathogenesis of marrow failure due to drugs or chemicals is not well understood.[88] Chloramphenicol produces two types of marrow suppression. The first is a toxic suppression that is dose-related and occurs in any patient receiving large doses of the drug for more than 7 to 10 days. This type is associated with vacuolization of blood-cell precursors, and occasionally with ringed sideroblasts in the marrow. It is reversible upon discontinuation of the drug.[89] On the other hand, 1 out of 10,000 patients taking chloramphenicol develops irreversible aplastic anemia and this idiosyncratic aplasia is unpredictable, not related to dose, and may occur months after the drug has been taken. A minority of patients with aplastic anemia of any etiology recover adequate marrow function, even when the offending agent is known and removed from the individual's environment. Death may result from hemorrhage due to thrombocytopenia or from infection due to neutropenia.[90]

Myelophthisic Anemias

Myelophthisic anemias are those associated with invasion of the marrow by carcinoma or hematologic malignancies (leukemia, myeloma), nonneoplastic granulomas, as in miliary tuberculosis, or fibrosis, as in myelofibrosis with myeloid metaplasia. The anemia is due in part to simple replacement of normal marrow by disease tissue, but its pathogenesis may be more complex. It is frequently associated with a leukoerythroblastic peripheral blood smear consisting of teardrop red cells, nucleated red cells and immature myeloid cells.

Iron-Deficiency Anemia

Iron deficiency is probably the most common cause of anemia in nontropical countries, and it usually responds rapidly to oral iron therapy. An understanding of the mechanism of production of the iron deficiency is crucial because only be removing or correcting the underlying cause can recurrence be prevented.

Extensive ferrokinetic studies utilizing radio-iron have vastly increased knowledge concerning iron metabolism.[91,92,93] Some of the more important features are presented schematically in Figure 28-3. Food iron, present mostly in the ferric state, is reduced in the stomach and upper intestine to the ferrous form. Absorption is most efficient in the duodenum, and decreases progressively as food moves caudally. The intestine plays an important role in adjusting the amount of iron that is absorbed. The amount of iron varies in accordance with the needs of the body. A current concept is that the amount of iron stored as ferritin in the columnar epithelial cells of the small intestine regulates the amount of iron absorption. When there is little or no ferritin in the mucosal cells, iron is rapidly transported across the cells and delivered into the capillaries. In the normal state, the mucosal cell contains

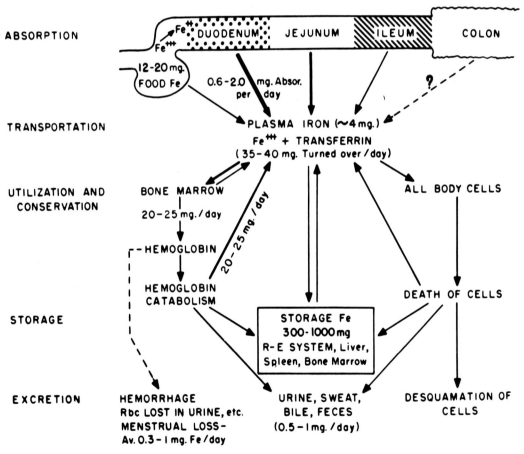

Fig. 28-3. Schematic outline of iron metabolism in the human adult. (Moore CV: Iron deficiency anemia. In Beeson PB, McDermott WB: Cecil–Loeb Textbook of Medicine, 12th ed. Philadelphia, WB Saunders, 1967)

iron (as ferritin) supplied from the body stores. This minimizes transport of iron from the gut to the capillaries. The ferritin in a mucosal cell is lost into the gut when the cell sloughs on reaching senescence.[94] Iron absorption is enhanced in iron-deficiency states and it is minimal when the serum iron is normal.

Iron is transported in the blood bound to transferrin, which is a β_1 globulin. The total amount of transferrin, or total iron-binding capacity of normal adults is usually between 300 mcg/dl and 360 mcg/dl, with an extreme normal range of 250 mcg/dl to 400 mcg/dl. Normally, about one third of the transferrin is bound to iron. The total amount of iron in the body of an adult man is 3 g to 5 g, of which approximately 55% is in hemoglobin, 25% in storage depots, 15% in myoglobin, and the remainder in tissue (cytochrome) enzymes. Only the hemoglobin iron and the storage iron are available for synthesis of new hemoglobin.

There is a striking conservation of iron by the body. The amount of iron lost from the healthy human body through desquamated skin and intestinal mucosa, sweat, urine, and bile is between 0.5 mg and 1 mg per day. There are 12 mg to 20 mg of iron in the normal adult diet in the United States (or about 6 mg/1000 calories) of which approximately 5% to 10% is absorbed. If one averages these figures, the mean amount of iron absorbed per day is about 1.2 mg, only slightly more than the normal daily loss. Normal menstrual blood loss varies from 25 ml to 60 ml, or about 10 mg to 30 mg of iron per menstrual period, which, if distributed over the entire month, would amount to between 0.35 mg and 1 mg per day. Pregnancy places a further heavy, but variable, strain on the ability of the mother to maintain iron balance. Iron is required for the fetus and for the milk if the baby is nursed. This means that 30 mg to 170 mg are lost in the placenta and cord as well as an estimated 90 mg to 310 mg loss owing to hemorrhage at the time of delivery. It has been estimated that 9 months of pregnancy plus 6 months of lactation would increase the total iron loss for this period by an average of 1 mg to 2.5 mg per day over the above basal losses.

From these data it is apparent that in adult males there is a modest favorable iron balance, whereas in infants and women during the menstrual and reproductive years, the balance is very precarious indeed. The ability of the intestinal mucosal cells to transport more iron into the blood when the serum iron begins to fall prevents hypochromic microcytic anemia from developing more often than it does. However, any protracted excessive menstrual blood loss can be expected to exhaust the iron stores eventually.

The time required for hypochromic microcytic anemia to develop is dependent on the amount and duration of blood loss and on the adequacy of iron stores in the body. Reserve iron is stored primarily in reticuloendothelial cells, mainly in the liver, spleen, and bone marrow. The total iron in storage depots is less in women than in men, and averages about 300 mg to 1000 mg. This is readily available, and equals the normal iron loss over a period of 1 to 5 years, which explains the long delay required for hypochromic microcytic anemia to develop when iron loss due to bleeding is only slightly in excess of iron absorption.

The most common causes of iron-deficiency anemia are excessive menstrual bleeding and chronic gastrointestinal hemorrhage. If excessive menstrual bleeding and multiple pregnancies can be excluded, and careful questioning fails to uncover any history of known blood loss, a gastrointestinal neoplasm or other source of chronic occult gastrointestinal blood loss should be considered. Innumerable lesions other than tumors can cause occult, as well as frank, chronic blood loss from the gastrointestinal tract, including esophageal varices, peptic ulcer, diverticulosis, intestinal parasitic infestation, regional enteritis, ulcerative colitis, vascular malformations, and hemorrhoids.

Less common causes of iron-deficiency anemia are improper diet (including diets low in iron content and diets that contain substances that interfere with iron absorption), and impaired absorption due to gastrointestinal disease. In order for iron deficiency to develop because of a low iron content in the diet, the diet must be grossly deficient and very low in animal protein. The constant eating of clay, particularly by women and children, is common among economically deprived people. Clay reduces iron absorption by chelating the metal, or precipitating it as insoluble compounds in the gut. Phytates and phosphates (in cereals) also convert iron into insoluble compounds.

Mechanisms contributing to reduced iron absorption include specific abnormalities of the small intestinal mucosa which are associated with reduced iron absorption (celiac disease, nontropical sprue), and absence of gastric acid (gastrectomy, atrophic gastritis with achlorhydria) which interferes with absorption of iron from some foods but not others.

In chronic iron deficiency anemia, the red blood cells are microcytic and hypochromic, the leukocyte level is normal, and the platelet count is normal or increased.[95] The serum bilirubin is normal or reduced, and the fecal urobilinogen is reduced. The serum iron level is below normal (i.e., less than 40 g/dl), the plasma iron-binding capacity is elevated, and transferrin, the iron-binding protein, is less than 15% saturated. The serum ferritin level is below normal. Bone marrow slides stained with special iron stains show an absence of iron in normoblasts and reticuloendothelial cells.

ANEMIAS RESULTING FROM DEFECTIVE MATURATION OF RED CELLS

Megaloblastic Anemias

Macrocytes are red cells with an increased mean corpuscular volume (MCV). They may be seen in either of 2 hematologic situations, reticulocytosis and megaloblastic anemias. Reticulocytes are round, have a larger internal volume than mature red cells and often are polychromatophilic on Wright's stained blood smears. Therefore, an increase in the percentage of reticulocytes in the blood due to acute blood loss or hemolysis, or during the recovery phase of any underproduction anemia may result in an increased MCV. In contrast, in the megaloblastic anemias, the mature red cell is often macrocytic and oval, and the MCV is increased roughly in proportion to the severity of the anemia.[96] Macrocytes must be distinguished from target cells which are seen in liver diseases or after splenectomy.[97] Although target cells appear large on blood smear, their MCV is normal and their appearance is due to increased membrane surface area.[98] Moreover, target cells survive normally in the circulation and their presence alone is not associated with anemia.

Ninety-five percent of megaloblastic anemias are due either to vitamin-B$_{12}$ or folic-acid deficiency. Less common causes include preleukemia and erythroleukemia, various cancer chemotherapeutic agents that affect DNA synthesis, and several very rare inherited disorders of DNA synthesis.[99,100]

Certain pathophysiological features are common to all megaloblastic anemias. Pancytopenia is often present and there is ineffective production of neutrophils and platelets, as well as of red cells. The peripheral blood smear is characterized by hypersegmentation of polymorphonuclear leukocytes and oval macrocytes. When anemia is severe, bizarre red-cell fragments, red cells with Howell-Jolly bodies, and nucleated red cells are seen. The most important and fundamental biochemical abnormality in both vitamin-B$_{12}$ and folic-acid deficiency is a block in nuclear DNA synthesis, whereas RNA synthesis appears to be normal.[101] This leads to the characteristic megaloblastic changes in the bone marrow, that include defective maturation of the nuclei of erythroid and myeloid precursors associated with reasonably normal maturation of the cytoplasm (nuclear-cytoplasmic dissociation). Similar morphologic changes are seen in other cells as well, including the gastrointestinal and vaginal mucosa. It should be emphasized that the metabolic cause of the neurologic abnormalities in pernicious anemia is unknown, but appears unrelated to the defect in DNA synthesis. Kinetic studies with radioactive iron reveal a rapid transit of injected iron to the marrow and increased incorporation of label into erythroid precursors, but decreased entry of red cells into the circulation.[102] Thus, an increased proportion of megaloblastic red-cell precursors die before leaving the marrow (ineffective erythropoiesis) and this increased but ineffective turnover accounts for the decreased reticulocyte count in the peripheral blood and increased levels of LDH and indirect bilirubin commonly seen in these disorders. Moreover, red cells which do enter the circulation have a reduced life span.

Specific Diseases Causing Vitamin-B$_{12}$ Deficiency. Vitamin-B$_{12}$ absorption requires binding of the ingested vitamin to intrinsic factor, a substance from gastric parietal cells, and the binding of this complex to mucosal cells of the distal ileum. The vitamin is ubiquitous in nature and there are sufficient stores in the human liver to last several years. Thus, dietary vitamin-B$_{12}$ deficiency is extraordinarily rare.[103] However, deficiency of vitamin B$_{12}$ may occur because intrinsic factor is lacking, as in pernicious anemia, after total gastrectomy, or because of diseases of the small intestine. Small intestinal diseases cause vitamin-B$_{12}$ deficiency by 2 mechanisms. First, bacterial, or parasitic, overgrowth and utilization of B$_{12}$ by the microorganisms occur with the blind loop syndrome, jejunal diverticulae, and disorders of intestinal motility or fish tape worm infestation. Second, diseases of the distal ileum (ileitis, ileal resection) may destroy the normal mucosal absorptive sites for vitamin B$_{12}$. Finally, a partial deficiency in vitamin-B$_{12}$ absorption may occur with chronic pancreatic insufficiency.[104] Vitamin-B$_{12}$ deficiency in the pediatric age group, although rare, may be due to classic pernicious anemia, to an inherited selective lack of intrinsic factor, or to selective ileal malabsorption of vitamin B$_{12}$.[105,106]

Pernicious anemia is the most common cause of vitamin-B$_{12}$ deficiency. It occurs most commonly in late adult life owing to a lack of intrinsic factor associated with atrophic gastritis. Inasmuch as gastric parietal cells also secrete hydrochloric acid, achlorhydria is a constant feature of pernicious anemia. The etiology and pathogenesis of the gastric disease is unknown, but genetic and immunologic phenomena are believed to be important.[107] In fact, antibodies to parietal cells and intrinsic factor are commonly found in the serum or gastric fluid of these patients.[108] An increased incidence of autoimmune thyroid disease is seen in patients with pernicious anemia and their families.[109]

Symptoms and signs of anemia are often late in appearance because of the anemia's insidious progression. Other clinical features of vitamin-B$_{12}$ deficiency include glossitis with a smooth, beefy-red tongue, anorexia, and diarrhea. The associated neurologic abnormality, subacute, combined degeneration of the spinal cord, initially involves the dorsal columns with pares-

thesia and diminished vibratory sensation. In more advanced cases ataxia and lateral column involvement occur, with paresis, spasticity, and Babinski signs. Impaired memory, disturbances of consciousness, and even psychoses are reported. All of these disturbances are reversible with parenteral vitamin-B$_{12}$ therapy, although neurologic deficits may not improve, particularly if present for a long period of time prior to therapy. In contrast, folic-acid therapy reverses most manifestations of pernicious anemia, but will not prevent progression of the neurologic disease.[110]

Specific Diseases Causing Folic-Acid Deficiency. Body stores of folic acid are small in comparison to the mean daily requirement of the vitamin; therefore, decreased dietary intake of the vitamin, the most common cause of folic-acid deficiency, results in megaloblastic anemia within 3 to 4 months.[111,112] Simultaneous ingestion of alcohol appears to accelerate this process.[113] Folic acid is absorbed predominantly in the jejunum. Intestinal disorders that affect large areas of this portion of the small intestine, such as non-tropical sprue and tropical sprue, are often associated with megaloblastic anemia.[114] Drug induced malabsorption of folate has been implicated in the occasional folic-acid-deficiency anemia associated with chronic intake of diphenylhydantoin or oral contraceptives, but other mechanisms may also be possible.[115,116] In addition, dietary folate lack is usually an etiologic factor in these cases. Increased folic-acid utilization occurs physiologically in infancy and pregnancy as well as in chronic hemolytic anemias.[117] Megaloblastic anemia may occur unless folate supplements are taken.

In any patient with megaloblastic anemia, it is crucial that the differentiation between folic-acid deficiency and vitamin-B$_{12}$ deficiency be made so that appropriate therapy is instituted and a rational approach is taken to delineate the precise cause of the deficiency. To this end, various laboratory tests are available, such as measurements of the concentration of vitamin-B$_{12}$ or folate in the serum or red cells, and the Schilling test, which allows differentiation of the gastric and intestinal causes of vitamin-B$_{12}$ deficiency. A rational sequence for the use of these tests has been recently reviewed.[118]

Sideroblastic Anemias

These are a heterogenous group of disorders that have in common the presence of ringed sideroblasts in the marrow. These are nucleated red cells with nonhemoglobin iron within the mitochondria. Prussian-blue staining of the marrow reveals iron (ferritin) arranged in a ring around the erythroid nucleus. The pathogenesis of ringed sideroblasts is unknown and may differ among the disease entities associated with these cells.

Inasmuch as iron normally combines with protoporphyrin to form heme, a defect in heme synthesis has been suspected, though none has been consistently demonstrated. Nonetheless, defective incorporation of iron into hemoglobin results in ineffective erythropoiesis and a hypochromic, microcytic anemia of variable severity. In some cases, particularly those acquired, a dimorphic red-cell morphology (microcytes and macrocytes) is present. Sideroblastic anemias may be hereditary (primarily sex-linked) or acquired.[119,120] The acquired forms may be idiopathic or associated with a number of other diseases, including alcoholism, drugs such as isoniazid and chloramphenicol, lead intoxication, and hematologic malignancies (leukemia, myeloma). A rare acquired form, pyridoxine-responsive anemia, responds completely to pharmacologic doses of pyridoxine.[121] All of the sideroblastic anemias are chronic, except those in which the offending agent (alcohol, drugs) is discontinued. Seven percent of patients with idiopathic-acquired sideroblastic anemia eventually develop acute myeloblastic leukemia.[122]

Thalassemia Syndromes

The thalassemias are a group of hereditary hemolytic anemias in which there is unbalanced hemoglobin synthesis, resulting in a hypochromic, microcytic anemia as well as variable degrees of ineffective erythropoiesis and hemolysis.[123] In the α-thalassemias there is decreased α-chain synthesis and normal β-chain synthesis, whereas in the β-thalassemias, β-chain synthesis is decreased and α-chain synthesis is normal. In contrast to the other hemoglobinopathies, the polypeptide chain produced in decreased amounts is normal in molecular structure. Defective synthesis of one or the other polypeptide chain of hemoglobin may be due to an absence of globin genes or to an absence of or a defective messenger RNA. In either case, the red cell is placed in double jeopardy: there is a hypochromic, microcytic anemia due to decreased total hemoglobin production and, at the same time, a relative excess of β-chains (in the case of α-thalassemias) or α-chains (in the case of the β-thalassemias). Excess or free polypeptide chains of hemoglobin are insoluble and precipitate within the cell. These precipitated chains, termed *Heinz bodies,* are capable of damaging the red cell membrane and limiting the degree to which red cells can deform in the microcirculation. They are primarily responsible for the ineffective erythropoiesis and intramedullary hemolysis observed in these disorders. Red-cell survival in the circulation is shortened as well, particularly in the more severe clinical forms of the disease. Indeed, thalassemias are often classified with the hemolytic anemias.

The β-thalassemias are particularly common in peoples from the Mediterranean Basin, Africa, Asia, and

the South Pacific. Alpha-thalassemia is found primarily among southern Asians and, in milder form, among American Blacks. A person inherits 2 genes regulating β-chain synthesis, 1 from each parent. The inheritance pattern for the β-thalassemias is autosomal codominant and the offspring of two parents, each heterozygous for β-thalassemia, may be normal (25% probability), heterozygous (50% probability) or homozygous (25% probability) for β-thalassemia. In general, the heterozygous state has minimal or moderate clinical manifestations and is referred to as either β-thalassemia minor or intermedia. The homozygous person has β-thalassemia major and is severely affected with the manifestations of severe chronic hemolysis (anemia, splenomegaly, jaundice, and organ damage due to iron overload). The genetic basis of the α-thalassemias is less well understood. There is considerable evidence that most normal individuals have 4 α-chain genes, 2 from each parent. If so, the 4 clinical types of α-thalassemia can be attributed to gene dosage. Thus, the silent carrier (asymptomatic, nonanemic) has 1 α-thalassemia gene; the person with α-thalassemia minor has 2 abnormal genes; the person with α-thalassemia intermedia (hemoglobin-H disease) has 3 abnormal genes; and the stillborn baby with α-thalassemia major has 4 abnormal genes. However, the genetics of some of the α-thalassemias, particularly in Blacks, may be more complex.

The diagnosis of the thalassemias should be considered in a patient with a hypochromic, microcytic anemia, evidence of ineffective erythropoiesis and hemolysis, and, in severe cases, evidence of chronic marrow compensation, such as reticulocytosis and marrow expansion to long bones and skull. In β-thalassemias, hemoglobin electrophoresis usually reveals increased levels of hemoglobin A_2 ($\alpha_2 \delta_2$) and often of hemoglobin F ($\alpha_2 \gamma_2$), with the non-α-chains (δ, γ) compensating to some degree for the deficiency of β-chains. In the α-thalassemias a relative excess production of non-α-chains can lead to the formation of hemoglobin Bart's (γ_4) in the newborn, and hemoglobin H (β_4) in children and adults. The Heinz bodies due to hemoglobin H are stable and may be seen with special stains in mature, circulating red cells.

HEMOLYTIC ANEMIAS

GENERAL CONSIDERATIONS

Red cells undergo premature destruction by 2 general mechanisms. First, they lyse in the circulation and release their contents directly into the peripheral blood (intravascular lysis). Second, and more commonly, they

are taken up by macrophages in the spleen and liver (mononuclear-phagocyte system) where they are destroyed and digested (extravascular lysis).

The spleen is capable of trapping and destroying red cells that have subtle abnormalities.[124] The liver lacks the spleen's fine discrimination and is unable to recognize these cells. However, because the blood flow to the liver is about sevenfold that to the spleen, the liver has a greater capacity for clearing red cells that have gross abnormalities. Phagocytosis of red cells induces a proliferative response in the spleen and, to a lesser extent, in the liver. This leads to hyperplasia, increased blood flow, and functional overactivity, thereby further augmenting the clearance of the abnormal red cells that instigated the process.[66]

The mononuclear-phagocyte system clears red cells from the circulation under 2 general conditions: first, when the surface of the red cell possesses chemical properties for which macrophages in the mononuclear-phagocyte system have specific receptors; and second, when the red cell possesses physical characteristics that limit its ability to traverse the filtering system of the spleen.

Extreme deformations of red-cell shape are required for the red cells to traverse orifices of diameters smaller than their own, as they must in the spleen filter. The discoid shape favors deformability, providing a surface area that is 60% to 70% in excess of the minimum necessary to encompass the red cell's contents, thus permitting a portion of the cell surface to accommodate changes in cell shape. The red-cell membrane bends readily; however, it strongly resists stretching.[125] The limits of deformability, therefore, depend on the surface area: volume ratio of the red cell.[126] Osmotic fragility is a useful test of this ratio. A modification of the structural properties of the red-cell membrane may also impair the cell's ability to flow through the mononuclear-phagocyte system. The fluid properties of the membrane depend on a fixed relationship between the amounts of cholesterol and phospholipid in the membrane.[3] The elastic properties of the red-cell membrane depend on the structure of certain proteins within the membrane and on the interaction of these proteins with ATP and calcium.[5,127] In addition, the flow properties of the red cells are strongly influenced by the nature of the red cell's contents. For example, a rise in internal viscosity appears to play a role in the destruction of red cells in persons homozygous for hemoglobin C, and a striking increase in intracellular viscosity also accompanies sickling in sickle-cell anemia. Finally, the passage of the red cells through the spleen filter is impeded by the presence of inclusion bodies that consist of precipitated globin within the red cell, as in the thalassemias, in deficiencies of enzymes in the hexose

monophosphate (HMP) shunt, and in the unstable hemoglobin hemolytic anemias.

Many, although not all, hemolytic processes are associated with a change in the morphologic appearance of red cells (Fig. 28-4). Spherocytes are the most common morphologic abnormality in hemolytic diseases. Small numbers of spherocytes occur in many disorders. They are most striking in patients with hereditary spherocytosis and patients with warm, antibody-induced, immunohemolytic disease. Fragmented red cells, called *schistocytes*, are a hallmark of shear stress or physical obstruction to red cells within the circulation. They are observed in prosthetic valve hemolysis, thrombotic thrombocytopenic purpura, and in disorders accompanied by intravascular fibrin deposition. Target-shaped red cells that are well-filled with hemoglobin occur in persons heterozygous for hemoglobin C (hemoglobin C trait), in sickle-cell anemia, and following splenectomy. However, the most common cause of target-shaped cells is liver disease of many etiologies. Target-shaped cells deficient in hemoglobin (hypochromic) are the hallmark of the thalassemia syndromes. Regularly-spiculated or crenated red cells occur in conjunction with uremia (burr cells) and are seen in small numbers following splenectomy, even in the absence of an underlying red-cell disorder.[128] Bizarrely spiculated red cells (acanthocytes) occur in abetalipoproteinemia in anorexia nervosa, and are a striking feature of spur-cell anemia.[129,130,131] Permanently sickled, crescent-shaped red cells are the hallmark of sickle-cell anemia. Modifications of their structure to a boat shape is a clue to the double heterozygous state of hemoglobin S and C (hemoglobin SC disease). The presence of both crescent-shaped red cells and hy-

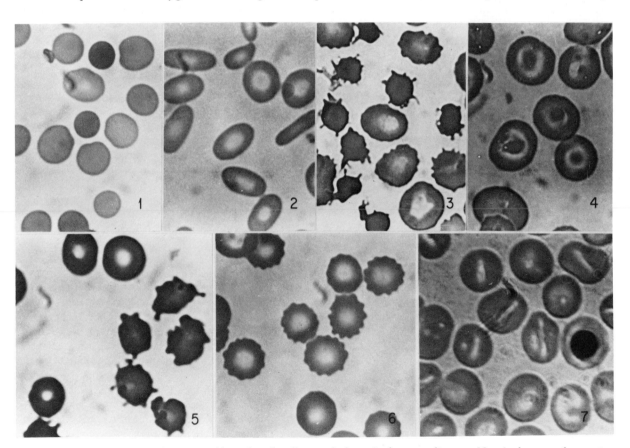

Fig. 28-4. Altered red cell morphology in human disease. No. 1 shows spherocytes (hereditary spherocytosis), No. 2 elliptocytes (hereditary elliptocytosis), No. 3 acanthocytes (abetalipoproteinemia), No. 4 target cells (liver disease), No. 5 spur cells (liver disease), No. 6 burr cells (uremia), and No. 7 stomatocytes (hereditary stomatocytosis). A nucleated red cell is also present (original magnification × 1000; reproduced from Cooper RA, Shattil SJ: The red cell membrane in hemolytic anemia. Mod Treat 8:329, 1971)

pochromic target-shaped cells on the same smear is suggestive of the doubly-heterozygous-state hemoglobin S and β-thalassemia.

EXTRINSIC CAUSES OF HEMOLYSIS

Splenomegaly

The unique ability of the spleen to filter mildly damaged red cells results from its unusual vascular anatomy.[132] The majority of blood circulating through the spleen flows directly from arterioles in the white pulp to venous sinuses in the red pulp, and then on into the venous system. In contrast, a minority of spleen-blood flow (1%-2% normally) leaves the arterioles of the white pulp to enter a nonendothelialized portion of the spleen, the marginal zone of the lymphatic white pulp. Although the reticuloendothelial cells that occupy this zone are not phagocytic, they serve as a mechanical filter hindering the progress of damaged red cells. As red cells leave this zone and enter the red pulp, they flow into narrow cords that end blindly, but which communicate with venous sinuses through small openings between the lining cells of the sinuses. These openings, averaging 3μ in diameter, test the ability of red cells to undergo a deformation of shape. Red cells that do not pass the stringent test imposed upon them by the spleen filter are engulfed by phagocytic cells and destroyed.

The normal spleen poses no threat to normal red cells. However, splenomegaly exaggerates the adverse conditions to which red cells are exposed. Causes of splenic enlargement may be considered in 3 broad categories: first, infiltrative diseases (such as amyloidosis, myeloproliferative diseases, and lymphomas) and storage diseases such as Gaucher's disease; second, systemic inflammatory diseases leading to splenic hypertrophy; and third, diseases in which the red cells' passage through the spleen is retarded owing to congestive splenomegaly. It is these latter 2 categories that are more likely to be associated with an increased hemolytic rate.

Red Cell Antibodies

Immune hemolysis in the adult occurs under 4 general conditions: first, alloantibodies that are acquired by blood transfusions or pregnancies are directed against transfused red cells; second, antibodies reactive at body temperature and directed against the patient's own red cells may be formed in the absence of other disease manifestations, or in association with another disease, commonly one related to the immune system; third, antibodies reactive at body temperature and directed against the patient's own red cells may be formed in response to the exposure to drugs; fourth, antibodies that are reactive in the cold and that are directed against

the patient's own red cells may be formed. As with warm antibodies, these last may occur in association with diseases of the immune system or with certain infections.

The Coomb's-antiglobulin test is the major tool for diagnosing these disorders. This test relies on the ability of antibodies prepared in animals and directed against specific human-serum proteins to agglutinate red cells if these human-serum proteins are present on the red-cell surface.[133] The serum proteins of particular interest are IgG and C3. The ability of heterologous or specific anti-IgG or anti-C3 antiserums to agglutinate the patient's red cells is referred to as a positive *direct Coomb's test.* There are times when it is advantageous to know whether there is antibody in the patient's serum that is reactive against other human red cells. This is important in crossmatching blood prior to blood transfusion and it is of prognostic significance in patients with warm antibody-hemolytic anemia. To determine this, an *indirect Coomb's test* is performed by incubating ABO-and Rh-compatible red cells with the patient's serum and subsequently performing a direct Coomb's test on these incubated red cells.

Warm reacting antibodies are usually of the IgG class. They induce a pattern of hemolysis that is acquired and that affects both the patient's own cells and normal transfused cells. Human red blood cells coated with IgG antibodies are bound to the surface of monocytes or splenic macrophages and undergo a spherical transformation.[134] This syndrome is frequently designated *autoimmune hemolytic anemia.* It is idiopathic in one third of cases but in approximately two thirds it occurs as a complication of an underlying disease affecting the immune system. The most common underlying diseases are chronic lymphocytic leukemia, non-Hodgkin's lymphomas, and systemic lupus erythematosus. The presentation and course of immunohemolytic anemia is quite variable. In its mild form, the only manifestation is a positive Coomb's test. A large fraction of patients with immunohemolytic anemia have a chronic, mild hemolytic state associated with spherocytosis, mild anemia, reticulocytosis, and splenomegaly. The direct Coomb's test is positive for IgG but not for C3, and the indirect Coomb's test is negative. A small number of persons may have immunohemolytic anemia and a negative Coomb's test.[135] In these cases, more sensitive techniques are required to detect antibody on the red-cell surface. Autoimmune hemolytic anemia may be more severe with marked spherocytosis, hemoglobin levels less than 7 g/dl, and reticulocyte counts of 30% or more. The Coomb's test is positive for IgG and frequently for C3 as well. This latter finding relates to the large number of antibody molecules per red cell, providing the opportunity for 2 molecules to be close enough together on the cell surface to fix complement.

The larger amount of antibody is also demonstrable by the indirect Coomb's test, which demonstrates antibody not only on the patient's red cells, but also in the patient's serum. In its most severe form, immunohemolytic anemia presents with a fulminant, overwhelming hemolysis and is associated with hemoglobinemia. Hemoglobinuria and shock is a syndrome that may be fatal.

Drugs have been directly related to immunohemolytic anemia by 3 mechanisms. First are drugs, such as alpha-methyldopa, that induce a disorder identical in almost every respect to the warm antibody immunohemolytic anemia described above. Second are drugs of the penicillin type that become associated with the red cell surface and induce the formation of an antibody, usually IgG, directed against the red cell–drug complex. Third are drugs, such as stibophen or quinine, that form a complex with plasma proteins against which an antibody forms; the drug-plasma protein antibody complex settles on red cells or platelets to involve them as innocent bystanders in a destructive process mediated by complement.[136]

Cold reactive antibodies induce hemolysis under 2 general conditions. First, in the syndrome of cold agglutinin disease, IgM antibodies are usually reactive with the I-antigen of red cells and less often with the i-antigen. These antibodies may occur spontaneously in the course of a lymphoproliferative disease, or as a complication of infectious mononucleosis or mycoplasma pneumonia. They bind to red cells in the cold and fix complement. They agglutinate red cells in the cold, but at body temperature they cause little or no hemolysis.[137] The agglutination *in vivo* in those portions of the body exposed to low temperature may cause acrocyanosis and even gangrene. Second, in paroxysmal cold hemoglobinuria, cold reactive antibodies of the IgG class may occur spontaneously or as a complication of syphilis or certain viral diseases. These antibodies fix complement and may lead to episodic, acute, severe hemolysis after cold exposure.

Microangiopathic Hemolysis

When red cells in the circulation are exposed to trauma, they fragment, resulting in red cells of bizarre shape.[138] This process occurs under 2 general conditions. First, red cells flowing across a pressure gradient created by an abnormal heart valve or valve prosthesis may undergo a shear stress that disrupts them.[139] Second, the deposition of fibrin or aggregated platelets in the microvasculature exposes red cells to a physical impediment that frequently cleaves them. Fibrin deposition appears to be the mechanism of microangiopathic hemolysis in disseminated intravascular coagulation and in vasculitides.[140] Intravascular platelet aggregates may form the physical impediment responsible for frag-

mentation hemolysis in thrombotic thrombocytopenic purpura. Intravascular hemolysis has also been observed when red cells flowing through small vessels over the surface of bony prominences were subject to impact trauma during such physical activities as marching, jogging, or congo drumming. In these situations, however, red cell fragments are not observed in the peripheral blood smear.

Toxins

A number of chemical and physical agents have a direct toxic effect upon red cells. A striking example is the fulminant hemolysis that may occur during septicemia with *Clostridium welchii*.[141] The phospholipase produced by this organism is capable of cleaving the phosphoryl bond of lecithin and lysing human red cells. Hemolysis may result from the direct action of snake and spider venoms on red cells.[142,143] Copper has a direct hemolytic effect on red cells and hemolysis has been observed following exposure of persons to copper salts such as during hemodialysis.[144] The transient episodes of hemolysis observed in patients with Wilson's disease are probably due to copper toxicity.[145]

The red-cell membrane is unstable at temperatures above 49°C. When studied *in vitro*, the red cell undergoes a process of budding, cleavage, and resealing above this temperature.[146] The same process is observed in patients who have suffered extensive burns. Hemoglobinemia and hemoglobinuria may accompany this process, and spherocytosis is common.

MEMBRANE DEFECTS (ACQUIRED)

Spur-cell Anemia. A moderate to severe hemolytic anemia characterized by irregularly shaped red cells with multiple spicules occurs in about 5% of patients with severe hepatocellular disease. Most patients with spur-cell anemia have advanced Laennec's cirrhosis, but it has also been reported in neonatal hepatitis.[131,147,148,149] Splenomegaly and jaundice are constant features. Hepatic encephalopathy is common. The surface membrane of spur cells contains 50% to 70% excess cholesterol, but its total phospholipid content is normal. In this way spur cells are distinct from the more usual target-shaped red cells in liver disease, which possess an excess of both cholesterol and phospholipid.[98,148] Cholesterol out of proportion to phospholipid decreases the fluidity of the spur-cell membrane, and there is an associated decrease in spur-cell deformability. These cells are removed and destroyed by the spleen.[3,150] Normal red cells acquire the spur abnormality when incubated in serum from affected patients. This results from the presence in serum of an abnormal, low-density lipoprotein with an increased

mole ratio of free (unesterified) cholesterol to phospholipid.

Paroxysmal Nocturnal Hemoglobinuria (PNH).

PNH is distinctive among hemolytic disorders in man because it is an acquired intracorpuscular defect. Although hemoglobinuria is the classic feature of this disease, it is intermittent in most patients, and never occurs in others. Hemosiderinuria is usually present. Mild granulocytopenia and thrombocytopenia are common. This disorder masquerades, often for several years, as a refractory anemia or a hypoplastic anemia. Red cells are normochromic and normocytic unless iron deficiency has occurred from the chronic loss of iron in the urine. Thromboses are a common complication of this disorder, and may also account for the abdominal pain and headache that are frequent complaints. The underlying abnormality which affects red cells, granulocytes, and platelets in PNH is an inordinate sensitivity of the membranes of these cells to complement. Careful analytic procedures have demonstrated 2, and in some cases, 3 separate populations of red cells with varying sensitivities to complement in patients with PNH.[151] The clinical manifestations relate directly to the proportion of the red cells most sensitive to complement that are produced. Although platelets share with red cells the sensitivity to complement, platelet survival is normal in PNH, and the frequent thrombocytopenia is due to decreased platelet production. The diagnosis is established by demonstrating the red cell's increased sensitivity to complement lysis by means of either the acid lysis test or the sucrose lysis test.[152]

Because it affects granulocytes, platelets, and red cells, but does not affect lymphocytes, this defect is thought to occur because of an acquired change in the stem cell that generates these cells. Acute myelogenous leukemia and PNH may be secondary manifestations of a primary bone marrow injury that is manifested initially as aplastic anemia. Moreover, a number of patients with PNH have subsequently developed acute myelogenous leukemia. Although the precise genetic locus has not been identified, it appears likely that PNH results from a mutation in the marrow stem-cell pool. The exact phenotypic representation on the red-cell membrane of this presumed mutation is not known.

MEMBRANE DEFECTS (HEREDITARY)

Hereditary Spherocytosis.

This is a disease of autosomal dominant inheritance in which intrinsically abnormal red cells are destroyed in the presence of an otherwise normal spleen. No family history can be obtained from 20% of patients and the genetic mutation in these appears to have arisen *de novo*.[153] The red-cell membrane in hereditary spherocytosis has a number of unusual characteristics. The surface area of these erythrocytes is decreased. This is due in part to a decreased amount of membrane lipid. The red-cell membrane is also more permeable to sodium than normal. Compensation is achieved by an increased rate of glucose metabolism to generate an increased amount of ATP with which the red cell extrudes this excess sodium. Thus, these red cells must remain metabolically active in order to maintain their integrity. In addition, the red-cell membrane is more rigid than normal, suggesting that it may have an abnormal interaction with ATP and calcium. It is assumed that these abnormalities relate to some basic defect in a structural membrane protein.

Their spheroidal contour and rigid structure impede the passage of hereditary spherocytes through the spleen. In the spleen, the red cells are exposed to an environment in which their increased metabolic rate cannot be sustained. The first injury inflicted upon them by the spleen is a further loss of surface membrane (conditioning), which produces a subpopulation of hyperspheroidal red cells in the peripheral blood. These are subsequently destroyed.

The major clinical features of hereditary spherocytosis are anemia, splenomegaly, and jaundice. Because of the increased bile-pigment metabolism, gall stones of the pigment type are common, even in childhood. Compensatory normoblastic hyperplasia of the bone marrow occurs with the extension of red marrow into the midshafts of long bones, and occasionally with extramedullary erythropoiesis. Because the bone marrow's capacity to increase erythropoiesis sixfold to tenfold exceeds the usual rate of hemolysis, anemia is only mild or moderate and often lacking in an otherwise healthy individual. Compensation may be temporarily interrupted by episodes of erythroid hypoplasia precipitated by infections, often of a minor nature. Hemolytic rate may increase transiently during systemic inflammatory diseases that induce further splenic enlargement.

The diagnosis of hereditary spherocytosis is supported by 2 laboratory tests, the osmotic fragility test and the autohemolysis test. In the osmotic fragility test, spherocytes have a decreased surface area per unit volume and they lyse more readily than do normal red cells when exposed to solutions of low salt concentrations.[154] The autohemolysis test is a measure of the amount of spontaneous hemolysis occurring after 48 hours of sterile incubation of hereditary spherocytes. In hereditary spherocytosis, about 10% to 50% of the red cells are lysed whereas less than 4% are lysed in normal red cells. Autohemolysis of these red cells is largely prevented by the addition of glucose prior to incubation.[155]

INTRINSIC CAUSES OF HEMOLYSIS

Enzyme Defects

Defects in the Embden–Meyerhof Pathway. Deficiencies of most of the enzymes in the Embden–Meyerhof pathway have been reported.[156] Many of these have only been encountered in isolated families. In general, all of the enzymopathies have similar pathophysiologic and clinical features. Patients present with a congenital nonspherocytic hemolytic anemia of variable severity. As a rule, the red cells are relatively deficient in ATP, considering their young age. As a result, these cells often have increased leakage of potassium ion out of the cell. In patients with pyruvate-kinase deficiency, bizarre erythrocytes are noted on the peripheral smear with large numbers of spicules. Spherocytes are usually few or absent. Hence, the term *congenital nonspherocytic hemolytic anemia* has been applied to these disorders. The red cells in these disorders are apt to be rigid and thus more readily sequestered by the monocyte-phagocyte system.

Among the reported defects of glycolytic enzymes, about 95% are due to pyruvate-kinase deficiency. The remainder are rare. Most of the glycolytic-enzyme defects are inherited in an autosomal recessive pattern. The diagnosis of this group of anemias depends upon specific enzymatic assays.

Defects in the Hexose-monophosphate Shunt. The normal red cell is well-endowed to protect itself against oxidant stress. Upon exposure to an offending drug or toxin, the amount of glucose that has metabolized during the hexose-monophosphate shunt is increased several fold. In this way, reduced glutathione is regenerated, protecting the sulfhydryl groups of hemoglobin, and perhaps the red cell membrane, from oxidation. Persons with an inherited defect in the hexose-monophosphate shunt are unable to maintain an adequate level of reduced glutathione in their red cells. As a result, hemoglobin-sulfhydryl groups become oxidized and the hemoglobin tends to precipitate within the red cells, forming Heinz bodies.

Among the congenital shunt defects, by far the most common is glucose-6-phosphate dehydrogenase (G6PD) deficiency. In fact, it is probably the most commonly encountered genetic disorder, affecting millions of people throughout the world. Over 100 G6PD variants have been described.[157] The normal form of G6PD is designated *B*. About 20% of Blacks have a G6PD variant (designated *A +*), which differs electrophoretically from *B* but is functionally normal. Among the clinically significant G6PD variants, the most common is the so-called *A − type*, encountered primarily in Blacks. G6PD *A −* has the same electrophoretic mobility as G6PD *A +* but it is unstable and has abnormal kinetic properties.[158] This variant is found in 15% of black men in the United States. Persons with the G6PD A − variant have a slightly shortened red-cell survival, but are not anemic. Clinical problems arise only when the affected red cells are subjected to some type of environmental stress. Most often, hemolytic episodes are triggered by viral or bacterial infections or by metabolic acidosis, but the precise mechanism by which these trigger hemolysis is unclear. Drugs or toxins that pose an oxidant threat to the red cell also cause hemolysis in G6PD-deficient persons. Of these drugs or toxins, antimalarials, and nitrofurantoins are most commonly incriminated.[157] The patient may experience an acute hemolytic crisis within hours of exposure to the oxidant stress. In severe cases, hemoglobinuria and peripheral vascular collapse can develop. Because only the older population of red cells, those most deficient in enzyme activity, is rapidly destroyed, the hemolytic crisis is usually self-limited, even if exposure to the oxidant continues.[159] The peripheral smear is often unimpressive, but on occasion spherocytes and fragmented red cells (bite cells) may be seen.[160] The demonstration of Heinz bodies requires the use of special stains. However, Heinz bodies are usually not seen after the first day or so because these inclusions are readily removed by the spleen.

A second relatively common G6PD variant has been discovered in peoples of the eastern Mediterranean area. Persons with this variant have a much lower level of enzyme activity than Blacks with the A − variant. As a result, they have more severe clinical manifestations. Some have a chronic hemolytic anemia, even in the absence of any exposure to oxidants. A minority of patients is extremely sensitive to fava beans and develops a fulminant hemolytic crisis following exposure. Sensitivity to fava beans is a poorly understood phenomenon that appears to be determined by a separate gene. It is not encountered with the A − variant.

A number of screening tests are available to establish the diagnosis of G6PD deficiency.[157] However, because the deficiency occurs primarily in older red cells, a false negative test may be seen during a hemolytic episode when there is a high proportion of young red cells. It may be necessary to repeat these diagnostic tests after the patient is recovered.

Hemoglobinopathies

Sickle-cell Anemia. About 0.15% of black children in the United States have this disease. The protean manifestations of this disorder can be attributed to a specific molecular lesion: the substitution of valine for glutamic acid at the sixth residue of the β-chain of hemoglobin.[161] Upon deoxygenation, a red cell containing hemoglobin S changes from a concave disc to

an elongated, crescent-shaped cell. Electron micrographs reveal the presence of fibers within the cytoplasm having diameters of about 150 A.[162] It is likely that each sickle fiber consists of a helical polymer with about 6 molecules of hemoglobin per cross-sectional area. Sickling, both within the intact red cell and in free solution is greatly affected by the presence of non-S hemoglobin.[163] For example hemoglobin C participates more readily than hemoglobin A in co-polymerization with hemoglobin S. Patients with SC disease may have a clinical syndrome similar to sickle-cell anemia whereas individuals with sickle trait (SA hemoglobin) are in general asymptomatic. In addition, hemoglobin F appears to inhibit sickling. Persons with sickle-cell anemia with a high percentage of hemoglobin F tend to have a milder clinical illness than do those with low levels of hemoglobin F.

As a red cell sickles, it becomes rigid and, as a result, may obstruct capillary blood flow. The deoxygenation of blood from patients with sickle-cell disease is associated with a marked increase in viscosity. It is likely that obstruction of flow leads to local tissue hypoxia. As a result, further deoxygenation takes place, leading to further sickling. This vicious cycle may result in the amplification of microscopic obstruction into a larger area of infarction.[164] The O_2-dependent sickle cycle is ordinarily reversible. However, the membrane of sickle cells may become sufficiently damaged so that the cells lose potassium and water, leading to the formation of irreversibly sickled forms.

Factors that lower the O_2 affinity of red cells enhance the formation of deoxyhemoglobin and, therefore, promote sickling. Thus, at any given O_2 tension, elevation of both intracellular 2,3-DPG and hydrogen-ion concentration results in increased numbers of sickled cells. In addition, sickling is highly dependent on hemoglobin concentration. Any pathophysiologic process that tends to pull water out of sickle red cells greatly increases their chance of sickling. Thus, the hypertonic environment of the renal medulla can cause local sickling and the formation of papillary infarcts, even in patients with sickle trait.[165]

Patients with sickle-cell anemia have a variety of clinical problems. Signs and symptoms usually do not appear until the sixth month of life, at which time most of the infant's fetal hemoglobin has been replaced by hemoglobin S. Among the constitutional manifestations is impairment of growth and development and a general failure to thrive. In addition, these patients have an increased tendency to develop serious infections owing to marked impairment of splenic function in childhood, and splenic infarction and fibrosis in adulthood.[166] Patients who suffer from sickle-cell anemia also have a deficiency of heat-labile opsonin, preventing effective coating of certain bacteria.[167]

These patients invariably have a severe hemolytic anemia and their hematocrit values range between 18% and 30%. The anemia becomes increasingly severe if erythropoiesis is suppressed. There are 2 main causes of aplastic crisis, infection and folic-acid deficiency. Morbidity and mortality of sickle-cell disease are due primarily to recurrent vaso-occlusive phenomena. Throughout their lives patients with sickle-cell disease are plagued by recurrent painful crises involving bones and abdomen. They often develop pleuritic chest pain with fever. An infiltrate may evolve on chest radiographs. The important differential is between pneumonia and pulmonary infarction. By the time patients reach adulthood, there is often evidence of anatomic or functional damage to various organs due to the cumulative effect of vaso-occlusive episodes. Almost any organ may be involved, but those organs most commonly involved are the lungs (hypoxia), the kidneys (isosthenuria, hematuria), and the liver (infarction, gallstones). The skeleton (aseptic necrosis, osteomyelitis), and the skin (leg ulcers) are also commonly involved.

The diagnosis of sickle-cell anemia and its differentiation from doubly heterozygous-sickling conditions such as SC disease or S-β-thalassemia involves analysis of red-cell morphology, screening tests for red-cell sickling, and hemoglobin electrophoresis. Often these studies must be performed on members of the patient's family as well. It should be stressed that a positive screening test for sickling, such as metabisulfite reduction or a solubility test, merely indicates the presence of hemoglobin S and does not distinguish between homozygous sickle-cell disease, sickle-cell trait, or double heterozygotes. Hemoglobin electrophoresis is necessary to establish the proper diagnosis. Patients with sickle-cell anemia have mild to moderate elevations of hemoglobin F and the majority of their hemoglobin is hemoglobin S.

Unstable Hemoglobin Hemolytic Anemias. The great majority of these variants are single amino-acid substitutions in the β-chain. A few are due to deletion of one or more amino acids within the β-chain. Patients present with a hemolytic anemia of variable degree. An autosomal dominant mode of inheritance can usually be established, although about 20% of cases appear to be spontaneous mutants. These variants have structural alterations at sites in the hemoglobin molecule that drastically affect its stability and solubility.[168] Many involve amino-acid substitutions in the portion of the subunit where heme is inserted. In such instances the heme may be displaced from the heme pocket. As a result, the solubility of the subunit is decreased, and the abnormal hemoglobin forms Heinz bodies. Red cells that contain this type of inclusion are

recognized by the mononuclear-phagocyte system and are either cleansed of their intracellular debris or destroyed. The displaced heme moiety is aberrantly catabolized, forming dipyrroles instead of bilirubin.[169] Pigmenturia is due to the excretion of dipyrroles rather than of hemoglobin. The degree of instability of these unstable hemoglobin variants, and, therefore, the extent of hemolysis varies considerably.

The diagnosis of hereditary, unstable hemoglobin is established as follows: (1) hemoglobin electrophoresis, revealing an abnormal component usually comprising less than 30% of the total hemoglobin; (2) Heinz bodies, demonstrated by incubating a freshly drawn sample of blood with a supravital stain; (3) instability of the hemoglobin, manifested by the presence of a significant precipitate when the hemolysate is incubated at 50°C or in the presence of 17% isopropanol.[170]

SUMMARY

Anemia is a decrease in the circulating mass of red blood cells leading to a reduction in the oxygen-carrying capacity of the blood. It can be asymptomatic or accompanied by mild to severe symptoms and physical signs related to the anemia itself, to the deleterious effect of anemia on various organs, and to the underlying disease responsible for the anemia. A rational approach to the diagnosis of the cause of anemia in a patient begins with the classification of the anemia as owing to (1) defective proliferation of red cells, (2) defective maturation of red cells, (3) increased destruction of red cells (hemolysis), or (4) acute blood loss. The patient's anemia is assigned to one of these categories with the aid of the peripheral blood smear, the reticulocyte count, an analysis of the stool for blood, and an analysis of the degree of erythroid cellularity of the bone marrow. With this approach, the underlying cause of the anemia is usually clarified. However, further specific tests to define the exact cause of the anemia may be necessary. An appreciation of the extent and duration of the symptoms and signs of the anemia as well as an understanding of its specific etiology are mandatory for optimal correction of both the anemia and its cause.

REFERENCES

1. **Cooper RA:** Lipids of human red cell membrane: Normal composition and variability in disease. Semin Hematol 7:296, 1970
2. **Steck TL:** The organization of proteins in the human red blood cell membrane. J Cell Biol 62:1, 1974
3. **Vanderkooi J, Fischkoff S, Chance B et al:** Fluorescent probe analysis of the lipid architecture of natural and experimental cholesterol-rich membranes. Biochemistry 13:1589, 1974
4. **Nicolson GL, Poste G:** The cancer cell: Dynamic aspects and modifications in cell-surface organization. N Engl J Med 295:179, 1976
5. **Evans EA, Hochmuth RM:** Membrane viscoelasticity. Biophys J 16:1, 1976
6. **Chen LT, Weiss L:** The role of the sinus wall in the passage of erythrocytes through the spleen. Blood 41:529, 1973
7. **Tosteson DC:** Sodium and potassium transport across the red cell membrane. In Jamieson GA, Greenwalt TJ (eds): Red Cell Membrane Structure and Function, p 291. Philadelphia, JB Lippincott, 1969
8. **Watkins WM:** Blood-group substances: Their nature and genetics. In Surgenor D, Mac N (eds): The Red Blood Cell, 2nd ed, Vol. 1, p 293. New York, Academic Press, 1974
9. **Harris JW, Kellermeyer RW:** The Red Cell. 2nd ed, p 460. Cambridge, Harvard University Press, 1970
10. **Perutz MF:** Molecular pathology of human hemoglobin. Nature 219:902, 1968
11. **Perutz MF:** Stereochemistry of cooperative effects in hemoglobin. Nature 228:726, 1970
12. **Riggs A:** Functional properties of hemoglobins. Physiol Rev 45:619, 1965
13. **Bunn HF, Jandl JH:** Control of hemoglobin function within the red cell. N Engl J Med 282:1414, 1970
14. **Fried W:** Erythropoietin. Arch Intern Med 131:929, 1973
15. **Emerson PM, Wilkinson JH:** Lactate dehydrogenase in the diagnosis and assessment of response to treatment of megaloblastic anemia. Br J Haematol 12:678, 1966
16. **Hillman RS, Finch CA:** Red Cell Manual, 4th ed, p 60. Philadelphia, F A Davis, 1974
17. **Bunn HF:** Erythrocyte destruction and hemoglobin catabolism. Semin Hematol 9:3, 1972
18. **Shattil SJ, Cooper RA:** Maturation of macroreticulocyte membranes in vivo. J Lab Clin Med 79:215, 1972
19. **Parsons CG, Wright FH:** Circulatory function in the anemias of children. Am J Dis Child 57:15, 1939
20. **Anderson NP:** Syndrome of spoon nails, anemia, cheilitis and dysphagia. Arch Dermatol Syph 37:816, 1938
21. **Pascher F, Keen R:** Chronic ulcers of the leg associated with blood dyscrasias. Arch Dermatol Syph 66:478, 1952
22. **Taylor ES:** Chronic ulcer of the leg associated with congenital hemolytic jaundice. JAMA 112:1574, 1939
23. **Torrence J, Jacobs P, Restrepo A et al:** Intraerythrocytic adaptation to anemia. N Engl J Med 283:165, 1970
24. **Lichtman MA, Murphy MS, Whitbeck AA et al:** Oxygen binding to hemoglobin in subjects with hypoproliferative anemia, with and without chronic renal disease: Role of pH. Br J Haematol 27:439, 1974
25. **Hjelm M:** The content of 2,3-diphosphoglycerate and some other phosphocompounds in human erythrocytes from healthy adults and subjects with different types of anemia. Forswars Medicine 5:219, 1969

26. Lenfant C, Torrance J, English E et al: Effect of altitude on oxygen binding by hemoglobin and on organic phosphate levels. J Clin Invest 47:2652, 1968

27. Huber H, Lewis SM, Szur L: The influence of anemia, polycythaemia and splenomegaly on the relationship between venous hematocrit and red cell volume. Br J Haematol 10:567, 1964

28. Wintrobe MM: The cardiovascular system in anemia. Blood 1:121, 1946

29. Bradley SE, Bradley GP: Renal function during chronic anemia in man. Blood 2:192, 1947

30. Roy SB, Bhatia ML, Mathur VS et al: Hemodynamic effects of chronic severe anemia. Circulation 28:346, 1963

31. Graettinger JS, Parsons RL, Campbell JA: A correlation of clinical and hemodynamic studies in patients with mild and severe anemia with and without congestive failure. Ann Intern Med 58:617, 1963

32. Fowler NO, Holmes JC: Blood viscosity and cardiac output in acute experimental anemia. J Appl Physiol 39:453, 1975

33. Escobar E, Jones NL, Rapaport E et al: Ventricular performance in acute normovolemic anemia and effects of beta blockade. Am J Physiol 211:877, 1966

34. Varat MA, Adolph RJ, Fowler NO: Cardiovascular effect of anemia. Am Heart J 83:415, 1972

35. Detweiler DK: The circulation. In Brobeck JR (ed): Best and Taylor's Physiologic Basis of Medical Practice, 9th ed, pp 3–158. Baltimore, Williams & Wilkins, 1973

36. Blumgart HL, Altshule MD: Clinical significance of cardiac and respiratory adjustments in chronic anemia. Blood 3:329, 1948

37. Rankin J, McNeill RS, Forster RE: The effect of anemia on the alveolar-capillary exchange of carbon dioxide in man. J Clin Invest 40:1323, 1961

38. Wales RT, Martin EA: Arterial bruits in anaemia. Br Med J 2:1444, 1963

39. Hardison JE: Cervical venous hum. N Engl J Med 278:587, 1968

40. Hunter A: The heart in anaemia. Q J Med 15:107, 1946

41. Goldstein B, Boas EP: Functional diastolic murmurs and cardiac enlargement in severe anemias. Arch Intern Med 39:226, 1927

42. Fowler NO: High cardiac output states. In Hurst JW (ed): The Heart, Arteries and Veins. 3rd ed, p 1508. New York, McGraw-Hill, 1974

43. Gonzales-de-Cossia A, Sanchez–Medal L, Smyth JF: Electrocardiographic modifications in anemia. Am Heart J 67:166, 1964

44. Scherf D, Klotz SD: Electrocardiographic changes after acute loss of blood. Ann Intern Med 20:438, 1944

45. Christ C: Experimentelle kohlenoxydvergiftung, herzmuskelnekrosen und electrokardiogramm. Beitr Pathol Anat 94:111, 1934

46. Yater WM, Hansmann GH: Sickle-cell anemia: A new cause of cor pulmonale. Am J Med Sci 191:474, 1936

47. Winsor T, Burch GE: The electrocardiogram and cardiac state in active sickle-cell anemia. Am Heart J 29:685, 1945

48. Whitaker W: Some effects of severe chronic anemia on the circulatory system. Q J Med 25:175, 1956

49. Friedberg CK: Diseases of the Heart, 3rd ed, p 1684. Philadelphia, W B Saunders, 1966

50. Oatway WH, Middleton WS: Correlation of lingual changes with other clinical data. Arch Intern Med 49:860, 1932

51. Darby WJ: The oral manifestations of iron deficiency. JAMA 130:830, 1946

52. Waldenström J, Kjellberg SR: The roentgenological diagnosis of sideropenic dysphagia (Plummer–Vinson's syndrome). Acta Radiol 20:618, 1939

53. Jacobs A: Epithelial changes in anemic East Africans. Br Med J 1:1711, 1963

54. Buckaleu VM, Someren A: Renal manifestations of sickle-cell disease. Arch Intern Med 133:660, 1974

55. Bradley SE, Bradley GP: Renal function during chronic anemia in man. Blood 2:192, 1947

56. Schwaber, JR, Blumberg AG: Papilledema associated with blood loss anemia. Ann Intern Med 55:1004, 1961

57. Földi M, Koranyi A, Szabo G: Über die Entstehung anämischer Odeme. Acta Med Scand 129:486, 1948

58. Marshall RA: A review of lesions in the optic fundus in various diseases of the blood. Blood 14:882, 1959

59. Goldhamer SM, Bethel FH, Isaacs R et al: Occurrence and treatment of neurologic changes in pernicious anemia. JAMA 103:1663, 1934

60. Grinker RR, Kandel E: Pernicious anemia: Results of treatment of neurologic complications. Arch Intern Med 54:851, 1934

61. Smithburn KC, Zerfas LG: The neural symptoms and signs in pernicious anemia. Arch Neurol Psychiatry 25:1110, 1931

62. Davidson S: Clinical picture of pernicious anemia prior to introduction of liver therapy in 1926 and in Edinburgh subsequent to 1944. Br Med J 1:241, 1957

63. Baird RL, Weiss DL, Ferguson AD et al: Studies in sickle-cell anemia. XXI. Clinico-pathological aspects of neurological manifestations. Pediatrics 34:92, 1964

64. Boggs DR, Frei E, III: Clinical studies of fever and infection in cancer. Cancer 13:1240, 1960

65. Panton PN, Maitland–Jones AG, Riddoch G: Pernicious anemia. An analysis of 117 cases. Lancet 1:274, 1923

66. Jacob HS, MacDonald RA, Jandl JH: Regulation of spleen growth and sequestering function. J Clin Invest 42:1476, 1963

67. Wintrobe MM, Beebe RT: Idiopathic hypochromic anemia. Medicine 12:187, 1933

68. Diggs LW: Siderofibrosis of the spleen in sickle-cell anemia. JAMA 104:538, 1935

69. **Muller–Eberhard U:** Hemopexin. N Engl J Med 283:1090, 1970

70. **Pimstone NR:** Renal degradation of hemoglobin. Semin Hematol 9:31, 1972

71. **Rowland LP, Penn AS:** Myoglobinuria. Med Clin North Am 56:1233, 1972

72. **Dacie JV:** The Haemolytic Anemias. Part I. The Congenital Anemias. 2nd ed, p 6. New York, Grune & Stratton, 1960

73. **Hillman RS, Finch CA:** Erythropoiesis: Normal and abnormal. Semin Hematol 4:327, 1967

74. **Hillman RS:** Characteristics of marrow production and reticulocyte maturation in normal man in response to anemia. J Clin Invest 48:443, 1969

75. **Erslev AJ:** Anemia in chromic renal disease. Arch Intern Med 126:774, 1970

76. **Hampers CL, Streiff R, Nathan DG et al:** Megaloblastic hematopoiesis in uremia and in patients on long term hemodialysis. N Engl J Med 276:551, 1967

77. **Eschbach JW, Adamson JW, Cook JD:** Disorders of red blood cell production in uremia. Arch Intern Med 126:812, 1970

78. **Stewart JH:** Haemolytic anemia in acute and chronic renal failure. Q J Med 36:85, 1967

79. **Cooper RA:** Pathogenesis of burr cells in uremia. J Clin Invest 48:22a, 1970

80. **Nathan DG, Schupak E, Stohlman F:** Erythropoiesis in anephric man. J Clin Invest 43:2158, 1964

81. **Cartwright GE, Lee GR:** The anemia of chronic disorders. Br J Haematol 21:147, 1971

82. **Ward HP, Kurnick JE, Pisarczyk GJ:** Serum level of erythropoietin in anemias associated with chronic infection, malignancy and primary hematopoietic disease. J Clin Invest 50:332, 1971

83. **Haurani FI, Burke W, Martinez EJ:** Defective re-utilization of iron in the anemia of inflammation. J Lab Clin Med 65:560, 1965

84. **Haurani FI, Young K, Tocantins LM:** Re-utilization of iron in anemia complicating malignant neoplasms. Blood 22:73, 1963

85. **Krantz SB:** Pure red cell aplasia. Br J Haematol 25:1, 1973

86. **Zaentz SD, Krantz SB:** Studies on pure red cell aplasia. VI. Development of two-stage erythroblast cytotoxicity method and role of complement. J Lab Clin Med 82:31, 1973

87. **Yunis AA, Bloomberg GR:** Chloramphenicol toxicity: Clinical features and pathogenesis. Prog Hematol 4:138, 1964

88. **Yunis AA:** Chloramphenicol-induced bone marrow suppression. Semin Hematol 10:225, 1973

89. **Weisberger AS:** Mechanism of action of chloramphenicol. JAMA 209:97, 1969

90. **Williams DM, Lynch RE, Cartwright GE:** Drug-induced aplastic anemia. Semin Hematol 10:195, 1973

91. **Bentler E, Fairbanks VF, Fahey JL:** Clinical Disorders of Iron Metabolism. New York, Grune & Stratton, 1963

92. **Beveridge BR, Bannerman RM, Evanson JM et al:** Hypochromic anemia: A retrospective study and follow-up of 378 in-patients. Q J Med 34:145, 1965

93. **Moore CV:** Iron metabolism and nutrition. Harvey Lect, 55:67, 1961

94. **Crosby WH:** The control of iron balance by the intestinal mucosa. Blood 22:441, 1963

95. **Schloesser LL, Kipp MA, Wenzel FJ:** Thrombocytosis in iron-deficiency anemia. J Lab Clin Med 66:107, 1965

96. **Wickramesinghe SN:** Kinetics and morphology of haemopoiesis in pernicious anemia. Br J Haematol 22:111, 1972

97. **Kilbridge TM, Heller P:** Determinants of erythrocyte size in chronic liver disease. Blood 34:739, 1969

98. **Cooper RA, Jandl JH:** Bile salts and cholesterol in the pathogenesis of target cells in obstructive jaundice. J Clin Invest 47:809, 1968

99. **Linman JW, Saarni MI:** The preleukemic syndrome. Semin Hematol 11:93, 1974

100. **Smith LH, Jr, Sullivan M, Hugneley CJ, Jr:** Pyrimidine metabolism in man. IV. Enzymatic defect of orotic aciduria. J Clin Invest 40:656, 1961

101. **Beck WS:** The metabolic basis of megaloblastic erythropoiesis. Medicine (Baltimore) 43:715, 1964

102. **Myhre E:** Studies on the erythrokinetics in pernicious anemia. Scand J Clin Lab Invest 16:391, 1964

103. **Smith ADM:** Veganism: A clinical survey with observations of vitamin B-12 metabolism. Br Med J 1:1655, 1962

104. **Toskes PP, Deren JJ, Conrad ME:** Clinical manifestations of pancreatic disease associated with vitamin B-12 malabsorption. Blood 40:944, 1972

105. **Miller DR, Bloom GE, Struff RR et al:** Juvenile "congenital" pernicious anemia: Clinical and immunological studies. New Engl J Med 275:978, 1966

106. **Imerslund O, Bjornstad P:** Familial vitamin B-12 malabsorption. Acta Haematol (Basel) 30:1, 1963

107. **Goldberg LS, Fudenberg HH:** The autoimmune aspects of pernicious anemia. Am J Med 46:489, 1969

108. **Samloff IM, Kleinman MS, Turner MD et al:** Blocking and binding antibodies to intrinsic factor and parietal cell antibody in pernicious anemia. Gastroenterology 55:575, 1968

109. **Doniach D, Roitt IM:** An evaluation of gastric and thyroid autoimmunity in relation to hematologic disorders. Semin Hematol 1:313, 1964

110. **Ellison ABC:** Pernicious anemia masked by multivitamins containing folic acid. JAMA 173:240, 1960

111. **Herbert V:** Megaloblastic anemias—mechanisms and management. In Dowling HF (ed): Disease-a-month, p 1. Chicago, Year Book Medical Publishers, August 1965

112. **Herbert V:** Experimental nutritional folate deficiency in man. Trans Assoc Am Physicians 75:307, 1962

113. **Sullivan LW, Herbert V:** Suppression of hematopoiesis by ethanol. J Clin Invest 43:2048, 1964

114. **Klipstein FA:** Folate deficiency secondary to disease of the intestinal tract. Bull NY Acad Med 42:638, 1966

115. **Klipstein FA:** Subnormal serum folate and macrocytosis associated with anticonvulsant drug therapy. Blood 23:68, 1964

116. **Streiff RR:** Folate deficiency and oral contraceptives. J Am Med Assoc 214:105, 1970

117. **Jandl JH, Greenberg MS:** Bone marrow failure due to relative nutritional deficiency in Cooley's hemolytic anemia. New Engl J Med 260:461, 1959

118. **Sullivan LW:** Differential diagnosis and management of the patient with megaloblastic anemia. Am J Med 48:609, 1970

119. **Mollin DL:** Sideroblasts and sideroblastic anemia. Br J Haematol 11:41, 1965

120. **Hines JD, Grasso JA:** The sideroblastic anemias. Semin Hematol 7:186, 1970

121. **Harris JW, Horrigan DL:** Pyridoxine-responsive anemias in man. Vitam Horm 26:549, 1968

122. **Kushner JP, Lee GR, Wintrobe MD et al:** Idiopathic refractory sideroblastic anemia. Clinical and laboratory investigation of 17 patients and review of the literature. Medicine 50:139, 1971

123. **Nathan DG:** Thalassemia. New Engl J Med 286:586, 1972

124. **Cooper RA, Shattil SJ:** Mechanisms of hemolysis—the minimal red cell defect. New Engl J Med 285:1514, 1971

125. **Rand RP, Burton AC:** Mechanical properties of the red cell membrane. I. Membrane stiffness and intracellular pressure. Biophys J 4:115, 1964

126. **Weed RI:** The importance of erythrocyte deformability. Am J Med 49:147, 1970

127. **Weed RI, LaCelle PL, Merrill EW:** Metabolic dependence of red cell deformability. J Clin Invest 48:795, 1969

128. **Turpin PF, LeBlond P, Gouffier E et al:** Acanthocytose acquise chez une femme splenectomisée pour sphérocytose héréditaire. Nouv Rev Fr Hematol 14:383, 1974

129. **Cooper RA, Gulbrandsen CL:** The relationship between serum lipoproteins and red cell membranes in abetalipoproteinemia: Deficiency of lecithin: Cholesterol acyltransferase. J Lab Clin Med 78:324, 1971

130. **Mant MJ, Faragher BS:** The hematology of anorexia nervosa. Br J Haematol 23:737, 1972

131. **Cooper RA:** Anemia with spur cells: A red cell defect acquired in serum and modified in the circulation. J Clin Invest 48:1820, 1969

132. **Weiss L:** A scanning electron microscopic study of the spleen. Blood 43:665, 1974

133. **Rosse W:** Correlation of in vivo and in vitro measurements of hemolysis in hemolytic anemia due to immune reactions. Prog Hematol 8:51, 1973

134. **LoBuglio AF, Cotran RS, Jandl JH:** Red cells coated with immunoglobulin G: Binding and sphering by mononuclear cells in man. Science 158:1582, 1967

135. **Gilliland BC, Baxter E, Evans RS:** Red cell antibodies in acquired hemolytic anemia with negative antiglobulin serum tests. New Engl J Med 285:252, 1971

136. **Worlledge SM:** Immune drug-induced hemolytic anemias. Semin Hematol 10:327, 1973

137. **Jacobson LB, Longstreth GF, Edgington TS:** Clinical and immunologic features of transient cold agglutinin hemolytic anemia. Am J Med 54:514, 1973

138. **Braun MC:** Microangiopathic hemolytic anemia. Ann Rev Med 21:133, 1970

139. **Marsh GW, Lewis SM:** Cardiac haemolytic anemia. Semin Hematol 6:133, 1969

140. **Bull BS, Rosenberg ML, Dacie JV et al:** Microangiopathic haemolytic anemia: Mechanisms of red cell fragmentation: In vitro studies. Br J Haematol 14:643, 1968

141. **Bennett JM, Healey PJM:** Spherocytic hemolytic anemia and acute cholecystitis caused by Clostridium welchii. New Engl J Med 268:1070, 1963

142. **Perkash A, Samp BM:** Red cell abnormalities after snake bite. J Trop Med Hyg 75:85, 1972

143. **Nance WE:** Hemolytic anemia of necrotic arachnidism. Am J Med 31:801, 1961

144. **Manzler AD, Schreiner AW:** Copper induced hemolytic anemia. A new complication of hemodialysis. Ann Intern Med 73:409, 1970

145. **Deiss A, Lee GR, Cartwright GE:** Hemolytic anemia in Wilson's disease. Ann Intern Med 73:413, 1970

146. **Ham TH, Shen SC, Fleming EM et al:** Studies on the destruction of red blood cells. IV. Thermal injury. Blood 3:373, 1948

147. **Smith JA, Lonergan ET, Sterling K:** Spur cell anemia. Hemolytic anemia with red cells resembling acanthocytes in alcoholic cirrhosis. New Engl J Med 271:396, 1964

148. **Cooper RA, Diloy–Purado M, Lando P et al:** An analysis of lipoproteins, bile acids, and red cell membranes associated with target cells and spur cells in patients with liver disease. J Clin Invest 51:3182, 1972

149. **Tchernia G, Navarro J, Becart R et al:** Anemic hemolytique avec acanthocytose et dyslipidemie au cours de deux hepatites neonatales. Arch Fr Pediatr 25:729, 1968

150. **Cooper RA, Kimball DB, Durocher JR:** The role of the spleen in membrane conditioning and hemolysis of spur cells in liver disease. New Engl J Med 290:1279, 1974

151. **Logue GL, Rosse WF, Adams JP:** Mechanisms of immune lysis of red blood cells in vitro: I. PNH cells. J Clin Invest 52:1129, 1973

152. **Hartmann RC, Jenkins DE, Jr:** The "sugar-water" test for paroxysmal nocturnal hemoglobinuria. New Engl J Med 275:155, 1966

153. **Dacie JV:** The Hemolytic Anemias. Part I. The Congenital Anemias. 2nd ed, Chap. 2, p 82. New York, Grune & Stratton, 1960

154. **Emerson CP, Jr, Shen SC, Ham TH et al:** Studies on destruction of red blood cells. IX. Quantitative methods

for determining the osmotic and mechanical fragility of red cells in the peripheral blood and splenic pulp. Arch Intern Med 97:1, 1956

155. **Selwyn JG, Dacie JV:** Autohemolysis and other changes resulting from the circulation in vitro of red cells from patients with congenital hemolytic anemia. Blood 9:414, 1954

156. **Valentine WN:** Deficiencies associated with Embden–Meyerhof pathway and other metabolic pathways. Semin Hematol 8:348, 1971

157. **Beutler E:** Abnormalities of the hexose monophosphate shunt. Semin Hematol 8:311, 1971

158. **Yoshida A, Stamatoyannopoulos G, Motulsky AG:** Biochemical genetics of glucose-6-phosphate dehydrogenase variation. Ann NY Acad Sci 155:868, 1968

159. **Dern RJ, Beutler E, Alving AS:** The hemolytic effect of primaquine. II. The natural course of the hemolytic anemia and the mechanism of its self-limited character. J Lab Clin Med 44:171, 1954

160. **Greenberg MS:** Heinz body hemolytic anemia. "Bite Cells"—a clue to diagnosis. Arch Int Med 136:153, 1976

161. **Pauling L, Itano HA, Singer SJ et al:** Sickle-cell anemia, a molecular disease. Science 110:543, 1949

162. **Bertles JF, Döbler J:** Reversible and irreversible sickling: A distinction by electron microscopy. Blood 33:884, 1969

163. **Bookchin RM, Nagel RL:** Interactions between human hemoglobins. Sickling and related phenomena. Semin Hematol 11:577, 1974

164. **Finch CA:** Pathophysiological aspects of sickle-cell anemia. Am J Med 53:1, 1972

165. **Perillie PE, Epstein FH:** Sickling phenomenon produced by hypertonic solutions: A possible explanation for the hyposthenuria of sicklemia. J Clin Invest 42:570, 1963

166. **Pearson HA, Cornelius EA, Schwartz AD et al:** Transfusion-reversible functional asplenia in young children with sickle-cell anemia. New Engl J Med 283:334, 1970

167. **Johnston RB, Newman SL, Struth AG:** Serum opsonins and the alternate pathway in sickle-cell disease. New Engl J Med 288:803, 1973

168. **Carrell RW, Lehmann H:** The unstable haemoglobin haemolytic anaemias. Semin Hematol 6:116, 1969

169. **Martelo OJ:** Diseases of disordered hemoglobin degradation. Adv Intern Med 20:345, 1975

170. **Carrell RW, Kay R:** A simple method for the detection of unstable hemoglobins. Br J Haematol 23:615, 1972

29

Nervousness and Fatigue
Sarah L. Minden
Peter Reich

Introduction
Clinical Approach to Assessment of Nervousness and Fatigue
  History
  Examination
  Formulation
Theoretical Explanations of Nervousness and Fatigue
  Pathophysiologic Explanations
    Overview
    Relevant Brain Anatomy
    Neurochemistry
    Stress
    Rest
  Psychological Explanations
    Overview
    Psychoanalytic Theory
    Learning Theory

    Ethological and Developmental Theory
    Other Phenomena
Differential Diagnosis
  Differential Diagnosis of Nervousness
    Normal Nervousness
    Psychological Disorders Presenting with Nervousness
    Physical Disorders Presenting with Nervousness
    Medications and Drugs of Abuse
  Differential Diagnosis of Fatigue
    Normal Fatigue
    Psychological Disorders Presenting with Fatigue
    Physical Disorders Presenting with Fatigue
    Medications and Drugs of Abuse
Summary

INTRODUCTION

Nervousness and fatigue are experienced by most people at some time in their lives, and they are among the most common complaints motivating people to seek medical help. These symptoms may reflect normal, foreseeable responses to a stressful situation, or they may indicate significant psychiatric or medical illness. The physician must distinguish between normal and pathologic symptoms and among the various causes of the abnormal. The diagnostic process is complicated, however, because of the many different, often idiosyncratic, words used by patients to convey their experiences of nervousness and fatigue and because of

the multiplicity of etiologies of these symptoms. For example, a young woman who describes the sudden onset of palpitations, shortness of breath, dizziness, tingling around her mouth and in her fingers, and the fear of dying or of losing her mind could be describing a panic attack, hyperventilation episode, cardiac arrhythmia, or pulmonary embolus. Many a patient who has presented with the most ominous signs and symptoms—crushing chest pain, inability to breathe, a choking sensation, tachycardia, rapid respirations, elevated blood pressure—has, after careful medical and psychiatric evaluation, been diagnosed as having anxiety neurosis.

Because of this confusing picture, physicians tend to

err on both sides, either missing diagnoses of serious medical illnesses or disregarding equally significant psychiatric disorders. In a large series of psychiatric outpatients, Hall and colleagues reported that 9.1% had undiagnosed medical disorders producing their psychiatric symptoms.[1] His review of the literature showed that physical illness caused psychiatric symptoms in 5% to 42% of cases, and in the majority these diagnoses were missed. Many studies support these findings.[2,3] On the other hand, Schwab points out that many patients with remediable psychiatric disorders—depressions, psychoses, anxiety states—are denied appropriate treatment because the psychiatric diagnosis is not made.

Despite the confusing nature of the clinical presentations, a thorough history, careful physical assessment, and a formal mental status examination often will point to the correct diagnosis, which may be confirmed or refuted by relevant laboratory studies.

CLINICAL APPROACH TO ASSESSMENT OF NERVOUSNESS AND FATIGUE

HISTORY

The key to a correct diagnosis is the history. The physician must understand precisely what each patient means when he speaks of nervousness and fatigue as he does, in his own terms. None of us talks like a physician or physiologist when it comes to our emotions, particularly when they are intense or frightening. The physician must translate what the patient says into the language of medicine.

All of us speak of both nervousness and fatigue in two quite different ways. We may use the language of the body and describe objective, somatic sensations. Or we may speak in terms of emotions and refer to subjective, inner experiences. In both cases, because these phenomena are difficult to describe, we tend to talk in metaphors, attempting to convey simultaneously a physical sensation and the emotional coloring with which we experience it. We may have "butterflies in our stomach," be "on edge," feel "keyed up," or be in a "bad mood." We may feel shaky, have "the jitters," complain of being sweaty and tense. One of us may say his heart is pounding or beating rapidly and that he feels breathless or about to choke. Another may experience blurred vision or ringing in his ears; still another complains of a lump in his throat or a heaviness in his chest. Some people have a tingling sensation and cold and clammy hands and feet, while others feel dizzy, light-headed, or faint. Still others complain of a dry mouth, diarrhea, constipation, or urinary fre-

quency. Sometimes there is no detectable change in bodily function but rather a heightened sense of processes that usually operate beyond conscious awareness.

We become preoccupied with these uncomfortable symptoms and may worry that something is physically wrong. We cannot concentrate, have trouble making decisions, and experience a sense of restlessness that interferes with completing tasks. We find it difficult to sort out the important from the trivial and to perceive phenomena accurately. We are irritable, short-tempered, and may have a sense of dread or a feeling that there is some danger lurking, although we cannot say what is alarming us. All in all, it is an unpleasant state.

Nervousness and anxiety are often used interchangeably. However, *nervousness* tends to be the more general and colloquial term for a state of excitability, tension, and jitteriness, and has a nonanatomic connotation of a physical disorder of "nerves." *Anxiety* is a more specific and clinical term for the same state and also places emphasis on a person's state of mind, signifying worry, apprehension, fear, or dread.

Fatigue has its own metaphors. We all complain of being "worn out," "all done in," "fed up," "disgusted." We say we are overworked, exhausted, apathetic, disinterested. In modern life, the medicine man with his tonics has been replaced by an array of stimulants and activities to jolt us out of our doldrums. Physically, people may say they are "weak all over," or point to weakness in particular muscle groups; they may say they lack strength and power or feel tired and faint.

The subjective experience is one of weariness, depletion, emptiness; we lack drive and ambition and are unable to find pleasure in anything.

But what does all this mean? What is the patient trying to say? Certainly he has indicated that something disagreeable is going on in *both* his mind and his body; it is up to the physician to decide which is the *primary* source of the problem in order to alleviate the discomfort. In trying to clarify the situation it is useful to have in mind what sorts of data to look for.

First, the symptoms need elaboration. When did they begin and how have they progressed? Are there any precipitating or relieving factors or other associated symptoms? Has this occurred at another time in the patient's life, and if so, under what circumstances? Do these symptoms run in the family? How do they interfere with the patient's life?

Second, medical conditions that cause nervousness and fatigue can be brought to light through the patient's responses to a methodical review of systems. Hall and colleagues found that four or more positive responses to a symptom checklist given to psychiatric

outpatients correlated highly with the presence of medical disease behind their psychiatric symptoms.[1] The most common physical complaints in order of frequency were sleep disturbance, severe weakness, extreme fatigue, inability to concentrate, memory loss, change in speech, chest pain, intermittent tachycardia, recent nocturia, recent onset of confusion, tremulousness, productive sputum, urinary frequency, dyspnea on exertion, and paresthesias. Most patients were unaware of their medical illnesses and had not sought medical attention.

Third, psychiatric disorders that present in this way can also be revealed by systematic review of a number of parameters. Are these symptoms acute or chronic? Are they related to a recent turn of events or do they seem part of the person's habitual way of coping with life, his character style? Does the precipitant seem to be "outside" the patient, requiring him to adjust to or deal with it in some way? Or do the symptoms have an autonomy from environmental events, seem to come from "inside," as in the case of an acute psychosis, a major depression, or an organic brain syndrome? The patient's past psychiatric history is often helpful in pointing toward these latter causes.

Situational or external precipitants tend to be of certain kinds:

Recent losses or changes such as the death of a close relative or friend, marriage or divorce, loss of a job, promotion or relocation, serious medical illness in the patient or family

Problems in relationships —tension, conflict—whether in the family, with friends, or at work

Developmental stages (adolescence, old age), which present new challenges and demands for adjustment

Unhurried answers to openended questions will provide a wealth of data about the patient's current situation. A sensitive, thoughtful inquiry that creates an atmosphere of support and trust enables physician and patient to work together toward clarifying the sources of the patient's symptoms.

Perhaps more important than any particular event itself is the way in which someone copes with it. The physician ought to develop a sense of what kind of person the patient is. Is this someone who usually deals with life well and is now overwhelmed for some reason? Or is the patient typically dependent, helpless, unable to manage the smallest discomforts and frustrations? One must take care that one's own biases and stereotypes do not interfere with an accurate assessment of the patient's personality. Attend to how the person relates to you: Is he hostile and defensive or open and trusting? Does he complain at length or sto-

ically minimize? Explore how he has handled difficult situations in the past. In this way a portrait may be sketched. It is often useful to talk with family members to get a broader perspective on how the patient's symptoms have affected his relationships, his ability to work and to enjoy life, and his self-esteem.

The feelings the patient evokes in the clinician serve as a barometer of distress: Severely depressed patients leave the interviewer feeling depleted, hopeless, while covertly resentful and bitter patients often induce feelings of anger and frustration.

EXAMINATION

The remainder of the clinical assessment involves a physical examination, mental status examination, and laboratory determinations. The physical examination may reveal the signs of autonomic arousal typical of nervousness: tachycardia, mild systolic hypertension, rapid respiratory rate, sweating, cold and clammy hands, coarse tremor, a tense facial expression, easy startle. But it may also show the stigmata of particular disease states that may be producing the nervousness and fatigue. The most common are cardiovascular, endocrine, nutritional and metabolic, infectious, and central nervous system (CNS) diseases.[3]

In the case of fatigue, there may be measurable diminution in the force of muscular contraction or in the capacity to perform work. But often there is only a subjective experience of "a discrepancy between the perceived effort and the outcome, [intuited] from something about fatigued muscles which can somehow be sensed by their owner even when they are not in use."[5]

The mental status examination is crucial in distinguishing between psychological and physical causes of these symptoms and in differentiating major psychiatric disorders from minor ones. If the symptoms result from psychosis, major affective disorders, or the organic brain syndromes, there will be telltale abnormalities on the exam. For instance, there may be evidence of a formal thought disorder with loose associations or flight of ideas and illogical thinking; there may be delusions, hallucinations, and deficits in attention, orientation, memory, and other cognitive functions. The patient may exhibit the psychomotor retardation or agitation of depression or the hyperactivity of mania; mood may be depressed or elated. A more detailed account of the distinguishing features of the different psychiatric disorders follows later in this chapter.

Laboratory data can be used to discriminate among the various causes of the nervousness and fatigue. Hall and colleagues found that of the patients with four

positive responses on his symptom checklist, "60% showed significant laboratory evidence of disease. . .[and] 77% of that group had illnesses that were previously unrecognized."[1]

FORMULATION

Following the history and examination, it will be necessary to pull together the material that has been gathered into a coherent account. While details follow in the sections on differential diagnosis, there will likely be one of four possible formulations:

1. *The nervousness and fatigue are understandable, "normal" responses to a particular situation*, and no medical or psychiatric disorder exists.
2. *A specific medical disorder exists*, the chief complaint of which is nervousness or fatigue.
3. *A psychiatric disorder exists* for which nervousness and fatigue are the presenting symptoms; in this case, nervousness is best spoken of as anxiety.
4. *A diagnosis cannot yet be made*, but the patient has real symptoms that deserve continuing observation and evaluation.

THEORETICAL EXPLANATIONS OF NERVOUSNESS AND FATIGUE

Our understanding of the pathophysiologic mechanisms of nervousness and fatigue is incomplete. Recent advances in neurochemistry and neurophysiology have pointed in new and exciting directions, but no comprehensive, unifying theory exists. Therefore, we often are unable to evaluate the relevance and importance of a particular experimental finding. Clinical application of what we have learned from the neurosciences is still rudimentary. Thus the explanations offered here are at times speculative and preliminary. Psychiatry over the past decade has made a marriage of sorts with the neurosciences: How successfully they will live together, complement one another, bring out the best in each other remains to be seen.

Central questions remain unanswered: How does thinking about something frightening produce a physical response? How does a neutral object stimulate fear in a phobic individual? Why does one person feel anxiety under circumstances that are not the least perturbing to another? Is emotion the result of the mind's perception of primary bodily changes, or do physiologic responses follow upon mental percepts?[6]

The study of nervousness as a state of mind is time honored, and purely psychological theories were all that existed until the past few decades. They have considerable explanatory power in their own realm and ought not to be disregarded as the neurophysiologic evidence accrues. The future may bring a comprehensive understanding that combines what is true and meaningful in all these accounts.

PATHOPHYSIOLOGIC EXPLANATIONS

Overview

Let us begin with a descriptive overview of a hypothetical mechanism for nervousness and follow with a more detailed account of its elements. Fatigue is less understood both conceptually and empirically; what is written here attempts to combine some disparate pieces of data and to offer one way of looking at the matter.

An event occurs. It is perceived by the sensory apparatus of the brain, and the information is relayed to the cerebral cortex and the reticular activating system (RAS) to compare it with memories and past experiences and to judge if it is unfamiliar or threatening (Fig. 29-1). If the stimulus is determined to be dangerous, the RAS creates a general state of arousal. The cerebral cortex is further stimulated (demonstrated by increased amplitudes on the electroencephalogram) and activates skeletal muscle through pyramidal and extrapyramidal pathways (measurable by electromyography). The limbic system structures are also aroused so that they, along with cortex and RAS, transmit to the hypothalamus the message of danger. The hypothalamus orchestrates the body's response to the danger. It activates the autonomic nervous system, particularly the sympathetic component, and it stimulates or inhibits the production of hormones by the pituitary. These hormones in turn will circulate to peripheral endocrine organs to cause them to release their hormones. The end result of combined neural and hormonal activity is the series of changes in the body organ systems that we have come to know as typical of acute anxiety or fear:

Cardiovascular changes include increases in heart rate, stroke volume, cardiac output, systolic blood pressure; and selective vasoconstriction and dilation to channel blood through vital organs and skeletal muscle

Pulmonary changes include increases in the rate and depth of respiration

Gastrointestinal changes include decreased peristalsis and secretion

Metabolic changes include increases in blood sugar and free fatty acids, and enhanced capacity for anaerobic metabolism

Pupil dilation

Increased sweating

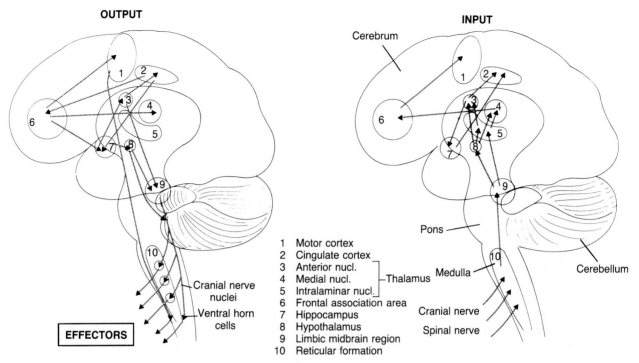

OUTPUT

INPUT

1 Motor cortex
2 Cingulate cortex
3 Anterior nucl.
4 Medial nucl.   ─Thalamus
5 Intralaminar nucl.
6 Frontal association area
7 Hippocampus
8 Hypothalamus
9 Limbic midbrain region
10 Reticular formation

Fig. 29-1. Circuitry in emotional brain. The hypothalamus receives input from all areas of the brain and activates the autonomic nervous system and stimulates the release of pituitary hormones, which in turn produce the physiologic changes characteristic of nervousness. (From Curtis BA, Jacobson S, Marcus EM: An Introduction to the Neurosciences, p 432. Philadelphia, WB Saunders, 1972)

There are a variety of secondary changes and effects:

Secondary cardiovascular changes include decreased blood flow to the brain with resulting light-headedness or even fainting. The increased rate and force of cardiac contractions are felt as palpitations.

Secondary pulmonary changes include hyperventilation, which decreases alveolar and arterial carbon dioxide tension, lowers blood *p*H, drives ionized calcium out of solution, and creates greater excitability in peripheral nerve endings, causing tingling in fingers and around the mouth and ultimately the carpopedal spasm of tetany. Dyspnea is the subjective experience of the excessive driving of the ventilatory apparatus.

If the stress is of short duration, the higher cortical centers will recognize an "all is well" state, call off the alert, and the system will begin to return to baseline. If the danger is perceived to persist or if the system cannot return to baseline for some other reason, then the state of hyperarousal continues. Initially this will be experienced simply as a state of chronic nervousness, but in time, with the "driving" of the body sys-

tems, there may be lasting alterations in organ structure and function.

It is plausible to think that when a system is driven long and hard it will eventually "wear down." Our understanding of fatigue presumably depends on greater knowledge of what goes on at the cellular level. But one can imagine that there are limits to the ability of single cells and organ-level aggregations to replenish energy substrates or to rebuild structural elements. There will be a critical state of depletion, with either opportunity to restore homeostasis if time for rest occurs, or with cell death if it does not. Many things drive the system: infection and the body's immune response to fight it, fever, emotional stress. Alternatively, the energy-producing apparatus may be consumed by cancer or chronic disease of any sort. Finally, there may not be sufficient nutrient input: For example, blood flow may be diminished by cardiovascular disease, oxygen supply may be insufficient owing to anemia or pulmonary disease, or nutrients may be unused (diabetes) or inadequately consumed (protein-, vitamin-, carbohydrate-deficiency states).

While the body's responses have been known in de-

tail for some time,[7] the interaction between cortex and end-organ has been clarified only recently. What remains for future study is how and where subjective or mental operations fit into the sequence.

An important breakthrough in understanding the mechanisms of nervousness and anxiety occurred when Pitts and McLure were able to produce panic attacks in those who suffered from them spontaneously, but not in normals, by intravenous infusions of lactate.[8] Perhaps even more significant was recognizing that this effect could be blocked by the monoamine oxidase inhibitor phenelzine[9] and by the tricyclic antidepressant imipramine.[10]

The blocking effects of these drugs pointed the way to the study of the CNS as one of the missing links in understanding nervousness and possibly fatigue. This involved combining the work of neuroanatomists, neurochemists, and neurophysiologists.

Relevant Brain Anatomy

Over the years, by selectively stimulating and ablating portions of brain in animals and man and watching for changes in behavior, neuroanatomists have been able to specify to a remarkable degree which areas of brain control which mental and somatic functions. The cortex of the frontal, parietal, temporal, and occipital lobes is now well mapped out and is known to be responsible for initiating voluntary movement, receiving and identifying somatic sensations, integrating and interpreting visual and auditory input, and producing speech. The cortex also remembers.

The prefrontal lobe or frontal association area is responsible for such intellectual functions as reasoning, planning, abstracting, judging. It is also involved in emotional control. The severance of its connections with other areas, particularly the limbic system, renders a person docile, unexcitable, free from anxiety, and unbothered by previously distressing events.[11]

The RAS, an extensive and diffuse network of ascending and descending tracts and nuclei forming the central core of the medulla, pons, and midbrain tegmentum, maintains arousal and level of attention. It participates in the comparison of incoming data with past experience and judges whether they are familiar or not—an important step in recognizing what is dangerous. It is important in the habituation to sensory stimuli and in sorting out what requires attention and what can be ignored. Danger, then, is first recognized as such by the cortex and RAS, which in turn activate the hypothalamus.

The limbic system or "emotional brain" was first described in 1937 by Papez as "a two way connexion in the nature of a circuit" for relaying information about emotion between hypothalamus and higher cortical centers. He pointed out that "emotional experience or subjective feeling" and the behavioral expression of emotion are quite separate, a notion that seems to be borne out in the phenomenology of both nervousness and fatigue.[12] Indeed, the more recent observations that propranolol, a β-adrenergic blocker, will prevent the somatic components of anxiety without affecting the psychological ones (except at very high doses), strengthens this bipartite view.[13]

The limbic system refers to a number of tracts and nuclei: the subcallosal, cingulate, and hippocampal gyri; the hippocampus itself; the temporal lobes; and the subcortical nuclei consisting of amygdala, septal nuclei, anterior thalamic nuclei, parts of the basal ganglia, and epithalamus. Possibly the most important region is the hypothalamus (see Figs. 29-1 and 29-4). This system acts as a unit in the regulation of "affective response to danger and the discrimination as to what is safe or dangerous."[14] Nevertheless, stimulation and ablation of its elements suggests that each part of the limbic system has a particular role to play in emotion. For example, the amygdala appears to excite emotion: Stimulation will produce a sense of danger and aggressiveness, while ablation causes placidity and lack of fear, rage, and aggression. The septal region in contrast seems to inhibit emotion: Stimulation results in relief from anger and frustration while ablation brings increased emotional reactivity, particularly rage and aggression. The hippocampus when stimulated is associated with hyperarousal and anxiety, whereas the cingulate gyrus causes a kind of alerting response.[11,14] All these behavioral effects are paralleled by the expected changes in cardiovascular and respiratory systems.

The functional center of emotional expression is the hypothalamus. Information is transmitted to it from other limbic structures and from all parts of the brain. It controls the operation of both the sympathetic and parasympathetic components of the autonomic nervous system. Parasympathetic effects include a decrease in heart rate, blood pressure, and respiratory rate, and an increase in salivation and gastrointestinal motility and secretion, pupillary constriction, and evacuation of bowels and bladder. The sympathetic effects that have already been enumerated result from direct innervation of particular organs or are mediated by the catecholamines epinephrine and norepinephrine, which are released from the adrenal medulla when it is stimulated by sympathetic neurons.

By secreting releasing factors [e.g. thyrotropin-releasing factor (TRF), somatostatin or growth hormone-releasing inhibiting hormone (SRIH), corticotropin-releasing factor (CRF)] into the hypothalamic-hypophyseal venous portal system, the hypothalamus induces

secretion of anterior pituitary hormones, adrenocorticotropic hormone (ACTH), thyroid-stimulating hormone (TSH), growth hormone (GH), and the gonadotropins [luteinizing hormone or interstitial cell-stimulating hormone (ICSH) and follicle-stimulating hormone (FSH), and prolactin]. These in turn act directly on cells (GH stimulates tissue growth and protein synthesis) or cause the production and release of those hormones (thyroid hormone, cortisol) that are the final effectors of many vital functions. By its dual control of neural and endocrine operations, then, the hypothalamus regulates cardiovascular and respiratory function; the metabolism of fat, carbohydrate, and protein; gastrointestinal function; and sexual activity. Because it synthesizes antidiuretic hormone (ADH) and

transfers it to the posterior pituitary for secretion, the hypothalamus controls body fluid and electrolyte balance. Finally, the hypothalamus is the major influence on the sleep cycle, temperature regulation, appetite and weight control.[11] In short, the hypothalamus evokes "the physiological changes associated with fear, anger, hunger, thirst, pleasure, and sex"[14] (Fig. 29-2).

Neurochemistry

Communication between neurons within the CNS has been clarified in recent years. The brain contains a vast number of amino acids, peptides, and proteins, which transmit impulses from one neuron to the next, regulate perception of pain, and act as hormones; they are intimately involved in the experience of emotion.

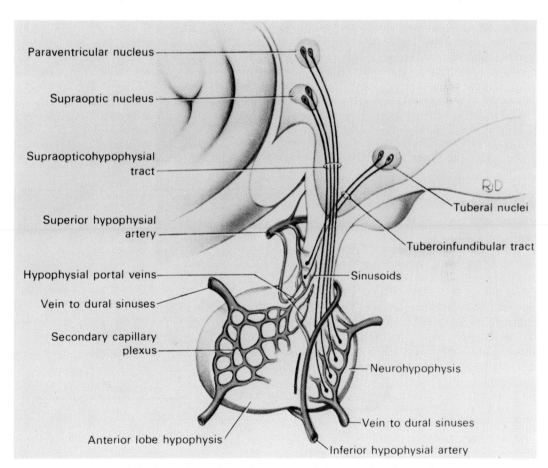

Fig. 29-2. Diagram of the hypophyseal portal system and the neural pathways between hypothalamus and pituitary. Hypothalamic releasing factors are secreted from the tubero-infundibular neurons into the capillaries of the portal vessels. They are then carried to the pituitary (hypophysis) where they stimulate the release of the pituitary hormones. Neurons from the supraoptic and paraventricular nuclei transmit antidiuretic hormone and oxytocin, respectively, directly into the posterior pituitary. (From Carpenter MB: Core Text of Neuroanatomy, p 177. Baltimore, Williams & Wilkins, 1972)

The neurotransmitters are a group of peptides and amino acids. The peptides include the catecholamines dopamine and norepinephrine, the indoleamine serotonin (5-hydroxytryptamine), and acetylcholine. Gamma-aminobutyric acid (GABA) is the best described of the amino acids. Transmission occurs between two synapsing neurons when one of these transmitters is released from the presynaptic neuron into the space between them, binds to a receptor protein on the postsynaptic neuron cell membrane, and thereby activates the second neuron. GABA inhibits cell firing (Fig. 29-3). Groups of neurons in discrete areas of the brain produce a single neurotransmitter. It is this fact that links structure and function in the CNS's control of emotion. For example, dopamine-producing neurons are found in the nigrostriatal tract, which originates in the substantia nigra and terminates in the corpus striatum (caudate and putamen); these neurons control fine motor activity; their destruction produces Parkinsonism. Dopamine-producing neurons also exist in the tuberoinfundibular tract, which begins in the arcuate nucleus and ends in the median eminence of the hypothalamus; these neurons are believed to control the release of hypothalamic-releasing factors. Dopaminergic neurons are prominent in limbic system structures. Based on the observation that drugs that block dopamine activity in the brain will reduce the symptoms of schizophrenia, it is hypothesized that an excess of dopamine causes these symptoms.

Norepinephrine is found in highest concentrations in the hypothalamus and the locus ceruleus which, if stimulated, produces anxietylike behavior in primates. By study of its chief metabolite, 3-methoxy-4-hydroxylphenyl glycol (MHPG), which is presumed to reflect central nonpinephrine activity, many researchers believe that levels of norephinephrine can "provide a biochemical criterion for distinguishing subtypes of depressive disorders."[15] Others suggest caution in interpreting such data as we do not yet know precisely what is "normal."[16]

Sweeney found that elevated MHPG levels are associated with anxiety, stress, and arousal.[17] This suggests a connection between anxiety and depression and may explain why antidepressants are useful in panic attacks. Serotonin is implicated in depressive states as well as in the regulation of sleep, appetite, temperature, and arousal (Fig. 29-4).

Concomitant with these hypotheses of alterations in

PRESYNAPTIC NEURON   POSTSYNAPTIC NEURON

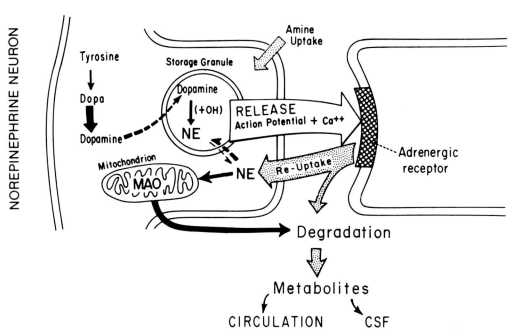

Fig. 29-3. Neuronal synapse showing synthesis of neurotransmitter, release, reuptake, and enzymatic degradation. (From Baldessarini RJ: Chemotherapy in Psychiatry, p 83. Cambridge, Harvard University Press, 1977)

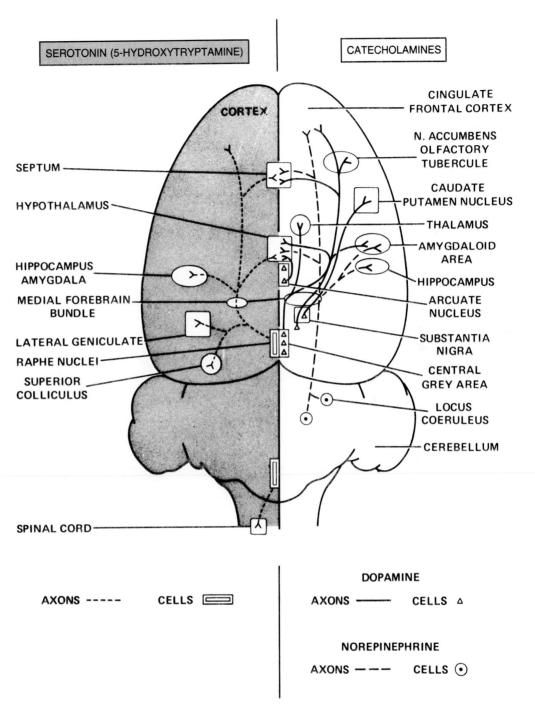

Fig. 29-4. Schematic representation of catecholamine and serotonin (5-hydroxytryptamine) pathways in the rat brain. (From Barchas JD, Berger PA, Ciaranello RD, Elliott GR: Psychopharmacology. From Theory to Practice, p 38. New York, Oxford University Press, 1977. Drawing courtesy of Dr. Stanley J. Watson)

levels of neurotransmitters are hormonal theories of emotion. Changes in the activity of neurotransmitters causes the release of hypothalamic and pituitary hormones. Hormonal changes have been most extensively studied in depression; however, since many endocrine diseases present with nervousness, it is possible that future research will demonstrate endocrine disturbances in anxiety states as well.

The following endocrine abnormalities have been found in depressed patients:

Hypersecretion of cortisol, absence of the usual diurnal variation, and failure to suppress the levels with administration of dexamethasone;[18,19]

Failure of GH levels to rise in response to insulin-induced hypoglycemia: Infants who have had maternal neglect (alternatively called Failure to Thrive and anaclitic depression) show inhibited GH secretion

Failure of TSH levels to rise in response to thyrotropin-releasing hormone (TRH) challenge[20,21,22]

GABA is an inhibitory transmitter concentrated in the substantia nigra, globus pallidus, and hypothalamus. Reduced levels of GABA in the basal ganglia are thought to be involved in Huntington's disease and also in anxiety. Recently, specific receptors for benzodiazepines, but not for other sedative-hypnotic drugs, have been found in the hippocampus, olfactory bulb, and thalamic nuclei. These receptors seem to have two components: binding of drug to one part of the receptor enhances the binding of GABA to the other.

Snyder proposes that anxiety occurs when particular neural pathways fire excessively.[23] There is a concomitant feedback signal for GABA release in order to inhibit neuronal firing; insufficient GABA results in continued discharge. When a benzodiazepine is present it binds to its portion of the receptor, enhances GABA-binding, and thereby potentiates the inhibitory effect. The theory goes on to explain tolerance and withdrawal symptoms: With continued intake of benzodiazepine, less GABA is needed, but as less will be produced or released, more benzodiazepine is required for the same inhibitory effect; hence, the development of tolerance. When the drug is stopped, there is insufficient GABA to inhibit neuronal firing, and a rebound hyperactivity occurs, producing withdrawal anxiety. Eventually the normal production and feedback mechanisms are restored.

Gray suggests that the particular site of action of the antianxiety drugs is the noradrenergic pathway from the locus ceruleus to the septohippocampal area where GABA-ergic neurons synapse on these neurons.[24]

The enkephalins and endorphins, discovered in 1975, are peptide neurotransmitters with opiatelike properties that mediate the response to pain. Found in hypo-thalamus and other limbic structures, these may be the source of the clinically well-known connection between pain and anxiety and depression. Indeed, there have been reports that endorphins have had some alleviating effects on the symptoms of depression and schizophrenia for brief periods of time.[25] Acetylcholine is widespread in the brain and has effects on behavior that have not yet been clarified.

Stress

Research on the effects of stress on animals and humans examines the conditions that evoke the responses we have been considering and measures the specific behavioral and physiologic changes that occur. *Stress* may be used to refer to "a characteristic of the environment, the response of the individual, or the *interaction* of an individual's perception of environment and his response, such that a particular situation is *stressful* for him."[26]

Changes in the levels of cortisol and the catecholamines epinephrine and norepinephrine have been studied under conditions of acute and chronic stress. Anticipating surgery, taking examinations, performing strenuous exercise, doing mental arithmetic under pressure, or relocating because of career demands all have been demonstrated to produce a rise in levels of these hormones. Individual differences in hormonal response, however, emphasize that it is a person's particular perception of an event as stressful rather than the event itself which underlies these changes. Studies of women undergoing biopsy for breast cancer[27] and parents of leukemic children[28] have shown that the presence of psychological defenses that protect the individual from being emotionally upset (denial, avoidance, isolation of affect) correlates with a lower level of stress-labile hormones, even though these defenses may be maladaptive by delaying contact with a physician or postponing the process of grieving. When such people are forced to confront the stressful situation and become clinically distressed, these hormones have been found to rise.

The stressful conditions that will cause an elevation in cortisol are typically unfamiliar, strange, unpredictable. If they are sustained or recreated, thus becoming familiar, cortisol levels do not rise and the pituitary does not secrete ACTH. Study of untrained and seasoned pilots and parachutists showed a significant cortisol rise only in the former. When subjects develop a successful coping response to a given stress they too show little hormonal change.[26]

This habituation of a hormonal stress-response for the corticosteroids is not true for the catecholamines. A study of mice housed under conditions of crowding

showed persistent increases in blood pressure, as well as in epinephrine and norephinephrine and the enzymes for synthesizing them.[29] Since the catecholamines are released as a result of direct neuronal stimulation of the adrenal medulla, these results are consistent with the hypothesis that sustained autonomic arousal, as in chronic anxiety, may be one of the many factors involved in a number of disease states. Classically, these are the psychosomatic or psychophysiologic disorders: peptic ulcer and dysfunction of intestinal motility and secretion; hypertension, coronary artery disease, and cardiac arrhythmias; asthma; rheumatoid arthritis and other immune system diseases; headache; frequency of micturition; and psychogenic vomiting. We can refer to only a few of the many studies in this area; the reader may consult a standard text for a more extensive summary.[30]

Taggart and colleagues studied the cardiovascular responses of public speakers (a "normal" anxiety-provoking situation) and found tachycardia ranging from 125 to 180 beats per minute and increased levels of plasma noradrenaline and free fatty acids.[31] In some with preexisting heart disease, ventricular and supraventricular ectopic beats and ST segment depression occurred. These changes could be blocked by β-blocking drugs, confirming the role of sympathetic arousal in producing these changes. While unproven, the implication is that the mobilized free fatty acids are then involved in the production of atheromatous plaques and hence in the narrowing of vessels that results in ischemia.

Type A behavior, with its "aggressiveness, competitiveness, ambition, drive for success, restlessness, impatience, devotion to work, a subjective sense of time urgency, abruptness of speech and gesture, and a tendency to hostility," has been shown in some studies to correlate with elevated plasma levels of triglycerides and cholesterol, increased diurnal secretion of norepinephrine, accelerated clotting, and extensive coronary artery narrowing.[32] While the causes of coronary artery disease are certainly multifactorial, such persistent autonomic arousal with its metabolic consequences may be significant.[33] Strong emotion, such as fear or anger, probably through the autonomically mediated increase in cardiac work and oxygen consumption, may be implicated in angina pectoris,[34] myocardial infarction, and various arrhythmias.[35–37] Psychological factors were present along with allergic and infective processes in 70% of asthmatic attacks in one study; contrary to popular belief they preceded alone only 1.2% of attacks.[38] There is also some evidence that intense emotion (anger, irritability, anxiety), especially if it remains unexpressed, may contribute to the onset of an attack.[39]

Some studies suggest that emotional stress is involved in rheumatoid arthritis and other disorders of immune system regulation, including cancer.[40]

Tension headache has been shown to be associated with anxiety in 50% to 80% of cases and with depression in 20% to 40%.[41]

The effects of stress remain incompletely understood.[42] The evidence is increasing that the role of anxiety, tension, and stress-related emotional responses is very complicated. In some cases, their presence seems to correlate with a better disease outcome, while in others they appear to have a direct and lasting negative impact on bodily function and integrity. These latter situations may be related to overwhelming stress or inadequate psychological adaptation.

Rest

The role of sleep deprivation in the etiology of fatigue is a complicated and insufficiently understood subject. Sleep is biphasic, with a peaceful, restful portion called *synchronized or S-sleep* (also non-rapid-eye-movement sleep or non-REM sleep) where there is a decrease in heart and respiratory rate, blood flow, and oxygen consumption; and an active, aroused portion called *desynchronized or D-sleep* (also rapid-eye-movement or REM sleep) where there is increased activity in all autonomically-mediated systems as well as a descending muscular paralysis.[43] The control of sleep onset and its phases appears to involve reciprocal activity and inhibition in the serotonergic and noradrenergic (sleep) systems, as opposed to the dopaminergic (arousal) system.

Studies of sleep deprivation have mixed results but do tend to suggest that a state of autonomic hyperarousal ensues with subjective reports of decreased alertness, decreased vigor, increased confusion, and increased fatigue. We hypothesize that sleep is a time of restoration and repair, but there are not conclusive data to establish this. It does seem clear that whatever interferes with sleep—anxiety, pain, illness—will lead to fatigue; when sleep is restored, fatigue will be lessened.

PSYCHOLOGICAL EXPLANATIONS

Overview

The pathophysiology of *what* happens to make us feel nervous and fatigued is increasingly clear. Buy *why* it should happen is not. To begin to answer the question of *why* someone is anxious and exhausted we must add a psychological dimension. Given the uncertainties of our current knowledge we are forced to view the psyche as if through a prism, from a variety of different perspectives, taking each facet in turn. The *psychodynamic*

point of view emphasizes the power of past experiences in determining present behavior and the role of intrapsychic conflict in disrupting mental equilibrium. *Learning theory,* on the other hand, looks at human behavior as a product of reinforced conditioning that conforms to certain laws derived from laboratory experimentation; behavior is independent of both conscious and unconscious wishes. *Ethologists* believe that certain regularities in human behavior are determined by species-specific inheritable repertoires that can be inferred from the naturalistic study of animals and men. Finally, many isolated observations, unconfined by any particular theory, exist to remind us of the power and autonomy of what we have for centuries simply called mind or will.

Psychoanalytic Theory

Sigmund Freud and his followers have theorized about anxiety in a number of ways but the most enduring is the notion of anxiety as a signal of danger.[44] Throughout life adults experience conflict between expressing their instinctual desires, aggression and sexuality, and conforming to the needs and wishes of society. Such conflict always produces anxiety. The mentally "healthy" solution is to recognize one's wishes, tolerate the anxiety, and find satisfactory mediating solutions.[45] In the neuroses exaggerated childlike fears of retaliation or disapproval persist and make a reasonable solution impossible. The anxiety increases and signals the ego to mobilize a set of defenses which, by subduing the primary impulse, more or less effectively contain the anxiety. These defenses include simply denying one's wishes or forgetting about them (repression), pretending one does not have them (reaction formation), or justifying them as more "reasonable" than they are (rationalization, intellectualization.)[46] However, the chronic reliance on these defenses distorts a personality and interferes with obtaining pleasure in life. Moreover, when these defenses prove inadequate because the impulse is too strong or the ego too weak, then the anxiety becomes overwhelming, and more serious symptoms are called into play to attempt to manage it. As Freud put it, "Each individual has in all probability a limit beyond which his mental apparatus fails in its function of mastering the quantities of excitation which require to be disposed of."[44] (See the discussion on post traumatic stress disorder, which follows later in this chapter.) Symptoms such as phobias or compulsions arise from attempts to avoid or escape from recognizing instinctual desires. For example, aggressive impulses, deemed unacceptable, may be denied and displaced onto an external object, such as an animal: "The animal is the aggressive one, not me; therefore I am afraid of *it*, not of my own impulses and desires, which would, if expressed,

make people disapprove of me." Neurasthenia, with its incapacitating fatigue, is the symptomatic escape from neurotic anxiety *par excellence,* a paralysis of energy and will that ensures that no impulse or desire at all be expressed.

There is an extensive psychoanalytic literature of anxiety that is beyond the scope of this chapter. One intriguing thought, however, is that raised by Compton.[47] Anxiety involves a time distortion: What is in actuality *not* occurring but imagined as possible to occur in the future (*e.g.,* the airplane will crash), is experienced *as if* it were occurring in the present. While he does not elaborate on this idea, it may be that it is this imaginary creation of a present danger that somehow sets into motion the neuroendocrine response we have described. Indeed, it is the restoration of the correct time frame—the forced recognition that the danger is in fact *not* presently occurring—that often serves to alleviate anxiety. The mind plays tricks on the body.

Learning Theory

Learning theorists postulate that *anxiety* is a learned response to particular stimuli acquired through the process of conditioning first outlined by Pavlov. A painful stimulus will produce a physiologic response in an animal. If the painful stimulus (unconditioned stimulus) is repeatedly presented with a neutral stimulus such as a bell or a light, the animal will come to be as afraid of the neutral stimulus (light) as he was of the painful one (shock). The light is considered the conditioned stimulus and the resulting fear is the conditioned response.

This theory has been used to explain phobias: During a forgotten traumatic experience in the past, a neutral stimulus (a dog) had been paired to a noxious stimulus and now independently elicits the fear response (animal phobia). This in turn compels the sufferer to do something to alleviate the fear: avoid dogs. Since this appears successfully to put an end to the anxiety, the avoidant behavior is reinforced. This process can be more complex. In cases where complaints of fatigue successfully permit avoidance of unwanted work or responsibility, or win longed-for attention, the fatigue will be reinforced.

Klein and others have pointed out the problems in learning theory's account of phobias:[48]

Because we usually cannot find the hypothetical original paired event, the theory does not explain why one person fears a certain situation and others do not, or why some objects, often in reality more threatening, such as traffic or weapons, tend not to become typical phobic objects.

Why does avoidant behavior spread to include other objects besides the original one?

Why do some phobias respond to flooding techniques, where the person is put directly into the frightening situation and permitted no escape? Theoretically this should strengthen the power of the neutral situation to elicit fear, as it is paired with such a massive anxiety response.

The use of biofeedback, relaxation exercises, and meditation have indicated that people can learn to modulate autonomically controlled phenomena such as blood pressure, heart rate, intestinal secretion and motility, thus supporting a place for classical conditioning in our understanding of both visceral and subjective aspects of anxiety.[49,50]

Ethological and Developmental Theory

Bowlby and others believe that infants are born with a biologically-determined and evolutionarily selected potential to behave in such a way as to attach their mothers to them: to cry, smile, babble, and gesture to induce reciprocal behaviors in the mother that will gratify their needs for food, nurturance, and protection.[51,52] Among these attachment behaviors are those for "emergencies," when the need for maternal help is great or some danger is perceived, particularly loss of or separation from the mother-figure. The infant's feeling state, presumably akin to anxiety, leads to dramatically compelling behaviors to re-establish the connection with the mother, literally to force her to return to care for him. When the child becomes mobile and wanders too far away, this separation anxiety serves as a signal to him to re-establish contact, whether by returning to her or calling out in some way for help.[53] The internal alarm is sounded when the degree or length of separation is too great for that particular child or when strange persons or situations appear (helplessness) or when illness, fatigue, or pain intervene. There is a complex interaction between the infant's innate capacity to tolerate anxiety and his ability to induce caring in others; the mother's ability accurately to perceive and appropriately respond to her infant's lures; the vicissitudes of life with its losses or separations that are handled well or badly—all of these determine a person's capacity to experience, tolerate, and find solutions to anxiety. At times of stress, illness, or loss, a person's ability to cope with the anxieties aroused by these situations—analogous to the infant's state—depends on how well his development has equipped him to create and maintain attachments with helping people. Research has borne out the central role of human relationships in exciting and soothing anxiety: "In adult life, increased anxiety has been related to disturbances in interpersonal relationships, and, in particular, to problems in marriage and companionship, problems at work, and problems for mothers in parenting. Fi-

nancial problems contribute to anxiety only when they reach severe levels. Social class and type of neighborhood have little bearing on the prevalence of anxiety."[54]

Klein applies ethological theories to understanding panic attacks:[48]

> I hypothesize that the protest-despair mechanisms have coevolved over our species history to deal with the regular evolutionary contingency of the lost toddler. Conceivably, the appearance of apparently spontaneous panic attacks or apparently spontaneous depressive episodes are due to a pathologically lowered threshold for release of these distressing affective regulatory states. If the threshold were lowered in that portion of the regulatory mechanism that controls protest, then spontaneous anxiety attacks occur, whereas if the lowered threshold occurs in the segment that regulates despair, then a phasic depressive episode results. I make the parsimonious hypothesis that the sole function of all antidepressants is simply to raise thresholds thoughout this apparatus (a far cry from the catecholamine deficiency theory). The beneficial effects on anxiety attacks and/or depression result from this normalization of function.

Other Phenomena

Cognitive factors are clearly powerful, for studies have shown that what a subject is told about an epinephrine injection can be more powerful in determining his response than the hormone itself.[55] Cannon's writing on voodoo death[56] and work on sudden cardiac death under conditions of emotional stress[57] point to the profound influence that psychological phenomena can have on the CNS and organism as a whole. How they do so remains to be elucidated.

Finally, there are some persons who seem to have a basic inability to describe their emotions, localize them in their bodies, distinguish among them, or to elaborate fantasies in association with them. These patients are believed by some to represent a discrete psychological entity called *alexithymia* (no words for feelings). While the observations appear valid, there is as yet no satisfactory explanation for the difficulty in labeling emotional experience.[58]

DIFFERENTIAL DIAGNOSIS

Nervousness and fatigue are nonspecific symptoms. In making a diagnosis one is most concerned to determine whether or not they reflect major psychiatric or medical disorders. One may approach the problem as suggested in the flow charts that accompany discussion of the specific symptom, where both physical and psychological illnesses are eliminated or accepted on the basis of specific criteria.[59] In most cases one can

rule out organic disease on the basis of history, review of systems, physical examination, and laboratory studies. Psychoses, major affective disorders, and organic brain syndromes are all detectable by history and mental status examination along with the rest of the evaluation. That leaves us with anxiety and somatoform disorders and with "normal" responses to situational stresses.

DIFFERENTIAL DIAGNOSES OF NERVOUSNESS

Normal Nervousness

Nervousness that has a recognizable cause that would similarly affect most people, that lasts only a "reasonable" amount of time, and that is not too intense, is not likely to be pathologic. What counts as "normal" is something that tends to be socially and culturally determined. Anxiety has positive value when it spurs us on to find new and better solutions to problems or to acquire the skills to deal more effectively with what at first seems overwhelming. In these cases it leads to greater competence and self-confidence. It is useful, too, when it propels us to leave or avoid situations that are best dealt with in that way: a young child first stops himself from walking into the street because of the anxiety aroused by imagining a parental "no."

We expect a person to be somewhat apprehensive when hospitalized, while awaiting surgery, or while confined to an intensive care unit.[60] Most people can deal with such situational anxiety by understanding why it occurs and by knowing that it will pass. Fear is a special case of "understandable" anxiety, when danger is real, present, or imminent. There is no difference in the physiologic sensations in nervousness and fear; the distinction lies in the fact that there is no *good* reason why the nervous person should be afraid. When this "fact" is recognized, the person begins to deal effectively with the distressing situation. When this does not occur, we enter the realm of psychological disorder. Figure 29-5 is a flow chart for the differential diagnosis of nervousness.

Psychological Disorders Presenting with Nervousness

Anxiety States. *Generalized anxiety disorder* is the paradigm of anxiety disorders and refers to a relatively persistent state of "motor tension, autonomic hyperactivity, apprehensive expectation, and vigilance and scanning."[59] The patient complains of constant or near-constant shakiness, jumpiness, muscle tension, fatigue. He feels "keyed up," appears tense, has darting eyes, startles easily, and restlessly fidgets or paces. There is an urgency to his complaints of discomfort and a pleading insistence on obtaining relief. He is convinced there is something wrong with his body or his mind. He can think of little else, feels under great pressure, is irritable, and exhausted. Sleep is fitful and provides no rest; he may drink alcohol or take tranquilizers to calm his "nerves." Neither you nor he can find anything to explain his condition; physical examination and laboratory studies reveal nothing beyond a mild sinus tachycardia, mildly elevated systolic hypertension, rapid breathing, mild tremor, and cold and clammy extremities. This is a chronic state where symptoms may subside for a while only to reappear when some external stress occurs. It has been estimated that 5% of the general population suffers significantly from anxiety, while among patients in a general medical practice the proportion rises to over 35%.[61] Twice as many women as men are affected.

We are using the term anxiety now as a diagnosis as well as a symptom. Such usage indicates that we are in the psychological realm and that no organic cause is known; if it were, we would speak instead of "nervousness" (as a symptom) or specify the nature of the anatomic arousal. The causes of generalized anxiety disorder and the other anxiety states described below are unclear, but current explanations include a disorder of neurotransmitters or of the autonomic nervous system; intrapsychic conflict where anxiety has broken through the usual ego defenses; or a biologic response to a definable stress. In the latter cases, the search for the conflict or the stress is the first step in treatment.

Panic disorder. This is a not uncommon disorder affecting 6.3 per 1000 population or two million Americans.[62,63] Panic attacks occur as discrete, unpredictable episodes of profound fear or dread, accompanied by physical sensations of dyspnea, dizziness, a lump in the throat, pain in the chest, palpitations, pounding in the head, sweating, shaking, tingling about the mouth and in the fingers. The patient is convinced he will die by choking or suffocating, is having a stroke or heart attack, or is about to pass out. The attack lasts a few minutes, but it may take hours to recover from this frightening experience. It comes "out of the blue," may recur often or never again.

The patient becomes tense and vigilant expecting "it" to happen again and so develops a secondary, ongoing anticipatory anxiety. He begins to fear going out of the house lest the attack occur and avoids places from which there is no escape or in which he cannot receive help should the attack recur (*e.g.,* tunnels, highways, crowds). Thus a phobic state develops. Such a patient can be strikingly incapacitated, never leaving home, unable to work or to find pleasure. Klein emphasizes that panic attack and agoraphobia are two discrete disorders: tricyclic antidepressants and monamine oxidase inhibitors will in many cases relieve the panic attacks (the primary disorder); but they have no effect

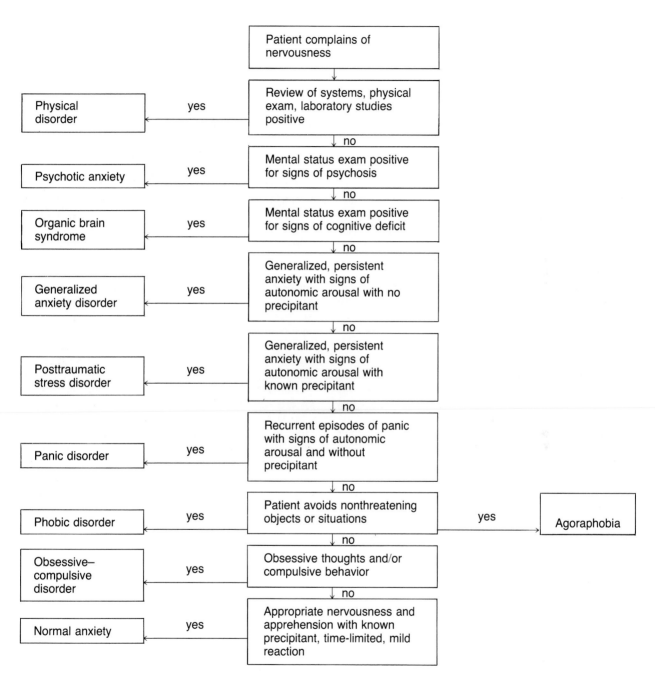

Fig. 29-5. Differential diagnosis of nervousness.

on the secondary avoidant phobic anxiety state, which requires psychotherapeutic measures.[48,64] Klein also believes there is a *forme fruste* of the panic attack such that "patients may have partial, rudimentary panic attacks, sufficiently uncomfortable to serve as an unconditioned stimulus. . ." to keep them at home; in this case the agoraphobia will be the presenting symptom, and there will be no history of panic attacks. He supports this notion with findings of "a continuously unstable level of skin conductance with subclinical spontaneous fluctuations in their level of autonomic discharge" in agoraphobes but not in normals.[48] The reason for the spontaneous occurrence of panic attacks is unknown, but neurophysiology may provide some answers.

Phobic disorders. "The essential feature is persistent and irrational fear of a specific object, activity, or situation that results in a compelling desire to avoid the dreaded object, activity, or situation (the phobic stimulus). The fear is recognized by the individual as excessive or unreasonable in proportion to the actual dangerousness of the object, activity, or situation."[59] Persons may fear social situations (social phobia) believing they will be scrutinized or do something embarrassing. They may have a single fear (simple phobia) of snakes, insects, heights, or airplanes. Or they may have the far more common agoraphobia described earlier. Phobic disorder affects less than 1% of the adult population. Animal and social phobias are quite common during childhood and adolescence, respectively. Psychoanalysis and learning theory offer the most trenchant accounts of these symptoms.

Posttraumatic stress disorder. This stands in sharp contrast to the anxiety states because of the readily identifiable precipitating event. There can be little doubt about the intimate connection between having been a helpless victim of a natural disaster (flood, earthquake) or a man-made horror, whether accidental (fire, explosion, automobile or plane crash) or intentional (rape, torture, death camps, war), and the symptoms that follow.[65–70] Characteristically, patients report intrusive, unwanted, vivid memories and thoughts of the trauma associated with painful waves of emotion; they are plagued by recurrent dreams and nightmares. Perhaps to prevent these intrusive thoughts and feelings, they experience a "numbness" or detachment from other people and situations. Typically, there is free-floating or panic anxiety, sleep disturbance, and a depressed or dysphoric mood. Patients avoid circumstances that might bring on memories or emotions and may use drugs or alcohol to try to block them out. Many feel guilty about having survived or about behaviors that permitted survival.

The diagnosis is not difficult when these symptoms occur in close temporal proximity to the trauma. However, they may not emerge for long periods of time, and occasionally the traumatizing event is forgotten or repressed, as with incestuous rape or torture. The syndrome may occur with less horrifying events and has been described after surgery and minor trauma.[71]

Prepsychotic and psychotic anxiety. The anxiety experienced by the person who is becoming acutely psychotic is of a magnitude and quality quite different from what we have been discussing. While a patient may find it hard to describe, he may experience uncanny feelings of intense dread, have terrifying sensations of his body disintegrating, and believe he is losing his mind. Nameless at first, these feeling states may come to be incorporated into delusional beliefs about the destruction of himself or others. When the diffuse fears are "explained" in this way, the panic seems to abate, perhaps because the world now seems less strange and unfamiliar. In both prepsychotic and psychotic anxiety, autonomic arousal is present. An adolescent who is nearly paralyzed with fear, who is convinced that his life is in danger and who is unable to put words on unique somatic and mental sensations, may be on the verge of a schizophrenic psychotic episode. A patient who has just undergone cardiac surgery may be terrified by the perceptual distortions and hallucinations that can be precipitated by the metabolic derangements of the postoperative state. Outward appearances may be misleadingly benign, but as the physician explores the nature of the patient's experience and the meaning it has for him, the enormity of this state will usually become apparent.

Depression. There is considerable interest at the present time in the relationship between anxiety and depression, prompted by the frequent (33%–50%) coexistence of depressive symptoms in patients with anxiety disorders and by the discovery that antidepressants (tricyclics and monoamine oxidase inhibitors) may relieve both kinds of symptoms.[72] Some feel that anxiety and depression represent two distinct syndromes,[73] while others believe that they represent two ends of a spectrum of a single affective disorder.[74,75] Still others feel that there are subgroups of anxiety disorders, namely those with and without secondary depression, and that these have different prognostic and genetic features.[72,76] Indeed, the secondary depression of alcoholism that results from "self-medication" often brings the patient to medical attention, rather than the anxiety. A detailed discussion of depression follows in the differential diagnosis of fatigue. The reader is referred to the previous discussion on the possible neurochemical links between the two disorders.

Common to the disorders just described above is the likelihood that the patient will in one way or another say, "I'm nervous." However, there are psychological

syndromes where the person is not really aware that he is anxious, although those around him might have no difficulty recognizing the state of arousal by the tense look on his face or the rigidity of his posture. Instead of overt anxiety the patient develops other kinds of symptoms, either of a purely mental nature, as in obsessive–compulsive disorder, or of a seemingly physical nature, as in the many somatoform disorders.

Obsessive–Compulsive Disorders. The obsessive patient is plagued by thoughts, images, and impulses that are recurrent, unshakable, and experienced as unwanted intrusions beyond his control. These thoughts are typically painful and distressing and may include guilty ruminations, self-doubts, impulses to do harm, and fears of being contaminated. The patient recognizes them as illogical and shameful but feels utterly captivated by them and forced to take them seriously. *Compulsions* are behavioral analogues to obsessions where the patient feels pressed to perform a certain act—handwashing, counting, checking—often in elaborately ritualistic ways, in order to ward off some per-

sistent worry that something dreadful will happen. There are varying degrees of consciously experienced anxiety depending on how effectively the symptoms are able to bind it. The more a patient attempts to resist the compulsions or to argue with the obsessing thoughts, the more likely it is that he will complain of anxiety; often there is a sense of mounting tension relieved only by giving in to the compelling act.

Somatoform Disorders. *Somatoform syndromes* have in common prominent physical symptoms for which no organic cause can be found.[77] The diagnosis is made on the basis of criteria that have been specified for each disorder and not merely on the failure to find a physical explanation (Fig. 29-6). The criteria are not as specific as one would wish, and a sizable percentage of patients who do fit them go on to develop (or reveal) actual medical illnesses.[78] What distinguishes this group of psychiatric disorders from those we have been discussing is the overriding insistence by the patient on somatic complaints and the minimization and denial of subjective experiences of anxiety or anxiety-related

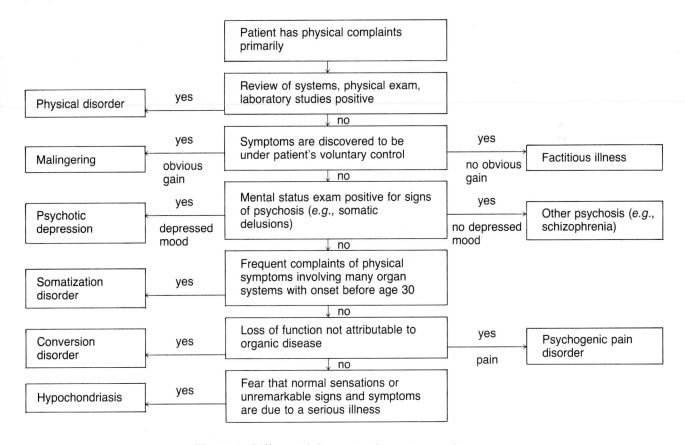

Fig. 29-6. Differential diagnosis of somatic complaints.

thoughts and concerns. We include them in a discussion of nervousness because the symptoms of somatization disorder and hypochondriasis often are similar to the somatic aspects of the anxiety states—indeed of any state of autonomic arousal.

Another somatoform disturbance—conversion disorder—is considered to represent the "conversion" of painful affects and unacceptable impulses into physical "equivalents." This process of symptom-formation simultaneously gives symbolic expression to feelings and wishes while still permitting them to remain outside of conscious awareness. Indeed, when the patient for some reason loses the symptom as an "outlet," the former *belle indifference,* that striking absence of concern and apprehension, is often replaced with intense anxiety. (See Chapter 30.)

Somatization disorder. These patients have, from the time of their teens or early twenties, complained of a great variety of physical symptoms that cannot be explained by physiologic processes despite searches for such causes in numerous medical evaluations. There is nothing to suggest voluntary production of these symptoms as in factitious illness or malingering. Anxiety and depression might be quite prominent or hidden behind the patient's dramatic, flamboyant, highly emotional presentation. Statistics indicate that most of these patients are women, although why this is so is not clear; female relatives may well have the same disorder while the males tend toward sociopathy and alcoholism. Although the patient may be quite seductive, she is often dependent and readily provoked to anger when her needs are not met; she shows an intense narcissistic preoccupation with herself and her discomforts. Somatization is distinguished from conversion disorder and anxiety states by its chronic course and by the variety and multiplicity of symptoms: Conversion and anxiety disorder generally present respectively with a single symptom or as a familiar symptom complex and involve predominantly the neurologic or cardiopulmonary systems.

Conversion disorder is discussed in detail in Chapter 30. We mention it here to remind the reader that the dissociation of painful affects, whether of anxiety per se or of sexual or aggressive feelings that would provoke anxiety were they to be consciously experienced, can lead to a representation of them disguised in somatic form. Furthermore, Lader and Sartorius found that while psychiatrists rated patients with conversion symptoms lower in anxiety than patients with manifest anxiety and phobias, the patients rated themselves higher, and the physiologic parameter of abnormal galvanic skin response supported the patients' own assessments.[79]

When the patient has only one or two symptoms such as dizziness, chest pain, lump in the throat, choking sensation (globus hystericus), or palpitations, the diagnostician should consider the possibility of conversion disorder instead of anxiety state. Confirmatory evidence includes a history of similar or other typical conversion symptoms in the past; a preceding situation that may have provoked internal conflict or offered a "model" for the particular symptom (as, when following the death of a parent from myocardial infarction, a patient develops incapacitating chest pain with no evidence of cardiovascular disease). The patient is unaware of any connection between the precipitating circumstances and his symptoms. There is often the secondary gain of avoiding noxious activities or relationships or of gaining attention without acknowledging dependent wishes. Finally, there may be a quality of indifference and an hysterical personality style.

Hypochondriasis. Nervousness constitutes both a mental and a somatic experience, a sense of fearful apprehension, and a variety of unpleasant bodily feelings. The patient with an anxiety disorder will tend to keep these two aspects quite separate, saying he feels troubled but he doesn't know why, and that he is *also* uncomfortable because of the symptoms in his body. The patient with conversion disorder will be aware only of the physical symptoms and may show little emotion about even the most incapacitating condition. With somatization disorder the mental state has found an explanation: "I am nervous *because* I have these physical symptoms." The extreme form of this is the hypochondriacal patient whose preoccupation with minor ailments or even normal bodily sensations (heart beat, breathing, peristalsis) may be so great as to block out any other human concern or interest. Such a patient presents to his physician a seemingly endless litany of complaints, described in vague, confusing, symbolic terms or in minute, exacting detail. Also extreme is the fear these symptoms produce in the patient: He is convinced (though not quite to delusional proportions) that the symptoms indicate some serious or life-threatening illness. Hence the urgency with which he states his case, the insistence that the physician "fix it," and his tendency to run from one caregiver to another seeking relief from his intolerable worry. Such a patient cannot be comforted or reassured by negative medical evaluation, no matter how often repeated. The usual experiences in life that most people consider suitable explanations for their nervousness—loss of a loved one or of a job, a major move—are unimportant to these patients; the only "reason" for their anxiety that they can imagine is that they are ill, and it will be only a matter of time and effort before the particular disease is discovered. Two dangers confront these patients:

first, the risk and expense of unnecessary tests and procedures; and second, the alienation of their physicians and families because of their tendency to arouse in others feelings of helplessness, frustration, anger, and impatience.

Physical Disorders Presenting with Nervousness

Many illnesses present with nervousness. There is little evidence that emotional states are involved in the onset or continuation of these disease processes. Indeed, it is a moot point whether we should be talking about "nervousness" at all rather than "symptoms of autonomic arousal"; but since we humans tend to use familiar words to describe unfamiliar somatic sensations, our patients will talk about "nerves" while we are thinking of neuroendocrine physiology. In other words, nervousness is the final stage of a common neural and endocrine pathway: Thyrotoxicosis and anxiety disorder simulate each other; the same symptoms may result from excess thyroxin from a hyperactive gland or pituitary, or from the complex, ill-defined chain of events we described earlier that typically begins with perceptions, thoughts, and memories.

The reasons for accurately distinguishing these disorders are obvious: Treatment is different in each case, and some of the illnesses can be life-threatening, particularly if not diagnosed and treated quickly. In most cases a thorough history and review of systems, a physical examination, and a mental status exam will point to the most likely diagnosis; laboratory studies are confirmatory.

Endocrine Disorders. *Thyrotoxicosis* due to an excess of thyroid hormone, whether from an overactive thyroid gland (Grave's Disease), or pituitary hypersecretion of TSH, or exogenous ingestion will cause patients to experience palpitations, dyspnea, heat intolerance, and increased sweating. Their appetites are increased, but they gain little or even lose weight. They may have more frequent bowel movements and menstrual irregularities or amenorrhea. They feel chronically tense, nervous, and "on edge"; they think less clearly, cannot concentrate, and are highly distractible. There is an inner sense of being "driven" or "turned on" despite profound fatigue and physical exhaustion. Older patients may have a quite different presentation: depression, fatigue, apathy.

Clinical signs include a diffusely enlarged gland; a fine tremor of the fingers and tongue; proximal muscle wasting; warm, moist, velvety skin; and fine, silky hair. Sympathetic overstimulation causes lid lag, infrequent blinking, and a wide-eyed stare. There may be exophthalmos and pretibial myxedema. One may find sinus tachycardia and atrial arrhythmias, systolic murmurs,

and elevated basal temperature. In the extreme state of thyroxtoxic storm, there may be malignant arrhythmias, heart failure, psychosis, and delirium, with progression to coma and death.

This "classical" picture, with an associated elevation of the serum thyroxine level, is not difficult to diagnosis. However, where the picture is more of apathy and inertia; or when signs are fewer and symptoms are milder; or when the patient emphasizes subjective and emotional phenomena, the diagnosis may be missed.

Anxiety states can be differentiated by the absence of the physical and laboratory findings of thyroid excess. In anxiety, extremities tend to be cold and clammy rather than moist and warm; weight loss is associated with anorexia and not increased appetite; and tremulousness is more coarse and irregular. In hyperthyroidism, the nervousness is unrelated to life events, although with today's psychologically minded patients, there is a tendency to "explain" physiologically-induced symptoms with psychological concepts (*e.g.* stress, repressed emotion, and so forth). The fatigue of simple anxiety lacks that sense of needing to keep moving and tends not to be present on awakening as it is in hyperthyroidism. Nevertheless, the possibility of hyperthyroidism should be considered in all anxious patients.

Corticosteroid excess. This may result from hyperfunction of the adrenal cortex or *Cushing's syndrome* (owing to bilateral adrenal hyperplasia and failure of feedback mechanisms on pituitary ACTH production, to an adrenal adenoma, or to carcinoma); ACTH-producing tumors, either in the pituitary or nonendocrine tumors such as oat-cell carcinoma of the lung or pancreatic carcinoma; and excessive exogenous ACTH or glucocorticoid intake. These conditions often begin with mental changes that vary a great deal from one patient to another but include depression, emotional lability, anxiety, agitation, difficulty with concentrating and short-term memory, and a more severe confusional state[81] or paranoid psychosis. With exogenous steroids euphoria is not uncommon. Patients complain of weakness and easy fatigability and of oligomenorrhea or amenorrhea.

Physical signs, when present, are unmistakable: "moon" facies, "buffalo" hump, truncal obesity with wasted extremities, and hirsutism. There may be measurable muscle weakness, hypertension, cutaneous striae, and easy bruising. Osteoporosis, vertebral body collapse, and pathologic fractures are evident on X-ray. Laboratory findings include elevated plasma and urinary 17-hydroxycorticoid levels with loss of the usual diurnal variation and failure to suppress with the administration of exogenous steroid (dexamethasone),

a mild neutrophilic leukocytosis, hypokalemia, hypochloremia, metabolic alkalosis, and glucose intolerance. Determination of the source of steroid excess can be made by a variety of laboratory tests. There is evidence that mood changes are more common when the primary disturbance is in the hypothalamic-pituitary system.[81]

Hypoglycemia. From any of its many causes, but depending on the rate and degree of drop in blood sugar and the particular sensitivity of a person's nervous system, hypoglycemia will activate the antonomic nervous system and produce an increase in circulating epinephrine. As a result the patient will experience all the signs and symptoms typical of anxiety. With decreased uptake of glucose by the brain, the patient may feel faint and light-headed or complain of fatigue, headache, blurred vision, and strange perceptual experiences. With persistent hypoglycemia there may be progressive confusion, agitation, bizarre behavior, and a gradual decline in the level of consciousness to stupor and coma. There may be focal and nonfocal neurologic signs and seizures. Repeated episodes of hypoglycemia or a single prolonged event can lead to permanent brain damage.

Correctly diagnosing episodic hypoglycemia and distinguishing it from panic attacks or genealized anxiety disorder is not hard when one knows that the patient suffers from diabetes mellitus and may be taking too much insulin or too little nourishment. However, in the early stages of diabetes, before symptoms of polyuria, polydipsia, and polyphagia with weight loss have developed, periods of hypoglycemia may occur spontaneously, and the physician should measure serum glucose two hours after a meal or perform a formal glucose tolerance test.

There are other causes of endogenous hypoglycemia. "Functional" or "reactive" hypoglycemia is diagnosed by the *simultaneous* occurrence of hypoglycemic symptoms and blood sugar levels of 30 mg to 40 mg per 100 ml two to three hours after a carbohydrate-rich meal. The etiology of this disorder is not understood. Hypoglycemia is currently popular as an explanation for chronic anxiety, fatigue, and depression, but these psychological states are in fact not part of the true syndrome, which should be narrowly defined by the two criteria mentioned above.

Other causes of hypoglycemia include insulin-secreting tumor of the pancreatic islet beta-cell, other endocrine disorders (*e.g.,* hypofunction of the anterior pituitary or adrenal cortex), alcoholism, severe liver disease, and inherited disorders of carbohydrate metabolism with onset in childhood. In all these cases, the attack will be relieved by the administration of glucose, a major differentiating feature from anxiety states. Insulinomas characteristically produce hypoglycemic attacks that become increasingly frequent and severe, and the history may suggest the typical association of attacks with exercise and fasting. The diagnosis is established by assays of insulin levels performed along with plasma glucose levels. The endocrine disorders will exhibit their own typical constellation of signs and symptoms, as will alcoholism and liver disease.

Hypocalcemia. When the parathyroid glands are inadvertently damaged or removed during thyroid surgery, the resulting decrease in the production of parathyroid hormone leads to decreased plasma levels of ionized calcium since there is less calcium mobilized from bone or absorbed from the intestines and kidneys. Hypocalcemia, especially in combination with alkalosis (*i.e.,* owing to hyperventilation), by destabilizing the nerve fiber membrane, characteristically produces discrete attacks of tetany, with carpopedal spasms, numbness and tingling of the extremities, palpitations, and muscle weakness. Many of these patients have mental symptoms including emotional lability, anxiety, depression, delirium, and psychosis.[82] Hypocalcemia also occurs in malabsorption syndromes, vitamin D deficiency, renal failure, hypoproteinemia, pancreatitis, and nutritional deficiency with hypomagnesemia. Hypocalcemia is most likely to be confused with the hyperventilation syndrome, which is described later in this chapter.

Premenstrual tension syndrome and menopausal symptoms are another cause of nervousness. Some women will complain of mood changes in the four or five days before their menstrual periods, especially nervousness, irritability, tearfulness, and fatigue. The prevalence of these complaints is unknown, as is their relationship to the affective disorders.[83] One study reported that while the majority of women experience a negative mood, less than one third find the problem severe enough to seek medical attention.[84] There may or may not be associated fluid retention with bloating and weight gain, pelvic discomfort, changes in appetite, headaches, and increased sweating. Alterations in hormonal balance are hypothesized to account for the mood change, but there is little that is documented about the exact nature of these changes. There is some suggestion that the mood changes may be related to changes in levels of endorphins and enkephalins.[85]

With the gradual cessation of menses in the middle of the fifth decade, many women experience considerable nervousness, tension, mood lability, irritability, weepiness, and depression. There may be associated somatic symptoms of hot flashes, headaches, and evidence of the loss of estrogen in the atrophic changes in vagina and vulva, osteoporosis, and elevated lipid levels. How hormonal alterations are involved in the mood changes has not yet been clarified. Whether or not these symptoms are experienced as distressing and

reason to seek medical help is quite variable and likely depends on a woman's prior psychological adjustment, sociocultural background, and her current adaptation to aging and role changes.

Neurologic Disorders. When spontaneous, neural discharge involves those regions of the brain known to control the expression of emotion—the temporal lobes and the limbic system—it will produce seizure phenomena of an emotional nature. While the manifestations of *temporal lobe epilepsy* (TLE) are highly variable, in some cases the ictal event or its aura may be a suddenly felt state of intense fear or panic. Patients may also have a sense of unreality that may be quite similar to the depersonalization and derealization that often occur in functional anxiety states. Recent work on the interictal personalities of these patients suggests that they experience their emotions more intensely and persistently than do most people and experience neutral events with considerable affective coloring. They tend toward temper outbursts, severe depression, and a general lability of mood. It has been suggested that the epileptic focus leads to the formation of more functional connections between limbic and cortical areas so that perceptions and thoughts are emotionally tinged.[86] The unusual manifestations of psychomotor epilepsy, including hallucinations, illusions, automatic behaviors, dreamy states, as well as the more enduring personality style of hyperemotionality, hyperreligiosity, hypergraphia, aggressivity, hyposexuality, and eccentricity, often result in these persons being considered "psychiatric" rather than neurologic patients. Some of these patients do go on to develop chronic paranoid psychoses.

TLE may be differentiated from panic attacks or other functional psychiatric disorders by the presence of an aura (often an olfactory or gustatory hallucination); by the stereotyped and recurrent nature of the behavior, no matter how bizarre. There may or may not be postictal clouding of consciousness and amnesia for the ictal event. A sleep-deprived EEG with nasopharyngeal leads supports the diagnosis, although a considerable percentage of patients will have repeatedly negative tracings.

Transient ischemic attacks owing to decreased cerebral blood flow resulting from narrowing of the carotid or vertebral–basilar arteries can be frightening experiences. If they involve the vertebral–basilar system and cause dizziness, visual disturbances, weakness, numbness, peculiar head sensations or feelings of body parts moving, and confused behavior, they may seem to mimic functional anxiety attacks. These attacks may be all the same or variable, may occur frequently, in clusters, or at long intervals. Typically, unless the person has had a stroke, there will be no persistent neurologic deficit, although there may be evidence of systemic or cerebrovascular disease or hypertension. The attacks occur in older persons, can last from a few seconds up to 12 hr but are usually between 5 min and 10 min in duration. Patients tend to exhibit other characteristic symptoms that point to either the carotid or vertebral–basilar system.

Following a head injury, some patients develop a posttraumatic nervous instability, called *postconcussive syndrome,* characterized by headache that is worsened by mental or physical activity; by giddiness; and by an intolerance of noise, crowds, or emotional excitement. Patients are tense, apprehensive, and worried; they are unable to concentrate or to consume a customary amount of alcohol. They are surprisingly intact intellectually.[87,88]

Brain tumors. These may present with changes in mental function, which include both emotional and cognitive elements. "A lack of persistent application to the tasks of the day, an undue irritability, emotional lability, a 'peculiar inertia,' faulty insight, forgetfulness, reduced range of mental activity, indifference to common social practices, and lack of initiative and spontaneity, all of which may be falsely attributed to worry, anxiety, or depression, are the usual symptoms. Much of this behavior is accepted by the patient with forbearance, and if he or she has any complaint, it is of being weak, tired, dizzy (nonrotational), or 'queer in the head.'"[89] Mental dullness tends to increase over time to the point of stupor, and headaches, vomiting, dizziness, seizures, and localizing signs and symptoms evolve. Behavioral symptoms likely reflect raised intracranial pressure rather than the type of tumor or its site, although tumors most likely to produce psychic changes are glioblastoma multiforme, astrocytoma, oligodendroglioma, metastatic carcinoma, meningioma, and primary reticulum cell sarcoma of the cerebrum. The diagnosis is made on the basis of a thorough neurologic examination, lumbar puncture, CT scan, and EEG.

Viral encephalitides may present with mental symptoms,[90] as may the vasculitides affecting the CNS.

Delirium and confusion. The early stages of an acute confusional state or delirium from any cause may include symptoms of nervousness, irritability, tremulousness, restlessness, insomnia, poor concentration, and bizarre behavior; this usually progresses to the more typical picture of clouded consciousness, inability to think clearly, and perceptual difficulty. These problems themselves—misperceptions, illusions, hallucinations, paranoid ideas, inability to maintain affective control—often produce a secondary anxiety as the patient struggles to comprehend what is going on within and around him. The causes of delirium are legion and include postoperative states and systemic illnesses (*e.g.,*

pneumonia), structural diseases of the brain, and metabolic disorders that interfere with neuronal functioning. These latter include drug intoxication and withdrawal, hypoxia and hypercarbia, hypoglycemia, uremia, hyperammonemia, electrolyte and acid-base disturbances, acute and chronic poisonings, and nutritional deficiencies. In all these cases there will be slowing, with or without focal elements, on the electroencephalogram and reversibility if the derangement is corrected promptly. While most of these abnormalities have a diffuse and general effect on the brain, in such disorders as herpes encephalitis or *Wernicke's syndrome* (thiamine deficiency), there is a known clinical–pathologic correlation between the behavioral symptoms and involvement of particular portions of the temporal lobes and limbic system.

Neuroendocrine Disorders. *Pheochromocytoma*, a tumor of chromaffin cells embryonically derived from neuroectoderm and producing norepinephrine and epinephrine, underscores the dual neural and endocrine basis of the signs and symptoms of nervousness. Usually located in the region of the adrenals but occasionally occurring elsewhere, the tumor synthesizes and releases catecholamines in episodic fashion, which causes paroxysmal headache, excessive sweating, and palpitations. There is often associated tremor, weakness, nausea, and sometimes epigastric discomfort. Less commonly, one finds chest pain, shortness of breath, light-headedness, blurred vision, and flushing. There are feelings of fear and apprehension. Whether they are due to hormonal effects on the CNS or simply represent a purely psychologic reaction to suddenly having such symptoms is unknown. The paroxysms are associated with hypertension in about one half of the cases, while in the others the hypertension is sustained or labile. The attacks occur spontaneously, although there are many known precipitants, including physical exertion, pressure on the abdomen, and emotional stress. Their frequency and duration are highly variable but tend to be the same each time for a given patient. Attacks may be severe enough to cause death from ventricular fibrillation, cerebral hemorrhage, or pulmonary edema. Necrosis or rupture of the tumor with massive catecholamine release results in cardiovascular collapse. The danger of misdiagnosing this tumor as anxiety neurosis is apparent, although when the symptoms are mild or if the hypertension is not suggestively paroxysmal, such an error is quite possible. Clues to the correct diagnosis include an association of the tumor with neurofibromatosis, hemangioblastoma, and thyroid cancer with or without parathyroid hyperplasia or adenoma, as well as with hypertension that can be provoked by smoking,

anesthesia, guanethidine, and ganglionic blocking agents.[92] The diagnosis is made finally on the basis of increased urinary and plasma catecholamines or their metabolites. (For a further discussion of pheochromocytoma, see Chap. 15, Arterial Hypertension.)

Cardiopulmonary Disorders. The relationship between nervousness and the cardiovascular and pulmonary systems is complex. While anxiety may itself produce organic dysfunction, chest pain and dyspnea cause fear and worry. The disorders discussed in the following pages represent an area where more work is needed to clarify the precise relationship between psychological and physiologic phenomena.

Hyperdynamic beta-adrenergic circulatory state is the most recent term in a long series of names given to a poorly defined disorder that is thought to result from an overactive sympathetic nervous system or hypersensitive beta-adrenergic receptors. It has also been called *DaCosta's syndrome, neurocirculatory asthenia, hyperkinetic heart syndrome, effort syndrome.* Some wonder if it is simply endogenous anxiety or panic disorder.[63] Patients develop attacks of palpitations, dyspnea, chest discomfort and tachycardia, and a preoccupying awareness of cardiac function. Symptoms begin in the early twenties, afflict women more than men, and run in families; patients may develop phobic avoidance of situations they believe provoke their symptoms. Medical evaluation tends to show normal physical exam and EKG both at rest and on exertion. Easton studied these patients and found that "cardiac index and heart rate were . . . notably elevated. Additionally, autonomic function was tested and shown to be normal by determining blood pressure and pulse rate, response to tilt, Valsalva maneuver, cold pressor test, carotid sinus massage, and response to administration of levarterenol bitartrate, tyramine, and atropine sulfate. The only significant abnormality noted was with an intravenous infusion of isoproterenol hydrochloride during which, at a rate of 3 μg/min, the heart rate increased more in the patients in a hyperdynamic beta-adrenergic state than in the normal subjects. This change in heart rate . . . was accompanied, in two-thirds of the patients, by a prompt, almost uncontrollable, hysterical outburst, reproducing the spontaneous attacks. These symptoms were reversed by intravenously administered propranolol, but not by placebo."[93] The author concludes that the problem lies in receptor hypersensitivity but acknowledges that a CNS mechanism has not been ruled out and that the relationship between the emotional and physiologic responses remains unclear. It is an interesting area for future research.[94]

Mitral valve prolapse (MVP) is a fairly common dis-

order affecting 5% to 10% of the population in which the mitral valve apparatus is structurally and functionally abnormal (myxomatous degeneration of the leaflet, attenuated or elongated chordae tendineae, abnormalities of the papillary muscles). The hemodynamic effects may be negligible or involve mitral regurgitation, ventricular dilatation, and fatal arrhythmias.[95] Auscultation reveals a mid- or late systolic click and late systolic murmur, and the EKG may show T-wave inversion in leads II, III, and aV_F. Echocardiogram shows the prolapsing mitral leaflet. Patients with this syndrome typically experience cardiac awareness, palpitations, dyspnea, nervousness, fatigue, and dizziness on either an acute or chronic basis. A number of studies have found that groups of patients with panic attacks have a higher incidence of mitral valve prolapse than the general population;[95] but since these are both common disorders, this may be a chance finding. MVP is another disorder that may ultimately teach us more about the interaction between anxiety and the autonomic nervous system.

Exercise and strong emotion will normally induce hyperventilation, but in some patients, the response may be quite extreme. Others for unknown reasons may begin to hyperventilate spontaneously, often without any awareness that they are doing so. Therefore they are unable to explain their feelings of lightheadedness and faintness, the ringing in their ears, the blurring of vision, the tingling around their mouths and in their extremities, the all-over-weakness, the carpopedal spasm. Some go on to complete loss of consciousness. Typically, the patient is frightened and gives no history of rapid breathing prior to these symptoms. No organic cause is found for the hyperventilation. It is generally felt that this is a disorder distinct from functional panic attacks and is called *hyperventilation syndrome*. The pathophysiology of the symptoms is understood: Overbreathing drives down the plasma carbon dioxide, *p*H rises, and a respiratory alkalosis results. In the acute situation there is insufficient time for the kidneys to compensate by increasing bicarbonate excretion. Oxygen becomes more tightly bound to hemoglobin and less easily released to the tissues; ionized calcium may pass out of solution rendering neural membranes less stable and permitting the depolarization that accounts for paresthesias and tetany (although the alkalotic state itself may be responsible for this).[96] Reduction in $PaCO_2$ produces widespread vasoconstriction that will reduce blood flow to the brain and coronary arteries. This may cause a faint, or it may cause increased heart rate, cardiac output, and angina. The syndrome may be confused with functional disorders, such as panic attacks; with other medical causes of acute onset of respiratory alkalosis or hyperventilation, such as pulmonary edema or embolus or pneumothorax; or with other causes of loss of consciousness, such as seizures, Stokes–Adams attacks, or cardiac arrhythmias. Hyperventilation syndrome, however, can be reproduced by having the patient breathe deeply and rapidly, and it can be interrupted by his rebreathing carbon dioxide (from a paper bag).

Diseases with Symptoms but No Signs. We have been describing disorders in which the patient's symptoms can easily be mistaken for functional anxiety. There are others in which patients do not complain of typical autonomic arousal but rather present a variety of somatic symptoms that are vague and hard to describe. These patients are often misdiagnosed as having "hysteria" or "hypochondriasis." The resulting demoralization, apprehension, and feelings of being misunderstood lead to a secondary anxiety and depression. In the early stages of multiple sclerosis (MS) and myasthenia gravis, typically, there are no objective findings to correlate with the patient's experience of transient motor, sensory, and visual disturbances, in the one instance, or with the easy fatigability of proximal and bulbar muscles in the other. Only later in the course of MS will there be sufficient demyelination to produce spasticity, Babinski signs, tremor, optic disc pallor, and abnormalities in the cerebrospinal fluid and in evoked potentials. With myasthenia gravis (a disorder of neuromuscular transmission), there may be considerable delay before weakness (typically, ptosis, diplopia, dysarthria, proximal muscle weakness) is unequivocally demonstrated to occur after exercise or to be relieved by the administration of edrophonium chloride (tensilon test).[97] Similarly, Huntington's chorea,[98] Wilson's disease, and combined systems disease[99] present with a variety of unusual complaints or manifest psychiatric symptoms before the characteristic features show themselves: chorea, ataxia, psychosis, and dementia with Huntington's chorea; tremor, rigidity, gait disturbance, cirrhosis, and evidence of abnormal copper metabolism with Wilson's disease; hyperreflexia and flexor spasm followed by hyporeflexia and flaccid paralysis, loss of position and vibratory sensation, and macrocytosis with combined systems disease.

While it is unwise and often fruitless to perform extensive tests in all these patients, the history is usually pertinent, and the best approach is to follow the patient over time. Care should be taken not to make a psychiatric diagnosis when criteria are absent simply because no physical disorder can be defined.

Acute intermittent porphyria, a disorder of porphyrin metabolism, inherited as an autosomal dominant trait, is another illness in which patients have

many vague somatic complaints with chronic anxiety and moodiness. The patient is typically a woman in her twenties or thirties who gives a history of periodic attacks of severe abdominal pain accompanied by nausea and vomiting reminiscent of renal colic or acute appendicitis. Neurologic manifestations range from neuralgias to paresthesias to paraplegias and may simulate encephalitis, poliomyelitis, or heavy metal poisoning. During an attack, which may be precipitated by barbiturates, sulfonamides, estrogen (menstruation and pregnancy), or alcohol, the patient may be confused or psychotic. The diagnosis is made by measurement of porphobilinogen in the urine or the activity of uroporphyrinogen I synthetase in erythrocytes.

Medications and Drugs of Abuse

A vast number of medications and "street" drugs produce the symptoms typical of nervousness—either as regular and expectable side-effects (*e.g.,* terbutaline), as untoward reactions in susceptible individuals (*e.g.,* corticosteroids), or as part of more complex intoxication and withdrawal syndromes (*e.g.,* delirium tremens). In studying 9000 patients with over 90,000 drug exposures, the Boston Collaborative Drug Related Programs found that over 200 patients "experienced moderately severe symptoms, such as agitation, bizarre and unusual feelings, depersonalization, anxiety, depression, fatigue, nervousness, malaise, and nightmares. The two agents most apt to produce psychiatric disturbance were prednisone, where ⅙ of the reactions that occurred were psychiatric in nature, and Isoniazid, where nearly ⅓ were neuropsychiatric."[100]

Intoxication. *Caffeinism* refers to the state of acute or chronic toxicity that occurs with intake of over 250 mg to 500 mg of caffeine daily. It represents an extreme form of the usual pharmacologic actions of this drug. To put this into perspective, 20% to 30% of Americans consume more than 500 mg of caffeine daily in coffee, tea, cola drinks, cocoa, and over-the-counter medications. One estimate of the prevalence of caffeinism is 10%. "Five cups of coffee, two headache tablets, and a cola drink amount to a daily intake of about 700 mg."[101] Caffeine's actions on the CNS have been studied and may shed light on some of the mechanisms of anxiety production. There is an increase in norepinephrine excretion; inhibition of the breakdown of cyclic AMP; increased sensitivity of postsynaptic catecholamine receptors, especially those for dopamine; possible alterations in acetylcholine and serotonin functions; changes in calcium metabolism; and enhancement of cyclic GMP.[101] During the intoxication phase people experience nervousness, irritability, agitation, tremulousness, easy startle, sensory disturbances, tachypnea, and

a paradoxical fatigue with very large doses. On withdrawal there is a typical headache, poor concentration, lethargy, and emotional instability. With intoxication there may also be palpitations, tachycardia, arrhythmias, nausea, diarrhea, and diuresis. The diagnosis is made by watching for the resolution of the symptoms with cessation of usage and their precipitation with reinstatement of the drug. Related drugs like aminophylline and theophylline may produce similar symptoms.

Amphetamines, whether taken as diet pills, for the treatment of depression or minimal brain dysfunction, or for recreational purposes, may cause restlessness, agitation, and anxiety often to a state of panic. There is hypervigilance, grandiosity, and, in some cases, a paranoid psychosis. Associated with this are tachycardia, elevated blood pressure, insomnia, perspiration or chills, nausea, and vomiting. On withdrawal there is a profound fatigue, lethargy, anxiety, irritability, confusion, and depression, along with headaches, muscle and abdominal cramps, and hot and cold sensations. *Cocaine* produces similar activating and withdrawal effects but to a milder degree. Other drugs like ephedrine, phenylephrine, phenylpropanolamine, and pseudoephedrine have similar stimulating properties.

In addition to the usual autonomic arousal, *phencyclidine* (PCP) in large doses can produce marked agitation, emotional lability, and grandiosity to a delusional degree. It also causes nystagmus, hypalgesia, ataxia, and dysarthria. Patients have perceptual distortions, may hallucinate, and may become unpredictably violent. This common street drug is taken alone or may be consumed inadvertently when it has been mixed in other preparations.[102]

Hallucinogens (LSD, mescaline) produce perceptual changes, typically visual distortions, illusions, or hallucinations. Depending on the context in which the drug is taken and a person's particular sensibility, there may be attendant anxiety or depression, fears of losing one's mind, or paranoid ideas. Physiologic effects are those of autonomic stimulation. Cannabis can cause an anxiety reaction, paranoia, and impaired judgment, but generally the effects tend to be milder.

Withdrawal. Alcohol and sedative-hypnotics (barbiturates and benzodiazepines) produce withdrawal states that begin with nervousness, irritability, restlessness, weakness, malaise, nausea, vomiting, tremulousness, tachycardia, and elevated blood pressure. These may progress to a state of delirium (delirium tremens) with confusion, hallucinations, and marked elevation of temperature, pulse, and blood pressure. There may be convulsions (usually preceding the delirium) and cardiovascular collapse.

Opiate withdrawal produces nervousness , along with the more specific findings of lacrimation, rhinorrhea, dilated pupils, piloerection, sweating, yawning, diarrhea, muscle cramps, and tremors. In midwithdrawal period (18 hr–24 hr), there also may be nausea, vomiting, and symptoms of autonomic arousal. Nicotine (tobacco) withdrawal typically causes irritability, nervousness, and restlessness, along with a craving for the drug.

Corticosteroids. Large doses of corticosteroids (the equivalent of over 40 mg of prednisone daily) can produce a highly variable psychiatric picture including labile mood, anxiety, depression, psychosis, or delirium.[103,104] "Seventy-five percent of patients who experience significant psychiatric reactions have received more than 40 mg of prednisone a day. The incidence of adverse psychiatric effects in patients taking less than 40 mg a day is 1 percent, as compared to 18 percent in patients taking 80 mg a day or more."[105]

Others. The following drugs have been known to cause nervousness and agitation as part of a larger constellation of psychiatric symptoms: lidocaine and propranolol; ethosuximide and primidone; salicylates and other nonsteroidal anti-inflammatory agents; adrenergic (sympathomimetic) drugs such as epinephrine and isoproterenol; cholinergic-blocking (parasympatholytic) agents such as atropine, trihexyphenidyl, benztropine mesylate, and over-the-counter sleeping and cold preparations containing scopolamine; thyroid preparations; estrogens; antihistamines; vitamin B complex; levodopa.[104]

DIFFERENTIAL DIAGNOSIS OF FATIGUE

In a recent study of patients presenting with fatigue as an isolated symptom, Morrison found that 39% had associated physical diagnoses, 41% had associated psychological diagnoses, and 12% had both physical and psychological diagnoses. Only 8% had no discernible explanation for their fatigue. The three most common associations were depression (31 of 176 patients), viral syndrome (27 of 176), and anxiety (19 of 176).[106] In Jerrett's series, while 37.7% of patients with lethargy had a readily detectable organic disease, the other two thirds had normal examinations and laboratory assessments. "Searching histories in these [latter] cases revealed probable causes in different lifestyles, eating habits, psychosexual problems, bereavement, various reactions to stresses, lack of arousal and varying degrees of depression." Jarrett takes the position that "if the history and physical examination are negative for organic disease there is no point in doing any routine investigation, even full blood count and urine testing,

because they are most unlikely to accomplish anything apart from reassuring the doctor—but they may have the opposite effect on an already over-anxious patient."[107]

Following is a description of both the psychological and physical disorders that have fatigue as one of their presenting symptoms, as well as some of the characteristics by which to differentiate them diagnostically (Fig. 29-7).

Normal Fatigue

Fatigue is normal, and indeed essential, when we have exerted ourselves and are in need of rest for repair and restoration. It may even be a not-unpleasant sensation, and after we have rested we feel refreshed and prepared to go on with our usual activities. Similarly, we expect weariness in the person who is grieving, in someone who has been acutely injured or ill, or in the sufferer with a chronic disease. But when we cannot explain adequately why a person is so exhausted and inactive, we look for psychological causes.

Psychological Disorders Presenting with Fatigue

Depression. Depression is a common disorder that may affect 15% to 30% of people at some time in their lives, although less than one quarter of those who are depressed seek professional help.[108] Fatigue may be the presenting complaint of a patient who ultimately is diagnosed as having depression, or it may be just one of the many symptoms that burden him. Depression is a psychiatric disorder for which there are strict diagnostic criteria; it should not be chosen as a diagnosis of exclusion when all others prove unfounded. It is a treatable disorder and should be actively considered in any patient presenting with fatigue.

The third edition of *The Diagnostic and Statistical Manual of Mental Disorders* of the American Psychiatric Association lists the following criteria for the diagnosis of Major Affective Disorder, Depressed Type, whether it occurs as part of a unipolar or bipolar picture when the patient also exhibits episodes of mania:

> Dysphoric mood or loss of interest or pleasure in all or almost all usual activities and pastimes. The dysphoric mood is characterized by symptoms such as the following: depressed, sad, blue, hopeless, low, down in the dumps, irritable. The mood disturbance must be prominent and relatively persistent, but not necessarily the most dominant symptom, and does not include momentary shifts from one dysphoric mood to another dysphoric mood, *e.g.*, anxiety to depression to anger, such as are seen in states of acute psychotic turmoil.[59]

Four of the following must be present daily for at least two weeks: poor appetite with significant weight loss

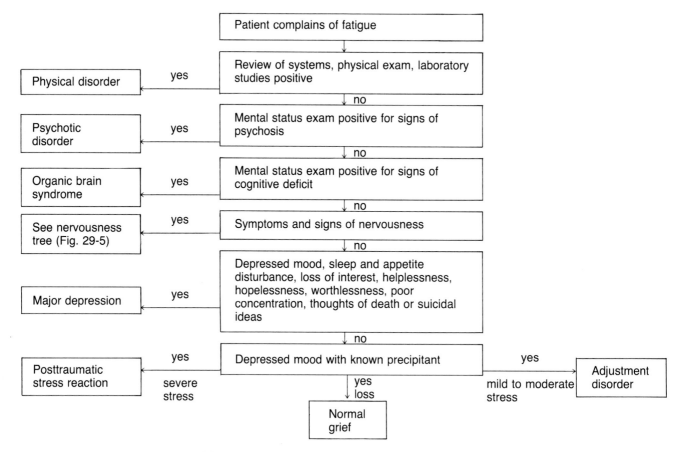

Fig. 29-7. Differential diagnosis of fatigue.

or increased appetite with significant weight gain; insomnia or hypersomnia; anxiety, restlessness, psychomotor agitation, or retardation; loss of usual interest or pleasure in usual activities, or decrease in sexual drive; loss of energy and fatigue; feelings of worthlessness and guilt; poor concentration, slowed thinking, indecisiveness; suicidal ideas or attempts; preoccupying thoughts of death. As well, patients may have multiple somatic complaints and may use alcohol or other drugs to deaden their emotional pain.

When this classic picture is present, the diagnosis is not difficult. However, it often requires considerable persistence, skill and sensitivity in interviewing, and discussions with family members to elicit the data to make such a diagnosis. This is particularly true when fatigue or other somatic complaints predominate and the patient is unaware of a dysphoric mood, or when the depression is chronic, as is the case in 15% of depressive disorders.[109] Depressed adolescents typically present with acting-out behavior or somatic complaints. Many elderly patients who appear to be de-

mented are in fact depressed and respond well to antidepressant medication.

One of the major distinguishing features of the fatigue in depression as compared to that in a physical disorder—though this by no means always holds—is that the depressed person awakens exhausted and unrefreshed but gradually over the course of the day feels somewhat better. The medically ill person is liable to fatigue as the day's activities progress. In addition, one can usually—again not always—elicit a history of dysphoric mood preceding the fatigue state in the depressed person, and his symptoms seem to be unaffected by events in the environment. Sick people tend not to feel worthless nor do they eschew the company of others. They still desire their former pleasures even though they may be physically unable to have them and are "cheered up" by improvement in their health or positive environmental changes.

Anxiety States. All of us are familiar with the sense of depletion that follows the "pent up" anxiety state

experienced prior to an examination and with the feeling of being drained after a sudden fright when the danger passes. Chronic, unremitting anxiety, whether from generalized anxiety disorder, from the anticipatory anxiety secondary to panic attacks, or from posttraumatic anxiety, invariably produces fatigue. *Neurasthenia* is the older term that captures the prominence of fatigue in the anxiety states.

Somatoform Disorders. Fatigue is often one of the somatic complaints of patients with somatization disorder or hypochondriasis. The absence of activity—a kind of paralysis—could also be a conversion symptom. The reader is referred to discussions of these disorders earlier in this chapter.

Grief. Fatigue and weariness are central experiences in the normal grief process. People tend to feel as if all their energy is taken up with thoughts and memories of the deceased, with nothing left to invest elsewhere. Sighing, feelings of emptiness, disinterest, listlessness are typical; as the grief abates the person feels a return of energy and involvement in living.

Physical Disorders Presenting with Fatigue

All illnesses, whether acute or chronic, produce fatigue. The mechanisms vary: Inflammatory processes and the host's own immune response are hypermetabolic states in which substrates and the capacity to replace them are depleted. Endocrine disorders may involve either a similar hypermetabolic state or inadequate production of the hormones that stimulate energy and growth. Finally, the cells may not receive the nutrients they require to carry out their energy-producing activities either because of inadequate intake, impaired utilization, or failure to transport them through the circulation. Drugs may create an energy-depleting hyperactivity or have toxic effects at the cellular level.

Infections. The most common cause of fatigue as a presenting symptom is a viral syndrome (influenza, infectious mononucleosis, and viral hepatitis). Indeed, the listlessness may be experienced well in advance of other more specific symptoms. Chronic infections like tuberculosis, brucellosis, malaria, chronic urinary tract infections, and subacute bacterial endocarditis often have fatigue as their only or most prominent symptom. A good history and physical examination, with appropriate laboratory studies, will lead to the correct diagnosis. In acute infections the fatigue is of short duration, and there will usually be signs and symptoms of the infectious process.

Endocrine Disorders. We have already indicated that hyperthyroidism can lead to a state of fatigue associated with the autonomically "driven" state and the myopathy common to this disease. *Hypothyroidism* results from the insufficient production of thyroid hormone owing to chronic thyroiditis (Hashimoto's disease), inherited defects in the biosynthesis of the hormone, iodine deficiency, ablation by surgery or radioactive iodine, or pituitary or hypothalamic dysfunction. The earliest symptoms are lethargy and easy fatigability, along with cold intolerance, constipation, and menstrual abnormalities. The patient's skin is dry and his face looks puffy, hair is sparse and coarse, and deep tendon reflexes have a delayed relaxation. Untreated, there is a gradual progression to the myxedematous state of hypothermia and stupor, possibly a delirium ("myxedema madness"), with cardiomegaly and adynamic ileus. The diagnosis is made on the basis of a low serum T4 and elevated TSH (unless hypothalamic or pituitary dysfunction is the cause).

Panhypopituitarism, resulting from postpartum thrombosis of the pituitary (Sheehan's syndrome), pituitary tumors, basilar meningitis, head injuries, or granulomatous diseases, leads to a failure of secretion of pituitary hormones (GH, luteinizing hormone, prolactin, adrenocorticotropin, TSH, and FSH), and consequently to the failure of the target endocrine organs. As a result, one or all of thyroid, adrenal, and gonadal insufficiency appear. The onset is often insidious, and the symptoms are variable and vague: fatigue, diminished libido, lethargy, cold intolerance. More specific findings of failure to lactate or menstruate, loss of axillary or pubic hair and of secondary sex characteristics, bradycardia, and hypotension may make the diagnosis easier. Laboratory findings will show low T4 and low TSH, low plasma cortisol and ACTH, low urinary 17-ketosteroids, 17-hydroxycorticosteroids, and 17-ketogenic steroids.

Fatigue is also the hallmark of *adrenal cortical insufficiency* (Addison's disease). It is initially brought on by exertion and stress but later becomes more severe and persistent. The fatigue follows from the low levels of cortisol and aldosterone that result from bilateral destruction of the adrenal glands (idiopathic, tuberculosis, autoimmune). One also finds anorexia, nausea, vomiting, weight loss, hypotension, and skin pigmentation. The diagnosis is confirmed by the failure of blood cortisol and aldosterone levels to rise with the administration of ACTH.

Other endocrine disorders discussed earlier, such as diabetes and Cushing's disease, may also produce a state of fatigue.

Cardiopulmonary Disorders. When body tissues do not receive sufficient nutrients and oxygen for any reason, fatigue results. Thus, failure of the heart to pump adequately (congestive heart failure, ischemic heart

disease, valvular heart disease, chronic atrial fibrillation); failure of the lungs to oxygenate the blood and the increased work of ventilation with "stiff lungs" (chronic obstructive or restrictive pulmonary disease); and anemia below 10 g/dl hemoglobin will all produce chronic lethargy and fatigue in addition to the symptoms characterizing the primary disorder.

Chronic Disease. All chronic diseases have fatigue as a prominent feature. This seems related to the illness state itself, distinct from whatever depression or demoralization results from being chronically sick. Chronic renal and liver disease, rheumatoid arthritis, systemic lupus erythematosis, multiple sclerosis, myasthenia gravis, and Parkinson's disease all produce a significant weariness. Cancer, often before it is detected, may cause an unexplained lassitude: This is particularly true of cancer of the pancreas and retroperitoneal tumors. Nutritional deficiencies (folate, iron, niacin, vitamin B_{12}, pyridoxine, thiamine) are additional important causes of fatigue, as are chronic electrolyte disturbances.

One study of postoperative fatigue found that it reached its maximum at 4 or 5 days after surgery and had in almost all cases resolved by two weeks. The authors attributed the fatigue to the combined effects of starvation, anesthesia, and sleep deprivation. Normal volunteers at bed rest alone did as badly on tests of psychomotor performance as the patients, suggesting inactivity and the supine position are important factors.[110]

Neurologic Disorders. One must distinguish muscle weakness from fatigue. Except for myasthenia gravis, fatigability is not a characteristic of muscle disease, which instead shows diminished strength of the contracting muscle. Also, the weakness resulting from a stroke or peripheral neuropathy will be focal and correspond to the innervation of the CNS or peripheral nervous system.

Sleep deprivation from any cause—anxiety, sleep apnea, narcolepsy, nocturnal myoclonus, and drug-induced deprivation of REM sleep—will result in fatigue.

Finally, the apathetic, passive, psychomotorically retarded appearance of the patient with dementia or frontal lobe pathology may be mistaken for tiredness and lethargy.

Medications and Drugs of Abuse

A variety of drugs and medications produce fatigue and depression. We have already mentioned that withdrawal from caffeine, alcohol, sedative-hypnotics, and amphetamines can be associated with significant exhaustion. Fatigue in particular is associated with antitubercular agents, digitalis, clonidine, methyldopa, antimalarials, and the succinimides. Depression may occur with a great many drugs but is most characteristic of antihypertensives, oral contraceptives, alcohol, and sedatives.[104,111]

SUMMARY

Nervousness and fatigue are familiar to all of us. When they arise under conditions that generally would be expected to produce these responses in anyone, they are considered normal. However, when the experience is too intense, too long-lasting, and cannot be explained in an ordinary way, people seek medical attention. In these cases nervousness and fatigue are usually found to be nonspecific symptoms reflective of either a psychiatric disorder or a medical illness. Sometimes no definitive diagnosis can be made, although the correct explanation—whether psychological or physical—tends to become clear over time.

Both nervousness and fatigue have two components: They are felt in the body in highly specific, measurable ways, and they are experienced in the mind as thoughts and fantasies of a typical sort. The term anxiety suggests that the symptoms are viewed as most likely psychological in origin. Despite the universality of these sensations and emotions, each patient will present his distress in unique terms. While a patient may emphasize either the physical or the mental aspects, the physician can make a diagnosis by understanding precisely what the patient is describing and by evaluating the psychological and social context along with his overall medical condition.

Why people become nervous and fatigued has troubled philosophers and scientists for centuries. Observations and experimental data are increasing, but as yet we do not have a comprehensive theory that can account for all kinds of nervousness and fatigue under all sorts of circumstances. Our theories tend to be tied to particular phenomena, and while they may offer compelling explanations of those situations, they usually cannot be more universally applied. For example, the neurosciences have much to tell us about the processes in the brain that seem to produce anxiety responses, but they do not indicate why, for example, a person may become fearful of a nonthreatening object. Psychoanalysis and learning theory usefully address some of these questions but leave many others unanswered.

Clinically, it is most important that the physician discover the source of the patient's complaints because in most cases there are specific treatments available. A thoughtful, persistent search for both medical and psychological explanations is usually rewarded. Even when the answers are not readily at hand, a patient's phys-

ical and emotional distress can be made more bearable by the physician's genuine concern to understand his complaints and pursue their cause: The anxiety and discouragement that come from having unexplained symptoms and from the worry that they are not seen as real thus may be minimized. The physician, too, will not feel at such a loss in the face of these universal human experiences.

REFERENCES

1. **Hall RCW, Popkin MK, Devaul RA et al:** Physical illness presenting as psychiatric disease. Arch Gen Psychiatry 35:1315–1320, 1978

2. **Koranyi EK:** Morbidity and rate of undiagnosed physical illnesses in a psychiatric clinic population. Arch Gen Psychiatry 36:414–419, 1979

3. **La Bruzza AL:** Physical illness presenting as psychiatric disorder: Guidelines for differential diagnosis. J Operational Psychiatry 12, No 1:24–31, 1981

4. **Schwab JJ:** Psychiatric illness in medical patients: Why it goes undiagnosed. Psychosomatics 23, No 3:225–229, 1981

5. **Editorial:** Human muscle fatigue. Lancet 2:729–730, 1981

6. **Cannon WB:** The James–Lange theory of emotion: A critical examination and an alternative theory. Am J Psychol 39:106–124, 1927

7. **Lader MH:** Psychophysiological aspects of anxiety. In Lader MH (ed): Studies of Anxiety (Br J Psychiatry, Spec Publ No 3). Ashford, Kent, Headley Brothers, 1969

8. **Pitts FN Jr, McClure JN Jr:** Lactate metabolism in anxiety neurosis. N Engl J Med 277:1329–1336, 1967

9. **Kelly D, Mitchell–Heggs N, Sherman D:** Anxiety and the effects of sodium lactate assessed clinically and physiologically. Br J Psychiatry 119:129–141, 1971

10. **Klein DF, Fink M:** Psychiatric reaction patterns to imipramine. Am J Psychiatry 119:432–438, 1962

11. **Curtis BA, Jacobson S, Marcus EM:** An Introduction to the Neurosciences. Philadelphia, WB Saunders, 1972

12. **Papez JW:** A proposed mechanism of emotion. Arch Neurol Psychiatry 38:725–743, 1937

13. **Noyes R:** Beta-blocking drugs and anxiety. Psychosomatics 23, No 2:155–169, 1982

14. **Kaplan HI, Sadock BJ:** Neurophysiology of behavior. In Kaplan HI, Freedman AM, Sadock BJ (eds): Comprehensive Textbook of Psychiatry, 3rd ed, pp 189–211. Baltimore, Williams & Wilkins, 1980

15. **Schildkraut JJ, Orsulak PJ, Schatzberg AF et al:** Toward a biochemical classification of depressive disorders. Arch Gen Psychiatry 35:1427–1433, 1978

16. **Hollister LE, Davis KL, Overall JE et al:** Excretion of MHPG in normal subjects. Arch Gen Psychiatry 35:1410–1415, 1978

17. **Sweeney DR, Maas JW, Heninger GR:** State anxiety, physical activity, and urinary 3-methoxy-4-hydroxyphenethyleneglycol excretion. Arch Gen Psychiatry 135:1418–1423, 1978

18. **Carroll BJ, Feinberg M, Greden JF et al:** A specific laboratory test for the diagnosis of melancholia. Standardization, validation, and clinical utility. Arch Gen Psychiatry 38:15–22, 1981

19. **Traksman L, Tybring G, Asberg M et al:** Cortisol in the CSF of depressed and suicidal patients. Arch Gen Psychiatry 37:761–767, 1980

20. **Sternbach H, Gerner RH, Gwirtsman HE:** The thyrotropin releasing hormone stimulation test: A review. J Clin Psychiatry 43, No 1:4–6, 1982

21. **Baldessarin RJ:** A summary of biomedical aspects of mood disorders. McLean Hospital J 6, No 1:1–34, 1981

22. **Winokur A, Amsterdam J, Caroff S et al:** Variability of hormonal responses to a series of neuroendocrine challenges in depressed patients. Am J Psychiatry 139, No 1:39–44, 1982

23. **Snyder SH:** Benzodiazepine receptors. Psychiatric Annals (Suppl) 11:19–23, 1981

24. **Gray JH:** Anxiety as a paradigm case of emotion. Br Medical Bull 37, No 2:193–197, 1981

25. **Klein NS:** The endorphins revisited. Psychiatric Annals 11, No 4:137–142, 1981

26. **Rose RM:** Endocrine responses to stressful psychological events. Psychiatr Clin North Am 3, No 2:251–276, 1980

27. **Katz JL, Weiner H, Gallagher TF et al:** Stress, distress and ego defenses. Arch Gen Psychiatry 23:131–142, 1970

28. **Wolff CT, Friedman SB, Hofer MA et al:** Relationship between psychological defenses and mean urinary 17-OHCS excretion rates: I. A predictive study of parents of fatally ill children. Psychosom Med 26:576–691, 1964

29. **Henry JP, Stephens PM, Axelrod J et al:** Effect of psychosocial stimulation on the enzymes involved in the biosynthesis and metabolism of noradrenaline and adrenaline. Psychosom Med 33, No 3:227–237, 1971

30. **Kaplan HI, Freedman AM, Sadock BJ (eds):** Comprehensive Textbook of Psychiatry, 3rd ed. Baltimore, Williams & Wilkins, 1980

31. **Taggart P, Carruthers M, Somerville W:** Electrocardiogram, plasma catecholamines and lipids, and their modification by oxprenolol when speaking before an audience. Lancet 2:341–346, 1973

32. **Lipowski ZJ:** Cardiovascular disorders. In Kaplan HI, Freedman AM, Sadock BJ (eds): Comprehensive Textbook of Psychiatry, 3rd ed, pp 1891–1907. Baltimore, Williams & Wilkins, 1980

33. **Jenkins CD:** Recent evidence supporting psychologic and social risk factors for coronary disease. N Engl J Med 294, No 19:1033–1038, 1976

34. **Medalie JH, Goldbourt U:** Angina pectoris among 10,000 men. Am J Med 60:910–921, 1976

35. **Lown B, De Silva RA, Lenson R:** Roles of psychologic stress and autonomic nervous system changes in provocation of ventricular premature complexes. Am J Cardiol 41:979–985, 1978

36. **Engel GL:** Psychologic stress, vasodepressor (vasovagal) syncope, and sudden death. Ann Intern Med 89:403–412, 1978

37. **Reich P, De Silva RA, Lown B et al:** Acute psychological disturbances preceding life-threatening ventricular arrhythmia. JAMA 246:233–235, 1981

38. **Williams DA, Lewis–Faning E, Rees L et al:** Assessment of the relative importance of the allergic, infective, and psychological factors in asthma. Acta Allergol (Kbh) 12:376–395, 1958

39. **Knapp PH, Nemetz SJ:** Acute bronchial asthma: Concomitant depression with excitement and varied antecedent patterns in 406 attacks. Psychosom Med 22:42–56, 1960

40. **Solomon GF, Amkraut AA, Kasper P:** Immunity, emotions, and stress. Ann Clin Res 6:313–322, 1974

41. **Dhopesh VP, Herring CL, Anwar R:** Tension headache in emergency department patients. Psychosomatics 21, No 8:631–635, 1980

42. **Weiner H:** Psychobiology and Human Disease. New York, Elsevier, 1977

43. **Hartmann E:** Sleep. In Kaplan HI, Freedman AM, Sadock BJ (eds): Comprehensive Textbook of Psychiatry, 3rd ed, pp 165–177. Baltimore, Williams & Wilkins, 1980

44. **Freud S:** Inhibitions, symptoms, and anxiety. In Standard Edition of the Complete Psychological Works of Sigmund Freud, Vol 20, pp 77–175. London, Hogarth Press, 1962

45. **Zetzel ER:** Anxiety and the capacity to bear it. In The Capacity for Emotional Growth, pp 33–52. New York, International Universities Press, 1970

46. **Freud A:** The Ego and the Mechanisms of Defense, rev ed. New York, International Universities Press, 1966

47. **Compton A:** A study of the psychoanalytic theory of anxiety, III. A preliminary formulation of the anxiety response. J Am Psychoanal Assoc 28:739–773, 1980

48. **Klein D:** Anxiety reconceptualized. Compr Psychiatry 21, No 6:411–427, 1980

49. **Jacob RG, Kraemer HC, Agras S:** Relaxation therapy in the treatment of hypertension: A review. Arch Gen Psychiatry 34:1417–1427, 1977

50. **Miller NE, DiCara LV, Solomon H et al:** Learned modifications of autonomic function: A review and some new data. Circ Res (Suppl 1) 27:3–11, 1970

51. **Bowlby J:** The nature of the child's tie to his mother. Int Psychoanal 39, No 5:350–373, 1958

52. **Ainsworth MDS:** Object relations, dependency, and attachment: A theoretical review of the infant–mother relationship. Child Dev 40:969–1025, 1969

53. **Mahler M:** On Human Symbiosis and the Vicissitudes of Individuation. Infantile Psychosis. New York, International Universities Press, 1968

54. **Hoehn–Saric R:** Anxiety: Normal and abnormal. Psychiatric Annals 9:11–24, 1979

55. **Schachter S, Singer JE:** Cognitive, social and physiological determinants of emotional state. Psychol Rev 69:379–399, 1962

56. **Cannon WB:** Voodoo death. Am Anthropol 44:169–181, 1942

57. **DeSilva RA, Lown B:** Ventricular premature beats, stress and sudden death. Psychosomatics 19, No 11:649–653, 1978

58. **Nemiah JC:** Alexithymia and psychosomatic illness. J Continuing Education Psychiatry, 39, No. 10:25, 37, 1978

59. **American Psychiatric Association,** Diagnostic and Statistical Manual of Mental Disorders, 3rd ed, p 213. Washington, DC, American Psychiatric Association, 1980

60. **Cassem NH, Hackett TP:** Psychiatric consultation in a coronary care unit. Ann Intern Med 75:9–14, 1971

61. **Lader MH, Marks I:** Clinical Anxiety. New York, William Heinemann Medical Books, 1971

62. **Sheehan DV:** Current concepts in psychiatry: Panic attacks and phobias. N Engl J Med 307, No 3:156–158, 1982

63. **Sheehan DV, Ballenger J, Jacobson G:** Treatment of endogenous anxiety with phobic, hysterical and hypochondriacal symptoms. Arch Gen Psychiatry 37:51–59, 1980

64. **Muskin PR, Fyer AJ:** Treatment of panic disorder. J Clin Psychopharmacol 1, No 2:81–90, 1981

65. **Titchener JL, Kapp FT:** Family and character change at Buffalo Creek. Am J Psychiatry 133:295–316, 1976

66. **Lindemann E:** Symptomatology and management of acute grief. Am J Psychiatry 101:141–148, 1944

67. **Burgess AW, Holstrum L:** The rape trauma syndrome. Am J Psychiatry 131:981–986, 1974

68. **Krystal H:** Trauma: Considerations of its intensity and chronicity in psychic traumatization. In Krystal H, Niederland WG (eds): Psychic Traumatization. Aftereffects in the Individual and Communities, pp 11–28. Boston, Little, Brown, 1971

69. **Friedman MJ:** Post-Vietnam syndrome: Recognition and management. Psychosomatics 22, No 11:931–943, 1981

70. **Horowitz MJ, Wilner N, Kaltreider N et al:** Signs and symptoms of posttraumatic stress disorder. Arch Gen Psychiatry 37:85–92, 1980

71. **Kaltreider NB, Wallace A, Horowitz MJ:** A field study of the stress response syndrome. Young women after hysterectomy. JAMA 242, No 14:1499–1503, 1979

72. **Dealy RS, Ishiki DM, Avery DH et al:** Secondary depression in anxiety disorders. Compr Psychiatry 22, No 6:612–618, 1981

73. **Roth M, Gurney C, Garside RF et al:** Studies in the classification of affective disorders: The relationship between anxiety states and depressive illnesses. Br J Psychiatry 121:147–161, 1972

74. **Gersh FS, Fowles DC:** Neurotic depression: The concept of anxious depression. In Depue RA (ed): The Psy-

chobiology of the Depressive Disorders: Implications for the Effects of Stress, pp 81–104. New York, Academic Press, 1979

75. **Woodneff RA, Guze SB, Clayton PJ:** Anxiety neuroses among psychiatric outpatients. Compr Psychiatry 13:165–170, 1972

76. **Clancy J, Noyes R, Hoenk PR et al:** Secondary depression in anxiety neurosis. J Nerv Ment Dis 166:846–850, 1978

77. **Nemiah JC:** Somatoform disorders. In Kaplan HI, Freedman AM, Sadock BJ (eds): Comprehensive Textbook of Psychiatry, 3rd ed, pp 1525–1544. Baltimore, Williams & Wilkins, 1980

78. **Slater ETD, Glithero E:** A follow-up of patients diagnosed as suffering from ''hysteria.'' J Psychosom Res 9:9–13, 1965

79. **Lader MH, Sartorius N:** Anxiety in patients with hysterical conversion symptoms. J Neurol Neurosurg Psychiatry 31:490–497, 1968

80. **Smith CK, Barish J, Correa J, Williams RH:** Psychiatric disturbance in endocrinologic disease. Psychosom Med 34, No 1:69–83, 1972

81. **Ettigi PG, Brown GM:** Brain disorders associated with endocrine dysfunction. Psychiatr Clin North Am 1:117–135, 1978

82. **Denko JD, Kaelbling C:** The psychiatric aspects of hypoparathyroidism. Acta Psychiatr Scand (Suppl 164) 38:1–70, 1962

83. **Endicott J, Halbreich U, Schacht S et al:** Premenstrual changes and affective disorder. Psychosom Med 43, No 6:519–529, 1981

84. **Sommer B:** Stress and menstrual distress. J Human Stress 4:5–11, 1978

85. **Halbreich U, Endicott J:** Possible involvement of endorphin withdrawal or imbalance in specific premenstrual syndromes and postpartum depression. Med Hypotheses 7:1045–1058, 1981

86. **Bear DM, Dedio P:** Quantitative analysis of interictal behavior in temporal lobe epilepsy. Arch Neurol 34:454–467, 1977

87. **Mersky H, Woodforde JM:** Psychiatric sequelae of minor head injury. Brain 95:521–528, 1972

88. **Miller H, Stein G:** The long-term prognosis of severe head injury. Lancet 1:225–228, 1965

89. **Adams RD, Hochberg F, Webster H deF:** Neoplastic disease of the brain. In Isselbacher KJ, Adams RD, Braunwald E et al (eds): Principles of Internal Medicine, pp 1951–1960. New York, McGraw–Hill, 1980

90. **Wilson LG:** Viral encephalopathy mimicking functional psychosis. Am J Psychiatry 133, No 2:165–170, 1976

91. **O'Connor JF, Musher IM:** Central nervous system involvement in systemic lupus erythematosus. Arch Neurol 14:157–164, 1966

92. **Holland OB:** Pheochromocytoma. In Isselbacher KJ, Adams RD, Braunwald E et al (eds): Principles of Internal Medicine, pp 1736–1741. New York, McGraw–Hill, 1980

93. **Easton JD, Sherman DG:** Somatic anxiety attacks and propranolol. Arch Neurol 33:689–691, 1976

94. **Frohlich ED, Taraz RC, Dustan HP:** Hyperdynamic beta-adrenergic state: Increased beta receptor responsiveness. Arch Intern Med 123:1–7, 1969

95. **Pariser SF, Jones BA, Pinta ER et al:** Panic attacks: Diagnostic evaluation of 17 patients. Am J Psychiatry 136:105–106, 1979

96. **Missri JC, Alexander S:** Hyperventilation syndrome: A brief review. JAMA 240, No 19:2093–2096, 1978

97. **Tollefson GD:** Distinguishing myasthenia gravis from conversion. Psychosomatics 22, No 7:611–621, 1981

98. **James WE, Meffard RB, Kimball I:** Early signs of Huntington's chorea. Dis Nerv Syst 30:550–559, 1969

99. **Hall RCW:** Anxiety. In Hall RCW (ed): Psychiatric Presentations of Medical Illness: Somatopsychic Disorders, pp 13–35. New York, SP Medical & Scientific Books, 1980

100. **Boston Collaborative Drug Related Programs:** Psychiatric side effects of non-psychiatric drugs. Semin Psychiatry 3:406–420, 1971

101. **Greden JF:** Caffeine and tobacco dependence. In Kaplan HI, Freedman AM, Sadock BJ (eds): Comprehensive Textbook of Psychiatry, Vol III, pp 1645–1651. Baltimore, Williams & Wilkins, 1980

102. **Mirin SM:** Drug abuse. In Bassuk EL, Schoonover SC (eds): The Practitioner's Guide to Psychoactive Drugs, pp 235–300. New York, Plenum Medical Book, 1977

103. **Goolker P, Schein J:** Psychic effects of ACTH and cortisone. Psychosom Med 15:589–613, 1953

104. **Hall RCW, Stickney SK, Gardner ER:** Behavioral toxicity of non-psychiatric drugs. In Hall RCW (ed): Psychiatric Presentations of Medical Illness: Somatopsychic Disorders, pp 337–406. New York, SP Medical & Scientific Books, 1980

105. **Boston Collaborative Drug Surveillance:** Acute adverse reactions to prednisone in relation to dosage. Clin Pharmacol Ther 13:694–698, 1972

106. **Morrison JD:** Fatigue as a presenting complaint in family practice. J Fam Pract 10, No 5:795–801, 1980

107. **Jerrett WA:** Lethargy in general practice. Practitioner 225:731–737, 1981

108. **Klerman GL:** Affective disorders. In Nicholi AM (ed): The Harvard Guide to Modern Psychiatry, pp 253–281. Cambridge, Belknap Press of Harvard University Press, 1978

109. **Weissman MM, Klerman GL:** The chronic depressive in the community—unrecognized and poorly treated. Compr Psychiatry 18, No 6:523–531, 1977

110. **Edwards H, Rose EA, Schorow M et al:** Postoperative deterioration in psychomotor function. JAMA 245, No 13:1342–1343, 1981

111. **Whitlock FA, Evans LEJ:** Drugs and depression. Drugs 15:53–71, 1978

30

Conversion Symptoms George L. Engel

Definitions
Incidence, Prevalence and Variety
**Mechanisms of Conversion Symptoms and
    Conversion Complications**
  How Bodily Symptoms Originate from an Idea or
    Fantasy
  Psychic Requirements for Conversion
  Determinants of the Choice of a Conversion
    Symptom
  Mechanisms of Conversion Complications
Clinical Diagnosis
  Interview Technique
  Diagnostic Criteria
    Suggestive Criteria
    Confirmatory Criteria
Common Conversion Symptoms:
  Pain
  Hyperventilation Syndrome
  Syncope, Stupor, Coma
  Seizures
  Weakness, Paralysis, Contractures, and Gait
    Disturbances
  Movement Disorders, Tremors, Tics
  Weakness and Fatigue (Pseudomyasthenia
    Gravis)
  Cutaneous Sensory Disturbances
  Visual Disturbances (Amaurosis and
    Amblyopia)
  Hearing Loss
  Anorexia, Nausea, Vomiting
  Dysphagia
  Globus Hystericus
  Dysphonia and Aphonia
  Nongaseous Abdominal Bloating
  Pruritis Vulvae and Ani
  Urinary Urgency, Frequency and Retention
  Concurrent Conversion and Physical Symptoms
  Hysterical Epidemics
**Differentiation from Other Psychosomatic
    Symptoms**
  Psychophysiologic Symptoms
  Hypochondriacal Symptoms
  Somatic Delusions
  Malingering and Factitious Illness

Psychosomatic symptoms have received much attention in recent years. Under conditions of emotional upset, patients may experience head pain, chest pain, or belly pain; nausea, vomiting, and epigastric distress; or palpitation, sweating, and muscle tension. Such symptoms may be brought about by a variety of mechanisms. Sometimes such symptoms reflect psychophysiologic changes that accompany affects, such as the nervousness, tremulousness, palpitation, and sweating of anxiety; or the fatigue, weakness, and anorexia of the depressive affects. Sometimes such symptoms are the result of organic disorders precipitated or exacerbated by emotional disturbances, such as peptic ulcer, angina pectoris, or migraine. But commonly such symptoms are the result of a psychic mechanism referred to as *conversion*, whereby an idea, fantasy, or wish is expressed in bodily terms rather than in words and is experienced by the patient as a physical rather than a mental symptom. Because conversion as a mechanism of symptom formation is so prevalent and because the variety of bodily systems that may be implicated is so great, conversion has been called the great

623

imitator of organic disease (Table 30-1). In 1873 Sir James Paget proposed the term *nervous mimicry*.[1]

Known to the ancients, conversion symptoms have been ascribed to many different mechanisms, perhaps the most influential being "wandering of the uterus"; hence, the term *hysteria* and the erroneous assumption that conversion symptoms are peculiar to females.[2,3] Appreciation of a psychological origin began in the early 19th century, whereas modern understanding was ushered in by Breuer and Freud's classic *Studies on Hysteria*, in 1893.[4] Freud was the first to propose the concept of conversion as an explanation for the somatic symptoms of hysteria, but subsequent writers have shown that, although conversion symptoms are more common among persons with psychological characteristics of hysteria, they may occur in virtually anyone, regardless of sex and personality type.[5,6]

DEFINITIONS

In ordinary clinical usage, the term *symptoms* refers to what the patient experiences and reports as manifestations of illness. Thus, symptoms are subjective (psychological) in the sense that the patient can report only what he is aware of. Patients tend to classify symptoms as *bodily*, (somatic, physical) or *mental* (psychological, emotional), according to what they perceive to be the source of the symptom. Nausea, pain, shortness of breath, and paralysis are ordinarily interpreted by the patient as indicating some bodily disorder, whereas anxiety, depression, hallucinations, crying, and memory loss are usually considered as evidence of an emotional or mental disturbance. In reality, however, bodily symptoms may occur in the absence of any underlying somatic disorder, and mental symptoms may derive

Table 30-1. *Conversion Symptoms*

Motor system
Generalized weakness (pseudomyasthenia gravis), fatigue
Paralysis, contractures and gait disturbances. (hemiplegia, hemicontracture, monoplegia, paraplegia, acroparalysis, acrocontractures, single muscle group contractures of the trunk, camptocormia, astasia abasia, dysbasia)
Movement disorders, tremors, tics
Aphonia (mutism), dysphonia, whispering dysphonia
Occular fixation, ptosis, blepharospasm, blinking

Sensory systems
Pain, aching, pressure, burning, fullness, hollowness, pruritus
Anesthesia, hypesthesia, dysesthesia, hyperesthesia
Sensations of dizziness, swaying, falling
Sensations of coldness, localized or generalized
Sensations of warmth, localized or generalized.
Blindness, ambylopia, clouding of vision, tubular vision, scotomata, monocular diplopia, polyplopia
Deafness
Loss of taste, bitter taste, burning tongue, burning mouth, orolingual pain
Anosmia

Level of consciousness
Fugue, amnesia
Stupor, coma
Convulsions, seizures
Syncope
Dizziness, lightheadedness, faintness, giddiness
Sleepiness

Respiratory system
Cough, tickle, hoarseness
Dyspnea, choking, suffocation, smothering, inability to breathe, hyperventilation
Sighing, yawning
Wheezing
Breath holding
Hiccups
Pain in chest, upper or lower respiratory passages

Cardiovascular system
"Pain in the heart"
Palpitations
Dyspnea, orthopnea

Gastrointestinal system
Sensation of dryness, burning, "acid" in mouth or throat
Anorexia
Bulimia
Thirst, polydipsia
Dysphagia, lump in the throat (globus)
Nongaseous abdominal distention, bloating
Pain, burning, fullness, and other abdominal sensations
Diarrhea, frequent bowel movements, tenesmus, constipation
Anorectal sensation—fullness, burning, pruritus ani

Urinary system
Retention, incontinence, urgency, frequency, dysuria, pain

Genital system
Anesthesia, parasthesia, pain, pruritus, fullness, and other sensations
Dyspareunia, vaginismus
Pseudocyesis

---

directly from a pathologic somatic process (*e.g.,* hallucinations with a brain tumor). The conversion symptom is the paradigm of the bodily symptom not based on concurrent somatic pathology.

Conversion symptoms originate as mental experiences but are perceived by the patient as bodily sensations. They derive from memories, fantasies, mental elaborations, and concepts of the body and its functions, which the patient unconsciously uses to express symbolically wishes or feelings in body language rather than verbally. Hence, the conversion symptom is entirely intrapsychic in nature. In contrast, symptoms of somatic origin derive from awareness of actual physical processes taking place in the body.

To illustrate, shortness of breath as a conversion symptom originates in the memory of some past respiratory experience, which is being used to express symbolically some fantasy, as, for example, that of being smothered or of smothering someone else. The fantasy of smothering reactivates a memory of feeling unable to breathe, which leads to the sensation (symptom) of breathlessness and the response of hyperventilation. Shortness of breath as a symptom of congestive heart failure, in contrast, originates in an awareness of the increased effort of breathing required to achieve ventilation in the face of pulmonary congestions. The sensation of being unable to breathe and the concomitant ideas of breathlessness and smothering derive from the neural and psychological processing of pathologic events involving the respiratory system.

Psychophysiologic processes, such as may be experienced during expression of emotions, may also give rise to bodily symptoms, such as the palpitations, diarrhea, and sweating of anxiety, the nausea of disgust, the blush of shame, and the anorexia and constipation of depression. For the most part, these symptoms derive from the patient's awareness of the bodily concomitants of affects (*e.g.,* the physiologic reactions to catecholamines secreted during anxiety), and constitute symptoms of somatic origin, in contradistinction to conversion. The differentiation of conversion symptoms from hypochondriacal symptoms, somatic delusions, and malingering, is discussed later in this chapter.

Distinction must be made among conversion as a process, conversion symptoms, and conversion complications. The term *conversion* refers to the intrapsychic processes whereby an unacceptable idea or fantasy is experienced and expressed symbolically as (*i.e.,* "converted" to) a bodily sensation or feeling.

The term *conversion symptoms* refers to the fantasized bodily sensations and behavioral or physiological reactions that occur in response to those sensations (*e.g.,* the sensation of nausea may lead to vomiting or a feeling of weakness may be displayed as paralysis).

The term *conversion complications* refers to the biochemical or physiologic processes set in motion by conversion symptoms. Nausea and vomiting as conversion symptoms may lead to metabolic alkalosis. Shortness of breath and hyperventilation may lead to respiratory alkalosis. The symptoms of alkalosis, light-headedness, paresthesias, and tetany, are somatogenic, not psychogenic, in origin; they have no primary psychologic meaning and in no way express symbolically the fantasy underlying the conversion vomiting or hyperventilation. A list of conversion complications is found in Table 30-2.

INCIDENCE, PREVALENCE, AND VARIETY

No accurate figures on the incidence or prevalence of conversion symptoms are available. Ljungberg estimates the prevalence of hysterical reactions in the general population of Sweden as 5%, whereas Farley gives a figure of 33% in a consecutive series of 100 postpartum women.[7,8] Among the population of 500 consecutive psychiatric outpatients, 24% had a history of one or more conversion symptoms.[54] One study based on

Table 30-2. *Conversion Complications*

Conversion Symptom	Conversion Complications
Paralysis and contractures	Muscle atrophy, sweating, coldness, cyanosis, bone demineralization
Localized cutaneous pain, burning, dysesthesia	Localized flushing, swelling, purpura, vesicles, dermatoses
Dyspnea, choking, smothering, suffocation, panting (hyperventilation)	Respiratory alkalosis with secondary symptoms (lightheadedness, paresthesia, tetany)
Anorexia, nausea, vomiting, dysphagia	Weight loss, inanition, electrolyte or nutritional deficiencies, alkalosis
Bulimia	Weight gain, obesity
Thirst	Polyuria, nocturia

data from psychiatric case registers yielded a rate for hysterical neurosis, conversion type, of 22 per 100,000 per year at Monroe County, New York, and of 11 per 100,000 per year in Iceland. These are undoubtedly minimum incidences because the survey included only patients referred to psychiatrists and recorded in a register.[64] Patients with conversion symptoms consult all varieties of medical specialists, but rarely psychiatrists. This is because they consider their complaints to have a physical origin. Psychiatric confirmation of a diagnosis is therefore infrequent, making prevalence figures unreliable. Among psychiatric consultations, about 15% are reported as manifesting a conversion reaction.[22] It is my impression, formed as a result of my experience as both an internist and psychiatrist, that as many as 20% to 25% of patients admitted to a general medical service have manifested conversion symptoms at one time or another in their lives. Conversion symptoms are considered to be appreciably more common among women than men, but this may well be due to the widespread bias that conversion is peculiar to women, the diagnosis often not even being considered in men. Conversion is common in the military, in Veterans Administration facilities, especially during wartime. It is also common in industry, especially after trauma. There is no clear support for the contention that conversion symptoms are more prevalent among the uneducated and unsophisticated.

In general, the forms assumed by conversion symptoms are much influenced by the prevailing beliefs and attitudes of the culture in which the patient grows up. In our present-day, biomedically oriented Western culture, conversion symptoms are likely to be consonant with widely disseminated notions of physical illness and therefore are often not recognized as such by physicians who are themselves products of the same culture. More easily recognized conversions are those displayed by persons from less familiar cultures and subcultures. These conversions are commonly colored by indigenous religious or folk beliefs, thus striking the physician as more bizarre and obvious.

Under conditions of social unrest, especially when groups are swept by emotion, epidemics of conversion symptoms may occur.[9,47,55] Fainting of teenagers in a crowd listening to a singing idol, or hyperventilation attacks among students in a girls' school upon the rumor of the pregnancy of a class member, are typical of such epidemics.[8]

Conversion symptoms may be noted at every age, though they are rare in children younger than 7 or 8 and probably never occur in youngsters under 4. Some patients begin to manifest conversion symptoms in adolescence, thereafter displaying multiple and changing symptoms throughout their lives.[25] Other patients

exhibit symptoms occasionally and transiently, usually during a period of stress. A single symptom or a complex of symptoms may persist unremittingly for months or years, or it may reappear periodically, like an old friend. A large proportion of the population periodically experiences minor conversion symptoms, which they accept as "natural," not calling for any medical investigation.

The great variety of conversion symptoms is illustrated by Table 30-1. Conversion complications appear in Table 30-2. Specific diagnostic features are discussed in a later section.

MECHANISMS OF CONVERSION SYMPTOMS AND CONVERSION COMPLICATIONS

HOW BODILY SYMPTOMS ORIGINATE FROM AN IDEA OR FANTASY

At first glance, it is difficult to grasp how such physical symptoms as pain, nausea, blindness, or paralysis may be expressions of ideas or fantasies rather than the result of some bodily change. Yet it is not unusual for some body activity to be used to express ideas. Gesture and pantomime are the most familiar. In the well-known game of charades, the performer may close his eyes or act blind to express the notion that something is invisible or should not be looked at. Everyday language, particularly metaphors, contains many instances of ideas being expressed in body terms, such as "It took my breath away," "I'm fed up," "I can't bear it." The person who speaks metaphorically of "keeping anger in," of something being "rammed down my throat," or "falling by the wayside," clearly is using body imagery to express himself.[10] Such expressions remind us that before the infant becomes capable of expressing his feelings and wishes in words, he uses his body. Furthermore, his first knowledge of his surroundings is formed in his bodily reactions and sensations in response to the environment.[11] Such metaphors as "I can't swallow that," "That leaves a bad taste," and "I could eat you up" doubtless have their roots in the body memory of that period in infancy when mouthing, tasting, and biting were major means of differentiating edible from inedible and desirable from undesirable. The distinction between good and bad in terms of what is taken into the mouth and what is rejected is one of the infant's earliest cognitive generalizations. It continues to be exhibited in adulthood by the pinching of the lips tightly together to express rejection, even though nothing is to be taken into the mouth.

The dream is the most common mental activity in which wishes, fantasies, and ideas are expressed in such nonverbal terms as visual imagery, body sensations, and even physical symptoms. As Freud first showed, and as is now being confirmed in current dream research, the content of dreams reflects the dreamer's continuing preoccupation with the problems of his waking life.[12] Cut off in sleep from the reality of the external environment and deprived of the possibility of action, the dreamer falls back on modes of thinking characteristic of the unconscious mental processes of the preverbal period of childhood. Aside from its patent illogic, the dream is marked by the tendency to express complex fantasies or ideas in symbolic forms derived from earlier body experiences and sensations. Especially relevant to the problem of conversion are dreams in which one is sick or disabled or is suffering such symptoms as blindness, weakness, paralysis, dyspnea, or pain. Analysis of such dreams reveals that sometimes the symptom is a direct symbolic expression in its own right (*e.g.,* blindness symbolizes the wish to see something forbidden or the failure to recognize or face something). At other times, the symptom derives from memories of a symptom that the dreamer had once before experienced or that he had observed or imagined some other person to suffer. Thus, shortness of breath or a sensation of suffocation in a dream may rise from a childhood memory of being pleasurably smothered by mother's embrace or from the recollection of a panting athlete at the moment of triumph. The symptom thereby expresses, symbolically, a regressive wish to be reunited with the mother or to be like the triumphant athlete. Shortness of breath may also originate in memories of a childhood attack of croup or of a parent's asthmatic attack, symbolically expressing the wishes or concerns that marked that original experience.

The occurrence of symptoms in dreams is commonplace, and readers will have no difficulty recalling from their own dreams how real such symptoms may seem at the time. This demonstrates that the capability to express ideas or wishes symbolically through the modality of a bodily symptom is a normal mental phenomenon. What needs to be considered now is how this may come about in the waking state.

PSYCHIC REQUIREMENTS FOR CONVERSION

Conversion symptoms characteristically develop under conditions of deprivation or frustration. They constitute a regressive way both of gratifying an unfulfilled need and of relating to others. The choice of the particular symptom is based on its suitability to represent symbolically the particular wish or fantasy that cannot

be fulfilled.[13] In this regard, the mechanism underlying conversion symptoms has much in common with the mechanism responsible for the form taken by the dream.[12] In both instances, the frustration encourages regressing to earlier modalities of expression and relating as substitute modes of gratification. This in turn mobilizes buried (unconscious) wishes or fantasies, which cannot be permitted access to consciousness except in a disguised form. In the dream, the unrecognizable symbolic representation of the fantasy permits the dreamer to enjoy his dream and sleep peacefully; should the disguise be threatened and the dream become unpleasant, the dreamer may awaken. With the conversion symptom, the patient's conviction that he is suffering from a physical disorder similarly keeps him from recognizing the unacceptable fantasy symbolically represented by the symptom. The following is an example:

> A man involved in a conflict with his partners dreams that he is playing golf with four or five men. They all have golf clubs and are hitting the ball skillfully. He has only a broomstick and is hitting at a pile of leaves when he suddenly realizes that he has been beating a squirrel cowering underneath. He awakens feeling anxious. Later in the day, shortly before he is to meet with his partners, he develops a severe aching pain over his back and shoulders and is obliged to go home. This was a conversion symptom.
>
> The dream clearly expressed the patient's feeling of inferiority to his partners, and in only a thinly disguised manner his rage toward them, displaced to the helpless squirrel. The conversion backache symbolically expressed the same aggressive fantasy, now turned on himself as punishment. The patient, however, was conscious only of a physical discomfort, which obliged him to leave work, and thereby incidentally to avoid a confrontation with his partners. In their eyes, as in his own, his pain identified him as sick and therefore entitled to the privileges of the sick role.

As the example indicates, the conversion symptom develops in relation to the internal (intrapsychic) conflict that is mobilized by the frustrating or threatening life situation. The emergence of a wish or fantasy toward which the person feels strong disapproval is met by repression, preventing it from becoming conscious. The ensuing conversion symptom has four aims: (1) to permit expression of the forbidden wish (although in a disguised form), recognizable neither by the patient nor by the person toward whom it is intended; (2) to impose punishment through suffering and disability for entertaining, even unconsciously, such a wish, and thereby to atone for guilt; (3) to remove the patient from the threatening or disturbing life situation; and (4) to provide a new mode of relating, namely, the sick role, which is sanctioned by society. Thus, the con-

version symptom is a compromise solution, and, as such, serves an adaptive function for the patient.

The symptom is the lesser of two evils because, if successful, the sufferer is at least spared the anxiety, guilt, shame, or helplessness that would otherwise have been engendered by the frustrating or dangerous life situation, as well as by the unacceptable fantasy. This constitutes the *primary gain*. At the same time, he achieves a *secondary gain* by virtue of the sick role.

The effectiveness of this adaptation is measured by the presence or absence of unpleasant affects or of other disturbances. The patient for whom a conversion symptom is serving its purpose is likely to manifest little anxiety or depression and is likely to be relatively indifferent to the symptom (*la belle indifference*), although he is required to act like a patient in order to fulfill the sick role. When the conversion symptom does not effectively defend against the emergence of the threatening fantasy, suffering from the symptoms and more insistence on the need for help are displayed. The patient also experiences more anxiety, guilt, shame, or depression.

> A relatively successful conversion symptom, bilateral ptosis and blepharospasm, is illustrated by a 45-year-old bachelor farmer in whom the sudden development of symptoms dramatically prevented him from shooting a bull tethered to a fencepost. From that point on he was unable to raise his lids. Although he was no longer able to care for the farm, he exhibited surprisingly little concern, especially considering how disabling the symptom was. Only after a year of persistent urging from his family did he consent to consult a physician. The symptom, it turned out, had developed on the anniversary of the death of his father, an irascible, alcoholic widower who owned the farm and for whom the son worked. Dominated and abused by the father, he had never succeeded in emancipating himself.
>
> Indeed, he could only say nice things about his father. On the day of the father's death, the son was horrified to come upon his body lying dead in a pool of blood (from a massive hematemesis), his eyes wide open and staring. The son became nauseated, vomited, and then fled in horror. Thereafter, he had many frightening dreams of the father staring at him accusingly, and he upbraided himself for not having at least lowered the lids of the dead man. The decision one year later to slaughter the bull, his father's prize possession, was an impulsive one for which he could give no adequate explanation. With the development of the conversion symptom, the frightening dreams ceased and his depression ameliorated. However, when the examining physician forcibly elevated his lids, the patient abruptly became anxious, broke out in a cold sweat, and fainted (vasodepressor syncope). As he was losing consciousness, he saw eyes staring at him.

In this case the inability of the patient to see and to open his eyes condensed a number of elements related to the rage toward his father that he was unable to acknowledge to himself. Most obvious was his feeling that his failure to lower his father's lids after death was a disrespectful and timid act for which he then berated himself. His own closed eyes symbolically expressed his unacceptable hostile fantasies and his reactive guilt. The impulsive decision to slaughter the father's prize bull on the anniversary of his death only disguised his unconscious hostility to his father, a symbolic act which in fact was thwarted by the development of the symptom. The patient's casual attitude toward his symptom documents its effectiveness in shielding him from the discomfort of dealing with his fantasies. The psychological defense afforded by conversion was temporarily interrupted when the physician manually elevated his lids, whereupon the patient experienced acute anxiety.

DETERMINANTS OF THE CHOICE OF A CONVERSION SYMPTOM

The raw materials for a conversion symptom are body sensations experienced in the past, that is, the memories of body sensations. Thus, any body parts or functions that can give rise to sensations or have mental representation can be implicated in the development of a conversion symptom.[14,15] Physiologic processes that are not felt cannot provide information for conversion. Thus, contractions of the stomach giving rise to cramps may contribute to a memory trace later used for conversion, whereas increased secretion of gastric acid, a silent physiologic process, cannot.

Whether such memories can be used for conversion depends on whether they have contributed or can contribute to the formation of cognitive structures (*i.e.*, ideas, wishes, or fantasies). If so, they are then available to represent the wish or fantasy when it cannot be entertained or expressed in words. A patient's choice of a particular conversion symptom, (*e.g.*, a sticking pain in the right cheek, a feeling of being unable to breathe, or blurred vision) thus depends on his personal, often idiosyncratic, past cognitive experience of the underlying sensation.

> A woman suffered aching pain in her arms after her second baby was stillborn. She rationalized that the baby might be better off dead because it may have been damaged by her toxemia, yet blamed herself for the death. In speaking on how much she missed the baby, she said, "My arms just ached to hold her." Her first baby had been difficult and fussy and she often felt obliged to carry her about even though "I was so tired my arms ached." The experienced sensation, an ache, condensed both desire and burden and was a conversion symptom.

Some sensations common to infancy and early childhood have a high potential for conversion use by virtue

of constituting preverbal body experiences that contributed to language formation. This has already been discussed in respect to the use of metaphors and other body imagery for expression. Other sensory experiences qualify for conversion utilization by virtue of being chronologically associated with strong feelings. Such experiences may include not only actual sensations originating from one's own body, but also sensations induced by imagining how someone else feels.

A woman whose conversion manifestations consisted of shaking chills (without fever) and pain in her face, "as if it had been scraped along the ground," had been involved in an auto accident when 11-years-old. In the darkness she was thrown into a snow pile where she shivered unnoted for what seemed an interminable period; her mother was dragged along the pavement by the car, her face scraped and bloodied. The patient remembered her hospitalization as the only time in her life when her mother was affectionate to her. The conversion symptoms developed when her marriage, which her mother strongly disapproved of, was breaking up.

The sensation of being cold and shivering expressed symbolically her yearning for her mother's affection, whereas the face pain symbolized her rage toward the mother who was so frustrating. We can imagine that the little girl took some grim satisfaction in her mother's injury, only to feel guilty when her mother was so kind to her.

The phenomenon of taking on another's symptom exemplifies an important determinant of symptom choice. Moved by strong feelings of guilt toward another person, a patient may impose upon himself the same symptoms that he imagined the other person to suffer. In so doing, he follows the primitive law of the talion, "an eye for an eye, a tooth for a tooth." In effect, he responds to the other's symptoms as if he were responsible for them and must therefore suffer in kind. This is a primitive form of thinking, characteristic of unconscious mental activity.

Ordinarily, the probability of a particular body experience being utilized for conversion is reinforced by numerous associations over years. Thus, a single symptom may effectively condense and express simultaneously a number of different motifs, another characteristic of unconscious mental activity. Hidden in such associations are numerous graifying fantasies or experiences of the past, sometimes quite remote from the conflict immediately underlying the symptom.

Attacks of breathlessness and hyperventilation in a 24-year-old woman had as their immediate provocation the stertorous breathing of her comatose dying mother-in-law at whose bedside she sat for 5 days.

In the background of her childhood, however, were memories and fantasies of (1) the heavy breathing of her father when he was angry at her or quarreling with her mother; (2) the sounds of the breathing of her parents engaged in sexual intercourse in the bedroom next to hers; (3) holding her breath so that she could better hear what was going on in the next room, only suddenly to become terrified that she might not herself be able to take another breath; (4) feeling suffocated as she was held by her father while being anesthesized for a minor surgical procedure; and (5) pleasant early childhood memories of inhaling the fragrance of her mother's bosom, later replaced by a fear that the mother might smother her against her breasts. Through all these associations the sensation of being unable to breathe and the response of hyperventilating successfuly expressed many different childhood fantasies of love and hate, along with the fantasies immediately linked with her current ambivalent feelings about her mother-in-law.

The various examples of conversion cited thus far also serve to emphasize the extent to which human relationships are involved in determining which body sensations become the representatives of the repressed wish or fantasy. Just as the original body experiences somehow were implicated in the sharing of feelings with the other person, so too the conversion symptom is meant to communicate a message and elicit a response from those for whom the repressed wish or fantasy is intended. It is both a disguised communication and a technique of relating, an unconscious game of charades, so to speak. Indeed, to the patient, it often appears to be the only satisfactory way of relating and expressing himself. Hence the patient conspicuously displays his symptom even when the symptom itself is of no great concern to him. Accordingly, conversion symptoms are usually more pronounced when the patient is with persons significant rather than casual for him. Although patients with symptoms of somatic origin may feel ashamed of or frightened by the symptoms, this is virtually never the case with a conversion symptom. For some patients, relating through conversion manifestations may even become a way of life, long after the original unresolved conflict has ceased to be an active issue.

MECHANISMS OF CONVERSION COMPLICATIONS

In the conversion process, a physical sensation from memory is used to represent an idea and is endowed with the quality of current reality. The sensation ordinarily evokes corresponding and usually appropriate motor and physiologic responses because it is perceived and processed as real by the interpretative systems of the brain. For example, conversion tickle in the throat induces coughing and conversion nausea induces vomiting. Occasionally, such physiologic responses set in motion a chain of events that give rise to further symptoms. We refer to these as *conversion complications*.[14] For example, if the conversion sensa-

tion is feeling unable to breathe, the response is to increase ventilation. So imperative may such a message be that negative feedback transmitted through chemoreceptors is ignored, and CO_2 is blown off to the point of respiratory alkalosis. The symptoms (*i.e.*, lightheadedness, paresthesia, and tetany) derive from the metabolic effects of hypocapnea on the central and peripheral nervous systems and in this sense constitute complications of conversion.

Similarly, a conversion involving a fantasy of injury may initiate physiologic responses to injury at the site implicated in the fantasy. This process is mediated through a neurosecretory mechanism involving antidromic activity along afferent nerves, with the secretion at the nerve terminals of polypeptides of the kinin group.[15,16] In some instances, local lesions, including ecchymoses, allergic dermatitis, and urticaria, may develop at such sites, presumably by virtue of interaction with other pre-existing pathogenic factors.[17,18,19] It is conceivable that the stigmata of certain religious mystics may be explained by such a mechanism.[20,21] In such cases, conversion is responsible for the location and time of onset of the lesions, but not for its pathologic nature or its subsequent course.[14]

CLINICAL DIAGNOSIS

In most cases, the diagnosis of conversion can be established on the first examination. To do so calls for understanding the mechanism of conversion, familiarity with the diagnostic criteria, and a style of interviewing that yields the relevant psychological data. The diagnosis cannot be based merely on the exclusion of organic disease because patients with conversion symptoms may have coexisting organic disease, the conversion presenting as an additional symptom or as an exaggeration of the organic symptom.[22] More often than not, the problem is to establish which symptom is based on conversion and which on a somatic process rather than merely to rule out one or the other. Extended followup indicates that symptoms most often misdiagnosed as conversion involve slow degenerative conditions affecting skeletal, muscular, and connective tissues, the spinal cord, and the peripheral nerves.[63]

INTERVIEW TECHNIQUE

Because conversion symptoms are commonplace and readily confused with symptoms of somatic origin, the physician is well advised to approach every bodily symptom with the possibility in mind that it might be a conversion symptom. This is best accomplished by always using an interview style that elicits social and psychological data concurrently with the physical symptomatology. Actually, such an approach is economical and efficient in the evaluation of any illness because it insures fuller understanding of those personal, family, and social circumstances that are most relevant to the understanding of the illness and the care of the patient. The details of such an interview approach are presented elsewhere.[23]

In considering conversion, the interview technique must take into account the fact that, although conversion symptoms are triggered by some circumstance of the patient's life, the patient is unaware of the association. This precludes direct questioning as a means of discovering such relationships. The patient who insists that he is not aware of anything upsetting him, unless it be the symptom itself, is being honest. This is because a function of the conversion is to protect him from the distress that he would otherwise experience were he to face his conflicts directly. Accordingly, the responsibility to recognize the connection between life events and symptoms rests solely on the physician, who listens for associations which the patient brings up spontaneously without recognizing their connection with the symptom. To do this requires that every new area being investigated be initiated with open-ended, nondirective questions, so that the patient is induced to respond in his own words and to provide his own associations. More specific questions are then developed on the basis of the information obtained. For example, the open-ended query "Tell me what the problem has been," enables the patient to respond in his own way while the interviewer notes what is of main concern to the patient and how he spontaneously relates elements of his illness and his life. The patient is then invited to elaborate on whatever detail of the story the interviewer deems pertinent (*e.g.*, "Tell me more about the pain"), following which he explores with more specific questions what the patient has related, until the particular subject has been fully characterized. Each area is investigated in this manner until all the details have been clarified and the full history has been obtained.

In order to uncover relationships between life events and symptoms, both must be explored simultaneously rather than as independent categories. This is accomplished by inquiring carefully into all the circumstances surrounding the onset of the symptom, as well as indicating interest each time the patient makes reference to his life circumstances. For example, when the patient passingly mentions his work, his wife, or his neighbors; or that he was home asleep, on the job, on vacation, or expecting a visit from his mother-in-law when the symptoms began, the interviewer promptly inquires about the item brought up. "What is your

work?", "What were you doing at that point?", or "Who was with you?" Sometimes merely an echoing question will suffice; "Your wife?"; "Your mother-in-law?" This approach is based on the principle that a patient is more likely to elaborate on personal matters when he, rather than the physician, introduces the subject. To many patients, a formal inquiry by the physician into "social history" or "family history" seems irrelevant, if not intrusive. Furthermore, the relevance of the life circumstance to the symptom is more readily clarified when both are considered in the context in which the patient introduced the theme. Often the patient with a conversion betrays the connection through his choice of words, gestures, or slips of the tongue. On other occasions, the sequence of the symptom developing immediately after or on an anniversary of a life event provides the clues. The interviewer takes care not to reveal to the patient that he suspects a connection, for this may only block further associations. Hence, the physician does not dwell on the personal data beyond what the patient seems willing to discuss. Should the patient show reticence, the doctor resumes exploring symptoms. The reader is referred elsewhere for fuller discussion of this patient-centered interview approach.[23,57]

DIAGNOSTIC CRITERIA

Suggestive Criteria

Ideally, to diagnosis conversion calls for elucidation of the unconscious meaning of the symptom, clarification of the intrapsychic conflict for which it is an attempted solution, and disappearance of the symptoms upon resolution of the conflict. In practice, however, certain unusual features of the symptom and the manner in which the patient reports his illness are what usually first arouse the physician's suspicion that the diagnosis may be conversion. These constitute *suggestive criteria*.

The Manner in which the Symptom is Reported. Because of the psychological value of the symptom to the patient, his manner of reporting is ambivalent. On the one hand, he is likely to display suffering and disability, sometimes in a dramatic manner. On the other hand, he subtly betrays attachment to, and even pleasure in, the symptom. Hence, a conversion etiology may be suspected for a variety of reasons: the patient appears relaxed, even smiling, as he describes a distressing symptom; he appears unconcerned about the effect on his life of such disabling symptoms as blindness or paralysis (*la belle indifference*); he gratuitously insists that the symptom must have an organic origin; or he emphasizes his own ability to tolerate the suf-

fering, while describing the terrible effect it is having on his family. The language used in describing a conversion symptom may be rich in imagery, often conveying the hidden psychological meaning.

> A man reported a sudden severe pain in his back. "I was just starting to sit down when I got this shot in the back. Boy, I come up quick, just bang! Felt like something going through a hole, like a pencil." The pain lasted only a second. A few days earlier he had attempted to rape the wife of an acquaintance, but was interrupted before he could complete the act. He fled from the back door imagining that the husband was pursuing him with a gun. The pain occurred when he heard a radio report that the assailant had been identified. The patient's choice of words neatly condensed the imagery of both the sexual attack and being shot.

Because of the central role of repression in the mechanism of conversion, patients are likely to be vague and imprecise in describing a conversion symptom and the circumstances surrounding its development. This may contrast with their ability to describe the details of a symptom of somatic origin. In effect, the repression encompasses not only the pathogenic conflict, but associated events as well. Accordingly, one may find patients with otherwise good memories for dates and events unable to remember the details of even striking events that happen to be associated with the development of the conversion symptom.

Inconsistency with Somatic Processes. The form of the conversion symptom is determined by the psychological needs it is intended to meet, not by the anatomic or physiologic properties of the body part involved. Hence, the possibility of conversion should be entertained in the following circumstances: whenever the symptom does not make sense in anatomic or physiologic terms (*e.g.,* inability to perceive vibration over one half of the sternum, or a pain that radiates from the occiput to the groin); when expected physical signs or laboratory findings are absent (*e.g.,* normal vital signs, color, and EEG during syncope or active corneal reflex with hemianesthesia of the face); when the clinical characteristics or course are inconsistent (*e.g.,* intermittent amblyopia with mild nonprogressive exophthalmos, or dyspnea and precordial pain, unaffected by exertion).

Hysterical Personality Features. Susceptibility to conversion symptoms is not limited to any personality type or psychiatric entity, but is decidedly greater among persons with hysterical personality traits. Superficially, such traits are not only commonplace in the general population, but are even considered attractive to the extent that they seem to reflect a capacity for warmth, sensitivity, sympathy, intuition, imagination,

and colorful emotional expression. More critical scrutiny, however, demonstrates that, appearances notwithstanding, hysterics are in fact conspicuously deficient in their capacity to communicate effectively and to establish lasting and emotionally gratifying human relationships. This renders them vulnerable to repeated frustration and disappointment and limits their effectiveness in coping with the vicissitudes of life and achieving realistic life goals. Throughout history, culturally determined male-oriented biases have tended to characterize many hysterical traits as typically feminine, so much so that such cultural influences may contribute to susceptible women hysterics displaying a caricature of the male society's idea of femininity. Hence, men showing the same basic character traits are less likely to be designated hysterical unless they also conform to the prevailing notion of femininity. More commonly, men hysterics are classified among antisocial or sociopathic personalities, with attention focused on their aggressiveness and other so-called masculine characteristics. In actuality, most of the features listed below as characterizing hysterical personality are independent of gender.

Many of the salient elements of the hysterical personality also involve psychological processes that are implicated in the conversion process. These include especially the use of body behavior for nonverbal expression and communication of needs and wishes and for mediation of human relationships, along with a propensity to resonate and identify with the feelings and bodily expressions of others (sympathetic feelings). These psychological qualities enhance the tendency to develop conversion symptoms, especially under circumstances where verbal expression and action are blocked.

The diagnostic criteria for the hysterical personality include the following:

1. *Colorful and dramatic expression, language and appearance.* The hysteric needs to attract attention to himself and to affect others. Indeed, many hysterics behave as if their own personal sense of vitality and identity depended on the kind of emotional reaction they arouse in others. They do so by their manner of dress and grooming and by being charming, entertaining, winsome, appealing, and sometimes frankly provocative or seductive. Verbal content often has the idiom of aggression and violence among men and flirtatious coquetry among women. The style of behavior is characteristically exaggerated, whether it be as the shy, innocent little girl, the teasing, seductive woman, the charming flamboyant man-about-town or the inhibited, timid young man. In keeping with this, the manner of presenting the history is typically dramatic, exaggerated, and self-centered.

2. *Role playing.* An unusual ability to put themselves in the place of others and to play their roles makes hysterics born actors and mimics. Further, they readily shift from one role to another as the occasion demands. This chameleon like quality contributes to the impression of the hysteric being dramatic, colorful, charming, entertaining, and, above all, unpredictable. Thus, such a person may in a few moments change from the apparently desperately ill patient to the charming hostess who puts the physician at his ease, only to resume the wan, languid look of illness as soon as the doctor focuses on the symptoms. Hysterical personalities may fail to recognize the implications or impact of their own behavior, reacting with surprise or disappointment when their intentions are misinterpreted.

3. *Use of body language and expression.* Hysterics characteristically make much use of their bodies for expression. Their language is replete with metaphoric body references. Their descriptions are typically supplemented by demonstrations, sometimes startlingly dramatic.

A mother, describing her child's attack of croup, not only began to speak in a high-pitched, whining tone of voice, but also sighed, gasped, choked, clutched her throat, and rolled her eyes about, dramatically re-enacting the little boy's attack, while at the same time exhibiting her own helplessness, fear, and anger. Her conversion manifestation was choking and hyperventilation.

4. *Demanding dependency.* Hysterical people are hungry for attention, admiration, and support. Hence, they are quick to solicit an emotional involvement with the physician. They have an intuitive ability to sense what will be most appealing to the doctor, but their basic narcissism proves difficult to gratify, and is ultimately frustrating to both the physician and the patient. Physicians often eventually become impatient, while the patient, in turn, typically responds by becoming even more manipulative, demanding, and angry, until he finally changes doctors. This sequence of overvaluation and disillusionment with each doctor is sufficiently typical as to have diagnostic value. A similar sequence often characterizes other relationships in everyday life as well.

5. *Suggestibility.* Hysterical patients are highly suggestible and readily take on the symptoms of others, whether it be a family member or the patient in the next bed. In groups with strong emotional ties this may assume epidemic proportions.[9,47,55] The physician may unwittingly suggest new symptoms or modify old ones simply by implying that he expects a symptom to be present or by appearing especially interested in a particular symptom. The person with

these personality characteristics may readily respond with symptoms to the details of informed consent. The open-ended interview approach, by not revealing what the doctor has in mind, minimizes such distortions.

6. *Manifest sexual problems.* Hysterical women, although commonly attractive and seductive, usually are, in fact, frigid, anesthetic, or dyspareunic. They may be shy, inhibited, and fearful of sexual activity, or they may be promiscuous. Solicitation of sexual activity may, in fact, be primarily a means of satisfying a wish to be held, cuddled, and nurtured, rather than a means of obtaining sexual pleasure. Hysterical men may be colorful and flamboyant, or shy and inhibited. They often have sexual fantasies; but a relatively ineffectual sex life, separations, divorces, and extramarital relations are common.

7. *Global, diffuse, impressionistic style of thinking.* When presented with an intellectual task, hysterical personalities tend to use hunches and inspiration, to gather impressions rather than facts, to resort to guesses rather than to serious concentration, and to act on impulse rather than on a well-thought-out plan. They belong to the larger category of "feelers," rather than "thinkers." Their evaluations, judgments, and decisions are more readily based on what is immediately impressive, striking, or obvious. They are influenced strongly by emotion and are especially susceptible to suggestions and pressures from others, even against their own will.

8. *Previous history of multiple conversion symptoms.* Many hysterical patients experience their first conversion symptoms in adolescence. Purtell has identified a group of chronic hysterical patients who present a dramatic or complicated medical history beginning before age 35 and marked by as many as 25 conversion symptoms persisting over a period of years.[25] They go from doctor to doctor, and by midlife usually have been subjected to many diagnostic and surgical procedures, occasionally with transient relief of a symptom, but more often with unexpected complications, persistence of old symptoms, or the appearance of a new symptom. Usually these symptoms are reported in traditional medical terms (*e.g.*, pleurisy, kidney stones, or gall bladder attacks). Hence, their conversion origin is likely to be overlooked by the physician who does not carefully review the symptomology for its consistency with such disorders. Abdominal pain of conversion origin is so frequently misdiagnosed as appendicitis in young women that the history of an appendectomy performed between the ages of 14 and 22 should always be carefully investigated to be sure the reported illness indeed fits the picture.[26,27]

9. *Psychiatric symptoms.* Hysterical patients are also prone to phobias, dissociative states, fugues, and amnesia. Episodes of depression are common, as are suicide gestures with drug overdosage or wrist slashing (often revealed by scars). Excessive dependence on medication is common.

Confirmatory Criteria

Any of the foregoing criteria only suggest the diagnosis of conversion. All are equally compatible with a somatic diagnosis as well. To make a certain diagnosis, all of the following *confirmatory criteria* must be fulfilled. If some, but not all, of the confirmatory criteria are met, conversion may be regarded as a probable diagnosis, and additional study is required.

Precipitation of Symptoms by Psychological Stress. Psychological stress is a necessary but hardly sufficient criterion for the diagnosis of a conversion illness because any illness, somatic as well as psychological, may develop in a setting of psychological stress.[28,29,46] However, the patient with a conversion illness is typically oblivious to any connection between his life situation and the symptoms, whereas a somatically ill patient often suggests the relationship himself. In fact, a patient's insistence on a psychic origin for a somatic symptom strongly favors a somatic rather than a conversion etiology.

Many stressful circumstances may induce conversion symptoms. In general, the more blatantly hysterical the individual, the more subtle may be the stimulus precipitating the conversion symptom; for example, a faintly suggestive remark may provoke conversion syncope in an inhibited hysterical girl struggling with sexual fantasies. The more usual settings include real or threatened losses and separations, acute grief, interpersonal conflicts, and sexual threats or temptations, to which the individual responds with a sense of frustration and helplessness. Such feelings may be fleeting or prolonged, but disappear and often are forgotten when the conversion symptom develops. Because the patient does not consciously connect the situation with the symptom, the interviewer must carefully note the dates and the sequence of events. Especially important are symptoms developing on the anniversary of significant events.

The farmer cited earlier, who developed blepharospasm and ptosis on the first anniversary of his father's death, is a case in point. This information emerged not when he was describing his symptom, but when he was telling how he had acquired his farm. The coincidence with the anniversary had not occurred to him.

Quite often the psychological stress of a physical illness provides the setting for a conversion symptom, especially among patients facing surgical or diagnostic procedures and patients with chronic disease, puz-

zling or undiagnosed illness, or illnesses of uncertain prognosis. These are all situations in which a patient is likely to feel helpless and frightened, vulnerable to vivid fantasy, and extremely dependent upon his physician.

> A patient recovering from a very severe myocardial infarction developed a hyperventilation attack on the day of discharge; a woman facing cystoscopy found herself unable to void; a diabetic who learned about gangrene of the toes from a fellow patient in his doctor's waiting room developed pain and numbness in his foot when his doctor went on vacation.

Such conversion symptoms are usually short-lived if the physician recognizes their origin and responds to the patient's underlying concerns. They may become quite intractable if approached as evidence of somatic illness.

Demonstration of the Determinants of the Symptom Choice.
This is the most valuable confirmatory criterion. There are four possible determinants of the choice of the symptom, any one or combination of which may be implicated.

1. *Body language.* The conversion manifestation may be selected by virtue of its ability to express in body terms the unconscious fantasy and the punishment for it, such as a pain in the chest being a "heartache," a paralyzed hand representing an inhibition of a wish to masturbate or to strike someone, or morning nausea indicating a pregnancy fantasy. However, the mere fact that a symptom can be translated into such parallels is not sufficient to establish its relevancy; it is also necessary to produce supporting evidence. It must be demonstrated that the patient with chest pain is relating the term *heartache* to a real situation in his life; that the man with the paralyzed hand has some basis for a wish to masturbate or hit someone; and that the woman with morning nausea has some evident concern about pregnancy. Further, the patient remains unaware of the real meaning of the symptom. When a patient volunteers that perhaps he is paralyzed because he wanted to hit someone, either that is not the real basis for the conversion, or the symptom has an organic etiology. He may simply be parroting, but without conviction, what another doctor had told him.

2. *A physical symptom previously experienced by the patient.* Past illnesses must be carefully explored, not only as to details of the symptoms, but, even more importantly, with respect to the surrounding circumstances. Experiences of illness, especially those of childhood, that involved a great deal of secondary gratification or were used to manipulate or control others, are especially likely to provide the basis for future conversion symptoms. Replication of the symptoms of an earlier illness then becomes the means of recreating a more gratifying life situation and averting current frustrations.

3. *Symptoms observed in someone else.* This is a common determinant of symptom choice. It involves identification with another person with whom the patient is or has been in conflict or in relationship to whom he is currently suffering frustration. The uncovering of the connection with the other person's symptom usually comes about in the course of eliciting information about the illness of family members and others. Here, the patient's idea of what the other person's symptoms were like is more important than the actual diagnosis. Sometimes, patients ascribe symptoms to the other person that are not ordinarily part of the alleged illness. For example, the lay person may just assume that the victim of acute pulmonary edema or of an asthmatic attack is suffering pain in the chest; or that the pain of myocardial infarction is located in the region of the left nipple. Sometimes one manifestation dominates in the patient's mind, as exemplified in the staring eyes of the dead father serving as the basis for the conversion blepharospasm of the farmer described earlier. The more closely the patient's description of the other person's symptoms corresponds with his own, the more likely it is that they were the model for the conversion. Careful attention to dates and sequences is necessary to establish that the patient's symptom did indeed develop after he learned of the other person's symptom. The relationship with the person whose symptom provided the model for the conversion usually is a close but ambivalent one. He is usually a family member or close friend, but may also be someone who merely resembles or can represent the more important person, as a fellow employee or the patient in the next bed.

> A woman suddenly developed a sharp pain in her lower right thigh. The involved area soon thereafter becoming ecchymotic; one week earlier, she saw a neighbor youth bleeding from a gunshot wound in the same location. In her mind he had a close resemblance to her brother. The location and timing of the lesion was determined by conversion mechanisms; the lesion was a conversion complication, psychogenic purpura.[21]

Identity of location is an important diagnostic requirement, but sometimes patients claim inability to recall the exact location of the other person's symptom. It may then be noted while protesting ignorance, the patient is at the same time unwittingly indicating the location of his own symptom.

A woman who mentioned in passing that her father had lost an eye in a shooting accident could not remember which eye, yet while trying to recall, she placed her finger to her left eye, the site of her symptoms (pain, blurring of vision, and twitching of the lids) which ultimately proved to be due to conversion.

4. *Symptoms wished on someone else.* The curses of everyday language (*e.g.*, "drop dead," "I wish he'd break his neck") may be translated into conversion symptoms when they evoke conflict and guilt. Thus a person may faint or develop a pain in the neck rather than entertain, much less utter, the terrible (for him) thought. Here the wish is felt as equivalent to the deed, and the patient inflicts the curse upon himself rather than upon his intended victim. Often the wish is more personal, such as the infertile woman, envious of her sister's pregnancy, who developed lower abdominal cramps as a conversion symptom rather than persist in her secret wish that the sister abort. Sometimes the symptom is based on an actual incident earlier in life.

A middle-aged, unmarried woman developed a "sticking pain" in her left cheek soon after her roommate of many years got married. They had been "like sisters." As a child she had, in a fit of anger, thrown an open safety pin, which lodged in her sister's left cheek. She never again permitted herself to feel angry, even when she felt deserted by her roommate.

Primary and Secondary Gains. *Primary gain* refers to the effectiveness of the conversion symptom in providing a satisfactory symbolic expression for the repressed wish, thereby averting underlying frustration. It is measured by the degree to which the conversion mechanism appears to be protecting the patient from the emotional distress that accompanied (or would accompany) an open conflict. Thus, the primary gain may be considered maximal when the patient is free of anxiety or depression and has little or no concern about the symptom. The serene woman with conversion paralysis, "resigned to God's will," who says she has come to the doctor only because of the insistence of the family, exemplifies a high degree of effectiveness of the conversion. *Secondary gain* refers to the advantages conferred on the patient by being ill. While any patient may derive some social gain from any illness, the patient with conversion symptoms typically uses the conversion illness to communicate wants and needs, to influence and manipulate, to gain sympathy and attention, to strengthen interpersonal bonds, to promote closeness, to evoke feelings of distress, and even to induce anger or sexual feelings. Such behaviors are especially likely to be reserved for the people with whom the patient is closely bound or with whom the patient

is in conflict. In contrast to the malingering patient, who is quite deliberate in his objectives, the conversion patient is largely unaware of how he uses symptoms and illness to affect others (see section on malingering later in this chapter). Thus, both primary gain and secondary gain serve to render the symptoms and the sick role desirable for the patient, the displayed suffering notwithstanding. Even when protesting determination to be rid of the symptom, the discerning physician will detect a resistance by the patient to any approach that might reveal the underlying psychological motives.

COMMON CONVERSION SYMPTOMS

Most patients present with more than one conversion symptom, sometimes in the form of complex syndromes, sometimes as apparently unrelated symptoms. Only occasionally is the conversion monosymptomatic. Combinations of symptoms commonly simulate familiar illness patterns. The history of multiple conversion symptoms generally favors a conversion explanation for the new symptom; however, the diagnostic criteria noted above must be fulfilled before a definite diagnosis is justified.

Pain

Pain is the conversion symptom seen most commonly today.[30,31,49,50] It may involve any part of the body, the head, back, and abdomen being the most frequently involved. Pain in the abdomen and face is more common among women, in the back and heart region among men. Conversion pain may exist in conjunction with other conversion symptoms, simulating a syndrome, such as abdominal pain, nausea, and vomiting. It may occur in addition to the symptoms of a somatic disorder, such as in the patient with coronary insufficiency who may have conversion chest pain in addition to the typical angina of effort or of coronary spasm, usually at different times and under different circumstances.

That the conversion symptoms should be pain rather than some other symptom derives mainly from the psychological links between pain on the one hand and aggression, guilt, punishment, and atonement on the other (see Chap. 3). Hence, conversion pain syndromes occur most commonly among persons who are struggling with underlying feelings of aggression and guilt, which they attempt to deal with through atonement by self-inflicted pain. Unacceptable feelings of anger directed toward a deceased person, for example, may be symbolically represented by pain, the site of which is often based on a pain that the deceased had suffered. In this way, expression of aggression is

averted, and feelings of guilt are assuaged. The "pain" of grief may be felt physically as "heartache," pain in the throat, or in the pit of the stomach.

Certain persons are excessively prone to suffer pain, especially conversion pain.[30] Such *pain-prone* persons are dominated by conflicts around issues of aggression, guilt, self-punishment, and atonement. Typically, they have a histories of repeated painful disorders, accidents, injuries, or operations, usually with uncertain diagnoses and indifferent treatment results. Often, no sooner is one pain problem resolved than another develops. The pain is commonly described with vivid imagery, portraying injury, torture, and mutilation (e.g. "like being stabbed with a red-hot poker", "like a bullet going through me", "like my flesh is being torn"). Some patients parade their suffering; others display the patient resignation of martyrs. Still others insist there are no problems or stresses in their lives, not even related to their pain and disability—a claim usually not supported by the family. In their backgrounds is often a history of violence and brutality; parents who fought, cruel punishments, an abusive alcoholic father, or alternation between angry, recriminating relationships, and cold, distant relationships. In such families, acts of aggression may constitute the dominant modality of interpersonal relating, physical punishment inflicted by the parent being experienced by the child as evidence of the parent caring. Display of parental affection and remorse following a beating not only tends to entrench such an association but to give it an erotic flavor as well. Pain-prone patients may recount with relish the hardships of punishments and the extent of their victimization and exploitation as children at the hands of parents. Occasionally, they report a childhood marked by uninterrupted love, peace, and serenity—a picture actually too good to be true.

> A woman with multiple conversion pains described her childhood in idyllic terms. Further inquiry, however, revealed that her loving relationship with her father consisted of regularly administered whippings, following which he would tearfully embrace his little girl and plead with her not again to misbehave. She solicited the punishment by confessing her misdeeds of the day.

Pain-prone women characteristically emphasize hardships, difficulties, defeats, and humiliations. Paradoxically, they appear to have solicited such situations rather than to have sought to avoid or overcome them.[30] They report bad marriages to abusive inconsiderate husbands, mistreatment by neighbors or employers, dirty, demeaning jobs, and just plain bad luck. Actually their bitter lives are reported with a certain relish, suggesting masochism. An inverse relationship

may exist between the occurrence of pain and the difficulties of the life situation. Parodoxically, when under stress, when life is treating them badly, they may become pain free; when they have a success or prospect of relief, pain may develop. Evidently, when the environment does not impose sufficient suffering to appease guilt, they inflict punishment upon themselves in the form of pain. Frequent solicitation of and submission to surgery and to painful diagnostic procedures is commonplace among pain-prone women.

Pain-prone men are less masochistic and more sadistic in their orientation.[31] They struggle with intense hostility, sometimes of homicidal character, which they attempt to control by relative isolation from others or by involvement in dangerous, often solitary, risk-taking activities, as hunting, fast driving, and scuba diving. Such men are decidedly accident-prone. They show a delicate balance between pain and acts of aggression; pain inhibits aggressive activity, whereas controlled aggressive behavior with a high risk of self-injury sometimes relieves the pain.

> A man with periodic anterior chest pain of conversion origin became infuriated when the hospital orderly directed him to return to bed. He raised his fist to punch him, but before he could do so he was seized with such intense pain that he collapsed on the bed.
>
> Another man could relieve his excruciating head pain by breaking up furniture or by raping his wife.

A less severe and usually socially better adjusted group of pain-prone men present themselves as hypermasculine individuals who place great premium on strength, courage, daring, and endurance. They fear being weak or passive and may greatly overestimate their own potential. The pain syndrome may develop when they suffer a defeat or loss or are thrust into a position of too great responsibility. An accident on the job may be the final step precipitating the chronic pain, permitting the patient to rationalize his defeat and subsequent inactivity. Some industrial compensation cases fall into this group. Among middle-aged men, pain in the heart region (pseudoangina) is a particularly common form, perhaps fostered by the notion that the heart attack is the price of success and overwork. Its differentiation from the pain of coronary spasm (Prinzmental's variant) may be difficult.

Not all psychogenic pain is based on conversion. Chronic pain may also involve hypochondriacal and delusional mechanisms or may be based on excessive preoccupation with an otherwise mild pain. Pain may also derive from psychophysiologic mechanisms as has been discussed (*e.g.*, muscle tension). Finally, pain originating from a conversion mechanism may persist as a behavior pattern and way of life long after its original purpose has been served.[49]

Hyperventilation Syndrome

A common conversion manifestation, hyperventilation occurs in response to conversion sensations involving difficulties in breathing.[33,34] Hence the syndrome is a complex of conversion symptoms and conversion complications. More often than not, the patient is not aware of hyperventilating. What the patient reports instead are the symptoms of hypocapnia and respiratory alkalosis (*i.e.,* lightheadedness, dizziness, buzzing in the head, numbness and tingling of the lips and fingertips, and rarely, tetany). The breathing difficulties that may be reported are choking sensations, suffocation, or inability to take a deep breath, though these usually are only revealed on direct inquiry. Although dizzy and lightheaded, they rarely actually lose consciousness. Examples of hyperventilation syndrome are cited earlier in this chapter.

Patients with the hyperventilation syndrome sigh frequently, especially when sensitive topics are being explored in the interview. They are prone to use imagery of breathing (*e.g.,* "It took my breath away," "I just gasped when. . .") and to display inspiratory and expiratory exclamations (*e.g.,* "Oh!" "Ah". The symptoms may be reproduced by having the patient overbreathe for 1 minute. Although most persons easily tolerate the hypocapnic symptoms induced by 2 to 3 minutes of overbreathing, the patient with the hyperventilation syndrome is highly sensitive and often cannot perservere beyond 30 seconds without experiencing severe symptoms identical with the spontaneous attacks. To avoid suggestion, the patient should be asked "What did you feel?", or "Have you ever felt like this before?", rather than "Was it like your symptoms?"

Hyperventilation may also occur as a concomitant of anxiety, in which case it is more properly designated as a psychophysiological syndrome.

Syncope, Stupor, and Coma

Conversion syncope, sometimes called hysterical syncope, is more common among women than men.[34,35] Typically, the faint occurs in the presence of others, the patient sliding or slumping to the ground, rarely suffering any injury. The appearance and claim of unconsciousness may last from seconds to many minutes and may fluctuate. Loss of consciousness often is not complete, the patient reporting being able to hear people speaking, but their voices sound as if coming from a distance. During the faint there are no changes in vital signs or color, and no sweating, unless the patient is also hyperventilating, which occasionally occurs. While "unconscious," the lids may flutter and the patient may moan, mutter, or move about. If the patient's arm is held above the face by the examiner and allowed to fall back, it will be deflected away from striking the face. A sharp command may terminate the attack. Sometimes the examiner may provoke a faint by having the patient hyperventilate or by a strong suggestion that a particular manipulation (*e.g.,* massaging the neck) will induce an attack. At times, the periods of apparent unconsciousness last long enough to be classifed as *stupors* or *comas.* Such episodes may be ushered in by a period of sleepiness or confusion and may last days at a time. Usually the patient can be aroused to cooperate in eating or toiletting, although he appears dazed and confused. Pupillary and corneal reflexes remain intact. Deviation of the eyes toward the side on which the patient is lying has been proposed as a physical sign indicating psychological mediation and normal cortical function.[61] Consciousness may return abruptly, the patient claiming amnesia for the period. The electroencephalogram (EEG) obtained during conversion unconsciousness is always normal. In all types of syncope and coma involving some interference with cerebral metabolism, the EEG is abnormal, usually slow, during the period of unconsciousness.[34,36] Patients with conversion stupors or comas are also prone to fugues and dissociative states.

Seizures

In contrast to the stereotyped sequence of *grand mal epilepsy,* the conversion (hysteric) seizure is marked by an unpredictable course, with clutching, grasping, pulling, struggling, tearing at the clothes, rolling from side to side, bizarre postures and expressions, and sometimes blatantly coital movements.[51,56,58,66] They tend to occur in public and may last from minutes to hours and often can be influenced by suggestion. Some fits have a tantrum like character. Tongue biting, injury, and incontinence are infrequent, but may occur. Consciousness may not be completely lost, the patient sometimes being able to report details of the seizure. Corneal, pupillary, and deep reflexes are present, and attempts to open the eye are resisted. Postictal confusion and somnolence are unusual.

A normal EEG during, or the first minute or so following, the seizure strongly favors conversion.[51,66] Because some epileptic patients have conversion convulsions in addition to true epileptic convulsions, an abnormal interseizure EEG does not rule out conversion. A valuable differentiating test during the seizure is deep, sustained pressure in the sternum. The patient with a conversion spell may experience this as unpleasant and attempt to grab the hand or push it away. Such a maneuver will not alter a true seizure.

Conversions seizures tend to be more common among adolescents, especially girls. An association with forced incestuous relationships with the father has been demonstrated in some cases.[58]

Weakness, Paralysis, Contractures, and Gait Disturbances

The great variety of pareses, paralyses, contractures, and gait disturbances of conversion origin are noted in Table 30-1. Conversion motor disturbances characteristically tend to fluctuate with repeated examination and suggestion and do not conform to known anatomical and physiological principles.[48,62] Though such symptoms may develop "out of the blue," many are posttraumatic, as with accidents, military combat, and natural disorders. The nature of the motor disturbance often reflects body positions or restrictions noted among the dead and injured or imposed on the victim himself by the accident or disaster. Hence, a detailed reconstruction of the patient's recollection of the incident is valuable. Such posttraumatic symptoms may appear as soon as the victim recovers from the shock or only after several days. Some may have suffered minor injury of the involved part; others are totally unscathed. Or the conversion manifestation may emerge during or after recovery from a more serious injury.

In conversion hemiplegia, the upper extremity is often more afflicted than the lower, usually hanging beside the body, incapable of any voluntary movement. A patient may have flaccid arm and a spastic leg. Weakness and paralysis are more pronounced peripherally, in contrast to the proximal distribution of organic hemiplegia. When attempting to move the paralyzed limb, the patient may contract the antagonistic muscles as well as the prime movers. As a result a limb will transiently hold its position after support for it has been removed. The weak or paralyzed arm held over the patient's face by the examiner and then released suddenly not only hovers a few seconds but also will fall safely to the side of the head, thereby avoiding injury. Instructed to flex the arm at the elbow against resistance, the arm of the patient with organic paralysis is easily extended by the examiner whereas with conversion, as in the normal, sudden release is followed by involuntary flexion of the stretched muscle. Observations of patients while they eat, dress, perform other activities, or sleep, will reveal an ability to use the limb in ways not possible if the patients were truly paralyzed. When walking, the point of the paralyzed foot is dragged along the ground and the trunk is bent. Weight is thrown on to the limb affected by the paralysis at each step, in contrast to the circumduction characteristics of hemiparesis of upper motor neuron origin. Reflexes are unimpaired and lower facial weakness is not present. Pains, aches, paresthesias, hyperesthesia, and anesthesia are commonplace and usually of inconsistent distribution (see Cutaneous Sensory Disturbances). Conversion hemicontracture typically develops

suddenly, without the phase of flaccid paralysis characteristic of organic hemiplegia.

Monoplegia is more often flaccid in the arm and spastic in the leg. In the flaccid type, paralysis is likely to be complete, the arm hanging down and swinging as an inert body beside the trunk when the patient walks. The hand is extended with outstretched and adducted fingers. The spastic arm or leg may be in flexion or extension. In contrast to organic contractures, which can be overcome, rigidity increases as the examiner intensifies his efforts to move the spastic limb.

The Hoover sign is especially valuable in differentiating organic from conversion paralysis of the leg.[67] Normally, when one elevates one leg above the plane of the bed while lying supine, the other leg is firmly pressed against the mattress to provide additional leverage. With organic paralysis, the good leg is used for leverage, but the paralyzed leg is not. With conversion paralysis, the "paralyzed" leg is used for leverage, while the "good" one is not, a demonstration that the paralysis is at the level of motivation (will), not of the motor system (Fig. 30-1). When the patient "wills" to elevate his good leg, he remains unaware that the opposite (paralyzed) leg is participating in the process. This may be tested by placing the hand under each heel in succession and noting whether the patient presses down when asked to raise the other leg against the resistance imposed by the examiner holding down the opposite knee. One may also observe whether the paralyzed limb is lifted from the bed as the patient attempts to raise himself to the sitting position with his arms folded and his legs separated. With conversion the affected leg will remain firmly on the bed. In the thigh-adduction test, the supine patient is instructed to adduct his good leg against resistance by the examiner. With conversion paralysis, the adductors of the paralyzed leg will be felt contracting, which does not happen with organic paralysis.

Conversion paraplegia is usually flaccid but may also be in spastic extension with the two limbs adducted and drawn together. The flaccid limbs can be moved passively with the greatest ease, whereas the spastic limbs go into more intense contracture. If the flaccid paraplegic can be made to walk while supported, it will be seen that the lower limbs execute the necessary movements, though feebly, and that apparently paralyzed muscles contract normally during the automatic act of walking.

The hand paralyzed on a conversion basic usually hangs limp and flaccid, forming a right angle with the forearm, ostensibly paralyzed at the wrist. Yet when asked to make a fist, the hand will extend. A coarse tremor may develop as the result of contraction of antagonistic muscles if the patient is asked to make some

Thigh adduction test

1. Patient is instructed to adduct "good" leg against resistance by examiner

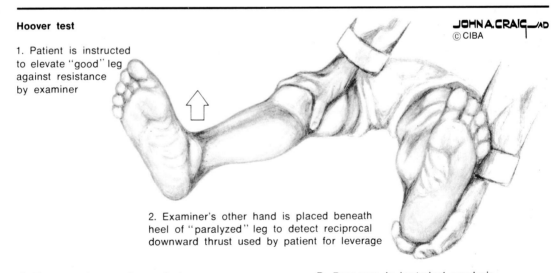

Adduction

2. Examiner's other hand is placed against "paralyzed" thigh to detect contraction

A. Response in organic paralysis

Patient can accomplish adduction with no contralateral adduction palpable in paralyzed leg

B. Response in hysterical paralysis

In adduction of "good" leg, patient involuntarily adducts "paralyzed" leg

Hoover test

JOHN A. CRAIG—AD
© CIBA

1. Patient is instructed to elevate "good" leg against resistance by examiner

2. Examiner's other hand is placed beneath heel of "paralyzed" leg to detect reciprocal downward thrust used by patient for leverage

A. Response in organic paralysis

Patient is able to elevate good leg without concomitant downward thrust of paralyzed leg

B. Response in hysterical paralysis

Elevation of "good" leg is accompanied by downward thrust of "paralyzed" leg

Fig 30-1. Tests for weakness in lower extremity. (From Weintraub MI: Hysteria: A clinical guide to diagnosis. © Copyright 1977, CIBA Pharmaceutical Company, Division of CIBA-GEIGY Corporation. Reprinted with permission from CLINICAL SYMPOSIA, illustrated by John A. Craig, M.D. All rights reserved)

movement. In the foot, the equinovarus position is assumed, with "steppage" when walking.

When conversion paralysis or contracture are of long standing, muscle atrophy and bone demineralization may take place and the skin may become cold, loose, sweaty and cyanotic, further examples of conversion complications (see Table 30-2).

Peculiar contractures may involve the hand, the foot, the sternomastoid and trapezius muscles (conversion torticollis), the neck muscles (pseudotetanus, pseudomeningitis), and the trunk (camptocormia, bent-back). In the trunk contractures, the body is bent forward at the hips, holding the trunk almost horizontal, the neck is extended and held rigidly with the eyes looking upward, and the arms hang loosely. The patient may walk easily and without a limp. The abnormal posture may disappear when the patient lies supine. Pain in the back is a common complaint.[59]

Occupational cramps serve to impair a specific learned motor skill. There is great variability, but generally one finds disabling muscular spasm, incoordination, and discomfort variously described as fatigue, weakness, stiffness, or pain, rendering performance of the skill difficult or impossible. Characteristically, for functions other than the particular skill, symptoms ameliorate or disappear. Virtually any occupational skill may be involved. Writer's cramp is probably the most familiar.[53]

Astasia-abasia is the classic conversion gait disturbance. When examined lying down, the patient may exhibit no motor difficulty; all movements, muscular power, and reflexes are normal. However, when placed in the upright position, he either collapses on his flaccid lower limbs or these limbs are shaken by a rapid tremor culminating in indefinite treading movement. In other cases, the lower limbs go into contracture preventing any walking. Other difficulties in walking of conversion origin (dysbasia) are characterized by incoordination, awkward postures, and modes of progression that actually require complex muscular coordination to prevent falling, indicating a remarkable ability to make rapid and appropriate postural adjustments quite incompatible with neurologic impairment. Some mimic how one might walk under special conditions (e.g., tight-rope, sticky surface, "zombie," struggling against the tide). As with other conversion symptoms, such peculiar gaits may derive from the circumstances of the actual traumatic situation as well as from fantasy.

Movement Disorders, Tremors, Tics

The conversion movement disorders are particularly difficult to distinguish from those due to brain lesions. Sudden onset and rapid development, association with local contractures, lack of usual neurologic findings, and characteristics resembling a meaningful gesture are suggestive of conversion disorders. A woman who unexpectedly lost her daughter developed an involuntary periodic head movement, facial expression, and clucking sound that suggested the familiar nod and sound of disbelief. Another patient spasmodically turned her head to the left and closed her eyes; this replicated her response when her daughter, sitting to her right, told her she was pregnant out of wedlock.

Weakness and Fatigue (Pseudomyasthenia Gravis)

Conversion myasthenia differs from myasthenia gravis in that weakness occurs throughout the waking hour, is unrelieved by rest or sleep, and is not directly related to severity of exercise or the muscle group used.[37] The weakness may be intensified at special times, such as while eating or during a headache. Inconsistencies of muscle strength are apparent when tested neurologically and functionally (e.g., during position holding, deep knee bends, or stair climbing). True ptosis does not occur, although a profound sense of tiredness may be expressed in such ways as "I couldn't hold my eyes open." Symptoms usually persist chronically over a period of years, and are not progressive.

Cutaneous Sensory Disturbances

Conversion hemisensory disturbance commonly involves an entire half of the body, including the head and the face, the line of demarcation being exactly at the midline.[62] Patchy sensory disturbances, hypesthetic or hyperesthetic, which vary from day to day and are inconsistent with patterns of innervation, are likely to be of conversion origin. The margins of sensory impairment in conversion are usually sharply defined, with borders at joints, skin creases, or the midline. They are not graded as with nerve lesions, and do not follow neural or dermatomal distribution. Rather, the area of involvement corresponds with the patient's image of his body and its functions (e.g., the entire half of the body from crown to toe; the hand below the wrist or the arm from shoulder down; or the exposed area). Usually all modalities of sensation are involved equally, resulting in the psychophysiologically illogical finding of diminished appreciation of vibration over the upper but not the lower portion of the tibia, or over one half of the sternum or skull. In contrast to patients with organic brain dysfunction, who feel double simultaneous stimulation only on the unimpaired side, patients with conversion sensory defects may respond normally even in the area hypesthetic to single stimulation.[52] It is noteworthy that patients professing complete loss of sensation but no motor impairment may have no difficulty with the finger-to-nose or heel-

to-knee and can still execute small movements for which intact superficial sensation is indispensable, such as picking up a pen or buttoning the jacket with eyes closed. Total anesthesia or analgesia may disappear during deep sleep, as demonstrated by the patient's withdrawal movements when the anesthetic area is noxiously stimulated.

Visual Disturbances (Amaurosis and Ambylopia)

The sudden onset of total blindness (amaurosis) as a conversion symptom may be dramatically verbalized with phrases such as "Why have the lights been turned off?" or "A curtain suddenly descended." Monocular conversion blindness is relatively less common.[32] Conversion amblyopia is especially common in school-age children. Initially, children typically complain of blurred vision and difficulty seeing the blackboard at school, but have no difficulty watching TV or playing sports. An important contributor to the development of conversion amblyopia may be an inadequately concealed family secret, something the child should not "see" (know about). In general, adults with conversion amblyopia or amaurosis report more severe symptoms and have greater social dysfunction than do children. They may need to be led by the hand, have difficulty walking, and clumsily bump into doors. Previous trauma to the eye, fear of eye disease, a history of eye disease in the family, and other preoccupations with vision may be important.

The diagnosis of conversion is suggested when measured visual activity is found to fluctuate, sometimes even within the same day, and when the patient hesitates as much over the large print as over the smaller print of the Snellen chart. Visual field testing on the tangent screen may reveal no enlargement of the field as the distance from the screen is increased (tubular vision). Further, the conversion visual field typically is circular, with no normal temporal enlargement, and is the same size whether obtained by a 5 mm object or a large sheet of white paper. With conversion visual problems, the subject may be able to see better through one color lens than another.

With monocular conversion blindness, both direct and consensual pupillary responses to light remain intact. The application of a highly refractive magnifying lens or prism over the patient's good eye will be interpreted by the patient as improving rather than distorting vision. That is because he unwittingly is using the affected eye. With the red glass test, the patient is asked to read a line of alternating red and black letters, with a red glass placed over the seeing eye. Because red letters are invisible when viewed through a red glass, their successful identification means that the patient is reading with the supposedly blind eye.

With bilateral conversion blindness, important negative findings include normal electroretinogram, electrooculogram, and visual evoked response. With the complaint of total blindness, the occurrence on the EEG of normal interruption of alpha rhythm upon opening the eyes favor conversion. Sparing of pupillary responses is a valuable sign but may also occur in the syndrome of cortical blindness due to extensive occipital lobe infarction.

Hearing Loss

Conversion deafness is relatively uncommon. The hearing loss disappears during sleep. If the sleeping patient is startled when exposed to a sudden loud noise, hearing is revealed to be present. The demonstration of K-complexes on the sleep EEG confirms intact pathways.

Anorexia, Nausea, Vomiting

Conversion anorexia is likely to be expressed as distaste for food or dislike of eating rather than as lack of appetite. Anorexia, nausea, or vomiting may be provoked by certain foods and not by others, especially foods conducive to fantasy, as fluid egg white, scum on milk, or raw meat. Such symptoms may occur before or after eating, on the sight of food, or only in certain settings or with certain people. A good appetite may abruptly be replaced by nausea at mealtime, only to return as soon as the meal is over. Commonly, food is taken into the mouth gingerly, in small morsels, and delayed in the forepart of the mouth, the act of swallowing threatening to evoke a gag. Vomiting, unless it occurs soon after a meal, is likely to consist only of mucus or a small amount of bile-stained gastric juice. However, it can be copious enough to lead to alkalosis and electrolyte imbalance. Morning nausea, gagging, and vomiting may indicate unconscious pregnancy fantasies in men (the *couvade syndrome*) as well as women.[68] Similar symptoms occurring at night may reflect an unconscious wish for and rejection of an oral sexual experience. The rejection of any repugnant idea may be expressed by anorexia, nausea, or vomiting.

Dysphagia

Conversion dysphagia is typically intermittent, nonprogressive, and referred to as a sensation of sticking in the throat or high in the esophagus. When observed eating, the patient may be noted to pucker his face and act as if it is difficult to move the bolus into the esophagus. The symbolic meaning of the food is more important than its consistency, with some solid foods being swallowed with ease, and with some soft or liquid foods producing discomfort.

Globus Hystericus

Globus hystericus is the feeling of a lump in the lower part of the neck or behind the upper part of the sternum, comparable to that experienced during crying (choked up). It more often occurs between meals. Not only does it usually not interefere with swallowing, but it may be relieved by drinking or eating. The symptom is intermittent in character, usually recurring over a period of years, and never progressing. Schatzki believes the sensation to arise as a physiologic response to frequent swallowing without adequate saliva formation, suggesting as the basis an underlying unconscious wish to swallow.[38]

Dysphonia and Aphonia

Dysphonia presents as whispering or a high-pitched expiratory or inspiratory stridor; Aphonia presents as a complete inability to utter any word at all.[39,40] There is sometimes an accompanying sensation of tightness in the throat or the chest. A normal voice may unexpectedly reappear when the patient is startled or when the patient speaks in his sleep. If the patient who can only whisper is asked to cough and the cough is loud and normal in sound, it indicates that the vocal cords can be approximated. In true cord paralysis, the cough is booming in quality. The vocal cords move properly, approximate accurately, and are free of lesions. In more extreme cases of mutism, the patient emits no sound, makes no movement of his lips, and indicates by gestures that he is incapable of speaking. He may be unable to move his tongue on command yet movements of mastication are preserved. Conflicts about speaking or revealing secrets are prominent.

Nongaseous Abdominal Bloating

Nongaseous abdominal bloating occurs almost exclusively among hysterical women with intense longings to be pregnant.[41] The marked abdominal protuberance is brought about by simultaneously relaxing the abdominal musculature and thrusting the lumbar spine forward, often so much so that the hand may easily be passed beneath the spine of the reclining patient. Though seemingly well-relaxed, the patient is unable to make her abdomen flatten by conscious effort. However, the protuberance can sometimes be reduced by turning the patient on her side and quickly and forcibly bringing the knees up to the chest. The enlargement may develop within a few minutes, but more often reaches a peak only by the end of the day. It disappears during sleep.

Pruritus Vulvae and Ani

A conversion origin of pruritus vulvae and pruritus ani may be suspected when there is evidence of sexual frustration and conflict, such as among widows, spinsters, and wives of impotent husbands.[42] Scratching may be a substitute for masturbation. Commonly, there is perineal or perianal factitious injury from scratching, with mild infection, lichenification, and other secondary changes, often misinterpreted as the primary cause. Conversion pruritus ani is more common among men, and often reflects an unconscious homosexual conflict. Such men may show paranoid features as well.

Urinary Urgency, Frequency, and Retention

Urinary urgency, frequency, and retention are commonly associated with unconscious sexual or pregnancy fantasies.[60] The urge to urinate may be intense and entirely unrelieved by emptying the bladder, yet the patient may not report nocturia. Urinary findings are minimal, considering the intensity of the symptoms. Inability to pass urine may be total, with enormous distention of the bladder requiring catheterization for relief. It may occur intermittently or it may be chronic. The urethral meatus ordinarily appears normal, with the sphincter firmly closed. Evidence of superficial irritation may prove to be secondary to trauma inflicted by the patient.

Concurrent Conversion and Physical Symptoms

Conversion and physical symptoms may occur together. Sometimes the conversion is based on some special meaning to the patient of the physical symptom or the circumstances of its occurrence. Thus, peculiar patterns of hypesthesia, pain, paralysis, or contracture may complicate the course of recovery from an injury or from surgery. Not infrequently, conversion symptoms develop during diagnostic study, especially when there is uncertainty or serious concern about the outcome, or in the context of disturbances in the relationship with the doctor.

> A young woman who was making an excellent recovery from a severe bout of ulcerative colitis abruptly developed nausea and vomiting, peculiar in that it involved primarily dietary items and oral medications prescribed by her physician. After two days with no relief, she requested that ileostomy and colectomy be performed, a procedure which she and her doctor had already rejected as no longer indicated. The patient then abashedly acknowledged that she had been having romantic fantasies about her doctor, stimulated by reading a novel in which a doctor falls in love with his patient and poisons his wife. Following the confession, symptoms ceased as abruptly as they had begun.

Particularly challenging is the diagnostic problem posed by the hysterical patient with a life-long pattern of multiple conversion symptoms who develops a physical illness. The alert physician will note that the

patient's description of the new physical symptoms sound different. It is often better defined and communicated with more genuine concern. An especially valuable clue is when the patient ascribes the new symptoms to psychological causes, a radical departure from the characteristic insistence on a physical cause.

A 36-year-old polysymptomatic hysteric woman experienced the sudden onset of a new symptom complex characterized by occipital headache, nausea, vomiting, and dizziness, all intensified by turning the head and flexing the neck. She flat-footedly ascribed the symptoms to having for the first time in her life blown up at her mother, the symptom onset coinciding precisely with her having turned her head sharply to confront her mother, who was seated behind her in the car. Uncharacteristically, she strenuously resisted the diagnostic study, which ultimately documented a posterior fossa tumor.

HYSTERICAL EPIDEMICS

Mass outbreaks of conversion symptoms typically occur in groups already bound together by some shared, often secret, danger or concern.[9,47,56] Among adolescent girls, especially in a restrictive environment, sexual fantasies are often at the root. During periods of social unrest, wartime, or threat of epidemic illness, a rumor or an actual illness may set in motion a wave of symptoms among persons who almost always already share some emotional bond. The epidemic usually begins with the rapid dissemination of rumors about a mysterious gas, an industrial poison, radiation, an infectious agent, or some disease-carrying insect. The reported or observed symptoms of the first victim provide the model for new cases which develop in rapid succession. Dizziness, weakness, fainting, falling, convulsions, shortness of breath, hyperventilation, coughing, hoarseness, aphonia, nausea, vomiting, pruritus, abdominal pain, and headache are among the more common symptoms. In any epidemic of an infectious disease, especially in institutions, there is virtually always a certain incidence of concurrent, conversion-based simulated illness as well.

DIFFERENTIATION FROM OTHER PSYCHOSOMATIC SYMPTOMS

Psychophysiologic Symptoms

Psychophysiologic symptoms result when psychologic defense and coping mechanisms, including conversion, are ineffectual or fail. Under such conditions, more primitive neurobiological systems of defense and adaptation are invoked, involving mainly autonomic neuroendocrine outflow systems. These include mechanisms to prepare the organism for flight, struggle, and defense against injury (the flight-fight pattern) or for conservation of resources and insulation against trauma (the conservation-withdrawal pattern).[11]

The failure of mental mechanisms to maintain adjustment is experienced by the patient in terms of unpleasant affects, such as anxiety, fear, anger, sadness, helplessness, or hopelessness, whereas the activation of biological systems involves such demonstrable physiologic changes as tachycardia, sweating, vasoconstriction, or hyperperistalsis. The patient's awareness of such physiologic processes results in such symptoms as palpitation, sweating, cold hands and feet, diarrhea, and fatigue. In this respect, although remotely induced by psychological processes, the psychophysiologic symptom itself is of organic origin, deriving as it does from the patient's awareness of actual bodily changes. In contrast to the conversion symptom, it has no primary symbolic meaning and serves no psychological function.

The basic difference between symptoms of conversion and those of psychophysiologic origin is perhaps best highlighted by the clinical observation that, when the conversion mechanism is failing in its adaptive function, the patient may become anxious or depressed and manifest psychophysiologic changes and symptoms; conversely, the development of a conversion symptom may terminate such symptoms. The farmer with conversion ptosis and blepharospasm, mentioned earlier, who became acutely anxious and fainted when his lids were held open, illustrated this inverse relationship.

Hypochondriacal Symptoms

The hypochondriacal patient displays an obsessive kind of preoccupation with physical symptoms or bodily processes. He appears to be unusually aware of even the most trivial sensation to which he ascribes the potential of grave consequences. Minor aches and pains, intestinal gas, borborygmi, cough, flushing, sweating, premature ventricular contractions, indeed virtually any perceptible physiologic change, may become the object of intense concern; so too may the discovery of a minor skin blemish, a palpable lump, or a visible arterial pulsation. The patient's concerns generally are couched in terms of fear of some serious or fatal disease. No amount of reassurance, no matter how soundly based, gives more than transient relief. Futhermore, any suggestion that the feared disease may indeed be present intensifies the patient's concern. This contrasts with the behavior of the patient with a conversion symptom, who does not view his symptom with such intense alarm and indeed may even seem relieved when

an organic diagnosis is proposed. Resignation to suffering, as is sometimes encountered with conversion symptoms, is never associated with the hypochondriacal symptom. Most confusion arises from the hysteric patient with chronic conversion symptoms whose efforts to gain the attention of the physician are misinterpreted as hypochondriacal concern. Anxious and depressed patients may amplify bodily sensations which are then reported as symptoms.[65] This may be a means to avoid acknowledging psychological distress or to gain admission to a health-care system that rejects patients with emotional or mental problems.

Somatic Delusions

Somatic delusions are psychotic manifestations and may be observed in patients with schizophrenia, paranoid states, psychotic depression, and delirium, dementia, or drug-induced psychoses. Although also originating in the mind, they differ from conversion symptoms by virtue of their palpably bizarre character. Thus, patients may believe that internal organs are shriveling up or disappearing, that the nose is misshapen or enlarged, that the genitals are deformed or missing, that a foreign object is in the rectum, abdominal cavity, uterus, or gullet, that insects are crawling under the skin, or that an extremity is enlarged or shruken. Although most such patients present no difficulty in diagnosis, an occasional patient whose delusions have been challenged in the past succeeds in couching the complaint in terms that suggest conversion or an organic process. However, when encouraged to elaborate, the patient who may have first defined his symptom as pain will eventually introduce the bizarre features that establish the delusional quality of the symptom.

Malingering and Factitious Illness

Physicians often are quick to accuse patients with conversion symptoms of malingering, especially because many of the diagnostic physical findings are identical in the two conditions (*e.g.,* a positive Hoover test). Hence, the differentiation must be based on psychological and social criteria. In actuality, malingering, the conscious simulation of disease, is rare in the general practice of medicine. Most cases occur in settings in which there is an immediate and usually obvious gain to be achieved by being sick, such as in penal institutions, the military, or when litigation is involved. Some unscrupulous individuals simulate for dishonest purposes, but they ordinarily avoid medical contacts lest they be unmasked. Children and some immature adults may make clumsy, amateurish efforts to play sick in order to avoid a difficult situation, but these are easily identified by virtue of the naivete of their notions of

illness. Among children, such malingering may hide a school phobia. More difficult to identify as malingering are patients who seek to prolong convalescence by simulating continuing symptoms of an illness, or who are receiving compensation or facing a lawsuit.

The ability to malinger successfully requires intellectual knowledge of and a familiarity with disease pictures. Hence successful malingerers are often drawn from persons who have worked in medical institutions or who have undergone extended periods of hospitalization.

The determinants of malingering are complex. Prominent are intense needs to be taken care of or to suffer. Some patients merely report and act out the symptoms of disease, whereas others fake fever by heating the thermometer, or bleeding by putting blood in sputum or urine. Some go so far as to injure themselves by inducing bruising or abscesses, introducing foreign bodies, or taking such drugs as digitalis, coumadin, atropine, insulin, diuretics, or thyroid hormones. The distribution of self-inflicted lesions is ordinarily limited by the patient's reach and handedness. Such self-destructive behavior may carry over into everyday life in the form of accident-proneness and masochistic relationships in which they are physically abused.

Not all patients who injure themselves are properly classified as malingerers. Occasionally, individuals secretly indulge in impulsive, compulsive, or bizarrely ritualistic bloodletting procedures, producing bleeding from skin or mucous membranes, especially urinary and genital tracts. Although such acts have complex psychodynamic origins, the patients themselves are not necessarily conspicuously deranged. On the contrary, the act may sometimes have the characteristics of a secret perversion in an otherwise adequately functioning person. When bleeding so induced is discovered in the course of medical examination, the patient is ashamed to acknowledge its cause, a different basis for dissembling than in the malingerer.

The so-called *Munchausen syndrome* refers to a group of illnesses manifested by chronic factitious symptomatology.[43,44] The diagnostic features include: (1) the dramatic presentation of medical complaints, suggesting a major emergency; (2) factitious evidence of disease; (3) evidence of many previous hospital experiences, particularly laparotomy scars and cranial burr holes; (4) eager submission to painful diagnostic and therapeutic procedures; (5) pathologic lying and false elaboration of the symptoms that intrigue the listener (pseudologia fantastica); (6) a history of signing out of hospitals against medical advice and wandering from hospital to hospital across the country (hospital hoboes); and (7) aggressive, unruly, truculent behav-

ior. Like the imposter, these patients know they are acting, but they cannot stop; their bizarre behavior has become a way of life.

The differentiation between malingering and conversion is at times difficult. In general, the malingerer is aloof, suspicious, hostile, secretive, unfriendly, and appears concerned about his symptom; the patient with conversion is more dependent, appealing, clinging, and, although clearly acting out the sick role, shows less than the expected concern about the symptom. Because the skillful malingerer applies his intellectual knowledge of the disease in the simulation, the end result is more likely to resemble the real thing. Careful observation, especially when the patient is unaware that he is being observed, will often reveal that the patient is not as disabled as he claims. Unlike the patient with a conversion, the malingerer must work hard to maintain his ruse. Hence, he cannot always resist the temptation to relax the deception, especially when he believes himself to be alone. Amelioration of symptoms with the establishment of an effective relationship with the physician is more characteristic of conversion than of malingering. Indeed the malingerer, because he is consciously involved in a deception, is unlikely to relate well. Nothing interferes more with a relationship than keeping secrets. The malingerer may be reluctant to cooperate in diagnostic procedures that may unmask him; the conversion patient is eager for confirmation of a somatic explanation for his symptom.

Deliberate deception of patients by physicians, such as with the use of placebos or sterile hypos, is of little diagnostic value and indeed may irrevocably damage the relationship with the patient. It is a far better method for the physician to try to understand the psychological reason for the symptom, whether it be based on conversion or on conscious simulation.

REFERENCES

1. **Paget J:** Nervous mimicry. In Paget J (ed): Clinical Lectures and Essays, pp 78–144. New York, D Appleton, 1975

2. **Veith I:** Hysteria. The History of a Disease. Chicago, University of Chicago Press, 1965

3. **Abse DW:** Hysteria and Related Mental Disorders. Baltimore, Williams & Wilkins, 1966

4. **Freud S:** Studies on hysteria (with Breuer, J.) 1893. Vol. 2. London, Hogarth Press, 1955

5. **Freud S:** Fragment of analysis of a case of hysteria (1905). Vol. 7, p 3–122. London, Hogarth Press, 1954

6. **Chodoff P:** The diagnosis of hysteria: An overview. Am J Psychiatry 131:1073–1078, 1974

7. **Ljungberg L:** Hysteria. A clinical prognostic, and genetic study. Acta Psychiatr Neurol Scand (Suppl 112) Vol. 32, 1957

8. **Farley J, Woodruff RA, Guze SB:** The prevalence of hysteria and conversion symptoms. Br J Psychiatry 114:1121, 1968

9. **Small GW, Nicholi AM:** Mass hysteria among school children. Early loss as a predisposing factor. Gen Psychiatr 39:721–724, 1982

10. **Sharpe EF:** Psychophysical problems revealed in language: An examination of metaphor. Int J Psychoanal 21:201, 1940

11. **Engel GL, Schmale AH:** Conservation-withdrawal: A primary regulatory process for organismic homeostasis. In Porter R, Knight J (eds): Physiology, Emotion and Psychosomatic Illness, pp 57–85. CIBA Foundation Symposium. Amsterdam, Elsevier–Excerpta Medica, 1972

12. **Palombo SR:** Dreaming and Memory. A New Information Processing Model. New York, Basic Books, 1978

13. **Fenichel O:** Conversion. In Fenichel O (ed): The Psychoanalytic Theory of Neurosis, pp 216–235. New York, Norton, 1945

14. **Engel GL:** A reconsideration of the role of conversion in somatic disease. Compr Psychiatry 9:316, 1968

15. **Chapman LF, Ramos AO, Goodell H et al:** Neurohumoral features of afferent fibers in man, their role in vasodilation, inflammation, and pain. Arch Neurol 4:617, 1961

16. **Chapman LF, Ramos AO, Goodell H et al:** Evidence for kinin formation resulting from neural activity evoked by noxious stimulation. Ann NY Acad Sci 104:258, 1963

17. **Barchilon J, Engel GL:** Dermatitis: An hysterical conversion symptom in a young woman. Psychosom Med 14:295, 1952

18. **Seitz PFD:** Symbolism and organ choice in conversion reactions. Psychosom Med 13:254, 1951

19. **Seitz PFD:** Experiments in the substitution of symptoms by hypnosis. Psychosom Med 15:405, 1953

20. **Lifschutz JE:** Hysterical stigmatization. Am J Psychiatry 114:527, 1957

21. **Ratnoff OD, Agle DP:** The psychogenic purpuras: A review of autoerythrocyte sensitization, autosensitization to DNA, "hysterical" and factitial bleeding and the religious stigmata. Semin Hematol 17:192–213, 1980

22. **McKegney FP:** The incidence and characteristics of patients with conversion reactions. I. A general hospital consultation service sample. Am J Psychiatry 124:542, 1967

23. **Morgan WL, Engel GL:** The approach to the medical interview. In Morgan WL, Engel GL (eds): The Clinical Approach to the Patient, pp 26–79. Philadelphia, W B Saunders, 1969

24. **Mayou R:** The social setting of hysteria. Br J Psychiatry 127:466–469, 1975.

25. **Perley J, Guze SB:** Hysteria—the stability and usefulness of clinical criteria. A quantitative study based on a follow-

up period of six to eight years in 39 patients. N Engl J Med 266:421, 1962

26. **Hardy HE:** A notable source of error in the diagnosis of appendicitis. Br Med J 2:1028, 1962

27. **Barraclough BM:** Appendectomy in women. J Psychosom Res 12:231, 1968

28. **Schmale AH:** Relationship of separation and depression to disease. Psychosom Med 20:259, 1958

29. **Schmale AH:** Giving up as a final common pathway to changes in health. In Lipowski ZJ (ed): Psychosocial Aspects of Physical Illness, pp 20–40. Basel, S Karger, 1972

30. **Engel GL:** "Psychogenic" pain and the pain-prone patient. Am J Med 26:899, 1959

31. **Tinling DC, Klein RF:** Psychogenic pain and aggression. The syndrome of the solitary hunter. Psychosom Med 28:738, 1966

32. **Rada RT, Meyer GG, Kellner R:** Visual conversion reaction in children and adults. J Nerv Ment Dis 166:580–587, 1978.

33. **Engel GL, Ferris EB, Logan M:** Hyperventilation: Analysis of clinical symptomatology. Ann Intern Med 27:683, 1947

34. **Engel GL:** Fainting, 2nd ed, pp 149–158. Springfield, IL, Charles C Thomas, 1962

35. **Romano J, Engel GL:** Studies of syncope. III. Differentiation between vasodepressor and hysterical fainting. Psychosom Med 7:3, 1945

36. **Engel GL, Romano J:** Delirium, a syndrome of cerebral insufficiency. J Chronic Dis 9:260, 1959

37. **Fullerton DT, Munsat TL:** Pseudomyasthenia gravis: A conversion reaction. J Nerv Dis 142:78, 1966

38. **Schatzki R:** Globus hysteria (globus sensation). N Engl J Med 270:676, 1964

39. **Kalman TP, Granet RB:** The written interview in hysterical mutism, Psychosomatics 22:362–366, 1981

40. **Barton RT:** The whispering syndrome of hysterical dysphonia. Ann Otolaryrgol 69:156, 1960

41. **Alverez WC:** Hysterical type of nongaseous abdominal bloating. Arch Intern Med 84:217, 1949

42. **Rosenbaum M:** Psychosomatic factors in pruritus. Psychosom Med 7:52, 1945

43. **Stern TA:** Munchausen's syndrome revisited. Psychosomatics 21:329–336, 1980

44. **Justus PG, Kreutziger S, Kitchens CS:** Probing the dynamics of Munchausen's syndrome. Ann Intern Med 93:120–127, 1980

45. **Engel GL, Schmale AH:** Psychoanalytic theory of somatic disorder: Conversion, specificity, and the disease onset situation. J Am Psychoanal Assoc 15:344, 1967

46. **Adamson JD, Schmale AH:** Object loss, giving up and the onset of psychiatric disease. Psychosom Med 27:557, 1965

47. **Kerckhoff AC, Back KW:** The June Bug. A Study of Hysterical Conversion. New York, Appleton-Century-Crofts, 1968

48. **Roussy G, Lhermitte J:** The Psychoneuroses of War, pp 1–65. London, University of London Press, 1918

49. **Steinback RA:** Pain Patients. Traits and Treatment. New York, Academic Press, 1974

50. **Blumer D:** Psychiatric considerations in pain. In Rothman RH, Simeone FA (eds): The Spine, Vol. 2, Chap 18, pp 871–906. Philadelphia, W B Saunders, 1975

51. **Ramani SV, Quesnez LF, Olson D et al:** Diagnoses of hysterical seizures in epileptic patients. Am J Psychiatry 137:705–709, 1980

52. **Green MA, Fink M:** Simultaneous tactile perception in patients with conversion sensory deficits. Mt Sinai J Med 41:141–143, 1974

53. **Moldofsky H:** Occupational cramp. J Psychosom Res 15:439–44, 1971

54. **Guze SB, Woodruff RA, Clayton PJ:** A study of conversion symptoms in psychiatric outpatients. Am J Psychiatry 128:643–646, 1971

55. **Lemkau PV:** On the epidemiology of hysteria. Psychiatrie Forum 3:1–14, 1973

56. **Gross M:** Pseudoepilepsy: A study in adolescent hysteria. Am J Psychiatry 136:210–213, 1979

57. **Reiser DE, Schroder AK:** Patient Interviewing, the Human Dimension. Baltimore, Williams & Wilkins, 1980

58. **Goodwin J, Simms M, Bergman R:** Hysterical seizures: A sequel to incest. Am J Orthopsychiatry 19:698–703, 1979

59. **Ballenger JD:** A case of camptocornia occurring in psychotherapy. J Nerv Ment Dis 162:291–294, 1976

60. **Barrett DM:** Psychogenic urinary retention in women. Mayo Clin Proc 51:351–356, 1976

61. **Henry JA, Woodruff GHA:** A diagnostic sign in states of apparent unconsciousness. Lancet 2:920–921, 1978

62. **Weintraub MI:** Hysteria. A clinical guide to diagnosis. Clin Symp 29, No. 6: 1977

63. **Watson CG, Buranen C:** The frequency and identification of false positive conversion reactions. J Nerv Ment Dis 167:243–247, 1979

64. **Stefansson JJ, Messina JA, Meyerowitz S:** Hysterical neurosis, conversion type: Clinical and epidemiological considerations. Acta Psychiatr Scand 53:119–138, 1976

65. **Barsky AJ, III:** Patients who amplify bodily sensations. Ann Intern Med 91:63–70, 1979

66. **Desai BT, Porter RS, Penry JK:** Psychogenic seizures. A study of 42 attacks in six patients, with intensive monitoring. Arch Neurol 39:202–209, 1982

67. **Hoover C:** A new sign for the detection of malingering and functional paresis of the lower extremities. JAMA 51:746–747, 1908

68. **Lipkin M, Lamb GS:** The couvade syndrome: An epidemiologic study. Ann Intern Med 96:509–511, 1982

31

Coma and Convulsion

James L. O'Leary
William M. Landau

Historical Résumé
Neural Basis of Consciousness
  Contribution of Studies upon Sleep
  Unconsciousness in Brain-Stem Lesions in
    Humans
**Abnormal States of Consciousness and Their
    Etiologies**
  Head Trauma
  Neoplasm and Brain Abscess
  Meningitis and Encephalitis
  Cerebrovascular Disease

Brain Metabolism and Metabolic Coma
Syncopal Attacks
Alcohol, Drugs, and Poisons
Hysteria
Convulsive Disorders
  Classification of Brain Waves
  Spectrum of Convulsive Disorders
  Generalized Seizures
  Focal Seizures
Narcolepsy
Summary

Coma and convulsion, outstanding symptoms of cerebral disorder, occupy the extremes of an excitability gradient that extends from a zone of hypoexcitability at one end of the normal range to one of hyperexcitability at the other. Coma develops as the state of neural excitability enters either of these end zones. Suspension of consciousness can occur either during a generalized epileptic attack (hyperexcitability) or when trauma, anoxia, infection, systemic metabolic disturbance, a toxin, poison, or drug markedly depresses neural functioning (hypoexcitability).

We digress to discuss certain rudiments of neurophysiology. The human brain contains some 10 billion nerve cells arranged in an intricate communication network roughly analogous to a telephone system or a computer, but infinitely more intricate than either. Each single-cell component functions both as a receiver-transmitter (cell body and dendrites) and as a conductor (axon). The axon terminals of one nerve cell are applied to the cell body or dendrites of others to pro-duce circuits of varying complexity. Information is propagated along axons in the form of variations in the spacing between a quick succession of all-or-none impulses. At the synapses, the digital all-or-none information carried by axons is transformed into an analogical, graded process. Two basic kinds of information are thus transmitted—excitatory and inhibitory. It is the excitatory processes upon which the nervous system depends chiefly for its operations. The inhibitory processes either prevent overaction or slow or stop action in progress. The richness of the interconnections between neurons makes for ready distribution of coded information through the neural net. However, inhibitory controls restrict normal activity to purposive channels. Under conditions of exalted excitability (*i.e.,* epileptic states), distribution of information is far too permissive, particularly when inhibitory brakes are also ineffective. In such circumstances, a few neurons discharging at frequencies up to 800 per second (a speed not uncommon at the site of epilep-

togenic lesions) may transmit impulses that rapidly infiltrate neighboring neurons poised on the threshold of discharge, drawing them into the orbit of excessive firing. Thus, a convulsion may avalanche across wide areas of the cerebral gray matter.

The depressed functioning of the hypoexcitable state is occasioned by elevation of the synaptic threshold and subnormal responsiveness of the membrane that invests the nerve cell, the former being one specific expression of the properties of the latter.

The important functions of synaptic transfer and impulse propagation depend upon the relative reactivity of the membrane: impaired excitability of the membrane greatly slows the operations of the system as a whole. Such slowing may cause an abnormal scarcity of circulating impulses within the neural net and an abolition of all but the most vital activities, resulting in unconsciousness.

The state of hyperexcitability, a prelude to convulsion, is manifested by low resistance at the synaptic bridges and a high tide of irritability. This leads to the discharge of spurts of impulses of excessive length and of astonishingly high frequency. This has the effect of overloading the system with circulating signals; through resultant overaction, this suspends the logistics of normal functioning and interrupts consciousness. The impulses discharge outward through avenues of diminished synaptic resistance, massively invading the nerve routes that lead to skeletal muscle. This produces the overt signs of convulsion. Because the nervous system depends largely upon energy sources transported by the blood supply, the time is relatively brief during which the chaotic overaction of convulsion can be maintained. As a result, it is more likely than not that a convulsion will terminate with the brain in a depressed state. However, the termination of seizure is not the result of depletion of energy substrates, but of complex mechanisms of change in neuronal-membrane excitability. During and after a generalized seizure, the accompanying unconsciousness can occur in two stages, the first that of overactivity associated with the convulsion proper, and the second (postictal parasomnia) with terminal underactivity.

By *unconsciousness* we mean a void of consciousness. The range of consciousness extends from the alert wakefulness (vigilance) of the expectant mind, through clouding (obtundity) and stupor, to precoma and coma. Any measure of loss implies the prior existence of a state of normal consciousness, which is the introspective yardstick that the experienced observer uses to estimate the severity of the loss. The definition of normal consciousness is most difficult. Its meanings are obscured by a haze of metaphysics. Brain has pointed out that to different savants it can mean six different things: forms of behavior by which we distinguish the unconscious person from the conscious person; psychological terms used to describe conscious states such as sensory and perceptual experiences; consciousness as related to the activity of the nervous system; the role of consciousness in the biological functions of the living organism; the logical terms that can be applied to conscious experience; and the metaphysical status of consciousness.[1] The notion of distinguishing between *content of consciousness* and the *state of awareness* in which it exists is also prevalent, the phrase *spontaneity of consciousness* being used for the latter. Sartre, for example, alludes to consciousness as a *pure spontaneity*, "confronting the world of things which is sheer inertness."[2] James appeared to challenge its very foundations in his essay, "Does Consciousness Exist?"[3]

HISTORICAL RÉSUMÉ

Efforts to understand the relation of physical states to mental states date back some 2400 years. One outcome of so many endeavors is the knowledge that speculations born of erroneous ideas concerning the brain or other body parts may be accepted as fact and persist unchallenged over a period of centuries.

It would seem that in early antiquity some crude but possibly accurate knowledge existed concerning brain structures. Those ancients may have been aware that the ventricles contained fluid instead of *pneuma* (air); several terms applied to brain parts were hydraulic in implication (*e.g.,* pons, aqueduct, and valve). It is conjectured that the erroneous view that the ventricles contained a *pneuma* replaced a correct one as a result of a decline in careful dissection, which caused a reliance on the scientifically unverified spoken or written word passed from one generation to another. That erroneous idea continued to be accepted until the 19th century, when Magendie (1825) showed that the ventricles of recently dead bodies contained fluid.

Apart from Aristotle, who viewed the seat of animal spirits as existing in the heart, the Greeks believed the ventricles to be the seat of sensation and motion. This erroneous idea was not discredited until the 16th century, when it was taught instead that sensation and motion were generated in brain substance. Modern anatomy and physiology begin in the 18th century with Prochaska, who laid the groundwork for reflexology.[4] Magendie and Bell shared the discovery that the dorsal roots of the spinal nerves were sensory and the ventral ones motor. Pierre Flourens, as well as discovering the respiratory center in the hindbrain, divided other brain functions between cerebrum and cerebellum (the cerebrum receiving and controlling

sensations, the cerebellum coordinating bodily movements). His views on the cerebrum were strictly non-localizationist ones, and were in opposition to those of the phrenologists, Gall and Spurzheim. Gall and Spurzheim were careful dissectors of the brain; they attempted to localize 30 or more faculties in various regions of the brain, and presumed that any well-developed character trait would require a corresponding local growth of nervous structure that would be reflected in a protuberance on the skull. Their theory proved markedly erroneous, as did the nonlocalizationist view of Flourens. Broca (1861), who reported a case in which a patient with chronic loss of speech was shown to have a localized lesion on the lateral side of the left frontal lobe, gave a clear impetus to the development of concepts of cerebral localization in man. A decade later, Fritsch and Hitzig, experimenting on dogs, demonstrated the motor control of the cerebral hemisphere over the opposite side of the body, as well as cerebral electrical excitability. Earlier, control of the cerebral hemisphere over motor functions had been denied by Flourens and others of his period.

For our purposes, consciousness is definable as a generalized product of the functioning of the waking brain, and is recognizable only through introspection. It is divisible into a state of awareness and a changing mental content, to which we attend. The content includes items of both primary and subsidiary import and is evident either in present perception or, after recall, in the memory of past events. Phylogenetically, its origin is said to lie in feeling.

The term *coma*, derived from the Greek *koma*, meaning deep sleep, designates a state of unconsciousness from which the subject cannot be aroused. The state of impaired consciousness that gradually develops into coma leads through obtundation (a state of drowsiness, indifference, and apathy, in which the threshold of arousal is significantly increased), through stupor (requiring vigorous, sometimes continuous, stimulation to maintain arousal), to deep coma, in which both the psychological and motor responses to stimulation are lost. Pupillary reactions, ocular motility, and abnormalities of respiration are valuable guides to the etiology of coma and, if structurally caused by a brainstem lesion, point to the probable site of severe impairment. Irreversible coma is a the sign of a permanently nonfunctioning brain.[61]

The advent of organ transplants has led to the reevaluation of the criteria for irreversible coma. A comprehensive definition has been provided by an ad hoc committee of the Harvard Medical School appointed to examine the criteria of brain death.[60] Those criteria include: (1) total unawareness of externally applied stimuli and of inner need, and complete unrespon-

siveness; (2) no movements or breathing; (3) no reflexes; (4) a flat or isoelectric electroencephalogram (EEG) with the presumptions that the personnel conducting the recording were competent, that the sensitivity of the equipment was adequate, and that the apparatus was operating normally. For this last criterion, they recommend the use of one channel for EEG and another for a noncephalic lead to pick up extraneously derived artifacts and identify them. The Cornell group has shortened the 24-hour period of no-observed-functions to 12 hours because no patient who had met their listed criteria of brain death for even 6 hours had ever survived. Controversy is still active as to whether EEG studies are necessary, or whether metabolic-circulation studies (arteriography, radionuclide brain scan) are indicated.

NEURAL BASIS OF CONSCIOUSNESS

CONTRIBUTION OF STUDIES UPON SLEEP

The vagueness of our concept of consciousness was alluded to previously, as was the behavioral significance of awareness or vigilance as an expression of the state, if not the content, of the mind. Any stimulus that usurps the attention of animal or man simultaneously produces vigilance and "activates" the scalp- or brain-recorded EEG; that is, it converts the usual spontaneous rhythm of the waking brain into an irregular tracing of low voltage in which no remainder of usual activity is evident. From that change we deduce the importance of the sensory paths to the cortex in the maintenance of awareness. Sensory monotony, or deprivation, has the opposite effect, lending itself to sleep.

In animals, a brain-stem severence at the mesodiencephalic junction, which permanently deprives the cerebral cortex of a sensory inflow, leads to perpetual slumber and the ocular and EEG manifestations of sleep.[6] Analysis of the phenomena of normal sleep in animals and humans has aided tremendously in the neurologic appraisal of consciousness and unconsciousness. It is recognized, of course, that the mental operations of animal and humans are most similar in sleep. Hereafter, we examine sleep as a prelude to matters that concern the pathologic suspension of consciousness.

The notion of a *sleep center* did not originate with von Economo, the German neurologist who is credited with describing the form of encephalitis called *sleeping sickness*. However, he did give it a strong impetus by concluding that a wakefulness center existed in the hypothalamic wall of the third ventricle because the

destructive lesions of encephalitis are centered there.[7] He also described a sleep center situated just in front of that area, verging upon the preoptic region. Lesions at the latter site were characterized by wakefulness (asomnia), and von Economo theorized that this sleep center produced sleep by inhibition of the remainder of the brain. Between them, these halfcenters were presumed to establish the diurnal sleeping-waking cycle. Later, W. R. Hess, stimulating a corresponding region of the ventral-most thalamus with slowly repetitive electrical pulses of long duration, also produced sleep.[8] He, too, proposed a more posteromedially situated wakefulness center.

Bremer is credited with replacing this older static view of a sleep center with the more dynamic one that sleep is due to an interruption of a continuous stream of afferent impulses that flows past the mesodiencephalic junction upwards and outwards to the cerebral cortex.[6] He believed the lemnisci to be the channels of flow. Later workers describe instead a collateral path (derived from the lemnisci) that filters more gradually through the in-lying brain stem tegmentum to connect at the level of the center median thalamic nucleus with a diffuse thalamocortical system.

Bremer showed that severance of the brain stem at the mesodiencephalic junction produced a state closely akin to sleep. The severance also replaced usual waking frequencies of the EEG with diffusely slow (delta) activity interrupted by spindles closely similar to those recorded in human EEG sleep tracings. Dempsey and Morison proved the origin in the mid-line thalamus of a fiber system which distributes diffusely to the cortex.[9] Through repetitive electrical stimulation at the thalamic source, they produced generalized wave sequences (recruiting response) in the cortex that closely resemble the spontaneously repetitive spindles of light sleep. Later, Moruzzi and Magoun showed that rapidly repetitive stimulation in the brain stem tegmentum can convert the sleep-type EEG with spindles (such as is produced during barbiturate anesthesia) to the low-voltage, desynchronized tracing characteristic of a just awakened, alert animal.[10] Tonic drive feeding into the diffuse thalamocortical system of Dempsey and Morison is presumed responsible for the maintenance of the waking state. When the tonic drive is interrupted, sleep intervenes—hence the term *reticular activating system* used by the followers of Moruzzi and Magoun.

For a long time, deepest sleep was associated with very slow delta-EEG activity and spindles, as observed by Bremer in his animals with brain stem transection. It came as a surprise, therefore, when a still deeper stage of sleep was recognized in the cat (Dement, Jouvet).[11,12] It was dubbed *paradoxical sleep* because the EEG closely resembled that of the awake, alert animal.

Irregular, continuous conjugate eye movements and occasional, irregular limb movements are conspicuous associated behavioral phenomena. If the cat is stimulated during paradoxical sleep, it reverts to the stage of sleep with slow waves and spindles, not to full awakening. It is known that the nervous system is peculiarly sensitive to auditory arousal. Thus, it is not surprising that responses of single tegmental neurones to auditory clicks are reduced during usual deep sleep and are practically absent during paradoxical sleep. However, the spontaneous activity of the same neurone is greatest during paradoxical sleep.[13] It has been shown recently that usual sleep, with slow waves and spindles, depends upon the integrity of cerebral mechanisms, whereas paradoxical sleep requires the operation of rhombencephalic mechanisms. Jouvet has suggested that paradoxical sleep is controlled by a noradrenergic system originating in the locus ceruleus in the pons, whereas slow-wave sleep is controlled by near-midline structures of the brain stem projecting rostrally through a serotinergic system.[14] Paradoxical sleep has been now demonstrated in many species, including humans. It has also been shown that dreaming is associated with this sleep phase. Also, in both animals and humans it has been shown that cerebral metabolic rate and circulation increase in paradoxical sleep, while there is no change from the waking state in slow-wave sleep.

Out of modern studies of sleep and activation has come a renewed interest in a mesodiencephalic center of consciousness. Penfield theorizes that the highest level of integration in the human brain, "to which all the sensations are carried and from which all motions spring," is situated in the mesodiencephalic region.[5,15] Penfield incorporates into his hypothesis much of the evidence just presented as well as other data based upon the evaluation of the unconscious state associated with brain lesions in humans. Walshe has reviewed the Penfield evidence critically and expresses the strong view that such localization is unwarranted.[16] His easily accessible account should be read by everyone interested in the problems of the study of the mind and brain.

UNCONSCIOUSNESS IN BRAIN-STEM LESIONS IN HUMANS

Much has been learned of the site of origin of comatose states from study of patients with lesions of the brain stem or the superstructure. One important source has been observations upon anencephalic and hydrocephalic infants.[17,18]

It appears that such mesodiencephalic subjects sleep and wake, react to hunger, loud sounds, and crude visual stimuli by movement of eye, eyelids, and facial

muscles. Such an infant may see, hear, taste, and smell. He may reject the unpalatable and accept such foods as it likes, utter sounds, show displeasure when hungry, and pleasure when sung to. He may also perform crude limb movements spontaneously. All this might perhaps be described as rudimentary awareness, or indeed as crude consciousness, if we could somehow make ourselves aware of its content.

Cairns analyzed the effect upon consciousness of lesions at lower and upper brain-stem levels. The latter include involvement of thalamic centers.[19] He found that a disturbance of the medulla or the pons can produce sudden loss of consciousness, ordinarily with associated disturbance of breathing and circulation. The question arises as to whether anoxia resulting from the cardiorespiratory deficit might not be the cause of coma in lower brain stem lesions. However, in some instances, loss of consciousness has been shown to precede the drop in blood pressure and respiratory change. Howell analyzed the case histories of 6 patients who showed foraminal impaction of the brain stem at postmortem.[20] He found the most common feature of this syndrome to be the hydrocephalic attack, consisting in its mildest form of a brief, agonizing headache (often lasting only a minute or two) with or without transitory confusion, deafness, or amaurosis. Inconstant features were bilateral cranial nerve palsies (involving nerves 7 to 10 inclusively), neck rigidity, and sustained hydrocephalus, which developed insidiously. Between attacks, patients were found to be alert, in contrast to the global impairment of consciousness seen with upper brain stem compressions. In fact, Howell states that global impairment is not part of this syndrome, and that, with medullary compression, a patient alert one moment may be dead the next. When coma occurred, it lasted a minute in one case, several hours in three others, with possible upper brain stem compression as well.

Two varieties of loss of consciousness occur in upper brain-stem and thalamic lesions, one intermittent and the other continuous.[19] The former is exemplified by petit mal epilepsy, the latter by coma with decerebrate rigidity, hyperthermia, hypersomnia, and akinetic mutism. In hypersomnia, persistent unconsciousness may resemble sleep, with quiet breathing, muscular relaxation, and loss of the expression that characterizes the waking state. The patient can be aroused temporarily, and the EEG is of the sleep type with diffuse delta activity, as is also true with other kinds of unconsciousness. In akinetic mutism, the eyes may follow the observer about, but the patient is otherwise unresponsive.

Because of their acute development, the signs of coma associated with downward pressure from supratentorial mass lesions may be significantly more dramatic.

Two possible sequences of brain stem dysfunction may accompany such conditions.[20] In one, the signs of uncal herniation occur, including third-nerve involvement and lateral midbrain compression. The other reflects bilateral diencephalic impairment, Cheyne-Stokes respiration, oculocephalic ("doll's head") eye movements, and bilateral motor involvement.

Howell, whose study upon brain stem and foraminal impaction has already been mentioned, examined some 150 cases of upper brain-stem compression. He reports that the main features of the syndrome are sufficiently constant for it to be distinguished from other conditions that cause coma. Increased headache, vomiting, and stiffness of the neck develop at the onset. The most constant feature is a global impairment of all mental functions, progressing rapidly or slowly from lethargy to a semicomatose state. Patients in this series might die before they become fully comatose. Thus, death could only be attributed to coma when severe aspiration or hypostatic pneumonia develop. Bradycardia occurs less frequently than tachycardia. Hyperpyrexia is common. In rapidly developing compression, sudden respiratory arrest might be seen. This could follow a phase of slow, shallow, grunting respiration. Loss of pupillary light reflex is very constant, although it might not be observed until compression is far advanced. Dilation of the pupil is usual, but it may remain small or even contracted. Decerebrate rigidity is common; it is exceptional not to detect extensor spasm of the limbs in response to painful stimulation at some stage of the illness.

Plum and Posner view abnormalities of pupils, respiration, and the oculocephalic and oculovestibular reflexes as having important localizing value in brain-stem lesions.[61] It is the combinations of these abnormalities that produce the important syndromes recognized by neurologists and opthalmologists as pointing to the probable site of disorder. In progressive involvement extending rostrocaudally, one combination of deficit may replace another in a manner indicative of the descent of the impairment. Associated cranial nerve deficits may confirm the site of the pathology.

Among respiratory abnormalities, Cheyne-Stokes respiration occurs most frequently in association with alterations deep in the cerebral hemispheres. Central neurogenic hyperventilation (sustained, regular, rapid, and deep hypernea) occurs in certain patients with involvement of the brain-stem tegmentum having lesions situated between lower midbrain and lower pons. Apneustic breathing (inspiratory cramp) is indicative of damage to the respiratory controls situated at mid- or caudal-pontine levels. Ataxic breathing may at times be confused with Cheyne-Stokes respiration. It retains its burst rhythmicity, but is completely irregular within the bursts. The use of respiration abnormalities for lo-

calization was not completely supported by North and Jennett, who recorded breathing patterns by impedance pneumography and other tests in 227 patients of a neurosurgical unit, most of whom had recent head injury, intracranial tumor, or ruptured aneurysm.[21] Abnormal respiratory patterns were recorded at some time in 60% of the patients. All subjects of lesions in the medulla had abnormal patterns. Medullary-and pontine-lesions cases frequently showed irregular breathing. However, only gross irregularity of breathing was found to have localizing value. Tachypnea (frequently above 25 respirations per min) and hyperventilation (arterial pressure of CO_2 less than 30 torr) were associated with poor prognosis when combined.

Mention of a few of the more common pupillary abnormalities will illustrate their localizing value.[22,61] In midbrain damage, nuclear lesions may interrupt both sympathetic and parasympathetic ocular circuits, leaving the pupil in midposition and fixed to all stimuli. Pontine lesions produce bilaterally small pupils, and lateral medullary lesions produce an ipsilateral Horner's syndrome with slight ptosis.

In examining ocular motility, reliance is chiefly placed upon the state of the eyes at rest and upon components of oculocephalic and oculovestibular reflexes. The oculocephalic reflex is produced by brisk rotation of the head from side to side and up and down. The oculovestibular reflex is produced by caloric (ice water) stimulation. In light coma, the oculocephalic reflexes can be demonstrated consistently, and caloric stimulation produces tonic lateral deviation. With greater cortical depression, which leaves brain-stem mechanisms relatively intact, both reflexes become very brisk. There are two principal intrinsic deficits in optic motility having localizing value. One, a conjugate-gaze paralysis, points to the pontine tegmentum; the other, paralysis of adduction, called *internuclear ophthalmoplegia*, is a disconjugate gaze paralysis due to involvement of the median longitudinal fasciculus between the vestibular and III-nerve nuclei.

"Drop attacks" occasionally signal a susceptibility to transient brain-stem ischemia.[62] The attack occurs while the subject is standing or walking, and comes on abruptly without warning. It is produced by a transient loss of strength in the lower extremities. Characteristically, there is no alteration of consciousness; vision, hearing, and speech remain intact.

Ingvar and Lundberg recorded EEG and ventricular fluid pressure (VFP) simultaneously in patients showing increased intracranial pressure associated with brain tumor.[23] Paroxysmal variations in the VFP were observed in the forms of large, suddenly appearing plateau waves with peaks of 100 torr and rhythmically recurring VFP variations showing a frequency of 1 to 2 per minute. It is important to note that high plateau waves can be accompanied by loss of consciousness and tonic-clonic movements. Only subtle EEG changes are found to accompany plateau waves. The onset of such a wave can be accompanied by the arousal-type EEG change; its termination with hyperventilation shows an increase in slow activity. However, despite the loss of consciousness and obvious tonic-clonic movements, no convulsive activity appears in the EEG. They conclude that the convulsive phenomena observed resulted from brain-stem seizures.

The term *locked-in syndrome* has been used to characterize a unique behavioral state that occurs following infarction of the efferent pyramidal tracts in the base of the pons and which, although irreversible, may persist over a period of time. The subjects are tetraplegic and mute, yet fully awake, with variable preservation of ocular movements, by which they are able to communicate. Decerebrate posturing can be evoked by noxious stimulation. The EEG may remain normal. One such patient who remained in good general condition over a 2-year period learned to communicate by Morse code using eye blinks and jaw movements.[24]

The evidence from organic lesions of brain stem and thalamus points to there being a crude form of consciousness in this region. This means that the cerebral cortex is essential for manifestation of higher levels of consciousness, even though a healthy cerebral cortex cannot of itself maintain the conscious state. Massive bifrontal lesions in man, for example, have been shown not to disturb crude consciousness, but instead to impair will, initiative, foresight, and judgment.[19]

ABNORMAL STATES OF CONSCIOUSNESS AND THEIR ETIOLOGIES

Figure 31-1 presents a scheme of the relationships of the waking state to normal sleep and to coma of a variety of etiologies.

In a 1933 survey of comatose patients who entered Boston City Hospital, alcohol was held responsible for 50% of the cases, trauma for 13%, and cerebrovascular disorders for 10%.[25,26,27] Other causes, each accounting for 3% or fewer of the cases, were poisoning, epilepsy, diabetes, meningitis, pneumonia, cardiac decompensation, exsanguination, central nervous system (CNS) syphilis, uremia, and eclampsia. Those causes in which prompt diagnosis and emergency treatment were imperative were diabetes, hyperinsulinism, poisoning, traumatic shock, exsanguination, subdural hematoma, brain tumor, abscess, meningitis, and eclampsia. History was of immediate importance in 60% of the cases, and ambulance drivers were instructed to bring in a relative or other witness, whenever possible, to facilitate obtaining a history. The depth of the coma, the

CAUSES OF UNCONSCIOUSNESS

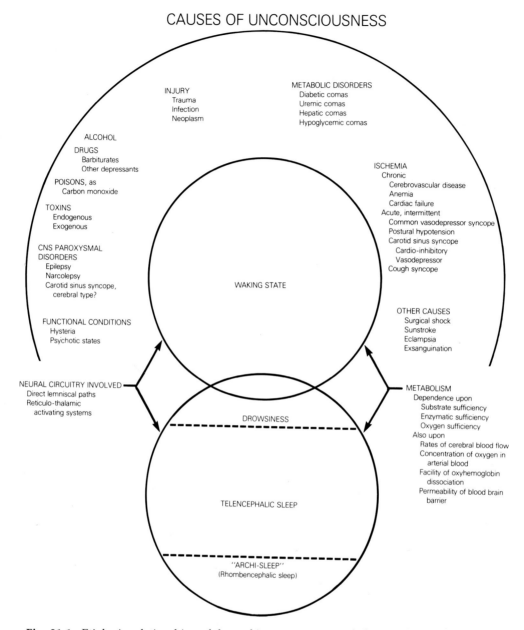

INJURY
Trauma
Infection
Neoplasm

METABOLIC DISORDERS
Diabetic comas
Uremic comas
Hepatic comas
Hypoglycemic comas

ALCOHOL
DRUGS
Barbiturates
Other depressants
POISONS, as
Carbon monoxide
TOXINS
Endogenous
Exogenous
CNS PAROXYSMAL
DISORDERS
Epilepsy
Narcolepsy
Carotid sinus syncope,
cerebral type?
FUNCTIONAL CONDITIONS
Hysteria
Psychotic states

ISCHEMIA
Chronic
Cerebrovascular disease
Anemia
Cardiac failure
Acute, intermittent
Common vasodepressor syncope
Postural hypotension
Carotid sinus syncope
Cardio-inhibitory
Vasodepressor
Cough syncope

OTHER CAUSES
Surgical shock
Sunstroke
Eclampsia
Exsanguination

WAKING STATE

NEURAL CIRCUITRY INVOLVED
Direct lemniscal paths
Reticulo-thalamic
activating systems

METABOLISM
Dependence upon
Substrate sufficiency
Enzymatic sufficiency
Oxygen sufficiency
Also upon
Rates of cerebral blood flow
Concentration of oxygen in
arterial blood
Facility of oxyhemoglobin
dissociation
Permeability of blood brain
barrier

DROWSINESS

TELENCEPHALIC SLEEP

"ARCHI-SLEEP"
(Rhombencephalic sleep)

Fig. 31-1. Etiologic relationships of the waking state to normal sleep and coma (see text).

state of reflexes, and the pupils were not found to be of great diagnostic importance, although, of course, neurologic signs ordinarily depended upon the depth of the coma. Tables 31-1 and 31-2, from Solomon and Aring, provide excellent summaries of physical and laboratory observations helpful in the differential diagnosis of coma and of the conditions in which it occurs.[26] To this list must be added the cranial CT scan, which has become an exceptionally powerful tool in the emergency room setting, often providing definitive diagnosis of gross structural lesions.

Hereafter, we outline the salient features of a variety of conditions that cause coma. The discussion is necessarily far from complete.

HEAD TRAUMA

The best possible history and neurologic appraisal are always obtained. For future reference, Symonds advises us to distinguish between patients who are never unconscious, those unconscious for but a few moments, and those who exhibit prolonged periods of

Table 31-1. *Physical Changes Helpful in the Diagnosis of Coma and the Conditions in Which They Occur*

Odor of breath
  Alcohol..alcoholism
  Acetone .... diabetes, uremia
  Illuminating gas .... carbon monoxide poisoning

Color of skin and mucous membranes
  Hyperemic....................................alcoholism
  Cherry red..................... carbon monoxide poisoning
  Cyanosis.............. cardiac decompensation, pneumonia
  Pallor......................hemorrhage, pernicious anemia
  Jaundice .... cholemia

Local signs of injury ......trauma, burns, hemorrhage, epilepsy,
                erysipelas

Temperature
  Increased .... pneumonia, meningitis, encephalitis
  Decreased............. carbon monoxide poisoning, diabetes

Pulse
  Rapid........... diabetes, pneumonia, meningitis, eclampsia
  Irregular ....cardiac decompensation
  Slow .... Stokes-Adams disease

Respiration
  Kussmaul... diabetes
  Increased .... pneumonia

Hemiplegia .... cerebral vascular lesions

Observation of convulsions..................epilepsy, cerebral
                vascular lesions, central nervous
                system syphilis, alcoholism

Vomiting .... cerebral hemorrhage, poisoning
Stiffness of the neck ....meningitis, cerebral vascular lesions
Kernig's leg sign positive....meningitis, cerebral vascular lesions

Chest signs
  Consolidation .... pneumonia
  Fluid ....empyema, ruptured aortic aneurysm
Pulmonary congestion ....ascites, enlarged liver, distended neck
                veins, cardiac decompensation

Distention and spasticity of the abdomen ...ruptured esophageal
      varix, carcinomatous erosion of the gastrointestinal tract,
      ruptured ectopic pregnancy, miliary tuberculosis
Muscular twitchings .... uremia
Abdominal tumor................................eclampsia
Bulging fontanels................................ meningitis
Soft eyeballs .... diabetes
Wounds or scars on the tongue .... epilepsy
Vaginal examination abnormal ......pelvic malignancy, ruptured
                ectopic pregnancy

Blood pressure
  Increased ....cerebral vascular lesions, uremia, eclampsia
  Decreased.. trauma

(Courtesy of Solomon P, Aring CD: The differential diagnosis in patients entering the hospital in coma. JAMA 105:7, 1935)

unconsciousness.[28] Patients with cerebral contusion may show focal neurologic signs. Those with severe head injury (as in automobile accidents) who come to postmortem often show severe laceration of the orbital surfaces of the frontal lobes and of the tips of the temporal lobes.[29] In middle meningeal hemorrhage (epidural hematoma) a brief interval of unconsciousness following the accident may be succeeded by lucidity, after which a rapidly deepening coma may develop several hours later. Subdural hematoma may be acute or chronic. In the latter instance, gradually increasing coma and progressive paralysis may develop even when there is no history of an accident. In all cases of head injury, proven or suspected, a careful watch should be made for changes in behavioral responsiveness as well as in both brain stem and spinal reflexes. Signs of increased intracranial pressure include slowing of pulse, respiratory abnormalities of several types (see above), and, usually very late, elevated blood pressure. An excellent brief survey of posttraumatic epilepsy is available.[30]

In prolonged unconsciousness due to head injury with brain-stem impairment, it is important not to discuss prognosis in the presence of the patient, who may recover and remember what went on about him.

NEOPLASM AND BRAIN ABSCESS

Either neoplasm or abscess may cause coma, with or without paralysis. The history is that of progressive neurologic deficit of variable duration. Important data include a history of headaches, vomiting, convulsions, paralysis, incoordination with failing vision, and personality change. Papilledema is an important sign. In the event of possible abscess, inquiry should be made into past lung, ear, or sinus diseases, with or without operative intervention. A history of skull fracture may also be important. Fever is often lacking, and when present may be attributable to active pyogenic infection in a locus from which the brain infection derives by hematogenous or direct extension. In tumors, suddenly developing coma may result from tentorial or foramen-magnum herniation or, rarely, from secondary hemorrhage.

MENINGITIS AND ENCEPHALITIS

In meningitis, severe headache may develop, closely followed by loss of consciousness. The important diagnostic signs are nuchal rigidity, and Kernig and

Brudzinski signs. Disconjugate ocular movements, pupillary abnormalities, convulsion, and focal neurologic signs may be seen. Tuberculous meningitis is gradual in onset, and isolated cranial nerves may be affected.

There are several types of encephalitis, any one of which may show hypersomnia as an acute symptom. However, lethargic encephalitis is outstanding for producing hypersomnia. Demyelinating encephalitides are associated with vaccinia, smallpox, measles, and antirabies treatment. Dissociated eye movements may be a feature of viral encephalitis. Diagnosis of specific viral etiology may be sought through neutralization and complement-fixation tests. These may be done on successive serum samples, seeking a rise in titer, obtained during the course of the illness.[31] Hemagglutination of cells is used in the case of arthropod viruses. It may be possible to isolate virus from the spinal fluid.

Slow viruses recently have been recognized as opening new possibilities of explanation for some of the less protracted dementias that may eventuate in comas. In such virus infections, evidence of disease may not appear until months or years after the virus enters the body. Kuru, a familial degenerative disease of the nervous system occurring in the highlands of New Guinea, evidently has been transmitted to chimpanzees, and transmission from chimpanzee to chimpanzee also was effected, with shortening of the incubation period.[63] Brain biopsy material from a patient having Creutzfeldt-Jakob disease with severe status spongiosus has also been inoculated into the champanzee; after 13 months the animal developed a clinical course remarkably similar to that of the patient and died. Neuropathologic findings were also very similar.[64]

CEREBROVASCULAR DISEASE

Coma may occur at the onset of cerebral hemorrhage, but more often it develops gradually. It is uncommon with cerebral thrombosis. Associated hemiplegia is frequent. Sudden loss of consciousness in cerebral hemorrhage is due to massive explosive injury to the cerebrum and to accompanying neural shock. Cerebral embolism also shows a sudden onset, but loss of consciousness is far less likely than with cerebral hemorrhage. Subarachnoid hemorrhage is distinguished by sudden onset of intense headache, often following exertion. Coma may come on more gradually. The pulse may be slowed, and meningeal signs are observed. Gross subarachnoid bleeding is evident in the CT scan; less intense bleeding may have to be ascertained by cautious lumbar puncture. Coma also may develop in hypertensive encephalopathy, either with or without convulsions; there is usually a history of severe hypertension.

Table 31-2. *Laboratory Observations Helpful in the Diagnosis of Coma and the Conditions in Which They Occur*

Lumbar puncture
  Spinal Fluid Pressure
    Increased.... cerebral vascular lesions, meningitis, trauma, central nervous system syphilis
    Decreased .... diabetes
  Bloody fluid .... cerebral vascular lesions, trauma
  Purulent fluid................................ meningitis
  Organisms by smear and culture .... meningitis
  Sugar
    Low .... meningitis
    High.. diabetes
  Protein high ..... meningitis; central nervous system syphilis
  Spinal fluid Wassermann positive.... central nervous system syphilis

Blood examination
  Sugar
    High.. diabetes
    Low .... insulin shock
  Nonprotein nitrogen high......................... uremia
  Wassermann test positive.... central nervous system syphilis
  Low red blood count, abnormal smear ... pernicious anemia, leukemia
  Culture positive......... pneumonia, meningitis, septicemia
  Spectroscopy .... carbon monoxide poisoning, methemoglobinemia

Urine examination
  Sugar .... diabetes
  Gross albuminuria .... eclampsia, uremia, cardiac decompensation

Gastric lavage
  Examination of gastric contents....................poisoning
Roentgenogram
  Skull.............. fracture across middle meningeal artery in extradural hemorrhage
  Lungs...........pneumonia, empyema, miliary tuberculosis
  Heart.............................cardiac decompensation
Electrocardiogram .... heart block, cardiac decompensation

(Courtesy of Solomon P, Aring CD: The differential diagnosis in patients entering the hospital in coma. JAMA 105:7, 1935)

Acute cerebellar hemorrhage or infarction typically presents with severe nausea and vomiting, headache, ataxia, and nystagmus. Early suspicion of these conditions is important, because early neurosurgical intervention may be life-saving. The CT scan is the procedure of choice to ascertain the diagnosis of acute cerebral bleeding with hematoma.

Acute cerebral infarctions may not be evident in the CT scan, even with iodine contrast infusion; manifest lesions may take several days to evolve.

When occlusive vascular lesions involve the lesser brain-stem vessels, such as the branches of the vertebrobasilar system, localizing signs and symptoms commonly occur without loss of consciousness, unless the lesion is hemorrhagic. However, symptoms of attacks of vertebrobasilar and carotid insufficiency may appear

as the prodrome of a massive cerebral thrombosis with unconsciousness. For that reason we list below principal symptoms of the two main types of insufficiency drawn from a United States Public Health Service (USPHS) cerebrovascular survey report.[32]

Vertebrobasilar Insufficiency

Dizziness
Diplopia
Blurred vision
Blindness
Pupillary change
Memory lapses
Confused behavior
Unilateral or bilateral numbness
Unilateral or bilateral weakness
Dysarthria
Dysphagia
Impaired hearing
Numbness of face
Staggering gait
Hiccuping

Carotid System Insufficiency

Unilateral weakness or numbness
Dysphasia
Confusion
Ipsilateral monocular blindness
Homonymous field defects
Headache
Possibly focal epileptic seizures

Ingvar and associates had the opportunity to examine hemispheric blood flow in a 60-year-old man who had suffered an acute vascular lesion of the brain from which he remained unconscious and unresponsive over an 8-month period.[65] The EEG was depressed, showing a low voltage delta pattern. The cerebral arterial pattern was essentially normal and air study revealed only moderate cerebral atrophy. In spite of these findings, hemispheric blood flow, as determined by ^{85}Kr, showed an average flow of about one quarter of the normal flow, and a cerebral oxygen consumption that was reduced proportionately. A biopsy of frontal cortex presented normal findings with no evidence of neuron loss or gliosis. The case illustrates the marked reduction of cerebral metabolism and circulation that can occur after a lesion of the upper brain stem with permanent coma.

BRAIN METABOLISM AND METABOLIC COMA

Under normal conditions, the brain derives most of its energy from the oxidation of glucose. It can metabolize other substrates, but they provide poor substitutes because the blood-brain barriers prevent them from en-

tering the brain in sufficient quantity to maintain a normal metabolic rate.[61] Each 100 g of brain takes up 5.5 mg of glucose per minute, and all but about 15% of this substrate is used in combustion with O_2 to form CO_2 and energy as adenosine triphosphate (ATP). Only one third is metabolized rapidly; the rest is incorporated into amino acids, proteins, and lipids. A continuous supply of O_2 is also required. Without it, some glucose can evidently still be metabolized to lactic acid, providing some energy, but this minor source cannot fulfill the requirements of the adult human brain for more than a few seconds.

The adult brain (which comprises only 2% of total body mass) utilizes 20% of the total O_2 and 65% of the total glucose consumed by the body. It requires 15% to 20% of the total blood circulation per minute to deliver the high requirements for O_2 and glucose. Thus, when supplies of one or both are cut off, neural function fails with disastrous rapidity.[33] It has been estimated that the cerebral blood flow of a recumbent normal man is 750 ml per minute. At any moment the blood circulating through the brain contains 7 ml of O_2, an amount sufficient to supply its needs for less than 10 seconds. However, under conditions of reduced systemic blood pressure, as little as one third of the normal 54 ml of blood per minute per 100 g of brain can maintain consciousness. In experiments of Rossen, Kabat, and Anderson, in which the human brain was deprived of O_2 by sudden and complete arrest of cerebral circulation, consciousness was lost in 6 seconds.[34] Restoration within 100 seconds was followed by rapid return of consciousness without objective evidence of brain injury.

When evaluating metabolic coma, the state of consciousness, respiration, pupillary reactions, eye movements, and biochemical blood data are important in distinguishing metabolic coma from structural brain disease and psychogenic unresponsiveness. Plum and Posner point out important distinguishing criteria.[61] The state of consciousness is particularly important in the subtle manifestations that can be detected as a warning signal in disease conditions known to feature coma as a complication. Hyper- or hypoventilation with coma may have different meanings, depending upon whether one or the other is a response to or compensation for, primary respiratory stimulation. Thus, in defining acidosis or alkalosis, biochemical data become of paramount importance. In deep coma, the state of the pupils is very important in distinguishing between metabolic and structural conditions. Preserved pupillary light reflexes with caloric unresponsiveness in the presence of either decerebrate rigidity or motor flaccidity, suggest metabolic coma. Early in coma, the eye movements are of a roving character; later, in deep coma, they are

directed forwards. In light coma, the response of the eyes to cold caloric stimulation may still produce conjugate deviation toward the stimulated side, whereas minimal if any response is elicited in deep coma.

Diabetic Coma. Diabetic coma is usually attributed to the gradual accumulation of acetoacetic and β-hydroxybutyric acids in the blood. However, Fazekas and Bessman note that in diabetic coma, cerebral O_2 consumption is greatly depressed, although cerebral blood flow, vascular resistance, and O_2 delivery may be normal and glucose supply may be far greater than normal.[35] They attribute the condition to inhibition of cerebral enzymatic activity, adding that they find no support for the contention that diabetic coma is due to the accumulation of ketone bodies, or to changes in water or electrolyte metabolism. Others point to the difficulty in assigning a primary enzymatic cause. Brain tissue acidosis, as determined by the cerebrospinal-fluid *p*H measurement, may be a critical factor in determining the comatose state.[36] Plum and Posner, in addition to discussing the more common diabetic acidosis with ketonemia, describe a lactic acidosis occurring especially in those diabetics treated with oral hypoglycemic agents.[61] In the latter, ketonemia is lacking.

Hypoglycemic Coma. Arteriovenous O_2 differences in the brain are closely related to the blood-sugar level. Intense hypoglycemia causes severe impairment of O_2 uptake by the brain. The almost sole dependence of the brain upon the constant delivery of glucose makes it particularly vulnerable to hypoglycemic states. Although it has other causes, hypoglycemic coma commonly presents in those with a history of insulin treatment for diabetes. It may present as a delirium, as a coma with accompanying facets of brain-stem dysfunction, as a strokelike illness, or as an epileptic attack with postictal coma. Whereas the neurologic deficits incurred may be reversible, the longer the hypoglycemia lasts, the more likely it is that neuronal loss is irreversible. The mechanism of the depressed metabolic state is not obvious. Study of experimental hypoglycemia shows that brain energy reserves are not reduced.[37]

Uremic Coma. Uremic coma is due to the accumulation of noxious substances as a result of impaired excretory and detoxifying mechanisms, as well as to disturbances in water and electrolyte metabolism.[35] Laboratory determinations do not delineate clearly the cause of the coma because the renal failure in which it occurs is accompanied by complex biochemical changes, and the azotemia varies in those with equally serious symptoms.[66] The best hypothesis is the existence of a toxin of small molecular size.

Hepatic Coma. Depth of hepatic coma is to some extent related to blood-ammonia level. Ammonia is produced in the intestine by bacterial action and conveyed to the liver by the portal vein. In the presence of either liver failure or extensive collateral circulation, such as develops in hepatic cirrhosis, ammonia accumulates in the blood in increasing amounts.[38] The slowing of the EEG correlates well with the extent of neurologic and mental disturbance. Reduction of dietary protein and administration of neomycin for gut sterilization may improve the character of the EEG and of the clinical state. Increasing protein intake or administering methionine or ammonium chloride causes the EEG to deteriorate.[39] When the liver is unable to eliminate the ammonia, either because it is bypassed or diseased, coma or death may ensue.

Clinically, full coma rarely develops suddenly unless there has been overwhelming liver damage or massive gastrointestinal hemorrhage. Blood ammonia is almost always elevated above 50 mg/dl, and nearly all patients have respiratory alkalosis. Hume and associates have described treatment by colectomy, which can reduce blood ammonia levels and normalize the EEG, paralleling improvement in clinical status.[67]

Pulmonary Disease. Profound hypoventilation can develop because of lung failure and lead to serious CO_2 retention along with hypoxemia and acidosis, which aggravate the situation. The neurologic symptomatology to be observed correlates well with CO_2 acidosis of spinal fluid, and, perhaps, with intracellular acidosis as well (Posner, Swanson, and Plum).[68] Such patients hypoventilate and can become cyanotic. Where there is obstructive emphysema as well, the patient wheezes, gasps, or puffs.[61] Headache is a common feature of the symptomatology, and this can be accompanied by slowly developing drowsiness, stupor, or coma. The pupils are often small and reactive to light, and the ocular movements are normal. Papilledema may occur with brain swelling due to CO_2 accumulation. Seizures are rare; myoclonus is common.

Endocrine Conditions. Coma can occur with myxedema with an onset that is rapid and subacute. Hypothermia and other evidences of severe, prolonged hypometabolism should be evident (*e.g.*, hair loss, thick, dry skin). Diagnosis can be confirmed by tests of thyroid function.

Coma may also develop in addisonian crises. Such patients may have flaccid weakness with hypoactive or absent tendon reflexes, resulting presumably from hyperkalemia. Generalized convulsions may also occur, attributable perhaps to hyponatremia and water intoxication.

Electrolyte Disturbances. Lesser variations in either the potassium or the sodium level of plasma are said not to affect the brain-wave tracing.[40] However, in hypokalemia with familial periodic paralysis, the EEG has been reported to be normal in some instances and disordered in others. Severe sodium depletion also has been said to slow the EEG and produce sleepiness, leading to coma.[41] Calcium deficit leads to convulsions and also produces EEG slowing. Excessive hydration in combination with sodium depletion can lead to convulsions and also slows the EEG, or transforms it into a convulsive pattern. Impaired consciousness can also result. Uncomplicated acidosis does not produce an unusual EEG effect, although that occasioned by inhalation of CO_2 brings about some increase in background fast activity and lowers the voltage of the EEG. Temporary alkalosis, as produced by hyperventilation, slows the EEG trace and produces amplitude buildup, especially in the frontal leads. More prolonged alkalosis (from vomiting, for example) occasions clouding of consciousness and produces runs of high-voltage, rhythmic, slow activity.[40]

SYNCOPAL ATTACKS

The pathophysiology of fainting (syncope) is discussed in Chapter 30, and is correlated with the many clinical conditions in which it may occur.

Pathophysiologic factors in the various kinds of faints have been systematized by Engel, who classifies them under broad categories of peripheral circulatory inadequacy, cardiac arrhythmias, and respiratory or pulmonary disorders.[42] Such brief periods of unconsciousness can be brought about in one of three ways: by cerebral ischemia, localized or generalized; by a change in composition of the blood; by a reflex cerebral dysfunction.[43]

Ischemia is the most important of these, and the site most vulnerable is believed to be the upper brain stem, a locus already discussed with respect to brain lesions, which are prone to cause sudden unconsciousness in the experimental animal or man. With prompt restoration of blood supply, such consciousness loss is readily reversible. The EEG is a very sensitive indicator of anoxia, and the rapidity with which a slow delta pattern replaces usual background activity during an attack of cerebral ischemia is intimately related to the abruptness of onset of unconsciousness. If ventricular standstill occurs (as may happen in Adams-Stokes attacks), brain-wave slowing can be closely related to alterations in pulse and blood pressure. Under these circumstances, the pulseless period that precedes the onset of unconsciousness may be variable, extending from a few to 10 or more seconds.

Vasodepressor syncope is the most common form of fainting, and can be precipitated by fear, anxiety, pain, or injury.[42] It practically never occurs except in the erect posture, and symptoms usually are relieved by lying down. At the onset of an attack, pulse and blood pressure may be somewhat elevated, blood pressure falling thereafter, systolic more rapidly than diastolic. Ordinarily, recovery is rapid. Slowing of the EEG has been observed as consciousness is lost. An important factor is said to be the shunting of blood from brain to muscle by vasodilation mediated by the cholinergic vasodilator system.

Postural hypotension can develop in several ways, the common denominator being the repeated occurrence of fainting upon a rise from bed. Limited capacity for postural adjustment is important, and micturition or postmicturition syncope occurring in the middle-aged person who arises from a deep sleep to hurry to the bathroom may have this precipitating base. In chronic orthostatic hypotension, the classical form of postural hypotension, blood pressure falls rapidly upon assumption of the erect posture. Both systolic and diastolic pressures fall, but there is little or no pulse alteration.[42] Consciousness also is lost rapidly, and is restored rapidly upon correction of the precipitating postural change. Diffuse disease of the autonomic nervous system is often held responsible.

Micturition syncope has long been believed to be due to a combination of orthostatic tension and the reflex action of a distended bladder. Tudor has concluded that the syndrome results from a cerebral hypoxia due to reflex cardioinhibitory and vasodepressor mechanisms triggered by emptying of the bladder.[69]

Adams-Stokes syndrome is the most widely known of the episodic syncopal attacks that occur in cardiac conditions. Such instances are divisible into two categories, one associated with permanent, complete heart block and slow pulse (Adams-Stokes syndrome), and the other rising from reflex or metabolic factors, with or without structural changes.[42] In Adams-Stokes syndrome, the attacks of syncope are believed to be due to a decrease in cerebral blood flow resulting from ventricular standstill, tachycardia, or fibrillation. The duration of asystole may be long, and convulsion caused by cerebral hypoxia may occur. High-voltage, slow EEG activity occurs during asystole, and if the standstill persists, the tracing may flatten out. Among the instances that arise in individuals with reflex or metabolic factors are those with transient and paroxysmal heart block. Afferents of vagal reflexes arising from the upper gastrointestinal tract, respiratory tract, mediastinum, and external auditory canal may contribute to causation, as may afferent paths arising in the eye or nasopharynx and carried in trigeminal and glosso-

pharyngeal nerves.[42] Increased activity of the vagus nerves resulting from such heightened afferent impulses may cause sinoatrial standstill or atrioventricular block. This is true especially if associated with metabolic or organic changes affecting the mechanisms controlling the origin and conduction of the stimulus to the heart beat. Reflex cardiac standstill and syncope can occur in patients with intense paroxysmal pain in the glossopharyngeal distribution (glossopharyngeal neuralgia).

Hypersensitivity of the carotid sinus is associated with syncope that utilizes an afferent arm that passes over a branch of the glossopharyngeal nerve. In this disorder, the specific nerve endings in the carotid sinus may be the major source of activation, but summate with overly sensitive afferents from other sources, which augment vagal outflow. Significantly more persons show carotid sinus hypersensitivity to massage than ever show spontaneous fainting of this origin. Engel advocates demonstration of identity between induced (by massage) and spontaneous faints, differentiation between massage of the sinus and of the carotid below it, and abolition of the hypersensitivity by atropine as criteria for establishing the carotid sinus as the source of troubles.[42] He points out that the sinus region in such cases is usually extremely sensitive to stimulation. Aside from prolonged asystole, there is a vasodepressor type of response in which the fall of blood pressure is independent of change of heart rate. According to Wayne, that fall of blood pressure is only abolished by epinephrine administration.[43]

A cerebral type of carotid-sinus syncope is also described in which fainting is not related to change in blood pressure or pulse and is not influenced by either atropine or ephedrine.[44] Gurdjian and associates believe this form to be misinterpreted.[45] They believe it to result instead from partial or complete occlusion involving components of the contralateral arterial supply. They believe, of course, that a carotid-sinus-inhibitory reflex may be associated with the ischemic response. Engel has contraverted this evidence using the criteria set forth above. He has found that the cerebral type of carotid-sinus reflex may be elicited by very gentle and brief nonocclusive stimulation of the sinus. Reese, Green, and Elliott have reported a case in which the features of the cerebral type of hypersensitivity were observed, and yet panarteriography failed to show significant disease of the cervical arteries.[46]

Cough syncope is prone to occur in robust, middle-aged men. Severe cough from any cause, may, if sufficiently strenuous and repetitious, cause loss of consciousness. The faint is caused by rapidly repeated inspiration, incomplete expiration, and rapidly repeated, very forceful expiratory effort against a closed glottis. Increased intrathoracic pressure results, which obstructs the return of blood to the right atrium and thus may reduce cardiac output to a critical degree.

In *Pickwickian syndrome,* the association of obesity with hypersomnolence, hypoventilation, and polycythemia occurs. In this instance, attention is directed to somnolence instead of to syncope. Drachman and Gumnit showed by intensive investigation of a single case, that lack of oxygen was the predominant factor in driving respiration and in awakening the subject from the somnolent state that she might otherwise fall into.[47]

ALCOHOL, DRUGS, AND POISONS

Alcohol is by far the most frequent cause of hospital admissions for coma. The signs and symptoms of acute alcoholism are too well known to need emphasis here. For clinical and medicolegal purposes, the concentrations of alcohol in blood or exhaled air can be determined. As in other kinds of unconsciousness, brain rhythms are slowed by alcohol, the degree of slowing being roughly related to the severity of intoxication.

About 20% of hospital admissions for acute drug intoxication are for barbiturate poisoning. When the subject is discovered in acute poisoning, deep sleep or coma is characteristic. Cyanosis may be prominent and Cheyne-Stokes respiration may occur. The involvement of superficial and deep reflexes relates to the degree of central depression. Extensor toe signs may be obtained. Pupils tend to be somewhat constricted, although they may dilate late in the course of the poisoning. The EEG shows the high-voltage slow delta activity that is a general characteristic of brain activity in comatose patients. Identification can be made of barbiturates in the stomach contents, blood, and urine. For treatment, Plum and Swanson believe that there is no substitute for the direct physiologic treatment of depressed respiration or circulation.[48] They found that the use of analeptic drugs provided little additional help. The immediate dangers to the patient admitted in a comatose state generally are respiratory. The airway must be cleared scrupulously and adequate intake of O_2 must be ensured. Circulatory treatment should include starting venoclysis at the time of admission to provide an immediate route if plasma expanders or vasopressor drugs become necessary. If cardiorespiratory and renal function are carefully maintained, complete recovery may be expected to occur, even though the coma lasts from several days to even a week or more. Unless renal function is impaired, supportive dialysis measures are not indicated.

In recent years a high proportion of coma cases associated with suicide attempts and accidental ingestion by children is being caused by newer sedatives, anti-

depressant drugs, neuroleptics, and minor tranquilizers. A urinary screening test for toxic agents is most helpful in arriving at an accurate diagnosis. Aggressive support of cardiorespiratory function is essential.

Opium, morphine, and other opium derivatives should also be remembered as possible causes of coma. Diacetylmorphine (heroin) is five times as potent as morphine and is especially apt to cause addiction. A variety of "street drugs" self-administered by addicts may cause both pharmacologic coma and contaminant infections of the brain. Not uncommonly salicylate poisoning may occur (especially in children) and may need consideration in differential diagnosis.

Among the poisonous gases causing coma, carbon monoxide is important.[49] Automobile exhaust or gases used in the home or produced in industry are the major sources of carbon monoxide. Skin, lips, and nail beds may be a cherry-red color, the pupils may be dilated, the temperature may be subnormal, and respirations may be irregular, rapid, or shallow. Blood chemistry studies for carbon monoxide and for methemoglobin may be diagnostic.

Dinitro-ortho-cresol, a weed killer, should be considered where poisoning is suspected as should pesticides which are diiosoprophyl fluorophosphate (DFP) congeners.

HYSTERIA

Considered as a cause of unconsciousness, hysteria usually occurs in women with chronic, multiple system complaints, often starting at adolescence. By age 30, such women frequently have had several surgical operations. When periods of unconsciousness are of brief duration, they may have been preceded by difficulty in breathing at a time of emotional stress with subsequent hyperventilation and respiratory alkalosis (with numbness, muscle cramps, and anxiety symptoms). (See Chapter 30, Conversion Symptoms.)

CONVULSIVE DISORDERS

The convulsion, describable for the generalized attack as a violent, involuntary contraction (tonic, then clonic), or as series of massive contractions of the voluntary musculature, is what gives the arresting appearance to the epileptic event. However, it needs to be understood that there is no single kind of epileptic event. The *seizure*, as an epileptic event is often referred to descriptively, may involve only brief episodes of staring, as in the *petit mal* (or absence attack) of childhood. It may be myoclonic, consisting of quick, contractile muscle bursts, which may be a single or repetitive.

Akinetic seizures present brief losses of muscle tone instead of contractions and may resemble the drop attacks described previously. There are also a variety of partial seizures, which point to a focal origin within the cerebral hemispheres and relate to the pattern of cerebral localization. Of these, jacksonian seizures develop in an orderly progression, commencing with a signal contraction in a local area of the musculature and sometimes progressing to a full-fledged generalization convulsion. Finally, there are focal seizures, which present with automatisms or a complex sequence of automatisms, such as is ordinarily referred to as a *psychomotor attack* (also called *partial complex seizures*). The common denominator for all of these kinds of attack is the occurrence of paroxysmal electrical disturbances of unique form and high voltage in the EEG. They are the sign of excessive synchronization in neuronal discharge such as occasions a seizure. Repetitive spike and spike and wave discharges are the principal kinds. They and others are depicted in the EEG classification presented in Figure 31-2. In generalized seizures of any consequence, an associated interval of unconsciousness is invariable, and stupor or sleep may extend the coma into the postictal period.

CLASSIFICATION OF BRAIN WAVES

The EEG is the most important diagnostic adjunct available in clinical appraisal of convulsive states. Brain waves recorded through the skull and scalp, as in the EEG, are field potentials largely generated by nerve-cell dendrites and somata, rather than axons. Tracings of unit activity have been recorded in experimental animal epilepsy and also during the surgical exploration of epileptogenic foci in humans.[50] There "epileptic" neurons may produce spontaneous discharges of 200 to 500 per second in bursts lasting for a fraction of a second and recurring many times per second. Neighboring normal cells can be recorded from the vicinity of such a focus, which is not exclusively epileptogenic.

In general, we believe that refractoriness to anti-convulsant drugs correlates positively with excessive, persistent disorders of brain rhythm. Certain types of seizures known to respond effectively to one medication but not to another often can be identified from the unique characteristics of a disordered EEG when other bases of clinical appraisal leave the issue in doubt. Examples are the 3 per second generalized spike-wave EEG of petit mal epilepsy and, in infants, asynchonous spikes that arise from a background of suppression (called *hypsarrhythmia*). In adults, when an aura or signal symptom (see Fig. 31-2) points to a focal seizure originating at a particular site on one side of the brain, the EEG may confirm the supposition in an intersei-

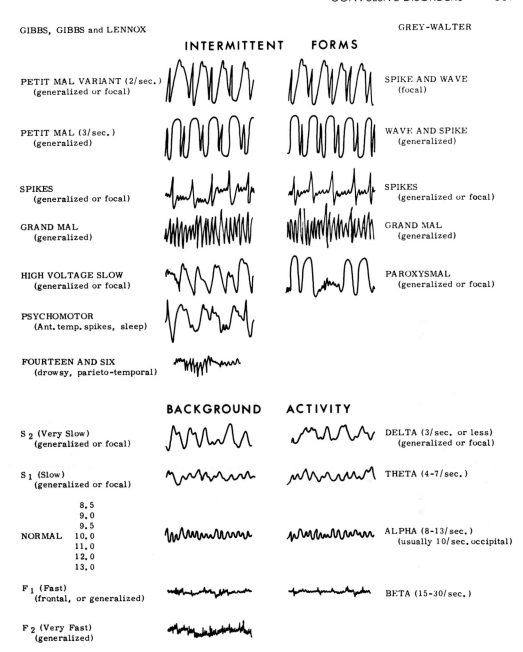

Fig. 31-2. EEG classifications.

zure interval by producing evidence of an associated spike or slow wave focus. For these reasons, it is profitable to consider EEG rhythms and their classification as a prelude to discussion of the pathophysiology of seizure.

Background Activity. The first recordings of spontaneous brain rhythms in animals were obtained long before the electronic era produced a technology capable of coping with the clinical aspects of electrical recording. Berger is credited with the first indubitable records of human brain activity. His clinical success activated a universal interest in brain recording. At the start, Adrian and Buytendijk were able to show that the isolated brain stem of the goldfish gives forth a rhythm that has the same frequency as the movement of the gills in the intact fish.[51] Ever since, spontaneous rhythms have been accepted as another manifestation

of the essential rhythmicity that sustains many of life's processes. Adrian also confirmed Berger's interpretation of the 10 per second adult alpha rhythm, which is recorded from the parieto-occipital scalp area in the relaxed subject who has his eyes closed. A variety of other electrical manifestations of the activity of the human brain also can be recorded through scalp electrodes. Differences appear among awake persons and asleep persons, and at different stages of life from infancy to old age. At birth, the EEG shows only low, slow waves of 4 per second or waves of a lower frequency. For the first year of life, these slow patterns increase in amplitude and are then replaced by intermediate slow frequencies at 4 to 7 per second. Finally (in a small percentage of infants beginning as early as the 10th month), the precursor of the alpha rhythm in turn replaces the intermediate frequencies as the principal background pattern of the human. In old age, neuronal degeneration and the ravages of cerebral vascular disease relate to the reappearance of slow activity. As with animals rhythm at 1 per second characterizes the human brain asleep. It is also the principal pattern associated with pathologic loss of consciousness for whatever reason. This rhythm (called *delta* and assigned limits of 1 to 4 per second) also appears focally as a pathologic process over sites of cerebral infarct, contusion, abscess, or tumor.

Intermittent Forms Characteristic of Convulsive States. In addition to the spontaneous background activity described above, intermittent wave patterns also occur. Often, these show a voltage 4 to 20 times greater than that of the background activity. They signify abnormally synchronized electrical disturbances of unique wave form that have a very high correlation with seizure state, and can be recorded in interseizure traces. Such intermittent forms can occur as single wave complexes, or can repeat the identical wave shape continuously over intervals extending from seconds to minutes. When diffusely recorded from the scalp (that is, showing no localization), they are presumed to signify a generalized cortical disturbance synchronized, but not necessarily triggered, from a limited central region. This is the mesodiencephalic origin of the diffuse thalamic projection system. Grand and petit mal seizure discharges of the usual idiopathic variety belong to this category, and Penfield and Jasper would list them as *centrencephalic seizures.*[52] In the case of repetitive spike-wave disturbance, it is important that brief runs lasting 4 to 6 seconds can occur without either a petit mal seizure or lapse of consciousness intervening. Such are called *subclinical or electrical seizures.* When closely repetitive large spikes occur at 12 to 24 per second, they correlate with grand mal seizures and

complete loss of consciousness. Such an occurrence is difficult to record during an attack because electrodes are easily torn off. However, very adequate records have been obtained by use of immobilizing drugs. There are also other unique, intermittent wave forms, such as single spikes or spike waves, which appear focally over an underlying epileptogenic focus of the brain. Such indicators of the site of the focal seizure often may be recorded in the interseizure period. Thus, they are a valuable asset to the electroencephalographer, because he does not have to depend upon recording a seizure. Presumably, when a seizure spreads widely from such a focus, these spikes become a confluent series that spreads as an avalanche to the remotest areas of the brain, producing generalized seizure manifestations.

It is important to understand that EEG classifications developed simultaneously in several different parts of the world. Those of Gibbs, Gibbs, and Lennox and Grey-Walter are in most common use (see Fig. 31-2).[53,54] They agree in general principles, but differ in details of subclassification of both background and intermittent forms. In interpretation, one must understand that even when intermittent types of activity that have a high correlation with convulsive state are lacking, the degree of departure of background activity from the expected norm for the age of the subject is useful in establishing an unknown EEG, such as one obtained from a subject with a convulsive disorder. Thus, the S-2 (very slow) pattern of the adult EEG occurs 20 times as frequently in epileptics as it does in normal controls.[53] By contrast, a mildly slow tracing occurs only twice as often.

During sleep, several unique intermittent (convulsive) features can appear which are not evident in the waking state. Outstanding among these are the anterior temporal spikes, which derive from the tips of the temporal lobes in psychomotor epilepsy.

SPECTRUM OF CONVULSIVE DISORDERS

Convulsions are of common occurrence. They occur in one of every 200 military draftees; incidence is significantly higher among still younger persons. Attacks are far more diversified than can be encompassed under the combined symptoms of loss of consciousness and massive generalized spasm. The term *epilepsy* also includes a variety of focal seizure patterns in which consciousness is either not lost at all or (at most) is altered, as well as other seizure patterns which show fleeting but complete interruption of consciousness attended by a minimum of rhythmic movement. Features common to all attacks are episodic occurrence, brief duration, and coincidence in the EEG of the unique

wave forms mentioned in the last section. The inseparable accompaniments of the epileptic attack, and their occurrence as brief interludes of the interseizure EEG trace, caused Gibbs, Gibbs, and Lennox to refer to epilepsy as *paroxysmal cerebral dysrhythmia*.[53] There may be instances in which seizure develops without concomitant scalp-recorded EEG change. However, if it does, its site of origin is either at a considerable distance from the scalp leads through which it might be recorded, or it is so extremely small as not to spread to even a nearby electrode.

The causes of epileptic attacks are multiple and can be systematized in a number of ways. One classification sets generalized against focal attacks. The origin of a focal attack is ascribed to one discrete area of the brain; the sequence of development of the seizure somehow exemplifies the function attributed to the parts through which it spreads. Focal seizures are usually symptomatic of an organic brain lesion and fall into the group called *symptomatic epilepsy*. Thus, only secondarily do they signify a pathophysiologic process. By contrast, generalized seizures of the kind referred to as *idiopathic* (or by Penfield as *centrencephalic*) represent a primary pathophysiologic process arising through some predisposition, genetically determined or otherwise. It is important to remember that instances of symptomatic epilepsy are not infrequent among generalized seizures. The perinatal period particularly abounds in contributory causes. Among these causes are changes in the uterine environment which predispose to congenital malformations such as viral or bacterial infections of the mother, kernicterus, anoxia, and mechanical birth trauma. Encephalitis and meningitis occurring in the postnatal period also take a significant toll, and postnatal trauma is the precipitating cause of some instances. In later life, the residuals of CNS-infectious processes, cerebrovascular disease, and neoplasm precipitate the condition. Thus, the relative proportion of the remainder of generalized seizures attributable to genetic predisposition remains moot. Lennox estimated that in a group of 2000 epileptics, a family history was obtained in about 20%.[55] However, the same writer has pointed out the similarity in detail of spike and wave discharges as they occur in uniovular twins. As in other disorders of paroxysmal recurrence, heredity and environment are not mutually exclusive determinants, but interact considerably.

GENERALIZED SEIZURES

We restrict the term generalized to seizures in which there is an interruption of consciousness, however fleeting, and in which the EEG discharge appears simultaneously or successively from leads over the two hemispheres.

Grand Mal. Onset is usually sudden and may be ushered in by an expulsion of air through a partially closed glottis, giving rise to an epileptic cry. Ordinarily the convulsion is of the tonic-clonic type. Loss of control of bladder or bowels and biting of the tongue are common. During and immediately following a seizure, the pupils may be fixed and pathological toe signs may be found. Postictal drowsiness is usual and therefore of important differential diagnostic value. Although repetitive spike activity of the type called *grand mal* is the most common seizure finding, tracings from young children may show a high-amplitude, synchronized slow pattern instead.

Petit Mal. A momentary stare or blank look (indicative of a suspension of consciousness) is the minimal finding, and often such lapses occur for some time before being discovered by teacher or parent. The episodes may be called spells, blackouts, trances, daydreaming, even thinking, by distracted parents. They are of abrupt onset and ending, often occur very frequently, and are of brief duration. The term *petit mal status* refers to longer lapses of consciousness. Status attacks sometimes last for many seconds or even several minutes, without a fall or convulsion. Gibbs and Gibbs detected a history of status in approximately one quarter of their petit mal cases.[56] The diagnosis can be established by detection of the classical 3 per second spike and wave pattern in the EEG. When such sequences are more than a few seconds long, they invariably are accompanied by a typical lapse. Hyperventilation producing alkalosis, ingestion of a large amount of alkali, hydration, anoxia, hypoglycemia, or emotional disturbance may precipitate attacks. Facial twitches and jerks of the limbs may accompany a lapse, individual twitches correlating in time with the spikes of the spike-wave pattern. Sometimes there also are minor automatisms such as licking the lips or shuffling the feet. The subject remains erect if standing.

Other seizure types related to petit mal by the similar occurrence of generalized spike and wave activity are myoclonic attacks, ranging from small jerks to mass spasms and falling spells sometimes called *akinetic epilepsy*.

Psychomotor Seizures. There is confusion among authorities about the exact limits of psychomotor seizure phenomena as well as about terminology for, and site of origin of, the seizures. Attacks with which they may be confused are automatisms of frontal or temporal lobe origin, uncinate attacks, and psychic equivalents of temporal lobe origin (as *déjà vu* and *déjà pensée*).[52] It

would appear that a nuclear pattern of automatism can attach to a variety of reported psychic experiences, including those of fear, rage, and the dream state. We are concerned, however, with the pattern of attack associated with anterior temporal spikes in the sleep EEG. That is best described by Gibbs and Gibbs.[56] For hours or days before a seizure the patient may be irritable. A seizure commences with a wild look, an inappropriate phrase, or a peculiar gesture. The movements during an attack may appear to be purposeful, but are poorly co-ordinated. To a degree, the movements are automatic and repetitive. They may consist of simple acts like lip smacking, hand wringing, or clutching or plucking at objects. In some cases they consist in more elaborate posturing or movements which have the appearance of being purposive, such as undressing or sweeping with a broom. Content of speech is commonly affected, and may be rambling or tangential. Inability to recollect events points toward a sufficient suspension or diversion of the stream of consciousness to mark the seizures as generalized. EEG traces that we have recorded during such seizures also show bilateral disorder, even though interseizure spiking during sleep may be principally unilateral.

FOCAL SEIZURES

It is the sensory aura or the motor signal symptom (Fig. 31-3) that lends distinctive character to a focal seizure. In the case of the *jacksonian motor seizures* there are 3 predominant foci in the motor cortex: movements of thumb and the index finger, the angle of the mouth, and the hallux (great toe). All such attacks spread from these parts in an ordered progression of convulsion, which as a rule corresponds fairly closely with the localization of motor control in the cortex.[57] However, the progression need not invariably follow the points indicated upon the familiar charts of cerebral localization. A jacksonian motor seizure, of course, may spread from an exquisitely localized source, such as the thumb or hallux, and become generalized. Other seizures with more massive signal symptoms derive from other areas of the frontal lobe. For example, the *frontal adversive seizure,* combining head and eye turning toward the opposite side, derives from the premotor territory. The *supplemental motor seizure,* which is initiated by the assumption of a posture in which the contralateral arm is raised and the head turned toward the arm, derives from frontal marginal cortex extending posteriorly to the paracentral lobule and inferiorly to the cingulate gyrus.[58]

Seizures of sensory origin present a variety of auras, each suggestive of a site of origin in one of the major sensory receiving areas of the cortex. Among them are auditory, visual, olfactory (uncinate), and somatosensory jacksonian types (see Fig. 31-3). The last is the sensory replica of the motor jacksonian seizure with progression, arising instead in the general sensory cortex just behind the major central sulcus, which divides the frontal from the parietal lobes. Spread of the disturbance from any one of these may eventuate in a generalized motor seizure. Other focal seizure types are the masticatory and the aphasic (of which speech arrest is one kind), arising, respectively, from temporal and frontal regions of the brain. Evaluation of the epileptic significance of episodic psychic aberrations rests upon uncertain ground unless indisputable neurologic concomitants occur. Such seizures pass through an intervening shadowland into mental experiences that would often engage the attention of a psychiatrist.

On occasion, sensory stimuli are known to precipitate seizures; instances of such activation by touch, pain, smell, noise, and music have been recorded. *Reading epilepsy* is a special variety of the latter, about 20 cases having been reported to date.[59] Seizures occur while the subject is reading and are precipitated by intermittent, brief, involuntary movements of the jaw. Several types of EEG abnormalities have been observed in such cases.

NARCOLEPSY

In cases in which narcolepsy occurs with all of its commonly related symptoms, recurrent attacks of sleepiness are associated with cataplexy (attacks of tonelessness), sleep paralysis and hallucinatory phenomena. The etiology of the disturbance is unknown, but it is believed to center in the sleep areas of the hypothalamus, if such exist. Sleep attacks may occur without warning many times a day. Ordinarily they happen when the subject is sitting quietly in a chair or lying in bed. The attack occurs without warning and may last up to a half an hour. Normal persons experience a fragment of a cataplectic episode every time their "knees become weak" through fear. Laughter, anger, fright, or surprise can bring on an attack. Besides the tonelessness of the somatic musculature, the voice may grow weak and the eyelids droop. After about a minute, recovery occurs. "Sleep paralysis" is a corresponding state of tonelessness that occurs when the subject is falling asleep or awakening. Frightening hallucinations also occur in some narcoleptics.

Rechtschaffen and associates examined the nocturnal sleep and eye movements of narcoleptics as compared with those of normal persons.[70] Seven of the

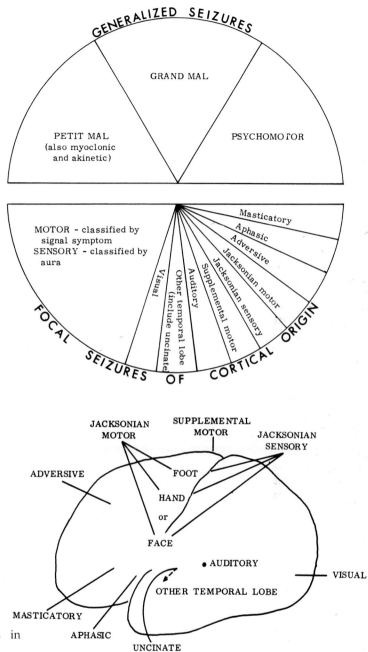

Fig. 31-3. Spectrum of convulsive disorders in relation to focal sites of onset.

nine narcoleptics showed a distinctive phenomenon unknown in pathologic conditions or in normal persons. They presented stage-I rapid-eye-movement periods (paradoxical sleep) at sleep onset rather than approximately 90 minutes thereafter, as normal subjects do. The authors suggested that the narcoleptic is susceptible to precocious triggering of the pontine reticular substance.

SUMMARY

The chapter commenced with a review of the pathophysiology of coma and convulsion. Sleep was used to illustrate a normal, reversible kind of unconsciousness that has its pathologic counterpart in lesions that destroy the rostral brain-stem tegmentum. Coma may also result from a sufficient general depression of brain

metabolism. The brain is almost entirely dependent for its energy upon the delivery of O_2 and glucose across the blood-brain barrier. For example, at any moment the blood circulating through the brain carries only enough O_2 to sustain functioning for a matter of 10 seconds. Even a brief failure of delivery of these important energy sources through ischemia (for example, in common vasodepressor syncope, or in an Adams-Stokes attack) can produce a corresponding suspension of consciousness. Disordered systemic metabolism may produce a more prolonged, although less drastic, effect upon the brain than does arrest of circulation. Uremia, diabetes, hypoglycemia, and liver disease can produce coma through interference with the delivery of glucose, or by suppression by toxins of the cerebral enzymatic activity necessary to convert glucose and O_2 to energy.

Coma also accompanies generalized seizures. In fact, a brief suspension of consciousness is the outstanding symptom in one type of generalized seizure called *petit mal*. In another type, called *grand mal* seizure, loss of consciousness is of longer duration and is accompanied by massive tonic-clonic spasm of the somatic musculature. In a third type, a diversion of the stream of consciousness occurs, coupled with an episode of automatism (psychomotor). EEGs of these three principal types have distinguished characteristics that are very useful diagnostically.

A variety of focal seizures also occur. These arise at a spot of cortical damage that results from invasion of neoplasm, anoxia, or scarring due to injury. The seizure process is the same as in the generalized seizure, and the focal attack may spread to produce one. It is the sensory aura or the motor-signal symptom that lends a distinctive character to a focal seizure, pointing to the site of origin in the plan of cerebral localization. Seizures of sensory origin present a variety of auras, each suggestive of a site of origin in one of the major sensory receiving areas of the cortex. Among these seizures are auditory, visual, olfactory, and sensory jacksonian types. Focal motor seizures commence in the motor cortex ahead of the central sulcus, such as in jacksonian motor seizures, with signal symptoms in thumb and index finger, hallux, or side of mouth. Other types of focal motor seizure are *adversive* and *supplemental motor*, which arise from other areas of the frontal lobe. In all instances, it is important to discover the etiology of a focal seizure, because it may be caused by a surgically remediable condition.

REFERENCES

1. **Brain R:** The physiological basis of consciousness. Brain 81:426, 1958

2. **Sartre JP:** Imagination. A psychological critique. Williams F (trans): Ann Arbor, University of Michigan Press, 1962

3. **James W:** A pluralistic Universe. New York, Longmans, Green & Co, 1932

4. **Prochaska G:** Dissertation on the Functions of the Nervous System. Laycock T (ed and trans): London, Sydenham Society, 1851

5. **Richerland A:** Elements of Physiology, de Lys GJM (trans): Philadelphia, Dobson, 1813

6. **Bremer F:** Cerveau isolé et physiologie du sommeil. Compte Rend Soc Biol (Paris) 118:1235, 1935

7. **von Economo CJ:** Sleep as a problem of localization. J Nerv Ment Dis 71:249, 1930

8. **Hess WR:** The Functional Organization of the Diencephalon. New York, Grune & Stratton, 1957

9. **Dempsey EW, Morison RS:** The production of rhythmically recurrent cortical potentials after localized thalamic stimulation. Am J Physiol 135:293, 1942

10. **Moruzzi G, Magoun HW:** Brain stem reticular formation and activation of EEG. Electroencephalog Clin Neurophysiol 1:455, 1949

11. **Dement W:** The occurrence of low voltage, fast, electroencephalogram patterns during behavioral sleep in the cat. Electroencephalog Clin Neurophysiol 10:291, 1958

12. **Jouvet M:** Telencephalic and rhombencephalic sleep in the cat. In Wolstenholme GEW, O'Connor M (eds): The Nature of Sleep. Boston, Little, Brown, 1960

13. **Huttenlocher PH:** Evoked and spontaneous activity in single units of medial brain stem during natural sleep and waking. J Neurophysiol 24:451, 1961

14. **Jouvet M:** The states of sleep. Sci Am 216:62–72, 1967

15. **Penfield W:** Centrencephalic integrating system. Brain 81:231, 1958

16. **Walshe FMR:** The brain stem conceived as the "highest level" of function in the nervous system; With particular reference to the automatic apparatus of Carpenter (1850) and to the "centrencephalic integrating system" of Penfield. Brain 80:510, 1957

17. **Puetsch P, Guilly P, Fischgold H et al:** Un cas d'anencephalie hydrocéphalique. Rev Neurol (Paris) 79:117, 1947

18. **Nielsen JM, Sedgwick RP:** Instincts and emotions in an anencephalic monster. J Nerv Ment Dis 110:387, 1949

19. **Cairns H:** Disturbances of consciousness with lesions of the brain stem and diencephalon. Brain 74:109, 1952

20. **Howell DC:** Upper brain stem compression and foraminal impaction with intracranial space-occupying lesions and brain swelling. Brain 82:525, 1959

21. **North JB, Jennett S:** Abnormal breathing patterns associated with acute brain damage. Arch Neurol 31:338–344, 1974

22. **McNealy DE, Plum F:** Brain stem dysfunction with supratentorial mass lesions. Arch Neurol 7:10, 1962

23. **Ingvar DH, Lundberg N:** Paroxysmal symptoms in intracranial hypertension, studied with ventricular fluid pressure recording and electroencephalography. Brain 84:446, 1961

24. **Feldman MH:** Physiological observations in a chronic case of "locked-in" syndrome. Neurology 21:517–525, 1971

25. **Solomon P, Aring CD:** The causes of coma in patients entering a general hospital. Am J Med Sci 188:805, 1934

26. **Solomon P, Aring CD:** The differential diagnosis in patients entering the hospital in coma. JAMA 105:7, 1935

27. **Solomon P, Aring CD:** A routine diagnostic procedure for the patient who enters the hospital in coma. Am J Med Sci 191:357, 1936

28. **Symonds CP:** Concussion and contusion of the brain and their sequelae. In Brock S (ed): Injuries of the Skull, Brain and Spinal Cord, 4th ed. Baltimore, Williams & Wilkins, 1960

29. **Courville CB:** Pathology of the Central Nervous System. Mountain View, CA, Pacific Press, 1937

30. **Walker AE:** Posttraumatic Epilepsy. Springfield, Charles C Thomas, 1949

31. **Robbins FC:** The clinical and laboratory diagnosis of viral infections of the central nervous system. In Fields WS, Blattner RJ (eds): Viral Encephalitis. Springfield, Charles C Thomas, 1958

32. **Cerebrovascular Study Group, Institute of Neurological Diseases and Blindness:** Survey Report, rev. ed. Bethesda; St Louis, National Institutes of Health.

33. **Tower DB:** Neurochemistry, Report of an Extramural Survey and Program Committee, Neurological & Allied Science. Bethesda; St Louis, US Public Health Service, 1960

34. **Rossen R, Kabat H, Anderson JP:** Acute arrest of cerebral circulation in man. Arch Neurol Psychiatry 50:510, 1943

35. **Fazekas JF, Bessman AMP:** Coma mechanisms. Am J Med 15:804, 1953

36. **Plum F, Posner JB:** Spinal-fluid pH and neurologic symptoms in systemic acidosis. N Engl J Med 277:605–613, 1967

37. **Ferrendelli JA, Chang MM:** Brain metabolism during hypoglycemia. Arch Neurol 28:173–177, 1973

38. **McLagen NF:** The biochemistry of coma. In Biochemical Aspects of Neurological Disorders. Oxford, Blackwell Scientific Publications, 1959

39. **Parsons–Smith BG, Summerskill WHJ, Dawson AM et al:** The electroencephalogram in liver disease. Lancet 2:867, 1957

40. **Kiloh LG, Osselton JW:** Clinical Electroencephalography. London, Butterworths, 1961

41. **Moyer CA:** Fluid Balance. Chicago, Year Book Medical Publishers, 1953

42. **Engel GL:** Fainting. Springfield, Charles C Thomas, 1962

43. **Wayne HH:** Syncope. Am J Med 30:418, 1961

44. **Weiss S, Baker JP:** The carotid sinus reflex in health and disease. Its role in the causation of fainting and convulsions. Medicine 12:297, 1933

45. **Gurdjian ES, Webster JE, Hardy WG et al:** Nonexistence of the so-called cerebral form of carotid sinus syncope. Neurology 8:818, 1958

46. **Reese CL, Green JB, Elliott FA:** The cerebral form of carotid sinus hypersensitivity. Neurology 12:492, 1962

47. **Drachman DB, Gumnit RJ:** Periodic alteration of consciousness in the "Pickwickian" syndrome. Arch Neurol 6:471, 1962

48. **Plum F, Swanson AG:** Barbiturate poisoning treated by physiological methods with observations on effects of betamethylglutarimide and electrical stimulation. JAMA 163:827, 1957

49. **Polson CJ, Tattersall RN:** Advances in clinical toxicology. Practitioner 187:549, 1961

50. **Calvin WH, Ojemann GA, Ward AA:** Human cortical neurons in epileptogenic foci. Comparison of the interictal firing patterns to those of epileptic neurons in animals. Electroencephalog Clin Neurophysiol 34:337–351, 1973

51. **Adrian ED, Buytendijk FJ:** Potential changes in the isolated brain stem of the goldfish. J Physiol 71:121, 1931

52. **Penfield W, Jasper H:** Epilepsy and Functional Anatomy of the Brain. Boston, Little, Brown & Co, 1954

53. **Gibbs FA, Gibbs EL, Lennox WG:** Electroencephalographic classification of epileptic patients and control subjects. Arch Neurol Psychiatry 50:111, 1943

54. **Grey–Walter W:** Normal rhythms—their development, distribution and significance. In Electroencephalography, a Symposium on its Various Aspects. London, MacDonald, 1950

55. **Lennox WG:** Epilepsy and Related Disorders, Vol. 1. Boston, Little, Brown & Co, 1960

56. **Gibbs FA, Gibbs EL:** Atlas of Electroencephalography, Vol. 2. Cambridge, MA, Addison-Wesley, 1952

57. **Walshe FMR:** On the mode of representation of movements in the motor cortex with special reference to "convulsions beginning unilaterally." Brain 66:104, 1943

58. **Ajmone Marsan C, Ralston BR:** The Epileptic Seizure: Its Functional Morphology and Diagnostic Significance. Springfield, Charles C Thomas, 1957

59. **Bickford RG, Whelan JL, Klass DW et al:** Reading epilepsy: Clinical and electroencephalographic studies on a new syndrome. Trans Am Neurol Assoc, 81st Meeting, pp 100–102, 1956

60. **Ad Hoc Committee, Harvard Medical School:** Report to examine the definition of brain death. JAMA 205:337, 1968

61. **Plum F, Posner JB:** Diagnosis of Stupor and Coma, Contemporary Neurology Series. Philadelphia, FA Davis, 1966

62. **Kubala MJ, Millikan CH:** Diagnosis, pathogenesis and treatment of "drop attack." Arch Neurol 11:107, 1964

63. **Gajdusek DC, Gibbs CJ, Jr, Alpers M:** Transmission and passage of experimental Kuru to chimpanzees. Science 155:212, 1968

64. **Gibbs CJ, Gajdusek DC, Asher DM et al:** Creutzfeldt–Jakob Disease (Spongiform encephalopathy): Transmission to the chimpanzee. Science 161:388, 1968

65. **Ingvar DH, Haggendal E, Nilsson NJ et al:** Cerebral circulation and metabolism in a comatose patient. Arch Neurol 11:13, 1964

66. **Plum F:** Metabolic encephalopathies. In Conn HF, Clohecy RJ, Conn RB (eds): Current Diagnosis. Philadelphia, WB Saunders, 1966

67. **Hume HA, Erb WH, Stevens LW et al:** Treatment of hepatic encephalopathy by surgical exclusion of the colon. JAMA 196:593, 1966

68. **Posner JB, Swanson AG, Plum F:** Acid-base balance in cerebrospinal fluid. Arch Neurol 12:479, 1965

69. **Tudor I:** Sincopa la mictiure. Neurologija 11:229, 1966

70. **Rechtschaffen A, Wolpert EA, Dement WC et al:** Nocturnal sleep of narcoleptics. Electroencephalog Clin Neurophysiol 15:599, 1963

32

Disturbances of Movement

William M. Landau
James L. O'Leary

Impaired Movement
  Muscular Dystrophy
  Polymyositis
  Metabolic Myopathies
  Periodic Paralysis
  Myasthenia
  Peripheral Neuropathy
  Anterior Horn Cell Disease
  Upper Motor Neuron Syndrome
Distortions of Movement and Posture
  Spasticity
  Parkinsonian Rigidity
  Myotonia
  Ataxia

  Dystonia
  Athetosis
Spontaneous Movement
  Fibrillation
  Fasciculation
  Spasm
  Tremor
  Chorea
  Ballism
  Oculogyric Crises
  Torticollis and Tic
  Palatal Myoclonus
  Clonic Convulsive Movements
Summary

Because the distribution of activity in the neuromuscular system is appraised readily by visual inspection, manipulation, and palpation, both in spontaneous behavior and reflex activation, clinical observation alone has proved to be a remarkably successful analytic method. By 1900, most of the major disorders mentioned in this chapter were well described, and in many cases correlated with neuropathologic findings. Most of the groundwork had been laid during the time that Cajal and Sherrington were developing our modern concepts of the neuron doctrine, the synapse, the reflex, and the final common path. In fact, many of the important early studies in neuroanatomy were derived from clinical material. In physiology, as Walshe has pointed out, the experiments demonstrating the elec-

trical excitability of the motor cortex in animals were based upon the clinical observations and inferences of Hughlings Jackson.

The fact that Jackson's early studies upon the natural experiments of disease proved accurate and valid warrants more than an historical footnote; the integrative theory of nervous functioning that he developed remains important. These ideas are the philosophical premises of most modern thinking and investigation in neurology (not of the motor system alone) and, although not often admitted, of experimental neurophysiology and psychology as well.

Here, as a framework for discussion of the pathophysiology of movement, we have space only to assert principles. For a better understanding of their deriva-

tion, the interested reader is referred to Walshe's review, and thence to some of the classical studies upon the subject.[1]

Disturbances of muscle activity may result from the following:

Primary muscle disorders
General body conditions affecting muscles
Disorders affecting the neuromuscular junction
Peripheral nerve disorders
Central nervous system disorders
General body conditions, which may affect the peripheral nerves, the central nervous system (CNS), or both.

Table 32-1 summarizes the conditions causing muscular weakness and outlines the major signs and symptoms associated with each category.

Symptoms may be due solely to the lack of function following a destructive lesion, such as when a muscle is completely paralyzed by transection of its motor nerve. In contrast, a discharging lesion is one in which diseased elements are abnormally active, such as when the anterior horn cells fire spontaneously in fasciculation, or the motor cortex, in convulsion.

There are both negative and positive results of CNS lesions. The negative aspect of a lesion in the motor cortex may be the loss of skilled movement, whereas a positive aspect would be the organization of remaining neural tissue into activity patterns that produce simpler, less variably adaptive movements and hyperactive reflexes. This is also called release of function. It is inferred that neural connections that become hyperactive are normally controlled and regulated by the damaged regions. Whether this regulation includes direct inhibition is seldom clear.

Jackson emphasized the view that both normal and injured nervous systems perform adaptive functions as an integrated whole. This does not mean that functional analysis is impossible or that all regions are equipotential. It means rather that behavioral function can be analyzed best in terms of levels of complexity. The nervous system clearly is not like a system of electrical relays, the higher triggering the lower. Rather, it is the ultimate organ of adaptation: its flexibility and variability of response are functions of the available multiplicity of connections. Jackson put it most simply, "the more gray matter, the more movements."

This leads to his concept of levels of neural integration. The lowest level of representation of movement in Jackson's language is the anterior horn cell and the local segmental reflex connections. This stump of the nervous system is capable of mediating stereotyped protective and ambulatory movements. A higher level of adaptive response in organized behavior is possible when the organism has available brain-stem and motor-cortical connections. The highest level of behavior is available with the complete nervous system.

A specific example of the levels of CNS dysfunction may be presented for the tongue. If the motor nerve is damaged, there is complete paralysis. If the pyramidal tract and brain-stem connections are damaged, the motoneuron and the muscle remain intact and can be activated in some reflexes, but most complex organized movement is not possible. If the motor cortex is relatively spared, the tongue may move quite well in complex movements of swallowing and purposeful movements of the tongue upon command. But if the region around the left sylvian fissure is damaged, the patient is aphasic and still unable to use the tongue in the most complex movements of speech.

Many movement disorders have several aspects of malfunction. Thus, their arbitrary assignment in the classification that follows is only for convenience of presentation.

IMPAIRED MOVEMENT

MUSCULAR DYSTROPHY

The primary symptom of muscle disease is the weakness in the movements of affected muscles. Clinical definition depends upon the distribution and the course of impairment. Distortions of movement may result from compensatory efforts to overcome weakness.

There are several varieties of progressive muscular dystrophy.[2,3] The majority have their onset early in life, with progression slow over a period of years. The impairment of the proximal musculature is early and most severe. The most common type is inherited as a sex-linked recessive trait. It probably occurs only in boys, begins during the first few years of life, and leads to severe disability before maturity. The early symptoms are difficulty in climbing stairs and in rising from the recumbent position. The patient uses his extremities in order to overcome the weakness of his trunk and pelvic girdle muscles. There is usually a swayback posture. The gait is waddling because of gluteal weakness. Stretch reflexes and response to direct muscle percussion are decreased. The calf muscles are prominently spared early in the course of the disease and may be enlarged by increased size of muscle fibers. However, true pseudohypertrophy due to fatty infiltration, with or without weakness, is rare.

Other varieties may affect either sex and may be inherited as dominant or recessive characters. They usually start in the first to third decades, progress less rapidly, and may affect primarily the face and shoulder

Table 32-1. Signs and Symptoms of Conditions Causing Muscular Weakness

Disease	Distribution	Atrophy	Fasciculation	Tendon Jerks	Tone	Direct Myotatic Response	Plantar Reflex	Associated Sensory Loss
Myopathy	Usually proximal	Usual except hypertrophic calves	None	Decreased	Decreased	Decreased	Normal	None
Myasthenia gravis	Eye and throat, variable in limbs	Rare	None	Normal or fatigable	Normal	Normal	Normal	None
Periodic paralysis	Ascending	None	None	Absent	None	None	None	None
Root or nerve disease	In root or nerve innervation	Present	Rarely evident	Decreased	Decreased	Increased or normal ⟍	Normal or depressed	Often in nerve or root distribution
Lower motor neuron syndrome	Usually distal; can be generalized	Prominent	Present	Decreased	Normal or decreased	Increased or normal	Normal or depressed	None
Upper motor neuron syndrome (chronic)	Movements of distal parts more affected	Minimal, if any	None	Increased	Spasticity	Normal	Extensor	Sometimes as a result of other cerebral damage
Parkinsonism	Generalized hypokinesia	None	None	Normal	Rigidity; often cogwheeling	Normal	Normal	None
Cerebellar disease	Ataxia, most prominent in limbs; weakness is mild	None	None	Normal (pendular)	Hypotonic	Normal	Normal	None

girdles or both limb girdles. There are families afflicted with dystrophy of distal limb muscles, but this is rare. Hereditary extraocular muscle dystrophy presents symptoms in adult life.

The most common cause of distal myopathy in early adult life is myotonic dystrophy. In addition to slowly progressive involvement of the forearms and legs along with the diagnostic myotonic phenomenon (see below), there are prominent atrophy of the sternomastoid and facial muscles, baldness, early lenticular cataract, gonadal atrophy, and other endocrine hypofunction.

The hypotonic, floppy infant is a complex diagnostic problem.[3,4] Many such patients suffer from diffuse brain damage, either congenital or progressive, and generally are severely retarded. When such processes are excluded, the most common disease of floppy babies is infantile motoneuron disease (Werdnig-Hoffman disease). Also progressive is an infantile variety of progressive muscular dystrophy. Recent muscle biopsy studies, using electronmicroscopy and histochemical techniques, have defined several varieties of rare, genetically determined myopathies associated with clinical pictures of nonprogressive or very slowly progressive weakness and hypotrophy. Infantile varieties of polyneuritis, polymyositis, and myasthenia gravis also may occur.

POLYMYOSITIS

Polymyositis is one of the collagen diseases. When there is associated skin or gastrointestinal involvement, it is called *dermatomyositis.* The disease may develop at any age but most commonly appears in adulthood and is often associated with a malignant neoplasm. Symmetrical muscle wasting and weakness, usually in a proximal distribution, develop over periods of weeks to years. Muscle tenderness and pain may occur, but are relatively uncommon. The clinical and biopsy findings may be quite similar to those of hereditary dystrophy, and only the age of onset, the clinical course, and the absence of family history may be distinctive.[5] Because many cases respond well to steroid therapy, clinical distinction is of practical importance. The electromyogram (EMG) often shows fibrillation potentials and small motor units. Several serum enzymes may also be increased. Rare causes of localized or diffuse myositis are sarcoidosis and trichinosis.

METABOLIC MYOPATHIES

Myopathy is rarely related to endocrine malfunction. Weakness usually is diffuse, but sometimes is more prominent proximally or distally.

Hyperthyroid myopathy may be proximal or general. Fasciculation, bulbar weakness, and eye muscle involvement may occur with wasting. Thus, there may be confusion with motoneuron disease or with myasthenia gravis; indeed, myasthenia gravis may also be present. Hypothyroidism is characterized by weakness and a unique, slowed relaxation due to abnormality of the contractile mechanism. Muscle enlargement may also occur. Slowed relaxation may be clinically evident in the tendon jerks. A proximal or diffuse weakness and wasting has been reported with hyperparathyroidism.

A proximal or generalized myopathy may occur in Cushing's syndrome, either spontaneous or induced. Myopathy in Addison's disease is associated with joint contractures thought to be related to primary affection of fascial tissue.

Hyperinsulinism may produce a distal, or less often proximal, muscle impairment. Evidence for both primary myopathy and neuropathy has been recorded. There is controversy concerning the occurrence of a primary myopathy in diabetes mellitus.

Congenital deficiency of muscle phosphorylase (McArdle) results in inability to metabolize muscle glycogen. The patient suffers painful muscle cramping leading to muscle contracture and weakness when he attempts to exercise beyond a minimum rate. These patients also may have myoglobinuria following excessive exercise. Muscle wasting is not conspicuous. In this and other enzymatic disturbances that prevent normal glycogen degradation (glycogenoses), a useful screening test is the absence of normal elevation of lactate in venous blood derived from ischemically exercised muscle.[46] The specific defect may then be defined by biochemical and histochemical studies of biopsy material.

PERIODIC PARALYSIS

Normal muscle membrane resting potential is determined primarily by the relative concentrations of the K^+ inside and outside the cell. The resting membrane is relatively impermeable to Na^+ and the K^+ concentration gradient is maintained by a metabolically active pump that extrudes Na^+. The K^+ thus diffuses inward to maintain ionic equilibrium; there is evidence that K^+ is also actively pumped inward by linkage with the Na^+ pump mechanism.

Secretion of acetylcholine at the end-plate results in a drastically increased membrane conductance for both Na^+ and K^+. The propagated action potential is then sustained by a transient regenerative and explosive increase in Na^+ conductance and inward flux, resulting in a transient reversal of membrane potential. With

inactivation, the restoration of Na^+ impermeability and the rapid diffusion of K^+ out of the cell, accelerated by a transient increase in K^+ conductance, return the membrane to the resting level. The sarcolemma-conducted action potential is thought to extend into the muscle fibre through the transverse tubule system, resulting in the activation of a process involving Ca^+ release that causes the actin and myosin protein fibrils to slide together, thus shortening the muscle. There is evidence that depression of resting potential augments the ionic-pump maintenance mechanism. Combined microelectrode, biochemical, and metabolic studies are beginning to explore the possible disturbances of these complex processes that may occasion the symptoms of the conditions under consideration here.

Periodic paralysis is a recurrent, acute familial syndrome of severe weakness leading to paralysis that comes on over a period of minutes to hours. Each episode lasts from a few hours to a day or more. The originally described periodic paralysis is usually associated with hypokalemia during attacks that may be reversed by potassium therapy. The paralysis is characteristically ascending and tends to spare the respiratory muscles.

Attacks of familial periodic paralysis occur during exercise or following a rest, often at night, and may be provoked by the administration of glucose or insulin, or both, and sometimes by adrenalin. An association is suggested between the movement of glucose into cells, the movement of K^+, and a related effect on Na^+ conductance or an effect on K^+ and Na^+ transport. Microcystic lesions are seen within muscle fibers during attacks. Especially among Japanese, the condition may be associated with hyperthyroidism and may be cured by treatment of the hyperthyroidism. A unique pathophysiologic feature of periodic paralysis is the electrical inexcitability of affected muscles (and, of course, of their motor nerves) during an attack. Muscle membrane potentials have been shown to be normal at this time. Potassium and acetazolamide therapy may help. Gamstorp has described a familial periodic paralysis associated with hyperkalemia or normokalemia. Attacks usually follow shortly upon exercise, and yet sometimes may be worked off by resuming activity. They may be provoked by administration of K^+ and often may be prevented by acetazolamide. Muscle fibers are significantly depolarized during attacks, and the affected muscles and motor nerves are electrically inexcitable.[47]

When diabetes mellitus is treated vigorously with insulin, especially when high insulin doses are used in the treatment of diabetic acidosis, extracellular K^+ enters cells with glucose; serum K^+, initially high, may fall to subnormal levels and muscle weakness may become a striking symptom.

Subnormal K^+ in extracellular fluids is associated with muscular weakness or paralysis in many conditions other than the rare familial periodic paralysis. These include high K^+ loss through the renal route from any cause (rapid, heavy, or prolonged diuresis, K^+ losing nephropathies, steroid hormone effects with renal K^+ loss and Na^+ retention such as in Cushing's syndrome, hyperaldosteronism, hyperadrenocorticism, steroid therapy) and high K^+ loss through the gastrointestinal route (vomiting, diarrheal diseases, excessive cathartics).

Paradoxically, a periodic weakness may also occur with potassium intoxication. Potassium metabolism is discussed in Chapter 35.

Paramyotonia congenita is an hereditary disease related to myotonia in which symptoms of stiffness and paralysis occur spontaneously or are provoked by exposure to cold. Several authors think that this is essentially the same as Gamstorp's disease.

A subacute syndrome of generalized weakness may be due to poisoning of the neural portion of the muscle end-plate by botulinus toxin. The toxin secreted by some species of ticks produces progressive paralysis by poisoning of the motor neuron fiber. Removing the tick reverses the paralysis.

MYASTHENIA

Myasthenia gravis is the archetype of disease at the muscle end-plate. Classically, this has been considered to be a disorder of neuromyal transmission, analogous to poisoning by competitive acetylcholine blocking agents like curare.

The neuromuscular junction consists of a complexly folded motor end-plate structure of the muscle fiber and the terminal fibers of the motor nerve that innervate it. The nerve fibers and muscle membrane are not in direct contact, but are separated by a small gap. When the propagated motor nerve impulse reaches its terminal, synaptic vesicles of acetylcholine are released; extracellular calcium is necessary for transmitter ejection to occur. The acetylcholine in the synaptic cleft then binds with the end-plate membrane of the muscle fiber. This results in a drastic increase in the muscle membrane permeability to both Na^+ and K^+, which in turn triggers a propagated impulse along the sarcolemma membrane of the muscle fiber, the muscle action potential, which through the transverse tubular system triggers muscular contraction. The acetylcholine survives only a few milliseconds. That which is not bound to the muscle membrane is destroyed rapidly by the enzyme cholinesterase which is normally present at the end-plate.

Because in this disease individual muscles vary in

their degree of clinical and pharmacologic impairment, it was postulated early that there is a localized defect in acetylcholine metabolism or end-plate structures.[6,7] Later, electrophysiological studies with microelectrodes concluded that there was a presynaptic defect in the amount of acetylcholine delivered into the cleft by the terminal nerve fiber.[8,48,49] That hypothesis has been abandoned now as a convergent flood of clinical and animal-model investigations have established that the proximate cause of symptoms is damage to the postsynaptic end-plate structure as shown by electron microscopy. The evidence is now overwhelming that this is an autoimmune disease in which the acetylcholine receptor protein of the muscle fiber end-plate is the antigen. Specific antibodies can be detected in the serum of most patients and an animal model of the syndrome can be produced by sensitization with the receptor protein.[9,10] Neuromuscular conduction reaches threshold level or fails because of deficiency of receptor binding sites.

The hallmark of the clinical picture is fatigability, particularly affecting the extraocular and bulbar muscles. Symptoms of diplopia, dysarthria, and dysphagia typically become worse later in the day. Limb muscles are involved in the more severe, generalized cases. Stretch reflexes are intact although sometimes fatigable, and muscle wasting occurs only rarely in chronically severely affected muscles. Characteristically, there are spontaneous exacerbations and remissions. There is an increased incidence of the disturbance in patients with other autoimmune diseases and hyperthyroidism. There is also frequent association with malignant tumors of the thymus.

For many years it was suspected that a curare-like humoral agent existed in the blood because of the occurrence of transient neonatal myasthenia in the offspring of affected mothers. This condition now seems to be well explained by exposure of the fetus to the mother's circulating antibody to receptor protein.

Severe generalized weakness with respiratory paralysis is called *myasthenic crisis*, which at one time led to a mortality rate for myasthenia gravis as high as 30%. With modern techniques for respiratory support, antibiotics for associated respiratory infections, and better long-term management, most patients can be saved.

Clinical diagnosis is established by the improvement or alleviation of the symptoms by increasing the amount of acetylcholine available in the synaptic cleft. This is accomplished by the administration of anticholinesterase drugs that combine directly with the cholinesterase, thus preventing the destruction of acetylcholine in the cleft and permitting it to saturate the postsynaptic receptors. This test is most conveniently performed with intravenous edrophonium (Tensilon), which improves the symptoms for several minutes without eliciting the spontaneous muscle fasciculations that the drug produces in normal subjects. When limb or facial muscles are affected, objective diagnostic evidence can be adduced in the clinical EMG laboratory. In normal subjects, supramaximal stimulation of the motor nerve at 3 per second elicits an integrated muscle electrical potential of constant amplitude. In a muscle affected by myasthenia gravis, the response diminishes rapidly from the first. This failure of a large portion of the end-plate population to respond can then be corrected by edrophonium injection.

Direct treatment of these symptoms can be attained with longer acting anticholinesterase drugs, especially neostigmine (Prostigmine) and pyridistogmine (Mestinon). With large doses, atropine-like drugs must be added to prevent visceral side effects, especially on the intestine.

Most authorities now agree that the most effective long-term strategic approach to therapy is to suppress the autoimmune process. Surgery for thymic tumors is, of course, always indicated, but there is good evidence that removal of the non-neoplastic thymus and long-term corticosteroid treatment are very effective. There may be a transient worsening of symptoms at the onset of corticosteroid administration. Refractory cases have also been treated with azathioprine (Imuran) and plasmapheresis.

A myasthenic syndrome (Lambert-Eaton), usually but not always associated with carcinoma, especially "oat-cell" lung cancer, presents with weakness and fatigability that affect limb musculature more prominently than cranial nerves.[11] A characteristic feature demonstrated by motor nerve stimulation at rapid rates (20 to 40 per second) is a dramatically increased response to successive volleys. At low frequencies (3 per second), transmission may be increasingly blocked, as is typically seen in myasthenia gravis. The augmentation phenomenon of the myasthenic syndrome may be apparent clinically as increasing strength of persistent voluntary grasp and by a striking, though transient, postexercise facilitation of strength. Microelectrode studies indicate normal amplitude of miniature (spontaneous) end-plate potentials (MEPPs), but a deficiency in the ability of nerve endings to eject acetylcholine.[50] As with anticholinesterase drugs, guanidine has specific therapeutic value in augmenting transmitter ejection, perhaps in relation to the sensitivity of the nerve endings to Ca^{++} and Mg^{++} concentrations. The fact that neomycin and botulinus-toxin polypeptides also interfere with transmitter release suggests that some cancer cells may secrete a similar substance.

A slight degree of neuromuscular block may occur

also in motor neuron disease, somehow related to disturbed function of the diseased neurons.

PERIPHERAL NEUROPATHY

The basic motor symptom of peripheral nerve disease is weakness. Following section of the nerve, the motor axons become electrically inexcitable in a few days and undergo wallerian degeneration. The muscle fibers supplied by the nerve undergo atrophy, and gross muscle atrophy may be apparent in 2 to 3 weeks. Affected muscles are flaccid, and although stretch reflexes are absent, myotatic response to direct muscle percussion may be increased. Sensory impairment and distortion of sensation are appropriate to the superficial distribution of mixed motor and sensory nerves.

If the gross nerve structure remains intact, or after surgical anastomosis when the nerve is severed, the central motor axons grow out toward the denervated muscles at a rate of 1 mm to 3 mm a day. If reinnervation occurs, the muscle mass may be restored to a varying degree. Functional recovery may be diminished if some nerve axons grow back into muscles other than those they originally supplied.

Acute contusion of a nerve may produce a physiologic block for a period of days to weeks without degeneration of the distal axons. The distal axons remain electrically excitable, there is no significant muscle wasting, and recovery is usually excellent. Even when a lesion in continuity is severe enough to produce degeneration of the distal axons, the recovery is usually better than that following surgical anastomosis because the nerve sheath relationships that guide axon growth are better preserved.

Chronic trauma may be produced by compression in several entrapment syndromes, the most common of which is carpal-tunnel compression of the median nerve. In addition to symptoms of pain and sensory loss or distortion, there may be weakness and wasting in the muscles of the thenar eminence. In many cases there is a significant delay of conduction of nerve impulses under the compressed region when the motor nerve is stimulated electrically.[12] This test is of diagnostic value; the physiologic explanation of delay is uncertain, but it is probably due to inactivation of one or more nodes of Ranvier or to segmental demyelinization.

Other commonly vulnerable loci are the peroneal nerve at the fibula (as affected in habitual leg crossing), the ulnar nerve at the elbow, and the brachial plexus at the first rib. Spinal roots are commonly compressed by herniated intervertebral disks near the intervertebral foramina. The anatomic distribution of muscle involvement defines the level at which a population of motoneurons is affected. Mononeuropathies are particularly prone to occur with trivial mechanical insult when there is systemic disturbance, such as alcoholism, malnutrition, or diabetes.

Neuropathies of systemic disease (toxic, metabolic, nutritional, genetic) may be due primarily to disturbed function of the axon itself, which degenerates from its distal extent back toward the cell body—the dying-back phenomenon. In other neuropathies (e.g., those produced by diphtheritic toxin), the primary disturbance is in the myelin sheaths and Schwann cells. Multifocal degeneration of the sheath cells, segmental demyelination, occurs over the full length of the axon. Theoretically, in dying-back neuropathies conduction velocity is unaffected so long as conduction occurs, whereas marked slowing and physiologic block characterize segmental demyelination. However, except for certain model neuropathies, it is probable that both axons and sheath cells are affected in most of the neuropathies seen clinically.

Multiple mononeuritis may occur in diabetes, polyarteritis nodosa, and other conditions. The more common polyneuritis is a syndrome of diffuse involvement of those motor and sensory axons that extend farthest from their cell bodies. Thus, weakness, wasting, loss of stretch reflexes, and proprioception usually are most marked in a diffuse distal pattern, particularly in the legs and the feet. The time course of neuropathies may vary from months and weeks in metabolic disturbances to an acute or subacute picture in toxic, porphyric or postinfectious polyneuritis, lupus erythematosus, and so on.

Predominant motor impairment is particularly characteristic of porphyric and chronic lead intoxication neuropathies. The earliest symptoms of subacute combined-system disease, like pernicious anemia related to vitamin-B_{12} deficiency, indicate mixed sensory and motor peripheral nerve impairment. Central involvement also affects the dorsal column spinal projection of sensory neurons, pyramidal tracts, optic nerves, and even general cerebral functions.

ANTERIOR HORN CELL DISEASE

Amyotrophic lateral sclerosis is a disease of adults in which there is a progressive degeneration of anterior horn cells in the spinal cord along with the homologous cranial motor neurons, excepting those to the extraocular muscles. In addition, there is an ascending degeneration of pyramidal tract fibers, the symptoms of which overlap those of the lower motor-neuron process. Thus, instead of the decreased stretch reflexes that might be expected with the muscle wasting and weakness of motoneuron damage, there are paradox-

ically increased stretch reflexes (as long as some motoneurons survive) and often extensor plantar responses (see below). Hyperirritable surviving mononeurons fire spontaneously, resulting in muscle fasciculation. The clinical picture is defined by the diffuse craniospinal involvement. An infantile variety of anterior horn-cell disease (Werdnig-Hoffman) is not associated with corticospinal tract involvement. A slowly progressive hereditary motor neuron degeneration (Kugelberg-Welander) may be confused with limb-girdle muscular dystrophy.

UPPER MOTOR NEURON SYNDROME

Upper motor neuron syndrome is an expression generally used in reference to the corticospinal tract because this is the largest single efferent internuncial pathway. Polemical controversy about which effects of upper motor neuron lesions are pyramidal, and which, if any, are exclusively extrapyramidal, is tending toward resolution by recent physiologic studies in monkeys. Predominant effects of pyramidal lesions upon fine movements may be attributed to the finding that the most potent motor cortex projections, long known (as in the Penfield homunculus pictures) to be directed to distal extremity muscles, are mediated by direct corticomotoneuronal synaptic connections, whereas proximal and axial musculature are reached only indirectly by interneuronal relays.[51] But the pyramidal tract is not the only important effector pathway arising from motor cortex. Grossly somatotopic movements may still be elicited by stimulation of the motor cortex after section of the medullary pyramids in the baboon.[52] In other experiments, a significant repertory of fine limb movements that survives pyramid section is seriously impaired by the additional destruction of the lateral brain stem and cord extrapyramidal tracts in the same animals, whereas axial and proximal limb movements are impaired only by medial extrapyramidal tract lesions.[53] Naturally occurring lesions in humans are practically never limited to the pyramidal tract. However, it may be that the upper motor neuron syndrome should be attributed to destruction of the most direct paucisynaptic pathways to motor neurons, most of which are carried in the corticospinal tract.

Spinal shock is a condition of severe reflex depression in the distal spinal cord following acute transection. This lasts for several weeks in humans, with gradual recovery of both nociceptive and stretch reflexes. The former, although they are polysynaptic, recover first, and may be present in depressed form immediately after the lesion is made. At this time, the two-neuron stretch reflex is severely depressed. Yet the same motoneurons can be excited by electrical stimulation of stretch receptor nerve fibers (H reflex). This suggests that depression occurs at the stretch receptor end-organs, which are less sensitive because of temporarily decreased activity in the fusimotor (gamma efferent) system.[13]

The shock phenomenon seems to be reasonably explicable on the basis of the sudden diminution of synaptic barrage at both interneuron and motoneuron synapses. The recovery of reflexes, not only to the normal level but also to the hyperactive state, has not been explained satisfactorily. It has been suggested that postsynaptic membranes, thus partially denervated, become hyperexcitable to the transmitter substance from surviving presynaptic terminals.[14] Another explanation of the development of increased reflexes over a long period of time is that dorsal root neurons develop additional collateral branches that increase the number of synaptic connections in the reflex pathways.[15] It is clear that there is monosynaptic reflex hyperexcitability at the motor neuron in human hemiplegia, and recent evidence indicates that increased fusimotor tone augments the excitability of the stretch receptors themselves.[16,54,55]

A transient period of hyporeflexia with flaccid paralysis also occurs with massive lesions of the upper motor neuron in the cerebral hemisphere. This is thought to be homologous to spinal shock, but less severe and prolonged because of the larger proportion of surviving efferent connections.

The classical model of chronic upper neuron lesion is the condition evolving from a lesion of the internal capsule. If the lesion develops slowly, the hyperreflexic state evolves continuously without the initial depressed phase of acute lesions. The paralysis is characterized by being most severe in the fine dexterous movements of the extremities. Thus, finger movement is more impaired than forearm movement, and forearm movement more than shoulder movement. Muscle strength is usually reduced, but severe disability may be present even with good strength of individual muscles because the repertoire of performance is greatly limited. Thus the hemiplegic patient may be limited to movements including flexion of the fingers, the wrist, and the elbow, and protraction and elevation of the arm, regardless of which movement of the fingers he is attempting to perform.

Beevor long ago showed that trunk muscles may be functionally weak for postural maintenance in one position in space and quite strong in another.[17] Thus, with a right hemispheral lesion, the sitting patient falls to the left, and the right paraspinal muscles are weak in the effort to sit up straight. The same muscles are quite strong in abducting from the upright position toward the right. Conversely, the left trunk muscles

are strong in adduction from right to midline and weak in continuation of the movement to abduction from midline toward the left. Beevor concluded that the motor cortex is concerned primarily in contralateral movements, not simply related to contralateral muscles in the fashion of marionette strings.

After an acute capsular lesion, the phasic stretch reflexes (tendon jerks) on the affected side are slightly decreased or normally active for several days. They then become more and more hyperactive. When the hyperactivity becomes extreme, a steady stretch stimulus applied to the muscle results in 4 to 7 rhythmic contractions per second, each followed by a silent period and a renewed stretch response.

The pathophysiologic basis for this clonus is increased motor-neuronal excitability and also some increase in stretch receptor excitability due to increased fusimotor tone. The first stretch-evoked afferent burst causes a brisk twitch contraction that unloads the muscle spindles that are anatomically parallel to the main muscle. This shutting off of excitatory input results in the silent period, which ceases when renewed passive stretch again excites a volley from the muscle spindles. This unloading-phenomenon silent period may be produced by the same mechanism if the load against which a steady voluntary contraction is exerted is suddenly removed—the unloading reflex. Increased resistance to passive limb movement manifests spasticity (see below).

Associated with the development of hyperactive reflexes is a functional recovery of behavioral movement conditioned by proprioceptive stimuli. If movement evolves toward complete recovery, there is also return of the stretch reflexes toward the normal level and, according to Twitchell, the grasp reflex may appear transiently as evidence of the facilitatory influence of contactual stimuli.[18]

The plantar reflex elicited by nociceptive stimulation of the lateral planta normally produces a reflex withdrawal of the foot from the stimulus. The prime movement is plantar flexion of the hallux with dorsiflexion of the ankle and irregular flexion of the hip and the knee. When the upper motoneuron is damaged, this reflex becomes hyperactive in a very special way: the extensor hallucis longus, which is silent in the normal plantar reflex, becomes by reflex irradiation a synergic cocontractor of the neighboring ankle dorsiflexors, tibialis anticus, and extensor digitorum longus. As a result, the hallux dorsiflexes even though there is active contraction of the hallux flexors. This is the *extensor toe sign of Babinski* (Fig. 32-1).[19]

The pathologic reflex usually has a lower threshold for response than the normal reflex; increased excitability also is indicated by the spatial irradiation of the afferent arc, so that stimuli applied elsewhere on the extremity than the lateral planta may be effective. On the efferent side, the extensor reflex tends to recruit a more vigorous generalized limb muscle synergy than does the normal flexor pattern.

The plantar reflex has great clinical value because it often becomes abnormal early in the course of disease before other signs or symptoms of pyramidal tract damage are apparent. Extensor toe signs may occur in transient conditions of cortical depression and coma.

In progressive paraparesis due to spinal cord disease, hyperreflexia in the extensor muscles is more

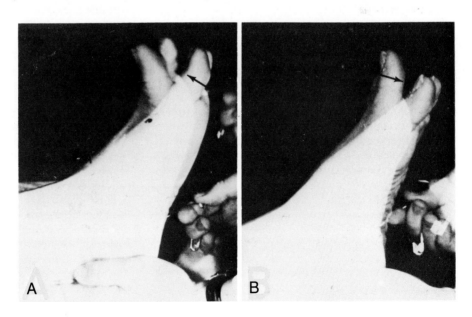

Fig. 32-1. Extensor plantar reflex (Babinski sign). (*A*) Superimposed motion picture frames showing dorsiflexion of the hallux along with dorsiflexion of the foot. (*B*) Same subject after block of the peroneal nerve, which paralyzes foot and toe dorsiflexors. The prime movement of hallux plantar flexion is apparent. In (*A*) this movement is overcome by the contraction of extensor hallucis longus.

prominent; the resting posture is one of extension. With progression, this commonly evolves into paraplegia in flexion in which the lower extremities tend to remain flexed at the hip, the knee, and the ankle. This is also the end stage of the phasic hyperactive-flexion reflex or flexor spasm, an exaggerated plantar reflex. The paraplegic limb may respond with vigorous transient flexion to a slight movement of the bed sheets, to the stimulation of trophic skin lesions, or (apparently) spontaneously. Because it has been possible to maintain patients with complete cord transection for an indefinite period of time, it has been found that some remain in extension most of the time, and some in flexion, without a significant relationship to the level of the cord lesion. Flexor spasms may occur in either circumstance. There is no clear understanding of why some patients with complete section assume one posture and others another posture.

A transient upper motor-neuron paralysis (Todd's paralysis) may be associated with the period immediately following a focal convulsive seizure. Although it has usually been assumed that this represents postconvulsive fatigue and decreased tonic activity in the appropriate motor cortex, critical analysis indicates that there may also be an element of active inhibition.[20]

Highest level paralysis occurs with cortical lesions in the motor region and is called *apraxia*. Here the patient may have preserved the capacity to use muscles in complex coordination for automatic or associated movements and yet be unable to perform a skilled act purposefully, such as using a key, a fountain pen, or a comb. The grasp reflex and instinctive grasp reactions generally are correlated with frontal or diffuse cortical lesions.

DISTORTIONS OF MOVEMENT AND POSTURE

SPASTICITY*

The tendon jerk is the most sensitive measure of stretch reflex excitability, because the synchronous activation of muscle-spindle stretch receptors results in temporal summation at the spinal cord. Spasticity is evident when the reflex synapses are so sensitive that even asynchronous afferent impulses, ineffective in a normal subject, result in muscle contraction.[54] Thus, when excitability is high, even slow, passive extension of a muscle results in reflex contraction that increases in intensity as the stretch increases, and then suddenly gives way (lengthening reaction). This whole reaction is the *clasp-knife phenomenon*, which, by definition, is clinical spasticity. The release of the clasp-knife tension is attributed to the autoinhibitory action of high tension on the muscle tendon (Golgi) stretch receptors and to the unloading of excitatory muscle-spindle stretch receptors by the contraction of the muscle.

Between the stage of increased tendon jerks and that of fully developed spasticity, varying degrees of incremental-decremental plastic resistance to passive movement may be observed. In human subjects, these tend to be variable and are often difficult to distinguish from poor cooperation in voluntary relaxation. True spasticity never occurs except in association with the hyperactive phasic-stretch reflexes. In spite of the reflex hyperexcitability, spastic muscles are flaccid and electrically silent when the limb is positioned so that there is no passive muscle stretch.

Although such terms as *spastic hemiparesis* are in common usage, the disturbance of movement is more the result of loss of control (negative effect) than it is a manifestation of increased stretch reflexes (positive-release effect). To be sure, in hemiparesis, the flexed posture of the upper extremity and the extended posture of the lower extremity reflect the effect of stretch reflexes. But the shoulder-arm synergy of the upper extremity and the coarse circumducting movement of the lower extremity in walking, accomplished largely with the proximal musculature, are essentially the same regardless of the degree of hyperreflexia. The tendency of the extremities to cross in the gait of upper neuron paraparesis does indicate a disability due to exaggeration of the stretch reflex in the thigh adductors.

Decerebrate rigidity in animals was originally defined by Sherrington as a state of hyperactivity of antigravity (extensor) stretch reflexes in all limbs resulting from midbrain transection. The homologous condition of hyperreflexia in humans with lesions of the corticospinal tract (probably, parallel descending pathways, too) is called *spasticity*; spasticity and decerebrate rigidity are physiologically synonymous.

There is much misunderstanding of the pathophysiology of decerebrate rigidity or decerebrate posturing in humans. A widely held view among clinicans is that brain-stem transection in humans produces a steady state of marked extensor posture of the lower extremities, with associated extension and hyperpronation of the upper extremities. This is contrasted with a putative condition of decorticate rigidity, attributed to up-

*The terms *flaccid* and *spastic* are confusing because they denote different methods of observation. Muscle tone is determined by evaluating the resistance to passive stretch. In normal, relaxed subjects, this resistance is slight but significant as compared with the hypotonia of severe neuropathy, myopathy, or cerebellar disease. Hypertonia in spasticity, as well as in some other conditions, is due to muscle contraction induced by the act of passive muscle lengthening. *Flaccidity is an observation of visual inspection and palpation of the muscle at rest*; this term properly contrasts with contraction. Thus, a muscle affected by tetanus toxin or parkinsonism shows activity at rest by inspection and palpation, which also can be shown by passive joint movement.

per motoneuron lesion at a forebrain level and manifested by similar lower extremity posture with flexion of the upper extremity.

Clinical studies and the results of animal experiments indicate that "decerebrate posture" is a transient state evoked by a strong noxious stimulus or by a central pathologic process (hypoxia or compression) that could produce direct brain-stem irritation. Experiments with monkeys performed by Feldman show that complete transection of the primate midbrain produces a flaccid animal with increased tendon jerks.[56] What Feldman calls the *reactive extensor postural synergy* (decerebrate posturing) can then be evoked by noxious stimulation, neck extension, or transient hypoxia. Related clinical studies affirm the view that spontaneous evolution of decerebrate posturing indicates an active irritative process of the CNS. The concept of a diagnostically significant "decorticate posture" is unsupported by the clinical and experimental studies.

PARKINSONIAN RIGIDITY

The pathologic basis of Parkinsonian rigidity is still controversial, although many authors believe that lesions in the substantia nigra are the most significant ones. There are also lesions of the basal ganglia, particularly the pallidum, and Denny–Brown emphasizes the damage to corticopallidal and striopallidal fibers.[21] There are two major aspects of the clinical syndrome: (1) constant innervated contraction of most of the musculature at rest, and (2) generalized weakness and difficulty in starting movements (hypokinesia). The abnormal resting tone sometimes may be relaxed by careful positioning of limbs, but it is practically always present in the waking state and is much exaggerated by emotional stress or attention. Although the generalized rigidity seriously interferes with motor activity, fine movements of the fingers may be relatively well preserved as compared with the syndrome of the upper motoneuron. Afflicted patients move slowly with stooped posture, short steps, and a lack of associated movements in the upper extremities. In some patients the symptoms at onset are limited to the limbs on one side of the body. Careful clinical examination distinguishes the syndrome from upper motor neuron hemiparesis (see above).

Passive movement at affected joints reveals a continuous resistance throughout the excursion tested. Most often this rigidity has a rhythmic phasic quality (cogwheeling), which is clearly related to the tremor (paralysis agitans) that many patients have. Rigidity is partially sustained by proprioceptive reflex drive because desensitization of muscle stretch receptors by anesthetic block of fusimotor fibers can abolish the hypertonicity.[22] An abnormality of fusimotor tone is unlikely. Although there is controversy about the relationship between rigidity and tremor, we think it most probable that tremor represents a reciprocal organization at the spinal level of the increased tonic neural drive from above, somehow released by the primary lesions. (see Tremor, below).[57]

The syndrome may occur in manganese poisoning and as a toxic effect of the therapeutic use of reserpine and phenothiazine drugs (rarely with permanent effect). Occasionally, such agents produce instead a choreic picture. These observations have suggested localized differences in neural transmission mechanisms in the affected regions of the forebrain.

Biogenic amines are decreased in affected substantia nigra and striatum of parkinsonian brains, a finding that was inferred to reflect the destruction of neurons containing the amines. Administration of large doses of the dopamine transmitter substance precursor, dihydroxyphenylalanine (DOPA, the L-form of which is the active agent), may produce dramatic improvement of symptoms, including hypokinesia.[58] Indeed, L-Dopa is now the most potent drug of choice for treatment of parkinsonism. Interesting neurologic side-effects may include psychologic changes and, with excessive dosage, choreic movements. Whether the therapeutic effect has any relationship to the mechanism of pathologic cell changes remains to be seen.

A currently popular but likely too simplistic hypothesis is that a normal balance of dopaminergic and cholinergic synapses in the basal ganglia systems is thrown out of balance in movement disorders. Thus, it is postulated that a relative decrease of dopaminergic system potency and increase of cholinergic system potency accounts for parkinsonian symptoms; these are remedied by either cholinergic blocking agents or increased supply of dopamine. The converse mechanism has been postulated for choreic symptoms.

MYOTONIA

Myotonia is a hereditary disturbance of muscle excitability and structure in which individual fibers are hyperirritable and may fire repetitively and produce prolonged contraction in response to physiologic activation by montoneurons or mechanical stimulation by percussion.[23] In addition, myotonic muscle continues to contract throughout the flow of threshold stimulation by direct electrical current, instead of firing only when the cathodal current is turned on, as in normal muscle. EMG recording indicates that individual muscle fibers may even go into high-frequency activity without any apparent triggering stimulus. Intracellular recording has shown spontaneous oscillations of mem-

brane potential similar to those seen in experimentally hypersensitive membranes, like that of hypocalcemic nerve.[24] A specific depression of membrane chloride permeability in myotonic muscle may be the proximate basis for the abnormal excitability. Recent biochemical evidence suggests that the primary genetic defect is in the structure of cell membranes, including even red blood cells.

Involuntary muscle contraction after a handgrasp or percussion may last 10 to 30 seconds. Associated with this hindrance to normal movement there may be innervated contraction of both the primary affected and associated muscle (afterspasm). Myotonia may be produced in normal animals and humans by the administration of desmosterol, which presumably becomes structurally incorporated into the muscle membrane so that its excitability characteristics are changed.[59]

In *myotonia congenita*, the stiffness of the proximal muscles of the lower extremities results in an unusual stiff gait, resembling that associated with hip joint disease. The myotonic phenomenon usually improves with exercise (warming-up) and may be helped to some degree by quinine or procainamide therapy.

In *dystrophia myotonica*, similar myotonia is seen in adults. The gait is disturbed by myotonia; moreover, weakness and atrophy of the quadriceps and the dorsiflexors of the feet are striking and further interfere with walking. There is often wasting and myotonia of the facial muscles, the sternomastoids, and the muscles of the forearm. Most patients with this condition are unaware of the muscle stiffness and come to medical attention because of the distal muscle wasting and weakness.

ATAXIA

Irregular failure of coordination in purposeful movement generally is attributed to disease of the cerebellum or its tracts. Except for their temporal course, the symptoms are qualitatively indistinguishable, whether lesions are confined to the tracts of the cerebellar peduncles, as in hereditary degenerations, to the cortex, as in degeneration due to distant carcinoma or other toxic effect (*e.g.*, excessive phenytoin medication), to single focal lesions, such as tumor or infarction, or to scattered lesions of the cerebellum and its brain-stem tracts, as in multiple sclerosis.

Limbs affected by cerebellar lesions have some degree of hypotonia and weakness, and difficulty in maintaining a stable position against gravity. When the hand is directed toward a target, the movement tends to decompose into oscillations toward either side of the target with a crescendo increase of amplitude, finally arrested to greater or less degree when the target is reached. This is called intention tremor. Similar

dysfunction in respiratory and bulbar musculature produces explosive, scanning, dysarthric speech.

Stretch reflexes are normal in amplitude, but the hypotonic state may be seen in pendulous oscillations following the initial contraction. This is particularly evident for the knee jerk.

Although Sherrington defined the cerebellum as the head ganglion of the proprioceptive system, more recent studies have shown that afferent pathways from skin, ear, and eye also project to the cerebellum. Patients with cerebellar lesions have no sensory loss, and the function of these projections is unknown.

Recent electrophysiologic analysis of cerebellar circuitry indicates a complex series of predominately inhibitory mechanisms in cerebellar cortex finally impinging through the cortical Purkinje cell output as inhibition of the cerebellar nuclei, which have an excitatory projection rostrally to the red nucleus and thalamus. Thus, it is proposed that cerebellar modulation of movement is primarily an inhibitory phenomenon.

It is of related interest, because major cerebellar projections are rostrally directed, that in waking monkeys conditioned to perform repetitive simple motor tasks, movement-correlated neuronal discharge in cerebellar nuclei slightly precedes that in motor cortex.

Walshe has emphasized that cerebellar symptoms are not present when there is superposed affliction of the cerebrospinal pathways.[25] This has also been shown when a pyramidal tract lesion is superposed on a cerebellar lesion in monkeys.[26] In the monkeys, improvement is reported following lesions of the pallidum, and in humans, following contralateral thalamic lesions.[27] Thus, the cerebellum is implicated in motor behavior in relation to forebrain projection rather than directly in organization at the spinal level. The theory that cerebellar symptoms are due to fusimotor hypotonia has not been confirmed.[22] Some current theories of the mechanism of cerebellar symptoms reduce to the absurd position that the function of the normal cerebellum is to prevent cerebellar ataxia. No more satisfactory explanation has been brought forward.

There is some degree of somatotopic localization of the cerebellum in that midline lesions of the vermis tend to be related to instability and ataxia of the trunk, whereas lesions of the medial anterior lobe produce predominance of lower extremity symptoms. The upper extremities may be involved by more lateral posterior lesions. If the dentate nucleus is spared, large ablations of neocerebellum may produce very little disability. Because the major cerebellar afferent paths and its efferent tract in the superior peduncle as far as the midbrain are uncrossed, unilateral cerebellar lesions produce ipsilateral ataxia.

Behavior resembling cerebellar symptomatology may occur in other conditions. The fact that frontal lobe

tumors may simulate contralateral cerebellar lesions has not been explained satisfactorily. The fact that ablation of the frontal lobe does not produce such symptoms has led to the argument that the phenomenon is due to distortion of brainstem structures by the mass of the tumor. Occasionally, a cerebral lesion that affects both precentral and parietal regions, associated with loss of position and localization sense, may also result in ataxia, whether the eyes are open or closed.

Severe proprioceptive loss, such as occurs most typically with degeneration of large nerve fibers in dorsal roots and dorsal columns in tabes dorsalis (due to syphilis), may result in a movement ataxia that is exaggerated when visuomotor control is removed by closing the eyes. Other signs of dorsal root affection include shooting pains and absent muscle stretch reflexes. Occasionally, too, the weakness associated with neuropathy affecting the motor nerves, or even a debilitating systemic disease, may cause ataxia.

DYSTONIA

Dystonia, a term indicating disordered muscle tone, usually is used more specifically to define conditions like *dystonia musculorum deformans,* in which there are severe tonic distortions of posture and movement most conspicuously affecting truncal, neck, and proximal limb musculature. Jung and Hassler have called the dystonic syndrome *proximal athetosis*.[28] Denny–Brown uses the term in a more literal and general sense as a relatively fixed attitude, emphasizing early distortions of limb movement as the disease develops.[21] Degenerative lesions seem to be primarily but not exclusively in the putamen, with thalamic and cortical involvement. However, it must be noted that in dystonia musculorum deformans, no neuropathologic findings of significance have been described; a pathophysiologic dysfunction must be assumed. Dystonic rigidity may be the major finding in juvenile and preterminal patients with Huntington's chorea, in which the most impressive degeneration is the caudate nucleus. The pathophysiology of dystonia is poorly defined. Denny–Brown believes that this released activity is a common feature of the advanced stages of the other basal ganglia conditions, and that it represents released contactual reflexes.

The increased motor-neuron activity level probably represents a release effected at an internuncial level of spinal cord or brain stem, as in parkinsonism, rather than at the final common path, as in spasticity.[60]

ATHETOSIS

Denny–Brown has defined athetosis in relation to its literal meaning of lack of fixation or stability of position, but it is used generally to define a condition with bizarre, wormlike distortions of movement, particularly affecting the hands, distal limb segments, and face. When affected extremities are quiet, there is no resistance to passive movement. The abnormal movements are usually irregular and tend to be stereotyped (*e.g.,* hyperextension of the fingers with hyperflexion at the wrists). Lesions affect the putamen predominantly. Denny–Brown believes that the instability represents the competition for expression of an approach reaction to cutaneous stimulation released by lesions of the precentral cerebral system, with avoidance reaction released by lesions of the parietal lobe system. Usually the symptoms are present from birth, although the condition rarely develops progressively. Athetosis is often associated with the spontaneous movements of chorea.

Tabetic athetosis is associated with severe loss of proprioceptive sense due to dorsal root and dorsal column disease. Irregular small movements of the distal extremities, particularly the fingers, occur during posture maintenance, and sometimes at rest. It has been suggested that the phenomenon represents denervation sensitization of motoneurons.[29]

SPONTANEOUS MOVEMENT

FIBRILLATION

Spontaneous, often rhythmic, contractions of individual muscle fibers constitute *fibrillation*.[30,31] Because normal muscle fibers are less than one tenth of a millimeter in diameter, and because atrophied fibers are even smaller, it is obvious that these contractions are not usually visible. Occasionally, fine vermicular movements can be seen when the affected muscle is in the tongue or underlies thin skin over portions of the hand. Elsewhere, they are detected by EMG as brief (1 msec), low-voltage potentials uninfluenced by voluntary effort.

The most common cause of fibrillation is separation of muscle fibers from their motoneuron, whether the lesion occurs at cord, root, or peripheral nerve. The orphaned muscle fibers undergo progressive atrophy for a month or more, during which there are also progressive physiologic changes. Instead of the normal localized sensitivity to acetylcholine at the end-plate, the fiber becomes equally sensitive over its entire surface.[32] There are also changes in the electrical characteristics of the membrane, so that adaptation to a continuous, stimulating electric current does not occur. Whereas normal muscle fibers contract only at the onset of a continuous threshold current, denervated fibers fire repetitively throughout the flow of current

and at lower threshold. There is also an increase in mechanical excitability; fibrillations are stirred up readily by movement of an EMG recording needle electrode. They are diminished by cooling. Although they may persist for many years after nerve section, they may not be present if there is excessive fibrosis. When motor axons grow back to form effective contact, threshold for electrical stimulation rises and fibrillation disappears before spontaneous innervated movement occurs.

Increased muscle fiber irritability and frank persistent fibrillation are seen sometimes in primary myopathies, particularly those that develop very rapidly, such as polymyositis.[33] The diffuse inflammatory reaction may produce direct changes in muscle-membrane irritability and also may effectively produce denervation by the destruction of muscle fiber segments between motor end-plates and surviving segments. Fibrillations are observed quite rarely in muscular dystrophy. Disappearance of previously observed fibrillations in polymyositis may serve as a measure of therapeutic clinical improvement.

FASCICULATION

Fasciculation is defined as the spontaneous isolated contraction of individual motor units. The muscle fibers supplied by a single motoneuron produce a brief twitch of a muscle fascicle, the size being larger in large muscles. Normal motor units in limb muscles may include many hundreds of muscle fibers, whereas those of the extraocular muscles contain only a few. Fasciculations usually occur irregularly at slow frequencies, ranging from once every several seconds to 2 or 3 a second.

Fasciculations are most notorious as a sign of diffuse motoneuron disease in amyotrophic lateral sclerosis. Curiously, these patients practically never complain of fasciculation and come to medical attention because of muscle weakness. By EMG the fasciculation units in this disease are often several-fold larger and more polyphasic than normal.[34] This seems to be because surviving motoneurons put out collateral axon branches to reinnervate orphaned muscle fibers. The hyperexcitability of the motoneuron in this condition extends beyond the cell body. Fasciculations have been observed to persist when the motor nerve is blocked or even severed. This hyperirritability, plus that related to newly growing axonal sprouts, may explain why muscle percussion is a useful technique for bringing out latent fasciculation.

Fasciculations also occur with other varieties of spinal cord disease. They may be seen associated with the early inflammatory reaction of poliomyelitis, or chronically, when the cord is damaged by neoplasm, compression, or scar.

Benign fasciculation commonly is seen in normal subjects, often when they are tense, anxious, or overfatigued. Neurologists in a medical schools are accustomed to visits from medical students who become concerned about themselves after hearing a lecture about amyotrophic lateral sclerosis. In middle age and beyond, benign fasciculations of the calf muscles are common. Benign twitches are not intrinsically different from those seen with motoneuron disease, except that the giant, more irregularly shaped fasciculation potentials are not seen in the EMG. Nor are there muscle fibrillations, atrophy, or weakness.

Nerve root compression may give rise to localized fasciculation more often than does peripheral-nerve compression. These fasciculations may be single, or they may be a brief tetanus of 2 to several action potentials at a rate of 60 to 100 per second. These fasciculations may appear more prolonged to visual inspection than do the usual single twitches.

Myokymia is a benign condition of unknown mechanism in which the patient may complain of spontaneous muscle twitching that characteristically occurs in the multiple high-frequency pattern.[35] This symptom is usually present in the calf muscles, but it may be generalized.

The involuntary muscle contraction of shivering looks like, and is by definition, fasciculation, although the discharge rate is faster. Thus it is important that the patient be examined for pathologic fasciculation in a warm environment. Fasciculations often are seen with electrolyte disturbance in toxic states like uremia. Contraction fasciculation is purposeful movement in muscles reduced to a very few motor units by a disease process.

SPASM

Spasm is a marked, if not violent, contraction of a muscle or group of muscles which is often but not always painful. The most common variety is common muscle cramp. It may occur in normal subjects when a muscle is contracted maximally, especially if it is in the shortened position as when the triceps surae is strongly contracted with the foot plantar-flexed. Once the cramp is set up, it cannot be stopped by relaxation, but may be resolved by massage and passive extension. The EMG during cramp shows high frequencies of unit discharge, several times the 20 to 30 per second seen in normal movement.[36] Cramp may occur more readily after excessive exercise, in patients with peripheral vascular disease, and in patients with motoneuron disease. Its mechanism is not known.

The spasm of tetany occurs predominantly in the distal extremities (carpopedal spasm), with the characteristic flexion of fingers and hands and flexion of toes with inversion of feet. It is due to low concentration of Ca^{++} in the serum. Low blood calcium may be caused by hypoparathyroidism, in which characteristic tetany develops spontaneously. Hyperventilation from any cause may produce respiratory alkalosis, with resultant lowering of Ca^{++} concentration and associated tetany, even when the total serum calcium is normal. Excitability of isolated nerve fibers is increased in a medium containing subnormal Ca^{++} concentration. Synaptic responsiveness of neuron somata likewise is exaggerated and may be manifested clinically as convulsions.

The diagnosis of tetany may be suggested by revealing latent tetany when it is not overtly present. Increased mechanical irritability is shown by the twitching of facial muscles evoked by tapping the cheek over the facial nerve (Chvostek's sign). Irritability is exaggerated by the metabolic effects of ischemia, as shown by carpal spasm following occlusion of forearm circulation by a cuff (Trousseau's sign).

Tetany in hypoparathyroidism follows primary elevation of serum phosphorus, with consequent fall in Ca^{++}. Renal disease (glomerular insufficiency) may produce similar hyperphosphatemia and hypocalcemia with tetany, as may excessive phosphorus ingestion. Other possible causes of symptomatic hypocalcemia include low calcium intake, high intestinal-calcium loss (vitamin-D deficiency, sprue, diarrhea), high urinary loss of calcium (essential hypercalciuria, renal tubular acidosis).

Tetanus toxin may provoke localized, sustained muscle contraction, in the beginning only as a prolongation of normal movement, later as sustained contraction. Such a condition may last for many days. Systemic spread of the toxin affects the muscles of mastication early and produces trismus. In addition to the increased neuromuscular excitability, there may be similar effects within the spinal cord attributable to block of synaptic inhibition of motor neurons.

A condition of unknown etiology with some clinical similarity to tetanus is persistent, involuntary muscle contraction (the stiff man syndrome). The mechanism of the often dramatic improvement with diazepam administration is also unknown. An even rarer similar condition, in which the disturbance has been localized to irritability of motor axons, responds remarkably to phenytoin.[61]

Postdenervation muscle spasm most commonly affects the facial musculature after nerve regeneration from Bell's palsy. There may be background activity of single motor units in the multiple fasciculation pattern of myokymia along with intermittent high-frequency bursts of one or more units associated with the clinical spasm. Here, as in nerve-root compression, one suspects a primary hyperirritable state in the proximal portion of the motor axon.

Generalized recurrent muscle spasm may be seen in many varieties of diffuse neuronal irritation, such as virus infection (rabies), strychnine poisoning, and various subacute degenerative neuronal diseases.

TREMOR

The term *tremor* implies a relatively continuous state during which individual muscle contraction varies in a rhythmic pattern. Parkinsonian tremor (paralysis agitans) is characteristically a tremor of rest. There is a regular contraction at 4 to 7 per second, which is most prominent in the upper extremities, producing the characteristic pill-rolling movement in the hand with spread to involve proximal muscles. Less often, tremor may involve the lower extremities and the facial muscles. During active movement, the silent periods between motor unit bursts may be filled in by contraction of the same and other motor units as the tremor becomes less evident or disappears, only to reappear as the limb comes to a new resting position.[37] However, sometimes this filling in does not occur, and movement may be produced by increased amplitude of tremor bursts. In most cases there is reciprocal relaxation of antagonistic muscles. However, there may be overflow contraction in the antagonists that is a handicap to movement. Thus, muscle contraction may occur in agonists and antagonists without gross movement. Cogwheel rigidity with passive movement in parkinsonian patients reflects a basic tremor, regardless of whether it is visually apparent. Tremor may increase during active movement, and may vary spontaneously, or even independently, in antagonistic muscles.

As noted previously, we believe that resting tremor is essentially a segmental phenomenon of reciprocal reaction to a tonic efferent discharge released by forebrain lesions.[57] The rhythm and reciprocal relationships are like those of clonus released by corticospinal tract damage. Unlike clonus, the stretch reflexes are not increased, but stretch receptor function is essential for the maintenance of both conditions because both are stopped by local anesthetic block of fusimotor fibers and consequent desensitization of muscle spindles, or by dorsal root section.[22] Shivering provides a useful physiologic model because the involuntary hypothalamic discharge produced by cooling leads first to diffuse muscle contraction and then to alternating reciprocal clonus.[38] Liberson has shown that when the

median nerve is stimulated electrically in a patient with parkinsonian tremor, the hand tremor rhythm is reset so that the next burst after the shock comes at the same interval as that between preceding and succeeding spontaneous bursts.[39] This resetting could hardly occur if the tremor pattern were established elsewhere than in the segmental level concerned. Moreover, although tremor may be affected by stimulation of various deep brain structures, no gross ganglionic tremor rhythms have been recorded from them. Tremor rhythm has been detected in single neurons of thalamic nucleus ventralis lateralis, but there is no basis for believing that this represents anything other than the normal afferent activity triggered by the tremor itself.[62]

Denny–Brown has observed in some patients with hepatolenticular (Wilson's) disease the evolution of less regular athetosis into regular tremor.[21] He believes that tremor, like athetosis, represents antagonistic movement patterns released by deranged forebrain mechanisms. He also believes that tremor primarily relates to lesions of the inner globus pallidus. However, concerning neuropathologic findings in parkinsonism, it is fair to say that there is no widely accepted correlation of symptoms with specific lesions. It is certain that parkinsonian symptoms may be associated with various degrees and distributions of pathologic findings among several basal forebrain structures.

Parkinson himself observed that resting tremor disappears in the limbs affected by hemiplegia, only to return if there is sufficient recovery of voluntary movement. Thus, it may be presumed that some pyramidal tract tonic activity is necessary for the maintenance of the abnormal movement. Indeed, Bucy suggests that therapeutic lesions aimed at the globus pallidus or thalamus to relieve tremor do so by inadvertent damage to the internal capsule.[40] Lesions in the thalamus seem more likely to produce good results. Whatever the mechanism, it is not specific to resting tremor. Symptoms of dystonia, chorea, essential tremor, and ataxic intention tremor also are said to be improved by the same lesion.[41,42,43,44] When the underlying disease process is progressive, relief of symptoms by brain lesions is usually transient.

Purdon–Martin believes that the pallidum is released to excessive activity by lesions of the substantia nigra, that the pallidum is the major efferent path of the basal forebrain neuronal complex, and that this explains why lesions of the pallidum may be helpful.[27,45]

Although some workers have reported that monkeys with ventral midbrain lesions simulate parkinsonian resting tremor, the results are inconstant and difficult to relate anatomically to the human condition. Thus, there is no convenient experimental model. The ventralis lateralis nucleus of the thalamus, which seems to

be the most effective target for therapeutic lesions, is a site of convergence of pathways ascending from the cerebellum and basal ganglia to the motor cortex.[63] Obviously, neural activity leading to behavioral movement must descend from the cortex by both pyramidal and extrapyramidal routes, and probably from other brain structures as well. Carman's concepts of "state of balance" of motor pathways, an origin of tremor rhythm in the thalamus, "imbalance or deficiency in the total input," a special central control of the fusimotor system, or the provision to cortex of "inappropriate information" from the thalamus, are unsupported by or are contradictory to facts, or else they are so vague that they have no operational significance that is subject to test.[63] The paradoxical relative preservation of voluntary movement as abnormal movement is suppressed by thalamic lesions remains a tantalizing problem.

Senile tremor may be related to the parkinsonian variety. Head tremor is conspicuous and the hand tremor may be exaggerated by movement. It is seldom disabling, and rigidity is not significant. Essential or heredofamilial tremor usually becomes evident in adolescence. There is a regular alternating tremor of the outstretched hands, usually somewhat faster than that of parkinsonism, but not present at rest. The tremor may be exaggerated during movement, diminishing at termination. Patients afflicted with this condition often can do remarkably fine work in spite of the tremor during limb transit. The condition usually is not progressive and there is no rigidity. Pathologic and physiologic bases are unknown. Propranolol has been reported to produce therapeutic improvement. Alcohol also helps. Flapping, or wing-beating, tremor of the outstretched hands in hepatolenticular degeneration (Wilson's disease, due to toxic accumulation of copper in the liver and brain as a result of genetic metabolic disorder) is slower than parkinsonian tremor, is less prominent or absent at rest, but has both clinical and pathologic features related to parkinsonism and athetosis. The lesions are most prominent in the putamen.

The liver flap, first described in other varieties of severe liver disease, is called *asterixis*. It also has been seen in other severe metabolic disorders, renal or pulmonary. Affected patients have clinical and EEG evidence of diffuse encephalopathy. Irregular lapses of muscle contraction shown by EMG are manifested clinically as an irregular 4 to 10 per second metabolic tremor or by sudden lapse of posture in the outstretched hands when the silences are prolonged (asterixis).[64] The symptom seems to indicate a limited capacity of the toxic brain to maintain a steady state of motor outflow.

Tremor attributed to midbrain lesions has features

relating to both the parkinsonian and cerebellar syndromes.[21] The resting tremor tends to be variable and includes pronation and supination of the forearm and protraction of the shoulder. With movement, the tremor may resemble the intention pattern of cerebellar disease.

The tremor of hyperthyroidism is irregular, rapid, and fine; it is maintained by tonic contraction of active muscles. It is not easily confused with those tremors due to neurologic lesions. The tremor of anxiety states may be similar or more coarse, but it is faster than parkinsonian tremor, and usually does not show the parkinsonian alteration in antagonists. The tremulousness seen in various chronic alcoholic conditions is manifest during movement, is irregular, unsteady, and slow, but not ataxic in the usual sense. It is probably related to asterixis.

CHOREA

The name of this symptom is derived from the Greek word for dance. Involuntary movements at rest are irregular, jerky, and highly varied; a finger or hand may twitch or flick in any direction. Often, minor movements are covered up by the patient's concealing them beneath some quasi-purposeful movement like scratching. Irregular twitching movements of the tongue, the face, and the lower extremities are usual. In advanced cases the movements involve whole extremities, and the patient may be bedridden.

Symptomatic relief may be obtained from reserpine, phenothiazine and benzodiazapine derivatives, which can produce the parkinsonian syndrome. Haloperidol is considered the drug of choice. Sedatives also may be helpful.

In hereditary chorea (Huntington) there is progressive degeneration of the striatum, particularly the caudate nucleus, but degeneration is also more widespread. Muscle tone and the ability to move purposefully between abnormal movements are normal, as are the reflexes. Denny–Brown emphasizes a continual flow of motion in chorea, but this is not present in early cases. He proposes that choreic movement, like athetosis, is a manifestation of conflicting movement biases triggered by sensory input, and released by the striatal lesions. Others propose damage to an inhibitory system with consequent release of abnormal function. The possibility of a discharging lesion is not excluded.

In rheumatic chorea (Sydenham) the pathologic findings that have been described are quite diffuse and nonspecific. The choreic symptoms are possibly due to anoxia related to rheumatic arteritis or to an autoimmune process. Some authors believe that the movements of this disease can be distinguished from Huntington's chorea. Chorea or parkinsonism may result from carbon-monoxide poisoning.

Chorea sometimes develops in the older age group without a family history. The lesions are thought to be similar to those of the hereditary variety . Hemichorea may occur following a vascular lesion in the internal capsule region. As the patient recovers from hemiparesis, the permanent lesion of the striatum manifests itself in the abnormal movements.

BALLISM

Ballism is usually present unilaterally following a contralateral lesion in or near the subthalamic nucleus of Luys.[27,45] Affected extremities undergo extreme flinging movements with such vigorous involvement of proximal muscles that the patient may injure other portions of his body or head. There may be slight weakness. Purposeful movement can be carried out between the abnormal ones. Whether these movements differ more than in degree from those of Huntington's chorea has been debated. Denny–Brown emphasizes the rotatory movements in ballism, together with internal rotation at elbow and wrist.[21] This syndrome can be reproduced by experimental lesions in the monkey and, as in humans, it can be relieved by secondary lesions in the pallidum or thalamus. Such movements also are diminished by motor cortex or pyramidal tract lesions.[26] Again, the symptoms are explained as a manifestation of released inhibitory control.

OCULOGYRIC CRISES

Oculogyric crises are involuntary tonic upward movement of the eye that may last from minutes to hours. The patient may be able to look downward briefly, but the abnormal movement soon overcomes his effort. The condition is seen in postencephalitic parkinsonism and also in the parkinsonian syndrome due to phenothiazine drugs. It is presumably due to a disorder of upper brain-stem function.

TORTICOLLIS AND TIC

Localized movements of the neck musculature and twitching movements of limbs, face, and tongue are probably related to pathophysiologic disturbances of basal ganglia even though examples of clinicopathologic correlation are exceptional. The concept that they are psychogenic is poorly supported by facts, and psychotherapy is notoriously not helpful. The tics and coprolalia of the probably genetically determined Gilles de la Tourette syndrome are often alleviated by haloperidol.

PALATAL MYOCLONUS

This is a regular rhythmic elevation of the palate at a frequency of 1 to 2 per second, persisting even during sleep in many cases. Concomitant synchronous or asynchronous movements may occur in facial, extraocular, and respiratory muscles. Lesions of various etiologies have been associated, but always in the brainstem region bounded by the inferior olivary nucleus, dentate nucleus, and red nucleus. The mechanism is unknown.

CLONIC CONVULSIVE MOVEMENTS

Focal motor seizures most often affect the thumb and fingers, the great toe, or the perioral region, presumably because the motor cortex has powerful direct corticomotoneuronal connections to these distal muscles.[51] The strong muscle contractions are brief tetani, rhythmic or irregular, and are impossible to control by effort. The movements are produced by sudden bursts of high-frequency discharge into the pyramidal tract. In general, such seizures connote abnormal discharge in the motor cortex rather than in subcortical regions. Clonic jerks may sometimes build up into tonic prolonged contractions, usually with spread to other areas (jacksonian seizure).

Short rhythmic bursts of muscle jerks (myoclonus), at the brain-wave rhythm of 2 to 3 per second, may involve whole limbs or parts of limbs in children with convulsive disorder. Such myoclonic seizures occur with diffuse neuronal disease at any age.

SUMMARY

Disturbances of function of striated muscle are related to disease of muscle, the motoneurons, the spinal cord, or the brain. Varieties of dysfunction include weakness, distortions of posture, movement, and coordination, abnormal reflexes, distortions of muscle tone, and spontaneous movements. Pathophysiologic analysis must include consideration of the function of uninjured tissue when normal structures are destroyed or become pathologically overactive. In many areas, pathophysiologic understanding lags far behind clinicopathologic correlation.

REFERENCES

1. **Walshe FMR:** Contributions of John Hughlings Jackson to neurology. A brief introduction to his teachings. Arch Neurol 5:119, 1961
2. **Walton JN, Nattrass FJ:** On the classification, natural history and treatment of the myopathies. Brain 77:169, 1954
3. **Adams RD, Denny–Brown DE, Pearson CM:** Diseases of Muscle. A Study in Pathology, 2nd ed. New York, Hoeber–Harper, 1962
4. **Greenfield JG, Cornman T, Shy GM:** The prognostic value of the muscle biopsy in the "floppy infant." Brain 81:461, 1958
5. **Greenfield JG, Shy GM, Alvord EC et al:** An Atlas of Muscle Pathology in Neuromuscular Diseases. London, Livingstone, 1957
6. **Grob D, Johns RJ, Harvey AM:** Studies in neuromuscular function. IV. Stimulating and depressant effects of acetylcholine and choline in patients with myasthenia gravis and their relationship to the defect in neuromuscular transmission. Bull Johns Hopkins Hosp 99:153, 1956
7. **Churchill–Davidson HC, Richardson AT:** Neuromuscular transmission in myasthenia gravis. J Physiol 122:252, 1953
8. **Dahlback O, Elmqvist D, Johns TR et al:** An electrophysiologic study of the neuromuscular junction in myasthenia gravis. J Physiol 156:336, 1961
9. **Aharonov A, Abramsky O, Tarrab–Hazdai R et al:** Humoral antibodies to acetylcholine receptor in patients with myasthenia gravis. Lancet 7930:340–341, 1975
10. **Drachman DB:** Myasthenia gravis. N Engl J Med 298:136, 186, 1978
11. **Eaton LM, Lambert EH:** Electromyography and electric stimulation of nerves in disease of motor unit. Observations on myasthenic syndrome associated with malignant tumors. JAMA 163:1117, 1957
12. **Lambert EH:** Clinical Examinations in Neurology, Chap 15. Philadelphia, WB Saunders, 1957
13. **Weaver RA, Landau WM, Higgins J:** Fusimotor function. II. Evidence of fusimotor depression in human spinal shock. Arch Neurol 9:127, 1963
14. **Teasdall RD, Stavraky GW:** Responses of deafferented spinal neurons to cortico-spinal impulses. J Neurophysiol 16:367, 1953
15. **McCouch GP, Austin GM, Liu CM et al:** Sprouting as a cause of spasticity. J Neurophysiol 21:205, 1958
16. **Meltzer GE, Hunt RS, Landau WM:** Fusimotor function. III. The spastic monkey. Arch Neurol 9:133, 1963
17. **Beevor C:** Remarks on paralysis of the movements of the trunk in hemiplegia, and the muscles which are affected. Br Med J 1:881, 1909
18. **Twitchell TE:** The restoration of motor function following hemiplegia in man. Brain 74:443, 1951
19. **Landau WM, Clare MH:** The plantar reflex in man, with special reference to some conditions where the extensor response is unexpectedly absent. Brain 82:321, 1959
20. **Efron R:** Post-epileptic paralysis: Theoretical critique and report of a case. Brain 84:381, 1961
21. **Denny–Brown DE:** The Basal Ganglia and Their Relation to Disorders of Movement. London, Oxford University Press, 1962
22. **Landau WM, Weaver RA, Hornbein TV:** Fusimotor nerve function in man: Differential nerve block studies in nor-

mal subjects and in spasticity and rigidity. Arch Neurol 3:10, 1960

23. **Landau WM:** The essential mechanism in myotonia. An electromyographic study. Neurology 2:369, 1952

24. **Norris FH, Jr:** Unstable membrane potential in human myotonic muscle. Electroencephalog Clin Neurophysiol 14:197, 1962

25. **Walshe FMR:** The significance of the voluntary element in the genesis of cerebellar ataxy. Brain 50:377, 1927

26. **Carpenter MB:** Brainstem and infratentorial neuraxis in experimental dyskinesia. Arch Neurol 5:504, 1961

27. **Martin JP:** Further remarks on the functions of the basal ganglia. Lancet 1:1362, 1960

28. **Jung R, Hassler R:** The extrapyramidal motor system. In Handbook of Physiology, Vol. 2, Sect. 1, Chap 35, p 863. Washington DC, American Physiological Society, 1960

29. **Moldaver J:** Contribution at l'étude de la regulation réflexe des movements. Arch Intern Med Exp 11:405, 1938

30. **Denny–Brown D, Pennybacker J:** Fibrillation and fasciculation in voluntary muscle. Brain 61:311, 1938

31. **Landau WM:** Synchronization of potentials and response to direct current stimulation in denervated mammalian muscle. Electroencephalog Clin Neurophysiol 3:169, 1951

32. **Thesleff S:** Effects of motor innervation on the chemical sensitivity of skeletal muscle. Physiol Rev 40:734, 1960

33. **Lambert EH, Sayre GP, Eaton LM:** Electrical activity of muscle in polymyositis. Trans Am Neurol Assoc 79:64, 1954

34. **Erminio F, Buchthal F, Rosenfalck P:** Motor unit territory and muscle fibre concentration in paresis due to peripheral nerve injury and anterior horn cell involvement. Neurology 9:657, 1957

35. **Denny–Brown D, Foley JM:** Myokymia and the benign fasciculation of muscular cramps. Trans Assoc Am Physicians 61:88, 1948

36. **Norris FH, Jr, Gasteiger EL, Chatfield PO:** An electromyographic study of induced and spontaneous muscle cramps. Electroencephalog Clin Neurophysiol 9:139, 1957

37. **Bishop GH, Clare MH, Price J:** Patterns of tremor in normal and pathological conditions. J Appl Physiol 1:123, 1948

38. **Denny–Brown D, Gaylord JB, Uprus V:** Note on the nature of the motor discharge in shivering. Brain 58:233, 1935

39. **Liberson WT:** Monosynaptic reflexes and their clinical significance. Electroencephalog Clin Neurophysiol [Suppl] 22:79, 1962

40. **Bucy PC:** The cortico-spinal tract and tremor. In Pathogenesis and Treatment of Parkinsonism, p 271. Springfield, Charles C Thomas, 1958

41. **Cooper IS:** Neurosurgical Alleviation of Parkinsonism. Springfield, Charles C Thomas, 1956

42. **Cooper IS:** Neurosurgical alleviation of intention tremor of multiple sclerosis and cerebellar disease. N Engl J Med 263:441, 1960

43. **Cooper IS:** Heredofamiliar tremor abolition by chemothalamectomy. Arch Neurol 7:129, 1962

44. **Cooper IS:** Dystonia reversal by operation on basal ganglia. Arch Neurol 7:132, 1962

45. **Martin JP:** Remarks on the function of the basal ganglia. Lancet 1:999, 1959

46. **Salter RH:** The muscle glycogenoses. Lancet 1:1301, 1968

47. **Brooks JE:** Hyperkalemic periodic paralysis. Intracellular electromyographic studies. Arch Neurol 20:13, 1969

48. **Thesleff S:** Acetylcholine utilization in myasthenia gravis. Ann NY Acad Sci 135:195, 1966

49. **Desmedt JE:** Presynaptic mechanisms in myasthenia gravis. Ann NY Acad Sci 135:209, 1966

50. **Elmqvist D, Lambert EH:** Neuromuscular transmission in patient with the myasthenic syndrome sometimes associated with bronchogenic carcinoma. Mayo Clin Proc 43:689, 1968

51. **Phillips CG:** Corticomotoneuronal organization. Projection from the arm area of the baboon's motor cortex. Arch Neurol 17:188, 1967

52. **Lewis R, Brindley GS:** The extrapyramidal motor map. Brain 88:397, 1965

53. **Lawrence DG, Kuypers GJM:** The functional organization of the motor system in the monkey. II. The effects of lesions of the descending brain-stem pathways. Brain 91:15, 1968

54. **Landau WM, Clare MH:** Fusimotor function. Part VI. H reflex, tendon jerk, and reinforcement in hemiplegia. Arch Neurol 10:26, 1964

55. **Dietrichson P:** Phasic ankle reflex in spasticity and parkinsonian rigidity. The role of the fusimotor system. Acta Neurol Scand 47:22–51, 1971

56. **Feldman MH:** The decerebrate state in the primate. Arch Neurol 25:501–525, 1971

57. **Landau WM, Struppler A, Mehls O:** A comparative electromyographic study of the reactions to passive movement in parkinsonism and in normal subjects. Neurology 16:34, 1966

58. **Cotzias GC, Van Woert MH, Schiffer LM:** Aromatic amino acids and modification of parkinsonism. N Engl J Med 276:374, 1967

59. **Winer N, Martt JM, Somers JE et al:** Induced myotonia in man and goat. J Lab Clin Med 66:758, 1965

60. **Landau WM, Clare MH:** Pathophysiology of the tonic innervation phenomenon in the foot. Arch Neurol 15:252, 1966

61. **Wallis WE, Van Poznak A, Plum F:** Generalized muscular stiffness, fasciculations, and myokymia of peripheral nerve origin. Arch Neurol 22:430, 1970

62. **Jasper HH, Bertrand G:** Thalamic units involved in somatic sensation and voluntary and involuntary movements in man. In Purpura DP, Yahr MD (eds): The Thalamus, pp 364–390. New York; London, Columbia University Press, 1966

63. **Carman JB:** Anatomic basis of surgical treatment of Parkinson's disease. N Engl J Med 279:919, 1968

64. **Leavitt S, Tyler HR:** Studies in asterixis. Arch Neurol 10:360, 1964

33

Fainting (Syncope) Roger B. Hickler
John P. Howe, III

Definition
Etiological Classification
Pathogenesis
Acute Reduction in Cerebral Blood Flow
  Cardiac Disorders
  Vascular Obstruction
  Failure of Venous Return
  Loss of Peripheral Vascular Tone
    Etiology and Anatomic Level of Defect
    Physiologic and Pharmacologic Tests
    Clinical Considerations
    Cholinergic As Well As Adrenergic Neural
      Deficits

  Cerebrovascular Disease
Disturbance in Composition of Blood Flowing to
  the Brain
  Hypoglycemia
  Hypocapnia
  Hypoxia
Neurophysiologic Factors
  Nonconvulsive Seizures
  Conversion Reaction—Hysteria
  Cerebral Type of Carotid Sinus Syncope
Summary

DEFINITION

Fainting and *syncope* are terms commonly used interchangeably to describe a transient loss or near loss of consciousness caused by reversible disturbances in cerebral function from (1) transient ischemia, (2) changes in composition of blood perfusing the brain, and (3) nonconvulsive changes in the pattern of central nervous system activity. Syncope should be distinguished from the following disorders: epilepsy, cataplexy, strokes, vertigo, and bouts of episodic weakness (*e.g.,* myasthenia gravis, and periodic familial paralysis).

ETIOLOGICAL CLASSIFICATION

I. Acute Reduction in Cerebral Blood Flow
  A. Cardiac disorders
    1. Disorders of cardiac rate and rhythm—Morgagni, Adams–Stokes attacks, ventricular fibrillation, cardioinhibitory attacks as in cardiac type of carotid sinus syncope and so forth
    2. Valvular heart disease "Effort syncope" associated with aortic stenosis and regurgitation, pulmonic stenosis, obstruction of mitral valve orifice owing to ball-valve thrombus or myxoma of the left atrium, and so forth
    3. Myocardial disorders Infarction, subaortic stenosis, and so forth
    4. Congenital heart disease
  B. Vascular obstruction
    1. Primary pulmonary hypertension
    2. Acute pulmonary embolism
    3. Acute aortic dissection
  C. Failure of venous return
    1. Increased intrathoracic pressure—Valsalva maneuver, cough, "fainting lark," breath-holding, and so forth

2. Decreased blood volume
   a) Rapid internal losses
      (1) Blood—massive hematoma; bleeding into lumen of bowel, thorax, abdomen; and so forth
      (2) Fluid—allergic reactions; septicemia; ascites (peritonitis, pancreatitis); dumping syndrome; and so forth
   b) Rapid external losses
      (1) Blood—hemorrhage (laceration, gastrointestinal, and so forth)
      (2) Fluid—third-degree burns, extensive dermatitis, vomiting, diarrhea, polyuria (*e.g.*, diabetic, and so forth)
3. Increased venous capacity
   a) Large varicosities, especially of the saphenous system
   b) Venomotor paralysis from drugs, especially nitrites-nitrates (*e.g.*, nitroglycerin, nitroprusside).
D. Loss of Peripheral Vascular Tone
   1. Vasodepressor syncope—active dilitation of resistance vessels
      Many conditioning and sensory afferent precipitating factors such as sensitive carotid sinus, fear, fatigue and debilitation, prolonged standing, instrumentation (such as venipuncture), removal of large volumes of fluid from body cavities (such as micturition and thoracentesis), and so forth
   2. Orthostatic hypotension owing to failure of baroreflex arc at any level
      a) Visceral afferents from baroreceptors—tabes dorsalis and as part of a polyneuropathy (*e.g.*, diabetic)
      b) Brain, especially hypothalamus and brainstem—tumors, multiple infarcts, drugs (*e.g.*, chlorpromazine, L-dopa)
      c) Visceral efferents from the brain
         (1) Spinal cord (intermediolateral column)—pernicious anemia, Shy-Drager syndrome
         (2) Paravertebral ganglia—familial dysautonomia, thoracolumbar sympathectomy, ganglionic blocking agents
         (3) Peripheral efferents—polyneuritis-polyneuropathy (*e.g.*, diabetic, amyloid, porphyric, toxic)
         (4) Sympathetic nerve-ending failure—idiopathic
      d) Unresponsive microvasculature—adrenergic blocking agents, prolonged bed rest, advanced age

E. Cerebrovascular Disease
   1. Extracranial obstruction of cerebral vessels associated with transient ischemic attacks
   2. Subclavian steal syndrome
II. Disturbance of Composition of Blood Flowing to the Brain
   A. Hypoglycemia
      Insulinomas, functional diseases (reactive, alimentary, and so forth)
   B. Hypocapnia
      Hyperventilation
   C. Hypoxia
      Low atmospheric oxygen tension, pulmonary disease, anemia, anoxemia of cyanotic congenital heart disease, as in tetralogy of Fallot and so forth
III. Neurophysiologic
   A. Nonconvulsive seizures
   B. Conversion reaction (hysteria) other than vasodepressor syncope
   C. Cerebral type of carotid sinus syncope

PATHOGENESIS

Underlying all forms of syncope is a sudden and reversible alteration of cerebral function, leading to a diminution in or loss of consciousness and postural muscle tone. The individual so afflicted will fall if unsupported in an obtunded or unresponsive mental state. Such an alteration is most commonly related to transient cerebral ischemia but may also relate to an altered chemical composition of blood flowing to the brain or to a self-limited, nonconvulsive change in cerebral function in the absence of identifiable circulatory or metabolic factors.

The change in cerebral cellular metabolism leading to the reduced level of consciousness and postural tone in the typical syncopal attack may have several determinants, depending on the precipitating factor. Normal cerebral function requires a fairly constant blood supply and oxygen delivery. Total interruption of the cerebral circulation leads to unconsciousness within 10 sec, and a cerebral oxygen content of less than 2 ml/ 100 g tissue leads to obtundation. Further, the brain has an obligatory dependence on a constant supply of glucose for its energy requirements. The cerebral vascular bed has a comparatively low resistance to flow and is uniquely dependent on its perfusion pressure. A fall below 70 torr in systolic pressure leads to syn-

cope by exceeding the lower limit of cerebral autoregulatory capacity.[1] Systemic arterial hypotension is the common denominator in all forms of syncope owing to cerebral ischemia except when related to focal cerebrovascular obstruction. In the upright posture the anatomic position of the brain above the heart adds to its vulnerability to cardiovascular derangements. While both autonomic reflex and local metabolic factors are involved in the regulation of cerebral blood flow, the predominant appear to be the latter, the most important being O_2 and CO_2 capillary tension.[2] With a reduction in cerebral arterial perfusion pressure, cerebral flow is protected by an attendant vasodilation ("autoregulation") in direct response to the associated fall in O_2 and rise in CO_2 tension. The increase in cerebrovascular resistance and resultant reduction in flow during hyperventilation syncope probably relates to the direct effect of the associated fall in CO_2 tension.

The precise nature of the hemodynamic alteration leading to cerebral ischemia and syncope in any given instance may be less obvious than one might suppose. Thus, in hyperventilation syncope, the ischemia results from a rise in cerebrovascular resistance in the presence of a normal cardiac output and arterial pressure. In vasodepressor syncope, the ischemia results from arterial hypotension owing to a drop in arteriolar resistance, often in the presence of a normal resting cardiac output. In orthostatic hypotension owing to failure of sympathetic tone, the hypotension leading to the ischemia relates to a reduction of *both* arteriolar resistance and cardiac output. In cardiac syncope owing to Adams-Stokes attacks or atrial ball-valve thrombus, the ischemia relates to hypotension from a depressed cardiac output in the presence of a normal peripheral vascular resistance. Finally, in cardiac syncope owing to physical effort in the presence of aortic or pulmonic stenosis, the hypotension leading to syncope may relate to a failure of cardiac output to rise appropriately in theface of an appropriately reduced arteriolar resistance.

The underlying metabolic aberration in the several forms of neuropsychologic syncope may be obscure. While a paroxysmal disturbance in cerebral electrical rhythm may be identified as the precipitating factor (as in nonconvulsive seizures associated with transient unconsciousness), this may not be apparent (as in hysterical fainting). This should be distinguished from the secondary changes in electrical activity that are the invariable consequence of syncope owing to cerebral ischemia—namely, the sudden appearance on the electroencephalogram of large-amplitude, slow-wave activity, starting in the occipital leads and spreading anteriorly.

ACUTE REDUCTION IN CEREBRAL BLOOD FLOW

CARDIAC DISORDERS

Disorders of Cardiac Rate, Rhythm, and Conduction. Rate, rhythm, and conduction disorders are the most common causes of cardiac syncope. Ventricular standstill, including asystole (Morgagni–Adams–Stokes attacks) and ventricular fibrillation, is the most frequent underlying arrhythmia. However, extremes of rate with bradycardia and tachycardia also precipitate loss of consciousness. Reflex bradycardia secondary to heightened vagal activity, as seen with carotid sinus diseases and glossopharyngeal neuralgia, will be discussed later.

The electrophysiologic mechanisms of these disorders may be grouped into three categories: first, failure of normal atrial and atrioventricular escape pacemakers to emerge after atrial standstill, complete heart block, or shift to a lower pacemaker site with chronic complete heart block; second, paroxysmal ventricular tachycardia, with or without complete heart block; third, supraventricular tachycardias and bradycardias. Ventricular standstill may follow cessation of tachycardias in the third category from delay in automaticity of suppressed pacemakers.[3,4]

These disorders have common hemodynamic consequences. The sudden shift in pacemaker activity induces a prompt fall in cardiac output. Depending on the status of the cerebral vascular system, loss of consciousness appears within 20 sec and seizures within 45 sec.[5]

Well-recognized clinical settings may herald the appearance of syncope from these disorders. Bifascicular block (right bundle branch block with left anterior hemiblock, right bundle branch block with left posterior hemiblock, and left bundle branch block) often precedes complete atrioventricular block. Of patients with right bundle branch block and left anterior hemiblock, 5% to 10% may progress to complete atrioventricular block,[6] which is commonly accompanied by syncope.[7] However, syncope also occurs with bifascicular block without this progression. Dhingra and associates prospectively documented that 16% of patients with chronic bifascicular block had syncope; of this group only 20% had syncope secondary to block progression.[8] Twenty-four hour ambulatory monitoring[9] and electrophysiologic studies (measurement of AH and HV intervals and response to atrial pacing)[10] are useful in determining which of these patients is at greatest risk for syncope. In the absence of conduction abnor-

malities, other causes, such as orthostatic hypotension, seizure disorders, and paroxysmal ventricular tachycardia must be considered.

Mobitz Type II second-degree atrioventricular block is associated with third-degree atrioventricular block and syncope.[11] Waugh and associates[12] reported that survivors of acute myocardial infarction complicated by this lesion are in a high-risk group; 45% had sudden death or syncope within 12 months of discharge. A slow, lower-level pacemaker focus activated by usually irreversible interruption of the conduction system is seen with this block.

Bradycardia alternating with supraventricular tachycardia, usually paroxysmal atrial flutter or fibrillation, is reported with syncope,[5] in the so-called bradycardia-tachycardia[13] or sick sinus syndrome.[14,15]

Syncope can appear upon slowing of an existing bradycardia.[16] Lower pacemakers, atrial and atrioventricular, fail to assume rhythmicity, which may lead to prolonged atrial and ventricular asystole and syncope.

Tachyarrhythmias alone may alter the diastolic filling period, decrease cardiac output, and lead to syncope.[17] Patients with Wolff–Parkinson–White syndrome become symptomatic with one of two arrhythmias: a reciprocating supraventricular tachycardia or atrial fibrillation with a rapid ventricular response.[18] The latter rhythm occasionally degenerates to ventricular fibrillation.[19] Recurrent ventricular tachycardia, particularly with underlying coronary heart disease, causes syncope and, in some instances, sudden cardiac death.[20]

Prolonged Q-T intervals, in patients with or without congenital deafness, can be a prelude to syncope. Patients with the Jervell and Lange–Nielsen syndrome[21] or the Romano-Ward syndrome[22] frequently have ventricular fibrillation precipitated by emotional and physical stresses. Clinically the syndrome may be recognized by alternating T-wave morphology produced by the same stimuli that precipitate syncope.[23] Prolongation of the repolarization by atrioventricular block sinus, bradycardia hypokalemia, and drugs must be excluded. The pathogenesis is not well understood. Heightened sympathetic activity is suggested by the nature of the precipitant, stress, and the reduction in mortality with β-blocking agents.

Drug-induced arrhythmias can predispose to syncope. Patients receiving therapeutic doses of propranolol may present with syncope, secondary to bradycardia and heart block.[24] The arrhythmias are probably secondary to the quinidinelike effects rather than to the β-blocking effects of propranolol. Both sinus node automaticity and ectopic foci may be suppressed; conduction velocity at all levels of the conduction system is diminished.[25] Verapamil may produce asystole and

syncope.[26] This effect has been most frequently observed after intravenous use, in the presence of β-blocking agents.

Syncope in the setting of quinidine therapy for chronic atrial arrhythmias is precipitated by paroxysmal ventricular tachycardia or fibrillation.[27,28] It may be seen with relatively low doses of quinidine and rarely, with the usual toxic effects of the drug. Diminished conduction may facilitate reentry pathways, while prolongation of refractoriness may lead to prolongation of the vulnerable period. The ventricular arrhythmia, "les torsades de pointes," may lead to syncope in the presence of delayed myocardial repolarization owing to both congenital and acquired causes.[29] This tachyarrhythmia has been precipitated by the usual suppressing drugs (e.g., quinidine, procainamide, and disopyramide), as well as by hypokalemia and liquid protein diets.

Pacemaker syncope is produced by one of two types of pacemaker malfunction: sensing failure, resulting in a competition between patient and pacemaker pacing and causing a decrease in cardiac output; or pacing failure, exposing the patient's underlying, unstable rhythm and leading to syncope.[30–32] Many patients who require pacing also use antiarrhythmic agents; syncope owing to a drug-induced arrhythmia must be considered before making the diagnosis of pacemaker syncope.

Valvular Heart Disease. All forms of valvular aortic stenosis (e.g., congenital, rheumatic, and calcific) predispose to syncope. Syncope, along with angina pectoris and left ventricular failure, is a clinical correlate of critical narrowing of valve area, usually to less than 0.5 cm^2.[4,33] Increased left ventricular work combined with limited coronary perfusion probably explains this association, although the exact mechanism for syncope is not clear.

Syncope has been attributed to sudden arrhythmias, secondary to decreased vascular supply of the conduction system.[34,35] However, Schwartz and associates documented that arrhythmias may appear well after the onset of syncope.[36] Syncopal seizures of short duration (20 sec–40 sec) were associated with regular sinus rhythm. Only with syncope lasting longer than 40 sec were ventricular standstill and fibrillation noted.

An alternate explanation is an abnormal cardiovascular response to exercise.[37,38] Wood suggested that these patients lack the ability to appropriately increase cardiac output.[39] Flamm and associates demonstrated that an increase in cardiac output does occur; however, at the onset of near-syncope, both cardiac output and arterial pressure fall.[40] Systemic vascular resistance fails to increase during the fall in arterial pressure, although

an increase would be expected if the hypotension were caused by left ventricular failure.

This explanation is supported by the observation that forearm vasoconstrictor responses to leg exercise are abnormal in these patients.[38] Forearm blood flow is increased, and forearm vascular resistance is decreased. This vasodilator response is not seen in severe mitral stenosis; it reverts to vasoconstriction after aortic valve replacement. These findings suggest that, in the presence of increased left ventricular pressure, ventricular baroreceptors are triggered by exercise, which leads to reflex vasodilation and precipitates syncope. These events may also explain the syncope of aortic regurgitation.

Mitral valve prolapse is occasionally associated with syncope. Recurrent supraventricular or complex ventricular arrhythmias appear to be the underlying mechanisms; there is no convincing evidence for obstruction to flow by either redundant chordae or distorted leaflets.[41,42]

Left atrial myxoma can present with a vivid form of syncope.[43] Clinical features include the sudden onset of positional syncope with normal sinus rhythm. Variations in blood pressure and heart rate may be induced by changes in posture.[44] The myxomas are usually attached to the atrial septum near the fossa ovalis by a stalk, which allows the mass to prolapse into the mitral orifice during diastole. Near-total obstruction may preclude diastolic filling of the left ventricle and effective stroke volume. A dysfunctioning prosthetic ball valve may lead to a similar clinical presentation.

Myocardial Disease. The appearance of syncope in ischemic heart disease was noted by Heberden in his original descriptions of angina pectoris.[45] In the presence of normal conduction on the resting electrocardiogram, it correlates with the angiographic findings of severe three vessel or left main coronary obstruction.[46] Arrhythmias and failure to respond to an increased output demand may explain loss of consciousness in angina and acute myocardial infarction.[47] Variant or Prinzmetal's angina can present with spontaneous pain, palpitations, and syncope. Continuous monitoring has shown ventricular fibrillation to be the precipitant in some patients with this syndrome.[48]

Idiopathic hypertrophic subaortic stenosis is frequently complicated by syncope. In contrast to aortic stenosis, its presence does not necessarily imply an ominous prognosis. It often appears after exercise when outflow obstruction is greatest. Braunwald and associates have suggested that syncope may be precipitated by the resulting decreased cardiac output.[49]

Abolition of syncope after ventriculomyotomy, with or without myectomy, supports this mechanical explanation.[50] Although the incidence of arrhythmias is low, some consider it the most likely explanation for syncope.[51,52] Ventricular tachycardia and fibrillation, as well as bradycardia with asystole, have been documented precipitants of syncope.

Congenital Heart Disease. Exercise also induces syncope in some forms of congenital heart disease. Valvular pulmonic stenosis and aortic stenosis are associated with effort syncope. Frank loss of consciousness at rest occurs with aortic disease. In contrast to aortic stenosis,[53] syncope as a harbinger of death is unusual with pulmonic stenosis.[54] Syncope occasionally complicates congenital heart block; predisposing factors include slow heart rates, inadequate rate response to exercise, and wide QRS morphology on standard ECG recordings.[55]

Syncope with tetralogy of Fallot appearing with stimuli of emotion and exercise may be secondary to a different mechanism.[56,57] An increased cardiac output and right-to-left shunt precipitated by these stimuli presents blood with high pCO_2 to cerebral chemoreceptors, which in turn leads to hyperpnea. The hyperpnea is followed by a further increase in cardiac output and in the magnitude of the right-to-left shunt. This increases the degree of anoxemia of blood circulating to the brain, and syncope ensues. This finding is rarely seen after early childhood.

Syncope and sudden death are not commonly seen with pulmonary hypertension associated with patent ductus arteriosus, ventricular septal defect, and atrial septal defect. Although exercise tends to increase the right-to-left shunt, the absence of pulmonic stenosis or infundibular contraction presumably precludes the degree of shunting, which leads to syncope in patients with tetralogy of Fallot.[58]

VASCULAR OBSTRUCTION

Primary Pulmonary Hypertension. Syncope with primary pulmonary hypertension is usually precipitated by exercise.[59] Palpitations, cyanosis, and precordial pain may be premonitory findings.[60] With exercise peripheral vascular resistance decreases, which results in a drop in arterial pressure. The heart cannot compensate with an increased output, as the narrowed pulmonary arterial vasculature prevents increased diastolic filling of the left ventricle for maintenance of an appropriate stroke volume; acute right heart failure and syncope ensue.[61] Typical vasodepressor syncope may be observed,[62] and a vasomotor reflex beginning in the

pulmonary artery and traveling over the vagus pathways has been proposed. James found segmental arteriopathy of the sinoatrial and atrioventricular nodal arteries in patients with primary pulmonary hypertension, which was not seen in similar arteries of patients with severe secondary pulmonary hypertension.[63] He postulated that his findings might explain the noted prevalence of atrial arrhythmias and heart block in this disease and, thereby, the syncope.

Acute Pulmonary Embolism. One seventh of patients with acute pulmonary embolism have been reported to have syncope as a presenting clinical finding.[64] Clinical correlates include hypotension, tachycardia, and acute cor pulmonale by physical examination or electrocardiogram. Most of these patients have obstruction of greater than 50% of the pulmonary circulation. In the presence of right ventricular failure, manifested by elevated end-diastolic pressure and diminished stroke volume, cardiac output is decreased. The transient nature of the clinical findings may be explained by early partial resolution of the embolic obstruction.

Acute Aortic Dissection. The hallmark symptom of acute dissection of the thoracic aorta is the abrupt onset of intense chest pain.[65,66] However, 20% of patients also experience syncope, often associated with bleeding into the pericardium.

FAILURE OF VENOUS RETURN

A critical balance between the blood volume and capacity of the circulation determines the quantity of blood available for cardiac filling in the form of venous return. An uncompensated decrease in the volume or increase in the capacity of only 3% would diminish cardiac output to zero.[67] Because of their large diameter, the veins and venules contain approximately 75% of the blood volume. The movement of blood from the venous end of the capillary to the right atrium depends on this differential in volume and capacity, which is expressed as the pressure gradient between these points, normally about 10 torr in the recumbent position. Factors increasing the pressure in the intrathoracic and intra-abdominal portion of the venae cavae (as with forced expiration against a closed glottis) or decreasing the pressure in the peripheral veins (as with diminished blood volume or failure of venomotor tone), will diminish this critical pressure gradient, and therefore, the venous return and cardiac output. The arterial pressure will fall to the extent that this decrease in cardiac output is not compensated for by a reflex increase in peripheral arteriolar resistance. Below a critical point, despite an adaptive decrease in cerebral vascular resistance, cerebral perfusion will be inade-

quate to sustain consciousness, and syncope will result.

With passive positioning of an adult into the upright posture, approximately 500 ml of blood will be trapped in the distensible venous system in dependent parts owing to the gravitational factor, and the hydrostatic effect adds an additional 70 torr to the pressure in veins of the foot. Reflex venomotor activity is required to move blood centrally to protect the venous filling pressure of the right heart. The associated fall in cardiac output by some 25% indicates the incompleteness of this defense. Active contraction of the musculature of the extremities can completely counteract this hydrostatic effect in peripheral veins and normalize the cardiac output. The gravitational effect on venous return (and hence cardiac output) emphasizes the critical importance of the upright position in predisposing to *all* forms of syncope relating to cerebral ischemia. The normal hemodynamic response to passive upright positioning is depicted in Fig. 33-1. The peripheral pooling of blood is compensated for by an almost instantaneous baroreceptor reflex, increasing peripheral vascular resistance (sympathetically induced arteriolar vasoconstriction) and partially buffering the fall in cardiac output (sympathetically induced venoconstriction and an increase in cardiac rate and contractile force). Once equilibrium is established, the pulse pressure is slightly narrowed by a fall in systolic and rise in diastolic pressure (each by a few torr) associated with a rise in pulse rate by a few beats per min. How-

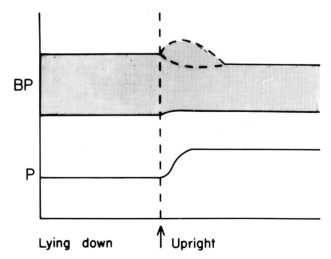

Fig. 33-1. Normal hemodynamic response to head-up tilting. (Reproduced with permission from Hickler R B: Diagnosis and management of orthostatic hypotension. In Weekly Update: Cardiology 1:1, 1979. Published by Biomedia, Inc, Princeton)

ever, mean arterial pressure remains unchanged, such that cerebral perfusion is defended and syncope is obviated. As an indicator of the increased sympathetic tone, plasma norepinephrine and renin concentrations will more than double within 30 min of upright positioning.[68]

Increased Intrathoracic Pressure. The pressure against the outer wall of the intrathoracic and intra-abdominal veins can be increased to 45 torr by forced expiration against a closed glottis (the Valsalva maneuver). This force is sufficient to collapse these great veins and to negate completely the pressure gradient favoring venous return from the periphery. If sustained, this will lead to syncope. There are a number of situations in which this appears to be the mechanism for fainting. Examples are straining at stool, lifting a heavy object, breath-holding, prolonged coughing spell ("tussic syncope"), tracheal or laryngeal obstruction (forced expiration), and "fainting lark" (the schoolboy trick of compressing a friend's chest while he voluntarily holds the air in his chest after a maximal inspiration). An important factor contributing to the syncope besides the diminished venous return in this general group may be the transmission of the increased intrathoracic pressure to the cerebral spinal fluid through the venous drainage system from the brain, with resultant compression and emptying of the intracranial capillary bed. In tussic syncope a concussive effect with each cough against the cerebrospinal fluid may augment this phenomenon.[69] Friedberg emphasizes that serious reflex cardiac dysrhythmia may be induced in the setting of a sudden increase in intrathoracic pressure and contribute to the cerebral ischemia and syncope.[70]

Decreased Blood Volume. The causes of hypovolemia are numerous (see the etiological classification). Hemorrhage, both internal and external, is a prime example. Other examples are simple dehydration, salt and water loss from gastrointestinal and renal disease, and plasma loss (as in extensive burns and paracentesis). A unique example has been described in some diabetics, who, in the absence of neuropathy, manifest orthostatic hypotension from volume contraction owing to a reduction in red cell mass.[71] Whatever the origin, tachycardia, hypotension, light-headedness, and often syncope on assuming the upright posture are cardinal features of this disorder. The pathophysiology is basically the same. A disparity between vascular capacity and distending volume on the venous (capacitance) side of the circulation leads to a fall in venous filling pressure and hence cardiac output and arterial pressure. A critical fall in the latter to below 70 torr systolic is likely to lead to syncope. Hypotension evokes a series of compensatory reflexes. The following is a description (shown schematically in Fig. 33-2) of the baroreceptor reflex:

> The primary pressoreceptors are the carotid sinus pressoreceptors, located in the walls of the internal carotid arteries slightly above the carotid bifurcation, and the aortic baroreceptors, located within the walls of the

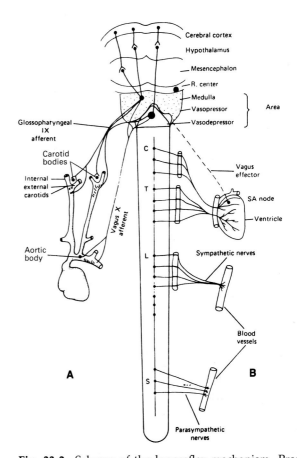

Fig. 33-2. Schema of the baroreflex mechanism. Pressoreceptors in carotid sinus and aortic arch and afferent nerves IX and X receive pressure stimulus and carry it to vasodepressor area (triangular and medial). Note connections from cerebral cortex and hypothalamus, which may also send stimuli to vasodepressor or vasopressor centers. (*A*) Chemoreceptors from carotid and aortic bodies receive and respond to changes in pCO_2 (increase) and pO_2 (decrease) and transmit response through nerves IX and X to vasopressor area. (*B*) Responses to stimuli from vasodepressor and pressor area may be traced from centers through spinal cord, through appropriate sympathetic ganglia and nerves, and vagus nerve to heart and blood vessels in lumbar (*L*) and sacral (*S*) areas. Two IX nerves are shown, but only one X nerve (in *A*), all afferent. (From Sturkie, PD: Circulation. In Basic Physiology, p 207. New York, Springer-Verlag, 1981. Reproduced with permission)

aortic arch. Stimulation of the pressoreceptors occurs by the stretching of the arterial wall consequent to the pressure within the arteries, and the pressoreceptor impulses are transmitted to the medulla of the brain by appropriate nerves; carotid pressoreceptor impulses are transmitted by the Hering nerve, a branch of the glossopharyngeal nerve, and aortic pressoreceptor impulses are transmitted through the vagus nerve. In general, the pressoreceptor impulses inhibit sympathetic stimulation of the entire circulatory system and enhance parasympathetic stimulation of the circulatory system.[72]

A fall in pressure causes an increase in sympathetic and a decrease in parasympathetic tone, resulting in an increase in heart rate and peripheral vascular resistance. Stretch-sensitive receptors with vagal afferents from the cardiopulmonary region have also been identified; they exert a tonic inhibition on the vasomotor center, causing tachycardia and increased peripheral vascular resistance under conditions of volume contraction.[73] The extent to which venous constriction partakes in these circulatory reflexes is controversial, although it is generally felt to occur.[74] Muscle veins are nonreactive to neural stimulation and are devoid of adrenergic nerve endings. In contrast, cutaneous and splanchnic veins are richly innervated and probably participate in the baroreceptor response by a decrease in capacitance, moving blood centrally to compensate for a hypovolemic-induced fall in cardiac output. Some 65% of blood expelled from the splanchnic region is due to passive, elastic recoil of the venous wall in response to a decrease in distending pressure under conditions of a normal central venous pressure. The latter relates to a decrease in venous inflow in response to reflex arteriolar vasoconstriction.[75] The remaining 35% is expelled by active venoconstriction. Passive as compared with active emptying of veins would become even more important under conditions of volume depletion associated with a lowered central venous pressure because of the geometry of the capiacitance system. However, the increment in venous pressure and return from these compensatory mechanisms is minimized by the enormous capacitance (distensibility) of the venous system (18 times that of the arterial). This serves to emphasize the vulnerability of cerebral circulation to the upright posture in the volume-depleted state.

Increased Venous Capacity. There may be a failure of venous return when the capacity of the venous system is enlarged without a corresponding increment in volume. The pathophysiology of syncope in this disorder, particularly in the upright posture, is identical with that just described for hypovolemia. A classical example is extensive varicose veins. The syndrome of dizziness and syncope under conditions of orthostatic stress with large varicosities in the saphenous system has been reported.[76] Vasoactive agents, such as the ganglionic blocking agents, guanethidine, and the nitrite-nitrate group, have a major relaxing effect on the smooth muscle of post-resistance vessels and produce postural hypotension, which may lead to syncope in the upright posture. Nitrite can produce postural syncope in relatively small doses, and its predominant effect on the cardiovascular system as a direct-acting vascular smooth muscle relaxant has been well described. While nitrite relaxes all vessels, the net effect on arterioles is relatively less than that on capacitance vessels.[77] As a consequence, central venous pressure is decreased, and cardiac filling and output fall. This, coupled with a relaxation of resistance vessels, produces a fall in arterial pressure, predominantly in systolic, with narrowing of pulse pressure and rise in heart rate. The accentuation of the venous pooling in the upright posture can lead to a typical "fainting reaction." The marked bradycardia, regularly observed just prior to unconsciousness, is evidence of the vagal component of a massive autonomic nervous system outpouring in response to cerebral ischemia. This reaction will be described in detail in the section on vasodepressor syncope, which nitrite syncope mimics closely in all its clinical aspects.

The hemodynamic response to the upright posture (orthostatic stress) common to all forms of a failed venous return prior to the superimposition of vasodepressor syncope is depicted in Fig. 33-3. It is characterized by a sharp reduction in cardiac output in the presence of a maximally working baroreflex mechanism. This produces a precipitous fall in systolic and mean arterial pressure, associated with a large increase in heart rate. The diastolic pressure fall is initially buffered by a maximal reflex arteriolar vasoconstrictive response. Pallor and light-headedness are regular sequellae.

LOSS OF PERIPHERAL VASCULAR TONE

Loss of peripheral vascular tone may be due to an active dilatation of resistance vessels, as in vasodepressor syncope (the common faint), or to a failure of constrictive (sympathetic) activity on resistance vessels, as in baroreflex failure. In either event, a decrease by 50% in arteriolar resistance will produce a comparable fall in mean aortic pressure, which is sufficient to cause syncope. Cerebrovascular resistance would have to fall proportionately if cerebral blood flow were to be preserved under such a degree of arterial hypotension. This appears to pertain for mean arterial pressures as low as 60 torr but in the range for syncope (30

torr–40 torr) cerebral vascular resistance cannot compensate, and cerebral blood flow becomes significantly reduced.[78] Normal supine cerebral blood flow is in the range of 50 ml/100 g brain; a decrease (in the upright position) to a critical value of 30 ml/100 g brain is indicative of imminent syncope in the adult human.[79]

An augmentation of venous return and cardiac output would be one mechanism for offsetting such a dramatic reduction in systemic arterial pressure and cerebral flow. Drugs, such as hydralazine, which have as their primary effect a relaxation of arteriolar smooth muscles, may decrease peripheral resistance by as much as 75%. Because reflex adrenergic mechanisms on the veins and heart are intact, cardiac output and heart rate may increase by 50% to 75%, and the hypotensive effect is minimized.[80] Postural hypotension and syncope are not important side effects. Thus, the severe hypotension and syncope observed in the upright posture in vasodepressor syncope and baroreflex failure, relating to a drop in arteriolar resistance equivalent to that produced by a drug such as hydralazine, indicate a failure of these compensatory mechanisms, which is *critical to the production of the faint*. In vasodepressor syncope the predominant site of active arteriolar dilatation is the musculature, where the venous system is uniquely devoid of sympathetic innervation;[81] further, the increased vagal tone on the heart compromises cardiac function through marked bradycardia and decreased contractile strength.[82] In baroreflex failure the generalized loss of sympathetic activity of the cardiovascular system accounts for the deficiency of these compensatory reflex mechanisms on venous return and cardiac function.[83,84]

Vasodepressor Syncope. On the subject of vasodepressor syncope Weissler and Warren have stated the following:

> Vasodepressor syncope, or the common faint, is the most frequently encountered clinical form of syncope. This form of fainting may occur as a response to sudden emotional stress or in a setting of real, threatened, or fantasied injury. The reaction is not infrequently brought on by venepuncture or the sight of blood, and is also observed after sudden painful experiences such as may occur during surgical manipulations or following severe tissue injury. It is particularly likely to occur in certain environmental settings, such as in a hot and crowded room, especially if the individual is fatigued, hungry or ill or has experienced recent blood loss. The common faint is usually encountered when the patient is in the upright or sitting posture but may rarely occur while the patient is recumbent.[62]

More specific precipitating factors may be cited, such as carotid sinus hypersensitivity (as evoked by a tight collar or turning of the head),[85] sudden emptying of a

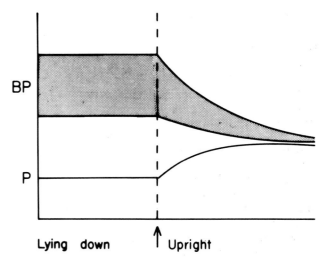

Fig. 33-3. Hemodynamic response to head-up tilting in orthostatic hypotension caused by failure of venous return. (Reproduced with permission from Hickler RB: Diagnosis and management of orthostatic hypotension. In Weekly Update. Cardiology 1:2, 1979. Published by Biomedia, Inc, Princeton)

distended urinary bladder ("micturition syncope"),[86] removal of large quantities of fluid during a chest or abdominal tap, esophageal spasm ("vagovagal syncope"),[87] glossopharyngeal neuralgia,[88] and ocular compression (oculovagal syncope).[89] Cerebral ischemia from any of the causes detailed previously in this report may directly trigger the vasodepressor reaction. Regardless of which of a large number of stimuli acting on the central nervous system, either directly as in cerebral ischemia, or indirectly through afferent neural pathways, is involved in a given instance of vasodepressor syncope, each results in a *common* efferent response with identical clinical and pathophysiologic features. It is indicative of a generalized, progressive, automatic discharge. The response may be divided into two phases, as elicited from tiltboard studies: The first consists of a gradual decrease in arterial pressure followed by the second, which consists of a sudden bradycardia associated with a precipitious fall in arterial pressure and unconsciousness. Throughout the first phase, which may last for many minutes, a number of premonitory signs and symptoms appear that can be attributed either to cerebral ischemia or to automatic discharge. The former consist of visual blurring, diminution of hearing, restlessness, and finally, clonic movements of the body just prior to loss of consciousness. The latter may be divided between adrenergic and cholinergic components. The adrenergic are tachycardia, pallor, hyperventilation, and pupillary dilatation. The cholinergic are perspiration, increased

peristaltic activity, nausea, and salivation. The brady-cardia, superimposed on the tachycardia just prior to the faint, is evidence of a vagal-cholinergic response that overwhelms the previously "appropriate" sympathetic stimulation of the heart.[90]

Forearm blood flow may increase as much as eight to ten times during the faint, largely relating to a profound drop in arteriolar resistance in the musculature, a response that is to a certain extent dependent on the cholinergic vasodilator system.[91] This system is anatomically part of the sympathetic nervous system and confined to muscle. The sustained nature of the active vasodilation and its incomplete blocking with atropine suggest an additional chemical mediator. Its precise nature is not understood, but the release of skeletal muscle adenosine, which is a potent vasodilator and produced only in the vicinity of blood vessels, is a possibility.[92] The identification of the purinergic (probably adenosine triphosphate) vasodilator component of the autonomic nervous system in recent years raises interesting possibilities in this regard,[93] although its potential relationship to the phenomenon of vasodepressor syncope remains to be determined. There is suggestive evidence that such fibers may reach the smooth muscle of peripheral vessels through the dorsal route of the spinal cord. Bradykinin and histamine do not seem likely candidates.[94] Some 15% to 20% of resting cardiac output goes to muscle, and an eightfold to tenfold increment in muscle flow during syncope indicates that almost the entire output is transiently diverted in this direction. Thus, flow is decreased in the cerebral, renal, and mesenteric vasculature despite a fall in the vascular resistance of these regions.

In animal studies Uvnäs has identified regions in the anterior cingulate gyrus of the brain that on stimulation produce vagal bradycardia, hypotension, and a profound decrease in vascular resistance and increase in flow to skeletal muscle.[95] Additionally, there is a loss of skeletal muscle tone, and the response, remarkably akin to human vasodepressor syncope, has been considered a defense mechanism called the "playing dead reaction." Atropinization fails to prevent this reaction, just as it may fail to prevent vasodepressor syncope, again pointing to the existence of an unidentified mediator that augments the sympathetic cholinergic vasodilation.

Weissler and colleagues have described the cardinal point: *The entire syncopal reaction can occur in the absence of a significant reduction in cardiac output*, emphasizing that the final hemodynamic aberration is the failure of cardiac output to *increase* appropriately to compensate for the precipitious fall in peripheral resistance.[96] Baroreflex-mediated cutaneous venoconstriction does occur during the faint, and central venous pressure

remains unchanged.[97] However, as indicated previously, muscle veins are not innervated, and inotropic and chronotopic cardiac activity are depressed by increased vagal tone, which must account for this failure. In the final analysis, then, the cerebral ischemia and syncope relate to a diminished proportion of an unchanged cardiac output flowing to the brain because of a precipitously depressed resistance and increased flow in the vasculature of skeletal muscle, which cannot be compensated for by an equivalent fall in cerebrovascular resistance or by venomotor and cardiac rate and contractile responses. The importance of vagal depression of heart rate in the evolution of the faint is indicated by the reported therapeutic efficacy of a permanent demand cardiac pacemaker in a patient with hypersensitive carotid sinus syncope.[98] A subnormal rise in plasma renin activity has been observed in the period just prior to the faint in individuals who manifest vasodepressor syncope on upright positioning, the significance of which remains to be elucidated.[99]

It is to be emphasized that the *initial* hemodynamic defense against gravitational stress in individuals who faint on the tiltboard is *normal*. Appropriate hemodynamic reflex activity is indicated by a rise in diastolic pressure and heart rate, narrowed pulse pressure, and well-preserved mean pressure associated with a normal (or supranormal) rise in plasma and urinary catecholamines.[100] It is only after a number of minutes that the described pathophysiologic events supervene. Figure 33-4 depicts the hemodynamic sequence in vasodepressor syncope attending the upright posture.

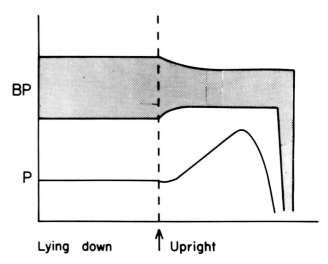

Fig. 33-4. Hemodynamic response to head-up tilting in vasodepressor syncope. (Reproduced with permission from Hickler RB: Diagnosis and management of orthostatic hypotension. In Weekly Update. Cardiology 1:2, 1979. Published by Biomedia, Inc, Princeton)

Finally, it should be mentioned that, in rare instances of vasodepressor syncope owing to irritable carotid sinus, bradycardia may be absent, the syndome relating purely to the peripheral vascular events. The latter may be so precipitous that syncope can occur without time for the evolution of the usual premonitory events (*e.g.,* sweating and pallor).

Baroreflex Failure—Pathophysiology. The fundamental disturbance in syncope owing to baroreflex failure, irrespective of the clinical background, is a failure of reflex adrenergic cardiovascular activity to prevent hypotension when the effective blood volume is sharply decreased in the upright posture because of gravitational venous "pooling" below the right heart. In healthy individuals the hypotension attending the 25% reduction in cardiac output that normally attends quiet standing after recumbency is compensated for by an equivalent baroreflex-mediated increase in peripheral vascular resistance, such that mean aortic pressure and cerebral perfusion are preserved. In orthostatic hypotension the adrenergic deficiency obviates this defense, and besides the primary failure of arteriolar vasoconstriction, failure of venomotor[101] and cardiac inotropic response augment the hypotensive response to upright positioning. In a study of eight patients with this disorder, Ibrahim and colleagues found that plasma volume was only minimally reduced (90% of normal); a major defect in cardiac contractility was indicated by a slow left ventricular ejection rate, which was implicated in the abnormally low (75% of normal upright) cardiac output on passive ventrical positioning.[84] The heart rate may[82] but usually does not[102] increase appropriately, depending on the extent and distribution of the autonomic defect. The pathognomonic hemodynamic response to upright positioning in orthostatic hypotension is depicted in Figure 33-5: (1) a prompt and progressive fall in both systolic and diastolic pressure, with marked narrowing of pulse pressure; (2) a pulse rate rise that is usually small for the degree of hypotension present.[90] This is differentiated from orthostatic hypotension owing to failure of venous return (Fig. 33-3) by the supranormal rise in heart rate in the latter.

Etiology and Anatomic Level of Defect

As outlined in the etiological classification, the anatomic level of the defect (and related pathology) leading to an interruption of the baroreflex arc is quite varied. Thus, in tabes dorsalis and in some cases of polyneuritis-polyneuropathy (*e.g.,* diabetic), it may be located in the visceral afferent nerves between the baroreceptor and the brain.[103] It may be in the brain, particularly the hypothalamus and brain stem, because of tu-

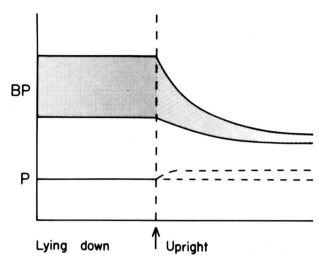

Fig. 33-5. Hemodynamic response to head-up tilting in orthostatic hypotension caused by baroreflex failure. (Reproduced with permission from Hickler RB: Diagnosis and management of orthostatic hypotension. In Weekly Update. Cardiology 1:2, 1979. Published by Biomedia, Inc, Princeton)

mors,[104] cerebrovascular disease,[105] or drugs.[106] Diseases interrupting the autonomic efferents in the spinal cord (intermediolateral columns) have long been known to produce postural hypotension: transverse myelitis, pernicious anemia and so forth; while the primary (idiopathic) neuronal wasting of the Shy–Drager syndrome is widespread (olivopontocerebellar and striatonigral), it includes a major defect in the intermediolateral columns.[107] The paraventebral ganglia are the level of block in thoracolumbar sympathectomy and with blocking agents; they are one of the foci of neuronal wasting in the postural hypotension attending familial dysautonomia.[108] The peripheral sympathetic efferents may also be the locus, as in postural hypotension associated with polyneuritis-polyneuropathy (diabetic, amyloid, porphyric, toxic,[109] and so forth), as noted in numerous reports. Clearly, a *mixed* state may pertain, involving several levels of the reflex arc simultaneously. Finally, while the term "idiopathic orthostatic hypotension" has been used to designate cases with the Shy–Drager syndrome, it probably should be limited to patients with an identified norepinephrine depletion at sympathetic nerve terminals in the absence of other demonstrable defects.[110] An important differentiating point is the finding of a normal supine level of circulating norepinephrine in Shy–Drager, contrasting with a uniquely low level in the latter.[111] The failure of patients in both instances to show an increase in plasma norepinephrine concentration on postural stress is common to all forms of orthostatic hypoten-

sion owing to baroreflex failure, except in the last cited group with an unresponsive microvasculature. The ultimate level of baroreflex arc failure is the microvasculature itself, which can become unresponsive to an intact neuroadrenergic discharge owing to the use of α-adrenegic blocking agent, prolonged bed-rest, or advanced age.

Physiologic and Pharmacologic Tests

A variety of physiologic and pharmacologic tests have been applied to determine the presence and level of the baroreflex failure. Some of the physiologic tests are detailed in Table 33-1. The integrity of the entire baroreflex system, including cardiac pacemaker and vascular smooth muscle, is determined by the blood pressure and heart rate response to passive upright positioning and the Valsalva maneuver (post-Valsalva response). When abnormal, the defect may be further localized to a point distal to the afferent pathway by finding an abnormal pressure and pulse response to such maneuvers as hyperventilation, the cold pressor test, and mental stress (*e.g.* loud noise, mental arithmetic). Finally, an abnormal reflex sweat test would point to a disorder in the autonomic outflow at a point *between* the vasomotor centers and the effector sites (heart and blood vessels). A summary of pharmacologic testing is presented in Table 33-2. Atropine should produce cardiac acceleration if the pacemaker mechanism is intact. Phenylephrine as a direct α-adrenergic

receptor stimulator should increase the blood pressure if the microvasculature is intact; in response to that increase, the heart rate should slow if the baroreceptor-afferent and central vagal-cardiac mechanism is intact. Tyramine, acting as an indirect-acting sympathomimetic, will discharge norepinephrine stored in sympathetic nerve endings, producing a rise in blood pressure. The absence of such a rise is indicative of a postganglionic sympathetic defect in the axon or nerve terminal characteristic of certain peripheral autonomic neuropathies and idiopathic orthostatic hypotension of the peripheral type. Similarly, a supranormal pressure response to nonepinephrine is characteristic of nerve terminal catecholamine depletion (Cannon's law of hypersensitivity of a denervated organ to its neurotransmitter). Leveston and colleagues have described another approach involving the response of plasma norepinephrine concentration to the stimulation of sympathetic ganglia with the cholinergic drug endrophonium.[112] An absent or blunted rise was indicative of postganglionic neuropathy (diabetic), whereas a normal rise was found in those patients with more centrally located (preganglionic) defects (Shy–Drager, brain stem infarct). However, among the complex of neurologic defects originally described by Shy and Drager was degeneration of the sympathetic ganglia,[113] and Davies and colleagues have found physiologic changes in patients with the Shy–Drager syndrome supposedly specific for patients with orthostatic hy-

Table 33-1. *Physiologic Testing of the Baroreflex System*

Test	Normal Response			Tests Integrity Of
	Blood Pressure	*Heart Rate*	*Generalized Sweating*	
Passive head-up tilt—60°	↔	↑		Total baroreflex system (Sensory afferent and motor efferent pathways)
Valsalva maneuver Post-Valsalva response after 10 sec–15 sec against 40 torr	↑	↓		
Hyperventilation—15 sec	↓	↑		Total motor efferent pathway Vasomotor center Sympathetic efferents—spinal cord and peripheral (adrenergic) Vascular smooth muscle Cardiac pacemaker
Cold pressor—ice to forehead for 1 min	↑	↑		
Mental stress Loud noise, mental arithmetic, and so forth	↑	↑		
Reflex sweat test Trunkal heating—radiant heat cradle for 30 min			+	Peripheral motor efferent pathway Sympathetic efferents—spinal cord and peripheral (cholinergic)

Table 33-2. *Pharmacologic Testing of the Baroreflex System*

Drug (Adult Doses)*	Abnormal Response	Tests Integrity Of
Atropine (1 mg–1.5 mg IV)	Absent or subnormal rise in heart rate	Cardiac pacemaker
Phenylephrine (20 μg–25 μg IV)	Absent or subnormal rise in BP Failure to produce cardiac slowing in response to rise in BP	Vascular smooth muscle Afferent and central vagal-cardiac mechanism
Tyramine (1 mg–2 mg IV/min)	Absent or subnormal rise in BP	Sympathetic nerve endings—
Norepinephrine (5 μg–10 μg IV/min)	Supranormal rise in BP	norepinephrine stores
Edrophonium (10 mg IV)	Absent or blunted rise in plasma norepinephrine concentration	Postganglionic sympathetic nerves

*References in text.

potension owing to postganglionic defects (low-plasma norpinephrine concentration and suprasensitivity to intravenous norepinephrine).[114] Therefore, it would be advisable to avoid an overly simplistic interpretation of the various tests in attempting to make such distinctions.

Clinical Considerations

In the clinical approach to the problem, the first question is to determine if the baroreflex failure is associated with somatic as well as autonomic neurol defects. In affirmative, then the problem is likely to fall into one of two subgroups: (1) that relating to an identifiable neurologic disease with involvement (central or peripheral) of the autonomic and somatic nervous systems (tabes, diabetes, and so forth), or (2) that related to one of several expressions of idiopathic neuronal failure that have a distinct clinical pattern, such as the Shy–Drager syndrome (orthostatic hypotension associated with urinary and rectal incontinence, loss of sweating, iris atrophy, external ocular palsies, rigidity, tremor, loss of associated movements, impotence, and amyotrophy).

If, on the other hand, there are no associated somatic neurologic deficits, then one must consider that the disorder is limited to the autonomic nervous system, the second major category with two subgroups. The baroreflex-autonomic failure would be a manifestation of either an early phase of Shy–Drager syndrome (prior to the appearance of somatic neural dysfunction, which frequently "follows the onset of autonomic dysfunction by some four years or less")[115] or a manifestation of an idiopathic defect that is, and will remain, limited to the peripheral autonomic nervous system. About 50% of patients presenting with orthostatic hypotension that cannot be classified as secondary to an iden-

tifiable category have no associated somatic neural dysfunction,[116] and it is unknown what proportion will or will not eventually develop such progressive changes beyond the autonomic nervous system.

There is good evidence that idiopathic orthostatic hypotension owing to an isolated defect of the peripheral autonomic nervous system deserves to be regarded as a separate entity from the Shy–Drager syndrome (without somatic neural deficits) on clinical grounds. It generally manifests a longer and more benign clinical history, although the presence of cholinergic defects (*e.g.,* constipation, heat intolerance), as well as adrenergic defects, is equally common in both.[111] Indeed, the prognosis in Shy-Drager is rather poor; death occurred on an average of seven to eight years after the symptomatic onset of the disease in one large series.[115]

Cholinergic as Well as Adrenergic Neural Deficits

In the great majority of cases, irrespective of etiology, cholinergic function (including cranial and sacral parasympathetic outflow) is also involved in the pathologic process and shows major deficiencies. Thus, the findings of adrenergic failure (*e.g.,* postural hypotension and low basal metabolic rate) are usually associated with, and often *preceded* by, evidence of cholinergic failure (*e.g.,* anhidrosis, impotence, and loss of bladder and bowel control). When cerebral ischemia leads to syncope in the upright posture, it occurs without the characteristic autonomic prodromata of the common vasodepressor faint, the latter including both hyperadrenergic and hypercholinergic features, as previously described. A specific exception would be following the administration of adrenergic blocking drugs (*e.g.,* guanethidine or phenoxybenzamine).

In all patients with Shy–Drager sndrome given de-

tailed neuropathologic examination, there has been degeneration of the dorsal nucleus of the vagus nerve; ciliary ganglionic degeneration is responsible for the characteristic loss of cholinergic pupillary function in postural hypotension associated with familial dysautonomia.

The parasympathetic lesion leading to bladder and bowel dysfunction (characteristic of the majority of patients with neurogenically determined orthostatic hypotension) has not been identified as yet owing to the complexity of the sacral outflow.

CEREBROVASCULAR DISEASE

Extracranial obstruction of cerebral vessels associated with transient ischemic attacks may lead to syncope. This is encountered in both carotid and vertebral-basilar artery obstruction (partial or complete) in the neck. In this setting anything leading to hypotension (e.g., hemorrhage, arrhythmia, upright posture) can produce transient ischemia in the distribution of the cerebral circulation served by the occluded vessel. The associated neurologic signs depend on that distribution (e.g., transient amblyopia, hemiparesis), the more global signs being dizziness, weakness, and on occasion, syncope. Compression of one carotid artery in the presence of contralateral carotid occlusion may produce syncope and, if prolonged, may result in a stroke. Transient ischemia attacks may also relate to small emboli of fibrin and platelets from the surface of an atherosclerotic plaque commonly found in the internal carotid artery just above its bifurcation in the neck.[117] Insufficiency in the carotid system characteristically produces episodes of dimness of vision or blindness on the side of the occlusive disease (amaurosis fugax) and hemisensory loss contralaterally. Insufficiency of the vertebral-basilar system characteristically produces episodes of occipital headache, bilateral visual disturbances and cranial nerve dysfunction, and "drop attacks" (sudden collapse without unconsciousness). However, such pat formulations frequently do not pertain, owing to the collateral nature of the cerebral circulation through the circle of Willis. Syncope in the setting of any such transient, focal neurologic signs should point to the extracranial circulation in the neck as the likely origin of the faint, and careful auscultation for associated arterial bruits should be performed.

A unique cause of transient ischemic attacks relates to occlusive disease of the subclavian artery just proximal to the origin of the vertebral artery and has been called the subclavian steal syndrome.[118] Syncope occurs in about 30% of symptomatic cases.[119] The cerebral arterial insufficiency relates to a reversal of flow in the vertebral artery distal to the subclavian occlusion, frequently in a setting of arteriolar dilatation in the arm musculature on exercise.

DISTURBANCE IN COMPOSITION OF BLOOD FLOWING TO THE BRAIN

HYPOGLYCEMIA

Hypoglycemia may develop in a number of clinical settings (e.g., insulin overdose, insulinoma or islet cell tumor, extensive liver disease, and in functional diseases—reactive, alimentary, and so forth). Irrespective of etiology, mild degrees of hypoglycemia through stimulation of the release of adrenomedullary catecholamines can produce tremor, anxiety, tachycardia, and "sympathetic" sweating. More severe hypoglycemia can lead directly to central nervous system changes, relating to the obligatory metabolic requirement of the central nervous system for glucose as a substrate for energy. These may be hunger, weakness, emotional instability (including psychotic behavior), and finally, loss of consciousness.

HYPOCAPNIA

Hyperventilation, which is usually hysterical in nature, may lead to a constriction of cerebral vessels owing to the direct effect of a low pCO_2 at the capillary level, as described earlier. The ensuant cerebral ischemia quite regularly leads to transient unconsciousness. Other symptoms directly attributable to the respiratory alkalosis are numbness and tightening of the face and extremities, confusion, and light-headedness. The faint may have all the features of a vasodepressor reaction as triggered by the cerebral ischemia.

HYPOXIA

As previously emphasized the cerebral cortex and "consciousness centers" have the highest vulnerability to hypoxia of any tissue in the body. Ten seconds of complete cerebral anoxia produces unconsciousness. It is not surprising that the wide variety of clinical states compromising cerebral oxygenation, besides those directly involved in the arterial circulation, have syncope and unconsciousness and conspicuous clinical features. Examples of this are inhalation of oxygen at low tension (e.g., high altitude), pulmonary disease with disordered ventilatory function, severe anemia, anoxemia (e.g., carbon monoxide poisoning), and right-to-

left shunts in certain forms of cyanotic congenital heart disease (*e.g.*, tetralogy of Fallot). As with syncope relating to a reduction of cerebral blood flow, irrespective of etiology, syncope relating to cerebral hypoxia may present the picture of a typical vasodepressor reaction.

NEUROPHYSIOLOGIC FACTORS

NONCONVULSIVE SEIZURES

Certain forms of nonconvulsive seizure, characterized by cerebral dysrhythmia and transient disturbance in consciousness in the absence of typical epileptiform motor activity may be confused with the several forms of syncope previously described. The akinetic form of petit mal is an example. The differentiation may require a careful historical account to establish evidence of a primary cerebral dysrhythmia (aura and postictal phenomena), in conjunction with evidence of an electroencephalographic abnormality preceding the faint.

CONVERSION REACTION—HYSTERIA

While vasodepressor syncope frequently occurs in individuals with a hysterical personality structure, there is a form of conversion reaction associated with syncope in emotionally disturbed individuals in which the typical features of a vasodepressor reaction are absent. The individual will slump to the floor, unresponsive to verbal stimulation, but apparently not totally unconscious. The reaction may be protracted in time, throughout and following which there are no signs or symptoms to point to a pathophysiologic event other than the unresponsive nature of the patient.

CEREBRAL TYPE OF CAROTID SINUS SYNCOPE

Syncope owing to irritable carotid sinus of the peripheral type (vasodepressor) and cardiac type (cardioinhibitory) have been described previously, the reaction frequently having both cardiac and peripheral components simultaneously in a given individual. In his classic description of carotid sinus syncope, Weiss and colleagues included a third variant: the *cerebral type*.[85] This accounted for instances of syncope upon carotid sinus stimulation in which neither peripheral (hypotension) nor cardiac (bradycardia) manifestations appeared. The implication is that the unconsciousness results from a direct effect of carotid sinus stimulation on cerebral consciousness centers. Carotid arterial occlusive disease must be carefully excluded before such a diagnosis should be entertained.

SUMMARY

Fainting (syncope) relates to an ischemic, metabolic, or neuropsychologic disturbance in cerebral function leading to transient unconsciousness. The most prevalent variety is due to cerebral ischemia, secondary to a disordered function at any level in the circulation with or without associated structural disease. The faint itself is transient, and complete recovery from the episode is the rule, irrespective of etiology. It may be symptomatic of no identifiable disease (as with idiopathic vasodepressor syncope) or evidence of a major pathologic condition of the cardiovascular system (*e.g.*, aortic stenosis, carotid occlusion). The patient's historic account is of supreme value in sorting out which of a large number of clinical possibilities pertains in any given instance.

REFERENCES

1. **Strandgaard S:** Autoregulation of cerebral blood flow in hypertensive patients. Circulation, 53:720, 1976
2. **Cook P, James I:** Drug therapy: Cerebral vasodilators. N Engl J Med 305:1508, 1981
3. **Buzzi A, Yraola L:** Transient ventricular standstill following low ventricular tachycardia as a cause of Morgagni-Adams-Stokes syndrome. Acta Cardiol 14:643, 1959
4. **Easley RM, Jr, Goldstein S:** Sino-atrial syncope. Am J Med 50:166, 1971
5. **Pomerantz B, O'Rourke RH:** The Stokes–Adams syndrome. Am J Med 46:941, 1969
6. **Rosenbaum MB, Elizari MV, Lazzari JO:** The Hemiblocks, p 131. Oldsmar, Tampa Tracings, 1970
7. **Kulbertus H, Collignon P:** Association of right bundle branch block with left superior or inferior intraventricular block. Its relation to complete heart block and Adams–Stokes syndrome. Br Heart J 31:435, 1969
8. **Dhingra RC, Denes P, Delon W et al:** Syncope in patients with chronic bifascicular block. Ann Intern Med 81:302, 1974
9. **Boudoulas H, Schaal SF, Lewis RP et al:** Superiority of 24-hour outpatient monitoring over multi-stage exercise testing for evaluation of syncope. J Electrocardiol 12:103, 1979
10. **Boudoulas H, Schaal SF, Lewis RP:** Electrophysiologic risk factors of syncope. J Electrocardiol 11:339, 1978
11. **Zipes DP, McIntosh HD:** Cardiac arrhythmias. In Conn HL, Horowitz O (eds): Cardiac and Vascular Diseases, Vol. 1, p 360. Philadelphia, Lea & Febiger, 1971
12. **Waugh R, Wagner G, Haney T et al:** Immediate and remote prognostic significance of fascicular block during acute myocardial infarction. Circulation 47:765, 1973

13. **Cheng TO:** Transvenous ventricular pacing in the treatment of paroxysmal atrial tachyarrhythmias alternating with sinus bradycardia and standstill. Am J Cardiol 22:874, 1968

14. **Lown B:** Electrical reversion of cardiac arrhythmias. Br Heart J 29:469, 1967

15. **Scarpa WJ:** The sick sinus syndrome. Fundamentals of clinical cardiology. Am Heart J 92:648, 1976

16. **Leitner ER Von, Meyer V:** His electrocardiogram during atrial stimulation in 50 patients with transient cerebral symptoms. Adv Cardiol 19:273, 1977

17. **Durme JP Van:** Tachyarrhythmias and transient cerebral ischemic attacks. Annotations. Am Heart J 89:538, 1975

18. **Gallagher JJ, Pritchett ELC, Sealy WC et al:** The preexisting syndromes. Prog Cardiovasc Dis 20:289, 1978

19. **Klein GJ, Bashore TM, Sellers TD et al:** Ventricular fibrillation in the Wolff–Parkinson–White syndrome. N Engl J Med 301:1080, 1979

20. **Tominaga S, Blackburn H:** Prognostic importance of premature beats following myocardial infarction. Experience in the coronary drug project. JAMA, No. 10, 223:1116–1124, 1973

21. **Jervell A, Lange–Nielsen F:** Congenital deafmutism, functional heart disease with prolongation of the Q-T interval and sudden death. Am Heart J 54:59, 1957

22. **Romana C, Gemme G, Pongiglione R:** Aritmie cardiache rare deli' eta pediatrica. Clinica Pediatrica 45:656, 1963

23. **Swartz PJ, Periti M, Malliani A:** The long Q-T syndrome. Am Heart J 89:378, 1975

24. **Niarchos AP:** Propranolol-induced bradycardia and syncope. Acta Cardiol 27:504, 1972

25. **Davis LD, Temte JV:** Effects of propranolol on the transmembrane potentials of ventricular muscle and Purkinje fibers of the dog. Circ Res 22:661, 1968

26. **Benaim ME:** Letter to the Editor, Asystole after verapamil. Br Heart J 15 April, p 169, 1972

27. **Selzer A, Wray HW:** Quinidine syncope. Circulation 30:17, 1964

28. **Reynolds EW, Vander Ark CR:** Quinidine syncope and delayed repolarization syndromes. Mod Concepts Cardiovasc Dis 45:117, 1976

29. **Smith WM, Gallagher JJ:** "Les Torsades de Pointes": An unusual ventricular arrhythmia. Diagnosis and treatment. Ann Intern Med 93:578, 1980

30. **Sowton E, Hendrix G, Roy P:** Ten-year survival of treatment with implanted cardiac pacemaker. Br Med J 20 July, p 155, 1974

31. **Leung FW, Oill PA:** Ticket for admission: Unexplained syncopal attacks in patients with cardiac pacemaker. Annals of Emergency Medicine 9:527, 1980

32. **Furman S:** Cardiac pacing and pacemakers VI. Analysis of pacemaker malfunction. Appraisal and reappraisal of cardiac therapy. Am Heart J 94:378, 1977

33. **Gorlin R, McMillan RR, Medd WE et al:** Dynamics of the circulation in aortic valve disease. Am J Med 18:855, 1955

34. **Leake D:** Effort syncope in aortic stenosis. Br Heart J 21:289, 1959

35. **Cobbs BW, Jr:** Clinical recognition and medical management of acquired valvular diseases. In Hurst JW, Logue RB (eds): The Heart, Arteries and Veins, 2nd ed, p 836. New York, McGraw-Hill, 1970

36. **Schwartz LS, Goldfischer J, Sprague GJ et al:** Syncope and sudden death in aortic stenosis. Am J Cardiol 23:647, 1969

37. **Johnson AM:** Aortic stenosis, sudden death, and the LV baroreceptors. Br Heart J 33:1, 1971

38. **Mark AL, Rioschols JM, Abboud FM et al:** Abnormal vascular responses to exercise in patients with aortic stenosis. J Clin Invest 52:1138, 1973

39. **Wood P:** Aortic stenosis. Am J Cardiol 1:553, 1958

40. **Flamm MD, Branniff BA, Kimball R et al:** Mechanism of effort syncope in aortic stenosis. Circulation 35:109, 1967

41. **Devereux RB, Perloff JK, Reichek N et al:** Mitral valve prolapse. Circulation 54:3, 1976.

42. **Swartz MH, Teichholz LE, Donoso E:** Mitral valve prolapse. A review of associated arrhythmias. Am J Med 62:377, 1977

43. **Yufe R, Karpati G, Carpenter S:** Cardiac myxoma: A diagnostic challenge for the neurologist. Neurology 26:1060, 1976

44. **Ghahramani AR, Arnold JR, Hildner FJ et al:** Left atrial myxoma. Am J Med 52:525, 1972

45. **Herberden W:** Some account of a disorder of the breast. M Tr Roy Coll Physicians (London) 2:59, 1772.

46. **Irving JB, Kifchin AH:** Syncopal attacks as symptom of severe coronary artery disease. Br Med J 1:555, 1975

47. **Cookson H:** Fainting and fits in cardiac infarction: Br Heart J 4:163, 1952

48. **Levi GF, Proto C:** Ventricular fibrillation in the course of Prinzmetal's angina pectoris. Br Heart J 35:601, 1973

49. **Braunwald E, Lambrew CT, Rochoff SD et al:** Idiopathic hypertrophic subaortic stenosis. A description of the disease based upon analysis of 64 patients. Circulation (Suppl 4) 30:3, 1964

50. **Ross J, Braunwald E, Gault JH et al:** The mechanism of the intraventricular pressure gradient in idiopathic hypertrophic subaortic stenosis. Circulation 34:558, 1966

51. **Maurice P, Ben–Ismail M, Pentner PH et al:** Les myocardiopathies obstructives. 1. Étude clinique et radiologique Arch Coeur 59:375, 1966

52. **Joseph S, Balcon R, McDonald L:** Syncope in hypertrophic cardiomyopathy due to asystole. Br Heart J 34:974, 1972

53. **Glew RH, Varghese PH, Krovetz LJ et al:** Sudden death in congenital aortic stenosis. Am Heart J 78:615, 1969

54. **Perloff JK:** Clinical recognition of congenital heart disease. p 141. Philadelphia, WB Saunders, 1970

55. **Nakamura FF, Nadas AS:** Complete heart block in infants and children. N Engl J Med 270:1261, 1969

56. **Wood P:** Attacks of deeper cyanosis and loss of consciousness (syncope) in Fallot's tetralogy. Br Heart J 16:387, 1954

57. **Morgan BC, Guntheroth WG, Bloom RS et al:** A clinical profile of paroxysmal hyperpnea in cyanotic congenital heart disease. Circulation 31:66, 1965

58. **Perloff JK:** Clinical Recognition of Congenital Heart Disease. p. 360. Philadelphia, WB Saunders, 1970

59. **Dressler W:** Effort syncope as an early manifestation of primary pulmonary hypertension. Am J Med Sci 223:131, 1952

60. **Schaefer H, Blain JM, Ceballos R et al:** Essential pulmonary hypertension: A report of clinical-physiologic studies in three patients with death following catheterization of the heart. Ann Intern Med 44:505, 1956

61. **Maycock RL, Hyde RW:** Pulmonary heart disease. In Conn HL, Jr, Horowitz O (eds): Cardiac and Vascular Diseases, Vol. 2, pp 1167–1188. Philadelphia, Lea & Febiger, 1971

62. **Kuba H:** Primary pulmonary hypertension. In Hurst JW, Logue RB, Rackley CE (eds): The Heart, Arteries and Veins, 5th ed, pp 1223–1224. New York, McGraw-Hill, 1982

63. **James NN:** On the cause of syncope and sudden death in primary pulmonary hypertension. Ann Intern Med 56:252, 1962

64. **Thames D, Alpert JS, Dalen JE:** "Syncope due to massive pulmonary embolism." JAMA 238:2509–2511, 1977

65. **Dalen JE, Howe JP, III:** Dissection of the aorta. Current diagnosis and therapeutic approaches. Clinical cardiology. JAMA 242:1530, 1979

66. **Wheat MW, Jr:** Acute dissecting aneurysms of the aorta: Diagnosis and treatment—1979. Fundamentals of clinical cardiology. Am Heart J 99:373, 1980

67. **Green JH:** An Introduction to Human Psychology, 2nd ed, p 47. London, Oxford University Press, 1972

68. **Morganti A, Lopez–Ovejero JA, Pickering TG et al:** Role of the sympathetic nervous system in mediating the renin response to head-up tilt. Am J Cardiol 43:600, 1979

69. **Kerr A, Jr, Eich RH:** Cerebral concussion as a cause of cough syncope. Arch Intern Med 108:138, 1961

70. **Friedberg CK:** Syncope: Pathological physiology: Differential diagnosis and treatment (I), Mod Concepts Cardiovasc Dis 40:55, 1971

71. **Tohmeh JF, Shah SD, Cryer PE:** The pathogenesis of hyperadrenergic postural hypotension in diabetic patients. Am J Med 67:772, 1979

72. **Guyton AG, Jones CE, Coleman TG:** Circulatory Physiology: Cardiac Output and Its Regulation. 2nd ed, p 317–319. Philadelphia, WB Saunders, 1973

73. **Thoren PN, Donald DE, Shepherd JT:** Role of heart and lung receptors with nonmedullated vagal afferents in circulatory control. (Suppl II) Circ Res 38:2, 1976

74. **Shepherd JT:** Role of the veins in the circulation. Circulation 33:484, 1966

75. **Brooksby GA, Donald DE:** Dynamic changes in splanchnic blood flow and blood volume in dogs during activation of sympathetic nerves. Circ Res 31:105, 1972

76. **Chapman EM, Asmussen E:** On the occurrence of dyspnea, dizziness and precordial distress occasioned by the pooling of blood in varicose veins. J Clin Invest 21:393, 1942

77. **Nickerson M:** Vasodilator drugs. In Goodman LS, Gilman A (eds): The Pharmacologic Basis of Therapeutics, 4th ed, p 746. New York, Macmillan, 1970

78. **James IM, Millar RH, Purves MJ:** Observations on the extrinsic neural control of cerebral blood flow in the baboon. Circ Res 25:77, 1969

79. **McHenry LC, Jr, Fazekas JP, Sullivan JF:** Cerebral hemodynamics of syncope. Am J Med Sci 241:173, 1961

80. **Koch–Weser J:** Medical intelligence: Drug therapy-hydralazine. N Engl J Med 295:320, 1976

81. **Fuxe K, Sedvall G:** The distribution of adrenergic nerve fibers to the blood vessels in skeletal muscle. Acta Physiol Scand 64:25, 1965

82. **Levy MN, Imperial ES, Zieske H, Jr:** Ventricular response to increased outflow resistance in absence of elevated intraventricular end-diastolic pressure. Circ Res 12:107, 1963

83. **Goodall McC, Harlan WR, Jr, Alton H:** Noradrenaline release and metabolism in orthostatic (postural) hypotension. Circulation 36:489, 1967

84. **Ibrahim MM, Tarazi RC, Dustan HP et al:** Idiopathic orthostatic hypotension: Circulatory dynamics in chronic autonomic insufficiency. Circulation 34:288, 1974

85. **Weiss S, Capps RB, Ferris EB et al:** Syncope and convulsions due to a hyperactive carotid sinus reflex: Diagnosis and treatment. Arch Intern Med 58:407, 1936

86. **Coggins CH, Lillington GA, Gray CP:** Micturition syncope. Arch Intern Med 113:14, 1964

87. **Kopald HH, Roth HP, Fleshler B et al:** Vagovagal syncope. Report of a case associated with diffuse esophageal spasm. New Engl J Med 271:1238, 1964

88. **Kong Y, Heyman A, Entman ML et al:** Glossopharyngeal neuralgia associated with bradycardia, syncope and seizures. Circulation 30:109, 1964

89. **Mallinson EB, Coombes SK:** A hazard of anesthesia in ophthalmic surgery. Lancet 1:574, 1960

90. **Hickler RB, Hoskins RG, Hamlin JT, III:** The clinical evaluation of faculty orthostatic mechanisms. Med Clin North Am 44:1237, 1960

91. **Blair DA, Glover WE, Greenfield ADM et al:** Excitation of cholinergic vasodilator nerves to human skeletal muscles during emotional stress. J Physiol 148:633, 1959

92. **Rubio R, Bere RM, Dobson JG, Jr:** Site of adenosine production in cardiac and skeletal muscle. Am J Physiol 225:938, 1973

93. **Campbell G:** Autonomic nervous supply to effector tis-

sues. In Bülbring E, Brading AF (eds): Smooth Muscle, pp 451–495. London, Arnold, 1970

94. **Ruch TC, Patton HD:** Physiology and Biophysics II—Circulation, Respiration and Fluid Balance. 12th ed, p 193, 203. Philadelphia, WB Saunders, 1974

95. **Uvnäs B:** Sympathetic vasodilator outflow. Physiol Rev 34:608, 1954.

96. **Weissler AM, Warren JV, Estes EH, Jr et al:** Vasodepressor syncope: Factors influencing cardiac output. Circulation 15:875, 1957

97. **Epstein SE, Stampfer M, Beiser GD:** Role of the capacitance and resistance vessels in vasovagal syncope. Circulation 37:524, 1968

98. **Von Maur K, Nelson EW, Holsinger JW, Jr et al:** Hypersensitive carotid sinus syncope treated by implantable demand cardiac pacemaker. Am J Cardiol 29:109, 1972

99. **Oparil S, Vassaux C, Sanders CA et al:** Role of renin in acute postural homeostasis. Circulation 41:89, 1970

100. **Hickler RB, Wells RE, Tyler HR et al:** Plasma catechol amine and electroencephalographic responses to acute postural change. Am J Med 26:410, 1959

101. **Page EB, Hickam JB, Sieker HO et al:** Reflex venomotor activity in normal persons and in patients with postural hypotension. Circulation 11:262, 1955

102. **Botticelli JT, Keelan MH, Jr, Rosenbaum FF et al:** Circulatory control in idopathic orthostatic hypotension (Shy–Drager syndrome). Circulation 38:870, 1968

103. **Sharpey–Schater EP, Taylor EP:** Absent circulatory reflexes in diabetic neuritis. Lancet i: 559, 1960

104. **Thomas JE, Schirger A, Love JG et al:** Postural hypotension as the presenting sign in craniopharyngioma. Neurology 11:418, 1961

105. **Appenzeller V, Descarrier L:** Circulatory reflexes in patients with cerebrovascular disease. N Engl J Med 271:820, 1964

106. **Cohen IM:** Complications of chlorpromazine therapy. Am J Psychiatry 113:115, 1956

107. **Johnson RH, Lee de J, Oppenheimer DR et al:** Autonomic failure with orthostatic hypotension due to intermediolateral column degeneration. Q J Med (New Ser) 35:276, 1966

108. **Pearson J, Axelrod F, Dancis J:** Current concepts of dysautonomia: Neuropathological defects. Ann NY Acad Sci 228:288, 1974

109. **Benowitz NL, Byrd R, Schambelan M et al:** Dihydroergotamine treatment for orthostatic hypotension from vacor rodenticide. Ann Intern Med 92:387, 1980

110. **Kontos HA, Richardson DW, Norvell JE:** Norepinephrine depletion in idiopathic orthostatic hypotension. Ann Intern Med 82:336, 1975

111. **Ziegler MG, Lake CR, Kopin IJ:** The sympathetic nervous system defect in primary orthostatic hypotension. N Engl J Med 296:293, 1977

112. **Leveston SA, Shah SD, Cryer PE:** Cholinergic stimulation of norepinphrine release in man. Evidence of a sympathetic postganglionic axonal lesion in diabetic adrenergic neuropathy. J Clin Invest 64:374, 1979

113. **Shy GM, Drager GH:** A neurological syndrome associated with orthostatic hypotension: A clinical-pathologic study. Arch Neurol Psychiatry 2:511, 1960

114. **Davies G, Sudera D, Mathias C et al:** Letter to the Editor, Beta-receptors in orthostatic hypotension. N Engl J Med 305:1017, 1981

115. **Thomas EJ, Schirger H:** Idiopathic orthostatic hypotension. Arch Neurol 22:289, 1970

116. **Schatz IJ, Padolsky S, Frame B:** Idiopathic orthostatic hypotension, JAMA 186:537, 1963

117. **Meyer JS:** Occlusive cerebrovascular disease; Pathogenesis and treatment. Am J Med 30:577, 1961

118. **Reivich N, Holling HE, Roberts B et al:** Reversal of blood flow through the vertebral artery and its effort on cerebral circulation: N Engl J Med 265:878, 1961.

119. **Wheeler HB:** Surgical treatment of subclavian-arterial occlusion. N Engl J Med 276:711, 1967

34

Vertigo and Dizziness— Disorders of Static and Dynamic Equilibrium Alfred D. Weiss

Introduction
Functional Organization of the Systems
  The Vestibular System
  The Oculomotor System
  The Vestibulosomatic System
Principles of Neurologic Lesion Localization
  The Cranial Nerves
  Disturbances of Brain Stem
  The Cervical Spine
Clinical Significance of Vertigo and Dizziness
  General Considerations
  Diseases of the Ear
  Diseases of the Eighth Nerve
  Brain Stem and Cerebellum

Neoplastic Diseases
Degenerative Diseases
Malformations
Demyelinative Diseases
Infectious Diseases
Nutritional Diseases
Hydrocephalus
Head Injuries
Drug Effects
The Cervical Spine
Ocular Dizziness
Dizziness in Epilepsy
Psychogenic Dizziness
Summary

INTRODUCTION

Vertigo and dizziness are among the more common distressing symptoms that afflict mankind. Yet the words used by patients to describe complaints relating to disturbances in the systems associated with static and dynamic equilibrium are surprisingly vague. They range from complaint of blurring of vision, double vision, blacking-out, light-headedness, faintness, passing-out, falling, being off balance, and weakness to fairly accurate description of a hallucination of movement of self or environment, either rotatory or linear, spontaneous, movement-provoked or position-related. Some patients are able to provide a fairly accurate description on careful questioning; other patients seem unable to do so but may, in the course of the examination, especially during caloric testing or during positional testing, exclaim that the sensation induced is the sensation of which they complain.

In eliciting the patient's history, it is extremely important to obtain as clear an idea as possible of the time and other characteristics at the onset of the symptoms, the duration, the accompaniment of other symptoms, their recurrence, and other aspects of the evolution of the illness. A neurologic symptom review then may serve to elicit additional aspects of the present illness or of related illnesses. Past medical history may reveal important clues to the possible nature of the

present illness. Of particular importance are questions relating to head injuries, the details of which must be obtained; previous severe illnesses, either systemic or localized, such as in the ear; previous history of tumors; significant systemic diseases; medications received; and noise exposure. The reciting of the family history should include the question of whether any close member of the family has had symptoms similar to those of which the patient complains. The symptom review often provides clues to the probable localization of lesions. The evolution of illness, past medical history, and family history often provide clues as to the etiology of the problem. The neurologic and otologic examinations may provide confirmation of the suspected loci of disturbances and may reveal additional unsuspected loci. The decision must then be made as to what further tests are necessary to confirm or disprove the formulation of lesion localization. The most important of these in the area of otoneurology are the audiometric battery and the electronystagmogram (including bithermal calorics). A wide range of additional tests are available of the sort normally employed in neurologic and otologic practice, as well as those of more general medical nature. Some tests are relatively harmless to the patient, while others carry significant risk. Almost all are expensive in varying degree. Consequently, testing should not be employed as casting a finely meshed net widely, but rather in terms of providing the most precise answers possible to the most specifically formulated questions possible. The clinician must always question how a positive or negative result of any given test will affect his formulation, as well as the probabilities of true and false positives and negatives in relationship to the questions asked, insofar as such statistics are available. The making of the decision to perform a given test is also complicated by the balancing of the risks of doing the test versus the risks of not doing it and thereby missing an important diagnosis, especially a diagnosis of a disease that has a much more favorable prognosis for the patient when treatment is rendered earlier rather than later.

FUNCTIONAL ORGANIZATION OF THE SYSTEMS

The specifications for the systems producing static and dynamic equilibrium in the human organism are peculiarly complex. The static postures range from the rather stable position of lying down to the rather unstable one of standing up, a position akin to that of an inverted pendulum. A person might lie prone or supine; he might stand with head bowed, turned, tilted, or thrown back, and yet he is stable in all of these positions. A person might crawl, walk, run, jump, balance on spare footing, swing on ropes or trapezes, dive under water, ride a bicycle, drive a car, or fly a plane. Throughout, he must maintain his desired orientation in space, stability of vision, coordination of limbs. It seems almost incredible that he does it so well. But how?

Let us begin by drawing the picture in broad strokes. The human organism consists of a torso, to which are attached four limbs and a neck with head. The limbs, back, and neck are multiply jointed, with each joint having rather well-defined types and ranges of movement. Active movement at the joints is due to muscle contractions, which are produced by firing of the peripheral motor nerves. The programming and command of movements, from the simplest to the most complex, is in the central nervous system (CNS), which then "knows" the position of joints and members from the command signal it issued, from proprioceptive and kinesthetic sensory inflow, from visual and tactile inflow, and from vestibular inflow under some circumstances. The sensory information may then be used as feedback for error correction in command signals. This implies the choice of a specific movement from a repertory of many possible movements, which introduces the psychological construct of "set." There is a vast flood of potential and actual sensory information impinging on the peripheral sensors. Set nerves sort and limit the sensory input to the CNS, assigning priorities, designating routes and levels of transmission, and processing.

In most normal human organisms, for any given set, information inflow, processing, and command outflow seem to occur in fairly well standardized patterns. The observer suspects the presence of pathology when the pattern deviates significantly from the range of normal variation, as defined either by statistical or by the observer's subjective criteria. The inference of clinical significance of such a finding depends on many factors but chiefly on the finding of corroborative evidence.

THE VESTIBULAR SYSTEM

The main sensor of equilibrium is the vestibular system. The vestibular labyrinths lie in the petrous temporal bones. They are organized functionally into three pairs of semicircular canals, a pair of utricles, and a pair of saccules (Fig. 34-1). The utricles are sensors of linear acceleration, of which the gravity vector is the single most important. They are omnidirectional, although the thresholds and gains are probably not uniform in all directions. The bilateral symmetry of the two utricles would, however, provide for functional symmetry of the lateral vectors. The function of the saccules may be similar but is less well understood.

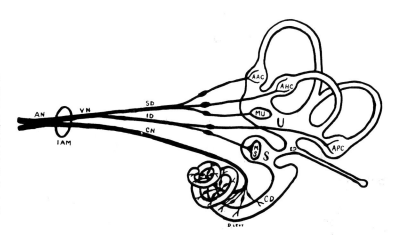

Fig. 34-1. Diagram of membranous labyrinth showing nerve distribution. AN = acoustic nerve; IAM = internal auditory meatus; VN = vestibular nerve; SD = superior division of vestibular nerve; ID = inferior division of vestibular nerve; CN = cochlear nerve; AAC = ampulla of anterior semicircular canal; AHC = ampulla of horizontal semicircular canal; APC = ampulla of posterior semicircular canal; U=utricle; MU = macula utriculi; S = saccule; MS = macula sacculi; CD = cochlear duct; ED = endolymphatic duct.

The semicircular canals are sensors of angular acceleration. Functionally they are paired as two lateral (or horizontal) canals, and the superior canal of either side is paired with the contralateral inferior canal. Each pair of canals lies in a plane that is at right angles to the planes of the two other pairs. This orthogonal arrangement permits the sensing of head rotation in any plane during positive or negative acceleration. The sensitive element of each canal is at its ampulla, which functions like a pressure transducer. A branch of the vestibular nerve passes to the ampulla of each semicircular canal, where it terminates in a receptor organ called the *crista*. In the absence of an effective stimulus to the semicircular canals, there is a constant flow of afferent impulses in the vestibular nerve. Stimulation of a semicircular canal produces modulation of the afferent impulses in the nerve, increasing or decreasing their frequency, depending on the direction of the stimulus. For example, if the stimulus is to turn the head to the right, the effect on the right horizontal canal will be to increase the rate of discharge in the right vestibular nerve, while the effect on the left horizontal canal will be the opposite. A similar effect—a modulation of afferent firing—can be achieved in one ear at a time by means of caloric stimulation, the degree of effect being a function of the effective strength of the stimulus. It follows then that the sudden loss of function of a semicircular canal or its nerve alters the pattern of afferent inflow and produces effects akin to those of a strong stimulus. The vestibular nerve traverses the internal auditory canal, together with the cochlear, facial, and interstitial nerves, and the internal auditory artery and veins. It crosses the cerebellopontine angle to enter the rostral medulla and terminates in the vestibular nuclei and portions of cerebellum. The vestibular nuclei are much more than simple relays of vestibular input but are complex processors of several sources of sensory input concerned with postural and ocular control; they also issue commands to these systems. Vestibular stimulation affects the movements of the eyes, head, neck, and limbs, as well as attitude of the body in space. A summary of the reflex connections of the cristae, the utricle, and the saccule is shown in Figures 34-2, 34-3, and 34-4.

THE OCULOMOTOR SYSTEM

The oculomotor system has a rather clearly specified relationship to the vestibular system in certain respects, which makes it a very convenient indicator of the effects of stimulation on the vestibular system, as well as an indicator of the presence of pathology in the vestibular system. In the latter connection, however, it is important to remember that the oculomotor system may reflect pathologies both within itself and in a number of systems of which the vestibular system is but one. In the normal, alert individual with his eyes open, the eyes move synchronously and in the same direction at all times except when convergence occurs. Each eye is moved by three pairs of muscles. It is a useful approximation to state that each pair of muscles moves the eyes in a plane parallel to the plane of one pair of semicircular canals. Stimulation of a pair of semicircular canals or of a semicircular canal will move the eyes parallel to that plane if the eye is deviated so that the line of sight is parallel to the plane of the canal. Restated another way, if the eyes look straight ahead, stimulation of the horizontal canals will move the eyes horizontally. If the eyes are deviated 45° towards the left, stimulation of the left superior and/or right inferior semicircular canals will produce vertical movement of the eyes. If the same canals are stimulated with the eyes deviated 45° in the other direction, or effectively 90° from the plane of the canals being stimulated, a purely rotatory movement of the eyes is produced. Again, stimulation of the same canals with the

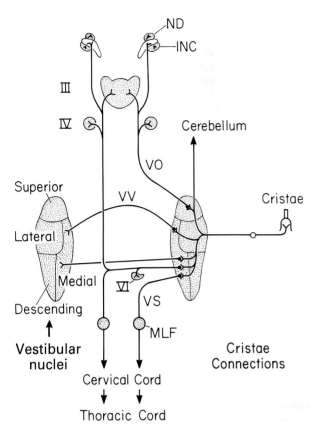

Fig. 34-2. Summary of the reflex connections of the cristae. III = oculomotor nucleus; IV = trochlear nucleus; VI = abducens nucleus; VO = vestibulo-ocular projection; VV = vestibulovestibular projection; VS = vestibulospinal projection; MLF = medial longitudinal fasciculus; ND = nucleus of Darkeschewitsch; INC = interstitial nucleus of Cajal. (From Gacek RR: Neuroanatomical correlates of vestibular function. Ann Otol Rhinol Laryngol 89:2–5, 1980)

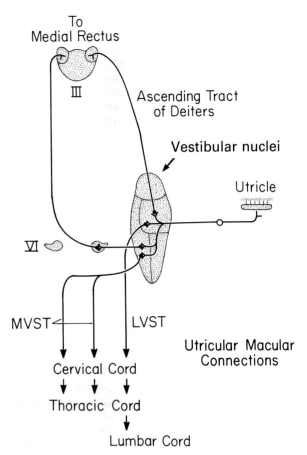

Fig. 34-3. Summary of the reflex connections of the utricle. MVST = medial vestibulospinal tract; LSVT = lateral vestibulospinal tract. (See Fig. 34-2 for additional abbreviations.) (From Gacek RR: Neuroanatomical correlates of vestibular function. Ann Otol Rhinol Laryngol 89:2–5, 1980)

eyes pointed straight ahead will produce a mixture of vertical and rotatory movement of the eyes. It appears that the function of the semicircular canals *vis-à-vis* the eyes is to stabilize visual fixation while the head is moving. Thus, if the person is walking with his head bobbing up and down somewhat, the eyes bob down and up in compensatory fashion in order to permit stabilization of vision. A passive turning of the head (*e.g.*, towards the right) will produce compensatory movement of the eyes to the left. If the head continues to move towards the right beyond the ability of the eyes to compensate by turning left, one of two things may occur: The eyes may continue to be forced in extreme left deviation without being able to move further, or the eyes may return rapidly towards or past the neutral forward position and then resume turning

towards the left once again. Such alternation of slow deviations with rapid saccades or resets is called *nystagmus*. Under normal conditions, when there is no visual target fixation and the patient is instructed to look forward, the eyes are deviated somewhat in the direction of the turn by the saccade, the slow phase bringing the eyes back to or just past the midline.

Definition of Nystagmus. Strictly speaking, nystagmus should consist of a rhythmic, reciprocating motion, in which the velocity in one direction is distinctly faster than that in the other direction. Usage has introduced terms such as *pendular nystagmus* in which the velocity is the same in both directions, but I prefer to apply the term *ocular oscillations* to this phenomenon. Nystagmus may be subclassified as spontaneous, positional, and induced. Spontaneous and positional nystagmus are never normal, although the clinical sig-

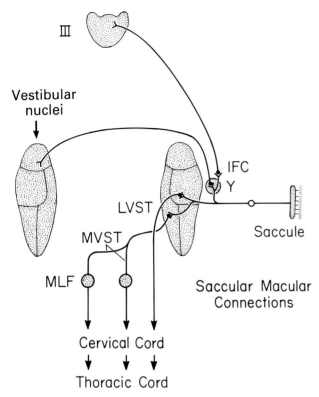

Fig. 34-4. Summary of the reflex connections of the saccule. IFC = infracerebellar nucleus; Y = Group-Y nucleus. (See Figs. 34-2 and 34-3 for additional abbreviations.) (From Gacek RR: Neuroanatomical correlates of vestibular function. Ann Otol Rhinol Laryngol 89:2–5, 1980)

nificance may vary. Induced nystagmus is usually a normal phenomenon, unless the degree or quality of the response is other than that normally expected.

Electronystagmography. The description in measurement of nystagmus has been improved tremendously in recent years by the introduction of electrical recording techniques called *electronystagmography* (ENG) or *electro-oculography.* This technique makes use of the fact that the eye is an electrical dipole. Placing electrodes at the opposite sides of the eye permit the recording of ocular deviations because of the relative shifts in polarity at the two electrodes. One may thus measure horizontal movements of the eyes, either both eyes together or each eye separately, and vertical movements of either eye.

ENG has become a very powerful tool in the analysis of eye movement and in the diagnosis of disturbances in the postural control system. It has a number of distinct advantages over visual observation alone. It permits the examination for spontaneous nystagmus to be made with eyes open in darkness as well as with eyes

closed, neither of which can be done readily by direction observation. Since it has been estimated that only about 10% of spontaneous nystagmus is visible to direct observation, failure to use ENG will lead to failure to observe this important pathologic sign in 90% of the cases in which it is present. The same is true for positional nystagmus.* Similarly, perrotatory nystagmus asymmetries and abnormal provoked nystagmus following short rotations cannot be seen in most instances by direct observation with eyes open in the light. Nor is it possible to tell by direct observation whether the spontaneous nystagmus seen with eyes open in the light is enhanced or abolished by eye closure, the two phenomena having completely different implications as to the localization of the lesion. Furthermore, with ENG, optokinetic nystagmus and calorically induced nystagmus may be quantified, permitting estimates not only of duration but also of slow- and, if necessary, fast-phase velocities, both with eyes open and with eyes closed.

For technical reasons, it is desirable to record horizontal and vertical eye movements concurrently on separate channels, since this reduces the likelihood of mistaking blinks for nystagmus or of misreading as vertical nystagmus a horizontal nystagmus present with eyes offset from neutral with eye closure.

Purely rotatory nystagmus cannot be recorded with current ENG techniques.

Another system of measurement called *photoelectric nystagmography* or *oculography* can be used only with eyes open either in light or darkness.

Spontaneous Nystagmus. Spontaneous nystagmus with eyes open should be looked for with visual fixation at approximately a meter, with eyes straight ahead, and with eyes deviated 30° to the right, left, upwards, and downwards. It is important to note the direction of nystagmus, conventionally designated by the direction of the rapid component, and a description as to whether the nystagmus is mainly linear or rotatory in nature. It must be noted if the two eyes move synchronously in deviation and in nystagmus. Nystagmus elicited only at the extremes of gaze deviation are not significant and are designated end-point nystagmus. The convention is to speak of nystagmus as being first degree if it is seen only when the eyes are deviated 30° in the direction of the rapid component, to call it second-degree nystagmus if the nystagmus is visible also with the eyes in a straight-ahead position, and to designate it third-degree nystagmus when it is present even when the eyes are deviated 30° away from the

*The use of Frenzel glasses (15 diopter positive lenses in an illuminated frame), which reduces fixation, will increase the detection of nystagmus with eyes open to about 20%. Eye closure is thought to be physiologically different than the mere abolition of fixation with eyes open.

rapid component. It is important to differentiate a third-degree nystagmus from a bidirectional first-degree nystagmus, since the latter almost always is of brain stem origin while the former is more commonly of peripheral origin. Vertical nystagmus in the eyes-forward position is usually of central origin, except in the presence of bilateral peripheral vestibular disease. It is important also to note if the nystagmus changes in character as gaze is deviated from one side to the other, since an unchanging rotatory nystagmus would tend to indicate a brain stem disorder, while a change from rotatory to vertical depending on direction of gaze would tend to implicate one of the vertical semicircular canals. This is true also of nystagmus seen during positional testing. Spontaneous nystagmus should be looked for with the patient seated in the erect position.

Positional Nystagmus. Testing for positional nystagmus is performed by beginning with a patient in the erect position with eyes fixed straight ahead at about a meter. The observer may provide the fixation point with his hand at arm's length. The patient is then moved briskly into a supine position with the hand hanging over the edge of the table as far as his neck will permit, again with eyes fixated at the examiner's arm's length. The examiner looks for nystagmus, counting off time as he does so. He should note the time of onset of nystagmus, the time of its cessation, its character, and some idea of its intensity, noting as well whether or not the patient complains of dizziness or vertigo. Should no nystagmus occur within 15 sec of the assumption of the position, the patient is moved to the next position. Should nystagmus occur, the position is maintained until nystagmus ceases or until 60 sec have elapsed, whichever occurs first, at which point the patient is moved to the next position. After head hanging, the next position is upright, followed by a position in which the head is turned to the right, and then the patient is moved into the supine position with the right ear hanging well over the edge of the table. After this, the patient returns to the upright seated position, is then moved to the left-ear-down position, and is then moved upright once again. If ENG is available, a similar procedure with eyes closed should follow, the order of testing usually being erect to supine, right-ear-down position, supine, left-ear-down position, supine, and upright. With eyes closed, each position is maintained for 1 min.

A number of classifications of positional nystagmus are in use. One of the simpler is that which divides positional nystagmus into three types. Type I consists of direction-changing persistent nystagmus. In this, nystagmus in any one or more positions persists for more than 60 sec from the time that the position is assumed. Nystagmus must be present in more than one direction, either during one position or in different positions. Type II positional nystagmus is direction-fixed persistent, which means that nystagmus persists for over 60 sec in any position from the time that the position is assumed but beats in only one direction when it is present. Type III positional nystagmus is direction-fixed or changing and transient, the nystagmus in any position always lasting less than 60 sec.

Caloric Testing. The best method available currently for testing the response of the vestibular system of each ear separately is the caloric test. It is performed by positioning the patient with the head elevated approximately 30° from the supine position so that the line from the external canthus of the eye to the external auditory meatus lies in the vertical. This line is approximately in the same plane as that of the horizontal semicircular canals. The temperature of the external auditory canal is then altered by flushing the canal with air or water of a predetermined temperature, usually 44°C or 30°C. Since the body temperature is usually 37°C, this introduces a temperature gradient of 7°C, which is transmitted to the middle ear and then to the horizontal semicircular canal. This induces a convection current within the horizontal semicircular canal, which produces a pressure change at the ampulla, stimulating that sensor. The 30°C stimulus produces nystagmus normally towards the opposite side, and the 44°C stimulus produces nystagmus towards the stimulated side. By stimulating each ear in turn with each of the two temperatures, it is possible to compute a comparison of responses between the two ears, as well as a comparison of the strength of directionality of response. This provides measures of reduced vestibular response, which may be due to disturbances of the inner ear, the vestibular nerve, or vestibular nuclei. A directional preponderance may reflect disturbances anywhere within the vestibular system, from labyrinth to nerve to brain stem to temporal lobe. (For accuracy, it is important that both tympanic membranes be intact and accessible to irrigation by the fluid and that there be a normal air space within the middle ear.) A number of different measures of response are used: duration; slow-phase velocity; fast-phase velocity; or beat frequency of nystagmus, as measured with eyes open or with eyes closed. Because normal responses vary with different techniques, each laboratory must provide its own standard of normal limits. Marked ocular deviation may be noted during the course of the response. A perverted response may also be noted, in which the response direction is different from that normally expected. This usually implicates brain stem. In the normal individual, both eyes move synchronously, while

35

Dehydration and Edema
Cecil H. Coggins

Anatomy and Definitions
Water Balance
  Normal Intake and Output
  Normal Regulation of Solute Concentration
    The Osmoreceptor
    The Antidiuretic Hormone
    The Renal Concentrating Mechanism
    Renal Response to the Antidiuretic Hormone
    Nonosmotic Stimuli for Antidiuretic Hormone
    Interrelations of Osmotic and Circulatory Stimuli
Dehydration—Simple Water Loss
  Signs and Symptoms of Dehydration
  Causes of Dehydration
    Impaired Fluid Intake and Nonrenal Loss
    Renal Water Loss
  Approach to the Dehydrated Patient
  Hypothalamic Diabetes Insipidus
  Polyuria Unresponsive to Antidiuretic Hormone
    Osmotic Diuresis
    Renal Disease
    Metabolic Disturbances
    Sickle Cell Disease
    Postobstructive Diuresis
    Drugs
Water Excess
  Artifactual Hyponatremia

  Impaired Circulation
  Circulation Possibly Impaired
  Normal Circulation
Salt Balance—The Regulation of Volume
  Distribution of Water Among the Body Fluid Compartments
  Regulation of Salt Balance
  Control of Salt Excretion
    Glomerular Filtration
    Proximal Tubule
    Henle's Loop
    Distal Tubule
    Collecting Tubule
Salt Lack—Extracellular Volume Depletion
  Signs and Symptoms
  Causes of Salt Lack
    Renal Salt Loss
    Diuretics
    Nonrenal Salt Loss
  Approach to the Patient
Salt Excess—Edema
  Definition
  Mechanisms of Edema Formation
    Capillary Mechanisms
    Renal Mechanisms
  Approach to the Patient with Edema
Summary

ANATOMY AND DEFINITIONS

The water content of a normal thin male is approximately 60% by weight. Females and obese persons have less water, and very young children have more. This water is distributed throughout the body in the cells (intracellular compartment), between the cells (interstitial compartment), and within the blood vessels (intravascular compartment) (Fig. 35-1). The interstitial and intravascular spaces together form the extracellular compartment. A small amount of additional fluid is present in the urinary spaces, the gastro-intestinal tract, the cerebral spinal fluid, the eyes, inner ears, and so forth. Normally about two thirds of the body water is intracellular. Of the one third that is extracellular, about one-fifth is intravascular (the plasma volume) and the rest interstitial. Thus, in a thin, 70-kg man, the total body water would be 42 liters, the intracellular fluid 28 liters, and the extracellular fluid 14 liters, of which about 11 liters is interstitial and 3 liters is intravascular plasma. The cell membranes and the capillary walls form the boundaries of these spaces and are freely permeable to water. This permeability ensures that the total solute concentration in each space is equal to that in the others, for if a difference in solute concentration

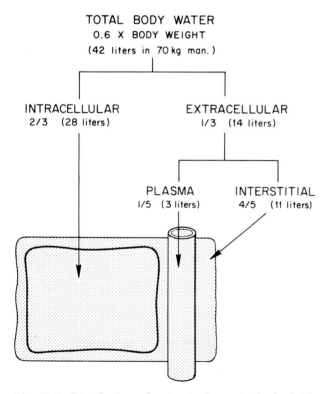

Fig. 35-1. Distribution of water in the major body fluid compartments.

occurred, water would flow across the osmotic gradient until the concentrations were again equal. The total solute concentration is measured in terms of the *milliosmol*—the osmotic pressure exerted when a solution containing 1/1000 of a mol of solute particles per kg of water is separated from pure water by an ideal semipermeable membrane. Normal plasma, interstitial fluid, and intracellular fluid all have an osmolality of about 285 mOsm per kg. Dehydration is a loss of water (*i.e.*, a loss of volume) from one or more of the body fluid compartments.

WATER BALANCE

NORMAL INTAKE AND OUTPUT

The normal daily intake of fluid varies widely depending upon the availability of water, the type of diet, and the preferences or habits of the individual. The output in turn normally can be adjusted over a wide range to assure constancy of total body water. The typical individual not engaged in strenuous work and not living in a hot, humid climate (Fig. 35-2) might have an intake of about 2200 ml of water each day, made up of 1500 ml ingested as fluid, 500 ml contained in solid food, and 200 ml produced in the body when the food is oxidized. A corresponding output would total 2200 ml, including 1200 ml of urine, 50 ml in stool water, 100 ml in sweat, and 700 ml evaporated from the lungs. As will be discussed, fluid loss by these routes may be remarkably increased in abnormal circumstances and may lead to negative fluid balance.

NORMAL REGULATION OF SOLUTE CONCENTRATION

Since the total solute concentrations or osmolalities of all the body fluid compartments are equal, control of the osmolalities of all of the compartments can be accomplished by regulation of any one of them. Osmotic regulation is accomplished by control of the body's intake and output of water. When water is lost from the body (by respiratory or skin losses, for example), a slight increase in the solute concentration of the body fluid leads normally to an increased thirst and intake of water and a diminished renal excretion of water until the fluid deficit is corrected and the osmolality returns to normal. Conversely, a dilution of the body fluids leads to decreased intake and increased rate of excretion of water. The mechanism by which these are accomplished involves (1) an osmotic sensor, (2) the production and release into the circulation of antidiuretic hormone, (3) the kidney's ability to concentrate urine, and (4) the sensation of thirst.

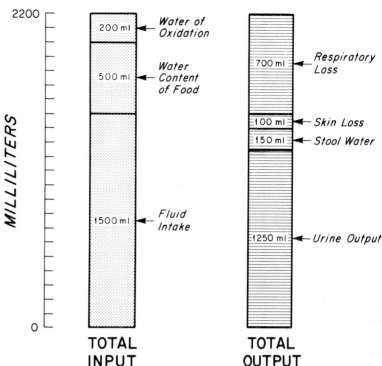

Fig. 35-2. Routes of water intake and loss for a typical individual living in a temperate climate. Wide variations may occur normally.

The Osmoreceptor

In the supraoptic and paraventricular nuclei of the anterior hypothalamus are cells responsive to changes in the solute concentration of the blood that perfuses the area (Fig. 35-3).[1] In these nuclei the hormone arginine vasopressin (which is the antidiuretic hormone in man and most other mammals) is produced and bound to a protein, neurophysin,[2] with which it travels down the supraoptico-hypophysial tract to be stored in the posterior pituitary. An increase in the osmolality of the blood perfusing the hypothalamus (perhaps by shrinking the cells as water moves out in response to the osmotic gradient) leads to increased synthesis of the hormone and transmission of nerve impulses down the axons of the tract releasing the hormone from the posterior pituitary. The same stimulus leads to the conscious sensation of thirst and increased water intake.

The Antidiuretic Hormone

Arginine vasopressin is a peptide hormone containing eight amino acids with a molecular weight of 1030 (Fig. 35-4). It differs from oxytocin, a hormone produced and stored in the same hypothalamic and pituitary areas, by only two amino acids; and from vasotocin, an "ancestral" pituitary hormone found throughout most vertebrates other than mammals, by only one. Vasopressin circulates in the blood unbound, or only loosely bound, in extremely low concentrations of approximately 1 pg to 5 pg per ml (about $1-4 \times 10^{-12}$ molar) with an apparent volume of distribution equal to the extracellular fluid space and a half-time in the circulation of about 20 min.[3] It appears to be degraded in large part by the liver, as well as by the kidneys.[4]

The Renal Concentrating Mechanism

As each renal tubule courses through the cortex of the kidney, the Henle's loop dips down, between the proximal and distal tubules, into the renal medulla (Fig. 35-5). In particular, the Henle's loop of the tubules whose glomeruli are located deep in the cortex travel far down through the medulla into the renal papilla. Specific characteristics of cells lining the ascending limb of these loops lead to the ability of the mammalian kidney to produce concentrated urine. The cells actively transport chloride from the tubular fluid into the interstitial fluid of the medulla, and the sodium ions appear to follow passively. This cell layer is impermeable to water, so the outward transport of sodium chloride produces a progressive dilution of the tubular fluid as it rises toward the cortex and an increase in the salt concentration of the surrounding medullary interstitial fluid. The resulting interstitial fluid hypertonicity can exist without dissipation in this location, unlike other areas of the body, because it is effectively isolated by the countercurrent arrangement of tubules and blood

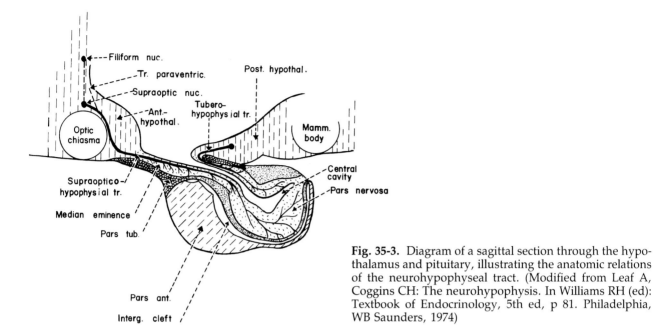

Fig. 35-3. Diagram of a sagittal section through the hypothalamus and pituitary, illustrating the anatomic relations of the neurohypophyseal tract. (Modified from Leaf A, Coggins CH: The neurohypophysis. In Williams RH (ed): Textbook of Endocrinology, 5th ed, p 81. Philadelphia, WB Saunders, 1974)

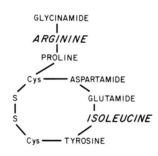

ARGININE VASOTOCIN

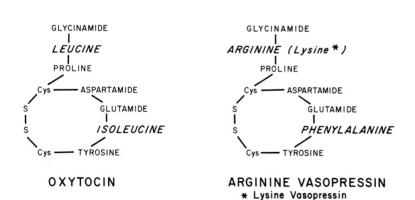

OXYTOCIN

ARGININE VASOPRESSIN
* Lysine Vasopressin

Fig. 35-4. Arginine vasopressin (ADH), oxytocin, and vasotocin have an identical amino-acid sequence except in two positions. Lysine vasopressin is the unique antidiuretic hormone in the pig family. (Leaf A, Coggins CH: The neurohypophysis. In Williams RH (ed): Textbook of Endocrinology, 5th ed, p 82. Philadelphia, WB Saunders, 1974)

728

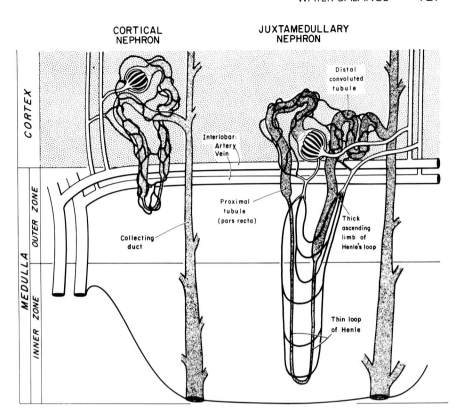

CORTICAL
NEPHRON

JUXTAMEDULLARY
NEPHRON

Distal
convoluted
tubule

Interlobar:
Artery
Vein

Proximal
tubule
(pars recta)

Thick
ascending
limb of
Henle's loop

Collecting
duct

Thin loop
of Henle

CORTEX

MEDULLA OUTER ZONE

INNER ZONE

Fig. 35-5. Juxtamedullary nephrons dip deeply into the hypertonic medulla. (Leaf A, Cotran R: Renal Pathophysiology. London, Oxford Press, 1976)

vessels supplying the renal medulla. In contrast with the normal blood osmolality of about 285 mOsm/kg, the interstitial fluid in the renal papilla may have an osmolality of 1000 mOsm or 1200 mOsm/kg as a result of the sodium chloride transport in the ascending limb of Henle's loops. At the same time this sodium chloride transport results in a dilution of the tubular fluid to about 150 mOsm/kg as it ascends within the loop back to the renal cortex.

Renal Response to the Antidiuretic Hormone

In the absence of vasopressin, this dilute tubular fluid is allowed to pass through the collecting duct and out into the renal pelvis, thus producing a large quantity of dilute urine. When vasopressin is present, however, the cell layer lining the collecting duct becomes permeable to water. As the tubular fluid flows through the collecting duct, water moves out of the duct by osmosis into the hypertonic interstitium and the urine becomes small in volume and highly concentrated. The collecting tubule cells have receptors on their surfaces, which are capable of binding vasopressin even in its extremely low circulating concentrations and of initiating a series of reactions that involve the activation of the enzyme adenylate cyclase. The resulting formation of cyclic AMP in the cell ultimately results, by

mechanisms not well understood, in an increased permeability of the tubular membrane.[5,6,7] Thus, the normally functioning kidney can switch from the production of copious dilute urine to a state of water conservation by means of a single permeability change induced by antidiuretic hormone (Figs. 35-6, 35-7).

At the same time that the kidneys are induced to conserve water, increased thirst leads to water intake, thus restoring the body's water balance and keeping serum osmolality within the narrow range of normal.

Nonosmotic Stimuli for Antidiuretic Hormone

The vasopressin mechanism responds to small changes in osmolality and is the means by which a normal concentration of solutes in the body fluids is maintained (Fig. 35-8). The hormone can also be released in response to circulatory stimuli (Fig. 35-9) and other nonosmotic stimuli.[8-10] When the circulation is impaired, as in shock or dehydration, baroreceptors in the aortic arch, carotid body, and left atrium respond to reduced pressure by stimulating the release of the antidiuretic hormone and thus the conservation of water. Severe heart failure may also induce reflex release of the hormone. This antidiuretic response may serve as a useful means of expanding blood volume and restoring circulation, though at the expense of the abnormalities in

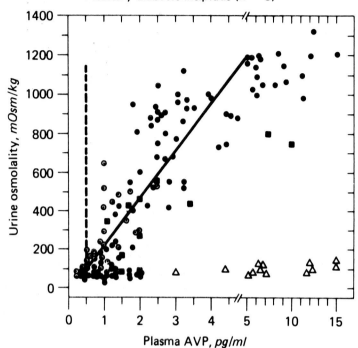

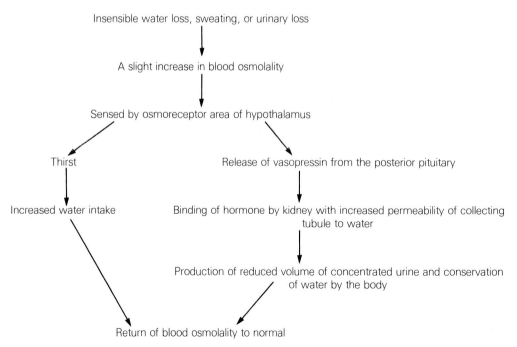

- ● Normal subjects (N = 23)
- ■ Primary polydipsia (N = 2)
- △ Nephrogenic diabetes insipidus (N = 2)
- ⊙ Pituitary diabetes insipidus (N = 8)

Fig. 35-6. The relationship of urine osmolality to plasma vasopressin in healthy adults and patients with different types of polyuria. (Robertson GL, Shelton RL, Athar S: The osmoregulation of vasopressin. Kidney Int 10:25, 1976)

Insensible water loss, sweating, or urinary loss

A slight increase in blood osmolality

Sensed by osmoreceptor area of hypothalamus

Thirst

Release of vasopressin from the posterior pituitary

Increased water intake

Binding of hormone by kidney with increased permeability of collecting tubule to water

Production of reduced volume of concentrated urine and conservation of water by the body

Return of blood osmolality to normal

Fig. 35-7. Sequence of water loss leading to water conservation in the normal subject.

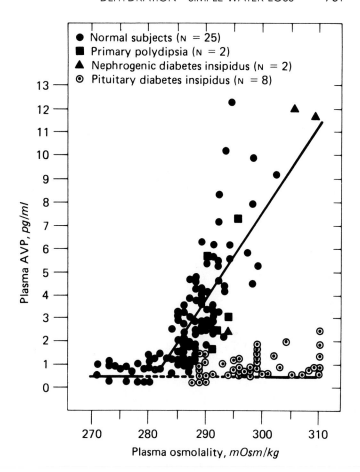

Fig. 35-8. The relationship of plasma vasopressin to plasma osmolality in healthy adults and patients with different types of polyuria. (From Robertson GL, Shelton RL, Athar S: The osmoregulation of vasopressin. Kidney Int 10:25, 1976)

osmolality that might result. In addition, strong circulatory stimuli (such as hemorrhagic shock) may produce circulating levels of vasopressin that are far higher than those released in response to severe hypertonicity. At high concentrations, vasopressin, as its name implies, is a direct pressor agent and may contribute to the maintenance of blood pressure through an increase in peripheral vascular resistance.

Interrelations of Osmotic and Circulatory Stimuli

As both osmotic and circulatory stimuli cause the release of vasopressin, one might expect to find, instead of a single fixed concentration of hormone resulting from a particular serum osmolality, a series of concentrations reflecting also the circulatory state. When the circulatory stimulus is strong, as in severe heart failure, vasopressin may be released and water retained despite the development of increasing degrees of hypotonicity and hyponatremia (Fig. 35-10).

DEHYDRATION—SIMPLE WATER LOSS

When water is lost from the body without the accompanying loss of large quantities of solute (sodium or potassium salts, for example), the loss of fluid volume affects all the body fluid compartments, and the solute concentration is increased therefore in each of them (Fig. 35-11). This rise in osmolality of all body fluids is reflected in an increased sodium concentration in the plasma and interstitial fluid.

SIGNS AND SYMPTOMS OF DEHYDRATION

The first signs and symptoms of lack of water in the body are thirst and the production of highly concentrated urine in reduced volumes. When the dehydration is more severe the mucous membranes are dry, sweat is absent, skin turgor is reduced, anorexia, fatigue, and fever may be present. Still more extreme degrees of dehydration, in which the extracellular and

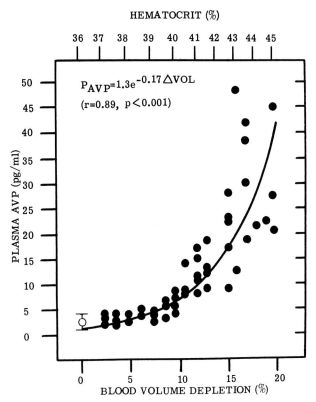

Fig. 35-9. Plasma volume was reduced in rats by the intraperitoneal injection of polyethylene glycol. Plasma osmolality was unchanged. Plasma AVP increased with the hypovolemia. (Dunn FL, Brennan TJ, Nelson AE et al: Relationship of osmolality and volume in controlling AVP in rats. J Clin Invest 52:3212, 1973)

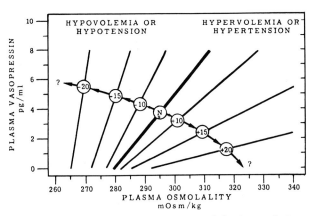

Fig. 35-10. Schematic representation of the interrelationship between osmotic and volume stimuli on vasopressin secretion. The numbers inside the circles indicate the magnitude of the volume changes required to shift the corresponding regression line. (Robertson GL, Shelton RL, Athar S: The osmoregulation of vasopressin. Kidney Int 10:25, 1976)

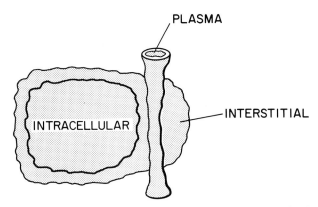

Fig. 35-11. When water is lost from the body, all body fluid compartments have reduced volume and increased osmolality. (Compare with Fig. 35-1.)

vascular fluid compartments are seriously compromised, produce postural hypotension and finally shock or renal failure (Table 35-1).

Weight loss, of course, accompanies dehydration. Loss of 4% to 5% of the body weight can ordinarily be tolerated without marked circulatory abnormalities, but a loss of a greater amount brings an increasing danger of circulatory collapse.

CAUSES OF DEHYDRATION

Impaired Fluid Intake and Nonrenal Loss

Dehydration occurs when intake of water fails to keep up with the rate of water loss from the body. Intake may be reduced when impaired consciousness limits either the sensation of thirst or the ability of the patient to take in water. Rarely, impaired thirst sensation accompanies disease or damage to the hypothalamus itself. The loss of water through the skin is accelerated by high environmental temperature, fever, heavy exertion, or as the result of burns. Hyperventilation leads to increased respiratory losses of water. With diarrhea, gastrointestinal losses may become massive and particularly serious in small children.

Renal Water Loss

Dehydration may also occur as a result of excessive renal loss of water. This failure to conserve water may result from a lack of antidiuretic hormone or an inability of the kidneys to respond to it.

Polyuria—Differential Diagnosis. The patient who cannot produce concentrated urine has *polyuria* (large volumes of dilute urine), and is in danger of becoming dehydrated unless his intake is also appropriately increased. The differential diagnosis of polyuria involves distinguishing between (1) a normal response to over-

Table 35-1. *Signs and Symptoms of Dehydration*

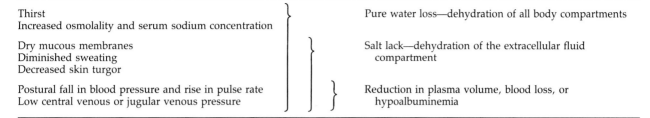

Thirst Increased osmolality and serum sodium concentration	Pure water loss—dehydration of all body compartments
Dry mucous membranes Diminished sweating Decreased skin turgor	Salt lack—dehydration of the extracellular fluid compartment
Postural fall in blood pressure and rise in pulse rate Low central venous or jugular venous pressure	Reduction in plasma volume, blood loss, or hypoalbuminemia

hydration and (2) an inability to concentrate urine. This inability may be the result of either lack of antidiuretic hormone or inability of the kidneys to respond to the hormone. In some instances it is easy to rule out the possibility of overhydration because signs of dehydration are clearly present. Often, however, it is extremely difficult. Overhydration might occur in a patient who received excessive intravenous fluids during surgery or who may have continued drinking fluids during a transient period of renal failure. Or it might be seen in a patient who for some unexplained reason continues to have strong thirst sensations even when normally hydrated (*psychogenic polydypsia*). Intake and output records are rarely accurate enough to be sure of a positive fluid balance; insensible losses are hard to estimate, and accurate weights are usually not available. Because the body solute concentration is maintained by a two-limbed control system, including both thirst and the antidiuretic hormone, either one of these mechanisms may be defective and the other one will keep the solute concentration within normal limits. Therefore, measurement of the serum osmolality or sodium concentration usually fails to distinguish whether polyuria is the normal response to overhydration or an abnormal defect in urine concentration. To identify the primary abnormality, it is often necessary to perform a dehydration test.

Dehydration Test. The dehydration test consists of measuring the patient's response to a controlled deprivation of water and to administered antidiuretic hormone. For the patient hospitalized for polyuria after neurosurgery, for shock, or for the relief of a urinary obstruction, this can be done by replacing fluid at a rate approximately 1 liter less each day than the estimated daily total losses until either the urine flow rate decreases or signs of dehydration begin to appear. If dehydration occurs while urine fails to become concentrated and urine flow rates remain high, then antidiuretic hormone is administered to test the kidneys' ability to concentrate using the following procedure: If an ambulatory patient is complaining of polyuria (after diabetes mellitus has been ruled out), the physician

may first ask the patient to dehydrate himself overnight and bring the first morning urine for measurement of concentration. An osmolality of 600 or more, or an accurate specific gravity of 1.022 or more, would indicate at least moderate concentrating ability.

If this is not achieved, hospitalization for a formal dehydration test is advisable. A useful test is one modified from a procedure described by Miller and associates.[11] Early in the morning weigh the patient carefully and begin fluid deprivation. Measure serum sodium concentration and total osmolality (if possible) in a *plasma* sample. Try to obtain blood without the prolonged use of a tourniquet. Urine should be voided hourly and its concentration measured (preferably by osmometer, although careful specific gravity measurements may suffice). The period of dehydration should be continued until

A plateau of urine concentration is reached, with each successive hour's sample increasing by no more than 30 mOsm/kg or 0.001 specific gravity as compared to the previous hour, or
Weight loss is in the range of 4% to 5% of the initial body weight, or
Signs of significant dehydration occur (marked fall in blood pressure and increase in heart rate when standing).

These signs may be reached in only 4 hours to 5 hours in a patient with marked polyuria, or it might take 18 or so hours for them to appear in a normal or only mildly affected patient.

At the end of this period another blood sample is obtained for measurement of sodium concentration and osmolality, and 5 units of aqueous antidiuretic hormone are injected subcutaneously. A final urine specimen is collected 60 minutes after the injection, and its concentration is again measured. Pitressin tannate, 10 units intramuscularly, may be used alternatively and the urine collected for 2 hours instead.

Test results can be interpreted as follows:

1. A concentrated urine at the end of the test (>700 mOsm/kg H_2O) with no significant increase in con-

centration after the administration of antidiuretic hormone indicates a normal ability of the hypothalamus to release the hormone and a normal ability of the kidneys to respond to it. This result is consistent with the diagnosis of psychogenic polydipsia or other causes of overhydration.

2. When the urine is less than 700 mOsm/kg at the end of the test, and the concentration increases significantly (>5%) after the antidiuretic hormone, a defect in endogenous hormone production or release has been demonstrated. This is consistent with the diagnosis of complete or partial hypothalamic diabetes insipidus. In complete diabetes insipidus the urine after the period of hydration usually has an osmolality less than 300 (or specific gravity <1.008), and it increases more than 100% after administration of antidiuretic hormone.

3. If the urine is not maximally concentrated after dehydration (<700 mOsm) and osmolality does not increase significantly after antidiuretic hormone, then a failure of the kidneys to respond to the hormone has been demonstrated, consistent with nephrogenic diabetes insipidus or other renal diseases. Moderate impairment may be associated with very mild renal disease or old age, and only with maximal osmolalities of less than 300 to 400 would significant polyuria be likely.

The causes of polyuria are summarized in Table 35-2.

APPROACH TO THE DEHYDRATED PATIENT

The information gained from taking the history, performing a physical examination and, if necessary, conducting the dehydration test described above allows the physician, through understanding the pathophysiology of the dehydration, to take appropriate measures for its correction and prevention.

If the cause of the dehydration is no longer present, replacement of water is the only therapy necessary. This can be most safely done by having the patient drink fluids guided by his own thirst. If he is unable to do this because of either gastrointestinal disease or neurologic impairment, fluids may be administered by the physician in the form of 5% dextrose and water given intravenously. The quantity required to return the fluids to normal may be calculated by the fractional change in solute concentration in the body fluids. Thus, if serum sodium has increased by 5% from its normal value (assuming no appreciable gain or loss of solute from the body), 5% of the original total body water must have been lost. In practice one would not plan to correct the total loss this way without rechecking serum sodium concentration as a guide.

Table 35-2. *Causes of Polyuria*

Overhydration
  Iatrogenic—surgery, intravenous infusion
  Psychogenic polydipsia

Lack of antidiuretic hormone
  (Partial or complete diabetes insipidus)
    Idiopathic
    Secondary to pituitary or hypothalamic damage

Unresponsive to antidiuretic hormone
  Osmotic diuresis—diabetes mellitus, mannitol, glycerol, tube-feeding, radiographic dyes
  Renal disease, especially tubular or medullary disease including nephrogenic diabetes insipidus
  Hypercalcemia or potassium depletion
  Sickle cell disease or trait
  Postobstructive diuresis, which includes elements of overhydration, osmotic diuresis, and tubular damage
  Drug-related—diuretics, lithium, demeclocycline, methoxyflurane

Beyond the correction of the water deficit, however, it is important for the physician to direct his attention to the cause of the dehydration so that he might prevent its recurrence.

HYPOTHALAMIC DIABETES INSIPIDUS

The patient who does not respond normally to the period of dehydration but who is able to concentrate his urine when antidiuretic hormone is administered has either complete or partial hypothalamic diabetes insipidus. This may be either idiopathic or may result from damage or disease of the hypothalamus or pituitary.[12] Approaches to therapy include the following:

No therapy. With an intact thirst center the patient drinks the appropriately large quantity of water he requires. Although this results in the inconvenience of waking frequently at night to drink fluids and of planning the day's activities within the constraints imposed by polyuria, no real danger results, and some patients prefer to remain untreated.

Chlorpropamide therapy (investigational for this use). This sulfonylurea drug, primarily used in the treatment of diabetes mellitus, has for many patients the ability to reduce urine volumes dramatically. It appears to augment or amplify the effect of small quantities of antidiuretic hormone and thus may be most useful in patients who retain a small but insufficient amount of hormone themselves.[13] The major potential complication of this therapy is hypoglycemia, and it is wise to warn the patient of hypoglycemic symptoms and to check blood glucose concentrations soon after beginning the drug and when high-dose levels are

required. Since chlorpropamide has a long duration of action (half-life of 24 hours–36 hours), the drug may be given in a single daily dosage, and several days at a given dosage should be tried before increasing it. Oral dosages as low as 100 mg/day may be effective, but occasionally as much as 500 mg/day is required. An occasional patient continues his high fluid intake despite a better controlled urine output; hence the physician should be alert for signs of water intoxication, and if in doubt, should check serum sodium concentration.

Replacement therapy—injection. Antidiuretic hormone (vasopressin) is available in an impure but clinically effective form as Pitressin. In the rapidly acting aqueous form, 0.25 ml (5 units) may be given subcutaneously or added to a slow intravenous drip (investigational) for temporary control of diabetes insipidus during surgery, following head injury, or for test purposes. The long-acting Pitressin tannate in oil is more useful for continued management. An intramuscular injection of 0.5 ml (2.5 units) or 1 ml (5 units) usually reduces urine volumes for from 24 hours to 48 hours or occasionally longer. Since the active hormone settles to the bottom of the oil in the ampules, it is extremely important to warm the suspension gently and shake it vigorously before drawing it into the syringe for injection. It is convenient for the patient to receive his injection in the evening so that control of urine volumes is likely to continue for two good nights' sleep. It is wise to allow an unmistakable increase in urine output and thirst (indicating a fall in level of antidiuretic hormone) to occur before administering the next dose, thus allowing for the excretion of any excess water that may have accumulated during the period of antidiuresis. In those rare patients in whom brain injury has impaired thirst as well as the ability to release antidiuretic hormone, management may be extremely difficult and requires careful twice-a-day weights, measurements of fluid intake and output, and periodic check of serum sodium level as an index of hydration.

Nasal spray. As an adjunct to extend the duration of the injections, or used by itself to achieve more limited periods of control of urine volumes, vasopressin may be administered as a nasal spray. The use of synthetic lysine vasopressin (Diapid) is preferable for this purpose to solutions or powders of crude posterior pituitary extract because it avoids some of the irritation and sensitization frequently seen with the latter. A synthetic analog of vasopressin, DDAVP (1-desamino-8-arginine vasopressin), has a long duration of action and administered nasally has now become the major therapy for diabetes insipidus.[14]

Patients with hypothalamic diabetes insipidus may also benefit from the methods described in the following sections.

POLYURIA UNRESPONSIVE TO ANTIDIURETIC HORMONE

Osmotic Diuresis

The renal excretion of large quantities of osmotically active solute increases the urine volume in two ways:[15]

1. However concentrated the urine is, the excretion of additional solute requires additional accompanying water to keep the solute concentration the same.
2. The passage of large volumes of fluid through the renal tubules during an osmotic diuresis itself reduces the medullary hypertonicity upon which concentration of the urine depends. Therefore, the maximal concentration of urine is also impaired. The most commonly encountered solutes producing osmotic diuresis are glucose (in diabetes mellitus); mannitol or glycerol, used therapeutically as osmotically active agents; radiographic dyes; and large blood urea loads following high protein feedings or the relief of urinary tract obstructions. Therapy consists of reducing the osmotic load and of supplying sufficient water to replace that lost in diuresis.

Renal Disease

Renal disease as a cause of impaired concentrating ability may often be suspected by history, elevated blood urea nitrogen (BUN), or creatinine or abnormal urinalysis. Nephrogenic diabetes insipidus is a sex-linked hereditary disease in which the kidneys are unresponsive to antidiuretic hormone but capable of essentially all their other normal functions.[16,17] The affected male infants are in danger of severe dehydration unless large quantities of water are supplied.

Metabolic Disturbances

Metabolic disturbances leading to polyuria include hypercalcemia, which can produce severe unresponsiveness to antidiuretic hormone with maximum urine osmolalities as low as 200 mOsm/kg and urine output of several liters per day. Potassium depletion also limits renal concentration, but not so severely, and it is not usually a cause of marked polyuria. Detection of these abnormalities requires measuring serum calcium and potassium levels.

Sickle Cell Disease

The low pH and pO_2 that characterize the renal medulla provide optimum conditions for the sickling of cells containing hemoglobin S, with resulting impairment of medullary circulation and hence reduced energy

supply for the transporting cells responsible for medullary hypertonicity. A limitation of concentrating ability is one of the few abnormalities measurable in a heterozygous carrier of sickle disease—one who has only sickle cell trait.

Postobstructive Diuresis

Urine output may be very large and concentrating ability limited in a patient following the relief of urinary tract obstruction, as in a patient with prostatic hypertrophy and obstruction following the insertion of a urethral catheter. The cause of the diuresis usually includes elements of overhydration resulting from continued fluid intake during the period of obstruction, osmotic diuresis from the accumulation of urea, and tubular damage resulting from pressure transmitted from the overfilled bladder.[18,19] Appropriate therapy is to increase intake to match output during the period that the blood urea level is rapidly falling, then to supply only 2 liters to 3 liters a day unless signs of dehydration appear.

Drugs

Drugs that are commonly associated with inability of the kidneys to produce normally concentrated urine include diuretics, lithium,[7] the antibiotic demeclocycline[20] and the anesthetic methoxyflurane.[21]

WATER EXCESS

Excess water intake ordinarily leads to a brisk urine output (polyuria) but no appreciable increase in total body water. In fact, normally the kidneys can excrete 25 to 30 or more liters per day without any severe degree of water retention in the body. When total body water is increased, therefore, it is clear that some abnormality in the kidneys' ability to excrete water must be present. When excess water is retained in the body it distributes itself throughout the fluid compartments, diluting the solute in each. Thus, a low serum osmolality and hyponatremia (unless artifactual) is diagnostic of impaired water excretion (Table 35-3). This impairment may involve elevated circulating levels of antidiuretic hormone or intrinsic renal impairment or both.

ARTIFACTUAL HYPONATREMIA

The body regulates the concentration of sodium in the plasma *water*. The laboratory reports the concentration of sodium in whole plasma. Plasma normally contains about 93% water, the remaining 7% being made up largely of proteins and lipids. In severe hyperlipidemia

Table 35-3. *Hyponatremia Associated with Water Excess*

Artifactual
Hyperlipemia
Severe hyperglycemia
Severe hyperproteinemia

Impaired Circulation
Salt loss
Dehydration
Hypovolemia
Heart failure
Hypotension
Nephrotic syndrome
Liver failure

Circulation Possibly Impaired
Diuretics with potassium depletion
Myxedema
Addison's disease

Circulation Normal
Inappropriate antidiuretic hormone syndrome (SIADH)
Acute and severe chronic renal failure
Various drugs (chlorpropamide, oxytoxin, nicotine, morphine, β-adrenergic drugs, cyclophosphamide, clofibrate)

(diabetic, nephrotic, idiopathic) or hyperproteinemia (macroglobinemia, occasional myeloma) the water content of plasma may be unusually low. In this circumstance, although sodium concentration in plasma water may be normal, the concentration in total plasma is low. This artificial abnormality of course does not represent a defect in salt or water metabolism, and serum osmolality remains normal.

IMPAIRED CIRCULATION

With circulatory insufficiency, hyponatremia is a common laboratory finding. The cause of the impaired circulation may be as obvious as severe congestive heart failure or as subtle as might occur with the contraction of plasma volume accompanying salt depletion.[22,23] As discussed under nonosmotic stimuli for antidiuretic hormone, both hypertonicity of the blood and hypovolemia or hypotension are stimuli for the release of antidiuretic hormone. If the circulation is severely impaired, antidiuretic hormone is released even in the absence of an osmotic stimulus, and water retention leading to hypotonicity and hyponatremia results. This is probably the main mechanism by which the hyponatremia of heart failure, liver failure, or nephrotic syndrome occurs. It has also been demonstrated, however, that with severe circulatory failure, water is retained even in the absence of antidiuretic hormone as a result of intrinsic renal abnormalities in water excre-

tion.[24] It is not clear to what extent this nonantidiuretic hormone mechanism contributes to water retention in these common diseases.

CIRCULATION POSSIBLY IMPAIRED

Addison's disease[25] (specifically glucocorticoid deficiency) and myxedema are both well known as causes of water retention. It is not clear to what extent this represents elevated antidiuretic hormone concentrations and to what degree intrinsic renal impairment of water excretion takes place, nor is it certain whether minor degrees of circulatory impairment contribute to these abnormalities. Diuretic use is frequently associated with hyponatremia. In some instances this clearly reflects volume depletion following excessive diuretic effect. In other cases, especially when associated with potassium depletion, volume depletion is not clearly demonstrable. Increased antidiuretic hormone is thought to be present, but the stimulus for its release is not well understood.[126]

NORMAL CIRCULATION

Some patients with hyponatremia clearly appear to have unimpaired circulation. These may include patients with acute or severe chronic renal failure in whom renal function is so severely impaired that adequate water excretion is impossible or patients who have taken a variety of drugs that are thought to stimulate excessive release of antidiuretic hormone.[27,28] Within this category also is the syndrome of inappropriate antidiuretic hormone (SIADH).[29] In this condition antidiuretic hormone is either released in excessive quantities from its normal storage sites in the posterior pituitary or is released from abnormal sites elsewhere in the body. Rarely, patients may appear to have "reset osmostats," in which the capacity to excrete and conserve water appears to be normal but the plasma osmolality is regulated at an abnormally low level.[30] Other patients appear to have insensitive antidiuretic hormone responses to changes in plasma osmolality and large changes in serum sodium concentration accompanying changes in fluid intake (Fig. 35-12).[31] The stimuli for intracranial release may include tumors, infections, metabolic abnormalities, or trauma of the central nervous system. Extracranial sites most commonly include undifferentiated "oat cell" tumors of the lung but also a variety of other tumors and occasionally infectious processes involving the lung. A characteristic of SIADH that is diagnostically useful is the presence of sodium in the urine, whereas the conditions with impaired circulation described above are generally characterized by salt retention as well as water reten-

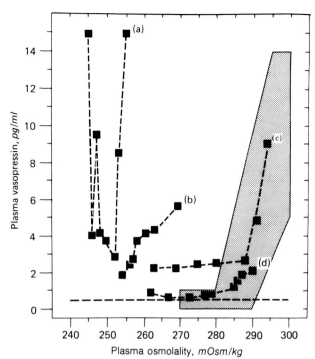

Fig. 35-12. An illustration of the relationship between osmolality and AVP in four types of SIADH. In (*a*) the high levels of hormone appear to bear no relation to osmolality. In (*b*) there is variation of AVP with osmolality, but the hormone suppresses at an abnormally low osmolality ("reset osmostat"). In (*c*) the relationship is normal except for a failure of the hormone to "shut off" completely at low plasma osmolality. In (*d*) the relationship appears completely normal, raising the question of abnormal renal sensitivity to AVP or of the presence of some other antidiuretic mechanism. (Robertson GL, Shelton RL, Athar S: The osmoregulation of vasopressin. Kidney Int 10:25, 1976)

tion and hence have low urinary sodium values. In SIADH all sodium taken in by the patient is promptly excreted. This is not only diagnostically useful but makes fruitless any attempt to correct the hyponatremia by administering salt. Volume expansion is a stimulus for salt excretion, and so only a reduction in volume expansion through a severe restriction of water intake results in sodium retention and correction of the severe hyponatremia.

SALT BALANCE—THE REGULATION OF VOLUME

DISTRIBUTION OF WATER AMONG THE BODY FLUID COMPARTMENTS

As already mentioned, thirst and the antidiuretic hormone system controlling urine concentration maintain

a constant osmolality of the blood. Since water moves freely among blood, interstitial fluid, and intracellular fluid, the osmolality remains the same in all these compartments. The volume of each compartment, therefore, reflects the quantity of solute that is within it. If a fluid compartment has certain solutes that are not free to move into other spaces, the volume of that compartment can be regulated by controlling the quantity of its specific solute. Sodium salts are the predominant osmotically active particles present in the extracellular fluid. They are largely excluded from most cells by the same type of active transporting mechanisms that limits potassium salts to a predominantly intracellular location. Therefore, regulation of the volume of the extracellular space can be accomplished by adjusting the quantity of sodium salts present in the body. Sodium, potassium, and other salts are not actively transported across, nor limited in movement through, the permeable wall of the capillaries. Therefore, none of them is limited in distribution to the intravascular space or useful in controlling the volume of the intravascular space. Those intravascular solutes that cannot penetrate the capillary wall and hence can exert an osmotic force to maintain intravascular volume are the plasma proteins, particularly albumin (see discussion on edema).

REGULATION OF SALT BALANCE

Regulating the quantity of salt in the body controls the volume of the extracellular fluid compartment. Although water balance has a double control system in which intake is regulated by thirst and output by antidiuretic hormone, there is no comparable, well-developed "salt hunger" to regulate salt intake in man. Therefore, the salt content of the body must be controlled by regulation of its renal excretion.

CONTROL OF SALT EXCRETION

Normal salt intake in man varies widely with cultural differences in diet and individual preferences. Typical American or European diets may contain 100 mEq to 300 mEq/day. The urinary excretion of salt approximates the average daily intake, with only small losses owing to sweating and fecal loss. The kidneys have remarkable flexibility in varying the sodium output in response to changes in intake or body content, and urine sodium may normally vary from about one milliequivalent per day during intense salt conservation to several hundred milliequivalents during salt diuresis. Since salt is freely filtered at the renal glomerulus, the salt concentration at the glomerular filtrate is about the

same as it is in plasma water. With approximately 150 liters of glomerular filtrate formed each day, about 150 liters × 145 mEq/liter or 21,750 mEq of sodium are filtered each day. It is thus apparent that most of the filtered sodium is reabsorbed back into the blood during the passage of the glomerular filtrate to the renal tubules. The fractional reabsorption ranges from close to 21,749/21,750 or 99.99% during salt conservation to 98% during salt diuresis. Changes in salt excretion and hence regulation of the salt content of the body are accomplished in the kidney by changing the amount reabsorbed between these limits.

Nearly all the anatomic segments of the renal tubule participate in reabsorption of sodium and chloride, although by different mechanisms. In most segments it appears that the amount of reabsorption can be varied in response to the needs of the body. The major segments of the renal tubule are the proximal tubule, Henle's loop, the distal tubule, and the collecting tubule. Knowledge of the nature of salt reabsorption in these segments has come largely from micropuncture experiments, in which small quantities of tubular fluid are sampled from tubular segments located on the surface of the kidneys of experimental animals or from experiments in which small segments of tubules are dissected out from the kidney and perfused with fluid resembling tubular fluid. We may use the information derived from these studies to estimate what must happen in human kidneys to control the rate of salt excretion.

Glomerular Filtration

The quantity of salt filtered at the renal glomerulus is the first factor affecting the rate of salt excretion. When the body contains an excess of salt, the interstitial fluid and plasma volumes are expanded, cardiac output and renal blood flow are elevated, and glomerular filtration rate is increased. Conversely, in salt depletion, glomerular filtration rate is low, and less salt is filtered into the renal tubules. This variation in the quantity of filtered salt helps to regulate salt excretion, but since the vast proportion of filtered salt is reabsorbed, changes in reabsorption can be expected to have a much more powerful effect on salt excretion regulation.

Proximal Tubule

Since the capillary walls in the glomerulus are permeable to water and salts, the concentration of sodium chloride in the proximal tubule fluid is about the same (allowing for the effects of the volume and electrical charge of plasma proteins, which are not filtered) as they are in the plasma. The epithelial cells of the prox-

imal tubule actively remove about 60% of the sodium ions during the passage of fluid through the proximal tubule.

Since this epithelium allows the free passage of water, a comparable fraction of water follows the sodium out of the tubular lumen into the peritubular space and into the peritubular capillaries. Both the reabsorbed fluid and the remaining tubular fluid are thus *isotonic* with plasma. This isotonic reabsorption is not fixed at a constant 60% but may vary, increasing in states of volume contraction and decreasing following salt loads. The control of this varying rate of reabsorption is at least partly accomplished by changes in the Starling forces (hydrostatic and plasma protein oncotic pressure) in the peritubular capillaries. For example, an increase in salt intake results in expansion of the plasma volume, leading to both a dilution of plasma protein concentration and an increase in capillary hydrostatic pressure. Each of these changes reduces the rate at which fluid moves into the peritubular capillaries and hence the rate at which it moves out of the proximal tubule lumen.[32] There may be additional control mechanisms involving hormones,[33] the sympathetic nervous system,[34,35] a feedback between the macula densa of the early distal tubule and the glomerulus of the same nephron, or a redistribution of the renal blood flow between inner and outer nephrons. Each has been suggested as an important control mechanism for the proximal tubule or other parts of the nephron, but at the present time no one of these has unequivocally been shown to be an important factor.

Henle's Loop

An active *chloride* transporting system leads to the removal of sodium chloride as tubular fluid rises through the thick ascending limb of the Henle's loop.[36] Since this tubular membrane is rather impermeable to water, the tubular fluid becomes more dilute as it rises, while the peritubular interstitial fluid becomes hypertonic. By the end of this segment of tubule, the sodium concentration of the tubular fluid is about 50 mEq/liter, compared with about 145 mEq/liter of the plasma or glomerular filtrate, and the sodium concentration of the interstitial fluid near the bend of Henle's loop may reach very high levels (600 mEq/liter in the hamster[37]). About 30% of the total filtered sodium and 10% of the water is reabsorbed in the loop. The descending limb of the loop is permeable to water, so water is reabsorbed from the tubular fluid as it descends to enter the medulla where the interstitium is hypertonic.

When increasing loads of tubular fluid are delivered from the proximal tubule into the loop, the active transporting "pumps" are capable of increasing the rate of removal of sodium chloride so that the fluid leaving the loop and entering the distal tubule, though larger in volume, still has about the same low sodium concentration of approximately 50 mEq/liter. There is no strong evidence at present for primary control mechanisms for sodium excretion acting in the loop.

Distal Tubule

About 5% of the filtered sodium is reabsorbed in the distal convoluted tubule. The fraction reabsorbed varies under the influence of the hormone aldosterone and is clearly one of the important control mechanisms by which the excretion of salt is regulated. The control is mediated through renin and angiotensin in the following way:[38] The circulation of blood to the glomeruli is monitored by the juxtaglomerular apparatus, a group of specialized myoepithelial cells located where the afferent arteriole enters the glomerulus. When pressure or flow is low, the enzyme renin is released into the circulation and perhaps also locally into the kidney. In the plasma, renin catalyzes the formation of angiotensin I from an inactive precurser, and this in turn is converted to the extremely active pressor agent, angiotensin II. In addition to increasing peripheral vascular resistance directly, angiotensin II stimulates the adrenal cortex to produce the steroid hormone aldosterone, which has a powerful effect on the renal distal convoluted tubule, accelerating the rate of sodium reabsorption. Thus, in salt depletion, when blood pressure and cardiac output are reduced, aldosterone is increased and more salt is retained in the body, tending to correct the circulatory impairment.

Collecting Tubule

By the time the tubular fluid reaches the collecting tubule, about 95% of the filtered salt has already been reabsorbed. The variation in reabsorption of the remaining salt is of great importance in determining the rate of salt excretion from the body, and there is evidence that under differing experimental conditions as little as 30% or as much as 80% of the presented load may be reabsorbed.[39] Unfortunately, there is as yet very little information about the mechanisms that control this variation.

In summary, then, variability in the rate of filtration of salt and varying rates of reabsorption in different segments of the renal tubule determine the final rate of salt excretion from the body. Control of the rate of excretion seems to be determined by adequacy of the circulation through several mechanisms, some well understood, some unknown.

SALT LACK—EXTRACELLULAR VOLUME DEPLETION

Since salt is primarily located in the extracellular fluid compartment, a lack of salt results primarily in a reduction in extracellular solute (Fig. 35-13). Since water moves freely between the fluid compartments and since the antidiuretic hormone control mechanisms tend to maintain a constant normal osmolality, the loss of salt is accompanied by excretion of water and hence reduction in volume of the extracellular fluid compartment. The loss of this volume of salt water is indeed a *dehydration*, but unlike the dehydration that results from primary loss of water, in which all the fluid compartments of the body share, this dehydration is limited to the extracellular fluid, which includes the intravascular and interstitial spaces, and serum osmolality and sodium concentration remain normal or somewhat low.

SIGNS AND SYMPTOMS

Dehydration of the interstitial space results in *poor skin turgor* in which a fold of skin, gently pinched and lifted, often remains for a moment above the level of the surrounding skin. Dryness of the skin and mucous membranes and absence of perspiration are also features. Dehydration (hypovolemia) of the intravascular space means reduced plasma volume and is evident first by postural changes in pulse and blood pressure, later by low jugular or central venous pressure and hypotension.

CAUSES OF SALT LACK

Lack of intake is generally *not* a cause of salt deficiency. The body's mechanisms of conserving salt, developed

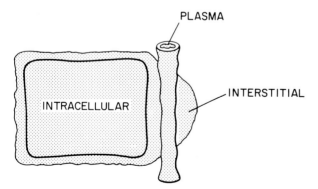

Fig. 35-13. Lack of salt results in reduction in the volume of the extracellular fluid compartment, including plasma and interstitial fluid, without an increase in osmolality. (Compare with Fig. 35-1.)

at an evolutionary time when salt was not as ubiquitous in food as at present, can reduce output to 1 mEq to 2 mEq per day—a very small quantity indeed.

Renal Salt Loss

When salt deficit is found, routes of excessive loss should be sought. The normal ability to conserve salt can be lost either as a result of disease or through the use of drugs.

Renal Disease. Many chronic renal diseases, especially by the time they progress to renal failure, interfere to some extent with the kidneys' ability to conserve salt. Typical obligatory salt losses might average 40 mEq to 80 mEq/day (about 1 g–2 g sodium or 2.5 g–5 g salt), but they are often much less if heart failure is superimposed on renal failure. Diseases affecting the tubules and renal interstitium are likely to produce greater salt losses than those primarily of the glomeruli, and a rare patient with medullary or tubular disease will have a true "salt-losing nephritis" that requires dietary supplements to avoid salt depletion.

Aldosterone Deficiency. This hormone is lacking in *Addison's disease*, in which the diffusely damaged adrenal cortex is incapable of synthesizing the hormone even in the presence of normal stimuli (chiefly angiotensin II, hyperkalemia, and hyponatremia).[40] Adrenal insufficiency resulting from hypopituitarism is *not* likely to lead to serious salt loss, because ACTH is not the major stimulus for aldosterone production. *Isolated hypoaldosteronism*, in which the production of adrenal glucocorticoids remains normal, has been reported in a variety of clinical settings that include hyperkalemia and a degree of salt-wasting.[41,42] Occasionally (especially in infants) this has been associated with a specific metabolic defect in the adrenal cortex resulting in failure to synthesize aldosterone, but more frequently the defect results from a lack of renin. Patients with this condition often have moderate renal failure from various causes, often including diabetes mellitus, but it is not clear what specific defect of the juxtaglomerular apparatus is involved. Occasionally the defect may include the production of an abnormal "big" renin with limited activity in producing angiotensin.[43] Patients with isolated hypoaldosteronism resulting from renin insufficiency do not generally have severe degrees of salt-wasting, perhaps because rising serum potassium levels provide a substitute stimulus for aldosterone production.

Diuretics

Enhancing the loss of salt through the kidneys is the purpose of diuretics. It is not surprising that excessive

diuretic effect leads to salt depletion. The powerful "loop" diuretics, such as furosemide and ethacrynic acid, are most likely to have an excessive effect.

Nonrenal Salt Loss

Fluid from the small intestine has appreciable sodium concentration, so diarrhea can lead to severe sodium depletion. Sodium bicarbonate as well as sodium chloride is lost by this route, so patients may become acidotic as well as salt-depleted from diarrheal fluid losses. Sweating, when severe, also leads to salt loss. As adaptation to a hot environment occurs, the salt concentration of sweat falls, so that severe salt depletion is more apt to occur during exertion in hot environments by unacclimated individuals.

APPROACH TO THE PATIENT

When poor skin turgor, dry mucous membranes, thirst, and postural hypotension and tachycardia occur, it is clear that contraction in volume (or dehydration) of the extracellular space is present. To determine whether this results from a primary loss of water from all compartments of the body or rather reflects a primary salt loss with hypovolemia limited to the extracellular compartment, it is necessary to measure serum osmolality or serum sodium concentration, which is ordinarily a good index of osmolality. When water loss is primary, the osmolality and sodium concentration are elevated, and replacement of water is the appropriate therapy. If salt loss is primary, the osmolality and sodium concentration are normal or somewhat low and the logical treatment is replacement of salt as well as water. This can often be done by adding salt to the diet if the condition is mild or chronic. If acute and more severe extracellular volume depletion is present (from cholera, for example), intravenous infusion of salt-containing solutions may be necessary. If the volume depletion is so severe that the intravascular hypovolemia is causing hypotension, it may be wise to begin the volume replacement with fluid that is distributed more specifically to the intravascular part of the extracellular space. This can be done by administering salt solutions that also contain albumin (5% albumin in saline) until normal blood pressure is restored. This principle holds even when the dehydration cause is pure water lack.

Later, or at the same time as salt is replenished, attention can be given to the cause of the salt lack, and the diarrhea can be treated, the diuretic stopped, the patient removed from the hot environment, and so on. If aldosterone deficiency is present and the underlying disease is not treatable, a mineralocorticoid substitute such as fludrocortisone may be chronically administered.

SALT EXCESS—EDEMA

The predominant clinical state in which a large excess of salt is present in the body is edema.

DEFINITION

Edema is a localized or generalized abnormal expansion of the interstitial space. Clinically, edema is identified as the visible, palpable swelling resulting from this expansion. The interstitial space must be expanded by several liters before generalized edema first becomes clinically apparent. Generalized edema is a common manifestation of congestive heart failure, cirrhosis of the liver, nephrotic syndrome, or malnutrition. Localized edema is frequently seen in burns, trauma, allergic reactions, inflammation, or obstruction of the flow through veins or lymphatics.

MECHANISMS OF EDEMA FORMATION

A localized area of edema requires that fluid move from the intravascular space in the capillaries, outward across the capillary wall, and into the interstitial space. Generalized edema requires both the abnormal movement of fluid out of the capillaries of the vascular system *and* retention of salt water by the kidneys. This can be seen to be true when it is realized that there may be only about 3 liters of plasma in the entire vascular tree, while patients frequently have 10 or more liters of edema fluid. We shall consider the capillary and the renal mechanisms separately, although they function simultaneously in practice.

Capillary Mechanisms

Normal. The distribution of water between the plasma and interstitial space is governed by the Starling forces balancing hydrostatic and osmotic pressure differences (Fig. 35-14). The hydrostatic pressure in the capillary that tends to force water out through the capillary walls is governed by the rate of flow of blood through the capillary, the pre- and postcapillary resistances, and the hydrostatic pressure in the veins into which the capillaries are emptying. This hydrostatic pressure is not the same in all capillaries of local network, since some vessels tend to be dilated with high flows and some constricted with low flows at any given time. The hydrostatic pressure at the arteriolar end of a capillary is, of course, higher than that at the venous end, since a pressure drop accompanies the resistance to the flow of blood along the length of the capillary. The average hydrostatic pressure within the capillary then is determined by (1) the flow within the capillary, (2) the length of the capillary and the resistance it presents to flow,

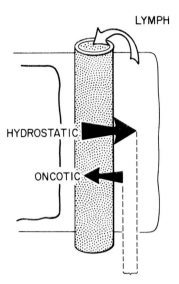

Fig. 35-14. Diagram of forces affecting movement of fluid between capillaries and interstitial fluid. The arrows represent the hydrostatic and oncotic pressure gradients across the capillary membrane. Normally there is a slight imbalance between hydrostatic and oncotic pressure, producing a net loss of fluid from the capillary. This fluid is returned to the circulation as lymph.

(3) the postcapillary resistance, and (4) the venous pressure. It is influenced by the variability of flow within a capillary network. The hydrostatic force gradient across the capillary wall is also influenced by the hydrostatic pressure of the interstitial space, which is much less than that within the capillary. This pressure has proved difficult to measure, and it is not certain whether it is positive or negative with respect to atmospheric pressure.

This hydrostatic force, which moves fluid out of the capillaries, is opposed by an osmotic force, which is attributable to solute particles within the plasma that cannot move freely through the capillary membrane. These osmotically active particles are the plasma proteins and some associated charged ions, the movement of which is restricted because of the electric charge on the protein molecules. The resulting osmotic pressure, which resists filtration and promotes reabsorption of fluid into the capillary, is called *oncotic pressure*. Albumin is by far the most important contributor to oncotic pressure by virtue of its greater abundance (about 5 g/100 ml plasma) and smaller molecular size (more particles per gram) than other plasma proteins.

The protein concentration of the interstitial fluid is much less than that of plasma, and so there is a net gradient of oncotic pressure tending to return fluid from the interstitial space to the capillary. This pressure gradient is about the same at the arteriolar and venous ends of the capillary. Although the osmotic force generated by the intravascular proteins is small compared to the total serum osmolality (about 1 mOsm compared with 280), it is capable of opposing the normal capillary hydrostatic pressure to maintain the plasma volume. Normally, there is an imbalance between the capillary hydrostatic and oncotic pressures, leading to a slight average movement of fluid out of the capillaries. This fluid is returned to the circulation as lymph.

Abnormal. The interstitial fluid space would be expected to expand abnormally—producing edema—if an imbalance in the Starling forces favored an increased outward movement of fluid from the capillary or if the return of lymph to the circulation were impaired. Clinical circumstances in which this edema formation often occurs include the following:

1. *Increased hydrostatic pressure* (Fig. 35-15). This occurs when there is increased hydrostatic pressure in the venous bed draining the capillary network. It may result from increased right ventricular end-diastolic pressure in heart failure; impaired venous flow as the result of thrombosis or external pressure on the veins; or with prolonged standing or incompetent valves when gravity produces increased pressure in the veins of the feet and legs. *Localized* increase in capillary hydrostatic pressure may occur with infection or inflammation when increased blood flow

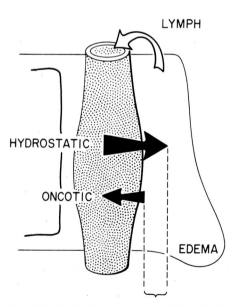

Fig. 35-15. An increase in capillary hydrostatic pressure can lead to increased loss of fluid from the capillary, with resultant edema.

through a capillary network occurs. No matter which of these causes increased capillary hydrostatic pressure, it will imbalance the forces across the capillary wall and lead to outward movement of fluid and gradual accumulation of edema.

2. *Decreased serum albumin and the resulting decrease in plasma oncotic pressure* (Fig. 35-16). This may result from urinary losses of protein (nephrotic syndrome); decreased synthesis of albumin (liver disease, protein malnutrition); or rarely, loss of protein from the gastrointestinal tract. The imbalance again leads to outward movement of fluid with the gradual accumulation of edema.

3. *Abnormal permeability of the capillary wall to protein* (Fig. 35-17). This can be caused by burn, trauma, inflammation, or allergic reaction. As the wall becomes increasingly permeable to proteins, these molecules are no longer able to generate an effective osmotic force across the capillary membrane. They leak into the interstitial space, raising its oncotic pressure.

4. *Obstruction of the lymphatics* (Fig. 35-18), leading to the accumulation of the fluid and small quantities of protein that are normally filtered. Lymphatic obstruction may result from tumors, surgery, or inflammatory or parasitic disease. The edema of heart failure results from impaired lymphatic flow because of elevated venous pressure in the thoracic duct outlet at the left subclavian vein, as well as from elevated capillary hydrostatic pressure.

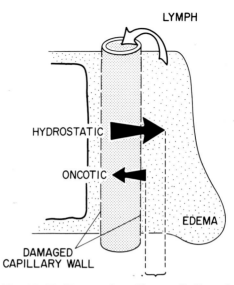

Fig. 35-17. Damaged capillary wall allows loss of protein from the capillary and reduced oncotic pressure gradient across the capillary membrane.

At what point will this increasing expansion of the interstitial space stop? As the interstitial space expands with the formation of edema, the hydrostatic pressure within it increases, thereby reducing the hydrostatic pressure gradient across the capillary membrane. The imbalance in Starling forces, therefore, is corrected and a new steady state achieved. In most clinical states in

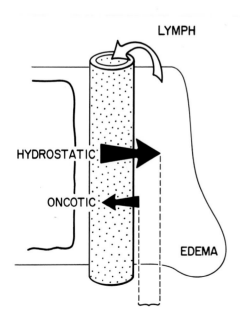

Fig. 35-16. Diminished oncotic pressure owing to hypoalbuminemia leads to increased loss of fluid from the capillary and edema.

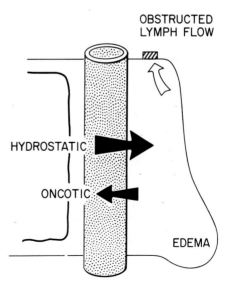

Fig. 35-18. Even when hydrostatic and oncotic pressure gradients are initially normal, obstruction of the lymphatics leads to accumulation of edema.

which edema occurs, the resultant net outward movement of fluid remains higher than normal, and hence lymph flow is increased. Of course, if obstruction of the lymphatics is itself the cause of the edema, interstitial pressure and protein concentrations ultimately reach those of the capillaries, and net filtration ceases.

Renal Mechanisms

When edema is generalized the expansion of the interstitial space by several liters implies a large increase in total body content of salt and water. This means that renal mechanisms must have been responsible for increased retention of salt and water. In a normal person volume deficit leads to the prompt reduction of salt excretion by the kidney so that dietary salt is retained and with it water, correcting the deficit rapidly. The retention of salt, as described above, involves some reduction in the amount of salt filtered at the glomerulus and a marked increase in the reabsorption of salt in the renal tubules. In a normal person salt deficit leads to a mild circulatory insufficiency, which stimulates a prompt reduction of salt excretion by the kidney. In this way dietary salt is retained and with it water, so that the deficit is rapidly corrected. The circulation then becomes normal, and the rate of salt excretion again rises to equal intake. In the patient with edema, however, the circulatory deficit which results from heart failure, liver disease, nephrotic syndrome, or other illness, persists despite the retention of salt and despite the massive expansion of the interstitial space. The perfusion of the kidney remains abnormal, and reabsorption of salt throughout the kidney remains intense.

APPROACH TO THE PATIENT WITH EDEMA

Successful therapy of the edematous patient requires identification of the primary abnormality leading to the expansion of the interstitial space. The physician must decide whether the abnormality at the capillary level is increased hydrostatic pressure, reduced plasma oncotic pressure, damaged capillary wall, or obstructed lymphatics. Similarly, the prime causes of the renal salt and water retention should be identified. This often includes evaluating the jugular or central venous pressure; the arterial blood pressure; the possibilities of cardiac, renal, or hepatic disease; local abnormalities of veins and lymphatics; and measurement of the serum protein concentration. The most effective treatment of edema is the reversal of the primary cause. If this is impossible, diuretic drugs (which block sodium reabsorption) may be used with the forewarning that while they mobilize edema, they may actually aggravate its underlying cause.

SUMMARY

Water is distributed throughout the body in the cells (intracellular compartment), between the cells (interstitial compartment), and within the blood vessels (intravascular compartment). The interstitial and intravascular spaces together form the extracellular compartment. Normally, about two thirds of the body water is intracellular. Of the one third that is extracellular, about one fifth is intravascular (the plasma volume) and the rest interstitial. Total solute concentration (osmolality) in each space is equal to that in the others because the cell membranes and capillary walls, which form the boundaries to these spaces, are freely permeable to water.

Normal regulation of solute concentration is accomplished by control of the body's intake and output of water. The mechanism by which this is accomplished involves (1) an osmotic sensor, (2) antidiuretic hormone, (3) the renal-concentrating mechanism, and (4) the sensation of thirst. When water is lost from the body in excess of solute, dehydration results. The rise in osmolality in body fluids is reflected in an increased sodium concentration in the plasma and interstitial fluid. Causes of dehydration include impaired fluid intake, nonrenal water loss, and renal water loss. When excess water is retained in the body, an abnormality in the kidneys' ability to excrete water is present; hyponatremia and a low serum osmolality result.

Normal regulation of the volume of extracellular space is accomplished by adjusting the quantity of sodium salts in the body. Salt excretion is controlled by the kidney. In the dehydration of extracellular volume (interstitial space) depletion, water and salt are lost in concert, and serum osmolality and serum sodium remain normal or somewhat low. The predominant clinical state in which a large excess of salt is present in the body is edema. Edema is the visible, palpable swelling resulting from localized and generalized abnormal expansion of the interstitial space. Both capillary and renal mechanisms play a part in the formation of edema.

Disturbances in osmoregulation and derangements in volume and distribution of body fluids are not isolated entities and generally occur as manifestations of underlying illnesses, producing profound disturbances of body physiology. In turn, fluid disturbances of themselves produce systemic derangements. A knowledge of the signs and symptoms of dehydration

and edema and of the regulatory mechanisms needed to maintain normal water and salt balance is necessary to understand the pathophysiology of the underlying disease process and its treatment.

REFERENCES

1. **Zimmerman EA et al:** Neurohypophyseal peptides in the bovine hypothalamus. Endocrinology 95:931–936, 1974

2. **Hope DB, Pickup JL:** Neurophysins. Handbook of Physical Endocrinology IV—Part 1, p 173–190. 1974

3. **Maxwell D et al:** The effect of distribution and clearance on plasma vasopressin in man. Clin Res 24:407A, 1976

4. **Lauson HD:** Metabolism of the neurohypophyseal hormones. Handbook of Physical Endocrinology IV—Part 1, p 287–394, 1974

5. **Handler JS, Orloff J:** Mechanism of action of antidiuretic hormone. Handbook of Physiology—Renal Physiology, p 791–814, 1973

6. **Hays R, Levine SD:** Vasopressin. Kidney Int 6:307–322, 1974

7. **Dousa TP:** Cellular action of antidiuretic hormone in nephrogenic diabetes insipidus. Mayo Clin Proc 49:188–199, 1974

8. **Dunn FL, Brennan TJ, Nelson AE et al:** Relationship of osmolality and volume in controlling AVP in rats. J Clin Invest 52:3212–3219, 1973

9. **Robertson GL, Athar S:** The interaction of blood osmolality and blood volume in regulation of plasma vasopressin in man. J Clin Endocrinol Metab 42:613–620, 1976

10. **Schrier RW, Berl T:** Nonosmolar factors affecting renal water excretion. N Eng J Med 292:81–88, 141–145, 1975

11. **Miller M et al:** Recognition of partial defects in antidiuretic hormone secretion. Ann Intern Med 73:721–729, 1970

12. **Coggins CH, Leaf A:** Diabetes insipidus. Am J Med 42:807–813, 1967

13. **Moses AM, Miller M:** Drug-induced dilutional hyponatremia. N Engl J Med 291:1234–1239, 1974

14. **Robinson, AG:** DDAVP in the treatment of central diabetes insipidus. N Engl J Med 294:507–511, 1976

15. **Gennari FJ, Kassirer JP:** Osmotic diuresis. N Engl J Med 291:714–720, 1974

16. **Williams RH, Henry C:** Nephrogenic diabetes insipidus. Ann Intern Med 27:84, 1947

17. **Bode HH, Crawford JD:** Nephrogenic diabetes insipidus—the Hopewell hypothesis. N Engl J Med 280:750–753, 1969

18. **Harris RH, Yarger WE:** The pathogenesis of post-obstructive diuresis. J Clin Invest 56:880–887, 1975

19. **Sonnenberg H, Wilson DR:** Role of the medullary collecting ducts in postobstructive diuresis. J Clin Invest 57:1564–1574, 1976

20. **Singer I, Rotenberg D:** Democlocycline—induced nephrogenic diabetes insipidus. Ann Intern Med 79:679–683, 1973

21. **Cousins MJ, Mazze RI:** Methoxyflurane nephrotoxicity. JAMA 225:1611–1666, 1973

22. **McCance RA:** Experimental human salt deficiency. Lancet 1:823–830, 1936

23. **Demarret JL et al:** Coma due to water intoxication in beer drinkers. Lancet ii:1115–1117, 1971

24. **Harrington AR:** Hyponatremia due to sodium depletion in the absence of vasopressin. Am J Physiol 222:768–774, 1972

25. **Boykin J et al:** Mechanism of effect of glucocorticoid deficiency on renal water excretion in the conscious dog. Clin Res 24:269A, 1976

26. **Fichman MP et al:** Diuretic-induced hyponatremia. Ann Intern Med 75:853–863, 1971

27. **Moses AM, Miller M:** Drug-induced dilutional hyponatremia. N Engl J Med 291:1234–1239, 1974

28. **DeFronzo RA et al:** Water intoxication in man after cyclophosphamide therapy. Ann Intern Med 78:861–869, 1973

29. **Bartter FC, Schwartz WB:** The syndrome of inappropriate secretion of antidiuretic hormone. Am J Med 42:790–806, 1967

30. **DeFronzo R, Goldberg M, Agus ZS:** Normal diluting capacity in hyponatremic patients. Ann Intern Med 84:538–542, 1976

31. **Robertson GL, Shelton RL, Athar S:** The osmoregulation of vasopressin. Kidney Int 10:25–37, 1976

32. **Daugherty TM, Ueki IF, Nicholas DP et al:** Comparative renal effects of isoncotic and colloid-free volume expansion in the rat. Am J Physiol 222:225–234, 1972

33. **Klahr S, Rodriguez J:** Natriuretic hormone. Nephron 15:387–408, 1975

34. **Slick GL, Aguilera AJ, Zambraski EJ:** Renal neuroadrenergic transmission. Am J Physiol 229:60–65, 1975

35. **Bello–Reuss E, Trevino DL, Gottschalk CW:** Effect of renal sympathetic nerve stimulation on proximal water and sodium reabsorption. J Clin Invest 57:1104–1107, 1976

36. **Burg MB, Green N:** Function of the thick ascending limb of Henle's loop. Am J Physiol 224:659–668, 1973

37. **Marsh DJ, Azen SP:** Mechanism of NaCl reabsorption by hamster thin ascending limb of Henle's loops. Am J Physiol 228:71, 1975

38. **Laragh JH, Sealey JE:** The renin–angiotensin–aldosterone hormonal system of regulation of sodium potassium and blood pressure homeostasis. Handbook of Physiology—Renal Physiology, Chap 26, pp 831–908. Washington, DC, American Physiological Society, 1973

39. **Stein JH, Reineck HJ:** The role of the collecting duct in the regulation of excretion of sodium and other electrolytes. Kidney Int 6:1–9, 1974

40. **Cohen JJ et al:** The critical role of the adrenal gland in

the renal regulation of acid-base equilibrium during chronic hypotonic expansion. J Clin Invest 58:1201–1208, 1976

41. **Schambelan M, Sebastian A, Biglieri EG:** Prevalence, pathogenesis and functional significance of aldosterone deficiency in hyperkalemic patients with chronic renal insufficiency. N Engl J Med 287:573–578, 1972

42. **Michelis MF, Murdaugh HV:** Selective hypoaldosteronism. Am J Med 59:1–5, 1975

43. **deLeiva A, Christlieb AR, Melby JC et al:** Big renin and biosynthetic defect of aldosterone in diabetes mellitus. N Engl J Med 295:639–643, 1976

36

Acid Base Regulation Norman S. Lichtenstein

Terminology
Acid Production
Body Buffers
  Response to Acid or Alkaline Load
  Responses to Changes in pCO_2
Respiratory Regulation
Renal Regulation
  Bicarbonate Reabsorption
  Titratable Acid Excretion
  Ammonium Excretion
  Urine pH
Metabolic Acidosis
  Causes
  Increased Anion Gap (Normocholoremic)
    Metabolic Acidosis
    Chronic Renal Failure
    Ketoacidosis
    Lactic Acidosis
    Ingestion of Toxins
  Normal Anion Gap (Hyperchloremic) Metabolic
    Acidosis
    Administration of Ammonium Chloride,
      Calcium Chloride, Arginine · HCl, Lysine ·
      HCl, and IV Hyperalimentation
    Gastrointestinal Losses
    Renal Causes
    Acetazolamide Ingestion

  Renal Tubular Acidosis
  Respiratory Compensation
  Signs and Symptoms
  Treatment
Metabolic Alkalosis
  Causes
    Loss of Gastric Contents
    Diuretics
    Post-hypercapneic State
    Congenital Chloridorrhea
    Ingestion of Excessive Alkali
    Mineralocorticoid Excess
  Respiratory Compensation
  Signs and Symptoms
  Treatment
Respiratory Acidosis
  Causes
  Compensation
  Signs and Symptoms
  Treatment
Respiratory Alkalosis
  Causes
  Compensation
  Signs and Symptoms
  Treatment
Mixed Disorders
Summary

This chapter deals with the regulation of the H^+ concentration of the body fluids. While acid-base metabolism is not in itself a sign or symptom, this section is included for two reasons: (1) the consequences of disordered acid-base metabolism can result in many signs and symptoms; and (2) the fundamentals of acid-base metabolism are essential for the understanding of other subjects discussed in this text. Within the last several years there have appeared several monographs and books on the basic physiology and clinical disorders of acid-base regulation, and these should be consulted for greater detail.

TERMINOLOGY

According to the Brönsted–Lowry definition, an *acid* is a donor of H^+; H_2CO_3 or $HC1$ would be acids. A *base* is an acceptor of H^+, as for example HCO_3^- or $C1-$. A *buffer* is the combination of a weak acid and its salt or a weak base and its salt. An example of the former would be the $H_2CO_3 - HCO_3^-$ pair, and an example of the latter would be the $NH_3 - NH_4^+$ combination. A buffer can accept or give up H^+ in a way that minimizes changes in *pH*. The change in *pH* with addition of H^+ is curvilinear, and the buffer is most effective at its *pK*, that *pH* at which the buffer is 50% dissociated.

The dissociation constant, *K*, for a weak acid, $HA \rightleftarrows H^+ + A^-$, is given as follows:

$$K = \frac{[H^+] \times [A^-]}{[HA]}$$

This can be rearranged to

$$[H^+] = K \times \frac{[HA]}{[A^-]}$$

The logarithm of both sides may be taken

$$\log [H^+] = \log K + \log \frac{[HA]}{[A^-]}$$

Or

$$-\log H^+ = -\log K - \log \frac{[HA]}{[A^-]}$$

Substituting *pH* for $-\log (H^+)$ and *pK* for $-\log K$, the equation may be rearranged as follows:

$$pH = pK + \log \frac{[A^-]}{[HA]}$$

In this form it is called the Henderson–Hasselbalch equation. For the major buffer system of the extracellular fluid of the body the equation reads

$$pH = pK + \log \frac{[HCO_3^-]}{[H_2CO_3]}$$

H_2CO_3 represents carbon dioxide gas dissolved in solution. Therefore, the denominator can be replaced by pCO_2 and the two quantities equated by the use of a constant, α, equal to 0.03:

$$pH = 6.1 + \log \frac{[HCO_3^-]}{\alpha pCO_2}$$

With a normal blood HCO_3^- of 24 mEq/liter and a normal pCO_2 of 40 torr, the equation may be written as

$$pH = 6.1 + \log \frac{24}{0.03 \times 40}$$

$$pH = 6.1 + \log \frac{24}{1.2} = 7.4$$

The Henderson–Hasselbalch equation will be referred to time and again and is the constant reference point for acid-base discussion. Although the equation is expressed in terms of the most prevalent buffer in the extracellular space, the $HCO_3^- - H_2CO_3$ pair, in fact it refers to the *pH* of other buffer pairs as well because of the isohydric principle. This states that when several buffers exist in the same solution they are in equilibrium with the same H^+ concentration. Thus, examination of just one buffer pair—for example, the $HCO_3^- : H_2CO_3$ ratio in the extracellular fluid—allows a prediction of the salt to acid ratio of all the other buffers in that compartment.

The normal *pH* of body fluids is 7.40, a H^+ concentration of $4 \times 10^{-8}M$ or only 0.04 mM/liter, which is three orders of magnitude smaller than the concentrations of the common ions Na^+, Cl^-, and HCO_3^-. The extremes of H^+ concentration compatible with life range between *pH* 6.8 and 7.8.

ACID PRODUCTION

When the carbohydrate and fat of normal diets are completely oxidized, CO_2 and water are formed. The amount of CO_2 produced is huge, approximating 15,000 mM to 20,000 mM per day. This CO_2 is eliminated completely by the lungs, resulting in no net addition of H^+ to the body. CO_2 is itself not an acid, but it may combine with water to form a weak acid, H_2CO_3. The H^+ produced that is *not* volatile, such as H_2SO_4 or H_3PO_4, must be excreted by the kidneys. This H^+ arises from three sources. The major source is the oxidation of the sulfur-containing amino acids methionine, cystine, and cysteine, which are especially high in meats. The complete oxidation of proteins containing these three amino acids yields H_2SO_4:

$$Methionine + O_2 \rightarrow urea + CO_2 \\ + H_2O + SO_4^= + 2H^+$$

A second source is phosphoproteins and phospholipids, which on complete oxidation yield H_3PO_4. A third and smaller source comes from the incomplete oxidation of fats and carbohydrates:

$$Glucose + O_2 \rightarrow 2 \; lactate^- + 2H^+$$
$$Triglycerides + O_2 \rightarrow acetoacetate^- + H^+$$

The total daily production of nonvolatile H^+ varies with the diet. A heavy meat consumer may produce one to two hundred milliequivalents of acid per day; a vegetarian, whose diet contains excessive potassium citrate, may produce no net acid at all and may even excrete HCO_3^- in the urine:

$$RCOO^- \; K^+ + O_2 \rightarrow urea + CO_2 + K^+ + HCO_3^-$$

On an average diet approximately 40 mEq to 80 mEq of nonvolatile H^+ are produced per day.

The lines of defense against changes in H^+ activity may be divided into three areas: (1) the body buffers; (2) the respiratory system, which controls the level of $p\mathrm{CO}_2$; and (3) the kidneys, which control the level of serum HCO_3^-.

BODY BUFFERS

Buffers are present throughout the extracellular as well as intracellular compartments. Their role is to mitigate changes in pH when H^+ is added to or removed from the body. The major buffers present vary depending upon the body fluid compartment sampled. In extracellular fluid the major buffer is the HCO_3^-–H_2CO_3 pair. By contrast, in intracellular fluid there is little HCO_3^-, and the major buffers are phosphates and proteins. In urine the two major buffers are phosphate and the NH_3 - NH_4^+ pair. In bone, the buffer is hydroxyapatite, a crystalline salt of Ca^{++}. When acid is added to the extracellular fluid, buffering begins immediately and takes about 1 hour to be completed. Intracellular buffering takes longer—about 2 hours to 4 hours to complete.

RESPONSE TO ACID OR ALKALINE LOAD

It is of interest to know the relative proportion of extracellular and intracellular buffering when an acute acid load is presented to the body. To answer this question Pitts nephrectomized dogs and then gave them large, acute acid loads (9.5 mEq H^+/kg). The distribution between intra- and extracellular fluids is shown in Figure 36-1. Approximately one half was buffered intracellularly and one half extracellularly. Extracellular HCO_3^- participated as follows:

$$NaHCO_3 + HCl \rightarrow NaCl + H_2CO_3 \rightarrow NaCl$$
$$+ CO_2 + H_2O$$

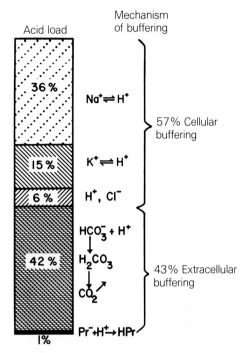

Fig. 36-1. Mechanisms of buffering of strong acid infused intravenously in the dog. (From Pitts RF: Physiology of the Kidney and Body Fluids, 3rd ed. Chicago, Year Book, 1974)

Intracellular buffering was accomplished by phosphates and proteins (Pr^-), including hemoglobin in red blood cells:

$$NaPr + HCl \rightarrow HPr + NaCl$$
$$KPr + HCl \rightarrow HPr + KCl$$

Thus, the negatively charged intracellular proteins, with the counterions K^+ and Na^+, accepted H^+ and in turn released K^+ and Na^+ into the extracellular fluid. A recent study has shown that in *very* severe metabolic acidosis (serum $HCO_3^- < 5$ mEq/liter) the proportion of intracellular buffering becomes even greater, accounting for up to 85% of the total buffering. Because of these ion shifts during acute mineral acid-induced acidosis, the serum K^+ (normally 3.5 mEq/liter–5 mEq/liter) may rise by several milliequivalents per liter and lead to K^+ toxicity. Since the serum Na^+ is much higher (135 mEq/liter–145 mEq/liter), the shift of a few milliequivalents of Na causes but a slight change in serum Na^+ concentration.

Similar experiments with large acute alkaline loads resulted in two thirds of the load being buffered extracellularly and one third being buffered intracellularly (Fig. 36-2). The $H^+ \rightleftarrows Na^+$ and $H^+ \rightleftarrows K^+$ exchanges with the proteins are the same reactions as shown for the acid load, but in the opposite direction. As a result

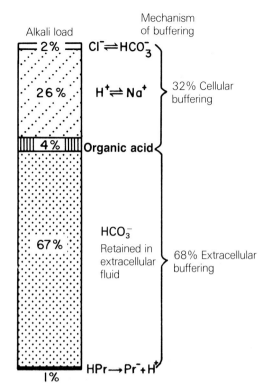

Fig. 36-2. Mechanisms of buffering of base infused intravenously in the dog. (From Pitts RF: Physiology of the Kidney and Body Fluids, 3rd ed. Chicago, Year Book, 1974)

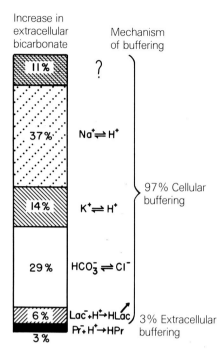

Fig. 36-3. Mechanisms of buffering of CO_2 in respiratory acidosis in the dog. (From Pitts RF: Physiology of the Kidney and Body Fluids, 3rd ed. Chicago, Year Book, 1974)

of these ion shifts the serum K^+ falls following an acute alkaline load.

RESPONSES TO CHANGES IN pCO_2

With acute CO_2 retention there is very little extracellular buffering, since HCO_3^-, the predominant buffer of this compartment, cannot buffer much additional H_2CO_3. As shown in Figure 36-3, 97% of the added CO_2 is buffered intracellularly by two major mechanisms:

1. There is $H^+ \rightleftarrows Na^+$ and $H^+ \rightleftarrows K^+$ exchange, occurring approximately one third with hemoglobin and two thirds with other intracellular proteins.
2. In red blood cells there is a $HCO_3^- \rightleftarrows Cl^-$ exchange mechanism by which HCO_3^- leaves and $Cl-$ enters the cells.

The mechanism for buffering a reduced pCO_2 concentration is shown in Figure 36-4. Again, virtually all the buffering occurs within cells by three mechanisms.

1. Intracellular proteins dissociate their H^+ and take up Na^+ and K^+.

2. Again, the $Cl^- \rightleftarrows HCO_3^-$ exchange occurs in red blood cells.
3. Low pCO_2 or decreased intracellular H^+ stimulates glycolysis, causing an increased production of lactic and pyruvic acids, which enter the blood to assist in buffering.

RESPIRATORY REGULATION

The respiratory system can respond to changes in pH, pCO_2 (and pO_2) by altering the rate and depth of respiration.

There are two groups of receptors:

1. *The peripheral chemoreceptors*, which are located at the bifurcation of the common carotid arteries and in the arch of the aorta, are stimulated by a decrease in pH and an increase in pCO_2 of the blood.
2. *The central chemoreceptors*, located near the ventral surface of the medulla, are stimulated by a decrease in pH and an increase in pCO_2 of the cerebrospinal and interstitial fluid of the brain. Response to changes in H^+ concentration (with pCO_2 held constant) occurs primarily through the peripheral receptors. Response to changes in pCO_2 occurs through both the central and peripheral receptors.

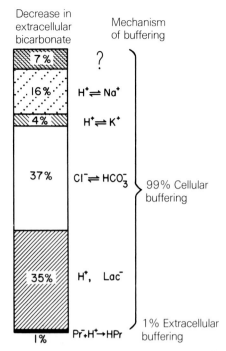

Decrease in extracellular bicarbonate   Mechanism of buffering

Fig. 36-4. Mechanisms of buffering of CO_2 in respiratory alkalosis in the dog. (From Pitts RF: Physiology of the Kidney and Body Fluids, 3rd ed. Chicago, Year Book, 1974)

The ability to respond to small decreases in HCO_3^- concentration by decreasing pCO_2 and to small increases in HCO_3^- by increasing pCO_2 makes the HCO_3^-–H_2CO_3 buffer pair very efficient in mitigating changes in pH. The time course for complete response varies from minutes to several hours, making the respiratory system intermediate in response time between the body buffers and the kidneys.

RENAL REGULATION

The kidney actively secretes H^+ into the tubular fluid or urine by three mechanisms: (1) HCO_3^- reabsorption, (2) titratable acid excretion, and (3) NH_4^+ excretion.

BICARBONATE REABSORPTION

The first mechanism, HCO_3^- reabsorption, is depicted in Figure 36-5. If the diet has been acidic and the need is to excrete an acid urine, the first process that must be accomplished is the reabsorption of the entire filtered load of $NaHCO_3$, since any loss of HCO_3^- is equivalent to the retention of H^+. The Na^+ passes across the luminal border of the tubular cell by facilitated diffusion and is then actively pumped out of the cell and into the peritubular blood. The HCO_3^- is reabsorbed by a more circuitous route. With CO_2 and water present in abundance in the cell, H_2CO_3 is formed (accelerated by the presence of the catalyst carbonic anhydrase), and then H^+ and HCO_3^- are generated. The HCO_3^- is absorbed from the cell into the blood, while H^+ is actively secreted into the lumen where it combines with the filtered HCO_3^- to form H_2CO_3, which, in the presence of carbonic anhydrase, then dissociates into CO_2 and water. It is evident that the reaction within the lumen is the reverse of that occurring within the cell and that active H^+ secretion has resulted in the regeneration of HCO_3^- in the blood.

The HCO_3^- reabosorption mechanism is quantitatively the most important part of renal H^+ secretion. With a stable blood HCO_3^- level of 24 mEq/liter and a normal glomerular filtration rate of 150 liters/day, the amount of HCO_3^- reabsorbed in 24 hours is

$$24 \text{ mEq/liter} \times 150 \text{ liter/day} = 3600 \text{ mEq/day}$$

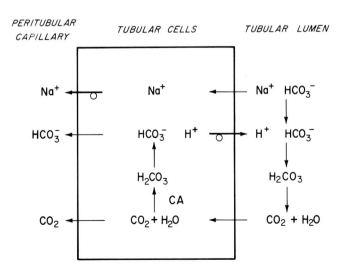

Fig. 36-5. Mechanism of bicarbonate reabsorption by the renal tubular cell. CA is carbonic anhydrase.

The 3600 mEq/day of H^+ secretion necessary to accomplish this HCO_3^- reabsorption is far in excess of the amunt of H^+ secreted by the titratable acid and the NH_4^+ mechanisms. The reabsorption of HCO_3^- is 85% to 90% completed in the proximal tubule, while the remaining 10% to 15% occurs in the distal tubule.

Below is a list of the factors that increase the rate of HCO_3^- reabsorption.

1. *Decreased extracellular fluid volume* (decreased Cl^-)
2. *Increased pCO_2*
3. *Decreased K^+*
4. *Increased adrenal steroids*
5. *Decreased parathyroid hormone*

At plasma HCO_3^- levels less than 22 mEq/liter, all filtered HCO_3^- is normally reabsorbed. Above this level or threshold a portion of the filtered HCO_3^- is not reabsorbed. Earlier studies purported to show that a tubular maximum (T_m) existed—a level above which all filtered HCO_3^- was rejected. It is now evident that these *maximum values* were artifacts of volume expansion. The middle curve in Figure 36-6 shows that infusion of hypertonic $NaHCO_3$, which produces a mild degree of expansion, causes an apparent T_m. If the infusion is isotonic HCO_3^-, the bottom curve is seen, but if during the HCO_3^- infusion, volume expansion is prevented by controlled hemorrhage or fluid removal, then HCO_3^- reabsorption continues to increase and does not reach a plateau. Thus, the apparent T_m is an artifact—the increase in HCO_3^- reabsorption with increased filtered load being opposed by a decrease in HCO_3^- reabsorption because of volume expansion.

When there is volume contraction, the body attempts to control and preserve volume by the reabsorption of all the filtered Na^+ presented to the tubules. (See Chapter 35.) Figure 36-7 demonstrates that Na^+ may be reabsorbed by one of two mechanisms: either together with an anion such as Cl^- or in exchange for cations, such as H^+ or K^+. Normally both mechanisms occur. However, in states of volume depletion (which can also be considered Cl^- depletion since $NaCl$ is the predominant extracellular electrolyte), there is less Cl^- available for reabsorption with Na^+, and hence a greater proportion of the Na^+ is reabsorbed in exchange for H^+ and K^+. It is evident from the earlier discussion that the process of H^+ secretion into the tubular lumen results in the addition of an equivalent amount of HCO_3^- into the blood. Hence, with Cl^- depletion there is increased HCO_3^- reabsorption.

Elevated pCO_2 causes an increase in the rate of HCO_3^- reabsorption by supplying more of the substrate CO_2 to the renal tubule cells. The reaction is pushed toward the formation of more H^+ and HCO_3^-, resulting in additional H^+ secretion and increased HCO_3^- reabsorption.

Elevated pCO_2 and decreased extracellular fluid volume are the two major determinants of increased HCO_3^- reabsorption. However, there are three other mechanisms that have a quantitatively smaller but still important effect on HCO_3^- reabsorption: serum K^+, adrenal steroids, and parathyroid hormone.

Decreased serum K^+ causes K^+–H^+ shifts, with K^+ leaving and H^+ entering cells. Thus the intracellular acidosis of the renal tubular cell may be the signal for causing H^+ secretion into the lumen and HCO_3^- regeneration in the blood. Adrenal steroids promote K^+ loss, which is mainly responsible for the increased HCO_3^- reabsorption. When K^+ losses are consistently

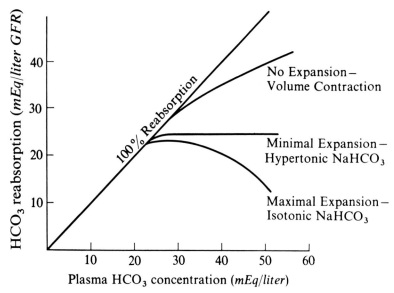

Fig. 36-6. Effect of extracellular volume on bicarbonate reabsorption. (From Seldin DW, and Rector FC: The generation and maintenance of metabolic acidosis. Kidney Int 1:306, 1972)

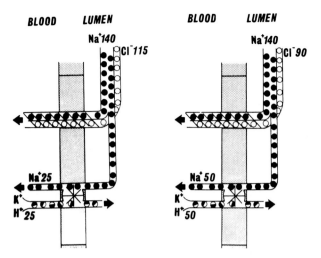

Fig. 36-7. Schematic representation of the influence of hypochloremia on renal transport mechanisms. (From Kassirer JP, Schwartz WB: The response of normal man to selective depletion of hydrochloric acid. Am J Med 40:10, 1966)

replaced, adrenal steroids alone cause minimal elevations in serum HCO_3^-. The mechanism by which parathormone reduces HCO_3^- reabsorption remains under investigation.

Each of the five factors that increases HCO_3^- reabsorption will, when acting in the opposite direction, cause a *decrease* in the rate of HCO_3^- reabsorption.

TITRATABLE ACID EXCRETION

Titratable acid is defined as the amount of H^+ excreted in combination with urinary buffers. It is determined by titration of the urine sample with a strong base such as NaOH. The number of milliequivalents of NaOH required to raise the urine pH from its initial value up to a pH of 7.4 equals the number of milliequivalents of H^+ added by the kidney to produce the titratable acid in that sample. The major component of titratable acid is the $H_2PO_4^-$–$HPO_4^=$ buffer pair, which has a pK of 6.8. At lower urinary pHs, other buffers such as creatinine, lactic acid, and β-hydroxybutyric acid, which have pKs of 4 to 5, will also contribute to the titratable acidity. Normally, titratable acid accounts for approximately 20 mEq to 40 mEq of H^+ excretion per day. With acidosis there can be a moderate increase in this amount, but only to the extent of the availability of urinary buffers and the limit to which urine pH can be lowered.

The mechanism by which titratable acid is excreted is shown in Figure 36-8. Na_2HPO_4, for example, is presented in the lumen, and Na^+ is actively reabsorbed. H^+ and HCO_3^- are generated intracellularly by the same mechanisms as shown previously. The H^+ is actively secreted into the lumen, titrating the Na_2HPO_4 to NaH_2PO_4. In this way extra H^+ may be added to phosphate and excreted into the urine.

AMMONIUM EXCRETION

The mechanism of NH_4^+ excretion is shown in Figure 36-9. In this instance, Na^+, together with an anion such as $SO_4^=$, is presented to the lumen. The H^+ and $SO_4^=$ together equal H_2SO_4, an acid that cannot exist within the milieu of the lumen because it requires a pH lower than the kidney is capable of producing. Therefore, the secreted H^+ combines with NH_3 to form NH_4^+, which is trapped in the lumen and excreted in

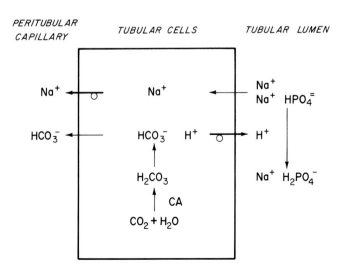

Fig. 36-8. Mechanism of titratable acid secretion by the renal tubular cell.

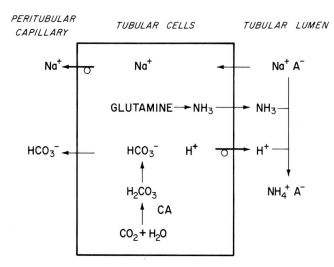

Fig. 36-9. Mechanism of NH_4^+ secretion by the renal tubular cell.

the urine as $(NH_4)_2 SO_4$. Amino acids, especially glutamine, are the major source of the NH_3.

$$Glutamine \rightarrow glutamic\ acid \rightarrow \alpha\text{-ketoglutaric}\ acid$$
$$+ NH_3 \qquad\qquad + NH_3$$

The rate of NH_4^+ excretion is affected by the four factors listed below:

1. *Urine pH*
2. *Chronicity of systemic acidosis*
3. *Rate of urine flow*
4. *Total number of nephrons*

Figure 36-10 illustrates the first two factors. As the urine pH becomes more acid, the rate of NH_4^+ excretion is increased. Also, if there has been a prior state of acidosis, then for any given urine pH, more NH_4^+ will be excreted. Systemic acidosis enhances glutamine metabolism, perhaps by acting on a rate-limiting step in glutamine metabolism or by facilitating glutamine entry into mitochondria. The rate of urine flow also influences the rate of NH_4^+ excretion, as more rapid flow permits more NH_3 to diffuse into the urine. Finally, the importance of the total number of nephrons becomes manifest only when they are deficient, as in chronic renal failure. The NH_4^+ mechanism is the main adaptive response to chronic acidosis. While normally 30 mEq to 60 mEq of NH_4^+ are excreted per day, in the presence of severe chronic acidosis, several hundred milliequivalents per day may be excreted after 4 days to 5 days of adaptation.

URINE pH

The H^+ activity, which is measured routinely when obtaining a urine pH, reflects only a trivial amount of

free H^+. For example, at a maximal urinary pH of 4.5, the H^+ concentration is less than 0.1 mEq/liter. However, the reason why this tiny amount is so important is that the urinary pH, which reflects the degree of acidity of the urine, directly infuences the amount of H^+ excreted with buffers. Thus, the more acidic the

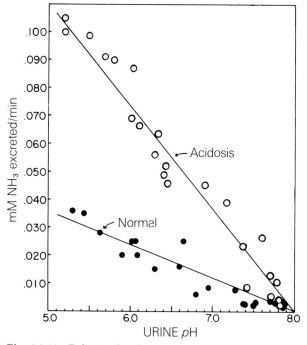

Fig. 36-10. Relationship between urine pH and ammonia excretion under conditions of normal acid-base balance and chronic acidosis. (From Pitts RF: The renal excretion of acid. Fed Proc 7:418, 1948)

urine becomes the greater will be the amount of NH_4^+ and titratable acid excreted in the urine.

H^+ secretion and excretion should be differentiated. The total H^+ *secretion* refers to the number of H^+ secreted per day to accomplish the process of HCO_3^- reabsorption, NH_4^+ secretion, and titratable acid secretion; it equals approximately 4000 mEq/day. *Net acid excretion* refers to the amount of H^+ eliminated from the body and equals NH_4^+ excretion, plus titratable acid excretion, minus HCO_3^- lost in the urine. On an average diet the nonvolatile H^+ produced equals 40 mEq to 80 mEq/day and, in the steady state, the amount of net acid excretion also equals 40 mEq to 80 mEq/day.

METABOLIC ACIDOSIS

In metabolic acidosis there is increased H^+ activity in the extracellular fluid, the primary disturbance being the addition of nonvolatile acid or the loss of base.

$$\downarrow pH = pK + \log \frac{HCO_3^- \downarrow}{pCO_2 \downarrow}$$

The primary event is a decrease in HCO_3^- ($\downarrow$), the compensation is hyperventilation to effect a decrease in pCO_2 ($\downarrow$), and the result is a decrease in pH ($\downarrow$), but to a level that is not as low as would have occurred without the respiratory compensation.

CAUSES

A method of categorizing the causes of metabolic acidosis is to note the effect of the acidosis on the anion gap. The anion gap may be defined as the serum (Na^+ + K^+) minus (HCO_3^- + Cl^-) and equals approximately 16 mEq/liter. Since the K^+ contribution is small, it may be omitted from the calculation, and then the anion gap is

$$Na^+ - (Cl^- + HCO_3^-) = 12 \text{ mEq/liter.}$$

Of course, electroneutrality requires that cations and anions balance each other precisely. The *gap* is a matter of terminology only and consists predominantly of the negative charges on albumin and other proteins, plus $SO_4^=$, phosphate, and organic acid anions, which are measured less frequently.

Focusing on the anion gap should not obscure the fact that the cause of the acidosis in every case is an increase in H^+ activity. The division into normal or increased anion gap serves only to categorize and aid in the clinical recognition of types of metabolic acidosis. Table 36-1 lists the causes of metabolic acidosis.

Table 36-1. *Causes of Metabolic Acidosis*

Increased anion gap (normochloremic)	Chronic renal failure
	Ketoacidosis
	Diabetic
	Alcoholic
	Starvation
	Lactic acidosis
	Ingestion of toxins
	Salicylates
	Methyl alcohol
	Ethylene glycol
	Paraldehyde
Normal anion gap (hyperchloremic)	Adminstration of HCl or its equivalent
	NH_4Cl, $CaCl_2$, arginine·HCl
	Lysine·HCl, hyperalimentation
	Intestinal losses
	Diarrhea
	Ureterosigmoidostomy
	Renal losses
	Early renal insufficiency
	Acetazolamide
	Proximal RTA
	Distal RTA
	Hypoaldosteronism

INCREASED ANION GAP (NORMOCHLOREMIC) METABOLIC ACIDOSIS

Chronic Renal Failure

The metabolism of a normal acid diet generates the equivalent of H_2SO_4, and the reaction with body buffers may be represented as

$$H_2SO_4 + 2\ NaHCO_3 \rightarrow Na_2SO_4 + 2\ H_2O + 2\ CO_2$$

The H^+ combines with HCO_3^-, causing a reduction in HCO_3^- and producing Na^+ plus an anion such as $SO_4^=$ or phosphate. A normal person easily excretes these anions. In the patient with renal failure and markedly reduced glomerular filtration rate, the normal rate of production of $SO_4^=$ and phosphate exceeds the ability of the kidneys to filter and clear these anions. Thus, there is retention of the anions, but the resultant increase in the anion gap is not in itself responsible for the acidosis.

The kidney attempts to regenerate HCO_3^- by using the three familiar mechanisms of NH_4^+ excretion, titratable acid excretion, and HCO_3^- reabsorption. Although each surviving nephron in chronic renal failure adapts remarkably well and secretes as much as five times the amount of NH_4^+ per nephron as normal, nevertheless at some point there are simply insufficient numbers of renal tubular cells remaining to secrete the needed amount of H^+ and NH_3. Titratable acid excretion proceeds but is somewhat diminished

because the total amount of phosphate filtered through the kidneys is reduced. The third mechanism, HCO_3^- reabsorption, is also partly at fault, since these patients may have a mild HCO_3^- "leak," which may be structural or related to the excess parathormone present. Of the three mechanisms, all of which are impaired, quantitatively it is the failure of adequate NH_4^+ excretion that contributes most to the acidosis. However, the ability to excrete a maximally acid urine is retained. Lastly, there is constant buffering of acid in the bone, where hydroxyapatite provides a large reserve of alkali to serve for chronic buffering of H^+, but at the expense of dissolution of bone calcium salts and production of osteomalacia and osteopenia.

Ketoacidosis

Lack of insulin in the diabetic patient results in the incomplete oxidation of fats and the accumulation of β-hydroxybutyric acid and acetoacetic acid.

$$\beta\text{-hydroxybutyrate}^- \ H^+ + NaHCO_3 \rightarrow$$
$$Na^+ \ \beta\text{-hydroxybutyrate}^- + H_2O + CO_2$$

The HCO_3^- is depleted by reaction with H^+, and sodium β-hydroxybutyrate and sodium acetoacetate accumulate and cause the increase in the anion gap. The presence of these anions can be demonstrated in urine or blood by the simple ketone tablet test (which, however, measures only acetoacetate and acetone, not β-hydroxybutyrate). Levels of all three ketone bodies are elevated, with the β-hydroxybutyrate being the predominant one. When insulin and fluids are supplied, this reaction proceeds in reverse, and HCO_3^- is regenerated. Therefore, except for severe ketoacidosis (pH < 7.10), exogenous administration of HCO_3^- is not necessary, since the body will produce its own HCO_3^- once insulin and fluids are supplied.

Ketoacidosis may also be seen in two other states in the absence of any diabetes—alcoholism and starvation.

Lactic Acidosis

Lactic acid is formed during the anerobic metabolism of glucose. The following reaction shows the relationship between pyruvic acid and lactic acid:

$$\begin{array}{ccc} O & & OH \\ \parallel & & \mid \\ CH_3C\!-\!COOH + NADH_2 & \rightleftharpoons & CH_3CH\!-\!COOH + NAD \\ \text{Pyruvic acid} & & \text{Lactic acid} \end{array}$$

The normal lactate level is 1 mEq/liter and the pyruvate level 0.1 mEq/liter. In states of hypoxia and increased $NADH_2$ the reaction is driven to the right with the formation of increased amounts of lactic acid. Lactic acidosis is seen in many conditions, with the common

denominators being a state of shock, poor perfusion, or hypoxia. In these conditions there is diminished delivery of O_2 to the tissues, which favors the formation of lactate from pyruvate. Despite administration of massive amounts of HCO_3^-, there may be little improvement because the rate of formation of lactic acid remains high. The treatment is to attempt to improve the circulation and O_2 delivery. Other states that may be associated with lactic acidosis are leukemia, diabetes mellitus, phenformin use, and ethanol ingestion. When no underlying cause can be found, the condition of idiopathic or spontaneous lactic acidosis exists. The etiology is unknown, but again local tissue hypoxia has been postulated. The mortality associated with this condition is very high.

Ingestion of Toxins

Salicylate intoxication can cause two different effects on pH. Initially there is hyperventilation leading to a decrease in pCO_2 and respiratory alkalosis. Subsequently, salicylate interferes with carbohydrate metabolism to cause the accumulation of organic acids, including lactic acid, β-hydroxybutyric acid, and acetoacetic acid. Therefore, the pH may reflect either respiratory alkalosis, metabolic acidosis, or a mixed disorder.

Methyl alcohol is metabolized to formic acid and probably results in the formation of other organic acids as well.

Ethylene glycol is converted to oxalic acid and other organic acids. In addition to causing acidosis, oxalate is itself toxic to the kidneys and may lead to renal failure. Both ethylene glycol and methyl alcohol intoxication may be treated with a cautious infusion of ethyl alcohol, which competitively inhibits the enzyme alcohol dehydrogenase, slows the metabolism of ethylene glycol and methyl alcohol, and allows for their excretion in the urine.

Ingestion of paraldehyde leads to accumulation of acetic acid as well as other organic acids.

NORMAL ANION GAP (HYPERCHLOREMIC) METABOLIC ACIDOSIS

Administration of Ammonium Chloride, Calcium Chloride, Arginine·HCl, Lysine·HCl, and IV Hyperalimentation

The administration of NH_4Cl is the equivalent of HCl because of the following reaction in the liver:

$$NH_4Cl \rightarrow NH_3 + HCl$$

Then

$$HCl + NaHCO_3 \rightarrow NaCl + CO_2 + H_2O$$

The HCO_3^- concentration is lowered, and Cl^- is increased, producing a hyperchloremic acidosis without any other retained ion.

The ingestion of $CaCl_2$ produces the following reaction in the alkaline intestinal fluids:

$$CaCl_2 + NaHCO_3 \rightarrow CaCO_3 + HCl + NaCl$$

$CaCO_3$ is insoluble and is eliminated in the stool, while HCl is absorbed into the body.

Certain intravenous hyperalimentation fluids have a relative excess of cationic amino acids such as arginine, lysine, and histidine. When these are metabolized, H^+ is formed, as in the following reaction:

$$R\text{–}NH_3^+ \ Cl^- + O_2 \rightarrow urea + HCl + CO_2 + H_2O$$

The use of arginine·HCl and lysine·HCl causes a similar release of H^+.

Gastrointestinal Losses

The intestinal fluids contain HCO_3^- in concentrations of 25 mEq to 50 mEq/liter. Thus, with diarrhea or loss of pancreatic fluids by drainage or fistula, excessive $NaHCO_3$ is lost without retention of any unmeasured anions.

A similar problem can result from ureterosigmoidostomy. When cystectomy is necessary for neurogenic bladder or bladder carcinoma, implanting the ureters into the sigmoid colon provides a method of urinary diversion. However, there is a metabolic price to be paid, because the urine that is formed remains in contact with the colonic mucosa for several hours at a time. The colon has an active Cl^-–HCO_3^- exchange pump by which Cl^- is absorbed from the lumen into the blood and HCO_3^- is secreted from the blood into the lumen. Thus, the "urine" remaining in the sigmoid can become rich in HCO_3^-, and with evacuation there is a net loss of HCO_3^-. Furthermore, the colon will reabsorb NH_4^+, which contributes to the acidosis. An alternative surgical procedure, the ileal loop, is designed as a conduit rather than a reservoir. Here urine is in contact with a much smaller bowel surface area for a much shorter period of time. These modifications reduce, but may not entirely eliminate, the complication of metabolic acidosis.

Renal Causes

As already discussed, patients with chronic renal failure and severely depressed glomerular filtration rate develop metabolic acidosis with an increased anion gap because of retention of phosphate, $SO_4^=$, and other anions. However, some patients with early renal dysfunction (creatinine 2 mg/dl–4 mg/dl), often owing to chronic pyelonephritis or obstruction, may develop a hyperchloremic acidosis. In these cases there is a disproportionate abnormality in tubular function as compared to glomerular filtration, resulting in a large reduction in H^+ secretion, while glomerular filtration is only mildly impaired.

Acetazolamide Ingestion

Acetazolamide is a diuretic that inhibits the enzyme carbonic anhydrase. Since reabsorption of HCO_3^- is partially dependent upon carbonic anhydrase, inhibition of the enzyme results in a loss of HCO_3^- into the urine. Typically, these patients stabilize with a serum HCO_3^- of 15 mEq to 20 mEq/liter. Although this diuretic is seldom used now for the control of edema or hypertension, it still retains an important place in the treatment of patients with glaucoma.

Renal Tubular Acidosis

All renal acidosis is "tubular" in the sense that any deficit of H^+ secretion and HCO_3^- reabsorption is the result of a tubular abnormality. Thus, the acidification defects of chronic renal failure described earlier can be considered tubular in origin. However, the name *renal tubular acidosis* (RTA) is reserved for a group of diseases in which there is usually little decrease in glomerular filtration (at least initially) but in which there is an inability to lower the urinary *p*H appropriately in the presence of a mild acidosis. Arbitrarily, this is taken to mean a failure to lower the urinary *p*H to less than 5.3 when the serum HCO_3^- is normal to slightly reduced (22 mEq/liter) and arterial *p*H is slightly acid.

In proximal RTA, the derangement is in the proximal tubules, such that the capacity to reabsorb HCO_3^- is reduced to a variable degree. The defect is analogous to the one produced after the administration of acetazolamide, which causes a leakage of HCO_3^- into the urine. Although the distal nephron, which normally reabsorbs 10% to 15% of the filtered HCO_3^-, increases its rate or reabsorption, the magnitude of the leak is such that it overwhelms the capacity of the distal nephron, and bicarbonaturia ensues. After a variable amount of HCO_3^- has been lost, a new steady state is reached at a lower serum HCO_3^- level. At this new level, *less* HCO_3^- is now being filtered—an amount just equal to that which the proximal and distal tubules can handle—and no more HCO_3^- appears in the urine (Fig. 36-11). At this point a urine with *p*H of less than 5.3 can be produced.

The defect in distal RTA is entirely different. Reabsorption of HCO_3^- is normal in the proximal and distal convoluted tubules. However, the collecting duct is unable to generate a maximal H^+ gradient. When stimulated by acidosis, H^+ gradients as high as nearly 1000:1 (blood *p*H 7.4, urine *p*H 4.5) can be achieved. In distal

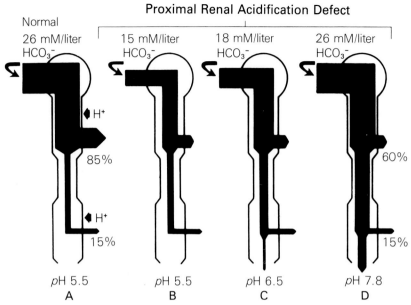

Proximal Renal Acidification Defect

Fig. 36-11. Schematic representation of the renal acidification defect in proximal RTA. (*A*) Normal. (*B*) Filtered bicarbonate is severely below normal, and urinary excretion is nil. (*C*) Filtered bicarbonate is moderately below normal but exceeding the capacity of the proximal tubule, and bicarbonate appears in the urine. (*D*) Filtered bicarbonate is at normal serum levels, and massive bicarbonaturia ensues. (From Morris RC, Sebastian A, McSherry E: Renal acidosis. Kidney Int 1:322, 1972)

RTA (more correctly the defect appears to be in the collecting ducts), there is impaired H^+ secretion or increased back diffusion of H^+; therefore, regardless of how low the serum HCO_3^- level drops, a urine pH of less than 5.3 is *never* achieved.

The diagnosis of RTA should be considered when in the presence of metabolic acidosis the urine pH is greater than 5.3 (provided infection with a urea-splitting organism, which raises urinary pH, is excluded). Administration of either the standard acute oral loading dose of NH_4Cl (0.1 g/kg) or the 3-day prolonged course of NH_4Cl will intensify the stimulus to acidify the urine. At some point the patient with proximal RTA will lower his urine pH to less than 5.3, whereas the patient with distal RTA will always have a pH greater than 5.3. A handy short test is simply to measure the urine pH on arising in the morning, when it is already likely to be quite acid. Patients with distal RTA usually have urine pHs greater than 6 at this time.

Table 36-2 summarizes the differences between uremic acidosis, proximal RTA, and distal RTA.

In chronic renal failure the major defect is a decrease in the absolute amount of NH_4^+ excretion because of the lack of a sufficient number of nephrons. There are also minor decreases in the rate of titratable acid excretion and HCO_3^- reabsorption. The ability to excrete a maximally acid urine is retained. In proximal RTA, the major defect is reduced ability to reabsorb HCO_3^- at normal serum HCO_3^- levels. When a new steady state is reached at a lower serum HCO_3^- level, HCO_3^- reabsorption is "normal" and urine pH is less than 5.3. In distal RTA the major defect is an inability

to decrease urine pH to less than 5.3, regardless of the degree of systemic acidosis. Although there is no defect in titratable acid or NH_4^+ secretion *per se*, the relatively high urine pH prevents the maximal titration of these buffers.

The causes of proximal RTA are numerous and may be grouped into several categories: (1) primary RTA, unassociated with any systemic disease; (2) genetic diseases, such as hereditary fructose intolerance, cystinosis, and Wilson's disease; (3) drugs, such as outdated tetracycline; and (4) a miscellaneous group of causes, including renal transplantation and medullary cystic disease. Proximal RTA syndromes are sometimes associated with multiple dysfunction of the proximal tubule—the Fanconi syndrome—which includes urinary

Table 36-2. *Pathophysiology of Renal Acidoses*

	Uremia	Proximal RTA	Distal RTA
During acidosis			
Urinary pH	<5.3	<5.3	>5.3*
NH_4^+ excretion	↓ *	N	↓
TA excretion	↓	N	↓
HCO_3^- reabsorption	N	N to ↓	N
At normal serum HCO_3^- level			
HCO_3^- reabsorption	N to ↓	↓ *	N

*Denotes the major defect.

loss of glucose, amino acids, phosphate, potassium, and uric acid.

The causes of distal RTA may be grouped similarly: (1) a primary form unassociated with any systemic disease: (2) genetic diseases, such as Fabry's disease and sickle cell anemia; (3) drugs, such as amphotericin B, toluene, and lithium; (4) autoimmune disorders, such as hypergammaglobulinemia, cryoglobulinemia, and lupus erythematosus; (5) nephrocalcinosis from hyperparathyroidism or hyperthyroidism; and (6) a miscellaneous group of causes including transplantation, obstructive uropathy, and cirrhosis.

RESPIRATORY COMPENSATION

The first line of defense against metabolic acidosis is the body buffer system. Acidosis also stimulates the peripheral chemoreceptors and brain medullary center to cause an increase in the respiratory rate and tidal volume. For example, an increase of 0.1 pH unit causes the respiratory rate to double. This hyperventilation reduces the pCO_2, blunting the pH change that would otherwise have occurred. For every decrease in HCO_3^- concentration of 1 mEq/liter there is normally a corresponding reduction in pCO_2 of 1.2 torr. A pCO_2 that is either more or less than expected is evidence for a mixed (more than one type) acid-base disorder.

SIGNS AND SYMPTOMS

The signs and symptoms in the patient depend in part on the primary disease causing the metabolic acidosis. In addition, there may be symptoms referrable to the acidotic state *per se* that can effect the respiratory, cardiac, neurologic, and other systems:

1. *Deep (Kussmaul) respirations occur as the lungs blow off CO_2* in an attempt to compensate for the decreased HCO_3^-. However, this sign may be subtle, and substantial increases in minute ventilation may occur without being perceptible to the observer.
2. *Severe acidosis, with pH less than 7.10, adversely affects cardiac function.* There may be decreased myocardial contractility, decreased response to catecholamines, hypotension, and a predisposition toward arrhythmias.
3. *Lethargy, confusion, and even coma may occur,* in part related to the acidosis in the cerebrospinal fluid.
4. *Acute acidosis tends to cause hyperkalemia,* with symptoms like muscle weakness and cardiac arrhythmias. Chronic acidosis leads to K^+ depletion and associated symptoms of polyuria, polydipsia, inability to concentrate the urine, muscle weakness, ileus, and cardiac arrhythmias (especially in the presence of digitalis).

5. *With chronic acidosis H^+ is buffered in bone,* leading to bone dissolution, osteomalacia, rickets, and retarded growth in children.
6. *In distal RTA the chronic acidosis leads to nephrocalcinosis and nephrolithiasis* because of a combination of three factors: bone dissolution from H^+ buffering, which causes hypercalciuria; decreased concentration of urinary citrate; and a relatively high urine pH. These factors, acting together, promote the precipitation of Ca^{++} in the urine and the formation of stones.

TREATMENT

In the therapy of metabolic acidosis attention should be directed first to the underlying disorder. For example, in diabetic ketoacidosis the most important initial measure in correcting the acidosis is to give insulin. Similarly, in lactic acidosis, an attempt to restore perfusion and oxygenation is of prime importance.

In addition, it may be necessary to give alkali, best done with $NaHCO_3$. Sodium lactate, acetate, and gluconate are metabolized milliequivalent for milliequivalent into $NaHCO_3$, but there are occasional patients who are unable to accomplish this conversion, and hence it is safer simply to use $NaHCO_3$.

In a hypothetical situation in a patient with a serum HCO_3^- of 9 mEq/liter, a pCO_2 of 22 torr, and a pH of 7.23, how much HCO_3^- should be administered? The apparent volume of distribution of HCO_3^- approximates 50% of body weight. Therefore, the HCO_3^- deficit in a 70-kg man would equal

$$(24 - 9) \text{ mEq/liter} \times 50\% \text{ of } 70 \text{ kg or}$$

$$15 \text{ mEq/L} \times 35 \text{ liter} = 525 \text{ mEq total}$$

One should take the calculated deficit as only a rough guide to therapy for three reasons:

1. The HCO_3^- space of 50% of body weight is a gross estimate only. In states of very severe acidosis, where the serum HCO_3^- is much less than 5 mEq/liter, the HCO_3^- space approximation increases and may equal up to 100% of body weight.
2. The calculation ignores the fact that a steady state may not be present. For example, even while HCO_3^- is being administered in a case of severe lactic acidosis, there may be large ongoing rates of acid production.
3. In most cases it is necessary to make only a partial correction initially in order to rescue the patient from dangerous levels. In the example just described, one might give one quarter of the calculated deficit over the first 6 hours and then remeasure the HCO_3^- and pH. Additional correction could be accomplished

more slowly over the next 6 hours to 48 hours. Furthermore, as metabolism improves in ketoacidosis or lactic acidosis, the patient begins to use his own "potential HCO_3^-," present as β-hydroxybutyrate and lactate, and metabolize it into HCO_3^-.

There are dangers in giving too much HCO_3^- too quickly. Neurologic symptoms may worsen because, while the arterial pH improves, the cerebrospinal fluid pH may paradoxically become more acidotic. With the addition of HCO_3^-, arterial pH rises and has an inhibitory effect on the peripheral and brain receptors, lessening the amount of hyperventilation. CO_2 crosses the blood–brain barrier much more rapidly than does HCO_3^-, and hence the cerebrospinal fluid pH will actually fall. Another adverse effect of rapid correction of pH is that the increase in arterial pH shifts the oxygen hemoglobin dissociation curve to the left, increasing the affinity of hemoglobin for O_2 and reducing O_2 delivery to tissues. If large amounts of $NaHCO_3$ must be given when circulatory overload is present, peritoneal or hemodialysis may be needed to remove excess fluid.

For treatment of distal RTA adults need approximately 1 mEq $NaHCO_3$ per kg body weight per day—enough to make up for the deficient H^+ production by the kidneys and to neutralize the total daily net H^+ production. Children require 3 mEq to 6 mEq HCO_3^- per kg body weight per day—the higher dose being necessary because of the large amount of H^+ produced as a result of bone growth. When $NaHCO_3$ is given, symptoms of hypokalemia such as polyuria and polydipsia are alleviated, bone pain decreases, osteomalacia heals, growth resumes, urinary calcium decreases, and the frequency of stones declines. In proximal RTA the magnitude of HCO_3^- loss may necessitate extensive HCO_3^- replacement, but treatment goals may be more limited.

METABOLIC ALKALOSIS

In metabolic alkalosis there is decreased H^+ activity in the extracellular fluid, the primary disturbance being the loss of acid or addition of base.

$$\uparrow pH = pK + \log \frac{HCO_3^- \uparrow}{pCO_2 \uparrow}$$

There is an increase in HCO_3^- ($\uparrow$), the compensation is hypoventilation to increase pCO_2 ($\uparrow$), and the result is an alkaline pH ($\uparrow pH$).

CAUSES

The causes of metabolic alkalosis are listed in Table 36-3. The major cause, probably accounting for 95% of

Table 36-3. *Causes of Metabolic Alkalosis*

Volume (Cl⁻) depletion	Loss of gastric contents
	Diuretics
	Post chronic hypercapnea
	Congenital chloridorrhea
Ingestion of excessive alkali	
Mineralocorticoid excess	Primary aldosteronism
	Cushing's syndrome
	Congenital adrenal hyperplasia
	Renin-secreting tumors
	Bartter's syndrome
	Excess licorice ingestion (glycyrrhizic acid)
	Carbenoxolone
"Saline resistant" (extreme K⁺ deficiency)	

cases of metabolic alkalosis, is a contraction of extracellular fluid volume owing to loss of gastric contents or the use of diuretics.

Loss of Gastric Contents

Ordinarily, HCl is secreted by the stomach, neutralized by $NaHCO_3$, and reabsorbed by the small bowel. However, when there is vomiting or when gastric fluid is removed by nasogastric suction, there is a net loss of HCl from the body. Even in patients whose gastric secretions contain little acid and the main electrolyte present is NaCl, its removal also causes a metabolic alkalosis. The kidney can be thought of as having two choices: It may excrete $NaHCO_3$ into the urine and thereby preserve a normal systemic pH at the expense of still further volume depletion, or it may retain $NaHCO_3$ in order to protect the body's volume status, but at the expense of a persistent alkalosis. Confronted with this choice, it jealously guards volume and reabsorbs all the filtered HCO_3^-. The Na^+ is avidly reabsorbed in exchange for H^+ and K^+, thus perpetuating the alkalosis and the K^+ depletion.

Diuretics

The use of diuretics is the most common cause of metabolic alkalosis. While acetazolamide causes a metabolic acidosis, the other commonly employed diuretics such as the thiazides, furosemide, and ethacrynic acid all tend to cause a metabolic alkalosis. They inhibit either active Na^+ or active Cl^- transport in various segments of the nephron. The net result is a loss of NaCl from the body, a shrinkage of the extracellular fluid volume, and a relative increase in HCO_3^- concentration. Along with the diuretic the patient is often on a low NaCl diet and hence does not replenish his salt

losses, which is the intent of therapy. The kidney's defense once again is to try to preserve the contracted volume by retaining $NaHCO_3$, but alkalosis and K^+ depletion will persist.

Post-hypercapneic State

In the process of adjusting to chronic elevation of pCO_2, the kidney retains HCO_3^- and excretes Cl^- in order to lessen the change in pH. However, if the compensated patient is placed on a ventilator and his pCO_2 brought down rapidly from high to normal levels, the chronically elevated HCO_3^- remains and the patient is left with a metabolic alkalosis. Since in the process of adaptation HCO_3^- was retained while Cl^- was excreted, this patient on the ventilator remains in a Cl^--depleted state, and only by repletion with Cl^- will the alkalosis be corrected.

Congenital Chloridorrhea

Congenital chloridorrhea is an extremely rare condition diagnosed soon after birth in which there is acidic diarrhea. There is a specific defect in active Cl^- reabsorption in the ileum that results in large amounts of Cl^- (together with Na^+ and K^+) appearing in the stool.

Ingestion of Excessive Alkali

The ingestion of absorbable alkali is a rare cause of metabolic alkalosis because of the excessive amounts required. This is illustrated by the following calculation: To raise the serum HCO_3^- level chronically to a mildly alkalotic level of 30 mEq/liter from a normal of 24 mEq/liter when the glomerular filtration rate is a normal 150 liters per day would require 900 mEq (150 liters/day × 6 mEq/liter) of HCO_3^- per day. This would mean taking 130 tablets (0.6 g each) of $NaHCO_3$ or 18 level tsp of ordinary baking soda every day. However, the kidney is so adept at excreting excess HCO_3^- that metabolic alkalosis from this cause rarely occurs. However, in the presence of renal disease, when the glomerular filtration rate is reduced, ingestion of excess HCO_3^- could more easily produce a metabolic alkalosis. In fact, underlying renal disease is an important factor in the development of alkalosis in the milk–alkali syndrome.

Mineralocorticoid Excess

In the previously described causes of metabolic alkalosis there has been volume depletion. By contrast, with mineralocorticoid excess, there is expansion of the extracellular fluid volume. This syndrome may be seen in primary aldosteronism; Cushing's syndrome; congenital adrenal hyperplasia; renin-secreting tumors; following excess licorice ingestion (which contains a steroid, glycyrrhizic acid); and following use of the drug carbenoxolone (used in ulcer patients to de-

crease stomach acid production). In the earlier causes of alkalosis, Cl^- had been lost from the body as a primary event. The kidney filtered and reabsorbed all the remaining Cl^-, and virtually none was found in the urine. Addition of NaCl corrected the alkalosis. In states of mineralocorticoid excess, steroids act on the distal nephron to accelerate Na^+ - H^+ exchange as a primary event. There is volume expansion, and Cl^- is partially rejected by the nephron and appears in the urine. Therefore, additional Cl^- intake merely increases the Cl^- in the urine without affecting the alkalosis. Correction of the alkalosis follows removal of the primary source of steroid production.

There is one other rare, nonsteroid type of "saline-resistant" alkalosis. It occurs in patients with profound K^+ depletion—total body K^+ deficits often in excess of 1000 mEq and serum K^+ less than 2 mEq/liter. If the K^+ deficit is partially replaced in these patients, they regain responsiveness to NaCl and the alkalosis may then be corrected in the usual way with the addition of NaCl.

RESPIRATORY COMPENSATION

The first line of defense against metabolic alkalosis is the body buffer system. Next, hypoventilation occurs in an attempt to increase the pCO_2 and bring the pH toward normal. For every increase in HCO_3^- concentration of 1 mEq/liter, there is an increase in pCO_2 of 0.7 torr. A pCO_2 value significantly different from this would suggest a mixed disorder—an additional superimposed respiratory acidosis or alkalosis. The development of hypoxemia acts as a stimulus to ventilation and can limit the amount of hypoventilation that might otherwise occur as a compensatory mechanism. It is rare for the pCO_2 to be higher than 60 torr merely on a compensatory hypoventilation basis alone.

SIGNS AND SYMPTOMS

There may be symptoms directly related to the primary disease process causing the metabolic alkalosis. Because of the elevated pH, symptoms of paresthesias and even tetany may be seen. From the usual accompanying volume-depletion, symptoms of weakness, muscle cramps and postural hypotension may occur. Since hypokalemia is a frequent accompaniment of metabolic alkalosis, there may also be polyuria, polydipsia, paresthesias, weakness, ileus, and cardiac arrhythmias.

TREATMENT

In the usual type of Cl^- depletion, alkalosis treatment consists of giving NaCl; and since there is invariably

K$^+$ depletion as well, KCl should also be given. Acidifying salts such as NH$_4$Cl, arginine·HCl, or lysine·HCl may be used. HCl itself may be given through a central venous line, although in the presence of normally functioning kidneys, NaCl alone is just as efficacious, since the body retains the NaCl and excretes the excess HCO$_3^-$. However, when metabolic alkalosis occurs in the setting of renal failure, the kidneys may be unable to excrete the excess HCO$_3^-$, and the cautious administration of HCl in this situation is appropriate.

RESPIRATORY ACIDOSIS

In respiratory acidosis there is increased H$^+$ activity in the body, the primary disturbance being an excess of CO$_2$ in the body fluids. The severity of the acidosis depends upon the amount of retained CO$_2$, the buffering capacity of the body fluids, and the amount of HCO$_3^-$ generated by the kidneys as compensation.

$$\downarrow pH = pK + \log \frac{HCO_3^- \uparrow}{pCO_2 \uparrow}$$

CAUSES

The causes of respiratory acidosis are enumerated in Table 36-4. In respiratory acidosis there is an inability to regulate normally the alveolar pCO_2, which may be due to disorders of lung, chest muscle, chest wall, or central nervous system. A variety of lung lesions—emphysema, asthma, pulmonary edema, and others—may impair gas exchange. Myopathies or myasthenia gravis decrease respiratory muscle function. Occasionally the chest muscle weakness from K$^+$ depletion may be severe enough to prevent proper ventilation. Kyphoscoliosis distorts the chest wall and restricts normal ventilation. Central nervous system lesions such as tumors or vascular accidents may affect the medullary respiratory center to cause hypoventilation. Drugs, even mild sedatives that are easily tolerated by the normal person, may cause additional respiratory depression in patients with chronic lung disease and should therefore be used cautiously in these patients.

COMPENSATION

The response to acute increases in pCO_2 is buffering:

$$CO_2 + H_2O \rightleftharpoons H_2CO_3 \rightleftharpoons H^+ + HCO_3^-$$

The buffering reaction occurs within cells, and there is very little HCO$_3^-$ added to the extracellular space. Figure 36-12 shows that the rise in HCO$_3^-$ concentration is small—for every increase in pCO_2 of 10 torr, there is an increase in serum HCO$_3^-$ of only 1 mEq/liter. Thus the body's defense against acute respiratory acidosis is quite limited.

With chronic increases in pCO_2 the renal compensation is most important. The generation of HCO$_3^-$, which becomes maximal after 4 days to 5 days, is such that for every rise in pCO_2 of 1 torr there is an increase in HCO$_3^-$ concentration of 0.33 mEq/liter.

SIGNS AND SYMPTOMS

Mild CO$_2$ retention may produce headache, weakness, and fatigue. Greater degrees of retention can cause drowsiness, blurred vision, confusion, tremor, and asterixis. Severe CO$_2$ retention (pCO_2 greater than 80 torr) may even lead to coma. The severity of the symptoms varies with the rapidity of development of the CO$_2$ elevation, as well as with the absolute level of pCO_2.

Many of these symptoms are related to the acidosis in the cerebrospinal fluid. CO$_2$ crosses the blood–brain barrier readily, while HCO$_3^-$ crosses it poorly. Therefore, for the same systemic pH, respiratory acidosis causes a greater fall in cerebrospinal fluid pH than metabolic acidosis and is associated with more neurologic signs and symptoms.

With respiratory acidosis there may also be some of the symptoms described earlier for metabolic acidosis—decreased cardiac contractility, arrhythmias, decreased response to catecholamines, and hyperkalemia. An additional finding may be hypoxemia, with its accompanying symptoms.

TREATMENT

As with the other disorders the primary treatment is to attempt to reverse the underlying disorder. Assisted

Table 36-4. *Causes of Respiratory Acidosis*

Pulmonary disease	Emphysema
	Asthma
	Pulmonary edema
Chest muscle disease	Myasthenia gravis
	Myopathies
	Severe K$^+$ depletion
Chest wall disease	Kyphoscoliosis
	Obesity (pickwickian syndrome)
CNS impairment	Lesions in respiratory center of medulla
	Drugs—sedatives, narcotics, anesthetics, alcohol

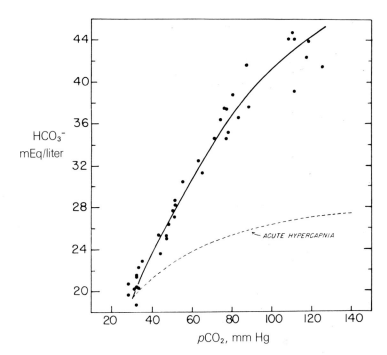

Fig. 36-12. Steady-state relationship between plasma bicarbonate concentration and pCO_2 during hypercapnia of increasing severity, chronic (*solid line*) and acute (*dashed line*). (From Schwartz WB, Brackett NC, Cohen JJ: The response of extracellular hydrogen ion concentration to graded degrees of chronic hypercapnia: The physiologic limits of the defense of pH. J Clin Invest 44:291, 1965)

ventilation may be needed, but if the chronically elevated pCO_2 is reduced too quickly to a "normal" of 40 torr, the elevated HCO_3^- remains, and now, in the presence of a normal pCO_2, gives rise to a metabolic alkalosis. Therefore pCO_2 should be lowered gradually and Cl^- given to permit excretion of HCO_3^- (the reverse of the body mechanism that established this compensation).

RESPIRATORY ALKALOSIS

In respiratory alkalosis there is decreased H^+ activity in the extracellular fluid, the primary disturbance being increased ventilation and decreased pCO_2 in the body fluids. The severity of the alkalosis depends upon the degree of lowering the pCO_2, the buffering capacity of the body fluids, and the amount of HCO_3^- excreted by the kidneys as compensation:

$$\uparrow pH = pK + \log \frac{HCO_3^- \downarrow}{pCO_2 \downarrow}$$

CAUSES

The cause of respiratory alkalosis are listed in Table 36-5. In responding to hypoxemia, which may come from pulmonary or cardiac disease or from residence at high altitudes, there is hyperventilation in an attempt to raise the pO_2, which at the same time lowers the pCO_2.

Central nervous system disorders, whether organic or drug-induced, may cause hyperventilation. A variety of metabolic disorders acting by unknown mechanisms may also lower pCO_2.

COMPENSATION

With acute hyperventilation the body buffers respond by releasing H^+ into the extracellular fluid. The source of the H^+ are the cell buffers and increased lactic acid from alkalosis-induced acceleration of glycolysis. In the acute response there is little time for renal compensation to occur, and the pH defense is meager.

Table 36-5. *Causes of Respiratory Alkalosis*

Hypoxemia	Pulmonary disease, atelectasis, pulmonary emboli
	Heart disease—congenital (right-to-left shunts), congestive heart failure
	Residence at high altitudes
CNS disorders	Organic
	Drugs—salicylates
Psychogenic hyperventilation	
Assisted ventilation	
Miscellaneous	Fever, sepsis
	Thyrotoxicosis
	Cirrhosis
	Anemia

By contrast, when the pCO_2 is chronically decreased the kidney can readily excrete HCO_3^- and defend systemic pH, with full adaptation taking 3 days to 4 days. For every decrease in pCO_2 of 1 torr, the HCO_3^- concentration is lowered by 0.5 mEq/liter.

SIGNS AND SYMPTOMS

An increased rate of respiration occurs, although at times a substantial decrease in pCO_2 may be present while signs of hyperventilation remain quite subtle. The symptoms produced are primarily neurologic—paresthesias of the hands, feet, and mouth; carpopedal spasm; light-headedness; and altered consciousness. These result from the effects of decreased H^+ and decreased ionized Ca^{++} on membrane excitability.

TREATMENT

Primary therapy should be directed at recognizing and treating the underlying disease. If the symptoms of respiratory alkalosis are severe, the inspired pCO_2 can be raised by breathing 5% CO_2 or rebreathing air in a paper bag. Rapid treatment of chronic alkalosis, if it raises the pCO_2 to normal, may "uncover" a metabolic acidosis (what was formerly a "compensation"), but the adminstration of alkali will rarely be necessary.

MIXED DISORDERS

The published information on normal compensations for single acid-base disorders has been compiled by several investigators and that of Goldberg is shown in Figure 36-13. If a pH, pCO_2 and HCO_3^- value falls within a shaded area (representing 95% confidence limits), it is compatible with the single acid-base disorder. If it is outside these areas, a mixed disorder may be present.

There are four possible combinations of dual disorders, and examples of each follow:

1. *Metabolic acidosis and respiratory acidosis*—a patient with chronic renal failure and emphysema
2. *Metabolic acidosis and respiratory alkalosis*—a patient with chronic renal failure and sepsis
3. *Metabolic alkalosis and respiratory acidosis*—a patient with nasogastric suction and emphysema
4. *Metabolic alkalosis and respiratory alkalosis*—a patient with nasogastric suction and sepsis.

It is even possible for three acid-base disorders to coexist simultaneously in one patient.

Recognition of mixed disorders can be aided by (1) knowledge of the expected compensation for each single disorder, either from the rules of thumb given earlier or by the use of a nomogram; (2) examination of anion gap, with an increased gap pointing toward a

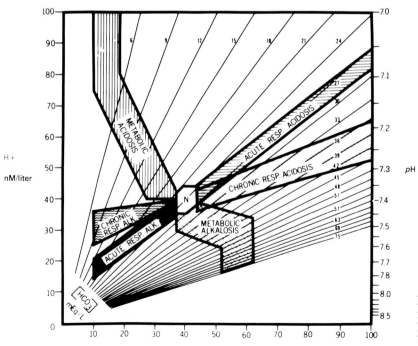

Fig. 36-13. Acid base map. Area of normal values is labeled N. (From Goldberg M, Green SB, Moss ML et al: Computer-based instruction and diagnosis of acid-base disorders. JAMA 223:269, 1973)

metabolic acidosis that may be "concealed" within the other disorders; and (3) study of the history, physical examination, and laboratory tests, which may give clues to additional complicating disorders.

Treatment of only one part of a mixed disorder may worsen the clinical situation, and therefore it is vital to recognize whether a single or mixed disorder exists in order to give proper therapy.

SUMMARY

The pH of arterial blood and interstitial fluid is usually maintained close to 7.4 despite wide variations in dietary intake of acid or alkali. The pH range over which cardiac function, metabolic activity, or central nervous system functions can be maintained is narrow; the widest range of pH values compatible with life is from 6.8 to 7.8, only one pH unit.

The body produces acid through the oxidation of carbohydrates, fats, phospholipids, and phosphoproteins. On an average diet, the body produces approximately 40 mEq to 80 mEq of nonvolatile H^+ per day. The lines of defense against changes in H^+ activity are (1) the body buffers; (2) the respiratory system, which controls the level of pCO_2; and (3) the kidneys, which control the level of serum HCO_3^-.

Body buffers are present throughout the extracellular as well as intracellular compartments. In extracellular fluid, the major buffer is the $HCO_3^- - H_2CO_3$ pair. In intracellular fluid, the major buffers are phosphates and proteins. In urine, the two major buffers are phosphate and the $NH_3 - NH_4^+$ pair. In bone, the buffer is hydroxyapatite, a crystalline salt of Ca^{++}.

The respiratory system responds to changes in pH and pCO_2 by altering the rate and depth of respiration, which changes the ratio of the $HCO_3^- - H_2CO_3$ buffer pair to maintain pH.

Renal regulation of acid-base regulation is modulated by changes in the rates of HCO_3^- reabsorption, titratable acid excretion, and NH_4^+ excretion in the kidney.

Acute or chronic metabolic alterations may produce acidosis or alkalosis. In metabolic acidosis there is increased H^+ activity in the extracellular fluid, with the primary disturbance being the addition of nonvolatile acid or the loss of base. In metabolic alkalosis there is decreased H^+ activity in the extracellular fluid, with the primary disturbance being the loss of acid or the addition of base.

Diseases of the respiratory system also cause acid-base disturbances. In respiratory acidosis, there is increased H^+ activity in the body, with the primary disturbance being an excess of CO_2 in the body fluids. In respiratory alkalosis there is decreased H^+ activity in the extracellular fluid, with the primary disturbance being increased ventilation and decreased pCO_2 in the body fluids.

The causes of these conditions and the compensatory mechanisms brought into play by the body to correct them are discussed in detail. A thorough knowledge of these compensatory mechanisms will lead to a better understanding of the pathophysiology and the signs and symptoms of disturbances in acid-base balance.

BIBLIOGRAPHY

Adrogue HJ, Madias NE: Changes in plasma potassium concentration during acute acid–base disturbances. Am J Med 71:456, 1981

Arbus GS: An in vivo acid–base nomogram for clinical use. Can Med Assoc J 109:291, 1973

Arruda JAL, Kurtzman NA: Mechanisms and classification of deranged distal urinary acidification. Am J Physiol 239:F515–F523, 1980

Berger AJ, Mitchell RA, Severinghaus JW: Regulation of respiration. N Engl J Med 297:92, 1977

Carter NW: Intracellular pH. Kidney Int 1:341, 1972

Cogan MG, Rector FC, Seldin DW: Acid–Base disorders. In Brenner BM, Rector FC (eds): The Kidney, 2nd ed, Vol 1, p 841. Philadelphia, W B Saunders, 1981

Davenport HW: ABC of Acid–Base Chemistry, 6th ed. Chicago, University of Chicago Press, 1974

Emmett M, Narins RG: Clinical use of anion gap. Medicine 56:38, 1977

Garella S, Chang BS, Kahn SI: Dilution acidosis and contraction alkalosis: Review of a concept. Kidney Int 8:279, 1975

Garella S, Dana CL, Chazan JA: Severity of metabolic acidosis as a determinant of bicarbonate requirements. N Engl J Med 289:121, 1973

Goldberg M, Green SB, Moss ML et al: Computer-based instruction and diagnosis of acid–base disorders. JAMA 223:269, 1973

Hills AG: Acid–Base Balance: Chemistry, Physiology, Pathophysiology. Baltimore, Williams & Wilkins, 1973

Kassirer JP: Serious acid–base disorders. N Engl J Med 291:773, 1974

Kurtzman NA: Regulation of renal bicarbonate reabsorption by extracellular volume. J Clin Invest 49:586, 1970

Leusen I: Regulation of cerebrospinal fluid composition with reference to breathing. Physiol Rev 52:1, 1972

McCurdy DK: Mixed metabolic and respiratory acid–base disturbances: Diagnosis and treatment. Chest 62:35S, 1972

Madias NE, Adrogue HJ, Horowitz GL et al: A redefinition of normal acid-base equilibrium in man; Carbon dioxide tension as a key determinant of normal plasma bicarbonate concentration. Kidney Int 16:612, 1979

Makoff DF: Acid–base metabolism. In Maxwell MH, Kleeman CR (eds): Clinical Disorders of Fluid and Electrolyte Metabolism, 2nd ed. New York, McGraw–Hill, 1972

Malnic G, Steinmetz PR: Transport processes in urinary acidification. Kidney Int 9:172, 1976

Mitchell JH, Wildenthal K, Johnson RL: The effects of acid–base disturbances on cardiovascular and pulmonary function. Kidney Int 1:375, 1972

Narins, RG, Emmett M: Simple and mixed acid–base disorders; A practical approach. Medicine 59:161, 1980

Pitts RF: Physiology of the Kidney and Body Fluids, 3rd ed. Chicago, Year Book Medical Publishers, 1974

Posner JB, Swanson AG, Plum F: Acid–base balance in cerebrospinal fluid. Arch Neurol 12:479, 1965

Rector FC: Renal acidification and ammonia production; chemistry of weak acids and bases: Buffer mechanisms. In Brenner B, Rector FC: The Kidney. Philadelphia, W B Saunders, 1976

Rector FC, Carter NW, Seldin DW: The mechanism of bicarbonate reabsorption in the proximal and distal tubules of the kidney. J Clin Invest 44:278, 1965

Relman AS: Metabolic consequences of acid–base disorders. Kidney Int 1:347, 1972

Rodman JS, Heinemann HO: Parathyroid hormone and the regulation of acid–base balance. Am J Med Sci 270:481, 1975.

Rose BD: Clinical Physiology of Acid–Base and Electrolyte Disorders. New York, McGraw–Hill, 1977

Siesjo BK: The regulation of cerebrospinal fluid pH. Kidney Int 1:360, 1972

Schrier RW: Renal and Electrolyte Disorders 2nd ed. Boston, Little, Brown & Co, 1980

Schwartz WB, Cohen JJ: The nature of the renal response to chronic disorders of acid-base equilibrium. Am J Med 64:417–428, 1978

Steinmetz PR: Cellular mechanisms of urinary acidification. Physiol Rev 54:890, 1974

Swan RC, Axelrod DR, Seip M et al: Distribution of sodium bicarbonate infused into nephrectomized dogs. J Clin Invest 34:1795, 1955

Swan RC, Pitts RF: Neutralization of infused acid by nephrectomized dogs. J Clin Invest 34:205, 1955

Tannin RL: Relationship of renal ammonia production and potassium homeostasis. Kidney Int 11:453, 1977

Valtin H: Renal Function. Mechanisms Preserving Fluid and Solute Balance in Health. Boston, Little, Brown & Co, 1973

METABOLIC ACIDOSIS

Arruda JAL, Carrasquillo T, Cubria A et al: Bicarbonate reabsorption in chronic renal failure. Kidney Int 9:481, 1976

Buckalew VM, Purvis ML, Shulman MG et al: Hereditary renal tubular acidosis. Medicine 53:229, 1974

Ditella PJ, Brynandin S, McCreary J et al: Mechanism of the metabolic acidosis of selective mineralocorticoid deficiency. Kidney Int 14:466, 1978

Fulop M: The ventilatory response in severe metabolic acidosis. Clin Sci 50:367, 1976

Fulop MF, Hoberman HD: Alcoholic ketosis. Diabetes 24:785, 1975

Kreisberg RA: Diabetic ketoacidosis: New concepts and trends in pathogenesis and treatment. Ann Intern Med 88:681, 1978

Morris RC, Sebastian A, McSherry E: Renal acidosis. Kidney Int 1:322, 1972

Oliva PB: Lactic acidosis. Am J Med 48:209, 1970

Park R, Arieff AI: Lactic acidosis. Adv Intern Med 25:33–68, 1980

Pierce NF, Fedson DS, Brigham KL et al: The ventilatory response to acute base deficit in humans. Ann Intern Med 72:633, 1970

Posner JB, Plum F: Spinal-fluid pH and neurologic symptoms in systemic acidosis. N Engl J Med 277:605, 1967

METABOLIC ALKALOSIS

Garella S, Chazan JA, Cohen JJ: Saline-resistant metabolic alkalosis or "chloride-wasting nephropathy". Ann Intern Med 73:31, 1970

Kassirer JP, London AM, Goldman DM et al: On the pathogenesis of metabolic alkalosis in hyperaldosteronism. Am J Med 49:306, 1970

Kurtzman NA, White MG, Rogers PW: Pathophysiology of metabolic alkalosis. Arch Intern Med 131:702, 1973

Madias NE, Ayus JC, Adrogue HJ: Increased anion gap in metabolic alkalosis. The role of plasma protein equivalency. N Engl J Med 300:1421, 1979

Schambelan M, Slaton PE, Biglieri EG: Mineralocorticoid production in hyperadrenocorticism. Am J Med 51:299, 1971

Schwartz WB, Van Ypersele de Strihou C, Kassirer JP: Role of anions in metabolic alkalosis and potassium deficiency. N Engl J Med 279:630, 1968

Seldin DW, Rector FC: The generation and maintenance of metabolioc alkalosis. Kidney Int 1:306, 1972

RESPIRATORY ACIDOSIS

Bleich HL, Berkman PM, Schwartz WB: The response of cerebrospinal fluid composition to sustained hypercapnia. J Clin Invest 43:11, 1964

Brackett NC, Cohen JJ, Schwartz WB: Carbon dioxide titration curve of normal man. Effect of increasing degrees of acute hypercapnia on acid–base equilibrium. N Engl J Med 272:6, 1965

Goldstein MB, Gennari FJ, Schwartz WB: The influence of graded degrees of chronic hypercapnia on the acute carbon dioxide titration curve. J Clin Invest 50:208, 1971

Polak A, Haynie GD, Hays RM et al: Effects of chronic hypercapnia on electrolyte and acid–base equilibrium. I Adaptation. J Clin Invest 40:1223, 1961

Schwartz WB, Hays RM, Polak A et al: Effects of chronic hypercapnia on electrolyte and acid–base equilibrium. II. Recovery, with special reference to the influence of chloride intake. J Clin Invest 40:1238, 1961

Van Ypersele De Strihou C, Gulyassy PF, Schwartz WB: Effects of chronic hypercapnia on electrolyte and acid–base equilibrium. III. Characteristics of the adaptive and recovery process as evaluated by provision of alkali. J Clin Invest 41:2246, 1962

RESPIRATORY ALKALOSIS

Arbus GS, Hebert LA, Levesque PR et al: Characterization and clinical application of the "significance band" for acute respiratory alkalosis. N Engl J Med 280:117, 1969

Cohen JJ, Madias NE, Wolf CJ et al: Regulation of acid–base equilibrium in chronic hypocapnia. J Clin Invest 57:1483, 1976

Gennari FJ, Goldstein MB, Schwartz WB: The nature of the renal adaptation to chronic hypocapnia. J Clin Invest 51:1722, 1972

Gladhill N, Beirne GJ, Dempsey JA: Renal response to short-term hypocapnia in man. Kidney Int 8:376, 1975

Gougoux A, Haehny WD, Cohen JJ: Renal adaptation to chronic hypocapnia: Dietary constraints in achieving H^+ retention. Am J Physiol 229:1330, 1975

37

Obesity
Aldo A. Rossini
George F. Cahill, Jr.

Definition
Methods for Estimating Obesity
Importance of Obesity
Differential Diagnosis
Physiology of Obesity
Fed State
Fasted State
Multifactorial Etiologies and Complications of Obesity
Inputs or Roots
Hereditary Basis of Obesity
Metabolic Basis of Obesity
Emotional and Psychological Factors

Cultural and Social Factors
Pathophysiologic Complications
Metabolic-Diabetes-Lipid
Cardiac Abnormalities
Pulmonary Abnormalities
Gastrointestinal Complications
Musculoskeletal Complications
Renal Complications
Cancer
Psychological Implications of Obesity
Exercise
Current Treatments of Obesity
Reasonable Approach to the Patient with Obesity

DEFINITION

Obesity refers to an accumulation of excess fat that is associated with physical or emotional morbidity. By some criteria over 45% of adult Americans are obese, a grim statistic in the light of epidemic starvation elsewhere in the world.[1] To the layman, corpulence is primarily a cosmetic problem that leads to bias and prejudice. To the physician, it may mean anything from an expression of poor self-discipline to a syndrome or disease with serious physical sequelae. For centuries, it has been the focus of humor and ridicule.

Among the first attempts to deal with obesity scientifically were attempts to classify individuals by body build. The endomorph was small-boned and fat; the ectomorph was tall and skinny with little muscle or fat; the mesomorph was the muscular, heavy-boned individual. The ectomorph rarely became obese; the me-somorph in midlife often developed obesity; the endomorph was predestined to obesity. These descriptive concepts strongly implied genetic determination. They were quite fatalistic and left little room for environmental considerations or therapy. The somatotype concept is still of some descriptive use, but it has little pathophysiologic meaning.

How can obesity be defined? To say simply that it is too much fat lacks objective quantification. Most commonly, an increase in body weight of 15% to 20% above an arbitrary optimal weight derived from a population mean according to age, height, and sex has been used. Because this process fails to define the percentage fat of the individual, appropriate corrections for small, medium, or large "frame" have been applied (Tables 37-1, 37-2). Adiposity, on the other hand, may be defined as normal weight, but the proportion of the body weight composed of fat is excessive.

769

TABLE 37-1. *Desirable Weights for Men 25 Years of Age or Older*

Height (with shoes on— 1-in heels)		Small Frame	Medium Frame	Large Frame
Feet	Inches			
5	2	112-120	118-129	126-141
5	3	115-123	121-133	129-144
5	4	118-126	124-126	132-148
5	5	121-129	127-139	135-152
5	6	124-133	130-143	138-156
5	7	128-137	134-147	142-161
5	8	132-141	138-152	147-166
5	9	136-145	142-156	151-170
5	10	140-150	146-160	155-174
5	11	144-154	150-165	159-179
6	0	148-158	154-170	164-184
6	1	152-162	158-175	168-189
6	2	156-167	162-180	173-194
6	3	160-171	167-185	178-199
6	4	164-175	172-190	182-204

(From Metropolitan Life Insurance Company, Statistical Bureau)

TABLE 37-2. *Desirable Weights for Women 25 Years of Age or Older*

Height (with shoes on— 2-in heels)		Small Frame	Medium Frame	Large Frame
Feet	Inches			
4	10	92-98	96-107	104-119
4	11	94-101	98-110	106-122
5	0	96-104	101-113	109-125
5	1	99-107	104-116	112-128
5	2	102-110	107-119	115-131
5	3	105-113	110-122	118-134
5	4	108-116	113-126	121-138
5	5	111-119	116-130	125-142
5	6	114-123	120-135	129-146
5	7	118-127	124-139	133-150
5	8	122-131	128-143	137-154
5	9	126-135	132-147	141-158
5	10	130-140	136-151	145-163
5	11	134-144	140-155	149-168
6	0	138-148	144-159	153-173

(From Metropolitan Life Insurance Company, Statistical Bureau)

METHODS FOR ESTIMATING OBESITY

Precise methods for estimation of fat mass are difficult. The most accurate is carcass analysis. A kind of "gold standard," it has been used to validate other methods.[2] A research procedure applicable in the clinic is the use of skinfold calipers. By pinching subcutaneous tissue in specific sites at a given pressure and then measuring the thickness, an estimate of the extent of the subcutaneous fat can be made. Assuming it to be proportional to the size of the other fat depots, total fat mass can then be estimated.[3] A thickness of over 20 mm in the triceps or infrascapular region in the male or over 26 mm in the female signifies excess lipid accumulation. Standard tables for these estimates are available.[4] Another simple clinical technique is to take body weight in kilograms, subtract the height in centimeters, and add 100:

$$\text{Body weight (kg)} - \text{height (cm)} + 100$$

If the number is positive the person is overweight.

Other research methods include radioisotope dilution to estimate total cell mass and body water. Body fat mass can then be calculated after appropriate corrections for mineral mass.[5] Gases soluble in fat, such as cyclopropane, have also been used to determine total fat mass, but the procedure is expensive, cumbersome, and inaccurate.[6] Underwater weighing to determine specific gravity is another cumbersome and expensive research procedure that requires exact correction for air trapped in lung and the gastrointestinal tract to provide any degree of accuracy.[7] For general purposes, the best clinical test to diagnose is the use of standard tables with a rough estimate of body frame.

IMPORTANCE OF OBESITY

Certain diseases, particularly diabetes, respiratory and cardiovascular diseases, osteoarthritis, and gallbladder disease, are correlated with obesity. Between ages 20 and 30, mortality rates increase from 142% of expected for the moderately obese to 179% for the markedly obese.[8] Of note, at one end of the spectrum are the spectacularly obese, such as Mr. H. who weighed 1069 pounds and died of uremia at age 32. Another gentleman died of coronary thrombosis at age 34 after breaking through the floor of his cabin.[9]

In middleclass America, obesity is socially and emotionally unacceptable. However, certain socioeconomic groups cherish obesity in children and adult females as evidence of financial and emotional security. Surveys in New York showed a prevalence of obesity in over 50% of adults of both sexes in lower economic groups. In contrast, the prevalence was 15% in males and 5% in females in the highest economic strata.

Historically, obesity was cherished and, without question, at times mandatory. Primitive man, confined

to a cave for the winter or about to set sail across the Pacific on a raft, was far likelier to survive if obese. It is not surprising therefore that the cyclicity of man's caloric homeostasis can be overridden by his thought processes. This contrasts with lower forms of life whose obesity cycles are seasonally dictated and thus innate. Hippocrates in Aphorism 35 noted that it is bad to be thin; thinness meant poor health and death. In the middle ages, obesity in royalty was flaunted as an expression of wealth. Henry VIII of England, for example, was portrayed at the banquet table with a rack of meat in his corpulent hand. In today's society, clothing, jewelry, automobiles, and a Florida suntan have all displaced obesity as signs of station, and obesity has become socially déclassé.

The prejudice against obesity touches all parts of life. A New York employment agency for senior executives noted only 9% of men in the higher income brackets were 10 or more pounds overweight, whereas 39% in the middle income group were fat. They even calculated that each pound cost up to $1000 in lost annual salary.[10] One of the authors served on an admission committee of a graduate school for 5 years and noted that it was four times more difficult for an obese student to gain admission, quite possibly because of prejudice and bias in interviews and recommendations. In certain positions, such as those of airline stewardess, receptionist, and certain sales personnel, obesity excludes the applicant from consideration.

DIFFERENTIAL DIAGNOSIS

In the process of cellular differentiation, fat cells or their analogs appear in various areas, including subcutaneous tissue, omentum, the perinephric space, and other less obvious areas, such as between the buccal muscles and in the retro-orbital and intra-articular areas. In general, these latter depots are not insulin-sensitive and therefore (fortunately) do not participate in the increases and decreases in total body lipid that occur in obesity on one hand and emaciation on the other. In fact, the last fat to be lost is that in the buccal and retro-orbital areas, as seen in the hippocratic facies of the individual with terminal carcinomatosis. Acting on this distribution of mesenchymal cells destined to be adipocytes are the sex hormones. The mammary, thigh, and buttock areas appear to undergo greater hypertrophy with female hormones, and, conversely, the protuberant abdomen (pot or baywindow) distribution is more indicative of androgenic control. Whether these loci undergo hypertrophy or hyperplasia of the fat cells as obesity occurs in each sex has yet to be determined, but most evidence suggests that it is hypertrophy. An

interesting correlation between truncal obesity and diabetes in females has just been reported,[11] and it now awaits corroboration by other studies.

The correlation of obesity and imbalance of sex hormones is also an important association. The association of menstrual irregularities and infertility has been documented. In a large study there was a significant correlation of obesity (30 lb) and hirsutism in women with anovulatory cycles compared to women with no menstrual irregularities.[14a] Furthermore, seven times as many women in the most obese group have evidence of polycystic ovary disease (Stein-Leventhal syndrome). The hyperandrogenic and hyperestrogen states exist owing to the conversion of androstendione to estrone. It is not clear how the elevated hormone levels cause increased food intake, but the hormonal imbalance is strongly related to obesity.

Other fat depots appear to be glucocorticoid-sensitive, as seen in Cushing's syndrome. In this instance, peripheral subcutaneous fat is diminished, and accumulations of lipid appear in the interscapular area (the buffalo hump), the abdomen, and the face (the moon facies). Thus, there is an overall centripetal distribution of the fat. Similarly, the grafting of ACTH-secreting tumors in animals has been shown to produce centripetal obesity in the recipient.[12] Conversely, virilizing tumors of the adrenal or ovary may result in the loss of estrogen-sensitive fat in breasts, thighs, and buttocks with a resultant angular, masculine appearance. In mixed tumors producing both glucocorticoids and androgens, mixed syndromes may occur. In any case, gross obesity is seldom seen with primary endocrine disease, except in children in whom hyperglucocorticoidism may initially present as generalized obesity.

In 1901, Fröhlich described obesity in young males with marked or moderate hypogonadism and attributed these findings to a lesion in the hypothalamic-pituitary areas.[13] The relatively common finding of delayed adolescence in fat boys with gynecoid fat distribution and even with some mammary hyperplasia has been loosely termed "Fröhlich's syndrome." The vast majority of these patients achieve normal male adolescence, albeit 2 to 3 years later than their contemporaries. Occasionally, true organic disease is associated with delayed or absent maturity and excessive obesity with organic lesions, such as cysts or tumors in the hypothalamic area,[14] but most of these show other neural deficits, such as mental retardation and abnormalities in other hypothalamic-pituitary functions.

In hypothyroidism, there may be increased weight, and obesity may become apparent and may be indistinguishable from that seen in the euthyroid obese person. Although the differential diagnosis may be difficult, clinical signs usually alert the physician to the

hypothyroid state: dry skin; slow mentation; delayed relaxation phase of reflexes; brittleness of nails; thick, coarse hair; deep, nasal-sounding, hoarse voice; and cold intolerance. However, florid myxedema is usually not accompanied by obesity, and the increased weight in these patients is usually fluid accumulation. The fluid contains a mucopolysaccharide, as was shown by Plummer many years ago.[15] Hypothyroidism and obesity are common problems whose appearance together in one person is usually coincidental. Correction of thyroid disease usually results in a weight loss of less than 10 lb. No clear-cut data suggest that thyroid diseases accounts for obesity.[58]

Another endocrine disorder rarely associated with obesity is a tumor of the β-cell in the pancreatic islets of Langerhans. Hypoglycemia can lead to increased hunger and food intake and occasionally to obesity. The vast majority of patients with islet tumors do not experience this sequence of events, however. Instead, they have intermittent, more severe hypoglycemia episodes with confusion or unconsciousness relieved by food or glucose.

Although these endocrinopathies must be included in the differential diagnosis of obesity, a careful history and physical examinations are usually all that is necessary to exclude them. If doubt remains, laboratory tests (see appropriate references) may be indicated. Sometimes they are necessary to convince the doubting patient that rare "hormonal" explanations do not account for their obesity problem. Less than 1% of all obesity has some identifiable, underlying endocrine etiology.

PHYSIOLOGY OF OBESITY

A normal 70-kg adult male has approximately 10 kg of fat (13%); a normal 60-kg female has 14 kg of fat (23%). Of the nonfat carcass in both, 75% is water. The remainder is protein, carbohydrate, and mineral. Carbohydrate is stored in tissue as aqueous glycogen. Each gram of glycogen is associated with 3 g to 4 g water, yielding per gram of total tissue only about 1 Cal. Protein is stored in the same way: 1 g protein with 4 g water; it yields less than 1 Cal/g total tissue. Fat, in contrast, is stored in a nearly anhydrous state and supplies 9 Cal/g of tissue. Triglyceride accumulation is thus essential to survival since its caloric yield is nearly an order of magnitude greater than that obtainable from stored carbohydrate or protein. Every calorie man accumulates in excess of that expended, no matter what the source of these calories, is converted to triglyceride and stored in adipose tissues.

Adipose tissue serves functions other than simple caloric storage. In the buttocks and buccal cheek pads

its protective role is obvious. In subcutaneous tissues it provides insulation. In man, the accumulation of fat in the mammary region, both in primitive and sophisticated societies, serves as a sexual stimulant. Adipose tissue accumulation in the buttocks is epitomized by the steatopygia of Hottentot women and represents to them a sign of great beauty and attractiveness.

FED STATE

During digestion of a meal, complex carbohydrates are hydrolyzed to simple sugars, mainly glucose, and transported to the liver. Under the influence of insulin, glucose is metabolized to glycogen, as well as to CO_2 to provide for immediate energy needs. Glucose in excess of energy and glycogen requirements is used for long-chain fatty acid synthesis, again thanks to an increase in insulin levels. The long-chain fatty acids are incorporated, three at a time, into triglyceride and then exported into blood as very low density lipoprotein (VLDL) or pre-β lipoprotein for eventual incorporation into adipose tissue. Other sites of glucose removal include the brain, which needs approximately 100 mg glucose/min to meet its energy needs. This process appears to be independent of insulin and proceeds as long as there is an adequate concentration of glucose. Muscle, including heart muscle, uses glucose as fuel but requires an increased level of insulin. Finally, some glucose gains access to adipose tissue where, as in liver, it is metabolized to intermediates, which are used for fatty acid synthesis. In this way, a fuel that can be stored only in a low caloric density form, glucose, is converted into an efficient fuel of high caloric density, lipid.

Protein in the meal is hydrolyzed into amino acids, which enter the portal circulation. The liver removes many of these, particularly the glucogenic amino acids. Others are carried to the periphery where muscle protein is synthesized to replace that catabolized since the last meal. Should amino acids be in excess, particularly branched-chain amino acids, they are taken up by adipose tissue and, like glucose, are used for fatty acid synthesis. Again, the excess calories derived from dietary protein are made into fat and stored accordingly. Of course, the synthesis of urea, to dispose of nitrogen, requires about one fourth of the original energy of the protein; this loss, the *specific dynamic action*, is one reason why protein diets may be more efficacious than other diets in weight-reduction programs.

The third component of the diet, the fat, is absorbed after partial hydrolysis and synthesis in the intestinal epithelium. These cells secrete triglyceride as particulate aggregates of lipid and lipoprotein called *chylomicrons* into the intestinal lymphatics. With adequate insulin, chylomicra are hydrolyzed in the capillaries of

adipose tissue. The constituent fatty acids are resynthesized into triglyceride inside the fat cell cytoplasm.

It can be seen that, no matter what the food source, when glycogen and body protein stores have been adequately expanded, any excess calories are converted into fat and stored as such.

Once a fatty acid has been made, it can be cleaved to its constituents: glycerol and fatty acids. Ultimately, the fatty acids yield molecules of acetate, but there is no major biochemical pathway whereby aminoacids or carbohydrate substrates can be remade. The only metabolic route for acetate is oxidation to CO_2. In simplest terms, once fat is synthesized and stored, it can yield only energy, not new protein or new carbohydrate. Fat cannot be rubbed off by exercise machines nor heated off in a sauna. Unless a surgeon cuts it off, a decrease can only be achieved by a negative caloric balance.

FASTED STATE

During fasting, fuel must be mobilized from storage tissues in order to keep the body going. The body proceeds through an orderly sequence of events to diminish utilization of glucose and protein and augment lipid mobilization. The first phase, that which occurs between meals, involves hepatic glycogen breakdown to provide glucose for brain consumption. The remainder of the body begins to reduce glucose utilization. After an overnight fast, muscle is metabolizing primarily free fatty acids released from adipose tissue. A low insulin level is the signal for hepatic glycogenolysis, adipose tissue lipolysis, and decreased muscle utilization of glucose. As glycogen stores are depleted, amino acids released from muscle protein serve as gluconeogenic precursors for hepatic glucose synthesis. The signal for muscle proteolysis likewise appears to be a low insulin level. Thus, early in starvation, the brain uses glucose and the remainder of the body free fatty acids.

With more prolonged starvation, levels of ketoacids in blood increase, and even the brain diminishes glucose utilization as it switches to utilization of ketoacids. The net effect is an even greater use of calories derived from fat and further sparing of body nitrogen, which otherwise would have been consumed in the process of gluconeogenesis. Totally fasted, man uses about 150 g to 180 g of triglyceride per day, less than ½ lb, an important fact for anyone trying to lose weight.

MULTIFACTORIAL ETIOLOGIES AND COMPLICATIONS OF OBESITY

A pictorial scheme for discussing obesity is presented in Figure 37-1. The inputs are depicted as the roots and the sequelae as the branches of a tree. The trunk is obesity itself.

INPUTS OR ROOTS

Hereditary Basis of Obesity

That obesity tends to occur in families has been known for centuries. Statistics reveal that fat children occur 10 times more frequently in the families of fat parents than in the families of lean parents. Gurney observed that if both parents are obese, obesity was present in 73% of offspring. If one parent is obese, a 40% prevalence was found; if both parents are lean, 9% of the offspring were obese.[17] Similar data have been reported by many other authors.[18,19] A strong genetic input in man has been supported by studies by Biron, who evaluted 120 natural children and 379 adopted children in 274 families.[20] Blood pressure and obesity tended to be independent of the family of rearing but correlated well with genetic background. Thus, if the biologic parents are obese and the child is brought up in a house where the parents are lean, the probability that the child will be obese is greater than for a child of lean biologic parents brought up in the same household.

In experimental animal models such as mice, obesity can be shown to be transmitted by various modes of inheritance. Obesity is an autosomal dominant trait in the yellow mouse. The KK mouse, the New Zealand Obese (NZO) mouse, and the Wellesley hybrid mouse are all examples of polygenic inheritance.[22,23] On the other hand, *db/db* and *ob/ob* mice are examples of autosomal recessive expressions of a single allele. Thus, many types of inheritance exist in experimental animals, but how these relate to human obesity is conjectural.[24] Genetic diseases, such as the Prader–Willi syndrome (hypotonia, mental deficiency, and hypogonadism) or Laurence–Moon–Bardet–Biedl syndrome (mental retardation, hypotonia, retinitis pigmentosa, and polydactylism) are examples in which gross human obesity is transmitted genetically, but the mode of inheritance is unclear.

Metabolic Basis of Obesity

The metabolic aspects of obesity can be subdivided into three major categories: (1) hypothalamic control, (2) the control exerted by the intestine and various hormones, and (3) the influence of adipose cell size and number.

The hypothalamus is an area of the diencephalon that clearly influences food intake. In experimental animals, a feeding center has been localized to the lateral hypothalamus.[25] Satiety signals appear to originate in the ventromedial nucleus of the hypothalamus.[26] Other structures, including cortex, amygdala, hippocampus, preoptic area, and septal area may also be involved in feeding.[27] The reticular system, which is involved with sleep and wakefulness, may also be important. The

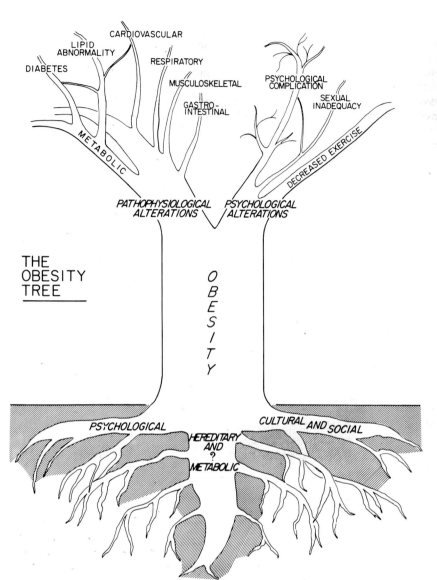

THE
OBESITY
TREE

Fig. 37-1. The multifactorial etiologies and complications of obesity.

exact role of these various structures and their relationship to the hypothalamus in the regulation of food intake is unknown.[28] When the lateral hypothalamus is selectively destroyed in an animal, it eats less. When the ventromedial hypothalamus is damaged, the animal overeats.[29] Similarly, when this area is chemically injured by gold thioglucose given to the animal, it rapidly puts on weight. The amount of hyperphagia and weight gain depend on the extent of the injury and the strain of the animal.[29] Mayer has postulated that it is the glucose level in blood that affects the ventromedial or satiety center and hence the selective destruction by gold thioglucose. In these animals, glucose has no effect in decreasing appetite. Mayer's glucostat

theory has since been shown to be an oversimplification, with many other factors not known to contribute to hunger and satiety.[24] One factor has been the role of neurochemical mediators in the hypothalamus. Administration of norepinephrine to the ventromedial hypothalamus stimulates food intake, while pretreating with α-blockade reduces food intake.[30]

In lower animals, such as the crab, removal of the brain results in a preparation that continues to eat until the stomach bursts.[31] In the white leghorn chicken, destruction of the ventromedial nucleus produces an animal in which food intake is not continuous but is related to intestinal contents.[32] Many studies in man and rats, particularly those by Panskepp in rats, have

shown reduction in food intake when various substrates are placed directly into the stomach.[33] This inhibition occurs whether the food is carbohydrate, fat, or protein. In other studies, bulk alone in the stomach depresses voluntary food intake. Thus, there is clearly a gastrointestinal servomechanism that is capable of altering eating behavior. This will be described subsequently in greater detail.

Another hypothesis regarding the regulation of food intake has been suggested by Kennedy, who claims that the primary function of the ventromedial nucleus of the hypothalamus is to sense and maintain fat stores.[34] Thus, the hypothalamus adjusts food intake in response to the size of the fat depots.[35] For example, when intact cockerels are force-fed approximately twice their voluntary food intake, they soon cease to eat voluntarily. With cessation of force-feeding, the birds do not eat spontaneously for 7 days to 10 days, or until the excess fat has been metabolized.[36] Similarly, in man, Sims and his colleagues in Vermont force-fed volunteers up to 5000 Cal per day. Afterward, the individuals markedly decreased their food intake until their weight decreased.[37,38]

What are the set points about which a person maintains weight? Normal man maintains his weight very accurately. His weight changes little each year despite his consumption of 10 to 20 times more calories than are stored in his body as adipose triglyceride. This implies the existence of a *set point* for body weight. Such set points may be fixed or may change. Many examples of resetting the size of body fuel depots are found in the animal kingdom, particularly in migratory birds. During the premigration period, the birds appear to establish a new set point, eating vigorously (premigratory hyperphagia) to achieve sufficient adipose tissue for the extra caloric needs of the flight. What is the mechanism that allows this animal to increase its weight for its migration? It appears to be a combination of seasonal changes, temperature, the ratio of the day-night light cycle, and the effects of pituitary and gonadal hormones.[39]

Another mechanism regulating food intake relates to the gastrointestinal tract. Mechanical factors, such as distention of the stomach, play an important role in inhibiting food intake, as exemplified in dog and rat experiments.[40,41] However, the effect is very small and transient. If isotonic glucose is introduced into the jejunum, no effect on food intake is observed. However, if hypertonic solutions are given, the animals become anorectic.[42] Chronic jejunal feedings can produce anorexia in a dog, but after vagotomy the animals again eat, suggesting that inhibition of food intake is mediated at least partly through peripheral neural mechanisms.[43] Hormonal factors have also been observed to influence food intake. Enterogastrone has been found to inhibit food intake in the mouse,[44] and cholecystokinin-pancreozymin has been found to suppress food intake in the rat.[45] Other anorectic agents have also been purported to exist.[46]

An interesting experiment was devised by Lepkovsky and colleagues at the University of California. The intestinal tracts of parabiotic rats were crossed. The proximal end of the duodenum of one parabiont was connected to the pylorus of its partner, and vice versa. Food eaten by one animal entered the stomach, and instead of entering its own duodenum, entered the duodenum of its counterpart. It was, therefore, possible to study oropharyngeal and gastric factors. The rat whose stomach emptied first would eat; the recipient of its gastric chyme did not eat. In other experiments, the animals were force-fed the same amount of food at the same time. The stomachs of the "eater" rats were practically empty, whereas those of their partners were full of food. These results suggest that gastric chyme affected both emptying of the gastric contents and food intake.[47]

The roles of taste and nutritional demands have also been very important in regulating dietary intake. Animals deficient in vitamins (thiamine, for instance) seek diets in which the vitamin is present. If a thiamine-deficient rat has the choice of two foods, identical except for the absence or presence of thiamine, the animal preferentially consumes the food in which thiamine is present.[48] The ability of the animal to differentiate the diets must depend in some way on sensory input, but the nature of this signal is unknown.

In other studies, rats fed a diet *ad libitum* either low or devoid of a single amino acid lost weight owing to a diminished intake of the diet. If the deficient amino acid was injected intraperitoneally, or in very small doses directly into the cerebrospinal fluid, the animal would resume eating the diet lacking that amino acid. Thus, the influence of amino acids on the neural regulation of food intake is important.[49] The relationship in the human of the hypothalamus and neural or hormonal influence on dietary intake is unknown, but the higher centers (cerebral cortex) appear to influence markedly the more primitive regulatory systems.[50]

As mentioned previously, obesity is a disorder in which there is an excess accumulation of adipose triglyceride. This could be due to either increased fat per cell (*hypertrophy*) or to an increased number of fat cells (*hyperplasia*) or a combination of the two. The development of relatively reliable methods to determine triglyceride content of single fat cells in isolated pieces of adipose tissue obtained by biopsy has been of help to our understanding of obesity. Knittle and Hirsch have identified two critical periods in the development

of fat cells: one from birth to 2 years and the other from 8 years to 12 years.[51] The number of fat cells appears to be fixed by the end of the growth period, and further weight gain after this time is accomplished by enlarging existing fat cells.[52] In rats, Hirsch and his colleagues found that caloric intake during neonatal life changes the adipose cell number, which then persists throughout the life of the animal, and this is associated with a permanent alteration in both body weight and adiposity.[53] However, more recent data suggests that hyperplasia may occur at later ages. It is important to remember that genetic factors also influence the final morphologic character of the adipose tissue. Thus, the avoidance of overnutrition and obesity at an early stage of development is evident. It has also been suggested that the newborn infant has or develops an appetite-control mechanism that appears to be related to the constitution of breast milk.[54] Identifying such biochemical factors is the subject of current research.

As mentioned previously, obesity is an accumulation of excess calories as fat. The laws of thermodynamics state that energy intake must exceed energy expenditure for obesity to be present. Various research laboratories have studied possible alterations of metabolism and thermogenesis in obese people. In one study of ouabain binding to sodium-pumping units (sodium-potassium ATPase) in red blood cells from obese subjects, binding was found to be lower than that in the red cells of normal subjects.[55] This study suggested that obese subjects did not have as many of these energy-consuming enzyme units as did normals and could not dissipate calories as efficiently as normal subjects. Although this finding has been disputed in subsequent studies, the possibility remains as a potential hypothesis.[56,57]

Emotional and Psychological Factors

The next root of the obesity tree relates to emotional and psychological factors. Freud postulated that when people are frustrated, they may revert to a primitive stage of oral gratification, and obesity ensues. It was also proposed by Renshaw that obesity may form a defensive shell against threatening sexual changes. Oral gratification replaces sexual gratification, and food is used to distract the self and to relieve tension. It is interesting that obesity, particularly in the male, is correlated with decreased libido and sexual activity.[59] Depression has been shown to cause altered eating behavior. Not uncommonly depressed people will have abnormal food cravings. The exact relationship between depression and obesity is not understood, but the physician should be aware of the sudden onset of obesity in depressed individuals. A more detailed de-

scription of these factors may be obtained in more specialized reviews.

Cultural and Social Factors

The final root of the obesity tree relates to the cultural and social background of the individual. In many cultures, obesity was a desirable and acceptable condition, particularly in females and children. As mentioned before, obesity could be a sign of wealth, importance, health, and the capacity to overcome famine and infection. In certain societies, constant urging of children to eat and to gain weight is evident, particularly in certain Mediterranean and Semitic cultures. These tendencies are seen, though to a lesser degree, even in second and third generation Jewish and Italian families.

In our society, definite social influences on body build are found. The beginning may be manifested when the newborn is brought home from the hospital. During the first night when the child cries, the first reaction of both parents is to give food. As the child grows, new experiences are found and related to food intake. Achieving the second year of life, the word "no" is frequently used throughout the day by the child. Because of the embarrassment put upon the parents and because of their own frustrations, the child often finds that a reward for not using the word "no" may be a cookie or other food reward. Thus, the child learns that the reward and punishment are related and reinforced with food intake. As the child grows and is further influenced by such things as radio, television, and conversations with other people, food achieves an even greater role. By watching most television programs, we are exposed to a continuous caloric stimulation through food advertisement. As the child grows into teenage and young adulthood, a major part of culture demands peer interrelationships centered around food. Restaurants, movie theaters, candy machines, ice cream stores, and pizza parlors are examples of reinforced associations to which the individual is exposed. Similarly, reinforcements around food are found in supermarkets, where foods are displayed in unique ways to tantalize the individual to make a purchase. The individual is constantly exposed in so many ways throughout the day that it is surprising that obesity is not even more common than it is.

PATHOPHYSIOLOGIC COMPLICATIONS

The following is not an exhaustive summary of the consequences of obesity, although the authors have attempted to highlight some of the complications. A more comprehensive review of the concomitants of obesity can be obtained in other works.[92]

Metabolic-Diabetes-Lipid

Of all the abnormal sequelae of obesity, diabetes is the best documented. Of patients with maturity-onset diabetes, 80% are obese, and 60% of grossly obese individuals are carbohydrate-intolerant.[60,61] Observations in obese preadolescents reveal that 20% have diabetes, markedly elevated basal plasma insulin levels, and exaggerated insulin response to various insulinogenic stimulants independent of the ages.[63,64] The hyperinsulism of obesity may be due to peripheral insulin resistance.[65] For as yet unexplained reasons, peripheral insulin resistance is associated with adiposity, and the correlation is linear.[66] Two hypotheses have been proposed. Roth and colleagues have shown a decreased number of insulin receptors on cell membranes of obese animals and man,[67] whereas Lockwood and Cuatrecasas[68] have postulated a decrease in the responsitivity of the enzyme inside the cell to insulin's action. This resistance has been shown in man in all tissues studied, including adipose tissue, muscle, liver, and circulating mononuclear cells.

Should diabetes be due to deficient β-cell release of insulin, it is obvious that the increased insulin load of the obese could unmask a previously latent mild diabetic. The fascinating problem is the physiologic mechanism whereby increased adiposity signals other cells in the body to alter their responses to insulin, be it at the receptor or at a site inside the cell. One might speculate that if muscle and liver, for example, can sense the degree of adiposity, so can the hypothalamus. Insulin resistance appears to correlate more closely with fat cell size than number.[69] However, dietary factors (high-carbohydrate diet) also appear to be related to the insulin antagonism.[70] With weight reduction insulin resistance diminishes much more rapidly than does body fat. Additional explanatory mechanisms, such as a diret effect of daily calorie flux, have been invoked.[71] This is the basis for the common observation that a mildly diabetic 250-lb person may develop normal glucose tolerance with a weight loss of 15 lb to 20 lb. In fact, the major improvement is frequently noted with loss of only a few pounds.

Other hormonal disturbances with obesity include increased cortisol secretion by the adrenals, leading to elevated 24-hr 17-hydroxycorticoid excretion.[72] Plasma cortisol levels are normal, and there is normal suppression with exogenous glucocorticoids and normal 24-h urine-free cortisol excretion, differentiating simple obesity from adrenal hypercorticism.

Gonadal function is also altered with obesity. In the male there is decreased libido and sexual activity. In the female there may be irregular menses, anovulatory cycles, and amenorrhea.[73] It is interesting that the same sequence may occur with marked loss of weight as in anorexia nervosa,[74] and again one wonders how the hypothalamus is able to sense the caloric status of the body.

Other hormonal alterations in obesity include deficient growth hormone release to many stimuli, including hypoglycemia.[75] Adipose tissue also is not only resistant to the action of insulin but also to lipid-mobilizing agents such as norepinephrine. Again, all of these return to normal with weight reduction.[78]

Another metabolic abnormality associated with obesity is hyperlipidemia, and levels of both cholesterol and triglycerides are increased.[77,78] It has been hypothesized that the hyperinsulinism of obesity increases fat synthesis and formation and release of very low density lipoprotein by the liver. Also, the excess calories ingested by themselves would increase exogenous fat derived from the gut, the chylomicrons. The possible causal relationship between elevated lipids and accelerated atherosclerosis leading to coronary artery disease, stroke, and peripheral vascular insufficiency has been much discussed, but it is beyond the scope of this text.[79]

Cardiac Abnormalities

The incidence of hypertension in obesity is greater than that in comparable individuals of lower weight. As is well known, increased blood pressure is a major risk factor in coronary artery disease.[80] The obese patient also experiences physiologic heart enlargement proportionate to the increase in body mass. Thus, the heart may perform increased work and experience increased oxygen consumption even at rest. Finally, there may even be triglyceride infiltration of the heart itself, but the physiologic effect of this phenomenon on function is not known.[81]

Pulmonary Abnormalities

Emphysema is frequently associated with prolonged obesity. There may be permanent reduction of vital capacity even after weight loss.[82] In extreme obesity, the Pickwickian syndrome may present with marked ventilatory insufficiency, intermittent periods of anoxia and hypercapnea, and episodes of somnolence, muscle-twitching, and cyanosis. Eventually, secondary polycythemia, cardiac hypertrophy, and right ventricular failure develop.[83] Ventilation/perfusion abnormalities causing reduction in expiratory reserve volume and reduction in arterial oxygen tension during resting tidal ventilation have been observed in obese subjects.[84] The obstructive sleep-apnea syndrome, however, is not more common in the obese than in those of normal weight, as once was believed.

Gastrointestinal Complications

Markedly obese patients have functional and structural abnormalities of the liver.[85] Fatty infiltration is common but occasionally leads to frank hepatic failure and death. Cholecystitis and cholelithiasis are common in obese patients. Colitis and peptic ulcer disease have also been found to be slightly increased in the obese individual.[86,87]

Musculoskeletal Complications

The obese obviously place much greater stress on bone and other supportive tissues. They are more prone to osteoarthritis and other degenerative problems, such as periarthritis, which may be severe.[86] The patient who is obese also has higher levels of circulating uric acid and an increased incidence of gout.[88] Increased urinary creatine has been observed in obese patients. It is believed to be both muscle and nonmuscle in origin.[88]

Renal Complications

A significant correlation between nephrosis and obesity has been reported.[89]

Cancer

The interrelationship between cancer and obesity, if any, is controversial. Some data suggest morbidity and mortality from cancer are increased in the presence of obesity. Hertig and Sommers found a 30% greater incidence of endometrial cancer in overweight women.[90] In addition, their prognosis was worse than that of nonobese women with the same disease.[91]

PSYCHOLOGICAL IMPLICATIONS OF OBESITY

Patients who are obese usually have distinct, recognizable lifestyles. In our society, they have difficulties and are often criticized for corpulence. Obese patients may be scolded and may suffer indignities from parents, siblings, spouses, friends, employers, teachers, and even doctors. Frequently, they are viewed as incorrigible debauchers, practitioners of the cardinal sin of gluttony. Often they are ridiculed and made cruel objects of fun. These persons are often suspicious, resentful, withdrawn, and depressed. Unfortunately, this environment and its hostility and insecurity initiate a vicious cycle with increasing weight gain. In personality studies of obese individuals, they were found to be immature, suspicious, and rigid.[93,94] Immaturity was often expressed in the failure to resist impulses, particularly to resist eating.

EXERCISE

As obesity develops, the desire and ability to exercise diminishes. Studies have shown that the obese individual is much more inactive than a normal-weight counterpart doing similar tasks.[95] In studies performed with motion pictures evaluating the exact activity of obese and thin girls playing tennis or swimming, it was found that the obese patient's inactive periods were much greater.[96] Similar results were found in office procedures, such as letter-filing, which fat secretaries did with less physical activity. As activity decreases, so does calorie expenditure, and another vicious cycle is initiated. Studies by Sims showed that normal weight volunteers who were force-fed to gain weight diminished their daily physical activity.[97] The obese individual is, therefore, both physically and emotionally less inclined to exercise. Although exercise is really not a very efficient means of weight reduction, it does help in calorie utilization, and also it must be remembered that when one exercises, one does not eat.

CURRENT TREATMENTS OF OBESITY

The current treatments of obesity may be categorized under four major headings: diet, drugs, surgery, and behavioral modification.

Diet. A middleaged 70-kg man has a daily basal requirement of approximately 1800 Cal. If a person increases his caloric needs because of increased activity, caloric intake must be increased accordingly. For instance, were he to do moderate work or exercise, daily caloric needs might be 2500 to 3500. It is not unusual for an obese patient to ingest an average of 2800 to 3000 Cal per day. To lose weight it is obviously necessary to decrease the caloric intake below that amount. A 1000-Cal/day deficit (7000 cal/week) would result in a 2-lb loss of fat (3500 Cal/pound of triglyceride).

The general format for this diet would be a balanced diet of 2000 Cal divided into three meals and perhaps in-between meal snacks. These are usually determined by a dietician who has completely evaluated the nutrient value of the food and has correlated it with the lifestyle and cultural background of the patient. It contains essential vitamins and minerals. This type of caloric restriction is very helpful, and the patient loses weight without the weakness that occurs with a more severe caloric deficit. The problem with this diet is that the patient usually will comply for only a short period of time. During special occasions he may overindulge and go off the diet and because of guilt and frustration

will return to the previous style of eating, and the program fails. Another problem that occurs with these low caloric diets is the dietary indiscretions that the patient himself may start. For example, he may skip meals and then make up the "lost" calories in certain other items, usually overshooting the deficit markedly. This prototype is the gorger who may be aiming for a caloric deficit of 7000 Cal/week and maintains this until the weekend; then, through heavy dietary indiscretions, he will eat a very large quantity of food. Thus, in one day, the loss of calories throughout the week has been totally nullified. Another category of patients has been classified as the nibbler. This person will supplement his restricted diets with small amounts of nibbling of food throughout the day. He rationalizes his intake by stating that the calories are small; however, he often consciously or unconsciously forgets the accumulated large quantities of food ingested. Again, frustration is produced in this group. An untoward response to reduction treatments has been recently reviewed, and a significant degree of depression has been observed. Thus, further care is needed in treating these patients.[98]

The question, even in the normal nonobese person, as to whether to eat one meal a day or to eat multiple meals remains controversial. In rats force-fed their total daily intake in two meals, more fat and less protein were deposited as compared to animals allowed to nibble throughout the day. Similarly, in studies in humans comparing the consumption of one, three, or six meals per day, it was observed that the subjects who ingested six meals per day had less elevation of either cholesterol or triglycerides compared to those subjects who ate either three or one meal per day.[99] Thus, it would be more beneficial for a person to eat small quantities of food throughout the day rather than to stuff calories into one occasion. However, the frequency of meals does not change the rate of weight loss.[100] The typical obese subject usually skips breakfast and occasionally lunch but eats large quantities of food for dinner.

Diets using liquid calories (e.g., Metrecal) have been attempted, but most who go on this diet usually continue it for only a short time because of the desire to eat solid foods, which they will add as supplements to the liquid diet. Low-calorie meals made up primarily of protein have been popularized and have been shown to have beneficial effects in losing weight, compared to similar caloric equivalents of low-protein intake.[101,102] Other popularized diets using this principle will be discussed later. Other manipulations of the diet, such as the use of a grapefruit before eating meals or imbibing large quantities of water prior to ingestion of meals, are of little true physiologic rationale and effectiveness except for their placebo effect in altering behavior.

Complete starvation has been used on occasion, either in short, intermittent episodes[103] or in a single, prolonged fast (6 weeks–10 weeks).[104] It is recommended that a fast be initiated in a hospital setting since various complications can arise. Complications in total starvation include cardiovascular manifestations, such as myocardial ischemia or low output owing to hypovolemia and leading to orthostatic hypotension;[105] gout; hyperuricemia;[106] Wernicke's encephalopathy;[107] lactic acidosis;[108] and polyneuritis. In complete caloric withdrawal, patients lose about ⅓ lb to ½ lb of fat per day. Initial weight loss may be 4 lb to 5 lb per day, but this is due to excretion of salt and water in the urine, a physiologic phenomenon resulting from withdrawal of carbohydrate from the diet. After this diuresis has passed, total daily weight loss is about 1 lb, one half of which is lean tissue and its accompanying water and protein. The major, real advantage of this type of program is the removal of the patient from the influences of his environment, as well as a large loss of weight in a short period of time, which is most helpful in his obtaining a new outlook. A major contraindication is the amount of lean tissue lost, and thus this regime is mainly for obese but otherwise healthy individuals.

Another method which has been given some consideration has been the use of roughage diets with high-fiber content.[109] It has been shown from various studies, especially from Africa, that populations on unrefined foods rarely become obese.[110] Similarly, when these individuals are exposed to foods of the western civilizations (e.g., concentrated, refined foods), they increase their weight, and obesity becomes evident.

Fad diets have achieved great notoriety, particularly the Atkins and Stillman regimes. They have been used by thousands of obese people, especially in the United States. The basic principle of the Atkins or "ketogenic" diet is provision of calories from high-fat content. The conversion of the high-fat diet into ketones by the liver and loss of these in the urine, as well as the stimulation of lipid-mobilizing factors, has been the selling point. Unfortunately, the energy lost in the urine in a 24-hr period amounts to only 50 or 75 Cal, an insignificant quantity. Also, the fat-mobilizing hormone purported to be increased is of questionable importance, if it even exists as a physiologic entity, of which there is some doubt. The major appetite-depressing activity of the diet is due to the production of the ketones, which are anorexigenic. A problem with this diet is the ingestion of fat, which leads to increased levels of cholesterol and triglycerides in the circulation and may be an im-

portant precursor to atherosclerosis. Also, the mild acidosis may contribute to other problems, such as osteoporosis.

Another dietary manipulation that has been popularized is the use of the Stillman diet, which consists of a high-protein, low-carbohydrate intake. In this diet, the protein serves as the anorexigenic agent, in addition to which about one fourth of the protein calories are metabolically unavailable for body energy as they are used to rid the body of the ingested nitrogen in the form of urea. The significance of this extra energy loss owing to protein has been recently questioned.[111] It must be remembered that most fad diets are so abnormal that the patient sooner or later abandons the program and returns to his former eating habits. This finding is best exemplified in a 14-year follow-up of 27 patients of an original 38 patients who were given dietary treatments: Only 5 successfully kept their weight down.[112]

Medications. Medications have been used in an attempt to curb dietary intake for many years. The most widely used were the amphetamines, which have been shown to augment weight loss when used in conjunction with diet for periods of up to several months.[113] Studies for more prolonged periods (1 or 2 years) have not been performed, nor have the long-term ill effects of the drugs been fully evaluated. Complications include habituation as well as hypertension, elevation of heart rate, and pulmonary hypertension.[114] Prolonged usage frequently leads to altered mental state and, sometimes, frank psychosis. The Food and Drug Administration has banned the use of amphetamines in the treatment of obesity.

Another category of allegedly anorexigenic compounds has been used in adult-onset diabetics: the hypoglycemic agents, the biguanides. However, in the controversial large Multicenter University Group Project Study, the reported side effects of increased heart rate and elevated blood pressure precluded their usefulness. In addition, occasional fatal lactic acidosis led to the total withdrawal of biguanides in the United States.[115] Other compounds, such as fenfluramine, have low potential for abuse and are now being used and studied. They have been found effective in large, carefully controlled studies.[116] However, the weight loss in those on the drug compared to those on placebo is only 1 lb to 2 lb greater after 2 months to 3 months. As with amphetamines, chronic use leads to the development of tolerance.

Filler compounds of the methylcellulose type act by a distention of the stomach. They produce a pseudofull sensation. These compounds also are of questionable value, however. Their use in synthetic low-calorie foods is still being evaluated. Another recent compound that has been given consideration for use is phaseolamin.[117] The effect of this compound is said to interfere with the action of amylase, which converts starches to glucose in the intestine. The theory is to allow patients to eat starches *ad lib.* Without hydrolysis to glucose these carbohydrates are not absorbable. However, as would be anticipated, the patient has severe diarrhea and flatulence and is subject to all the problems of malabsorption since the starches are metabolized by flora in the large intestine.

Another pharmacologic approach to obesity has been the use of thyroid hormone. In some studies, obese individuals were found to have low-thyroid indices suggesting "hypometabolic" obesity.[118] Other studies have revealed normal functions.[119] Studies have suggested that the administration of thyroid hormones potentiates weight loss in obese patients, while other investigators have not been able to observe this effect.[120] The administration of a large dose would produce the potentially dangerous condition of hyperthyroidism.

Another approach has been the use of multiple medications or "rainbow" drugs. The combination of digitalis, diuretics, and thyroid hormone has been used. Since the diuretic augments loss of weight as water and electrolyte, the digitalis acts as an anorectic, and the thyroid produces hypermetabolic effects, the patient is expected to experience dramatic and joyful results. However, the consequences of such therapy are occasionally found in the emergency rooms where patients have entered with cardiac arrhythmias, dehydration, hyponatremia, hypokalemic alkalosis, or signs and symptoms of hypermetabolism. Unfortunately, even deaths have been reported.[122]

Another fad is the use of chorionic gonadotropin (HCG), originally popularized by Simeons, who rationalized its use since patients with hypogonadism were obese and HCG was effective in treating these patients. This compound, which is expensive, is given by frequent intramuscular injections, and well-documented clinical studies indicate lack of affect.[4]

A multiplicity of other compounds have been used. Vitamins, such as E, A, C, and D have been proposed, as well as secret remedies with sucrose or lactose as the main constituent. The obese individual is tantalized by these and other nostrums, and the end-results are the same: frustrations, anxiety, guilt. But now financial loss is also added to the list, since all of these are simply fraudulent attempts to prey on the fat person's wallet.

Surgery. The surgical approach has included the use of *panniculectomy,* or removal of segments of fat and

the overlying skin. However, the proportion of fat removed is insignificant. Following the surgery, the patients replace the fat very rapidly elsewhere and infection and lymphedema at the operative site are frequent complications. Other surgical procedures such as "jaw-wiring" have been attempted. Although these procedures are radical, their effectiveness is poor and potentially dangerous.

At the present time, jejunoileal bypass is in decline. This surgical procedure consists of anastomosing a short segment of the jejunum to a terminal segment of the ileum.[125] The rationale for its effectiveness is to reduce the jejunal and ileal absorptive surface so that food will hve less transit time in the intestine as well as exposure to a smaller absorptive surface, thus wasting the excess food rather than absorbing it. Dramatic loss of weight in many obese subjects has been encouraging. However, the complications of this surgery preclude its effectiveness. Some of the frequent complications are outlined in Table 37-3. Gastric bypass surgery may replace jejunoileal bypass for patients who respond to no other therapy. Initial results are encouraging.

Behavior Modification. Behavior modification has been used in treating obese subjects with fair results. One of the first modifications is exercise, but this alone will never be successful in reducing weight unless it is combined with dietary control. In a study by Gwinup, weight loss paralleled length of time walking exceeding 30 minutes daily in obese women.[126] The consumption of 200 Cal (24-oz beer) necessitate a person to run for 15 min, swim for 20 min, walk for 1 hr, or sing an opera for 3 hr. Thus, the use of exercise alone is, at best, a minimally effective method of losing calories.

Other types of behavior modification may be helpful for the obese patient. Group participation is one that has been popularized (*e.g.,* Tops, Weight-Watchers) and found to be very helpful in giving the obese person a sense of camaraderie analogous to that found in Alcoholics Anonymous. Positive reinforcement when weight is lost is an example of the psychotherapeutic advantage of these groups. Other behavior modifications include such methods as recording daily food intake as well as the time, amount, and the circumstances of eating. With a food list, the patient becomes more aware of the quantity and environmental and psychological situations associated with eating. Other approaches modify the external stimuli: Eating snacks in one location or room and eating at only certain times of the day may aid the obese patient in becoming more aware of dietary indiscretions. Other examples of behavior modifications, such as chewing food thoroughly before continuing to eat or allowing a 2-min

Table 37-3. *Jejunoileal Bypass*

Indications	Complications
Premorbid obesity	Mortality of surgery
Pickwickian	Postoperative complications
Severe heart	Long-term complications
disease	Fluid and electrolyte deficiency
Liver—	Diarrhea
Kidney—	Anemia
Diabetes	Vitamin deficiency
Psychological	Oxalate kidney stone
	Liver failure
	Orthostatic hypotension
	Lipid abnormality
	Ulcer
	Intussuception
	Gallbladder disease

interruption of the meal, may be useful techniques in the obese patient. Further reviews of behavior modification methods by Stunkard[127] and Bruno[128] are recommended for more detailed information. In summary, these methods try to alter the environment that leads to the caloric intake into an uncomfortable milieu. Other modifications, such as deprivation of sleep, have been used in an attempt to curtail the appetite.

REASONABLE APPROACH TO THE PATIENT WITH OBESITY

A reasonable approach to the patient with obesity can be summarized with the following program: A complete evaluation on admission to the clinic or office should include a medical history with a detailed description of caloric intake and a history of body weight and eating habits. Other pertinent information, such as social, cultural, and family weight, and a categorization as to eating habits (nibbler or gorger) should be documented. Many of these questions can be answered by the patient in a questionnaire form.

The current treatments of obesity may be categorized into four major groups: diet, drugs, surgery, and behavioral modification. Bray has compared all of the weight reduction programs, and summarized the success of the various methods (Fig. 37-2). Formal educational sessions should be set up with or without other patients in an attempt to educate the subject in basic energy physiology and to help the obese people to understand their problem and how they may modify it. Many patients may find interaction with other obese patients helpful, as in groups similar to Alcoholics Anonymous. Patients should maintain daily records of their food intake and record their moods, as has been

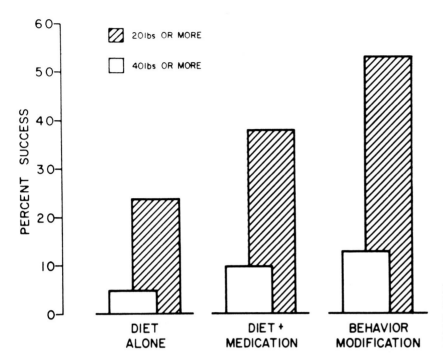

Fig. 37-2. Percent of patients achieving success with various treatments of obesity. (From Bray GA: The Obese Patient. Philadelphia, WB Saunders, 1976)

recommended by Stunkard.[127] This accomplishes two purposes: The patient obtains a true realization of his total intake per day, and he discovers how his moods influence his intake. Behavioral modifications are also recommended so that slight changes in daily habits may be helpful in altering daily eating habits. Recommendations such as chewing the food 20 times prior to swallowing, eating high-roughage foods when hungry (celery, carrots, and so forth), having less food available at the table, or eating only at set times of the day are useful. The patients should be encouraged to exercise, albeit not as a means of losing calories but rather as a health promotor and a diversion from food. Finally, frequent follow-ups and positive reinforcement should be encouraged with the physician as well as the dietician, nurse, and others involved in the program. The patients may have pictures taken demonstrating their accomplishments, and records of weights can be kept in bold print in the chart. Thus, there is a positive approach to the patient rather than a continuous negative approach, which produces feelings of despair and guilt.

The use of a high-protein diet supplemented with vitamins should be outlined with the aid of a dietician. The use of anorectic agents should be avoided if at all possible. Finally, if all else fails, the possible use of gastric bypass might be considered.

For rapid "crash" programs, such as for the obese patient who is a candidate for elective surgery, a diet of almost pure "lean" protein composed of fowl, fish,

or lean meat (*e.g.*, veal), is able to maintain muscle mass with selective loss of fat. This meat, supplemented by fruit and leafy vegetables or oral vitamins, may amount to not more than 1 lb daily in portions of 300 Cal to 400 Cal. After 2 or 3 months of this regimen, 30 lb to 40 lb of fat may be lost without the degree of muscle loss that would have occurred with total starvation.

At the present time, education, diets, and behavior modification are only aids. Of utmost importance is the prevention of obesity from birth, and further research into the etiology and possible reversal of the pathologic obese state is needed.

REFERENCES

1. **US Public Health Service, Division of Chronic Disease:** Obesity and Health: A Source Book of Current Information for Professional Health Personnel. Public Health Service Publication No. 1485. Washington, DC, US Government Printing Office, 1966

2. **Widdowson EM:** Chemical analysis of the body. In Brozek J (ed): Human Body Composition, Approaches and Applications. Oxford, Pergamon Press, 1965

3. **Seltzer CC, Mayer J:** A simple criterion of obesity. Postgrad Med 38:101–107, 1965

4. **Bray GA:** Obesity in Perspective. A conference sponsored by the John E. Fogarty International Center for Advanced Study in the Health Services. National Insti-

tutes of Health, Bethesda, MD, DHEW Publication No. NIH-75-708, pp 84–85, 1973

5. **Moore FD, Olesen KH, McMurrey JD et al:** The Body Cell Mass and Its Supporting Environment: Body Composition in Health and Disease. Philadelphia, W B Saunders, 1963

6. **Lesser GT, Deutsch S, Markofsky J:** Use of independent measurement of body fat to evaluate overweight and underweight. Metabolism 20:792–804, 1971

7. **Keys A, Grande F:** Body weight, body composition and calorie status in modern nutrition in health and disease. In Wohl MG, Goodhart RD (eds): Diet Therapy. Philadelphia, Lea & Febiger, 1968

8. **Society of Actuaries:** Build and Blood Pressure Study, Vols I and II. Chicago, Society of Actuaries, 1959

9. **McWhirter N, McWhirter R:** Guiness Book of Records. Heaviest Man, pp 20–21. New York, Sterling, 1975

10. **Editorial:** Obesity: Race, Creed, Sex and Fat. Med World News 25:5, 1974

11. **Kissebah AH, Vydelingum N, Murray R et al:** Relation of body fat distribution to metabolic complications of obesity. J Clin Endocrinol Metab 54:254–260, 1982

12. **Mayer J:** Obesity: Physiologic considerations. Am J Clin Nutr 9:530–537, 1961

13. **Fröhlich A:** Ein fall von tumor der hypophysis cerbri ohne akromegalie. Wien Klin Rundsch 15:883–886, 906–908, 1901

14. **Bray GA:** The Obese Patient. Philadelphia, W B Saunders, 1976

15. **Plummer WA:** Body weights in spontaneous myxedema. Trans Am Assoc Study Goiter pp 88–98, 1940

16. **Murray L (ed):** Obesity: Tracing psychoendocrine clues. Sexual Medicine Today 5, No. 10:6–12, 1981

17. **Gurney R:** The hereditary factor in obesity. Arch Intern Med 57:557–561, 1936

18. **Fellows HH:** Studies of relatively normal obese individuals during and after dietary restrictions. Am J Med Sci 181:301–312, 1931

19. **Thomas CB, Cohen BH:** Familial occurrence of hypertension, coronary artery disease, obesity and diabetes. Ann Intern Med 42:90–127, 1955

20. **Biron P, Mongeau JG, Bertrand D:** Familial aggregation of blood pressure in adopted and natural children. Circulation (Suppl) 3:49–50, 1974

21. **Danforth CH:** Hereditary adiposity in mice. J Hered 18:153–162, 1927

22. **Bray GA, York DA:** Genetically transmitted obesity in rodents. Physiol Rev 51:598–646, 1971

23. **Cahill GF, Jr., Jones EE, Lauris V et al:** Studies on experimental diabetes in the Wellesley hydrid mouse: II. Insulin levels and response of peripheral tissue. Diabetologia 3:171–174, 1967

24. **Mayer J:** Genetic factors in human obesity. Ann NY Acad Sci 131:412–421, 1965

25. **Mayer J:** Regulation of energy intake and body weight: The glucostatic theory and the lipostatic hypothesis. Ann NY Acad Sci 63:13–15, 1955

26. **Anand BK:** Nervous regulation of food intake. Physiol Rev 41:677–708, 1961

27. **Jansen GR, Hutchison CF:** Production of hypothalamic obesity by microsurgery. Am J Physiol 217:487–493, 1969

28. **Rogers AR, Leung PMB:** The influence of amino acids on the neuroregulation of food intake. Fed Proc 32:1709–1919, 1973

29. **Brecher G, Waxler SH:** Obesity in albino mice due to single injections of gold thioglucose. Proc Soc Exp Biol Med 70:498–501, 1949

30. **Leibowitz SF:** Reciprocal hunger regulating circuits involving alpha and beta adrenergic receptors located respectively in the ventromedial and lateral hypothalamus. Proc Nat Acad Sci USA 67:1063–1070, 1970

31. **Wiersmo CAG:** Reflexes and central nervous system. In Waterman TH (ed): The Physiology of Crustsacea, Lense, Organs, Integration and Behavior, p 241. New York, Academic Press, 1961

32. **Lepkovsky SO, Bortfeld P, Dimick MK et al:** Role of upper intestines in the regulation of food intake in parabiotic rats with their intestines 'crossed' surgically. Isr J Med Sci 7:639–646, 1971

33. **Panksepp J:** Is satiety mediated by the ventromedial hypothalamus? Physiol Behav 7:381–389, 1971

34. **Kennedy GC:** The role of depot fat in the hypothalamic control of food intake in the rat. Proc R Soc Med 140:578–592, 1953

35. **Mu JY, Semes B, Yin TH et al:** Variability of body fat in hyperphagic rats. Yale J Biol Med 41:133–142, 1968

36. **Lepkovsky S, Furuta F:** The role of homeostasis in adipose tissue upon the regulation of food intake of white leghorn cockerels. Poultry Sci 50:573–577, 1971

37. **O'Connell M, Danforth E, Jr., Horton ES et al:** Experimental obesity in man: III. Adrenocortical function. J Clin Endocrinol Metab 36:323–329, 1973

38. **Sims EAH, Horton ES, Salans LB:** Inducible metabolic abnormalities during development of obesity. Annu Rev Med 22:235–250, 1971

39. **King JR, Farner DS:** The relationship of fat deposition to Zugunruke and migration. Condor 65:200, 1933

40. **Janowitz HD, Hollander F:** The time factor in the adjustment of food intake to varied caloric requirements in the dog: A study of the precision of appetite regulation. Ann NY Acad Sci 63:56–67, 1955

41. **Miller NE, Kesson ML:** Reward effects of food via stomach fistula compared with those of food via mouth. J Comp Physiol Psychol 45:555–564, 1952

42. **Hill RG, Ison EC, Jones WW et al:** The small intestine as a factor in regulation of eating. Am J Physiol 170:201–25, 1952

43. **Holinger PH, Kelley EH, Ivy AG:** The vagi and appetite. Proc Soc Exp Biol Med 29:884–885, 1932

44. **Schally AV, Redding TW, Lucien HW et al:** Entero-

gastrone inhibits eating by fasted mice. Science 157:210, 1967

45. **Glick Z, Thomas DW, Mayer J:** Absence of effect of injections of the intestinal hormones secretin and cholecystokinin-pancreozymin upon feeding behavior. Physiol Behav 6:5, 1971

46. **Garrattini S, Saminin R:** Anorectic Agents: Mechanisms of Action and Tolerance. New York, Raven Press, 1981

47. **Lepkovsky S:** Newer concepts in the regulation of food intake. Am J Clin Nutr 26:271–284, 1973

48. **Harris LJ, Clay J, Hargreaves FJ et al:** Appetite and choice of diet: The ability of the vitamin B-deficient rat to discriminate between diets containing and lacking the vitamin. Proc R Soc Med 113:151–190, 1933

49. **Rogers QR, Leung PMB:** The influence of amino acids on the neuroregulation of food intake. Fed Proc 32:1709–1719, 1973

50. **Kennedy GC:** Appetite and obesity. Medical Press 243:211–214, 1960

51. **Hirsch J, Knittle JL:** Cellularity of obese and non-obese human adipose tissue. Fed Proc 29:1516–1521, 1970

52. **Salans LB, Horton E, Sims EAH:** Experimental obesity in man: Cellular character of the adipose tissue. J Clin Invest 50:1005–1011, 1971

53. **Knittle JL, Hirsch J:** Effects of early nutrition in the development of rat epididymal fat pads: Cellularity and metabolism. J Clin Invest 47:2091–2098, 1968

54. **Hall B:** Changing composition of human milk and early development of an appetite control. Lancet 1:779–781, 1975

55. **Deluise M, Blackburn GL, Flier JS:** Reduced activity of the red-cell sodium–potassium pump in human obesity. N Engl J Med 303:1017–1022, 1980

56. **Bray GA, Kral JG, Bjorntorp:** Hepatic sodium–potassium–dependent ATPase in obesity. N Engl J Med 304:1580–1582, 1981

57. **Mir MA, Charobambous BM, Morgan K et al:** Erythrocyte sodium–potassium ATP-ase and sodium transport in obesity. N Engl J Med 305:1264–1268, 1981

58. **Danforth E:** Thermogenesis, obesity and thyroid hormones. Thyroid Today. 4, No. 6, 1981

59. **Renshaw DC:** Sexuality and depression in infancy, childhood and adolescence. Medical Aspects of Human Sexuality 9:24–25, 1975

60. **Bierman EL, Bagdade JD, Porte D, Jr:** Obesity and diabetes: The odd couple. Am J Clin Nutr 21:1434, 1968

61. **Smith M, Levine R:** Obesity and diabetes. Med Clin North Am 48:1387–1397, 1964

62. **Chiumello G, Del Guerci MJ, Canelutti M et al:** Relationship between obesity, chemical diabetes and beta pancreatic function in children. Diabetes 18:238–243, 1969

63. **Drash A:** Relationship between diabetes mellitus and obesity in the child. Metabolism 22:337–344, 1973

64. **Karam JH, Grodsky GM, Forsham PH:** Excessive insulin response to glucose in obese subjects as measured by immunochemical assay. Diabetes 12:197–204, 1963

65. **Rabinovitz D, Zierler KL:** Forearm metabolism in obesity and its response to intra-arterial insulin. Characterization of insulin resistance and evidence for adaptive hyperinsulinism. J Clin Invest 41:2173–2181, 1962

66. **Salans LB, Knittle JL, Hirsch J:** The role of adipose cell size and adipose tissue sensitivity in the carbohydrate intolerance of human obesity. J Clin Invest 47:153–165, 1968

67. **Archer JA, Gordon P, Roth J:** Defect in insulin binding to receptors in obese man. J Clin Invest 55:166–174, 1975

68. **Livingston JN, Cuatrecasas P, Lockwood DH:** Insulin insensitivity of large fat cells. Science 177:626–628, 1972

69. **Jacobsson B, Smith U:** Effect of cell size on lipolysis and antilipolytic action of insulin in human fat cells. J Lipid Res 13:651–656, 1972

70. **Grey N, Kipnis DM:** Effect of diet composition on the hyperinsulinemia of obesity. N Engl J Med 285:827–830, 1971

71. **Jackson IMD, McKiddie MT, Buchanan KD:** Effect of fasting on glucose and insulin metabolism of obese patients. Lancet 1:285–287, 1964

72. **Dunkelman SS, Fairhurst B, Player J, Waterhouse C:** Cortisol metabolism in obesity. J Clin Endocrinol Metab 24:832–841, 1964

73. **Frisch RE, McArthur JW:** Menstrual cycles: Fatness as a detminant of minimum weight for height necessary for their maintenance or onset. Science 185:949–951, 1974

74. **Lundberg DO, Walinder J, Werner I et al:** Effects of thyrotropin-releasing hormone on plasma levels of TSH, FSH, LH and GH in anorexia nervosa. Eu J Clin Invest 2:150–153, 1972

75. **Beck P, Koumans JHT, Winterling CA et al:** Studies of insulin and growth hormone secretion in human obesity. J Lab Clin Med 64:654–667, 1964

76. **El–Khodary AZ, Ball MF, Stein B et al:** Effects of weight loss on the growth hormone response to arginine infusion in obesity. J Clin Endocrnol Metab 32:42–51, 1971

77. **Albrink MJ, Meigs JW:** The relationship between serum triglycerides and shinfold thickness in obese subjects. Ann NY Acad Sci 131:673–683, 1965

78. **Mann GV, Teel K, Hayes O et al:** Exercise in the disposition of dietary calories. Regulation of serum lipoprotion and cholesterol levels in human subjects. N Engl J Med 253:349–355, 1955

79. **Wilens SL:** Bearing of general nutritional state on atherosclerosis. Arch Intern Med 79:129–147, 1947

80. **Levy RL, White PD, Stroud WD et al:** Overweight, its prognostic significance in relation to hypertension and cardiovascular–renal disease. JAMA 131:951–953, 1946

81. **Short JJ, Johnson HJ:** The effect of overweight on vital capacity. Life Extension Examiner, New York Proceedings 1:36–41, 1939

82. **Kerr WJ, Lagen JB:** The postural syndrome related to

obesity leading to postural emphysema and cardiorespiratory failure. Ann Intern Med 10:561–595, 1936

83. **Ward W, Kelsey W:** The Pickwickian syndrome. A review of the literature and report of a case. J Pediatr 61:745–750, 1962

84. **Holley HS, Milic-Emili J, Becklake MR et al:** Regional distribution of pulmonary ventilation and perfusion in obesity. J Clin Invest 46:475–481, 1967

85. **Zelmans, S:** The liver in obesity. Arch Intern Med 90:141–156, 1952

86. **Armstrong DB, Dublin LI, Wheatley GM et al:** Obesity and its relation to health and disease. JAMA 147:1007–1014, 1951.

87. **Solomon N:** The study and treatment of the obese patient. Hosp Prac 90–94, 1969

88. **Thorsten S, Nolan S, Sun A et al:** The increased creatinuria of obesity. Cur Med Dig 1026–1031, Oct. 1972

89. **Weisinger JR, Kempson RL, Eldrige FL et al:** The nephrotic syndrome: A complication of massive obesity. Ann Intern Med 81:440–447, 1974

90. **Hertig AT, Somers SC:** Genesis of endometrial carcinoma. Cancer 2:946–959, 1949

91. **Hildreth RC:** Obesity—A complication in carcinoma cervix uteri. J Mich Med Soc 49:1175–1178, 1950

92. **Cahill GF, Jr, Aoki TT, Rossini AA:** Metabolism in obesity and anorexia nervosa. In Wurtman RJ, Wurtman JJ (eds): Nutrition and the Brain. Vol 3. New York, Raven Press, 1979

93. **Goldblatt PB, Moore ME, Stunkard AJ:** Social factors in obesity. JAMA 192:1939–1044, 1965

94. **Moore ME, Stunkard A, Srole L:** Obesity, social class, and mental illness. JAMA 181:962–966, 1962

95. **Chirico AM, Stunkard AJ:** Physical activity and human obesity. N Engl J Med 263:935–940, 1960

96. **Bullen BA, Reed RB, Mayer J:** Physical activity of obese and non-obese adolescent girls appraised by motion picture sampling. Am J Clin Nutr 14:211–223, 1964

97. **Sims EAH, Horton ES:** Endocrine and metabolic adaptation to obesity and starvation. Am J Clin Nutr 21:1455–1470, 1968

98. **Stunkard AJ, Rush J:** Dieting and depression reexamined. Ann Intern Med 81:525–533, 1974

99. **Young CM, Scanlon SS, Topping CM et al:** Frequency of feeding weight reduction and body composition. J Am Diet Assoc 59:466–472, 1971

100. **Gwinup G, Byron RC, Roush WH et al:** Effect of nibbling versus gorging, on serum lipids in man. Am J Clin Nutr 13:209–213, 1963

101. **Reinberg A, Appelbaum M, Assan R:** Chronophysiologic effects of a restricted diet (220 cal/24 hr as Casein) in young healthy but obese women. Int J Chronobiol 1:391–404, 1973

102. **Appelbaum M, Reiberg A, Assan R et al:** Hormonal and metabolic circadian rhythms before and during a low protein diet. Isr J Med Sci 8, No. 6:867–873, 1972

103. **Duncan GG, Jenson WK, Fraser RI et al:** Correction and control of intractable obesity: Practical application of intermittent periods of total fasting. JAMA 181:309–312, 1972

104. **Drenick EJ et al:** Prolonged starvation as treatment of severe obesity. JAMA 187:100–105, 1964

105. **Blood WL, Mitchell W, Jr:** Salt excretion of fasting patients. Arch Intern Med 106:321–326, 1960

106. **Drenick EJ:** Hyperuricemia, acute gout, renal insufficiency and urate nephrolithiasis due to starvation. Arthritis Rheum 8:988–997, 1965

107. **Drenick EJ, Javen CB, Swendseid ME:** Occurrence of acute Wernicke's encephalopathy during prolonged starvation for the treatment of obesity. N Engl J Med 274:937–939, 1966

108. **Cubberley PT, Polster SA, Schulman CL:** Lactic acidosis and death after the treatment of obesity by fasting. N Engl J Med 272:628–631, 1965

109. **Heaton KW:** Food fibre and as obstacle to energy intake. Lancet 1:1418–1421, 1973

110. **Trowell H:** Fibre and obesity. Lancet 1:95, 1974

111. **Bradfield RB, Jourden MH:** Relative importance of specific dynamic action in weight reduction diets. Lancet 2:640–643, 1973

112. **Sohar E, Sneh E:** Follow-up of obese patients: 14 years after a successful reducing diet. Am J Clin Nutr 26:845–848, 1973

113. **Patel N, Mock DC, Jr, Hagans JA:** Comparison of benzphetamine, phenmetrazine d-amphetamine and placebo. Clin Pharmacol Ther 4:330–333, 1963

114. **Martin WR, Sloan JW, Sapira JD et al:** Physiologic, subjective and behavioral effects of amphetamines, methamphetamines, ephedrine phenmetrazine and methylphenidate in man. Clin Pharmacol Ther 12:245–258, 1971

115. **Knatterud G, Klimt CR, Osborne RK et al:** A study of the effects of hypoglycemic agents on vascular complications in patients with adult-onset diabetes. Evaluation of Phenformin Therapy. Diabetes 24:65–184, 1975

116. **Fenfluramine:** Med Lett 15, No. 8:33–34, 1972

117. **Fawcette G:** Our new age, pass the phaseolamin. Boston Globe, December 29, 1974

118. **Scriba PC, Richter J, Horn et al:** Zur frage der schlddrusenfunktion bei adipositos. Klin Worchenschr 45:323–324, 1967

119. **Glennon JA, Brech WJ:** Serum protein bound iodine in obesity. J Clin Endocrinol Metab 25:1673–1674, 1965

120. **Gordon ES, Goldberg M, Chesy GJ:** A new concept in the treatment of obesity. JAMA 186:156–166, 1969

121. **Goodman NG:** Triiodothyronine and placebo in the treatment of obesity. Medical Annals of the District of Columbia 38:658–662, 1969

122. **Jelliffe RW, Hill D, Tatter D et al:** Death from weight control pills. JAMA 208:1843–1847, 1969

123. **Asher WL, Harper HW:** Effect of human chorionic

gonadotrophin on weight loss, hunger, and feeling of well-being. Am J Clin Nutr 26:211–218, 1973

124. **Hirsch J:** The treatment of obesity. Am J Clin Nutr 26:1039–1044, 1973

125. **Payne JH, Dewind L, Schwab CE et al:** Surgical treatment of morbid obesity: Sixteen years experience. Arch Surg 106:432–437, 1973

126. **Gwinup G:** Effect of exercise alone on the weight of obese women. Arch Intern Med 135:676–680, 1975

127. **Stunkard AJ:** New Treatments for Obesity: Behavior Modifications in Treatment and Management of Obesity, pp 103–116. Bray GA, Bethune JE (eds). Hagerstown, MD, Harper & Row, 1974

128. **Bruno FJ:** Think Yourself Thin. Los Angeles, CA, Barnes & Noble, 1973

38

Undernutrition
Richard S. Rivlin
Robert J. McConnell
Martha Osnos

Introduction
Perspective of Nutrition Problems
Weight Loss or Subnormal Body Weight as Symptoms
Maternal Undernutrition and Child Development
  Undernutrition and Low Birth Weight
  Undernutrition and Brain Development
  Extreme Forms of Undernutrition in Childhood
  Anemia in Pregnancy
  Breast Versus Artificial Feeding
  Child Abuse
Undernutrition Resulting from Drug Administration
  Some Signs and Symptoms of Undernutrition Resulting from Drug Administration
  Drug Effects Upon Some Specific Nutrients
  Undernutrition Produced by Certain Drugs
Undernutrition in Cancer

Weight Loss and Anorexia
Mechanisms of Weight Loss
Undernutrition and Tumor Growth
Undernutrition and Cancer Causation
Undernutrition and Aging
  Animal Investigations on Food Consumption
  Nutrition and Longevity in Man
    Physiologic Changes with Aging and their Implication for Nutrition
    Undernutrition in the Elderly Owing to Psychosocial Factors
Undernutrition and Hormones
  Growth Hormone
  Thyroid Hormones
  Adrenal Cortical Hormones
  Insulin
  Gonadal Hormones
Summary

INTRODUCTION

Nutritional status is often not considered sufficiently when a patient is being evaluated. The typical student case history describes patients only as either "well nourished" or "poorly nourished," with little attention to specific characteristics. In many disorders, nutritional factors are important in etiology, in determining the course of the illness, and in governing the response to therapy.

Undernutrition may result not only from inadequate dietary intake, but also from inability to metabolize nutrients normally or from increased loss of nutrients from the body. Deficiency of one nutrient may precipitate or exacerbate deficiencies of other nutrients. Symptoms and signs of undernutrition are often difficult to appreciate at the bedside unless they are extreme. These considerations suggest that the physician should scrutinize the patient more carefully from a nutritional point of view, obtaining a careful history of dietary intake, and should consider those features of the patient's illness that relate to nutritional status.

The perspective of nutritional problems worldwide was well summarized by MacBryde in the previous edition of this volume[1] and is reprinted here.

PERSPECTIVE OF NUTRITION PROBLEMS

There is quite properly, though belatedly, a great recent upsurge in the attention paid to nutrition in the United States and throughout the world. Active workers in the field have long known that widespread malnutrition exists even in the most "advanced" and relatively "affluent" areas, despite great progress in our nutritional knowledge in the last few decades. Delivery to all people of the practical results of scientific knowledge and of technological achievements is now becoming an active concern not only of the health professions, but also of governments and of the general public.

Two obstacles have prevented good nutrition from extending to many populations and individuals—poverty and ignorance. In many countries the poor and uneducated constitute the great majority of the population. They are often unable to purchase an optimal diet. Sometimes distribution problems preclude access to the best foods. Perhaps even more commonly, although proper foods may be economically and physically obtainable, they are not chosen. Many persons, often large groups or even whole tribes, choose poor diets because of lack of information, misinformation, convenience, habit, locale, or religious or ethnic customs. In the United States, one might mistakenly think from reading nutrition manuals that we are all Anglo-Saxon in our eating habits. The truth is instead that our people are heterogeneous in racial and social backgrounds and customs; food choices differ widely in various groups and localities. The foods that are considered pleasing to the palate are often widely different among Spanish-Americans, Chinese-Americans, Italo-Americans, Afro-Americans, Anglo-Saxon Americans, Jewish-Americans, and so forth, and even among different generations of the same family. Some encourage young children to abandon milk early and to drink wine regularly at meals. Some, even with free choice in a modern supermarket, select chiefly "white meat" (fat pork), greens, and cornmeal.

Even in the United States, considered highly fortunate among nations because of the economic adequacy of the great majority and because of the wide availability of education, about one person in eight is inadequately nourished. There are no nationwide surveys, but partial surveys permit this estimate. Thus, of the present population of 210 million, about 26 million persons are believed to be inadequately nourished. The majority of these are children. The most common cause of malnutrition in the United States is poverty, as it is in many other countries.

The United States has available the resources and technology to produce and distribute all nutrients necessary for all our people (plus much more for export), but this has not yet been accomplished.

About 10% of the population is obese (15% or more over ideal weight). This 10%, plus the 12% estimated to be undernourished, makes the startling total of about 22% believed to be improperly nourished or malnourished in our country.*

Some students of nutrition estimate that 75% of human beings subsist on diets providing inadequate calories and insufficient protein.

WEIGHT LOSS OR SUBNORMAL BODY WEIGHT AS SYMPTOMS

The symptoms of weight loss or subnormal body weight may not be emphasized by the patient or the family, but unless there is an obvious explanation, they always should receive serious consideration by the physician. With or without weight loss, lack of energy, weakness, and easy fatigue are usually associated symptoms of an inadequate supply of calories. When not only the energy principle (calories) but certain other essential nutrients are lacking, there may be a wide variety of symptoms, according to the specific food elements involved.

In the absence of weight loss or subnormal body weight, the evidences of undernutrition may be easily overlooked in the history or physical examination unless they happen to be striking. One of the primary purposes of this chapter is to describe the chief symptoms of malnutrition (of which weight loss is only one) and to discuss the mechanisms of their development. The protean symptomatic manifestations of nutritional deficiencies require constant alertness to permit their detection in early or mild stages. It is, of course, in these early stages that diagnosis is of the greatest importance, for by the time florid signs have appeared, correction may be difficult or irreparable damage may have been done.

MATERNAL UNDERNUTRITION AND CHILD DEVELOPMENT

Maternal nutritional status is of vital importance to the growth and development of the human infant. The human fetus increases its weight 6 billion times during gestation; during the last 6 months of gestation, fetal weight increases 100 times.[2] Maternal blood supplies the fetus with many macro- and micro-nutrients, including nucleic acids, minerals, and vitamins.[3-5]

---

*Present estimates in 1983 are higher than these.

Therefore, the fetal environment is dependent upon the medical and general care given to the mother and upon the socioeconomic status of the entire family.

UNDERNUTRITION AND LOW BIRTH WEIGHT

Approximately 15% of successful pregnancies result in low birth weight (LBW) infants (less than 2500 g at delivery).[6] This includes those born before completion of 37 weeks of gestation and those born at full-term who have suffered intrauterine growth retardation. Studies conducted among urban poor in the United States have identified maternal undernutrition as a prime cause of intrauterine growth retardation.[7] Furthermore, fetal malnutrition may account for up to 6% of all neonatal deaths.[8]

In industrial societies, although strongly associated with small initial maternal size and low weight gain during pregnancy, LBW usually is attributable to specific pathologic conditions such as maternal hypertension, heavy maternal cigarette smoking, multiple pregnancies, or fetal malformations.[9–12] Maternal malnutrition combined with infection further adversely affects fetal growth.[13] Surviving LBW babies are a tremendous burden on society, since they are usually mentally retarded. The cost of upkeep of such an individual throughout his lifetime has been estimated to exceed $100,000, whereas $100 spent towards supplementation of the maternal diet during the last 4 weeks of pregnancy would probably do much to reduce the incidence of intrauterine growth retardation.[14] Indeed, recent studies have shown that an adequate food supply during the last 4 weeks of pregnancy increases the birth weight by about 300 g.[15] Extensive studies performed in preindustrialized countries, including India, Indonesia, Mexico, Colombia and Guatemala, confirm that improvement in nutritional status during pregnancy decreases the incidence of LBW and perinatal infant mortality.[15,16]

Undernutrition in pregnant women may spring not only from unfortunate socioeconomic conditions but also from misguided concepts of nutrition and excessive dieting.[17,18] Excessive dieting leads to lack of essential amino acids, vitamins,[19,20] and metals, including copper,[21] zinc,[22] and magnesium.[23] The National Academy of Sciences currently recommends that weight gain during pregnancy should average 24 lb, with a range of 20 lb to 25 lb.[24]

UNDERNUTRITION AND BRAIN DEVELOPMENT

The effects of undernutrition on brain development and intellectual competence are numerous and complex.[25–27] Furthermore, the environmental deprivations of poverty, ignorance, poor sanitation, and recurrent infections may act with nutrition to affect adversely the development of the central nervous system (CNS).[28,29]

Since two thirds of the brain cells of the adult human being are present at birth, and the remaining one third develops within the first 12 months of extrauterine life, the timing of undernutrition is of critical importance to brain development.[30,31] In marasmic infants dying within the first year of life, brain weight, total protein, total RNA, total cholesterol, total phospholipid, and total DNA content are proportionally reduced.[32,33] Therefore, there is a slowed rate of DNA synthesis and cell division, resulting in a decreased number of brain cells in the cerebrum, cerebellum, and brain stem.[34] Animal investigations have demonstrated that the sensitive cortex may be more adversely affected by undernutrition than is the brain as a whole.[35] Such undernutrition occurring early in life, during the hyperplastic stage of brain growth, results in a reduced number of brain cells—the size, lipid, and RNA contents of which are normal. Persistence of undernutrition beyond 8 months to 12 months of age results in a smaller number of cells with reduced size and lipid content.[36]

Recent investigations have dealt with the role of trace metals in the development of the CNS. Copper-deficient suckling rats show decreased whole brain and cerebellum growth, with reduction in the extent of myelination.[37] Parallels have been drawn between this experimental model and Menkes' kinky hair disease, a sex-linked recessive disorder characterized by growth retardation and cerebral and cerebellar degeneration owing to copper malabsorption. Prenatal[38] and postnatal[39] zinc deficiency results in decreased brain weight, DNA, RNA, and protein content, and in impaired psychological development.

In a manner similar to the effects on biochemical development, the timing and severity of undernutrition are important to intellectual development.[40–42] Severe undernutrition within the first 6 months of life has been shown to retard intellectual development,[41] whereas undernutrition occurring late in life does not seem to have as adverse an effect on intelligence.[36] Similarly, infants rehabilitated from undernutrition during the first 4 months of life have a much better chance of normal development than those rehabilitated later in infancy.[36]

EXTREME FORMS OF UNDERNUTRITION IN CHILDHOOD

Undernutrition in childhood may vary from a mild disorder to a critical, life-threatening illness. The extreme forms of undernutrition in childhood generally have been classified as being of two types: marasmus and

kwashiorkor. By definition, *marasmus* is a condition caused by markedly low intake of both calories and protein, resulting in tissue-wasting and growth failure. The condition is usually observed in very young children who have been weaned very early or who have never been breast fed. Because of the growth failure, they often seem to be younger than their chronologic age. Curiously, the biochemical indices of undernutrition, such as the serum protein concentrations, are generally not markedly abnormal. A child with marasmus is shown in Figure 38-1.

Kwashiorkor, in contrast to marasmus, is due to deficient protein intake with maintenance of generally adequate caloric intake. This condition is usually observed following weaning when the protein intake is sharply curtailed. These children exhibit growth fail-

ure, edema, hair loss, change in hair color to a blond or reddish hue, and fatty liver. There are profound decreases in the serum albumin concentrations and other indices of malnutrition. An example of kwashiorkor is shown in Figure 38-2.

ANEMIA IN PREGNANCY

Anemia occurs often in pregnancy generally as a result of iron and folic acid deficiency, either singly or in combination. In many women not previously suspected of being iron-deficient, the hemoglobin concentration remains below normal for as long as a year after delivery. The total depletion of iron owing to childbirth and lactation for 6 months amounts to approximately

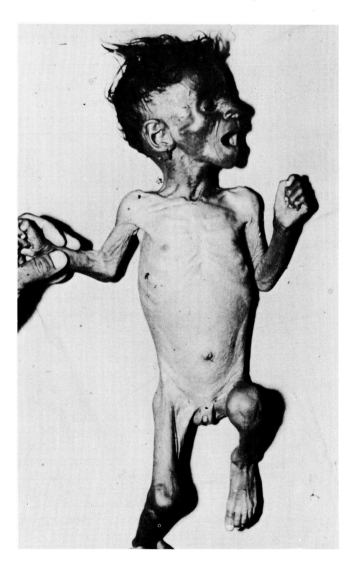

Fig. 38-1. Photograph of a child with marasmus, illustrating the extreme degree of tissue wasting and inanition. (From Winick M: Malnutrition and Brain Development, p 169. New York, Oxford University Press, 1975)

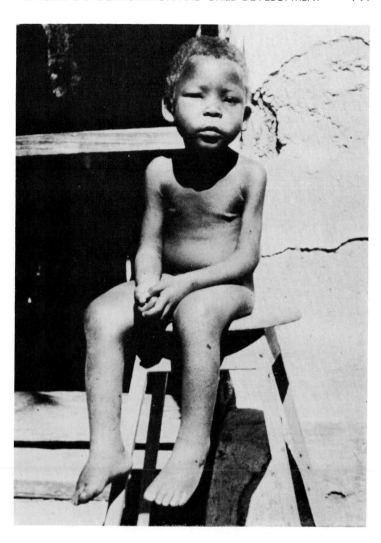

Fig. 38-2. Photograph of a child with kwashiorkor, illustrating the facial, abdominal, and ankle edema and lethargy. (From Winick M: Malnutrition and Brain Development, p 8. New York, Oxford University Press, 1975)

905 mg.[43] Deficiency of folate is also extremely common. In Finland, 50% of samples of serum and 25% of samples of bone marrow from pregnant women show evidence of folate deficiency.[44] It is important to note that iron stores in women receiving both iron and folic acid during pregnancy were better preserved than in those women for whom iron alone was prescribed.[44] Iron deficiency results from poor nutrition prior to pregnancy, and additionally because of poor absorption towards the end of pregnancy.[45–49] Folic acid and iron therapy during pregnancy are highly recommended and are widely used in modern medical practice.[50]

BREAST VERSUS ARTIFICAL FEEDING

A basic question pertaining to postnatal nutrition is whether there are advantages of breast over artificial feeding. Breast feeding is the oldest method and in many ways the most satisfying from nutritional and psychological points of view. In agrarian and nomadic societies, there is virtually no substitute available for breast feeding. In industrial societies, a major drawback to breast feeding exists for mothers working away from home.[51]

A variety of formulas has been developed, which permits adequate nutritional intake for bottle-fed infants. Even seriously ill infants may respond well to mixtures of L-amino acids, dextrose, and other nutrients.[52] Satisfactory formulas may be prepared using soya protein, medium-chain triglycerides, polyunsaturated fatty acids, and glucose.[53] Many medical scientists believe that breast feeding is superior to artificial feeding, that there should be a ban on the advertising of formulas, and that formulas should be available only by prescription.

Breast feeding might be practiced more widely in industrialized countries if the period of hospitalization for delivery were not so short. It might be necessary to provide 10 to 15 days of experienced and encouraging support before a successful pattern of milk production and feeding by the mother is ensured.[54] Breast-fed babies often have a greater initial weight gain than do bottle-fed babies, particularly if solid food supplementation is made before 4 months of age. While rapid weight gain may be advantageous in a variety of circumstances, it must be pointed out that obesity in adult life is strongly correlated with breast feeding during infancy.[55]

In considering the influence of the postnatal period upon the nutrition of the newborn, one should not neglect its effect upon the nutrition of the nursing mother. The energy cost of lactation is considerable, and milk production of 840 ml per day requires a maternal daily caloric intake of 1000 kcal containing 40 g protein.[51] Where the mother has had marginal dietary intake during pregnancy, the process of nursing may compromise her medical status even further.

After weaning, maternal influences upon the child's nutritional intake remain strong.[56-59] The mother's attitudes toward eating, her own habits and patterns, her body weight, and her knowlege or ignorance of the entire subject of nutrition have profound effects upon the growing child with respect to both physical and mental development.[60]

CHILD ABUSE

A special form of undernutrition that is being recognized increasingly as a national problem is that due to child abuse and neglect. It has been estimated that at least 200,000 children a year die in the United States as a result of some form of child abuse. The physical abuse given children attracts wide attention, but systematic starvation and refusal to feed them properly are often hidden from public view. The late consequences of such actions may be profound.[61]

UNDERNUTRITION RESULTING FROM DRUG ADMINISTRATION

Untoward drug reactions that are dramatic and rapid in onset, such as anaphylaxis, leukopenia, or rash, promptly gain the attention of the practicing physician. Less obvious signs and symptoms of drug usage often go unnoticed. The nutritional complications of drug usage are usually subtle, seemingly nonspecific, and protracted in course. It is only recently that these complications have come under careful and systematic scrutiny.[62-65]

It is important to recognize that drugs may cause undernutrition first by reducing food intake. This commonly occurs when the drug produces anorexia. Loss of appetite is such a common symptom in clinical medicine that physicians often fail to search for an underlying mechanism. When nausea and vomiting are produced by drugs, food intake is reduced further, and the fluid and electrolyte loss may be enormous. Often drugs may limit food intake by causing a reduction or loss in taste acuities. A good example of this type of agent is penicillamine, which may cause loss of taste acuity by binding zinc and removing it from the body.[66] When food seems bland and tasteless, there may be little impetus to eat, at least in a given short-term period. Drugs may also cause loss of interest in eating by a central mechanism when the patient becomes anxious, depressed, withdrawn, or develops a more severe psychiatric disorder.[67]

Drugs may produce undernutrition by a wide variety of other mechanisms. These include interfering with intestinal absorption, binding to plasma proteins, transport across cell membranes, peripheral utilization, intracellular transformations, storage, turnover, elimination, or excretion.[62-65]

The signs and symptoms of undernutrition owing to specific drugs are determined in large part by the specific nutrients that are affected. Individuals whose dietary intake of nutrients is of marginal adequacy for economic or other circumstances would obviously be more susceptible to the effects of drugs. Special attention needs to be directed toward elderly patients, both because they constitute the largest group of drug users and also because of the likelihood that their rates of drug inactivation and excretion may be reduced.

SOME SIGNS AND SYMPTOMS OF UNDERNUTRITION RESULTING FROM DRUG ADMINISTRATION

Anorexia, as noted above, is commonly caused by drugs and should always be kept in mind as an indication of drug effects when a patient reports decreased food intake or unexpected weight loss. Questioning the patient about associated symptoms and obtaining a careful history of temporal relationships to the initiation of drug therapy may prove useful in arriving at a diagnosis.

Weight loss can be produced by a variety of other mechanisms. Malabsorption, as for example that produced by cathartics, can limit utilization of essential nutrients and accelerate their loss through the gastrointestinal tract.[68,69] Fever of "unknown origin" is frequently caused by drugs.[70] If protracted, fever would be expected to increase nutritional requirements, resulting in loss of weight if food consumption is not increased. Thyroid hormones given in large amounts

as drugs induce loss of weight that is composed predominantly of nitrogen and calcium.[71] The final common path in the pathogenesis of weight loss due to drugs is generally protein-calorie undernutrition. In children, weight loss caused by drugs is often associated with growth retardation.

Anemia is often produced by drugs, and its origins may be multifactorial. Amethopterin (methotrexate), a folic acid antagonist used in the treatment of a number of neoplasms, produces a megaloblastic anemia.[72] Drugs such as hydralazine, cycloserine, and isoniazid, which interfere with the metabolism of pyridoxal phosphate (vitamin B_6), may produce a hypochromic, microcytic anemia which is sideroblastic in form.[73] Pyridoxal phosphate is required for activity by δ-aminolevulinic acid synthetase, a critical enzyme involved in the formation of heme.[74] Drugs may produce deficiency of vitamin B_{12}, resulting in anemia virtually identical in appearance to that resulting from deficiency of folic acid. Drugs that interfere with the absorption of vitamin B_{12}, and hence its availability in the bone marrow, include cholestyramine, neomycin, para-amino salicylic acid, colchicine, and biguanide derivatives.[75] Drugs that interfere with the absorption or metabolism of vitamin K, such as cholestyramine, and anticonvulsants and aspirin,[76] promote hemorrhagic tendencies that led to blood depletion. Anemia may also result from a variety of other mechanisms. Prolonged protein-caloric shortages induced by drugs are also of critical importance in the development of anemia.

Dermatitis is a symptom that is frequently due to deficiencies of vitamin C or of one or more of the B vitamins. Scaly skin lesions occurring in areas exposed to light are suggestive of niacin deficiency.[77] In general, however, the skin lesions owing to deficiencies of the B vitamins are not specific or characteristic.[78] Rash, particularly a pruritic rash, is a frequent side effect of many drugs, and excoriated skin lesions may confuse recognition of an underlying nutritional etiology.

Dermatitis, cheilosis, and angular stomatitis are frequently seen as symptoms of deficiency of one or more of the B vitamins, particularly niacin, riboflavin, or B_6. In patients with marginal dietary intake of the B vitamins, these skin abnormalities could be produced by drugs that interfere with vitamin metabolism. Soreness and redness of the tongue may be observed with drugs that induce deficiencies of folate or B_{12}.

Diarrhea is another symptom that may be caused by drug administration. Often the mechanism is not clearly defined. In some instances, malabsorption is an accompaniment of diarrhea. The losses of fluids, electrolytes, and other nutrients may be enormous with prolonged, drug-induced diarrhea.

Symptoms and signs owing to malabsorption of a specific nutrient may be produced by a variety of mechanisms. For example, mineral oil, commonly used as a laxative, dissolves vitamins A, D, and K and leads to dietary deficiencies of these vitamins.[68,79] Cholestyramine, a drug used to lower serum cholesterol in cases of hypercholesterolemia or to treat pruritus in patients with liver disease, binds bile salts and other nutrients to yield deficiencies of fat-soluble vitamins, B_{12}, and iron.[80] Phenformin, an oral agent used in the management of adult-onset diabetes, is a competitive inhibitor of B_{12} absorption from the small intestine.[81]

DRUG EFFECTS UPON SOME SPECIFIC NUTRIENTS

Niacin. Deficiency of niacin in an extreme form leads to pellagra, with its classical symptom complex of dermatitis, diarrhea, dementia, and death. Lesser degrees of deficiency produce weakness, general malaise, and gastrointestinal dysfunction. Niacin is unusual among the vitamins in that it can be synthesized by the body: Tryptophan is converted by a series of reactions to niacin.[77] When niacin intake is marginal, adequate tryptophan in the diet prevents niacin deficiency from occurring. The conversion of tryptophan to niacin requires pyridoxine. In patients receiving chemotherapy for tuberculosis with isoniazid, a pyridoxine antagonist, symptoms of niacin deficiency may result. In this fashion, deficiency of one vitamin produced by a drug may lead to deficiency of an additional vitamin.[82]

Riboflavin. Riboflavin deficiency is generally observed in association with deficiencies of other B vitamins. Signs and symptoms of riboflavin deficiency are not pathognomonic and include soreness and burning of the lips, mouth, and tongue; photophobia; lacrimation; cheilosis; angular stomatitis; seborrheic dermatitis; glossitis; and superficial vascularization of the cornea.[78]

In experimental animals riboflavin deficiency can be specifically produced by administration of boric acid. This agent forms a one-to-one complex with riboflavin with high affinity, removes the vitamin from the circulation, and increases its excretion.[83] The effect of acute ingestion of boric acid upon increasing the urinary excretion of riboflavin is shown in Figure 38-3. These findings raise the possibility that chronic use of boric acid therapeutically, or toxicity owing to boric acid, could precipitate a state of riboflavin deficiency in man.

Iron. Symptoms and signs of iron deficiency are due largely to the production of anemia and to the epithelial changes that occur secondarily in the skin, nails, mouth, and gastrointestinal tract. Iron deficiency typically results either from a reduction in oral intake or from acceleration of iron loss. Drugs may produce iron deficiency by both of these mechanisms. Sodium

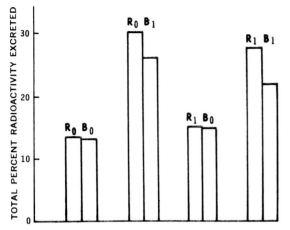

Fig. 38-3. Total percentage of $2\text{-}^{14}\text{C}$-riboflavin excreted in rat urine after two injections in rats on a diet deficient in riboflavin (R_0) or supplemented with riboflavin (R_1), without (B_0) and with (B_1) boric acid. The addition of boric acid to the diet increased the excretion of radioactive riboflavin in both the riboflavin-deficient and riboflavin-supplemented animals. (Adapted from Roe DA, McCormick DB, Lin RT: Effects of riboflavin on boric acid toxicity. J Pharm Sci 61:108, 1972)

bicarbonate administered to experimental animals reduces the rate of iron absorption.[84] If enough gastric acid is neutralized, dietary iron absorption is impaired. Gastric acid appears to be involved in facilitating the reaction of dietary iron with low molecular weight ligands to form soluble complexes that can be easily absorbed. In the absence of sufficient gastric acid, iron is polymerized and precipitated rather than absorbed.[85] Because gastric acid production declines with age, sodium bicarbonate therapy would be of particular relevance in older patients as a potential cause of iron deficiency.

Acceleration of iron loss from the body occurs frequently as a result of gastrointestinal bleeding. An important drug to be considered here is aspirin. Certain patients with preexisting gastric disorders, such as peptic ulcer and alcoholic gastritis, may be unusually susceptible to the effects of small doses of aspirin. Of even greater concern is the fact that daily doses of approximately 1 g to 3 g are likely to produce some degree of blood loss even in normal subjects.[86] In most cases, blood loss is occult, but the potential for major loss of blood is always present. The etiology of the blood loss owing to aspirin is probably related both to direct effects upon the gastric mucosa and to systemic effects upon blood coagulation.

Zinc. Deficiency of zinc may result in a variety of clinical manifestations including disturbances in vitamin A metabolism, delay in wound healing, loss of taste sensation, impairment of function of certain key metalloenzymes, and possible growth and reproductive failure. As noted above, zinc deficiency may result from the administration of penicillamine, a chelating agent used to remove excess copper from the body in patients with Wilson's disease.[66] A number of individuals treated with penicillamine have reported disturbances of taste, which appear to be due to the binding and removal of zinc by this drug. Thus, a drug employed to remove a toxic amount of one metal may result in signs and symptoms owing to depletion of a second metal.

Magnesium. Deficiency of magnesium is being recognized more frequently in daily clinical practice. Symptoms and signs resulting from deficiency include anorexia, muscle weakness, nausea and vomiting, seizures, and other metabolic and behavioral abnormalities. An example of drug-induced deficiency of this metal is that produced by long-term use of diuretics. The excretion of magnesium is increased by thiazide diuretics, ammonium chloride, and mercurial diuretics.[87] Loss of magnesium is probably related both to the dosage employed and to the duration of therapy. No doubt patients with borderline stores of magnesium would be especially sensitive to the effects of diuretics. If therapy with diuretics were sufficiently protracted, magnesium deficiency would probably be demonstrable in many subjects with previously normal magnesium stores.

UNDERNUTRITION PRODUCED BY CERTAIN DRUGS

Diphenylhydantoin. Folic acid deficiency is a well-recognized complication of therapy with diphenylhydantoin alone or in combination with other anticonvulsant drugs. In one study, serum folate levels lower than normal were detected in half of a large group of patients receiving diphenylhydantoin; low levels were noted most often in patients who had undergone a prolonged period of treatment.[88] A megaloblastic bone marrow and macrocytosis on peripheral smear may be observed prior to the development of symptomatic anemia. It is impressive that folate-deficient anemia may be a complication of drug therapy even in patients who are apparently eating an adequate diet.

The mechanisms of folate deficiency under these circumstances have been the subject of considerable study. Diphenyhydantoin was initially thought to reduce folate absorption from the gastrointestinal tract by inhibiting conjugase activity.[89] It now appears more likely that the drug increases pH within the gastrointestinal tract and that this effect accounts for reduced folate

absorption.[90] In addition, diphenylhydantoin may interfere with the conversion of folic acid into its more metabolically active form, 5-methyltetrahydrofolate. In any event, the clinician caring for epileptic patients who require long-term therapy with anticonvulsants should follow the hematologic status closely and should consider giving supplemental folic acid.

It should be recalled that folic acid deficiency is not the only form of undernutrition produced by diphenylhydantoin. There is increasing evidence that bone disease in the form of rickets or osteomalacia may also be complications of long-term therapy with this drug. Serum calcium levels may be reduced and serum alkaline phosphatase activities elevated in as many as one fourth of patients receiving therapy. Reduced calcium content of bone has been demonstrated by several techniques, and abnormalities, initially subtle but later more obvious, may be visible on radiologic examination.[91] In the past when epileptic patients sustained bone fractures, they were attributed to injuries during the periods of uncontrolled movements. The contemporary physician now has to consider the likelihood that the bones were weak initially and therefore more susceptible to traumatic injury.

Oral Contraceptives. The metabolic effects of oral contraceptives, such as worsening glucose tolerance and elevating blood lipid concentrations, have been increasingly recognized. Folate deficiency is now regarded as another important complication of therapy. Women receiving oral contraceptive drugs have lower serum and blood cell folate concentrations and higher urinary excretions of forminimoglutamic acid (FIGLU) than do normal controls.[92] These abnormalities are most pronounced in women with dietary inadequacies.[93] Within 3 months of discontinuation of therapy, folate concentrations can be restored to normal. The exact mechanisms accounting for folic acid deficiency are unknown but are probably multiple, involving changes in intestinal absorption, metabolism, binding, and excretion.

A large number of other nutritional effects of oral contraceptives have been described recently, and the list will probably continue to increase.[62,94] The urinary excretion of thiamine and riboflavin was reported to increase in certain groups of women and the plasma concentrations of pyridoxal phosphate to diminish.[95] That oral contraceptive drugs may alter the storage and distribution of vitamin A is suggested by the observation in experimental animals that plasma levels of the vitamin are increased but hepatic concentrations are markedly reduced. Reductions in the plasma concentrations of vitamins C, B_{12}, riboflavin, and pyridoxine have been observed in drug users.[96] Vitamin C

concentrations were noted to decrease both in serum and in platelets.[97] Zinc concentrations were increased in red cells but decreased in plasma. By contrast, plasma concentrations of copper were increased.[98]

The physiologic significance of these findings is currently under study, and it is apparent that they have important implications for therapy of women in high socioeconomic groups but particularly for those in impoverished circumstances.

UNDERNUTRITION IN CANCER

WEIGHT LOSS AND ANOREXIA

Unexplained weight loss is one of the classic symptoms of cancer. A patient may report to his family physician that despite apparently maintaining his usual dietary intake and exercise patterns, his weight has gradually decreased over a period of time. Frequently the exact time of onset of the weight loss is unclear to the patient, perhaps because he is otherwise well. Should cancer be searched for in such a patient, one might find a solitary coin lesion on chest radiograph, or a polyp on radiographic examination of the gastrointestinal tract. These small, innocent-looking lesions hardly seem likely to be responsible for the extensive amount of weight loss that the patient may demonstrate in the early stages of his disease, and yet, time after time, weight loss has been the initial, presenting complaint of a patient with cancer.

Other individuals with cancer have weight loss that seems to occur concomitantly with other clinical manifestations as a part of a major severe illness. In very advanced cancer, several factors may contribute to weight loss, including anorexia, nausea, and vomiting. In some neoplastic diseases, particularly lymphoma, there is diminished intestinal absorption, leading to impaired utilization of dietary nutrients. When hemorrhage occurs, the body is depleted of iron, electrolytes, and protein. Ulceration and necrosis of tissues lead to further loss of nutrients. When infection occurs, the nutritional reserves are strained additionally. Hypoalbuminemia may be the result of disturbances in hepatic metabolism as well as of dietary inadequacy.[99,100]

The pattern of weight loss in cancer is variable. In some patients who have a myopathy in association with cancer, specific muscle groups, usually the proximal muscles, may become atrophic and account for some of the weight loss. In the usual patient with myopathy, the weakness is far out of proportion to the degree of muscle atrophy demonstrable.[101] The patient often has a gaunt or haggard appearance owing to the loss of the temporalis muscles. There are a variety of histo-

logic findings in these cases; one observation is that in patients with cancer of the breast or colon, biopsies have revealed a marked decrease in the fat content within muscle.[102] Usually there are no signs of a specific vitamin deficiency, and cheilosis, angular stomatitis, and dermatitis are distinctly uncommon.

Anorexia must also be regarded as a classic symptom of cancer, and its origin is usually obscure. Many patients report that they do not feel like eating, and others report smaller appetites. Some patients say that food does not taste very good to them and that they have a persistently bad taste in their mouths. This symptom complex has recently come under investigation, and a report[103] suggests that distortions of taste occur in some patients with cancer. The role of taste and smell in cancer needs to be investigated more fully, because defects of these sensations could explain some of the anorexia and could possibly be treated. This problem is under active investigation in a number of laboratories at present. Thus, nutritional factors are involved both in cancer prevention and treatment.[104–106]

In experimental animals bearing transplanted tumors, food consumption patterns are altered. The amount of food consumed gradually diminishes with increasing size of the tumor.[107] Normally, if the nutrient density of the diet offered to an animal is reduced, the animal increases its bulk intake so that the total intake of nutrients is kept relatively constant. During the growth of Walker 256 carcinosarcoma, Sprague–Dawley rats progressively lose their ability to increase bulk intake in response to reduced nutrient density of the diet, and nutritional intake therefore falls. Frequency and duration of feeding appear to decrease early in the course of tumor growth.[102] It will be of interest to determine whether disturbances in the recognition of dietary signals may be a feature of early cancer in man.

Chemotherapy further intensifies the undernutrition that may be present in the cancer patient. Anorexia, nausea, and vomiting become more prolonged and severe. Fever, by increasing the metabolic rate, increases the caloric requirement. Certain drugs, such as amethopterin (methotrexate), produce a deficiency of folic acid.[108] Other drugs, such as actinomycin D, inhibit RNA synthesis and have complex effects upon protein metabolism.[109] The nutritional state of the patient is profoundly altered by chemotherapy. Several considerations also suggest that the response to chemotherapy may depend upon the vitamin status of the patient prior to treatment.[110,111]

MECHANISMS OF WEIGHT LOSS

The mechanisms of weight loss in the uncomplicated cancer patient remain obscure. An early view, and one which still may have some relevance, is that tumors function as "nitrogen traps," taking up and retaining amino acids from the blood and depleting the host tissues.[112,113] The term *trap* implies that uptake into the tumor is accelerated, whereas in fact protein metabolism is disturbed at numerous sites in intermediary metabolism, including synthesis of enzymes, endocrine control of enzyme activity, turnover of substances, and so on.[114] What is apparent is that the growth of the tumor tissue is generally more resistant to dietary deprivation than that of normal tissues.

Tumors also appear to be relatively more resistant than host tissues to vitamin deficiency. When hepatomas are grown experimentally in the riboflavin-deficient rat, the concentrations of the coenzymes flavin mononucleotide and flavin-adenine dinucleotide are markedly depleted in the host liver. By contrast, in samples of hepatoma from riboflavin-deficient rats, flavin mononucleotide concentrations are only slightly reduced and those of flavin adenine dinucleotide reduced not at all.[115,116] The extent to which these and other mechanisms are operative in human cancer is under study at present.

From time to time, humoral agents, which may be implicated in producing undernutrition in the host, have been extracted from tumors. In one such report,[117] mouse Ehrlich ascites carcinoma cells were fractionated with ammonium sulfate after homogenization. One of the fractions was injected into recipient mice, with a resulting fall in the serum albumin concentration within 24 hr. The physiologic significance of this observation is uncertain, especially since extracts prepared similarly from liver and spleen of normal animals also lowered serum albumin concentrations. The search continues in man for humoral substances that could produce cachexia.

UNDERNUTRITION AND TUMOR GROWTH

It is apparent that tumors produce complex disturbances in the nutritional status of the host and that once these disturbances occur, tumors generally seem better able to cope with them than do the host tissues. One may then ask whether undernutrition modifies tumor growth and proliferation. Evidence from animal experiments suggests that it does.

When tumors are transplanted into an animal in which caloric intake has been curtailed, the rate of growth of the tumor is greatly reduced compared to the rate of growth in normal animals. Dietary restriction decreases the incidence not only of transplanted tumors but also of spontaneous tumors and of tumors induced by carcinogens. These effects have been demonstrable with a wide variety of tumors and in several experimental animal species.[118–123]

For example, the frequency with which spontaneous mammary carcinomas appeared in a certain strain of mice was greatly reduced when the mice were subjected to severe caloric restriction.[124] Similarly, underfeeding of mice reduced the incidence of spontaneous lymphoid leukemia in a strain that has an otherwise high incidence of this spontaneous tumor.[125] In addition to reducing the incidence tumors, caloric restriction also delays the time at which lesions are first detectable.

These points are illustrated in Figure 38-4. The total numbers of sarcomas and skin tumors, induced by benzo(a)pyrene, as well as of naturally occurring mammary carcinomas in DBA mice, which were detected during observation periods of 24 weeks to 86 weeks, were less than one fourth in animals subjected to caloric restriction than in those permitted to feed *ad libitum*. The greatest effect of reduced caloric intake was on the appearance of mammary tumors.[126]

Restriction of the dietary supply of a specific vitamin or other nutrient similarly retards the development of spontaneous or induced tumors in animals. For example, in riboflavin-deficient animals, as recently summarized,[116] mammary tumors, lymphosarcoma, and Walker carcinoma exhibit reduced rates of growth. The effects of nutritional deprivation are probably operative at several stages of carcinogenesis. Both activation and inactivation of carcinogens may be altered by specific nutritional factors.[116,120]

Dietary fat and protein have also been implicated as factors that influence the growth rate of tumors. In rats, feeding a diet high in beef fat content greatly accelerated the development of intestinal tumors induced by azoxymethane.[127] Diets low in protein appear to reduce the incidence of tumors produced by certain carcinogens, but diets high in protein may also inhibit carcinogenesis, most notably that induced by 4-dimethylaminoazobenzene (DAB).[120]

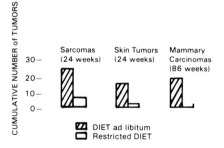

Fig. 38-4. The effect of restricted caloric intake in DBA mice on the incidence of sarcomas and skin tumors induced by benzo(a)pyrene, and of mammary tumors occurring naturally. (Adapted from Tannenbaum A: The genesis and growth of tumors. II. Effects of caloric restriction *per se*. Cancer Res 2:460, 1942)

If caloric restriction in experimental animals retards the development of tumors, should we make this recommendation for patients with established cancer, or as a measure for preventing cancer in the general population? The incidence of certain types of cancer in man—those of the endometrium, breast, gallbladder and possibly uterus—is in fact higher in obese than in lean individuals.[119] In a very provocative report,[128] forced feeding of a high-caloric diet in cancer patients may have accelerated tumor growth. It is apparent from these results that nutritional influences are complex and that no simple formulation of their effects on tumor growth can be made at present.

UNDERNUTRITION AND CANCER CAUSATION

The relation of diet and nutrition to cancer prevalence has become a subject of enormous popular interest. At a recent conference on this subject, it was estimated that as many as one half of all cancers in woman and one third of all cancers in men could be related to nutritional factors.[129] Several examples of these relationships are considered here briefly.

The prevalence of cancer of the colon shows very striking geographic variations, being very high in the United States and Western Europe and very low in the developing countries.[130] The diets consumed by these populations are obviously very different from one another, and attention has been focused on several characteristics of diets and their effects upon the gastrointestinal tract. In western countries, there is consumption of large quantities of fat and protein with carbohydrate supplied in the form of simple sugars. The western diet is, in fact, deficient in complex sugars, bran, and dietary fiber when compared to that of the developing countries. The fecal volume in the western countries is relatively small, its consistency relatively firm, and the transit time of ingested substances (the time required for substances to pass from mouth to anus) is markedly prolonged.[131] If transit time were prolonged, any carcinogens in the diet or generated by bacterial flora would have a more extended period of time in contact with the intestinal mucosa, thereby increasing the likelihood of carcinogenesis. Dietary fiber adds to the bulk of the stool, decreases the transit time, and appears to exert a protectve effect upon the development of colon cancer.

It is important to mention in this connection that carcinoma of the colon is not the only disease that has been related to deficiency of dietary fiber; others include chronic constipation, diverticulosis, cholelithiasis, hiatus hernia, and hemorrhoids. For years clinicians have been prescribing low-residue diets for elderly patients who have chronic constipation and diverticulosis with the expectation that stools would

become softer, bulkier, and less troublesome. It now appears more likely that these objectives can be obtained by feeding a high-residue diet, which contains large amounts of bran and fiber.

The pathogenesis of colon cancer in terms of nutrition is multifactorial, and it is likely that deficiency of dietary fiber interacts with other variables. Bile acids are now believed to be involved in the production of colon cancer, probably by their being degraded by bacteria within the lumen to carcinogenic phenanthrene derivatives. The incidence of colon carcinoma in several population groups is proportional to the total fecal content of dihydroxycholanic acid.[132] Feeding fiber to patients may modify the pattern of bile salt metabolites in the direction of less active carcinogens. Dietary fiber, in addition, binds bile salts. These two actions of fiber may have additional benefits in protecting against colon cancer.[133-135]

Many other nutritional factors are currently under study to determine their possible roles in the causation of human cancer. Much interest is currently being directed towards vitamin A deficiency in man as a possible factor in carcinogenesis, and vitamin A administration as a protective factor against cancer development.[136] This direction of research derives much of its impetus from renewed attention paid to early observations, such as those by Orten and associates that vitamin A deficiency in rats increased the incidence of odontomas.[137]

In addition, the high incidence of gastric cancer in Japan and its recent decline,[138] together with evidence that Japanese moving to western countries have a reduced incidence of this neoplasm, constitute a strong case for dietary factors being involved in gastration. Nitrites derived from dietary nitrates may be one of the relevant factors here, and the concentrations of nitrates in the soil and nitrites added as a preservative in foods are coming under increased scrutiny.[123]

UNDERNUTRITION AND AGING

Undernutrition in the aged population is a serious problem largely because the aged are often impoverished, isolated, and neglected. In addition, many of the physiologic changes that occur with age impair the utilization of dietary nutrients. With an increased number of aged persons in contemporary society, greater attention needs to be directed towards their specific nutritional problems.

Any systematic approach to investigating undernutrition in the elderly must face the problem of defining which changes in metabolism are physiologic and which are pathologic. Do the findings in a group of 90-year-

olds represent the last stages in a particular process, or are they the very qualities that have enabled the individuals to survive for so long? Only by a series of long-term prospective analyses can these questions be answered.[139]

ANIMAL INVESTIGATIONS ON FOOD CONSUMPTION

Research on nutrition in the elderly may be handicapped by the difficulty in finding a suitable animal model. The rat, for example, unlike man, does not have an adolescent growth spurt but continues to grow throughout its lifetime. Nevertheless, one has to study experimental animals in the hope that they will provide insights into the aging process in man. Research on aging requires definition of an animal model system with respect to both genetic and environmental variables and needs meticulous observations on the animals during their full natural lifetime.[140]

One interesting approach to studying nutrition in the experimental animal has been to correlate the quantity of food consumed with life expectancy. While excessive food restriction is detrimental in many ways, overindulgence also limits life expectancy. Studies in laboratory rats permitted to feed *ad libitum* have clearly shown that those animals that choose larger amounts of food to eat have considerably shorter survival times than those animals that choose smaller amounts to eat.[141] Results of some of the experiments are shown in Figure 38-5. Animals that ate 24 g of food per day survived an average of less than 500 days, compared to nearly

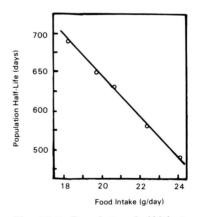

Fig. 38-5. Population half-life in days as a function of amount of food consumed by male rats during the 100–199-day age interval when allowed to feed *ad libitum*. Population half-life was estimated from the percent survival curves. (Adapted from Ross MH: Nutrition and longevity in experimental animals. In Winick M (ed): Current Concepts in Nutrition, Vol 4, Nutrition and Aging, p 45. New York, John Wiley & Sons, 1976)

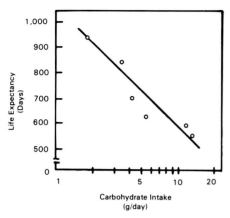

Fig. 38-6. Life expectancy in days expressed as a function of mean daily intake of carbohydrate in male rats fed either *ad libitum* or restricted amounts of three complete purified diets differing only in their protein:carbohydrate ratio. The regimens were maintained throughout life beginning at 21 days of age. (Adapted from Ross MH: Nutrition and longevity in experimental animals. In Winick M (ed): Current Concepts in Nutrition, Vol 4, Nutrition and Aging, p 45. New York, John Wiley & Sons, 1976)

700 days for rats whose food consumption was 25% less. Animals seem to establish their patterns of food intake relatively early in life, and it is in the period of 100 days to 200 days after birth that caloric intake has its greatest influence on the eventual life span. At ages later than these, the amount of food consumed correlates poorly with the span of life.[142] Early and rapid growth of the animal appears to be associated with failure to achieve the maximum life span.

The quality of the diet also has an important influence on the life expectancy: the greater the carbohydrate intake per day, the shorter the life expectancy. This point is illustrated in Figure 38-6. In animals fed *ad libitum* whose carbohydrate intake was approximately 12 g per day, mean life expectancy was slightly greater than 500 days. By contrast, in animals subjected to restriction of carbohydrate intake to 2 g per day, mean life expectancy was greater than 900 days.[143]

The central question about these studies is how relevant they are for man and the extent to which they should form the basis for establishing nutritional guidelines for our elderly population.[144]

NUTRITION AND LONGEVITY IN MAN

There recently was a great deal of interest in certain specific areas of the world where a number of the inhabitants were reported to live to extreme old age, including some who lived to well over 100 years. Unfortunately, it now appears that these three popu-

lation groups are not as old as originally thought, but the research still provides interesting insights into the relationship between nutrition and longevity.

These locations were (1) a village in Ecuador, (2) a district in the Caucasus Mountains in Russia, and (3) the Hunza province in Kashmir—regions that are distinct from one another geographically and genetically.[145] Food practices were studied, and it was estimated that the elderly Russians consume an average of 1800 kcal per day and that the population in the Hunza province about 1900 kcal per day. These figures are generally about 25% lower than the caloric intake recommended for the elderly United States population and are certainly suggestive of some degree of voluntary caloric restriction. In Ecuador, mean caloric intake has been estimated to be only 1200 kcal per day.

The nature of the diet eaten by the elderly population of the three regions is obviously of great interest. In Ecuador, the community is agricultural, raises its own vegetables and grain, and the diet is almost exclusively vegetarian. The population in Hunza also consumes a vegetarian diet with only tiny quantities of animal fat and protein. Symptoms and signs of malnutrition have apparently not been prominent in any of these groups, and teeth are frequently in remarkably good condition. What is striking about the type of diet consumed by the aged in the Caucasus mountains, in contrast to that of the other two groups, is that their consumption of animal fats and proteins is very high, including liberal amounts of milk, cheese, and yogurt.

Obviously much needs to be learned about these isolated population groups before generalizations applicable to the world population as a whole can be made. One feature that seems to characterize the lifestyles of all three population groups is a high degree of physical activity, which extends throughout their entire lifetimes. This includes strenuous work and long walks in difficult terrain. Many of the elderly continue a full day's work in the farm and field that is equal to the work of younger laborers.

Physiologic Changes with Aging and Their Implication for Nutrition

In aged animals and in elderly people, protein stores and lean body masses are reduced below levels found in the young,[146,147] especially with respect to the muscle mass.[148] It has generally been thought that the reduction in lean body mass is a progressive process that occurs as the individual ages. In support of this view is the evidence that the total amount of protein synthesized per day decreases in elderly individuals.[149]

Recently this concept has been challenged by the findings in a longitudinal study in rats.[150] While it was true that the older rats as a group had lower lean body

masses than the group of younger rats, those animals that were studied at several different ages showed no significant changes in their lean body mass. That is, the elderly survivors consisted of the animals that had relatively low lean body mass when they were younger. These results suggest that longevity may be greater in animals that have a low lean body mass during the period of their rapid growth and development rather than that lean body mass declines with age. It is important to determine the nature of any alterations in body protein metabolism with aging in order to define appropriately the amino acid and protein requirements for elderly persons.

The physiologic changes that occur with age are complex and involve virtually every organ system. These have recently been reviewed in a comprehensive fashion.[151-153] Attention needs to be directed towards several specific mechanisms that could account for undernutrition in the elderly and could produce symptomatology. Gastric acid production decreases with age. This could be a significant factor in the etiology of iron deficiency in the elderly. The incidence of achlorhydria may be as high as 20% to 30% in the population over 60 years of age.[154] In addition, digestive secretions decrease with age.[155] This may be a factor resulting in diminished efficiency of digestion, although it is difficult to quantitate the magnitude of the effect. The excretion of D-xylose in urine after an oral load, a measurement of the absorptive capacity of the small intestine, apparently remains virtually unchanged until after the age of 80.[156] Thus, malabsorption of dietary nutrients might not occur until extreme old age. The fact that calcium absorption across the small intestine diminishes with aging[157] suggests a possible factor involved in the development of osteoporosis. The pathogenesis of osteoporosis remains controversial. Recent findings in experimental animals indicate that in addition to calcium balance, one must also consider phosphorus balance, since an excess in the phosphorus-to-calcium content of the diet may accelerate loss of bone.[158] One problem with contemporary American diets is that the processed cheeses, snack foods, and soft drinks contain extremely high quantities of phosphorus.[159]

The signs and symptoms of osteoporosis are largely familiar. One theory is that periodontal disease may be a manifestation of osteoporosis and is often one of the earliest symptoms to appear. Loss of teeth is not necessarily a nonspecific feature of aging but rather may be due to weakening of bone in the supporting tooth structures. Clinically and histologically, the process consists of areas of demineralization in the alveolar bone of the mandible.[160] With progressive damage to these structures, infection and hemorrhage develop. It appears likely that periodontal disease may

respond to therapy with calcium, and the effect of calcium therapy on the reversal of osteoporosis is currently under active study. All authorities have agreed on the necessity for making an early diagnosis of osteoporosis if therapy is to be maximally effective. Once compression fractures of the spine have occurred, it is possible that the disease process can be halted, but it is unlikely that it can be reversed. Prevention of osteoporosis may be even more important. The etiology of osteoporosis is complex, but several considerations suggest that nutritional factors (calcium, protein, fluoride, vitamin D, and vitamin A) may play a role in prevention.[61,62]

The points briefly discussed here are only a few of the many ways in which the diet of the elderly influences their nutritional status and their health. Atherosclerosis and its relation to dietary cholesterol and lipid intake is a major subject in itself. Some degree of voluntary undernutrition to the extent of preventing obesity doubtless would be beneficial, inasmuch as obesity appears to worsen glucose tolerance, increase cholesterol production, and elevate serum triglyceride levels.[163,164]

Undernutrition in the Elderly Owing to Psychosocial Factors

Undernutrition in elderly individuals probably is derived less from physiologic than from psychosocial factors. The elderly frequently live and eat alone, subsisting on a fixed income, with limited physical mobility and little impetus to care for themselves. Economies in the quality and quantity of foods consumed must, of necessity, be made.

Evidence that undernutrition is widespread in the elderly has been obtained in a wide range of studies. In one recent investigation of the nutritional status of elderly persons in Tennessee of varying educational and social backgrounds, a spectrum of differences in the adequacy of dietary intake was documented. In black females, protein intake was only 70% of that considered satisfactory according to the recommended dietary allowances of the National Research Council. In this group, calcium intake was 58% of that considered satisfactory, and the intakes of iron, vitamin A, thiamine, and riboflavin were only 23% to 46% of satisfactory levels. Black males consumed slightly greater amounts of each of these items than did black females, but no item was entirely adequate in amount. Dietary inadequacies were enormously more common in those persons with no formal education than in those with a college degree.[165] Other recent studies confirm dietary inadequacies in the older population.[166,167]

This study clearly focuses upon the magnitide of the nutritional problems in the elderly population of the

United States and suggests that supervised food distribution in a socialized environment would be most beneficial.

UNDERNUTRITION AND HORMONES

GROWTH HORMONE

One of the earliest features of protein-calorie malnutrition (PCM) is retardation of growth.[25] The relationship between this growth retardation and growth hormone production has been a subject of considerable controversy in the literature. Studies of the pathology of the pituitary gland have revealed a decrease in the number of anterior lobe acidophils in severely malnourished children.[168] Experimental work has suggested that there is a reduction in the growth hormone content of the anterior pituitaries of protein-deficient animals,[169] possibly owing to a lack of stimulation by the hypothalamic growth hormone releasing factor.[170] Furthermore, weight gain and concomitant nitrogen, potassium, and phosphorus retention have been reported in malnourished infants during the administration of exogenous growth hormone, suggesting that adequate pituitary stimulation of peripheral tissues may have been lacking in the untreated patients.[171]

By contrast, high-plasma levels of growth hormone (HGH) have been found in most children with kwashiorkor.[172] These elevated levels of HGH are not suppressed by glucose loading as in normal individuals and may in fact be paradoxically increased by this maneuver.[173] Insulin-induced hypoglycemia has resulted in scattered responses,[174] and glucagon has caused an increased HGH secretion in undernourished children.[175] Arginine loading generally produces a normal elevation of HGH in children with PCM, but some blunted responses have been recorded.[176]

On the whole, basal HGH levels tend to be elevated in kwashiorkor, are poorly suppressible by hyperglycemia, and can be further raised by a variety of stimuli, suggesting that there is a normal pituitary reserve of the hormone. Protein refeeding returns HGH levels to normal in children with kwashiorkor,[172] indicating that protein deficiency may play a major role in the disordered HGH homeostasis of this condition. In marasmus, basal HGH levels are lower, and pituitary reserves less, than in kwashiorkor.

Since the tissue actions of HGH are mediated by a group of insulinlike hormones called the *somatomedins*,[177] studies have been made of somatomedin activity in PCM.[178,179] Despite the normal or even elevated levels of HGH in growth-retarded children with PCM, serum levels of somatomedin activity are low[178] but return to normal after several weeks of nutritional supplementation.[179]

The elevated serum levels of HGH often found in PCM may, however, play a part in some of the metabolic derangements characteristic of this disorder. HGH is known to be diabetogenic,[180] and raised HGH levels may therefore contribute to the glucose intolerance of PCM.[181] The elevated levels of free fatty acids demonstrated in PCM may be accounted for by the lipolytic effect of HGH.[181] Finally, the lowered catabolic rate of albumin seen in PCM may be due to high HGH levels,[182] since this hormone has been shown to slow albumin catabolism.

THYROID HORMONES

Thyroid hormones are needed for normal growth and development, especially in the young.[183] Not only do tissues respond to hypothyroidism in a manner similar to that in undernutrition, but there may be a concomitant reduction of food intake owing to abnormalities in taste and smell.[184] Similarly, some of the catabolic features of hyperthyroidism, such as weight loss, decreased glycogen synthesis, creatinuria, ketosis, and negative nitrogen balance, may reflect inadequate caloric intake in the face of hyperstimulation of metabolism by excess thyroid hormones.[185]

Thyroid gland hypoplasia has been reported in both human[186] and experimental PCM.[187] Tests of thyroid function have also been reported to be lowered in malnutrition, including serum total and free thyroxine,[188] thyroxine secretory rate,[189] thyroid-to-serum radioiodide concentration,[190] ^{131}I-uptake,[191] oxygen consumption,[191] and extrathyroidal conversion of T_4 to T_3.[192] Since thyroid-stimulating hormone (TSH) levels in PCM tend to be normal or low,[193] thyroid hypofunction in PCM has been attributed mainly to decreased stimulation of the thyroid by the pituitary. Some evidence, including thyrotropin-releasing hormone (TRH) stimulation tests, has implicated defects within the thyroid gland itself.[194] Recent work has suggested that low serum levels of T_4 may be ascribed to depressed serum concentrations of TBG in kwashiorkor but not in marasmus.[193]

Abnormalities in thyroid function tests also occur in the self-imposed starvation of patients with anorexia nervosa. Peripheral conversion of T_4 to T_3 is impaired, although basal and TRH-stimulated TSH levels are usually normal.[196]

Not only does the state of nutrition influence the synthesis and release of thyroid hormones, but thyroid

hormones, in turn, influence nutrition through their regulation of various metabolic processes.

Experimental evidence indicates that the effect of thyroid hormones on protein metabolism is biphasic. In hypothyroid animals, low doses of thyroxine increase protein synthesis and decrease nitrogen excretion, whereas larger doses inhibit protein synthesis and increase the concentration of free amino acids in muscle, liver, and blood.[197] The control of cytoplasmic protein metabolism by thyroid hormones may be mediated through the synthesis of nuclear and ribosomal RNA.[198]

Thyroid hormones also exert biphasic effects on glucose and glycogen metabolism. Low doses of hormones promote increased glycogen synthesis in muscle and liver,[199] probably by enhancing intestinal absorption of glucose and by stimulating gluconeogenic enzyme systems in the target organs.[200] High doses of hormones increase the activity of hepatic glucose 6-phosphatase,[201] resulting in decreased rates of glucose uptake and glycogen synthesis in the liver.

Most aspects of lipid metabolism are enhanced by thyroid hormones, including synthesis, degradation, and mobilization. In general, degradation prevails, and thyroid hormone excess results in a decrease in the tissue stores and blood levels of triglycerides, phospholipids, and cholesterol. Conversely, deficiency of thyroid hormones produces an increase in the levels of these substances.

Administration of thyroid hormones increases lipolysis in adipose tissue through a direct stimulation of the adenylcyclase-cyclic adenosine monophosphate (AMP) system[202] and by enhancing the lipolytic response to other agents, such as ACTH, glucocorticoids, glucagon, HGH, and catecholamines.[203] Oxidation of free fatty acids (FFA) is also increased,[204] which may contribute to the thermogenic action of thyroid hormones.

Hepatic production of triglycerides is stimulated by thyroid hormones,[205] presumably because of an increased availability of FFA and glycerol mobilized from fat depots and an increase in hepatic enzyme content.[206] Removal of triglycerides peripherally is accelerated, probably because of an increased activity of liproprotein lipase.[205]

Thyroid hormones commonly lower serum cholesterol concentration as the end result of a series of actions. Synthesis of cholesterol is enhanced through stimulation of the rate-limiting enzyme β-hydroxy-β-methylglutaryl-CoA reductase.[207] Catabolism of cholesterol is facilitated by thyroid hormones through an increased fecal excretion of endogenous neutral steroids and a smaller increase in conversion to fecal bile acids.[208] Furthermore, excess thyroid hormones can lead to malabsorption of dietary fat.[209]

ADRENAL CORTICAL HORMONES

Histologic examination of tissues from malnourished children[168] and experimental animals[187] has suggested an increased activity of the adrenal cortex in PCM. Clinical studies of children[210] and adults[211] with PCM have revealed elevated plasma levels of cortisol and diminished urinary excretion of 17-hydroxycorticoids and 17-ketosteroids. Furthermore, cortisol binding to plasma proteins is diminished, resulting in an increased concentration of plasma free cortisol.[212,213] The elevated plasma levels of both total[210] and free cortisol[212] fall with recovery from the malnourished state.

Stimulation testing done with ACTH[210] and metyrapone[211] has produced appropriate adrenal and pituitary responses in malnourished individuals. Administration of dexamethasone has resulted in incomplete suppression of plasma cortisol in the same subjects. Recently, the metabolic clearance rate of cortisol has been shown to be reduced in PCM.[211]

Studies in malnourished women with anorexia nervosa have shown abnormalities in cortisol metabolism similar to those observed in PCM. Patients with anorexia nervosa have elevated mean plasma cortisol levels, although the normal circadian variation is preserved.[214] The elevated cortisol levels are probably due to a decrease in the metabolic clearance rate.

The high circulating levels of adrenal steroids may contribute to some of the metabolic derangements characteristic of PCM. The increased hepatic concentrations of fat and glycogen,[215] impaired glucose tolerance,[181] and depressed cell-mediated immunity[216] seen in malnourished patients may be related to a state of functional hyperadrenalism.

INSULIN

Abnormal oral and intravenous glucose tolerance tests have been demonstrated in malnourished infants.[217–219] Although the glucose intolerance of PCM is most likely due to impaired insulin secretion,[219] diminished sensitivity to insulin has also been suggested.[220]

Fasting levels of insulin are usually low in PCM and rise with treatment.[181] After stimulation with oral or intravenous glucose, the insulin secretion of malnourished infants is blunted. Although this defective insulin secretion may persist for months after treatment with an optimal diet,[221] it eventually shows improvement in the vast majority of patients.[219] Deficient insulin responses to glucagon[181] and arginine[222] also occur in PCM.

Abnormalities in the shape of the insulin secretory curve have been reported in untreated PCM.[223] Com-

monly, this occurs as a delayed and sustained insulin response to an oral glucose load but an early peak response to intravenous glucose in the same patient. After treatment, there is often a greater improvement in the insulin response to oral as opposed to intravenous glucose administration. These observations suggest that there may be impairment of gut insulinotrophic factors[224] in the untreated state that recovers on treatment.[225] Potassium deficiency may also contribute to the abnormalities of insulin release in PCM.[225] Recent evidence indicates that a glucoreceptor system of the pancreatic β-cell may be impaired during starvation and induced by the fed state.[226] Such a mechanism might explain the blunted response of the β-cell to glucose that occurs during starvation and its rapidly restored response during refeeding.

GONADAL HORMONES

Under certain conditions, food intake may be related to gonadal function. In normally menstruating rhesus monkeys, food is rejected at midcycle, a time when ovulation normally occurs. In pregnant monkeys, food is rejected during the third to fifth week of the pregnancy.[227] The fact that both of these time periods are associated with known alterations in the secretory rates of luteinizing hormone (LH) follicle-stimulating hormone (FSH), estrogen, and progesterone raises the possibility of important hormonal influences on the pattern of food consumption.

Gonadal function in turn is sensitive to alterations in nutritional status. It is well known that severe reduction in food intake both in experimental animals and humans results in cessation of menstrual cycles. Pituitary and ovarian weights, as well as plasma LH and FSH concentrations, are reduced in rats maintained on half their normal food consumption.[228,229] In women with anorexia nervosa, a disorder in which 25% or more of body weight may be lost, plasma and urinary gonadotropin concentration and serum estradiol concentrations are markedly reduced. Sherman and colleagues have reported the LH response to gonadotrophin-releasing hormone to be impaired and that of FSH normal in anorexia nervosa,[230] whereas others have observed normal release of both pituitary hormones.[231] Recent studies suggest that the secretory pattern of LH in anorexia nervosa reverts to a form observed in prepubertal or early pubertal girls in which serum levels are reduced and no peaking of LH secretion occurs synchronous with sleep.[232] The hormonal disturbances that are observed in anorexia nervosa generally return to normal with remission of the disease and attainment of normal weight. Menses generally return, but at variable time intervals, after weight gain is achieved.[233]

In men who have undergone PCM, libido and potency are markedly diminished. There is clinical evidence of hypogonadism, and plasma testosterone levels are reduced. The fact that under these conditions LH and FSH levels are elevated rather than depressed below normal levels[234] suggests that hypogonadism is of testicular rather than hypothalamic-pituitary origin. Further evidence for this point of view is the finding that plasma levels of testosterone were not stimulated normally by human chorionic gonadotropin (HCG) administration.[234] Serum levels of zinc were generally normal. This point is of interest because zinc deficiency has been proposed as a possible etiology for the short stature and hypogonadism observed in the Middle East.[235]

SUMMARY

Undernutrition may be due both to diminished dietary intake and to decreased utilization of dietary nutrients. Chronic illness and drug therapy, particularly if prolonged, may compromise nutritional status in a vulnerable patient and convert a marginal deficiency into an overt one. During the initial periods of early life, both somatic and mental development are strongly influenced by nutrition; both the timing and the severity of undernutrition determine the degree of impairment. The nutritional status of pregnant patients is dependent to a large extent upon the intake of key nutrients, such as iron, prior to pregnancy. Breast feeding has many advantages for infant feeding both in industrial and in preindustrial societies.

Drugs may produce undernutrition by causing anorexia, nausea, vomiting, or diarrhea. Some drugs cause a specific loss of taste acuity. Other mechanisms of undernutrition caused by drugs include interference with intestinal absorption of specific nutrients, binding of nutrients to plasma proteins, their transport across cell membranes, peripheral utilization, intracellular transformations, storage, turnover, and elimination or their excretion. Certain categories of pharmacologic agents, such as diuretics, laxatives, and analeptics, may be particularly likely to cause drug-induced nutritional deficiencies.

Malnutrition in cancer is variable in degree, multifactorial in etiology, and often intensified by the type of therapy, whether surgery, radiation, or chemotherapy. Anorexia and early satiety appear to be classic symptoms of cancer and are of unknown origin. There is some evidence that tumors may be more resistant than host tissues to vitamin deficiency. Undernutrition in general and deficiencies of such nutrients as zinc and riboflavin in particular have major effects upon

tumor growth. The role of certain nutrients, including vitamin A, fat, nitrates, fiber, and others, upon cancer prevalence in man is under active study at the present time.

Undernutrition in aging is of growing importance as the elderly population increases. In experimental animals, caloric restriction has been shown to prolong life span and delay the emergence of several illnesses. Major physiologic changes occur with aging that may compromise intake and utilization of dietary nutrients. These changes include loss of teeth, loss of gastric acid, diminished intestinal absorption, changes in body composition, and other factors. The elderly are particularly susceptible to drug-induced nutritional deficiencies because they are the largest users of drugs, have multiple drug needs, and are likely to require prolonged therapy for a chronic condition.

Hormonal factors may produce undernutrition and undernutrition, in turn, regulates hormone release. Human growth hormone levels tend to be elevated in kwashiorkor and may possibly mediate some of the metabolic alterations observed, such as elevated serum levels of free fatty acids. Thyroid hormones are particularly sensitive to undernutrition; the peripheral conversion of thyroxine to triiodothyronine is markedly impaired and may account at least in part for the fall in metabolic rate that occurs with starvation. Abnormalities in cortisol metabolism are regularly observed in undernutrition, and there is diminished insulin response to a glucose challenge. Amenorrhea and diminished libido are classic findings in undernutrition.

Thus, undernutrition arises in a variety of ways, and it is essential for the physician to consider the underlying mechanisms when determining etiology and when devising a therapeutic plan.

The work of Robert J. McConnell was supported by Training Grant #IT-32-HD-07000-01.

Research was supported by NIH grants 5P01 CA 29502, 5T32 CA 09427, CM 15735, and by grants from the Stella and Charles Guttman Foundation, the National Dairy Council, the National Live Stock and Meat Board, the William H. Donner Foundation, the United States Brewers Association, the Fairchild Foundation, the Richard Molin Memorial Foundation, the Sperry Corporation, and Hoffmann-La Roche, Inc.

REFERENCES

1. **MacBryde CM:** Weight loss and undernutrition. In MacBryde CM, and Blacklow RS (eds.): Signs and Symptoms, 5th ed, p. 872. Philadelphia, J.B. Lippincott, 1970

2. **Widdowson E:** How the foetus is fed. Proc Nutr Soc 28:17, 1969

3. **Naismith DJ:** Maternal nutrition and the outcome of pregnancy, a critical appraisal. Proc Nutr Soc 39:1, 1980

4. **Pitkin RM:** Nutritional influences during pregnancy. Med Clin North Am 61:3, 1977

5. **Bell EF, Filer LJ, Jr:** The role of vitamin E in the nutrition of premature infants. Am J Clin Nutr 34:414, 1981

6. **Metcoff J:** Biochemical markers of intrauterine malnutrition. In Winick M (ed.): Nutrition and Fetal Development, New York, John Wiley, 1974

7. **Naeye RL, Diener, MM, Hancke HT, et al:** Relation of poverty and race to birth weight and organ and cell structure in the newborn. Pediatr Res 5:17, 1971

8. **Usher RH:** Clinical and therapeutic aspects of fetal malnutrition. Pediatr Clin North Am 17:169, 1970

9. **Sinclair JC, Saigal S:** Nutritional influences in industrial societies. Am J Dis Child 129:549, 1975

10. **Brooke OG:** Food and foetus in the neonate. Proc Nutr Soc 39:17, 1980

11. **Church M:** Dietary factors in malnutrition: Quality and quantity of diet in relation to child development. Proc Nutr Soc 38:41, 1979

12. **Witter F and King TM:** Cigarettes and pregnancy. Prog Clin Biol Res 36:83, 1980

13. **Beisel W:** Synergistic effects of maternal malnutrition and infection on the infant. Am J Dis Child 129:571, 1975

14. **Editorial:** Maternal nutrition—What price? N Engl J Med 292:208, 1975

15. **Lechtig A, Delgado H, Lasky R et al:** Maternal nutrition and fetal growth in developing countries. Am J Dis Child 129:553, 1975

16. **Lyengar L:** Effects of dietary supplements late in pregnancy on the expectant mother and her newborn. Indian J Med Res 55:85, 1967

17. **Stewart AL, Reynolds EOR, Lipscomb AD:** Outcome for infants of very low birth weight. Survey of world literature. Lancet 1:1038, 1981

18. **Rosso P:** Maternal nutrition, nutrient exchange and fetal growth. Curr Concepts Nutr 5:3, 1977

19. **Turchetto E:** Alimentazione infantile e vitamin C. Acta Vitaminol Enzymol (Milano) 28:138, 1974

20. **Schreier K:** Ernährung und geistige Entwicklung. Monatsschr fur Kinderheilk 121:554, 1973

21. **Cordano A:** Copper requirements and actual recommendations per 100 kilocalories of infant formula. Pediatrics 54:524, 1974

22 **Sandstead H:** Zinc nutrition in U.S. Am J Clin Nutr 26:1251, 1973

23. **Caddell J:** On the role of magnesium depletion in severely malnourished children. J Pediatr 84:781, 1974

24. **Committee on Maternal Nutrition, Food and Nutrition Board, National Research Council:** Maternal Nutrition and the Course of Pregnancy. Washington, DC, National Academy of Sciences, 1970

25. **Winick M:** Malnutrition and Brain Development p. 169. New York, Oxford University Press, 1975

26. **Naeye RL, Blanc W and Paul C:** Effects of maternal nutrition on the human fetus. Pediatrics 52:494, 1973

27. **Jones DG:** The vulnerability of the brain to undernutrition. Sci Prog 63:483, 1976

28. **Winick M, and Coombs J:** Nutrition, environment, and behavioral development. Annu Rev Med 23:149, 1972

29. **Anderson GD:** Nutrition in pregnancy. South Med J 72:1304, 1979

30. **Martin HP.:** Nutrition: Its relationship to children's physical, mental, and emotional development. Am J Clin Nutr 26:766, 1973

31. **Zamenhof S, Van Marthens E, Grauel L:** DNA (cell number) and protein in rat brain. Nutr Metab 14:262, 1972

32. **Winick M, Rosso P:** The effect of severe early malnutrition on cellular growth of human brain. Pediatr Res 3:181, 1969

33. **Ross P, Hormazabal J, Winick M:** Changes in brain weight, cholesterol, phospholipid, and DNA content in marasmic children. Am J Clin Nutr 23:1275, 1970

34. **Brasel JA, Winick M:** Maternal nutrition and prenatal growth. Arch Dis Child 47:479, 1972

35. **Clark GM, Zamenhof S, Van Marthens E et al:** The effect of prenatal malnutrition on dimensions of the cerebral cortex Brain Res 54:397, 1973

36. **Chase HP:** The effects of intrauterine and postnatal undernutrition on normal brain development. Ann NY Acad Sci 205:231, 1973

37. **Prohaska JR, Wells WW:** Copper deficiency in the developing rat brain: A possible model for Menkes' Steely–Hair Disease. J Neurochem 23:91, 1974

38. **Sandstead HH, Fosmire GJ, McKenzie JM et al:** Zinc deficiency and brain development in the rat. Fed Proc 34:86, 1975

39. **Fosmire GJ, Al Ubaidi YY, Sandstead HH:** Some effects of postnatal zinc deficiency on developing rat brain. Pediatr Res 9:89, 1975

40. **Editorial:** Cellular growth in infantile malnutrition. Nutr Rev 29:6, 1971

41. **Lloyd–Still JD, Hurwitz I, Wolff PH et al:** Intellectual development after severe malnutrition in infancy. Pediatrics 54:306, 1974

42. **Lloyd–Still JD Shwachman H:** Intelligence after malnutrition. Lancet 1:679, 1974

43. **Editorial:** Current practice. Iron and folate supplement in pregnancy. Br Med J 1:415, 1967

44. **Castren O, Levanto A, Rauramo L et al:** Preventive iron and folic acid therapy in pregnancy. Ann Chir Gynaecol Fenniae (Suppl) 7:382, 1968

45. **Goltner E:** Quarter of pregnant patients are anemic. Med Clin 75:491, 1980

46. **Oski FA:** Nutritional anemias, Semin Perinatol 3:381, 1979

47. **Stockman JA:** Anemia of prematurity. Clin Perinatol 4:239, 1977

48. **Varadi S:** Iron and folic acid deficiency in pregnancy. Br Med J 1:656, 1965

49. **Theuer R:** Iron undernutrition in infancy. Clin Pediatr 13:522, 1974

50. **Fleming AF, Martin YD, Hahnel R et al:** Effects of iron and folic acid antenatal supplements on maternal haematology and fetal well being. Med J Aust 2:429, 1974

51. **Hartouche J:** The importance of breast feeding. J Trop Pediatr 16:133, 1970

52. **Alvear DT, Somers LA:** Parenteral nutrition in seriously ill neonates. Am J Surg 127:696, 1974

53. **Rondini G:** The dietotherapeutic effect of an integrally formulated milk. Minerva Pediatr 26:1843, 1974

54. **Isbister J:** Breast feeding. Med J Aust 2:625, 1972

55. **Collip P:** Nutrition of the fetus, infant, and child. Am J Dis Child 126:558, 1973

56. **Brown RE:** Weaning foods in developing countries. Am J Clin Nutr 31:2066, 1978

57. **Mata L:** Breast feeding: Main promoter of infant health. Am J Clin Nutr 31:2050, 1978

58. **Jackson RL:** Long term consequences of suboptimal nutritional practices in early life. Some important benefits of breast feeding. Pediatr Clin North Am 24:63, 1977

59. **Hueheman R:** Environmental factors in preschool obesity. J Am Diet Assoc 64:480, 1974

60. **Owen G, Lippman G:** Nutritional status of infants and young children in the U.S.A. Pediatr Clin North Am 24:211, 1977

61. **Holmes M, Topper D:** Child Abuse and Neglect; The View from the Literature and the View from the Field. Washington, DC, Government Printing Office, 1976

62. **Roe D:** Drug Induced Nutritional Deficiencies. Westport CN, AVI Press, 1976

63. **Hathcock JN, Coon J (eds):** Nutrition and Drug Interrelations. New York, Academic Press, 1978

64. **Redmond GP:** Effect of drugs on intrauterine growth. Clin Perinatol 61:5, 1979

65. **Basu TK:** Interaction of drugs and nutrition. J Hum Nutr 31:449, 1977

66. **MacFarlane MD:** Penicillamine and zinc. Lancet 2:962, 1974

67. **Aiache JM:** Effects of diet on the absorption of drugs. Pharm Acta Helv 55:210, 1980

68. **Cummings JH, Sladen GE, James OFW:** Laxative-induced diarrhea: A continuing clinical problem. Br Med J 1:537, 1974

69. **Weser E:** Nutritional aspects of malabsorption. Short gut adaptation. Am J Med 67:1014, 1979

70. **Petersdorf RG, Beeson PB:** Fever of unexplained origin. Report of 100 cases. Medicine 40:1, 1961

71. **Rivlin RS:** Therapy of obesity with hormones. N Engl J Med 292:26, 1975

72. **Hryniuk WW, Bertino JR:** Treatment of leukemia with large doses of methotrexate and folinic acid: clinical biochemical correlates. J Clin Invest 48:2140, 1969

73. **Horrigan DL, Harris JW:** Pyridoxine-responsive anemias in man. In Vitamins and Hormones, Vol 26, p. 549. New York Academic Press, 1968

74. **Harris JW, Horrigan DL:** Pyridoxine responsive anemia—Prototype and variations on the theme. Adv Intern Med 12:103, 1964

75. **Roe DA:** Drug-induced deficiency of B vitamins. N.Y. J Med 71:2770, 1971

76. **Fausa O:** Salicylate-induced hypoprothrombinemia. Acta Med Scand 188:403, 1970

77. **Horwitt MK:** Niacin. Goodhart RS, Shils ME (eds.): In Modern Nutrition in Health and Disease, 6th ed, p 204. Philadelphia, Lea & Febiger, 1980

78. **Goldsmith GA:** Riboflavin deficiency. In Rivlin RS (ed): *Riboflavin*, p 221. New York, Plenum Press, 1975

79. **Curtis AC, Bollmer RS:** The prevention of carotene absorption by liquid petrolatum. JAMA 113:1785, 1939

80. **Hashim SA, Berger SS, Jr, Van Itallie TB:** Experimental steatorrhea induced in man by bile acid sequestrant. Proc Soc Exp Biol Med 106:173, 1961

81. **Tomkin GH:** Malabsorption of vitamin B_{12} in diabetic patients treated with phenformin: A comparison with metformin. Br Med J 3:673, 1973

82. **DiLorenzo PA:** Pellagra-like syndrome associated with isoniazid therapy. Acta Derm Venereol (Stockh) 47:318, 1967

83. **Pinto J, Huang YP, McConnell RJ et al:** Increased urinary excretion resulting from boric acid ingestion. J Lab Clin Med 92:126, 1978

84. **Benjamin BI, Cortell S, Conrad ME:** Bicarbonate-induced iron complexes and iron absorption: One effect of pancreatic secretion. Gastroenterology 53:389, 1967

85. **Jacobs A:** Digestive factors in iron absorption. Prog Gastroenterol 2:221, 1970

86. **Weiss HJ:** Aspirin—A dangerous drug? JAMA 229:1221, 1974

87. **Shils ME:** Magnesium, calcium and parathyroid interactions. In Levander OA, Cheng L (eds): Micronutrient Interactions: Vitamins Minerals and Hazardous Elements. Ann NY Acad Sci 355:165, 1980

88. **Klipstein FA:** Subnormal serum folate and macrocytosis associated with anticonvulsant drug therapy. Blood 23:68, 1964

89. **Hoffbrand AV, Necheles PF:** Mechanisms of folate deficiency in patients receiving phenytoin. Lancet 2:528, 1968

90. **Benn A, Swann CHJ, Cooke WT et al:** Effect of intraluminal pH on the absorption of pteroylmonoglutamic acid. Br Med J 1:148, 1971

91. **Bowden AM:** Anticonvulsants and calcium metabolism. Dev Med Child Neurol 16:214, 1974

92. **Shojania AM, Hornady GJ, Barnes PH:** The effect of oral contraceptives on folate metabolism. Am J Obstet Gynecol 111:782, 1971

93. **Wood JK, Goldstone AG, Allan NC:** Folic acid and the pill. Scand J Haematol 9:539, 1972

94. **Webb JL:** Nutritional effects of oral contraceptive use. J Reprod Med 25:150, 1980

95. **Prasad AS, Lei KY, Oberleas D et al:** Effect of oral contraceptive agents on nutrients: II. Vitamins Am J Clin Nutr 28:385, 1975

96. **Briggs M, Briggs M:** Oral contraceptives and vitamin nutrition. Lancet 1:1234, 1974

97. **Kalesh DG, Mallikarjuneswara VR, Clemetson CAB:** Effect of estrogen-containing oral contraceptives on platelet and plasma ascorbic acid concentrations. Contraception 4:183, 1971

98. **Prasad AS, Oberleas D, Lei KY et al:** Effect of oral contraceptive agents on nutrients: I. Minerals. Am J Clin Nutr 28:377, 1975

99. **Theologides A:** Pathogenesis of cachexia in cancer. A review and a hypothesis. Cancer 29:484, 1972

100. **Shils ME:** Nutritional problems induced by cancer. Med Clin North Am 63:1009, 1979

101. **Croft PB, Wilkinson M:** The incidence of carcinomatous neuromyopathy with special reference to carcinoma of the lung and breast. In Brain R, Norris FH, Jr (Eds): The Remote Effects of Cancer on the Nervous System, p 44. New York, Grune & Stratton, 1965

102. **Morrison SD:** Origins of nutritional imbalance in cancer. Cancer Res 35:3339, 1975

103. **DeWys WD:** A spectrum of organ changes that respond to the presence of cancer. Abnormalities of taste as a remote effect of a neoplasm. Ann NY Acad Sci 230:427, 1974

104. **Newell GR, Ellison NM:** Nutrition and Cancer: Etiology and Treatment. New York, Raven Press, 1981

105. **Reddy BS, Cohen LA, McCoy GD et al:** Nutrition and its relationship to cancer. Adv Cancer Res 32:237, 1980

106. **Gori GB:** Role of diet and nutrition in cancer cause, prevention and treatment. Bull Cancer (Paris) 65:115, 1978

107. **Mider GB, Tesluk J, Morton JJ:** Effects of Walker carcinoma 256 on food intake, body weight and nitrogen metabolism of growing rats. Acta Unio Intern Contra Cancrum 6:409, 1948

108. **Bertino JR, Booth BA, Cashmore A et al:** Studies of the inhibition of dihydrofolate reductase by the folate antagonists. J Biol Chem 239:479, 1964

109. **Young CW:** Actinomycin and antitumor antibiotics. Am J Clin Pathol 52:130, 1969

110. **Bertino JR, Nixon PF:** Nutritional factors in the design of some selective antitumor agents. Cancer Res 29:2417, 1969

111. **DiPalma JR, McMichael R:** The interaction of vitamins with cancer therapy. CA 29:280, 1979

112. **Henderson JF, LePage GA:** The nutrition of tumors: A review. Cancer Res 19:887, 1959

113. **Mider GB:** Some aspects of nitrogen and energy metabolism in cancerous subjects. Cancer Res 11:821, 1951

114. **Weber G, Lea MA:** The molecular correlation concept of neoplasia. In Weber G (ed): Advances in Enzyme Regulation, vol 4, p 115. Oxford, Pergaman Press, 1966

115. **Rivlin RS, Hornibrook R, Osnos M:** Effects of riboflavin deficiency upon concentrations of riboflavin, flavin mononucleotide and flavin adenine dinucleotide in Novikoff hepatoma in rats. Cancer Res 33:3019, 1973

116. **Rivlin RS:** Riboflavin and cancer: A review. Cancer Res 33:1977, 1973

117. **Ueki H, Tsunemi S, Tanaka M et al:** Biochemical studies on cachexia due to cancer. 11. Extraction of hypoalbuminemic substances from Ehrlich Ascites Carcinoma cells and from tissues of mice. Yakagaku Zasshi 94:143, 1974

118. **Tannenbaum A, Silverstone H:** Nutrition in relation to cancer. Adv Cancer Res 1:451, 1953

119. **Editorial:** An update on nutrition, diet and cancer. Dairy Council Digest 51:5, 1980

120. **Young, VR, Newberne PM:** Vitamin and cancer prevention: Issues and dilemmas. Cancer 47:1226, 1981

121. **Masek J:** Nutrition, diet and cancer. Bibl Nutr Dieta 29:48, 1980

122. **Alderson MR:** Nutrition and cancer: Evidence from epidemiology. Proc Nutr Soc 40:1, 1981

123. **Rivlin RS:** Nutrition and cancer: State-of-the-art. Relationship of several nutrients to the development of cancer. J Am Coll Nutr 1:75, 1982

124. **Visscher MB, Ball ZB, Barnes RH et al:** The influence of caloric restriction upon the incidence of spontaneous mammary carcinoma in mice. Surgery 11:48, 1942

125. **Saxton JA, Boon MC, Furth J:** Observations on the inhibition of development of spontaneous leukemia in mice by underfeeding. Cancer Res 4:401, 1944

126. **Tannenbaum A:** The genesis and growth of tumors. II. Effects of caloric restriction *per se*. Cancer Res 2:460, 1942

127. **Nigro ND, Singh DV, Campbell RL et al:** Effect of dietary beef fat on intestinal tumor formation by azoxymethane in rats. J Natl Cancer Inst 53:453, 1974

128. **Terepka AR, Waterhouse C:** Metabolic observations during the forced feeding of patients with cancer. Am J Med 20:225, 1956

129. **Wynder EL:** Introductory remarks. Cancer Res 35:3238, 1975

130. **Haenzel W, Correa P:** Cancer of the colon and rectum and adenomatous polyps. A review of epidemiological findings. Cancer 28:14, 1971

131. **Burkitt DP:** Epidemiology of cancer of the colon and rectum. Cancer 28:3, 1971

132. **Hill MJ, Draser BS, Aries VC et al:** Bacteria and the etiology of cancer of the large bowel. Lancet 1:95, 1971

133. **Hill MJ:** Metabolic epidemiology of dietary factors in large bowel cancer. Cancer Res 35:3398, 1975

134. **Levine RA:** An overview of fiber and gastrointestinal disease. In Kurtz RC (ed): Contemporary Issues in Clinical Nutrition, Vol 1, p 1. Nutrition in Gastrointestinal Disease. New York, Churchill–Livingstone, 1981

135. **Sherlock P, Lipkin M, Winawer SJ:** The prevention of colon cancer. Am J Med 68:917, 1980

136. **Peto R, Doll R, Buckley JD et al:** Can dietary beta-carotene materially reduce human cancer rates? Nature 290:201, 1981

137. **Orten AU, Burn CG, Smith AH:** Effects of prolonged chronic vitamin A deficiency in rat, with special reference to odontomas. Proc Soc Exp Biol Med 36:82, 1937

138. **Hirayama T:** Epidemiology of cancer of the stomach with special reference to its recent decrease in Japan. Cancer Res 35:3460, 1975

139. **Rivlin RS:** Nutrition and aging: Some unanswered questions. Am J Med 71:337, 1981

140. **Gibson DC (ed):** Development of the rodent as a model system of aging. DHEW Publication, No. (NIH) 72-121. Washington, DC, US Government Printing Office, 1972

141. **Ross MH:** Nutrition and longevity in experimental animals. In Winick M (ed): Current Concepts in Nutrition; vol 4, Nutrition and Aging, p. 45. New York, John Wiley, 1976

142. **Ross MH:** Length of life and caloric intake. Am J Clin Nutr 25:834, 1972

143. **Ross MH, Bras G:** Influence of protein under- and overnutrition on spontaneous tumor prevalence in the rat. J Nutr 103:944, 1973

144. **Rockstein N, Sussman ML:** Nutrition, Longevity and Aging. New York, Academic Press, 1976

145. **Leaf A:** Unusual longevity-the common denominators. Hosp Prac p 75, October, 1973

146. **Novak LP:** Aging, total body potassium, fat-free mass, and cell mass in males and females between ages 18 and 85 years. J Gerontol 27:438, 1972

147. **Forbes GB, Reina JC:** Adult lean body mass declines with age: Some longitudinal observations. Metabolism 19:653, 1970

148. **Young VR:** Nutrition and aging. Adv Exp Biol Med 97:85, 1978

149. **Young, VR, Perera WD, Winterer JC et al:** Protein and amino acid requirements of the elderly. In Winick M (ed): Current Concepts in Nutrition; vol 4, Nutrition and Aging, p 77. New York, John Wiley, 1976

150. **Lesser GT, Deutsch S, Markofsky J:** Aging in the rat: Longitudinal and cross-sectional studies of body composition. Am J Physiol 225:1472, 1973

151. **Masoro EJ:** Physiological changes with aging. In Winick M (ed): Current Concepts in Nutrition; vol 4, Nutrition and Aging, p 61. New York, John Wiley, 1976

152. **Masoro EJ, Yu BP, Bertrand HA et al:** Nutritional probe of the aging process. Fed Proc 39:3178, 1980

153. **Hsu J, Davis R:** Handbook of Geriatric Nutrition. Park Ridge, NJ, Noyes Publications, 1981

154. **Ham TH (ed):** A Syllabus of Laboratory Examinations in Clinical Diagnosis. Cambridge, MA, Harvard University Press, 1956

155. **Kohn RK:** Principles of Mammalian Aging. Englewood Cliffs, NJ Prentice Hall, 1971

156. **Guth PH:** Physiologic alterations in small bowel function with age. The absorption of D-xylose. Am J Dig Dis 13:565, 1968

157. **Bullamore JR, Wilkinson, R, Gallagher JC et al:** Effect of age on calcium absorption. Lancet 2:535, 1970

158. **Laflamme GH, Jowsey J:** Bone and soft tissue changes with oral phosphate supplements. J Clin Invest 51:2834, 1972

159. **Lutwak L:** Periodontal disease, In Winick M (ed): Current Concepts in Nutrition; vol 4, Nutrition and Aging, p 145. New York, John Wiley, 1976

160. **Krook L, Lutwak L, Whalen JP et al:** Human periodontal disease. Morphology and response to calcium therapy. Cornell Vet 62:32, 1972

161. **Avioli LV:** What to do with "postmenopausal osteoporosis"? Am J Med 65:881, 1978

162. **Riggs BL, Hodgson SE, Hoffman DL et al:** Treatment of primary osteoporosis with fluoride and calcium. JAMA 242:446, 1980

163. **Fredrickson DS, Levy RI, Lees RS:** Fat transport in lipoproteins—an integrated approach to mechanisms and disorders. N Engl J Med 276:273, 1967

164. **Hall Y, Stamler J, Cohen DB et al:** Effectiveness of a low saturated fat, low cholesterol, weight-reducing diet for the control of hypertriglyceridemia. Atherosclerosis 16:389, 1972

165. **Todhunter EN:** Life style and nutrient intake in the elderly. In Winick M (ed): Current Concepts in Nutrition; vol 4, Nutrition and Aging, p 119. New York, John Wiley, 1976

166. **Beauchene RE, Davis TA:** The nutritional status of the aged in the U.S.A. Age 2:23, 1979

167. **O'Hanlon PD, Kohrs MB:** Dietary studies of older Americans. Am J Clin Nutr 31:1257, 1978

168. **Tejada C, Russfield AB:** A preliminary report on the pituitary gland in children with malnutrition. Arch Dis Child 32:343, 1957

169. **Srebnik HH, Nelson MM:** Anterior pituitary function in male rats deprived of dietary protein. Endocrinology 70:723, 1962

170. **Meites J, Fiel N:** Effect of starvation on hypothalamic content of somatotropin releasing factor and pituitary growth hormone content. Endocrinology 77:455, 1965

171. **Monckeberg F, Donoso C, Oxman S et al:** Human growth hormone in infant malnutrition. Pediatrics 31:58, 1963

172. **Pimstone B, Becker D, Kernoff L:** Growth and growth hormone in protein calorie malnutrition. S Afr Med J 46:2102, 1972

173. **Alvarez LC, Dimas CO, Castro A et al:** Growth hormone in malnutrition. J Clin Endocrinol Metab 34:400, 1972

174. **Godard C, Zahnd GR:** Growth hormone and insulin in severe infantile malnutrition. 1. Plasma growth hormone response to hypoglycemia. Helv Paediatr Acta 26:266, 1971

175. **Milner RDG:** Metabolic and hormonal responses to glucose and glucagon in patients with infantile malnutrition. Pediatr Res 5:33, 1971

176. **Beas F, Contreras I, Maccioni A et al:** Growth hormone in infant malnutrition: The arginine test in marasmus and kwashiorkor. Br J Nutr 26:169, 1971

177. **Philips LS, Vassilopoulou–Sellin R:** Somatomedins. N Engl J Med 302:371,438, 1980

178. **Grant DB, Hambley J, Becker D et al:** Reduced sulphation factor in undernourished children. Arch Dis Child 48:596, 1973

179. **Hintz RL, Suskind R, Amatayakul K et al:** Plasma somatomedin and growth hormone values in children with protein-calorie malnutrition. J Pediatr 92:153, 1978

180. **Daughaday WH:** The Adenohypophysis. In Williams RH (ed): Textbook of Endocrinology, 5th ed, p 31. Philadelphia, WB Saunders, 1974

181. **Milner RDG:** Hormonal and metabolic interrelationships in malnutrition. Arch Dis Child 45:276, 1970

182. **James WPT, Hay AM:** Albumin metabolism: effect of the nutritional state and dietary protein intake. J Clin Invest 47:1958, 1968

183. **Brasel JA, Winick M:** Differential cellular growth in the organs of hypothyroid rats. Growth 34:197, 1970

184. **McConnell RJ, Menendez CE, Smith FR et al:** Defects of taste and smell in patients with hypothyroidism. Am J Med 59:354, 1975

185. **Carter WJ, Shakir KM, Hodges S et al:** Effect of thyroid hormone on metabolic adaptation to fasting. Metabolism 24:1177, 1975

186. **Kinney TD, Follis RH (eds):** Nutritional disease. Fed Proc (Suppl 2) 17, 1958

187. **Platt BS, Stewart RJC:** Experimental protein–calorie deficiency: histopathological changes in the endocrine glands of pigs. J Endocrinol 38:121, 1967

188. **Krieger I, Taqi Q:** Free serum thyroxine level and basal metabolic rate. Am J Dis Child 129:830, 1975

189. **Singh DV, Anderson RR, Turner CW:** Effect of decresed dietary protein on the rate of thyroid hormone secretion and food consumption in rats. J Endocrinol 50:445, 1971

190. **Cowan JW, Margossian S:** Thyroid function in female rats severely depleted of body protein. Endocrinology 79:1023, 1966

191. **Beas F, Monckeberg F, Horwitz I et al:** The response of the thyroid gland to thyroid stimulating hormone (TSH) in infants with malnutrition. Pediatrics 38:1003, 1966

192. **Chopra IJ, Smith SR:** Circulating thyroid hormones and

thyrotropin in adult patients with protein–calorie malnutrition. J Clin Endocrinol Metab 40:221, 1975

193. **Graham GG, Baertl JM, Claeyssen C et al:** Thyroid hormonal studies in normal and severly malnourished infants and small children. J Pediatr 83:321, 1973

194. **Pimstone B, Becker D, Hendricks S:** TSH response to synethetic thyrotropin-releasing hormone in human protein-calorie malnutrition. J Clin Endocrinol Metab 36:779, 1973

195. **Miyai K, Yamamoto T, Azukizawa M et al:** Serum thyroid hormones and thyrotropin in anorexia nervosa J Clin Endocrinol Metab 40:334, 1975

196. **Beumont PJV, George GCW, Pimstone BL et al:** Body weight and the pituitary response to hypothalamic releasing hormones in patients with anorexia nervosa. J Clin Endocrinol Metab 43:487, 1976

197. **Ness GC, Takahashi T, Lee YP:** Thyroid hormones on amino acid and protein metabolism. I. Concentration and composition of free amino acids in blood plasma of the rat. Endocrinology 85:1166, 1969

198. **Tata JR, Windell CC:** Ribonucleic acid synthesis during the early action of thyroid hormones. Biochem J 98:604, 1966

199. **Battarbee HD:** The effects of thyroid state on rat liver glucose-6-phosphatase activity and glycogen content. Proc Soc Exp Biol Med 147:337, 1974

200. **Bottger I, Kriegel H, Wieland O:** Fluctuation of hepatic enzymes important in glucose metabolism in relation to thyroid function. Eur J Biochem 13:253, 1970

201. **Orunesu M, Fugassa E, Pranzetti P:** Liver glycogen metabolism in the hyperthyroid rat. Ital J Biochem 18:327, 1969

202. **Krishna G, Hynie S, Brodie BB:** Effects of thyroid hormones on adenyl cyclase in adipose tissue and on free fatty acid mobilization. Proc Natl Acad Sci USA 59:884, 1968

203. **Challoner DR, Allen DO:** An *in vitro* effect of triiodothyronine on lipolysis, cyclic AMP-C^{14} accumulation and oxygen consumption in isolated fat cells. Metabolism 19:480, 1970

204. **Diamant S, Gorin E, Shafrir E:** Enzyme activities related to fatty-acid synthesis in lever and adipose tissue of rats treated with triiodothyronine. Eur J Biochem 26:553, 1972

205. **Nikkila EA, Kekki M:** Plasma triglyceride metabolism in thyroid disease. J Clin Invest 51:2103, 1972

206. **Roncari DAK, Murthy VK:** Effects of thyroid hormones on enzymes involved in fatty acid and glycerolipid synthesis. J Biol Chem 250:4134, 1975

207. **Guder W, Nolte I, Wieland O:** The influence of thyroid hormones on β-hydroxy-β-methylglutaryl-coenzyme A reductase of rat liver. Eur J Biochem 4:273, 1968

208. **Miettinen TA:** Mechanism of serum cholesterol reduction by thyroid hormones in hypothyroidism. J Lab Clin Med 71:537, 1968

209. **Middleton WRJ, Thompson GR:** The mechanism of steatorrhea in induced hyperthyroidism in the rat. J Lab Clin Med 74:19, 1969

210. **Alleyne GAO, Young VH:** Adrenocortical function in children with severe protein-calorie malnutrition. Clin Sci 33:189, 1967

211. **Smith SR, Bledsoe T, Chhetri MK:** Cortisol metabolism and pituitary–adrenal axis in adults with protein–calorie malnutrition. J Clin Endocrinol Metab 40:43, 1975

212. **Leonard PJ, MacWilliam KM:** Cortisol binding in the serum in kwashiorkor. J Endocrinol 29:273, 1964

213. **Aboul–Dahab YKW, Zaki K, Wishadi et al:** Plasma cortisol, total bound and unbound in severe malnutrition in children. J Egypt Med Assoc 55:89, 1972

214. **Boyar RM, Hellman LD, Roffwarg H et al:** Cortisol secretion and metabolism in anorexia nervosa. N Engl J Med 296:190, 1977

215. **Waterlow JC, Weisz T:** The fat, protein and nucleic acid content of the liver in malnourished human infants. J Clin Invest 35:346, 1956

216. **Schonland MM, Shanley BC, Loening WEK et al:** Plasma-cortisol and immunosuppression in protein–calorie malnutrition. Lancet 2:435, 1972

217. **Bowie MD:** Intravenous glucose tolerance in kwashiorkor and marasmus. S Afr Med J 38:328, 1964

218. **Baig HA, Edozien JC:** Carbohydrate metabolism in Kwashiorkor. Lancet 2:662, 1965

219. **Becker DJ, Pimstone BL, Hansen JDL et al:** Insulin secretion in protein–calorie malnutrition. I. Quantitative abnormalities and responses to treatment. Diabetes 20:542, 1971

220. **Alleyne GAO, Trust PM, Flores H et al:** Glucose tolerance and insulin sensitivity in malnourished children. Br J Nutr 27:585, 1972

221. **James WPT, Coore HG:** Persistent impairment of insulin secretion and glucose tolerance after malnutrition. Am J Clin Nutr 23:386, 1970

222. **Graham GG, Cordano A, Blizzard RM et al:** Infantile malnutrition: Changes in body composition during rehabilitation. Pediatr Res 3:579, 1969

223. **Becker DJ, Pimstone BL, Hansen JDL et al:** Patterns of insulin response to glucose in protein–calorie malnutrition. Am J Clin Nutr 25:499, 1972

224. **Elrick H, Stimmler L, Hlad CJ et al:** Plasma insulin response to oral and intravenous glucose administration. J Clin Endocrinol 24:1076, 1964

225. **Pimstone B, Becker D, Weinkove C et al:** Insulin secretion in protein–calorie malnutrition. In Gardner LI, Amachen P (eds): Endocrine Aspects of Malnutrition: Marasmus, Kwashiorkor, and Psychosocial Deprivation, p 289. Santa Ynez, CA, Kroc Foundation, 1973

226. **Permutt MA, Kipnis DM:** Insulin biosynthesis and secretion. Fed Proc 34:1549, 1975

227. **Czaja JA:** Food rejection by female Rhesus monkeys during the menstrual cycle and early pregnancy. Physiol Behav 14:579, 1975

228. **Howland BE:** Gonadotrophin levels in female rats subjected to restricted feed intake. J Reprod Fert 27:467, 1971

229. **Howland BE:** Effect of restricted feed intake on LH levels in female rats. J Anim Sci 34:445, 1972

230. **Sherman BM, Halmi KA, Zamudio R:** LH and FSH response to gonadotropin-releasing hormone in anorexia nervosa: Effect of nutritional rehabiliatation. J Clin Endocrinol Metab 41:135, 1975

231. **Wiegelmann W, Solbach HG:** Effects of LH–RH on plasma levels of LH and FSH in anorexia nervosa. Horm Metab Res 4:404, 1972

232. **Boyar RM, Katz J, Finkelstein J et al:** Anorexia nervosa.

Immaturity of the 24-hour luteinizing hormone secretory pattern. N Engl J Med 291:861, 1974

233. **Crisp AH, Stonehill E:** Relation between aspects of nutritional disturbance and menstrual activity in primary anorexia nervosa. Br Med J 2:149, 1971

234. **Smith SR, Chhetri MK, Johanson AJ et al:** The pituitary–gonadal axis in men with protein–calorie malnutrition. J Clin Endocrinol Metab 41:60, 1975

235. **Sandstead HH, Shurkry AS, Prasad AS et al:** Kwashiorkor in Egypt. I. Clinical and biochemical studies, with special reference to plasma zinc and serum lactic dehydrogenase. Am J Clin Nutr 17:15, 1965

39

Skin Color in Health and Disease

Harold Jeghers
Leon M. Edelstein

Factors Involved in Normal Skin Pigmentation
Methods of Analysis of Skin Color
Sources of Skin Color
Patterns of Normal Skin Color
Basic Pattern and Individual Variation
Racial Variations
Sex Differences and the Effects of the Sex
Hormones
Skin Color Changes After Exposure to Sunlight
Increased Pigmentation of the Skin
Yellow Pigmentation
Hemoglobin Pigmentation
Melanin Pigmentation (Melanosis)
Metabolism of Melanin
Screening by Melanin
Causes of Melanosis
Clinical Picture in Melanosis
Metallic Pigmentation

Dermal Pigmentation—Blue Coloration
(Ceruloderma)
External Pigmentation of the Eye
Nail Pigmentation
Miscellaneous Pigmentations
Decreased skin Pigmentation
Anemia
Decrease in Melanin Pigmentation
Albinism
Vitiligo
Other Hypopigmentary Disorders
Edema of the Skin
Diminished Blood Flow to the Skin
Scar Tissue
Macerated or Desquamating Skin
**Value of Colored Illustrations in Medical
Education**
Summary

FACTORS INVOLVED IN NORMAL SKIN PIGMENTATION

The living human skin normally contains pigments responsible for skin color. Abnormal skin pigmentation can be appreciated only when the range and the many modifying factors of normal skin coloration are thoroughly understood. Consequently, a considerable portion of our presentation of skin pigmentation will be devoted to the normal skin color.

METHODS OF ANALYSIS OF SKIN COLOR

At the very beginning of his examination, the physician discovers much of importance by noting the color of his patient's skin. In optical terms, we say that the eye has been stimulated by light reflected from the skin. When properly interpreted, the message carried by this reflecting light can prove helpful in appraising the clinical status of the patient.

Observation of skin color of patients admitted to a

hospital at night should be repeated later in bright daylight. Many hospital rooms and offices are too dark, even during the day. Examination must be done in good daylight or with artificial light approximating sunlight, to permit proper inspection of the body surface. In addition to the skin, note should also be made of the color of the mucous membranes of the oral cavity and eyes, of the finger- and toenails, of each iris, and of the hair. These specific body areas may not only have color changes helpful in interpreting skin color but at times a diagnostic color specificity of their own.

More attention should be paid to the pathogenesis of abnormal skin coloration in courses in applied physiology and physical diagnosis. Properly interpreted, abnormal skin color provides much useful diagnostic information of systemic disease as well as skin disease.

Light impinging on the skin is not simply reflected from the very surface. The human skin is translucent. Light penetrates the various layers of the epidermis, the dermis, and even the more superficial strata of the subcutaneous tissue (Fig. 39-1). We may think of these layers as a series of colored screens, since normally each contains some pigment. The term *pigment* is used here to denote any colored material present in the skin—whether deposited in the tissue proper or present in the blood passing through the skin—and not merely melanin, too often thought of as the only important skin pigment. This broad concept of skin pigment is necessary to understand properly normal and abnormal skin color. As the light strikes each layer of the skin, a portion is absorbed, some is transmitted, and some is reflected. Of each portion transmitted, some will be reflected from a deeper layer. Thus, each reflected portion returns to the surface modified by the pigment of the complex skin structure. The reflected light carries two varieties of information: In its aggregate, it can be appreciated as skin color; and by analysis of the reflected light, one can determine the contributions of the various pigments to the color.

The human eye is an admirable instrument for the first type of information—color *per se*. Even this function is poorly performed at times because of the prevalence of poor color sensitivity, as well as the rarer forms of color blindness. Moreover, it is impossible to

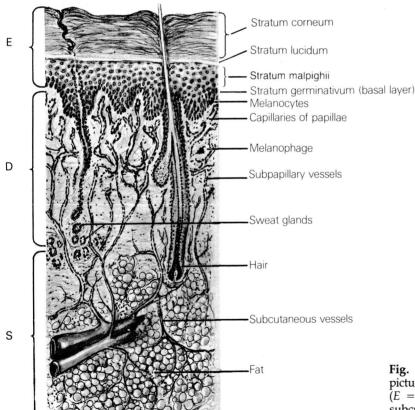

E

Stratum corneum

Stratum lucidum

Stratum malpighii
Stratum germinativum (basal layer)
Melanocytes
Capillaries of papillae

Melanophage

D

Subpapillary vessels

Sweat glands

Hair

S

Subcutaneous vessels

Fat

Fig. 39-1. Composite (semidiagrammatic) picture of the histologic appearance of the skin. (E = extent of epidermis; D = dermis; S = subcutaneous tissue) (E. A. Edwards, as modified by L.M. Edelstein)

record or to tell others the color of a skin area in any fashion that is qualitatively reproducible. This difficulty is resolved to a certain extent by the use of color comparators, such as color charts or color tops.

An entirely objective measurement and recording of color is possible through the use of the spectrophotometer, a technic first used in 1926 by Sheard, Brown, and Brusting for the analysis of skin color.[1,2,3,4] The highly accurate Hardy recording spectophotometer, introduced in 1935, was used by Edwards and Duntley and their associates,[5,6,7,8] by Buckley and Grum,[72,74] and by many others[75–79] for additional and expanded studies not previously possible. Further simplification of this approach for use of skin reflectance has permitted large-scale anthropologic studies of the skin color in humans and others.[111–116] As a result of such investigations, analysis of skin color has been placed on a rational basis and is now explainable in both quantitative and qualitative terms. The use of these instruments must still be looked upon as a research procedure and not directly utilizable for clinical practice, but much that is applicable to medicine has been learned through their use. The objective measurement of color is expressed in terms synonymous with those used by physicists. Thus, the physicist expresses color in terms of *dominant wave length, relative brightness,* and *excitation purity* to correspond with *hue, brightness,* and *saturation.*

Lerner and his coworkers have developed a relatively simple quantitative method for measuring skin color by photography and reflectance measurements, which is a useful additional method of study.[93,94]

The eye is inaccurate and may fail entirely in appreciating the second variety of information contained in the skin reflectance: the identity and relative quantity of the pigments contributing to the color. It is particularly for this kind of information that spectrophometry has been so useful. Infrared photography has been successfully used to study certain aspects of skin color changes not readily visible to the eye, such as vascular patterns in the skin[121] and erythema in heavily melaninized skin.[122] Wood's lamp (ultraviolet or black light) accentuates areas of epidermal pigmentation not readily visible to the unaided eye and also helps distinguish between epidermal and dermal pigmentations.[123]

Recently, photographic methods comprising a variation of light spectra have been used to differentiate the depth of pigment in the skin with special regard to melanin. This work was carried out by Morikawa and colleagues using ultraviolet, visible, and infrared wave lengths.[314] The determination of pigment depth correlated well with corresponding histologic analysis. It was found that for epidermal melanin, ultraviolet photography was the most informative. For dermal melanin, infrared photography was very effective. For hypopigmentation (as in vitiligo), ultraviolet photography demonstrated the lesion most clearly.[314]

A material is a pigment by virtue of absorbing some particular wave lengths in the visible spectrum. A pure white substance has absorption entirely outside the visible spectrum. A substance is pure black in color because of complete absorption of all light rays within the visible spectral range. Gray color of a substance is due to partial but uniform absorption of all visible spectral rays; light gray representing less absorption than dark gray. Any color is produced by absorption of some and reflection of other light rays from the visible spectrum. The total light reflected from the skin contains the absorption bands of each pigment in the skin, identifiable by spectrophotometry. In the accompanying reproduction of curves obtained by the use of the Hardy instrument (see Figs. 39-3, 39-6–39-8, and 39-10–39-13), the reflectance values of the skin, or transmission values of solutions of pigments, are shown for all wave lengths from the violet limit of visibility at 400 mμ to the red limit at 700 mμ.* Each pigment has a zone or zones characteristic of it which are known as its *absorption bands.* The finding of such bands in the curve indicates the presence of the corresponding pigments. Moreover, since the extent of light absorption is proportional to the amount of pigment present, one can give an estimate of the quantity of pigment.[5,6]

Analysis of human skin color by means of spectrophotometry is indicative of the importance of the science of physics to medical research.[11] However, in actual practice, physicians judge skin color by total visual impression. With a proper understanding of basic science concepts, this provides considerable useful information for clinical diagnosis.

Color photography is useful to supplement visual impressions, particularly if a permanent record is desired to document some unusual or diagnostic pattern or increases or decreases in skin color. Many large hospitals provide facilities for this. Photographs should depict the portion of the body where color changes are most evident (if not generalized). Use of the palms to show increased melanin or carotene is a good example. A published example in color shows how effective this technic can be.[9]

Another helpful method is to compare the patient's present skin color with photographs (preferably in color) taken in the past when he was in good health. A published example strikingly depicts this.[10]

Nanometers is the current designation for the measure of the wavelength of light. The older terminology, millimicrons (mμ), was in use when the illustrations in this chapter were published originally. The chapter text, therefore, uses this terminology to avoid confusion.

SOURCES OF SKIN COLOR

Figure 39-1 gives, in semischematic form, the characteristic histologic appearance of a section of the skin with emphasis upon the components important in skin color.

On the surface of the skin is the keratinized layer (stratum corneum). Beneath this is a clear zone (stratum lucidum) most evident on the palms and soles. However, using the modified congo red stain, recent studies have demonstrated the presence of the stratum lucidum throughout the body integument.[12] Beneath the stratum lucidum is the stratum granulosum characterized by large blue (H & E stain) keratohyalin granules. The epithelial cells that occupy the largest volume of the epidermis, that is, the area between the stratum lucidum and the dermoepidermal junction, comprise the stratum malpighii. Although previously called prickle cells, these epithelial cells are now more specifically referred to as keratinocytes, since their primary function is the synthesis of keratin.[189] Melanization of the epidermis is carried out by the epidermal-melanin unit.[59] This is made up of the epidermal melanocyte population, which is present for the most part in the basal layer, plus the associated keratinocyte population. It has been estimated that there are 36 keratinocytes associated with each dendritic melanocyte constituting the epidermal-melanin unit.

The basal layer of the epidermis contains conical indentations of dermis that contain terminal capillary loops derived from the superficial subpapillary blood vessels. This portion of the dermis is termed the *papillary dermis*. The dermis normally contains cells called melanophages,* which phagocytize, as well as dermal melanocytes.[54,55] The subcutaneous tissue contains hair follicles and shafts and fat cells, all of which play their role in skin color.

Ordinarily, melanin is present in melanocytes, located chiefly at the dermoepidermal junction, as well as in epithelial cells throughout the epidermis, including the stratum corneum. Carotone is also present in the stratum corneum.

Four pigments and the additional optical effect called *scattering* have been found to be responsible for normal skin color.[5] Whether the sweat glands contribute to color, however, is not clear. Melanin is the main pigment of the epidermis. The main pigments of the dermis are oxyhemoglobin and reduced hemoglobin present in the papillary capillary projections and su-perficial subpapillary vascular plexuses. The pigments of the subcutaneous layer include carotene in the fat and oxyhemoglobin and reduced hemoglobin in the deeper vascular plexuses.

Scattering consists of a rearrangement of light as it passes through a turbid medium whereby the reflected light shows a preponderance of the lower wave lengths (blue colors).[5] In other words, the light is rendered "more blue" or "less red." All of the skin pigments are yellow or red in hue. Spectrophotometrically, brown is a yellow of low purity. The skin is turbid, particularly in the basal layers of the epidermis. The resultant scattering offsets to some extent the otherwise extreme redness of the pigments (Plate 5) and gives a composite color, which we appreciate as "flesh color."

Scattering additionally accounts for the blue color shown by heavy masses of pigment of whatever nature lying deeply within or beneath the skin (Plate 5). Rare exceptions occur, such as the red color of cinnabar and green color of chromate tattooing. The heavy mass of pigment absorbs almost all of the red light rays penetrating to it. The major part of the light reflected from such an area is that scattered from the turbid basal epidermis and is therefore predominantly blue. This subject will be discussed in further detail later.

Melanin. In the epidermis, melanin is formed by specialized cells (melanocytes) located chiefly in the basal layer.[142] The melanin granules (melanosomes) are transmitted to the adjacent and overlying epidermal cells. In the process of keratinization, as the epidermal cells advance toward the surface, the pigment granules that they contain proceed with them. An occasional melanocyte also can be visualized proceeding toward the keratin layer.[88]

A congenital inability to form melanin is seen in albino individuals. The formation of melanin is a vital process. As the basal cells are pushed superficially in the growth of the epidermis, the cells become progressively lifeless and the granules of melanin disintegrate. In a fair-skinned person, melanin granules are not only fewer in number but smaller in size and occupy one or two lower layers of epithelium. In persons of darker complexion melanin granules are larger in size and more numerous, occupying somewhat more rows of cells. Edwards and Duntley noted that the disintegration of melanin gives rise to a diffuse derived pigment, which they termed *melanoid*.[5] It appears to have an absorption band in the visible violet at 400 mμ and to give the skin a yellowish, sallow appearance if present in excess. Others feel that melanin in fine particulate form occurring in the stratum corneum, in conjunction with strong hemoglobin absorption bands in the 400 mμ to 420 mμ range, could account for the

---

*The change in the terminology of pigment-producing cells was decided at the Third Conference on the Biology of Normal and Atypical Pigment Cell Growth.[54,55] Under this terminology an adult melanin-producing cell is called a *melanocyte* instead of a *melanoblast* and a cell engulfing melanin a *melanophage* instead of a *chromatophore*.

changes noted in the skin reflectance curve in this range.[95]

Although present in the skin in particulate form, melanin behaves spectrophotometrically as though in solution. It shows its greatest absorption in the ultraviolet, yet is has strong absorption in the visible spectrum, too, with fair transmission only toward the red.

The basic or primary melanin formation of an individual is unrelated to exposure to sunlight and follows a definite pattern (Fig. 39-2). *Eumelanin* is the most common biopolymeric pigment derived from tyrosine.[62] It is a random polymer that has an absorption capability in the range of 200 mμ to 2400 mμ and is found in skin, hair, and eyes. In the skin, it is concerned with *constitutive skin color*,[59]—the degree of melanin pigmentation that has been genetically programmed and is unrelated to influences such as solar radiation or melanocyte stimulating hormone (MSH). Secondly, it is concerned with *facultative skin color*, which

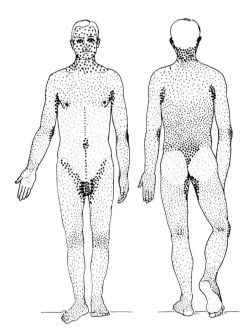

Fig. 39-2. The bodily distribution of melanin. Note primary areas of accentuation in the eyelids, the axillae, the nipples, the areolae, the nape of the neck, the umbilicus, the linear nigra, and the genitoanal region. Accentuation on the face is due to sunlight exposure and at the elbows and knees to friction. Note the small amount of melanin on the palms and soles.

With the exception of the eyelids, the ears, the axillae, the perineum, and the penis, the data were derived from spectrophotometry. The scale was omitted from consideration. (From Edwards EA, Duntley SQ: Pigments and color of living human skin. Am J Anat 65:1, 1939)

is that component of increased melanin synthesis directly related to stimulation by ultraviolet radiation, MSH, ACTH (*i.e.*, Addison's Disease), and the state of pregnancy or pseudopregnancy (*i.e.*, birth control pill).[27,59] This portion of melaninization is reversible and therefore potentially controllable.

Szabo has painstakingly studied the melanocyte population in different regions of the body and in different layers of the skin. He has demonstrated that there is a normal population of dermal melanocytes that can be stimulated with ultraviolet irradiation and that their response is similar to that of basal melanocytes.[87]

Melanin is a powerful pigment, and when much is present, as after tanning or in the dark races, it effectively obscures the other pigments in the skin. In such people, observations of color change are possible only in regions primarily poor in melanin, as in palms, soles, and certain mucous membranes.[95]

Melanin may give rise to blue effects, through scattering, when massed deep in the dermis. Normally this occurs in the eyelids and axillae, in which the material is present in dermal melanophages, or in a hairy area that has been shaved, as in the male cheek, where melanin is present in the deep-lying hair bulbs.[80]

Melanin appears to be the main pigment of the hair, although some additional pigments have been discovered recently.[80]

Pheomelanin is a less common form of melanin and is found most commonly in red or yellow hair follicles.[117] It differs from eumelanin by its solubility in dilute alkaline solutions, whereas eumelanin is insoluble in most solvents and quite resistant to harsh chemical digestion. Pheomelanin is found within the appropriate melanosomes in a similar fashion to eumelanin. Although not completely understood, it appears that the pheomelanin polymer is developed as a modification of the eumelanin pathway involving the chemical reaction of cysteine with dopaquinone forming 5-S-cysteinyl-dopa. This then becomes one of the polymerizing subunits in addition to the standard indole semiquinone. Furthermore, glutathione, an analogous sulfhydryl compound, may be included in the polymer in a similar fashion to cysteine. These sulfur-containing moieties apparently alter the absorption characteristics of the melanin polymer producing shades of red and yellow.

The third form of melanin, *neuromelanin*, is the main constituent of the pigmented cytoplasmic bodies found in the nervous system, liver, and cardiac and skeletal muscle. This pigment is found in lysosomes in these tissues and to a great extent is derived from oxidation products within the catecholamine pathway. This form of melanin does not appear to affect skin color.

Variations in hair color correspond to differences noted in varying dilutions of melanin.

Oxyhemoglobin and Reduced Hemoglobin. The constant perfusion of the cutaneous and subcutaneous tissues by blood compels one to consider the pigments of the blood as cutaneous pigments. The vessels penetrated by light and thus contributing to skin color are arranged in three beds: (1) vessels of the dermal papillae, mainly capillaries; (2) the subpapillary plexus, made up predominantly of veins; and (3) the subcutaneous vessels, in which only the large veins are prominent visually. The subpapillary venous plexus presents the largest surface area of the three vascular beds. The subcutaneous veins show up mainly as blue, through the phenomenon of scattering. It is apparent, then, that the blood pigments exert their effect on skin color chiefly by their presence in the papillary and subpapillary networks.

What are the pigments involved? Those of the blood plasma, yellow in color but usually quite pale, are without much effect on normal skin color. Hemoglobin constitutes the important pigment material. *Hemoglobin exists in the red cells in both the reduced (deoxygenated) and the oxidized form.* Each has a distinct absorption spectrum and color. *Oxyhemoglobin,* the more brilliantly red of the two, is especially characterized in the spectrum by absorption bands at 542 mμ and 576 mμ. *Reduced hemoglobin (deoxyhemoglobin)* is darker and less red, or (one might say) more blue. Its curve shows a single band at 556 mμ replacing the two bands of oxyhemoglobin. The proportion of hemoglobin that is oxidized varies with the class of vessel under scrutiny. Thus, in arteries, the quantity of oxidized hemoglobin is from 90% to 95%; in the veins it is about 50%; whereas in the capillaries, the value lies between the arterial and venous levels. The subpapillary venous plexus has a larger surface area than the papillary capillary network. This is the main reason why the oxyhemoglobin bands in most areas of the skin are considerably replaced by those of reduced hemoglobin. In some areas, the fine veins are usually prominent, whereas the capillaries are poorly developed. Such areas of venous preponderance are to be found in the lower trunk and on the dorsa of the feet (Fig. 39-3). In certain areas, on the contrary, the arterial flow and capillary perfusion are comparatively great, with a corresponding prominence of oxyhemoglobin. This is especially true in the head and neck, the palms, the soles, and in the skin over the ischial tuberosities. To the eye, these areas are considerably redder than the surrounding skin (Fig. 39-4).

The overall contribution of hemoglobin to skin color will vary with the total quantity of that material, as in anemia or polycythemia. *Rapid changes in skin color are entirely due to changes in vessel caliber, in blood flow, and in the degree of hemoglobin oxidation* (Fig. 39-5). Arterial dilation results in an increased capillary perfusion with reddening of the skin, because of the presence of more hemoglobin, whereas arterial constriction or obstruction induces the opposite effect—a pale skin, because of a reduction in the quantity of hemoglobin viewed and a diminution in the degree of its oxidation. The capillaries are probably not capable of change in caliber independent of such changes in the arteries or veins. Interference with venous outflow depends upon posture, venous constriction, or obstruction. Under these circumstances, both the quantity and ratio of reduced hemoglobin (deoxyhemoglobin) are increased (Fig. 39-6). A comparison of visual analysis of vascular change with spectrophotometric examination demonstrates that the eye appreciates quite well the increase in quantity and ratio of reduced hemoglobin under these circumstances.

An obstruction to venous outflow may exist simultaneously with either arterial constriction or dilation, adding the bluer hue of reduced hemoglobin to the paleness of the arterial constriction or to the ruddiness of arterial dilation.

Cyanosis is appreciated when reduced hemoglobin is present in concentrations of 5 g or more per 100 ml

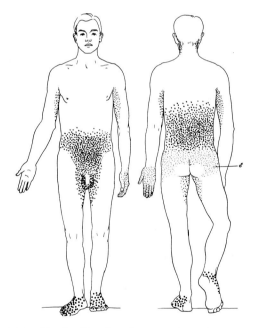

Fig. 39-3. The bodily distribution of predominantly venous blood. Areas not included here or in Fig. 39-4 show no special predominance, except that investigation was not made of the regions noted in Fig. 39-2. (From Edwards EA, Duntley SQ: Pigments and color of living human skin. Am J Anat 65:1, 1939)

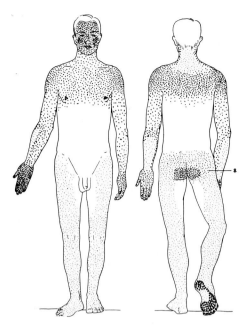

Fig. 39-4. The bodily distribution of predominantly arterial blood. Areas not included here or in Fig. 39-3 show no special predominance, except that investigation was not made of the regions noted in Fig. 39-2. (From Edwards EA, Duntley SQ: Pigments and color of living human skin. Am J Anat 65:1, 1939)

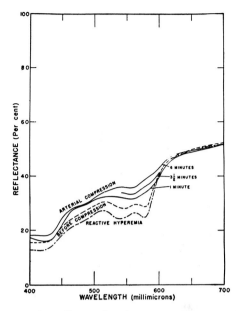

Fig. 39-5. The effects of ischemia in changing the appearance of the palm. A manometer cuff on the arm was quickly inflated above systolic pressure. In 1 minute, the curve has lost its evidence of oxyhemoglobin, and the general shape of the curve shows this to be due mainly to an increase in the reduced form.

As ischemia continues, the 3½- and 6-minute curves show less and less absorption by reduced hemoglobin (deoxyhemoglobin), indicating a progressive diminution of blood in the skin. Vasoconstriction of cutaneous vessels may be responsible. In these relatively bloodless curves, the absorption band of carotene at 482 mμ, previously obscured, now becomes evident. Upon deflation of the cuff, reactive hyperemia is evidenced by the greatly increased absorption, with strong evidence of oxyhemoglobin. (Courtesy of E.A. Edwards)

of blood. Cyanosis may be general (because of insufficient aeration) or local (because of obstruction to the venous flow).

An intensely red skin does not necessarily mean arterial dilation and increased capillary flow. The hands and feet occasionally may be cold but still bright red, with evidence of highly oxygenated hemoglobin. Such findings suggest the lack of utilization of oxygen by the tissues. This is seen when the part is subjected to *extreme cold*, because very little oxygen exchange takes place at low temperature levels. It may be that lowered tissue utilization of oxygen when it exists in other conditions, such as lowered metabolism, may influence skin color. In other instances, such a change would appear to depend upon the opening of the normal arteriovenous communication of the hands or feet. Of course, it may be seen also in the presence of abnormal arteriovenous fistulae as well, especially when the fistulae are multiple and small.

Carotene. Carotene is the yellow pigment of the subcutaneous fat. The term is used here to include a group of related carotenoids. It is found likewise in the cornified superficial layer of the epidermis and in the sebaceous glands, as well as in the blood plasma in a slight and variable amount.[5]

Carotene shows absorption bands at 455 mμ and 482 mμ (Fig. 39-7). Its color in concentrated form is a golden yellow. Spectrophotometric analysis of skin color has shown that carotene is an important normal skin color component. It shows regional variations in quantity closely resembling the pattern of arterial preponderance (Fig. 39-8). Carotene, being lipid-soluble, is present maximally in lipid-rich subcutaneous areas (buttock and breast) and in those areas where surface lipid is high either from sebum secretion (face) or from lipids released in areas of most active keratinization (*i.e.,* palms and soles).

The human subject obtains carotene mainly through the ingestion of fruits and vegetables. Intestinal absorption of carotene requires the presence of dietary fat, pancreatic lipase, and bile salts. Conversion of most of the carotene to vitamin A takes place in the wall of

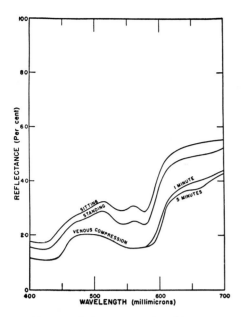

Fig. 39-6. Venous distention in the skin in response to posture and to venous compression. The palm becomes darker with the subject standing and the hand dependent. The increased absorption is caused by the presence of more hemoglobin, but the slight blunting of the twin bands of oxyhemoglobin and the general shape of the curve show this to be due mainly to an increase in the reduced form.

Compression of the arm by a manometer cuff inflated below diastolic pressure gives a further increase in the amount of reduced hemoglobin (deoxyhemoglobin) present. With continued compression, the amount of reduced hemoglobin increases for about 5 minutes, at which time the veins seem to have reached their limit of distensibility. The portion of the curve shown reveals further reduction of the hemoglobin present but no increase in total amount. Fatigue of the veins with further distensibility undoubtedly would occur with greatly prolonged compression. The absorption band at 660 mμ in the 5-minute curve is unexplained. (Courtesy of E.A. Edwards)

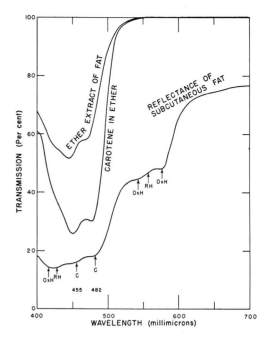

Fig. 39-7. The reflectance of the removed subcutaneous fat from a cadaver compared with the transmission of its ether extract and with a known solution of carotene in ether. The absorption of carotene at 455 mμ and 482 mμ is evident in all three curves. Only the band at 482 mμ is pronounced in the curves of living skin. Absorption bands of hemoglobin are noted in the fat specimen. Some of the pigment has been oxidized by exposure to the air. (From Edwards EA, Duntley SQ: Pigments and color of living human skin. Am J Anat 65:1, 1939)

Normal Sweat and Sebum. Sweat and sebum have not been found to affect skin color appreciably. When allowed to accumulate excessively, the secretion may obscure the skin's surface. However, sebum contains a little carotene, and when intake of this substance is unusually high, areas of much sebaceous secretion may appear to be yellow. This accounts in part for the characteristic localization of the yellow color to the greasy portion of the face in carotenemia.

PATTERNS OF NORMAL SKIN COLOR

BASIC PATTERN AND INDIVIDUAL VARIATION

Classifications of patterns of skin pigmentation are to be mentioned in reference to race, sex, and age. It is important to emphasize, however, that the particular skin colors of any two persons falling into the same category as far as these factors are concerned always will show some difference. It is often unsafe to make

the upper small intestine and duodenum during its absorption.[97] Enzymatic conversion to vitamin A may also take place in the liver. Excess carotene is either destroyed metabolically or excreted in sebum and possibly, to some minor degree, in the urine.

More than 30 pigments constitute the lipochrome or carotenoid group of pigments widespread in nature in plants and some animal substances. The majority have a yellow color; others are yellow to red in hue. Only four of these (α-carotene, β-carotene, γ-carotene, and cryptoxanthine) have provitamin A activity, and these collectively or separately are the ones commonly known as carotene and are the carotenoid pigments most important in skin color in man.

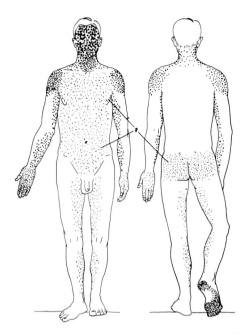

Fig. 39-8. The bodily distribution of carotene. With the exception of the regions listed under Fig. 39-2, which were not examined, the unshaded areas were particularly poor in carotene. (From Edwards EA, Duntley SQ: Pigments and color of living human skin. Am J Anat 65:1, 1939)

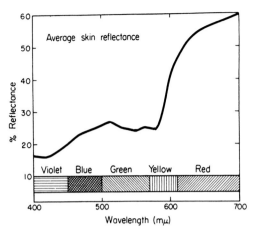

Fig. 39-9. Reflectance curve: average skin, left cheek. Note the dips at approximately 415 mμ, 542 mμ, and 575 mμ. These are due to oxyhemoglobin. They are blunted when there is more reduced hemoglobin, which has a band at 555 mμ. The absorption slope from 465 mμ to 510 mμ is due to carotenoids, which have a maximal absorption band at 480 mμ. In general, more red and yellow are reflected and less green, blue, and violet. This explains the visual appearance of normal skin. (From Buckley WR, Grum F: Reflection spectrophotometry: Use in evaluation of skin pigmentary disturbances. Arch Dermatol 83:249–261, 1961)

deductions of variation in color by comparing one subject with another. It is much safer to compare differences in color of one area with another in the same person, or of the same area at different times. The spectrophotometric reflectance of normal skin of the cheek and the explanation for its red-yellow rather than blue-violet visual appearance is given in Figure 39-9.

Age. It is apparent that skin color is considerably influenced by age. Darkening of the areas of constitutive melanin occurs in both sexes with puberty.[59a] In general, the skin darkens with age. At times a distinct melanosis is seen in aged individuals. This seems to be due to a progressive increase in melanin deposit. Evidence suggests that the younger skin also shows a more active circulation and a greater quantity of carotene. Definitive spectrophotometric analysis of age changes in skin color are not available.

Regional Distribution of Pigments. It is apparent that different regions of the body vary in skin color because of their particular content of the pigments (see Figs. 39-2–39-4 and 39-8 for the original distribution of the different pigments). Differences in thickness of the skin are also of undoubted importance, because a heavy epidermis will cause more scattering. Thickening of the cornified epidermis may add greater quantity of

carotene, and possibly melanin. Areas in which the stratum corneum is thinnest, such as mucous membrane surfaces, accentuate the hemoglobin pigments.

Rapid variations in color because of changes in blood vessel caliber and flow are particularly marked in the hands, the feet, and the face. One should attempt to approximate basal conditions before giving much weight to changes in color in these regions.

RACIAL VARIATIONS

Spectrophotometry has confirmed histologic evidence that variations in the content of melanin are alone responsible for the differences in color of the various races.[5,95]

Gates and Zimmerman have correlated racial coloration with melanin in the epidermis, but not with the sparse amounts of the pigment in the melanophages of the dermis.[56] Shizume and Lerner have found approximately the same level of pituitary MSH in blacks as in whites.[57] There are racial differences in melanogenesis before and after ultraviolet light stimulation as demonstrated by ultrastructural studies.[118–120]

The colors of the skins of the races can be arranged in a series conforming to the graduations of color in solutions of melanin of varying strength (Fig. 39-10).[5] No evidence has been found to support the theory

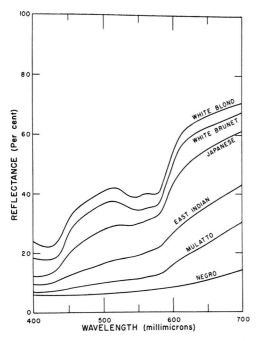

Fig. 39-10. Comparison of readings from the buttocks of males of different racial groups. This area was chosen as one in which pigment content would be minimally disturbed by exposure to sunlight. The curves vary only in their melanin content. Note how readily the oxyhemoglobin and carotene absorption bands can be seen in the spectral reflection curve in the white blond and how they are obliterated by the increased melanin in the skin of those more heavily pigmented. (From Edwards EA, Duntley SQ: Pigments and color of living human skin. Am J Anat 65:1, 1939)

(which has been occasionally stated) that the pigmentation of the dark races is due to pigment not normally found in the white race or to an increase of the ordinary pigments other than melanin.

The heavy melanin deposit of the dark races, especially of blacks, considerably obscures the other pigments.[95] Nevertheless, regions of the body with the least melanin deposit, such as the palms and soles, still may furnish valuable information regarding skin color.

SEX DIFFERENCES AND THE EFFECTS OF THE SEX HORMONES

Spectrophotometry indicates that the ruddier appearance of the male is caused by the presence in the skin of more blood (hemoglobin) and melanin than in the female. Contrariwise, the female possesses more carotene than does the male.

The regional patterns of pigment distribution differ somewhat between the two sexes. Females show stronger areas of primary melanization in the nape of the neck, the linea nigra, and axilla than do males. The contrast in amount of melanin deposit between areas richly supplied and those poorly supplied is more marked in the female than in the male. The buttocks of the female shows a slight arterial preponderance, rather than a venous one as in the male. Finally, females show good evidence of carotene in the breast, abdomen, and buttocks, regions that are poor in carotene in the male.

Study of castrated men and ovariectomized women gives evidence that much of the sex difference in color is genetic and not subject to complete disappearance, or reversal, upon removal of the gonads. This is not to gainsay that the gonads affect skin color considerably through their hormones. It is noteworthy that reactions to these sex hormones take place in the entire skin of the human, rather than in specialized zones as in other animals. A possible exception is the areolar hyperpigmentation resulting from direct application of estrogen cream.

Effects of Castration in the Male. From visual observations, it was believed that the pale sallow skin of the male castrate was due to a deficiency in melanin, but spectrophotometry indicates that melanin production in the castrate or eunuchoid individual is only slightly diminished.

The factor mainly responsible for the abnormal color of the castrate is a pronounced reduction in cutaneous blood flow, the hemoglobin being reduced in quantity and in the degree of oxidation. Areas characterized by a large venous bed showed evidence of venous dilation and stagnation, with a real increase in reduced hemoglobin.

Carotene is substantially increased in the skin of the castrate and could be a factor in giving the sallow appearance to these individuals.

All of the changes enumerated can be reversed by the administration of male sex hormone.

The Hormonal Control of Skin Color in the Female. The effects of the sex hormones are well shown in the female by the changes after ovariectomy, as well as those incident to the menstrual cycle.

As in the male, removal of the gonads causes a diminution in superficial cutaneous blood flow, with a lowered amount of hemoglobin and a relative increase in its reduced form (Fig. 39-11). Administration of estrogen is followed by an increased blood flow and an increase in oxyhemoglobin. Progestin increases the degree of oxidation and hemoglobin but does not consistently increase the total hemoglobin present. The simultaneous administration of both products gives the

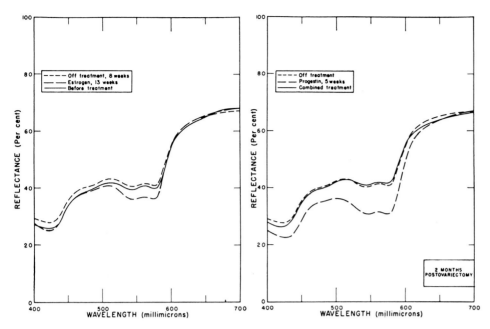

Fig. 39-11. Spectrophotometric curves of the deltoid region of an ovariectomized subject. On the left, the pretreatment curve is low in hemoglobin content, and with dominance of the reduced form. After treatment with estrogen, the curve shows a real increase in oxyhemoglobin. With cessation of treatment, the curve reverts to its pretreatment character.

On the right, the administration of progestin produces a marked increase in oxyhemoglobin. The combined use of progestin and estrogen diminishes the hemoglobin content, causing the curve to revert to its off-treatment level. (From Edwards EA, Duntley SQ: Cutaneous vascular changes in women in reference to the menstrual cycle and ovariectomy. Am J Obstet Gynecol 57:501, 1949)

parodoxical result of a diminution of the quantity of hemoglobin with a predominance of the reduced form. The spectrophotometric evidence available fails to show any changes in melanin attributable to variations in estrogen or progestin levels. However, certain women, either during pregnancy or after ingesting oral contraceptives (which simulate pregnancy hormone changes), will develop melasma.[109,110,199,285,297]

It will be recalled that, contrary to the situation in the male, the output of the sex hormones in the female fluctuates widely in different times of the menstrual cycle. Early, before ovulation, neither estrogen nor progestin is present in appreciable quantity. At this time the woman's skin resembles that of the ovariectomized subject. After midcycle there is greatly increased superficial blood flow, with a maximum in the premenstrual period. This is consistent with the high estrogen production of the proliferative stage, during ovulation, and the immediate postovulatory period. Progestin is produced in the presecretory phase leading up to the premenstrual period, and the combined

effect of the two hormones finally lowers the cutaneous circulation to the level observed at the beginning of the cycle (Fig. 39-12).

SKIN COLOR CHANGES AFTER EXPOSURE TO SUNLIGHT

Skin color changes after exposure to sunlight depend as much on blood vessel effect as on melanin synthesis. Edwards and Duntley followed these changes after a single heavy exposure (Fig. 39-13).[7] The initial hyperemia and redness increased to a maximum 11 hours after exposure. An increase in melanin was apparent in 2 days and reached its maximum on the 19th day. The early hyperemia was followed by a venous enlargement and stasis, which contributed considerably to the darkness of the tanned skin.

Since all persons are customarily exposed to sunlight, with much variation in the potency of actinic rays as well as in the area of skin exposed, the effect of sunlight exposure always must be considered by physicians in their evaluation of skin color.[27]

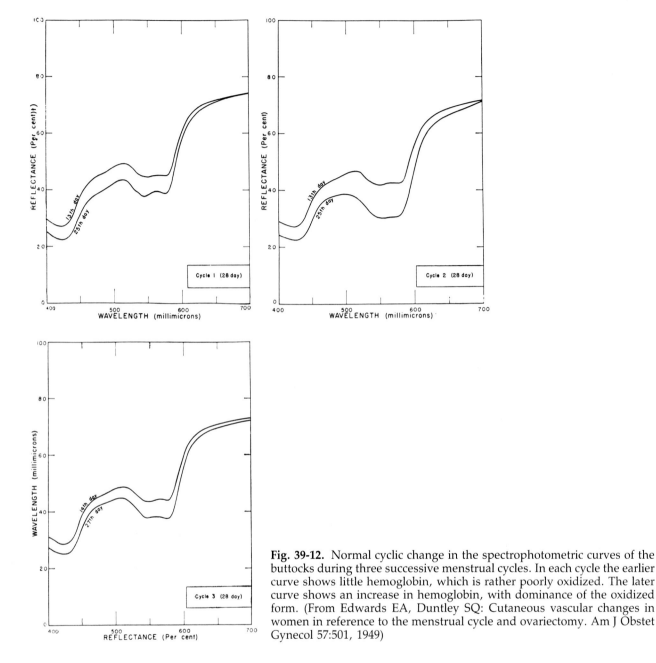

Fig. 39-12. Normal cyclic change in the spectrophotometric curves of the buttocks during three successive menstrual cycles. In each cycle the earlier curve shows little hemoglobin, which is rather poorly oxidized. The later curve shows an increase in hemoglobin, with dominance of the oxidized form. (From Edwards EA, Duntley SQ: Cutaneous vascular changes in women in reference to the menstrual cycle and ovariectomy. Am J Obstet Gynecol 57:501, 1949)

Fortunately, the changes in skin color resulting from exposure to sunlight produce a surface pattern area that usually can be recognized (e.g., shape of the bathing suit, sleeve length, neckline, and so forth).

Findlay has shown that vasoconstriction and vasodilation affect production of melanin by ultraviolet light.[98] This may in part explain the difference in skin color described previously because of hormonal influence on blood flow. It is now generally appreciated that longer wave ultraviolet light and even ordinary artificial light may play an appreciable role in melanin darkening and production.[99,104]

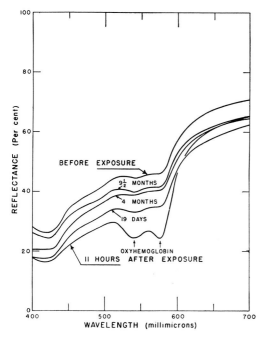

Fig. 39-13. Spectrophotometric curves of the skin after a single exposure to sunlight. Hyperemia (oxyhemoglobin bands at arrows) is maximum at 11 hours, melanin at 19 days, and melanoid at 4 months. Blood stagnation, as registered by evidence of reduced hemoglobin (blunting of oxyhemoglobin bands and depression of peak between them), persists from the early disappearance of the hyperemia for the entire duration of the experiment. (Edwards EA, Duntley SQ: Analysis of skin pigment changes after exposure to sunlight. Science 90:235, 1939)

INCREASED PIGMENTATION OF THE SKIN

Increased pigmentation of the skin may involve hemoglobin, melanin, or carotene, physiologically normal pigments (but present in excess amounts), or other pigments of endogenous or exogenous origin. Table 39-1 contains a classification of increased pigmentation of the skin modified slightly from material presented by Jeghers in detail elsewhere.[13] The reader is referred to this source for more complete clinical descriptions and for a detailed bibliography on this subject to that date.

YELLOW PIGMENTATION

By curious coincidence, almost all of the causes of increased skin pigmentation not resulting from hemoglobin, melanin, or metallic pigmentation produce a yellow color and can be grouped together under the designation "yellow pigmentation."[13] The most im-

Table 39-1. *Classification of Pigmentation of the Skin*

Normal Pigmentation of the Skin
  Skin color in health is produced by a composite of the four following pigments in normal amounts plus the optical effect of scattering phenomenon
    Carotene
    Melanin
    Oxyhemoglobin
    Reduced Hemoglobin

Increased Pigmentation of the Skin
    Yellow pigmentations (see Table 39-2)
    Hemoglobin pigmentations (see Table 39-3)
    Melanin pigmentations (see Table 39-4)
    Metallic pigmentations (see Table 39-5)
    Dermal pigmentations (see Table 39-6)
      produced by excess of normal or presence of abnormal pigments in the dermis
    Miscellaneous pigmentations

Decreased Pigmentation of the Skin
    Diminished amount of hemoglobin (anemia)
    Decreased or absent melanin
    Edema of the skin
    Diminished blood flow to the skin
    Scar tissue
    Macerated or desquamating skin

portant ones and their clinical characteristics are listed in Table 39-2.[13] These possibilities should be investigated in any patient presenting a predominantly yellow color of the skin.

Jaundice. *Jaundice* (icterus) is the most common cause of a yellow skin color and usually indicates a disease with a potentially serious prognosis. The general pathophysiologic aspects of jaundice are provided in detail in Chapter 24. This section is concerned only with the influence of bile pigments on color change in the skin and mucous membranes.

A small amount of *bilirubin*, usually 0.3 mg to 1 mg/100 ml of serum is usually present in the blood in free form, and as such, does not readily stain the skin and mucous membrane. It is not detectable even spectrophotometrically in normal skin color. The serum bilirubin must reach 2 mg to 4 mg/100 ml before jaundice can be clinically recognized on a routine physical examination. Elevation of serum bilirubin without visible jaundice is called *latent jaundice.* It is believed that when jaundice is developing, tissue staining, detectable upon clinical observation, lags behind plasma staining, as indicated by an elevation of the serum bilirubin; the reverse is often true when jaundice is subsiding. Even if deep, jaundice is readily overlooked in most types of artificial light. Only bright daylight or artificial light

Table 39-2. *Differential Characteristics of Yellow Pigmentations of the Skin*

Clinical Condition	Pigment Responsible	Skin Color	Comparative Range of Intensity of Skin Color*	Characteristic Localization	Mechanism of Production	Specific Aids to Diagnosis	Comment
Carotenemia	Carotene	Canary yellow Lemon yellow Orange yellow	X to XX	Palms, soles, alae nasi; occasionally diffuse; absent in bulbar conjunctivae and mucous membranes	Excess ingestion of carotenoid foods. Low BMR (?); absorbed from gut without conversion to vitamin A	Three-layer test of serum; specific blood levels increased	Often a factor in skin color in Simmonds' disease, the male castrate, and so forth; see text
Jaundice (hemolytic)	Bilirubin	Lemon yellow with pallor	X to XXX	Bulbar conjunctivae, mucous membrane, and diffuse skin	Hemolysis of blood with bilirubin retention	Quantitative test for bilirubin; lack of bile in urine	Modified by pallor of anemia
Jaundice (hepatic and obstructive)	Bilirubin and biliverdin	Light yellow, dark yellow, orange, saffron, or yellowish-green	X to XXXX	Bulbar conjunctivae, mucous membrane, and diffuse skin	Regurgitation of bile pigments into blood	Quantitative tests for bilirubin and biliverdin; bile in urine	Melanosis may develop when jaundice is chronic
Myxedema	Carotene	Sallow yellow, old-ivory tint	X	Palms, soles, and face	Diminished metabolism impairs utilization of carotene	Low BMR; normal serum bilirubin	Skin color modified by myxedematous condition of skin and anemia
Ingestion quinacrine hydrochloride	Quinacrine hydrochloride	Yellow to greenish-yellow	X to XXX	Diffuse skin—accentuated in exposed portion and body folds; minimal or absent in bulbar conjunctivae and mucous membrane	Direct staining of epidermis of skin	History; specific urine tests for the medication	Blue spots owing to scattering phenomenon or to pigment deposited in corium or in cartilage; noted rarely

Condition	Pigment/Substance	Color	Distribution	Intensity*	Mechanism	Diagnosis	Comments
Chronic uremia	Lipochromes (urochromes) Carotene Diminished hemoglobin Melanin	Yellowish-pallor Yellowish-tan Buckwheat tint	Accentuated in skin exposed to light; absent in bulbar conjunctivae or mucous membrane	X	Retention of urinary chromogen with deposition in tissues; oxidized to yellow color on exposed surfaces	Blood chemistries and urinalysis	Melanosis stimulated in most instances
Industrial staining	Various yellow chemicals	Yellows of various hues	On exposed skin (face, hands, ankles, and hair); absent in bulbar conjunctivae or mucous membrane	X to XXXX	External staining of exposed skin and hair	Occupational history; rarer with preventive measures	Some yellow chemicals produce liver damage and true jaundice as well as staining skin directly
Picric acid ingestion (simulated jaundice)	Picric acid and break-down derivatives	Yellow	Bulbar conjunctivae, mucous membrane, and diffuse skin	X to XX	Picric acid and derivatives deposited in skin and mucous membrane	Urine orange to red in color; specific tests of urine for picrates; history	May also occur with use of picric acid ointments; of historical interest
Generalized plane xanthomatoses of skin	Cholesterol and cholesterol esters	Golden yellow Chamois yellow	Patchy on skin even when diffuse; none in bulbar conjunctivae or mucous membrane	X to XX	Deposition of lipoids in skin	Biopsy of skin shows local lipoids	Characteristic color seen best in the common xanthomata palpebrarum
Local discolorations of old ecchymosis, Cullen's sign Grey Turner's sign, and so forth	Initially hemoglobin, later bilirubin and derivatives	Initially blue because of dermal location of blood; later greenish-yellow to yellow	At site of trauma; Cullen's sign at umbilicus or in abdominal scars; Grey Turner's sign on left flank	X to XXX	Breakdown of blood or hemorrhagic fluid in tissues	Clinical observation only	Depends on local formations of bilirubin, biliverdin, and derived pigments
Lycopenemia	Lycopene	Orange yellow	Skin diffusely involved; most marked on palms and dorsa of hands, forearms, face, and soles	X to XX	Excess ingestion of tomatoes	History; increased serum carotenoids with spectro-photometric confirmation of lycopene	Specific histologic and histochemical changes in liver

*X indicates skin color is barely detectable clinically. XX, XXX, XXXX indicates marked change in skin color.

approximating sunlight are satisfactory for clinical observation of skin and eye color.

The color change in jaundice is usually detected most readily and earliest in the bulbar conjunctivae. Elastic tissue has a great affinity for bilirubin and is called *bilirubinophilic*.[196] It is believed that the characteristic distribution of jaundice, with its accentuation in the bulbar and palpebral conjunctivae; in the mucous membranes of the oral cavity (especially the lips, hard palate, and under the tongue), and in certain portions of the skin about the neck and upper part of the body, reflects the greater amount of elastic tissue that these areas contain.[196,197] Prominent hemoglobin color may interfere with the early clinical detection of jaundice in mucous membranes. This factor may be minimized by examination of the lips through a glass slide pressed against the mucous membrane to squeeze capillary blood from the field of observation. This strikingly enhances the detection of the bilirubin pigmentation. When severe and chronic, the entire skin eventually appears jaundiced.

Observations of the eyes for "scleral" icterus to detect jaundice is a routine part of every physical examination. Recent reports of postmortem studies (histologic and gross) of globes removed from patients jaundiced at death show the bile pigments deposited mainly in the conjunctivae and almost none in the sclera.[125,126] In fact, removal of the bulbar conjunctiva from the globe revealed a "white" sclera that clearly serves primarily to provide a "white background" to highlight the yellow pigments in the conjunctival vessels and stromal tissue. "Conjunctival icterus" or "icteric conjunctivas," rather than "scleral icterus," has been proposed as the preferred term.[125,126]

Bilirubin is the important pigment causing the yellow skin color recognized as jaundice.[195,197] The color of the skin in jaundice is variable and has been described as faint pale yellow through deep yellow, orange, saffron, yellowish green, or, rarely, even a dominant green. A bronze or dark brown color, if present in addition to a yellow tint, suggests some degree of melanosis. Scratching from pruritis and avitaminosis, both commonly present with long-persistent jaundice are possible causes. That irritation from scratching can cause this is shown by the report of melanosis in all body areas except a butterfly-shaped area over the upper back (the *butterfly sign*), a skin region not readily reached to scratch.[200]

The yellow to orange colors are attributed to bilirubin and the green hue to biliverdin. Watson and associates show clearly that biliverdin, an oxidation product of bilirubin, is often present in jaundiced persons and gives a green tint to the yellow skin when the biliverdin content exceeds 0.3 mg/100 ml of serum.[14,15] *Biliverdinemia* is a feature of regurgitation jaundice and when marked is almost always indicative of neoplastic obstruction of the biliary tract.[201] A lesser degree is common in liver disease. Rarely, it is the dominant color in hepatitis.[124,198] It occurs occasionally in benign biliary obstructions.[15] However, only in cancer or cancer obstruction did it exceed 1 mg/100 ml. These findings are in accord with the clinical impression that strongly evident biliverdin (green) jaundice indicates a serious prognosis because of its frequently cancerous etiology. More recent and improved spectrophotometric studies of blood in green jaundice appear to indicate that mesobilirubin and other green pigments (in addition to biliverdin) appear to contribute to the green tint noted.[201] Another observation of note was that a green tint may be clinically evident with very low biliverdin levels even in the presence of very high bilirubin levels.

It is significant that biliverdinemia is not observed with jaundice of a purely hemolytic origin.[15] Perhaps the absence of biliverdin accounts for the pale lemon yellow color of hemolytic (retention) jaundices and the fact that free bilirubin does not penetrate tissue as readily as the conjugated form. Anemia also adds an element of pallor.

A yellowish-blue or greenish color of the skin has been described as resulting from a combination of the yellow of jaundice and the purplish-blue of cyanosis, a situation noted with the cardiac lesion of tricuspid insufficiency.[202] Jaundice and cyanosis may also occur simultaneously in other conditions and also influence the color of bilirubin.

Jaundice may rarely present in unusual skin patterns, sometimes of diagnostic value. For example, areas of edema[16,17] or paralysis,[197] if already present, may not become pigmented with bile pigments in jaundice. Meakins showed clearly that jaundice could not be detected in skin areas already edematous from cardiac failure.[16,17] This curious phenomenon explains the mechanism of unilateral jaundice, as evidenced in a report of cardiac failure and hemiplegia. Edema appeared only on the paralyzed side whereas jaundice appeared on the other side.[50]

The reverse of this phenomenon is the report by Conn of unilateral edema and jaundice after portacaval anastomosis owing to bilirubin bound to albumin in ascitic fluid dissecting subcutaneously through the incision to produce a dependently localized area of subcutaneous edema.[205] Jaundice was evident in the edematous area but not elsewhere. This paper presents an excellent discussion of the pathophysiologic principles involved in this unique clinical situation in addition to explaining the lack of jaundice in cardiac edema.

Jaundice in individuals with one artificial eye presents, at first glance, the impression of unilateral jaundice.[13] Resolving subconjunctival hemorrhage in one eye, local staining in one eye owing to prolonged use of certain local medications, or following choroidal hemorrhage are possible reasons for unilateral conjunctival icterus.[204] With systemic jaundice, both eyes are involved equally.

The center of large urticarial skin lesions or wheals produced by histamine injections may manifest jaundice before it is evident in the surrounding tissue or to a greater degree than the generally jaundiced skin.[17] The yellowish line bordered by two lines formed by streaking the skin lightly (*yellow dermographia*) is a similar phenomenon.[207] All these contrast with persons with vitiligo, where jaundice in the depigmented patches is less evident than the surrounding pigmented skin.[206] The mechanism is not established but may be an optical effect of contrast of the vitiligo areas with pigmented skin.

Early detection of jaundice in the newborn and during the neonatal period is vitally important, since bilirubin encephalopathy (kernicterus) can lead to serious brain damage if not treated promptly. Physiologic jaundice is frequent and not to be confused with the many pathologic causes of jaundice at this time. To avoid repeating invasive measures to secure blood for bilirubin levels, attention has been directed to multiple daily examinations of the skin for jaundice. Helpful to this approach has been the demonstrations by Kramer[208] and others[209,210] that progressive hyperbilirubinemia in the newborn is manifested by skin icterus, which advances in a cephalopedal direction from the face, the trunk, and the extremities to the palms and soles and that each zone evidences a higher bilirubin concentration. A predictable direct relationship between bilirubin levels and each cephalopedal level was demonstrated.

Detectable skin jaundice required a level of 4 mg/per 100 ml or more with a progressive upward range for each zone. All infants manifesting icteric hands and feet had bilirubin levels greater than 18 mg/100 ml. Of interest is the observation that infants require a much higher level of plasma bilirubin to produce clinically detectable jaundice than do adults.[196]

Cephalopedal progress ceased when the bilirubin level stabilized. It often progressed more rapidly with underweight premature infants. All skin areas cleared simultaneously as the bilirubin level diminished. Bedside observation for jaundice was thus put on a rational basis. The ruddy hemoglobin color could be minimized by diascopy (observation of skin through glass or clear plastic to blanch the skin over a bony prominence and squeeze out the hemoglobin color).

Using this basic knowledge, various noninvasive devices have been developed to study bilirubin levels by study of skin icterus. These vary from the diascopic technic of comparing blanched jaundiced skin against graded color standards to more elaborate methods using skin spectral reflectance measurements.[209,211–214]

Two other types of abnormal colors in the newborn deserve brief comment. Rarely, the skin may have a green discoloration at birth, owing to meconium staining of recent origin or, more commonly, a yellow discoloration from a more chronic presence of meconium in the amniotic fluid.[215] Both can simulate but be readily distinguished from jaundice. The other, a rare occurrence, is an adverse but reversible reaction to phototherapy for jaundice in the newborn, believed to be due to photodecomposition of bilirubin, which produces a bronze discoloration of the skin and serum (the *bronze baby syndrome*).[216,217]

Carotenemia. *Carotenemia* results clinically when an excess of carotene (carotenoid pigments) stains the serum and skin.[13,18,218,251] The term *carotenoderma* is used at times to indicate excess tissue staining with carotene.[13,18] The color of carotenemia (canary or lemon yellow in hue) is best detected where the skin has a heavy layer of stratum corneum (palms and soles) and in areas of the face (forehead, tip of the nose, nasolabial folds) that are rich in sebaceous gland activity and well keratonized. Areas subject to repeated pressure (elbows, knees, outer malleoli) become keratinized and accentuate the yellow color also. Carotene may also be noted in areas normally rich in subcutaneous fat (the breasts, buttocks, and abdomen). It is often evident behind the ears and over the knuckles. It is absent in the bulbar and palpebral conjunctivae[96] and in mucous membranes of the mouth, areas normally with neither fat nor keratin, and in the scrotum, which lacks subcutaneous fat. Rarely, subconjunctival fat, if present, may be yellow from carotene and may simulate the appearance of conjunctival icterus. This overall distribution pattern of yellow color is essentially an exaggeration of the skin distribution of carotene in normals (see Fig. 39-8). A reliable bedside test for the detection of carotenemia is the comparison of the physician's palm, if normal in color, with the palms (or soles) of the person suspected of being carotenemic.[18,219]

Carotenemia results from prolonged excess ingestion of foods rich in carotene; its use as medication[220,221] (*e.g.*, its use as a protection for the photosensitivity of erythropoietic protoporphyria); lowered body metabolism (*e.g.*, myxedema, cretinism, panhypopituitarism, and so forth), which hinders conversion of carotene to vitamin A; diminution of androgenic hormonal activity (*e.g.*, the male castrate); and renal failure[228,229] and the

nephrotic syndrome.[218] Being fat-soluble, excess caro-tene may occur in hyperlipemic states. A mild degree is physiologic in the normal skin color of women as compared with men.[5] Carotenemia was at one time common in diabetic patients but is less so at present. It probably resulted from the high lipochromic diet for-merly used, although some thought it was due to di-minished conversion of carotene to vitamin A. A recent study comments on yellow skin color in diabetes mel-litus.[222]

Theoretically, severe liver disease could cause caro-tenemia by preventing conversion of carotene to vita-min A. However, if jaundice were marked, it would mask the detection of carotenemia. Laboratory proce-dures can separate carotene and bilirubin for identifi-cation in the serum, if both are present. Of much interest have been reports of carotenemia owing to an inborn error of metabolism with failure of enzymic cleavage of carotene to vitamin A.[223,224] Carotenemia has been repeatedly noted in anorexia nervosa.[225,226,235] This diagnosis should be strongly considered in those who are carotenemic and notably underweight. Release of xanthophyll from depot fat as it is mobilized because of severely reduced caloric intake is one possible ex-planation.[227]

Generally, carotenemia *per se* is considered harmless and gradually disappears when excess intake or un-derlying metabolic causes are corrected. However, some believe carotenemia itself may be the cause of clinical changes. Current knowledge of carotenemia has been the subject of a recent helpful and detailed review by Lascari.[218]

This subject is one of special interest to pediatricians in that a benign and self-limiting carotenemia may oc-casionally occur in normal children during the ages of approximately 6 months to 18 months.[230] Children are said to develop carotenemia more readily than adults. Carotene is present in breast milk whereas bilirubin is not, a possible rare cause of carotenemia in a nursing infant.[18] Levels in newborns are low, since passage through the placenta is limited.[218]

The exact role of the xanthophylls as a group in con-tributing to normal or abnormal yellow color of the skin is not clear. Elevated levels have been noted in hypothyroidism, nephrotic syndrome, and hyperli-pemic xanthomatoses. The spectral absorption curve for xanthophyll is somewhat similar to that of β-caro-tene.

Lycopene, the familiar orange-red pigment of toma-toes, is a carotenoid pigment, which, when ingested in excess, may produce a pigmentary syndrome known as *Lycopenemia.*[81,203] It differs from carotenemia in the source of the carotenoid pigment, the presence of ele-vated lycopene levels in the serum, a deeper orange skin color, and specific histologic changes in the liver.

Chemicals and Drugs. A large number of *yellow chem-icals used in industry* can stain externally the exposed portions of the skin and even the hair a distinct yellow color.[13,249,250] This characteristic color distribution, ab-sence of staining of mucous membranes and bulbar conjunctivae, and the occupational history make the diagnosis easy. Persons with this syndrome are often referred to as *industrial canaries.* The yellow color in certain instances is accentuated upon exposure to light.[13,249,250]

The importance of knowing about this condition lies in the fact that exposure to some of these industrial chemicals also may damage the liver with resultant true jaundice and thus confuse the clinical problem.

There has been increasing attention over the years to prevention of such occupational exposure. There is a paucity of reports in the current literature as com-pared to the past, suggesting the effectiveness of pre-ventive and protective measures.

A number of medications, yellow in color, may pro-duce a yellow skin color if taken in dosages beyond the ability of the body to metabolize or excrete them, if taken in normal dosages if excretory body functions are impaired by disease, or if taken for a longer dura-tion than customary. Only a few comments on this problem will be made here. Details can be found in review articles.[13,231] Being rare, most of these medica-tions are not well known and for that reason this man-ifestation is very likely to be initially misdiagnosed as jaundice.

Some drugs are of historical interest only, such as *dinitrophenol,* which was widely used in the 1930s for treatment of obesity because of its metabolic stimulat-ing properties and withdrawn when its toxic proper-ties became known.[13,232] This drug could discolor plasma, skin, and mucous membranes to simulate jaundice. Current interest in dinitrophenol concerns the use of its derivatives in agriculture (*e.g.,* insecti-cides, herbicides, and so on) and in industry with the potential of poisoning, as evidenced by a recent case report.[73] It should be considered in persons with yel-low skin staining, unexplained fever, profuse sweat-ing, weight loss, and so forth, with known exposure to these substances.

Ingestion of *picric acid* or its absorption from oint-ments applied to open wounds can simulate jaundice closely by the ability of this yellow chemical to stain both the skin and mucous membranes.[13,233] Simulation of jaundice in this fashion was apparently a common means of malingering by soldiers in some armies dur-ing World War I.[233] This substance is toxic and occa-sionally produces liver disease with true jaundice. This is another cause of historical interest.

Quinacrine hydrochloride, a drug used at times in the therapy of amebiasis, tapeworm infestation, and ma-

laria, is the best-known example of a medication that may produce a striking yellow skin pigmentation after a week or so of continuous use.[234] It became well known during World War II from its use for malaria. It produces a diffuse yellow skin color as a result of direct staining of tissues, usually easily distinguished from jaundice by absence or minimal staining of the bulbar conjunctivae (more marked in the areas exposed to sunlight).[19] Rarely, pigmentary changes in the deeper layers of the skin, nail beds, or mucous membrane may be produced by this drug, causing a blue color by staining these deeper tissues.[19,105] There are rare reports of simulation of jaundice by its use.[13]

Rarely, *phenazopyridine*, used as a urinary tract analgesic, has been reported to stain the skin and mucous membranes a yellowish-orange color simulating jaundice in the presence of impaired renal function.[245]

Rifampin is an antibiotic that may produce a transient orange pigmentation of skin and mucous membrane in therapeutic doses. With massive overdose, the skin is a deeper orange, or even a bright red (*"the red man syndrome"*).[246,247] A unique feature, helpful in the diagnosis, is pigmented sweat, which can be wiped off the skin with a cloth. The urine, vomitus, and stool are also similarly pigmented.

Sodium fluorescein, intravenously administered, has been used to detect gastrointestinal bleeding, in ophthalmology, and in plastic surgery. It produces a yellowish staining of the skin and mucous membrane that persists for 24 hours to 48 hours.[127,248] It not only simulates jaundice but has been reported to mask true jaundice.[248]

Yellow pigmentation of the teeth induced by *tetracycline* has been reported in a high percentage of young children who received this antibiotic for control of pulmonary infections associated with cystic fibrosis.[107] The offspring of a woman who received tetracycline therapy for cystic acne during pregnancy also showed yellow-brown pigmentation of the teeth.[108]

Uremia. Patients with *chronic uremia* often manifest a skin color that has a distinct pale yellow or yellowish-tan hue.[13,238] The pallor can be explained readily by the severe anemia so common in this condition. The yellowish skin discoloration has been attributed to retention in the skin of chromogens ordinarily excreted in the urine and responsible for its normal amber or yellow color. Excretion of a pale urine is characteristic of long-standing renal failure. The oxidation influence of light on the skin tends to accentuate the yellowish color on the exposed portions of the skin. Retention of carotenoid pigments also has been postulated as a cause for a yellowish skin color in uremia.

Recent important biochemical studies of uremic patients by Tsaltas demonstrated that the pigmentation is due in part to increased lipid-soluble pigment (lipochromes and carotenoids) in the plasma, epidermis, and subcutaneous fat.[228,229] These pigments in the plasma in laboratory studies darken in sunlight as compared to plasma kept in the dark. Plasma pigments diminish with dialysis and renal transplantation. Skin pigmentation can also lighten with restored renal function. It darkens with sun exposure.

At times, chronic uremia also appears to lead to an increase in melanin pigmentation. Malnutrition and trauma from scratching may be responsible. Studies by others demonstrated high plasma levels of immunoreactive β-melanocyte stimulating hormone (β-MSH) in uremia without elevated adrenocorticotropic plasma levels.[236,237,238] This suggests a metabolic reason for the melanosis in addition to the previously mentioned etiologic factors.

Xanthomata. Xanthomas of the skin are yellowish to yellowish-brown in color. Xanthelasma palpebrarum most commonly exists as a benign local skin manifestation of the eyelid but may appear, more rarely, along with other skin types (xanthoma tuberosum, xanthoma papulo-eruptivum, xanthomata tendinea, and xanthoma striatum palmare), which occur in various combinations or anatomic locations, as cutaneous markers of various inborn metabolic errors and acquired disorders of lipoprotein metabolism.[239–241] Diffuse normolipemic plane xanthoma occurs rarely, manifested by extensive macular skin involvement.[242,243] At times the diffuse yellow skin color simulates jaundice but can be easily differentiated. About 50% of cases in one review of generalized plane xanthoma were associated with diseases of the reticuloendothelial system, mostly multiple myeloma.[242]

Diseases of the Skin. There are a number of dermatologic disorders characterized by yellow color of a local lesion.[20,21] They are not likely to be confused with the type of skin discoloration discussed in this section.

The lesions of urticaria pigmentosa may give a yellow color.[20] At times, freckles look yellowish-tan. The skin at times in the male castrate and in subsiding suntan may manifest a sallow, yellow appearance.[5,7] However, melanin ordinarily does not produce a striking yellow skin color. Its closest approximation is to give a yellowish-brown or tan.

Diffused Blood. Blood diffused through the subcutaneous tissues, in the nature of an ecchymosis, hematoma, suffusion, and so forth, causes at first a purplish-blue or blue discoloration owing to its dermal location. As the blood pigment breaks down locally in this site, biliverdin, bilirubin, and other similar pigments are formed. Therefore, diffuse blood in skin tissues can produce localized areas of yellowish-green discolora-

tion (biliverdin and bilirubin) changing to yellowish discoloration (bilirubin). The most common example is the well-known "shiner" resulting from trauma to the soft tissue about the eye. Examples of this color change helpful in diagnosis are *Cullen's sign*, which consists of this type of discoloration about the umbilicus or scars in the abdominal wall and is highly suggestive of ruptured tubal pregnancy or of hemorrhagic pancreatitis; and the *Grey Turner's sign*, a similar discoloration in the left flank which suggests hemorrhagic pancreatitis or retroperitoneal hematoma, as from a ruptured aneurysm.[13] These represent, in a sense, localized areas of jaundice (biliverdin and bilirubin discoloration).

HEMOGLOBIN PIGMENTATION

As explained previously, reduced hemoglobin (deoxyhemoglobin) and oxyhemoglobin in the small blood vessels of the superficial and especially of the deeper subpapillary plexuses play an important role in the normal skin color. Many deviations from this normal pattern are seen in clinical practice as a result of changes in the nature of hemoglobin from normal. These conditions are tabulated in Table 39-3.[13]

All of the hemoglobin pigmentations have in common the feature that the color change is detected most readily upon clinical observation in the portions of the body in which the keratinized layer of the epidermis is thinnest or absent and stratum mucosum is most superficial. These are the lips, the palpebral conjunctivae, the fingernails, and the mucous membranes of the mouth. Abnormal hemoglobin colors are accentuated in the areas shown in Figure 39-4 in which oxyhemoglobin is normally predominant. Abnormal

hemoglobin colors also are conditioned by the physiologic factors governing circulation in the superficial capillaries. Patients with carcinoid syndrome may have a periodic bright red to reddish-purple flush, which may be in the "blush areas" or generalized. It is probably the result of vasodilation or vasodilation with stasis.

Melanin pigment in skin, if sufficient in amount, may effectively screen out the specific absorption pattern of any hemoglobin color change and prevent its clinical recognition. A representative example is the difficulty of detecting erythema or cyanosis in the skin of a black.

The palms and the soles, the fingernails, the lips, the palpebral conjunctivae, and the tongue should be inspected for hemoglobin color change in the darker racial groups because of the minimal or absent melanization in these areas.

Cyanosis results when the reduced hemoglobin (deoxyhemoglobin) blood reaches 5 g/dl. Apparently this is an average value, since Comroe and Botelho have shown by the use of an oximeter for standardization that even trained observers (anesthetists, cardiologists, and so forth) vary greatly in the ease with which they detect its presence by clinical observation in experimental subjects exposed to progressively increased degrees of anoxia.[22]

Several groups in later studies stressed the importance of proper lighting in detecting cyanosis by clinical inspection, checking their results against laboratory analysis of proper blood samples. Ear lobes, conjunctivae, and nailbeds are unreliable areas to detect cyanosis. The lips and buccal mucosa are reliable as detection sites, with good correlation with laboratory values. In one study, the tongue was considered the most sensitive site to detect cyanosis clinically.[253–255]

Table 39-3. *Classification of Hemoglobin Pigmentations*

Type	*Skin Color Produced*	*Clinical Significance*
Predominance of reduced hemoglobin (deoxyhemoglobin)	Varies from purplish-blue to heliotrope	Clinically recognized as cyanosis
Predominance of oxyhemoglobin	Red	Color characteristic of blush, flush, erythema, inflammation, arteriolar dilation, and so forth
Increased amount of hemoglobin	Reddish-blue	Caused by polycythemia vera; blood contains normal amount of oxygenated hemoglobin as well as increased amounts of reduced hemoglobin
Methemoglobinemia	Chocolate blue	Various causes; see Ref. 23
Sulfhemoglobinemia	Lead or mauve-blue	Various causes; see Ref. 23
Carboxyhemoglobinemia	Cherry red	Carbon monoxide poisoning
Cyanhemoglobinemia	Bright red	Seen as bright red spots in persons dead from hydrocyanic poison
Nitricoxide-hemoglobinemia	Bright red	Seen on exposure to nitrate explosion in closed space

The blue color of cyanosis varies in tone and hue from deep purplish-blue to heliotrope and is influenced by numerous clinical factors. The purplish-blue hue is likely to be seen with carbon dioxide retention (which dilates vessels) accompanies anoxia. Cyanosis owing to suffocation is a representative example. The ashen gray color of a person in peripheral vascular collapase represents the sum of pallor owing to poor blood profusion of the skin plus the increased extraction of oxygen by the tissues. A false impression of cyanosis occasionally may be gained by inspection of the lips. The vermilion border may be quite blue because of dermal melanin in dark-skinned people, particularly of Mediterranean origin. For a detailed discussion of the mechanism and classification of cyanosis see Chapter 20.

Predominance of oxyhemoglobin explains almost all clinical situations characterized by a red skin color. In most instances the explanation is simply an increase in number or dilation of the superficial skin vessels or an increase in rapidity of superficial skin blood flow so that the red color of oxyhemoglobin dominates the total skin color to a greater degree than normal. For example, inflammation can increase the size and number of superficial capillaries.

While the color is the same in various disorders, such things as the etiology, the mechanism responsible, the skin color pattern (and its body location and type of spread) may vary enough to indicate a specific diagnosis. For example, *flushing* is due to either transient vasodilatation owing to direct action on a vascular smooth muscle or to mediation by vasomotor nerves.[256] It produces transient vasodilatation with reddening of the face and at times the neck and other upper body areas. Causes can vary from menopause to alcohol ingestion, carcinoid syndrome, or other reasons. This contrasts sharply from the *generalized erythematous* rash of scarlet fever, which is caused by an erythrogenic toxin with a generalized persistent vasodilatation. A study of the skin in this type of rash by magnification, shows numerous, separated, red spots, each resulting from dilated terminal capillary loops derived from the superficial subpapillary blood vessels and each in its own conical indentation of dermis up to the basal layer of the epidermis. Without magnification, the enlarged "red dots" appear to the naked eye as a diffuse red rash. Pressure on the skin by two separate fingers squeezing blood out of the superficial vessels produces a blanched area in the shape of the fingers.[257] A study of Figure 39-1 helps to understand the anatomy involved.

Fever can cause a flushed skin. Repeated application of heat for chronic pain to an area of the skin can produce a persistent, reticular, red-colored area known as *erythema ab igne* and may lead to hemosiderin and melanin in the dermis with production of a mottled pigmented skin pattern.[258] Heat application for chronic pain owing to pancreatic disease is a specific example.[260] The red color in a variety of skin rashes owing to drug reactions or infectious diseases represent other examples of oxyhemoglobin predominance. Some rashes may involve leakage of hemoglobin from vascular lesions. These may vary from red to purplish-blue. In other words, they are of a purpuric nature. Small petechial hemorrhages represent leakage from small vessels in the dermal papillary projection into the epidermis causing them to be small, separated from other petechiae, and red in color, as the hemoglobin is near the skin surface. An ecchymosis, by contrast, represents leakage from the subpapillary plexus, is larger in area having no anatomic barrier to limit spread, and purplish-blue to blue in color, characteristic of hemoglobin pigment in the dermal area.

Exanthemata owing to viral diseases have a varied pathogenesis.[259,261] Some diseases produce enanthemata also. Hemoglobin plays a role in their color.

The flushed red skin of fever is well known. Curiously, accidental hypothermia may prevent tissue utilization of oxygen, so the skin may be bright red and at times edematous. With death from hypothermia, postmortem lividity is red, and with rapid death, cyanosis may be lacking in hypostatic areas.[262]

The tongue looks beefy red in a deficiency glossitis (papillary atrophy) because of desquamation of the superficial, opaque, whitish, avascular filiform papillae (analogous to the stratum corneum of the epidermis), with resultant more superficial position of capillaries just below the lingual mucosa and in the papillary projections.

A rare oxyhemoglobin (red) dominant color is the *harlequin color phenomenon* in the newborn, characterized by an exact midline demarcation of the body into a pale half and a flushed half.[263–265] It is attributed to a transient vasospastic reaction in the hypothalamus, where unilateral control of the tone of the skin vessels is located.

Rarely, a red skin color, not owing to oxyhemoglobin, may result from massive overdose of a medication, such as rifampin, producing "the red man syndrome."[246,247] There are other causes recorded.

Patients with true polycythemia appear to have a flushed, slightly cyanotic appearance, which is called *erythremia* or *erythrosis*.[252,253] It is a common belief that this represents the full effect of the red oxyhemoglobin tinted with the blue of an increased amount of reduced hemoglobin because of the body's incapacity to oxygenate the hemoglobin increment in this condition. However, oxygen unsaturation (reduced hemoglobin)

may be normal, and the color may be more reddish than blue. Peripheral capillary stasis further exaggerates these color changes, which are particularly evident in the tongue.

Persons exposed to carbon monoxide fumes develop *carboxyhemoglobinemia,* characterized by a peculiar cherry-red color quite unlike the red of oxyhemoglobin. It disappears within half an hour after cessation of the exposure. In cases with fatal issue, the color persists.[13] The bright red skin spots occasionally seen with *cyanhemoglobinemia* resulting from hydrocyanic poison also persist after death.[13] The oxyhemoglobin of normal pink skin color disappears after death, and instead one notes the bluish blotches and mottling of unoxygenated hemoglobin in dependent areas, to which the blood moves because of gravity.

Whereas a clinically recognizable cyanosis requires the presence in the blood of 5 g of reduced hemoglobin per 100 ml of blood, a comparable skin color results from 1.5 g of methemoglobin and less than 0.5 g of sulfhemoglobin.[23] Methemoglobinemia produces a chocolate-blue skin color and sulfhemoglobinemia a mauve-blue one. Because of the small amount of these abnormal hemoglobin pigments necessary to produce cyanosis, individuals so affected are often quite comfortable and without symptoms, in contrast with the distress frequently noted when true cyanosis is present. This is especially true if the underlying condition is benign, as in idiopathic methemoglobinemia. These abnormal hemoglobins and other aspects of cyanosis are discussed in detail in Chapter 20.

Although cyanosis ordinarily is related to hemoglobin changes in red blood cells, it may also occur after hemolysis, in which methemoglobin and metalbumin are present in the plasma.[23] Methemalbuminemia may cause cyanosis and suggests such diagnoses as intravascular hemolysis, hemorrhagic pancreatitis, and others.[286]

MELANIN PIGMENTATION (MELANOSIS)

Melanosis is a term commonly used to denote increased melanin pigmentation of the skin. Inasmuch as this pigment is an important component of skin color normally, it becomes clinically significant only when increased or markedly decreased in amount. Any increase in the degree of melanization is relative, since the degree of melanization normal for a person of one complexion or racial group may be abnormal for another.

Melanin pigmentation in any individual can be judged best by contrasting it with its previous intensity (sometimes readily done from old photographs), by comparing one area of the body to another, and by comparison with other members of the same family of

like basic complexion. Frequently the relatives have noticed and commented on a change in the person's complexion.

Fitzpatrick, Seiji, and McGugan have proposed a clinically useful classification of disturbances in human melanin pigmentation caused by decreased or increased amounts.[82] Table 39-4 contains this classification. Mosher, Fitzpatrick, and Ortonne have recently expanded the clinical detail in this classification, which, along with their text material, provides an excellent and authoritative resource for any reader interested in additional information on the clinical aspects of melanosis.[300]

Inasmuch as all normal persons have melanocytes in their skin, everyone has the potential for developing melanosis if affected with any of the systemic diseases listed in this classification. Only the albino, with his generalized defect of melanin formation in the skin, remains unable to develop melanosis.

Metabolism of Melanin

Melanin is a normal endogenous body pigment.[142] Over the years, many of the older controversial aspects of the mechanism of its formation and its biochemistry have become clarified. For a more detailed discussion of the metabolism of melanin and for a complete bibliography, the reader is referred to the important papers by Lerner and Fitzpatrick;[25] Fitzpatrick and Lerner;[58] Lorincz;[67] Lerner;[68] Okun, Edelstein, and colleagues;[188–191] and Fitzpatrick and associates.[59,128]

Aside from the metabolism of melanin, however, there have been several recent advances in the field of pigment cell biology that may enlarge the spectrum of the tyrosine (tyrosinase?)-phenol oxidase system in the melanocyte. Demopoulos has shown that the melanoma obtains a greater portion of its energy from the tyrosine-phenol oxidase system rather than from glycolysis or the cytochrome oxidase system[129–132] and that this phenol oxidase system may be linked to ATP generation.[192] In these studies the copper oxidase, tyrosinase, seemed to be the enzyme involved. However, recent studies of Okun, Edelstein, and associates[138,139,140,316,317] indicate that a peroxidase, not tyrosinase, may be the key enzyme in initiating melanin synthesis from tyrosine. On the other hand, tyrosinase appeared to be a substrate specific dopa-oxidase, with no significant ability to use tyrosine in melanin synthesis. Thus, peroxidase may be involved in an alternate ATP-energy-generating system not unlike that described by Demopoulos. In addition, the ability of peroxidase to oxidize tyrosine to melanin raises the possibility that this enzyme also may have a role in catecholamine formation, since the oxidation of tyrosine to dopa is the common initial step in both mel-

Table 39-4. *Disturbances of Human Melanin Pigmentation**

Type	Decreased Pigmentation	Increased Pigmentation	
	White (or Lighter Than Normal)	*Brown or Black*	*Gray, Slate, or Blue†*
Genetic or Nevoid	ALBINISM, oculocutaneous‡ Albinism, localized cutaneous Vitiligo (may be diffuse) Phenylketonuria (hair and iris) Infantile Fanconi's syndrome (hair)	Neurofibromatosis (*café au lait*) Polyostotic fibrous dysplasia (Albright's syndrome) Ephelides (freckling) Xeroderma pigmentosum Acanthosis nigricans (juvenile type) GAUCHER'S DISEASE‡ NIEMANN-PICK DISEASE‡	Oculodermal melanocytosis (nevus of Ota) Dermal melanocytosis (mongolian spot)
Metabolic		HEMOCHROMATOSIS‡ HEPATOLENTICULAR DISEASE (Wilson's disease)‡ PORPHYRIA (congenital & cutanea tarda)‡	HEMOCHROMATOSIS‡
Nutritional	Kwashiorkor (hair)	Kwashiorkor Pellagra (may be diffuse) Sprue (may be diffuse)	Chronic nutritional insufficiency
Endocrine	HYPOPITUITARISM‡ Addison's disease (vitiligoid)	ACTH- and MSH-PRODUCING PITUITARY TUMORS‡ ACTH THERAPY‡ Pregnancy (may be diffuse) ADDISON'S DISEASE‡ Estrogen therapy (nipple)	
Chemical	Arsenical intoxication Hydroquinone, monobenzyl ether Chloroquin and hydroxychloroquin (hair) Guanonitrofurazone Chemical burns (with loss of melanocytes)	ARSENICAL INTOXICATION‡ BUSULFAN‡ Photochemical (drugs, tar)	Fixed drug eruption Quinacrine toxicity
Physical	Thermal burns (with loss of melanocytes) Trauma (with loss of melanocytes)	Ultraviolet light Heat Alpha, beta, and gamma radiation Trauma (for example, chronic pruritus)	
Infections & Inflammations	Pinta Leprosy§ Fungous infextions§ Postinflammatory§ (atopic dermatitis, drug eruptions, and so forth)§ Vogt-Koyanagi syndrome	Postinflammatory (dermatitis, exanthems, drug eruptions)	Pinta (exposed areas)
Neoplasms	Leukoderma acquisitum centrifugum (halo nevus) In sites of melanoma after disappearance (therapeutic or spontaneous) of tumor	Uticaria pigmentosa Adenocarcinoma with acanthosis nigricans	MALIGNANT MELANOMA advanced (generalized dermal pigmentation syndrome, with melanuria)‡
Miscellaneous	Scleroderma (circumscribed & systemic types)§ Canities (hair) Alopecia areata (hair)	SCLERODERMA, SYSTEMIC‡ CHRONIC HEPATIC INSUFFICIENCY‡ WHIPPLE'S SYNDROME‡ Melasma (chloasma)	

*This classification includes disorders of interest to physicians in general; many pigmentary disorders not listed are of special interest to the dermatologist.
†Gray, slate, or blue color results from the presence of *dermal* melanocytes, or phagocytized melanin in dermis.
‡Small capital type indicates that pigmentary change is diffuse, not spotty, and there are no identifiable borders.
§Usually *partial* loss of pigmentation; viewed with the Wood's light, the lesions are not chalk white, as in vitiligo.
(From Fitzpatrick TB, Seiji M, McGugan AD: Medical progress: melanin pigmentation. New Engl J Med 265:328, 1961)

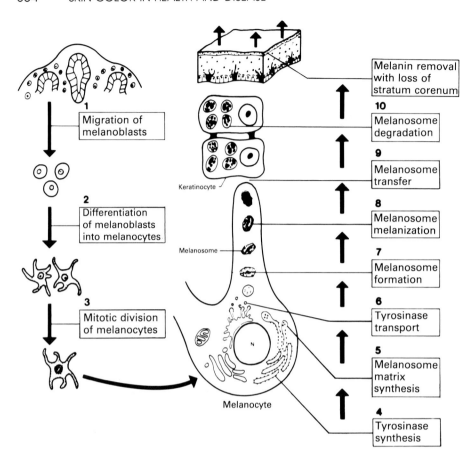

Fig. 39-14. Morphologic and metabolic pathway of epidermal melanin pigmentation. (From Dermatology in General Medicine, 2nd ed, by Fitzpatrick TB, Eisen AZ, Wolff K et al. New York, McGraw-Hill, 1979. Used with permission of McGraw-Hill Book Company.)

anin and catecholamine biosynthesis. Thus, peroxidase may be the enzyme involved in the synthesis of visceral neuromelanin seen in brain,[133–136] liver, heart, adrenal and testis, and gastrointestinal tract (melanosis coli). Such knowledge should lead to a better understanding of the physiologic and pathophysiologic role of tyrosinase and peroxidase in cell growth and function and possibly may shed additional light on subcellular factors controlling skin color.

The morphologic and metabolic pathway concerned with epidermal melanin pigmentation is outlined in Figure 39-14.[59] Here it is seen that the melanocytes[24,25,58,82] are derived from blast cell precursors developed within the embryonic neural crest (1).* These cells are termed *melanoblasts*. Once formed within the developing embryo, they migrate throughout the body, finally resting on such tissues as the skin, wherein they complete their differentiation into the functional melanocyte (2). After basal melanocytic epidermal migration and differentiation have been completed (2), the

melanocytic population undergoes mitotic division in order to reach the appropriate and necessary cell density for optimal melanin production (3). With the establishment of a stable epidermal melanocytic population, melanogenic oxidase enzyme synthesis (4) is then initiated. The enzymes involved include peroxidase[189] and L-dopa oxidase (tyrosinase).[59] During the formation of the melanogenic enzymes, there is also the synthesis of structural proteins. These structural proteins are assembled to form the melanosome matrix (5) The *melanosome*[193] is the specialized cytoplasmic organelle of the melanocyte, which has an important function: the synthesis of the final melanin polymer. After melanosome matrix synthesis has been completed, melanogenic oxidase transport is then carried out (6). The combination of melanosome matrix protein and melanogenic enzymes produce the complete melanosome (7). Once formed, melanosome melanization normally occurs (8). After melanization, the melanosome is ready for transfer (9) to the epidermal keratinocyte. The structural and functional integration of the melanocyte and the keratinocyte is termed by Fitzpatrick and colleagues the *epidermal melanin unit*.[59]

*Numbers 1 through 10 refer to those seen in the flow diagram (Fig. 39-14).

One of the important functions of the epidermal melanin unit is the transfer of melanosomes from the melanocyte population to the keratinocyte population of the epidermis. The epidermal melanin unit is comprised of an epidermal melanocyte functioning in conjunction with approximately 36 keratinocytes. The mechanism of melanosome transfer from the melanocyte to the keratinocytes involves a cytophagic process. This refers to the phagocytosis of the distal portion of the melanocytic dendrite by the keratinocyte. Within this portion of the dendrite may exist one or more melanized melanosomes. Once the melanosomes have been transferred to the keratinocyte, they may exist as single, nonaggregated particles or as aggregates of two or more particles within membrane-bound vesicular bodies. These bodies are similar to phagolysosomes (secondary lysosomes), which are commonly found in macrophages. The melanosomes within the keratinocytes are gradually degraded into small, electron-dense particles during the upward migration of the keratinocytes into the stratum corneum. This melanosomal degradation process (10) is followed by melanin removal resulting from the loss of the stratum corneum. At least one control mechanism of epidermal melanization relates to feedback control involving the delicate balance between epidermal melanin loss and melanosomal synthesis and transfer.[59]

Variations in racial pigmentation appear to relate, at least in part, to the size, density, and degrees of aggregation and melanization of the melanosomes within the keratinocyte population.[59] Thus, for example, minimally pigmented Caucasoids have fewer highly melanized melanosomes within their melanocytic dendrites than Caucasoids who are more heavily pigmented. On the other hand, Mongoloids and Negroids have progressively greater numbers of more heavily melanized melanosomes within their keratinocyte population. In addition to the degree of melanization of the melanosome is the significant difference in distribution and size of the melanosomes among these races. For example, in the Caucasoid, the melanosomes tend to be smaller and more widely spaced within a limiting membrane (complex melanin granule) than in the Mongoloid, whereas, in the Negroid, the melanosomes are much larger and singly dispersed (rather than membrane-enclosed) when compared with the Caucasoid and Mongoloid. Consequently, the greater intensity of skin color involves a greater absorption of ultraviolet and visible light by the larger, highly melanized, and more numerous singly dispersed melanosomes within the keratinocyte population.[59]

It is conceivable that dermal melanocytes may be more numerous in the regions of the eyelids and axillae to account in part for the greater darkness of the skin noted in these areas in some persons.[118–120] Melanin is absent in the epidermis of albinos, present in the least amount in blonds, somewhat more abundant in brunets, and still more in the darker racial groups.[13]

Melanin in humans is formed from the amino acid tyrosine, which acts as the physiologic substrate in a complex enzymatic action. Lerner and Fitzpatrick reviewed the evidence for the present belief that the enzyme tyrosinase (a copper-protein complex) is a single enxyme with two activities: catalyzation of the oxidation of the amino-acid tyrosine to dopa and the oxidation of dopa in turn to melanin.[25] It is important to emphasize that a complex series of chemical reactions constitutes the intermediate stages of this reaction, and thus the formation of melanin is subject to a variety of controlling factors other than the basic enzymatic reaction itself. These reactions as schematized by Fitzpatrick and colleagues are shown in Figures 39-14 and 39-15.[82] The metabolic requirements for tyrosine are satisfied by conversion of phenylalanine to tyrosine by enzymatic action in the liver, and to a lesser extent, by dietary tyrosine (Fig. 39-16).

Melanin is excreted from the skin by desquamation and by drainage through the lymphatics to the blood stream and through the kidney. The amount in the urine is at times grossly visible (melanuria), a condition most likely to result from extensive metastases from melanotic tumors.

Originally, Lerner and Fitzpatrick listed the many biochemical factors regulating the formation of melanin.[25] Some substances (e.g., dopa) catalyze the tyrosine-tyrosinase reaction. Other substances (e.g., sulfhydryl compounds) inhibit tyrosinase by their ability to bind the copper necessary for this enzymatic action or by their ability to inhibit the oxidation reaction directly (e.g., reducing agents such as ascorbic acid).[144] If the sulfhydryl groups are oxidized, the inactivated copper is released with increased tyrosinase reaction. A pH higher than the optimal range prolongs the induction period of tyrosine oxidation, whereas at lower values of pH tyrosinase activity is reduced. The tyrosine-tyrosinase reaction increases with limited rise in temperature. The redox (oxidation-reduction) potential, if high, is associated with a long tyrosine induction period. The amount of the physiologic substrate tyrosine is naturally important. Lastly, oxidation is important; melanin is light-colored in reduced form and darker (black) in oxidized form (Fig. 39-16).[58,59]

Screening by Melanin

Melanin in the skin protects against excessive exposure to sunlight or other sources of ultraviolet rays. It may prevent harmful effects. Some understanding of the mechanism of screening by melanin has been ad-

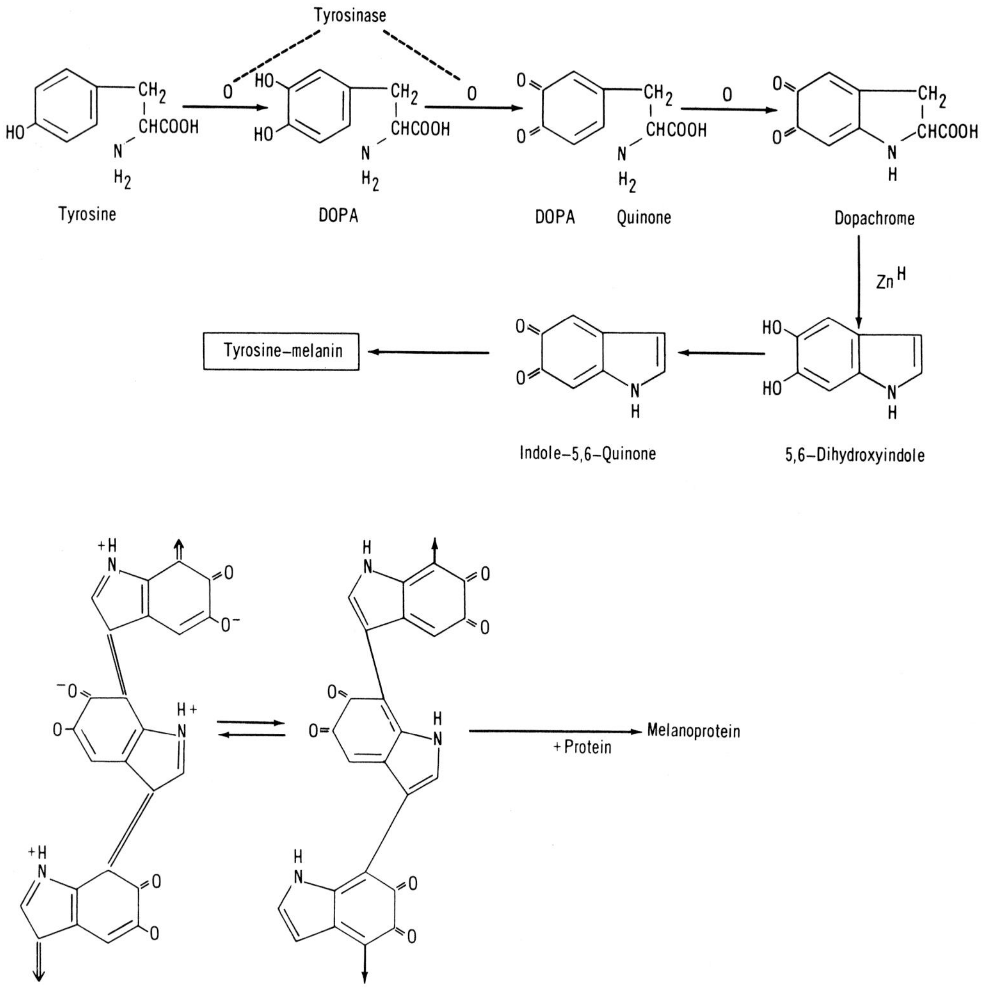

Fig. 39-15. Biosynthesis of tyrosine melanin. (From Fitzpatrick TB, Seiji M, McGugan AD: Medical progress: Melanin pigmentation. N Engl J Med 265:328, 1961)

vanced recently by Seiji[193] and others. The proposed mechanism by which melanin functions as a photoprotective polymer is complex. However, the screening effect is concerned with its ability to absorb radiation, attenuate it by scattering, dissipate the energy as heat, and act as a stable free radical in the process. By means of this, melanin may act as a biologic electron exchange polymer protecting the cells and tissues against reducing or oxidizing conditions, which might release reactive free radicals, thus causing alterations in cell metabolism. In addition, melanin in its usual perinuclear position then may absorb high-energy photons and create harmless free radicals within the polymer; it thus may protect a radiosensitive nucleus and its functional DNA.[143]

Causes of Melanosis

External (Physical) Causes. In many instances of melanosis, the factor responsible is the external application of a physical agent to the skin.[26]

Because of the ubiquity of exposure to sunlight, melanosis from ordinary exposure is accepted as a component of normal skin color and called *tan.* Only when the exposure is excessive is the increase of melanization likely to be noticed. Tanning has no clinical significance unless confused with melanosis resulting from internal causes. Exposure to some artificial source of ultraviolet radiation acts in the same way as does exposure to natural sunlight. Persons with light complexions (blond) tan less readily and to a lesser degree than those with dark complexions (brunet). Melanin

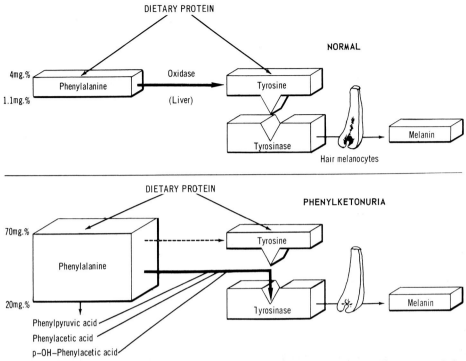

Fig. 39-16. Pathogenesis of decreased melanin pigmentation in phenylketonuria. Inhibition of tyrosine-tyrosinase mechanism by phenylalanine and other aromatic metabolites. (From Fitzpatrick TB, Seiji M, McGugan AD: Medical progress: Melanin pigmentation. N Engl J Med 265:328, 1961)

resulting from ultraviolet exposure is deposited only in the epidermis and never in the dermis and therefore is of a brownish hue.[26]

The skins of albinos and the vitiliginous areas of otherwise normal skins manifest erythema and serious burning upon exposure to ultraviolet radiation because of failure of melanization in skin with these defects.

The skin may be *photosensitized* to actinic rays by application of certain substances externally and possibly by their presence internally. After sensitization, marked melanosis may develop with only very limited exposure to sunlight. The deposition of melanin pigment in such induced hypersensitive states occurs in the upper dermis as well as the epidermis, with a resultant grayish-brown color.[26] This type of pigmentation may persist much longer than the ordinary melanosis owing to actinic rays. Dihydroxyacetone is a topical agent able to produce a bronze appearance in the skin to simulate suntan. It apparently combines with material in the outer keratin layer and is removed as the keratin is normally shed in a few days. The pigmented compound has not been characterized chemically, but it is definitely not melanin. It does not have the protective

activity against sunburning that melanin possesses.

The alpha rays of thorium-x and to a lesser degree beta and gamma radium rays stimulate melanization. In dark brunets, this may occur without a preceding erythema, although usually it follows an erythema.[26]

The application of heat to the skin in any form sufficient to produce prolonged or repeated erythema leads to melanosis of the areas so exposed. The classic clinical example is the reticular pattern of melanin pigmentation that follows *erythema caloricum* (erythema ab igne) because of repeated application of hot water bottles to the abdomen for pain.[258,260] Melanosis from heat is attributed to an increase in the rate of sulfhydryl oxidation, which releases bound copper, and to an increase in the tyrosinase reaction, as well as direct acceleration of the enzymatic oxidation of tyrosine.[25]

Application of any of these physical agents to a degree sufficient to destroy skin (second and third degree burns) destroys the melanocytes, so that the resultant scar tissue has less pigment (both melanin and hemoglobin) than normal and by contrast appears whiter or less pigmented than normal skin.

Irritation of the skin by application of caustic chem-

icals may stimulate melanization through the production of severe erythema.

Mechanical irritation of the skin, if long continued, may produce local erythema and eventually melanosis. Classic examples clinically are melanized areas in the groin from a truss and in the axillae from crutches.

An interesting example of melanosis predominantly of external origin, commonly seen in every hospital receiving indigent and neglected patients, is so-called *vagabonds' disease* or *beggars' melanosis*.[13] The pigmentation characteristically is more marked on covered than on exposed portions of the body and is especially noticeable over areas in which clothes chafe. Lack of bathing, failure to remove dirty clothes, and presence of body pediculi with resulting irritation, increase in heat in body folds, and scratching are the main factors. However, such persons are usually malnourished so that internal factors may contribute to the melanization.

Severe pruritus is common in chronic uremia, chronic obstructive jaundice, and Hodgkin's disease. It is likely that continual scratching by the patients with these diseases acts as a form of constant mechanical irritation and contributes to the melanosis occasionally seen in these conditions. It is characteristic of all forms of melanosis resulting from external physical agents that the degree of melanization gradually diminishes when the exciting factor is removed.

Internal (Systemic) Causes. The types of melanosis of chief importance in clinical practice are those that result from internal causes. No attempt will be made here to discuss all of the dermatologic disorders with melanosis, although some may be of systemic origin. Beerman and Colburn[90] have reviewed them concisely and Cowan[89] has reviewed the ocular pigmentary disturbances. This chapter is concerned primarily with mechanisms of melanosis in conditions that are of prime interest in internal medicine (Table 39-4). The following several paragraphs will attempt to group and explain present concepts of such mechanisms according to the basic physiologic disturbances responsible rather than to discuss them purely from the viewpoint of their presence in a wide variety of apparently unrelated diseases.[25] In most instances, the origin of melanosis involves nutritional, endocrine, nervous, or dermal causes, or some combination of these.

Melanosis of Nutritional Origin. There seems little doubt that many instances of melanosis can be explained on the basis of metabolic disturbance of nutritional origin. At the end of World War II, it was noted that pigmentation was common in persons held for long periods in prison or concentration camps under starvation regimens.[25,29,30] The mechanism of the melanosis here is difficult to evaluate, since nutritional deficiency in humans is invariably of complex origin. An interesting speculation has centered about the possibility that the predominantly vegetable diets of these starved people contained proportionally less sulfhydryl amino acids (cystine and methionine), which normally inhibit melanin formation, than the amino-acid melanin precursors phenylalanine and tyrosine.

In addition, there is a strong possibility that the malnutrition may have been associated with deficiency of certain factors in the diet or that inadequacy of total caloric content may have secondarily produced abnormalities of endocrine function.

Melanosis is common in pellagra (niacin deficiency) and occurs both with the low-grade chronic variety and following the subsidence of an acute pellagrous dermatitis. The mechanism for this melanosis is considered to be similar to that which follows the various types of erythematous reactions resulting from physical agents, as described previously.[25] This is probably true for the type following the acute phase of pellagrous erythema. In low-grade chronic pellagra, hyperkeratosis and pigmentation of pressure areas without much erythema are at times prominent features. Release of sulfhydryl inhibition of melanin formation may be a factor.

Pigmentation is at times a prominent feature in scurvy (vitamin-C deficiency). Both melanosis and hemosiderosis (resulting from purpura in the skin) must be considered to explain changes in skin color in this disorder.[25] General malnutrition might also play an important role in some instances.

Although extremely rare in the United States, melanin pigmentation has been noted in the skin of patients with vitamin-A deficiency.[13] It exhibits a peculiar localization to the site of the hyperkeratotic follicular lesion so characteristic of this disease.

Lerner and Fitzpatrick attribute the pigmentation in all three of these vitamin deficiencies to the release in the epidermis of normal sulfhydryl inhibition of tyrosinase, with the reason for the production of the decrease in sulfhydryl group different in each of them.[25] In pellagra, the mechanism is one characteristic of any postinflammatory variety; in vitamin-A deficiency, it is diversion of sulfhydryl for increased keratin formation; and in scurvy, it is the deposition of iron and copper in the skin as a result of the hemorrhagic tendency.

Melanosis of Hormonal Origin—Pituitary and Adrenal. The generally accepted clinical impression that the endocrine system plays a major role in the control of melanin metabolism finds increasing experimental and scientific support in the medical literature.[83,85,86,91,92] The pituitary gland seems to play the

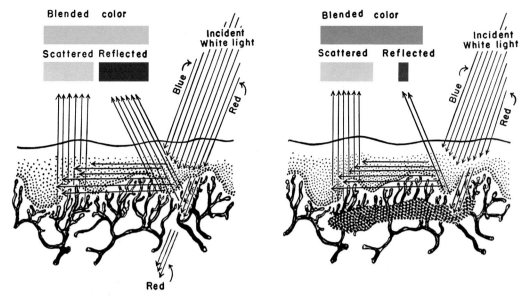

Plate 5. (*Left*) Incident white light (composed of spectral rays—violet, indigo, blue, green, yellow, orange, and red) strikes the skin with differential absorption, transmission, and reflectance at each layer. Note the reflection of some red rays from the hemoglobin in papillary capillaries and the transmission of other red rays through living tissue to give the red color of transillumination. The turbidity of the lower layers of the epidermis scatters the blue rays back to the surface. The composite of reflected red and scattered blue light blended gives to normal skin its "flesh-color" appearance.

(*Right*) The large mass of pigment present in the dermis absorbs most of the red spectral light rays, permitting reflection or transmission of only a small portion of them. Blue spectral light rays are scattered not only from deeper layers of the epidermis (as is true normally) but also from the pigment mass, resulting in a marked increase in the amount of blue light returned to the skin surface. The composite of the increased scattered blue light and minimal reflected red light gives the skin over the pigment mass a blue color. The mass in the dermis represents any of the types of pigment described in the text under Dermal Pigmentation, Blue Coloration. (Courtesy of Edward A. Edwards)

dominant role, followed in importance by the adrenals, leaving estrogen and progesterone and other endocrine substances a lesser but not well-established significance.

The often-confirmed observations of the darkly pigmented appearance of the acromegalic and the characteristic pallor of hypopituitarism (Simmonds' disease) give firm clinical support to the idea that the pituitary gland in humans is concerned in some way with melanin metabolism. The concept of a separate melanophore hormone, produced in the pars intermedia of the pituitary gland, has been accepted for lower forms of animal life.[13]

The presence of MSH in man is now well-documented.[83] This concept received renewed interest with reports of melanosis developing in a white male receiving ACTH; the pituitary extract was found to contain a significant amount of melanophore hormone (intermedin).[25,34] Such contamination could explain pigmentation reported from use of other pituitary preparations.[25] Previous evidence suggested that MSH, present as a contaminant, was responsible in earlier reports of increased melanin pigmentation with ACTH preparations. Lerner and McGuire showed that chemically pure ACTH in very large doses has skin-darkening properties.[94]

Lerner and associates in excellent reviews discuss the polypeptide nature and separate identity of α-MSH and β-MSH secreted by the intermediate lobe of the pituitary.[68,83,84] The reader is referred to these papers for a detailed background of this subject. This secretion has been described for many years as intermedin, melanophore-dilating principle, melanophore hormone, and so forth and generally is accepted as significant in the pigmentation of fish and amphibia. Recent studies have now determined the presence of MSH in human blood and urine. The highly active biologic effect of MSH in humans is indicated by the ability of a few micrograms to influence melanocytes with a prompt detectable increase in skin pigmentation, then with diminution to previous skin color a few weeks after cessation of its use.[66]

The pattern of secretion and activity of MSH resembles that of other pituitary hormones, as Calkins had postulated previously.[35] Thus, the level of its urinary excretion is raised when adrenal cortical activity is low, as in Addison's disease or after adrenalectomy. Of interest was the observation of a greatly increased MSH production during pregnancy, a period when melanization of the eyelids, the nipples, and the aerolae of the breast is increased and the linea nigra of the abdomen appears.[57,66] The level of MSH production is low in panhypopituitarism, which correlates with the pale skin color associated with this disorder.

Several products of the adrenal are antagonistic to the action of MSH. Epinephrine and norepinephrine have an inhibiting action and appear to block its action on the melanocyte. This is in accord with clinical observation that, in instances of Addison's disease in which the adrenal medulla is destroyed along with the cortex, the cutaneous pigmentation is greater than with the presence of only cortical insufficiency. Cortisone and hydrocortisone diminish melanin production,[66] possibly through inhibition of MSH production.

Hall, McCracken, and Thorn have studied skin pigmentation in relation to adrenal cortical function by means of the Hardy spectrophotometer.[53] They found that a great diminution in cutaneous blood flow accompanied the melanization of Addison's disease or surgical adrenalectomy.

Recently there have been reports of MSH-like and ACTH-like peptides produced by various malignant tumors of the lung (including oat-cell and carcinoid types) and of the pancreas (including undifferentiated carcinoma and islet-cell tumors). This suggests possibly a genetic expression of biosynthetic pathways not found in normal cells of these organs. Thus, when general hyperpigmentation is found in association with adrenal cortical hyperactivity (e.g., Cushing's syndrome), the physician should search for possible extrapituitary sites of malignant neoplastic secretion of these hormonelike peptides.[144] Occasionally, in Cushing's syndrome, diffuse depigmentation of the hands and feet has been seen and is thought to be related to high serum cortisol levels, resulting in decreased synthesis of MSH by the pituitary.[194]

Cortisone caused a lowering of melanin skin content in patients with intact adrenals. Darkening of the skin with use of ACTH apparently depends upon increase in cutaneous blood flow as well as on melanin formation. The latter effect may be due to some other product of the pituitary accompanying the ACTH as a contaminant,[53] possibly MSH.

The almost invariable presence of melanosis in Addison's disease has served to center considerable attention on the relation of the adrenal glands to melanin metabolism. A voluminous literature attests to the various theories and extensive research concerning this problem.[13,25]

It is believed generally that the adrenal hormones inhibit melanization under certain circumstances, as evidenced by the striking hyperpigmentation that occurs in animals following adrenalectomy, or in humans following surgical removal of adrenal cortex or the destruction or atrophy of the adrenal gland from disease.[25]

There are various theories to explain melanosis in Addison's disease, including the following:[13,25,36,37]

1. Loss of sympathetic nervous inhibition of melanization occasioned by failure of the adrenal stimulation
2. Failure of the diseased adrenal gland to use the precursor of epinephrine, which results in its conversion to melanin
3. Diminished storage in the adrenals of vitamin C, which normally has an inhibiting effect on melanin formation
4. Depression of blood level of sodium from adrenal cortical failure, with resultant increased oxidation of ascorbic acid and diminution of its concentration, leading, in turn, to loss of its inhibitory influence on melanin formation
5. Possible influence of the adrenal gland in regulating the metabolism of sulfhydryl compounds, with resultant decrease in their concentration in the skin and loss of their inhibiting effect on melanin formation[25]
6. Loss of control of melanogenesis by a pituitary-adrenal axis, in which normally the adrenal hormones inhibit release of MSH or its peripheral action on melanocytes.[25,37,57,66]

The last theory (No. 6) best explains the known facts and was discussed in more detail previously. Figure 39-17 clearly presents this concept in a diagrammatic fashion.[66]

Both clinical observations and laboratory studies have established clearly that primary adrenal cortical insufficiency causes melanosis, whereas adrenal cortical insufficiency secondary to hypopituitarism does so only rarely.[13,25,66]

It is interesting to note that a syndrome consisting of melanosis associated with atrophic bronchitis and generalized cytologic dysplasia has been reported in patients on busulfan therapy for chronic granulocytic leukemia. Pigmentation was comparable to that of adrenocortical deficiency, but urinary steroid secretion was normal.[145]

The frequent observation of vitiligo in Addison's disease, with deep melanosis and marked patchy depigmentation irregularly distributed, is striking.

Gonads. We have mentioned already the influence of the gonads in determining the color of the skin in the normal male and female, the deviations from normal that occur in castrated men and ovariectomized women, and the reversibility of each of these with the appropriate sex hormone therapy. The gonads normally control skin color, not only through their influence on melanization, but also by regulating the skin content of hemoglobin and carotene.[5,6,8]

Oral administration of estrogen in women prior to the menopause has been reported as increasing the degree of melanization in the nipples, aerolae, and linea nigra.[31] Similar hyperpigmentation is said not to develop when estrogens are used after the menopause, perhaps because of diminished functional activity of the pituitary gland at this time of life. Application of estrogen-containing ointment to the skin has been reported as producing areas of increased melanization. The influence of estrogen and progesterone on human melanization requires more study for final clarification.

Melanosis of some degree occurs in almost every pregnancy. It is manifested as pigmentation of the face and accentuation of the areas of primary melanization (namely, the nipples and areolae, the linea nigra, and the vulvar areas), as well as by a generalized increase.[13,31] Occasionally the facial pigment is accentuated over the cheeks, the bridge of the nose, and the forehead in a pattern known as *chloasma gravidarum*,[13] or more recently called *melasma gravidarum* or simply *melasma*. "Mask of pregnancy" is another term. The probable factors involved in melanosis of pregnancy are presented in graphic form in Figure 39-17. As a general rule, termination of pregnancy leads to a marked diminution in the degree of the pigmentation, but some sequelae are left in the form of permanent residue in the nipples, the areolae, the linea nigra, and elsewhere. These are commonly accepted as presumptive clinical evidence of a past pregnancy.[13]

Oral contraceptive drugs containing both estrogens and progestins occasionally may produce melasma.[297] Upon cessation of their use, the pigmentation may persist longer than that seen with pregnancy.

Further influence of the gonads is noted in the darkening of primary areas of melanization in both sexes at puberty and the interesting observation that benign nevi rarely become malignant before puberty.[32]

Numerous examples of *in vitro* and *in vivo* experiments in animals are on record that demonstrate the influence of the sex hormones on melanin metabolism.[13,25,33] Arrhenoblastoma, the masculinizing tumor of the ovary, has been reported as producing darkening of the skin. Apparently both estrogens and androgens increase melanin skin pigmentation. However, the biochemical nature of this action is still obscure.

Thyroid. There is also the possibility that the thyroid gland is concerned with melanin metabolism, as suggested by the common occurrence of melanosis in hyperthyroidism—especially when chronic.[13] Lerner has surveyed the present status of this endocrine gland in relation to melanin pigmentation.[68]

It is of considerable interest that the precursor of melanin, tyrosine, is also the precursor of the thyroid hormones, thyroxine and tri-iodotyrosine.

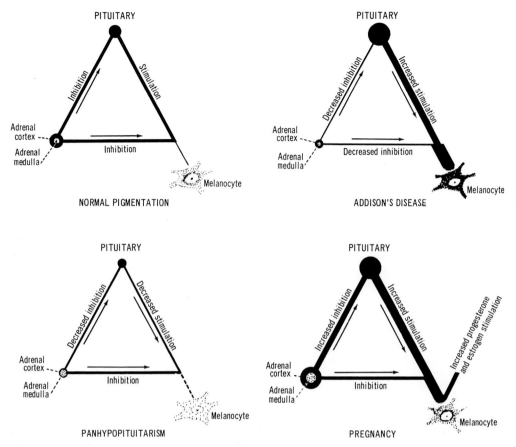

Fig. 39-17. (*Upper left*) Normal pigmentation. Hydrocortisone inhibits the output of MSH by the pituitary gland. Noradrenalin and adrenaline inhibit the action of MSH on the pigment-forming cells. (*Upper right*) Addison's disease. MSH output is increased because hydrocortisone inhibition of the pituitary is decreased. If the adrenal medulla is destroyed, the inhibition of MSH by adrenaline and noradrenalin is removed. (*Lower left*) Panhypopituitarism. MSH output is decreased because of decrease in pituitary function. (*Lower right*) Pregnancy. MSH output, progesterone, and estrogens are increased. Progesterone may have a direct MSH-like action. (From Lerner AB, Shizume K, Bunding I: The mechanism of endocrine control of melanin pigmentation. J Clin Endocrinol 14:1463, 1954)

Melanosis of Neurogenic Origin. There are a number of clinical and a few experimental observations that strongly suggest that melanization of the skin in humans may be subject (at least in some degree) to neurogenic control.[13,25] It is believed by some that imbalance in the activity of the autonomic nervous system may be important, with skin pigmentation being stimulated by parasympathetic predominance and inhibited by sympathetic predominance. Further evidence for the role of the nervous system in pigmentation is the occasional occurrence of vitiligo along the distribution of a cutaneous nerve. Similarly, repigmentation of a vitiliginous limb has been observed following accidental

servering of that nerve, whereas the vitiligo of the contralateral limb remained the same.

Lerner and Fitzpatrick, although unable to explain the mechanism, indicate the possible role of certain neurogenic factors in controlling melanogenesis in human skin.[25] They cited in support of this belief experiments reported by Haxthausen wherein normally pigmented skin gradually depigmented when grafted to an area of vitiligo, whereas vitiliginous skin gradually repigmented when grafted to normal skin. They also comment on the fact that the pigmentation of acanthosis nigricans, which in adults may be due to an abdominal visceral carcinoma (especially of the

stomach), often develops when the lesion involves the celiac plexus or chromaffin system.

Melanosis is common in neurofibromatosis.[13] The congenital neurocutaneous syndrome of melanosis of the skin and central nervous system and the tendency for a skin pigment spot or a tuft of hair to localize over a spina bifida occulta are examples of the curious association of nervous lesions with melanosis.[13] Other types have been described.[13,25,68] Meningeal melanosis may occur in patients with giant pigmented nevi. A cerebral melanoma should be suspected if signs of an intracranial-space-occupying lesion become evident.[147] Free melanin or melanin-containing cells have been noted in the cerebrospinal fluid in these two situations.

Melanosis with Skin Disease. A variety of skin diseases are known to produce melanosis.[24] Any dermatologic disorder that produces an inflammatory response may be followed by melanosis, for reasons previously discussed.

It is likely that certain systemic diseases with end-organ response in the skin may produce melanosis by changes in skin metabolism of a localized nature. Arsenic apparently produces melanosis by its deposition in the skin with resultant binding of epidermal sulfhydryl substances, which results in removal of the inhibition of the tyrosinase enzyme.[25] Arsenic also may act to produce skin inflammation. The melanosis seen with scleroderma and dermatomyositis probably results from local changes in the skin that occur in these conditions.

The reader is referred elsewhere for further information on skin pigmentation in dermatologic diseases.[24,28,90]

Clinical Picture in Melanosis

Melanin normally present in the skin is not of uniform intensity over the entire body but is accentuated in certain areas called primary zones (see Fig. 39-2). These include the eyelids, the axillae, the nipples, the areolae, the umbilicus, the linea nigra, the genital region, the nape of the neck, and the anal region. In women the nape of the neck, the linea nigra, and the axillae are more heavily melanized than these areas in the male. Szabo has shown marked variations in the number of melanocytes in the epidermis in different regions of the body.[87]

Likewise, the pattern of melanosis is not one of uniform increase in intensity over the entire skin but is subject to accentuation in certain areas, which vary with the disease responsible or with exposure to external factors influencing melanin metabolism.

Although derived from the Greek word meaning *black,* melanin in the epidermis ordinarily produces a yellowish-tan, tan, or brown color, although it may occasion-

ally appear black. When melanin is present in melanophores in the upper dermis without much in the epidermis, it produces a slate-gray color; when present deep in the dermis it produces a blue color.[5,13,24]

In most instances the abnormal melanosis shows accentuation in the groin, the axillae, under the breasts, between the buttocks, in skin folds, and so forth—all areas of higher than average skin temperature. It is well known that increased temperature accentuates melanin formation. Friction from belts, trusses, buttons, waistbands, and garters, as well as areas of chafing, may likewise predispose to local areas of accentuation. Still another pattern is for the accentuation to occur in the normally accentuated primary zones of melanization, such as the nipples, the areolae, the linea nigra, the genital areas, and the anal areas. Another common pattern is preponderant melanosis of portions of the skin exposed to sunlight. Pigmentation of the face may be uniform or accentuated in areas, as in the "mask of pregnancy." At times the eyelids becomes heavily melanized. The hair may rarely participate by darkening, but patients with Addison's disease have been observed with prematurely white hair. Not uncommon is the development of melanization of the mucous membranes of the oral cavity and, at times, of the eye and of the vagina. Even the nail bed may show melanosis.

With a few exceptions (*e.g.*, acanthosis nigricans, arsenic poisoning, and so forth), the melanoses of internal origin generally have a similar histologic picture consisting of an increase in the number and density of melanin particles (melanosomes). For the most part, therefore, a skin biopsy in melanosis tells only that the pigment is melanin, as was usually surmised from the history and clinical inspection.

A few diseases produce a melanotic skin picture which, upon clinical inspection, is characteristic of or at least suggestive of the basic systemic disease responsible. These include the "rain drop" appearance and hyperkeratosis of arsenic poisoning; the wrinkled, velvety, and often papillomatous pigmentation of the neck, axillae, and groin seen in acanthosis nigricans; the ocular pingueculae and melanosis of Gaucher's disease; the blue cartilaginous areas of the ears and nose, the sclerae, and eardrums, of ochronosis; the facial mask and nipple-areolae accentuation of pregnancy, chloasma uterinum, and estrogen therapy of young women; the perifollicular skin and ocular localization of vitamin-A deficiency; and so forth.

As a general rule, however, the pattern of melanosis is not distinctive of the underlying disease. The degree and pattern of melanosis from the same disease may vary greatly from one person to the next, including, at times, the ordinarily distinctive ones mentioned pre-

viously. The melanosis of certain localized hyperpigmented lesions is often distinctive enough to be readily recognized on clinical inspection (*e.g.,* neurofibromatosis, Albright's syndrome, xeroderma pigmentosum, Peutz-Jeghers syndrome, and so forth). In reference to xeroderma pigmentosum, it has been found that the dermal fibroblasts of these patients are unable to repair their own DNA after ultraviolet radiation (with resultant thymine dimer formation) when compared with dermal fibroblasts of normal skin. These studies were carried out by use of technics of tissue culture and autoradiography.[148]

Freckles (ephelides) are the most common of the localized hyperpigmented lesions of melanosis. The pigmentation is in the form of clearly demarcated yellowish-brown to tan areas, varying in size and shape but predominantly small and most prevalent on the exposed parts of the body. They are absent in infancy, appear in childhood, never occur on the palms, soles, or inside the mouth, are more prominent in summer and tend to fade in late adult life. The tendency to develop freckles is an inherited dominant characteristic. Except for occasional confusion with melanosis resulting from disease, their main significance is cosmetic.

Except possibly albinos, all persons have the potential to develop a melanotic neoplasm. Aside from the color of the local lesion and its metastases, persons with neoplasm in an advanced stage often have melanuria and may rarely develop a generalized darkening of the skin because of the release from the tumor of precursors of melanin that are oxidized to this pigment in the epidermis.[60] This is one of the few instances in which melanin not produced locally by melanocytes can darken the skin;[25] it likewise occurs in ochronosis, in which an intermediate product of the catabolism of tyrosine—homogentisic acid—accumulates in the extracellular fluid and is deposited and darkens in cartilage, an area in which melanocytes do not occur.[13,25,58]

Mongolian spots[313] (aggregates of dermal melanocytes) are blue in color and most commonly located over the sacral areas, but they may occasionally occur elsewhere. They are most common in certain of the darker races but are seen infrequently in white babies. Such spots persist for a variable number of years after birth and eventually disappear.[13,39] Of special current interest is their ability to simulate traumatic ecchymoses or the "battered-child" syndrome.

The common pigmented nevus varies from flesh color to brown to blue-black, depending upon the amount and depth of pigment-laden nevus cells.

The tendency for the skin pigmentation in Albright's syndrome to occur in unilateral irregularly marginated patchy areas in roughly the same body location as the bone lesion is a distinctive clinical pattern. Also easily recognizable are the smoothly marginated café-au-lait[149] spots and axillary freckling[150] so commonly associated with neurofibromatosis. Such clean differentiation by visible skin patterns may not always be possible. Sometimes skin biopsies in melanotic conditions are helpful. Studies have shown that the melanotic macules in Albright's syndrome and in neurofibromatosis may be distinguished clearly by means of histologic examination of split-skin preparations of basal melanocytes, which show giant melanosomes in the latter condition. This is not generally seen in Albright's syndrome.[151]

The pigmentation pattern characteristically associated with the generalized form of intestinal polyposis (Peutz-Jeghers syndrome) occurs as small melanin spots distributed in an acral fashion inside and about the mouth, on the face, more prominent on the lower than the upper lip, and occasionally on the fingers and toes.[52] This pigmentation has thus far not been associated with polyposis limited to the stomach, the large bowel, or the rectum.

Melanin Pigmentation of Mucous Membranes. Histologic observations have shown that melanin-producing cells (melanocytes) are present in the oral mucosa of most white persons. Grossly visible melanized areas in the mouth (*melanoplakia*) are normally unusual in white persons of light complexion, are occasionally noted in those of dark complexion, and are very frequently observed in blacks. Therefore, melanoplakia has the most diagnostic significance if seen in a person of light complexion or if it develops in a person in whom the mouth is known to have been clear of melanin spots by previous examination. In the darker racial groups, melanosis of the tongue rather than of the buccal mucosa proper may be suggestive of disease. The melanocytes in the mouth are subject to the same internal stimuli as those in the skin, so that melanoplakia occurs frequently in diseases that produce marked melanosis of the skin (Table 39-4). It is possible that the melanocytes in the oral mucosa may react to local physical factors in the mouth very much as do those of skin. Heat, chemical irritation, and friction may be important in this regard.[13,40,41] Also, benign and malignant tumors can arise from these oral melanocytes.[152,153]

In highly melanized human populations physical examination may reveal diffuse or mottled melanin pigmentation of the normal gingiva as well as the skin. Melanin is heavily deposited in the lower third of the surface epithelium. It is important to be familiar with normal variations in pigmentation so that significant deviations from this baseline may be detected as related to chemicals and irritants and specific disease

states. This subject has been reviewed in detail by Dummet[152,153] and others,[283] and the reader is referred to these sources. Several of the more important pigmentary changes within the oral cavity include developing nevi and freckles, seen as brown to black macules, in addition to malignant melanoma, usually presenting as a black nodule. Oral melanin spots can be seen with systemic diseases such as Peutz–Jeghers syndrome, and these lesions remain indefinitely. On the other hand, in Addison's disease diffuse tan-to-brown melanin pigmentation is found involving gingival mucosa. In contrast to these hyperpigmented lesions, areas of hypopigmentation may also occur.[69] These white spots may be seen as oral manifestations of vitiligo and albinism.

Another dark pigment, to be distinguished from melanin, can be found in oral tissues. Hemosiderin may be present, usually as a result of trauma but rarely, as an oral manifestation of Shamberg's disease.[154]

As discussed elsewhere in this chapter, the oral mucous membranes are pigmented by metallic pigments (as in argyria), by bilirubin (as in jaundice), and by certain yellow medications. Lead and bismuth may produce a line at the gum edge. Primarily they reflect hemoglobin colors, normal and abnormal.

It is of interest that melanocytes have also been demonstrated in the conjunctiva. At times, diseases that produce skin melanosis also result in an external ocular melanosis. However, this is less frequent than melanoplakia.

METALLIC PIGMENTATION

Under certain conditions, abnormal skin color results from the deposition in skin of a group of pigments (not normally present), which have in common the fact that all are metallic. The various skin pigmentations resulting can be classified as metallic pigmentation and are presented in tabular form in Table 39-5.

Most metallic pigments responsible for skin pigmentation are exogenous in origin. The important exception is hemosiderin, an iron-containing pigment that results from local or general increased destruction of blood or from some defect in endogenous iron metabolism. The term *hemosiderosis* has been used in a general sense to depict deposition of this substance in body tissue.

Idiopathic Hemochromatosis. Basically, idiopathic hemochromatosis (IH) is characterized by a hereditary defect in endogenous metabolism of iron with deposition of hemosiderin in certain visceral and endocrine organs as well as in the skin. It is manifested clinically by cirrhosis, skin pigmentation, diabetes, cardiac failure, arthropathy, hypogonadism, and other features.

Of interest here is the skin pigmentation present in over 90% of patients and the buccal mucosa pigmentation present in about 10% to 20%. Often noted in the skin also are icthyosis-like changes, atrophy, and partial loss of body hair. Koilonychia is another common finding.[266,267]

The pathogenesis of cutaneous hyperpigmentation in IH is still considered to be unknown. However, the possibilities include the following:

1. Pituitary or adrenal iron overload causing increased MSH release and resultant epidermal synthesis. Specific MSH studies in IH apparently have not been done to date.
2. Direct iron stimulation of melanogenesis (Fenton reaction).
3. Iron deposition and hemosiderin within eccrine sweat glands.

The slate gray color component in 50% of patients with IH appears to relate to the quantity of cutaneous iron, since with therapy it resolves in many cases. However, the residual brown color component appears to relate to melanin deposition within the epidermis and does not resolve parallel to therapy. In patients with IH the biopsy of the skin can be diagnostic if iron deposition can be demonstrated within the eccrine sweat glands using standard stains for hemosiderin.

Usually, melanin pigmentation predominates and has the characteristic color of melanosis.[267] Dermal pigment contributes a grayish color. If both are present, a bronze appearance may be noted, with the term *bronze diabetes* applied when diabetes is prominent owing to pancreatic involvement.

Exogenous Hemochromatosis. There are a number of well-established etiologic mechanisms for this type of hemochromatosis. It can result from injection of an excess of blood in the form of repeated transfusions.[43] Dietary iron excess or iron excess when cirrhosis of the liver is present, certain hemolytic anemias, and other rarer conditions may be responsible. To date, it appears that cutaneous hyperpigmentation is not a major problem in these forms of the disease.

Hemosiderosis of the Lower Legs. Extravasation of blood in the skin of the lower legs, particularly if repeated or of chronic duration, leads to deposition of hemosiderin in the dermis and stimulation of melanin formation with production of a tan, brown, copper, or sepia skin color. This type of pigmentation is limited to the area below the knees and above the upper level at which the shoe exerts a protective pressure and is more marked anteriorly than posteriorly. The pigmentation may be diffuse or localized to small areas, particularly about ulcers or areas of trauma. The most

Table 39-5. *Classification of the Metallic Pigmentations*

Type	Pigment Responsible	Where Deposited	Skin Color	Circumstances for Its Causation	Clinical Significance
Idiopathic hemochromatosis	Melanin and hemosiderin	Generalized in epidermis and dermis	Tan; slate gray; bronze	Inherited endogenous defect in iron metabolism; see text for discussion of pathogenesis	Skin pigmentation characteristic of this disease and rarely absent; usually both melanin and hemosiderin are present
Exogenous hemochromatosis	Hemosiderin; melanin secondary	Generalized in dermis	Tan; slate gray; bronze	As a result of repeated blood transfusion, hemolytic anemias, excess iron intake, and rare causes	Quite rare; suspect with use of many blood transfusions, hemolytic anemia, excess iron intake, and so forth
Hemosiderosis of the lower legs	Hemosiderin; melanin secondary	Deeper epidermis and dermis of legs	Brownish-copper hue; sepia	Limited to legs below knee and above shoe line; results from increased hydrostatic pressure in legs plus local capillary or blood hemolytic factor	Seen most commonly in venous stasis of leg veins, leg trauma, sickle-cell disease, chronic purpuric eruptions, congenital hemolytic jaundice, Mediterranean anemia, Gaucher's disease, Cushing's syndrome and some rare dermatologic disorders (see Ref. 13)
Argyria	Silver	Generalized in dermis	Gray to blue	Deposited in skin regardless of route of entry to body; color exaggerated by exposure to the sun	Chiefly of cosmetic importance; closely simulates cyanosis
Bismuthia	Bismuth	Generalized in dermis	Gray to blue	Deposition in skin over diffuse area	A rare cause of generalized skin pigmentation
Bismuth line	Bismuth sulfide	Gums near teeth	Black	Deposited in gums of persons receiving bismuth, especially if tartar deposits on teeth are present	Diagnostic of bismuth treatment location limited to the mouth (rule out lead exposure)
Chrysiasis	Gold	Upper dermis predominantly	Gray, grayish-blue to bluish-green	May follow prolonged use of gold therapy; concentrated in areas exposed to the sun	Cosmetic; gold more toxic than silver
Hydrargyria	Mercury	Epidermis and dermis of local areas	Brown or slate gray; red-cinnabar	Of local origin; produced by rubbing mercury creams on skin, especially the face and neck	Chiefly cosmetic; simulates systemic causes of facial pigmentations; rare sensitization
Lead line	Lead sulfide	Gums near teeth	Black	Deposition in gums of lead sulfide; local mechanism is similar to bismuth line	Lead does not pigment the skin; lead line in gums is diagnostic of lead poisoning
Iron pigmentation	Basic ferric acetate	Dermis	Brown	Produced by tattoo of dermis, when iron salts are used on skin lesion lacking epidermal covering	Local areas only; of cosmetic importance
Chromium	Chromium oxide	Dermis	Green	Tattoos	Local areas only; of cosmetic importance; rare sensitization

[845]

characteristic example seen clinically is the pigmentation noted in association with varicose veins, especially if ulceration occurs. Hemorrhagic diathesis, venous stasis in the leg veins, increased capillary fragility, and changes in tissue pressure are all predisposing factors. Some of the more common diseases responsible are listed in Table 39-5. Because of the many local causes of hemosiderosis in the legs, this area should never be used for biopsy study for hemochromatosis. Tan-colored spots, localized mainly over the anterior tibial region (pigmented pretibial patches), are common in diabetes.[155,156,268] Upon histologic examination, these spots show moderate telangiectasis of dermal vessels and hemosiderin deposits in dermal macrophages; thus, the skin pigmentation is associated with a chronic vasculitis yet is possibly related to trauma or diabetic alteration of small arteries or arterioles in the dermis and subcutaneous tissue.

Metal Ions in the Skin.[282,315] Any silver compound that enters the body, regardless of the route of administration, results in deposition of silver in the dermis of the skin; when a sufficient threshold is reached, it becomes clinically visible and is known as *argyria*.[270,274] The localization of this pigment to the dermis and about the sweat glands, and its absence in the epidermal layer, produces a skin color of slate gray, blue-gray, bluish, or lead color. Melanin in dermis is stimulated also. The deposition is uniform and generalized but accentuated in areas exposed to solar and artificial ultraviolet light. Fingernails and toenails early manifest bluish lunulae, most marked at their distal edge and darker in the fingers than toes because of greater sunlight exposure of the former.[271] Conjunctivae and oral mucosa are involved as well as the skin. Exposure to sunlight must be strictly avoided. Clinically, argyria is of importance because of the disagreeable lifelong skin color and the ease with which it is confused with cyanosis.[269,298] It often leads to a needless workup for heart or lung problems. The early fingernail changes and the inability to squeeze the "color" out of the skin by finger pressure (as in hemoglobin pigments), along with the history, can suggest the diagnosis.

Chrysiasis is skin pigmentation produced rarely from a gold preparation used parenterally for a long period.[276,277] The metal deposits in the dermis produce a gray or grayish-blue color, limited to sun-exposed areas and less striking in mucous membranes.

Much more rarely than with silver, prolonged use of bismuth may produce a generalized, persistent skin discoloration resembling argyria which is known as *bismuthia*.[275] The conjunctivae and oral mucosa, as well as skin, are involved. Its great rarity should be stressed. Much more commonly, bismuth sulfide may produce

a black line, similar to a "lead line," along the gums near the teeth.[299]

Of historical interest are older reports of the former use of mercury in preparations used on the face and neck, with resultant production of mercury pigmentations, which were accentuated in skin folds and resembled argyria in appearance.[272,273]

Arsenical melanosis may be diffuse, but more often it is of "rain drop" appearance owing to many small, nonpigmented areas.[279] Dermal involvement may produce a grayish-brown or slate color. Presence of palmar and plantar keratoses and Mees' stripe of the fingernails suggests the diagnosis.

Metallic iron can pigment the skin as a tattoo if it reaches the dermis through a defect in the epidermis, but it cannot act systemically to influence skin color. The red or green tattoos are due to mercury (cinnabar) and chromium, respectively.

Lead poisoning often produces a lead-line at the gum edge near poorly kept teeth, owing to formation of lead sulfide.[280] It is similar to the bismuth line formed by bismuth sulfide.

The excellent reviews by Granstein and Sober on heavy-metal-induced hyperpigmentation can be consulted for more detail.[231,315]

DERMAL PIGMENTATION—BLUE COLORATION (Ceruloderma)*

As previously explained, normal "flesh" color of the skin is dependent upon the fact that scattering adds a blue component to offset the predominant red color reflected from the hemoglobin (Plate 5). It has been mentioned also that the same phenomenon explains the blue color seen over a heavy mass of pigment in the dermis of whatever nature.

Scattering accounts for the blue color of a surprisingly wide variety of conditions encountered in medical practice.[13] The blue color of a large superficial subcutaneous vein is perhaps the best-known example. The mass of blood within the lumen of the vein, although dark red in color by reflected light if seen outside of the body (Plate 5), acts as a deep pigment substance to absorb the light reaching it. The light reflected from the tissues overlying the blood mass is scattered in the turbid vein wall and the deep part of the epidermis, to emerge as a blue color.

Findlay's interpretation of his more recent biophysical data obtained using a Hardy reflectance spectrom-

---

*Fitzpatrick and colleagues have recently termed dermal pigmentation (blue coloration) *ceruloderma*.[311] The reader is referred to their definitive and highly informative treatise for a collation of data presented at the Proceedings of the International Conference on Dermal Pigment Biology and Disorders (Scientific Session of the International Conference of Dermatology and Cosmetic Science) held in Tokyo on October 8th and 9th, 1980.[309]

eter and a Nikon epi-illuminator significantly lessened the importance of *light scatter*,—red-brown transmission colors of melanin and the optics of the epidermis—in the development blue skin color.[100] Findlay offers an alternative explanation, which he terms *subtractive color mixing*. This refers to the reflection of blue light by dermal collagen fibers, which are superficial, with absorption of the light between green and red by the more deeply positioned dermal melanin. When the collagen was effectively removed, the blue color disappeared. The presence or absence of the epidermis seemed to make no difference in the development of the blue skin color.

However, some investigators believe that light scattering remains an important factor in the determination of skin color.[101–103] In terms of blue skin, there is general agreement that this is determined by reflection of blue wavelengths by superficial collagenous connective tissues with absorption of green through red wavelengths by a more deeply situated dermal pigment such as melanin or hemoglobin.

The biophysical mechanism of blue coloration (ceruloderma) of skin has been reviewed recently in great depth by Anderson.[310] The reader is referred to this treatise for a concise and helpful discussion.

Dermal melanocytosis is one common cause of blue skin and is represented by conditions such as mongolian spots, blue nevus, nevus of Ota, nevus of Ito, and more recently, dermal melanocyte hamartoma.[278,312,313] These deeply situated melanocytes may produce abundant melanin within the dermis presenting as an ideal biologic model of Findlay's subtractive color mixing concept.

The tattoo artist produces a blue color in the skin by the use of black ink, the degree of blue produced being proportional to the amount of black ink and depth in the dermis at which the needle deposits the particles. The blue color of the skin that results from road accidents in which dark-colored dirt is scraped into the skin and the color that results from powder marks from explosion are other examples. A curious type of blue atrophic skin spots is seen in drug addicts who flame the hypodermic needle for sterilization purposes; injections produce blue tattoo marks by depositing carbon soot particles in the dermis or subcutaneous tissues. At times hypodermic injections of medication do the same thing. Similar spots have been noted from bites of pubic pediculi.

The blue sclerae associated with fragilitas ossium are explained by the greater transparency of the sclerae in this condition which allows white light to penetrate to the pigmented coat of the eye with resultant absorption there, and greater preponderance of blue wavelengths in the reflected light rays scattered in the sclera itself. Greater transparency of the sclerae at birth may account for their tendency to blueness in the newborn. Rarely, individuals are born with their melanocytes located in the deep dermis instead of the lower epidermis over part or even most of their skin. Such persons exhibit a striking blue skin color in such areas. This unusual condition is only of cosmetic importance, since the skin is otherwise normal. A more common variety is the so-called *mongolian spot*, localized commonly but not exclusively over the sacral area at birth.[313] It is due to a collection of functioning dermal melanocytes in this area which tend to lose their activity as the child develops, with gradual return of normal skin color. The blue phase of pinta has been demonstrated to be due to deposition of melanin in the dermis. The blue color of the ears and nose, or even the skin, in ochronosis is due to pigment deposited in the cartilage of the ear or nose, or at times deep in the skin.[11,13,244] During World War II, use of quinacrine hydrochloride for malaria rarely was noted to produce areas of blue color over the nose, fingernails, palate, and so forth, apparently the result of deposition of this substance or stimulation of some other pigment deep in the dermis.[19] A syndrome mimicking ochronosis has been described after prolonged local use of a preparation containing resorcin in the treatment of chronic leg ulcer.[106] The patient had dark urine containing black resorcin polymers.

There are other types of drug-induced bluish scatter pigmentation. A remarkable example is that caused by deposition in the skin of polymers of the oxidation products of chlorpromazine. Occasionally a patient on long-term therapy with chlorpromazine may have widespread deposition of the pigment: in the deep dermis, in the reticuloendothelial system, and in the parenchymal cells of liver, myocardium, kidney, brain, and lung. The pigment is actually brown, but because of the scattering effect, the skin has a purple color, and affected persons have been referred to as "*purple people*."[157] Formation of melanin in the skin may be provoked by this drug, as suggested by Van Woert.[158] He has demonstrated *in vitro* that there is great increase in tyrosinase activity induced by phenothiazine compounds.[159]

The blue or purplish color of a deep ecchymosis due to a collection of pigment mass (free blood) in the subcutaneous tissue is another example.

The blue color of hematomas and the blue appearance of the umbilicus or of thin abdominal scars when the peritoneal cavity contains free blood are still other examples.

Fitzpatrick, Montgomery, and Lerner discuss other disorders that produce a dermal pigmentation capable of producing a blue skin color. The excellent classifi-

cation proposed by these authors is given in Table 39-6.[60] A more detailed classification has recently been published by Fitzpatrick and colleagues.[311]

The bluish discoloration occasionally noted about the eyelids and in the axillae may be because these areas in some normal people contain melanin in the dermis as well as the epidermis. The blue sheen of the shaven cheek or axillae of a person with dark hair results from scattering because of the darkly pigmented hair shafts in the deep dermis.[5,13] The reader is referred elsewhere for reference to the literature on this subject and for a key to available published color plates.[13] Those not familiar with this form of skin color will profit greatly from a study of such colored illustrations.

External Pigmentation of the Eye

Abnormal color change of the various external membranes of the eye—the eyelids, palpebral conjunctivae, bulbar conjunctivae, the sclerae, and cornea—may be related to various skin pigmentations and is of considerable clinical interest and diagnostic importance. These structures should be carefully evaluated, along with the skin, as to abnormal color. Although not external, each iris should also be observed for color. This subject is complex and only brief comment will be made here. Details can be found in journal literature and monographs. The following discussion provides some representative examples.

Eyelids. The classic "shiner" (ecchymosis) may be due to trauma or it may be a manifestation of a disease causing purpura. Dark circles around the eyes may represent dehydration, perhaps weight loss, and so forth. Melanin hyperpigmentation is often hereditary and believed also at times to be of biliary or renal origin.[287–290]

Conjunctivae. Bilirubin, melanin, and metallic pigmentations are well known and discussed elsewhere in this chapter.

Sclera. The blue sclerae of osteogenesis imperfecta,[13] the blue color of areas of scleromalacia,[291] changes as-

Table 39-6. *Classification of Dermal Pigmentation (Blue Coloration—Ceruloderma)*

Genetic	Blue nevus
	Mongolian spot (abnormally placed melanocytes in the dermis)
	Nevus of Ota
	Racial (in the eyelids, axillae, and nails of certain normal individuals)
	Incontinentia pigmenti
Chemical	Mercury (contained in face creams)
	Heavy metal intoxication (silver, bismuth, gold, lead)
	Carbon particles (tattoo, accidental pencil implant, drug addicts)
	Fixed drug eruption
Nutritional	Chronic malnutrition (splotchy, slate-gray pigmentation noted in prisoners of war and in experimental human starvation)
Metabolic	Hemochromatosis (owing to hemosiderin particles in the dermis)
	Ochronosis (polymerized homogenitisic acid in the dermis)
Neoplastic	Primary melanoma arising from blue nevus and nevus of Ota
	Metastatic malignant melanoma nodule in the dermis
	Malignant melanoma with melanuria and dermal pigmentation
	Pigmented basal-cell carcinoma
	Glomus tumor
	Hemangioma and hemangiosarcoma
	Neurofibromatosis*
Infectious and inflammatory	Pinta
	Chronic inflammatory dermatoses
	Pediculosis pubis (maculae ceruleae)
Circulatory	Purpura and hemosiderosis
	Cyanosis
	Methemoglobinemia
	Sulfhemoglobinemia

*Presently considered as genetic in origin (see Table 39-4)
(Classification from Fitzpatrick TB, Montgomery H, Lerner AB: Pathogenesis of generalized dermal pigmentation secondary to malignant melanoma and melanuria. J Invest Dermatol 22:163, 1954)

sociated with connective disease, ochronotic[292] pigment spots, Gaucher's disease, and so forth are representative of this group.

Irides. Although within the eye, the color of each iris can be observed readily by clinical inspection. There is a surprisingly extensive literature on changes in its color related to systemic disease.[293,294] Iris color is controlled by heredity (blue recessive to brown), metabolism of melanin, and cervical sympathetic stimulation. All the colors of the iris (blue, green, gray, brown, and so forth) are due to melanin. With brown color, all layers of the iris have melanin pigment; with blue color, melanin is present only in the inner layer. Other shades of color depend on varying degrees of melanization between these two perimeters. With total albinism, the irides are pink in color.

Heterochromic iridis means the iris color in one eye is different from the other or one iris has areas of different color. Heterochromic iridis is associated with a wide variety of diseases or syndromes. Typical examples are the congenital form of Horner's syndrome, cervical neuroblastoma, nevus of Ota, Waardenburg's syndrome, and others. Details can be found in helpful reviews.[293,294]

Lisch spots (multiple pigmented nodules in the iris) may be noted in neurofibromatosis.[295] Brushfield's spots of the iris are much more frequent in Down's syndrome than in normals.[296]

These limited examples (which exclude the cornea) indicate how helpful evaluation of the color of each external structure of the eye can be.

Nail Pigmentation

Abnormal color of fingernails and toenails may have a diagnostic specifity of its own or aid in the evaluation of skin color. Comparison of fingers and toes may indicate whether the color change is solar-accentuated, since the fingers almost always have greater sunlight exposure. This is characteristic of the metallic pigmentations, especially argyria. Each substructure of the nail should be evaluted; these include the lunula, nail matrix, nail bed, and nail plate. Systemic diseases may manifest color changes in one or more of these substructures. For example, certain diseases discolor the lunula early. Argyria, which has been discussed elsewhere in this chapter, produces a blue or azure lunula.[271] One specifically distinctive lunula is noted in Wilson's disease.[301] Several diseases cause a red lunula.

Melanocytes are present in the nail bed, as indicated by the frequent presence of band melanin pigmentation in blacks.[42,302] This is rare in whites. However, diffuse melanosis of nails is rare in any racial group

and, if present, is suggestive of systemic disease such as Addison's disease, adverse effects of chemotherapeutic agents, and so forth. The distal brown arc of chronic renal failure is another variant.

Examples of a distinctive change in the nail plate are single or multiple white lines across the nail known as *Mees' lines* (owing to arsenic and various other causes). The yellow nail syndrome is another.[304]

The pink portion of the nail reflects hemoglobin color (*i.e.,* cyanosis, pallor, and so forth), but not in the presence of poor peripheral circulation (shock). A large number of medications, cancer chemotherapy agents, irradiation, and bacterial and fungus infections can cause color changes.

White discoloration (leukonychia) has many causes; Muehrcke's lines, owing to hypoalbuminemia, is one that is well known.[303]

It is beyond the scope of this chapter to provide adequate detail on nail pigmentation. There is an extensive journal literature that can be approached through review articles[305,307] and monographs.[306,308] A broad understanding of nail color and its abnormalities is a useful asset in clinical diagnosis.

MISCELLANEOUS PIGMENTATIONS

There are a few conditions capable of producing abnormal pigments not readily classified in one of the preceding groups. Most of these are of academic interest and only rarely affect skin color to a degree to be of clinical importance. A few which come to mind are hematin in malaria, methemalbumin, porphyrins, and so forth. In the group would fall also the skin discolorations produced by the injection or ingestion of medicinal or testing substances. These will not be discussed.

Much detail on drug-induced skin pigmentation can be found in the excellent reviews by Levantine and Almeyda[281] and Granstein and Sober.[231] Space does not permit their coverage in this chapter.

DECREASED SKIN PIGMENTATION

Most commonly, abnormal skin color reflects an increase of normal pigments or the presence of abnormal pigments. However, abnormal skin color at times may result from the diminution of the amount of one or more of the normal pigments or modification of their appearance by some anatomic or physiologic factor. Such changes may be just as indicative of disease as increase in skin pigmentation and fit usually into one of the following categories.

ANEMIA

The degree of pallor produced by anemia is ordinarily proportional to the hemoglobin content of the blood. As with any color values affected by amounts of chemical types of hemoglobin, the pallor of anemia is most readily detected in nonmelanized areas (the lips, the palpebral conjunctivae, and the transparent fingernails). Skin color in anemic patients varies for reasons other than diminution of hemoglobin alone. Hemolytic anemia may produce a combination of pallor and jaundice, as exemplified by the lemon-yellow pallor of severe pernicious anemia. Certain anemias may be associated with the skin deposition of hemosiderin. Vitiligo is not uncommon in anemia. Modern descriptions of hypochromic anemia in adolescent girls no longer include a greenish-yellow pallor. Melanin skin pigmentation occurs in refractory normochromic anemias, some cases of idiopathic microcytic hypochromic anemia, pernicious anemia,[9] anemia resulting from folic acid deficiency,[284] and certain erythroblastic types of anemia. It may hide skin pallor and be associated at times with a spotty type of melanin pigmentation of the oral mucosa. The yellow pallor of certain hemolytic anemias may be modified by the presence of hemoglobinemia and methemoglobinemia.

DECREASE IN MELANIN PIGMENTATION

The great attention ordinarily paid in clinical practice to increased melanin pigmentation of the skin has overshadowed to a considerable degree the appreciations that there are many biochemical factors that inhibit melanin formation rather than increase it, leading to a decrease in skin pigmentation. Lerner and Fitzpatrick have reviewed the many inhibitors of melanin formation.[25] Most of these are of importance *in vitro* or *in vivo* in animals. Some, however, have been shown to be significant as melanin inhibitors in humans, and others appear to have the theoretical potential to become inhibitors. The implications of this phase of melanin metabolism have received little attention in regard to its relation to skin color in disease.

Albinism

Albinism results not, as formerly believed, from the inherited absence of melanocytes in the skin and the eyes, but rather from the inability of the melanocytes to convert tyrosine to melanin, the defect being genetically controlled.[58] Melanocytes are said to be present in albino skin in numbers comparable to those in normal white skin.[61] There is no lack of the substrate tyrosine. The defect is therefore an inherited enzymatic abnormality. This has been pictorially presented by Fitzpatrick and colleagues.[82] Albinism can occur in any racial group. The entire skin, eyes, and hair of such persons are completely lacking in melanin. The skin appears to be pale or a whitish-pink, the hair white, and the irides pink in color.

Inherited hypomelanotic diseases have been reviewed in a clear and concise fashion by Witkop, Fitzpatrick, and Quevedo,[70] and by Nordlund.[71] For a detailed review of the many subsets of albinism and albanoidism, one is referred to these sources. Briefly, *albinism* is defined as those depigmentary conditions that are associated with nystagmus, photophobia, and decreased visual acuity. However, *albanoidism* is defined as those diseases with generalized cutaneous hypopigmentation of the skin or eyes but lacking photophobia and nystagmus. If hearing loss is present, it is usually associated with localized cutaneous hypopigmentation rather than a diffuse form of hypomelanization. The classic form of albinism reveals no clinically or biochemically detectable melanin in the skin, hair, or eyes and a complete absence of the melanogenic enzyme system.

Partial albinism also occurs. It is controlled by a dominant gene, with lack of pigment being limited to part of the skin or hair, but with the eyes (as a rule) being normally pigmented.[44] This type can be confused easily with vitiligo. History will usually reveal that in albinism the lesion has been present since birth.

There are other forms of partial albinism such as piebaldism and Waardenberg's syndrome, in which a white forelock is present. These may be associated with other neurocutaneous genetic defects.

Another genetic disease of the melanocyte causing cutaneous hypopigmentation or depigmentation is the Chediak-Higashi syndrome. This is concerned with a hereditary gigantism of cytoplasmic organelles and involves not only melanosomes but also lysosomes of circulating leukocytes, especially granulocytes. Thus it seems that the disease is one of general membrane alteration rather than just a problem in the synthesis of an enzyme (tyrosinase). These patients typically have blond hair, pale skin, and photophobia owing to decreased uveal pigment. They have anemia and leukopenia and are highly prone to infection. If the child lives to the age of 10 or so, he frequently develops a lymphomalike terminal illness. The disease is inherited as a single autosomal recessive trait. The detailed membrane biochemistry has not been elucidated as yet.[160]

Vitiligo

Vitiligo (leukoderma) represents an acquired loss of melanin pigmentation in one or more areas of the skin. It is readily recognized by its patchy distribution and,

although extensive in some persons, almost never covers the entire body. It is more noticeable in persons normally heavily melanized (*e.g.*, blacks) and at times is readily overlooked in light blonds. Paradoxically, patches of vitiligo not uncommonly occur in the midst of skin areas of hyperpigmentation owing to systemic diseases, or they may be seen adjacent to hyperpigmented patches.

Vitiligo may result from (1) a variety of skin diseases that anatomically involve the melanocytes, (2) systemic disturbances that inhibit melanin formation biochemically, (3) nervous influence, or (4) autoimmune antibody formation.[161] It has been proposed that vitiligo involves autoantibodies directed against the melanocyte, melanosome, or melanin itself, but studies to determine these possibilities have not been definitive as yet.

The most informative and conceptual source reviews are found in the reports and investigations of Lerner[68,163,170–172] and Nordlund.[164–169]

Vitiligo appears to be an autosomal dominant hereditary disease, for in the studies of Nordlund and Lerner[165,168] and El-Mofty,[175] approximately one third of their patients had vitiligo. This is a disfiguring disease of hypomelanization either localized in macular patches or diffuse throughout the integument. The word *vitiligo* stems from the Latin word *vitelius,* which means calf.[174] It was first used in the second century because the white spots of the disease resembled the white patches on the coat of the calf. The macular, milk-white areas of cutaneous depigmentation are most commonly found on the exposed surfaces of the body such as the face, upper chest, and dorsal portions of the hands. Other frequent areas of involvement include axillae, groin, penis, and the skin about the eyes, nose, mouth, ears, nipples, and umbilicus.

Vitiligo is an important disease of cutaneous discoloration because (1) it affects one to two million Americans as well as 1% of the world's population; (2) moderate to severe psychological disturbances may result from its bizarre appearance; and (3) it is frequently associated with systemic autoimmune diseases or diseases that are related to an abnormal immune system. There are three theories suggested as explanation for the destruction of the melanocytes in vitiligo. The first theory proposes that penolic and quinonoide compounds of the melanin biosynthetic pathway may be toxic to the basal melanocytes under certain circumstances. The rationale for this relates to the many workers in the rubber and plastic industries whose exposure to analogous phenolic and quinonoide compounds results in industry-related vitiligo.

The second theory suggests a neurologic cause for melanocytic degeneration, possibly related to catechol toxicity derived from norepinephrine. This would explain the segmental distribution of vitiligo in some patients.

Finally, the third theory, and currently the most widely accepted, concerns the autoimmune destruction of melanocytes. Suggestive evidence for this theory includes the following:

1. Approximately one fourth of the vitiligo population has some form of autoimmune endocrinopathy such as Addison's disease, diabetes mellitus, or thyroiditis.[173] In addition, patients with lymphoid neoplasia such as mycosis fungoides, Hodgkin's disease, and multiple myeloma may develop diffuse generalized vitiligo during the course of their malignancy.
2. Recently, Nordlund and Lerner examined 350 melanoma patients and found 29 of these had vitiligo. Curiously, each of these 29 patients had some form of metastasis, and their survival varied from 5 years to 20 years. This data led these investigators to a new therapy for malignant melanoma: the induction of vitiligo by certain chemicals and the comparison of this melanoma population with one receiving standard forms of chemotherapy and immunotherapy. Their preliminary results indicate that this therapy is as effective as the standard therapy.
3. Complement-fixing antimelanocyte antibodies have been demonstrated in the serum of some patients with mucocutaneous candidiasis and vitiligo.[173]

A common form of vitiligo occurs in persons otherwise healthy; it appears to be functional in nature, simulating in many ways the pattern of alopecia areata. This type may disappear as readily as it develops or may persist indefinitely; it may change in location with recurrence or recur in identical areas.

Vitiligo is common in hyperthyroidism and may be due to increased sympathetic activity in this disease,[13] or to increased conversion of the melanin precursor tyrosine to thyroxine.[25] Areas of vitiligo have been noted in a black patient who was being treated with thiouracil.[45] This drug is known to act as an inhibitor of melanin *in vitro* by combining with the copper of the copper-tyrosinase complex. Thiouracil taken orally resulted in normal urine color in a patient with marked melanuria associated with metastatic melanoma.[46]

There is a sevenfold increase in the incidence of vitiligo in older patients with diabetes mellitus as compared with that in the general population.[176] Vitiligo is also common with pernicious anemia.[177] Because of this known association, an investigation of B_{12} absorption was done by the Schilling test in a large group of patients with vitiligo. There was definitely subnormal absorption (less than 3%, as compared to normal 8%–10%) in 20% of these patients.[178] Recent appearance of unex-

plained vitiligo should alert the physician to the possible presence of an associated systemic disease. Especially to be considered are Addison's disease, hyperthyroidism, diabetes mellitus, and pernicious anemia.

Chemical Depigmentation. An occupational vitiligo has been described in which depigmentation occurred in areas in contact with rubber wear containing *p*-benzylhydroquinone.[47] Apparently this substance acts as a melanin inhibitor not only *in vitro* but also locally by penetration when applied to human skin. The vitiliginous areas usually remelanized slowly with cessation of application of this chemical to the skin. Hydroquinone added to diets of certain experimental animals has produced depigmentation of the hair, with return of hair pigmentation when normal diet was resumed.[48]

Studies by Lerner and Fitzpatrick indicate that monobenzyl ether of hydroquinone in ointment can be used locally to lighten hyperpigmented skin areas such as freckles, lentigines, melasma of pregnancy, and so forth.[63] Occasionally, marked contact-type dermatitis from this substance has been reported. More recently it has been noted that hydroquinone itself can be used effectively with lower incidence of skin sensitization. This substance can diminish the pigmentation of the normal skin of black persons as well as hyperpigmentation of skin in white persons but does not affect normal white skin color nor the color of the eyes and hair. Applied to the skin of a pregnant black woman to produce depigmentation, it caused no change in skin color of her fetus *in utero,* a point verified at the time of delivery. This substance apparently acts through the ability of hydroquinone to interfere with enzyme reactions. Regeneration of skin color may require two or more months after cessation of its use. Other compounds such as the mercaptoamines have also been found to produce depigmentation, and their mechanism of action has been reviewed.[179,180]

Chemical Repigmentation in Vitiligo. Some interesting studies of therapeutic interest with regard to vitiligo have centered on the observation that 8-methoxypsoralen used systemically, followed by exposure to solar or artificial ultraviolet radiation, may bring about remelanization.[64,65] Some investigations have suggested that a psoralen-tanned skin has a two-fold protection against the sun, because in addition to increased basal melanogenesis, there may be prolonged presence of melanin in the stratum corneum.[181-183]

It is apparent that functions of melanocytes in some areas of normal skin can be inhibited metabolically by one mechanism with formation of vitiligo, while simultaneously those in other areas are stimulated, with resultant melanosis.

Other Hypopigmentary Disorders

Aside from vitiligo and albinism, hypopigmentary disorders have been clearly divided into four categories by Klaus according to the area in the pigmentation sequence that is defective.[162] *The first category deals with a developmental defect of the epidermal melanin unit* wherein the latter is poorly developed. An example of this would be piebaldism. This is characterized by a white forelock and large hypopigmented areas of the integument. Microscopically, the depigmented areas reveal sparse, malformed, or absent melanocytes, and these are replaced by Langerhans' cells.

The second category concerns defects in melanin synthesis best demonstrated in patients with severe malabsorption syndromes such as kwashiorkor or chronic pancreatitis. This defect is characterized by diffuse hypopigmentation of hair and skin with hyperkeratosis. Histologically, the melanocytes are normal in number but smaller and with the poorly formed dendrites associated with a marked decrease in dopa-staining of the cytoplasmic granules.

The third category includes disturbances associated with damage to or loss of melanocytes. This is best exemplified by the halo depigmentation seen about halo nevi and halo melanoma. In the black melanoma patient population, according to Klaus, vitiligolike areas can also be found in up to 25% of those studied. In view of the host's immune response seen histologically in halo nevi and halo melanoma, it has been suggested that there may be an autoimmune destruction of basal melanocytes in such areas.

The fourth category relates to abnormalities in the melanosome transfer process. This is best demonstrated by the reversible hypopigmentation seen in various stages of eczema and psoriasis. In eczema, histologically, although the melanocytes appear normal, electron microscopy has confirmed that there are significantly reduced numbers of melanin granules in the keratinocytes. Klaus suggests that the epidermal inflammation in eczema in some way interferes with the melanosome transfer process. On the other hand, in psoriasis, the hypopigmented areas that form within psoriatic plaques in black patients and in a perilesional fashion in whites undergoing Goeckerman therapy show very few melanin granules within the keratinocytes. Here, in the absence of significant epidermal inflammation, it is thought that the accelerated epidermal turnover (that is, the rapid transepidermal migration of keratinocytes related to their high rate of proliferation) does not allow sufficient time for melan-

ocyte-keratinocyte interaction. This would then interrupt melanosome transfer.

Nevi and Depigmentation. A vitiliginous area may develop about a nevus, producing the "halo nevi." Ultrastructural studies of the biology of this tumor reveal degeneration of both basal melanocytes and nevus cells with invasion by the large number of lymphocyte-like cells. This would be compatible with an autoimmune process.[184,185] Hypopigmented nevi have been reported as an early sign of tuberous sclerosis.[186]

Generalized Diminution of Melanin Pigment of the Skin. A number of systemic disorders produce a generalized decrease in melanization of the skin, which may become clinically recognizable as pallor.

Paleness of the skin is characteristic of the male castrate. This is only in part due to diminished melanization.

Lack or diminution of melanin skin pigmentation has been noted commonly in Simmonds' disease, a disorder attributable to a destructive process of the anterior lobe of the pituitary gland.[38] This clinical finding is of great differential value in distinguishing between true Addison's disease and its simulation of secondary adrenal failure owing to hypopituitarism.[13,25,38] Hypothyroidism is characterized by pallor, even in the absence of edema or anemia. There is poor circulation to the skin and decrease in melanization.

Comment has been made that children with the rare disease phenylketonuria have pale or light-colored skin, which fails to tan upon exposure to sunlight. It is due to an inborn error of metabolism in which the essential amino acid phenylalanine cannot be converted into tyrosine. *In vitro*, phenylalanine exerts an inhibitory effect on tyrosinase. Dietary restriction of phenylalanine in these cases results in increase of pigmentation toward normal.[72] This concept has been admirably schematized by Fitzpatrick and his associates (Fig. 39-16). Dietary source of tyrosine alone may not be adequate for melanin synthesis.[25,58]

Edema of the skin diminishes the intensity of melanin pigmentation as well as the color of hemoglobin.[13]

Black babies have a rather light skin color at birth and show a progressive degree of melanogenesis until a peak is reached in the sixth to eighth postnatal week.[51]

Depigmentation of many test animals, including cattle, results from the use of copper-deficient diets.[25] The counterpart of this in humans has not been reported but is theoretically possible. As previously mentioned, copper is necessary for the tyrosine-tyrosinase enzyme reaction.[25]

Diets deficient in the filtrate factors of the vitamin-B complex readily produce depigmentation of the hair in many test animals.[25] Gray hair and skin depigmenta-

tion have been reported in children on vitamin-deficient diets, with return to normal pigmentation after adequate treatment.[49]

A number of studies indicate that the pigmentation of Addison's disease has been markedly diminished in intensity by the administration of ascorbic acid in large doses.[13] Ascorbic acid inhibits melanin formation and may also act to reduce the amount of melanin already present in the skin.[25,28]

EDEMA OF THE SKIN

Edema of the skin is associated with pallor. The structural elements of the integument are rendered more distant from each other, separated as they are by fluid. Light penetrating the skin path thus meets a diminished quantity of pigment. Fewer rays are absorbed and more reflected; the skin therefore appears paler than normal. To this effect may be added the changes in the transmissibility of the tissues and perhaps significant reactions of the blood vessels, which may aid in producing the whiteness of the skin.

The characteristic white pallor of edematous skin is best shown in a child with nephrosis. Pallor is striking even though the red blood cell count may be almost normal.

Edema also hides melanin, as shown by the apparent partial loss of pigmentation noted in a subject with Addison's disease made edematous by deoxycorticosterone therapy.[13]

Jaundice cannot be detected in skin edematous prior to its onset. Unilateral body edema may occur as a tropic phenomenon in certain types of cerebrovascular disease. If jaundice then occurs in such a person, it may be limited unilaterally to the nonedematous side.[50] This explains the mechanism of unilateral jaundice.

The characteristic white color of an intracutaneous skin wheal is another example of the ability of fluid in the skin to raise it away from elements that cause color, or to dilute or separate them. The result is apparent depigmentation; the skin may be very pale.

It is evident that edema of the skin may influence its color strikingly. Therefore, *one must use caution in evaluating skin color in edematous areas.*

DIMINISHED BLOOD FLOW TO THE SKIN

One notes a striking pallor of the skin, if, for any reason, blood flow to the capillaries of the papillary porjections and the superficial subpapillary plexuses is temporarily diminished. This serves to minimize the hemoglobin component of normal skin color. This is seen during syncope, early in Stokes–Adams syn-

drome, early in arterial emboli or other types of arterial obstruction, in peripheral circulatory constriction, and so forth.

Some persons (even though their hemoglobin content is normal) appear pale because of the inadequacy of the papillary and subpapillary vascular network or the flow of the blood through these areas. That the pallor of the skin of a castrate results in part from such inadequate blood flow has already been discussed.

Inadequate blood flow in the tissues, if persistent, leads to stasis cyanosis, often mottled, so that one notes blotchy blue areas against a pale background. The characteristic ashen-gray color of peripheral circulatory constriction (shock) can be attributed to the combination of the pallor of poor capillary circulation of the skin combined with some degree of cyanosis of peripheral stasis origin.

SCAR TISSUE

Scar tissue when new is vascular and pink and when completely formed and healed is avascular and white. The white color is indicative in part of the minimal amount of melanin and hemoglobin pigment that it contains. Its optical characteristics resemble edematous tissue, and it even more strikingly reflects white light—with little differential absorption or reflection of the light rays within the visible spectrum.

MACERATED OR DESQUAMATING SKIN

Areas of the skin with these changes, similar to scar tissue, appear to have less than the normal amount of pigmentation and are white in color.

The coated tongue looks white because the filiform papillae, which have thickened and become opaque, along with debris collected between them, hide the deeper pigments and reflect white light without differential light ray absorption. With desquamation of the white filiform papillae, the mucosa with its prominent capillary projections is exposed, and one then sees the red color of a smooth atrophic tongue.

VALUE OF COLORED ILLUSTRATIONS IN MEDICAL EDUCATION

The old proverb that "one picture tells more than a thousand words" is even more true when changed to read "one *colored* picture. . . ." Word descriptions of color of the skin have distinct limitations. Most helpful in teaching students the color appearance of the skin in disease is actual observation of patients. Unfortunately, patients suitable for depicting a particular con-

dition are available only sporadically in any given institution. Next most useful would be movies, lantern slides, and photographs in color. The great expense of preparation has limited the number of colored photographs or illustrations published in monographs and medical journals, and those that have been printed are widely scattered. There is considerable educational value in systematically studying those available in the literature. For this purpose the reader is referred elsewhere for a guide to many of the colored plates available in the journal literature prior to 1944 depicting abnormalities in the color of the skin in systemic disease.[13] Other good color illustrations can be found by perusal of standard texts and systems of medicine. (See Chapter 7 on Sore Tongue and Sore Mouth in this book.)

SUMMARY

Careful inspection of the color of the skin and mucous membranes yields significant information in a large number of disorders.

The normal skin color depends upon various factors, chief among which are the proportion of the light that is reflected to that which penetrates, and the depth of penetration; the amounts and proportions of the various pigments (melanin, oxyhemoglobin and reduced hemoglobin, and carotene); and the phenomenon of scattering.

In health, skin coloration varies greatly among races and greatly among persons of the same race; with age and sex; with tanning from sunlight; with relative vascularity of the skin and vasomotor phenomena (flushing, vasoconstriction and so forth); and in different regions of the body. An understanding of the factors influencing normal skin coloration is necessary to permit interpretation of possible deviations from normal.

Abnormally increased pigmentation can be classified as due to (1) increased yellow components, (2) increased hemoglobin pigment of various types, (3) increased melanin, (4) increased content of metal deposits, or (5) effects of certain chemicals and drugs. Recognition of the specific cause of the abnormal increase may be of great diagnostic value, and observation of alterations in the degree of pigmentation may allow deductions concerning the result of therapy, the prognosis, and so forth in many conditions. The influence of dermal pigmentation on skin color is discussed in detail.

Decreased skin pigmentation occurs in partial or complete albinism, in vitiligo, in anemia, in certain endocrine states, in edema, and in skin with diminished blood supply. Proper interpretation of the pathologic physiology resulting in such losses of skin coloration is of great medical importance.

This chapter summarizes present knowledge concerning normal and abnormal skin pigments, methods of recognizing and measuring them, and the mechanisms and significance of abnormalities and alterations in skin coloration.

The authors acknowledge the contributions of Edward A. Edwards, M.D., coauthor of this chapter in the early editions, and Herbert Mescon, M.D., coauthor in the fourth edition.

REFERENCES

1. **Sheard C, Brown GE:** The spectrophotometric analysis of the color of the skin. Arch Intern Med 38:816, 1926

2. **Sheard C, Brunsting LA:** Color of skin as analyzed by spectrophotometric methods; I. Apparatus and procedures. J Clin Invest 7:559–574, 1929

3. **Brunsting LA, Sheard C:** Color of skin as analyzed by spectrophotometric methods; II. Role of pigmentation. J Clin Invest 7:575–592, 1929

4. **Brunsting LA, Sheard C:** Color of skin as analyzed by spectrophotometric methods; III. Role of superficial blood. J Clin Invest 7:793–813, 1929

5. **Edwards EA, Duntley SQ:** Pigments and color of living human skin. Am J Anat 65:1–33, 1939

6. **Edwards EA, Hamilton JB, Duntley SQ et al:** Cutaneous vascular and pigmentary changes in castrate and eunuchoid men. Endocrinology 28:119–128, 1941

7. **Edwards EA, Duntley SQ:** Analysis of skin pigment changes after exposure to sunlight. Science 90:235–237, 1939

8. **Edwards EA, Duntley SQ:** Cutaneous vascular changes in women in reference to the menstrual cycle and ovariectomy. Am J Obstet Gynecol 57:501–509, 1949

9. ***Ogbuawa O, Trowell J, Williams JJ et al:** Hyperpigmentation of pernicious anemia in blacks. Arch Intern Med 138:388–389, 1978

10. ***Lawrence GD, Bravo E, Bartter FC:** Hyperpigmentation on cortisone after adrenalectomy for primary aldosteronism. Arch Intern Med 134:734–737, 1974

11. **Jeghers H:** Skin color in health and disease. Med Phys 2:984–988, 1950

12. **Edestein LM, Jhung JM, Brookman D et al:** Congo red: A simple stain for the stratum lucidum. Journal of Medical Technology 40, No 1: 1–4, 1974

13. **Jeghers H:** Pigmentation of the skin. N Engl J Med 231:88–100, 122–136, 181–189, 1944

14. **Watson CJ:** Bile Pigments. N Engl J Med 227:665, 705, 1942

15. **Larson EA, Evans GT, Watson CJ:** A study of the serum biliverdin concentration in various types of jaundice. J Lab Clin Med 32:481–488, 1947

16. ***Meakins JC:** Distribution of jaundice in circulatory failure. J Clin Invest 4:135–148, 1927

17. **Meakins JC:** Jaundice in congestive heart failure. Mod Concepts Cardiovasc Dis 18:37–38, 1949

18. **Jeghers H:** Skin changes of nutritional origin. N Engl J Med 228:678, 714, 1943

19. ***Lutterloh CH, Shallengerger PL:** Unusual pigmentation developing after prolonged suppressive therapy with quinacrine hydrochloride. Arch Dermatol Syph 53:349–354, 1946

20. **Weidman FD:** Pathology of yellowing dermatoses; 1. Nonxanthomatous (jaundice, carotinemia, blood pigmentation, melanin, colloid degeneration and elastic degeneration). Arch Dermatol Syph 24:954–991, 1931

21. **Montgomery H:** Cutaneous manifestations of diseases of lipoid metabolism. Med Clin North Am 24:1249–1261, 1940

22. **Comroe JH, Jr, Botelho S:** Unreliability of cyanosis in recognition of arterial anoxemia. Am J Med Sci 214:1–6, 1947

23. **Finch CA:** Methemoglobinemia and sulfhemoglobinemia. N Engl J Med 239:470–478, 1948

24. **Becker SW, Obermayer ME:** Modern Dermatology and Syphilology, 2nd ed. Philadelphia, J B Lippincott, 1940

25. **Lerner AB, Fitzpatrick TB:** Biochemistry of melanin formation. Physiol Rev 30:91–126, 1950

26. **Becker SW:** Skin: Melanin pigmentation produced by physical agents. Med Phys 1:1430–1433, 1944

27. **Fitzpatrick TB, Lerner AB, Calkins E, Summerson WH:** Mammalian tyrosinase; melanin formation by ultraviolet irradiation. Arch Dermatol Syph 59:620, 1949

28. **Becker SW:** Pigmentary diseases of the skin. Clinics 3:886–922, 1944

29. **Keys A:** Caloric undernutrition and starvation, with notes on protein deficiency. JAMA 138:500–511, 1948

30. **Burger G, Sandstead H, Drummond J:** Starvation in western Holland. Lancet 2:282–283, 1945

31. **Davis M, Boynton J, Ferguson J et al:** Studies on pigmentation of endocrine origin. J Clin Endocrinol 5:138–146, 1945

32. **Pack GT, LeFevre R:** Age and sex distributions and incidence of neoplastic diseases at Memorial Hospital, New York City, with comments on "cancer ages." J Cancer Res 14:167–294, 1930

33. **Hamilton JB:** Influence of the endocrine status upon pigmentation in man and in mammals. In The Biology of Melanomas, Vol 4, p 341. New York Academy of Sciences, 1948

34. **Sprague RG, Power MH, Mason HL et al:** Observations on the physiologic effects of cortisone and ACTH in man. Arch Intern Med 85:199–258, 1950

35. **Calkins E, quoted in Becker SW, Obermayer ME:** Modern Dermatology and Syphilology, 2nd ed. Philadelphia, J B Lippincott, 1940

*Indicates medical journal article containing a color plate not readily available elsewhere.

*Includes color plate.

36. **Lea AJ:** Influence of sodium chloride on the formation of melanin. Nature 155:428, 1945

37. **Sodeman WA:** Addison's disease. Am J Med Sci 198:118–132, 1939

38. **Sheehan HL, Summers VK:** The syndrome of hypopituitarism. Q J Med 18:319–378, 1949

39. **MacFarlane E:** The sacral spot in Bengal. Science 95:431, 1942

40. **Monash S:** Normal pigmentation of oral mucosa. Arch Dermatol Syph 26:139–147, 1932

41. **Laidlow GF, Cahn LR:** Melanoblasts in gum. J Dent Res 12:534, 1932

42. **Monash S:** Normal pigmentation in nails of Negro. Arch Dermatol Syph 25:876–881, 1932

43. **Schwartz SO, Blumenthal SA:** Exogenous hemochromatosis resulting from blood transfusions. Blood 3:617–640, 1948

44. **Macklin MT:** Genetic aspects of pigment cell growth in man. In The Biology of Melanomas, Vol 4, p 144. New York Academy of Sciences, 1948

45. **Hellerstein HK:** In Becker SW, Obermayer ME: Modern Dermatology and Syphilology, 2nd ed. Philadelphia, J B Lippincott, 1940

46. **White AG:** Effect of tyrosine, tryptophane and thiouracil on melanuria. J Lab Clin Med 32 (part 2):1254–1257, 1947

47. **Oliver EA, Schwartz L, Warren LH:** Occupational leukoderma. Arch Dermatol Syph 42:993, 1940

48. **Martin GJ, Ansbacker S:** Confirmatory evidence of the chromotrichial activity of p-aminobenzoic acid. J Biol Chem 138:441, 1941

49. **Gillman T, Gillman J:** Powdered stomach in the treatment of fatty liver and other manifestations of infantile pellagra. Arch Intern Med 76:63–74, 1945

50. **Page IH:** Ipsolateral edema and contralateral jaundice associated with hemiplegia and cardiac decompensation. Am J Med Sci 177:273–276, 1929

51. **Zimmerman AA, Cornbleet T:** The development of epidermal pigmentation in the Negro fetus. J Invest Dermatol 11:383–395, 1948

52.***Jeghers H, McKusick VA, Katz KH:** Generalized intestinal polyposis and melanin spots of the oral mucosa, lips and digits. N Engl J Med 241:993, 1031, 1949

53. **Hall TC, McCracken GH, Thorn GW:** Skin pigmentation in relation to adrenal cortical function. J Clin Endocrinol 13:243–257, 1953

54. **Gordon M (ed):** Pigment Cell Growth: Proceedings of the Third Conference on the Biology of Normal and Atypical Pigment Cell Growth, New York, 1951, p 365. New York, Academic Press, 1953

55. **Fitzpatrick TB, Lerner AB:** Terminology of pigment cells. Science 117:640, 1953

56. **Gates RR, Zimmerman AA:** Comparison of skin color with melanin content. J Invest Dermatol 21:339–348, 1953

57. **Shizume K, Lerner AB:** Determination of melanocyte stimulating hormone in urine and blood. J Clin Endocrinol 14:1491, 1954

58. **Fitzpatrick TB, Lerner AB:** Biochemical basis of human melanin pigmentation. Arch Dermatol Syph 69:133, 1954

59. **Fitzpatrick TB, Szabo G, Seiji M et al:** The melanin pigmentary system. In Fitzpatrick TB, Eisen AZ, Wolf K, Freedberg IM, Austin KF (eds): Dermatology in General Medicine, 2nd ed, pp 131–157. New York, McGraw–Hill, 1979

60. **Fitzpatrick TB, Montgomery H, Lerner AB:** Pathogenesis of generalized dermal pigmentation secondary to malignant melanoma and melanuria. J Invest Dermatol 22:163–172, 1954

61. **Becker SW, Jr, Fitzpatrick TB, Montgomery H:** Human melanogenesis: Cytology of human pigment cells. Arch Dermatol Syph 65:511, 1952

62. **Ambani LM, Jhung JW, Edelstein LM et al:** Quantification of melanin in hepatic and cardiac lipofuscin. Experientia 33:296, 1976

63. **Lerner AB, Fitzpatrick TB:** Treatment of melanin hyperpigmentation. JAMA 152:577–582, 1953

64. **Lerner AB, Denton CR, Fitzpatrick TB:** Clinical and experimental studies with 8-methoxypsoralen in vitiligo. J Invest Dermatol 20:299–314, 1953

65. **Kanof NB:** Melanin formation in vitiliginous skin under the influence of external applications of 8-methoxypsoralen. J Invest Dermatol 24:5–10, 1955

66.***Lerner AB, Shizume K, Bunding I:** The mechanism of endocrine control of melanin pigmentation. J Clin Endocrinol 14:1463–1490, 1954

67. **Lorincz AL:** Pigmentation. In Rothman S (ed): Physiology and Biochemistry of the Skin, pp 515–562. Chicago, University of Chicago Press, 1954

68. **Lerner AB:** Melanin pigmentation. Am J Med 19:902–924, 1955

69. **Witkop CJ:** Depigmentation of the general and oral tissues and their genetic foundations. Ala J Med Sci 16, No. 4:331–343, 1979

70. **Witkop CJ, Fitzpatrick TB, Quevedo WD:** Albinism. In Stanbury JB, Wyngaardin JB, Fredrickson DS (eds): The Metabolic Basis of Inherited Disease, 4th ed, pp 283–316. New York, McGraw–Hill, 1978

71. **Nordlund JJ:** Basis of pigmentation and the disorders of pigmentation. In Ackerman AB (ed): Pathology of Malignant Melanoma. New York, Masson, 1981

72. **Buckley WR, Grum F:** Reflection spectrophotometry: I. Use in evaluation of skin pigmentary disturbances. Arch Dermatol 83:249–261, 1961

73. **Leftwich, RB, Floro JF, Neal RA et al:** Dinitrophenol poisoning: A diagnosis to consider in undiagnosed fever. South Med J 75:182–184, 1982

74. **Buckley WF, Grum F:** Reflection spectrophotometry: III. Absorption characteristics and color of human skin. Arch Dermatol 89:170–176, 1964

*Includes color plate.

*Includes color plate.

75. **Monash S:** Skin color: A correlation of reflectance measurement and clinical appearance. Arch Dermatol 84:654–659, 1961

76. **Edwards EA, Finklestein NA, Duntley S:** Spectrophotometry of living skin the ultraviolet range. J Invest Dermatol 16:311–321, 1951

77. **Post PW, Krauss AN, Waldman S et al:** Skin reflectance of newborn infants from 25 to 44 weeks gestational age. Hum Biol 48:541–557, 1976

78. **Krauss AN, Post PW, Waldman S et al:** Skin reflectance in the newborn infant. Pediatr Res 10:776–778, 1976

79. **Toda K, Pathak MA, Fitzpatrick TB et al:** Skin color: Its ultrastructure and its determining mechanism. In Riley V (ed): Pigment Cell, Vol 1, pp 66–81. Basel, S Karger, 1973

80. **Fitzpatrick TB, Brunet P, Kubita A:** The nature of hair pigment. In Montagna W, Ellis RA (eds): The Biology of Hair Growth. New York, Academic Press, 1958

81. **Reich P, Schwachman H, Craig JM:** Lycopenemia: A variant of carotenemia. N Engl J Med 262:263–269, 1960

82. **Fitzpatrick TB, Seiji M, McGugan AD:** Medical progress: Melanin pigmentation. N Engl J Med 265:328, 374, 430, 1961

83. **Lerner AB, McGuire JS:** Effect of alpha- and beta-melanocyte stimulating hormones on the skin color of man. Nature 189:176, 1961

84. **Rees LH:** ACTH, lipotrophin and MSH in health and disease. Clin Endocrinol Metab 6, No. 1: 137–153, 1977

85. **Brown JD et al:** Pituitary pigmentary hormones. JAMA 240:1273–1278, 1978

86. **Nakanishi S, Inoue A, Kita T et al:** Nucleotide sequence of cloned cDNA for bovine corticotropin-B-lipotropin precursor. Nature 278:423–427, 1979

87. **Szabo G:** Quantitative histological investigation on melanocyte system of human epidermis. In Gordon M (ed): Pigment Cell Biology, pp 44–125. New York, Academic Press, 1959

88. **Birbeck MSC, Breathnach AS, Everall JD:** An electron-microscope study of basal melanocytes and high level clear cells (Langerhans cells) in vitiligo. J Invest Dermatol 37:51–64, 1961

89. **Cowan A:** Ocular pigment and pigmentation; 18th annual de Shweinitz lecture. Arch Ophthalmol 55:161–173, 1956

90. **Beerman H, Colburn HL:** Some aspects of pigmentation of the skin. Am J Med Sci 231:454–475, 1956

91. **Deutsch S, Mescon H:** Melanin pigmentation and its endocrine control. N Engl J Med 257:222–226, 268–272, 1957

92. **Lerner AB:** Hormonal control of pigmentation. Annu Rev Med 11:187–194, 1960

93. **Lerner AB, McGuire JS:** Effect of alpha- and beta-melanocyte stimulating hormones on the skin color of man. Nature 189:176–179, 1961

94. **Lerner AB, McGuire JS:** Melanocyte-stimulating hormone and adrenocorticotrophic hormone: Their relationship to pigmentation. N Engl J Med 270:539–546, 1964

95. **Buckley WR, Grum F:** Reflection spectrophotometry: III. Absorption characteristics and color of human skin. Arch Dermatol 89:110–116, 1964

96. **Abrahamson IA Sr, Abrahamson IA Jr:** Hypercarotenemia. Arch Dermatol 68:4–7, 1962

97. **Lascari AD:** Carotenemia: A review. Clin Pediatr 20:25–29, 1980

98. **Findlay GH:** Cutaneous vasoconstrictors, primary pigmentation and the grey-blue reaction. Br J Dermatol 73:238–243, 1961

99. **Pathak MA, Riley FC, Fitzpatrick TB:** Melanogenesis in human skin following exposure to long-wave ultraviolet and visible light. J Invest Dermatol 39:435–443, 1962

100. **Findlay GH:** Blue Skin. Br J Dermatol 83:127–134, 1970

101. **Dawson JB, Barker DJ, Ellis DJ et al:** A theoretical and experimental study of light absorption and scattering by in vivo skin. Phys Med Biol 25, no. 4:695–709, 1980

102. **Gilchrest BA, Fitzpatrick TB, Anderson RR et al:** Localization of melanin pigmentation in the skin with Wood's lamp. Br J Dermatol 96:245–249, 1980

103. **Toda K, Pathak MA, Fitzpatrick TB et al:** Skin color: Its ultrastructure and its determining mechanism. In Riley V (ed): Pigment Cell, pp 66–81. Basal, S Karger, 1973

104. **Monash S:** Immediate pigmentation in sunlight and artificial light. Arch Dermatol 87:686–690, 1963

105. **Tuffanelli D, Abraham RK, Dubois E:** Pigmentation from antimalarial therapy: Its possible relationship to the ocular lesions. Arch Dermatol 88:419–426, 1963

106. **Thomas AE, Gisburn A:** Exogenous ochronosis and myxedema from resorcinol. Br J Dermatol 73:378–381, 1961

107. **Sternberg TH, Bierman SM:** Unique syndromes involving the skin induced by drugs, food additives and environmental contaminants. Arch Dermatol 88:779–788, 1963

108. **Madison JF:** Tetracycline pigmentation of teeth. Arch Dermatol 88:58–59, 1963

109. **Esoda ECJ:** Chloasma from progestational oral contraceptives. Arch Dermatol 87:486, 1963

110.***Jelinek JE:** Oral contraceptives and the skin. Am Fam Physician 4:68–74, Nov 1971

111. **Weiner JS:** A spectrophotometer for measurement of skin color. Man 253:152, 1951

112. **Weiner JS, Harrison GA, Singer R et al:** Skin color in southern Africa. Hum Biol 36:294–307, 1964

113. **Wasserman HP:** The colour of human skin: Spectral reflectance versus skin colour. Dermatologica 143:166–173, 1971

114. **Harrison GA:** Differences in human pigmentation: Measurement, geographic variation, and causes. J Invest Dermatol 60:418–426, 1973

*Includes color plate.

115. **Lees FC, Byard PJ:** Skin colorimetry in Belize. 1. Conversion formula. Am J Phys Anthropol 48:515–522, 1978

116. **Post PW, Rao DC:** Genetics and environmental determinants of skin color. Am J Phys Anthropol 47:399–402, 1977

117. **Prota G, Nicolaus RA:** On the biogenesis of phaeomelanins. In Montagna W, Hu F (eds): Advances in Biology of Skin, Vol 8, pp 323–328. London, Pergamon Press, 1967

118. **Szabo G, Gerald A, Pathak MA et al:** Racial differences in human pigmentation of the ultrastructural level. J Cell Biol 39:132a–133a, 1968

119. **Szabo G, Gerald A, Fitzpatrick TB et al:** Racial differences in melanogenesis before and after ultraviolet stimulation and electronmicroscope study. J Invest Dermatol 50:268, 1968

120. **Szabo G, Gerald A, Pathak MA et al:** Letter to the Editor: Melanosomes behave differently in different races. Nature 222:1081, 1968

121. **Gibson HL, Buckley WR, Whitmore KE:** New vistas in infrared photography for biological surveys. J Biol Photogr Assoc 33:1, 1965

122. **Kaufman HS, Sulsberger MB:** Infrared thermometry for reading reactions on darkly pigmented skin. JAMA 202, 109–111, 1967

123. **Gilchrest BA, Fitzpatrick TB, Anderson RR et al:** Localization of melanin pigmentation in the skin with Wood's lamp. Br J Dermatol 96:245–248, 1977

124. **Fenech FF, Bannister WH, Greech JL:** Hepatitis with biliverdinaemia in association with indomethacin therapy. Br Med J 3:155, 1967

125. **Gordonson LL:** Letter to the Editor: Scleral icterus. N Engl J Med 271:913, 1964

126. **Tripathi RC:** Letter to the Editor: Conjunctival icterus; Not scleral icterus. JAMA 242:2558, 1979

127. **Pittman FE:** The fluorescein string test: An analysis of its use and relationship to barium studies of the upper gastrointestinal tract in 122 cases of gastrointestinal tract hemorrhage. Ann Intern Med 60:418, 1964

128. **Fitzpatrick TB, Miyamoto M, Ishikawa K:** The evolution of concepts of melanin biology. In Montagna W, Hu F (eds): Advances in Biology of Skin, Vol 8, pp 1–30. London, Pergamon Press, 1967

129. **Demopoulos HB:** Effects of reducing the phenylalanine uptake of patients with advanced malignant melanomas. Cancer 19:65, 1964

130. **Demopoulos HB, Gerving MA, Bagdoyan H:** Selective inhibition of growth and respiration of melanomas by tyrosinase inhibitors. J Natl Cancer Inst 35:823, 1965

131. **Demopoulos HB, Kaley G:** Selective inhibition of respiration of pigmented S91 mouse melanomas by phenyl lactate, and the possible related effects on growth. J Natl Cancer Inst 30:611, 1963

132. **Demopoulos HB:** Effects of low phenylalanine-tyrosine diets on S91 mouse melanomas. J Natl Cancer Inst 37:185, 1966

133. **Van Woert MH, Prassad KN, Borg DC:** Spectroscopic studies of substantia nigra pigment in human subjects. J Neurochem 14:707–716, 1967

134. **Van Woert MH, Bowers MG, Jr:** Aromatic amino acid metabolism during L-dopa therapy of Parkinson's disease. In Barbeau A, McDowell FH (eds): L-dopa and Parkinsonism. Proceedings of Laurentian Research Conference on L-dopa, Montreal, Quebec, 1969. Philadelphia, F A Davis, 1970

135. **Cotzias GC, Van Woert MH, Schiffer LM:** Aromatic amino acids and modification of Parkinsonism. N Engl J Med 276:374–379, 1967

136. **Van Woert MH:** Reduced nicotinamideadenine dinucleotide oxidation by melanin: Inhibition by phenothiazines (33275). Proc Soc Exp Biol Med 129:165–171, 1968

137. **Okun MR:** Histogenesis of melanocytes. J Invest Dermatol 44:285–299, 1965

138. **Okun MR, Edelstein LM, Niebauer G et al:** The histochemical tyrosine: Reaction for tyrosine and its use in localizing tyrosinase activity in mast cells. J Invest Dermatol 53:39–45, 1969

139. **Okun MR, Edelstein LM, Or N et al:** The role of peroxidase vs the role of tyrosinase in enzymatic conversion of tyrosine to melanin in melanocytes, mast cells, and eosinophils: An autoradiographic-histochemical study. J Invest Dermatol 55:1–12, 1970

140. **Okun MR, Edelstein LM, Or N et al:** Histochemical studies of conversion of tyrosine and dopa to melanin mediated by mammalian peroxidase. Life Sci 9:491–505, 1970

141. **Mason HS, Ingram DJE, Allen B:** The free radical property of melanin. Arch Biochem 86:225, 1968

142. **Mason HS:** The structure of melanin. In Montagna W, Hu F (eds): Advances in Biology of Skin, Vol 8, pp 293–312. London, Pergamon Press, 1967

143. **Pathak MA:** Photobiology of melanogenesis: Biological aspects. In Montagna W, Hu F (eds): Advances in Biology of Skin, Vol 8, pp 397–420. London, Pergamon Press, 1967

144. **Hallwright GP, North KAK, Reid JD:** Pigmentation and Cushing's syndrome due to malignant tumor of the pancreas. J Clin Endocrinol 24:496–500, 1964

145. **Ward HN, Konikov N, Reinhard EH:** Cytologic dysplasia occurring after busulfan (Myleran) therapy. Ann Intern Med 63:654, 1965

146. **Resnick S:** Melasma induced by oral contraceptive drugs. JAMA 199:601–606, 1967

147. **Morris LL, Danta G:** Malignant cerebral melanoma complicating giant pigment naevus: A case report. J Neurol Neurosurg Psychiatry 31:628–632, 1968

148. **Reed WB, Landing B, Sugarman G et al:** Xeroderma pigmentosum: Clinical and laboratory investigation of its basic defect. JAMA 207:2073–2079, 1967

149. **Crowe FW, Schull WJ:** Diagnostic importance of cafe-au-lait spot in neurofibromatosis. Arch Intern Med 91:758–766, 1953

150. **Crowe FW:** Axillary freckling as a diagnostic aid in neurofibromatosis. Ann Intern Med 61:1142–1143, 1964

151. **Benedict PH, Szabo G, Fitzpatrick TB et al:** Melanotic macules in Albright's syndrome and in neurofibromatosis. JAMA 205:618–626, 1968

152. **Dummett CO, Barens G:** Pigmentation of the oral tissues: A review of the literature. J Periodontol 38:369–378, 1967

153. **Dummett CO:** Pigmentation and depigmentation: Biology, systemic disease, and oral manifestation. Ala J Med Sci 16, no. 4:261–289, 1979

154. **Harris DC:** Oral manifestations associated with Shamberg's disease. Oral Surg 19:304–308, 1965

155. **Danowski TS, Sabeh G, Sarver ME et al:** Shin spots and diabetes mellitus. Am J Med Sci 251:570–575, 1966

156. **Fisher ER, Danowski TS:** Histologic, histochemical, and microscopic features of the shin spots of diabetes mellitus. Am J Clin Pathol 50:547–554, 1968

157. **Nahum LH:** The purple people syndrome. Conn Med 29:332, 1965

158. **Van Woert MH:** Isolation of chlorpromazine pigments in man. Nature 219:1054–1056, 1968

159. **Van Woert MH:** Activation of tyrosinase by chlorpromazine. In Reilly V (ed): Proceedings of the 7th International Pigment Cell Conference, Seattle, Washington. New York, Appleton–Century–Crofts, 1970

160. **Weary PE, Bender AS:** Chediak–Higashi syndrome with severe cutaneous involvement. Arch Intern Med 119:381–386, 1967

161. **Bor S, Feiwel M, Chavarin I:** Vitiligo and its aetiological relationship to organ-specific autoimmune disease. Br J Dermatol 81:83–88, 1969

162. **Klaus SN:** The biologic basic of eight unusual hypopigmentary disorders. Ala J Med Sci 16(4):290–304, 1979

163. **Charcot–Turner ML, Lerner AB:** Physiologic changes in vitiligo. Arch Dermatol 91:390–396, 1965

164. **Nordlund JJ:** Disorders of hypopigmentation. Conn Med 42, no. 4:227–230, 1978

165. **Norlund JJ, Lerner AB:** In Demis J, Crounse R, Dobson R, McGuire J (eds): Clinical Dermatology, pp 1–14. New York, Harper & Row, 1979

166. **Nordlund JJ, Lerner AB:** Vitiligo—Its relationship to systemic disease. In Dermatology Update, pp 411–432. Amsterdam, Elsevier, 1979

167.***Nordlund JJ, Todes–Taylor N, Albert DM et al:** Prevalence of vitiligo and poliosis in patients with uveitis. J Am Acad Dermatol 4:528–537, 1981

168. **Lerner AB, Nordlund JJ:** Vitiligo: Loss of pigment in the skin, hair, and eyes. J Dermatol (Tokyo) 5:1–8, 1978

169.***Nordlund JJ et al:** Halo nevi and the Vogt–Koyanagi–Haradi Syndrome: Manifestations of vitiligo. Arch Dermatol 116:690–692, 1980

170. **Lerner AB:** On the etiology of vitiligo and gray hair. Am J Med 51:141–147, 1971

171. **Lerner AB, Nordlund JJ, Albert DM:** Pigment cells of the eyes in people with vitiligo. N Engl J Med 296:232, 1977

172.***Lerner AB, Nordlund JJ:** Vitiligo. What is it? Is it important? JAMA 239:1183–1187, 1978.

173. **Betterle C, Del Prete GF, Peserico A et al:** Autoantibodies in vitiligo. Arch Dermatol 112:1328, 1976

174. **McBurney EI:** Vitiligo: Clinical picture and pathogenesis. Arch Intern Med 139:1295–1297, 1979

175. **El–Mofty AM:** Vitiligo and Psoralens. Oxford, Pergamon Press, 1968

176. **Dawber RPR:** Vitiligo in mature-onset diabetes mellitus. Br J Dermatol 80:275, 1968

177. **Allison JR, Jr, Curtis AC:** Vitiligo and pernicious anemia. Arch Dermatol Syph 72:407–408, 1955

178. **Bleifeld W, Gehrmann G:** Vitamin B_{12} absorption in vitiligo. German Med Monthly 12:273, 1967

179. **Bleehan SS, Pathak MA, Hori Y et al:** Depigmentation of skin with 4-isopropylcatechol, mercaptoamines and other compounds. J Invest Dermatol 50:103–117, 1968

180. **Frenk E, Pathak MA, Szabo G et al:** Selective action of mercaptoethylamines on melanocytes in mammalian skin. Arch Dermatol 97:465, 1968

181. **Becker SW, Jr:** Psoralen phototherapeutic agents. JAMA 202:422, 1967

182. **Pathak MA:** Mechanism of psoralen photosensitization and in vivo biological action spectrum of 8-methoxypsoralen. J Invest Dermatol 37:397, 1961

183. **Pathak MA, Fitzpatrick TB:** Relationship of molecular configuration to activity of furocoumarins which increase cutaneous responses following long wave ultraviolet radiation. J Invest Dermatol 32:255, 1969

184. **Swanson JL, Wayte DM, Helwig EG:** Ultrastructure of halo nevi. J Invest Dermatol 50:434–437, 1968

185. **Jacobs J, Edelstein LM, Snyder LM et al:** Ultrastructural evidence of melanocytic tumor cell destruction in halo nevus. Cancer Res 35:352, 1975

186. **Gold AP, Freeman JM:** Depigmented nevi: The earliest sign of tuberous sclerosis. Pediatrics 35:1003–1005, 1965

187. **Hughes JD, Wooten RL:** The orange people. JAMA 197:730, 1966

188. **Okun MR, Edelstein LM, Hamada G et al:** Peroxidatic tyrosinase activity of mast cells, eosinophils and melanoma cells. In Reilly V (ed): Proceedings of the 7th International Pigment Cell Conference, Seattle, Washington. New York, Appleton–Century–Crofts, 1970

189.***Okun MR, Edelstein LM:** Gross and microscopic pathology of the skin. In Okun MR, Edelstein LM (eds): Enzymatic Basis of Melanogenesis, pp 906–910. Boston, Dermatopathology Foundation Press, 1976

190. **Edelstein L:** Melanin: A unique biopolymer. In Ioachim H (ed): Pathobiology Annual, p 309. New York, Appleton–Century–Crofts, 1971

---

*Includes color plate.   *Includes color plate.

191. **Riley PA:** Melanins and melanogenesis. In Ioachim HL (ed): Pathobiology Annual, Vol 10, pp 223–251. New York, Raven Press, 1980

192. **Demopoulos H, Regan MAG, Regan D:** The vital respiratory role of tyrosinase in pigmented melanomas. In Reilly V (ed): Proceedings of the 7th International Pigment Cell Conference, Seattle, Washington. New York, Appleton–Century–Crofts, 1970

193. **Seiji M:** Subcellular particles and melanin formation in melanocytes. In Montagna W, Hu F (eds): Advances in Biology of Skin, Vol 8, pp 189–222. London, Pergamon Press, 1967

194. **Brooks VEH, Richards R:** Depigmentation in Cushing's syndrome. Arch Intern Med 117:677, 1966

195. **With TK:** On the occurrence in human serum of yellow substances different from bilirubin and carotenoids. Acta Med Scand 122:501–512, 1945

196. **With TK:** The pathogenesis and different forms of jaundice. Acta Med Scand 128:25–41, 1947

197. **Sherlock S:** Jaundice. In Diseases of the Liver and Biliary System, 5th ed, pp 234–259. Oxford, Blackwell Scientific Publications, 1975

198. **Fenech FF, Bannister WH, Grech JL:** Hepatitis with biliverdinaemia in association with indomethacin therapy. Br Med J 2:155–157, 1967

199. **Resnik S:** Melasma induced by oral contraceptive drugs. JAMA 199:601–606, 1967

200.***Reynolds TB:** The "butterfly" sign in patients with chronic jaundice and pruritus. Ann Int Med 78:545–546, 1973

201. **Greenberg AJ, Bossenmaier I, Schwartz S:** Green jaundice: A study of serum bilirubin, mesobilirubin and other green pigments. Am J Dig Dis 16:873–880, 1971

202. **Wearn JT:** Combination of Jaundice and Cyanosis as Helpful Diagnostic Sign in Tricuspid Valvulitis, pp 60–65. Baltimore, Waverly Press, 1936

203. **Hughes JD, Wooten RL:** The orange people. JAMA 197:138–139, 1966

204. **Tolentino FI, Brockwurst RJ:** Unilateral scleral icterus due to choroidal hemorrhage. Arch Ophthalmol 70:358–360, 1963

205. **Conn HO:** Unilateral edema and jaundice after portacaval anastomosis. Ann Intern Med 76:459–461, 1972

206. **Neering H:** Vitiligo and jaundice. Br J Dermatol 93:229, 1975

207. **Derbes VJ, Engelhardt HT:** Yellow dermographia. Arch Dermatol Syph 48:310–311, 1943

208. **Kramer LI:** Advancement of dermal icterus in the jaundiced newborn. Am J Dis Child 118:454, 1969

209. **Hegyi T, Hiatt IM, Gertner I:** Transcutaneous bilirubinometry: The cephalocaudal progression of dermal icterus. Am J Dis Child 135:547, 1981

210.***Gorten MK:** Detection of neonatal jaundice. GP 26:101–104, 1964

211. **Culley PE, Waterhouse JAH, Wood BSB:** Clinical assessment of depth of jaundice in newborn infants. Lancet 1:88, 1960

212. **Gosset IH:** A perspex icterometer for neonates. Lancet 1:87–89, 1960

213. **Hannemann RE, DeWitt DP, Wiechel JF:** Neonatal serum bilirubin from skin reflectance. Pediatr Res 12:207–210, 1978

214. **Yamanouchi I, Yamanchi Y, Igarashi I:** Transcutaneous bilirubinometry: Preliminary studies of non-invasive transcutaneous bilirubin meter in the Okayama National Hospital. Pediatr Res 65:195–202, 1980

215.***Cochran WD:** Colors of the newborn. Postgrad Med 49:206–211, 1971

216.***Kopelman AE, Brown RS, Odell GB:** The "bronze" baby syndrome: A complication of phototherapy. J Pediatr 81:466, 1972

217. **Sharma RK, Ente G, Collipp PJ et al:** A complication of photo therapy in the newborn: The "bronze baby." Clin Pediatr 12:231, 1973

218. **Lascari AD:** Carotenemia: A review. Clin Pediatr 20:25–29, 1981

219.***Mandell F:** I am curious yellow. JAMA 217:1551, 1971

220. **Pollitt N:** Beta-carotene and the photodermatoses. Br J Dermatol 93:721–724, 1975

221. **Matthews-Roth MM, Pathak MA, Fitzpatrick TB et al:** B-carotene as an oral photoprotective agent in erythropoietic protoporphyria. JAMA 228:1004–1008, 1974

222. **Hoerer E, Dreyfuss F, Herzberg M:** Carotenemia, skin color and diabetes mellitus. Acta Diabetol Lat 12:202–207, 1975

223. **Sharvill DE:** Familial hypercarotinaemia and hypovitaminosis A. Proc R Soc Med 63:605–606, 1970

224. **McLaren DS, Zekian B:** Failure of enzymic cleavage of B-carotene: A cause of vitamin A deficiency in a child. Am J Dis Child 121:278–280, 1971

225. **Crisp AH, Stonehill E:** Hypercarotenaemia as a symptom of weight phobia. Postgrad Med J 43:721–725, 1967

226. **Popo MA, Schwabe AD:** Hypercarotemia in anorexia nervosa. JAMA 205:121–122, 1968

227. **Lord Cohen of Birkenhead:** Letter to the Editor: Hypercarotenemia in anorexia nervosa. JAMA 206:2318, 1968

228. **Tsaltas TT:** Studies of lipochromes (urochromes) in uremic patients and normal controls. I. The elimination of plasma lipochromes by hemodialysis. Trans Am Soc Artif Intern Organs 15:321–327, 1969

229. **Tsaltas TT:** Studies of lipochromes in uremic patients and normal controls II: Isolation and identification of carotenoids and lipochromes and their oxidation products in plasma. Trans Am Soc Artif Intern Organs 16:272–279, 1970

230. **O'Neil RR:** Letter to the Editor: Benign carotenemia of infancy. Pediatrics 31:692, 1963; and **Lowe CU:** Letter to

the Editor: Benign carotenemia. Pediatrics 31:692–693, 1963

231.*Granstein RD, Sober AJ: Drug- and heavy metal-induced hyperpigmentation. J Am Acad Dermatol 5:1–18, 1981

232. Simkins S: Dinitrophenol and dessicated thyroid in treatment of obesity: Comprehensive clinical and laboratory study. JAMA 108:2110–2117, 2193–2199, 1937

233. Editorial: Jaundice produced artificially by picric acid. Lancet 2:209, 1917

234. Kyle RA, Bartholomew LG: Variations in pigmentations from quinacrine: Report of case mimicking chronic hepatic disease. Arch Intern Med 109:134–138, 1962

235. Robboy MS, Sate AS, Schwabe AD: The hypercarotenemia in anorexia nervosa: A comparison of vitamin A and carotene levels in various forms of menstrual dysfunction and cachexia. Am J Clin Nutr 27:363–367, 1974

236. Gilkes JJH, Eady RAJ, Rees LH et al: Plasma immunoreactive melanotrophic hormones in patients on maintenance haemodialysis. Br Med J 1:656–657, 1975

237. Smith AG, Shuster S, Thody AJ et al: Role of the kidney in regulating plasma immunoreactive beta-melanocyte-stimulating hormone. Br Med J 1:874–876, 1976

238. Smith AG, Shuster S, Comaish JS et al: Plasma immunoreactive B-melanocyte-stimulating hormone and skin pigmentation in chronic renal failure. Br Med J 1:658–659, 1975

239. Pedace FJ, Winkelmann RK: Xanthelasma palpebrarum. JAMA 193:121–122, 1965

240.†Polano MK, Paes H, Hulsmans HAM et al: Xanthomata in primary hyperproteinemia: A classification based on the lipoprotein pattern of the blood. Arch Dermatol 100:387–400, 1969

241. Frederickson DS: "The case of the yellow palms" and other syndromes in need of detection. Med Ann District Columbia 36:207–211, 1967

242. Lynch PJ, Winkelmann RK: Generalized plane xanthoma and systemic disease. Arch Dermatol 93:639–646, 1966

243.*Altman J, Winkelmann RK: Diffuse normolipemic plane xanthomata: Generalized xanthelasma. Arch Dermatol 85:115–122, 1962

244. Goldston M, Steele JM, Dobriner K: Review—Alcaptonuria and ochronosis: With a report of three patients and metabolic studies in two. Am J Med 13:432–452, 1952

245. Eybel CE, Ambruster KFW, Ing TS: Skin pigmentation and acute renal failure in a patient receiving phenazopyridine therapy. JAMA 228:1027, 1974

246. Broadwell RO, III, Broadwell SD, Comer PB: Suicide by rifampin overdose. JAMA 240:2283–2284, 1978

247. Newton RW, Forrest ARW: Rifampicin overdosage: The "red man syndrome." Scott Med J 20:55–56, 1975

248. Miller LS: Letter to the Editor: Fluorescein discoloration of eyes, masking insidious onset of hepatitis. JAMA 229:137, 1974

249. Schwartz L: Occupational pigmentary changes in the skin. Arch Dermatol Syph 56:592–600, 1947

250. Schwartz L: Dermatitis from explosives. JAMA 125:186–190, 1944

251. Patel H, Dunn HG, Tischler B et al: Carotenemia in mentally retarded children: Incidence and etiology. Can Med Assoc J 108:848–852, 1973

252. Lundsgaard C: Erythrosis, or false cyanosis. J Exp Med 30:295–297, 1919

253. Lin YT: Pathophysiology of general cyanosis: Graphic analysis. NY State J Med 77:1393–1396, 1977

254. Morgan–Hughes JO: Lighting and cyanosis. Br J Anaesth 40:503, 1968

255. Medd EW, French EW, Wyllie V McA: Cyanosis as a guide to arterial desaturation. Thorax 14:247, 1959

256. Wilkin JK: Flushing reactions: Consequences and mechanisms. Ann Intern Med 95:468–476, 1981

257.*Dick GF, Dick GH: Scarlet Fever, p 36. Chicago, Year Book Medical Publishers, 1938

258. Shahrad P, Marko R: The wages of warmth: Changes in erythema ab igne. Br J Dermatol 97:179–186, 1977

259. Lerner AM, Klein JO, Cherry JD et al: New viral exanthems. N Engl J Med 269:678, 1963

260.*Butler ML: Erythema ab igne, a sign of pancreatic disease. Am J Gastroenterol 67:77–79, 1977

261. Mims CA: Pathogenesis of rashes in virus diseases. Bacteriol Rev 30:739–760, 1966

262. Mant AK: Autopsy diagnosis of accidental hypothermia. J Forensic Medicine 16:126, 1969

263.*Birdsong McL, Edmunds JE: Harlequin color change in the newborn. Report of a case. Obstet Gynecol 7:518–521, 1956

264. Pearson HA, Cone TE, Jr: Harlequin color change in a young infant with tricuspid atresia. J Pediatr 50:609–612, 1957

265. Neligan GA, Strang LB: A "harlequin" colour change in the newborn. Lancet 2:1005–1007, 1952

266. Chevrant–Breton J, Simon M, Bourel M et al: Cutaneous manifestations of idiopathic hemochromatosis: A study of 100 cases. Arch Dermatol 113:161–165, 1977

267. Cawley EP, Hsu YT, Wood BT et al: Hemochromatosis and the skin. Arch Dermatol 100:1–6, 1969

268. Bauer MF, Levan ME, Frankel A et al: Pigmented pretibial patches: A cutaneous manifestation of diabetes. Arch Dermatol 93:282–286, 1966

269. Rich LL, Epinette WW, Kasser WK: Argyria presenting as cyanotic heart disease. Am J Cardiol 30:290–292, 1972

270.*Pariser RJ: Generalized argyria: Clinicopathologic features and histochemical studies. Arch Dermatol 114:373–377, 1978

*Includes color plate.

†Includes illustration of various types of xanthomata.

*Includes color plate.

271. **Whelton MJ, Pope FM:** Azure lunules in argyria. Arch Intern Med 121:267–269, 1968

272.* **Lamar LM, Bliss BO:** Localized pigmentation of the skin due to topical mercury. Arch Dermatol 93:450–453, 1966

273.* **Burge KM, Winkelmann RK:** Mercury pigmentation— An electron microscope study. Arch Dermatol 102:51–61, 1970

274. **Bleehan SS, Gould DJ, Harrington CI et al:** Occupational argyria: Light and electron microscopic studies and x-ray microanalysis. Br J Dermatol 104:19–26, 1981

275.* **Lueth HC, Sutton DC, McMullen CJ et al:** Generalized discoloration of the skin resembling argyria following prolonged use of bismuth: A case of "bismuthia." Arch Intern Med 57:1115–1124, 1936

276. **Jeffery DA, Biggs DF, Percy JS et al:** Quantitation of gold in skin in chrysiasis. J Rheumatol 2:28–35, 1975

277. **Cox AJ, Marich KW:** Gold in the dermis following gold therapy for rheumatoid arthritis. Arch Dermatol 108:655–657, 1973

278.* **Burkhart CG:** Dermal melanocyte hamartoma: A distinctive new form of dermal melanocytosis. Arch Dermatol 117:102–104, 1981

279. **Ayres JR, Anderson NP:** Cutaneous manifestations of arsenic poisoning. Arch Dermatol Syph 30:33–43, 1934

280. **ten Bruggenkate CM, Lopes Cardosa E, Maaskant P:** Lead poisoning with pigmentation of the oral mucosa: Review of the literature and report of a case. Oral Surg 39:747–753, 1975

281. **Levantine A, Almeyda J:** Drug reactions XXII—Drug induced changes in pigmentation. Br J Dermatol 89:105–112, 1973

282.* **Granstein RD, Sober AJ:** Drug- and heavy metal-induced hyperpigmentation. J Am Acad Dermatol 5:1–18, 1981

283. **Hedin CA, Larsson A:** Physiology and pathology of melanin pigmentation with special reference to the oral cavity. Swed Dent J 113–129, 1978

284. **Downham TF II, Rehbein HM, Taylor KE:** Hyperpigmentation and folate deficiency. Arch Dermatol 112:562, 1976

285. **Resnik S:** Melasma induced by oral contraceptive drugs. JAMA 199:601–606, 1967

286. **Drysdale HC:** Methaemalbuminaemia as a cause of cyanosis. Br Med J 1:962, 1978

287. **Henkind P, Friedman AH:** External ocular pigmentation. Int Ophthalmol Clin 11:87–111, 1971

288. **Winkelmann RK:** Dark circles under the eyes. JAMA 193:161, 1965

289. **Maururi CA, Diaz LA:** Dark circles around the eyes. Cutis 5:979–982, 1969

290. **Goodman RM, Belcher RW:** Periorbital hyperpigmentation: An overlooked genetic disorder of pigmentation. Arch Dermatol 100:169–174, 1969

291. **Williams GT, Rosenthal JW:** Scleromalacia perforans as a complication of rheumatoid arthritis: Report of a case and observations concerning therapy. Ann Intern Med 51:801–805, 1959

292. **Smith JW:** Ochronosis of the sclera and cornea complicating alkaptonuria: Review of the literature and report of four cases. JAMA 120:1281–1288, 1942

293. **Gladstone RM:** Development and significance of heterochromia of the iris. Arch Neurol 21:184–192, 1969

294. **Jaffe N, Cassady R, Filler RM et al:** Heterochromia and Horner syndrome associated with cervical and mediastinal neuroblastoma. J Pediatr 87:75–77, 1975

295.† **Holt JF:** Neurofibromatosis in children. Am J Roentgenol 130:615–639, 1978

296.‡ **Solomons G, Zellweger H, Jahnke PG et al:** Four common eye signs in Mongolism. Am J Dis Child 110:46–50, 1965

297.* **Jelinek JE:** Oral contraceptives and the skin. Am Fam Physician 4:68–74, 1971

298. **Parker WA:** Argyria and cyanotic heart disease. Am J Hosp Pharm 34:287–289, 1977

299. **Robinson HM:** An evaluation of the bismuth blue line. J Invest Dermatol 18:341–363, 1952

300.* **Mosher DB, Fitzpatrick TB, Ortonne Jean–Paul:** Abnormalities of pigmentation. In Fitzpatrick TB, Eisen AZ, Wolff K, Freedberg IM, Austen KF (eds): Dermatology in General Medicine, 2nd ed, pp 568–654. New York, McGraw–Hill, 1979

301.* **Bearn AG, McKusick VA:** Azure lunulae—An unusual change in the fingernails in two patients with hepatolenticular degeneration (Wilson's disease). JAMA 166:903, 906, 1958

302. **Leyden JJ, Spott DA, Goldschmidt P:** Diffuse and banded melanin pigmentation. Arch Dermatol 105:548–550, 1972

303.§ **Muehrcke RD:** The finger-nails in chronic albuminemia: A new physical sign. Br Med J 1:1327, 1956

304.* **Hiller E:** Pulmonary manifestation of the yellow nail syndrome. Chest 61:452–458, 1972

305. **Sheam MA:** Nails and systemic disease. West J Med 129:358–361, 1978

306. **Samman PD:** The Nails in Disease, 3rd ed, p 197. Chicago, Year Book Medical Publishers, 1978

307. **Daniel CR III, Osment LS:** Nail pigmentation abnormalities: Their importance and proper examination. Cutis 25:595–607, 1980

308. **Zaias N:** The Nail in Health and Disease, p 260. Jamaica, NY, Spectrum Publications, 1980

309.* **Fitzpatrick TB, Kubita A, Morikawa F et al (eds):** The Biology and Diseases of Dermal Pigmentation, pp 1–379. Tokyo, University of Tokyo Press, 1981

*Includes color plate.

†See p. 617 for illustration of Lisch spots

‡Includes illustration of Brushfield spots

§Includes a special illustration

*Includes color plate.

310. **Anderson RR:** The physical basis of blue skin color. In Fitzpatrick TB, Kubita A, Morikawa F et al (eds): The Biology and Diseases of Dermal Pigmentation, pp 5–6. Tokyo, University of Tokyo Press, 1981

311. **Fitzpatrick TB, Ishihara M, Toda K et al:** Classification of dermal pigmentation (ceruloderma)—Blue skin. In Fitzpatrick TB, Kubita A, Morikawa F et al (eds): The Biology and Diseases of Dermal Pigmentation, pp 65–66. Tokyo, University of Tokyo Press, 1981

312. **Kubita A, Hori Y, Ohhara K et al:** Nevus of Ota. In Fitzpatrick TB, Kubita A, Morikawa F et al (eds): The Biology and Diseases of Dermal Pigmentation, pp 67–76. Tokyo, University of Tokyo Press, 1981

313. **Kikuchi: I, Inoue S:** Circumscribed dermal melanocytosis (Mongolian Spot). In Fizpatrick TB, Kubita A, Morikawa F et al (eds): The Biology and Diseases of Dermal Pigmentation, pp 83–94. Tokyo, University of Tokyo Press, 1981

314. **Morikawa F, Nakayama Y, Iikura T et al:** The application of photographic techniques for the differentiation of the location of melanin pigment in the skin. In Fitzpatrick TB, Kubita A, Morikawa F et al (eds): The Biology and Diseases of Dermal Pigmentation, pp 231–244. Tokyo, University of Tokyo Press, 1981

315. **Sober AJ, Granstein RD:** Chemical and pharmacologic agents causing dermal pigment. In Fitzpatrick TB, Kubita A, Morikawa F et al (eds): The Biology and Diseases of Dermal Pigmentation, pp. 117–126. Tokyo, University of Tokyo Press, 1981

316. **Shapiro H, Edelstein LM, Patel R et al:** Inability to demonstrate hydroxylation of tyrosine by murine melanoma "tyrosinase" (L-dopa oxidase) using tritiated water assay technique. J Invest Dermatol 72:191, 1979

317. **Okun M, Schley L, Ziegelstein H:** Oxidation of tyrosine to dopachrome by perioxidase isolated from murine melanoma. Physiol Chem Phys 14:8, 1982

40

Itching (Pruritus)

Harley A. Haynes
Sylvia Christine Johnson

Mechanisms of Itch
  Mediators
  Nerve endings, receptors, and pathways
  Factors affecting perception of itch
Pruritus Resulting from Systemic Disease
  Renal disease
  Hepatobiliary disease
  Pregnancy
  Endocrine disorders
    Diabetes mellitus
  Thyroid disease
  Malignant disease
  Benign hematologic disorders
Pruritus Not Resulting from Systemic Disease
  Pruritis without diagnostic skin lesions
  Pruritus with diagnostic skin lesions
Pruritus Ani and Pruritus Vulvae
Approach to the Patient with Pruritus
Summary

Pruritus is an important symptom not only because it is the most common subjective manifestation of cutaneous disease, but also because it may reflect systemic disease. This discussion will focus on the mechanism of itch, pruritus secondary to systemic disease, environmental causes of itch, and localized pruritic dermatoses. The pathophysiology of pruritus has recently been reviewed.[1] It is fair to say that this subject is still very incompletely understood.

MECHANISMS OF ITCH

MEDIATORS

The first evidence that proteases can mediate itch came from work by Shelley and Arthur on the tropical plant *Mucuna pruriens*.[2] This plant contains barbed spicules of cowhage, which for centuries have been known to cause itching. It was previously presumed that the itching was due to mechanical pricking of the spicules, but in 1955 Shelley and Arthur analyzed the itch-pro-ducing principle and found it had the characteristics of an endopeptidase. They subsequently showed that other endopeptidases, such as trypsin, chymotrypsin, and papain, caused pruritus when superficially introduced into the skin. Itch elicited by trypsin and chymotrypsin is probably to some extent mediated by histamine released by dermal mast cells, whereas papain causes itching without a wheal and flare reaction and is active in an area previously depleted of histamine by agents such as compound 48/80, dextran, and polymyxin. Histamine appears to act directly on nerve endings to cause pruritus without the necessity of any cutaneous alterations.[3]

The role of kinins in itch has been a subject of conflicting reports in the literature.[4–6] Intradermal injections of bradykinin and kallikrein produce itch.[6] Bradykinin induces a flare reaction, while kallikrein does not. Itch induced by bradykinin is inhibited by an antihistamine, while kallikrein-induced itch is not. Thus bradykinin itch is probably mediated by histamine, whereas kallikrein, like papain, is a protease that evidently does not cause histamine release.

Histamine has been favored as a physiologic stimulus for pruritus, since very small amounts of histamine will produce itching. After histamine is injected there is a latent period of about a half-minute before itch is perceived. Itching occurs before a wheal forms and subsides before the wheal disappears.[7] Antihistamines can block both the itch and the wheal from histamine but have little effect beyond a sedative effect on pruritus not mediated by histamine.

Prostaglandins are important in many biologic processes, and they may have a role in itching as well. Prostaglandin E_1 has been demonstrated to lower the threshold for pruritus evoked by both histamine and papain.[8,9] It is suggested that prostaglandins synthesized locally in inflamed skin, though not themselves pruritogenic, may sensitize the nerve receptors to the effect of other mediators. Aspirin sometimes is an effective antipruritic. We might speculate that it acts by suppression of prostaglandin synthesis.

NERVE ENDINGS, RECEPTORS, AND PATHWAYS

The site of itch perception seems to be a finely arborizing aggregate of nerve endings at the dermal-epidermal junction. Shelley and Arthur showed that cowage spicules were most effective in eliciting itch if their tips were inserted just to the dermal-epidermal junction.[10] Spicule application after removal of the epidermis by cantharidin or by superficial shaving still elicited pruritus, indicating that the epidermis itself was not critical in the production of itching by this protease. The earlier view that itching is an epidermal phenomenon was probably based on work that removed both the epidermis and the closely adherent subepidermal neural receptor unit. Whether or not intraepidermal nerves exist is controversial.[11]

In addition to the free nerve endings, specialized nerve end-organs exist beneath the epidermis. These are Merkel's disks, mucocutaneous end-organs, Meissner's corpuscles, the Vater-Pacini corpuscles, Krause's organs, and Ruffini's endings. It was previously thought that each of these receptors mediated specific sensory modalities (touch, temperature, pressure, pain, and so forth), but the modern concept is that these morphologic divisions do not imply specialized physiologic function. Each type of nerve ending probably responds preferentially, but not exclusively, to a particular stimulus.[12] In favor of a de-emphasis on specialized nerve function is Weddell's observation that the human cornea contains no specialized nerve endings but can perceive multiple types of sensory stimuli.[13]

Shelley and Arthur classified cutaneous sensory nerves into groups according to diameter, degree of myelinization, and conduction velocity.[10] From their experiments they concluded that itching is mediated by the fine, unmyelinated, slowly conducting C fibers. More recent discussions indicate a contribution by the myelinated δ-fibers of the A group as well.[14] While these fibers also conduct pain, there is some functional difference. Morphine is very effective in relieving pain but may intensify itching. Conversely, heating the skin to 40°C to 41°C quickly abolishes itch but intensifies burning pain.[15]

In an investigation to determine whether there was a central nervous system (CNS) effect of opiates on pruritus, it was found that in normal human subjects pretreatment with the opiate antagonist naloxone hydrochloride significantly increased the itch threshold to intracutaneous injections of histamine while not affecting the wheal and flare reaction locally.[15a] This study suggests that opiate receptors in the brain might well be involved in the perception of itch from a variety of causes, as well as from opiate administration.

Itching has been divided into protopathic and epicritic types. The origin of these terms dates to 1905 when Head studied regenerating nerve fibers.[16] *Protopathic* refers to the crude and primitive sensory experiences that are the earliest ones to return. The more finely developed and discriminatory sensation that returns later is referred to as *epicritic*. Rothman elaborated on this view of sensation.[17] Protopathic itching is poorly localized, uncomfortable, and persists after stimulation has ceased. Epicritic itching, on the other hand, is better localized, more pleasant, arises spontaneously, and is not associated with skin disease. In chronic dermatoses, persistent scratching may injure the cutaneous nerves and produce a state analogous to protopathic itching. There is some evidence that δ-A fibers carry epicritic itch, while C fibers mediate protopathic itch.[14] The neuronal pathway for the perception of itch is diagrammed in Figure 40-1. The fibers ascend in the contralateral anterolateral spinothalamic tracts to the posterior lateral ventral nucleus of the thalamus and then course through the internal capsule to the sensory area of the posterior central gyrus of the cortex.[18]

The mechanism whereby scratching relieves itch, albeit temporarily, is not clear. The sensory stimulus from scratching may distort the neuronal input so that itch is not perceived at the same time. Scratching often appears to work by generating a mild pain, which is more tolerable than the preceding itch. Some patients develop a masturbatory equivalent and scratch until a sense of satisfaction, almost orgasmic in quality, occurs. This is followed by a period of time in which the itch is not perceived. It is possible that changes in the

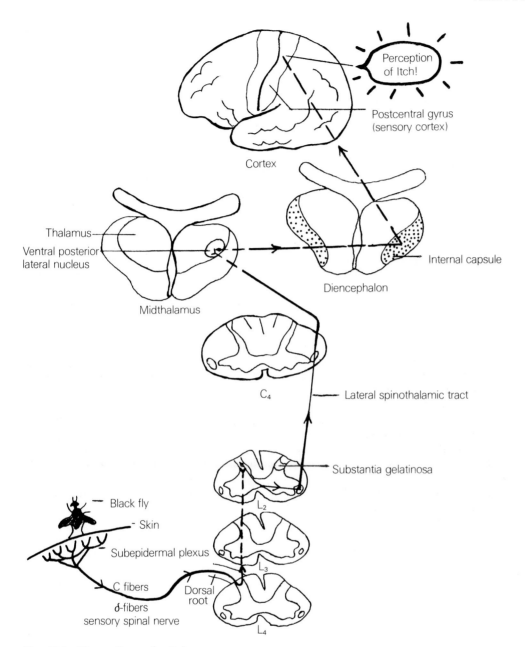

Fig. 40-1. The pathway for itch.

CNS function are very important in altering or abolishing the itch sensation. A gate-control theory has been advanced by Melzack and Wall. Sensory input itch through large A fibers arrives first and tends to interrupt summation of sensations of itch arriving through the small C fibers of slower conductive velocity.[19,20]

FACTORS AFFECTING PERCEPTION OF ITCH

Intradermal injection of histamine has been used experimentally to study itch. Itch threshold to intradermal histamine has been found to be lower at night, with vasodilatation, with increased skin temperature, and during psychic stress.[21,22] These factors are clini-

cally quite important in treating the patient with pruritus of nearly any etiology. Intrinsic factors may affect the perception of itch as well. Patients with atopic dermatitis clinically are found to develop itch more easily, more severely, and of longer duration than other people. Intracutaneous injection of trypsin causes itch that lasts longer in involved and uninvolved skin of patients with atopic dermatitis than in patients with other eczemas and psoriasis.[23]

Acquired pruritic dermatoses may also alter the perception of itch, but it is difficult to be sure which is cause and which is effect. When pruritus was induced by administering electric current to the flexor wrists with noninvasive electrodes, subjects who had a previous pruritic dermatosis had a lower itch threshold than patients with a negative history of prior skin disorder.[24] The effect of a pruritic disorder upon the itch threshold may account for the common clinical problem of a stimulus-initiating itch causing scratching and various types of skin damage, which themselves cause itch. This vicious cycle may continue even after removal of the initiating stimulus.

Even sleep does not necessarily eliminate itch. Scratching in various pruritic dermatoses has been recorded during the stages of sleep and has been found to correlate with changes in CNS excitability as judged by other criteria such as the threshold of response to auditory stimuli.[25,26,27]

PRURITUS RESULTING FROM SYSTEMIC DISEASE

Generalized pruritus without skin lesions sufficient to explain this symptom may be due to underlying systemic disease. The systemic diseases most commonly associated with pruritus are as follows:

Chronic renal failure
Obstructive hepatobiliary disease
Pregnancy
Hyperthyroidism
Hypothyroidism
Malignant disease
  Lymphoma
    Hodgkin's disease
    Mycosis fungoides
    Other non-Hodgkin's lymphomas
    Multiple myeloma
  Leukemia
  Visceral carcinomas
  Carcinoid syndrome

Hematologic disease, benign
  Polycythemia rubra vera
  Mastocytosis
  Iron deficiency
Intestinal and tissue parasitosis
Drug allergy

Experimental data suggesting probable mechanisms of itching exist for pregnancy, hepatobiliary disease, and renal disease. The pathogenesis of pruritus in thyroid disease is largely speculative, and why malignancy may cause itching is almost completely unknown.

When should the physician evaluate an itching patient for systemic disease and how extensive should the workup be? Any patient who presents with pruritus without a skin eruption must be considered a suspect for systemic disease, as must be the patient whose only skin lesions are the excoriations that are produced by scratching (Figs. 40-2–40-4) or the lichenification produced by rubbing (Fig. 40-5). Causes of pruritus such as thyroid disease and hepatobiliary disease can often be suspected on the basis of signs and symptoms that are easily detected by the history and physical examination. A malignancy, on the other hand, may be occult and not apparent unless specifically sought.

RENAL DISEASE

The pathophysiology of the pruritus in chronic uremia is not clear, but the symptom can be one of the most annoying and difficult for the uremic patient. The intensity of pruritus in renal failure does not correlate well with the level of blood urea nitrogen (BUN); dialysis improves pruritus in some, but not all, uremic patients. Relief of uremic pruritus with sauna baths to induce perspiration has been observed, but the mechanism of relief is not understood.[28] The hypothesis can be offered that some pruritogenic chemical is excreted through the sweat; alternatively, one could evoke an effect of heat on the cutaneous sensory nerves, since heating the skin to 40°C to 41°C blocks the sensation of itch.[15] Ultraviolet light treatments have also controlled pruritus in uremic patients.[29] More recent studies found that it was the sunburn spectrum (290 nm–320 nm) of ultraviolet light, known as UVB, which was effective. Moreover, treatment of only one half of the skin surface produced relief from pruritus over the entire skin surface, suggesting some systemic effect of the phototherapy. Some patients sustain a long remission (over 10 months) without additional phototherapy.[30] Further evidence that some circulating compounds may cause the pruritus in uremia is the relief from pruritus observed in some patients treated with oral cholestyremine or with oral activated char-

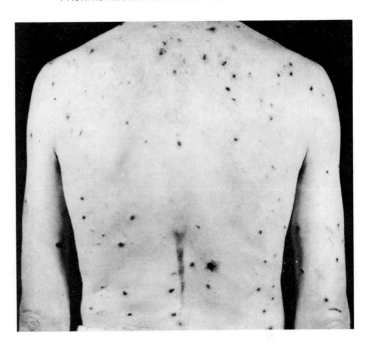

Fig. 40-2. Neurotic excoriations.

coal.[31,32] One must assume that both the cholestyramine and the charcoal act to bind some chemical or chemicals unknown in the intestinal tract and cause them to be excreted in the feces.

Secondary hyperparathyroidism is a frequent complication of uremia and may at times play a role in uremic pruritus. Although the exact relationship of pruritus and secondary hyperparathyroidism has not been fully elucidated, several workers have observed relief of pruritus immediately following subtotal parathyroidectomy.[33,34] The severity of pruritus does not consistently correlate with parathormone levels, how-

ever,[34,35] and no change in elevated parathormone levels occurred in some patients whose pruritus responded to oral charcoal.[32] Parathormone can induce mast cell proliferation in rats, and it has been observed that the number of mast cells may be increased in uremic patients and that elevated serum histamine may contribute to pruritus.[36,37] The serum calcium level has also been implicated as a factor in uremic pruritus.[34]

Intravenous xylocaine gives very transient relief of pruritus during dialysis,[38] but this is assumed to be a result of some sensorineural blockade and not any alteration of the basic pathogenesis of uremic pruritus.

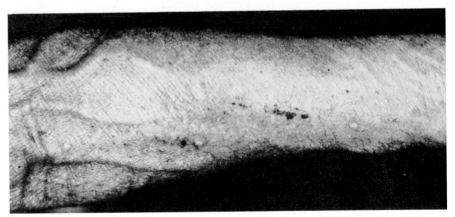

Fig. 40-3. Linear scratch marks and epidermal thickening in chronic dermatitis.

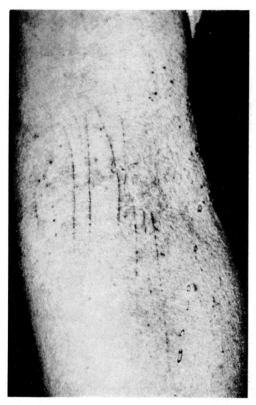

Fig. 40-4. Linear scratch marks in flexural eczematous dermatitis.

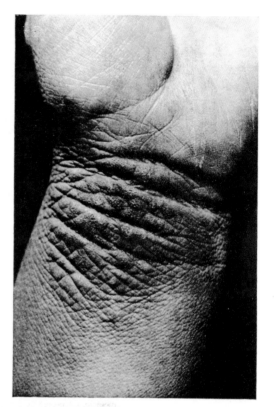

Fig. 40-5. Lichenification in eczematous dermatitis.

HEPATOBILIARY DISEASE

Obstructive biliary disease, especially primary biliary cirrhosis, may be associated with pruritus. It is not jaundice *per se* that causes the itch, since itching does not occur in jaundice secondary to hemolytic disease. Present evidence suggests that bile salts may be partly responsible for the pruritus. Numerous efforts have attempted to define the relationship between bile salts and itching. Skin levels of bile salts correlate with pruritus better than serum levels.[39] Patients with hepatobiliary disease and pruritus have a higher skin content of bile acids than do normals or patients with hepatobiliary disease without itch. Schoenfield studied serum and skin surface bile acids serially in five patients with obstructive jaundice, two given cholestyramine and three surgically drained.[40] Pruritus disappeared when the bile acids in the skin were normal, even if serum bile acids were still increased. In one patient pruritus persisted despite normal serum bile acids; skin bile acids were elevated. Another careful study has shown that the pruritus of cholestasis is not directly related to the skin tissue concentration of any of the major bile acids,

although a relationship to a particular form of bile acid could not be excluded.[41]

Varadi presented the first direct evidence that bile acids can produce pruritus in human skin.[42] He incorporated crude human bile plus the unconjugated salts of bile acids into cold cream and applied them to areas of skin from which the stratum corneum had been stripped. Dihydroxy salts caused pruritus, but the mono- and trihydroxy derivatives did not. Kirby and colleagues produced itching by application of bile salts to the erosions produced by cantharidin blisters in volunteer subjects, and again the dihydroxy salts were the most effective.[43]

The mechanism whereby bile salts induce pruritus is still speculative. One hypothesis is that bile salts release a mediator within the skin. The evidence is against histamine being that mediator: Antihistamines do not alleviate the pruritus associated with hepatobiliary disease, and vascular dilation and whealing do not accompany this type of itching. Herndon suggests that lysosomal proteases may be an important mediator.[44] Two observations support this contention:

1. *Patients with primary biliary cirrhosis* may develop a pruritic papulovesicular eruption. It is known that

in vitro injection of proteases may cause the formation of vesicles.[45]

2. *Patients with primary biliary cirrhosis and other chronic diseases associated with itching (e.g.,* Hodgkin's disease and chronic renal failure) may become hyperpigmented. Proteolytic enzymes, by splitting off a peptide, may convert inactive protyrosinase to tyrosinase, thereby activating melanin formation.[46]

In spite of the pathogenetic uncertainties, symptomatic therapy for itching owing to hepatobiliary disease is usually aimed at decreasing bile salt concentration. The anion exchange resin cholestyramine may relieve pruritus, sometimes without significantly changing the serum concentration of bile acids.[47] In this regard it is interesting that cholestyramine binds the dihydroxy more than the trihydroxy derivatives. A small number of patients with chronic cholestasis and intractable pruritus had good relief of pruritus by plasma perfusion through charcoal-coated glass beads.[48] The relief lasted up to 5 months, even though bile salts return to pretreatment levels in 3 days to 5 days. This finding suggests pruritogens other than bile acids alone. Albumin infusion may temporarily relieve itching by binding serum bile salts. Phenobarbital[49] and a diet rich in polyunsaturated fatty acids[50] have successfully treated the pruritus of cholestatic jaundice, both apparently acting by increasing fecal bile salt excretion. The observations most contrary to a prime role of bile acids are the efficacy of 17 α-substituted androgens, such as methyltestosterone, in relieving the pruritus while often causing a rise in serum bile acids and a worsening of cholestasis.[51,52]

PREGNANCY

Pruritus that occurs during pregnancy is sometimes due to intrahepatic cholestasis apparently caused by estrogen. Estrogen produces hyperplasia and hypertrophy of bile ducts in mice,[53] but light microscopy of the liver in pregnant women with pruritus gravidarum has shown only bile stasis of a mild degree without cellular damage.[54,55] Electron microscopy has revealed dilatation of bile ducts and flattening and distortion of microvilli.[54,55]

Once pruritus occurs in a pregnancy it usually recurs in all subsequent full-term pregnancies.[54,56] It may be accompanied by jaundice or be the only manifestation of hepatic dysfunction. Bilirubin is usually elevated but may be normal, with total bilirubin rarely exceeding 5 mg/dl.[56] The other usual liver function test abnormalities are elevated alkaline phosphatase, hypoalbuminemia, and elevated cholesterol, all of which return to normal after delivery.[54] Similar clinical and laboratory abnormalities have been observed with use of oral contraceptives.[57,58]

ENDOCRINE DISORDERS

Diabetes Mellitus

Although diabetes is commonly listed as a cause of pruritus, the only study that was specifically directed at this association was done in 1927.[59] Only 33 of 500 patients surveyed at the Joslin Clinic had pruritus at the time of study or in the past. Only half of these, or about 3% of the total, had generalized pruritus. As a rule, generalized pruritus is not likely to be due to diabetes. There may be an increase in localized, pruritic anogenital candidiasis and tinea in diabetics, but these local infections must be distinguished from generalized pruritus.

Thyroid Disease

Itching has been reported as a manifestation of both hypo- and hyperthyroidism. Asteatosis ("dry skin") is the presumed mechanism in the former. In hyperthyroidism the vasodilated state may contribute to pruritus by lowering the itch threshold. Ergotamine has been shown to relieve the pruritus of hyperthyroidism, probably by contracting the usually dilated blood vessels. Sympathetic blockade has also been reported to relieve itching owing to hyperthyroidism.[60] Pruritus consistently disappears with treatment of hyperthyroidism by any therapeutic modality.[50,61] Urticaria, which is pruritic, has been reported to occur with hyperthyroidism, an association that may be fortuitous, but the urticaria also cleared with control of the hyperthyroid state.[62]

MALIGNANT DISEASE

Most authorities consider pruritus to be present in about 25% of patients with Hodgkin's disease,[63] although this figure is probably high now that the disease is more often diagnosed in the early stages. Such pruritus clears after remission of Hodgkin's disease. The cause of pruritus in Hodgkin's disease is unknown. One study has shown elevated levels of IgE in such patients; both the pruritus and the levels of IgE responded to successful treatment of the lymphoma.[64] In one case pruritus resolved after removal of a cavitary pulmonary lesion representing Hodgkin's disease.[65] Other non-Hodgkin's lymphomas may cause pruritus as well. Well-differentiated lymphocytic lymphoma or lymphosarcoma is particularly likely to have associated pruritus[66] (Fig. 40-6). Paraproteinemia may present with pruritus.[67] Mycosis fungoides, a T-cell lymphoma trophic to

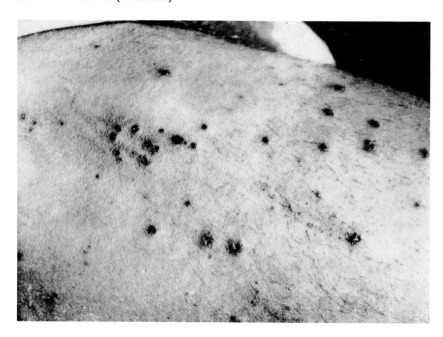

Fig. 40-6. Prurigolike eruption in lymphosarcoma. In contrast with neurotic excoriations, the edges of the lesions are infiltrated.

skin, may have an early phase lasting a decade or more with pruritus but displaying only very subtle skin lesions. Eventually, obvious infiltrated plaques and tumors appear (Figs. 40-7, 40-8). Leukemic patients do not commonly have pruritus, but when present, it is more common in chronic than acute leukemia and in lymphocytic than in granulocytic forms.[68] The mechanism of this pruritus is unknown except for one patient with basophilic leukemia, which resulted in high serum levels of histamine.[69] Possibly, various mediators of inflammation might be increased in some leukemias and result in pruritus. In addition, carcinoma of any internal organ can cause pruritus, but the frequency of this manifestation is very low, and the pathophysiology is unknown. Malignancies with prodromal pruritus have been reported in breast, stomach, uterus, prostate, thyroid, and lung.

Carcinoid syndrome may be accompanied by severe pruritus. Tumor-produced serotonin is implicated as the causative agent for the pruritus, its vasodilatory action on the skin capillaries lowering the threshold for itching. In one case a serotonin antagonist (cyproheptadine) relieved the pruritus in carcinoid syndrome.[70]

BENIGN HEMATOLOGIC DISORDERS

It is well known that pruritus following a hot bath or shower may be a symptom of polycythemia vera in approximately one third of patients. Although the itching in these patients sometimes responds to allopurinol, the mechanism is unclear, since serum uric acid is not always elevated nor does the level correlate with the intensity of pruritus.[71] Even more difficult to explain is the response of pruritus of polycythemia vera to oral cholestyramine, but presumably some pruritogenic substance is thereby excreted through the intestinal tract.[72]

Mastocytosis has pruritus as its most frequent symptom. It may present with pruritus without obvious skin lesions, although brown-to-pink papules that urticate on being firmly stroked are usually present. The symptoms in mastocytosis are all thought to be secondary to the release of unphysiologic quantities of histamine from the mast cells. Symptoms in addition to pruritus are flushing (36%), gastrointestinal tract symptoms (23%), duodenal ulcer (4%), tachycardia (18%), and various neuropsychiatric symptoms such as fatigue, headache, and malaise (12%).[73] These symptoms were markedly improved by oral disodium cromoglycate in several patients. This drug acts by stabilizing mast cell membranes and thus reducing histamine and other mediator release. Histaminuria in these patients persisted during therapy and raises the possibility that disodium chromoglycate may act by other mechanisms in this condition.[74]

Iron deficiency can cause pruritus that is very responsive to iron replacement therapy.[75] The mechanism is unknown, but this cause should be sought in a workup of a pruritic patient. Some additional uncommon causes of pruritus are mentioned in a review.[76]

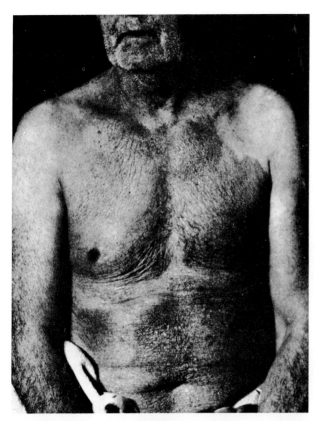

Fig. 40-7. Mycosis fungoides. Intensely pruritic arciform erythematous premycotic lesion.

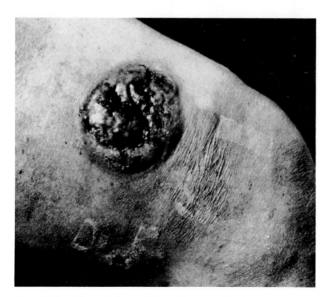

Fig. 40-8. Mycosis fungoides. Nonpruritic tumor.

PRURITUS NOT RESULTING FROM SYSTEMIC DISEASE

PRURITUS WITHOUT DIAGNOSTIC SKIN LESIONS

Xerosis ("dry skin") is a common cause of pruritus, particularly in older people in the winter. Prolonged exposure to refrigerated air-conditioning has been reported to have caused "winter itch" during the summer in 18 patients in Texas.[77] These situations seem to be due in large part to dehydration of the stratum corneum to a point where it becomes brittle, the resultant microscopic fissures causing low-grade irritation and inflammation that itches. If xerosis is felt to be the etiology of pruritus, it is wise to initially treat the patient with only topical agents (such as emollients) and avoid giving oral antipruritic agents, because the latter may mask a more serious cause of itching.

A benign cause of itching that may be obscure because of the absence of a skin eruption is that due to contamination of clothing with fiberglass, usually from curtains washed in the same machine or tub. Clues to the diagnosis are the sudden onset of pruritus with a prickling quality in several family members following wash day.[78,79] The fiberglass particles can be detected by microscopic examination of cellophane tape that has been applied to affected skin or by scrapings treated with potassium hydroxide.

Pruritus is a feature of heroin addiction, which should be suspected in a patient with periorbital edema and redness who tends to rub his face. Amphetamine abuse also may cause itching. Pruritus without other skin manifestations occasionally occurs as a presumed allergic reaction to a variety of therapeutic drugs. Ordinarily, however, either an exanthematous eruption or urticaria appear as a cutaneous manifestation (Figs. 40-9, 40-10).

Comings and Comings have reported an unusual form of pruritus, benign in nature, and localized to the lower scapula in eight members of one family.[80] The only visible lesion was on the clothes: a small ragged spot overlying the area of pruritus. X-linked or autosomal dominant inheritance is suggested.

Psychogenic pruritus, so-called neurotic excoriations (see Fig. 40-2) may present in a fashion to cause the physician to suspect an underlying disease process. In fact, there is no easy way to distinguish this entity from the specific disease-related states and all such patients should have a thorough medical evaluation.

PRURITUS WITH DIAGNOSTIC SKIN LESIONS

Itching is a prominent symptom of many dermatoses. Among these are allergic contact dermatitis (Fig. 40-11), atopic dermatitis (Fig. 40-12), lichen simplex

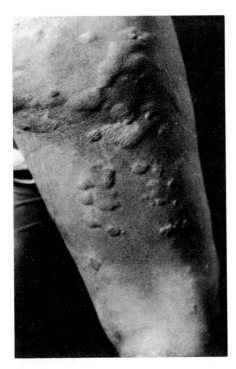

Fig. 40-9. Urticarial type of allergic reaction. This reaction is most commonly seen in hypersensitivity to drugs or foods.

chronicus, urticaria (see Fig. 40-9), drug eruption (see Fig. 40-10), lichen planus, tinea, candidiasis, dermatitis herpetiformis, scabies (Fig. 40-13), and pediculosis. These conditions should be diagnosed by physical examination, with confirmation, when indicated, by skin biopsy or microscopic examination of scales for yeast, fungi, or parasites.

PRURITUS ANI AND PRURITUS VULVAE

Anal and vulvar pruritus often present difficult problems for the physician. The anogenital area is particularly susceptible to pruritus because of the local environmental conditions and the rich innervation of the tissue (Fig. 40-14). Often no specific cause of such itching can be found, and scrupulous hygiene after defecation often relieves perianal pruritus.[81,82] It is possible that bile salts or other fecal constituents might be responsible for many of the cases of perianal pruritus.

Specific disease entities that commonly cause itching in the perianal and perivulvar region are fissures, seborrheic dermatitis, psoriasis, condyloma acuminata, candidiasis, tinea, contact dermatitis, parasitic infestation with *Enterobius vermicularis* (pinworm) or *Pedic-*

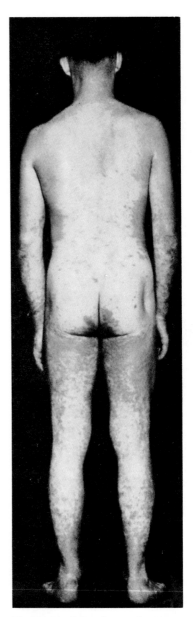

Fig. 40-10. Macular erythematous eruption caused by hypersensitivity to diphenylhydantoin.

ulus pubis, and erythrasma.[83,84] Less common causes of anogenital pruritus are lichen sclerosus et atrophicus, Bowen's disease, and extramammary Paget's disease. An abnormal vaginal discharge should be evaluated and treated appropriately. Estrogen deficiency with atrophy of the mucosa of the external genitalia may be associated with pruritus, but whether replacement hormonal therapy alleviates this problem is debatable.[84]

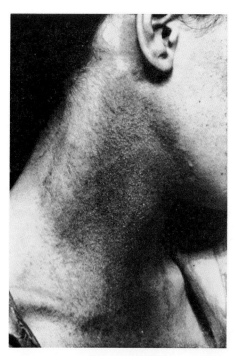

Fig. 40-11. Eczematous type of allergic reaction with intraepidermal vesicle formation. The allergen in this case was resorcinol.

APPROACH TO THE PATIENT WITH PRURITUS

If a patient has itching that is neither localized to a discrete area, nor explained by diagnostic skin lesions, serious consideration must be given to an extensive workup to evaluate the presence or absence of underlying disease of which the pruritus is a symptom. The older patient often has "dry skin," which is a tempting explanation for the itch. If increasing the environmental humidity and the topical application of emollients clears this symptom, no further investigation is warranted unless specific clues are uncovered by the history and physical examination. If itching persists, then further evaluation is indicated. When a patient requires such evaluation of the cause of pruritus, the following tests should be included:

A thorough physical examination, including a pelvic and
   rectal examination, with a pap smear and a stool test
   for occult blood
Chest film
Complete blood count
Differential count
Serum iron test
Liver, thyroid, and renal function tests

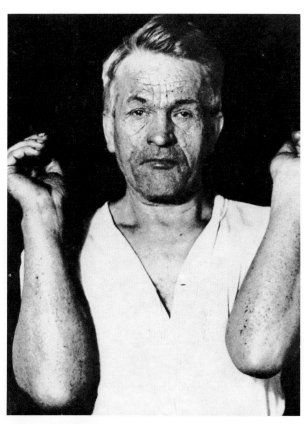

Fig. 40-12. Atopic dermatitis with reaction to pollen. It is difficult to decide whether the punctiform lesions are dried crusts of broken vesicles or scratch marks.

Additional tests such as a sedimentation rate, serum protein electrophoresis, serum calcium, and extensive radiologic survey for occult neoplastic disease are indicated when the physician feels these are appropriate.

If a specific, treatable disease is found, the therapy will usually cure the pruritus. When, as in uremia or carcinoma, curative therapy is not always possible, then symptomatic management becomes essential. There are no medications for itch that are as effective or specific as those for pain. Antihistamines, particularly hydroxyzine, are often most helpful, mostly because of their sedative effect.[85,86,87] Aspirin, at times, is very helpful but should not be used in urticaria as it is a histamine releaser.[88] Local applications of soothing emollients, perhaps with 1% phenol and ¼% menthol, may bring much relief. Simple application of cold, moist towels is often very helpful. One should avoid those chemical, mechanical, thermal, and psychic stimuli that appear to exacerbate the pruritus. The topical application of antihistamines (such as diphenhydramine) is

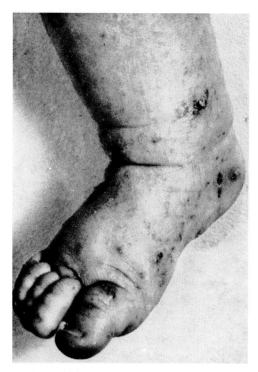

Fig. 40-13. Scabies. Excoriated burrows on medial aspect of heel.

generally to be avoided as they are not very effective topically and often are potent sensitizers. Topical corticosteroids are antiinflammatory, vasoconstrictive, and antipruritic, but their use over large surface areas for prolonged periods can cause adrenal suppression. The potent, fluorinated corticosteroids often cause dermal atrophy with resultant telangiectasia, striae, and easy bruising. Topical 1% hydrocortisone alcohol or acetate is free of these side effects and is recommended for use in these locations.[89]

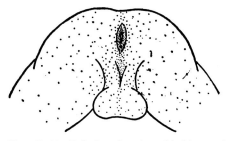

Fig. 40-14. Relative density of itching points in the male anogenital region. (Longo V: Sulla topografia della sensibilitá pel (prurito). Archivio di Fisiologia 36:197, 1936)

SUMMARY

Itching is one of the major important and common symptoms, but its pathophysiology is incompletely understood. That which is known of the pathophysiology is described in this chapter and is related insofar as possible to clinical entities. Unless pruritus is caused by a cutaneous disorder with diagnostic skin lesions, its etiology will not be discernible upon physical examination of the skin. A schema is presented organizing pruritus into that resulting from systemic diseases and that not resulting from systemic diseases, the latter subdivided into pruritus with, and pruritus without, diagnostic skin lesions. In addition, the special problems related to pruritus ani and pruritus vulvae are discussed separately. Finally, a rational clinical approach to the patient with pruritus is presented.

REFERENCES

1. **Herndon JH, Jr:** The pathophysiology of pruritus. Int J Dermatol 14:465–484, 1975
2. **Shelley WB, Arthur RP:** Studies on cowhage (Mucuna Pruriens) and its pruritogenic proteinase, mucunain. Arch Dermatol 72:399–406, 1955
3. **Scuka M:** Analysis of the effects of histamine on the endplate potential. Neuropharmacology 12:441, 1973
4. **Cormia FE, Dougherty JW:** Proteolytic activity in development of pain and itching. Cutaneous reactions to bradykinin and kallikrein. J Invest Dermatol 35:21–26, 1960
5. **Keele CA:** Chemical causes of pain and itch. Annu Rev Med 21:67–74, 1970
6. **Hagermark O:** Studies on experimental itch produced by kallikrein and bradykinin. Acta Derm Venereol (Stockh) 54:397–400, 1974
7. **Rothman S:** Pathophysiology of itch sensation. In Montagna W (ed): Advances in Biology of Skin, Vol 1, pp 189–201. New York, Pergamon, 1960
8. **Greaves MW, McDonald–Gibson W:** Itch: Role of prostaglandins. Br Med J 3:608–609, 1973
9. **Lovell CR, Burton PA, Duncan EH:** Prostaglandins and pruritus. Br J Dermatol 94:273–275, 1976
10. **Shelley WB, Arthur RP:** The neurohistology and neurophysiology of the itch sensation in man. Arch Dermatol 76:296–323, 1957
11. **Bourlond A:** Cutaneous innervation. J Invest Dermatol 67:106–109, 1976
12. **Iggo A:** Cutaneous and subcutaneous sense organs. Br Med Bull 33:97–102, 1977
13. **Lele PP, Weddell G:** The relationship between neurohistology and corneal sensibility. Brain 79:119–154, 1956
14. **Lorinca AL:** Neurophysiologic reactions of the skin: Pathophysiology of pruritus. In Fitzpatrick TB, Eisen AZ,

Wolff K et al (eds): Dermatology in General Medicine, 2nd ed, pp 221–224. New York, McGraw–Hill, 1979

15. **Keele CA, Armstrong D:** Substances Producing Pain and Itch, p 289. London, Edward Arnold, 1974

15a. **Bernstein JE, Swift RM, Sultani K et al:** Antipruritic effect of an opiate antagonist, naloxone hydrochloride. J Invest Dermatol 78:82–83, 1982

16. **Head H:** Studies in Neurology, Vol Z. London, Oxford University Press, 1920

17. **Rothman S:** Beiträge zur physiologie der juckempfindung. Arch Dermatol Syph 139:227–234, 1922

18. **Bishop GH:** The relation of nerve fiber size to modality of sensation. In Montagna W (ed): Cutaneous Innervation p 88. Oxford, Pergamon, 1960

19. **Melzack R, Wall PD:** Pain mechanisms: A new theory. Science 150:971, 1965

20. **Melzack R, Schecter B:** Itch and vibration. Science 147:1047, 1965

21. **Cormia FE:** Experimental histamine pruritus, I. Influence of physical and psychological factors on threshold reactivity. J Invest Dermatol 19:21–34, 1952

22. **Cormia FE, Kuykendall V:** Experimental histamine pruritus. II. Nature; physical and environmental factors influencing development and severity. J Invest Dermatol 20:429–446, 1953

23. **Rajka G:** Itch duration in the uninvolved skin of atopic dermatitis. Acta Derm Venereol (Stockh) 48:320–321, 1968

24. **Edwards AE, Shellow WVR, Wright ET et al:** Pruritic skin disease, psychological stress and the itch sensation. Arch Dermatol 112:339–343, 1976

25. **Felix R, Shuster S:** A new method for the measurement of itch and the response to treatment. Br J Dermatol 93:303–312, 1975

26. **Savin JA, Paterson WD, Oswald I:** Scratching during sleep. Lancet 11:296–297, 1973

27. **Savin JA, Paterson WD, Oswald I et al:** Further studies of scratching during sleep. Br J Dermatol 93:297–302, 1975

28. **Snyder D, Merrill JP:** Sauna baths in the treatment of chronic renal failure. Transactions of the American Society for Artificial Internal Organs 12:188–192, 1966

29. **Saltzer EI:** Relief from uremic pruritus: A therapeutic approach. Cutis 16:298–299, 1975

30. **Gilchrest BA, Rowe JW, Brown RS et al:** Ultraviolet phototherapy of uremic pruritus. Long-term results and possible mechanism of action. Ann Intern Med 91:17–21, 1979

31. **Silverberg DS, Jana A, Reisin E et al:** Cholestyramine in uremic pruritus. Br Med J 1:752–753, 1977

32. **Pederson JA, Matter BJ, Czerwinski AW et al:** Relief of idiopathic generalized pruritus in dialysis patients treated with activated oral charcoal. Ann Intern Med 93:446–448, 1980

33. **Hampers CL, Katz AI, Wilson RE et al:** Disappearance of "uremic" itching after subtotal parathyroidectomy. N Engl J Med 279:695–697, 1968

34. **Massry SG, Popovtzer MM, Coburn JW et al:** Intractable pruritus as a manifestation of secondary hyperparathyroidism in uremia. N Engl J Med 279:697–700, 1968

35. **Young AW, Sweeney EW, David DS et al:** Dermatologic evaluation of pruritus in patients on hemodialysis. NY State J Med 73:2670–2674, 1973

36. **Neiman RS, Bischel MD, Lukes RJ:** Uremia and mast cell proliferation. Lancet I:959, 1972

37. **Rockhoff SD, Armstrong JD:** Parathyroid hormone as a stimulus to mast cell accumulation in bone. Calcif Tissue Res 5:49–55, 1970

38. **Tapia L, Cheigh JS, David DS et al:** Pruritus in dialysis patients treated with parenteral lidocaine. N Engl J Med 296:261–262, 1977

39. **Schoenfield LJ:** Bile acids on the skin of patients with pruritic hepatobiliary disease. Nature 213:93–94, 1967

40. **Schoenfield LJ:** The relationship of bile acids to pruritus in hepatobiliary disease. In Schiff L, Carey JB, Dietschy J (eds): Bile Salt Metabolism, pp 260–261. Springfield, Ill, Charles C Thomas, 1969

41. **Ghent CH, Bloomer JR, Klatskin G:** Elevations in skin tissue levels of bile acids in human cholestasis: Relation of serum levels and pruritus. Gastroenterology 73:1125–1130, 1977

42. **Varadi DP:** Pruritus induced by crude bile and purified bile acids. Arch Dermatol 109:678–681, 1974

43. **Kirby J, Heaton KW, Burton JL:** The pruritic effect of bile salts. Br J Dermatol (Suppl 10) 91:11–12, 1974

44. **Herndon JH:** Pathophysiology of pruritus associated with elevated bile acid levels in serum. Arch Intern Med 130:632–637, 1972

45. **Kahl FR, Pearson RW:** Ultrastructural studies of experimental vesiculation: I. Papain. J Invest Dermatol 49:43–60, 1967

46. **McGuire JS:** Activation of epidermal tyrosinase. Biochem Biophys Res Commun 40:1084–1089, 1970

47. **Datta DV, Sherlock S:** Treatment of pruritus of obstructive jaundice with cholestyramine. Br Med J 1:216–219, 1963

48. **Lauterberg BH, Pineda AA, Burgstaler EA et al:** Treatment of pruritus of cholestasis by plasma perfusion through USP-charcoal-coated glass beads. Lancet 2:53–55, 1980

49. **Stiehl A, Thaler M, Admirand WH:** The effects of phenobarbital on bile salts and bilirubin in patients with intrahepatic and extrahepatic cholestasis. N Engl J Med 286:858–861, 1972

50. **Van Itallie TB, Hashim SA, Crampton RS et al:** The treatment of pruritus and hypercholesteremia of primary biliary cirrhosis with cholestyramine. N Engl J Med 265:469–474, 1961

51. **Lloyd–Thomas HGL, Sherlock S:** Testosterone therapy for the pruritus of obstructive jaundice. Br Med J 4:1289–1291, 1952

52. **Alva J, Iber FL:** Relief of pruritus of jaundice with methandrostenolone and speculation on the nature of pruritus in liver disease. Am J Med Sci 250:60–65, 1965

53. **Gardner WV, Allen E, Smith GM:** Hyperplasia and hypertrophy of the mucosa of larger biliary ducts in mice receiving estrogens. Proc Soc Exp Biol Med 46:511–513, 1941

54. **Eliakim M, Sadovsky E, Stein O et al:** Recurrent cholestatic jaundice of pregnancy. Arch Intern Med 117:696–705, 1966

55. **Mistilis SP:** Liver disease in pregnancy with particular emphasis on the cholestatic syndromes. Australasian Annals of Medicine 17:248–260, 1968

56. **Sadovsky E, Eliakim M, Schenker JR:** Pruritus gravidarum of hepatic origin. Isr J Med Sci 6:540–543, 1970

57. **Boake WC, Schade SG, Morrissey JF et al:** Intrahepatic cholestatic jaundice of pregnancy followed by enovid-induced cholestatic jaundice. Ann Intern Med 63:302–308, 1965

58. **Orellana–Alcalde JM, Dominguez JP:** Jaundice and oral contraceptive drugs. Lancet II:1278–1280, 1966

59. **Greenwood AM:** A study of the skin in 500 cases of diabetes. JAMA 89:774–776, 1927

60. **Eliakim M, Rachmilewitz M:** Pruritus: A neglected symptom in thyrotoxicosis. Isr Med J 18:262–268, 1959

61. **Barnes HM, Sarkany I, Calnan CD:** Pruritus and thyrotoxicosis. Transactions of the St. Johns Hospital Dermatological Society 60:59–62, 1974

62. **Isaacs NJ, Ertel NH:** Urticaria and pruritus: Uncommon manifestations of hyperthyroidism. J Allergy Clin Immunol 48:73–81, 1971

63. **Bluefarb SM:** Cutaneous Manifestations of the Malignant Lymphomas, p 534. Springfield, Ill, Charles C Thomas, 1959

64. **Amhot PL, Green LA:** Atrophy and immunoglobulin E concentrations in Hodgkin's disease and other lymphomas. Br Med J No. 6109:327, 1978

65. **Dhingra HK, Flance IJ:** Cavitary primary pulmonary Hodgkin's disease presenting as pruritus. Chest 58:71–73, 1970

66. **Rosenberg SA, Diamond HD, Jaslowitz B:** Lymphosarcoma: A review of 1269 cases. Medicine 40:31, 1961

67. **Zelicovici M, Cahane P, Bianu G:** Pruritus as a possible early sign of paraproteinemia. Isr J Med Sci 5:1079–1081, 1969

68. **Winkelmann RK, Muller SA:** Pruritus. Annu Rev Med 15:53–65, 1964

69. **Youmans JD, Taddeini L, Cooper T:** Histamine excess symptoms in basophilic chronic granulocytic leukemia. Arch Intern Med 131:560, 1973

70. **Kehil ME, Brown H, Fred HL:** The carcinoid crisis. Arch Intern Med 114:26–28, 1964

71. **Lyell A, Vera P:** The itching patient. Scott Med J 17:334–347, 1972

72. **Chanarin I, Szur L:** Relief of intractable pruritus in polycythemia rubra vera with cholestyramine. Br J Haematol 29:669–670, 1975

73. **Demis DJ:** The mastocytosis syndrome: Clinical and biological studies. Ann Intern Med 59:194–206, 1963

74. **Soter NA, Austen KF, Wasserman SI:** Oral disodium chromoglycate in the treatment of systemic mastocytosis. N Engl J Med 301:465–469, 1979

75. **Vickers CFH:** Nutrition and the skin: Iron deficiency in dermatology, pp 311–315. Proceedings of the Tenth Symposium on Advanced Medicine, London. Royal College of Physicians, 1974

76. **Botero F:** Pruritus as a manifestation of systemic disorders. In Callen JP (ed): Cutaneous Aspects of Internal Disease, pp 627–633. Chicago, Year Book Medical Publishers, 1981

77. **Chernosky ME:** Pruritic skin disease and summer air conditioning. JAMA 179:1005–1010, 1962

78. **Peachey RDG:** Glass–fibre itch: A modern washday hazard. Br Med J 2:221–222, 1967

79. **Fisher BK, Warkentin JD:** Fiber glass dermatitis. Arch Dermatol 99:717–719, 1969

80. **Comings DE, Comings SN:** Hereditary localized pruritus. Arch Dermatol 92:236–237, 1965

81. **Eyers AA, Thompson JPS:** Pruritus ani: Is anal sphincter dysfunction important in aetiology. Br Med J 2:1549–1551, 1979

82. **Parrish JA, Gilchrest BA, Fitzpatrick TB:** Between You and Me: A sensible and Authoritative Guide To The Care and Treatment of Your Skin, p 47. Boston, Little, Brown & Co, 1978

83. **Hudson CN:** Pruritus vulvae. Br Med J 1:656, 1971

84. **Pillsbury DM:** Chronic anal and vulvar pruritus. In Moschella SL, Pillsbury DM, Hurley HJ (eds): Dermatology, pp 318–322. Philadelphia, W B Saunders, 1975

85. **Fischer RW:** Comparison of anti-pruritic agents administered orally. JAMA 203:418–419, 1968

86. **Cook TJ, MacQueen DM, Wittig HJ et al:** Degree and duration of skin test suppression and side effects with antihistamines. J Allergy Clin Immunol 51:71–77, 1973

87. **Rhoades RB, Leifer KN, Cohan R et al:** Suppression of histamine-induced pruritus by three antihistaminic drugs. J Allergy Clin Immunol 55:180–185, 1975

88. **Hagermark O:** Influence of antihistamines, sedatives, and aspirin on experimental itch. Acta Derm Venerol (Stockh) 53:363–368, 1973

89. **Arndt KA, Clark RAF:** Principles of topical therapy. In Fitzpatrick TB, Eisen AZ, Wolff K et al (eds): Dermatology in General Medicine, 2nd ed, pp 1753–1758. New York, McGraw-Hill, 1979

Index

Page numbers followed by f and t refer respectively to figures and tabular material. The letter n represents footnotes. In general, entries are grouped by the descriptive anatomical adjective rather than by the noun signifying the condition. For example, conditions relating to the adrenal gland can be found by looking under *adrenal* rather than under *hypercorticism* (adrenal hypercortism) or *hyperplasia* (adrenal hyperplasia).

"Abdominal angina"
  arteriography in diagnosis of, 172
  pain of, 169
Abdominal lymph nodes, 511–517
  anatomy of, 511–513
  clinical significance of, 513–515
  intra-abdominal syndromes, 516–517
Abdominal pain, 165–178
  abdominal lymphadenopathy and,
      513, 514
  "acute," 177–178
  in acute hemolytic anemia, 570
  in alcoholic hepatitis, 424
  in allergic purpura, 545
  anatomy and physiology of, 166
  arteriography, 172
  biliary tract origins, 175–176
  biopsies, 172
  in calcified-lymph-node syndrome,
      516
  of cardiac origin, 158
  computed tomography, 172
  as conversion symptom, 633–635
  endoscopic examination, 171–172
  esophogeal origins, 173
  etiologic classification of, by organ
      system, 173–177
  extra-abdominal, causes, 173
  gastric origins of, 173
  genitourinary tract origins, 176–177
  hepatic origins, 175–176
  historical perspective, 165–166
  history of study of, 165–166
  intensity, factors influencing, 169
  intestinal origins, 173–175
  jaundice with, 424–425
  laparoscopy, 172–173
  from liver, 175, 176
  location, 168
  miscellaneous causes, 170
  neurologic pathways, 166–167
  onset, 169
  pancreatic origins, 175–176
  in paroxysmal nocturnal hemoglobi-
      nuria, 582
  patient history, 168

percutaneous transhepatic cholangiog-
      raphy and, 171–172
  due to peritonitis, 176
  physical examination, 170–171
  due to pleural effusion, 177
  due to pneumonia, 177
  quality, 168–169
  radioisotopic scanning for, 172
  reduction of, factors influencing, 169
  referred, 168
  in sickle-cell anemia, 584
  somatic, deep, 167–168
  due to spinal cord and vertebral le-
      sions, 177
  temporal features, 169
  ultrasonography, 172
  visceral, 167
  within the abdomen, causes of, 173
Abdominal rigidity, in acute myocardial
      infarction, 156
Abdominal tap and vasodepressor syn-
      cope, 697
Abetalipoproteinemia (Bassen-Korn-
      zweig syndrome), 97
  red cell morphology in, 579f
Abscess
  amebic, 429
  appendiceal, 171
  brain, and coma, 652, 654
  cranial, and headache, 78
  liver, 176, 206, 456
  lung, 323–324
  perinephric, 185, 188
  psoas, 170, 235
  renal cortical, 188
  retropharyngeal, 480, 481
  subdiaphragmatic fever in, 453
    right, referred shoulder pain from,
        206
  subpectoral, 503–504, 507
  tuberculosis of spine and, 199
Absorption bands, definition of, 813
Acanthocytes, 579
Acanthocytosis, 382, 384
Acanthosis nigricans, 841–842
Acetaminophen and jaundice, 424

Acetazolamide (Diamox)
  and intraocular pressure, 87
  and metabolic acidosis, 757
  for pseudotumor cerebri, 79
Acetylcholine, 600
  in migraine, 68
Achilles tendon, monoarticular pain
      and, 221
Achlorhydria in diseases associated with
      atrophic glossitis, 127
Achondroplasia, 21, 32
Achylia gastrica with atrophic glossitis,
      127
Acid accumulation in pain mechanism,
      140
Acid–base regulation, 748–765
  acid production, 748–749
  body buffers, 749–750, 749–751f
  definition of terms, 748
  metabolic acidosis, 755–760
  metabolic alkalosis, 760–762
  mixed disorders, 764–765
  by renal system, 751–755
  by respiratory system, 750–751
  respiratory acidosis, 762–763
  respiratory alkalosis, 763–764
Acidosis. *See also* Ketoacidosis; Metabolic
      acidosis; Renal tubular acidosis;
      Respiratory acidosis
  coma and, 656–658
  from diarrhea, 741
  from "ketogenic" diet, 780
  pulmonary disease and, 657
Acoustic neuroma, 718, 719
  bilateral, 719
Acoustic trauma, 111, 716
Acromegaly
  hypertrophic osteoarthropathy vs.,
      249
  melanosis in, 839
  somatomedin and, 30
Actinomycin D, 796
Actinomycosis, 324
  clubbing and, 253
  oral lesions in, 133
"Acute abdomen," 177–178

Adams-Stokes syndrome, 314, 658–659, 718, 722
  blood flow and pallor in, 853–854
  syncope in, 691
  vertigo in, 720
Addisonian crises, coma and convulsions in, 657
Addisonian pernicious anemia, 126
Addison's disease (adrenal cortical insufficiency), 617, 853
  aldosterone deficiency in, and salt loss, 740, 741
  anorexia, nausea, and vomiting in, 370
  depigmentation in, 853
  and erythropoietin, 573
  fatigue in, 617
  general lymph node enlargement in, 522
  hunger and, 363
  melanosis in, 815, 839–840, 841f, 844, 849
  myopathy in, 672
  and pseudotumor cerebri, 78
  vitiligo with, 851, 852
  water retention in, 737
Adenitis
  inguinal, 504–506
  mesenteric, 481
Adenocarcinoma, 171
"Adenoid facies," 109
Adenoiditis, age changes in lymphoid tissue and, 480
Adenoids
  middle ear infection and, 109
  serous otitis and, 109
Adenolymphoma, 501
Adenoma
  bronchial, 326
  hemoptysis in, 333
  villous, 382, 385
Adenosine, skeletal muscle, 698
Adenosine diphosphate (ADP), 537, 542, 543f, 550
Adenosine 5'-phosphate, 121–122
Adenosine monophosphate (AMP), 538, 539
Adenosine triphosphate (ATP), 537, 539, 565, 698
Adenovirus in acute hemorrhagic cystitis, 190
Adhesive capsulitis, 219
  shoulder pain in, 240
Adiposity
  definition of, 769
  physiology of, 772–773, 775–776
Adolescence. See also Puberty
  nutritional deficiency in, 120
Adrenal cortical hormones in undernourishment, 802

Adrenal cortical insufficiency. See Addison's disease
Adrenal function
  contralateral spread of cancer, 472
  heart rate and, 299
  and melanin metabolism, 839, 840, 841f
  in pubertal process, 35
  in sexual precocity, 39
Adrenal hypercorticism, obesity vs., 777
Adrenal hyperplasia and metabolic alkalosis, 761
Adrenal hypertension, 281–284
Adrenergic drugs, 615
Adrenergic system
  and baroreflex failure, 701–702
  in vasodepressor syncope, 697
Adrenocorticotropic hormone (ACTH), 596–597
  adverse reactions to, 12
  and corticosteroid excess, 609
  and hypothermia, 446
  and melanization, 815, 839
  for retrobulbar neuritis, 94–95
  stress and, 600
Adson's test, 242
Adult celiac disease and lymphoma, 516
Aerobacter cloacae, 459
Afferent nerves, 44, 45f, 46f
Afibrinogenemia, 554
African trypanosomiasis, 497
  lymphadenopathy in, 497
Afterpain (hyperpathia), 55
Aging
  sensory-neural hearing impairment and, 110
  undernutrition and, 798–801
Agoraphobia, 604, 606
Agranulocytic angina, 129
Agranulocytosis, drug-induced, 569
Air-condition testing, 715
Akinetic mutism, brain-stem lesions and, 651
Akinetic seizure, 660, 663
  dizziness in, 722
Albanoidism, 850
Albinism, 814, 843, 850
  irides in, 849
  oculo-cutaneous, 550
  ultraviolet radiation and, 837
Albright's syndrome, melanosis in, 843
Albumin, 738, 742, 743
Albuminuria
  as complication of fever, 451
  jaundice with, 429
Alcohol
  and cluster attacks, 70, 71
  coma from, 652, 659
  depression from, 618
  dizziness from, 722

  and fetal growth, 19
  and folic-acid deficiency, 577
  and gouty arthritis, 222
  and headache, 77
  hypertension and, 285
  ingestion of, vomiting from, 368
  nutritional deficiency and, 119, 120
  as therapeutic in tremor, 684
  tolerance of, in post-traumatic syndrome, 75
  and vestibular system, 718
  withdrawal from, 614
Alcoholic hepatitis, 423, 424, 428
Alcoholism, 10, 13
  esophagitis and, 149
  hematemesis and melena due to, 399, 411
  ketoacidosis in, 756
  and pancreatitis, 175
  and polyneuropathy, 238–239
  sideroblastic anemia and, 577
  tremulousness in, 685
  and vitamin deficiencies, 126–127, 129
Aldosterone deficiency and salt loss, 740, 741
Aldosteronism, primary
  hypertension in, 272, 282–283
  and metabolic alkalosis, 761
Alexithymia, 663
Alkali ingestion, 761
  and petit mal, 663
Alkalosis. See also Respiratory alkalosis
  coma and, 656, 658
  hypocalcemia with, 610
  metabolic, 609–610, 760–762
  vomiting and, 367
Allergies
  to anesthetic, and postoperative fever, 457
  as cause of fever, 457
  cough in, 326
  dermatitis as conversion complication, 630
  edema in, 741, 743
  oral lesions in, 131
  pruritic skin reactions, 873–874, 874–875f
  purpura, 545–547
  and serous otitis, 109
Alpha-granule deficiency, 550
Alpha heavy chain disease, 516
Alpha-methyldopa, and immunohemolytic anemia, 581
Alpha rhythm, 662
Alveolar proteinosis, 327
Amaurosis, conversion, 641
Amblyopia, conversion, 641
Amebic abscess, leukocyte count in, 429
Amebic dysentery, 377
  clubbing and, 249, 253

Amenorrhea
    anemia and, 569
    in anorexia nervosa, 367
    obesity and, 777
Amethopterin (methotrexate), 119
    and folic-acid deficiency, 125–126, 796
    and megaloblastic anemia, 793
Amino acids
    deficiency of, from excessive dieting
        in pregnancy, 789
    and emotions, 597–598
    growth failure and, 33
Aminoglycosides, fever from, 458
Aminophylline intoxication, 614
Amitriptyline and temperature, 458
Ammonia, blood, hepatic coma and,
    657
Ammonium chloride and metabolic aci-
    dosis, 756–757
Ammonium excretion, renal, 753–754
Amnesia in conversion patient, 631, 633
Amphetamines
    addiction to, 13
    anorexia induced by, 368
    itching from, 873
    poisoning by, 614
    in treatment of obesity, 780
Amphotericin B and renal tubular aci-
    dosis, 759
Ampulla of Vater, tumors of, 426, 430,
    431f
Amylase function, phaseolamin and, 780
Amylase level
    acute abdomen and, 178
    in pancreatitis, 175
Amyl nitrite for angina pectoris, 156
Amyloidosis, 385
    factor-X coagulopathy and, 557
    familial Mediterranean fever with, 455
    general lymph node enlargement and,
        522
    neuropathy of, 239
    and pathologic bleeding, 547
    pulmonary, 334
    and splenomegaly, 580
Amyotrophic lateral sclerosis, 675–676
    fasciculation in, 682
    oral lesions in, 131
Amyotrophy in Shy-Drager syndrome,
    701
Amytal narcosis, fever from, 458
Anabolic steroids and jaundice, 424
Anaclitic depression. See Failure to
    thrive
Anaerobic threshold, 336
Anal fissure, 170
Anal itching, as reaction to antibiotics,
    131
Analgesia, conversion, 641
Androgens and melanosis, 840

Anemia(s). See also Pernicious anemia
    apathy due to, 566
    aplastic. See Aplastic anemia
    arterial murmur in, 428
    and atrophic glossitis, 126–128
    in bone marrow disease, 573
    cardiovascular symptoms, 567–569
    characteristics, 566
    in Chediak-Higashi syndrome, 850
    in chronic inflammatory disease, 573
    classification, 571–573, 572t
    congestive heart failure and, 568
    definition of, 563
    drug-induced, 793
    dyspnea in, 336, 341, 344
    electrocardiographic changes in, 568
    erythropoietin lack, 573
    fever and, 454
    folic-acid deficiency and, 577
    genitourinary symptoms, 569
    hemolytic. See Hemolytic anemia(s)
    hepatomegaly in, 570
    hypoplastic hemoptysis in, 333
    immunohemolytic, 580–581
    iron-deficiency, 574–575
    jaundice in, 570–571
    lethargy and fatigue in, 618
    lymph node enlargement in, 570
    in malignancy, 573
    megaloblastic, 576–577
        and atrophic glossitis, 126–127
        Dilantin-induced, 130
    myelophthistic, 574
    myocardial infarction and, 569
    neurologic symptoms, 569–570
    pallor due to, 566–567
    pernicious. See Pernicious anemia
    in polymyalgia rheumatica, 224
    in pregnancy, 790–791
    and pseudotumor cerebri, 78
    in rheumatoid arthritis, 223
    sideroblastic, 577
    sickle-cell anemia and, 568
    skin changes due to, 566–567, 850
    splenomegaly in, 570
    spur cell, 581–582
    thalassemia syndromes, 577–578
    vitamin B_{12} deficiency and, 576
    vitamin C deficiency and, 129
    weakness and fatigue due to, 566
Anesthesia
    as cause of hyperthermia, 457–458
    conversion, 638, 641
Anesthesia dolorosa,
    reflex sympathetic
        dystrophy vs., 237
Aneurysms, 272
    abdominal pain from, 169
    of aorta, 160, 161, 325
        hemoptysis caused by, 333

    and headache, 78
        subarachnoid hemorrhage, 79
    ruptured, hematemesis and melena
        from, 397, 399, 410
    saccular, referred back pain, 206
Angina pectoris, 151
    anemia and, 568
    effects of chilling on, 155
    emotions and, 601
    hyperthyroidism and, 299
    origin of pain in, 140
    pain of, 151, 155–156, 157f, 160
        nature of, 53, 55, 57
    rheumatic pains distinguished from, 215
    syncope and, 693
Angiodysplasia, 414
Angiofollicular lymph node hyperplasia,
    484, 509
    retroperitoneal involvement in, 513
Angiography
    coronary, 151–152, 156
    fluorescein, 92, 93f, 95
    in hematuria, 187, 188
    selective celiac, 404
Angioimmunoblastic lymphadenopathy,
    484
Angiopathy in urinary tract malignancy,
    187
Angiotensin, 739, 740
Angle-closure glaucoma, 92–94
Angular stomatitis
    in B-complex deficiencies, 124, 125, 126f
    vitamin deficiencies and, 793
Anion gap, definition of, 755
Ankle joint pain, 221
    innervation and, 215
Ankle pain from trauma, 216
Ankylosing spondylitis
    and apophyseal joints, 200
    back pain from, 199
Ankylosis, 81
    in hypertrophic osteoarthropathy, 248,
        253
Anorectic agents
    administration of, 780, 782
    hormonal, 775
Anorexia, 361
    alcoholism and, 424
    as conversion symptom, 641
    defined, 363
    in dehydration, 731
    drug-induced, 368, 792
    in endocrine disorders, 370–371
    in giant cell arteritis, 80
    in herpangina, 132
    in intra-abdominal disorders, 368–370
    malnutrition causing, 371
    in motion sickness, 371
    neurologic factors in, 366–367
    nutritional deficiency and, 119

Anorexia (*continued*)
  pancreatic carcinoma and, 176
  psychic and neurologic factors in, 366–367
  and vitamin deficiencies, 123, 129
  and weight loss, in cancer, 795–796
Anorexia nervosa, 366–367
  carotenemia in, 828
  cortisol metabolism in, 802
  gonadal function in, 777, 803
  thyroid function in, 801
Anovulatory cycles, obesity and, 777
Anoxia, skin color in, 830–831
Anterior auricular lymph nodes, 493–494, 495
Anterior horn cell disease, 675–676
Anterior tibial compartment syndrome, 243
Anthrax, 517
  lymph node suppuration in, 521
Antibiotics. *See also specific drugs*
  fevers and hyperthermias from, 458
  and methotrexate toxicity, 125–126
  and nutritional deficiency, 119
  reactions to, 131
  and vitamin-K deficiency, 555
Antibodies
  anticoagulant, 557–558
  to factor VIII in hemophilia, 553
  platelet, 548
  red-cell, and hemolysis, 580–581
Anticholinergic drugs
  and body temperature, 458
  constipation caused by, 379
Anticholinesterase drugs, 674
Anticoagulants
  adverse reactions to, 12
  endogenous. *See* Inhibitors
  and hematuria, 187
  hemoptysis caused by, 334
  and lymph-node enlargement, 484
  and vitamin K, 554–555
Anticonvulsant drugs and vitamin K, 793
Antidiuretic hormone (arginine vaso-pressin; ADH), 597, 727–731
  characteristics, 727
  in dehydration test, 733–734
  and metabolic acidosis, 757
  nonosmotic stimuli for, 729–730, 732f, 736–737
  polyuria unresponsive to, 735–736
  for postlumbar-puncture headache, 79
  renal response to, 729, 732
  in replacement therapy, 735
  syndrome of inappropriate antidi-uretic hormone, 737
Antihistamines, 615
  fever from, 458

Antihypertensive drugs, depression in-duced by, 618
Antimalarial drugs
  fatigue from, 618
  and G6PD-deficiency, 583
Antineoplastic agents
  adverse reactions to, 12
  fever induced by, 458
Antinuclear antibody in lupus erythema-tosus, 130
Antitubercular drugs, fatigue from, 618
Anxiety. *See also* Nervousness
  depression and, 606
  hyperventilation with, 637
  hypochondriasis and, 644
  in hypoglycemia, 702
  nervousness distinguished from, 592, 594, 604
  in post-traumatic syndrome, 75, 76
  psychological explanations of, 601–603
  psychotic, 606
  sore tongue and mouth and, 119
  stress and, 600–601
Anxiety neurosis, 591
  pheochromocytoma vs., 612
Anxiety states, 604–607
  conversion disorder vs., 608
  endocrine disturbances and, 600
  fatigue in, 615–617
  somatization vs., 608
  thyrotoxicosis vs., 609
  tremor in, 685
Aortic aneurysm
  clubbing and, 253
  cough caused by, 320, 325
  hemoptysis caused by, 333
  referred back pain from, 206, 207
  ruptured, hematemesis caused by, 397, 399, 410
Aortic dissection, syncope in, 694
Aortic pain, 150, 160–161
  atherosclerosis and, 242
  characteristics of, 161
  mechanism of, 160
  ostalgic, 142
Aortic regurgitation, syncope of, 693
Aortic stenosis, syncope in, 691, 693
Aortic valvular disease, 154
Apathy, anemia and, 567
Aphasia
  language development and types of, 114, 115t
  in sickle-cell anemia, 570
Aphoria, 113
  conversion, 642
Aphthous stomatitis, 133
Aplastic anemia, 547, 573
  fever from, 454

and paroxysmal nocturnal hemoglobi-nuria, 582
  retinal hemorrhage in, 570
Apneustic breathing, brain-stem lesions and, 651
Apophyseal joints, pain in, 200
Appendiceal abscess, 171
Appendicitis
  age changes in lymphoid tissue and, 480, 481
  anorexia, nausea, and vomiting in, 369
  as cause of peritonitis, 176
  pain in, 167–170, 174–175, 177–178
  retrocecal
    referred back pain from, 207
    ureteral pain in, 185
Appendix, role in lymphoid system, 468, 470
Appetite, 364–365
  regulation of, 773–776
Apprehension in vocal cord paralysis, 113
Apraxia, 678
Arachnoiditis and nerve root pain, 235
Arginine vasopressin. *See* Antidiuretic hormone
Argyria, 845t, 846, 849
Ariboflavinosis. *See* Riboflavin defi-ciency
Arm. *See also* Extremity *entries*
  conversion symptoms, 638
  pain, 240–242
Arnold-Chiari malformation, 721
Arreflexia in polyneuritis and poly-radiculitis, 240
Arrhenoblastoma, melanosis in, 840
Arrhythmias. *See also specific arrhythmias*
  in metabolic acidosis, 759
  in metabolic alkalosis, 761
  in mitral valve prolapse, 297
  as psychosomatic disorder, 601
  from "rainbow" treatment of obesity, 780
  in respiratory acidosis, 762
  and syncope, 691–693
Arsenical melanosis, 842, 846
Arsenic polyhemopathy, 239
Arterial anoxemia and clubbing, 256
Arterial obstruction, pallor of skin in, 853–854
Arterial pain, systolic impulse and, 56
Arterial–venous fistula, 547
Arteriography in abdominal pain, 172, 178
Arteriosclerosis
  of gastric vessels, 410
  muscle pain secondary to, 230
  retinal changes in, 273–274

Arteriovenous malformations (AVM), and headache, 78
Arteritis, headache and, 79–80
Artery(ies). *See specific arteries*
Arthralgia
    in Crohn's disease, 170
    in giant cell arteritis, 80
    and hypertrophic osteoarthropathy, 248
    in lupus erythematosus, 130
    steroid fever and, 455
Arthritis. *See also* Gouty arthritis; Osteoarthritis; Psoriatic arthritis; Juvenile rheumatoid arthritis; Rheumatoid arthritis
    aseptic, febrile episodes with, 455
    Behçet's syndrome and, 133
    "extended lumbar sympathectomy" in, 215
    of hip, back pain from, 205
    infectious, 215, 217
        chronic clubbing vs., 246
        joint pain in, 222
    in lupus erythematosus, 130
    "migratory," in rheumatic fever, 222
    mimicked by entrapment neuropathy, 237
    tuberculous, 217
Arthropathy. *See also* Joint *entries*
    idiopathic hemachromatosis and, 844
Articular pain. *See* Joint pain
Articulation
    definition of, 112
    disorders of, 113–114
Asbestosis, lymphadenopathy in, 509
Ascaris infestations, clubbing and, 253
Ascending cholangitis, 453
Ascites, 170, 176, 430
    abdominal lymphadenopathy and, 513, 514
    constipation and, 380
    and peritonitis, 176
Ascitic fluid, 428
Ascorbic acid. *See* Vitamin C
Aseptic arthritis, febrile episodes in, 455
Aseptic necrosis, sickle-cell anemia and, 584
Ashy cyanosis, referred cardiac pain and, 158
Asomnia, 650
Aspergillosis, 324
Aspergillus fumigatus, 321, 325
Aspirin, 10
    for acute muscle contraction headache, 72
    as antipruritic, 866
    and eighth cranial nerve, 111
    hematemesis and melena caused by, 410–411

and iron loss from gastrointestinal bleeding, 794
    and jaundice, 424
    and qualitative platelet defect, 549
    and vitamin K, 793
Astasia-abasia, 640
Asteatosis in thyroid disease, 871
Asterixis, 684, 685
    from CO_2 retention, 762
Asthenia, neurocirculatory, 296–297, 302, 612
Asthma. *See also* Bronchial asthma
    cardiac, 344
    dyspnea in, 336, 341, 342
    hypoxia in, 353
    as psychosomatic disorder, 601
    and respiratory acidosis, 762
Astrocytomas, 234, 611, 720
Asystole, and syncope, 691–693
Ataxia, 680–681
    from cerebellar lesions, 713
    in malformations, 720–721
    in pernicious anemia, 570
    vitamin-B_{12} deficiency and, 577
Ataxic breathing, 651
Ataxic intention tremor, neurosurgical alleviation of, 684
Atelectasis
    cough in, 320
    hypoxia in, 353
    mediastinal lymph node enlargement and, 510
    and postoperative fever, 456, 457
Atherosclerosis
    of aorta, 242
    and central retinal vein, 89–90
    of cerebral vessels, 272
    elevated lipids and, 777
Athetosis, 681
    evolution into tremor, 684
Atkins diet, 779–780
Atopic dermatitis, 868, 873, 875f
Atrial ball-valve thrombosis, syncope in, 691
Atrial fibrillation, 295, 297, 298
    characteristics, 307
    diagnosis, 309
    etiology, 308
    hyperthyroidism and, 299–300
    lethargy and fatigue from, 617
    mechanism, 307–308
    prognosis, 310
    symptoms, 308–309
Atrial flutter, 295, 297, 306–307
Atrial septal defects, 308
Atrioventricular block
    paroxysmal atrial tachycardia with, 305–306
    syncope from, 691–692

Atrophic gastritis
    and iron absorption, 575
    pernicious anemia and, 576
Atrophic glossitis, 126–128
Atropine, 615
    fever from, 458
    tachycardia due to, 302
    in testing of baroreflex failure, 700, 701t
    and vasodilation in syncope, 698
Attachment, theory of, 603
Audiometry, 714–715
Audiometry-battery testing, 708
Auditory apparatus. *See also* Ear(s); Hearing; *and related entries*
    anatomy and physiology of, 107–108
    injury from whiplash, 717
    localization of lesions, 714–715
Auditory meatus, lymphadenopathy and, 495
Auditory responses, 102, 103–105t
Autoantibodies, thrombocytopenia due to, 548–549
Autohemolysis test, 582
Autoimmune disorders
    fever in, 457
    and renal tubular acidosis, 759
Autoimmune hemolytic anemia, 580–581
    generalized lymphadenopathy, 522
Autoimmune thrombocytopenia, 549
Autoimmune thyroid disease, pernicious anemia and, 576
Autonomic hyperreflexia and headache, 77
Autonomic nervous system
    anxiety and, 604, 606, 609, 613
    cluster headaches and, 71
    and melanization, 841
    and postural hypotension, 658
Avitaminosis and melanosis in jaundice, 826
"Axial streaming," 256
Axillary lymph nodes, 501–504
    anatomy, 501–502
    Burkitt's lymphoma and, 487
    cancer and blockage of, 509
    cancer metastasis and, 518–519
    in cat-scratch disease, 518
    clinical significance, 502–503
    subpectoral abscess of, 503–504
    xeroradiography and, 492
Azotemia
    with anemia, 569
    growth failure and, 33
    following hematemesis and melena, 395–397
    jaundice with, 429
    in uremic coma, 657

Babinski's sign, 240, 677, 677f
  in pernicious anemia, 570
Bacillary dysentery, 377
  clubbing and, 253
Bacillus ducreyi, 521
Bacillus tularensis, 496
Back pain, 195–208
  abdominal lymphadenopathy and,
    513, 514
  anatomic and physiological aspects of,
    195–196, 197f
  causes of, 198–207
    body mechanics, 205, 206f
    joints and intervertebral disks,
      202–204, 242
    lesions of thoracic, abdominal, and
      pelvic organs, 206–207
    ligaments, fascia, and muscles,
      204–205
    psychogenic factors, 207
    spinal column disorders, 198–200
    spinal cord meninges, 205
  as conversion symptom, 635, 640
  with foot pain, 221
  in hemolytic anemia, 570
  nerve supply in, 196–198
  from osteoarthritis, 220
Back strain (back sprain), 204
Bacteremia
  in anthrax, 517
  in iliac lymphadenitis, 507
  lymph node function and, 468
Bacterial endocarditis
  clubbing in, 252, 253
  fatigue in, 617
  and leukocytoclastic vasculitis, 545
  subacute, and clubbing, 249
Bacterial infections. *See also specific organisms*
  and purpura, 545
  of urinary tract, 189–190
Bacterial lipopolysaccharides, 480
Bacterial mastoiditis, dizziness in, 721
Bacterial peritonitis, 176
Bacteriuria, 188–191
Bainbridge reflex, 301
Ballism, 685
Banti's syndrome, 408
  anemia and, 570
Bárány noise box, 715
Barbiturates
  addiction to, 13
  coma from, 659
  dizziness from, 722
  fever from, 458
  for postlumbar puncture headache, 79
Barium in acute abdomen, 178
Baroreflex system, 696, 697
  failure of
    anatomic level of defect, 699–700

cholinergic and adrenergic neural
    deficits in, 701–702
  clinical approach, 701
  etiology of, 699–700
  pathophysiology of, 699
  tests, 700–701, 700t
  normal mechanism of, 694–696
  physiologic and pharmacologic testing
    of, 700–701
Basal cell carcinoma, anterior auricular
    lymphadenopathy and, 495
Base. *See also* Acid–base regulation
  definition of, 748
Base angle in clubbing, 246, 247f
Basilar artery migraine, 64, 67
Basilar meningitis, 721
Basilar pleura, right shoulder pain from,
    219
Basilar pneumonitis, pain in, 168
Bassen-Kornzweig syndrome. *See* Abe-
    talipoproteinemia
Bayliss effect, 262
B-cell islet tumor, hunger and, 363
B cells, 479, 480, 487
  diseases resulting from defects in
    maturation of, 482
  in Hodgkin's disease, 484
  in inflammatory lymph-node reac-
    tions, 482, 483
BCG vaccine
  and axillary lymphadenopathy, 503
  and inguinal lymphadenopathy,
    506–507
Beggars' melanosis, 838
Behavior modification in obesity, 781,
    782
Behçet's syndrome, 133
Belching, abdominal lymphadenopathy
    and, 514
Belle indifférence, la, 608, 628, 631
Bell's palsy, 683, 721
"Benign postoperative fever," 456–457
Bent-back, 640
Benzene
  and aplastic anemia, 573
  and polyneuropathy, 239
Benzodiazepines, 600
  for chorea, 685
Benztropine mesylate, 615
P-Benzylhydroquinone, 852
Berger's disease, skin changes in, 228
Beri-beri heart disease, 569
Bernard Soulier syndrome, 537, 550
Berylliosis, 483
Beryllium granulomatosis, 326
Beryllium intoxication, lymphadenopa-
    thy in, 509
Beta-blocking agents and drug-induced
    syncope, 692

Beta thromboglobulin (BTG), 537
Bezold's sign, 109
Bicarbonate reabsorption, renal, 751–753
Bicipital tendinitis, 219
Bifascicular block and syncope, 691–692
Biguanides, 780, 793
Bilateral ptosis as conversion symptom,
    628
Bile acid toxicity, 382, 385
Bile salt disorders, 383–384
Biliary cirrhosis
  clubbing and, 253
  liver function tests and, 529
  serum lipids in, 429
  splenomegaly in, 428
Biliary colic, 168, 170, 175
Biliary disease(s). *See also specific condi-
    tions*
  malabsorption from, and vitamin-K
    deficiency, 555
  pruritus in, 870–871
  vomiting in, 369, 370
Biliary tract. *See also* Common bile duct;
    Common duct stone
  accidental injury to, and jaundice,
    424
  congenital malformation of, 425
  obstruction of, 430
    and jaundice, 423, 425
    liver function tests and, 429, 430
  pain from, 169
  radionuclide imaging of, 172
  retrograde endoscopic cannulation
    and, 171
  as source of abdominal pain, 175
  tumor(s) of, 435f, 437f
    biliverdinemia, 826
    jaundice, 423, 425, 427–428
Bilirubin
  and hemolytic anemias, 571
  and jaundice, 423, 429, 823–827
  and skin color from diffused blood,
    823–830, 824–825t
  steroids and, 423
Bilirubinophilic tissue, 826
Biliverdin, 826
  and skin color from diffused blood,
    829–830
Biofeedback, 603
Biopsy
  needle, of liver, 423, 431–433
  percutaneous, 172
  peroral, 172
  scalene lymph node, 499–500
Biopsychosocial model, 43
Biotin deficiency, 125
Birth control pills. *See* Oral contraceptives
Bismuthia, 845t, 846
Bismuth poisoning, oral lesions in, 130

Bladder. *See also specific conditions*
  anatomical role of, 181
  calculi in, 187
  cancer of, contralateral spread of, 472
  innervation of, 184
  localization of pain from, 185
  neurogenic dysfunction of, and uri-
    nary tract infection, 190
  pain from, 177
  as source of hematuria, 186, 187
  tumors of, 187
  washout techniques, 189
Blast cells. *See* Lymphocytes
Blastomycosis
  North American, 324
  oral lesions in, 133
Bleeding. *See also* Hemorrhage; Patho-
    logic bleeding
  into respiratory tract. *See* Hemoptysis
  systemic, with hematuria, 187
Bleeding-time test, 542, 544
Bleomycin, fever from, 458
Blepharospasm as conversion symptom,
    628
Blind-loop syndrome, 126, 385
  and vitamin-B$_{12}$ deficiency, 576
Blindness. *See also* Visual loss
  in classic migraine, 66
  of conversion origin, 641
  giant cell arteritis and, 224
  in sickle-cell anemia, 570
Blink reflex electromyography (EMG), 714
B lymphocytes, *See* B cells
Bloating
  abdominal lymphadenopathy and, 514
  from enzyme deficiency, 174
  in lactase deficiency, 169
Blood and thunder, 89–90
Blood disorders. *See specific conditions*
Blood flow, diminished
  pallor in, 853–854
  and syncope. *See* Syncope, from re-
    duced cerebral blood flow
Blood poisoning, 517
Blood pressure. *See also* Hypertension;
    Hypotension
  in anemia, 567
  generation of, 261–263
  in treatment of occluded central reti-
    nal artery, 87
Blood transfusion
  dilutional factor loss from, 557
  and hepatitis, 424
  and thrombocytopenia, 549
Blood urea nitrogen (BUN) in jaundice,
    429
Blood volume in anemia, 567
Blue coloration of skin. *See* Dermal pig-
    mentation

Blue nevus, 847
"Blush areas," 830
Body buffers, 749–750, 749–751f
Body computed tomography (BCT) of
    lymph nodes, 492
Body fat. *See also* Obesity
  age and, 29f
  measurement of, 26
  sex differences and, 26
  storage of, physiology of, 772–773,
    775–776
Body imagery, 626, 629
Body language of conversion patient,
    632, 634
Body size. *See* Growth
Body temperature, 442–447. *See also* Fever
  in children, 445–446
  in elderly, 446
  limits of, 446–447
  menstruation and, 446
  physiological mechanisms and,
    442–444
  in pregnancy, 446
  variability of, in health, 444–446
Body types, theories of, 769
Body water. *See also* Dehydration;
    Edema; Water balance, normal
  normal distribution of, 726, 737–738,
    744
Body weight. *See* Obesity; Weight;
    Weight loss
Boeck's sarcoid, scalene node biopsy
    and, 499–500
Bone disease(s). *See also specific disorders*
  phenylhydantoin and, 795
Bone dissolution in metabolic acidosis,
    759
Bone marrow hypoplasia, 547, 548
Bone maturation, 21–25, 25f, 26f
  in hypothyroidism, 25, 31
Bone pain, 56
  in clubbing and osteoarthropathy, 249
  pathophysiology of, 229
  in sickle-cell anemia, 584
  thoracic, 142
Bone scans, 229
Bone tenderness in acute leukemia, 570
Bone tumors and monoarticular pain,
    216
Borderline hypertension, 270
Bordetella pertussis, 322
Boric-acid ingestion, 793, 794f
Borrelia recurrentis, 458
Bottle vs. breast feeding, 791–792
Botulism, 453, 673
Boutonneuse fever, 517–518
Bowel. *See also specific disorders*
  abdominal pain from inflammation of,
    170

abnormal distension of, 170
anemia and infarction of, 566
Bowel sounds, 170
Brachial arteriovenous aneurysm, club-
    bing and, 253
Brachial plexus
  neuritis of, 219, 241
  pain originating in, 235
  scalenus anticus syndrome, 241–242
Bradycardia
  in cluster headache, 70
  provoked by cough, 328
  and syncope, 691–693
  vomiting and, 365, 366
Bradycardia-tachycardia, 311, 692
Bradykinin peptides, 44
Brain. *See also* Cerebellar, Cerebral, *and
    related entries*
  abscess of, and coma, 652, 654
  edema of, and headache, 77
  historical concepts of, 648–649
  infarction of, and anemia, 566
  maternal undernutrition and develop-
    ment of, 789
  mechanism of nervousness and,
    594–597
  metabolic functioning of, 656
    in coma, 656–658
  tumor(s) of
    coma, 652, 654
    EEG and VFP findings, 652
    mental changes in presentation of,
      611
Brain damage, fever and, 453
Brain death, 649
Brain stem
  intrinsic tumor of, 720
  lesions of
    coma from, 654–656
    localization of, 714, 715
    and unconsciousness, 650–652
  migraine and ischemia of, 67
  vertigo in vascular disorders of,
    719–720
  viral diseases and, 721
Brain waves. *See also* EEG
  classification of, 660–662
Brawny arm, 474
Breast
  male, pubertal changes in, 35
  pain in, 143–144
  premature development of, 39, 40
Breast vs. artificial feeding, 791–792
Breast cancer, 472
  diagnosis of, 487–488
  lymphatic metastases, 474, 502–503,
    511, 518–520
  myopathy with, and weight loss, 796
  pain in, 143, 144

Breathing. *See also* Respiration; *and specific respiratory conditions*
  difficulty in, as conversion symptom, 625, 627, 629–630
  in severe hepatic disease, 426
  in sore tongue and mouth, 119
Bronchial adenoma, 326, 333
Bronchial asthma
  cough in, 321, 326
  pneumomediastinum in, 328
Bronchial cancer
  clubbing and, 252
  pain in, 144
  and superior vena caval obstruction, 511
Bronchial obstruction, mediastinal lymphadenopathy and, 509–510
Bronchial pain, 144–145
Bronchiectasis, 321, 323
  clubbing and, 252
  hilar lymphadenopathy and, 509
  in pertussis, 322
  saccular, hemoptysis in, 333
Bronchioalveolar cell carcinoma, 326
Bronchiolitis, 321
  hypoxia in, 353
Bronchiolitis obliterans, 325
Bronchitis
  chronic, 322–323
    dyspnea in, 341
    cough fractures in, 327
    hemoptysis in, 333
    hypoxia in, 353
Bronchoesophageal fistula, 511
Bronchogenic carcinoma
  cough in, 326
  fever in, 453
  hemoptysis in, 333
Broncholithiasis, calcified lymph nodes and, 510
Bronchomediastinal trunk, anatomy of, 474
Bronchopneumonia, 323
  congestive heart failure with, 456
  in pertussis, 322
Bromides, fever from, 458
Bronze baby syndrome, 827
Bronze diabetes, 844
Brucellosis
  axillary lymphadenopathy and, 502
  fatigue in, 617
  fever in, 450, 451
  and generalized lymphadenopathy, 522
  granulamatous lymphadenopathy and, 483
Brudzinski's sign, 235, 654–655
Bruises. *See also* Ecchymoses
  in factor-V deficiency, 554

Bruits
  in abdominal lymphadenopathy, 513, 515
  in anemia, 568
Brushfield's spots of iris, 849
Bruton agammaglobulinemia, 482
Bubonic plague
  inguinal lymphadenopathy and, 506
  as lymph node syndrome, 517
Buccal mucous membrane. *See also* Tongue and mouth
  normal morphology and physiology of, 118–119
Buccinator lymph nodes, 494f, 500
Buffalo hump, 771
Buffers. *See also* Body buffers
  definition of, 748
Bulging flanks in ascites, 170, 176
Bunion formation, 221
Burkitt's lymphoma, 485f, 486–487
  retroperitoneal involvement in, 513
Burns
  edema in, 741, 743
  gastric erosion in, 415–416
  and hemolysis, 581
Burr cells, 579
Bursae, pain in, 56
Bursitis, 215
  elbow pain from, 218
  mimicked by entrapment neuropathy, 237
  monoarticular pain from, 217
  of shoulder, 218–219
  trochanteric, 211, 217, 220
Busalphan therapy, melanosis from, 840
Butterfly sign, 826
Buttock pain in atherosclerotic disease of aorta, 242
Byssinosis, 341–342

Cachexia, constipation and, 380
Café-au-lait spots, 843
Caffeine
  headache from withdrawal of, 77
  sinus tachycardia due to, 302
Caffeinism, 614
Calcification of lymph nodes, 510
  axillary, 503
  intra-abdominal, 516
  in tuberculous mesenteric lymphadenitis, 516
Calcific bursitis, 218
Calcific tendonitis, 218–219
Calcium
  heart rate and, 299
  in normal platelet function, 538, 539
Calcium chloride administration, 756–757

Calcium serum
  in acute pancreatitis, 178
Calculous cholecystitis, 425
Calculus(i)
  and hematuria, 187
  ureteral pain from, 184–185
Calf pain, 243
Callus formation on foot, 221
Caloric testing, 712–713
Calories
  and lactation, 792
  and longevity, 798–799
  and marasmus, 790
  obesity and, 773, 776, 778–779, 781, 782
Camptocormia, 640
Cancer. *See also* Metastasis(es); *and specific forms*
  anemia in, 573, 574, 577
  biliverdinemia in, 826
  emotional stress and, 601
  en cuirasse, 520
  and jugulodigastric lymphadenopathy, 496
  lassitude in, 618
  metastasis to head and neck lymph nodes, 501, 502f
  neuropathies and, 239
  obesity and, 778
  in occipital lymph nodes, 495
  pruritus in, 872
  supraclavicular lymph nodes and, 498–499
  and thrombocytopenia, 548
  undernutrition in, 795–798
Cancerophobia, 132
Candida albicans, 325
Candidiasis, 873–874
Canker sore, 133
Cannabis intoxication, 614
Cannon's law of hypersensitivity, 700
Capillary fragility and hemosiderosis, 846
Capillary lymphangioma, 473
Capillary lymphangitis, 473
Capillary mechanisms in edema formation, 741–743
Capital femoral epiphysis, hip pain and, 219
Carbenoxolone, 761
Carbohydrate, 772
  malabsorption of, 384
  nutritional deficiency and, 121–122
Carbon dioxide
  exchange, 357–358
  retention of, in respiratory acidosis, 762
  in treatment of occluded central retinal artery, 87

Carbon monoxide and eighth cranial nerve, 111
Carbon monoxide poisoning
and chorea or Parkinsonism, 685
coma in, 660
Carboxyhemoglobinemia, 563
Carcass analysis, 770
Carcinoid, gastric, 410
Carcinoid syndrome
pruritus in, 872
skin color in, 830
Carcinoma. See Cancer; and specific sites
Cardiac arrest, emotional stress and, 603
Cardiac arrhythmias. See Arrhythmias; and specific conditions
Cardiac decompensation, 652
Cardiac disease(s). See also specific conditions; Heart entries
and clubbing, 246–249, 252–254, 254f, 255f
congenital, growth deficiency in, 33
cyanosis in, 352, 355
dyspnea in, 343–344
fever in, 456
syncope in, 691–693
vascular ectasias and, 415
vomiting in, 371
Cardiac edema, jaundice and, 826
Cardiac function in metabolic acidosis, 759
Cardiac neurosis, 295–296
Cardiac output
in anemia, 567–568
insufficient, and vertigo, 720
Cardiac pain, 51–54, 57, 151–161
characteristics of, 155–158
acute myocardial infarction, 156–157
angina pectoris, 155–156, 157f
precordial ache and tenderness, 157–158
conversion, 53, 634–636
coronary blood flow and, 151–155
angiography, 152
history of treatment, 151
tracts and reference of, 157t, 158–160
Cardiac tumors, clubbing and, 253
Cardiomegaly, anemia and, 568
Cardiophrenic lymphadenopathy, 509
Cardiopulmonary disorders, fatigue in, 617–618
Cardiospasm (spasticity of the cardia), 149
Cardiovascular disorders. See also Specific conditions
cough in, 325
fasting and, 779
hemoptysis in, 333
nervousness and fatigue from, 593, 612, 613

obesity and, 770, 777
Cardiovascular system
anemia and, 567–569
hypertension and, 272–273, 275–277
in mechanism of nervousness, 594, 595
Carditis in rheumatic fever, 222
Caroli's disease, 425
Carotene, 814, 817–818
definition of, 817, 818
as medication, 827
and vitamin A, 817–818, 827, 828
Carotenemia, 818, 827–828
Carotene pigmentation
bodily distribution of, 817, 819f, 827
sex differences and, 820, 828
Carotenoderma, 827
Carotid artery
in cluster headache, 70–71
syncope, 702, 703
Carotid sinus hypersensitivity, vasodepressor syncope and, 697
Carotid sinus reflex episodes, dizziness in, 720
Carotid sinus syncope, 659, 691, 698, 699
Carotid system insufficiency, 655–656
Carpal-tunnel compression of median nerve, 675
Carpal tunnel syndrome, 241
Carpopedal spasm, 683
in respiratory alkalosis, 764
Cartilage proliferation, 21
Caseation of hilar nodes, 510
Castleman's disease, 484
Castration and skin color, 820, 854
Cataplexy in narcolepsy, 664
Cataracts, 95–96
Catarrhal choledochitis, 425
Catecholamines, 596, 598, 599f, 603
and body temperature, 449
central pain mechanisms and, 63
decreased response to
in metabolic acidosis, 759
in respiratory acidosis, 762
in hypoglycemia, 702
in pheochromocytoma, 612
stress and, 600–601
and thyroid storm, 455
Cathartic drugs
abuse, 387
and undernutrition, 792
"Catheter fever," 459
Cat-scratch disease
acute lymphadenitis with, 483
anterior auricular lymphadenopathy and, 496
axillary lymphadenopathy and, 502

epitrochlear lymphadenopathy and, 504
and extremity-lesion-and-lymphadenopathy syndrome, 518
and generalized lympadenopathy, 522
oropharyngeal lesion and, 518
and suppuration of lymph nodes, 521
Cauda equina
anatomy of, 231, 232f
"claudication" of, 204
Causalgia, 237
Cavernous lymphangioma, 473
Celiac disease, 384, 390
abdominal discomfort in, 174
and iron absorption, 575
Celiac preaortic lymph nodes
anatomy of, 511, 512f
clinical significance, 514
Celiac sprue, peroral biopsy and, 172
Cell-mediated immunity, 479
Cellular clearance mechanisms and coagulation, 541–542
Cellular component of hemostasis. See Platelets
Cellular nutrition, defective, 32–33
Cellulitis
of breast, pain from, 144
lymphangitis with, 473
Central cyanosis, 352–353
Central nervous system (CNS)
control of movements by, 708
and decerebrate posturing, 679
extremity pain originating in, 231
hypertension and, 272
in pathophysiology of nervousness, 596, 598
in post-traumatic headache, 76
and thermoregulation, 442–444, 448
undernutrition and growth of, 789
Central nervous system disorders
bleeding, 548
from allergic purpura, 545–547
in disseminated intravascular coagulation, 556
in hemophilia, 553
from vitamin-K deficiency, 555
as cause of fever, 453
coma from syphilis, 652
hyperventilation from brain-stem lesions, 651
infectious, and epilepsy, 663
of movement, from lesions, 670
nervousness and fatigue in, 593
and respiratory acidosis, 762
and respiratory alkalosis, 763
Central retinal artery occlusion, 86–88
Central retinal vein occlusion, 89–90
Central serous retinitis, 93f, 94
Central serous retinopathy, 93f, 94, 98

Centrencephalic seizures, 662, 663
Cerebellar disease
  ataxia from, 680–681
  and muscular weakness, 671t
  tremor and, 684–685
Cerebellar hemorrhage, 655
Cerebellar infarction, 655
Cerebellar lesions, Romberg test and, 713
Cerebellar signs, evaluation of, 713, 715
Cerebellar tumors, 720
Cerebellar vermal ataxia, 713
Cerebello-pontine-angle (c-p-a) lesions, 110
Cerebral disorders. *See also* Coma; Convulsive disorders
  anoxia and headache, 77
  carotid sinus syncope, 703
  contusion and coma, 654
  embolism, 655
  giant cell arteritis, 80
  hemorrhage and coma, 655
  ischemia and syncope. *See* Syncope, from reduced cerebral blood flow
Cerebral thrombosis, 655–656
Cerebrospinal fluid (CSF)
  in postlumbar puncture headache, 79
  in pseudotumor cerebri, 78
Cerebrovascular disease
  coma in, 652, 655–656
  and epilepsy, 663
  syncope from, 702
  fever in, 453
Cerebrum–cerebellum distinction, 648–649
Ceruloderma. *See* Dermal pigmentation
Cervical chylous effusions, 476
Cervical cytopathology, 187
Cervical lymph nodes, 494–498
  Burkitt's lymphoma and, 487
  cancerous metastases, 501, 502f
  in keratoconjunctivitis, 496
  nasopharyngeal carcinomas and, 484
  oculoglandular syndrome and, 496
  oropharynx lesions and, 518
  pharyngoconjunctival fever and, 496
  tuberculosis of, 518
Cervical neuroblastoma, heterochromic iridis in, 849
Cervical rib syndrome, 241
Cervical spine in assessment of dizziness and vertigo, 715
Cervical spine disease
  muscle contraction headache in, 74
  dizziness in, 722
Cervical spondylosis, pain referred to shoulder in, 240
Cervical tuberculous lymphadenitis with supportive scrofula, 521

Cervix, carcinoma of, and lumbosacral plexus, 235
Chagas' disease, 496
  megacolon in, 379
Chagas-Romana sign, 496
Chancroid, 506
  genital lesion with groin lymphadenopathy, 578
  oculoglandular syndrome and, 496
  and suppuration of lymph nodes, 521
Charcot-Bouchard aneurysm, 272
Charcot-Marie-Tooth syndrome, 239
Charcot's biliary fever, 175, 453
Chediak-Higashi syndrome, 548, 850
Cheilosis, 793
  in B-complex deficiencies, 123–125, 127
  iron-deficiency anemia and, 569
Chemicals, 123, 124
  cough from, 321
  eye injury from, 99
  headaches from, 77
  peritonitis from, 176
  purpura from, 545
Chemotherapy
  and nail-color changes, 849
  nausea and vomiting induced by, 368
  and undernutrition of cancer, 796
Chesapeake hemoglobin, 357
Chest deformities and clubbing, 253
Chest muscle disease and respiratory acidosis, 762
Chest pain. *See also* Thoracic pain
  from cervical spondylosis, 240
  as conversion symptom, 634–636
  mediastinal lymphadenopathy and, 511
  in sickle-cell anemia, 584
Chest radiograph in evaluation of hypertension, 276–277
Chest tap and vasodepressor syncope, 697
Chest wall disease
  lymphoma involving sternal nodes, 511
  and respiratory acidosis, 762
  tumor and clubbing, 252
Chest wall pain, 141–144. *See also* Thoracic pain
  from breast, 143–144
  from dorsal root, 142–143
  from intercostal nerve, 141
  from myalgia, 141–142
  from ostalgia, 142
Cheyne-Stokes respiration, 344, 345, 651
  in barbiturate poisoning, 659
Chickenpox and herpes zoster, 141
Child abuse, undernutrition from, 792
Chill phase of fever, 450

Chills
  in acute hemolyte anemia, 570
  in acute pyelonephritis, 191
  jaundice and, 425
Chlamydia, 133
Chloasma gravidarum, 840
Chloral hydrate, dizziness from, 722
Chlorambucil, fever from, 458
Chloramphenicol, 131
  and aplastic anemia, 573
  fever from, 458
  and sideroblastic anemia, 577
Chloridorrhea, congenital, 761
Chlorpromazine
  for hypothalamic diabetes insipidus, 734–735
  induction of hypothermia by, 446
  and lupus inhibitor, 558
  and purple skin coloration, 847
Cholangiography, percutaneous transhepatic, 171–172
Cholangiolytic cirrhosis, clubbing and, 253
Cholecystitis, 431
  abdominal pain in, 175
  friction rub in, 427–428
  obesity and, 778
  pain of, 167, 168
  radionuclide imaging and, 172
  renal-ureteral pain from, 185
  ultrasonography in diagnosis of, 172
Cholecystography, 430–431
Cholecystokinin-pancreozynin, 775
Choledochal cyst, 425
Cholelithiasis, 430
  dietary-fiber deficiency and, 797
  obesity and, 778
Cholera, 382, 385
Cholestasis, serum bilirubin in, 429
Cholestatic jaundice, 871
Cholestatic syndrome, 425
Cholesteatoma, middle ear infections with, 716
Cholesterol
  "ketogenic" diets and, 779–780
  obesity and, 777, 800
  thyroid hormones and, 802
Cholestyramine, 793, 891
  and vitamin K, 793
Cholinergic blocking agents, 615
Cholinergic system
  and baroreflex failure, 701–702
  and movement disorders, 679
  in vasodepressor syncope, 697–698
Choluria
  in anemia, 571
Chondrocalcinosis, 223
Chorea, 685
  athetosis and, 681

dopaminergic and cholinergic systems and, 679
neurosurgical alleviation of, 684
in rheumatic fever, 222
Chorionic gonadotropin (HCG), 780
Chorioretinitis, 98
Christmas disease, 552–553
Chromatin body, 17–18
and growth impairment, 32
Chromium pigmentation, 845t, 846
Chromosomes and growth, 17–19, 30t, 32
Chronic obstructive pulmonary disease, 321, 323
Chronic paroxysmal hemicrania (CPH), 69, 70
Chrysiasis, 845t, 846
Chvostek's sign, 683
Chylomicra, 772–773, 777
Chylothorax, 476
in lymphangiomyoma, 509
Chyloperitoneum
abdominal lymphadenopathy and, 513, 574
Chylous ascites (chyloperitoneum), 476
Chylous effusions, 475–476
Chyluria, 476
Chymotrypsin, 865
Circulatory tree, 261–263
Circulatory tumor antigen–antibody complexes, 249
Cirrhosis, 428. See also Biliary cirrhosis
blood urea nitrogen (BUN) in, 429
clubbing and, 253
cyanosis in, 356
edema in, 741
eyes in, 426
hypersplenism in, 549
idiopathic hemochromatosis and, 844
jaundice and, 423
melena and hematemesis in, 393, 397, 400, 407–409
postnecrotic, 129
pruritus in, 425
and renal tubular acidosis, 759
sex and incidence of, 426
skin in, 426
temperature in, 456
vascular spiders in, 426
and vitamin deficiency diseases, 126–127, 129
Cisterna chyli, 475
Clasp-knife phenomenon, 678
"Claudication of the cauda equina," 204
Clay, eating of, and iron-deficiency anemia, 575
Cleft lip, GH deficiency and, 31
Cleft palate
GH deficiency and, 31

speech and, 114
Clomaphine, 37, 40
Clonic convulsive movement, 686
Clonic movements in vasodepressor syncope, 697
Clonidine, fatigue from, 618
Clonus, resting tremor vs., 683
Clostridium welchii, 581
Clubbing, 245–257
associated underlying diseases and, 249–250, 252–253
clinical features of, 246–250
definition of, 245
hereditary, 252
laboratory findings in, 250
pathogenesis of, 253–257
pathology of, 253
radiographic findings in, 250–252
relationship to hypertrophic osteoarthropathy, 245–246, 248, 252
Cluster headache, 69–72
accompaniments of, pathophysiology of, 71–72
autonomic nervous system and, 71
biochemical aspects, 71
classification, 69
clinical features, 69–70
hormones and, 71
medical history and, 70
vascular aspects, 70–71
Cluster migraine, 69
Cluster-tic syndrome, 69
Cluster vertigo, 69
Cluttered speech, 114
Coagulation. See also Hemostasis
inhibitors of, 557–558
in normal hemostasis, 536f, 539–542
laboratory approach to, 542–543, 544f
Coagulation cascade, 540f
Coagulation disorders, 543, 551–558
classification of, 546t
factor deficiencies, 551–557
acquired, 554–55
congenital, 554
consumption, 555–556
VIII, 552–554
loss, 556
IX, 552–554
functional classes of, 539–542
inhibitors (anticoagulants) and, 557–558
Coagulation factors, 539–558
antibodies to, 557–558
characteristics of, 539t
deficiencies, 551–557
disturbances of, and hematuria, 187

high-molecular-weight kininogen (HMWK), 539–541, 554, 555
prekallikrein, 539, 541, 554, 555
Coarctation of aorta, hypertension and, 272, 284
"Cobblestone tongue," 124
Cocaine, 13, 164
Cocci in pyelonephritis, 189
Coccidioidomycosis, 324
and calcification of lymph nodes, 510
mediastinal lymph node enlargement in, 509
suppuration of lymph nodes from, 521
Cochlear lesions, localization of, 714, 715
Cogan's disease, 718
Cogwheel rigidity in Parkinsonism, 679, 683
Colchicine, 793
Cold abscess in tuberculous mesenteric lymphadenitis, 516
Cold-reactive antibodies and hemolysis, 581
Cold sore. See Herpes simplex
Colic, intestinal, 169
Colitis, obesity and, 778
Collagen
abnormalities of, and pathologic bleeding in vascular disorders, 547
platelet adherence to, 537, 550
Collagen diseases. See also specific conditions
coronary artery disease and, 152
fever in, 449
growth failure in, 33
and mediastinal lymphadenopathy, 509
neuropathies associated with, 239
oral lesions in, 129–130
reactive lymphadenopathy in, 483–484
Collateral circulation, 153–154
Collecting system, tumors of, 187
Colon disease(s)
cancer
clubbing and, 253
diet and, 797–798
myopathy with, and weight loss, 796
perforated carcinoma, 175
low back pain from, 207
neoplastic, 170
perforated ulcer and peritonitis, 176
Colonic diverticular disease, 410, 414
Colon pain, 174
Colonoscopy, fiberoptic, 171, 172
Color. See also Skin color
measurement of, 512–513
Color photography and skin color, 813, 854

Coma, 647–666
  brain-stem lesions and, 650–652
  from CO_2 retention, 762
  as conversion symptom, 637
  in convulsive states, 660, 666
  definition of, 647, 649
  etiologies of, 652–660
    alcohol, drugs, and poisons, 659–660
    cerebrovascular disease, 655–656
    head trauma, 653–654
    hysteria, 660
    laboratory observations, summarized, 655t
    meningitis and encephalitis, 654–655
    metabolic coma, 656–658
    neoplasm and brain abscess, 654
    physical changes, summarized, 654t
    relationship to wakefulness and sleep, 653f
    syncopal attacks, 658–659
  in giant cell arteries, 80
  hepatic, hematemesis preceding, 409
  irreversible, 649
  in metabolic acidosis, 759
  neurophysiology of, 647–648
  in sickle-cell anemia, 570
  sleep studies and understanding of, 649–650
Combined headache, 66
Combined systems disease, early mental symptoms of, 613
Common bile duct, 436f
  obstruction of, 428. See also Common duct stone
  stricture of, jaundice from, 425
Common cold, cough in, 322
Common duct stone, 432f
  age and, 426
  jaundice and, 423, 425, 429
  tests for, 429
Communicative set, 112
Competition, chemical, and nutritional deficiency, 119
Complicated migraine, 64, 67
Compression fracture of vertebral body, 199
Compulsions, 602, 607
Computed tomography (CT)
  cranial, 653
  in hepatobiliary and pancreatic disorders, 172
  in jaundice, 423, 431, 437f
  of lymphoid system, 488, 490, 492–493
Computers, 2
Concussion, fever in, 453
Conductive hearing impairment, 107–109
  in external ear, 108
  in middle ear, 108–109

Confusion
  from CO_2 retention, 762
  mental symptoms of, 611
  in metabolic acidosis, 759
  in migraine equivalents, 67
  in niacin deficiency, 123
Congenital heart disease
  cyanosis in, 355
  and hypertrophic osteoarthropathy, 247–249, 252–254, 255f
  syncope in, 693
Congenital nonspherocytic hemolytic anemia, 583
Congestive heart failure, 731, 736, 742–744
  anemia and, 568, 569
  clubbing and, 253
  cyanosis in, 352
  edema in, 741
  fever from, 456
  hypertrophic osteoarthropathy vs., 249
  lethargy and fatigue in, 617–618
  tachycardia in, 302–303
  vomiting with, 371
Conjugate-gaze paralysis, 652
Conjunctivae, pigmentation of, 848
Conjunctival icterus, 826
  unilateral, 827
Conjunctival injection
  in cluster headache, 70, 71
  in riboflavin deficiency, 125
Conjunctival melanosis, 844
Conjunctivitis
  anterior auricular lymphadenopathy and, 495–496
  in Behçet's syndrome, 133
  in common cold, 322
Connective tissue
  lymph formation in, 469, 470, 472
  reticular, in lymph nodes, 477
Connective tissue disorders. See also specific disorders
  blue sclerae in, 848–849
  pathologic bleeding in, 547
Consciousness
  abnormal states of. See Coma, etiologies of
  definition of, 648
  loss of. See Syncope
  neural basis of, 649–652
  in subarachnoid hemorrhage, 79
  vitamin-B_{12} deficiency and, 577
Constipation, 375–380, 392
  abdominal lymphadenopathy and, 513, 514
  abdominal pain with, 170
  definition of, 376–377
  dietary-fiber deficiency and, 797–798

  in hypothyroidism, 566
  from laxative abuse, 379
  low back pain with, 207
  mechanical basis of, 380
  in niacin deficiency, 123
  in postganglionic disorders, 379
  psychological factors in, 378
  spinal cord lesions and, 378
  from weakness of voluntary muscles, 380
Constitutive skin color, 815
Contractures, conversion, 638–640
"Contre-coup" hearing impairment, 111
Convection in body-heat elimination, 442
Conversion pain, 57
  location of, 53
  temporal aspects of, 55
Conversion symptom(s), 608, 623–645
  anorexia, nausea, vomiting, 641
  aphonia, 642
  choice of, 628–629, 634
  clinical diagnosis of, 630–635
    diagnostic criteria, 631–635
    interview technique, 630–631
  complications of, 625t
  defined, 625
  mechanisms, 629–630
  contractures, 638–640
  cutaneous sensory disturbances, 640–641
  definition of terms, 624–625
  differential diagnosis of
    vs hypochondriacal symptoms, 643–644
    vs malingering and factitious illness, 644–645
    vs psychophysiologic symptoms, 643
    vs somatic delusions, 644
  differentiation of, from other psychosomatic symptoms, 625, 636, 643–645
  dysphagia, 641
  dysphonia, 642
  epidemic of, 643
  fatigue, 640
  gait disturbances, 638–640
  globus hystericus, 642
  hearing loss, 641
  hyperventilation syndrome, 637
  incidence of, 625–626
  malingering vs., 635, 644–645
  mechanisms of, 626–629
  movement disorders, 640
  nongaseous abdominal bloating, 642
  pain, 635–636
  paralysis, 638–640
  physical symptoms concurrent with, 642–643

pruritus vulvae and ani, 642
seizures, 637
syncope, stupor, and coma, 637, 703
tics, 640
tremors, 640
urinary urgency, frequency, and retention, 642
visual disturbances, 641
weakness, 638–640
Convulsions
fever and, 451
in sickle-cell anemia, 570
Convulsive states, 660–666
Addisonian crisis, 657
from calcium deficit, 658
definition of, 647, 660
EEG classification of, 660–662
focal seizures, 664, 665f
generalized seizures, 663–664, 665f
in meningitis, 655
neurophysiology of, 647–648
spectrum of, 662–663
Todd's paralysis following, 678
Coomb's-antiglobulin test, 580
Copper deficiency
and CNS development, 789
and depigmentation, 853
from excessive dieting in pregnancy, 789
Copper exposure and hemolysis, 581
Coprolalia, 685
Coronary artery disease, 152–154
anemia and, 566, 569
atrial fibrillation in, 308
atrial flutter in, 307
cluster headache and, 70
extrasystoles in, 298
mitral valve prolapse in, 297
as psychosomatic disorder, 601
Coronary blood flow, 151–155
angiography and, 151–152
Coronary insufficiency, conversion chest
pain with, 635
Coronary spasm, pseudoangina vs., 636
Coronary thrombosis
atrial fibrillation in, 308
after gastroduodenal hemorrhage, 406
Cor pulmonale, 568
Cortical necrosis, 187
Corticosteroids, 31–32
and compression fracture of vertebral
body, 199
excess of, 609–610
and growth impairment, 31–32
for polymyalgia rheumatica, 224
and psychiatric disturbances, 614, 615
for reflex dystrophy in extremity, 231
for retinal arteritis, 88
Corticotropin-releasing factor (CRF),
596–597

Cortisol
anorexia nervosa and, 802
hypersecretion of, 600
obesity and secretion of, 777
stress and, 600
Cortisone
and hypothermia, 446
and melanin production, 839
and methotrexate toxicity, 125–126
Coryza, 114
Cosmetics, reactions to, 11
Costen's syndrome, 134
Cotton dust fever, 459
Cough, 317–329
in acute otitis media, 108
in allergic disorders, 326
in cardiovascular disorders, 325
characteristic types of, 321
complications of, 327–328
hemoptysis following, 331
inflammations causing, 320, 322–324
and intercostal muscle pain, 142
mechanisms of, 318–320
in mediastinal lymph node enlargement, 509
from mediastinal tumor, 149–150
neoplasms causing, 326
in paroxysmal nocturnal dyspnea, 344
postinfarction, 157
in spontaneous pneumothorax, 146
stimuli producing, 320–321
tracheobronchial pain and, 144
treatment of, 328–329
Cough headache, benign, 77
Cough syncope, 659
Coumarin anticoagulants, 554–555
Courvoisier's law, 428
Couvade syndrome, 641
Coxsackie virus, 132–133
polymyositis secondary to, 230
Cranial CT scan, 653
Cranial inflammation, headache due to,
79–80
Cranial nerve palsy
serous otitis and, 109
in sickle-cell anemia, 570
Cranial nerves, localization of lesions in,
713–715
Cranial structure diseases, headache
and, 80
Cranial vasculature in migraine, 67
Creatine, urinary, obesity and, 778
Creatinine, urinary, as growth indicator,
27
Crepitus
in osteoarthritis, 223
in rheumatoid arthritis, 223
Cretinism (congenital hypothyroidism),
31

and carotenemia, 827
thyroid hormone and, 19, 26f
U:L ratio in, 20–21
Creutzfeldt-Jakob disease, 655
Crigler-Najjar syndrome, 429
Cristae, function of, 709, 710f
Crohn's disease, 170, 483
examination for, 171
Croup, 321
Cryoglobulinemia
and leukocytoclastic vasculitis, 545
and renal tubular acidosis, 759
retinal hemorrhage and, 89
Cryptococcosis, 324
Cryptococcus neoformans, 325
Cryptorchidism, 31
Cullen's sign, 830
"Curving" of fingernails, 246, 247f
Cushing's syndrome, 31–32
corticosteroid excess from, 609
hypertension in, 272, 283
melanin metabolism in, 839
and metabolic alkalosis, 761
myopathy in, 672
Na+ retention in, 673
obesity in, 771
purpura in, 547
Cutaneous circulation, 351–352
Cutaneous sensory disturbances, conversion, 640–641
Cyanosis, 349–359
argyria vs., 846
in cardiovascular disease, 355
central, 352–353
cutaneous circulation and, 351–352
definition of, 349
effects of O_2 on, 358–359
in hemoglobin abnormalities, 356–357
O_2 transport and, 349–351
peripheral, 352
in Pickwickian syndrome, 777
in pulmonary disorders, 353–354
relationship to CO_2 exchange, 357–358
skin color in, 816–817, 830–831
Cyclic fever, 455
Cyclic vomiting, 367
Cyclo-oxygenase deficiency, 551
Cycloserine, 793
Cystic fibrosis, hemoptysis in, 334
Cystic hygroma, 473
Cystic mastitis, 144
Cystinosis, 758
Cystitis
clinical picture of, 191
in diabetes mellitus, 191
and hematuria, 187
hemorrhagic, 190
pain of, 177
pyelonephritis vs., 189

Cytomegalovirus (CVM), 325, 456, 483
Cystoscopy, 190
Cytopathology, 187, 188
Cytoplasmic enzymes, 565

DaCosta's syndrome, 612
Deafness. *See also* Hearing—impairment
    as conversion syndrome, 641
Decerebrate rigidity, 678–679
    in metabolic coma, 656
    brain-stem lesions and, 651
"Decorticate rigidity," 678–679
Defervescence phase of fever, 450–451
Degenerative joint disease, monoarticu-
    lar pain in, 216
Dehydration, 731–736
    approach to patient in, 734
    causes of, 732–734
    of extracellular space, 740–741
    and hematuria, 186
    from "rainbow" treatment of obesity,
        780
    signs and symptoms of, 731–732, 733t
    from thoracic-duct injury, 475
    vomiting and, 367
Dehydration fever, 455
Dehydration test, 733–734
Dejerine-Sottas disease, 236, 239
"Delayed speech," 114
Delirium
    causes of, 611–612
    fever and, 451
    in giant cell arteritis, 80
    mental symptoms of, 611
    in niacin deficiency, 123
    somatic delusions in, 644
Delirium tremens, 614
Delta-granule deficiency, 550
Delta rhythm, 662
Demanding dependency in hysterical
    personality, 632
Demeclocycline and concentration of
    urine, 736
Dementia
    and coma, 655
    fatigue vs., 618
    somatic delusions in, 644
Demyelinative diseases, dizziness in,
    721
Dengue, temperature curve in, 453
Dense lymphoid tissue, 477
Dental development, 25, 27t
Dental infections and cervical lymphade-
    nopathy, 497
Deoxycortisone therapy, 853
Deoxyhemoglobin. *See* Reduced-hemo-
    globin pigmentation

Deoxyribonucleic acid. *See* DNA
Depersonalization in classic migraine, 66
Depression, 593
    abdominal pain with, 170
    anorexia in, 366
    anxiety and, 606
    catecholamines and, 603
    clinical picture of, 615–616
    drug-induced, 618
    eating behavior and obesity in, 776
    endorphins and, 600
    hormonal changes in, 600
    hypochondriasis and, 644
    in hysterical patient, 633
    muscle contraction headache and, 73
    pancreatic carcinoma and, 176
    in post-traumatic syndrome, 75, 76
    psychogenic dyspnea in, 342
    serotonin and, 598
    tension headache and, 601
Depressor reflex, 301
DeQuervain's syndrome, 217
Dermal melanocyte hamartoma, 847
Dermal pigmentation (ceruloderma),
    814, 846–848
    drug-induced, 847
Dermatitis
    atopic, itching in, 868, 873, 875f
    in Behçet's syndrome, 133
    from vitamin deficiencies, 793
        B-complex, 124–125
Dermatitis herpetiformis, 390, 873–874
Dermatalogic disorders, melanosis in,
    838, 842
Dermatomes, 44, 45f, 46f
Dermatomyositis, 230, 672
    generalized lymphadenopathy in, 522
    melanosis with, 842
Dermographia of mastocytosis, 390
Dermoid tumors, 234
Dermopathic lymphadenopathy, 483
Desmoids, 230
Desmosterol, myotonia from, 680
Desquamating skin, pigmentation of, 854
Development. *See also* Growth; Sexual
        development
    of communication skills, 102,
        103–106t, 114, 115t
    psychosocial, pain and, 45–50
Diabetes insipidus
    in eosinophilic granuloma, 327
    hypothalamic, 734–735
    nephrogenic, 730f, 731f, 735
Diabetes mellitus
    acute abdomen and, 178
    carotenemia in, 828
    and cataracts, 95, 96
    coma in, 657
        incidence of, 653

coronary artery disease and, 152
    growth impairment and, 31
    hunger and, 363
    hypoglycemia in early stages of, 610
    idiopathic hemochromatosis and, 844
    ketoacidosis in, 756
    lactic acidosis in, 756
    lacunes and, 720
    mononeuropathy in, 238
    mucormycosis in, 325
    multiple mononeuritis in, 675
    muscle weakness from insulin treat-
        ment in, 673
    myopathy in, 672
    obesity and, 770, 771, 777
    orthostatic hypotension in, 695
    and polyneuropathy, 238
    pruritis in, 871
    radicular pain from, 275
    retinopathy in, 90–92, 93f
    skin changes in, 228
    tan-colored spots in, 846
    urinary tract infections and, 190–191
    vitiligo with, 851, 852
Diabetic ketoacidosis, 370
    abdominal pain in, 177, 178
    fever in, 455
Diabetic neuropathy, 241
    femoral, 243
Diacetylmorphine. *See* Heroin
Diamox. *See* Acetazolamide
Diaphragm, neurogenic tumor of, club-
        bing and, 253
Diaphragmatic pain, 146–147
Diarrhea, 375–376, 380–392
    abdominal lymphadenopathy and, 513
    abdominal pain with, 170
    in acute gastroenteritis, 175
    in appendicitis, 175
    causes of, 381t
    characteristics of, 380
    definition of, 377
    and dehydration, 732
    diagnostic assessment of, 389–391
    drug-induced, 793
    from enzyme deficiency, 174
    hypocalcemia from, 683
    inflammatory basis of, 388–389
    in lactase deficiency, 169, 172
    malabsorption resulting in, 380–387,
        516
    mechanical basis of, 388
    and metabolic acidosis, 757
    in migraine equivalents, 67
    neuromuscular origins of, 387–388
    in niacin deficiency, 123, 124
    in pernicious anemia, 566
    as reaction to antibiotics, 131
    sodium depletion from, 741

Diastasis recti, 380
Diastolic hypertension, 270–271
Diastolic murmurs in anemia, 568
Diazepam for stiff man syndrome, 683
Diet. See also Undernutrition; and specific
      nutritional deficiencies
   and aging, 798–801
   as cause of nutritional deficiency, 119,
      120
   and folic-acid deficiency, 577
   and iron deficiency, 575
   in treating obesity, 778–782
   and vitamin-B_{12} deficiency, 576
Dietary-fiber deficiency, 797–798
Dieting, excessive, in pregnancy, 789
Diffuse fibrosing alveolitis, 327
Diffuse lymphomas, 486
   lymphocytic, 509
      epitrochlear node involvement in,
         504
Diffused blood, skin color from, 829–830
DiGeorge's syndrome, 482
Digestive disturbances, abdominal
      lymphadenopathy and, 513
Digital-nerve entrapment, 243
Digitalis
   adverse reactions to, 12
   in cardiac failure, 155
   fatigue from, 618
   and fever, 458
   tachycardia caused by, 312
   in treatment of obesity, 780
Dihydrostreptomycin, 718
Dihydroxyacetone, 837
Diiosoprophyl fluorophosphate poison-
      ing, 660
Dilantin. See Diphenylhydantoin
Dilutional anemia, 563
Dilutional thrombocytopenia, 549
Dinitro-ortho-cresol poisoning, 660
Dinitrophenol (DNP), 828
   and temperature, 458
Diphenylhydantoin (Dilantin)
   and folate malabsorption, 577
   gingivitis induced by, 130
   macular erythematosus eruption from,
      874
   and undernutrition, 794–795
Diphtheria, 453
   pharyngitis in, 322
Diphtheria antitoxins, brachial plexus
      neuritis from, 241
Diplophonia, 113
Diplopia
   in giant cell arteritis, 80
   oculomotor system, 714
   in pseudotumor cerebri, 78
Direct immunofluorescence, 189
Direct oxidative pathway, 122

Disconjunctive ocular movements in
      meningitis, 655
Disks. See Intervertebral disks
Dislocations, chronic, 81
Dissecting aortic aneurysms, 160, 161
Dissociative states in hysterical personal-
      ity, 633
Distal myopathy, 672
Diuresis
   high K^+ loss from, 673
   postobstructive, 736
Diuretic drugs
   and concentration of urine, 736
   and edema, 744
   and metabolic alkalosis, 760–761
   for obesity, 780
   and salt depletion, 740–741
Diurnal variation in body temperature,
      445
Diverticulitis
   of colon, abdominal pain in, 175
   pain of, 168
Diverticulosis
   dietary-fiber deficiency and, 797–798
   jejunal, 385–386, 576
      hematemesis and melena from,
         410
Diverticulum, perforated, and peritoni-
      tis, 176
Dizziness
   in c-p-a tumor, 110
   clinical approach to, 707–708, 716
   clinical significance of, 715–723
      cervical spine, 722
      demyelinative diseases, 721
      drug effects, 722
      ear diseases, 716–719
      eighth-nerve diseases, 719
      epilepsy, 722
      infectious diseases, 721
      intrinsic brain-stem tumors, 720
      malformations, 720–721
      nutritional disease, 721
      ocular disturbance, 722
      psychogenic etiology, 723
      vascular disturbance, 720
   neurologic lesion localization in as-
      sessment of, 713–715
   postural, in anemia, 568
   in pseudotumor cerebri, 78
   streptomycin administration and, 111
DNA, 17–18
   endogenous pyrogen and, 449–450
   synthesis of, 479
      folic acid and vitamin B_{12} deficiency
         and, 128
      and marrow hypoplasia, 548
      maternal undernutrition and, 789
      and megaloblastic anemia, 576

Dopamine, 598, 599f
   central pain mechanisms and, 63
Dopaminergic system and movement
      disorder, 679
Dorsal column lesions with loss of pro-
      prioception, 713
Dorsal column–medial lemniscal tract,
      46–47
Dorsal root pain, 142–143
Down's syndrome, 32
   Brushfield's spots in, 849
Dreams, 627
Drop attacks, 652, 718
   dizziness in, 722
Drowsiness
   in anemia, 569–570
   from CO_2 retention, 762
   in pulmonary disease, 657
Drug addiction. See also specific drugs
   nutritional deficiency and, 120
Drug fevers, 458
Drugs. See also specific drugs
   conditions induced by. See specific con-
      ditions
   and fetal growth, 19
   generalized lymphadenopathy and,
      522
   in patient's history, 10, 13
   overdose of, hypoxia in, 353
   prescription, dangers of, 11–12
   toxicity of
      and cataracts, 95
      and tunnel vision, 96
Drumstick fingers, 245, 247. See also
      Clubbing
Dry cough, 318
Dubin-Johnson syndrome, 423, 424
Duodenal drainage, 423, 430
Duodenal pain, 57
Duodenal ulcer
   back pain from, 206–207
   clubbing and, 253
   melena and hematemesis in, 393, 400,
      402, 406
   pain of, 173–174
Dupuytren's contracture, 428
Dying-back neuropathies, 675
Dysautonomic cephalagia, post-trau-
      matic, 75, 76
Dysbasia, 640
Dysentery
   amebic, 377
      clubbing and, 249, 253
   definition of, 377
Dysesthesia
   in cervical rib syndrome, 242
   in polyneuritis, 240
   in thalamic pain syndrome, 231
   vitamin B_{12} deficiency and, 239

Dysfibrinogenemias, 554
Dysphagia, 511
    conversion, 641
    in esophageal disease, 149
    in herpangina, 132
    from iron deficiency, 569
Dysphonia, conversion, 642
Dysplasia, oral, 133
Dyspnea, 335–347
    in alveolar proteinosis, 327
    in anemia, 344, 566, 568
    in cardiac disease, 342–344
    in chronic pulmonary disease, 341–342
    in lymphangiomyoma, 509
    from mediastinal tumor, 149–150
    nature of, 335–336
    neuroanatomic pathways in, 339–340
    in neurologic disease, 344–346
    postinfarction, 157
    psychogenic, 342
    settings precipitating, 336
    in spontaneous pneumothorax, 146
    theories of, 340
    in vocal cord paralysis, 113
Dysproteinemia, 558
    angioimmunoblastic lymphadenopa-
        thy with, 484
Dyssebacea, nasolabial
    in niacin deficiency, 123
    in riboflavin deficiency, 125
Dystonia, 681
    neurosurgical alleviation of, 684
Dystonia musculorum deformans, 681
Dystrophia myotonica, 680
Dysuria
    in acute pyelonephritis, 191
    bladder pain and, 185

Ear(s). See also Hearing; Vestibular en-
        tries; and specific conditions
    anatomy and physiology of, 107–108
    pain in
        in acute otitis media, 108
        common causes of, listed, 111–112
        noise-induced hearing loss and, 111
    vertigo and dizziness from diseases
        of, 716–719
        external ear disturbances, 716
        labyrinthine disturbances, 717–719
        middle ear disturbances, 716–717
Ecchinococcal disease, 325
Ecchymoses
    in coagulation-factor deficiency, 553
    as conversion complication, 630
    in disseminated intravascular coagula-
        tion, 556
    of eyelids, 848

    in hemostatic failure, 543, 544
    in idiopathic thrombocytopenic pur-
        pura, 549
    simulated by Mongolian spots, 843
    skin color in, 831, 847
    from vitamin-K deficiency, 555
Eclampsia, coma from, 652
Ectodermal dysplasias, mitral valve pro-
        lapse in, 297
Ectopic pregnancy, pain from, 171, 177
Eczema, pruritis in, 868, 870f
Edema, 741–744
    abdominal lymphadenopathy and,
        513, 514
    in anemia, 568
    approach to patient in, 744
    of brain, headache and, 77
    in hypertrophic osteoarthropathy, 248,
        249
    lymphatic, 473–474, 743–744
    mechanisms of, 741–744
        abnormal, 742–744
        capillary, 741–744
        renal, 744
    melanin screening by, 853
    pulmonary, 325
        cyanosis in, 352
        dyspnea and, 342–343
        hemoptysis in, 333
        and respiratory acidosis, 762
    skin color in, 853
    and skin pattern of jaundice, 826
Effort syncope, 693
Effort syndrome, 612
Ehler-Danlos syndrome, 547
Ehrlich's test of urinary porphobilino-
        gen, 178
Eighth-nerve disease, 719, 720
Elastin abnormalities and pathologic
        bleeding, 547
Elbow
    diagnosis of rheumatoid arthritis and,
        223
    pain in, 218, 241
        tennis elbow (lateral epicondylitis),
            211, 218
    ulnar-nerve entrapment at, 241
Electric shock and sudden visual loss, 99
Electrical seizures, 662
Electrocardiograph (ECG)
    in anemia, 568
    in evaluation of hypertension, 275–276
Electrocochleography, 715
Electroencephalogram (EEG)
    in appraisal of convulsive states,
        660–662
    brain-stem lesions and, 652
Electrolyte disturbances
    coma in, 658

    fasciculation in, 682
    fatigue from, 618
Electronystagmography (ENG), 707, 708,
        711, 712, 714
Electroretinogram, 97
Elephantiasis, 473, 474
Elliptocytosis, 579f
Embden-Meyerhof pathway, defects in,
        583
Embolism
    fever from, 454
    in posterior circulation, 720
    pulmonary, hemoptysis in, 333
    syncope in, 694
Emotional brain, mechanism of nervous-
        ness and, 594–597
Emphysema, 323, 657
    clubbing and, 253
    constipation and, 380
    dyspnea in, 336
    obesity and, 77
    partial bronchial obstruction by lymph
        nodes and, 510
    and respiratory acidosis, 762
    subcutaneous, 328
Empyema, clubbing and, 246, 252
Encephalins, central pain mechanisms
        and, 63
Encephalitis
    coma in, 655
    and epilepsy, 663
    and premature puberty, 39
    sleep center and, 649–650
Encephalomyelitis, Behçet's syndrome
        and, 133
Encephalopathy, hypertensive, 272
Endocarditis
    bacterial. See Bacterial endocarditis
    fever in, 456
    gonococcal, fever in, 452–453
    mimicked by left-atrium myxomas,
        456
Endocrine disorders. See also specific con-
        ditions
    anorexia, nausea and vomiting in,
        370–371
    coma in, 657
    and erythropoietin, 573
    in myopathy, 672
    obesity and, 771–772, 777
    presenting with fatigue, 617
    presenting with nervousness, 600,
        609–611
    pruritis in, 871
Endocrine system. See also Hormones;
        and specific hormones and glands
    in adolescence, 33–35
Endogenous pyrogen (EP), 448–450, 452,
        454, 455

Endometrial cancer, obesity and, 778
Endometriosis, 187
  of lung, 334
Endorphins, 48–49, 63, 600
Endoscopic retrograde cholangiopan-
    creatography (ERCP), 423, 431,
    434f
Endoscopy
  fiberoptic, 171
  gastrointestinal, 402, 404–405
Endosteum, bone pain and, 142
Endotoxins
  endothelial damage by, 545
  and fever, 454
  in Jarisch-Herxheimer reaction, 458
  and proliferation of lymphocytes,
    480
Endrophonium in testing of baroreflex
    failure, 700, 700t
Enkephalins, 600
Enteric fever, 450
Enteritis
  oral lesions in, 133
  regional. See Regional enteritis
Enterococci in pyelonephritis, 189
Enterogastrone, 775
Entrapment
  of peripheral nerve, 236
  of suprascapular nerve, shoulder pain
    from, 240
Entrapment syndromes, 675
  forearm and hand pain in, 241
  in lower extremities, 243–244
  meralgia paresthetica, 242–243
Enzyme deficiency, abdominal pain
    from, 174
Enzymopathy, hemolytic anemia and,
    583
Eosinophilia and hepatitis, 429
Eosinophilic granuloma, 327, 485f
Ependymomas, 234
Ephedrine intoxication, 614
Ephelides (freckles), 829, 843
Epicondylitis, lateral, 211, 217
Epicritic itch, 866
Epidemic vestibular neuritis, 718
Epidermal melanin unit, 834–835, 852
Epidermoid cysts of bony phalanges,
    246
Epidermoid tumors, 234
Epidural hematoma, coma in, 654
Epigastrium, burning sensations in,
    from niacin deficiency, 123
Epilepsy, 652, 660–666. See also Convul-
    sive disorders
  causes of, 663
  definition of, 660, 662
  dizziness in, 722–723
  EEG classification of, 660–662

generalized vs. focal, 647, 663–664,
    665f
  post-traumatic, 654
Epinephrine, 596, 615
  and body temperature, 458
  and melanocyte-stimulating hormone,
    839
  and platelet adhesion, 550
  stress and, 600–601
  tachycardia due to, 302
Episodic cluster headache, 69
Epistaxis
  in factor-V deficiency, 554
  in idiopathic thrombocytopenic pur-
    pura, 549
  from tooth extraction, 553
  from vitamin-K deficiency, 555
Epithelial inclusion cysts, 503
Epitrochlear lymph nodes, 504
  systemic syphilis and, 945
Epstein-Barr virus, 483
Equilibrium. See also Dizziness; Vertigo
  oculomotor function and, 709–713
  vestibular function and, 708–709,
    709–711f
  vestibulosomatic function and, 713
Ergonovine and spasm of arteries, 152
Ergotamine, 67
  in headache, 75
  headache from withdrawal of, 77
Erysipelas, 471, 474
  anterior auricular lymphadenopathy
    and, 495
Erysepeloid of Rosenbach, 517
Erysipelothrix rhusiopathia inoculation,
    517
Erythema
  melanosis and, 837, 838
  palmar, 129, 428
Erythema ab igne, 831
Erythema caloricum, 837
Erythema chronicum migrans, 518
Erythema multiforme, oral lesions in,
    129–130
Erythema nodosum
  in Crohn's disease, 170
  mediastinal lymphadenopathy in, 509
  oral lesions in, 129
Erythremia (erythrosis), 831–832
Erythrocytes. See Red blood cells
Erythropoiesis, 479, 565–566, 571
Erythropoietin lack, 573
Erythroprotein, 565
Escherichia coli, 189
  in osteomyelitis of spine, 199
Esophageal carcinoma, 149
Esophageal reflex, 399–400
Esophageal spasm and vasodepressor
    syncope, 697

Esophageal temperature, 445
Esophageal varices, 407–409, 426
  diagnosis of, 399, 400, 402
  jaundice and, 429
Esophagitis
  erosive, 399, 400, 409–410
  peptic, 169
  phlegmonous, 149
Esophagus
  pain from, 57, 149, 150f
  as source of abdominal pain, 173
  traction diverticulum of, 510
Essential thrombocythemia, platelet dys-
    function and, 551
Essential tremor, 684
Estradiol in sexual development, 34f
Estrogen
  and body temperature, 446
  child's ingestion of, 39
  and food consumption, 803
  and intrahepatic cholestasis, 871
  and migraine, 68
  overproduction of, 39
  and recurrent fever, 456
  and skin color, 820, 821f, 838, 840,
    841f
Estrogen preparations, 615
Estrogen-protein preparations in control
    of height, 33
Ethacrynic acid, 111
  ototoxity of, 718
Ethanol ingestion and lactic acidosis,
    756
Ethmoid sinus infection, serous otitis
    and, 109
Ethological theory, 602, 603
Ethosuximide, 615
Ethyl alcohol. See Alcohol
Ethylene glycol ingestion and metabolic
    acidosis, 756
Etiocholanolone, 456
Eumelanin, 815
Eunochoidism, 37, 38
  skin color in, 820
Eustachian tubal function
  dizziness and, 716–717
  and serous otitis, 109
Evaporation in body-heat elimination,
    442
Exanthemata, skin color in, 831
Exercise
  and hematuria, 186
  hypertension and, 284
  obesity and, 778, 781
Exogenous hemochromatosis, 844, 845t
Exsanguination, coma from, 652
Extensor toe sign. See Babinski sign
External ear, conductive hearing impair-
    ment in, 108

Extracellular fluid
  buffering mechanisms, 749–750,
    749–751f
  definition of, 726, 744
  depletion, 740–741
Extraocular muscle dystrophy, 672
Extrasystoles, 298
Extremities, 227–244. *See also specific body parts*
  athetosis, 681
  conversion symptoms, 638–640
  lesions of, and regional lymphadenopathy syndrome, 517–518
  in pernicious anemia, 566
Extremity pain
  in hemolytic anemia, 570
  in intervertebral disk lesions, 202–203
  pathophysiology of, 228–240
    brachial and lumbosacral plexuses, 235
    central nervous system, 231
    joints, 230–231
    muscle, 229–230
    peripheral nerve, 235–240
    radicular pain, 231–235
    skin, 228–229
  in regional syndromes, 240–244
Eye closure and nystagmus, 711
Eyelids
  edema of, in oculonodal complex, 496
  oculoglandular syndrome vs. tumor of, 496
  pigmentation of, 848
Eye movements in coma, 655–657
Eye(s). *See also* Vision; Visual loss
  direct trauma of, 98–99
  external pigmentation of, 848–849
  in jaundice, 426
  pain in
    angle-closure glaucoma, 92–94
    retrobulbar neuritis, 94–95
    in transient visual loss, 97
Eyestrain and muscle contraction headache, 74

Fabry's disease, 482
  and renal tubular acidosis, 759
Face, conversion pain in, 635
Facial flushing in cluster headache, 70
Facial lymph nodes, 494f, 500
  oculoglandular syndrome and, 496
Facial nerve, lesion localization and, 714
Facial weakness in cerebello-pontine-angle tumor, 110
Factitious fever, 451
Factitious illness, 607f, 608
  conversion symptoms vs., 644–645
Factitial proctitis, 474

Factors. *See* Coagulation factors
Facultative skin color, 815
Fad diets, 779–780
Failure to thrive
  growth hormone in, 600
  in sickle-cell anemia, 584
Fainting. *See* Syncope
"Fainting lark," 695
Falsetto, 113
Familial Mediterranean fever, 455
Familial periodic paralysis, 672–673
Family history, taking of, 12
Fanconi syndrome, 547
Fantasies and conversion symptoms, 623, 625–630
Fascia and back pain, 204–205
Fasciculation, 682
Fascitis, 230
Fasted state, physiology of, 773
Fasting in treatment of obesity, 779
Fatigue, 591–604, 615–619
  in anemia, 566
  in chronic pyelonephritis, 191
  clinical assessment of, 592–594
  from CO_2 retention, 762
  as conversion symptom, 640
  defective posture and, 205
  in dehydration, 731
  differential diagnosis of, 603–604, 615–618
    flow chart, 616f
    normal fatigue, 615
    medications and drugs of abuse, 618
    physical disorders, 617–618
    psychological disorders, 615–617
  in niacin deficiency, 123
  pathophysiologic explanations, 594–601
    brain anatomy, 596–597
    neurochemistry, 597–600
    rest, 601
    stress, 600–601
  in pseudotumor cerebri, 78
  psychological explanation of, 601–603
Fat. *See* Body fat; Obesity
Fat-mobilizing hormone, 779
Fats, dietary, 772–773
  malabsorption of, 382–383
Fatty liver, serum lipids and, 429
Fava-bean sensitivity, 583
Febrile states. *See* Fever
Felons, 246
Felty's syndrome, hypersplenism in, 549
Femoral nerve mononeuropathy, 243
  diabetic, 238
Fenfluramine, 780
Ferritin, 255
Fetal development, 19

maternal nutrition and
  brain development and, 789
  low-birth-weight and, 789
  maternal anemia and, 790–791
Fever, 446–461
  abdominal lymphadenopathy and, 513, 514
  in acute appendicitis, 174
  in acute myocardial infarction, 156
  in acute otitis media, 108
  in acute pyelonephritis, 191
  albuminuria with, 451
  in allergic purpura, 545
  in allergy, 457
  with anesthesia, 457–458
  beneficial effects of, 451–452
  in blood diseases, 454
  "catheter," 459
  in central nervous system diseases, 453
  chemotherapy for cancer and, 796
  clinical causes of, reviewed, 452–458
  clinical features of, 450–451
  in common duct stone, 425
  complications of, 451
  convulsions with, 451
  cotton dust, 459
  in Crohn's disease, 170
  in cystitis, 191
  definition of, 442, 447
  in dehydration, 731
  delirium with, 451
  drug-induced, 458–459
    and undernutrition, 792
  in embolism and thrombosis, 454
  factitious, 451
  in fluid balance disturbance, 455
  in giant cell arteritis, 80
  habitual, 459
  in heart diseases, 456
  in heat stroke, 454–455
  in heavy sedation, 458
  hematemesis and melena and, 397
  in hematologic disease, 570
  in herpangina, 132
  herpes simplex lesions with, 451
  in iliac lymphadenitis, 507
  in infections, 452–453
  jaundice and, 425
  limit of, compatible with life, 446–447
  in liver diseases, 456
  in meningitis, 79
  metal fume, 459
  "milk," 459
  in neoplasms, 453–454
  nutritional deficiency and, 119
  pathogenesis of, 448–450
  in peptic ulcer, 457
  in perforated carcinoma of colon, 175
  in polymyalgia rheumatica, 224

postinfarction, 157
postoperative, 456–457
psychogenic, 459–460
in "pyrogens," 458–459
in rheumatoid arthritis, 223
in sarcoid, 456
in serum sickness, 457
in skin abnormalities, 457
skin color in, 831
steroid, 455–456
tachycardia and, 298, 302
teething, 459
in temporal arteritis syndrome, 88
thermoregulation during, 447–448
in thrombotic thrombocytopenic purpura, 549
in thyroid disease, 455
in tissue trauma, 456–457
types and terminology, 447
of unknown origin (FUO), 460
vomiting and, 370
"Fever blisters," 451. See also Herpes
simplex
Fever headache, 77
Fever therapy
and herpes, 451
in neurosyphilis, 451
Fiber, dietary, 797–798
Fiberglass contamination of clothing, 873
Fibrillation, 681–682
Fibrin clot formation, chemistry of,
539–542. See also Coagulation
Fibrin deposition and hemolysis, 581
Fibrinogen
in coagulation, 539, 540, 543
congenital deficiency of, 554
in normal platelet function, 537, 539
Fibrin(ogen) degeneration products
(FDP), 542, 543, 556–558
Fibrinolysis
in disseminated intravascular coagula-
tion, 555–557
in liver disease, 555
Fibrinolytic system, 541, 542
Fibrinous pleurisy, 143–144
Fibroblasts, reticular cells vs., 476
Fibroid pulmonary tuberculosis, 252
Fibrolipomatosis, 488–490
Fibromyositis, 142
Fibrosing alveolitis, dyspnea in, 336
Fibrositis, 204–205, 224
Filaria sanginis hominis, 474
Filiariasis, 878
inguinal lymphadenopathy and, 506
Finger joint pain, 217–218
Fingernails
in arsenical melanosis, 846
in diagnosis of clubbing, 246, 247f
Fingers, clubbed. See Clubbing

Fish tapeworm infestation, 126
and vitamin B_{12} deficiency, 576
Fistula(s). See specific type
Fitzgerald-factor deficiency, 554
Fixed hypertension, 270
Flaccidity, definition of, 678n
Flank pain in pyuria, 191
Flatulence, lactase deficiency and, 172
Fletcher-factor deficiency, 554
Flexion contracture of knee joint, 221
Flooding techniques, 603
Floppy infants, 672
Fludrocortisone, 741
Fluid balance. See also Water balance,
normal
fever from disturbance of, 455
Fluorescein angiography, 92, 93f
in macular degeneration, 95
Flushing, 830
in cluster headache, 70
Focal myositis, 230
Focal seizures, 660, 664, 665f
clonic convulsive movements of, 686
Todd's paralysis and, 678
Folate deficiency and thrombocytopenia,
548
Folic acid
biochemical role of, 122, 123, 126–127
deficiency of, 125–126
and anemia, 573, 576, 577, 790–791
and atrophic glossitis, 126–127
diphenylhydantoin and, 794–795
diseases causing, 577
oral contraceptives and, 795
Follicle-stimulating hormone (FSH), 33,
34f, 596–597
deficiency of, and sexual precocity, 39
and food consumption, 803
Follicular hyperplasia, 483
Follicular lymphoma, 486
Folliculitis, occipital lymphadenopathy
and, 494–495
Foot. See also Extremity entries
conversion contractures of, 640
pain in, 243–244
monoarticular, 221
from trauma, 216
Foraminal inpaction of brain stem, 651
Forearm pain, 241–242
Foreign bodies in lungs, hemoptysis
caused by, 332
Formulas, infant, 791
Fractures
cough, 327
fever after, 456
of lower tibia, ankle joint and, 221
pathophysiology of pain from, 229
of spine, nerve root compression
from, 234

Fragilitas ossium, 847
Franconi syndrome, 758–759
Freckles, 829, 843
Freiberg-Kahler's disease, 221
Frenzel glasses, 711n
Friction rub
in hepatoma, 170
and splenic infarct, 170
Friedrich's ataxia, 718
"Frölich's syndrome," 771
Frontal adversive seizure, 664
Frontal lobe pathology, fatigue vs., 618
Frostberg's reversed-3 sign, 430, 431f
"Frozen shoulder," 219, 240
Fructose intolerance, 758
Functional disorders, defined, 14, 15
Fungus infection
and calcification of lymph nodes, 510
of lungs, 324–325
hemoptysis in, 332–333
Furunculosis and hearing impairment in
external ear, 108
Fusimotor hypotonia, cerebellar symp-
toms and, 680
Fusospirochetal infection, pharyngitis
due to, 322

Gain
in differential diagnosis of somatic
complaints, 607f
from malingering, 644
primary vs. secondary, 628, 635
Gait
cerebellar vs. vestibular lesions and,
713, 715
conversion disturbances of, 640
in cerebello-pontine-angle tumor, 110
in hydrocephalus, 721
Gait ataxia in Wernicke's encephalopathy, 721
Gallbladder
carcinoma of, 426
examination of, 426–428
jaundice and previous surgery on,
423, 425
pain from, 57
perforated, ascitic fluid and, 428
radionuclide imaging of, 172
reference of pain from, 158–160
ruptured, and peritonitis, 176
Gallbladder disease
obesity and, 770
referred shoulder pain from, 206, 219
tumors, 430
[67]Gallium-citrate scan, 172
Gallstones, 430, 431, 432f
abdominal pain and, 175

Gallstones (*continued*)
  in hereditary spherocytosis, 582
  and pancreatitis, 175
  postoperative, 423, 425
Gamma-aminobutyric acid (GABA), 598, 600
"Ganglion," 218
Ganglionic blocking agents and postural hypotension, 696
Gangrene
  in polymyalgia rheumatica, 224
  in Raynaud's disease, 228
Gas gangrene, 453
Gases, irritant, cough due to, 325
Gastrectomy
  and iron absorption, 575
  and vitamin-B_{12} deficiency, 576
Gastric acid production and iron deficiency, 800
Gastric bypass, 781, 782
Gastric cancer
  dietary factors in, 798
  hematemesis and melena in, 393, 395, 399, 400, 402, 407
Gastric carcinoid, 410
Gastric neoplasm, abdominal pain and, 170
Gastric ulcer, pain of, 173–174
Gastritis
  atrophic, 575, 576
  hematemesis and melena in, 393, 399, 400, 404, 409–410
  peptic, 169
Gastroenteritis
  pain in, 169, 174, 175
  stool inspection for, 171
Gastrointestinal bleeding. *See also* Hematemesis; Melena
  and anemia, 574, 575
  fever in, 457
  and iron loss, 794
  in vitamin-K deficiency, 555
Gastrointestinal disorders
  in diseases associated with atrophic glossitis, 127
  high K^+ loss from, 673
  and hypertrophic osteoarthropathy, 252, 253
  and nutritional deficiencies, 119
  obesity and, 778
  psychophysiological, 169, 170
Gastrointestinal function
  food-intake regulation, 775
  in mechanisms of nervousness, 594
  sore tongue and mouth and, 119
Gastrointestinal lesions, referred back pain from, 206
Gastrointestinal losses and metabolic acidosis, 757, 760

Gastrointestinal pain, physiologic factors in, 57
Gastrointestinal system
  anemia and, 569
  innervation of, 361–363
  mechanical obstruction of, 368–369
Gate-control theory of pain, 43–49
Gaucher's disease, 482
  blue sclerae in, 848–849
  general lymph node enlargement in, 522
  hypersplenism in, 549
  melanosis in, 842
  and splenomegaly, 580
Generalized anxiety disorder, 604
Generalized lymphadenopathy, 521
Generalized seizures, 663–664, 665f
Genetic factors
  in clubbing, 256
  in growth, 17–19, 30t
Genital lesion and groin lymphadenopathy, syndrome of, 518
Genitourinary schistosomiasis, 187
Genitourinary system. *See also* Urinary *entries*
  anemia and, 569
  as source of abdominal pain, 176–177
  tuberculosis of, and hematuria, 187
Gentamycin, ototoxicity of, 718
Geographic tongue, 134
German measles. *See* Rubella
Ghon pulmonary complex, 517
Giant cell (temporal) arteritis (GCA), 80
  in polymyalgia rheumatica, 224
Giant mediastinal node hyperplasia, 484
Giant nodal hypertrophy with sinusoidal histiocytosis, 483
Giddiness. *See also* Dizziness
  in vascular disorders, 720
Gigantism, 33
Gilbert's syndrome, 423, 424, 429
Gilles de la Tourette syndrome, 685
Gingival bleeding
  in idiopathic thromocytopenic purpura, 549
  in scurvy, 547
Gingival melanosis, 843–844
Gingivitis, Dilantin-induced, 130
Gingivostomatitis
  birth control pills and, 131
  herpetic, 132–133
Glanders, oculoglandular syndrome and, 496
Glanzmann's thrombasthenia, 551
Glass tongue, 130
Glaucoma
  acute, 92
  angle-closure, 92–94
  central retinal vein occlusion and, 90

muscular contraction headache in, 74
  tunnel vision and, 96
Glioblastoma multiforme, 611
"Glitter cells," 188
Globus hystericus, 642
Glomerular filtration of salt, 738–739
Glomerular insufficiency and tetany, 683
Glomerulonephritis, 272
  from allergic purpura, 545
  and hematuria, 187
Glomus in pathogenesis of clubbing, 254–255
Glomus tumor of middle ear, 716
Glossitis
  atrophic, 126–128
  in B-complex deficiencies, 124, 125, 576
  Dilantin-induced, 130
  median rhomboid, 134
  in periarteritis nodosa, 130
  syphilitic, 130
Glossitis areata exfoliativa, 134
Glossopharyngeal nerve, 715
Glossopharyngeal neuralgia, 57
  syncope in, 659
  and vasodepressor syncope, 697
Glucocorticoids
  deficiency of, water retention in, 737
  for idiopathic thrombocytopenic purpura, 549
  and purpura, 547
Glucose in nutrition of nerve cells, 238
Glucose tolerance, obesity and, 800
Glucose-6-phosphate-dehydrogenase (G6PD) deficiency, 583
Glutathione (GSH), 565
Gluten enteropathy, 127
Glycogen degradation, 672
Glycogen metabolism, thyroid hormones and, 802
Glycolytic-enzyme defects, 583
Glycoproteins
  deficiency of, in Glanzmann's thrombasthenia, 551
  in normal red-cell function, 565
  in platelet adherence, 549–550
  in platelet reactions, 537
Glycyrrhizic acid, 761
Golgi complex, 476, 479
Gonadal dysgenesis (Turner's syndrome), 18, 32
Gonadal hormones. *See* Sex hormones; *and specific hormones*
Gonadotropins, 596–597. See *also* Human chorionic gonadotropin
  ectopic production of, and sexual precocity, 39
  premature release of, 39
  selective deficiency in, 39

Gonococcal arthritis, 222
Gonococcal endocarditis, fever in, 452–453
Gonococcal inguinal adenitis, 518
Gonococcal perihepatitis, 428
Gonococcal peritonitis, 176
Gonorrhea
    extragenital, with regional lymphadenopathy, 517
    genital lesion with groin lymphadenopathy, 518
    penile lesions in, 506
    septic joints and, 216
Goodpasture's syndrome
    and hematuria, 187
    hemoptysis in, 334
"Gooseflesh" in chill phase of fever, 450
Gout
    cause of fever in, 449
    fasting and, 779
    obesity and, 778
Gouty arthritis, 215, 217, 222–223
    ankle or hindfoot pain in, 221
    foot pain in, 221, 222
Gram-negative infections
    and disseminated intravascular coagulation, 556
    endothelial damage and, 545
Grand mal epilepsy, 661f, 662, 663, 665f, 722
    conversion seizures vs., 637
Granular leukocytes in lymph nodes, 478
Granulocytes as source of pyrogen, 448
Granulocytopenia in paroxysmal nocturnal hemoglobinuria, 582
Granuloma
    eosinophilic, 327
    post-stapedectomy, 717
Granuloma inguinale and infectious lymphadenitis, 506
Granulomatous disease of childhood, 521
Granulomatous lymphadenopathy, 483
Granulopoiesis, 479
Grasp reflex, 678
Graves' disease, 609. See also Hyperthyroidism
    cervical lymph node enlargement in, 498
Gray platelet syndrome, 550
Greater petrosal nerve, 71
Grey Turner's sign, 830
Grief
    conversion pain from, 636
    fatigue in, 617
"Griping" pain, 169
Growth, 17–33
    chemical indication of, 26–27

comparing parameters of, 25, 26f
dental, 25, 27t
excessive, 33
genetic endowment and, 17–19
hormonal regulation of, 28–30
impairment of
    from chronic acidosis, 759
    clinical causes of, 30–33
    drug-induced weight loss, 793
    functional classification of, 30t
    in sickle-cell anemia, 584
    somatomedins, 801
maternal undernutrition and, 788–792
measurement of, 19–26
    body proportions, 20–21, 23t, 24t
    height, 19–20, 20–22, 23t, 24t
    normal, and age, 23t, 24t
    value of charts in, 19–20
    weight, 23t, 24t, 25–26, 28f, 29f
prenatal, 19
pubertal, 20, 21f, 22f
skeletal, 21–25, 25f, 26f
thyroid hormones and, 801
Growth hormone (GH)
    corticosteroids and, 32
    deficiency of, 30–31
    and depression, 600
    and excessive growth, 33
    and fetal development, 19
    hypothalamus and, 596–597
    non-growth effects of, 28–30
    and penile development, 34
    regulation of growth by, 28
    tissue unresponsiveness to, 32
    and undernutrition, 801
Guanethidine and postural hypotension, 696
Guillain-Barré syndrome, 235, 239, 240
Guilt feelings, pain and, 49–50
Gums, 118. See also Tongue and Mouth
    in niacin deficiency, 124
    in vitamin-C deficiency, 128
Gynecomastia, 35, 256, 428

H⁺, secretion vs. excretion of, 755
H⁺ concentration. See Acid–base regulation
Hageman trait, 554
Hair
    in anemia, 567
    color of, 816
Hairy cell leukemia, 485f, 487, 522
Hallucinations in narcolepsy, 664
Hallucinogens, 614. See also specific drugs
Hallux limitus, 221
Hallux rigidus, 216, 221
Halo depigmentation, 852

Haloperidol
    for chorea, 685
    for Gilles de la Tourette syndrome, 685
Halothane, 457
    hepatotoxicity, 424
Hampton technique, 402
Hand. See also Clubbing; and Extremity entries
    abnormalities associated with congenital cardiovascular defects, 252
    conversion symptoms, 638–640
    "osteoarthritis" in, 224
Hand, foot and mouth disease, 132–133
Hand-Schüller-Christian disease, 485f
Hannot's cirrhosis, clubbing and, 253
Hardy reflectance spectrometer, 813, 846–847
Harlequin color phenomenon, 831
Hashimoto's disease, 617
Hay fever, cough in, 326
Head
    lymph nodes of, 493–501
        cancerous metastasis, 501, 502f
        diagram, 494f
    trauma to
        coma from, 652–654
        fever from, 453
        hearing impairment from, 109
        and sensory-neural hearing loss, 111
        and sudden visual loss, 98–99
        vertigo and dizziness in, 708, 716–719, 722
Headache, 61–80. See also Migraine
    in abscesses, 78
    in allergic purpura, 545
    in aneurysms, 78
    in arteriovenous malformations, 78
    in arteritis and phlebitis, 79–80
    in anemia, 569–570
    chemicals and, 77
    classification of, 63–64
    cluster, 69–72
    CO₂ retention and, 762
    as conversion symptom, 635, 636
    in c-p-a tumor, 110
    in cranial inflammation, 79–80
    in cranial and neck structure diseases, 80–81
    drug-induced, 77
    food and, 77
    general pathophysiology of, 62–63
    hematoma and, 78
    hypertension and, 77, 271–272
    hypoxia, 77
    incidence of, 62
    intracranial, 77–79
    in meningitis, 79

Headache (*continued*)
  muscle contraction (MCHA), 72–76
  in paroxysmal nocturnal hemoglo-
      binuria, 582
  physical causes of, 77–81
  postlumbar puncture, 79
  post-seizure, 77
  post-traumatic, 74–77
  in *pseudotumor cerebri*, 78–79
  psychosomatic, 601
  in pulmonary disease, 657
  in sinusitis, 80
  steroid fever and, 455
  in subarachnoid hemorrhage, 79
  in systemic infection, 77
  temporomandibular joint syndrome
      and, 80–81
  tumors and, 77–78
  understanding of pain and, 63
  vascular, 77
  vasomotor, nasal, 77
Hearing, 101–111
  assessment of, in children, 102–106
  impairment of, 106–111
      auditory-apparatus anatomy and
          physiology, 107–108
      in brain-stem vascular disorders, 719
      in external ear, 108
      in Menière's disease, 717–718
      in middle ear, 108–109
      misdiagnosis of, in children, 106
      otologic examination, 106–107
      sensory-neural, 110–111
      in vasodepressor syndrome, 697
  normal developmental expectancies
      in, 102, 103–105t
Heart. *See* Cardiac *and related entries; and
      specific conditions*
Heart block provoked by cough, 328
"Heartburn," 173
Heart failure. *See* Congestive heart fail-
      ure
Heart murmurs in anemia, 568
Heart surgery, febrile reaction to, 456
Heat cramp, 454
Heat exhaustion, 454
Heat stroke, 454–455
Heavy chain disease, γ-chain form of,
      and generalized lymphadenopa-
      thy, 522
Heavy metal poisoning
  neuropathy from, 239
  oral lesions from, 130
Heavy work, 338
Heberden's nodes, 224, 246, 247f
  osteoarthritis associated with, 217
Hectic fever, definition of, 447
Height
  excessive, 33

measurement of, 19–20, 20–22f, 23t,
      24t, 26f
  short stature. *See* Growth, impairment
      of
Heimlich maneuver, 319
Heinz bodies, 577, 583
  in unstable hemoglobin hemolytic
      anemias, 584–585
Hemachromatosis, 844, 845t
Hemangioma(s)
  hemoptysis in, 333
  multiple, of jejunum, 410
Hemarthroses
  in congenital factor-deficiency disease,
      553
  in hemostatic failure, 543
Hematemesis, 393–418
  azotemia following, 395–397
  in cirrhosis, 407–409
  endoscopy and selective angiography
      for, 402, 404–405
  in esophagitis, 409–410
  etiology of, 397, 399
  fever and, 397
  in gastritis, 409–410
  in hiatal hernia, 410
  history and physical examination for,
      399–400
  in peptic ulcer disease, 405–407
  radiographic examination for, 400, 402
  severity of hemorrhage in, 394
  sources of hemorrhage in, 393
  in stomach cancer, 407
Hematocrit
  in anemia, 566
  normal range of, 563, 564t
Hematogenous osteomyelitis, back pain
      from, 199
Hematoma
  headache in, 78
  and chest muscle pain, 142
  riboflavin deficiency and, 796
  skin color in, 847
  in subarachnoid hemorrhage, 79
Hematuria, 185–188
  abdominal lymphadenopathy and, 514
  definition of, 185–186
  free hemoglobin in urine vs., 571
  in hemophilia, 553
  in idiopathic thrombocytopenic pur-
      pura, 549
  site of origin of, 186–187
  undiagnosed, 188
  from vitamin-K deficiency, 555
Hemianopsia, 97–98
  in classic migraine, 66
Hemichorea, 685
Hemic murmurs, 568, 569
Hemicontracture, conversion, 638

Hemiparesis
  and hemichorea, 685
  in migraine, 66
  "spastic," 678
Hemiplegia
  coma and, 655
  conversion, 638
  and resting tremor, 684
  shoulder pain in, 240
  in sickle-cell anemia, 570
Hemiplegic migraine, 64, 66
Hemobilia, 412–413, 426
Hemochromatosis, 223
  sex and incidence of, 426
  skin in, 426
Hemodynamic response to upright pos-
      ture, 694–696, 698
  in vasodepressor syncope, 698f, 699
Hemodynamics, 263–265
Hemoglobin
  abnormalities of, 356–357
  in normal red-cell function, 565
  O₂ affinity of, and anemia, 567
Hemoglobin concentration
  in anemia, 566
  normal range of, 563–564
Hemoglobinemia
  immunohemolytic anemia with, 581
  and red-cell recovery from burns, 581
Hemoglobinopathy(ies), 583–585. *See
      also* Sickle-cell anemia; Thalasse-
      mia(s)
  in acute abdomen, 178
Hemoglobin pigmentation, 814, 816,
      817, 819, 823f, 830–832
  classification of, 830t
  and detection of jaundice, 826
  diminished blood flow and, 853–854
  in nails, 849
  and pallor of anemia, 850
  sex differences and, 820–821, 822f
Hemoglobin saturation and partial pres-
      sure of O₂, 565f
Hemoglobinuria and red-cell recovery
      from burns, 581
Hemolysis, microangiopathic, 581
Hemolytic anemia(s), 578–585
  ankle ulcers in, 567
  autoimmune, 522, 580–581
  characteristics, 578–580
  constitutional signs in, 570–571
  enzyme defects and, 583
  fever in, 454
  hemolysis in
      microangiopathic, 581
      due to red cell antibodies, 580–581
      due to splenomegaly, 580
      due to toxins, 581
  hereditary spherocytosis, 582

membrane defects (acquired), 581–582
membrane defects (hereditary), 582
paroxysmal nocturnal hemoglobinuria (PNH), 582
pathophysiologic classification of, 571, 572t
serum bilirubin in, 429
sickle-cell, 583–584
skin color in, 850
spur-cell, 581–582
thalassemia syndromes, 577–578
in thrombotic thrombocytopenic purpura, 549
unstable hemoglobin, 584
Hemolytic jaundice, congenital, 424
skin color in, 826
Hemolytic-uremic syndrome, 549
Hemopexin, 571
Hemophilia
fever in, 454
gastrointestinal bleeding in, 399
and hematuria, 187
hemoptysis in, 333
retinal hemorrhage and, 89
Hemophilia A, 552–553
Hemophilia B, 552–553
Hemopoiesis
lymph nodes and, 469
lymphoid cells and, 479
Hemoptysis, 331–334
causes of, 332–334
localization of bleeding site in, 331–332
mediastinal lymphadenopathy and, 510
pathophysiology of, 331
sputum studies in, 332
Hemorrhage. See also organ or area involved
gastrointestinal. See Gastrointestinal bleeding; Hematemesis; Melena
inappropriate. See Pathologic bleeding
into knee joint, 220
pulmonary. See Hemoptysis
tachycardia and, 302
in factor deficiency, 554
Hemorrhagic cystitis, 190
Hemorrhagic diathesis and hemosiderosis, 846
Hemorrhagic disease of brain stem, 720, 722
Hemorrhagic disease of newborn, 555
Hemorrhagic disorders, fever in, 454
Hemorrhoids
dietary-fiber deficiency and, 797
rectal bleeding from, 170
Hemosiderin, 844–846
in anemia, 850
Hemosiderinuria in paroxysmal nocturnal hemoglobinuria, 582

Hemosiderosis, 844
pulmonary hemoptysis in, 333
of lower legs, 844–846
in scurvy, 838
Hemostasis, normal, 535–542
cellular (platelet) component of, 536–539
failure of. See Pathologic bleeding
laboratory evaluation of, 542–543
plasmatic (coagulation) component of, 536f, 539–542
three components of, 536f
vascular component of, 535–536
Henderson-Hasselbalch equation, definition of, 748
Henle's loop, normal function of, 739
Hennebert's sign, 717
Henoch-Schönlein syndrome, 545–547
Heparin, 543
and migraine, 68
Hepatic. See also Liver
Hepatic artery, aneurysm of, 410
Hepatic cirrhosis. See Cirrhosis
Hepatic coma, 657
Hepatic ducts, iatrogenic stenosis of, 431, 435f
Hepatic encephalopathy in spur-cell anemia, 581
Hepatic foetor, 426
Hepatic lymph, 469
Hepatic metastases
friction rub and, 170
pain from, 169
Hepatitis
age and sex and, 426
anorexia in, 369
drug-induced, 423–425
halothane, 457
fatigue in, 617
jaundice from, 423–425
liver function tests and, 429, 430
neonatal, 581
palpability of spleen in, 428
polyarticular pain in, 221
post-transfusion, 424
testicular atrophy and gynecomastia in, 428
tests for, 429
Hepatobiliary disease, pruritis in, 870–871
Hepatocellular disease, jaundice and, 426
Hepatolenticular disease, athetosis and tremor in, 684
Hepatoma
arterial murmur in, 428
ascitic fluid in, 428
friction rub in, 170
sex and incidence of, 426

Hepatomegaly
abdominal pain from, 175–176
alcoholism and, 424
anemia and, 570
clubbing and, 253
in neuropathy of amyloidosis, 239
Hepatosplenomegaly in lepromatous leprosy, 522
Hereditary hemorrhagic telangiectasia (HHT), 547
Hereditary nephritides and hematuria, 187
Heredofamilial tremor, 684
Hermansky-Pudlak syndrome, 550
Hernia. See also Hiatal hernia
pain from, 169
strangulated, 380
umbilical, 170
ventral, 380
Herniated intervertebral disk, 234
radicular pain from, 242
Heroin (diacetylmorphine), 13, 660
coma from, 660
and generalized lymphadenopathy, 522
and pruritis, 873
Herpangina, 132, 133
Herpes
encephalitis, mental symptoms in, 612
opportunistic lung infection with, 325
Herpes genitalis, 506
Herpes simplex
as complication of fever, 451
gingivostomatitis in, 132
labyrinth involvement in, 717
Herpes zoster
intercostal pain in, 141
nerve root infection, 233, 234
oral lesions in, 132
peripheral nerve involvement, 238
Ramsay-Hunt syndrome, 495
Herpes zoster ophthalmicus, anterior auricular lymphadenopathy in, 495
Herpes zoster oticus, 717
brain-stem involvement of, 721
localization in eighth nerve, 719
Herxheimer reaction, 518
Heterochromatic bead (chromatic body), 17–18
Heterochromic iridis, 849
Hexose-monophosphate (HMP) shunt, 122
enzyme defects in, 578–579, 583
Hiatal hernia, 147
dietary-fiber deficiency and, 797
hematemesis and melena in, 399, 410
HIDA scan in jaundice, 423, 431
High-molecular-weight kininogen (HMWK), 539–541, 554, 555

Hilar adenitis from lung infection, 509
Hilar lymph nodes, 508
    Boeck's sarcoid and, 500
    lymphadenopathy in, 509–511
Hip disease, knee pain from, 221
Hip joint pain, 211, 216, 219–220, 242–243
    arthritic, lumbar sympathectomy and, 215
    in degenerative joint disease, 216
    physiology of, 214, 215
Hiroshima hemoglobin, 357
Hirschsprung's disease, constipation in, 379
Histamine
    in cluster headache, 70, 71
    and itch, 865–868
    in migraine, 68
Histidine and metabolic acidosis, 757
Histiocytic lymphomas, 486, 487
Histiocytic medullary reticulosis, 485f, 486
    and generalized lymphadenopathy, 522
Histiocytic proliferation, 483
Histiocytosis, malignant, 486
Histiocytosis X, 485f, 487
Histoplasmosis, 324, 483
    and calcification of lymph nodes, 510
    mediastinal lymph node enlargement in, 509
    oral lesions in, 133
    right middle lobe syndrome in, 327
History, taking of, 1–4, 6–10, 12–13
HLA-B27 histocompatibility antigen, 200
Hoarseness, 112–113
    in hypothyroidism, 566
    from mediastinal lymph node enlargement, 511
Hodgkin's disease, 484–486
    abdominal, clubbing and, 253
    abdominal lymphadenopathy and, 514, 515
    calcification of lymph nodes in, 510
    cough in, 320
    difficulty of diagnosis of, 481
    epitrochlear node involvement in, 504
    fever in, 454, 455f
    and herpes zoster, 141
    histiocytic proliferation and, 483
    lymphoma, 496
    mediastinal lymphadenopathy in, 150, 509
    melanosis in, 838
    ostalgia in, 142
    pruritis in, 871
    and vitiligo, 851
Hoffman's sign, 240
Home visits, 7

Hoover test, 638, 639f
    in malingering, 644
Hormones. See also Endocrine entries; and specific hormones and glands
    in cluster headache, 71
    and "emotional brain," 595f, 596–597, 599–600
    in fetal development, 19
    and food-intake regulation, 775
    in genesis of migraine, 68
    genetic factors in tissue unresponsiveness to, 32
    and melanosis, 838–840, 841f
    psychological defenses and, 600
    regulation of growth by, 28–32
    and stress, 600–601
    undernutrition and, 801–803
Horner's syndrome
    heterochromic iridis with, 849
    with superior sulcus tumors, 235
Horse serum and neuritis of brachial plexus, 235
Human chorionic gonadotropin (HG)
    and puberty failure, 37
    in sexual development, 33–35
Humoral immunity, 479
Humoral changes and migraine, 68
Hunger, 363–364. See also Starvation
Huntington's chorea, 685
    ballism vs., 685
    dystonic rigidity in, 681
    early psychiatric symptoms of, 613
    GABA levels in, 600
Hydantoin-type anticonvulsant drugs, lymphadenopathy from, 522
Hydralazine, 697, 793
    and lupus inhibitor, 558
Hydrargyria, 845t, 846
Hydration and petit mal, 663
Hydroencephalus, 651
    gait problems in, 721
    in meningitis, 79
    ophthalmic nerve and, 714
    projectile vomiting and, 367
Hydrocortisone and melanin production, 839, 841f
Hydronephrosis, iliac lymphadenopathy and, 514
Hydroquinone, 852
Hydrostatic pressure in edema formation, 741–744
Hydroxyproline, urinary, as growth indicator, 27, 29f, 31
Hyperadrenocorticism, 673
    and growth failure, 31–32
Hyperaldosteronism, 673
Hyperalgesia
    in peritonitis, 174
    referred pain and, 166, 168

Hyperalimentation, intravenous, 757
Hyperbilirubinemia
    ineffective erythropoiesis and, 565
    of newborn, skin icterus in, 827
Hypercalcemia in pancreatitis, 370
Hypercalciuria, 683
Hypercapnea in obesity, 777
Hyperchloremic metabolic acidosis, 756–759
Hypercortisolism, 547
Hyperdynamic beta-adrenergic circulatory state, 612
Hyperemesis gravidarum, 370
Hyperesthesia
    conversion, 638
    in polyneuritis, 240
    of soles of feet, 570
Hyperexcitability, cerebral, 647, 648
Hypergammaglobulinemia and renal tubular acidosis, 759
Hyperglobulinemia and hematuria, 187
Hyperglycemia
    diabetic neuropathy and, 238
    in pancreatic cancer, 425
Hyperinsulinism
    coma from, 652
    muscle impairment from, 672
    obesity and, 777
Hyperkalemia
    isolated hypoaldosteronism in, 740
    in respiratory acidosis, 762
Hyperkeratosis
    in arsenic poisoning, 842
    in pellagra, 838
Hyperkinetic heart syndrome, 612
Hyperlipidemia
    carotenemia in, 828
    labyrinthine disturbance and, 719
    obesity and, 777
    plasma water in, 736
Hypermenorrhea, 566
Hypermetabolism
    and nutritional deficiency, 120
    from "rainbow" treatment of obesity, 780
Hypernephroma
    chills and, 450
    fever in, 453, 454
Hyperparathyroidism, 27
    anorexia, nausea and vomiting and, 370–371
    and cataracts, 95
    distal renal tubular acidosis in, 759
    hypertension in, 272, 284
    pancreatitis and, 370
    in uremic pruritis, 869
Hyperpathia (afterpain), 55
Hyperphagia, 366
Hyperphosphatemia and tetany, 683

Hyperplasia, 81
    follicullar, 483
    giant mediastinal node, 484
    lipomelanotic reticular, 522
    oral, 133
    paracortical, 483
Hyperpnea, 335
    brain-stem lesions and, 651
    in cardiac disease, 343
Hyperproteinemia, plasma water in, 736
Hyperreflexia
    in spasticity, 678
    in upper motor neuron syndrome,
        676–678
Hypersomatotropism, 33
Hypersomnia, 651
    in encephalitis, 655
Hypersomnolence in Pickwickian syn-
        drome, 659
Hypersplenism, 549
    in hairy cell leukemia, 487
    jaundice from, 429
Hypertension, 261–289
    adrenal, 281–284
    amphetamines and, 780
    atrial fibrillation and, 308
    atrial flutter and, 307
    benign intracranial, 78–79
    biguanides and, 780
    borderline, 270
    and central retinal vein occlusion, 90
    consequences of, 265–267
    diastolic, 270–271
    and dissecting aneurysms, 160
    essential, 277–278
    evaluation of patient with, 271–277
    fixed, 270
    hemodynamics of, 263–265
    hemoptysis caused by, 334
    labile, 270
    lacunes and, 720
    malignant, and hematuria, 187
    oral contraceptives and, 278–279
    obesity and, 777
    in pheochromocytoma, 612
    portal, 400
    psychosomatic, 601
    pulmonary
        amphetamines and, 780
        syncope with, 693–694
    pulmonary venous dyspnea and, 343
    renal, 279–281
    secondary, 277–278
    systolic, 270–271
    treatment of, 284–288
        goal of, 271
        lifestyle changes, 284–285
        pharmacologic, 285–286
        rationale for, 267–270

    renin-antiotensin system and,
        286–288
Hypertension headache, 77
Hypertensive emergencies, 288–289
Hypertensive encephalopathy, 77
    coma in, 655
Hyperthermia. See also Fever
    anesthesia and, 457–458
    brain-stem lesions and, 651
    fever distinguished from, 442, 447, 448
    habitual, 459
    malignant, 457–458
    neurogenic, 453
Hyperthyroidism
    anxiety and, 609
    atrial fibrillation in, 308
    circulatory response to, 299–300
    diarrhea in, 387
    distal renal tubal acidosis in, 759
    and erythropoietin, 573
    fatigue in, 617
    general lymph node enlargement in,
        522
    melanosis in, 840
    and nutritional deficiency, 119
    periodic paralysis and, 673
    and polyneuropathy, 238
    pruritis in, 871
    from thyroid hormone administration,
        780
    tremor of, 685
    vitiligo in, 851, 852
    vomiting in, 371
Hyperthyroid myopathy, 672
Hypertonicity of blood and antidiuretic
        hormone release, 736
Hypertrophic osteoarthropathy, 245–257
    associated underlying diseases and,
        249–250, 252–253
    clinical features of, 246–250
    definition of, 245
    laboratory test findings in, 250
    pathogenesis of, 253–257
    pathology of, 253
    radiographic findings in, 250–252
    relationship to clubbing, 245–246, 248,
        252
Hyperuricemia
    fasting and, 779
    and gouty arthritis, 222
Hyperventilation, 335
    in anemia, 344
    brain-stem lesions and, 651, 652
    in cardiac disease, 343
    with coma, 656
    as conversion symptom, 625, 629, 632,
        637
    and dehydration, 732
    neurogenic, 345

    and petit mal, 663
    psychogenic, 343
    and respiratory alkalosis, 763, 764
    and syncope, 691, 702
    in vasodepressor syncope, 697
Hyperventilation syndrome, 613
    hypocalcemia vs., 610
Hypnotics, withdrawal from, 614
Hypoalbuminemia, 849
    in cancer, 795
Hypoaldosteronism, isolated, 740
Hypocalcemia, 610
    and tetany, 683
Hypocapnia, syncope from, 702
Hypochlorhydria in diseases associated
        with atrophic glossitis, 127
Hypochondriasis, 607f, 608–609
    conversion differentiated from,
        643–644
Hypoesthesia, stocking, 570
Hypoexcitability, cerebral, 647, 648
Hypoglycemia, 610
    from chlorpropamide therapy, 734–735
    diabetic neuropathy and, 238
    hunger and, 363
    and obesity, 772, 777
    and petit mal, 663
    placental deprivation and, 19
    symptoms of, 702
Hypoglycemic agents, 780
Hypoglycemic coma, 657
Hypogonadism
    hypothalamic tumors and, 39
    idiopathic hemochromatosis and, 844
    malnutrition and, 803
    and obesity, 771, 773
    in puberty failure, 37–38
    U:L ratio in, 21
Hypogonadotropism, 37–38
Hypokalemia
    coma and, 657, 658
    in metabolic alkalosis, 761
    perioidic paralysis and, 673
    in primary aldosteronism, 272
Hypokalemic alkalosis from "rainbow"
        treatment of obesity, 780
Hypokinia
    in Parkinsonian rigidity, 679
"Hypometabolic" obesity, 780
Hyponasality, 114
Hyponatremia, 731
    circulatory insufficiency and, 736–737
    coma and, 657
    from "rainbow" treatment of obesity,
        780
    water excess and, 736
Hypoparathyroidism
    and pseudotumor cerebri, 78
    tetany in, 683

Hypophyseal portal system, hypothalamic releasing factors and, 596–597

Hypopituitarism
bone development in, 25
dental development and, 25
growth hormone deficiency and, 30–31
pallor in, 839

Hypoplasia, megakaryocytic, 547–548

Hypoplastic anemia
hemoptysis in, 333
mouth in, 129

Hyporeflexia in upper neuron lesion, 676

Hypotension. *See also* Orthostatic hypotension; Postural hypotension
in acute abdomen, 178
dizziness and, 720
in metabolic acidosis, 759
referred cardiac pain and, 158
as stimulus for antidiuretic hormone, 736
and syncope. *See* Syncope, from reduced cerebral blood flow

Hypothalamic diabetes insipidus, 734–735

Hypothalamus
and cluster headache, 71
in emotional-brain circuitry, 595f, 596–597, 599f
and obesity, 771, 773–775
in pubertal process, 34
and sexual precocity, 39
in thermoregulation, 443–444, 447–448, 458
tumors of, 771
anorexia and, 367

Hypothermia
in elderly, 446
limit of, compatible with life, 446
in myxedema with coma, 657

Hypothyroidism, 566
bone development and, 25, 31
congenital. *See* Cretinism
dental development and, 25
diagnosis of, 617
and erythropoietin, 573
heart rate in, 300
labyrinthine disturbance in, 719
muscle impairment in, 672
obesity in, 771–772
pallor in, 853
pruritis in, 871

Hypotonia, 773

Hypotonic infant, 672

Hypotonicity of blood, circulatory failure and, 736

Hypoventilation
with coma, 656
in Pickwickian syndrome, 659
in pulmonary disease, 657

Hypovolemia
and antidiuretic hormone, 736
from fasting, 779
in salt lack, 740
and syncope, 695–696

Hypoxemia, 352, 553
in pulmonary disease, 657
in respiratory acidosis, 762
and respiratory alkalosis, 763
vomiting and, 367

Hypoxia, 352–354
and syncope, 702–703

Hypoxia headache, 77

Hypsarrhythmia, 660

Hysteria. *See also* Conversion symptoms
hyperventilation in, 702
tunnel vision in, 96
unconsciousness in, 637, 660
use of term, 624

Hysterical epidemics, 626, 643

Hysterical personality features, 631–633

"Icteric conjunctivitis," 826

Icterus. *See* Jaundice

Icterocyanosis, 352

Ichthyosis, 457

Idiopathic atrophic gastritis, 127

Idiopathic hemachromatosis (IH), 844, 845t

"Idiopathic hematuria," 188

Idiopathic steatorrhea, 174

Idiopathic thrombocytopenic purpura (ITP), 548–549

IGF-I, 30, 32

IgM secretion in lymphomas, 487

Ileitis, regional. *See* Regional ileitis

Ileus, 170
in metabolic acidosis, 759
in metabolic alkalosis, 761
renal pain and, 184
resection of, and vitamin-B_{12} deficiency, 576
ureteral pain and, 185

Iliac lymph nodes
anatomy of, 511–513
clinical significance of, 514, 515

Iliac lymphadenitis, 507

Imipramine
blocking of anxiety by, 596
and temperature, 458

Immune response, lymphoid cells and, 479–480

Immunoblastic lymphadenopathy, 522

Immunodeficiency diseases, hereditary, 481–482
normal maturation and, 482t

Immunoglobulin(s), 478–480
as inhibitor of coagulation, 558
in lymphoid system, 469

Immunohemolytic anemia, 580–581

Immunologic destruction of platelets, 548–549

Immunologic disorders
and fetal growth, 19
psychosomatic, 601

Immunologic injury, vascular, 545–547

Immunosuppressive therapy
and herpes zoster, 141
and susceptibility to infection, 216

"Impingement syndrome," 219

Impotence in Shy-Drager syndrome, 701

Impulse propagation, 648

Inanition fever, 455

Incontinence in Shy-Drager syndrome, 701

Indanedione anticoagulants, 554–555

Indomethacin and tumor-related fevers, 453–454

"Industrial canaries," 828

Infantile motoneuron disease, 672

Infectious diseases. *See also specific conditions*
axillary lymphadenopathy and, 502
dizziness in, 721
edema formation in, 742–743
of mother, and epilepsy, 663
nausea and vomiting in, 368
nervousness and fatigue in, 593, 617
postoperative fever from, 457

Infectious mononucleosis
adult-acquired toxoplasmosis vs., 522
combined paracortical and follicular hyperplasia in, 483
fatigue in, 617
and generalized lymphadenopathy, 522
and mediastinal lymphadenopathy, 509
as lymph node syndrome, 518

Inferior deep lymph nodes, 497–498

Inflammatory disorders. *See also specific conditions*
anemia in, 573
cough in, 320, 322–324
diarrhea in, 382
edema in, 741–743
growth failure and, 33
hemoptysis in, 332–333
intra-abdominal, 369–370
of lymph nodes, 482–484

of lymphoid system, lymphadenopathy and, 490
and splenomegaly, 580
Influenza
fatigue in, 617
fever in, 451
tracheobronchitis in, 322
Influenza virus and acute hemorrhagic cystitis, 190
Infraclavicular lymphadenitis, 503–504
Infraorbital lymph nodes, 494f, 500
occuloglandular syndrome and, 496
Infrapatellar fat pad, injury to, 220
Infrared photography and skin color, 813
Ingravescent pain in migraine, 65, 66
Inguinal adenitis, 504, 506
Inguinal lymph nodes, 484, 504–507
Burkitt's lymphoma and, 487
Inhibitors (anticoagulants), 539, 541–543
and coagulation disorders, 551, 557–558
Innominate-artery aneurysm, clubbing and, 253
Inoculation
and axillary lymphadenopathy, 502, 503
extremity lesion and regional lymphadenopathy from, 517–518
and generalized lymphadenopathy, 522
inguinal adenitis from, 506–507
and neuritis of brachial plexus, 235
Inoculation lymphoreticulosis. See Cat-scratch disease
Inoculation tuberculosis
axillary lymphadenopathy and, 502
epitrochlear lymphadenopathy and, 504
Insect bites
abdominal pain from, 177
and hemolysis, 581
Insecticides, neuropathies from, 239
Inspiratory cramp, brain-stem lesions and, 651
Insulin
adverse reactions to, 12
in malnourishment, 802–803
Intention tremor, 680
Intercostal muscles in referred cardiac pain, 158
Intercostal nerve pain, 141
"Intercurrent gout," 222
Interleukin-1 (IL-1), 450
Intermittent claudication, 230
Intermittent (Pel-Ebstein or relapsing) fever, 451, 453, 454, 455f
abdominal lymphadenopathy and, 514
definition of, 447

Interstitial cell-stimulating hormone (ICSH), 596–597
Interstitial fluid
definition of, 726, 744
dehydration of, 740–741
in edema, 741–744
Interstitial hypertrophic neuropathy, 239
Interstitial nephritis, and hematuria, 187
Intertracheobronchial lymph nodes, 508
Intervertebral disks
disease of
osteoarthritic, 224
shoulder and arm pain in, 219, 240
herniated, 234
radicular pain from, 242
lesions of, back pain from, 200–204
protrusion of, in lumbar spinal stenosis, 204
Interview, patient–physician, 1–6, 630–631
Intestinal blind-loop syndromes, 126, 385, 576
Intestinal colic, 169
Intestinal disorders. See also specific disorders
abdominal pain from, 173–175
low back pain from, 207
psychosomatic, 601
Intestinal lipodystrophy, 127
Intestinal lymphangiectasis, 172
Intestinal lymphoid aggregations, 468, 470
Intestinal obstruction
abdominal lymphadenopathy and, 513, 514
and acute abdomen, 177
history of, and abdominal pain, 170
pain of, 167, 169, 174
renal-ureteral pain from, 185
vomiting due to, 369
Intestinal trunk, anatomy of, 474–475
Intestinal tuberculosis, clubbing and, 253
Intestine. See Large intestine; Small intestine
Intoxication. See also specific agents and conditions
nervousness from, 614
Intra-abdominal lymph nodes
anatomy of, 511–513
clinical significance of, 513–515
clinical syndromes, 516–517
Intracellular fluid
buffering mechanisms and, 749–750, 749–751f
definition of, 726, 744
Intracerebral hematoma, 79
Intracranial (traction) headache, 77–79

Intracranial hemorrhage in hemophilia, 553
Intracranial injury, 76
Intracranial pain, 57
Intracranial pressure
behavioral symptoms of, 611
in cerebello-pontine-angle tumor, 110
EEG and VFP findings in, 652
signs of, 654
Intracranial vasoconstriction in migraine, 67
Intraocular pressure. See also Glaucoma
treatment of occluded central retinal artery and, 87
Intrathoracic pressure and syncope, 695
Intravascular fluid, definition of, 726, 744
Intravenous hyperalimentation, 757
Intravenous urography, 187
Intrinsic factor, 126
and vitamin-B_{12} deficiency, 576
Intussusception, 380
from allergic purpura, 545–547
mesenteric lymphadenitis and, 517
retrograde jejunogastric, 412
Iodides, fever from, 458
Iridocyclitis, 133
Iris
atrophy in Shy-Drager syndrome, 701
color changes in, 849
Iritis, 94
Iron deficiency, 120, 574–575, 793–794
and anemia in pregnancy, 790–791
and atrophic glossitis, 127
chronic renal disease and, 573
in elderly, gastric acid production and, 800
gastrointestinal symptoms in, 569
pruritis in, 872
Iron excess, 844
Iron metabolism, 574–575
Iron pigmentation, 845t, 846
Irritability
in anemia, 569–570
in niacin deficiency, 123, 124
in post-traumatic syndrome, 75
in riboflavin deficiency, 124
Irritable bowel syndrome, 170, 174, 387, 390
Irritant gases, cough due to, 325
Ischemia. See also specific conditions
in anterior tibial compartment syndrome, 243
of calf muscles, 243
cerebral. See Syncope, from reduced cerebral blood flow
cutaneous changes from, 228
skin color and, 816–817

Ischemic attacks, headaches and, 77
Ischemic heart disease, lethargy and fatigue in, 617–618
Islet tumors and obesity, 772
Isoantibodies, thrombocytopenia due to, 549
Isoniazid
    and anemia, 793
    and factor-XIII inhibition, 558
    fever from, 458
    and jaundice, 424
    and niacin deficiency, 793
    psychiatric disturbances from, 614
    and sideroblastic anemia, 577
Isoproterenol, 615
Isothenuria, sickle-cell anemia and, 569
Itard-Cholewa's sign, 109
Itching. See Pruritis

Jacksonian seizures, 661, 664
Jarisch-Herxheimer reaction, 458
Jaundice (icterus), 423–433
    abdominal findings in, 427f
    abdominal lymphadenopathy and, 513–515
    anemia and, 570–571
        spur-cell, 581
    classification of, 423–424
    clinical approach to, 424–430
        duodenal drainage, 423, 430
        history, 424–426
        liver profile, 429–430
        minilaparotomy, 430
        physical examination, 426–429
        prothrombin response to vitamin K, 430
        routine tests, 429
    cyanosis and, 352
    definition of, 423
    hematemesis and melena and, 400
    in hereditary spherocytosis, 582
    in infectious hepatitis, 221
    melanosis in, 838
    needle biopsy of liver in, 423, 431–433
    neonatal, 827
    in pancreatic carcinoma, 170
    in pancreatitis, 175
    percutaneous transhepatic cholangiography in, 171–172
    radiologic procedures in, 430–433, 431–437f
    retrograde endoscopic cannulation in, 171
    simulated by effects of chemicals and drugs, 828–829
    skin color in, 823–827
    unilateral, 826–827, 853

Jaw claudication in giant cell arteritis, 80
"Jaw-wiring," 781
J-Cape Town hemoglobin, 357
Jejunal diverticulosis, 385–386
    hematemesis and melena from, 410
    and vitamin B_{12} deficiency, 576
Jejunoileal bypass, 781
Jejunum
    and food-intake regulation, 775
    multiple hemangiomas of, 410
Jervell and Lange-Nielsen syndrome, 692
Joint capsule
    anatomy of, 211–213
    pain sensitivity of, 214
Joint hemorrhage in hemophilia, 552–553
Joint (and periarticular) pain, 56, 211–225, 229. See also specific joints
    in allergic purpura, 545
    altered function from neuropathy and, 236, 237
    anatomic considerations in, 211–214
    ankle, 221
    apophyseal, 200
    definition of, 211
    degenerative joint changes and, 223–224
    diagnostic considerations in, 215–216
    elbow, 218
    finger, 217–218
    foot, 221
    gouty arthritis and, 222–223
    hip, 219–220
    in hypertrophic osteoarthropathy, 248
    in infectious arthritis, 222
    knee, 214, 215, 220–221
    monoarticular, 216–221
    in nonarticular rheumatism, 224–225
    and pain in extremities, 230–231
    pathogenesis of, 215
    physiologic considerations in, 214–215
    polyarticular, 221–224
    rheumatic fever and, 222
    rheumatoid arthritis and, 223
    sacroiliac, 200
    shoulder, 218–219
    systemic disease and, 221
    systemic disorders and, 221
    unexplained, 224–225
Joints in hypertrophic osteoarthropathy, 253
Jugular trunks, anatomy of, 474
Jugulodigastric lymph node (main tongue node), 496, 498
Jugulo-omohyoid lymph nodes, 494, 498
Juvenile rheumatoid arthritis (Still's disease), 223
    change in sacroiliac joints in, 200

fever in, 457
generalized lymphadenopathy in, 522
jaundice and history of, 424

Kala-azar, 453
Kallman's syndrome, 38
Kanamycin, 111
    ototoxicity of, 718
Kansas hemoglobin, 356
Kaposi's sarcoma, 521
Karyotype, 18
Kawasaki's disease, 498
Kayser-Fleischer rings, 426
K^+ depletion
    chronic acidosis and, 759
    and respiratory acidosis, 762
    and "saline-resistant" alkalosis, 761
Kempsey hemoglobin, 357
Kenya typhus, 517–518
Keratinization, 814
Keratinocytes, 814, 834–835
Keratitis, 125
Keratoconjunctivitis, oculoglandular syndrome from, 496
Keratoderma blenorrhagica, 133
Keratoses in arsenical melanosis, 846
Kernicterus, 827
    and epilepsy, 663
Kernig's sign, 205, 235
    in meningitis, 654–655
Ketoacidosis
    as cause of metabolic acidosis, 756
    diabetic. See Diabetic ketoacidosis
    nausea and vomiting in, 370
"Ketogenic" diet, 779–780
Ketonemia, 178
Kidneys. See also Renal entries
    anatomical role of, 181
    blood urea nitrogen and, 429
    innervation of, 181–184
    pain from, 57
        localization of, 184, 185
        referred, 207
    sickle-cell anemia and, 584
    as source of hematuria, 186–187
    total obstruction of, and pyuria, 188
Kidney disease(s). See also specific conditions
    contralateral spread of cancer, 472
    neoplasms, 187
Kinins
    in inflammatory process, 215
    and itch, 865
    and migraine, 68
    in pain mechanism, 55, 63, 166
Klebsiella-Enterobacter-Serratia bacilli, 189
Klinefelter's syndrome, 35

Knee joint pain, 220–221
    lumbar sympathectomy and, 215
    physiology of, 214, 215
    sensitivity of menisci, 214
Knee pain, 243
Koilonychia
    in anemia, 567
    in idiopathic hemochromatosis, 844
Kugelberg-Welander disease, 676
Kuru, 655
Kussmaul respirations in metabolic aci-
        dosis, 759
Kwashiorkor, 789–790, 791f
    defective melanin synthesis in, 852
    growth hormone in, 801
    pancreatic insufficiency and, 383
Kyphoscoliosis
    hypoxia in, 353
    and respiratory acidosis, 762
Kyphosis, 199, 205, 206f

Labile hypertension, 270
Labyrinth
    membranous, 709f
    pathology of
        middle ear disturbances and, 716
        vertigo and dizziness and, 717–719
Labyrinthine concussion, 716, 717
Lacrimal gland enlargement, 496
Lactase deficiency, 384
    pain from, 169, 174
    peroral biopsy and, 172
Lactate
    anxiety induced by, 596
    and coronary disease, 151
Lactation, nutrition and, 119, 120, 792
Lactic acid in ischemic pain, 140
Lactic acidosis
    biguanides and, 780
    as cause of metabolic acidosis, 756
    fasting and, 779
Lactic dehydrogenase (LDH), 565
Lacunes, 720
Laennec's cirrhosis, 408
    spur-cell anemia and, 581
Lalling, 114
Lambert-Eaton syndrome, 674
Langerhans' cells, 487
Langer's arch, 503
Language, 101. See also Speech
    comprehension and use of, 112, 114
    development of
        normal expectancies in, 102,
            103–106t
        stages of, and types of aphasia, 114,
            115t
    of hysterical personality, 632

metaphorical, and conversion, 626,
        631
Laparoscopy in abdominal pain, 172
Laparotomy
    in abdominal pain, 172–173
    exploratory, in jaundice, 423
Large intestine as source of abdominal
        pain, 173–175. See also Colon entries
Laryngeal function, phonation disorders
        and, 112–113
Laryngeal hypoplasia, 31
Laryngitis, acute, 322
Lasègue's sign, 205
Laser treatment
    of central serous retinopathy, 98
    in diabetic retinopathy, 91
    in macular degeneration, 95
Lassitude. See Lethargy
Lateral epicondylitis (tennis elbow), 211,
        217
Lateral sinus thrombosis, 367
Lateral tracheobronchial lymph nodes,
        508
Laurence-Moon-Bardet-Biedl syndrome,
        773
Laxative abuse, 379
L-dopa (levadopa), 615, 679
Lead line, 845t, 846
Lead poisoning
    abdominal pain from, 177
    and eighth cranial nerve, 111
    motor impairment in, 675
    oral lesions in, 130
    sideroblastic anemia and, 577
Lean body mass, 26, 28f
    aging and, 799–800
Learning theory, 602
    on anxiety, 602–603
Left atrial myxoma, syncope in, 693
Leg. See also Extremity entries
    conversion symptoms, 638, 639f
    pain in, with foot pain, 221
    ulcerations of
        from deep venous system failure,
            228
        sickle-cell anemia and, 584
Leiomyoma, gastric, 400, 402
Leishmaniasis
    hematuria in, 187
    localized to lymph nodes, 522
Lemniscal system, 46–47
Leprosy
    granulomatous lymphadenopathy
        and, 483
    lepromatous
        generalized lymphadenopathy in,
            522
        histiocytic proliferation in, 483
        lymph node suppuration in, 521

Leptospirosis, 425
    age and, 426
    eyes in, 426
    and hematuria, 187
    tests for, 429
Lethargic encephalitis, 655
Lethargy. See also Fatigue
    anemia and, 567
    in giant cell arteritis, 80
    incidence of organic disease in pa-
        tients presenting with, 615
    in metabolic acidosis, 759
Letterer-Siwe disease, 485f
Leukemia
    bone tenderness in, 570
    fever in, 454
    and generalized lymphadenopathy,
        522
    hairy cell, 485f, 487, 522
    hemoptysis in, 333
    joint pain in, 221
    lactic acidosis and, 756
    lymphocytic, 454, 580
    methotrexate toxicity and, 125–126
    monoblastic, mouth in, 129
    myelogenous, 551, 582
    myelophthisic anemia and, 574
    organ enlargement in, 570
    ostalgia in, 142
    pallor in, 567
    pruritis in, 872
    Raynaud's phenomenon in, 228
    retinal hemorrhage in, 570
    sideroblastic anemia and, 577
    ulcerated and necrotic lesions of, 569
Leukemic infiltrates and hematuria, 187
Leukemic reticuloendotheliosis, 485f,
        487
Leukocyte endogenous mediator (LEM),
        452
Leukocytes. See also B cells; T cells
    granular, 478
Leukocytoclastic vasculitis (LCV), 545
Leukocytosis
    in alcoholic hepatitis, 424
    in appendicitis, 174
    in clinical pictures of pyuria, 191
    in iliac lymphadenitis, 507
    in jaundice, 429
    in myocardial infarction, 156
    in perforated carcinoma of colon, 175
    in perforated colon, 175
    in rheumatoid arthritis, 223
    with steroid fever, 455
    tachycardia and, 302
Leukonychia, 849
Leukopenia
    in Chediak-Higashi syndrome, 850
    in lupus erythematosus, 130

Leukoplakia, 133
Levodopa (L-dopa), 615, 679
Leydig cells, 33–34
Libido
    loss of, in anemia, 569
    obesity and, 776, 777
    protein-calorie malnourishment and,
        803
Lichen planus, 873–874
    oral lesions in, 130
Lichen simplex, 873–874
Licorice ingestion, 761
    hypertension due to, 283–284
Life expectancy, food consumption and,
    798–800
Lidocaine, 615
Ligaments
    and back pain, 204–205
    of Cooper, 519–520
    pain sensitivity of, 214
Lightheadedness
    as conversion complication, 630
    in muscle contraction headache, 73
    in post-traumatic syndrome, 75
    in respiratory alkalosis, 764
"Lightning" pains of tabes dorsalis, 234
Light scatter and skin color, 814, 815,
    846–847
Light work, definition of, 337–338
Limb ataxia, 715
Lipase, serum, in acute abdomen, 178
Lipid metabolism
    carotene and, 817
    thyroid hormones and, 802
Lipid-mobilizing agents
    "ketogenic" diet and, 779
    obesity and, 777
Lipodystrophy, intestinal, 127
Lipoma
    cancerous lymphadenopathy vs., 501
    of sucking pad, 500
Lipomelanic reticulosis, 483
Lipomelanotic reticular hyperplasia of
    lymph nodes, 522
Lipopolysaccharides, bacterial, 480
Lips
    cancer of, 472
        hemimandibulectomy in, 501
    lymphangiectasis in, 473
    morphology and physiology of,
        118–119
Liquid-calorie diets, 779
Lisch spots, 849
Lithium
    and concentration of urine, 736
    and renal tubular acidosis, 759
Liver. See also Hepatic entries
    abscess of
        fever from, 456

perforated, and peritonitis, 176
    referred shoulder pain from, 206
carcinoma of, fever from, 453
coagulation-factor production in, 540,
    555
disease(s) of. See also specific diseases
    carotenemia in, 828
    and clubbing, 252, 253
    edema in, 436, 741, 743, 744
    fatigue from, 618
    obesity and, 778
    pathologic bleeding and, 555
    red-cell morphology in, 579f
    right shoulder pain from, 219
    temperature in, 456
    tumors, 430
    examination of, 426–428
    extravascular lysis in, 578
    needle biopsy of, 423, 431–433
    new diagnostic procedures and, 171–172
    and nutritional deficiency, 119
    pain from, 57
    percussion of, 171
    sickle-cell anemia and, 584
    as source of abdominal pain, 175, 176
Liver flap, 684
Liver function tests, 423, 429–430
"Liver tongue," 129
Lobar pneumonia, 323
Locked-in syndrome, 652
Long tract signs in cervical spondylosis,
    240
Longevity, food consumption and,
    798–800
Lordotic posture, 186
Low birth weight (LBW) maternal un-
    dernutrition and, 789
Lower motor neuron syndrome, 671t
Lumbago, 205
Lumbar lordosis, 205, 206f
Lumbar puncture
    and headache, 77, 79
    for pseudotumor cerebri, 78
Lumbar spiral stenosis, 201, 204
"Lumbar sympathectomy," 215
Lumbar trunks, anatomy of, 475
Lumboperitoneal shunting in pseudotu-
    mor cerebri, 79
Lumbosacral plexus, pain from lesions
    of, 235
    foot, 242
    hip and thigh, 242
Lung(s). See also Pulmonary entries; and
        specific conditions
    abscess of, 323–324
        clubbing and, 252
        hilar lymphadenopathy and, 509
        hypertrophic osteoarthropathy and,
            249

cancer of
    hypertrophic osteoarthropathy and,
        247–249, 252, 253, 256
    Lambert-Eaton syndrome, 674
    lymphatic drainage of lung and,
        508–509
    metastatic, 326
    scalene node biopsy and, 499–500
    SIADH and, 737
fungal infections of, 324–325
opportunistic infections of, 325
Pancoast's tumor of, 150, 235, 253
parasitic diseases of, 325
referred back pain from, 206
and respiratory acidosis, 762
sickle-cell anemia and, 584
Lung-thorax system, maximal pressure-
    volume of, 318, 319f
Lupus cell phenomenon, 130
Lupus erythematosus
    autoimmune thrombocytopenia and,
        549
    disseminated
        generalized lymphadenopathy in,
            522
        oral lesions in, 129, 130
    fatigue in, 618
    fever in, 457
    and hematuria, 187
    hypothermia in, 446
    hypoxia in, 354
    and immunohemolytic anemia, 580
    jaundice and history of, 424
    and leukocytoclastic vasculitis, 545
    lupus inhibitor in, 558
    platelet autoantibodies in, 548
    and pseudotumor cerebri, 78
    and renal tubular acidosis, 759
    tachycardia in, 312
Luteinizing hormone (LH), 33, 34f,
    596–597
    in cluster headache, 71
    deficiency of, 39–40
    and food consumption, 803
Lycopenemia, 828
Lymph
    composition of, 469–470
    filtration of, 468, 478
    formation of, 469
    transport of, 471
    uncommon pathways in flow of, 472
    volume of, 471–472
Lymphadenitis, 468
    acute, 483
    of axillae and groin, 503
    iliac, 507
    infraclavicular, 503–504
Lymphadenography, 488. See also Lym-
    phography

Lymphadenopathy, 468, 480–523. *See also under specific conditions*
  age differences and, 480–481
  anemia and, 570
  Burkitt's lymphoma, 486–487
  classification of causes of, 481t
  cystic hygroma vs., 473
  diagnostic methods, 488–493
  diffuse lymphomas and, 486
  hairy cell leukemia, 487
  hereditary causes of, 481–482
  histiocytic medullary reticulosis, 486
  histiocytosis X, 487
  Hodgkin's disease and, 484–486
  immunodeficiency diseases and, 481–482
  inflammatory causes of, 482–484
  due to inflammatory reactions in lymph nodes, 482–484
  lysosomal storage diseases and, 482
  metastatic neoplasm and, 487–488
  mycosis fungoides, 487
  due to neoplastic diseases, 484–488
  nodular lymphomas and, 486
  non-Hodgkin's lymphoma and, 486
  regional, 493–516. *See also specific nodes*
    abdominal nodes, 511–517
    axillary nodes, 501–504
    epitrochlear nodes, 504
    head and neck nodes, 493–501
    inguinal nodes, 504–507
    mediastinal nodes, 507–511
    popliteal nodes, 505f, 507
  Sézary's syndrome, 487
  syndromes, 517–522
    breast cancer, 518–520
    extremity lesion, 517–518
    generalized lymphadenopathy, 521–522
    genital lesion, 518
    oropharynx lesion, 518
    suppuration, 520–521
  Waldenström's macroglobulinemia, 487
Lymphangiectasis, 473, 474
  intestinal, 172
Lymphangiography, 483, 488. *See also* Lymphography
Lymphangioma, 473, 509
Lymphangiomyoma, retroperitoneal involvement in, 513
Lymphangitis, 468, 470, 472–473
  clubbing and, 253
  and obstruction of lymphatic vessels, 474
Lymphangitis carcinomatosum, 487
Lymphatic capillaries, 469–470. *See also* Lymphatic vessels
  anatomy of, 470–471

  dilatation of, 473
  in lymphangitis, 473
Lymphatic drainage, 471
  of abdominal cavity, 511–513
  areas lacking, 472
  of lower extremity, genitalia, and lower abdomen, 504–507, 512f
  of lungs and mediastinum, 500, 508–509
  of mammary gland, 519f
  of submaxillary nodes, 497
  of upper extremity, 501–502, 503f, 504
Lymphatic edema, 473–474, 741, 743–744
Lymphatic nevus, 473
"Lymphatic system," 468
Lymphatic vessels, 470–476. *See also* Lymphatic drainage
  anatomy of, 468, 474–475, 508f, 512f
  chylous effusions, 475–476
  dilatation of, 473
  lymphography of, 488–492
  main categories of disease affecting, 468
  normal structure and function of, 468, 470–472
  obstruction of, 473–474
  uncommon pathways of lymph flow, 472
Lymph nodes. *See also* Lymphadenopathy; *and specific nodes*
  age and change in, 480–481
  anatomy of, 476–478
  biopsy of, 481, 499–501
  calcification of, 503, 510, 516
  cervical, in serous otitis, 109
  functions of, 468–469, 478
  hamartoma of, 484
  histology of, 468–469, 478–480
  major categories of disease affecting, 468
  as source of lymphocytes, 470
  in tubular lymphangitis, 473
Lymphoblasts, 478–480
Lymphoceles, 473
Lymphocyte-activating factor (LAF), endogenous pyrogen and, 450, 452
Lymphocyte-depleted disease, 485, 486
Lymphocyte-predominant tumors, 485
Lymphocytes, 468–469, 478–480. *See also* B cells; T cells
  sources of, 470
  thoracic-duct injuries and loss of, 475
Lymphocytic-histiocytic tumors, 486
Lymphocytic leukemia
  fever and, 454
  and immunohemolytic anemia, 580
Lymphocytic lymphomas, 486, 487
  abdominal lymphadenopathy and, 514, 515

  and generalized lymphadenopathy, 522
Lymphogranuloma venereum, 380
Lymphography, 488–492
Lymphoid cells, 468–469, 478–480
Lymphoid system, 468–523. *See also* Lymph *and* Lymph- *entries*
  definition of, 468
Lymphoid tissue, age and, 480–481
Lymphoid tumors, vitiligo and, 851
Lymphoma(s), 484–487
  angioimmunoblastic lymphadenopathy and, 484
  cervical, 496–497
  chills and, 450
  diarrhea caused by, 385
  diminished intestinal absorption in, 795
  enlarged supraclavicular node vs., 499
  epitrochlear involvement, 504
  evolution of classification of, 485f
  fever in, 449, 454, 455f
  hypersplenism in, 549
  intra-abdominal, and malabsorption, 516
  and jugulodigastric lymphadenopathy, 496
  lymphocytic, 486, 487, 514, 515, 522
  lymphography and, 490
  parotid, 501
  pruritis in, 871–872
  scalene node biopsy and, 499–500
  and splenomegaly, 580
  and vitamin deficiencies, 127
Lymphopathia venereum, 496, 506
  acute lymphadenitis with, 483
  genital lesion with groin lymphadenopathy, 518
  and periproctitis, 507
  suppuration from, 521
Lymphorrhea, 473
Lymphosarcoma
  fever in, 454
  ostalgia from, 142
Lymph sinuses, 477
Lypodystrophy, intestinal, 385
Lysergic acid diethylamide (LSD), 13, 614
  and body temperature, 458
Lysine and metabolic acidosis, 757
Lysosomal storage diseases, 482

Macerated skin, pigmentation of, 854
Macrocheilia, 473
Macrocytes, 576
Macrocytic anemia
  with atrophic glossitis, 127
  vitamin-C deficiency and, 129

Macroglobulinemia
  general lymph node enlargement in,
    522
  plasma water in, 736
Macroglossia, 473
Macrophages
  in lymph nodes, 478–480
    inflammatory reactions, 483
  lysosomal storage diseases and, 482
  as source of endogenous pyrogen,
    448, 449
Macula in retinal detachment, 88, 89
Macular degeneration, 95
Magnesium deficiency, 794
  from excessive dieting in pregnancy,
    789
Main tongue lymph node. See Jugulo-
    digastric lymph node
Malabsorption, 119, 120, 380–387, 516
  aging and, 800
  and atrophic glossitis, 127
  in bile salt disorders, 383–384
  from biliary disease, and vitamin-K
    deficiency, 555
  of carbohydrates, 384
  drug-induced, and undernutrition,
    792, 793
  of fat, 382–383
  pathophysiology of, 380, 382
  secondary syndromes, 385–387
  of water, 384–385
Malaise
  in acute hemolytic anemia, 570
  in giant cell arteritis, 80
  in temporal arteritis syndrome, 88
Malaria
  chronic, and clubbing, 253
  fatigue in, 617
  fever in, 450, 453
Malformations, dizziness and vertigo in,
    720–721
Malignant histiocytosis, 486
Malignant hyperthermia, 457–458
Malingering, 607f, 608
  conversion vs., 635, 644–645
Mallory-Weiss syndrome, 411
Malnutrition. See also Undernutrition
  anorexia induced by, 371
  and delayed puberty, 37, 38
  edema in, 741, 743
  middle ear infection and, 109
  and polyneuropathy, 238
Malum coxae senilis. See Osteoarthritis
Mammary gland. See Breast
Manganese poisoning, Parkinsonian
    rigidity in, 679
MAO inhibitors
  and body temperature, 458
  and headache, 77

Marasmus, 789–790
  binding-globulin disorders in, 801
  growth hormone levels in, 801
March fracture, 221
Marfan's syndrome, 21, 547
  mitral valve prolapse in, 297
Marie-Strümpell disease. See Ankylosing
    spondylitis
Marijuana, 13
Marital history, 12
Marrow disease and anemia, 573–574
Marrow injury and paroxysmal noctur-
    nal hemoglobinuria, 582
"Mask of pregnancy," 840, 842
Mastectomy, lymphadema from, 474
Mastocytosis, pruritis in, 872
Mastodynia, mammary pain in, 144
Mastoid cortex in acute otitis media, 109
Mastoiditis
  bacterial, dizziness in, 721
  posterior amicular lymphadenopathy
    and, 495
Maternal deprivation syndrome, hypo-
    somatotropism and, 30
Maternal neglect. See Failure to thrive
May-Hegglin anomaly, 548
"McBurney's point," 174
MCHA. See Muscle contraction head-
    ache
Measles
  lymph node response in, 484, 522
  tracheobronchitis in, 322
Measles virus vaccine, and inguinal
    lymphadenopathy, 507
Measurements. See Growth, measure-
    ment of
Mechanical stimuli, cough produced by,
    320
Meckel's diverticulum, 410
Median nerve
  carpal tunnel syndrome, 241
  reflex sympathetic dystrophy and, 237
Median rhomboid glossitis, 134
Mediastinal emphysema, 150
Mediastinal lymph nodes, 507–511
  biopsy of, 500
  Burkitt's lymphoma and, 487
  cancer metastasis and, 519
Mediastinal pain, 57, 142, 147, 148f,
    149–151
Mediastinal tumors
  clubbing and, 249, 252
  cough due to, 326
  pain from, 142
  referred back pain from, 206
Mediastinitis, 510
Mediastinoscopy, 500
Meditation, 603
Mediterranean lymphoma, 516

Medium work, 338
Medullary lesions
  dyspnea and, 346
  and unconsciousness, 652
Medullar sponge kidney and hematuria,
    187
Medullary necrosis, 191
Medulloblastomas, 720
Mees' stripe of fingernails, 846, 849
Megacolon, 379
Megakarocytes, 536
  immunologic destruction of platelets
    and, 548
Megakarocytic hypoplasia, 547–548
Megaloblastic anemia(s), 576–577
  and atrophic glossitis, 126–127
  Dilantin-induced, 130
Melanin, 814–816
  bodily distribution of, 815
  chlorpromazine and, 847
  decreased, 833t, 850–853
  definition of, 812, 814
  hemoglobin color change screened out
    by, 830, 831
  increased. See Melanosis
  metabolism of, 832–835, 836f, 837f,
    850
  measurement of, 812–813
  racial differences and, 819–820, 830,
    831
  screened by edema, 853
  screening function of, 835–836
  sex differences and, 820, 821
  sunlight and, 815, 821–822, 823f
Melanocytes, 814, 832, 834–835
Melanocyte-stimulating hormone
    (MSH), 815, 839, 840, 841f
  and idiopathic hemachromatosis, 844
  race and, 819
Melanoid, 814
Melanophages, 814
Melanoplakia, 843
Melanosis, 832–844. See also Melanin
  in anemia, 850
  from argyria, 846
  causes of, 836–842
    external (physical), 836–838
    hormonal, 838–840, 841f
    internal (systemic), 838
    neurogenic, 841–842
    nutritional, 838n
    skin diseases, 842
  classification of disturbances, 832, 833t
  clinical picture in, 842–844
  definition of, 832
  of external membranes of eye,
    848–849
  in idiopathic hemochromatosis, 844
  in jaundice, 826

of nails, 849
oral-tissue, 238
uremia and, 829, 838
Melanosomes, 814, 834–835
abnormalities in transfer of, 852–853
Melanotic neoplasm, 843
Melanuria, 835
Melasma. *See also* Melanosis
oral contraceptives and, 821
Melasma gravidarum, 840
Melena, 393–418
abdominal lymphadenopathy and, 513
abdominal pain and, 170
azotemia following, 395–397
characteristics of, 394
in cirrhosis, 407–409
color of stools in, 394
endoscopy and selective angiography for, 402, 404–405
etiology of, 397, 399
fever and, 397, 398f
without hematemesis, 393–394
in hiatal hernia, 410
history and physical examination for, 399–400
in idiopathic thrombocytopenic purpura, 549
in peptic ulcer disease, 405–407
radiographic examination for, 400n, 402
sources of hemorrhage in, 393
in stomach cancer, 407
from vitamin-K deficiency, 555
Membranous labyrinth, 709f
Memory impairment
in post-traumatic syndrome, 75
vitamin V$_{12}$ deficiency and, 577
Menarche and pseudotumor cerebri, 78
Ménière's disease, 717–718
nausea and vomiting in, 371
sensory-neural hearing impairment in, 110
Meningeal melanosis, 842
Meningioma, 234, 611
Meningismus, 79
meningeal lesions and, 205
Meningitis
back pain and, 205
coma in, 652, 654–655
dizziness in, 721
and epilepsy, 663
headache in, 79
labyrinthine vertigo in, 717
meningococcal, herpes simplex in, 451
and nerve root inflammation, 235
projectile vomiting and, 367
in pulmonary cryptococcosis, 324
in tuberculosis of spine, 199
tuberculous, 655

Meningococcal meningitis, herpes simplex in, 451
Meningococcal septicemia, polyarticular pain in, 222
Meningococcemia, 453
Meningoencephalitis in giant cell arteritis, 80
Menkes' kinky hair disease, 789
Menopause, 610–611
oral symptoms of, 131
Menorrhagia
anemia and, 569
in idiopathic thrombocytopenic purpura, 549
Menstruation
anemia and, 569, 575
in anorexia nervosa, 803
backache from, 207
body temperature in, 446
and cluster headache, 71
endometriosis and, 187
iron metabolism and, 575
migraine and, 68
"mittelschmerz" and, 169
obesity and, 777
onset of, 35, 36
premenstrual tension syndrome, 610
pseudotumor cerebri and, 78
and skin-color changes, 821, 822f
Mental deficiency and hereditary obesity, 773
Mental lymph nodes, 494f, 500
Meralgia paresthetica, 242–243
Mercaptoamines, 852
Mercurials, fever from, 458
Mercury poisoning, oral lesions in, 130
Mescaline, 614
Mesenteric adenitis, 481
Mesenteric lymphadenitis syndrome, 516–517
Mesenteric lymphatics, 471
Mesenteric lymph nodes
anatomy of, 511, 512f, 513
clinical significance of, 514–517
Mesentery-vessel occlusion, pain from, 169, 174, 177
Mesobilirubin, 826
Metabolic acidosis, 755–760
causes of, listed, 755t
increased anion gap (normochloremic), 755–756
normal anion gap (hyperchloremic), 756–759
signs and symptoms of, 759
treatment of, 759–760
Metabolic alkalosis, 609–610, 760–762
Metabolic coma, 656–658
Metabolic disorders. *See also specific conditions*

nervousness and fatigue from, 593
and polyneuropathy, 238, 239
and polyuria, 735
Metabolic myopathies, 672
Metal fume fever, 459
Metallic pigmentation, 844–846
Metaphors, body and, 626, 629, 632
Metastasis(es), 472, 611
abdominal lymphadenopathy and, 514–515
breast cancer, 474, 502–503, 511, 518–520
facial lymph nodes and, 500
head and neck lymph nodes and, 501, 502f
to hilar lymph nodes, 509
inguinal nodes and, 505
to lung, 326
hemoptysis in, 333
lymphatic neoplasms, 487–488
lymphography, 490, 491f
mental node and, 501
of skin neoplasms in axillary nodes, 502–503
supraclavicular lymph nodes and, 498–499
of testicular tumors, 506, 512f
Metatarsal pain, 221
Methemoglobinemia, 357, 563
Methotrexate. *See* Amethopterin
Methoxyflurane and concentration of urine, 736
3-Methoxy-4-hydroxylphenol-phenyl glycol (MHPG), 598
Methyl alcohol ingestion and metabolic acidosis, 756
Methylcellulose filler compounds, 780
Methyldopa
fatigue from, 618
fever from, 458
and jaundice, 424
Metrecal, 779
Microangiopathic hemolysis, 581
Microcirculation, decreased strength of, 547
Microlithiasis, pulmonary, 334
Micropenis, 31, 34
Micturition, frequent, as psychosomatic disorder, 601
Micturition syncope, 658, 697
Midbrain lesions, dyspnea and, 345
Middle ear
conductive hearing impairment in, 108–109
infections of, vertigo and dizziness and, 716–717
lesions of, localization of, 714
surgery to, traumatic labyrinthine vertigo from, 717
tumor of, 109

Middle lobe syndrome, 510
Middle meningeal hemorrhage, coma in, 654
Migraine, 64–68
    classic, 64, 66, 67
    cluster symptoms with, 69
    common, 64, 66
    muscle contraction headache with, 73
    visual aura (scintillating scotoma) of, 66, 97
    vomiting and, 367
Migraine equivalents, 64, 67
Miliary tuberculosis
    myelophthisic anemia and, 574
    nature of fever in, 451
"Milk fever," 459
Milk intolerance, lactase deficiency and, 172
Milliosmol, definition of, 726
Milroy's disease, 473
Mineralocorticoid excess, 761
Mineral oil, 793
Minilaparotomy in jaundice, 423–424, 430
Miosis in cluster headache, 70–72
Miotic agents in angle-closure glaucoma, 92
Mitral stenosis
    atrial flutter in, 308, 397
    dyspnea in, 342, 343
    hypertension and, 272
    tachycardia in, 304
Mitral valve prolapse (MVP), 157–158, 297, 612–613
    syncope in, 693
Mitral valvulotomy, complications of, 456
"Mittelschmerz," 169
Mixed-cellularity disease, 485–486
"Moeller's glossitis," 123
Molar gland cyst, facial lymphadenopathy vs., 500
Mold infections, oral lesions in, 133
Monge's disease, clubbing and, 253
Mongolian spots, 843, 847
Moniliasis, antibiotics and, 131
Monoamine oxidase enzyme and migraine, 68
Monoamines and body temperature, 449
Monobenzyl ether of hydroquinone, 852
Monoblastic leukemia, mouth in, 129
Monocytes as source of endogenous pyrogen, 448, 449
Mononeuropathy
    ischemic, 238
    multiplex, 238, 239
    peripheral-nerve pain in, 235–236
Mononucleosis. See Infectious mononucleosis

Monoplegia, conversion, 638
Monoradicular syndromes, 233t
Monosodium glutamate and headache, 77
Monosomy X. See Turner's syndrome
Moon facies, 771
Morgani-Adams-Stokes attacks, syncope and, 691
Morphine, 48
    in acute myocardial infarction, 156
    coma from, 660
    fever from, 458
Morquio's disease, 21
Mortality, neonatal, 789
Morton's metatarsalgia, 221
Morton's neuroma, 221, 243
Motion sickness, 371
Motoneuron disease
    fasciculation in, 682
    hyperthyroid myopathy vs., 672
    muscle cramp in, 682
    neuromuscular block in, 674–675
Motor disturbances, conversion, 624t, 638–640
Motor flaccidity in metabolic coma, 656
Mountain sickness, clubbing and, 249, 253
Movement disorders, 669–670. See also under specific conditions
    anterior horn cell disease, 675–676
    ataxia, 680–681
    athetosis, 681
    ballism, 685
    chorea, 685
    clonic convulsive movements, 686
    conversion, 640
    dystonia, 681
    fasciculation, 682
    fibrillation, 681–682
    metabolic myopathies, 672
    muscular dystrophy, 670–672, 682
    due to muscular weakness, signs and symptoms of, 671t
    myasthenia, 673–675
    myoclonic, palatal, 686
    myotonia, 679–680
    neuropathology and, 669–670
    oculogyric crises, 685
    Parkinsonian rigidity, 679
    periodic paralysis, 672–673
    peripheral neuropathy, 675
    polymyositis, 672
    spasm, 682–683
    spasticity, 678–679
    torticollis and tic, 685
    tremor, 683–685
    upper motor neuron syndrome, 676–678
Mouth. See Tongue and mouth

Mouth breathing in serous otitis, 109
Mucociliary clearance of lungs, 318
Mucocutaneous lymph node syndrome, 498
Mucormycosis, 324–325
Mucoviscidosis, 383
Mucous membranes
    in anemia, 566–567
    bleeding
        in disseminated intravascular coagulation, 556
        in hemophilia, 553
        in von Willebrand's disease, 554
    buccal, 118–119. See also Tongue and mouth
    dryness of
        in dehydration, 731
        in salt lack, 740
    melanin pigmentation of, 843–844
    in niacin deficiency, 123–124
    in riboflavin deficiency, 124–125
    in serous otitis, 109
Muehrcke's lines, 849
Müller maneuver, 402
Multifocal atrial tachycardia, 310–311
Multiple mononeuritis, 675
Multiple myeloma
    anemia and, 569
    back pain from, 199
    fever in, 454
    inhibitors in, 558
    ostalgia in, 142
    and vitiligo, 851
    xanthomas with, 829
Multiple sclerosis (MS)
    dizziness in, 721
    early mental symptoms in, 613
    fatigue in, 618
    labyrinth involvement in, 718
    localized in eighth nerve, 719
    retrobulbar neuritis in, 94
Mumps, labyrinth involvement in, 717
Munchausen syndrome, 644–645
Muscle contraction headache (MCHA), 72–74
    post traumatic, 74–76
Muscle guarding, 168
    in acute gastroenteritis, 175
    in acute myocardial infarction, 156
    examination for, 170
Muscle membrane resting potential, 672–673
Muscle-phosphorylase deficiency, 672
Muscle(s). See also specific conditions
    atrophy, as conversion complication, 640
    cramps of, 682
        in metabolic alkalosis, 761
    flaccidity of, in pernicious anemia, 570

hemorrhage of, in hemophilia, 552–553
ischemia of, acid accumulation and, 140
lesions of, in back pain, 204–205
pain in
in chest wall, 141–142
in extremities, pathophysiology of, 229–230
in fibrositis, 224
rigidity of
in acute abdomen, 177
in appendicitis, 174
in biliary colic, 175
from peritonitis, 174
spasm of, 682–683
in ankylosing spondylitis, 200
in compression fracture of vertebral body, 199
intervertebral disk disease and, 201–202
meningeal lesions and, 205
in perforated carcinoma of colon, 175
in spinal column lesions, 204
in tuberculosis of spine, 199
and thermoregulation, 442, 444
twitching of, in Pickwickian syndrome, 777
weakness of
conditions causing, summarized, 671t
fatigue vs., 618
and impairment of movement, 670–672
in metabolic acidosis, 759
in myasthenia gravis, 674
in Parkinsonian rigidity, 679
periodic paralysis, 672–673
peripheral neuropathy and, 675
upper motor neuron syndrome, 676–677
Muscular dystrophy, 670–672
fibrillation in, 682
Muscular rheumatism, 204–205
Musculoskeletal disorders, obesity and, 778
Myalgia. See also Muscle(s), pain in
back pain and, 204
in giant cell arteritis, 80
steroid fever and, 455
Myasthenia gravis, 113
conversion, 640
early mental symptoms in, 613
fatigue in, 618
hyperthyroid myopathy vs., 672
hypoxia in, 353
and impairment of movement, 671t, 673–675

infantile, 672
and respiratory acidosis, 762
Myasthenic crisis, 674
Mycobacterial infections, 325
atypical, granulomatous lymphadenopathy and, 483
Mycoplasma pneumonia, 323
Mycosis fungoides, 485f, 487
and generalized lymphadenopathy, 522
pruritis in, 871–872, 873f
and vitiligo, 851
Myelofibrosis
fever in, 454
myelophthisic anemia and, 574
platelet dysfunction and, 551
Myelogenous leukemia
paroxysmal nocturnal hemoglobinuria and, 582
platelet dysfunction and, 551
Myeloma. See also Multiple myeloma
and myelophthisic anemia, 574
plasma water in, 736
Raynaud's phenomenon in, 228
Myelophthisic anemias, 574
Myelophthisis, 548
Myeloproliferative disorders, 551
and splenomegaly, 580
Myocardial contractivity, reduced,
in metabolic acidosis, 759
in respiratory acidosis, 762
Myocardial function
and angina pectoris, 151, 156
coronary blood flow and, 151–155
impaired, in neuropathy of amyloidosis, 239
Myocardial infarction, 151–153
anemia and, 568, 569
congestive heart failure with, 456
emotions and, 601
fever in, 454
pain of, 140, 152, 156–157
syncope and, 692, 693
tachycardia in, 312
vomiting with, 371
Myocardial ischemia
anemia and, 566
from fasting, 779
pain location in, 51–53
Myocarditis in lupus erythematosus, 130
Myoclonus, 686
Myofascial pain–dysfunction syndrome, 80
Myoglobinuria
free hemoglobin in urine vs., 571
in muscle-phosphorylase deficiency, 672
Myofibrositis, 204–205
Myokymia, 682, 683

Myopathy(ies), 671t
in cancer and weight loss, 795–796
distal, 672
fibrillation in, 682
metabolic, 672
and respiratory acidosis, 762
Myositis, 230
pain of, 142, 204
Myotonia, 679–680
and distal myopathy, 672
Myotonia congenita, 680
Myxedema
carotenemia in, 827
clubbing and, 253
coma with, 657
hypothyroidism and, 617
and water retention, 737
weight increase in, 772
Myxoma
of lower esophagus, clubbing and, 253
of left atrium, 456

Nails. See also Fingernails
in anemia, 567
pigmentation of, 846, 849
Nalidixic acid, 78
Naloxone, 48
Narcolepsy, 664–665
Nasal blockage
in acute otitis media, 108
in serous otitis, 109
Nasal sinusitis, 80
Nasal stuffiness in cluster headache, 70, 71
Nasal vasomotor headache, 77
Nasopharynx
adenoid tissue of, 480
carcinoma of
and cervical node enlargement, 484
posterior cervical lymph involvement, 497
serous otitis and, 109
tumors of, clubbing and, 253
Nausea, 361, 365
abdominal lymphadenopathy and, 513
in acute appendicitis, 174
in alcoholic hepatitis, 424
in angle-closure glaucoma, 92
cancer and
chemotherapy, 796
weight loss, 795
in cholecystitis, 175
with conversion pain, 635
as conversion symptom, 625, 641
with cystitis, 191
drugs and toxic agents inducing, 367–368
undernutrition and, 792

Nausea (*continued*)
 in endocrine disorders, 370–371
 history of, and abdominal pain, 170
 in intra-abdominal disorders, 368–370
 in local ototic infection, 111
 in Ménière's syndrome, 110, 371
 and migraine, 65, 66
 in migraine equivalents, 67
 in motion sickness, 371
 with muscle contraction headache, 73
 in post-traumatic dysautonomic
    cephalalgia, 75
 in pregnancy, 370
 in pseudotumor cerebri, 78
 psychic and neurologic factors in,
    366–367
 in pyuria, 191
 referred cardiac pain and, 158
 renal pain and, 184
 ureteral pain and, 185
 in vasopressor syncope, 697–698
Neck
 contractures of, conversion, 640
 diseases of, headache and, 80–81
 disk disease of, shoulder pain from,
    219
 lymph nodes of, 493–501
    cancerous metastasis to, 501, 502f
    cervical,
       deep, 496, 497–498
       superficial, 497
    diagram, 494f
    scalene, 499–500
    submental, 497
 pain in, from cervical spondylosis, 240
 stiff (nuchal rigidity)
    in meningitis, 79, 654
    in sickle-cell anemia, 570
    in subarachnoid hemorrhage, 79
Necrotizing papillitis (medullary necro-
    sis), 191
Necrotizing pneumonia, hemoptysis in,
    332
Neomycin, 111, 793
 ototoxicity of, 718
Neonatal hepatitis, spur-cell anemia in,
    581
Neonatal jaundice, skin in detection of,
    827
Neonatal mortality, fetal malnutrition
    and, 789
Neoplasia, 81
Neoplasms. *See* Tumors
Neospinothalamic tract, 46, 47
Nephritis
 in lupus erythematosus, 130
 interstitial, and hematuria, 187
 postradiation, and hematuria, 187

Nephrocalcinosis
 from chronic acidosis, 759
 and hematuria, 187
 and renal tubular acidosis, 759
Nephrogenic diabetes insipidus, 730f,
    731f, 735
Nephrolithiasis from chronic acidosis,
    759
Nephropathies, K^+ loss from, 673
Nephrosis
 obesity and, 778
 pallor in, 853
Nephrotic syndrome
 carotenemia from, 827–828
 edema in, 741, 743, 744
 factor deficiencies and, 557
Nerve entrapment. *See* Entrapment; En-
    trapment syndromes
Nerve injury and post-traumatic head-
    ache, 76
Nerve roots, 671t
 anatomy of, 231, 232f
 compression of, 234–235
    and fasciculation, 682
 pain of. *See* Radicular pain
Nervous lesions and melanosis, 841–842
Nervous mimicry, 624
Nervousness, 591–615, 618–619
 anxiety distinguished from, 592, 594,
    604
 clinical approach to assessment of,
    592–594
 differential diagnosis of, 603–615
    flow chart, 605f
    medications and drugs of abuse,
       614–615
    normal nervousness, 604
    physical disorders, 609–614
    psychological disorders, 605–609
 in niacin deficiency, 123
 pathophysiologic explanations of,
    594–601
    brain anatomy, 596–597
    rest, 601
    neurochemistry, 597–600
    stress, 600–601
 psychological explanations of, 601–603
Nervous system. *See* Autonomic
    nervous system; Central nervous
    system (CNS)
Neuralgia, 55, 57
 hyperpathia in, 55
 mimicked by entrapment neuropathy,
    237
Neurasthenia, 602, 617
Neuritides, postinfectious, 235
Neurocirculatory asthenia, 296–297, 302,
    612

Neuroendocrine disorders presenting
    with nervousness, 612
Neuroenteritis, 94
Neurofibromatosis
 Lisch spots in, 849
 melanosis in, 842–843
"Neurokinin," 68
Neurologic disorders. *See also specific dis-
    orders*
 dyspnea in, 344–346
 fatigue and, 618
 presenting with nervousness, 611–612
 vomiting and, 367
Neuromas and peripheral nerve pain,
    236
Neuromelanin, 815
Neuropathic joint disease, 217
Neuropathy. *See also specific disorders*
 ataxia from, 681
 with carcinoma, 239
 and muscular weakness, 671t
 peripheral-nerve pain, 235–240
Neurophysin, 727
Neuropsychologic syncope, 691, 703
Neuroses. *See* Psychoneuroses
Neurosyphilis, fever therapy in, 451
Neurotic excoriations, 869f, 873
Neurotransmitters, 597–600
 in migraine, 68
Neurovascular function in migraine,
    67–68
Neutropenia
 in aplastic anemia, 573
 mouth in, 129
Nevus(i)
 and depigmentation, 852, 853
 lymphatic, 473
Nevus of Ota, 847
 heterochromic iridis with, 849
Niacin
 biochemical action of, 121–122
 deficiency of, 120, 123–124, 127, 132
    drug effects and, 793
    melanosis in, 838
    and polyneuropathy, 238
    skin lesions from, 793
Nicotine withdrawal, 615
Niemann-Pick's disease, 482
 general lymph node enlargement in,
    522
Night blindness, 96, 97
Night sweats in giant cell arteritis, 80
Nitrates and headache, 77
Nitrite–nitrate syncope, 696
Nitrites
 in diet, 798
 and headache, 77
 tachycardia due to, 302

Nitrofurantoins
  and G6PD deficiency, 583
  and pseudotumor cerebri, 78
Nitroglycerin
  in angina pectoris, 156
  and headache, 77
    cluster headache, 70, 71
Nitrogen retention, growth hormone
    and, 31, 32
Nocardiosis, 324
Nociceptive-nocifensive system. *See*
    Pain, neural organization of
Node of Cloquet, 504, 505f, 512f
Node of Stohr, 497
Nodosa allergic purpura, and hematu-
    ria, 187
Nodular conjunctivitis, 496
Nodular lymphomas, 486
  lymphocytic, 504
Nodular sclerosing disease, 484–486
Noise-induced hearing impairment,
    110–111
Nonconvulsive seizures, 703
Nongaseous abdominal bloating, 642
Non-Hodgkin's lymphoma, 486, 496
  and immunohemolytic anemia, 580
  pruritus in, 871, 872f
Norepinephrine, 596, 598, 599f
  and melanocyte-stimulating hormone,
    839
  in migraine, 68
  obesity and, 777
  and spasm of arteries, 152
  stress and, 600–601
  in testing of baroreflex failure,
    700–701
  in thermoregulation, 458
Norethandrolone, 425
Normochloremic metabolic acidosis,
    755–756
Normochromic anemia in pyelonephri-
    tis, 191
Normocytic anemia, vitamin-C defi-
    ciency and, 129
Normokalemia, periodic paralysis and,
    673
North American blastomycosis, 324
Nuchal rigidity. *See* Neck, stiff
Nucleus pulposus, displacement and
    herniation of, 201–202
Nutrition
  and fetal growth, 19
  and hematuria, 186
  weight as indicator of, 25–26
Nutritional deficiency diseases, 119–129.
    See also Undernutrition; *and spe-
    cific disorders*
  atrophic glossitis in, 126–128

  depigmentation in, 853
  etiology of, 119–120
  from excessive dieting in pregnancy,
    789
  fatigue from, 618
  incidence of, 120
  multiple deficiency, 123
  pathophysiology and chemistry of,
    120–123
  and tumors, 796
Nutritional disorders. *See also* Obesity;
    and specific disorders
  edematous, hypertrophic osteo-
    arthropathy vs., 249
  and melanosis, 838
  and polyneuropathy, 238–239
Nystagmus, 710–712
  in albinism, 850
  drug-induced, 722
  labrinthine pathology and, 717, 718
  localization of vestibular lesions, 714
  in middle-ear infection, 716
  in sickle-cell anemia, 570

O_2 transport, 349–351
Oat cell tumors
  and Lambert-Eaton syndrome, 674
  syndrome of inappropriate diuretic
    hormone and, 737
Obesity, 769–782
  and back pain, 205, 206f
  breast feeding in infancy and, 792
  childhood, 33
  constipation and, 380
  cultural and social factors in, 776
  current treatments of, 778–781, 782t
  definition of, 769
  differential diagnosis of, 771–772
  in elderly, 800
  emotional and psychological factors
    in, 776
  heredity and, 773
  hip pain in, 216
  hypertension and, 284
  hypoxia due to, 353
  importance of, 770–771
  incidence of, 788
  measurement of, 770
  metabolic basis of, 773–776
  pathophysiologic complications of,
    776–778
  physiology of, 772–773
  in Pickwickian syndrome, 659
  pseudotumor cerebri and, 78
  psychological implications of, 778
  reasonable approach to, 781–782

  and respiratory acidosis, 762
  "tree" of, 774f
Obsessive-compulsive disorders, 607
Obstipation, 174, 380
  abdominal pain and, 170
Obstructive pulmonary disease
  chronic, 323
  cough in, 321
Obstructive sleep-apnea syndrome, 777
Obstructive uropathy and renal tubular
    acidosis, 759
Obtundation, 649
Occipital lymph nodes, 493–495
Occupational activity, physical tolerance
    in, 337–338
Occupational cramps, 640
Occupational history, 13
Ochronosis, 843
  blue coloration in, 847
Ochronotic pigment spots, 848–849
Ocular disturbances and Crohn's dis-
    ease, 170
Ocular dizziness, 722
Ocular melanosis, 844
Ocular oscillations, 710
Ocular palsies in Shy-Drager syndrome,
    701
Ocular phoria, 714
Oculocephalic eye movements, brain-
    stem lesions and, 651
Oculocephalic reflexes, 651, 652
Oculo-cutaneous albinism, 550
Oculoglandular syndrome, 495–496
  infraorbital node and, 500
Oculogyric crises, 685
Oculomotor nerve palsy, 79
Oculomotor system, 709–713
  functional operation of, 709–710
  lesion localization and, 714
  nystagmus, 710–713
Oculonodal complex, 496
Oculosympathetic paralysis in post-trau-
    matic headache, 75
Oculovagal syncope, 697
Oculovestibular reflexes, 651, 652
Ohm's law, 262
Oil of chenopodium and eighth cranial
    nerve, 111
Olecranon bursitis, 218
Olfactory nerve, lesion localization in,
    714
Oligodendroglioma, 611
Oncotic pressure in edema formation,
    741–744
Ophthalmic nerve, lesion localization in,
    714
Ophthalmoplegia, internuclear, 652
Ophthalmoplegic migraine, 64, 66, 78

Opiates
  coma from, 660
  constipation due to, 379
  nystagmus from, 722
  and perception of itch, 866
  withdrawal from, 615
Opioid mechanisms (endorphins),
    48–49, 63, 600
Opportunistic infections of lungs, 325
Oral contraceptives
  depression induced by, 618
  and gingivostomatitis, 131
  hypertension and, 272, 278–279
  and jaundice, 424
  and melanin, 815, 821, 840
  and migraine, 68
  nausea and vomiting induced by, 370
  and pseudotumor cerebri, 78
  and undernutrition, 795
Oral gratification and obesity, 776
Oral lesions. See Mouth and tongue
Oral temperature, normal range of, 445
Oral-tissue melanosis, 843–844
Oral tuberculosis, 497
Orange peel skin (peau d'orange), 474, 487
  mammary gland, 520, 520f
Orf virus, 518
Organic disease, definition of, 14, 15
Organic solvents and peripheral neu-
    ropathy, 239
Organ transplants
  post-operative fever in, 456
  and renal tubular acidosis, 759
Orgasmic cephalgia, 77
Oropharynx lesion with cervical lymph-
    adenopathy, syndrome of, 518
Orthopnea, 336
  in cardiac disease, 343, 344
Orthostatic hypotension, 658
  dizziness in, 720
  fasting and, 779
  Shy-Drager symptom differentiated
    from, 701
  syncope in, 691, 696, 697f, 699–701
Osgood-Schlatter disease, 220
Osler-Rendu-Weber disease, 399, 400,
    401f
Osmolality. See Solute concentration
Osmotic diuresis, 735
Osmotic fragility test, 582
Osmotic regulation, 726–731, 732f
Ossicular displacement in middle ear, 716
Ostalgia. See Bone pain
Osteitis deformans, 142
Osteoarthritis
  appearance of, in hemochromatosis,
    223
  degenerative disk disease and, 219,
    224

in first metatarsophalangeal joint, 221
  foot damage from, 221
  with Heberden's nodes, 224
  hypertrophic, hypertrophic osteoar-
    thropathy vs., 248
  obesity and, 770, 778
  pain in, 216, 217, 220–221, 223–224
    dorsal root, 142
  rheumatoid arthritis vs., 223–224
  of spine, 200–201
Osteoarthropathy, hypertrophic, 245–257
Osteochondritis of femoral head, hip
    pain from, 219
Osteogenesis imperfecta, 547
  blue sclerae in, 848–849
Osteomalacia
  in chronic acidosis, 759
  phenylhydantoin and, 795
Osteomyelitis
  with amyloidosis, clubbing and, 253
  fever in, 453
    intermittent, 451
  pain in, 142, 229
  sickle-cell anemia and, 584
  vertebral, back pain from, 199
Osteopenia and back pain, 199
Osteophyte production in lumbar spinal
    stenosis, 204
Osteoporosis, 800
  from "ketogenic" diet, 780
Ostium secundum defect, mitral valve
    prolapse in, 297
Otitis externa, 108
  dizziness and vertigo and, 716
Otitis media, 108–109
Otologic evaluation, 106–107
Otosclerosis, 109
  dizziness with, 717
Oval window, post-stapedectomy gran-
    uloma or fistula of, 717
Ovarian cancer, contralateral spread of,
    472
Ovarian cyst
  abdominal pain in, 171
  pain from torsion of, 177
Overweight. See Obesity
Ovulation, pain associated with, 169
Oxidant stress and G6PD deficiency, 583
Oxyhemoglobin pigmentation, 814, 816,
    817f, 830, 831. See also Hemoglo-
    bin pigmentation
  sex differences and, 820–821, 822f
  sunlight and, 823f
Oxytocin, 727, 728f

Pacemakers and syncope, 691, 692
Paget's disease, 27. See also Hyperpara-
    thyroidism

labyrinth investment in, 717
  pain in, 229
Pain, 41–59, 63. See also specific body sys-
    tems, organs, and conditions
  basic characteristics of, 41–43
  clinical interpretation of, 50–59
    associated physiologic aspects, 52t,
      56–57
    behavioral and psychosocial as-
      pects, 52t, 57–59
    classification of sources of input, 51,
      52t
    qualitative aspects, 52t, 55–56
    quantitative aspects, 52t, 53–54
    report of "pain" or "no pain", 50
    temporal aspects, 52t, 54–55
    topographic aspects, 51–53
  congenital insensitivity to, 54
  deep, types of, 167–168
  link with anxiety and depression, 600
  mechanism of, 140
    in MCHA, 74
    tissue tension, 140
  neural organization of, 43–49
    central control (cognitive) system,
      43–44, 47–48
    central (opioid and monopioid)
      modulating systems, 48–49
    four levels of, 43–44
    modulating (gating) spinal cord sys-
      tem, 43, 45–46
    motivational-affective (action) sys-
      tem, 43–47
    receptors and afferent fibers, 44–45,
      45f, 46
    sensory-discriminative system, 43,
      46–47
  psychological aspects of, 42, 43, 47,
    49, 50–51, 52t, 57–59. See also
    Conversion symptoms
  psychosocial development, 49–50
  radiating, 53
  referred, 166, 168
    abdominal, 166
    cardiac, 158–160
  suffering vs., 227
  understanding of, and headache, 63
  visceral vs. somatic, 140–141
Pain-proneness, 636
Palatal abnormalities, middle-ear infec-
    tion and, 109
Palatal myoclonus, 686
Paleospinothalamic tract, 47
Pallidum, therapeutic lesions in, 684,
    685
Pallor
  in anemia, 566–567, 850
  from decreased melanization, 853
  diminished blood flow and, 853–854

in edema of skin, 853
in leukemia, 567
in vasodepressor syncope, 697
Palmar erythema, 129, 428
Palmar keratoses, 846
Palpitation, 295–299
in anemia, 566, 568
in mitral valve prolapse, 297
in neurocirculatory asthenia, 296–297
organic heart disease and, 297–298
tachycardia and, 298–299, 303
Pancoast's tumor, 150
clubbing and, 253
Horner's syndrome with, 235
Pancreas
ascites of, 428
cancer of, 425, 428
abdominal pain from, 169, 170, 175, 176
and back pain, 207
fatigue from, 618
jaundice from, 426, 429
right subclavicular lymph node and, 498
sex and incidence of, 426
temperature in, 453, 454f
venous thrombi in, 428–429
diseases of
vomiting in, 369
and peritonitis, 176
pain from, 57
retrograde endoscopic cannulation and, 171
as source of abdominal pain, 175–176
tumors of, 430
jaundice from, 430, 431, 432f, 434f, 437f
and vitamin-B$_{12}$ deficiency, 576
Pancreatic-fluid loss, 757
Pancreatitis, 434f
abdominal pain in, 169, 175–176
acute abdomen from, 178
back pain from, 207
defective melanin synthesis in, 852
steatorrhea in, 382
vomiting in, 370
Pancytopenia, 547
in hairy cell leukemia, 522
Panendoscopy, 171
Panhypopituitarism, 617
in anorexia nervosa, 367
and carotenemia, 827
Panic attacks
hyperventilation syndrome vs., 613
and mitral valve prolapse, 613
Panic disorder, 604–606
hyperdynamic beta-adrenergic state vs., 612
Panniculectomy, 780–781

Pansinusitis, 721
Pantothenic acid. See also Vitamin B-complex
biochemical role of, 122
deficiency of, 125
and polyneuropathy, 238
Papain, 865, 866
Papillary necrosis and hematuria, 187
Papilledema, 93f, 94
in anemia, 570
in brain abscess, 654
ophthalmic nerve, 714
in pseudomotor cerebri, 78
in pulmonary disease, 657
Papillitis, 94, 133, 191
Para-amino salicylic acid, 793
Para-aortic lymph nodes
anatomy of, 511, 512f, 513
clinical significance, 513–515
Paracortical hyperplasia, 483
Paradoxical sleep, 650
in narcolepsy, 664–665
Paragonimiasis, 325
Paraldehyde ingestion and metabolic acidosis, 756
Paraplegia, conversion, 638
Paralysis(es)
conversion, 638–640
periodic, 671t, 672–673
in polyradiculitis, 240
and skin pattern of jaundice, 826
Paralysis agitans, 679, 683–684
Paralytic ileus, vomiting due to, 369
Paramyotonia congenita, 673
Paranoid states
conversion pruritus ani and, 642
psychomotor epilepsy and, 611
somatic delusions in, 644
Paraproteinemia, 558
pruritus in, 871
Parasitic diseases
of lungs, 325
hemoptysis in, 333
lymphedema from, 474
polymyositis secondary to, 230
Parasympatholytic agents, 615
Parathyroid fever, 452
Paravascular fibers, 44
Pareses, conversion, 638–640
Paresthesia(s)
in carpal tunnel syndrome, 241
in cervical rib syndrome, 241–242
conversion, 630, 638
in metabolic alkalosis, 761
in pernicious anemia, 570
in polyneuritis and polyradiculitis, 240
in respiratory alkalosis, 764
in sickle-cell anemia, 570
in ulnar-nerve entrapment, 241

vitamin B$_{12}$ deficiency and, 239, 576–577
Parietal lymph nodes. See Retroperitoneal lymph nodes
Parietal peritoneum, pain from, 57
Parietal pleura, pain in, 145–146
Parinaud's syndrome, 495–496
Parkinsonism, 598
drug-induced, 685
fatigue in, 618
and muscular weakness, 671t
rigidity of, 679, 683
tremor in, 679, 683–685
Paronchychia, chronic, 246, 247f
Parotid enlargement, 428
Parotid lymph nodes, 494f, 500–501
Paroxysmal atrial tachycardia (PAT), 303–305
with atrioventricular block, 305–306
Paroxysmal junctional tachycardia, 310
Paroxysmal nocturnal dyspnea, 343–344
Paroxysmal nocturnal hemoglobinuria (PNH), 548, 582
Paroxysmal ventricular tachycardia, 312–313
Paroxysmal vertigo of childhood, in migraine equivalents, 67
Parrot-beak nails, 245, 247. See also Clubbing
Partial complex seizures, 660
Partial thromboplastin time (PTT) test, 542–544
Pathologic bleeding, 543–559
in amyloidosis, 547
approach to patient, 543–545
in chemical injury, 545
classification of causal hemostatic disorders, 546t
coagulation disorders and, 546t, 551–558
factor deficiency(ies)
accelerated destruction, 555–557
accelerated loss, 557
production defect, 552–555
inhibitors, 557–558
diagnosis based upon routine screening tests, 551t
in hereditary hemorrhagic telangiectasia, 547
in heritable diseases of connective tissue, 547
in hypercortisolism, 547
in immunologic injury, 545–547
with microorganisms, 545
due to physical injury, 545
platelet disorders and, 547–551
acquired dysfunction, 549–551
congenital dysfunction, 549–551
thrombocytopenia, 547–549

Pathologic bleeding (*continued*)
  due to scurvy, 547
  due to senile purpura, 547
  vascular disorders and, 545–547
    decreased mechanical strength of
      microcirculation, 547
    direct, 545–547
Pathophysiologic diseases, definition of,
    14, 15
Pathophysiology, basic groups in, 14
Patient–physician relationship, 2–6
Peau d'orange, 474, 487
  mammary gland, 520, 520f
Pediculosis, 873–874
Pediculosis capitis
  occipital lymphadenopathy and,
    494–495
  posterior cervical lymphadenopathy
    and, 497
  and suppuration of lymph nodes, 521
Pediculosis pubis, 506
Pel-Ebstein fever. *See* Intermittent fever
Pellagra. *See also* Niacin, deficiency of
  melanosis in, 838
Pelvic examination in abdominal pain,
    171
Pelvic inflammatory disease, pain of,
    177
  abdominal, 171
  renal-ureteral, 185
Pelvic organs, referred back pain from,
    207
Pendular nystagmus, 710
Penicillamine
  and undernutrition, 792
  zinc deficiency from, 794
Penicillin
  adverse responses to, 12
  fever caused by, 458
  hypersensitivity to, tongue and mouth
    and, 131
  and immunohemolytic anemia, 581
Penis
  cancer of, as lymph node syndrome,
    518
  lesions of, and lymphadenitis, 506
Peptic esophagitis, 169
Peptic gastritis, 169
Peptic ulcer
  cluster headache and, 70
  constipation from drug treatment of,
    379
  fever in, 457
  jaundice from, 429
  melena and hematemesis in, 394, 400,
    402, 404–407
    azotemia following, 395
    BUN level with, 397
  obesity and, 778

pain in, 169, 173–174
  abdominal, 170
  referred back pain, 206
pancreatitis and, 370
perforation of
  ascitic fluid in, 428
  acute abdomen from, 178
  and back pain, 207
  and peritonitis, 176
  as psychosomatic disorder, 601
  pyloric obstruction in, 369
Peptides and emotions, 597–600
Percutancous biopsy, 172
Percutaneous transhepatic cholangiogra-
    phy (PTC), 171–172, 423, 431,
    432–433f, 435f
Perianal disease
  and Crohn's disease, 170
  examination for, 171
Periaqueductal gray (PAG), stimulation
    of, and pain relief, 48
Periarteritis nodosa
  hematemesis and melena in, 410
  oral lesions in, 129, 130
  skin changes in, 228
Periarthritis, obesity and, 778
Periarticular pain. *See* Joint pain
Pericardial effusion, 149
  in lupus erythematosus, 130
Pericardial pain, 147–149
Pericardiotomy, complications of, 456
Pericarditis
  following myocardial infarction, 157
  tuberculous, 149
Perihepatitis, gonococcal, 428
Perineal cancer, 472
Perinephric abscess, 170
  pyuria and, 188
  shoulder pain from, 185
Periodic fever, 455
Periodic paralysis, 671t, 672–673
Periodontal disease, 800
Periosteum, bone pain and, 142
Periostitis, pain in, 229
Peripheral circulatory constriction. *See*
    Shock
Peripheral cyanosis, 352
Peripheral nerves
  compression of, fasciculation from,
    682
  dermatome vs. innervation by, 231–233
  pain originating in, 235–240
    bone lesions, 229
    in diabetes mellitus, 238
    from entrapments, 236–237
    from multiple causes, 238–240
    referred to skin, 228
    from reflex sympathetic dystrophy,
      237–238

from single nerve, 235–236
  from trauma, 236
  in B-complex deficiency, 125
  in giant cell arteritis, 80
Peripheral neuropathy, 235–236, 238–240
  hyperpathia in, 55
  hypertrophic osteoarthropathy and, 249
  impaired movement from, 670, 675
  in pernicious anemia, 570
Peripheral vascular tone, loss of, and
    syncope, 696, 702
Periproctitis from lymphopathia vener-
    eum, 507
Peristaltic activity in vasodepressor syn-
    cope, 697–698
Peritoneal carcinoma, 428
Peritoneal effusions in lupus erythema-
    tosus, 130
Peritoneal tap in acute abdomen, 178
Peritonitis
  ascitic fluid and, 428
  febrile episodes with, 455
  from lymph node suppuration, 517
  muscle guarding in, 170
  pain from, 168–170
    abdominal, 174, 176
    renal and ureteral, 185
  in tuberculous mesenteric lymphaden-
    itis, 516
Perivascular plexus, 44
Perlèche, 124
Permanent threshold shift (PTS) in hear-
    ing, 111
Pernicious anemia, 565–567, 576
  and atrophic glossitis, 126, 128
  gastrointestinal symptoms of, 569
  neurologic manifestations of, 239, 570
  peripheral neuropathy in, 675
  and postural hypotension, 699
  skin color in, 850
  vitiligo with, 851, 852
Peroneal muscular atrophy, 239–240
Peroneal-nerve entrapment, 243
Peroral biopsy, 172
Peroxidase and melanin synthesis,
    832–833
Persistent jugular lymph sac, 498
Pertussis, 322
  characteristics of cough in, 321
  pneumomediastinum in, 328
  tracheobronchitis in, 322
Petechiae
  in disseminated intravascular coagula-
    tion, 556
  facial, from vomiting, 545
  in hemostatic failure, 543, 544
  in idiopathic thrombocytopenic pur-
    pura, 549
  perifollicular, in scurvy, 547

Petit mal epilepsy, 660, 661f, 663, 665f
    brain-stem lesions and, 651
    nonconvulsive seizure vs., 703
Petit mal status, 663
Peutz-Jeghers syndrome, 400
    melanosis and, 843, 844
Peyer's patches, in lymphoid system,
        468, 470
Phagocytosis of antigens in lymph
        nodes, 468, 470, 478
Phantom pain, 49
Pharyngeal tonsil, 480
Pharyngitis, acute, 322
Pharyngoconjunctival fever, 496
Pharynx in neutropenia, 129
Phaseolamin, 780
Phasic-stretch reflexes in spasticity, 678
Phenazopyridine, yellow skin from, 829
Phencyclidine (PCP) intoxication, 614
Phenelzine, blocking of anxiety by, 596
Phenformin, 793
    and lactic acidosis, 756
Phenothiazines
    addiction to, 13
    and body temperature, 458
    for chorea, 685
    dizziness from, 722
    and melanin formation, 847
    and Parkinsonism, 679, 685
    and pseudotumor cerebri, 78
Phenylbutazone
    and aplastic anemia, 573
    fever from, 458
    in testing of baroreflex failure, 700,
        701t
Phenylephrine, toxicity of, 614
Phenylethylamine, 68
Phenylketonuria, 853
Phenylpropanolamine intoxication, 614
Phenytoin
    and ataxia, 680
    fever from, 458
Pheochromocytoma, 458, 612
    headache associated with, 77
    hypertension and, 272, 281–282
Pheomelanin, 815
Phlebitis, headache and, 79–80
Phlebotomy for clubbing, 250
Phlegmonous esophagitis, 149
Phobia, 606
    in hysterical personalities, 633
    in panic disorder, 604–606
    in post-traumatic syndrome, 75
    psychological theories of, 602–603
Phonation
    definition of, 112
    disorders of, 112–113
Phonophobia and migraine, 65
Phospholipid, antibodies to, 558

Phosphorus
    and eighth cranial nerve, 111
    and tetany, 683
Photoelectric nystagmography, 711
Photophobia
    in albinism, 850
    in Chediak-Higashi syndrome, 850
    in meningitis, 79
    in migraine, 65, 66
    in muscle contraction headache, 73
    in post-traumatic headache, 75
    in subarachnoid hemorrhage, 79
Physical tolerance
    in occupational activity, 337
    in recreational activity, 338
Physician–patient relationship, 2–6
Physiologic jaundice of the newborn, 31
Picric acid, yellow skin from, 828
Pickwickian syndrome, 659, 777
    and respiratory acidosis, 762
Piebaldism, 850, 852
Pigmentation. See also Skin color; and
        specific pigmentations
    classification of, 823t
    of conjunctivae, 848
    definition of, 812
    dermal (ceruloderma), 814, 846–848
        drug-induced, 847
    of desquamating skin, 854
    eye, 848–849
    hemoglobin. See Hemoglobin pigmen-
        tation
    measurement techniques, 812–813
    nail, 849
Pigmented pretibial patches, 846
Pinta, blue phases of, 847
Periformis syndrome, 243
Pitch of voice, 112, 113
Pitressin, 735
Pituitary diabetes insipidus, 730f, 731f
Pituitary dwarfism
    growth hormone and, 31
    somatomedin and, 30, 31
Pituitary function
    abnormal, clubbing and, 253
    disorders of. See Hypopituitarism
    and fetal development, 19
    and melanin metabolism, 839, 840, 841f
Pituitary gigantism, 33
Pituitary growth hormone. See Growth
        hormone (GH)
PL^A1 antigen, 549
Placebo effect, 49
Plague
    and generalized lymphadenopathy,
        522
    and suppuration of lymph nodes, 521
Plantar keratoses, 846
Plantar reflex, 677

Plantar tendonitis, 221
Plant lectins, 480
Plasmablasts, 479
Plasma cells, 478–480
    defective state of, 482
Plasma proteins, 738, 742
Plasmatic component of hemostasis. See
        Coagulation
Plasma volume
    definition of, 726
    experimental depletions of, 732f
    in salt lack, 740
Plasminogen activator, 536, 542, 555
Plateau phase of fever, 450
Platelet aggregation
    and chest pain, 155
    congenital platelet disorders based
        upon, 549, 550t
    defective, 551
    tracing, 542, 543f
Platelet antibody tests, 545
Platelet coagulant activity (PF₃) defect,
    551
Platelet count, 542, 544, 545. See also
        Thrombocytopenia
Platelet-derived growth factor (PDGF),
        537
Platelet disorders, 543, 547–551
    classification of, 546t
    qualitative, 549–551
        adhesion defect, 549–550
        aggregation defect, 551
        coagulant activity deficiency, 551
        release defect, 550–551
    quantitative, 547–549
        immunologic destruction, 548–549
        megakaryocytic hypoplasia, 547–548
        nonimmunologic thrombocytopenia,
            549
        thrombopoiesis, ineffective, 548
Platelet factor 3 (PF₃), 536
    defect of, 551
Platelet factor 4 (PF₄), 537
Platelets
    morphology of, 536–537
    in normal hemostasis, 536–539
    laboratory approach to, 542, 543f
Platybasia, 721
"Playing dead reaction," 698
Pleural effusion
    cough in, 320
    in lupus erythematosus, 130
Pleural pain, 57, 145–146
Pleurisy
    diaphragmatic, 147
    after myocardial infarction, 157
    pain in, 145–146, 169
Pleuropulmonary sources of abdominal
        pain, 177

Plummer-Vinson's syndrome, 569
Pneuma, concept of, 648
Pneumococcal septicemia, polyarticular
    pain in, 222
Pneumoconioses, 325–326
    clubbing and, 253
    lymphadenopathy in, 509
Pneumocystis carinii, 325
Pneumomediastinum, 328
Pneumonia
    abdominal pain from, 177, 178
    atrial fibrillation in, 308
    bronchiectasis in, 323
    chronic lipoid, 334
    coma in, 652
    cough in, 321
    hemoptysis in, 332
    herpes simplex in, 451
    hilar lymphadenopathy and, 509
    hypoxia in, 353
    interstitial, in pertussis, 322
    irritant gases causing, 325
    lobar, 323
    nature of fever in, 450
    necrotizing, hemoptysis in, 332
    primary influenza virus, 322
    in tuberculosis, 324
Pneumonitis
    clubbing and, 252–253
    after myocardial infarction, 157
Pneumothorax
    in eosinophilic granuloma, 327
    hypoxia in, 353
    in lymphangiomyoma, 509
    and mediastinal emphysema, 150
    pain of, 145, 146
Podagra, 221
Poisoning. *See also specific agents*
    coma from, 652, 659–660
Poliomyelitis
    back pain from, 205
    fasciculations in, 682
    hypoxia in, 353
Polyarteritis
    fever in, 457
    and hematuria, 187
Polyarteritis nodosa
    hemoptysis in, 334
    and leukocytoclastic vasculitis, 545
    multiple mononeuritis in, 675
Polychromatophilia, 566, 572t
Polycystic ovary disease, 771
Polycystic renal disease, and hematuria,
    187
Polycythemia
    erythremia in, 831–832
    obesity and, 777
    in Pickwickian syndrome, 659
Polycythemia vera

and hematuria, 187
    pruritis in, 872
Polydactylism, 773
Polydipsia
    in metabolic acidosis, 759
    primary, 730f, 731f
    psychogenic, 733
Polymer fumes, 459
Polymorphous ventricular tachycardia,
    312
Polymyalgia in temporal arteritis syn-
    drome, 88
Polymyalgia rheumatica, 80, 142,
    204–205, 224
Polymyositis, 230, 672
    back pain from, 204
    carcinoma-related neuropathy and,
        239
    fibrillation in, 682
    infantile, 672
Polyneuritis, 240
    fasting and, 779
    infantile, 672
    and polyneuropathy, 238, 240
Polyneuritis–polyneuropathy, baroreflex
    failure in, 699
Polyneuropathy of peripheral nerves,
    238–240
Polyposis of colon and esophagus, club-
    bing and, 253
Polyradiculitis. *See* Guillain-Barré syn-
    drome
Polyuria
    causes of, 734t
    differential diagnosis of, 732–733
    in hypothalamic diabetes insipidus,
        734–735
    in metabolic acidosis, 759
    in metabolic alkalosis, 761
    in renal response to antidiuretic hor-
        mone, 729, 730f
    plasma vasopressin and plasma osmo-
        lality in, 731f
    unresponsive to antidiuretic hormone,
        735–736
Pompe's disease, 482
Pontine lesions
    dyspnea and, 346
    and unconsciousness, 651, 652
Popliteal lymph nodes, 505f, 506, 507
Porphyria
    acute intermittent hypertension and,
        272
    cause of fever in, 449
    intermittent, 613–614
        abdominal pain in, 177
    neuropathy associated with, 239
Portal cirrhosis, clubbing and, 253
Positional nystagmus, 712

Positional vertigo in labyrinthine pathol-
    ogy, 717
Position sense, loss of, in pernicious
    anemia, 570
Postconcussive syndrome, 611
Postdenervation muscle spasm, 683
Posterior auricular lymph nodes, 493, 495
Posterior cervical lymph nodes, 494, 497
    in rubella, 495
Posterior tibial nerve, entrapment of,
    243–244
Posthypercapneic state, 761
Post–lumbar puncture headache, 79
Postnasal discharge
    in acute otitis media, 108
    serous otitis and, 109
Postnatal trauma and epilepsy, 663
Postnecrotic cirrhosis, 129
Postobstructive diuresis, 736
Postoperative fatigue, 618
Postoperative fevers, 456–457
Postpartum infections, intermittent fever
    in, 451
Postradiation nephritis, and hematuria,
    187
Postseizure headache, 77
Post-transfusion purpura, 549
Post-traumatic conversion symptoms,
    638
Post-traumatic epilepsy, 655
Post-traumatic headache, 74–77
    MCHA as, 74–76
Post-traumatic stress disorder, 606
Post-traumatic syndrome, 75–77
Postural hypotension, 658, 696–702
    in dehydration, 731–732
    in extracellular volume depletion, 741
    in metabolic alkalosis, 761
Posture
    and back pain, 205, 206f
    distortions of, 678–681
        ataxia, 680–681
        athetosis, 681
        dystonia, 681
        myotonia, 679–680
        Parkinsonian rigidity, 679
        spasticity, 678–679
Potassium, heart rate and, 299
Potassium 40 as index of cellular meta-
    bolic mass, 26
Potassium intoxication, periodic weak-
    ness from, 673
Potency, protein-calorie malnourishment
    and, 803
Pott's disease, back pain in, 199
Prader-Willi syndrome, 773
Preaortic lymph nodes
    anatomy of, 511, 512f
    clinical significance, 513, 514

Precordial pain, 157–158
    in angina pectoris, 155
Prednisone, psychiatric disturbance
        from, 614, 615
Pre-excitation syndrome, 304
Pregnancy
    backache in, 207
    body temperature during, 446
    and cluster headaches, 71
    constipation in, 380
    desirable weight gain in, 789
    and iron balance, 575
    megaloblastic anemia of, 126
    and melanization, 815
    melanin metabolism in, 839, 840, 841f
    nutritional deficiency in, 119, 120
    pruritus in, 871
    undernutrition in, 788–792
    vascular spiders in, 426
    vomiting of hematemesis in, 411
    urinary tract infection and, 190
Pregnancy fantasies, conversion symp-
        toms and, 641, 642
Prekallikrein, 539, 541, 554, 555
Premenstrual tension syndrome, 610
Prepsychotic anxiety, 606
Presbycusis, 110
    dizziness and, 718–719
Primary gain, 628, 635
Primidone, 615
Printzmetal's angina, 314
    pseudoangina vs., 636
    syncope in, 693
Procainamide for lupus inhibitor, 558
Procaine for "intolerable angina pecto-
        ris," 156–157
Proenzymes. See Zymogens
"Profile sign" in clubbing, 246, 247f
Progesterone
    and body temperature, 446
    and food consumption, 803
    and melanosis, 839, 840, 841f
    and migraine, 68
Progestin and skin color, 820–821
Projectile vomiting, 367
Prolactin, 596–597
Promyelocytic leukemia and dissemi-
        nated intravascular coagulation,
        556
Pronunciation, 112, 113
Propranolol, 596, 615
    in headache, 75
    and syncope, 692
    and tremor, 684
Proprioception
    and movement ataxia, 681
    Romberg test for lesions, 713, 715
    in tabetic athetosis, 681
Prostacyclin (PGI₂)

deficiency of, in thrombotic thrombo-
        cytopenic purpura, 549
    in normal platelet function, 536, 538
Prostaglandin(s)
    in congenital platelet release defects,
        550–551
    and fever, 449
    and itch, 866
    in migraine, 68
    in normal platelet function, 537–539
    and pain, 44, 140
Prostate
    carcinoma of, and lumbosacral plexus,
        235
    examination of, 171
    hyperplasia of, and hematuria, 187
    pain from, 177, 207
Prostatitis
    clinical picture of, 191
    and hematuria, 187
Prostration
    in acute hemolytic anemia, 570
    with cystitis, 191
Protein
    deficiency of, in marasmus and
        kwashiorkor, 789–790
    dietary, 772
    loss of
        in edema formation, 743
        following thoracic-duct injury, 475
Protein C, 541
Protein-calorie malnutrition (PCM), hor-
        mones and, 801–803
Protein malnutrition and erythropoietin,
        573
Proteus vulgaris, 189
Prothrombin, 540–541
Prothrombin response, 430
Prothrombin time (PT) test, 542–544
Protopathic itch, 866
Proximal athetosis, 681
Pruritic dermatosis, lymphadenopathy
        and, 522
Pruritis (itching), 865–876
    approach to patient in, 875–876
    jaundice and, 425, 826
    mechanisms of, 865–868
    and melanosis, 826, 838
    non-systemic causes of, 873–874
    in pancreatic cancer, 425
    as reaction to antibiotics, 131
    from systemic disease, 868–872
        benign hematologic, 872
        diabetes mellitus, 871
        hepatobiliary, 870–871
        malignant, 871–872
        pregnancy, 871
        renal, 868–869
        thyroid disease, 871

Pruritus ani, 874, 876f
    conversion, 642
Pruritus vulvae, 874
    conversion, 642
Pseudoangina, 636
Pseudoariboflavinosis, 133–134
Pseudoephedrine intoxication, 614
Pseudogout, 222
Pseudohemophilia. See von Willebrand's
        disease
Pseudohypertropic muscular dystrophy,
        clubbing and, 253
Pseudomeningitis, 640
Pseudomonas in osteomyelitis of spine,
        199
Pseudomyasthenia gravis, 640
Pseudopregnancy and melanization,
        815, 821
Pseudotetanus, 640
Pseudotumor cerebri, 78–79
Pseudoxanthoma elasticum, 400, 402f,
        410, 413–414, 547
Psoas abscess, 170
    and lumbar plexus, 235
Psoas muscle spasm in iliac lymphadeni-
        tis, 507
Psoriasis
    oral lesions in, 130
    pruritus in, 868
Psoriatic arthritis, 200, 223
    changes in sacroiliac joints, 200
Psyche vs. soma, 8
Psychiatric disorders, misdiagnosis of
        medical illnesses as, 591–593
Psychoanalytic theory, 602
Psychodynamic point of view,
        601–602
Psychogenic cough, 321
Psychogenic dizziness, 723
Psychogenic fever, 459–460
Psychogenic vomiting, 366, 367
Psychological defenses, hormone levels
        and, 600
Psychomotor attacks, 611, 660, 663–664,
        665F
Psychoneuroses, 14
    habitual hyperthermia and, 459
    oral symptoms in, 132
    psychoanalytic theory of, 602
Psychosis(es), 14
    amphetamines and, 780
    constipation and, 378
    somatic delusions in, 644
    vitamin-B¹² deficiency and, 577
Psychosomatic disorders, 14, 601
    differentiation of conversion and, 625,
        636, 643–645
Psychotic anxiety, 606
Psychotic depression, 644

Ptosis
  bilateral, 628
  in cluster headache, 70–72
  conversion, 640
Puberty, 33–40
  body changes of, 35–36, 37t
  delayed, 36–38
  endocrinology of, 33–35
  growth and, 20, 21f, 22f
  hypothyroidism and, 31
  premature, 38–40
  time of occurrence of, 36, 38f
Pulmonary disorders. See also specific conditions
  asterixis in, 684
  clubbing and osteoarthropathy and, 246–249, 252–253
  coma in, 657
  cyanosis in, 353–354
  nervousness and, 612, 613
  presenting with fatigue, 618
Pulmonary edema
  acute, 325
  cyanosis in, 352
  dyspnea and, 342–343
  hemoptysis in, 333
  and respiratory acidosis, 762
Pulmonary embolism
  hemoptysis in, 333
  syncope in, 694
Pulmonary fibrosis, cough in, 320
Pulmonary hemangioma, clubbing and, 253
Pulmonary hypertension
  amphetamines and, 780
  syncope with, 693–694
Pulmonary infarction, 325
  congestive heart failure with, 456
  cough in, 321
  pain in, 146
Pulmonary lymph nodes, 508
Pulmonary tuberculosis, 324
  clubbing and, 252
Pulmonic stenosis, syncope in, 691
Pupillary abnormalities
  brain stem lesions and, 651, 652
  in meningitis, 655
  in metabolic coma, 656
Pupillary changes in sickle-cell anemia, 570
Pupillary dilation
  in nervousness, 594
  in post-traumatic headache, 75
  in vasodepressor syncope, 697
Pupillary reactions in pulmonary disease, 657
Pupillary reflex, 87
  in vitreous hemorrhages, 89
Purinergic system, 698

"Purple people," 847
Purpura, 544, 545
  allergic, 545–547
  decreased strength of microcirculation and, 547
  in eyelid, 848
  factitious, 545
  psychogenic, 634
  thrombocytopenic, 454, 548–549
Purpuric disorders. See Platelet disorders; Vascular disorders
Pyelitis, 191
Pyelonephritis, 272
  anemia in, 473
  fever in, 453
  and hematuria, 187
  hyperchloremic acidosis in, 757
  nature of fever in, 451
  obstructive disorders and, 190
  pain of, 176
  pyuria and, 188–191
Pyloric carcinoma, clubbing and, 253
Pyloric obstruction, 369
Pyoderma, 390
Pyogenic staphylococci in lymphangitis, 473
Pyonephrosis, iliac lymphadenopathy and, 514
Pyopneumothorax, osteoarthropathy and, 249
Pyorrhea and scurvy, 128, 129
Pyrexia. See also Fever
  definition of, 447
Pyridoxal phosphate, 122
Pyridoxine (vitamin B₆). See also Vitamin-B complex
  biochemical role of, 122
  deficiency of, 123, 125, 793
    and polyneuropathy, 238
  drugs and, 793
Pyridoxine-responsive anemia, 577
Pyriform sinus, 501
Pyrogens, 447–450, 452, 455–456
  contamination of biologic preparations by, 458–459
  "spontaneous" release of, 454
Pyuria, 188–191
  bacterial etiology of, 189–190
  definition of, 188
  hematuria with, 187
Pyruvate-kinase deficiency, 583

Questionnaire, patient, 4–5
Quinacrine hydrochloride, 847
  yellow skin from, 828–829
Quinidine
  fever from, 458
  and syncope, 692

Quinine
  and eighth cranial nerve, 111
  and immunohemolytic anemia, 581
  toxicity of, and tunnel vision, 96
Quotidian fever, definition of, 447
Q–T intervals and syncope, 692

Rabies, muscle spasm in, 683
Rademacher's disease, 522
Radial nerve entrapment, 241
Radiating pain, 53
Radiation in body-heat elimination, 442
Radiation enteritis, 385
Radiation exposure, 11, 19
  from radiography, 22
  and lymphadema, 474
Radicular (nerve root) pain, 57
  in ankylosing spondylitis, 200
  from disk herniation, 201–203, 242
  in extremities, 231–235
    monoradicular syndrome, 233–234
    polyradicular syndrome, 234–235
  in forearm and hand, 241
  from lumbar disk disease, 243
  osteophytic pressure and, 201
Radiculitis, 142
  hyperpathia in, 55
Radiography
  in acute abdomen, 178
  of bone maturation, 21–22
  and bone pain, 229
  in clubbing, 250, 250–251f
  in differential diagnosis of jaundice, 430–433, 431–437f
  gastrointestinal, 400, 402
  lumbosacral neuritis from, 235
  radiation exposure from, 22, 474
Radioisotopic scanning in abdominal pain, 172
Radionuclide imaging, 172
  of urinary tract, 187
"Rainbow" therapy for obesity, 780
Rainier hemoglobin, 357
Ramsay-Hunt syndrome, 495
Rapid-eye-movement (REM) sleep. See Paradoxical sleep
Rash(es). See also specific disorders
  in Crohn's disease, 170
  drug-induced, 458, 522, 793
  and histocytic proliferation, 483
  oxyhemoglobin and red skin color in, 831
  in rickettsialpox, 518
  in rubella, 221
  in scrub typhus, 517
Rat-bite fever, 453
  inguinal lymphadenopathy and, 506
  as lymph node syndrome, 518

Raynaud's disease, 228, 255
Reaction formation, 602
Reactive extensor postural synergy, 679
Reading epilepsy, 664
Rebound tenderness
    peritoneal, 170, 185
    in renal pain, 184
    in ureteral pain, 185
Receptor organs, 44
Recreational activity, physical tolerance
    in, 338
Rectal examination
    in abdominal pain, 171
    in appendicitis, 174–175
Rectal incontinence in Shy-Drager syndrome, 701
Rectal neoplasm, 170
"Rectal shelf," 171
Rectal temperature, 445
Rectal tenesmus, ureteral pain with, 185
Rectocele, 380
Rectosigmoid, carcinoma of, 235
Rectum disease, low back pain from, 207
Red blood cell casts, 186, 187
Red blood cells. See also Anemia; Hemolytic anemia
    and classification of anemias, 571, 572t
    disease-specific morphologic changes
        in, 579f
    normal, 563–564
        cytoplasm of, 565
        life span, 565–566
        membrane of, 564–565
    in urine. See Hematuria
Red cell antibodies, 580–581
"Red man syndrome," 831
Reduced hemoglobin and erythemia, 831–832
Reduced-hemoglobin pigmentation, 814, 816–817, 830. See also Hemoglobin
    pigmentation
    sex differences and, 820–821, 822f
Reflex cardiac standstill and syncope, 659
Reflex sympathetic dystrophy, 231, 237–238, 242
Reflex tympanometry, 714
Reflux esophagitis, 399–400
Refsum's disease, 718
Regenerating nerve, pain of, 236
    reflex sympathetic dystrophy vs., 237
Regional enteritis, 383, 385, 390
    clubbing and, 253
    growth failure in, 33
    pain of, 168, 169, 174
Regional ileitis, 127
    clubbing and, 249
    and nutritional deficiency, 119

Regurgitation in esophageal disease, 149
Reiter's syndrome, 133, 223
    changes in sacroiliac joints, 200
Releasing factors, 596–597
Relapsing fever. See Intermittent fever
Relaxation therapy, 603
Remittent fever, definition of, 447
Renal acid–base regulation, normal, 751–755
Renal artery embolism, 187
Renal blood flow, anemia and, 569
Renal calculi, 187
Renal colic, 168–170, 176–177
Renal cortical abscess, 188
Renal disease(s). See also specific conditions; Kidneys
    acute abdomen and, 178
    arteritis in, 684
    fatigue from, 618
    hypertension and, 272, 279–281
        evaluation of, 276–277
    and impaired concentrating ability, 735
    and metabolic alkalosis, 761
    in neuropathy of amyloidosis, 239
    obesity and, 778
    pruritis in, 868–870
    and salt loss, 740
    tetany in, 683
    and water retention, 736–737
"Renal epistaxis," 188
Renal-erythropoietic factor, 565
Renal failure
    from allergic purpura, 545–547
    and anemia, 573
    carotenemia from, 827
    from dehydration, 731–732
    and hyperchloremic metabolic acidosis, 757
    melena and hematemesis and, 396–397
    nail color in, 849
    and normochloremic acidosis, 755–756
    and retinal detachment, 89
    in thrombotic thrombocytopenic purpura, 549
    uremic coma in, 657
Renal function
    and edema formation, 741, 744
    in normal osmotic regulation, 727–729
    salt excretion, 738–741
Renal insufficiency
    with anemia, 569
    oral lesions in, 131
Renal parenchyma
    hypertension and, 279
    as origin of hematuria, 186, 187
    tumors of, 187
Renal tuberculosis, hematuria in, 187

Renal tubular acidosis (RTA), 757–759
    growth failure and, 33
    hypocalcemia from, 683
Renal vein thrombosis and hematuria, 187
Renal water loss, 732–734
Renin, 739, 740
Renin-angiotensin system, 286–288
Renin-secreting tumors, 761
Renovascular hypertension, 279–281
Repression, psychological, 602, 631
Reserpine
    for chorea, 685
    and Parkinsonian rigidity, 679
Resonance (speech function), 112
Resorcin, 847
Resorcinol, allergic skin reaction to, 875f
Respiration
    in speech, 112
    in vocal cord paralysis, 113
Respiratory acid–base regulation, normal, 750–751
Respiratory acidosis, 762–763
    buffering mechanism in, 750
Respiratory alkalosis, 763–764
    buffering mechanisms in, 750, 751f
    conversion and, 625, 629–630, 637
    in hyperventilation syndrome, 613
    and tetany, 683
Respiratory compensation
    in metabolic acidosis, 759
    in metabolic alkalosis, 761
    in respiratory acidosis, 762
    in respiratory alkalosis, 763–764
Respiratory disease. See also Pulmonary
        entries; and specific disorders
    brain-stem lesions and, 651–652
    obesity and, 770, 771
Respiratory paralysis in myasthenia
    gravis, 674
Resting tremor, 679, 683–684
Restlessness
    in anemia, 569–570
    in niacin deficiency, 124
    in vasodepressor syncope, 697
Retching, 366
Reticular activating system (RAS), 594, 596
Reticular cells, 476–477
Reticular fibers, 476
Reticular lymphangitis, 473
Reticular system, 47
Reticulocytes, 565–566
Reticulocytosis, 576
    in immunohemolytic anemia, 580
"Reticuloendothelial system," 468
Reticuloendotheliosis, leukemic, 485f, 487
Reticulosis, lipomelanic, 483

Reticulum cell sarcoma of cerebrum, 611
Retina
    central serous retinitis, 93f, 94, 98
    changes in, hypertension and,
        273–275
    chorioretinitis, 98
    detachment of, 88–89
    diabetes mellitus and, 90–92, 93f
    hemorrhages of, 89–90
        in anemia, 570
    occlusion of central artery, 86–88
Retinitis pigmentosa, 95–97, 773
Retrobulbar neuritis, 94–95
Retrograde endoscopic pancreatic and
        biliary duct cannulation, 171
Retrograde jejunogastric intussuscep-
        tion, 412
Retrograde ureteropyelography, 187
Retroperitoneal (parietal) lymph nodes
    anatomy of, 511–513
    Burkitt's lymphoma and, 487
    clinical significance, 513–515
    iliac nodes as, 507
Retroperitoneal tumors, 618
Retropharyngeal abscess, 480, 481
Reversed-3 sign, 430, 431f
Rhabdomyosarcoma, 230
Rhegmatogenous retinal detachment, 88
Rheumatic chorea, 685
Rheumatic disease(s). See also specific dis-
        orders
    back pain from, 204–205
    systemic
        and foot damage, 221
        polyarticular pain in, 221–224
Rheumatic fever
    atrial fibrillation in, 308
    congestive heart failure with, 456
    hypertension and, 272
    jaundice and history of, 424
    joint pain in, 211, 215, 222
    nature of fever in, 451, 457
    vs. rheumatoid arthritis, 223
Rheumatic heart disease, 569
Rheumatism, nonarticular, 217, 224–225
Rheumatoid arthritis, 81
    anemia in, 573
    ankylosing spondylitis vs., 200
    axillary lymphadenopathy and, 502
    brevity of acute attacks of, 222
    epitrochlear lymphadenopathy and,
        504
    fatigue from, 618
    generalized lymphadenopathy in, 522
    hypertrophic osteoarthropathy and,
        248
    inflammation in, 215
    juvenile. See Juvenile rheumatoid ar-
        thritis

and leukocytoclastic vasculitis, 545
    metatarsal pain in, 221
    osteoarthritis vs., 223–224
    pain of, 216
        monoarticular or pauciarticular, 217
        polyarticular, 223
    as psychosomatic disorder, 601
    reactive lymphadenopathy in, 483–484
    tetraethylammonium and, 215
Rheumatoid factor, 223
Rheumatoid spondylitis. See Ankylosing
        spondylitis
Rhinitis
    in common cold, 322
    vasomotor cough in, 326
Rhinorrhea
    in cluster headache, 70, 71
    in otitis media, 108
Rib cartilages, slipping, 141
Riboflavin
    biochemical role of, 121–122
    deficiency of, 120, 124–125, 127, 793,
        794f
    and hematoma, 796
Ribonucleic acid. See RNA synthesis
Rickets
    and acidosis, 759
    phenylhydantoin and, 795
Rickettsial infections, 517–518
    and purpura, 545
Rifampin
    orange skin from, 829
    and "red man" syndrome, 831
Right lymphatic duct, anatomy of, 474
Right middle lobe syndrome, 327
    hemoptysis in, 333–334
Right subdiaphragmatic abscess, re-
        ferred shoulder pain from, 206
Rigidity
    Parkinsonian, 679, 683
    in Shy-Drager syndrome, 701
Ringworm
    of scalp, 494–495
    between toes, 506
Rinne test, 715
Ristocetin, 550, 552
    platelet aggregation induced by, 554
RNA synthesis, 479
    actinomycin D and, 796
    endogenous pyrogen and, 449–450
    vitamin B$_{12}$ and folic acid deficiency
        and, 128
Role playing in hysterical personality,
        632
Romano-Ward syndrome, 692
Romberg's sign, 570
Romberg test, 713, 715
Rostrocaudally, 651
Rotational testing, 713

Rotatory nystagmus, 717
Rotor's syndrome, 423, 424
Roughage diets, 779
Rubella (German measles)
    auricular lymphadenopathy in, 495,
        522
    and fetal growth, 19
    labyrinth involvement in, 717
    polyarticular pain in, 221
Rutin, 255

Saccular aneurysms, referred back pain
        from, 206
Saccular bronchiectasis, hemoptysis in,
        333
Saccules, function of, 708, 709, 711f, 713
Sacroiliac joints, pain from, 200
"Sacroiliac sprain," 200
Salicylates, 615, 660
    analgesic mechanism of, 140
    fever from, 458
    and metabolic acidosis, 756
    ototoxicity of, 718
    for rheumatic fever, 222
"Saline-resistant" alkalosis, 761
Salivary glands, 497
Salivation in vasodepressor syncope,
        697–698
Salt balance, 737–739
Salt excess. See Edema
Salt lack, 740–741
"Salt-losing nephritis," 740
Sarcoidosis, 483, 510, 672
    cough in, 327
    dyspnea in, 336
    fever in, 456
    mediastinal lymph node enlargement
        in, 509
    reactive proliferation of lymph nodes
        in, 522
Sarcoma, ostalgia from, 142
Scabies, 873–874, 876f
Scalene lymph nodes, 494, 499–500
Scalenus anticus syndrome, 241
Scalp infections
    lymph nodes and, 494–495
    posterior cervical lymphadenopathy
        and, 497
Scalp muscles. See Muscle contraction
        headache (MCHA)
Scarlet fever
    fever in, 453
    lymph node response in, 522
    oral lesions in, 130
    skin color in, 831
Scar tissue
    formation of, and post-traumatic
        headache, 75, 76

painful, reflex sympathetic dystrophy vs., 237
  skin color in, 854
Scattering and skin color, 814, 819, 846–847
Schistocytes, 579
Schistosomiasis, 325
Schizophrenia
  dopamine and, 598
  endorphins and, 600
  somatic delusions in, 644
Schmorl's nodule, 199
School phobia, 644
Schwannoma, 234
Sciatic nerve
  diabetic mononeuropathy and, 238
  entrapment of, at sciatic notch, 243
  intervertebral disk disease and, 201–202
  palpation of, in herniated disk, 242
  reflex sympathetic dystrophy and, 237
Scintigraphy, 493
Scintillating scotoma, 97
  in classic migraine, 66
Sclerae, blue coloration in, 847–849
"Scleral" icterus, 826
Scleroderma, 385
  inguinal lymphadenopathy and, 506
  melanosis with, 842
  Raynaud's phenomenon in, 228
Scleromalacia, 848–849
Sclerosing carcinoma of bile ducts, 425
Sclerosing cholangitis
  jaundice and, 423, 425, 433f
  sex and incidence of, 426
Sclerosing glossitis, 130
Scoliosis
  back ache and, 199, 205
  childhood spine pain from, 234
Scopolamine, 615
Scratching and pruritus, 866–867
"Scrotal" tongue, 118
Scrub typhus, 517
  inguinal lymphadenopathy and, 506
Scurvy. See Vitamin C, deficiency of
Sebaceous cysts, cancerous lymphadenopathy vs., 501
Seborrhea, nasolabial
  in niacin deficiency, 123
  in riboflavin deficiency, 125
Seborrheic dermatitis in B-complex deficiency, 125
Sebum, 817, 818
Secondary gain, 628, 635
Sedatives
  adverse reactions to, 12
  and depression, 618
  fever due to, 458
  withdrawal from, 614

Sedentary work, definition of, 337
Sedimentation rate
  in polymyalgia rheumatica, 224
  in rheumatoid arthritis, 223
Segmental demyelination, 675
Seizures. See also Convulsive states; Epilepsy; and specific disorders
  conversion, 637
  definition of, 660
Self-injury, 644
Seminal vesicles
  referred low lumbar and sacral pain from, 207
  and renal-ureteral pain, 185
Senile purpura, 547
Senile tremor, 684
Sensation loss, pain from, 236, 237
Sensory disturbances, conversion, 624t, 640–641
Sensory-neural hearing impairment, 110–111
Sentence formation. See Language
Sentinel node, 498
Septic arthritis of hip joint, 220
Septicemia
  chills in, 450
  fever patterns in, 453
  joint pain due to, 222
  lymphatics and, 468, 473
  mesenteric lymphadenitis and, 517
  from subpectoral abscess, 504
Septic fever, definition of, 447
Septic joints, monoarticular pain in, 216
Septic thrombophlebitis, 454
Septoptic dysplasia, 31
Serotonin, 598, 599f
  and body temperature, 449
  central pain mechanisms and, 63
  in cluster headache, 71
  and MCHA, 74
  in migraine, 68
  and platelet function, 537
  in thermoregulation, 449, 458
Serotonin antagonists, 550
Serous otitis (media), 109
Serous retinal detachment, 89
Serpent's head fingers, 245, 247. See also Clubbing
Serum glutamic oxaloacetic transaminase (SGOT) level, 429–430
Serum glutamic pyruvic transaminase (SGPT) level, 429–430
Serum sickness, 457
  and generalized lymphadenopathy, 522
Set point for body weight, 775
Sex chromosomes, 17–19
Sex hormones. See also specific hormones
  in adrenal dysfunction, 39
  in control of height, 33

delayed puberty and, 36–38
  exogenous sources of, and sexual precocity, 39
  and food consumption, 863
  and obesity, 771, 777
  partial pubertal syndromes and, 39–40
  premature puberty, 38–39
  in pubertal development, 33–35
  and skin color, 820–821, 840, 841f
Sexual activity, obesity and, 776, 777
Sexual development, 33–40
  body changes in, 35–36, 37t
  disturbances of pubertal mechanism, 36–40
  endocrinology of, 33–35
  precocious, excessive growth and, 33
  radiation exposure and, 19
Sexual problems in hysterical personality, 633
Sézary's syndrome, 485f, 487
  and generalized lymphadenopathy, 522
Shamberg's disease, 844
Shifting dullness in peritonitis, 171, 176
Shiftman syndrome, 683
Shivering, 683
  in chill phase of fever, 450
  fasciculation vs., 682
  hypothalamus and, 444, 447–448
Shock
  in acute hemolytic anemia, 570
  in dehydration, 731–732
  nail appearance in, 849
  pallor of, 854
  tachycardia in, 302
Short stature, genetic, 32
Shoulder girdle muscle pain, 142
Shoulder-hand syndrome, 156, 231, 237
Shoulder pain, 218–219, 240–241
  in arthritis, 218
  referred, 206
Shy-Drager syndrome, 699–702
SIADH (syndrome of inappropriate antidiuretic hormone), 737
Sickle-cell disorders, 583–584
  abdominal pain in, 177
  ankle ulcers in, 567
  cardiovascular aspects of, 568
  concentrating ability in, 735–736
  differential classification of, 584
  fever in, 454
  genitourinary system and, 569
  and hematuria, 187
  intracellular viscosity in, 578
  neurologic manifestations of, 570
  Raynaud's phenomenon in, 228
  and renal tubular acidosis, 759
  retinal hemorrhage and, 89
  spleen in, 570
  target cells in, 579

Sickle-cell hemoglobin, 356
Sickle-cell trait, 584
  hematuria and, 569
Sick sinus syndrome, 692
Sideroblastic anemias, 577
Signal node, 498
Signs. *See also* Symptoms
  definition of, 1
Silicone lymphadenopathy, 503
Silicosis, 509
  of mediastinal lymph nodes, periph-
    eral calcification in, 510
  scalene lymph node and, 500
Simmonds' disease, 839, 853
Sinus histiocytosis with massive lymph-
    adenopathy (SHML), 498
Sinusitis
  headache in, 80
  middle-ear infection and, 109
Sinus tachycardia, 297, 302–303
Site-of-injury headache, post-traumatic,
    75, 76
Skeletal growth, 21–25, 26f
Skeletal muscles
  pain in, 56
  tone of, and vasodepressor syncope,
    698
Skin. *See also specific conditions*
  conversion complications of, 640
  diseases of, fever in, 457
  histological appearance of, 812f, 814
  in jaundice, 426
  lesions of
    in allergic purpura, 545
    in lupus erythematosus, 130
    in vitamin deficiencies, 123, 793
  obstruction of lymphatic vessels and,
    473–474
  pain and, 56, 228–229
  peau d'orange, 474, 487, 520, 520f
  salt lack and, 740
  sickle-cell anemia and, 584
  turgor of
    in dehydration, 731
    in salt lack, 740, 741
  ulcers of, in rheumatoid arthritis, 223
Skin color, 811–855
  in anemia, 566–567, 850
  classification of pigmentation, normal
    and abnormal, 823t
  colored pictures in study of, 813, 854
  dermal pigmentation (blue colora-
    tion—ceruloderma), 814, 846–848
  diminished blood flow and, 853–854
  external pigmentation of eye, 848–849
  hemoglobin pigmentation, 814,
    816–817, 819, 823f, 830–832
    classification of, 830t
    detection of jaundice, 826

sex differences, 820–821, 822f
in macerated or desquamated skin, 854
melanin pigmentation, 814–816,
    832–844. *See also* Melanin; Mela-
    nosis
metallic pigmentation, 844–846
methods of analysis of, 811–813
miscellaneous pigmentations, 849
nail pigmentation, 849
normal patterns of, 818–822
  age and, 819
  race and, 819–820, 835
  sex and, 820–821, 822f
  sunlight and, 815, 821–822, 823f,
    835–837
scar tissue and, 854
in skin edema, 853
sources of, 814–818
yellow, 823–830
  carotene and, 817–818, 827–828. *See
    also* Carotene
  from chemicals and drugs, 828–829
  in dermatologic disorders, 829
  differential characteristics of,
    824–825t
  diffused blood and, 829–830
  in jaundice, 823–827
  in uremia, 829
  in xanthomata, 829
Skinfold calipers, 770
Skull fractures, eighth-nerve trauma in,
    719
Sleep
  itch during, 868
  paradoxical, 650
    in narcolepsy, 664–665
  studies of, and understanding of con-
    sciousness, 649–650
  waking state and coma vs., 653f
Sleep centers, 649–650
Sleep deprivation and fatigue, 601, 618
Sleep EEG, 662
Sleeping sickness, 649
Sleep paralysis, 664
"Slouch back," 205, 206f
Small intestine
  disease of, and vitamin B_{12} deficiency,
    576
  as source of abdominal pain, 173–175
  tumors of, 410
Small lymphocyte, 478–480
Smallpox vaccination, reactions to, 483
Smoking, 10
  bronchogenic carcinoma and, 326
  and central serous retinopathy, 98
  cough caused by, 320, 321, 323
  cough syncope and, 327
  esophagitis and, 149
  and fetal growth, 19

hypertension and, 284
oral lesions from, 133
Snake bites
  abdominal pain from, 177
  and hemolysis, 581
Snellen chart, 85
Snoring, serous otitis and, 109
Social history, taking of, 12–13
Sodium
  hypertension and, 285
  renal regulation of, 738–739
Sodium bicarbonate and iron deficiency,
    793–794
Sodium fluorescein, yellow skin from,
    829
Solitary lymph cyst, 473
Solute concentration (osmolality)
  in dehydration, 731, 732f
  measurement of, 726
  normal regulation of, 726–731, 732f
  and salt balance, 737–738, 741
Soma vs. psyche, 8
Somatic delusions, conversion symp-
    toms vs., 644
Somatic vs. true visceral pain, 166–168
Somatoform (somatization) disorders,
    607–609
  fatigue in, 617
Somatomedins, 28–30
  corticosteroid therapy and, 32
  diabetes and, 31
  dwarfism and, 30, 31
  in pituitary gigantism, 33
  in protein-calorie malnutrition, 801
  tissue unresponsiveness to, 32
Somatostatin, 28
Somatostatin-releasing inhibiting hor-
    mone (SRIH), 596–597
Somatotropin, 30–31
Somatotype concept, 769
Somnolence in Pickwickian syndrome,
    777
Sore throat
  in acute otitis media, 108
  in scarlet fever, 130
Sound-conduction mechanism of ear,
    107–108
South African tick bite fever, 517–518
South American trypanosomiasis, 379
Space-occupying intracerebral lesions,
    hypertension and, 272
Space of Disse, 469–470
Spasm. *See* Muscle, spasm of
Spastic coronary disease, 152, 155
"Spastic hemiparesis," 678
Spasticity, 677–679
"Spastic" pain, 514
Specific dynamic action, 772
Spectrometry, 846–847

Spectrophotometry, 813, 817–822f
Speech, 101–102, 112–114
   basic functions in, 112
   disorders of phonation, 112–114
   normal developmental expectancies
      in, 102, 103–106t
Spermatic cord, pain from, 177
Sphenopalatine ganglion in cluster
      headache, 71
Sphereocytosis, 579
   hereditary, 582
   in immunohemolytic anemia, 580
   and red-cell recovery from burns, 581
Sphincteric disturbances in pernicious
      anemia, 570
Spider hemangiomas, 129
Spiller's neuritis, 241
Spina bifida occulta, 842
Spinal accessory nerve, removal of pos-
      terior cervical nodes and, 497
Spinal cord
   degeneration of, vitamin B$_{12}$ and,
      576–577
   diseases of
      cervical spondylosis, 240
      fasciculations in, 682
   injury to, fever in, 453
   lesions of
      abdominal pain from, 177
      back pain from, 205
      constipation and, 379
      dyspnea and, 345–346
      extremity "pain" from, 231
      radicular pain and, 57, 231–235
Spinal root lesions, pain from, 169
Spinal shock, 676
Spine. See also Back pain; Intervertebral
      disks
   malignant tumors of, 199–200
   stenosis of, congenital, 204
Spirillum minus, 453, 518
Spirillum recurrentis, 453
Splanchnic (true visceral) pain, 166, 167
Spleen
   enlarged. See Splenomegaly
   examination of, 170, 426, 427f, 428
   extravascular lysis in, 578
   impairment of, in sickle-cell anemia,
      584
   infarct of, friction rub in, 170
   in lymphoid system, 468
   pain from, 57
Splenic artery, aneurysm of, 410
Splenic flexure syndrome, 387
Splenomegaly, 428
   anemia and, 570
   causes of, 580
   in hairy-cell leukemia, 522
   and meolysis, 580

   in hereditary spherocytosis, 582
   hypersplenism and, 549
   in immunohemolytic anemia, 580
   in spur-cell anemia, 581
   thrombocytopenia with, 548
Spondylitis. See also Ankylosing spondy-
      litis
   of psoriatic arthritis, 200
Spondylolisthesis, back pain from, 199
Spondylosis, muscular contraction head-
      ache in, 74
Spontaneous movement, 681–686
   ballism, 685
   chorea, 685
   clonic convulsive movements, 686
   fasciculation, 682
   fibrillation, 681–682
   oculogyric crises, 685
   palatal myoclonus, 686
   spasm, 682–683
   torticollis and tic, 685
   tremor, 683–685
Sporotrichosis
   lymphadenopathy and, 517
      axillary, 502
   oculoglandular syndrome and, 496
   and suppuration of lymph nodes,
      521
Sprue
   abdominal discomfort in, 174
   and atrophic glossitis, 127
   clubbing and, 249, 253
   hypocalcemia from, 683
   and iron absorption, 575
   and megaloblastic anemia, 577
Spur-cell anemia, 581–582
Spur cells, 579
Sputum, 328
   in hemoptysis, 332
Squamous cell carcinoma
   anterior auricular lymphadenopathy
      and, 495
   cervical lymph node metastases of,
      496–497
Stance. See also Posture
   cerebellar vs. vestibular lesions and,
      713, 715
Staphylococcal infections
   bronchopneumonia, 509
   of joints, 216
   lymphadenitis, 521
      iliac, 507
   in osteomyelitis of spine, 199
   septicemia, 446
   urinary-tract, 189, 190
Starling forces, 741–744
Starvation
   and erythropoietin, 573
   gouty arthritis from, 222

   ketoacidosis in, 756
   melanosis in, 838
   and polyneuropathy, 238
   in treatment of obesity, 779
Stasis cyanosis, 854
Steatorrhea, 382
   in bile salt disorders, 383–384
   and lymphoma, 516
Stein-Leventhal syndrome, 771
Stem-cell maturation, 481–482
Sterile pyuria, 189
Sternberg-Reed giant cells, 485
Sternomastoid contracture, conversion,
      640
Steroid fever, 455–456
Steroids. See also Corticosteroids
   adverse reactions to, 12
   in carpal tunnel syndrome, 241
   in clubbing, 250
   in giant cell arteritis, 80
   and pseudotumor cerebri, 78, 79
   renal K$^+$ loss from, 673
   for retrobulbar neuritis, 94–95
   serum bilirubin and, 423
Stevens-Johnson syndrome, 129
Stibophen and immunohemolytic ane-
      mia, 581
Stiff neck. See Neck, stiff
Stigmata, religious, 630
Stillman diet, 779, 780
Still's disease. See Juvenile rheumatoid
      arthritis
"Stitch," 147
Stocking hypoesthesia, 570
Stokes-Adams syndrome. See Adams-
      Stokes syndrome
Stomach
   carcinoma of, bleeding in, 407
   pain from, 57, 173
Stomatitis
   in B-complex deficiencies, 124, 125
   in heavy metal intoxication, 130
Stool
   blood in. See also Melena
      with abdominal pain, 170
      inspection for, 171
   in jaundice, 426, 429
Storage pool disease, 550
"Strawberry tongue," 130
Streptobacillus moniliformis, 453, 518
Streptococcal infections
   and allergic purpura, 545
   axillary lymphadenopathy and, 502
   iliac lymphadenitis, 507
   in lymphangitis, 473
   in peritonitis, 176
   and rheumatic fever, 222
   of wounds, and lymph node syn-
      drome, 517, 521

Streptococcus hemolyticus, 517
Streptococcus pneumoniae, 323
Streptomycin
  and factor-V inhibition, 558
  fever from, 458
  ototoxicity of, 718
  sensory-neural hearing loss caused
    by, 111
Stress, 600–601
  hypertension and, 284
  MHPG levels and, 598
  post-traumatic, 606
  in precipitation of conversion symp-
    toms, 633–634
Stretch reflexes
  in anterior horn cell disease, 675–676
  in ataxia, 680
  in clonus vs. tremor, 683
  in peripheral neuropathy, 675
  in spasticity, 678
  in upper neuron syndrome, 676–677
Stridor, 113
Stroke in giant cell arteritis, 80
Stroma of lymph nodes, 476–477
Structural disorders, definition of, 15
Strychnine poisoning, muscle spasm in,
    683
Stupor
  as conversion symptom, 637
  definition of, 649
  in pulmonary disease, 657
  in sickle cell anemia, 570
Stuttering, 114
Stypven time test, 543, 544f
Subaortic stenosis, syncope and, 693
Subarachnoid aneurysm, 272
Subarachnoid hemorrhage, headache
    from, 79
Subclavian-artery aneurysm, 253
Subclavian steal syndrome, 702
  dizziness in, 720
Subclavian trunk, anatomy of, 474
Subclinical seizures, 662
Subdiaphragmatic abscess, fever in, 453
Subdural hematoma, coma from, 652,
    654
Subinguinal lymph nodes, lymphogra-
    phy of, 489f, 491f
Sublingual mumps, 497
Submaxillary lymph nodes, 494, 495, 497
  in keratoconjunctivitis, 496
  in oculoglandular syndrome, 496, 497
  oculonodal complex and, 496
  pharyngoconjunctival fever and, 496
Submaxillary salivary glands, 497
Submental lymph nodes, 494, 497
  cancer and, 498
Subpectoral abscess, 503–504
  external iliac lymphadenitis vs., 507

Subphrenic abscess, 147
Substance-P, 63
Substantia gelatinosa (SG) cells, 45–46
Substernal oppression, 158
Subtractive color mixing, 847
Succinimides, 618
Sucrase deficiency, 384
Sudeck's atrophy, 237
Suffering, pain distinguished from, 227
Suggestibility in hysterical personality,
    632–633
Suicide attempts in hysterical personal-
    ity, 633
Sulfhydryl inhibition of melanin forma-
    tion, 838, 842
Sulfonamides, fever from, 458
Sunlight and skin pigmentation, 815,
    821–822, 823f, 835–837
Superficial cervical lymph nodes, 494,
    496–497
Superficial cubital lymph nodes, 504
Superior deep cervical lymph nodes,
    494, 496
Superior mediastinal lymph nodes,
    507–508
Superior sulcus tumor. *See* Pancoast's
    tumor
Superior vena caval obstruction, 511
Supplemental motor seizure, 664
Suppuration of lymph nodes
  from acute mesenteric lymphadenitis,
    517
  peritonitis from, 517
  syndrome of, 520–521
Suppurative infraclavicular lymphadeni-
    tis. *See* Subpectoral abscess
Supraclavicular lymph nodes, 494,
    498–499
Supratrochlear lymph nodes, 504
Supraventricular tachycardia, 297, 304,
    310
Swamp fever, 506
"Sway-back," 205
Sweat glands, congenital absence of, 457
Sweating
  absence of
    in dehydration, 731
    in heat stroke, 454
  in clubbing, 246, 247
  in defervescence phase of fever,
    450–451
  hypothalamus and, 444, 447–448
  in nervousness, 594
  referred cardiac pain and, 158
  salt loss from, 741
  in Shy-Drager syndrome, 701
  and skin color, 818
  "sympathetic," in hypoglycemia, 702
  in vasodepressor syncope, 697

"Swimmer's ear," 108
Swiss-type combined deficiency,
    481–482
Sydenham's chorea, 685
Sympathetic block
  for reflex dystrophy in extremity, 231
  in reflex sympathetic dystrophy, 237
Sympathetic nervous system, heart rate
    and, 301–302
Sympathomimetic drugs, 615
  headache from withdrawal of, 77
Symptomatic epilepsy, 663
Symptoms, 1–15. *See also specific symp-
    toms*
  analysis and interpretation of, 4–10,
    13–15
  as "buffer," 10
  definition of, 1, 624–625
  environmental hazards and, 10–12
  family history and, 12
  marital history and, 12
  occupational history and, 13
  patient–physician interview and, 1–6
  social history and, 12–13
Synaptic transfer, 648
Syncope, 689–703
  in anemia, 568–570
  blood flow and pallor in, 853–854
  as conversion symptom, 633, 637
  cough, 327–328
  definition of, 689
  from disturbance in composition of
    blood to brain, 702–703
  etiological classification of, 689–690
  neuropsychologic factors in, 703
  pathogenesis of, 690–691
  pathophysiologic classification of,
    658–659
  in post-traumatic syndrome, 75
  from reduced cerebral blood flow,
    658, 691–702
    cardiac disorders, 691–693
    failure of venous return, 694–696,
      697f
    loss of peripheral vascular tone,
      696–702
    vascular obstruction, 693–694
Syndrome, definition of, 9
Syndrome of inappropriate antidiuretic
    hormone (SIADH), 737
Synovitis
  produced by urate crystals, 222
  in rheumatic fever, 222
Synovium
  anatomy of, and joint pain, 211–213
  pain sensitivity of, 214
Syphilis
  aortitis in, 152, 160
  bone pain in, 229

epitrochlear lymphadenopathy and
systemic phase of, 504
and fetal growth, 19
hepatic, 428
Jarisch-Herxheimer reaction to drug
therapy in, 458
of lung, clubbing in, 249, 253
lymphadenopathy and, 495
generalized, 522
genital lesion with, 518
granulomatous, 483
oculoglandular syndrome and, 496
oral lesions in, 130, 133
perilabyrinthitis from, 717
polyneuropathy and, 240
Syphilitic chancre
anterior auricular lymphadenopathy
and, 495
axillary lymphadenopathy and, 502
extragenital
lymphadenopathy and, 504
regional lymphadenopathy with, 517
oral, with regional neck lymphadenopathy, 518
of penis, 506
and submaxillary lymphadenopathy,
497
Syringobulbia, 721
Syringomyelia, oral lesions in, 131
Systolic bruit in hepatoma, 170
Systolic hypertension, 270–271
Systolic murmurs in anemia, 568

Tabes dorsalis, 57, 234, 240
baroreflex failure in, 699
and movement ataxia, 681
Tabetic athetosis, 681
Tachycardia, 299–314
in anemia, 568
in anxiety, 601
bradycardia and, 311n
and chemical control of heart, 299–300
in extracellular volume depletion, 741
in fever, 456
hypoglycemia and, 702
in mitral valve prolapse, 297
multifocal atrial, 310–311
nausea and, 365
and nervous control of heart, 300–302
in neurocirculatory asthenia, 297
palpitation and, 298–299
paroxysmal atrial, 303–305
with atrioventricular block, 305–306
paroxysmal junctional, 310
paroxysmal ventricular, 312–313
sinus, 302–303
and syncope, 691–693, 697, 698

Tachypnea, 335
brain-stem lesions and, 652
T cells, 470, 479, 480, 487
diseases resulting from defects in
maturation of, 481–482
in Hodgkin's disease, 484
in inflammatory lymph node reactions, 482, 483
Tearing in cluster headache, 70, 71
Technetium-99, 172, 229
Teeth
development of, 25, 27t
tetracycline-induced yellow pigmentation of, 829
vitamin-B complex diseases and, 124
Teething and fever, 459
Telangiectasia
hereditary, 410
hemorrhagic, 333
of Osler-Rendu-Weber syndrome, 400
Temperature. See Body temperature; Fever
Temporal arteritis syndrome, 87–88
Temporal lobe epilepsy (TLE), 611
Temporary threshold shift (TTS) in hearing, 110–111
Temporomandibular joint disorders and
muscular contraction headache,
74
Temporomandibular joint syndrome
(TMJ), 716
headache in, 80–81
Tenderness of palpation
in abdominal pain, 170, 171
in ureteral pain, 185
Tendonitis
shoulder pain from, 218–219
trochanteric, 220
Tendon jerks and spasticity, 678
Tendon reflexes in pernicious anemia,
570
Tendons, pain in, 56
Tenesmus, 185
Tennis elbow (lateral epicondylitis), 211,
217
Tenosynovitis, 215, 218
in infectious arthritis, 222
in rheumatoid arthritis, 218
Tension headache, 72
anxiety and depression and, 601
Terbutaline, 614
Terminal ileitis, 517
Testicular feminization, 40
Testes
atrophy of, 428
cancer of
contralateral spread of, 472
lymphadenopathy and, 515
pain from, 177

tumors of, 506
and common bile duct, 436f
Testosterone
in cluster-headache patients, 71
overproduction of, 39
refractoriness to, 40
in sexual development, 34f
Tetanus, 453
muscular effects of, 683
Tetanus antitoxins, brachial plexus neuritis from, 241
Tetany, 683
as conversion complication, 630
in metabolic alkalosis, 761
Tetracycline
fever from, 458
and pseudotumor cerebri, 78
reactions to, 131
and renal tubular acidosis, 758
and vitamin B_{12} absorption, 127
yellow pigmentation of teeth from,
828
Tetralogy of Fallot
dyspnea in, 344
syncope in, 693
Thalamic lesions
therapeutic, 684, 685
and unconsciousness, 651
Thalamic pain syndrome, 231
Thalassemia(s), 565, 577–578
and hemolytic anemia, 577–578
retinal hemorrhage and, 89
splenomegaly and, 570
α-Thalassemia, 577–578
β-Thalassemia, 577–578
S-β-Thalassemia, 584
Thalidomide, 19
Thelarche, premature, 40
Theophylline intoxication, 614
Thermal stimuli, cough produced by, 321
Thermoreceptors, 443, 444
Thermoregulatory center (TRC), 448, 449
Thermoregulatory system, 442–444. See
also Body temperature; Fever
Thiamine
in alcoholic neuropathies, 238–239
biochemical role of, 121–122
deficiency of, 120, 125. See also Wernicke's syndrome
dizziness in, 721
and polyneuropathy, 238
Thiazide diuretics, 223
Thigh adduction test, 639f
Thigh pain, 242–243
Thiouracil, 458, 851
Thirst
in dehydration, 731
impaired sensation of, 732
psychogenic, 733

Thoracic duct
   anatomy of, 475
   anomalous, and lymph flow, 472
   composition of lymph of, 469–470
   results of injury to, 475–476
Thoracic outlet syndrome, 241
Thoracic pain, 139–161
   aortic, 160–161
   cardiac. See Cardiac pain
   chest wall, 141–144
   diaphragmatic, 146–147
   esophageal, 149, 150f
   mediastinal, 147, 148f, 149–151
   origin of stimuli in, 139–141
   pericardial, 147–149
   pleural, 145–146
   tracheobronchial, 144–145
Thorax as source of abdominal pain,
      171, 177, 178
Thorazine, 424
Three-glass test, 189
Thrombin, 540–542
Thrombin time (TT) test, 543, 544
Thrombocytopenia, 129, 547–549
   accelerated destruction, utilization or
      loss of platelets, 548–549
   in aplastic anemia, 573
   classification, 546t
   deficient thrombopoiesis, 547–548
   in disseminated intravascular coagula-
      tion, 556
   in hairy-cell leukemia, 487
   and hematuria, 187
   hemoptysis in, 333
   laboratory evaluation of, 542. See also
      Platelet count
   in paroxysmal nocturnal hemoglo-
      binuria, 582
   storage-pool-like platelet deficiency
      and, 550
Thrombocytopenic purpura, 454,
      548–549
Thrombophlebitis
   congestive heart failure with, 456
   fever in, 453
   hypertrophic osteoarthropathy vs.,
      249
   septic, 454
Thrombopoiesis
   deficient, 547–548
   ineffective, 548
Thrombosis
   aseptic, fever and, 454
   paroxysmal nocturnal hemoglobinuria
      and, 582
   pulmonary, hemoptysis in, 333
Thrombotic thrombocytopenic purpura
      (TTP), 549
   fragmentation hemolysis in, 581

Thrush, 133
Thymus
   in lymphoid system, 468, 470
   tumors of, clubbing and, 252
Thyroidectomy and clubbing, 253
Thyroid function, 31
   disorders of. See Hypothyroidism
   and melanin metabolism, 840
   nutritional factors in, 801–802
Thyroid hormone, 615
   and fetal growth, 19
   for obesity, 780
   and undernutrition, 801–802
   and weight loss, 792–793
Thyroiditis, vitiligo with, 851
Thyroid-stimulating hormone (TSH)
   in depression, 600
   in malnutrition, 801
Thyroid storm, 455
Thyrotoxicosis, 59, 609
   atrial flutter in, 307
   dyspnea in, 336
   fever in, 455
   palpitation in, 298
   tachycardia in, 302, 304
Thyrotropin-releasing factor (TRF),
      596–597
Thyroxine-binding globulin, 801
Tibial tubercle, partial separation of, 220
Tic, 685
   as conversion symptom, 640
Tinea, 873–874
Tinea crurum, inguinal, 506
Tinel's sign, 236, 241, 243
Tinnitus
   in anemia, 569–570
   in brain-stem vascular disorders, 719
   in sensory-neural hearing impairment,
      110, 111
   in middle-ear disturbances, 716
   in otosclerosis, 109
Tissue anoxia and clubbing, 255, 256
Tissue responsiveness and growth, 32,
      33
Tissue tension, 140
Tissue trauma, fevers after, 456
Titratable acid excretion, renal, 753
T lymphocytes. See T cells
Tobacco. See Smoking
Todd's paralysis, 678
Toes, clubbing of, 247, 248
Toluene, 759
Tongue and mouth, 117–134. See also
      specific conditions
   cancer of, 472, 498
      hemimandibulectomy in, 501
   local lesions of, 132–134
   lymphangiectasis in, 473
   lymph nodes of, 494, 496, 498

   medical history, 119
   morphology of, normal, 118–119
   nonnutritional systemic processes
      and, 129–132
   physical examination of, 119
   physiology of, normal, 118–119
   soreness
      due to allergy, 131
      due to antibiotics, 131
      due to aphthous stomatitis, 133
      due to cirrhosis, 129
      due to "collagen" diseases, 129–130
      due to Dilantin gingivitis, 130
      due to enteritis, 133
      due to erythemas, 129–130
      due to geographic tongue, 134
      due to granulomas, chronic, 133
      due to heavy metal intoxication, 130
      due to herpetic gingivostomatitis,
         132–133
      due to hyperplasia and dysplasia,
         133
      due to hypoplastic anemia, 129
      idiopathic and drug-induced neutro-
         penia, 129
      due to isolated simple papillitis, 133
      due to leukemia, 129
      due to leukoplakia, 133
      due to lichen planus, 130
      due to local trauma, 133–134
      due to menopause, 131
      due to neurologic lesions, 131
      due to nutritional deficiency dis-
         eases, 119–129
         atrophic glossitis, 126–128
         vitamin B complex, 120–122,
            123–126
         vitamin C, 122–123, 128–129
      in pernicious anemia, 566, 569
      due to psoriasis, 130
      due to psychoneurosis, 132
      due to scarlet fever, 130
      due to syphilis, 130
      due to systemic infections, 130
      due to thrombocytopenia, 129
      due to tumors, 133
      due to uremia, 130
      due to Vincent's stomatitis, 132
Tonsilitis
   age changes in lymphoid tissue and,
      480
   in lymphoid system, 468, 470, 494,
      496
   middle ear infection and, 109
   in neutropenia, 129
Tophaceous gout, 222
Torsades de pointes, 312, 314
   and syncope, 692
Torticollis, 685

conversion, 640
    spine pain from, 234
Touch sensation, impaired
    in pernicious anemia, 570
Touraine-Solente-Golé syndrome, 252
Tourniquet test, 542
Toxemia, 473
Toxic shock syndrome, 453
Toxoplasmosis
    adult-acquired, generalized lymphade-
        nopathy in, 522
    cervical lymphadenopathy with, 518
    and chorioretinitis, 98
    histiocytic proliferation in, 483
Tracheobronchial lymph nodes, 507, 508
Tracheobronchial pain, 57, 144–145
Tracheobronchitis, 322
    acute, 322
    hemoptysis in, 332
Trachoma, 495
Traction diverticulum of esophagus, 510
Traction headache, 77–79
Transverse myelitis, 699
Trapezius contracture conversion, 640
Trauma. See also under specific body parts
    hematuria from, 187
    hemoptysis caused by, 332
    in predisposition to urinary tract in-
        fections, 190
Traumatic shock, coma from, 652
Tremor, 683–685
    from CO_2 retention, 762
    as conversion symptom, 640
    hypoglycemia and, 702
    Parkinsonian rigidity and, 679, 683
    in Shy-Drager syndrome, 701
Trenchmouth, 132
Trepopnea, 336
Trichinosis, 204, 672
    and chest muscle pain, 142
    polymyositis secondary to, 230
Trichloroethylene, 239
Tricyclic antidepressants, 458
Tricuspid disease, 352
Trigeminal nerve
    and cerebello-pontine-angle tumor,
        110
    lesion localization in, 714
Trigeminal neuralgia, 55, 57
    in cluster-tic syndrome, 69
    oral discomfort in, 134
Trigger points, 55, 57
Triglycerides, 772–773, 775
    obesity and, 777, 800
    "ketogenic" diet and, 779–780
    thyroid hormones and, 802
Trigone, 186
Trihexyphenidyl, 615
Trismus, 683

Trisomy 21. See Down's syndrome
Trochanteric bursitis, 211, 217
    "hip pain" and, 220
Trochanteric tendonitis, 220
Troisier's node, 498–499
Tropical sprue, 384
Trousseau's sign, 683
True visceral pain, 166, 167
Trunk contractures, conversion, 640
Trypanosomiasis, South American, 379
Trypsin, 865, 868
Tryptophan, 793
    deficiency of, 124
Tubercle bacillus, lipid coat of, 480
Tuberculosis, 324
    ascitic fluid and, 428
    calcification of lymph nodes in, 510
    cough in, 320
    fatigue in, 617
    and generalized peripheral lymphade-
        nopathy, 522
    granulomatous lymphadenopathy
        and, 483
    hemoptysis in, 332
    hilar lymph node involvement, 509
    hip pain and, 216, 219
    inoculation, 502, 504
    intestinal, clubbing and, 253
    laryngitis in, 322
    and mediastinitis, 150
    miliary, 451, 574
    monoarticular, 216–217
    oculoglandular syndrome and, 496
    oral lesions in, 133, 497
    posterior cervical lymphadenopathy
        and, 497
    pulmonary, clubbing and, 252
    renal, hematuria in, 187
    right middle lobe syndrome in, 327
    in sacroiliac joint, 200
    scalene node biopsy and, 499–500
    of spine, 199
    and vitamin deficiencies, 127
Tuberculosis inoculation, extremity le-
        sion and lymphadenopathy syn-
        drome from, 517
Tuberculous cervical adenitis, 497
Tuberculous elbow, epitrochlear node
        involvement in, 504
Tuberculous lymphadenitis, 516
    mesenteric, 516
    suppuration from, 527
Tuberculous lymphadenopathy, general-
        ized epitrochlear involvement, 504
Tuberculous meningitis, 655
Tuberculous pericarditis, 149
Tuberculous peritonitis, 176, 428
Tubo-ovarian abscess, renal-ureteral
        pain in, 185

Tubular lymphangitis, 468, 473, 521
Tubular necrosis, 187
Tularemia, 483, 496
    axillary lymphadenopathy and, 502
    epitrochlear lymphadenopathy and,
        504
    and generalized lymphadenopathy,
        522
    and suppuration of lymph nodes, 521
    ulceroglandular, as lymph node syn-
        drome, 517
Tumarkin's otolithic catastrophe, 718,
        722
Tumor(s). See also under specific organs
    of bone, pain from, 229
    and brachial plexus, 235
    of breast, pain from, 144
    as cause of fever, 449, 453–454
    cough due to, 326
    of eighth nerve, 719
    and epilepsy, 663
    and headache, 77–78
    and hematuria, 187
    hemoptysis caused by, 333
    inguinal lymphadenopathy and, 505,
        506
    of liver
        alcoholic hepatitis distinguished
            from, 424
        pain of, 425
    of lymph nodes, 484–488
        Hodgkin's disease, 484–486
        lymphoma
            Burkitt's, 486–487
            diffuse, 486
            hairy cell leukemia, 487
            histiocytosis X, 487
            histiocytic medullary reticulosis,
                486
            malignant, 484
            mycosis fungoides, 487
            nodular, 486
            non-Hodgkin's, 486
            Sézary's syndrome, 487
            Waldenström's macroglobuline-
                mia, 487
        metastatic neoplasms, 487–488
    malignant. See Cancer; and specific con-
        ditions
    mediastinal, 149–150
        bone pain from, 142
    and monoarticular pain, 216
    of muscle, primary, 230
    nerve root compression and pain
        from, 234
    obstipation caused by, 380
    and parietal pleura, 146
    polymyositis and, 230
    of tongue and mouth, 133

Tunnel vision, 96–97
Turner's syndrome (gonadal dysgenesis), 18, 32
Tussive syncope, 695
    dizziness in, 720
Tympanic membrane
    anesthesia (Itard-Cholewa's sign), 109
    deformities of, 108
    in otitis media vs. otitis externa, 108–109
    perforation of, 716
    in serous otitis, 109
    temperature of, 445
Tympanometry, 714, 715
Tympanosclerosis, 109
Type A behavior, 601
Typhoid fever, 452
    and herpes, 451
    histiocytic patterns in, 483
    tracheobronchitis in, 322
Thyphus fever, 452
    and herpes, 451
Tyramine, 68, 77
    in testing of baroreflex failure, 700, 701t
Tyrosinase and melanin synthesis, 832–835, 836f, 837f
    heat and, 837

U:L ratio. See Growth, measurement of
Ulcer. See specific type
Ulcerative colitis, 170, 390
    clubbing and, 249, 253
    growth failure in, 33
    jaundice with, 425
Ulnar nerve
    entrapment at elbow, 241
    reflex sympathetic dystrophy and, 237
Ultrasonography
    in abdominal pain, 172
    in jaundice, 423, 431, 436f
    and lymphoid system, 492
    of urinary tract, 187, 188
Ultraviolet photography and skin color, 813
Ultraviolet radiation. See also sunlight
    exposure to, 836–837
    and melanization, 815
    and repigmentation in vitiligo, 852
    for uremic pruritis, 868
    visual loss from, 99
Umbilical hernia, 170
    hypothyroidism and, 31
Umbilicus
    infection of, and lymphadenitis, 503
    in jaundice, 428

Unconsciousness. See also Coma; Consciousness; Syncope
    in brain-stem lesions, 650–652
    definition of, 648
Undernutrition, 787–804. See also Nutritional deficiency diseases and specific deficiencies
    and aging, 798–801
    in cancer, 795–798
    in childhood
        breast vs. artificial feeding, 791–792
        child abuse, 792
        extreme forms, 789–790, 790f, 791f
    from drug administration, 792–795
    and hormones, 801–803
    maternal, and child development, 788–792
    worldwide perspective on, 787–788
Unsteadiness, sensory-neural hearing impairment and, 111
Unilateral jaundice, 826–827, 853
Upper motor neuron syndrome, 671t, 676, 678
Upper respiratory infection, 106–108
Uremia
    abdominal pain in, 177
    coma from, 652
    and detached retina, 88
    fasciculation in, 682
    melanosis in, 829, 838
    nausea and vomiting in, 370
    oral lesions in, 131
    and platelet adhesion defect, 550
    pruritis in, 868–869
    red-cell morphology in, 579
    skin color in, 829
Uremic acidosis, 758
Uremic coma, 657
Ureter(s)
    anatomical role of, 181
    calculi of, 187
    catheterization of, 189
    innervation of, 181–184
    localization of pain from, 184–185
    as source of hematuria, 186, 187
    total obstruction of, and pyuria, 188
    tumors of, 187
Ureteropyelography, retrograde, 187
Urethra
    catheterization of, and urinary tract infection, 190
    innervation of, 184
    pain from, 176, 177, 185
    as source of hematuria, 186
Urethritis
    in Behçet's syndrome, 133
    and hematuria, 187
Urinalysis, 185

Urinary incontinence in Shy-Drager syndrome, 701
Urinary tract. See also specific conditions
    abdominal lymphadenopathy and, 513, 514
    conversion symptoms of, 642
    infections of
        fatigue in, 617
        nausea and vomiting in, 370
    neoplasms of, 187
    pain in, 181–192
        anatomic and physiological conditions of, 181
        hematuria, 185–188
        modes of expression of, 184–185
        nerve supply and, 181–184
        pyuria, 188–191
Urine
    blood in. See Hematuria
    in jaundice, 425–426, 429
Urine concentration. See Polyuria
Urine pH, 754–755
Urography, 185
    intravenous, 187
Urticaria, 873–874
    as conversion complication, 630
    in hyperthyroidism, 871
    visible jaundice in, 827
Urticaria pigmentosa, 390
    yellow skin of, 529
Uterus
    bleeding from, 554
    displacement of, 207
Utricles, function of, 708, 709, 710f, 713
Uveitis, 390
    in Crohn's disease, 170

Vaccination. See Inoculation
Vagabonds' disease, 838
Vagina
    itching of, as reaction to antibiotics, 131
    ulcers of, in Behçet's syndrome, 133
"Vagovagal syncope," 697
Vagus nerve, heart rate and, 300–301
Valsalva maneuver, 402, 498, 695
    and baroreflex system, 700
Valvular heart disease
    lethargy and fatigue in, 617–618
    and syncope, 692–693
Variant angina, syncope in, 693
Varicella, labyrinth involvement in, 717
Varices, esophageal, 399, 400, 402, 430f, 407–409
Varicose veins
    hemosiderosis with, 846
    syncope from, 696

Vascular component of hemostasis, 535–536
  laboratory approach to, 542
Vascular contraction, mechanisms of, 535–537
Vascular disorders, 543, 545–547. *See also specific disorders*
  classification of, 546t
  vertigo and dizziness in, 719–720
Vascular ectasias, 414–415
Vascular endothelium, 536
Vascular headache. *See also* Migraine
  muscle contraction headache with, 73
  physical causes of, 77
  post-traumatic, 75, 76
Vascular insufficiency of small intestine, 169
Vascular obstruction, and syncope, 693–694
Vascular spiders, 400, 426
Vasculitis
  Behcet's syndrome and, 133
  and rheumatoid arthritis, 223
Vasoconstriction in regulation of body temperature, 443, 444, 450
Vasodepressor material (VDM), 255
Vasodepressor syncope, 658, 691, 697–699
  in pulmonary hypertension, 693
Vasodilation
  in defervescence phase of fever, 450–451
  in regulation of body temperature, 443, 447–448
Vasomotor function
  in muscle contraction headache, 74
  in post-traumatic headache, 76
Vasomotor rhinitis, 77
  cough in, 326
Vasopressin. *See* Antidiuretic hormone
Vasospasm in subarachnoid hemorrhage, 79
Vasotocin, 727, 728f
Vegan syndrome, 126
Venous capacity, increase, and syncope, 696, 697f
Venous disease(s). *See also specific conditions*
  lower extremity pain from, 243
Venous obstruction
  edema in, 741–743
  muscle pain from, 230
  skin color and, 816–817
Venous return, syncope in failure of, 695–696, 697f
Venous stasis
  and hemosiderosis, 846
  hypertrophic osteoarthropathy vs., 249

Venous thrombosis
  in jaundiced patient, 428–429
  muscle pain from, 230
Ventricles, historical conceptions of, 648
Ventricular fibrillation, 313–314
  and syncope, 691, 692
Ventricular fluid pressure (VFP), brain-stem lesions and, 652
Ventricular flutter, 313–314
Ventricular phonation, 113
Ventricular premature contractions, 297
Ventricular standstill, 658
  syncope from, 691–693
Ventricular tachycardia, 297
Ventriculomyotomy, 693
Verapamil, 692
Verbal output, 166t. *See also* Language; Speech
Vertebral body fractures, 199
Vertebral lesions, abdominal pain from, 177
Vertebrobasilar insufficiency, 655–656
Vertigo
  in anemia, 569–570
  clinical approach to, 707–708, 716
  clinical significance of, 715–723
    cervical spine, 722
    drug effects, 722
    ear diseases, 716–719
    eighth-nerve diseases, 719
    epilepsy, 722–723
    intrinsic brain-stem tumors, 720
    malformations, 720–721
    psychogenic etiology, 723
    vascular disorders, 719
    viral diseases, 721
  in cerebello-pontine-angle tumor, 110
  in Ménière's syndrome, 110
  neurologic lesion localization in assessment of, 713–715
  in post-traumatic syndrome, 75
Very heavy work, definition of, 338
Vesico-ureteric reflux, 190
Vestibular disorders. *See also* Dizziness; Vertigo
  stance and gait in, 713
Vestibular labyrinth. *See* Labyrinthine pathology
Vestibular-nerve tumors, 719
Vestibular neuritis, 718
Vestibular neuronitis
  brain-stem involvement in, 721
  eighth-nerve involvement in, 719
Vestibular nuclei, ischemia and, 719–720
Vestibular system
  caloric testing of, 712–713
  functional organization of, 708–709
  lesion localization in, 714–715

  oculomotor system and, 709
  rotational testing of, 713
Vestibulosomatic system, 713
Vibratory sense, loss of
  in pernicious anemia, 570
  vitamin B_{12} deficiency and, 576–577
Vidian nerve, 71
Villous adenoma, 382, 385
Vincent's stomatitis, 132
Viomycin, 111
Viral infections. *See also specific disorders*
  acute lymphadenitis with, 483
  blebs of tympanic membrane in, 109
  dementia and coma in, 655
  encephalitis, 655
  fatigue with, 615, 617
  intermittent fever in, 451
  of muscle, 230
  muscle spasm in, 683
  and neuritis of brachial plexus, 235
  in pneumonia, 323
  polyneuritis and, 240
  and purpura, 545
  and sudden sensory-neural hearing impairment, 110
Virchow's node, 497–499
Virilization. *See also* Puberty
  adrenal dysfunction and, 39
Visceral lymph nodes. *See* Intra-abdominal lymph nodes
Visceral pain, 57. *See also* Abdominal pain
  history of study of, 165–166
  true, 167
Viscus
  perforated, renal-ureteral pain, 185
  rupture of, pain from, 169
Visual loss, 85–100
  acute, 86–95
    angle-closure glaucoma, 92–94
    with diabetes mellitus, 90–92, 93f
    occlusion of central retinal artery, 86–88
    retinal detachment, 88–89
    retinal hemorrhages, 89–90
    retrobulbar neuritis, 94–95
  chronic, 95–97
    cataracts, 95–96
    macular degeneration, 95
    tunnel vision, 96–97
  cerebello-pontine-angle tumor and, 110
  distorted vision with blurring, 98
  in giant cell arteritis, 80
  hemianopsias, 97–98
  locations of pathologic processes in, 86
  measurement of, 85
  sudden traumatic, 98–99
  transient, 97

Vision
  disturbances of
    in anemia, 569–570
    from CO$_2$ retention, 762
    conversion, 641
    in pseudotumor cerebri, 78, 79
    in vasodepressor syncope, 697
  loss of. *See* Visual loss
  and proprioception, 713
Vitamin antagonists, 125
Vitamin A
  carotene and, 817–818, 827, 828
  deficiency of
    and carcinogenesis, 798
    melanosis in, 838
  for retinitis pigmentosa, 97
  thoracic-duct injury and absorption of, 475
  toxicity of, and pseudotumor cerebri, 78
Vitamin B complex. *See also specific B-complex vitamins*
  biochemical action of, 120–122
  deficiency of, 123–126, 128, 129, 793
    atrophic glossitis and, 127
    geographic tongue, 134
  preparations, 615
Vitamin B$_{12}$
  biochemical action of, 122, 127–128
  deficiency of, 793
    and anemia, 576–577
    and atrophic glossitis, 126–128
    diseases causing, 576–577
    drug-induced, 793
    neurologic effects of, 239, 570
    in pernicious anemia, 566, 569
    and pseudotumor cerebri, 78
    and thrombocytopenia, 548
  drug effects on, 793
Vitamin C (ascorbic acid)
  biochemical action of, 120, 122–123
  deficiency of (scurvy), 128–129, 793
    and atrophic glossitis, 127
    and dermatitis, 793
    fever in, 454
    and hematuria, 187
    pathologic bleeding from, 547
    skin color in, 838
Vitamin D
  deficiency of, and hypocalcemia, 683
  mineral oil and, 793
  thoracic duct injury and absorption of, 475
Vitamin deficiencies. *See* Nutritional deficiency diseases; *and specific vitamins*
Vitamin K
  deficiency of
    clinical picture of, 555

    coagulation factors and, 552, 554–555
    drugs and, 793
    prothrombin response to, 430
    and synthesis of coagulation factors, 540, 541
Vitiligo, 827, 850–852
  in Addison's disease, 840
  in anemia, 850
  local, ultraviolet radiation and, 837
  neurogenic factors and, 841
Vitreous hemorrhages, 89
Vocabulary growth, 106t. *See also* Language; Speech
Vocal cord paralysis, 113
Voice disorders. *See* Phonation, disorders of
Voice production. *See* Speech
Volvulus, 380
Vomiting, 361, 365
  abdominal lymphadenopathy and, 513
  act of, 365–366
  in alcoholic hepatitis, 424
  in angle-closure glaucoma, 92
  in appendicitis, 174
  in biliary colic, 175
  of blood. *See* Hematemesis
  in calcified-lymph node syndrome, 516
  in cardiac disease, 371
  chemotherapy of cancer and, 796
  in cholecystitis, 175
  with conversion pain, 635
  as conversion symptom, 625, 641
  with cystitis, 191
  drugs and toxic agents inducing, 367–368
    undernutrition and, 792
  in endocrine disorders, 370–371
  and facial petechiae, 545
  in gastroenteritis, 175
  history of, and abdominal pain, 170
  in intestinal obstruction, 174
  in intra-abdominal disorders, 368–370
    inflammation, 369–370
    mechanical obstruction of gastrointestinal tract, 368–369
  in local ototic infection, 111
  in Ménière's syndrome, 110, 371
  and migraine, 65, 66
  in migraine equivalents, 67
  in motion sickness, 371
  with muscle contraction headache, 73
  and nutritional deficiency, 126, 129
  in perforated carcinoma of colon, 175
  physiology of, 365
  in post-traumatic headache, 75
  in pregnancy, 370
    and megaloblastic anemia, 126

    psychic and neurologic factors in, 366–367, 601
  in pyuria, 191
  referred cardiac pain and, 158
  renal pain and, 184
  ureteral pain and, 185
  and weight loss, in cancer, 795
von Recklinghausen's disease, 110, 235, 719
von Willebrand's disease, 537, 543, 549, 550, 552–554
von Willebrand factor (vWF), 536, 537
Voodoo death, 603

Waardenburg's syndrome, 849, 850
Wakefulness center, 649–650
Waking state, relationships to sleep and coma, 653f
Waldenstrom's macroglobulinemia, 485f, 487
Waldeyer's ring, 496, 501
Warthin-Finkeldy giant cells, 484
Warthin's tumor, 501
Watch-glass nails, 245, 247. *See also* Clubbing
Water
  distribution in body of, 726, 737–738, 744
  excess of, 736–737
  loss of. *See* Dehydration
  malabsorption of, 384–385
Water balance, normal, 726–731
  intake and output, 726, 727f
  regulation of solute concentration, 726–731, 732f
Weakness, 592. *See also* Fatigue; Muscle(s), weakness of
  alcoholism and, 424
  in anemia, 566
  in calcified-lymph-node syndrome, 516
  CO$_2$ retention, 762
  as conversion symptom, 638, 640
  in giant cell arteritis, 80
  in metabolic alkalosis, 781
  in niacin deficiency, 124
  sore tongue and mouth and, 119
  from thoracic-duct injury, 475
Weber's test, 715
Wegener's granulomatosis
  cough in, 327
  and hematuria, 187
  hemoptysis in, 334
  and leukocytoclastic vasculitis, 545
Weight. *See also* Obesity
  desirable, 770t
  in measurement of growth, 23t, 24t, 25–26, 28f, 29f

subnormal, as symptom in undernutrition, 788
Weight gain in pregnancy, 789
Weight loss. *See also* Undernutrition
  alcoholism and, 424
  associated with abdominal pain, 170
  in cancer, 795–796
    pancreatic, 176, 425
  in dehydration, 732
  drug-induced, and undernutrition, 792–793
  in giant cell arteritis, 80
  in rheumatoid arthritis, 223
  as symptom of undernutrition, 788
  from thoracic-duct injury, 475
Weil's disease, 518
Wernicke's encephalopathy
  dizziness in, 721
  fasting and, 779
Wernicke's syndrome, 612
Werdnig-Hoffman disease, 672, 676
Wet cough, 318
Wheezing, 149–150
Whiplash injury, 717
Whipple's disease, 382, 384
  peroral biopsy and, 172
Whisper speech, 113
White blood cell casts, 188
White blood cell count in acute abdomen, 178
White blood cells in urine. *See* Pyuria

Wickott-Aldrich syndrome, 548
Wilson's disease, 424, 426, 581, 684
  early psychiatric symptoms of, 613
  lunula in, 849
  and renal tubular acidosis, 758
Winterbottom's sign, 497
Withdrawal syndrome
  diarrhea in, 387
  nervousness in, 614–615
Wolff-Parkinson-White syndrome, 304
Wood's lamp, 813
Word formation. *See* Language
"Work hypertrophy," 570
Wrist
  diagnosis of rheumatoid arthritis, 223
  "ganglion," 218
  median nerve entrapment at, 241
Writer's cramp, 640

Xanthomata, 426
  yellow pigmentation in, 829
Xanthophylls, 828
X chromosomes, 17–19
  and growth impairment, 32
  and hemophilia, 552, 553
  sexual infantilism in girls and, 37
Xeroderma pigmentosum, 843
Xeroradiography, 492
Xerosis, pruritis from, 873

Xerostomia, oral sensations in, 134
Xiphisternal crunch, 328
X-rays. *See* Radiography

Yakima hemoglobin, 357
Y chromosomes, 17–19
Yeast infections, oral lesions in, 133
Yellow dermographia, 827
Yellow pigmentation. *See* Skin color, yellow
Yellow rounded digit, 253
Yersinia enterocolitica, 516–517
Yersinia infections, 133, 483, 516–517
Yersinia pseudotuberculosis, 516–517

Zieve's syndrome, 429
Zinc deficiency, 794
  from excessive dieting in pregnancy, 789
  and growth, 32–33
  and hypogonadism, 803
  pre- and postnatal effects of, 789
Zinc oxide fumes, 458
Zirconium, reactions to, 483
Zollinger-Ellison syndrome
  diarrhea in, 387
Zymogens, 539–541

ENCYCLOPEDIA OF 20TH-CENTURY ARCHITECTURE

Board of Advisors

Diana Agrest
Agrest and Gandelsonas Architects

Nezar AlSayyad
University of California, Berkeley

Eve Blau
Harvard University

Robert Bruegmann
University of Illinois-Chicago

William Brumfield
Tulane University

Jeffrey Cody
Chinese University of Hong Kong

Nnamdi Elleh
University of Cincinnati

Stephen Fox
Rice University

Kenneth Frampton
Columbia University

Diane Ghirardo
University of Southern California

Michael Graves
Michael Graves and Associates

Renata Holod
University of Pennsylvania

Steven Izenour†
Venturi, Scott Brown, and Associates

Richard Longstreth
George Washington University

Christian F. Otto
Cornell University

Michèle Picard
Montreal, Quebec

Beth Savage
National Register of Historic Places

Franz Schulze
Lake Forest College

Denise Scott Brown
Venturi, Scott Brown, and Associates

Helen Searing
Smith College

Joseph Siry
Wesleyan University

Martha Thorne
The Art Institute of Chicago

Dell Upton
University of California, Berkeley

ENCYCLOPEDIA OF 20TH-CENTURY ARCHITECTURE

Volume 3
P–Z
Index

R. Stephen Sennott, Editor

Fitzroy Dearborn
New York   London

Editorial Staff
Sponsoring Editor: Marie-Claire Antoine
Development Editor: Lynn M. Somers-Davis
Editorial Assistant: Mary Funchion
Production Editor: Jeanne Shu

Published in 2004 by
Fitzroy Dearborn
An imprint of the Taylor & Francis Group
29 West 35th Street
New York, NY 10001

Published in Great Britain by
Fitzroy Dearborn
An imprint of the Taylor & Francis Group
11 New Fetter Lane
London EC4P 4EE

Copyright © 2004 by Taylor & Francis Books, Inc.
Fitzroy Dearborn is an imprint of the Taylor & Francis Group.

All rights reserved. No part of this book may be reprinted or reproduced or utilized in any form or
by any electronic, mechanical, or other means, now known or hereafter invented, including
photocopying and recording, or in any information storage and retrieval system, without permission
in writing from the publisher.

10 9 8 7 6 5 4 3 2 1

Library of Congress Cataloging-in-Publication Data

Encyclopedia of 20th-century architecture / R. Stephen Sennott, editor.
     p. cm.
Includes bibliographical references and index.
    ISBN 1-57958-243-5 (set : alk. paper) — ISBN 1-57958-433-0 (vol. 1 :
alk. paper) — ISBN 1-57958-434-9 (vol. 2 : alk. paper) — ISBN 1-57958-435-7
(vol. 3 : alk. paper)
   1. Architecture, Modern—20th century—Encyclopedias.   I. Title:
Encyclopedia of twentieth-century architecture. II. Sennott, Stephen.
   NA680.E495 2004
   724'.6'03—dc22

                                               2003015674

ISBN   1–57958–243–5 (Set)

Printed in the United States on acid-free paper.

CONTENTS

Advisory Board Members   ii

Acknowledgments   vii

Introduction   ix

Entry List   xiii

Thematic List of Entries   xxv

Entries A–Z   1

Notes on Contributors   1471

Index   1483

P

PAIMIO SANATORIUM

Designed by Alvar Aalto and Aino Aalto;
completed 1933
Paimio, Finland

The Tuberculosis Sanatorium in Paimio, Finland, the contract won in competition by Finnish architects Alvar and Aino Aalto in 1929, completed in 1933, synthesized two potent modernist agendas. First, the design embraces modernism's utopian social commitment and its deep confidence in rational design processes. Second, the building expresses explicitly the elemental organizational tactics of functionalist architecture and its concomitant machine imagery. Metaphorically, if Le Corbusier's Villa Savoye was a machine for living in, the Aaltos' Paimio Sanatorium was a machine for becoming healthier in.

Following World War I, avant-garde architects proclaimed the emergence of a spirited and vital new, modern age. This was to be a more orderly and healthy age, brought forth by applying the lessons of modern industrial technique and rational thinking to the outlived historicism of prewar architecture as well as to the disorder and squalor of existing urban environments. Rooted in a strong sense of social commitment and relying on the effectiveness of serial production and rational processes as design strategies, modern architects sought a better, healthier world. The Aaltos' Tuberculosis Sanatorium at Paimio was both a symbol of the social role of the new architecture and a potent visual paradigm of the new world that modern architecture intended to bring into being.

Sun. Light. Fresh air. The physical presence of these natural elements informed the basis of building design and engendered the qualities of good health associated with modernist social thinking. Moreover, as a polemic, sun, light, and fresh air were vital images of the modern, healthier world. Few other building types were as convincing a symbol of modern architecture as was the sanatorium. The actual medical treatment for tuberculosis at the time—lots of sun, light, and fresh air—provided a strong image base for the design of the building and coincided with the metaphor of "health" central to modernist thought.

The completion of the Paimio Sanatorium acknowledged Alvar Aalto's prominent place among the modern architects of the day because it bore witness to his understanding and mastery of modernism's social as well as compositional tenets. However, the sanatorium was not the Aaltos' first modernist work. Having fostered connections to the international avant-garde in the mid-1920s, they moved their office to the city of Turku in 1927 and completed two important "functionalist" works. "Functionalism" was the term used by Finnish architects to label the new, modern architecture. The first important work was the Standard Apartment Building in Turku (1929), and the second was the *Turun Sanomat* Newspaper Building (1927), which was the first work in Finland to incorporate Le Corbusier's "Five Points of a New Architecture," setting the Aaltos apart from their contemporaries. During this period, the Aaltos were active advocates and propagandists for Finnish functionalism.

Conceptually, the Paimio Sanatorium is a straightforward modernist composition: an articulated but linked set of relatively discrete functional elements expressed in both plan and volumes. The building complex is functionally zoned, with each element placed in the landscape according to its requirement for sun and view. The primary functional elements include the patient's wing, comprised of an elongated suite of rooms with an open-air terrace extension, and the communal dining and assembly areas. These two pieces are linked by a seven-story volume, the entry, and control area, which houses the vertical circulation. A circulation passage connects through these elements to the service area—with its expressed water tank, smokestack, and staircase—which in turn joins the garage. The housing units for both the doctors and the staff are separated from the main building, being located in the surrounding forest. We have, then, the rational and orderly composition of differing human activities rendered into a highly visible and expressed set of spaces and forms.

The Aaltos employed the material vocabulary that came to be associated with the modernist machine aesthetic: concrete, white stucco, steel, and glass. The overall image of the building comes from its concrete frame rendered in white stucco. The whiteness not only stands in contrast to the fir forest setting in which it is located but also provides an image of cleanliness and healthiness. Each activity volume incorporates a different glazing pattern to articulate its particular function, further reinforcing the elemental nature of the organization. The industrial glazing, with its steel sash and serially produced image, complements the pipe-rail balustrades painted in primary colors; the bright,

colorful awnings; and other machined elements that give the building a somewhat nautical quality.

Despite its mechanistic appearance, Paimio went beyond the conventions of modernist elemental composition. Volumetrically and in plan, its discrete elements are not unified geometrically or orthogonally, as in Gropius's more regularized Bauhaus building (1926), but form a more haptic pattern: a chain of architectural pieces in the landscape. Eschewing the modernist tendency to place buildings as isolated elements on the landscape, Paimio appears as a dialogue between the internal world of space and activity and the exterior concerns of context and form. For example, the patient wing and communal areas splay away from each other to form a *cour de hounor*, allowing the entry court with its undulating canopy to gain more spatial prominence. Although the white, rational image stands in contrast to the deep green forest, the sanatorium is actually a sun trap. The patient wing, facing southeast, provides each patient with morning sunlight. The open-air terraces at the east end of the wing have been rotated further south to catch more sun. The dining and lounge area is oriented, with equal care, to receive the sun at different times during the day.

Paimio is not without precedent, for the Aaltos were traveling throughout Europe, meeting with the avant-garde architects and artists during the period of its design. Influences from the Dutch architect Jan Duiker and his Zonnestraal Sanatorium (1926–28), the French architects Andre Lurçat and Le Corbusier, and Russian constructivism are evident in the work. Yet it was the Aaltos' ability to meld these influences into an independent synthesis that is extraordinary. Moreover, their entry for the earlier Kinkomaa Sanatorium competition (1927) used a similar elemental composition strategy, whereas their later competition entries for the Kälviä Sanatorium (1929) and the Zagrev Central Hospital (1931) demonstrate further refinement of the ideas seen in Paimio. The sanatorium stands as witness to the Aaltos' mastery of modernist design canons and social programs, and its functionalist expression placed their name with those of Gropius, Mies van der Rohe, and Le Corbusier, among others, in the international scene of the day.

The development of detail in Paimio is extraordinary. Attention was paid to the venting of the windows, panel heating elements, nonsplash washbasins, and light fixtures that did not cast light into a bedridden patient's eyes. The suite of furnishings developed for Paimio—chairs and tables incorporating continuously curved, bentwood frames and backs and made of laminated, molded birch—represent the culmination of a series of furniture studies and wood experiments that began in 1927. In the Paimio furniture, the Aaltos combined serial production with Finnish laminated plywood technology. The free-form quality of these pieces informed his buildings immediately following the sanatorium and signaled their movement away from functionalist tenets toward the more personal style that emerged in the late 1930s.

WILLIAM C. MILLER

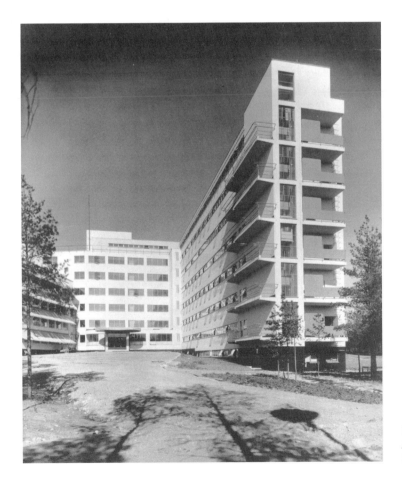

Paimio Tuberculosis Sanatorium, elevation, designed by Alvar Alto and Aino Alto (1933)
Photo © G. Welin/Alvar Aalto Archives

See also **Corbusier, Le (Jeanneret, Charles-Édouard) (France); Finland; Gropius, Walter (Germany); Villa Savoye, Poissy, France**

Further Reading

Over the course of Alvar Aalto's 50-year career (Aino Aalto died in 1949), much has been published on his architecture. The year 1998 marked the celebration of the centenary of his birth, and a number of new interpretive works have appeared. In most publications addressing the larger spectrum of his career, great emphasis is placed on the significance of the Tuberculosis Sanatorium at Paimio to Alvar and Aino Aalto's overall development. The references listed below include those that have important or interesting discussion or documentation of the Sanatorium.

Aalto, Alvar, *Paimio 1929–1933* (bilingual English-Finnish edition), Jyväskylä: Alvar Aalto Museo, 1976

Fleig, Karl and Elissa Aalto (editors), *Alvar Aalto: The Complete Works*, volume 1, London: Alec Tiranti, and Scarsdale, New York: Wittenborn, 1963; 5th edition, Zurich: Artemis, 1990 (volume 1 contains material on the Sanatorium)

Miller, William Charles, *Alvar Aalto: An Annotated Bibliography*, New York: Garland, 1984

Pearson, Paul David, *Alvar Aalto and the International Style*, New York: Whitney Library of Design, 1978; London: Mitchell, 1989

Quantrill, Malcolm, *Alvar Aalto: A Critical Study*, London: Secker and Warburg, and New York: Schocken Books, 1983

Reed, Peter (editor), *Alvar Aalto: Between Humanism and Materialism*, New York: Museum of Modern Art, 1998

Ruusuvuori, Aarno (editor), *Alvar Aalto, 1898–1976*, Helsinki: Museum of Finnish Architecture, 1978; 5th edition, 1990

Schildt, Göran, *Moderna tider: Alvar Aalto's möte med funktionalismen*, Helsinki: Soderstrom, 1985; as *Alvar Aalto: The Decisive Years*, New York: Rizzoli, and Keuruu, Finland: Otava, 1986

Schildt, Göran, *Alvar Aalto: The Complete Catalogue of Architecture, Design, and Art*, New York: Rizzoli, and London: Academy Editions, 1994

Schildt, Goran, *The Architectural Drawings of Alvar Aalto, 1917–1939*, 11 vols., New York and London: Garland, 1994 (see especially volume 4)

Tuomi, Timo, Kristiina Paatero, and Eija Rauske (editors), *Alvar Aalto in Seven Buildings: Interpretations of an Architect's Work: Alvar Aalto in sieben Bauwerken: Interpretationen des Lebenswerks eines Architekten* (bilingual English-German edition), Helsinki: Museum of Finnish Architecture, 1998

Weston, Richard, *Alvar Aalto*, London: Phaidon, 1995

PALACE OF THE SOVIETS COMPETITION (1931)

The 1931 competition for the Palace of the Soviets in Moscow represents a turning point in Soviet architecture. The competition prefaced the gradual demise of the Soviet avant-garde movement known as Constructivism and the rise of a more historically attuned approach to architecture that dominated in the Soviet Union up to and beyond the Cold War. More specifically, the competition rejected the modernist aesthetic in favor of a new architectural language, which was officially endorsed in 1937 at the First Conference of Soviet Architects and was known as "socialist realism."

Ostensibly, the Palace of the Soviets was intended to celebrate the anticipated completion of the first Five Year Plan (to occur in 1933). The Palace of the Soviets competition was also a deliberate Soviet response to the international competition for the headquarters of the League of Nations, held in Geneva four years earlier. The project was influenced heavily by the government and implemented by the Palace Construction Council, a subsidiary of the Party Central Committee. The competition brief for the building, which was developed by the Construction Council, called for a range of cultural and political spaces. The primary function of the Palace was to house the nation's highest governing body, the elected assembly of the Supreme Soviet. In addition, it was also intended to support Revolutionary festivals, conferences and musical and theatrical productions. The building included two large halls (one seating 15000 people, the other 6000), two smaller halls each seating 500 people, and two more seating 200 people. The brief called for a new relationship between form and content that was capable of representing socialist doctrine, class struggle, and the dominance of the proletariat. The site chosen for the competition was on the Moskva River in Moscow, and it was decided that the Cathedral of the Christ-Savior (built between 1838 and 1880 to celebrate the Russian defeat of Napoleon) would be demolished to create a new site southwest of the Kremlin for the Palace.

Initially, in February 1931, 12 Soviet architects were invited to submit proposals for a preliminary closed round of the competition. The prominent Soviet modernist and Constructivist schools of SASS (formally OSA), ASNOVA, and ARU as well as the rival school of VOPRA all submitted team proposals (at the request of the Construction Council). Individual entries from Alexei Shchusev, Nikolai Ladovsky, Alexander Nikolsky, Boris Iofan, Genrikh Liudvig, and Daniil Fridman were also submitted.

On 18 July 1931, the competition was extended into a more open event and the already commissioned designs (exhibited in August 1931) were included in this later stage. Further to this, 12 architects were invited to submit proposals for this round, including nine international architects such as Le Corbusier, Auguste Perret, Walter Gropius, Erich Mendelsohn, and Hans Poelzig. The three Soviet architects invited, Zholtovski, Iofan, and Krasin, were all experienced professional architects. In total, this revised competition drew 160 entries, with 24 from foreign architects. A further 112 "noncompetitive" entries were received from ordinary Soviet citizens, which, although not being considered for the competition, received considerable attention in the press. Among the individual soviet entries were schemes by leading figures at the time such as Konstantin Melnikov, Ivan Leonidov, Moisei Ginzburg, and the Vesnin brothers.

Of the first-round entries, the majority belonged to the modernist or Constructivist school of thinking. Many of the schemes, both local and international, borrowed heavily from machine forms and industrial imagery. Of the international entrants, Le Corbusier's generated the most interest because of its dynamic exposed roof structure. However, it was his functional and symbolic representation of each of the elements of the brief, and the manipulation of traffic to emphasize entry points, that most characterized his project. In the context of architectural history, Le Corbusier's scheme remains the most influential of the entrants. In contrast, Mendelsohn's scheme used the natural fall of the site to arrange a compact but less expressive arrangement, and Gropius adopted a circular configuration, connecting the two halls through a central circulation core. Of the Soviet

schemes, the project submitted by Ginzberg included a large sphere that anchored an otherwise rectilinear composition. The scheme proposed by the Vesnins was composed of a circular and rectilinear form, with a statue of Lenin situated above a tower. Among the more original entries was that of Melnikov, who rejected both the classical and modernist approaches, attempting instead to provide an architectural representation of the achievements of the Revolution. The eventual form he proposed evoked the proletariat symbol of an inverted cone that had been split apart by the forces of revolution.

At the end of this stage, the jury members (including Maxim Gorky among others) awarded two first prizes to the strongly historical designs of the Soviet architects Iofan and Zholtovsky. An additional first prize was awarded to an American architect, Hector Hamilton, with the majority of the remaining prizes being awarded to Soviet architects. Even before awarding the prizes, the Construction Council announced that "the monumentality, simplicity, integrity and elegance of architectural conception of the Palace of Soviets was not found in totally acceptable form" in any of the entries. The jury demonstrated particular dissatisfaction with the modernist proposals that it maintained were too industrial. Le Corbusier's scheme was cited as representing "a complicated machine," which, in its over emphasis on function, was seen as detrimental to the symbolism required by the brief.

On 5 May 1933, following two more stages in the competition that contained only invited Soviet architects (and mostly with a bias toward Russian Revivalism), the ultimate prize was awarded to the neoclassical design of Boris Iofan. Iofan's scheme was over 220 meters in height and consisted of a series of colonnaded tiers stacked on each other and finally culminating in a statue of "the liberated proletariat." A few days after the winning entry was announced, Stalin proposed that the statue should be enlarged four times in size to a height of 75 meters and made in the image of Lenin. This was the beginning of what Kruschev would later denounce as Stalin's "Cult of Personality." The intervention of the war in 1941 prevented Iofan's building ever being realized, despite the completion of documentation by Iofan in collaboration with the academics Shchuko and Gelifreikh. In spite of this, the legacy of the project in not only Soviet but also international architectural circles is immense. Most notably, it announced the end of the energetic architectural avant-garde in the Soviet Union and ushered in a new age of architecture, dominated by political personalities, rather than architectural creativity.

MICHAEL CHAPMAN

See also **Constructivism; Exhibition Building; Ginzburg, Moisei (Russia); Melnikov, Konstantin (Russia); Mendelsohn, Erich (Germany, United States); Russia/Soviet Union; Vesnin, Alexander, Leonid, and Viktor (Russia)**

Further Reading

Cooke, Catherine and Igor Kazus, *Soviet Architectural Competitions, 1920s–1930s*, London: Phaidon Press, 1992

Cunliffe, Antonia, "The Competition for the Palace of the Soviets in Moscow, 1931–1933," *Architectural Association Quarterly*, 11/2 (1979)

De Jong, Cees and Erik Mattie (editors), *Architectural Competitions; Architektur-Wettbewerbe; Concours d'architecture* (trilingual English–German–French edition), 2 vols., Cologne: Taschen, 1994

Lizon, Peter, "Quest for an Image to Serve a Revolution: Design Competitions for the Palace of the Soviets," *Journal of Architectural Education*, 35/4 (Summer 1982)

Lizon, Peter, *The Palace of the Soviets: The Paradigm of Architecture in the USSR*, Colorado Springs, Colorado: Three Continents Press, 1992

PALAIS STOCLET, BRUSSELS

Designed by Josef Hoffmann; completed 1911
Brussels, Belgium

The Palais Stoclet is a villa designed by Josef Hoffmann in Brussels and built between 1905 and 1911 for the Belgian millionaire Adolphe Stoclet and his wife. Although built in Belgium, the Palais is one of the finest examples of Viennese Art Nouveau, or Jugendstil, and is the most comprehensive realization of the design goals of the Vienna workshops. The building represents an elaborate example of the synthesis of architecture, interior design, and garden design that the Viennese movement accomplished. The Palais is a design *Gesamtkunstwerk*, or total work of art—an important aesthetic goal of Central European art that had, in addition to architectural design, important influences in opera (Wilhelm Wagner) and painting (Wassily Kandinsky). *Gesamtkunstwerk* design sought to create an aesthetic union of all components of a building. To achieve this, a single artist would design all aspects of the building and its furnishings, as in work by Peter Behrens and Henry van de Velde. The Palais, however, represented a collaborative effort involving the full resources of the Vienna workshops. Led by Hoffmann as architect and project coordinator, some 50 craftsmen contributed to the design, execution, and decoration of the entire villa, including its furniture, artwork, light fixtures, wall coverings, bathroom tiles, and cutlery. All aspects of Viennese modernism came together in the Palais Stoclet.

Stylistically, the building represents the Viennese version of Art Nouveau, or what is sometimes referred to as "secession-style," because the forms are geometrical rather than vegetative curves. Brussels had already been the home of Art Nouveau buildings by Victor Horta and Henri van de Velde. The addition of the Palais Stoclet made Brussels one of the few cities where organic and geometrical forms of Art Nouveau were successfully combined.

The son of a wealthy Belgian banker, Stoclet lived in Vienna for about 18 months in 1903–04 and was planning to build a home in the city. Impressed by the proportions of a villa in Vienna's suburbs built for the painter Carl Moll, the Stoclets learned that Josef Hoffmann was the architect and approached him about building a villa. The Stoclets originally intended to build in Vienna, but following the death of Stoclet's father, they returned to Brussels. The Stoclets gave Hoffmann carte blanche with the design and building costs, which used only the finest and costliest materials. Construction took six years, and each time something failed to please either Stoclet or the designers, it was disassembled, redesigned, and rebuilt without regard to

the mounting expense. The Palais was to be a perfectly realized artistic dwelling, and its final cost never has been revealed.

The Palais stands in a suburb of Brussels at Avenue de Tervueren 279–281. The building consists of two parts: a large residential block, and a service wing with a garage and workshop for Stoclet, who was an auto enthusiast. The residential block has three floors, plus a basement and an attic. The service wing had only a single floor. The strong horizontal movement of the main structure balances the tall, vertical lines of the stairwell tower. Four human figures sculpted by Franz Metzner crown the tower; they surround a dome of gilded vegetation, similar to Olbrich's Secession building. Figures of Hercules, Apollo, Athena, and the Hindu god Ganesha also adorn the building.

Despite the use of rich materials, the building's effect is serene rather than pompous. The Palais was built of reinforced concrete and brick that was faced with plates of white Norwegian marble. The exterior has a monumental quality created by the elegant use of geometric forms and white surfaces punctuated by regular fenestration. Gilded bronze bands unify the various elements and provide a counterpart to the generally white exterior of the building.

The combination of volumes projecting from a basic rectangular prism was admired widely in art circles, leading to comparison with baroque use of volumes; it created formal drama and the illusion of even greater use of space. The gradual ascension of formal elements was an attempt to blend the building into the countryside. Gardens complement the house.

The interior of the Palais Stoclet was intended for an affluent lifestyle. Most rooms have lavish proportions: the main bedroom is 30 by 18 feet, and Mme Stoclet's dressing room is 20 by 20 feet. Designers and patrons chose luxurious treatments for the public rooms, featuring polychrome marble, rosewood, and parquet floors. The main dining room is especially opulent, with an inlaid mosaic frieze designed by Gustav Klimt that is artistically significant in its own right. The frieze's themes are expectation and fulfillment, amusing choices for a dining room. They were Klimt's only opportunity to actualize his painted mosaics.

The entire household was designed and created as a unit. In an extravagant prefabrication, each room was completely assembled in Vienna for approval before being dismounted and shipped to Brussels for installation. The utensils, furnishings, and architecture were intended to complement one another in total harmony, like an organic system. Subtle relationships reflected the *Gesamtkunstwerk* concept; for example, chairs in the public rooms had backs that were exactly as high as the bronze bands on the exterior of the building. The rooms and

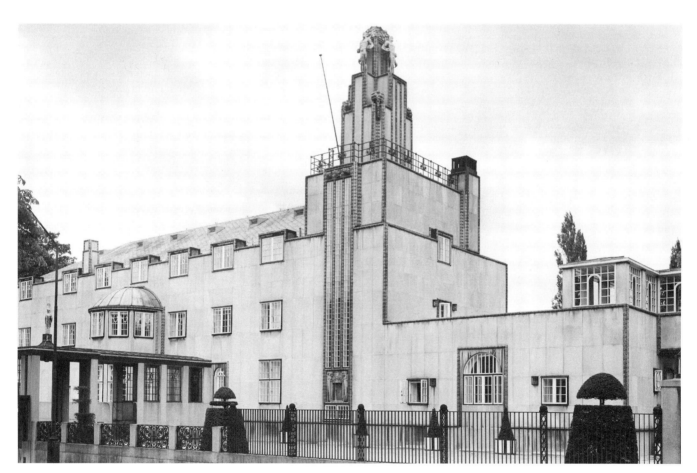

Palais Stoclet, Brussels, designed by Josef Hoffmann (1905–11)
© Wayne Andrews/Esto

arrangement also were intended to showcase the Stoclets' art collection, but other than the art collection, no preexisting furnishings or decorations were used.

Virtually every figure associated with the Vienna Workshops became involved in the project. Klimt's cartoons for the dining room mosaic were executed by the Vienna workshops using inlay of white marble, gold, silver, enamel, coral, and other semiprecious stones. The painters and designers Koloman Moser, Carl Otto Czeschka, and Leopold Forstner contributed to the furniture and other design elements. Bertold Löfler and Michael Powolny designed the ceramic decorations. Franz Metzner created the exterior sculpture as well as an animal frieze for the nursery. From the wallpaper and draperies to the garden terraces, trellises, and garden furniture, the Palais Stoclet is the supreme achievement of the collaborative ideals of Hoffmann and the Vienna workshops.

TIMOTHY PURSELL

See also **Art Nouveau (Jugendstil); Hoffman, Josef (Austria)**

Further Reading

Kallir, Jane, *Viennese Design and the Wiener Werkstätte*, New York: Braziller, 1986

Nebehay, Christian, *Vienna, 1900: Architecture and Painting*, Vienna: Brandstätter, 1983

Schweiger, Werner, *Wiener Werkstätte: Design in Vienna, 1903–1932*, New York: Abbeville Press, 1984

Sekler, Eduard, *Josef Hoffmann: The Architectural Work*, Princeton, New Jersey: Princeton University Press, 1985

Sterner, Gabriele, *Wiener Werkstätte: 1903–1932*, New York: Taschen, 1995

Varnedoe, Kirk, *Vienna, 1900: Art, Architecture, and Design*, New York: Museum of Modern Art, 1986

Vergo, Peter, *Art in Vienna, 1898–1918: Klimt, Kokoschka, Schiele, and Their Contemporaries*, Ithaca, New York: Cornell University Press, 1975

PALLASMAA, JUHANI 1936–

Architect, Finland

Juhani Pallasmaa (born 1936 in Hämeenlinna, Finland) is a Helsinki-based architect, exhibition designer, and town planner. Pallasmaa is also a prolific essayist and the former director of both the Finnish Museum of Architecture and the architecture program at Helsinki University of Technology, where he graduated in 1966.

Pallasmaa's modest oeuvre of built work belies his substantial influence in Finland and abroad. His first project was characteristically intellectual and architectural: Moduli 225, developed in 1969 with Kristian Gullichsen. The stick-built system of prefabricated building components is based on a 75-by-225-cm module and sought a practical outlet for the 1960s interest in proportional systems, as standardization offered not only economies of scale but also the possibility of relating a module of construction directly to a module of proportion. Roughly 50 houses were built. The domestic scope of Moduli 225 characterizes it as both a reinterpretation of traditional Japanese construction as well as a reworking of Finnish architect Alvar Aalto's postwar inquiry into standardized dwellings.

However, Pallasmaa's subsequent teaching and research persuaded him that modern cities suffered more from standardization than they gained. Writing in 1983 that "probably the greatest shortcoming of the Modern Movement is that it has not been able to transform itself into a positive vernacular tradition," Pallasmaa set out to diagnose the causes of this failure as well as to attempt to explain what a "positive vernacular" might be. This ongoing inquiry has involved stitching together psychological, phenomenological, and architectural observations into broad themes while maintaining concern for the social milieu or individual experience. These broad themes—already in play with Moduli 225—center on two poles: a concern for the ordinary (the role of traditional and quotidian in architecture) and the question of architectural and cultural modernism.

Pallasmaa's interest in mute, harmonious proportions is paired with the ideal of an unprepossessing, modest, even anonymous architecture, characterized by unheroic forms and materials. A limited material and formal palette is typically deployed in contrasts: open versus closed, hand-made versus machine-made, edge versus surface. In his buildings and installations, the juxtaposition of disparate materials constitute Pallasmaa's efforts to appeal to the multiple senses—his built work is "experiential" rather than cerebral. Also, the deployment of ordinary materials represents Pallasmaa's own interest in vernacular traditions, albeit as reinvented for a modern age.

Adopting poet Joseph Brodsky's dictum that beauty can only be achieved by working with the every day, Pallasmaa's first important building, the Rovaniemi Art Museum (1986) recycles a former postal depot into a gallery. The long masonry building was originally reconstructed with bricks salvaged from war-destroyed Lapland; Pallasmaa's retrofit exposes these reclaimed bricks throughout the interior, providing a quiet, poignant backdrop to the art mounted therein. On the exterior, Pallasmaa's interventions are subtle and deliberate: A new entrance threshold of glass and steel projects from the facade, fronted by five columns of different granites, marking the entrance and contrasting with the delicate entry pavilion behind.

Pallasmaa has also reworked the idea of the granite column entrance for the installation "Driveway Square" at the Cranbook Academy (1994), where the columns play a role as part of a cosmic marker. Another project in Lapland, the Sámi Museum and Northern Lapland Visitors Center (1998), inserts a minimalist building of modest scale into an arctic fells landscape, with a sympathetic installation of Sámi cultural artifacts inside.

Anonymity and harmony are hallmarks against which Pallasmaa measures contemporary society and its architectures. Pallasmaa's critical output in the 1980s asserted that Postmodern architecture represented neither reforms of modern architecture nor new "positive" vernaculars. A 1988 essay, "Tradition and Modernity," revisits the modernist canon using criteria different from formal innovation. Pallasmaa constructs an archaeology of modernism with his 1996 text *The Melnikhov House* (with Andrei Gozak)—an analysis of the modern house the Russian architect Konstantin Melnikhov built for himself in Moscow. The contradictions between the house's platonic interlocking cylinders and its complicated, organic construction suggest traditional precedents for Melnikhov's otherwise unorthodox, Platonic home. Pallasmaa evokes Melnikhov's complicated milieu via an examination of materials and details.

Indeed, the idea of home is central to Pallasmaa's thinking. Before 1986 nearly all his built work was housing, including a

summer atelier for Tor Arne (1970). His studies concerning the idea of "home" are careful to avoid cliché, including the sentimental or kitsch. Instead, Pallasmaa has relied on the work of French philosopher Gaston Bachelard (*La poétique de l'espace [The Poetics of Space], 1958*) to construct a practical phenomenology of architecture against the tactile and sensual poverty of modern construction. Pallasmaa's work also extends to the scholarly, and his comprehensive survey of Aalto's furniture as well as a monograph of the Villa Mairea, Aalto's own domestic *Gesamtkunstwerk* (total work of art), reflects his expansive approach to domestic architecture.

Timo Lindman

See also **Aalto, Alvar (Finland); Finland; Gullichsen, Kristian (Finland); Helsinki, Finland; Melnikov, Konstantin (Russia); Villa Mairea, Noormarkku, Finland**

Biography

Winner of the Finnish State Architecture Award, Professor Pallasmaa teaches at the Helsinki University of Technology and maintains an architectural office in Helsinki. He lectures widely and has been a visiting professor in Ethiopia and the United States.

Selected Works

Atelier for Tor Arne, Vänö Island, 1970
Rovaniemi Art Museum, Rovaniemi, Finland, 1986
Sámi Museum and Northern Lapland Visitors Center, 1998

Selected Publications

Alvar Aalto Furniture, 1987
Hvitträsk—Home as a Work of Art, 1987
Language of Wood: Wood in Finnish Sculpture, Design, and Architecture, 1987
"Tradition and Modernity: The Feasibility of Regional Architecture in Postmodern Society," *The Architectural Review* (1988)
Mailmassaolon taide (The Art of Being in the World), 1993
Pallasmaa, Juhani and Teppo Järvinen (editors), *Architecture du Silence*, 1994
The Eyes of the Skin: Architecture and the Senses, 1996
Pallasmaa, Juhani and Andrei Gozak, *The Melnikhov House: Moscow (1927–1929)*, 1996
Alvar Aalto: Villa Mairea 1938–39, 1998

Further Reading

Helander, Vilhelm and Simo Rista, *Suomalainen rakennustaide; Modern Architecture in Finland* (bilingual Finnish–English edition), Helsinki: Kirjayhtymä, 1987
Korvenmaa, Pekka, "From House Manufacture to Universal Systems" in *Rakennettu Puusta; Timber Construction in Finland* (bilingual Finnish–English edition), Helsinki: Museum of Finnish Architecture, 1996
Nikula, Riitta, *Architecture and Landscape: The Building of Finland*, Helsinki: Otava, 1993
Norri, Marja-Riitta, Elina Standertskjöld, and Wilfried Wang (editors), *Finland* (exhib. cat.), Munich and New York: Prestel, 2000
Poole, Scott, *The New Finnish Architecture*, New York: Rizzoli, 1992
Quantrill, Malcolm, *Finnish Architecture and the Modernist Tradition*, London and New York: E and FN Spon, 1995

PAMPULHA BUILDINGS
BELO HORIZONTE, BRAZIL
Designed by Oscar Niemeyer; completed 1942

Scattered around the Pampulha artificial lake in what was then the northern edge of the city of Belo Horizonte, the four buildings by Brazilian architect Oscar Niemeyer (completed in 1942) represent a landmark of Brazilian modern architecture.

In 1941 the city's mayor, Jucelino Kubitchek (who would be the president to build Brasília 15 years later), commissioned the young Niemeyer to design a series of buildings around the Pampulha lake, inaugurating a partnership that would change the architectural and urban face of the country. The designs for the four Pampulha buidings—Capela da Pampulha, Casino, Iate Clube, and Casa do Baile—became the paradigm for Brazilian architectural modernism as well as an international icon.

The Capela da Pampulha, or Chapel of Saint Francis of Assisi, is an intimate chapel built on a small peninsula in a curved piece of land between the lake and its encircling road. The chapel's entire back wall, which faces the street, is covered by a mural of *azulejos* (painted ceramic tiles) by the artist Candido Portinari. *Azulejos* is a Portuguese technique widely used on Brazilian modernist buildings. Gardens by Roberto Burle Marx guide visitors around the chapel to the *adro* (open area in front of churches used as transition space) that spreads between the entrance and the lake edges. The floor is designed in an amoeboid pattern in white marble and black granite that penetrates the chapel and unites inside and outside. From the *adro*, one can see the whole form—its parabolic vaults covered by small ceramic tiles (*pastilhas*), the glazing and *bris-soleil* at the facade, and the inverted bell tower and its inclined canopy—uniting the tower with the main door that marks and defines the entrance.

The Casino was also built on a peninsula between the lake and the road, this time with the entrance to the main cubic volume facing Burle Marx's gardens and the driveway. Elements of the entrance, such as its free-form canopy supported by thin steel columns and the continuous glass wall on the facade, would be exhaustively replicated all around postwar Brazil. Inside the cubic main volume, the ramp dominates, and the round concrete columns punctuate the rhythm of the interior space. At the back, closer to the lake, an elliptical dance hall is integrated with the main volume by another ramp, and its continuous glass wall brings the lake landscape inside the building. Kenneth Frampton (1980) exalted that the "Niemeyer genius reached its height in 1942" at the Casino, where he "reinterpreted the Corbusian notion of *promenade architecturale* in a spatial composition of remarkable balance and vivacity."

For the Iate Clube, Niemeyer experimented with the inverted roof to maximize the view of the lake for those using the main upper hall. This roof form would become a trademark of Brazilian modernism.

In the Casa do Baile (dance hall), a small cylindrical building houses the bar, restaurant area, and stage. Attached to this cylinder is a meandering canopy supported by rounded columns that provide shelter and define the space. The volumes are covered with painted ceramic *azulejos*. The canopy is the highlight of the building and, following the curves of the lake, defines the external space for those under it and frames the view for those passing by the road.

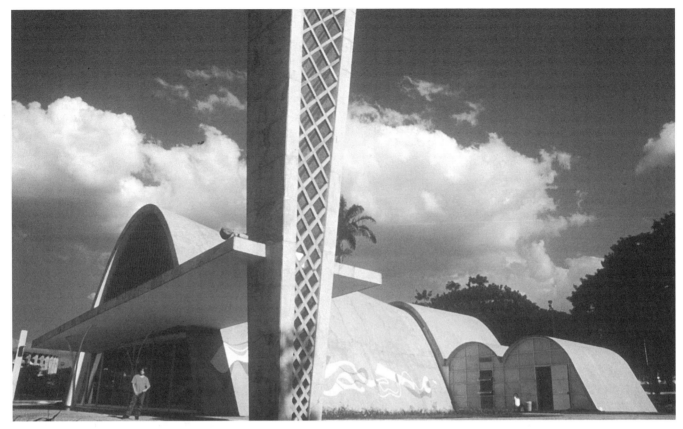

Church of St. Francis of Assisi, Pampulha, Brazil, designed by Oscar Niemeyer (1942)
© Roberto Segre

At Pampulha, Niemeyer (now working alone) produced an architecture that was, for the first time, distanced from the Le Corbusian syntax of his early influence and that was certainly more mature and personal than his designs for the Brazilian Pavilion at the New York World's Fair (1939) or the Hotel (1940) in Ouro Preto. If Niemeyer was applying the Le Corbusian idea of spatial promenade, he was also challenging the Le Corbusian idea of the "Five Points of a New Architecture," especially at the Capela. The Pampulha buildings masterfully solve the conflict between local versus international references, representation versus abstraction, and industrialization versus artisan construction.

The relevance and originality of the Pampulha buildings resonated in Brazil and abroad even before the buildings were completed. In 1942, as part of the good-neighborhood policy toward South America, an exhibition was being organized at the Museum of Modern Art in New York City. The "Brazil Builds" exhibition included works by Lúcio Costa, Affonso Reidy, Rino Levi, and the young Niemeyer, who was represented by the Pampulha buildings, still under construction. The international debate of the following decade would embrace the work, with Nikolas Pevsner labeling Pampulha as subversive work, Reyner Banham discussing it as the first national style in modern architecture, and Gino Dorfles defining it as neobaroque. In this sense, Pampulha defined the conceptual foundation of what would be the best Brazilian architecture of the 20th century.

FERNANDO LARA

See also **Burle Marx, Roberto (Brazil); Church of St. Francis of Assisi, Brazil; Costa, Lúcio (Brazil); Niemeyer, Oscar (Brazil)**

Further Reading

Bruand, Yves, *Arquitetura Contemporânea no Brasil*, São Paulo: Perspectiva, 1981

Frampton, Kenneth, *Modern Architecture: A Critical History*, New York: Oxford University Press, 1980

Lemos, Carlos A.C., *Arquitetura Brasileira*, Sao Paulo: Melhoramentos, 1979

Segawa, Hugo, "The Essentials of Brazilian Modernism," *Design Book Review* (1994)

Underwood, David, *Oscar Niemeyer and the Architecture of Brazil*, New York: Rizzoli, 1994.

PANAMA-PACIFIC INTERNATIONAL EXPOSITION, SAN FRANCISCO (1915–16)

The Panama-Pacific International Exposition, the great world's fair held in San Francisco in 1915–16 to celebrate the completion of the Panama Canal, is remembered primarily for Bernard Maybeck's Palace of Fine Arts, his majestically overscaled rotunda. As noteworthy as Maybeck's structure is, the exposition

should also be remembered for its innovative site planning and its carefully considered use of color.

The completion of the Panama Canal was an event of such significance that it was considered fitting that the United States should host a world's fair in commemoration. Although New Orleans was the early favorite, influential politicians from the Pacific Coast ensured that San Francisco was eventually chosen to showcase both the canal and the city's reconstruction after the earthquake and fire of 1906. Planning for the exposition began in 1911, when the Harbor View site (now the Marina) was selected for its views of the bay and for its location at the termination of then-fashionable Van Ness Avenue. The exposition's physical layout was determined by an architectural commission that was headed by Willis Polk and then George Kelham and included prominent California architects and several eastern practitioners of national reputation, including Thomas Hastings, Henry Bacon, and the firm of McKim, Mead and White. The Board of Architects chose to develop Ernest Coxhead's so-called court scheme, as developed by Chicagoan Edward H. Bennett; this arrangement best unified the various exhibition buildings and controlled the cold winds that blew off the bay by adopting an introverted ground plan in which most facilities were surrounded by a high ornamented wall. Every structure was to be in some way subordinate to the whole. As Polk put

it, "The serene goddess of harmony" was to be given her due by imposing a strict architectural unity on the exterior of the general exhibition buildings—color, texture, and landscape were to be tightly controlled.

The courts were designed around specific themes, such as "The Court of the Four Seasons" or "The Court of Abundance." The centerpiece of this circulation spine, McKim, Mead and White's Court of the Universe, focused on a pair of monumental triumphal arches and was bounded by Corinthian colonnades on an elliptical plan that was intended to recall Bernini's Piazza at St. Peter's Basilica. Despite this significant gesture to the Western classical tradition, the architectural board thought of the complex as a sprawling Islamic citadel, what Willis Polk called "an Aladin's Palace, facing the azure harbor and the mountains beyond." This aesthetic sensibility was retained by many of the exposition architects as they developed their individual projects, most of whom employed a tower or a dome in one way or another. Carrère and Hastings' signature building, the Tower of Jewels, sported Byzantine details and 50,000 glass jewels, fabricated in five colors by Austrian workshops. Louis Christian Mullgardt's Court of the Ages was modeled on Moorish prototypes such as the Alhambra, whereas the exposition halls themselves were designed largely by another local architect, William B. Faville, in a "Hispano-Moorish" style that employed

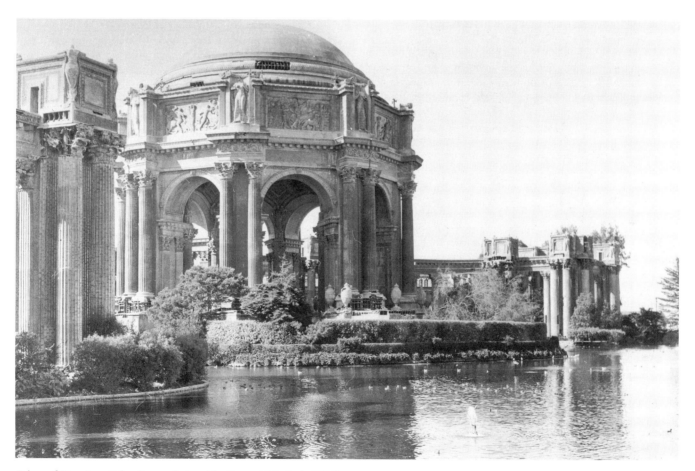

Palace of Fine Arts, Baker Street, designed by Bernard Maybeck (1915)
© Historic American Buildings Survey/Library of Congress

Roman classical motifs. Bakewell and Brown's Palace of Horticulture was reminiscent of the Blue Mosque in Constantinople with its enormous glass dome, spiky minarets, and cascading semidomes (although it sported French baroque ornament).

Color was a distinguishing hallmark of the exposition. Unlike the use of white at the Chicago, Buffalo, and St. Louis expositions, color was deemed to be an important actor in setting the exotic mood of the exposition grounds. The architectural renderer Jules Guerin was commissioned as the chief of decoration. He established a palette dominated by a warm faux travertine, a russet red, a burnt orange, and sea-foam green. Whereas some critics were concerned that the wide use of color obscured the detailed ornament of the architecture, most observers were enchanted by nightly illuminations and the shimmering fields of color encountered when viewing the site from one of San Francisco's many hills.

The exposition's most acclaimed building was Bernard Maybeck's Palace of Fine Arts. As chairman of the architectural commission, Polk had been given the assignment to design the Palace of Fine Arts, which stood at one end of the primary axis. Because Polk was busy with his other duties, he held an in-house competition to make a preliminary design deadline. Maybeck made a quick charcoal sketch of a Roman ruin that met with immediate acclaim and won him the role as architect of the building. Maybeck chose the forms of ruined antiquity for his palace, but he freely mixed different periods and styles of classical architecture. Unfortunately, contemporary writers and critics could not take it for what it was and insisted on classifying every column, frieze, and architrave. Yet anyone who analyzed the palace from a historical perspective was missing the entire point of the building. Maybeck did not sketch a building as much as an emotion. As Maybeck explained in a pamphlet issued at the exposition, the proper attitude with which one should view art was "that of sadness modified by the feeling that beauty has a soothing influence . . . to make a Fine Arts composition that will fit this modified melancholy, we must use those forms in architecture and gardening that will affect the emotions in such a way as to produce this modified sadness." For Maybeck, Roman ruins, French picturesque parks, and the engravings of Piranesi all evoked the desired emotion. Although he does not use the term, he might well have been referring to notions of the sublime.

The lagoon and all the other landscape elements were an integral part of the scheme. Maybeck and John McLaren worked closely together to ensure this synthesis. The lagoon reflected the palace in the water and forced the viewer to move around it, observing the rotunda from many different angles and in many different lights. On reaching the colonnades, the viewer was then swept along their lengths, appreciating the sculpture placed in the intercolumnations and above on the capitals and looking out again toward the rotunda, where the iconographic sculptural program of the palace was best revealed. On reaching the rotunda, one paused and was drawn toward the lagoon into its space, where the murals in the distended coffers of the dome were best appreciated. At the water's edge, Maybeck designed an alter to art, adorned with Ralph Stackpole's *Venus*, which was framed by great hedges planted by McLaren.

The landscape, colonnades, and rotunda were simply window dressing for the exposition hall, which was simply a decorated shed of steel three-hinged arches lashed together inside hollow tile walls and fitted out with frame partitions and numerous skylights. Like the other buildings at the exposition, the colonnades and rotunda were constructed out of timber and staff. Maybeck seriously proposed allowing the building to rot so that children of the future might find bits of ornament and sculpture or a wondrous ruin of a previous generation. Unique among the structures of the exposition, the Palace of Fine Arts was spared the wrecker's ball, but by the 1950s the structure was decomposing. By the end of the decade, a movement to rebuild the structure in concrete was begun, and in 1960 a sponsor was found. Today, the rebuilt palace is the backdrop for numerous community activities, television commercials, and weddings.

The exposition included more than just the walled city. Numerous state and international pavilions accompanied the thematic exposition halls. The international pavilions were usually designed in a National Romantic mode or in a traditional national style, whereas the state pavilions took on Beaux-Arts classical forms or replicated a historic structure associated with the state, such as Massachusetts's replica of Bulfinch's statehouse or Virginia's faux Mount Vernon. Perhaps the most memorable state pavilion was Oregon's redwood-log temple, "reminiscent of the Parthenon in Athens." The entertainment midway, known as The Zone, contained the usual array of rides, sideshows, and ethnographic exhibits but also featured replicas of the Grand Canyon and Yellowstone Park, sponsored by the Santa Fe and Union Pacific Railroads, respectively. The most visited attraction, however, was L.E. Myers's five-acre scale model of the Panama Canal, which visitors toured from a 1200-seat moving platform.

Although the celebratory mood of the exposition was dampened by World War I, the directors and exhibitors at the exposition did their best to present an optimistic, progressive view of human social and political development. Perhaps San Francisco itself was the best object lesson in the tenacious desire of the human spirit to overcome natural and political disaster. In nine years, the City by the Bay not only reconstructed itself from the ashes of the 1906 earthquake and fire but also constructed on the rubble of the old city the evanescent city of the Panama-Pacific International Exposition, a powerful expression of the Progressive Era.

JEFFREY THOMAS TILMAN

See also Carrère, John Mervin, and Thomas Hastings (United States); Exhibition Building; Maybeck, Bernard R. (United States); McKim, Mead and White (United States)

Further Reading

"An Early Glimpse of the Panama-Pacific Exposition Architecturally," *The Architect and Engineer of California*, 30/3 (October 1912)

Barry, John Daniel, *The City of Domes: A Walk with an Architect about the Courts and Palaces of the Panama-Pacific International Exposition*, San Francisco: J.J. Newbegin, 1915

Burke, Katherine Delmar, *Storied Walls of the Exposition*, San Francisco: Katherine Delmar Burke, 1915

Cardwell, Kenneth H., *Bernard Maybeck: Artisan, Architect, Artist*, Santa Barbara, California: Peregrine Smith, 1977

Denivelle, Paul E., "Texture and Color at the Panama-Pacific Exposition," *Architectural Record*, 45/11 (November 1915)

James, Juliet Helena Lumbard, *Palaces and Courts of the Exposition: A Handbook of the Architecture, Sculpture, and Mural Paintings*

with Special Reference to the Symbolism, San Francisco: California Book, 1915

Maybeck, Bernard R., *Palace of Fine Arts and Lagoon, Panama-Pacific International Exposition, 1915*, San Francisco: Paul Elder, 1915

McCoy, Esther, *Five California Architects*, New York: Reinhold, 1960

Mullgardt, Louis Christian (editor), *The Architecture and Landscape Gardening of the Exposition*, San Francisco: Paul Elder, 1915

Pierson, William H., Jr. and William H. Jordy (editors), *American Architects and Their Buildings*, 5 vols., Garden City, New York: Doubleday, 1970–76

Starr, Kevin, *Americans and the California Dream, 1850–1915*, New York: Oxford University Press, 1973

Woodbridge, Sally, *Bernard Maybeck: Visionary Architect*, New York: Abbeville Press, 1992

Woollett, William L., "Color in Architecture at the Panama-Pacific Exposition," *Architectural Record*, 45/5 (May 1915)

PARIS, FRANCE

In terms of their phenomenal size and scale, in the use of iron, glass, or concrete for their construction, or in the novelty of their form, many buildings of the 19th century in Paris established an outstanding tradition of architectural innovation in the city that was influential in the development of modern architecture all over the world. Architects such as Anatole de Baudot, Henri Labrouste, and Louis-Auguste Boileau were at the forefront in the use of new materials, and engineers such as Gustave Eiffel and Victor Contamin designed structures of unprecedented height and span for the international exhibition of 1889.

From the beginning of the 20th century to its end, no decade (other than the period 1940–50, of World War II and its aftermath) in Paris passed without seeing the building of major landmarks in the progress of architectural design.

One of the most densely populated cities in Europe, roughly circular and bisected from east to west by the Seine River, central Paris is today encircled by the *périphérique*, the eight-lane motorway within which live some 1.6 million people in an area of great historical importance, containing major Roman remains, great medieval buildings, and narrow medieval streets traversed by wide, 19th-century boulevards. The whole city is dominated by large-scale 17th-, 18th-, and 19th-century squares, gardens, palaces, and public buildings. It is therefore not surprising that refurbishment is one of the main 20th-century themes; re-use is another, and yet another has been the relocation of museums, libraries, and administrative offices in new buildings. New housing is a constant focus of activity.

The city began the century with a huge international exhibition for which many temporary and some permanent buildings were erected. Two large exhibition halls, built for the Exposition Universelle of 1900, were the Grand Palais by Henri-Adolphe-Auguste Deglane, Louis-Albert Louvet, and Albert Thomas and the Petit Palais by Charles Girault, both still standing in what is now the Avenue Winston-Churchill. The Grand Palais as well as the adjacent Pont Alexandre III (the first bridge to cross the Seine in one span, designed by the engineers Résal and Alby) are, like the Petit Palais, flamboyant in their neobaroque style, but they are also openly expressive of the iron structure to which they owe their form.

An antihistoricist movement had already by then made its mark in Paris and was encouraged by the opening of Samuel Bing's *Maison de l'Art Nouveau* in the rue de Provence in 1895.

Using exposed ironwork, reinforced concrete, or masonry, buildings in the short-lived style known as Art Nouveau are remarkable for their curved and undulating lines; their organic, floral decoration; and their studied avoidance of motifs associated with the past. Important Art Nouveau buildings in Paris by Hector Guimard include the apartment building Castel Béranger (1894–98) and the entrances to many Métro underground railway stations (1899–1903). Some of these designs were still being carried out as late as 1914. For his own house in the avenue Mozart (1909–12) and the synagogue in the rue Pavée (1913), Guimard remained faithful to the Art Nouveau after it had fallen from general favor. The Samaritaine department store (1905) by Franz Jourdain was characteristic of the movement, in that exposed structural ironwork is combined with lavish polychrome faience decoration.

At the same time, significant buildings were being designed with little or no decoration at all. Following the pioneering systems of reinforced concrete devised by Hennebique, Coignet, and Considère, the brothers Auguste and Gustave Perret were the first architects to make extensive use of this constructional technique in all their buildings. The apartment house at 22 rue Franklin (1902–03), the garage in the rue Pontieu (1905–06, demolished ca. 1969), the Théâtre des Champs-Elysées (1910–13), and the church of Nôtre Dame, Le Raincy (1922–23), are well-known examples of buildings revealing their structure and with minimal or no decorative features. Henri Sauvage designed two influential apartment houses: the *Maison à Gradins* in the rue Vavin (1911–12) and the *Immeuble d'appartements* (1924–26) in the rue des Amiraux explore the setting back of each successive floor, with full-length balconies and the use of white-tiled facades to bring light to the apartments and to the street.

An elegant reinforced-concrete structure was designed for a cardboard factory at Lancey near Paris by the Swiss engineer Robert Maillart (1872–1940), and a pair of spectacular 300-meter-long aircraft hangars (destroyed 1939–45) at Orly in the form of 62.50-meter-high parabolic arches were commissioned by the French government in 1916 from Eugène Freysinnet (1879–1962).

The work of such architects and engineers as Perret, Maillart, and Freysinnet were among the sources of inspiration to the Swiss-born Charles-Edouard Jeanneret (Le Corbusier), who settled in Paris in 1917 and who built his first Parisian building, the Villa Ker-Ka-Re (1922–23), at Vaucresson in the western suburbs. This house, with its asymmetrical facade, had smooth, white, cement-rendered walls; horizontal and vertical strips of windows; and a flat roof. Its design reflected the close interest the artist had in Cubist painting. A studio house in the avenue Reille for the painter Amédée Ozenfant was completed in 1924. Le Corbusier was subsequently to design a number of celebrated and influential buildings in and near Paris, including the Maison Roche/Jeanneret (square du Docteur Blanche, 1923–24), the Maison Planeix (boulevard Masséna, 1924–28), the suburban villa Stein/de Monzie (Les Terrasses, 1926–28) at Garches, and the dazzling Villa Savoye (Les Heures Claires, 1928–29) at nearby Poissy.

Other important Parisian houses of this period characterized by their pure, white, cubic forms were the Maison Tzara

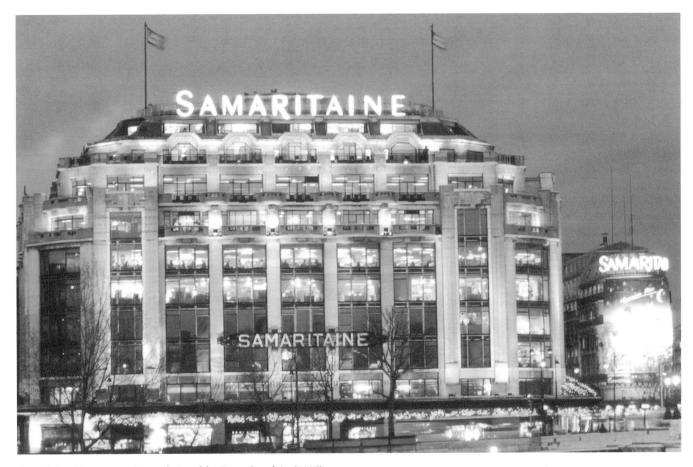

Samaritaine Department Store, designed by Franz Jourdain (1905)
© Charles Jean Marc/CORBIS SYGMA

(1925–27) by the Viennese architect Adolf Loos (although the ground floor is of coursed rubble), the Villa Seurat (1924–26), and the Maison Guggenbuhl (1927) by André Lurçat and the group known as the Cité Mallet-Stevens (1926–27) by Robert Mallet-Stevens. The unique Maison de Verre (1929–31) by Pierre Chareau has, by contrast, a sheer wall of glass as its facade.

In 1937 the Exposition des Arts et Techniques was the occasion for the erection of a number of monumental public buildings that continue to impose on the modern appearance of Paris: the Palais de Chaillot (Place du Trocadéro, by Carlus, Boileau, and Azéma) and the twin Musées d'Art Moderne (Palais de Tokyo, by Dondel, Aubert, Viard, and Dastugue) nearby on the Avenue de New York. Both are stone-clad reinforced-concrete structures epitomizing the stripped neoclassicism in vogue in the more conservative circles at the period.

Meanwhile, Le Corbusier continued to contribute buildings of fundamental importance to the Modern movement in architecture: the Asile Flottant (1929), a converted barge moored on the Quai d'Austerlitz to shelter vagrants, and the Cité de Refuge de l'Armée du Salut (1929–33) were commissioned by the Salvation Army. The Swiss Pavilion (1932) at the Cité Internationale of the Cité Universitaire is a hostel for Swiss students. This building clearly differentiates its component parts, with its ground-hugging curved lobby, its staircase tower, and its long,

rectangular, curtain-walled dormitory slab raised on in situ cast stilts, or *pilotis*. In many respects, it established themes that were to be developed by Le Corbusier and countless other architects for the rest of the century.

During World War II and the Occupation, there was no significant architectural activity, and the economy took until the 1950s to recover sufficiently for serious new buildings to be financed. Le Corbusier designed the twin Maisons Jaoul (1952–56) in Neuilly, which, although of low cost and very modest in scale, were widely influential on many architects: their use of simple, shuttered concrete forms and segmental vaults resting on exposed brickwork walls heralded a new roughness and primitivism. In 1959 Le Corbusier, with Lucio Costa, designed a new pavilion for Brazilian students at the Cité Universitaire. Only 200 meters from the Swiss Pavilion and, like it, essentially consisting of a dormitory slab raised on *pilotis*, straddling the ground-floor communal spaces, the Brazilian Pavilion is by contrast rough, heavy, and vigorous in its concrete forms. An overall grid of *brise-soleil* projecting balconies and screens extends over the facade.

The Headquarters of UNESCO (1953–58) was one of the first large-scale undertakings of the period, an eight-story building, in plan a curved Y shape, by Marcel Breuer (United States), Bernard Zehrfuss (France), and Pier Luigi Nervi (Italy). It was

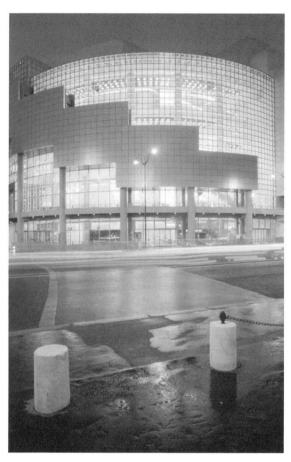

France Opéra de la Bastille, designed by Carlos Ott (1989)
© Charles Jean Marc/CORBIS SYGMA

designed to respect the form of the Place Fontenoy, behind the École Militaire, and to fit in with one of the most complex and important axial sequences of the city. A splendid program of commissions from leading artists of many nationalities was inaugurated to embellish the interior and its exterior site.

One of the largest buildings of the complex around the Place de la Défense, which closes the axis of the avenue de la Grande Armée to the west of the Etoile, was the CNIT, Palais des Expositions (1957–58), by Camelot, de Mailly, Zehrfuss, and Esquillan. Triangular in plan and covered with a continuous fluted concrete-shell roof rising from three points on the ground, the Italian Pier Luigi Nervi was the engineer, and the veteran pioneer of metal cladding, Jean Prouvé, designed the vast elliptical curtain walls of glass and steel on each side.

With the hostility felt by General de Gaulle and his government to the Montparnasse Tower block, which rose above the southern skyline of Paris in the 1960s, skyscrapers were banned from the central area, and the Défense, which is beyond the *périphérique*, was the first area to develop a cluster of tall buildings.

A restrained but powerful, moving, and effective memorial to those who died in concentration camps is the Mémorial de la Déportation (1961–62) by Henri Pingusson It is situated at the tip of the Ile de la Cité. The visitor descends a steep and narrow staircase to a small open courtyard from which nothing can be seen but the sky above and the parting of the waters of the river through a low metal grille ahead. An underground space behind has the names of the camps and a tunnel of thousands of tiny lights stretching as far as the eye can see.

With the establishment of the cultural Centre Georges Pompidou, or Beaubourg, the era of "Grands Projets" began for Paris, in which successive presidents of France committed the state to an astonishing series of monumental additions to the city. The design of a London-based Anglo-Italian architectural practice, Renzo Piano and Richard Rogers, the Pompidou Center (1970–77) is at once a realization of the ideas current in the Archigram Group in London during the 1960s and a worthy successor to the Parisian tradition of novel metal-and-glass buildings. Alongside a new square, or piazza, under which there is a parking lot, rises the rectangular steel-framed block, with open floors internally—all clear of any vertical structural supports. All services, heating, ventilation, electricity, water, and drainage are on the exterior, making an until-then-unprecedented exposure of all the technology required in a modern public building. Close by, IRCAM (1977), an institute for interdisciplinary research into music, was designed by Piano and Rogers as a network of spaces under the new Place Igor Stravinsky; in 1989, Renzo Piano added to it a 25-meter tower aboveground. Since 1970 vast areas have been developed underground in Paris. The remarkable 19th-century iron-and-glass market pavilions of the Halles Centrales (by Victor Baltard and Félix Callet in 1869) were demolished during the 1970s, and in their place, following gigantic excavations, an underground shopping area, the Forum, was designed by Penchreac'h and Manoilesco. The subterranean complex also contains a busy new RER/Métro transport interchange and, 20 meters down, an Olympic-size swimming pool, a gymnasium, and a *vidéothèque* (1985) by Paul Chemetov.

Two outstanding new museums were created in the mid-1980s, both inserted into old buildings. One, the Musée d'Orsay (1986), in the disused Gare d'Orsay (1900, Victor Laloux), was designed by the Italian architect Gae Aulenti with monumental but open galleries and towers under the vault of the giant railway station nave. The Musée Picasso (1985) was, by contrast, a transformation by Roland Simounet of a 17th-century house in the Marais district, the Hotel Salé (Hôtel Aubert de Fontenay). Simounet inserted into the ancient fabric of the building a brilliant sequence of well-lit spaces and volumes while respecting, where they had survived near dereliction, details of the original architecture.

The Cité des Sciences et de l'Industrie, a very large science and technology museum, was created in a conversion of the former slaughterhouses of La Villette by Adrien Fainsilber in 1986. In 1988 the Archives Nationales were moved from the Hôtel de Soubise to a new building by Stanislas Fiszer, and in 1989 the Ministère de l'Economie aet des Finances was rehoused in a building featuring a spectacular bridge over the Quai de la Rapée (P. Chemetov and B. Huidboro), having been moved to clear the Richelieu wing of the Louvre for yet another Grand Projet.

The Opéra de la Bastille (1989) by Carlos Ott was built on the site of the old Bastille station. This was the first of President Mitterand's projects, designed to bring opera to mass audiences, leaving the old Opéra of Charles Garnier to concentrate on ballet. It is a roughly triangular building in plan, with a vast backstage complex of machinery to facilitate rapid scene changes

and an ambitious succession of operas throughout the year. The main entrance, at the blunt apex of the plan, is rounded to counterpoint the curved plan of the Place de la Bastille. The 1980s also saw the construction of the Institut du Monde Arabe (1987, Jean Nouvel, Pierre Soria, and G. Lezenne), with its remarkable curtain wall of 30,000 light-sensitive diaphragms that open and close irises to admit or to exclude light, a reinterpretation of the latticework screens of the *Moucharabieh*.

Perhaps the most prominently visible addition to the cityscape of the period was the Grande Arche de la Défense by the Danish architect Johann-Otto von Spreckelsen, a giant 110-meter open cube that now frames the termination, at La Défense, of the great seven-kilometer axis that begins at the Louvre and runs through the Arc de Triomphe.

These grand projects continued in the 1990s. The massive reorganization of the whole of the Louvre and its new subterranean concourses is signaled by its new entrance, the Grande Pyramide (1993). This and other major additions were by the American architect I.M. Pei. The new Bibliothèque de France (1995) by Domique Perrault, the largest building of the Mitterand era, is the enormous focus of the Seine-Rive Gauche redevelopment area, a project that will continue for the next 15 years and that will include a new university campus. The Cité de la Musique (1991–94) by Christian de Portzamparc, incorporating a museum, houses the Conservatoire National Supérieur de Musique et de la Danse, and Kenzo Tange's first European building, Le Grand Ecran, was commissioned by President Jacques Chirac for audiovisual production and projection. Its 55-meter-high open steel campanile on the Place d'Italie is transfixed by a striking Constructivist composition of giant metal cubes and beams by Thierry Vide. Jean Nouvel's Fondation Cartier pour l'Art Contemporain (1994) is partly concealed by freestanding screens of metal and glass on a monumental scale aligned with the boulevard Raspail, so that the building is hidden and revealed by a complex interplay of foliage, transparency, and reflections.

In the last decade of the 20th century, Paris has seen the creation of large new parks, among them Le Parc André Citroën (1992) by Patrick Berger and others and Le Parc de la Villette (1993) by Bernard Tschumi. Superb new sports stadiums have been built; for example, the Stade Sébastien-Charléty (1994) by Henri and Bruno Gaudin and the Stade de France (1998) at Saint-Denis by Macary, Zublena, Régembal, and Costantini. Ambitious new hospitals have been built, such as the Hôpital Robert Debré (1997) by Pierre Riboulet, a long, curved building that follows the slope of a large site in the 19th Arrondissement.

The 1990 project of the Ministère de la Poste to build 1500 dwellings on its sites has already resulted in a number of attractive and imaginative new buildings, such as those in the Place Jeanne d'Arc (Dubus and Richez) or in the rue Oberkampf (1993, Borel).

A constant program of restoration, new housing, new facilities, and refurbished street furniture has improved the city in almost every quarter, a good example being the enormous program of improvements made to the avenue de l'Italie during 1999–2000.

The municipality of Paris set up enlightened agencies such as the RIVP (Régie Immobilière de la Ville de Paris) and the designation of areas of the city as ZACs (Zones d'Aménagement Concertées, such as those at Reuilly, 1987–97, or Bercy, 1993–

36) as key elements of the continuing restructuring, repair, and embellishment of the urban fabric of this great city.

ALAN WINDSOR

See also **Art Nouveau (Jugendstil); Breuer, Marcel (United States); Corbusier, Le (Jeanneret, Charles-Édouard) (France); Grande Arche de La Défense, Paris; Horta, Victor (Belgium); Maillart, Robert (Switzerland); Maison de Verre, Paris; Mallet-Stevens, Robert (France); Metro Station, Paris; Notre Dame, Le Raincy; Nouvel, Jean (France); Pei, I.M. (United States); Perrault, Dominique (France); Perret, Auguste (France); Pompidou Center, Paris; Tschumi, Bernard (France); Villa Savoye, Poissy, France**

Further Reading

Campbell, Barbara-Ann, *Paris: A Guide to Recent Architecture*, London: Ellipsis and Cologne: Könemann, 1999

Collins, Peter, *Concrete: The Vision of a New Architecture: A Study of Auguste Perret and His Precursors*, London: Faber and Faber, and New York: Horizon Press, 1959

De Witt, Dennis J. and Elizabeth R. De Witt, *Modern Architecture in Europe: A Guide to Buildings since the Industrial Revolution*, London: Weidenfeld and Nicholson, and New York: Dutton, 1987

Hitchcock, Henry-Russell, *Architecture, Nineteenth and Twentieth Centuries*, London and Baltimore, Maryland: Penguin, 1958; 4th edition, London and New York: Penguin, 1977; reprinted, New Haven, Connecticut: Yale University Press, 1987

Hoyet, Jean-Michel, *L'Architecture Contemporaine à Paris; Contemporary Architecture in Paris* (bilingual French–English edition), translated by Bernard Wooding, Paris: Techniques and Architecture, 1994

Middleton, Robin and David Watkin, *Neoclassical and 19th Century Architecture*, 2 vols., New York: Abrams and London: Academy Editions, 1980

Whittick, Arnold, *European Architecture in the Twentieth Century*, 2 vols., London: Lockwood, 1950; New York: Philosophical Library, 1950–

PARK HOTEL, SHANGHAI

Designed by Laszlo Hudec; completed 1934
Shanghai, China

The Park Hotel (1934), also known as the Guoji Fandian (or the International Hotel), was designed by Hungarian architect Laszlo Hudec (1893–1958) in Shanghai with the aid of Chinese and European architects and assistants in his firm. Since its completion in 1934, this skyscraper hotel has been a major landmark on the horizon of this enormous city. At 284 feet, the Park Hotel stood as the tallest building in Shanghai until the 1980s. Its value to the history of architecture lies in the circumstances of its origin, as witnessed by a young I.M. Pei, who cites his exposure to the hotel's construction as the reason that he decided to become an architect. The hotel is a significant vector where the steady streams of European and American ideas and technology spreading around the world after World War I intersected with the self-conscious aspirations of certain Chinese groups to a global culture.

Shanghai before World War II was a cosmopolitan city that had seen tremendous growth since the first Europeans settled in it in the early 19th century. As one of several areas conceded to Britain in the aftermath of the Opium War in 1842, what had been a small but prosperous trading center strategically located at the mouth of the Yangtze River quickly changed through the influx of foreigners. By the 1930s, there were people of 56 different nationalities living in the city. Foreigners and Chinese alike were attracted by the city's unique opportunities for economic success afforded by the autonomous and liberal city regulations granting foreigners rights beyond those of the vast majority of Chinese inhabitants. Many Chinese living in Shanghai had fled civil strife throughout the century of Shanghai's "glory days." In this enclave of international trade within Chinese borders, Chinese of different regional groups established bonds that evolved into powerful economic, political, and social organizations.

It was from a group of successful Chinese bankers that the bank owning the Park Hotel evolved in 1923. The Joint Savings Society (JSS) was one of the ten largest modern banks in China by 1928, modeled on Western-style commerce by Chinese businessmen with an overseas education. They were from the coastal provinces of Zhejiang and Kiangsu, and some rose to a position where their advice—and their money—was sought by Chiang Kai-shek's government. This group's political and underworld associations are complex and unclear. However, as part of an elite group of financiers who believed that China's future lay in the participation of a global culture, they instituted new types of services, such as the China Travel Agency and modern banks based on Western models. The Park Hotel was operated by International Hotels Ltd., a Chinese company that also ran the new International Hotel School as part of the hotel.

The hotel rose over the racecourse, the most important social center for the international community, and participated tangibly in Shanghai's symbiotic relationship with foreign capital. It was the most visible structure on Nanking Road, a street famous for its culture of consumption. Nanking Road has been called the source of the transformation of the Chinese way of life. For many Chinese, who by a large margin held the majority in a city famous for its international composition, the street's shops, with Western goods advertised by blazing neon signs, held out hopes of status and success and symbolized impossible dreams of happiness.

At the time of its construction, local media praised the Park Hotel as a modern enterprise in every aspect that made use of modern technology to provide up-to-date services. Its Otis elevators were of the same model and speed installed in the Empire State Building only three years earlier. Publications on

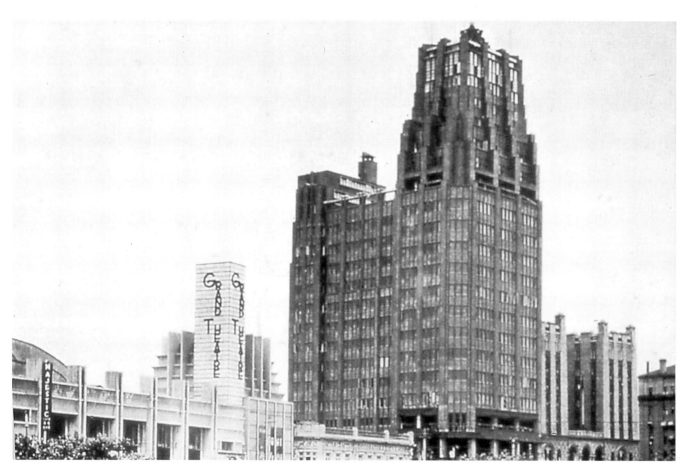

Park Hotel, Shanghai, designed by Laszlo Hudec (1934)
© Lenore Hietkamp

the hotel in European, American, and Shanghai trade journals of the 1930s reveal an appreciation for the use of new technology in air conditioning, sprinklers, and steel manufacture as well as an acknowledgement of the growing trade of Western building products in China.

The hotel is evidence of the creative opportunities available to Shanghai's architects not seen elsewhere in the world. The convergence in this city at this time of practitioners and wealthy patrons from many different countries, as well as evolving or nonexistent building codes in which to experiment, meant that architectural ideas from around the world found unique expression in Shanghai. The unusual dual function of the Park as hotel and bank clearly reflected its origins in the JSS. From the second to the 19th floor, it was a hotel with all the latest modern amenities and a private suite for one of its board of directors. The bank and its vaults occupied the first floor and basement.

The Park was an apartment hotel skyscraper in a streamlined Art Deco style, a building type then popular in American cities and, when urban dwellings became fashionable for their ability to represent sophisticated and progressive ideals, in Shanghai.

Hudec traveled widely to both Europe and the United States. In 1927–28 he sketched skyscrapers and hotels in New York and California. This architect cited the work of Raymond Hood as his principal source of inspiration in the Park Hotel and suggested that, like Hood's misunderstood skyscraper designs, the Park Hotel was innovative in its solution to the problem of tall building design.

The hotel's dark, brooding appearance can be attributed to the architect's Central European heritage. The creation of regional styles, a topic under close scrutiny at the time of Hudec's Beaux-Arts training in Budapest from 1911–14 continued to be of interest to Hudec in Shanghai. Much of this architect's work, observed in close proximity to a widely diverse body of architectural styles in Shanghai, carries associations with Central or Northern European architecture, especially through surface decoration and general sensibility.

The hotel's architect, Laszlo Hudec, is acknowledged in Shanghai today as a significant contributor to the city's historic architecture. His work is virtually unknown outside Shanghai because China's 20th-century culture avoided the close scrutiny of Western scholars until the 1990s. The unusual architectural opportunities of this dynamic city provided fertile proving ground, and Hudec's own architectural office was well established by 1925, with a peak period of production between 1925 and 1934.

Like many other structures of note during the early 20th century, the Park Hotel illustrates its architect's concern with evolving an architecture that represented the dynamic developments in technology as well as a growing awareness of the meaning of architecture in society. Modern technology, American apartment hotel typology, and hybrid skyscraper design easily convey sentiments of a humanity's heroic and sophisticated presence on earth, just as other skyscrapers in the United States did. However, the message is carried to further depths with this highly visible structure on what continues to be China's symbolic street of capitalist enterprise. The human achievements acclaimed by the building of the Park Hotel were that of an elite group of Chinese who firmly believed that the attainment of a global culture was the hope for China's future. It is a message that once again finds expression in the current architectural climate of Shanghai.

LENORE HIETKAMP

Further Reading

Hietkamp, Lenore, "The Park Hotel, Shanghai (1931–1934), and Its Architect Laszlo Hudec: 'Tallest Building in the Far East' as Metaphor for Pre-Communist China" (Master's thesis), University of Victoria, Canada, 1998

Johnston, Tess and Tung-Ch'iang Erh, *A Last Look: Western Architecture in Old Shanghai*, Hong Kong: Old China Hand Press, 1993

Johnston, Tess and Tung-Ch'iang Erh, *The Last Colonies: Western Architecture in China's Southern Treaty Ports*, Hong Kong: Old China Hand Press, 1997

Neyer, W.S., Q.L. Dao, and F.L. King, *The Memorial Supplement for the Construction of 22-Storied Building for the Joint Savings Society–Shanghai, Built by Voh Kee Construction Co.*, Shanghai: Voh Kee Construction, 1934

Shipley, William S., "China Modernizes," *Scientific American*, 150 (April 1934)

Yeh, Wen-hsin, "Shanghai Modernity: Commerce and Culture in a Republican City," *China Quarterly*, 150 (June 1997)

PARKING GARAGE

The development of the parking garage in the 20th century was a direct consequence of the automobile's unprecedented disruption of the 19th-century city. Whereas traditional urban areas had been constrained by pedestrian speed and the centralizing logic of the railroad station, the automobile's omnidirectional movement, its mass availability, its high speeds, and its sheer physical size all demanded greater decentralization and dispersal. In the friction between these two paradigms of city organization, the parking garage emerged in the middle part of the century as a form of suture. Inside it, the enormously scaled automobile-oriented urbanism of the strip and the freeway would brush against that of the shopping arcade, the village green, and the office building. In one side came a driver and his heavy cloak, and out the other emerged a pedestrian.

The roots of the parking garage typology begin in the closing years of the 19th century with the invention of the motorcar. From the very beginning, it was understood that these new machines were not fit to be left outdoors. Besides simply being expensive and vulnerable to theft, most were too mechanically temperamental to be left to the vagaries of the climate. The majority of their wealthy owners simply adapted their existing coach houses to accommodate these new "horseless carriages." Those without the room and presumably without more reputable choices found space for rent in existing livery stables. Such makeshift accommodation continued into the early 1920s, by which time some underutilized warehouse facilities were also being pressed into service for automobile storage. In the relatively rare cases in which these buildings made use of their upper floors, vertical transport of the automobiles was easily handled by the preexisting freight elevators.

Unfortunately, all these patchwork adaptations and accommodations were soon overwhelmed by the enormity of the automobile's crescendoing effect. Whereas at the beginning of the

century the total number of passenger cars was less than 10,000, by 1920 there were eight million autos in use. By 1930, that number had tripled to 23 million. By 1950, despite the Great Depression and the rationing of World War II, the number had nearly doubled again to 40 million. Between 1950 and 1960, two million additional cars were added each year.

Compounding the congestion generated by the sheer number of these vehicles, all requiring roadways on which to drive and spaces in which to park, was an irrefutable geometric dilemma. Whereas a person at a baseball game sat comfortably in about five square feet and an office worker was comfortable in about 50, a parked Cadillac required almost 200 square feet. This meant that in densely used areas where crowds gathered in large numbers—places such as office buildings, shopping malls, hotels, airports, or downtown department stores—there was simply no room to store all their cars. Making matters worse was the commonplace observation that no person arriving by car was willing to walk more than a few hundred yards to get where he needed to go. The only way to store that many cars that close to their final destinations was to stack them on top of one another, thereby formalizing the notion of the multitiered automobile warehouse. These new buildings, totally subservient to the spatial needs and mechanical capacities of the automobile, were nevertheless named with an exotic word of French origin: *garages*.

Given a consensus by the late 1920s on the need for some sort of formalized structure in which to store all these new cars but without strong typological or historical precedents from which to work, the early parking garages were amazingly varied, with solutions ranging from the prosaic to the utterly fantastic.

The most straightforward garages had floor plates, which were joined by a system of ramps that the automobile would navigate under its own power. The simplest schemes, such as Victor Gruen and Krummeck Associates' Milliron's Department Store in Los Angeles (1949), continued an existing surface lot up a ramp onto the roof of a building. Slightly more complex and certainly more elegant was Paul Schneider-Esleben's use of a ramp in his freestanding Haniel Parking Garage in Düsseldorf (1953), which externally suspended two straight ramps alongside four enclosed floors of parking. In Miami architect Robert Law Weed's unnamed garage (1948) opted for an unenclosed "split-level" plan that incorporated small and discontinuous half-level ramps within it.

Other designers preferred to use curved ramps. Venice's famous Autorimessa (late 1930s) designed by Eugeio Miozzi, often called Europe's first major parking garage, could store 2500 cars arriving from the mainland on seven rectangular floor plates connected by two one-way helical (corkscrew) ramps. Toulouse's Victor Hugo Parking Garage designed by Cabinet Genard Architects (1959) also had two cylindrical ramp towers, but each of these was composed of two intertwining ramps in a double helix arrangement. Architects Albert C. Martin and Associates did away with all ramps for the May Company Department Store on Wilshire Boulevard in Los Angeles (1953), elegantly folding three parking levels so that each touched the existing grade independently. Other designers developed what is now considered the most efficient solution to the ramp-deck dichotomy and designed parking garages like the Rupert Street Multi-Story Car Park in Bristol (R. Jelinek-Karl, 1960) in which one

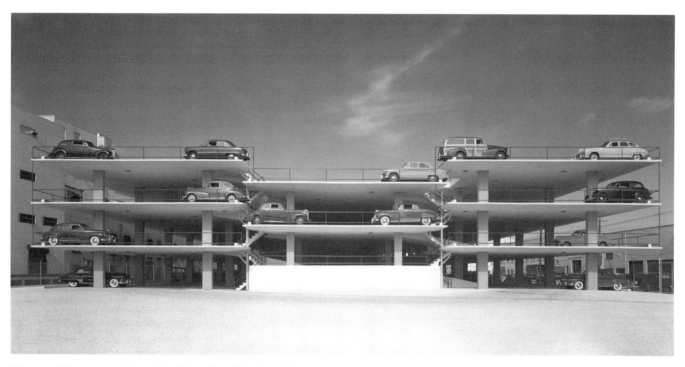

Miami parking garage, designed by Robert Law Weed (*c.*1949)
© Esto. All rights reserved. Ezra Stoller

continuously coiled floor plate is used for both ascent and parking simultaneously.

For locations in which ramped garages were not feasible, more fantastic solutions were tried. For example, in densely developed downtown cores, where aesthetic discomfort about unfamiliar parking garages dovetailed with the high value of real estate, the difficulties of subterranean parking seemed worth contemplating. San Francisco was the first city to donate the land under its Union Square Park for a privately run garage (1941), but it was copied in Los Angeles (1951), Chicago (1954), Bern (1957), and Dresden (1961) to name just a few places.

For other valued locations where even underground parking was not possible, enormous building-scaled hoisting machines were built to store automobiles in giant three-dimensional cubbyholes. By mechanizing the means of ascent and storage, these structures minimized non-parking areas, such as ramps, lanes, and even door-opening stall widths, thereby squeezing the absolute maximum storage capacity out of a parcel of land. In Chicago, for example, Thielbar and Fugard's Jewelers Building (1926) incorporated a mechanical car parking system inside the skyscraper's core, reaching 40 stories high. Two popular proprietary technologies were the "Bowser" overhead crane system (Parking Facility #1, 1955, Chicago, by Shaw, Metz, and Dolio Architects) and the totally automated, push-button "Pigeon-Hole" system (Park-O-Mat, 1951, Washington, DC). Even more fantastic schemes were studied as prototypes, including the extremely narrow "Speed-Park" forklift system (20 feet of street frontage required), a revolving "ferris-wheel garage," and the "Point-Lift System," in which a central elevator tower was surrounded by rotating floor plates.

Given that the form of the parking garage was so fluid during this midcentury period of invention, it should be no surprise that the functional program was equally in flux. Many early garages billed themselves as complete auto-service facilities and included refueling pumps, service stations, valet parking attendants, and car-washing equipment. Others incorporated restaurants and lounges. The most foresighted designers began to reconceive the links between the parking garage and its surrounding contexts. In the simplest cases, this meant a bridge or covered walkway that joined two adjacent structures (Ford Administrative Building Garage, Dearborn, Michigan, by Skidmore, Owings and Merrill). More developed schemes include Bertrand Goldberg's 1962 Marina City in Chicago. Goldberg rejected a stand-alone garage in favor of a design that integrated the necessary parking structure within the massing of the tower's adjacent planta. Taken to extremes, this tendency to combine the parking garage into a larger architectural program gave rise to a fantastic collection of hybrid buildings—a walk-up/drive-through/parking garage bank (American National Bank, mid-1950s, Austin, Texas, by Kuehne, Brooks, and Barr, Architects), a department store in which conveyor belts linked parking spaces to retail counters (Foley's Department Store, mid-1950s, Houston, by Kenneth Franzheim, Architect), and LeRoy Warner's mythologized park-at-your-desk office building (Cafritz Building, 1954, Washington, DC).

By the end of century, most of these radical experiments in form and organization had ended, and the parking garage began to be seen as a commonplace, utilitarian, and predictable sort of building without great aesthetic or architectural significance. Probably this was in part the result of a lingering memory of the parking garage's utilitarian origins in the warehouse and livery stable. Furthermore, the maturation of the typology necessarily dimmed the exoticism and inventive wonder that had infused so many of the earlier experiments. Finally, and most significant, the parking garage remained hostage to the continuing friction between a traditional notion of the city and the rise of the automobile. As a consequence, all too often garage designers had motivations that were as much defensive as anticipatory, seeking bulwarks against the unwelcome automobile rather than new models for architectural inhabitation and use. By the mid-1960s, for every majestic and visionary project such as Paul Rudolph's Temple Street Parking Facility (1962) in New Haven, Connecticut, there were dozens of unimaginative disappointments—cheap, ugly, and banal in every respect. Sadly, no designer seemed able to realize the complex and redemptive vision imagined by Louis Kahn in his "Dock Complex" plan (1956) for Philadelphia, in which a "street becomes a building" and the parking garage assumed its rightful place as an integrated, complex, and celebrated typology in the modern city.

RONN M. DANIEL

See also **Automobile**

Further Reading

The Klose catalog is the best international record of the early monuments and typological experiments within the history of parking garage design, whereas Baker and Funaro offer a more selective overview of developments in the United States. The extended *Architectural Forum* article ("Garages Grow Up") provides a fascinating glimpse into the professional discourse in the midcentury years.

Baker, Geoffrey Harold and Bruno Funaro, *Parking*, New York: Reinhold, 1958

"Garages Grow Up," *Architectural Forum*, 98 (February 1953)

Harris, Neil, "Parking the Garage" in *Cultural Excursions: Marketing Appetites and Cultural Tastes in Modern America*, Chicago: University of Chicago Press, 1990

Klose, Dietrich, *Parkhäuser und Tiefgaragen; Multi-Story and Underground Garages* (bilingual English–German edition), Stuttgart, Germany: Hatje, 1965; as *Metropolitan Parking Structures: A Survey of Architectural Problems and Solutions*, translated by E. Rockwell, New York: Praeger, 1965; as *Multi-Story Car Parks and Garages*, London: Architectural Press, 1965

Sennott, R. Stephen, "Forever Inadequate to the Rising Stream: Dream Cities, Automobiles, and Urban Street Mobility in Central Chicago" in *Chicago Architecture and Design, 1923–1993: Reconfiguration of an American Metropolis*, edited by John Zukowsky, Munich: Prestel Verlag, and Chicago: Art Institute of Chicago, 1993

Vahlefeld, Rolf and Friedrich Jacques, *Garagen und Tankstellenbau: Anlage, Bau, Ausstattung*, Munich: Callwey, 1953; 2nd edition, 1956; as *Garages and Service Stations*, translated by E.M. Schenk, London: Leonard Hill Books, 1960

PARKWAYS

Parkways played an important role in the development of the modern landscape. As the first comprehensively designed limited-access public motorways, parkways paved the way for the expressways and interstate highways that transformed the American landscape in the second half of the 20th century. As symbols of progress and modernity, parkways embodied con-

temporary conceptions of modern design, efficiency, and technological progress. At the same time, their naturalistic landscaping and historical allusions suggested that modern technologies and modernist principles could be harmonized with traditional values and aesthetics.

Parkways long predated the automobile. Frederick Law Olmsted and his partner Calvert Vaux introduced the term "park-way" to describe the attractive approaches they proposed for Brooklyn's Prospect Park in 1868. The idea of connecting suburban parks with urban centers and elite residential developments by means of attractively landscaped parkways soon became a key element of American city planning. Parkways were seen as means of spreading the benefits of parks throughout the urban area, as verdant corridors that enabled pleasure seekers to escape the dangers and disruptions of ordinary city streets, and as powerful economic stimulants that enhanced property values and encouraged high-class residential development. As the connecting fabric of metropolitan park systems, parkways helped transform the focus of American city planning from isolated developments to large-scale comprehensive improvements. Olmsted and other planners, such as Horace Cleveland, Harland Bartholomew, John Nolen, George Kessler, John C. Olmsted, and Frederick Law Olmsted, Jr., went on to design notable parkway and boulevard systems for cities such as Buffalo, Boston, Chicago, Kansas City, Minneapolis, Seattle, St. Louis, and Washington, DC.

The first parkways resembled contemporary boulevards. Brooklyn's formally landscaped Eastern Parkway consisted of a central pleasure drive bordered by tree-lined park strips that were flanked by additional roadways for commercial vehicles and access to abutting properties. The series of drives and bordering parkland that Olmsted planned for Boston's Muddy River in the 1880s, now known collectively as "The Emerald Necklace," redefined the basic parkway concept from an attractively landscaped but essentially urban avenue to a winding roadway ensconced in an elongated, informal park. The project represented a middle stage in the evolution from traditional boulevard to modern limited-access parkway in circulation terms as well. Park development constrained access on the stream side of the main roadway, but turning and entering traffic from the urban side of the parkway remained a source of danger and disruption.

The proliferation of private automobiles in the first quarter of the 20th century rendered 19th-century parkway and boulevard systems obsolete, creating a demand for a new type of parkway geared toward the social, spatial, and technological demands of the automobile age.

The first public parkway designed solely for automobile use was the Bronx River Parkway, which was completed in 1925 and stretched for 15 miles from the Bronx Zoo to the Kensico Reservoir in central Westchester County. The design team of engineer Jay Downer and landscape architects Herman Merkel and Gilmore Clarke employed all the features that would come to identify the classic mid-20th-century motor parkway. These elements included the segregation of the main parkway drive in a broad, landscaped corridor that provided ample room for broadly curving roadway alignments and aesthetic enhancements while screening out incompatible development; the elimination of access from abutting properties; a significant reduction in the number of intersecting roadways, most of which were carried over the main parkway drive on attractively designed grade sepa-

rations; construction through largely undeveloped locations to minimize costs and maximize design flexibility; and a prohibition on slow, dangerous, and unsightly commercial traffic. The Bronx River Parkway included several short landscaped medians, but fully divided motorways did not make their appearance until the mid-1930s. The driveways were laid out with gentle grades, ample sight lines, and broad, sweeping, subtly banked curves. Careful attention was paid to harmonizing the roadway with the surrounding terrain to enhance the impression of gliding effortlessly through the landscape, where traditional picturesque compositions were simplified for easy appreciation at modern speeds.

The Bronx River Parkway proved tremendously successful as a scenic pleasure drive and commuter thoroughfare. Motorists, landscape architects, and planners quickly recognized that this new style of parkway was not only more attractive than conventional roadways but also safer, faster, and more efficient. The Bronx River Parkway's popularity spurred a parkway building boom that lasted through the 1930s, as planners sought to answer pressing demands for recreational amenities, transportation improvements, and suburban recreational development. Westchester County constructed numerous additional parkways, including the Saw Mill River, Hutchinson River, and Cross County. New York public works czar Robert Moses oversaw construction of the Northern and Southern State Parkways and their various offshoots to provide access to suburban homes and new state parks on Long Island. The nation's capital also embarked on an ambitious parkway-building program. Although the general outlines of the Washington parkway system antedated the Bronx River Parkway, Rock Creek and Potomac Parkway, Mount Vernon Memorial Highway, and George Washington Memorial Parkway employed similar design strategies.

By the late 1930s, rising speeds and traffic volumes made it increasingly difficult to combine efficient highway design with traditional park values. Connecticut's 1938 Merritt Parkway was popular with commuters but lacked the aesthetic sophistication and recreational amenities of earlier parkways. New York's Belt and Henry Hudson Parkways were also devoted more toward traffic movement than scenic appreciation, as was Los Angeles's Pasadena Freeway, which was conceived originally as the Arroyo Seco Parkway but was renamed before its completion in 1940. Highway engineers soon realized that they could appropriate the basic circulation features that made parkways safe and efficient without incurring the expense of elaborate landscaping and recreational development. This recognition led to the proliferation of minimally landscaped freeways, expressways, and interstate highways that came to dominate the post–World War II American landscape.

Attractive parkways continued to be constructed during the expressway era. The National Park Service (NPS) pressed on with the development of long-distance recreational parkways initiated as public works projects during the Depression. The Blue Ridge Parkway, stretching for 469 miles between Shenandoah and Great Smoky Mountains National Parks, was completed in 1987 and stands as the paragon of the parkway builder's art. The 1954 Baltimore–Washington Parkway and postwar sections of the George Washington Memorial Parkway demonstrated the appeal of independently aligned roadways separated by broad, landscaped medians. New Jersey's 1956 Garden State Parkway posed a striking contrast to the neighboring Turnpike,

and New York's Taconic State Parkway (1931–63) received widespread praise as the ultimate manifestation of the modern, multiuse motor parkway. Although largely completed by the 1960s, the Natchez Trace Parkway through Tennessee, Alabama, and Mississippi remains unfinished and will extend classic parkway development into the 21st century.

The sylvan surroundings and dynamic streamlined ribbons of mid-20th-century motor parkways captured the imagination of contemporary designers, critics, and everyday motorists. Sigfried Giedion hailed parkways as supreme embodiments of the space–time ethos of modern design. Lewis Mumford proclaimed the Taconic State Parkway on par with any artistic creation of the modern age. The "magic motorways" of Norman Bel Geddes's popular Futurama exhibit at the 1939 World's Fair were predicated on parkway design principles, and Nazi engineers studied the Westchester and Washington-area parkways before designing the Autobahns, which eventually supplanted the slower-speed parkways as paradigms for modern motorway design. By the 1960s, however, the excesses of postwar expressway development prompted calls for a return to parkway-style landscape aesthetics, which have found their way into some of the more attractive late-20th-century interstate highways.

TIMOTHY DAVIS

Further Reading

The best comprehensive treatments of the U.S. parkway were written by contemporary observers. Several monographs have traced the evolution of individual parkways and a few recent studies of 20th-century design, planning, and technology have touched briefly on parkway development.

Caro, Robert A., *The Power Broker: Robert Moses and the Fall of New York*, New York: Knopf, 1974

Giedion, Sigfried, *Space, Time, and Architecture*, Cambridge, Massachusetts: Harvard University Press, and London: Oxford University Press, 1941; 5th edition, Cambridge, Massachusetts: Harvard University Press, 1967

Jolley, Harley E., *The Blue Ridge Parkway*, Knoxville: University of Tennessee Press, 1969

McShane, Clay, *Down the Asphalt Path: The Automobile and the American City*, New York: Columbia University Press, 1994

Newton, Norman T., *Design on the Land: The Development of Landscape Architecture*, Cambridge, Massachusetts: Harvard University Press, 1971

Nolen, John and Henry V. Hubbard, *Parkways and Land Values*, Cambridge, Massachusetts: Harvard University Press, 1937

Radde, Bruce, *The Merritt Parkway*, New Haven, Connecticut: Yale University Press, 1993

Snow, W. Brewster (editor), *The Highway and the Landscape*, New Brunswick, New Jersey: Rutgers University Press, 1959

Tunnard, Christopher and Boris Pushkarev, *Man-Made America: Chaos or Control? An Inquiry into Selected Problems of Design in the Urbanized Landscape*, New Haven, Connecticut: Yale University Press, 1963

Wilson, Richard Guy, Dianne H. Pilgrim, and Dickran Tashjian, *The Machine Age in America: 1918–1941*, New York: Brooklyn Museum, 1986

PARLIAMENT BUILDING, CHANDIGARH, INDIA

Designed by Le Corbusier; completed 1960

In 1963, at the inauguration ceremony for Le Corbusier's Parliament building in Chandigarh, Prime Minister Nehru described the design as "symbolic of the freedom of India, unfettered by the traditions of the past . . . an expression of the nation's faith in the future." Few man-made structures of any era evoke the same timeless, dignified, and otherworldly presence of Le Corbusier's Parliament. This monumental composition of abstract concrete forms draws its inspiration from solar geometry and from the physical and spiritual impact of the sun on the people of India. The end result of this approach to design is a building that is as rich in symbolism as it is in composition and texture. However, the origins of the Parliament building are terrestrial, not cosmic, and its function and existence are predicated on political rather than transcendental forces.

Following the partition of the new state of Pakistan from India in 1947, the province of Punjab was effectively split into two parts. With the primary Punjab city of Lahore now in Pakistan, there was a strong political imperative to create a new capital city for the Indian Punjab in the Ambala district north of New Delhi. This new city was to be sited between two rivers on a vast plateau at the base of the Himalayas and was to be known as Chandigarh. In 1950 a team of four architects—Le Corbusier, Maxwell Fry, Jane Drew, and Pierre Jeanneret—was commissioned to undertake the design of the city and its major public buildings. In February 1951 the team proposed that Chandigarh be founded on a modernist street grid with the commercial district at its center and with its political structures clustered together at its top (the northeast). It was these political structures, collectively known as the "Capitol," that were to occupy much of Le Corbusier's attentions until his death in 1965.

The Capitol is an almost classical composition of buildings, monuments, artificial landforms, and vast geometric piazzas, all viewed against the backdrop of the Himalayas. To the top, or the northeastern extent, of the Capitol, Le Corbusier designed the Governor's Palace (unbuilt) as a "crown" for the central public square. To the right of this square (southeast) is the High Court (1956), or Palace of Justice, and to its left, directly facing the High Court across the central square, is the Parliament, or Assembly, building. Farther to the left, beyond the Parliament, is Le Corbusier's Secretariat (1956), which houses the ministries of the government in a single nine-story building that echoes his earlier Unité d'Habitation (1953) in Marseilles.

The Parliament, which was not only the last completed building in the Capitol complex but also the cheapest, was conceived by Le Corbusier as possessing a distinctive profile. The silhouette of the Parliament is a direct result of the ingenious composition of four discrete volumes. The largest of these volumes is three stories high at the piazza level, is roughly square in plan, and in elevation is presented as a horizontal, rectilinear form. Three of the sides of this volume are lined with the blades of Le Corbusier's *brises-soleil* (sunscreens for the offices inside), whereas the fourth facade, which faces the High Court and the central piazza, is shielded by a large freestanding portico. Prominently positioned in this facade is a centrally pivoted ceremonial door. This door is covered in a brightly colored enamel collage by Le Corbusier that depicts a range of iconic signs (including traces of Le Corbusier's Modulor and solar path diagrams). The portico, which shelters both this door and the entire facade, is covered with a heavy scooped roof and is supported on eight concrete walls that are perforated with rounded holes, as if to belie their structural function. The ceremonial entrance through this portico is flanked by twin pools of water that provide reflections of

the Parliament's distinctive hyperbolic and pyramid roof forms. The larger of these roof forms, a hyperbolic shell with a truncated apex, was inspired by the industrial cooling towers of Ahmedabad. The base of this form is situated within the main square volume, from which it rises through the latter's roof. The hyperbolic shell houses the assembly chamber for the Parliament at its base and a variety of special-purpose viewing galleries at upper levels. The fourth and final form is the council chamber, which is similarly located within the greater square volume and is designated with a lopsided pyramid that also protrudes above the main roof. Adjacent to this pyramid is a service tower to allow access, via a steel bridge, to the roof of the assembly chamber. Both the pyramid and the truncated hyperbolic shell contain elaborately sculpted skylights to partially illuminate the spaces below and to celebrate the relationship among the sun, the building, and the people. Within the original square volume, both chambers are surrounded by a regular grid of three-story-high concrete columns and a series of ramp and mezzanine levels. This space, which is called the Forum, is lit by clerestory windows and possesses a weight and majesty that few 20th-century buildings have been able to emulate. Both internal and external surfaces are finished in rough concrete (a necessity of construction in India at that time) and openly display a dense patina of age. Enigmatic bas-reliefs in the concrete walls serve only to amplify the curiously spiritual character of the building.

Paradoxically, it is this character of spiritual otherness that has attracted the majority of the criticisms leveled at the building. The Parliament is unashamedly overpowering in its scale, finish, and appearance. Much of this is the result of Le Corbusier's fascination with global issues: the passage of the sun, the weathering of materials, and what it means to live so closely with the environment. All these preoccupations have produced a building that is attuned more to the elements than to the government and the people of India. This is both the building's strength and its weakness.

MICHAEL J. OSTWALD

See also **Chandigarh, India; Corbusier, Le (Jeanneret Charles-Édouard) (France)**

Further Reading

The design and construction of the Parliament and the Capitol are documented in volumes 5, 6, and 7 of the complete works of Le Corbusier and Pierre Jeanneret. Evenson produced the classic scholarly description of the design of Chandigarh and the Capitol.

Le Corbusier, *Chandigar—Capitole*, 3 vols., New York: Garland, and Paris: Fondation le Corbusier, 1983

Le Corbusier, *Chandigarh: City and Musée*, New York: Garland, and Paris: Fondation le Corbusier, 1983

Le Corbusier, *Le modulor: essai sur une mesure harmonique a l'echelle humaine applicable universellement a l'architecture et la mécanique*, Boulogne: Éditions l'architecture D'aujourd'hui, 1950; as *The Modulor: A Harmonious Measure to the Human Scale, Universally Applicable to Architecture and Mechanics*, translated by Peter de Francia and Anna Bostock, London: Faber and Faber, 1954; 2nd edition, Cambridge, Massachusetts: Harvard University Press, 1954

Le Corbusier and Pierre Jeanneret, *The Complete Architectural Works*, edited by Willy Boesiger, 7 vols. (trilingual English-French-German edition), Zurich: Editions d'Architecture Erlenbach, and London: Thames and Hudson, 1965 (see especially vols. 5–7)

Curtis, William J.R., *Le Corbusier: Ideas and Forms*, New York: Rizzoli, and Oxford: Phaidon, 1986

Evenson, Norma, *Chandigarh*, Berkeley: University of California Press, 1966

Futagawa, Yukio (editor), *Chandigarh, the New Capital of Punjab, India, 1951–*, Tokyo: Edita, 1974

PATKAU, PATRICIA AND JOHN

Architects, Canada

The work of Patricia and John Patkau can be characterized by a very particular reference to site and by its discretely tectonic character. In developing their approach to design, this young Canadian practice has sought to search out the particular and, in doing so, avoid the generalized solutions that are so pervasive in modern architecture and especially so in North America. Patricia and John Patkau founded their practice in 1978 in Edmonton, Alberta. Their early work consisted of houses and educational buildings on the prairies. Six years later, they relocated to Vancouver, British Columbia, and during the last 16 years, working from a studio in a loft in the heart of the city, they have designed a series of private houses and public buildings for sites not only on the west coast but across Canada as well.

Their winning competition design for the Canadian Clay and Glass Gallery (1986) in Ontario marked a significant point in the development of their work. The construction of this project was delayed by a lack of funding, but when it was eventually completed in 1992, the Gallery also established an important landmark in contemporary Canadian architecture.

John Patkau studied at the University of Manitoba and graduated with a Master of Architecture degree in 1972, whereas Patricia Patkau (b. 1950) graduated from Yale University after completing her undergraduate studies at the University of Manitoba. Working together and with their colleague Michael Cunningham, they have developed one of the most significant architectural practices in Canada. The Patkaus scrutinize the site, construction, and materials in the settings in which they work so as to reveal the special characteristics of the place. This concern for the nature of place, which they have characterized as "investigations into the particular," has significantly shaped their approach to design. In 1988 they designed a new school for the Seabird Island Band—a Salish community at Agassiz in the Pacific Northwest. Organized to consider alternatives to the institutional and prefabricated school building that were customarily provided by government for remote First Nation communities, this project was developed by the Patkaus, who worked in close collaboration with the Salish people to design a new school, built by the community. The zoomorphic form of the building created some construction problems, but despite this, the new school was well constructed by its community builders in a government-sponsored scheme.

The Patkaus continue to receive private commissions; many of these have been within areas of outstanding natural beauty. In sharp contrast to the long-established and densely built landscapes of Europe, these buildings have frequently represented the first acts of settlement on a site. This first settlement on a site has fundamentally influenced the development of the residential architecture of the Patkaus. The Barnes House, for example, which was completed in 1994, is located at the edge of rocky outcrop overlooking the Straits of Georgia in British Columbia

and sited in a depression in the rock, but with the main living room on the upper floor turned to focus the long view to the ocean. The house not only is embedded in the site but also serves to focus a view onto the landscape. Their designs are derived from the topography and detail of the landscape. However, they also relish the constructional detail and explore a heterogeneity in ways that are reminiscent of Alvar Aalto's work.

The design of new public buildings—a library at Newton, Strawberry Vale School on the outskirts of Victoria, new facilities for the Emily Carr College of Art and Design in Vancouver, as well as a new community school on the waterfront in Toronto—has ensured that the architecture of Patricia and John Patkau has not been isolated within private worlds or remote sites. These public buildings have been significant not only because of their complexity and public presence but also because they embody elusive and original qualities that make reference to the culture of Canada. In this respect, the work can again be viewed alongside that of Aalto, an architect whose work became an important part of the construction of a new nation. Canada can be viewed as a social democratic nation that emerged from the British Commonwealth anxious to define itself and to seek out differences that distinguish it from its expansive neighbor, the United States. In the last few years, the architecture of the Patkaus has played a role in this process.

Increasingly, the work of Patkau Architects has been seen on the international stage. Since 1994 their work has been shown extensively in Europe and North America, and in 1999 they were selected to represent Canada in the Venice Biennale. This notice has also brought their work to the attention of the promoters of major national and international architectural competitions. Invitations to compete for several significant design projects have resulted in successful submissions for new buildings in the United States, and at present they are designing new student residences for the University of Pennsylvania in Philadelphia as well as for the Grande Bibliotheque du Québec in Montreal.

These young Canadian architects have stated that they see their work as "only at the beginning of the issues of heterogeneity that we are interested in—the variety, the difference and differentiation, the irregularity juxtaposed to regularity." As they move into the design of large civic buildings set within different urban contexts, it will be revealing to see how their declared desires for the buildings that they design—to "become more differentiated, more irregular, more various"—are made manifest.

BRIAN CARTER

See also Aalto, Alvar (Finland)

Selected Works

Canadian Clay and Glass Gallery, Ontario, 1986
School for Seabird Island Band, Agassiz, British Columbia, 1988

Further Reading

"An Interview with John Patkau," *Fifth Column*, 9/2 (1996)
"Barnes House Nanaimo, British Columbia," *Progressive Architecture*, 74/1 (January 1993)
"Canadian Clay and Glass Gallery in Waterloo, Ontario, Canada," *Architectural Record*, 183/1 (January 1995)
"Patkau Architects," *Architectural Design*, 68/3–4 (March–April 1998)
"Residential Condominium," *Progressive Architecture*, 62/1 (1981)
"Strawberry Vale School, Victoria, Canada," *Techniques and Architecture*, 437 (1998)
"Tectonic Craftsmanship: Critique: Canadian Clay and Glass Gallery; Waterloo, Ontario; Patkau Architects," *Canadian Architect*, 40/4 (April 1995)

PAUL, BRUNO 1874–1968

Designer and Architect, Germany

Bruno Paul was born in the village of Seifhennersdorf in rural Saxony in 1874. His father was an independent tradesman, craftsman, and dealer in building materials. When he was 12 years old, Paul left Seifhennersdorf for Dresden, where he attended the Gymnasium and entered a teacher's training school. By 1892 he was determined to pursue a career in the arts. He learned to draw while working in the office of a local architect. In 1893, he was accepted as a student at the Saxon Academy of Fine Arts.

In 1894 Paul moved to Munich, the artistic capital of Wilhelmine Germany. He enrolled at the Munich Academy as a student of the painter Paul Höcker, one of the founding members of the Munich Secession who provided Paul's introduction to the city's circle of progressive artists. In 1896 Paul left the Academy and began a career as an illustrator. He was a regular contributor to *Jugend* and, from 1897, a member of the staff of the satirical journal *Simplicissimus*. Paul's weekly contributions to *Simplicissimus* between 1897 and 1906 won him international acclaim.

In 1898 Paul began working as an applied artist. He was a leading figure in the development of Jugendstil and quickly established himself as the premier designer for the *Vereinigte Werkstätten für Kunst im Handwerk*, a maker of artistic housewares in Munich. The Jugendstil Hunter's Room he designed for the *Vereinigte Werkstätten* in 1900 received a gold medal at the Paris International Exposition and was the first of a series of prestigious commissions that won widespread professional admiration. In 1906 Paul designed a festival decoration for a barracks in Munich, his first commission on an architectural scale. His design impressed Kaiser Wilhelm II and facilitated his appointment to the vacant directorship of the School of Applied Arts in Berlin.

Paul's appointment in Berlin was integral to the program of educational reforms promoted by Hermann Muthesius and Wilhelm von Bode. Paul, who was a member of the Munich Secession and the Berlin Secession as well as being one of the 12 artists who founded the German Werkbund, proved a committed reformer. He revised the curriculum of the School of Applied Arts to promote practical craftsmanship as the basis of artistic education. He emphasized the training of designers for the applied arts industries. Only the most dedicated and talented students progressed to classes in architecture, painting, or sculpture. Paul implemented the full scope of his program of reforms in 1924, when the School of Applied Arts was merged with the Art School of the Prussian Academy. The new institution, the United State Schools for Fine and Applied Arts, provided a coherent educational program that encompassed every technical and creative aspect of artistic endeavor. Until Paul was removed

from the directorship of the combined schools in 1933 for his perceived antipathy to the Nazi government, he led an institution regarded by Nikolaus Pevsner as one of the two most important in Germany—an honor shared with the Bauhaus (Pevsner, 1936). In terms of the scope of its curriculum and the number of its students, Paul's school in Berlin far surpassed its contemporary in Dessau.

As a designer, Paul provided more than 2000 furniture patterns to the *Vereinigte Werkstätten*. He also designed furniture for the *Deutsche Werkstätten* in Dresden as well as designing ship interiors for the *Norddeutscher Lloyd*, pianos for *Ibach*, and streetcars for the city of Berlin. Paul's most significant design was the *Typenmöbel* of 1908, the first example of modern, unit furniture conceived to allow an unlimited number of combinations of standardized, machine-made elements. Like much of his work, the *Typenmöbel* was widely published in contemporary professional journals.

Paul's architecture was closely related to his designs for furnishings and interiors. Before World War I, he was best known as a residential architect whose houses were simple and elegant, efficiently planned, and devoid of superfluous ornament. His favored vocabulary, an abstracted classicism, had a profound influence on the work of his students and apprentices, who included Ludwig Mies van der Rohe, Paul Thiersch, Edwin Redslob, and Adolf Meyer. In 1914 Paul designed a model house and two restaurants for the Werkbund exhibition in Cologne. His buildings reflected the prevailing tone of the exhibition and underscored the extent to which his prewar work reflected the harmonious culture advocated by the Werkbund.

After 1918 Paul's architecture reflected the changing economic and social conditions of the Weimar Republic. In 1924 he designed the *Plattenhaus Typ 1018* for the *Deutsche Werkstätten*, a prefabricated-concrete dwelling developed in response to the pressing need for affordable housing. Although the stark, prismatic volumes of the *Plattenhaus* reflected the vocabulary of the *Neue Sachlichkeit* (New Objectivity), the elegant detailing was typical of Paul's prewar designs. By the end of the decade, he was completing large commercial projects throughout Germany. In 1928 he was working on a department store for the *Sinn* company in Gelsenkirchen, the *Dischhaus* office building in Cologne, and the *Hochhaus am Kleistpark*, the first skyscraper in Berlin. All these buildings demonstrated Paul's mastery of the emerging International Style. Although Paul's projects of the 1920s were frequently innovative, their carefully considered proportions and practical detailing clearly derived from his earlier work. When Paul relinquished his directorship in 1933, he returned to private practice and continued working as an architect through the 1950s.

As a teacher, designer, and architect, Paul was one of the progenitors of the Modern movement. His work embodied one of the most significant and frequently overlooked directions in the history of progressive design in Europe: that of a pragmatic modernism attuned to the needs and desires of the middle class. Nikolaus Pevsner credited his work with effecting a fundamental change in popular taste (Pevsner, 1936, p. 200). Paul's mature designs embodied simplicity and clarity of form, stylistic abstraction, and functional elegance. By promoting these ideals through his involvement with the Werkbund, his leadership of the School of Fine and Applied Arts in Berlin, and his prolific work as a designer, Paul facilitated the popular acceptance of modernism as the characteristic style of the 20th century.

W. OWEN HARROD

See also **Mies van der Rohe, Ludwig (Germany); Pevsner, Nikolaus (England); Werkbund Exhibition, Cologne (1914)**

Further Reading

Ahlers-Hestermann, Friedrich, *Bruno Paul: oder, Die Wucht des Komischen*, Berlin: Gebr. Mann, 1960
Günther, Sonja, *Interieurs um 1900*, Munich: Fink, 1971
Günther, Sonja, *Bruno Paul, 1874–1968*, Berlin: Gebr. Mann, 1992
Pevsner, Nikolaus, "Post-War Tendencies in German Art Schools," *Journal of the Royal Society of Arts* (1936)
Popp, Joseph, *Bruno Paul*, Munich: Bruckmann, 1916
Schäfer, Jost, *Bruno Paul in Soest: Villen der 20er Jahre und ihre Ausstattung*, Bonn: Habelt, 1993
Ziffer, Alfred (editor), *Bruno Paul, Deutsche Raumkunst und Architektur zwischen Jugendstil und Moderne*, Munich: Klinkhardt und Biermann, 1992
Ziffer, Alfred and Christoph De Rentiis (editors), *Bruno Paul und die Deutschen Werkstätten Hellerau*, Dresden: Hellerau, 1993

PEACE MEMORIAL AND MUSEUM

Designed by Kenzo Tange; completed 1955
Hiroshima, Japan

The Hiroshima Peace Memorial and Museum not only marked the grisly ending of World War II but also skillfully expressed the challenges that Japan's architects faced in the new era.

In 1949, when Kenzo Tange's proposal took first place in a competition for the design of the Peace Park, he was already widely known for successful entries in two wartime competitions: a commemorative building (1942) for the Greater East Asia Coprosperity Sphere and the Japan-Thai Culture Center (1943). Today, most texts on Tange ignore these projects, but they demonstrate the evolution of generating ideas ultimately consummated in Hiroshima. In each, Tange's solutions subsumed individual buildings to a sweeping axial gesture that extended symbolically into the landscape. A central plaza served to unite these compositions at the scale of the site; Tange had spent much of the war researching urban design, and he embraced several models not found in Japan, including the Greek agora, the Roman forum, and Capitoline Hill by Michelangelo. These precedents also served to make the postwar design of Peace Park particularly fitting; in an era when the American occupation forces were actively promoting democracy and public assembly, the design called for a remarkable plaza, able to accommodate 50,000 people.

In the case of Tange's Peace Park, the axis extended through the ruins of the 1914 Prefectural Industrial Promotion Hall, now generally referred to as the Atomic Dome—the only competition proposal to incorporate this building, which is now a World Heritage site. In the postwar master plan for the reconstruction of Hiroshima, also by Tange, this axis continued, linking the Peace Park with zones devoted to children, sports, and culture. Although he was commissioned to design a children's library, ultimately these areas were completed without reference to Tange's master plan and without any linkage to the Peace Park.

The earlier competitions also established a direction for Tange's stylistic approach, responding to fascist ideology by explicitly welding Japan's architectural traditions to modern expression and material use. In particular, Tange referred to Ise Shrine in these projects; by the time of the Peace Park, he also drew on Katsura Imperial Villa for inspiration. When postwar propaganda efforts concentrated on shifting the perception of Japan from its *bushido* roots to the arts, Tange's work was widely acclaimed for its "Japanese" character. However, Tange was equivocal on this point. In his presentation of the Peace Park to CIAM (Congrès Internationaux d'Architecture Moderne) in 1951, he noted, "The role of tradition is that of a catalyst, which furthers a chemical reaction but is no longer detectable in the end result. . . . We Japanese architects, in our endeavors to resolve the problems facing modern Japan, have devoted a great deal of attention to the Japanese tradition, and have, in the end, arrived at the point which I have sought to elucidate for you. If, however, there can be detected a trace of tradition in my works or in those of my generation, then our creative powers have not been at their best, then we are still in the throes of evolving our creativity."

Tange later described the imprint of history in the Peace Park as twofold: Yayoi traditions were elegant and intellectual, and the Jomon was vigorous and creative. The delicate treatment of the louvered facade on the central Memorial Museum might be said to reveal Yayoi influences, whereas the primitive strength of the buildings and the plasticity found in the *pilotis* reflected Jomon influences. By embracing these "Jomon" characteristics, he made a virtue of one of the challenges of postwar construction: because wartime demands for steel had brought domestic building to a standstill, the labor and experience needed for refined construction were unavailable, even in the case of reinforced concrete, which was suddenly widely employed. Furthermore, despite the maturity of the design, Tange had little experience in construction supervision, as this was his first built work. Critics praised the "correct degree of roughness" found in the execution of the Peace Park's buildings.

Tange did not have complete control of the Peace Park's execution. He was ultimately responsible for only two of the three main buildings in the complex: the Memorial Museum (1952) and the Community Center (1955) to the east. A third building, an international conference center located to the west of the museum, was constructed using donations from the people of Hiroshima, and it was felt that a local architect would be more suitable. Although the building generally conformed to the master plan in both massing and the use of a module, Tange made a point of repudiating it.

At the heart of the Peace Park is a centograph that stands as a memorial to victims of the atomic bomb. In the competition proposal, it was to have been the largest structure on the site, an arch (inspired by Le Corbusier's 1931 proposal for the Palace of the Soviets) visible from the Inland Sea. Later, Tange came to the conclusion that this piece should in fact be much smaller, more a sculptural piece than an architectural one, and he invited the Japanese-American sculptor Isamu Noguchi to propose a solution. Because government officials felt that having an American involved in the project was unacceptable, in the end Noguchi was commissioned to design two bridges flanking the park to the north and south. Tange's centograph, a concrete saddle vault, was built instead; in 1985 this was replaced with a granite version

as part of a complete refurbishment, begun in 1983 and supervised by Tange's office.

The results of the remodeling are unfortunate; both buildings flanking the Memorial Museum were replaced. The new buildings conform superficially to the original massing and column/beam organization of the earlier facades, but the detailing and use of materials are contemporary and lack the power of the originals. Furthermore, the three buildings have been physically linked with a second-floor passageway, and granite cladding was added to some areas of the facade of the Memorial Museum. Tange's office is also supervising construction of a new building, the "National Hall Dedicated to Mourning Hiroshima's Atomic Bomb Fatalities," to be located east of the centograph, further altering the park.

Although it remains possible to have some sense of the original character of the complex, much has been lost. The Peace Park continues to hold symbolic importance as ground zero of the bombing of Hiroshima. In its current state, however, it can no longer be said to hold the importance that it once commanded in architectural circles.

DANA BUNTROCK

See also **Tange, Kenzo (Japan)**

Further Reading

A detailed bibliography of Japanese sources is available in Kurita, with a somewhat more limited but easily accessible bibliography of primary and secondary sources in the more contemporary Bettinotti. Bettinotti alone shows the current character of the complex.

Bettinotti, Massimo (editor), *Kenzo Tange: 1946–1996, Architecture and Urban Design; Architettura e disegno urbano* (bilingual English-Italian edition), Milan: Electa, 1996

Boyd, Robin, *Kenzo Tange*, New York: Braziller, and London: Prentice Hall, 1962

Kultermann, Udo (editor), *Kenzo Tange: Architecture and Urban Design, 1946–1969*, Zurich: Verlag für Architektur Artemis, New York: Praeger, and London: Pall Mall Press, 1970

Kurita, Isamu (editor), *Tange Kenzo*, Tokyo: San'ichishobo, 1970

Stewart, David B., *The Making of a Modern Japanese Architecture: 1868 to the Present*, Tokyo and New York: Kodansha, 1987

Tange Kenzo: Kenchiku to Toshi [Kenzo Tange: Architecture and the City], Tokyo: Sekai Bunka-Sha, 1975

PEI, I.M. 1917–

Architect, United States

I.M. Pei is one of the last and certainly the most accomplished of the architects trained by Walter Gropius and Marcel Breuer at Harvard University's Graduate School of Design. (The best known of the others are Edward Larrabee Barnes, Philip Johnson, and Paul Rudolph.) In a career spanning more than half a century, Pei has won virtually every award of any significance in his profession, from the Gold Medal of the American Institute of Architects to the Pritzker Prize. The durability of his prominence, however, has much to do with his ability to grow as an artist as well as his skills in creating one of the most respected firms in American architectural history.

Pei's achievement is the more remarkable in light of his background. He was born in 1917 in Canton, China, the son of a prominent banker, and received his early schooling in Shanghai. He came to the United States in 1935 to study, first at the

University of Pennsylvania and then at the Massachusetts Institute of Technology, where he concentrated in engineering.

After completing his degree, Pei went on to Harvard in 1940 to pursue architecture during the heady days of Gropius and Breuer, who had brought with them the avant-garde theories and practices they had developed at the Bauhaus in Germany. Pei received his Master's degree in 1946 and briefly served on the Harvard faculty.

Despite his training under European émigrés, Pei has always retained a recognizably Chinese sensibility to nature, art, and time. (Pei's thesis under Gropius was a design for an art museum in China.) This sensibility was developed during childhood visits to his family's villa in the ancient city of Suzhou, not far from Shanghai. There, Pei was exposed to the culture of "rock farming," the traditional practice of selecting rocks in nature and setting them aside to be eroded in lakes and rivers into ornamental elements for the gardens of scholars and the wealthy.

Following his Harvard years, Pei was obliged to subsume his design sensibilities to issues of planning and development when he went to work in 1948 for William Zeckendorf as head of the New York real estate magnate's in-house architectural team. There, Pei oversaw schemes for the redevelopment of such cities as Denver, Philadelphia, and Washington, DC, acquiring a sense of large-scale planning as well as an appreciation of finance and management.

With the financial decline of the Zeckendorf firm, Pei set out on his own in 1955. He took with him several colleagues and went on with them to create I.M. Pei and Partners, which was to become one of the most respected architectural teams in the nation. Many of the buildings that the partners were to design were mundane, however well engineered and detailed, but many were of extremely high quality, and each partner was allowed to pursue projects in a semiautonomous fashion. The shared affinity in the office for abstract forms in concrete and glass often made it difficult to identify the lead designer for a particular project, but Pei, who has been responsible for roughly one-third of the firm's nearly 200 buildings and urban design projects, can claim most of the best.

Pei's first major achievement was the National Center for Atmospheric Research (NCAR), finished in 1967, outside Boulder, Colorado. NCAR was a boldly sculptural composition that sought to integrate the scientific needs of scientists with a form that was visually sympathetic to the Rocky Mountains that rose behind it.

The success of the Colorado building contributed heavily to Pei's selection in 1964 by Jacqueline Kennedy Onassis as architect for the John F. Kennedy Memorial Library. Originally intended for a site in Cambridge, Massachusetts, adjacent to Harvard University, the project fell prey to local politics and was

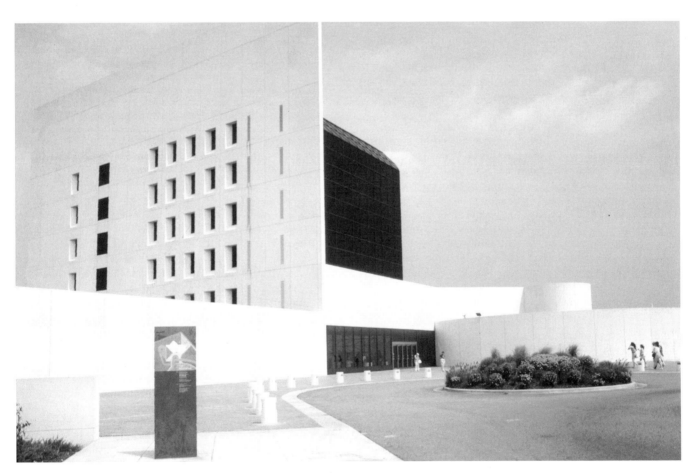

John F. Kennedy Library, Columbia Point, Massachusetts (1979)
Photo © Mary Ann Sullivan

eventually transferred to a site on Boston Harbor. Although the combination of crisp, abstract geometry with a large glassed-in atrium overlooking the water was characteristic of the developing Pei aesthetic, in the end the extended delays and design changes that were imposed on the original made the building a disappointment, as the architect himself has conceded publicly.

Nevertheless, the momentum created for the firm by the Kennedy commission raised I.M. Pei and Partners to national prominence. That momentum nearly stalled, however, when the windows of the John Hancock Building, a sleek office tower completed by the firm in 1976 in Boston, began to break and fall out. The designer of the building was Pei's partner, Henry Cobb, but the crisis affected the entire firm, and although the cause of the failure was eventually attributed to the manufacturer of the glass, the negative publicity slowed new commissions to a trickle.

The firm began its slow return to health largely on the strength of Pei's work in art museums, most notably the Everson Museum of Art (1968) in Syracuse, New York, and the Johnson Museum (1973) at Cornell University. These were hard-edged, late modernist geometric compositions in concrete but with interiors that were both dramatic and sensitive and judged to be superior settings for their collections.

The enthusiastic reception of these buildings led to Pei's selection as architect of the East Building of the National Gallery of Art in Washington, DC, completed in 1978. Key to the success of the building was the client, Paul Mellon, whose father had paid for the original National Gallery (1941), designed by John Russell Pope. The East Building was a full-fledged expression of Pei's enduring affection for abstract form, yet it was inflected on the interior with a skill at manipulating light to soften the effect of the hard materials, primarily marble and glass, and organizing the movement of visitors to create added visual interest.

In 1979, following the reopening of relations between the United States and China, Pei accepted an invitation to design a hotel on the outskirts of Beijing. Pei hoped to develop a modern architectural form for his native country, which had sunk into grim utilitarianism, while maintaining traditional Chinese architectural themes. Although the building enjoyed considerable critical success, it was neglected by its government owners and failed to spark the stylistic progress that Pei had contemplated.

However, the pains of Fragrant Hill, completed in 1982, were minimal compared to those of the Louvre museum in Paris, the first phase of which was completed in 1989. French President François Mitterrand asked Pei to undertake a fundamental renovation and reorganization of the museum, and Pei responded with a proposal that was as much urban planning as architecture, redistributing the collection by emptying portions of the palace formerly occupied by government agencies and creating a system of underground access. However, the attention of the public was concentrated on the glass pyramid that Pei inserted at the center of the composition. The initial reaction was outrage that a non-French architect would have the temerity to tamper with what is arguably the most sacred site of French culture. However, on completion of the pyramid itself, the reception changed dramatically. Pei had hoped to minimize the effect of a new structure on the existing historic architecture but ended up creating a landmark that rapidly began to compete with the Eiffel Tower as a symbol of Paris itself.

The year 1989 saw a host of other openings in addition to the Louvre Pyramid, including the Meyerson Symphony Center in Dallas and several smaller commissions. All were distinguished by a softening of Pei's austere modernist palette. The Meyerson in particular displayed an almost Romantic use of curves that modulated the architect's familiar formal rigor to powerful effect. Even the 70-story Bank of China tower in Hong Kong (his only true skyscraper design), with its irregular stepped shaft, displayed a compositional delicacy that had been absent from many of Pei's earlier works.

By no means were all of Pei's commissions of this period uniformly good. The Rock 'n' Roll Hall of Fame in Cleveland, Ohio, recalled the lifelessness of the Kennedy Library and for some of the same reasons. Pei's best work has always resulted from a close personal relationship with a wealthy and powerful client, such as Paul Mellon or François Mitterrand, and in the case of Rock 'n' Roll, the instability of the funding and disagreements among the backers aggravated Pei's understandably limited familiarity with the musical history that the building was meant to celebrate.

In 1989 Pei had already begun a gradual separation from his firm, by then named Pei, Cobb, Freed, and Partners (in recognition of his longtime collaborators Henry Cobb and James Freed), and while maintaining an office in the same building and still calling on the organization's staff, began to practice even more independently. The projects of this period included the Shinji Shumeikai bell tower (1990) for a religious organization in Shiga, Japan; the Regent (now Four Seasons) Hotel (1992), in New York City; and projects for art museums in Athens and Luxembourg.

However, what might prove to be Pei's last major work is the Miho Museum outside Kyoto, Japan, completed in 1998. Designed for the religious organization that had commissioned the Shiga bell tower, the museum was built on a remote site in a nature preserve near Kyoto. To reduce the effect of the building on the natural surroundings, the entire top of a small mountain was removed, the museum inserted, and the mountain—including many of the original trees—restored. Access was provided by an elegant suspension bridge and a tunnel, both designed by the architect, working with the structural engineer Leslie Robertson, who was the engineer on the Bank of China tower, among other Pei projects.

The museum is characterized by Pei's familiar elegant detailing in glass and steel, but its greatest success lies in the combination of crisp modernist forms with classic Japanese architectural tradition rendered in contemporary materials. In that, the Miho Museum represents a fulfillment of Pei's most fundamental affections—for nature, for elegant abstract form, and for the display of fine works of art.

CARTER WISEMAN

Biography

Born Ieoh Ming Pei in Guangzhou, China, 26 April 1917; immigrated to the United States 1935; naturalized 1948. Received bachelor's degree in architecture from the Massachusetts Institute of Technology, Cambridge 1940; master's degree in architecture from the Harvard Graduate School of Design, Cambridge 1946. Married Eileen Loo 1942: 4 children. Served on

Bank of America (formerly NationsBank) Corporate Center and
    Founders Hall, Charlotte, North Carolina, 1992
Hakata Bay Oriental Hotel and Resort, Fukoka, Japan, 1995
New North Terminal, Washington National Airport, Washington,
    D.C., 1997
Petronas Towers, Kuala Lumpur, Malaysia, 1998
Zurich Tower, The Hague, Netherlands, 1999
Tuassig Cancer Center, Cleveland, Ohio, 2000
International Finance Center, Hong Kong, 2000

Selected Publications

"Skyscrapers," *Perspecta: The Yale Architectural Journal* (1982)
"Architectural Form and the Tradition of Building," Tokyo: *A + U*
    extra edition, (July 1985)
"Pieces of the City," *Architectural Digest* (August 1988)
"Four Buildings Responsive to their Critical Surroundings," Tokyo:
    A + U (January 1993)
Observations for Young Architects, New York: Monacelli, 1999

Further Reading

Cesar Pelli: Selected and Current Works, Mulgrave, Victoria: Images,
    1993
Crosbie, Michael J., *Cesar Pelli: Recent Themes*, Basel and Boston:
    Birkhäuser, 1998
Gray, Lee Edward, *Pattern and Context: Essays on Cesar Pelli*,
    Charlotte: University of North Carolina, 1992
Futagawa, Yukio (editor), *The Commons and Courthouse Center,
    Indiana, 1971–74; Pacific Design Center, Los Angeles, California,
    1972–76; Rainbow Mall and Winter Garden, Niagara Falls, New
    York, 1975–77*, Tokyo: A.D.A. Tokyo, 1981
World Architecture Review (1998) (special issue on Cesar Pelli)

PENNSYLVANIA STATION, NEW YORK

Designed by McKim, Mead and White;
completed 1911
New York, New York

Pennsylvania Station (1902–11) was a landmark New York City
railroad station designed by McKim, Mead and White for the
Pennsylvania Railroad. A "monumental gateway" to the city, its
construction was made possible by the very latest engineering
technology, although its neoclassical style was reminiscent of
ancient Roman baths. Recognized in its time as among the top
architectural achievements of 20th-century American architecture, this famous terminal survived only half a century before it
was demolished.

In 1900 New York was served by Grand Central Station,
owned by the New York Central Railroad, which controlled all
railways north and east of the city and was reaching west to
Chicago. The Pennsylvania Railroad, trying to gain New York
traffic, had completed a right of way as far east as Jersey City,
directly across the Hudson River from New York, but had not
yet found a way to cross the river. Tunneling attempts in the
1870s had been disastrous, and a bridge proposal failed. By
1900, however, technological advances, such as the introduction
of electric traction railways at the new Gare d'Orsay (1897–
1900) in Paris and the availability of stronger electric locomotives and heavier tunneling equipment, had revived possibilities
for the Hudson crossing. Pennsylvania Railroad president Alexander Cassatt visited Paris to see the new system and returned

home ready to proceed, hiring the prominent firm of McKim,
Mead and White.

The new Pennsylvania Railroad extension would run east
over the Hackensack Meadows, tunnel beneath the Hudson,
and then continue underground to a majestic new terminal at
Eighth Avenue and Thirty-third Street. A newly acquired interest in the Long Island Railroad meant that the tunnels would
then cross Manhattan and the East River to connect to Long
Island.

Of the firm's three namesake partners, Charles Follen McKim
(1847–1909) was most responsible for Pennsylvania Station's
design. His work, inspired by classical and Renaissance Roman
architecture, was noted for its monumentality and elegant restraint. He worked closely with Pennsylvania Railroad chief executive officer Samuel Rea and chief engineer William H. Brown.
He was also assisted by two associates, William Symmes Richardson and Tenuis Van der Bent. As McKim's health gradually
failed, his associates took over primary responsibility for the
work, and both he and Cassatt died before the project was completed.

Design work began in 1902. Cassatt had proposed a "grand
portal" that included a high-rise European-style hotel, but
McKim rejected that idea. Historian Leland Roth speculates that
this decision doomed the station years later, as a multipurpose
structure would have been more adaptable to changing times.
Construction began in 1904, and although the station opened
in the fall of 1910, it was not completed until a year later.

Occupying two full city blocks, the finished Pennsylvania
Station was a functional and critical success; this New York
landmark was widely published and admired in the United
States, England, and Europe. With its neighbor, Grand Central,
Pennsylvania Station did much to establish the classical form as
the standard for large train stations of the time. Even in 1924,
Sir Charles Reilly praised the firm's body of work, including
Pennsylvania Station, as having "that sublime quality which
makes great buildings akin to the permanent works of nature."

The pink granite exterior was a restrained classical composition, with Doric-columned porticoes and pilasters delineating
each of its facades. It departed from traditional train station
architecture in its low primary roofline, as its trains were entirely
underground and did not need the height of a train shed. The
interior reflected McKim's deep admiration of Roman architecture, but its superstructure was modern steel, and the soaring
spaces within were made possible by this latest engineering element. From the Seventh Avenue main entrance, one proceeded
through a portico and an arcade of shops and then descended
a staircase into the majestic groin-vaulted main waiting room,
lined in warm buff travertine. This room, with an elaborate
coffered ceiling supported by Corinthian columns and lit by
thermal windows, was the centerpiece of the design, a direct
reference to both the *tepidarium* of the Baths of Caracalla and
the vast space of St. Peter's in the Vatican. Adjoining it was the
equally dazzling concourse, with arched steel ribs and airy lat-
ticed columns supporting a groin-vaulted glass roof that echoed
the great European train sheds. With its staircases cascading
down to the underground platforms, the concourse provided
what Richardson called a transition "from the monumental side
of the station to the utilitarian."

Traffic flow within the building was carefully planned. The
station covered a fan of 21 parallel tracks 45 feet underground

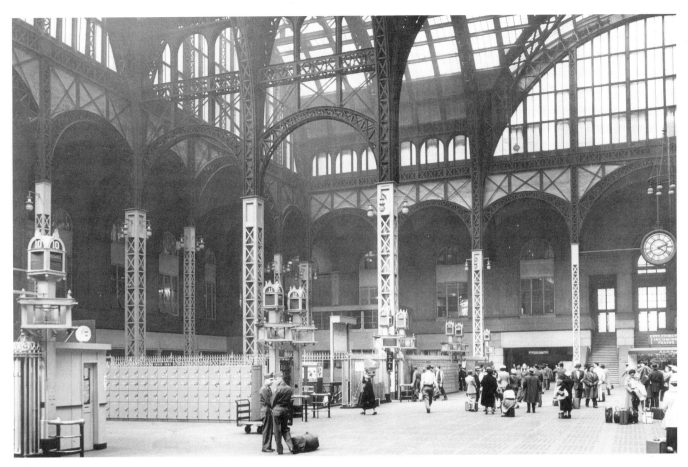

Pennsylvania Station, interior, designed by McKim, Mead and White (1911)
© Museum of the City of New York Print Archives

and a network of service tunnels at multiple levels. A special concourse with direct street access served commuters, whose trains ran on the three northernmost tracks, and was connected to nearby subway lines. The station's concourses could be entered at numerous points from surrounding streets, and two ramped driveways, entered from Seventh Avenue on both sides of the arcade, allowed a sheltered and efficient means to drop off and pick up both passengers and baggage by automobile or taxicab.

As time went on, the taste for monumental classicism dissipated, rail travel declined, and Pennsylvania Station aged poorly. Increasing neglect, grime, and insensitive architectural intrusions, most notably a glaring plastic shell covering a modern ticket counter, diminished the station's worth in its owners' eyes. In the early 1960s, Pennsylvania Railroad announced plans to demolish Pennsylvania Station and replace it with an entirely subterranean modern terminal above which would be a new Madison Square Garden arena and an office skyscraper. Outraged architects, historians, and critics, including Ada Louise Huxtable and Lewis Mumford, railed publicly against the proposal, even offering a counterproposal that would generate income while preserving the building; however, their efforts were in vain. Between 1963 and 1965, Pennsylvania Station was torn down, and only a few statues were saved. Its lovely stonework was dumped into New Jersey marshes as landfill. However, Pennsylvania Station's loss

galvanized the historic preservation movement across the United States and led to federal, state, and local laws protecting important structures from callous demolition.

Most critics agree that the second Pennsylvania Station, designed by Charles Luckman, is grim and mediocre, even judged solely on its own merits. At present, architect David Childs plans to renovate the nearby Farley Post Office Building as a third incarnation of Pennsylvania Station.

KATHERINE LARSON FARNHAM

See also **McKim, Mead and White (United States)**

Further Reading

A more extensive bibliography can be found in the Historic American Building Survey's record of Pennsylvania Station (HABS No. NY-5471) housed in the Prints and Photographs Division of the Library of Congress, Washington, DC. This bibliography includes journal articles pertaining to its demolition. Also see Roth, page 428, for sources.

Couper, William (editor), *History of the Engineering, Construction, and Equipment of the Pennsylvania Railroad Company's New York Terminal and Approaches*, New York: Blanchard, 1912

Diehl, Lorraine B., *The Late, Great Pennsylvania Station*, New York: American Heritage, 1985

McKim, Mead and White, *The Architecture of McKim, Mead, and White in Photographs, Plans, and Elevations*, New York: Dover, 1990

Middleton, William D., *Manhattan Gateway: New York's Pennsylvania Station*, Waukesha, Wisconsin: Kalmbach Books, 1996

Muschamp, Herbert, "An Appreciation: Style and Symbolism Meet in Design for Penn Station," *New York Times* (16 May 1999)

Reilly, Charles Herbert, *McKim, Mead, and White*, New York: Blom, 1972

Roth, Leland M., *McKim, Mead, and White, Architects*, New York: Harper and Row, 1983

Wilson, Richard Guy, *McKim, Mead, and White, Architects*, New York: Rizzoli, 1983

PERKINS AND WILL

Architecture firm, United States

Perkins and Will was formed in 1935 by two Cornell University classmates, Lawrence Bradford Perkins (1907–97) and Philip Will, Jr. (1906–85). Part of a new generation of young architects innovating in the years between the world wars, these men brought new ideas and idealism to post–World War II building needs, particularly in the area of school design. Their work is marked by the study of the program that the proposed structure intends to solve by looking at the way in which people use buildings. This humanistic approach was influenced to some extent by their collaboration with Eliel and Eero Saarinen. According to Lawrence Perkins, it is one of the qualities that has set their firm's brand of modernism apart from that of the more severe International Style modernists, such as Mies van der Rohe, which was attractive to many young firms after World War II.

Specifically, Perkins and Will's practice and promotion of progressive, functional school design in the 1940s and 1950s had a tremendous influence on American architecture in the last half of the 20th century. It was natural for Lawrence Perkins to participate in the design of schools; his father, the well-known Chicago architect Dwight Perkins, designed nearly 40 schools in the early part of the 20th century and served as the Chicago Board of Education architect. After moving to Chicago in 1933, Philip Will, Jr., was responsible for the necessarily simplified, modern design of prefabricated houses for Howard Fisher's firm General Houses, Inc. He worked directly on the company's Steel House for the 1933 Chicago Century of Progress Exposition.

Soon after forming their firm in 1935, the two architects were joined by E. Todd Wheeler, and the firm was known as Perkins, Wheeler, and Will until 1946. The first significant commission that the architects received was the Crow Island School (1940) in Winnetka, Illinois. The eager young architecture firm combined with an enlightened school superintendent, Carleton Washburne, and the respected modern visionaries Eliel and Eero Saarinen, making for a highly successful and influential new school building that provided major direction to the new firm.

Perkins thoroughly researched and rethought the school's uses with an eye to providing a new kind of educational facility. He interviewed grade-school children, teachers, and administrators in the planning stages. As Perkins explains, "The program . . . said that that classroom was to be a place for a fully rounded learning and living experience at each age group; that each room was to be a colorful, flexible, child-scaled work space where the learning activity of childhood could be channeled effectively and pleasantly . . . color, warmth, and a place in which

to work and act vigorously—these were keynotes of the earliest program" (Perkins and Cocking, 1949).

As a result, Perkins and Will, along with the Saarinens, produced a very sensitively designed school. One of the more striking aspects is the auditorium with progressively smaller molded-plywood seating toward the front so that the children would be in seats proportionate to their own sizes. The architects designed a new type of L-shaped classroom with large window walls on two sides, allowing for more and better natural light. Other innovations include individual bathrooms in each classroom, a separate activity area, and round tables instead of marching desks. In addition, the trend was toward a more healthful environment, and each class had a private courtyard, expanding the possibilities for classroom activity.

Perkins published many of the revolutionary ideas employed in Crow Island School in his book *Schools* (1949), written with school superintendent Walter Cocking. This publication served a similar function in promoting progressive design for schools, as George Nelson and Henry Wright's *Tomorrow's House* (1945) did for promoting the postwar homes. For example, Perkins and Cocking pointed out that Greek and Roman architecture were modern in their own time yet inappropriate for today's American needs. Changing philosophies regarding education, they held, meant rethinking school's functions. They argued for the functional reasons for the existence of features such as continuous banks of windows, trying to relieve the stigma associated at the time with the widespread acceptance of modern architecture. They illustrated *Schools* with contemporary schools by famous architects, such as Richard Neutra and William Lescaze, to prove the benefits of such well-considered schemes. In 1957 Perkins followed up with *Workplace for Learning*, which featured many of the success stories of the ten years since *Schools* was published. This included Perkins and Will's Heathcote School (1954) in Scarsdale, New York, which Perkins considered more successful than Crow Island because of its complete interaction with nature on the site, aided by its numerous glass corridors punctuated with lively colored panes.

Perkins and Will provided notable solutions to corporate building types, also conceived around the people who were to use them. The Scott, Foresman, and Company Headquarters (1965) in Glenview, Illinois, a campus planned for a publisher of educational materials, was undoubtedly informed by the firm's many educational buildings. Here a series of interlinked glass and concrete pavilions housing different aspects of the company were designed to give a sense of community on a 44-acre site. Trees and fountains mix with walkways between the buildings to create a flow while simultaneously reinforcing a sense of repose.

Another example of the firm's well-considered design solutions influenced later generations of architectural form givers in the urban setting. The First National Bank of Chicago (1966) was an anomaly on the Chicago skyline when it was constructed, as it eclipsed most of the Loop buildings, helping to set a precedent for the new, taller skyscrapers that became ubiquitous in American cities in the decades to follow. This building, too, was a specific and inspired design solution to a complex program. The bank had to enclose all its various activities in one building, as the State of Illinois at that time forbade branch banking. Therefore, the 60-story-tall structure flares at the base to accommodate the numerous public banking facilities, and the building

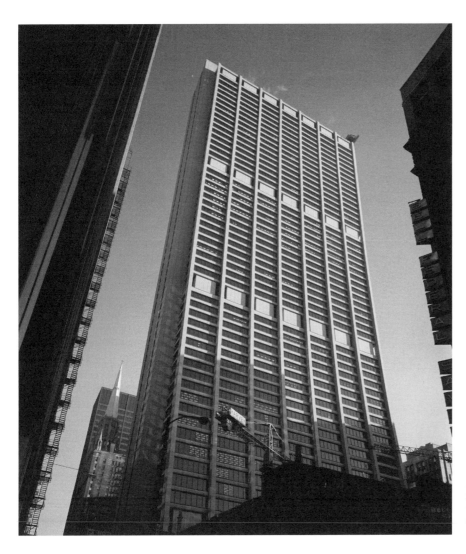

First National Bank of Chicago, designed by Perkins and Will (with C.F. Murphy Associates), 1966
© G.E. Kidder Smith/CORBIS

tapers upward to house offices from there. Vertical steel supports gesture up, housing the curving glass wall that has been likened to "a huge ribbed sail caught in the Chicago wind" (*Architectural Record* 148 [September 1970]).

Over the decades, Perkins and Will has grown to include engineering and design services. It remains one of the largest architectural firms in the nation, with offices in Chicago, Atlanta, Charlotte, Los Angeles, Miami, Minneapolis, New York, and Paris, carrying on the work of the firm's principals. The firm continues to specialize in educational facilities and other areas in which the founding principals innovated.

JENNIFER KOMAR OLIVAREZ

Biography

Lawrence B. Perkins

Born in Evanston, Illinois, 12 February 1907; son of Prairie School architect Dwight Perkins. Attended the University of Wisconsin, Madison 1924–25; studied at Cornell University, College of Architecture, Ithaca, New York 1926–30; bachelor's degree in architecture 1930. Married 1) Margery Isabella Blair 1932 (died 1981): 4 children; married 2) Joyce Ellen Sandlerin 1982. In private practice, Chicago from 1935; founding partner, Perkins, Wheeler, and Will 1935–46; partner, Perkins and Will, later Perkins and Will Partnership, 1946–70; chairman of the board, 1970–73, director, from 1973, Perkins and Will Architects. Adjunct professor of architectural design, University of Illinois, Chicago 1974–82; visiting professor, University of Illinois, Urbana from 1982. Member, 1945–65, chairman, 1948–54 and 1963–65, Evanston Planning Commission; fellow, American Institute of Architects 1953; chairman, advisory board, Cook County Illinois Building Codes Commission 1963–66; director, Adlai Stevenson Institute of International Affairs, Chicago 1965–75, member, advisory committee, Cook County Forest Preserves from 1963. Died in Evanston in 1997.

Philip Will, Jr.

Born in Rochester, New York, 15 February 1906. Studied at Cornell University, College of Architecture, Ithaca, New York 1924–30; bachelor's degree in architecture 1930; married Caroline Elizabeth Sinclair 1933: 2 children. Architectural draftsman, Gordon and Kaelber Architects, Rochester 1928–29; architectural draftsman, Shreve, Lamb, and Harmon, New York 1930–

33; associate architect, General Houses Incorporated, Chicago 1933–34; associate architect, South Park Gardens, Chicago 1934. Founding partner, Perkins, Wheeler, and Will 1935–46; partner, Perkins and Will, later Perkins and Will Partnership, 1946–70; senior vice president, 1970–71, vice chairman, 1970–73, director, 1973–83, chairman, 1975–83, Perkins and Will Architects. Director, Illinois council, American Institute of Architects 1947–49; director, 1947–51, second vice president, 1951–52, president, 1952–54, American Institute of Architects, Chicago chapter; fellow, American Institute of Architects 1951; chairman, Citizens of Greater Chicago 1954; president, Alumni Council of the College of Architecture, 1954–56, trustee, 1963–73, chairman, trustee committee on buildings and grounds, 1966–73, Cornell University; second vice president, 1956–58, first vice president, 1958–60, American Institute of Architects; member, 1959–64, chairman, 1965, City of Evanston, Illinois, Planning Commission; chairman, Committee on the Performance Concept, Building Research Advisory Board, Washington, DC 1965; honorary fellow, Royal Architectural Institute of Canada; honorary fellow, Philippine Institute of Architects; honorary member, Society of Mexican Architects; honorary member, Society of Architects of Peru. Died in Venice, Florida, 22 October 1985.

Perkins and Will

Founded as Perkins, Wheeler, and Will, Chicago 1935–46 by Lawrence B. Perkins, E. Todd Wheeler, and Philip Will, Jr.; became Perkins and Will, Chicago 1946–64; renamed Perkins and Will Partnership 1964–70; renamed Perkins and Will Architects from 1970; branch offices opened in New York 1951 and Washington, DC 1962.

Selected Works

Crow Island School, Winnetka, Illinois (with Eero and Eliel Saarinen), 1940
Heathcoate Elementary School, Scarsdale, New York, 1954
United States Gypsum Building, Chicago, 1963
Scott, Foresman, and Company Headquarters, Glenview, Illinois, 1965
First National Bank of Chicago (with C.F. Murphy Associates), 1966

Selected Publications

Schools (with Walter D. Cocking), 1949
Workplace for Learning, 1957
"The Perkins and Will Partnership," *Building Construction* (April 1969)

Further Reading

This selection represents the most significant writings by the firm and about Crow Island School, the firm's most notable commission, along with an unpublished source (Blum) with much biographical information on Lawrence Perkins.

Blum, Betty, *Oral History of Lawrence Bradford Perkins, F.A.I.A* (unpublished transcript of interviews), 1986
Clarke, Jane, "Philosophy in Brick," *Inland Architect*, 33/6 (November/December 1989)
Hudnut, Joseph, "Crow Island School, Winnetka, Illinois," *Architectural Forum*, 75 (August 1941)
Perkins, Lawrence B. *Workplace for Learning*, New York: Reinhold, 1957
Perkins, Lawrence B. and Walter D. Cocking, *Schools*, New York: Reinhold, 1949

PERRAULT, DOMINIQUE 1953–

Architect, France

Dominique Perrault is the principal and founder of the architectural practice Perrault Projects, established in Paris in 1981. He achieved international recognition in 1989, when at the age of 35 he was awarded the commission for perhaps the grandest of French President Mitterand's projects, the National Library of France in Paris, completed in 1995. Perrault's approach could be seen as part of a European trend, loosely defined as Supermodernism, including the work of Norman Foster, Renzo Piano, Jean Nouvel, and Rem Koolhaas. In Perrault's architecture, technological expression is tempered by a minimalist aesthetic, often making use of bold geometric forms at a monumental scale combined with subtle tectonic qualities, material textures, and lighting effects.

The practice built its early reputation on a series of large-scale industrial commissions, such as the Traffic Control Centre for the Peripherique in Paris (1984); the University for Electric Engineering, Marne-la-Vallée, Paris (1987); and the Water Purification Plant, Ivry-sur-Seine (1987, completed in 1993). Each of these projects deploys a complex range of geometric forms, but it was the monumental simplicity of the Hotel Industriel Jean-Baptiste Berlier (1990) in Paris that directed Perrault's later work. This bold glass rectangular slab containing ten stories of open-plan workspace stands out alongside a chaotic edge-city context of highways and railroad tracks. The sleek external skin contrasts with the concrete and stainless-steel interior, and the whole building displays a quiet monumentality that sets it apart from its unpromising surroundings.

The Center for Book Treatment, Bussy St. Georges, France (1995), the Olympic Velodrome and Swimming Pool, Berlin (1999), and the Media Library, Venissieux, France (2001), display a similar combination of pure geometry and smooth external surface treatment. The Olympic Velodrome and Swimming Pool project's dramatic sunken landscape setting also hints at another source of inspiration for Perrault, who has written of his interest in the work of Earthworks artists such as Walter de Maria and Richard Long. Another touchstone for this more recent preoccupation with the relationship between architecture and landscape—or as Perrault describes it, a concern with geography rather than history and a wish to create places as opposed to buildings—is the house he designed for himself and his partner on the Normandy coast in the north of France. Sunk into the ground along its northern side, the house seems little more than a wall with a large opening framing a view of the garden, and it is the desire to dissolve the building into the landscape design that characterizes two of the more substantial recent projects. His mysterious, almost evanescent installation/house project titled Kolonihavehus, Copenhagen, and designed for the Copenhagen as European Capital of Culture Exhibition (1996) sits like a minimalist cube in a quiet forested landscape.

The redevelopment of the Uni Metal planning project in Caen (1995) and the Plant APLIX (1999) in Nantes also adopt a landscape strategy comprising gridded territories to define areas for building. A more extreme case of this deference to context can be seen at the Conference Center Usinor-Salicor at Saint-Germain-en-Laye (1991), where an underground space is created beneath an existing villa and roofed with a flat glass disk sur-

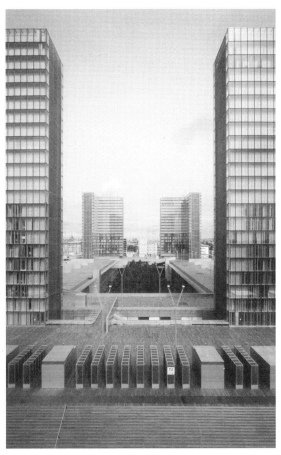

National Library of France, Paris, designed by Dominique Perrault (1995)
© Perrault and Partners

rounding the historic structure. In addition to these and other built projects, Perrault has also undertaken a number of competitions and studies, most notably Library Kansai Khan, Kyoto (1996), the Museum of Modern Art, New York (1997), and the Cultural Center, Santiago de Compostela (1999).

In 1997 he was awarded the Mies van der Rohe Foundation prize for his National Library, deservedly the practices' most widely regarded project, particularly for its effect at the urban scale. The building consists of four 22-story L-shaped towers containing the book storage spaces and administrative offices, sheathed in a double skin of timber shutters and an outer curtain-wall of full-height glazing. The towers sit at the four corners of a colossal elevated rectangular platform, which is covered in simple timber decking and surrounded by steps leading up from the street level. The effect of this "ziggurat," which contains the reading areas, is to create a grand ceremonial space above—somewhat isolated from everyday life—that increases the sense of ritual in approaching the building. This is reinforced by the enormous central garden into which the visitor descends toward the two main entrances, and once inside, a similarly monumental scale is maintained through the smooth surfaces and minimal detailing. The most dramatic of the interior finishes involves the use of woven metal textiles, which produce varying

effects of translucency that Perrault has experimented with on other projects.

JONATHAN A. HALE

See also **Contextualism; Foster, Norman (England); Koolhaas, Rem (The Netherlands); Nouvel, Jean (France); Piano, Renzo (Italy); Supermodernism**

Biography

Born 1953 in Clermont Ferrand, France. Earned architecture degree (1978) and certificate in town planning (1979), Ecole nationale des Ponts et Chaussées; earned postgraduate degree in history (1980), Ecole des Hautes Etudes in Social Sciences. Opened Paris office, Dominique Perrault and Partners 1981; winner of the Programme for New Architecture (PAN XII) 1983; winner of Album of Young Architecture, Ministry of Culture, Paris, France 1983. Won international competition for National French Library, Paris 1989; won competition for Olympic Velodrome and Swimming Pool, Berlin 1992; opened Berlin office 1992; won competition for the Court of Justice of the European Community in Luxembourg 2000; subsequently opened third office in Luxembourg 2000. Recipient of numerous awards and prizes including Great National Prize of Architecture, France 1996; Mies van der Rohe Prize 1997; World Architecture Award, Hong Kong 2001. Chevalier of the Legion of Honour; member of German Association of Architects, British Institute of Royal Architecture; served as President, French Institute of Architects 1998–2001. Lives and works in Paris, France.

Selected Works

Traffic Control Centre for the Peripherique, Paris, 1984
University for Electric Engineering, Marne-la-Vallée, Paris, 1987
Hotel Industriel Jean-Baptiste Berlier, Paris, 1990
Conference Center Usinor-Salicor at Saint-Germain-en-Laye, 1991
Water Purification Plant, Ivry-sur-Seine, 1993
The Center for Book Treatment, Bussy St. Georges, France, 1995
Uni Metal (urban planning project), Caen, France, 1995
Kolonihavehus, Copenhagen (project for the Copenhagen as European Capital of Culture Exhibition), 1996
National Library of France (Bibliothèque de France), 1996
Olympic Velodrome and Swimming Pool, Berlin, 1999
Plant APLIX, Nantes, France, 1999
Media Library, Venissieux, France, 2001

Selected Publications

Dominique Perrault, Zürich: Artemis, 1994
Dominique Perrault Architect, Basel: Birkhauser Verlag, 1999
Dominique Perrault: progetti e architecture, edited by Laurent Stalder, Milano: Electo, 2000

Further Reading

Ferré, Albert and Frédéric Migayron (editors), *Dominique Perrault, arcquitecto* (exhib. cat.), Barcelona: Actar, 1999
Jacques, Michel and Gaëlle Lauriot (editors), *Bibliothèque nationale de France 1984–1995: Dominique Perrault, Architecture*, Paris: Artemis with Arc en Reve centre d'architecture, 1995
Marcos, Javier Rodriguez and Anatxu Zabalbeascoa (editors), *Dominique Perrault: Small Scale*, Barcelona: Editorial Gustavo Gili, 1998

PERRET, AUGUSTE 1874–1954

Architect, France

Auguste Perret occupied a pivotal position in the development of the use of reinforced concrete in modern architecture, a tradition extending from Hennebique to de Baudot. Contemporary French concerns—on the one hand, an intense interest in new constructional methods, and on the other, a desire for traditional, formalist systems of proportioning and ordering—find eloquent and convincing confluence in Perret's work. Born in Brussels, Perret attended the École des Beaux-Arts, where he was influenced by rationalist theorists Gaudet and Choisy, who belonged to a tradition stemming from Viollet-le-Duc and Laugier. Perret combined Gaudet's classical compositional principles and Choisy's simple and direct structural solutions with the basics of building construction acquired with his brother Gustave in their father's firm.

The apartments in the Rue Franklin (1904) were the first to exploit the constructional possibilities of reinforced concrete to gain a greater openness of plan, which was later to influence Le Corbusier's *plan libre* (free plan), and larger windows on a restricted site. The external framework is emphasized and covered, partly for practical reasons, by ornamental tiles that follow the structural contours. The angular effect contrasts with contemporary Parisian Art Nouveau apartments.

Decorative elements are eschewed in the Garage Ponthieu (1905), which Perret called "the world's first experiment in aesthetic reinforced concrete." The concrete frame of the interior, with its large spans and thin supports, allowed considerable flexibility in accordance with the function of the building. The formal aspects include the strongly geometric facade with classical resonances in its arrangement, the upper attic story, and the two cylindrical, nonconstructional pillar supports of the main entrance. The Théâtre des Champs-Elysées (1913) in Paris, originally planned by Henri van de Velde but carried out to Perret's designs, shows a contrast between the ingeniously delicate framework of the building designed to allow uninterrupted views and the heavy walls, pilasters, and cornices of the facade that betray Perret's classical sympathies.

The church of Notre Dame at Le Raincy (1923) near Paris marks a departure from, and yet a logical culmination of, Perret's pre–World War I work. A building of high technical innovation, this memorial church established him as the leading exponent of this architectural system. The structure demonstrates the way in which a modern material such as reinforced concrete could be used to reinterpret traditional ecclesiastical typologies while maintaining a visual connection with established forms. The outer walls constructed from prefabricated components create perforated concrete screens that allow the light to filter into the interior. These combine with the nave, aisles, and slim columns carrying low-arching vaults to create a light and graceful interior. Traditional principles, both classical and Gothic, are invoked, and yet the building denies adherence to either.

After the war, Perret further pursued the neoclassical elements of simplicity and clarity exhibited so clearly in the Théâtre des Champs-Elysées. His command of the essentials of classicism is well represented in designs for the competitions for the Palace of the League of Nations (1927) in Geneva and the Palace of the Soviets (1931) in Moscow. Perhaps the best expression of

Perret's doctrine was the Hôtel du Mobilier National (1934) in Paris, which addressed the problem of combining diverse practical requirements in one building and the problem of a sloping site. The Musée des Travaux Publics (1932) in Paris served as a museum for large engineering models, and so the internal columns were minimal. The tide of opinion among the international avant-garde was indifferent to the classical affinities of these buildings despite their structural novelty and ingenuity.

Special interest attaches to the apartment building (1932) built speculatively at 51–55 rue Raynouard in Paris. Perret occupied an apartment at the top, and a spiral staircase gave access to the firm's offices on the lower level. Perret accommodated the challenges of the corner triangular site by building nine stories above the level of the rue Raynouard and 12 above the level of the rue Berton. The structure introduced a radical approach in that all the posts and beams were poured in place and the in-fills precast in bare concrete.

Perret's most important postwar commission was the reconstruction of Le Havre (1956), destroyed during the war. With a group of disciples, he developed a master plan that serves as a model of 20th-century neoclassical town planning. Perret designed the plaza that housed the new city hall as well as the church of St. Joseph (1957). He was the first president of the Ordres des Architectes and was elected to the Institut de France.

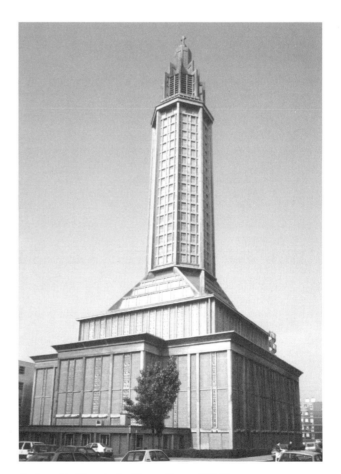

St. Joseph's Church, Le Havre, France (1957)
Photo © Mary Ann Sullivan

After receiving numerous international distinctions, he was named president of the International Union of Architects. He died in 1954 in his rue Raynouard apartment.

HILARY J. GRAINGER

Biography

Born in Brussels, 12 February 1874; son of a stonecutter with a building business and brother of architect Gustave Perret. Studied at the École des Beaux-Arts, Paris 1891–95. Married Jeanne Cordeau 1902. Worked for father's construction firm, Paris 1897–1905; the firm became Perret et Filis 1896; by the turn of the century the firm moved into architecture and contracting. On their father's death, the Perret brothers divided the firm: A.G. Perret Architects, established 1905 by August and Gustave; Perret Frères, established 1905 and managed by third brother, Claude. Inspector-General of Public Works and National Palaces. Professor, École des Beaux-Arts, Paris. Member, French National Committee for the Reconstruction. Gold Medal, Royal Institute of British Architects 1948; Gold Medal, American Institute of Architects 1948. Died in Paris, 25 February 1954.

Selected Works

Apartments, 25 bis rue Franklin, Paris, 1904
Garage, rue Ponthieu, Paris, 1905
Théâtre des Champs-Elysées, Paris, 1913
Notre Dame, Le Raincy, near Paris, 1923
Apartment Building, 51–55 rue Raynouard, Paris, 1932
Museum of Public Works, Paris, 1932
Mobilier National Building, Paris, 1934
Le Havre Reconstruction, 1956
Church of St. Joseph, Le Havre, 1957

Selected Publications

Contribution à une théorie de l'architecture, 1952
Architectes Français, 1874–1954, 1876–1952 (exhib. cat.; with G. Perret), edited by J.B. Ache, 1976

Further Reading

Collins provides the most comprehensive consideration of Perret's work in reinforced concrete.

Champigneulle, Bernard, *Perret*, Paris: Arts et Métiers Graphiques, 1959
Collins, Peter, *Concrete: The Vision of a New Architecture*, London: Faber and Faber, and New York: Horizon Press, 1959
Jamot, Paul, *A.-G. Perret et l'architecture du béton armé*, Paris and Brussels: Vanoest, 1927
Mayer, Marcel, *A. et G. Perret: 24 Phototypies*, Paris: Cercle d'Études Architecturales Librairie de France, 1928
Rogers, Ernesto Nathan, *Auguste Perret*, Milan: Il Balcone, 1955

PERRIAND, CHARLOTTE 1903–99

Furniture and interior designer, France

Charlotte Perriand, typically remembered as Le Corbusier's privileged assistant, remains not only one of the most significant figures of French modernism but also one of the most influential French interior designers. Her artistic activity spans over three quarters of the 20th century. Trained between 1920 and 1925 at the École Centrale des Arts Décoratifs under traditional French *décorateurs* committed to an Art Deco concept of modernity, her first exhibition as an independent professional took place at the 1926 Salon d'Automne, where she presented a *coin de salon* in a conventional French *art décoratif* manner. Her radical turn toward machine-derived furniture, however, occurred at the 1927 Salon d'Automne with a *bar sous le toit*, which brought her instant notoriety. She was almost immediately invited to join Le Corbusier and Pierre Jeanneret's office and was soon to become, at age 25, their main furniture and interior designer. In association with Le Corbusier and Pierre Jeanneret, she furnished the villa Laroche in 1928, the villa Church at Ville-d'Avray in 1929, the Swiss pavilion at the Cité Universitaire in 1932, and the Cité Refuge of the Salvation Army in 1932.

Her early modernist work, oriented primarily to demonstrating the viability of industrial materials and forms for elite purposes, was characterized by lightweight furniture made of bicycle tubes enhanced with leather seats and a wealth of highly reflective, chrome-plated and glazed surfaces evoking the glittery automobile wheels, windshields, fenders, and hoods that were taking over the metropolitan landscape. Early on, Perriand's interest in mechanical metaphors broadened to include movement and transformability, as her dining chairs began to rotate on ball bearings, similar to those she wore around her neck; her tables expanded or shrank along rolling, rubber surfaces.

Although adopting Le Corbusier's concept of furniture as "home equipment," Perriand's contribution both to the Le Corbusier-Jeanneret office repertoire and to Le Corbusier's own development in respect to interior design was considerable. She brought to the office a distinctly new orientation, associated with a novel sense of the *art de vivre*.

Through a more personal and expressive rendition of modernism, Perriand introduced an understanding for "total design" enhanced with lavish comfort and whimsical sophistication. Perriand's radical, comprehensive aesthetic approach to modern interiors was complemented by Le Corbusier's programmatic concept of *équipement* as opposed to *décoration*. This self-proclaimed functionalist approach to interior design dominated the first common exhibition of the Perriand–Le Corbusier–Jeanneret trio at the 1929 Salon d'Automne. The exhibits presented under Thonet's sponsorship were dedicated to the *Equipement de l'habitation: des casiers, des sièges, des tables*—all characterized by standardization and modular deployment, resulting in what became known as the Le Corbusian concept of *objet type*. A characteristic example of such type-object in Perriand's production was her 1928 rotating dining chair—erroneously attributed to Le Corbusier—that she re-used over the years in different contexts.

Passionately involved with radical leftist groups among artists, Perriand joined in 1932 the Association des Ecrivains et Artistes Révolutionaires (AEAR), sponsored by the Communist Party, and participated in the activities of the Maison de la Culture led by Louis Aragon. She viewed this activity as a logical extension of her role in the 1930 creation of the Union des Artistes Modernes (UAM).

Informed by her social and political commitments, which included two trips to the Soviet Union and projects for the Front Populaire government, in 1936 Perriand presented at the Third Housing Exhibition of the Salon des Arts Ménagers inexpensive,

mass-produced home fittings, such as her innovative *chaise pliable et empilable*. She combined with her own furniture standard Flambo metal shelving that could meet the needs of a small worker's apartment necessarily oriented toward multifunctional, transformable spaces. Along with her new interest in affordable, industrially produced house equipment, she increasingly turned to an *art brut* in which wood and natural forms replaced metal, and artisanal objects took over designs emblematic of the machine.

Consistent with a newfound essentialism, Perriand explored further through photography the aesthetic potential of "accidental" forms, whether natural or industrial. Her first, 1938 *tables en forme*, replaced furniture boasting mechanical motion with static objects shaped to fit the movement of the human body, thus providing metaphors for her new organicism.

In 1940, three months before the Nazi invasion of France, Perriand accepted Japan's invitation to assume the position formerly held by Bruno Taut as industrial design adviser to the government. Japan's efforts at modernization without jeopardizing its intricate cultural heritage met successfully with Perriand's own efforts to achieve a seamless symbiosis between the industrial and the artisanal, the fabricated and the natural. She found in the everyday life of the Japanese house some principles that she had tried to apply in her work with Le Corbusier: the influence of the environment on modes of inhabitation and the liberation of the interior space through the absorption of household equipment into the walls of the dwelling. This concept emulated the Zen Buddhist understanding of the Void as "stimulating emptiness" rather than sterile absence. Perriand reinvented for Western needs the relationship between space and motion by adapting to modern life the Japanese view that harmonious human movement is possible only within emptiness. Her exhibitions for the Takashimaya department stores played a significant role in adapting Western modern techniques to fit the Japanese traditional spirit and were just the beginning of a series of similar exhibitions held simultaneously in France and Japan after the war.

Ultimately, Perriand's contact with Japan and its distinctive classicism—recognized as germane to Western modernism at least since Frank Lloyd Wright and French *Japonisme*—helped purify her own *art brut* into a postwar sophistication reminiscent, in some respects, of her early modernist phase. Her 1950 adaptation of the chaise longue, in which bent bamboo stems replaced the metallic tubular supports, is an example of this transformation. In general, the Japanese lesson emerged in her work through the reintroduction of simple, plain wood; sliding translucent panels that open widely on natural environments; low, horizontal furniture; and transformable modular storing devices. An example of such interiors were her kitchens for Le Corbusier's Unité d'habitation in Marseille or the so-called street interiors of Air France lobbies around the world that encompassed both the exclusive and the mass produced and remain examples of the best French design of the postwar era. Never severing her cultural ties to Japan, in 1993 she designed a teahouse for UNESCO in Paris. In December 1997, at age 94, she came for the first time to the United States, where she received the Brooklyn Museum of Art's Modernism Design Award for Lifetime Achievements.

DANILO UDOVICKI-SELB

Biography

Born in Paris, 24 October 1903. Studied design at the École de l'Union Centrale des Arts Décoratifs, Paris 1920–25; attended the life-classes of Bernard Boutet de Monvel and André Lhôte, Académie de la Grande Chaumière, Paris 1924–26; pursued decorative arts studies with Paul Follot and Maurice Dufrène. Married Jacques Martin 1943: 1 child. In private practice, Paris from 1927; set up a studio in the Place Saint Sulpice 1927–30 and the Boulevard de Montparnasse 1930–37; associate in charge of furniture and fittings, studio of Le Corbusier and Pierre Jeanerret, Paris 1927–37; member, editorial board, *L'architecture d'aujourd'hui* 1930–74; worked with Jean Prouvé, Pierre Jeanerret, and George Blanchon, Paris 1937–40; established office for prefabricated building research, Rue Las Cases, Paris 1940; Industrial Design Consultant to the Japanese Ministry of Commerce and Industry, Tokyo 1940–41; independent designer in Tokyo 1941–44 and Indochina 1943–46; worked in Tokyo 1953–56 and 1962–68; worked in Rio de Janeiro and Latin America 1969–76. Member, Salon des Artistes Décorateurs, Paris 1927; member, CIAM 1928; founding member, Union des Artistes Modernes, Paris 1930; member, Association des Etudiantes et Artistes Révolutionnaires, Paris 1931; consultant to the École Régionale des Beaux-Arts et des Arts Appliqués, Besançon, France 1966–68; jury president, International Office Furniture Competition, Paris 1983–84. Gold Medal, French Academy of Architecture 1978; Commandeur, Ordre National de Mérite 1978; Chevalier, Ordre des Arts et Lettres 1981; Chevalier, Légion d'Honneur 1983. Died in 1999.

Selected Works

Examples of Perriand's furnishings can be seen at the Musée des Arts Décoratifs, and the Fondation Le Corbusier in Paris.

Coin de salon, Salon des artistes décorateurs, 1926
Living room objects, Salon des artistes décorateurs, 1927
Bar sous le toit, Salon d'Automne, 1927
Dining room with mechanical table and rotating chairs, Salon des artistes décorateurs, 1928
Villa Laroche *équipement* (Le Corbusier-Jeanneret, architects), 1928
Villa Church at Ville-d'Avray (Le Corbusier-Jeanneret, architects), 1928–29
Equipement de l'habitation, in collaboration with Le Corbusier and Pierre Jeanneret, at the Salon d'Automne, *Chassis porte-coussin* armchair and modular storing furniture built by Thonet, 1929
Editor's office, *La semaine à Paris*, 1930
Studies for a *Maison minimum*, 1930
Chaise longue à position variable, Cologne International Exhibition (with Le Corbusier and Pierre Jeanneret), 1931
Interior furnishings of the public spaces of the Swiss Pavilion, Cité Universitaire, Paris (Le Corbusier-Jeanneret, architects), 1930–32
Interior furnishings of the Salvation Army's Cité Refuge (*crèche* and dormitories) (Le Corbusier-Jeanneret, architects), 1932
Le home du jeune homme, Brussels International Exhibition (with Le Corbusier and Pierre Jeanneret), 1935
Pavilion of the Agriculture Ministry, Paris International Exhibition, 1937
Photography with Fernand Léger and Pierre Jeanneret, exploring an *Art brut*, 1936–38
Tables en forme, one table made with rough pine-tree posts for the Temps Nouveaux Pavilion, office desk for Jean-Richard Bloch, editor of the daily *Ce Soir*, 1938
Hotel addition, Saint-Nicolas-de-Véroce Alpine Valley, 1939

Portable, prefabricated aluminum cabins (with Jean Prouvé and
   Pierre Jeanneret), 1940
"Tradition, Selection, Creation" (exhibition) for the Takashimaya
   department stores, Tokyo-Osaka, 1941
Furniture for a *Maison familiale minimum* (with architects
   P. Nelson, R. Gilbert, and Ch. Sebillote), presented at the Grand
   Palais international exhibition, 1947
Memorial Saint-Lô Hospital (collaboration with Paul Nelson), 1947
Design for a standardized, minimum modular storage element—the
   drawer, and its various accessories; patented in various materials
   and mass produced for the BHV department store, 1948–55
Open kitchen for Le Corbusier's *Unité d'habitation*, Marseille, 1950
Bathroom in the Japanese tradition for the Salon des Arts Ménagers,
   Formes utiles section, 1952
"Suspended" toilet bowl, 1952
Rooms for the Tunis Pavilion, Cité Universitaire, Paris (Jean Sebag,
   architect), 1952
Brazzaville Air France building furnishings (with Jean Prouvé), 1952
Maison d'étudiants, Paris (with Jean Prouvé), 1953
Interior furnishings, Hotel de France, Conakry (Lagneau and Weill,
   architects), 1953
Air France lobby, London (P. Bradok, architect), 1957
House in the Sahara for oil drilling workers, Salon des Arts
   Ménagers, 1958
Furnishings for the Brasil Pavilion, Cité Universitaire, Paris (Lucio
   Costa, architect), 1959
Air France lobby in Tokyo (J. Sakakura and Ren Suzuki, architects),
   1959
Chalet at Mirabel-les-Allues, Savoie, France, 1960
Apartment, Rio de Janeiro (with architect Maria Elisa Costa), 1962
Furniture for the Musée National d'Art Moderne, Paris, 1965
Residence for the Ambassador of Japan, Paris (Sakakura and
   Reidberger, architects), 1966
Modernization of the Geneva United Nations Headquarters (with
   Beaudouin and Carlu), 1959–70
Perriand apartment, Montparnasse, Paris, 1970
Interior furnishings, Station des Arcs, 18,000-bed hotel facilities in
   the Alps, 1967–82
Teahouse Pavilion, UNESCO, Paris, 1993

Selected Publications

"Monologue in a London Flat," *Architect and Building News*
   (October 1930)
"Habitation familiale: son développement économique et social,"
   L'architecture d'aujourd'hui, 6/1 (January 1935)
"L'art d'habiter," *Techniques et architecture*, 9–10 (1950) (special
   issue edited by Perriand)
"Japon: une tradition vivante," *L'architecture d'aujourd'hui*, 65 (May
   1956) (special issue edited by Perriand)
"La maison japonaise," *Aujourd'hui: art et architecture*, 12 (April
   1957)
Charlotte Perriand: une vie de création, 1997

Further Reading

"The Apartment Interior," *Architectural Record*, 80 (October 1936)
"Charlotte Perriand, la plus célèbre décoratrice de France," *La
   tribune de Lausanne* (16 February 1964)
Charlotte Perriand: Un art de vivre (exhib. cat.), Paris: Musée des
   Arts Décoratifs, and Flammarion, 1985
Henriot, Gabriel, "Le XVIIIe salon des artistes décorateurs au Grand
   Palais," *Mobilier et décoration*, 8 (1928)
Holme, C. Geoffrey, *Decorative Art: The Studio Year Book*, London:
   Studio, 1931 (see especially the essay by Maurice Dufrène,
   "Interior Decoration in Europe and America")

*Le Corbusier, Charlotte Perriand, Pierre Jeanneret: la machine à
   s'asseoir* (exhib. cat.), Rome: De Luca, 1976
"Le Home du Jeune homme," *L'architecture d'aujourd'hui*, 6/10
   (October 1935)
McLeod, Mary, "Charlotte Perriand: Her First Decade as a
   Designer," *Architectural Association Files*, 15 (1987)
Mihailovic, Cécile, "Entre le rêve et l'objet" in *Créer un produit*,
   Paris: Centre du Création Industrielle, Centre Georges
   Pompidou, 1983
"Rencontre avec Charlotte Perriand," *Modulo*, 46 (July-August-
   September 1977)
Renous, Pascal, *Portraits de décorateurs*, Dourdan, France: Vial, 1969
Sakakura, J. and Charlotte Perriand, *Contact with Japanese Art:
   Selection, Tradition, Creation*, Tokyo: Kujiokayama, 1941
Sert, José-Luis, "Charlotte Perriand," *Aujourd'hui: art et architecture*,
   7 (March 1956)
Winternitz, Lonia, "Einwohnraum: von Le Corbusier in
   Zusammenarbeit mit Pierre Jeanneret und Charlotte Perriand,"
   Innen-Dekoration, 41/6 (June 1930)

PETRONAS TOWERS, KUALA LUMPUR
Designed by Cesar Pelli; completed 1996
Kuala Lumpur, Malaysia

Claiming the title of the tallest buildings in the world at the
time of their completion, the Petronas Towers were designed
by Cesar Pelli and completed in 1996. Built in Kuala Lumpur
City for the Petronas Company, the national petroleum company of Malaysia, the twin towers are part of an enormous commercial development that contains the headquarters of Petronas
as well as a hotel and leased office space. Dominating the central
part of the city, the twin towers were the first phase of a "city
within the city"—an 18 million-square-foot complex located on
the grounds of what was formerly a horse-racing track.
   Pelli's Petronas Towers exemplify the never-ending quest to
build taller structures—a quest that inspired the building of the
Tower of Babel, the city of San Gimignano, Gothic cathedrals,
and the modern skyscraper. The skyscraper building type
emerged in the United States in the late 19th century, with
Chicago and New York competing to have the tallest building
in the world. Made possible by the invention of the elevator,
improved fireproofing technology, and metal structural cages,
skyscrapers of the Chicago School became important civic and
corporate status symbols. Some of the earliest examples of this
type include the Home Insurance Building (1885) by William
LeBaron Jenny; Reliance Building (1894) by Burnham and
Root; and Guaranty Building (1895) by Sullivan and Adler.
Petronas Towers joins a list of buildings that have held the title
of the tallest building in the world: Masonic Temple (1892) by
Burnham and Root in Chicago; the Woolworth Building (1913)
in New York City by Cass Gilbert; the Empire State Building
(1931) in New York City by Shreve, Lamb and Harmon; the
World Trade Center (1972–73, destroyed in 2001) in New York
City by Minoru Yamasaki; and the Sears Tower (1974) in Chicago by Skidmore, Owing and Merrill. The Petronas Towers
bested the Sears Tower by nine meters, standing at 452 meters
to the tip of the spire. There was some controversy about which
building was actually higher, since the Sears Tower has a higher
occupiable floor, but Petronas reaches a higher overall height.
Although Petronas Towers will someday be eclipsed as the tallest

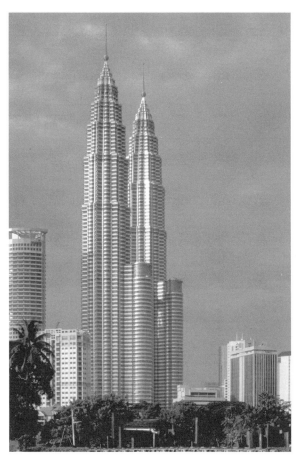

Petronas Office Towers, designed by Cesar Pelli
© Jeff Goldberg/ESTO. Photo courtesy of Cesar Pelli and Associates

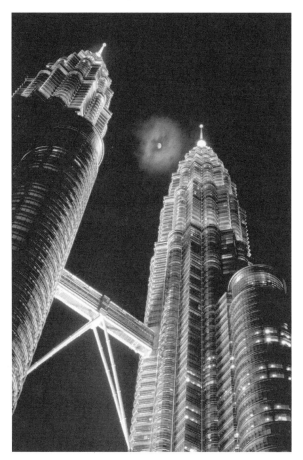

Petronas Office Towers, designed by Cesar Pelli
© Jeff Goldberg/ESTO. Photo courtesy of Cesar Pelli and Associates

in the world, it will remain the tallest concrete frame structure for many years to come.

After an international competition, the architectural commission for the towers was awarded to Cesar Pelli Associates, a firm that had executed several tall buildings noted for their rich palette of materials and elegant skyscraper profiles. The U.S. firm of Thornton-Tomasetti Engineers with their Malaysian counterpart Ranhill Bersekutu undertook the challenge of engineering the high-strength concrete frame. In addition to the technical demands of these towers, the high profile of the project, and the nationalistic nature of the program caused unusual stipulations to be placed on the design. The technology to build the towers, while developed with international expertise, had to be transferable to the Malaysians working on the project. The subcontractors were required to develop fabrication plants in Malaysia and to train local workers, both of which would have longterm benefits for the Malaysian economy.

Each of the two main towers stands 88 stories tall, with a slimmer "bustle" tower at 44 stories. The twin towers are joined with a skybridge at levels 41 and 42. The massing of the towers is relatively slender with setbacks at levels 60, 73, 82, 85, and 88, terminating in a 49-meter stainless-steel spire. The glass and stainless-steel skin of the building is faceted as a result of the complex geometry of each tower's plan.

The eight-pointed star created by two interlocked squares is one of the fundamental geometries underlying Islamic design. The basic square represents the earth and its four cardinal points, or heaven and its four rivers. The development of simple forms into complex geometry reflects the incomprehensibility of God. In the case of the Petronas Towers plan, eight small circles were superimposed at each intersection, creating a multifaceted floor plate. This result satisfied a programmatic desire for multiple corner offices, each taking advantage of the complex's park-like setting.

This geometry also dictated a structural solution that allowed the floor plates to be apparently column-free. In addition to a central concrete core, there are 16 perimeter columns, each 2.4 meters in diameter, arrayed in a 46-meter diameter circle. A ring beam, haunched to allow mechanical systems to pass underneath, connects the columns. At the setbacks, columns were engineered for a slight slope to eliminate transfer beams. Cantilevers framed in steel create the triangles and arcs that make up the points of the star.

Steel was the dominant structural material for tall buildings for most of the 20th century, and the decision to depart from this norm was made early in the Petronas Towers design process. High-strength concrete became the preferred material partially because of its compressive strength and partially because of the

government's incentive to use materials that could be fabricated domestically. Another advantage is that the concrete's mass stabilizes the towers so that movement is not a significant problem.

The site chosen for the towers, however, posed significant challenges. The nature of the soil was extremely unpredictable, and in fact an underground cliff was discovered. Master-plan changes had to be made to accommodate found conditions, and the excavation for each "barrette pile" (concrete friction element) had to be surveyed to an average depth of 80 meters.

The steel-framed connecting skybridge that attached to the towers at their midpoint was another major technical challenge. A clear space between the towers was very important in the design and massing of the building, and therefore the connector piece had to be light and relatively transparent. The connector bridge was braced against each tower with a pair of split "V" legs, each slender element containing a tuned mass damper. Each set of legs was attached to its tower with a fully rotating ball joint that allowed for movement up to 500 millimeters. The connector was prefabricated by a Korean manufacturer and was raised over several days after a ceremonial celebration.

RENÉE CHENG

See also **Chicago School; Empire State Building, New York; Pelli, Cesar (Argentina and United States); Sears Tower, Chicago; Skyscraper; Woolworth Building, New York; World Trade Center, New York**

Further Reading

Dupré, Judith, *Skyscrapers*, New York: Black Dog and Leventhal, 1996

Jodidio, Philip, *New Forms: Architecture in the 1990s*, Cologne and New York: Taschen, 1997

Kamin, Blair, "Duel in the Sky," *Chicago Tribune Magazine* (6 February 1994)

Mujica, Francisco, *History of the Skyscraper*, Paris and New York: Archaeology and Architecture Press, 1929; reprint, New York: Da Capo Press, 1977

"The Petronas Towers," *Architectural Design*, 65/7 (1995)

"Petronas Towers," *Architecture*, 95/9 (1996)

Petroski, Henry, *Remaking the World: Adventures in Engineering*, New York: Knopf, 1997

Post, Nadine, "Malaysia Cracks Height Ceiling as It Catapults into Future," *Engineering News-Record* (15 January 1996)

Van Leeuwen, Thomas, "The Skyward Trend of Thought: Some Ideas on the History of the Methodology of the Skyscraper" in *American Architecture: Innovation and Tradition*, edited by David G. De Long, Helen Searing, and Robert A.M. Stern, Rizzoli: New York, 1986

Zaknic, Ivan, Matthew Smith, and Dolores Rice (editors), *100 of the World's Tallest Buildings*, Mulgrave, Victoria: Images, London: Hazar, and Corte Madera, California: Gingko Press, 1998

PEVSNER, SIR NIKOLAUS 1902–83

Architecture historian and critic, England

Nikolaus Pevsner transformed the discipline of architectural history in Britain. More than any other single individual, architect, or critic, he molded the taste of English architects throughout the 1940s and 1950s and developed public awareness and appreciation of architecture in Britain for an even longer period. He was a naturally gifted teacher, an indefatigable researcher, and a highly opinionated critic. Before he arrived in Britain as a refugee from Nazi Germany in 1933, architectural history and criticism in Britain was very largely a dilettante activity taken up by gentleman architects and university professors. By the time he died, 50 years later, British scholarship in the fields of architectural theory and history was second to none: vigorously disciplined, genuinely enlightening and innovative, and securely based in higher academic institutions.

This transformation was not effected by Pevsner alone, of course. His fellow countryman Sir Ernst Gombrich, the noted art theorist and historian, achieved as much in academic circles. However, among architects, architectural students, and the general public in Britain, Pevsner's achievements and influence stand head and shoulders above any other. He achieved this status through his prolific writings, which were scholarly yet popular; through his editorship (1942–45) and long association with the *Architectural Review*, Britain's most prestigious monthly architectural journal; and through his many years of teaching architectural history (as professor of history of art at Birkbeck College, University of London, 1942–69, and as Slade Professor of Fine Art at the University of Cambridge, 1949–55, and at the University of Oxford, 1968–69). Many generations of architectural students have grappled with the question he asked in the introduction to his book, *An Outline of European Architecture* (1942), "What is architecture?" and disputed his answer, "A bicycle shed is a building; Lincoln Cathedral is a piece of architecture." In the late 1930s and throughout the 1940s, they were convinced by him of the intellectual validity and inevitable victory of the Modern movement in architecture through reading his *Pioneers of the Modern Movement from William Morris to Walter Gropius* (1936).

Modest and unassuming in manner, Pevsner had an iron will and determination. He persuaded Sir Allen Lane, founder of Penguin Books, to embark on Penguin's most ambitious, extensive, and financially uncertain project: the publication in 46 volumes, eventually, of a series, The Buildings of England. This was to consist of a series of scholarly and entertaining catalogs of the most important, and the more interesting, buildings, archaeological sites, urban neighborhoods and ensembles, towns, and villages—historic, traditional-vernacular, and modern—country by country. The early volumes were entirely researched and written by him. In later volumes, he was more dependent, both in research and in the actual writing, on the assistance of others—many his former students at Birkbeck College. However, when the series was finally completed in 1974, the series was unmistakably his—his vigorous scholarship, acute observation, and idiosyncratic likes and dislikes were evident in every volume—and, not content with England, he persuaded Penguin to commission volumes on the countries of Wales and Scotland.

The Buildings of England series made Pevsner a household name in Britain. Few families would embark on a motor tour or a provincial holiday in England without packing the appropriate volumes of The Buildings of England to take with them. As the volume and extent of heritage tourism grew in Britain throughout the 1960s, 1970s, and 1980s, so did sales of these particular books. He was a popular broadcaster as well, delivering the Reith Lectures of 1955 on BBC radio on the subject "The Englishness of English Art."

Pevsner's intellectual formation was rigorously academic. Born in Leipzig, Germany, he was educated in Leipzig, Munich, Berlin, and Frankfurt and was destined for a career in art history. He joined the staff of the Dresden Gallery in 1924 while engaged in research for his doctorate. His doctoral dissertation was published, as Leipziger Barock, in 1929. In the same year, he joined the staff of Göttingen University. He visited England in 1930, developed an interest in English 19th-century design, and emigrated to England in 1933.

During the 1930s, as an "enemy alien" in World War II, life in England was not easy for Pevsner but, rather, was precarious and insecure. It was not until after the war, under a progressive government and with a tenured teaching appointment at London University, that he could feel secure. In 1946 he became a naturalized British citizen. He acquired a house, in Hampstead Garden Suburb, in which to bring up his family.

Responsibilities and honors were showered on Pevsner: the responsibilities he welcomed and bore diligently, whereas the honors sat highly on his slightly bowed shoulders. He was appointed to the Royal Fine Arts Commission, the Historic Buildings Council, and similar organizations and was chairman of the Victorian Society, which he was largely instrumental in founding, from 1958 to 1976. He was made a Commander of the British Empire (CBE) in 1953 and a Fellow of the British Academy (FBA) in 1965 and was awarded the Royal Institute of British Architects (RIBA) Royal Gold Medal in 1967 and knighted in 1969. In the same year, his native land honored him with the award of the Grand Cross of the Order of Merit of the Federal Republic of Germany.

Pevsner was a prolific writer and published many books and articles in learned journals. For Sir Allen Lane, he edited the series King Penguins from 1941 and persuaded his patron to publish the Pelican History of Art series, which was launched in 1953 with *Painting in Britain 1530 to 1790* by Ellis Waterhouse and *The Art and Architecture of India* by Benjamin Rowland. Among his later books are *Sources of Modern Architecture and Design* (1968), *Some Architectural Writers of the Nineteenth Century* (1972), and *A History of Building Types* (1976). He remained intellectually active until the end of his life, although the onset of Parkinson's disease in the early 1970s limited his mobility and caused him and his many friends and colleagues considerable distress. He died in 1983.

ANTHONY D.C. HYLAND

Biography

Born in Leipzig, 30 January 1902. Studied at the University of Leipzig, Munich, Berlin, and Frankfurt am Main. Art historian, the Gemäldegalerie, Dresden; editor, *Architectural Review*, London 1942–45. Lecturer in art and architectural history, University of Göttingen 1929–35; lecturer 1942–69, chair 1959–69, Birkbeck College, University of London; lecturer, University of Cambridge 1949–55; lecturer, University of Oxford 1968–69. Member, later chair and president, Victorian Society from 1958. Royal Gold Medal, Royal Institute of British Architects 1967; knighted 1969. Died in London, 18 August 1983.

Selected Publications

Pevsner was a prolific writer. He contributed regularly to learned journals in English, German, and French and was widely translated into

Spanish and Italian. Several of his more popular books ran to several editions and were published in both Britain and the United States. The select Pevsner bibliography included in *Concerning Architecture*, edited by John Summerson (1968; see listing under "Further Reading"), contains almost 300 entries up to the end of 1967 and does not claim to be comprehensive. The list below contains only his more important books and a few key journal articles.

Leipziger Barock, Die Baukunst det Barockzeit in Leipzig, 1928
Pioneers of the Modern Movement from William Morris to Walter Gropius, 1936; 2nd edition, as *Pioneers of Modern Design from William Morris to Walter Gropius,* 1949; revised and partly rewritten edition, 1960
An Enquiry into Industrial Art in England, 1937
An Outline of European Architecture, 1942
The Leaves of Southwell, 1945
"The Architecture of Mannerism" in *The Mint,* edited by Geoffrey Grigson, 1946
"Richard Payne Knight," *The Art Bulletin,* 31/4 (1949)
"Building with Wit: The Architecture of Sir Edwin Lutyens," *Architectural Review,* 109/4 (1951)
High Victorian Design: A Study of the Exhibits of 1851, 1951
The Buildings of England, 46 vols., 1951–74
"Johannesburg: The Development of a Contemporary Vernacular in the Transvaal," *Architectural Review,* 113/6 (1953)
The Englishness of English Art, 1956
"Roehampton: LCC Housing and the Picturesque Tradition," *Architectural Review,* 126/7 (1959)
Les sources du Vingtieme siècle (with Jean Casson and Emile Langui), 1961; as *The Sources of Modern Art,* translated by K.M. Delavenay and H. Leigh Farnell, 1962; as *Gateway to the Twentieth Century: Art and Culture in a Changing World,* 1962
The Penguin Dictionary of Architecture (with John Fleming and Hugh Honour), 1966
Sources of Modern Architecture and Design, 1968
Some Architectural Writers of the Nineteenth Century, 1972
A History of Building Types, 1976

Further Reading

Summerson, John (editor), *Concerning Architecture: Essays on Architectural Writers and Writing Presented to Nikolaus Pevsner,* London: Allen Lane, and Baltimore, Maryland: Penguin, 1968

PHILADELPHIA, PENNSYLVANIA

Philadelphia began the 20th century as the third-largest city in the United States, after New York and Chicago. It was an economically prosperous manufacturing center and a significant port that attracted many immigrants from the poorer areas of Eastern Europe, southern Italy, and the southern United States. Although it had lost its position as America's political, financial, and cultural capital to Washington, DC, and New York, Philadelphia was a thriving industrial metropolis at the turn of the 20th century.

The epitome of Philadelphia's confidence at this time can be seen in its City Hall (1871–1901), designed by John McArthur, Jr., and Thomas Ustick Walter in an ornately decorative Second Empire style with sculptures by Alexander Calder. This imposing and monumental structure fills a massive square block broken only by pedestrian passages that continue Philadelphia's axes of Broad and Market Streets into its center courtyard. In addition, City Hall's tower, with clock and sculpture of founder William

Penn, prominently stands out from all parts of the city. This was especially so before Helmut Jahn's Liberty Place (1987), when there was an unwritten "gentleman's agreement" not to build higher than City Hall's tower.

During the 20th century, Philadelphia gradually moved away from its 19th-century manufacturing history and developed into a service economy with the building of office buildings, hotels, department stores, apartment buildings, banks, and cultural buildings.

Daniel Burnham's Land Title Buildings (1897 and 1902) introduced to Philadelphia the practice of downsizing the presence of a building's steel frame behind external ornament and a curtain wall. (City Hall is constructed with load-bearing stone approximately 22 feet thick at its base.) This practice continued into the 20th century, most notably with the Art Deco–style East Penn Square (1930) by Ritter and Shay. The first Philadelphia building to break away from this tradition was George Howe and William Lescaze's Philadelphia Savings Fund Society (PSFS) Building (1932), one of the first International Style skyscrapers in the United States and a daring architectural statement by a conservative institution such as a bank.

The convention of expressing a tall building's steel frame continued as modernism flourished in the decades after World War II. The Penn Center development (1953–82), proposed by Edmund Bacon and Vincent Kling, was made possible by the construction of Suburban Station (1924–29) and 30th Street Station (1927–34), both by Graham, Anderson, Probst and White, and the 1953 demolition of Broad Street Station (1892–93) and its elevated railroad tracks. Penn Center is worthy of mention if only because of its integration of transportation, retail, and office facilities. Other notable buildings in this area west of City Hall include the pyramid-topped Mellon Bank Center (1990) by Kohn Pederson Fox and the electric-razor-like Bell Atlantic Tower (1991) by the Kling-Lindquist Partnership.

Befitting a city with money to spend, Philadelphia produced a considerable amount of large department stores and retail centers in the 20th century. The Lit Brothers Store (1891–1907), Strawbridge and Clothier Department Store (1890s–1920s), and Gimbel's Department Store (1890s–1900, demolished 1980) were all major retail outlets around the vicinity of Eighth and Market Streets composed of assorted buildings that were built or converted as was needed. In contrast, Burnham's John Wanamaker Department Store (1902–11), a blocky Renaissance *palazzo* on the outside with an impressive atrium on the inside, was purposely built to be a self-contained shopping experience.

Philadelphia's last big foray into retail in the 20th century came between 1974 and 1983 with the development known as "The Gallery" by Bower and Fradley (phase 1) and Bower Lewis Thrower (phase 2). Basically an urban shopping mall, The Gallery can be commended for its integration with the street grid

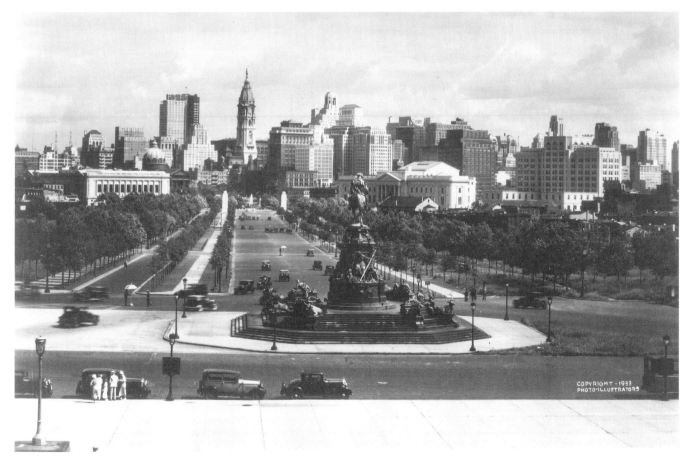

View of the city looking towards the Philadelphia Museum of Art, ca. 1933
© Library of Congress

of Philadelphia and also with the underground Market East Train Station (1985). The Gallery cannot be commended, however, for its typical and banal shopping mall appearance and for the way it stole the street life away from nearby Chestnut Street, which had been pedestrianized in 1973.

Prominent bank buildings in 20th-century Philadelphia include the Girard Trust Company (1905–08), a brilliantly white Ionic temple by McKim, Mead and White. The Federal Reserve Bank (1931–35) by Paul Phillipe Cret is a bit more stripped down in its classicism. The previously mentioned PSFS Building was internally innovative in the way its banking hall was located on an upper floor of its sleek polished-granite base, with street level given over to retail.

The major cultural project of the early 20th century was the creation of the Benjamin Franklin Parkway (1907–41), a spacious boulevard modeled after Paris's Champs-Elysées, which cuts through Philadelphia's street grid to connect City Hall with Fairmount Park. The idea for the Parkway was first inspired by the World's Columbian Exhibition of 1893 in Chicago, which promoted broad avenues with gleamingly white neoclassical buildings under the guise of the City Beautiful Movement.

The Parkway itself was officially designed and planned by Jacques Grabér and Paul Philippe Cret, but its crowning glory is the Philadelphia Museum of Art (1916–28) by Horace Trumbauer, especially in the way it mediates Fairmount Park and the city. Along the Parkway are other neoclassical civic buildings, such as the Rodin Museum (1927–29), also by Grabér and Cret; the Franklin Institute Science Museum (1932–34) by John Windrim; and the Philadelphia Free Library (1917–27) by Trumbauer and its near twin, the Philadelphia County Courthouse (1938–41), based on a design by Windrim.

The second half of the 20th century produced two stars of the international architectural scene from Philadelphia: Louis Kahn and Robert Venturi. Kahn's Philadelphia masterpieces include the Margaret Esherick House (1960) in Chestnut Hill, a private residence that beautifully makes use of natural light to enhance the interior, and the University of Pennsylvania's Richards Medical Research Laboratory (1957–61) whose "served" and "service" spaces influenced a generation of architects. Venturi was born in Philadelphia and briefly worked for Kahn before establishing his own practice with John Rauch in 1964 and Denise Scott Brown in 1967. His Philadelphia masterpieces include the Vanna Venturi House (1962), a private residence for his mother, and the Guild House (1960–63), an apartment house for the elderly both of which have been mistakenly credited as the foundation of Postmodernist architecture.

After World War II, the character of Philadelphia began to change. Beginning in 1948, under the good intentions of creating space around Independence Hall (the location of the signing of the Declaration of Independence and the writing of the Constitution), many buildings were cleared to form empty strips of land called Independence Mall and Independence Park. For the United States' bicentennial celebrations in 1976, all this space began to make sense, especially coupled with the Liberty Bell Pavilion (1976) by Mitchell/Giurgola, a glass box that displays the icon of Philadelphia tourism. After the bicentennial, however, these areas became an empty wasteland. In brilliant opposition to the fakeness of Independence Mall, Robert Venturi designed his Franklin Court (1976) as a tubular steel outline of Benjamin Franklin's former house, putting the actual exhibits underground.

The tourist-world of Independence Mall is in the process of being reconstructed to include an Independence Visitor Center and a National Constitution Center. In addition, a new home for the Liberty Bell, designed by Bohlin Cywinski Jackson, that allows views of Independence Hall without a background of skyscrapers will open in 2003. The view of the city as a museum piece was especially reinforced after the construction of the Pennsylvania Convention Center (1994) by Thompson, Ventulett, Stainback, and Associates, which converted the Reading Terminal train shed (1891–93) for part of its facilities after its redundancy following the construction of the Market East Train Station. With the anticipation of thousands of different visitors every week, hotel speculation went rampant, with many office buildings converted into hotels, including the seminal PSFS Building. Along with the hotels also came the tourist-traps that could be located anywhere and not necessarily particular to Philadelphia—namely a Hard Rock Café and a planned Disney Quest "family entertainment center." Conversely, the Kimmel Center for the Performing Arts (2001) by Rafael Viñoly Architects, part of a planned arts district on South Broad Street, rises above the anonymity of the subsequent Convention Center development and sets a good example for future development like a proposed entertainment complex with tram across the Delaware River and a new downtown baseball stadium.

CHRISTOPHER WILSON

See also **Burnham, Daniel H. (United States); City Beautiful Movement; Cret, Paul Philippe (United States); Graham, Anderson, Probst, and White (United States); Howe, George, and William Lescaze (United States); International Style; Jahn, Helmut (United States); Kahn, Louis (United States); Kohn Pederson Fox (United States); McKim, Mead and White (United States); Office Building; Vanna Venturi House, Philadelphia; Venturi, Robert (United States); Wanamaker Store, Philadelphia**

Further Reading

Bacon, Edmund, *Design of Cities*, New York: Viking, and London: Thames and Hudson, 1967; revised edition, 1974

Brownlee, David B., *Building the City Beautiful: The Benjamin Franklin Parkway and the Philadelphia Museum of Art*, Philadelphia: Philadelphia Museum of Art, 1989

Gallery, John Andrew (editor), *Philadelphia Architecture: A Guide to the City*, Cambridge, Massachusetts: MIT Press, 1984; 2nd edition, Philadelphia: Foundation for Architecture, 1994

Lukacs, John, *Philadelphia: Patricians and Philistines: 1900–1950*, New York: Farrar Straus Giroux, 1981

Morrone, Francis, *An Architectural Guidebook to Philadelphia*, Layton, Utah: Gibbs-Smith, 1999

Rybczynski, Witold, *City Life: Urban Expectations in a New World*, New York: Scribner, 1995

Saidel, Jonathan, et al., *Philadelphia: A New Urban Direction*, Philadelphia: St. Joseph's University Press, 1999

Teitelman, Edward and Richard W. Longstreth, *Architecture in Philadelphia: A Guide*, Cambridge, Massachusetts: MIT Press, 1974

Wurman, Richard S., *Philadelphia Access*, New York: Access Press, 1994; 3rd edition, 1998

PHOENIX CENTRAL LIBRARY

Designed by Will Bruder (bruderDWLarchitects);
completed 1995
Phoenix, Arizona

The Phoenix Central Library was the first major commission for Will Bruder (1946–), an artist and self-trained architect who lives and works in New River, Arizona, in the desert north of Phoenix. Opened in 1995, the building has earned critical acclaim from the architectural profession for its poetic and economical integration of everyday materials, natural lighting, and environmental technologies as well as for its local and regional specificity, achieved without recourse to historical pastiche. Planned in close collaboration with the library's professional staff, the building also received in 1997 an Award of Excellence in a library building award program cosponsored by the American Institute of Architects and the American Library Association.

The campaign for a new central library in Phoenix began in the early 1980s, but the project began in earnest only in 1988, when the city passed a $1.2 billion bond issue to finance the construction of several new cultural institutions. In the summer of 1989, the city issued a request for proposals for the library, and by the end of the year a selection committee had picked Bruder's firm (known as bruderDWLarchitects) from a pool of five finalists that also included Antoine Predock and Ricardo Legorreta. In the first half of 1990, the design team (led by Bruder and Wendell Burnette) refined the building program by conducting interviews with the entire library staff (including city librarian Ralph Edwards, central library director Rosemary Nelson, and president of the library board of trustees Elinor Green Hunter) and by holding 28 citizen meetings. The basic design concepts were in place by November 1990. Despite some resistance to the initial design (fueled in part by Bruder's description of the building as a "kinetically energized arrival pavilion"), the city council approved the plan in early January 1991.

As a library, the Phoenix building owes a great deal to postwar developments of the building type and particularly to the concept of the modular library. Using a planning module based on the standard dimensions and spacing of bookshelves, this system allowed bookshelves to be placed anywhere in the library and facilitated the integration of reading and book storage areas. Such buildings typically had large, square (or nearly square) footprints; uniform ceiling heights; and flat ceilings to conceal the requisite air-handling equipment and artificial lighting. At the Phoenix Central Library, a skeleton of concrete columns in the main body of the building rises from a planning module 32 feet, 8 inches square, creating a nearly square footprint approximately an acre in area at the upper floors. On the first four floors, these columns carry a precast T ceiling system that houses the east-west chases for lighting fixtures, air ducts, and power and data lines; concealed behind slightly concave aluminum panels, these chases are in turn served by aluminum-covered soffits, called "power bellies," which run north-south just inside the main body of the building. Flexibility—the watchword of postwar library planning—is here enhanced by housing ancillary and service functions in "saddlebags" (the architects' term for the curved, copper-clad elements that flank the main body of the building along its east and west sides) and extended to computer terminals that can be located anywhere in the library.

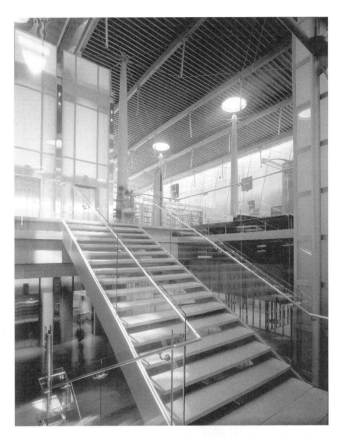

Phoenix Central Library (1995), grand staircase leading to Reading Room
© Bill Timmerman. Photo courtesy William P. Bruder Architects

While the Phoenix Central Library updates the technology of the modular library, it also moves beyond the monotonous interiors that characterized libraries in the postwar period. In part, this is achieved by glazing the north and south walls and providing natural lighting and dramatic views of the city and surrounding mountains. Computer-controlled mechanical louvers on the building's south side adjust continuously to block the strong desert sun, and on the north side Teflon-covered sails prevent glare. Natural lighting is also brought into the core of the building through the "crystal canyon," a five-story skylit atrium surrounded on three sides by glass and on the fourth by glass-encased elevators.

The Phoenix Central Library also updates the postwar type with the reintroduction of a monumental public reading room. In this case, the room is on the fifth floor, where it can take advantage of substantially taller ceiling heights and dramatic views; mechanical systems at this level are laid beneath a raised floor deck. Dominated by 30-foot-tall columns that taper from two feet at the base to ten inches at the top, this room has been compared to the great reading room in Henri Labrouste's Bibliothèque Nationale (1858–68) in Paris and to hypostyle halls of ancient Egyptian temples. Above each column is a skylight of laminated glass seven feet in diameter; in each, a hole in the blue interlayer provides clear glass opening four inches in diameter, calculated to allow the sunlight of the summer solstice to "light" the candlestick columns. (The library sponsors

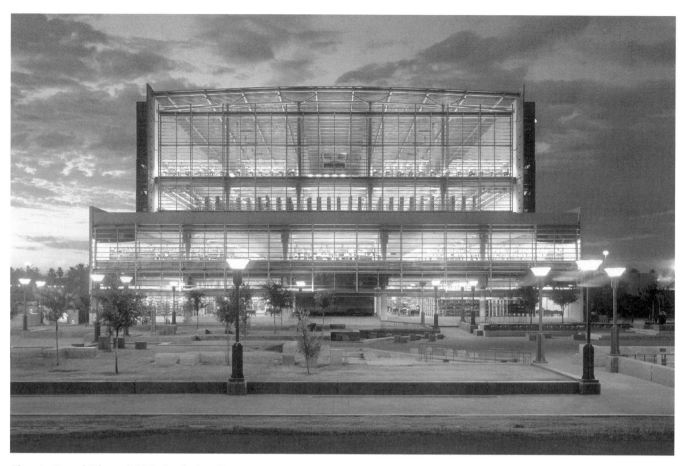

Phoenix Central Library (1995), South elevation
© Bill Timmerman. Photo courtesy William P. Bruder Architects

a solstice event each year, which has brought as many as 1500 people to witness the effect.)

These skylights also call attention to the fact that the columns stop short of the ceiling, which seems to float overhead. The ceiling is, in fact, supported by a "tensegrity" structure developed by Michael Ishler, an engineer with Ove Arup and Partners. Anchored to the steel caps bolted to the top of the columns, steel cables support vertical struts that in turn support the north-south purlins of the galvanized-steel roof deck. The roof deck also stops short of the walls on the east and west sides of the room, allowing daylight to wash down their concrete surfaces.

The Phoenix Central Library is noteworthy also for its regional character. Bruder, for example, drew on a number of regional metaphors in the process of refining the initial design concept. In addition to the crystal canyon and the saddlebags mentioned previously, Bruder has compared the building itself to a man-made mesa, its scaleless mass rising abruptly from the desert floor. The building also acknowledges its locale through its attention to the power of the desert sun. The 12-inch concrete walls, which separate the main body of the building from the saddlebags to the east and west, insulate those facades and allow the air conditioning to function smoothly. The experience of the main reading room—where the glazing of the north and south walls is most apparent and where sunlight washes the east and west walls—is particularly affected by the time of day and the time of year.

The library's regional specificity is also evident in the choice of materials: copper used to clad the steel-frame saddlebags is one of Arizona's most important natural resources (although copper sheets of the size needed here could be found at a competitive price only in Germany). Striations in the copper are the result of roll forming, a technique normally used to construct metal grain silos. Its use here is both expressive (in that it links the library to the industrialized agribusiness that sustains the state) and practical: because of the rigidity of the corrugation that it achieves, the technique allowed the use of an exceptionally thin gauge copper that cost only $1 more per square foot than the stucco often used in the Southwest to imitate adobe. In the end, the library cost less than $100 per square foot, demonstrating Bruder's commitment to an architecture in which "both pragmatism and poetry are served with equal passion" (Bruder, quoted in Ojeda, 1999).

ABIGAIL A. VAN SLYCK

See also **Arup, Ove (England); Historicism; Library**

Further Reading

Barreneche, Raul A., "High Heat, High Tech," *Architecture*, 84/10 (October 1995)

Brawne, Michael, *Library Builders*, London and Lanham, Maryland: Academy Editions, 1997

"Bruder DWL Architects: Phoenix Central Library," *GA Document*, 46 (February 1996)

Curtis, William, "William Bruder en Arizona," *L'architecture d'aujourd'hui*, 307 (October 1996)

Ojeda, Oscar Riera (editor), *Phoenix Central Library*, Gloucester, Massachusetts: Rockport, 1999

PIANO, RENZO 1937–

Architect, Italy

Renzo Piano, born in 1937 in the Mediterranean harbor city of Genoa, has been one of the most influential architectural personalities since the 1980s. He was strongly influenced by Franco Albini and Ernesto Rogers, who were his professors at the Polytechnical University in Milan. Jean Prouvé, Pierluigi Nervi, and the work of Buckminster Fuller also exerted a strong influence on the architect.

After Piano ended his academic career at the Polytechnical University, he founded Studio Piano, his first architectural office (1964–70). During this period, Piano also worked with Louis I. Kahn in Philadelphia and Z.S. Makowsky in London. He first gained international recognition when he went into partnership with English architect Richard Rogers from 1971 to 1977, emphasizing technology in architecture. From 1977 to 1981, he partnered with engineer and humanist Peter Rice (1935–92), who influenced Piano's work significantly with his focus on structural systems. After the death of Rice, Piano founded the Renzo Piano Building Workshop. The innovative and experimental character of Piano's work is based on team workshops that are filled with young talent from around the world. Like only a handful of architects, Piano has planned and realized a broad range of projects on a worldwide basis.

For Piano architecture is a creative process of communication and participation in which architectural solutions follow a process of diagnosis, design, realization, and documentation. This procedure was developed during the UNESCO-Workshop in Otranto, Italy (1978). A mobile display and communication box covered with a tent structure offered a central public forum. Piano created an environment allowing direct verbal confrontation and active participation of the community in the search for respectful restoration methods.

Piano and Rogers's Georges Pompidou Center (1978) is located in a sensitive urban environment in downtown Paris. Against considerable public and political resistance, Piano and Rogers designed a cultural forum in the form of a highly visible machine. Approximately 25,000 visitors participate daily in all sorts of cultural events on the inside as well as on the rectangular plaza in front of the Pompidou Center. Visitors enter the building through a transparent escalator that is attached to the external structural framework, which opens to a multilevel, open spatial layout. The floor plan is flexible and non–load bearing.

In 1982 Piano produced the space of the Palazzo a Vela in Turin, Italy, for the exhibition of the works of Alexander Calder. He put a stage installation together that incorporated the play of light, space, and temperature. Piano was able to create an open environment that liberated the boundaries of materiality. The dark and cool space offers a dimension where the mobile structures of Calder have a maximal effect on their observer.

Piano's work often experiments with the use of materials, which was especially evident in the IBM Traveling Pavilion (1986). The 48-meter-long tube was designed to display new forms of communication technology. The modular and transparent exhibition space is remarkable in its unusual combination of old and new materials and their connecting techniques.

In Turin Piano was engaged with the reorganization of a historical industrial monument, the Lingotto (1995). In the 1920s, engineer Matté Trucco designed a 500-meter-long and five-story-high industrial complex for the car manufacturer Fiat. At its time, the structure followed the requirements of functionalism. Piano transformed this highly visible sign of the industrial revolution into a "multifunctional service and research center." He placed a large auditorium space for cultural events into the existing structure. An inner courtyard was transformed into a public garden that reflected the Mediterranean character of Turin, and a rooftop, bubble-formed conference room located close to a helicopter platform became a new symbol of innovation for the city.

For the 500-year anniversary of Columbus's discovery of America, Piano completed in 1992 his first large-scale urban project. His hometown, Genoa, commissioned Piano to permanently reorganize the old harbor to revitalize the abandoned maritime area. Piano was confronted with the difficult task of linking the industrial harbor with the historic town structure by overcoming a division marked by an elevated major arterial road. Piano demolished no buildings but, rather, carefully implemented new functions in restored historical buildings or added new ones. His gentle revitalization concept helped to develop the old harbor into a vital cultural and recreational center of Genoa.

Piano and Rice built the San Nicola sports stadium (1990) in Bari, Italy, for the soccer world championship. The project requirements demanded that 60,000 people could enjoy the game and that standards for security not be ignored. They focused on optimal visibility, modular separation of fan masses, and an unusually high number of exit systems. Staircases between the seating sections also enhanced the vertical and horizontal cross ventilation. Piano and Rice created an elliptical floral-like stadium, expressing the plasticity of reinforced concrete in the manner of Pier Luigi Nervi.

The 220 low-income apartments (1991) in the Rue de Meaux in Paris were Piano's first housing complexes in which he proved that architectural and spatial quality do not always depend on large budgets. The facade demonstrates Piano's passion to reinvent the application of traditional and new materials. Glass, terra-cotta, and fiber-reinforced concrete exude Piano's interpretation of Le Corbusian rationality.

Piano's final project with Rice was the design and construction of the Kansai International Airport (1994) in Osaka, Japan; a steel building of simple geometry in which most internal structural elements were left visible. A physical site literally did not exist, as the proposed location of the airport was in the oceanic bay of Osaka. An artificial island on stilts first had to be built under extreme engineering demands. Piano envisioned a 1.7-kilometer-long building whose form derived from precise mathematical calculations following the laws of aerodynamics.

Piano unifies science and architecture in his work. Punta Nave, the Renzo Piano Building Workshop in Genoa-Vesima (1991), also serves as a UNESCO laboratory for climate and

the use of natural light in architecture. The transparent building is located on a significant slope, accessible only by cable car. The workshop building is organized in sections that step topographically down hills, providing most workspaces with a view to the Mediterranean Sea. The glass roof is partially covered with solar-controlled louvers that interact automatically with changing daylight conditions. With this rather small project, Piano was able to create a productive team space in which architects and scientists are able to explore architectural solutions in tune with their environment. Among others, this building exemplifies Piano's methods and ideas pertaining to sustainable architecture.

In Switzerland, Piano realized the Fondation Beyler Museum (1997) in Riehen/Basel. Similar to the Menil Collection, his most important building material was the natural light that he physically enclosed with sandstone, steel, and glass. The strict and rectangular building is covered by a glass roof and opens on three sides to a park. Like few other architects, Piano understands how to dissolve the barriers between inside and outside. One is reminded of Mies van der Rohe's Barcelona Pavilion in the way that Piano connects exhibition space on the inside and water ponds on the outside. The museum is extended into a space continuum that finds a symbiosis between art and architecture.

At the very end of the 20th century, Piano's most significant project was the new multifunctional development of the Potsdamer Platz (1999) in Berlin. The Potsdamer Platz was one of Europe's most important centers of cultural life in the 1920s. For Piano it meant that he had to redevelop what years ago was either destroyed by World War II or erased by postwar city planners. Under the leadership of Piano, internationally renowned architects, such as Arata Isozaki, Hans Kohlhoff, Lauber and Wöhr, Rafael Moneo, and Richard Rogers, have transferred the Postdamer Platz from a deserted empty historical space back into a lively part of downtown Berlin. New architectural developments range from shopping centers, theater, cinemas, restaurants, offices, and corporate headquarters to apartment houses. Surrounded by the water of the nearby Spree River, Piano designed eight of the 19 buildings of the Postdamer Platz. His buildings have the double-layered terra-cotta facade to formally unify the large area as a whole. As the core project, he created a new piazza between Potsdamer Strasse and Kulturforum as a metaphoric intersection between the former East and West German cultures.

Piano's projects are difficult to place in a particular category, but he is certainly one of the most exceptional architects of the 20th century. He constantly tries to liberate his design intentions from formal constricting preoccupations as he unifies art and technique. For Piano, the design process is not a linear progression to the final product. Piano's architecture develops out of a circular process in which presolutions are constantly reevaluated. For that reason, the team workshops develop a countless number of models on an extraordinary high level of craftsmanship. His architecture often applies the latest technology but is never dominated by it. As a result, most of his buildings appear rich in details but often seem so light as to lift up in the wind. Stability is achieved by their flexibility—an intelligent relationship to dominant cultural, historical, and environmental facts.

RICHARD KÖCK

See also **Cultural Centre Jean Marie Tjibaro-Noumia, New Caledonia; Fiat Works, Turin; Kahn, Louis (United States); Kansai International Airport Terminal, Osaka; Menil Collection, Houston, Texas; Pompidou Center, Paris; Rogers, Richard (England)**

Biography

Born in Genoa, Italy, 14 September 1937, son of a builder. Studied at Milan Polytechnic School of Architecture with Ernesto Rogers, Jean Prouvé, and Franco Albini (1959–64). Studied two years at the University in Florence. Married first wife Magda Arduino in Milan; 3 children: Carlo, Matteo, and Lia. Opened first architectural office (1964–70) in Milan, with additional work with Louis Kahn in Philadelphia and Z.S. Makowky in London. First major commission in 1969, the Italian Industry Pavilion at Expo 1970 in Osaka, Japan. In partnership with Richard Rogers (Piano & Rogers, 1971–77). Later worked with Peter Rice in partnership (Atelier Piano & Peter Rice, 1977–81). Established Renzo Building Workshop with offices in Genoa and Paris, with about 100 employees (1980). Since 1992, married to E. Rossato. Awarded numerous international prizes: International Union of Architects Prize, Mexico City (1978), Honorary Fellow American Institute of Architects (1981), Honorary Fellow Royal Institute of British Architects (1985), Royal Gold Medal for Architecture/Royal Institute of British Architects (1989), Honorary Doctorate Stuttgart University, Germany (1990), Honorary Doctorate University of Delft, the Netherlands (1991), Goodwill Ambassador for Architecture, UNESCO (1994), Pritzker Architecture Prize (1998).

Selected Works

Pavilion of the Italien Industry for the Expo in Osaka, Japan, 1970
Office building for B&B, Como, Italy, 1973
Pompidou Center, Paris, France, 1977
IRCAM, institute for acoustic research, Paris, France, 1977
Rehabilitation project for historical centers, Otranto, Italy, 1979
VSS experimental vehicle for FIAT, Turin, Italy, 1980
Calder retrospective exhibition, Turin, Italy, 1982
Musical space for Prometeo opera by L. Nono, Venice, Italy, 1984
Office building for Lowara factory, Vicenza, Italy, 1985
IBM Travelling Exhibition in Europe, 1986
Museum for the Menil Collection, Houston, Texas, 1986
San Nicola football stadium, Bari, Italy, 1990
Housing for the City of Paris, Paris, France, 1991
Renzo Piano Building Workshop, Punta Nave, Italy, 1991
Columbus International Festival, Aquarium and Congress Hall, Genoa, Italy, 1992
Reorganization Lingotto for Fiat, Turin, Italy, 1994
Kansai International Airport, Osaka, Japan, 1994
Cité Internationale, Lyon, France, 1995
Museum of Science and Technology, Amsterdam, Netherlands, 1996
Museum of the Beyeler Foundation, Riehen/Basel, Switzerland, 1997
Debis Tower, Potsdamer Platz, Berlin, Germany, 1997
Cultural Center Jean Marie Tjibaou, Nouméa, New Caledonia, 1998

Selected Publications

Renzo Piano and Building Workshop, Buildings and Projects, 1971–1989, New York: Rizzoli International Publications, 1989

Renzo Piano: progetti e architetture 1987–1994, Boston: Birkhäuser Verlag, 1994

The Renzo Piano Logbook, London: Thames and Hudson, 1997

Fondation Beyeler: A Home for Art, Boston: Birkhäuser Verlag, 1998

Renzo Piano: Sustainable Architecture, Barcelona: Corte Madera, Gingko Press, 1998

Architekturen des Lebens (Architecture of Life), Ostfildern/Ruit: Hatje Cantz Verlag, 2000

Further Reading

Buchanan, Peter, *Renzo Piano Building Workshop: Complete Works*, 4 vols., London: Phaidon Press, 1993–

Dini, Massino (editor), *Renzo Piano: Progetti e architetture, 1964–1983*, Milan: Electa, 1983; as *Renzo Piano: Projects and Buildings, 1964–1983*, New York: Electa/Rizzoli, and London: Electa/Architectural Press, 1983

Lepik, Andres (editor), *Renzo Piano: Architekturen des Lebens* (exhib. cat.), Ostfildern, Germany: Hatje Cantz, 2000

PIETILÄ, REIMA (1923–93) AND RAILI (1926–)

Architects, Finland

In the 1960s, Reima and Raili Pietilä became the leading architects of Finland by proposing an organic architecture as opposed to the uniform, prefabricated architecture of that time, an approach that related their work to that of Alvar Aalto. The roots of Pietiläs' architecture lie partly in the tradition of European Expressionism of the 1920s; partly in the theoretical influence of Aulis Blomstedt, the founder of the study group Le Carré Bleu; and partly in the awareness of the genius loci. They created a theory of imitating nature with architecture, and their design approach can be described as being natural and intellectual at the same time.

Although Reima and Raili Pietilä adressed issues such as language, literature, philosophy, and art on the theoretical level, the formal approach of their architecture is often directly related to the landscape and to the natural conditions of the building site. Lasting until 1969, their most creative period began in 1958, when Reima won the competition for the Finnish Pavilion at the Brussel's World's Fair.

After graduating in architecture from the Helsinki Institute of Technology, Reima Pietilä was first employed by the Master Planning Department of Helsinki City. In 1957 he set up his own private practice, having won the 1956 competition for the Finnish Pavilion, a monument to the Finnish sawmill industry. The wooden modular structuralism of the exhibition building was based on a symbiosis of local features and a strictly abstract composition, much in the spirit of the Le Carré Bleu group aesthetics. In 1960 he was joined in his practice by his wife, Raili, who had also graduated from the Helsinki Institute of Technology the year before and who had worked for a while at Aalto's office. The Kaleva church in Tampere, sited on an open hill, was their first project together. The competition was won in 1959 and the building completed in 1966. The floor plan is composed of U-shaped concrete curves that mark the outline of a Christian fish symbol. The section is very simple, with a flat roof: the plan was extruded to derive the interior space, a high volume with long, vertical window slits. The sculptural monumentality of the interior with its mystical light choreography was intended to recall organ music and was much indebted to the sculptural space concept of Umberto Boccioni.

The Pietiläs' Dipoli student and conference center (1966) at Otaniemi is reminiscent of Aalto's habit of opposing a geometric form with an organic shape. The site where Dipoli was built was given character by its large, exposed, granite shield originating from the glacial era. The roofline is a simulation of the microgeography of the site while also being a reptilian metaphoric image. The idea was to work against any tradition and preconceived styles but to let the building become part of the forest. More than any other project of the Pietiläs, it is not architecture in the traditional sense but, rather, part of the environment.

The modular strategy appears again in the Suvikumpu Housing Project (1969), a mixed development of 162 apartment units sited on a steep, wooded hillside in Espoo that was planned in 1962 with some additions made in 1983. To avoid the monotony of massing, the apartments are connected along a line, following the form of the central hill. The landscape is reflected in the varying vertical and horizontal masses of the building. The facades are composed of white plaster and dark wooden surfaces that invoke the region's bright sunlight and respond to the changing patterns of light and textures of the surrounding woods.

After this project was realized, the Pietiläs did not receive any important commissions in Finland, except for two minor projects, until 1975. This period certainly had a negative effect, as their later work did not achieve the strength of the earlier projects. Reima Pietilä was nominated a professor of arts, and from 1973 to 1979 he taught at the University of Oulu, initiating the Oulu School—an architectural trend rich in form—and applying regional and international features. In 1973 the Pietiläs received the commission for building the offices of the Ministry of Foreign Affairs (1982) at the Sief Palace in Kuwait, and in 1975 they won the competition for the Hervanta Congregational, Leisure, and Shopping Center (1979) in a suburb of Tampere. In 1978 they won the competition for the Tampere Main Library ("Metso"), which was finished in 1986. In these projects, the Pietiläs moved toward an early kind of Postmodernism. In the Sief Palace, they combined environmental elements, such as sun baffles, with local cultural traditions and metaphorical statements, such as fountains in the shape of coral flowers of the reef below the building. For the Hervanta shopping center, the formal influence of railway stations and the turn-of-the-century mall in Tampere was most important. However, the architects make references to the ruins of the Forum Romanum, and the adjacent congregational center of Hervanta suggests a forest fable. The Tampere Main library grew out of two images: a male wood grouse and a mollusk shell. This representational approach seems to follow the tradition of organic-shaped library buildings that Aalto had established. Indeed, the curved roof of the Metso recalls typical Aalto designs.

In their late works, the Pietiläs returned to the design concepts of Dipoli: to create a "naturalized" building. There is no longer any ambition to imitate natural forms but, rather, one to set up a dialogue with nature. In the Finnish Embassy (1985) in New Delhi, the roof patterns viewed from above simulate the geomorphology of Finland, with its parallel furrows and hills,

strip lakes, and islands. From the side, the eaves are shaped like snow sculptured by the wind. The chimneys on the roof of Mäntyniemi (1987), the residence of the Finnish president in Helsinki, resemble a burnt forest, as a simulation of a possible or fictional Stone Age scenery, and the elevations take their cue from the landscape as well.

DÖRTE KUHLMANN

See also **Aalto, Alvar (Finland); Finland; Helsinki, Finland**

Further Reading

Connah, Roger, *Writing Architecture: Fantômas Fragments Fictions: An Architectural Journey through the Twentieth Century,* Cambridge, Massachusetts: MIT Press, 1989

Norri, Marja-Riitta and Roger Connah (editors), *Pietilä modernin arkkitehtuurin välimaastoissa; Pietilä: Intermediate Zones in Modern Architecture* (bilingual English–Finnish text), Helsinki: Museum of Finnish Architecture, 1985

Quantrill, Malcolm (editor), *One Man's Odyssey in Search of Finnish Architecture: An Anthology in Honour of Reima Pietilä; Suomalaisen arkkitehtuurin etsijä: Omistettu Reima Pietilälle* (bilingual English–French text), Helsinki: Building Information Institute, 1988

Quantrill, Malcolm, *Finnish Architecture and the Modernist Tradition,* New York and London: E and FN Spon, 1995

PILGRIMAGE CHURCH AT NEVIGES

Designed by Gottfried Böhm; completed 1968
Neviges, Germany

After World War I, the Catholic Church began to change its position concerning restraints between worship and the physical architecture of the church. By the end of World War II, the evenly proportioned synagogue-style or basilica plan of the past, where the programmatic and visual thrust of the church centered on the sanctuary, was being replaced by spaces conceived from individual congregational requirements. The technological development of steel girders and concrete combined with relaxed church regulations moved church building away from traditional ecclesiastical architecture.

Mary, Queen of Peace, the Pilgrimage Church (1968) at Neviges, Germany, that is today a quarter of the city of Velbert, is the oldest pilgrimage church north of the Alps associated with the "Immaculata." Built by Gottfried Böhm, it was a response to the increased number of pilgrims of the 1950s.

The object of the pilgrimages is a 17th-century etching of the Virgin owned by the monks at Dorsten, Germany. Mary is reported to have spoken through the picture directly to one of the Franciscan clerics, instructing him in the art of healing. In 1680 the engraving was moved for protection to the fortified, baroque church of Neviges. This building housed the artwork until 1968, when it was moved to Böhm's new pilgrimage church.

Böhm, a third-generation architect and the son of the respected builder of Roman Catholic churches, Dominikus Böhm, had designed a variety of buildings ranging from museums to public housing when he was commissioned. Before the Neviges project, Böhm had built an important church in Kassel, Germany, an assignment that introduced many of the problems and solutions that he successfully integrated later at the Pilgrimage Church.

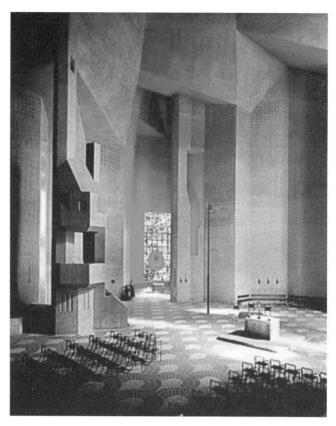

Interior, Pilgrimage Church at Neviges, Germany (1968)
© Inge and Arvid von der Ropp

An estimated 10,000 pilgrims make the annual visit to view the miraculous engraving of Mary and the expressionistic church that houses it. They arrive by train, bus, or automobile. All modes of transportation set the pilgrim on his or her journey at the Elberfelder road. From here, the pinnacles of Böhm's Pilgrimage Church can be glimpsed from time to time as the traveler makes his way through the historic village of Neviges. Böhm intended that the tantalizing glimpses of the church should be gained as the pilgrim processes through the half-timbered, slate-roofed town. Eventually, the old baroque church is reached, as is the monastery. Then time and architecture take a great leap forward as the initial stages of the goal are reached. Böhm presents a gentle-stepped polychromed stairway organically hugging the natural contours of the site. Workstations as well as modular units of the pilgrim's house containing welfare services and sleeping cells are on the left; temporary tent-like coverings can be stretched over the slight steps to accommodate outdoor activities. Then, as one passes beyond the last pod of the pilgrim's house, the church thrusts upward like a prism reflecting the steep pitched roofs of Neviges and the evergreen clad mountains in the background.

The Pilgrimage Church roof is constructed of a concrete skin 25 centimeters thick. Therefore, the interior is a negative of the exterior; the form of the building is plastic and boundless. The church is impossible to accurately measure, although approximate dimensions are listed as 37 meters wide by 50 meters in

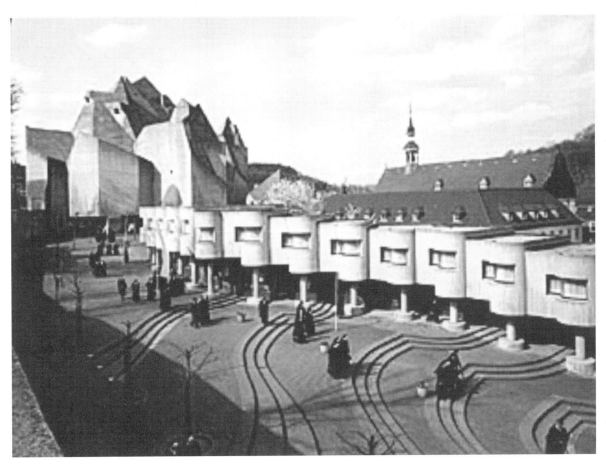

Exterior, Pilgrimage Church at Neviges (1968)
© Inge and Arvid von der Ropp

length. The exterior walls measure between ten and 20 meters, with the apex of the uppermost creased plane computed at 34 meters. No right angles exist, and the form is totally asymmetrical. The floor is a multicolored design extrapolation of the outside steps and sweeps the visitor into the structure, past loggias that are reminiscent of the cellular administration pods directly outside. Quite simply, Böhm brings the pilgrim to the village, the village to the administration buildings, and the administration buildings to the Pilgrimage Church. Only in the sanctuary is the processional stopped.

The altar, unlike the synagogue-style church, is not fixed; it is movable, dependent only on the function of the changing activity of the church. The chairs are likewise not secured to one specific place. Like the village macrocosm Böhm's structure imitates, the pilgrim is at liberty to move about, to explore the ecclesiastical environment and reflect on the architecture, the world, and the spirit.

Massive, vertical stained glass windows touch the muted concrete interior with pink and burgundy light. The glass is designed with the traditional symbols associated with Mary; however, the execution is anything but conventional. The outsized scale is sometimes overwhelming. A single crimson rose burns in a window, the symbol of the Virgin's sacrifice; an emerald interlace evoking Hiberno-Saxon manuscripts uncoils along the steps.

The Pilgrimage Church (Mary, Queen of Peace) is important in that it breaks completely with the symmetrical designs of ecclesiastical architecture. It redefines the concept of pilgrimage church and brings it into contemporary existence as conference center, hostel, and spiritual focus.

ALLISON HOUSTON SAULS

See also **Böhm, Gottfried (Germany); Church**

Further Reading

Emanuel, Muriel (editor), *Contemporary Architects*, New York: St. Martin's Press, and London: Macmillan, 1980
Raèv, Svetlozar (editor), *Vorträge, Bauten, Projekte*, Stuttgart: Krämer, 1988; as *Gottfried Böhm: Lectures, Buildings, Projects*, translated by Peter Green, Stuttgart: Krämer, 1988
Trachtenberg, Marvin and Isabelle Hyman, *Architecture, from Prehistory to Post-Modernism: The Western Tradition*, New York: Abrams, 1986

PLAN OF CANBERRA, AUSTRALIA

Designed by Walter Burley Griffin; completed 1911

The plan of Australia's capital city of Canberra, as designed in 1911 by the Chicago architect Walter Burley Griffin (1876–

1937), is one of the major examples of a 20th-century planned capital and the only one whose design was selected in competition. The 12 sheets of drawings, as rendered by Marion Mahony Griffin (1871–1961) and her assistants and presently housed in the National Archives of Australia, record one of the most significant chapters in the history of modern urban planning.

The need for an Australian national capital arose when the six separate British colonial states on the continent were federated in 1901 to provide a mechanism for dealing with one another and with the outside world. From the Australian perspective, this need for a new capital city was not great; the competition for its creation was announced only a decade later. The decision to locate the new Australian Capital Territory between Melbourne in Victoria and Sydney in New South Wales—the capitals of the two most populous states and notorious rivals—was more political than practical and produced the only major inland Australian city.

The competition for a capital city with an initial population of 25,000 was announced on 30 April 1911 with a closing date of 31 January 1912. By that time (or at least by early March, when the actual judging began), the Department of Home Affairs had received 137 submissions. Although these included designs from around the world, British and Australian architects had boycotted the competition because of the makeup of the adjudicating committee as well as the Australian government's position that the winning design would not necessarily be implemented.

On 23 May 1912, the committee unveiled the winning designs and, in the presence of reporters, ceremoniously cut open the envelopes, revealing the identities of the winners. Walter Burley Griffin of Chicago was awarded first prize; second prize went to Eliel Saarinen of Helsinki, Finland; and third prize was given to Alf Agache of Paris.

The selection of Griffin, a youthful 35 years of age, came as a complete surprise to nearly everyone. Raised in Chicago's western suburbs, Griffin studied architecture at the University of Illinois (1895–99); drafted for Dwight Perkins and Robert Spencer, two members of the emerging Prairie School; and between 1901 and 1906, worked for Frank Lloyd Wright as landscape designer, office manager, and site superintendent. Between 1906 and 1914, Griffin practiced independently in Chicago before resettling in Australia to supervise the construction of Canberra. His experience as federal capital director was fraught with difficulties, and he resigned in 1920. Although Canberra was officially dedicated in 1927 and has subsequently grown to a population of more than 300,000, it bears only a general resemblance to Griffin's original design.

Griffin's career encompassed the three separate disciplines of architecture, landscape architecture, and urban planning. Many of his most satisfying projects, like Canberra, combine all three. Because nothing remains of his reputed plan for enlarging Shanghai, China (ca. 1905–06), his earliest surviving urban scheme appears to be the small town of Idalia, Florida, designed around February to March 1911, only a few months before the official announcement of the Canberra competition. Griffin later recalled, however, that he had known of the impending need for an Australian capital city for many years and was eager to contribute to its success. As he explained in 1913 to King O'Malley, head of the competition committee, "I . . . entered this Australian event to be my first and last competition, solely because I have for many years greatly admired the bold radical steps in politics and economics which your country has dared to take . . . yours is the greatest opportunity the world has afforded for the expression of the great civic ideal." As James Weirick has explained, Canberra "was intended to express in its physical form, the true nature of the democratic experience" (Weirick, 1998).

The site was composed of a rolling valley surrounded by hills and bisected by the wide streambed of the intermittent Molonglo River. Griffin created a design whose basic format was determined by this landscape. The axis defined by the crown of the nearest high hill, Mount Ainslie north of the river (and just outside the city limits), to the most prominent point in town, Kurrajong to the south, became the generating line of the entire plan. Griffin termed this the Land Axis. At the point where this line crossed the Molonglo, Griffin defined a perpendicular Water Axis, to be given expression by damming the river to create a series of lakes, the central three of which would be formal and geometric and the outer two left irregular and "natural."

Griffin ordered the landscape by separating areas according to use: civic, cultural, political, economic, and residential. He divided the city into hexagonal, octagonal, and circular subcenters, connected by major boulevards that radiated from the subcenters. The scheme was subtly configured to the changing topography while remaining part of a clearly defined geometric diagram originating from Kurrajong.

Although the competition guidelines had called only for the general placement of some 38 public buildings, most entries included perspective renderings that attempted to give a corresponding architectural image to the proposed city. Although Mahony's perspectives at first glance suggest that this was also the case with Griffin's entry, in fact Griffin went beyond this, making complete designs for the group. By combining the footprints on the plans with the elevations and section that appear on the various axial drawings, it is possible to re-create the individual buildings. Griffin added another structure not listed in the competition precis: atop Kurrajong Hill, he placed a design labeled as the Capitol building, a stepped ziggurat that was to serve as a kind of national focal point, what Griffin called "the figurative embodiment of the spirit of the Commonwealth" (Griffin, 1923, quoted in Weirick, 1989).

Griffin intended his plan to provide a legible cipher of the interrelationships among the political, economic, cultural, and spiritual forces at work in a progressive, democratic nation. The very placement of the public buildings in the great triangle descending from the Capitol to the central lake revealed the relative positions of the branches of government.

The sources for Canberra are wide and varied. Griffin drew on such city plans as Christopher Wren's 1666 scheme for rebuilding London; Pierre L'Enfant's plan for Washington, DC (1790), and its reintroduction as the Senate Park Commission's plan of 1901; the City Beautiful movement, especially Daniel Burnham and Edward Bennett's Plan of Chicago (1906–09); and the English Garden City movement. There is no real precedent, however, for the hierarchies of building placement, the configurations to subtle changes in topography, and the unity of landscape to urban design found in the plan of Canberra.

PAUL KRUTY

See also **Griffin, Walter Burley, and Marion Mahony Griffin (United States)**

Further Reading

Harrison, Peter, *Walter Burley Griffin, Landscape Architect*, edited by Robert Freestone, Canberra: National Library of Australia, 1995

Johnson, Donald Leslie, *Canberra and Walter Burley Griffin: A Bibliography of 1876 to 1976 and a Guide to Published Sources*, Melbourne and New York: Oxford University Press, 1980

Reps, John W., *Canberra, 1912: Plans and Planners of the Australian Capital Competition*, Carlton South, Victoria: University of Melbourne Press, 1997

Van Zanten, David, "Walter Burley Griffin's Design for Canberra, the Capital of Australia" in *Chicago Architecture, 1872–1922: Birth of a Metropolis*, edited by John Zukowsky, Munich: Prestel-Verlag, and Chicago: The Art Institute of Chicago, 1987

Weirick, James, "Don't You Believe It: Critical Response to the *New Parliament House*," *Transition*, 27/28 (Summer/Autumn 1989)

Weirick, James, "Spirituality and Symbolism in the Work of the Griffins" in *Beyond Architecture: Marion Mahony and Walter Burley Griffin: America, Australia, India*, edited by Anne Watson, Sydney: Powerhouse Publishing, 1998

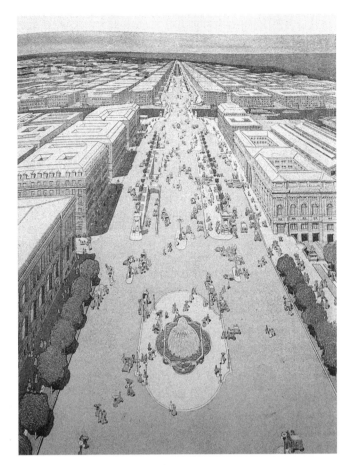

Plan of Chicago
© Dennis Gale

PLAN OF CHICAGO

The Plan of Chicago, developed mainly by architect Daniel H. Burnham (1846–1912) and his assistant Edward H. Bennett (1874–1954), was the first master plan for an American city and its region in the 20th century. Burnham developed ideas for the plan from 1894 on, though his consistent work on the project for Chicago's Commercial Club began in late 1906. The plan was published as a book in 1909 with renderings by Jules Guérin (1866–1946), when its drawings were exhibited at The Art Institute of Chicago. Although the city's form was discussed for decades after the Great Chicago Fire of 1871, the plan was largely motivated by success of the World's Columbian Exposition of 1893 in Chicago, for which Burnham had served as chief of construction and that had posited a neoclassical model for urban design that integrated public buildings and parks. The Plan of Chicago also owed much to Burnham's work as head of the MacMillan Commission, charged by the U.S. Congress with the planning of central Washington, DC, in 1901–02, and to his plans for Cleveland (1903), San Francisco (1905), and Manila (1905). The Plan of Chicago was also based on Burnham's systematic consultation with local experts and citizens, a process that helped to ensure its acceptance and partial implementation.

Burnham's earlier urban plans featured a central focal group of neoclassical public buildings linked to each other and to the surrounding city with broad, tree-lined avenues. This idea was central to the Plan of Chicago, which featured large new railroad passenger terminals and a cultural and civic center on the city's near West Side, dominated by a tall, domed city hall. Architecturally, the plan included recommendations for common cornice heights for buildings and generous street widths, aiming to create a visually unified cityscape on the model of Second Empire Paris. Burnham requested plans of pre- and post-Haussmann Paris, along with information on over 20 American and 30 European cities. As Burnham wrote: "the city has a dignity to be maintained; and good order is essential to material advancement. Consequently, the plan provides for impressive groupings of public buildings and reciprocal relations among such groups." Burnham saw his city some 70 years after its founding in 1833 as having reached a stage of development that called for permanent monumentality in civic buildings and landscapes.

The Plan of Chicago was to both enable and present an image of ordered economic growth. In this it went further than many essays in the City Beautiful Movement by proposing to consolidate Chicago's extensive and varied rail traffic network, including tracks of common width, and a shared system for handling freight. Presented in the same year that the Model T Ford was introduced, the Plan of Chicago featured a regional highway system for automobiles, including both radial arteries and circumferential ring roads within a 60-mile radius of the city's center to connect it with its suburbs and to link suburbs to each other. The future city was to be an efficient transportation network for the facilitation of commerce, with extensions of an ordered plan out into the surrounding region. As Burnham wrote: "The plan frankly takes into consideration that fact that the American city, and Chicago pre-eminently, is a center of industry and traffic. Therefore attention is given to the betterment of commercial facilities; to methods of transportation for persons and for goods; to removing the obstacles which prevent or obstruct circulation; and to the increase of convenience." Toward this end, the plan proposed routing different types of motor traffic on double-decker streets connected by ramps, with pleasure vehicles above freight trucks. Water transport was to

be improved by straightening the Chicago River and by building windbreaks stretching a mile into Lake Michigan to protect new harbor facilities.

The plan included an inland park system that vastly extended Chicago's earlier parks with connecting carriage boulevards designed by Horace Cleveland and Frederick Law Olmsted. Perhaps most important for the city's future development, the plan proposed a comprehensive treatment of 23 miles of lakefront parks for public recreation, including lagoons for rowing, and numerous playgrounds, especially for the city's poorer classes who had little access to green space inland. As Burnham wrote, "When a citizen is made to feel the beauty of nature, when he is lifted up by her to any degree above the usual life of his thoughts and feelings, the state of which he is a part is benefited thereby." The plan's aim was to promote good citizenship at a time when 1.3 of Chicago's 1.7 million residents were foreign born and when the deplorable working and living conditions of the city's poor were as described in Upton Sinclair's *The Jungle* (1906). The plan aimed to create an ideal built environment that would educate citizens' tastes and shape social norms according to bourgeois models and in the service of capitalist interests. Burnham wrote: "It is realized, also, that good workmanship requires a large degree of comfort on the part of the workers in their homes and their surroundings, and ample opportunity for that rest and recreation without which all work becomes drudgery." Although aimed at improving the quality of life for all, the plan included no provisions for publicly funded housing.

The Plan of Chicago directly influenced the subsequent development of the city from the mayor's appointment of an official planning commission in late 1909 through the financial crash of 1929. Major improvements of these 20 years based on the plan included the widening and enhancement of Michigan Avenue north of the Chicago River, the landfills and development of Grant Park on the central lakefront and lakefront parks to the north and south, and the construction of Wacker Drive along the Chicago River. The Plan of Chicago had rapid influence beyond the city, first in inspiring the German Kaiser to appoint a commission in 1912 to replan the capital of Berlin. The Plan of Chicago was also a point of reference for developing the Regional Plan of New York City and its environs of 1929.

JOSEPH M. SIRY

See also **Burnham, Daniel H. (United States); Chicago (IL), United States; City Beautiful Movement**

Further Reading

Art Institute of Chicago, *The Plan of Chicago: 1909–1979*, Chicago: The Art Institute of Chicago, 1979
Bluestone, Daniel, *Constructing Chicago*, New Haven: Yale University Press, 1991
Burnham, Daniel H. and Edward H. Bennett, *Plan of Chicago*, 1909, edited by Charles Moore, with a new introduction by Kristen Schaffer, New York: Princeton Architectural Press, 1993
Ciucci, Giorgio, Francesco Dal Co, Mario Manien-Elia, and Manfredo Tafuri, *The American City: From the Civil War to the New Deal*, Cambridge, Massachusetts: MIT Press, 1979
Draper, Joan E., "Paris by the Lake: Sources of Burnham's *Plan of Chicago*" in *Chicago Architecture 1872–1922: Birth of a Metropolis*, edited by John Zukowsky, Munich: Prestel Verlag, 1987

Field, Cynthia R., "The City Planning of Daniel Hudson Burnham" (Ph.D. dissertation), Columbia University, 1974
Hines, Thomas S., *Burnham of Chicago: Architect and Planner*, Chicago: The University of Chicago Press, 1974/1979
Mayer, Harold M. and Richard C. Wade, *Chicago: Growth of a Metropolis*, Chicago: The University of Chicago Press, 1969
McCarthy, Michael P., "Chicago Businessmen and the Burnham Plan," *Journal of the Illinois State Historical Society* (Autumn 1970)
Moore, Charles, *Daniel H. Burnham: Architect, Planner of Cities*, 2 vols., 1921, New York: DaCapo Press, 1969
Schaffer, Kristen, "Daniel H. Burnham: Urban Ideals and the *Plan of Chicago*" (Ph.D. dissertation), Cornell University, 1993
Wilson, William H., *The City Beautiful Movement*, Baltimore: Johns Hopkins University Press, 1989
Wolner, Edward W., "Daniel Burnham and the Tradition of the City Builder in Chicago: Technique, Ambition, and City Planning" (Ph.D. dissertation), New York University, 1979

PLAN OF NEW DELHI

At an imperial durbar in 1911 hosted outside the walled city of Shahjahanabad (later called Old Delhi), King George V announced plans to transfer the seat of the government of India from Calcutta to a new imperial capital to be built in the vicinity of that very spot. It was to become the "New" Delhi. The aim was to present the British Raj as the legitimate successor of the Mughal Empire precisely at a time when British rule was being challenged by Indian nationalists. Near Shahjahan's old capital, amid the ruins of a score of erstwhile capital cities and far from the tumultuous nationalist politics of Calcutta, a new imperial British capital was hoped to capture the fiction of peaceful and benevolent domination of an alien people. The historic importance of the site of Delhi was to be revived after a century of neglect to serve as a necessary counterpoint to the demonstration of British power.

By early 1912, a Delhi Town Planning Committee was organized, comprising Edwin L. Lutyens, an architect then known mostly for his design of country houses; John A. Brodie, city engineer of Liverpool; and George S.C. Swinton, chairman-elect of the London County Council. Henry V. Lanchester, who had a well-established architectural practice in London, was appointed as an external consultant. Among them, only Swinton had any previous firsthand knowledge of India. The committee's responsibility was to suggest a suitable site for the new capital and to formulate a general plan for the city. From the very beginning, two assumptions were made clear. First, the new capital would be used only as the government's winter residence, with the customary annual migration to Shimla during the summer months. Second, the centerpiece of this plan would be the Government House (later called the Viceroy's Palace, presently the Rashtrapati Bhavan), the residence of the head of the British administration, the viceroy. Designed as the center of government and not a commercial city, the imperial capital was to physically represent the administrative and power hierarchy of the British Raj, complete with its class and racial stratification.

At the initial stages, two different sites and two types of plans were proposed. One of the sites was to the north of Shahjahanabad near the British Civil Lines and Durbar Grounds; the other was to the south of the existing city between Raisina Hills and

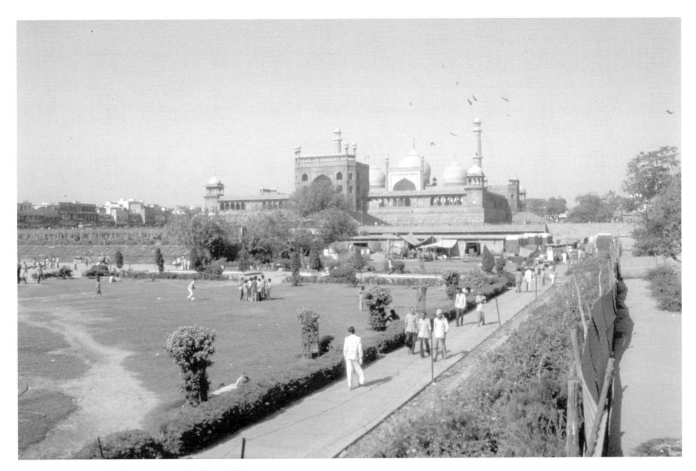

Green spaces around the Jami Masjid, New Delhi
© Aga Khan Trust for Culture

the Jamuna River. The Town Planning Committee favored the spacious southern site as more suitable for their exaggerated monumental vision of the city and the ease with which one could make visual reference to the historic monuments that were located on the southern and eastern limits. The principal feature of the committee's early plan was a ceremonial avenue with closely packed government buildings terminating at the Government House and opening up a vista to the Jami Masjid, the largest Mughal mosque in the existing city; the rest of the new capital was conceived on a rectangular matrix of roads. The monotony of the plan raised questions, and Lanchester attempted to improve on the committee's scheme by suggesting replacing the rectangular pattern with a series of radial streets. At the crossing of the ceremonial avenue and these radial arteries, he proposed a plaza around which to arrange the Secretariat buildings. When the committee was again asked to reconsider the northern site, their revised plan took some hint from Lanchester's layout. They proposed a more tightly knit ensemble of government institutions headed by the monumental place of the Government House and deviated from the rectangular pattern by making the peripheral roads adjust to the topography.

When officially "opened" in 1930, the city was planned for a maximum population of 65,000, covering an area of 3200 acres. The final plan, which underwent many subsequent adjust-ments, was based on a revised treatment of the southern site that retained several ideas from the preceding plans. The Government House, or Viceroy's Palace, was still the focal point. It was perched on Raisina Hills and connected by straight avenues to the Purana Qila on the west, to the railway station on the northwest, and to Safdarjung's tomb on the south. The scheme borrowed from the principles of Beaux-Arts planning as well as from new notions of the garden city but ultimately conformed to the hierarchical planning pattern of British cantonments in India. By the time the final plan was reached, Herbert Baker, an architect who had acquired a reputation for his work in South Africa, was brought into the team and the specific architectural treatment of the monuments were being prepared. Lutyens was awarded the design of the Viceroy's Palace and Herbert Baker the Secretariat and Council House. It was the monumental classical architectural vocabulary, which Lutyens had rehearsed long before he was given the building commission, that gave specific meaning to the plan that ultimately developed. The appliqué of Indian decorative elements on this imperial classicism at a later stage only enhanced the symbolic logic of the plan, which was meant to unambiguously subordinate the "old" city and the Indian population to the new capital and its British denizens.

A long, processional 440-feet east–west parkway, named King's Way (presently Rajpath) and a cross-avenue named

Queen's Way (presently Janpath) formed the central armature of a multinode hexagonal plan. Traveling along King's Way from the Purana Qila, the visitor encountered a series of monuments along the Central Vista—a wide expanse of green space accentuated by water channels. Anchored by the monumental canopy that once housed the statue of King George V and, on the west, the War Memorial, the parkway led to the "cultural" node, which was meant to house four colonial institutions at the four corners of the crossing of King's Way and Queen's Way—the Imperial Museum, the Oriental Institute, the Imperial Library, and the Imperial Record Office (presently the National Archives, the only building constructed before Indian independence). Then a dense arrangement of imperial symbols prepared the visitor for the principal focus of the plan—the Secretariat Blocks on raised platforms on either side framing the centrally located Viceroy's Palace, which dipped from view as one approached the Secretariat Plaza, only to emerge later in its full regalia once one reached the top of the plaza. This vanishing vista was the result of a controversial miscalculation of the street gradient. The Viceregal Estate, the entry to which was guarded by a series of Britannia lions and anchored with the Jaipur column, covered approximately two-thirds of a square mile and housed, in addition to the main palace and integral council chamber, the symmetrically arrayed staff quarters and the elaborate "Mughal" garden. The rotund Council House (included in the plan in 1919, presently the Parliament Building) played a subsidiary role in the imperial administration and was located off the main axis to the north of the Secretariat Blocks. Radial avenues from the Council House and War Memorial, as well as Queen's Way, converged on Connaught Place—the principal commercial node—before leading to the railway station. Residential space was allocated according to a strict sociospatial taxonomy based on site elevation, proximity to the Viceroy's Palace, dwelling and plot size, and most important, segregation along occupational and racial lines. The houses of the members of the Executive Council were located closest to the seat of power, whereas gazetted officers were allocated space to the south of the Central Vista near the lavish and exclusive green recreational space of racecourse and parks. Indian princes were encouraged to purchase land to the east, whereas European clerks were assigned space to the north. Indian and Anglo-Indian clerks and "menial" staff were situated on the periphery of the new city in separate enclaves. The separation between the new and the old city was physically completed with a surrounding wall (demolished in 1950) and a 100-yard-wide and mile-and-a-half-long green space around the old city.

Obsessed with the demonstration of imperial power, the planners created an infrastructure of inequity that would pose both physical and ideological problems when, at midcentury, the city became the capital of a new democracy. Defined on the basis of unequal access to resources and glaring population differentials between the old city and the new, it was neither amenable to public transportation nor anticipatory of a significant population increase and its attendant need for schools, shopping, and housing.

SWATI CHATTOPADHYAY

Further Reading

Robert Irving's book provides a detailed description of the planning process. For critiques of the imperial ideology embodied in the city plan, consult the works of Anthony King, Thomas Metcalf, and Hosagrahar Jyoti.

Evenson, Norma, *The Indian Metropolis: A View toward the West*, New Haven, Connecticut: Yale University Press, 1989

Irving, Robert Grant, *Indian Summer: Lutyens, Baker, and Imperial Delhi*, New Haven, Connecticut: Yale University Press, 1981

Jyoti, Hosagrahar, "City as Durbar: Theater and Power in Imperial Delhi" in *Forms of Dominance: On the Architecture and Urbanism of the Colonial Enterprise*, edited by Nezar AlSayyad, Aldershot, Hampshire, and Brookfield, Vermont: Avebury, 1992

King, Anthony, *Colonial Urban Development: Culture, Social Power, and Environment*, London and Boston: Routledge and Paul, 1976

Metcalf, Thomas R., *An Imperial Vision: Indian Architecture and Britain's Raj*, Berkeley: University of California Press, 1989

PLASTICS

At no time in history has a material developed so rapidly and became interwoven in the fabric of our daily lives as have plastics. In fact, today's styles of living would be unimaginable without their existence. Less than 200 years old, these materials have become part of almost every facet of our daily lives. Plastics have played a variety of roles in the building and construction industry, but especially so in the 20th century.

Although the invention of many forms of plastic has origins in the 19th century, their practical application for consumer products and other industrial uses came about in the 20th century. For example, a major milestone was achieved in the evolution of plastics when John Wesley Hyatt, an American, invented Celluloid in 1866 by adding camphor (a derivative of the laurel tree) to nitrated cellulose. This was the first thermoplastic in the sense that it could be molded under heat and pressure to form a shape and that it would retain that shape after the heat and pressure were removed. In 1891 Louis Marie Hilaire was trying to produce man-made silk in Paris when he modified nitrated cellulose to form rayon. In 1907 Leo Baekeland, a New York chemist, discovered the first completely synthetic man-made substance, which he called Bakelite. This liquid resin is considered the first thermoset plastic ever produced because once it hardened, it would never change. Later, in 1913, Dr. Jacques Edwin Brandenberger, a Swiss textile engineer, produced viscose (now known also as rayon), which led to his invention of cellophane, the first true waterproof wrapping material. After the use of cellophane spread worldwide, DuPont's laboratories, under Wallace H. Carothers, developed Fiber 66, which was later named nylon. This fiber replaced animal hair in toothbrushes and silk stockings. In fact, nylon stockings enjoyed great public acceptance when unveiled in 1939, and reinforced nylon fabrics were being used in air-supported structures. At B.F. Goodrich, Waldo Semon, an organic chemist, developed an inexpensive, fire-resistant, and easily formable substance named polyvinyl chloride (PVC), or vinyl, which became the base material for thousands of household products, from garden hoses to records. Meanwhile, in Germany, H. Staudinger discovered the molecular structure of plastics, and Carothers, in turn, realized that by adding and replacing elements into the chainlike molecules of plastics, one could produce many types of new compounds. This particular discovery gave the plastics industry its prolific nature vis-à-vis the many useful polymers introduced since then, such as nylon, acrylics, neoprene, SBR (Styrene Butadiene Rubbers),

saran, polyethylene, Velcro, Teflon, Spandex, Nomex, and Kevlar, all of which replaced, at one time or another, materials typically supplied by nature. The most widely utilized polymer, however, has been polyethylene, a thermoplastic first discovered in 1933 by Fawcett and Gibson. At present, polyethylene is the largest-volume plastic in the world, with such uses as milk jugs, soda bottles, grocery and dry-cleaning bags, food storage containers, packaging, and in the construction industry as a reliable source of water proofing.

After World War II, plastic products were everywhere. Inventors were continuously filing patents for new plastics, and the American public's view of the image of such products became increasingly negative. In reality, polymers had two main disadvantages. First, they had relatively low stiffness, and as such they were rendered nonviable where structural integrity was required. Second, they degraded rapidly when exposed to heat and ultraviolet (UV) radiation. Consequently, plastic products were thought of as cheap, nonenduring, fake, and environmentally unfriendly. The U.S. military, however, noted the desirable characteristics of polymers. As such, it was military applications in the mid-1950s and 1960s that carried the torch for the plastics industry. In aerospace applications, higher rigidity and lighter weight led to a landmark development in the evolution of plastics, and fiber-reinforced polymers were born. By combining the relative flexibility of some thermosetting plastics, such as epoxies, and the high rigidity of fibrous materials, such as graphite, aramid, and boron, new and far superior materials were created and dubbed advanced composites. The notion that embedding fibers, short or long, in a binding medium to create a new and improved plastic manifested itself in different forms and led to the creation of such materials as ceramic/metal composites and braided Kevlar. These superior plastics were used in applications ranging from armored personnel suits and gear to intercontinental ballistic missiles and the space shuttle.

Plastics and the Construction Industry

All the desirable qualities of 1950s plastics did not escape the watchful eyes of the construction industry, which has always been on the lookout for more competitive building materials to replace existing ones. Plastics appeared as vinyl siding and as foam insulation in homes and buildings, making them much more energy efficient and comfortable for their occupants. Plastics were also used in underground storage tanks and in pipe systems. There were even a few adventurous attempts by individuals and companies to construct all-plastic houses intended as showcases only and not for mass production. A primary early example was the Monsanto House of the Future (1957–68) at Disneyland in Anaheim, California. This structure was envisioned at the Massachusetts Institute of Technology and assembled for Disneyland in 1957 using structural fiberglass-reinforced polyester elements. Other attempts during the 1950s to build houses out of plastics were made, but they never quite presented the construction industry with any serious alternatives. The only notable effort to mass-produce affordable plastic housing was made by Ionel Schein when he presented his *Maison Plastique* (Plastic House) in a housing exhibition in 1956. The Bucharest-born designer used 15 different plastics and three colors—yellow, red, or blue—in all 70 prototypes he produced.

In 1974 the higher prices of raw materials, resulting from the oil embargo and more competitive concrete and steel industries, put an end to Schein's production of plastic houses.

In the late 1970s and in response to the stabilization of oil prices as well as emerging environmental concerns for conserving natural resources, most manufacturing industries made serious and successful attempts at incorporating plastics into their design and materials selection processes. Once again, plastics were gaining an excellent reputation for superior and cost-effective performance in applications where their beneficial characteristics can be best employed. The construction industry was not immune to this movement. Plastics were recyclable, and as such they reduced construction waste; their use in construction is environmentally responsible, conserves natural resources, and is consistent with the concept of sustainability; in addition, their ease of fabrication, transportation, and erection resulted in a relatively lower life-cycle cost. As a result, they started appearing in many applications, such as glass-reinforced plastic (GRP) moldings to replace cast-iron work, as cladding and roofing materials in multistory buildings, as corrugated translucent sheeting (e.g. indoor swimming pools), as replacement of metals for electrical insulation purposes (e.g. ladders, man lifts, light and telephone poles, special hospital structures, CB radio antennas, radar and military facilities, airport control towers, transmission and electrical power towers, and power plant structures), as structural and nonstructural elements in water/wastewater treatment and desalination plants, as agricultural and irrigation equipment and structures (e.g. manure filters, weirs, barn structures, and watergate guides), as cooling towers (e.g. housing units), as industrial chimneys, and as waterfront and offshore structures (e.g. oil rigs and marine risers).

Architecturally, plastics presented the designer with the advantage of controlling the texture, color, and the shape of any designed element. This inherent quality of manufacturing plastics allowed for greater design flexibility in such issues as shading, form flow, and patterns repetition, all the while maintaining lower costs and faster erection time than other conventional materials. Examples of such cases include but are not limited to cladding panels for the Olivetti Training Centre (1972) in Haslemere, Surrey, England; 50-meter-diameter roofing domes at the Sharjah International Airport (1977) in the United Arab Emirates; and the access ramps to Terminal 2 (1978) at Heathrow Airport in London. A more widespread use of FRPs (Fiber-Reinforced Plastics) in construction was hindered for three main reasons. First, there was still a prevalent lack of knowledge in the general design philosophy, behavior, and limitations of such materials, including their relative low stiffness and heat- and UV-light-resistive capabilities. Second, there existed other competitive, long-established, and more familiar construction methods and materials. Third, building and design codes dealing with the design specifications and testing methods of plastics did not exist at the time. All these reasons made it difficult for designers and builders to shift into unknown and untested building materials. As such, during the 1970s and early 1980s, the usage of FRPs remained limited to specific applications in which they were the only choice for the conditions under which a specific structure existed.

Since the mid-1980s, the world has witnessed an unprecedented reliance on and use of plastics in construction. The integration of plastics into the building industry proliferated so rap-

idly that in 1998 more than 20 percent of all plastic resin sales in North America were used for fixed construction. In fact, about two-thirds of all thermosetting polymers (mainly polyesters and vinylesters) produced today are consumed by the building and construction industry. There were six main reasons for that remarkable growth: environmental concerns increased regarding the sustainability, conservation, and recycling of used materials; the prices of raw materials for producing plastics had dropped significantly while costs of lumber soared; with much improved fire retardancy and heat and UV resistance, FRPs had proven by then, through research and actual field-performance track records, that they were solid substitutes for typical construction materials; there were significant advances in the technology of producing polymers, in improving their qualities, and in manufacturing their fiber-reinforced components; the end of the Cold War allowed for a tremendous amount of information and expertise about high-performance plastics (i.e. advanced composites) to migrate from the military and aerospace industry into the construction world; and finally, a worldwide deterioration of some infrastructures (i.e. bridges and highways) demanded the immediate attention of governments worldwide and forced them to look for alternative construction materials. As a testament to the energy-absorption capabilities and strength of fiber-reinforced plastics, the California Department of Transportation approved, after the 1994 Northridge earthquake, the use of plastics for seismic retrofitting of reinforced-concrete highway decking and column systems. In addition, the versatility of improved polymers allowed inventors to come up with such structural elements as glue-laminated timber members (glu-lams) and fiber-reinforced glu-lams. These elements allow for larger load-carrying and spanning capabilities, less natural wood to be used, and lower cost when compared with lumber members. In addition, polymers were being used to produce plastic lumber and polymer concretes, which, when reinforced with glass fibers, produced members with exceptional strength and rigidity and of lighter weight and smaller dimensions.

As confidence and knowledge about plastics in the world of construction increased, designers and contractors found themselves routinely adding them to their repertoire of available options for building materials. Plastics have been successfully used in such projects as the FRP Turret Sun Bank Building (1988) in Orlando, Florida; the Nations Bank Tower (1989) in Atlanta, Georgia; and as window/door lintels (1993) at Pennsylvania State University in University Park, Pennsylvania. Realizing the potential of plastics in construction, government agencies supported collaborative academic and industrial research efforts to further the understanding of the nature and characteristics of fiber-reinforced plastics. A landmark result of such efforts was the plastic industrial building constructed at Weston, West Virginia, in November 1995. This 12.31-meter-long, 6.45-meter-wide, 4.31-meter-high structure was the result of a joint research-and-development effort between the U.S. National Science Foundation, the West Virginia Department of Transportation, and the Constructed Facilities Center at West Virginia University headed by Professor Hota GangaRao. Perhaps the most salient structural building achievement for plastics to date is the Eyecatcher (1999). This is the first five-story residential/office building constructed completely out of fiber-reinforced plastic (glass and polyester) pultruded structural profiles. Fiberline Composites of Denmark unveiled the Eyecatcher Project during the Swissbau '99 Fair in Basel, Switzerland. After the exhibition, the ten-meter-wide, twelve-meter-long, fifteen-meter-high building was disassembled and brought to its new and permanent location at Münchensteinerstrasse 210, Basel. The Eyecatcher, which opened in 1999 as an office building, will require absolute minimal maintenance over the next 50 years and will have a life expectancy of 100 years.

The Future

Today, with more than six billion human beings living and building on this planet, environmental consciousness is at its peak, and the efforts of aggressive recycling programs and conservation of our natural resources are at an all-time high. Plastics are playing a major role in these conservational endeavors in the building industry, where plastics are competing in the main arena of conventional construction materials and in structurally demanding applications. Given their remarkably short history, the prolific nature of their industrial evolution during the 20th century, and the inherent likelihood of accidental discoveries in their field, one could only conclude that the use of plastics in general, and in the building and construction industry in particular, will experience an even larger proliferation in the new millennium. As such, the 20th century will always be remembered as the dawn of the plastics age.

ZOUHEIR A. HASHEM

Further Reading

Elias, Hans-Georg, *An Introduction to Plastics*, New York: VCH, 1993

Fenichell, Stephen, *Plastic: The Making of a Synthetic Century*, New York: HarperBusiness, 1996

Hollaway, Leonard, *Glass Reinforced Plastics in Construction*, Glasg: Surrey University Press, 1978, and New York: Wiley, 1978

Meikle, Jeffrey L., *American Plastic: A Cultural History*, New Brunswick, New Jersey: Rutgers University Press, 1995

Mosallam, Ayman and Zouheir Hashem, "Structural Applications of Pultruded Composites" in *Advanced Composites Materials*, edited by Hosny, Mosallam, Rizkalla, Mahfouz, Sharm El-Shaikh, Egypt: Egyptian Society of Engineers, 1996

Mossman, Susan, *Early Plastics: Perspectives, 1850–1950*, London and Washington, DC: Leicester University Press, 1997

Wilson, Forrest, "Plastics, Past and Future," *Architecture*, 77/4 (April 1988)

Witcher, Daniel, "Application of Fiber Reinforced Plastics in New Construction and Rehabilitation of the Infrastructure" in *Fiber Composites in Infrastructure*, edited by H. Saadatmanesh and M.R. Ehsani, Tuscon, Arizona: Dept. of Civil Engineering and Engineering Mechanics, University of Arizona, 1996

PLATE GLASS

Glass is an unusual material created from the basic components of earth-sand, soda, and lime. In buildings, glass can be the source of both intriguing delight and distress. Used as fenestration in building envelopes, it creates the well-balanced and skillful face of a building, the facade. Glass allows light to enter, warms interior spaces in the winter, and is capable of establishing a flowing relationship to the outside. Glass can contribute like

no other building material to the enjoyment of architecture; it encloses, protects from the environment, and visually connects at the same time.

The origins of glass and glassmaking can be traced back to Phoenician times, around 5000 B.C. Sailors, lacking stones on which to place their cooking pots, used as an alternative the soda carried as cargo by their ships. As the fire's heat increased, the sand and soda turned into molten glass. The public baths in ancient Pompeii were among the first usages of plate glass; records indicate that a single sheet of glass measuring 3 by 4 feet (800 by 1100 millimeters) was used as a window, an extraordinary achievement at the time.

Between the 10th and 15th centuries, the small island of Murano near Venice was the unchallenged center of glassmaking, although the technology quickly spread via France to Germany, Belgium, and England. Other techniques to produce high-quality building glass included the blowing of glass cylinders that were then split, reheated, allowed to flatten, and then rolled on a flat surface.

In the early 18th century, larger and relatively inexpensive pieces of glass increasingly entered the building trade in Europe. It cannot be denied that the quality of the product had much improved from the humble beginnings of Venetian glass manufacturing, yet one area remained where the glass quality was insufficient: the making of mirrors. Mirrors, more than regular glass panes, required a much higher surface quality, free of distortion. The goal to create a high-quality glass material to be used in mirrors led to the invention of plate glass. The casting of mirrors was developed in France by Abraham Thevart around 1688 and led to the founding of the St. Gobain glassworks, which was at the time the major glass-producing center in the world.

Because of milestone inventions of the industrial age at the end of the 19th century, such as steam machines and electricity, plate glass and thus mirrors became commonplace. Waterpower, steam engines, and electrical machines made the polishing and grinding of the glass plate material easier and faster: plate glass became affordable. At the end of the 19th century, storefronts and the facades of commercial buildings in the metropolitan centers of the Western world used vast quantities of plate glass.

Because plate glass has a rough surface, as opposed to sheet glass (the Libbey Owens Glass Company developed continuous sheet glass production in the United States in 1905 in Charleston, West Virginia), which is transparent as it is formed, it needs to be manually ground flat and then polished with coarse, sand-based abrasives. Through manual grinding and polishing, one surface was first treated, followed by the reverse side. The result of this time-consuming process was a glass with almost perfect optical quality, nearly free of distortion (depending on the quality of the mixture of base materials), and of an unprecedented size.

After being monopolized in France, Belgium, and Germany, in 1895 the Pittsburgh Plate Glass Company (PPG) became the first successful manufacturer of plate glass in the United States. The company was founded in 1883, with the first glass production plant in Creighton, Pennsylvania, near Pittsburgh. The company produced plate glass in varying thickness, generally between one-quarter and one-and-one-quarter inches. The be-

ginning of the 20th century brought further development in the area of glass production, mainly because of improved polishing and grinding techniques. In 1925 the company of Pilkington Brothers in Doncaster, England, developed the technology of continuous grinding and polishing. By 1937 the plate of glass was horizontally moved through a double roller and then ground and polished in the same line of production—with both sides handled simultaneously (twin grinding).

Large panes of polished plate glass allowed the initial floors of commercial buildings to be opened up to the eager and curious eyes of "window shoppers," a term that described a significant change in the behavior of consumers to view and select merchandise without crossing the threshold of the respective enterprise. The first four floors of the 14-story Reliance building were designed in this manner in 1890 by Charles B. Atwood of Daniel Burnham's office and the structural engineer E.C. Shankland: all perimeter bay windows were filled with plate glass.

Between 1930 and 1940, glass products moved forward in importance as new uses of glass were suggested. The all-glass door appeared and was soon widely favored. The glass door, without structural elements obstructing the view to the inside of stores, reduces the visual barrier that formerly prevented potential customers from entering. Advertisements by the glass in-

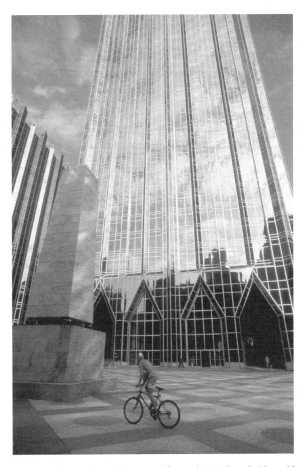

Plaza and PPG Place Skyscraper (formerly Pittsburgh Plate Glass Company, PPG Industries, Inc.), Philip Johnson and John Burgee (1979–84)
© Richard Bickel/CORBIS

dustry in architectural magazines of the time noted, "Today store fronts of large plate glass try to make sure that passers-by won't pass them by!" (Pittsburgh Plate Glass advertisement in *Progressive Architecture*, 1946). Large display windows made of structural plate glass successfully competed with other, more traditional materials. Designs for large stores by the architect Morris Lapidus in the 1950s turned storefronts into eye-catching, gigantic, and glittering display cases made of plate glass.

Not only in the area of storefront design did plate glass try to establish new records. In 1950 the UN Board of Design Consultants, under the directorship of Wallace K. Harrison and the contracting firm of Fuller-Turner-Walsh-Slattery Inc., designed and built on the island of Manhattan in New York "the world's largest window," a window wall made of heat-absorbing plate glass with dimensions of 280 by 500 feet. The UN Headquarters also boasts 5400 individual plate-glass windows and large numbers of opaque spandrel glass elements.

In 1961 Libbey-Owens-Ford developed new testing methods for large plate-glass elements with a thickness of a quarter inch. Tests indicated that thickness rather than the ratio of width to length is the important factor governing the strength of plate glass for larger panes.

Plate glass also became more and more favored in residential design in the 1950s and 1960s. The Case Study Houses, commissioned by John Entenza and published in his influential magazine *Arts and Architecture*, formed the cutting edge of design in America and abroad in the postwar period. In these designs for progressive residences by Richard Neutra, Pierre Koenig, Rudolph R.M. Schindler, and others, plate-glass walls extend from floor to ceiling, creating a tall interior space, with the transparent walls allowing a spatial flow between the interior and exterior. The crisp, pure geometry of these house designs, using large panes of polished plate glass and the interweaving of interior and exterior spaces, became hallmarks of the International Style in residential architecture. The horizontal roof planes of these Californian residences, which were largely copied in other parts of the world, seem to float without gravity on large surfaces of vertical plate glass.

Plate glass was also used in school designs of the time to add a feeling of spaciousness; designers also selected plate glass because of its ease of maintenance. With glass being widely used, it was more than natural that issues of solar heat gain, glare, and safety of the material became more necessary to consider than any other building material issue. Tinting of plate glass to reduce the large heat gain of uninterrupted glass walls was developed in the early 1950s; the trade names Solargrey, Solarbronze, and Solex, for example, described the color in which the surface of plate glass was treated to reduce thermal conductivity. Safety issues were addressed by the development of tempered plate glass, mainly used for doors. An excellent late example of the use of green-tinted plate glass is the Lever House in New York by architect Gordon Bunshaft of Skidmore, Owings and Merrill.

In the United States and most other industrialized nations, plate glass is no longer produced. It was superceded by float glass, the most recent advancement in glass manufacturing.

RALPH E. HAMMANN

See also **Bunshaft, Gordon (United States); Burnham, Daniel H. (United States); Glass; Harrison, Wallace K., and Max** **Abramovitz (United States); Lever House, New York; Neutra, Richard (Austria); Schindler, Rudolph M. (Austria and United States); Skidmore, Owings and Merrill (United States); Skyscraper**

Further Reading

Hamon and Perrin provide a historical overview and a socioeconomic analysis of the living and working conditions in the village of Saint Gobain, France, the center of 18th-century European glass manufacturing. Godfrey traces the background of medieval glassmaking, the political and legal battles related to the manufacturing process, the glass manufacturing monopoly, and production and technological aspects of glassmaking in England. Dreppaerd includes a glossary of terms as well as the history of the glass industry, drinking glasses, bottles, and other vessels. Palmer catalogs table glasses for beverages, glass for serving food, accessories, lamps, bottles, and flasks and includes illustrations of the manufacturing process of early building glass. Allen offers a reference source for construction methods and contains a detailed section about glass and glazing. A detailed illustrated guide to the use of glass and glazing in building construction is provided by Amstock.

Allen, Edward, *Fundamentals of Building Construction: Materials and Methods*, New York and Chichester: Wiley, 1985; 3rd edition, New York: Wiley, 1999

Amstock, Joseph S., *Handbook of Glass in Construction*, New York: McGraw Hill, 1997

Drepperd, Carl W., *ABC's of Old Glass*, Garden City, New York: Doubleday, 1949

Godfrey, Eleanor S., *The Development of English Glassmaking, 1560–1640*, Chapel Hill: University of North Carolina Press, 1975

Hamon, Maurice and Dominique Perrin, *Au coeur du XVIIIᵉ siècle industriel: Condition ouvrière et tradition villageoise à Saint-Gobain*, Paris: Éditions P.A.U., 1993

Palmer, Arlene, *Glass in Early America: Selections from the Henry Francis du Pont Winterthur Museum*, Winterthur, Delaware: Henry Francis du Pont Winterthur Museum, and London: Norton, 1993

PLATT, CHARLES ADAMS 1861–1933

Architect, United States

Charles Adams Platt was one of the leading American domestic architects and landscape architects of the early 20th century. He was born in 1861 in New York City, where he eventually established his practice as an architect and landscape designer. His father was a corporate lawyer and his mother a member of the Cheney family, important silk-mill owners from Manchester, Connecticut. He began his artistic education during summer vacations in Manchester, where two uncles were artists. While still in his teens, he became an early member of the Etching Revival, learning to etch from the Philadelphia artist Stephen Parrish. Platt trained briefly in painting at the National Academy of Design and the Art Students League before going to Paris in 1882 for further study at the Académie Julian. While in Paris, he met architecture students at the École des Beaux-Arts and discussed with them his emerging interest in this art. In 1886 he married a New Yorker, Annie C. Hoe, while in Europe; she died the following year, losing twin daughters in childbirth. While slowly recovering from this tragedy, Platt continued to paint and spent the summer of 1890 with artist friends in Cor-

nish, New Hampshire. He would continue to summer in the Cornish art colony, where the quality of the landscape and the collegiality of sympathetic friends remained an important force throughout his life.

In 1892 Platt invited his brother William, then an apprentice in the landscape architect office of Frederick Law Olmsted, to accompany him on a tour of the gardens of Italy. Charles Platt used the sketches and photographs they made of approximately 25 gardens from throughout the Italian peninsula to illustrate two articles for *Harper's* magazine in 1893. He expanded these articles into a book, *Italian Gardens*, published in 1894. This modest volume was one of the first illustrated publications in English depicting the gardens of Renaissance Italy, and it heavily influenced the emergence of a formal garden style in America.

Platt turned from this book to a career as a designer of gardens and then as an architect, both without any academic training or apprenticeship. He had begun to experiment with architecture in his own summerhouse and garden at Cornish in 1890. He expanded and refined the gardens for his house, following the lessons learned from his travels in Italy. In the summer of 1893, he married Eleanor Hardy Bunker, the widow of his Paris friend and fellow painter Dennis Miller Bunker.

Throughout the 1890s, Platt's Cornish neighbors commissioned him to design informal residences and geometric gardens, all influenced by what he had seen in Italy. Among these early clients was the architectural critic Herbert Croly, who became an important promoter of Platt's architectural and landscape architectural talents in his articles for *The Architectural Record*. By the late 1890s, he was executing significant commissions as a garden designer for patrons beyond Cornish. Most important among these early designs were his plans for Faulkner Farm, the Charles F. Sprague estate (1897–98), and for Weld, the Larz Anderson estate (1901), both in Brookline, Massachusetts. These projects illustrate Platt's adaptation of the Renaissance villa garden to American conditions. By the turn of the century, he had established himself as an architect, producing mainly designs for country houses and gardens. He relied in these early days on the advice of a wide circle of artistic friends in New York City and in Cornish, including the architect Stanford White. Platt's associates at the Century Association, the private club for professionals and amateurs in literature and the arts, proved invaluable as advisers and clients. Having no formal training in horticulture or engineering, he often worked in collaboration with other landscape architects, including the Olmsted Brothers, Warren Manning (1860–1938), and Ellen Biddle Shipman (1869–1950), his Cornish neighbor and most frequent collaborator. He developed a small office in New York from which he executed commissions throughout the country, relying on the professional expertise of younger men and carefully controlling the design solutions of the firm. By 1904, when Herbert Croly published a review article on Platt's work for *The Architectural Record*, he had established a recognized style in planning and design of domestic architecture. Commissions for "Platt houses" and their landscapes annually grew in number and scale.

Among the most influential of Platt's designs for country houses and gardens were those for Maxwell Court, the Francis T. Maxwell House (1903) in Rockville, Connecticut; Gwinn

(1908), the William G. Mather place near Cleveland, Ohio; the Manor House (1911), the John T. Pratt estate in Glen Cove, New York; and Villa Turicum (1918), the immense country estate of Harold and Edith Rockefeller McCormick in Wake Forest, Illinois. Platt's work was frequently illustrated and discussed in architectural and landscape magazines, including *The Architectural Record* and *Country Life in America*. In 1913 he became the subject of the first commercially produced monograph on a living American architect or landscape architect. In addition to his work on country houses, he designed a series of elegant tall office buildings and apartment houses in New York City throughout his career. Institutional designs monopolized much of his time in the 1910s and 1920s. He became recognized as a leading architect for art museums, which included the Freer Gallery of Art (1923) on the Mall in Washington, DC, and an unrealized proposal for a National Gallery of Art (1924). He also gained national recognition as an architect and planner for schools and colleges, especially the master plans he prepared for Phillips Academy in Andover, Massachusetts, between 1922 and 1930 and the plans for the University of Illinois, Urbana, that he prepared between 1921 and 1933. He designed numerous buildings for both campuses and other schools and universities throughout the country.

Platt was a careful student of history and applied the lessons he learned to the needs of contemporary buildings, pleasure gardens, and public spaces. In all his work, Platt emphasized careful planning, evident in the meticulous axial relationships of rooms or the integration of exterior and interior space through the use of architectonic garden components and strong vistas. Although he almost never wrote about his own work, his designs were frequently published and exerted a strong influence on his generation.

KEITH N. MORGAN

Biography

Born in New York, 16 October 1861. Attended the National Academy of Design, New York and the Art Students League, New York 1878–82; studied painting independently 1882–83 and under Jules Lefèvre at the Académie Julian, Paris 1883–87; Julian toured Italy 1892. Married Annie C. Hoe, 1886; she died 1887. Married Eleanor Hardy Bunker (widow of painter Dennis Miller Bunker) 1893: 4 children. Designed and built a studio in Cornish, New Hampshire 1890. In private practice, New York from 1898. Died in Cornish, 12 September 1933.

Selected Works

Platt House and Studio, Cornish, New Hampshire, 1890
Gardens, Faulkner Farm, Charles F. Sprague estate, Brookline, Massachusetts, 1898
Gardens, Larz Anderson estate, Brookline, 1901
Gardens, Francis T. Maxwell House, Rockville, Connecticut, 1903
Herbert Croly House and Garden, Cornish, 1904
Studio Building, New York City, 1906
William G. Mather House and Garden, Cleveland, Ohio, 1909
John T. Pratt House and Garden, Glen Cove, New York, 1913
Villa Turicum, estate of Harold and Edith Rockefeller McCormick, Wake Forest, Illinois, 1918

Freer Gallery, Washington, DC, 1923
Campus Design, Phillips Academy, Andover, Massachusetts, 1930
Campus Design, University of Illinois, Urbana, 1933

Selected Publications

Italian Gardens, 1894
Monograph of the Work of Charles A. Platt, 1913

Further Reading

For a catalogue raisonné of Platt's work, see Morgan (1985); Morgan (1995) contains a bibliography of writings by and about Charles A. Platt.

Croly, Herbert, "The Architectural Work of Charles A. Platt," *Architectural Record*, 15 (March 1904)
Hewitt, Mark Alan, *The Architect and the American Country House*, New Haven, Connecticut: Yale University Press, 1990
Morgan, Keith N., *Charles A. Platt: The Artist as Architect*, New York: Architectural History Foundation, and Cambridge, Massachusetts: MIT Press, 1985
Morgan, Keith N. (editor), *Shaping an American Landscape: The Art and Architecture of Charles A. Platt*, Hanover, New Hampshire: University Press of New England, 1995

PLAZA

The term *plaza* is a Spanish word for an open space in the city. It is cognate with the French and English *place*, which are ultimately derived from the Greek word *plateia*, meaning "broad street." The Italian-word equivalent is *piazza*. The contemporary American term is *square*, although the terms *park* and *green* are also utilized. In all cases, the terms mean an urban space (which might be paved or landscaped) surrounded by streets and defined by buildings on one or more sides. They vary highly in both size and geometric configuration. A plaza is inextricably related to the architectural frame that defines it, as it is the functions in these buildings and their density that directly influence its use and design.

Plazas are the public open spaces in a city whose primary purpose is to provide a gathering place for the people to foster the creation of community. They are sometimes called urban living rooms, places of formal and informal socialization. They are also places of spatial focus providing orientation, repose, and historical continuity.

Plazas can also accommodate specific activities, such as markets, performances, celebrations, protests, and recreation. The traditional use of public spaces for political activity waned in the 20th century in democratic countries but remains alive in socialist countries, as evidenced by the recent incidents at Wenceslas Square in Prague and Tiananmen Square in Beijing. The use for markets also waned during this century in the industrialized cities of the world. The other uses remain current.

Virtually all Western historical cities, planned and unplanned, were formed around one or more urban plazas. The vast majority of these cities throughout the world were founded before the 20th century. Thus, the primary design activity of this century has been preservation with only modest changes. Many cities have renovated their primary plazas. This is most evident in Savannah, Georgia, with its integrated pattern of historical squares.

In cities where there has been dramatic change in density and transportation, the plazas have changed in design. This occurred in the 20th century primarily in the United States, Canada, and Australia. The most common response has been to build a parking garage beneath the plaza and concomitantly redesign it. This occurred first at Union Square in San Francisco in 1942.

Existing plazas in some cities needed to be redesigned in the 20th century to correct design deficiencies. Bryant Park behind the New York Public Library at Fifth Avenue and 42nd Street had become the turf of drug dealers because of its physical and visual separation from the surrounding streets. Landscape architects Hanna/Olin produced a highly acclaimed scheme that took out the perimeter hedge and widened the entry points. They also provided abundant seating and luxuriant plantings.

In other cities, the plaza had to be redesigned because of a changed context. This is the case with Boston's Copley Square, which has been the subject of periodic design competitions since 1893. The 1966 design treated the square as a terraced Italian piazza, windswept and inhospitable and lacking pedestrian amenities. The battle to preserve its scale was essentially lost with the construction of the 60-story John Hancock Building on a corner of the square. It overwhelms the two masterpieces of historical architecture on the square: Trinity Church and the Boston Public Library. Another design competition in 1984 resulted in a scheme based on a village green. Now, increased pedestrian traffic from surrounding development threatens the survival of the soft landscape in this small but precious public place.

In Barcelona, Spain, more than 150 open spaces have been rebuilt in an effort to revitalize the city after the neglect during the Spanish civil war. These range from neighborhood parks to urban plazas, many featuring large sculptural works. All are designed as multiuse gathering spaces. Their designs are a dialectic between formal and informal geometries taking advantage of circumstantial opportunities. The Mediterranean tradition of paved places has been continued with judicious use of trees and planting. For the 1992 Olympics, the port was reconstructed as an urban plaza defined by shops and restaurants featuring twin high-rise towers.

In Italy there is a great urban tradition of the piazza as the social and spatial focus of a town. Some of these have been artistically redesigned to foster new vitality. Redesigned piazzas in Cormans, Vilanova, Pirano, and Santa Severina are abstract minimalist compositions of paving geometry and urban elements that create new perceptions of these places as they relate to the historic buildings that define them.

Some cities have had to create plazas where none existed. This occurred in Portland, Oregon, because of the need for a true central civic place. A design competition in 1980 resulted in a highly contextual scheme created by a design team led by architect Willard Martin. The resulting Pioneer Square is almost completely paved in brick, an unusual condition in the United States, which favors green, open spaces. To ensure the successful use of this square, a private association programs 300 events throughout the year, including dinners, dances, concerts, exhibits, and fairs. This draws 2.5 million people annually to a city whose population is only 500,000.

New squares in Boston and Toronto were created in conjunction with new city halls. The Boston City Hall Plaza (1962–

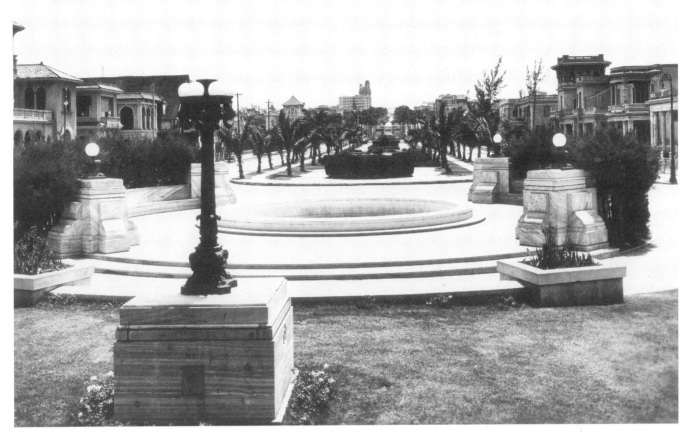

Avenue de los Presidentes, El Vedado, Havana, Cuba
© Library of Congress, courtesy Archive of Hispanic Culture Collection

68) is a large, tiered, brick-paved space reminiscent of the Campo in Siena, Italy. Nathan Phillips Square in Toronto is formed around a large pool and fountain that becomes an ice-skating rink in winter.

Most new plazas designed and built in the 20th century in the United States, Canada, and Australia have been in conjunction with real estate developments. The modern era of the developer plaza begins with the design and construction of Rockefeller Center (1931–39) on three blocks in Manhattan. John D. Rockefeller, Jr., wanted to create an appealing complex of buildings around an urban space to make his development succeed during the 1930s Depression era. The team of architects created a design that brought pedestrians through a garden from Fifth Avenue to a sunken plaza in the middle of the complex. The sunken urban space connected the street-level shops to an extensive underground concourse system, creating pedestrian links between all the buildings. The plaza reflects the change of seasons, being an ice-skating rink in winter and an outdoor cafe with a fountain in summer. What started as a real estate venture has developed into one of the best social spaces in New York City.

Corporations have often built plazas in conjunction with new urban headquarters. One of the first of this type was the Seagram Building (1958) on Park Avenue in Manhattan designed by Ludwig Mies van der Rohe. This flat, elevated, granite-paved plaza was intended to showcase the modern office tower that was set back from the street. The only features are two shallow pools of water, surrounded by ledges that separate the plaza from the side streets. Inadvertently, this plaza has become one of high pedestrian use because of its direct physical and visual connection to Park Avenue.

There are now dozens of corporate plazas in Manhattan alone, including Union Carbide, Chase Manhattan Bank, and Marine Midland Bank. Perhaps the bleakest is at the World Trade Center: five acres of paving with an overscaled fountain to match the overscaled 110-story buildings. Chicago has the Sears Tower, San Francisco the Bank of America, and Los Angeles the Wells Fargo Bank, each with its own plaza. Every large American city has its share of corporate plazas. Usually, these are windswept expanses of paving with token landscaping and few if any pedestrian amenities. Many have been created through zoning bonuses that allow taller and/or bigger buildings if plazas are provided. The research of William H. Whyte has been instrumental in making these plazas more pedestrian friendly.

There is an extensive legacy of urban open spaces in the cities of the world. In some countries, these are still utilized for traditional purposes. In other countries, they are languishing in use because of changing cultural norms and dispersal of the population. The suburban shopping mall has become the most

ubiquitous substitute for the urban plaza. The primary question for the 21st century will be whether historic urban places can be preserved, redesigned, and utilized.

MICHAEL J. BEDNAR

Further Reading

Kostof, Spiro, *The City Assembled: The Elements of Urban Form throughout History*, Boston: Little Brown, and London: Thames and Hudson, 1992

Moughtin, Cliff, *Urban Design: Street and Square*, Oxford and Boston: Butterworth Architecture, 1992; 2nd edition, Boston: Architectural Press, 1999

Webb, Michael, *The City Square*, London: Thames and Hudson, 1990; as *The City Square: A Historical Evolution*, New York: Whitney Library of Design, 1990

Whyte, William H., *The Social Life of Small Urban Spaces*, Washington, DC: Conservation Foundation, 1980

Zucker, Paul, *Town and Square: From the Agora to the Village Green*, Cambridge, Massachusetts: MIT Press, 1959

PLEČNIK, JOŽE 1872–1957

Architect, Yugoslavia

An old modest house, located at No. 4 Karunova Street in the Trnovo district to the northeast of Ljubljana's core, has remained as Jože Plečnik's modest legacy; he was undoubtedly one of the most significant 20th-century Slovenian architects and a prominent pioneer of modern architecture in Central Europe.

Plečnik's house is characterized by frugality and an elegant, albeit monastic, ambience. The search for an identity for Slovenian architecture; the fascination with folk traditions; craftsmanship; the interest in the classical world, particularly the Renaissance and Mannerist periods; and a devotion to the sacred are among the themes that characterize Plečnik's oeuvre.

His architectural career unfolds from the last quarter of the 19th century to the mid-20th century. Vienna, Prague, and Ljubljana became the geographic areas of the architect's activities, each one coloring a phase of his production. In 1891 Plečnik's father passed away, a circumstance that contributed to Plečnik's decision to move to Vienna as opposed to returning to Ljubljana to take over his father's woodworking workshop.

The following year, with assistance from the architect Leopold Theyer, who procured him employment with the firm K.K. Hof-Bau und Kunsttischelerei J.W. Müller, Plečnik finally moved to Vienna. His arrival in the capital of the Austro-Hungarian Empire was timely as it coincided with the transformation of the imperial city into one of the centers of world architecture. The architectural and urban efforts of Otto Wagner and several of his followers were decisive contributions to the transformation of this city's infrastructure and physiognomy. In 1894 Plečnik met Wagner, who accepted him as a student at the Academy of Fine Arts. This was a definitive period in the formation of the future architect, who became a devoted adherent of Wagner's ideals. Wagner gave primacy to technique over form and to innovation over tradition and emphasized a positive Rationalist position, thus anticipating many of the critical themes developed later as part of the Modern movement.

In 1898 Plečnik graduated third in his class after Josef Hoffman and Jan Kotera. His efforts earned him a bursary that al-

lowed him, from 1898 to 1899, to travel to Italy with short incursions into France and Spain. Although the death of his mother prompted the young architect to put an abrupt end to this Grand Tour, the rich extant correspondence and drawings from the period show Plečnik as a very sensitive and keen observer of architecture and art.

Plečnik's Viennese period, marked by an initial devotion to Wagner's rational aesthetic, also reflects the architect's involvement with the Vienna Secession movement, founded in 1897 by architects Joseph Hoffman and Joseph Maria Olbrich and painter Gustav Klimt. Plečnik worked on projects for the Secession, which included designs for contemporary furniture and household furnishings. His first important commission, the Zacherl House (1903–05) in central Vienna, dates from this epoch. Undoubtedly the architect's early masterpiece, the Zacherl House is innovative in the use of concrete technology for the structural support.

Plečnik's interest in sacred art, a theme that would pervasively appear throughout the architect's career, also emerged during the early years of the 20th century. His Church of the Holy Spirit in Ottakring (1910–13), the first reinforced-concrete church in Vienna, is an excellent example of the expressive use of materials.

The second period of Plečnik's professional career began in Prague in 1911. With the help of his friend Jan Kotera, he was appointed to a teaching position at the Prague School of Applied Arts. Plečnik's stay in the Czech city, which included many visits to Vienna until the outbreak of World War I, permitted him to distance himself from the strong German nationalism then emerging in Vienna and to concentrate on the study of Slavic art, a theme that would shape his later work.

The search for Wagner's replacement as a director of the Academy of Fine Arts in Vienna during the early 1910s gave Plečnik the hope for a return to the city that he considered his home. Although Plečnik was the faculty's choice for the post, the students protested the appointment, and after two years the position was given to Léopold Bauer instead. Disillusioned by this turn of events, Plečnik discarded any plans to return to Vienna.

The second decade of the century saw Plečnik actively involved in teaching in Prague. This phase was distinguished by a lack of built production that was nonetheless counteracted by a return to a preoccupation with craft—particularly metalworking—through his teaching activities. During this period, the architect often traveled to Slovenia, beginning a process of reacquaintance with his family and native land that greatly contributed to his desire to return to Ljubljana.

In the early 1920s, Plečnik concluded his academic activities at the Prague School of Applied Arts and returned to Slovenia, where he began teaching activities at the Polytechnic School of Ljubljana. However, before his departure for Slovenia, he received the offer from the newly elected president of the Czech republic, Tomás Masaryk, to become the architect of the Prague Castle. This important commission, through which Masaryk intended to transform Prague's highly visible historical royal compound into the architectural symbol of the new democracy, became Plečnik's obsession throughout a great part of this period. He returned to Prague each year until 1935—the year Masaryk abdicated—to supervise the work. Other significant buildings from this period include his restoration of the Presi-

dent's summer residence in Lány (1921–23) and the Sacred Heart Church in Prague (1928–32).

Ljubljana marks the last, and undoubtedly most productive, period in the architect's career. After the return to his homeland, Plečnik devoted himself to an architectural and cultural campaign that produced significant buildings raging from sacred architecture to institutional projects and urban interventions, transforming the architectural fabric of that city. The buildings from this phase clearly express the architect's search for a national Slovenian language, idiosyncratic nonetheless, but craftily executed and based on Mediterranean rather than Nordic precedence. This period includes the Church of Saint Francis of Assisi, Siska (1925–31); Saint Michael's Church, Barje (1937–38); and the renovation of the Chamber of Commerce, Craft, and Industry (1925–27), the Headquarters of the Vzanjemna Insurance Company (1928–30), the National University Library (1936–41), and the Central Funerary complex at the Zale Cemetery (1938) in Ljubljana. The Ljubljana oeuvre epitomizes the syncretic amalgam of themes and motives, influenced by classic, neoclassic, and vernacular imagery that persistently nourished the production of Plečnik—without doubt one of the significant, yet overlooked, figures of modern architecture.

RICARDO CASTRO

Biography

Born in Lujbljana, 23 January 1872, third of four children, son of a woodworker; studied woodworking, Technical School in Graz 1888–92; while there met architect Leopold Theyer, his first mentor. Met Otto Wagner (1894), with whom he studied at the Academy of Fine Arts, Vienna 1895–98; graduated in 1898. Traveled on scholarship to Italy, France, and Spain 1898–99. Returned to Vienna and began to work in Wagner's studio 1899–1900. Moved to Prague in 1911; appointed to faculty of Prague School of Applied Arts; taught at the trade school in Prague 1911–20; designed alterations at Prague Castle. Settled in Ljubljana (1920), where he taught at Ljubljana University until his death in Trnovo, Ljubljana, 7 October 1957.

Selected Works

Villa Weidmann, Vienna, 1901
Loos Residence, Vienna, 1901
Zacherl House, Vienna, 1905
Church of the Holy Spirit, Ottakring, Vienna, 1913
National Gallery of Art, Ljubljana, 1913
Headquarters for Vzanjemna Insurance Company, Ljubljana, 1930
Church of Saint Francis of Assisi, Siska, Ljubljana, 1931
Sacred Heart Church, Prague, 1932
Central Funerary complex, Zale Cemetery, Ljubljana, 1938
St. Michael's Church, Barje, Ljubljana, 1938
National University Library, Ljubljana, 1941

Further Reading

Burkhardt, Francois, Claude Eveno, and Boris Podrecca (editors), *Arhitekt Jože Plečnik, 1872–1957: Razstava v Ljubljani 1986*, Ljubljana, Slovenia: Enotnost, 1986; as *Joze Plecnik, Architect, 1872–1957*, translated by Carol Volk, Cambridge, Massachusetts: MIT Press, 1989

Lukeš, Zdenek, Damjan Prelovšek, and Tomáš Valena, *Josip Plečnik: Architekt Prazského hradu*, Prague: Správa Prazského hradu, 1996; as *Josip Plecnik: An Architect of Prague Castle*, Prague: Prague Castle Administration, 1997

Polano, Sergio, *Lubiana: L'opera di Joze Plecnik*, Milan: Clup, 1988

POELZIG, HANS 1869–1936

Architect, Germany

Hans Poelzig was an important exponent of German Expressionism. Together with Walter Gropius, Adolf Meyer, and Peter Behrens, he was one of the most important German architects before 1914.

From 1889 to 1894, Poelzig studied architecture with the renowned Gothic Revivalist Karl Schäfer at the Technical University (Technische Hochschule) in Berlin-Charlottenburg. From 1899 to 1916, he taught at the Academy of Fine and Applied Arts (Akademie für Kunst und Kunstgewerbe) in Breslau (now Wroclaw), first as professor of style (Fach Stilkunde) and after 1903 as director of the academy. From 1916 to 1920 he also served as city architect (Stadtbaurat) in Dresden and visiting lecturer at the Dresden Technical University. In 1920, he moved to Berlin, where he had a master workshop at the Prussian Academy of Arts. In 1923 he was appointed professor at the Berlin Technical University. In 1933 he succeeded Bruno Paul as director of the U.S. School for Free and Applied Arts in Berlin, only to be stripped of all his academic offices shortly thereafter by the National Socialists. In 1936 he accepted a professorship in Ankara, Turkey; however, he died before being able to begin work in this émigré position. Poelzig was a member of the "Novembergruppe" and the Workers' and Soldiers' Council for Art, the presiding officer of the German Werkbund (1919–21), and a member of the governing council of the League of German Architects (Bund Deutscher Architekten, 1926–33).

Poelzig was passionate about the arts generally, and he also created large-format paintings. His contemporaries considered him to be an unpredictable, temperamental creative force. In addition to being an innovative architect, Poelzig was an influential teacher whose concepts and ideas reached a large audience. Especially during his tenure in Breslau, he promoted a program of cooperative effort between handicrafts and art, and thus—years before the Bauhaus program was formulated—he represented a similar, pathbreaking position.

Unlike many of his contemporaries, Poelzig was less rooted in Jugendstil and more inspired by new concepts of living and house design, such as those formulated by Alfred Lichtwark and Hermann Muthesius. He was also significantly influenced by rationalist ideas about style based on an honest use of building materials. Fundamental traits such as these are apparent even in early works, such as his own house near Breslau/Wroclaw (1906), the Zwirners house in Löwenberg/Lwówek Slaski (1909–10), and the house for the Breslau Art and Crafts Exhibition (1904). Ever more pronounced, Poelzig had a strong interest in deriving plastic architectonic forms from the chosen building materials, a practice that he had given theoretical form in his 1899 study *Materialstillehre* (Lessons in Materialist Style). Alongside his designs for country houses, his industrial designs bear this trademark. The first such work of importance was the water tower (*Oberschlesienturm*) in Posen/Poznan (1911, partially destroyed) with its crystalline features, which was built as an exhibition pavilion in conjunction with a mining exhibit.

The exterior featured an exposed iron skeleton open to the elements into which he placed brick niches that were clearly meant only to fill in the gaps in the exposed frame.

Poelzig also used building materials symbolically. Rather than rely on ornament borrowed from historicist or Jugendstil models, he allowed the special character of the building materials to determine the decorative shape of a building's interior and exterior. In this way, he composed visual confrontations based on the innate qualities of the materials. In his design for the Werdermühle in Breslau (1906–08), facade portions in glass contrast with massive brick walls. Similarly, in an office building (1912) on Breslau's Junkernstrasse, he juxtaposed steel-framed concrete construction reminiscent of half timbering with horizontal bands of windows running unbroken around the rounded corners of the building. In this way, even before World War I, he created a design motif that was frequently used by the rationalistic architecture of the 1920s and 1930s and that for him was suggested by the plastic potential of glass, steel, and brick.

Poelzig successfully combined diverse elements into harmonious architectural designs. In many projects, he wanted to decrease the monotony of large industrial complexes and administrative buildings. Into such designs, he incorporated a variety of architectural forms to artistically balance large-scale architectural masses and expressive construction. A good example of his use of these principles is found in the avant-garde, pseudo-objectivist buildings for a chemical factory (1911–12) in Luban. There, Cubist forms blended into each other. Round-arched windows set flush with the masonry contrast sharply with rectangular windows. To show off the design's engineering, rectangular windows were specifically chosen for the parts where load-bearing steel beams visible in the facade made such windows possible. Occasionally, he punctuated such rationalist, material-derived effects with purely decorative elements; for example, Gothic-inspired stepped gables.

Poelzig's work after World War I was rooted in the Expressionist movement, particularly his practice of overplastering plastic architectonic elements to heighten their effect. He began a series of crystalline structures, including his design for the House of Friendship (1916) in Istanbul, the plans for a Town Hall (1917) in Dresden, and the Festival Hall (1920) in Salzburg. These projects show how he moved toward an ever more individualistic treatment of design elements and materials. He combined new architectural concepts with an extremely personal interpretation of formal traditions.

These developments culminated and were most demonstratively realized in his best-known building, the Grosses Schauspielhaus (1918–19), a transformation of the Schumann Circus in Berlin undertaken for Max Reinhardt as an experimental theater. In the theater's vaulted auditorium, he created a famous cavelike effect by covering the domed ceiling with a sheath of stalactite forms. The room's organic appearance was in part the result of his use of a post-and-lintel system. Poelzig's use of light as an aesthetic element in giving form to the space was innovative, creating a total spatial effect based on an elaborate conception of color—his "light architecture," or *Lichtarchitektur*. The theater's exterior was flat, with little surface decoration, although decidedly monumental in appearance. Together with the simply delineated and sparsely decorated structure of the I.G. Farben administrative building (1930) in Frankfurt am Main, the exterior of the Grosses Schauspielhaus pointed the way to the International Style of the 1930s.

The Radio House in Berlin (Haus des Rundfunks, 1929–30) likewise stands in this path of development. It was the first German broadcasting building to be built. Based on a triangular floor plan, Poelzig articulated a brick-masonry facade with colored ceramic plates, creating a fenestration of high plasticity that, in pillar fashion, emphasizes the perpendiculars of the three wings of the building, each of which reaches over 150 meters.

Simple yet striking articulation of the volumes typifies Poelzig's subsequent sketches, designs, and buildings. These include the Capitol Cinema (1925) in Berlin, the Mosaic Fountain (1926) in Dresden, the competition designs for the expansion of the Reichstag (1929) in Berlin, the new plan for the Luxemburg Platz (1929), proposed designs for numerous gas stations (1927), and Poelzig's participation in the competition for the new Reichs Bank building (1932). Poelzig's late work shows increasing neoclassical tendencies; for example, in his contest entries for a theater (1935) in Dessau. In addition to his activity as an architect, Poelzig designed scenery for the theater and films, notably for *The Golem* (1920) and other films by P. Wegener.

STEPHAN BRAKENSIEK

Biography

Born in Berlin, 30 April 1869. Studied under Karl Schäfer at the Technische Hochschule, Berlin 1889–94. City architect, Dresden 1916–20. Professor of style 1899–1903, director 1903–16, Akademie für Kunst und Kunstgewerbe, Breslau; visiting lecturer, Technische Hochschule, Dresden 1916–20; master workshop, Prussian Academy of Arts, Berlin from 1920; professor, Technische Hochschule, Berlin from 1923; director, U.S. School for Free and Applied Arts, Berlin from 1933; stripped of academic offices by National Socialists 1934; accepted position as professor in Ankara, Turkey, but died before starting. Member, Novembergruppe; member, Workers' and Soldiers' Council for Art; president, German Werkbund 1919–21; member of governing council, Bund Deutscher Architekten 1926–33. Died in Berlin, 14 June 1936.

Selected Works

House, Breslau Arts and Crafts Exhibition, 1904
Poelzig House, Leerbeutel, Germany, 1906
Werdermühle, Breslau, 1908
Zwirners House, Löwenberg, Germany, 1910
Water Tower (partially destroyed), Posen, Germany, 1911
Office Building, Junkernstrasse, Breslau, 1912
Milch Chemical Factory, Luban, Germany, 1912
House of Friendship (competition project), Istanbul, 1916
Town Hall, Dresden, 1917
Grosses Schauspielhaus, Berlin, 1919
Festival Hall, Salzburg, 1920
Capitol Cinema, Berlin, 1925
Mosaic Fountain, Dresden, 1926
Reichstag Expansion (competition; unexecuted), 1929
I.G. Farben Headquarters, Frankfurt am Main, 1930
Radio House, Berlin, 1930

Selected Publications

"Werkbundaufgaben. Rede auf der Stuttgarter Werkbundtagung 7.9.1919" in *Mitteilungen des Deutschen Werkbundes*, 1919
"Bau des Grossen Schauspielhauses" in *Das Grosse Schauspielhaus. Die Bücher des Deutschen Theaters*, 1920

"Festspielhaus in Salzburg" in *Das Kunstblatt*, 1921
"Vom Bauen unserer Zeit" in *Die Form*, 1922
"Architekturfragen" in *Das Kunstblatt*, 1922
"Festbauten" in *Das Kunstblatt*, 1926

Further Reading

Biraghi, Marco, *Hans Poelzig: architettura ars magna, 1869–1936*, Venice: Arsenale, 1991

Feireiss, Kristin (editor), *Hans Poelzig: ein grosses Theater und ein kleines Haus*, Berlin: Galerie für Architektur und Raum, 1986

Hans Poelzig: Haus des Rundfunks, Berlin: Ars Nicolai, 1994

Heuss, Theodor, *Hans Poelzig: Bauten und Entwürfe: das Lebensbild eines deutschen Baumeisters*, Berlin: Wasmuth, 1939

Killy, Herta Elisabeth, *Poelzig, Endell, Moll und die Breslauer Kunstakademie, 1911–1932* (exhib. cat.), Berlin: Akademie der Künste und Wissenschaften Berlin, 1965

Marquart, Christian, *Hans Poelzig: Architekt, Maler, und Zeichner*, Tübingen, Germany: Wasmuth, 1995

Mayer, Birgit, "Studien zu Hans Poelzig: Bauten und Projekte der 20er Jahre" (Ph.D. dissertation), Munich University, 1986

Meissner, Werner, Dieter Rebentisch, and Wilfried Wang (editors), *Der Poelzig-Bau: vom I.G. Farben-Haus zur Goethe-Universität*, Frankfurt: Fischer, 1999

Posener, Julius (editor), *Hans Poelzig: gesammelte Schriften und Werke*, Berlin: Mann, 1970

Posener, Julius, *Hans Poelzig: Reflections on His Life and Work*, edited by Kristin Feireiss, Cambridge, Massachusetts: MIT Press, and New York: Architectural History Foundation, 1992

Reichmann, Hans-Peter (editor), *Hans Poelzig: Bauten für den Film*, Frankfurt: Deutsches Filmmuseum, 1997

Schirren, Matthias (editor), *Hans Poelzig: die Pläne und Zeichnungen aus dem ehemaligen Verkehrs- und Baumuseum in Berlin* (exhib. cat.), Berlin: Ernst, 1989

POLSHEK, JAMES STEWART 1930–

Architect, United States

James Stewart Polshek has restored to late-20th-century practice one of the most admirable legacies of modernism—its belief that architecture is wedded to ethics, that the primary concern is not the creation of personal monuments but of functional and structurally sound buildings that answer the evolving programmatic and economic needs of the time. By extending that notion to embrace the vital importance of context as a key ingredient of such responsibility, Polshek mediates the dogmatic utopian oversimplifications that often flawed modernist practice. Thus, his works are not isolated icons of style but rather buildings that defer to both the site and the people who inhabit them.

Born in 1930 in Akron, Ohio, Polshek entered the premedical program at Case Western Reserve University in Cleveland, but an introductory course in architectural history led to a dramatic change in plans. He transferred to the School of Architecture for his fourth and final year and in 1951 entered Yale University's graduate program, receiving a master of architecture degree with honors in 1955. After a brief stint under I.M. Pei at Webb and Knapp developers in New York City, in January 1956 he accepted a Fulbright scholarship in Copenhagen that allowed him to observe firsthand the making of sound and economically viable buildings in a socially progressive country while permitting him to travel to see the work of such early heroes as Le Corbusier and Alvar Aalto.

On returning to New York City in 1957, Polshek accepted a position in the office of the Harvard-trained Ulrich Franzen, but in 1962 he embarked on a remarkable odyssey for a young man: the commission for two major buildings in Japan for the Teijin Textile Company. He lived in Japan until 1964, absorbing the lessons not only of modern masters such as Kenzo Tange and Kunio Maekawa but also of traditional Japanese architecture. The two concrete behemoths for Teijin, in the Brutalist idiom then current, received awards in Japan and the United States, and Polshek's career was launched. One measure of his growing visibility was the invitation in 1968 to design the Quinco Mental Health Center in that town of trophy works by leading architects, Columbus, Indiana. Set in a wooded area, Quinco's *béton brut* planes create a "bridge" over an existing creek, incorporating the structure into its natural surroundings.

Subsequently, Polshek received a broad range of commissions to include master plans for cities, campuses, colleges, and cathedrals, designs for public housing, corporate headquarters, sewage treatment plans, embassies, theaters, convention centers, museums, libraries, and apartment houses. Polshek undertook domestic commissions (such as private homes for individuals) as well, although his preference for community architecture prevailed, including projects involving preservation, restoration, and adaptive re-use. Especially noteworthy are the reconstructions of such landmarks as Carnegie Hall (1978–87), Cass Gilbert's U.S. Customs House, the American Museum of Natural History, and the Cooper-Hewitt Museum of Design, all in Manhattan, and Delano and Aldrich's Sage Hall, Smith College, in Northampton, Massachusetts.

A particular triumph of what Polshek terms "reinforcement" is 500 Park Tower in New York City (1980): the sleek aluminum, glass, and stone surfaces of the 40-story residential and commercial tower, the massing of which is inspired by the PSFS building in Philadelphia, form a bold but empathetic backdrop to the former Pepsi-Cola headquarters of 1959 by Gordon Bunshaft, which Polshek has restored. His "Cinderella wand" has endowed even modest relics with new lives as stunning images and functional ensembles: at the Seamen's Church Institute in New York's South Street Seaport (1991), which houses as many different kinds of spaces as an ocean liner—offices, a navigation training laboratory, dining services, an art gallery, and a chapel, among others—a nautical note is struck by the upper floors, clad in white enameled steel, which rise dramatically but compatibly from the base of the resurrected 18th-century brick facade. Such opportunities profoundly influenced Polshek's architectural vocabulary no less than his design philosophy. Asked to insert a new building into an existing configuration or to expand or alter structures from various stylistic periods, he responds with a nuanced sensitivity while avoiding historical pastiche. Through the devices of abstraction and the selection of materials, he transforms references to traditional details into contemporary solutions.

Polshek relishes commissions for entirely new buildings, which he handles with a similar gusto for resolving complex programs that must be embodied symbolically as well as served practically. Whether starting from scratch or renewing, a number of favorite motifs appear repeatedly, in particular the figure of the square, which he learned to appreciate in Japan. It is a means of both proportioning spaces and organizing planes: square tiles articulate brick walls, and gridded windows and screens shield

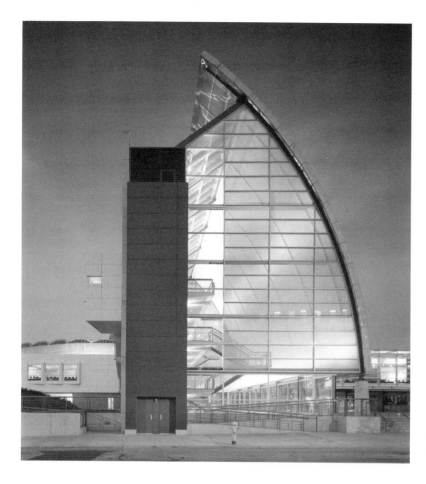

Inventure Place, Inventors Hall of Fame, Akron, Ohio, designed by James S. Polshek, James G. Garrison, Joseph L. Fleischer, D.B. Middleton, Don Weinreich, Jihyon Kim, Joanne Sliker, and Gaston Silva (1995)
© Jeff Goldberg/Esto

interior volumes. Characteristic as well are metallic structures and surfaces: steel, zinc, chromium, bronze, copper, and corrugated aluminum (often painted in bright colors) are cherished for their elegance and brio alongside the more familiar masonry, wood, and stucco materials. Reminiscences of admired exemplars from earlier avant-garde movements, such as De Stijl and Constructivism, and of works by architects such as Louis Kahn, Frank Lloyd Wright, George Howe, and Pierre Chareau are skillfully assimilated to leave a delicate but intriguing residue.

The inspired Rose Center for Earth and Space at the New York Museum of Natural History, which Polshek began renovating and expanding in 1995, opened to great acclaim in February 2000. A pure sphere encased in a meticulously detailed glass box, the design brings together the modernist geometry that Polshek loves—the Phileban solids employed by late-18th-century precursors like Claude-Nicholas Ledoux and Etienne Boullee—with the current search for symbolic meaning in architecture, for the sphere embodies the universe as it discloses its secrets. The year 2000 as well saw Polshek embarking on the commission for the William Clinton Presidential Library in Little Rock, Arkansas.

The way in which Polshek has organized his successive partnerships is key to his philosophy. He understands that collaboration is the essence of architectural achievement. The client is an indispensable member of the design team along with the members of his office, whose various contributions Polshek encourages and scrupulously credits. The size of the office has varied from 30 to more than 100 over the years and represents at once a model of the American large architectural practice and an exception in the camaraderie and collegial interchange among participants.

In 1972 Polshek became dean of the Graduate School of Architecture, Planning, and Preservation at Columbia University where he served for 15 years, assembling an unprecedented diverse faculty and shaping the curriculum to respond to the complex needs of the last quarter of the 20th century. He also transmitted his vision of the professional architect as urbanist, who must cope with the megascale of complexes that engage entire portions of cities no less than the individual building, and as preservationist, who must patiently repair the rifts in the urban fabric. By example, he continues to teach that architects should not aim for the instantly identifiable individual statements of dubious practical utility that tend to be glorified by the media and that they can responsibly fulfill their social and professional responsibilities while making works that communicate and bring sensual pleasure and intellectual delight to their viewers.

HELEN SEARING

See also **Aalto, Alvar (Finland); Adaptive Re-Use; Bunshaft, Gordon (United States); Chareau, Pierre (France); Corbusier, Le (Jeanneret, Charles-Édouard) (France); Howe, George, and William Lescaze (United States); Kahn, Louis (United States); Wright, Frank Lloyd (United States)**

Biography

Born in Akron, Ohio, 1930. Undergraduate at Case Western Reserve University, Cleveland, B.S., 1951. Master of Architecture. Yale University 1955. Fulbright Fellow, Royal Academy of Fine Arts, Copenhagen, Denmark 1956–57. Worked for Webb and Knapp (under I.M. Pei) 1955, Ulrich Franzen 1957–60, and Westerman and Miller 1960–61. Practiced in Japan 1962–63. Independent practice 1963–70. Founder, James Stewart Polshek and Associates 1970–79; James Stewart Polshek and Partners 1980–93, Polshek and Partners 1994–98, and the Polshek Partnership 1999. Taught at Cooper Union, New York City 1965–66, and Yale University Graduate School of Architecture 1966–68. Dean, Graduate School of Architecture, Planning and Preservation, Columbia University 1972–87. Elected Fellow of the American Institute of Architects 1972. Numerous design awards from the American Institute of Architects, national, state, and local chapters (including the Medal of Honor from the New York Chapter in 1986), the Institute for Urban Design, the National Endowment for the Arts, the Art Commission of the City of New York, the New York Landmarks Conservancy, The City Club of New York, National Trust for Historic Preservation, among others. AIA Firm of the Year Award 1992.

Selected Works

Oster House, Stony Point, New York (with L. Schniewind), 1959
Teijin Central Research Institute, Tokyo, Japan, 1963
New York State Bar Center, Albany, New York City (restoration and addition), 1968
Quinco Mental Health Center, Columbus, Indiana, 1969
Twin Parks East Housing, New York City, 1969
Physical Education Building, State University of New York, Old Westbury campus, 1975
Rochester Riverside Convention Center, Rochester, New York, 1980
500 Park Avenue (renovation) and 500 Park Tower, New York City, 1980
Liberty House, Battery Park City, New York, 1982
Stroh River Place Master Plan, Detroit, Michigan, 1983
Washington Court Apartments and Shops, New York City, 1984
Bard College Student Residence, Annandale-on-Hudson, New York, 1985
Barnard College Student Residence, New York City, 1985
Schenectady Downtown Plan, 1986
Residential Condominium, Battery Park City, New York, 1986
Brooklyn Museum of Art Expansion plan (with Arata Isozaki), 1986
Carnegie Hall, New York (renovation/reconstruction of the auditorium; cafe, museum, reception room expansions), 1987
U.S. Embassy Chancery, Muscat, Oman, 1989
Seamen's Church Institute, New York City, 1991
Center for the Arts Theater, Yerba Buena Gardens, San Francisco, California, 1993
Skirball Institute of Biomolecular Medicine and Residence Tower, New York University Medical Center, New York City, 1993
Inventure Place, National Inventors Hall of Fame, Akron, Ohio, 1995
The New York Times Printing Plant, Queens, New York, 1996
Jerome L. Green Hall, Columbia University Law School, New York City (renovation and addition), 1996
Santa Fe Opera Theater, Santa Fe, New Mexico, 1998
Queens Borough Public Library, Flushing, New York, 1998
Mashantucket Pequot Museum and Research Center, Mashantucket, Connecticut, 1998
Iris and B. Gerald Cantor Center for Visual Arts, Stanford University Museum of Art, Stanford, California, 1999
Rose Center for Earth and Space, American Museum of Natural History, New York City, 2000

Further Reading

A + U, 242 (November 1990)
Bartolucci, Marisa, "Citizen Architect," *Metropolis*, 63 (June 1995)
Polshek, James Stewart, *James Stewart Polshek: Context and Responsibility*, New York: Rizzoli, 1988
Stephens, Suzanne, "Architectural Ethics," *Architecture* (March 1992)
"The Works of James Stewart Polshek," *Space Design* (July 1978)

POMPIDOU CENTER

Designed by Renzo Piano and Richard Rogers;
completed 1977
Paris, France

From the moment the results of the open international competition for a new cultural center in Paris were announced in 1971, the Pompidou Center attracted both strong praise and fierce criticism. Designed by architects Renzo Piano and Richard Rogers together with structural engineers Ted Happold and Peter Rice of Ove Arup and Partners, the winning scheme was conceived as an antimonumental democratic palace of culture. Since opening in 1977, the Pompidou Center—also known simply as Beaubourg, the name of the site where it is located—has proved to be immensely successful in fulfilling the ambition of its designers, becoming both a focus of the contemporary visual arts in France and one of the most popular tourist destinations in Europe.

The competition, initiated by French President Georges Pompidou, attracted 681 entries. The nine-person jury included four architects of international distinction: Jean Prouvé (president of the jury), Philip Johnson, Oscar Niemeyer, and Jørn Utzon. In the event, Utzon was ill and unable to participate in the selection process. The winning scheme, selected in the first round of deliberations by a vote of 8 to 1, caused controversy when it was discovered that the designers were young and relatively unknown and that they were not French.

The building offered a bold vision of a new kind of monument that, instead of being pompous and elitist, would be populist and fun. Its thinking reflected a number of influences: Le Corbusier's principles of *pilotis* (Stilts), the free plan, and the occupiable roof; the provocative avant-garde visions of Archigram and Cedric Price; and ideas about prefabricated systems buildings as advanced by architects including Jean Prouvé and Ezra Ehrencrantz. The architects organized the building as a disarmingly simple rectangular volume overlooking an enormous new public square. Pushing structure, services, and circulation to the exterior created vast open floors—each providing 7500 square meters of column-free space—that fulfilled the internal flexibility required by the competition brief. The envelope itself, inspired by a famous unbuilt scheme for the Maison de la Publicité (1935) on the Champs Élysées by the German architect Oscar Nitzchke, was to be an information machine animated by changing images and text.

The completed building, built under political pressure and to an extremely fast timetable, is remarkably faithful to the com-

petition scheme. It is one of the outstanding achievements of the century and of the movement that subsequently would be called High Tech. A fastidious attention to detail that far surpassed conventional building technology of the time complements the building's formal simplicity, setting new standards for both the architectural profession and the building industry.

Like the Eiffel Tower built a century earlier, the Pompidou Center uses technology to capture the spirit of the time. Happold and Rice were determined to use cast steel for the structure of the building. Although cast iron had been widely used in the 19th century, it had been supplanted by steel alloys that were less brittle and by rolling processes that were more efficient. Marrying 19th-century techniques with 20th-century knowledge of fracture mechanics, Rice was particularly interested in using cast steel as a way of reintroducing the human imprint of craft into techniques of industrial mass production.

A single row of columns along the east and west facades carries enormous castings called gerberettes, named in honor of Heinrich Gerber, a 19th-century German bridge engineer who developed the cantilever principle that defines the structural concept of the building. The gerberettes, connected to the columns with giant steel pins, are rotating arms with the inboard end shaped to carry 44.8-meter clear spanning steel trusses on seated connections without welds or bolts. To counterbalance these loads, "sputnik" bosses at the outer ends of the gerberettes are tied to the foundations with a series of tension rods. The gerberettes are shaped to reflect structural forces and, appropriately in view of Rice's intentions, also have been described as strongly anthropomorphic.

The 95,000-square-meter building—which includes a mix of art galleries, design centers, libraries, theaters, cinemas, and restaurants—was constructed in just four-and-one-half years. To compress the construction program, the steel superstructure, like many of the building components, was prefabricated during the 26-month period when the cast-in-place concrete foundations, mechanical plant rooms, and parking floors were built below grade. Following a diplomatic intrigue, the steel contract controversially was awarded to the German firm Krupp. The steel was brought to Paris by rail and, because of its enormous scale, transported to site at night on specially designed trucks. The contractors assembled the superstructure in vertical slices without scaffolding. With an astounding 1500 tons of steel erected per month, it took just eight months to complete both frame and floors. Like the primary structure, the enclosure and secondary systems of the building were all designed as prefabricated kits of parts.

In the public imagination, the Pompidou Center is embodied in the color-coded vertical services risers and mechanical plant

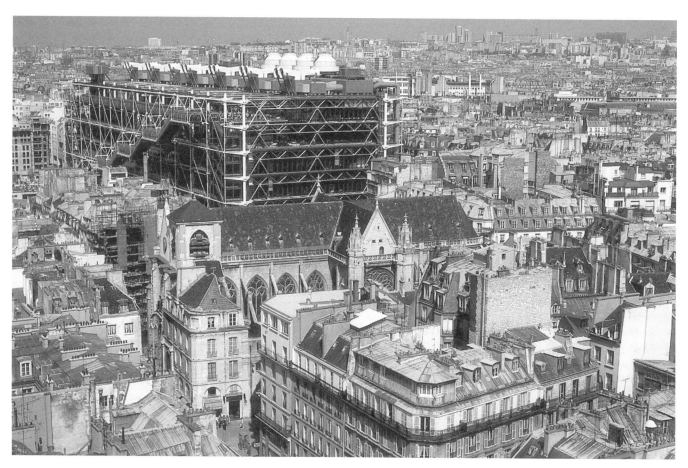

Pompidou Center, Paris
Designed by Renzo Piano and Richard Rogers (1977)
© Michael Dedandcé

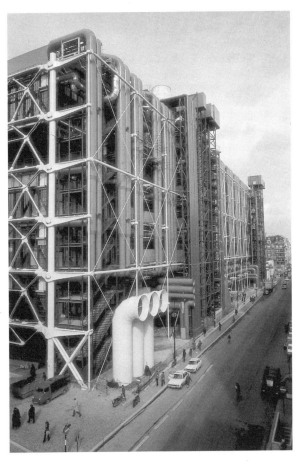

Pompidou Center, aerial view from a distance
© Gianni Berengo Gardin

that define the east facade and the public escalators that are hung in clear plexiglass and steel tubes along the west facade. Viewed from the narrow medieval streets that surround the site, the services—characterized as irreverent, strident, and playful—express the radical spirit of the building. Although the envelope was not realized as an information machine, the escalators and public circulation galleries animate the west facade, making it an extension of the square. The public promenade rises far above the rooftops of the surrounding historic quarter to reveal spectacular panoramic views of Paris.

Following the completion of the Pompidou Center and an adjacent building for the Institute for Research and Coordination of Acoustics and Music (IRCAM) in 1977, the partnership of Piano and Rogers ended. Propelled to international prominence by the success of the Pompidou Center, each went on to achieve a distinguished reputation in his own right. Their subsequent individual collaborations with Peter Rice, ended by Rice's untimely death in 1992, produced a number of distinguished buildings noted for both the advancement and humanization of technology.

ANNETTE W. LECUYER

See also **Plano, Renzo (Italy); Rogers, Richard (England)**

Further Reading

A + U Extra Edition (December 1988) (special issue titled "Centre Culturel d'Art Georges Pompidou, Paris, 1971–1977")
"Centre Pompidou," *The Architectural Review*, 161/693 (May 1977)
Cruickshank, Dan, "Centre Pompidou: Paris, 1977–1997," *RIBA Journal*, 104/4 (April 1997)
Davies, Michael, Laurie Abbott, and Alan Stanton, "Centre Pompidou," *Architectural Design*, 47/2 (1977)
Demoraine, Helen and Francois Barre, "Beaubourg: Le C.N.A.C. Georges Pompidou," *L'architecture d'aujourd'hui*, 189 (February 1977)
Piano, Renzo, *Du plateau Beaubourg au Centre Georges Pompidou*, Paris: Éditions du Centre Pompidou, 1987
Rice, Peter, *An Engineer Imagines*, London: Artemis, 1994; 2nd edition, London: Ellipses, 1996
Silver, Nathan, *The Making of Beaubourg: A Building Biography of the Centre Pompidou, Paris*, Cambridge, Massachusetts: MIT Press, 1994

PONTI, GIO 1891–1979

Architect and designer, Italy

One of the most accomplished and prolific Italian architects of the 20th century, Gio (Giovanni) Ponti was not only an architect but also a poet, painter, ceramist, graphic artist, and designer of exhibitions, theater costumes, glassware, tableware, furniture, lighting fixtures, and ocean-liner interiors.

Ponti graduated with a degree in architecture from the Milan Polytechnic in 1921. That same year, he set up a studio with architects Mino Fiocchi and Emilio Lancia. Later, he went into partnership with Lancia—forming Studio Ponti-Lancia (1926–33)—and then with engineers Antonio Fornaroli and Eugenio Soncini—forming Studio Ponti-Fornaroli-Sancini (1933–45). This became Studio Ponti-Fornaroli-Rosselli in 1952, when Alberto Rosselli became a partner. After Rosselli's death in 1976, Ponti continued work with Fornaroli.

Ponti's early works, such as the house he designed for himself and his wife (née Giulia Vimercati) at no. 9, Via Randaccio (1925), in Milan; Villa Bouilhet, Garches (1926), in Paris; and the furnishing for Palazzo Contini-Bonacossi (1931), in Florence reflect the *Novecento Italiano*'s neoclassic revivalism that was prevalent at the time.

The creation of the *Movimento Italiano per l'Architettura Razionale* (Italian Movement for Rational Architecture) in 1927 presented Italian architects with the opportunity to discard their reliance on the classical effects of arches and columns for a new approach to architecture, one that took into account new developments in building technology. Through his architectural work, his writings in *Domus* magazine (which he founded in 1928), and his involvement with the Triennial Exhibitions of Milan, Ponti promoted a renewal of Italian architecture and decorative arts and transformed the "classic" language into a rationalist vocabulary. In his articles and books, such as *La Casa all'Italiana* (1933; House Italian Style), he imparted his conviction that architecture must always preserve some national characteristics.

In the 1930s, Ponti produced the *Domuses*, or "typical houses" (1931–36) in Milan; the Universal Exhibition of the Catholic Press (1936) in Vatican City; and the first Montecatini Building (1936) in Milan. In these projects, he gradually abandoned the neoclassical conventions and replaced them with a

rationalist system of aesthetics. The first Montecatini building also marks his first integrated project. Here he designed not only the building but also the fittings, appliances, and furniture.

During the 1940s, Ponti's efforts were dedicated to writing, painting, and industrial design, but during the 1950s, Ponti was very productive architecturally. He traveled to Brazil, Mexico, Venezuela, the United States, and the Middle East. He carried out a series of projects in some of these countries, such as Villa Planchart (1955) and Villa Arreaza (1956) in Caracas, an auditorium on the eighth floor of the Time and Life Building (1959) in New York, and a building for government offices (1958) in Baghdad.

It is during this decade that Ponti produced his most renowned building: the Pirelli Skyscraper (1955–58) in Milan. An office block of over 30 stories, it was at one time the tallest building in Europe and still is one of the world's most refined and elegant tall buildings. Lessons inherent in the design of this building have been absorbed all over the world. Pier Luigi Nervi, acting as structural engineer, contributed to the building's elegant stature by designing a structure based on two full-width reinforced-concrete diaphragm walls that reduce in size toward the top. The thickness of the floors was dispensed with by making them taper at the edge. This allowed Ponti to design a facade that does not have the arbitrary repetitiveness of curtain walling

but, instead, one that emphasizes the finiteness of the building and creates the illusion of lightness.

The quest for lightness in mass was an underlying element in Ponti's architecture. The concept of using walls as screens to give a sense of transparency first appeared in his competition project for the Palace of Water and Light at the "E42" Exhibition (1939) in Rome. The idea was further developed in the Pakistan House Hotel (1963) in Islamabad, the Church of San Francesco (1964) in Milan, the Church for the Hospital of San Carlo (1966) in Milan, and the facade of the INA building at no. 7 Via San Paolo (1967) in Milan. It culminated in the Taranto Cathedral (1970) and the Denver Art Museum (1971) in Denver, Colorado, where the walls are purely an enclosure surrounding the volume within.

Ponti's 60-year architectural practice was paralleled by a host of other activities. Commencing with his public debut at the Biennial Exhibition of the Decorative Arts in Monza in 1923, Ponti became involved in the organization of the subsequent Triennial Exhibition (known as the Ponti Triennale) in Milan as a member of the executive committee. From 1923 to 1930, he worked at the *Manifattura Ceramica Richard Ginori* in Milan and Sesto Fiorentino, changing the company's whole output. From 1936 to 1961, he was professor on the permanent staff of the Faculty of Architecture at the Milan Polytechnic. In 1941

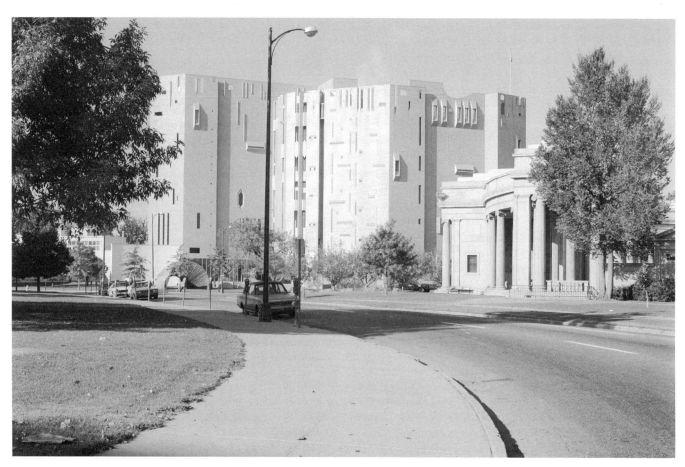

Denver Art Museum, designed by Gio Ponti (1971)
© G.E. Kidder Smith/CORBIS

he resigned as editor of *Domus* and set up the magazine *Stile*, which he edited until 1947. In 1948 he returned to *Domus*, where he remained editor until his death. He also wrote an article in every one of the 560 issues of the magazine. He designed fabrics for the Jsa factory from 1950 to 1958. In 1957 he created the *Superleggera*, or Ponti-chair, for Cassina. Light enough to be lifted with one finger, the *Superleggera* chair has become a universally classic feature.

Ponti's vitality was proverbial among those who knew him. He worked relentlessly to promote Italian culture and over the years produced work that maintained the freshness of experiment and influenced generations of Italian designers and architects.

HAGIT HADAYA

Further Reading

Hoffer, Peter, "Gio Ponti: 1892–1979," *Architectural Review*, 166/944 (1979)

La Pietra, Ugo (editor), *Gio Ponti*, Milan: Rizzoli; New York: Rizzoli, 1996

Ponti, Lisa Licitra, *Gio Ponti: The Complete Work, 1923–1978*, Cambridge, Massachusetts: MIT Press, and London: Thames and Hudson, 1990

Veronesi, Giulia, "Ponti, Gio," in the *Encyclopedia of Modern Architecture*, edited by Wolfgang Pehnt, New York: Harry N. Abrams, 1964

POPE, JOHN RUSSELL 1873–1937

Architect, United States

After World War I, John Russell Pope's neoclassical architecture helped define an American national image as the United States took on grandiose powers and managerial confidence. Pope sought to create a nationally recognized American architecture along conservative Roman and Greek classical design. From his earliest proposals for the Lincoln Memorial and the proposal requested by Assistant Secretary of the Navy Franklin D. Roosevelt to romanize Alfred Mullett's State, War, and Navy Building to his completed plans for the National Gallery of Art, Scottish Rite Temple, Constitution Hall, Pharmaceutical Building, National Archives, and Jefferson Memorial, no one else would so successfully dominate the look and space of the U.S. capital.

Pope studied architecture under William Robert Ware at the Columbia University College of Mines. After graduating from Columbia in 1894, he won both the McKim Traveling Fellowship and the first student award granted by the American School of Architecture in Rome (later the American Academy in Rome). After a year and a half in Rome, Pope attended the École des Beaux Arts in Paris. These experiences marked Pope's architecture for the rest of his career. The influence of the Beaux Arts school as well as his personal connection to Charles Follen McKim set Pope on a path of large-scale public buildings of neoclassical design that relied on a wide range of classical tropes. These ideas, as well as landscape, art, and writing, created a sense of reflection for the visitor. Also of some significance to Pope's early career and future success was his marriage to Sadie Jones, the stepdaughter of Henry Walters, a cousin of the Delano family—a fact not lost on Franklin Delano Roosevelt.

Pope apprenticed with Bruce Price, an architect notable for his domestic Shingle style. In 1905 Pope opened his own office. During this time, his chief intellectual mentor, Charles Follen McKim, became the architectural adviser on the Senate Park Commission, where he designed the dome for the first building the Senate Park Commission built on the north side of the National Mall, the United States National Museum, which is now the Natural History Museum. Along with Daniel Burnham, McKim played a central role in the creation of a planned monumental core for Washington, D.C., that followed the neoclassical design of the Capitol and James Hoban's White House. McKim and Burnham were picked by Senator James McMillan of Michigan, chairman of the Senate Committee on the District of Columbia, to be the architectural advisers for the Senate Park Commission. The Senate Park Commission's plan to memorialize Abraham Lincoln became one of the most significant design programs of the National Mall. In 1911 Congress appropriated money to create the Lincoln Memorial Commission, which began an 11-year process of designing and locating the monument to Lincoln. The commission requested that Pope and Henry Bacon, both protégés of McKim, prepare designs for the memorial, but the commission finally chose Bacon's beautiful adaptation of the Parthenon for the western end of the Mall.

Pope's work was to come later. During the first two decades of the 20th century, he designed classically inspired mansions: the Robert and Katharine McCormick House, the John R. McLean House, and the Henry White House, all in Washington, D.C. In 1929 he contributed a classical addition to the Constitution Hall and designed the National City Christian Church. This work, along with his work on the Baltimore Museum of Art (1929) and connections to Roosevelt, made him the preeminent architect for the nation's capital during the third decade of the 20th century.

Pope's American Pharmaceutical Association Building (1933) was so cleanly designed that it received some praise from modernists for its compatibility with Bacon's Lincoln Memorial. However, his other projects would not receive such positive notices from the modernists. In 1937 Frank Lloyd Wright attempted to convince Franklin Roosevelt that Washington, D.C., needed to represent a distinctly American architecture and not just repeat the historicist styles of Europe. No one was more responsible than Pope for the miles of columns in the national capital.

Pope's most successful building is generally agreed to be the National Gallery of Art (1936–41), in which he revised the Roman Pantheon as a Beaux Arts temple of art. The exterior view of the building is designed to prepare the visitor for entry to the building. The exterior volumes of the building express the plan and elevation of the building. Andrew Mellon, the major art donor to the national collection, selected pink Tennessee marble for the exterior. The color of the solid blocks of marble gradually lightens toward the top of the walls to keep the large scale of the walls from being perceived as overwhelming.

Built at the same time, the Jefferson Memorial was one of Pope's least successful buildings and provoked Wright to compose another letter to President Roosevelt expressing his disdain for what he characterized as an "arrogant insult to the memory of Thomas Jefferson." Although the open monument, also inspired by the Roman Pantheon, can appear as a restful gazebo from some vistas—mostly when viewed from across the tidal

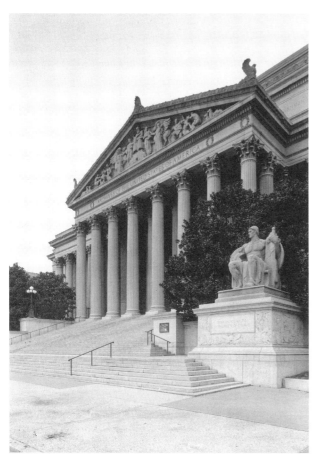

National Archives building, Washington, DC (1935)
© Historic American Buildings Survey/Library of Congress

basin or the Potomac River—it fails to work as successfully as Bacon's Lincoln Memorial. Like the National Gallery of Art, it is a model example of Beaux Arts design, in which architecture, sculpture, and engraved inscriptions are organized to create a sense of balance and harmony.

Pope was consistently able to create monuments and buildings that captured the popular taste of many Americans during the first half of the 20th century. Remarkably, they retained a great deal of their appeal and presence during the changes of the second half of the century, and that accomplishment has a lot to do with his architectural language of classicism, which continues to speak to Americans about themselves and their place in the world.

CHAR MILLER

See also **Classicism; Lincoln Memorial, Washington, DC; McKim, Mead and White (United States); Wright, Frank Lloyd (United States)**

Selected Publications

Yale University: A Plan for Its Future Building, New York: Cheltenham Press, 1919
The Architecture of John Russell Pope, with introduction by Royal Cortissoz, New York: Helburn, ca. 1924

Plan and Design for the Roosevelt Memorial in the City of Washington, New York: Pynson Printers, 1925
University Architecture, New York: Helburn, 1937

Further Reading

Bedford, Steven McLeod, *John Russell Pope: Architect of Empire*, New York: Rizzoli, 1998

PORTLAND PUBLIC SERVICE BUILDING

Designed by Michael Graves; completed 1982
Portland, Oregon

After its completion in 1982, Michael Graves's Portland Public Service Building quickly became a major icon of Postmodernism, notable for its references, symbolism, and ornament. With its stylized pilasters, rusticated surfaces, oversize keystone motif, and strong colors, Graves's design was clearly a turn away from modernism. Almost immediately, Graves's design became an icon representing the reinvented eclecticism of Postmodernism, and soon it became both an emblem and a target. For supporters of Postmodernist aesthetics and approaches to architecture, the Portland Building (Portland Public Services Building) became an emblem of a renewal of architectural vitality. Graves's design represented an alternative to a fussy, intellectualized, and overly complicated modernism that spoke to no one but the architectural elite. With the Portland Building, architecture regained the symbols and syntax from past historical styles, thus allowing the architect to communicate with a larger segment of the public. In contrast, modernists, including Pietro Belluschi, attacked the design of the Portland Building and the Postmodernist approach that it represented. Standing apart from its neighboring buildings, the Portland Building represented a return of revivalist eclecticism—with a new twist—that they had fought so valiantly to overcome in the early decades of the 20th century.

In June 1979, the City of Portland sponsored a competition for the design of the Portland Building. This new building was to house city offices and commercial offices on the upper floors and to provide space for retail businesses at the street level. Philip Johnson and his architectural partner John Burgee were appointed advisers to a committee of jurors drawn from local political and business circles. In January 1980, three competition finalists were chosen: Michael Graves, Arthur Erickson, and Mitchell/Giurgiola. Graves's design was declared the winner, but the city council, unready to accept that design, called for a second competition between Graves and Erickson. Graves was again declared the winner. Graves's victory was in part the result of his strict adherence to the stated budgetary restriction placed on the project. The competition called for 362,000 square feet of interior space for just over $22 million, or $51 per square foot. Graves's plan was the only one that met these budgetary goals.

The decision to award Graves first prize was clearly influenced by Philip Johnson, who was sympathetic to Postmodernist objectives. Portland's city council had specified that it wanted an excellent and exciting design that would symbolize civic pride and responsible government.

Thus, the Portland Building focused the attention of the architectural and popular media on Portland. When the building

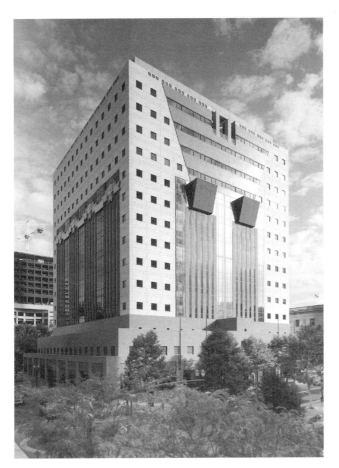

Portland Public Services Building, designed by Michael Graves (1982)
© Proto Acme Photo. Michael Graves and Associates

Service Building in uneasy unity" (see Macrae-Gibson, *The Secret Life of Buildings*, 1985). Macrae-Gibson admired Graves's juggling act that provides active balance of forms and symbols. In referring to the three finalists for the competition, Philip Johnson exclaimed, "It was perfectly clear as we opened the submissions that only one spoke of genius" (Jencks, 1983). Susan Doubilet, on the other hand, found fault with the lack of integration with the park across Fourth Avenue to the east of the structure. Belluschi asserted, "So they demolish the hated glass box and erect the enlarged juke box or the oversized beribboned Christmas package, well-knowing that on completion it will be out-of-date" (Bosker). A supporter of Michael Graves, Charles Jencks, provides a more balanced response: "The Portland [Building] still is the first major monument of Post-Modernism, just as the Bauhaus was of Modernism, because with all its faults it still is the first to show that one can build with art, ornament and symbolism on a grand scale in a language the inhabitants can understand" (Jencks, 1983).

DOUGLAS G. CAMPBELL

Further Reading

The books by Charles Jencks and Michael Graves provide the most useful information. Doubilet's interview contains Graves's responses to criticisms of the project.

Doubilet, Susan, "Conversation with Graves," *Progressive Architecture*, 64 (February 1983)
Graves, Michael, *Michael Graves: Buildings and Projects, 1966–1981*, edited by Karen Vogel Wheeler, Peter Arnell, and Ted Bickford, New York: Rizzoli, 1982
Jencks, Charles, *Kings of Infinite Space: Frank Lloyd Wright and Michael Graves*, New York: St. Martin's Press, 1983; revised edition, London: Academy Editions, and New York: St. Martin's Press, 1985
Olson, Kristina Marie, *Living with It: Michael Graves' Portland Building* (Master's thesis), State University of New York at Stony Brook, 1988

was opened in October 1982, the response was mixed. Certainly, this is the norm for any architectural design that breaks with tradition. In the instance of the Portland Building, Postmodernism is expressed through a colorful exterior with dark red-brown verticals and blue-green base contrasted with cream-colored walls while two-dimensional garlands ornament the facades on the north and south sides. On the east and west facades, large pilaster-like vertical bands of windows and wall topped with massive, projecting capitals support a keystone-shaped segment made up of alternating bands of windows and bands of painted concrete. Graves plays with color, spatial illusion, and architectural elements from the classical canon to provide associations with past traditions of ornament. He also suggested that a large symbolic sculpture be placed above the main entrance on Fifth Avenue. Although omitted originally because of cost, a 25-foot-tall hammered copper statue, *Portlandia*, by Michael Kaskey, was eventually added to the structure, giving additional prominence to the main entrance. The design has been both criticized and praised by architects and critics.

Praise comes from Gavin Macrae-Gibson: "It is not the cosmic harmony of the Renaissance, the Nature of the Enlightenment, or the machines of Utopian modernism but the nature of the new sublime that holds the fragments of the Portland

PORTMAN, JOHN C., JR. 1924–

Architect, United States

John Portman's self-declared mission as an architect was to create an architecture for people. He combined his skills as entrepreneur, developer, architect, and real estate manager to reinvigorate downtown Atlanta, a city that at the time Portman began his practice in 1953 had not built a high-rise building since 1930. If Portman did little to house Atlanta's citizens, he was intent on designing better environments for work: functional marketplaces for buying and selling and attractive hotels for tourists, conventioneers, and traveling businessmen. His Atlanta Merchandise Mart (1961) initiated the development of Peachtree Center, where he would continue to build for nearly 40 years. Perceiving the city as fundamentally an economic and social entity, Portman resolved to return the historic agora to modern Atlanta.

It was there, at the Hyatt Regency (1967), that Portman introduced the modern atrium hotel, transforming the urban hotel, as traditionally found in dense congested downtowns, to a new, experiential structure. The old form was re-created, traditionally enclosed spaces opened out in order to create active internal public environments promoting social interaction and

positive human response. Multistoried, ivy-clad balconies oriented hotel rooms and corridors inward to a 21-story atrium. The hotel lobby became a piazza, with a textured floor inspired by European cobblestone streets and patterned sidewalks. Natural light, water, and trees softened concrete surfaces, and the free movement of pedestrians animated the urban space perceived as an internal park or oasis within the city. Portman gave further expression to the life of the space through the dynamic vertical movement of space-age style, glass-enclosed elevator cabs rocketing through the skylight overhead to a rotating rooftop restaurant called Polaris.

Portman enlarged the Hyatt in subsequent years and added two more hotels to Peachtree Center: the Westin Peachtree Plaza (1976) and the Marriott Marquis (1985). The latter was a theatrical demonstration of architectural space-making that broadened the hotel atrium at its base (to dramatize the interior effect) and extended the volume upward to a staggering 50 stories in height. Office slabs as well as enlarged and newly built exhibition and market structures continued a coordinated expansion of Peachtree Center throughout the 1970s and 1980s until Portman crowned the complex in 1993 with the 60-story office tower, One Peachtree Center.

In addition to Peachtree Center, Portman's other multiuse urban centers included Renaissance Center (1976) in Detroit and the Embarcadero Center (1974, 1976) in San Francisco. He has applied his concepts about livable environments for work, market, and hotel to suburban sites in Atlanta at Riverwood (1989) and Northpark Town Center (1986, 1989). Northpark projected an 18-year, edge-city development to incorporate office towers, hotels, and nearly one million square feet of shopping mall, but the project was cut short by the recession of the early 1990s, by which time only two office towers had been constructed. Portman's Marina Square hotels and shopping mall (1987) in Singapore and his Shanghai Center (1990) in China spread his ideas internationally.

Portman's architectural language embodied an eclectic modernism. His influences range from such disparate figures as Louis Kahn (whose monumental geometry, exquisitely surfaced concrete, and use of light Portman admired) to Edward Durell Stone (to whose bourgeois ornamentalism and stylizing Portman could not always remain immune). When competing markets forced Portman in 1986 to redesign the lobby of his 1976 Westin Peachtree Plaza Hotel, he adopted the artificial historicism of Postmodernism and transformed the lobby into a classical masquerade, a stage-set of architectonic props of the kind Charles Jencks has decried as the carnivalesque. Portman's remodeling was an effort to redress a constricted concrete-encased hotel lobby that was originally little more than the leftover space

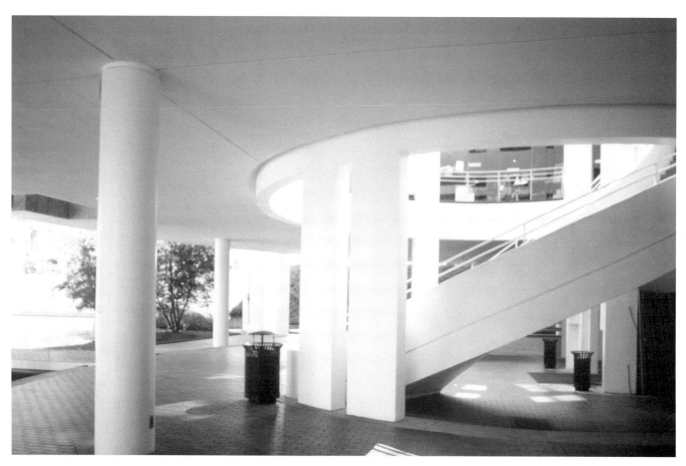

Portman, John C., Jr. (United States)
R. Howard Dobbs University Center, Emory University, the Asbury Circle entrance (1986)
Photo © Mary Ann Sullivan

around the elevator core. Portman took a lesson from the Mediterranean bazaar and crowded into the lobby an assemblage of elongated arcades, pedimented pavilions, and glittering lights; attracted by published images of a now upscale hotel, the people returned.

One of Portman's most successful projects outside the arena of commerce and trade was the Emory University Student Center (1986) in Atlanta, sited on an axis with his earlier Physical Education Center (1983). Portman preserved the exterior facade of architects Ivey and Crook's dining hall (1926) as a backdrop for a theatrical interior space enclosed by a semicircle of terraced balconies reminiscent of theater loges, dress circles, and balconies. The classicism of the integrated dining hall elevation appears to be onstage, and the whole calls to mind Andrea Palladio's Teatro Olimpico (1580) in Vicenza, Italy. This referential focal point is set against elements of Le Corbusier–inspired white modernism outside, where *pilotis* and interpenetrating ramps join a formal geometry shaping the main entry. The travertine-like surface richness of the exterior walls and trim references as well the marble cladding were perhaps inspired by Kahn and Emory's earlier architecture.

The quintessential Portman project is the beach house he designed for himself on Sea Island, Georgia—a 22,000-square-foot retreat named Entelechy II (1986). It was one of Portman's most controversial projects but was unquestionably his most personal. Although it embodied Portman's life experiences and public work, it also expressed in very personal ways his various interests in art, including his own painting and sculpture, and it reveals Portman as a modernist who is open to a wide range of eclectic possibilities in design. The name Entelechy is inspired by the Aristotelian concept of "becoming," and the beach house followed Portman's creation of Entelechy I (1964), the architect's suburban home in north Atlanta. Entelechy I was the early progenitor of Portman's fundamental vocabulary. It was the first significant project to generate Portman's forms, architectural conceits, and environmental design devices—including "exploding columns," water and plantings, and a geometric ordering in plan—and to employ art objects as appointments—all features later evidenced in his hotel and urban center complexes. In the same way, Entelechy II recapitulated and embodied in visual form a life enriched by travel, reading, observing, and studying art.

Entelechy II was a synthesis of house and museum, studio and retreat, weekend vacation home and monumental mega-structure. The house provided enclosed garden settings, poolside terraces, courtyards, lawns, and traditional rooms in which to display sculpture and paintings that its architect-owner admired, including reduced-scale maquettes of sculptural forms that adorn major public spaces in Portman's urban projects. At the same time, the studio-retreat was a workplace for Portman's own production of art. Since the mid-1980s, Portman has expanded his artistic range by creating art in other media: abstract expressionist paintings filled with the colors and light of the South; metal, stone, and bronze figural sculptures; furniture (including his delightful Rickshaw Chair [1985] made for the poolside at Sea Island); and large-scale abstract, yet referential, pop sculptures inspired by such disparate personalities as Mickey Mouse, Dolly Parton, and Cyclopes Polyphemus.

This Pop side of Portman's work suggests that as a popular modernist in architecture, his kindred spirits extend from the heroic form-makers of the 1950s and 1960s to such commercial stylists as Morris Lapidus. Despite his thoughtful introspection about his work, the public admires him not for the intellectual content of his work but for his inherent romanticism. His travel experiences in the East and West have been as rich as those of the most cosmopolitan of his contemporaries. His intention always has been to gather these disparate forces, influences, and stimuli in service to the creation of environments for life and work—architectural spaces embodying human values and promoting social interchange. If his buildings may be said to display a signature, it is reflected in their references to fundamentals: to nature, to art, and to an architectural beauty based in humanistic and organic principles.

ROBERT M. CRAIG

See also **Historicism; Hotel; Kahn, Louis (United States); Lapidus, Morris (United States); Postmodernism; Stone, Edward Durell (United States)**

Biography

Born in Walhalla, South Carolina, 4 December 1924. Attended the United States Naval Academy, Annapolis, Maryland 1944; studied at the Georgia Institute of Technology, Atlanta; bachelor's degree in architecture 1950. Married Joan Newton 1944: 6 children. Served in the United States Naval Reserve 1942–44. Employed by Ketchum, Gina and Sharp, H.M. Heatley Associates, New York and Atlanta 1945–49; worked for Stevens and Wilkinson, Atlanta 1950–53. Private practice, Atlanta from 1953; partner, Edwards and Portman 1956–68; president, John Portman and Associates from 1968; president, Central Atlanta Progress 1970–72. National Advisory Board Member, Georgia Institute of Technology, Atlanta 1975–78; director, Atlanta High Museum of Art 1982. Principal, Portman Properties; chairman of the board, Portman Barry Investments Incorporated; chairman of the board, Atlanta Market Center; president, Peachtree Center Management Company; chairman of the board, Peachtree Purchasing; chairman of the board, Portman Hotel Company; principal, Project Time and Cost; director, Citizens and Southern Bank; director, Commerce Club; trustee, Atlanta Arts Alliance; advisory council member, Agnes Scott College, Decatur, Georgia; trustee, National Jewish Hospital and Research Center; trustee, Scottish Rite Children's Hospital; trustee, Georgia Technology Foundation. Honorary consul of Denmark in Atlanta; fellow, American Institute of Architects; member, Royal Order of the Knights of Dannenborg, Denmark 1975; officer, first class, Royal Belgian Order of the Crown 1983.

Selected Works

Atlanta Merchandise Mart, Atlanta, 1961
John Portman House (Entelechy I), Atlanta, 1964
Hyatt Regency Hotel, Peachtree Center, Atlanta, 1967
Levi Strauss, Two Embarcadero Center, San Francisco, 1974
Westin Peachtree Plaza Hotel, Peachtree Center, Atlanta, 1976
Three Embarcadero Center, San Francisco, 1976
Renaissance Center, Detroit, phase I, 1976
Westin Bonaventure, Los Angeles, 1977
Atlanta Apparel Mart, 1979
George Woodruff Physical Education Center, Emory University, Atlanta, 1983

Marriott Marquis Hotels, Atlanta and New York, 1985
Northpark Town Center, Atlanta, phase I, 1986; phase II, 1989
R. Howard Dobbs University Student Center, Emory University,
    Atlanta, 1986
Entelechy II, Sea Island, Georgia, 1986
Marina Square, Singapore, 1987
Peachtree Center Athletic Club, Atlanta, 1989
INFORUM, Atlanta, 1989
Riverwood, Atlanta, 1989
Shanghai Center (project), 1990
One Peachtree Center, Peachtree Center, Atlanta, 1993

Selected Publications

The Architect as Developer (with Jonathan Barnett), 1976
"An Architecture for People and Not for Things," *Architectural
    Record*, 161/1 (January 1977)
"The Architect and the American Dream," in *The American Dream:
    A Collection of Essays*, edited by Claire A. Downey, 1983
John Portman (with Paolo Riani and Paul Goldberger), 1990
John Portman: An Island on an Island (with Robert M. Craig and
    Aldo Castellano), 1997

Further Reading

Portman's *The Architect as Developer* (1976, with Jonathan Barnett)
and *John Portman* (1990, with Paolo Riani and Paul Goldberger) offer
the best overviews of Portman's work. The first focuses on his joint
role as developer and architect (as does the 1969 *Architectural
Forum* article on Atlanta's downtown development); the second includes color
photographs of Portman's major projects. Saxon treats Portman's prototypical atrium hotels historically as well as from the viewpoint of design,
fire safety, construction, and other technical perspectives. "Back to Babylon" discusses the prototypical atrium hotel masterpiece, the Regency
Hyatt House (Hotel) in Atlanta. Leitner's *Art in America* essay and
Portman's 1977 *Architectural Record* essay (see under Selected Publications) articulate the architect's philosophy of designing for people.
Craig's 1988 *Southern Homes* essay and his article in *John Portman*
consider Portman's Entelechy I, while Entelechy II (the beach house)
is the focus of Goldberger's *Architectural Digest* essay as well as the major
1997 monograph on the house by Portman, Craig, and Castellano. The
1997 monograph moves beyond descriptive discussion to analytical and
critical appraisal of Portman's design and publishes furniture, sculpture,
and paintings by the architect and others adorning this museum-beach
house. Barkin-Leeds's exhibition catalog essay discusses major themes
observable in Portman's paintings and sculpture. Finally, Craig's *Journal
of American Culture* essay considers Portman among popular modernists
in Atlanta.

"Atlanta," *Architectural Forum* (April 1969)
"Back to Babylon," *Interiors* (July 1967)
Barkin-Leeds, Temme, *John Portman: A Retrospective Exhibition*,
    Atlanta, Georgia: Sun Trust Bank, 1999
Craig, Robert M., "Making Modern Architecture Palatable in
    Atlanta: POPular Modern Architecture from Deco to Portman to
    Deco Revival," *Journal of American Culture*, 11/3 (1988)
Craig, Robert M., "Mythic Proportions: The Portman Home,"
    Southern Homes, 7/1 (January/February 1989)
Goldberger, Paul, "Architecture: John C. Portman, Jr.," *Architectural
    Digest* (December 1987)
Leitner, Bernhard, "John Portman: Architecture Is Not a Building,"
    Art in America (March 1973)
"Metropolitanizing Atlanta: John Portman's Continuing Peachtree
    Center Program Weaves Intimate Human Amenities into a
    Major Urban Core," *Interiors* (November 1968)
Saxon, Richard, *Atrium Buildings: Development and Design*, New
    York: Van Nostrand Reinhold Company, and London:
    Architectural Press, 1983; 2nd edition, 1987

PORTOGHESI, PAOLO 1931–

Architectural historian and Architect, Italy

Paolo Portoghesi, an architectural historian in Italy, single-
handedly revived interest in baroque architecture in the 1960s,
leading to important contributions to Postmodern design and
theory. A series of books and articles include *Guarino Guarini*
(1956), *Borromini nella cultura europea* (1964), *Roma barocca*
(1966), *Bernardo Vittone* (1966), *Francesco Borromini* (1967),
and *Borromini, architettura come linguaggio* (1967; Borromini,
Architecture as Language). Every historian of Italian baroque
architecture acknowledges Portoghesi for generating interest in
this area. Subsequently, during the 1970s and 1980s, Portoghesi
was a leading figure in the Postmodern movement in Italy and
beyond, both as a historian and as an architect. In the 1990s,
Portoghesi has been a leading figure in the Architecture and
Nature movement in Italy. He is a prodigious architect as well
as a prolific writer and is recognized internationally as an articulate critic of architecture and urban projects.

Portoghesi was born in Rome in 1931 and graduated from
the University of Rome in 1957. From 1962 to 1966, he taught
the history of criticism at the Faculty of Architecture in Rome.
He was also professor of the history of architecture at the Milan
Polytechnic from 1967 to 1979 and the dean there from 1968
to 1976. In 1966 he was elected a member of the Accademia
di San Luca, Italy's most prestigious arts academy. Since 1979
he has been the director of the architecture section at the highly
important Venice Biennale. There he received great praise for
making important progress in the advancement of Italian architectural culture. He currently teaches architecture at the University of Rome. He recently moved his studio from Viale Aventino
in Rome to Calcata, a medieval *borgo* 30 miles north of Rome,
where he lives in a house that he restored.

Portoghesi's other books include *Infanzia delle macchine*
(1968; The Infancy of Machines), *Victor Horta* (1969), *Le inibizioni dell'architettura moderna* (1974; The Inhibitions of Modern
Architecture), *Dopo l'architettura moderna* (1980), and *Postmodern, L'architettura nella società post-industriale* (1982). In 1997
he published an exhibition catalog called *Arte e natura*, and a new
book, *Natura e Architettura*, was published in 1999. Important
architectural projects include the Casa Balsi (1961), the Casa
Bevilacqua (1973), the Church of the Holy Family in Salerno
(1974), and the Mosque and Islamic Cultural Center (1984) in
Rome. Whereas many architectural historians and architects
have learned from Portoghesi's writings about baroque architecture and contemporary architecture, several writers have in turn
made Portoghesi the subject of their own books and articles.
The long list of authors includes Francesco Moschini, Mario
Pisani, Carlo Argan, and Christian Norberg-Schulz, a conclusive
testimony to Portoghesi's importance to 20th-century architecture.

As a historian, Portoghesi was influenced mainly by the methods of Carlo Argan and Rudolf Wittkower. Like them, he has
always seen architecture as a language, with a particular vocabulary and syntax. This approach has dominated his analyses of
architecture in its historical context and its relevance to contemporary practice. He even went so far as to classify the various
design motifs incorporated by Francesco Borromini as language
tropes to explain the architecture in terms of language itself. A

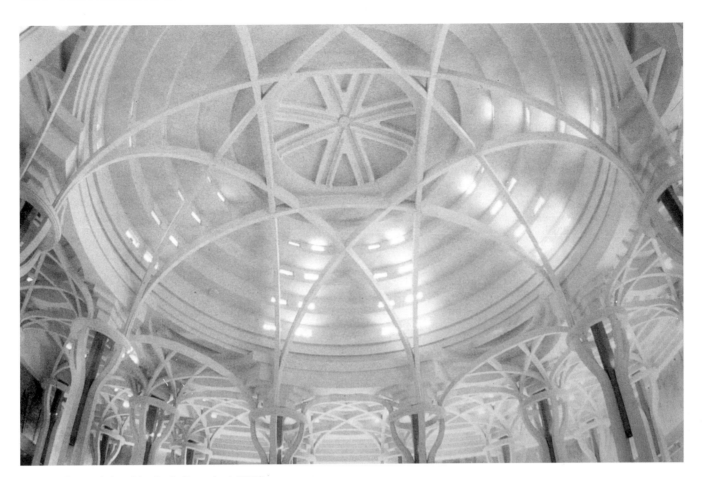

Mosque, Rome, designed by Paolo Portoghesi (1984)
© John Hendrix

freedom from restraint can be seen as common to Portoghesi's career: the baroque, the Postmodern, and art and nature all suggest his theoretical interests in an architecture that embraces discipline and spontaneity in its study of the past.

Throughout his career, Portoghesi's architecture reflects his preoccupations as a historian. His early work is based on the appropriation and reinvention of baroque forms. A historical consciousness is present in all his designs, especially those of the Postmodern period, in which he sought, both as a historian and as an architect, a new language of architecture. His most successful designs contain the presence of history, yet they are free from the restraints of the formalized systems of 20th-century architecture and modernism. In the Postmodern movement, Portoghesi found sympathy in the work of Philip Johnson, Michael Graves, and Stanley Tigerman, among others, which he introduced to a receptive Italian audience in his book *Postmodern*. The themes from this book evolved to include Portoghesi's more recent concern with the relation between architecture and nature. In this ageless relationship, he seeks to develop and explain architecture as a natural organism, an "architecture born of architecture." According to Portoghesi, the architect is seen as an element in a great biological process in which architecture is seen as an instrument for understanding this process. Portoghesi's architecture, for example, has been characterized as "crystallized music." For inspiration, Portoghesi has looked to the work of Frank Lloyd Wright and Louis Kahn, among others, who brought a profound understanding of nature and architecture to the architectural profession. As always, Portoghesi continues to search for new languages of architecture, new forms of expression, always rooted in the study and lasting memory of history.

JOHN HENDRIX

Biography

Born in Rome, 2 November 1931. Attended the University of Rome; graduated with a degree in architecture 1957, and a degree in art history 1958. Opened his own architecture office 1958. Taught history of criticism at the Faculty of Architecture in Rome 1962–66; professor of the history of architecture 1967–79, and dean 1968–76, Architecture Faculty of Milan Polytechnic; professor of the history of architecture, University of Rome 1982–. Elected member of the Accademia di San Luca 1966, and Academy of Arts and Design of Florence 1978. Director, *Dizionario enciclopedico di architettura e urbanistica* (Encyclopedia of Architecture and City Planning) 1968; director, *Controspazio* (magazine) 1969–83; director, *Eupalino* (magazine)

1983–; director, *Materia* (magazine) 1990–. Director, Architecture Section at the Venice Biennale 1979–82, and President 1983–. Currently lives in Calacata, a medieval *borgo* 30 miles north of Rome.

Selected Works

Casa Bevilacqua, Gaeta, Italy, 1973
Church of the Holy Family, Salerno, Italy, 1974
Mosque and Islamic Cultural Center, Rome, 1984

Selected Publications

Guarino Guarini, 1956
Borromini nella cultura europea, 1964
Roma barocca, 1966; as *Roma Barocca: History of an Architectonic Culture*, translated by Barbara Luigia La Penta, 1970
Bernardo Vittone, 1966
Francesco Borromini, 1967
Borromini, architettura come linguaggio, 1967; as *The Rome of Borromini: Architecture as Language*, translated by Barbara Luigia La Penta, 1968
Dizionario enciclopedico di architettura e urbanistica, 1968
Infanzia delle macchine, 1968
Victor Horta, 1969
Roma del Rinascimento, 1970; as *Rome of the Renaissance*, translated by Pearl Sanders, 1972
Le inibizioni dell'architettura moderna, 1974
Dopo l'architettura moderna, 1980; as *After Modern Architecture*, translated by Meg Shore, 1982
Postmodern: L'architettura nella società post-industriale, 1982; as *Postmodern: The Architecture of the Postindustrial Society*, 1982
Natura e architettura, 1999; as *Nature and Architecture*, translated by Erika G. Young, 2000

Further Reading

Argan, Carlo, *Paolo Portoghesi*, Roma: Gangemi, 1993
Moschini, Francesco (editor), *Paolo Portoghesi: Progetti e disegni, 1949–1979; Paolo Portoghesi: Projects and Drawings, 1949–1979* (bilingual English–Italian edition), Florence: Centro Di, and London: Academy Editions, 1979; New York: Rizzoli, 1980
Norberg-Schulz, Christian. *Alla ricered dell'architettura perduta*, Roma: Officina, 1975
Norberg-Schulz, Christian, *Architettura di Paolo Portoghesi et Vittorio Gigliotti*, Roma: Officina, 1982
Pisani, Mario, *Dialogo con Paolo Portoghesi: Per comprendere l'architettura*, Rome: Officina, 1989
Pisani, Mario, *Paolo Portoghesi, opere e progetti*, Milan: Electa, 1992
Pisani, Mario (editor), *Paolo Portoghesi*, Rome: Gangemi, 1993
Priori, Giancarlo, *L'architettura ritrovata: Opere recent di Paolo Portoghesi*, Rome: Kappa, 1985
Priori, Giancarlo, *Paolo Portoghesi*, Bologna, Italy: Zanichelli, 1985

POST OFFICE SAVINGS BANK, VIENNA

Designed by Otto Wagner; completed 1904

Designed by Viennese architect Otto Wagner, the Post Office Savings Bank was completed in 1904. A member of the Viennese Secession, Wagner was educated at the Weiner Technische Hochschule, or Polytechnique (a program modeled on the Paris L'École Polytechnique), and the prestigious Bauakademie in Berlin, where he was influenced by members of the Schinkelschule.

Wagner's approach to architecture at the turn of the century was essentially an amalgamation of the rationalism of the Schinkelschuler (members of the so-called Schinkel School, so named after the 19th-century German architect Karl Friedrich Schinkel) and the 19th-century "architects of the Ringstrasse" (Gottfried Semper and Karl von Hasenauer). Yet Wagner's polytechnical education also made him aware of the significance of technology and impending social change for architecture. Like his predecessor Gottfried Semper, his awareness led him to formulate an antiacademic position—one against the stodgy rule-based and tradition-bound education of the Vienna Academy of Fine Arts. Supported by Wagner, architects Josef Maria Olbrich (Wagner's chief assistant) and Josef Hoffman (his most prized student) joined with two prominent Viennese artists, Gustav Klimt and Koloman Moser, to form the Viennese Secession in 1897. Under the skilled leadership of Klimt, the Secession group developed a new vision for architecture, inscribing *Ver Sacrum*, a publication devoted to the aims and ideas of the Secessionists, with works and ideas expressive of their revolutionary approach to the arts and architecture. The Secessionist claims and actions were indeed revolutionary. Wagner stood as an elder statesman of the group, supporting not only the program of the Viennese Secession but also its leaders and adherents through his pedagogy and his works of architecture.

A principal example of Wagner's embrace of Secessionist ideas for architecture is his design for the Imperial and Royal Vienna Post Office Savings Bank, known as the Postsparkasse. The building, completed in two phases (1904–06 and 1910–12), is regarded as one of the primary examples of early modern architecture. Although Wagner's Secessionist colleagues—Klimt, Moser, and to some degree Olbrich and Hoffman—were caught up in esoteric and utopian visions, Wagner remained attentive to contemporary technical and social developments and their effect on architecture in a similar manner to those architects who understood the nature of building in their own context as well as the context of the history of architecture. In an essay titled "Die Qualität des Baukünstlers" (The Quality of the Building-Artist) in 1912, Wagner argued that "the ultimate goal of the architecture of his day was to add a building from our own time to the symphony of monumental buildings of all times" (Mallgrave, 1996). Yet he did not discount the symbolist aspects of the Secessionist movements; elaborate and diverse material and structural details adorn the building's exterior and interior.

The essential form of the building is trapezoidal, with the main hall—the public area of the building—axially placed in almost equal measure between the two major wings extending perpendicularly from the building's main facade. Programmed as large work spaces that could be partitioned as necessary, the bank administration, postal offices, and mailrooms are located in these wings.

The exterior of the building is sheathed in thin sheets of Sterzing marble, the details of which Wagner obsessively manipulated to produce an undulating plane along the projected face of the long, horizontal main facade. The building's foundation is faced with granite, and the bolts holding the granite slabs are countersunk, giving them even greater prominence on the facade. Wagner also used aluminum—a material that only since the mid-19th century could be mined in great quantities—to refine certain details on the facade. The acroteria—an ornamental aluminum "structure" and details by the Viennese artist

Othmar Schimkowitz—crowns the building. The liberal and pointed use of aluminum signals both Wagner's embrace of advanced technologies and materials and, in his accentuated use of materials and ornamental detailing, his adoption of Secessionist ideas.

Wagner continues his essay on the use of technology and materials throughout the entrance sequence and interior of the main public hall. The main facade, fronting a fairly narrow street, opens out to the Ringstrasse across a public square that focuses the main entry and extends slightly into the urban space. Immediately on crossing the building threshold, the space of the city is compressed into a stair hall of elaborate plasticity. Flowing forms and animated light stancheons reduce the scale of the space even further, lending it an aura of mystery. The stair—reminiscent of Michelangelo's stair leading into the Laurentian Library or perhaps, more directly, similar to Schinkel's elaborate orchestration of public and private space in the entry of the Altes Museum—leads through a cross axis of discrete secondary circulation just beyond the view of the public. The entire procession—from the Ringstrasse through the square into the projected face of the main entry—attenuates both time and the usual sense of separation accorded thresholds; in this case, the movement from the scale of the city into a series of zones or chambers suggests a new kind of threshold where one side (the public) borrows and extracts from the other (the private) and vice versa. Accordingly, the spaces produce a quizzical, even aporetic form of experience, a kind of "intimate urbanism"—a scenario that

Fritz Neumeyer suggests is akin to a railroad car or an "economical, efficient modern *mask*" (Mallgrave, 1996). Wagner's expressive use of form and materials on the interior furthers the building's sense of intimacy, in particular where the interior spaces are punctuated by animated figures choreographed within dynamic, rarified spaces. With great discipline, Wagner engages every available design opportunity, and stancheons, details, light, and materials together engage the range of bodily senses. The light of the public spaces, in particular the triple-naved counter space covered by the horizontal lights of the etched glass ceiling and the glass-and-steel floor, suggests mysterious activities just beyond that which can be seen. Distinctions between artificial and natural light are blurred to this effect, and the concrete structure and mechanical systems, both designed with contemporary technological advances in mind, only add to Wagner's conflation of symbolist ideas and built form.

Throughout the interior, Wagner continued to fashion the spaces and furniture in accordance with the tactility of the materials used (marble, glass, aluminum, ceramic tile, and iron), pervasive diffuse light, and the animated details that constitute a seamless marriage of function and ornament. In so doing, he wedded what were generally regarded as two separate domains of architecture: urbanism and interior (private) space. The sensuousness of the building's interiors, suggested by the erotic attention to detail on the exterior, promoted the unmasking of bourgeois sensibilities and restraint that defined fin-de-siècle Viennese society—one of the primary aims of the Secessionists.

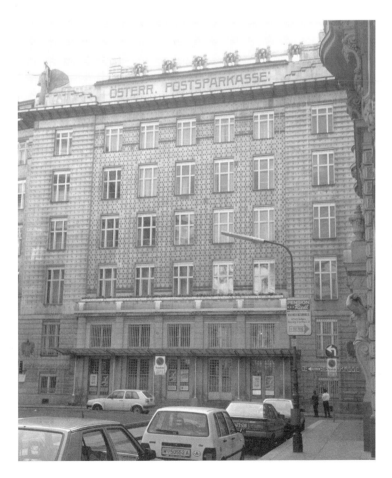

Post Office Savings Bank, Vienna, designed by Otto Wagner (1904)
© Howard Davis/GreatBuildings.com

Thus, Wagner's architecture was motivated by social and cultural aims; he understood that buildings must strive to communicate significant cultural ideals, in particular those that embraced change and development. Yet Wagner also affirmed another deeply held belief for modern architects: the need to embrace modern technologies, materials, and constructional methods. The marriage of both in the Vienna Postal Savings Bank—social and cultural responsibility and technological—marks an important step for the nascent Modern movement in architecture.

ELIZABETH BURNS GAMARD

See also **Art Nouveau (Jugenstil); Vienna Secession; Wagner, Otto (Austria)**

Further Reading

Geretsegger, Heinz and Max Peintner, *Otto Wagner, 1841–1918: The Expanding City and the Beginning of Modern Architecture*, London: Pall Mall Press, 1970

Janik, Allan and Stephen Toulmin, *Wittgenstein's Vienna*, Chicago: Ivan R. Dee, Inc., 1996

Schorske, Carl E., *Fin-de-Siècle Vienna: Politics and Culture*, New York: Random House, 1981

Wagner, Otto, *Modern Architecture: A Guidebook for His Students to This Field of Art*, translated by Harry Francis Mallgrave, London: Oxford University Press, 1996

Wagner, Otto, *Otto Wagner: Reflections on the Raiment of Modernity (Issues & Debates)*, edited by Harry Francis Mallgrave, Julia Blumfield, and Thomas Reese, Los Angeles: Getty Center for Education in the Arts, 1996

POSTMODERNISM

Postmodernism became an intellectual buzzword within architectural circles in the 1980s and 1990s. Traced to literary theory, where Postmodernism was used to refer to new modes of fiction characterized by self-reflexivity, linguistic play, and the use of referential frames within frames (the "Russian doll" effect), the term rapidly entered other fields, such as the visual arts and architecture, to end up as a common denominator to describe the cultural climate of the last decades of the 20th century. The precise content of the term has always been elusive—the more it was in vogue, it seemed, the less precise its meaning. In architecture, however, Postmodernism has been understood to refer to a formal language that could clearly be distinguished from its modernist predecessor because of its free use of historical, vernacular, or populist references. A closer look, however, reveals that also in architecture, the confusing connotations and paradoxical overtones of the term "Postmodernism" often gain the upper hand.

Important Publications and Exhibitions

Charles Jencks, in his widely influential *The Language of Postmodern Architecture* (1977), argued that modern architecture had run its course. He even provided a precise "death" of modernity: in St. Louis, Missouri, on 15 July 1972, at 3:32 p.m., when several of the 14-story slab blocks that together formed Pruitt Igoe, a prize-winning social housing scheme designed by Minoru Yamasaki and built only 20 years before, were demolished—the

final proof, thought Jencks, that modern architecture could not live up to its promises and failed to provide its users with a liveable environment. Lacking in modern architecture, Jencks stated, was communication: modern architecture did not conceive of buildings as conveyors of meaning and did not treat architecture as a language. Modern architecture's ideals of purity, transparency, and functional efficiency (elements of the established International Style) failed to relate to a general public. A Postmodernism characterized by meaningful architecture that was sensitive to its urban context would provide the substitute. For Jencks the most important feature of this new architecture was its "double coding": Postmodernist buildings communicate on two levels at once—they convey a specific meaning to a minority public of experts (other architects, art historians, and the like), who recognize formal references to historical styles, innovations, or ironic gestures, while at the same time they communicate with a larger public by invoking images that satisfy feelings of nostalgia and continuity. Whereas modernism rejected all popular references as kitsch, Postmodern architecture would rather embrace the input of mass culture.

The criticism of modern architecture formulated by Jencks was not completely new. In the 1960s, there had been a growing literature that critiqued modern architecture and urbanism for their abstract and anonymous character, their paternalistic attitudes, and their negation of history. In 1961 Jane Jacobs published her widely influential book *The Death and Life of Great American Cities*, in which she attacked modern urbanism for failing to design liveable and safe environments. She argued that modern architecture's hatred of the street was especially noxious, for it led to the creation of monotonous, monofunctional, utterly boring, and even unsafe dwelling environments in which social interaction was hampered rather than stimulated. Robert Venturi complained in his 1966 *Complexity and Contradiction* that modernist ideals such as purity or directness led to a kind of order that was rigid and stereotypical, whereas the complexity and contradictions of ambivalent formal languages, such as mannerism, were much more capable of evoking a continuing interest. Instead of the puritanically moral language of orthodox modern architecture, he preferred "hybrid" rather than pure elements, compromising rather than clean, distorted rather than straightforward, and ambiguous rather than articulated.

Aldo Rossi, in *L'architettura della città* (1966; The Architecture of the City, 1982), claimed that the modernist precept "form follows function" was naïve. Study of the history of the city reveals a persistence of historical forms rather than constant innovation: urban forms tend to endure, even if their functions wither; this persistence gives rise to the emergence of new functions. For Rossi the city (and context) is a crucial phenomenon at the heart of architecture. A contemporary architecture, therefore, has to base itself on the morphotypological study of the city (morphology referring to the historical development of the form of the city, typology to the study and classification of types in their relationship to the urban form).

The books of Jacobs, Venturi, and Rossi are some of the earliest significant publications that analyzed a nascent Postmodernism. Other publications, such as Sibyl Moholy-Nagy's *Matrix of Man* (1968), Peter Blake's *Form Follows Fiasco* (1977), and Colin Rowe's and Fred Koetter's *Collage City* (1978) exerted influence. For Rowe and Koetter, it was clear that modern architecture's utopian beliefs had grown outdated. They proposed a

"collage city," in which the modernist technique of collage would bring together several urban fragments stemming from different traditions. The collision of these fragments would lead to an amalgam of simultaneous order and disorder that would allow for diverging interpretations, thus opening up the city for choice and freedom, as well as multiplicity and ambiguity.

Another important impulse during the 1960s and 1970s concerned the interest in popular and vernacular architecture. These populist architects criticized modern architecture for its paternalistic, bureaucratic, and antidemocratic character. Publications such as Sibyl Moholy-Nagy's *Native Genius in Anonymous Architecture* (1957), Bernard Rudofsky's *Architecture without Architects* (1964), or Amos Rapoport's *House, Form and Culture* (1969) provoked a genuine interest among a whole generation of architects for such factors as culture, site, climate, or conventions, which had been more or less neglected within modernism. John Turner (1968) pointed to squatter settlements as "an architecture that works" (p. 355), arguing that the housing problems in developing countries should be solved by a bottom-up approach, relying on the experiences of self-builders in squatter settlements, rather than by the top-down approach favored by large-scale modernist housing programs. Advocacy planning and participatory design gained influence in the United States as well as in Europe. At the same time, there was a growing interest in built products such as Levittown, New York, or Las Vegas. This trend culminated in Venturi, Scott Brown, and Izenour's *Learning from Las Vegas* (1972), a book in which they pleaded for the ordinariness of everyday life.

That Postmodern architecture also sought a different relation with history was evidenced at the 1980 Venice Biennale *The Presence of the Past*, organized by Paolo Portoghesi, who characterized the evolution away from modernist orthodoxy as "the end of prohibition." The exhibition featured work by Venturi, Charles Moore, Hans Hollein, and Ricardo Bofill, as well as Aldo Rossi's Teatro del Mondo, a small wooden theater, built on a ship, echoing the shape of the monuments of the San Marco basin where it was temporarily moored. Another important, dually sited exhibition—"Revision der Moderne" (Frankfurt, 1984) and "Nouveaux Plaisirs d'Architectures" (Paris, 1985)—included the work of Peter Eisenman, Frank Gehry, Rem Koolhaas, Oswald M. Ungers, Hollein, Moore, Rossi, and Venturi. Curator Heinrich Klotz argued that Postmodern architecture meant not a rejection but rather a revision of modern architecture, thus aiming at a third way between reaction and rupture. For Klotz, Postmodernism embraced fiction alongside function: a building is not just an instrument but also a work that involves representation, poetics, and metaphor.

Tendencies within Postmodernism

A dominant distinguishing strand of Postmodernism is that of the vernacular, relying on popular images and references. Robert Venturi's first building, the house for his mother, Vanna Venturi (Philadelphia, 1962), cleverly played with the archetype of the house. Its front facade looks appealingly conventional, but a closer look reveals that the interior layout is quite complex and that what at first appears as a rather large chimney in fact hides a shifted stair and a small extra room. The house features ornamental strips, mullion windows, and arches—elements that were banished from any modernist building.

Charles Moore, Michael Graves, and Robert Stern have contributed a great deal to Postmodern architecture in the United States. Moore's Piazza d'Italia (New Orleans, 1979) is without doubt one of the most influential projects exemplary of a populist and pluralist approach. The Piazza was commissioned to reflect the identity of the Italian community in New Orleans. Moore combined several references to Italy in the design, such as columns in an Italian order, a raised platform in the form of the Italian boot, and a fountain. At the same time, the design was built in a highly unusual combination of materials, using not only marble and stainless steel but also neon and cardboard. Michael Graves's Portland Public Service Building (1982) in Portland, Ohio, and his Humana Tower (1985) in Louisville, Kentucky, show how a Postmodernist language can be applied to the facades of office buildings that in terms of program and plan differ only slightly from their modernist predecessors. Stern did a similar exercise with his Point West Place (1984) in Framingham, Massachusetts, but is also capable of reinterpreting more faithfully historical languages, such as the Shingle style (e.g., Bozzi Residence, 1983, East Hampton, Long Island).

Whereas in the United States the populist tendency relies on play with formal elements, the best-known examples of participatory design are found in Europe; namely, Lucien Kroll's building for the Medical Faculty of the Catholic University of Louvain (Brussels, 1974) and Ralph Erskine's Byker housing project (Newcastle upon Tyne, 1981). Kroll's "La Mémé," as it is affectionately called, provides its student inhabitants with the possibility of continuously redesigning the distribution of its interior spaces. The building's facades appear as hybrid collages bringing together a surprising diversity of styles and references, implying that behind these walls a similar diversity of students has found shelter. Erskine's housing project in Newcastle resulted from a laborious design process involving the future inhabitants. Where the project faces a highway at its northern side, it features a very high wall with only a few openings. It shows a much more friendly face toward the other side, sprinkling the facade with a multitude of balconies made of wood and painted in bright orange and blue.

Throughout the 1980s, however, in Europe the neorationalist tendency became eclipsed by the populist model. Following the theoretical lead of Rossi's *Architecture of the City*, neorationalism favored an urban architecture imbued with analyses of historical urban fabrics and forms. Instead of inventing new prototypes, neorationalists argued, new contributions to the city should be based on the rational transformation of existing types in accordance with their historical and urban context. This approach has been highly successful in the work of Aldo Rossi, Giorgio Grassi, Rafael Moneo, and Oswald Ungers. For example, Rossi's Modena Cemetery (1985) combines multiple references to urban forms and to symbols of life and death with an abstracted language to convey a feeling of melancholy. Moneo designed the impressive Roman Museum (1983) in Merida, where he included archaeological findings in the foundations of the building and managed to provide the whole with a magnificent sense of Roman grandeur. Ungers's highly regarded Deutsches Architektur Museum (Frankfurt am Main, 1985) reinterpreted the tradition of the urban villa by including in a bourgeois residence alongside the Main River a house within a house, thus evoking

a fundamental architectural theme appropriate for a museum of architecture.

Whereas the neorationalists saw their work as the continuation and transformation of a progressive historical genealogy, there were other protagonists of the so-called reconstruction of the city who advocated a straightforward return to classicism. Authors such as Demetri Porphyrios, Maurice Culot, and Leon Krier—with the occasional support of England's Prince Charles—argued that only a faithful reproduction of 18th-century typologies and formal idioms would be capable of providing a true sense of urbanity. According to such critics, industrialization and modernization had deprived architecture and the city of their very essence, turning architecture into a soulless repetition of the same and the city into a loose conglomerate of freestanding buildings without any streets or squares in which public life could unfold. The desire for a return to preindustrial forms has led to various built projects in Brussels (the complex in the Lakense Straat [1994] designed by different architects commissioned by the Archives d'Architecture Moderne), London (Richmond Riverside [1988] by Quinlan Terry), and elsewhere. Its most successful exponent might well be the increasingly influential movement of New Urbanism in the United States, which combines urbanist ideas similar to those of Léon Krier and Culot with an architectural imagery that refers to the American colonial tradition of small towns.

A classicist revival can also be recognized in the work of the Belgian Charles Vandenhove, who built in Belgium, Holland, and France. Vandenhove began his career developing an eloquent modernist language in a series of individual houses and larger projects, gradually transforming this language toward a more classicist idiom. Vandenhove's Theatre des Abesses complex (1996) in Paris faithfully finishes the urban block it is part of, looking as if it has always been there. The buildings facing the street are inconspicuous, built in the Parisian idiom familiar since the mid-19th century. The theater, lying in the back, is more outspoken, featuring a Palladian entrance with a fronton and a vestibule with pillars.

In the United States, Philip Johnson has, with his partner John Burgee, occasionally designed projects that were faithful replicas of historical examples (e.g., his College of Architecture [1985], Houston, Texas, a replica of a project by Claude-Nicholas Ledoux), but his Postmodernist stage is rather characterized by a free and informal use of historical references (such as his AT&T Building [1984], New York).

There are also many architects whose work is clearly Postmodernist but who cannot be categorized straightforwardly in any of the previously mentioned classifications (populist, neorationalist, or classicist). Ricardo Bofill of Spain, for example, is well known for his unorthodox use of classicist elements (columns, pilasters, pediments, cornices, and moldings) within social housing schemes. James Stirling combined classicist references with highly populist elements in his Neue Staatsgalerie (1984, with Michael Wilford) in Stuttgart, a building that can be seen as exemplary of Postmodernism's multiple references, urban sensitivity, and witty connotations. Austrian Hans Hollein's Abeitburg Museum (1982) in Mönchengladbach, Germany, sensitively interacts with its urban context, reinterpreting several building types and combining these into a difficult whole that nevertheless has a clear signature. In Japan and in Southeast Asia, an eclectic attitude has been especially prolific, as exemplified in the work of Arata Isozaki. His Tsukuba Civic Center (Tsukuba, Japan, 1983) features a replica of Michelangelo's Campidoglio that is sunk under a plaza among other Western sources.

Such examples underline Jencks's initial characterization of Postmodernism as a radical eclecticism. Postmodern architects are free to borrow elements from the context, from the past, from classicism, from popular culture, and from the architectural language and concepts of modernism. The latter makes up for a confusing connotation, for it means that sometimes the work of architects such as Richard Meier or Rem Koolhaas has been labeled Postmodernist, although it clearly continues a modernist tradition (be it with ironic or even cynical overtones).

The Postmodern Condition

The common element among the different strands of Postmodernism in architecture seems to be the rejection of the narrow focus on functionality and efficiency that characterized modernism. Postmodernity is brought about by the loss of the grand narratives of modernism: the modernist ideal of an increasing rationality that would result in progress and emancipation for all mankind has lost its validity and is seen as an illusion. In this sense, Jencks's diagnosis of Postmodernism in architecture corresponds with the French philosopher Jean-François Lyotard's interpretation of *La Condition Postmoderne* (1979; The Postmodern Condition). According to Lyotard, the main feature of the Postmodern condition is that the grand narratives (in literature, history, art, and philosophy) have come under scrutiny. Grand narratives are collectively shared ideas and convictions that are communicated by repeatedly told stories that grant legitimacy to institutions and values that form the basis of society. Such grand narratives, Lyotard argues, have lost their self-evident character, and their importance tends to become devalued in the minds of the people to whom they are addressed. Hence, there is a general loss of shared ideals that can act as guidance for decisions about future developments in our society.

This, however, is about as far as the correspondences between Jencks and Lyotard can be stretched. Jencks describes Postmodernism as that which chronologically succeeds modernism, whereas Lyotard discerns much more complex relations between the modern and the Postmodern. In his later essays on Postmodernism, Lyotard claims that the relationship between modern and Postmodern can never be simply chronological because the modern includes in a certain way the Postmodern: modern is what is new, but this means that it always follows on the previous thing, which was new (Lyotard, 1991). Jencks, moreover, stresses the aspect of communication and symbolism: Postmodernism treats architecture as a language, capable of conveying meanings, although he does not question how cultures navigate such communication. One of the arguments raised by Lyotard is precisely that the power of the grand narratives rests on their presumed comprehensibility by all, whereas it has become clear to him that societies, generations, and classes do not share a universal "metalanguage."

Criticizing Postmodernism

One of the earliest critics of Postmodernism in architecture was Jürgen Habermas (1980, 1981). Habermas blamed Post-

modernism for hiding a conservative attitude behind a seemingly progressive mask. For him, Postmodernists have given up the project of modernity, the project of emancipation, to seek refuge in nice and pleasant but socially irrelevant formal games. Americans David Harvey (1990) and Fredric Jameson (1991) elaborated similar criticisms. According to Harvey, the post-Fordist version of capitalism produces a need to express social distinctions among people and classes. This need brings forth the fascination for ornaments and decorations, which are seen as codes and symbols expressing social distinction. At the same time, these codes are not clearly legible but, rather, tend to dissimulate the real geography of social unevenness by piling up a series of images and reconstructions that act as costume dramas, rendering invisible the tragedies going on behind the screens. Jameson also sees Postmodernism as a discourse generated by the economic necessities of late capitalism in which the commodity consumption has usurped modernity's critique of those very forms and processes.

Kenneth Frampton (1980) has most rigorously criticized Postmodernism's tendency toward superficiality and sheer visual attractiveness. He pleads for a critical regionalism that would uphold modernism's longing for authenticity and critical responsibility while at the same time respecting local factors of site, climate, and materials. Diane Ghirardo (1991) blamed Postmodernist and other star architects for the fact that their return to art and their interest in issues of appearance had diverted attention away from the toughest issues in land development and the building process toward trivial matters of surface.

HILDE HEYNEN

See also **AT&T Building, New York; Bofill, Ricardo (Spain); Deconstructivism; Eisenman, Peter (United States); Erskine, Ralph (England); Frampton, Kenneth (United States); Gehry, Frank (United States); Graves, Michael (United States); Hollein, Hans (Austria); Isozaki, Arata (Japan); Jacobs, Jane (United States); Johnson, Philip (United States); Neue Staatsgalerie, Stuttgart; New Urbanism; Portland Public Services Building, Portland, Oregon; Portoghesi, Paolo (Italy); Regionalism; Rossi, Aldo (Italy); Scott Brown, Denise; Stern, Robert A.M. (United States); Stirling, James (England); Ungers, Oswald Mathias (Germany); Vanna Venturi House, Philadelphia; Venturi, Robert (United States)**

Further Reading

Jencks (1977) wrote the publication introducing the term Postmodernism in the architectural discourse. Jencks has later published a lot more on Postmodern architecture. Of these later publications, the lavishly published book from 1987 is most interesting, as in this publication Jencks narrows down Postmodernism to new classicism. Good surveys of Postmodernism in architecture can be found in Klotz 1988 and Ghirardo 1996. Portoghesi 1983 rather focuses on theoretical issues. Tzonis and Lefaivre 1976 is especially recommended for giving an overview of participatory and populist tendencies. General introductions into Postmodernist culture at large, also covering other fields (philosophy, visual arts, performance art, film, television, and so on) are Connor 1997 and Woods 1999, and both also offer very helpful bibliographies. Docherty 1993 is a very good reader collecting key texts in different fields. An early critique is formulated in several essays in Foster 1983, with influential texts by A.O. Habermas, Frampton, Crimp, and Baudrillard. Harvey 1990 and Jameson 1991 analyze Postmodernist culture from a point of view that is informed by neo-Marxist analytical tools and that stresses the links between cultural phenomena and the economic realities of late capitalism. Larson 1993 focuses on the links between architectural culture, economy, and the struggle for professional excellence. Watson and Gibson 1994 is a very interesting reader, collecting materials from architecture, urbanism, and geography.

Blake, Peter, *Form Follows Fiasco: Why Modern Architecture Hasn't Worked*, Boston: Little, Brown and Company; Toronto: Little, Brown and Company, 1977

Connor, Steven, *Postmodernist Culture: An Introduction to Theories of the Contemporary*, Oxford: Blackwell; Malden, Massachusetts: Blackwell, 1989; 2nd edition 1997

Dethier, Jean (editor), *Nouveaux plaisirs d'architectures: les pluralismes de la création en Europe et aux Etats-Unis depuis 1968 vus à travers les collections du Deutsches Architekturmuseum de Francfort*, Paris: Centre Georges Pompidou/CCI, 1985

Docherty, Thomas (editor), *Postmodernism: A Reader*, Brighton: Harvester Wheatsheaf, 1993

Foster, Hal (editor), *The Anti-Aesthetic. Essays on Postmodern Culture*, Seattle, Washington: Bay Press, 1983; reprinted in Britain as *Postmodern Culture*, London: Pluto, 1985

Frampton, Kenneth, "Towards a Critical Regionalism," in *The Anti-Aesthetic*, edited by Hal Foster, Seattle, Washington: Bay Press, 1983, pp. 16–30

Ghirardo, Diane (editor), *Out of Site: A Social Criticism of Architecture*, Seattle, Washington: Bay Press, 1991

Ghirardo, Diane, *Architecture after Modernism*, London: Thames and Hudson; New York, Thames and Hudson, 1996

Habermas, Jürgen, "Modern and Postmodern Architecture" in *Architecture Theory since 1968*, edited by K. Michael Hays, Cambridge, Massachusetts, and London: MIT Press, 1998

Habermas, Jürgen, "Modernity—An Incomplete Project" in *The Anti-Aesthetic*, edited by Hal Foster, Seattle, Washington: Bay Press, 1983

Harvey, David, *The Condition of Postmodernity*, Oxford: Blackwell, 1990

Heynen, Hilde, *Architecture and Modernity: A Critique*, Cambridge, Massachusetts, and London: MIT Press, 1999

Jacobs, Jane, *The Death and Life of Great American Cities*, New York: Vintage Press, 1961

Jameson, Fredric, *Postmodernism or, The Cultural Logic of Late Capitalism*, Durham, North Carolina: Duke University Press, 1991

Jencks, Charles, *The Language of Post-modern architecture*, London: Academy Editions, 1977

Jencks, Charles, *Post-Modernism: The New Classicism in Art and Architecture*, New York: Rizzoli, and London: Academy Editions, 1987

Klotz, Heinrich (editor), *Revision der Moderne: Postmoderne Architektur 1960–1980*, München: Prestel Verlag, 1984

Klotz, Heinrich, *The History of Postmodern Architecture*, translated by Radka Donnell, Cambridge, Massachusetts: MIT Press, 1988

Larson, Magali Sarfatti, *Behind the Postmodern Façade*, Berkeley: University of California Press, 1993

Lyotard, Jean-François, *The Inhuman: Reflections on Time*, Cambridge: Polity Press, 1991

Lyotard, Jean-François, *The Postmodern Condition: A Report on Knowledge*, translated by Geoff Bennington and Brian Massumi, Manchester: Manchester University Press, 1984

Lyotard, Jean-François, *The Postmodern Explained: Correspondence 1982–1985*, Minneapolis: University of Minnesota Press, 1992

Moholy-Nagy, Sibyl, *Native Genius in Anonymous Architecture*, New York: Horizon, 1957

Moholy-Nagy, Sibyl, *Matrix of Man: An Illustrated History of Urban Environment*, New York: Praeger, 1968

Portoghesi, Paolo, Francesco Cellini, and Thomas Becker, *The Presence of the Past: 1st International Exhibition of Architecture, the Corderia of the Arsenale*, London: Academy Editions, 1980

Portoghesi, Paolo, *Postmodern: The Architecture of the Postindustrial Society*, New York: Rizzoli, 1983

Rapoport, Amos, *House, and Culture*, Englewood Cliffs, New Jersey: Prentice-Hall, 1969

Rossi, Aldo, *The Architecture of the City*, translated by Diane Ghirardo and Joan Ockman, Cambridge, Massachusetts, and London: MIT Press, 1982

Rowe, Colin and Fred Koetter, *Collage City*, Cambridge, Massachusetts, and London: MIT Press, 1978

Rudofsky, Bernard, *Architecture without Architects: A Short Introduction to Non-Pedigreed Architecture*, Albuquerque: University of New Mexico Press, 1964

Turner, John, "The Squatter Settlement: An Architecture that Works," *Architectural Design*, 38/8 (1968)

Turner, John, *Housing by People: Towards Autonomy in the Built Environment*, London: Marion Boyars, 1976

Tzonis, Alexander and Liane Lefaivre, "In the Name of the People," *Forum*, 25/3 (1976)

Venturi, Robert, *Complexity and Contradiction in Architecture*, New York: The Museum of Modern Art, 1966

Venturi, Robert, Denise Scott Brown, and Steven Izenour, *Learning from Las Vegas*, Cambridge, Massachusetts, and London: MIT Press, 1972

Watson, Sophie and Keith Gibson (editors), *Postmodern Cities and Spaces*, Oxford: Blackwell, 1994

Woods, Tim, *Beginning Postmodernism*, Manchester and New York: Manchester University Press, 1999

POWER PLANT

Energy consumption is directly related to gross national product, and the expansion of the world market due to industrialization has accelerated the demand for energy. Originally, small electrical generators were built by factory owners in Europe and the United States for their own manufacturing, but in the 20th century the proliferation of electric lights and appliances required the construction of centralized stations. Throughout most of the century, power plants were icons of progress, but since the last quarter of the century, the power plant has come to embody the threat of environmental degradation. The high-tech exoskeletal aesthetic organic to many steam-generated power plants has been borrowed and modified by architects such as Richard Rogers (England) and Eric Owen Moss (United States). Curiously, however, power plants themselves have received almost no attention, remaining virtually invisible features in the landscape unless identified as an environmental hazard.

Power plants come in a variety of types and forms, but ultimately they do the same thing: spin a turbine connected to an electric generator, thus producing electricity. One type is distinguished from another by the mechanism used to spin the turbine. Power plants are large-scale machines converting kinetic energy into electrical energy, usually by transforming thermal energy into kinetic energy first. The form of a power plant often expresses this process by architecturally compartmentalizing the stages of transference in distinct structures connected by plumbing and other conveying systems. Some types are spread across the landscape, however, taking advantage of the energy stored in local meteorological phenomena, such as wind blowing through a pass, a river propelled downstream by gravity, or the sun's energy after it filters through the earth's atmosphere.

Steam-Generated Power Plants

Most power plants use steam to generate electricity, and the first public electric-generating stations were built in Europe and the United States in the late 1880s. Boilers of increasing size and complexity were developed in the 20th century, fired successively by wood, coal, oil, and natural gas and then by nuclear, solar, and geothermal energy.

In steam-powered electricity generators, water is pumped into a steel chamber called a boiler, where it is heated by the consumption of the fuel (e.g., the burning of coal). The resulting steam is then channeled to nozzles that inject the steam against the fins of a turbine, forcing it to spin. Coal-fired plants are the most common, and a typical coal-burning plant will produce 600 megawatts of energy in this process. The steam is then condensed back into water and returned to the boiler or expelled for cooling either in a cooling tower or in artificial ponds. Cooling towers are perhaps the largest and most architecturally distinctive features of power plants, usually constructed of reinforced concrete and parabolically tapered from a broad base to a narrower top. Although condensed steam is clean, if discharged prior to cooling in such a tower (or in its horizontal equivalent, a cooling pond), its high temperature can disturb and even kill fish and other wildlife. Waste from fuel, especially coal and oil, must also be expelled. Chimney stacks, like boilers, became increasingly complex throughout the century, and a system of scrubbers and filters have been developed to reduce levels of sulfuric dioxide, which creates acid rain. By the 21st century, a coal-fired steam-generating electrical plant could be expected to have three principal structures: the multistory boiler, the precipitator or scrubber, and the chimney stack (the streamlined character of the chimney belies the complex machinery inside its tapered conical form).

Non–Fuel-Burning Power Plants

There are two types of active solar power electric-generating plants, and both are rare compared to fuel-burning plants. The first reflects the sun's rays by the use of hundreds of reflectors arrayed in a field. The reflectors, called heliostats, are mechanically tilted to follow the sun's arc and to reflect light onto a parabolic receiver located approximately 50 meters atop a tower to the south. Water is pumped to the receiver, where it is boiled by the reflected thermal energy, thus producing steam. The experimental Eurelios plant at Adrano, Italy, built in the 1980s, utilizes this process and produces 1 megawatt of electricity. The second type of solar plant uses semiconductors called solar cells to directly transform the sun's energy into electricity. Like the first type, a solar field consists of hundreds of panels mechanically aligned to track the sun's trajectory. The first plant of this variety was built in Hysperia, California, in 1982 and produces as much electricity as the Eurelios plant and occupies the same land area, approximately 1,000 square meters.

Hydroelectric plants skip the steam-generating process, using the force of water to spin the turbines. Dams are the best-known

hydroelectric generators and the most monumental, but water may also be pumped to a high point (a hill or a tower) and then allowed to rush down to the turbines. Wind farms utilize the kinetic energy of air currents to produce electricity, and a typical farm consists of thousands of steel windmills 30 to 50 meters high, each installed with an electrical generator behind the propeller. The surreal landscape of the wind farm is highly visible since they are often sited in passes where the flow of air is funneled and where civil engineers are likely to situate highways. The 6,500-turbine wind farm at Altamont Pass, California (1986), for example, generates only 300 megawatts (at maximum capacity, which it rarely reaches). By comparison, Hoover Dam (1936) generates 650 megawatts, while the Volta Dam (1965) in Ghana generates 750 megawatts (and nuclear power plants typically generate nearly 900 megawatts). Although these two types of plants do not pollute the environment like fuel-burning plants do, they still have an impact on the landscape. Dams, especially when built in a series called a cascade (such as those in the Tennessee Valley in the United States or on the Dnepr River in the former Soviet Union), often raise the water table in areas on the upstream side of the reservoir, even flooding basements in urban areas. Farms along rivers can be inundated, impacting local economies and ecologies. Even windmills can have adverse environmental effects since the siting of wind farms on migration routes seriously disturbs the nesting and foraging habits of birds.

Geothermal power plants have been constructed since the last third of the 20th century in Ireland, the United States, and parts of Europe. These plants, or fields, consist of a scattering of wells several kilometers deep, each well comprised of two bores. The objective is to tap in to the heat generated in the earth's core and stored in the earth's mantle. Water is pumped into the first bore and heated by the magma or dry rock at the bottom of the well. It is then pumped back out the second bore as steam, at temperatures of 200 degrees Celsius or greater. The steam is then used to power the electric-generating turbines.

Nuclear Power Plants

Nuclear power was hailed in the third quarter of the 20th century as a clean source of energy, and the first power plant was constructed in 1956 at Calder Hall in Great Britain. With core meltdowns in the United States (Three Mile Island in 1979) and the Soviet Union (Chernobyl in 1986), however, the former, optimistic view has been substantially revised.

In nuclear plants, a steel-encased core consisting of thousands of fuel rods (usually uranium, sometimes plutonium) encased in zircaloy creates heat via fission. Discovered in 1938, fission is the splitting of uranium or plutonium atomic nuclei, a process that creates energy in the form of heat. The fuel rods are cooled by either water (at high pressure), gas, or liquid steel, which circulates through the core before it is pumped into another steel container called a heat exchanger. There, the heated coolant is circulated in pipes inside a secondary water supply that in turn becomes heated, thus producing steam. In some cases, the heat exchanger is omitted, and water circulates directly from core to turbine. More so than in other steam-generating systems, nuclear power plants require an elaborate network of plumbing and instrumentation to monitor the flow of coolant. Because radioactivity is generated during fission, the core and its coolant are extremely hazardous, and containment structures are usually constructed around the reactor and the heat exchanger. If too little coolant is present in the reactor core, fission accelerates, and heat is increased to the point of meltdown. This is what happened at both Three Mile Island and Chernobyl, and in the case of the latter, the remaining water in the core became so hot under pressure that a steam explosion blew the roof off the reactor, exposing the core to the atmosphere. The reactors at Chernobyl were not enclosed in a containment building. After the catastrophe, the Soviets encased the dangerous reactor in a steel-reinforced concrete bunker dubbed "the tomb," an allusion to the 10,000-year half-life of the contaminated material buried inside.

JERRY WHITE

See also **Factory/Industrial Town Planning**

Further Reading

Donahue, John M. and Barbara Rose Johnston (editors), *Water, Culture, and Power: Local Struggles in a Global Context*, Washington, D.C.: Island Press, 1998

Downing, Richard A. and D.A. Gray (editors), *Geothermal Energy: The Potential in the United Kingdom*, London: HMSO, 1986

Gretz, J. et al. (editors), *Thermo-Mechanical Solar Power Plants*, Dordrecht, The Netherlands: Reidel, 1984

Hart, David, *The Volta River Project: A Case Study in Politics and Technology*, Edinburgh: Edinburgh University Press, 1980

Hay, Duncan, *Hydroelectric Development in the United States, 1880–1940*, 2 vols., Washington, D.C.: Edison Electric Institute, 1991

Hills, Richard L., *Power from Steam: A History of the Stationary Steam Engine*, Cambridge and New York: Cambridge University Press, 1989

Markvart, Tomas (editor), *Solar Electricity*, Chichester, West Sussex, and New York: Wiley, 1994; 2nd edition, 2000

Medvedev, Zhores, *The Legacy of Chernobyl*, New York: Norton, and Oxford: Blackwell, 1990

Righter, Robert W., *Wind Energy in America: A History*, Norman: University of Oklahoma Press, 1996

Rybach, L. and L.J. Patrick Muffler (editors), *Geothermal Systems: Principles and Case Histories*, Chichester, West Sussex: Wiley, 1981

Shannon, Robert H., *Handbook of Coal-Based Electric Power Generation*, Park Ridge, New Jersey: Noyes, 1982

Walker, John F. and Nicholas Jenkins, *Wind Energy Technology*, Chichester, West Sussex: Wiley, 1997

PRAGUE, CZECH REPUBLIC

The Vltava River (Moldau), a natural axis of the settlement basin surrounded by hills, forms a favorable area for habitation. The city of Praha (Prague) was established in the 8th and 9th centuries, when the center of the then-Slavonic state was transferred to Bohemia (Czech lands). The old town of Prague, with its narrow, winding streets along with the churches, monasteries, and palaces, was built in the Romanesque period. The new town, built as a medieval city, was established in 1348 by a royal edict issued by Charles IV. At that time, the city, adorned by more than 100 churches and chapels with a population of 50,000, was larger than London or Paris. Today, Prague holds more than 1.5 million people. The epithet given to Prague—the Hundred Spire City—is more than deserved, and this ancient character continues to define Prague's 20th-century urban setting.

In the middle of the 19th century, architecture became an instrument to obtain a political autonomy from the Habsburg monarchy. One building in particular, the National Theater, had been a political and cultural symbol for the rise and culmination of the Czech national revival. Built from the national collection, the original theater, designed by Josef Zitek, was located on the prominent Vltava riverfront and was completed in 1881. Three months later, however, it burned down, only to prompt another collection to rebuild the burned building. The theater, rebuilt by Josef Schulz, an associate of Zitek's, was constructed in 1883. Thus, the patriotic Czechs have been very emotional regarding their National Theater and any changes with it or its surroundings.

Ever since 1918, when Prague became the capital of the new republic of Czecho-Slovakia, proposals were made to modernize and enlarge the theater. Shortly after World War II, it was determined that both the exterior and the interior of the National Theater needed reconstruction and that the operation and running of the theater needed more space for expansion. Two national design competitions were held, and a number of design studies were made on the subject of expansion. The design submitted by the Brno architect Bohuslav Fuchs was selected as the winner. However, reservations about the decision-making process slowed down the design development of the project. After the death of Fuchs in 1972, the team resigned from the project commission. The necessity of the reconstruction overshadowed the expansion project. After seven years of work, in 1983 the reconstruction and addition to the National Theater in Prague was completed in time to mark the centennial. Although the result of the arduous effort is there, the polemic is continuing. The relationship between old and new remains a topic of debate among citizens of the city and the nation alike.

At the turn of the 20th century, historicism was countered by Jan Kotera (1871–1923), Pavel Janak (1882–1956), Josef Gocar (1880–1945), and Otakar Novotny (1880–1959). In the midst of Art Nouveau, these architects were characterized by rationalism. The first important Art Nouveau design by Kotera, the Peterka House (1899–1900) on Wenceslas Square, clearly expresses the different building uses on the street elevation. The Mozarteum (Urbanek Department Store, 1912–13) is a symmetrical composition with the ground-floor commercial storefront and second-floor ribbon-window fenestration. The upper residential consists of three progressively upward-recessed bays of brick in-fill framed into stepped concrete verticals. This dynamic facade predates Kotera's later Cubist period.

The Jan Stenc Publishing House (1909–11) by Novotny, finished in patterned bricks of different colors, features a functional layout. Daylight pours into the printing press halls through the large expanses of glass. Janak was at first the ideological leader who later designed fine Functionalist buildings, relying on Cubist forms. The stately Reuinone Adriatica Insurance Company building (1923–25) of a late Cubism, referred to as Rondo Cubism, has a dominating presence on the busy Narodni Trida (the Nation's Avenue). However, the key buildings of Prague's Cubism are Grocar's House at the Black Madonna (1912) and the Josef Chochol's (1880–1956) tenement and single-family houses (1912–14) below Vysehrad Hill. Side chairs, armchairs, tables, desks, dressers, and sofas were designed in Cubist language by Chochol, Gocar, Janak, and Novotny as well as Vlastimil Hofman (1884–1964), Jiri Kroha (1893–

1974), Antonin Prochazka (1882–1945), and Rudolf Stockar (1886–1950).

The 1918 foundation of the democratic Republic of Czechoslovakia gave the intelligentsia a new platform of liberal ideology. In 1920 an avant-garde group of artists, writers, architects, musicians, and actors started a society called the "Devetsil" (the Nine Powers). The group published a journal and organized lectures and exhibitions. The ARDEV (the Architects of Devetsil) members produced studies of different housing types. The "Purist Four"—Jaroslav Fragner (1898–1967), Karel Honzik (1900–66), Evzen Linhart (1900–47), and Vit Obrtel (1901–88) with Josef Havlicek—were instrumental in founding the ARDEV. In 1932 the art critic and theorist Karel Tiege, the leader of Devetsil, published housing studies in the book *Nejmensi byt* (The Smallest Flat). The ideas of communal housing came from the socialist ideas of Soviet Constructivism. Novotny, on the other hand, was active in the "SVU (Society of the Fine Artists) Manes." The building for this important institution, which housed a gallery, meeting rooms, and a restaurant, was designed in 1927–30 by Novotny. Straddling the Vltava River and executed in a clear modern idiom, the Manes has held shows of trendsetting artists and architects of Prague ever since.

To demonstrate new ideas of modern dwelling, Prague architects organized a housing exhibition with goals similar to the Weissenhofsiedlung in Stuttgart (1927–29) or the New House in Brno (1928). Master planned by Janak, the Baba Housing (1928–32) single-family homes were designed by Gocar, Janak, Jan E. Koula, and Linhart. The family living was extended outdoors by means of large window openings, balconies, verandas, and roof terraces. A new type of office building was defined in the Pensions Institute (1929–34), designed by Havlicek and Honzik. The architects employed here the quintessential elements of functionalist architecture: a uniform structural modular system, expressed vertical circulation, ribbon windows bringing maximum daylight into a free-plan interior, and a roof terrace.

Following the 1938 Munich Treaty, then the devastation of World War II, the Communist takeover in 1948, the invasion of Czechoslovakia by the Red Army in 1968, and the political and social changes brought about by these events, Prague suffered many setbacks. During the 41 years of the Communist Party totalitarian regime, architects were expected to design in a government-dictated style called socialist realism. Functionalism was condemned as an expression of bourgeois cosmopolitanism. The November 1989 "Velvet Revolution" marked the fall of the Communist government, and free Prague emerged again.

In the last quarter of the 20th century, despite the totalitarian regime's restriction of free expression and the imposition of Moscow-style aesthetics, several new buildings stand out as important contributions to 20th-century Prague architecture. These include the Department Store "Maj" (1973–75) on the Narodni Trida by Miroslav Masak (1932–), Martin Rajnis (1944–), and Johnny Eisler (1946–); the Tennis Stadium (1986–89) on Stvanice Island by Jana Novotna (1946–) and Josef Kales (1934–); and the Retirement Home (1983–89) at Chodov by Jan Lynek (1943–), Vladimir Milunic (1941–), Tomas Kulik (1954–), and Jan Louda (1949–). The husband-and-wife team of Jan Sramek (1924–78) and Alena Sramkova (1929–) designed a key transportation hub of the Main Train Station (1972–79) and the CKD Building (1976–83) on the Narodni Trida. The Vltava riverfront has been complemented by the National Netherlands Building (1992–95), known as the "Fred and Ginger," by Frank Gehry with Vladimir Milunic.

PETER LIZON

See also **Art Nouveau (Jugendstil); Czech Republic/Czecho-slovakia; Weissenhofsiedlung, Deutscher Werkbund (Stutt-gart 1927)**

PRAIRIE SCHOOL

The Prairie School was an indigenous Midwestern phenomenon. Beginning in the Chicago suburbs during the 1890s, it spread outward through the entire region in the first two decades of the 20th century. Many of its most distinctive achievements were in small towns, such as Mason City, Iowa, and Owatonna, Minnesota. Unquestionably, the spiritual leader of the movement was Louis Sullivan (1856–1924), who developed a philosophy that emphasized the organic quality inherent in a successful building. In his buildings, by his writings, and by the force of his charismatic personality, he passed this philosophy on to a group of young architects who became his disciples. Without doubt, the most gifted of these was Frank Lloyd Wright, who was with Adler and Sullivan for six years prior to his departure to found his own office in 1893. Wright saw the provision of well-designed houses for the newly affluent Midwestern upper-middle class as a great opportunity. His clients did not possess great fortune but were generally technological entrepreneurs. Many had a taste for music. Wright gave them dwellings that responded to the vision of Sullivan and that at the same time went beyond that vision to achieve a synthesis very much his own. For the next 15 years, he pursued his goals with remarkable vigor and great success. The first executed houses in which the new style was fully visible were the Bradley house (1900) in Kankakee, Illinois, and the Ward Willits house (1901) in Highland Park, Illinois. In the next few years, there followed a number of important works, notably the Davenport, Dana, Heurtley, Huntley, and Thomas houses, all finished by 1904. These houses had important elements in common: flowing interior space, directional or centrifugal lines, generous low roofs with pronounced overhangs, broad chimneys, reduced floor heights, rows of casement windows, geometric leaded glass, and an intimate relationship to the site. The interiors featured furniture and sometimes fabrics designed by the architect. Wright's objective was to control every aspect of the architectural experience. All were designed on a unit system, meaning that they were based on a single module with a length equal to some specific architectural element, often, as in the Willits house, the distance between center lines of window mullions. None of these houses show any hint of historicism. Although most were located in suburbs, with varying kinds of topography, all reflected the horizontal lines of the prairie.

The sources of these designs, for Wright and for the gifted young men and women in his Oak Park studio, were mixed. They owed something to the earlier Shingle style, and they owed much to the contemporary English Arts and Crafts movement. The houses of Voysey and the theoretical writings of C.R. Ashbee were discussed as they appeared in the pages of *The Studio*. In addition, they owed a debt to Japanese art, which most of them knew through prints (Hokusai and Hiroshige were familiar names). After 1904, the year of the St. Louis World's Fair, there was a bit of influence from Germany and Austria. All these influences, however, were melded by Wright and the staff of his studio into a distinctive Midwestern and American expression.

Among Wright's studio apprentices, the most important were Marion Mahony, Walter Burley Griffin, William Drummond, and Barry Byrne. All were substantially influenced by Wright, and all in later years made substantial contributions of their own. Their contemporaries spoke of a "New School of the Midwest." Outside the studio, Hugh Garden, Robert Spencer, and George Maher, at different times in their careers, produced excellent designs in the Prairie School manner.

In Minneapolis the firm of Purcell and Elmslie developed its own distinctive version of the style. By 1910 it was generally recognized in the nation's architectural press that the most progressive tendencies in American architecture were in the Midwest. Wright's own series of articles in *The Architectural Record* titled "In the Cause of Architecture" (1909) were perhaps the clearest evidence of this evaluation. International recognition came with the publication of the famous Wasmuth folio on his work (Berlin, 1910) and with the influential articles of Hendrik Berlage for the *Schweizerische Bauzeitung* in 1911. These publications had substantial impact on the Modern movement in Europe.

For Wright the climax of his Prairie period came with the great houses of 1908–09, particularly the Robie (1908) and Coonley (1909) houses, the first in Chicago and the second in Riverside, Illinois. Among public buildings, his major achievements were Unity Temple (1904–05) in Oak Park and the headquarters for the Larkin Company in Buffalo, New York, done in the same years. The Prairie School idiom, however, was not one that lent itself easily to large public buildings and industrial structures. There are a few of these. In the latter category, Hugh Garden made some noteworthy contributions with the Grommes and Ullrich Building (1901), the Schoenhofen Brewery (1905), and the Dwight Building (1910), all in Chicago. The last structure was for a printing company and was framed in flat-slab concrete. The Prairie School architects also did a few churches. Of these, Sullivan's Methodist Episcopal Church (1910) in Cedar Rapids, Iowa, with a contribution by George Elmslie, is perhaps the finest. On the whole, however, the Prairie School aesthetic lent itself to houses and small commercial buildings, and it is these building types by which its practitioners should be judged.

Prairie School architects attempted almost every problem in the decorative arts, and they had great success with chairs, tables, case furniture, fabrics, and perhaps most important of all, leaded glass; their achievements would have been impossible without the cooperation of cabinetmakers such as John W. Ayers and glass studios such as Giannini and Hilgart and the Linden Glass Company; and for Wright, the assistance of the Milwaukee interior decorator George Niedieken was vital in such large commissions as the Robie and Coonley houses and the May house (1909) in Grand Rapids, Michigan. The architects saw building as a cooperative process in which client, designer, and artisan all had important roles to play. Among themselves, they deplored the tendency of Wright to claim all the credit for their achievement, as he commonly did after 1913–14.

In certain respects, the Prairie School style can be understood as an idiom that could be employed by architects who had little or no contact with Wright, Sullivan, or Chicago. For the central figures—Wright, Sullivan, Griffin, and Purcell and Elmslie—architectural design was an act of faith, an optimistic faith in the liberal ideals of American democracy. They liked to think

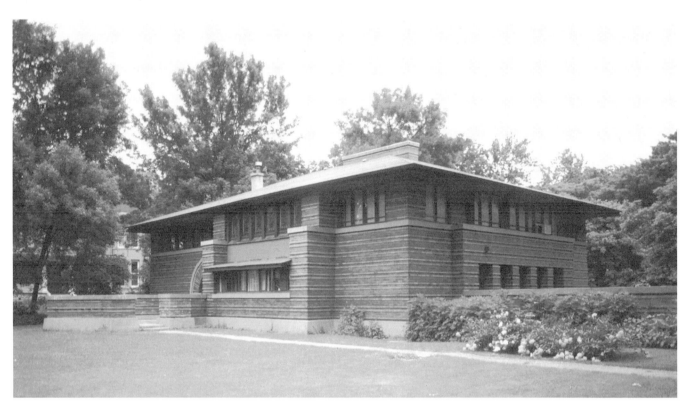

Arthur Heurtley House, Oak Park, Illinois, designed by Frank Lloyd Wright (1902)
Photo © Mary Ann Sullivan

of their architecture as "progressive" and strongly disliked the academic traditionalism of McKim, Mead and White and their Eastern contemporaries. In fact, they viewed it as a rehash of outworn European forms. The Prairie School manner, however, was sufficiently attractive that it was sometimes employed by architects who had relatively little sympathy with the ideals of the leaders. Thus, Osgood and Osgood in Grand Rapids, a firm that was essentially eclectic, did two houses in a distinctly Prairie School manner. These dwellings might well have been responses to client demand. Sidney Robinson and Richard Guy Wilson have shown that Iowa is dotted with buildings that have Prairie School elements. The same kind of demonstration could easily be made for Minnesota, Wisconsin, and Illinois. Wilson and Robinson also argue that the Prairie School had two distinct and separate phases. The first has been identified as from 1900 to about 1920. They date the second from Wright's return to the Midwest in the 1930s and cite his later Iowa houses and the work of Alfred Caldwell in Dubuque. This position is arguable, and it has recently received support in *Frank Lloyd Wright and Colleagues: Indiana Works* (Michigan City, Indiana, 1999). This exhibition catalog also includes certain projects by the landscape architect Jens Jensen, whose stature in his field is comparable to that of Wright in the building arts. Jensen certainly had a prominent role in the development of the Prairie symbolism.

The gradual decline of the original Prairie School after 1914 was the result of several broad historical factors. For a variety of reasons, the supply of clients willing to accept the innovations advocated by the architects dwindled considerably. Women were

becoming increasingly important in American society, and as Thomas Tallmadge pointed out, wives now received their education from magazines edited in Boston and New York. In 1910 *House Beautiful*, which had always been sympathetic to the Prairie School architects, moved its offices to New York. The last prairie houses appeared in its pages in 1914. The story of *Country Life in America* is similar. Its last mention of a prairie house was in January 1914, when it featured a dwelling in Seattle by Andrew Willatzen, who had worked in Wright's office and absorbed some of his thought. The general shift of the publishing industry to New York had enormous consequences for the cultural life of the entire nation, as it meant a homogenization of American culture. The Prairie School had flourished as a healthy type of regionalism, and regionalism became unfashionable.

The architects themselves withdrew from the Midwestern scene. Wright's personal life was chaotic, and he spent much of the decade of World War I in Japan. Sullivan, the philosophical leader of the group, was able to build only a handful of small banks and gradually descended into poverty and alcoholism. Walter Burley Griffin and Marion Mahony, two of Wright's most talented apprentices, went to Australia in 1913 and spent most of their careers in that country. Purcell went to Philadelphia in 1918 to enter the advertising business and in 1922 moved to the West Coast because of ill health. Nonetheless, the achievement of the Prairie School was substantial, and it left the Midwest a great legacy in the form of a large number of buildings that are sought out and admired to this day.

LEONARD K. EATON

See also **Chicago, (IL), United States; Griffin, Walter Burley, and Marion Mahony Griffin (United States); Larkin Building, Buffalo, New York; National Farmers' Bank, Owatonna, Minnesota; Purcell, William Gray, and George Grant Elmslie (United States); Robie House, Chicago; Sullivan, Louis (United States); Taliesin West, near Phoenix, Arizona; Unity Temple, Oak Park, Illinois; Wright, Frank Lloyd (United States)**

Further Reading

The drawings of Frank Lloyd Wright are held by the Taliesin Foundation in Scottsdale, Arizona. The Northwest Architectural Archives at the University of Minnesota holds the Purcell and Elmslie Collection, whereas the Prairie Archives at the Milwaukee Art Museum holds those of George Niedecken. The Burnham Library at the Chicago Art Institute and the Avery Library at Columbia University also have many drawings relating to the Prairie School.

Art museums across the United States own examples of Prairie School work in the decorative arts including the Chicago Art Institute, Milwaukee Art Museum, and Minneapolis Art Institute, Minnesota. The Metropolitan Museum of Art in New York has the important triptych of windows from the Coonley Playhouse and has restored the living room of the Francis Little house (Wayzata, Minnesota, 1913). Both of these are works by Frank Lloyd Wright. Several of Wright's prairie houses have been restored. The most notable ones are the Susan Lawrence Dana house (Springfield, Illinois, 1902) and the Meyer May house (Grand Rapids, Michigan, 1909). A restoration of the Robie house (Chicago, 1908) is in process.

The literature on Frank Lloyd Wright is enormous and continues to expand. Aside from the important but often misleading *An Autobiography* (New York and London: Longman Green, 1932), the most significant comprehensive works for Wright's prairie period are:

Ausgefuhrte Bauten and Entwurfe von Frank Lloyd Wright, Berlin: Wasmuth, 1910; reprint, Tubingen: Wasmuth, 1986; as *Studies and Executed Buildings*, London: Architectural Press, and New York: Rizzoli, 1986
Brooks, Harold Allen, *The Prairie School: Frank Lloyd Wright and His Midwest Contemporaries*, Toronto: University of Toronto Press, 1972; New York: Norton, 1976
Hitchcock, Henry-Russell, *In the Nature of Materials, 1887–1941: The Buildings of Frank Lloyd Wright*, New York: Duell Sloan and Pierce, and London: Elek Books, 1942
Hoffmann, Donald, *Frank Lloyd Wright's Robie House: The Illustrated Story of an Architectural Masterpiece*, New York: Dover, 1984
Hoffmann, Donald, *Frank Lloyd Wright: Architecture and Nature*, New York: Dover, 1986
Hoffmann, Donald, *Understanding Frank Lloyd Wright's Architecture*, New York: Dover, 1995
Hoffmann, Donald, *Frank Lloyd Wright's Dana House*, Mineola, New York: Dover, 1996
The Life-Work of the American Architect Frank Lloyd Wright, edited by H.-T. Wijdeveld, Santpoort, Holland: C.A. Mees, 1925; reprint, New York: Horizon Press, 1965
Manson, Grant Carpenter, *Frank Lloyd Wright to 1910*, New York: Reinhold, 1958; London: Van Nostrand Reinhold, 1979
Storer, William Allin, *The Frank Lloyd Wright Companion*, Chicago: University of Chicago Press, 1993
Van Zanten, David T. (editor), *Walter Burley Griffin: Selected Designs* (Palos Park, Illinois: Prairie School Press, 1970)

The files of *The Prairie School Review* published by Bill and Marilyn Hasbrook of Park Forest, Illinois, from 1964 to 1972 is another invaluable source of information. Particularly notable are the articles by Joseph Griggs on Iannelli (2, 4, 1965), David T. Van Zanten on Marion Mahoney Griffin (3, 2, 1966), Donald Hoffman on Parker Berry (4, 1, 1967), and Robert E. McCoy on Griffin's work at Mason City (5, 3, 1968). Through the Prairie School Press, the Hasbroucks have also made available reprints of many important Prairie School documents such as the original publication on Purcell and Elmslie in *The Western Architect*. In the end, however, the most important documentation of the Prairie School is the buildings themselves. They stand as the legacy of an era in which the Midwest, in no uncertain terms, challenged the traditional cultural leadership of the East. As the years pass, the challenge looks increasingly significant.

PRECAST CONCRETE

Precast construction typically refers to concrete that is manufactured in a factory rather than at the site. Poured-in-place concrete, in contrast, is a process where formwork and reinforcing bars are set and the wet concrete and its aggregates poured in the precise position that they are to occupy in the completed building. Poured-in-place construction allows contractors to tailor the various components of a building and more easily compensate for minor discrepancies discovered during the course of a project. In many cases, however, precast construction offers both technical and cost advantages. Precast components are manufactured in factories, transported to the site, and then assembled and fastened together on the job. They may or may not be reinforced, but if so, they are usually prestressed.

The technical advantages of forming reinforced-concrete components in a factory first involve environmental factors. Heat and humidity influence the length of time that concrete requires to set and cure as well as its load-bearing strength. The factory environment allows manufacturers to control these atmospheric variables far better than at a site. Precast structural members are often designed at higher strength than most on-site counterparts (which are designed typically for 3,000 pounds per square inch, 28 days after pouring). Temperature can be raised in a factory, accelerating the amount of time that concrete requires to cure. Also, reinforcing can be more precisely set into place, and the tolerances and coverage of concrete around the reinforcing steel can be more accurately controlled, thus producing more efficient structural components. Complex rebar configurations and more accurate lapping of one rebar over another can be more easily managed and inspected in a factory, where the movement of laborers and technicians is not inhibited by on-site obstacles. Site conditions are also rarely conducive to the pretightening of steel tendons, and thus prestressed structural sections are far easier to construct in a factory setting. Prestressing is a process where steel cables called tendons are anchored to the ends of formwork and tensioned before concrete is poured. After the concrete hardens and gains sufficient strength, the cables are released. This internally applies a precompressive stress, which potentially reduces or minimizes undesirable tensile stresses created by the structural member's own weight as well as the load that it will have to support once installed in the building. Prestressing tends to minimize cracking as well as de-

flections. Finally, factory conditions also tend to allow better control over the finished appearance of concrete, including surface sheen, aggregate density, and color.

The cost advantages of precast construction derive from an economy of scale. Factory settings are economical when manufacturing multiple copies of the same component. Poured-in-place construction requires assembling the formwork for components on-site, setting the rebar, pouring the concrete, and then removing the formwork for reassembly at the next pour, usually requiring more time and labor than manufacturing the equivalent part in a factory. This is important because it can have a significant impact on the overall cost and length of time to complete a building project.

Precast construction comes with inherent limits, however, dictated primarily by the problem of transportation. Manufactured components must be transported from the factory to the building site via ship, train, or truck and sometimes by a combination of means. Consequently, components must not be so long or heavy that they prohibit transportation. Generally, components longer than 30 feet are impractical. Weight is an especially crucial factor in transportation, and it is common for engineers to anticipate the problem of transport by incorporating steel hooks or loops anchored in the concrete for the purpose of lifting and lowering by crane. The cost-effectiveness of precast construction can be compromised by building sites located in remote areas or in regions where infrastructure is insufficient. A mountainous site, for example, may be a poor choice for precast construction if existing roads twist and turn at radii that a large truck cannot negotiate.

The ramifications of precast construction affect both engineering and aesthetics. Construction schedules must be carefully planned so that needed components arrive on-site when needed. Since some parts may be built on-site and others manufactured in a remote factory, and in many cases precast components may be manufactured in separate factories miles apart, the interface between components is a crucial concern of engineers and architects. A kit-of-parts approach to construction encourages the manufacturing of standardized parts that can fit together in a variety of configurations. Generally, irregular building designs can be problematic, while modularity tends to be advantageous in precast construction.

The most common precast structural components tend to be linear: beams, ribbed beams (also called T beams), inverted T beams, solid flat slabs, hollow-core slabs, and tilt-up wall panels. Unreinforced-concrete components include wall panels with specific finishes either poured or applied as veneer. Unlike poured-in-place reinforced concrete, precast construction lacks the structural advantage of continuity, where rebar segments can be lapped in a series the entire length of a structure. This is why connections between components require great care. Slip-slab construction is a hybrid method where floor slabs are poured on grade at the site, then lifted into place by jacks secured to building columns. This process is cost-effective for multistory buildings with repetitive floor configurations since the forms do not need to be moved from one floor to the next. However, the connection between floor slabs and columns requires the same expertise as precast construction connections.

JERRY WHITE

Further Reading

Nawy provides an excellent technical analysis of the material and its potential, while Merritt's prescriptive discussion gives practical construction information and addresses the important issue of interfacing with other systems. Ching and Adams, however, is the best source for illustrated information.

Ching, Francis D.K. and Cassandra Adams, *Building Construction Illustrated*, New York: Van Nostrand Reinhold, 1975; 3rd edition, New York: Wiley, 2001

Merritt, Frederick S. (editor), *Building Construction Handbook*, New York: McGraw-Hill, 1958; 6th edition, as *Building Design and Construction Handbook*, edited by Jonathan T. Ricketts, 2000

Nawy, Edward G., *Reinforced Concrete: A Fundamental Approach*, Englewood Cliffs, New Jersey: Prentice-Hall, 1985; 4th edition, 2000

Precast Concrete Institute, *Architectural Precast Concrete*, Chicago: PCI Institute, 1989

Precast Concrete Institute, *PCI Design Handbook, Precast and Prestressed Handbook*, Chicago: PCI Institute, 1971; 5th edition, 1999

PREDOCK, ANTOINE 1936–

Architect, United States

The architectural vision of Antoine Predock is spiritual, environmental, and symbolic. His work, grounded in ideas derived from the varied landscapes of the American Southwest, returns to architecture a mysterious connection with place and human feeling that many believe has been eroded by 20th-century life. A key element in his approach to design is context. For Predock, however, context goes beyond contextualism to embrace the site and all that will happen there over time. Predock has applied his architectural vision to a variety of building types, but his ideology is most vivid in his institutional works—such as the Spencer Theater for the Performing Arts (1998) in Alto, New Mexico; the Arizona Science Center (1997) in Phoenix; and the American Heritage Center Art Museum (1993) at the University of Wyoming, Laramie—and in his designs for domestic space, including the Venice House (1991) in Venice, California; the Rosenthal House (1993) in Manhattan Beach, California; and the Hotel Santa Fe (1992) at Euro Disney, outside Paris.

Predock's work is affected by all his life experiences, ranging from a visit to the Egyptian pyramids to a ride on his motorcycle. He received his bachelor of architecture degree from Columbia University in New York City in 1962 after beginning his education at the University of New Mexico in Albuquerque in 1957. While a student in New York, he became involved in the art of dance. Predock translated the movement of the body in dance into spatial elements within his architecture as both a strong processional component and a focus on an accumulation of viewpoints. Through the many different buildings of the complex, the Nelson Fine Arts Center (1989) at Arizona State University in Tempe architecturally offers a number of processional choices that are further multiplied by the transition from daytime to nighttime. The complex can also be interpreted as a piece of performance art with its numerous balconies, arcades, loggias,

and steps, each providing a different stage for the user to engage and act on.

Predock's early work was relatively modest in scale. After working for three years as a designer in the offices of I.M. Pei and Partners in New York City and Gerald McCue Associates in San Francisco, Predock founded his own firm in Albuquerque in 1967. The four-person office built its reputation on houses and institutional buildings that blended comfort with the vernacular Southwest image, depicted by Predock in the employment of natural desert colors and contextual materials in a tough, defensive architecture. The 1986 completion of the Fuller House in Scottsdale, Arizona, marked the national and international recognition of his bold, abstracted, and original style. The house is deeply set into the earth and oriented with respect to the east–west axis, which provides the potential heating and cooling properties of each room. Nature is brought into the design through the inclusion of a sunrise terrace and a sunset tower separated by a circular pool, which acts as the terminus of the water channel that runs parallel to the east–west axis of the house.

Inspired by architects such as Louis I. Kahn and Frank Lloyd Wright, Predock included with his regional sensibility the ele-ments of the modern in his 1993 design of the Turtle Creek House in Dallas, Texas. Giant limestone ledges recall the geologic setting of Dallas, and the great glass wall recalls architecture of the International Style. The house, surrounded with trees and plantings, provided a specialized setting for the patrons who were avid bird-watchers. Not only do the plantings welcome the birds but also the siting of the house along the major north–south migratory flyways greets the feathered creatures. This same axis also became the dominant processional path through the house.

Predock's interpretation of the Tucson, Arizona, environment dictated the design of the Ventana Vista Elementary School (1995). From a distance, this "city for children" nestles into the landscape and color palette of the desert site. At the heart of the complex, Predock placed a large white tent, reminding the children of the larger environment and imparting his notion that life in the desert was not always so predictable or sedentary. The fourth- and fifth-grade neighborhood is located on the highest part of the site. The walls of this neighborhood's classrooms are easily opened up to the exterior by large rolled-up garage doors. The second- and third-grade neighborhood revolves around spaces for reading, such as the sorcerer's terrace, and

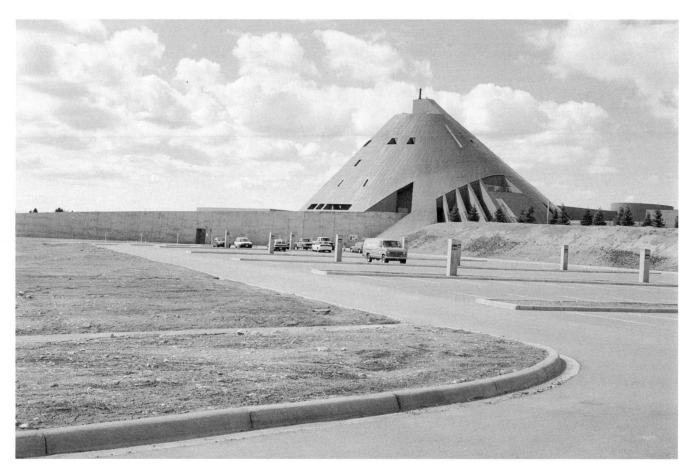

American Heritage Center and University Art Museum, University of Wyoming, Laramie, designed by Antoine Predock (1993)
© G.E. Kidder Smith/CORBIS

spaces for contemplation and dreaming, including the desert kaleidoscope, where children can peer through cylindrical skylights into a shallow dome and out to the sky. The sense of discovery continues for all children on the path to the celestial realm and the solstice wall, the apertures of which not only frame distinct views of the landscape and sky but also align with the sun during the summer and winter solstices. Spy holes in the classroom walls enable children to catch a glimpse of their classmates at work.

Predock's firm continues to receive outstanding commissions, including the San Diego Padres Park at the Park in San Diego, California, and the Cornerstone Arts Center at Colorado College in Colorado Springs. Underway at the University of Minnesota in Minneapolis is the Gateway Center, a granite-clad geode attached to two parallel copper boxes. Its architectural distinctiveness draws from Minnesota themes, particularly in the 90-foot-high granite geode that evokes Lake Superior's north shore. Fissures of glass, allowing natural light in during the day and bathing the surrounding area with projected light at night, crisscross the granite planes. The Gateway Center illustrates Predock's fascination with engineering and architecture, developed early in his career at the University of New Mexico under the tutelage of his mentor, Don Schlegel.

Predock's creative and insightful work has won numerous worldwide awards and has been the subject of many architectural exhibitions. His projects, invigorated by the form and spirit of the place, including its environment, rituals, and culture, have brought to architecture a soul and character unknown in the work of many of his contemporaries. Although his buildings are not easily copied in the formal sense, the ideology of his design provides an exciting model for those practicing today. For Predock, architecture is more than a fleeting moment in a designer's mind. A building has a life all its own, one that takes on a magical quality from things that come before, during, and after its original conception. As Predock has stated, "We remind ourselves that we are involved in a timeless encounter with another place, not just a little piece of land. All of the readings that have accumulated and been assimilated there, that are imagined there, that may happen there in the future—all of these collapse in time and become the raw material with which we interact."

VICTORIA M. YOUNG

Biography

Born in Lebanon, Missouri, 24 June 1936. Attended the University of New Mexico, Albuquerque 1957–61; bachelor's degree in architecture 1962; studied at Columbia University, New York on a traveling fellowship. In private practice, Albuquerque from 1967. Kea Distinguished Professor, University of Maryland, School of Architecture 1981–82; visiting professor, Arizona State University 1982–83 and 1983–84; visiting professor, Southern California Institute of Architecture 1984 and 1990; visiting professor, Harvard University, Cambridge, Massachusetts 1987; architect in residence, California State Polytechnic University, Pomona 1988; distinguished visiting professor, Clemson University, South Carolina 1988; distinguished visiting professor, University of Genoa 1988. Fellow, American Institute of Architects.

Selected Works

Fuller House, Scottsdale, Arizona, 1986
Nelson Fine Arts Center, Arizona State University, Tempe, 1989
Venice House, California, 1991
Hotel Santa Fe, Euro Disney Theme Park, near Paris, 1992
Turtle Creek House, Dallas, Texas, 1993
Rosenthal House, Manhattan Beach, California, 1993
American Heritage Center Art Museum, University of Wyoming, Laramie, 1993
Ventana Vista Elementary School, Tucson, Arizona, 1995
Arizona Science Center, Phoenix, Arizona, 1997
Spencer Theater for the Performing Arts, Alto, New Mexico, 1998

Selected Publication

Italian Sketchbooks, 1985

Further Reading

Information about Predock's work is available in all genres of media. A select yet highly comprehensive bibliography, as well as a complete list of his designs and awards, can be found in *Antoine Predock, Architect* and *Antoine Predock, Architect 2*.

Baker, Geoffrey Howard, *Antoine Predock*, Chichester, West Sussex: Academy Editions, 1997
Predock, Antoine, *Antoine Predock, Architect,* compiled by Brad Collins and Juliette Robbins, New York: Rizzoli, 1994
Predock, Antoine, *Architectural Journeys*, compiled by Brad Collins and Elizabeth Zimmerman, New York: Rizzoli, 1995
Predock, Antoine, *Antoine Predock, Architect 2*, edited by Brad Collins and Elizabeth Zimmerman, New York: Rizzoli, 1998
Predock, Antoine, *Turtle Creek House: Antoine Predock*, New York: Monacelli Press, 1998
Zabalbeascoa, Anatxu (editor), *Antoine Predock: Architecture of the Land*, Barcelona: Gili, 2000

PREFABRICATION

Buildings are traditionally constructed by assembling materials and components of the building trades according to an approved set of design drawings and specifications on a given site. Having a smooth and timely pace for erecting buildings is highly dependent on the quality and steadiness of supplies, the availability of qualified labor, a safe and conflict-free working environment, and, last but not least, the weather. Because all these more or less controllable variables pose substantial risks, the desire to standardize the design and to relocate the production process into a highly controllable, productive factory environment is an old dream of builders and clients alike. The technique dates back to the early stages of industrialization, at the turn of the 20th century, with prime examples being London's Crystal Palace, built in 1851 for the Great Exhibition in Hyde Park, London, by Joseph Paxton, and cast-iron building facades created for commercial structures in the fire hazard–prone early metropolitan areas of our times.

The term "prefabrication" in architecture normally describes the assembly of buildings or their components at a location other than the building site. With the help of this method, the risk-creating variables of cost control, weather, and a dependable and, because of repetition, experienced workforce helps to optimize the use of materials and time in a controlled environment.

Prefabricated units can range from singular building parts that later find their way into a conventional on-site construction project, such as doors, windows, and roof trusses, to room-size elements, from bathrooms to entire buildings. Prefabrication can also take place on-site if the scope of the project is very large, as in the case of housing developments of the 1960s, 1970s, and 1980s in Eastern Europe, the former Soviet Union, and Scandinavia.

Historically, the main materials for prefabrication are wood, iron, and concrete. Early traces of wood for prefabrication date back to the 1848 gold rush in the United States; experiments with prefabricated housing units made of wood in Great Britain, Germany, and Sweden were conducted between the two world wars. In 1850 in New York, complete wooden houses where shipped as building kits to California in response to the huge demand in the West. Several hundred housing units made of other materials, such as corrugated galvanized iron, were imported from Manchester, England, completely fitted with wallpaper, water closets, and furniture to satisfy the demand for housing in California, where an established building industry was not yet available. Patented plantation and camp buildings produced by lumber dealers in New York and Boston consisted of a number of interchangeable parts and could be erected in hours. In Germany the company of Christoph and Unmack, founded in 1882, produced load-bearing wood panels for cabins and camp buildings that were shipped in very large quantities to many parts of the world. The oldest known U.S. firm specializing in prefabrication was founded in Boston in 1892. Ernest F. Hodgson manufactured dwellings of wood, which the firm labeled in a patent, dating back to 1861, "the portable house." Other derivatives of early prefabrication in the United States are so-called mail-order houses. Companies such as Sears, Roebuck, and Company (Newark, New Jersey), Montgomery Ward (Chicago, Illinois), Aladdin Company (Bay City, Michigan), Gordon-Van Tine Company (Davenport, Iowa), and many others produced "precut" timber kits of parts, designed for owner erection. Many might consider the system of precutting not to be a true prefabrication process. The enormous number of produced units, the industrialized process of factory-controlled cost estimating, the purchasing and cutting of wood products, numbering industrialized quality control, and packaging all were carried out in a efficient factory-assembly-line manner. Between 1908 and 1940, customers ordered some 100,000 houses from Sears, Roebuck, and Company alone. The designs could be selected from a catalog, ordered by mail, and shipped by rail. Approximately 450 ready-to-assemble designs covered almost every style, from cottage to mansion. Beside Sears's brick and concrete masonry unit homes, the traditional wood frame erected on a wooden platform was used as the standard method of construction.

Industry in the United States also experimented with concrete and iron as prefabrication methods. In 1920 story-height precast reinforced-concrete stone elements were produced under trade names such as "Armostone," "Moore Unit," and "Tee-Stone." Frank Lloyd Wright designed a precast system in 1920 that consisted of two precast-element walls: one interior wall and one outside, reinforced and connected with tie-rods and separated by an insulating air space. The large sizes of concrete elements made handling on a conventionally equipped, small-scale construction site difficult. Smaller-scaled precast units, such as 16-by-8-by-8-inch concrete blocks, were, and still are today, more widely accepted.

Early experiments of prefabrication in Great Britain with elements made of iron date to Victorian times, when numerous prefabricated buildings were shipped from Britain to every corner of the world. British settlers on the Australian west coast could order corrugated-iron cottages from the Phoenix Iron Works in Glasgow, Scotland, and from the firm of Richard Walker. Other requests from Australia called for the shipment of "portable" churches, temporary metal structures to replace the hastily improvised timber structures of the early days. In Melbourne alone, 19 metal churches were erected with kits shipped from the homeland between 1836 and 1851. When it was packed and ready for shipment to the colonies, a church weighed about 50 tons; the cost in the second half of the 19th century was £1000, and the building was ready to be used in five weeks. Before shipment to foreign coasts, it was common practice to fully assemble the structure on the grounds of the factory as a final quality check, which always attracted public attention. The lighthouse in Gibb's Hill, Bermuda, is a sturdy, prefabricated iron structure shipped from England in 1857; the so-called Gordon's Lighthouse in Barbados, a fully prefabricated-metal construction, stood for 112 years. The Iron Palace for King Eyambo on the banks of the Calabar River in Nigeria, erected in 1843, was built by the foundry of Laycock, Liverpool, "a composite structure of plate and panels of iron upon a wooden skeleton merely," as the *Liverpool Times* described it.

Besides prefabricated galvanized sheet-metal elements, cast iron contributed to a large degree to the importance of metal prefabrication techniques. James Bogardus is more identified with the advances of cast-iron prefabrication than any other inventor. Already holding numerous patents for metal fabricating tools and mills, Bogardus conceived the idea of taking cast iron beyond its already widely accepted role as a decorative building material to a multistory structural system. His first building would be his own factory in New York City, for which he tried to associate with other veteran iron makers to raise the necessary funds. Bogardus's system consisted of basic elements: a hollow column with flanged sides, a C-shaped hollow beam, a spandrel panel, and a diversity of decorative cast-iron elements, such as cornices, entablatures, window elements, cornerstones, and Medusa-head keystones, the trademark of the Bogardus Ironworks. With these decorative elements, which suited the Victorian taste of the time, a variety of designs could be created. The buildings were assembled by bolted connections, hidden on the inside of every element, forming rigid moment connections between columns and beams. Bogardus was granted a patent for his "building system" in 1850. It did not take long for numerous commercial buildings with cast-iron facades to surface, and other founders and builders created competition. It was also clear that the new technique would not be confined to New York but instead would spread to every major commercial center in the United States. Stove makers, founders of cook pots, and hardware manufacturers soon entered the field of cast-iron architecture. Part of the attraction of cast iron as a building material was its fire resistance. Despite Bogardus's claim that his own factory was made entirely out of metal, many cast-iron buildings used a significant amount of timber and stone building materials. Many of Bogardus's own designs, both in Baltimore (1904) and

in Chicago (1871), were consumed by fire. At the end of the Victorian period, the material and the associated prefabrication techniques fell out of favor. Despite early hopes, they were not fire safe, nor could they resist strong winds, as shown by the entirely demolished cast-iron warehouses in Havana, Cuba—destroyed in 1906 by a hurricane.

Neither fire safety nor resistance against wind is a major concern for reinforced precast concrete. With the invention of heavy trucks in the 1930s, reinforced precast concrete elements could be transported to almost every construction site. The first modern use of precast concrete was in the Notre Dame du Haut Cathedral in Raincy, France, by the architect-engineer Auguste Perret in 1922. The main structural systems of the church still show a largely in situ concrete system, yet the wide use of precast elements for in-fill walls and partitions led the way for the industry. Such is the case with iron: prefabricated structures in concrete can be distinguished as load-bearing elements, such as columns, beams, and floor slabs, and in-fill materials and components, such as windows, panels, and utility cores. Yet concrete lends itself to a few interesting new techniques, developed in the years before World War II and employed in the years after the war, that are uncommon in any other prefabricated process. The technique of a "lift slab" casts the reinforced-concrete slabs of a multistory building on grade, one over the other, with sleeves designed for slab connections to previously erected columns. After the curing process is completed, the "stack" of slabs is lifted into place and bonded to the connections with the vertical structural member, the column. Volumetric steel forms with a high degree of precision and built-in heating equipment to accelerate the curing process can produce U-shaped "tunnel forms" stacked on top of each other. It was mostly building types with a high degree of equally sized room cells, such as hotels and apartment buildings, that were erected with this method. Advantages to prefabrication methods employing concrete are an organized, orderly supply and storage of aggregates at a different place than the site of erection; a clean construction site; the multiple re-use of expensive formwork; and the improved surface quality of the finished product. Despite these advantages, the prefabrication of entire room cells (or "big boxes") or ceiling-height big panels never caught on in the United States. In Europe, South America, and the former Soviet Union, including most of its allies, a significant number of housing projects were carried out with prefabricated-concrete panels. Notable innovations in the technique originated in Scandinavia and France and were paralleled by extensive large-scale developments in East Germany, Yugoslavia, and the Soviet Union. Most of the panel systems in these cases were based on the full wall-size big panels. Despite the large number of projects executed, big panels proved to be expensive overall, called for multitude of joints that had to be made in the field, and seldom permitted the degree of prefinishing and shop incorporation of utilities as originally anticipated.

Today, prefabricated "architectural" precast concrete is widely used in the United States and worldwide mainly as building components (not as a primary structural material), either for enclosure or highly repetitive elements, such as staircases. The surface quality of architectural precast concrete produced in developed countries is high compared with the beginnings of the industry. Because of the advantages in thermal properties over glass, mainly because of thermal mass inertia, precast concrete for building envelopes has the chance to become a prime material in times of increased energy costs.

RALPH HAMMANN

See also **Concrete; Notre Dame, Le Raincy; Precast Concrete; Reinforced Concrete**

Further Reading

Bruce, Alfred and Harold Sandbank, *A History of Prefabrication*, New York: John B. Pierce Foundation, 1945

Dietz, Albert G.H. and Lawrence S. Cutler (editors), *Industrialized Building Systems for Housing*, Cambridge, Massachusetts: MIT Press, 1971

Freedman, Sidney (editor), *Architectural Precast Concrete*, Chicago: Precast Prestressed Concrete Institute, 1973; 2nd edition, 1989

Gayle, Margot *Cast-Iron Architecture in New York*, New York: Dover, 1974

Gayle, Margot and Carol Gayle, *Cast-Iron Architecture in America: The Significance of James Bogardus*, New York: Norton, 1998

Gibb, Alistair G.F., *Off-Site Fabrication*, Latheronwheel, Scotland: Whittles, and New York: Wiley, 1999

Herbert, Gilbert, *Pioneers of Prefabrication: The British Contribution in the Nineteenth Century*, Baltimore, Maryland: Johns Hopkins University Press, 1978

The International Prefabricated Housing Design Competition, Tokyo: Misawa Homes Institute of Research and Development, 1973

Kelly, Burnham, *The Prefabrication of Houses*, Cambridge, Massachusetts: MIT Press, and New York: Wiley, 1951

Sackett, James, *Modular Housing: An Introduction to Building Using a Factory Approach*, Arlington, Massachusetts: Cutter Information Corporation, 1990

Segre, Roberto, *Arquitectura y urbanismo de la revolución Cubana*, Havana: Editorial Pueblo y Educación, 1989

Stevenson, Katherine Cole, *Houses by Mail: A Guide to Houses from Sears, Roebuck, and Company*, Washington, D.C.: Preservation Press, 1986

Vale, Brenda, *Prefabs: A History of the UK Temporary Housing Programme*, London: Spon, 1995

Waite, Diana S. (editor), *Architectural Elements*, Princeton, New Jersey: Pyne Press, 1972

White, R.B., *Prefabrication: A History of Its Development in Great Britain*, London: HMSO, 1965

PRIMITIVISM

Primitivism is a set of ideas arising in Western Europe during the 18th century, a period of unprecedented European colonial expansion. Primitivism does not name a group of artists or architects or a style arising at a particular moment but, rather, encompasses the various responses produced by contact between Western and non-Western societies during the colonial period. It has three primary meanings: a belief in the superiority of a simple life close to nature, a belief in the superiority of non-industrial society to that of the present, and a valorization of the art and architecture of primitive peoples or primitive creators. All three definitions indicate that primitivism is a critical attitude toward present society, culture, and art and a preference for societies, cultures, and art from simpler times, states of evolution, or mentalities. It is also used to indicate the art and architecture of primitive peoples or cultures, although this is not a correct usage, as primitivism is a phenomenon of Western culture, not the product of "primitive" peoples. The word *primitivism*

(*primitivisme*) was used first in France in the 19th century; William Rubin traces its appearance to the *Nouveau Larousse* between 1897 and 1904, meaning "imitation of primitives." The term *primitive* has a wide range of meanings, including original, primeval, little evolved, elemental, natural, naïf, characteristic of an early stage of development, and produced by a relatively simple people or culture or a self-taught artist. This term is generally used to designate societies considered to have a lower level of evolutionary development than Western societies.

There are two tendencies in primitivism: a search for origins in the classical, exemplified by the primitive hut of Enlightenment theories, and the valorization of peasant, vernacular, or non-literate culture as a means for producing a more primal art or architecture. This latter meaning is used extensively in the history of modern art but applies to modern architecture as well. In his groundbreaking book of 1938, *Primitivism in Modern Painting*, Robert Goldwater defined "primitivism" as a search among Western artists for something below the surface of things—further back in time, psychology, or geography—that is simpler and more profound, valuable, or powerful because of its simplicity. The primitivists assumed that delving beneath the surface would reveal this basic quality. This search for simplicity unites the disparate primitivist movements, but the nature of "simplicity" varies with the goals of the seeker. Primitive art is usually, according to Goldwater, a stimulus or catalyst to modern art, not directly borrowed from or the direct cause of primitive qualities in that art. The primitive helped Western artists and architects formulate their own goals and methods and served as a referent, not a direct source. Colin Rhodes, historian of primitivism in modern art, points to an equivocal issue at the heart of primitivism: although artists used the primitive as a support and justification for cultural or social change, their efforts were directed toward change expected to emerge within the West. There was no question of the comprehensive substitution of Western culture, or its unacceptable aspects, by the primitive.

Enlightenment primitivism was motivated by a search for origins, a "higher" source, and a belief in the superiority of a simple life close to nature, exemplified by Montaigne's and Rousseau's valorization of the savage who lived in a more natural, less corrupt state of being. Enlightenment theories of architecture posited a primal architectonic form, the primitive hut, from which all forms of architecture derived. The glorification of the "noble savage," as Peter Collins notes, contributed to the 19th-century revivals of Greek and Gothic architecture and the valorization of such styles as primitive, pure, and natural. In the mid-19th century, artists and architects sought a lost, relatively simple style that was part of their tradition. This form of primitivism demonstrates a preference for non-industrial society to that of the present. A.W.N. Pugin, John Ruskin, and William Morris shared a distaste and distrust for the mechanization and materialism of the industrial age. They called for the revival of medieval art and architecture as a way of healing society and people, who had become extensions of machines rather than whole beings. Their theories stimulated the Gothic Revival, illustrated by Charles Barry and Pugin's Houses of Parliament (1836–51) in London and the Arts and Crafts movement. The Mission Revival in the United States merged Arts and Crafts sensibility with a primitivist vision of early California under the Spanish missionaries (Charles Lummis, El Alisal, Los Angeles, begun 1898).

In the 19th century, the search for primitive origins converged with Darwinism and the "discovery" of primitive civilizations by Western colonizing powers to produce a hierarchy of races and cultures, with Europe and the United States at the apex. Colonization was justified, in part, by reference to the crude technology and material culture of the colonized peoples, seen as a sign of their innate evolutionary inferiority. Certain figures, such as Paul Gauguin, resisted the characterization of non-European culture as inferior; instead, they championed primitive cultures as an alternative to the overcivilized art and intellect of Western society. Primitivist artists appreciated archaic and non-Western styles for their sincerity, vigor, and expressive power, qualities that these artists and architects missed in the official art of their day. Whereas bourgeois society prized the virtuosity and finesse of academic realism and classicism, some artists and architects began to value the simple and naïf and even the crude and raw. Primitivism in this sense is a comparative concept, a theory of difference, and an implicit challenge to the assumption that Western culture was superior to the primitive. The Greene brothers, for example, emulated Japanese architecture in their Gamble House (1908) in Pasadena, California. They took the craftsmanship of the Eastlake and Craftsman styles and combined them with Japanese influences to create a freer attitude toward the organization of spaces and an integrated system of woodwork, stained glass, and custom furniture. Frank Lloyd Wright drew on Japanese and Mayan architecture, recreations of which he saw at the World's Columbian Exhibition of 1893 in Chicago. The effect of Japanese architecture asserted itself in the horizontal lines, unpainted wood, and delicate colors of Wright's Prairie-style work. In his concrete, textile block houses of the 1920s, such as La Miniatura (1923) in Pasadena, Wright may have been inspired by Mayan sculpture and massing.

Art Nouveau, Jugendstil, or Style Liberty was heavily influenced by primitive sources. The "new art," which flourished from about 1893 to 1905, was so called because it rejected historical precedent, academic regulation, and static convention. Art Nouveau borrowed from Japanese decorative art and Mycenaean art and was motivated by a primitivist intent to create a more direct, less refined art by means of light, sinuous ornament and materials. Victor Horta, in Belgium, combined the emphasis on structure of the Gothic Revival, new materials such as iron and plate glass, and the inspiration of natural forms from the Arts and Crafts. Horta's first important Art Nouveau work was the Tassel House (1892–93) in Brussels, in which the twisting iron columns and ornament united with painted decoration to create a total environment of serpentine forms. He used iron without stone cladding along with materials and vocabulary derived from industrial and public buildings, such as railway stations.

By this time, according to Goldwater, the search for beginnings had shifted from cultural to physical–emotional and became a search for "lower" rather than "higher" origins. In the 20th century, exotic, indigenous arts and those made by children and madmen were valued for expressing emotional intensity. Expressionism exhibits this tendency toward emotional primitivism. Expressionist architects in the Netherlands and Germany, such as Michel de Klerk (Eigen Haard, 1917–20, in Amsterdam) and Hans Poelzig (Chemical factory, 1911–12, in Luban), explored highly individualistic, expressive form. Modern architects looked to the primitive as a source of artistic and architectural

stimulus that was not regulated by the norms of European civilization and that would provide the means for a more primal architecture. Bruno Taut wrote several visionary books in the 1910s and 1920s, including *Stadtkrone* (1919), in which he imagined agrarian, craft-based settlements reminiscent of Morris's vision of medieval society. Each city had a crystalline "city crown" (*Stadtkrone*), a religious and spiritual center, designed in pyramidal form like a Gothic cathedral, that acted as a symbol of the community spirit uniting the city's dwellers. The Bauhaus was, at its foundation, based on similar utopian ideals of community and the cooperation of all the arts under architecture. It was a social project for the future, realized through educating a new guild of craftsmen. Architecture would be the one unifying element in society, according to the ideals of the Bauhaus founders. They chose to emulate the Gothic cathedral because all the people of the cathedral towns had participated in building these monuments and because they unified sculpture, painting, weaving, and the other arts within one structure. The Glass Chain participants—Walter Gropius, Bruno and Max Taut, the Luckhardt brothers, Hans Scharoun, and others—explored free, unconscious form, an extension of utopian Expressionism, as an alternative to rational, machine-based design.

Le Corbusier passed through the three types of primitivism during his career. His early work in La Chaux-de-Fonds was part of a regional Arts and Crafts movement, creating design founded on natural forms and vernacular buildings (Villa Stotzer, 1907). After his Voyage d'Orient (1911), Le Corbusier became a staunch advocate of universal, classical language, translated into the undecorated, machine vocabulary that he believed was appropriate for the times (Villa Savoye, 1929, in Poissy). In his later work, he employed vernacular types and emphasized less finished materials, such as brick arches and stone (Maisons Jaoul, 1954–56, in Neuilly). This "peasantism" influenced younger architects, especially members of Team X and the New Brutalists in Britain.

In the post–World War II period, there was a shift toward a universalizing view of humanity: the Family of Man. The earlier emotional primitivism continued, manifested in psychosocial references to primal qualities, such as shelter, enclosure, and place. Bernard Rudofsky's *Architecture without Architects* (1964) devalued professional training and "designed" form in favor of organic, natural architecture produced by indigenous peoples in non-industrialized countries. The New Brutalism, which took its name from Dubuffet's *art brut*, attempted to create a simpler, more immediate architecture that expressed a new aesthetic of coarseness and the primitive. Allison and Peter Smithson's proposal for Golden Lane housing (1952) in London was illustrated with images of Greek islands, working-class backyards, Casbahs, and other dwellings expressive of a place and a way of life. Dutch architect Aldo van Eyck referred to the settlements of the Dogon in Africa and the Pueblos in the southwestern United States to create a more socially responsive architecture, as in his Orphanage (1957–62) in Amsterdam. In Italy the firm BBPR revived elements of the medieval *palazzo* tower in the Torre Velasco (1956–58) in Milan, rendered in concrete. Bruce Goff used an extravagant naturalism in the Bavinger House (1950) in Norman, Oklahoma, as Dell Upton notes, that connects to a wider anti-artificial primitivism. Upton links American primitivism to European trends, with the difference being that the noble savage was the Indian in American mythology.

Postmodernism contains primitivism as a return to high-classical origins and a search for "low" origins in vernacular or popular sources. The rigorous classicism of Quinlan Terry, for example, revived a universal, timeless classical language; by contrast, Charles Moore employed forms derived from such vernacular sources as northern California barns (The Sea Ranch, 1965) and Italian hill towns (Kresge College, University of California, Santa Cruz, 1974). Frank Gehry's appropriation of the ephemeral, vernacular constructions of southern California—lifeguard stations, chain-link fences, plywood walls, and strip-mall stucco (Gehry House, 1977 and 1992, Santa Monica)—exhibits a primitivism of low building sources.

The issue of "primitivism" in Third World countries challenges its definition as a purely Western phenomenon. Work by Western-trained architects such as Hassan Fathy, Luis Barragán, Balkrishna Doshi, and Geoffrey Bawa combines local materials and traditional building forms with modern programs and systems. This postcolonial architecture confounds the hierarchies and patronizing attitude established by social Darwinism, imperialism, and primitivism. Instead of a search for origins in a distant time, place, or culture, these architects produce hybrids of modernism and indigenous forms responsive to particular local conditions. The classical primitive hut has been abandoned in favor of other traditions.

PATRICIA MORTON

Further Reading

Alofsin, Anthony, *Frank Lloyd Wright—The Lost Years, 1910–1922: A Study of Influence*, Chicago: University of Chicago Press, 1993

Collins, Peter, *Changing Ideals in Modern Architecture, 1750–1950*, Montreal: McGill University Press, and London: Faber and Faber, 1965; 2nd edition, Montreal: McGill University Press, 1998

Goldwater, Robert John, *Primitivism in Modern Painting*, New York and London: Harper, 1938; enlarged edition, as *Primitivism in Modern Art*, Cambridge, Massachusetts: Belknap Press, 1986

Harrison, Charles, Francis Frascina, and Gillian Perry, *Primitivism, Cubism, Abstraction: The Early Twentieth Century*, New Haven, Connecticut: Yale University Press, 1993

Montaigne, Michel de, "Des cannibals" in *Les essays*, Paris: Angelier, 1595; as "On the Cannibals" in *Michel de Montaigne: The Complete Essays*, Screech, translated by M.A. New York: Penguin, 1993

Rhodes, Colin, *Primitivism and Modern Art*, New York: Thames and Hudson, 1994

Rousseau, Jean Jacques, *Du contrat social, ou, Principes du droit politique*, Amsterdam: Rey, 1762; as *The Social Contract*, translated by Maurice Cranston, New York: Penguin, 1968

Rubin, William Stanley (editor), *Primitivism in 20th Century Art: Affinity of the Tribal and the Modern*, 2 vols., New York: Museum of Modern Art, 1984

Rykwert, Joseph, *On Adam's House in Paradise: The Idea of the Primitive Hut in Architectural History*, New York and London: Museum of Modern Art; 2nd edition, Cambridge, Massachusetts: MIT Press, 1981

Taut, Bruno, *Die Stadtkrone*, Jena: Diedrichs, 1919; reprint, Nendeln, Lichtenstein: Kraus, 1977

Upton, Dell, *Architecture in the United States*, Oxford and New York: Oxford University Press, 1998

PRISON

The prison is an ancient building type and has always served essentially the same purpose of involuntary detention. The pris-

on's status among architects has varied over time: in the 19th century, the creative possibilities opened by the reinvention of the building type occupied many of architecture's recognized leaders, and hopes for the reform of society through architectural means were widely shared. However, as most of today's experts affirm, this first period of inventiveness generated most of the major ideas in prison architecture: the broad outlines of debate have stayed the same since that time. Private prisons, "direct supervision," and other contemporary preoccupations are simply refinements and restatements of century-old strategies that have come in and out of favor over the years. For most of the 20th century, the construction of prisons was a healthy industry but had relatively little to offer to, or gain from, the architectural imagination.

One of the key principles in the development of modern prison architecture was the attempt to render imprisonment in itself neutral. Other than the deprivation of liberty for a certain length of time according to the offense, the prisoner was, at least theoretically, to suffer no other punishment. This generated a new need for self-contained buildings that could provide for a relatively complete range of human needs and behaviors. The cell in particular stimulated early experiments in central plumbing and heating. Some of the seminal ideas in both architectural and judicial reform were stated by the utilitarian philosopher Jeremy Bentham in his *Panopticon*, first published in 1787. At once an architectural and a social project, the proposed building consisted of a stacked ring of cells open toward a shuttered surveillance tower in the center. Although strict copies of this project were rare, such ideal geometries of surveillance were taken up in a significant number of projects, built and unbuilt, that followed.

Early debates over round-the-clock confinement led to reformers' taking sides between the "Pennsylvania" and "Auburn" systems. The former and more radical of the two had been developed from the 1780s by Quaker reformers, finding its definitive statement in William Haviland's Eastern State Penitentiary, opened in Philadelphia in 1829. Each cell, arranged in double-loaded cell blocks radiating from a central hub, was equipped with complete furnishings for solitary life and work, including a small individual courtyard. Although developed in the United States, the system was much more widely adopted in Europe. The Auburn system, named after a New York State prison completed in 1816 (W. Britten and J. Cray), provided a combination of individual cells for sleeping and spaces for collective—but silent—work by day. Perhaps because it was less expensive to operate, it became the norm in the United States for the next century and a half, and elements of the system are still embraced all over the world. The architecture of the Auburn-style prison placed cells back to back in long, rectangular volumes, separated by a galleried surveillance space from the exterior wall. The main cell block at Alcatraz, completed in 1912 (and now part of a popular national park site), is an example of this approach, which quickly took advantage of advances in reinforced-concrete and steel technology. Here, cells could be smaller and simpler than under the Pennsylvania system, as they were to be used only for sleeping.

The first decades of the 20th century essentially prolonged the 19th century's debate over solitary confinement and its variants. The cell remained the heart of the system, and it continued to be designed as a single-occupancy space, even though popula-tion pressures were such that very few remained so for long. After the radial plans associated with the Pennsylvania system, the barracks-like rectilinear arrangements of the Auburn system, and a few experiments with courtyard and Panopticon-type cylindrical arrangements, all of which had been explored in the 19th century, the 20th century began with a new enthusiasm for what became known as the "telephone-pole" prison. The principle, first seen at Fresnes Prison (1898, F.-H. Poussin) near Paris, was the symmetrical distribution of rectilinear cell blocks along a covered security corridor—the "pole" of the arrangement. This arrangement, like radial plans, put an emphasis on efficient and secure circulation but without the difficulties linked to the use of the triangular outdoor spaces left over.

Beginning in the 1920s and continuing to the present, some city jails on limited sites have been built as high-rise buildings, although these pose special security problems. Not long after, on the eve of World War II, some minimum-security prisons began to be conceived according to a so-called campus or open arrangement, where buildings representing different services would be scattered across a relatively open site plan and where only the perimeter was definitively secured. Like the (physically) similar forced-labor camps found notably in the Soviet Union and Germany at the same time, the architecture inside was less specialized—and less expensive—than that of the high-security institutions. However, as this provocative comparison indicates, the human relations component of incarceration became more central, with corresponding possibilities, as the direct preventive role of the architecture diminished.

Since the 1970s, cell blocks have become "housing units," and surveillance is often deemphasized through the use of less "institutional," but no less carefully placed, guard stations. Indeed, as with hospitals and hotels, the size of new projects is measured in beds, not prisoners or cells. Some experts contend that as such efforts to normalize prison life intensify, the prison itself will dissolve into the community, with only a vestigial presence in the form of decentralized services provided to the inmates. Others predict the increasing dominance of wholly electronic means of surveillance, already in partial and experimental use in several parts of the world. However, apart from an apparent tendency to rely more and more on private subcontractors, most modern states maintain an extensive prison system—led by the United States and Russia, where per capita imprisonment is reaching historic high levels. "Correctional architecture," as prison design is now known, will likely remain an important and lucrative, if somewhat obscure, specialty field in architecture.

DAVID VANDERBURGH

Further Reading

Evans is an excellent analysis of historical and formal issues in prison architecture; although limited to the 19th century, many of the arguments are applicable to the present. Di Gennaro et al. is still probably the most thorough single source for 20th-century projects. Spens surveys some of the most recent realizations, some stylistically ambitious.

Di Gennaro, Giuseppe et al., *Prison Architecture: An International Survey of Representative Closed Institutions and Analysis of Current Trends in Prison Design*, London: Architectural Press, 1975
Evans, Robin, *The Fabrication of Virtue: English Prison Architecture, 1750–1840*, Cambridge and New York: Cambridge University Press, 1982

Foucault, Michel, *Surveiller et punir: Naissance de la prison*, Paris: Galliniard, 1975; as *Discipline and Punish: The Birth of the Prison*, translated by Alan Sheridan, New York: Pantheon, and London: Lane, 1977; 2nd edition, New York: Vintage, 1995

Hopkins, Alfred, *Prisons and Prison Building*, New York: Architectural Book, 1930

Johnston, Norman Bruce, *The Human Cage: A Brief History of Prison Architecture*, New York: Walker, 1973

Spens, Iona (editor), *Architecture of Incarceration*, London: Academy Editions, 1994

Vanderbilt, Tom, "Prison Architecture," available at http://www.stim.com/Stim-x/7.1/Architect/Architect.html.

PRITZKER ARCHITECTURE PRIZE

The Pritzker Architecture Prize, established in 1979 and awarded annually, is a major international prize for architecture given to a living architect for a body of work. Created by Jay and Cindy Pritzker and funded by the Hyatt Corporation through the Hyatt Foundation, the prize is intended to "honor a living architect whose built work demonstrates a combination of those qualities of talent, vision, and commitment, which produced consistent and significant contributions to humanity and the built environment through the art of architecture." From its inception, the prize was intended to increase public awareness of both individual architects and the profession. The high standards for selection, the open nominations procedure, and the independence of the international jury have led to the prize being referred to as the "Nobel Prize" of architecture, after which many of the procedures are modeled. Laureates receive a $100,000 grant, a formal citation certificate, and (since 1987) a bronze medallion. Before 1987 a limited edition Henry Moore sculpture was given to each winner. Although the award is a form of competition, there is no commission for a project to build; rather, the winner receives the honor of being recognized as one of the best in the profession.

There is an open nomination process for the Pritzker Architecture Prize, continuous from year to year, with more than 500 architects under consideration annually. The executive director accepts nominations from any licensed architect and also seeks them actively from critics, the jurors, past prizewinners, professionals in related disciplines, and academics—in short, from anyone interested in advancing the profession of architecture. The nomination procedure closes every January and is followed by jury deliberations in the early part of the year that include site visits to as many projects as possible. These site visits to experience the buildings in context are considered an integral part of the jury process because winners are judged primarily by their built works, not by publications, theoretical ideas, portfolios, or other means. An international jury makes the final selection, and all the jury deliberations and voting are done in secret. A decision and its official announcement are made annually in the spring, followed in May or June by an awards ceremony with a dinner for several hundred members of the architecture and art communities.

The jury consists of eight people on average and has been chaired from the beginning by J. Carter Brown, director emeritus of the National Gallery of Art in Washington, D.C., and chairman of the United States Fine Arts Commission. Jurors are selected for their extensive and broad knowledge of the field, professional integrity, and capacity for unbiased judgment. The Pritzker family participates neither in the selection of the jury nor in the selection of the winner. Jury members have included Cesar Pelli, architect and former dean of the Yale University School of Architecture; Giovanni Agnelli, chairman of Fiat of Torino, Italy; Ada Louise Huxtable, American author and architectural critic; and architects Frank Gehry, Philip Johnson, Arata Isozaki, Ricardo Legorreta, Fumihiko Maki, and Charles Correa. Although the composition of the jury has changed gradually over the course of the prize's first 21 years, its purpose and procedures remain relatively constant.

Although the Pritzker Architecture Prize has achieved its stated goals of making the public more aware of the discipline of architecture and the work of the laureates, some of the weaknesses in the structure of the profession are reflected in the juries' selections. For example, as of the year 2000, no women have been awarded the prize. In addition, because the prize is awarded to a body of work, most of the winners are already established architects. The award has not been a vehicle for the discovery of younger architects, and in general, the juries have historically avoided the avant-garde. Furthermore, the winner's contribution to the discipline and effect on the profession do not always seem to be considered in the decision-making process. In some cases, such as Christian de Portzamparc (1994) and Tadao Ando (1995), the prize was awarded to an architect whose work has not had a significant effect on their peers, whereas more influential architects, such as Jørn Utzon of Denmark, have been overlooked. In the history of architectural awards, the Pritzker is still relatively young, and the extent of its lasting effect remains to be seen.

The Pritzker Architecture Prize laureates to date are Philip Johnson of the United States (1979), Luis Barragán of Mexico (1980), James Stirling of Great Britain (1981), Kevin Roche of the United States (1982), I.M. Pei of the United States (1983), Richard Meier of the United States (1984), Hans Hollein of Austria (1985), Gottfried Boehm of Germany (1986), Kenzo Tange of Japan (1987), Gordon Bunshaft of the United States and Oscar Neimeyer of Brazil (1988), Frank O. Gehry of the United States (1989), Aldo Rossi of Italy (1990), Robert Venturi of the United States (1991), Alvaro Siza of Portugal (1992), Fumihiko Maki of Japan (1993), Christian de Portzamparc of France (1994), Tadao Ando of Japan (1995), Rafael Moneo of Spain (1996), Sverre Fehn of Norway (1997), Renzo Piano of Italy (1998), Sir Norman Foster of the United Kingdom (1999), and Rem Koolhaas of the Netherlands (2000).

LINDA HART

Further Reading

Thorne, Martha (editor), *The Pritzker Architecture Prize: The First Twenty Years*, New York: Abrams, 1999

PRUITT IGOE HOUSING

Designed by Minoru Yamasaki; completed 1954–76
St. Louis, Missouri

Pruitt-Igoe was an early and important post–World War II public housing project. Built on the near north side of St. Louis as

part of a massive urban-renewal program, Pruitt-Igoe was one of the largest public housing complexes in the United States. With 33 buildings rising through 11 stories and towering over 57 acres of the city, it was hailed in the early 1950s as an innovative application of modernist design principles to the problem of chronic urban-housing shortages. At its peak, it housed some 14,000 people in 2870 apartments. Yet by the early 1970s, the project was crumbling and nearly derelict, its residents plagued by crime, isolation, and persistent poverty. Pruitt-Igoe was not only the worst housing project in the city but also one of the most glaring failures of federal housing provision in U.S. history. For many architects, planners, and critics, the demolition of three Pruitt-Igoe buildings in 1972 symbolizes the death of architectural modernism.

Pruitt-Igoe emerged as one piece in a larger postwar urban-renewal program. As with most northern and midwestern cities, World War II had taken a toll on St. Louis, as large numbers of southern black and white migrants streamed into already dense inner-core neighborhoods in search of industrial work. Returning soldiers and their burgeoning families further exacerbated a widespread strain on housing and municipal services. To provide cities with the legal and fiscal tools to cope with deepening urban problems, Congress passed the 1949 Housing Act, which enabled municipalities to create redevelopment authorities with broad powers to assemble land parcels for clearance and "urban renewal." The St. Louis urban-renewal program, overseen by veteran city engineer Harland Bartholomew, made full use of the federal provisions. Bartholomew and his protégé, Charles Farris, working for a succession of Democratic-machine mayors, undertook an unprecedented transformation of St. Louis through a program of slum clearance, zoning application, expressway construction, and public housing development.

As prerequisites for improving their city, planners and politicians viewed the eradication of blighted neighborhoods and the reorganization of the urban landscape into modern, efficient land uses. Thus, the St. Louis public housing program developed both as a catchment system for urban residents displaced through slum clearance and as a way to funnel federal largesse into a visible showcase of modern municipal action. In 1950 the city was ready to translate this "city-efficient" vision into reality with federal backing for 5800 units of public housing. Disposed toward large-scale project design and development, Bartholomew and then-Mayor Joseph Darst allocated nearly half of these units to one public housing development: Pruitt-Igoe.

Designed by Minoru Yamasaki of Hellmuth, Yamasaki, and Leinweber, the Pruitt-Igoe plan called for a Le Corbusier–like "*ville radieuse*" of garden apartments and high-rise edifices interspersed with broad tree-lined and landscaped plazas. Innovative skip-stop elevators would open onto every third floor, enabling a broad gallery to stretch for 85 feet across the front of the building. Not only would the skip-stop elevators reduce costs, architects argued, but the galleries would provide space for "vertical neighborhoods" to replace the streets and sidewalks of the low-rise city. Here, above the noise and congestion of the old neighborhoods, children could play, and adults could gather without fear for their safety.

In an attempt to ameliorate both white residents and segregationist political interests, the project was divided on the drawing board into racially distinct clusters. Officials designated the Wendell Olliver Pruitt Homes for black families and the James Igoe Apartments for white families. However, Pruitt-Igoe was completed in 1954, in the wake of the *Brown vs. Board of Education* decision, and the project had to be integrated on settlement. As a result, most white families dropped off the rolls, leaving the project desegregated by law while segregated in fact.

Meanwhile, federal cost-cutting measures eliminated many of the best features of Yamasaki's design, such as scattered low-rise units, landscaping, playgrounds, and recreation facilities, while increasing the density from 30 to 50 units per acre. Federal officials also insisted on the elimination of ground-floor bathrooms and most recreational facilities. With little foresight, they ordered an increase in the number of two-bedroom apartments at the expense of spaces for larger families, which led to overcrowding and structural strain.

Despite these problems, most families that initially settled the project regarded their move into Pruitt-Igoe as an improvement in their housing conditions. Many enjoyed indoor toilets and laundry facilities for the first time, and the project did eventually boast a number of amenities, including a playground, recreation center, public library branch, Boy Scout troop, day care center, and health clinic. Families managed to carve out new networks within the project and to raise children amid difficult circumstances. Many residents were involved in tenant organizing and civil rights campaigns through the 1960s. Today, many former residents remember Pruitt-Igoe not simply as the desolate landscape of media and scholarly accounts but as home—the place where they grew up and where they experienced many important life events.

Statistics collected by the St. Louis Housing Authority show that Pruitt-Igoe residents were similar in nearly all respects to residents of other public housing projects—at least in the first five years. Over time, however, they came to differ in one crucial respect: the high percentage of female-headed households. Many better-off families left the project for market-rate housing in the increasingly depopulated neighborhoods around the project, creating an irreversible occupancy crisis. The Housing Authority tried to maintain occupancy by filling Pruitt-Igoe with very poor, single-parent, female-headed families. The relative absence of black male adult residents, sociologists have argued, left women and children more vulnerable to crimes of property and violence. By the mid-1960s, Pruitt-Igoe was regarded as the most dangerous public housing project in the city. Firefighters routinely refused to answer alarm calls, and mail carriers and other service agents avoided the project. A series of highly publicized murders and snipings sealed the project's fate as a symbol of inner-city urban decay and crime.

As the personal safety and morale of residents declined with an alarming rapidity, the physical structure of Pruitt-Igoe deteriorated as well. Shoddy construction had already resulted in constant problems with doors, locks, windows, cabinets, heaters, and electric wiring. However, rising vacancy rates in the project left dwindling funds for maintenance and upkeep, placing the Housing Authority in a severe financial strain. The skip-stop elevators frequently malfunctioned, and the dim stairwells and galleries became gauntlets of crime that residents had to run on a daily basis. Plumbing systems that were poorly installed and maintained frequently froze and burst, causing widespread water damage. Without ground-floor bathrooms, children constantly urinated in the stairwells and elevators. Ongoing disagreements between the Housing Authority and the City of St. Louis over

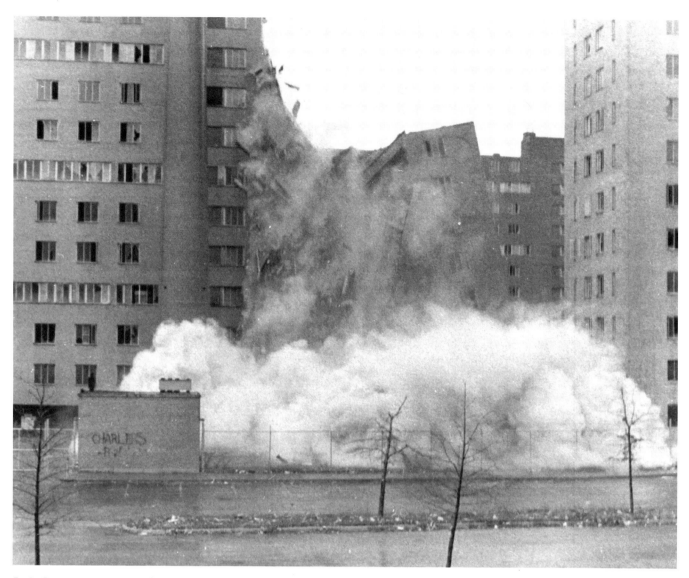

Pruitt Igoe Housing Project, designed by Minoru Yamasaki, April 21, 1972 demolition
Photo by Richard Moore © Missouri Historical Society

trash pickup and project maintenance resulted in an environment littered with refuse and garbage.

Numerous attempts were made in the mid- to late 1960s to improve the project. Pruitt-Igoe happened to exist in a city with a renowned collection of urban sociologists and political scientists who were loosely connected through Washington University's Urban Research Institute and Social Sciences Institute. Scholars such as Alvin Gouldner, Eugene Meehan, Roger Montgomery, Lee Rainwater, George Wendel, and William Yancey lent their talents to the study of Pruitt-Igoe and to the implementation of intervention strategies. The project was part of a Model Cities target area, and a variety of urban poverty programs and tenant control strategies came and went in an effort to reverse the decline. Pruitt-Igoe tenants themselves joined other public housing residents in a citywide rent strike that drew national attention to their plight. The strike dramatized the physical and mental stress of life in the projects and called attention to the civil rights and social justice issues involved.

Yet no interventions proved successful in the long term. By 1972 Pruitt-Igoe had become such an embarrassment to the city government and the Housing Authority that they decided to demolish it. Even the residents themselves were divided over the fate of the project: some favored partial demolition, whereas others favored low-rise retrofitting. Between 1972 and 1976, however, the project was detonated, leaving a 57-acre empty lot in the middle of the city. Aside from a small elementary school built on the southwest corner in 1992, the site remains empty.

Over the years, scholars and critics have grappled with the causes of the project's failure. Architectural critics generally hold that design is at the heart of the matter. Oscar Newman's widely read manifesto *Defensible Space* argues that high-rise public housing projects such as Pruitt-Igoe fail because they preclude spatial

regulation and defense by tenants, leaving them vulnerable to crime. Colin Rowe and Fred Koetter argue in *Collage City* that the spatial organization of Le Corbusier–influenced landscapes reveals a deep-seated authoritarian impulse toward social engineering inherent in modernist design. Both Charles Jencks (*The Language of Post-Modern Architecture*) and Peter Blake (*Form Follows Fiasco*) use Pruitt-Igoe as a metaphor for the failure of modernist architecture. Jencks argues that the modern design idiom abolishes history and ignores the contexts of place—attributes that had long governed architectural practice. Blake presses Pruitt-Igoe into a broad attack on CIAM (Congrès Internationaux d'Architecture Moderne) design principles, arguing that they result in sterile, inhuman environments. Each of these critics regard the 1972 detonations as a clarion call for a new era of architecture, one sensitive both to the weight of history and to the contingencies of local environments.

Social scientists, on the other hand, hold that Pruitt-Igoe's failure has less to do with design and more to do with structural conditions of racism and poverty. Lee Rainwater's now classic *Behind Ghetto Walls*, derived from lengthy interviews with Pruitt-Igoe residents in the mid-1960s, demonstrates that racial segregation, joblessness, and chronic poverty result in socioeconomic isolation and anomie among public housing residents. Eugene Meehan's definitive policy analysis *The Quality of Federal Policy Making* holds that public housing was doomed to failure from the outset because it never addressed the root causes of poverty and inadequate housing. Rather, the provision of public housing was always an ambivalent goal, hamstrung by fiscal austerity and lack of commitment. Roger Montgomery's concise article "Pruitt-Igoe: Policy Failure or Societal Symptom?" shows how problems endemic to the St. Louis housing market led to the decline of the city's public housing program. He rejects the prevalent view among politicians and journalists that Pruitt-Igoe failed because of inadequate design or liberal welfare policies, arguing instead that the project unraveled because of declining land values, increased housing options in neighborhoods depopulated by "white flight," persistent racism, and inner-city poverty.

More recent research by historians and urban analysts supports this latter view. Although design was clearly a factor in the decline of Pruitt-Igoe, scholars such as Mary Comerio and Kate Bristol demonstrate that it was not the cause. In fact, Bristol argues that the decline-by-design thesis is a rhetorical strategy common among architects and critics, one that serves to bolster the power of the profession by inflating the role that architects actually play in housing policy. Architects, Bristol argues, deceive themselves with their own rhetoric because they fail to grasp the basic fact that design cannot by itself compensate for drastic social inequalities. Moreover, Pruitt-Igoe itself was never the example of modernist hubris that its critics claim. Contrary to standard memory, Pruitt-Igoe won no architectural awards, and its own designers were critical of the high-rise form as a strategy for mass housing. Their designs were merely constrained by criteria dictated in advance by the Housing Authority, which favored high-rise, high-density public housing.

Mary Comerio's research takes the onus off design and places Pruitt-Igoe's failure within the broader historical context of urban renewal and redevelopment, industrial relocation and economic restructuring, "white flight," and the dwindling urban tax base. Pruitt-Igoe, she argues, and the larger public housing

program in the United States were caught up in entrenched historical processes over which architects—and even, to an extent, planners and municipal officials—had little control. Moreover, treating public housing as an issue of design obscures the social realities of race and class in urban environments and distracts critics from the deeper political and economic structures within which designers and planners operate.

In the end, Pruitt-Igoe reflects a federal capital investment of $50 million, a relatively small portion of the postwar federal housing chest. Tens of thousands of people found themselves directly involved with the project, whether as designers, planners, politicians, builders, residents, social workers, librarians, or police. This is a small number when compared with the tens of millions of Americans affected by the federal underwriting of suburban expansion and home building. However, the power that Pruitt-Igoe continues to exercise over the practices of architecture, policymaking, and planning is disproportionately great. For better or worse, and with more passion than accuracy, Pruitt-Igoe will long stand as a symbol of flawed urban design ideals, municipal redevelopment schemes, and federal housing policies.

JOSEPH HEATHCOTT

Further Reading

While there is an extensive literature on Pruitt-Igoe, much of it is dispersed through scholarly and trade journals, edited collections, occasional papers, and conference presentations. Three book-length monographs from the 1970s use Pruitt-Igoe as a backdrop for research on social issues such as black family life and structure, welfare programming, and public housing policy. Most of the literature falls within either social science, policy analysis, or architectural criticism. Only recently have scholars outside of these fields turned attention to Pruitt-Igoe and to its history as an urban place.

Blake, Peter, *Form Follows Fiasco: Why Modern Architecture Hasn't Worked*, Boston: Little Brown, 1977

Bristol, Kate, "The Pruitt-Igoe Myth," *Journal of Architectural Education*, 44/3 (1991)

Comerio, Mary Catherine, "Pruitt-Igoe and Other Stories," *Journal of Architectural Education*, 34/4 (1981)

"Four Vast Housing Projects for St. Louis: Helmuth, Obata, and Kassabaum, Inc.," *Architectural Record*, 120/2 (1956)

Heathcott, Joseph, "Pruitt-Igoe: Lives, Liberalism, and the Urban Landscape in Postwar America" (Ph.D. dissertation), Indiana University, 2000

Jencks, Charles, *The Language of Post-Modern Architecture*, London: Academy Editions, 1972; New York: Rizzoli, 1977; 6th edition, 1991

Meehan, Eugene, *Public Housing Policy: Convention versus Reality*, New Brunswick, New Jersey: Center for Urban Policy Research, Rutgers University, 1975

Meehan, Eugene, *The Quality of Federal Policy Making: Programmed Failure in Public Housing*, Columbia: University of Missouri Press, 1979

Montgomery, Roger, "Pruitt-Igoe: Policy Failure or Societal Symptom?" in *The Metropolitan Midwest: Policy Problems and Prospects for Change*, edited by Barry Checkoway and Carl V. Patton, Urbana: University of Illinois Press, 1985

Newman, Oscar, *Defensible Space: Crime Prevention through Urban Design*, New York: Macmillan, 1972; as *Defensible Space: People and Design in the Violent City*, London: Architectural Press, 1973

Rainwater, Lee, *Behind Ghetto Walls: Black Families in a Federal Slum*, Chicago: Aldine, 1970; London: Allen Lane, 1971

Rowe, Colin and Fred Koetter, *Collage City*, Cambridge, Massachusetts: MIT Press, 1978

Schmandt, Henry J. and George D. Wendel, "Pruitt-Igoe: Sozialwohngau in St. Louis, 1954–1976," *Werk Archithese*, 64 (May 1977)

PUBLIC HOUSING

Often used loosely, the term *public housing* describes several very different categories of housing. In a narrow sense, particularly in the United States, public housing tends to refer to dwellings funded by the national government and owned and operated by a local authority. In a broader interpretation, public housing consists of those units whose occupants cannot afford housing available on the so-called free market and who benefit, according to income-linked criteria, from some form of public assistance, extended either directly to the tenants or to developers or owners, who in turn provide discounted rent. Finally, one may argue that all housing targeted for any type of public subsidy is public housing, regardless of who owns it.

This last perspective would indicate that in the United States and many other countries most housing is, in fact, subsidized with public funds. This is so because its cost to private owners is lowered by national, state, and local governments through tax expenditures (for example, the deduction of mortgage interest and property tax from personal taxable income, amounting to more than $65 billion annually) and the provision of public infrastructure (such as roads), among other subsidies. Indirect subsidies of this type are not tenure neutral (they benefit owners much more than renters), and they are also highly regressive (they benefit households with high incomes much more than those with low incomes).

These distinctions and their implications are highly significant in the debates that help shape housing policies and programs in the United States and elsewhere. However, it is not possible here to engage the full scope of this discussion. This brief article focuses mainly on U.S. public housing in the more conventional, narrower definition.

Historical Background

Public housing is a means-tested, non–cash transfer program. Only households with incomes below specified levels are eligible. At present, they pay 30 percent of income for rent. Initially authorized by the (Wagner Steagall) Housing Act of 1937, public housing in the United States was meant to house families who were temporarily poor as a result of the economic depression. Its establishment came after a hard-fought, lengthy battle in which the National Association for Real Estate Boards, the U.S. Savings and Loans League, and the U.S. Mortgage Bankers Association opposed "socialist" government intervention in the housing market. The compromise that was reached has been seen by many as more an effort to boost the construction industry and reduce unemployment than to provide affordable housing.

After World War II, the Housing Act of 1949 declared the goal of "a decent home and suitable living environment for every American family." It called for the construction of 810,000 public housing units in six years. However, production fell far short, and private commercial interests succeeded in appropriating funds that had been tied to residential redevelopment. In the following decades, the U.S. commitment to public housing steadily declined, and in January 1973 President Richard Nixon imposed a moratorium on all federal housing assistance. The moratorium was lifted the following year with the enactment of legislation oriented to demand-side subsidies.

Subsequent significant changes in housing policy included a shift away from large projects (scattered-site approach), a trend toward privatization (e.g. in management and sale of units), and especially an increased use of the existing housing stock through a system of allowances and vouchers that reduced the cost of housing to tenants. Today, few new units are built. The total number of public housing units is, in fact, declining at present, as large problem projects are being torn down and replaced by higher-quality redevelopments built at lower densities.

Profile and International Scope

Public housing in the United States provides homes to about 3.3 million people, accounting for about 1.5 percent of all occupied dwelling units. The percentage is also relatively low in other countries that have traditionally relied heavily on the private-sector supply to meet housing demand: Australia (6 percent), New Zealand (5 percent), and Canada (5.5 percent), to name three. In Japan, which has also favored a minimal role for government in housing provision, public housing for low-income households similarly constitutes 5 percent of the total stock. These figures contrast sharply with those in regions where national government has played an active role in creating a relatively large postwar social housing sector, such as Israel (13 percent), France (18 percent), Germany (20 percent), Denmark (24 percent), Britain (31 percent), Sweden (36 percent), The Netherlands (45 percent), Hong Kong (50 percent), and Singapore (86 percent). Privatization trends have more recently resulted in a decline of some of these figures, although they remain high in comparison. Countries in Eastern Europe and Russia have long had a very large housing sector controlled by the central state. During the 1990s, their economies underwent a process of transformation oriented to a more market-based organization of society. Nonetheless, at the end of the 20th century, after significant sell-offs to tenants against nominal prices, diminished but still significant public housing stocks remained in, for example, Russia (49 percent), Poland (25 percent), and Hungary (13 percent).

In the United States, the popular image of public housing conjures up mass-produced high-rises and superblocks built at high densities with low-quality construction materials according to bad designs and situated in undesirable locations. Undeniably, many projects fit that description. The Department of Housing and Urban Development estimates that about 100,000 units are "severely distressed," that is, physically deteriorated and with high vacancy and unemployment rates. However, such units constitute a minority of public housing, concentrated in a few large cities, and they are not representative. In fact, the largest proportion of public housing developments in the United States, 38 percent, comprises two- or three-story walk-ups; 34 percent are single-family attached or detached dwellings. Only 28 percent consist of buildings of four or more stories, a share that is dwindling under the HOPE VI program. Public housing in the United States includes many examples of fine designs, and some of the most recent developments incorporate design concepts

strikingly similar to some of the earliest public housing in the country.

Initially, U.S. public housing was intended as temporary housing for poor households expected to work their way up to private-market housing. However, increasingly it became a last resort for people with no prospects for other housing options. As a result, over time, public housing has become residualized. Many residents are dependent on welfare (over 50 percent) and social security or disability payments (25 percent). About 75 percent of households are headed by a single adult, usually an elderly person or a single parent. A majority are nonwhite.

In western and northern Europe after World War II, many governments embarked on large-scale housing programs to meet pent-up demand and make up for housing stock destroyed in the war. More than 5 million units were built. Most of this construction occurred in the form of high-rises built on peripherally located estates. By the mid-1970s, the absolute shortages had been eliminated. Demand fell. Households with rising incomes moved out, leaving behind those without choice. Vacancies rose, revenues declined, and conditions quickly deteriorated. Since then, local authorities and nonprofit landlords, oriented to providing and managing social housing, have increasingly faced social welfare challenges engendered by economic, political, and demographic trends in the larger society.

In eastern Europe, national governments controlled property rights and financial resources. Central planning produced a mass-housing sector owned and operated by state agencies and state-run industries. Large estates comprising prefabricated dwelling units in multistory buildings became home to 170 million people. Access to housing was a legislated entitlement, and since wages were low, households spent only a small proportion of their income on rent (often around 3 percent). Limited rent revenues and subsidies insufficient for operating and maintenance needs, often combined with low-quality building materials and fast construction, caused the housing to fall into disrepair quickly. Responsibilities for upkeep and repair became a salient issue in the transition of the former state socialist systems into more market-oriented societies.

In the developing countries, with a few exceptions, public housing has constituted only a minute portion of housing production. Typically, self-help and other informal processes of housing provision have been much more important. Insofar as scarce resources were used for the building of public housing, the beneficiaries have usually been civil servants rather than the poorest segments of the population. Current efforts are generally directed toward enabling housing markets to work, although it remains to be seen whether this approach will extend access to housing to the lowest-income groups.

Design in Context

In terms of architecture and project layout, there have been three stages in the evolution of public housing in the United States. In the 1930s and the early 1940s, semienclosed courts with walk-up buildings dominated, aligned with the streets but with entries usually from the interior of the site. Open areas between lines of row houses or walk-ups or around widely spaced elevator high-rises placed at an angle to the street or in closed streets were more characteristic of projects built from the 1940s through the 1960s. From the late 1970s onward, public housing designs more typically include private yards and semi- or fully enclosed courts for row houses and low-rises with entrances reoriented to front the streets. The different designs have been seen as the enactment of prevailing belief systems concerning the place of public housing and its residents in the surrounding community and society at large.

Illustrative of the broader context of design is the Pruitt-Igoe project in St. Louis, which opened its doors to the first tenants in the early 1950s amid high praise for its design. When it was dynamited scarcely 20 years later, many critics decried design features, such as the lack of semipublic space and the mismatch between the social and physical environment (for example, large families in high-rise apartments), attributing to them the project's failure. Others, however, have downplayed the significance of design in the demise of Pruitt-Igoe and similar projects, instead emphasizing the role of insufficient budgets and discriminatory policies.

Current Approaches

Public housing remains a valuable resource. It is home to millions of households who cannot afford market housing. Maintaining this resource requires that extant challenges be effectively met. Current approaches fall into two categories. The first is tenant based, primarily under the Section 8 program. It seeks to ameliorate the concentration of poverty by portable subsidies, such as vouchers and allowances, aimed at increasing household mobility, and sometimes provides additional supports, such as job training. The second, area-based, supply-side approach focuses on the housing estates themselves in an attempt to address problems in a comprehensive manner. The latter approach is multipronged (incorporating more accountable forms of management, providing programs and services in support of resident needs, attracting mixed-income tenant populations, and carrying out research-based design) and seeks to avoid past mistakes that led to higher rates of vandalism and crime. HOPE VI funding has stimulated improved architecture and site planning to foster neighborly interactions and promote safety (crime prevention through environmental design). In addition, examples are growing of public housing that integrates programs to assist residents in becoming economically more self-reliant (for example, Project Self-Sufficiency) and that provides services that facilitate independent functioning (such as Section 202).

The problems facing U.S. public housing—problems of design, siting, maintenance, and population composition—are often attributable to oppositional economic and political forces rather than to causes inherent in the public subsidy of housing. Smaller schemes that use individual street addresses rather than project names and that are woven into the fabric of the surrounding community by integrating services and mixing different income groups will make public housing less distinguishable from private housing. Indeed, evidence links the emergence of successful public housing to the dissolution of its standout image and to its being an integral part of a comprehensive approach to housing.

WILLEM VAN VLIET

See also **Apartment Building; Pruitt Igoe Housing, St. Louis, Missouri**

Further Reading

Cisneros, Henry, *Defensible Space: Deterring Crime and Building Community*, Washington, D.C.: U.S. Department of Housing and Urban Development, 1995

Fisher, Robert Moore, *20 Years of Public Housing*, New York: Harper, 1959

Franck, K. and M. Mostoller, "From Court to Open Space to Street: A History of Site Design of U.S. Public Housing," *Journal of Architecture and Planning Research*, 12/3 (1995) (special issue on public housing transformation)

Goering, John, Ali Kamely, and Todd Richardson, *The Location and Racial Composition of Public Housing in the United States*, Washington, D.C.: U.S. Department of Housing and Urban Development, 1994

Marcuse, P., "Mainstreaming Public Housing" in *New Directions in Urban Public Housing*, edited by David P. Varady, Wolfgang F.E. Preiser, and Francis P. Russell, New Brunswick, New Jersey: Center for Urban Policy Research, 1998

Power, Anne, *Hovels to High Rise: State Housing in Europe since 1850*, London and New York: Routledge, 1993

Power, Anne, *Estates on the Edge: The Social Consequences of Mass Housing in Northern Europe*, London: Macmillan, and New York: St. Martin's Press, 1997

Priemus, Hugo and Niels L. Prak (editors), *Post-War Public Housing in Trouble*, Delft, The Netherlands: Delft University Press, 1985

Rainwater, Lee, *Behind Ghetto Walls: Black Families in a Federal Slum*, Chicago: Aldine, 1970

Schnapper, Morris Bartel (editor), *Public Housing in America*, New York: Wilson, 1939

PUIG I CADAFALCH, JOSEP 1867–1956

Architect, Catalonia

Josep Puig i Cadafalch was one of the leading architects of the *modernisme* movement that flourished in the Spanish region of Catalonia during the first decades of the 20th century. In many ways, Puig moved elegantly between the organic extravagance of *modernisme* and the ordered geometry of *novecentismo*. This was in part because of the fact that he was much younger than Antoni Gaudí i Cornet and Lluís Domènech i Montaner, the leading architects of the first movement, and somewhat older than the next generation. Puig drew inspiration from 15th-century Catalan Gothic architecture, a style that was decidedly different from classic High Gothic. Despite his almost religious zeal for regional historical traditions, he also looked outside Spain for inspiration. Puig traveled widely throughout Europe, especially Germany and Austria, and wrote approvingly of the work of Henry-Clement Van de Velde, Josef Maria Olbrich, and Otto Wagner. He particularly admired Olbrich's designs for buildings at the Darmstadt artist's colony. The English Arts and Crafts also had an enormous effect on his architectural style.

Puig rigorously examined and studied the historical architecture of Catalonia, eventually publishing several leading scholarly texts. He rejected monumentalism and classical forms in favor of a style firmly rooted in Catalan culture and society. Puig abhorred classical styles, declaring that they had little to do with native tradition and were simply another non-Catalan fashion imposed by the central government in Madrid. In his own work, Puig attempted to combine the folk traditions of rural Catalonia with the deliberate artistry and modern materials of urban society. In all his structures, he combined a commitment to local tradition and history with a strong faith in modernity and internationalism.

Puig emphasized simple volumes that echoed the traditional floor plans of Catalan farmhouses. These areas had an organic layout with spaces that gently flowed together. His interiors became known for their remarkable sense of intimacy and warmth produced through diffuse lighting and lavish use of wood as decoration. A strong sense of nationalism and history led him to encourage local craft techniques, including woodworking, ceramics, stained glass, and sgraffito. Puig's structures emphasized a richness of detail combined with a simplicity of form. The exteriors often faced the street with large, planar facades of stucco or unadorned brick punctuated with almost baroque-like stone oriels and decoration. The specific decorative elements ranged from organic flowers and animals to heraldic devices, shields, and symbols of nobility.

His first major work was the Casa Martí (1896) in Barcelona's Gothic quarter. The hulking building recalled a feudal manor house of the medieval Catalan past. The exposed brick walls combined with stonework decoration to give the structure an artisanal feel. The interior contained large spaces covered by wood beams and illuminated by delicate iron chandeliers. This illustrated Puig's deliberate combination of traditional form with modern ornament. It was this interior that, a year after completion of the structure, housed a cafe called the Els Quatre Gats (the Four Cats). The building soon became the social gathering place of Pablo Picasso, Miquel Utrillo, Ramon Casas, and

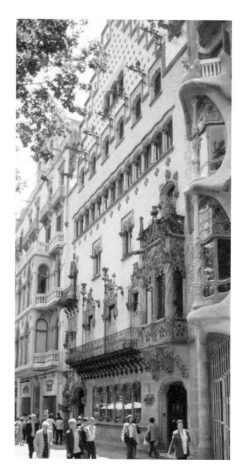

Puig i Cadafalch, Josep (Catalan) (1990) designed by Casa Antoni Amatller, facade
Photo © Mary Ann Sullivan

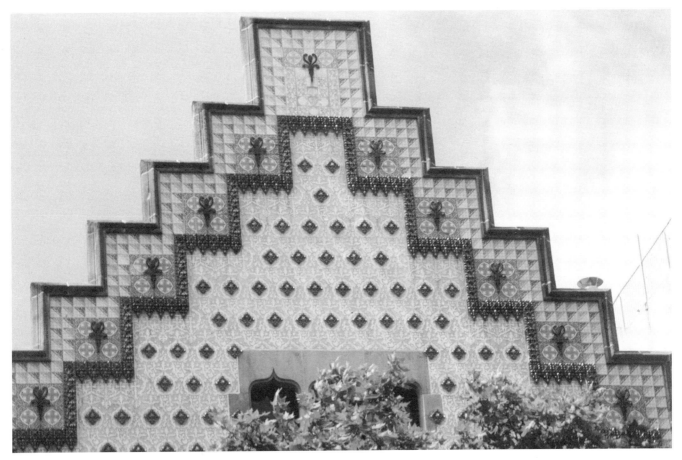

Puig i Cadafalch, Josep (Catalan) designed by Casa Antoni Amatller, detail
Photo © Mary Ann Sullivan

Santiago Rusinyol, artists who would soon bring Catalan *modernisme* an international reputation.

The politics of Catalan nationalism, combined with a growing class of wealthy patrons, led to a series of important commissions during the period 1900–05. It was with these houses that the architectural style of Puig found its greatest expression. The first, constructed for a wealthy chocolate maker, was the Casa Amatller (1900). Puig designed the house to be a jewel of individuality set within what he viewed as the rigid conformity of Ildefons Cerdá's gridlike urban plan for Barcelona. He wished to express the opulence and power of his wealthy clients through extravagant use of rich materials and symbolism. The plan exhibited the characteristics typical to rural Catalan homes, with a large central courtyard and a central stair rising to the main public room of the first floor. The interior was richly appointed in wood and plaster. The public rooms contained ornate columns, and the highly decorated wooden ceiling beams recalled traditional Spanish *mudéjar* ornamentation. The flat wall facing the street, however, revealed that Puig was not simply blindly following the ancient tenets. Instead, the wall was peppered with sgraffito and topped by an ornate pediment decorated with brightly colored tiles. The outline of the structure resembled the stepped triangular rooflines of Northern European homes. In addition to the tiles, the architect decorated the front of the structure with both whimsical and pious sculpture. Saint George, the patron saint of Catalonia, shared space with rats, pigs, and frogs. Eventually, Domènech built the Casa Lleó Morera to the left, and the building on the right was replaced by Gaudí's Casa Batlló, making the short block one of the single greatest concentrations of modernist architecture in the entire city.

A second home designed for a wealthy patron was the Casa Terrades (1905), better known as the "Casa de les Punxes" (House of the Points). The nickname came from the building's four small round turrets and a large main tower topped by sharp spires. It again demonstrated Puig's affection for Northern European designs. A series of profusely decorated doorways and window openings punctuated the plain brick walls. The decorative sculpture again included a large ceramic plaque dedicated to St. George. The choice of decoration illustrated the ostentatious religiosity of the wealthy bourgeoisie and also their nationalism.

In addition to being a practicing architect, Puig had a second career as an architectural historian. He employed a scientific approach that emphasized observation and measurement. Puig was convinced of the connections between all aspects of a region's culture, including language, art, and architecture. He thought of architecture as a communal art form created by peoples and nations rather than individuals and that historic forms had been dictated by the particular needs and traditions of the

region. Although exiled following the Spanish civil war, Puig's theory and practice continued to influence Spanish architecture. The emphasis on regional design elements and quality decoration was later taken up by members of the loosely organized School of Barcelona, which included Ricardo Bofill, Oriol Bohigas, and Studio Per.

BRIAN D. BUNK

Biography

Born in Mataró, Spain, 15 October 1867. Graduated from the Escuela Superior de Arquitectura, Barcelona in 1891. Municipal architect, Mataró 1891–97. In private practice as an architect, Barcelona from 1897; made important contributions to the study of Catalan Romanesque architecture. Professor, Escuela Superior de Arquitectura, Barcelona from 1897. Died in Barcelona, 24 December 1956.

Selected Works

Casa Martí, Carrer de Montsió, Barcelona, 1896
Casa Garí, El Cros, Argentona, Spain, 1898
Casa Amatller, passeig de Gràcia, Barcelona, 1900
Casa Terrades (Casa de les Punxes), Avinguda Diagonal, Barcelona, 1905
Casa Serra, Rambla de Catalunya, Barcelona, 1907
Casa Companys, Barcelona, 1911
Casarramona Factory, Barcelona, 1911
Casa Pich i Pon, Barcelona, 1921

Selected Publications

L'arquitectura romànica a Catalunya, 3 vols., 1909–18
Le premier art roman: l'architecture en Catalogne et dans l'occident méditérranien aux Xe et XIe siecles, 1928
La geografía y els origens del primer art romànic, 1930

Further Reading

Specific works dedicated solely to Puig i Cadafalch are generally unavailable in English. Bohigas et al. (1990) treat Puig in the context of general architectural histories. Bohigas's *Arquitectura modernista* is also a general survey of the entire *modernisme* movement and contains important information on, as well as illustrations of, Puig's work. Bassegoda Nonell, Cirici, and Jardí are thorough treatments in Spanish and Catalan of Puig as an architect, politician, and historian. Hughes's book is a readable introduction to the cultural and historical milieu of Barcelona and contains a brief discussion of Puig and his work.

Bassegoda Nonell, Juan, *Puig i Cadafalch*, Barcelona: Ediciones de Nou Art Thor, 1985
Bohigas, Oriol, *Arquitectura modernista*, Barcelona: Editorial Lumen, 1968
Bohigas, Oriol, Peter Buchanan, and Vittorio Magnago Lampugnani, *Barcelona, arquitectura y ciudad, 1980–1992*, Barcelona: Gili, 1990; as *Barcelona, City and Architecture, 1980–1992*, New York: Rizzoli, 1991
Cirici, Alexandre, "La arquitectura de Puig i Cadafalch," *Cuadernos de arquitectura*, 63 (1966)
Hughes, Robert, *Barcelona*, New York: Knopf, and London: Harvill, 1992
Jardí, Enric, *Puig i Cadafalch: Arquitecte, polític, i historiador de l'art*, Esplugues de Llobregat, Spain: Editorial Ariel, 1975

PURCELL, WILLIAM GRAY, AND GEORGE GRANT ELMSLIE

Architecture firm, United States

The partnership of William Gray Purcell (1880–1965) and George Grant Elmslie (1871–1952) was remarkable in the annals of architecture. It lasted from 1909 until 1922. During these years, the two men made a major contribution to the Prairie School and created some of its finest buildings.

Born on a farm in northeastern Scotland, Elmslie attended the famous Duke of Gordon School in Huntly. His education included a strict Presbyterianism along with a consciousness of the mysticism that is a strong feature of the Scottish heritage. With his family, Elmslie immigrated to the United States in 1884. They settled in Chicago, where his father was already working. After a brief period in business school, Elmslie followed the suggestion of his parents and began the study of architecture in the office of Joseph Lyman Silsbee, where George Maher and Frank Lloyd Wright were already working. When Wright left Silsbee in 1889 to join Adler and Sullivan, he asked Elmslie to come with him. The offer was accepted, with momentous consequences for both Sullivan and Elmslie. When Wright left the office in the mid-1890s, Elmslie became Sullivan's chief draftsman, a position that he held for 15 years. During this period, Elmslie learned thoroughly the principles of organic architecture and became adept at designing ornament in the Sullivan manner. He detailed nearly all the exterior ornament for the Wainwright Building (1890) in St. Louis, designed the ironwork entrance for the Carson Pirie Scott Store (1901–03) in Chicago, and had a major share in the design of the National Farmers Bank (1908) in Owatonna, Minnesota. By 1909 business in the Sullivan office had declined to such an extent that Elmslie was open to the offer of a partnership from William Gray Purcell, a young Minneapolis architect whom he had known since 1903.

Purcell had grown up in Oak Park, Illinois, in comfortable circumstances. He was educated in its excellent schools, at a liberal private academy, and at Cornell University, where he took an architectural degree in 1903. The academic curriculum was profoundly distasteful to Purcell. (In correspondence with this writer, he always referred to it contemptuously as "Bozart.") Nonetheless, he mastered conventional drafting techniques and, after graduation, was briefly in Sullivan's office, an experience that stayed with him for the rest of his life. He also worked in Berkeley for John Galen Howard and in Seattle. Then, in 1906, at the suggestion of his father, Purcell departed for a yearlong odyssey in Europe in company with his Cornell classmate George Feick. The two young men not only visited the classical sites in Greece and Italy and the French cathedral towns but also called on such progressive leaders as Hendrik Berlage in the Netherlands, Martin Nyrop in Denmark, and Ferdinand Boberg in Sweden. On their return to the United States, Feick convinced Purcell that there was room for a new kind of architectural firm in Minneapolis. They opened an office in February 1907. Elmslie joined them in 1909, and in 1913 Feick withdrew. Although Purcell moved to Philadelphia in 1916, he continued his association with Elmslie until 1922.

The great years for Purcell and Elmslie and for the other Prairie architects were those immediately preceding World War I. Elmslie brought with him much domestic work from clients who wanted progressive houses but could no longer endure the difficulties of working with Sullivan. These clients included

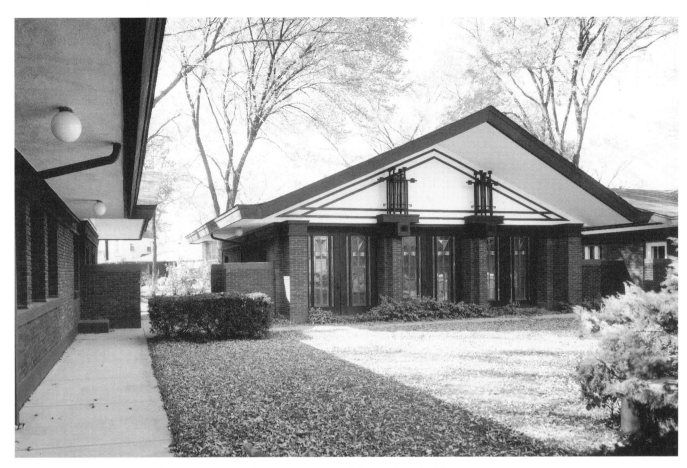

Babson Stable and Service building, inner court showing east elevation of garage Riverside, Illinois
(*c.*1916 additions and alterations to the 1908 original Babson House by Louis Sullivan)
© Historic American Buildings Survey/Library of Congress

Henry Babson, the Cranes, and the Bradleys. For Babson there were several additions to his estate in Riverside, Illinois, and for the Bradleys there was the much-admired "bungalow" (1913) at Cape Cod. There were other important domestic commissions as well: the Powers House (1910) in Minneapolis, the Decker House (1913) at Lake Minnetonka, the E.S. Hoyt House (1915) at Red Wing, and an exquisite small house on Lake Place in Minneapolis for Purcell himself in the same year. This last dwelling has been beautifully restored and is today the property of the Minneapolis Institute of Arts. All these houses had in common an open plan, beautiful proportions, a knowing choice of materials, and where the budget allowed, furniture and leaded glass in a highly individualized manner. Superficially, they resemble the contemporary Prairie houses of Frank Lloyd Wright, whose work Purcell and Elmslie had earlier admired. The houses of Purcell and Elmslie, however, were usually lighter in feeling and often more livable.

The other great specialty of the firm was the small-town bank. Encouraged by the success of the Sullivan-Elmslie Bank (1908) for Carl K. Bennett at Owatonna, Minnesota, the new partnership actively sought similar omissions throughout the Midwest. Happily, they found a number of similar progressive-minded bankers. Their banks in Leroy, Grand Meadow, and Adams, Minnesota, and in Rhinelander, Wisconsin, are particularly fine. These banks stand like jewel boxes in hamlets that are reminis-

cent of Gopher Prairie in the novels of Sinclair Lewis. The largest of their banks, a superlative creation, is the Merchants' Bank (1912) of Winona, Minnesota. For this building, the firm used pier-and-lintel framing with steel girders set on brick piers to define the cubic form of the banking room, thus relieving the walls of support function so that they could be opened up for large panes of leaded glass. There was also a great deal of terracotta ornament, and the chairs and the other furniture were designed to match the architectural elements, all in keeping with Prairie School principles.

The largest building to be constructed by Purcell and Elmslie was the Woodbury County Courthouse for Sioux City, Iowa, done in association with William L. Steele. Steele won the commission in 1916 and then asked Elmslie to develop a plan expressing the agricultural wealth of the region and the sturdy population of its inhabitants. Despite opposition from several quarters, the Elmslie concept was carried through. It featured an amazing amount of terra-cotta ornament and a series of massive friezes by Alfonso Iannelli, who had earlier worked with Wright at the Midway Gardens. About 60 percent of the designing was done by Elmslie, who moved to Sioux City for the duration of the job. The remainder came through the Minneapolis office. The courthouse is a building of an almost indigestible richness.

Design procedures in the office of Purcell and Elmslie were essentially democratic, with both partners contributing at differ-

ent stages to the finished project. In a profound sense, the two men were necessary to each other. Elmslie had a deep understanding of the organic principles underlying the architecture of Louis Sullivan, but at times his preoccupation with the role of ornament could degenerate into decorative efflorescence. Purcell, equally convinced of organic and democratic principles but more cautious by nature, was a restraining influence and at the same time was stimulated by his partner to explore the essential nature of design. Elmslie tended to think graphically. Purcell was happy with verbal expression and in later years wrote a column of architectural criticism for *The Minnesota Architect*. Both were committed to social progress and to experimentation with the low-cost dwelling. Their work can generally be distinguished from that of Wright and the other Prairie School architects by its generally axial order and frequently by a whimsical touch. Spatially, they were not as adventurous as Wright, but in many ways they were more humane. Although Wright did his best to denigrate Purcell and Elmslie, their achievement has been largely recovered by a later generation of architectural historians. Today, it is generally recognized that they made a major contribution to the Prairie School and to the American architecture of their period.

LEONARD K. EATON

Biographies

George Grant Elmslie

Born in Huntly, Scotland, 20 February 1871; family moved to Chicago 1884. Educated in Chicago public schools. Joined the office of J. Lyman Silsbee, Chicago 1888; joined firm of Adler and Sullivan, Chicago 1889; became head draftsman when Frank Lloyd Wright left the firm 1893. Partner, with William Gray Purcell and George Feick, Purcell Feick and Elmslie, Chicago 1909–13; partner, Purcell and Elmslie, Chicago 1913–22. Continued working in Chicago from 1922. Died in Chicago, 23 April 1952.

William Gray Purcell

Born in Wilmette, Illinois, 2 July 1880. Studied architecture, Cornell University, Ithaca, New York; graduated 1903. Worked in the office of Henry Ives Cobb, Chicago 1903; worked in the office of Louis Sullivan 1903; worked for John G. Howard, Berkeley, California 1904; worked for Charles H. Bebb and Leonard L. Mendel, Seattle, Washington 1904. Established, with George Feick, Purcell and Feick, Minneapolis, Minnesota 1907; partner, with Feick and George Grant Elmslie, Purcell Feick and Elmslie, Chicago 1909–13; partner, Purcell and Elmslie, Chicago 1913–22. Private practice, Portland, Oregon from 1922. Died in Pasadena, California, 11 April 1965.

Purcell and Elmslie

Established as Purcell Feick and Elmslie, Chicago 1909; became Purcell and Elmslie, Chicago 1913–22; major architects of the Prairie movement; most active between 1913 and 1920.

Selected Works

The Art Institute of Chicago and the Minneapolis Art Institute hold examples of the furniture and architectural ornamentation of Purcell and Elmslie. The Minneapolis Art Institute also holds the title to Purcell's Lake Place Home (1913). It may be visited by arrangement. The extensive Purcell papers are at the Northwest Architectural Archives, University of Minnesota. These archives also hold many of the firm's drawings.

Powers House, Minneapolis, 1910
Merchants Bank of Winona, Minnesota, 1912
Edna S. (William Gary) Purcell House, Minneapolis, 1913
Decker House, Holdridge, Minnesota, 1913
Edison Shop, Chicago, 1913
Bradley House, Woods Hole, Massachusetts, 1913
First State Bank, LeRoy, Minnesota, 1914
Capitol Building (unbuilt), Canberra, Australia, 1914
E.S. Hoyt House, Red Wing, Minnesota, 1915
Babson Stable and Service Building, Riverside, Illinois, ca. 1916
    (with Louis Sullivan)
Woodbury County Courthouse, Sioux City, Iowa (with William L.
    Steele), 1917
Factories, Alexander International Leather and Belting Corporation,
    Philadelphia, 1918
First National Bank, Adams, Minnesota, 1920

Selected Publications

Purcell was a prolific writer as well as an accomplished graphic designer. The three articles in *The Western Architect* of 1913–15 are the best contemporary summaries of the work of the firm.

William Gray Purcell
"Expressions in Church Architecture" *The Continent* (29 June 1911)
"Walter Burley Griffin, Progressive," *The Western Architect*, 18/12
    (September 1912)
"Made in Minnesota," *The Minnesotan*, 1/9 (April 1916)
St. Croix Trail Country, 1967

William Gray Purcell and George Grant Elmslie:
"The American Renaissance?" *The Craftsman*, 21/4 (January 1912)
"H.P. Berlage, the Creator of a Democratic Architecture in
    Holland," *The Craftsman*, 21/5 (February 1912)
"The Statics and Dynamics of Architecture," *The Western Architect*,
    19/1 (January 1913)
"Work," *The Western Architect*, 21/1 (January 1915)
"Work," *The Western Architect*, 22/1 (July 1915)

Further Reading

A good evaluation of the achievement of Purcell and Elmslie in a broad context is found in Brooks. The exhibition catalog essay by Hammons is thus far the most comprehensive treatment of the work of Purcell and Elmslie and contains a commission list of their executed works and projects.

Brooks, H. Allen, *The Prairie School: Frank Lloyd Wright and His
    Midwest Contemporaries*, Toronto: University of Toronto Press,
    1972; New York: Norton, 1976
Gebhard, David S., "William Gray Purcell and George Grant
    Elmslie and the Early Progressive Movement in American
    Architecture from 1900 to 1920" (Ph.D. dissertation), University
    of Minnesota, 1957
Hammons, Mark I., "Purcell and Elmslie, Architects" in *Minnesota,
    1900: Art and Life on the Upper Mississippi, 1890–1915*, edited
    by Michael Conforti, Newark: University of Delaware Press,
    1994

R

RAILROAD STATION

The railroad station as a building type was born in the early 19th century, when vehicles that traveled on their own "railroads" began to be used for the transportation of not only goods but also humans. The primary reason for such a building was the basic need to shelter both trains and people. However, the railroad station fulfilled a psychological need as well. Before the widespread use of railroads, traveling was an arduous and extended affair consisting of a series of gradual transitions from one place to another. By means of the railroad (and later the airplane), traveling became an easier task consisting of merely embarking and disembarking a vehicle, with no stops in between. For the industrial city, the railroad station became what the city gate had been for the medieval city—that special in-between transitional location, the first and last view of a city, the physical and psychological location of entrance and exit.

The architectural history of the railroad station suggests a dialogue between the building and its train tracks. Buildings were first placed alongside of the tracks, as is still the case in many suburban and rural train stations. Those on both sides of the tracks were sometimes linked with naturally lit steel-and-glass atriums, or train sheds. Those stations that terminated a train line, usually in large urban metropolises, tended to screen both tracks and shed from view by means of either a separate construction, as in Euston Station (1839, Philip Hardwick, demolished 1962) in London, or a third building that linked shed and buildings either side, as in Gare de l'Est (1852, François Duquesney) in Paris. The shed and buildings of St. Pancras Station in London, although touching, were designed and built separately by engineer William H. Barlow (1868) and architect Sir George Gilbert Scott (1876). Toward the end of the 19th century, the size of a railroad station's train shed became its qualifying criterion, and a contest began to see who could build the largest. Broad Street Station (1893, Joseph and John Wilson, demolished 1953) in Philadelphia reached a limit with its ingenious 300-foot three-hinged wrought-iron shed.

By the turn of the 20th century, the areas around such large urban terminals were no longer on the outskirts of town in unwanted industrial areas. Instead, the city had usually grown up around them, and they found themselves on valuable real estate. To take advantage of this, some train tracks, originally at street level or elevated, were buried below ground, and their land was sold for development. A new station building, not just shed and facade, could then be built on top of these sunken tracks. The main characteristic of this new type of station was its central hall or concourse—large enough to accommodate huge numbers of people and lofty enough to present itself as the center of the city, if not the whole world. Such is the case with Pennsylvania Station (1910, McKim, Mead, and White, demolished 1964) in New York; Union Station (1907, D. H. Burnham and Company) in Washington, D.C.; and Grand Central Station (1913, Warren and Westmore and Reed and Stem) in New York.

In Chicago, the acknowledged railroad city of the early 20th century, Daniel H. Burnham and Edward H. Bennett gave lengthy consideration to the location, multimode functions, and style of the modern railroad terminal in their influential Plan of Chicago (1909). For the next decade or so, City Beautiful architects and planners often made a new railroad terminal one of the chief urban forms.

By hiding the tracks from view, the concourse-type railroad station eliminated the previously mentioned design problem of separate buildings and train sheds. This elimination of separate building and shed is also characteristic of modernist railroad stations where train tracks and their roof covering, instead of being hidden below ground, became integrated into a complete design. Helsinki Station (1910–20, Eliel Saarinen), which does not rely on any 19th-century Gothic, Doric, or Moorish eclecticism for its decoration, is an early example of this. The main station in Florence, Italy (1934–36, Giovanni Michelucci), was one of the first International Style railroad stations, integrating its building and shed so easily perhaps because steel and glass were part of the whole building's palette.

Because of the increased usage of the automobile and the airplane, there were not many new railroad stations built after World War II, with the exception of those rebuilt because of war damage. Stazione Termini (1951, Montuori and Calini) in Rome, although newly built, was a prototype followed by most rebuilt stations: long, flat, and unarticulated facades, attempting to unify both building and shed into one composition.

A general period of railroad station decline occurred in the 1960s and 1970s, as many were abandoned and even de-

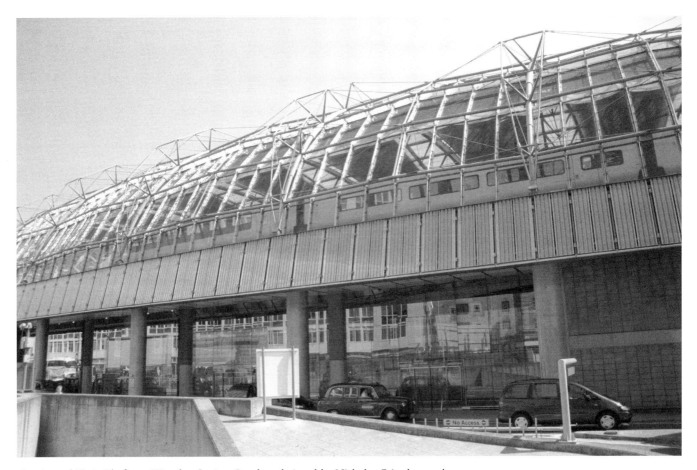

Continental Train Platform, Waterloo Station, London, designed by Nicholas Grimshaw and Partners (1993)
© Don Barker/GreatBuildings.com

molished, particularly in the United States. During the 1980s, a small railroad station renaissance occurred as existing stations were enlarged and appended to become home to shopping malls, restaurants, office space, and other non–rail-related functions. In this way, railroad stations became more of a place to visit and stay rather than just a place to pass through. Charing Cross Station in London had its 1906 train shed removed and replaced with an office building (1984, Terry Farrell). Similarly, Union Station in Washington, D.C., turned its concourse into a giant shopping mall by pushing back its platforms (1988, Benjamin Thompson Architects).

Newly built railroad stations at the end of the 20th century were mostly constructed in response to increased high-speed train lines or the creation of city-center links to out-of-town airports. Atocha Station in Madrid turned its central hall into a palm-treed shopping mall, and another station was built next door to handle a new Madrid–Seville express (1984–92, Rafael Moneo). Waterloo Station in London was appended with a contemporary reinterpretation of a 19th-century train shed to accommodate a high-speed service under the English Channel to continental Europe (1993, Nicholas Grimshaw and Partners). Roissy Station at Charles de Gaulle Airport in Paris cleverly joined high-speed and regional train lines with not only the airport but also a hotel (1994, Paul Andreu). Finally, the form of the Lyon-Satolas Station for Lyon Airport (1996, Santiago Calatrava) in France uses bird-in-flight imagery similar to the TWA Terminal (1962, Eero Saarinen) in New York.

The future of the building-type railroad station in the 21st century obviously depends on the future of rail travel. However, as indicated by the French examples cited previously, a new and faster means of transportation, such as the airplane, does not necessarily mean the decline of new railroad stations and facilities.

CHRISTOPHER WILSON

See also **Calatrava, Santiago (Spain); City Beautiful Movement; Grand Central Station, New York City; Grimshaw, Nicholas (England); Helsinki Railway Station, Finland; Moneo, Rafael (Spain)**

Further Reading

Binney, Marcus, *Great Railway Stations of Europe*, London: Thames & Hudson, 1984
Binney, Marcus, *Architecture of the Rail: The Way Ahead*, London: Academy Editions, 1995
Davey, Peter, "Places of Transition," *Architectural Review* (February 1995), pp. 4–5

Dethier, Jean, *All Stations: (Les Temps du Gares)—A Journey through 150 Years of Railway History*, London: Thames and Hudson, 1981

Edwards, Brian, *The Modern Station: New Approaches to Railway Architecture*, London: E & FN Spon, 1997

Grow, Lawrence, *Waiting for the 5:05—Terminal, Station and Depot in America*, New York: Universe Books, 1977

Kern, Stephen, *The Culture of Time and Space 1880–1918*. Cambridge, Massachusetts: Harvard University Press, 1983

The Lilly Library, *From the Donkey to the Jet: Man's Experience with Travel*, Bloomington: Indiana University Press, 1978

Meeks, Carroll, *The Railroad Station: An Architectural History*, New Haven, Connecticut: Yale University Press, 1956

Pevsner, Nikolaus, *A History of Building Types*, Princeton, New Jersey: Princeton University Press, 1970

RAMSES WISSA WASSEF ARTS CENTRE

Designed by Ramses Wissa Wassef, completed 1989
Harrania, Egypt

The School and Arts Centre at Harrania, which bears his name, is the magnum opus of Ramses Wissa Wassef (1911–74), a prominent Egyptian architect and educator. Convinced of the value of and the need for training and practice in arts and crafts and in the educational and cultural development of young children, he began teaching weaving to a small group of children who attended a primary school that he had designed in Old Cairo in the 1940s. The satisfaction and benefit that those children gained from his devoted teaching and the high quality of the work they produced persuaded Wissa Wassef to establish a school specifically for training children in the arts and crafts.

In 1951, he and his wife bought a plot of land at Harrania, a small village near Giza, for that purpose. There was no precise brief. Wissa Wassef was his own client, and the demand for the sort of school he had envisioned was unknown, unproven; initially, it would have to be funded solely from his own resources. It would have to be built economically, and it must not alienate the community of *fellahin* (peasant farmers and farm laborers) among whom, in the village of Harrania, he had settled. He would use only local materials—the silty brown earth of the narrow fertile plain between the Nile and the desert escarpment to the west—and he would design and build in the vernacular tradition. From the field study visits that he had made with his architectural students to Upper Egypt, he had discovered the quality and the beauty of the Nubian villages; his colleague at the School of Fine Arts, Hassan Fathy, had recently embarked on the planning and design of a new village, in the Nubian vernacular tradition, on the west bank of the Nile near Luxor in Upper Egypt. Encouraged by Hassan Fathy's example and fired with enthusiasm by his own discovery of Nubian architecture, Wissa Wassef described his decision to build in the traditional way:

> I had just visited Aswan, where I had been struck by the beauty of the Nubian houses in the villages of the area, I learnt that it was still possible to find bricklayers who could make vaulted roofs for houses. I felt a strange excitement when I thought that these same methods had existed since the first dynasties of the Pharaohs. They had survived throughout Egyptian, Coptic and Islamic history, and

were still used in popular architecture. I decided to make use of some these bricklayers from Aswan, and turn their experience to account in building vaults for my school. (de Stefano, n.d.)

The school grew slowly. Village children were enrolled to learn weaving, and they were encouraged to assist the Nubian builders in making mud bricks and building adobe walls for the school buildings: weaving workshops, storerooms, and display spaces. Later, Wissa Wassef introduced the teaching of pottery: kilns, pottery workshops, and storerooms were needed. By the late 1950s, tapestries and carpets designed and made by the students were being exhibited internationally—in the United States, Switzerland, Germany, and Sweden—and money earned from the sale of the students' work was shared between the weavers themselves and the school. The pace and scale of building increased; by 1970, the first phase of building was complete.

In the early 1970s, his daughters Suzanne and Yoanna joined Wissa Wassef and his wife, Sophie, in teaching at the school. The small ceramic sculpture museum was designed and built and named after Sophie's father, the sculptor Habib Gorgy. In 1973, Suzanne married the architect Ikram Nosshi, one of her father's former students at the School of Fine Arts. After Wissa Wassef's unexpected death in 1974 at the age of 63, Nosshi continued the architectural development of the school under the direction of Sophie Habib Gorgy, Wissa Wassef's widow. She expanded and extended the scope of the school, acquiring more land, encouraging the building of houses on the site for her daughters and their families, and creating the Ramses Wissa Wassef Museum, which houses the permanent collection of the Arts Centre and traces the development of tapestry weaving, ceramics, and all the crafts taught there since the early days of its foundation. Completed in 1989, the museum, designed by Nosshi, forms the culmination of the complex and, although designed by a different hand, fits perfectly into the environment created by Wissa Wassef and his wife.

On entering the main gate of the Arts Centre, one enters a new world. The immediate environment is bleak; the village of Harrania has grown out of all recognition since the 1950s, when the Wissa Wassefs began to realize their vision, and has become a peri-urban suburb of greater Cairo. Within the boundary walls, the naturally rendered adobe walls, roof terraces, vaults, and domes of the congeries of buildings are linked by arcaded verandas, courtyards, brick-paved passageways, open staircases, and small shady gardens, all planned in an organic and apparently spontaneous way. The whole complex is surrounded by an extensive garden, planted with a wide variety of trees and shrubs, and has the appearance of an old, established rural community. Internally as well, the various working spaces, large and small, and the museums and galleries for displaying the tapestries, carpets, textiles, batiks, pottery, and ceramics are comfortably cool and appropriately lit with tiny skylights set into domes and vaults, clerestory windows, and simply designed perforated screen walls. The whole place is an oasis of calm and peace and at the same time an ever-flowing spring of creativity. In 1983, its merits were internationally recognized by winning the Aga Khan Award for Architecture. In the award citation, the project was commended "for the beauty of its execution, the high value of its objectives and the social impact of its activities, as well as its influence as an example . . . for its role as a centre of art and

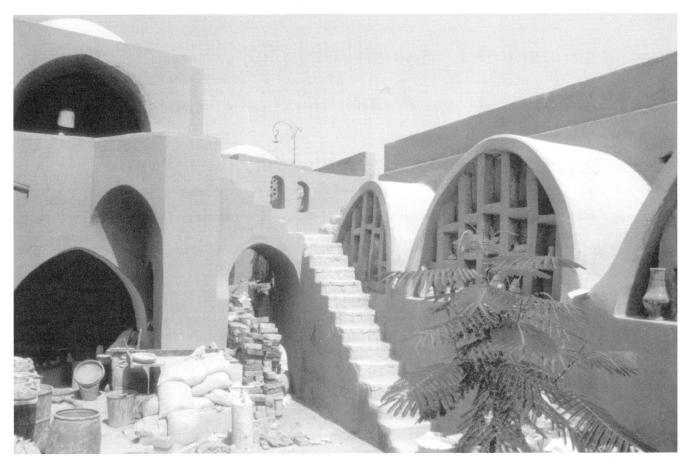

Pottery Studio in Courtyard, Ramses Wissa Wassef Arts Centre
Photo by Charles Avedissian © Aga Khan Trust for Culture

life and for its endurance, its continuity and its promise" (quoted in de Stefano, n.d.).

At the dawn of the 21st century, the Arts Centre has become an icon of "green architecture," a model of holistic design for architects around the world; and for Egyptians, trying to cope with the environmental pollution and population pressure of peri-urban greater Cairo, it has become a beacon of hope.

ANTHONY D.C. HYLAND

See also **Wassef, Wissa (Africa)**

Further Reading

de Stefano, E.A., *Threads of Life: A Journey in Creativity: Ramses Wissa Wassef Arts Centre Giza*, Harrania, Egypt: Ramses Wissa Wassaf Art Centre, n.d.
Holod, Renata and S. Rastorfer (editors), *Architecture and Community: Building in the Islamic World Today: The Aga Khan Award for Architecture*, New York: Aperture, 1983

RANCH HOUSE

After World War II, the American ranch house replaced the bungalow and the Cape Cod cottage as the preeminent American house type. Because housing costs had doubled in the 1940s, most architects designed flexible, multiuse spaces emphasizing both function and convenience, including the ranch house. However, because of both the Depression and wartime materials shortages, most consumers could fulfill dreams of a new house only with glossy magazines and corporate-sponsored scrapbooks. The end of World War II brought an enormous demand for new housing. The wartime development of new materials and new manufacturing methods enabled merchant builders to meet postwar consumer demand, which was subsidized by new federal loan programs. Concurrently, consumer magazines, merchant builders, and museum exhibitions promoted the ranch house as affordable shelter for the newly informal, family-oriented, and frequently suburban American lifestyle. Consumers embraced the ranch house as the paradigm for new, modern, and convenient housing, a preference endorsed by consumer magazines, an architectural pedigree that included Frank Lloyd Wright, and the unprecedented growth of suburbia after World War II.

The postwar ranch house is characterized by spaciousness facilitated by new building techniques, new materials, and interior design. The single-story house typically featured three zones: an open-plan common space, a centralized service core, and a cluster of private bedrooms. The open plan emphasized the flow of space between rooms, modulated by pass-throughs, open shelving, and built-in storage units. Indoor-outdoor living areas and large expanses of glass promoted the interpenetration of interior and exterior space. The rambling plan, horizontal em-

phasis, and low-pitched roof ideally integrated the ranch house into the landscape. Although the single-story ranch house proved prototypical, both the split level and the raised ranch abounded. Architects and merchant builders tailored the plan, exterior facings, and features such as appliances to the home owner's means. For example, in 1959, *American Home* featured a 1040-square-foot ranch house for $12,950 (including lot), and the *House Beautiful* Pace Setter House boasted 3100 square feet for $51,500 (including indoor pool and air conditioning).

Ranch house designers drew on numerous sources, including Spanish colonial architecture, Frank Lloyd Wright's Usonian houses, and California modernism, to create a distinctly American house type. Architect Cliff May traced the postwar ranch house to the 19th-century Spanish colonial rancho in the West. Arguing that form followed function, May claimed that the casual, outdoor-oriented "California life" of a small population of wealthy ranchers had generated the rambling, open-plan, single-story, adobe house with a *corredor*, or porch, instead of a hallway. The 20th-century suburban ranch house retained its associations with California casualness, indoor-outdoor living, and the notion of a putatively native architectural heritage.

Designers also adapted Frank Lloyd Wright's Usonian houses, first realized in the Herbert Jacobs House (1937). The Jacobs House used the L-shaped, "pollywog plan." The head of the pollywog contained both common spaces and the service core, including kitchen, bath, and other utilities. The interior expressed Wright's notion of organic architecture consisting of an open-plan space subdivided by ceiling levels, lighting effects, and built-in furniture. Private rooms, such as bedrooms, the study, and the workshop, formed the tail of the pollywog. Generous eaves, natural materials, and a horizontal silhouette integrated house and landscape. Wright's rhetoric also commended his domestic architecture to postwar readers of magazines such as *House Beautiful*, which promoted Wright as an American genius whose vision of American individualism embodied by the single-family home not only accorded with Cold War ideology but also affirmed the postwar development of suburbia.

Wright's reorientation of the kitchen, or "work space," from backstairs to the ideological and spatial center of the Usonian house proved fundamental to the postwar ranch house. The kitchen served as the control center, allowing the homemaker physical, visual, and even verbal access to the entire house, such as that afforded by the intercom system, one of a new array of appliances that facilitated the self-sufficiency of the postwar family. Whereas previously even working-class women had hired help to do laundry and heavy cleaning, the postwar economy dictated that most women labored alone, assisted by appliances rather than servants.

Both Wright and California modernists, such as Richard Neutra, used large expanses of glass—including picture windows, window walls, and sliding-glass doors—to integrate interior and exterior space. Similarly, *Sunset* promoted the "total combination of indoor-outdoor space" created by ground-level access to outdoor living areas as the ideal situation for casual living and informal entertaining. The low rambling profile, overhanging eaves, and features such as planter boxes integrated into the facade further unified house and landscape. Exterior adornment drew on both vernacular tradition and architectural design, at times simultaneously. A ranch house might combine the scalloped bargeboards of the Swiss chalet with geometric arrange-

ments of facing materials indebted to modernists such as Edward Durell Stone.

The open plan essential to the ranch house not only maximized space on a limited budget but also promoted American political and cultural values. In a series of articles written during the 1950s, *House Beautiful* associated the open plan with Wright's organic architecture, American sociability, and democratic freedom of choice. Similarly, the ranch house served as a vehicle for American nationalist ideology at the American National Exposition in Moscow in 1959, where exhibits of domestic technology included a "six-room, ranch-type house, completely furnished, within the price range of [the] average US worker" sectioned like a dollhouse and dubbed "Splitnik" (" 'Made in U.S.A.'—In Red Capital," *U.S. News & World Report* 47 [3 August 1959]). Despite the frequent association of the ranch house with the American way of life, critics such as John Keats noted that the open plan, often curtailed by restricted budgets, actually prohibited the gracious living promised by consumer magazines.

Ultimately, the postwar American ranch house catered to traditional families who not only craved comfort and convenience on a limited budget but also anticipated the American lifestyle promised by consumer magazines, television, and merchant builders' plan books. The postwar popularity of the ranch house eroded regional architectural differences, replacing local traditions with a national archetype. The ranch house embodied the American dream of planned suburban communities populated by city commuters and housebound homemakers who graciously entertained with an array of convenience foods consumed in the spacious confines of the open-plan, indoor-outdoor living area.

KRISTIN U. FEDDERS

Further Reading

Clark, Clifford Edward, Jr., *The American Family Home, 1800–1960*, Chapel Hill: University of North Carolina Press, 1986

Dyal, Donald H., *Sun, Sod, and Wind: A Bibliography of Ranch House Architecture*, Monticello, Illinois: Vance Bibliographies, 1982

Keats, John, *The Crack in the Picture Window*, Boston: Houghton Mifflin, 1956

Mason, Joseph B., *History of Housing in the U.S., 1930–1980*, Houston, Texas: Gulf, 1982

May, Cliff et al., *Sunset Western Ranch Houses*, San Francisco: Lane, 1946; reprint, Santa Monica, California: Hennessey and Ingalls, 1999

Young, Alfred Joseph, "The Suburban Ranch House: A Case Study of the Democratization of Modernism" (M.Arch. thesis), Georgia Institute of Technology, 1990

RASMUSSEN, STEEN EILER 1898–1990

Architect, architectural historian, and critic, Denmark

Steen Eiler Rasmussen's broad range of talents were manifest in his activities as an architect, town planner, educator, historian, and critic. Although he exerted influence in all these areas in his native Denmark, his ideas were disseminated to a wider audience via his translated books and his work as a visiting scholar in England, Turkey, Australia, and the United States. Born in

Copenhagen in 1898, Rasmussen entered the two-year preparatory course at the Royal Danish Academy of Fine Arts at the age of 18 and, on completion, joined the office of Carl Brummer. During his first year at Brummer's office, he collaborated with Knud Christiansen on three first prizewinning competition entries for the renewal of the Prinsensgade Quarter in Copenhagen and town plans for Ringsted and Hirtshals. Rasmussen was elected as a member of the Academic Council of the Royal Danish Academy of Fine Arts in 1922 and two years later was appointed as its first lecturer in town planning. In 1938, he was promoted to professor of architecture, a post that he held until 1968. During this period, he also served as a member of the Copenhagen Building Commission and the Copenhagen Traffic Commission and as chairman of the Danish Planning Laboratory and the Regional Planning Committee for Copenhagen.

The early inclination toward town planning would continue to occupy Rasmussen throughout his life. His most significant work in this area is undoubtedly "The Finger Plan of 1948," which was an attempt to produce an overall regional plan for greater Copenhagen. Conceived in collaboration with a team headed by Peter Bredsdorff, the plan called for the city to grow along a series of "fingers" marked by railway lines extending radially from the center. The area between these transport corridors was intended for forests and agricultural lands. According to Rasmussen, no one was to live farther than a 10-minute walk to a station, and those living in the outermost areas should be able to reach the center of the city within 30 to 45 minutes. Although the plan was never accorded legal status, the main structure of the plan was carried out in principal at local levels. The significance of the "Finger Plan" lies in the fact that although many other European cities sought to limit the growth of the town and establish "satellite towns," Rasmussen devised a means by which the city could remain a singular entity and extend outward in a controlled manner.

Rasmussen's interest in the city was not confined to his town-planning proposals but also extended to his work as a historian and critic. In 1927, he was afforded the opportunity to serve as a guest lecturer at the Architectural Association in London. Struck by the differences between life in Copenhagen and life in London, Rasmussen began to record the observations made during his initial period of residence and many subsequent visits and compiled the material into the book titled *London: The Unique City*, which was published in 1934. Although the book was almost immediately translated into English and has appeared in a number of editions, Rasmussen experienced disappointment because the book did not fulfill his intention of initiating a debate among legislators and politicians. Speaking of his disappointment in his foreword to the 1973 revised edition of the book, he stated that he had learned that one could not provoke discussion with a large book, but only with short, concentrated attacks in periodic publications. Rasmussen's commitment to debates regarding the quality of the physical environment are clearly seen in the numerous published articles in Danish newspapers and in his work as editor of the journal *Arkitekten* from 1927 to 1933.

In addition to his book on London, two more of Rasmussen's books have been translated into English: *Experiencing Architecture* and *Towns and Buildings*. Both works can be described as primers that provide a clear and cogent introduction to architecture and town planning, and they represent Rasmussen's range

of interest and breadth of knowledge. Soon after publication of the English editions of his books, Rasmussen was invited as a guest professor to various schools throughout the world, including the Massachusetts Institute of Technology; Yale University; the University of California, Berkeley; the Royal College of Art; and the University of New South Wales.

Rasmussen described himself as an "unsuccessful" architect as the result of many of his town-planning proposals not being carried through to an acceptable level of resolution because of a lack of commitment by municipal authorities. However, he was involved in a number of architectural projects that demonstrate both his aptitude as an architect and his adherence to the tenets of functionalism as they were expressed in Denmark at the time. Of particular note are Rasmussen's own residence (1937), an extension to the hotel Hornbaekhus (1942), the Rungsted School (1953), and the "Blanche" hostel (1961) in central Copenhagen. Two multifamily housing projects, "Skovgaarden" (1958, 1961) and "Banehegnet" (1962), serve as examples of how Rasmussen's ideas about town planning and architecture could be realized.

Speaking on his teaching methods that were developed over a career that spanned more than 60 years, Rasmussen stated that it was not his wish to tell students how problems should be solved but merely to get their minds working. A survey of his work reveals that his most significant contribution to 20th-century architecture came about not through his architectural and town-planning projects but through acute observations that continue to instruct his readers that architecture and town planning are not ends in themselves.

KEVIN MITCHELL

Biography

Born in Copenhagen, 2 February 1898. Graduated from the Copenhagen School of Architecture 1918. Arranged exhibit *Britisk Brugskunst*, Danish Museum of Decorative Arts, Copenhagen 1932; chair, planning committee for the Copenhagen area 1945–58; cooriginator, Finger Plan for Copenhagen 1947. Lecturer on urban planning, 1924–38, professor of architecture, 1938–68, Royal Academy of Art, Copenhagen. Died in Copenhagen, 19 June 1990.

Selected Works

Rasmussen House, Copenhagen, 1937
Hotel Hornbaekhus (addition), Copenhagen, 1942
"The Finger Plan of 1948," Town Plan, 1948
Rungsted School, Copenhagen, 1953
"Skovgaarden" Housing Project, 1958, 1961
"Blanche" Hostel, Copenhagen, 1961
"Banehegnet" Housing Project, 1962

Selected Publications

London, 1934; translated as *London: The Unique City*, 1937
Byer og Bygninger, 1949; translated as *Towns and Buildings*, 1951
Om at Opleve Arkitektur, 1957; translated as *Experiencing Architecture*, 1959
København, 1968

Further Reading

Published architectural and town-planning projects appeared in the journal *Arkitekten* between 1919 and 1960. For a good introduction to the range of Rasmussen's work, see Heath.

Heath, Ditte (editor), *Steen Eiler Rasmussen: Architect, Town Planner, Author* (exhib. cat.), Copenhagen: The Foundation for the Publication of Architectural Works, The School of Architecture in Aarhus, 1988

Langberg, Harald (editor), *Hvem byggede hvad: Gamle og nye bygningen i Danmark*, 3 vols., Copenhagen: Politikens, 1952; 2nd revised edition, 1968

Rasmussen, Steen Eiler, *København 1950*, Copenhagen: Nyt Nordisk Forlag, 1950

Slente, Finn (editor), *Bibliografi over Steen Eiler Rasmussens forfatterskab*, Copenhagen: Kongelige Bibliotek, Strube, 1973

RATIONALISM

The Rational School in mid-nineteenth century was an amorphous body of architects who held that architecture was ornamented construction, essentially structural form, however refined or adorned. Found in the philosophy that reason is the source and test of knowledge and best served by deductive inquiry, and as an extension of the Enlightenment, it was French in tradition as bequeathed by master masons of the so-called Middle Ages. It was differentiated from the British empirical tradition that ultimately was popularized as the picturesque, a distinction to exist well into the 20th century. Yet French and German architects consistently applied the theory to classical buildings; an early epitome was J.G. Soufflot's Church of St. Geneviève (Panthèon), Paris, 1757, a building to lead into Romantic Classicism. Academic design rituals were then perpetuated by the École des Beaux-Arts, Paris, followed by its many imitators in North America 1890–1940.

But the *École* had devolved to *classique* formalism, much to the chagrin of committed rationalists such as Jean-Baptiste Rondolet, who in 1802 argued that architecture derives from construction and is not an imaginative art. Or those impressed by the influential books of J.N.L. Durand, Rondolet's contemporary. Proposing that architecture be conditioned—as his fellow revolutionaries insisted—by social demand, that style be the "visible expression of its functioning parts," axial symmetry and classical forms in simple geometry were Durand's aesthetic preferences. As a planning methodology, he used a square grid to order structure and explain plan. It was a type of orderliness that post–1850 attracted theorist and architect E.E. Viollet-le-Duc. But Durand's obsession was French Gothic with its constructional clarity of parts, not just expressed but plainly exposed. His written expositions on modernism (that is, speculation as to an appropriate architecture for his day), on the use of new materials and technologies, on reasoned "principles, as opposed to rules" or imitative forms, on buildings as organisms, on style rather than the styles, and so on, remains highly persuasive.

Traditionally, the architecture of rationalism tended toward classicism, thereby emphasizing its foundation in 18th-century mathematics (measurable truth), therefore geometry plays a significant role. More lately this can be seen, for instance, in the early works of Frank Lloyd Wright, those post–1937 by a disciplined Ludwig Mies van der Rohe, and those beginning in the 1960s by Louis I. Kahn and his intelligent follower Mario Botta. From their individualistic variety we also can see that there is no coherent rationalistic style.

It is generally held that Rationalism arrived in the United States *c.*1800 through French emigrant architects such as Joseph J. Ramée, Maximilian Godefroy, and Benjamin H. Latrobe. But it was swamped by Jeffersonian Romanticism and formalism. The counter was found first in the words of Ralph Waldo Emerson and then in the might of industrialization and concomitant technical and engineering developments.

Emersonian nature and utility and inspired sculptor Horatio Greenough, who praised monumental buildings that addressed the "sympathies, the faith, or the taste of a people." He wrote Emerson that architecture was: "A scientific arrangement of spaces and forms to functions and to sit, . . . features proportioned to their graduated importance in function." The expression of functionality was the demonstration of reason. (The philosopher, whose tool is words, would refer to positivism.) Borrowing from American architect Louis Sullivan, who drew from Kant, Emerson, Greenough, and others, Wright was inspired by the "form follows function" aphorism, extending it by reflection on his family's love of Emerson, who urged a link with those "pertinent object lessons nature so readily furnishes," as Wright said. Is there anything in nature that does not function correctly, wondrously? Rationalism easily becomes entangled with the notion of utility and nearly synonymous with functionalism. But nature was the perfect teacher.

The application of rationalism reached a practical epitome beginning in the 1880s with the frighteningly tall buildings in New York City and Chicago. They had adopted structural systems evolved by engineers and building contractors and contained utilitarian features and technical innovations within a variety of facades. The expression of stacked spaces (to the Romantic), of stacked floors (to the rationalist), and vertical systems (water, people, structure, waste, etc.) was—and is—the architectural problem.

Although many were inspired by Viollet-le-Duc's words Wright made them contemporary and vital by speaking of an organic architecture for America's modern society and by producing works of an articulated (functional) clarity. The demonstration is the Darwin Martin house of 1904–05, and the Larkin Administration building (1903–06), both in Buffalo and both a rationalist's paradigm for differing building types.

Many of Wright's buildings possessed what he referred to as "picturesque" characteristics as he interpreted them from the English Arts and Crafts movement. His persuasion had a marked influence on European theory post–1910. Thus Wright and many of those founding modernists who were inspired by his words (not necessarily by his romantic designs), such as Walter Gropius, Le Corbusier, even Louis Sullivan (from whom Wright had drawn much nationalistic and transcendentalist fervor), and by Albert Kahn's industrial architecture, extracted intellectual sustenance from 19th-century theory and speculation.

In 1902 Sullivan wanted to impress on his audience "the simple truth—immeasurable in power of expansion—of the subjective possibilities of objective things." The architect's role was to interpret those things. In Europe Hendrik P. Berlage wrote about the "pure art of utility" and believed his Amsterdam Exchange buildings (1897–1903) followed principles espoused by Viollet-le-Duc. Auguste Perret was perhaps France's most ardent

classical rationalist so dramatically expressed in concrete structures and axial symmetry from 1903–25; consider Notre-Dame Le Raincy (1922–24). Up to the 1960s Le Corbusier was France's most versatile structural rationalist, as a comparison of Monzie house, Garches (1927), and the monastery of Le Tourette, Lyon (1957–60) patently reveal. Yet his three-dimensional compositions are also picturesque in manners that baffle rigid theorists.

When in the 1920s the central Europeans, in particular the Germans, absorbed the visual aspects of the rationalism inherent in Albert Kahn's industrial architecture (where primary considerations were daylight, production process, functionality, money, construction time, and structure), they elected for a reductive, chaste, plain interior and exterior aesthetic constructed in glass, concrete, or steel, usually exposed. Wright and others (such as the Dutch) worried that such an architecture might lead to a rejection of its traditional role as a social art to become merely utilitarian, rationalized rather than rational. In the 1920s the Modern movement was driven by rationalism until its industrial style was found to be a useful expression for internationalism as promoted by the political left. Mies van der Rohe in the 1920s, for example, took much from Wright (and others) to generate a dynamic architecture based on American industrial buildings. By the late 1930s he settled for what is best classified as a severe classicism, appearing rational but in fact it was prescriptively formal and abstract. Thus the reasons for Kahn's industrial aesthetic were abandoned by the Germans when they accepted an aesthetic that claimed to be expressively functional but was in fact a style applied to all building types, regardless of all other considerations.

In the late 1920s seven architects launched the Italian Rationalist Movement, announcing that a "[n]ew architecture, true architecture, must emerge from a strict adherence to logic, to rationality." Their buildings and projects, supposedly born in Italy's traditions (and in opposition to the bustling but defunct futurists) and in fascism were widely diverse in appearance, many with structural clarity while immodestly betraying the influence of Russian Constructivists, Le Corbusier, and the Bauhaus. Giuseppe Terragni was their more expert apostle through the 1930s.

Then in 1941, a theoretical work was released on antecedents of 20th-century architecture by Siegfried Giedion, *Space Time and Architecture*. It was a faithful rationalist document in praise of functionalism. Giedion's intention was to concentrate on "the interrelations with other human activities . . . [on] architecture, construction, painting, city planning, and science" (1954). This was followed in 1948 by his second seminal study, *Mechanization Takes Command*, whose title reveals all.

In the decades after midcentury, rationalism became both clarified and distorted. Louis Kahn believed that a building had measurable qualities, that there were ordinate and subordinate spaces with natural hierarchies, that these functional aspects wanted to be defined by their unique form, and that perceptual awareness of architecture was in the orderly arrangement of forms. Supported by his poetic philosophy, these relationships were vigorously exploited by simple volumetric geometry, notably his A.N. Richards Laboratories, Philadelphia (1957–61), the second paradigm of 20th-century rationalism. If we accept that architectural form is shaped by programmatic functions, and this should include social and economic conditions, or by the spirit of its time, or by timeless principles, then the two extremes

at midcentury were Kahn's romantically, picturesquely ordered forms and Mies van der Rohe's internally preordered forms classically composed. The reaction was the exploitation of form over function and hierarchies that were so apparent in 1950s sensualism and later the work of Arata Isozaki and Morphosis, to cite two examples.

A new neorationalism arose in the 1960s, again in Italy and composed by Fabio Reinhart and Aldo Rossi, among others, who rejected their predecessors. Soon there was the Madrid School, then in Germany architects Mathias Ungers and J.P. Kleihus, and in the United States, architects such as the New York Five, of whom the prolific Richard Meier has since remained the most faithful to original tenets. Again, these architects produced a wide variety of characteristics, none architectonically related, all distinct yet often claiming a mix of rationalistic and existential foundations.

Much of neorationalism was a theoretical twist with the attempt to relate architecture to political theories (usually Marxist) or to social theories, particularly through semiotics, which recognizes that buildings carry meanings (signs) and symbolic overtones, more often than not because of cultural continuity or history. Much of its theory was derived from or instituted in linguistics. Therefore one can understand that the problem of analogies with the complexities of architecture are many, not the least that semiotics (and the earlier structuralism) is evaluative, tending to operate postmortem, therefore only clumsily relevant to the processes inherent in creating architecture let alone to design methodology.

There is something strangely romantic in the architectonic application of those socioeconomic theories. Perhaps this reflects the continuing debate between rationalism and Romanticism, between the ongoing search for objective principles of design with universal application (regardless of complexity or culture, all functions are naturally similar throughout history), and the personal freedom that followed the collapse early in the century or generally agreed principles: witness Expressionism in the 1920s or sensualism in the 1950s or the independent Oscar Niemeyer and Frank O. Gehry.

The house in Riva San Vitalo, Italy (1972–73), by Mario Botta, should send shivers of joy through a rationalist because of its precisely extended square, obvious structure and responding use of materials, consistent vertical organization, functional expression, deceiving formality and careful proportions, all providing a modern clarification of Viollet-le-Duc's ideas, of Wright's organic song, and a sensible adaptation of Louis Kahn's functional geometry.

DONALD LESLIE JOHNSON

See also **Botta, Mario (Switzerland); Brutalism; Classicism; Constructivism; Corbusier, Le (Jeanneret, Charles-Édouard) (France); Futurism; Giedion, Sigfried (Switzerland); Modernism; Kahn, Albert (United States); Kahn, Louis (United States); Mies van der Rohe, Ludwig (Germany); Notre Dame, Le Raincy; Perret, Auguste (France); Skyscraper; Structuralism; Sullivan, Louis (United States); Terragni, Giuseppe (Italy); Wright, Frank Lloyd (United States)**

Further Reading

Collins (1965), Middleton and Watkin, and Gelernter describe or interpret historical, theoretical, and practical parameters. Lesnikowski dis-

cusses ideas and illustrates buildings *c.*1800 to the present, Banham nicely outlines the transition period *c.*1910, and Frampton the century's varied courses up to the 1980s. Each of the foregoing contains a discussion about rationalism and/or its proponents. Delevoy et al. display verbally and pictorially the transition from Louis Kahn to the so-called neorationalists; antihumanist proposals and baroque fantasies abound. Langmead and Johnson and Collins (1959, on Perret) outline two individual cases, one about Atlantic cross currents prior to *c.*1950.

Architectural Design. "Eugène-Emmanuel Viollet-le-Duc 1814–1879," 50, no. 3/4 (1980)

Architectural Design. "From Futurism to Rationalism," and Peter Dickens, "The Hut and the Machine," 51, no. 1/2 (1981)

Banham, Reyner, *Theory and Design in the First Machine Age,* London: Architectural Press, 1960

Collins, Peter, *Changing Ideals in Modern Architecture 1750–1950,* London: Faber, 1965

Delevoy, Robert, et al., *Rational Architecture the Reconstruction of the European City,* Bruxelles: Archive d'Architectures Modern, 1978

Frampton, Kenneth, *Modern Architecture, a Critical History,* 2nd ed., London: Thames and Hudson, 1985

Gelernter, Mark, *Sources of Architectural Form: A Critical History of Western Design Theory,* Manchester: Manchester University Press, 1995

Giedion, Siegfried, *Mechanization Takes Command,* New York: Oxford University Press, 1948

Giedion, Siegfried, *Space Time and Architecture, the Growth of a New Tradition,* Cambridge, Massachusetts: Harvard University Press, 1941, 3rd ed., 1954

Hearn, M.F. (editor), *The Architectural Theory of Viollet-le-Duc Readings and Commentary,* Cambridge, Massachusetts: MIT Press, 1990

Hoffmann, Donald, "Frank Lloyd Wright and Viollet-le-Duc," *Journal of the Society of Architectural Historians* 28 (October 1969)

Langmead, Donald and Donald Leslie Johnson, *Architectural Excursions. Frank Lloyd Wright, Holland and Europe,* Westport, Connecticut: Greenwood, 2000

Lesnikowski, Wojciech G., *Rationalism and Romanticism in Architecture,* New York: McGraw-Hill, 1982

Middleton, Robin and David Watkin, *Neoclassical and Nineteenth Century Architecture,* New York: Abrams, 1980

Summerson, John, *Heavenly Mansions,* New York: Norton, 1963

RAYMOND, ELEANOR 1887–1989

Architect, United States

Eleanor Raymond was one of a minority of women architects practicing in the United States in the early 20th century and was a significant figure in the history of American modernism. After several years of work in Boston's settlement houses, participation in the suffrage campaign, and an internship in the office of Boston landscape architect Fletcher Steele, Raymond entered the newly founded Cambridge School of Architecture and Landscape Architecture for Women in the summer of 1916. Directed by Harvard University professor and architect Henry Atherton Frost, the Cambridge School offered women a unique opportunity to master a Beaux-Arts–inspired curriculum within an all-female environment. However, enduring discrimination in the architectural profession and the Cambridge School's lack of accreditation remained obstacles for many graduates. After Raymond's completion of the program in 1919, she was made a partner in Frost's Cambridge firm, where she remained until opening her own practice in Boston in 1935.

Trained solely in the practice of domestic architecture, Raymond completed nearly 100 houses in her 50 years as an architect. She is best known for several projects that reflect her early interest in European modernism; most notably, the Rachel Raymond House in Belmont, Massachusetts (1931), and a studio for Boston sculptor Amelia Peabody in Dover, Massachusetts (1933). Much of Raymond's work, however, was firmly rooted in the still popular period styles of the Colonial Revival—a fact partially explained by the relatively conservative taste of New England clients and Raymond's own reservations about modernism.

Her early work was influenced in massing and in ornamental detail by the domestic architecture of colonial and early 19th-century New England. The planning of these houses, however, reflected a new concern for economy, efficiency, and the up-to-date amenities requested by her upper-middle-class suburban clients. In 1923, Raymond built her own house out of a partially demolished townhouse on Charles Street on Boston's Beacon Hill. Designed to be in keeping with the red brick Federal architecture of this historic neighborhood, 112 Charles Street (1923) was also home to several other single women involved in the design profession, including Raymond's longtime companion Ethel Power. Power, who served as editor of *House Beautiful* magazine from the early 1920s until the mid-1930s, was an important promoter of Raymond's work. The women of 112 Charles Street often collaborated on projects, creating a valuable network of female colleagues and clients.

During a 1928 trip to Paris and a 1930 trip to Germany, Raymond and Power viewed the work of European modernists such as Le Corbusier and Walter Gropius. The Rachel Raymond House in Belmont, Massachusetts (1931), designed for Raymond's sister, an interior decorator, reflected her interest in creating a regional modernism on her return to Boston. Built of a traditional wood frame with rough-sawed cedar cladding, the house differed in materials from the concrete and stucco monuments of the International Style. However, the house's rectilinearity and its flat roofs and upper-story terraces recall Gropius's housing for the faculty of the Bauhaus, which Raymond had visited in the fall of 1930. The interior continues these themes; an L-shaped, combined living room and dining room embodies the open planning principles of European modernism, whereas the retention of a central hall plan and the inclusion of decorative wood trim and antique Chinese hardware on the built-in cupboards disavow the machine age aesthetic. This merging of European and American sources significantly pre-dates the house that traditionally is credited with introducing modernism to the United States, Walter Gropius's house in Lincoln, Massachusetts (1937).

Raymond's clientele included a number of notable women who shared her professional aspirations and unmarried status. Most prominent was Amelia Peabody, a Boston sculptor and philanthropist who commissioned 16 projects between 1933 and 1972. Many of these commissions exemplified Raymond's interest in modernism and advanced building technologies. For example, the three-room studio that she designed for Peabody on her farm in Dover, Massachusetts (1933), featured easily cleaned cinder block walls, factory-ordered windows, a streamlined sitting room, and an experimental forced hot air system of heating.

Raymond's Dover Sun House (1948), a house designed around Hungarian chemist Maria Telkes's pioneering solar heating system, was also funded by Peabody. The heat collectors, which ran along the length of the attic story of the southern facade, stored a five-day supply of solar heat for the small two-bedroom house. Internationally recognized, the Dover Sun House was listed as one of Raymond's greatest contributions to the development of domestic architecture in her successful nomination to the American Institute of Architects Fellowship in 1961.

Raymond's interest in preserving the building traditions of colonial New England is best represented by the compound that she designed in Gloucester, Massachusetts, for mining heiress Natalie Hays Hammond (1942). Perched on a dramatic shoreline site, the Hammond Compound consists of three residences and a central dining hall grouped around a central courtyard. The buildings' steeply pitched roofs, small-paned casement windows, and dark-stained clapboarding hearken back to the domestic architecture of 17th-century New England, reflecting Hammond's fascination with American and British history. Despite its conservative appearance, the Hammond Compound reflects progressive planning principles in its attention to the needs of three single professional women.

In addition to domestic projects, Raymond also designed several chapels, an addition to an airplane parts manufacturing plant, and numerous farm outbuildings. As is the case with many women architects, Raymond received relatively little critical attention during her lifetime, an omission attributed in part to the eclectic nature of her work, which defies the stylistic categories of conventional architectural history. The rise of the women's movement during the 1970s and 1980s brought with it several surveys and monographs that helped to recover Raymond's career; in 1981, Raymond was the subject of a one-woman exhibition at the Institute of Contemporary Art in Boston.

NANCY B. GRUSKIN

See also **Gropius House, Lincoln, Massachusetts; Gropius, Walter (Germany)**

Biography

Born in Cambridge, Massachusetts; first of three daughters to attend Wellesley College, graduated 1909. Died in Cambridge on 1989.

Selected Works

112 Charles Street, Boston, 1923
Rachel Raymond House, Belmont, Massachusetts, 1931
Amelia Peabody Studio, Dover, Massachusetts, 1933
Dover Sun House, Dover, Massachusetts, 1948
Hammond Compound, Gloucester, Massachusetts, 1942

Selected Publication

Early Domestic Architecture of Pennsylvania, 1931

Further Reading

The most complete collection of Raymond's professional and personal materials is held by the Frances Loeb Library of the Harvard Graduate School of Design. *House Beautiful* magazine between the years 1921 and 1934 also provides a number of informative articles about Raymond's work of the period.

Anderson, Dorothy May, *Women, Design, and the Cambridge School*, West Lafayette, Indiana: PDA, 1980
Campbell, Robert, "Eleanor Raymond: Early and Indomitable," *AIA Journal* 71 (1982)
Cole, Doris, *Eleanor Raymond, Architect*, Philadelphia, Pennsylvania: Art Alliance Press, 1981
Eleanor Raymond: Architectural Projects, 1919–1973 (exhib. cat.), Boston: Institute of Contemporary Art, 1981
Gruskin, Nancy Beth, "Building Context: The Personal and Professional Life of Eleanor Raymond, Architect (1887–1989)," Ph.D. diss., Boston University, 1997
Torre, Susanna (editor), *Women in American Architecture: A Historic and Contemporary Perspective*, New York: Whitney Library of Design, 1977

REGIONAL PLANNING

Regional planning began from the idea that the essential basis for planning should be geography, not municipal jurisdictional lines. Although today this idea is easily accepted in principle, its history has been that of a reasonable proposition often ignored and frequently difficult to implement.

The beginning of regional planning in the United States is marked by the publication of Patrick Geddes' *Cities in Evolution* (1915), which first noted the tendency of large cities to disperse as they grew because of the influence of the automobile and industrial power. Although the idea of regional planning and governance had been considered as early as 1909, when the National Municipal League had its annual conference, Geddes recognized that the concept of a "city line" was being transformed by the growth of metropolitan regions, which no longer stopped at the end of municipal jurisdictions but were stretching into vast, spread-out areas that he termed "conurbations." Geddes observed the dispersed growth of areas such as Pittsburgh, Chicago, and the entire region between New York and Boston and predicted that such growth was the wave of the future, where "millions of people" would congregate in a way that ignored the significance of city boundaries.

Geddes, a Scotsman, had a significant influence on a small group of idealistic planners, especially Lewis Mumford, who nourished his ideas, elaborated on them with the help of other innovative planning founders, and eventually put them into practice in the early 1920s. However, it was Geddes who established the idea of the geographic region as the proper object of the planner's focus.

Geddes was an eccentric man who conducted masques and pageants to recapture past civic life. His was a large vision of not only how cities should be planned but also how the world must be transformed from the rule of technology and money into a new utopia. This transformation would take place, he maintained, by the creation of a "neotechnic" order that evolved through the public conservation of resources, eventually replacing the present of "more and more of worse and worse."

According to Geddes, the regional environment was the appropriate locale for this evolution because it contained the seeds for ideal human growth. Thus, his famous maxim "Survey before plan" meant that attention should be focused on the natural geographic characteristics of a region, such as its river basins, watersheds, and geology, and its social and cultural composition as well. Without naming it, he described urban sprawl as a dan-

ger to community life ("Towns must now cease to spread like expanding ink stains and grease spots."). Geddes was certain that the remedy could be found by understanding the varied organic composition of regional settlements and planning for growth by integrating nature into towns that grow "botanically."

These ideas were a shock to the system of early 20th-century urban planners, most of whom were firm in the embrace of the City Beautiful movement, with the girded, formal, symmetrical orthodoxy it entailed. A diverse group of unconvinced planners and architects, however, sought a different direction. The group, which included Lewis Mumford, Clarence Stein, Benton Mackaye, and Charles Harris Whitaker, came under the influence of Geddes and concocted a scheme that led to the Regional Planning Association of America (RPAA).

In 1923, the RPAA published a five-part program that set forth the principles for regional planning that included the development of new garden city types of communities over the next few years. The group elaborated on the need for regional planning as an antidote to the type of cities such as New York, Chicago, Philadelphia, and Boston that were turning into "dinosaurs" because of the dispersed urbanization that was being created by the automobile. Mumford termed this development the "fourth migration," the result of a technological revolution that was turning the movement of population centers outward for the first time. The goal of the RPAA was to lead it into "new channels" by developing a national plan that would define regions by unified geographic characteristics consisting generally of climate, soil, vegetation, industry, and culture.

Part of the RPAA's argument was economic. Stuart Chase contended that regional planning could achieve vast improvements over the inefficiencies of transport and energy that existed without it. Another part of the argument was based on the conservation of resources ("Regional planning is the new conservation," said Mumford), recognizing that a regional focus can treat "people, industry and the land" as single unit so that the population is distributed in a way that is compatible to its resources. Finally, the argument rested on the issue of attaining a "fuller quality of life" through regional planning by developing new communities that harmonized with the natural environment. These communities were not suburban housing tracts but rather "garden cities" that took their influence from Ebeneezer Howard and strengthened "indigenous America" against the tide of disbursed, thoughtless development.

The RPAA's diagnosis of the direction of urbanization in the United States was nearly prophetic. Much of its interpretation of the endemic problems of what Mumford described as the fourth migration is heard from contemporary urban planners who are daily confounded by the effects and consequences of urban sprawl. Moreover, most of the current remedies that are proposed to combat sprawl are contained, at least in concept, within the proposals originally described by the RPAA. In terms of policy implementation, however, the RPAA's influence remains solidly within the realm of good ideas. The two major experimental communities directly linked to the RPAA—Sunnyside Gardens in Queens, New York, and Radburn, New Jersey—exist mainly as curiosities on the road to suburbanization, which in the years following the RPAA developed as such a powerful tide that regional planning, as envisioned by Mumford, Stein, and the rest of RPAA, was essentially pushed out of the picture.

If the RPAA comprised the formative idealists of regional planning, the planners who first conceived of the Regional Plan of New York in 1923 were sober pragmatists. The group, headed by Thomas Adams and brought together by the Russell Sage Foundation, set out to create a regional plan for New York that was rooted in achieving economic efficiencies for a growing concentration of economic activities in the New York area through a scheme of "recentralization" of business and industry.

The plan, which encompassed an area of more than 5000 square miles, proved to be widely influential in the evolution of the New York metropolitan area, mainly because of its congeniality to business investment and its grasp of emerging trends in population movement and industrial development. Many of its suggestions for highways, bridges, and tunnels were eventually brought to realization by the power broker Robert Moses. Distinctly nonutopian in outlook, the plan called for new roads, parks, and beaches at the same time that it designated the last significant open space near Manhattan—Hackensack Meadows in New Jersey—for commercial development and omitted any consideration of public housing. In addition, although it steered away from consideration of garden cities and ideal communities, it nevertheless included a section by Clarence Perry that described the development of "neighborhood units," which offered a significant alternative to the model of the suburban single-family house and a source for ideas on clustered development planning years afterward.

The Regional Plan of New York was the first attempt to address the needs of a metropolitan area outside its municipal boundaries. Without any regulatory power of enforcement, such as zoning, it relied on the power of good planning ideas to achieve its goals, which could ill afford to antagonize those engaged in business and investment. To Mumford, however, the plan was dreadfully misconceived. His criticisms of the plan and Thomas Adams's defense of it constituted one of the most famous dialogues in American planning history: Mumford proselytizing for the ideal, Adams for the obtainable.

One of the significant participants in the Regional Plan of New York was Frederic Delano, the uncle of Franklin Delano Roosevelt, who was receptive to the idea of regional planning well before he became president of the United States. While governor of New York, he proposed a state commission ("cooperative planning for the common good") in rural homes and frequently spoke supportively of regional planning as a means to relieve congestion in the cities and redistribute population and industry more equitably and responsibly. At about the same time (1930), the National Municipal League described municipal boundaries as "obsolete" and called for expanded jurisdictional lines to "give reality to the work of planning principles."

In June 1933, shortly after taking office, President Roosevelt pushed a $25 public works bill through Congress that included funds to establish a resettlement administration, which was set up to plan a series of experimental greenbelt towns on the periphery of large metropolitan areas. However, the Resettlement Administration's creator, Rexford G. Tugwell, soon came into conflict with Congress, which considered this effort at regional planning by the federal government the bulwark of socialism. Within months, Tugwell and the Resettlement Administration were put out of business, although three greenbelt towns were eventually built (Greenbelt, Maryland, near Washington, D.C.;

Greenhills, near Louisville, Kentucky; and Greendale, Wisconsin, near Milwaukee).

The most shining symbol of New Deal regional planning was the Tennessee Valley Authority (TVA), which was the last direct federal involvement by the federal government before World War II. President Roosevelt described the project as an exercise in regional planning, but it was actually much more, as it included a massive flood control project on the 650-mile-long Tennessee River basin and a huge power-producing operation that by 1944 was generating half the nation's power. Originally, it was intended also as an armaments production facility, a proposal that President Roosevelt was successful at eliminating.

The period immediately following World War II saw a resurgence of interest in the idea of regional planning as the idea of reshaping local governments into regional jurisdictions was frequently debated. In 1950, Atlanta adopted its plan for improvement, which integrated the relationship of the City of Atlanta to Fulton County. In 1953, the Ontario Parliament approved the federated municipality of Metropolitan Toronto, reflecting what seemed to be the current tide of good planning. Numerous reports and studies in the early 1950s called for "intergovernmentalizing" services and frequently petitioned for new interjurisdictional initiatives to better coordinate policies and planning. Fueled by a surge in federal spending, these efforts generally sought to make capital planning on the municipal level more efficient and to coordinate the federal government's spending programs. When Congress passed the Housing Act of 1954, for example, it included direct federal assistance to regional and metropolitan planning agencies. Shortly thereafter, the National Municipal League responded by developing a so-called model state and regional planning law. In 1955, the Commission on Intergovernmental Relations, known as the Kestnbaum Commission, emphasized that metropolitan areas were the most critical "focal points" for dealing with urban needs.

Despite the increased attention to jurisdictional reform, local governments were reluctant to disturb traditional lines of authority. Efforts at metropolitan reorganization in, for example, Cleveland and St. Louis were ineffective. By 1959, the Advisory Commission on Intergovernmental Relations was forced to conclude that metropolitan reorganization, whether through consolidation or internal restructuring, faced an uphill battle because of strong local resistance. When voters were faced with public referendums, they were either indifferent or opposed. Jurisdictional reform held little appeal outside Washington, D.C., or among urban planners focusing on regional matters. By the early 1960s, the idea of jurisdictional reform—and with it regional planning and governance—had lost much momentum. The continued expansion of federal funding and the mounting complexity of urban problems, however, required that some new structural solution be found. The answer, for the most part inadvertently created, was the development of new area-wide organizations of locally elected officials, which soon came to be referred to as Councils of Governments (COGs).

A veritable nationwide COGs movement soon developed, nurtured by federal funds. It began with the creation of the Detroit-area Inter-County Supervisor's Committee in 1956, and by 1960 more than one half of 212 metropolitan areas had created new COGs. Areawide planning was gaining ground all across the nation. COGs provided a means to effectively address metropolitan problems, satisfying federal priorities for increased coordination of planning functions within the metropolitan region while avoiding the issue of jurisdictional reform. The federal preference for such planning was unambiguous. In the 1960s and 1970s, federal aid programs for highways, mass transit, and open space insisted on metropolitan planning as a funding requirement. By 1979, 39 separate federal programs required regional or metropolitan planning as a requirement for local participation.

Regional planning had found its home within the arms of COGs. Sustained by federal financial assistance in the form of Section 701 comprehensive planning grants, regional planning at long last gained institutional credibility as COGs joined with the National Association of Regional Councils. Regional planning commissions proliferated as never before by becoming COGs. At the same time, however, because of their voluntary nature, regional planning functions were separated from the idea of regional governance. The Miami Valley Regional Planning Commission, the Association of Bay Area Governments, and the Metropolitan Washington (D.C.) Council of Governments were examples of this type of structure. Although countless regional plans were developed, few were implemented in any meaningful way, and many suffered from overly general recommendations. Whatever their virtues, most of these plans had the problem of being politely ignored by local jurisdictions. The regional planning COGS settled into a comfortable existence of clearinghouses for federal grants, including those for water-quality planning, air-quality planning, solid-waste management, and the A-95 review process. Many were limited to information exchange, coordination, technical assistance, and the provision of some services.

In speaking about regional planning in the 1930s, the National Municipal League had warned that "to be of value plans must be executed." In the early 1960s, this advice seemed particularly relevant as the goals of regional planning became separated from regional governance through the establishment of COGs that had no real ability to implement their plans.

Although the COGS structure of regional planning has become the dominant one, there are significant exceptions. Since 1967, the Twin Cities Metropolitan Council has been a prime model for regional planning in a major metropolitan area that effectively combines planning, policies, and implementation. Significantly, it came into being as an action by the State of Minnesota, not a local referendum. It is distinctive because its role in making regional policy is authoritative rather than advisory. With its own political base, it has enjoyed a relatively productive history working with local municipalities within a seven-county area, particularly since passage of the Land Planning Act of 1976, an important effort in regional growth management.

Similarly, the Portland (Oregon) Metropolitan Area developed a regional approach to planning. Its evolution encapsulates both the weaknesses and the strengths of regional planning. In the early 1960s, Portland, like many metropolitan areas, established a voluntary association of governments to address areawide planning needs. The Columbia Region Association of Governments (CRAG) originally encompassed an area of four counties and 14 cities. CRAG emphasized intergovernmental cooperation to combat a number of regional problems, such as loss of farmland and the escalating public cost of spread-out development.

By the early 1970s, however, it became clear that CRAG's advisory influence was powerless to overcome conflicts among member jurisdictions. In 1973, in response to heightened environmental concern, the Oregon State Legislature passed a bill that significantly strengthened CRAG's role. It made local membership in CRAG mandatory and gave it authority to overrule local development plans within 27 participating jurisdictions that did not conform to the regional comprehensive plan. This bill, in conjunction with the passage of a state land use development law, eventually led to the Metropolitan Service District (METRO), a directly elected regional government with wide responsibilities. With strong land use powers, METRO became the rare bird of regional planning, an organization that came into being from broad public consensus that is able to address regional land use policies effectively.

Although the federal government retracted many programs fostering regional planning in the early 1980s, such as Section 701 comprehensive planning grants, other federal programs brought about new regional planning responsibilities. The most significant was the Coastal Zone Management Act of 1972, which provided grants to states to develop comprehensive programs for preserving coastal resources. The result was the establishment of state-run coastal programs in 18 coastal states that assumed regional planning responsibility and varying levels of land use control in waterfront areas.

However, the most significant helping hand that regional planning has received came about on the state level as a result of heightened interest in growth management programs. Numerous states have passed some sort of growth management (or "smart development") controls in the last two decades. Usually, state growth management strategies have relied on regional planning agencies that came out of COGs, strengthened with additional funding and new authority. In general, these regional planning agencies implement state growth management goals by identifying valuable regional resources and developing regional growth management plans. In Florida, for example, eleven regional planning councils were established to develop plans and review local jurisdiction plans for consistency. Even states in which regional councils do not exist within a strict government framework with regulatory authority, such as Florida, Georgia, Vermont, and Maine, nonetheless have regional statutory authority over local plans.

Most growth management strategies are concerned with directing development to appropriate regions within a regional environment—to limit urban sprawl in favor of preserving open space and balancing service capacities. In Oregon, this effort has relied on the establishment of regionally drawn urban service boundaries, which attempt to attain a regional balance between compact development and protection of natural resources. In all cases, regional planning councils are concerned with identifying the greater-than-local planning issues that must be dealt with through an integrated growth policy. Increasingly, the recognition that a problem such as urban sprawl requires a comprehensive area-wide solution has reinvigorated the role of regional planning.

RICK ADAMS

See also **Mumford, Lewis (United States)**

Further Reading

Further readings on Regional Planning begin with its roots in English Utopian Planning and extend through its appeal to urban theorists such as Lewis Mumford and more recent ecological planners. The distance between these theories and actual implementation of regional plans rounds out one of the most influential planning stories in the 20th century.

Boyer, Christine M., *Dreaming the Rational City: The Myth of City Planning*, Cambridge, Massachusetts: MIT Press, 1983

Geddes, Sir Patrick, *Cities in Evolution*, London: Williams and Northgate, 1915

Hall, Peter, *Cities of Tomorrow*, Oxford, England and Cambridge, Massachusetts: Blackwell Publishers, 1996

Le Corbusier, *The City of To-morrow and Its Planning*, translated by Frederick Etchells, London: J. Rodker, 1929

Mumford, Lewis, *The Story of Utopias*, New York: Boni and Liveright, 1922

REGIONALISM

Regionalism in architecture is the desire to shape buildings according to the particular characteristics of a specific place. Regionalism aims to obtain a visual harmony between the building and its geographical setting, to connect with the culture and architectural traditions of the local area, and to manage the local climate as naturally and as efficiently as possible. Because regional buildings in a particular place respond to a similar set of local characteristics, they will possess a similar look that can often be described as a style like "Southwestern" or "Cape Cod," and as these characteristics vary from place to place, buildings in different regions will have distinctly different appearances relative to each other.

Regionalism is the oldest and most pervasive of all building ideas. In the prehistoric world, and in vernacular settlements throughout the world, builders used local materials because they were conveniently at hand. They also adapted their forms to the local climate in order to moderate temperature swings and to manage precipitation for comfort and survival. For example, buildings in hot, dry climates are often constructed of thick adobe walls, which first absorb heat during the hot days, providing a cool interior, and then radiate the heat into the building during the colder nights. Buildings in the wet climate of Northern Europe evolved steep roofs to shed rain and snow. Most regions of the world have similarly developed vernacular traditions of building that are well adapted to their particular geographical circumstances. Distinctive regional vernacular traditions include Greek fishing villages, Italian hill towns, and the adobe of Santa Fe. Even today, a great deal of the mass-produced built environment may be seen as regional in character. Houses in the suburbs of London look different from those in Switzerland, which look different from those in Thailand. When builders are not self-conscious about style or fashion, regional tendencies are most likely to emerge because they make practical sense and derive from successful traditions in the area.

In the world of high-style or high-status architecture, however, the concept of regionalism has had a more complex history. For buildings like temples, public monuments, palaces, and corporate headquarters, clients and their designers often seek to express power, status, or philosophical outlooks that are not about the practical realities of dealing with the local climate or geography. These statements are usually about abstractions and

are often meant to apply more universally than to a particular location. For example, ancient temples were designed as appropriate homes for deities whose powers transcended a local place and time. These buildings therefore employed a rigorous orthogonal geometry that was thought to be more universal and timeless in character than the more casual geometries that adapted themselves to the peculiarities of the local site. More recently, proponents of the International Modernist movement between the World Wars used a similar palette of industrial forms and materials for buildings in widely diverse geographical areas, because they wanted to express a universal view of modern life and industrialization that transcended individual places.

These two ideas—regionalism and the universal—are not necessarily mutually exclusive. One might express a universal sense of beauty while still accommodating local conditions and traditions, for example. But many times in the history of Western architecture, the one has been pursued at the expense of the other and vice versa. Builders sensitive to regional practicalities may scoff at higher aesthetic concerns and meanings, whereas high-fashion designers may disparage regional concerns as parochial or inconsequential in relation to bigger philosophical issues. From the Renaissance on, for example, many architects transplanted ancient Roman Classical forms to other regions to express their connection with the high civilization of Rome, even

though the shallow roofs that were originally designed for the Italian climate did not work as well in the wetter climates of northern Europe or the east coast of America.

To understand the history of regionalism in high-status Western architecture in the 20th century, one must look back to the end of the 18th century. Until then, high-status architecture was dominated by various versions of Roman Classical architecture applied irrespective of the local conditions. But several broad cultural movements in Europe and America led to a renewed appreciation of different regions and their possibilities for design. Namely, the Romantic movement in the arts drew attention to the raw and varied beauty of nature and to picturesque vernacular villages and cottages that appeared to live in harmony with nature. Second, as people began to identify more with their cultural groups than with the kingships that had often transcended cultural boundaries, they began to look for the special qualities of their own nationality and place, including the indigenous architectural traditions that they could claim as their own. Third, the rapidly expanding Industrial Revolution created manufactured goods of such variable quality that many began to call for a revival of handcraft by skilled craftspeople. Crafts were distinctly regional in character, which encouraged a renewed look at local traditions.

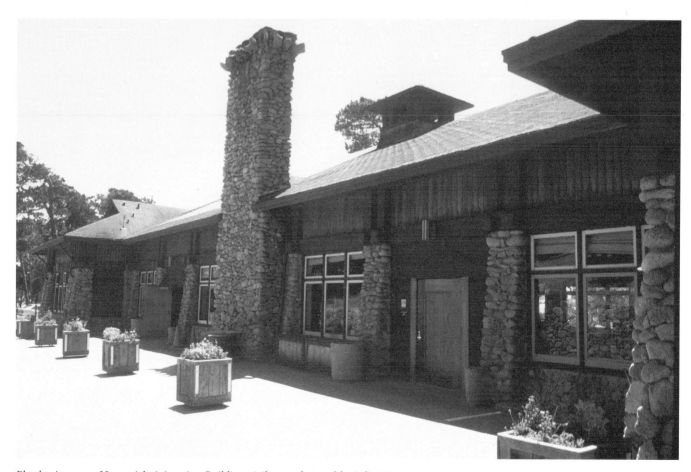

Phoebe Apperson Hearst Administration Building, Asilomar, designed by Julia Morgan
Photo © Mary Ann Sullivan

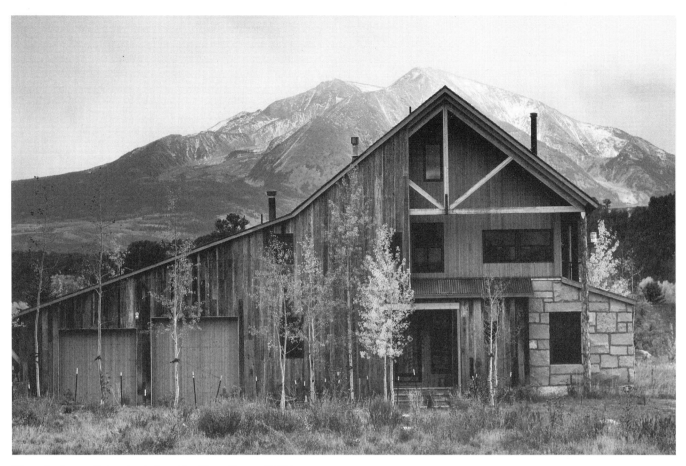

House in Aspen, Colorado, designed by Harry Teague (1997)
Photograph © Robert Millman

All of these combined in the Gothic Revival movement in the first decades of the 19th century, which in turn led to the Arts and Crafts Movement in the latter half of the 19th century and the first decades of the 20th. The Arts and Crafts architects in Britain revived the medieval vernacular traditions of building in their local regions, which they believed fitted the local culture and climate while embodying good craftsmanship. Charles Rennie Macintosh derived a number of his forms from Scottish Baronial castles, Sir Edwin Lutyens drew on medieval house forms in the southern English county of Surrey, and Charles Annesley Voysey stripped down medieval house forms to their underlying essences, leading to some of the first simplified modernist architectural forms that nonetheless still exuded a regional sense of place.

This new focus on regionalism invaded the École des Beaux Arts, the school of architecture and art in Paris that had become the world center for teaching the principles of ancient Roman Classicism. The professor of theory at the École at the turn of the century, Julien Guadet, taught that a building in the city should be different from one in the country, just as one at the seaside must be different from one in the mountains. This helped inspire a movement later named Academic Eclecticism by the historian Richard Longstreth, which among other things attempted to fuse the regional with the universal. These architects derived their ideas from traditional architectural styles that they believed embodied timeless and universal principles of design, but at the same time they chose their precedents to fit the particular geographical setting.

The Arts and Crafts tradition and aspects of Academic Eclecticism influenced Frank Lloyd Wright, who became America's most influential spokesperson for the regionalist idea. Borrowing the phrase "organic architecture" from Louis Sullivan and drawing on Japanese design sensibilities, Wright insisted that buildings should harmonize with nature and sensitively address the local geology and site conditions. While living in Chicago in the first decades of the 20th century, he developed the Prairie School, whose low, horizontal lines he said captured the essence of America's Midwestern plains. The buildings that he later designed for the Arizona desert looked distinctly different from the ones he designed in Wisconsin, as each responded to the particular local characteristics.

Wright's contemporary, Bernard Maybeck, also pursued the regionalist implications of Academic Eclecticism and the Arts and Crafts movement. After moving to the Bay Area of San Francisco before the turn of the century, he began to develop a distinctive style for the area that was based in part on medieval vernacular German forms and in part on the Shingle Style that had enjoyed a brief popularity in the northeast seacoast resort

towns several decades earlier. Despite these disparate and remote sources, Maybeck fused them into an organic whole that inspired other architects, including Julia Morgan, and that still defines much of the special character of the East Bay area today.

In the first two decades of the 20th century, many other builders and architects followed this pattern of adapting and combining various architectural traditions to fit a particular location. The Greene brothers Henry and Charles combined Arts and Crafts and Japanese traditions for their distinctive version of the Craftsman style in Pasadena. Their shallow roofs, open sleeping porches, and casual assymetric forms suited well the moderate climate and emerging southern California culture.

Regionalism faded in popularity for high-status buildings after the Second World War. The mood in America and Europe had changed to favor an international outlook and a positive view of industrialization, and these were best expressed with the ahistorical, technological, and non-regional forms of Modernism. In the 1970s, however, the mood changed again. As the world economy became more pervasively global in character and universal in taste, and as generic office buildings and chain retail stores began to make London look like Los Angeles or Houston, many people began to seek again a special quality in their particular place. Out of this grew the Historic Preservation movement, which sought to save historic buildings and districts for their local character, rather than risk another blandly generic redevelopment.

A number of architects have sought regional expressions from the 1980s, including Robert Venturi in Philadelphia, Robert Stern in New York, Antoine Predock in New Mexico, Harry Teague in Colorado, and Glenn Murcutt in Australia. Like their regionalist predecessors before World War II, most of these new regionalists have explored aspects of the traditional styles and vernacular forms that might provide clues to appropriate design qualities in their region; but in most cases, their Modernist roots have led them to find fresher or more contemporary expressions of the traditional ideas.

For example, a traditional Colorado barn form inspired Harry Teague's design for a vacation home in Aspen, Colorado. This sensitively expresses the forms of the landscape and the traditions of the area, whereas the uninterrupted space within supports the casual life-style of living in one large great-room. On closer inspection, however, one can see that the architect has stripped away the outer skin on part of the façade to reveal the inner structure and a recessed wall of windows that carefully frames external views. The modifications to the traditional form are Modernist in spirit, and the materials, massing, siting, and connections between inside and outside unmistakably link this building to its local context.

MARK GELERNTER AND VIRGINIA DUBRUCQ

See also **Arts and Crafts Movement; Contextualism; Craftsman Style; Environmental Issues; Greene, Henry M. and Charles S. (United States); Historicism; Historic Preservation; Lutyens, Edwin (England); Mackintosh, Charles Rennie (Scotland); Maybeck, Bernard (United States); Morgan, Julia (United States); Prairie School; Stern, Robert A. M. (United States); Sullivan, Louis (United States); Sustainability and Sustainable Architecture; Voysey, Charles F. A. (England); Wright, Frank Lloyd (United States)**

Further Reading

Regionalism as it applies to vernacular building traditions is covered in books too numerous to mention here and in fields including anthropology, architectural history, construction, and cultural history. For just a few examples, see Carver's *Japanese Folkhouses* and Nabokov and Easton's *Native American Architecture*. Also see Fletcher's *History of Architecture* for a good overview of the various cultural and environmental forces that shaped architecture in regions throughout the world. Books on regionalists in the 20th century can often be found under the name of the architect; for example, Woodbridge's *Bernard Maybeck*.

Boutelle, Sara Holmes, *Julia Morgan, Architect*, New York: Abbeville Press, 1988

Carver, Norman F., *Japanese Folkhouses*, Kalamazoo, Michigan: Documan Press, 1984

Collins, Brad, and Elizabeth Zimmermann, *Antoine Predock, Architect 2*, New York: Rizzoli, 1998

Davey, Peter J., *Architecture of the Arts and Crafts Movement*, New York: Rizzoli, 1980; as *Arts and Crafts Architecture*, London: Phaidon Press, 1995

Fletcher, Banister, *A History of Architecture for the Student, Craftsman, and Amateur: Being a Comparative View of the Historical Styles from the Earliest Period*, London: Batsford, and New York: Scribner, 1896; as *Sir Banister Fletcher's A History of Architecture*, 20th edition, edited by Dan Cruickshank, Oxford and Boston: Architectural Press, 1996

Fluckinger, Dan (editor), *Lake/Flato*, Rockport, Massachusets: Rockport, 1996

Frampton, Kenneth, "Towards a Critical Regionalism: Six Points for an Architecture of Resistance," in *The Anti-Aesthetic: Essays on Postmodern Culture*, edited by Hal Foster, Port Townsend, Washington: Bay Press, 1983; reprint, as *Postmodern Culture*, London: Pluto, 1985

Gelernter, Mark, *A History of American Architecture: Buildings in Their Cultural and Technological Context*, Hanover, New Hampshire: University Press of New England, and Manchester: Manchester University Press, 1999

Longstreth, Richard W., *On the Edge of the World: Four Architects in San Francisco at the Turn of the Century*, New York: Architectural History Foundation, and Cambridge, Massachusetts: MIT Press, 1983

Nabokov, Peter, and Robert Easton, *Native American Architecture*, New York: Oxford University Press, 1989

Rudofsky, Bernard, *Architecture without Architects: A Short Introduction to Non-Pedigreed Architecture*, New York: Museum of Modern Art, and London, Academy Editions, 1964

Woodbridge, Sally Byrne, *Bernard Maybeck: Visionary Architect*, New York: Abbeville Press, 1992

REICHSTAG, BERLIN

Initially designed by Paul Wallot, completed 1894; redesigned by Sir Norman Foster, completed 1999
Berlin, Germany

Built at the end of the war-ravaged 20th century, the new German Parliament building is significant for the refurbishing of a tarnished image—not of the Reichstag itself, but of German national identity. The conversion of the Reichstag by Sir Norman Foster, completed in 1999, was the building's most optimistic incarnation of its troubled history. The Reichstag always had symbolized a democratic German forum, although it was not until 1999 that a fairly elected democratic body convened within its chambers.

In 1871 the German Parliament, operating under the strict control of Kaiser Wilhelm and Chancellor Bismarck, had very limited power. Traditionally convened at the convenience of the emperor, the appointed parliament was finally allowed to have a meeting place of its own in 1882. After two competitions, the design was awarded to Paul Wallot, a little-known German architect. The neo-Renaissance building was constructed between 1884 and 1894 after many design compromises negotiated between the Kaiser, Bismarck, and the parliamentarians.

The building was a gift from the Kaiser to his people, but he actively hated it—reluctantly inscribing *Dem Deutschen Volke* ("to the German people") over the entry in 1916, while privately referring to it as *Reichsaffenhaus* ("the imperial monkey house"). The seating arrangement reflected the emperor's power—his ministers and officials sat on a raised rostrum at the end of the room, presiding over the members. Members could only address the body formally; interruptions and debate were rare.

A fire, rumored to be an act of arson by the Nazis, devastated the building in 1933. The scarred building was then shelled and vandalized by the Russian army in 1945, leaving it a ruin. A poorly executed partial renovation in 1961 restored the building's functionality, but parliamentary sessions were not held due to political opposition by Russia and England—two of the four occupying forces in then-divided Berlin. Existing in the shadow of the Berlin Wall, the Reichstag was the backdrop of several historic takeovers, protests, speeches, and concerts.

In 1991, two years after the fall of the Berlin Wall and reunification of West and East Germany, the Bundestag narrowly approved a move of the capitol from Bonn back to Berlin. It was a controversial decision; the wrecked and ill-regarded Reichstag was chosen over the popular provisional Parliament Building then nearing completion.

A competition for converting the Reichstag was held in 1992. In the second stage of the competition, Foster and Associates were awarded the commission. Reconstruction began in 1995 after a dramatic wrapping of the building by the environmental artists Christo and Jean-Claude. Work was completed in 1999, and the first parliamentary session was held on 19 April 1999.

The competition's winning scheme called for a light steel and glass roof hovering over the entire Reichstag. This proposal could be seen as similar in spirit to the elegant wrapper Foster designed for the Carré d'Art in Nimes (1984–93). As the design of the master plan of the surrounding area evolved, the huge glass cover was eliminated. Design emphasis was shifted to a new dome that would become a lantern for the building.

From the exterior, the renovation was restrained. The sleek interiors of metal and glass were visible behind the old masonry colonnade. The gigantic dome, mostly glass and striated by spi-

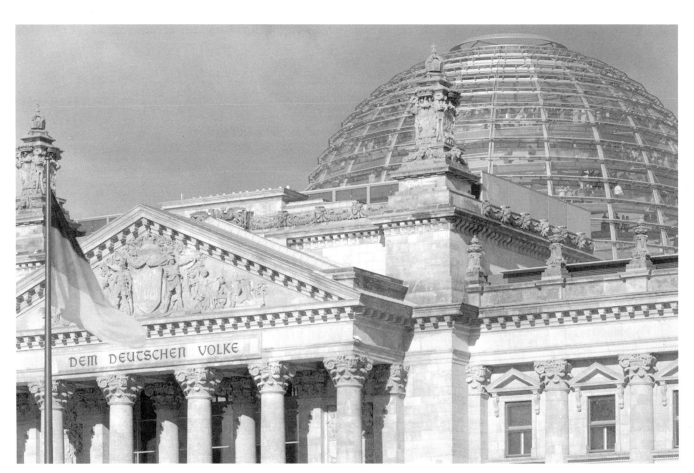

Reichstag building showing Wallot's Facade and Norman Foster's dome
Photo © Dennis Gilbert/VIEW

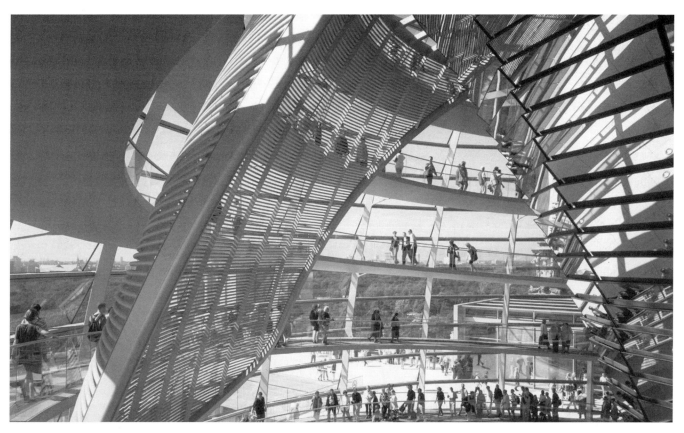

Reichstag, interior of the dome
Photo © Nigel Young/Foster and Partners

raling ramps, was the most visible change to the 19th-century facade.

Internally, the old and new materials were clearly separated and placed in dialogue. Exposing layers of history found during the renovation became part of the design strategy. Marks of the masons, 19th-century decorative moldings, Russian bullet holes, and graffiti all were framed by fresh plaster walls.

The main organization of the original building was preserved—a central parliament chamber flanked by two exterior courts. The chamber was semi-circular and gently raked with a concentric public viewing gallery cantilevered from the second floor. In a notable departure from the 19th-century room, the ceiling of the chamber followed the geometry of the dome above. Light was distributed evenly through a series of mirrors and filters. A central reflective element formed the hub of a bicycle-wheel cable system anchored at the spring point of the dome. Light and airy, the room's focus was an enormous eagle, an icon moved from Bonn.

Circulation in the building was organized to reflect a genuine democracy. Citizens, lawmakers, and visitors all entered through the same portal and used the grand stair. The formality of the original plan was restored, removing the many small revisions from the 1960s renovation that had obscured the secondary axes. Most of the massive masonry walls were retained, but a new transparency was gained through skillful manipulation of natural and artificial light.

At the end of the public sequence was the spectacular glass dome with intertwining double helical ramps. The structure of the 40-meter dome, along with ramps and central mirror, all are hung from the original masonry walls. This required the construction of a significant temporary structure and the use of a 40-meter crane (one of only four in Europe at the time).

From the dome, visitors gained a panoramic view of the city as well as a limited view down to the parliamentary chamber illuminated beneath. In the middle of the dome was a mirrored sculptural element that had multiple functions: it directed light, which was diffused by a shade, to the chamber below; it reflected focused artificial light beams across the city at night; and it acted as a heat chimney, exhausting hot air from the chamber below.

Appropriate to Germany's innovative environmental legislation in the latter part of the 20th century, the Reichstag followed many sustainable building practices. The building adapted the original 19th-century heating and cooling strategy, relying on two existing aquifers. These underground lakes were used to store heated or cooled water, which then flowed into radiators in the floors or ceilings. Power was generated by burning vegetable and seed oils, renewable resources that burned with minimal waste.

RENÉE CHENG

See also **Foster, Norman (England); Berlin, Germany; Berlin Wall, Berlin; Memorial**

Further Reading

Cullen, Michael, "Reichstag Revisited," *Architectural Review* 193, no. 1153 (March 1993)

Davey, Peter, "Democracy in Berlin," *Architectural Review* 206, no. 1229 (July 1999)

Gregotti, Vittorio, "A Lost Opportunity," *Casabella* 601 (May 1993)

Jones, Peter, "Parliamentary Precedents," *Architectural Review* 193, no. 1153 (March 1993)

Taylor, Ronald Jack, *Berlin and Its Culture: A Historical Portrait*, New Haven, Connecticut: Yale University Press, 1997

REINFORCED CONCRETE

Several European engineers, working independently, developed reinforced concrete throughout the 19th century. Francios Hennebique of France was one of many to patent his experimental work (1887), and in the last two decades of the 19th century, he devised a coherent system of reinforced concrete. By 1917, Hennebique's international firm had completed a staggering 17,000 contracts, forging a worldwide industry. Although the use of this type of construction was widespread in Europe, North Africa, and North America at the turn of the century, most builders were interested in its fireproofing characteristics, and few understood the tensile potential inherent in the reinforcing. The notion that steel and concrete could function monolithically had already been demonstrated on paper and in practice by many engineers, but the structural ramifications of that fact required time to disseminate. Some early experiments erroneously failed to demonstrate that iron embedded in concrete could withstand a greater load than iron without concrete.

Swiss engineer Robert Maillart was one of the first designers to break from the masonry past by using steel-reinforced concrete in forms and configurations appropriate to its technical properties. The monolithic potential of this new material offered great advantages in weight and labor, and with new theories of structural analysis emergent in the early 20th century, standards for both the design and the construction of reinforced concrete were adopted in several countries as early as 1902. These standards were ultimately invested with quasi-legal status, incorporated into building codes later in the century.

Reinforced concrete is the union of two materials: concrete, which is strong in compression, and steel, which is strong in tension. Without reinforcing, concrete's tensile strength is typically only 10 per cent of its compressive strength. This tensile strength is so minimal, in fact, that it is typically omitted from structural calculations. Steel comes in the form of bars ranging from 3/8 inch to nearly 3 inches in diameter. Placed into formwork before the concrete is poured, the steel reinforcing bars, or rebars, are typically located where engineers expect stress due to tension to be greatest, referred to as the tensile zone (in the case of a simply supported beam, the tensile zone occupies the bottom half of the beam). Because steel is also strong in compression, rebars are employed even when tension is not expected to be severe, such as in axially loaded columns. One of the advantages of reinforced concrete is that the concrete insulates the steel during a fire. Another is that concrete and reinforcing steel expand at approximately the same rate during fluctuations of temperature. This is important because if the embedded steel were to expand at a greater rate than the surrounding concrete, stress and possible failure may result.

The embedment of the rebar requires care, however, because several factors can spoil the advantages of its use. Proper concrete mixes are required so that the steel and the concrete bond and thus work as one unit. Also, the concrete must protect the rebar from corrosion, although corrosion in limited quantity actually increases bonding. Pouring the concrete also presents opportunity for error because efforts to force the wet concrete and its aggregates to fill the formwork can dislocate rebars from their intended position.

This is also true for wire-mesh reinforcement, which is often used instead of rebar in slab-on-grade applications, such as sidewalks, driveways, and floor slabs. Welded strands of steel formed in a gridlike mesh are often used to resist light tensile stress or to prevent concrete from cracking because of temperature changes. This form of reinforcing is sometimes used to resist more severe stresses, such as the conical shaped wire mesh used in the columns of Frank Lloyd Wright's Johnson Wax Company Administration Building (1939) in Racine, Wisconsin. Twenty-two-foot-tall columns were supported by a base only 9 inches in diameter, tapering lotuslike at the ceiling. When a test column was axially loaded on the site, the concrete and its welded wire-mesh reinforcing supported 60 tons, five times the anticipated load.

Generally, there are two ways that a reinforced-concrete structure can fail, namely, excessive compressive stress or tensile stress. Engineers typically design reinforced concrete to fail in tension rather than compression by underdesigning the rebar. Most codes require this because steel fails gradually by yielding before reaching its ultimate capacity. When a reinforced-concrete structure fails because of tensile yielding, deflection gradually increases and becomes visually detectable. Compressive failure, on the other hand, is often sudden and sometimes drastic and even explosive.

Because concrete is poured rather than cut, rolled, or extruded, designers sometimes can afford the liberty of shaping structural elements to take special advantage of reinforced concrete's inherent properties. Roof slabs, for instance, can be made 6 inches thick and folded or curved in dynamic forms. Rebar can be stretched taut in its forms before the concrete is poured, thus prestressing the structural member and allowing for lighter and thinner and thus more efficient structural elements. Reinforcing tenons may also be stretched after concrete has set, in a system called post-tensioning, which also increases the reinforced concrete's ability to carry loads. As analytical and mathematical sophistication has increased, engineers can often anticipate where the most severe lines of stress are likely to develop in a given structure. The pattern of reinforcing can therefore be superimposed over those same lines, called isostatic lines, which is exactly how Italian engineer Pier Luigi Nervi devised his dramatic scheme for a factory in Rome (Gatti Wool Factory, 1951). The underside of the factory's floor slabs were articulated with an irregular grid of reinforced beams radiating out from columns and crisscrossed by circles of beams concentrically ringing out from those same columns. This irregular, nearly curvilinear waffle pattern is a classic example of what advocates would call beauty derived from pure structure. However, it was a structural solution that may have been efficient in its use of concrete and reinforcing, but the irregularity of the grid pattern required ex-

tremely elaborate formwork, thus reducing the solution's cost-effectiveness. For this reason, as well as the analytical complexity of determining the pattern of stress, Nervi's isostatic-inspired slabs were rarely emulated. Waffle stab systems, however, where reinforced beams intersect one another at right angles, forming square voids rather than irregular voids and thus becoming more amenable to repetitive formwork, have been widely used.

JERRY WHITE

Further Reading

Nawy, although technical, is an excellent overall source. Ching and Adams is the best first source. Peters, however, gives an excellent historical analysis of reinforcing, in context with other technical and industrial systems.

Billington, David P., *Robert Maillart and the Art of Reinforced Concrete*, Cambridge, Massachusetts: MIT Press, 1990

Ching, Francis D.K. and Cassandra Adams, *Building Construction Illustrated*, New York: Van Nostrand Reinhold, 1975; 3rd edition, New York: Wiley, 2001

Louis de Malave, Florita Z., *Work and Life of Pier Luigi Nervi, Architect*, Monticello, Illinois: Vance Biographies, 1984

Nawy, Edward G., *Reinforced Concrete: A Fundamental Approach*, Englewood Cliffs, New Jersey: Prentice Hall, 1985; 4th edition, 2000

Peters, Tom F., *Building the Nineteenth Century*, Cambridge, Massachusetts: MIT Press, 1996

RENAULT DISTRIBUTION CENTRE

Designed by Sir Norman Foster; completed 1983
Swindon, England

Foster and Partners designed the Renault Distribution Centre in Swindon, England, on a 16-acre sloping site at the western edge of the town. Renault needed a distribution facility for spare parts for the car dealers in England, office space, exhibition space, and a cafeteria. Being a fairly rural area, the town planners and Renault were concerned with making a visually interesting building that would enhance the surroundings.

With its sea of yellow steel masts, the Distribution Centre has come to embody the essence of the work of the often-called High-Tech architecture, which, although it explores new materials and their highly technological capacities, is also an "appropriate technology," with its lightweight and flexible metal structure, for the automotive industry.

As an alternative to the ubiquitous "big box" or factory-in-a-shed—as are many of Richard Foster's buildings, such as the Willis Faber and Dumas offices (1975) in Suffolk—the Centre is inventive and expressive of a second machine age of architecture. The unique suspension structure is exposed as a bridge, and it exemplifies the collaboration between architect and engineer in fabricating nonstandardized parts for a building rather than employing off-the-shelf products. Although the metal parts are produced with the help of the computer, they are customized to the specific structure of the building. The architects, with the engineers Ove Arup and Partners, developed a repeatable single-story module to be built over the site with a lightweight roof suspended from a mast structure with an interior filled with natural light. It successfully continues the idea of modular construction and the machine aesthetic as exemplified in the Reliance Controls Center (1967), also in Swindon, designed by Team 4, and Foster's Modern Art Glass Factory (1973) in Kent.

Foster's design began with a building module 24 square meters, 7.5 meters high at the edges, and up to 9.5 meters at the center, suspended from a 16-meter-high tubular steel mast to create an open network. Forty-two of these modules were then erected in a 9-by-4-meter grid with 36 modules housing the warehouse space laid out in a two-directional grid for easy access to the parts and equipment. Six additional modules comprise the distribution and office spaces, a car showroom, a training school, workshops, seminar rooms, and a cafeteria. The entrance is composed of one module left open at the sides like a canopy. The building can be expanded by continuing the same modular system.

The modules are constructed of diverse metal components in a portal frame. Steel beams faceted into an arch are supported from the top of the prestressed circular rolled hollow steel masts by thin steel tension rods at 45-degree angles. The tension rods reach the beams and continue beneath the roof and with supports from below to join with the next beam. The beam-and-mast system creates an umbrella shape that supports each other, and the steel ties at each mast provide the moment connection. The steel beams have holes to reduce the weight but also to provide an aesthetic lightness that is clearly visible in the way the circular holes are lined up from roofline to roofline.

Tubeworkers Limited developed the rods and their bolts and pin joints in a custom-made system originally developed for sailing rigging, but here in a spheroidal graphite cast iron, which has a low melting point for shaping and the tensile properties of cast steel. This was the first time the product was used for a building.

The facades are a combination of steel panels and glass. A Pilkington system of 10-millimeter-thick flatbed armor-plated glass in 4-by-2-meter sheets is suspended on bolts countersunk into the glass and held in place with special steel spider legs. Lightweight steel transoms span between the mullions with the same spider-leg fastener.

The insulated steel wall panels are custom made by a caravan company with a 4-meter-long horizontal span between the steel mullions, placed on edge fastened by flanges at the back. The few interior wall divisions are the same lightweight steel panels or glass for visibility between spaces. The exterior walls are recessed from the roofline, bringing the structure to the fore. The end modules, each with a corner mast, are tied down with tension rods and stabilized on concrete foundations.

The roof is one PVC membrane with insulation secured by metal disks that seal the openings from the penetrations of the masts and vents. Twenty-seven trapezoidal-shaped roof lights at the point of each module are held in place by 6-millimeter bolts at the top of each plate. The roof lights, recalling early 20th-century factories, provide views, natural sunlight, and smoke ventilation.

A fascia seals the wall and the roof connection with a flexible neoprene-coated nylon fabric often used for hovercraft skirts, and the fastenings are those used for truck trailer covers. Foster also designed office furniture for the complex that he had used in other Renault projects.

The Distribution Centre is a flexible building, not a static monument, but one that reflects the ever-changing automotive technologies. The building bespeaks customized standard sys-

tems for its own construction, specific to its own needs yet is fully adaptable, a feature that is also visible in Foster's Hong-kong and Shanghai Bank Headquarters (1986). The vertical yellow masts on the horizontal landscape have been compared to sailing ships or umbrellas basking in the sun, and the building has become an identifiable trademark for Renault in England.

NINA RAPPAPORT

See also **Arup, Ove (England); Foster, Norman (England)**

Further Reading

Foster, Norman, *Norman Foster: Selected and Current Works of Foster and Partners*, Mulgrave, Victoria: Images, 1997
Lambet, Ian (editor), *Norman Foster, Foster Associates: Buildings and Projects*, 3 vols., Hong Kong: Watermark, 1989
Sudjic, Dejan, *Norman Foster, Richard Rogers, James Stirling: New Directions in British Architecture*, London: Thames and Hudson, 1986; New York: Thames and Hudson, 1987

REPRESENTATION

"At the End of the Century: One Hundred Years of Architecture," the traveling exhibition organized by the Museum of Contemporary Art in Los Angeles, offered a vast array of architectural representation, from the 1914 Sant'Elia Italian futurist drawings to the working model of Gehry's 1997 Bilbao Guggenheim Museum. Although the futurists did not produce any built work, Sant'Elia's depictions of an imagined architecture befitting the new machine age have become part of the canon of modern architecture; eloquent and seductive, the drawings constitute the most radical architectural proposition that gave expression to a modern city driven by agile transportation systems. Whereas in Sant'Elia's work the drawings became the architecture, in Gehry's Guggenheim new means of representation begot a new architecture. The building's insistence on irregular forms challenged the traditional orthogonal architectural drawing conventions of plans and sections, and both design and construction had to rely greatly on the latest computer-modeling technology.

Architectural representation provides the visualizing context in which architects think through a design. Drawings, models, sketches, cross sections, axiometric views, and most recently computer-generated walk-throughs are where architecture is initially conceived and displayed. If developments in materials and technology make possible new construction methods, it is through the different means and uses of representation that architects configure the idea and desire for the new building's iterations; representation ceases to be merely the communication of design and becomes instead an architectural manifestation as potent and valid as the built results. In some cases, as with the Italian futurists, there is no built outcome, yet the visualization of a dynamic new architecture in Sant'Elia's drawings that posited itself firmly against the historicism of the 19th century was an influential reference for modern architects. In others, as in Gehry's Guggenheim, new ways of building are directly reliant on means of representation that allow the visualization of new formal configurations. To many theorists, critics, and architects, architecture rests as much in representation as it does in the built form itself.

Differences in the means of representation are often indicative of the biases of the architecture. The importance of the plan in the works of Frank Lloyd Wright, Ludwig Mies van der Rohe, and Le Corbusier was in part what pitted modern architecture against the historicism that preceded it. The new plans proposed a radically new arrangement and delineation of rooms, but more important, positing the plan as the building's critical generator implied that its corresponding elevation, or what the building might look like, was directly borne out of it and not arbitrarily applied as one might have applied architectural styles in the 19th century. The elevation regained importance later in the Postmodern architecture of Robert Venturi, Michael Graves, Charles Moore, Robert Stern, and others, whose designs relied substantially on the representation of architectural signs and languages. Reacting against simplistic interpretations of modern architecture principles after World War II, they imbued their work with allusive, recognizable imagery and symbolism, calling on and reinterpreting classical or vernacular forms. Although plans and elevations are two-dimensional drawings, architects see their three-dimensional buildings through them.

In their 1978 classic, *Collage City*, Colin Rowe and Fred Koetter used not a particular drawing but rather a manner of making as a metaphor for an urban-planning idea. As modern architecture developed in the first decades of the 20th century, the Cubists probed the nature of painting and two-dimensional representation by breaking with perspectival conventions in place since the Renaissance. Instead, they created innovative paintings that simultaneously represented three dimensions and called attention to the two-dimensionality of the canvas. One work by Picasso, *Still Life with Chair Caning* (1911–12), was used in the book to illustrate a composite approach to the design of urban environments. Rowe and Koetter proposed treating the found urban fabric minutiae of old cities and the newly made sweeping urban-renewal schemes of modern architecture as the colliding pieces with which to compose a multivalent collage city, much like Picasso had used the found-chair-caning print and applied paint strokes to make a harmonious composition. There is wit, they argued, in finding linkages between two seemingly unlike pieces by virtue of their carefully orchestrated adjacency, and collage was proposed as a way of thinking in the design of architecture and cities. A comparison to painting also calls attention to the dual nature of cities as two-dimensional entities as seen from airplanes and on architects' boards and as three-dimensional environments.

The ability to think about a building through its representation does not end at its construction. Photography, as it represents and conjures architecture, offers additional ways to understand and interpret built forms, and this ultimately affects one's understanding of it. The early acknowledged master in the eloquent use of photography to convey architectural ideas is Le Corbusier, who composed the photographic representations of his buildings as carefully as if the photographs were the buildings themselves. Since the last decades of the 20th century, the dominance of glossy pictures in magazines and books as the purveyors of architecture has raised the objection of some pundits, who fear that this reliance on the photograph for one's understanding of a building is not conducive to great architecture. It is true that carefully framed photographs can raise expectations about a building not fulfilled at the site visit and that the great architectural spaces of Louis Kahn are notoriously difficult to photograph. Ultimately, however, we must remember Susan Sontag's important 1977 book, *On Photography*, in which she argues that

the photograph is too malleable a medium to be merely a record of reality but that it becomes instead a reality all its own, as valid as its unmediated counterpart.

Advances in digital media have cast anew the question of what constitutes a truthful depiction of reality, architectural or otherwise. It has become increasingly facile to simulate the continuous sequence of views through an environment generated entirely in a computer. These immersive environments are reminiscent of Walt Disney in their promise of habitation, albeit mediated, in an imaginary world. Theme parks are fictions, the way in which a painting and a film are fictions or something like full-scale representations of an idealized world. They are three-dimensional theatrical sets with which one interacts as both spectator and participant. For both, their potency lies not in how closely they approximate reality but in the believability of their illusory reality. As with other forms of representation, some architecture today remains exclusively in digital form. As such, it is reduced to a system of three-dimensional coordinates inside the computer and is infinitely malleable. However, even when it becomes manifest in physical reality, the medium radically changes the nature of the architecture, as in Gehry's previously mentioned Guggenheim project, in which a direct connection between digital configurations and manufacturing processes allowed formal configurations that had proved impossible to visualize through traditional drawing methods.

MARIA SIEIRA

See also **Guggenheim Museum, Bilbao**

Further Reading

Koshalek, Richard, Elizabeth A.T. Smith, and Russell Ferguson (editors), *At the End of the Century: One Hundred Years of Architecture*, Los Angeles: Museum of Contemporary Art, and New York: Abrams, 1998

Mitchell, William J., *The Reconfigured Eye: Visual Truth in the Post-Photographic Era*, Cambridge, Massachusetts: MIT Press, 1992

Naegele, Daniel J., "Le Corbusier's Seeing Things: Ambiguity and Illusion in the Representation of Modern Architecture" (Ph.D. dissertation), University of Pennsylvania, 1996

Panofsky, Erwin, *Perspective as Symbolic Form*, translated by Christopher S. Wood, New York: Zone Books, 1991

Rowe, Colin and Fred Koetter, *Collage City*, Cambridge, Massachusetts: MIT Press, 1978

Sontag, Susan, *On Photography*, New York: Farrar Straus and Giroux, 1977; London: Penguin, 1978

Venturi, Robert, Denise Scott Brown, and Steven Izenour, *Learning from Las Vegas*, Cambridge, Massachusetts: MIT Press, 1972; revised edition, as *Learning from Las Vegas: The Forgotten Symbolism of Architectural Form*, 1996

RESEARCH CENTER

A research center consists of a building or complex of buildings devoted to the service of scientific inquiry that include astronomical observatories and biological, chemical, medical, and physical laboratories as well as buildings for related demands. As a modern building type, these facilities share their appearance with the institutionalization of Western science that occurred during the 17th and 18th centuries but that took a recognizable form only after the middle of the 19th century. As the value of science began to make itself felt on the progress of technology during the last half of the 19th century, and as a career in the sciences was seen as the best hope of improving the life of the common individual, distinctive buildings devoted to teaching and the development of each scientific discipline emerged.

At the beginning of the 20th century, the dominant location of research centers was to be found on university campuses. Of the various scientific disciplines, buildings for chemistry generally presented the largest capital investment and the most difficult architectural problems. Laboratory siting was commonly downwind of the campus center because of the increased production of unhealthy fumes, corrosive chemicals, water pollution, and occasional mishaps. Daylighting and natural ventilation strategies were paramount in the development of plans and building massing of which the Chandler Chemical Laboratory (1884) at Lehigh University in South Bethlehem, Pennsylvania, by Addison Hutton, was perhaps the dominant model of this period. Solid construction and excellent materials typify these facilities.

At the beginning of the 1920s, powered ventilation systems were introduced to this type. One of the first laboratories to solely employ powered systems was the Sterling Chemistry Building (1923) at Yale University in New Haven, Connecticut, by Delano and Aldrich. Located on the northern edge of the campus, the building was finished in a Collegiate Gothic style with engaged pilasters and ornamented terra-cotta chimney flues. More important, however, the building was massed as a block. Using the crawl space beneath the main floor of the building as a flue, similar to a Roman hypocaust (an underground furnace system), the building was to be continuously flushed with fresh air with a single motorized fan.

In contrast, industrial laboratories begin to appear during the 1930s and were usually sited adjacent to their manufacturing counterpart. Freed from the architecturally sensitive environment of university settings, laboratory designs were either a singly or a double-loaded corridor type and usually limited to three stories in height because of the efficiency of the mechanical systems. Their construction was typical of industrial buildings.

The most striking and progressive design of this era appeared in 1938, when Russian-born and British-educated architect Serge Chermayeff was commissioned to design a laboratory for the Dyestuff's Division of the Imperial Chemical Industries in Blackley, England. The building form was massed as a series of long, narrow fingers several hundred feet in length and roughly 24 feet in width. The form was a result of a rationalized examination of ergonomic and physical factors to achieve the maximum daylight penetration for bench-top experiments and the most effective mechanical ventilation system layout. The confidence in the mechanical system at this time permitted the laboratory ceilings to be lowered, reducing total building volume, cost, and equipment size. Fusing scientific research with a futuristic image, this is perhaps the earliest example in which the design of the building structure became a secondary consideration to the mechanical and related building systems. This new approach to laboratory design of systems first and structure second came to be the recommended approach for this building type by the end of the 1950s. Typical examples from this era include the Chemistry Laboratory (1947) of the Illinois Institute of Technology in Chicago by Mies van der Rohe and the Science and

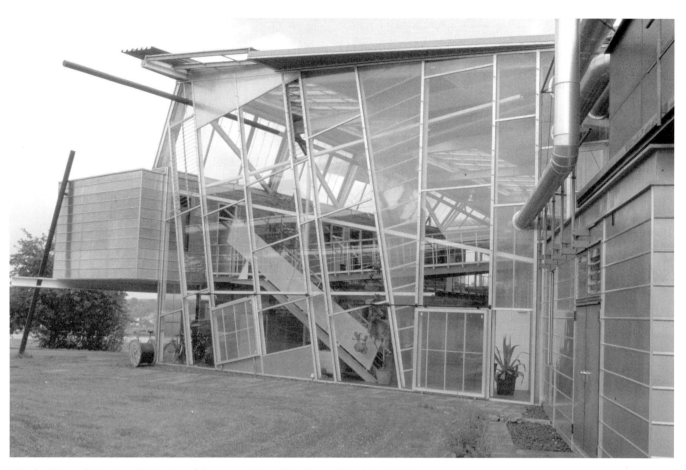

Hysolar Research Institute, University of Stuttgart, designed by Gunter Behnisch (1987)
© Donald Corner and Jenny Young/GreatBuildings.com

Pharmacy buildings (1947) at Drake University in Des Moines, Iowa, by Saarinen, Swanson and Saarinen. The form has remained a cost-effective approach into the 21st century.

Recent efforts at trying to provide an improved research facility have led to several striking laboratory designs. The Patscenter (1982) in Princeton, New Jersey, by Peter Rice of Ove Arup and Partners, resulted in a masted tensile structure supporting a rigid roof with an externally exposed mechanical system in an effort to integrate the mechanical systems with building structure and produce a clean interior environment. Similarly, the Schlumberger Cambridge Research Center (1985) in Cambridge, England, by Michael and Patty Hopkins, was based on a masted tensile structure with a Teflon-coated fabric membrane. However, relying on the use of advanced structural systems that produce a high-tech expression has not resulted in an innovation to laboratory design that has been widely accepted.

In the decade following World War II, the representational question posed by scientists to architects became the promotion of a humanistic face for science. New laboratories were expected to improve the negative social image of science that producing weapons of mass destruction had in part created. The new labs were to also provide creative environments in which scientists were encouraged to interact and remain sensitive to the larger human condition. Notable examples based on these ideas are

the Richards Medical Research Center (1962) at the University of Pennsylvania in Philadelphia and the Salk Institute (1967) in La Jolla, California, both by Louis Kahn. Of the two projects, however, it is the Salk Institute, with its romantic siting, full-height interstitial service spaces above each laboratory for maximized flexibility, and the originally intended housing and conference support facilities, that has proven to be an inspiring model for an institutional research community.

Although Kahn's approach proved more costly, the extra flexibility to meet changing demands is a more effective solution in the long run for medical and biochemical research centers. Prominent examples of this type are the E.R. Squibb and Sons, Inc., World Headquarters (1972) in Princeton, New Jersey, by Hellmuth, Obata and Kassabaum, which has remained the preeminent corporate research complex. Comprised of interconnected modules with labs and offices at the perimeter and support instruments at the plan core, it has become a well-accepted solution. Another excellent example of the interstitial approach arranged as an urban campus is the Fred Hutchinson Cancer Research Center (1993) in Seattle, Washington, by Zimmer Gunsul Frasca Partnership, with laboratory planner McLellan and Copenhagen, Inc. Although these designs were approached from differing architectural points of view, they managed to

succeed in balancing the difficult technical, social, and representational demands that accompany this building type.

Large-scale government team research methods contributed greatly to global transformation initiated by science in the last half of the 20th century. Resulting from the lessons learned in two world wars, plus the ever-growing cost and scale of research complexity, by the end of the century research centers came to be dominated by government programs and corporate facilities. National laboratories, such as Argonne, Los Alamos, and Oak Ridge, date from World War II and are small-scale cities in their own right. Large-scale corporate research complexes, such as those of IBM, Kodak, and Microsoft, now serve every major industry. Typically removed from an industrial environment, these facilities can occur in a pastoral setting coupled to an administrative center to form a corporate headquarters that announces a global presence. The most prominent at midcentury was the General Motors Technical Center (1946–54) in Michigan by Eero Saarinen and Associates. Recent prominent examples include the Panasonic Information and Communications Systems Center (1992) in Tokyo by Nikken Sekkei, and the Max Planck Institute for Chemical Ecology and Biogeochemistry (2000) on the Beutenberg Campus in Jena, Germany, by Ottow, Marx, Bachmann. Conflicting issues of security, seclusion, and public and environmental safety versus unbounded exploration, complex technical demands, and maximum building flexibility remain key factors that impact this building and campus form.

RANDY SWANSON

See also **Hopkins, Michael and Patty (England); Kahn, Louis (United States); Saarinen, Eero (Finland); Saarinen, Eliel (Finland); Salk Institute, La Jolla, California; Schlumberger Cambridge Research Centre, England**

Further Reading

Ashbrook, Peter C. and Malcolm M. Renfrew (editors), *Safe Laboratories: Principles and Practices for Design and Remodeling*, Chelsea, Michigan: Lewis, 1991

Braun, Hardo, et al., *Bauen für die Wissenschaft: Institute der Max-Planck-Gesellschaft; Building for Science: Architecture of the Max Planck Institutes* (bilingual German-English edition), Basel and Boston: Birkhäuser, 1999

Braybrooke, Susan (editor), *Design for Research: Principles of Laboratory Architecture*, New York: Wiley, 1986

Bronowski, Jacob, *Science and Human Values*, New York: Harper, 1956

Cardwell, D.S.L., "Science, Technology, and Industry," in *The Ferment of Knowledge: Studies in the Historiography of Eighteenth-Century Science*, edited by G.S. Rousseau and Roy Porter, Cambridge and New York: Cambridge University Press, 1980

Crow, Michael M., *Limited by Design: R and D Laboratories in the U.S. National Innovation System*, New York: Columbia University Press, 1998

Greene, Jay, *Major Medical Research Centers: Planning and Design*, Washington, D.C.: The American Institute of Architects, 1994

Griffin, Brian, *Laboratory Design Guide: For Clients, Architects, and Their Design Team: The Laboratory Design Process from Start to Finish*, Oxford and Boston: Architectural Press, 1998

Laboratories and Research Facilities: New Concepts in Architecture and Design (bilingual English-Japanese edition), Tokyo: Meisei, 1996

Nuffield Foundation, Division for Architectural Studies, *The Design of Research Laboratories*, London and New York: Oxford University Press, 1961

Smith, Herbert L., Jr. (editor), *Buildings for Research*, New York: Dodge, 1958

RESORT HOTEL

The resort hotel is an outgrowth of its 19th-century counterparts, including the spas and seaside resorts of Great Britain and the United States and the mountain resorts of Switzerland. The importance of the natural setting makes the relationship between architecture and site a key component of resort hotel development that continues throughout the 20th century. The hotel building grouped with associated recreational facilities and outbuildings seeks to enhance the experience of natural landscape features, such as mountains and bodies of water. For instance, the Suvretta House (1912, Karl Koller) in St. Moritz, Switzerland, is closely linked to the adjacent ski slopes, while Hotel Negresco (1910–13, Edouard-Jean Niermans) in Nice, France, features water-based activities. In comparison to urban commercial hotels, resort hotel architecture emphasizes linking interior spaces with the outdoors using balconies, verandas, and courtyards. This emphasis descends from the horizontal forms and rambling porches of 19th-century resort hotels.

Otherwise, resort hotel architecture addresses many of the functional needs that other hotels do. The architect must carefully blend elegant public spaces, efficient service spaces such as kitchens and laundries, and comfortable guest rooms. With the expansion of tourism in the 20th century, many new resort hotels are constructed in places such as the Caribbean, the South Pacific, and southern and western portions of the United States, making these landscapes newly accessible to tourists traveling by bus, automobile, airplane, or train.

Improved railroad transportation during the late 19th and early 20th centuries encouraged tourism and the development of resort hotels. Railroad companies built and operated many resort hotels to encourage travel to western Canada or the southwestern United States from eastern locations. At the time, these resorts offered the only modern facilities in ruggedly beautiful locations, thereby providing a tamed adventure for travelers. These ventures could be highly profitable but also risky. Resort hotels linked to the railroads failed when newer, competing resorts opened nearby; when transportation patterns changed to favor the automobile; or when other locations became more fashionable.

With the growth of tourism in the early 20th century, particularly in the United States during the boom years of the 1920s, resort hotels became accessible to a wider economic range of guests. Many famous resorts, such as the Greenbrier in White Sulphur Springs, West Virginia, remain exclusively upper-class playgrounds, but places such as Coney Island, Atlantic City, the Poconos, and the Catskills offer resort facilities for middle- and prosperous working-class urban residents. This proliferation of resorts in the 20th century represents the expansion of leisure culture across class lines.

Resort hotels often feature eclectic and evocative design motifs to attract guests. Creative adaptations of regional motifs and historic architectural features give resort hotels a distinctive ap-

pearance and sense of place. A good example is Old Faithful Inn (1902–03, Robert C. Reamer), built by the Great Northern Railway at Yellowstone National Park. Materials such as boulders, logs, and peeled branches create an oversized, romantic version of a frontier cabin combined with a Swiss alpine resort. This theme is echoed in other park structures in the West, such as the Canyon Hotel (1910–11), also designed by Reamer for Yellowstone, or the Lake McDonald Lodge (1913–14, Cutter and Malgram) in Glacier National Park, Montana. Despite the rustic motifs, these examples are full-service resort hotels dedicated to guest comfort. In each case, the hotel is situated to provide guests with spectacular views of the natural landscape.

Another noteworthy resort idiom that developed during the first half of the 20th century was a modified Spanish mode popularized by the resorts of Florida, California, and the southwestern United States. The work of architect Addison Mizner in Palm Beach and Boca Raton typifies the use of fanciful Spanish motifs to create an exotic regional look promoting Florida as a tourist destination. Mizner's Cloister Inn (1925–26) in Boca Raton is a prime example, featuring the pale pink stucco and red-tiled roof that was typical of Florida architecture and resort landscape. A carefully asymmetrical plan arranged around a series of courtyards deliberately invokes the history and incremental development of Old World buildings.

Resort hotels in the southwestern United States and California use another variation on Spanish motifs that emphasize the plainer tradition of Spanish Colonial missions in the region. The Mission Inn (1902–03, Arthur B. Benton) in Riverside, California, is an important early example that combines artistic use of white stucco and red tile with selective copying from extant missions. Resort hotel architecture frequently promotes a romanticized sense of place for visitors while providing modern accommodations and comforts.

After the upheaval of World War II, tourism resurged in the 1950s, inspiring the construction of a new generation of resort hotels. A key figure during this period is Morris Lapidus, a set designer turned architect who created the most influential resort hotels of the 1950s. Lapidus's Fontainebleau Hotel (1953) in Miami Beach was wildly popular among the public and criticized by the architectural profession for its hybrid of International Style and updated French Renaissance motifs. The sleek elegance of Lapidus's high-rise resort hotels influenced resort hotel design in many of the newly developing resort locations, such as Hawaii, Tahiti, Mexico, and South America. Inexpensive air travel allowed increasingly large numbers of tourists from around the world to reach faraway vacation places.

In the second half of the 20th century, the resort setting became secondary to the theatricality of the architecture itself, as signaled by Lapidus's hotels. This new trend is most evident in places such as Las Vegas and Orlando, where the location is virtually unimportant compared to the grandiose stage set of the resort hotel. The element of fantasy and play inherent in resort architecture is exaggerated as hotels using a variety of regional and historical themes coexist in their competitive efforts to attract guests. In the late 20th century, the resort hotel employs a wide variety of forms while still sharing a set of functional purposes. These trends and variations reinforce the creativity and luxury inherent to the best resort hotel development throughout the 20th century.

LISA DAVIDSON

See also **Disney Theme Parks; Hotel; Lapidus, Morris (United States)**

Further Reading

Denby, Elaine, *Grand Hotels: Reality and Illusion: An Architectural and Social History*, London: Reaktion Books, 1998

Donzel, Catherine, Alexis Gregory, and Marc Walter, *Palaces et grand hôtels d'Amerique du Nord*, Paris: Flammarion, 1989; as *Grand American Hotels*, New York: Vendome Press, and London: Thames and Hudson, 1989; as *Grand Hotels of North America*, Toronto: McClelland and Stewart, 1989

Düttmann, Martina, and Friederike Schneider, editors, *Morris Lapidus: Architect of the American Dream*, Basel and Boston: Birkhäuser, 1992

Limerick, Jeffrey, Nancy Ferguson, and Richard Oliver, *America's Grand Resort Hotels*, New York: Pantheon Books, 1979

Mizner, Addison, *Florida Architecture of Addison Mizner*, New York: Helburn, 1928; reprint, New York: Dover, 1992

Root, John Wellborn, "Hotels and Apartment Hotels," in *Forms and Functions of Twentieth-Century Architecture*, volume 3: *Building Types: Buildings for Residence, for Popular Gatherings, for Education, and for Government*, edited by Talbot Hamlin, New York: Columbia University Press, 1952

RESTAURANT

Of all the structures, signs, and symbols that stream by the automobile window, none appears more suggestive than the orange roofs, golden arches, and smiling faces of the contemporary restaurant-scape. Here, the designs suggest, is a secret code revealing Americans' most basic desires and needs. As Americans have become more and more reliant on their automobiles, the early tendency of eating a meal of convenience in a luncheonette has grown into a consistent alternative to eating at home. Initially, though, the desire for restaurants needed no automobile.

Eat-and-run cuisine took shape following the Civil War. The Civil War encampment, the chuck wagon of the American West, and the railroad dining car each helped to introduce Americans to fast cooking and fast eating. Industrial workers, with a bit of discretionary income and very limited time, became some of the first consumers of meals—particularly lunch—at establishments called beaneries, greasy spoons, and stool lunches. By the end of the 19th century, the expansion of commercial cities into white-collar labor combined with mass transportation's creation of the commuter to further American interest in eating out. Cafeterias designed specifically for the luncher on a timetable allowed customers to move along a line while selecting from a display of daily items. Delicatessens provided sandwiches, and stores such as Woolworth's installed lunch counters.

Between 1910 and 1927, the estimated number of restaurants grew by 40 percent. In New York City, the number of eating establishments grew from 7500 in 1915 to 17,000 in 1925. Scholars suggest many factors for this change in American behavior: a greater number of men and women working a way from home, a decline in the use of domestic help to prepare meals, and Prohibition, which eliminated bars and the social life that accompanied them. There were also technological advances that facilitated this type of food preparation, including, refrigeration, shipping, storing, packing, and so forth. At this point, the propensity to eat out met its mate for the rest of the 20th century: the automobile.

As the automobile became more familiar in everyday American life after 1920, planners and developers formalized refueling stations for the human drivers. Tearooms were one of the earliest way stations designed to support family travel. The term conjured an obviously safe establishment during the era of the speakeasy. With a limited menu, based around afternoon tea, ice cream, cold drinks, and standard lunches or dinners, packaging was critical for the first time in the industry. Owners used quaint names such as Copper Kettle, Wishing Well, Pine Cone, or Silver Spring to reinforce their family image. Most often, such establishments could be found along major tourist routes to resorts. This was the model followed by one of the industry great entrepreneurs.

Beginning in 1925, Howard D. Johnson took the form of the tearoom to develop the nation's first great restaurant chain. During his family's own travels, Johnson realized that the new highways of the Northeast were almost entirely without food services for the traveler. After opening a few restaurants, Johnson expanded his operation in 1935 by permitting individual investors (called agents rather than franchisees) to build their own Howard Johnson's. The restaurants combined all the aspects of the tearoom with the first recognizable, roadside architectural form: the orange roof combined with a colonial motif. In doing so, Johnson married the familiar with striking oddity. By 1940, the chain included 125 restaurants, and Johnson had secured exclusive access to the nation's greatest expressway: the Pennsylvania Turnpike. Details from colonial architecture were used by Johnson as well as by the Dutchland Farms chain to add dignity to restaurants. Along the highway, such restaurants loomed like a colonial mansion, often with trappings of farm or country life added as well. After World War II, Howard Johnson's and other similar restaurants would abandon colonial detail to become bastions of modernist design. In many ways, such restaurant design defines the postmodern landscape that we call the "strip."

No structure reflected the connection between modern design and eating-out like the American diner. First manufactured as lunch-cars in the early 1900s, the metal, self-contained diner could be set down and wired up almost anywhere. Offering low cost and instant gratification for purchasers, the diner quickly became a standardized form on the American roadway. This provided owners with a bit of recognition without the central control demanded from Johnson and other chains. After World War II, many diners could not compete with the newer fast-food chains. The survivors often exaggerated their Modern detail, abandoning the resemblance to a rail car for a wider form—still pre-fabricated steel—that could seat family diners. The competitors, however, were not slowing down.

From the earliest days of auto travel, food stands informally provided refreshment in rapid, accessible fashion with no thought toward image or ambience. Convenience defined such locations, though there was variation within the fast-food form. White Castle hamburgers (1921) combined the food stand with the restaurant to create a restaurant that could be put almost anywhere. Drive-in restaurants would evolve around the idea of quick service, often allowing drivers to remain in their automobile. Fast food as a concept, of course, derives specifically from Ray Kroc and the McDonald's concept that he marketed out of California (1952). Clearly the idea of providing service to automobile drivers had created an entire offshoot of the restaurant industry.

The design of such establishments quickly became part of the attraction. Most important, each of these types accentuated its contemporariness by incorporating modern design, including heavy use of glass, metal, and neon lighting. Kroc was one of the first restaurateurs to understand the importance of the physical structure. He required each franchise to duplicate the standard building design—the now-famous structure with its overhanging slanted roof, visual front, wall panels decorated in striped tile, and flanking golden arches. The form would, of course, change with consumption patterns. For instance, restaurants would eventually incorporate drive-through windows into the overall design. The standardization of such structures defined American eating patterns along the "strip" through the end of the 20th century.

Although each restaurant and shopping mall bore its own design and architecture, planners and developers synched the entire composite into a design referred to as the commercial strip. Restaurants led the way from Main Street and downtown into the suburban regions. The trend toward automobility demanded a new organization to the landscape and restaurants had already pointed toward planned areas outside of urban or town centers. Fast food became the anchor of such "strips," with McDonald's or Burger King generally acting as the first wave of commercial development. Design has followed this trend while adding a dash of the amusement park: postmodern designs such as those of Taco Bell cartoon bone fide architectural styles such as Mission to distinguish themselves from the rest of the strip. Although diners have largely been squeezed out of the market, new family dining restaurants such as TGIFridays have created a homogenized form that is somewhere between fast food and a "sit-down" restaurant. The strip is the home for each, as it is for most contemporary restaurants.

In urban areas, the restaurant landscape has continually evolved to meet the demands of changing tastes and needs. Although dining rooms for the wealthy established themselves by the middle of the 19th century, these were often luncheonettes or inns and taverns. Demographic trends (including residential patterns in ethnicity and economic class) significantly influenced the overall development of restaurants for other classes of patrons. In urban areas, restaurants, with department stores, theaters, and hotels, were made more viable and widely available by the introduction of electricity during the 1890s. Entire shopping and eating districts could now be open into the evening; most important, restaurants were no longer stifled by the limitations of midday meals or overnight patronage. This new opportunity was seized by many entrepreneurs.

Between 1910 and 1930, Americans began to consider eating out a much more viable option. Most important, many more men and women were working away from home and required the convenience of available dining. This trend coincided with a drop in available domestic helpers to assist in making meals and Prohibition, which eliminated barrooms between 1919 and 1933. This, of course, created a social void for many Americans. Finally, technological developments such as refrigeration and food packing and shipping made it much more conceivable to produce meals for many customers at once.

In the early 1900s, efforts to differentiate restaurants as well as the growing diversity of American population stimulated the growth of ethnic eateries. In urban areas, ethnic cuisine became a way of sharing cultural enclaves with patrons from other ethnic

groups. For instance, Chinatowns became well defined at least partly through the restaurateur. This diversity has only grown more obvious. From barbecue pits in the Southeast and beef houses in the Great Plains to fish houses in the Pacific Northwest, regional cuisines have become a terrific indicator of cultural plurality, which the U.S. began to achieve after 1980. Although mass communications has flattened out much of the dining experience nationally, diverse opportunities in dining allow Americans in many urban areas to choose from as many as 100 different cuisines.

Although ethnicity continues to be a driving force in the distribution and selection of restaurants, other patterns are also observable in the demographics of the restaurant business. Technologies such as the automobile allowed restaurants to move outside of urban areas. This trend placed a priority on modern design elements such as signage and the use of windows, each of which suggested the streamlining trend of modern design.

BRIAN BLACK

Further Reading

Belasco, Warren, *Americans on the Road: From Autocamp to Motel, 1910–1945*, Baltimore: Johns Hopkins, 1997
Belasco, Warren, *Appetite for Change: How the Counterculture Took on the Food Industry*, Ithaca, New York: Cornell University Press, 1993
Jakle, John A., and Keith A. Sculle, *Fast Food: Roadside Restaurants in the Automobile Age (The Road and American Culture)*, Baltimore: Johns Hopkins, 1999
Liebs, Chester H., *Main Street to Miracle Mile: American Roadside Architecture*, Baltimore: Johns Hopkins, 1995

REVELL, VILJO GABRIEL (also Rewell) 1910–1964

Architect, Finland

When Viljo Revell was born in 1910 in the Finnish coastal town of Vaasa, his homeland was nearing the end of almost eight centuries of its being a pawn in the political and economic struggles between Sweden and Russia. The 20th century would prove to be one of Finland's most tumultuous, and the political and economic climate of the country had an irrefutable impact on the design and construction industry during the period when Viljo Revell practiced architecture.

During the Napoleonic Wars, Russia successfully invaded Finland in 1809 and to appease the Finns established the Grand Duchy of Finland, leaving intact the traditions of the subject nation. Early in the 20th century, attempts to "Russify" Finland resulted in the formation of numerous resistance movements. Furthermore, the unstable political situation in Russia and Europe indirectly deflated the resource and agrarian economy of the entire region. Even though Russia finally accorded to Finland its independence late in 1917, competing domestic interests manifested themselves in the Red and White Armies, which embarked upon a brutal, class-based civil war.

The 1920s saw the brief emergence of an architecture that responded to Finland's independence, a national romanticism characterized by a prevalence of wooden materials used in Finnish vernacular building. Classicism inspired the symmetrical

floor plans and exterior elevations, as well as the building ornament—garlands, medallions, columns, and arched porticoes. However, this style was quickly superseded by the practical economies of the functionalist movement, which was evolving in continental architecture and city planning. Stressing that purpose and function should determine form, these buildings were characterized by a spartan simplicity and utilitarian decoration. By the mid-1920s, Scandinavian journals reviewed the concepts proposed by Le Corbusier, a proponent of this new design philosophy, and innovative young architects visited the Continent to see concrete examples. Admired for its vitality and honesty, its airiness, light, and soundness, functionalism appeared in Finland and Sweden during the late 1920s, just as Viljo Revell was embarking on his architectural education at Helsinki's Institute of Technology, where he studied until 1937.

Finland's slow recovery from the repercussions of World War I and the ensuing Civil War was further hampered by the effects of the depressed world economy of the 1930s. Nonetheless, Viljo Revell's first building was constructed during this period on the site of an abandoned Russian military barracks building in central Helsinki. Initially conceived in 1933 by a five-student team as a temporary bazaar structure, the design was expanded to include a bus coach station and a commercial building with a cinema, restaurants, and shops. To the astonishment of the local architectural community, the city council supported Revell's proposed new design over that of the city's own architect. The final project design for the Lasipalatsi Building (1936), or Glass Palace, was completed by a trio of students: Viljo Revell, Niilo Kokko, and Heimo Riihimäki.

The Lasipalatsi Building was definitely outside the bounds of the prevailing classically inspired or Jugend style buildings, and it initially aroused public criticism. A swath of large windows extended along the entire two-story street frontage, wrapping around the curved corners and lending to the white-plastered structure a modern quality that heralded future architectural innovations. Above the main entrance a multistoried glass wall canted out over the street. The state-of-the-art Bio-Rex Cinema was housed in a large cubic form, set well back from the street behind a one-story section with a roof terrace. The complex also contained the HOK restaurant, its 700-person capacity making it the country's largest public dining facility. Lasipalatsi was constructed according to functionalist precepts: bright and light open spaces with attention given to hygienically smooth textures of the finishing materials. Technical ingenuity was evident in the ferroconcrete structure and in the latest kitchen equipment and cinema projection systems. Brightly colored blinds controlled the sunlight, and neon lights advertised the businesses within. Artisans coordinated the interior decor with the overall building architecture. Separate from the building and to the rear, near the bus loading area, was an iconographic smokestack, clock, and light tower marking the underground heating and power plant for the complex. Designed for a ten-year life span, the Lasipalatsi Building has survived in the hub of the capital city, and it was recently restored in 1998 to reflect the structural, functional, and ideological intentions of its original designers.

The international conflict precipitated by Germany in 1939 resulted in strategically situated Finland being caught in the midst of a battle between the Soviets and Germany. Unwilling to transfer any territories to the Soviets, the Finnish mounted a valiant resistance to their invading troops along the Mannerheim

Line. The resultant peace agreement in March 1940 ceded or leased substantial territory to the Soviet Union, forcing the expulsion of all Finnish occupants and land owners. In order to regain these lands, the Finnish government permitted Germany to use Finland as a military staging base for attacks on Norway and the Soviet Union. When the Soviets retaliated in June 1941, Finland felt justified in declaring war on this Western ally. Ensuing diplomatic negotiations proved fruitless, and in 1944 the Soviets regained much of the territory previously lost to Finnish and German troops.

In 1936, Revell had worked briefly in the office of Alvar Aalto, assisting with the Finnish Pavilion for the 1937 Paris International Exhibition. He then designed a small commercial building for his hometown of Vaasa, but the outbreak of war halted the construction industry until the Finnish Association of Architects established a Bureau for Reconstruction in 1942. Revell was named to head this institution, and for the next seven years his energies were devoted to conducting research into the development of standards for new construction materials and techniques, the modular systematization of buildings, and methods for prefabrication. Revell's first large-scale project did come out of this era, nonetheless. The Romantic style of his vocational school for the Liperi Rehabilitation Centre for War Consumptives (1948) was indicative of the nostalgia that briefly developed after World War II, as Finland renounced modernism and reverted to the Romantic Nationalism that had dominated the early decades of the century.

After entering private practice, Revell's first successful competition entry was for the Industrial Centre and Teollisuuskeskus Building, also known as the Palace Hotel (1952), overlooking the Helsinki harbor and market. Designed in collaboration with Keijo Petäjä, the Palace Hotel was one of many design projects in which Revell was quite content to share the limelight with others, even those with less experience than himself. His unprejudiced attitudes and his ability to encourage innovative design solutions became a trademark of Revell's approach to architectural practice, and because of this, he attracted young and talented newcomers to his studio.

The floor plan for the Palace Hotel forms an asymmetrical "H," with the rooms opening off corridors whose widths corresponded with anticipated circulation loads. In a Le Corbusian manner, the mass of the building was elevated on two-story-tall columns, or pilotis. Revell's logical approach to design was evident in the hotel's clearly articulated circulation patterns and floor plans. His attention to details, particularly noticeable in the fashionable Grill Restaurant, was evident throughout.

Postwar conditions had a tremendous impact on the Finnish economy, and beginning in the 1950s, the government's policy of reconciliation and declared state of neutrality saw Finland precariously balanced between the Soviet Union and Western Europe. Revell's Reconstruction Agency was just one aspect of the social-welfare system that Finland adopted to care for war survivors and to establish a thriving industrial sector in what had previously been an agricultural economy. With the 1953 Housing Production Act, the government embarked on two decades of intensive construction programs to provide subsidized housing for the over 400,000 refugees who had arrived from the Soviet territories. Severely restricted funding often resulted in sterile and boring apartment blocks and row houses, suburban developments, and new towns. Occasionally, some were interna-

tionally recognized for the excellent quality of their design, but more often they became bleak dormitory villages for newly uprooted migrants, isolated far from essential services and lifestyle amenities. Revell's architectural commissions attempted to find suitable solutions for these issues, and his systematic approach enabled him to become a master of conservative, yet innovative, use of space, materials, and energy resources.

In 1952 construction began on Tapiola, the internationally admired garden-city suburb of Helsinki. Revell's office designed five standardized apartment buildings and a school during the community's first and second development phases. Typical of government-supported projects of this era, the apartment sizes were strictly limited, and whenever these were exceeded, Revell had to compensate by making other apartments even smaller. For these projects, Revell experimented with using prefabricated elements, at the time a novel application for residential construction in Finland.

Revell was also able to apply his rational approach to smaller scale housing, such as the Kärjensivu Rowhouse (1955), sited on a rocky hillside fronting a bay near Helsinki. To minimize costs and maximize comfort, he selected the row house form, putting all living spaces on the upper level and utility rooms, garage, sauna, and entrance on the ground floor. Movable partitions and modular cupboards enabled occupants to customize the interiors. Radiant floor heating provided evenly distributed warmth at minimum cost. Energy expenses were also addressed by constructing the entire wall overlooking the bay of fixed triple-glazed windows, thus creating Finland's first glass-walled building.

In conjunction with community and residential projects, Revell's office applied the systematic process to the design of several schools. The Meilahti Primary School (1953) in Helsinki was designed with Osmo Sipari. Classrooms were arrayed in a sinuous line, part of which curved protectively around an outdoor play area, sheltering the students from the winds and reflecting the sun's warmth. The school's design was adapted to the landscape, its plan being clearly separated into distinct functional modules, which along with the outdoor play areas stepped up the sloping terrain.

The postwar peace treaty negotiated between Finland and the Soviet Union also included reparations in the form of "goods in kind" to be paid to the Soviet Union until 1952, and in order to meet these obligations, Finland undertook industrial development on a massive scale. Many architectural practices designed factories with workers' accommodations, and the competition for the Hyvon-Kudeneule hosiery factory and employee housing (1955) near Hanko was won by Viljo Revell and Osmo Lappo. Primary attention was given to planning an efficient assembly process, minimizing energy consumption, and reducing operational costs. Revell specified a combination of prefabricated and cast-in-place reinforced concrete elements, as well as corrugated anodized aluminum sheets for finishing the exterior walls. To visually unify the complex, all buildings contained a limited variety of materials and structural forms. The designs of such industrial complexes were a natural expression of Revell's functional design talent.

Revell's work was not confined to utilitarian projects, however. In 1958, he completed a private commission for the Danish-born entrepreneur and art collector Gunnar Didrichsen—a villa on the Helsinki island of Kuusisaari. Revell used the

hilltop site to advantage, creating a two-story wall of triple-glazed windows overlooking the water. The flat roof with its thick parapet extended out over the window walls, but the central portion of the roof was raised, and clerestory windows let natural light flood the central portion of the house. Revell also designed the built-in furnishings and architectural hardware. In the wooded surroundings the Didrichsens installed a sculpture garden that included, at Revell's request, the Archer by Henry Moore. To house their growing art collection, a new wing was added in 1965, and the villa now functions as the Didrichsen Art Museum, Viljo Revell's architecture being a major theme.

Given the international renown of Finnish architects Alvar Aalto and Eero Saarinen and the provocative urban development projects, the outside world began to take note of this small northern country. In 1958, Revell was prompted to enter the competition for a new city hall in Toronto, Canada, and from among a field of over 500, the jury selected his proposal. Revell worked in association with the large Canadian modernist firm of John B. Parkin Associates. His design for the Toronto City Hall (1965) included two towers of unequal height rising facing each other above a multistoried plinth. Between the towers, the saucer-shaped council chamber was a discrete element supported on slender piers. The elliptically shaped floor slabs of the office towers cantilevered out from the massive rear walls, creating open floor areas that would provide maximum flexibility for interior layouts. The building group created by these three elements was fronted by an open plaza (Nathan Phillips Square) containing a large reflecting pool spanned by elliptical arches, an elevated walkway around the perimeter, and a massive rendition of Henry Moore's sculpture, the Archer. As with many publicly funded projects, the issue of cost overruns soon came to the fore, and Revell was constantly forced to compromise his unique design, even after construction was well underway. Massive columns soon interrupted the open interior spaces, the council chamber was supported on an immense concrete cylinder that overwhelmed the interior spaces below, and building finishes were frequently modified. In the view of several critics of the day, Revell's bold and innovative concept was altered to such a degree that construction of the City Hall should not have proceeded. In spite of the controversy, the Toronto City Hall became a well-loved nexus for the city's inhabitants, and as an international landmark of Modern architecture, it garnered an international reputation for Viljo Revell. Unfortunately, Revell's health seriously declined during this period, and close friends ascribed his premature death to the turmoil surrounding this project.

While living in North America, Revell designed a lakeside cottage (1960) for the H.F. Johnsons in northern Wisconsin. The cottage, with its sauna overhanging the water's edge, was built using traditional, load-bearing timber construction methods. The horizontal emphasis and open planning concepts of modernism provide a counterpoint to the natural materials.

When the World Health Organization held a competition for the design of their new Geneva Administrative Headquarters in 1960, Revell was one of the 15 architects invited to participate. The collaborative entry, submitted by Revell and three other Finnish colleagues, garnered an Honourable Mention. They adhered to modernist principles, elevating the low-rise building above a broad terrace. Recognizing that employees would be from many countries, the designers minimized the use of long, isolating office corridors. They created a triangular-shaped central volume containing an open hall, council chamber, and museum, which connected the three projecting wings.

In 1962, Revell worked on his final project submission with a team of Finnish architects and engineers. Although never constructed, the design of the office tower for Peugeot in Buenos Aires displayed an innovative use of concrete and steel technology. The competition drawings described a pedestrian plaza and massive underground parking garage at the base of the building, surmounted by a skyscraper, which was subdivided into three groups of 12 to 14 floors. Each group was separated by three-story-high concave beams spanning between tapering pairs of structural piers located at each corner of the tower. Each cluster of concrete floor slabs was supported by internal prestressed cables and exterior cable nets, suspended from the centrally located services core and the massive tie beams.

In hindsight, the architectural community has realized that Finland produced several talented designers during the postwar decades although they were, at the time, eclipsed by the greater reputations of Aalto and Saarinen. In achieving national and international recognition, Viljo Revell is considered a leader of this group. Revell did not limit his modernist ideals to a particular genre of architecture, and his designs covered the architectural spectrum from customized luxury homes to mass housing projects, industrial plants, commercial centers, and educational and institutional buildings. Revell's untimely death in midcareer terminated the ascent of a talented modern architect.

RHODA BELLAMY

See also **Aalto, Alvar (Finland); Bauhaus; Blomstedt, Aulis (Finland); Concrete; Helsinki, Finland; Toronto City Hall**

Further Reading

Recently published English-language resources devoted to Viljo Revell are limited, so the following list includes an older survey of his work, edited by Ålander Kyösti, and still available in libraries. The more recent work, *Heroism and the Everyday, Building Finland in the 1950s*, edited by Nikula Riitta, was published as a catalogue for an exhibition describing the work of several architects whose designs contributed to the emergence of Finland's international architectural reputation—naturally, Viljo Revell is among them. Furthermore, Revell's work and the manner in which it contributed to the development of Finland is frequently discussed in general surveys of the modernist tradition in the Scandinavian countries. Such historical overviews, as well as discussions of the legacy of earlier 20th-century architectural styles, assist us in understanding the environmental context for Revell's designs and the contribution that he made toward the architectural landscape that is particular to Finland.

Ålander, Kyösti (editor), *Viljo Revell, Works and Projects / Bauten und Projekte*, translated by Jonathon Fleming, Fred Fewster and Kingsley A. Hart, New York: Praeger, 1966
Lane, Barbara Miller, *National Romanticism and Modern Architecture in Germany and the Scandinavian Countries*, Cambridge and New York: Cambridge University Press, 2000
Nikula, Riitta (editor), *Heroism and the Everyday, Building Finland in the 1950s*, Helsinki: Museum of Finnish Architecture, 1994
Norri, Marja-Riitta, Elina Standertskjöld, and Wilfried Wang (editors), *20th Century Architecture: Finland*, Helsinki: Museum of Finnish Architecture and Frankfurt am Main: Deutsches Architektur-Museum, 2000
Quantrill, Malcolm, *Finnish Architecture and the Modernist Tradition*, London: E & FN Spon, 1995

REWAL, RAJ 1934–

Architect, India

Despite his rigorous education and training in modernist design aesthetics, Raj Rewal remains rooted in the culture of his native India. As Rewal himself noted, "Our generation has been trying to discover the common thread in which the fabric of Indian architecture has been woven in the past and its significance for our times."

Rewal's concern is with understanding the architectural history of India (especially of the Mughal period) and forms such as the *haveli* (or urban courtyard house) of the Rajasthan region; the attention to materials and climatic design mark each of his projects. Most of the architect's buildings have been erected in the public sector, mainly institutional complexes and low- to middle-income housing. Most of his buildings are in New Delhi, the Indian capital, although since the 1980s he has built more widely, including outside the country.

Rewal's early project for the French Embassy Staff Residences (1967–69) reveals his preoccupation with concrete as a structural material with brick-and-stone in-fill. The clustering of the low-rise units and their orientation to the sun and wind are a prototype for his later, larger housing schemes. This is taken to much greater heights in his Permanent Exhibition Complex (1970–74) at Delhi's trade fairgrounds, consisting of the Hall of Nations and the Hall of Industries—large single-volume spaces—the largest of which spans 78 meters and is 34 meters high. The structures are articulated as precast-concrete space frames. This experimentation, with the engineer Mahendra Raj, translates the use of steel and concrete, adapting the technology for local conditions and labor-intensive building skills.

Rewal's consistent use of concrete structure with block in-fill, usually clad in the beige and red sandstone used in many historic buildings, gives his architecture a signature quality. The sense of stability and mass in his works are, to some extent, offset by their verticality and cantilevering of forms, as is evident in his office building, Engineers India House (1979–83) and Standing Conference of Public Enterprises (SCOPE) office building (1980–89), both in New Delhi. In the latter project, the fragmentation of volumes and the series of interlocking polygonal structures with their deep recessed opening and sunscreens help to modulate his "metabolic Brutalism." This form of expression was continually refined until he produced his elegant World Bank Building (1993), built around a central square courtyard.

In another of Rewal's preoccupations—that of housing—he tries, usually successfully, to reconcile a rationalist sense of function, structure, and fabrication with typologies abstracted from the past. His Sheikh Serai Housing (1970–82), with its cruciform site plan and large central public square connected by pathways, keeps parking in central areas surrounded by housing clusters. The notion of pedestrian streets and the grouping of low-rise units was further developed in the elegant Asian Games Village (1980–82). Comprised of 500 units, the Village is clustered in groups around courtyards, separated by "gateways" and connected internally by a series of open spaces and paths reserved for pedestrians. It provides an insight into his strategy for dense low-rise (up to four stories) development.

Rewal's notion of the "living unit" as a combination of indoor and outdoor flexible space and patterns of growth that can be multiplied in numerous combinations is taken to new heights in his CIDCO mass-housing scheme (of which 1048 units were built by 2000) in Belapur, New Mumbai, as part of a much larger settlement. The units (each an average of 40 square meters) on a site of 19 acres achieve a density of 55 units per acre. The units are organized in seven neighborhoods, each defined by a system of peripheral roads built along contours of the site. Here, as in all his works, Rewal's attention to open landscaped (planted and hard) areas is an integral part of his conception of space and movement through the project.

Rewal is perhaps best known for his institutional projects. These complexes respond to the hot, dry climate and urban environment, providing interlocking spaces, streets, pavilions, terraces, and gardens surrounded by buildings. As the architectural critic Razia Grover noted, "[They] are meshed in a system that responds to climate as well as the pragmatic requirements of each scheme." For example, the National Institute of Immunology (1983–90) uses the rocky site and central courtyard around which to organize the building. Again in the Central Institute of Educational Technology (CIET; 1986–89), the courtyard generates the spatial complexity of the building.

With the Parliament Library (1989–2001) and the World Bank Building (1990–93), both in New Delhi, and the Ismaili Centre in Lisbon, there is a shift in Rewal's architecture to a concern with what one might term a "symbolic ethos" that reflects the essence of culture in building. Rewal's term for this is *rasa* (literally, "the juice of the core"). The Library, won through a major competition, forms part of Lutyn's Capitol Complex in Delhi. In response to the built surroundings and the climate, the building is essentially depressed under a plaza forming its roof, with parts visible above this plane. This formal contextual gesture is a success. The World Bank also reveals a similar introspective stance and attention to detail with a resolution seldom found in contemporary Indian buildings. This synthesis of classicism with modern sensibilities evokes a feeling that the architect has been able to draw on what the anthropologist Claude Lévi-Strauss called the "deep structure" of society without having to resort to using imagery of the past.

A departure from Rewal's more familiar imagery, materials, and technology was made in a social and religious complex, the Lisbon Ismaili Center (1995–99). The garden court is surrounded by an expressive steel structure, clad in stone, marble, and more steel, in a more fragmented and Western version of his buildings in India. Here, too, there is a concerted effort to come to terms with the local climate, culture, and built environment.

The vocabulary of interlocking spaces, expression of structure, use of materials and technology, attention to detail, and craftsmanship define the contemporary sensibility that identifies Rewal's buildings as his work. His work is like a tectonic puzzle that, once solved, reveals the nature and essence of time and place to the people who experience it.

HANSAN U. KHAN

Biography

Born in Hoshiarpur in the Punjab, India, 1934; studied architecture in New Delhi (1951–54) and Brixton School of Building (1955–61) in London. Worked in Paris for Michel Ecochard (1962–64); married in 1962; returned to New Delhi to set up his own practice (1964–72). Opened a second office in Tehran,

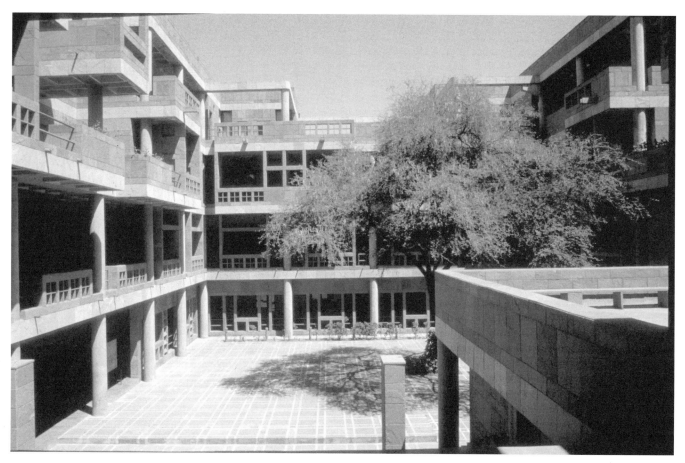

Central Institute of Educational Technology, Main courtyard for open-air studios and performances (1987)
Photo by Ram Rahman © Aga Khan Award for Architecture

Iran (1974); in 1985 founded the Architectural Research Cell with Ram Sharma; curated "The Traditional Architecture of India" for Festival of India, Paris (1986). Received the Gold Medal of the Indian Institute of Architects and the Sir Robert Mathew Award from the Commonwealth Association of Architects (both in 1989); awarded by the Indian Institute of Engineers for the Housing at Belapur, Mumbai, and the J.-K. Trust's Great Masters Award for Lifetime Contribution to Architecture in the Post-independence Era (1995). Associate of the Royal Institute of British Architecture (RIBA), Indian Institute of Architects (IIA); made an Honorary Member of the Mexican Association of Architects (1993). Lives and works in New Delhi.

Selected Works

(All works are built and in New Delhi unless otherwise indicated. Dates of completion noted here.)

French Embassy Staff Quarters, 1969
Nehru Pavilion, 1972
Permanent Exhibition Complex (Hall of Nations and Hall of Industries), 1974
Arbita Housing, Tehran, 1977
National Institute of Public Finance and Policy, 1980
Sheikh Serai Housing, 1982
Asian Games Village, 1982

Hall of States at the Permanent Exhibition Complex, 1982
Engineers India House, 1983
National Institute of Immunology, 1983–90
Zakir Hussain Housing, 1984
State Trading Corporation, 1986
Standing Conference of Public Enterprises (SCOPE), 1989
Central Institute of Education Technology (CIET), 1989
City and Industrial Development Corporation of Maharashtra Ltd. (CIDCO), mass housing—1048 units built, Belapur, New Mumbai, 1988–99
International Centre for Genetic Engineering & Biotechnology, 1989–97
World Bank (Regional Mission) Building, 1993
Ismaili Centre, Lisbon, Portugal, 1999
Housing for the British High Commission, 1999
Parliament Library, 2001

Selected Publications

"The Relevance of Tradition in Indian Architecture" in *Architecture in India* (exhib. cat.), 1985
"The Relevance of Tradition in Architecture Today" in *Contemporary India: Essays on the Uses of Tradition*, edited by Carla M. Borden, 1989; as *Contemporary Indian Tradition*, 1989
Humane Habitat at Low Cost: CIDCO, Belapur, New Mumbai, New Delhi: Architectural Research Cell, 2000

Further Reading

Ahuja, Sarayu, "Doing History Proud: Architectural Features of Raj Rewal's Institute of Immunology," *Indian Architect and Builder* (May 1988)

"Asian Games Village," *A + U*, 148 (January 1983)

Bhatia, Gautam, "A Sandstone Citadel," *Inside Outside* (October/November 1987)

Chemetov, Paul, *La modernité: Un projet inachevé: 40 architects,* Paris: Éditions du Moniteur, 1982

"CIET," *Techniques et architecture,* (August/September 1989)

Cruickshank, D., "Rewal Rasa," *The Architectural Review* (January 1990)

Curtis, William J.R., "Modernism and the Search for Identity," *The Architectural Review* (August 1987)

Curtis, William J.R., "Modern Architecture: Indian Roots: Raj Rewal," *Architecture + Design,* 5/5 (March–April 1989)

Dalal, Abhimanyu, "Interpretations, Tradition, and Modernism in Three of Raj Rewal's Recently Completed Projects," *Architecture + Design,* 5/5 (March/April 1989)

"Engineer's India House, New Delhi," *Mimar,* 18 (October–December 1985)

"French Embassy Quarter," *Architecture d'aujourd'hui* (October 1979)

Gottwald, Sylvia, "India's Intricately Woven Fabric of Housing, Streets, and Spaces," *Architecture* (September 1984)

Grover, Razia, "Raj Rewal" in *Contemporary Architects,* edited by Muriel Emanuel, London: Macmillan, and New York: St. Martin's Press, 1980; 3rd edition, New York: St. James Press, 1994

Jain, Jyotindra et al., *Raj Rewal: Library for the Indian Parliament,* New Delhi: Architectural Research Cell/Roli Books, 2002

Khan, Hasan-Uddin, "Rewal's Asian Games Housing, New Delhi," *Mimar,* 7 (January–March 1983)

Sen, Geeti, "Raj Rewal: Architect Extraordinary," *Inside Outside,* 8 (August/September 1979)

Singh, Patwant, "Traditional Elements in Contemporary Form," *Design* (April/June 1982)

Taylor, Brian Brace, *Raj Rewal,* London: Mimar, and Ahmedabad, India: Mapin, 1992

RICOLA STORAGE BUILDING, LAUFEN, SWITZERLAND

Designed by Herzog and de Meuron, completed 1987

Designed and constructed in 1986–87, the Ricola Storage Building in Laufen, Switzerland, is an important example of Jacques Herzog and Pierre de Meuron's architectural work. Their effect has been felt by theoreticians and practitioners in equal measure, in large part because of the essential idea that lies behind the Herzog and de Meuron's views on the discipline of architecture. This idea, what the architects refer to as *Architektur Denkform,* supports the notion that the discipline of architecture cannot be split neatly into the two poles of theory and practice but is instead based on the recognition that architecture constitutes a seamless whole in which theory and practice are reconciled and inclusive of each other. This approach is an idea that translates roughly as "architecture as built thought," "architecture as a form of thought," or, even more reductively, "architecture as thought." This approach is consistent with a long-standing search for alternatives to Enlightenment ideals in architecture, a search that in the 20th century resulted in the adaptation of phenomenological ideals to architecture-philosophical ideals that Herzog and De Meuron, in both building and codifying their idea of *Architektur Denkform,* attempt to carry to a logical conclusion in works such as the Ricola Storage Building.

The Storage Building, an addition to Ricola's existing administrative and factory offices, is located in a former limestone quarry and functions as the area for products and materials used in the manufacture of herbal sweets. Like many of Herzog and De Meuron's projects, the circumstances and conditions of the site and program provide the initial foundation for the architectural idea, an idea that is quickly modified according to a suggested use of materials, structure, and the mechanics of the construction process. As a result, the building is understood as "a part of the sequence of events, of a dynamic process and not a static one" (Wang, 1992). Site and program, coupled with materials, structure, and constructional means, provide the visual and intellectual organization.

The final result is an exceptionally rigorous project that, although encapsulating the architects' highly reflexive approach to architecture, deserves further elaboration. The Storage Building is constructed of simple building components: a steel-frame structure surrounded by a cladding assembly. The external envelope comprises a system of interwoven horizontal and vertical elements made of wooden battens, wood-cement (*Eternit*) panels, and sheet metal. In maintaining the identity of each component part, the building details express the nature and process of construction, exposing the "thinking" of the building process. The *Eternit* panels, their width expanding as they ascend the facade, are largest at the top of the cladding system. Furthering the sense of identity accorded each building component, each vertical member is supported by numerous individual foundations. A kind of "constructed parapet," the cantilevering timber construction projecting from the top, serves to expose the building's internal constructional system, thereby suggesting the qualities associated with an assemblage.

Accordingly, the building's internal system, a galvanized sheet-metal box that serves as an inner liner or container, is again revealed externally on the inner facade at the connection to the original administration building, where it is detailed with extraordinary precision. According to Wang, the use of exposed timber construction, coupled with the delineated exposure of the cladding materials, "enables visual references to the stacking of sawn timber boards around the numerous saw mills in the area as well as to the limestone quarry in which the building sits." Thus, the building is known for only what it is: a building for storage. Herzog and De Meuron's recognition of the mechanics of the building's construction as a significant aspect of the architectural form—enunciated by the formal and material nature of the various systems—creates a woven tapestry of resonating, highly reflexive relationships. These relationships, arrayed through the multiple elements provided by the processes and materials of site, construction, function (use), and materials, embody a "unified field theory of architecture," a Zenlike restfulness.

Herzog and De Meuron consistently abide by their self-described ideology of *Architektur Denkform* in all aspects of their architectural production, a conceptual apparatus that deserves further explanation. Unlike traditional methods of design, the architects do not begin with a formal idea (what is sometimes referred to as a *parti* or, in contemporary terms, diagram); rather,

the "beginning" of architecture is actually a series of beginnings, each re-informing the others in turn. By revealing particular facets of design, the mixed media record of sketches, drawings, photographs, and models assume a heightened level of importance as well, as much for the results yielded by the various techniques as for the information gathered for further study. Hence, the elements of design and building, garnered through the activity of design process, are not isolated from other components of the building process; rather, they act as equivalent elements within a field of elements, all of which are informed and adjusted by their consequent relations to one another. As has been the case with most if not all of their architectural projects over the past two decades, *Architektur Denkform* aptly describes Herzog and De Meuron's approach to the design and construction of the Ricola Storage Building. Decisions regarding the use of materials and structure, the means of construction, and the circumstances of the project's siting provide the complex primary ground for the design, a process that bears all of the building's attributes at all stages of the design process. "Materialized thought," the resulting architecture is a constructed gestalt, a unified entity or work of art that requires no explanation other than or beyond itself.

ELIZABETH BURNS GAMARD

See also **Factory; Herzog, Jacques, and Pierre de Meuron (Switzerland)**

Further Reading

Mack, Gerhard, *Herzog and de Meuron: Das Gesamtwek; The Complete Works* (bilingual German–English edition), 2 vols., Basel and Boston: Birkhäuser Verlag, 1996

Wang, Wilfried, *Herzog and de Meuron*, Zurich: Artemis, 1992; 3rd enlarged edition, Boston: Birkhäuser, 1998

Zaugg, Remy, et al., *Herzog et de Meuron: Une exposition*, Paris: Les Presses du Réel, 1995; as *Herzog and de Meuron: An exhibition*, Ostfildern bei Stuttgart, Germany: Cantz, 1996

RIETVELD, GERRIT THOMAS 1888–1964

Architect and furniture designer, the Netherlands

Gerrit Thomas Rietveld was a prolific designer of furniture and architecture whose two most famous works, the Red-Blue Chair (1918) and the Schröder-Schräder House (1924), are considered icons of early modern architecture and design. Rietveld's career spanned more than 40 years and included numerous designs for buildings and furniture as well as a number of published articles. An important figure in the De Stijl movement, Rietveld was concerned primarily with the experience of architectural space. Through the articulation of component parts, scale, and structure, he created designs that, although not monumental, provided a setting that elevated the life of the occupant.

Born on 24 June 1888 in Utrecht, Rietveld left school at age 11 to work in his father's furniture maker's shop. He left his father's shop in 1906 to work as a draftsman in the jewelry studio of C.J. Begeer in Utrecht, simultaneously pursuing architecture and drawing courses in the evening. In 1911, Rietveld established his own furniture maker's shop in Utrecht and continued his evening architectural studies under the architect P. Houtzagers. During this time, he designed several shops and

a collection of furniture commissioned by H.G.J. Schelling, an architect for Dutch Rail.

The first design for which Rietveld received recognition was the Red-Blue Chair. Originally of unfinished wood, Rietveld added the color to articulate the individual components. Two planes set at an angle to each other create the seat and back and rest on a composition of horizontal and vertical rails. Extension of the wooden rails and planes beyond their intersection points accents the open quality of the composition. An early version of the chair had side panels that were later removed to create a greater feeling of openness. The cross section of the rail, emphasized with the bright yellow paint, establishes a modular system for the chair. The Red-Blue Chair was followed by other pieces of furniture, including a buffet, in a similar style of horizontal and vertical rails.

In 1921, Truus Schröder-Schräder commissioned Rietveld to design a study in the house she shared with her husband and three children. This small commission was the beginning of a collaboration and friendship that continued for many years and resulted in his most famous design: the Schröder-Schräder House. Considered to be the preeminent architectural manifestation of the De Stijl movement, the house is the creation of a total living environment based on Mrs. Schröder-Schräder's ideas about modern living and Rietveld's spatial explorations. Rietveld saw in De Stijl an alignment with his own interest in the study of new definition of architectural space. Both the Red-Blue Chair and the Schröder-Schräder House were prominently featured in the publication *De Stijl*, edited by Theo van Doesburg.

In 1928, Rietveld was a founding member of the first CIAM (Congrès Internationaux d'Architecture Moderne) in Switzerland and was a deputy delegate in the 1930 CIAM in Frankfurt with Mart Stam. Rietveld's interest in modernism included the role of industrialization and mass production in architecture and design. In 1929, he proposed the "core" house in which vertical circulation, plumbing, and heating were condensed into a prefabricated core around which the house would be built. Presented in a 1929 exhibition in Utrecht, the concept was well received, but none was ever built. Rietveld designed a number of housing projects, many in conjunction with Truus Schröder-Schräder, including a series of row houses across from the Schröder-Schräder House. In 1930, Rietveld designed, on invitation, five row houses for the 1930–32 Werkbund Siedlung in Vienna.

This interest in industrialization can also be seen in a series of designs for economical furniture by Rietveld and produced by Metz & Co. These included a line of "crate" furniture (1934), easily assembled from precut parts, and the famous Zig-Zag Chair (1934), a single bent plane of wood. Industrialization for Rietveld provided a means by which good design could be made accessible as well as having the ability to eliminate the repetition of tasks required in hand production. Although economy was key in terms of both cost and manufacture, Rietveld was equally concerned with the function and flexibility of an item.

Despite his early successes, however, it was not until the 1950s that Rietveld began to receive larger commissions. Prior to that time, he had produced small commercial and residential designs, some in a distinctly vernacular character. In 1954, Rietveld received the commission for the Netherlands Pavilion for the Venice Biennale, where he used the architecture to create a distinct yet subdued exhibition space through the integration of natural light. Also in 1954, and initially intended as a temporary

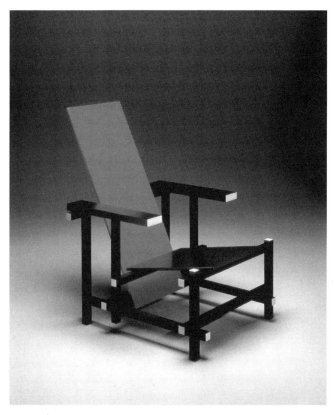

Gerrit T. Rietveld, Red and Blue Armchair, designed 1918
© Mario Carrieri. Photo courtesy Cassina S.p.A.

structure, was the Sonsbeek Pavilion in Arnhem, which was later reconstructed in Otterlo. As in the Schröder-Schräder House, Rietveld explored the layering of spaces through the dissolution of boundaries. The Pavilion is a composition of seemingly independent horizontal and vertical planes creating a series of spaces that are simultaneously redefined by glass walls. Rietveld manipulated economical materials, such as concrete block stacked on its side so that the holes are visible, wood, and glass, to create an interpenetration of space similar to the work of Mies van der Rohe's Barcelona Pavilion.

Rietveld began designs for two prominent art academies, as well as for the De Ploeg Textile Factory (1956), that exemplify his later works. In 1961, he entered into a successful partnership with the architects Johan van Dillen and Johan van Tricht and received a number of larger commissions, some of which, such as the Rijksmuseum Vincent van Gogh (1963–72) in Amsterdam, were completed by the partners after Rietveld's death.

Rietveld received a number of awards and honors during his life, including the Crown Order of Belgium, the Order of Oranje-Nassau, and the Sikkens Prize. He was recognized by his peers with the Bond van Netherlandse Architecten and an honorary degree from the Technische Hogeschool in Delft. Although Rietveld did ultimately receive recognition for his contribution to modern architecture, no single other work was to have the impact of his early designs: the Red-Blue Chair and the Schröder-Schräder House.

KATHERINE WHEELER BORUM

Biography

Born in Utrecht, 24 June 1888; son of a cabinetmaker. Studied drawing at the Municipal Evening School, Utrecht 1906–08; studied architectural drawing with P. Houtzagers, Utrecht 1908–11; studied architecture with P.J. Klaarhamer, Utrecht 1911–15. Worked in father's business, Utrecht 1899–1906; draftsman, C.J. Begeer's Jewelry Studio, Utrecht 1906–11. In private practice as a cabinetmaker, Utrecht 1911–19; private architectural practice, Utrecht 1919–60; collaborated with Mrs. Truus Schröder-Schräder, Utrecht from 1921; partner, Rietveld, van Dillen, and van Tricht from 1960. Instructor in industrial and architectural design, Academie voor Bëeldende Kunsten, Rotterdam and the Hague and the Academie voor Baukunst, Amsterdam 1942–58. Member, De Stijl 1919–31; founding member, CIAM 1928; Dutch delegate, CIAM conference, Frankfurt 1929; honorary member, Bond van Nederlandse Architecten 1963. Died in Utrecht, 25 June 1964.

Selected Works

Red-Blue Chair, 1918
C. Begeer Shop, Utrecht, 1920
Hartog House Interior, Maarssen, 1920
Hanging Lamp, 1920
G.Z.C. Jewelry Store, Amsterdam, 1922
Berlin Chair, 1923
Wessels Shop, Utrecht, 1924
Schröder-Schräder House, Utrecht, 1924
Van Huffel Chemist's Shop, The Hague, 1924
P. Ketting Study, Interior, Utrecht, 1925
Dr. Muller Nursery, Utrecht, 1925
Dr. Harenstein Living Room, Interior (with Truus
    Schröder-Schräder), Amsterdam, 1926
Weteringschans Bedroom, Interior (with Truus Schröder-Schräder),
    Amsterdam, 1926
Lommen House, Wassenaar, 1927
Birza House Interiors, Utrecht (with Truus Schröder-Schräder),
    1927
Normaal Housing (with Truus Schröder-Schräder), 1927
One-Piece Moulded Chair, 1927
Garage and Chauffeur's Quarters, Utrecht, 1928
Zaudy Shop, Weisel, Germany, 1928
Klep House, Breda, 1931
Row Houses, Werkbund Seidlung, Vienna, 1932
Row Houses, Robert Schumannstraat, Utrecht, 1932
House and Music School, Zeist, 1932
Metz and Company Shop, The Hague (with W. Penaat), 1933
Row Houses, Erasmuslaan (with Truus Schröder-Schräder), 1934
Szekley House, Santpoort, 1934
Zig-Zag Chair, 1934
Hondius Crone House Interiors, Bloemendaal, 1935
Hillebrand House, Blaricum, 1935
Vreeburg Cinema, Utrecht (with Truus Schröder-Schräder), 1936
Smedes House, Den Dolder, 1936
Mees House, The Hague, 1936
Hypothecair Crediet Bank, The Hague, 1939
Brandt-Corstius Vacation House, Petten, 1939
Verrijn-Stuart Summer House, Breukelerveen, 1941
One-Piece Stamped Chair, 1942
Smit House, Kinderdijk (unbuilt), 1949
Van Ommeren House, Elst, 1949
Stoop House, Velp, 1951
Home for Children, Curacao, 1951
Klausen House, Den Dolder, 1952

Bicycle Shed, 1953
Netherlands Pavilion, Biennale, Venice, 1954
Sonsbeek Park Sculpture Pavilion, Arnhem, 1954; rebuilt Otterlo, 1965
Van Ravensteijn-Hintzen House, Laren, 1954
Driessen House, Arnhem, 1954
Juliana Hall and Entrance, Trade Fair, Utrecht, 1956
Visser House, Bergeyk (with H. Schröder), 1956
De Ploeg Textile Factory, Bergeyk, Netherlands, 1956
Blaha House, Best, 1957
Housing, Hoograven (with H. Schröder and van Grunsven), 1957
Van Daalen House, Bergeyk, 1957
UNESCO Press Room, Paris, 1957
Schrale Breton Offices, Zwolle, 1958
Gerrit Reitveld Exhibition at the Centraal Museum, Utrecht, 1958
Housing, Utrecht, 1959
Van Doel House, Ilpendam, 1959
Ket Shop, Leeuwarden, 1959
Gemeentelijk Lyceum School, Doetinchem (with van Tricht), 1959
De Zonnehof Exhibition Hall, Amersfoort, 1960
Koot House, The Hague, 1960
Design Center Showroom, Amsterdam, 1962
Mado Shop, Utrecht, 1963
Academie voor Beeldende Kunst, Arnhem, 1963
Van Sloobe House, Heerlen, 1964
Miners' Housing, Limburg, 1964
Primary School, Badhoevedorp, 1964
Savings Bank, Dedemsvaart, 1965
Church, Uithoorn (with van Tricht), 1965
Hoofdorp Cemetery Auditorium, 1966
Steltman Jewelery Shop Interior, The Hague, 1967
Engelhard House, Amstelveen, 1967
Instituut voor Kunstnijverheidsonderwijs (now known as Gerrit Rietveld Academy), Amsterdam, 1968
Rijksmuseum Vincent van Gogh, Amsterdam, 1972
Centraal Museum extensions (with van Dillen), 1972

Selected Publications

Nieuwe zakelijkheid in der nederlandse architektur, 1932
Over kennis en kunst, lezing-cyclus over stedebouw, 1946
Rietveld 1924—Schröder Huis, 1963

Further Reading

Most of Rietveld's writings have not been translated into English; the few that have may be found in the books by Brown (1958) and Küper.

Baroni, Daniele, *I mobili di Gerrit Thomas Rietveld*, Milan: Electa, 1977; as *The Furniture of Gerrit Thomas Rietveld*, Woodbury, New York: Barrons, 1978; as *Gerrit Thomas Rietveld Furniture*, London: Academy Editions, 1978
Berg, E. and H. Bak, "Rietveld and His Museum Buildings," *Arkitekten* (12 March 1974)
Brown, Theodore, *The Work of G. Rietveld, Architect*, Utrecht: Bruna, and Cambridge, Massachusetts: MIT Press, 1958
Brown, Theodore, "Rietveld's Egocentric Vision," *Journal of the Society of Architectural Historians*, 24 (1965)
Buffinga, A., *G.Th. Rietveld*, Amsterdam: Meulenhoff, 1971
Casciato, Maristella, "Family Matters: The Schröder House, by Gerrit Rietveld and Truus Schröder" in *Women and the Making of the Modern House: A Social and Architectural History*, edited by Alice Friedman, New York: Abrams, 1998
Doumato, Lamia, *Gerrit Thomas Rietveld, 1888–1964*, Monticello, Illinois: Vance Bibliographies, 1983
G. Rietveld, Architect (exhib. cat.), Amsterdam: Stedelijk Museum, 1971; London: Arts Council of Great Britain, 1972
Jaffé, H.L.C., *De Stijl, 1917–1931: The Dutch Contribution to Modern Art*, Amsterdam: Meulenhoff, and London: Tiranti, 1956
Küper, Marijke and Ida van Zijl, *Gerrit Th. Rietveld, 1888–1964: The Complete Works*, Utrecht, the Netherlands: Centraal Museum, 1992
Mulder, Bertus and Ida van Zijl, *Rietveld Schröder House*, Bussum, the Netherlands: V and K, and New York: Princeton Architectural Press, 1997
Overy, Paul, *De Stijl*, London: Studio Vista, 1969
Overy, Paul, "Carpentering the Classic: A Very Popular Practice: The Furniture of Gerrit Rietveld," *Journal of Design History*, 4/3 (1991)
Overy, Paul et al., *Het Rietveld Schröder Huis*, Houten, the Netherlands: De Haan, 1988; as *The Rietveld Schröder House*, Houten, the Netherlands: De Haan, Cambridge, Massachusetts: MIT Press, and London: Butterworth Architecture, 1988
Rond, Dennis and Annemiek Testal, *Rietveld in Amsterdam: alle uitgevoerde en niet uitgevoere projekten; Rietveld in Amsterdam: All Executed and Not Executed Projects* (bilingual Dutch-English edition), Rotterdam: Uitgeverij, 1988
Slothouber, Erik (editor), *De Kunstnijverheidsscholen van Gerrit Rietveld; The Artschools of Gerrit Rietveld* (bilingual Dutch-English edition), Amsterdam: de Balie, 1997
St. John Wilson, Colin, "Gerrit Rietveld: 1888–1964," *Architectural Review*, 136 (1964)
Troy, Nancy, *The De Stijl Environment*, Cambridge, Massachusetts: MIT Press, 1983
Yee, R., "A Touch of De Stijl," *Progressive Architecture* (March 1975)

RIO DE JANEIRO, BRAZIL

The city of Rio de Janeiro was founded on the margins of Guanabara Bay in 1556 and remained a small village until the 17th century, when it developed into an important commercial port. In 1763, Rio became the capital of Brazil, and in 1808 it was named the capital of the whole Portuguese Empire when the king and the nobility moved there, fleeing Napoleon. The city remained the capital of the Brazilian Empire after independence in 1822 and entered the 20th century as the capital of the Brazilian Republic (proclaimed in 1889) until the federal government moved to Brasilia in 1960. From 1930 to 1960, Rio was the core of Brazilian modernism while *carioca* (native of Rio) architects reshaped the whole country. Fortunately, inspired by the fantastic natural beauty of the city, this generation of modernist architects was able to give Rio some of the finest buildings of the 20th century.

Brazilians entered the 20th century under strong influence of positivism and sanitary engineering, and the city of Rio de Janeiro, being the capital of the republic and the intellectual center of the country, was dominated by such ideas. The republic adopted French eclecticism as the appropriate language to affirm its power and convey technological advancement. The 1900s would be marked in Rio by the urban reformations of Pereira Passos, with avenues being opened and slums being displaced with civic buildings in French neoclassical style taking their place (Teatro Nacional, 1906). A few years later, another plan by French urbanist Alfred Agache (1927) would be the structure for Rio's main transformations of the first half of the century. Still, in the second decade of the century, Rio would experiment with issues of local identity and their relationship to interna-

tional images, with the arrival of Art Deco on one hand and the development of neo-Colonial styles on the other. The Deco tradition left landmarks such as the Cristo Redentor statue over Corcovado hill, and the neo-Colonial movement, led by José Mariano Filho, would battle against the modernist avant-garde ideas throughout the 1920s and 1930s. In 1929, the high points of this debate would be a series of conferences by Le Corbusier when, visiting Rio for the first time, he produced the famous sketches of an elevated highway along the shore.

In 1930, in what would be one of the key moments of Brazilian architecture, Lúcio Costa was named director of Rio's ENBA (National School of Beaux-Arts). As soon as he was named, Costa began a radical reformation of the art and architecture curriculum, based on the Bauhaus pedagogy and Le Corbusier's ideas. The strong reaction against these proposed changes led to Costa's substitution, but the ideas that he installed flourished with a generation of students known later as the *carioca* school: Oscar Niemeyer, Roberto Burle Marx, Affonso Raidy, Jorge Moreira, Milton Roberto, and Luis Nunes, among others.

Also in the 1930s, young architects such as the Roberto brothers (Milton and Marcelo) built the ABI building (Brazilian Press Association headquarters, 1935) and the Santos Dumont Airport (completed 1944). Atílio Correa Lima designed the Seaplane station (1940), and Niemeyer designed a nursery (Obra do Berço, 1937) and his own house (1939) at Lagoa.

In 1936, Le Corbusier was invited as a supportive consultant for the team of architects commissioned to design the new building for the Brazilian Ministry of Education and Health (MES). The invitation of Le Corbusier served as a support for canceling the previous competition, as the government considered the winning design incompatible with the modern image that they were trying to establish. The MES building would inspire a whole generation of young architects and artists with the murals by Candido Portinari, sculptures by Bruno Giorgi, and gardens by Burle Marx around the architecture developed by Lucio Costa, Carlos Leão, Jorge Moreira, and Oscar Niemeyer, all a result of Le Corbusier's visit.

During the 1940s, many important modernist buildings were developed and designed by the *carioca* generation. The Roberto brothers were using precast concrete in industrial projects, Niemeyer designed the Boavista Bank (1946), and Jorge Moreira was designing the University Campus at Ilha do Fundão (1949). Meanwhile, Afonso Reidy completed the Pedregulho residential complex (1947), a curvilinear apartment building that reflected the terrain's contours.

The architecture of the 1950s is still considered a high point in Brazilian modernism. For example, Affonso Raidy's Museum of Modern Art (1952) is an exposed-concrete structure disposed horizontally at the Flamengo seashore in order not to disturb the landscape. Burle Marx was responsible for the gardens that surround the museum and the whole Flamengo park shore. The 1950s would also witness fascinating buildings by Sergio Bernardes (House for Lota M. Soares and Elizabeth Bishop, 1952), Henrique Mindlin (Avenida Central building, 1957), and Francisco Bolonha (Joseph Bloch school, 1960). In a time of accelerating industrialization and urbanization, housing lies at the core of the 1950s debate and practice, led by Carmen Portinho at the municipal office. One of the best apartment buildings of this time is the Parque Guinle complex (Bristol and Caledônia buildings, 1950) by Lucio Costa.

After the 1950s boom, Rio de Janeiro would suffer with the transfer of the federal government to Brasilia in 1960. A general loss of investments and decreasing construction activities led not only to fewer buildings but also to problematic changes in the municipal codes that would allow faster construction to bring profits. The quality of the 1950s was lost, and after the military coup in 1964, few interesting buildings or projects appeared in Rio.

The military regime exiled architects such as Niemeyer and repressed schools of architecture that were a focus of cultural and political discussion on the 1960s. The 1970s experienced accelerating wealth disparity, with architecture losing its social commitment in favor of apartment buildings, hotels, and financial institutions for the wealthy classes. The Petrobras building (state oil company, 1968) by Gandelfi and Assad and the Coca-Cola headquarters (1972) by Edison and Edmundo Musa represent the paradigm of those times. Costly apartment buildings with security devices dominated the architectural scene at Barra da Tijuca, Lagoa, and Ipanema. The major public buildings of the military period in Rio include the State University Complex (1968) by Luis Paulo Conde and the Copacabana sidewalks (1970) by Roberto Burle Marx.

With the redemocratization of the 1980s, a series of public buildings by Oscar Niemeyer was built in Rio. The CIEPSs, a full-time school program built in modulate precast concrete, were scattered around the peripheral areas of the city, serving the needy communities. In downtown Rio, the Sambódromo, a half-mile-long open walkway for the samba schools' carnival parades, ends in a elegant plaza dominated by a sculpture designed by Niemeyer. Across the bay in Niterói, the Museum of Contemporary Art (1996) was also designed by the 90-year-old Niemeyer.

In the 1990s, an extensive project of urban design, public facilities, and renovation was put forward by architect Luis Paulo Conde, first as municipal secretary of urbanism (1992–96) and then as mayor (1996–2000). Rio Cidade (downtown urban design renovations) and Favela-bairro (improvements and infrastructure at the shanty hills) are among the successful cases of good architecture serving the public at the end of the century, reshaping and improving the already astonishing landscape of Rio de Janeiro.

FERNANDO LARA

See also **Bò Bardi, Lina (Brazil); Brasilia, Brazil; Brazil; Burle Marx, Roberto (Brazil); Costa, Lúcio (Brazil); Favela; Niemeyer, Oscar (Brazil); Pampulha Buildings, Belo Horizonte, Brazil**

Further Reading

Bruand, Yves, *Arquitetura Contemporânea no Brasil*, São Paulo: Perspectiva, 1981

Lemos, Carlos A.C., *Arquitetura Brasileira*, Sao Paulo: Melhoramentos, 1979

Meade, Teresa, *"Civilizing" Rio: Reform and Resistance in a Brazilian City, 1889–1930*, University Park: Pennsylvania State University Press, 1997

Mindlin, Henrique, *Modern Architecture in Brazil*, New York: Reinhold 1956

Segawa, Hugo, "The Essentials of Brazilian Modernism," *Design Book Review* (1994)

Segawa, Hugo, *Arquiteturas no Brasil 1900–1990*, Sao Paulo: Edusp, 1998

Underwood, David, *Oscar Niemeyer and the Architecture of Brazil*, New York: Rizzoli, 1994

Xavier, Alberto (Org), *Arquitetura Moderna no Rio de Janeiro*, Sao Paulo: Pini, 1991

RIYADH, SAUDI ARABIA

The city of Riyadh (plural of *rawdhah*, oasis) was founded on the ruins of several communities around 1740. Although it was chosen as the capital of the second Saudi state in 1824, it came to prominence only after its independent governor, Abdulaziz Al-Saud, began a campaign to consolidate modern Saudi Arabia in 1902. The speed and scale of Riyadh's transformation since, particularly during the 1970s, has had few parallels. From a walled city of less than 1 square kilometer in 1920, it has grown into a sprawling modern capital of 1,500 square kilometers. Its population has increased from an estimated 14,000 in 1902, to 666,480 in 1974, to more than 2.8 million in 1992, to an estimated 3.5 million by 1998.

The physical transformation of Riyadh began in the mid-1930s with King Abdulaziz's decision to build a large palace and administrative complex two kilometers north of the existing city. Known as al-Murabba', it covered an area of 16 hectares and was linked to the town by a paved stone road. The complex was complemented in the late 1940s by a new residential quarter, al-Futah, to the west of the road, where palatial mansions were built for the king's younger sons. Abdulaziz's building program had several lasting impacts on the form of the city: it stretched its size, it set a northerly direction for its future growth, it showed that the old walls could no longer be considered a barrier to growth, and it introduced a new means of transportation—the private motor vehicle. Architecturally, the buildings of al-Murabba' relied on traditional processes, techniques, and materials adapted by local craftsmen to a new scale and new requirements. The result was a magnificent Najdi style.

Transformation of the city continued after World War II with construction of an airport and a railway. Railroad tracks were laid between Riyadh and the Persian Gulf city of Dammam, with a station built 4 kilometers east of the old city in 1951. In 1952, a terminal building and mosque were constructed 7 kilometers north of the city at a landing strip that had been in use since 1946. In 1951, Crown Prince Saud also built a palace at the garden plot of Nasiriyyah northwest of the city. These three projects necessitated the city's first major road-building program. Nasiriyyah was linked to Murabba' Palace and the town, with a branch leading to the railway station. Another road was built connecting the airport to the city center. The early 1950s also brought the end of the old city as an intact physical entity. Its walls were removed, the old governor's palace and main mosque were rebuilt, and streets were widened to provide access for motor vehicles.

After succeeding to the throne in 1953, King Saud made three decisions directly bearing on the future of Riyadh. He transferred all government agencies from Mecca and began a program of building new ministries to the west of the airport road; he ordered construction of al-Malaz, a new suburb 4 kilometers northeast of the city, to house transferred government

employees; and he expanded and rebuilt his palace at Nasiriyyah. By 1957, seven ministry buildings, designed by the Egyptian architect Sayid Krayim, were complete. Nasiriyyah had been expanded to cover 250 hectares, employing a grid pattern of boulevards, gardens, and modern structures, and al-Malaz was well on the way toward a goal of providing 750 villas, 180 apartment units, buildings for a new university, and support facilities. These projects brought new conceptions of space, street patterns, building types, and materials to the city, and together they came to be known as New Riyadh (although al-Malaz, in particular, acquired this name). Al-Malaz would have a particularly important impact because it introduced the grid as a street pattern and the villa as a house type, forms that would become pervasive in the future development not only of Riyadh but also of every city and town in Saudi Arabia.

As Riyadh continued growing through the 1950s and into the early 1960s, other neighborhoods were built, and apartment buildings appeared along al-Thumairi, al-Wazir, and al-Khazan Streets. Distinct among these were the Fahd bin Moh'd building (late 1950s), the Moh'd bin Saud building (1959), the al-Riyadh building (1960), and the Zahrat al-Riyadh building (1968). Two larger noteworthy projects were also initiated in the late 1960s. These were the Riyadh Intercontinental Hotel and Conference Center (1971) by Trevord Dannat, which avoided the faceless style typical of the time by adopting indigenous architectural elements, and the King Faisal Specialist Hospital (1974), designed by Hospital Design Partnership.

A new phase of Riyadh's urban growth arrived in the late 1960s, when the Saudi government contracted with Doxiadis Associates of Athens to prepare a master plan for the capital city. The plan, approved in 1973, called for a supergrid of boulevards 2 kilometers apart, a major commercial and civic spine extending north to south with an administrative area perpendicular to it, and residential districts extending on both sides of the spine. Among other important effects, the plan confirmed the role of the private automobile as the primary mode of transportation in the city. To implement the plan, the government created a technical committee chaired by the Riyadh governor that would later form the nucleus for the Arriyadh Development Authority (ADA). Since its inception in 1974, this government authority has guided Riyadh's development and carried out large-scale building and renovation projects in the city center, the al-Murabba' district, and elsewhere in the metropolitan area.

Great changes arrived in Riyadh following the oil boom of the early 1970s, leading some critics to describe the city as the biggest construction site in human history. In terms of design excellence, three major projects stand out from the late 1970s: the General Organization for Social Insurance (GOSI) Headquarters (1978), the Saudi Arabian Monetary Agency Towers (1978), and the Saudi Fund for Development (SFD) Headquarters (1980). The GOSI Headquarters, designed by Nabil Fanous and Basim Al-Shihabi, is a graceful modern composition of interlocking Cubistic volumes reminiscent of the Boston City Hall. Its 1987 extension, also by Al-Shihabi (Omrania: Architects, Planners and Engineers), today provides a stark contrast to the original design by using reflective glass on a six-story triangular block to mirror the older building. In his design for the Saudi Arabian Monetary Agency, Minoru Yamasaki employed two massive ten-story towers, identical in structure and facade. In the SFD Headquarters, Urban Coile International took a different

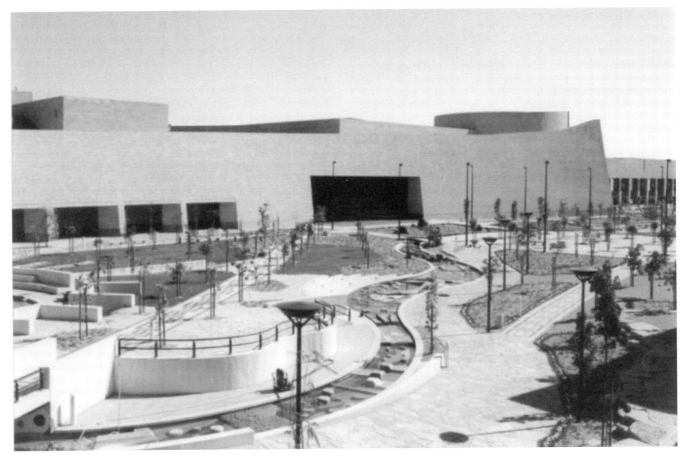

King Abdulaziz Historic Center (1998), Beeah Group Consultants and Rasem Badran
© Saleh Al-Hathloul

approach, attempting to create a modern office building with local roots. Its use of old Diriyyah buildings as a point of reference for exterior expression and its interior arrangements around a covered courtyard have since been emulated by a number of other projects.

Distinctive projects in the 1980s included al-Khairia Center (1982) by Kenzo Tange, the Institute of Public Administration (1982) by The Architects Collaborative and M. al-Sabiq, and the King Khalid International Airport Terminal Complex (1983) by HOK. Today, the twin, triangular 14-story office towers of al-Khairia Center provide a landmark for the northern areas of the city. By choosing a cylindrical shape for the dome of the center's mosque and an elegant square column for its minaret, Tange also introduced new forms into mosque architecture. The structure of the King Khalid Terminal, located 35 kilometers north of the city, consists of four equilateral triangles arranged in a linear form, providing the shortest possible walking distance from curbside or parking to departure and arrival gates. The triangular forms also provide an ample area for security controls while allowing open space to penetrate through to the arrival floor.

Another important 1980s addition to Riyadh was King Saud University (1984), designed and engineered by HOK + 4 consortium. The master plan for this 20,000-student campus by

United Planner Schwanzer GMBH Vienna called for individual buildings to be compactly clustered and interconnected by a system of "spines" serving both as pedestrian "streets" on the main level and as service ways at ground level. Courtyards were used on the upper level for climate control, and windows and other openings were kept small to minimize the intrusion of harsh sunlight.

Since the mid-1980s, local architects have assumed an increasingly important role in the design of the city, and individual buildings have attempted to become more sensitive to local tradition. These trends are especially evident in the work of two local design teams: Basim Al-Shihabi of Omrania, whose most impressive projects have been Tuwaiq Palace (1985), the General Organization for Social Insurance (GOSI) Headquarters Building (1978, 1987), and the Gulf Cooperation Council Headquarters (1987); and Ali Shuaibi and Abdulrahman Al-Hussaini (of Beeah Group Consultants), particularly their designs for al-Kindi Plaza (1986). International architects have also become more responsive to local conditions. One excellent example is King Fahad International Stadium (1987) by Ain Friezer and Partners, a masterpiece of tent architecture. Another is Imam Moh'd Bin Saud Islamic University (1988). The master plan and design for this 15,000-student campus was produced by Techni Beria using a compact organic plan and a system of

courtyards repeated throughout the academic buildings to provide human scale and shorten walking distances.

Especially noteworthy designs in the 1990s have included the Ministry of Interior (1992) by Mousalli, Shaker, Mandily and Archi-System, whose inverted pyramid form produced an instant landmark; the Ministry of Municipal and Rural Affairs (1995) by Zuhair Fayez, which takes the form of an oasis in the middle of the city; the Al-Jazirah Newspaper Headquarters (1995) by Suter and Suter and al-Shathri; and the King Fahad Cultural Center (1991) by Widle Plan.

Since 1974, the ADA has also undertaken a number of large-scale building and renovation projects. One of the most important has been development of the Diplomatic Quarter (DQ). A 586-hectare site was allocated for this project 8 kilometers northwest of the city center after the Saudi government decided to transfer foreign diplomatic missions from Jeddah to Riyadh in 1975.

The master plan for the DQ was by Speerplan, Regional Und Stadtplaner GMBH; its central area urban design was by Beeah of Riyadh, and the layout of its residential districts was by Farah Tashkandi. The DQ may one day hold as many as 120 embassies and 30,000 inhabitants. Today, more than 51 embassies and more than 40 other public or service-sector projects have been completed. Many of the embassies have been designed by well-known architects from their respective countries, including the Japanese Embassy (1985) by Kenzo Tange; the Canadian Embassy (1985) by Sanky Partnership; the Tunisian Embassy (1987) by Mimita, Bin Mahmoud and Faraj; and the French Embassy (1988) by Guy Naizot. Three other DQ projects have won international awards: Al-Kindi Plaza (1986) by Beeah; DQ Landscaping (1986) by Bödeker, Boyer, Wagenfeld and Partners; and Tuwaiq Palace (1985) by Atelie Otto, Büro Happold, and Omrania.

Four other ADA initiatives have been extremely important to the overall design of the city. One was the Ministry of Foreign Affairs (1984) by Henning Larsen and its attendant Staff Housing (1983) by Speerplan Regional Und Stadtplaner GMBH and CRS (with the involvement of Ali Shuaibi as ADA adviser). This successful housing project, employing dwelling clusters around cul-de-sacs with exterior access and an auto-free recreational spine, has now been emulated in the al-Hamra neighborhood (1994) of Riyadh, in Medina, and elsewhere in Saudi Arabia.

Also important has been ADA's rebuilding of Qasr al-Hukm, the Justice Palace District, including the entire old walled city and an additional area to its west. The first redevelopment plan here was by Franco Albini (1978); the second was by Beeah (1983), subsequently revised by ADA staff. Individual building projects have included the Governorate, Municipality, and Police Department buildings (1985) by Albini; the Great Mosque and Redevelopment of the Old City Center (1992) by Rasem Badran; the al-Migliyah Commercial Center (1992); the al-Ta'meer Center-1 (2000) by Dar Al-Mimar (Abdulhalim and Badran) with Arrow, Inc., and Site International; and the Riyadh Court Complex (2000) by M. Makkiyah and Saud Consult.

Finally, ADA has recently been involved in the redevelopment of al-Murabba', known as the King Abdulaziz Historic Center (1998). The urban design for this project was by Beeah and Rasem Badran, and it has subsequently involved the renovation or new construction of a series of buildings designed by several architects. This project represents a return to the city's roots. Located on the old Murabba' site, its completion marks the centennial of the beginning of the process that led to Saudi Arabia's unification. Its high-quality urban spaces, magnificent architecture, and well-thought-out linkages of traditional and modern forms create a complementary focal point to Qasr Al-Hukm in the center of the city.

SALEH AL-HATHLOUL

See also **Ministry of Foreign Affairs, Riyadh, Saudi Arabia; Mosque; Saudi Arabia**

Further Reading

Of the following works cited, Facey provides a detailed history of Riyadh from its origins until the 1950s, including references to primary and secondary sources. Good overviews of the city's urban development are provided by al-Angari, al-Hathloul, and Daghistani. A record of the city's architecture since the late 1970s appears in the architecture magazine *Albenaa*. *Architecture for a Changing World* includes good coverage of several winning projects from Riyadh.

al-Angari, Abdulrahman Bin Mohammed, "The Revival of the Architectural Identity: The City of Arriyadh," Ph.D. diss., University of Edinburgh, 1997
al-Bina'; Albenaa (bilingual, bimonthly Arabic-English journal)
al-Hathloul, Saleh, *Tradition, Continuity, and Change in the Physical Environment: The Arab-Muslim City*, Riyadh: Dar al-Sahan, 1996
Architecture for a Changing World, Seville, Spain: FISA (Fundación Internacional de Síntesis Arquitectónica), and Geneva: Aga Khan Trust for Culture, 1996
Daghistani, Abdal-Majeed Ismail, *Arriyadh: Urban Development and Planning*, Jeddah: Kingdom of Saudi Arabia, 1985
Facey, William, *Riyadh: The Old City*, London: Immel, 1992
King, Geoffrey R.-D., "Some Examples of the Secular Architecture of Najd," *Arabian Studies* 6 (1982)
Mousalli, Mohammad Said, Farid Amin Shaker, and Omar Abdullah Mandily, *An Introduction to Urban Patterns in Saudi Arabia: The Central Region*, London: Art and Archaeology Research Papers, 1977
Othman, Zahir, "The Role of Planning Authorities in Urban Development: A Case of Arriyadh Development Authority" in *Urban Development in Saudi Arabia*, edited by Saleh al-Hathloul and Narayanan Edadan, Riyadh: Dar al-Sahan, 1995
Philby, John B., "Riyadh: Ancient and Modern," *Middle East Journal* 13, no. 2 (1959)
Riyad: The City of the Future, Riyadh: Arab Urban Development Institute, 1984

ROADSIDE ARCHITECTURE

Roadside architecture, the bastard offspring of the automobile, had a pervasive effect on the American landscape during the 20th century. Often denounced for crassness and monotony yet irresistibly convenient to a population getting around on four wheels, roadside architecture was both the bane of the aesthetically sensitive and a boon to motorists looking for food, fuel, and lodging.

When the century opened, the automobile had been in existence just seven years, and only 8000 sputtering, self-propelled vehicles plied the streets and roads. The promise of freedom of movement proved so compelling, however, that the number of registered automobiles reached 458,000 by 1910, surpassed eight million by 1920, and exceeded 23 million by 1930. New

automobile-oriented building types, such as filling stations, motels, and drive-in movie theaters, arose. Older building types, such as restaurants, banks, and grocery stores, gradually changed form.

A mere seven per cent of the nation's roads were hard surfaced by 1904, but many organizations, such as the Lincoln Highway Association, were formed in the 1910s and 1920s to lobby localities, state governments, and federal authorities to construct reliable, all-weather roads. Filling stations dispensing motor oil and gasoline were among the first automobile-oriented facilities to crop up as the roads improved. In urban districts, it was not uncommon for a two-story or taller building containing stores, offices, and apartments to be razed so that its site could be occupied by a diminutive gas station, surrounded by pavement, Chester Liebs observes in *Main Street to Miracle Mile*. The traditional urban practice of placing buildings shoulder to shoulder, right up to the sidewalk, gave way to a looser, more discontinuous pattern, with each building standing alone, farther back from the street.

Because gas stations soon invaded settled residential districts and desirable business areas, petroleum companies felt pressure in the 1910s and 1920s to design stations whose appearance would be seen as an asset rather than an eyesore. In Indianapolis in 1927, for instance, the Ohio-based Pure Oil chain introduced an English cottage-style station that skillfully drew from the romantic house designs popular at the time. Scholars such as Liebs have viewed the styles employed by roadside businesses as "sales costumes," donned with salesmanship and appeasement of popular taste in mind. John A. Jakle and Keith A. Sculle, two leading scholars of roadside architecture, have attributed much of the character of roadside architecture to the concept of "place-product-packaging," in which all the physical aspects of an enterprise, including signs, logos, uniforms, architecture, lighting, and landscaping, are part of a carefully coordinated effort to establish a strong corporate identity. The consistent identity links all the units in a chain and reassures the customers, thereby helping the chain outsell local competitors.

However, the best roadside architecture sprang not only from hardheaded marketing calculations but also from imaginative and occasionally even idealistic impulses. Pure Oil adopted the English cottage-style station not only because it would ease the station's acceptance but also because the station's architect, Carl A. Petersen, regarded the design, with its "Romantic Suburb" connotations, as the most beautiful and appropriate choice, a judgment heartily shared by the company's president, Henry M. Dawes. Similarly, when Howard Johnson was establishing his Massachusetts-based restaurant chain in the latter 1930s and early 1940s, his chief architect, Joseph G. Morgan, produced balanced, dignified compositions that far surpassed the public's usual expectations for eating along the road. Morgan adapted the traditional architecture of New England churches and town halls to the visibility requirements of highway commerce—covering the roofs of Howard Johnson's outlets with conspicuous shiny orange tiles, just as Petersen had clad Pure Oil's roofs with fade-resistant blue tiles—but he gave the buildings pleasingly set-back wings, a carefully detailed row of dormers, a deftly proportioned rooftop lantern, and other touches that bespoke a concern for quality.

Diners, which evolved from lunch wagons that first appeared in Providence, Rhode Island, in 1872, were popular-priced restaurants that for many years resembled streetcars or railroad dining cars. By the end of the 1910s, a number of manufacturers were making diners in factories and shipping them to their sites, first in urban locations, later along outlying highways. Over the years, they increasingly adopted a machine aesthetic, refined through the extensive use of stainless steel. By 1940, the streamlined diner, a striking product of American industrial design, had made its debut.

In the West, the California coffee shops of the 1940s and 1950s by Los Angeles designers such as John Lautner, Douglas Honnold, and Martin Stern wowed motorists with an energetic modernism characterized by large sculpted roofs, expansive walls of glass, and dramatic lighting effects. Some critics dismissed the coffee shops as excessively flamboyant, labeling them "googie," a put-down inspired by the Googie's restaurant that Lautner designed in West Hollywood (built in 1949). However, architectural historian Alan Hess has argued that the expressive modernism of southern California chains such as Biff's, Ship's, Norm's, and Tiny Naylor's—an approach spread nationwide in the 1950s and 1960s through designs by the Los Angeles firm of Armet and Davis for chains such as Denny's and Bob's Big Boy—represented an important instance of modernism becoming broadly popular, a kind of modernism for the common man. Because some designers of "googie," such as Lautner, produced houses and other buildings that commanded respect within the profession, Hess argued that no clear-cut boundary existed between serious architecture and many buildings that served everyday commercial purposes.

There had, of course, been a streak of amateurism and in some cases humorous literalism in some roadside buildings from the beginning of the century through the 1930s. In 1931, along Route 25 in Riverhead, New York, poultry grower Martin Maurer built "The Big Duck," a 20-foot-high, 30-foot-long structure of wood, galvanized wire, and cement, shaped to look like the Long Island Peking ducks that he sold inside it. Its eyes were taillights from a Model T Ford. Giant fish, hot dogs, teapots, chili bowls, root beer barrels, and other objects were common in the 1920s and 1930s. This was especially so in the Los Angeles area, where a Brown Derby restaurant was built in the shape of a hat in 1926, ice cream was dispensed from The Igloo beginning in 1928, the Zep Diner was built in the shape of a Zeppelin in 1930, and many other giant objects were created. One of the most noted chains in that vein was Wigwam Villages, which began in Horse Cave, Kentucky, in 1933 and eventually grew to seven locations scattered from Orlando, Florida, to San Bernardino, California. Wigwam Villages featured lunchrooms and overnight lodging in buildings shaped like tepees.

A variety of new building types appeared as the car became central to American life. In 1933 in Camden, New Jersey, Richard M. Hollingshead, Jr., built the first drive-in theater, allowing people to watch movies while sitting in their cars. About 50 drive-in theaters were in operation throughout the country by the outbreak of World War II. After the war, their numbers grew rapidly, to more than 1700 by 1950, according to Liebs. The tall, wide tower supporting the drive-in's screen became a roadside landmark, sometimes interestingly stylized. The popularity of outdoor theaters peaked in 1958, after which came a long decline.

Drive-in restaurants started to appear in the early 1920s, beginning with the first Pig Stand drive-in, on the Dallas–Fort

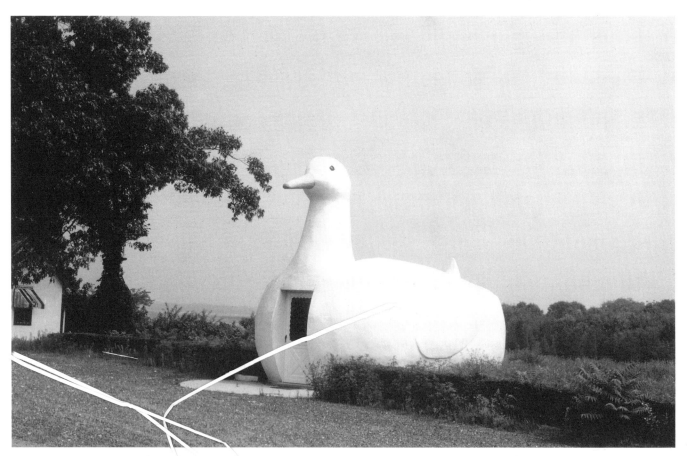

"The Big Duck" (1931); originally on Route 25, Riverhead, Long Island, NY; moved in 1936 to Flanders, NY
© Philip Langdon

Worth Highway in Texas in 1921. Tray boys and tray girls, later known as carhops, brought food and beverages to customers, who ate in their cars. At many drive-ins, a canopy extended above the cars, supplying midday shade. For visual interest, the canopy could take a variety of shapes, from undulating to angular. Some drive-ins, especially in California, gained visual excitement by having a circular or octagonal central building from which a tall illuminated pylon rose. At round or octagonal drive-ins, the cars clustered, nose in, all the way around the building. Drive-ins flourished nationwide in the 1950s and began declining in the 1960s because of community reaction against their noise, trash, and rowdiness and because of growing competition from other kinds of restaurants, especially coffee shops, which were comfortable no matter what the weather, and fast-food establishments, whose self-service method got the food to the customers cheaply and more quickly.

By the 1920s, the demand for overnight lodging along the roads gave birth to the motel, which typically took the form of a continuous one-story structure with the rooms opening directly to the parking area, thereby eliminating the formal spaces and corridors associated with hotels. "Motel" was a contraction of "motor" and "hotel" and has been traced as far back as 1926, when Arthur Heineman opened the Milestone Mo-tel in San

Luis Obispo, California. The generally modest buildings sometimes formed an "L" or a "C" around a central lawn or a swimming pool.

Roadside commercial buildings usually borrowed structural and stylistic ideas from other types of buildings; they were popularizers rather than pioneers. However, they were quick to adopt modern materials. The Wichita, Kansas–based White Castle System of Eating Houses in 1928 commissioned the first use of porcelain-enameled steel panels for the cladding of an entire building. The interchangeable steel panels were secured with a locking device that eliminated the use of rivets or bolts, thus making it easier to take the structure apart and move it. Superb for projecting an image of cleanliness, white porcelain-enameled panels became standard not only for the White Castle hamburger restaurants but for many companies' gas stations in the 1940s and 1950s. The most famous gas station design using white panels on a crisp, boxlike building was Walter Dorwin Teague's prototype for Texaco, introduced in the mid-1930s. The design integrated an office, rest rooms, and service bays into a sleek, flat-roofed structure clad in white panels that could be hosed down to restore their sparkle.

As retailers built new stores along suburban roads, they frequently used a facade with glass from floor to ceiling to put the

interior on display, give a glimpse of their merchandise, and show that they were open. Although many retailers occupied stand-alone buildings, there was demand for collections of stores that could conveniently serve customers arriving by car. From this developed the shopping center, a linked series of storefronts that usually faced a parking area shared by all the center's stores. Shopping centers, bringing architectural unity to a row of stores set back from the street, have been traced by Liebs all the way back to a development in Baltimore in 1907, when the customers came in carriages. Shopping centers proliferated in the 1920s and 1930s, serving people arriving by car. By the 1950s, these small centers were ubiquitous, and the next stage in the evolution of roadside retailing was at hand: the enclosed, inward-focused, climate-controlled shopping mall. The first complete example was the Southdale mall, designed by Victor Gruen and Associates and built in Minneapolis in 1956.

Commercial development of the American roadside periodically resulted in eruptions of hostility from a public fed up with billboards, bright lights, primary colors, and clashing architectural forms. Peter Blake's 1964 jeremiad *God's Own Junkyard*, which declared most highways to be "hideous scars on the face of this nation" (109), voiced repulsion at the crassness and ugliness that afflicted much of the roadside environment. Lady Bird Johnson led a campaign for roadside beautification in the mid-1960s, and municipalities increasingly used design control regulations to tranquilize roadside architecture—discouraging unusual forms, forbidding flashing lights and revolving signs, requiring landscaping, and generally insisting on a softer, more subdued look. Such regulation was rarely welcomed by avant-garde architects such as Robert Venturi, Denise Scott Brown, and Steven Izenour, whose 1972 book *Learning from Las Vegas* valiantly searched for virtue among the dross. The Big Duck, cited in *God's Own Junkyard* as an example of what is bad about roadside architecture, was celebrated by the Venturi group. However, by the 1970s the "vitality" of Las Vegas, where casinos were willing to invest in enormous outdoor displays, had little in common with most stretches of American road, which were dominated by aesthetic dullards such as McDonald's and Wendy's. The golden arches, which burst through the roof of the McDonald's prototype that Stanley C. Meston created for Richard McDonald in 1952, had been reduced to a sign and logo in front of a pseudo-mansard-roofed building that lacked the pleasurable detail and proportions exhibited by the prewar Howard Johnson's and also lacked the exuberance and spontaneity of the "googie" 1950s Big Boy.

In 1977, the Society for Commercial Archeology (SCA) was founded to document and preserve worthy examples of 20th-century commercial design, especially the nation's rapidly disappearing roadside sights. In the years since, pleas from organizations such as the SCA have averted the demolition of a number of buildings, including the oldest surviving McDonald's, which had been serving hamburgers and shakes beneath pulsating neon in Downey, California, since 1953. Roadside architecture in the final three decades of the century became soullessly formulaic. Motorists who hoped for something quirky and full of character looked to "blue highways" (minor roads, often colored blue on road maps) or sought out old thoroughfares, such as the National Road. There, remnants of history remained, testifying to the imagination of the automobile age.

PHILIP LANGDON

See also **Automobile; Gruen, Victor David (United States); Shopping Center; Suburban Planning**

Further Reading

Belasco, Warren James, *Americans on the Road: From Autocamp to Motel, 1910–1945*, Cambridge, Massachusetts: MIT Press, 1979

Blake, Peter, *God's Own Junkyard: The Planned Deterioration of America's Landscape*, New York: Holt Rinehart and Winston, 1964

Hess, Alan, *Googie: Fifties Coffee Shop Architecture*, San Francisco: Chronicle Books, 1986

Jakle, John A. and Keith A. Sculle, *The Gas Station in America*, Baltimore, Maryland: Johns Hopkins University Press, 1994

Jakle, John A. and Keith A. Sculle, *Fast Food: Roadside Restaurants in the Automobile Age*, Baltimore, Maryland: Johns Hopkins University Press, 1999

Jakle, John A., Keith A. Sculle, and Jefferson S. Rogers, *The Motel in America*, Baltimore, Maryland: Johns Hopkins University Press, 1996

Jennings, Jan (editor), *Roadside America: The Automobile in Design and Culture*, Ames: Iowa State University Press, 1990

Langdon, Philip, *Orange Roofs, Golden Arches: The Architecture of American Chain Restaurants*, New York: Knopf, 1986

Liebs, Chester, *Main Street to Miracle Mile: American Roadside Architecture*, Boston: Little Brown, 1985

Venturi, Robert, Denise Scott Brown, and Steven Izenour, *Learning from Las Vegas*, Cambridge, Massachusetts: MIT Press, 1972

Witzel, Michael Karl, *The American Drive-In*, Osceola, Wisconsin: Motorbooks International, 1994

ROADWAY SYSTEMS

Although the road preceded the automobile, it was the invention of the motorcar that transformed meandering muddy paths into functional roadways. The first 20 years of the 20th century marked a transportation revolution that began with the automobile and that brought about a new national system of roadways. In 1905, only one in every 1078 Americans owned an automobile; by 1920, one in every 13 Americans had become proud owners of the century's most remarkable invention.

Although the automobile was a French invention dating to as early as the 1860s (witness such French words as *garage, chassis, chauffeur,* and of course, *automobile*), the North American adaptation of the motorcar in the early 20th century was distinctly non-European. Instead of expensive motorcars designed for the wealthy, American auto designers concentrated on affordable, mass-produced vehicles, such as Ransom E. Olds' 1900 horseless buggy. By 1910, more than two dozen companies were producing unpretentious low-cost vehicles, including Henry Ford's 1908 Model T. Their affordability countered the warning that Woodrow Wilson had made in 1906 when he cautioned that the popularity of the motorcar would lead to socialism by stirring dangerous envy of the rich.

As a practical vehicle for the average American, the automobile needed to be more than a curiosity for display. Its utility depended on reliable roadways. As the proud motorist ventured into the realm of travel, limited by a top speed of four miles per hour and requirements that he be preceded by a man with a red flag so as not to scare the horses, the need for improved roadways became strikingly apparent.

The first public organizations to get involved in road improvements were municipalities, many of which had grown weary of the problems of the automobile's predecessor: the horse. Horses cost cities large amounts of money to remove manure and haul away abandoned carcasses. Many municipalities welcomed the automobile as a cleaner, more trouble free alternative. Thus, the first decades of the 20th century marked a change in many cities from cobblestones to more even road surfaces, built at public expense. The cobblestones had kept horses from slipping since the Middle Ages, but for the automobile, new smooth and quiet road surfaces, such as macadam (a form of crushed stone), were required. As traffic increased, tougher surfaces were applied, such as asphalt and eventually concrete—all initiated before the 1920s.

By the middle of the 1920s, smooth road surfaces had significantly enhanced the utility of the automobile, speeding its way into the future at faster and faster speeds. Road building became a major function of local governments, which were prodded by a collection of pressure groups that included automobile manufacturing, oil companies, and tire manufacturers who lobbied intensely for new roadways. Others were also quick to see the economic dividends attached to highway building, such as real estate speculators who argued in front of city councils for new roads as a basis for increasing property tax revenues in new areas.

At a pace, new thoroughfares were built as an emblem of modernity and forward thinking. Following the lead of William K. Vanderbilt's Long Island Motor Parkway, the first limited-access thoroughfare opened in 1911, and roadways were built for higher speeds and greater efficiency. The Bronx River Parkway, in New York's Westchester County, featured limited access and landscaping when it was completed in 1923. The first thoroughfares accentuated the scenic qualities of the roadside. The use of "parkway" in their names implied their primary use for pleasure driving. The Hutchison River Parkway in 1928, the Saw Mill River Parkway in 1929, the Cross County Parkway in 1931, and the Henry Hudson Parkway along the West Side of Manhattan in 1934 all exemplified the scenic qualities of the new roadways. However, it was not long before this idea of roadways for recreation was replaced by the utility of commuter expressways.

By 1929, New Jersey began construction of a 13-mile expressway between Elizabeth and Jersey. In Boston, two new expressways were completed at opposite sides of the city. Chicago opened Wacker Drive, a new, elevated bilevel motorway that was designed for a daily commute of 60,000 vehicles. In Los Angeles, the Arroyo Silo Parkway was opened in 1940 after nearly 40 years of planning. Backed by downtown department stores, the new freeway became an instant success, but instead

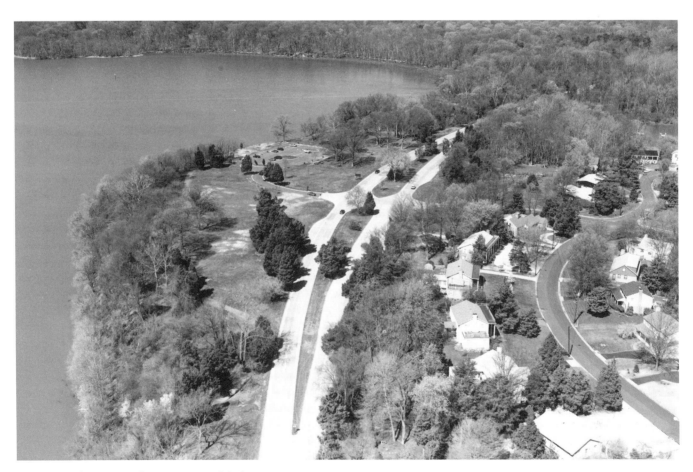

Aerial view of George Washington Memorial Parkway, 1992
© Jack Boucher, Historic American Engineering Record)/Library of Congress

of funneling shoppers into the downtown area, it launched a massive suburban migration that powered the development of the nation's most elaborate freeway system.

From the beginning, public subsides advanced the development of new roadways. The Federal Road Act of 1916 founded new highway departments, and a 1921 reenactment created the Bureau of Public Roads and provided matching funds for more than 200,000 miles of roads. State gasoline taxes, starting in 1919, provided another source of road-building funds, enabling the value of highway construction projects to surpass $1 billion by 1925.

By 1943, the enormous economic potential of road building had become obvious not only to suburban land developers but also to a diverse group of oil and tire manufacturers, construction industrialists, and automobile manufacturers who united as the American Road Builders Association. Spearheaded by General Motors, the group's largest contributor, the association became exceedingly influential, second only to the munitions industry. Their influence, along with a campaign by Cold War scientists to attain "Defense Through Decentralization," led to the Interstate Highway Act of 1956, which called for a 42,000-mile system of federally funded limited-access thoroughfares at a cost of $26 billion.

The influence of the Interstate Highway Act has ranged broadly across American society, transforming it into a suburban nation. With this expansion, architects designed a range of building types suited to automobile commuters and travelers, including hotels, shopping malls, office campuses, and others. With the advent of air travel, architects designed large and distinctive airports, all linked to their nearby cities by expressways. With each completed link of the nationwide system of high-speed, limited-access roadways, the population has spread farther from abandoned urban cores to satellite cities and low-density suburbs. To be sure, other factors abetted this extraordinary migration, such as federal mortgage subsidies and home ownership tax credits, but the Interstate Highway Act paved the way. As the nation has been increasingly consumed by highways, traffic jams, and endless commutes, the conventional wisdom of highway building has been challenged. Led by numerous "freeway revolts" that began in California in the 1960s, opposition to "more and more of worse and worse" has mounted, sometimes halting highway construction projects or seriously modifying their size. Efforts to develop public transportation alternatives have increased, even in Los Angeles, where the freeway was once seen as the spine of life. Still, overall, no unanimously accepted alternative has gained precedence over the drive of highway expansion.

RICK ADAMS

See also **Automobile; Parkways; Suburban Planning; Urban Planning**

Further Reading

Banham, Reyner, *Los Angeles: The Architecture of Four Ecologies*, Harmondsworth, England: Penguin, 1973
Jackson, J.B., *Discovering the Vernacular Landscape*, New Haven: Yale University Press, 1984
Jackson, Kenneth, *Crabgrass Frontier: The Surbanization of the United States*, New York: Oxford University Press, 1985
Mumford, Lewis, *The City in History*, New York: MJF Books, 1997
Venturi, Robert, Denise Scott-Brown, and Steven Izenour, *Learning from Las Vegas: The Forgotten Symbolism of Architectural Form*, Cambridge, Massachusetts: MIT Press, 1974

ROBIE HOUSE

Designed by Frank Lloyd Wright; completed 1910
Chicago, Illinois

When Frederick Robie went to Frank Lloyd Wright in the winter of 1908 for a house on fashionable Woodlawn Avenue at the corner of Fifty-eighth Street in Chicago, Robie worked with his father, who among other things was a supplier of parts to the growing automobile industry. Like Wright, Robie was fascinated with the new machine and even planned to open his own automobile factory. This surely explains the three garages (and no stable) that Wright incorporated into Robie's house. Preliminary plans for Robie House were completed in November 1908, with working (or contract) drawings following in March 1909. Construction began in the spring of 1909 and ended in the early winter of 1910. The house was furnished between September 1909 and May 1910.

Because Wright turned his business over to architect Herman Von Holst in September 1909 and went to Europe for a year, completion of the house was left to Marion Mahony, long an associate of Wright, whom Von Holst had hired to complete Wright's unfinished commissions. It is likely that she designed the art glass of the house and iron gates of the auto court, as these had not been detailed before Wright left for Europe. George Niedecken, an interior architect from Milwaukee, already at work in the house before Wright's departure, continued to have furniture and furnishings made according to Wright's plans until they ran out, then designed additional furniture himself, mostly for the living room.

Wright's brick house for Frederick Robie is the most monumental of his Prairie houses having the main living space on the second floor. Although Wright wrote frequently in a rationalist vein about his distaste for dank basements and cluttered attics, his real reason for wanting to eliminate basements and attics was both visual and psychological. As a place of shelter and refuge, he felt that the home ought to be wedded visually to the earth, which to him meant relatively low structures spreading out horizontally, anchored by massive chimneys at the center and protected by overhanging hip roofs of low pitch. Typical 19th-century houses elevated above partially exposed basements with rooms having high ceilings and crowned by massive hip or gable roofs were anathema to him. Early photographs of Robie House looking north show just such a house behind it.

Although in later years Robie thought that it was he who had inspired Wright to design for him a house with the visual and functional characteristics that mark Robie House, Wright had actually developed the design over a ten-year period for other clients with different tastes and requirements. The first house of this type was erected in Chicago in 1899 for Joseph Husser. Except for having many details of late 19th-century origin, the Husser house was remarkably like Robie House, even to having its entrance halfway down the left side, a common practice in Chicago for siting large houses on the deep but narrow lots of that city. For example, Robie House stands on a

parcel 60 feet wide by 180 feet deep. The result of thus reviving for Robie House the plan of the Husser house, which was not built on a corner and had residential lots on either side of its narrow front, has been to cause both laypersons and academicians to suppose that the right side of Robie House facing on Fifty-eighth Street is actually its front rather than Woodlawn Avenue, which is its address. This confusion has fostered the myth that Wright intended when designing the house to lead the observer slowly and inevitably around the house from its Fifty-eighth Street side to the Woodlawn Avenue front, where at last he would discover the entrance door sequestered in shadow at the end of a long walk.

Another residence, designed in 1905 and built of stucco on frame in Riverside, Illinois, for Frederick Tomek, served as the intermediary for translating the late 19th-century forms of the Husser house into the mature Wrightian style of Robie House. In fact, Wright has stated that the Tomek house served as a model for Robie House. Originally, the entrance to the Tomek house was to have been halfway down its right side, just the reverse of the Husser and Robie houses. However, before construction began, the entrance was moved to its left side, which faced the street. Both the Tomek and the Robie house consist of a lower floor at grade with the main living floor above it. The latter is devoted primarily to a large living and dining room connected through a passageway illuminated by a continuous bank of windows, actually French doors at Robie House. The living room opens onto a porch. A partial third floor, looking something like a low tower or "belvedere," as Wright termed it, contains the bedrooms.

By 1905, when Wright designed the Tomek house, his style had become highly abstract and rectilinear in character. Almost invariably, he built his residences after 1902 of rectangular masses, piers, and panels. These were sometimes solid, as for walls and piers, and sometimes transparent, as for doors and windows, the latter always casements grouped in horizontal banks. When possible, Wright carried the geometry of the exterior into the interior, where he applied it with equal vigor to walls, piers, screens, furniture, and furnishings.

In fact, it is the slope of the hip roofs of Robie House that deny for it the logical and final next step in Wright's aesthetic development, complete rectilinearity, a goal already achieved by him through his use of the overhanging flat roof for Unity Temple and the Yahara Boat Club, both designed in 1905, and for the proposed Fireproof House of 1907. It was not until 1909, however, that Wright first built a residence in which he abandoned the hip in favor of the flat roof. This was the thoroughly rectilinear house that he erected for Laura Gale in Oak Park, Illinois. As a result, Robie House, despite its unrelenting rectilinear geometry and horizontal massing, remains a transitional work

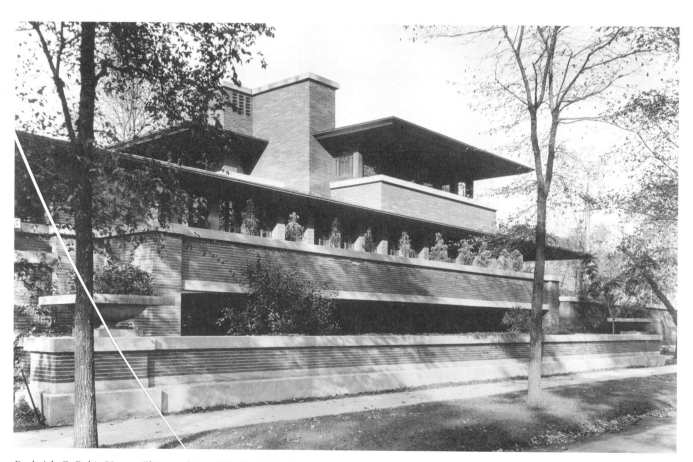

Frederick C. Robie House, Chicago, designed by Frank Lloyd Wright (1910)
© James Reber. Photo courtesy The Frank Lloyd Wright Archives

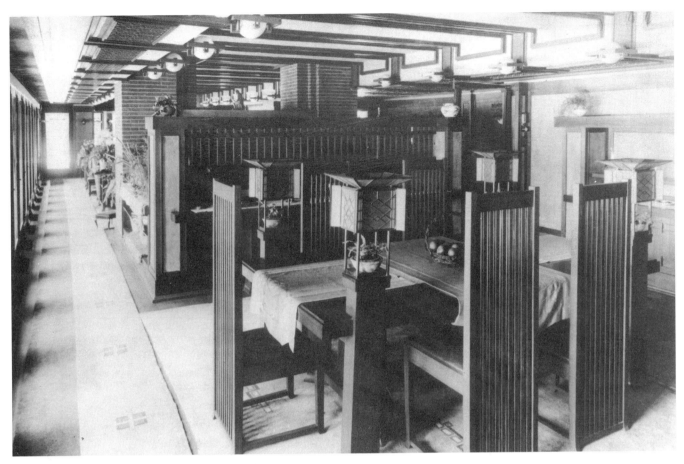

Interior dining room, designed by Frank Lloyd Wright (1910)
© James Reber. Photo courtesy The Frank Lloyd Wright Archives

along with Wright's great Coonley House of 1907 because of the dissonant angularity of its overspreading hip roofs.

Given the abstract geometry here and there in Wright's work from the Winslow house of 1894 onward, one might suppose that the European avant-garde was somehow affected by this aspect of his work. Certainly, Wright was aware of developments in Europe through European publications and from his visits to the St. Louis Exposition in 1904. Yet, except for a few European architects who passed through Chicago before 1910 and who might have returned with illustrations of Wright's work, the only important presentation of Wright's architecture did not appear until March 1908, when the *Architectural Record* featured his work. In it, Europeans would have seen the massive abstract geometries of the Larkin Building and Unity Temple along with those of the Fireproof House. However, as Robie House was not completed until early 1910, its potential for effecting the evolution of European architecture had to wait until 1911, when it appeared in the German publications of Wright's work by Wasmuth. As a result, if Wright's abstract style did inspire European architects to move in that same direction, Robie House could not have played a part until after 1911.

Robie House does relate, however, to developments in European modernism going back to the 1890s and earlier. Certain aspects of Wright's style, especially his extensive use of casement

windows, presumably derive from the English Victorian Gothic and probably more directly from the use of such windows by Voysey, Baillie Scott, and other English architects in the 1890s. Wright's continuing interest in creating artistic interiors for his houses whenever he found a pliable client with sufficient resources and in the art furniture with which he furnished those houses also surely goes back to the English Arts and Crafts movement of the 1860s to 1890s. That Wright also sought to devise a style of his own, one no longer derived from the historic styles, also served to align him with Europe's avant-garde architects.

Unfortunately, Robie got to live in his house for little more than a year. His wife left him in April 1911, and he sold the house to another family in December of that year. After the new owner died suddenly in 1912, the house passed to a third family, who occupied it until 1926, when they sold it to the Chicago Theological Seminary for use as a dormitory. In 1957, a preservation battle erupted when the seminary proposed demolishing the house. Fortunately, Robie House was saved by developer William Zeckendorf and eventually became the property of the University of Chicago. It is now being restored and maintained by the Frank Lloyd Wright Home and Studio Foundation and is a historic site of the National Trust for Historic Preservation.
PAUL SPRAGUE

Further Reading

Nearly everything the reader will want to know about the Robie house is contained in two copiously illustrated books published in 1984, Connors and Hoffmann.

Bolon, Carol, Robert Nelson, and Linda Seidel (editors), *The Nature of Frank Lloyd Wright*, Chicago: University of Chicago Press, 1988

Connors, Joseph, *The Robie House of Frank Lloyd Wright*, Chicago: University of Chicago Press, 1984

Hoffmann, Donald, *Frank Lloyd Wright's Robie House: The Illustrated Story of an Architectural Masterpiece*, New York: Dover, 1984

ROCHE AND DINKELOO

Architecture firm, United States

Kevin Roche (1922–) and John Dinkeloo (1918–81) met in 1950 when they joined the office of Eero Saarinen and Associates at Bloomfield Hills, Michigan, where they worked for 11 years along with Robert Venturi, Chuck Bassett, Tony Lumsden, Gunnar Birketts, and Cesar Pelli. After Saarinen's sudden death in 1961, Roche and Dinkeloo formed a partnership in Hamden, Connecticut, to complete the projects that were under way at that time. The nascent partnership saw not only the successful completion of ten international projects but also went on to receive many other important commissions. Roche and Dinkeloo practiced together until 1981, and during that 20-year period they designed a number of outstanding buildings for a diverse group of corporate and institutional clients.

The ten buildings that Roche and Dinkeloo inherited from Saarinen were projects that they had been centrally involved in designing and included some of the most significant American buildings of the period, sharing innovative approaches to technology and new materials: the Gateway Arch, St. Louis, Missouri; the TWA Terminal, New York City; Dulles International Airport, Washington, D.C.; the Headquarters for John Deere and Company in Moline, Illinois; and the CBS Headquarters in New York.

The first project awarded to the new practice was the Oakland Museum (1961–68) in California. Eero Saarinen had been on the original list of architects being considered for the project, and Roche Dinkeloo, who asked to be considered after his death, was selected from a group of 35 architects. Their award-winning museum design included landscaped roofs that created a new park at the heart of the city. Over the next 20 years, the practice grew to become one of the most vital American offices of that era, designing a wide range of different building types for both civic and corporate clients.

The most significant buildings designed by Roche Dinkeloo include a series of university facilities, the office tower (1965–69) for the Knights of Columbus together with the neighboring Coliseum (1965–72) in New Haven, and arguably the most important, the Headquarters for the Ford Foundation (1963–68) in New York. These monumental buildings made innovative use of novel materials such as glass, advanced glazing systems, and self-rusting steel while at the same time exploiting the potential of structural forms as large-scale ordering systems. Projects such as the factories and offices for Cummins Engine in Darling-

ton, England (1963–65), and later at Columbus, Indiana (1970–73), developed these ideas in ways that improved the industrial working environment, whereas a series of designs for corporate headquarters for Richardson-Merrell Inc. (1970–74), Union Carbide (1976–82), and General Foods (1977–82) explored the needs of large new office buildings sited in green-field sites by integrating offices and parking within the landscape.

In 1967, Roche Dinkeloo began work on the renovation and extension of the Metropolitan Museum of Art in New York, a project that would extend over more than 30 years. In addition to a new gallery wing and a bookshop, a series of glassy pavilions were designed for the Robert Lehman Collection in 1974 and subsequently for the Temple of Dendur.

Since Dinkeloo's death, Roche has directed the practice with a group of associates and continued the design for the Metropolitan Museum of Art, creating new galleries and restoring the existing building. The work of Roche's office has become increasingly preoccupied with formal issues and the development of a historicist eclecticism.

Roche and Dinkeloo were the recipients of numerous honors and awards. In 1974, they received the Architectural Firm Award from the American Institute of Architects (AIA), and eight years later Roche was awarded the Pritzker Architecture Prize. In

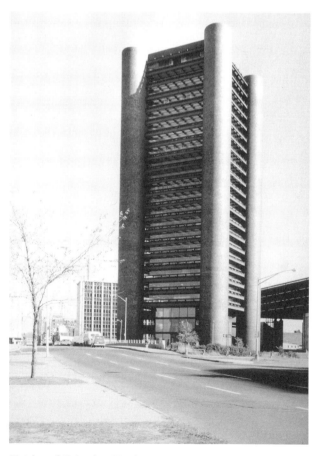

Knights of Columbus Headquarters, New Haven, Connecticut (1969)
© G.E. Kidder-Smith, courtesy of Kidder Smith Collection, Rotch Visual Collections, M.I.T.

1995, the Ford Foundation Headquarters received the AIA's Twenty-Five-Year Award for an outstanding building of distinction.

BRIAN CARTER

See also **Brutalism; Dulles International Airport, Chantilly, Virginia; Gateway Arch, St. Louis, Missouri; Saarinen, Eero (Finland); TWA Airport Terminal, New York**

Biographies

Kevin Roche

Born in Dublin, 14 June 1922; emigrated to the United States 1948; naturalized 1964. Attended the National University of Ireland, Dublin 1940–45; bachelor's degree in architecture 1945; pursued postgraduate studies at the Illinois Institute of Technology, Chicago 1948–49. Designer with Michael Scott and Partners, Dublin 1945–46 and 1947–48; architect, the firm of Maxwell Fry and Jane Drew, London 1946; architect in the United Nations Planning Office, New York 1949; associate, Eero Saarinen and Associates, Bloomfield Hills and Birmingham, Michigan and Hamden, Connecticut 1950–66; principal associate in design 1954–61. Member, Board of Trustees, American Academy in Rome 1968–71; member, Woodrow Wilson International Center for Scholars, Smithsonian Institution, Washington, DC 1969–71; member, Commission of Fine Arts, Washington, DC from 1969; academician, National Academy of Design; member, Royal Institute of British Architects; member, Académie d'Architecture, France; member, Accademia Nazionale di San Luca, Italy; honorary fellow, Institute of Architects of Ireland. Kevin Roche, John Dinkeloo and Associates has continued under the direction of Roche.

John Gerard Dinkeloo

Born in Holland, Michigan, 28 February 1918. Attended Hope College, Holland 1936–39; studied at the University of Michigan School of Architecture, Ann Arbor 1939–42; bachelor's degree in architectural engineering 1942. Designer, 1942–43, chief of production 1946–50, the firm of Skidmore, Owings and Merrill, Chicago; head of production, Eero Saarinen and Associates, Bloomfield Hills, Michigan 1950–56; partner, Eero Saarinen and Associates, Bloomfield Hills and Birmingham, Michigan 1956–61 and Hamden, Connecticut 1961–66. Trustee, Hope College. Died in Fredericksburg, Virginia, 15 June 1981.

Roche and Dinkeloo

Partnership established in Hamden, Connecticut 1966 as Kevin Roche, John Dinkeloo and Associates; received the Grand Gold medal, French Academy of Architects 1977 and the Pritzker Prize 1982.

Selected Works

Cummins Engine Company Components Plant, Darlington, Durham, England, 1965
Oakland Museum, California, 1968
Ford Foundation Headquarters, New York City, 1968
Knights of Columbus Headquarters, New Haven, Connecticut, 1969
Veterans Memorial Coliseum, New Haven, Connecticut, 1972
Cummins Engine Company Sub-Assembly Plant, Columbus, Indiana, 1973
Richardson-Merrell Corporation Headquarters, Wilton, Connecticut, 1974
Union Carbide Corporation World Headquarters, Danbury, Connecticut, 1982
General Foods Corporation Headquarters, Rye, New York, 1982
Metropolitan Museum of Art (master plan and additions), New York City, 1985

Further Reading

Cook, John W. and Heinrich Klotz, *Conversations with Architects*, New York: Praeger, and London: Lund Humphries, 1973 (includes an interview with Kevin Roche)
Futagawa, Yukio, *Kevin Roche, John Dinkeloo, and Associates, 1962–1975*, Tokyo: A.D.A. Edita, and Fribourg: Office du Livre, 1975; New York: Architectural Press, 1977
Heyer, Paul, *Architects on Architecture: New Directions in America*, New York: Walker, 1966; London: Allen Lane, 1967; new enlarged edition, New York: Walker, 1978
Scully, Vincent, *Modern Architecture*, New York: Braziller, 1956; London: Prentice Hall, 1961; revised edition, New York: Braziller, 1974
Scully, Vincent, *American Architecture and Urbanism*, New York: Praeger, and London: Thames and Hudson, 1969; revised edition, New York: Holt, 1988
Tafuri, Manfredo and Francesco Dal Co, *Architettura contemporanea*, Milan: Electa, 1976; as *Modern Architecture*, translated by Robert Erich Wolf, New York: Abrams, 1979

ROCKEFELLER CENTER, NEW YORK

Designed by Raymond Hood, completed 1940
New York City

Rockefeller Center is widely considered to be a handsome commercial building complex, and it has been the model for other groups of structures dedicated to a mix of business and entertainment. The Center comprises 30 buildings (although some are connected), with another being planned as of 1999. They extend from Fifth Avenue toward Seventh Avenue, between 48th and 52nd Streets, although the original and most famous structures were limited to most of the three blocks between 48th and 51st Streets, Fifth to Sixth Avenues.

The original group, planned and built from 1929 to 1940, was erected on land that belonged primarily to Columbia University. John D. Rockefeller, Jr., who leased the Columbia properties, bought several additional lots on Sixth Avenue as plans progressed. At first, the blocks were intended for bulky office towers on three sides of a large open square. A new Metropolitan Opera House was to occupy the fourth side, at the west, extending toward Sixth Avenue. When the stock market crash of 1929 made this plan unworkable, Rockefeller requested new plans for high and low commercial buildings around a smaller plaza. Most were to be office buildings with shops at ground level and along a subterranean concourse connected to a subway line that replaced a noisy elevated railway on Sixth Avenue. Other buildings, at the west end near the noise, were windowless, soundproof theaters; of the two originally there, only Radio City Music Hall has survived. A cinema was introduced later in the middle of the north block. The leasing program was focused on broadcasting (later television) and film industry tenants, and on individually owned international shops. Travel and airline offices,

foreign consulates, the U.S. passport agency, and auxiliary services such as passport photographers, restaurants, pharmacies, and a post office completed the primary rental program. The adaptability of the owner and his professional colleagues, the targeting of tenant groups, and the refined, varied design in handsome materials helped to ensure the project's eventual profitability and public esteem, although, in its early years, the project suffered financially as a result of the Depression.

Only the central one of the three original blocks was designed and executed according to a fixed plan. Here, twin low buildings flank a path adorned with plants, fountains, and small statues. The path leads to the central plaza, depressed so as to allow commercial premises around the perimeter. Zoning regulations made it impossible to build ground-level shops and restaurants, because just west of the plaza, a 66-story tower rises, taking up most of the bulk and height allowed under the zoning rules then in force. On the north block, Radio City Music Hall and an office building above it were determined at the start, whereas the high International Building along Fifth Avenue, with additional low wings for shops and offices, was added in the mid-1930s. The south block contained the Center Theater along Sixth Avenue, now replaced by an office tower. Buildings for the Associated Press and Eastern Air Lines, among others, were added as tenants appeared and as they could be fitted into the space permitted by zoning rules.

The appealing aspects of the Center include the plaza, which accommodates a restaurant in summer; an ice rink in winter; flying flags of the United Nations; statues, including Paul Manship's *Prometheus* overlooking the plaza and Lee Lawrie's *Atlas* on Fifth Avenue; relief sculptures by Lawrie, Isamu Noguchi, and Carl Milles; landscaping; and public seating. Connoisseurs of architectural detailing admire the metalwork in the focal tower and the frames of the original shop windows. Urbanists praise the extra street added west of the plaza, the underground concourse with its subway access and connections among the Center's buildings, and the provision of public space in a private enclave. The combination of low and high structures shows that aesthetic considerations, and not exclusively financial ones, were present in the minds of the owner, John D. Rockefeller, Jr., the property developers he employed (Todd, Robertson and Todd), and the architects (Reinhard and Hofmeister; Corbett, Harrison and MacMurray; Hood, Godley, and Fouilhoux; of these, L. Andrew Reinhard, Harvey Wiley Corbett, Wallace K. Harrison, and Raymond Hood were the principal designers).

In the years between 1947 and 1973, several new buildings were added, primarily by Harrison and his later partner, Max Abramovitz. Most interesting are their buildings across Sixth Avenue, starting with the Time-Life Building (1957–60), an example of technological expression of supports and ducts. The three blocks south of this contain visually coordinated single towers, completed by 1973. The two central ones have large plazas, mandated by revised zoning rules but realized with more plants, seats, and other public amenities than were customary at the time. West of these buildings are additional small public parks. In these years and later as well, various architects remodeled some of the lobbies and other spaces that were not protected from change by the Center's designation as a city landmark in 1985.

In 1999, the Landmarks Preservation Commission permitted the new owners to enlarge windows on the facades of the four low buildings on Fifth Avenue and to make alterations in the central plaza. Less-controversial changes include the introduction of a facade for the Christie's auction house in the center of the original south block, and repaving of the original private street introduced into the project to increase the number of offices with street frontage.

Through assiduous maintenance, upgrading of technical features, and expert public relations, the Center has managed to retain its position as a premier location for business and as a popular tourist attraction in midtown, an area that the Center itself helped to establish as the heart of the city.

CAROL HERSELLE KRINSKY

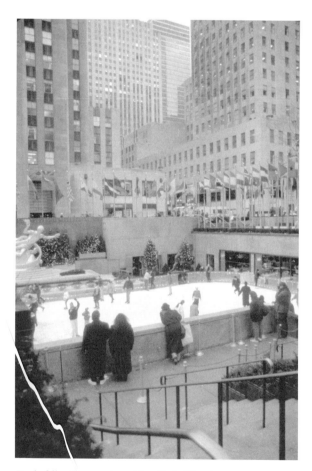

Rockefeller Center plaza, New York City
© GreatBuildings.com

See also **Harrison, Wallace K., and Max Abramovitz (United States); Hood, Raymond (United States); New York (NY), United States; Office Building; Plaza; Skyscraper**

Further Reading

Balfour, Alan, *Rockefeller Center: Architecture as Theater*, New York: McGraw-Hill, 1978

Jordy, William, "Rockefeller Center and Corporate Urbanism" in *The Impact of European Modernism in the Mid-Twentieth Century*, by Jordy, Garden City, New York: Doubleday, 1972

Krinsky, Carol Herselle, *Rockefeller Center*, New York: Oxford University Press, 1978

New York (N.Y.) Landmarks Preservation Commission, *Rockefeller Center Designation Report*, New York: Landmark Preservation Commission, 1985

"Rockefeller Center: The Decision," *Village Views* 8, no. 2 (1999)

"Rockefeller Center: The Proposed Alterations," *Village Views* 8, no. 1 (1998)

Stern, Robert A.M., Gregory Gilmartin, and Thomas Mellins, *New York, 1930: Architecture and Urbanism between the Two World Wars*, New York: Rizzoli, 1987

Tafuri, Manfredo, in *La città americana dalla guerra civile al New Deal*, by Giorgio Ciucci et al., Rome: Laterza, 1973; as "The Creation of Rockefeller Center," in *The American City: From the Civil War to the New Deal*, translated by Barbara Luigia La Penta, Cambridge, Massachusetts: MIT Press, 1979; London: Granada, 1980

ROGERS, RICHARD 1933–

Architect, England

Richard Rogers was born in Florence in 1933 of British parents. He received his architectural education at the Architectural Association School in London and at Yale University, where he held a Fulbright Scholarship. At Yale, he heard lectures by Paul Rudolf and Louis Kahn and also met his British contemporaries, Norman Foster and James Stirling.

He began work by designing a family house at Creek Vean in Cornwall, with white walls and large windows, a house of impeccable modernity that still appears fresh after nearly half a century. His career took off when he designed a factory, in partnership with Sue Rogers and Norman and Wendy Foster, a double husband-and-wife group that set up under the name of "Team 4." The Reliance Controls Ltd. Factory at Swindon (1967) became well known as an example of industrial architecture that makes its impact from the visual quality of its structural system, in this case a clear succession of rectangular bays stiffened by tensioned diagonal braces.

Rogers has become increasingly devoted to the architecture produced by structural tours-de-force. Of these, the Pompidou Center in Paris (1971–77, with Renzo Piano) is the most famous. As with Reliance, the building is essentially a shed, and the main elevation is similarly marked by a clear succession of rectangular bays overlaid by diagonal tension cables. The designs for Lloyds in the City of London and for Inmos at Newport South Wales both continue to gain their principal effect from the display of structure and service elements on the exterior. Rogers (like Foster) has therefore become a principal proponent of a "true" functionalist architecture, going beyond Louis Kahn in the analysis of form and mechanism, in an attempt to eliminate the arbitrary and willful character of facade making.

Through this development, modernism was pushed closer to the machine, but also closer to sculpture: Rogers's work emerges from this conjunction. He was also influenced by Archigram, for whom expression was as important as technology. Disciples of the Archigram group, in fact, as employees of Piano and Rogers, realized the design development and working drawings for the Pompidou Center, so that it became the nearest thing we have to a completed Archigram building. But it is also the building that most completely expresses Rogers's attitude to architecture: for it has no hint in it, as has the Lloyds Building, of a conventional interior dominated by ancient tribal rituals, but is entirely the product of an intellectual movement toward the "real" sources of functional truth: the exposure of the bones and guts along with devotion to the principles of change and indeterminacy in use, of which the prophet was the Archigram guru, Reyner Banham.

From 1977 Rogers's work has had the benefit of a multidisciplined approach, with the formation of the Richard Rogers Partnership, bringing in the collaboration of John Young, Marco Goldschmied, and Mike Davies, and improved access to in-house engineering services. With this improved organization, the firm has become something of an icon of the High-Tech aspect of modern architecture.

It is not that the High-Tech architect eschews beauty. But the beauty to be uncovered has to be identified with necessity, the result of applying reason along with engineering principles. The method of construction becomes an artistic strategy and hence an end in itself. In the Tokyo Forum Project of 1991, for example, the spaces of use are first enclosed in a gleaming semitransparent shell, then suspended from a metal armature, then approached by a complex of escalators. The object becomes a symbol of its own otherworldliness, a chapel to progress.

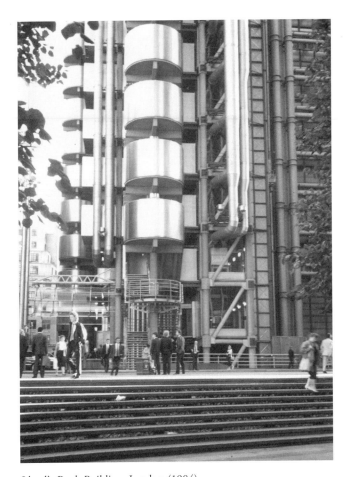

Lloyd's Bank Building, London (1984)
© GreatBuildings.com

A more balanced approach is envisaged in the design for the European Court of Human Rights (1989–94) at Strasbourg. Here the elements into which the complex is broken down are not the service elements as such, but spaces of use; they stand on the ground, forming a composition that is less obsessively analytical and more expressive of human habitation and intercourse, whereas the building takes its scale and shape from its context on the curve of a river and from its situation within the city. This increased sensitivity toward the city is also evident in the very elegant project for the Alcazar, in Marseilles (1988). Within a seven-story height limit (surely a donné for the French city) he inserted a wedge-shaped volume closely into the texture of the adjoining blocks. Service elements are still lined up on one side, office space on the other, with between them, a "spine," which at ground level becomes a pedestrian route linking the frontage on the Cours Belsunce to the quiet contained space of the Place de la Providence. The way the building draws back to allow the space of this quiet square to be drawn into the scheme, the way it curves gently to make an entrance from the Cours Belsunce, show a distinct sensitivity not only to an analytical idea of urban form but also to the sense of civic propriety. In France, where Rogers has many projects under consideration, there are several that seem to open up a less machine-oriented perspective, such as the master plans for Dunkirk Neptune (1990) and Port Aupec (1990) and schemes for Bussy St. Georges (1989–) and Sextius Mirbeau (1990). In all of these there is a distinct element of contextual relevance.

Rogers has been accepted as a master of modern design, to judge by his creation as a Chevalier de l'Ordre National de la Légion d'Honneur in 1985 and in his own country, too, as is evident from his election to the Royal Academy in 1978, the award of the Royal Gold Medal of the RIBA in 1985, his knighthood of 1991 for services to architecture, and his peerage of 1996, the latter giving him a role that could strongly influence in political and therefore in practical terms the future of architecture within Britain. He will, of course, go down to posterity as the principle author of the Millennial Dome at Greenwich, a tour de force in which a tent suspended from steel gantries is given the spread and authority of an immense domed space. His designs continue to exploit the cutting edge of architectural technology, as with the Headquarters for the Lloyd's Register of Shipping and the new Terminal 5 at Heathrow Airport.

In 1995 Rogers was invited by the BBC to give the Reith Lectures, and he chose to build his lectures around the theme of the dense modern city. In his argument, although the city has in the past been a major pollutant, this is not necessarily so: It can be rethought scientifically so that it contributes to a sustainable environment while preserving the social vivacity that makes a society vital.

ROBERT MAXWELL

See also **Archigram; Foster, Norman (England); Kahn, Louis (United States); Piano, Renzo (Italy); Pompidou Center, Paris**

Selected Publications

Architecture—a Modern View, New York: Thames and Hudson, 1990
Richard Rogers and Partners, Architectural Monographs. London: Academy Editions, 1983

Further Reading

Richard Rogers: Interview with Dennis Sharp, *Building* (London) (April 1979)
Powell, Kenneth (editor), *Richard Rogers*. Zurich, London, Munchen: Artemis, 1994

ROMAÑACH, MARIO 1917–1984

Architect, Cuba

Mario Romañach excelled among the vanguard professionals of 1950s modern Cuban architecture, including Frank Martínez, Nicolás Quintana, Manuel Gutiérrez, Emilio del Junco, Joaquín Cristófol, Humberto Alonso, Nicolás Arroyo, Eduardo Montelieu, Alberto Beale, and Antonio Quintana. Although Romañach's work is still under studied, his oeuvre constituted a model of contemporary design adapted to the material and environmental conditions of the tropic, an example soon to be followed by the new generations of Caribbean architects. On graduation from the University of Havana in 1945, Romañach designed collaboratively with Silverio Bosch until 1955, when he began to work independently.

He collaborated with Antonio Quintana in the competition for the main building of the College of Architects (1943) and the Havana Regulatory Plan (1944). Afterward, Romañach, Quintana, and Pedro Martínez Inclán received the commission to design the Workers' Neighborhood of Luyanó (*Barrio Obrero de Luyanó*, 1944–48), the first Cuban structure to use modern blocks for residential housing. Concurrently, he developed friendships with Walter Gropius, Richard Neutra, and José Luis Sert, who visited the School of Architecture in Havana, where Romañach was a professor from 1951 to 1952. His introverted character kept him at the margins of the student political struggles that grew in reaction to Fulgencio Batista's dictatorship (1952–58). Nonetheless, Romañach defended the progress of the Modern movement; he participated in ATEC (Tectonic Group for Contemporary Expression) and ARCA (Renovating Association of the College of Architects). Between 1945 and 1955, he designed and built 58 works including private homes, apartments, and various public buildings. Early in his career, Romañach's houses possessed a commercial and functionalist character, fulfilling the aesthetic requirements of the traditionalist Cuban middle class. Despite its relative conservatism, the Julia Cueto de Noval House (1948) in Havana achieved a clear and volumetric organization. However, the innovative residence built for the son, José Noval Cueto (1949), was less well received. This house marked the apex of Cuban and perhaps Antillean rationalism, integrating precise compositional structure, smooth white façades, the articulation of functional spaces, and structural regularity. Organized within a rectangular box supported by beams and divided into two blocks joined by open circulation galleries (after the model of Marcel Breuer's bipolar house) the house's interior included a pool and a tropical garden. Thus, through a system of transparencies, double façades (real and virtual), and shaded spaces, Romañach adapted the formal models of Mies van der Rohe, Walter Gropius, and Le Corbusier, issuing from Europe and the United States to the tropical environment.

Works built in the 1950s express Romañach's experimentation with the individual and collective dwelling and arrive at a

particular type that is defined as Cuban "modern regionalism," an elaboration of the influences of Richard Neutra and traditional Japanese architecture. The Havana house of Luis H. Vidaña (1953), the residence of Ana Carolina Font (1956), and the mansion of Rufino Álvarez (1957) mark Romañach's maturation. In these innovative works, he designed walls of refracting colored bricks cement blocks, created a system of canopy ceilings that appear almost suspended in air, explored the use of natural wood, and achieved sophisticated spatial articulations with the organization of transparent and shaded environments.

The buildings for the Territorial Company of La Sierra in Miramar (1956) and the Company for the Investment of Private Goods and Bonds (1958) display the innovative and illuminating spatial treatments found in Romañach's apartment buildings and private homes. These effects achieve a monumental dimension in the "Las Palmas" Presidential Palace (1956) that he designed with José Luis Sert and Gabriela Menéndez for the dictator Fulgencio Batista as part of a governmental commission that also hired Wiener, Sert, and Schulz, Town Planning Associates.

As Chief of the Havana Plan of the National Planning Group (1955), Romañach developed several urban projects that were never executed in La Coronela, La Habana del Este, and the proposed Satellite City of Columbia, intended to house 10,000 inhabitants. With the arrival of Fidel Castro's government (1959), Romañach immigrated to the United States to teach at Harvard University at the invitation of Sert. He developed innumerable public and private projects in his Philadelphia office. Even though some of his works received significant prizes (such as Chatam Towers in New York City, 1967) they were lacking, along with the work of other architects who had emigrated from Cuba, the poetic depth and creativity that characterized his works in Havana.

ROBERTO SEGRE

See also **Breuer, Marcel (United States); Corbusier, Le (Jeanneret, Charles-Édouard) (France); Mies van der Rohe, Ludwig (Germany); Sert, Josep Lluís (United States); Regionalism; Urban Planning**

Biography

Born in Havana, in 1917 (date unknown); son of a local architect; graduated from the School of Architecture, University of Havana (1945). Collaborated with Antonio Quintana for the competition for Cuban Society of Architects building (1943); employed by the Ministry of Public Works, Havana (1944). Received the Gold Medal from the Cuban National Society of Architects (1949); taught at the Havana School of Architecture (1951–52); joined ATEC (Tectonic Group for Contemporary Expression), ARCA (Renovating Association of the College of Architects); became chief of the Havana Master Plan (JNP, National Planning Group) working with Eduardo Montelieu, Nicolás Quintana, Jorge Mantilla, and José Luis Sert (1955). Immigrated to the United States in 1960 with his family; established architecture practice (Perkins and Romanach) in Philadelphia (1960); collaborated with his daughter, architect María Cristina Romañach. Visiting professor, School of Architecture at Harvard University (1959), Yale and Columbia Universities (1961–73); associate professor, Cornell University (1960–67), and chairman

(1971–74) and full professor (1963–84), University of Pennsylvania, Philadelphia. Honorary degree (University of Pennsylvania, 1971); Fellow, American Institute of Architects, 1978; member, National Academy of Design, 1980. Died in Philadelphia on 3 March 1984.

Selected Works

Havana Regulatory Plan (with Antonio Quintana), 1944
Miramar Houses, Havana, 1946
Workers' Neighborhood of Luyanó (with Quintana and Pedro Martínez Inclán), Havana, 1948
Julia Cueto de Noval House, Havana, 1948
José Noval Cueto House, Havana, 1949
Luis H. Vidaña House, Havana, 1953
Evangelina Aristigueta de Vidaña House, Havana, 1955
Ana Carolina Font House, Havana, 1956
"Las Palmas" Presidential Palace (with José Luis Sert and Gabriela Menéndez), Havana, 1956
Rufino Álvarez Residence, Havana, 1957
Chatam Towers in New York City, 1967

Further Reading

Carley, Rachel, *Cuba. 400 Years of Architectural Heritage*, New York: Whitney Library of Design, 1997
De Soto, Emilio, *Álbum de Cuba*, Volumes I–VI, Havana: Colegio de Arquitectos de Cuba, 1950–1956
Quintana, Nicolás, "Evolución histórica de la arquitectura en Cuba," in *La Enciclopedia de Cuba*, edited by Vicente Báez, Volume 5, Madrid: 1/112, Playor, 1975
Rodríguez, Eduardo Luis, *La Habana. Arquitectura del siglo XX*, pictures by Pepe Navarro, Barcelona: Blume, 1998
Rodríguez, Eduardo Luis, "La década incógnita. Los cincuenta: modernidad, identidad y algo más," *Arquitectura Cuba* (1997)
Segre, Roberto, *América Latina Fim de Milênio. Raízes e Perspectivas da Sua Arquitetura*, São Paulo: Studio Nobel, 1991
Segre, Roberto, *Arquitectura y Urbanismo de la Revolución Cubana*, Havana: Editorial Pueblo y Educación, 1995
Zequeira, Martín, María Elena, and Eduardo Luis Rodríguez, *La Habana. Guía de Arquitectura*, Sevilla: Junta de Andalucía, and Havana: Ciudad de La Habana, 1998

ROMANIA

At the beginning of 20th century, Romania was much indebted to Western European architectural currents. The recently created national style had only a feeble impact on the public.

Foreign architecture, mainly Neoclassicism and Romanticism, was progressively introduced in the principalities of Wallachia and Moldavia during the 19th century as a consequence of the process of opening up to Western European civilization. The two principalities, vassals of the Ottoman Empire, sought a model for emancipation and also political assistance, aspiring to create an independent unified state. After this state was founded in 1859, and particularly after it obtained its independence in 1878, its first institutions embraced foreign architectural currents as a sign of modernization. At this time, the most widespread was the ecclecticism of the École des Beaux-Arts in Paris, which eventually became the official style of the Romanian kingdom. French architecture was practiced not only by French nationals but also by the first Romanian architects, who were themselves trained at the École.

Some of these young architects trained in France, where they came in contact with the theories of E.E. Viollet-le-Duc, the French archaeological school, and the innovative concepts of Guadet. Once home, they relentlessly worked to create a new Romanian architecture based on the local tradition. Among them, the most fervent was Ion Mincu, the father of this new style called either "national" or "Romanian," which mirrored the national ideology that animated the Romanian intelligentsia of the time.

Yet the first decade of 20th century was still strongly dominated by French ecclecticism, which maintained its status of official architecture and was also very in vogue for the rich residencies. The Beaux-Arts style was displayed in a variety of forms, going from classic solemnity (the Palace of the Chamber of Deputies, 1907, by Dimitrie Maimarolu in Bucharest) to a light elegance (the Casino, 1913, by Petre Antonescu in Sinaia) or to flamboyant fantasies (the town hall of Iasi, 1907–26, by Ioan D. Berindey). If the Beaux-Arts style was perfectly assimilated, Romanian architects were less familiar with other currents, such as Art Nouveau, one of the rare examples of which is the Casino in Constanta (1910) by Daniel Renard. In contrast, Art Nouveau was very popular in Transylvania, where it radiated from Central Europe. A province of the Austro-Hungarian Empire until 1918, Transylvania adopted the multiple facets that the inventive vocabulary of Art Nouveau developed on the vast territory of the empire: the aesthetic of Lechner's Art Nouveau, as in several works of Jakab Deszö and Marcel Komor, including the "Black Eagle building," 1907–09, in Oradea and the Palace of Culture, 1913, in Tîrgu-Mures; the researches of a new Hungarian national image of the "Young Architects," including the Museum, 1911, by Karoly Kos, in Sfîntul Gheorghe; and compositions inspired by Sezession and Jugendstil, including the work of E. Thoroczkai-Wigand in Tîrgu-Mures.

Starting in 1906, the date of the General National Exposition in Bucharest (Stefan Burcus and Victor Stefanescu), which celebrated 40 years of reign of King Carol I, the national style gained an important place on the architectural scene of Romanian kingdom. The exposition, with its multitude of pavilions, brought recognition for this style. In their quest for an expression of the Romanian specificity, the exponents of the national style sought relevant examples in local tradition that they referred to as both major art history monuments and folk art. Among the chief promoters of the national style were Petre Antonescu, Paul Smarandescu, Statie Ciortan, Toma T. Socolescu, and Nicolae Ghika-Budesti.

As its doctrine responded perfectly to the aspirations of national unity and as its aesthetic satisfied the taste for picturesque dispositions, the new style was progressively embraced in several architectural programs. First adopted in residential architecture, it spread progressively to administrative buildings, schools, and post offices, some of the most significant examples of this period being the Prefecture of Galati (1906) by Ion Mincu, the Prefecture of Craiova (1912–13) by Petre Antonescu, and the town hall of Constanta (1913) by Victor Stefanescu. At the creation of greater Romania, by the unification of the ancient kingdom with Transylvania, Bessarabia, and Bukovina at the end of World War I, the national style was unsurprisingly appropriated as an official architecture. The establishment of the new state generated a period of prosperity and of economic as well as cultural effervescence, which explains the unprecedented growth of architecture. The sustained building campaign obviously benefited the national style, which now covered all the architectural programs and all the territory of Romania. To mention the huge operation of rising orthodox churches in Transylvania, the construction of oversize churches, called "cathedrals," was a symbolic act of recuperating a territory released from Catholicism.

Whereas the national style responded to the new context of the acknowledged national spirituality, modernism expressed the opening toward European culture and the efforts of synchronizing Romanian culture with European tendencies. The architect and artist Marcel Iancu played an important role in the introduction and assimilation of the principles of Modern architecture. He contributed to the initiation to modernism through a sustained publishing campaign, writing numerous articles in the style of the avant-garde manifestos in the magazine *Contimporanul* from 1924 to 1930. The diffusion of modernism was encouraged by the commands of the intellectual milieu, opened not only to the new architectural trends, but also by the prosperous members of the middle classes as well as by several societies, institutions, and industries that appropriated Modern architecture as the emblem of their efficiency. After 1930, the period of early modernism in Romania, the incontestable center of new trends was Bucharest. However, several examples, remarkable by their perfect adherence to the formal vocabulary of modernism, were erected in other areas of the country. These examples belong less to the housing program (except for the villas executed by I. Boceanu in Cîmpina or the villa Tataru in Cluj, designed in Gio Ponti's studio) than to the field of public buildings. It was an architecture that advanced the idea of autonomy from the geographic environment—such as the sanatoriums in the mountain zones (Toria, 1933–34, by Grigore Ionescu in Ciuc and Bucegi, 1934, by Marcel Iancu in Predeal) and the hotels in the seaside resorts (Belona, 1933, by G.M. Cantacuzino in Eforie)—and that underscored the expressive potential of the reinforced-concrete structure—such as the Central Market in Ploiesti (1931–33) by Toma T. Socolescu. The industrial buildings of the 1930s exclusively adopted the vocabulary of modernism, employing vigorous structures with large openings in reinforced concrete (the IAR Industries building, 1933, by G.M. Cantacuzino in Brasov) and emphasizing the expressiveness of the volumes and the materials, particularly brick (the Banloc Plants, 1937–38, by O. Doicescu and the Astra Plants, 1936–37, by Costinescu in Brasov).

Parallel to the boom of modern architecture and obviously influenced by its principles, the national style developed a new expression that adopted the formal simplicity and functionality of modernism. Not only was this new image a transgression of a clear decline of the style (the result of an epigonic production), but it also brought a change of vision. Instead of the historic examples, sometimes quoted in a historicist manner, tradition was now understood as the essence of Romanian spirituality through the perspective of folk art values. The new expression found adepts among the old exponents of the national style (Andrei Saguna Orthodox College, 1938–39, by George Cristinel in Sibiu), but it was particularly popular with young architects (the Military Club by C. Iotzu in Brasov and the numerous villas designed by H. Delavrancea-Gibory at the seaside).

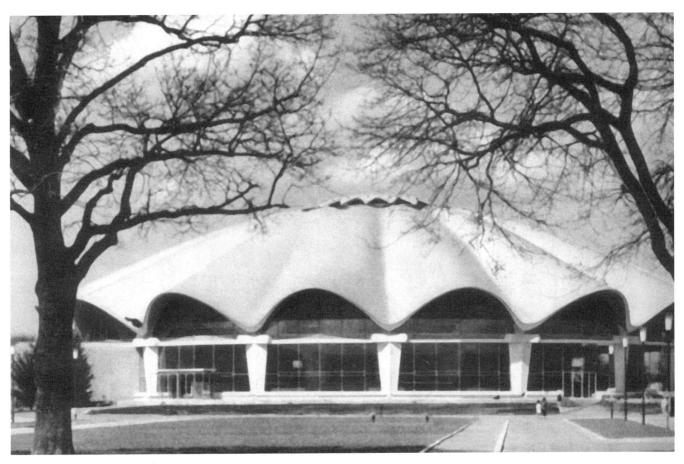

The State Circus (1960), Bucharest, Romania. Designed by Nicolae Porumbescu and Constantin Rulea.
© Carmen Popescu

The second half of the 1930s was a time of increased authoritarian politics, which culminated in the dictatorship of King Carol II and was followed at the beginning of the 1940s by the creation of the military state. The adoption of the new classicism perfectly mirrored this shift in the state politics. Frequently called "the style Carol II," this tendency became the symbol of the official architecture and was developed mainly in the capital.

The important political changes that followed World War II and that culminated in the installation of the Communist regime on 30 December 1947 brought a radical transformation for the development of architecture. The state established almost total control over architecture and urbanism, which became dependent on the strictly centralized economic and social politics. The evolution of postwar architecture was decisively conditioned by the dominance of standardized plans and of serialized industrial methods of construction, by the reduction in investment costs, and by the replacement of theoretical and critical discourse with the authoritarian intervention of the party ideology. However, this pattern was transgressed in particular cases, as when requested by the importance of representation. This representation emphasized either the regime itself or its ideology, either the urban role of the building or the uniqueness of its function—in the city or in the whole country.

The regime exercised a progressive control over architecture that was reflected in each phase of this period. The first part of 1950s was marked by the so-called realist-socialist architecture of Soviet influence. In these years, housing developments were built in numerous cities in Romania, as were plants and the infrastructure for the International Youth Festival, which took place in 1953 in Bucharest. The utmost symbol of this architecture remains Casa Scînteii (House of the Spark, 1950–51, by architects H. Maicu, L. Staadecker, M. Alifanti, N. Badescu, and others in Bucharest), a local reproduction of the Soviet models, where the forms, mainly classical, were adorned with details inspired partly by national tradition. Parallel to that, the old generation of architects continued to use the vocabulary of the interwar rationalism that was present in Romanian architecture until the end of the decade. The most relevant examples are the Clothing Industries APACA building (1948) by M. Alifanti, I. Ghica Budesti, and others and the Palace of the National Broadcasting (1960) by T. Ricci, L. Garcia, and M. Ricci, both in Bucharest.

The most interesting period of evolution in Romanian architecture started in the 1960s and lasted until the mid-1970s against the background of an apparent ideological liberalization. Functionalist architecture became official, and the urbanist prin-

ciples of the Athens Charter were conclusively adopted. The dormitory districts built in almost all Romanian cities, with their impersonal architecture and huge dimensions (up to hundreds of thousands of inhabitants), were erected according to these principles of the Athens Charter. Starting at the end of the 1960s, the Black Sea littoral became the experimental ground for both New Urbanism and Modern architecture. The necessity of modern public equipment in the cities brought the opportunity for various architectures, some of them of an incontestable value, to be employed. Among the most significant buildings of this period are a series of hotels (particularly at the Black Sea in the resorts Neptun, Olimp, and Aurora and in the mountain resorts, such as Poiana Brasov), theaters (the National Theater, 1972–74, by Al. Iotzu in Craiova), cultural centers (such as those built in 1968 by N. Porumbescu in Suceava and in 1975 in Baia Mare, where he employed a stylized interpretation of the traditional decorative patterns), and higher-education institutions and administrative centers (the Administrative Center 1972, by M. Alifanti in Baia Mare is considered one of the most valuable works of the period). The Catholic church (1976) by I. Fackelman in Orsova is unique in the whole postwar period.

The years following the devastating earthquake of 1977 coincided with the emphasis of the totalitarian and nationalistic ideology of the Communist regime. This mutation in the official ideology had dramatic consequences for architecture. Although numerous cities were affected by rapid degradation because of the demolitions of their historical downtowns (increasing the damage caused by the earthquake), the tentative decision to rebuild urbanlike villages, according to controlled planning, threatened to destroy the environment of traditional life. The architectural structures that replaced the demolished edifices, often reorganized as new civic centers, reflected the strict application of the regime ideology, resulting in a schematic and simplistic vocabulary. The control over architecture harshened, and a reduction in the quality of architecture became evident. Official architecture clearly was oriented to a rhetoric of monumentality that was specific to dictatorships, the most significant example being the Pharaonic complex of the House of the People in Bucharest by Anca Petrescu and collective. This enormous architectural complex concentrated the most important part of the state investments, a fact that drastically diminished the construction activity, and only a few buildings succeeded in escaping the anonymity of a common architecture. This explains why the Postmodernism of the 1980s did not produce noteworthy experiments.

Starting in 1990, after the fall of the Communist regime, Romanian architecture entered a new period of intense researches and the rediscovery of former local marks and of integration in the contemporaneous international movement. Unlike previous periods, Bucharest is no longer the only center of architectural experiments. Several other cities have developed such experiences, the most significant example being the city of Timisoara for the refined architecture of Serban Sturdza, I. Andreescu and V. Gaivoronschi, R. Mihailescu, and others.

CARMEN POPESCU AND NICOLAE LASCU

Further Reading

Centenar Horia Creanga 1892–1992, Bucuresti, Romania: Editura UAR, 1992

Constantin, Paul, *Arta 1900 in Romania* (Art 1900 in Romania), Bucuresti: Meridiane, 1972

Echilibrul uitat. Timisoara 1991–1996; as *Romanian catalogue at the Venice Biennial*, Bucuresti, Romania: Simetria, 1996

Ionescu, Grigore, "Arhitectura romaneasca dupa al doilea razboi mondial," *Arhitectura* no. 3–4 (1991)

Ionescu, Grigore, *Arhitectura pe teritoriul Romaniei de-a lungul veacurilor*, Bucuresti, Romania: Editura Academiei, 1982

Machedon, Luminita and Ernie Schoffham, *Romanian Modernism: The Architecture of Bucharest 1920–1940*, Cambridge, Massachusetts and London, England: MIT Press, 1999

Union of Romanian Architects, *Bucuresti, anii 1920–1940: între avangarda si modernism*; as *Bucharest in the 1920s–1940s, between avant-garde and modernism*, Bucuresti, Romania: Simetria, 1994

ROME, ITALY

In the history of the city of Rome, it was not just the Church that appropriated and used art and architecture for political or propagandistic purposes. From the city's annexation to the kingdom of Italy in 1870, Rome became a space of contest in which the contrasting discourses of the classical Roman Empire, the papacy of a universal Church, and the secular Savoyard monarchy were articulated. Such discourses affected and often reshaped the urban landscape. One of the best examples is constituted by the Vittorio Emanuele II monument (or Vittoriano), built between 1885 and 1911 to honor the memory of the first king of united Italy. Some 80 meters high, it irrevocably changed the cityscape, throwing out of scale the capitol itself. The architect, Giuseppe Sacconi, winning an international competition, employed a dazzling white "bottocino" marble from Brescia that further emphasized the monument with respect (or disrespect) to its surroundings. The Vittoriano was constructed in the Beaux Arts architectural style, which was popular at the time as appropriately "imperial" for urban monuments throughout all the major European capitals. Interestingly, both Liberal and Fascist governments between the wars emphasized the Vittoriano's centrality within the city's space and Italian territory. Mussolini in particular used the monument to promote an imperial spatiality through his performative rhetoric, which often unfolded while facing the monument in the adjacent Piazza Venezia.

The advent of Fascism had quite an effect on the architectural history of Rome. In the early 1930s, the population of Rome had grown from 244,000 to over a million. The practical necessity to provide a modern infrastructure in terms of public transport and utilities and to boost the regime's image in Italy and abroad threatened to put Fascism on a conflicting course both with the papacy (some 18 churches and Church buildings were destroyed from 1928 to 1939) and with the city's own classical heritage (many archaeological sites were disrupted to build those grand avenues that had to host the regime's parades and other mass events). It soon appeared evident that the key issues of planning in the city had to deal with finding a feasible compromise between the conflicting double logic of conservation or demolition. It has been convincingly argued that the three principal laws that informed Fascist design, architecture, and urban planning were the law of health (hygienic reasons were often at the basis of many interventions in the city), the law of speed (in the sense of both fast execution and, from a futurist perspective, active traffic, light, and air), and the Roman law, with its insistence

on the grandiose in the sense of the imposing and powerful. From Mussolini's early years in power, his ideas on monumental interventions in the city center reflected such laws. One of the best examples in this sense is the plan to free the Mausoleo di Augusto (or Augusteo). According to the project devised by the architect Vittorio Morpurgo, new porticoed buildings of the National Fascist Institute of Social Insurance were to define the piazza in which the Mausoleo stands on the north and east sides. A wide street piazza was created between the churches of San Girolamo and San Rocco. Moreover, a reconstruction of the *Ara Pacis* was located in glazed protective building (an example of rationalist architecture in sharp contrast with its classical content) between Via Ripetta and il Lungotevere. Quite different from the works around the Augusteo is the EUR project (also known as E 42). In this case, the plan was to build a new Rome, a modern one but with the same characters of monumentality and universality, on a hilltop five miles south of piazza Venezia. The EUR was meant to house the World Exhibition of Rome in 1942; thus, the task was to create a city of representation that conjugated the scenographic and artistic necessities of a world exhibition with the practicalities of a real city. Although the first plan was not extremely original, it must be said that it lacked the usual iconography of fasces, eagles, statues, or epigraphs that would come later. However, Romanità and modernity, monumentality and rationalist aspirations could not coexist, so it happened that the more advanced projects were relegated to the temporary exhibitions buildings, whereas the permanent buildings had a neoclassical style. The EUR was not completed because of the war; still, what is left proves wrong the widespread misconception that after Bernini and Borromini, little of significance was built in Rome.

EUR lies to the south of the city, toward the sea, in an area that had been open countryside until only a few years before. The building project was entrusted to the top architects of the day, who sought to blend the principles of ancient classical architecture with European rationalism. One fine example of this composite style is the Palazzo della Civiltà del Lavoro, familiarly known as the "square colosseum." The defining features of this original zone are the broad avenues and wide-open squares.

The Fascist era also saw the building of another major example of this type of architecture: the Foro Italico. Formerly named after Mussolini, the Foro Italico is a large sports complex that encloses several facilities, including an indoor swimming pool decorated with mosaic work. It also contains the Stadio dei Marmi, a stadium encircled by 60 marble statues of athletes donated by towns and cities around the country. A sphere measuring three meters in diameter rests in the forecourt.

The Dora zone, completed in 1926, offers a unique example of Roman architectural eclecticism from the early years of the 20th century. A large, decorated arch leads rather unexpectedly into a remarkable area designed by Gino Coppedè, whose surname provides the popular name for the zone. Every building has its own special ornamentation, though Art Nouveau and mock-medieval motifs stand out in the rich mix of styles.

After the war, the Italian architects who had best represented the cause of modern architecture were dead: G. L. Banfi, G. Pagano, E. Persico, and G. Terragni. However, a new sensation started influencing Italian culture: that of making contact with reality in a new way, seeing reality with new eyes. It was this sensation that gave rise to Neorealism, which became widely known thanks to the films of Roberto Rossellini and Vittorio De Sica but that influenced the arts and architecture as well. The best example of the latter is the architecture of Ridolfi at Terni and the Tiburtino district in Rome in the early 1950s. To the design of the Tiburtino district, a sort of manifesto of architectural neorealism, C. Aymonino, C. Chiarini, M. Fiorentino. F. Gorio, M. Lanza, S. Lenci, P. Lugli, C. Melograni, G. Menichetti, L. Quaroni, and M. Valori also contributed.

Neorealism, particularly for the architects of the Roman School (Ridolfi, Quaroni, and Fiorentino), is characterized by a concern for everyday reality, a preference for popular forms, an interest for one's immediate environment, and the rejection of any abstraction. Such concerns were already evident in the design for the Stazione Termini (1947), the new Rome railway station, by Quaroni, Ridolfi, and Fiorentino. Between 1950 and 1954, Ridolfi also designed what was a nucleus of innovative tall houses on the Viale Etiopia, the so-called African quarter. In the years between 1954 and 1962, three different plans were prepared for Rome while architects were facing a cultural and political debate that included the status of a new town-planning discipline and a new legal ruling on building land. In the 1962 plan, inspired by Quaroni and Piccinato, a multifunctional axis girdling the east zone of the city was due to connect up with the national superhighway system. In addition, the plan included the creation of three areas of expansion that would deploy some of the functions of the congested city center. Unfortunately, the Rome plan was not realized, mainly because of administrative deficiencies.

For the Olympic Games in 1960, the Palazzo and Palazzetto dello Sport and the Flaminio Stadium were built by Vitellozzi and Pier Luigi Nervi; these structures combined technological inventions with neomonumental organisms. In the 1960s, the EUR came to prominence again by developing into an efficient business district and a residential area for the upper-middle class. It became the only real administrative pole of the capital at a time when Italy was in the midst of a real economic miracle. Also noticeable are the new magistrates' courts, designed by the Perugini-Monteduro group between 1959 and 1969, on Piazzale Clodio; the Vitellozzi's project (1959–67) for the Biblioteca Nazionale at castro Pretorio; the RAI-TV office building (1963–65) on Viale Mazzini by Berbarducci and Fioroni; and Albini's Rinascente department store in the area of Piazza Fiume/Via Veneto. Also worth mentioning is the residential complex (1973–82) in Corviale (Rome), which contained new building types and was realized with advanced techniques of prefabrication.

From 1975 to 1984, while Rome had a left-wing administration, there were plans for rehabilitating the most derelict districts (*borgate*), building new public housing, acquiring more green space, and recovering historical buildings. The projects implemented after the national *Roma Capitale* law have given rise to 445 projects, mainly relating to road improvements and public facilities.

In the early 1980s, the Italian architect Paolo Portoghesi launched a style that has been designated postmodern and is characterized broadly by a taste for citation, pastiche, and free association. Portoghesi's only projects in Rome are the mosque and the cultural Islamic center in Via Magnani and the City of Science for the site of the old slaughterhouse in Testaccio.

The sprawling metropolis that now extends all over the *Agro romano* has its roots in the idea of a centralized Italian state, and its development as a bureaucratic city has been plagued by an army of land speculators and builders. Since its annexation to the kingdom of Italy, architects working in Rome have often been caught in an inextricable web of bureaucratic and political difficulties. In the past 30 years, the city has changed remarkably, yet the contrast between a dominant center and a subaltern periphery is still a sharp one. Rome is only recently starting to live up to what is expected of it given its exceptional past.

ANNA NOTARO

See also **Fascist Architecture; Gregotti, Vittorio (Italy); Moretti, Luigi (Italy); Nervi, Pier Luigi (Italy); Portoghesi, Paolo (Italy); Sant'Elia, Antonio (Italy); Terragni, Giuseppe (Italy)**

Further Reading

Adam, Robert, *Classical Architecture: A Complete Handbook*, London and New York: Viking, 1990

Benevolo, Leonardo, *Storia dell'architettura moderna*, 2 vols., Bari, Italy: Laterza, 1960; as *History of Modern Architecture*, 2 vols., translated by H. J. Landry, London: Routledge and Kegan Paul, and Cambridge, Massachusetts: MIT Press, 1971; see especially vol. 2, *The Modern Movement*

Cederna, Antonio, *Mussolini urbanista: Lo sventramento di Roma negli anni del consenso*, Rome and Bari, Italy: Laterza, 1979

Clark, Roger H., and Michael Pause, *Precedents in Architecture*, New York: Van Nostrand Reinhold, 1984; Wokingham, Berkshire: Van Nostrand Reinhold, 1985; 2nd edition, New York, 1996

Galardi, Alberto, *Architettura italiana contemporanea*, Milan: Edizioni di Comunità, 1967; as *New Italian Architecture*, translated by E. Rockwell, New York: Praeger, and London: Architectural Press, 1967

Kostof, Spiro, *The Third Rome, 1870–1950: Traffic and Glory*, Berkeley, California: University Art Museum, 1973

Millon, Henry A., and Linda Nochlin (editors), *Art and Architecture in the Service of Politics*, Cambridge, Massachusetts: MIT Press, 1978

Norberg-Schulz, Christian, *Architettura barocca*, Milan: Electa, 1971; as *Baroque Architecture*, New York: Abrams, 1971; London: Academy Editions, 1972

Norwich, John Julius (editor), *Great Architecture of the World*, London: Beazley, and New York: Random House, 1975; revised and expanded, as *The World Atlas of Architecture*, Boston: G.K. Hall, and London: Beazley, 1984

Partridge, Loren W., *The Art of Renaissance Rome, 1400–1600*, London: Calmann and King, and New York: Abrams, 1996

Trachtenberg, Marvin, and Isabelle Hyman, *Architecture: From Prehistory to Post-Modernism: The Western Tradition*, New York: Abrams, and London: Academy Editions, 1986

Yarwood, Doreen, *The Architecture of Europe*, New York: Hastings House, and London: Batsford, 1974

ROSSI, ALDO 1931–97

Architect, Italy

Aldo Rossi was an influential architect, designer, teacher, and theoretician whose works emphasized historical types and memories as poetic elements in architectural design. Working primarily in Italy, his later work was designed and constructed for cities in the United States, Germany, Argentina, and Japan.

Rossi's representations of architecture, from the scale of furniture to that of urbanism, were reminiscent of Giorgio de Chirico's metaphysical paintings and the Enlightenment-era projects of Étienne-Louis Boullée. Rossi's design sketches contain haunting irregularities of scale and typology, disciplined and refined in their final construction. Rossi's timeless vocabulary of forms remained relatively constant throughout his career, although the scale, material, and functions shift across projects. His works synthesized pure repetition, modern space, and remembered forms into a singular vision that he named "analogous architecture," and the frequent return to the questions of cultural meaning and signification in architectural forms permeated his writings, images, and buildings.

Rossi's professional education at the Milan Polytechnic brought him into close contact with Marxist critical theory and the revolutionary potentials in architecture under the influence of Italian Neorealism in the arts. These sources influenced his work as a writer and editor of the journal *Casabella-Continuita* (1961–64). Although his early written and built work was sympathetic to the ascetic modernism of the Viennese architect Adolph Loos (1870–1933), he moved far from this position in his later career.

In 1966, Rossi published his influential book on urban theory titled *L'Architettura della citta* (The Architecture of the City). Identifying building typology and urban morphology as inseparable and always saturated with history, the city is conceived as a political construct. Written from a rationalist perspective indebted to the Enlightenment, the text places politicized humanist concerns over the orthodoxy of modernist functionalism and forms. Monuments and housing types are saturated with unique social and political meanings and cannot be considered purely functionalist forms. This reconceptualization of the historically structured meanings of cities operated as the foundation for his and others subsequent designs.

Rossi's later writings and projects moved from an ascetic architecture of concrete to rich metaphoric constructions invoking memories of cities (as fragments). It was a progression from ideological concerns to questions of memory and a revival of humanist referents, an attempt to recuperate what modern urbanism had eliminated. Rossi's works were a deeply personal examination and reconstruction of architecture's own history. Rossi did not copy or imitate existing models but proposed reduced typological elements to allow cultural and personal meanings to be projected into them. Relying on a limited number of significant classical types and anonymous vernacular forms that are immediately familiar, Rossi's architecture animated memories of these architectural forms to create a strong visual and spatial effect of timelessness.

Rossi's architecture communicated simultaneously personal and archetypal concepts, much like a visual language. He frequently described this method as "analogous architecture," which he derived from the work of psychologist Carl Jung, who described analogous thought as "sensed yet unreal, imagined yet silent . . . it is archaic, unexpressed, and practically inexpressible in words." Analogous architecture draws on the dialogue between the real and representation (as in photography or theater) to communicate meaning through nonlinguistic associations, fusing past and present into experience and remembering.

Rossi examined the limits of analogous architecture at a large urban scale in his later works and specifically through drawing

in the hypothetical designs for an Analogous City (1976) and an invited entry to the Roma Interrotta (1977). Given the original segment of Nolli's map of Rome containing the Baths of Caracalla, Rossi proposed a historically self-conscious architecture that was to be "borrowed, converted, and invented," a habitual urban strategy examined in his text *Scientific Autobiography* (1981). In this text, he stated, "The construction of a logic of architecture cannot omit the relationship with history."

Rossi's design projects originated in a Loosian search for reductive, rational, and precise architectural expression but then involved distinct Platonic shapes found in books of perspectival drawing and stereometrics. In his many designs for urban spaces, he situated autonomous and enigmatic monuments in the voids of public space to make their haunting presence and silence obvious. Their timelessness was animated only by cast shadows. The competition project (1962) for a Monument to the Resistance in Cuneo, Italy, offers a cube with a slit framing the distant battlegrounds. The built iron bridge (1962) for the Milan Triennale and the Monument de la Piazzetta Manzoni (1988–90) in Milan continue to develop this language of concrete form without any scale or material references, as if they were childhood memories. The unbuilt Piazza del Municipio (1965) in the Segrate district of Milan appears as a fusion of monument and tomb, the two aspects of architecture that Loos identified as belonging to art. These dematerialized but visually heavy forms invoke political and historical associations between modernism and Fascism as inevitable and fated.

Rossi's first built large-scale project, the urban housing project Gallaratese (1969–73) in Milan, was a fusion of high-modernist housing typology within an attenuated form nostalgic for premodern Milanese urban housing, galleries, or barracks. As a representation and inventory of earlier precedents, they are built in the grammar of the early monuments and plazas. A relentless repetition of panel-like columns is punctuated only by two massive round columns in the center of this arcade, marking a small crevice in the form above. These support the undifferentiated flats in an extended linear schema. The circulation is arranged as corridors or elevated private streets unseen from the ground plane. Each housing unit appears identical, with identical fenestration, and the overall stark and simplified result implies that there is no individuality in a social class.

Rossi completed two schools that evoked a concern with childhood memories through his emergent vocabulary. The elementary school (1972–76) at Fagnano Olana, Italy, and a secondary school (1979) at Broni, Italy, are both organized around a dominant central courtyard containing individualized central elements as in the early plaza designs. The public space is defined spatially by a strong perimeter boundary created by the repetition of identical classrooms. This classical ordering schema appears in most later projects when the functional program contains a diversity of spaces.

The role of timeless forms and historical memories in architecture is evident in Rossi's competition-winning design for the addition to the Cemetery of San Cataldo (1971–84 in phased construction) in Modena, Italy. Rossi fuses monument and tomb within a larger concept of the cemetery as a city of the dead, designed to evoke memories of urban conditions through its volumes and plazas. Other funerary architecture is distributed axially as diverse object-types through the center space like scaleless volumes or districts. The communal graveyard is inside and beneath a cone-shaped form, marking one end of the axis. The opposite end holds the shrine to the war dead. This monumental metaphysical object is constructed as an orange cube perforated with square openings, its insides containing unadorned metal balconies arranged like fire escapes. It is a disturbing house of the dead, roofless and windowless. Between these two object-types, more ossuaries are arranged in a riblike diminishing pattern of linear construction, forming a triangular district articulated as a labyrinth or mandatory path. The cemetery complex draws heavily on visual and historical references to history, memory, and death through Rossi's remembered archetypal forms.

During San Cataldo's construction, Rossi's written and drawn works began to attract significant international recognition, defining a place for the reemergence of history in the postmodern period. Contemporaneous with San Cataldo, Rossi's architecture began to include increasingly differentiated materiality (pattern, color, and textures) and overt references to nostalgic memories of historic precedents. Timeless historical types become specific to their unique sites and contexts. Rossi's early interest in cinema and theater became a dominant analogy in the theoretical and urban projects that followed.

The Teatro del Mondo (Theater of the World), created for the Venice Biennale (1979), was a floating pavilion enclosing a centralized theater space. The steel frame of its octagonal wood form was welded to a functioning barge that traveled the seas of Italy, creating a transitory object that combined building, barge, and folly. Its echoes of historical theaters in the round and its toylike appearance showcased Rossi's personal rediscovery of the Renaissance relationship between theater and architecture, first explored in his furniture-size theoretical project the Little Scientific Theater (1978). In the Carlo Felice Theater (1983–89) in Genoa, Italy, a unique historical precedent became the site of construction for "civil architecture." Barbarino's prior neoclassical theater facing the ducal palace was reborn as a large, 2000-seat balconied theater. A chimney-like cone, used in earlier projects, distributes light by penetrating through the internal public spaces. A stone-clad tower block rises above the theater, and the entrance to the theater acts as a filter between city and spectacle.

In 1981, Rossi submitted the winning housing scheme for the international design competition for urban renewal in the former West Berlin (IBA). Finished in 1988, the perimeter-block housing project exhibits a wide range of materials and scale. Although housing is supported by an arcade as in Gallaratese, the vertical circulation towers facing the interior courtyard, pitched spires over elevators, and gridded glass facades between masonry housing blocks materially differentiate each element of the project, creating the impression of linkages between identical small buildings. Only the oversize columns at both ends of the project recall his earlier works. Other works in Berlin included the smaller apartment building (1983) in Berlin-Tiergarten on Rauchstrasse and an unbuilt competition design (1978) for the Museum of German History.

In the 1980s, Rossi turned his methodology toward commercial institutions within urban contexts. The Commercial Center of Fontivegge (1982–89) in Perugia, Italy, is a U-shaped complex of shops and offices framing a multistory house form on exaggerated piers. The Commercial Center "Centro Torri" (1985–88) in Parma, Italy, adopts the typology of Renaissance market stalls to recuperate commerce as "the center of human

life." Ten brick towers mark the dominant central arcade that holds the stores together. The office building (1984) for Officine GFT in Turin and the unbuilt Edificio Techint (1984) in Buenos Aires, Argentina, turned back from normative modernism to three-dimensional assemblages of historical elements. In 1989, the Il Palazzo Hotel and Restaurant Complex in Fukuoka, Japan, drew on Roman construction forms, presenting a blank public facade of travertine with exquisitely detailed, disengaged columns separated by iron banding at each floor level. Constructed on a raised public plaza, this project translates premodern urban gestures into a frenetic high-tech context, offering the qualities of serenity, silence, and eternity that Rossi pursued in all his works.

Rossi's earliest passions and vocabulary remained a constant referent throughout his career, reemerging and slowly transforming into more sophisticated compositions, all with increasing sensitivity to materiality and related connections. Virtually every project can be read as an examination of the historical essence of architectural form and an interrogation of the city as a historical force. His highly personal approach placed the human condition at the conceptual and physical center of the works, and by offering unique memories of historical forms, he created an architecture that invites the projection of individual meanings on the constructed forms. His widely disseminated writings, drawings, and buildings encouraged the turn away from dehistoricized modern urbanism in Europe and elsewhere.

THOMAS MICAL

Biography

Born 3 May 1931 in Milan. Graduated from the degree program in architecture Milan Politecnico in 1959. Editor of *Casabella-Continuita* (1961–64). Published the influential text *The Architecture of the City* (1966); taught at the Milan's Politecnico, ETH Zurich, Cooper Union, and the Venice Instituto Universitario di Architettura. Awarded the Pritzker Prize in Architecture (1990). Died in Milan, 4 September 1997.

Selected Publications

L'architettura della città, Padua, Italy: Marsilio, 1966; 2nd edition, 1970; as *The Architecture of the City*, translated by Diane Ghirardo and Joan Ockman, Cambridge, Massachusetts: MIT Press, 1982
Autobiografia cientifica, Barcelona: Gili, 1981; as *A Scientific Autobiography*, translated by Lawrence Venuti, Cambridge, Massachusetts: MIT Press, 1981

Further Reading

Adjmi, Morris (editor), *Aldo Rossi: Architecture, 1981–1991*, New York: Princeton Architectural Press, 1991
Adjmi, Morris, and Giovanni Bertolotto (editors), *Aldo Rossi: Drawings and Paintings*, New York: Princeton Architectural Press, 1993
Aldo Rossi, Tokyo: A + U, 1982
Aymonino, Carlo, et al., *Carlo Aymonino, Aldo Rossi: Housing Complex at the Gallaratese Quarter, Milan, Italy, 1969–1974*, Tokyo: A.D.A. Edita, 1977
Arnell, Peter, and Ted Bickford (editors), *Aldo Rossi, Buildings and Projects*, New York: Rizzoli, 1985
Frampton, Kenneth (editor), *Aldo Rossi in America: 1976 to 1979*, New York: Institute for Architecture and Urban Studies, 1979

Hyatt Foundation, *The Pritzker Architecture Prize 1990, Presented to Aldo Rossi*, Los Angeles: Hyatt Foundation, 1990
Richardson, Sara, *Aldo Rossi: Surrealist Vision*, Monticello, Illinois: Vance Bibliographies, 1987

ROTTERDAM, THE NETHERLANDS

Descriptions of Rotterdam, in the province of South Holland, abound in quantitative superlatives: the world's largest port, Europe's densest metropolis (more than 4,000 people per square kilometer), one of the country's most industrialized areas, the Dutch town most grievously destroyed during the German occupation of 1940–1945, and also the tallest, boasting many more skyscrapers than any other city in the Netherlands. Moreover, even in a country renowned for creating itself from land won from the sea, Rotterdam stands out, aggressively reclaiming portions of *Maasvlakte* (Maas Flats; the Maas is the major river) for its expanding terminals, chemical plants, and petroleum refineries as well as for satellite towns. A thoroughly 20th-century city in which remarkably few buildings from previous periods survive, Rotterdam enters the new millennium with a vigorous architectural and urbanistic growth that bids fair to surpass other Dutch contenders.

The population of almost 600,000 (more than 1 million live in adjacent municipalities) makes Rotterdam second in size only to Amsterdam (*c.*728,000), and comparisons are instructive no less than inevitable. Both were chartered in the early 1300s on sites that began as a dam on a river (the Rotte and the Amstel, respectively), but thereafter their fortunes diverged. Amsterdam rose to power in the Golden Age of the 17th century; Rotterdam, based more exclusively on shipping-related activities, began its economic challenge only after 1872, when the opening of the New Waterway (*Nieuwe Waterweg*), which connected the port city directly with the North Sea, set it on the path to eventual maritime dominance. Urbanistically Rotterdam followed at a somewhat later date a trajectory similar to Amsterdam's: the late 19th century brought severe overcrowding in the inner city, unplanned speculative growth on the outskirts, and the gradual adoption of municipal codes and extension plans to counter these problems. Although both cities are water-girt, Rotterdam's aqueous bodies are larger and more intrusive; instead of picturesque canals, it offers major rivers and harbors spanned by imposing bridges very different in size from those of Amsterdam. Although Amsterdam's new construction is mainly outside the inner city, Rotterdam's heart is one huge construction site constantly in transition. That makes it dynamic if a bit unsettling, oriented to the future with little fidelity to the past. Rotterdam has also been more hospitable to foreign firms: Marcel Breuer (De Bijenkorf Department Store, 1955–57, with Dutchman A. Elzas), and Skidmore, Owings and Merrill (the three Europoint 24-story towers, 1971–75) have worked there, and in the 1990s it has been the first to welcome such international figures as Norman Foster, Renzo Piano, and Helmut Jahn.

Architecturally the contrast was noted already in 1923, in the oft-quoted letter by Erich Mendelsohn describing Rotterdam as analytic in danger from the deadly chill in its veins and Amsterdam as visionary, threatened by the fire of its own dynamism. The claim may be somewhat exaggerated, but its basic premise about the distinct characters of each city touches on a truth that

has obtained throughout much of the century. Rotterdam was the stronghold of Dutch functionalism, the *Nieuwe Bouwen*, which exalted usefulness over aesthetics. Until recently, its major monuments were almost exclusively for practical ends—housing, commercial, and industrial structures rather than cultural buildings—and the stunning elegance that several attained was a by-product of efficiency and economy; speed and size took precedence over beauty.

During the fin-de-siècle, Rotterdam was overshadowed artistically by The Hague, its near neighbor and the seat of government, and followed it in favoring the Franco-Belgian variant of the Art Nouveau, unlike Amsterdam, where the more sober, indigenous, and enduring version of *Nieuwe Kunst* prevailed. The major work during this period is the *Witte Huis* of 1897–98 (one of the few buildings in the center to have survived the firebombing), the first Dutch, indeed European, skyscraper. Designed by W. Molenbroek, the mansard-roofed, 138-foot-high, 11-story office building with load-bearing walls of stone and white brick was prophetic of Rotterdam's future as the dominant skyscraper city of the Netherlands. Henry Hobson Ricardson's work (one of its stylistic influences) was familiar in Holland through the teachings of H.P. Berlage, who, regrettably, found few opportunities in Rotterdam. A workers cooperative (1906–07) and an insurance company (1911; destroyed) were his only executed works; his grand redesigns of the Hofplein square (1921 and 1926), commissioned by the municipality, were rejected. The most conspicuous public building of the first two decades was the neo-Northern Renaissance Town Hall by Henri Evers (1855–1929), professor at Rotterdam's Academy of Fine Arts and Technical Sciences from 1887–1902. Subject of an invited competition of 1912, the choice of Evers's ecclectic design, an anachronism before it was completed in 1920, indicated the city's conservatism, for it might have chosen the much more original entry by Willem Kromhout (1864–1940).

Kromhout, whose work was akin to Berlage's but more playful and exotic, left a distinguished career in Amsterdam as architectural leader and teacher to move in 1910 to Rotterdam to teach at the academy and reestablish his practice. If earlier he had inspired the Amsterdam School, now among his students were future leaders of the *Nieuwe Bouwen* such as J.J.P. Oud, Cor van Eesteren, and Leendert van der Vlugt. Kromhout's own free style retained allusions to architecture from the early Christian, Byzantine, and medieval periods laced with Arabic and Art Nouveau motifs, the whole transformed by a unique imagery that expressed the individual program.

In 1920 Kromhout, who had been president of the Amsterdam club, Architectura et Amicitia, was instrumental in founding, with Michiel Brinkman (1873–1925), a new association, *De Opbouw*, dedicated to architectural debate. It would attract various factions, including representatives of De Stijl, theosophists (the universalist philosophy popular with many Dutch cultural leaders), and dedicated functionalists, who brought in avant-garde architects from Germany and the Soviet Union and rejected the aesthetic priorities of other members, in part as a response to the urgent task facing architects and city officials—creating inexpensive housing.

In 1916 Rotterdam established a Municipal Housing Service, which embarked on constructing extensive new residential quarters outside the center. Among the most acclaimed are the blocks (1919–21) by Brinkman on Justus van Effenstraat in Spangen,

a new worker's neighborhood, which provide housing for 270 families and community facilities—a bathhouse, a laundry, and a children's play space—in the generously sized interior courtyards. The first two stories are composed of flats; those at ground level have modest private gardens. Portals provide access to the interior terrain where the entries to most of the dwellings are located. Comprising the top two stories are *maisonettes*, the doors of which open onto a continuous gallery wide enough to permit delivery vans and provide exercise space for children.

Spangen also is home to the first municipal housing by Oud, city architect from 1918–1933; I & V (1918–20), and VIII & IX (1919–20). These necessarily sober brick perimeter blocks are enlivened by abstract sculptural effects at the corners and over entryways and windows, which reveal, however tenuously, the impact of De Stijl, to which Oud briefly belonged but felt obliged to leave when he took the municipal job, believing that social projects precluded its formal tactics. More obviously indebted to that movement was the red, yellow, and blue temporary superintendent's office of 1923 (recently reconstructed) belonging to the *Witte Dorp* (white village) in Oud-Mathenesse, another worker's quarter. The modest one-and-a-half story row houses, intended as semipermanent, remained in use until the 1990s. Oud's most mature housing project in Rotterdam, Kiefhoek (1925–29), is a canonical example of the International Style, with its continuous strip windows and taut, white-stuccoed surfaces.

One of the most justly celebrated examples of the *Nieuwe Bouwen* is the Van Nelle Factory and Administration Building, by Johannes Andreas Brinkman (1902–1949) and L.C. van der Vlugt (1894–1936) assisted by Mart Stam. The architects exploited all the possibilities of transparency and dynamic movement in this interconnected complex in which each of the varied functions is signaled by the contrasts of curved with rectilinear volumes, and rendered stucco planes with large sheets of glass. The structure, which includes novel mushroom-shaped columns, and the skin are skillfully distinguished in the prescribed manner of the International Style.

Another functionalist active chiefly in Rotterdam is Willem van Tijen (1894–1974), who shares responsibility—and fame—for two groundbreaking blocks of flats: Bergpolder (1932–34) and Plaslaan (1937–38), the former in association with Brinkman and Van der Vlugt, the latter with H.A. Maaskant (1907–77), who became his partner in 1937. Both were erected at the behest of the company NV Volkswoningbouw Rotterdam, established on the initiative of the municipal planner, A. Plate, to experiment with new construction techniques. Each stands discretely in a parklike setting, reflecting the tenets of Congrès Internationaux d'Architecture Moderne (CIAM), which was very influential in Dutch planning circles and was headed from 1930 to 1947 by Van Eesteren. Bergpolder, the first high-rise housing slab in the Netherlands, has balconies facing west and, on the eastern side, a gallery at each of its nine levels. The steel skeleton was enclosed with numerous prefabricated elements, still a rarity in the Netherlands at the time. The ten-story Plaslaan has a concrete frame and is more luxurious, with larger flats for the middle class. Orientation is reversed for views; the galleries are on the west. It has a roof terrace and at ground floor a laundry space, the concierge's dwelling, a few guest rooms, a shop, and storage space.

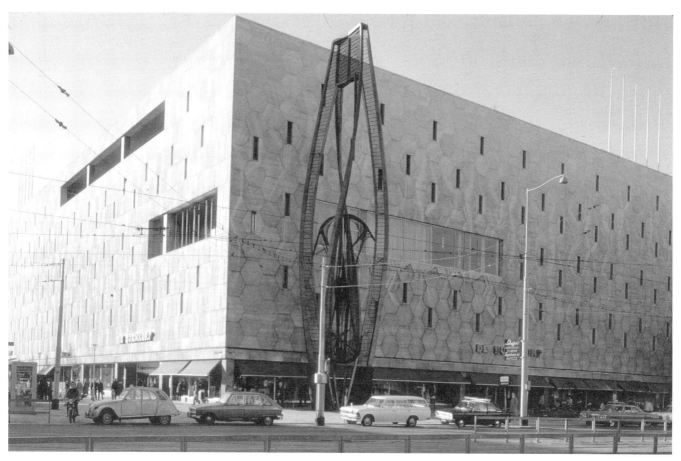

De Bijenkorf, Rotterdam (1957), by Marcel Breuer
© Greatbuidings.com

Represented also in Rotterdam is the most conservative movement in the Netherlands, the Delft School, comprised mainly of Roman Catholics and nationalists who believed in building according to the timeless Dutch tradition of load-bearing brick. The garden village Vreewijk, by Marinus Granpré Molière (1883–1972), with its pitched-roofed low-rise row houses is a significant example. So is the Museum Boymans-Van Beuningen of 1928–35, by A. van der Steur (1893–1953), city architect from 1931–39, who adapted the round arches and brick-and-stone vernacular worshiped by this school to the rare institutional building found in Rotterdam in this period. Yet a third way appeared in the singular architecture of Rotterdam native (and from 1915 to 1959 designer in various capacities for the National Dutch Railways), Sybold van Ravesteyn (1889–1983), who in the 1930s abandoned the functionalist route to introduce baroque themes and moderne decoration, as demonstrated in his various stations in Rotterdam (Beurs, Delftse Poort, and Feyenoord, 1934–37) and elsewhere and in the delightful Blijdorp Zoo (1937–41). In 1957, after many alterations from his first proposals of 1941, Van Rayestevn's Central Station for Rotterdam was completed.

On 14 May 1940, to force the Netherlands to capitulate, Nazi planes made a terrifying example of Rotterdam's inner city. Reconstruction after 1945 was as pedestrian as it was expedient,

in part because of the attempt by municipal and national planners to negotiate a compromise between modern functionalists and the Delft School. One thoroughly functionalist project to receive international approbation was De Lijnbaan (1949–53), arguably the first car-free shopping precinct in the modern world. What made it particularly successful was its mixture of boutiques, offices, and housing, each in its own container (i.e., functions were combined not in a single building but in a single urban district). The two-story rows of shops are accessed on the front from pedestrian streets, with deliveries made in the rear via service streets that also serve the blocks of flats and offices behind. The concrete frame that structures the shops allows internal flexibility according to the needs of each retailer. Kiosks, plantings, and handsome paving articulating the module that governs the proportions are palliatives to the rather bland architecture. The apartments are by H. Maaskant and others, the shopping center by the firm of Van den Broek (J.H.; 1898–1978) and J.B. Bakema (1914–1981), which garnered innumerable commissions, and not just in Rotterdam, in the sixties and seventies.

Rotterdam has continued to expand its boundaries to create huge housing districts on the periphery. In 1974 the city again embarked on an aggressive policy of renewal, which as well as restoration of existing areas included new construction like the

549-unit superblock by Carel Weeber (b.1937), *De Peperklip* (1978–82), named for its unusual footprint. Its multicolored, tile-faced, prefabricated concrete panels acknowledge the Dutch fondness for polychromy, and its mix of apartment types is heir to the spatial ingenuity frequently encountered in this densely populated land. Exciting new developments are occurring as well on the Southern Tip, which besides housing includes commercial and government buildings such as Cees Dam's Central Tax Bureau and Wilhelmina Tower (1997–99), their strong cubic, curving and prow-shaped volumes boldly contrasting with each other.

A healthy shift began in the later '80s when institutional structures took their place beside the more practical building types. In the Rotterdam Schowburg (theater; 1982–88), Wim Quist (b. 1930) was asked by the municipality to provide for a complex program including opera, ballet, and different kinds of theatrical performances; it is a serious and sober building with an intricately sectioned interior that respects the functionalist tradition. More striking and lucid are the Deconstructivist Kunsthal (1988–92) by Rem Koolhaas and the Office of Metropolitan Architecture, and the Erasmus Bridge (1990–96) by UN Studio, headed by Ben van Berkel (b. 1957). Affectionately dubbed the baby-blue Monster, the 139-meter concrete and metal sky-colored bridge that spans 800 meters over the Maas challenges the skyscrapers in height and functions simultaneously as a thoroughfare for cars, cycles, pedestrians, and trams and as urban stage, lighted at night to reveal the dematerialized reflection of its daytime self.

Rotterdam's architectural position has been ratified by the fact that it now is the home of two prime institutions, both of which have moved from Amsterdam: first the Netherlands Architectural Institute (NAi), which in 1995 was installed in its remarkable polychrome and polytextured intertwined series of buildings by Jo Coenen (b. 1949), and the Berlage Institute, an internationally recognized educational facility established in 1990, that in 2000 relocated to the former bank building at Botersloot 25 (1951) by Oud. Further, Rotterdam takes pride in the fact that it resembles a giant construction site that is never fixed in place. It has embraced with unparalleled enthusiasm the new pluralism manifest during the last decade of the 20th century and, as European Design City of 2001, is determined to retain its uniqueness in the new millennium.

HELEN SEARING

See also **Amsterdam; Amsterdam School; Art Nouveau (Jugendstil); Berlage, Hendrik Petrus (the Netherlands); Breuer, Marcel (United States); De Stijl; Duiker, Johannes (the Netherlands); Foster, Norman (England); International Style; Jahn, Helmut (the Netherlands); Koolhaas, Rem (the Netherlands); Mendelsohn, Erich (Germany); Netherlands; Oud, J.J.P. (the Netherlands); Piano, Renzo (Italy); Skidmore, Owings and Merrill (United States); Team X, the Netherlands; Van Nelle Factory, Rotterdam**

Further Reading

Unlike Amsterdam, which has an extensive reading list in English, Rotterdam thus far has been examined chiefly in Dutch. Particularly useful for the English-speaking reader for the period when Rotterdam first gained attention as an architectural leader is *Rotterdam 1920–1960*, a catalog published on the occasion of five exhibitions on the *Nieuwe Bouwen*. Although it covers far more territory than Rotterdam alone, Rem Koolhaas's runaway favorite, *Small, Medium, Large, Extra-Large*, casts a fascinating and provocative light on the city and should be read by all who wish to fathom Rotterdam's character as manmade artifact. Although a general book on contemporary architecture and theory, *10 × 10* includes many projects executed in Rotterdam. For further references, see bibliography under the Netherlands.

Barbieri, Umberto (editor), *De Kop van Zuid*, Rotterdam: Rotterdamse Kunststichting Uitgeverij, 1982

Beerne, Wim, Rob Dettingmeijer, Frank Kauffmann, Ton Idsinga, and Jeroen Schilt, *Rotterdam: 1920–1960*, Delft: Delft University Press, 1982. Text in English and Dutch

Brinkman, J.A., J.H. van den Broek, W. van Tijen, and H. Maaskant, *Woonmogelijkheden in het nieuwe Rotterdam*, Rotterdam: W.L. and J. Brusse, 1941

Constantinopolous, Vivian, and Iona Baird (editors), *10 × 10*, London: Phaidon, 2000

Grinberg, Donald, *Housing in the Netherlands, 1900–1940*, Rotterdam: Nijgh-Wolters-Noordhoff Universitaire, 1977

Ibelings, Hans (editor), *Van den Broek en Bakema 1948–1988, architectuur en stedenbouw*, Rotterdam: Netherlands Architectural Institute, 2000

Jacobs, Brian, *Strategy and Partnership in Cities and Regions: Economic Development and Urban Regeneration in Pittsburgh, Birmingham and Rotterdam*, London: Macmillan Press and New York: St. Martin's Press, 2000

Jonge, Alle de (editor), *Alexanderpolder: New Urban Frontiers*, Bussum: Thoth, 1993

Koolhaas, Rem, with Bruce Mau and Jennifer Sigler, *Small, Medium, Large, Extra-Large*, Rotterdam: 010 Publishers, 1995

Nieuwenhuis, Jan, *Mensen Maken een Stad, 1855–1955*, Rotterdam: Dienst van Gemeentewerken, 1955

Ruiter, Fred de, Marijke Meijs, Ad Habets (editors), *Stadsvernieuwing Rotterdam 1974–1984*, 3 vols. Rotterdam: i 10, 1984

Traa, C. van (editor), *Rotterdam, der Neubau einer Stadt*, Rotterdam: A. Donker, 1957

Wentholt, R., *De binnenstadsbeleving in Rotterdam*, Rotterdam: A. Donker, 1968

Wonen-TA/BK: Architectuurgids Rotterdam 53/6 (1980)

ROW HOUSE

The row house, also known as a town house in the United States or a terrace house in England, is a ubiquitous feature of Western urban landscapes. It is defined as one unit of a series of attached houses that shares at least one common wall with its neighbor. The traditional urban row house front is parallel to the street and shares sidewalls with its neighbors, giving it a narrow, rectangular footprint and only two facades. Generally, it is one or two rooms wide but varies in depth and height.

Certain features of the row house are timeless. It has housed the entire socioeconomic spectrum and thus ranges from luxurious in size and appointments to small and functional. Although it remained essentially a static, relatively rigid form until this past century, it has been affected by changes in architectural styles and societal needs in ways similar to freestanding homes. It is cheaper to build and easier to maintain, and its street access keeps residents attuned to their neighborhood. Its efficient land use and sense of private space make it an attractive alternative

to higher-density apartment blocks. It has consistently fought the idea that attached housing is less desirable than freestanding housing and in the final decades of the 20th century has experienced a renaissance as a solution to many housing issues in historic and newly developing cities around the world.

Formerly, row houses were built by individual owners or in groups by small-scale speculators. Twentieth-century row houses, however, were most commonly built in entire blocks or complexes by developers who included community facilities as part of the complex. Row houses were designed not as individual entities but as component parts of a larger whole and were seen in relation to the community at large. Despite this emphasis on the whole, market-driven builders still attempted to make attached houses individualized and private by varying the facades, building materials, floor plans, and home sizes from unit to unit and minimizing intrusions from neighbors. There was increased attention to row house surroundings as well. It became universal to provide each unit with private outdoor living spaces, such as patios, balconies, and gardens, and landscaping became a crucial part of town house design. Access to services and private garages was provided by alleys linked to the urban street grid.

The form of the 20th-century row house had infinite variations defined by local or regional preferences or characterized by broader architectural design trends. Those built as urban in-fill often attempted to blend in by echoing older houses in scale, materials, and orientation, but architects emphasized individuality by varying the facades or staggering the houses by height or setback. As many were built in suburban areas, the row house form was liberated in these more expansive settings from the gridlike plots of city streets. Traditional straight rows continued, but circles, clusters, steps, and curves were common as well. Groups of houses were often designed to follow the topography of their location, rising up hillsides or curving along a shoreline, as seen in San Francisco or Miami. The shape of each house unit itself varied widely, from a plain gabled block to such extremes as a trapezoid or even a tilted cube, as in Piet Blom's Pole Houses (1978–84) near Rotterdam. The widespread adoption of central heating and electricity enabled open floor plans designed to meet the needs of different populations. Interior space was greatly expanded by the use of split-level floor plans. Large windows and glass walls brought in more air and light than ever before. Another universal change was the addition of the garage, as convenient parking was a much-desired amenity after the automobile was made affordable to the middle classes. Initially, the garage was tucked under or behind the house, but more recently it has become part of the ground-level facade. In terms of style, eclecticism was mixed with pure form; 20th-century row houses expressed all the major architectural trends of the century and admixtures thereof and were designed by idealistic architects and profit-minded developers alike.

Twentieth-century changes in society and land use have had an immeasurable impact on the row house, which diverged dramatically from its constricted plan and adapted itself to both city and suburban lifestyles with astonishing flexibility. Initially, its popular image was negative, as older row house neighborhoods became slums and the attached house seemed to connote an undesirable ethic. The vast spread of suburbs and commuter culture led to the building of millions of detached homes across the countryside while row houses were left behind in the cities to deteriorate. Although innovative row house designs were explored in prewar Europe and working-class row houses were still built in growing cities, the form was obsolete elsewhere. Urban-renewal efforts in the 1960s led to the razing of entire row house neighborhoods in favor of high-rise public housing, seen as the best way to house the inner-city poor. By the 1980s, however, social reformers concluded that this housing type bred crime, misery, and a sense of isolation, and soon many cities began tearing down the high-rise projects and replacing them with new row houses.

The rediscovery of the row house was not limited to public housing, however. By the 1970s, faced with environmental conservation efforts and rising land costs, developers began to reconsider town houses as a commercially viable option. The row house lent itself nicely to the concept of a condominium development, which gave it a more upscale image, and increasing concerns about sprawl have made town house communities a popular option. Greater appreciation of historic town houses has added to the appeal of new ones. Vacation homes have become another force behind the row house revival, as many resort developments were restricted in size because of land conservation and higher-density attached housing was needed to shelter increasing numbers of vacationers.

Finally, changes in the traditional family unit also supported town house developments, with increasing numbers of single people, divorced parents, childless couples, and retirees seeking smaller-sized homes. For many members of these groups, a row house fulfills the need for one's own house and garden while providing certain amenities not found in a detached home. Increased security, decreased maintenance, lower costs, and a feeling of community among neighbors are common motivations. Many architects designed successful town house communities by targeting these demographic groups, adapting the once-inflexible row house to meet highly specific needs.

KATHERINE LARSON FARNHAM

Further Reading

Most relatively recent books about 20th-century row houses study them in conjunction with other forms of conjoined or community housing and view them through both architectural and sociological lenses. The following resources document and critique numerous examples of row houses and their uses worldwide.

Architectural Record, *Apartments and Dormitories*, New York: Dodge, and McGraw-Hill, 1958; new edition, as *Apartments, Townhouses, and Condominiums*, New York: McGraw-Hill, 1975

Binney, Marcus, *Town Houses: Urban Houses from 1200 to the Present Day*, New York: Whitney Library of Design, 1998; as *Town Houses: Evolution and Innovation in 800 Years of Urban Domestic Architecture*, London: Mitchell Beazley, 1998

Mackay, David, *Multiple Family Housing: From Aggregation to Integration*, London: Thames and Hudson, and New York: Architectural Book, 1977

Murray, James A. and Henry Fliess, *Family Housing: A Study of Horizontal Multiple Housing Techniques*, Ottawa: Canadian Housing Design Council, 1979

Nolon, John R. and Duo Dickinson, *Common Walls/Private Homes: Multiresidential Design*, New York: McGraw-Hill, 1990

Peters, Paulhans, *Häuser in Reihen: Mehrfamilienhäusen, Kettenhäusen, Häusegruppen*, Munich: Callwey, 1973

Vance, Mary A., *Row Houses: A Bibliography*, Monticello, Illinois: Vance Bibliographies, 1988

ROWE, COLIN 1920–99

Architecture historian and critic, England

Colin Frederick Rowe was born in 1920 in Rotherham, Yorkshire. He studied architecture at the Liverpool School of Architecture and wrote a thesis on the unpublished drawings of Inigo Jones under Rudolf Wittkower at the Warburg Institute. His studies with Rudolf Wittkower led to his coming into a Palladian inheritance, but his fascination with Palladio was not that of an art historian but that of an architect who saw in Palladio's use of harmonic proportions a series of clues that could be exploited to imbue all plans with intellectual qualities.

In 1951, Rowe was awarded a Fulbright Scholarship for study in the United States and at Yale University was able to work with Henry Russell Hitchcock. Hitchcock raised his interest in the transformations by which modernism developed out of 19th-century architecture. He also communicated his enthusiasm for walking in the city, whether it was New York or London, examining the evidence as it presented itself to the eye. This immediacy had a lot to do with Rowe's appeal, and it is also represented in both his writing and his lecturing style, which tended toward the conversational.

Between 1952 and 1953, Rowe traveled in the United States and worked in Vancouver with Sharp, Thompson, Berwick and Pratt on the Blue Cross Building and on Bakersfield Junior College in Los Angeles; he also traveled in Mexico and between 1953 and 1956 was at the University of Texas, Austin, where he taught for five semesters, collaborating with the design teacher Bernhard Hoesli and creating an entirely new framework for teaching architectural design. His brief intervention at Austin created the legend of the Texas Rangers, a band of teachers who saw a way of teaching modernity consistent with traditional architectural principles.

Between 1958 and 1962, Rowe was a lecturer at Cambridge University. There, Peter Eisenman fell under his spell and was induced to study Terragni closely and to become interested in Italian mannerism. Rowe's enthusiasm for the inherent contradictions that made Italian mannerism, allied to frequent trips to Italy, created something of a legend, and when he came to inhabit the Palazzo Massimi during a spell running the Rome program of Cornell University, it seemed perfectly appropriate, a personal apotheosis.

From 1962, Rowe was professor of architecture at Cornell, took up residence in Ithaca, and remained there as a teacher until his retirement. Under his influence, a whole generation of students at Cornell learned about the social nature of city space, well before it became a new orthodoxy, the inspiration for New Urbanism. For example, in the Manhattan Project of 1966, organized by Peter Eisenman's Institute for Architecture and Urban Studies, Rowe suggested that the city would be better approached not as a series of individual object buildings but as a basic ground—the city fabric—like a field of standing corn waiting to have spaces made in it. His approach was undoubtedly influenced by his experience of Italian cities, where the still-vital tradition of the *passagiatta* continued to represent the popular appeal of city space. This acute sense of the space as social conferred on Rowe's whole view of architecture an important freedom from the traditional art-historical approach.

It was Rowe's peculiar virtue to imbue the present moment of creation with an excitement derived from past moments of creation, and students were often sent to the library to check out the plan of a Palladian villa before drawing up their plan for a secondary school. In his very personal method of analyzing architecture as a sourcebook of new ideas, Rowe imbued Le Corbusier with a style that he hardly deserved. By the same token, architecture of any period could be scrutinized for its potential as idea. He never lost his sense of architecture as a unique form of mental activity: a story of how thought and feeling can imprint themselves on inert material. Without adopting any fashionable theory, he drew attention to the psychological dimension in architectural form, and without ever managing his career, he conveyed possibilities that have changed the course of architecture in England and in America.

Rowe was attracted by the openness of American society (he became an American citizen in 1984) and by the extraordinary effect that this freer horizon had on architectural models imported from Europe. During his five semesters at the University of Texas, Austin, he not only revolutionized the teaching of architectural design by bringing in European models but also alerted Americans to their own heritage by his praise for the city of Lockhart and generally by pointing to the continuity in the American revitalization of the classical and the dynamic quality of American settlements.

Rowe's life as a scholar was bent on the discoveries that come only through close reading. A master of hermeneutics, he was not intimidated by cultural studies and preferred to ignore "the whole semiology thing." His first essay, "The Mathematics of the Ideal Villa" (*Architectural Review*, 1947), remains in some ways his best, but all his writing was tremendous in showing how modern architecture, just as clearly as classical architecture, can be understood through the subtleties of form that it employs. In this way, he established a crucial continuity in architectural culture.

In 1981, Rowe was awarded the American Institute of Architects' Topaz Award for services to teaching. In 1985, he was awarded the Andrew Dickson White Professorship in architecture at Cornell and became emeritus in 1990. After retirement, he resided for a time in London, bemoaning the death of James Stirling, whose "education" he had intended to complete. Bereft of old friends, he returned to Washington. In 1995, he received the Royal Institute of British Architect's Gold Medal. His books include *The Mathematics of the Ideal Villa, and Other Essays* (1976), *Collage City* (1978, with Fred Koetter), *The Architecture of Good Intentions* (1994), and *As I Was Saying* (three volumes, 1996). He died in 1999 in Washington, DC.

ROBERT MAXWELL

See also **Hitchcock, Henry-Russell (United States); Institute for Architecture and Urban Studies; Stirling, James (Great Britain)**

Selected Publications

"Introduction" in *Five Architects: Eisenman, Graves, Gwathmey, Hejduk, Meier*, 1975
The Mathematics of the Ideal Villa, and Other Essays, 1976

Collage City (with Fred Koetter), 1978
"Introduction" in *James Stirling, Buildings and Projects*, by Peter
    Arnell and Ted Bickford, 1984
The Architecture of Good Intentions, 1994
As I Was Saying, 3 vol., 1996

Further Reading

Caragonne, Alex, *The Texas Rangers: Notes from the Architectural
    Underground*, Cambridge, Massachusetts: MIT Press, 1995

ROYAL INSTITUTE OF BRITISH ARCHITECTS (RIBA)

The Royal Institute of British Architects (RIBA) began its life
in 1834 under the name "Institute of British Architects." After
a Royal Charter was obtained from William IV in 1837, the
term "Royal" was added, and the purpose of the RIBA was clearly
expressed: "(for) the general advancement of Civil Architecture
and for promoting and facilitating the acquirement of the knowledge of the various Arts and Sciences connected therewith."

During the period from 1834 to 1900, most of the structure
and workings of the 20th-century RIBA were put into place.
Its Register of Architects, Architectural Library and Drawings
Collection, Competitions Committee, Professional Practice
Committee, Qualification Examinations, Scale of Charges, Code
of Professional Conduct, membership rules, and publication of
building contracts were all established during this time.

Architectural examinations became a compulsory condition
of RIBA membership in 1882, but it was not until 1905 that the
RIBA adopted the policy of statutory (rather than discretionary)
registration of architects. This policy move was brought on by
pressure from the Society of Architects, a body formed in 1884
by dissatisfied RIBA members. The Society of Architects and
the RIBA later merged in 1925.

In 1931, a competition was held to design the national headquarters of the RIBA on Portland Place in London. This competition was won by George Grey Wornum (1888–1957), and the
building opened in 1934. The building's appearance is very
much a product of its time period: not quite completely modernist—instead, a rather stripped-down classicism bordering on Art
Deco in its subtle usage of a limited palette of materials, generous
proportions, and low-relief sculpture. The RIBA's London
Headquarters, however, does befit a building representing a
professional body: it is prominently located on the corner of
Portland Place and Devonshire Street and contains the RIBA's
library, a large auditorium, a bookshop, several sizes of gallery
spaces, and the RIBA's administrative offices, all organized
around a central main stairway.

One of the most significant changes to the RIBA in the 20th
century was the Architects' Registration Act, which came into
force on 1 January 1932. This took the responsibility for the
architects' register away from the RIBA and gave it to a newly
formed Architects Registration Council of the United Kingdom
(ARCUK). This separation of duties came about because the
RIBA was beginning to be seen by the government less like
the representative body of the profession and more as merely a
"gentleman's club." It was thought that if the register were kept
separately from the RIBA, then the public's interests would be
better served.

The RIBA, however, still maintained control over professional examinations and the schools of architecture that were
accredited to conduct them. This division of labor is completely
opposite to the situation in the United States, where the National
Council of Architectural Registration Boards (NCARB) is responsible for architectural examinations and the American Institute of Architects (AIA) for professional registration. Membership in the RIBA (of which registration with ARCUK is
mandatory) gives an architect the right to call him- or herself a
"chartered architect," whereas registration with the ARCUK allows only for the title "registered architect."

The years following World War II saw a large increase in the
number of architects in England to match the increased amount
of construction, especially in the area of public housing. A widening of architects' responsibilities also occurred. In addition
to the traditional roles of building designer and construction
manager, British architects began to take leading roles in processes from large-scale town planning to smaller-scale furniture
design. During this time, the RIBA focused its attention mainly
on influencing the way that architects functioned and were
treated. Topics such as fee scales, salaries, government interference, economic fluctuations, and the promotion of "good" architecture were addressed and attempted to be regulated.

In 1969, three separate companies owned by the RIBA were
formed to provide additional services for RIBA members above
those provided by membership fees. RIBA Publications Ltd is-
sues legal and professional documents used by architects and the
construction industry and also runs the RIBA Bookshops in
London, Manchester, Leeds, Birmingham, and Belfast. RIBA
Services Ltd provides technical and other services, such as the
RIBA Product Selector, Office Library Service, Conference and
Exhibition Service, Appointments (Employment) Bureau, and
RIBA-approved Building Site Signboards. Finally, National
Building Specifications Ltd publishes specification documents
to be used in conjunction with professional contracts. The own-
ership of these companies was transferred to a holding company,
RIBA Companies Ltd, in 1985.

The British economic boom of the 1980s, combined with
government policies that decreased social architecture expenditure, saw many British architects move away from jobs with local
government authorities and into the private sector. During this
same time period, the RIBA was forced by the Thatcher government to change its standard fixed-percentage scale of charges
from "mandatory" to "recommended." The result was a more
competitive atmosphere in which architects began undercutting
each other in hopes of a commission—devaluing the knowledge,
skill, and experience that a professional architect possesses.

During the 1990s, the RIBA endeavored to become more
open to its members and the general public. The most physical
result of this campaign was renovating and restyling its London
headquarters; incorporating a privately run cafe, a new bookstore, additional gallery space, and handicapped access; and
founding an Architecture Center open to the public. In 1995,
the RIBA introduced a program of compulsory Continuing
Professional Development for its members, similar to the AIA's
Continuing Education System (CES), in which members must
periodically update their knowledge of professional and technical
issues to keep abreast of new developments.

In 1993, a report to the Department of the Environment
recommended abolishing architects' statutory registration with

ARCUK and ending the protection of the title "architect." These recommendations did not come to be. Instead, in 1997, ARCUK was changed to the "Architects Registration Board" (ARB), a majority of whose council members are external lay members (nonarchitects). The consequences of this on the RIBA is yet to be seen in the 21st century.

CHRISTOPHER WILSON

Further Reading

Kaye, Barrington, *The Development of the Architectural Profession in Britain: A Sociological Study*, London: Allen and Unwin, 1960

Royal Institute of British Architects, *The RIBA: Organisation and Functions*, London: RIBA Publications, 1992

Saint, Andrew, *The Image of the Architect*, New Haven, Connecticut: Yale University Press, 1983

RUDOLPH, PAUL 1918–97

Architect, United States

The American architect Paul Marvin Rudolph is best known for his large-scale, rough-surfaced concrete buildings of the 1960s. His architecture, inspired by the postwar work of Le Corbusier and Frank Lloyd Wright, is often confused with the Brutalism practiced by the Smithsons and theorized by Reyner Banham. Along with Eero Saarinen, Philip Johnson, Edward Durell Stone, and Minoru Yamasaki, Rudolph rejected functionalism in favor of a highly expressionist architecture based on historical precedents. He turned away from the Bauhaus-derived values that he had learned from Walter Gropius at Harvard University's Graduate School of Design in an attempt to reconcile Wright and Le Corbusier to produce a monumental, urban architecture. Rudolph's architecture is one of the most complete expressions of the humanistic and often heroic ambitions of postwar American architecture.

During the late 1950s and early 1960s, Rudolph was internationally acclaimed as one of the most imaginative heirs to the first generation of modernists. He was widely emulated for his boldly graphic drawing style, which emphasized the section, and for the rugged surfaces of his buildings. Rudolph accomplished a great deal in a short period of time, but by the early 1970s his highly ambitious works had fallen out of favor with the rise of Postmodernism, and he received little notice afterward.

As chairman of Yale University's architecture department (1958–65), Rudolph made it one of the most important American architectural schools of the decade. He was well regarded as a teacher, attracted top students, and fostered an Anglo-American axis that introduced such important figures to the United States as James Sterling, Colin St. John Wilson, and the Smithsons to serve as critics and teachers at Yale. Most remarkably, he was the architect of his own school, Yale's Art and Architecture Building (1958–64), which is among the most controversial of the large-scale concrete buildings of the 1960s.

Born in 1918 in the small town of Elkton, Kentucky, to the family of a Methodist minister, Rudolph spent his formative years not far from the public works projects of the Tennessee Valley Authority in the mountainous region where Alabama, Kentucky, and Tennessee intersect. He excelled in music and art. A formative experience was seeing Frank Lloyd Wright's Usonian Rosenbaum House (1939) in Florence, Alabama. As an undergraduate from 1935 to 1940, Rudolph studied architecture at the Alabama Polytechnic Institute (now known as Auburn University), where he received a Beaux-Arts education and first noted the potential that the regional buildings of the Deep South had for modern architecture. Rudolph's talents were recognized, and he received a scholarship from Harvard's Graduate School of Design, newly reorganized under Joseph Hudnot and Walter Gropius.

Before matriculating at Harvard in 1941, in 1939 Rudolph journeyed south to see Wright's Florida Southern College in Lakeland, Florida, which would inform many of his later campus designs. In Florida, Rudolph met Ralph Twitchell, an architect who was building beach houses in nearby Sarasota based on Wright's Usonian designs. Rudolph worked briefly with Twitchell before leaving for Harvard in the fall of 1941. There, he studied under Walter Gropius and Konrad Wachsman and made the acquaintance of students who would become his lifelong colleagues, such as I.M. Pei and, most significant, Philip Johnson.

Rudolph spent most of World War II supervising ship construction in the Brooklyn Navy Yards, where he recognized the significance of the new wartime materials and developed his unique drawing style. After the war, Rudolph completed his degree in just one semester (1947), traveled to Europe on a prestigious Wheelwright Fellowship (1948–49) from Harvard, and entered into a partnership with Ralph Twitchell in Florida. In Sarasota, Rudolph's design talents complemented Twitchell's salesmanship to produce between 20 and 30 eloquent, structurally expressive beach houses. These houses received international attention, mainly because of Rudolph's innovative graphic presentation. His pen-and-ink chiaroscuro-like style was instantly recognizable and easily reproduced in architectural journals. Twitchell and Rudolph's best-known house was the Cocoon, or Healey Guest House (1948), which used cocoon—a preservative plastic spray used to mothball ships in the Brooklyn Navy Yards—to create a dramatic catenary roof.

Always intensely individualistic, Rudolph began his own practice in 1952. At the same time, he renounced Gropius's concept of "teamwork" and the functionalism that he had been taught at Harvard. He lectured extensively in architecture schools throughout the United States and soon formulated a philosophy that reacted against functionalism in favor of the expressionism that he would adhere to for life. In his 1956 lecture and article, "The Six Determinants of Architectural Form," Rudolph said that in addition to function, architects should consider the importance of environment (by which he meant surroundings rather than a concern for nature), regionalism, materials, psychology, and spirit of the times.

An early advocate of urbanism, Rudolph attempted to integrate his buildings into the preexisting conditions of the site, as in his first major public commission, the Mary Cooper Jewett Arts Center (1958) in Wellesley, Massachusetts. His early efforts were often classed with the formalist or eclectic work of Philip Johnson, Minoru Yamasaki, and Edward Durell Stone. The Jewett Center featured screens in the manner of Stone and received widespread acclaim for the sensitive manner in which it dealt with the problem of inserting a modern structure into a historic campus. Before the project was completed, Rudolph was named chairman of Yale's architecture department at the age of 39.

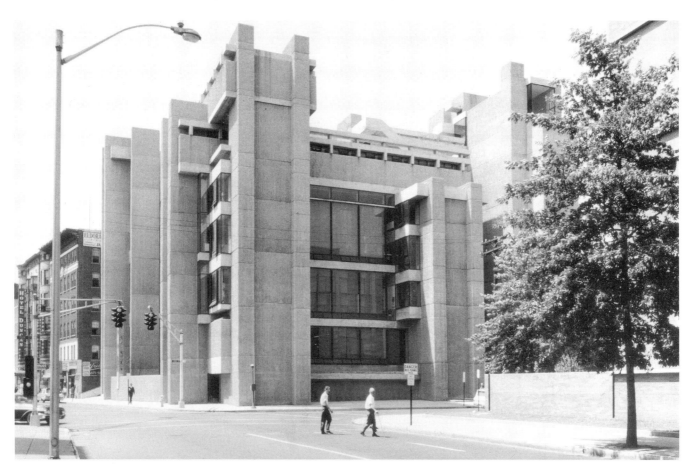

Yale University Art and Architecture Building, New Haven, Connecticut. Designed by Paul Rudolph (1964)
© G.E. Kidder-Smith, courtesy of Kidder Smith Collection, Rotch Visual Collections, M.I.T.

Soon after, Rudolph received the commission for Yale's Art and Architecture Building (1958–64), a building that would unite the teaching of the arts in one monumental structure in fulfillment of many of Rudolph's developing ideas about urbanism. The building was a monumental gateway marking the western edge of the campus. It was the culmination of a processional that led the pedestrian from the New Haven Green past Yale's earlier arts building, among them Louis Kahn's Yale University Art Gallery (1955). The rough-edged, corduroy-like exterior was achieved by first pouring the concrete into forms and then breaking the ridged edges with a bush hammer to create an irregular outline that would cast an ever-changing play of shadows across the facade. Although it was similar to Le Corbusier's *beton brut*, this method was actually derived from the precisely rendered parallel lines in Rudolph's pen-and-ink drawings. The building resembled both Le Corbusier's La Tourette (1955) and Wright's then recently demolished Larkin Building (1903).

However, in violation of the established norms of modernism, the labyrinthine interior seemed to have little relation to the exterior. The 36 or so different levels were arranged in a pinwheel-like form around two double-height central spaces containing a drafting room and jury pit. The building was topped by a glamorous penthouse that housed visiting lecturers

and critics overnight. The sublimely gloomy, cavernous interior spaces disconcerted many who thought that they were more like a glimpse into the maker's unconscious than a rational design for a school for the arts. Rudolph carpeted the building in a startling bright orange and decorated the interior with works of art, including a curtain by the abstract expressionist artist Willem de Kooning.

Critics such as Nikolaus Pevsner, who still upheld the Bauhaus as the norm, warned students in a dedication speech not to emulate so individualistic a building. Charles Jencks labeled the building "camp"—the exaggerated homosexual style first theorized by Susan Sontag in her 1961 essay, "Notes on 'Camp.'"

Camp, however, was precisely the point. With its intricate interiors and decorative use of Beaux-Arts plaster casts and ornamental fragments from demolished Louis Sullivan buildings, the interior of the building can be interpreted as a product of the homosexual camp, also practiced by Philip Johnson at this time, that reacted against the normative conditions enforced by postwar modernism and society. Most remarkably, the rough-edged concrete surfaces found both inside and out gave the building an aura of aggression that had as much to do with the hypermasculinization of postwar homosexual culture (e.g. the interest

in bodybuilding and male figures of rebellion, such as James Dean and Marlon Brando) as it did with anything found in the culture of architecture. Vincent Scully said that the roughened surfaces were sadomasochistic. "The building repels touch: it hurts you if you try," he wrote in *Architectural Review* in 1964. Rudolph intended his surfaces to be a statement in favor of decoration and expression—qualities long repressed by the Modern movement—and against the alienation and corporate conformity of the slick, glass-walled structures of the International Style.

Although it was soon called "Brutalist," the building's highly aestheticized values were in fact the diametric opposite of the British Brutalism practiced by the Smithsons. In fact, Banham said that the Art and Architecture building had nothing to do with his definition of Brutalism. The building was actually the culmination of the monumental, heroic humanism of the 1950s practiced in the United States. It was the final project of Yale President A. Whitney Griswold's campaign to create for Yale a museum of modern architecture with buildings by Eero Saarinen, Philip Johnson, and others that would defend the liberal arts against the sciences and mass culture.

The accidental burning of the building in 1969 at the height of student unrest and the apocrypha that this has generated has unfortunately overshadowed Rudolph's other achievements. Leaving Yale in 1965 for private practice, Rudolph began a series of campus buildings and master plans in a similar vein, among them the Charles Dana Arts Center (1963–66) at Colgate University in Hamilton, New York; the chapel and master plan for the Tuskegee Institute (1958–69) in Tuskegee, Alabama; the Boston Government Services Center (1962–71); and the master plan for a campus that he regarded as the most complete expression of his ideas: the University of Massachusetts (1963–72) in Dartmouth. An idea for which Rudolph is rarely given credit was the development of a rough-surfaced, mass-produced concrete block ubiquitous in American construction during the 1970s that economically imitated the effects of his bush hammer construction.

By the early 1970s, Rudolph's monumental projects had fallen out of favor with clients who thought that they were expensive and impractical and with a younger generation that now saw them as representing the Establishment. A casualty of state politics, the University of Massachusetts campus was taken away from Rudolph and completed by others, and the Boston Government Services Center—intended to house the health, education, and welfare bureaucracy of the Great Society—was never completed. This virtual ruin became a symbol of the demise of the liberal idealism of the 1960s after the political and economic disarray of the early 1970s. The chorus of critical voices that had begun to turn against Rudolph culminated with the publication in 1972 of Robert Venturi, Steven Izenour, and Denise Scott Brown's unfavorable comparison in *Learning from Las Vegas* between his Crawford Manor Housing for the Elderly (1962–66) in New Haven, Connecticut, and Venturi and Rauch's Guild House (1960–63) in Philadelphia, Pennsylvania. Ironically, Rudolph had hired Venturi to teach at Yale, and there were many similarities between their ideas.

During the 1970s and 1980s, Rudolph returned to practicing architecture in an austere, almost 19th-century atelier-like environment. He maintained rigorous control of his drawings as the key to his creativity and produced two important private works:

the Bass House (1970–72) in Fort Worth, Texas, a large villa that combined elements of Wright's Fallingwater with the lightweight architecture of the 1920s and 1930s, and his own multilevel private penthouse apartment (1977–97) on Manhattan's Beekman Place, a sybaritic fun house of multiple layers and transparent Plexiglas surfaces derived from his drawing methods and designed to accommodate his roving, homoerotic gaze.

In the 1980s, Rudolph embarked on an ambitious new career in Southeast Asia as the designer of a series of startling sculptural skyscrapers in Hong Kong, Singapore, and Jakarta. These buildings were infrequently published and seen by few in the West, thus giving rise to the myth that Rudolph was inactive. By the late 1980s, however, Rudolph had developed a devoted following among critics such as Michael Sorkin, who saw Rudolph as the last holdout against Postmodernism at a time when many of his contemporaries had turned their backs on their modernist past. Few acknowledged that Rudolph's reaction against functionalism and the International Style had in fact informed Postmodernism, particularly the branch theorized by Venturi.

Rudolph died in 1997 just at the moment when his architecture was undergoing a reappraisal by subsequent generations. He left behind a remarkably varied group of students in the United States and Britain who have become the leading practitioners of the last quarter of the century: Stanley Tigerman, Robert A.M. Stern, Charles Gwathmey, Der Scutt, Sir Norman Foster, and Richard Rogers.

TIMOTHY M. ROHAN

Biography

Born in Elkton, Kentucky, 23 October 1918, the son of a Methodist minister. Attended Alabama Polytechnic Institute (now Auburn University) 1935–40; studied under Walter Gropius at the Graduate School of Design, Harvard University, fall 1941. War years were spent as a lieutenant supervising ship construction in the Brooklyn Navy Yards. Returned to Harvard and received master's degree in 1947. Winner of a Harvard Wheelwright Fellowship for travel 1948–49. Chairman Yale University's School of Architecture 1958–65: pupils included Stanley Tigerman, Robert A.M. Stern, Charles Gwathmey, Der Scutt, Sir Norman Foster, and Richard Rogers. Partners with Ralph Twitchell, Sarasota, Florida, 1947–52. Independent practice, 1952–97. Died in New York, 8 August 1997.

Selected Works

Rudolph's extensive archive of drawings and papers is now housed in the Library of Congress, Architecture, Design and Engineering Collection in the Division of Prints and Photographs. Rudolph gave several important drawings to the Museum of Modern Art, New York, as well.

Healey Guest House/Cocoon House, Siesta Key, Florida (with Ralph Twitchell), 1948
Mary Cooper Jewett Arts Center, Wellesley College, Wellesley, Massachusetts, 1958
Yale Art and Architecture Building, Yale University, New Haven, Connecticut, 1964
Crawford Manor Housing for the Elderly, New Haven, Connecticut, 1966
Charles A. Dana Creative Arts Center, Colgate University, Colgate, Massachusetts, 1966

Chapel and master plan for the Tuskegee Institute, Tuskegee, Alabama, 1969
Boston Government Services Center, Boston, 1971
Master plan and humanities building for the University of Massachusetts, Dartmouth, 1972
Bass House, Fort Worth, Texas, 1972
Paul Rudolph residence, Beekman Place, New York, 1977–97
Colonnade Condominiums, Singapore, 1987
Office headquarters for Dharmala Sakti, Jakarta, 1988
Bond Centre Office Towers, Hong Kong, 1988
Concourse Offices and Condominiums, Singapore, 1992

Selected Publications

"Walter Gropius—the Spread of an Idea," *L'architecture d'aujourd'hui* (February 1950) (special issue devoted to the work of Gropius and his students in the United States)
"The Six Determinants of Architectural Form," *Architectural Record* 120 (October 1956)
The Architecture of Paul Rudolph, with introduction by Sibyl Moholy-Nagy, captions by Gerhard Schwab, and comments by Paul Rudolph, 1970
"From Conception to Sketch to Rendering to Building" in *Paul Rudolph: Architectural Drawings*, edited by Yukio Futagawa, 1972

Further Reading

Banham, Reyner, *New Brutalism: Ethic or Aesthetic?* New York: Reinhold, 1966
Jencks, Charles, *Modern Movements in Architecture*, New York: Anchor, 1973; 2nd edition, London and New York: Penguin, 1985
Paul Rudolph: Drawings for the Art and Architecture Building at Yale, 1959–1963 (exhib. cat.), New Haven, Connecticut: Yale School of Architecture, 1988
Pevsner, Nikolaus, "Address Given at the Opening of the Yale School of Art and Architecture, 1963" in *Studies in Art, Architecture, and Design*, by Pevsner, volume 2, Princeton, New Jersey: Princeton University Press, New York: Walker, and London: Thames and Hudson, 1968; as *Studies in Art, Architecture, and Design: Victorian and After*, Princeton, New Jersey: Princeton University Press, and London: Thames and Hudson, 1982
Scully, Vincent, "Art and Architecture Building, Yale University," *The Architectural Review*, 135 (May 1964)
Smith, Charles R., *Paul Rudolph and Louis Kahn: A Bibliography*, Metuchen, New Jersey, and London: Scarecrow Press, 1987
Sorkin, Michael, "The Invisible Man" in *Exquisite Corpse: Writings on Buildings*, by Sorkin, London and New York: Verso, 1991
Stern, Robert A.M., "Yale, 1950–1965," *Oppositions*, 4 (October 1974)
Stoller, Ezra, *The Yale Art and Architecture Building*, New York: Princeton Architectural Books, 1999
Venturi, Robert, Denise Scott Brown, and Steven Izenour, *Learning from Las Vegas*, Cambridge, Massachusetts: MIT Press, 1972

RUSSIA AND SOVIET UNION

The origins of 20th-century Russian architecture derive not only from technological advances in construction at the turn of the century but also from a reaction to 19th-century Western eclectic styles that architects in St. Petersburg and Moscow applied profusely to the facades of apartment houses and commercial buildings. By the 1870s, there arose a national style based on decorative elements from medieval Muscovy as well as on motifs from folk art and traditional wooden architecture. Major examples of the Russian style in Moscow include the Historical Museum (1874–83), built on the north side of Red Square to a design by Vladimir Shervud (1833–97), and the Upper Trading Rows (1889–93) by Alexander Pomerantsev (1848–1918), assisted by the construction engineer Vladimir Shukhov (1853–1939). The influence of this historicism continued through the early 1900s as the "neo-Russian" component of the style moderne. Painters such as Viktor Vasnetsov (1848–1926), who created the entrance building at the Tretiakov Gallery (c.1905), and Sergei Maliutin (1859–1937) were particularly active in using traditional Russian decorative arts as part of a new architectural aesthetic.

The "new style," or style moderne, that arose in Russian architecture at the turn of the century included among its diverse sources the Arts and Crafts component of the Russian Revival style as well as Art Nouveau and the Vienna School. Its main emphasis was on the innovative use of materials such as glass, iron, and glazed brick in functional yet highly aesthetic designs. The style flourished above all in Moscow, where its leading practitioner was Fedor Shekhtel (1859–1926). Shekhtel worked primarily for patrons among Moscow's entrepreneurial elite, such as the extended Riabushinsky family. His most notable work was a mansion (1900–02) for Stepan Riabushinsky, which is rivaled by his more modernist design for the Alexandra Derozhinsky mansion (1901). Shekhtel also designed a number of commercial buildings and public buildings in Moscow, such as the Yaroslavl Railway Station.

Other leading architects of the early 20th century in Moscow include Lev Kekushev (1863–1919), Adolf Erikhson, and William Walcot (1874–1943). All three were involved in the prolonged construction of one of the largest and most significant moderne buildings in Russia: the Hotel Metropole (1899–1905). Like Shekhtel, both Kekushev and Walcot produced major examples of the modern style in the design of private houses for wealthy clients.

In St. Petersburg, the style moderne appeared primarily in the design of apartment complexes by architects. (St. Petersburg's relatively compact urban plan impeded the construction of detached private houses.) Yet, despite the rapid expansion of apartment space, the lack of adequate housing, particularly for workers, remained a major social problem. The style moderne also appeared in St. Petersburg's commercial buildings, such as the Singer Building (1902–04) on Nevsky Prospekt by Pavel Siuzor (1844–c.1919).

After 1905 the style moderne began to merge with a form of modernized classicism, known in Russia as *neoklassitsizm*. Architects in St. Petersburg were especially receptive to the neoclassical revival, and they applied it to almost every major structural type, including banks, department stores, apartment buildings, and private houses. One of the most accomplished and versatile architects in this style was Fedor Lidval (1870–1945), designer of the Hotel Astoria (1911–12).

In Moscow the most accomplished revivalist was Roman Klein (1858–1924), architect of the Museum of Fine Arts (1897–1912; known since 1937 as the Pushkin Museum) and the Muir and Mirrielees department store (1906–08). Although less prolific than Klein, other architects distinguished themselves in a more austere variant of the neoclassical revival for major office buildings in Moscow's commercial center. In contrast to

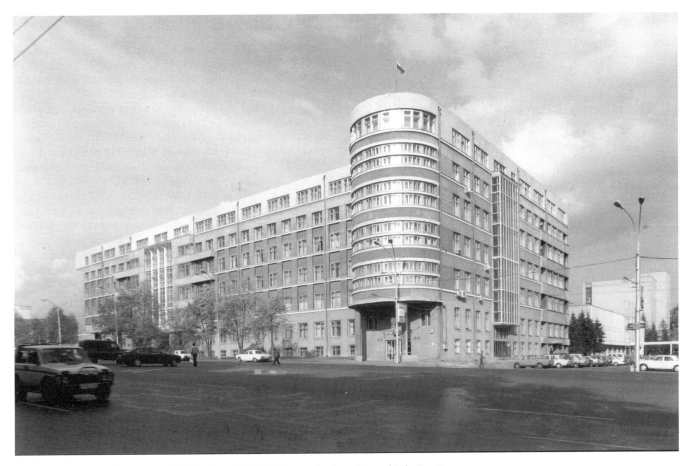

Territorial Executive Committee Building, by A.D. Kriachkov and others, Norosibirsk, Russia
© William C. Brumfield

their American contemporaries, Russian architects made little use of the skeletal frame in the design of large buildings, but they frequently applied new techniques of reinforced-concrete construction.

Russia's rapidly developing industrial base lay in a shambles after a war, a revolution, and a civil war; technological resources were extremely limited in what was still a mainly rural nation; and Moscow's population—poorly housed before the war—increased dramatically as the city became in 1918 the administrative center of a thoroughly administered state. One of the USSR's earliest edicts, in August 1918, repealed the right to private ownership of urban real estate. Even as the country plunged into civil war, groups of architects in Moscow and Petrograd (formerly St. Petersburg) designed workers' settlements that represent an extension of the Garden City movement which had already tentatively appeared in Russia during the decade before World War I.

The prerevolutionary building boom had established a viable foundation, in both architectural theory and practice, for urban development on a large scale. Furthermore, the Russian architectural profession was relatively intact after the emigration that decimated other areas of Russian culture after the revolution. In addition, the most prominent art and architectural schools in Moscow and Petrograd were capable of providing a base for the development of new cadres despite sometimes sweeping changes in the composition of the faculty. Nonetheless, there were enormous problems in resuscitating these institutions, of allocating resources for new construction, and of devising a plan for coordinating further development.

With the gradual recovery of the economy in the 1920s, bold new designs—often utopian in concept—brought the USSR to the attention of modern architects throughout the world. The assumption that a revolution in architecture (along with the other arts) would inevitably accompany a political revolution was soon put to the test by social and economic realities. The brief history of the Soviet avant-garde in architecture was marked by theoretical debates and factional disputes, such as that between rationalism and Constructivism. At the same time, the role of artists such as El Lissitzky, Kazimir Malevich, Vladimir Tatlin, and Nikolai Punin in defining new approaches to volume and structure had a profound impact on the conceptualization of avant-garde architecture.

Constructivism, the most productive modernist movement, adopted a rigorously functional approach to design that rejected "bourgeois" decorative effects and concentrated on clearly defined geometric volumes articulated on a monumental scale that expressed the ethos of the new state. Ironically, the backward condition of Soviet building technology in the 1920s often re-

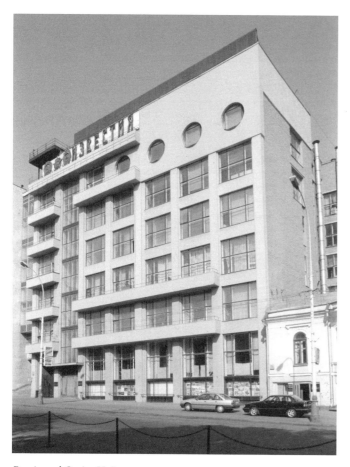

Russia and Soviet Union
Izvestiia Building, designed by Grigory Barkhin, Moscow (1925–27)
© William C. Brumfield

sulted in a primitive realization of those Constructivist projects that reached the stage of implementation.

In Moscow leading Constructivist architects and theoreticians included Moisei Ginzburg (1892–1946), whose most notable building was the apartment house (1928–30) for the People's Commissariat of Finance; Grigory Barkhin (1880–1969), designer of the Izvestiia Building (1925–27); Ilya Golosov (1883–1945), architect of the Zuev Workers' Club (1927–29); Panteleimon Golosov (1882–1945), author of the Pravda Building (1930–35); and the Vesnin brothers, Leonid (1880–1933), Viktor (1882–1950), and Alexander (1883–1959), architects of a number of major projects, such as the Likhachev Palace of Culture (1931–37), built for the workers of a large automobile factory.

These and other Constructivist projects in Moscow set a standard for functional design in administrative and apartment buildings as well as social institutions, such as workers' clubs. Another prominent modernist active during the same period but not a part of the Constructivist movement was Konstantin Melnikov (1890–1974), known for his designs for exposition pavilions, a number of workers' clubs (most notably the Rusakov Club, 1927–28), industrial structures such as the Leyland Bus

Garage (1926–27), and his own house (1927–29) in the Arbat district of Moscow.

Important projects by Constructivist architects also appeared in other Soviet cities, such as Leningrad, Kharkov, Gorky (Nizhnii Novgorod), Sverdlovsk (Ekaterinburg), and Novosibirsk. Notable examples in Leningrad include the Kirov District Soviet complex (1930–35), whose overall design was entrusted to the architect Noi Trotskii (1895–1940). Beginning in 1928, the five-year plans, with their emphasis on the rapid expansion of heavy industry, led to the massive rebuilding of industrial centers. In Kharkov, a massive complex of several buildings known as the State Industry Building (Gosprom, 1926–28) was designed by an architectural team headed by Sergei Serafimov (1878–1939). In Sverdlovsk, whose entire city center was redesigned with the participation of architects such as Moisei Ginzburg, a model housing development known as "Chekists' Village" (1929–38) was designed by I. Antonov, V. Sokolov, and A. Tumbasov. Industrial architecture also received much attention, as foreign architects such as Ernst May, Erich Mendelsohn, Hannes Meyer, and Albert Kahn collaborated with Soviet architects and engineers in creating mammoth industrial complexes. Theoreticians such as Ivan Leonidov (1902–59) developed concepts of the "linear city" for new industrial centers.

During the 1930s, more conservative trends asserted themselves in major buildings sponsored by the bureaucratic apparatus, as designs inspired by classical, Renaissance, and other historicist models received the party's approval. Prominent traditionalists, trained in the prerevolutionary neoclassical revival, included Ivan Zholtovskii (1867–1959), Aleksei Shchusev (1873–1949), and Noi Trotskii (1895–1940). Despite the formal break with Constructivism, earlier work by Shchusev and Trotskii belongs to the Constructivist movement, and other connections with the architecture of the 1920s continued throughout the 1930s. The grandomania of prewar Stalinist architecture is best expressed by the project for the Palace of the Soviets (1933–35) in Moscow, designed by Boris Iofan (1891–1976), Vladimir Gelfreikh (1885–1967), and Vladimir Shchuko (1878–1939). The structure was to be built on the site of the massive Cathedral of Christ the Savior (demolished in 1931), but the project was canceled in the late 1940s.

After World War II, architectural design became more firmly locked in traditional, often highly ornate eclectic styles, epitomized by the postwar skyscrapers in Moscow and other Soviet cities. Of the seven such towers in Moscow, the largest is the building of Moscow State University (1949–53) by Lev Rudnev (1885–1956), Pavel Abrosimov (1900–61), and Alexander Khriakov (1903–76). On this, as on several other projects during the Stalinist period, much of the construction was done by prison labor.

In the period following Stalin's death, in March 1953, a reassessment of priorities, particularly in regard to the housing crisis, led to a functionalism that had been among the goals of Soviet design and planning during the 1920s. Teams of engineers and architects began to produce standardized plans that could be applied with relatively simple technology, and the pursuit of a historical framework for architectural style was largely discarded, as indicated by the abolition of the Academy of Architecture in the early Khrushchev era. The acceleration of standardized construction achieved an impressive volume, first with five-story apartment buildings that appeared throughout the

country and subsequently with mass-produced buildings as high as 20 stories and, in rare cases, even higher.

The industrialization of building and the curbing of decorative pomposity produced a different set of problems. Apart from the general monotony of design, creative projects were constrained by the processes of standardized, "industrial" construction based on prefabricated modules or precast-concrete forms assembled on-site. The seams and cracks that resulted from such methods of assembly gave many buildings a shoddy appearance. Whatever the project type, Soviet architects were usually faced with a narrow range of options limited by mass-construction methods and meager financial resources.

Even showcase projects with considerable support shared in the general monotony. The most prolific practitioner of postwar Soviet modernism was Mikhail Posokhin (1910–89), who had collaborated in the design of a Stalinist apartment tower on Insurrection Square but shifted adroitly into the new functionalism of the Sputnik era. His design for the Kremlin Palace of Congresses (1959–61, in collaboration with A. Mndoiants and others) had the appearance of a modern concert hall of huge proportions, whose marble-clad rectangular outline was marked by narrow pylons—also faced with white marble—and multi-storied shafts of plate glass. The main virtue of its style was how relatively unobtrusively the large structure stood among the historic Kremlin ensemble, part of which had been destroyed in the 1930s.

Not all Soviet architecture of the modern period descended to nondescript conformity. Futuristic construction technology appeared in the Ostankino Television Tower (1967, N. Nikitin, L. Batalov, and others), a reinforced-concrete monolith of impressive design and engineering. The ferroconcrete shaft, 385 meters in height (on a foundation of only four meters), supports a steel-frame antenna superstructure that rises another 150 meters. Technological ingenuity also characterizes the design of many contemporary sports arenas, which, like television, served the regime's propaganda interests. Large stadium complexes began to take shape even in the late Stalinist period, such as Leningrad's Kirov Stadium (1950, A. Nikolskii and others) on Krestovskii Island and culminating with the Luzhniki stadium complex (1955–56, A. Vlasov and others) in south Moscow. The emphasis on the culture of sports, which reached a crescendo in the preparations for the 1980 Summer Olympics, produced some of the most interesting forms in contemporary Russian architecture. An example notable for its high technology and sweeping lines is the Velotrek bicycle racing stadium (1978–79, Natalia Voronina and others) in the west Moscow suburb of Krylatskoe, with a bifurcated roof composed of rolled-steel membranes four millimeters thick stretched between a pair of tilted elliptical arches supported by a truss frame system.

With the demise of the Communist system in the USSR, the revival of private practice in architecture seems likely to change the face of the profession, even as new problems arise in zoning, housing, and resource allocation. Foreign investment has encouraged the assimilation of Western commercial architecture, from modernism to postmodernism to deconstructivism. At the same time, historicist elements from Russian and even Stalinist architecture are being recycled in new projects for cities such as Moscow in order to achieve a distinctive, colorful urban environ-

ment. It would be premature to comment on the success of these efforts, but Russian architecture is rapidly regaining the variety that characterized it at the beginning of the 20th century.

WILLIAM C. BRUMFIELD

See also **Art Nouveau (Jugendstil); Constructivism; Golosov, Ilya (Russia); Leonidov, Ivan Ilich (Russia); Melnikov, Konstantin (Russia); Moscow, Russia; Shekhtel, Fedor (Russia); St. Petersburg, Russia; Vesnin, Alexander, Leonid, and Viktor (Russia)**

Further Reading

Modern Russian architecture and particularly the early Soviet avant-garde have received considerable attention from Western scholars, as well as from Russians. The following list is a sample of some of the more prominent works.

Barkhin, M.G., et al. (editors), *Mastera sovetskoi arkhitektury ob arkhitekture* (Masters of Soviet Architecture on Architecture), 2 vols., Moscow: Iskusstvo, 1975

Bliznakov, Milka, "The Realization of Utopia: Western Technology and Soviet Avant-Garde Architecture," in *Reshaping Russian Architecture: Western Technology, Utopian Dreams*, edited by William C. Brumfield, Cambridge and New York: Cambridge University Press, 1991

Borisova, Elena A., and Tatiana P. Kazhdan, *Russkaia arkhitketura kontsa XIX–nachala XX veka* (Russian Architecture of the End of the 19th Century and the Beginning of the 20th), Moscow: Izd-vo "Nauka," 1971

Brumfield, William C., *The Origins of Modernism in Russian Architecture*, Berkeley: University of California Press, 1991

———, *A History of Russian Architecture*, Cambridge and New York: Cambridge University Press, 1993

Cohen, Jean-Louis, *Le Corbusier et la mystique de l'USSR*, Brussels: Mardaga, 1987; as *Le Corbusier and the Mystique of the USSR*, translated by Kenneth Hylton, Princeton, New Jersey: Princeton University Press, 1991

Cooke, Catherine, *Russian Avant-Garde: Theories of Art, Architecture, and the City*, London: Academy Editions, 1995

Ginzburg, Moisei IAkovlevich, *Stil i epokha*, Moscow: Gosudarstvennoe Izdatelstvo, 1924; as *Style and Epoch*, translated and edited by Anatole Senkevitch, Jr., Cambridge, Massachusetts: MIT Press, 1982

IAralov, IUrii Stepanovich, compiler, *Zodchie Moskvy* (Architects of Moscow), edited by S.M. Zemtsov, 2 vols., Moscow: Moskovskii Rabochii, 1988

Khan-Magomedov, Selim O., *Pioneers of Soviet Architecture: The Search for New Solutions in the 1920s and 1930s*, translated by Alexander Lieven, edited by Catherine Cooke, New York: Rizzoli, and London: Thames and Hudson, 1987

Khazanova, V.E., *Sovetskaia arkhitektura pervykh let Oktiabria, 1917–1925 gg.* (Soviet Architecture of the First Years of October, 1917–1925), Moscow: Nauka, 1970

Lissitzky, El, *Russland: Architektur für eine Weltrevolution*, Berlin: Ullstein, 1965; as *Russia: An Architecture for World Revolution*, translated by Eric Dluhosch, Cambridge, Massachusetts: MIT Press, 1970

Lodder, Christina, *Russian Constructivism*, New Haven, Connecticut: Yale University Press, 1983

Riabushin, A.V., and N.I. Smolina, *Landmarks of Soviet Architecture, 1917–1991*, New York: Rizzoli, 1992

Starr, S. Frederick, *Melnikov: Solo Architect in a Mass Society*, Princeton, New Jersey: Princeton University Press, 1978

S

SAARINEN, EERO 1910–61

Architect, Finland

Eero Saarinen shared the same date of birth with his famous architect father, Eliel (20 August 1873 and 1910); both the elder and the younger Saarinen were and are very likely to remain the only father-son duo recipients of the Gold Medal of the American Institute of Architects.

The younger Saarinen was born in Kirkkonummi (Kyrksläte), Finland (then Russia) and grew up in the secluded retreat of "Hvitträsk," the home/studio where Eliel Saarinen entertained many of Finland's intellectuals and artists and produced ideas in architecture and planning. Saarinen attended high school at a special progressive school housed within the University of Michigan's School of Education (then nearby Baldwin High School in Birmingham, Michigan) and apprenticed in the Cranbrook architectural office from 1928 to 1931, taking eight months in Paris, France, beginning in late 1929 to study sculpture at the Académie de la Grande Chaumière. After his return to Cranbrook, Saarinen developed furniture designs from 1930 to 1931 that concurrently embraced a conscious variety of styles, from handicraft to an industrial aesthetic. He entered Yale University in the fall of 1931 and completed Yale's five-year program in three years.

With the award of a traveling fellowship, Saarinen visited Europe and the Near East and then worked in Finland, where he came in more direct contact with European modernism. Thus began his own synthesis of historic architecture and the progressive trends of technological innovation and its expression. On his return to the United States in 1936, Saarinen entered into a partnership with his father separate from Cranbrook (Eliel Saarinen and Eero Saarinen, 1936–42). Through small commissions, independent competition entries, and collaborations, he achieved national recognition for his American modernism. He briefly worked as a designer for the office of Norman Bel Geddes on the General Motors "Futurama" building for the 1939 New York World's Fair. In buildings such as the Kleinhans Music Hall (1938–41, with Kidd and Kidd) in Buffalo, New York, and Crow Island School (1940, with Perkins, Wheeler and Will of Chicago) in Winnetka, Illinois, as well as first place in the 1939 national competition for the Smithsonian Art Gallery (unexecuted), the Saarinens became synonymous with a progressive style free of the radical overtones of the International Style.

Charles Eames was among the younger designers with whom Eero collaborated, and their molded-plywood furniture designs for the "Organic Design in Home Furnishings" competition and exhibition at the Museum of Modern Art (1941) established their position among a new generation of modernists. World War II saw a number of transformations in their practice, changes that also represented the gradual independence of the son from the aesthetic dispositions of his father. It was at the end of this period that Eero's entry in the 1948 competition for the Jefferson National Expansion Memorial (St. Louis, Missouri) was awarded first prize (both father and son submitted designs under the firm name, resulting in a brief confusion as to the winner). Presenting a "Gateway to the West," its abstract 630-foot-high catenary-arch form combined symbolism with technological daring and structural innovation.

Saarinen's aesthetic took on its own character during the 1940s with buildings such as the suspended tensile-roof structure of the "Demountable Space"/Community House project (1941, with Ralph Rapson) for the United States Gypsum Company, the "Unfolding House" project (1943–44) based on trailer/containers, and the "Serving Suzy" restaurant project (1944) featuring a mobile food service for the Pittsburgh Plate Glass Company. Built works included the Opera-Concert Hall and Berkshire Music Center at Tanglewood (1940–41) in Stockbridge, Massachusetts (a structure that employed laminated wood arches and tensile rod–suspended roofs); the steel Case Study House #8 and #9 (1945–50, with Charles Eames; #9 built as John Entenza House) for *Arts & Architecture* in Pacific Palisades, California; and the lightweight Music Tent (1949, with Smith, Hegner and Moore, Associate Architects) for the Goethe Bicentennial Convocation Music Festival in Aspen, Colorado.

The most significant example of this evolution was the postwar, $100 million General Motors Technical Center (1951–56, designed with Smith, Hinchman and Grylls, Associate Architects) in Warren, Michigan. The initial scheme of 1945 combined familiar design motifs of Eliel Saarinen, such as the interplay between a horizontal space (the man-made lake) and the vertical accent of a water tower and the younger Saarinen's desire for industrial objects. After three years, a new scheme, influenced by Mies van der Rohe, was proposed. This included the use of a standard planning module and a new thin-skin technology for the building envelopes based on car-manufacturing techniques, including the innovation of neoprene gaskets for window installation, modeled on the system developed for car windshields. The GMTC plan formed the background of a portrait of Saarinen on the 2 July 1956 cover of *Time* magazine.

The 1950s saw work ranging from the reductivist, anonymous, and abstract, such as the visually neutral indeterminacy of the IBM Manufacturing Plant (1956–59) in Rochester, Minnesota, and the Bell Telephone Laboratories (1957–62) in Holmdel, New Jersey, to the evocative expressionism in the forms of the thin-shell Trans World Airlines (TWA) airport terminal (1956–62) in New York City and the suspended roof of the David S. Ingalls Hockey Rink (1956–59) at Yale University in New Haven, Connecticut.

Structure and construction were used to serve themes other than structure in Saarinen's search for form. Formal invention was paralleled by technical innovation, where technique and evocative imagery were often merged. Representation was manifested in metaphorical forms, most notably in the TWA terminal's evocation of a "bird in flight." The Ezra Stiles and Samuel F.B. Morse Colleges (1958–62) at Yale University consisted of injection-formed concrete walls that alluded to a medieval community of scholars. The campus of Concordia Lutheran Senior College (1953–59) in Fort Wayne, Indiana, represented a Scandinavian village. At the Massachusetts Institute of Technology in Cambridge, the Kresge Auditorium (1950–55) and MIT Chapel (1953–55) oppose the advanced thin-shell technology of the auditorium dome against the primal imagery of a closed brick cylinder placed in a circular moat for the chapel. His only tall building, the Columbia Broadcasting System Headquarters (1960–64) in New York City, was also the last design of his career. Its solid, masonry cladding proposed his first departure from the modernist glass box, where he alluded instead to the context of Manhattan.

PETER C. PAPADEMETRIOU

See also **Airport and Aviation Building; Concrete; Dulles International Airport, Chantilly, Virginia; Expressionism; Gateway Arch, St. Louis, Missouri; Saarinen, Eliel (Finland); Tensile Structures; TWA Airport Terminal, New York**

Biography

Born in Kikkonummi, Finland, 20 August 1910; emigrated to the United States 1923; naturalized 1940; son of architect Eliel Saarinen. Studied sculpture at the Académie de la Grand Chaumière, Paris 1929–30; studied architecture at Yale University, New Haven, Connecticut; bachelor's degree in fine arts 1934; received a Charles O. Matchum Fellowship for travel in Europe 1934–36. Worked in father's architectural practice, Ann Arbor, Michigan 1936–41; partner, with father and J. Robert Swanson, Saarinen, Swanson and Saarinen, Ann Arbor 1941–47; employed in the Office of Strategic Studies, Washington D.C. 1942–43; partner, Saarinen, Saarinen and Associates, Ann Arbor 1947–50. Principal, Eero Saarinen and Associates, Birmingham, Michigan from 1950. Fellow, American Institute of Architects; fellow, American Academy of Arts and Sciences. Gold Medal (posthumous), American Institute of Architects 1962. Died in Ann Arbor, 1 September 1961.

Selected Works

Smithsonian Institution Art Gallery (First prize, competition; unbuilt), Washington, D.C. (with Eliel Saarinen and J. Robert Swanson), 1939
Kleinhaus Music Hall, Buffalo, New York (with Eliel Saarinen), 1940
Crow Island School, Winnetka, Illinois (with Eliel Saarinen, Perkins, Wheeler and Will), 1940
Summer Opera House and Chamber Music Hall, Berkshire Music Center, Tanglewood, Massachusetts (with Eliel Saarinen), 1942
Kresge Auditorium and Chapel, Massachusetts Institute of Technology, Cambridge (with Anderson and Beckwith), 1955
General Motors Technical Center, Warren, Michigan (with Smith, Hinchman and Grylls), 1956
Concordia College, Fort Wayne, Indiana, 1958
IBM Manufacturing Plan, Rochester, Minnesota, 1959
Ingalls Hockey Rink, Yale University, New Haven, Connecticut, 1959
Samuel F.B. Morse and Ezra Stiles Colleges, Yale University, New Haven, Connecticut, 1962
Bell Laboratories, Holmdel, New Jersey, 1962
Dulles International Airport, Chantilly, Virginia (with Ammann and Whitney), 1962
Trans World Airlines Terminal, Idlewild (John F. Kennedy) Airport, New York, 1962
John Deere and Company Headquarters, Moline, Illinois, 1963
Jefferson National Expansion Memorial (First prize, 1948 competition), St. Louis, Missouri, 1964
Columbia Broadcasting System Headquarters, New York, 1964
St. Louis Arch, Missouri, 1968

Selected Publications

Eero Saarinen on His Work, edited by Aline B. Saarinen, 1962; revised edition, 1968

SAARINEN, ELIEL 1873–1950

Architect, Finland

Eliel Saarinen was a leading proponent of a humane approach to modernist architecture whose work was influential in bringing about a transition from the decorative obsession of Romantic Nationalist architecture to modernism. As designer and president of Cranbrook Academy (1932–50) in Bloomfield, Michigan, Saarinen had a significant impact on the teaching of architects and designers. Born in Rantsalami, Finland, the son of a highly educated and culturally aware Lutheran pastor, his early years were divided between rural towns and the city of Moscow. As a youth, Saarinen, who was impressed with the art of the

Hermitage in Moscow, was more devoted to painting than to his formal studies at the lyceum. In 1893, his devotion to painting led him to study painting at the University of Helsinki while simultaneously studying architecture at the Polytekniska Institutet (1893–97). In 1896, while still an architectural student, he formed a partnership with two fellow students, Herman Gesellius and Armas Lindgren. They quickly won first prize in the competition to build the Talberg Building (1897) in Helsinki. More significant prizes and commissions followed. A first prize in the competition to design the Finnish Pavilion for the Paris Exposition of 1900 brought the partnership critical acclaim in Europe. Compared with the pavilions of other nations, the Finnish Pavilion was simple in form and refined in its combination of restrained and appropriately Nordic ornamentation, including frescoes by Akseli Gallen-Kallela.

Saarinen's ability to spend the long hours necessary for solving complex architectural problems was the basis for his subsequent success. With his designs for the Helsinki and Viipuri Railroad Stations, he moved away from seeking a uniquely Finnish solution and toward International Style modernism, allowing function to play an ever-larger role in determining his architectural solutions. Never sacrificing functionality for avant-gardism, his urban planning designs for Helsinki, Canberra, and Chicago retained a concern for community and context. Although none of these large-scale plans was realized, Saarinen was able to put his planning skills to good use in his designs for Cranbrook Academy.

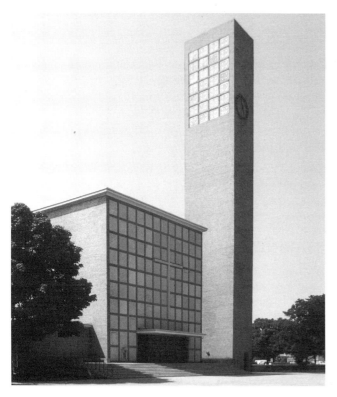

First Christian Church (originally the Tabernacle Church of Christ), (1942)
Photo © Mary Ann Sullivan

Saarinen's early architectural practice focused on defining and creating a Finnish style of architecture, giving focus to the notion of *Gesamtkunstwerk*, or the total work of art. Exteriors tended toward the rugged and plastically picturesque using local rusticated soapstone or granite. Interiors were richly detailed, with the partners attending to every detail, from the design of tiled stoves to decorative carvings, many of which were derived from Finnish culture or landscape. This interest in *Gesamtkunstwerk* led the firm to design and construct Hvitträsk (1901–03), a communal office and dwelling complex located 18 miles from Helsinki. At Hvitträsk, they emphasized a cultured rusticity with exposed-log interiors, copper fireplace hoods, exposed beams, and a functional approach to the arrangement of space. A log tower and effective placement on a sloping, dramatic site above White Lake (Hvitträsk) emphasized a romantic attachment to the wilderness of the northern forests. Even as Hvitträsk was under construction, the partnership, and eventually Saarinen on his own after the partnership began to dissolve in 1905, moved away from Romanticism toward greater simplicity of ornament and formal clarity. The rugged stone-and-log construction and informality of Hvitträsk gave way to the smoother stuccoed exterior and formality of the Molchow House (1905–07) in Mark-Brandenburg, Germany. Saarinen's designs for the Helsinki Railway Station provide an excellent opportunity to observe changes in his approach to design; the medieval-style tower and crenellations of his early drawings gave way to the simpler, more streamlined elevations of the final design. His final design for the Helsinki Railroad Station demonstrates his awareness of German architecture in general and the influence of Behrens in particular. Glass and concrete play a large role in his railroad station designs. At Viipuri, a large concrete barrel vault with minimal ornamentation dominated the interior of the station's main hall. Large windows above the main entrance created an overall feeling of openness and efficiency. Ornamented soapstone columns and oak furnishing balanced this emphasis on function with their tactility.

After the disruptions of the Russian Revolution and World War I, Saarinen's second-place finish in the competition for the Tribune Tower (1922) in Chicago brought him again into the architectural limelight. Shortly thereafter, he traveled to Chicago and was soon working on plans to develop the lakefront of Chicago. In 1924, Saarinen became a visiting professor of architecture at the University of Michigan. In 1925, he was asked by George G. Booth to develop educational plans for what would eventually include Cranbrook Academy. From 1925 to 1950, Saarinen was architect-in-residence, and in 1927 he became the chief architectural officer for Cranbrook. Designs for Cranbrook include the Cranbrook School for Boys (1926–30), the Saarinen Residence (1928–29), the Kingswood School for Girls (1929–30), the Institute for Science (1931–33), and the Museum and Library (1942–43). Saarinen's design for the Museum and Library structures connected by a peristyle exemplifies his later, more austere approach to design. Large functional spaces, straight lines, and geometric formal relationships and the wall of glass on the north face of the library connect Saarinen's design with the International Style. On the other hand, the choice of brick and stone, the abstract designs of the ceiling, the figurative sculpture of Carl Milles' *Orpheus Fountain* to the north of the peristyle, and attention to the relationship between landscaping

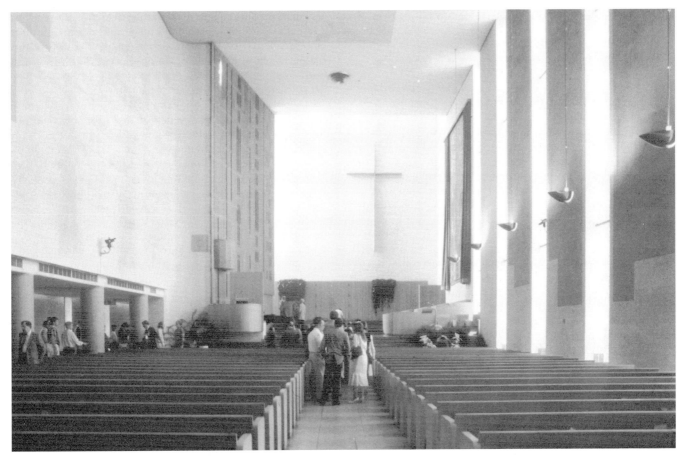

First Christian Church (originally the Tabernacle Church of Christ), interior (1942)
Photo © Mary Ann Sullivan

and structure maintain a humanity not always present in International Style architecture.

DOUGLAS CAMPBELL

See also **Finland; Helsinki Railway Station, Finland; International Style; Saarinen, Eero (Finland)**

Biography

Born in Rantasalmi, Finland, 20 August 1873; emigrated to the United States 1923; naturalized 1945. Studied painting at the University of Helsinki and architecture at the Polyteknista Institutet, Helsinki 1893–97; degree in architecture 1897. Married sculptor and weaver Loja Gesellius 1904: 2 children; son is architect Eero Saarinen. Partner, with Herman Gesellius and Armas Lindgren, Gesellius-Lindgren-Saarinen, Helsinki 1896–1905; partner, Gesellius-Saarinen, Helsinki 1905–07. Solo private practice, Helsinki 1907–23, Evanston, Illinois 1923–24, and Ann Arbor, Michigan 1924–27; collaborated with son, Ann Arbor 1937–41; partner, with son and J. Robert Swanson, Saarinen-Swanson-Saarinen, Ann Arbor 1941–47; partner, Saarinen, Saarinen and Associates, Ann Arbor from 1947. Visiting professor of architecture, University of Michigan, Ann Arbor 1924; director, 1925–32, president, 1932–50, director of the graduate department of architecture and city planning, 1948–50, Cranbrook Academy of Art, Bloomfield Hills, Michigan. Honorary member, Imperial Academy of Art, St. Petersburg 1906; honorary member, Deutsche Werkbund 1913; honorary member, Zentrale Vereinïgung der Architekten Österreichs, Vienna 1913; honorary member, Finnish Academy of Art 1920; honorary member, Society of Arts and Crafts, Budapest 1921; honorary member, Freie Deutsche Academie des Stadtebaues 1922; honorary member, Royal Institute of British Architects 1924; honorary member, Society of Finnish Architects 1930; honorary member, Architects' Society of Uruguay 1931; honorary member, Central Institute of Architects of Brazil 1931; chairman, City and Regional Planning Committee, American Institute of Architects 1935; fellow, American Institute of Architects 1944; academician, National Academy of Design, New York 1946. Commander First Class, Finnish Order of the White Rose 1925; Grand Cross, Finnish Order of the Lion 1946; Gold Medal, American Institute of Architects 1947. Died in Cranbrook Hills, 1 July 1950.

Selected Works

Tallberg Apartment Building (First prize, competition; with Herman Gesellius and Armas Lindgren), Helsinki, 1897

Finnish Pavilion, Paris Exposition (with Herman Gesellius and Armas Lindgren), 1900

Hvitträsk, Kirkkonummi (with Herman Gesellius and Armas Lindgren), 1903

Railway Station, Viborg, Finland, 1904

Molchow House, Remer Country Estate, Mark-Brandenburg, Germany (with Herman Gesellius), 1907

National Museum, Helsinki, 1912

Helsinki Railway Station, 1919

Tribune Tower (Second prize, competition), Chicago, 1922

Saarinen House, Bloomfield Hills, Michigan, 1929

Cranbrook School for Boys, Bloomfield Hills, 1930

Kingswood School for Girls, Cranbrook, Bloomfield Hills, 1930

Institute of Science, Cranbrook, Bloomfield Hills, 1933

Kleinhaus Music Hall, Buffalo, New York (with Eero Saarinen), 1940

Crow Island School, Winnetka, Illinois (with Eero Saarinen), 1940

Tabernacle Church of Christ, Columbus, Indiana (with Eero Saarinen), 1942

Museum and Library, Cranbrook Academy of Art, Bloomfield Hills, 1943

Selected Publications

Munksnas-Haga (with Gustaf Slerengall), 1915

The Cranbrook Development, 1931

The City: Its Growth, Its Development, Its Future, 1943

The Search for Form: A Fundamental Approach to Art, 1948; reprinted as *The Search for Form in Art and Architecture*, 1985

Further Reading

Eliel Saarinen: Projects, 1896–1923 provides extensive coverage of Saarinen's career prior to his move to the United States. Christ-Janer's book provides biographical material, catalogs his architectural works, and covers Saarinen's career as an architect and educator.

Christ-Janer, Albert, *Eliel Saarinen*, Chicago: University of Chicago Press, 1948; revised edition, as *Eliel Saarinen: Finish-American Architect and Educator*, 1984

Saarinen, Eliel, *The Saarinen Door*, Bloomfield Hills, Michigan: Cranbrook Academy of Art, 1963

Saarinen, Eliel, *Eliel Saarinen: Suomen-aika*, edited by Marika Hausen, Helsinki: Otava, 1990; as *Eliel Saarinen: Projects, 1896–1923*, translated by Desmond O'Rourke and Michael Wynne-Ellis, Cambridge, Massachusetts: MIT Press, 1990

Wittkopp, Gregory (editor), *Saarinen House and Garden: A Total Work of Art*, New York: Abrams, 1995

SAFDIE, MOSHE 1938–

Architect, Israel and Canada

An Israel-born and Canada-educated architect who has maintained practices in Jerusalem, Montreal, Boston, and elsewhere, Moshe Safdie is best known for his internationally recognized modern revisionist project, the Habitat housing experiment for the 1967 World's Exposition in Montreal.

The initial idea for Habitat came to Safdie when he was working on his student thesis concerning cellular housing, questioning the social, environmental, ethical, and tectonic ideas of modernist architecture. Safdie drew on his childhood memories of the Israeli settlements to create an unsentimental articulate structure based on these traditional forms. Habitat was one of the first prefabricated housing complexes built at the time and

was the forerunner of R. Buckminster Fuller's megastructure Triton City (1968). Fuller's project model introduced a floating city comprised of prefabricated cellular units, a flexible structure that was never realized. It was during the late 1960s that Safdie, like Fuller, began to believe in the promise of industrialization and prefabrication for low-cost and improved structures. The 1960s espoused various collective social agendas by architects as well as politicians; similarly, architects and urban designers were reassessing the urban and architectural ideas of the modernists. Expo '67's Habitat project proved to be too expensive, and many difficulties arose in its construction. Greatly reduced in size, Habitat proved to evoke Safdie's revisionist attitude, one that rejected the Le Corbusian and Miesian vertical models of Unite d'Habitation and the Lake Shore Drive Apartments in Chicago.

During the 1970s Safdie concentrated his efforts on massive urban design schemes that emphasized context. One of these schemes was a plan (1971) for a new town, Coldspring, close to Baltimore, Maryland. During this time, he also produced a number of urban projects in Israel including the Yeshivat Porat Joseph Rabbinical College (1971–79) in Jerusalem and the Desert Research Institute (and Ben Gurion Archives) (1974) in the Negev. The Rabbinical College, located in the center of the Jewish Quarter of the old city, combines a traditionally shaped structure with traditionally shaped domes of the region, using modern construction and materials. In this work, Safdie explored the use of natural lighting and its symbolic quality. This symbolic use of lighting played a key role in his later works. Corresponding to its site and its context within the city, the Rabbinical College marries tradition with modernist invention. Safdie's work in Jerusalem particularly corresponds with the indigenous architecture of the city, blending with its traditional geometric shapes and colors as well as with the site.

In 1982, Safdie was commissioned by the Canadian government to design the new National Gallery of Canada in Ottawa. The building was completed in 1988, when he was then asked along with the firm Belzile, Brassard, Gallienne, Lavoie, with Sungur Incesulu and Maurice Desnoyers, to offer a scheme for a competition held for the Quebec Museum of Civilization (1988). They won the commission, and Safdie used ideas from his Jerusalem projects concerning the importance of place and cultural traditions; only this time, the northern and French culture of Canada was considered in the design process.

Safdie's writings, including *Beyond Habitat* (1970) and *For Everyone a Garden* (1974), argue for a reevaluation of modernism that promotes the humanistic and ethical dimensions of architecture. Safdie is also dedicated to the idea of the importance of designing public buildings that are intertwined with city street life. *Beyond Habitat by Twenty Years* (1987) reviews the architectural, aesthetic, and political concerns of the 1960s, from Habitat project through Postmodernism of the 1980s. Safdie admonishes the postmodernist agenda of historical eclecticism that centers on architecture concerned mainly with stylization and detachment from site. Safdie's technological ideas (manifest in Habitat) are also viewed as a starting point for other projects concerned with high-volume housing construction. He remains committed to a practice of contextualized architecture that is achieved through locality, iconography of site, color, and building technologies found geographically. His work investigates the importance of place, history, cultural identity, tectonics, and materiality.

REBECCA DALVESCO

See also **Exhibition Building; Fuller, Richard Buckminster (United States); Habitat 1967, Montreal**

Biography

Born in Haifa, Palestine (now Israel), 14 July 1938; moved to Canada 1955; dual citizenship 1959. Studied under H. P. D. Van Ginkel at McGill University, Montreal 1955–61; bachelor's degree in architecture 1961. Married 1) Nina Nusynowicz 1959 (divorced 1981): 2 children; married 2) Michal Ronnen 1981: 2 children. Architect with Van Ginkel and Associates, Montreal 1961–62; architect with the office of Louis I. Kahn, Philadelphia 1962–63; section head, architect, and planner for the Canadian Corporation for the 1967 World Exhibition, Montreal 1963–64. Private practice, Montreal from 1964; private practice, Jerusalem from 1971; private practice, Boston from 1978; private practice, Toronto. Visiting professor, McGill University 1970; Davenport Professor of Architecture, Yale University, New Haven, Connecticut 1971; professor of architecture and director of the Desert Architecture and Environment Department, Desert Research Institute, Ben Gurion University, Beersheva, Israel from 1975; professor of architecture and urban design and director of urban design program, Harvard University Graduate School of Design, Cambridge, Massachusetts 1978–84; Ian Woodner Studio Professor of Architecture and Urban Design, Harvard University Graduate School of Design 1984–89. Fellow, Royal Architectural Institute of Canada; member, Ontario Association of Architects; member, Israel Institute of Architects and Engineers; member Royal Canadian Academy of Arts; member, American Institute of Architects. Order of Canada 1988.

Selected Works

Habitat Housing, World's Exposition, Montreal, 1967
Habitat Housing (unbuilt), New York, 1968, 1970
Habitat Housing, Israel, 1970
Town Plan, Coldspring, Maryland, 1971
Habitat Housing, Puerto Rico, 1972
Desert Research Institute and Ben Gurion Archives, Negev, Israel, 1974
Yeshivat Porat Joseph Rabbinical College, Jerusalem, 1979
Housing, Singapore, 1984
National Gallery, Ottawa (with Parkin), 1988
Museum of Civilization (First place, competition), Quebec (with Belzile, Brassard, Gallienne, Lavoie, Sungur Incesulu and Maurice Desnoyers), 1988
Khalsa Heritage Memorial Anandpur Sahib, Punjab, India, 1997–2005 (scheduled completion)
Hebrew College, Newton Campus, Massachusetts, 2000
Ben Gurion Airport, Tel Aviv, 2000
Exploration Place Science Center and Children's Museum, Wichita, Kansas, 2000

Selected Publications

Beyond Habitat, 1970
For Everyone a Garden, edited by Judith Wolin, 1974
Beyond Habitat by Twenty Years, 1987
The City after the Automobile (with Wendy Kohn), 1997

Further Reading

Gray, John (interviewer), *Habitat: Moshe Safdie*, Montreal, Quebec: Tundra Books, 1967

Kohn, Wendy (editor), *Moshe Safdie*, London: Academy Editions, 1996
Murray, Irena Zantovská (editor), *Moshe Safdie: Buildings and Projects, 1967–1992*, Montreal: McGill-Queen's University Press, 1996
Steiger, Gail (editor and producer), *Desert Cities 3 Phoenix/Jerusalem* (videorecording), Tempe: Arizona State University College of Architecture and Environmental Design, 2000
Watanabe, Jun (editor), *Moshe Safdie: Building in Context; Moshe Safudei: 1970 nen iko no kiseki* (bilingual English–Japanese edition), Tokyo: Process Architecture, 1985

SAINSBURY WING, NATIONAL GALLERY

Designed by Venturi, Scott Brown and Associates; completed 1991
London, England

The Sainsbury Wing by Venturi, Scott Brown, and Associates is the major 20th-century extension to England's premier art museum, the National Gallery, built in 1833–37 to the designs of William Wilkins (1778–1839). An addition by E. M. Barry was completed in 1876, and subsequently, galleries were added in piecemeal fashion in 1887, 1911, 1927, and 1970, but these are deferentially tucked behind the original building's main facade on Trafalgar Square. In contrast, the Sainsbury Wing confidently gestures toward its monumental urban setting and complements a building long perceived as awkward and compromised. The architects have cunningly mirrored the more pleasing stylistic features of Wilkins' Neoclassical structure while quietly serving practical needs by using the most sophisticated technology available in museum design.

The controversial history of this wing commenced in 1958, when the government acquired the site of the former Hampton's furniture store immediately to the west of the National Gallery. To encourage the government to raise funds to use these premises for museum purposes, the *Sunday Times* newspaper the following year mounted a competition that garnered an unmemorable group of proposals in the monolithic Brutalist style then dominating British architecture. Nothing came of the *Times*'s intervention, and plans to extend the National Gallery on this site languished until December 1981, when the government launched its own contest. However, the program, addressed to developers as well as architects, was tainted from the outset by the requirement, for financial reasons, that the galleries should form but a small part of a larger commercial enterprise. From 79 entrants to the first phase in April 1982, seven architectural firms, each with its own developer, were selected to pursue the project. After much debate, Ahrends, Burton, and Koralek won the opportunity to finalize their proposal, but their definitive scheme met with general public dismay, most poignantly encapsulated in the words of Charles, prince of Wales, who in 1984 likened it to a "vast municipal fire station" as well as a "monstrous carbuncle on the face of a much loved and elegant friend." The misguided brief was set aside, and in 1985 the Sainsbury brothers—Simon, John, and Timothy, owners of a thriving supermarket chain and generous donors to the arts—offered a munificent gift to make possible the erection of an extension solely at the disposal of the National Gallery.

A reformulated competition was then held in which four British firms—James Stirling and Michael Wilford, (Alan) Col-

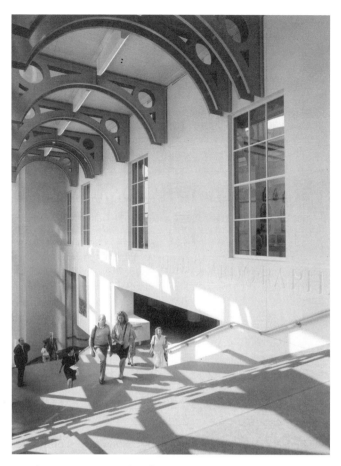

Sainsbury Wing, National Gallery, London
© Photo by Phil Starling, courtesy Venturi, Scott Brown and Associates

quhoun and (John) Miller, Jeremy Dixon, and Piers Gough of Campbell, Zogolovitch, Wilkinson, and Gough—were invited to submit entries. They were joined by the Americans Henry N. Cobb of I. M. Pei and Partners (today Pei, Cobb, and Freed) and Robert Venturi and Denise Scott Brown (at that time Venturi, Scott Brown, and Rauch). The choice in 1986 of Robert Venturi and Denise Scott Brown in the face of such a strong English showing was somewhat of a surprise, especially because Venturi, Scott Brown, while not inexperienced in museum additions, had not previously executed a building in Britain. However, the jury found their scheme the most sensitive to the scenography of London's most celebrated square. Although all six entries, unlike the aggressively modernist designs in the 1982 competition, incorporated some references to the classical vocabulary of Wilkins' building, it was Venturi, Scott Brown, and Associates's proposal that most skillfully integrated the new with the old rather than standing as a separate entity. Their dramatic but sympathetic resolution turns on a veritable cascade of the Corinthian order, which begins to the west of the main entrance as a fluted, fully engaged column faithfully reproducing those on Wilkins' original portico. Then the rhythm quickens as a crescendo of irregularly spaced Corinthian pilasters form a masonry screen of Portland stone that inflects toward the National Gallery before terminating along the side as prelude to a glazed

curtain wall, behind which lies the grand staircase. The concrete and steel frame facilitates the skillful composition of a complex variety of interior spaces.

Standing sentry at the entrance are slender, brightly painted metal columns reminiscent of John Nash (1752–1835) in an Egypto-Pompeiian mood. Within and immediately to the left is a large shop that also can be accessed directly from a side street. The foyer comprises a checkroom, an information desk, and an area sufficiently generous to accommodate informal concerts and performances. This space leads to the grand stairway, that icon of public architecture that has been strategically displaced from the center to the extremity of the wing, a *parti* used in other Venturi, Scott Brown institutional facilities, such as the Seattle Art Museum. The glazed envelope on the eastern side provides enticing views toward London's most famous square as well as to the original building. On the inner, more solid surface that defines the stair on the west, a limestone frieze, carved in early 19th-century lettering with the names of renowned artists, didactically enlivens the upward and descending journeys. The ceiling above the stair is punctuated by suspended metal arches that allude both to Renaissance structural systems and to Victorian iron architecture while reminding the visitor that subsequent building technologies and economies have rendered these arches a purely visual conceit.

At the topmost, fifth level lie the sixteen permanent galleries, comprising 1408 square meters and dedicated to the museum's European (notably Italian, northern, and English) masterpieces from 1260 to 1510. Because the pictures vary greatly in size, subject, and medium, providing a compatible home was a challenge but one that was met successfully by the firm in an appropriately contextual way. Each white-walled room, scaled to the works on display, is articulated by cool gray *pietra serena* moldings, doorframes, and Tuscan Doric columns, a combination beloved by the Florentine Filippo Brunelleschi. Another architect to whom homage is paid is Louis Kahn, whose museums gave Venturi, Scott Brown valuable lessons in circulation and lighting. Although a few British critics have faulted certain features of the Sainsbury Wing as being overly theatrical, eclectic, and mannered, the galleries have won widespread praise for their serenity and purity, qualities attained through the dignified details and the natural light that, purged of harmful ultraviolet rays and supplemented by artificial lighting, illuminates the Old Master pictures in a way that most favorably enhances their colors and textures. Clerestoried monitors, square or oblong according to the plan of their respective galleries, are set under a double-glazed roof that admits measured light via electronically controlled louvers. Passage through the collection may vary according to the visitor's preference, but enfilades give order to the spatial sequences. At this topmost level, the link to the main building provides an inviting vista toward the more richly colored and ornate older rooms.

Immediately below, on level 4, are restaurant facilities and other visitor services, including a unique computerized Micro Information Gallery. Level 3 contains the entrance foyer, and the auditorium and temporary galleries are located on the two lowest floors, beneath ground level, where daylight would inhibit the requisite flexibility. The galleries comfortably accommodate diverse types of exhibitions, whether monographic shows devoted to a single artist or epoch or thematic displays rich in objects and artifacts.

The historical references that enrich the architectural language of the Sainsbury Wing are particularly apposite to a museum, and allusions to Christopher Wren, medieval, Georgian and Victorian London, Italian masters of the Renaissance, and mannerist and baroque periods, as well as 20th-century heroes such as Sir Edward Lutyens, are discernible. One of the hallmarks of Venturi, Scott Brown, and Associates's variety of Postmodernism is the recognition that after modernism, one cannot return to history pure and simple; thus, they offer a piquant palimpsest rather than a revivalist copy, an interplay between past and present that is enriched by witty transpositions in scale, materials, and the putative functions of their sources and quotations.

HELEN SEARING

See also **Brutalism; Historicism; Kahn, Louis (United States); Lutyens, Edwin (England); Museum; Postmodernism; Venturi, Robert (United States)**

Further Reading

Amery, Colin, *A Celebration of Art and Architecture: The National Gallery Sainsbury Wing*, London: National Gallery, 1991

Dixon, John Morris, "Learning from London," *Progressive Architecture* 72, no. 8 (August 1991)

Moos, Stanislaus von, "Body Language and Artifice," *A + U* (July 1990)

The National Gallery, London and New York: Architectural Design Editions, 1986

Newhouse, Victoria, *Towards a New Museum*, New York: Monacelli Press, 1998

Venturi, Robert, "From Invention to Convention in Architecture," *Royal Society of Arts Journal* (January 1988)

Wilson, Michael, *A Guide to The Sainsbury Wing at the National Gallery*, London: National Gallery Publications, 1991

SALK INSTITUTE, LA JOLLA, CALIFORNIA

Designed by Louis Kahn; completed 1966

In 1959 the City Council in San Diego, upon learning of the Salk Institute's intention to build a research institute, offered a number of sites for the development including a unique piece of coastal land in La Jolla. The remoteness of the site and its relationship to the vast Pacific Ocean are often commented on in relation to the building's function, as a place of cutting-edge research with philosophical implications. In February 1960 Salk had a site meeting with Kahn, who soon began work on a master plan. The complex was to include the laboratories, as well as two unbuilt components—a meeting hall and residences to the extreme west of the site. Apparently due to over expenditure on the laboratories, design work on the unbuilt components was suspended in 1963. Meanwhile, the property was deeded to Salk in April 1960, and construction of the laboratories proceeded from June 1962 until 1965.

Stage one of the Salk Institute comprises two parallel laboratory buildings that delineate the long sides of a rectangular courtyard space. Each laboratory block contains a column-free space that is 60 feet wide by 240 feet in length. Significantly, Kahn's design allowed each of the laboratory spaces to be coupled with a service floor. This allows each block to consist of two laboratory and associated service levels above ground and another such coupling of levels below ground—light reaches the lower laboratories via sunken courtyards on either side. Although the structure of the Richards Building fails to provide a satisfactory "servant" space for pipes and ducts at ceiling level, the Salk laboratories are each "served"—to use Kahn's words—by nine-foot-deep service floors, or "pipe laboratories." At the time these spaces seemed to provide excessive room for pipes and ducts, but since that time much of the space has been filled. These service floors occupy the spaces between a series of Vierendeel trusses, which Kahn developed with August Komendant, his engineer and collaborator on this and many other projects.

In what would become a signature motif of his later work, Kahn rejected his contemporaries' rough handling of concrete, choosing instead to detail the off-form concrete for these laboratory blocks with great care and finesse. Like Le Corbusier's rough concrete *(béton-brut)*, which was made famous in his Unité d'Habitation (1952) in Marseilles and his Capitol Complex (1952–60) in Chandigarh, concrete at the Salk Institute is presented as unmanipulated. However, whereas Le Corbusier made a virtue of the often-unintentionally rough finish he achieved in his buildings in Marseilles and Chandigarh, Kahn's concrete at the Salk only displays the marks of carefully planned formwork and ties.

In the intermediate zone between the laboratory buildings and the central plaza are a series of small towers that comprise individual studies for the scientists. Each study features a 45-degree angled wall section providing oblique views of the Pacific Ocean to the west. The studies have weathered teak wall panels, providing the only moment of relief and counterpoint to the off-form concrete used elsewhere. Befitting their domestic scale, the study windows feature finely crafted glazing, insect screen, and sliding louver components, reminiscent of those found in Kahn's houses.

The Salk Institute's most memorable feature—its ascetic treeless plaza of travertine and concrete—was intended to feature two parallel rows of Italian cypress trees, until the laboratories were almost complete and Kahn began to have misgivings. Credit for the potent image that is so familiar today belongs to the Mexican architect Luis Barragan, who recommended to Kahn that the open space be left completely bare. Kahn conceived the resulting plaza as a "facade to the sky," with a central canal that marks the development's axis of symmetry. From the rear of the plaza, also known as the Theodore Gildred Court, the canal appears to extend to the ocean horizon; in fact, it spills into a series of pools below and to the west of the plaza.

According to Kahn, particular buildings of the same type share an archetypal counterpart, or form, which is seen in the mind's-eye as a vague idea that can only be represented by an *esquisse*-like diagram. The Salk Institute is important in this context because it provided Kahn with an ideal arrangement, or archetypal form, for a laboratory building and a model for subsequent laboratory proposals, such as the University of Virginia Chemistry Building (unbuilt). In its form it would also be an intimation toward what Kahn termed "the unmeasurable," a transcendent realm of inspiration with mystical and divine connotations.

STEVEN FLEMING

See also **Barragán, Luis (Mexico); Concrete; Corbusier, Le (Jeanneret, Charles-Édouard) (France); Kahn, Louis (United States); Modernism; Research Center; Rationalism**

Further Reading

Benedikt, Michael, "Between Beakers and Beatitudes," *Progressive Architecture*, 74:10 (1993)

Brownlee, David, "The Houses of Inspiration: Designs for Study," in *Louis I. Kahn: In the Realm of Architecture*, edited by David Brownlee and David DeLong, New York: Rizzoli, 1991

Crosbie, Michael J., "Dissecting the Salk/A Talk with Salk," *Progressive Architecture*, 74, no. 10 (1993)

Danto, Arthur C., "Louis Kahn as Archai-Tekt," in *Philosophizing Art: Selected Essays*, Berkeley: University of California Press, 1999

Friedman, Daniel S., "Salk Institute for Biological Studies," in *Louis I. Kahn: In the Realm of Architecture*, edited by David Brownlee and David DeLong, New York: Rizzoli, 1991

Kahn, Louis I., "Address," in *Louis I. Kahn: Writings, Lectures, Interviews*, edited by Alessandra Latour, New York: Rizzoli, 1991

Kahn, Louis, "Form and Design," *Architectural Design*, 31, no. 4 (April 1961)

SALMONA, ROGELIO 1929–

Architect, Columbia

The designs of Rogelio Salmona comprise over 70 projects built during the past 40 years and range from domestic to large housing complexes as well as institutional architecture. He is undoubtedly one of the most prolific and significant architects of Latin America.

Wanting to study fine arts but advised by his father to take a similar but more pragmatic route, Salmona entered the National University to study architecture in 1948. His first year of studies coincided with Le Corbusier's visit to Bogota, where he had been invited to develop an urban master plan. In 1948, Salmona's father decided to send his children to France in light of the increasing political unrest in Colombia. Salmona began working for the architect at the atelier de la rue de Sèvres 35, where he would stay for the next ten years. Under Le Corbusier, he would further develop his passion for drawing, thereby coming in direct contact with the pragmatic aspects of architecture though his work in projects such as the Jaoul and the Rob et Roq houses and in the projects for Chandigarh. At this same time, however, he began attending the lectures given by the art historian Pierre Francastel at La Sorbonne and developing a strong friendship with him. Francastel's social concerns and humanistic views deeply influenced Salmona's attitudes toward architecture and led him in particular to develop a sense for an architecture in tune with the Latin American reality and in opposition to both the precepts imparted by Le Corbusier and those emerging from the International Style.

From the onset, Salmona's preoccupations with craftsmanship infused his work with the tectonic aspects of architecture and a concern for its experiential qualities. His understanding of history, his intimate relation with the Colombian landscape, and his affinity for the use of brick (Bogota's local material par excellence) and concrete (with which he had worked extensively while at Le Corbusier's atelier) became his trademarks.

Three significant projects serve as a watershed in the career of the architect: the Torres del Parque residential complex (1967) in Bogota, the President's House for Illustrious Guests (1981) in Cartagena, and the National Archives of Colombia (1992) in Bogota. Las Torres del Parque is without doubt one of the most significant housing projects of its kind, built in the Americas at the precise moment at which the International Style precepts were being questioned. The project consists of three brick towers built on a steep plot at the northern edge of the Parque de la Independencia (Independence Park) at the beginning of the Monserrate foothills. Las Torres del Parque was designed to house some 1,500 dwellers in 300 units.

An architecture aligned neither to the vanishing ideals of the International Style nor to the emerging and multifaceted postmodern trends of the 1960s that replaced them, Las Torres is uncompromisingly fresh and vigorous, and it expresses a profound sympathy for a sense of urbanity, evocative of memorable places. In this project, Salmona also introduced a major choreography of urban places in which plant materials play a major role, giving a precise character to the outdoor zones of the project and integrating it with the adjacent park.

Salmona's President's House for Illustrious Guests in Cartagena is a careful intervention in the topography. While respecting and enhancing the silhouette of neighboring El Manzanillo fort, it creates a new landscape on what previously was a barren site occupied by ruins. To accomplish this, Salmona used simple pragmatic principles derived from the Spanish-Moorish tradition as well as from pre-Hispanic sources.

The President's House is a compound formed of seven courtyards. Quarters for the president, his guests, and accompanying personnel have been carefully arranged around these courtyards. Additional facilities include a living room, a dining room, meeting rooms, a library, and service areas. Throughout the house, the materials used in its construction are consistent: brick, tile, coral stone, concrete, and hardwood. Rooms vary in proportion according to their function, yet they maintain a continuous unity. Differentiation is evident everywhere, carried out with extreme subtlety. The President's House speaks clearly of solemnity and becomes a lesson in the restrained use of materials and forms.

In the General Archives of Colombia, site, history, and distance become integral elements of Salmona's form-making process. It is not accidental that Salmona, although alluding to the traditions of Colonial architecture in Colombia, reintroduces two important concepts evident in pre-Columbian buildings and poetry: the roof ambulation and the skewed access to precincts along diagonal lines. It is possible to experience both wandering and wondering on the Archives' roof, which has become the ludic area of the building occupied by a garden and areas adjacent to the cafeteria. Pedestrians on the roof can view and seize the entire surrounding urban panorama modulated by the distant landscape while observing the comings and goings of users traversing the building's great central cylindrical void. The central space of the Archives is undoubtedly a significant addition to the public spaces of Bogota. Acting as a sounding box that gathers the echoes, the light, and some of the landmarks of the city, it is, in every sense, a memorable place.

RICARDO L. CASTRO

See also **Corbusier, Le (Jeanneret, Charles-Édouard) (France); International Style; Parliament Building, Chandigarh**

Biography

Born in Paris, 28 April 1929. Studied at the Universidad Nacional de Colombia, Bogota 1948–49; apprentice to Le Corbusier, Paris 1949–57; attended the École des Hautes Etudes Sociales, Sorbonne, Paris 1949–57; studied at Metiers Art School, Paris 1953–54. Returned to Colombia in 1958; began a successful architectural practice in Bogota and started teaching at the Universidad de los Andes. Granted a professional degree in 1963 by the Universidad de los Andes.

Selected Works

Torres del Parque Apartments, Bogota, 1967
Colombian Architects Association Headquarters (First prize, competition), Bogota, 1967
Casa de Huespedes de Colombia, Cartagena, 1981
National Archives, Bogota, 1992

Selected Publications

"Reflections upon Latin American Architecture," in *Architecture and Body*, edited Scott Marble et al., 1988
"Casa para la memoria," *Revista de la Asociación Latinoamerica* 13 (1993)
"La Casa Cartagenera: ensueño y poesia," *Restauración* 5 (1993)

Further Reading

Full details of Salmona's biography appear in Téllez, which also includes illustrated critical analyses of the most significant buildings prior to 1991. Sixteen significant projects up to 1997 are discussed and illustrated in Castro.

Arango, Silvia, *Historia de la arquitectura en Colombia*, Bogotá: Universidad Nacional de Colombia, 1990
Castro, Ricardo L., "The Work of Rogelio Salmona: The President's Guest House in Cartagena, Colombia," in *Critical Regionalism: The Pomona Meeting Proceedings*, edited by Spyro Amourgis, Pomona: California State Polytechnic University, 1991
Castro, Ricardo L., "Thoughts at the Edge of Architecture: Solitude and the Marvelous-Real," *ARQ Architecture Québec* 67 (June 1992)
Castro, Ricardo L., "Architectural Criticism in the Chimeric Realm", *Design Book Review* 32/33 (1994)
Castro, Ricardo L., "Wet Architecture: Rogelio Salmona's Quimbaya Gold Museum," *The Fifth Column* 9, no. 2 (1996)
Castro, Ricardo L., *Rogelio Salmona*, Bogotá, Colombia: Villegas Editores, 1998
Castro, Ricardo L., "Site Resonance and Sense of Distances: Rogelio Salmona's Nueva Santa Fé Community Centre in Bogotá," *The Fifth Column* 10, no. 2–3 (1998)
Fonseca, Alberto and Alberto Saldarriaga, *Aspectos de la arquitectura contemporánea en Colombia*, Medellín: Editorial Colina, 1977
Gutiérrez, Ramon, "La persistencia y el cambio: Casa de Huéspedes Ilustres, Cartagena de Indias," *A and V* 48 (1994)
"Rogelio Salmona, Colombia," *Zodiac* 8 (1992)
Salmona, Rogelio and Germán Téllez, "The House of Illustrious Guests, Colombia, Cartagena de Indias," *A + U* 4, no. 331 (1998)
Téllez, Germán, *Rogelio Salmona: arquitectura y poetica del lugar*, Bogotá, Colombia: Facultad de Arquitectura, Universidad de los Andes, 1991

SANT'ELIA, ANTONIO 1888–1916

Architect, Italy

Sant'Elia attended a technical school in Como and graduated as master builder in 1906. He moved to Milan in 1905, where he worked as a draftsman for a canal company, then for the municipal engineering department. In 1909, his study for a villa appeared in the Milanese review *La Casa*, and he enrolled at the Brera Academy. Between 1911 and 1914, Sant'Elia participated in numerous competitions and exhibitions that would prepare him for the most significant project of his oeuvre: *La Città Nuova* (The New City). In 1914, he exhibited 60 drawings in the show of the group Nuova Tendenze, which he co-founded. Its catalogue contained his *Messaggio*, a text later transformed into the Manifesto, with six views of *La Città Nuova*. These, with the sketches, represent the peak of his graphic work. He probably met the Futurist Fillipo Tomaso Marinetti at this time.

When Italy entered the war in 1915, Sant'Elia was among the first to volunteer, joining the same regiment as Umberto Boccioni, Marinetti, and Mario Sironi, among other Futurists. He enjoyed a brief period of leave, but his relations with the Futurists were then interrupted. Conscripted and sent to the front again, as second lieutenant in the infantry during the ensuing attacks against enemy trenches between June and July 1916, he was wounded and decorated. At this time, Sant'Elia was commissioned to design a cemetery for the Arezzo Brigade at Monfalcone. It was still under construction when he fell during an assault, shot in the forehead by a machine gun bullet.

Before Futurism, there had been pragmatic solutions to the problems of urbanism through the use of new materials—steel, glass, and concrete—but without a radical renewal of architectural language. The symbolic and typological themes of the metropolis, skyscrapers, factories, residential and commercial complexes, power- and railway stations, had already been treated by Otto Wagner, Tony Garnier, and the Chicago School, but the first real urban vision of the future in Italy was presented by Sant'Elia in his *Messaggio* and drawings of *La Città Nuova*. Here he proposed, even if in utopian terms, the profound modifications that were needed to connect architecture to urban structure. The power and originality of his vision derives from an ability to interrelate, in all their complexity, the forms and volumes of his chosen elements. He shows an interconnected system of circulation and communication that is different from the American model of isolated skyscrapers. Though it would seem partly to derive from illustrations of futuristic American visions, he presents an architectural understanding of simultaneity derived not only from crisscrossing circulation but, above all, from a close relation between urban form and building type. The layered traffic suggests a new and mutual dynamism between building and circulation that may be understood by reference to the concepts that Umberto Boccioni had pioneered: fusion, all-embracing atmosphere, and a concept of space as a field. The radical innovation of his imagery, his conception of the city as flows, acceptance of the world of machinery, use of industrial types as models, and promotion of undecorated flat surfaces with brilliant hues are all original. Sant'Elia was concerned with showing how industrialization and the working city required new forms of art, thought, behavior, and language.

The Fascists tried to claim him as their national architect, but his work is without a consciously national character. In the postwar decade Futurism was seen as little more than an offshoot of Fascism, so the discovery of the *Messaggio* 42 years after it originally appeared offered hope of severing Sant'Elia from Futurism, and hence Fascism. Both documents were apparently ghost written, and despite the absence of the word "Futurism"

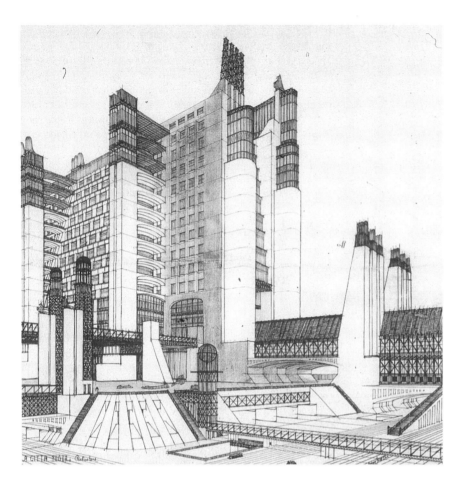

La Città Nuova, Apartment block with external elevators, tunnel, covered passage, on three traffic levels (tramway, road for cars, metal gangway), beacons and wireless telegraphy; ink and pencil on tracing paper
© Musei Civici, Como Italy. Photo courtesy Ross Jenner

in the *Messaggio*, in inspiration and form, both are under the pervasive influence of Marinetti and Boccioni. Saint'Elia never disclaimed the Manifesto, and if his designs show evidence of originality, it has to be proven that he was not also the principal source of the written ideas.

Provincial, untraveled, caught between modernity and tradition, Sant'Elia in his last works reveals a nostalgic return to the Viennese orbit under whose sway he began. The ideas that Sant'Elia developed before the war became ever more a part of the mainstream of Modern architecture but were never again so vigorously or freshly presented.

ROSS JENNER

See also **Città Nuova (1914); Fascist Architecture**

Biography

Born in Milan 30 April 1888; attended a technical school in Como and graduated as master builder in 1906; moved to Milan in 1905 to work as draftsman for a canal company, then for municipal engineering department; participated with Italo Paternoster on the international competition for Monza cemetery 1912; designed the rustic Villa Elisi near Como and with Paternoster went to Bologna, where he successfully took the entrance exam for the Academy of Fine Arts. Opened his own studio in Milan 1913; participated in competitions for offices for the Ve-

rona Savings Bank and in 1914 for a church in Salsomaggiore. Exhibited sketches in the "First Exhibition of Lombard Architects" in Milan 1914; exhibited 60 drawings at the seat of the "Artistic Family" in the show of the group Nuova Tendenze, co-founded in February by Sant'Elia. Enlisted in the Italian army in July 1915 and was killed by a machine-gun bullet on 10 October 1916 in Monfalcone.

Selected Works

La Città Nuova (project), 1914

Selected Publications

"Messaggio," English translations in Banham, R., *Theory and Design in the First Machine Age*, New York: 1970; and in Meyer, Esther da Costa, *The work of Antonio Sant'Elia: retreat into the future*, New Haven: Yale University Press, 1995
"Architettura Futurista," Manifesto, 1914. Included in Argan, G. C., et al., *Dopo Sant'Elia*, Milan, 1935. English translations in Carrieri, R., *Futurism*, Milan, 1963, pp. 150; and in *Futurist Manifestos*, Apollonio, Umberto (editor), New York: Viking Press, 1973, pp. 160–172

Further Reading

Maurizio Calvesi provides an important argument against separating Sant'Elia from Futurism. Alberto Sartoris examines an early book by the architect, containing the text of his "Manifesto." Reyner Banham provides perhaps the most ardent promotion of Sant'Elia in English.

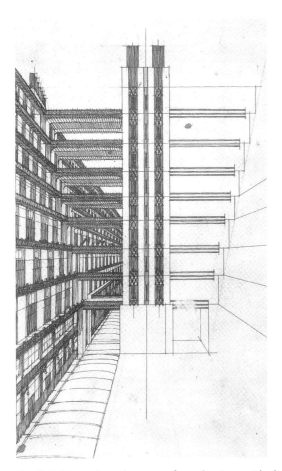

La Città Nuova, Secondary street for pedestrians, with elevators in the middle; ink and pencil on tracing paper
© Collection of Parade Acetti, Milan, Italy

Esther da Costa Meyer provides the most recent and comprehensive study of the architect, in any language

Antonio Sant'Elia: L'architettura disegnata (exhib. cat.), Venice: Marsilio, 1991
Argan, Giulio Carlo, "Il pensiero critico di Antonio Sant'Elia," *L'arte* 33, no. 5 (1930)
Ashton, Dore, and Guido Ballo (editors), *Antonio Sant'Elia* (exhib. cat.), Milan: Mondadori, 1986
Banham, Reyner, *Theory and Design in the First Machine Age*, New York: Praeger, and London: Architectural Press, 1970
Calvesi, Maurizio, "Il futurista Sant' Elia: Un'analisi del manifesto," in *Le due avanguardie: Dal futurismo alla pop art*, by Calvesi, Milan: Lerici, 1966
Caramel, Luciano, and Alberto Longatti, *Sant'Elia: L'opera completa*, Milan: Mondadori, 1987; as *Antonio Sant'Elia: The Complete Works*, New York: Rizzoli, 1988
Crispolti, Enrico, *Architettura futurista: Attraverso l'architettura futurista* (exhib. cat.) (bilingual Italian–English text), Modena, Italy: Galleria Fonte d'Abisso, 1984
Meyer, Esther da Costa, *The Work of Antonio Sant'Elia: Retreat into the Future*, New Haven, Connecticut: Yale University Press, 1995
Sartoris, Alberto, *L'Architetto Antonio Sant'Elia*, Milan: s.l., 1930

SANTIAGO, CHILE

The city of Santiago was founded in the 16th century, between two rivers at the base of a hill, following the Spanish grid plan for American cities. Until the 19th century, references in the skyline were churches and significant public buildings. In the 20th century, the city center included high-rise buildings of six to ten stories.

Parallel to the downtown area, a peripheral zone, unbounded from the city center, began to grow, separating the working activities from housing. Appearing toward the east, the communes of Providencia in 1897 and Las Condes in 1901, together with the city center, concentrate the best examples of 20th-century architecture in the city.

By 1900, the city of Santiago had emerged with clear recognition of its limits and structure because of the ideas of the intendant, Benjamín Vicuña Mackenna inspired himself in the French baron Haussman and the Spanish Idelfonso Cerdà, which later was further developed by the Austrian Carl Brunner, differentiating a center and four sections in a concentric scheme that was maintained well into the 20th century.

By the 1930s, the first manifestations of the leading urban and architectural trends prevailing in Europe and the United States appeared, introducing Art Nouveau and Art Deco expressions, followed by modernism and the International Style. In the 1950s, residential growth in the communes of Providencia and Las Condes, inspired by the Garden City movement, broke the urban scheme that had prevailed since colonial times. In the 1970s, a large commercial axis with high-rise buildings developed, connecting the center with these communes and transferring traditional business to new centers in these areas.

The primary architectural expression in Santiago remains the skyscraper. The first manifestations, built between 1920 and 1940, borrow their image from those prevailing in the United States and Europe, expressed as an eclectic mix of styles in rapid succession. Formally, the first examples of tall buildings use the *palazzo* model in its two versions, referring to the image of the *palazzo* itself or stretching the middle part up to the needed height. In the first case, classical elements are used: in the second, a variety of styles are adopted. Clear examples of the classical *palazzo* are the *Banco del Pac'fico* (Bank of the Pacific, 1921) by Shade, Oyarzún and Phillippi and the office building of the *Banco Hipotecario* (Mortgage Bank, 1925) by Siegel and Sons. Fine examples of the stretched *palazzo* are the *Edificio Ariztía* (Ariztía Building, 1921) by Alberto Cruz Montt and the Díaz Building (1925) by Valdivieso and de la Cruz.

Around 1927, the first Art Deco designs appear, with a nationalistic character showing local indigenous elements, such as the Merced 849 (1927) by Luciano Kulczewski or the Ministerio de Hacienda (Exchequer Ministry Building, 1930) by Smith Solar and Smith Miller. At the same time, the first rationalist designs appear, such as a streamlined version, an example being the Oberpauer Building (1929) by Sergio Larraín, today a national monument. Especially interesting in this period is the architecture of J. Martínez, with works such as the University of Chile's Law School (1934) and the Military School (1943), which suggests the Fascist architecture of the 1930s in Europe.

In a second stage of architecture in Santiago, between 1945 and 1960, rationalism precedes the International Style. Early

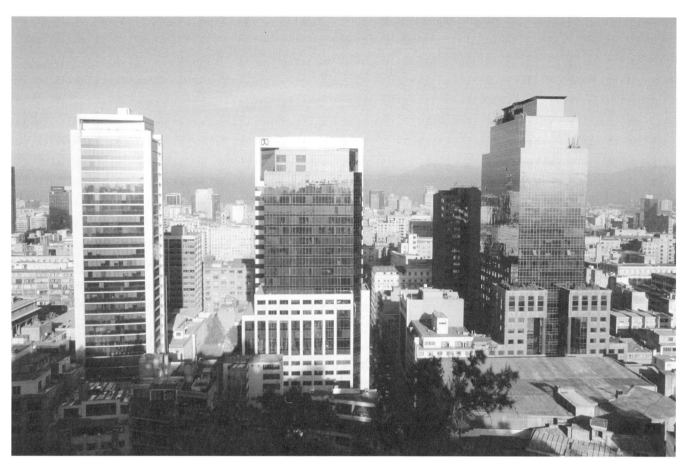

Downtown district of Santiago
© Hubert Stadler/CORBIS

examples include the Banco del Estado (State Bank, 1945) by Héctor Mardones and later the Plaza Italia Building (1956) by Santiago Roi. A fine Le Corbusier–inspired building is the Benedictine Church and Monastery (1954–65), by J. Bellalta, P. Gross, J. Swimburn, R. Irarrazaval, and Fathers M. Correa and G. Guarda.

From 1960 to 1980, the volume of the block disappears, and the isolated tower emerges with an open space, surely inspired by Mies' Lake Shore Drive Apartments or the Seagram Building. In this period, clearly the International Style is consolidated, producing buildings with volumetric purity and the use of curtain walls. Fine examples of this period are the Reval Building (1963) by Jorge Aguirre; the Costanera Building (1975) by Echenique, Cruz and Boisier; and the Torre Santa María, Santa María Tower (1977), by C.A. Cruz, J.M. Figueroa, J. Claude, Alemparte and Barreda. This period also sees the development of large complexes inspired by Le Corbusier that in some cases wiped out extended areas of the city. These include the *Remodelación San Borja* (San Borja Unit, 1960s) by the Ministry of Housing; the *Unidad Vecinal Providencia* (Providencia Neighborhood Complex, 1966) with its twin towers by Esquenazi and Barella; the *Torres de Tajamar* (Tajamar Towers, 1962–67) by Bresciani, Valdes, Prieto, Castillo, Lorca, Huidobro and Bolton;

and the *Villa Presidente Frei* (President's Frei Complex, 1965) by J. Larraín, O. Larraín, and D. Balmaceda. Other complexes also began to appear in the garden city communes toward the new areas farther east of the city, such as the *Remodelación San Luis* (San Luis Renovation, 1974) by Sandoval and Arancibia and the *Torres de Vitacura* (Three Towers of Vitacura, 1973) by Mauricio Despouy. An important Le Corbusier–inspired building is the Cepal Headquarters for Latin America (1963–68) by E. Duhart, R. Goycoolea, C. de Groote, and O. Santelices.

A fourth and final period of architectural development includes the last two decades of the 20th century, when several of the models used in the previous stage continued to prevail, such as the curtain wall–isolated high-rise, as demonstrated by the building Estado 10 (1982) by Borquez, Paredes and Sotomayor, or using the mirror glass wall as a covering, such as the *Edificio Catedral* (Cathedral Building, 1982) by Echenique, Cruz, Boisier and Dunner or the Shell Building (1989) by Asahi and Associates. Other interesting examples include the *Consorcio Nacional de Seguros-Vida* (Insurance Building, 1992) by B. Huidobro, E. Browne, and Judson (with European influences) and the CTC Building (1995) by M. Paredes, J. Iglesis, and L. Prat.

The Lever House (designed by Gordon Bunshaft, New York City, 1951) model continues its influence in the Crowne Plaza

Hotel (1981) by Alemparte and Barreda. Other examples increasingly use mirror glass. The interior galleries used in the past, penetrating the city block, are now rescued and reinterpreted in several fine examples, such as the Panorámico Building (1981) by San Martín, Browne and Wenborne, which is later renovated by Record-n and Sartori (1990), and the Edificio Plaza Lyon (1977) by Larraín, Murtinho and Associates and the Shell Building (1989) by Asahi and Associates.

New in the 1980s and 1990s is the presence of more local and contextual aspects that adhere to Postmodern currents. Examples include the use of pre-Colombian references in the Montolin Building (1988) by C. Fernández and Associates, Art Deco references in the Financo Building (1989) by Alemparte and Barreda, classical elements in the Codelco Building (1984) by Boza and Associates, and the CCT Building (1991) by G. Mardones and Associates, inspired in the old brick buildings of downtown Santiago.

The recognition of scale of place directed the design of the Fundación Building (1982) and the Americas Building (1990) by Boza and the Torre San Ramón (San Ramón Tower, 1988) by Flaño, Nuñez, and Tuca.

The use of color or the curve is also present as a strong plastic element applied to buildings, such as that located at Callao and Versalles Streets (1991) by Boza and Associates and the Banmedica Building (1998) by B. Huidobro and Associates.

At present, architects are reinterpreting famous existing buildings, such as the Simon Bolivar Building (1991) by Paredes and Associates, with a clear reference to the AT&T Building by Philip Johnson in New York, and the Cruz Blanca Building (1991) by G. Kreft, producing a bizarre reference to the Chrysler Building in New York. We leave the 20th century and enter the 21st with an increasingly eclectic architecture that, together with the mall culture, is slowly making our cities lose their local character in a world of globalization.

MARCELA PIZZI AND MARÍA PAZ VALENZUELA

See also **Chile**

Further Reading

Boza, Cristián, *100 Años de Arquitectura Chilena, 1890–1990*, Santiago: Editorial Gabriela Manzi Z., 1996

Eliash, Humberto, and Moreno, Manuel, *Arquitectura y Modernidad en Chile, 1925–1965*, Santiago: Ediciones Universidad Católica de Chile, 1989

Facultad de Arquitectura y Urbanismo de la Universidad de Chile, *150 años de Enseñanza de la Arquitectura en la Universidad de Chile 1849–1999*, Santiago: Ograma 1999

Strabucchi Chambers, Wren, *Cien Años de Arquitectura en la Universidad Católica 1984–1994*, Santiago: Ediciones ARQ, 1994

Universidad de Chile, Facultad de Arquitectura y Urbanismo y Ministerio de Vivienda y Urbanismo, *Guía de la Arquitectura de Santiago, Chile, 13 Recorridos*, Ograma S.A., 2000

De Toesca a la Arquitectura Moderna 1780–1950, Santiago: La Huella de Europa, 1996

SANTOS, ADÈLE NAUDÉ 1938–

Architect, South Africa

Adèle Naudé Santos' early design projects in southern Africa in collaboration with her first husband, Antonio de Souza Santos, included innovative private houses, apartment buildings, and low-cost workers' housing and facilities, including a church and school. Her early houses incorporated principles of planning the "house as a city," controlling space through section, and a process for analyzing site and social issues that would govern her design and teaching throughout her career. The most remarkable of these early projects were the five Molteno houses at Rowan Lane, Kennilworth, Cape Town (1973), fitted into an existing garden grove, and House Stekhoven (1972), a private residence that opened like a grand piano from a dull cul-de-sac of suburban houses dramatically toward Table Mountain, seen as the culmination of a private garden from carefully segregated family spaces through glazed walls and across shared walkways sheltered by an undulating *bris-soleil*.

Throughout her career as architect and educator, Naudé Santos treated practice as a component of research. "The work is usually designed experimentally, imagining space or spatial sequences," she wrote. "The cross-section is a design tool that often precedes the plan." Research projects have included urban design studies such as "Open Space Choice for Blighted Inner City Neighborhoods" (1985) and "Urban Design Strategy for Center City East, San Diego" (1993) as well as the development of housing prototypes for Misawa Homes, Tokyo (1989), and for the city of Kitakyushu, Japan (1992–94), where the Kadota and Dairi Nishi housing projects were built (1996).

In the 1980s, Naudé Santos often used entries in national and international design competitions as a means to further her research into contextualizing design. She won competitions of the Hawaii-Loa Pacific Center for the Media Arts (1986), the Los Angeles ArtsPark (1989), and the Perris California Civic Center (1991) and had premiated entries in competitions for In-fill Housing, Harlem, New York (1986) and Hillside Housing, Cincinnati (1985). In 1988, she also won an invited competition sponsored by the Museum of Contemporary Art, Los Angeles, and the Community Redevelopment Agency for New Case-Study Houses. Replacing dingbat models for low-cost housing with a "small-town" structure made up of courtyards linked by offset walkways, with 40 interlocking, variably functioned units with distinctive curved roofs and balconies, her winning Franklin-La Brea project, with revisions, was built (1995), nestled atop the intersection of Franklin and La Brea Avenues in Los Angeles.

Expanding her practice to Japan, Naudé Santos was commissioned to design a mixed-use building in Harajuku, Tokyo (1984), where she interlocked shared and private spaces for a joint family, ideas worked out further in a two-unit family house in Tokyo (1990). As Philip Arcidi wrote in *Progressive Architecture* (November 1990), "In this house, Santos's spatial strategy yields results that complement those of her public buildings. . . . She renders the interior an exceptional sequence of layered volumes, where Nature is encountered within an urban refuge."

Other major projects in Japan included a playful small office building of interlocking spaces, bringing light deep into a very constrained Ichiban-Cho urban site (1988), that has adjusted gracefully to changing uses since it was built; the Ohgimi Beach House (1988), a company lodge that "settles like a leaf" into a protected pine forest in exurban Ninomiya; and Tokyo Fantasia, an unbuilt atrium office building organized around a remarkable six-story garden stairway.

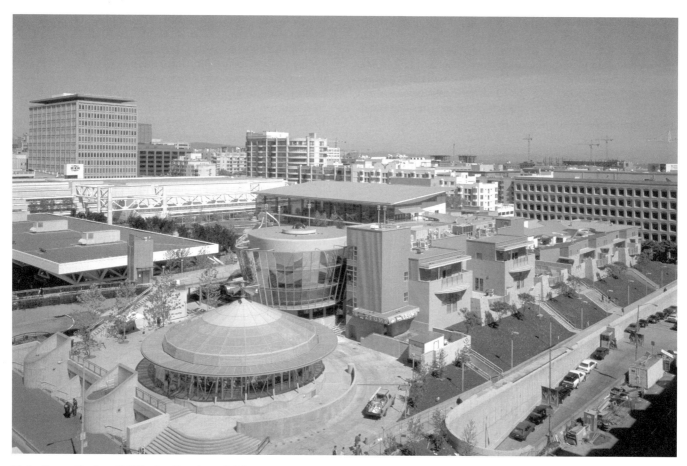

Yerba Buena Gardens (1998), San Francisco, California
Photo © Antonio Garbasso. Courtesy Adele Naude Santos and Associates with LDA Architects.

In the United States in the 1990s, Naudé Santos designed public spaces that interpenetrated spatially complex interiors with the variable light and nature of a variety of exterior landscapes, including the Institute of Contemporary Art, Philadelphia (1991); Albright College Center for the Arts, Reading, Pennsylvania (1991), a series of buildings that reshaped a campus around an open atrium-amphitheater that incorporated a collaboration sponsored by the National Endowment for the Humanities between Naudé Santos and the environmental artist Mary Miss; the Natatorium at Albright College (1990); and the unbuilt Perris California Civic Center. These public projects culminated in the Zeum and Rooftop Complex at Yerba Buena Gardens, San Francisco (1998), intertwining a children's museum, a child-care center, a glazed pavilion for an antique carousel, a bowling alley, a cafe, and an indoor ice-skating rink forming a subtle people's acropolis on top of the city's Moscone Convention Center.

Throughout her career, Naudé Santos explored housing in sociologically sensitive spatial terms, nowhere more experimentally than in a series of lofts, some for her own use in Boston (1980) and Philadelphia (1983) and others responding to San Francisco's demand for live-work units, as in the five lofts that she interwove around a shared court that she carved into the center of an old warehouse between Rich and Zoe Streets (1998). These issues of space, design, and society also governed her teach-

ing and formed a rigorous frame for the new curriculum that she and the formidable faculty whom she recruited had begun to frame for the new school that she conceived for the University of California, San Diego. As a final gift to that city, the school sponsored the production of an urban design strategy that the city adopted, as the school itself was being dismantled in 1994 during one of California's deep financial downturns and was able to graduate only a single class.

MICHAEL W. MEISTER

See also **Africa: Southern and Central Africa**

Biography

Born in Cape Town, South Africa, 14 October 1938; received British citizenship 1961; father was architect Hugo Naudé. Attended University of Cape Town; degree from the Architectural Association, London 1961; master's degree in urban design from Harvard University, Cambridge, Massachusetts 1963; master's degree in architecture and city planning from the University of Pennsylvania, Philadelphia 1968. Principal, Adèle Naudé Santos, Philadelphia from 1979; principal, Adèle Naudé Santos and Associates, San Diego and San Francisco; partner, Santos Levy and Associates, with Alan Levy, Philadelphia from 1990. Profes-

sor, Rice University, Houston 1973–79; professor, Graduate School of Design, Harvard University 1979–81; professor and chair of the architecture department, University of Pennsylvania, Philadelphia 1981–87; founder and first dean, School of Architecture, University of California, San Diego 1990–95; Thomas Jefferson Professor of Architecture, University of Virginia 1993–94; professor, University of California, College of Environmental Design, Berkeley from 1995. Exhibition of her work held at the Kitakyushu, Japan, Museum of Modern Art (1998).

Selected Works

Stekhoven House, Cape Town, 1972
Molteno Houses, Cape Town, 1973
Loft, Boston, 1980
Loft, Philadelphia, 1983
Mixed-Use Building, Tokyo, 1984
Hillside Housing (competition; unbuilt), Cincinnati, 1985
Hawaii-Loa Pacific Center for the Media Arts (First prize, competition; unbuilt), 1986
In-fill Housing (competition; unbuilt), Harlem, New York, 1986
Office Building, Ichiban-Cho, 1988
Ohgimi Beach House, Ninomiya, 1988
Tokyo Fantasia Office Building (1988; unbuilt)
Los Angeles ArtsPark (First prize, competition; unbuilt), 1989
Misawa Homes (prototype), Tokyo, 1989
Two-Unit House, Tokyo, 1990
Natatorium, Albright College, Reading, Pennsylvania, 1990
Institute of Contemporary Art, Philadelphia, 1991
Albright College Center for the Arts, Reading, 1991
Civic Center (First prize, competition; unbuilt), Perris, California, 1991
Franklin-La Brea Project (with revisions), Los Angeles, 1995
Kadota Housing project, Kitakyushu, Japan, 1996
Dairi Nishi Housing Project, Kitakyushu, 1996
Zeum and Rooftop Complex, Yerba Buena Gardens, San Francisco, 1998
Rich and Zoe Streets Lofts, San Francisco, 1998

Selected Publication

Urban Futures—A Vision for Centre City East (organizer), 1994

Further Reading

De Beer, Piet, "Adèle Naudé Santos, Sculptress of Space," *South African Architect* (September 1998)
Kloos, Maarten, *Architecture Now*, Amsterdam: Architecture and Natura Press, 1991
Lacy, Bill (editor), *100 Contemporary Architects: Drawings and Sketches*, New York: Abrams, and London: Thames and Hudson, 1991
Lenci, Ruggero, "Adèle Naudé Santos, ANS & A, Architectural Itinerary in Two Hemispheres," *L'architettura cronache e storia* 569 (March 2003)
Yee, Rendow, *Architectural Drawing: A Visual Compendium of Types and Methods*, New York: Wiley, 1997

SÃO PAULO, BRAZIL

The city of São Paulo, capital of the state with the same name and the industrial and financial center of Brazil, has been described since the last decades of the 19th to the 20th century as a locomotive. Unlike cities with outstanding natural beauty, such as Rio de Janeiro, São Paulo has been likened to a powerful engine, the product of human impact, altering and overcoming natural obstacles in favor of civilization.

São Paulo was founded by the Jesuits in 1554 as a mission center (the central colonial area called Patio do Colégio) on a plateau 760 meters (2,493 feet) above sea level, although only 72 kilometers (35 miles) from the Atlantic coast. It remained a small town for a long time and would have to wait until the 18th century to be chartered as a city (1711) and a further century and a half to experience unparalleled urban growth to become today one of the largest cities in the world, housing more than 15 million inhabitants in its metropolitan area.

Local pride had attributed the industriousness of São Paulo inhabitants ("Paulistas") to the "bandeirantes" who had the city as a base for their expeditions. They were explorers responsible for marking territory for the Portuguese crown while imprisoning or killing native Indians and searching for precious stones. However, it was the massive European immigration at the turn of the 20th century (Italian, Portuguese, Spanish, German, Syrian-Lebanese, and later Japanese), together with the coffee export boom and industrialization, that defined the modern city and its architecture.

As a result, if in 1895 São Paulo had 130,000 inhabitants, in 1900 its population had almost doubled. Disorderly growth was met with remarkable urban improvements, including the opening of avenues, lighting, gasworks, public transportation, and works for embellishment. Municipal commissions prepared reports on the living conditions of the working classes of the industrial neighborhoods of the city, especially Luz, Bom Retiro, Brás, and Mooca. Epidemics such as smallpox, Spanish flu, and yellow fever, as well as the moral and physical menace of slums, were to be avoided by sanitation, street planning, and drainage and channeling of rivers, all planned by the local administration and the newly created Engineering School (Escola Politécnica, 1894). The opening of Avenida Paulista (1891) and the building of Viaduto do Chá (1892), uniting the old center to new industrial areas, and of the São Paulo Railway Station (Estação da Luz, 1901) were seen as proof of progress.

Architecture was a major force behind these changes. The style chosen—ecclecticism—reflected European models and was considered to be the most civilized and appealing to bourgeois taste. It can be found at Carlos Ekman's Vila Penteado (rua Maranhão) and in the works of architect engineer Francisco de Paula Ramos de Azevedo (1851–1928), who studied in Belgium and planned a large number of private mansions and public buildings, such as the school Caetano de Campos (1894), the Palácio das Indústrias (Industry Palace, 1911–24, with Domiziano Rossi), and the Municipal Theatre (Teatro Municipal, 1895–1911, with associates).

In 1912, the City of São Paulo Improvements and Freehold Company (known as the "City") was established in London with the aim to develop distant suburban areas in São Paulo following the pattern of Ebenezer Howard's (1850–1928) garden cities. Raymond Unwin (1863–1940) and Barry Parker (1867–1941) were commissioned to develop the areas of Jardim América and City Lapa and to rearrange the Trianon Park at Avenida Paulista (1917–19). The growth of São Paulo and workers' unrest during the first decades of the century led Mayor Washington Luis to declare during the opening of São Paulo Industry Palace that the city was "Chicago and Manchester together in one."

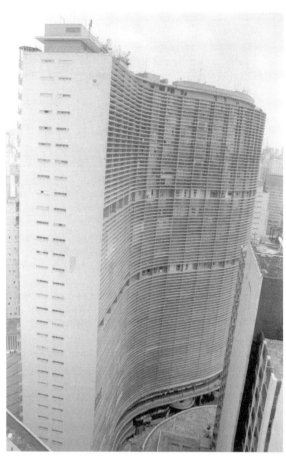

Copan Building (1957) designed by Oscar Niemeyer
© Eduardo Costa

During the 1922 São Paulo's Modern Art Week, spearheaded by the intellectuals Mário de Andrade and Oswald de Andrade, among others, there was an urgent cry for devising a national style in the arts and a modern aesthetics rooted on indigenous sources. Ecclecticism was substituted for a vigorous modern architecture and urban planning. Skyscrapers were built, and the Plano de Avenidas, an ambitious design of radial streets by the engineer Francisco Prestes Maia (1826–1965; twice mayor, nominated 1937–45, elected 1961–65), was partly executed.

Modern architecture in Brazil has created a regional version of the International Style. Although there are examples of the Art Deco style, such as Rino Levi's cinemas and skyscrapers of the 1920s (Columbus Building, Rino Levi, 1932, demolished; Martinelli Building, 1934, 105 meters and 26 floors, the largest ever built in South America at the time), São Paulo houses several examples of the local adoption of Le Corbusier's "five steps." Gregori Warchavchik (1896–1982) designed several residences, including his own (1928, rua Santa Cruz), a boxlike building based on geometry, symmetry, and standardization of building materials that was visited by Le Corbusier himself in 1929. The Esther Building (Praça da República, 1938) by Álvaro Vital Brazil (1909–97), with Ademar Marinho (1909–), featured a roof terrace, continuous window strips, and free facade composition in a residential and commercial building.

In the postwar period, with about two million inhabitants, São Paulo experienced huge and disorderly growth as a result of real estate speculation, clandestine housing, and lack of basic public services. Verticalization was regarded as a symbol of the city's economic power, beating its rival Rio de Janeiro. During his 1958 visit, Roger Bastide noted with astonishment, "Here the architect's hand replaced God's hand." The highlights of this period are the Masp Building (Modern Museum of Art, 1957–68) by Lina Bo Bardi (1914–92) and Niemeyer; several buildings, such as Copan, a lyrically curved residential and commercial building; the buildings of Ibirapuera Park and the park itself; and landscapist Burle Marx (1909–94). The park was conceived as a 1.6-million-square-meter green area inside the metropolis. Niemeyer's Memorial da América Latina (Latin America Memorial) was built only in 1988–89.

During the 1960s, São Paulo found in the architect Vilanova Artigas (1915–85) a voice of renovation. He created the architecture courses at the University of São Paulo and planned its building (1961–68), defending that design as a tool for political, social, and ideological emancipation. His engaged and revolutionary style cost him a serious persecution during Brazil's dictatorial rule but enabled him to open the road for a "Paulista School" against Rio de Janeiro's "Niemeyer School."

The Paulista Brutalism movement was soon to follow, with several examples in the houses built by Carlos Milan (1927–64). Among the new crop of architects, several stood out, such as Rodrigo Lefevre (1938–84), Paulo Mendes da Rocha (1928–), Fábio Penteado (1928–), Júlio Katinsky (1932–), Siegbert Zanetiini (1934–), Ruy Othake (1938–), Joaquim Guedes (1932–), and Sérgio Ferro (1938–).

The city's underground was built during 1973–79, a remarkable engineering work featuring an original use of reinforced concrete in all stations.

The last decades of the 20th century witnessed São Paulo stepping, perhaps too late, into the preservation era, listing several buildings and areas and sponsoring daring revitalization projects, such as the Pinacoteca do Estado (1998, Paulo Mendes da Rocha). At the same time, however, pollution and urban violence had worsened, social inequality had mounted, and urban growth continued at a chaotic pace. "Postmodern" architecture has had its share at Avenida Paulista, once the setting for the mansions of the local bourgeoisie and today a corridor of skyscrapers; the same happened at the Avenida Berrini skyscrapers for offices and banks, many of them the work of Carlos Bratke and his associates. These huge glass towers are a few steps away from one among several existing favelas (shantytowns). Housing problems have escalated, and about 2.5 million inhabitants live today in clandestine urban areas, constituting a parallel city inside São Paulo the size of the country's third-largest city in population.

CRISTINA MENEGUELLO

Further Reading

Artigas, João Batista Vilanova, *Caminhos da arquitetura*, São Paulo, Brazil: Livraria Editora Ciencias Humanas, 1981; 2nd edition, São Paulo, Brazil: Fundação Vilanova Artigas, 1986

Bacelli, Ronei, "A presença da cia city em São Paulo e a implantação do primeiro bairro Jardim, 1915–1940," Masters thesis, University of São Paulo, 1982

Bresciani, Maria Stella, "Images of São Paulo: Aesthetics and Citizenship," in *Cultura material e arqueologia histórica*, edited by Pedro Paulo A. Funari, Martin Hall, and Sian Jones, Campinas, Brazil: Instituto de Filosofia e Ciencias Humanas, Universidade Estadual de Campinas, 1998

Harris, David and Sebastiao Salgado, "São Paulo: Megacity," *Rolling Stone* (26 December 1996–9 January 1997)

Harvey, Robert, "São Paulo, São Paulo," *The Economist* 303 (25 April 1987)

Lemos, Carlos, *Ramos de Azevedo e seu escritório*, São Paulo, Brazil: Pini Editora, 1993

Porto, Antônio Rodrigues, *História urbanística da cidade de São Paulo, 1554–1988*, São Paulo, Brazil: Carthago and Forte, 1992

Segawa, Hugo, *Arquiteturas no Brasil: 1900–1990*, São Paulo, Brazil: Editora da Universidade de São Paulo, 1998; 2nd edition, 1999

Toledo, Benedito Lima de, *São Paulo: três cidades em um século*, São Paulo, Brazil: Livraria Duas Cidades, 1981; 2nd edition, 1983

Wirth, John and Robert L. Jones, *Manchester and São Paulo: Problems of Rapid Urban Growth*, Stanford, California: Stanford University Press, 1978

SARASOTA SCHOOL

The Sarasota School was the name given to a group of architects practicing from 1940 to 1960 in and around Sarasota, Florida, on the Gulf of Mexico. The Sarasota School was one of several regional interpretations of modern architecture in the United States to emerge in the years following the end of World War II, including the Bay Area School in San Francisco and the Case Study Houses group in Los Angeles. By comparison to these other regional movements, the Sarasota School was the least intentional, evolving as it did from Ralph Twitchell's fortuitous presence during one of Florida's building booms. From the very start of his Sarasota career in 1936, Twitchell's work exhibited a respect for the unique landscape and climate of the west coast of Florida, his interest in local vernacular building culture, and his desire to employ newly emerging construction materials and methods to appropriately house the particularly American version of a tropical lifestyle then being defined in Sarasota.

In 1941, Twitchell was joined by Paul Rudolph, who moved to Florida as a result of his interest in Frank Lloyd Wright's recent works, in particular Florida Southern College. Rudolph was a designer of remarkable ability, and the buildings and projects that resulted from this partnership were astonishing in their consistent high quality. In their designs, Rudolph and Twitchell endeavored to engage the landscape and to develop individual buildings that employed modernist concepts of spatial liberation framed by a complementary urban order. Their project for the Finney residence on Siesta Key (1947), a design that Rudolph had made the previous year while a graduate student at Harvard University, proposed a series of walls, bridges, and dredged inlets that allowed the house to be fully integrated with its site, acting to join remote bodies of land and water while remaining delicately suspended above the landscape. The Rudolph and Twitchell project for six linked residences on the Revere property in Siesta Key (1948) represents a remarkably prescient and constructive critique of postwar American suburban development. These six houses, of which only the Revere residence was built, opposed the typical suburban distribution of houses as freestanding objects, proposing instead a series of plastically interlocked walls and horizontal planes, providing a mix of shade and sun to open-air courts while weaving interior and exterior space to yield both increased privacy and significantly greater density.

The paradise-like settings of the Sarasota School houses, which today appear so lushly "natural," were in fact the result of a process of ruthless scalping, shaping, and dredging of the original mangrove-covered, water-saturated landscape to produce navigable canals and buildable sites. These newly created and virtually barren lots on the Gulf coast required the architects of the Sarasota School to design not only the houses but also their sites. The result was a series of buildings that subtly wove their sharp-edged geometric forms into the relentless horizontality of the Florida landscape, employing structural and constructional techniques developed for the local climate, economy, and available materials and providing their occupants varied seasonal experiences of sun-drenched interior and exterior spaces. The Healy "Cocoon House" (1950), built on the edge of a canal in Siesta Key, with its suspended rubberized roof secured with cable stays, exemplified the manner in which Twitchell's interest in engaging new building technologies complemented Rudolph's capacity to explore their liberative spatial possibilities.

Following the establishment of his individual practice in 1951, Rudolph began to receive significant national and international attention. His Revere model house was visited by more than 16,000 people during 1949. His working relationship with the architectural photographers Ezra Stoller and Joseph Steinmetz (Steinmetz Studio, Sarasota, 1947) was instrumental in Rudolph's ability to create his own publicity. Skillful photographs highlighted the crisp lines and thin planes of the Leavengood residence built in St. Petersburg (1951), the Sandeling Beach Club built in Siesta Key (1952), the Walker Guest House built on Sanibel Island (1952), and the Hiss "Umbrella House" built on Lido Shores (1953). When combined with Rudolph's signature perspective drawings of both built and unbuilt projects, these publications conveyed a sense of informality and naturalness of lifestyle while exhibiting an inevitability and precision in their architectonic resolution.

At its height, the Sarasota School included Mark Hampton, Victor Lundy, Tim Siebert, Jack West, Gene Leedy, Carl Abbott, Bert Brosmith, Joseph Farrell, William Rupp, and Ralph and William Zimmerman, many of whom began their careers working for Rudolph and Twitchell. Each of these architects developed his own distinct qualities of space and form, from Lundy's sweeping pagoda-like wood roofs (St. Paul's Lutheran Church, Sarasota, 1958) to Leedy's rhythmic lines of precast concrete beams (First National Bank, Cape Canaveral, 1963) to Abbott's elegantly articulated geometries (Weld Residence, Boca Grande, 1966). The variety of designs within such a small community defied the stereotypical representation of modern architecture as lacking richness and diversity.

After starting construction on his four final Florida masterworks—Riverview High School in Sarasota (1958), Sarasota High School (1959), the Deering residence in Casey Key (1959), and the Milam residence in Ponte Vedra (1960)—Rudolph in 1958 was appointed dean of the School of Architecture at Yale University, where among his first students were Norman Foster and Richard Rogers. With the exit from Sarasota in the 1960s of Rudolph, Lundy, Hampton, Rupp, Farrell, Brosmith, and Leedy, the Sarasota School ended.

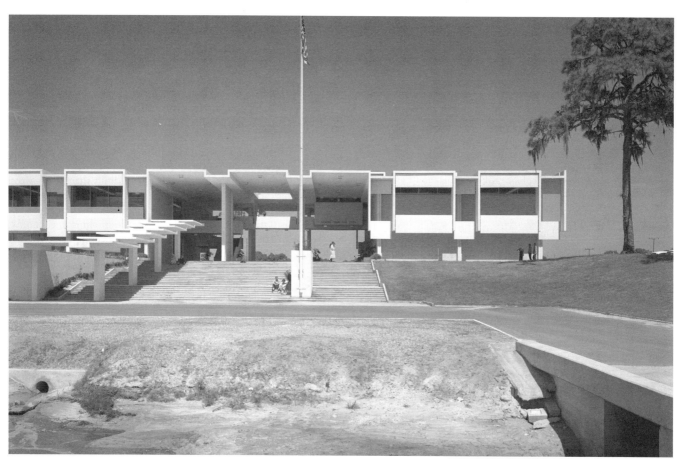

Sarasota High School, Sarasota, Florida, designed by Paul Rudolph (1959)
Ezra Stoller © Esto

Although the American architectural profession has been slow to recognize the quality of the work of the Sarasota School (having failed to award Rudolph the American Institute of Architecture Gold Medal at his death in 1997), it received extensive and immediate international attention. Typical is the experience of British architects and Team 10 founders, Alison and Peter Smithson, who, in their search for alternatives to the universal formula of the International Style in the early 1950s, were inspired by the works being built in Sarasota. The Sarasota School exemplified the concept of a regionally inflected modern architecture, true to the universal intentions of spatial liberation yet capable of engaging local climate, landscape, and building culture and demonstrating the significant benefits of an evolutionary rather than revolutionary development of modern architecture.

ROBERT MCCARTER

See also **Foster, Norman (England); Rogers, Richard (England); Rudolph, Paul (United States); Smithson, Peter and Alison (England); Team 10 (Netherlands)**

Further Reading

"Four Churches by Victor Lundy," *Architectural Record* 126.no.6 (December 1959)

Domin, Christopher; and Joseph King, *Paul Rudolph: The Florida Houses*, New York: Princeton Architectural Press, 2002

Hiss, Philip, "What Ever Happened to Sarasota?" *Architectural Forum* 126, no. 5 (June 1967)

Howey, John, *The Sarasota School of Architecture: 1941–1966*, Cambridge, Massachusetts: MIT Press, 1995

"Progress Report: The Work of Mark Hampton," *Progressive Architecture* 39, no. 6 (June 1958)

Rudolph, Paul, *The Architecture of Paul Rudolph*, New York: Praeger, and London: Thames and Hudson, 1970

Rudolph, Paul, *Paul Rudolph*, New York: Simon and Schuster, and London: Thames and Hudson, 1971

Rudolph, Paul, *Paul Rudolph: Drawings*, edited by Yukio Futagawa, Tokyo: A.D.A. Edita, 1972; as *Paul Rudolph: Architectural Drawings*, London: Lund Humphries, 1974

"Sarasota's New Schools: A Feat of Economy and Imagination," *Architectural Record* 125, no. 2 (February 1959)

"The Sarasota School of Architecture," *Florida Architect*, Convention Issue (September–October 1976)

West, Jack, *The Lives of an Architect*, Sarasota, Florida: Fauvre, 1988

SAUDI ARABIA

With a land area in excess of 2.2 million square kilometers, the kingdom of Saudi Arabia today covers most of the Arabian peninsula. The recent history of its architectural and urban development has been closely linked to its emergence as a modern nation and to the development of a powerful economy based

on the exploitation of natural resources. Saudi Arabia's opening to the international economy from the 1950s on introduced new building technologies and styles that have today largely replaced centuries-old traditional practices. However, since the 1980s, the maturation of native Saudi institutions and the work of Saudi designers, engineers, and planners has led to many successful projects that bridge modern design practices and technologies and still-valued traditional forms and lifestyles.

Climate has played a key role in urban form and architectural production in Saudi Arabia for centuries. The kingdom generally lies within one of the world's hottest and driest regions, with more than 50 percent of its land being desert. Yet within this dominant climatic milieu, local characteristics vary considerably. This relationship was long evident in the traditional approaches to the built environment in Saudi Arabia's four principal regions: the Central (*Najd*) and Northern region; the Western (*Hijaz*) region; the Eastern region along the Persian Gulf; and the Southern mountainous region.

In the extremely hot and arid areas of the Central and Northern region, the courtyard was long the main feature of any building. Courtyards traditionally acted as climatic moderators and allowed a unique private lifestyle to develop. In desert communities, built largely of adobe, open spaces generally only took the form of private courtyards and narrow, winding streets.

In the Western (*Hijaz*) region, with its hot and humid climate of Red Sea coastal communities, the basic traditional building type was the multistory row house built of coral stone and imported wood. The refined building art of this region was also influenced by an intermixing of cultures and the import of technological skills as the result of trade and pilgrimage. One distinct vernacular form that developed here was the *mashrabiyah*, a facade of transparent wooden screens, originally used in the houses of Jeddah to afford both ventilation and visual privacy. When this form gained popularity as a decorative element, it in turn influenced house design in the hot and dry inland cities of Mecca and Medina and in the upland city of Taif.

The Eastern Region along the Persian Gulf includes the cities of al-Ahsa, Qatif, Dammam, and Jubail and is characterized by a maritime inland desert climate. Here, two-story courtyard houses built of mud were the typical building type. Such dwellings often featured traditional *bagdir* or *malqaf*, wind catchers used to control ventilation.

The Southern region, which includes the Asir Mountains and extends from Taif through Baha to Abha, is characterized by a cooler climate with considerable seasonal rain. In its settlements, many located at altitudes greater than 2000 meters, buildings generally took the form of square, multistory towers. Four principal construction types developed based on the local microclimate and available materials: mud tower houses, stone rubble houses, stone apron houses, and mud and slate tower buildings. A particularly characteristic form of the Asir region was the *qasabah*, a freestanding tower of mud or stone used in isolated farming villages both for defense and to warn of the approach of raiders from other tribes.

Until the second half of the 20th century, these regional urban and architectural traditions responded well to local cultural and material conditions and allowed people to adjust their activity cycles to climatic variations. In more recent times, however, modern forms and patterns have been introduced that have largely replaced these traditional practices.

Two major building campaigns of the 1950s can today be judged as having initiated this process: the expansion of the holy mosques of Mecca and Medina and the huge program involved in transferring the nation's capital from Mecca to Riyadh. From 1951 to 1955, the government undertook a major effort to repair and expand the Prophet Mosque in Medina, with the result being a fourfold increase in the area for prayer; a second huge project from 1955 to 1974 expanded the holy mosque in Mecca, where the area available for prayer was increased from 29,127 to 193,000 square meters. The building program in Riyadh likewise spanned many years. Its first phase, in the mid-1950s, included construction of both a complex of ministry buildings on the airport road and a housing project for government employees in the Malaz area. Also a part of the early work were the rebuilding and expansion of the royal palace at Nasirriyah to cover 250 hectares, the rebuilding of the main mosque and government palace in the city center, and the widening of the two main streets leading into the city.

Coupled with the Aramco grid plans for al-Khobar and Dammam in 1947 and the Aramco Employees Home Ownership program launched in 1951, these government building campaigns laid a foundation for the development of contemporary building and planning practices in Saudi Arabia. However, the introduction of new processes, materials, and techniques was first carried out largely through the import of foreign expertise to the kingdom. From the early 1960s on, the gridded street pattern and the villa as a preferred house type assumed primacy in the development of most every city and town. Processes of urban change and expansion were given further impetus by the compensation given private property owners in Mecca, Medina, and Riyadh following the expropriation of their traditional city center houses to make way for government projects. Apartment buildings also first began to appear in Riyadh, Mecca, Medina, and Jeddah from the late 1950s on. In the mid-1950s, the government launched a national school-building program, which brought international-style design in reinforced concrete and cement block to the smallest towns and villages.

A further change in Saudi cities and towns in the 1960s was the introduction of high-rise construction. Distinct among the earliest such projects were the Saudi Arabian Airlines and the Saudi Radio Broadcasting buildings in Jeddah. However, the twenty-two-story Queen building (1972) in Jeddah represented the most radical break with tradition, and for many years it stood as a principal landmark on the city's skyline. Other notable projects in the early 1970s included the UPM Campus in Dhahran by CRS, whose design considered the natural terrain and employed an exposed-aggregate texture to blend with its surroundings; the Equestrian Club Building (1973) in Riyadh by Frank Basil, which responded effectively to climate using new architectural forms; and the Intercontinental Hotels and Conference Centers (1971) in Riyadh by Trevord Dannat and in Mecca (1973) by Rolf Gutbrod and Frei Otto, which emerged from international design competitions.

Following the oil boom of 1973, the new wealth had profound, wide-reaching consequences for Saudi cities and towns. This was particularly evident in campaigns of infrastructure development and in the design and construction of new universities, schools, hospitals, hotels, airports and seaports, factories, housing estates, and entire new towns. The oil boom also led to the establishment of the national Real Estate Development

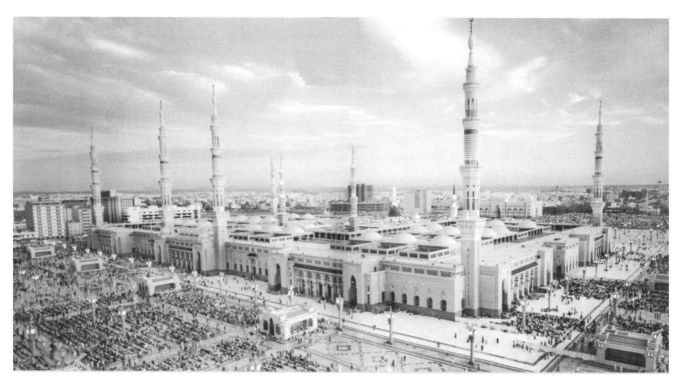

Holy Prophet Mosque of Medina (1950–55, first phase; 1983–1994, second phase)
© Saleh Al-Hathloul

Fund, offering individual Saudi citizens subsidized long-term loans to build private houses, apartments, and office buildings. Half the country's housing stock has been replenished through this program since its initatiation. Coupled with government land grants, available to every Saudi citizen 18 years of age or older, it has led to a several-fold expansion of most Saudi cities and towns.

Although most early modern architecture and planning in the kingdom was carried out by foreign-trained experts, from the 1980s onward, local architects, engineers, and planners began to assume an increasingly important role. For instance, Ali Shuaibi and Abdurrahman Al-Hussaini of Beeah Group Consultants have given special emphasis to sociocultural values, in particular to the desire to relate modern construction methods to the Islamic past. Their distinct planning work has included the al-Uqair Tourist Development Plan (1986), the Jubail Subregional Plan (1998), and the Strategic Comprehensive Plan (1998) for the Holy Environs and Mecca, which addressed the need to accommodate and transfer two million pilgrims between Mecca and the Holy Environs during the five-day pilgrimage. Beeah Group Consultants has also been known for such urban design work as its Central Spine, DQ (1980); the Qasr al-Hukm project (1983); and the King Abdulaziz Historical Center (1998), all in Riyadh. The continued value of seclusion and privacy in Saudi culture was evident in the design of al-Kindi Plaza (1986) in Riyadh, which won the Agha Khan Award for Architecture. Other important designs are the Saudi Embassy (1987) in Yemen, the King Saud Mosque (1992) in Riyadh, the SAPICO Headquarters (1992) in Islamabad, and the Municipality of Me-

dina Complex (2000), all of which combine past and present, a necessity in the perpetuation of culture.

Equally impressive projects have been designed by the team known as Basim al-Shihabi of Omrania. Their projects include the General Organization for Social Insurance (GOSI) Headquarters (1978); the Twaiq Palace (1985), an Agha Khan Award winner; the Gulf Cooperation Council building (1987); and the King Abdulaziz Archival building (al-Darah) (1998), all in Riyadh. The current direction of ideas that al-Shihabi originally synthesized in the 1970s are evident in the NNCI Headquarters building (1999) and the Kingdom Complex, which includes a 330-meter-high tower to be completed in 2001.

A third noteworthy Saudi architecture firm, Mohammad Al-Naim and Farahat Tashkandi of Al-Nai, has emphasized the importance of continuity in cultural traditions in a changing world. This theme can be seen in their neighborhood layouts and land subdivision projects for MOMRA (1993) and in layouts for the Namar and Uraid neighborhoods (1994) in Riyadh. The team's design for municipal prototype houses attempted to revitalize the traditional Arab house, not through formalistic adaptation but by reconstituting essential values in new forms. Other work has included the School of Environmental Design building, KAU (1987), in Jeddah and the College of Architecture and Planning, KFU (2000), in Dammam. Mohammad Al-Naim and Farahat Tashkandi's work on the Al Abbas Mosque (1995) in Riyadh won them an award for transforming traditional aesthetic values to a more modern look.

Ziad Zaidan of Idea Center is another firm whose distinction lay in the team's Master Plan and Urban Design schemes for

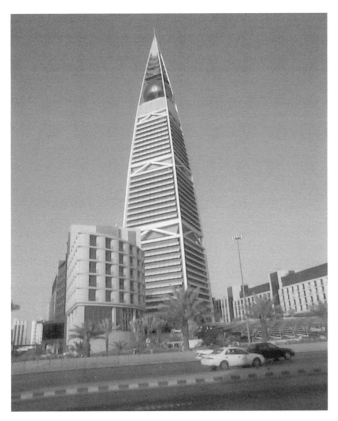

Al-Faisaliah Center (2000), designed by Norman Foster, in Riyadh
© Saleh Al-Hathloul

Yanbu Industrial City, a contemporary settlement for 150,000 people aimed at combining state-of-the-art technology with the principles of Islamic town planning. Ziad Zaidan is also known for its Umm al-Qura University campus (1995) in Mecca, in association with Perkins and Will, a carefully considered campus plan creating a harmonious synthesis of old and new. Other projects have included the Asir Governorate Complex (1995) in Abha, adapting elements of Asir architectural tradition with modern materials and technology, and Aramco's Western Region Headquarters (1989) in Jeddah, for which the team won the American Institute of Architects' Award for Excellence in Architecture. Zaidan also served as architectural consultant for the Institute du Monde Arabe (1987) in Paris, designed by Jean Nouvel and the Architecture Studio.

Abdulla Bokhari of Archi-Plan is a strong believer in the influence and importance of theories in design. Bokhari sees tradition as having no authority except as a platform for further transformation or as an ongoing experiment. This approach is best seen in his designs for the SANCST Cultural and Leisure Facilities Center (1989) and the UNDP Headquarters (2000), both in Riyadh.

Several regional architects have also produced important work in Saudi Arabia, including the contributions of Sami Anqawi, director of the Pilgrimage Research Center for many years and a practicing architect in Amar. His strong commitment to tradition is best reflected in the renovation of the Amar Office Building in Old Jeddah and in his design of the al-Yamani residence (1980s) in Mecca. Saleh Qadah's work in Asir is also worth noting for his ability to use traditional architectural features as part of modern designs. This was well demonstrated in Almiftah Village (1989) and in the Chamber of Commerce Building (1989), both in Abha.

In addition to these individual designers and design teams, the government-backed Arriyadh Development Authority (ADA) has also been a major contributor to the shaping of urban patterns and architecture styles in the kingdom. Among the most notable projects carried out by the ADA in the Riyadh area have been the development of the Diplomatic Quarter, a new town within the city; the MFA Staff Housing (1983); the development of the Justice Palace District (1985–2000); and the development of the King Abdulaziz Historic Center (1998). The award-winning quality of the ADA's projects is often demonstrated through magnificent architecture that marries traditional and modern forms.

In the political arena, Mohammad Said Farsi, the well-known mayor of Jeddah from the early 1970s to the mid-1980s, was also influential in the development of new trends in architecture and planning in the kingdom. An architect and planner, his efforts to preserve the old city and develop Jeddah's architectural tastes had wide-ranging effects on the architectural profession in Saudi Arabia.

In terms of architectural education, Ahmad Farid Moustafa was also extremely influential on the course of architecture and planning in the kingdom. Moustafa served as the first head of the Department of Architecture at King Saud University in the late 1960s. Later he was a founder and dean for the School of Architecture and Planning at King Faisal University. In these positions, he had a tremendous effect on the first generation of architectural students in Saudi Arabia. Adel Ismail and Mohammad Said Mousalli were others who played major roles in the development of architecture education, both through their teaching at King Saud University and through their involvement as advisers for government agencies.

Formal architecture education began in Saudi Arabia with the establishment of the Department of Architecture at King Saud University of Riyadh in 1967. Other schools followed: the College of Architecture and Planning at King Faisal University, Dammam (1975); the School of Environmental Design, King Abdulaziz University, Jeddah (1976); the College of Environmental Design, University of Petroleum and Minerals, Dammam (1979); and the Department of Islamic Architecture, Umm al-Qura University, Mecca (1983). Some of the first graduates of these universities in turn began teaching careers of their own in the 1980s. These have included Saleh Al-Hathloul, Mohammad Al-Hussayn, Mohammad bin Saleh, Tarik Al-Sulaiman, and Jameel Akbar. Such educators have had a broad effect on the field through teaching, writing, and involvement as jurors, reviewers, and evaluators of major projects.

The role of national professional organizations has also increased in importance. In 1982, the Engineering Committee was formed through the Chamber of Commerce to oversee and organize design and consulting practice. The Saudi Association for Architects and Planners (AL-UMRAN) was formed in 1989, and its membership now exceeds 1000. *Albenna* magazine, covering architectural and development issues, produced its first issue in February–March 1979.

In addition to these local influences, the work of international architects in Saudi Arabia has continued, and in recent years this has also become more responsive to local conditions. Among the many excellent examples of work by international design teams in Saudi Arabia have been the Haj Terminal (1982) at King Abdulaziz Airport in Jeddah by Skidmore, Owings, and Merrill, a 20th-century adaptation of traditional tent structures; the National Commercial Bank (1984) in Jeddah, also by Skidmore, Owings, and Merrill, a modern corporate headquarters successfully integrated into a traditional setting; the Ministry of Foreign Affairs (1984) in Riyadh by Henning Larsen, whose monumental formalism presents an intelligent response to changing opinions; and King Fahad International Stadium (1987) in Riyadh by Ain Friezer and Partners, a masterpiece of tent architecture.

Other examples include the Central Government Complex (early 1980s) in Taif by Leslie Martin, a complex that responds well to climatic requirements and blends with local architecture; Imam Moh'd Bin Saud Islamic University (1988) by Techni Beria; King Saud University, Al-Gassim Campus (1995), by Kenzo Tange Associates, K. Baytarian and Associates, and So-mait Engineering Services, a 10,000-student campus based on a hierarchy of open spaces; and the Nuzul Hotel (1995) in Skaka by John Lingly, which efficiently uses passive cooling systems and local design methods.

Many other projects from the last 25 years also deserve recognition: the Riyadh TV Tower (1981), designed by ADIT of France; the Council of Ministers Building (early 1980s) in Jeddah by Kenzo Tange; the King Khalid International Airport Terminal (1983) in Riyadh by Hellmuth, Obata, and Kassabaum (HOK); and the King Fahad International Airport Terminal (1993) in Dammam by M. Yamasaki, who was the designer for the Dhahran Airport Terminal (1961).

Also of note have been Al-Ta'meer Center I (1999), designed by Arrowstreet, Inc., in association with Dar Al-Mimar (Badran and Abdul Halim), a festival market in the heart of Riyadh incorporating sustainable-design elements; Al-Khaleej Village (1990) in Dammam, an earlier, influential model for a seaside resort city; Sultan bin Abdulaziz City for Humanitarian Services (2000) in Riyadh by the OEO/HLW design partnership, a hospital and training complex; and Al-Faisaliah Center (2000) in Riyadh by Norman Foster, a 300-meter-high skyscraper to complement al-Khairia Center (1982) by Kenzo Tange.

Since the late 1970s, urban renewal has also become an important trend in the kingdom. Such urban design schemes were first developed for downtown Riyadh by Albini (1978) and Beeah (1983) and were subsequently revised by the ADA's staff. The rebuilding of the al-Muraba area in Riyadh (1998), an urban design by Beeah and Badran, will also create a cultural and historic center to complement Riyadh's city center. Other major urban-renewal programs have concerned further recent expansions of the holy mosques in Mecca and Medina. In Mecca, an urban design scheme (1986) by Dar Al-Handasah takes the Ka'bah as its center and proposes the continuation of prayer space on the ground level up to the first Ring Road. In Medina, the whole area of the old city has been encompassed in the Prophet mosque extension (1994), and the surrounding area up to the first ring road has been transformed into a gridded plan.

Thus, it is evident that various climates, regional materials, local vernacular traditions, and economic and technological de-velopment have significantly directed architecture and its practice in 20th-century Saudi Arabia. The first half of the century reflected centuries of building habits and cultural needs, whereas the second half showed the immediate and large-scale effect of economic prosperity in an internationally important region that adapted new buildings types and modern urban planning to suit a variety of modern needs.

SALEH AL-HATHLOUL

See also **Jeddah, Saudi Arabia; Ministry of Foreign Affairs, Riyadh, Saudi Arabia; Riyadh, Saudi Arabia**

Further Reading

Of the works cited below, King, Hariri-Rifai, and Talib provide a good overview of Saudi Arabia's traditional architecture. The works by Eben Saleh and Alkokani and by Nomachi document the historic development and the extensions of the two holy mosques in Mecca and Medina and their effect on the urban structure of the two cities. A record of most architecture projects in Saudi Arabia since the late 1970s appears in *Albenna Architecture Magazine*. The Aga Khan Award for Architecture books include good coverage of winning projects from Saudi Arabia.

Abbas, Hamid, *Qissat al-Tawsiah al-Kubra*, Jeddah: Majmu'at Bin Ladin al-Su'udiyah, 1995

Albenna Architecture Magazine, nos. 1–118 (February 1979–June 2000)

Al-Hathloul, Saleh, and Aslam Mughal, "Makkah: Developing the Center of Islam District," *Urban Design International* (2000)

Davidson, Cynthia A., *Legacies for the Future: Contemporary Architecture in Islamic Societies*, London: Thames and Hudson, 1998; New York: Thames and Hudson, 1999

Eben Saleh, Mohammad Eben Abdullah, and Abdelhafeez Feda Alkokani (editors), *Proceedings of the Symposium on Mosque Architecture*, 10 vols., Riyadh: King Saud University, 1999; see especially vol. 1, *The Architecture of the Two Holy Mosques*

Khan, Hasan-Uddin, *Contemporary Asian Architects*, Cologne and New York: Taschen, 1995

King, Geoffrey, *The Traditional Architecture of Saudi Arabia*, London: Tauris, 1998

Kultermann, Udo, *Contemporary Architecture in the Arab States*, New York: McGraw-Hill, 1999

Nomachi, Ali K., *Al Madina al-Munawwarah*, Medina: Tharaa International, 1997

Hariri-Rifai, Wahbi, and Mokhless Hariri-Rifai, *The Heritage of the Kingdom of Saudi Arabia*, Washington, D.C.: GDG Publications, 1990

Steele, James, *Architecture for a Changing World: The Aga Khan Award for Architecture*, London: Academy Editions, 1992

Talib, Kaiser, *Shelter in Saudi Arabia*, London: Academy Editions, and New York: St. Martin's Press, 1984

SCARPA, CARLO 1906–78

Architect, Italy

For much of his career a figure isolated and detached from the mainstream, Carlo Scarpa was recognized only after his death as one of the great architects of the 20th century. His work does not fit easily into standard genealogical accounts of modernist architecture. It is characterized by a virtuosity of light, color, and texture; an extraordinary refinement of detail; and complex manipulations of materials and geometry.

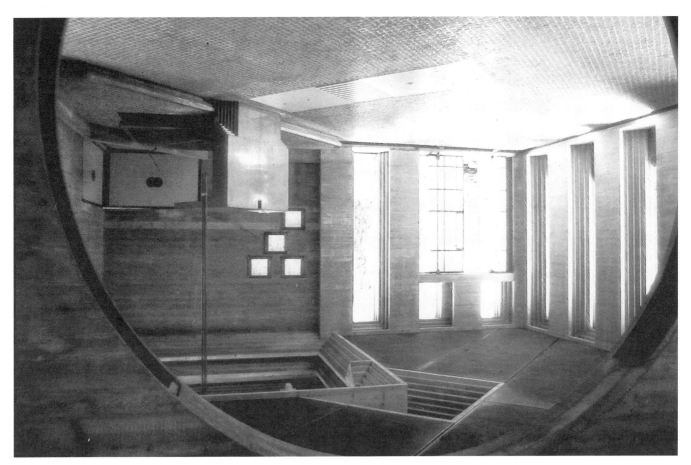

Chapel, Brion Tomb, San Vito d'Altivole, Italy (1972)
© Ross Jenner

Scarpa obtained a diploma as a teacher of architectural drawing from the Academy of Fine Arts in Venice in 1926, when he also began teaching at the Architectural Institute of Venice University. Before beginning his career as an architect, he gained an exceptional understanding of materials working as artistic director of Venini, one of the most prominent manufacturers of Venetian glass, from 1933 to 1947. He was influenced by Frank Lloyd Wright, but the sumptuous visual density of his work is rooted more in the traditions of Venetian craftsmanship and Viennese ornamentation, typified by Josef Hoffmann and the *Wiener Werkstätte*. Scarpa taught at the IUAV from 1926 until his death, becoming director in 1972.

Scarpa designed numerous exhibitions in London, Paris, Rome, and Milan. For over 30 years, beginning in 1942, he consulted for the Venice Biennale. A major break through in his career was the 1948 "Paul Klee" exhibition, followed by a book pavilion in 1950. Among his greatest contributions to post-war Italian architecture was the reconstruction of several historic buildings as museums, most notably the Palazzo Abatellis (Palermo, 1953–54), the Museo di Castelvecchio (Verona, 1956–64), and Quirini-Stampalia (Venice, 1961–63), where he elevated restoration to the level of art form. The restructuring of the Museo Correr (1953–60) and the Ca' Foscari (1954–56) in Venice received acclaim. At the same time, he undertook the layout and installation of the first six rooms of the Uffizi in Florence (1954–56, with Ignazio Gardella and Giovanni Michelucci) and planned the extension to the gypsum museum in Possagno (1955–57). Other outstanding works include the Olivetti Showroom (Venice, 1957–58), and the Gavina Showroom (Bologna, 1961–63). The Banca Popolare di Verona (1973–80), his last large work, posthumously completed, suggests the directions he might have followed had he not died prematurely. Among his domestic works, the Veritti House (Udine, 1955–61) and Ottolenghi House (Bardolino, 1974–) are most notable. It is, however, Brion-Vega Tomb and Cemetery (San Vito d'Altivole, 1970–72) that best typifies Scarpa's enigmatic quality and his tendency to realize form as a condition of process.

Rejecting the neutral spaces of mainstream modernism, Scarpa created settings highlighting the uniqueness of objects. Container and content interact across history, manifesting a new attitude to the past and a break with modernism's utopian teleologies. His architectural interventions create an overall artwork that embraces painting and sculpture dialogically. Historical objects and contexts are no longer simply assimilated, juxtaposed, or contrasted but rather interpreted by the architecture itself. At the Castelvecchio, for example, Scarpa hauntingly entangles the principal threads of circulation and lines of vision around the

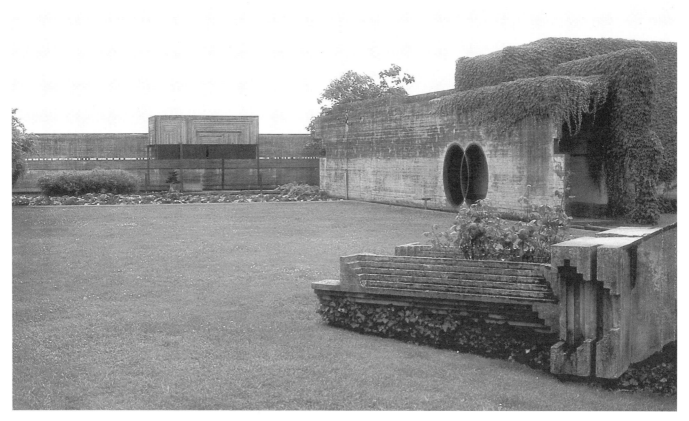

Entry and meditation pavilion, Brion Tomb, San Vito d'Altivole (1972)
© Ross Jenner

equestrian figure of the Cangrande. At other times, the engagement amplifies the displays: in the extension to the Possagno museum for Canova's plaster casts a refined arrangement admits the changing daylight through slots and cutout cubes of sky, vivifying the chalky prototypes and walls.

Scarpa tended to approach his projects without fixed concepts. Instead, they grew out of personal interactions with clients, craftsmen, artists, and preexisting contexts. Designs were developed as processes of making, particularly in his unique mode of drawing that proceeded, like the fabric of the final buildings, in strata and palimpsests, and with meticulous attention to the smallest detail. In this sense, the works were both occasional and decorative: They were befitting celebrations or commemorations of occasions and persons—alien to both contemporary functionalist and later neorationalist approaches, but located within a respect for tradition.

Scarpa's interest in the facade points to an acceptance of convention in architecture and a special attention to civic concerns, as in the Banca Popolare di Verona. His work is grounded in the specificities of place and region but without fixation on local identity. It is ornamental, arising from a complex poetics of differentiation and junction of nodes and seams. The sheer complexity of his compositions embraces encryption, numerology, astrology and mathematical games, the play of allusion, and

a diffusion of associations by the resonance of figures and motifs at multiple scales.

Scarpa was seen by many of his contemporaries as distanced from true modern architecture. His ways of working were regarded as archaic, as a reactionary indulgence in lost practices without future, obsessed with detail, precious materials, and luxurious artifice. The Venice Order of Architects sued him for unlawfully practicing as an architect, but he successfully defended the lawsuit. His nonchalance regarding the tasks of the contemporary world, the fact that he worked for museums, foundations, and private clients rather than for public administration, provoked ideological criticism. Although he enjoyed considerable respect as a designer and specialist in restoration and the interior design of museums and exhibitions, only Mazzariol and Zevi, his earliest defenders, promoted his importance as an architect.

Since his death nonmodern perceptions have highlighted and legitimized the metaphorical potential of Scarpa's work. Its dispersed, fragmentary nature and its perpetual capacity to defy geometric closure are acknowledged by Tafuri in his comparison with Umberto Eco's idea of the *opera aperta*. His composition by breaks and scattering anticipated the disjointed work of the deconstructivists. Detail has now become a source of interest to those concerned with ornament and tectonics alike—we are

perhaps closer to him today than his contemporaries were. Scarpa's influence on subsequent architecture has been diffuse but indirect; his work is too singular to be directly emulated.

ROSS JENNER

See also **Tafuri, Manfredo (Italy); Zevi, Bruno (Italy)**

Selected Publications

"Letter of the Venetian Rationalists," Published in *Il Lavoro Fascista*, 1931, *Carlo Scarpa: The Complete Works*

"A Thousand Cypresses," Lecture given in Madrid, 1978

The Other City: The Architect's Working Method As Shown by the Brion Cemetery in San Vito d'Altivole/Die andere Stadt: Die Arbeitsweise des Architekten am Beispiel der Grabanlage Brion in San Vito d'Altivole (bilingual English—German edition), Berlin: Ernst, 1989

Selected Works

Brion-Vega Cemetery and Brion Tomb, San Vito d'Altivole, Italy, 1972

Banca Populare di Verona, Verona, Italy, 1980

Further Reading

Albertini, Bianca and Alessandro Bagnoli, *Scarpa: L'architettura nel dettaglio*, Milan: Jaca Book, 1988; as *Carlo Scarpa: Architecture in Details*, translated by Donald Mills, Cambridge, Massachusetts: MIT Press, and London: Architecture Design and Technology Press, 1988

Beltramini, Guido, Kurt W. Forster, and Paola Marini (editors), *Carlo Scarpa: Mostre e musei, 1944–1976: Case e paesaggi, 1972–1978*, Milan: Electa, 2000

Crippa, Maria Antonietta, *Carlo Scarpa: Il pensiero, il disegno, i progetti*, edited by Marina Loffi Randolin, Milan: Jaca Book, 1984; as *Carlo Scarpa: Theory, Design, Projects*, translated by Susan Chapman and Paola Pinna, Cambridge, Massachusetts: MIT Press, 1986

Dal Co, Francesco and Giuseppe Mazzariol (editors), *Carlo Scarpa: Opera completa*, Milan: Electa, 1984; as *Carlo Scarpa: The Complete Works*, New York: Electa/Rizzoli, 1985

Detti, Edoardo, *Carlo Scarpa, 1906–1978: Histoires comme experience*, Marseilles: Éditions Parenthèses, 1986

Frascari, Marco, "A Heroic and Admirable Machine: The Theatre of the Architecture of Carlo Scarpa, Architetto Veneto," *Poetics Today* 10, no. 1 (1989)

Los, Sergio, *Carlo Scarpa*, Cologne: Taschen, 1993

Los, Sergio, *Carlo Scarpa: Guida all'architettura*, Venice: Arsenale Editrice, 1995; as *Carlo Scarpa: An Architectural Guide*, translated by Antony Shugaar, 1995

Mazzariol, Giuseppe, "Opere di Carlo Scarpa," *L'Architettura: Cronache e storia* 3 (1955)

Nakamura, Toshio (editor), *Karuro Sukarupa-Carlo Scarpa* (bilingual Japanese-English edition), Tokyo: A + U, 1985

Olsberg, R. Nicholas, et al., *Carlo Scarpa, Architect: Intervening with History*, New York: Monacelli Press, and Montreal: Canadian Centre for Architecture, 1999

Zambonini, Giuseppe, "Process and Theme in the Work of Carlo Scarpa," *Perspecta* 20 (1983)

SCHAROUN, HANS 1893–1972

Architect, Germany

Although born in Bremen, Germany, on 20 September 1893, Hans Scharoun grew up in the town of Bremerhaven, Germany's major port just west of the industrial city of Hamburg. Exhibiting a fascination with machines and architecture in his earliest sketches and drawings, Scharoun took careful notice of the rapid changes he saw in the world around him, changes even more exaggerated in the activities of the port. Bremerhaven, Germany's gateway to the world, felt the impact of cultures beyond Germany's borders and was thus more cosmopolitan than much of the country. It was also a place in which new forms of technology and transport drove the city's development; in this context, new theories involving space and time were not abstract but quite real, leaving an imprint on the port's infrastructure and, consequently, the city's architecture. As remarked by Peter Blundell-Jones, a noted scholar of Scharoun's work, Scharoun appeared to have received the imprint of these ideas as well, for his architecture and planning ideas were anything but sentimental. From his earliest attempts at architecture and urban planning, Scharoun engaged the dynamics of economic exchange and technological development directly. Yet Scharoun's concept for architecture, or *Baukunst* (at the time German architects pointedly used, after Schinkel, the term *Baukunst*, or "building art," rather than "architecture" to describe their work), was not simply utilitarian but sought an expression of the Modern era. Scharoun's vision, one he shared with several other members of his generation, espoused a kind of functionalism—although not the functionalism promoted by several of his contemporaries, including the *Sachlichkeit* architects Hannes Meyer and Ludwig Hilberseimer. Rather, Scharoun emphasized the spiritual foundation of organic form, where the formation of the interior generated the exterior form.

Scharoun was accepted as a student of architecture at the Technische Hochschule in Berlin-Charlottenburg in 1912 and became well versed in engineering technologies, the primary emphasis of the architectural course at the time. He also worked as an assistant in the Berlin office of Paul Kruchen, an assistant at the Technische Hochschule and Scharoun's first real mentor. While on holiday from his studies, the young architect worked as a bricklayer's apprentice. The curriculum of the Technische Hochschule did not engage his imagination; unlike contemporary architectural education, there was little focus on design in most German architectural programs at the time. Nonetheless, Scharoun took part in numerous competitions, seeing them as opportunities in which he could develop and exercise his architectural ideas. When World War I broke out, Scharoun voluntarily entered military service, where he was eventually assigned to assist Kruchen, who had by then become a military architect. His early reputation as an architect was in fact based on these competitions; in comparison with other competition entrants, Scharoun's work was exceptionally progressive. The most significant of these was his competition entry for the planning of the cathedral area in Prenzlau, a project that led to an association with the noted Expressionist architect Bruno Taut and the architectural critic Adolf Behne, both of whom resided in Berlin. Both Taut and Behne were active in the utopian group *Arbeitsrat für Kunst* (Work Council for Art), an association of architects, writers, and artists founded immediately after the November 1918 revolution. The group, reflecting the burgeoning socialist sentiments of many cultural figures during the Weimar Republic, sought to recover an art that was "for the people" and vice versa, a people energized by their creative actions. In so doing, many of them not only dispensed with the past but, in utopist

fashion, overlooked the difficulties of the present in favor of the possibility of future redemption. Seeing change and development as modern architecture's foundational premise, Scharoun quickly became an associate and advocate of the group, participating in Taut's "chain letters," a secretive, semianonymous correspondence known as the *Gläserne Kette* (Glass Chain). Scharoun's language and visionary sketches from the period, bursting with intense light, color, and contrasts and using Expressionist symbols, are infused with utopian visions shared by members of the group such as Wassily Luckhardt, Herman Finsterlin, and Walter Gropius. Typical Expressionist architectural programs, such as *Volkshaus* (House of the People) and *Stadtkrone* (Crown of the City or City's Crown), with titles such as "Monument to Joy" and "Crystal on the Sphere" (Luckhardt) and *Kultbau*, or "Cult-Building" (Scharoun), exposed the underlying influences of German nature mysticism and 19th-century German Romanticism. Although interested in fantasy and longing, Scharoun's legacy from the period centered around subtle aspects of architecture: daylighting (*Lichtführung*, literally "the control of daylight") and organic form.

Expressionism's resort to quasi-mystical (spiritual) issues and forms of nature was effectively subsumed into the development of functionalism in the 1920s. Ornament—the rendering of ideas in architecture through surface application and detail—gave way to the embrace of space and time, a shift dependent on changes in the ideas and methods of the physical and natural sciences. Accordingly, space—immaterial and implied—became the residence of Spirit (*Geist*), whereas form, perceived as plastic and mutable, was infused with references to organisms, growth, and change.

Scharoun's architectural work from this period mirrored his incorporation of these influences, and his associations with certain architects and artists (several of whom exhibited an interest in the a "constructed organicist" version of the post-Dada group *Neue Sachlichkeit*, or New Objectivity) grew. Among his closest associates were artists Kurt Schwitters, Hans Richter, and Theo van Doesburg, all of whom worked to sublimate the mechanics and demands of persistent change and spirit in their art. Scharoun's particular interest in painting and collage—at this time highly gestural and expressive, with a hint of attention to vernacular traditions—supported the architect's functionalist ethic. At the time, functionalism was both a method and a philosophy (or shared faith) whereby the spirit moves from within to without; accordingly, "form" is the result of spiritual expansion and expression moving out into the world. Scharoun's incorporation of fluid, complex forms and rhythms, coupled with his embrace of architecture's new technologies and materials, aided and abetted his general resistance to academic form. Rather than static works resting on the landscape hidden behind an ordered facade, Scharoun's architectural designs—his spaces and forms—remained fluid and organic, engaging the landscape directly in providing a place for the infusion of plant life within while extending space into the landscape itself.

Ironically, Hans Scharoun's reputation and significance as an architect increased just as political and social tensions led to the demise of the Weimar Republic and the rise of Fascism in Germany. In the mid-1920s, the "housing question" became a central focus for the development of modern architecture. Although a professor at the Kunstakademie in Breslau, Scharoun yearned for Berlin's cosmopolitan cultural arena, finally relocat-

ing to the city in 1927–28. It was a fortuitous move professionally, and he began to obtain various commissions (his association with Berlin developer Georg Jacobowitz was particularly fruitful). Scharoun also had the good fortune of participating with several of his former *Arbeitsrat* colleagues, collaborating on several planning and housing developments, including both the Modern Siemensstadt living/housing project (1928–31) and a single-family dwelling for the Weissenhofsiedlung Stuttgart, a housing exhibition organized by the Deutscher Werkbund, in 1927. Both projects, manifestos of "social housing," were "intended as . . . models for [a] new way of life." However, the die had been cast portending the rise of Fascism by the late 1920s, and options for further exploration of Modern cultural and social ideas diminished substantially.

Although he did not immigrate during the period—an option taken by many of his closest friends and associates—Scharoun suffered an internal exile throughout the late 1930s and 1940s. The last building of his "Weimar years," a house for industrialist Fritz Schminke on the border of Czechoslovakia built in 1933, showcases Scharoun's maturing architectural vision; light, material, structure, form, space, function, furniture, and landscape are fused into a seamless, organic whole. As German Fascism increased its hold, Scharoun's work went underground; exterior projections of his architectural ideas—formal and material play and movement—became hidden behind the mask of Nazism's mandated, antimodern "German vernacular." Nonetheless, Scharoun, in his design of small, residential projects, clearly maintains his developmental trajectory, exploring with even greater intensity the dynamics of interior space and light and exterior form. These projects—the Mohrmann House (1938) in Berlin-Lichtenrade and the Endell House (1939) in Berlin-Wannsee are primary examples—map the increasing internalization of his architectural work and effectively mirror Scharoun's internal exile.

Again ironically, it was during this same period that Scharoun's most significant intellectual relationship developed: Hugo Häring, 11 years Scharoun's senior, became Scharoun's principal mentor, a relationship that would continue until Häring's death. During the 1920s, Häring was known primarily for his architectural ideas and was, according to Blundell-Jones, considered more of a contemplative (theoretical) architect than a builder. During the years of fascist rule and World War II, Häring and Scharoun developed a close relationship—like Scharoun, he was also an internal exile—with the elder man fulfilling the role of mentor, Scharoun's "intellectual authority." Häring's architectural theories were quickly absorbed by Scharoun, who adopted them as explanations for his own architecture.

Immediately after the end of World War II, Scharoun was asked to help with the planning and rebuilding of Berlin and was appointed Berlin city architect until the city elections in 1946. Housing was a critical issue, and Scharoun began to work on numerous city-planning and apartment projects, including those associated with the Planungs-Kollektiv. His work in this area exhibited a concern for the entire built environment and its future viability. Incorporating the necessary functions of daily life within his planning schemes, Scharoun added public buildings, shopping areas, parks, schools, kindergartens, administrative offices, and cultural and recreational elements, including crafts workshops and spaces for weekly markets and provisions for small-scale industry and future growth. In addition, his intro-

duction of a wide range of transportation systems (with pedestrian access being the most important) underlined Scharoun's attention to the human dimension of architecture.

Scharoun was able to build many of his designs after the war, including apartment complexes, schools, and theaters—all building programs that directly engaged issues pertaining to the human dimension and, even more specifically, the quality of life. As one of the remaining architects of his generation still active in West Germany, Scharoun continued to explore architectural themes that had governed his work throughout his career: fluid space and change, program flexibility, technological advances, the primacy of the interior uses as a determinant of form, the dynamic interaction of landscape and form, and contextual response. Although there are numerous examples, notable housing projects include his design for apartments in Berlin, his "Romeo and Juliet" housing project (1954–59) in Stuttgart, Charlottenburg-Nord (1950s–1960s), and the Böblingen Flats (1965) near Stuttgart. Scharoun was extremely interested in the relationship between architectural program, order, form, space, and light and the learning processes associated with educational programs, and he designed several schools, such as the Geschwister Scholl (1958–62) in Lünen, where he adopted an aggressive color program, and the Volksschule (1960–71) at Marl in Westphalia. Scharoun's theaters included the Kässel (1952), Mannheim (1953), and Zürich (1964) theater projects. The Wolfsburg Theatre (1965–1973), completed after Scharoun's death on 25 November 1972, absorbs the energy of the earlier projects and stands today as a testament to Scharoun's architectural genius. This is also the case in his design for the German Maritime Museum (1969–75), a project commissioned by the State of West Germany and located in Bremerhaven, where his earliest visions for a new architecture first took root. Likewise, his most famous building, the Berlin Philharmonie (begun in 1968 and completed in 1987), sublates many of the ideas found in his earliest architectural work, becoming something of a refined exemplar of Expressionist architecture. The programs for the Philharmonie and the later Chamber Music Hall appear as instruments themselves—fluid arrangements of myriad systems that lend themselves to Scharoun's improvisational approach to the making of form.

Among Scharoun's last projects, a State Library (1964–79) and a Musical Instruments Museum and Institute for Musical Research (1969–84), both sited immediately adjacent to both the Berlin Philharmonie and Mies van der Rohe's masterful National Gallery in Berlin, display the full range of Scharoun's vision. The created context is thoughtfully nuanced, with the grouping of buildings open and responsive not only to one another but to the entire city of (West) Berlin as well—a studied contrast in the closed conditions presented by the city's isolated context at the time. Completed after Scharoun's death, they represent not only the sum of one architect's vision but also, in returning to the opening themes of the 1910s and 1920s, the culmination of a generation's vision, a generation that, from the beginning, saw architecture as a form of redemption, a form of life that engaged and affirmed the dynamics of social interaction.

As an architect, Scharoun was prolific. The number of projects designed amounts to more than 300, the majority (238) of which were built despite the intervening years of Fascist rule and the post–World War II economic difficulties. Scharoun's insistence on a dynamic, "organic" architecture, in particular an

architecture fully engaged in the rhythms of daily life, exhibits his concern for architecture as a form of life (*Lebensform*). This idea encapsulates the sense of play and the use of fluid ordering systems in Scharoun's work; architecture did not exist as an object but rather functioned as an organism, a viable, developmental, and flexible network of associations and interrelationships.

ELIZABETH BURNS GAMARD

See also **Berlin, Germany; Berlin Philharmonic Concert Hall; Deutscher Werkbund; Häring, Hugo (Germany); Taut, Bruno (Germany); Weissenhofsiedlung, Deutscher Werkbund, Stuttgart (1927)**

Selected Publications

Hans Scharoun: Bauten, Entwürfe, Texte, edited by Peter Pfankuch, Berlin: Akademie der Künste, 1974; new edition, 1993

Further Reading

Blundell-Jones, Peter, *Hans Scharoun*, London: Phaidon Press, 1995

SCHINDLER, RUDOLPH M. 1887–1953
Architect, Austria and United States

Rudolph M. Schindler practiced in the Los Angeles area from 1920 until his death, producing a series of houses and apartment buildings that explored new concepts of form, materials, and space. Critical of the reigning machine-oriented orthodoxy of most advanced European and American modernists that became known as the International Style, Schindler's work is highly personal and individualistic.

Born in Vienna, Schindler studied structural engineering at the technical university, architecture under Otto Wagner at the academy, and informally with Adolf Loos. Inspired by Frank Lloyd Wright's Wasmuth publications, Schindler immigrated to the United States in 1914, met Louis Sullivan, and after repeated attempts secured employment with Frank Lloyd Wright and worked on several projects, including the Imperial Hotel. Wright sent Schindler to Los Angeles to supervise work on the Barnstall residence, known as Hollyhock. Schindler contributed a number of designs to Wright's project (studio residence A is generally credited to Schindler).

Schindler's earliest work, from 1921 to 1928, initially contained certain Wrightian mannerisms, but he also explored the possibilities of concrete and southern California's sybaritic living. His King's Road, or Schindler-Chase House (1921–22) in Hollywood was designed for two couples who shared common living spaces but who each had their own room and an open sleeping porch. The house is a series of interlocked tilt-slab concrete forms (which he derived from the American architect Irving Gill) paired with large openings, originally covered in canvas and later with sliding glass. Built on a slab, the building was in a sense a neutral container for the life within and without, with large indoor and outdoor fireplaces.

The Lovell Beach House (1922–26) in Newport Beach was composed of five poured-in-place concrete frames that carried what Schindler described as "space trays." Constructed of wood, the trays are multilevel and project beyond the end of the frames,

creating a dynamic sense of space. With abstract forms that referred to pier pilings, Schindler's Lovell house was probably his best-known work.

Beginning around 1928, Schindler began to use the wooden stud frame; his architecture grew more cubic with flat, stucco-covered wall surfaces. Typically, his houses are enclosed on the street elevation and open to gardens or views. Fenestration is eccentric with varying shapes and sizes. With the C. H. Wolfe House (1928–29) on Catalina Island, Schindler posed the building as a series of boxes with open porches on a hillside, whereas the J. J. Buck House (1934) in Los Angeles spread across a lot as a series of interlocked stucco-covered forms. As with all of Schindler's work, the house was conceived as a total unit incorporating site, landscape, and furniture into the plan and the style.

Schindler's final phase, from 1935 on, becomes more expressionistic, with roofs and walls placed at eccentric angles, often resulting in radically dynamic space. The Guy C. Wilson House (1935–38) in Los Angeles has floor-to-ceiling glass walls poised 50 feet in the air and a butterfly roof that goes off at two angles. The S. T. Falk Apartment Building (1940) in Los Angeles, also on a steep site, features a series of overlapping geometries and bent forms; its volumes resemble precariously arranged boxes held in equilibrium. The Ellen Jansen (1949) and Adolphe Tishler (1950) houses in Los Angeles appear almost unfinished with their collision of planes, forms, and beams. Spatially, Schindler's late work defies verbal description, as color and a multiplicity of surfaces resound in different directions.

The eccentric character of Schindler's work, his bohemian demeanor, and the Los Angeles location led to a dismissive attitude by eastern critics, who refused to acknowledge his contributions to modern architecture. Schindler pursued lectures, exhibitions, and publications of his work and was largely successful up to around 1949, when he was diagnosed with cancer. Since the mid-1960s, Schindler studies have blossomed, and his current status probably outranks that of his contemporary, Richard Neutra. Although critics and historians have attempted to define his work with reference to Wagner, Wright, Loos, De Stijl, and other movements, Schindler's oeuvre escapes classification. Schindler's major effect came at least three decades after his death in the work of Frank Gehry, Thom Mayne, and the Santa Monica School.

RICHARD GUY WILSON

See also **Brutalism; Gill, Irving (United States); Loos, Adolf (Austria); Neutra, Richard (Austria); Wagner, Otto (Austria); Wright, Frank Lloyd (United States)**

Biography

Born in Vienna, 10 September 1887. Graduated with degree in structural engineering, Imperial and Royal Technical University, 1911, and diploma in architecture under Otto Wagner at the Academy of Fine Arts, 1913, both in Vienna. Worked for Mayr and Mayer architects 1911–1914 in Vienna. Arrived in New York March 1914; worked as draftsman and designer for Ottenheimer, Stern, and Reichert in Chicago until 1917. Toured New Mexico, Arizona, and California in 1915; worked for Frank Lloyd Wright at Oak Park Studio, Taliesin, and Los Angeles, 1917–ca. 1922. Married Sophie Pauline Schindler, 29 August 1919; one child Mark Schindler, born 20 July 1922. Moved to Southern California, December 1920; lived in Los Angles and later Hollywood; became part of Hollywood's avant-garde community, securing patrons. Entered partnership ca. 1926–ca. 1928 with Richard Neutra under the name of Architecture Group for Industry and Commerce. Remained in independent practice until death on 22 August 1953.

Selected Works

King's Road House (architect's house), West Hollywood, California, 1922
Lovell Beach House, Newport Beach, California, 1926
C. H. Wolfe House, Catalina Island, 1929
J. J. Buck House, Los Angeles, 1934
Guy C. Wilson House, Los Angeles, 1938
S. T. Falk Apartment Building, Los Angeles, 1940
Ellen Jansen House, Los Angeles, 1949
Adolphe Tishler House, Los Angeles, 1950

Further Reading

Gebhard, David, *Schindler*, New York: Viking Press, 1971; 3rd edition, San Francisco: William Stout, 1997
Giella, Barbara, *R. M. Schindler's Thirties Style: Its Character (1931–1937) and International Sources (1906–1937)*, Unpublished

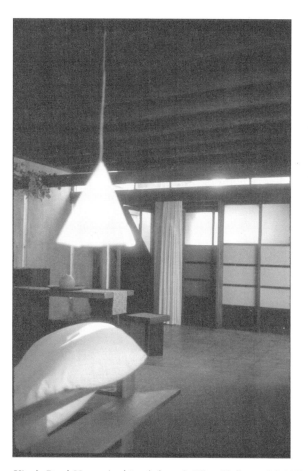

King's Road House (architect's house), West Hollywood (1922)
© GreatBuildings.com

Ph.D. dissertation, Institute of Fine Arts, New York University, 1987

Koulermos, Panos, and Stefanos Polyzoides, Five Houses of R. M. Schindler, *A + U* 75 (Nov. 1975), 61–126

March, Lionel, and Judith Sheine (editors), *R.M. Schindler: Composition and Construction*, London: Academy Editions, 1993

McCoy, Esther, *Five California Architects*, New York: Reinhold, 1960

McCoy, Esther, *Vienna to Los Angeles: Two Journeys*, Santa Monica: Arts + Architecture Press, 1979

Sarnitz, August, *R. M. Schindler Architect 1887–1953*, New York: Rizzoli, 1989

Sheine, Judith, *R. M. Schindler*, Barcelona: Editorial Gustavo Gill, 1998

Smith, Elizabeth, Michael Darling, and Richard Guy Wilson, *The Architecture of R. M. Schindler*, New York: Abrams, 2001

SCHLUMBERGER CAMBRIDGE RESEARCH CENTER

Cambridge, England
Designed by Michael Hopkins and Partners; Phase I completed 1985; Phase II completed 1993

The Schlumberger complex is located in a research park at the northwest edge of Cambridge, England. Schlumberger, a global company that provides technical services to support the exploration, drilling, and production of oil, is also a notable patron of architecture, having previously commissioned buildings by Philip Johnson and Renzo Piano. Michael Hopkins was selected for the Cambridge project from a shortlist of 20 international practices.

Phase I, commissioned in 1982 and completed in 1985, includes laboratories, offices for scientists, and a test station with a range of drilling pits used to simulate difficult and dangerous field conditions. Because of noise, dirt, and the risk of explosion, test stations traditionally had been isolated in separate buildings. However, both the preoccupations of Hopkins and the aspirations of Schlumberger led to a radically different approach. The test station is combined with a winter garden, which serves as both entrance hall and restaurant, to form a long north-south central spine that is flanked on the east and west by two slimmer bars comprised of laboratories overlooking the central space and offices with views out to the surrounding pastoral landscape. The natural slope of the site is utilized to sink the floor of the test station and service yard 2.5 meters below the winter garden. This lower level also provides an easily accessible services undercroft.

The efficient, rational plan gives little hint of the drama of the section. A tensile roof encloses the 24-meter-wide central zone, where a clear height of approximately 17 meters is provided above the drilling pits. Framed by an exposed steel structure of lattice columns and prismatic beams, raked booms and a network of tension rods support the translucent skin. The structure of the single-story offices and labs, a derivation of Hopkins's Patera system, is also exoskeletal but, in contrast with the central spine, is more restrained. Anthony Hunt Associates designed the steel structure, and the lightweight structures unit of Ove Arup and Partners designed the fabric roof.

A zoned servicing strategy supports the contrasting spatial and structural characters of the central spine and flanking wings.

The winter garden and test station, although weather tight, are conceived as quasi-external spaces; the labs are sealed spaces in which tightly controlled environmental conditions for research can be maintained; and the offices have opening windows and sunshading that can be adjusted by the occupants.

The building works as an icon in the heroic modernist tradition and, by addressing human needs, significantly advances the idea of the workplace. Transparency—with fully glazed walls between winter garden, test station, and labs and a glazed external envelope—creates a high degree of visual interaction both within the building and between the building and the outside world. An egalitarian workplace laced together by open meeting spaces and the generosity of the winter garden integrates disparate functions—clean and dirty, quiet and noisy, front and back of house. This social and programmatic integration is reiterated in the marriage of orthogonal and curvilinear geometries, of compressive and tensile structures, and of rational Miesian discipline with more exuberant expressionism.

This building for Schlumberger was Michael Hopkins's first use of a tensile fabric structure and the first large-scale architectural use of Teflon-coated fabric in the United Kingdom. Hopkins would further explore fabric structures in subsequent projects including the Mound Stand at Lord's Cricket Ground (1987), the amenity building and ventilation towers at Inland Revenue (1995), and the Younger Universe Pavilion in Edinburgh (1998).

As a product of systems-building thinking—inspired by the pioneering work of Ezra Ehrencrantz and developed in Hopkins's early association with Norman Foster—Hopkins designed Phase I as an open-ended, extendible system of prefabricated parts. However, oil research methods were changing rapidly. By the time Phase II was commissioned in 1990, Schlumberger was relying more on computer simulation, making the test station less central in its research program. Phase II is consequently a separate building that echoes Hopkins's 1988 Solid State Logic scheme near Oxford. Located to the south of Phase I, the extension plays the role of gatehouse, with two pavilions joined by an atrium that houses the reception area for the site and defines a central axial path to the winter garden. Each of the two-story pavilions is square in plan with offices for scientists at the perimeter surrounding labs, computer suites, conference rooms, and mechanical plant. Phases I and II are unified visually by similarly detailed glazed facades and conceptually by the integration of the rational and expressive sensibilities of Hopkins' work. However, the structure of Phase II, for which Buro Happold were consultants, is utterly different. The upper floor is prefabricated ferroconcrete used as permanent formwork for an in situ concrete slab. Recalling Pier Luigi Nervi's Gatti Wool Factory (1954) in Rome, the soffit is detailed to express clearly the patterns of structural stresses in the slab. An understated, light structure of air-filled pillows of clear PTFE (polytetra fluoroethylene) sheet spanning between simple steel beams encloses the central atrium.

The Schlumberger Cambridge Research Center is one of the emblematic projects of the so-called British High Tech movement led by Norman Foster, Richard Rogers, Nicholas Grimshaw, and Michael Hopkins. However, like other buildings designed by Hopkins during the same period—notably the David Mellor Cutlery Factory (1988), Bracken House (1992), Glyndebourne Opera House (1994), Inland Revenue, and the Emman-

uel College Music Room (1995) the ferroconcrete used in Phase II of Schlumberger signals a shift away from the light steel and glass buildings of Hopkins's early career and the application of systems thinking and prefabrication to heavier, more traditional materials and methods of construction.

Phase I received the *Financial Times* Architecture Award in 1985 and a Royal Institute of British Architects (RIBA) National Award, a Civic Trust Award, and a Structural Steel Award in 1988. In 1993, Phase II received an RIBA Regional Award and was a finalist for the *Financial Times* Award.

ANNETTE W. LECUYER

Further Reading

Davies, Colin, *Hopkins: The Work of Michael Hopkins and Partners*, London: Phaidon, 1993

Groák, Steven and Roger Barbrook, "A Cambridge Test: Hopkins for Schlumberger," *The Architects' Journal* 182, no. 38 (18 September 1985)

Herzberg, Henry, "High Flyer," *The Architects' Journal* 180, no. 43 (24 October 1984)

International Biennale of Architecture, *British Architecture Today: Six Protagonists*, Milan: Electa, 1991

Jenkins, David, *Schlumberger Cambridge Research Centre: Michael Hopkins and Partners*, London: Phaidon, 1993

Winter, John and Sarah Jackson, "Technology Stretching High-Tech," *The Architects' Journal* 196, no. 17 (28 October 1992)

SCHOOL

School buildings have undergone tremendous change in the course of the 20th century. In part, these changes were driven by a dramatic increase in school enrollments, as children in industrialized nations were driven out of the workplace by new technologies and protective labor legislation, and compulsory school attendance laws become more commonplace. Even more important to the form of school buildings were new pedagogical theories advanced at the turn of the century, notably by Maria Montessori in Italy, John Dewey in the United States, and Karl Popper in Germany. Building on the ideas of the 19th-century kindergarten movement, these thinkers popularized the concept that children learn best by doing, rather than through rote memorization. Montessori emphasized the importance of the Prepared Environment, in which furnishings were sized and arranged to enhance the autonomy of young children. Dewey was equally influential in arguing that high schools should prepare students for life, and not just for college.

Kindergartens were among the first educational environments affected by these new pedagogical theories. In the United States and England they tended to take the form of a specially shaped classroom attached to a primary school, while in Europe the kindergarten tended to be a distinct building type. Those associated with the Waldorf School Movement (which began in 1919 when Rudolph Steiner started Die Freie Waldorfschule, for the children of the workers at the Waldorf-Astoria cigarette factory in Stuttgart) tended to favor organic forms that seemed to support Steiner's emphasis on cultivating higher mental faculties through the total harmony of the senses. More common in the 1920s and 1930s were kindergartens designed in a modern idiom, like the 1934 nursery school on the outskirts of Zürich

where architect Hans Leuzinger provided direct access to the out-of-doors, ample daylighting, and light movable furniture scaled to young children.

Schools for older children took longer to address all of the implications of the new pedagogy. The regimented classroom (with chairs bolted into place facing the teacher's desk) remained the basic unit of school design, although educators and architects refined the arrangements of these rooms to insure that students could see the blackboard and hear the teacher's instructions. In the United States, the first architectural indication of the new educational theories involved the provision of facilities beyond the classroom: fully-equipped playgrounds, baths, gymnasia, art studios, scientific laboratories, shops for woodworking and handicrafts, and home economics classrooms. Auditoria and libraries were often included as well, to serve both students and the wider community. In order to make these amenities more affordable, the Gary, Indiana, school system introduced the platoon system (also called the Gary plan) in 1909. Aimed at using all school facilities at once, this system divided the student body into two platoons, each of which used conventional classrooms for academic subjects while the other was involved in special activities. Schools planned for this system typically included a large auditorium at the center of the building, with special classrooms grouped together on lower floors. After World War I, junior high schools (for grades 7–9) were also understood as a cost effective and developmentally appropriate means of providing adolescents with the manual training and home economics classrooms not used by students in the primary grades, where the focus remained on the acquisition of basic academic skills.

This new attention to the distinct needs of different age groups also extended to the architectural expression of early 20th-century schools in the United States. San Francisco school architect John J. Donovan, for one, argued that school architecture should anticipate the psychological responses of children; elementary schools "should reflect the spirit, quietness and refinement of a good home," while high schools "should have the character, repose, and presentation befitting the important work going forward within" (Donovan, 1921, 27–28). In practice, this meant that high schools retained a degree of monumentality, expressed in Colonial Revival or collegiate Gothic form in the late 1910s and 1920s, and later in Art Deco and Moderne styles associated with civic and commercial architecture. These two- and three-story buildings presented strongly symmetrical facades focused on a single main entrance set well above grade. In contrast, elementary schools minimized the building's scale. Not only did one-story buildings become more common, but many schools (like the Ashland School in St. Louis by William B. Ittner) provided two main entrances often at or near grade level. Articulated with Tudor Revival, Colonial Revival, or Mission Revival details, these buildings used historical vocabularies associated with domestic architecture to ease the child's transition from home to school.

In Europe, progressive educational reform often went hand in hand with attempts to bring students into closer communion with the natural landscape. Early in the twentieth century, open-air schools—with neither heating nor glazing—were built primarily for the tubercular children; the first of these was the Waldschule (Forest School) established in Charlottenburg, Germany in 1904. By the 1920s, however, open-air schools were recommended for non-tubercular children as well. In Frankfurt, Germany, architects working under the leadership of Ernst May

in the 1920s designed decentralized schools called *Pavilionschule* (pavilion schools) or *Freiflachenschule* (open plan schools) with one-story wings disposed over large open sites to increase light and air circulation; the Niederursel School designed by Franz Schuster in 1928, may be the first of this type. Although there were some French pavilion schools (notably the open-air school in Suresnes designed by Eugène Beaudouin and Marcel Lods), France retained a tradition of density, building multistory blocks with outdoor space provided on rooftop terraces.

By the late 1930s, architects and educators increasingly worked together to develop new approaches to school design. In England, for instance, Walter Gropius and Maxwell Fry designed Impington Village College (Cambridgeshire, 1940) to house a school that educator Henry Morris envisioned as an innovative community center with its assembly hall, workshops, library and recreational facilities available to adults. Its loose asymmetrical plan increased natural lighting, improved cross ventilation, and provided direct access to the out-of-doors from each classroom, while its flat roofs and modern detailing eschewed any reference to traditional school architecture. In a similar vein, Perkins, Wheeler, and Will designed Crow Island Elementary School (Winnetka, Illinois, 1940) in close collaboration with teachers, using asymmetrical planning, low (9-foot) ceilings, generous glazing, and direct outdoor access from each classroom to make the school welcoming to young pupils.

In the postwar period, architects embraced industrial production techniques developed during the war as the best way to meet an acute demand for schools fueled by the baby boom. In England, the effort was pioneered in the architectural office of the Hertfordshire County Council, under the direction of Stirrat Johnson-Marshall. There in the late 1940s, county architects designed informally planned primary schools, like the Monkfrith School in East Barnet (1950, Mary Crowley and Oliver Cox, job architects), where daylighting from contiguous sides, warm-air heating systems, dispersed seating at movable tables, and bright colors set new standards for child-centered classrooms.

Another effort to link prefabrication, modular planning, and school design was the SCSD (School Construction Systems Development) system spearheaded by Ezra Ehrenkrantz and implemented in high schools throughout California beginning in 1962. Based on the coordinated manufacture of modular components, the SCSD system was primarily intended to lower school construction costs. Educators, however, were drawn to the system's potential for providing spaces that could be quickly reconfigured for individualized or group instruction. The trend toward open-plan schools (whether built on the SCSD system

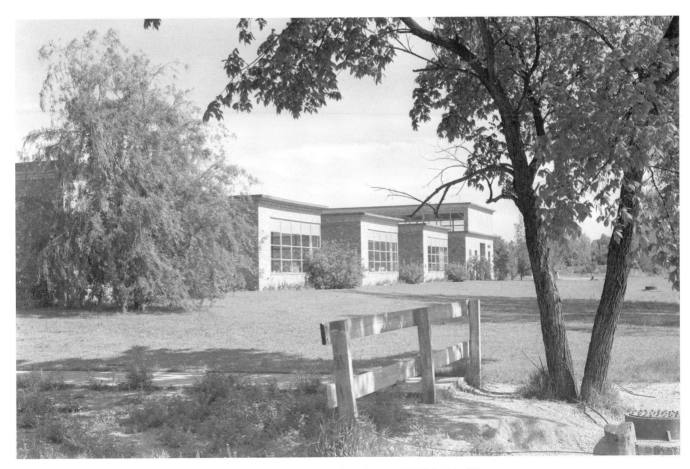

Crow Island School, Winnetka, Illinois, designed by Eliel Saarinen with Perkins and Will (1939–49)
© Johnson Architectural Images/GreatBuildings.com

or not) developed rapidly in the 1960s and early 1970s, affecting half of the all schools built in the United States between 1967 and 1969 and ten percent of all elementary schools in use in the United Kingdom in 1985. The Mt. Hope, New Jersey, Elementary School (Perkins and Will, 1971) displays several characteristics of the type: a large floor plate (maximizing the building's enclosed area in order to minimize costs and enhance flexibility), heavy reliance on florescent lighting, open classrooms grouped on an upper level (allowing fixed equipment required in the cafeteria and gymnasium to remain on the ground level), movable furnishings used as classroom partitions, and spatial continuity between classrooms and circulation space. Although such schools avoided the rigidity of conventional classrooms, they also sacrificed daylighting and direct access to the out-of-doors. Open plans also introduced new noise and discipline problems, while the systems approach to school construction could result generic buildings with little architectural character.

The last two decades of the 20th century saw a reaction against the open plan school. The self-contained classroom returned, albeit with greater attention to providing a variety of seating arrangements. Irregular planning also re-emerged, and for the same reasons it had been popular in the 1930s and 1940s: to enhance natural lighting, improve access to the out-of-doors, and decrease noise levels. Finally, the child's reaction to the qualities of place reappeared as an issue of concern to architects. At the same time, new programmatic requirements—the need to incorporate computer technologies, a new emphasis on project-based learning, renewed calls to integrate educational and community facilities—emerged to elicit new responses to this complex building type in the 21st century.

ABIGAIL A. VAN SLYCK

Further Reading

Branch, Mark Alden, "Tomorrow's Schoolhouse: Making the Pieces Fit," *Progressive Architecture* 75 (June 1994)

Challman, S. A. *The Rural School Plant*, Milwaukee, Bruce Publishing, 1917

Cohen, Ronald D., and Raymond A. Mohl, *The Paradox of Progressive Education: The Gary Plan and Urban Schooling*, Port Washington, N.Y., Kennikat Press, 1979

Dewey, John, *The School and Society*, Chicago, University of Chicago Press, 1899

Donovan, John J., et al., *School Architecture: Principles and Practices*, New York, Macmillan, 1921

Dudek, Mark, *Kindergarten Architecture: Space for the Imagination*, London, E & FN Spon, 1996

Graves, Ben E., *School Ways: The Planning and Design of America's Schools*, New York, McGraw-Hill, 1993

Gyure, Dale Allen, "A 'Child's World' and a 'People's Clubhouse': School Architecture and the Work-Study-Play System in Gary, Indiana, 1907–1930," *Arris: Journal of the Southeast Chapter, Society of Architectural Historians* 12 (2001)

Liscombe, Rhodri Windsor, "Schools for the 'Brave New World': R.A.D. Berwick and School Design in Postwar British Columbia," *BC Studies* 90 (Summer 1991)

Montessori, Maria, *The Montessori Method; Scientific Pedagogy as Applied to Child Education in "the Children's Houses" with Additions and Revisions by the Author*, 1912, trans., Anne E. George, Cambridge, Massachusetts, R. Bentley, 1965.

Perkins, Lawrence B., and Walter D. Cocking, *Schools*, New York, Reinhold Publishing, 1949

Rand, George, and Chris Arnold, "Evaluation: A Look at the '60's Sexiest System [SCSD]," *AIA Journal*, 68 (April 1979)

Saint, Andrew, *Towards a Social Architecture: The Role of School-Building in Post-War England*, New Haven, Yale University Press, 1987

"Schooling," *Architectural Review* 189: 1135 (September 1991)

von Vegesack, Alexander, Jutta Oldiges, and Lucy Bullivant, eds., *Kid Size: The Material World of Childhood*, Milan, Skira; [Weil am Rhein], Vitra Design Museum, 1997

SCHRÖDER-SCHRÄDER HOUSE

Designed by Gerrit Thomas Rietveld; completed 1924
Utrecht, Netherlands

The Schröder-Schräder House is an icon of early modern domestic architecture and is considered the greatest and most influential work of Gerrit Thomas Rietveld (1888–1964). Located in Utrecht at Prins Hendriklaan 50, the design is the result of the close collaboration between Rietveld and the client, Truus Schröder-Schräder (1889–1985), whose full contribution has only recently been recognized. They collaborated in 1921 in the design of a study for Mrs. Schröder-Schräder in her house on Biltstraat. In 1923, on the death of her husband, Frits Schröder, Mrs. Schröder-Schräder decided to build a small house for herself and her three children that would represent her ideas of a new, modern way of living.

Sitting at the end of a row of traditional Dutch houses, the Schröder-Schräder House is a balanced, asymmetrical composition of seemingly independent planes and lines. The ends of the elements slip past each other with balconies and roof planes also projecting from the body of the house as though not fully containing the space inside. Rietveld initially conceived of the house as constructed in concrete, and it was noted as such in some early publications. This proved to be too costly, and only the foundations and balconies are of concrete, and the walls are of traditional brick masonry with plaster. Both wood and steel are used for structural support, wood generally at the floors and steel for the balconies and flat roof.

Sheltered by the southeast balcony in the main entry to the house is a traditional Dutch door lacquered black. The ground floor is a composition of fixed walls in which essential functions have been carefully integrated into the design. Within the compact space of the entry hall, a coat closet, a telephone counter, and a place for mail delivery, as well as storage for the children's toys, are carefully composed and built-in. Also on the ground level is a small study with a built-in desk, bookshelves, and a door into the garden. Although the room behind the study was intended as a garage, Mrs. Schröder-Schräder never owned an automobile, and both Mrs. Schröder-Schräder and Rietveld periodically used this room as a studio. To the right of the entry hall is the kitchen with room for four people to dine. A small window and shelf for deliveries is built-in, as is a speaking tube to the living-dining area on the upper level. Accessed from the kitchen is a small cellar, and behind the kitchen is a maid's room. Mrs. Schröder-Schräder, however, never had a live-in servant, and this room was used primarily for reading. Closely linked to the site, the garage, kitchen, and study have their own doors to the garden, and spatial connections are made between the rooms with large transoms at the top of the walls.

Despite the fact that the drawings given to the building commission indicate the ground floor as the living area with the upper level noted as an "attic," this was never the intention. It is the upper level that most exemplifies Mrs. Schröder-Schräder's desire for an architecture to match her attitudes toward living. These ideas were manifested in an inherent freedom in the ability to change the layout to accommodate a variety of spatial configurations. A single, open room, the upper level can be divided by movable partitions that follow tracks in the floor and guides along the ceiling. Closing the partitions creates four smaller rooms that provided privacy for the children and Mrs. Schröder-Schräder and a shared living-dining area. The three bedrooms are equipped with built-in storage and a sink to promote self-sufficiency. A skylight above the stair provides access to the roof and fills the center of the upper level with light. The bath and toilet area along the party wall can be enclosed by movable partitions at the stair. Gerard van de Groenekan, Rietveld's assistant, constructed the built-in furniture; chairs and small tables were also of Rietveld's design. The living-dining area is a slightly larger space with a built-in table, storage, and a shelf for the children to do their homework. It was here that the lively discussions that Mrs. Schröder-Schräder envisioned occurred.

Rietveld created the interpenetration of spaces and the connection to the surrounding landscape by the dematerialization of boundaries either physically, as in the use of movable partitions, or through the use of color. Rietveld's offsetting of the support at the corner window in the living-dining room literally opens the space and creates a direct connection to the landscape. In turn, the colors of the floor and walls of the upper level define spaces not constricted by the placement of partitions.

The Schröder-Schräder House is often considered a quintessential example of De Stijl architectural principles. Theo van Doesburg, the founder of De Stijl, published the house several times in his journal *De Stijl*. However, the house was not initially acknowledged by the general Dutch press, despite its appearance in many influential European architecture magazines and Henry Russell Hitchcock's 1929 *Modern Architecture*. The 1950s brought a resurgence of interest in the house in conjunction with a growth in the popularity of Rietveld's work.

Rietveld moved to the house after the death of his wife and lived there until his own death in 1964. Over time, a number of changes were made to the house; a dumbwaiter was added from the kitchen to the upper living-dining area, and in 1935 a room was added on the roof to give Mrs. Schröder-Schräder more privacy from the many visitors who came to see the house. This room was later demolished. The original, rural context of the house also has changed with urban expansion and the construction of a bypass in 1964. Mrs. Schröder-Schräder established the Rietveld Schröder House Foundation in 1970 to assist in the maintenance and preservation of the house. Five years later, the foundation hired the architect Bertus Mulder to begin restoration of the interior and exterior of the house. The Schröder-Schräder House was opened to the public in 1987.

KATHERINE WHEELER BORUM

Further Reading

Banham, Reyner, *Theory and Design in the First Machine Age*, London: Architectural Press, and New York: Praeger, 1960; 2nd edition, 1967

Brattinga, Pieter (editor), *Rietveld, 1924: Schröder Huis*, Amsterdam: Steendrukkerij de Jong, 1963

Brown, Theodore, *The Work of G. Rietveld, Architect*, Utrecht: Bruna, and Cambridge, Massachusetts: MIT Press, 1958

Büller, Lenneke, Frank den Oudsten, and Truus Schröder, "Schröder House: The Work of Gerrit Rietveld, between Myth and Metaphor," *Lotus International* 60 (1989)

Casciato, Maristella, "Family Matters: The Schröder House, by Gerrit Rietveld and Truus Schröder" in *Women and the Making of the Modern House: A Social and Architectural History*, edited by Alice Friedman, New York: Abrams, 1998

Futagawa, Yukio and Ida van Zijl (editors), *Gerrit Thomas Rietveld: The Schröder House, Utrecht, Netherlands, 1923–24*, Tokyo: A.D.A. Edita, 1992

Mulder, Bertus and Ida van Zijl, *Rietveld Schröder House*, Bussum, The Netherlands: V and K, and New York: Princeton Architectural Press, 1997

Nagao, S. and Y. Tominaga, "The Schröder House, 1924," *Space Design* (March 1976)

SCOTT BROWN, DENISE 1931–

Architect and theorist, United States

Controversial both for her ideas and for her prominence as a female theorist and practitioner in a period when few women architects succeeded, Denise Scott Brown has exercised a powerful influence on architecture and urbanism since the 1970s. Reconnecting form to its social meaning and emphasizing architecture's position within its cultural environment, her concerns have coupled with Robert Venturi's interest in historical precedent to produce an inclusive interpretation of architecture's context that incorporates social, economic, historic, and formal dimensions. Along with a shared aesthetic of simplification, juxtaposition, and deadpan irony, their theories have been central to the development of Postmodernism and the advancement of the architectural profession generally.

Scott Brown was born in 1931 in Nkana, Zambia, into a well-to-do Jewish household of Lithuanian and Latvian ancestry. After architectural studies at the University of Witwatersrand, Johannesburg, she earned a diploma at the Architectural Association in London in 1955 and was registered in the United Kingdom in 1956. Her teachers included Arthur Korn, a Bauhaus émigré and coauthor of the MARS plan for postwar London who emphasized the connections between social structure and urban form, and historian John Summerson, whose preoccupations with mannerism and Georgian urbanism contrasted with contemporary CIAM (Congrès Internationaux d'Architecture Moderne) and "townscape" planning ideas. Peter and Alison Smithson's focus on advertising, everyday experience, and neighborhood "association" also stimulated her interest in pop art and ordinary urban environments. At the University of Pennsylvania, she obtained masters degrees in city planning and architecture in 1960 and 1965, studying under sociologist Herbert Gans, a "participant–observer" of Levittown, who defended the aesthetic validity of popular culture, and planner David Crane, an originator of advocacy planning. An early article, "The Meaningful City" (1965), adapted Crane's articulation of three levels of urban meaning—"heraldic," "physiognomic," and "locational"—to urban design. Her multifaceted education generated a sophisticated understanding of the interaction between architectural form and social forces as well as the conviction that

architects should foster rather than negate patterns of urban order arising from the aggregation of many individual social and economic decisions.

Scott Brown met Robert Venturi at the University of Pennsylvania in 1960. Sharing an anthropological attitude toward their aesthetic environment and an affinity for the local, the complex, and the irregular, they soon began collaborating, marrying in 1967 and formalizing their architectural partnership in 1968. Their visits to Las Vegas led to the publication of two seminal articles: "A Significance for A&P Parking Lots, or Learning from Las Vegas" (1968) and "Ugly and Ordinary Architecture, or the Decorated Shed, Parts I and II" (1971). Their studios on Las Vegas and Levittown at Yale in 1968 and 1970 employed interdisciplinary research and design methods and applied traditional categories of architectural analysis to everyday postwar urban forms. In *Learning from Las Vegas* (1972, with Steven Izenour), they argued that Las Vegas's extravagant signs and its large, low, generic buildings were extreme but informative models of current building practices, the avatars of a new, late Modern—or what was soon to be called Postmodern—vernacular. In an automobile-dominated culture, pedestrian-oriented, modernist "space" was less significant than "symbolism over vast space."

They invented two new terms—the *duck* and the *decorated shed*—to describe the operation of architectural symbolism. The duck's entire form was an image of an idea. The Las Vegas casino was a decorated shed: constructed conventionally and generically but with an ornamented, symbolic facade. In both, symbolic considerations dominated structural and functional ones. Drawing on linguistic theory as well as associational philosophy, Venturi and Scott Brown argued that architecture is understood by association to previous experience. Rather than emphasizing structural and functional "truth," therefore, buildings should make reference to what people already know: the conventions of vernacular as well as historical forms. Their insistence on the validity of the ordinary person's aesthetic choices contested modernism's belief that architecture should create both a better world and a "modern man" suited to live in it. Theorist and historian Kenneth Frampton's dispute with Scott Brown over this distinction between "is" and "ought" rested on a disagreement over the identity of architecture's audience: the worker to whom modern architecture had often been dedicated or the lower-middle class denizens of Gans's Levittown (Frampton, 1971; Venturi and Scott Brown, 1984).

Scott Brown's interest in the everyday environment also engendered a four-year investigation of the imagery of American

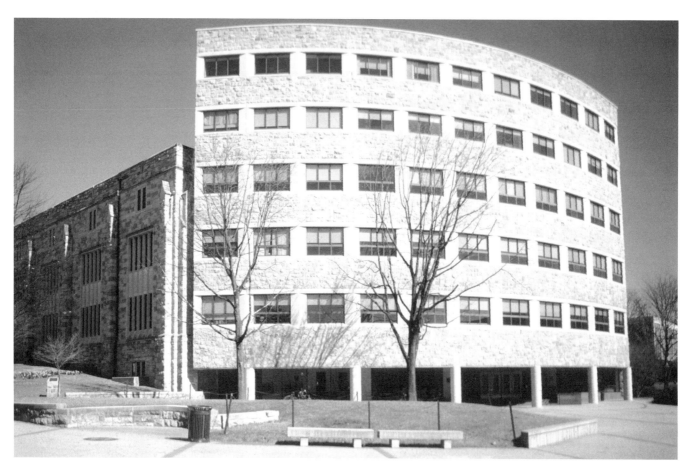

Carol M. Newman Library Renovation and Addition, Virginia Polytechnic Institute and State University (1971)
Photo © Mary Ann Sullivan

suburbs. This research culminated in "Signs of Life" (1976), an exhibition of suburban, strip, and city imagery mounted at the Smithsonian Institution's Renwick Galley in Washington, D.C. The exhibit consisted of three sections: the Home, three dioramas of typical American housing types; the Strip, neon signs and billboards, many especially constructed for the exhibit; and the Street, texts and images describing Main Street. Its deadpan presentation delighted the public but puzzled architects, who expected aesthetic judgments on American urbanism.

Scott Brown's writing, which often delineates the connection between the personal and the theoretical, encompasses architectural and urban theory, preservation, education, and critiques of the "star system" in architecture. Her role as partner in charge of planning at Venturi, Scott Brown and Associates is equally significant. Ranging from facilities programming to the design of urban districts, Scott Brown's work also includes important contributions to the firm's architectural projects. Her involvement in the Sainsbury Wing of the National Gallery (1991) in London is especially notable. In 1992, she and Venturi were awarded the Presidential Medal of the Arts. Her plans, the recipients of many awards, emphasize user participation, sensitivity to existing urban fabric, practicability, and what she calls a "feminist, darning and mending" approach to evolutionary change (Gabor, 1995). They have sometimes generated controversy with their insertion of "pop" elements into existing fabrics. Her Philadelphia Crosstown Community Plan (1968) restored a once-vital, center-city commercial neighborhood that had undergone a steep decline in the 1960s, suffering from both the loss of its middle-class population and the city's plan to cut a highway through it. Employing Edward Ruscha–style collages to illustrate existing character, her proposal mixed sensitive reuse with new construction and substituted one-way streets for the proposed expressway. Miami Beach's Art Deco District (1978) was a thriving but run-down area inhabited by Eastern European Jewish retirees and Cuban immigrants. Scott Brown's pragmatic approach, which included a color palette, inexpensive facade renovations, street furniture, and paving patterns, won a Progressive Architecture Urban Design Award in 1982.

Scott Brown's innovative approach to studio teaching has influenced many contemporary planners and architects. She has taught at the University of Pennsylvania, at the University of California at Berkeley and Los Angeles, and at Yale, Harvard, and Rice Universities. In 1996, she won the Association of the Collegiate Schools of Architecture and the American Institute of Architects Topaz Award for outstanding architectural educators, the first woman to receive this award.

DEBORAH FAUSCH

Biography

Born Denise Lakofski in Nkana, Zambia, 3 October 1931; emigrated to the United States 1958; naturalized 1967. Attended the University of Witwatersrand, Johannesburg, South Africa 1948–51; studied under Arthur Korn at the Architectural Association School, London 1952–55; AA Diploma and Certificate in Tropical Architecture 1956; studied at the University of Pennsylvania, Philadelphia, under Louis I. Khan 1958–60; master's degree in City Planning 1960; master's degree in Architecture 1965. Married (1) architect Robert Scott Brown 1955 (died 1959); (2) architect Robert Venturi 1967. Worked as a student architect with firms in Johannesburg and London 1946–52; architectural assistant to Enrö Goldfinger and Dennis Clarke Hall, London 1955–56; architectural assistant to Giuseppe Vaccaro, Rome 1956–57; architectural assistant to Cowin, DeBruyn, and Cook, Johannesburg 1957–58. Architect and planner, with Robert Venturi and John Rauch, Venturi and Rauch, Philadelphia 1967–80; partner, Venturi, Rauch and Scott Brown 1980–89; principal in charge of urban planning and design, Venturi, Scott Brown and Associates from 1989. Assistant professor, School of Fine Arts, University of Pennsylvania, Philadelphia 1960–65; visiting professor, School of Environmental Design, University of California, Berkeley 1965; associate professor, initiated urban design program, School of Architecture and Urban Planning, University of California, Los Angeles 1965–68; visiting professor in urban design, Yale University School of Architecture, New Haven, Connecticut 1967–70; visiting critic, Rice University, Houston, Texas 1969; member, Visiting Committee, School of Architecture and Urban Planning, Massachusetts Institute of Technology, Cambridge 1973–83; Regents Lecturer, University of California, Santa Barbara 1972; chair, Evaluation Committee for the Industrial Design Program, Philadelphia College of Art 1972; Baldwin Lecturer, Oberlin College, Ohio 1973; member, Advisory Committee, Temple University Department of Architecture, Philadelphia from 1980; member, Curriculum Committee, Philadelphia Jewish Children's Folkshul from 1980; visiting professor, University of Pennsylvania, School of Fine Arts, Philadelphia 1982 and 1983; Eliot Noyes Visiting Critic, Harvard University, Cambridge, Massachusetts 1989; member, advisory board, Department of Architecture, Carnegie Mellon University 1992–96; dean of the search committee, Department of Architecture, Washington University, St. Louis, Missouri 1992. Fellow, Morse College, Yale University 1970; member, Policy Panel, National Endowment for the Arts, Design Arts Program 1981–83; member, Board of the Society of Architectural Historians 1981–84; advisor, United States National Trust for Historic Preservation from 1981; Butler College Fellow, Princeton University, 1983; member, Capitol Preservation Committee, Commonwealth of Pennsylvania 1983–87; member, Board of Trustees, Chestnut Hill Academy 1985–89; member, Board of Directors, Central Philadelphia Development Corporation from 1985; member, Board of Directors, Urban Affairs Partnership, Philadelphia 1987–91; chair, American Institute of Architects 1993; member, Architectural Association, London; member, American Planning Association; member, Society of Architectural Historians; member, Society for College and University Planning; member, Royal Institute of British Architects. Commendatore, Order of Merit, Italy 1987.

Selected Works

Philadelphia Crosstown Community Planning Project, 1968
California City Planning and Urban Design Study, 1970
Polytechnic Institute and State University, Blacksburg, Virginia, 1971
Galveston Development Project for "The Strand," 1974
City Edges Planning Study, 1975
Jim Thorpe Mauch Chunk Historic District Study, 1977
Princeton Urban Design Planning Study, 1978
Washington Avenue Revitalization Plan (Art Deco District, Miami Beach, Florida), 1978
Hennepin Avenue Redevelopment Plan, Minneapolis, 1980
Republic Square District Master Plan, Austin, 1983

Memphis Center City Development Plan, 1987
Houston Museum of Fine Arts Master Plan, 1990
National Museum of the American Indian Museum Facilities
   Program of Requirements for the Smithsonian Museum, 1993
Dartmouth College Campus Plan, 1993
Denver Civic Center Cultural Complex Plan, 1995
Gateway Visitor Center and Independence Mall: Planning for
   Independence National Historic Park, 1996
Bryn Mawr College Concept Plan, 1997

Selected Publications

Many of Scott Brown's writings have been collected in *Venturi, Scott Brown and Associates on Houses and Housing* (1992), *Urban Concepts* (1990), and *A View from the Campidoglio* (1986).

"The Meaningful City," *AIA Journal* 43, no. 1 (1965)
"On Pop Art, Permissiveness, and Planning," *Journal of the American Institute of Planners* 35, no. 5 (1969)
"On Architectural Formalism and Social Concern: A Discourse for Social Planners and Radical Chic Architects," *Oppositions* 5 (1976)
"On Formal Analysis as Design Research," *Journal of Architectural Education* 32, no. 4 (1979)
"Architectural Taste in a Pluralist Society," *Harvard Architectural Review* 1 (1980)
"A Worm's Eye View of Recent Architectural History," *Architectural Record* 172, no. 2 (1984)
"Invention and Tradition in the Making of American Place," *The Harvard Architecture Review* 5 (1986)
"Learning from Brutalism," in *The Independent Group: Postwar Britain and the Aesthetics of Plenty*, edited by David Robbins, 1990
Urban Concepts: Architectural Design 60, no. 1–2 (1990)
"Talking about the Context," *Lotus International* 74 (1992)

With Robert Venturi

"A Significance for A&P Parking Lots, or Learning from Las Vegas," *Architectural Forum* 128, no. 2 (1968)
"Ugly and Ordinary Architecture, or the Decorated Shed," Part I, *Architectural Forum* 135, no. 4 (1971); Part II, *Architectural Forum* 135, no. 5 (1971)
"The Highway," *Modulus* 9 (1973)
A View from the Campidoglio: Selected Essays, 1953–1984, 1984

With Robert Venturi and Steven Izenour

Learning from Las Vegas, 1972; revised edition, 1977

With Robert Venturi and Virginia Carroll:

"Styling, or 'These Houses Are Exactly the Same. They Just Look Different,'" *Lotus International* 9 (1975)

With James Steele (coeditor)

Venturi, Scott Brown and Associates on Houses and Housing, 1992

Further Reading

Venturi and Scott Brown's archive is located at the University of Pennsylvania. Journal issues devoted to the firm's work include *A + U* 11 (1974); *Werk-Archithese* 64, nos. 7–8 (1977); *L'architecture d'aujourd'hui* 197 (1978); *A + U* 1 (1978); *A + U* extra edition, 12 (1981); *Quaderns d'arquitectura* 162 (1984); and *A + U* 6 (1990). The books by Von Moos provide a considered presentation of their work and ideas.

Barrière, Philippe and Sylvia Lavin, "Entre imagination sociale et architecture," *L'architecture d'aujourd'hui* 273 (1991)
Colquhoun, Alan, "Sign and Substance: Reflections on Complexity, Las Vegas, and Oberlin" in *Essays in Architectural Criticism: Modern Architecture and Historical Change*, by Colquhoun, Cambridge, Massachusetts: MIT Press, 1981
Cook, John W. and Heinrich Klotz, *Conversations with Architects*, New York: Praeger, and London: Lund Humphries, 1973
Fausch, Deborah, "Ugly and Ordinary: The Representation of the Everyday" in *Architecture of the Everyday*, edited by Deborah Berke and Steven Harris, New York: Princeton Architectural Press, 1998
Frampton, Kenneth, "America, 1960–1970: Notes on Urban Images and Theory," *Casabella* 35 (1971)
Gabor, Andrea, *Einstein's Wife: Work and Marriage in the Lives of Five Great Twentieth-Century Women*, New York: Viking, 1995
Von Moos, Stanislaus, *Venturi, Rauch, and Scott Brown: Buildings and Projects, 1960–1985*, New York: Rizzoli, 1987
Von Moos, Stanislaus, *Venturi, Scott Brown, and Associates: Buildings and Projects, 1986–1998*, New York: Monacelli Press, 1999

SCULLY, VINCENT, JR. 1920–

Historian, United States

One of the most inspirational and influential educators of the 20th century, Vincent Scully, Jr., has been widely recognized as a leader of architectural historians and critics of the United States.

When he was admitted to Yale College from New Haven's Hillhouse High School in 1936, he was only 15. At the time, his primary interests were literary criticism and French, which would teach him Cartesian clarity and rigor and guide his search for facts and the clearness of things. After graduating with a B.A. in 1940, he attempted to enlist in the Royal Canadian Air Force and the U.S. Army Air Force but ultimately went into the U.S. Marine Corps, serving in both Europe and the Pacific. At the end of World War II, Scully returned to Yale as a graduate student of art history. Within the next three years, he received his M.A. (1947) and Ph.D. (1949) degrees from Yale. With the exception of a year of study in Rome (1951–52) and another year of traveling in Greece (1957–58), he would never leave his alma mater, where he has taught continuously from 1947 to the present, even following his official retirement in 1991 as Sterling Professor Emeritus of the History of Art.

At Yale, Scully benefited first from the teaching and later the collegiate friendship of several outstanding scholars and teachers in the history of art, including George Kubler, Charles Seymour, Jr., and Sumner McKnight Crosby, all of whom had in turn studied under the preeminent French humanist Henri Focillon. Focillon's conception of style in the visual arts and of the structure and behavior of historical time, best described in his seminal book *Vie des Formes* (1934), translated into English by Kubler as *The Life of Forms in Art* (1942), must have attracted Scully's attention in particular. Above all, Focillon's singular ability to penetrate beyond superficial phenomena to grasp the deeper relationships would leave a lasting impression on him.

Scully's dissertation, titled "The Cottage Style," was a brilliant reassessment of 19th-century American architecture, not a popular topic at the time. In it, he argued convincingly that late 19th-century domestic architecture in the United States "had clearly begun to demonstrate positive characteristics of originality and invention"—most noticeable in the work of architects such as Bruce Price; McKim, Mead and White; Henry Hobson Richardson; and Frank Lloyd Wright. Published as *The Shingle Style* in 1955, the book became an instant classic, and after

multiple reprintings, it remains the definitive study on the subject. Not only would this work lead to a reevaluation of American domestic architecture between 1872 and 1889, but it would serve as a source of inspiration to 20th-century architects such as Robert A.M. Stern, Charles Moore, and Robert Venturi, whose domestic designs of the 1960s and 1970s marked a full-fledged revival of the American Shingle style.

Scully has covered an extraordinary range of topics in 19 books and some 200 articles, including chapters and essays in books, journals, and book reviews. Scully has explored the interaction of man, architecture, and the natural setting. Always considering architecture in its broadest sense as the creation by man of the built environment in relation to the natural environment, he examined ancient Greek architecture in *The Earth, the Temple, and the Gods* (1962), indigenous North American architecture in *Pueblo: Mountain, Village, Dance* (1975), and world architecture from prehistory to the present in *Architecture: The Natural and the Manmade* (1991).

His writings in recent years have deeply explored the theme of the preservation of the man-made in balance with the increasingly more fragile natural environment and the ways architecture must respond in a sensitive way to societal needs. Appropriately enough, when invited in 1995 by the National Endowment for the Humanities to deliver the Twenty-fourth Annual Jefferson Lecture in the humanities at the John F. Kennedy Center for the Performing Arts in Washington, D.C., his topic was "The Architecture of Community."

Even earlier, however, in *American Architecture and Urbanism* (1969), Scully had written critically about the ravages of urban renewal and the drama of poor neighborhoods that were so much affected across the nation during the 1950s and the following decades. As a witness to the destruction of important buildings in downtown New Haven, Scully wasted no time in becoming a spokesman for the cause of historic preservation. During many years, he has participated in preservation battles that have helped save important historic buildings. In 1999, his voice was a decisive factor in the reversed decision that stopped the demolition of four buildings at the rear of the Sterling Divinity Quadrangle of Yale.

Throughout his career, Scully has been the recipient of numerous awards and recognitions. Starting as a Junior Sterling Fellow while a graduate student at Yale, he was later also made Morse Fellow (1951–52), Senior Faculty Fellow (1962–63), and Paskus Fellow in History at Jonathan Edwards College (1955–68). As Fulbright Fellow, he traveled to Italy in 1951–52, and a Bollingen Fellowship allowed him to travel to Greece in 1957–58. He holds four honorary doctorate degrees, from the University of Hartford (1969), the New School for Social Research (1988), the University of Miami (1990) and Albertus Magnus College (1992). In 1986, he received the Association of Collegiate Schools of Architecture (ACSA)/(AIA) "Topaz" Award for Excellence in Architectural Education from the ACSA/American Institute of Architects (AIA) and in 1989 he was made an Honorary Fellow of the Royal Institute of British Architects. During the 1990s alone, he was honored with more than 15 major distinctions, including the "Golden Plate" Award from the American Academy of Achievement (1993), the American Academy of Rome Award (1994), the Lucy G. Moses Preservation Leadership Award from the New York Landmarks Conservancy (1994), the ACSA Tau Sigma Delta Gold Medal (1996), and

the Byrnes-Sewall Prize for Teaching Excellence in Yale College (1997).

Scully has maintained close relationships with leading contemporary architects who have respected him as a critic. Indeed, in his writings the distinction between historian and critic have become blurred. As he puts it most eloquently in *American Architecture and Urbanism*, "Art history must therefore be conservative, experimental, and ethical. It loves old and new things, and it demands value. The line between history and criticism should therefore be difficult to draw in any field; in the modern field, it must be almost nonexistent."

HUMBERTO RODRÍGUEZ-CAMILLONI

Selected Publications

The Architectural Heritage of Newport Rhode Island, 1640–1915 (with Antoinette Downing), 1952; 2nd edition, 1967

The Shingle Style: Architectural Theory and Design From Richardson to the Origins of Wright, 1955; new edition, as *The Shingle Style and the Stick Style: Architectural Theory and Design from Downing to the Origins of Wright*, 1971

Frank Lloyd Wright, 1960

Modern Architecture: The Architecture of Democracy, 1961; revised edition, 1974

The Earth, the Temple, and the Gods: Greek Sacred Architecture, 1962; revised edition, 1979

Louis I. Kahn, 1962

Arquitectura actual, 1967

American Architecture and Urbanism, 1969; new edition, 1988

Pueblo Architecture of the Southwest: A Photographic Essay (with William Current), 1971

The Shingle Style Today; or, The Historian's Revenge, 1974

Pueblo: Mountain, Village, Dance, 1975; 2nd edition, 1989

Wesleyan (with Philip Trager), 1982

The Villas of Palladio (with Philip Trager), 1986

New World Visions of Household Gods and Sacred Places: American Art, 1650–1914, 1988

"Introduction," in *The Architecture of the American Summer: The Flowering of the Shingle Style*, 1989

The Great Dinosaur Mural at Yale: The Age of Reptiles (with others), 1990

Architecture: The Natural and the Manmade, 1991

French Royal Gardens: The Designs of Andre LeNotre (with Jeannie Baubion-Mackler), 1992

Between Two Towers: The Drawings of the School of Miami (with others), 1996

Further Reading

Cohen, Susan, "Vincent Scully Shares His Views on Architecture," *Greenwich News* (14 January 1988)

Dean, Andrea Oppenheimer, "Siteseer," *Historic Preservation* 46, no. 5 (September/October 1994)

Feinberg, Gary, "Vincent Scully: Scholar in Our Midst," *South Beach* 1, no. 5 (May/June 1993)

Forgey, Benjamin, "The Architect's Civilizing Voice," *Washington Post* (13 May 1995)

Goldberger, Paul, "Selections from the Writings of Vincent Scully: Introduction," in *The Architectural League of New York Dinner in Honor of Vincent Scully*, New York: The Architectural League of New York, 1995

McCullough, David, "Architectural Spellbinder," *Architectural Forum* 111 (September 1959)

"Retiring Yale Professor Casts a Towering Shadow," *Journal Inquirer* (17 May 1991)

Stevenson, James, "Profiles: What Seas What Shores," *The New Yorker* (18 February 1980)

"Vincent Scully On Civilized Architecture," *M* 4, no. 1 (October 1986)

Whoriskey, Peter, "Miami as Art: A Legend Appraises Our Architecture," *Miami Herald* (29 January 1996)

SEAGRAM BUILDING, NEW YORK

Designed by Ludwig Mies van der Rohe; completed 1958
New York, New York

Of all the American monuments to the International Style, it is the Seagram Building by Mies van der Rohe that fully defines the aesthetic and time of high modernism, the era of postwar corporate and urban consciousness. In glass, steel, and bronze, the Seagram symbolizes the bricks and mortar and martinis that were the 1950s.

The Seagram, a 40-story slab skyscraper of amber glass within a grid of bronze I beams, rises above a fountained plaza on Manhattan's Park Avenue. The body of the building, in typical Mies fashion, is supported by a templelike entry that is reminiscent, within a thoroughly modern composition, of the earliest post-and-lintel roots of archaic architecture. The design is of interest not only for the glass slab that rises suavely above midtown Manhattan but also for the invention of the plaza fronting Park Avenue and the resulting relationship of urban architectural object to its opposition, void space, within the city grid.

Architectural historian William H. Jordy, in his definitive analysis of the building, spoke of the Seagram as modern expression of "the potential of structure to create noble order, in the sense in which it created noble order in the past" coupled with "truth of its time."

For modernism, the Seagram is an ideal, perhaps even a Platonic ideal, of perfection and purity of form. It symbolizes the type form of the gridded glass skyscraper, emblem of the 20th century. The building has always seemed the epitome of form and function united in its most integrated and reductive sense, the clearest expression of Mies' edicts that "form follows function" and that architecture is "almost nothing." It is émigré Mies' American sublime manifestation of his German utopian renderings.

Like its creator, the Seagram is both simple and complex. The simplicity is the gridded steel frame with glass-curtain wall as a modern extension of the archaic building. The complexity is inherent in the expression of that simplicity through the applied bronze I beams, which, although they symbolically stand for the meaning of structure, are themselves unstructural. Thus, the aesthetic of truth-in-structure is expressed through an untruthfully convoluted visual metaphor.

Over the four decades since its design, the Seagram has drawn architecture and urban planning into a number of problems. The primary problem is the truth-in-structure problem, but other, more prosaic problems also exist. Unlike the ideal typeform buildings of the past, such as the Parthenon and the Pantheon, the Seagram as a type form was created within the fastest paced civilization in history. Thus, the Modern type form engenders its own imitation and reaction within its lifetime. Thinking

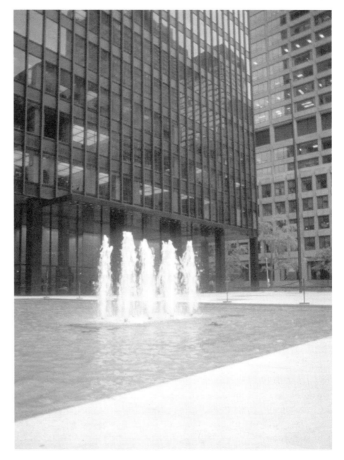

Seagram Building Plaza: New York City (1958)
Ezra Stoller © Esto

architects, after the Seagram, wrestled with the questions of, "Where can construction go after total reduction?" and "How can the art of architecture follow perfection of form?"

For the thoughtful architect, the Seagram has been inspirational, a standard against which tall buildings will always be judged. Less-gifted builders have simply lowered the standard set by Mies for the gridded glass-and-steel skyscraper. His work has been exploited, copied, and shortchanged as a standardized form by developers the world over, cheaply, in terms of both dollars and aesthetics. Thus, it is critical for an appreciation of early skyscraper design never to read the chronology of modern architecture backward, blaming the beautiful early type forms, such as the Seagram, for the debased works of later imitators.

A further problem engendered by the Seagram is inherent in the design of the slab versus the plaza. For this revolutionary design, revised zoning rules had to supersede the famous New York setback skyscraper law that had been passed to ensure that giant buildings would not block light and air within the crowded Manhattan grid. As the rules of the 1916 zoning law had dictated the aesthetics of the setback skyscraper, so now with the Seagram plan would new zoning standards allow for new forms in American architecture. The Seagram plan meant that skyscrapers could go straight up to higher elevations without setbacks, in giant continuous slabs. In exchange for height, the footprint of the

building would cover only a small percentage of the site, allowing an open plaza to be created.

The assumption of city planners was that a public urban amenity would thus be created and financed through private corporate funding. Although the concept of a plaza of negative space could be fully animated by Mies, by a less-deft planner the modern plaza has all too often proven to be no urban amenity. Poor imitation of the Seagram plaza has led to urban plazas that are not, as Mies's is, confined voids in an aesthetic dialectical relationship with the solid form of a building but rather simply voids of leftover space. Planners have learned that it is better to maintain a continuous street setback than to disrupt it arbitrarily.

It is possible that the Seagram's influence on architectural style has been even wider than Mies could have expected, for the perfection and reduction of this building perhaps engendered the reactionary excesses of Postmodernism. After working with Mies on the Seagram, architect Philip Johnson left Mies but continued to react to the Miesian influence for decades. Johnson's prolific later ornamental Postmodernism, the antithesis of his own International Style tenets, may be read as a reactionary comment on his own work on the Seagram Building.

These problems, of course, are latter-day events for which Mies should not be held responsible. It is not to his detriment that he sought, through his type form for the modern skyscraper, to create perfect architectural form; nor is it his fault that the imitators of architecture so rarely comprehended the meaning of his architectural ideals. Mies would not have concerned himself with such problems, for his concerns were solely with the significance of his *Baukunst*.

LESLIE HUMM CORMIER

Further Reading

The Mies van der Rohe Archives are in the Museum of Modern Art, New York City.

Jordy, William H., "The Laconic Splendor of the Metal Frame: Ludwig Mies van der Rohe's 860 Lake Shore Drive Apartments and His Seagram Building" in *The Impact of European Modernism in the Mid–Twentieth Century*, by Jordy, Garden City, New York: Doubleday, 1972

Schulze, Franz, *Mies van der Rohe: A Critical Biography*, Chicago: University of Chicago Press, 1985

SEARS TOWER, CHICAGO

Skidmore, Owings and Merrill; completed 1974
Chicago Illinois

The Sears Tower, today owned by a private investment firm and rented to a variety of office tenants, serves as a landmark and a symbol of the Chicago skyline. The building is seen from distant vistas in every direction in this flat, prairie-land city on the edge of Lake Michigan, thus creating the awareness of the dynamic presence of the Chicago skyline and urban environment.

During the period 1974–1997, the Sears Tower, at a height of 1454 feet and 110 stories, held the title of the world's tallest building encompassing 4.5 million gross square feet and 3.7 million square feet of net useable office space. In 1997 the Petronas Towers in Kuala Lumpur, Malaysia (designed by Cesar Pelli), although only 88 stories high, usurped that honor with a height of 1483 feet. The Sears Tower continues to provide the world's highest occupied floors.

The generation of the form and concept of the vertical tower is an interesting combination of client's program, site and technology. The Federal Aviation Administration who ruled that no building in Chicago could be higher than 2000 feet above sea level determined the height. The site is at an elevation of 546 feet and, thus, a final height of 1,454 feet was determined.

The initial goal was not to build the world's tallest building. Sears, Roebuck and Company determined that its floor space needs would eventually be 4.5 million gross square feet. Skidmore, Owings and Merrill (SOM), the architects, conducted a study that demonstrated the company could save 30% of walking time in a department if floor areas were stacked vertically and not arranged horizontally. Sears also determined that the ideal department size was 110,000 square feet and that its initial needs were for only 60 percent of the gross 4.5 million square feet. The remaining 40 percent would initially be rental space.

Following an initial concept of two separate towers, SOM began to develop a scheme that was a number of vertical buildings tied together to make one building. Fazlur Kahn, a structural engineer and partner in SOM, developed a system called "bundled tubes" for the Sears Tower. The solution was a system composed of nine structural bays each 75 feet by 75 feet in plan and independent of each other. Nine skyscrapers of varying heights are tied together in one building with the lateral wind loads resisted by the interlocked exterior tubes, cantilevered from the ground augmented by horizontal diaphragms. With this concept in place, it became possible to stop the tubes at any level without affecting the structural integrity. The result was a vertical form that is composed of a nine-tube base, floors 1 through 50; followed vertically by seven tubes on floors 51–65 where the northwest and southeast tubes were discontinued; followed vertically by floors 66–90, composed of five tubes in the shape of a cruciform in plan and finally the top floors 91–110 composed of two bundled tubes.

A building of this size and height is also strongly controlled by the vertical transportation system. In order to satisfy user expectations as to speed and comfort of movement, a point of density arrives wherein the ground floor elevators consume the entire entry floor. To facilitate the size and density of the Sears Tower, technologies involving double-deck elevators and high-speed express elevators were employed. The Tower's 103-cab system divides the building into three separate zones. Fourteen double-deck elevators carry passengers, non-stop to either the 33rd–34th floors or the 66th–67th floors where sky lobbies provide space for loading and unloading at two different floor levels. Once at these levels passengers can go to local floors via 63 single-deck elevator cabs. The 103rd floor is a public observation deck and serves large crowds by providing two express elevators, which connect the ground and top floors. These elevators travel at the rate of 1,800 feet per minute, reaching the summit in less than one minute.

The Sears Tower is the second in a series of three headquarters buildings for the company. The first building constructed in 1904 was located at Arthington and Homan Avenues in the Chicago West Side Lawndale community. It included a 14½-story tower and a campus of decentralized offices. It is still standing today. This environment produced a corporate culture

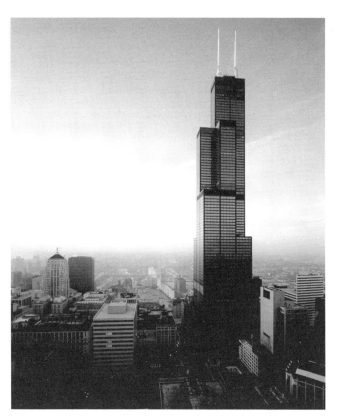

Sears Tower, Chicago (1974)
© Timothy Hursley. Photo courtesy S.O.M., Chicago

wherein a high degree of personal interaction occurred through chance meetings along daily pedestrian routes. The present Sears Tower replaced this earlier structure in 1974.

The downtown Sears Tower served the Sears Corporation until 1992 when a new headquarters was developed in Hoffman Estates in the Northwest suburbs of Chicago. This building, designed by Perkins and Wills, Architects, returned to the culture of the first building by creating a horizontal scheme that provided travel through atriums and public corridors to encourage informal conversations and relationships among employees and departments. The comparison of the three structures provides an enlightening overview of the direction and styles of corporate America as to office building design.

The exterior appearance of the tubes is a dark, uniform surface composed of black aluminum frames and bronze-tinted glare reducing glass. Although an aesthetic success on the Chicago skyline, it is much less attractive and inviting at ground level. Its great height is virtually imperceptible at its base. In 1985 to improve the relationship to the pedestrian and make it more inviting for those entering the building, a new atrium entry-way was created at the Wacker Street entrance and a new entry added at Jackson Boulevard. In 1992 when Sears Corporation moved to its new location in Hoffman Estates, the new owners determined to remodel the existing public spaces in a 70 million dollar project. The goal was to make the building more attractive to new tenants. New lobbies were added at the Franklin Street and Wacker Drive entrances.

Today the building is no longer the home of the Sears Corporation nor is it the world's tallest building, but it is still the dominant visual symbol on the Chicago skyline, a symbol of the spirit and style of this Midwestern community and an attraction to thousands of visitors each year.

JACK KREMERS

See also **Chicago (IL), United States; Petronas Towers, Kuala Lumpur; Skidmore, Owings, and Merrill (United States); Skyscraper**

Further Reading

Willis, Carol, *Form Follows Finance*, Princeton: Princeton Architectural Press, 1995
Graham, Bruce, "Sears Tower," in *Bruce Graham of SOM*, New York: Rizzoli, 1989
Saliga, Pauline A., "Sears Tower" in *The Sky's the Limit*, edited by Saliga, New York: Rizzoli, 1990

SEASIDE, FLORIDA

Seaside, Florida, is an 80-acre resort development on the Florida panhandle begun in 1981 by Robert and Daryl Davis. Unlike the conventional high-rises or apartment clusters lining the beach, Miami firm Andres Duany and Elizabeth Plater-Zyberk (DPZ) designed Seaside as a traditional, small southern town of private residences and public streets. Emblematic of what later became known as New Urbanism, Seaside's design was intended to produce a modest, mixed-income, mixed-use, pedestrian-oriented holiday community.

Although various postmodernist architects in the 1970s had been incorporating references to vernacular architecture into individual buildings and analyzing the figural relationships between public and private urban space, Seaside represented the first effort to reconfigure contemporary development in the form of a traditional American town. Its use of conventional suburban-planning tools—codes and master plans—for this purpose was unprecedented and has since stood as an alternative suburban development model to urban sprawl. Its popularity, ever-higher prices, and pronounced traditional styling have made it the subject of both tremendous praise and scorn. Along with later DPZ projects, Seaside's design revived interest among many allied disciplines in early 20th-century town-planning ideas, and its designers challenged the lack of attention to urbanism and public space in both conventional land-planning practices and contemporary avant-garde architectural design.

DPZ's interest in Team X ideas about using architecture to promote group social relations dovetailed with Robert Davis's desire not simply to develop the land he had inherited but to found a town and community that would be part traditional small town and part utopian social experiment. Together, the designers and the developer toured and measured traditional southern towns. In an effort to reproduce the towns' spatial quality and authentic variety, DPZ refrained from designing any of the buildings at Seaside themselves. Instead, through a *charrette* process, the firm developed a master plan and codes to direct individual property owners' design decisions. The design won a *Progressive Architecture* citation for urban planning in 1984.

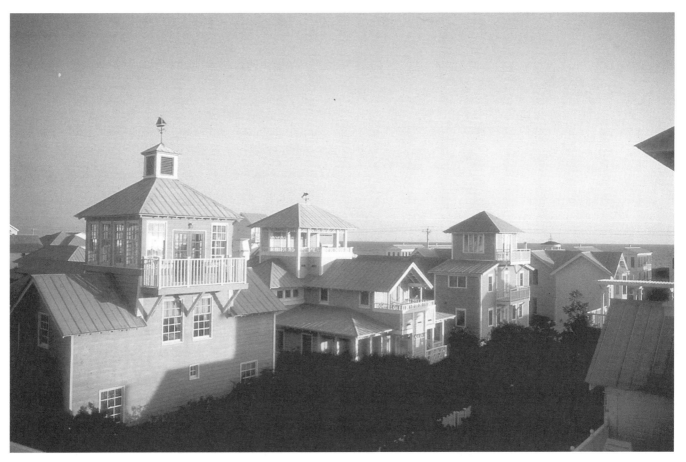

Town of Seaside, Florida
© Elizabeth Plater-Zyberk

The master plan extends the existing streets of neighboring Seagrove across the site, locates a central green in an existing gorge, and straddles the two-lane coastal highway with commercial activities. Its central focus and loose grid recall City Beautiful projects from the 1920s. Unlike most coastal resorts, development along the 2800 feet of beach is low and minimal, allowing water views to extend deep into the site and preserving public access to the beach. There are approximately 300 residential lots, all of which are within a five-minute walk of the center. A church, a school, a post office, and the resort's recreational amenities are prominently scattered throughout the site, where they visually terminate vistas and serve as public or semipublic focal points to the various neighborhoods. Private buildings, however, are visually unified through required build-to lines, picket fences, percentage of porch frontage, number of stories, and general building type.

Every lot on the master plan is keyed to one of eight different, regionally based building types visually displayed in an easy-to-understand one-page urban code. North–south streets call for relatively deep setbacks from the street and "Florida cracker" low, porch-fronted "bungalows" so as to maximize public views of the Gulf of Mexico. East–west streets, however, with no ocean view, offer smaller, more affordable lots, coded for versions of the Charleston "single house": taller and tight up to the street, with a side yard. A diagonal boulevard (located to preserve existing trees) has the largest lots, and "antebellum mansions" are able to serve as inns, apartments, or large single-family residences. Three- to five-story, mixed-use, arcaded party-wall buildings, similar to those found in New Orleans or Eufala, Alabama, line the central commercial area, whereas three-story townhouses above shops and workshops create another, quieter square behind it.

This diversity has been unified by a number of factors: the restriction of landscaping to indigenous plants, the encouragement of construction of rear cottages, the allowance of 215-square-foot towers, and an architectural code that allows for stylistic variation within strict limits. It establishes acceptable window proportions, roof pitches, materials, and a few mandatory construction details. Most of the homeowners have chosen to build in a more or less Victorian or classical style, although the overall emphasis on design has resulted in the commissioning of well-known contemporary designers including Steven Holl, Aldo Rossi, Machado & Silvetti, Mockbee and Coker, Deborah Berke, and Walter Chatham.

Counter to suburban privatization, Seaside consistently promotes the hierarchical importance of the public realm and com-

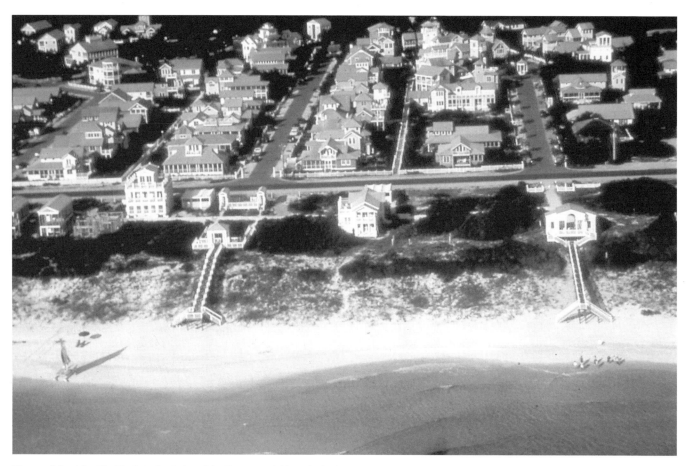

Town of Seaside, Florida (1979), designed by Duany and Plater-Zyberk
© Duany and Plater-Zyberk

munity building. The codes discipline the private buildings into spatially, visually, and socially defining the streets and squares as outdoor public rooms. Privileging the pedestrian over the car, they are narrow and brick paved. The provision of shops, office space, and a public junior high charter school in the town center has succeeded in encouraging walking. Front porches are required to be close enough to the street to allow for sociable interaction. There is a seasonal newspaper, and the Seaside Institute, a nonprofit educational organization, programs public events to engage the immediate community and the broader audience interested in New Urbanism.

The true community of Seaside however remains amorphous; there are very few year-round inhabitants at Seaside. Most of the homes are vacation properties rented out through the Seaside Rental Agency. Robert Davis argues that, as a resort, Seaside demonstrates to more visitors the virtues of living in a walkable community of small lots and shared public spaces. Critics point to Seaside as merely a simulation of community and public life as well as a commodified nostalgia for the sentimental past. To some critics, the seeming impossibility of dissent renders it a consensual tyranny rather than a democratic utopia, a point made in the 1997 film *The Truman Show*, which was shot on location in Seaside. Although such questions have in no way slowed the countless efforts to emulate Seaside, they point to

the continued controversy surrounding New Urbanism and the questions it raises.

ELLEN DUNHAM-JONES

See also **Duany and Plater-Zyberk (United States); New Urbanism; Suburban Planning**

Further Reading

Abrams, Janet, "The Form of the (American) City: Two Projects by Andres Duany and Elizabeth Plater-Zyberk," *Lotus International* 50 (1986)

Bressi, Todd (editor), *The Seaside Debates: A Critique of the New Urbanism*, New York: Rizzoli, 2002

Brooke, Steven, *Seaside*, Gretna, Louisiana: Pelican, 1995

Duany, Andres, and Elizabeth Plater-Zyberk, "The Town of Seaside," *The Princeton Journal* 2 (1995)

Duany, Andres, Elizabeth Plater-Zyberk, and Jeff Speck, *Suburban Nation: The Rise of Sprawl and the Decline of the American Dream*, New York: North Point Press, 2000

Harvey, David, "The New Urbanism and the Communitarian Trap," *Harvard Design Magazine* 1 (Winter/Spring 1997)

Krieger, Alex, and William Lennertz (editors), *Andres Duany and Elizabeth Plater-Zyberk: Towns and Town-Making Principles*, New York: Rizzoli, and Cambridge, Massachusetts: Harvard University Graduate School of Design, 1991

Langdon, Philip, *A Better Place to Live: Reshaping the American Suburb*, Amherst: University of Massachusetts Press, 1994

Mohney, David (editor), "Seaside and the Real World: A Debate on American Urbanism," *ANY: Architecture New York* 1, no. 1 (1993)

Mohney, David, and Keller Easterling (editors), *Seaside: Making a Town in America*, New York: Princeton Architectural Press, 1991

SEIDLER, HARRY 1923–

Architect, Australia

In his first published article in 1949, Harry Seidler laid out a philosophy incorporating relationships between modern European painting, the sculptural arts, and architecture. Its outline was derived from Walter Gropius's Harvard University Graduate School of Design program and directed almost exclusively to visual elements (mass, transparency, tension, polarity, and so on) that architecturally evolved in some measure from structural exploitation. Seidler's early houses were dedicated to these visual determinations but showed a noticeable diversity as a result of experimentations with structure knitted to easy formal architectonic considerations, such as plan and simple geometric shape.

The prize-winning house for his mother (1948–50) was first among works in the 1950s that immediately captured attention worldwide, notably in Europe and the Los Angeles magazine *Arts and Architecture*. They were recognized as an apogee of architectural refinement and dynamic sensibility as promoted by central European émigré designers.

With Gropius, Seidler discovered a language for architectural thought; with Josef Albers at Black Mountain College, he learned "to think in visual terms," and with Oscar Niemeyer he discovered form and mass, sun control, how to express structure, and attention to site conditions. His early work was derivative of Marcel Breuer (he does not apologize for this) but soon matured to reach a formal epitome in a block of apartments (1962) at Diamond Bay, Sydney.

A close collaboration with Italian structural engineer Pier Luigi Nervi beneficially changed Seidler's large and tall buildings designs. The Australia Square development (1962–67) in Sydney contains a round tower constructed of precast elements, repetitive floor to floor—a lesson in constructional efficiency that clarified expression by simplification. The tower stands on a stepped pedestrian plaza, open to but also partly screening surrounding streets and shared with a shorter rectangular office building sitting on giant sculpted piers. The Square set an urban design standard envied throughout the Western world.

Parallel to this experience, Seidler referred to the series of paintings by American postwar protominimalist painter Frank Stella that employed circular segments, and he reexamined Albers's free forms and the "richness" of Dutch-American Abstract Expressionist Willem de Kooning's nonobjective paintings. The result was the introduction of an overtly baroque character first explored tentatively for Condominium Apartments (1969–70) at Acapulco, Mexico.

The 1970s were an expansive period that saw the completion of a number of major commissions, including the Trade Group Office (1970–74) in Canberra, which employed Nervi's long-span, posttensional constructional system to a schemata based on the functional responses of Louis I. Kahn; the MLC Center (1971–75) in Sydney, a significant urban pedestrian precinct and office tower; and the Australian Embassy (1973–74) in Paris, with Breuer as local consultant, a bipartite scheme of conceptual maturity and constructional style that prevailed into the 1990s. Seidler maintained a variety of commissions ranging from medium-size houses to civic centers (such as Waverley, 1982–84, near Melbourne) to large urban-planning schemes. Of the latter, the QVI building (1987–91) in Perth, Western Australia, and Grosvenor Place (1982–88) in Sydney, with expansive pedestrian plazas and minimal site coverage by towers, are exceptional.

For the most part, Seidler's current architectural practice is directed to resolving formal and social issues raised by tall buildings in urban situations. Following on from the MLC Center, the most notable of these have been the lively Riverside Development (1983–86) in Brisbane, typical of his concrete structural system, sun control aesthetic, and the Albers-influenced two- and three-dimensional forms; the more angular Capita Center office tower (1984–89) in Sydney, with a full-height stepped central space open to the weather with occasional terraces landscaped with 20-meter-high trees; and the elegantly sophisticated Hong Kong Club and Office Building (1980–84), whose baroque plan and interior spaces meld perfectly with an expressive and exposed-concrete structural system. The exclusive club occupies the lower 4 floors with 17 above for rental. Seidler has said that his desire to

> instill an aura of timeless serenity and yet elegance and pleasure led to the use of curvilinear geometry and forms throughout. . . . The curved forms, however, are used within the geometric disciplines imposed by structural considerations [and] harks back to . . . the Baroque era of the 17th and 18th centuries

This building's "poetic geometry" suggests how his Hong Kong and Shanghai Banking headquarters might have appeared if he, rather than Norman Foster, had won the competitive commission.

For the Vienna city government, Seidler has designed a complex of about 800 apartments in a 35-story triangular tower (similar to Lincoln Centre, 1996–98, in Kuala Lumpur) and seven blocks of four to eight stories in a terraced garden (1993–c.2001), each with views across the Danube to the old town. Diagonals, curves, and swirls exaggerate structure and function and act as counterpoints to rectilinear elevations. They are a further elaboration of forms found earlier, including the Horizon Apartment Tower (1990–98) at Darlinghurst, Sydney, that provides a vigorous alternative response to the glossy glass towers rising everywhere.

It is reasonable to compare Seidler's work with that of a graduate student colleague at Harvard, I.M. Pei. Both exhibit clarity of concept, a high level of sophistication, a love of fluid geometry and plain forms, a certain monumentality, a correct and economical use of expertly detailed materials, and a preference to boldly express structure.

Not from memory of days with Niemeyer but appearing as a reflective homage to the nonagenarian Brazilian's present-day white free forms is Seidler's Berman house (1996–c.2001). Sitting proud above a rugged stone and bush landscape, it is distinctly fresh, from a young inquiring mind.

In the cause of architecture, Seidler has transcended earlier, merely visual precepts to extend modernism (logically he believes) to avoid "transient fashion" and " 'post-mod' cliches," as he puts it, and engage in a most lively, rational architecture. His honorary degrees, visiting teaching positions, and significant international awards attest to a continuing influence.

DONALD LESLIE JOHNSON

Biography

Born in Vienna, Austria, 25 June 1923; emigrated to Australia 1948; naturalized 1958. Attended the University of Manitoba, Winnipeg 1941–44; bachelor's degree in architecture 1944; studied at Harvard University under Walter Gropius and Marcel Breuer 1945–46; master's degree in architecture 1946; studied design under Josef Albers, Black Mountain College, Beria, North Carolina 1946. Chief assistant to Marcel Breuer, New York 1946–48; worked with Oscar Niemeyer, Rio de Janeiro 1948. Principal, Harry Seidler and Associates, Sydney from 1948; trustee, Art Gallery of New South Wales 1976–80. Visiting professor, Harvard Graduate School of Design 1976–77; councilor, University of New South Wales 1976–80; visiting professor, University of British Colombia, Vancouver 1977–78; Thomas Jefferson Professor of Architecture, University of Virginia, Charlottesville 1978; visiting professor, University of New South Wales, Sydney 1980; visiting professor, University of Sydney 1984. Honorary fellow, American Institute of Architects 1966; life fellow, Royal Australian Institute of Architects 1970; fellow, Australian Academy of Technical Sciences 1979; member, Académie d'Architecture, Paris 1982; academician, International Academy of Architecture, Sofia 1987. Officer, Order of the British Empire 1972; Companion, Order of Australia 1987.

Selected Works

Dates are from initiation of final design to completion of construction.

R. Seidler House, Turramurra, Sydney, 1948–50
Rose House, Turramurra, Sydney, 1949–50
Sussman House, Kurrajong Heights, New South Wales, 1951
Williamson House, Mosman, New South Wales, 1951
RAIA Convention Exhibition and Model House, Sydney, 1954
Horwitz Office Building, Sydney, 1954
Lend Lease House Office, Sydney, 1961
Australia Square, Sydney, 1962–67
Diamond Bay Apartments, Sydney, 1962
NSW Government Stores, Alexandria, 1964–65
Seidler House, Killara, 1966–67
Condominium Apartments, Acapulco, Mexico, 1969–70
Trade Group Offices, Canberra, 1970–74
Harry Seidler Offices, Milsons Point, Sydney, 1971–73; extension 1988–94
MLC Center, Sydney, 1971–75
Australian Embassy, Paris, France, 1973–74
Hong Kong Club and Offices, Hong Kong, 1980–84
Waverley Civic Center, Melbourne, 1982–84
Grosvenor Place, Sydney, 1982–88
Hannes House, Cammeray, New South Wales, 1983–84
Riverside Development, Brisbane, 1983–86
Hilton Hotel, Brisbane, 1984–86
Capita Center, Sydney, 1984–89
Shell Headquarters, Melbourne, 1985–89
Phoenix Tower project, Sydney, 1987
QVI Office Tower, Perth, 1987–91
Waverley Art Gallery, Melbourne, 1988–89
IBM Tower, Sydney, 1990–91
Horizon Apartment Tower, Darlinghurst, Sydney, 1990–98
Olympic Housing 2000 (competition project), 1992
Farrell House, Sydney, 1993
Wohnpark Neue Donau (housing), Vienna, Austria, 1993–c.2001
Grollo Tower, project for tallest in world, Melbourne, 1995
Berman House, Joadja, New South Wales, 1996–c.2001
Harrington Apartment Tower, Sydney, 1999–c.2001

Selected Publications

"Painting toward Architecture," *Architecture* (Sydney) 37 (October 1949)
Houses, Interiors, Projects, 1954
Harry Seidler, 1955–63, 1963
Australia Square, 1969
Planning and Building Down Under: New Settlement Strategy and Current Architectural Practice in Australia, 1978
"Afterword" in *The Australian Ugliness*, by Robin Boyd, 2nd edition, 1980
"A Methodology," *RIBA Transactions* 3, no. 1 (1983–84)
Internment: The Diaries of Harry Seidler, May 1940–October 1941, edited by Janis Wilton, translated by Judith Winternitz, 1986
"A Perspective of Planning and Architectural Directions," *Architect* (Sydney) 27 (April 1987)
Towers in the City, 1988
"Losing by the Rules," *World Architecture* 7 (1990)
Harry Seidler: Selected and Current Works, edited by Stephen Dobney, 1997

Further Reading

Since 1948 publications about Seidler have appeared worldwide in journals and books. Reports, project reports, and cassettes and videos of lectures and seminars given by Seidler are held in the Mitchell Library, Sydney, and the National Library, Canberra.

Abercrombie, Stanley, "Four by Seidler," *Interior Design* 61 (May 1990)
Blake, Peter, *Architecture for the New World: The Work of Harry Seidler*, Sydney: Horwitz, and New York: Wittenborn, 1973
Blake, Peter, *Harry Seidler: Australian Embassy; Ambassade d'Australie* (bilingual English-French edition), *Paris*, Sydney: Horwitz, and New York: Wittenborn, 1979
Boyd, Robin, *Australia's Home: Its Origins, Builders, and Occupiers*, Carlton, Victoria: Melbourne University Press, 1952; 2nd edition Ringwood, Victoria: Penguin, 1968
Drew, Philip, "Sydney Seidler," *Architectural Association Quarterly* 6, no. 1 (1974)
Drew, Philip, "Harry Seidler. Australian Embassy, Paris," *A + U* 100 (January 1979)
Drew, Philip, *Two Towers: Harry Seidler, Australia Square, MLC Centre*, Sydney: Horwitz, 1980
Farrelly, E.M., "Capita Center," *Architectural Review* 189 (August 1992)
Frampton, Kenneth and Philip Drew, *Harry Seidler: Four Decades of Architecture*, London and New York: Thames and Hudson, 1992
Frampton, Kenneth, "Structure and Meaning," *World Architecture* 7 (1990)
Frampton, Kenneth, *Riverside Center*, Sydney: Horwitz, 1988
Freeland, J.M., *Architecture in Australia*, Melbourne: Cheshire, 1968
Geran, Monica, "Harry Seidler," *Interior Design* 65 (January 1994)
Hohl, R., *Bürogebände: International Office Buildings*, Teufen, Switzerland: Niggli, 1968; as *Office Buildings: An International*

Survey, translated by E. Rockwell, London: Architectural Press, and New York: Praeger, 1968

Johnson, Donald Leslie, "Bauhaus, Breuer, Seidler: An Australian Synthesis," *Australian Journal of Art* 1 (1978)

Johnson, Donald Leslie, *Australian Architecture, 1901–05: Sources of Modernism*, Sydney: Sydney University Press, 1980

Odoni, Geovanni, "Harry Seidler: Rose Seidler House," *Abitare* 339 (April 1992)

Space Design 197 (February 1981) (special issue entitled "Seidler, 1948–1980")

Taylor, Jennifer, *Australian Architecture since 1960*, Sydney: Law Book, 1986; 2nd edition, Melbourne: National Education Division, the Royal Australian Institute of Architects, 1990

Towndrow, Jennifer, "Seidler's Poetic Geometry," *RIBA Journal* 96 (July 1989)

Tsakalos, Vasilios, "Vienna Housing," *Architecture Australia* 83 May (1994)

"Waverley Civic Center," *Architecture Australia* 77 (July 1988)

SEJIMA, KAZUYO 1956–

Architect, Japan

Kazuyo Sejima's works are cool-headed depictions of the social alienation of her generation. She was born in Ibaraki prefecture, Japan, in 1956 and studied at Japan Women's University, receiving an undergraduate degree from the Housing Department in 1979 and a master's degree in architecture in 1981. On completing her studies, she joined the firm Toyo Ito Architect and Associates, where she worked from 1981 until she established her own office in 1987. While with Ito, her most notable contributions were as the project architect for Pao (1985), a set of furnishings to accommodate the nomadic, consumerist lifestyles of contemporary Japanese women. Although Sejima now repudiates this project, the interpretation of society that it represents remains closer to the outlook in her subsequent work than to Ito's. In particular, Sejima continues to place an emphasis on emotionally unencumbered movement supported by functional flexibility.

Sejima also acknowledges Ito's influence in her material vocabulary, especially translucent films on glass, bright aluminum finishes, and attenuated steel structures. However, a concern with light and reflectance has led Sejima to experiment with wrapping buildings in a broader palette of unusual components and to using novel approaches toward materials. Examples include polycarbonate panels at Y House (1994), S House (1996), and M House (1997); patterned films applied to clear glass, with written characters at the N Museum (1997), leaflike patterns at the Koga Municipal Park Cafe (1998), or a rough striping referring to wood grain at the O Museum (1999); and reflective louvers intended to create a collage of images by mirroring the sky and the ground against the backdrop of interior activities at Hitachi Reflé (1998). Aesthetically, these materials combine with flat, white surfaces to create an architecture that is luminous and photogenic, contributing to her early recognition abroad.

Sejima's 1990 design for a corporate residence, the Saishunkan Seiyaku Women's Dormitory (part of a series of well-publicized projects in the "Kumamoto Artpolis"), brought her instantaneously to international attention. She impassively proposed an architectural embodiment of the disciplined communal lifestyles of the women employee residents, eschewing private space in favor of a polished, airy communal area. Limited sleeping areas for four are ordered with military precision behind frosted glass, after Sejima's earlier proposals for a single large sleeping space proved too shocking.

Residential work remains Sejima's most provocative. She describes herself as designing for a new genus of family, one not always blood relatives or having any sort of consistent structure or stability. Because of this, her designs lack sentimentality, studiously avoiding privileging a location that celebrates the family unit, such as the hearth or kitchen. Rather, her housing is organized in a way more reminiscent of corporate environments: members of the household come together mostly in corridors, while on the move, and individual private rooms, intended as bedrooms, have the uniformity and barrenness of offices. These rooms often have folding doors or pivoted shutters that allow the line between the common and private rooms to be adjusted. She thus further reduces the private character of individual rooms: the walls between sleeping spaces and more conventionally public areas are more or less permeable, as users like.

Critics fear that Sejima's unruffled celebration of homogeneity is coldly prescient. Less well recognized is that she mitigates these qualities by creating a defensive boundary between residents and the outside, an approach that she shares with other Japanese architects, such as Tadao Ando. In her work since 1993, this intention has been reflected in establishing a core living space with little connection to the exterior and has resulted in buildings where major spaces are below ground or where the exterior envelope is almost entirely translucent, cutting off any views beyond the building envelope. Although Westerners often see such designs as unusually harsh, they fit comfortably within conventional Japanese residential expectations. However, in recent nonresidential projects, Sejima has returned to an approach seen in her earliest residential designs, extending interior space into the landscape.

Much of Sejima's work to date has been commissioned by architects or clients associated with the arts community, and her museum and studio spaces are also notable. The Multi-Media Studio (1996) and N Museum have the same purity seen in Sejima's residential work, especially in their minimalism and contextual detachment. Sejima's proposal for an addition to the Sydney Museum of Art (1997) is her first overseas commission, although the project has stalled. (A theater and culture center for Almere, the Netherlands, designed in 1999, may ultimately be completed first.) Notably, in Sejima's oeuvre, retail and corporate facilities are unremarkable, in part because the strategies that make her residential work extraordinary are more commonplace in the building type.

Although sometimes described as ahistoric because of the abstraction of her work, Sejima identifies closely with modernism but intensifies its formal effects. Ito's work has been a crucial foil for her: the remarkable Platform I (1988) and Platform II (1990) seem to have been designed in response to Ito's Silver Hut (1984), whereas the Villa in the Forest (1994) builds on Ito's White U (1976). Notably, Silver Hut and White U were for Ito's family and among his most challenging early works, whereas Sejima was able to go further in her very first projects, with nonfamilial clients. Conventional prototypes also serve as inspiration: in the Gifu Kitagata Apartments (Phase I, 1998), a public housing complex, Sejima acknowledges the influence of Le Corbusier's Unite d'Habitation and Espirit Nouveau. Al-

though there are no direct connections, Sejima's abstraction also leads to her being identified with the Shinohara School.

Because Sejima emphasizes the intuitive side of her design process, the disciplined structural innovations found in her buildings are less often noted. In the Police Box at Chofu Station (1994), for example, Sejima worked with the eminent engineer Matsui Gengo, using a cylindrical room to create lateral stability while allowing for an uninterrupted glass surface running the length of the roof and opposite exterior walls. Her Koga Municipal Park Cafe is enclosed with a strikingly thin roof and nearly nonexistent walls, the result of recent collaborations with Mutsuro Sasaki. This project will perhaps begin to draw more attention to Sejima's structural sophistication.

Almost since the inception of the office, Ryue Nishizawa has worked closely with Sejima. Recently, the two architects have begun to characterize all projects since the beginning of the Multi-Media Studio in 1995 as the works of the firm Kazuyo Sejima and Ryue Nishizawa and Associates, although these have often been published only in Sejima's name. Although Sejima and Nishizawa intend to continue their collaborations, Nishizawa also established his own firm in 1998. Both have said that they will design projects independently of the partnership.

DANA BUNTROCK

Biography

Born in Ibaraki prefecture, Japan, 1956. Attended Japan Women's University, Tokyo; master's degree in architecture, 1981. Worked in the office of Toyo Ito Architect and Associates, Tokyo, 1981–87. In private practice, Kazuyo Sejima and Associates, Tokyo, from 1987; in collaboration with Ryue Nishizawa from 1995. Has served as lecturer at Japan Women's University and at the Technical Institute of Tokyo.

Selected Works

Platform I, Katsu'ura, Chiba prefecture, 1988
Platform II, Kita Koma (Gun), Yamanashi prefecture, 1990
Saishunkan Seiyaku Women's Dormitory, Kumamoto City, Kumamoto prefecture, 1991
Pachinko Parlor I, Hitachi, Ibaraki prefecture, 1993
Pachinko Parlor II, Hitachi Naka, Ibaraki prefecture, 1993
Villa in the Forest, Chino, Nagano prefecture, 1994
Police Box at Chofu Station, Chofu City, Tokyo, 1994
Pachinko Parlor III, Hitachi Ohta, Ibaraki prefecture, 1996
Multi-Media Studio, Oogaki, Gifu prefecture, 1996
S House, Okayama City, Okayama prefecture, 1996
N Museum, Nakahachi, Wakayama prefecture, 1997
M House, Shibuya Ward, Tokyo, 1997
K Head Office, Hitachi, Ibaraki prefecture, 1997
Gifu Kitagata Apartments, Phase 1, Motosu, Gifu prefecture, 1998
Koga Municipal Park Cafe, Koga, Ibaraki prefecture, 1998
Hitachi Reflé/Hitachi No'ushiku Station Facilities, Ushiku, Ibaraki prefecture, 1998
O Museum, Iida, Nagano prefecture, 1999

Selected Publications

Sejima's own writings are limited to brief formal descriptions of her works found in magazines and journals. One interesting exception is "Sejima Kazuyo—Nishizawa Ryue to no Taiwa" (A Conversation with Kazuyo Sejima and Ryue Nishizawa), *Kenchiku Bunka* 54, no. 632 (June 1999) (special issue entitled "Mutsuro Sasaki: Vision of Structure").

Further Reading

Sejima tends to speak simply of her work, emphasizing design strategies and formal resolution. In addition, she is still young, and so little is available on her work in any language. Japanese-language sources elaborate on her theoretical positions, while English-language sources are mostly based on photographs of her built work, in keeping with Sejima's own emphasis on execution over ideas.

Futagawa, Yukio (editor), *Sejima Kazuyo Dokuhon, 1998* (Kazuyo Sejima Reader, 1998), Tokyo: A.D.A. Edita, 1998
Hasegawa, Yuko, "Forms of Indeterminacy," *Casabella* 658 (July/August 1999)
"Kazuyo Sejima, 1987–1999, and Ryue Nishizawa, 1995–1999," *Japan Architect* 35 (Autumn 1999)
Kazuyo Sejima + Ryue Nishizawa: Gifu Apartments,
Sejima, Kazuyo, *Kazuyo Sejima, 1988–1996*, Barcelona, Spain: El Croquis, 1996
"Sejima Kazuyo, 1987–1996," *Kenchiku Bunka* 51 (January 1999)
Takamatsu, Shin, and Doi, Yoshitake, "Gendai kenchiku wo kangeru dai kyu kai: muruchi mediakou bou (Thinking about Contemporary Architecture: Ninth in a Series: Multimedia Studio)," *GA Japan* 24 (January/February 1997)

SERT, JOSEP LLUÍS 1902–83
Architect and urban planner, United States

The career of Josep Lluís Sert and the ascendancy of modern architecture enjoyed a fortunate simultaneity, for Sert emigrated to the United States just in time for the height of his career to be synchronized with the American building boom and European postwar rebuilding. Advancing the causes of the elder modernists who had preceded him, with a freedom of aesthetic expression that they had had to eschew for functionalism, Sert built buildings where they had often been confined to theorizing. True to his utopian modernist roots as an early member of the Congrés Internationaux d'Architecture Moderne (CIAM), Sert's oeuvre focused on the planning of public architecture for socially significant projects. For Sert, however, aesthetics were never secondary to functionalism, and thus the integration of the arts with architecture became an important tenet of his modernism.

Associated with liberal causes in Spain, Sert debuted internationally at the Paris World's Fair of 1937 with his design for the Pavilion for the Spanish Republic, housing Picasso's *Guernica*. As a Catalonian refugee, the youthful Sert then followed an itinerant life, renouncing his homeland; moving to Paris, where he worked with Le Corbusier, to New York; and eventually attending Harvard University, where he followed Walter Gropius as head of the design school, concurrently establishing his own firm of Sert, Jackson and Gourley.

Sert had thrown down the gauntlet of modern urban planning with his seminal text for the CIAM, *Can Our Cities Survive?* (1942), calling for the basic human rights to fresh air, sunlight, space, and healthful environs. His ability to quantify such quality-of-life issues set Sert at the apex of the fundamentals of modern urban planning, just as his emotional commitment to a humane environment, coupled with a very rationally applied methodology, made his the first really effective synthesis of the early modernists' theories. Sert's lifelong contribution was to fuse rationalism with humanity and creativity.

Sert built his first socially significant project, the Barcelona Anti-Tubercular Dispensary (1935, extant), to fight disease not only medically but also socially, for it provided a poor population with a small but restorative environment. The double-winged structure encloses a treed open courtyard, creating a miniature open space in a dense city sector. Sert's functional and imaginative solution raised the work to the level of oasis amid urban chaos.

If "oasis" is the ancient image recalled by Sert's modern urbanism, then "temple" reflects his architecture for art and human spirit, the first of which was his Spanish Pavilion (1937), a tent-like, lightweight structure appropriate to its ephemeral existence as exposition architecture. The simplicity of Sert's reductivist statement—post and lintel with stretched tent above—echoed richly of the archaic spiritual temple. Processional up the modern machined entrance ramp climaxed with Picasso's modern interpretation of the ancient tragedy of war, *Guernica*, deftly moving the viewer between abstraction and reality, from world's fair to world war.

With the Spanish Pavilion, Sert embarked on an artistic journey that increasingly drew his most intense personal expression. The integration of art, architecture, and spirit via the archaic experience of processional; the light and space hinted at in this early work; and the meditative possibilities of architecture would have their mature expression in Sert's late museums of art. His style evolved, retaining its Mediterranean roots for more than six decades: a thoughtful architecture of primary colors against pure white, agglomerative massing of cubic forms, functionally derived flat pattern, and intense interest in space and light.

Sert understood aesthetic dialectics, moving elegantly from art to architecture, from architecture to nature, and from vernacular materials to the modern machined world, always the modernist émigré drawn back to ancient echoes. In Sertian space, vacant walls of poured concrete are held in a striking aesthetic tension to his signature saturated colors, the solidity of his cubic forms is juxtaposed with the void space of courtyards, and silence is always at the center of action.

In major international works commissioned at the height of his American career, from the late 1950s into the early 1970s—the Fondation Maeght (1964, Provence, France), the Fondation Miró (1975, Barcelona, Spain), and the Center for the Study of World Religions (1958, Cambridge, Massachusetts)—Sert was able to give free rein at last to his innate artistic and spiritual nature.

Processional and vista are important in these late Sertian works for art and spirit. As if these were sacred sites, the Maeght and Miró museums are approached via long, winding hill roads, integrated with the natural topography, white cubes amid landscape. The Fondation Miró is vaulted, and the Fondation Maeght is topped by an inverted Le Corbusian roof, whose origins can also be traced back to Sert's own oeuvre in the white awning above his Spanish Pavilion. Each art museum is com-

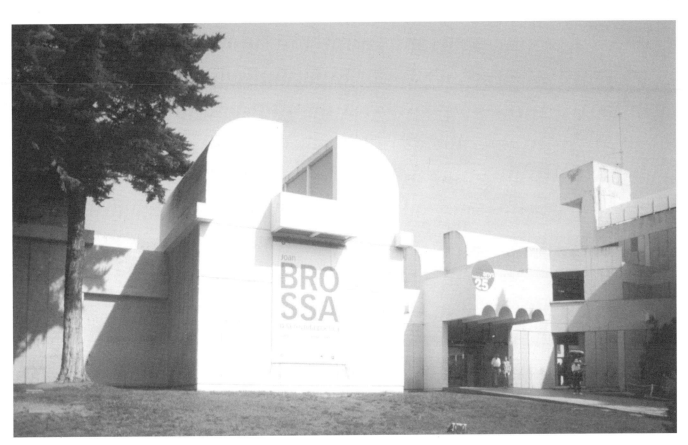

The Fundació Miró, (Joan Miró Center for the Study of Contemporary Art), Barcelona
Photo © Mary Ann Sullivan

posed of a series of masses of cubic forms, like an indigenous hill town, built of positive and negative spaces, in clusters resembling Iberian atrium houses. These modern compositions become visual meditations on the accretions of time, space, and stucco.

For Sert, the active and the contemplative, the sacred and the secular, and the integration of the arts with architecture were all significant pursuits of modernism. At Harvard University, Sert left a legacy of buildings and plans exploring these themes, in the Science Center (1970), Peabody Terrace (1964), an unrealized campus plan, and the Carpenter Center for the Visual Arts (1963), a project in which he was affiliated with his friend Le Corbusier.

The Harvard Center for the Study of World Religions, however, speaks most clearly of Sert the man and his vision. One room of this work might be considered a summation of Sert's oeuvre: the meditation room, the metaphorical center of the design. Here Sert planned for art, architecture, and spirit to be mutually enhancing in an empty room of blank white walls illuminated by a sole natural light source. In this silent statement of space, light, peace, and the universal imagery of spirit, Sert achieved a unity of beliefs with artistic form, of form with spirit. Here, in Sert's words, truly is "a different monumentality."

LESLIE HUMM CORMIER

Biography

Born in Barcelona, 1 July 1902; emigrated to the United States 1939; naturalized 1951. Studied at the Escuela Superior de Arquitectura, Barcelona; master's degree in architecture 1929. Assistant to Le Corbusier and Pierre Jeanneret, Paris 1929–31; established GATCPAC, a group of architects affiliated with CIAM 1930–36. Private practice, Barcelona 1931–37. Lived in Paris from 1937–39. Founder and partner with Paul Lester Wiener and Paul Schulz, Town Planning Associates, New York 1939–57; private practice, Cambridge, Massachusetts from 1957; partner, with Huson Jackson and Ronald Gourley, Sert, Jackson and Gourley 1958–63; partner, Sert, Jackson and Associates from 1963. Professor of city planning, Yale University, New Haven, Connecticut 1944–45; professor of architecture and dean of the Graduate School of Design, 1953–69, consultant to the Harvard Planning Office, 1956–69, emeritus professor, from 1969, Harvard University, Cambridge, Massachusetts; Thomas Jefferson Memorial Foundation Professor of Architecture, University of Virginia, Charlottesville 1970–71; member, Advisory Council, Princeton University School of Architecture and Urban Planning, New Jersey 1972–74. Member, board of directors and planning committee, Citizens Housing Council of New York 1945; president of CIAM 1947–56; chairman, Planning Board of Cambridge, Massachusetts 1957; chairman, American Institute of Architects Committee on the National Capital 1964; fellow, American Institute of Architects; member, National Institute of Arts and Letters; member, American Academy of Arts and Sciences; honorary member, Royal Architectural Institute, Canada; honorary member, Royal Society of Arts, London; honorary member, Royal Institute of British Architects; honorary member, Académie Royale, Belgium; honorary member, Akademie der Künste, Berlin; honorary member, Royal Academy of Arts, London; honorary member, Society of Architects, Mexico; honorary member; Institute of Urbanism, Peru;

honorary member, Académie d'Architecture, France; honorary member, Sociedad de Arquitectos, Columbia. Gold Medal, French Academy of Architecture 1975; Gold Medal, American Institute of Architects 1981. Died in Barcelona, 15 March 1983.

Selected Works

Central Anti-Tubercular Dispensary, Calle Torres Amat, Barcelona (with J. Torres and J. Subirana), 1935
Master Plan, Barcelona (with GATCPAC, Le Corbusier, and Pierre Jeanneret), 1935
Spanish Pavilion, World's Fair, Paris (with Luis Lacasa), 1937
Joan Miró Studio, Palma, Majorca, 1955
Center for the Study of World Religions, Cambridge, Massachusetts 1958
Carpenter Center for the Visual Arts, Harvard University, Cambridge, Massachusetts (with Le Corbusier), 1963
Maeght Foundation, Museum of Contemporary Art, Saint-Paul-de-Vence, France (with Bellini, Lizero, and Gozzi), 1964
Peabody Terrace for Married Students, Harvard University, Cambridge, Massachusetts, 1964
Undergraduate Science Center, Harvard University, Cambridge, Massachusetts, 1970
Joan Miró Center for the Study of Contemporary Art, Barcelona (with Anglada, Gelabert, and Ribas), 1975

Selected Publications

Solutions, 1942
Can Our Cities Survive? An ABC of Urban Problems, Their Analyses, Their Solutions, Based on the Proposals Formulated by the CIAM, 1942
The Heart of the City: Towards the Humanism of Urban Life (coeditor with Jaqueline Tyrwhitt and Ernesto Nathan Rogers), 1952
The Shape of Our Cities (coeditor with Tyrwhitt and Rogers), 1957
Cripta de la Colonia Güell de Antoni Gaudí, 1969

Further Reading

The Sert Archive at the Graduate School of Design, Harvard University, is the most complete view of Sert the man and the architect. The archive includes works of architecture and urban planning, professional and personal correspondence, and photographs. Particularly interesting are documents concerning Sert's circle of artistic friends, including Le Corbusier, Picasso, Braque, Miró, and Calder. Readers will note that the spelling of Sert's first and middle names varies throughout his career, as he chose to identify his name with either its Catalonian or Spanish roots at different times.

Bastlund, Knud, *Jose Luis Sert*, New York: Praeger, and London: Thames and Hudson, 1967
Gardner, Richard, *Josep Luis Sert: Architect to the Arts*, Cambridge, Massachusetts: The President and Fellows of Harvard College, 1978

SHANGHAI WORLD FINANCIAL CENTER

Designed by Kohn Pedersen Fox, to be completed in 2007
Shanghai, China

Designed by the American architectural firm Kohn Pedersen Fox in 1994 for the Japan-based Mori Building Development

Co., the Shanghai World Financial Center will rise to a projected height of 500 meters, making it the tallest building in the world by nearly 50 meters. The building is part of a global paradigm shift that has occurred over the last decade, resulting in the world's tallest buildings, traditionally located in Chicago or New York, now emerging in rapidly developing parts of Asia. Cesar Pelli's Twin Towers in Kuala Lumpar were the first to announce this trend, and the Shanghai World Financial Center (which is significantly taller than Twin Towers) is clearly destined to establish itself as China (and Asia's) tallest building.

Construction of the 94-story structure began in August 1997, and the first stage of construction, involving the structural groundwork, was completed in October 1998. The financial crisis that crippled Asian markets in the late 1990s forced a temporary halt to construction, during which time financial backing was secured to recommence construction of the tower. Following a range of delays, the tower, in a slightly modified form, is now to be completed by 2007 in time for the Beijing Olympics in the following year. Key changes to the design resulted in an increase in height from 460 meters to a new projected height of 500 meters.

The building occupies a site on Pudong Road adjacent to the recently completed Jin Mao Tower in the rapidly developing Lujiazhui financial and trade district in Pudong. This area has been dedicated to development by the Chinese government and is intended to become the Asian epicenter for international trade and banking. The Shanghai World Financial Center is the second of a planned trilogy of high-rise towers in the area. The program provides for a total of nearly 320,000 square meters of useable area, with a combination of ground-floor retail, commercial office space, hotel suites, and an observation deck at the top of the building.

The design of the tower represents a transition by Kohn Pedersen Fox from the extravagant Post-modern towers that characterized the firm throughout the 1980s toward the more streamlined and technological aesthetic that dominates their recent architecture. Such a shift demonstrates a nostalgia for the clean forms of modernism, diminishing the role of the façade of the tower in favor of more refined and monumental geometric forms. This is evident in the design of the tower, which takes the form of a chiseled wedge, carved by two sweeping arcs and punctuated dramatically at the apex by a circular void 50-meters in diameter. The diminishing proportion of the floor-plates formed by the tapered block allows for commercial office space at the lower levels and hotel suites above in the more longitudinally proportioned zones of the building. An observation deck is to be located on a bridge across the dynamic circular void at a height of 380 meters.

The tower is square at the base, tapering to a single line at the apex oriented along the diagonal of the ground-floor plate. The sweeping arcs give the tower a twisted, animated form providing unique views of the tower from different vantage points throughout the city. This is most noticeable from the historical Bund area on the opposite side of the Huang Pu River, which bends around the Pudong area and provides the primary sites for viewing the building in the skyline. The circular void that dominates the top of the tower is the same diameter as the sphere atop the nearby Oriental Pearl TV tower, initiating a solid-void dialogue with the adjacent landmark, which the twisting form of the tower addresses. The circular cutout is intended pragmati-

cally to reduce the considerable wind-loads on the building, especially significant in typhoon-stricken Shanghai. It also contains thinly veiled references to traditional Chinese architecture and the circular moon-gate that adorns many temples and gardens across China. The geometry of the square and the circle that is pervasive throughout the tower is intrinsic to Chinese philosophy, symbolic generally of the earth and the sky and ideas of unity and harmony.

Juxtaposed against the monolithic tower is a fractured podium, which responds to the disparate urban cacophony of Pudong, induced by several years of rampant development. Because of setback restrictions, the tower is confined to the center of the site, dissected by a triangular shaft that slices through the building at ground level and forms the entry to the lift-core. Based on the geometry of a perfect circle, from which the square floorplate of the tower projects, the podium wraps around the rear of the building, peeling back to reveal the intersection of the tower with the ground at the front, north-western edge of the site. This gesture addresses the main road of the Lujiazui district and contains a landscaped public space protected by an enveloping shield of trees. The southern and western sides of the tower are bounded by a landscaped public garden that links several parts of the urban Lujiazui district and connects the three projected towers. A large area of on-grade car parking is located on the southeastern side of the tower, screened from the parkland by a natural earth-berm.

The lower portions of the building are to be clad in a combination of smooth and heavily rusticated granite. This is juxtaposed against the lightly reflective glass and stainless steel of the tower, anchoring the composition at the base and celebrating the lightweight elegance of the glass and steel as it disappears into the sky. The original design called for a steel structure cased in concrete, using slender perimeter columns at 3.6-meter intervals to transmit lateral loads and the reinforced concrete core to transport loads to the ground. This was later rationalized to use steel-reinforced concrete perimeter columns of the same size and spacing but to bolster the structure with a second concrete tube around the central core. The columns are interconnected by horizontal steel trusses and diagonal perimeter bracing throughout the tower, which binds the columns vertically.

Until its completion, it is difficult to gauge the significance of the building within the broader architectural context. The design attempts to bridge the chasm between the latent forces of ancient Chinese culture and the volatile global economy of modern Asia through the understated clarity of late modernism. As a result, the tower announces a new phase in the architectural language of Kohn Pedersen Fox and a new direction in Asian high-rise construction, but judgment of the success of the building must wait until the completion of construction.

MICHAEL CHAPMAN

See also **China; Kohn Pedersen Fox; Skyscraper**

Further Reading

Pedersen, William, "Shanghai World Financial Center," in *KPF: Selected and Current Works*, edited by Stephen Dobney, Mulgrave: The Images Publishing Group, 1997, pp. 74–79

Pedersen, William, "Shanghai World Financial Center," *A + U* 309 (June 1996), pp. 56–65

Sullivan, Ann C., "Asia's Tallest Towers," *Architecture* (September 1996), pp. 159–163

SHAW, HOWARD VAN DOREN 1869–1926

Architect, United States

Howard Van Doren Shaw is best known for his eclectic yet sophisticated designs for country houses, churches, commercial centers, and residential developments in and around Chicago. An admirer of all things British, Shaw often combined elements associated with Gothic, Tudor, Georgian and Arts and Crafts architecture to provide buildings for such notable clients as Joseph Ryerson and Gustavus Swift. While Shaw knew and admired progressive architects like Frank Lloyd Wright, and even sometimes employed Prairie School motifs in his own work, he was inspired more by the works of contemporary British architects like Edwin Lutyens to fulfill the needs of Chicago's more conservative clientele.

Shaw was born into a family of considerable wealth and social prominence, and raised in Chicago's fashionable Prairie Avenue neighborhood. In 1890 he entered the Massachusetts Institute of Technology, the most distinguished school of architecture in the country at the time. At MIT Shaw was exposed to a curriculum modeled on the Ecole des Beaux Arts in Paris, which stressed the importance of adapting the rules and forms of classical and

medieval architecture to modern structures. Shaw completed the demanding two-year curriculum in only one year, returning to Chicago in 1891 to work in the office of Jenney and Mundie. The firm's principal partner, Major William Le Baron Jenney, best known as the architect of the first skyscraper, the Home Insurance Building of 1884, undoubtedly refined Shaw's knowledge of engineering and the design of tall structures.

Shaw's first major commission was for the Lakeside Press Building in Chicago (1897–99), the earliest of several structures Shaw would undertake for Chicago's printing and publishing industry. In most ways the seven-story building is a typical late 19th century "Chicago Style" skyscraper, though it was adorned with medieval English details and equipped with reinforced open-shell concrete floors and an innovative system of delivering water throughout the building in case of fire. The building's fire resistance and aesthetic success led to Shaw's selection to design the Henneberry Press Building in Chicago (1902), remarkable for its vast glass façade under a shallow pediment, and an impressive Beaux Arts style structure for Ginn and Company Publishers (1907). The culmination of Shaw works for Chicago's printing establishment was a massive Gothic style factory for R. R. Donnelley and Sons (1911–29).

While Shaw designed many other commercial structures, the bulk of his practice was centered on the production of fine coun-

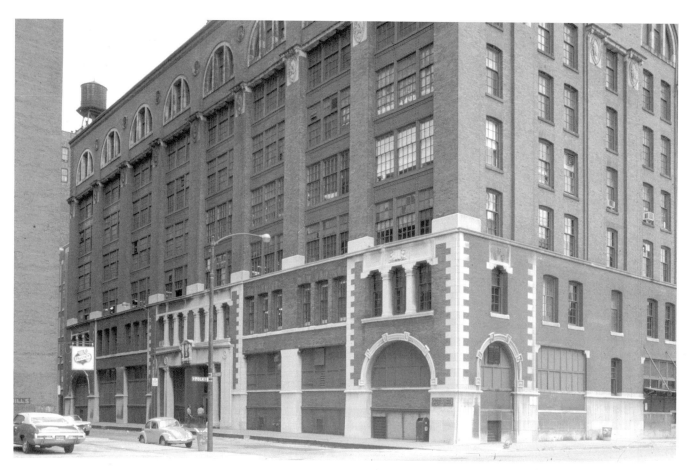

731 S. Plymouth Building (1897), Chicago, Illinois. Designed by Howard Van Doren Shaw.
Photo © GreatBuildings.com

try houses, especially for well-to-do clients in fashionable Lake Forest. Shaw built an extraordinary house there for himself, "Ragdale" (1898), a structure reflecting the architect's keen interest in the British Arts and Crafts work of C.F.A. Voysey. Passionate about details and quality construction, Shaw built much of Ragdale himself, proving in the process to be a skillful carpenter, mason, roofer, painter and landscape designer. Known for his insistence of high quality workmanship, Shaw designed and carefully supervised the construction of over twenty houses in Lake Forest alone by 1915. He employed mostly Tudor styles at first, as in the house for John Bradley (1898), and then Georgian, as in the house for A. A. Sprague (1907). But Shaw was also capable of building a Florentine palace, as he did for Edward Ryerson (1906), and a Mediterranean villa, like the one built for Donald McLennan (1912). Whatever the style, though, Shaw plans typically revealed his training in the methods of the Ecole des Beaux Arts: generously proportioned rooms were aligned along axes that extended to geometrically defined gardens and lawns.

In 1915 Shaw turned his attention to small-scale urban planning when he became part owner and sole architect for Market Square in Lake Forest. The first planned shopping center in the country, Market Square revitalized a dilapidated section of town by integrating commercial and residential quarters, coordinating both pedestrian and automotive traffic, and wedding various English, Dutch and German architectural motifs to create a charming "old world" village square. The idea of combining small-scale residential and commercial buildings around a common, landscaped square also served as the focus for Shaw's design of Marktown (1917), a residential development for the workers of the Mark Corporation of East Chicago, Indiana. With its creative mix of forty different English-style cottages, Marktown proved to be one of the most sophisticated adaptations of British Garden City Movement planning in America.

Even at the height of his career Shaw maintained a fairly small office of apprentices and draftsmen, most notably David Adler. Shaw was gracious in social situations, a member of several civic organizations, and noted for his sense of humor. Despite persistent ill health, he traveled frequently to Europe to collect ideas and artifacts for his clients. His love for the arts was manifested by his considerable devotion to the Chicago Art Institute, for which he served as a long-time trustee and part-time architect. Appropriately, his own house, Ragdale, has served since 1976 as home to the famous Ragdale Foundation of writers, artists, and composers.

Most of what remains of Shaw's letters, manuscripts, and drawings can be found today in the Chicago Art Institute's Ryerson and Burnham Libraries, which were designed by Shaw himself from 1919–22.

GAVIN EDWARD TOWNSEND

See also **Arts and Crafts Movement; Craftsman Style; Garden City Movement; Lutyens, Edwin (England); Voysey, Charles F.A. (England)**

Biography

Born in Chicago, Illinois, May 7, 1869. Son of Theodore Shaw, a successful dry goods wholesaler whose connections with Chicago's business community would lead to some of his son's later architectural commissions. Attended Harvard School for Boys in Kenwood, Chicago; left Chicago during his junior year to attend Yale University, received a Bachelor of Arts in 1890; studied architecture at the Massachusetts Institute of Technology, 1890–91. Worked in the Chicago firm of Jenney & Mundie, Traveled throughout Europe 1892–93. Left for Europe in 1892; spent a year sketching and photographing buildings in Spain, France, Italy, Germany and especially England; returned to United States in 1893; married Frances Wells, 20 April 1893 and established his own practice later that year. Trustee of the Art Institute of Chicago 1904–26. Served as second vice president of the Illinois chapter of the AIA in 1905 and was elected a Fellow of the AIA in 1907. Received the AIA Gold Medal in 1926 and died of pernicious anemia May 6, 1926.

Selected Works

Lakeside Press Building, Chicago, 1897–99
Howard Shaw House (Ragdale) Lake Forest, 1898
Henneberry Press, Chicago, 1902
Edward F. Swift House, Lake Geneva, WI, 1906
Prentiss Loomis Coonley House, Lake Forest, 1908
Durand Commons, Lake Forest College, Lake Forest, 1909
Finley Barrell House, Lake Forest, 1909
Walter D. Douglas House, 3900 Walden Rd., Deep Haven, Minnesota, 1909
R. R. Donnelley & Sons Co Building, Chicago, 1911–29
Fourth Presbyterian Church (with Cram, Goodhue and Ferguson), Chicago, 1911–37
Gustavus F. Swift Jr. House, Chicago, 1913
Market Square, Lake Forest, 1916
Marktown, East Chicago-Whiting, Indiana, 1917
Burnham Library, Art Institute of Chicago, Chicago, 1919
Quadrangle Club, University of Chicago, Chicago, 1920
University Church of the Disciples of Christ, Chicago, 1923
Kenneth Sawyer Goodman Memorial Theatre, Chicago, 1925

Further Reading

Eaton, Leonard K., *Two Chicago Architects and Their Clients: Frank Lloyd Wright and Howard Van Doren Shaw*, Cambridge, MA: MIT Press, 1969
Greene, Virginia A., *The Architecture of Howard Van Doren Shaw*, Chicago: Chicago Review Press, 1998
Tallmadge, Thomas, "Howard Van Doren Shaw," in *Dictionary of American Biography*, edited by Dumas Malone, New York: Scribners, 1950
Wilson, Richard Guy, *The AIA Gold Medal*, New York: McGraw-Hill, 1984

SHEKHTEL, FEDOR 1859–1926

Architect, Russia

Among Russian architects at the turn of the 20th century, Fedor Shekhtel is unique not only in the range of accomplishment over some three decades but also in the degree to which his work embodied the cultural aspirations of his era. As no other architect, Shekhtel enlarged and gave coherent expression to the creative possibilities of the modern style, yet after 1908 he retreated from modernism to a reworking of traditional forms in Russian architecture.

Shekhtel was born and raised in a middle-class environment in the Volga town of Saratov. His father was a civil engineer of

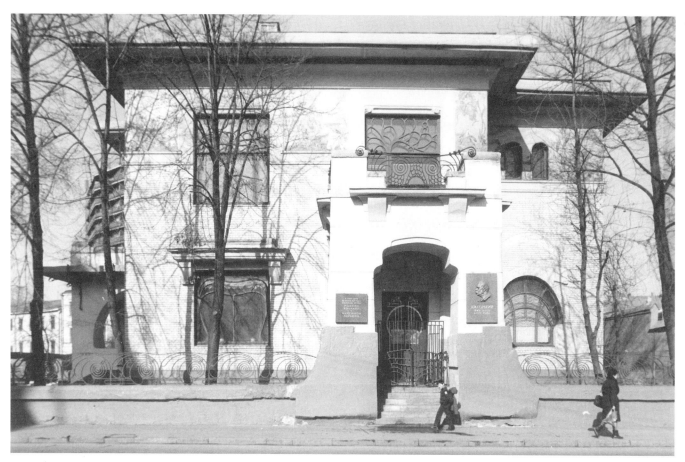

House for Stepan Riabushinskii (1902), designed by Fedor Shekhtel
© William C. Brumfield

German extraction, and his mother, Maria, came from a distinguished merchant family, the Zhegins, whose connections extended into the merchant elite of Moscow. After the death of his father, Shekhtel moved with his family to Moscow around 1875. Having spent a year (1876–77) in the third class at Moscow's School of Painting, Sculpture, and Architecture, he began private work that combined his love for architecture and theater with the design of sets for impresarios such as Mikhail Lentovskii.

During the 1880s, Shekhtel served his apprenticeship in the offices of Alexander Kaminskii and Konstantin Terskii, architects for Moscow's merchant elite in the 1870s. By the end of the 1880s, Shekhtel had designed and built his first independent projects, including the exuberantly eclectic mansion for S.P. von Dervis (1889) at the estate of Kiritsy near Riazan. In 1894, Shekhtel received certification as a "technician-builder" for his design of a large neo-Gothic townhouse for Zinaida Morozova, wife of the industrialist Savva Morozov. The design, which dates from 1893, was some three years in construction; and although both the interior and the exterior display the ostentatious striving for effect typical of that time, Shekhtel also used the style to explore the dynamic relation between interior space and its projection in the design of the exterior.

From this use of Gothic stylization as a path to structural innovation, Shekhtel moved to a radically modern idiom in his house for Stepan Riabushinskii (1902) near the Nikita Gates in central Moscow. Begun in 1900, the Riabushinskii house displays a stylistic affinity with houses designed by Olbrich at the Matildenhöhe community, yet it also incorporates the emphasis on decorative arts pioneered at Abramtsevo, the Arts and Crafts colony established in the 1870s on the country estate of railroad magnate Savva Mamontov. Shekhtel defined the exterior as a play of contrasting elements, angular and sinuous, precise in line and complex in decorative form. In designing the interior of the house, Shekhtel approached the limits of the free-form possibilities of the modern style. The central space, extending the entire height of the structure and containing the main stairway, serves as a core around which most of the rooms are grouped. The stairway itself is one of the most theatrical moments in Russian modernism, a frozen wave of polished gray aggregate cascading from the upper story to the bottom landing. His other major residence of the period, designed in 1901 for Alexandra Derozhinskaia, wife of a wealthy Moscow industrialist, represents a rejection of elaborate decoration in favor of a monumental definition of mass and space.

In public architecture, Shekhtel defined some of Moscow's most important spaces with buildings such as the Moscow Art Theater (1902), with its superb interior detailing, and the rebuilding of the Yaroslavl Railway Station (1902), with traditional decorative elements in a modernized interpretation known

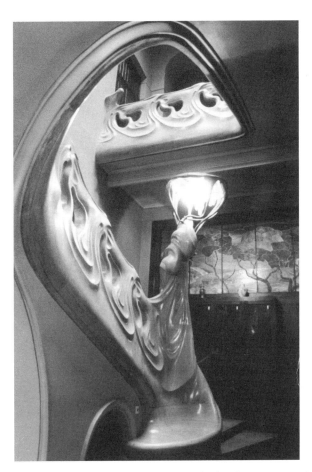

Detail of staircase, House for Stepan Riabushinskii
© William C. Brumfield

financial district and the office and printing works (1907) of the Riabushinskii newspaper *Utro Rossii* (Russia's Morning). The main facades of both consisted of a plate-glass grid with a surface of high-quality pressed brick and no ornament, although the corners are rounded and articulated—a characteristic feature of Shekhtel's large commercial projects, such as the building for the Moscow Merchants' Society (1909) and the Shamshin apartment building (1909).

In the final phase of his career, Shekhtel turned to new interpretations of retrospective styles, such as the neoclassical revival for his own house in Moscow (1909) and the museum dedicated to his close friend Anton Chekhov in Taganrog (1910). His design for the Old Believers Church (1910) in Balakovo (Samara province) is a sensitive fusion of traditional motifs within a modern structure.

In the union of modern form and function that characterized the main body of this work, Shekhtel suggested the spirit of a new economic order in Moscow. Although that order, as well as his professional practice, collapsed in the aftermath of war and revolution, Shekhtel remained in Moscow with his family and continued to teach until his death in 1926. A cautious revival of his legacy began in the 1960s, and he is now considered one of the leading cultural figures of Russia's "Silver Age."

WILLIAM C. BRUMFIELD

See also **Olbrich, Josef Maria (Austria); Russia and Soviet Union**

Biography

Born in Saratov, Russia, 16 July 1859. Studied in the faculty of architecture, Moscow College of Painting, Sculpture, and Architecture 1876–77. Worked as an illustrator and theater designer, did stage design for the Moscow Arts Theater. Taught composition, Stroganov School of Applied Arts, Moscow 1896–1917; taught at the Free Studios, Moscow (previously the Stroganov School) from 1918. President, Moscow Architectural Society 1908–22; jury member on early Soviet competitions, including the Palace of Labor 1922. Died in Moscow, 26 June 1926.

Selected Works

S.P. von Dervis Mansion, Kiritsky, Russia, 1889
Morozova House, Moscow, 1893
Kuznetsov Porcelain Store, Moscow, 1899
Arshinov Store, Kitai-gorod, 1899
Office for A.A. Levenson Printing Works, Moscow, 1900
Moscow Insurance Society Building, 1901
Russian Pavilion, Glasgow Exposition, 1901
Riabushinskii House, Moscow, 1902
Derozhinsky Mansion, Moscow, 1902
Moscow Art Theater, 1902
Yaroslavl Railway Station, Moscow, 1902
Riabushinskii Brothers Bank, Moscow, 1903
"Utro Rossii" Printing Works, Moscow, 1907
Moscow Merchants' Society Building, 1909
Shamshin Apartment Building, Moscow, 1909
Shekhtel House, Moscow, 1909
Anton Chekhov Museum, Taganrog, 1910
Old Believers Church, Balakovo, 1910

as the "neo-Russian" style. This style was prefigured by Shekhtel's designs for large wooden pavilions at the 1901 Glasgow Exposition.

In commercial architecture at the turn of the 20th century, Shekhtel developed the multi-storied arch, with spandrel beams and plate glass, as a defining tectonic element in two commercial structures: the headquarters for the Kuznetsov porcelain firm (1898–99) and the Arshinov Store in Kitai-gorod (1899), with its facade of glazed green brick. A more picturesque approach was adopted in his "chateau" style for the main office of the A.A. Levenson Printing Works on Mamontov Lane (1900), behind which was a printing plant in a modern, functional design.

On a much larger scale, Shekhtel's building for the Moscow Insurance Society on Old Square (1901) represents a shift from the Renaissance detail and arched facades of his earlier commercial buildings to an orthogonal, grid framework of brick and reinforced concrete. Although the Insurance Society building—more commonly known as "Boiars' Court," named after the hotel situated in the building—retains a number of stucco decorative devices, the rationalism of its design signaled the beginning of the modern era in Moscow's financial district.

The clearest expression of the new rationalist approach in Shekhtel's work occurred in commercial buildings such as the Riabushinskii Brothers Bank (1903) in the center of Moscow's

Selected Publication

"Skazka o trekh sestrakh: zhivopis, skulptura i arkhitektura (A Tale of Three Sisters: Painting, Sculpture, and Architecture)," in *Mastera sovetskoi arkhitektury ob arkhitekture* (Masters of Soviet Architecture on Architecture), edited by Mikhail G. Barkhin et al., vol. 1, 1975 (text of a lecture delivered by Shekhtel in 1919)

Further Reading

The most extensive examination in English of Shekhtel's work is Brumfield. For a comprehensive catalog of Shekhtel's architectural projects and commissions, see Kirichenko.

Borisova, Elena A., and Tatiana P. Kazhdan, *Russkaia arkhitektura kontsa XIX–nachala XX veka* (Russian Architecture of the End of the 19th Century and the Beginning of the 20th), Moscow: Izd-vo "Nauka," 1971

Brumfield, William C., *The Origins of Modernism in Russian Architecture*, Berkeley: University of California Press, 1991

Cooke, Catherine, "Fedor Shekhtel: An Architect and His Clients in Turn-of-Century Moscow," *Architectural Association Files* 5–6 (1984)

Kirichenko, Evgeniia Ivanova, *Fedor Shekhtel*, Moscow: Stroiizdat, 1973

Kirillov, Vladimir, *Arkhitektura russkogo moderna* (Architecture of the Russian Moderne), Moscow: Izd-vo Moskovskogo Universiteta, 1979

Sarabianov, Dmitrii Vladimirovich, *Stil modern: Istoki, istoriia, problemy* (Style Moderne: Sources, History, Problems), Moscow: Iskusstvo, 1989

SHINOHARA, KAZUO 1925–

Architect, Japan

Regularly described as a "philosopher of architecture," Kazuo Shinohara is as well known for his writing as he is for his designs. Despite producing barely 50 buildings in almost as many years, each of his works has been exquisitely crafted to express a particular philosophical position. Rather than discussing these buildings in isolation, Shinohara presents them as models of how he believes architecture should respond to the modern world. Through his writing and teaching, Shinohara influenced an entire generation of post–World War II Japanese architects, including Toyo Ito, Itsuko Hasegawa, and Issei Sakamoto, who were known collectively in the 1970s as the "Shinohara school."

Kazuo Shinohara was born in Shizuoka prefecture in Japan in 1925 and entered the Department of Architecture at the Tokyo Institute of Technology at the age of 22. Following graduation in 1953, Shinohara became an associate of the same institution, where he remained for the following 40 years, being appointed associate professor in 1962, professor in 1970, and professor emeritus in 1986. Shinohara completed a doctorate on spatial composition in traditional Japanese architecture in 1967. Ironically, it was after the completion of this research that he began to reject the ordered spaces of the Japanese vernacular that characterized so many of his early designs in favor of a more complex and technological approach to design.

Two themes, order and chaos, distinguish Shinohara's early architectural works and writings from his later ones. The shift between these two extremes, from a preoccupation with order toward a fascination with disorder, took place between 1967 and 1970, although traces of Shinohara's growing interest in chaos are apparent as early as 1964. Prior to 1967, Shinohara describes his designs, including such projects as the House in Kugayama (1954), the House in Chigasaki (1960), and the House in Komae (1960), as distinctly ordered and traditional. These projects, which are named after the locations in which they are sited, are characterized by largely symmetrical spatial compositions that are variants of historic Japanese house types.

Following these works, Shinohara began to refine his approach to geometry and structure to even greater levels of abstraction. This growth in design method is seen in the Umbrella House (1961), the House in White (1966), and the Suzusho House (1968), all of which feature simple geometric forms, white walls, and exposed-timber beams. Despite the success of these buildings, in the years that followed, Shinohara began to question the role played by the house in the city and the importance of order and symmetry. In the Incomplete House (1970) and the House in Itoshima (1976) on the Genkainada Sea, symmetry still governs the exterior of the dwelling, but inside the pure, hierarchical planning that distinguishes so many of his early works has been eroded. This shift is even more apparent in Shinohara's Uehara House (1976) in Tokyo, which features a stark concrete exterior perforated with irregularly spaced geometric windows. This house, which is supported on a system of Y-shaped concrete columns, is asymmetrical in both plan and section and does not possess the same polished finish of many of his early works. The Uehara House is one of Shinohara's first designs that expresses the dual desire to isolate the interior from the exterior and to recognize the complexity of modern life in the arrangement of spaces and forms. Shinohara describes these intermediate works as possessing a "savage" or "barbarous" quality that is a result not only of his use of raw concrete but also of his newly developed interest in the irregular geometry of nature.

For Shinohara, both the dream of utopia that preceded World War II and the influx of modern architecture in Japan that followed in its aftermath were doomed to failure because they did not take account of the need for complexity in urban space. It was only in modernism's aftermath that people began to see that cities such as Tokyo possess a natural complexity that is intrinsic to its vitality. Shinohara describes the urban chaos of Tokyo as being paradigmatic of "the beauty of progressive anarchy," a concept that for him relates to the sense of energy and disorder often encountered in urban spaces. The Ukiyo-e Museum (1982), Shinohara's first nonresidential building, attempts to capture this chimerical urban beauty in its facades through an irregular composition of squares, triangles, and arcs. Internally, the museum is a mixture of contrasts, smooth floors are juxtaposed against rough concrete walls, and natural finishes compete with vibrant red and green window frames.

By 1987, Shinohara had begun to openly argue that "chaos is a basic condition of the city" and that if architecture is to respond to this chaos, it must adopt a new guise that is informed by both technology and the sciences of complexity. He maintains that architects must focus their attention on machines (particularly computers, the F-14 fighter plane, and the *Apollo 11* lunar landing craft). Because modern machines are highly adaptable to complex environments, Shinohara proposes that they are suitable metaphors for design in an increasingly unpredictable world. Shinohara calls this approach to architecture, which

he documented in his 1988 article "Chaos and Machine," Modern-next. Although Shinohara has developed this philosophy of design in a number of projects, including the Hanegi Complex (1988) in Tokyo and the inverted triangle of the Police Station (1990) in Kumamoto, it is his Centennial Hall (1987) in Tokyo that has become iconic for the way in which it expresses his philosophy of design. Externally, the Centennial Hall is visually reminiscent of sections of an aircraft. The building is formed about a horizontal, metal-clad, half cylinder that intersects two rectangular blocks at a point high above the street level. The half cylinder is the literal evocation of the machine of Modern-next. The static silver, gray, and white rectangular prisms provide connection between the ground and the sky. The elaborate interlocking of these forms renders the overall building volume difficult to read against the chaos of the surrounding city. For Shinohara, this is the only way that architecture can capture the essential vitality of the modern world.

MICHAEL J. OSTWALD

Biography

Born in Shizuoka, Japan, 2 April 1925. Received a bachelor's degree in engineering from the Institute of Technology, Tokyo 1953; earned a doctorate in engineering 1967. Served in the Japanese Army, Japan and Korea 1945. In private practice, Tokyo from 1954; established a studio at the Tokyo Institute of Technology 1962. Instructor 1953–62, associate professor 1962–69, professor of architecture 1970–85, and professor emeritus from 1986, Tokyo Institute of Technology; visiting professor of architecture, Yale University, New Haven, Connecticut 1984; visiting professor of architecture, Technische Universität, Vienna 1986. Honorary fellow, American Institute of Architects 1988.

Selected Works

House in Kugayama, Tokyo, 1954
House in Chigasaki, Japan, 1960
House in Komae, Tokyo, 1960
Umbrella House, Tokyo, 1961
House in White, Tokyo, 1966
Suzusho House, Hayama, Japan, 1968
Incomplete House, Tokyo, 1970
House in Itoshima, Fukuoka prefecture, Japan, 1976
Uehara House, Tokyo, 1976
Ukiyo-e Museum, Matsumoto, 1982
Tokyo Institute of Technology Centennial Hall, Tokyo, 1987
Hanegi Complex, Tokyo, 1988
Kumamoto-kita Police Station, Tokyo, 1990

Selected Publications

Residential Architecture, 1964
Theories on Residences, 1970
Kazuo Shinohara: 16 Houses and Architectural Theory, 1971
Theories on Residences II, 1975
Kazuo Shinohara II: 11 Houses and Architectural Theory, 1976
Kazuo Shinohara (with Yasumitsu Matsunaga), 1982

Further Reading

Shinohara (1994) provides a thorough list of publications by and about Kazuo Shinohara. Shinohara's design philosophy is outlined in detail in his 1988 paper, "Chaos and Machine."

Shinohara, Kazuo, "Chaos and Machine," *Japan Architect* 63, no. 5 (May 1988)
Shinohara, Kazuo, *Kazuo Shinohara*, Berlin: Ernst, 1994
Shinohara, Kazuo, and Akio Kurasaka, "Kazuo Shinohara," *Space Design* no. 172 (January 1979)
Sinohara, Kazuo, and Hiroyuki Suzuki, "Architectural-Space Exploration," *Japan Architect* 54, no. 3(263) (March 1979)
Sinohara, Kazuo, and Hisako Watanabe, "Chaos and Order, in the Change of Technology" *Kenchiku Bunka* 43, no. 504 (October 1988)
Stewart, David, *Kazuo Shinohara: Centennial Hall, Tokyo*, Stuttgart, Germany: Edition Axel Menges, 1995
Taki, Koji, "Oppositions: The Intrinsic Structure of Kazuo Shinohara's Work," *Perspecta* no. 20 (1983)
Tange, Kenzo, and Kazuo Shinohara, "After Modernism; A Dialogue between Kenzo Tange and Kazuo Shinohara," *Japan Architect* 58, no. 11–12 (319–20) (November/December 1983)

SHOPPING CENTER

Two trends were crucial for the development and success of the shopping center: decentralization at the urban scale and increasingly sophisticated techniques of advertising and display that encouraged the purchase of goods. In this sense the department stores, such as the famous Bon Marché of Paris (ca. 1862) and the much larger Marshall Field's store of Chicago (ca. 1880) prefigured the 20th-century shopping center and its later manifestation, the shopping mall. The French example was particularly important because it was fashioned as a place of "democratic luxury," where goods were presented to the clientele in the exciting manner of world's fair displays. The shopping center did not become identifiable as a distinct building type, however, until the 1920s. The 18th- and 19th-century arcades, and the late 19th-century department stores were not the precedents of this building type, per se, although they certainly influenced retail architecture and the culture of consumption. Until the 1930s in the United States, where it first materialized, a shopping center was nothing more than a term denoting an assemblage of businesses, usually situated "downtown." In fact, downtown centers that sported a cluster of businesses, stores, and a department store were considered the definition of a shopping core. Outlying districts that offered shops and businesses might also have been considered a shopping center, but these types of gathered buildings and spaces were not coordinated or planned as one. By 1930, however, developers and architects created identifiable centers incorporating business factors as well as architectural issues. The premeditated nature of this new landscape intervention marks the shopping center's most salient characteristic as a distinct building type.

The typology developed out of a larger effort to decentralize the urban nucleus, a trend that originated in the previous century. The five-unit block built as an integral component of the residential community at Riverside, Illinois, in 1870 is perhaps a more useful precedent than, say, the Marshall Field's store. Just as Riverside was an early prototype of what would become a more powerful 20th-century movement to the suburb, so too was its store building. As cities in the second half of the 19th century grew in terms of density, land area, and pollution, the demand for neighborhoods in pseudopastoral settings increased. Streetcar lines made such suburban communities viable, as resi-

dents could maintain ties to the city while remaining in what they considered to be a healthy environment. As a method of enticing homebuyers, American developers found it necessary to build a retail facility as part of these new communities. For such early neighborhoods to be viable, residents had to feel many of their shopping necessities could be met without trekking downtown.

Market Square in Lake Forest, Illinois, was an important and early example, built in 1916 to cater to some of Chicago's wealthiest families. Designed by Howard Van Doren Shaw with the collaboration of real estate magnate Arthur Aldis, this was far more than a mere retail building. It was part of a larger commercial project that cost more than half a million dollars and was raised by investors as well as by bonds, resulting in twenty-eight stores, twelve office suites, thirty apartments, and sundry other community facilities. Built adjacent to existing merchants, the project was intended to offer a true center for shopping, one that proved financially profitable as well as aesthetically unobjectionable. The design team that matched a business mind with an architect went a long way to assuring the project's success and was largely responsible for the way the plan provided for automobile access and parking. The main street was widened to facilitate parking for the growing number of Lake Forest residents with automobiles. The collection of shops was U-shaped, and patrons could park their cars in the tree-lined open space of the U. No distinction was made between cars in motion and parked autos in this lot ornamented by a fountain, but delivery vehicles used separate rear-side courts for service. Lauded as an application of the City Beautiful movement to commercial architecture, Market Square proved influential.

Consumer culture and the display of goods were revolutionized during this same period, as architects like Morris Lapidus devised increasingly seductive techniques for displaying goods for sale. Storefront windows grew until the façade became one large display, signs were built overhead the size of entire buildings, and the scale of the storefront was increased to catch the eye of the motorist at a distance. Meanwhile, shopping had been a point of application for developments in psychoanalysis, as the task of the psychologist in the first half of the century resembled that of the advertising firm's attempts to divine the buying impulse. Eventually, these shopping complexes grew so large, and attendant parking lots were in turn so vast, developers and architects were forced to experiment with organizational plans. The scheme that proved most successful was a plan arranged around a pedestrian path often lined with grass and shaded by trees, so that consumers would leave their cars behind as they strolled along on a new interior shopping experience. Other schemes included the cruciform plan, a clustered or doughnut shaped plan, and circular plans where shops all faced a common green space. The pedestrian path was often punctuated with fountains or sculpture, whereas these shopping centers were surrounded by massive parking lots that wrapped around the backs of the stores in such a way that a customer could park near any given store. Perceptually disconnected from the street, this "mall" was an environment unto itself. As historian Richard Longstreth noted, "Once divorced from their cars and walking amid what seems like an entirely different world, customers tended to spend greater blocks of time meandering, meeting friends, having meals, and buying goods."

Northgate, built just outside Seattle in 1950, was one of the first malls to open in the United States. Its 800,000 square feet of shops, anchored by a large department store, were designed along a two-story, 1500-foot-long pedestrian path dubbed the "Miracle Mall." In 1956, a fully enclosed mall in Minnesota called Southdale opened. Designed by Victor Gruen, who believed that malls held the potential for restoring social space to a socially bankrupt society, the enclosure allowed for climate control so that shoppers would not be deterred by heat, cold, or snow. The success of these malls was profound, as by 1960 department store owners no longer had faith in the stand-alone branch store as a viable business proposition. The dominance of the mall also had an ironic effect on the role of the architect in the retail market, because such large-scale projects, financed and built in one swoop as one integrated building and under single ownership, handed the architect greater influence in the design process. After the 1970s, when the completely enclosed pedestrian path became standard, architects were allowed even greater design control over such projects.

The influence of American practices was also felt abroad. The first mall in Great Britain, for example, opened at Brent Cross in 1976. It was an 800,000-square-foot complex boasting 82 tenants, 4000 employees, and 3500 parking spaces. Site selection and planning began in 1959, and before its opening, the investment company negotiated a 125-year lease. For much of the century, the department store in Great Britain, once a native product in the early 19th century, had been influenced by American display techniques. These methods, coupled with the power of advertising, customer surveillance, and changes in departmental organization, proved to have an effect beyond the shopping center's precincts. The new space of consumption ascribed explicit cultural meaning to gender roles and greatly influenced the appropriate modes of heterosocial conduct. Although the gender of shopping changed in the last quarter of the century, as men proved as vulnerable as women to mass marketing and seductive advertising strategies, the truly remarkable aspect of the shopping center was the way social space was transformed into a consumer experience. By the end of the century, it was common for sites intended for other purposes to be reconfigured as consumer opportunities, such as railway stations, hotel lobbies, airports, and even museums that entice patrons to shop.

JERRY WHITE

See also **Chicago School; Gruen, Victor David (United States); Lapidus, Morris (United States); Shaw, Howard Van Doren (United States); Suburban Planning**

Further Reading

Richard Longstreth's *City Center to Regional Mall* is the best work on the origins of the shopping mall. Although it lacks an analysis of the culture of consumption, it is an excellent investigation of the architectural and business aspects of the Southern California shopping center. A whole host of works theorizing the consumer experience along lines of class, gender, and race can be had, and a useful revue of this work can be found in either Bill Lancaster's *The Department Store: A Social History*, or Miller's *Shopping, Place and Identity*.

Benson, John, and Gareth Shaw. *The Evolution of Retail Systems, 1800–1914.* New York: Leicester University Press, 1992.

Bowlby, R. *Shopping with Freud.* London: Routledge, 1993.

Kowinski, William Severini. *The Malling of America.* New York: William Morrow, 1985.

Leach, William. *Land of Desire: Merchants, Power, and the Rise of a New American Culture.* New York: Pantheon Books, 1993.

Longstreth, Richard. *City Center to Regional Mall: Architecture, the Automobile, and Retailing in Los Angeles, 1920–1950.* Cambridge: MIT Press, 1997.

Miller, Daniel, Peter Jackson, Nigel Thrift, and Beverly Holbrook. *Shopping, Place and Identity.* London and New York: Routledge, 1998.

Miller, Michael B. *The Bon Marché: Bourgeois Culture and the Department Store, 1869–1920.* Princeton: Princeton University Press, 1981.

Porter-Benson, Susan. *Counter Cultures, Saleswomen, Managers and Customers in American Department Stores, 1890–1940.* Urbana and Chicago: University of Illinois Press, 1988.

Reekie, G. *Temptations: Sex, Selling and the Department Store.* Sydney: Allen and Unwin, 1993.

SHRINE OF THE BOOK

Designed by Frederick Kiesler and Armand Bartos;
completed 1965
Jerusalem, Israel

The Shrine of the Book is a small, domed pavilion on the grounds of the Israeli Museum complex in Jerusalem. It was built by two architects living in the United States—Frederick Kiesler and his former student Armand Bartos—to house the Dead Sea Scrolls, seven ancient manuscripts dating from the era of the Jewish revolts against the Romans nearly 2,000 years ago. For Kiesler, who had achieved great prominence in New York as an artist and architectural theorist but who had completed only a handful of built commissions, the shrine provided an opportunity to construct his masterpiece.

The story of the discovery of the Dead Sea Scrolls is intimately tied up with the history of the establishment of the state of Israel. In the summer of 1947, a Bedouin shepherd boy stumbled into a cave near the town of Qumran and inside discovered clay jars containing parchments sewn together into long scrolls wrapped in linen. In November of that year, Dr. Elazar Sukenik, the head of Hebrew University's Department of Archaeology, was approached by an antiquities dealer eager to sell the newly discovered documents. Although the next day the United Nations was scheduled to vote on the partition of Palestine, Dr. Sukenik, realizing that the fragment he viewed through a barbed-wire fence was almost 1,000 years older than the oldest known, disregarded the violence around him and traveled to Bethlehem to make the purchase. As he studied the scrolls that night in his living room, the radio brought the news that the UN motion had carried and that the state of Israel was to be reborn.

All told, the Bedouin shepherd had discovered seven scrolls, of which Dr. Sukenik had purchased three. The remaining four scrolls were acquired by the metropolitan of the Syrian Orthodox Monastery of Saint Mark in the Old City of Jerusalem, who had shipped them to New York in search of a better price. Although Dr. Sukenik died believing them lost, his son, General Yigael Yadin, also an archaeologist, was on a 1954 speaking tour in the United States when a journalist called his attention to an obscure, seven-line classified advertisement in the *Wall Street Journal* offering "Four Dead Sea Scrolls for Sale." Yadin moved quickly to secure the scrolls from the vault of the Waldorf Astoria, purchasing them with the financial backing of New York industrialist Samuel Gottesman, Armand Bartos's father-in-law. Following Gottesman's death in 1956, the D.S. and R.H. Gottesman Foundation agreed to provide the funds for the construction of the Shrine of the Book in Jerusalem.

From its inception, the architectural program for the Shrine of the Book was symbolically overdetermined. First were the scrolls themselves, breathtaking in historical, archaeological, and religious significance. For Jews, often called "the people of the book," the discovery of a manuscript written so near to biblical times was theologically earthshaking. Second was the coincidence between the discovery of the scrolls and the founding of the state of Israel. Both the parchments and the nation had lain dormant from the fall of the second Jewish state until the resurrection of the third. The scrolls provided a link between those Jews whose revolt had been crushed by the Romans and those who founded a new nation, bathing legitimacy on their territorial claims. Third was Kiesler's own struggle to practice architecture in a manner consistent with his critiques of the then-dominant International Style. Against its ethos of rationalism and transparency, Kiesler unleashed his surrealist passions for the mythological, the sexualized, the poetical, and the primal. What better commission for Kiesler than a sacred shrine to ancient scrolls, scratched from the prehistoric earth, that awed "the somnolent religious world of cathedrals" and recounted a "war between the sons of light and the sons of darkness"?

Kiesler and Bartos flew to Jerusalem in October 1957 and met with Mazar Ben Zvi, the president of Hebrew University. As Kiesler recounts the events that followed in his journal *Inside the Endless House*, he persuaded the university to enlarge its ambitions and construct a monumental sanctuary for the shrine on the new Givat Ram Campus (then under construction). On the flight back to New York, using a pencil nub on the back of an envelope from his jacket pocket, Kiesler scratched a double-parabolic dome, "a plastic representation of 'rebirth.'"

By late December 1957, preliminary drawings of the dome were complete. The scheme called for a unified centralized chamber, partially buried in the ground, in which the manuscripts and related artifacts would be displayed. The dome would fill the lobby of the planned cubic library building, and its throat and tip would peek out of the roof. Predictably, the campus architects objected, and the Shrine of the Book was removed to a second site outside the library, to be entered via a subterranean corridor. By 1959, detailed drawings were completed for this scheme, but in the fall of that year, the site was moved again, this time to the new campus of the Israel Museum. Kiesler and Bartos's design process seems to have been essentially additive, and the dome and corridor were transferred to the new location. Because they no longer had the strong mass of the library to play against, the architects added a freestanding basalt wall to balance the composition. Some ancillary office and library space was also added. Although Kiesler is credited with the design sketches and poetic ideas, Bartos remained in Israel during most of the construction and provided the essential on-site refinements and supervision.

The Shrine of the Book is composed of five primary pieces arranged in a linear sequence. A visit to the shrine begins with a transverse walk across a stone entry plaza. To the right, the massive white-tiled dome hovers in a rectilinear pool of water,

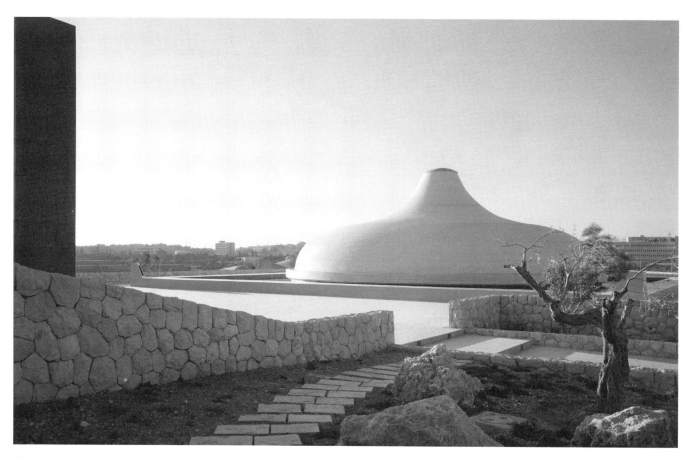

Shrine of the Book, Jerusalem, designed by Armand Bartos and Frederick Kiesler (1965)
Ezra Stoller © Esto

and to left, the black wall looms overhead. Walking between these dueling giants, the visitor turns and descends an open staircase to a sunken court. On one side of the court are supporting offices, and to the other is the entrance to the shrine. Once inside the lobby, the black wall reappears, but this time punctured with an opening at its base. As one passes through that opening and its tubular gates, a dark passage descends slowly through a sequence of asymmetrical arches. Display cases on the side walls provide the primary illumination. At the end of this hall, another staircase climbs upward into the ribbed open dome, which swings its concentrically corrugated surface from almost 80 feet at its base to just 6 at its throat. Desert sunlight pours down from a transparent monocular void at the apex. Surrounding the periphery are more display cases, and atop a central platform is a vertical shaft ringed with the unfurled "Book of Isaiah." Below is a subterranean corridor lined with rough-hewn stones, claustrophobic and cavelike, in which nontextual artifacts are entombed. A single passage leads out from the dome and back to the surface.

Not surprisingly, the double-parabolic dome proved difficult to build. Kiesler was adamant that the dome be both monolithic and homogeneous—one vessel programmatically, structurally, and aesthetically—and he vetoed all designs that had it resting atop some form of cylindrical base or that used a system of structural ribs. Although a difficult challenge for the shrine's

builder, Hillel Fefferman, Kiesler prevailed, and the dome was built as a cast-in-place single concrete shell. The ribbing on the interior prevented acoustical problems, and exterior tiles afforded its elegant white finish. A small exterior lip protrudes from the side of the dome just atop the reflecting pool, providing an illusion of buoyancy.

In accordance with Kiesler's invocations of the primal, the Shrine of the Book attempted to choreograph the four elements of the ancients. A literal penetration into the earth is expressed materially through strata of progressively roughening and darkening masonry. At the deepest point in the complex, an axis is opened through the eye of the dome, linking the depths of the archaeological past with the bright skies of the heavens. On the surface, a pool of water surrounds the dome, small jets sprinkle its exterior, and a trough of water encircles the base of the black wall. Plans for an even more dramatic jet of water that would have shot up from the central shaft and out of the dome's eye were abandoned when unexpected backsplash could not be solved. Similarly, Kiesler's plans for a flaming trough of fuel to cap the massive black wall were also abandoned, although torches were installed for the opening ceremonies in 1965.

The importance of the shrine was recognized even before its completion, and it was immediately seen to be Kiesler's long-delayed masterpiece, a triumphant success crowning a lifetime of deferred hopes and unrealized visions. It was awarded the

Gold Medal by the Architectural League of New York and is now considered by the Israeli government to be one of its national treasures. Still, perhaps the greatest testimony to Kiesler and to his lifelong struggle for poetic expression in architecture is the fact that the Shrine of the Book continues to demand to be interpreted symbolically. Some are compelled by the relationship to the scrolls themselves, reading the white dome as the lid of a pottery jar and the shrine as a great cave, engaged together in a battle of light against the darkness of the basalt wall. Others see the shrine as a symbol of rebirth; just as the Hebrew nation was reborn after 2,000 years of exile, bringing an ancient language and people back to Jerusalem, so, too, does the shrine emerge from the ground like a great dormant seed. Others are drawn to shrine's mysterious sexuality—seeing in the dome a female breast and traveling a dark passage into a great protective womb, violated only by the episodic sprays from the tall central shaft. Others draw parallels with the dream of Jacob's ladder, the staffs of the Jewish Torah, or the Roman Pantheon. Ultimately, the significance of the Shrine of the Book does not lie in the selection of one of these readings over another. Rather, by speaking mythologically, by simply opening up a field of symbolic interpretation, Kiesler's shrine sidestepped modern architecture's dilemma of the monument and created a sacred building as rewarding to, the heart, and the spirit as it is to the mind.

RONN M. DANIEL

Further Reading

An excellent introduction to the Dead Sea Scrolls appears in Pearlman. The best pictorial description of the Shrine is found in *The Shrine of the Book*, and the most complete history of the design's evolution is in Cohl. Also interesting are Kiesler's essays and poems on the Shrine.

Cohl, Alan, "The Shrine of the Book," *Architecture of Israel* 31 (Autumn 1997)
Feuerstein, Günter, "Kiesler's Dome of the Scrolls," *Daidalos* 53 (September 1994)
Kiesler, Frederick, *Inside the Endless House: Art, People, and Architecture: A Journal*, New York: Simon and Schuster, 1966
Pearlman, Moshe, *The Dead Sea Scrolls in the Shrine of the Book*, Jerusalem: Israel Museum, 1988; 3rd edition, 1992
Phillips, Lisa (editor), *Frederick Kiesler*, New York: Whitney Museum of American Art, 1989
The Shrine of the Book (exhib. cat.), Jerusalem: Israel Museum, 1991 (text in English, German, French, and Hebrew)

SIRÉN, HEIKKI (1918–) AND KAIJA SIRÉN (1920–)

Architects, Finland

The husband-and-wife partnership Arkkitehtitoimisto Kaija ja Heikki Sirén was established in Helsinki in 1949. In 1985, they retired, and their son Jukka Sirén took charge and continued the work of the firm. Heikki Sirén's father, Johann Sigfrid Sirén, designed the Parliament (1924–30) in Helsinki, which marked the climax of late Finnish classicism. Both Heikki (1918–) and Kaija (1920–) studied under Professor Sirén at Technical University in Helsinki. Born 20 years after Alvar Aalto, Heikki Sirén belonged to the next generation, which was equally inspired and, at the same time, overshadowed by Aalto.

The elder J.S. Sirén's disciplined academic classicism emphasized the importance of a clear plan as demonstrating the synthesis of the problem. The pair gained world recognition with the Chapel of the Technical University at Otaniemi, west of Helsinki, in 1957. No other single work ever matched the recognition that it achieved worldwide for its brilliant classical simplicity allied to a uniquely Finnish identification with trees and the forest. This concept echoed the primitive values of a forest people by its daring selection of a forest clearing outside the chapel as the core site of spirituality and redemption.

Its classicism was so well disguised beneath the chapel's vernacular references that it is easily missed. However, on closer analysis the clarity of plan is the secret foundation of the chapel's underlying simplicity and experiential impact. The modest mode of building in brick and timber exploited the Finnish tradition of wooden houses with their spacious yards. In one respect, the chapel's simplicity is confusing. The building derives its power from the synthesis of several sources, including the Finnish identification and rootedness in nature found in the medieval Finnish national epic the *Kalevala*, the Siréns' obvious admiration of anonymous indigenous architecture, and the notion that architecture creates the "stage" for human life.

The arrangement of an entry courtyard preceding the chapel separated the sacred from the profane. The chapel had its cross outside, a feature that is reminiscent of a proscenium theater with the glass wall replacing the proscenium arch and the forest clearing now reconstituted as a sacred stage. The cross set in the landscape was not new—Gunnar Asplund used it for his 1940 Forest Crematorium at Sockenvägen—but what is different in the Sirén version is the visual coupling of the cross with the chapel. Subsequently, Tadao Ando repeated the outside cross formula in his Church on the Water (1988) at Tomamu on Hokkaido.

Many people are attracted by the ultimate simplicity of the Siréns' architectural features. At the chapel, for example, the entry screen of horizontal timber poles in the courtyard permits the outside to be visible and thus transmits metaphysical ideas of considerable weight that mirror a Finnish identity linked at many levels to nature. Nature belongs to a pantheistic religious experience imbued by a kind of rich poverty.

Prior to the chapel, the small stage of the Finnish National Theatre (1954) in Helsinki had been the Siréns' first and most noteworthy work. It was completed as an annex to the theater building and the new auditorium and had a lobby and restaurant on the ground floor. The interior spaces were reflected on the outside in the openings formed in the dark clinker elevation, which provides a suitable backdrop to adjacent Kaisaniemi Park. The Kontiontie terrace houses (1954) at Tapiola were built with black-stained prefabricated wooden elevation units inserted between white blades of masonry to produce a starkly striking effect in the winter landscape.

From this time, the work of the pair includes the Students' Restaurant (1952) at Otaniemi, the Concert Hall (1954) at Lahti, and a multistory apartment house, Otaniemi (1956). Both the Aarnivalkea School (1957) at Tapiola and the school (1958) at Espoo employed a simple steel-frame and in-fill aesthetic in-

spired by Mies van der Rohe, but these were carried out with a flare for mating the cubic masses to their sites. The Town Hall (1967) at Kankaanpää and the Villa Punjo (1967) at Espoo testify to the Siréns' capacity to unite their buildings with forest settings by a simple juxtaposition of a finely tuned classical simplicity and rhythmic succession of masses.

The Siréns were unsuccessful when they entered architectural competitions. In 1974, they won the Linz Brucknerhaus Concert Hall competition and the 1978 competition for a Conference Palace (1984) for Baghdad, Iraq. The elegant radial arrangement of the Linz auditorium, with the foyer running around the circumference and overlooking the river, was reinforced by a warm timber interior of considerable elegance.

The Baghdad Conference Palace was faced in a bluish-glazed tile outside, selected out of respect for Babylonian tradition, with the parapet of the concrete-unit external wall curved inward so as to direct the hot outside air up between the glass-and-aluminium fenestration and behind the screening concrete blades. The planning of the three-story Conference Palace concentrated the auditoriums and foyers within a single compact rectangular volume that was plainly expressed outside. As a consequence, the focus is directed inside on the lobbies and foyers, all grouped around the large multiuse auditorium. One of the aims was to remove any suggestion of superficial regional ornamentation and, thus, to focus on such fundamental ideas as a disciplined floor plan and a monumentality for the overall massing.

The Siréns' holiday retreat (1966) on the island of Lingonsö exemplifies their respect for tradition. The cottage, sauna, and annex house are linked by raised walkways. These were built using an experimental prototype of prefabricated timber that was borrowed from a traditional solid-log sauna system. Wood was selected for its weathering properties to ensure that the buildings settled into the landscape gradually. In 1967, a sea chapel was added to the group for meditating, relaxing, and sunbathing. Mounted on an elementary horizontal timber platform on the bare shore rock, with round logs at the corners and overhanging beams to support the flat roof, the sea chapel at Lingonsö is an instance of a deliberately primitive yet highly refined temple beside the sea.

By remaining rooted in their Finnish heritage, the Siréns gained the confidence to explore other entirely different traditions without running into accusations of cliché or pastiche. This proves, as if any proof is required, the maturity and depth of their commitment to respecting and creatively drawing on the resources of their Finnish heritage.

PHILIP DREW

Biographies

Heikki Sirén

Born in Helsinki, 5 October 1918; son of architect J.S. Sirén. Studied under J.S. Sirén at the Technische Hochschule, Helsinki; degree in architecture 1946. Married Kaija Anna-Maija Helena Tuominen, architect, 1944: 4 children. Worked in the office of professor J.S. Sirén, Helsinki 1944–48. Partner, Arkkitehtitoimisto Kaija ja Heikki Sirén, Helsinki from 1949. Special teacher of architecture, Technische Hochschule, Helsinki 1957–

58; guest lecturer, Technische Hochschule, Trondheim 1960; director, architectural seminar, Technische Hochschule, Vienna 1966. Member, Finnish Academy of Technical Sciences 1971; foreign member, Académie d'Architecture, Paris 1983; honorary fellow, American Institute of Architects 1986; honorary member, Finnish Architects Association 1992.

Kaija Sirén

Born in Kotka, Finland, 12 October 1920. Studied under J.S. Sirén at the Technische Hochschule, Helsinki; degree in architecture 1948. Married Heikki Sirén, architect, 1944: 4 children. Partner, Arkkitehtitoimisto Kaija ja Heikki Sirén, Helsinki from 1949. Foreign member, Académie d'Architecture, Paris 1983.

Selected Works

Students' Restaurant, Otaniemi, 1952
Finnish National Theater, Helsinki, 1954
Kontiontie Terrace Houses, Tapiola, 1954
Concert Hall, Lahti, 1954
Multistory Apartment House, Otaniemi, 1956
Aamivalkea School, Tapiola, 1957
Chapel of the Technical University, Otaniemi, 1957
School, Espoo, 1958
The Siréns' Holiday Retreat, Island of Lingonsö, 1966
Town Hall, Kankaanpää, 1967
Villa Punjo, Espoo 1967
Conference Palace, Baghdad, 1984

Further Reading

The Sirens have suffered more than most from the general isolation of the Finnish language. For information on individual buildings, consult the Finnish magazine *Arkkitehti* (Helsinki) or the Paris journal *Architecture d'aujourd'hui*, which followed and published their work. As a general introduction consult Helander and Rista.

Borràs, Maria Lluïsa, *Arquitectura Finlandesa en Otaniemi: Alvar Aalto, Heikki Siren, Reima Peitilä*, Barcelona: Ediciones Polígrafa, 1967

Bruun, Erik and Sara Popovits (editors), *Kaija and Heikki Siren: Architects*, Helsinki: Otava, 1977

"Concert Hall, Linz, Austria," *Planen, Bauen, Wohnen* 58 (1974)

"Conference Centre, Baghdad," *A + U* (February 1984)

"Conference Hall, Baghdad," *Techniques et architecture* (February/March 1984)

"Conference Palace, Baghdad," *Space Design* (November 1983)

Helander, Vilhelm and Simo Rista, *Suomalainen rakennustaide; Modern Architecture in Finland* (bilingual Finnish-English edition), Helsinki: Kirjayhtmä, 1987

"Kaija and Heikki Siren, Architects," *Architettura* 29 (1958)

"The Art of Discrete Isolation: Siren's Holiday Retreat," *Design* 297 (September 1973)

"The Northern Architects Kauia and Heikki Siren," *Space Design* 10 (1975)

Schildt, Goran, "Finlande", *Architecture d'aujourd'hui* 31, no. 93 (January 1961)

Walden, Russell, *Finnish Harvest: Kaija and Heikki Sirens' Chapel in Otaniemi*, Helsinki: Otava, 1998

"Work of Heikki Siren," *Kindaikenchiku* 19 (1965)

SIZA, ÁLVARO 1933–

Architect, Portugal

Portuguese architect Álvaro Siza (Álvaro Joaquim Melo Siza Viera), is one of the best-known Portuguese architects of the

20th century. Although Siza produced numerous projects for clients in Portugal (houses, schools, and other institutions), it was not until the 1980s that he began to receive recognition through exhibitions and commissions in other European countries.

Siza's architecture is strongly rooted in the Modern movement, but incorporates a subjective approach to concept and design, seeking alternative interpretations of modernism. Siza has stated, "Architecture is increasingly a problem of use and reference to models. . . . My architecture does not have a pre-established language and does not establish a language. It is a response to a concrete problem, a situation in transformation in which I participate."

The geographic and climatic conditions of the place of Siza's architecture are of profound importance to this thinking in addition to cultural and social concerns. In Siza's oeuvre sensitivity to context does not result in nostalgic historicism or critical regionalism. It is rather a unique approach to a universal language transformed to respond to a local situation. His built works strive to integrate conflicting demands and affinities, often embodying points of tension that exist in a delicate balance.

For Siza, a building is at the same time autonomous and responsive, unified and diversified. He eschews using technology for technology's sake and employs local materials such as stucco, brick, and stone—all traditional building materials that he uses to create abstract compositions.

His swimming pools (1966) located in Leça de Palmeira, a small town near Porto, were his first projects to receive acclaim outside Portugal. These seaside pools easily make the transition from man-made concrete to the natural rock formations, creating sublime bathing pools. The changing rooms are in an unobtrusive pavilion of concrete with wood roofs that guide the visitor through a corridor-like space before opening on to the expansive sea.

The Pinto e Sotto Maior Bank (1974) in Oliveira de Azmeis, a small town in northern Portugal, is very representative of his early work. This small building does not adopt the formal architectural vocabulary of the place but rather creates a dialogue with its surroundings. The curved, glass facade looks out on to the square, however, creating a formal juxtaposition with the traditional forms of the square. Another bank building, the Borges and Irmao Bank (1986) in Vila do Conde, Portugal, takes a similar approach. It is both a separate entity and a participant in the townscape, respecting the scale of its surroundings. From the outside, little is revealed of the character of the interior. However, the space flows because of the visual connection between floors.

In 1977, following the revolution in Portugal, the local government of Evora commissioned Siza to plan a housing project in the rural outskirts of the town. It was to be one of several that he would do for the national housing association, consisting of 1,200 low-cost row houses, some one-story and some two-story units, all with courtyards. The layout of the new section gave order to an area at the periphery of the town while connecting it with existing housing areas.

During the 1980s, Siza was asked to undertake increasingly larger institutional projects, such as the School of Architecture (1992) at Porto University in Porto, the Teachers Training College (1991) at Setubal, and the Centro Galiziano (Museum of Modern Art, 1994) in Santiago de Compostela, Spain, located within the historical city.

This Centro Galiziano building fits into a complicated and historic site employing concepts of integration and contrast. The reductive, elongated form of the museum—produced by two adjacent wings—seeks to create classical order in an area that had suffered decline. The granite exterior contrasts with the stark white interior. Once again, Siza has approached the work with sensitivity to context without relinquishing the autonomy and strength of the new construction. Other notable museum projects include the addition to the Serralves Foundation and Museum in Porto (1999), the renovation and extension to the Stedelijk Museum in Amsterdam (1997), and the Manzana del Revellín Cultural Centre in Ceuta, Portugal (1997).

Other outstanding, widely published projects of Siza's include the Aveiro University Library at Aveiro, Portugal (1994); the Vitra Factory at Weil-am-Rein, Germany (1994); Schlesisches Tor Apartments at Kreuzberg, Germany (1983); the Portuguese Pavilion at Expo '98 in Lisbon, Portugal (1998); the Santa Maria Church in Marco de Canavezes, Portugal (1997).

MARTHA THORNE

See also **Tavora, Fernando (Portugal)**

Biography

Born in 25 June 1933 in Matosinhos, just north of Porto in Portugal. Studied architecture at University of Porto, School of Architecture (1949–55). Opened his own atelier in Porto (1954) and began his career by designing smaller works, mainly residences in the late 1950s–1960s. Collaborated with Portuguese architect Fernando Tavora (1955–58); began teaching at University of Porto (1966); became full professor (1976–present); has taught and lectured outside Portugal at Harvard University, the École Poytechnique of Lausanne, Switzerland, and Los Andes University of Bogota. Awarded the Pritzker Architecture Prize (1992).

Selected Works

Swimming pools, Leça de Palmeira, Portugal, 1966
Alves Santos House, Póvoa do Varzim, Portugal, 1969
Pinto e Sotto Maior Bank, Oliveira de Azmeis, Portugal, 1974
J.M. Teixeira House, Taipas Guimaraes, Portugal, 1980
Borges and Irmao Bank, Vila do Conde, Portugal, 1986
"Joao de Deus" Kindergarten, Peñafiel, Portugal, 1988
Residential complex Schilderswijk West, The Hague, Netherlands, 1988
School of Architecture, Porto University in Porto, 1992
Teachers Training College, Setubal, Portugal, 1991
Vitra Factory, Weil-am-Rein, Germany, 1994
Centro Galiziano (Museum of Modern Art), Santiago de Compostela, Spain, 1994
Manzana del Revellín Cultural Centre, Ceuta, Portugal, 1997
Architect's Office, Porto, 1998
Boavista Residential Complex, Porto, 1998
Serralves Museum and Foundation, Porto, 1999

Further Reading

Alvaro Siza 1954–1988. A + U Extra Edition Tokyo: A + U, (June 1989).

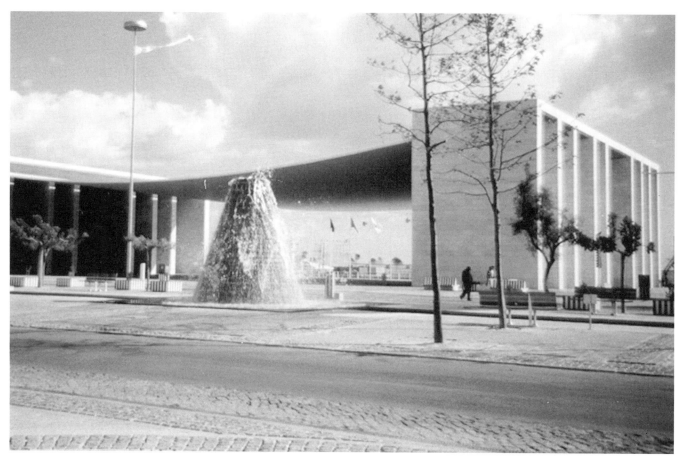

Pavilion of Portugal, Lisbon World Expo '98
© Dan Delgado *d2 Arch*

Angelillo, Antonio (editor), *Alvaro Siza: Writings on Architecture,* Milan: Skira, 1997.

Dos Santos, José Paolo, editors). *Alvaro Siza: Works and Projects, 1954–1992.* Barcelona: Gustavo Gili, 1994

Fleck, Brigitte. *Alvaro Siza.*, Basel and Boston: Birkhäuser, 1992

Frampton, Kenneth, *Alvaro Siza: Tutte le Opere,* Milan: Electa, 1999

Jodidio, Philip, *Alvaro Siza* (Architecture & Design Series), Koln and London: Taschen, 1999

De Llano, Pedro and Carlos Castanheira. *Alvaro Siza.* Madrid: Sociedad Editorial Electa España, 1995.

Siza, Alvaro, *Alvaro Siza, Arquitecto: Centro de Art Contemporanea de Galicia,* Galicia,Spain: Xunta de Galicia, 1993

Testa, Peter, *The Architecture of Alvaro Siza.* Cambridge, Mass.: M.I.T., 1984

Testa, Peter, *Alvaro Siza,* Basel and Boston: Birkhäuser, 1996

Wang, Wilfired, et al., *Alvaro Siza, City Sketches.* Basel and Boston: Birkhäuser, 1994

SKIDMORE, OWINGS AND MERRILL

Architecture firm, United States

An early proponent of the International Style, the architectural firm of Skidmore, Owings and Merrill (SOM) was best noted for its technical innovations in skyscraper design, especially during the 1950s, 1960s, and 1970s. The "glass box" aesthetic, derived from Mies van der Rohe, for SOM became an experiment in which, although the general style and form remained quite consistent and even somewhat bland, subtle modifications and structural enhancements were progressively undertaken. SOM's version of corporate architecture dominated the field of high-rise building during this period, even after competing up-and-coming firms introduced more progressive design concepts and seemingly left SOM a dinosaur living off past laurels. Yet owing to its vast resources, stability, and reputation, the firm was able to maintain a consistently strong position with corporate clients, even after the retirement of the founding partners and key designers.

Founded in Chicago in 1936, SOM emerged during troubled economic times and with few early building projects. Lawrenceburg, Indiana, native Louis Skidmore (1897–1962) graduated with an architectural degree from the Massachusetts Institute of Technology (MIT) in 1924. After working for Maginnius and Walsh for two years, Skidmore won the prestigious Rotch Traveling Fellowship in 1926 and spent the next three years in Europe. While in Paris, he met and married Eloise Owings, sister of his future partner Nathaniel Owings (1903–84). Owings, a

native of Indianapolis, had attended the architectural school at the University of Illinois at Urbana in 1921. After becoming ill and passing up an appointment to West Point, Owings eventually graduated with a bachelor of arts degree in architecture from Cornell University in 1927. The first major work of the brothers-in-law was for the 1933 Century of Progress International Exposition in Chicago, of which Skidmore was named assistant to the general manager. Their collaborative effort consequently led to the opening of a second office in New York in 1937, and a partnership strengthened by the addition in 1939 of another MIT graduate, John Merrill (1896–1975). Merrill, born in St. Paul, Minnesota, had attended the University of Wisconsin at Madison for two years before joining the U.S. Army during World War I. After his graduation from MIT, Merrill had worked in Chicago for Granger and Bollenbacher and had done some work for the U.S. Housing Administration.

Even though projects were few during the pre–World War II period, the firm's capability to skillfully provide both solid architectural and engineering design led to a major commission in 1942. SOM was chosen to plan and design on 60,000 acres in eastern Tennessee an entire community, Oak Ridge, as part of the U.S. government's secret nuclear production program. In this town, which eventually grew from a population of zero to 75,000 by its completion in 1946, the production of uranium for the Manhattan Project occurred. After the war, an increasing number of projects began flowing in, and the firm gained a reputation for proficient if not extraordinary design work. It was the personal and professional relationships developed by the founding partners during this era that led to substantial work later and wide recognition for their planning abilities. In that context, Owings was appointed chairman of the Chicago Plan Commission from 1948 to 1951.

The firm's reputation was elevated to a new level with its first major skyscraper commission, the highly acclaimed Lever House (1951) in New York City, designed by Gordon Bunshaft (1909–90) for the Lever Brothers Soap Company. The 24-story green glass curtain–walled and stainless-steel structure reflected in its design not only New York's changing zoning laws that now permitted slab skyscrapers without setbacks but also the emergence of corporate modernism in the United States. Here, the form of Le Corbusier met the surface treatment of Mies van der Rohe, resulting in a modestly scaled structure in sharp contrast with the solid masonry of its neighbors.

SOM followed up the Lever House with another corporate commission, the Inland Steel Building (1958) in Chicago, one of the first high-rise buildings constructed in the Windy City after the Depression. With Walter Netsch (1920–) as chief designer, this 19-story glass box with accompanying 25-story stainless-steel service tower exemplifies Miesian abstraction. The architects separated the service core from the office block through a stark contrast between metal and glass sheathing. Soon a trademark of SOM, it was repeated most notably in the Crown Zellerbach Building (1959) in San Francisco. The firm replicated the glass box skyscraper model in buildings of varying heights, including the Manufacturers' Trust Company (1954), the Union Carbide Building (1960), and Chase Manhattan Bank (1961), all in New York. In 1961, the awarding of the AIA's first Architecture Firm Award solidified SOM's position as a premier architectural firm.

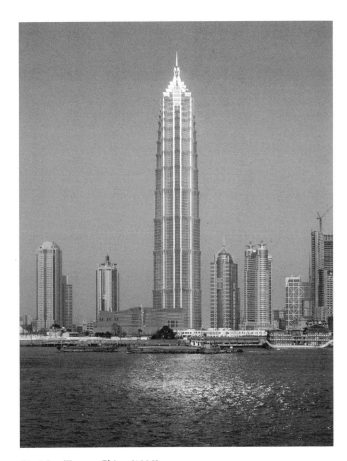

Sin Mao Tower, China (1998)
© China Jin Mao Group. Photo courtesy Skidmore, Owings and Merrill, Chicago

During the 1970s, the firm reacted to changing economic conditions that required multi-purpose megastructures, literally vertical cities in the sky. Two of its best-known structures of this type were constructed in Chicago, both designed by Bruce Graham (1925–) and engineered by Fazlur Khan (1929–82). The John Hancock Center (1970) is by far the most satisfying. This multi-purpose 100-story structure of black anodized aluminum with tinted bronze glass rises 1,107 feet as a single tapered shaft. It combines retail, commercial, and residential functions into one colossal building. In order to combat wind and gravity loads, large cross bracing was used on the building's exterior, a technique that had been employed slightly earlier by SOM in the Alcoa Building (1968) in San Francisco, although there to provide stability against seismic disturbances, not wind pressure. The cross bracing at the John Hancock Center became the building's decoration, its exoskeleton exploited in a very sculptural manner.

The Sears Tower (1974) in Chicago was for many years the tallest building in the world at 1,454 feet. The black aluminum sheathing and dark smoked glass, without the benefit of even the smallest degree of sculptural articulation, exhibits coldness and a lack of human scale or interaction. Still, the general aesthetic of both the Sears Tower and the John Hancock Center can be best understood within the context of contemporary min-

imalist sculpture and viewed as a continuation of SOM's exploration of Miesian ideals.

While the firm's skyscraper commissions progressively increased in the 1960s and 1970s, other types of projects also came its way, most significantly the campus design and buildings for the United States Air Force Academy (1962) in Colorado Springs. The school's Cadet Chapel offered SOM a rare opportunity to design a religious structure, and Netsch responded with a unique approach, constructing three chapels (one Protestant, one Jewish, and one Catholic, each of a varying aesthetic) under one roof. Certainly one of the most expressionistic and symbolic of SOM's works, the outward appearance abstractly references forms associated with aircraft and flying. Shortly after this commission, SOM began working on another campus plan, this time for the University of Illinois at Chicago Center (1965).

The firm was not restricted to skyscraper or campus planning projects. Indeed, SOM's work spanned the entire range of architectural forms. Some of its key designs include the technically sophisticated McMath Solar Telescope at Kitt Peak (1962) in Tucson, Arizona, where a cooled mixture of glycol and water circulates through a specially designed "skin" that absorbs the sun's rays and prevents the generation of disruptive thermal currents on the telescope's surface. The environmentally conscious Weyerhaeuser Headquarters (1971) in Tacoma, Washington, with its five long horizontal ivy-covered terraces, contains the same amount of square footage as a 35-story skyscraper, approximately 354,000 square feet. The Haj Terminal (1982) in Jeddah, Saudi Arabia, was designed using a Teflon-coated fiberglass membrane in forms that references the tents set up by the million-plus pilgrims passing through the airport during the yearly pilgrimage to Mecca. Bunshaft's three-story concrete Hirschhorn Museum and Sculpture Garden (1974) in Washington, D.C., devoted to housing modern art, appears as a modernist's response to Frank Lloyd Wright's Guggenheim Museum in New York, lifted up on massive *pilotis* as per the Le Corbusier model.

It is important to note that the firm's three founders actually designed few of SOM's hallmark buildings. They developed and led an architectural firm modeled on a corporate organization. Branch offices were opened in a number of cities with design principals in charge of each office. Instead of the more typical hierarchical arrangement of power, authority within SOM was arranged in a linear fashion, as each office head theoretically had equal voice in how the firm was run. A stipulation in the founding partners' agreement required retirement at age 65 for each principal, thus prompting a constant renewal of the firm's direction and focus.

With such an arrangement, it is not surprising that SOM's designs exhibit a good deal of diversity and quality, particularly during the 1970s and beyond. The firm grew to an immense size in terms of both employees and offices. In addition to the original Chicago and New York offices, a San Francisco office was opened in 1946 when the firm took on the design of Subic Bay Naval Base in the Philippines and the Monterey Naval Postgraduate School. In 1967, the Washington, D.C., office was established to handle the firm's work on the master plan of the Washington Mall. Other new offices were established in Los Angeles and Miami. Not all the new offices survived, however, as the firm constantly reacted to changing economic and building trends. Those offices founded in Denver, Portland, and Boston were eventually closed in 1987, Houston's closed in 1988, and new offices were opened in the late 1980s in London and Hong Kong, as construction boomed in those areas.

Netsch once bitingly complained that SOM in the 1980s was producing "Reagan architecture for Reagan times." The rejuvenation of design that the founding partners had intended thus did not always come to pass. In fact, once SOM had reached its pinnacle in the early 1970s with the visually satisfying John Hancock Center and the record-breaking height of the Sears Tower, the firm had the luxury of essentially sitting back and waiting for clients to come forward. Still, several fine structures were designed by SOM in the 1980s, including Bunshaft's postmodern National Commercial Bank (1984) in Jeddah, Saudi Arabia, and the United Gulf Bank (1987) in Manama, Bahrain.

Because of its huge size and ability to provide numerous services ranging from interiors to transportation planning, corporate SOM could easily service clients' needs and provide one-stop shopping. The size of the firm particularly suited the requirements of developers in the 1980s, as the focus moved from single high-rise structures to large-scale complex city developments, such as Rowes Wharf (1987) in Boston, World Wide Plaza (1989) in New York, and Canary Wharf (1991) in London. This trend continued into the 1990s, except that the location for building more often than not was in the Pacific Rim. Among SOM's more recent projects are the 88-story Jin Mao Tower (1998) in Shanghai and the Korea World Trade Center (1999) in Seoul. The firm also won a competition to design a master plan for Saigon South, a new community designed for one million inhabitants south of Ho Chi Minh City, Vietnam.

VALERIE S. GRASH

See also **Bunshaft, Gordon (United States); Corbusier, Le (Jeanneret, Charles-Édouard) (France); Glass; Glass Skyscraper (1920–21); Guggenheim Museum, New York City; Haj Terminal, Jeddah Airport; International Style; International Style Exhibition, New York (1932); Lever House, New York City; Mies van der Rohe, Ludwig (Germany); Sears Tower, Chicago; U.S. Air Force Chapel, Colorado Springs**

Biographies

Louis Skidmore

Born in Lawrenceburg, Indiana, 8 April 1897. Graduated from Bradley Polytechnic Institute (now Bradley University), Peoria, Illinois 1917; studied at the Massachusetts Institute of Technology, Cambridge 1921–24; bachelor's degree in architecture 1924; visiting scholar, American Academy, Rome 1927. Worked for Maginnius and Walsh, Chicago 1924–26; chief of design and assistant to the general manager, Century of Progress Exposition, Chicago 1929–35. President, New York Building Congress; chairman, advisory council of the School of Architecture, Princeton, New Jersey; consultant architect to the United Nations, New York; consultant architect, University of Michigan, Ann Arbor; fellow, American Institute of Architects. Awarded Gold Medal, American Institute of Architects 1957. Died in Winter Haven, Florida, 27 September 1962.

Nathaniel A. Owings

Born in Indianapolis, Indiana, 5 February 1903. Studied at the University of Illinois, Urbana 1921–22; attended Cornell University 1927. Chairman, Chicago Planning Commission 1948–51; vice-chairman, California Highway Scenic Roads Commission 1964–67; chairman, Temporary Commission on the Design of Pennsylvania Avenue, Washington, D.C. 1964–73; member, 1966–70, and chairman, 1970–72, United States Secretary of the Interior's Advisory Board on the National Parks, Historic Sites, Buildings, and Monuments, Washington, D.C.; chairman, Urban Design Concept Team for the United States Interstate Highway System 1967–70; member, Permanent Commission on the Design of Pennsylvania Avenue 1973–82; trustee, American Academy, Rome; fellow, American Institute of Architects. Awarded Gold Medal, American Institute of Architects 1983. Died in Santa Fe, New Mexico, 13 June 1984.

John O. Merrill

Born in St. Paul, Minnesota, 10 August 1896. Attended the University of Wisconsin, Madison 1914–16; studied at the Massachusetts Institute of Technology, Cambridge 1919–21; bachelor's degree in architecture 1921. Worked for Granger and Bollenbacher, Chicago; chief architect for the Midwest States, United States Housing Administration 1939. Director, Chicago Building Code Revision Commission 1947–49; fellow, American Institute of Architects; president, Chicago chapter, American Institute of Architects. Died in Chicago, 13 June 1975.

Skidmore, Owings and Merrill

Established as Skidmore and Owings in Chicago 1936; New York office opened 1937; became Skidmore, Owings and Merrill in 1939; branch offices in San Francisco, Los Angeles, Washington, D.C., Miami, London, and Hong Kong; the firm continues today under the same name.

Selected Works

Atom City, Oak Ridge, Tennessee, 1946
Lever House, New York, 1951
Manufacturer's Hanover Trust, New York, 1954
Inland Steel Company Headquarters, Chicago, 1958
Crown Zellerbach Corporation Headquarters, San Francisco, 1959
Union Carbide Building, New York, 1960
Chase Manhattan Bank, New York, 1961
United States Air Force Academy, Colorado Springs, 1962
McMath Solar Telescope, Kitt Peak, Tucson, Arizona, 1962
University of Illinois, Chicago Circle, 1965
Alcoa Building, San Francisco, 1968
John Hancock Center, Chicago, 1970
Weyerhaeuser Headquarters, Tacoma, Washington, 1971
Sears Tower, Chicago, 1974
Hirshhorn Museum and Sculpture Garden, Smithsonian Institution, Washington, D.C., 1974
Haj Terminal, King Abdul Aziz International Airport, Jeddah, Saudi Arabia, 1982
National Commercial Bank, Jeddah, 1984
United Gulf Bank, Manama, Bahrain, 1987
Rowes Wharf Multi-Purpose Complex, Boston, 1987
World Wide Plaza, New York, 1989
Canary Wharf Development, London, 1991
Jin Mao Tower, Shanghai, 1998
Korea World Trade Center, Seoul, 1999

Selected Publications

Architecture of Skidmore Owings and Merrill, 1950–1962, 1962
Architecture of Skidmore Owings and Merrill, 1963–1973, 1974
Nathaniel Owings:
The American Aesthetic, 1969
The Spaces Between: An Architect's Journey, 1973

Further Reading

Bush-Brown provides a *catalogue raisonné* of SOM's work. Important works on individual SOM designers are Graham and Krinsky, while Bruegmann treats an individual structure. Dean provides excellent insight into the organization of the firm.

Bruegmann, Robert, (editor), *Modernism at Mid-Century: The Architecture of the United States Air Force Academy*, Chicago: University of Chicago Press, 1994
Bush-Brown, Albert, *Skidmore, Owings and Merrill: Architecture and Urbanism, 1973–1983*, Stuttgart, Germany: Hatje, and New York: Van Nostrand Reinhold, 1983; London: Thames and Hudson, 1984
Dean, Andrea Oppenheimer, "Profile: SOM, a Legend in Transition," *Architecture* 78, no. 2 (1989)
Graham, Bruce, *Bruce Graham of SOM*, New York: Rizzoli, 1989
Krinsky, Carol Herselle, *Gordon Bunshaft of Skidmore, Owings and Merrill*, New York: Architectural History Foundation, and London: MIT Press, 1988

SKYSCRAPER

As the archetypal urban commercial building, the 20th-century skyscraper exhibited continual structural innovation and stylistic exploration. Historicism and eclecticism moved in and out of fashion throughout the century, interspersed with periods of a new "modern" aesthetic that exploited the pure form created by the steel-frame and glass curtain wall. In addition to concerns for ornamentation, constant competition to create taller structures not only demonstrated the desire of patrons and architects to physically outdo one another in creating a landmark structure but also reflected changing economic conditions and building patterns within particular cities. Importantly, not every skyscraper was constructed in an attempt to outdo its neighbor, and not every high-rise building exhibited innovation. Critically successful structures in terms of aesthetics were also not always profitable. Mitigating factors such as material and technical innovation, zoning regulations, economic climate, and the client's purpose for construction affected the skyscraper's success as much as the designer or engineer did.

In the 19th century, the earliest high-rise buildings tended to simply be mere enlargements of traditional forms, such as the tower, progressively adding stories and increasing height without adequately addressing the aesthetic of a tall structure. Designers such as Louis Sullivan, John Wellborn Root, and George B. Post eventually tackled this problem, theoretically and in practice, by considering the nature of skyscraper form itself as a new building type. When combined with advances in engineering and materials, the skyscraper thus became not only a monument to modern progress but also a symbolic link to the historical past, a past that the United States lacked and sought to evoke or, perhaps, to distance itself from.

Two perceived "schools" of skyscraper design embodied these purposes. The Chicago School, with its emphasis on structural rationality and economy, personified what was new about skyscraper design in the United States, breaking from historical ornament or form. Speculative commercial construction thrived in Chicago after the devastating fire of 1871 and dictated a simpler, more cost-effective method of exterior articulation as well as making the best use of available land for office space. On the other hand, in New York, corporate commissions had always demanded more ornamentation and more historical references, all in an attempt to present a landmark structure that would elevate and promote its occupants. Businesses such as insurance companies and newspapers employed elaborate styles that not only were self-promoting but also galvanized civic pride.

Although the Chicago School made an indelible impression on many American cities and especially on European modernists, it was the Beaux-Arts–inspired style popular in New York that dominated skyscraper construction as the 20th century dawned. Ironically, the World's Columbian Exposition of 1893 in Chicago, with its gleaming White City image personifying monumentality and strength, prompted this classical interest and, according to Louis Sullivan, set back architectural design by decades. Like the great mercantile princes of the Italian Renaissance, businessmen turned to Beaux-Arts–trained or–inspired architects to construct buildings that, by appropriating a classicized style, implied power and respectability. Not surprisingly, the most popular high-rise design firm at the beginning of the century was D.H. Burnham and Company, founded by the man responsible for the plan of the White City. Its successor firm, Graham, Anderson, Probst and White, continued this domination well into the 1910s.

A typical Beaux-Arts skyscraper consisted of either a simple yet ornamented tower block, such as Burnham's Flatiron Building (1903) in New York, or a basic office block aggrandized with an elaborate tower, such as Ernest Flagg's Singer Building (1908) in New York, with its Second Empire mansard roof that was dramatically lit at night, or Napoleon Le Brun's Metropolitan Life Insurance Company Building (1909) in New York, a direct but much taller copy of the campanile of St. Marco in Venice. Corporate commissions, such as the Singer and Met Life buildings, served as physical advertisements for the companies that commissioned them, even if those businesses occupied only a small amount of office space within each structure. Like the great medieval cathedrals of Europe, competition for prestige led companies to request towering structures that dominated their immediate environment as well as the city as a whole.

Cass Gilbert's Woolworth Building (1913) in New York turned appropriately enough to Gothic style for inspiration, a style that more naturally emphasized verticality. As the company was so decentralized, Woolworth actually used less than two stories of office space; thus, it was not functional need but rather advertising and ego that created this "Cathedral of Commerce," emphasized by the Napoleonic imagery in Woolworth's office and other ornamentation. Individual patrons such as Woolworth were replaced after World War II by corporate entities with far less interest in displaying so personal a building program. Instead, the building material and form more directly referenced the product sold by the company, such as the aluminum curtain walls of Wallace K. Harrison and Max Abramovitz's Alcoa Building (1953) in Pittsburgh and the plate-glass Gothic-inspired

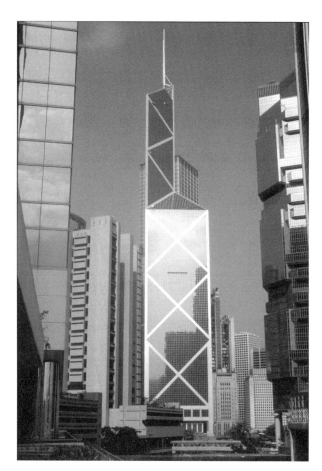

Bank of China Tower, by I.M. Pei, Hong Kong
© GreatBuildings.com

PPG Place (1984), also in Pittsburgh, by Philip Johnson and John Burgee.

In the first half of the century, two key moments in skyscraper design need to be mentioned. The first was Graham, Anderson, Probst and White's Equitable Building (1915) in New York, not for any innovation but rather for the impact that its massive scale and glut of office space had on New York. It was the stimulus for the famous 1916 zoning ordinance that necessitated setback construction, a requirement that other cities soon adopted and an aesthetic that was endorsed by architects through the 1920s and 1930s in the Art Deco and art moderne styles. The other event was the 1922 Chicago Tribune Building Competition, which brought forth all the design variety and visionary dreams of American and European architects regarding the skyscraper form.

European cities neither desired nor needed skyscrapers in the pre–World War II era; thus, European architects created paper dreams of skyscraper cities. Futurist Antonio Sant' Elia's Città Nuova project (1914) and German Expressionist Bruno Taut's Alpine Architektur (1919) embraced modern technology and materials, albeit in an impractical manner. Greater contributions were to be made later by Ludwig Mies van der Rohe, but his Friedrichstrasse Office Building project (1921) in Berlin revealed a logical conclusion to the Chicago School in design with its

honeycomb repetition of office stories and its lack of applied ornament. Even Russian Constructivists, such as the Vesnin Brothers in their Pravada Building project (1924) in Moscow, understood the underlying dictums of decorative purity based on technical form, not historical precedents.

When the *Chicago Tribune* newspaper staged an architectural competition to design "the most beautiful building in the world" for its headquarters, nearly 300 entries from 23 different countries were submitted. Entries ranged from the sublime (Walter Gropius' design revealing both an understanding of the Chicago School's functionality and the asymmetry of De Stijl) to the ridiculous (Adolf Loos' oversize Doric column). The winning entry, by Raymond Hood and John Mead Howells, continued the Gothic revival visible in the Woolworth Building, with the 1485 "Butter Tower" from Rouen Cathedral as a direct design source and flying buttresses used decoratively, not structurally, on the spire. Considering the winning entry, the clients apparently desired established aesthetics, not innovation. However, second-place winner Eliel Saarinen's design turned out to be vastly more influential than Hood and Howells' design, especially among Art Deco and art moderne designers of the 1920s and 1930s who appreciated his ziggurat approach in massing and the unbroken vertical emphasis in the building's line.

Theoretical works by Hugh Ferriss (The Metropolis of Tomorrow, 1929) and Claude Bragdon (The Frozen Fountain, 1932) lauded the setback style as visionary and dynamic, yet in practical application it simply became necessary. Cities such as New York, Los Angeles, Chicago, Pittsburgh, Boston, and others recognized the potential (and, as in the case of the Equitable Building, the very real) damage that out-of-scale skyscrapers caused to neighboring buildings and the business district as a whole. These problems were not limited to blocking light and creating cavernous environs but were related directly to economics, such as devaluating commercial office rental prices by creating an overabundance of office space. Thus, the setback style became an aesthetic reality in large part because of zoning regulations.

Considering the necessity of setbacks, American architects soon adopted and learned from Eliel Saarinen's *Chicago Tribune* design. Even Raymond Hood modified his Gothic decor into a setback style for his American Radiator Building (1924) in New York and eventually moved beyond medievalism in his McGraw-Hill Building (1930), also in New York. Whether "modernizing" forms of Gothic or exploring the stepped-back form and geometric patterns of pre-Columbian architecture, both Art Deco and art moderne were styles created with big business in mind. Visually engaging works, not austere corporate images, drew the public's attention and created landmark buildings. A perfect example of this phenomenon is William Van Alen's Chrysler Building (1930) in New York, with its modernized gargoyles resembling automotive hood ornaments and the great telescoping stainless-steel arches at its spire. The building visually represented the company as advertisement and, as it became the tallest structure in the world at 1048 feet, symbolized the company's strength through its dominance of the New York skyline.

Unfortunately, the Chrysler Building's claim to fame did not last for long, as Shreve, Lamb and Harmon's more restrained Empire State Building (1931) in New York soon outdistanced its competitor at 1250 feet in height. Not a corporate commission but rather a speculative construction, the Empire State Building was far less theatrical than the Chrysler Building. Still, its mere size guaranteed its landmark status. It also displayed an impractical but reverent appreciation for modern air travel, as its spire was fancifully designed to be a mooring dock for dirigibles. This romanticized vision of the skyscraper, in its ornamentation and form, reflected well the giddiness of the jazz age and the economic prosperity of American business, a situation that all too quickly ended in 1929 with the stock market crash and the beginning of the Great Depression.

In the 1930s, new construction of skyscrapers slowed and then virtually halted. Yet, with political upheaval and war brewing in Europe, architects who had only dreamed of skyscrapers arrived in the United States as exiles, including Walter Gropius, Le Corbusier, and Mies van der Rohe. Their theoretical European modernism took root in the architecture schools in which they taught, such as at Harvard University, the Massachusetts Institute of Technology, and the Armour Institute of Technology (later the Illinois Institute of Technology). A full rethinking of the skyscraper began by which its external form became expressive of its internal functions and the structure's form and materials became the ornamentation. The earliest expression of this new aesthetic was George Howe and William Lescaze's Philadelphia Savings Fund Society Building (1932) in Philadelphia, with its elevator core pulled out at the back of the building and its glass curtain wall, steel-framed office tower cantilevered above the entrance block. Traditional materials, such as polished granite, brick, and limestone, were used, but the look was entirely new and not necessarily welcomed by the architectural establishment. Nevertheless, the International Style had taken root and continued to strengthen through midcentury.

Modernism, as preached by Mies van der Rohe, was a reductive architecture with a strong underlying classical sensibility. Mies's maxim "Less is more" personified his belief that pure austere form should serve as all the necessary decoration. His Lake Shore Drive Apartments (1952) in Chicago, although not a commercial but a residential venture, demonstrated his tenets for high-rise construction. The black-painted prefabricated steel-frame and clear-glass windows simply encased the interior space without expressing internal function. There is no projecting cornice, no grand entrance, and no elements characteristic of the typical tripartite skyscraper design. He would repeat this formula in the corporate Seagram Building (1958) in New York, done with Philip Johnson, and in numerous commercial, residential, educational, and other high-rise designs.

Designers who came in contact with Mies, affected by his commanding personality and strength of convictions, embraced his tenets and adopted them in their own interpretations of the Miesian glass box. For example, Eero Saarinen's CBS Building (1965) in New York took a more sculptural approach to modernism, as the vertical granite piers projected out from the wall surface and all sense of human reference in scale was denied through the building's abstraction. The structure startlingly isolated itself from its environment yet worked well as pure design. However, not all designers were as talented as Saarinen was, and in the 1950s, 1960s, and 1970s, cities, towns, and college campuses were polluted with poorly constructed and downright ugly Miesian copies gone awry.

The most successful Miesian-inspired firm was Skidmore, Owings and Merrill. Their early masterpiece, Lever House

(1952) in New York, designed by Gordon Bunshaft, celebrated light and openness, revealing a significant influence of Le Corbusier as well, with the *pilotis*, or stilts, raising the main office tower off the humanly oriented space below. Eventually, the firm developed a more sculptural version of Miesian-inspired modernism, as visible in the John Hancock Building (1970) in Chicago, with its structural yet decorative external cross bracing and tapered form.

Their next major commission, the unsatisfying Sears Building (1974) in Chicago, fell victim to the ever-present corporate need to construct physically dominating, out-of-scale skyscrapers. At 1454 feet and 110 stories, the Sears Building became the tallest building in the world, yet its bundled setbacks, when combined with the Miesian aesthetic, resulted in a very bland structure. Minoru Yamasaki's 1350-foot-tall World Trade Center (1976) in New York had no more success, as its twin towers (which thankfully played off each other) appeared ready to capsize Manhattan, perched as they were on the edge of the island. Cesar Pelli's Petrona Towers (1998) in Kuala Lumpur, at 1483 feet, finally topped the massive heights attained by both these structures.

Not all architects or critics appreciated the International Style and modernism as preached by architects such as Mies van der Rohe and Skidmore, Owings and Merrill. The International Style could be, just as the term implied, a form used in any location because it had no cultural or historical ornamentation that would affect its contextual use. Frank Lloyd Wright in particular railed against "soulless" architecture that neglected cultural context or interaction with its direct urban environment. Concerned as he was for "small-town" development, Wright rarely attempted skyscraper design, and when he did, it was usually undersized, such as the 15-story Price Tower (1955) in Bartlesville, Oklahoma. Only once did Wright attempt the stratospheric proportions popular with corporate patrons: his 1956 project for a Mile High Skyscraper for Chicago, a soaring structure that was as impractical then as it is today. In his scheme, the skyscraper was not placed in competition with other high-rise buildings in an urban environment; rather, it rose isolated in the countryside. Ironically, Wright's vision of the dominance of suburban America was to become a reality as people increasingly migrated from the city center to suburban developments in the post–World War II era.

Business interests moved with them. Increasingly, corporate headquarters took the form of low, sprawling structures with green lawns and miles of employee parking lots. The trademark corporate skyscraper was increasingly becoming a thing of the past, yet those that did stay and built in the cities understood the need to contextualize their presence. Thus, the stark, crisp modernism of Hugh Stubbins Associates' Citicorp Center (1978) in New York and I.M. Pei and Henry Cobb's John Hancock Tower (1975) in Boston increasingly battled a Postmodernism aesthetic that reintroduced historicism and context. Plazas, gardens, and other public spaces became an important aspect of the design, as much as the buildings' materials, ornamentation, and form.

Begun in 1978, many consider Johnson and Burgee's AT&T Building (1984) in New York the first Postmodern skyscraper, with its broken pediment (Chippendale-like) top and emphasis on its pink-granite stone walls. The reintroduction of rich, colorful materials as well as the appropriation of a wide variety of historical forms characterized Postmodern design. It could be playful and fun, such as Michael Graves's Portland Building (1982) in Portland, Oregon, with its miniature Acropolis on top, demonstrating not only the abstract way in which history could be referenced but also the new emphasis on the skyscraper top lost during the modernist years. Postmodernism could also be elegant and austere, as represented by the work of Kohn Pedersen Fox, arguably the most successful skyscraper design firm of the late 1970s, 1980s, and 1990s. Their 333 Wacker Drive (1983) in Chicago responded to its site and surrounding environs with its curving green-glass curtain wall and specific design elements that alluded to nearby landmarks.

By attempting to integrate their buildings firmly into the urban environment, Postmodern architects brought back an appreciation for historicism and traditional materials that modernists had rejected in favor of pursuing pure form and modern materials. Both "schools" continued to exist at the end of the century and adapted to changing client needs, particularly in the 1980s, when skyscrapers increasingly became part of larger urban development plans with a wide variety of buildings clustered together. This usage differed from the traditional isolating nature of the skyscraper, which, whether corporate commission or speculative investment, had historically been multiuse structures themselves. They not only provided company headquarters but also housed financial institutions, retail establishments, offices for professionals, and residential units. Now those roles were being delegated to individual components within the greater complex.

The slanted focus on American skyscrapers during the 20th century accurately reflects where the most significant construction and designs were occurring, a situation that did change during the century's final two decades. Thriving economic markets in oil-rich Middle Eastern countries in the 1980s and in Pacific Rim countries during the 1990s led to a boom market in high-rise construction in those areas. Europe additionally presented increasing skyscraper opportunities for builders, particularly in Germany and other former Soviet-bloc countries after the collapse of the Berlin Wall and the USSR. Still, clients in these countries turned primarily to American architectural firms such as Skidmore, Owings and Merrill (National Commercial Bank, 1984, Jeddah, Saudi Arabia), I.M. Pei (Bank of China Tower, 1989, Hong Kong), Kohn Pedersen Fox (Westendstrasse 1/DB Bank Headquarters, 1993, Frankfurt), and Cesar Pelli.

It can be argued that in the 20th century, architects explored the full range of aesthetic, stylistic, material, and structural possibilities for the skyscraper form. The design tastes and innovations that dominated the earliest high-rise buildings in the 19th century either mutated into various expressions of historicism or evolved into pure form with the aid of European modernists. However, understanding these factors provides only a fraction of the skyscraper story. More specific studies of the economic and business climates of individual cities, particularly beyond Chicago and New York, and how that affected skyscraper design and construction have yet to be undertaken.

VALERIE S. GRASH

Further Reading

Some of the most innovative scholarship on skyscraper history, particularly with regard to the economic conditions that influenced design, may be found in Willis, Koolhaas, Agrest, and Leeuwen. Goldberger

represents the best attempt at an overall skyscraper history, while Hitchcock and Johnson, Robinson and Bletter, Klotz, and Jencks are the best works on individual movements. The best works on New York are Stern et al. (1987, 1995).

Agrest, Diana, "Architectural Anagrams: The Symbolic Performance of Skyscrapers," in *Architecture from Without: Theoretical Framings for a Critical Practice*, by Agrest, Cambridge, Massachusetts: MIT Press, 1991

Curtis, William J.R., *Modern Architecture since 1900*, Oxford: Phaidon, 1982; Englewood Cliffs, New Jersey: Prentice Hall, 1983; 3rd edition, London: Phaidon, and Upper Saddle River, New Jersey: Prentice Hall, 1996

Goldberger, Paul, *The Skyscraper*, New York: Knopf, 1981; London: Allen Lane, 1982

Hitchcock, Henry-Russell, Jr. and Philip Johnson, *The International Style*, New York: Norton, 1932; reprint, with a new foreword, New York and London: Norton, 1995

Huxtable, Ada Louise, *The Tall Building Artistically Reconsidered: The Search for a Skyscraper Style*, New York: Pantheon, 1984

The International Competition for a New Administration Building for the Chicago Tribune, MCMXXII, Chicago: Chicago Tribune, 1923; abridged reprint, as *Chicago Tribune Tower Competition*, New York: Rizzoli, 1980

Jencks, Charles, *The New Moderns: From Late to Neo-Modernism*, London: Academy Editions, and New York: Rizzoli, 1990

Klotz, Heinrich, *Moderne und Postmoderne*, Braunschweig, Germany: Vieweg, 1984; 3rd edition, 1987; as *The History of Postmodern Architecture*, translated by Radka Donnell, Cambridge, Massachusetts: MIT Press, 1988

Koolhaas, Rem, *Delirious New York: A Retroactive Manifesto for Manhattan*, London: Thames and Hudson, and New York: Oxford University Press, 1978; new edition, New York: Monacelli Press, and Rotterdam: 010 Publishers, 1994

Landau, Sarah Bardford and Carl W. Condit, *Rise of the New York Skyscraper, 1865–1913*, New Haven, Connecticut: Yale University Press, 1996

Leeuwen, Thomas A.P. van, *The Skyward Trend of Thought*, Amsterdam: AHA Books, 1986; Cambridge, Massachusetts: MIT Press, 1988

Robinson, Cervin and Rosemarie Haag Bletter, *Skyscraper Style: Art Deco, New York*, New York: Oxford University Press, 1975

Stern, Robert A.M., Gregory Gilmartin, and Thomas Mellins, *New York, 1930: Architecture and Urbanism between the Two World Wars*, New York: Rizzoli, 1987

Stern, Robert A.M., Thomas Mellins, and David Fishman, *New York, 1960: Architecture and Urbanism between the Second World War and the Bicentennial*, New York: Monacelli Press, and Cologne: Taschen, 1995; 2nd edition, 1997

Willis, Carol, *Form Follows Finance: Skyscrapers and Skylines in New York and Chicago*, New York: Princeton Architectural Press, 1995

SMITH, CHLOETHIEL WOODARD 1910–92

Architect and urban planner, United States

In her designs, Chloethiel Woodard Smith strove to combine functionalism and aesthetics. Her concerns with "quality over quantity" and "improving the collective neglect," as she described her goals, were strongly influenced by Lewis Mumford and her work for the Federal Housing Administration (FHA). Smith met Mumford during her undergraduate studies and corresponded with him until his 1990 death. After completing her

M.Arch. in 1933, Smith spent two years working for different architectural firms before accepting the position as chief of research at the FHA in 1935. She worked for that organization until 1939. Consequently, she spent most of her career in Washington, D.C., and was a significant force in shaping the American capitol in the 1950s and 1960s.

Her projects in Washington include the E Street Expressway, office buildings, and residential communities. Smith managed the unequaled feat of securing commissions from three different developers to build three of the four office buildings at a prominent intersection in a major American city: the corner of Connecticut Avenue and L Street in Washington, D.C. Although they are competent modernist designs, the three corporate structures at Chloethiel's corner, as it is affectionately known, do not reflect Smith's best work. Her most inspired designs and those for which she is best known are her residential communities. Among these are two that helped to revive southwest Washington: Capitol Park and Harbour Square.

Both Capitol Park and Harbour Square reflect Smith's determination to "add something more" to the urban environment through the use of varied designs, landscaping, control of automobile traffic, and providing support facilities instead of adhering to stylistic dogma. In Capitol Park (1965–67), designed in partnership with Nicholas Satterlee, Smith characteristically relied on landscaping and miniparks to connect the different building types to one another and their surroundings. The changes of scale within both the landscaping and the structures—five Le Corbusian high-rise apartment buildings and wood-framed townhouses—provide diversity within unity. To further avoid monotony, the facades of the high-rises are varied, and the exteriors of the townhouses are painted in different pastel colors. In order to accommodate the different types of housing, streets are not laid out along a grid pattern. They are arranged to allow easy access to the housing. The automobile is accommodated yet does not determine the plan. Smith also provided quality-of-life facilities, such as laundries and swimming pools. A 1964 promotional brochure for Capitol Park described it as "The New Town in the City." "New Town" was the phrase that Smith preferred for her urban-renewal projects such as Capitol Park.

Therefore, "New Town" was applied also to the 1966 Harbour Square development by Chloethiel Woodard Smith and Associates. Although similar support services were included, at Harbour Square Smith's approach to the integration of contemporary and traditional forms was different from the one she utilized in Capitol Park. Seven historic houses from the 1770s were incorporated into a row of new townhouses. These are balanced by high-rise apartment blocks. Smith placed all the new buildings on the ground to relate them to the historic structures. Automobiles are not allowed into Harbour Square, although access to the underground parking is convenient. Variety is provided through the use of different building types, courtyards, and landscaping. In Harbour Square, Smith again made the new development compatible with its surroundings by respecting the historic fabric and strategic landscaping.

Smith's innovative approach to the use of historic forms, her insistence that support services be included, and the automobile corralled contributed to the success of LaClede Township (1966–67) in St. Louis. In this federal housing project, two- and three-story wood-frame houses are arranged along streets

accentuated by traffic circles. Although Smith was strongly criticized for designing a housing project closely resembling the clutter of buildings that had been cleared for it, LaClede Town was truly an urban-renewal project, unlike Capitol Park and Harbour Square, which were urban-removal projects. LaClede demonstrates Smith's belief it is possible to provide affordable, quality, and pleasing housing despite the residents' income levels. As such, LaClede stands in direct contrast to the purely modernist design of another St. Louis housing project, Pruitt Igoe, by Minoru Yamasaki, which was completed in 1954 and demolished in 1972. Furthermore, in her reliance on traditional housing forms at LaClede, Smith was anticipating such New Urbanist towns as Seaside and Celebration, albeit for completely different residents. She understood that well-designed and well-built homes, support facilities such as the delicatessen, art gallery, and controversial pub, and links to the surrounding areas are more capable than high mortgages of instilling community pride. At LaClede, Smith strongly demonstrated well-designed public housing could provide a positive environment while meeting government regulations.

Smith's belief that good design resulted from many factors and not simple adherence to stylistic dogma manifested itself early in her career. For example, in 1939 she organized the exhibition "Washington, The Planned City without a Plan," in which she criticized the Washington Planning Commission for continuing to follow the L'Enfant and McMillan plans. She advocated that these plans were outdated and unable to meet the needs of a modern city. Her criticism was so shocking that the Washington chapter of the American Institute of Architects (AIA) Retracted its sponsorship. Less problematic were her articles about the spread of the International Style to South America. Instead of belittling South American architects for importing the European style, she discussed the positive aspects of South American modernism within its sociopolitical context.

These articles constitute one aspect of her international career. Although the majority of Smith's career was spent in Washington, she also lived and worked in Canada and Bolivia. Her familiarity with South America and her responsiveness to local conditions were instrumental in securing the commission for the American Embassy Chancery and Residence (1959) in Asunción, Paraguay.

Smith's international projects were well received, but her most critically acclaimed work was in the United States. She included the American Embassy in Paraguay and Capitol Park among her most successful designs and surprisingly did not list LaClede Town. It is difficult to understand by what criteria an architect judges her own work. As early as 1960, Smith's colleagues gave their approval by electing her a fellow to the AIA. Her colleagues were expressing their confidence in her unflinching commitment to good architecture and urban planning. They would not be disappointed. In 1960, Smith was slightly past the midpoint of her 49-year career, and her best work was yet to come.

LORETTA LORANCE

Biography

Born 2 February 1910 in Peoria, Illinois. B.Arch. with honors, University of Oregon, Eugene, 1932; M.Arch. in City Planning, Washington University, St. Louis, Missouri, 1933. Worked for architectural firms in New York, Seattle, and Portland, Oregon, 1933–35; chief of research and planning, Federal Housing Administration, Washington, D.C., 1935–39; organized exhibition "City for Living" in Montreal 1940–41; wrote articles, consulted, taught at University of San Andres, La Paz, Bolivia, 1942–45; received Guggenheim Fellowship to study modern architecture in South America, 1944; partner in Smith, Keyes, Satterlee and Lethbridge, Washington, D.C., 1951–56; partner in Satterlee and Smith, Washington, D.C., 1956–63; principal of Chloethiel Woodard Smith and Associates, Washington, D.C., 1963–82. Elected a fellow to the American Institute of Architects, 1960. Died in Washington, D.C., 1992.

Selected Works

"Washington, the Planned City without a Plan" (exhibition), Washington, D.C., 1939
"City for Living" (exhibition), Montreal, Quebec, 1941
Chesnut Lodge, Rockville, Maryland, 1955–75
American Embassy Chancery and Residence, Asunción, Paraguay, 1959
Channel Waterfront Master Plan, Washington, D.C., 1960
Capitol Park Apartments, Washington, D.C., 1967
Harbour Square, Washington, D.C., 1966
LaClede Township, St. Louis, Missouri, 1967
E Street Expressway, Washington, D.C., 1968
Harcourt, Brace and World Store and Executive Offices, New York City, 1968

Selected Publications

Smith's drawings are housed at the Prints and Drawing Collection in Washington, D.C. Her correspondence with Lewis Mumford is located at Van Pelt Library, University of Pennsylvania.

"South America: Colombia, Venezuela," *Architectural Forum* 85 (November 1946)
"South America: Argentina," *Architectural Forum* 86 (February 1947)
"Recent South American Building," *Architect's Yearbook* 3 (1949)
"Cities in Search of Form," *AIA Journal* 35 (March 1961)
"Esthetic Lion Taming in the City," *AIA Journal* 38 (November 1962)
"Public Works: Dominant Forms for the City," *AIA Journal* 39 (January 1963)
"The City and the Architect," *Home Builders* 20 (February 1963)
"The New Town: Concept and Experience," *Building Research* 3 (January–February 1966)
"Architects without Labels: The Case Against All Special Categories" in *Architecture: A Place for Women*, 1989

Written by CWS & Associates

This Is Capitol Park—The New Town in the City, 1964
*Chloethiel Woodard Smith & Associated Architects,
Georgetown Square: Miller-Evans Joint Venture*, 1976

Further Reading

The most comprehensive study of Smith's work to date is Jayne Doud's unpublished M.A. thesis. The American Institute of Architects Foundation included Smith in the 1979 exhibition *Two on Two at the Octagon: Design for the Urban Environment*. Although the focus of the exhibition was Smith's urban designs, the accompanying catalog provides a chronological survey of her work.

American Institute of Architects Foundation, *Two on Two at the Octagon: Design for the Urban Environment*, Washington, D.C.: Octagon, 1979

Berkeley, Ellen Perry, "LaClede Town: The Most Vital Town in Town," *Architectural Forum* 129 (November 1968)

Conroy, Sarah Booth, "Sketches of a Designing Woman," *Washington Post* (4 November 1989)

Doud, Jayne L., "Chloethiel Woodard Smith, FAIA: Washington's Urban Gem," M.A. thesis, University of Oregon, Eugene, 1994

"A Fresh Idea for Hillsides: Here Is How It Works," *House and Home* 14 (November 1958) "Two Story House Gives Flexibility for Big Families," *House and Home* 8 (October 1955)

"Washington Waterfront to Highlight Seafood, Strolling, Shopping," *Progressive Architecture* 43 (April 1962)

"Washington's Architect Smith: Leading Lady in Urban Renewal," *Look Magazine* 29 (September 1965)

SMITHSON, PETER, (1923–) AND SMITHSON, ALISON, (1928–93)

Architecture firm, England

Alison and Peter Smithson were, until 1993, principals of their own London-based architectural practice and together were responsible for some of the most influential writings and buildings in 20th-century British architecture. Their work is characterized by the breadth of their projects, which range from city planning to furniture design. Their involvement with the Pop art movement in 1950s London and, later, as cofounders of the influential Team X group that grew out of the Congrès Internationaux d'Architecture Moderne (CIAM), established their place within modern postwar architecture in Britain.

The firm built their early reputation on a winning competition design, the Hunstanton School (1954) in Norfolk, inspired by the early Chicago School buildings of Mies van der Rohe. This rectilinear pavilion in brick, steel, and glass became the first built landmark of a new movement known as the New Brutalism (or simply Brutalism) in England. The Economist Building (actually three buildings around a raised plaza built in concrete but faced in Portland stone) followed in London in 1964. The Smithsons then designed two buildings in disparate settings: student accommodations for St. Hilda's College, Oxford (1970), in essence a scaled-down version of one of the earlier Economist "towers" but sensitively contextualized, and the housing at Robin Hood Gardens (1970), sandwiched between highways in the east end of London and itself a fragment of their influential competition project for Golden Lane (1952).

A number of competition entries from the early 1950s established the Smithsons among a new avant-garde of architects eager to transcend the limits of the International Style without betraying the rationality and rigor of modernist principles. The Smithsons's solution was radical although contradictory: on the one hand, their work made reference to anthropological patterns of human association and settlement, and on the other, advocated the embrace of new industrial technologies.

The Smithsons' involvement with a movement of British Pop artists known as the Independent Group at the Institute of Contemporary Arts (ICA) provided an opportunity to present their work to an audience of avant-garde artists, curators, critics,

theorists, and other architects. The multimedia exhibitions "A Parallel of Life and Art" (ICA, 1953) and "This is Tomorrow" (Whitechapel Gallery, 1956) included the Smithsons' work. The latter included a primitive hut surrounded by a sand-covered protected territory, accompanied by a symbolic collection of relics, or "found objects"—reminders of human activity as well as machine-age technologies. The concept of the house as the focus of post-war domesticity and commodity fetishism provided the theme for the Smithsons' "House of the Future" entry constructed for the Ideal Homes Exhibition in London (1956). The Smithsons organic styling and built-in furniture, using molded plastic and fiberglass construction, produced a startling contrast to the traditional brick-and-timber palette of the prevailing residential architecture.

Other projects diverted from the individualism of the home to consider large-scale movement patterns in city centers. Like Golden Lane, the Smithsons' project for the Sheffield University competition (1953) used pedestrian circulation as its major ordering device. This strategy was extrapolated in the Berlin Hauptstadt competition (1958), in which an elevated pedestrian network bridges the existing roadways. This project represented the desire to imagine a new scale of urban architecture, one more suited to the increased speed of movement and the loss of engagement between inhabitants and their immediate surroundings. These goals dovetailed with the work and concerns of Team X, a group that included other European architects such as Ralph Erskine, Giancarlo di Carlo, and Aldo van Eyck. As editor of the *Team X Primer* (published initially in *Architectural Design* in 1962), Alison Smithson articulated statements of theory alongside diagrams and drawings of architectural projects that analyzed the crucial nature of architectural context and the continuity of historic living patterns. Nonetheless, the *Primer* illustrates proposals, such as the London Roads Study (1959), that appear to disregard existing buildings and topographies.

By the 1970s, a shift in the Smithsons's work acknowledged these earlier contradictions, most clearly manifest in the campus buildings at the University of Bath. The Smithsons defined the Bath architecture as Team X structures—through what they termed "mat-building"—with blocks arranged along a raised pedestrian deck above a ground-level service road. The inherent incompleteness of this extendable structure provided a challenge to the Smithsons's sensibility, demanding that they create at least a suggestion of stability and closure to an otherwise infinite system. The Bath buildings presented new themes not previously seen in their built work: the notion of "conglomerate ordering," referring to volumetric masses wrapped in a unifying skin; the building as "climate register," expressing its relation to the external environment; the concern for the sensory pleasure to be gained from concrete materials; and the sensitivity to inhabitation, making the building exquisitely appropriate to its function. All these notions find built expression, having been briefly outlined in their earlier writings, and thus, the Bath buildings represent a culmination of a long career of challenging and thoughtful practice.

JONATHAN A. HALE

See also **Brutalism; Team X (Netherlands)**

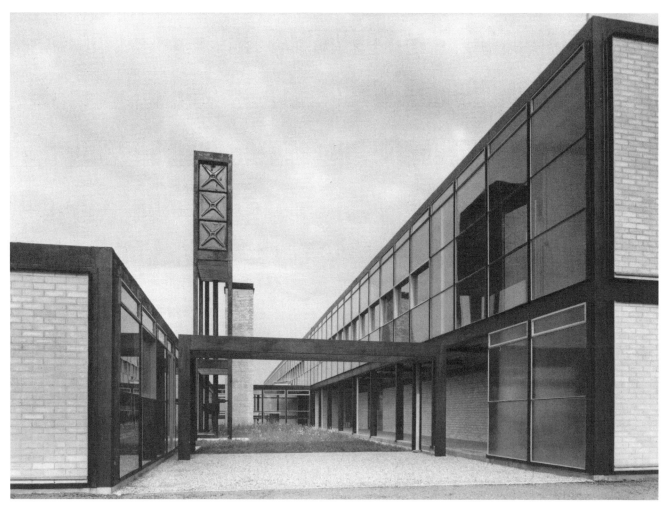

Hunstanton Secondary School (1954), Norfolk, England. Designed by Peter and Alison Smithson.
Photo © Royal Institute of British Architects (RIBA) Library Photographs Collection

Biographies

Peter Smithson

Born in Stockton-on-Tees, County Durham, England, 18 September 1923. Attended the University of Durham School of Architecture 1939–42 and 1945–47; studied at the University of Durham Department of Town Planning 1946–48; attended the Royal Academy Schools, London 1948. Married Alison Gill 1949: 3 children. Served in the British Army, India and Burma 1943–45. Temporary technical assistant, London County Council Architects Department 1949–50. Lecturer, Architectural Association, London. Founder and member, Independent Group, Institute of Contemporary Arts; associated with Team X.

Alison Smithson

Born Alison Margaret Gill in Sheffield, England, 22 June 1928. Studied at the University of Durham School of Architecture 1944–49. Married Peter Smithson 1949: 3 children. Temporary technical assistant, London County Council Architects Department 1949–50. Lecturer, Architectural Association, London. Founder and member, Independent Group, Institute of Con-temporary Arts; associated with Team X. Died in London, 16 August 1993.

Peter and Alison Smithson

Met in the University of Durham; established a partnership in London 1950.

Selected Works

Hunstanton Secondary Modern School (first place, competition), Norfolk, 1954
The Economist Building, London, 1964
Garden Building, St. Hilda's College, Oxford, 1970
Housing Development, Robin Hood Gardens, London, 1972
East Building, University of Bath, Avon, 1988
Entrance Hall, University of Bath, Avon, 1983
House of the Future (competition project), Ideal Homes Exhibition, London, 1956
Haupstadt Area Plan (competition project), Berlin, 1958
London Roads Study, 1959

Selected Publications

Uppercase, 1960
The Euston Architecture, 1968

Ordinariness and Light: Urban Theories, 1952–1960, and Their Application in a Building Project, 1963–1970, 1970
Without Rhetoric: An Architectural Aesthetic, 1955–1972, 1973
The Shift, 1982

Allison Smithson

Team X Primer (editor), 1962

Further Reading

Vidotto, Marco, *A + P Smithson: Pensieri, progetti, e frammenti fino al 1990*, Genoa: Sagep, 1991; as *Alison + Peter Smithson* (bilingual English–Spanish edition), translated by Santiago Castán and Graham Thomson, Barcelona: Gili, 1997

Webster, Helena (editor), *Modernism without Rhetoric: Essays on the Work of Alison and Peter Smithson*, London: Academy Editions, 1997

SOCIAL SECURITY COMPLEX, ISTANBUL

Designed by Sedad Hakkí Eldem; completed 1970
Istanbul, Turkey

The Social Security Complex, in the historic Zeyrek district of Istanbul, was commissioned by the Turkish Social Security Agency (Sosyal Sigortalar Kurumu, hereafter SSK), which is the public health care and retirement office for blue-collar workers. Rental offices and stores made up the bulk of the initial proposal, which also comprised a health clinic, a bank, and a restaurant in addition to a cafeteria and an unbuilt coffee kiosk. After winning an Aga Khan Award for Architecture in 1986, the complex gained international recognition as well.

Designed and built between 1962 and 1970 by Sedad Hakkí Eldem, the significance of the project comes primarily from its being, as stated in the Aga Khan jury report, one of the first examples of contextualist architecture, which combines local architectural and urban forms with the universal norms of modern architecture. It was an attempt for a synthesis of traditional Turkish architecture and modern materials and techniques without jeopardizing the requirements of a modern office building.

When the competition for the SSK was held in 1962, the monolithic, glass-sheathed block of the International Style was becoming susceptible to criticism because of its homogenizing qualities. Accordingly, quests for locally and contextually sensitive architectures were under way both in Turkey and elsewhere in the West. It should suffice to remember the "vernacular" shift that occurred in the work of someone such as Le Corbusier, who had earlier been a proponent of a universal machine civilization. Likewise, by the 1960s, especially in Italy, the potential contribution of the past to architectural production was being extensively meditated on by Franco Albini, Ignazio Gardella, and the BBPR, among others. Typological and morphological studies were also being undertaken on different urban sites, the pioneer of which was the work of Saverio Muratori on Venice.

In Turkey as well, typological studies of traditional residential architecture had already begun under the supervision of Eldem and a few others at the Academy of Fine Arts in Istanbul. Those researches would have intermittent but considerable impact on Turkish architecture. Eldem, while displaying different architectural tendencies during his remarkably long career, nevertheless maintained a lifelong interest in traditional architecture. In the 1960s, he was, together with Turgut Cansever, among the notable Turkish architects who were thinking on history and locale in relation to architecture.

The SSK project, instead of concentrating in one singular block, diffused the program to smaller units that are articulated around courtyards, streets, and bypasses. Its models are the traditional Ottoman *külliye*—mostly religious complexes in which different functions are fulfilled by separate buildings organized around open spaces—and the traditional urban residential pattern of Istanbul displayed by the very district where it was placed.

With its wooden houses, small mosques, *medreses*, and tombs, in addition to the Byzantine church of Pantocrator and the Roman aqueduct, the traditional organic fabric of the Zeyrek area had already been dented by the opening of Atatürk Boulevard, which cut through the district and was quickly flanked by concrete high-rises. By constituting an environmentally sensitive model, one of the objectives of the SSK project was to resist land speculation, which was threatening the destruction of the area. Given the threat that such historic areas are under in developing countries, that consciousness raising about Zeyrek's value is a crucial contribution of the SSK.

Situated on a steep triangular lot between Atatürk Boulevard and the Zeyrek slope, the complex aimed to harmonize with its physical context and topography. On the north, it responded to the organic urban tissue of Zeyrek, which reproduced the fragmentary form and the modest scale of its wooden houses. The southeastern facade, with its tall, cascading masses, was in accord with the high-rises of Atatürk Boulevard. At the northeastern tip of the lot, where the unrealized coffee kiosk would have been built, the boulevard is connected to the cobblestone slope by a skillful arrangement of steps that lead to a small square at the adjacent higher level. This small plaza, which utilizes an existing fountain, marks the end of an "inner street" that traverses the whole complex.

The project consists of blocks of different sizes, heights, and functions that are arranged around the two-level "inner street" running parallel to the boulevard. Each of the modular units, connected at lower levels and separate at the top—from the southwestern office-and-store block to the central bank-and-restaurant and clinic blocks to the northeastern cafeteria-and-store unit—displays its architect's lifelong interest in the traditional "Turkish house."

Based on solid lower levels, as in traditional residential architecture, and gradually projecting toward the top, the blocks repeat the same facade elements: rows of vertical windows modulated by short concrete pilasters (a characteristic of Eldem's architecture) and below them tile in-fill panels emphatically distinguished from the reinforced-concrete skeleton of the building. As in his other projects, Eldem, here as well, succeeds in lending the lightweight, slender appearance of timber, which is part of the image of traditional architecture, to his reinforced-concrete building. Likewise, he reconciles the flat-roof requirement of the brief with his interest in traditional forms by creating a historical expression through the wrapping of the roofs with large eaves.

The end product is a geometrically disciplined modern interpretation of tradition. In Atilla Yücel's words, "[The SSK] stands in between the spatial morphology of a spontaneously grown historic Istanbul quarter and the rigid architectonic discipline of an August Perret classicism."

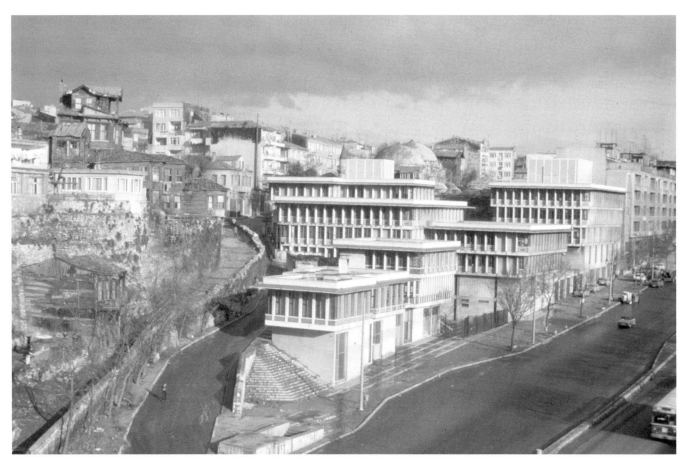

Social Security Complex, Istanbul, designed by Sedad Hakki Eldem (1970)
Photo by Mustafa Pehlivanoglu © Aga Khan Award for Architecture

The SSK stands out also within the oeuvre of its architect, who often reflects the results of his typological studies at the university in his architectural work. The "Turkish house" to which Eldem's architecture alludes is often seen as an idealized type based on the upper-class mansions of Istanbul and one that stands by itself, indifferent to its surroundings. At the SSK, as noted by Sibel Bozdogan, Eldem, for the first time, transcends the freestanding object and goes beyond building typology "into the realm of urban morphology."

Although the SSK had considerable influence on later Turkish architecture (as displayed by the Ziraat Bankasi in Bakirköy, among others), in time the context—the traditional urban tissue—with which the building tried to establish a dialogue disappeared, leaving the initial intentions of the architect irretrievably undercut. The original design was further weakened by the changes in the initial functions of the blocks and the conversion of the large part of the circulation spaces and stores into storages for a firm that rented the building.

BELGIN TURAN

Further Reading

Bozdogan, Sibel, "A Contextualist Experiment" in *Sedad Eldem: Architect in Turkey*, by Bozdogan, Suha Özkan, and Engin Yenal, London: Butterworth Architecture, 1989; New York: Aperture, and Singapore: Concept Media, 1987

Yücel, Atilla, "Contemporary Turkish Architecture," *Mimar* 10 (October–December 1983)

Yücel, Atilla, "Pluralism Takes Command: The Turkish Architectural Scene Today" in *Modern Turkish Architecture*, edited by Renata Holod and Ahmet Evin, Philadelphia: University of Pennsylvania Press, 1984

SOLAR ARCHITECTURE

The technique of passive solar design—the direct use of solar energy to provide heat and light in buildings—has a long history in building design. Its evolution during the 20th century began as a reaction to what Reyner Banham (1969) subsequently termed "a dark satanic century." Rapid urbanization during the 19th century brought with it polluted, unsanitary, and overcrowded conditions to the large industrial cities of Europe and North America. In England, as epidemics of disease threatened entire urban populations, liberal reformers reacted against a laissez-faire attitude to city development and instead promoted hygiene and sanitation as the founding principles of healthy urban planning.

By the beginning of the 20th century, the bactericidal properties of direct sunlight had been established, and countries such as England and Germany enacted laws ensuring sun rights for all citizens. In England, architects such as Raymond Unwin (1863–1940) began to systematically study solar geometry with the aim of maximizing solar access in and around buildings.

Throughout the 1920s and 1930s, the health benefits of sunlight remained a strong influence in European urban planning and building design. In Germany, large residential complexes, such as Siemensstadt (1929) in Berlin, master planned by Walter Gropius (1883–1969), utilized the *Zeilenbau* (row house) form. This functional and land-efficient arrangement, influenced by the spirit of the *Neue Sachlichkeit* (New Objectivity), consisted of high-density apartment blocks running north-south and set at precise distances to maximize the penetration of sunlight from the east and west. The addition of roof terraces or balconies provided further opportunities for occupants to soak up the sun.

During the 1930s, in response to the harsh economic conditions of the interwar period, the emphasis in passive solar design moved away from daylighting alone. Saving fuel, particularly that used for winter heating, became a design priority. By 1933, the Swiss solar community of Neubühl near Zurich consisted of rows of apartments oriented almost directly south with large areas of south-facing glazing to trap winter heat. However, as war loomed in Europe, the most significant developments in solar energy use for home heating occurred in America.

Chicago-based architect George Fred Keck (1895–1980) had recognized the potential of passive solar heating while working on the highly glazed "House of Tomorrow," built for the 1933 Century of Progress Exposition in Chicago. In 1940, following several years of experimentation with different passive solar configurations, Keck designed a house for Howard Sloan, a Chicago real estate developer. The detached house, situated in Glenview, Illinois, established what was to become the archetypal form of the passive solar house. All the necessary elements of the house—its walls, floors, roofs, and windows—were arranged to maximize the benefits of solar energy in the form of heat and daylight. The rectangular plan of the house was elongated along its east-west axis and arranged with the fully glazed living spaces facing directly south. Large monopitch roofs overhung the glazing to intercept high-angle summer sun to prevent the house from overheating in summer.

In America, Keck's designs received wide publicity, and the 1940s saw a growing market for energy-efficient, solar homes. This period also saw significant research and development into passive solar design by a group of engineers at the Massachusetts Institute of Technology who constructed and monitored a series of both passive and active solar homes. Despite these developments, by the 1950s a plentiful supply of cheap fossil fuels diminished economic incentives for solar energy. In both domestic and commercial buildings, mechanical heating, cooling, and ventilation technologies had become widely established, further reducing demand for solar alternatives.

During the 1960s and early 1970s, passive solar design enjoyed a limited rebirth inspired by two fundamental concerns. First, many had begun to question the technological optimism of modernism and the International Style. Architects such as Ralph Erskine (1914–) began to draw on preindustrial and indigenous building techniques as the basis of a climate-specific architecture that was both regionally and culturally appropriate.

Second, a more overtly political environmental movement grew critical of the social and environmental effects of industrial capitalism. By the early 1970s, a number of autonomous cooperative communities, such as Arcosanti (1970) in Arizona and The Centre for Alternative Technology (1973) in Wales, had been established. For those environmentalists such as Steve Baer, who chose to live this alternative lifestyle, the development of independent and renewable energy from sources such as the sun was essential. Baer's own house (1972) in New Mexico consisted of an L-shaped organic cluster of 11 "Zomes" arranged to collect solar energy through large areas of south-facing glazing and then store it as heat within the thermal mass of water-filled drums. At night, large insulated shutters were pulled up over the glass to retain heat.

By the late 1970s, passive solar design was no longer the sole preserve of environmentalists. The oil crisis of 1973 had generated political concerns about the long-term availability of fossil fuels and had resulted in widespread academic research into the use of solar energy. A number of passive solar buildings were constructed on both sides of the Atlantic. During the 1980s, these concerns for energy efficiency were extended to global climate issues under the rubric of sustainability. In Europe, architects such as Renzo Piano and Norman Foster and Partners began to utilize passive solar features in the form of daylight and shading in order to naturally air-condition large-scale buildings. Among many, Norman Foster and Partners' Commerzbank Headquarters (1997) in Frankfurt, Germany, successfully utilizes principles of solar design and sustainable architecture.

GRAHAM FARMER

See also **Arcosanti, Arizona; Century of Progress Exposition, Chicago (1933); Energy Efficient Design; Environmental Issues; Erskine, Ralph (England); Foster, Norman (England); Gropius, Walter (Germany); Piano, Renzo (Italy); Sustainability and Sustainable Architecture**

Further Reading

Banham, Reyner, *The Architecture of the Well Tempered Environment*, London: The Architectural Press, 1969.

Behling, Sophia and Behling Stefan, Sol Power, *The Evolution of Solar Architecture*, New York: Prestel-Verlag, 1996.

Butti, Ken and Perlin, John, *A Golden Thread: 2500 Years of Solar Architecture and Technology*, London: Marion Boyars Publishers, 1981.

Energy Research Group, *The Climatic Dwelling: An introduction to climate responsive residential architecture*, London: James and James, 1996.

Farmer, John, *Green Shift: Towards a Green Sensibility in Architecture*, Oxford: Butterworth-Heinemann, 1996.

Olgyay, Victor, Design with Climate: A Bioclimatic Approach to Architectural Regionalism, Princeton: Princeton University Press, 1963.

Pearson, David, *The Natural House Book*, London: Conran Octopus, 1991.

SOLERI, PAOLO 1919–

Architect, Italy

Paolo Soleri was born in 1919 in Turin, Italy, where he studied at the Polytechnic, receiving a doctorate in architecture in 1946.

From 1947 to 1948, he attended Taliesin West, Frank Lloyd Wright's famous architecture studio. After practicing in southern Italy and Turin in the early 1950s, he emigrated with his wife, Carolyn Woods, to the United States and settled in Arizona. Soleri devoted his life to the research of alternative urban development. His chief interest was in cities as a framework in which to combine human and natural resources and diversity of functions and events. This study moved him to explore a new concept, arcologies, environments that fused architecture and ecology.

His concern for the relationship between human-made objects and the earth is expressed in his early Dome house (1949) designed for Leonora Woods, his future mother-in-law. Located on a hillside at Cave Creek, Arizona, the house had retaining walls that were cast with red boulders and concrete, following Wright's technique. Soleri also explored thermal inertia resulting from a glazed dome above the living room and the excavated areas underground. The dome can be shaded or opened according to the seasons.

In 1951, Soleri moved with his wife to southern Italy and began his explorations in ceramics. His first major building, a workshop for Ceramica Artistica Solimene (1953) in Vietri-sul-mare, faces the Mediterranean on the Amalfi coast. It was built on reinforced concrete covered outside with pottery. Here, Soleri anticipates later explorations using materials from the area and relating engineering, site, and handicraft.

After returning to the United States in 1955, Soleri began his project for Cosanti (from the Latin "before things") on a five-acre site in Scottsdale, Arizona. The complex grew according to the needs of the community and the experience gained in construction techniques. Soleri explored here the technique of wash-away silt casting, using it in construction of cast-concrete architectural buildings, wind-bells, sculptures, and models. Cosanti consists of several units related with the site in an organic language of architectural form. The first structure was the Earth House (1956), inmersed in the site after the land was excavated. The ceramic studio (1956) consisted of a structure of ribbed reinforced concrete. Other spaces are the Cosanti Gallery, with a vault formed in a mound; a series of working spaces with solar devices, the piscine and canopy; and the foundation offices (1971). As a comprehensive site, Cosanti provided an array of architectural prototypes. This was Soleri's first experience relating craft, work, ecology, and life in one complex.

Soleri's chief aim was to keep the integrity of both the natural and the urban. He needed a large-scale laboratory to research and develop his model for how to inhabit cities in the future. To demonstrate how to improve urban conditions and to minimize the impact of destructive forces of suburbia on the environment, Soleri started Arcosanti in 1971. Still in the process of construction, Arcosanti is located in Cordon Junction, 70 miles north of Phoenix in the mesa country. Soleri defines Arcosanti as an urban laboratory, an instrument for research meant to accommodate up to 7,000 people. Mostly pedestrian oriented, this prototype arcology project will eventually rise up to 25 stories, covering only 13 acres and leaving open 860 acres.

Arcosanti is composed of a series of public and semipublic areas, private zones, and utilities, most of which rely on passive energy. The East Crescend Complex is considered the essence of arcology, combining living and working spaces. These include the Colly Soleri Music Center (1989), a semipublic area dedi-cated to studios and diverse types of private housing. Arcosanti also has two greenhouses, gardens, a small vineyard, a field, and an orchard.

Over the last three decades, Arcosanti has been built by thousands of volunteers, all sharing part of Soleri's approach and visionary ideas about the environment. In this setting, workers share a communal way of life based on production of craft, agriculture, and a healthy use and inhabitation of the land. Soleri calls this approach the ethic of the urban and speaks of the culture of the automobile as the instrument of isolation and segmentation. In his view, our cities will require planners not only to change cities physically but also to change the habits and principles of human interaction. Presently, about 70 individuals live and work in Arcosanti. The community hosts a music festival, exhibits, lectures, and seminars. Arcosanti remains, essentially, a laboratory for multiuse architecture based on pedestrian circulation, energy efficiency, and careful solar orientation.

One of Soleri's recurrent themes has been the notion of bridge cities, which were published by the Museum of Modern Art in *The Architecture of Bridges* (1948). A large exhibition of his drawings of bridges and ideas about arcology held at the Corcoran Gallery of Washington in 1970 introduced the public to his notion of miniaturization, concentration, and ecological balance. Soleri has written several books and lectures all over the world.

Although Arcosanti concentrated most of Soleri's energies and efforts, he also designed the University of Arizona Cancer Center Chapel (1986) in Tucson. The interior of the chapel, stylized as a tree, has a multitude of metal wind-bells cascading from the ceiling. He also designed the De Concini residence (1982) in Phoenix and produced urban studies for the development of Scottsdale (1992).

Soleri's experiences in Cosanti and Arcosanti inspired him to develop a meaningful and alternative urban theory. His notion of "evolutionary coherence" in the city argues that urban megastructures share some characteristics with the complex systems of nature. Soleri is critical of the explosive growth of some metropolitan areas, such as Phoenix and Los Angeles. His planning thesis is based on concentration and miniaturization. Soleri has been defined as a visionary architect, urban planner, and process philosopher, and his work and books have advanced a new spirituality of technology, science, habitat, and humankind. His life has been devoted to experimentation in urban planning, architecture, and the applied arts. His idealism and research on the relationship between inhabitation, life, and work constitute his fundamental contribution.

JOSE BERNARDI

See also **Arconsanti, Arizona**

Biography

Born in Turin, Italy, 21 June 1919; emigrated to the United States 1955. Studied at Turin Polytechnic 1941–46; degree in architecture 1946; fellow, Frank Lloyd Wright Foundation, Taliesin West, Arizona and Taliesin East, Wisconsin 1947–48. In private practice, Turin and Southern Italy 1950–55; president, Cosanti Foundation, Scottsdale, Arizona from 1956; organized the Minds for History series of dialogues and lectures, Arcosanti,

Arizona 1989. Distinguished visiting lecturer, Arizona State University College of Architecture, Tempe. Graham Foundation Fellowship 1962; Guggenheim grant 1964 and 1967.

Selected Works

Dome House, Cave Creek, Arizona, 1949
Ceramica Artistica Solimene, Vietri-sul-mare, 1953
Cosanti, Scottsdale, Arizona, 1955
Earth House, Scottsdale, Arizona, 1956
Ceramic Studio, Scottsdale, Arizona, 1956
Cosanti Gallery, Scottsdale, Arizona, 1971
Arcosanti (unfinished), Cordon Junction, Arizona, 1971
De Concini Residence, Phoenix, Arizona, 1982
University of Arizona Cancer Center Chapel, Tucson, Arizona, 1986

Selected Publications

Arcology: The City in the Image of Man, 1969
The Sketchbooks of Paolo Soleri, 1971
The Bridge between Matter and Spirit Is Matter Becoming Spirit: The Arcology of Paolo Soleri, 1973
Arcosanti: An Urban Laboratory? 1983
Paolo Soleri's Earth Casting: For Sculpture, Models, and Construction (with Scott M. Davis), 1984
Technology and Cosmogenesis, 1985

Further Reading

Burkhart, François, "Thirty-Five Years After: A Visit to Cosanti," *Domus* 812 (February 1999)
Cook, Jeffrey, "Paolo Soleri," Central Arizona Chapter of American Institute of Architects, *A Guide to the Architecture of Metro Phoenix*, Phoenix, Arizona: Phoenix Publishing, 1983
Mayne, David S. and Debra Giannini (producers), *Soleri's Cities: Architecture for Planet Earth and Beyond* (videorecording), Chicago: Home Vision, 1993
"Soleri's Arizona," *Domus* 812 (February 1999)
Wall, Donald, *Documenta: The Paolo Soleri Retrospective*, Washington, D.C.: Corcoran Gallery of Art, 1970

SOTA, ALEJANDRO DE LA 1913–96

Architect, Spain

Alejandro de la Sota is the maestro of many late 20th-century Spanish architects. On the one hand, he was an influential teacher at the school of architecture in Madrid from 1956 to 1972. On the other, he was a master builder whose projects set an example to be followed by his many disciples. It is unfortunate that his influence did not extend beyond the boundaries of Spain. He was recognized internationally only in the 1980s. Born in the Galician region in the northwestern part of Spain in 1913, he graduated from the school of architecture at the Polytechnic of Madrid in 1941. From 1942 to 1949, he worked for a central government housing and relocation agency, creating a series of rural housing developments for post–civil war Spain. Although the groupings relied on a rational plan and the repetition of forms, he adorned the houses with elements of vernacular architecture. With the exception of this first job, all his subsequent architecture was clearly modernist and characterized by its simplicity, rationalism, and abstract geometry. A follower of the Modern movement, de la Sota's building always seemed understated, although his genius was ever present. De la Sota,

who suffered from Parkinson's disease in his final years, died in Madrid in 1996.

In the buildings, projects, and furniture designs of de la Sota, the primary idea is paramount. The final design is the result of a process that eliminates, little by little, extraneous and unrefined aspects. In the end, what is left is pure, concentrated, but also poetic. The generating idea of a project does not always come from the same source. In some cases, it may be the structure, the site, a technological aspect, or a programmatic intention. Functional and technical concerns become the architectural language. The tectonic quality of the building is always present, as de la Sota's works make constant references to the materials of which they are constructed. Each project seems to start fresh from the new situation at hand. Once de la Sota remarked that there is no reason to do the same thing over and over again. He expressed the idea that each project should present a new challenge and a new opportunity for exploration. De la Sota practiced architecture for about 50 years, maintaining an atelier type of approach. His body of work, both built and unbuilt projects, is part of the rich heritage of Spanish architecture of the end of the 20th century.

In 1955, a single-family house was built in Madrid on Doctor Arce Street. The site exerted its influence on the final form. The required setbacks from the property lines encouraged a compact structure on the widest part of the side. The house, on a busy street, looks inward. The windows to the street facade are few and small. The facade toward the garden is the exact opposite, with its large windows creating a transparency between interior and exterior. The entire house is made of brick with uneven surfaces that catch the changing natural light. The plan is simple; the staircase, with its gentle curve, seems to push out the exterior wall of the house, creating a bulge in the facade.

The Civil Government Offices in Tarragona (1957), really the central government building in the province during Franco's regime, shows clearly the architect's evolving vocabulary. The building, for representation, administration, and housing, is the union of three blocks, each used for one purpose: The entrance is pushed underneath the main podium, which itself comprises the main government floors. The top of the podium forms a terrace that dominates the square in front. It also creates a break between the building used for government functions and the official residences located in the cube above. A modular system of 18 by 18 feet is the underlying principle of the composition. The residential cube is exactly three modules by three modules. The clear use of geometry and the play between voids and solids call to mind Le Corbusier and Mies van der Rohe. Terragni's name also surfaces with a comparison made to the Casa del Fascio. The main building material is cut and polished local marble.

The Maravillas Gymnasium (1965) had to respond to a very difficult site with limited financial resources. The narrow, trapezoidal site, about 90 feet wide, has a steep slope of about 36 feet. The solution is one of fitting the building into the void and occupying the entire site. An ingenious structural solution using 60-foot trusses set at right angles to the street span the gymnasium. On the upper level, the 18-foot spaces between the trusses are used for classrooms. Below is the gymnasium, with the benches on one side and light from the windows above flowing into the other. The materials used are few and grant an idea of the thin skin enclosing the space, which becomes lighter

and lighter as one goes up. At the lower level, the building faces a busy street and therefore has a rather closed facade at street level with brick. Higher up is glass, which seems to fold back and finally on top, surrounding the play space, is a wire fence.

The Post Office and Telecommunications Building (1984) in Leon, Spain, can be thought of as a functional building employing state-of-the-art technology. It is apparently a simple cube that allows work to be carried out efficiently while admitting that changes in use can occur over time. The structure is simple, and the interior is filled with light. The materials echo the intention of the building. It is clad in Robertson panels and uses glass, stainless steel, and straightforward fixtures.

The projects of de la Sota, from the early works, such as the TABSA Aeronautical Plant (1957) near Madrid, to his final ones, such the University Library (1993) in Santiago de Compostela, although always loyal to modernism, can also be seen as a quest for purity, order, and simplicity.

MARTHA THORNE

See also **Spain**

Further Reading

The majority of articles published on Alejandro de la Sota's work are in Spanish. However, the Pronaos publication, *Alejandro de la Sota*, was also translated to English.

Alejandro de la Sota, Architect, Madrid: Pronaos, 1989; 2nd edition, as *Alejandro de la Sota*, 1997
"Alejandro de la Sota, de la Sota's Chair," *Domus* 691 (February 1988)
Alejandro de la Sota: The Architecture of Imperfection, London: Architectural Association, 1997
Baldellou Santolaria, Miguel Angel, *Gimnasio Maravillas, Madrid, 1960–1962: Alejandro de la Sota*, Almería, Spain: Colegio de Arquitectos de Almería, 1997
Curtis, William, et al., *Alejandro de la Sota*, Madrid: Arquitectura Viva, 1997
De la Mata, Sara and Enrique Sobejano, "Alejandro de la Sota," *Arquitectura* 72, no. 283–284 (an interview)
"Josep Llinàs Carmona with Alejandro de la Sota: Restoration of the Civil Government Headquarters of Tarragona, Tarragona, Spain, 1985–1987," *A + U* 12 (December 1996)
Llano Cabado, Pedro de, *Alejandro de la Sota, o nacemento duhna arquitectura*, Pontevedra, Spain: Deputatción Provincial de Pontevedra, 1995
Thorne, Martha, "Entrevista a Alejandro de la Sota," *Quaderns d'arquitectura I urbanisme* 156 (1983)
Werk, Bauen + Wohnen 5 (May 1997) (special issue on Sota)

SOUTHEAST ASIA

The architecture of Southeast Asia is characterized by pitched overhanging roofs and elevated floor archetypes. It has developed in political entities with varying cultures and histories. North and South Korea, Singapore, Thailand, and Indochina (Vietnam, Laos, and Cambodia) were all influenced by Confucian, Buddhist, and Taoist traditions, whereas the Philippines incorporated Christian and some Muslim forms, and Malaysia, Brunei, and Indonesia were influenced by Hindu and Islamic architecture.

Colonialism and Western interventions in the 20th century, especially the introduction of modernism, wrought dramatic changes on the built forms of all these countries. The peoples of the area have nevertheless retained traditional cultural styles, sometimes expressed in their architecture. At the beginning of the 21st century, almost as a reflection of the global profusion of information and images, architecture in Southeast Asia has a wide range of pluralistic architectural expressions.

Colonial Architecture

Southeast Asia's colonizers brought different approaches to architecture and urban planning. In Malaysia/Singapore the British presence led to the development of the Indo-Saracenic style that began with Indian architecture, exaggerating it with a baroque overlay. British-run architectural firms sprang up and helped establish this style, including the influential firms of Thompson, McPherson and McNair and Palmer and Turner, who practiced in several countries. Although alternative models were provided by the Malay *kampung*, or village settlement, and by Chinese courtyard houses and shophouses, the British influence prevailed. The 1933 British town plan for Kuala Lumpur established the concept of the "orderly city," reflecting "civilised life," for British colonies worldwide, and Singapore began to expand quickly on this model.

In 18th-century Indonesia, the houses retained their indigenous inward orientation, with courtyards and gardens, but under Dutch Colonial influence were reinterpreted in a mix of Amsterdam architectures. This changed when the Dutch architect Henri Maclaine Pont studied the palace architecture of Java in the 1920s and incorporated climatic and cultural lessons into his own designs, as did architects such as Thomas Karsten and Notodiningrat. Three outstanding examples are the campus of the Institut Technologi Bandung (1920) by Maclaine Pont, Bandung's Government Complex (1925) by J. Gerber, and Karsten's design for the Semarang People's Theatre (1920s).

In Thailand, the only country in the region that was never colonized, the 20th-century kings introduced European design, leading to hybrid styles of architecture. The grand Victorian Government House (c.1905) in Bangkok was built according to drawings by Italian architect Annebale Rigotti in an Italianate classical style mixed with local Oriental features, which became the vogue. Another foreign-influenced work was the Khrom Phra Palace (c.1926) by the French architect Charles Bequelin; later, in the 1960s, the influence of modernist architecture is apparent. However, the critic Udo Kultermann notes: "An important fact to remember is that in Thailand the majority of clients were Thai and the choice of architectural language was theirs," (1986, p. 58).

The French governance of Indochina from 1858 to 1954 included a *mission civilisatrice*, which in its urban design and social planning can still be felt. A great effort was directed at the end of the 19th century toward the master plans and architecture of Phnom Penh, Hanoi, and Haipong. The new settlements were built apart from the traditional city—for example, in Hanoi, the oldest area, the "36 streets quarter," was left largely intact, and the colonial development was put on the other side of the lake.

Early public buildings often imitated those in France: the Opera House (1900) in Hanoi by Eugene Teston was a copy of the Paris Opera, as Saigon's Hotel de Ville (1908) by Fernand Gardes was a copy of the Paris town hall. However, when Ernest Hébard was called to Indochina as the first director of urbanism

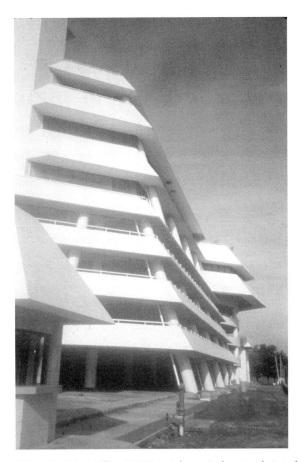

Dharmala Sakti Office (1986) in Jakarta, Indonesia, designed by
Paul Rudolph
Photo courtesy Paul Rudloph © Aga Khan Award for Architecture

in 1921, he studied the region's ancient past and, as Gwendolyn
Wright noted, "freely mixed elements from different countries,
in order to generate his ideal of an innovative, adaptive aesthetic"
(1991, p. 64). This approach is well illustrated by his Ministry
of Finance (1927) and the Louis Finot Museum (1931), both
in Hanoi.

Spain heavily influenced the Philippines, a Spanish colony
since 1521, in its ornate religious architecture. Under American
governance after 1898, it was perhaps the first country in Southeast Asia to embrace the International Style and Western planning; its architecture remained imitative of the West. Daniel
Burnham's Plan for Manila (1906) and William Parson's Manila
Hotel (1912) are good examples. The Manila Post Office (1926)
by Juan Arellano recalls Schinkel's Altes Museum in Berlin.

Between the World Wars the colonial powers began to sponsor Modern European architecture rather than the neoclassical
indigenous amalgam. As a prelude to modernism, some of the
finest Art Deco buildings can be found in Bandung, Indonesia.
Examples are the Grand Hotel Preanger (1932) by C.P. Wolff
Schoemaker and the "Denis" Gebouw (1935) by A.F. Aalbers.
Kallang Airport Terminal (1937) in Singapore by the PWD and
the Central Market (1936) in Kuala Lumpur by Y.T. Lee are
also Art Deco. However, the aftermath of World War II brought

with it the functionalism of the Modern movement and continuing Western cultural domination.

Independence, Nationalism, and Modernity

The nationalist movements brought the need to express freedom
from a colonial, foreign-dominated past and, beyond that, even
from local traditions. This rupture with the symbolic and visual
past was achieved partially through new building types, such as
airports, parliament complexes, and state mosques, expressing a
national and collective identity. From the late 1950s the International Style and, to some extent, Soviet monumentalism gained
adherents.

Local architects began to be influential in Malaysia and Singapore. An early modernist building of note is the Federal Hotel
(1957, with a 1969 addition) by Goh Hock Guan. Perhaps the
first truly local and most important firm, the Malaysian Architects Co-Partnership (1960–67), was founded by four Chinese
British-trained architects who also studied in the United
States—William Lim, Chen Voon Fee, Lim Chin See, and Lim
Chong Keat. Their modernist works include the Singapore Conference Hall (1965) and the Seramban Mosque (1967). Lim
Chong Keat went on to found Jurbina Bertiga (Team 3) and
undertook major projects including the tallest structure in Penang, the Komitar Complex, built between 1976–87. Other
important first-generation architects include Lai Lok Kun, Rus-
lan Khalid, and especially Hijjas Kasturi, whose Luth Building
(1986) and Lot 10 (1994), a metal-clad shopping center, are
good examples of contemporary mainstream architecture in
Kuala Lumpur.

Malay architects began to look back to the Malay house with
its pitched overhanging roofs for a contemporary Malaysian
identity. The earliest examples of this can be found in the Language and Literacy Agency Building (1959) by Y.T. Lee and in
the National Museum (1963) by the Singaporean firm Ho
Kwong Yew and Sons. Around the same time, Baharuddin Abu
Kassim and colleagues of the PWD were forging the expression
of a national Islamic identity through architecture as in the National Mosque (1965), a modern building that used a folded
concrete-plate parasol roof.

Chinese-Malay architects dominated Malaysian building
until the 1970s when indigenous architects, aided by an affirmative action program, began to compete more successfully in the
building boom. Newly established government entities such as
the Urban Development Authority promoted public-private
joint ventures. The 1980s begat a profusion of commercial
blocks and mass-housing and tall office buildings, such as the
35-story Dayabumi Office (1984) in Kuala Lumpur, designed
by the firms MAA and BEP.

A second generation of Malaysian architects includes Ha-
jeedar, who designed the Subang View Hotel (1980), and Shah-
roun bin Dato Haroun of Dimensa, whose Condominiums
(1987) are sited in Port Dickson. Ken Yeang of T.R. Hamzah
and Yeang designed the Plaza Atrium (1983) in Kuala Lumpur
and the 31-story MBF Tower (1993) in Penang. His own residence, Roof Roof House (1984), conceived as "an environmental filter," sparked a long-term concern with tropical architecture.

In Singapore after World War II, designers were both foreign
and Chinese. Palmer and Turner's 1954 Bank of China Building
and Ng Keng Siang's Asia Insurance Building (1954) are examples. After independence in 1965 modernist buildings predomi-

nated, including the Jurong Town Hall (1974) by Raymond Woo of Team 3 International. RDC, founded in 1974, undertook the Science Center (1975), while the Alfred Wong Partnership designed the National Theatre (1963) and Scotts Shopping Complex (1984).

Foreign architects designed a majority of the landmark buildings. I.M. Pei did the Overseas Chinese Banking Corporation (with BEP Architects in 1976), and Moshe Safdie designed the Habitat Singapore (1984). Australians Geoffrey Malone and Philip Conn of IPC designed the high-tech Crystal Court (1985). Kenzo Tange's works for years dominated the city skyline, including Overseas Union Bank Plaza (1983–93) and Tele-Tech Park (1994).

Asia's famous shopping centers began in Singapore with the Golden Mile Shopping Centre (1972) and Peoples' Park (1973) by Tay Kheng Soon and William Lim of DP Architects. Lim later left DP Architects to form a smaller, more experimental practice and designed many fine projects such as Unit 8 condominiums (1984), Tampines Community Center (1989), and the Design School (1995) at the LaSalle-SIA College of the Arts. Akitek Tenggara, Tay Kheng Soon's firm, designed Chee Tong Temple (1987) and the dramatic steel-and-concrete Institute of Technical Education (1993) in Bisham. A new generation of architects including Manop Architects, Richard Ho, and Tangguanbee produces innovative work, including the latter's playful Institution Hill Apartments (1988).

Government architects also play a major role in Singapore building. The PWD did the Central Provident Fund (1977) and Changi International Airport (1981 and 1990). Lee Kwan Yew, the country's long-serving president, set up government agencies for physical planning of the Central Business District and the New Towns. The Housing and Development Board (HDB, founded 1960) designed and built the large housing estates where more than 80 per cent of Singaporeans live. Liu Thai Ker, CEO of HDB until the 1990s, was perhaps the most influential planner–architect shaping the physical fabric of the country. The largely successful projects have made Singapore the epitome of the modern Asian city.

However, the desire to be modern led to the razing of old buildings and whole areas, such as Chinatown. It was only in the mid-1980s that the government realized that areas with character and identity were being destroyed in favor of blandness.

Korea's upheavals in the 20th century led to the division of the country. While North Korea followed the Soviet Union's monumental style of architecture, South Korea's rapid reconstruction in the 1960s was greatly influenced by European and American internationalism and the use of concrete, giving rise to what was referred to locally as the "simple-structure style," replacing country's traditional low-rise timber buildings with tiled roofs.

Until the 1980s foreign architects, such as Skidmore, Owings and Merrill, with their Lucky-Goldstar twin towers (1986), designed the major buildings. Western influence can be seen in the works of two major Korean architects who worked for Le Corbusier in Paris before returning to Seoul. Kim Swoo Geun returned in 1952; he and his practice, the Space Group of Korea, designed the National Assembly (1960) and the Gumi Arts Complex (1990). The second, Kim Chung-up, designed over 200 buildings, later returning to tradition and local crafts as in his last work, the Olympic Gate (1988).

The second generation of Korean architects began to appear in the 1990s. Kim Won of Kwang-Jang Architects designed the Sisters Convent of Korean Martyrs (1993) in Seoul, a brick-faced complex of clear geometric forms. His Gallery Bing and Zo Kunyong's X-Plus Building (1992), both in Seoul, are good examples of ultramodernist work. The 1998 Olympic Games provided a great impetus for architects such as Ilkum and Woo and Williams, who designed a large housing scheme for the Olympic Village. Kyu Sung Woo also designed the elegant Wanki Museum (1993) in Seoul.

In the Philippines, among the post independence (1946) architects were Pablo Antonio with the Gonzaga Building (1957) and Angel Napkil, the Werkbund Exhibition-like National Press Club (1958). The government under Ferdinand Marcos produced ambitious large-scale modernist monumental buildings, many of the best examples of their 20th-century architecture. The leading and most prolific architect was Leandro V. Locsin, who interpreted his heritage through abstraction. Among his works are the Chapel of the Holy Sacrifice (1955) in Quezon City, the Hyatt Regency Hotel (1967), Manila, and the Berguet Center (1984) in Manaluyong. His most important design is the Cultural Center in Manila (1969–76), of which the Theatre of the Performing Arts (1969) is perhaps his best building. Other influential Filipino architects are Gabriel Formoso, Alfredo Luz and Jorge Ramos, and the Manosa Brothers, with their San Miguel Building (1984), Manila. Francisco "Bobby" Manosa's work combines traditional materials, craftsmanship and forms with contemporary needs, as in his Tahanang Pilipino (1984), popularly known as the Coconut Palace due to its use of materials.

Under Soekarno Indonesia's "New Order" nationalism was expressed after independence in 1945 by Modern architecture and Soviet monumentalism. Examples in Jakarta are the National Mosque (1962) by Siliban, the National Monument, a tall stele topped by a golden flame (1945–66), and Gadjah Mada Complex (1977) by Anthony Lumsden. Later, President Soeharto favored architecture of traditional values to establish a unifying identity for the diverse archipelago, and in 1975 Taman Mini Indonesia (Indonesia in Miniature Park) was created to display all the country's vernacular architectural styles.

Firms such as Atelier 6, founded in 1969, designed both modernist buildings such as Lippi Headquarters (1982) in Jakarta and the vernacular-inspired Carita Beach Hotel (1993) in West Java. Additions to ITB (Bandung) in the early 1990s contained neovernacular buildings by Iwan Sudradjat. In 1986 a new University of Indonesia campus at Depok, near Jakarta, planned by The Lempaga Technologi-FTUI, was designed to reflect Javanese-Indonesian forms, with buildings such as the Rectorate Tower (1989) by Gunawan Tjahjono and the Mosque (1992) by Trianto Y. Hardjoko that clearly express this dictate.

Foreign architects continued to build in Thailand with John Carl Warnecke's 1956 U.S. Embassy, Robert-Mathew Johnson-Marshall's Asian Institute of Technology (1968), both in Bangkok, and Kisho Kurokawa's Japan Studies Institute (1985) in Rangsit. The most prominent Thai architect is the English-trained Sumet Jumsai, whose firm SJA + 3D was established in 1969—applying technological innovations to local architecture. Buildings that exemplify his approach are at the Campus of Thammasat University (1986), Rangsit. They are all based on a square grid; most of them are raised above ground or water

and are unified by prominent pitched roofs that lend traditional character. In a very different vein, he explores "high-tech aesthetic" in the Science Museum (1977) and a theory of "robot architecture" (reflecting interaction between humans and machines) in his controversial toy robot like Bank of Asia (1986) and the Nation Building (1991), all in Bangkok. The second important Thai architect is the American-trained Strabandhu Ongard. His later works, the Surijasat (1978) and Khun V. Ed (1983) houses and the Toshiba Headquarters (1986), present an amalgam of Thai and European architecture. Other prominent practitioners include CASA, Suriysat, Tiptus, and Plan Architects.

Elsewhere in the region, Brunei and Vietnam for example, contemporary architecture continues to be dominated by nonnative architects. In Bandar Seri Bagwan, the capital of Brunei, the symbolic Sultan Omar Ali Saifuddin Mosque (1958, architect unknown) expresses Islam, whereas the sultan's palace, Istana Nurul Iman (1984), by Locsin, is a monumental modernist complex. Kenzo Tange produced the new city center (1994) of Ho Chi Minh City and also the Master Plan for Brunei's capital in 1985. Vietnam now sees itself developing an architecture that is characterized by Chinese-influenced shophouses, French boulevards, Soviet housing, and Western-style commercial development. This sense of ecclecticism and overlay is common to much architecture in the region at the beginning of the 21st century.

Two topics provide a reading of the region's architecture today: one is the issue of identity as exemplified through hotel design, and the other is the form of the contemporary Asian city including the ubiquitous skyscraper.

Tourist hotels, which are economically vital for Southeast Asia, usually try to present the culture of the region. They take their clue from vernacular architecture, are built in beautiful settings, and include all comforts. They present an imagined authenticity, using replicated forms, and also stereotype the tourist's notions of the local culture. They are, however, an important modern building type that gives an image of regional homogeneity. Among the earliest is the Tandjung Sari (opened in 1962) in Sanur, Bali, conceived by its owner-operator, Wija Wawo Runtu; the Bali Hyatt (1973, renovated in 1994) also in Sanur, by Palmer and Turner out of Hong Kong; and the Tanjong Jara Beach Hotel (1973–80) on the east coast of Malaysia, by Wimberly, Whisenand, Allison, Tong and Goo of Hawaii. The entrepreneur Adrian Zecha, who with his architects established the "Bali style," has developed some of the most remarkable ones, the Aman Resorts. The American Ed Tuttle designed the Amanpuri (1987) on Phuket Island, Thailand, and the Australian Peter Muller the Amandari (1989) in Ubud, Bali. More recently, alternatives to the Bali style are provided by the ecological emphasis at the Pearl Farms Beach Resort (1994) on Samal Island, Mindanao, Thailand, by Bobby Manosa, and by the search for historical references at the neo–Art Deco hotel Chedi (1993) in Bandung, by Kerry Hill.

High-rise buildings adapted to the region's climate and local technology were developed in the 1980s, and Ken Yeang wrote about and built "bio climatic skyscrapers." Perhaps this is most successfully explored in his award-winning high-tech, metallic office building with its vertically spiraling planting, the Menara Mesiniaga (1992) in Selangor, near Kuala Lumpur, and by Paul Rudolph in his Dharmala Sakti Office (1986) in Jakarta, a tall concrete building of stacked roofs on *pilotis* (stilts) that allow for natural ventilation throughout the building. The skyscraper continues to be the most prominent image of progress and modernity; note Kuala Lumpur's twin Petronas Towers, designed by Cesar Pelli, which at 450 meters, were the tallest buildings in the world on completion in 1998.

Despite these glittering constructions, a majority of the urban population in Southeast Asia is poor and lives, sometimes as squatters, in sprawling settlements. Urban population distribution is distinguished by the presence of one major city—the primate city—of each country, characterized by rapid and uncontrolled growth, as in Jakarta, Bangkok, and Manila. A successful project that deals with the urban situation in Indonesia—the Kampung Improvement Program—was instituted by the government in the late 1970s. Since the 1990s private entrepreneurs have also developed new settlements, as in Lippo Karawaci, near Jakarta, a major urbanism that continues to expand.

The theory of buildings and human settlement in the tropics found its voice (among others in a multitude of disciplines) in architects Shlomo Angel, William Lim, Ken Yeang, and Tay Kheng Soon. Their concern with expressing an abstraction of a pan-Southeast Asian identity, instead basing it on regional or ethnic identity, has led to notions of a modern tropical city. It is likely that their ideas will find form in the 21st century. Tay's Development Guide Plan for Kampung Bugis (1989) and Yeang's JB2005 (1994) are excellent examples of this new thinking.

HASAN-UDDIN KHAN

See also **Petronas Towers, Kuala Lumpur; Tange, Kenzo (Japan)**

Further Reading

Anderson, Benedict and Richard O'Gorman, *The Spectre of Comparisons: Nationalism, Southeast Asia, and the World*, London and New York: Verso, 1998

Architecture and Identity: Proceedings of the Regional Seminar in the Series Exploring Architecture in Islamic Cultures, Singapore: Concept Media, 1983

Beamish, Jane and Jane Ferguson, *A History of Singapore Architecture: The Making of a City*, Singapore: Brash, 1985

Beng, Tan Hock, *Tropical Resorts*, Singapore: Page One, 1995

Broman, Barry Michael, *Old Homes of Bangkok: Fragile Link*, Bangkok: Siam Society, and DD Books, 1984

Jessup, Helen, "Netherlands Architecture in Indonesia, 1900–1942," Ph.D. diss., Courtauld Institute of Art, University of London, 1989

Jumsai, Sumet Chumsai Na 'Aytthaya, *Naga: Cultural Origins in Siam and the West Pacific*, Singapore and New York: Oxford University Press, 1988

Khan, Hasan-Uddin, *Contemporary Asian Architects*, Cologne and New York: Taschen, 1995

Khan, Hasan-Uddin "Architectural Agendas of Identity in Asia," in *Global Cultures and Placemaking in the 21st Century*, Lincoln: University of Nebraska Press, 2000

King, Anthony D., *Colonial Urban Development: Culture, Social Power, and Environment*, London and Boston: Routledge and Paul, 1976

Klassen, Winand W., *Architecture in the Philippines: Filipino Building in a Cross-Cultural Context*, Cebu City, Philippines: University of San Carlos, 1986

Koreana 3, no. 3 (1989) (special architectural issue)

Kultermann, Udo, *Architekten der Dritten Welt*, Cologne: DuMont, 1980

Kultermann, Udo, "Architecture in Southeast Asia," a series of articles in *Mimar: Architecture in Development*, Singapore, "1. Thailand" in *Mimar 20*, Apr. 1986; "2. Indonesia" in *Mimar 21*, Aug. 1986; "3. Singapore" in *Mimar 23*, Mar. 1987; "4. Malaysia" in *Mimar 26*, Dec. 1987

Kusno, Abidin, *Behind the Postcolonial: Architecture, Urban Space, and Political Cultures in Indonesia*, London and New York: Routledge, 2000

Lim, William Siew Wai, *Cities for People: Reflections of a Southeast Asian Architect*, Singapore: Select Books, 1990

Lim, William Siew Wai (editor), *Architecture and Development in Southeast Asia*, Manilla: Solidarity, 1991

Logan, William Stewart, *Hanoi: Biography of a City*, Seattle: University of Washington Press, 2000

Park, Sam Y., *An Introduction to Korean Architecture*, 2 vols., Seoul: Jungwoo Sa, 1991

Powell, Robert, *Innovative Architecture of Singapore*, Singapore: Select Books, 1989

Powell, Robert, *The Asian House: Contemporary Houses of Southeast Asia*, Singapore: Select Books, 1993

Seow, Eugene J., "Architecture in Malaysia," Ph.D. diss., Singapore National University, School of Architecture, 1974

Steinberg, David Joel (editor), *In Search of Southeast Asia: A Modern History*, New York: Praeger, and London: Pall Mall Press, 1971

Tay, Kheng Soon and Akitek Tenggara, *Line, Edge, and Shade: The Search for a Design Language in Tropical Asia*, Singapore: Page One, 1997

Wright, Gwendolyn, *The Politics of Design in French Colonial Urbanism*, Chicago: University of Chicago Press, 1991

Yeang, Ken, *Tropical Urban Regionalism: Building in a South-East Asian City*, Singapore: Concept Media, 1987

Yeang, Ken, *The Architecture of Malaysia*, Amsterdam: Pepin Press, 1992

Yoong, Chan Che (editor), *Post-Merdeka Architecture: Malaysia, 1957–1987*, Kuala Lumpur, Malaysia: Pertubuhan Akitek Malaysia, 1987

SOUTO DE MOURA, EDUARDO 1952–

Architect, Portugal

Among the vanguard of modern Portuguese architects, Eduardo Souto de Moura emerges from a recently revitalized architectural tradition that was singularly rich in the Renaissance and baroque periods. In the transition from the 15th to the 16th centuries, with astounding wealth accruing from a growing number of colonies, Portugal experienced a flourish of late Gothic building. This was the Manueline period, named for Manuel I (reigned 1495–1521) under whom colonies in southern Africa, the Indies, the Far East, and Brazil were discovered and settled. In the 18th century, with gold and diamonds flowing into the country from Brazil, the Portuguese baroque reached one of its most intense periods.

During most of the 20th century though, economically stagnant and politically authoritarian, the only "modern" construction of buildings in Portugal were scattered examples of a neoclassical block-like fascist structures. The impetus for modernist architecture in the Portuguese-speaking world came not from Portugal but from Brazil, primarily with the inauguration in 1960 of Brasília. That futuristic capital's signature structures, the presidential residence, the cathedral, the Congress, and the Foreign Office reflected the influence of Le Corbusier as interpreted with lyrical, tropical exuberance by Lúcio Costa and Oscar Niemeyer. Aesthetically Portugal itself only became free to follow this style after the democratic revolution of 1974. Financially it only became capable of supporting a significant increase in building after admission into the European Union and the consequent growth of its economy.

Souto de Moura was born in the north of Portugal on 25 July 1952 in the country's second-largest city, Porto (also referred to as Oporto). It was there from the *Escola de Belas Artes* that in 1980 he received his degree in architecture. He forms the third generation in the Portuguese architectural "School of Oporto."

This movement originated among young architects at the fine arts school in Porto during the decade of the 1960s, the waning years of the Salazar dictatorship and its debilitating colonial wars in Portuguese Africa. The Atlantic harbor of Porto, lying on the Douro River, is generally known to the outside world for the port wine named after it, which originates from the vineyards in the valley of the Douro. To those who live in Porto, however, the city is known for the industriousness of its small businessmen, merchants, and manufacturers. With the post–World War II growth of European and coastal Atlantic trade, its metropolitan area expanded to half a million people. This growth required much new construction together with significant remodeling of older buildings. Responding to these building and design needs were Portuguese architects trained in the School of Oporto.

The school began with the ideas of Fernando Távora (1923–), seeking in the late 1950s for a modernist building style that was socially responsible and allowed economy in the use of basic forms and materials. This led him to minimalism and Alvar Aalto's concepts regarding discrete yet organically integrated construction elements. The great disciple of Távora was Alvaro Siza Vieira (1933–), whose purist poetic style won him the 1992 Pritzker architecture award. One of the leading students and longtime colleagues of Siza Vieira has been Souto de Moura.

Like his predecessors, much of Souto de Moura's work has been in Porto and cities in the north of Portugal, particularly Braga and Évora. Throughout most of his career he has designed houses, among his most famous works, and commercial spaces. He has also done extensive restoration of historic and domestic structures. He has taught in Zurich and Lausanne, and beginning in the late 1980s his work assumed a more international projection, especially in Italy.

In Porto he has built or restored numerous houses and apartments, medical buildings, a library, a museum, and a customs building. Possessing his own minimalist style, the effectiveness of his work is borne by a subtle juxtaposition of elementary building materials: stone, wood, glass, and metal. He incorporates these elements in structures whose dramatic weight is often conveyed in basic geometric shapes of rectangles, squares, cubes, cylinders, and circles.

Two important early works were the plan for the city market in Braga (1980–84) and the "Casa das Artes" cultural center in Porto (1981–91). The city of Braga has now outgrown the former, and he is redesigning the area as a complex of shops and cafes. The cultural center projected a striking model that concentrated the accumulated design tradition of international modernism.

Most significant, though, was a small weekend home built in the Algarve (1984–89), in the south of Portugal. Its all-white

elements presented a subdued profile of long rectangular walls over which hovered the low silhouette of a dome and, varying with the angle of view, a triangle and cylinder. Occupying only one-fifth of the lot on which it lies, the structure establishes a balance of subdued tensions between itself and its setting.

Of further significance has been a series of residences he has built since the early 1980s in Nevogilde, a developing seaside neighborhood of Porto. On more restricted terrains, these houses also have demonstrated a style achieved through balancing subdued forces of contrast in structure and environment. However, they furthermore demonstrate his command of interiors, a spare equilibrium of the elements of space and light, and a progressive integration of a spectrum of structural elements, stone, wood, and glass, respecting principles of Mies van der Rohe. In Braga he built (1989–94) a two-story house that strikingly balances a stone environment on the lower floor with a glass one on the upper.

Among his more recent and significant challenges have been designing a civic center in Sicily, converting a monastery into a country inn, and redesigning the customs center of Porto. He has received numerous awards and honors in Portugal and abroad, including an Italian one for his use of stone. In 1998 he was the first architect to receive the coveted Portuguese cultural distinction, the Premio Pessoa. In the same year the Swiss-Italian city of Mendrisio mounted a retrospective exhibition of his work, emphasizing his skill for balancing structures in terms of their component parts and their placement within an environment.

EDWARD A. RIEDINGER

See also **Lisbon, Portugal; Malagueira Quarter, Evora, Portugal; Siza Vieira, Alvaro J.M. (Portugal); Tavora, Fernando (Portugal)**

Selected Publications

Temi di progetti; Themes for Projects, Milano: Skira, 1998
"The Art of Being Portuguese," in *On Continuity*, edited by Rosamund Diamond and Wilfried Wang, New York and Cambridge, Massachusetts: 9H, 1995
Souto de Moura, Barcelona: G. Gili, 1990

Further Reading

Allen, Isabel, *Structure as Design: 23 Projects that Wed Structure and Interior Design*, Gloucester, Massachusetts: Rockport, 2000
Angelillo, Antonio, et al., *Eduardo Souto Moura*, Lisbon: Blau, 1994
Ojeda, Oscar Riera (editor), *Ten Houses: Wheeler Kearns Architects*, Gloucester, Massachusetts: Rockport Publishers, 1999
The New Modernists: Six European Architects, VHS video, New York: Michael Blackwood Productions, 1997

SPACE FRAME

A distinctly 20th-century structural form, the space frame is a three-dimensional system that transfers gravitational and lateral loads through a network of interconnected structural elements. In this efficient system, the load path is completely controlled, utilizing mainly straight elements that are securely joined together to safely transfer applied loads to other structural subsystems. The effectiveness of their structural form comes from three factors. First, unlike other structural forms where entire members are sized on the basis of maximum stresses that occur at singular points along their elements, the peak stresses in lattice space structures are distributed more evenly through the use of members transferring mainly tension and compression forces and, as such, requiring smaller cross-sectional profiles. Second, the fact that they are highly indeterminate structures causes stress redistribution in the event of one member or more failing during the life expectancy of such frames. This fact allows for the increase in allowable design code stresses and leads to smaller members. Third, coupled with their structural efficiency, their simplified and repetitive assembly techniques afford them the versatility to take on either flat or curved forms, making them systems of choice for designers and builders.

Space frames are seen as an evolutionary step in the eternal quest for building and spanning more with less natural resources and increased cost-effectiveness. Earlier efforts to construct lighter-weight structural forms included Schwedler's fully triangulated framed domes in 1863. Even the famed Dr. Alexander Graham Bell experimented with such spatial structural forms when, in 1907, he illustrated their effectiveness as structural systems by building a tetrahedron-based frame that could be used for the construction of kites, airplanes, and building structures. In 1942, architect Charles Atwood developed the Unistrut system, consisting of steel elements bolted into a flat gusset plate to form a space frame.

However, the major innovation in space frames came about when Dr. Max Mengeringhausen introduced his Mero system in 1943. His system gave birth to today's space frame technology. Consisting of up to 18 hollow steel tubes that can be screwed into a steel ball at the same time to form a single joint, the system simply and expeditiously builds a huge network of solidly connected members to form a long span structure.

Later, during World War II, the military realized the mass-production and prefabrication potential of such systems and utilized them in such structures as radar domes. In the 1950s, designers such as Konrad Wachsmann were developing space frame systems similar to the Mero. An example of Wachsmann's tetrahedral tubular space frame system is a U.S. Air Force hangar that measured 240 by 155 meters with a 50-meter cantilevered roof extending in both directions. Buckminster Fuller also invented geodesic domes known as "tensegrity" structures that became very popular optimal building forms in the 1960s and 1970s and led to the publication of the do-it-yourself books *Domebook One* and *Domebook Two*.

Expo '67 in Montreal featured space frame structures that opened the eyes of designers and builders alike to the potential of such building forms. The 1970s witnessed an eruption of space frames being used for airplane hangars, huge roofing systems, and efficient building frames. The British Airways 01 hangar at Heathrow Airport, designed by professor Z.S. Makowski, is a primary example of large roofing construction. The hangar spans 135 meters, accommodates two jumbo jets at the same time, utilizes tubular hollow sections, and can be mechanically jacked up in anticipation of future larger aircraft. The Interfirst Bank Building (1981) in Dallas, Texas, designed by Skidmore, Owings and Merrill, is an example of the versatility in the form design of space frame, which matched the half-pyramid shape of the building itself.

The advent of faster and more accessible computational power to structural engineers allowed for an explosion in the

amount of shape complexity and design optimization of those structural forms. The Javits Convention Center (1987) in New York City, designed by I.M. Pei and Partners, is a primary example of how computer analyses allowed the creation of such complex building shapes.

The attractive properties of high strength-to-weight ratios and considerable torsional stiffness did not escape the ever-watchful eyes of the aerospace industry, which started utilizing the technology in their air-space frames. At the same time, the car manufacturing industries began as early as the 1950s utilizing space frames in their high-performance car chassis. Today, Audi's A8 luxury car uses a very sophisticated form of aluminum space frame for its chassis. The frame was designed in concert with Alcoa and required 40 patents, ten years, and seven new aircraft aluminum alloys.

The National Aeronautics and Space Administration also invested for decades in space frame research. The result is its U.S. Laboratory module for the International Space Station currently under construction at the Marshall Space Flight Center station manufacturing facility in Huntsville, Alabama. However, perhaps the epitome of computer and space frame construction technologies coming together is the Fremont Street Experience Light and Sound Show in Las Vegas, Nevada. A 90-foot-high steel space frame, completed in September 1995, provides a high-tech display canopy over a 1,400-foot stretch of the Fremont Street and serves also as a spectacular foyer for existing casino and hotel resorts in the Las Vegas downtown district. The frame is arched, being 5 feet deep and 44 feet in curved radius. The inside of the canopy contains 2.1 million light bulbs acting like television pixels and fully controlled by 21 computers generating animated images perfectly syncopated to sound. The computer-generated light and sound show is produced using concert-quality sound emanating from a system of 208 speakers capable of generating 540,000 watts. Unofficially, this space frame is considered to be the world's largest graphics display system.

Today, there are tens of thousands of space frames all over the world. The future likely will witness an even greater reliance on space frame construction for the simple reason that computer, materials, manufacturing, and construction technologies are constantly evolving and successfully thriving to reduce cost with improved products. As such, in the very near future, architects, structural designers, and builders will have the option of designing and building space frames out of materials that are far superior in strength and much lower in weight than any of the currently conventional materials and methods. Primary examples of such construction materials are fiber-reinforced plastic composites. Their industry is extremely prolific, and they are lightweight, corrosion resistant, and ideal for tailoring their fiber orientations to optimally resist principal stresses induced under any loading conditions.

ZOUHEIR A. HASHEM

Further Reading

Mainstone, Rowland J., *Developments in Structural Form*, London: Allen Lane, and Cambridge, Massachusetts: MIT Press, 1975; 2nd edition, Boston and Oxford: Architectural Press, 1998

Moore, Fuller, *Understanding Structures*, Boston and London: McGraw-Hill, 1999

Wilkinson, Chris, *Supersheds: The Architecture of Long-Span, Large-Volume Buildings*, Oxford and Boston: Butterworth Architecture, 1991; 2nd edition, 1996

Wilson, Forrest, "Space Frames" in *Encyclopedia of Architecture: Design, Engineering, and Construction*, edited by Joseph A. Wilkes and Robert T. Packard, vol. 4, New York and Chichester, West Sussex: Wiley, 1988

SPAIN

Spanish architecture of the 20th century has exhibited a dynamic eclecticism that is rooted in the country's turbulent political history and in the persistent individualism of its historically autonomous provinces. The Castilian capital of Madrid and the Catalonian capital of Barcelona were the epicenters of the nation's architectural achievement throughout much of the century, each having gained international recognition for both their architecture schools and their architects of distinction.

By the early 20th century, Barcelona's dramatic population growth prompted city officials to address its urban expansion through an international competition that was ultimately won by the French Beaux-Arts architect Léon Jaussely (1875–1932), whose scheme was modified for implementation in 1917. At the same time, Antoni y Cornet Gaudí's (1852–1926) idiosyncratic use of Art Nouveau, Gothic, and Moorish influences, evident in such projects as the Sagrada Familia (Expiatory Church of the Holy Family, 1882–1926), dominated Catalan *modernisme*, a regional movement characterized by an interest in aesthetic and political separatism coupled with a respect for traditional craftsmanship and a personalized vocabulary of ornamentation. His structural experimentation and militant interest in creating a distinctively regional form of architecture had a profound impact on his contemporaries, Lluís Domènech i Montaner (1849–1923) and Josep Puig i Cadafalch (1869–1957), as well as subsequent generations of Barcelonese architects.

Antonio Palacios y Ramilo (1876–1945) was the primary architectural force in the Spanish capital of Madrid. His grandiose Palacio de Correos y Communicaciones (1918) went beyond the city's Beaux-Arts classicism and its neo-Plateresque references in its free use of space and light as well as in its indebtedness to the Wagnerschule of Vienna. Palacios' role as a professor at the Escuela de Arquitectura de Madrid (ETSAM) and as an academician of the Real Academia de Bellas Artes de San Fernando ensured his impact on early 20th-century Madrileño architecture; his brand of Beaux-Arts eclecticism came to populate the Gran Vía, a major artery through the city's old slums that was created between 1910 and 1930.

Fernando García Mercadal (1895–1984), a 1921 graduate of ETSAM, led the group of young architects known as the "Generation of 1925" to embrace contemporary architectural avant-gardism after spending four years traveling on a Pensión de Roma (Rome Prize) study grant. His encounters with Peter Behrens (1920), Josef Hoffmann (1924), Le Corbusier (1925), and Adolf Loos (1927) led him to introduce certain rationalist tendencies in such projects as his small pavilion, the Rincón de Goya (1928, demolished in the Spanish civil war), in Zaragoza. In April of the same year, García Mercadal edited an issue of *La Gaceta Literaria* (The Literary Gazette) that was dedicated solely to the theme "New Art in the World: Architecture, 1928"

and that featured an illustrated survey of the Dessau Bauhaus, quoted passages by Henry Van de Velde and Ludwig Mies van der Rohe, as well as essays written by some of García Mercadal's leading contemporaries. The group's crowning achievement, the Madrid university campus (1936), reconciled avant-garde eclecticism with the new rationalism but was largely destroyed during the Spanish civil war (1936–39).

Bauhaus utopianism directly impacted the Spanish architectural scene of the 1930s after Mies van der Rohe inaugurated his German Pavilion at the Barcelona International Exhibition of 1929. Standing for less than eight months, this linchpin of 20th-century avant-gardism provided a fluid architectural space of glass, water, marble, and travertine and came to epitomize the precepts of the International Style.

The creation in 1930 of the *Grupo de Arquitectos y Técnicos Españoles para la Arquitectura Contemporánea* (GATEPAC) in Zaragoza was of significant importance to the promotion in Spain of utopian modernism by the *Congrès Internationaux d'Architecture Moderne* (CIAM) and the *Comité International pour la Réalisation des Problèmes d'Architecture Contemporaine* (CIRPAC). GATEPAC's rationalist aims, articulated in the magazine *A.C.* (1931–27) and manifested in the early works of the Catalonian Josep Lluís Sert (1902–83), came to be associated with the International Style and especially the architecture of Le Corbusier. The Catalonian group of GATEPAC forged direct connections with the Swiss visionary: at the Fourth CIRPAC Congress, Le Corbusier assisted the group in designing a new urban study for the city of Barcelona (Macià plan, 1935).

The rise of modernist architecture was stemmed by the Spanish civil war and the establishment of the Franco regime (1939–75), which ultimately resulted in the dissolution of GATEPAC and the exodus of many of the nation's leading architects, including Sert, who became dean of Harvard University's Graduate School of Design. Architects remaining in Spain were disconnected from the world's architectural community: access to documentation and foreign-language publications was minimized under Franco's censors, and much of the Madrid Architecture Library had been destroyed during the war years. Public building projects encouraged during the early years of the dictatorship were generally antimodernist, with autarchic tendencies gleaned from the classical architectural tradition in Spain, in which mimetic references to Rome's legacy on the Iberian peninsula and Philip II's El Escorial (1582, Juan Bautista Toledo and Juan de Herrera), the Renaissance palace and monastery outside Madrid, were highly desirable. The Catalan-born José Antonio Coderch y de Sentmenat (1913–84) was the most remarkable architect of the period. His ability to reconcile GATEPAC-era rationalism, the vernacular traditions of Mediterranean villa architecture, the Scandinavian organicism of Eric Gunnar Asplund and Alvar Aalto, and the austere outlines and creative spatial layouts of Bruno Zevi resulted in private seaside homes of great ingenuity. His use of local materials, in many instances brick and tile, along with a so-called deep plan, became characteristics of the later Barcelona School (e.g., Ugalde House, 1952, in Caldes d'Estrac; Apartment Building, 1954, in La Barceloneta).

During the early 1950s, Spain's autarchic isolationist philosophy dissipated; new interchanges were established with democratic nations, and Spain's economic system was bolstered by a new liberalism and a sizable monetary credit from the United States.

In Barcelona, "Group R" (1951–59) sought an imbrication of the regional Catalonian architectural tradition with the rationalist idiom of such exiled architects as Sert. Meeting formally for some eight years and organizing courses such as "Economics and Urban Development" and "Sociology and Urban Development," this group eventually transformed into the so-called Barcelona School. Studio Per, Josep Martorell Codina (1925–), Ricardo Bofill Levi (1939–), Oriol Bohigas Guardiola (1925–), and others were able to explore the Group R ideals of rationalism and "poetic realism" under the Franco regime primarily through commissions from the private sector (such as Editorial Gustavo Gili, 1961, Bassó and Gili; Argentona House, 1955, Martorell and Bohigas; and Meridiana Building, 1966, MBM). The Barcelona School came to reject the notion of a utopian industrialized society and sought to redefine local and traditional construction processes; as such, it was especially influenced by English New Brutalism and Italian neorealism.

Contemporary attempts to establish connections with international modernism remained isolated in Madrid and were dependent on the influx of translated versions of such authors as Zevi and Sigfried Giedion and the increasing ability for Spaniards to travel outside the Iberian peninsula. Historian Juan Daniel Fullaondo, inspired especially by the antirationalist leanings of Zevi, sought to create a new Madrid School around the peri-

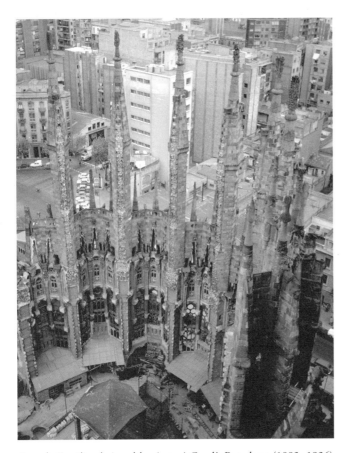

Sagrada Familia, designed by Antoni Gaudí, Barcelona (1882–1926)
© Donald Corner and Jenny Young/GreatBuildings.com

odical *Nueva Forma* (New Form), and the Galician architect Alejandro de la Sota (1913–) adopted an essentialist language far removed from the Franco regime's ideological framework of isolation and tradition (for example Gobierno Civil, 1957, in Tarragona). Nonetheless, it was not until José Antonio Corrales (1921–) and Ramón Vázquez Molezún (1922–) unified a simple geometric form on an irregular multileveled site at the Exposition Universelle et Internationale in Brussels that a new era of freedom in Spanish architecture was launched (Spanish Pavilion, 1958, World Expo).

From the 1960s on, as the urban fabric of Spain's leading cities continued to stretch along with the nation's economic expansion, many of its architects became increasingly engaged in solving problems associated with postindustrial urbanization, such as public housing, integration between architecture and landscape, and the design of transportation infrastructures. The cities of Barcelona, Madrid, and Bilbao became epicenters of public architecture with a social conscience as their perimeters burgeoned with shantytowns of displaced workers from the country's impoverished regions. A prominent advocate of the primacy of the individual in an urban context, Coderch devoted the last decade of his life to reconciling the autonomous apartment unit with the unified apartment block. After nearly three decades of isolation from the world scene, Spanish architecture as a whole became more widely disseminated in publications and exhibitions and more prominently recognized as an increasing number of the nation's architects began to gain international attention and acclaim.

General Franco's death in November 1975 propelled Spanish culture into a period of significant changes; especially marked was the change from an authoritarian regime to a constitutional monarchy and a democratic state as well as the partial restoration of the nation's historically autonomous provinces, which resulted in a renewed fervor to mark the built environment with an emphatically regionalist aesthetic. Additionally, the country's architecture schools notably underwent significant modifications: increased staffing by professional architects, greater specialization and diversification, and an interest in redefining the architectural school as an intellectual forum. In the early 1970s, the contemporary design theories of Aldo Rossi's *L'architettura della città* (1966; *Architecture and the City*) and Robert Venturi's *Complexity and Contradiction in Architecture* (1966) became available in Castilian translations, and a number of new Spanish architectural publications emerged, most notably the Italian-influenced *2C Construcción de la Ciudad* (1972–85; Construction of the City) and the more pragmatic Catalonian *Arquitectura Bis* (1974 and later).

Oriol Bohigas, who in 1981 became the director of urbanism for the City of Barcelona, promoted a regionalist urbanization program for the Catalonian capital. In the process, much of the city was redesigned, and its distinctive neighborhoods, or barrios, were revitalized with new plazas and parks. Helio Piñón (1942–) and Alberto Viaplana's (1933–) minimalist Plaça dels Països Catalans (1983, also called the Plaza de la Estación de Sants, designed along with Enric Miralles) was the first of a series of urban spaces called *plazas duras* ("hard" squares) created under Bohigas' administration that helped establish Barcelona as a leading center of modern urban renewal and the host for the 1992 summer Olympic Games.

In 1986, the Andalusian capital of Seville was officially proclaimed the site of the 1992 Universal Exposition commemorating the fifth centenary of the discovery of America. This selection, as in the case of Barcelona, prompted a large-scale urban-renewal program that included the redesign of the city's transportation and communication infrastructures and the renovation of the so-called La Cartuja district, a man-made "island" along the Guadalquivir River. Neorationalist adherent Rafael Moneo (1937–) sensitively designed the new airport to reflect its Sevillian roots, with austere Moorish-inspired arches and a series of blue domes illuminated by a central oculus. Moneo's former students Antonio Cruz Villalón and Antonio Ortiz García created the Santa Justa Railway Station, a project that aligned the new transportation hub with a distinctively Spanish Postmodernism.

The Franco regime's continued promotion of mimetic architectural historicism deterred many young Spanish architects of the 1980s from utilizing a postmodernist idiom; however, Bofill and Oscar Tusquets (1941–) adopted postmodern tendencies that are evident in the former's INEF Building (1991) and the latter's Más Abello Housing Complex (1990), both in Barcelona. A more expressive architectural language, the inheritor of the legacy of Antoni Gaudí, was adopted by the Valencia-born Santiago Calatrava (1951–), whose bridge and recent museum designs are neosurrealist versions of avian osteomorphic forms.

In the latter decades of the century, both public and private sectors have contributed significantly to the advance of innovative architecture by employing progressive young architects. Regions such as the Basque provinces, Andalusia, and Valencia—bolstered by the economic expansion correlated to the nation's acceptance into the European community in 1986—have promoted highly individualized and internationally recognized building projects, including Frank Gehry's titanium-sheathed Guggenheim Museum (1997) in Bilbao and Giorgio Grassi's University Library (1999) on the Nou-Campus in Valencia.

KELI E. RYLANCE

See also **Barcelona, Spain; Bofill, Ricardo (Spain); Calatrava, Santiago (Spain); Coderch y de Sentmenat, José Antonio (Spain); Gaudí, Antoni (Spain); Moneo, Rafael (Spain); Sert, Josep Lluís (United States)**

Further Reading

Baldellou, Miguel Ángel, and Antón Capitel, *Arquitectura española del siglo XX*, (Vol. 40 of Summa Artis), Madrid: Espasa Calpe, 1995.

Capitel, Antón. *Arquitectura española: años 50-años 80*, Madrid: MOPU Arquitectura 1986

Fernández Alba, Antonio. *La crisis de la arquitectura española, 1939–1972*, Madrid: Edicusa, 1972

Flores, Carlos, and Xavier Güell, *Arquitectura de España 1929/1996*, Barcelona: Caja de Arquitectos Fundación, 1996

Montaner, Josep Mª, *Después del movimiento moderno. Arquitectura de la segunda mitad del siglo XX*, Barcelona: Editorial Gustavo Gili, 1999

Ruiz Cabrero, Gabriel, *Spagna: architettura, 1965–88*, Milan: Electa, 1989

Saliga, Pauline, and Martha Thorne (editors), *Building in a New Spain: Contemporary Spanish Architecture*, Chicago: The Art Institute of Chicago, 1992

Solà-Morales, Ignacio, and Antón Capitel, *Birkhäuser Architectural Guide Spain 1920–1999*, Basel: Birkhäuser Verlag, 1998

Zabalbeascoa, Anatxu, *The New Spanish Architecture*, New York: Rizzoli, 1992

ST. PETERSBURG (LENINGRAD), RUSSIA

At the beginning of the 20th century, St. Petersburg was in the midst of a transformation of commercial and living space that had begun in the 1860s and would continue until World War I. Although the great imperial monuments remained standing, practically everything around them was rebuilt during this period in an eclectic array of architectural styles, including the style moderne. The densely constructed St. Petersburg environment consisted of buildings within a city plan that followed the straightedge wherever its deltaic terrain permitted. The city's height restrictions, which limited most construction at five or six stories, also encouraged perspectival uniformity.

In this setting, the plasticity of structure and material that characterized the style moderne in Moscow frequently assumed a two-dimensional form that depended on the texture and shaping of the facade of contiguous apartment buildings. Of the several hundred building projects undertaken in the city between 1898 and 1915, only a small fraction applied the new style in anything other than a fragmentary, decorative manner. There were, nonetheless, architects whose work defined a distinctive variant of the new style known as the "Northern moderne." Fedor Lidval (1870–1945) was the most productive among them, and his career ranged from the early moderne to the more austere neoclassical revival. Lidval's buildings—primarily large apartment houses and banks—also illustrate the developing links between large construction projects and private capital resources in St. Petersburg.

Among other architects active in the apartment construction boom, the work of Aleksei Bubyr is notable for its original approach to structure as a sculpted, textured block. A 1902 graduate of the Institute of Civil Engineering, Bubyr often collaborated with the architect Nikolai Vasilev, who also designed a number of large housing projects in St. Petersburg. Yet Bubyr himself developed a distinctive interpretation of the rationalist side of the style moderne, with equal attention to aesthetics and engineering. In the latter area, he was a pioneer in the use of reinforced concrete for the walls as well as the floor construction of apartment buildings, and this familiarity with new construction methods is reflected in the free style of even his largest structures.

The apartment house that Bubyr built in 1910–12 on the Fontanka Quay (no. 159) is striking not only for its lack of ornamentation but also for its massive outline, looming above the largest of St. Petersburg's canals. In constructing the facade, Bubyr resorted to the familiar device of unfinished granite on the lower surface, but only to the level of the first-floor window ledge. For the most part, the walls are covered with gray roughcast, yet the facade is framed by a top floor and corner bays of smooth, light stucco that produce a clarity of line and a bright exterior. Bubyr emphasized the tectonic character of the building with multistoried window bays that define the vertical lines of the facade and at the same time provide more light for the

main rooms of each apartment. The upper stories culminate in a complex line, beginning as a mansard roof with low, narrow dormers (in effect, a seventh story) and rising at the corners to high gables and a series of pyramidal forms covered by ceramic roofing tiles.

The style moderne also appeared in the design of public buildings for banking and commerce. The most notable landmark of early 20th-century commercial architecture is the headquarters of the Singer Sewing Machine Company (1902–04), at the corner of Nevskii Prospekt and the Catherine Canal. Its architect, Pavel Siuzor (1844–c.1919), had established a career remarkable not only for prodigious output (some 100 original projects and reconstructions, of which more than 60 are extant) but also for its success in adapting to stylistic and technical innovations. Among the technical advances in the Singer Building is the use of something approaching a skeletal structural system, although not the steel frame of the type widely used in the United States. The exterior facades are supported with a ferroconcrete and brick frame, and the interior floors (also reinforced concrete) rest on iron columns. By surfacing the arcade of the first two floors with rusticated blocks of polished red granite and using a lighter, gray granite for the upper stories, Siuzor created a visual base for the structure, which rises in granite-surfaced piers and glass window shafts that extend from the third to the sixth floor in a secondary arcade pattern. The culminating element of the building is the elongated metal-ribbed and glass cupola, which could be illuminated to advertise the Singer logo.

By 1910 the style moderne had yielded to various modernized forms inspired by classical and Renaissance motifs, such as the Azov-Don Bank (1908–09) and the Hotel Astoria (1911–12), both by Fedor Lidval; the Mertens Building (1922–12) by Marian Lialevich (1876–1944); the Guards' Economic Society department store (1908–09) by Ernest Virrikh (1860–after 1921), Stepan Krichinskii (1874–1923), and Nikolai Vasilev; the Vavelberg banking building (1910–12) by Marian Peretiatkovich (1872–1916); and various apartment buildings by Vladimir Shchuko (1878–1938) and Andrei Belogrud (1875–1933). Perhaps the most accomplished architect of the neoclassical revival was Ivan Fomin (1872–1936), who specialized in the design of private houses but also conceived of an enormous apartment development known as New Petersburg (1911–12), only a few buildings of which were completed before World War I.

After the outbreak of World War I, the overheated Russian economy led to a collapse of the construction industry. The monumental buildings that had been erected by the hundreds in the preceding decades could no longer be maintained. In addition, the terror of the 1918–21 civil war led to the almost total collapse of services and infrastructure in Petrograd, as the city was called after 1914. After the death of Lenin, the name was changed again, to Leningrad, in 1924.

Under the direction of Sergei Kirov, the city began to recover from its precipitous economic and political decline after the revolution. Although the historic central districts of the city remained largely intact by virtue of a comprehensive preservation policy and the limited resources of an abandoned capital, Constructivist architecture began to appear in the late 1920s in the design of administrative and cultural centers for the city's largest outer districts, where workers' housing was under construction. One of the earliest examples was Moscow-Narva District House

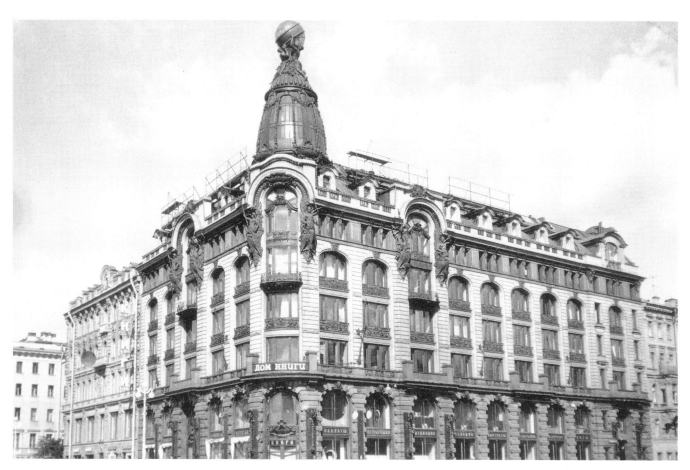

Singer Sewing Machine Company building, designed by Pavel Siuzor (1904)
© William C. Brumfield

of Culture (1925–27; later renamed the Gorkii Palace of Culture) by Alexander Gegello and David Krichevskii. Essentially a symmetrical structure designed around a wedge-shaped amphitheater of 1,900 seats, the compact building demonstrated the beginnings of a functional monumentality dictated by actual circumstances—circumstances that had been ignored in the earlier Workers' Palace and Palace of Labor competitions.

The construction of a number of model projects occurred in the same district, including workers' housing (1925–27), by Gegello and others, on Tractor Street; a department store and "factory-kitchen" (1929–30; to eliminate the need for cooking at home), built in a streamlined early Bauhaus style by Armen Barutchev and others; and the Tenth Anniversary of October School (1925–27), designed by Aleksandr Nikolskii, on Strike Prospekt. The centerpiece of the district (subsequently renamed Kirov) was the House of Soviets (1930–34), designed by Noi Trotskii. Its long four-story office block, defined by horizontal window strips, ends on one side in a perpendicular wing with a rounded facade and on the other in a severely angular ten-story tower with corner balconies.

A similarly austere, unadorned style emphasizing the basic geometry of forms was adopted by Igor Ivanovich Fomin and A. Daugul for the Moscow District House of Soviets (1931–35) on Moscow Prospekt. Yet the facade, composed of segmented windows of identical size, signifies the repetition of an incipient bureaucratic style rather than the streamlined dynamic of earlier Constructivist work. During the same period (1931–35), Igor Fomin and Evgenii Levinson designed an apartment complex for use by the Leningrad Soviet in the fashionable prerevolutionary Petrograd district, on the bank of the Karpovka River near Kamennoostrovskii Prospekt (subsequently renamed after Kirov). With an open passageway supported by granite columns in the center of the curved facade, the design echoes the work of Moisei Ginzburg and, especially, of Le Corbusier. A stylobate of gray granite provides a base for the rest of the structure, whose facade is coated in artistic concrete with a scored surface. The careful attention to such details of architectural and decorative design is unusual for this period and indicates the privileged status of the city bureaucrats for whom the structure was built.

The 1935 Leningrad city plan, devised by Lev Ilin and modified in the late 1930s by Nikolai Baranov, involved a shift from the historical central districts to a new grand avenue—Moscow Prospekt—leading to the south and to a proposed administrative complex centered on the House of Soviets. This building, and the plaza surrounding it, formed the most grandiose project of the 1930s (if one considers the Moscow Palace of Soviets to have been, in effect, utopian). Ultimately, the project was reduced in scale, and the outbreak of war curtailed construction still further,

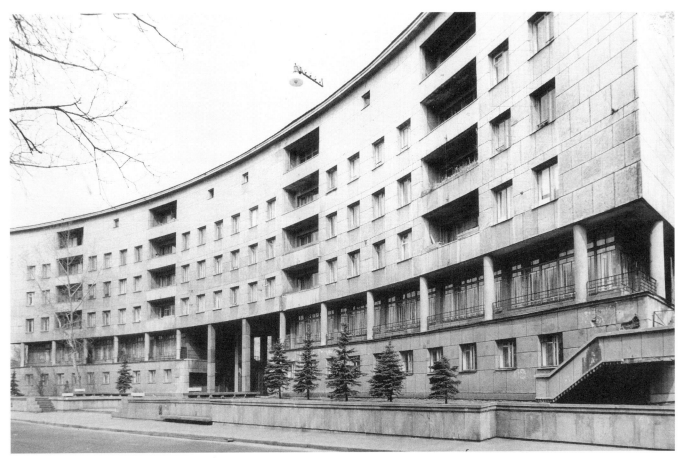

New Petersburg Apartment Building, by Ivan Fomin and E. Levenson (1912)
© William C. Brumfield

but the House of Soviets (1936–41), designed by an architectural collective headed by Noi Trotskii, was completed in the purest form of totalitarian monumentality: 220 meters long and 150 meters deep. The central facade is marked by 20 attached columns, above which is a massive frieze depicting scenes from the construction and defense of the socialist homeland. The design attempted to draw on the legacy of classical architecture and city planning in St. Petersburg with its open squares and monumental facades and at the same time to supersede that legacy by sheer exaggeration of scale.

The outbreak of World War II found Leningrad catastrophically unprepared. Surrounded by German and Finnish forces during the 900-day siege, the city was subjected to almost constant artillery bombardment. With the breaking of the siege in early 1944, architects and construction teams immediately began the process of restoring not only the great monuments but also the city's apartment buildings.

In the post-Stalinist period, most of the city's growth occurred in large housing projects of standardized design on the outskirts of the historic center, which itself remained relatively well preserved. Following the collapse of the Soviet Union in 1991, the decline in funding for city services led to a crisis in maintaining the many prerevolutionary apartment buildings that provide the city with its urban texture. In addition, eco-

nomic stagnation and lack of investment have hampered the development of innovative architectural concepts. Under these circumstances, the primary goal is to preserve and renovate the architectural legacy of a time when St. Petersburg was one of Europe's great capitals.

WILLIAM C. BRUMFIELD

See also **Ginzburg, Moisei (Russia); Russia and the USSR**

Further Reading

Brumfield, William C., *The Origins of Modernism in Russian Architecture*, Berkeley: University of California Press, 1991
———, *A History of Russian Architecture*, Cambridge and New York: Cambridge University Press, 1993
Ginzburg, Abram M., and Boris Kirikov, *Arkhitektory-stroiteli Sankt-Peterburga serediny XIX–nachala XX veka: Spravochnik* (Architect-Builders of St. Petersburg from the Middle of the 19th Century to the Beginning of the 20th), St. Petersburg: Piligrim, 1996
Kirichenko, Evgeniia Ivanova, *Russkaia arkhitektura, 1830–1910-kh godov* (Russian Architecture, 1830–1910), Moscow: Iskusstvo, 1978; 2nd edition, 1982 (summary in English)
Petrov, Anatoli Nikolaevich, et al., *Pamiatniki arkhitektury Leningrada* (Monuments of Architecture of Leningrad), Leningrad: Stroiizdat, 1958; 4th edition, 1975

Ruble, Blair, *Leningrad: Shaping a Soviet City*, Berkeley: University of California Press, 1990

Schlögel, Karl, *Jenseits des Grossen Oktober: Das Laboratorium der Moderne, Petersburg, 1909–1921*, Berlin: Siedler, 1988

STADIUM

Today, major cities heatedly debate the need for new structures for their most prominent inhabitants: their athletic teams. As sports have become primary generators of revenue for cities, the cutting-edge stadium has become an earmark of a city on the move. Hellmuth, Obata, and Kassabaum, Inc., Sports Facilities Group (HOK) has been the trendsetter in contemporary stadium design since 1983. With 1400 architects, the company now is building consistently enough to create divisions based around different sports, including hockey, basketball, baseball, football, and soccer. HOK, based in Kansas City, Missouri, is responsible for Oriole Park at Camden Yards, which defined a return in baseball to traditional ballparks. Perfectly suited to alternative agenda in the postmodern era, contemporary designers must walk careful lines between tradition and cutting-edge enhancements to the sports spectacle.

The first modern stadium appeared in Victoria, Britain, in the late 1890s. However, there was obviously a precedent even before this: The ancestral prototypes for modern facilities are the stadiums and hippodromes of ancient Greece. Here, Olympic and other sporting contests were staged, starting in the eighth century B.C. Greek stadiums, which could be found in many larger cities, were laid out in a U shape, with the straight end forming the starting line for races. Some also followed the model of theaters and were built into hillsides. Other forms during this early history included Roman amphitheaters and circuses.

In the late 1800s, designers began experimenting with more modern facilities, although they often relied on classical models. Ballparks for the nation's most popular sport, baseball, took shape in many cities. In the early 1900s, the ballparks in many cities were used separately by major-league players and Negro-league players. From the era of the smaller ballpark, the next epoch emerged in the form of great stadiums, such as New York's Yankee Stadium (1923), Philadelphia's Shibe Park (1909), Chicago's Wrigley Field (1926) and Comiskey Park (1910), and Boston's Fenway Park (1912), to name just a few. The forms that today are called stadiums, ballparks, or sports facilities would not appear until the 1940s. After World War II, a new wave of stadium building shifted to multipurpose facilities with partial

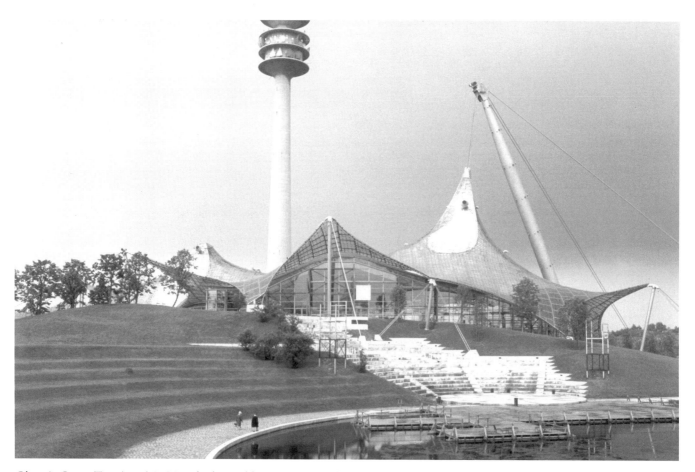

Olympic Games Tent (1972) in Munich, designed by Gunter Behnisch
© GreatBuildings.com

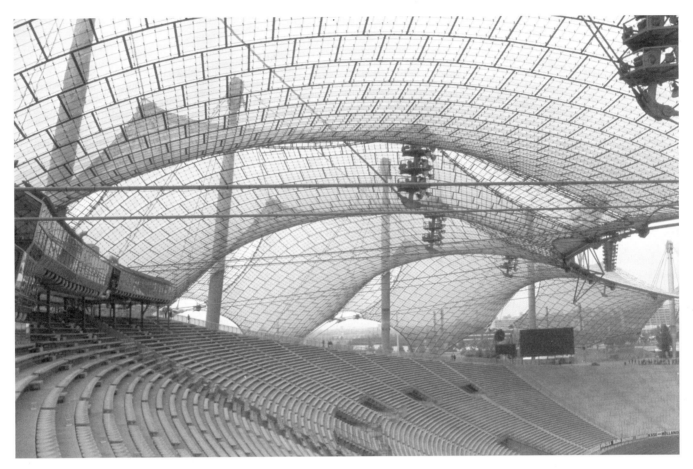

Detail of Munich Olympic Games tent (1972)
© GreatBuildings.com

roofs. The Oakland Coliseum, Shea Stadium, and others were often located in suburban areas and surrounded by acres of car parking. In addition to baseball, such stadiums could be used for football and public gatherings, such as concerts.

The multipurpose form of stadium had its origins in the enclosed dome. The originator of this form was the Houston Astrodome, which opened in 1964. Judge Roy Hofheinz, with the quirky idea of combining attending a sports event with going to a cocktail party, designed the dome around the idea of sky-boxes. These private boxes allowed high-paying clients to attend games without interacting with other fans. A young pitcher for the Houston Astros bounded into the stadium in April 1965, taking in the miracles of the dome: air conditioning, grass growing indoors (artificial turf would be laid in 1966), the translucent roof (greenhouse by day, a planetarium by night), and seating for 66,000.

Many traditionalists viewed attending baseball in air-conditioned splendor as a travesty. The players, however, were most critical of the roof, the panels of which created a glare that made it impossible to see the ball. The league tried changing the color of the ball, but to no avail. The team painted over the roof panels, banishing the sun and killing the grass—Tifway 419 Bermuda, which had been specially developed by scientists in Georgia. For the rest of the season, the Astros simply painted over the dead grass. Following the season, Monsanto's new artificial turf, renamed AstroTurf, was installed. By 1973, five more stadiums would have synthetic surfaces, and many others would follow.

Other domes would follow, including the Louisiana Super-dome, the largest dome when it was built in 1975, with a seating capacity of 76,800. Although traditionalists would wage war against domes and artificial turf, there was practical value to the controlled environment. Particularly when professional sports became more concerned with moneymaking, these technologies reduced the games' dependence on weather and made these events more appealing for family and business groups. The effort to reconcile these needs led to some significant innovations, including the retractable domed roof, which was first installed in the Toronto Skydome, designed by Canadian architects Rod Robbie and Michael Allen in 1989. As a site for concerts and other sports events, including Canadian Football League games, in addition to baseball, this stadium featured movable lower stands and a retractable AstroTurf surface that permits a baseball-to-football conversion in 12 hours' time. Large, domed sports stadiums continue to be built around the world, including Milwaukee's Miller Park (2001, HKS, Inc., Dallas; NBBJ of Los Angeles; and others) and the Osaka Dome (1997, Nikken Sekkei). From 1965, when the Houston Astrodome was opened,

PLATE liii

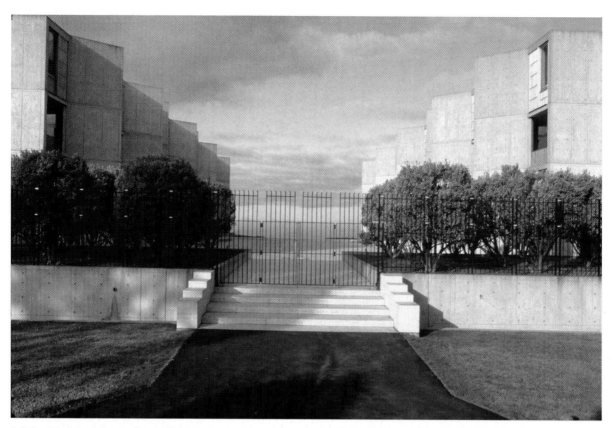

Salk Institute (1966), La Jolla, California
Designed by Louis I. Kahn (United States)
© GreatBuildings.com

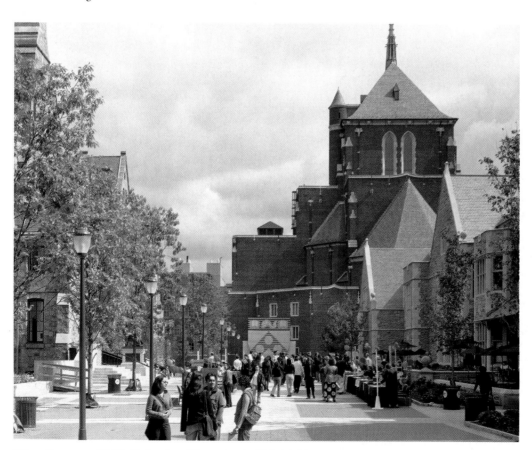

Wynn Commons (2000), University of Pennsylvania, Philadelphia
Designed by Denise Scott Brown of Venturi, Scott Brown and Associates (United States)
© Matt Wargo. Photo courtesy Venturi, Scott Brown and Associates

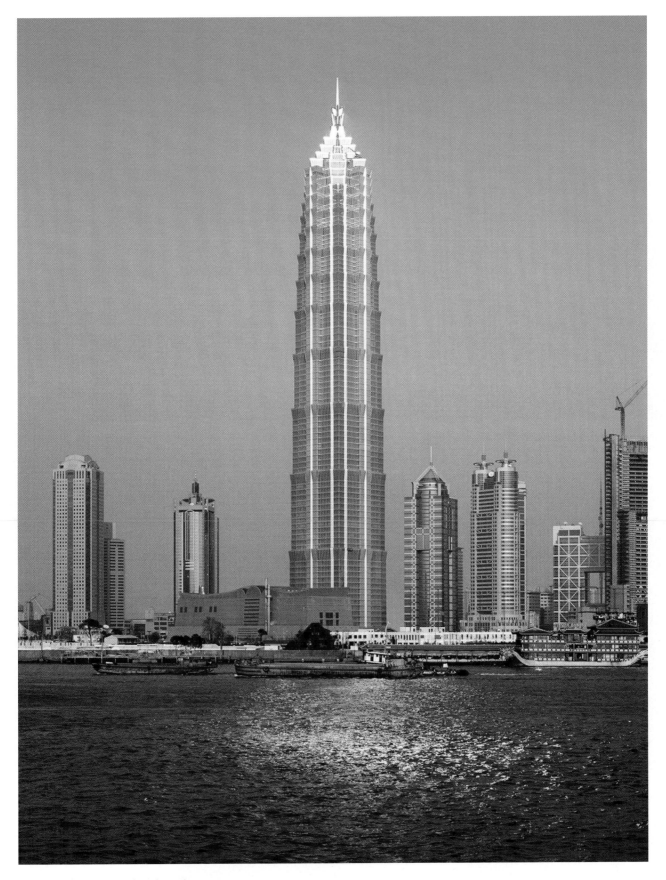

Jin Mao Tower (1998), Shanghai, China
Designed by Skidmore, Owings and Merrill (United States)
© China Jin Mao Group. Photo courtesy S.O.M., LLP, Chicago, Illinois

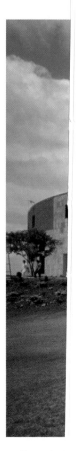

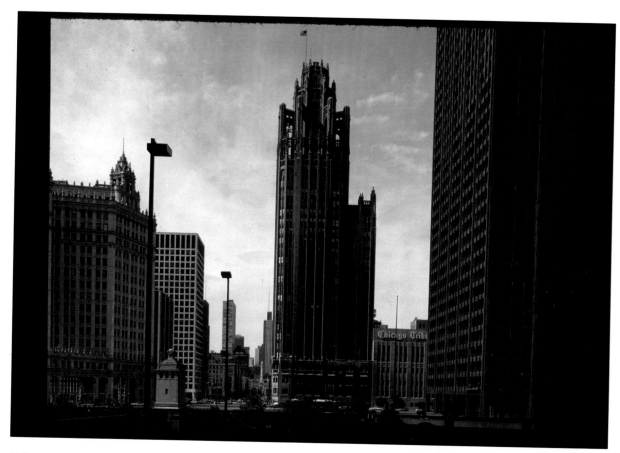

Vidhan Bhav
Designed by
© Aga Khan

Tribune Tower (1925), Chicago, Illinois
Designed by Raymond M. Hood and John Mead Howells (United States)
© GreatBuildings.com

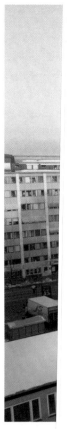

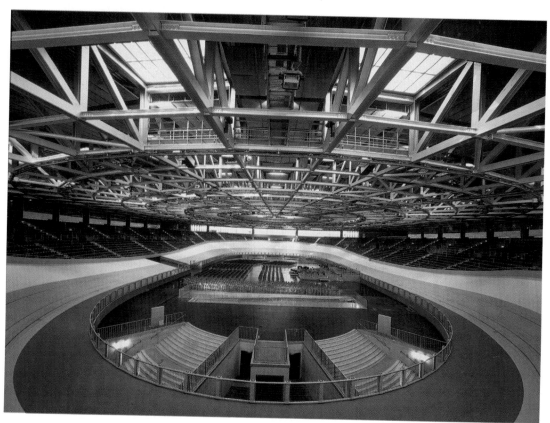

Stockholm
Designed b
© Lennart

Berlin Olympic Velodrome (1999), Berlin, Germany
Designed by Dominique Perrault (France)
© ADAGP, Paris. Photo by G. Fessy

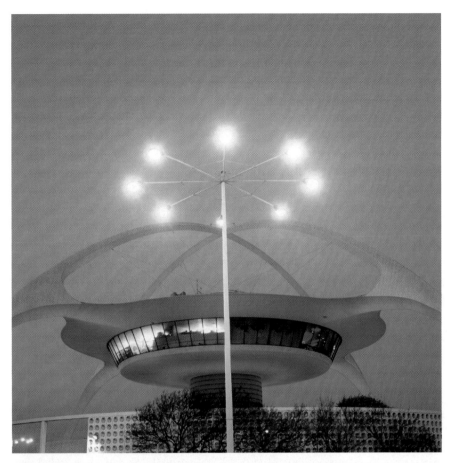

Theme Building at Los Angeles International
Airport (1961–65), Los Angeles, California
Designed by Paul Revere Williams, in collaboration
with Pereira & Luckman and Welton Becket
Associates (United States)
© Joseph Sohm, Chromo Sohm Inc. / CORBIS

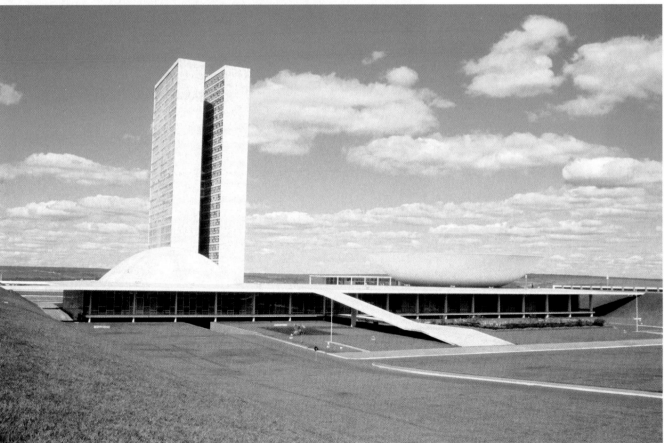

Vienn
Desig
© Ho

National Congress Complex (1958–60), Brasilia, Brazil
Designed by Oscar Niemeyer (Brazil)
© Bettmann / CORBIS

to 2000, nearly 30 significant domed sports stadiums were built, mostly in cities in the United States, Canada, and Japan. Importantly, several domed stadiums were built as part of a host city's preparations for the Olympic Games; these include the Amsterdam Arena (1996) and Paris architect Roger Tallibert's Le Stade Olympique (1976). The domes have fueled a return to the more traditional model of stadiums designed in the early 1900s. Clearly, many communities now idealize the ballparks that predated Yankee Stadium. The contemporary version of this early baseball park, however, is quite different in scale and amenities.

Many late 20th-century stadium projects have followed the 1992 model of Oriole Park at Camden Yards (HOK Sport, Kansas City, Mo.) in Baltimore and the new Comiskey Park, designed by Osborn Engineering Company in Chicago, as well as stadiums in Denver and Cleveland. Returning to the one-dimensional parks and often to natural bluegrass surfaces, these forms combine modern convenience with nostalgic detail. The postmodern fusion has been a universal success, functioning to attract entire families to baseball games and revitalizing aging urban centers. Many stadiums have included amusement and shopping facilities within the park for those less enamored with sports.

Twentieth-century stadiums often accommodate more than one sport and, thus, prolong their function and profitability beyond a single sport season that lasts a few months. During the last two decades of the 20th century, many major North American cities built sports stadiums for their home teams in hockey, basketball, and football. Among more recent American sports arenas, the Pepsi Center in Denver was designed in 1999 by HOK for the city's professional hockey and basketball teams and features luxury suites and a 300-seat restaurant overlooking the sports field.

The 20th-century stadium as a prominent and innovative building type has served more than just professional sports. As gathering places for national political events or other large-scale public or state-sponsored occasions, North Korea's May Day Stadium (capacity 150,000), Iran's National Stadium (capacity 128,000), and Pirouzi (capacity 128,000) represent the world's largest domed structures. Others include City Stadium Jornalista Mário Filho in Brazil (capacity 120,000) and East Bengal in India (capacity 120,000).

BRIAN BLACK

Further Reading

Benson, Michael, *Ballparks of North America: A Comprehensive Historical Reference to Baseball Grounds, Yards, and Stadiums, 1845 to Present*, Jefferson, North Carolina: McFarland, 1989

Cagan, Joanna, and Neil De Mause, *Field of Schemes: How the Great Stadium Swindle Turns Public Money into Private Profit*, New York: Common Courage Press, 1998

John, Geraint, and Rod Sheard, *Stadia: A Design and Development Guide*, Oxford and Boston: Butterworth-Architecture, 1994; 2nd edition, Oxford and Boston: Architectural Press, 1997

Klobuchar, Amy, *Uncovering the Dome: Was the Public Interest Served in Minnesota's 10-Year Political Brawl over the Metrodome?* Minneapolis, Minnesota: Bolger, 1982

Kuklick, Bruce, *To Every Thing a Season: Shibe Park and Urban Philadelphia, 1909–1976*, Princeton, New Jersey: Princeton University Press, 1991

Smith, Ron, and Kevin Belford, *Ballpark Book*, St. Louis, Missouri: Sporting News, 2000

Valavanes, Panos, *Hysplex: The Starting Mechanism in Ancient Stadia: A Contribution to Ancient Greek Technology*, Berkeley: University of California Press, 1999

STEEL

Steel is a material present in the structure of virtually all works of 20th-century architecture: in the connectors, plates, nails, bolts, and screws of timber floors and frames; in the deformed bars hidden within the cement and stone matrix of reinforced concrete; and in the hot-rolled wide-flange columns and beams characteristic of steel skeletal frameworks. Although its history as a building material can be traced back at least to the fifth century B.C., and although its potential to revolutionize the whole process and form of building was in many ways already evident in the 19th century, it is in the 20th century that the architectural expression of steel was most thoroughly explored.

Steel refers to any metal consisting primarily of iron, although the term is now commonly used in a more restrictive sense, reserved for the mild carbon steels that first appeared in the mid-19th century and the high-strength, corrosion-resistant ("weathering"), and stainless steels developed more recently. Cast- and wrought-iron products had been used extensively in building, especially in the 19th century, but were largely superseded by the beginning of the 20th century by hot-rolled steel members. The ultimate victory of steel over earlier forms of iron was the result of steel's superior structural properties along with an increasingly efficient manufacturing process—based on the innovations of Bessemer, Siemens, Thomas, and others—that dramatically reduced its cost while increasing its output. Stimulated first by the needs of the railway industry in the mid-19th century and later by a dramatic increase in large-scale building projects, construction in steel became inextricably linked with the accelerated pace of commercial and industrial development in the 20th century.

The economic and social changes accompanying this development met with mixed reactions. Chicago architect Louis Sullivan found a kind of spiritual poetry in the steel frame's aspiration for verticality; Italian futurist Sant'Elia proclaimed in 1914 that the steel bridges, railway stations, cars, and planes of the modern epoch already signaled a radical discontinuity with the traditional forms of the past; and Russian Constructivist Vladimir Tatlin's proposal for a spiraling steel monument to the Third International in 1920 provided a dynamic and optimistic visual image for the new technology. Yet other artists and critics saw only the negative social consequences of the 20th century's new steel-framed architecture: dark, canyonlike streets; anonymous, repetitive facades; and degrading or dangerous working conditions. Steel was not simply the material par excellence of the industrial revolution; at the dawn of the 20th century, it was also a potent symbol of economic power and monopolistic arrogance, personified in the legendary figures of Andrew Carnegie, J. P. Morgan, and Elbert H. Gary.

With the development of steel architecture, other formal and technical issues have emerged: reconciling requirements for fireproofing and corrosion protection with the desire for direct expression; exploiting the potential of standardization, prefabrication, and mass production; expressing the ideal of lightness and elegance or the tectonics of load and resistance; and incorpo-

rating the image of the machine (whether derived from industry, transport, or war) or the influence of other aesthetic tendencies (from Constructivism to deconstruction). These issues are subsumed within the following discussion, which is based on three critical 20th-century building types: the office building, the long-span "shed," and the house.

Chicago School architects pioneered the steel-framed office building in the late 19th century, and similarly important skyscrapers were designed in New York City and most major American urban centers. In New York, the 30-story Park Row Building (1898) was soon surpassed in height by a series of early-20th-century stone-clad, steel-framed towers, braced internally with diagonal trusswork or made rigid with riveted steel portal frames. The most influential of these buildings was the Woolworth Tower (1913). Designed by Cass Gilbert, it was the tallest building in the world at the time, having overtaken the 50-story Metropolitan Life Insurance Building (1909), designed by Nicholas Le Brun and Sons, which had just surpassed the 47-story Singer Building (1907), designed by Ernest Flagg. At the beginning of the Great Depression, two steel-framed structures in New York City took skyscraper design to new heights, both literally and metaphorically: the Chrysler Building (1929) by William Van Allen and the Empire State Building (1931) by Shreve, Lamb, and Harmon. The Chrysler Building is notable in this context for its crown of stainless-steel cladding, one of the first extensive building applications for the newly invented steel alloy.

Critics have argued about the architectural significance of these New York skyscrapers and whether their exuberant facades of stone and brick—reminiscent in many cases of medieval towers and Renaissance campanile—adequately express the nature of modern steel construction. Although their effect as cultural icons is unquestioned, in general it is the earlier-19th-century Chicago School buildings of Sullivan, Root, Burnham, and Jenney that are cited as exemplars of steel-framed building and precursors of modern design. After World War II, architects generally eliminated cornices and other traditional decorative elements derived from historic architectural styles in favor of the unornamented, rectilinear geometry associated with 20th-century modernism. Even so, the expression of steel framing remained problematic. For example, in Mies van der Rohe and Philip Johnson's Seagram Building (1958) in New York City, the actual steel structure is first encased in concrete fireproofing and then hidden behind a metal and glass curtain wall. Even with bronze I-beams applied on the facade to stiffen the vertical mullions, expression of the actual steel framework is, at best, indirect.

A more direct expression of steel structure is achieved by exposing the characteristic flanged shapes of actual painted or corrosion-resistant steel beams and columns or by celebrating the geometry of structural forms characteristic of steel—usually trussed or rigid frameworks evocative of steel industrial or civil engineering works. In the first case, Kevin Roche and John Dinkeloo's use of exposed and unpainted corrosion-resistant steel girders for the Knights of Columbus Headquarters (1969) in New Haven, Connecticut, and Skidmore, Owings, and Merrill's use of partially exposed painted steel girders (the flanges being covered for fire protection) in the U.S. Steel Building (1972) in New York City may serve as examples.

In the second case, the geometric form of truss or frame (rather than the shape of the individual elements) evokes steel structure. Three buildings by Skidmore, Owings, and Merrill illustrate this approach. The Inland Steel Building (1957) in Chicago expresses its welded-steel framework by locating the vertical elements of the framework outside the glass plane of the curtain wall, the Alcoa Building (1964) in San Francisco positions its triangulated steel bracing structure 18 inches in front of its glass curtain wall, and the Hancock Building (1970) in Chicago sets its steel trusswork into the plane of the facade. Two buildings in Hong Kong provide additional examples based on the same principle. The Bank of China (1990) by I. M. Pei selectively expresses the complex triangular geometry of its steel frame, suppressing the articulation of horizontal truss elements and thereby changing the apparent pattern of the framework on the facades from a series of Xs—which would have negative cultural connotations—to a series of diamonds. Norman Foster's Hongkong and Shanghai Bank (1986) employs a more explicitly machine-derived aesthetic, using tension elements to literally hang sections of the building—eight floors at a time—from steel trusses that in turn are cantilevered from mammoth steel columns. In these examples, the actual articulated steel structure is clad in sheet metal or, in the case of Pei's triangulated framework, stone veneer. Steel "exoskeletons" may also be unclad, as at the Foundation Cartier (1994) in Paris by Jean Nouvel, where abstract planar surfaces of parallel curtain wall screens are contrasted with exposed angular steel frames designed to provide structural stability.

The Shed

The use of steel for long-span roof structures has its roots in 19th-century bridges, train sheds, market halls, and exhibition spaces. Structures such as the Crystal Palace (1851) in London and the Galerie des Machines (1889) in Paris already showed the potential of iron (or steel, in the case of the Galerie). New functions requiring long-span roofs evolved in the 20th century, including hangars for airships and aircraft as well as single-level factories oriented toward the new flexible assembly-line production techniques pioneered in the automobile industry.

Long-span steel trusses, originating with 19th-century bridges (Benjamin Baker's steel-truss Forth Bridge in Scotland was the world's longest spanning structure at the time of its completion in 1890) were used in numerous factories and other building types to create large, column-free interior spaces. Albert Kahn's Glenn Martin Aircraft Plant (1937) in Middle River, Maryland, is of interest not only because its 300-foot (91-meter) trusses created the largest flat-roof span attempted up to that time but also because Mies van der Rohe used a photograph of its interior to construct his famous collaged image for a Concert Hall project, published in 1943. Additional representative examples in which steel parallel-chord, horizontal trusses are featured as important architectural elements include the New Haven Veterans Memorial Coliseum (1972) by Kevin Roche and John Dinkeloo, where exposed corrosion-resistant steel trusses carry a multilevel parking structure over the stadium below, and the McCormick Place Convention Center (1970) in Chicago by C. F. Murphy Associates, in which two perpendicular sets of

parallel trusses are used. An unusual multistory application of long-span steel trusses can be seen at the Georges Pompidou Center (1977) by Renzo Piano and Richard Rogers, where the truss span—and therefore the required depth of the structure—is reduced through the use of sophisticated cast-steel "gerberettes" cantilevered inward from water-filled tubular steel columns to support the trusses, the columns being expressed on the building's exterior along with tensioned steel rods and diagonal cross bracing.

Variations on steel-trussed arches and frames, providing lightweight and structurally efficient spans, can be seen in early-20th-century hangars for airships (zeppelins) and factory buildings, especially in Germany. An early example, influenced by the three-hinged steel arch forms of 19th-century bridge and exhibition structures, is Peter Behrens's AEG Turbine Factory (1909) in Berlin, in which hinges and vertical elements making up the repetitive steel arches are expressed on the exterior of the side facade. Norman Foster's Sainsbury Centre (1977) in Norwich, England, uses tubular steel-trussed rigid portal frames that contain the mechanical services for the building while providing a clear span for the display and academic functions within. A more complex three-hinged trussed arch appears in Nicholas Grimshaw's Waterloo International Rail Terminal (1994) in London. There, the required asymmetry results in steel tension elements of the truss—expressed as thin rods—being located first above and then below the roof structure, creating a form at once rational and counterintuitive. A final example is the International Exhibition Center (1996) in Leipzig by Ian Ritchie, in which arched trusses with cast-steel support arms form an exoskeleton supporting the vaulted Main Hall.

Polyhedral-based structures—three-dimensional versions of simple planar trusses—were pioneered by Alexander Graham Bell in 1907 and developed into more sophisticated space frames by Max Mengeringhausen in Germany in the 1940s and Konrad Wachsmann in the United States in the 1950s. Buckminster Fuller invented the geodesic dome, based on the triangulation of a spherical surface, in the late 1940s. Steel-lamella roofs, consisting of intersecting, offset systems of parallel ribs, have been used in hangars, stadiums, and other long-span applications. Later-20th-century versions of these forms include the Javits Convention Center (1986) in New York City by I. M. Pei, consisting of a steel space frame used for both walls and roofs; Fuller's geodesic dome for the U.S. Pavilion (1967) at the Montreal Expo; and the steel-lamella Louisiana Superdome (1975) by Sverdrup and Parcel Associates.

Long-span masted tension structures, inspired by 19th-century suspension bridge and 20th-century cable-stayed designs, use steel rods in tension to support horizontal roof surfaces. The Burgo Paper Mill (1962) in Mantua, Italy, by Pier Luigi Nervi quite literally mirrors the form of conventional suspension bridges to create clear-span spaces below its suspended roof. More recent masted steel structures exploit the same principles, although their forms have become less derivative of bridge design and more articulate in expressing the exposed-steel connections between tension rod, horizontal beam, and vertical mast. Notable examples by Richard Rogers include the Fleetguard Distribution Center (1979) in Quimper, France; the Inmos Microprocessor Factory (1982) in South Wales; and the PA Technology Laboratories (1985) in Princeton, New Jersey. Norman Foster's

Renault Distribution Center (1980) at Swindon, England, has a more complex geometry defined by perforated, tapered beams; masts; and tension rods. The Darling Harbour Exhibition Center (1988) in Sydney, Australia, by Philip Cox, Richardson, and Taylor makes reference, in its masted supports and steel outriggers, to the adjacent maritime harbor and its associated nautical motifs. The suppression of tension elements and the elaboration of the mast into compressive "treelike" structural forms—first systematically studied by Frei Otto—can be seen in several steel-framed projects by Santiago Calatrava, including the BCE Place Gallery (1992) in Toronto and the Oriente Station (1998) in Lisbon.

In tensioned-membrane structures, steel cables are combined with fabric membranes to create extremely lightweight, long-span structures. Frei Otto's tent structures for the German Pavilion (1967) at the Montreal Expo and for the Munich Olympics (1972) are landmarks in the development of these forms. Two late-20th-century long-span examples are the Georgia Dome (1992) in Atlanta, engineered by Weidlinger Associates and based on a patented "tensegrity" geometry defined by triangulated steel tension cables and floating steel compression struts, and the Millennium Dome (1999) by Richard Rogers in which the dome—historically a compressive structure—is transformed into a tensioned membrane by hanging the steel cable net defining its domical surface from an array of twelve inclined steel masts that penetrate the membrane. Lightweight domical surfaces can also be formed with membranes by mechanically increasing the interior air pressure, as in a balloon: An early example of such a pneumatic structure, contained by a net of steel cables, is the American Pavilion at the Osaka Expo (1970) by Davis Brody Associates.

With the development of welded connections—first invented in the late 19th century but not used in buildings until the 1920s—steel beams and frames could more readily be designed within the modernist syntax of interpenetrating line and surface, uninterrupted by gusset plates, bolts, or rivets. The buildings of Mies van der Rohe at the Illinois Institute of Technology in Chicago illustrate this type of abstract welded-steel expression, most dramatically in the exposed parallel portal frames of Crown Hall (1956). Later projects from the 1960s and 1970s, influenced by Mies's work, include Roche and Dinkeloo's Cummins Engine Company plant (1966) at Darlington, England; the Reliance Controls plant (1966) at Swindon, England, by Team 4 (including Norman Foster and Richard Rogers); and Skidmore, Owings, and Merrill's Republic Newspaper Plant (1971) at Columbus, Indiana. Functional requirements—for example, the need for daylighting in the immense new factory buildings of the steel, automotive, and aircraft industries—could also be addressed using welded-steel frames, angled or stepped to accommodate monitor skylights. Such bent frames can be found in Albert Kahn's Chrysler Half-Ton Truck Plant (1937) in Detroit and, more recently, in Helmut Jahn's Terminal One Complex for United Airlines (1987) in Chicago, the latter project using clusters of tubular steel columns supporting perforated steel beams that define skylit, linear public circulation spaces within the terminal. Curved, welded ribbed frames are used at an even more monumental scale in Rafael Viñoly's Tokyo International Forum (1996), defining an immense elliptical tied-arch roof

supported by two centrifugally spun steel pipe columns 400 feet (124 meters) apart.

The House

The use of steel in the construction of factories, train sheds, market halls, and office buildings parallels the development of 19th- and 20th-century industry and commerce. The use of steel in 20th-century residential design has less of an objective basis, despite Le Corbusier's famous aphorism defining the modern house as a "machine for living in." Although steel-based technology was critical to the production of cars, trains, airships, and airplanes, attempts to design mass-produced, prefabricated, standardized, and flexible kits of steel parts applicable to the production of houses were generally less successful. In fact, although at least one fireproof steel residence—the Reid House (1894) in Chicago by Beers, Clay, and Dutton—was constructed before the 20th century, ambivalence about the appropriateness of exposed steel within the domestic sphere, as well as its relatively high cost compared with traditional residential construction systems, delayed the first applications of steel framing to residential construction. An experimental steel-framed house was produced for the German Bauhaus Exhibition of 1923 by painter Georg Muche and Adolf Meyer, but this house, along with a subsequent design completed in 1927, had little lasting influence.

The first truly influential steel-framed houses, built on both sides of the Atlantic Ocean at the end of the 1920s, rely for their expressive power on the juxtaposition of steel framing with large surfaces of glass. Among the most important are Richard Neutra's Lovell Health House (1929) in Los Angeles; Pierre Chareau's Maison de Verre (1932) in Paris; Mies van der Rohe's Tugendhat House (1930) in Brno, Czechoslovakia; and Leendert Cornelis van der Vlugt's van der Leeuw House (1929) in Rotterdam. Whereas Chareau has made the specific character of rolled steel—the flanged column shapes and the bolted and riveted connections—an integral part of his architectural expression, Neutra's steel frame is integrated into a more abstract gridded composition of glass and cement, visible only on the exterior of the house, where the closely spaced vertical members of the steel framework are selectively exposed as window mullions or supports for projecting rooms and balconies. In Mies' Tugendhat House, similar in its detailing and expression to the better known German Pavilion (1929) designed for the World Exhibition at Barcelona the previous year, the actual bolted-steel framework is never truly revealed. Instead, only the grid of columns, clad in chromium-plated sheet steel and set didactically between abstract planes of floor and roof, can be seen. The van der Leeuw House is perhaps the most literally "machinelike" of all, boasting a whole array of electronic gadgetry and controls within a structure based on four parallel steel frames that penetrated the house from front to back.

A different tendency can be seen in the polygonal Dymaxion House (1927), designed by Buckminster Fuller, in which a rigorous analysis of functionality and structural efficiency is combined with an interest in mass production at low cost, unfettered by the aesthetic preoccupations of the European modernists. Fuller refined the design during the 1930s and 1940s and found manufacturers to build prototypes but was unable to implement the idea commercially on a large scale.

During the period immediately after World War II, especially in the United States, steel was vigorously promoted as a material suitable for residential construction. John Entenza's *Art & Architecture* magazine published a series of so-called Case Study houses, the most influential of which was designed by Charles and Ray Eames for themselves in Pacific Palisades, California. The Eames House (1949) pioneered an aesthetic derived from the assembly of off-the-shelf, mass-produced, standard steel elements: open-web steel joists, corrugated-steel decking, and rolled-steel-column sections.

Two non-Californian steel-framed houses designed in the late 1940s were also extremely influential. Mies van der Rohe's Farnsworth House (1951) in Plano, Illinois, and Philip Johnson's Glass House (1949) in New Canaan, Connecticut, evince less concern with issues of economy, standardization, and mass production and more interest in exploring the formal qualities of the rectangular glass box within a welded-steel frame. The Farnsworth House was designed with its horizontal steel-framed floor and roof planes cantilevered outward from within two rows of external steel columns, raising the house off the ground. Johnson, however, by placing his Glass House directly on the ground with no cantilevered elements and by positioning his black-painted steel columns inside the glass plane, has shifted the emphasis from the steel frame to the glass enclosure.

Many postwar steel houses combine in various degrees formal qualities associated with the work of Eames and Mies. Influential Californian Case Study houses, such as Raphael Soriano's Olds House (1950) in Pacific Palisades, Craig Ellwood's Bailey House (1958) in Los Angeles, and Pierre Koenig's Stahl House (1960) in Los Angeles, all are based on rectilinear grids of steel columns, with steel beams and corrugated-steel roof decks completing the framing schemes and largely defining the formal vocabulary. Beginning in the mid-1950s, modern steel houses began to be built in England as well, including Michael Manser's Capel Manor House (Kent, 1970), the Richard Horden house (Dorset, 1975), the John Winter house (1969) in London, and Ian Ritchie's Eagle Rock House (1982) in East Sussex. Soriano, in particular, has been an influential figure for both British and American architects building in steel. Having experimented with lightweight steel trusses, beams, and columns since the late 1930s, he lent a certain credibility to the well-publicized but still largely unrealized ideal of industrialized building based on modularity, standardization, and prefabrication.

Interest in industrialized building—for housing, schools, and other building types—has been a continuous current in architectural thought for most of the 20th century. Early research into the mass production of lightweight steel structures, on the model of automobile production, can be seen in the work of Jean Prouvé and Buckminster Fuller from the 1920s and 1930s. Several industrialized steel systems for schools were implemented in the period after World War II, most notably the Hertfordshire County Council and CLASP systems in Britain in the 1940s and 1950s and the School Construction System Development Program in California led by Ezra Ehrenkrantz during the 1960s. By the end of the century, industrialized products were routinely used in a variety of applications, ranging from metal building systems—consisting of heavy steel frames with corrugated-steel cladding—to complete "volumetric" steel-framed housing units, the latter accounting for a small but growing proportion of total new home construction in Japan.

Steel-based industrialized housing systems were developed in Britain, the United States, and France in the aftermath of World War II, including several designed by Prouvé in the 1940s based on his earlier use of bent steel sheet in his Pavillion Démontable (1939). Jerry Wells and Fred Koetter continued research into the potential of light-gauge, cold-formed sheet steel for modular housing (1971), as did Cedric Price in the same year. Other experimental steel-based building systems designed in the 1970s and 1980s include Helmut Schultz's "Team for Experimental Systems and Building Techniques" (TEST) at the University of California, Michael Hopkins's Patera System in Britain, Gunter Hübner and Frank Huster's prototype housing system in Germany, Renzo Piano's experimental houses in Italy, and Michiel Cohen and Jan Pesman's Heiwo system in the Netherlands. However, these industrialized building attempts were only partially successful, with houses produced often only as prototypes, occasionally in limited numbers, and sometimes not at all.

Notwithstanding the limited application of steel-framed industrialized building systems to housing, the use of prefabricated, industrial steel elements has had a notable effect on later-20th-century residential architecture. In particular, an ad hoc and idiosyncratic use of corrugated-steel panels for roofing and siding can be seen in the provocative residential work of Frank Gehry, beginning with his Davis Studio/Residence (1968–72) in Malibu, California, and including the first addition to his own house (1978) in Santa Monica, California. The Australian architect Glenn Murcutt has also used corrugated steel and steel framing as crucial elements in many of his residential designs, including the Marie Short House (1975) in New South Wales and the Ball-Eastaway House and Studio (1983) in Glenorie, Sidney. Where the raw, industrial quality of steel cladding in Gehry's work reinforces a sense of displacement already evident in the deliberately fragmented or truncated forms of his structures, Murcutt's use of the same material achieves an opposite effect, imparting what has been described as a sense of dignity to the corrugated surfaces.

Steel as Skin

Steel appears in architecture primarily as structure, but it is also used as nonstructural cladding, or "skin." Gehry's corrugated-steel panels and the Chrysler Building's stainless-steel crown have already been noted. Other representative examples include Jean Prouvé's innovative sheet-steel curtain wall for the Maison du Peuple (1939) at Clichy, France; Skidmore, Owings, and Merrill's stainless-steel mullions at Lever House (1953) in New York City; Harrison and Abramovitz's textured panels of stainless steel for the Socony Mobil Building (1955) in New York City; Richard Meier's gridded porcelain enamel steel panels at the Athenium (1979) in New Harmony, Indiana; and Frank Gehry's overlapping galvanized-steel sheet cladding at the California Aerospace Museum (1984) in Los Angeles.

The uniqueness of steel sheet and plate also manifests itself in a group of idiosyncratic structures not easily categorized by function or formal type but having in common a kind of sculptural presence in which distinctions between structure and skin become less clear. Eero Saarinen's 630-foot (190-meter)-high Gateway Arch (1965) in St. Louis uses a double layer of steel, with quarter-inch (six-millimeter) stainless-steel plate forming the outside layer, as both cladding and structure. Le Corbusier's pavilion for Heidi Weber (1967) in Zurich, based on his earlier steel project for the "Saison de l'eau" at the Exposition de Liegè (1939), contains an angular sheet-steel roof cantilevered from a series of steel piers and detached from but covering a rectilinear steel structure below. Bernard Tschumi's abstract, orthogonal sculptural "follies" and expressionistic "gallery" structures within the Parc de la Villette (1982) in Paris provide a final example based on the use of both painted and porcelain-coated sheet steel.

JONATHAN OCHSHORN

See also **Bank of China Tower, Hong Kong; Chicago School; Chrysler Building, New York City; Empire State Building, New York City; Farnsworth House, Plano, Illinois; Fuller, Richard Buckminster (United States); Gateway Arch, St. Louis, Missouri; German Pavilion, Barcelona (1929); Illinois Institute of Technology, Chicago; Mies van der Rohe, Ludwig (Germany); Monument to the Third International (1920); Skyscraper; Pei, I.M. (United States); Sullivan, Louis (United States); Tschumi, Bernard (France)**

Further Reading

An excellent history of steel houses in the 20th century is provided by Jackson; for an overview of long-span structures ("sheds"), see Wilkinson; for a history that includes the development of early-20th-century American skyscrapers, see Condit. The importance of engineers is discussed in Billington, Rice, and Thornton. A comprehensive overview of steel in relation to architecture can be found in Blanc.

Billington, David P., *The Tower and the Bridge: The New Art of Structural Engineering*, New York: Basic Books, 1983
Blanc, Alan, Michael McEvoy, and Roger Plank (editors), *Architecture and Construction in Steel*, London and New York: Spon, 1993
Condit, Carl W., *American Building Art: The Twentieth Century*, New York: Oxford University Press, 1961
Jackson, Neil, *The Modern Steel House*, London and New York: Spon, 1996
Landau, Sarah Bradford, and Carl Condit, *Rise of the New York Skyscraper, 1865–1913*, New Haven, Connecticut: Yale University Press, 1996
Rice, Peter, *An Engineer Imagines*, London: Artemis, 1994; 2nd edition, London: Ellipsis, 1996
Thornton, Charles H., et al., *Exposed Structure in Building Design*, New York: McGraw-Hill, 1993
Wilkinson, Chris, *Supersheds: The Architecture of Long-Span, Large-Volume Buildings*, Oxford: Butterworth Architecture, 1991; 2nd edition, Oxford: Architectural Press, 1996
Willis, Carol, *Form Follows Finance: Skyscrapers and Skylines in New York and Chicago*, New York: Princeton University Press, 1995

STEEL-FRAME CONSTRUCTION

This method of construction provides support by means of a closely knit structure of steel. Primary and secondary members compose the skeleton of the structure, to which a covering can be applied. With a steel frame, it is possible to enclose space with suspension structures. Steel framing is the counterpart to vaulting, in which the materials are in compression, and to pneu-

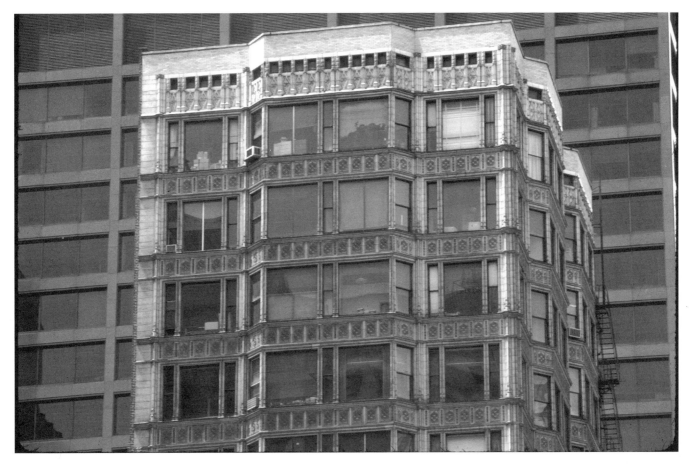

Reliance Building (detail, upper stories) Chicago, designed by Daniel Burnham (1895)
© Johnson Architectural Images/GreatBuildings.com

matic structures, in which the skins are held in place by air pressure.

The basic elements of the steel skeleton frame are vertical columns, horizontal girders that span the longer distance between columns, and beams that span shorter distances. The frame is reinforced to prevent distortion and possible collapse caused by uneven or vibratory loads. Lateral stability is provided by connecting the beams, columns, and girders and by diagonal bracing or rigid connections among columns, girders, and beams.

A frame composed of three end-connected members, more commonly known as a truss, cannot change its shape, even if its joints could act as hinges. Moreover, the principle of triangulation—attaching a horizontal tie beam to the bottom ends of two peaked rafters—can be extended indefinitely. Thus, spanning systems of almost any shape can be subdivided into triangles, the sides of which can be made of any appropriate material (most commonly steel or wood), and assembled using suitable end connections. Each separate part is then subject only to either compressive or tensile stress. The exterior skin, or curtain wall, that is placed over the steel frame can be made of metal (stainless steel, aluminum, or bronze), masonry (concrete, brick, or tile), or glass.

In the second half of the 19th century, builders in New York City and Chicago experimented with high-rise buildings. A valuable learning experience came with the construction of the Statue of Liberty (1886). Erected between 1883 and 1886, the statue is a copper-sheathed enclosure standing 151 feet, making it comparable in size, if not in weight, to the skyscraper of its day.

The sculptor of the Statue of Liberty, Frederic Auguste Bartholdi, posed a problem for his engineer Gustave Eiffel that was less one of supporting vertical loads and more one of resisting the force of wind on the extensive surface area surrounding the hollow interior. Eiffel's solution to the wind load problem involved several valuable innovations for American building. Most important, the diagonally braced frame inside the figure represented the most extensive system of wind bracing employed for any American structure to that time other than a bridge.

The braced and riveted steel skeleton was used in New York with the construction of Bruce Price's American Surety Building (1895) at Broadway and Pine Street. With a height of 20 stories, rising 303 feet above grade, a masonry wall was simply out of the question. For this height, a wall without supplementary columns inserted in the masonry would need to be at least seven and a half feet thick at the base. At this time, the Chicago architect Louis Sullivan, in his Wainwright Building (1890–91) in St.

Louis, Missouri; his Guaranty Building (1895) in Buffalo, New York; and his Carson Pirie Scott Department Store (1899–1904) in Chicago gave new expressive form to urban commercial buildings, known as the Chicago School. These buildings made a successful transition from the masonry-bearing wall to the steel frame, which assumed all the load-bearing functions.

By 1895, engineers and architects in Chicago had contributed several innovations to skyscraper construction. The engineer Corydon T. Purdy, in collaboration with William Holabird and Martin Roche, seems to have been the first to use portal arches as wind bracing when he designed the steel frame of the Old Colony Building (1893–94) in Chicago. In this system of bracing, deepening the ends of the girder into quarter-circular fillets gives the underside of the girder an arched profile.

The culmination of the Chicago School's contributions to steel-frame construction came with the Reliance Building (1894–95) after the plans of D. H. Burnham & Company and the engineer Edward C. Shankland. The steel frame of this slender tower is carefully braced in two ways: clinch-deep spandrel girders provide the usual portal bracing, and two-story columns erected with staggered joints increase the rigidity of the vertical members.

DENNIS RANDOLPH

Further Reading

Condit, Carl W., *American Building: Materials and Techniques from the First Colonial Settlements to the Present*, Chicago: University of Chicago Press, 1968; 2nd edition, 1982

Condit, Carl W., *The Chicago School of Architecture: A History of Commercial and Public Buildings in the Chicago Area, 1875–1925*, Chicago: University of Chicago Press, 1964; revised edition, as *The Rise of the Skyscraper*, Chicago: University of Chicago Press, 1952

Freitag, Joseph Kendall, *Architectural Engineering: With Special Reference to High Building Construction, Including Many Examples of Chicago Office Buildings*, New York: Wiley, 1895; 2nd edition, 1901

Hool, George A., and Nathan C. Johnson (editors), *Handbook of Building Construction*, 2 vols., New York: McGraw-Hill, 1920; 2nd edition, 1929

Kurtz, Max, *Comprehensive Structural Design Guide*, New York: McGraw-Hill, 1969

Mainstone, Rowland, *Developments in Structural Form*, Cambridge, Massachusetts: MIT Press, and London: Allen Lane, 1975; 2nd edition, Oxford and Boston: Architectural Press, 1998

Millais, Malcom, *Building Structures*, London and New York: E and FN Spon, 1997

Waddell, John Alexander Low, *De Pontibus: A Pocket-Book for Bridge Engineers*, New York: Wiley, and London: Chapman and Hall, 1898; 2nd edition, 1906

STEINER HOUSE, VIENNA

Designed by Adolf Loos; completed 1910
Vienna, Austria

The Steiner House is among the best known of Adolf Loos's early residential works. Loos designed the house in early 1910, at the same time he was working on the even more controversial Michaelerplatz Building, and the two projects bear a certain kinship despite their programmatic differences. Both works followed immediately in the wake of Loos's famed address, "Ornament und Verbrechen" (Ornament and Crime), first delivered in January of the same year, and as a result, they may be understood as exemplars of the antiornamental ideas he laid out in the talk. The Steiner House, however, which was completed by the end of 1910, more than a half year before the much-discussed Michaelerplatz Building, initially drew little public notice, no doubt in large measure because it was a private domicile in an inconspicuous residential neighborhood.

The clients, wealthy textile manufacturer Hugo Steiner and his wife, Lily, a graphic artist and painter, subsequently commissioned Loos to design the interiors of their elegant Knize tailor shops in Vienna, Paris, and Berlin. The house itself, by contrast, is rather modest in terms of both its scale and its detailing. The freestanding structure is roughly square in plan (13.5 by 14.5 meters). Seen from the front, it appears to consist of a single story with a high attic. In fact, the house has three stories, which are clearly visible from the rear garden. The most distinctive feature of the building, the curving sheet-metal roof, was Loos' reply to the local building codes, which required that the streetfronts of houses in the area be no more than one story, with a second-story mansard. Loos maximized the space by concealing not one but two stories in the attic and connecting the half-barrel vault in the front to a flat concrete roof covering the rear two-thirds of the structure. The resulting configuration, despite its somewhat peculiar profile, allowed Loos to make use of nearly the entire interior volume.

The front and rear facades of the house are symmetrically arranged, although the windows and doors have varying formats and dimensions. By contrast, the fenestration pattern on the two sides is irregular, and on the southeastern side is a projecting bay topped by a small balcony accessible from the second story. Unlike Loos' later residential works, with their complex interlocking volumes, the regular horizontal layering of the floors is maintained, but the rooms on the three levels are of different heights: the ceilings on the ground floor are 2.85 meters, those on the second floor 3 meters, and those on the uppermost floor 2.10 meters. The ground floor contains a large vestibule, a kitchen, and an adjoining living and dining room, which extend the length of the house's rear. On the second story were originally two bedrooms, a servant's room, a small children's room, and a studio for Lily Steiner (facing out to the street), and the third floor was taken up with a laundry room and other service spaces. In addition, the house also has a basement, which at the time of its completion housed a garage, another servant's room, a furnace room, and a coal storage space. As in all of Loos' residences, there is a clear distinction between the public and private domains and between the served and serving spaces. The principal living areas and the bedroom above are linked with a stair, but there is a second spiral staircase to allow the servants access to all four floors.

The original interior detailing was remarkably simple, combining white walls, dark-stained oak wainscoting, and beamed ceilings on the ground floor and painted white wainscoting and floral wallpaper in the upstairs bedrooms. A number of the rooms were also originally furnished with both built-in and freestanding furniture of Loos' own design, including chairs, benches, stools, and a buffet. In contrast to the exterior, with its associations to the Mediterranean vernacular, the interior evoked an air of contemporary Anglo-Saxon domesticity, a feel-

ing that was further enhanced by the flowing quality of the principal ground-floor spaces—living room, dining area, and music room—that Loos would further develop in his subsequent houses. Movement to and from these spaces, however, was limited to a conventional enclosed hallway, a strategy that Loos would later largely abandon.

In the early histories of modernism, much was made of the Steiner House's simple, planar walls and lack of traditional detailing, which seemed to directly presage the rise of the new purist architecture of the post–World War I period—an idea further advanced through views of the house's rear garden facade, which were juxtaposed with later works by Le Corbusier and others. Vincent Scully, writing in 1961, similarly noted the connection between "the obsessive puritanism" of Loos' prewar works and his polemical statements concerning the elimination of ornament. More recently, however, it has become clear that many of the features of the Steiner House, like Loos' other buildings of the time, derived as much from his attempt to find an appropriate modern language as from his belief in continuing the Viennese tradition. Indeed, both the house's sheet-metal roof and its smooth stucco finish draw directly on traditional local building practices, and the design must be seen not only in light of the turn-of-the-century Viennese interest in abstraction but also in that of the contemporary Biedermeier Revival. Loos' apparent rejection of ornament in this view is less an expression of a new functionalism than a reaffirmation of older ideas of bourgeois modesty and propriety, values that very much suited the house's first owners. The apparent contrast between the exterior and interior, which has also been repeatedly observed, may also be understood not as an inherent contradiction but as a reflection of Loos' notion of the difference between the public sphere, where propriety is paramount, and the private world, where a more relaxed attitude may prevail. Such an interpretation suggests not only the complexity of Loos' views but also the transitional nature of the house's design.

CHRISTOPHER LONG

Further Reading

Denti, Giovanni and Silvia Peirone, *Adolf Loos: Opera completa*, Rome: Officina, 1997

Gravagnuolo, Benedetto, *Adolf Loos: Theory and Works*, New York: Rizzoli, 1982

Kurrent, Friedrick (editor), *Adolf Loos, 1870–1933: 40 Wohnhäuser, Bauten und Projekte von Adolf Loos, Studienarbeiten an der Technischen Universität München*, Salzburg: Pustet, 1998

Lustenberger, Kurt, *Adolf Loos*, Zurich: Artemis, 1994

Münz, Ludwig and Gustav Künstler, *Der Architekt Adolf Loos*, Vienna: Schroll, 1964

Ottillinger, Eva B., *Adolf Loos: Wohnkonzepte und Möbelentwürfe*, Salzburg: Residenz Verlag, 1994

Rukschcio, Burkhardt (editor), *Adolf Loos*, Vienna: Graphische Sammlung Albertina, 1989

Rukschcio, Burkhardt and Roland Schachel, *Adolf Loos: Leben und Werk*, Salzburg and Vienna: Residenz Verlag, 1982; 2nd edition, 1987

Safran, Yehuda and Wilfried Wang (editors), *The Architecture of Adolf Loos: An Arts Council Exhibit*, London: The Council, 1985; 2nd edition, 1987

Scully, Vincent, Jr., *Modern Architecture: The Architecture of Democracy*, New York: Braziller, 1956; London: Prentice-Hall International, 1961; revised edition, New York: Braziller, 1974

Tournikiotis, Panayotis, *Loos*, Paris: Macula, 1991; as *Adolf Loos*, New York: Princeton Architectural Press, 1994

STERN, ROBERT ARTHUR MORGAN 1939–

Architect, United States

A brilliant polymath in command of a daunting array of talents, Robert Stern is perhaps the true successor to Philip Johnson, one of his mentors, as one of the prime figures in the American architectural world. In 1998, Stern was appointed dean of the school of architecture at Yale University, where he had earned a Master of Architecture degree (1965). He was coeditor of *Perspecta 9–10*, the first double issue of that distinguished periodical created by graduate architectural students at Yale. In 1970, he began teaching in the Graduate School of Architecture, Planning, and Preservation at his undergraduate alma mater, Columbia University (B.A., 1960), and in 1984 undertook a four-year term as first director of its Temple Hoyne Buell Center for the Study of American Architecture.

Stern's eclecticism and reliance on quotation in his architectural practice has been criticized, but as in the 19th century, exemplars are chosen according to their appropriateness to program or context. Furthermore, the often dazzling spatial strategies, as well as the techniques of collage and juxtaposition, are thoroughly of the 20th century. Initially a disciple of Robert Venturi, whom Stern launched (when in 1966 he curated "40 under 40," an important exhibition that brought a new generation of architects to public attention) on the national stage while still a student at Yale, gradually Stern moved in a more overtly historicizing direction. Nevertheless, the quality of wit and irony so important to postmodernists such as Venturi and Charles Moore also pervades Stern's work; their affinity for Pop art is mirrored in his amusing allusions that at times approach parody.

Stern's Postmodernism, a movement that he did much to foster, has many different sources, although he is particularly fond of the classical tradition (as explained in his book *Modern Classicism*), especially as represented in late 18th-century France (Poolhouse, Llewellyn Park, 1981, and Point West Place Offices, Framingham 1985 are both based on Claude-Nicolas Ledoux), Colonial (Residence in at Apaquogue, East Hampton, 1993), and Federal America (Observatory Hill Dining Commons, 1984, and Darden School of Business, 1996 both at the University of Virginia and therefore, predictably, transcriptions of Thomas Jefferson's work); his "Late Entry to the Chicago Tribune" (1980) marries Adolf Loos with Mies van der Rohe (each a classicist in his own right). However, Stern also is one of the most skillful manipulators of the late 19th-century Shingle style (houses on Martha's Vineyard, 1983), which he learned about firsthand from his Yale professor and later colleague Vincent Scully and from the frequent commissions in his early career that comprised extensions to authentic Shingle-style houses. When the building type demands it, he may turn to the Richardsonian Romanesque; thus, the Ohrstrom Library, 1991, at St. Paul's School is, in plan and elevation, an interpretation of Richardson's small-town libraries, complete with the eyebrow dormer windows, and Stern himself identifies Charles Rennie Mackintosh as a guide. Craftsman features, including touches

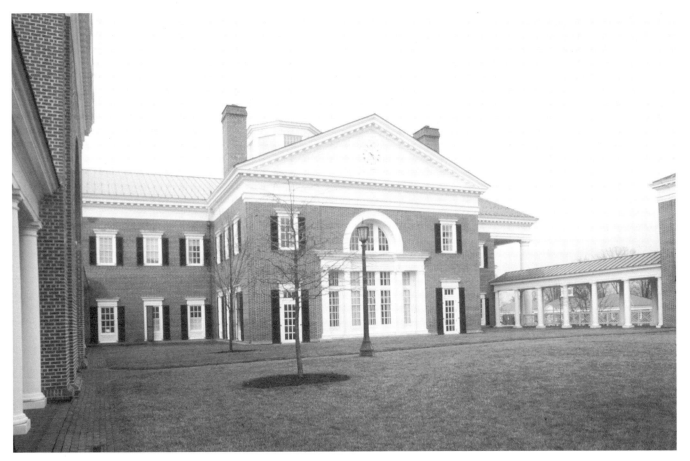

Darden Graduate School of Business Administration, University of Virginia (1996)
Photo © Mary Ann Sullivan

of Frank Lloyd Wright and Julia Morgan, inform the Roger Tory Peterson Institute, 1993, and the Columbus Regional Hospital, 1995, and Spanish Colonial contextualizes the Police Building, 1990, in Pasadena. Significantly, the five-story office building for Bancho House, 1989, does not look to Japanese architecture but to the classicizing style of the nearby British Embassy and other Westernized buildings in Tokyo. Further, as heroic modernism itself has passed into history, Stern is happy to emulate its most positive aspects; as his remodeled loft duplex (1999) in New Haven attests, he is especially fond of furniture produced under its banner, from Le Corbusier and Charlotte Perriand to Eames and Saarinen.

Stern's first executed work was the Wiseman House in Montauk (1967), an obvious bow to the Vanna Venturi residence, though altered to suit a family with children and incorporating elements from Le Corbusier. Houses of the next decade (including those done with John Hagmann, a Yale classmate who was a partner from 1969 to 1977), such as the Lang House in Washington, Connecticut, 1974, and the Beebe houses in Montauk, 1972, continued Venturi's lessons but revealed a penchant for interestingly varied sections and sensitive treatment of natural light and of views toward the land- and seascape. Stern has said that private houses are his obsession, and he has continued to

design them, although subsequently, more public building types have eclipsed the domestic side of his practice.

However, the dense urban matrix composed of commercial structures informs his work. His first job (1967–70) was with the New York Housing and Development Administration, and he has published an invaluable series of exhaustively researched books on New York City architecture. His firm has been responsible for many renovations and additions in New York City and has erected tall buildings in Boston as well as Manhattan. Yet small towns delight him, too: he has supported New Urbanists such as Andreas Duany and Elizabeth Plater-Zyberk and mirrored their insights in his planning, with Jacquelyn Robertson of Celebration, Florida, and other Disney sites. He also acknowledges studying his summer hometown of East Hampton in this connection. Stern even has affection for the much-maligned suburb, writing cogently on its virtues and making several ideal schemes that exploit its possibilities.

HELEN SEARING

See also **Celebration, Florida; Duany and Plater-Zyberk (United States); Johnson, Philip (United States); Moore, Charles (United States); Postmodernism; Venturi, Robert (United States)**

Biography

Born New York City, 23 May 1939. Bachelor of Arts Columbia University 1960. Master of Architecture, Yale University 1965. Married Lynn Solinger 1966 (divorced 1977): 1 child, Nicholas. Stern & Hagman Architects 1969–77; Principal, Robert A. M. Stern Architects from 1977. Worked in the office of Richard Meier 1966; from 1967–70, special assistant for Design, Housing and Development Administration of the City of New York. Teaching positions at Columbia University from 1969; Bishop Visiting Professor, Yale University 1979; Appointed Dean of the School of Architecture, Yale University 1998. Visiting critic at the Universities of Houston, Pennsylvania, North Carolina, Rice, at Mississippi State University, Rhode Island School of Design, North Carolina State University, Institute for Architecture and Urban Studies. First director, Temple Hoyne Buell Center for the Study of American Architecture, Columbia University 1984–88. President, Architectural League of New York 1973–77. Trustee, American Federation of the Arts 1967–79; Cunningham Dance Foundation 1969–73. FAIA. AIA National Honor Award 1980, 1985, 1990; New York Chapter of the AIA, Distinguished Architecture Award 1982, 1985, 1987, Medal of Honor 1984; John Jay Award, Columbia College 1991; Academy of Arts Lifetime Achievement Award, Guild Hall, East Hampton, NY 1999.

Selected Works

Wiseman House, Montauk, New York (with Stern and Hagmann), 1967
Beebe Residence, Montauk, 1972
Lang House, Washington, Connecticut (Robert A.M. Stern Architects), 1974
Residence and Poolhouse, Llewellyn Park, New Jersey, 1981
Residence, Martha's Vineyard, Massachusetts, 1983
Observatory Hill Dining Hall, University of Virginia, Charlottesville, 1984
Office Building, Point West Place, Framingham, Massachusetts, 1985
Kol Israel Synagogue, Brooklyn, New York, 1989
Urban Villas, Tegel Harbor, Berlin, 1989
Fine Arts Building, University of California, Irvine, 1989
Bancho House Office Building, Tokyo, 1989
Casting Center, Walt Disney World, Lake Buena Vista, Florida, 1989
Police Headquarters, Pasadena, California, 1990
Ohrstrom Library, St. Paul's School, Concord, New Hampshire, 1991
Tivoli Apartments, Tokyo, 1991
Norman Rockwell Museum, Stockbridge, Massachusetts, 1993
Roger Tory Peterson Institute, Jamestown, NY, 1993
Medical Center, Disney Town, Celebration, Florida, 1995
Columbus Regional Hospital, Columbus, Indiana, 1996
William H. Gates Computer Science Building, Stanford University, Palo Alto, California, 1996
Darden School of Business, University of Virginia, Charlottesville, 1996
Federal Court House, Beckley, West Virginia, 1999
Baron Estate, Dallas, 2000

Selected Publications

Forty under Forty: Young Talent in Architecture, 1966
George Howe: Toward a Modern American Architecture, 1975
New Directions in American Architecture, 1969; revised edition, 1977

The Architect's Eye: American Architectural Drawings from 1799–1979 (with Deborah Nevins), 1979
The Anglo American Suburb (with John Massengale), 1981
Raymond Hood (with Thomas P. Catalano), 1982
"One hundred years of resort architecture in East Hampton," in *East Hampton's Heritage: An Illustrated Architectural Record*, edited by Robert J. Hefner, 1982; 2nd edition, 1996
New York, 1900: Metropolitan Architecture and Urbanism, 1890–1915 (with Gregory Gilmartin and John Massengale), 1983
Pride of Place: Building the American Dream (with Thomas Mellins and Raymond Gastil), 1986
Pride of Place: Building the American Dream (videorecording), directed by Murray Grigor, 1986
New York, 1930: Architecture and Urbanism between the Two World Wars (with Gregory Gilmartin and Thomas Mellins), 1987
Modern Classicism (with Ray Gastil), 1988
New York, 1960: Architecture and Urbanism between the Second World War and the Bicentennial (with Thomas Mellins and David Fishman), 1995; 2nd edition, 1997
Robert A.M. Stern: Buildings, 1996
Robert A.M. Stern: Houses, 1997
New York, 1880: Architecture and Urbanism in the Gilded Age (with Thomas Mellins and David Fishman), 1999

Further Reading

Arnell, Peter, and Ted Bickford (editors), *Robert A.M. Stern, 1965–1980: Toward a Modern Architecture after Modernism*, New York: Rizzoli, 1981
Dixon, Peter Morris, *Robert A.M. Stern: Buildings and Projects, 1993–1998*, New York: Monacelli Press, 1998
Kraft, Elizabeth, *Robert A.M. Stern: Buildings and Projects, 1987–1992*, New York: Rizzoli, 1992
Nakamura, Toshio (editor), *The Residential Works of Robert A.M. Stern; Robato Sutan no jutaku, interia* (bilingual English–Japanese edition), Tokyo: A + U, 1982

STICKLEY, GUSTAV 1858–1942

Architect and designer, United States

Gustav Stickley remains one of the most well known figures of early 20th-century American architectural history, not because he was an architect creating revolutionary spaces or employing new materials or innovative structural systems but because he was perhaps the most influential designer of his generation. Stickley furniture and the Craftsman bungalow style established an appealing image that came to embody the honest and simple life of an unsophisticated, independent, democratic American. It is ironic that such an architectural influence would spring from a man who was not a trained architect but whose career as a furniture designer prompted a widespread change in domestic taste and residential design. Stickley's model houses influenced builders and home owners throughout the country to create whole neighborhoods of Craftsman bungalows as well as an interior aesthetic that personified home for an entire generation.

Elements inspired by English domestic architecture and an Arts and Crafts attitude toward craftsmanship especially informed the Stickley aesthetic. Inspired by the communal character of medieval great halls, Craftsman living rooms displaced formal parlors and opened to large dining rooms, creating gathering places for family and friends: the fireplace hearth and ample

dining room table encouraged conversation, intimacy, and conviviality, making the bungalow a place for social interaction as well as private comfort. Built-in bookcases, stenciled walls, and objets d'art brought a cultural enrichment and art into the lives of the inhabitant on a daily basis. Evidences of artisan craftsmanship abounded as sconces and chandeliers were handcrafted, linens and textiles ornamented tabletops and chests, and tilework enriched fireplace surrounds. The Craftsman interior was an artistic home in which art and life were synthesized, but not by means of sophisticated, dust-collecting bric-a-brac and the excessive ornamentation that had characterized Eastlake and Queen Anne interiors of the late Victorian Aesthetic movement, to which Stickley's simplified forms and restraint may be seen to be in reaction.

Gustav Stickley was the eldest son of a large family and one of the oldest of an emerging generation of American Arts and Crafts figures: born in Wisconsin in 1858, Stickley was two years younger than his archrival, Elbert Hubbard (b. 1856), founder of the Roycrofters, but four years older than Bernard Maybeck (b. 1862) and a decade older than Frank Lloyd Wright (b. 1867) and the Greene brothers (Charles Sumner Greene, b. 1868; Henry Mather Greene, b. 1870). Toward the end of the 1890s and following a series of enterprises in various furniture-making companies over about 15 years, Stickley traveled to England and the Continent, where he was exposed to Arts and Crafts ideals and the message of artisan handwork. William Morris (1834–96) had recently died, and John Ruskin (1819–1900) was too ill to receive visitors, but Stickley's affinity to their ideals and philosophy was indicated by his devoting the first issue of *The Craftsman* magazine (1901–16) to Morris and the second issue to Ruskin. Between Stickley's England visit and the establishment of *The Craftsman* in 1901, Stickley produced his first pieces of Craftsman furniture, rejecting the stylish and ecclectic furniture of his earlier business associations. As he began to make simpler Craftsman pieces, Stickley also experimented with proportions, refined forms, and developed a finish that would maintain the natural qualities of wood while protecting its surfaces and color.

Some 40 years earlier, when Philip Webb (1831–1915) completed Red House (1859) for William Morris, the client realized proper furniture and interior fittings were unavailable for his simple and "styleless" house, and so Morris looked to his artist and artisan friends to design pieces to ornament the house, establishing William Morris and Company to produce such furnishings for a wider audience and clientele. Stickley was faced with the reverse situation. He had developed a simplified, styleless furniture aesthetic and realized that late Victorian houses, particularly the popular Queen Anne domestic forms, were unsuitable for his simple, honest, and unadorned furniture, and thus the Craftsman bungalow was born.

The earliest designs for Craftsman houses were amateurish, and Stickley's first architects less competent, but following a brief association (1903–04) with Harvey Ellis, both the refinement of furniture and the quality of architecture improved. By the middle of the first decade of the 20th century, Stickley's Craftsman aesthetic had reached a maturity that stimulated a national craze. Both Craftsman furniture and Craftsman houses were marked by a frank structural expression that was strong and conspicuous in the elimination of carving, inlay, moldings, and ornament. Built-in furniture (bookcases and china cabinets) became part

architecture, part furniture, and even freestanding furniture, such as settles, thronelike armchairs, and large refectory-inspired dining room tables or writing tables and appeared architectonic in their four-square, virtually "trabeated" construction and form.

As Stickley first turned from the ecclectic historicism and revivalism of earlier aesthetics, the United States was experiencing a surge of Arts and Crafts interest. Elbert Hubbard had established his Roycrofter community in East Aurora, New York, in 1895 and was soon publishing *The Philistine* magazine and his *Little Journeys to the Homes of the Great* book series. Arts and Crafts societies were founded in Boston and Chicago in 1897, in Minneapolis in 1899, and in Grand Rapids, Michigan, in 1902. Frank Lloyd Wright was buying and making artisan fittings and furnishings, including Stickley furniture, for his home in Oak Park (built 1889 on), and he produced his own artisan prairie houses during the first decade of the 20th century. Charles Keeler (1871–1937) founded the Ruskin Club (1896) in Berkeley, California, and Bernard Maybeck was building "simple homes" in the San Francisco Bay Area "tradition" already at the turn of the century. Greene and Greene were building bungalows in southern California when Stickley visited there in 1904, and the Greene brothers soon took the Arts and Crafts aesthetic to an extraordinary level of refinement and richness in such "ultimate bungalows" as the Blacker House (1907) and the Gamble House (1908).

Throughout the period, Stickley's Craftsman empire was widening. In November 1903, *The Craftsman* magazine announced the Home Builder's Club, through which any subscriber could order free home plans for houses costing $2,000 to $5,000. By 1916, when the magazine folded, some 200 plans had been published, appearing monthly since 1904. By 1914 Stickley's Craftsman furniture was being sold by some 50 dealers.

In 1905 Stickley was headquartered in New York City, although he maintained his furniture factory earlier established at Eastwood (Syracuse), New York. In 1911 Stickley built the Craftsman Farms in Morris Plains, New Jersey, and two years later he took the dramatic step of leasing a small skyscraper in New York in which to consolidate his enterprises. The 12-story, 200-foot-deep Craftsman Building on 39th Street in New York City contained four lower floors of showrooms for furniture, draperies, and rugs; four middle floors housing the Craftsman Permanent Homebuilders Exposition, in which manufacturers rented space to display house and garden products and model rooms; and four top floors for various Stickley enterprises supporting the Craftsman movement: Craftsman workshops demonstrating crafts, Craftsman architects available to discuss house plans, and the editorial offices of *The Craftsman* as well as club rooms, lecture rooms, a library, and a restaurant, the latter serving meats, vegetables, and fruits homegrown on the Craftsman Farms in an ambiance in which restaurant patrons sat at Craftsman dinner place settings amidst Craftsman chairs, Grueby tiled fireplaces, and Craftsman fittings.

The whole was too much. Stickley had overextended, and by March 1915, The Craftsman Inc. was bankrupt. *The Craftsman* magazine published its last issue in December 1916 and merged with *Art World* in January 1917. Stickley left New York and soon returned to Syracuse for a brief but unsuccessful effort to work with his brothers in the furniture business (Stickley Associated Cabinetmakers, 1917–18). By 1918, Stickley was 60,

the country was at war, and his wife had died. Stickley moved back to his old Syracuse home, now owned by his daughter and her husband, and for 24 years lived in a third-floor suite with a small kitchen where he continued experimenting with wood finishes, still working with his hands in admiration of the natural properties of wood.

From the end of the 19th century until World War I, Stickley created a national empire of furniture and furnishings that inspired a national movement in architecture. When Midwest regional artist Grant Wood painted the tapered piers of a bungalow porch and called his picture "Main Street Mansion," he made an icon of Stickley's Craftsman bungalow for Everyman: a simple American house characterized by a direct structural expression of carpentry and joinery and an honest display of materials. The Craftsman house was the product of entrepreneurial enterprise, Arts and Crafts ideals, and Stickley's reverence for simplicity. Within the short period of a single generation and in the tradition of an Emersonian, self-reliant individualism, a furniture maker had become one of the most influential designers in the history of American domestic architecture: In the opening years of the 20th century, Stickley produced the quintessential house style for democratic America.

ROBERT M. CRAIG

See also **Arts and Crafts Movement; Bungalow; Greene, Henry M. and Charles S. (United States); House; Maybeck, Bernard (United States); Regionalism; Wright, Frank Lloyd (United States)**

Selected Publications

Craftsman Homes, New York: Craftsman, 1909; reprint, as *Craftsman Homes: Architecture and Furnishings of the American Arts and Crafts Movement*, New York: Dover, and London: Constable, 1979

More Craftsman Homes, New York: Craftsman, 1912; reprint as *More Craftsman Homes: Floor Plans and Illustrations for 78 Mission Style Dwellings*, New York: Dover, and London: Constable, 1982

The Best of Craftsman Homes, Santa Barbara, California: Peregrine Smith, 1979

Collected Works of Gustav Stickley, edited by Stephen Gray and Robert Edwards, New York: Turn of the Century Editions, 1981

Craftsman Bungalows: 59 Homes from "The Craftsman," New York: Dover, 1988

Further Reading

The standard biographical monograph on Stickley is Mary Ann Smith's *Gustav Stickley, The Craftsman. The Craftsman* magazine provides the largest collection of writings by Stickley and others espousing the Craftsman aesthetic. Anthologies of Stickley articles, house plans and views, and furniture and decorative arts essays are collected in *The Best of Craftsman Homes* (drawn from Stickley's *Craftsman Homes* and *More Craftsman Homes*). Various publishers have reissued Stickley furniture catalogs. Clay Lancaster's *The American Bungalow, 1880–1930* traces various Craftsman, California, Japanese, and Prairie variants on bungalow themes in a survey of the house style in the United States, whereas Anthony King's *The Bungalow* studies historic bungalow development in India, Britain, North America, Africa, and Australia, viewing it as a "production of global culture."

Bavaro, Joseph J. and Thomas L. Mossman, *The Furniture of Gustav Stickley: History, Techniques, and Projects*, New York: Van Nostrand Reinhold, 1982

Cathers, David M., "Introduction," in *Stickley Craftsman Furniture Catalogs: Unabridged Reprints of Two Mission Furniture Catalogs, "Craftsman Furniture Made by Gustav Stickley" and "The Work of L. and J.G. Stickley,"* by Gustav Stickley, New York: Dover, and London: Constable, 1979

Cathers, David M., *Furniture of the American Arts and Crafts Movement: Stickley and Roycroft Mission Oak*, New York: New American Library, 1981

The Craftsman 1–31 (1901–16)

Freeman, John Crosby, *The Forgotten Rebel: Gustav Stickley and His Craftsman Mission Furniture*, Watkins Glen, New York: Century House, 1966

King, Anthony D., *The Bungalow: The Production of a Global Culture*, London and Boston: Routledge and Kegan Paul, 1984; 2nd edition, New York and Oxford: Oxford University Press, 1995

Lancaster, Clay, *The American Bungalow, 1880–1930*, New York: Abbeville Press, 1985

Smith, Mary Ann, *Gustav Stickley, the Craftsman*, Syracuse, New York: Syracuse University Press, 1983

STIRLING, JAMES 1926–92

Architect, Scotland and England

James Frazer Stirling was born in Glasgow in 1926 but was rather proud of having been conceived on board a ship docked in Manhattan. His father was a marine engineer, and this might account for Stirling's love of tight, shipshape modern design. He studied architecture at Liverpool University, where the presence of Colin Rowe as a fellow student may help explain the classical and humanist tendencies seen in his later work.

In 1953 Stirling worked for Lyons Israel and Ellis in London, where he met James Gowan. They commenced practice together in 1956 and soon became known for a series of buildings that, although uncompromisingly modern, owed little to the then-dominant International Style. The principal works of the partnership were houses at Ham Common (1955–58); a competition project for Churchill College, Cambridge (1958); a project for Selwyn College, Cambridge (1959); and the Leicester University Engineering Building (1959–63), which achieved worldwide fame both for its dramatic contrast of red bricks and greenhouse glazing and for the audacity of its formal precision.

From 1964 to 1971, Stirling practiced alone. To this period belong many original designs, including the Cambridge University History Faculty Building (1964–67); residential units for students (1964–68) at St. Andrew's University; the projects for Dorman Long Headquarters (1965) in Middlesborough; the Florey Building (1966–71) for Queen's College, Oxford; housing for Runcorn New Town (1967–76); the Olivetti Training Centre (1969–72) at Haslemere; and projects for Siemens AG (1969) in Munich and for Derby Civic Centre (1970). In the two last projects, Leon Krier was assistant, and his hand may be detected in drawings made between 1968 and 1970. It seems that Stirling's work did not conform sufficiently to the current ethos, and almost ten years were to pass before he again received an important British commission—for the extension of the Tate Gallery in London (1986).

From 1971 to 1992, Stirling was in partnership with his associate Michael Wilford. Their more important work includes projects for the Olivetti Headquarters (1971) at Milton Keynes

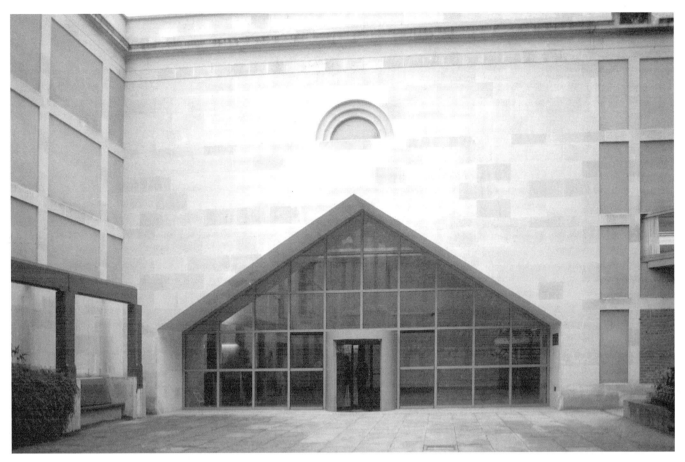

The Clore Gallery for the Turner Collection, Tate Gallery, London (1986)
Photo © Mary Ann Sullivan

and for an Arts Centre (1971) at St. Andrew's University, competition designs for the Kunstsammlung Nordrheim-Westfalen in Düsseldorf and the Wallraf-Richartz Museum in Cologne (both 1975), extensions to the Staatsgalerie Stuttgart (1977, opened 1984), and a new building for the Württenbergisches Staatstheater in Stuttgart.

After taking part in a competition for lower Manhattan in 1968 and serving as a visiting critic and professor at the Yale University School of Architecture from 1960, Stirling became well known in the United States. As a result, he received a number of commissions, including an extension to the Rice University School of Architecture (1979–81) in Houston; the Sackler wing of the Fogg Art Museum (1984), Harvard University, Cambridge, Massachusetts; and the Chemistry Department (1981), Columbia University, New York. The latter project was abandoned, but the Performing Arts Center for Cornell University in Ithaca, New York, was completed in 1988 and the Science Library for the University of California, Irvine, in 1996.

Some critics have seen Stirling's work after 1970 as taking on an increasingly formalist tendency. Works such as the Staatsgalerie Stuttgart and the Tate Gallery extensions have been referred to as Postmodern. Close examination, however, will show the underlying unity of all his work, although there is certainly an important shift (somewhat analogous to the shift in Le Cor-

busier's late work with the Chapel of Notre Dame du Haut in Ronchamp) in that, compared with his earlier buildings, a freer rein is given to expressive gestures. Stirling is always consciously experimental in his use equally of eclectic reference and formal structures. In freely admitting the premeditated nature of all artistic creation, he has liberated himself from the false determinism that plagued so much architectural production after 1945. The element of historicity in his work is no less self-conscious and willful than was the element of modernity in his early work. It is this candor and lack of preconception that perhaps makes his work so vital.

Some of Stirling's most interesting work remains in the form of projects, such as the superb design for a Public Library (1983) at Latina in Italy; the competition entries for the National Gallery Extension (1985) in London; the Thyssen Art Gallery (1986) in Lugano; a design for residential development (1988) at Canary Wharf, London; the Philharmonic Hall (1988) for Los Angeles; the Bibliothèque de France (1989); and the Tokyo International Forum (1989).

However, other larger commissions have matured, giving us the Research and Production Headquarters for Braun Pharmaceuticals (completed 1992) at Melsungen, near Frankfurt, with the collaboration of Walter Nägeli. Since Stirling's death in 1992, we have the Music Academy (completed 1995) at Stutt-

gart; the Science Library (completed 1996) for the University of California, Irvine; the Temesek Polytechnic University (1998) in Singapore; a mixed development at No. 1 Poultry (completed 1998) in the city of London; the mixed residential and offices building (completed 1999) in Carlton Gardens; and the Performing Arts Centre (under construction) at Salford, Lancashire.

Of these, the Braun Headquarters is especially remarkable for the expressiveness of its forms. The single line of conical capitals carrying the administration building is rendered immaterial in certain lights by the choice of materials, so that the building seems to float rather than bear down. It is as though the language of modern architecture had been taken into meditation and revised in the light of an inner vision.

All these works show a remarkable consistency in their conception and design, which is probably explained by the talent and the loyalty of the architects that Stirling and Wilford have employed. Since Stirling's unnecessary death in 1992, the control of the office has passed to his partner, Michael Wilford, who has affirmed his commitment to the sort of architecture that Stirling practiced: experimental, making use of technology but not allowing technology to impose its values alone, aiming always to extend and improve the city fabric, and communicating enjoyment to ordinary people. The working team remains largely intact, and the work continues in large measure to be imprinted with his genius. In 1992, just before going into the hospital for a routine operation, Stirling accepted a knighthood.

ROBERT MAXWELL

See also **Chapel of Notre-Dame-du-Haut, Ronchamp, France; Neue Staatsgalerie, Stuttgart**

Biography

Born in Glasgow, Scotland, 22 April 1926. Studied at the Liverpool School of Art 1942; attended the University of Liverpool School of Architecture 1945–50; exchange student in New York 1949; degree in architecture 1950; studied at the School of Town Planning and Regional Research, London 1950–52. Served in the British Army 1942–45. Worked as senior assistant for Lyons, Israel, Ellis and Gray, London 1953–56; partnership with James Gowan, London 1956–63. Private practice, London from 1964; partner, with Michael Wilford, James Stirling and Partner, later James Stirling, Michael Wilford and Associates, London 1971–92. Visiting lecturer, Architectural Association, London 1955; visiting lecturer, Regent Street Polytechnic, London 1956–57; visiting lecturer, Cambridge University School of Architecture 1958; Royal Institute of British Architects Lecturer 1965; Davenport Professor, Yale University, New Haven, Connecticut from 1967; visiting professor, Akademie der Künste, Düsseldorf from 1977; Banister Fletcher Professor, London University 1977; Architect-in-Residence, American Academy, Rome 1982. Associate, Royal Institute of British Architects 1950; honorary member, Akademie der Künste, Berlin 1969; honorary fellow, American Institute of Architects 1976; honorary member, Accademia delle Arti, Florence 1979; honorary member, Accademia Nazionale de San Luca, Rome 1979; fellow, Royal Society of Arts, London 1979; honorary member, Bund Deutscher Architekten, West Germany 1983. Gold Medal, Royal Institute of

British Architects 1980; Pritzker Prize 1981; knighted 1992. Died in London, 25 June 1992.

Selected Works

Low-rise Flats, Ham Common, London, 1958
Churchill College (competition project), Cambridge, 1958
Selwyn College (project), Cambridge, 1959
Engineering Building, Leicester University, 1963
Dorman Long Headquarters (project), Middlesborough, Yorkshire, 1965
History Faculty Building, Cambridge University, 1967
Student Housing, St. Andrew's University, Scotland, 1968
Siemens AG (project), Munich, 1969
Derby Civic Centre (competition project), 1970
Florey Building, Queen's College, Oxford, 1971
Olivetti Headquarters, Milton Keynes, Buckinghamshire, 1971
Arts Centre, St. Andrew's University, 1971
Olivetti Training Centre, Haslemere, Surrey, 1972
Kunstsammlung Nordrheim-Westfalen (competition project), Düsseldorf, 1975
Wallraf-Richartz Museum (competition project), Cologne, 1975
Low-cost Housing, Runcorn New Town, Cheshire, 1976
Staatsgalerie (extension), Stuttgart, 1977
Building for the Württenbergisches Staatstheater, Stuttgart, 1977
School of Architecture (extension), Rice University, Houston, 1981
Chemistry Department (unbuilt), Columbia University, New York, 1981
Public Library (project), Latina, Italy, 1983
Sackler Wing, Fogg Art Museum, Harvard University, Cambridge, Massachusetts, 1984
National Gallery Extension (competition project), London, 1985
Clore Gallery, Turner Collection, Tate Gallery, London, 1986
Thyssen Art Gallery (competition project), Lugano, 1986
Residential Development (competition project), Canary Wharf, London, 1988
Performing Arts Center, Cornell University, Ithaca, New York, 1988
Philharmonic Hall (competition project) Los Angeles, 1988
Bibliothèque de France (project), Paris, 1989
Tokyo International Forum (project), 1989
Research and Production Headquarters, Braun Pharmaceuticals, Melsungen, Germany (with Walter Nägeli), 1992
Music Academy, Stuttgart, 1995
Science Library, University of California, Irvine, 1996
Temesek Polytechnic University, Singapore, 1998
Mixed Development, No.1 Poultry, London, 1998
Mixed Development, Carlton Gardens, London, 1999

Selected Publications

James Stirling: Buildings and Projects, 1950–1974, 1975
James Stirling (with Robert Maxwell), 1983

Further Reading

Maxwell, Robert, "The Far Side of Modernity," *Architectural Review* 1150 (December 1992)
Maxwell, Robert, "[Introduction]" in *James Stirling, Michael Wilford and Associates, 1975–1992*, by Michael Wilford and Thomas Muirhead, London: Thames and Hudson, 1994
Rowe, Colin, "[Introduction]" in *James Stirling, Buildings and Projects*, by Peter Arnell and Ted Bickford, New York: Rizzoli, and London: Architectural Press, 1984

STOCKHOLM PUBLIC LIBRARY

Designed by Erik Gunnar Asplund; 1918–28; additions
1928–31
Stockholm, Sweden

The City Library (Stadsbiblioteket) in Stockholm, designed by
Erik Gunnar Asplund, is one of those unusual 20th-century
buildings that has had two lives. Design work began in 1918,
and the Library opened to widespread acclaim ten years later.
Its second life came in the late 1970s and the 1980s, when
architects and critics were looking afresh at early 20th-century
architects such as Asplund, whose work represented a form of
modernity that did not involve the adoption of modernist functionalism.

The commission of the City Library was prompted by a gift
from the Knut and Alice Wallenberg Foundation. Their dona-
tion of one million kronor (Swedish crowns) stipulated that
matching funds as well as land and all design costs be provided
by the Stockholm City Council. Carl Westman (1866–1936),
who had just completed the Rådhuset (1908–15), the municipal
courthouse in Stockholm, was invited to serve as architectural
consultant, but he declined, and an offer was made to Asplund,
then only 32 years old, who was appointed on 2 December 1918.
It was an important commission, not only for the prominence of
building and site but also for its uniqueness: It was the first
public library building in Sweden from which patrons themselves could remove books from the shelves.

The site chosen was the corner of Sveavägen and Odengatan,
slightly outside the center of the city, on a lot that included
the termination of the Brunkebergsåsen ridge, on which Carl
Hårleman had built an observatory (1746–53). The first plan
(published 1921) was to develop the entire lot, including a
school of economics and law faculty for the University of Stockholm as well as the Library and a market hall along Odengatan.
Work began initially on the Library program, and in May 1920
Asplund and the city librarian Fredrijk Hjelmqvist were sent to
the United States to study American libraries. Their journey
took them to the major cities on the East Coast and the Midwest,
and the visitors were particularly impressed by Cass Gilbert's
Main Library (1913–21) in Detroit, Michigan, which provided
a model for the centralized plan, second-story book room, and
upper-level down lighting later employed in Stockholm. Asplund was also impressed by the functionalist process by which
Americans studied libraries. "In America," he wrote in his travel
journal, "one gets an overwhelming impression of the extraordinary, almost scientific care with which the libraries are designed.
It is a continuously evolving development towards better result.
Experiences of earlier libraries are studied and utilized in every
new one."

Asplund was predisposed to a classically inspired solution for
the Library. His earliest sketches, possibly from 1919, employ
circular spaces that suggest that the original inspiration might
have been Palladio's Villa Rotunda in Vicenza. This kind of
source might have been expected for someone educated at the
Klara School (1910–11), where stripped-down classicism was
used to evoke modernity. Revisions (1921) to the original proposals, after the American trip, show a gridded facade with paired
columns and a truncated entablature that recalls, albeit much

simplified, Ivar Tengbom's contemporary Konserthuset (1920–
26). As part of this early scheme, a dome rises prominently from
the center of the block.

Changes were made by the time of construction. The building was raised to a broad plinth above street level to accommodate the irregular terrain, and the university buildings and market hall were suppressed. Along Sveavägen, shops were added,
and entry to the Library was placed on axis with the main door
along a ramplike flight of stairs through the (later) shopping
block. The Library itself is a square with a projecting cylinder
rather than a raised dome, as originally proposed, to mark the
circular reading room rotunda. Around the outside of the Library
is a low-relief Etruscan-Egyptian frieze, and the marble door is
Egyptian in style, with canted sides. From the marble entrance
lobby, a flight of narrow stairs between dark marble walls leads
directly to the reading room, a fact that is also revealed from
street level.

The central reading room is the heart of the plan. Three
levels of open-shelved books surround the central space. This
was Asplund's clear design preference, and he argued to the
program committee that in addition to its formal value, the
circular plan was more functional, allowing more space along
the walls for bookshelves and on the floor for desks, chairs, and
the librarians' station. The reading areas were furnished with
lights, tables, and chairs designed by Asplund. All other rooms
(for reading, study, and periodicals) are subservient to the central
space, located either in the surrounding square or, as light wells,
in the spandrels between the square and the rotunda. One of
the most noted rooms is a special section for children that was
decorated with a semicircular fresco by Nils Dardel depicting
the dream figure of John Blund and his umbrella. (Blund is a
kind of sandman who brings sleep and happy dreams to Scandinavian children.)

There has been much discussion of the nature of Asplund's
sources. Roman sources from the Pantheon to the Castel
Sant'Angelo (Rasmussen, 1940) and to the Tomb of Hadrian,
as illustrated by Fischer von Erlach (Donnelly, 1992), have been
the most commonly cited for the square plus cylinder. Caldenby
(1985) and others have suggested that the Library might depend
on Claude-Nicolas Ledoux's Rotonde de la Villette (1785–89),
one of his tollbooths for Paris. It has also been suggested that
Asplund knew Étienne Boullée's Cenotaph for Isaac Newton
(Wrede, 1980), an unlikely possibility, as Boullée's image was
generally available only later. A more conventional source, one
that is typologically appropriate, would have been Sidney
Smirke's rotunda (1854–57) for the British Museum in London.
Perhaps the initial idea for a dome came from Hårlemann's
observatory on the hill above. Finally, it cannot be forgotten
that the City Library stands at the north end Sveavägen, a street
that originates at Tessin's Royal Palace on Gamla Stan and that
provides justification for the monumental character of the building. Indeed, a specific recollection might be found in the ramplike entry, which recalls the approach to the Royal Palace up
Slottsbacken in addition to stairway sequences that had inspired
him during his Italian journey (1913–14), as has been observed
by Winter. Finally, the classicizing order of the building includes
decorative motifs: Egyptian, Etruscan, and Greek Revival, most
notably from Michael Gottlieb Bindesbøll at the Thorvaldsen

Museum in Copenhagen (1839–48), whose Egyptian-style portal seems to have been a specific inspiration.

The precise symbolic program of the Library remains elusive. Of course, the circle within the square and the dome recollect a heavenly universality. An early drawing (1921) shows a medallic portrait of a bald-headed man with a short beard in profile over the door, possibly a representation of an ancient philosopher. On the floor of the entry mosaic is the inscription (in Greek) "Know Thyself." In the entrance hall, the walls are reliefs by Ivar Johnson with scenes from Homer's *Iliad*. Somewhat at odds with this evocation of ancient myth and philosophy are the original door handles of the Library, now preserved on the second floor. They represent Adam eating the apple (inside handle) and Eve with the apple (outside handle), and both needed to be gripped and held, if briefly, by patrons entering and exiting the Library. Do they suggest the potential dangers of knowledge or a recognition that it is in human nature to eat from the tree of knowledge? Or are they prelapsarian guardians of a paradisaic place of knowledge?

The Library remains largely unaltered from its original construction. In 1974, a double flight of stairs was built to handle traffic to the upper gallery, elevators were installed, and building restoration was undertaken (1979–81) with the opening of a further light well. The original entrance doors were replaced, the furnishings were renovated, and the lighting was improved at that time. In 1994, the entire Library and terrace building was replastered and painted.

Following the completion of the Library, Asplund plunged into work on the Stockholm Exhibition of 1930 and began his brief functionalist period. Already, the reflecting pool (completed 1931) along Sveavägen evokes modernist architectural concerns as do the retail shops at street level and the small rear facade addition (1928–31). Indeed, the building was completed at a critical point in Swedish architectural history. Writing in the magazine *Byggmästaren* (1928), the architect Uno Åhrén declared, "New classicism is dead." The Library, he wrote, "stands at the border, not between two minor stylistic tendencies of Swedish architecture, as some suggest, but between two phases of fundamental difference in mentality." Åhrén was right to the extent that the succeeding years did not favor the classicizing references that Asplund deployed in the Library. Nonetheless, writers on Asplund, such as the Englishman Eric de Maré (1955), continued to praise the prefunctionalist phase of Asplund's career despite—or perhaps because of—its traditional nature.

In the 1970s, when Asplund became a focus of attention for a generation of Postmodernist architects "stalking," in the words of Treib (in Engfors, 1986), "the considered balance between modernity and tradition," the Library became a pilgrimage site. Architects such as Leon Krier looked to the Library as a model of geometric typology. In the United States and Italy, Romaldo Giurgola and Aldo Rossi helped revive interest in Asplund; Kenneth Frampton and Stuart Wrede (1980) were also influential in the United States, along with Michael Graves and Thomas Beeby, who were probably introduced to Asplund by the architectural critic Colin Rowe (see the essay by Parsons in Engfors, 1986).

NICHOLAS ADAMS

Further Reading

The standard works on Asplund by Caldenby and Hultin and Wrede provide the best overview. The brochure by Winter contains important information on the renovation and Asplund's contribution to the interior decorations.

Caldenby, Claes, "Time, Life, and Work: An Introduction to Asplund" in *Asplund*, edited by Caldenby and Olof Hultin, Stockholm: Arkitektur Forlag, 1985; New York: Rizzoli, 1986

Caldenby, Claes and Olof Hultin (editors), *Asplund*, Stockholm: Arkitektur Forlag, 1985; New York: Rizzoli, 1986

De Maré, Eric, *Gunnar Asplund: A Great Modern Architect*, London: Art and Technics, 1955

Donnelly, Marian C., *Architecture in the Scandinavian Countries*, Cambridge, Massachusetts: MIT Press, 1992

Engfors, Christina (editor), *Lectures and Briefings from the International Symposium on the Architecture of Erik Gunnar Asplund*, Stockholm: Arkitekturmuseet, 1986

Holmdahl, Gustav, Sven Ivar Lind, and Kjell Ödeen, *Gunnar Asplund, arkitekt, 1885–1940: Ritningar, skisser, och fotografier*, Stockholm: Tidskriften Byggmästaren, 1943; 2nd edition, 1981; as *Gunnar Asplund, Architect, 1885–1940: Plans, Sketches, and Photographs*, Stockholm: AB Tidskriften Byggmästaren, 1950; 2nd edition, 1981

Rasmussen, Steen Eiler, *Nordische Baukunst*, Berlin: Wasmuth, 1940

Winter, Karin, *Stockholm City Library: Architect Gunnar Asplund*, Stockholm: Stockholm Stadsbibliotek, 1998

Wrede, Stuart, *The Architecture of Erik Gunnar Asplund*, Cambridge, Massachusetts: MIT Press, 1980

STOCKHOLM, SWEDEN

The center of Swedish activity in architecture during the 20th century was Stockholm, its capital city. Not only was Stockholm the locus of political, financial, and cultural power, but it was also the site of the major architecture school in Sweden, the Kunigligan Teknikiska Högskolan.

The two most significant buildings in Stockholm at the beginning of the 20th century, the Nordiska Museum and the Town Hall, represent different aspects of national consciousness in architecture. With its prominent position on the island of Djürgården, Isak Gustaf Clason's (1856–1930) Nordiska Museum (1889–1907) was intended to be a temple for Swedish culture. Its towers recall the great castles of the Vasa period (Gripsholm, Vadstena, and Kalmar), and its gables recall the Trefaldighetskyrkan (1658) in Kristianstad. The entrance portal is in the form of a secular Gothic-style cathedral with Mother Svea and Odin. The use of stone from around Sweden and the naturalistic carving by local stonemasons recall principles enunciated by the English critic John Ruskin. At the center of the building is a great room, evoking both castle hall and ecclesiastical nave, and a monumental statue of Gustav Vasa by Carl Milles (1875–1955). In short, the building celebrates national culture through its great moments of history, both real and mythic, and representative examples of its geology.

By contrast, the Town Hall (1904–23), designed by Ragnar Östberg (1866–1945), is much less explicit in its sources; historic architecture is evoked through the lens of the native traditions of arts and crafts. Although made of brick, traditionally common in southern Sweden, its profile recalls an Italian communal palace rather than any Swedish building. Östberg has confected his

historical references: part Romanesque, part Gothic, and part Byzantine. The great top-lit hall at the center of the building, the so-called Blue Hall, is slightly out of square, deliberately recalling the craft traditions of the Middle Ages.

New influences arrived from the United States and from Germany in the 1910s and 1920s. Sweden was especially receptive to North American architecture as a result of emigration. Many architects and artists traveled to America, some to stay, some to profit on their return. Ferdinand Boberg, for example, took advantage of his visit to Chicago for the World's Columbian Exposition of 1893 to study American building practices, and Gustaf Wickman (1858–1916) and Carl Westman (1866–1936) visited the United States and were inspired by H.H. Richardson. With the construction of a pair of concrete skeleton-frame skyscrapers, North American influence became technological and urbanistic. Over 60 meters tall, the skyscrapers were part of the 1919 master plan. The new street, Kungsgatan, broke through the old ridgeline, leaving the old street as a flying bridge. The northern skyscraper, inspired by Louis Sullivan, was designed by Sven Wallander (1890–1968) and employed a tripartite division and vertical pilaster strips "to describe," as Wallander said, "the forces at work within." The southern tower, similar in form, was built by Ivar Callmander (1880–1951) in 1925. The urbanistic effect recalls the multilevel visions of New York in Moses King's *Views of New York* or even the most up-to-date American architecture at Grand Central Terminal in New York City, where the Park Avenue flyover had just been connected.

In this period, connections with Germany and Austria are decisive for the architecture of Stockholm, as can be seen in works such as the Liljevachs Konsthall (1913–16), built by Carl Bergsten (1879–1935) for the sawmill magnate C.F. Lilejevalch. It was built on a grid plan with concrete piers and brick screen in-fill. In its rationalism, it recalls the work of Peter Behrens and Heinrich Tessenow and thus marks a significant passage from Östberg's Town Hall. Like Östberg's Blue Hall in the Town Hall, the main gallery is lit by a clerestory window that encircles the room at the upper level, but the gray-concrete trim and columns alternate with the white of the walls to recall Behrens' favored Italianate sources, as the coffered ceiling and decorative details further reveal. Bergsten also built the church at Hjorthagen (1904–06), which recalls Wiener Werkstätte designs. Architects such as Ivar Tengbom (1878–1968) also employed a simplified Italianate classicism.

The figure that most effectively represents the advanced trends of architecture in this period in Stockholm is Gunnar Asplund (1885–1940). In the early phase of his career, he combined apparent opposites: the traditions of Östberg's folk architecture with the reductionist geometry of the Germanic countries. His Woodland Chapel (1920), for example, employed traditional materials (wrought iron, stone, and wood) but in rigid geometric order. In his designs with Sigurd Lewerentz (1885–1975), with whom he shared design responsibilities for the Woodland Cemetery (1915–40), these are integrated into the traditions of Swedish landscape made mythic with biblical references. Lewerentz's Chapel of the Resurrection (1925) is strongly classical in inspiration, and in the Skandia Cinema (1922–23) and City Library (1920–28), Asplund's classicizing tendencies emerge clearly.

Asplund soon moved in a new direction. In 1928, he was appointed chief designer for the Stockholm Exhibition organized by Slöjdföreningen (the Society for Arts and Crafts), which opened on 16 May 1930 on Djurgården. Asplund took on the task of shaping Swedish notions of European modernism. With his associates, notably Sven Markelius (1889–1972), Uno Åhrén (1897–1977), and Wolter B. Gahn (1890–1985), he provided a series of exhibition buildings decorated with flags, constructivist neon signs, nighttime floodlighting, and playful graphics to display new techniques of construction and new design approaches in housing, office design, and urbanism. With this group, which included Gregor Paulsson (1889–1977) and Eskil Sundahl (1890–1974), Asplund authored a manifesto of modern functionalism (1931) with the declarative title *acceptera*: "Accept the reality before you only through it do we have any prospect of mastering it, of coping with it so as to alter, and to create culture that is a handy tool for one's life." Swedish architects were receptive to the ideas of functionalism. With many architectural problems in need of solutions, notably in the field of housing, functionalism seemed to offer a logical path toward their resolution. The strip window, for example, which might need to be rationalized elsewhere, made perfect sense at 60 degrees north, where the sun barely moved beyond the horizontal much of the year. At another level, however, the success of functionalism reflected a broader cultural effort: 20th-century Swedes who wanted a modern Sweden based on values other than those of the state, the church, or bourgeois capitalism. The first public building in the functionalist style was Markelius and Åhrén's Kårhus (student center, 1928–30) at the Kunigligan Teknikiska Högskolan. Lewerentz's unadorned gridded facades for the Riksförsäkringsverket (1930–32), or national insurance board, is a significant early example of government-commissioned functionalism.

It was not until after World War II that significant architectural inroads were made into the old fabric of the city, although not always with happy results. The Hötorscity office and commercial complex, for example, was started in 1945 and recalls Gordon Bunshaft's Lever House in New York City. By David Helldén (1905–90), Anders Tengbom (1911–), Sven Markelius, Lars Erik Lallerstedt (1864–1955), and Backström (1903–92) and Reinius (1907–95), of the firm Backström and Reinius, Hötorscity consists of five multistoried slab blocks (with a significant pedestrian component). Construction was not completed until the mid-1950s. The development gave Stockholm an American-style architectural skyline. In 1971–73, Kulturhuset, a megastructure at Sergels Torg by the architect Peter Celsing (1920–74), inspired in part by Le Corbusier, provided a city-sponsored communal center with theaters, restaurants, meeting space, and exhibition space nearby. One of the most significant buildings of this period was Celsing's gridded facade to the Riksbanken (1976), behind Kulturhuset, which suggested greater acceptance of historical forms. In effect, Lewerentz's Riksförsäkringsverket grid of the 1930s was transformed into rusticated stone. Important church buildings by Celsing (Olaus Petrikyrkan, 1957–59) and Lewerentz (Markuskyrkan in Björkhagen, 1956–60) demonstrated a new attention to traditional materials.

By the 1970s, the era of large-scale city demolition was over. Protests in 1971 over the felling of a stand of elms in Kungsträdgården to make way for a subway station marked the change in public sentiment, although the last of the great reconstructions was still ongoing at the end of the century. Cityterminalen (1986–89) by Arken Arkitektur with Ahlqvist and Culjat, Ralph Erskine (1914–), and Tengboms Arkitektkontor is a mixed

public-private venture adjacent to the Normmalm shopping district designed to create a new business-conference center at Stockholm's transportation node (bus, subway, and train). Slowed by the downturn in the economy at the beginning of the 1990s, when completed the project will form a new, efficient business center near the heart of the old city.

Any survey of Stockholm in the 20th century must touch on housing. At the beginning of the century, more than 50 percent of living quarters consisted of one room plus a kitchen or less. There were various experiments: garden city–style suburban developments at Gamla Enskede (1907) designed by Per Olof Hallman (1869–1941) and Herman Ygberg (1844–1917), functionalist-style worker housing at Svarneholmen (1928–1930) designed by Olof Thunström (1896–1962) of the firm KFAI, and the founding in 1936 by the City of Stockholm of the Familjebostäder and Stockholmshem housing companies, both of which were responsible for the erection of large-family housing in areas such as Abrahamsberg, Åkeshov, Riksby, and Åkeslund. The first examples of collective housing were designed by Markelius at John Ericssonsgatan (1934–35).

The nature of housing construction changed after World War II. In 1941, the Stockholm City Council decided to build a new subway system, and construction began between Slussen and Hökarängen (1950) and Hötorget and Vällingby (1952). The two lines were linked at the main train station, T-Centralen, in 1957, and housing was developed along these lines. The plan was to build developments of between 10,000 and 15,000 inhabitants centered on a subway station with small commercial and service centers, a school, and playing fields within walking distance. Among the newly incorporated suburbs, Vällingby is among the best known and became an international model for new town construction. Planning began as early as 1940, and ground was broken in 1951. With its commercial center designed partially by Backström and Reinius, its adjacent subway station by Magnus Ahlgren (1918–), churches by Celsing and Carl Nyrén (1917–), and segregated pedestrian/cycle paths, it was model of efficiency. Around the center were large slab blocks of multistory apartments, and farther out were row houses. Farsta (1953–61) was a similar counterpart south of central Stockholm.

In 1965, the Swedish government sought to put an end to the housing shortage and developed the Miljonprogrammet (Million Dwelling Program), which also had an effect on Stockholm. In Rinkeby and Tensta, for example, huge anonymous apartment buildings were built, and although later examples improved this type at Norra Järva, Akalla, Husby, and Kista, they were not popular. Additionally, terrace housing on an American pattern—that is, without proximate public services and thus requiring the use of an automobile for all activities—was built in areas such as Kälvesta and Hässelby.

At the end of the 20th century, it is difficult to isolate projects that will have lasting architectural influence on the city. From a visual point of view, the Globen sports complex by Berg Arkitektkontor AB (1986–88) is the most important but is not universally welcome. The giant sphere looms over Södermalm like an escapee from a Walt Disney amusement park. More significant, Ralph Erskine's Aula Magna (1988–90) at Frescati represents the continuing engagement of Stockholm's urban architecture with its natural environment, and the Moderna Museet and Arkitekturmuseet (1990–98) by Rafael Moneo (1937–) on

Skeppsholmen and Ricardo Bofill's (1939–) Bågen Residence (1989–1991), a vast, crescent-shaped housing development at Södra station, are examples of the renewed influence of foreign architects, something not felt strongly in Stockholm.

NICHOLAS ADAMS

Further Reading

Caldenby, Claes, Jöran Lindvall, and Wilfried Wang, *20th-Century Architecture: Sweden*, Munich and New York: Prestel, 1998

Constant, Caroline, *The Woodland Cemetery: Toward a Spiritual Landscape: Erik Gunnar Asplund and Sigurd Lewerentz, 1915–61*, Stockholm: Byggförlaget, 1994

Hall, Thomas, *Huvudstad i omvandling: Stockholms planering och utbyggnad under 700 år*, Stockholm: Sveriges Radio, 1999

Hall, Thomas and Katarina Dunér (editors), *Den svenska staden: planering och gestaltning—från medeltid till industrialism*, Stockholm: Sveriges Radios Forlag, 1997

Hultin, Olof, et al., *The Complete Guide to Architecture in Stockholm*, Stockholm: Arkitektur Forlag, 1998

Rudberg, Eva, *The Stockholm Exhibition, 1930: Modernism's Breakthrough in Swedish Architecture; Stockholmsutstallningen, 1930: modernismens genombrott i Svensk arkitektur* (bilingual English-Swedish edition), Stockholm: Stockholmia, 1999

STONE

Stone has two distinct architectural faces: in monumental architecture, it stands for wealth, power, and permanence; on the other hand, especially when used at a domestic scale and based on local craft traditions, it appears as modest, forthright, and natural. These two aspects of stone correspond to the varying levels of effort and skill marshaled in its fabrication, transportation, and erection. Finely worked, accurately cut blocks, sometimes of exotic origin or polished to a jewel-like finish, characterize monumental architecture, while fieldstone, rubble, or roughly worked stone set in thick mortar beds is more often associated with modest works. Stone's symbolic content is not determined by these two traditions alone but also reflects the revolutionary changes brought about by industrialization and by the attitudes—ranging from ambivalence to outright hostility—with which those changes are greeted. Increasingly anachronistic from a purely functional standpoint, stone survives in 20th-century architecture largely as a medium through which these attitudes can be symbolically expressed.

At the beginning of the 20th century, monumental stone architecture is associated primarily with neoclassical and Gothic Revival styles. McKim, Mead and White's Pennsylvania Station (1910) and James J. Farley Post Office (1912), both in New York City, employ classical stone facades—Doric and Corinthian, respectively—coexisting with an infrastructure of glass and steel necessary to accommodate and express the realities of modern urban life. Ralph Adams Cram, America's leading Gothic Revivalist, also incorporates modern construction technologies—including various hidden reinforced-concrete decks, lintels, and bond beams—together with traditional limestone detailing in projects such as his Princeton University Chapel (1922) in Princeton, New Jersey.

At the same time, neoclassical monumentality was attacked from several points of view at the beginning of the 20th century. The Arts and Crafts movement, reacting to the social and physi-

cal fallout associated with industrialization, proposed a return to "honest" craft values. These values are expressed in the rough stone walls of W.R. Lethaby's All Saints' Church (1902) in Herefordshire, England, and the rounded rubble stone foundations of the John Bakewell Phillips House (1906) designed by the Greene Brothers in Pasadena, California. Edwin Lutyens' use of rubble stone in early 20th-century residential projects such as Grey Walls (1900) in Gullane, Scotland, is similarly rooted in an Arts and Crafts sensibility, although his monumental Viceroy's House (1931) in New Delhi, clad with finely worked red-and-buff-colored Dholpur sandstone, reaffirms the neoclassical tradition, albeit combined with vernacular elements.

The most radical of the reactions against traditional architectural styles was International Style modernism. Modernists invoked the idea of "truth to materials" to provide intellectual cover for the unsettling changes in the built environment associated with the industrial revolution—specifically, the rationalization of the building process to increase productivity and reduce costs. Eliminating gratuitous decoration (such as the ornamented stone facades of traditional monumental architecture) became a fundamental tenet of modernism. However, the use of stone as honest bearing wall or smooth-surfaced veneer was generally accepted.

Le Corbusier's Villa de Mme de Mandrot (1931) in Le Pradet, France, illustrates the use of undecorated stone walls within a modernist syntax, as does his earlier exploration of parallel masonry bearing walls in the Maisions Citrohan projects of the early 1920s. While such structural stone walls remained fairly common in domestic-scaled buildings—Frank Lloyd Wright's dramatic use of stone piers supporting horizontal cantilevers of reinforced concrete at Fallingwater (1938) in Bear Run, Pennsylvania, is a notable example—the development of steel and concrete frameworks rendered stone load-bearing walls virtually obsolete for larger institutional or commercial buildings. An exception is Kevin Roche's Creative Arts Center at Wesleyan University (1973) in Middletown, Connecticut, consisting of 14-inch-thick limestone bearing walls laid without mortar and capped by a reinforced-concrete roof structure. Roche uses a similar stone system in his additions to the Metropolitan Museum of Art (1974–80) in New York City.

Attitudes toward nonstructural cladding, articulated by 19th-century theorists such as John Ruskin, Carl Bötticher, and Gottfried Semper and adapted in the 20th century by European architect-theorists such as Otto Wagner and Adolf Loos, provided a theoretical basis for the "honest" expression of thin stone veneer. Wagner's Post Office Savings Bank (1906) in Vienna, although constructed with conventional brick bearing walls, is clad with thin marble panels visibly attached to the brick walls with aluminum-capped iron bolts. Adolf Loos used stone and other cladding materials to develop richly surfaced interior spaces that correspond not to the structure of his houses but to the logic of their social functioning. Loos' Müller House (1930) in Prague includes thin green-veined Cipollino marble panels on key interior surfaces, emblematic of wealth and refined taste but at the same time marked by a certain modern dissonance.

Stone cladding was often used to impart a kind of traditional legitimacy to otherwise modern buildings. Examples include Mies van der Rohe's Barcelona Pavilion (1929), Giuseppe Terragni's Casa del Fascio (1936; now Casa del Populo) in Como, Italy, Edward Durrell Stone and Philip Goodwin's Museum of Modern Art (New York City, 1939), and the United Nations Secretariat Building (New York City, 1953) by Wallace K. Harrison and others.

On the other hand, rough stone was used to impart a more domestic or natural feeling to modern buildings. Marcel Breuer and Walter Gropius' Hagerty House (1938) in Cohasset, Massachusetts, utilizes stone and stucco surfaces to create a picturesque though still modern formal composition. Eero Saarinen's IBM Facility (1956) in Yorktown, New York, contrasts roughly worked stone walls reassembled from existing pasture barriers on the site with modern glass curtain walls.

Still, stone use declined in the three decades following World War II in favor of more technologically advanced materials and curtain-wall systems. Within the modernist genre, stone was relegated to thin veneer without decorative embellishment, understated in its color and texture. Saarinen's CBS Building (1965) and Breuer's Whitney Museum of American Art (1966), both in New York City, are faced in a muted, thermal-finished granite cladding consistent with the minimalist aesthetic of the time. Other examples include Kevin Roche's Ford Foundation Building (1968) in New York City, with granite cladding defining the boundaries of its abstract cubic form, and I.M. Pei's East Wing of the National Gallery (1978) in Washington, D.C., similarly using stone veneer—in this case Tennessee marble matching the original stone used in the museum's West Wing—to define its abstract angular geometry.

The 1980s saw an explosion in the use of stone cladding, typical of postmodern exuberance, while advances in stone fabrication technology significantly reduced costs. The postmodern synthesis—combining the symbolic values of traditional architecture with the rational infrastructure of modernism—gained both notoriety and legitimacy with the construction of Philip Johnson's pink granite AT&T Building (1983) in New York City. Other notable examples within this genre include Michael Graves' Humana Headquarters Building (1985) in Louisville, Kentucky, covered with several varieties of exterior granites and interior marbles; Kohn Pedersen Fox's Procter and Gamble World Headquarters (1985) in Cincinnati, Ohio, clad in six-inch-thick buff-colored Indiana limestone panels spanning from floor to floor; and Cesar Pelli's World Financial Center (1985–88) in New York City, consisting of two million square feet of stone, primarily polished and thermal-finished granite.

Earlier attempts at such a synthesis can be seen in the abstracted monumental classicism promoted by Mussolini during the 1930s and 1940s. Guerrini, Lapadula and Romano's Palace of Italian Civilization (1942) in *Esposizione Universale di Roma* (EUR), just outside of Rome, is an example; its monumental cubic form, defined by rows of deep-set travertine arcades, mimics the stone arches and axiality of classical and baroque Rome while maintaining plain and unornamented surfaces. In the United States, a variant form of abstracted neoclassicism can be seen in the arched travertine facade of Wallace K. Harrison's Metropolitan Opera House (New York City, 1966).

Especially outside the United States, Postmodernism draws on the platonic geometries associated with such 18th-century visionary designers as Claude-Nicolas Ledoux and Etienne-Louis Boullée. The stone block or panel becomes important in this context not just for its symbolic resonance but also as the basic elemental unit to which the overall geometric form of the building is inextricably tied. Charles Correa's Jawahar Kala Kendra

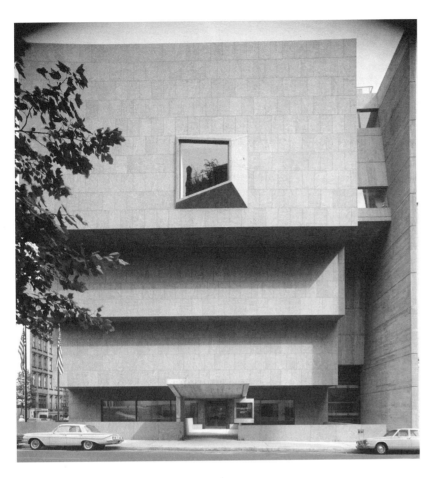

Whitney Museum of American Art (1966), New York City, designed by Marcel Breuer
Ezra Stoller © Esto

Museum (1990) in Jaipur, India, is based on a nine-square plan, with each square block symmetrically stepping down at the corners, consistent with the module of its red sandstone cladding; Aldo Rossi's Monument to Sandro Pertini (1990) in Milan, Italy, is a symmetrical cubic block clad in gray and pink marble into which a monumental stair is cut. Here, stone provides a historic link both to Milan's Duomo (whose stone was cut from the same quarry) and to the traditional rose granite street pavement removed for subway construction and reused by Rossi on the site.

A self-consciously critical, if not overtly ironic, attitude toward the use of stone can also be discovered in Postmodern architecture. Vittorio Mazzucconi's 22 Avenue Matignon (1976) in Paris juxtaposes fragments from an old stone facade within a new glass curtain wall. Francesco Venezia's Museum (1989) in Gibellina, Sicily, sets part of an earthquake-damaged stone building into a new stone structure in which the old and new are integrated yet clearly distinguished. Hans Hollein's Jewelry Shop (1974) in Vienna creates a deliberately "cracked" stone facade that challenges not only the modernist notion of honest expression but also the canonic meaning of stone as a signifier of wealth and permanence. Venturi, Scott Brown and Associates' Sainsbury Wing of the National Gallery (1987) in London takes a Corinthian pilaster motif from the existing museum's 19th-century neoclassical facade, carefully reproduces it in a new stone facade, and then incrementally transforms it into an increasingly abstract (modern) figure. Rem Koolhaas' Nexus World Kashii

(1991) in Fukuoka, Japan, features a curving wall whose concrete surface texture expertly simulates—and caricatures—the traditional stonework of Japanese castles. Examples of the deliberate and didactic juxtaposition of stone with more modern construction technologies include Álvaro Siza's Galician Center for Contemporary Art (1994) in Santiago de Compostela, where granite cladding rests on exposed steel channels and posts, and Jacques Herzog and Pierre de Meuron's Stone House (1982) in Tavole, Italy, in which a slatelike rubble in-fill wall is contrasted with a rigorously orthogonal exposed reinforced-concrete frame.

Stone has also been "reinvented" by several 20th-century architects who have developed wall systems combining aspects of stone masonry and concrete technology. Frank Lloyd Wright's "desert rubble masonry"—first used at Taliesin West (1937) in Scottsdale, Arizona—sets unworked stones tight against concrete formwork so that they become visible on the wall's surface. Similarly, Eero Saarinen's Norwegian-based system, adapted for his Stiles and Morse Colleges (1962) at Yale University, injects pressurized concrete into forms filled with rough stones. Peter Zumthor, for his Thermal Bath (1997) in Vals, Switzerland, created a composite concrete-masonry system in which locally quarried gneiss blocks defining the continuous cavelike internal spaces and external massing of the building are made integral with reinforced-concrete cores.

Finally, stone buildings have continued to be built in traditional ways throughout the 20th century. Quinlan Terry's Mait-

land Robinson Library (1993) in Cambridge, England, with its pemented stone facade, may serve as an example of the continuing interest in literal, neoclassical form. The use of stone based on local, vernacular traditions can be seen in numerous 20th-century projects: examples include Ricardo Bofill's Sanctuary of Meritxell (1978) in Andorra, faced with thick stone excavated from the site by Galician masons; Jan Olav Jensen and Per Christian Brynildsen's Hospital (1985) in Maharastra, India, featuring stone load-bearing walls built with local materials by local masons; and Raffaele Cavadini's Municipal Buildings (1995) in Iragna, Switzerland, faced with dry split stones detailed according to local tradition.

JONATHAN OCHSHORN

See also **AT&T Building, New York; Cram, Ralph Adams (United States); Herzog, Jacques, and Pierre de Meuron (Switzerland); McKim, Mead and White (United States); Postmodernism; Rossi, Aldo (Italy); Saarinen, Eero (Finland); Sainsbury Wing, National Gallery, London; Taliesin West**

Further Reading

The history of stone in 20th-century architecture can be pieced together from readings in general architectural histories and in the accounts of individual architects, but sections or chapters dealing specifically with stone are unusual. Exceptions include Sailer (1991), Goff (1997), and Patterson (1994). Detailed drawings illustrating stone construction in the works of architects such as Ralph Adams Cram, Adolf Loos, Edwin Lutyens, McKim, Mead and White, Mies van der Rohe, and Otto Wagner can be found in Ford (1990). Innovative late-20-century stone projects from around the world are featured in the periodical *A+U* (1998).

Allen, Edward, Fundamentals of Building Construction Materials and Methods, 3rd Edition, New York: John Wiley and Sons, 1999

"Architecture in Stone," *A + U*: Architecture and Urbanism, no. 4 (331) (1998)

Ford, Edward, The Details of Modern Architecture, Cambridge, Massachusetts and London, England: MIT Press, 1990

Goff, Lee, *Stone Built Contemporary American Houses*, New York: Monacelli Press, 1997

Patterson, Terry L, *Frank Lloyd Wright and the Meaning of Materials*, New York: Van Nostrand Reinhold, 1994

Sailer, John, *The Great Stone Architects: Interviews with Philip Johnson, John Burgee, Michael Graves, Cesar Pelli, Helmut Jahn, John Portman and Der Scutt*, Oradell, New Jersey: Tradelink Publishing, 1991

STONE, EDWARD DURELL 1902–78

Architect, United States

Edward Durell Stone was one of a handful of architects who introduced historicism and ornament into the modernist architecture of the 1950s and 1960s. In an era dominated by the modernist glass boxes of Mies van der Rohe and others, with abstract spaces united behind increasingly anonymous facades, Stone sought an ornamental and exotic version of modernism. Where some architects in this era explored a more expressive modernism, as did Eero Saarinen, Paul Rudolph, and Gordon Bunshaft, Stone, Minoru Yamasaki, and Philip Johnson inde-

pendently explored the combination of modernist forms and materials with classical motifs and elements. Although Stone began his career as an International Style modernist, the ornamental detailing of his U.S. Embassy building (1954) in New Delhi, India, exemplifies the stylistic characteristics of his mature style. From the mid-1950s on, Stone explored a fusion of classical and arabesque detailing with fundamentally modernist forms and materials, resulting in an architecture of elegance and luxury. This decorative modernism proved extremely popular with both the American public and his patrons, landing him a number of prominent commissions, including the American Pavilion (1958) at the World's Fair in Brussels and the John F. Kennedy Center for the Performing Arts (1971) in Washington, D.C. Regardless of his personal and professional success, architects, critics, and historians derided his work as formalist and derivative. However, Stone exerted a powerful influence on the everyday commercial and residential architecture of the 1950s, 1960s, and 1970s in America.

Born in Fayetteville, Arkansas, Stone briefly studied art at the University of Arkansas before moving to Boston (where his brother Hicks was an architect) in the early 1920s. Finding work as an office boy, Stone attended classes and lectures at the Boston Architectural Club. While continuing his studies in classical architecture, Stone joined the firm of Henry R. Shepley (a Boston Beaux-Arts architect) as a draftsman. In 1926, he won a scholarship to Harvard but, dissatisfied with its traditional curriculum, quickly transferred to the Massachusetts Institute of Technology (MIT) to study with Jacques Carlu (an early exponent of modernism). While at MIT, Stone won the Rotch Scholarship, then spent two years in Europe studying the monuments of antiquity and the works of the European modernists. Stone returned to New York in the inauspicious year of 1929 and eventually found work on Rockefeller Center's Radio City Music Hall (1932) under Wallace K. Harrison.

Following his work on Rockefeller Center, Stone came into his own as an architect with the design of the modernist Mandel House (1933) in Mount Kisco, New York. The house clearly evoked the major elements of European modernism as defined by the International Style Exhibition (which had opened the previous year in New York), including asymmetrical massing, smooth planar geometries, ribbon windows, and an open plan. In addition to a number of other modernist houses, Stone was responsible (along with Philip Goodwin) for the design of the Museum of Modern Art (1939) in New York. In the 1940s and 1950s, Stone continued to explore other modernist idioms, from the concrete grid of his El Panama Hotel (1946) in Panama City (reminiscent of the work of Le Corbusier) to a series of houses that explored organic materials and siting.

Regardless of the style or materials of Stone's architecture, his work was increasingly infused by a classical sense of massing and order. Although present in a number of his designs, Stone's predilection for classical symmetry and detailing reached its most elegant and compelling expression in his 1954 design for the U.S. Embassy in New Delhi. The building consists of a rectangular *cella* surrounded by a series of attenuated columns. Behind the colonnade is the building's most interesting feature: the screen wall that shelters the offices and the interior court from the searing heat.

Stone's design was part of a large-scale embassy-building program initiated by the U.S. government in 1954 that called for

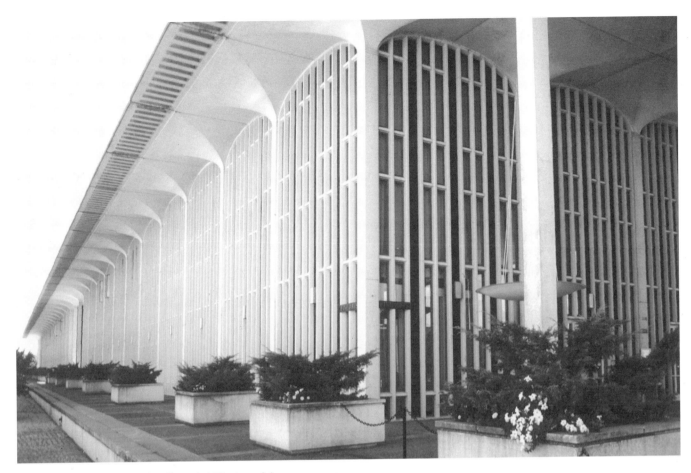

State University of New York, Albany (1962) view of the entrance
Photo © Mary Ann Sullivan

embassy designs that harmonized with the climate and historical context of the host country. The U.S. Embassy's screen wall (composed of patterned concrete terrazzo blocks) served both of these functions by filtering the heat and sun while evoking the patterned walls of mosques and mausoleums. Indeed, with its rigid classical symmetry, airy interior court, and arabesque screen walls, the embassy was praised as the new American Taj Mahal. Intended as an act of architectural diplomacy, Stone's willingness to appropriate Indian imagery into his modern design has been criticized by recent historians as an example of American cultural hegemony during the Cold War. Critics initially praised the design for its success in reintroducing monumentality into modern architecture while relieving the monotony of glass-and-steel modernism. Stone had borrowed much from the work of Mies van der Rohe and other modernists (e.g., cruciform columns, projecting horizontal slab roof, and recessed walls treated as abstract geometry), but his lavish use of materials and the richly patterned screen wall set him apart from his contemporaries.

Stone revisited the basic aspects of the U.S. Embassy with minor variations several times in the following decades, using the same concrete-block pattern at the Stuart Pharmaceutical Company (1956) Headquarters in Pasadena, California; a round version of the embassy for the United States Pavilion (1958) in

Brussels; and a rectilinear box with screen walls and attenuated columns at the campus of the State University of New York at Albany (1962) and the John F. Kennedy Center for the Performing Arts. Stone did depart from these screen walls on several occasions, notably in his design of skyscrapers, such as the General Motors Building (1968) in New York City.

Although Stone had served as a university professor (teaching at New York University between 1935 and 1940, as an associate professor at Yale University from 1946 to 1952, and as a visiting critic and professor at Princeton University, the University of Arkansas, and Cornell University), his most lasting contribution to American architecture was his decorative modernism. Although not popular with critics, Stone's influence can be felt throughout the popular vernacular both commercial and residential structures. By using the concrete-block motif seen on the U.S. Embassy, countless Americans were able to introduce modernism and exoticism into everyday architecture.

MATTHEW S. ROBINSON

Biography

Born in Fayetteville, Arkansas, 9 March 1902. Attended the University of Arkansas, Fayetteville 1920–23; apprenticed to

Henry R. Shepley, Boston 1923–25; studied at Harvard University, Cambridge, Massachusetts 1925–26; attended the Massachusetts Institute of Technology School of Architecture, Cambridge 1925–26; Rotch Traveling Scholar in Europe 1927–29. Served in the United States Air Force 1942–45. Worked with a consortium of architects designing Rockefeller Center, New York 1929–35. In private practice, New York from 1935; president, Edward Durell Stone and Associates, New York, with offices in Palo Alto, California, Los Angeles, and Chicago. Instructor in advanced design, New York University 1935–40; associate professor of architecture, Yale University, New Haven, Connecticut 1946–52; visiting critic, Princeton University, New Jersey 1953; visiting critic, University of Arkansas, Fayetteville 1955 and 1957–59. Trustee, American Federation of the Arts; director, American National Theater and Academy; director, Whitney Museum, New York; fellow, American Institute of Architects; member, National Academy of Design; member, National Institute of Arts and Letters. Fellow, American Academy of Arts and Sciences 1960; fellow, Royal Society of Arts, London 1960. Gold Medal, American Institute of Architects 1955. Died in New York, 6 August 1978.

Selected Works

Mandel House, Mount Kisco, New York, 1933
Museum of Modern Art, New York City (with Philip Goodwin), 1939
El Panama Hotel, Panama City, 1946
United States Embassy, New Delhi, 1954
Stuart Pharmaceutical Company Headquarters, Pasadena, California, 1956
United States Pavilion, World's Fair, Brussels, 1958
State University of New York, Albany, 1962
General Motors Building and Plaza, New York City (with Emerby Roth and Sons), 1968
Florida State Capitol Complex, Master Plan, Tallahassee (with Smith and Hills), 1969
John F. Kennedy Center for the Performing Arts, Washington, D.C., 1971

Selected Publications

The Evolution of an Architect, 1962
Recent and Future Architecture, 1967

Further Reading

The only monographs on Stone's work are autobiographical. To date there is not significant critical assessment of Stone's life or career in print; he has been largely ignored by critics and historians. Two recent studies of embassy buildings by Ron Robin and Jane Loeffler address the significance of the U.S. Embassy in New Delhi, as well as the larger cultural ramifications of its design. A significant part of Stone's importance lies in his popular appeal, and the cover story in *Time* magazine of 1958 is a typical example of his treatment in the popular media.

Loeffler, Jane C., *The Architecture of Diplomacy: Building America's Embassies*, New York: Princeton Architectural Press, 1998
"More than Modern," *Time* 61 (31 March 1958)
Robin, Ron Theodore, *Enclaves of America: The Rhetoric of American Political Architecture Abroad, 1900–1965*, Princeton, New Jersey: Princeton University Press, 1992

STRUCTURAL SYSTEMS

Structural systems are considered any collection of construction materials arranged in specific configurations for producing the most efficient medium that safely transfers applied gravity and lateral loads in any given structure. More specifically, structural systems can be categorized into four main groups: solid, framed, surface, and tensile. Typically, combinations of those groups, particularly the first three, which encompass a huge and highly competitive variety of systems available for the designer to choose from, are selected for the construction of any specific building project. In general, the bases of such selection are economy, special structural requirements, problems of design and construction, and materials and scale limitations. Realistically, however, in the majority of built projects the overriding criterion for selecting systems is that of economy.

Solid and monolithic elements of foundations include footings (strip and isolated), slab-on-grade, large piers, and abutments. They represent the last components of the load path in a structure. Their main purpose is to safely transfer all applied loads to the supporting soil.

Structural walls function either as supports for horizontal spanning systems (as bearing walls) or as stabilizing elements for the lateral bracing of structures (as shear walls). Depending on the way they are constructed, walls can be classified as either solid or framed elements. Examples of such systems can be found in any building project, such as supports for floor and roof structural subsystems. Examples of structural walls acting as lateral bracing elements also abound, but particularly notable are shear walls in skyscrapers. In 1976, architects Johnson and Burgee designed the 36-story Pennzoil Plaza in Houston, Texas, with a concrete core for wind load resistance.

The oldest and most basic manner in which a frame is constructed is based on the post-and-beam system. It is composed of two essential elements: the posts (typically vertical compression members) and the beams (typically horizontal elements transferring applied loads through shearing forces and bending moments). The degree of rigidity of the connections between those elements determines the amount of moment being transferred from the beams to the posts. The beams can be continuous over several posts (columns), creating a multibay arrangement. Similarly, columns can be vertically continuous, creating a multistory configuration. As such, this system can be expanded to form the three-dimensional skeletal frame of a building structure. Examples of such systems include the Empire State Building (New York City, designed by Shreve, Lamb and Harmon, 1931).

Other frame-based arrangements include such innovative systems as geodesic domes. Made famous by R. Buckminster Fuller in the 1960s, they utilize multiple stable triangularly shaped units that, when framed side-by-side, form a shell-like structure. Architects Murphy and Mackey in St. Louis, Missouri, implemented this framing concept in their design of the Climatron, a geodesic dome used in the Missouri Botanical Gardens.

Trusses

Perhaps the most efficient framing elements are trusses used for horizontal spanning in roofs and floors as well as for bridges. Trusses rely exclusively on straight members framed together through bolted, welded, or a combination type of joints. By

lining up the axes of the joined members and directing applied loads to the joints only, a truss will transmit tension and compression forces mainly through its members. The advantage of trusses lies in the openness of their structure, allowing required electrical cables/conduits and mechanical pipes/ducts to go through them without requiring additional dedicated space. Because of their relatively lightweight and rigid triangularly based framework, trusses are capable of spanning very large distances. There are many examples of truss structural systems, but perhaps the most visible are the ones used in bridge construction. The San Francisco–Oakland Bay Bridge, opened in 1936, is one such example, with a truss system connecting San Francisco to Treasure Island.

Arches and Vaults

The main objective of the arch is to span horizontally, utilizing a structural system that develops internal compression forces only. A temporary structure is erected in order to hold the arch solid elements (*voussoirs*) while being placed starting at the ends of the arch. Once both sides of the arch are completed, the last voussoir (keystone) is inserted in place and the temporary shoring removed. If expanded in one direction, arches form tunnel vaults. If crossed at 90 degrees, two vaults will produce a groin vault. Modern arches and vaults are being achieved using structural systems such as framed truss members forming the arch without resorting to solid elements. In 1998, Tate and Snyder architects employed steel trusses, formed into arches, to support the curved roofing system in the main lobby of Terminal D of McCarran International airport in Las Vegas, Nevada.

Plates and Shells

Classified as surface structures because of their very high surface-area-to-thickness ratio, plates and shells encompass slabs, panels, folded plates, and shells with various simple, as well as complex, geometric surface configurations (e.g., conical, spherical, and hyperboloidal). Architectural history in filled with cases of those forms. Notably, however, because of the vast repertoire of construction materials available to the designer in the 20th century, today's architects have found these forms very tempting. As such, there are many cases where plates and shells have been successfully incorporated into the architectural design. In 1997, the American architect Frank Gehry made use of the shell system concept to encapsulate his entire Guggenheim Museum in Bilbao, Spain, with curved titanium surfaces.

Tent and Cable-Suspended Systems

These systems act in an opposite way to the concept of arches and vaults, the difference being that the internal forces induced in cable-suspended or tent systems are tensile in nature. Engineers and builders have been successful in utilizing such systems whenever a large span is desired. Completed in 1999 and spanning 1,198 feet (365 meters), the Millennium Dome in Greenwich, London, is a contemporary example of the cable-suspended tent system.

Because of their elegant design and structural efficiency, cable-suspended constructions have also been mandatory when it comes to large-span bridges, for example in the Golden Gate Bridge (with a span of 1280 meters) in San Francisco (1937).

Another type of tent construction, air-inflated structures, has domelike roof structures and has become the preferred method of covering giant open-air public spaces. In 1988, architect Nik-

ken Sekkei and the Takenaka Corporation used an air-inflated membrane to cover the 660-foot (201-meter) span of the Tokyo Dome in Bunkyo Ward, Tokyo.

ZOUHEIR A. HASHEM

See also **Empire State Building, New York; Fuller, Richard Buckminster (United States); Guggenheim Museum, Bilbao**

Further Reading

Ambrose, James. *Building Structures*, New York: John Wiley & Sons, Inc., 1993.
Allen, E. and Iano, J. *The Architect's Studio Companion*, New York: John Wiley and Sons, 1989.

STRUCTURALISM

The term *structuralism* is generally applied to the work of a diverse group of French intellectuals working in the 1950s and 60s. Drawing on modern philosophy and the human sciences that arose in the 19th and early 20th centuries—linguistics and anthropology—and to a lesser extent on the hard sciences and mathematics, structuralism's influence continued long after its formal existence as a coherent movement. In the most general sense, structuralism was the search for the most elementary and universal patterns underlying cultural reality—patterns and structures that form the basis of social life in its most fundamental expressions: language, economy, science, and so forth. Less doctrine than method, the basic tenets of structuralism were adapted to virtually every discipline in the academy. Simply stated, these tenets were, first, individual phenomena (utterances, rituals, the formation of social institutions) only have significance when considered as part of a larger system; second, the huge variety of isolated phenomena that are discernible within the world or a given system are specific permutations of a very few general principles; and third, the structure or conceptual model constructed to chart these general principles (and the meaning of their individual manifestations) is just that—a conceptual model or structure that by definition cannot be empirically verified.

Even though generalizations like these can be identified, structuralism's significance lay in what it rejected as much as in what it adopted as its own method. By asserting the necessity of distinguishing between specific phenomena and their underlying principles, and placing the emphasis on the latter, structuralism leveled the cultural field to a certain extent, doing away with a Eurocentric model that would maintain a qualitative difference between, for instance, the social activities of modern and "primitive" societies. The fundamental rejection of the dichotomy modern/primitive, especially evident in the work of the anthropologist Claude Lévi-Strauss, was also a rejection of a century-and-a-half of Hegelian determinism, or the myth of cultural progress. In addition, by insisting on the syntactical consideration of phenomena—the relationships between them, as opposed to their individual significance—structuralism rejected metaphysical hermeneutics as well as phenomenology. This philosophical conflict was played out most dramatically in the debates between Lévi-Strauss and the existentialist/Marxist philosopher Jean-Paul Sartre in the pages of the journals *Les Temps*

Moderne, *L'Homme*, and *L'Express*. Whereas Sartre maintained the existence of conscious, human agency, Lévi-Strauss insisted on the importance of the underlying elements that gave meaning to human action. The climate in postwar France was much more conducive to Lévi-Strauss's approach, which seemed more objective than Sartre's—an important attribute during a time in which many academic disciplines sought grounding in the hard sciences and mathematics.

Lévi-Strauss's "structural anthropology" was not developed *ex nihilo*; it drew on the achievements of past ethnographers and, perhaps more important, on developments in the field of linguistics. Whereas some earlier ethnographers had recognized the importance of a comparative method, according to Lévi-Strauss they remained mired in empiricism, which prevented them from ascending beyond the level of the specific. Lévi-Strauss sought to do away with the endless observation and cataloguing of human behavior characteristic of ethnography and to implement a more conceptual comparative model that would establish underlying structural principles. For Lévi-Strauss, this gap was bridged definitively when he was exposed to the work of the Swiss linguist Ferdinand de Saussure.

Lecturing earlier in the century, Saussure had students whose notes were published as the *Course in General Linguistics*. The essential lessons of "the course" established Saussure as the founder of structuralism. By far the most significant idea in Saussure's teachings is the fundamental distinction he makes between the signifier and the signified. For Saussure, there is no determined or natural relationship between a word and what it represents—be it thing or idea. Rather, words are small units in a larger linguistic system—phonemes whose meaning arises solely from their syntax, or relation to one another. From this assertion, Saussure derived yet another important dichotomy—that between *langue* and *parole*, or the greater, underlying system of language and the individual instances of its utterance or speech. Thus, Saussure broke language off from the empirical world and established a method for studying it as an autonomous system. Moreover, this system was to be studied synchronically as opposed to diachronically or historically. The relational nature of the signifier meant that for any given word or phrase, the relation to the rest of the system had to be considered simultaneously. Thus, the entire structure is being studied at the same moment as an individual utterance. In the field of linguistics, this constituted a break with etymological studies of language, but for French structuralism, the emphasis on synchrony formed the basis for the later rejection of classical history.

Saussure became one part of a triad of great thinkers to whom the new generation of French intellectuals turned, the other two being Freud and Marx. Significantly, each of these figures asserted systems that made a fundamental distinction between specific, verifiable reality, and an underlying system: Saussure's *langue/parole* distinction, the Freudian unconscious/conscious construction, and the fundamental tenet of Marxism, the base/superstructure dichotomy.

Saussure's structuralist linguistic model allowed Lévi-Strauss to assert that like the system of language (*langue*), human cultural activity should also be analyzed relative to its underlying, relational structure. Lévi-Strauss's student thesis, *The Elementary Structures of Kinship*, published in 1948, had a wide influence, far beyond the disciplinary confines of anthropology. For supporters of Lévi-Strauss and structuralism, who were growing in number, *The Elementary Structures* suggested a methodological revolution that could bring all of the human sciences to the level of rigor and legitimacy of the natural sciences. Thus, the promise of structuralism was initially that of objectivity but was transformed as it disseminated throughout the academy.

The radical and highly influential psychoanalyst Jacques Lacan superimposed Saussure's structuralism onto the Freudian model. He asserted that the Freudian unconscious was in fact the system of language, whose structure is only partially discernible through its specific manifestations or through speech.

Roland Barthes adapted the Saussurian/structuralist model to semiotics, opening the gates of serious analysis to a huge array of cultural phenomena, from avant-garde literature to laundry detergent and the annual cycling race the Tour de France. For Barthes, these practices and products formed units within a semiotic system, analogous to words within a linguistic system. Instead of a "language," however, the popular cultural practices Barthes analyzed were specific instances of a system of cultural myth making geared toward providing the illusion of drama and meaning to a neutralized and modern quotidian existence.

Barthes's work was an early indication that although structuralism was meant to be the scientific redemption of the human sciences, its other aspect was cultural criticism. The idea that the system of cultural signs was itself a kind of production and system of exchange provided an attractive alternative to Marxism, which was plagued with ideological concerns in the postwar period. Marxists such as Henri Lefebvre showed a great deal of interest in structuralism, and Louis Althusser embarked on a rigorous structuralist re-reading of Marx's works.

As structuralism was disseminated throughout the academy, its critical aspects came to the fore. Determining the elementary structures within various disciplines meant casting off many old paradigms. As these models were "deconstructed," it became apparent that some were imbued with incredible ideological significance. Namely, structuralism initiated a new critique of several fundamental, modern concepts; diachronic history, western metaphysics and phenomenology, and the unified human subject were the most significant of these. Picking up on earlier critiques of occidental humanism and history, Michel Foucault, Jacques Derrida, and Gilles Deleuze and Felix Guattari ushered in a new phase of structuralism that some have dubbed poststructuralism.

Foucault refurbished Nietzschean genealogy to serve as a new historical method that he used to interrogate the humanist legacy of the enlightenment and the industrial age. His studies of the history of insanity and reason, law and punishment, and later of sexuality unveiled the underlying concerns of cultural institutions, namely the exercise of power. Derrida, following up on Martin Heidegger's critique of modern philosophy, conducted close, deconstructionist readings of seminal texts. He demonstrated the moments in which the western discourse of reason and categorization collapsed on itself or revealed weaknesses and lacuna within its own structure.

In a sense, structuralism predicated its own destruction: What began as an objective method for the human sciences ended with a critique of the very notion of objectivity and the objects of scientific study. Derrida read Saussure as critically as he read Kant. By the late 1960s, structuralism itself had been added to the list of institutions being assaulted by intellectuals and the popular press. Especially in the French context, where Charles

de Gaulle's Fifth Republic was so quick to institute modern methods of bureaucracy and city planning, the critique of technological modernity had deep implications. In May 1968, one of the many slogans students scrawled on walls and blackboards during the uprisings was "Structures do not march in the streets," indicating what was correctly perceived as structuralism's lack of social engagement.

Structuralism and Architecture

The exact effect of structuralism on architectural theory and practice is difficult to determine but should not be underestimated. However, it is clear that it was the semiotic aspects of structuralism that appealed to architects and critics much more so than the anthropological facet. However, the very ubiquity of structuralism, especially in Europe during the 1950s and 1960s, makes it possible to see connections even in cases in which direct influence is not apparent. For instance, one finds an emphasis on social infrastructure—explicitly opposed to architectural function—in the work of those architects associated with Team X, the youthful offshoot of CIAM (Congrés Internationaux d'Architecture Moderne): Alison and Peter Smithson, Aldo van Eyck, and the firm Candilis, Josic, Woods. For this vanguard, architecture was to provide a framework for the emergence of genuine social interaction—a conceptual model that parallels the notion of underlying structure and its specific manifestations, which is analogous to Saussure's *langue/parole* distinction. This lent to modernism a scientific and sociological dimension that had been lacking from the utopian functionalism of the 1920s.

However, it was the critical aspects of later structuralism and poststructuralism that appealed to architects and theorists, such as Barthes's critique of cultural mythology, Foucault's genealogies of institutional power, and Derrida's notion of deconstruction, the latter having evoked architecture as a foundational metaphor. Without exception, these three writers acknowledged the importance of architecture and urbanism within any semiology of modern society. Surprisingly, only a few notable architects and critics made serious attempts to acknowledge or incorporate their theories: Peter Eisenman, Bernard Tschumi, Diana Agrest and Mario Gandelsonas, and Manfredo Tafuri are examples of those who did. Although they are very different from one another, the work of these practitioners and theorists used concepts from structuralism and Marxism to question, analyze, and deconstruct the founding ideologies of architecture.

Though not strictly speaking structuralist, a much more widespread development is apparent in the 1960s and 1970s: an interest in semiotics and its Anglo-American equivalents, "communications theory" or semantics, all of which are related to "postmodernism" in architecture. The interest in architectural meaning, or language, and specifically the use of historicist elements such as classical ornamentation and devices is characteristic of this movement. Charles Jencks and Robert Venturi and Denise Scott-Brown were the foremost theorists of this tendency and called for the use of conventionalized, familiar architectural elements as a critique of a failed functionalist model.

Just as Lévi-Strauss's structural anthropology attacked the facile empiricism of his own discipline, architects have used structuralism to critique—more and less effectively—architecture's most basic assumptions and myths.

LARRY BUSBEA

See also **Deconstructivism; Postmodernism; Postructuralism**

Further Reading

Given the vastness of the topic, only the most general sources treating the topic of structuralism are listed here. In addition to these titles, readers should also pursue the works of the individual writers mentioned above.

Colquhoun, Alan, "Postmodernism and Structuralism: A Retrospective Glance," *Assemblage* 5 (February 1988)

Dosse, François, *Histoire du structuralisme*, 2 vols., Paris: Editions la Découverte, 1992; as *History of Structuralism*, 2 vols., translated by Deborah Glassman, Minneapolis: University of Minnesota Press, 1997

Jencks, Charles, and George Baird (editors), *Meaning in Architecture*, London: Barrie and Rockliff, the Cresset P., 1969; New York: Braziller, 1970

Lévi-Strauss, Claude, *Anthropologie Structurale*, Paris: Plon, 1958; as *Structural Anthropology*, translated by Claire Jacobson and Brooke Grundfest Schoepf, New York: Basic Books, 1963; London: Allen Lane, 1968

Macksey, Richard, and Eugenio Donato (editors), *The Languages of Criticism and the Sciences of Man: The Structuralist Controversy*, Baltimore, Maryland: Johns Hopkins University Press, 1970

Saussure, Ferdinand de, *Cours de linguistique générale*, edited by Charles Bally and Albert Sechehaye, Paris: Payot, 1916; as *Course in General Linguistics*, translated by Wade Baskin, New York: Philosophical Library, and London: Fontana, 1959

STUDIO PER

Architectural firm, Spain

Studio Per was a collaborative group formed in 1964 by Pep Bonet (1941–), Oscar Tusquets (1941–), Cristian Cirici (1941–), and Lluis Clotet (1941–). Primarily because of political considerations, Spanish culture remained relatively isolated from the main currents of Western European art. Therefore, critics in Western Europe and the United States largely ignored Spanish architecture. As Spain became more open, both politically and culturally, a new generation of architects began to attract international recognition. The four men of Studio Per came together in the burgeoning artistic climate of 1960s Barcelona and soon emerged as leaders of this movement. The designs of Studio Per and others provided the foundations for the development and consolidation of contemporary Spanish architecture. The work of this group continued into the postdictatorship period of democratic Spain, and they participated in the dramatic refurbishing of Spain's architectural reputation, both nationally and internationally. In general, their work can be characterized by a qualified acceptance of the International Style tempered with pragmatic revisions, including a legacy of the organic and an avoidance of unnecessarily utopian theory. They contributed to general currents of postwar architecture that rejected or modified the ideology of modernism.

All the men had been students of Federico Correa at the Escuela Técnica Superior de Arquitectura and inherited a tradition of Catalan architecture going back to Antoni Gaudí i Cor-

net, Josep Puig i Cadafalch, and Lluís Domènech i Montaner. The group was part of the newly recognized but loosely organized movement of Spanish architects, including Ricardo Bofill and Oriol Bohigas, known as the School of Barcelona. Although a single firm, Studio Per was actually the combination of two distinct tendencies: the Postmodernism of Clotet and Tusquets alongside the postrationalism of Bonet and Cirici. This singular combination enabled the group to produce multivalent works that featured a mixture of opposites. The group took inspiration from the architectural philosophies of Robert Venturi and Aldo Rossi. An emphasis on form and composition along with an unabashed faith in the value of historical tradition became important tenets of Studio Per's artistic philosophy. Despite this reverence for traditional forms, the architects avoided slavish devotion to past styles and always injected their projects with the very latest design elements and structural materials.

The work of Studio Per was characterized by a fine attention to detail and an honest pragmatism. They viewed each project as a unique problem and opportunity, and the group rejected adherence to rigidly programmatic solutions. The architects attacked basic problems of location, client wishes, and legal constraints with an eye toward simple, elegant solutions. The work of Studio Per questioned established norms and avoided the blind implementation of romantic ideals. Instead, the architects constructed synthetic designs aimed at achieving unorthodox yet convincing solutions. They often employed high doses of irony and a respectful misappropriation of the past.

The guiding principles of Studio Per's architectural philosophy can be seen in the Casa Regás and Belvedere Giorgina (1972). The project was designed as a summer home in the mountains near Girona, Spain. The site already contained the massive ruined foundation of an ancient dwelling. The architects chose to build on the antiquated walls while also constructing a new section of the house. This fusion of the traditional and modern, the existing and the new, is one of the most important legacies of Studio Per. The original home provided the location for the service elements of the household, whereas the new building contained the living quarters. A short while later, the client envisioned a second structure for the same site. In this project, the designers had to deal with an extremely small space of approximately 40 square meters. The solution was a single structure topped by a neoclassical belvedere. The work became somewhat controversial at the time for its ironic appropriation of classical elements.

The House on the Island of Pantelleria (1974) continued the elements seen in the Casa Regás and Belvedere Giorgina. The building is situated on a small island between Italy and Tunisia. The site was in a protected natural park, and this imposed limitations on new building. Clotet and Tusquets, the principal designers, chose to retain the ancient walls and foundations. They reconstructed the dwelling with local volcanic rock and formed simple volumes that echoed the modular form of traditional buildings on the island. The home extended over two levels, one containing the sleeping quarters and the other the kitchen and other service areas. The dual levels flow over the landscape, following the natural slope to the sea. The most innovative design elements are the open-air terraces, marked by rows of simple columns that again recall the island's traditional architectural elements. The house was a simple, elegant design that respected

local materials and forms while at the same time seeming modern.

In addition to being an architectural firm, Studio Per also constituted itself as an industrial design and furniture maker. A separate design studio, BD Ediciones de Diseño, was formed in 1972. As designers, they helped raise international awareness of the innovative artistic culture of both Spain and Barcelona in particular. The group achieved some success as furniture and industrial designers, winning numerous Spanish and international awards.

Although disbanded, the individual architects and designers of Studio Per have continued to exert a great influence on Spanish and international architecture and design. Tusquets and Clotet in particular played large roles in the 1980s rejuvenation of Spanish design and construction. The project culminated in the Olympic Games of 1992, for which Clotet designed apartment buildings in the Olympic Village and Tusquets a hotel.

BRIAN D. BUNK

Biography

Established in Barcelona, 1964 by: Josep Bonet Bertran (born 19 November 1941 in Barcelona); Lluis Clotet Ballús (born 31 July 1941 in Barcelona); Cristian Cirici Alomar (born 26 September 1941 in Barcelona); Oscar Tusquets Guillem (born 14 June 1941 in Barcelona). Until 1980, Clotet and Tusquets and Bonet and Cirici worked in pairs on separate projects. After 1980, each member followed his own course, but continued to belong to Studio Per.

Selected Works

Casa Fullà, Barcelona, 1969
Casa Bricall de Vilasar, Barcelona, 1969
Casa Regás and Belvedere Giorgina, Girona, Spain, 1972
Agancia de Viajes Aerojet, Barcelona, 1973
Casa Vittoria, Isla de Pantelleria, Spain, 1974

Selected Publication

"En Barcelona por una arquitectura de la evocación" (Lluis Clotet), *L'architecture d'aujourd'hui* 149 (1970)

Further Reading

A complete study of Studio Per is difficult to locate, especially in English. Mann contains a detailed discussion of two of the four partners and some of their most important works. Saliga and Thorne discuss the firm's work in the historical context of contemporary Spanish architecture. For more information, see Richardson.

Mann, Claudia Maria Alexandria, *Clotet/Tusquets*, Barcelona: Gili, 1983
Moix, Llàtzer, *La ciudad de los arquitectos*, Barcelona: Anagrama, 1994
Muntanola, Josep, *El Studio Per o los confines de la Arquitectura Actual*, Barcelona, 1976
Pehnt, Wolfgang (editor), *Encyclopedia of Modern Architecture*, London: Thames and Hudson, 1963; New York: Abrams, 1964; revised edition, as *Encyclopedia of 20th-Century Architecture*, edited by Vittorio Magnago Lampugnani, London: Thames and Hudson, 1985; New York: Abrams, 1986

Richardson, Sara S., *Lluis Clotet and Studio PER: A Bibliography*, Monticello, Illinois: Vance Bibliographies, 1988

Saliga, Pauline A., Martha Thorne, and Kenneth Frampton (editors), *Building a New Spain: Contemporary Spanish Architecture*, Barcelona: Gili, and Chicago: Art Institute of Chicago, 1992

STUTTGART, GERMANY

Stuttgart, capital of the German state of Baden-Württemberg, derives its architectural distinction from its remarkable geographical position: the city lies in a basin of the Neckar highlands and is almost completely surrounded by a high ridge. The only opening is a narrow pass on the northeast leading toward the Neckar.

The city that grew from a horse farm founded around 950 (hence the name, derived from *Stuten-Garten* or mares' garden) gained its charter in 1250 and was enlarged, especially during the 18th century, as the capital and princely residence of the counts and later dukes of Württemberg. The first systematic expansion plans occurred in 1832, just as industrialization began to affect the capital as it transformed into a metropolis.

After an uninspired period of construction in the second half of the 19th century, the 20th century brought exemplary architectural achievements to the city, making Stuttgart one of the most important centers of modern architecture in Germany.

One of the most influential buildings in the history of the new architecture in Stuttgart is the Central Station (1914–27) by Paul Bonatz and E. F. Scholer. In this monumental, cubical building clad in shell-limestone blocks, all of the amenities of a modern train station were cogently realized, from the passage of trains over optimal traffic and transport ways, to travelers' needs, to the Station Hotel and other functions. The architects made effective use of steel and concrete, using construction techniques inherent in these materials' properties. Despite this innovation, they were unwilling to use the same materials on the stone-clad façade that features a tall, columned hall facing the city center.

Another striking building that defines the cityscape is the newspaper headquarters, Tagblatt Tower (1928), designed by E. Otto Osswald as Stuttgart's first skyscraper. Originally planned as a counterweight to the Erich Mendelsohn's Schocken Department Store of 1928 (demolished 1960), the eighteen-floor, sixty-one-meter-high reinforced concrete construction of the press tower was an important symbol of the new architecture in Stuttgart and remains a milestone in the history of skyscraper construction in Germany.

Originally built in 1927 as part of an exhibition of the German Werkbund in the north of the city, the Weissenhofsiedlung represents one of the most decisive steps in the development of modern housing and constituted the high point of avant-garde architecture of the 1920s in the Württemberg capital. The Weissenhofsiedlung essentially created a model housing estate in which seventeen of the leading architects followed the design motto *Die Wohnung für den modernen Großstadtmenschen* (The Dwelling for the Modern Metropolitan Man) in designing innovative structures. Architects included Ludwig Mies van der Rohe (who designed the overall plan), J. J. P. Oud, Mart Stam, Victor Bourgeois, Le Corbusier, Josef Frank, Peter Behrens, Walter Gropius, Ludwig Hilberseimer, Hans Poelzig, Adolf Rading, Hans Scharoun, Bruno Taut, and Max Taut as well as the Stuttgart architects Richard Döcker and Adolf G. Schneck. The project pursued the programmatic goal of demonstrating ways in which rationalization was possible in housing construction and showing how planned development of affordable and reduced-cost housing could provide, in the words of Lord Mayor Dr. Karl Lautenschlager in 1925, an "improvement of total housing culture." Critics of the project claimed that although the small, affordable apartment stood in the foreground of conceptual interests, in reality—with the exception of the J. J. P. Oud—the architects did not design houses for the working class.

Approximately twenty-one individual buildings were finally constructed, with a total of sixty-three apartments. Generally using steel skeleton construction, the individual buildings showed a remarkable degree of uniformity manifest in their straight lines, absolutely unadorned and shimmering white facades, flat roofs, and the balcony treatment reminiscent of ship railings. Likewise, technical materials such as steel and concrete were used within the interiors. Technical apparatus such as pipes and heating units were not hidden but were placed demonstratively on the walls to underscore functionality. Textiles as well as conventional furniture were generally rejected. The walls had neither paneling nor molding, and the doors had neither frames nor curves.

After the Nazi seizure of power in 1933, the Weissenhofsiedlung was defamed as Stuttgart's eyesore (*Schandfleck*), its architects castigated as "cultural Bolsheviks." World War II left the project damaged from bombing and still unappreciated; the project was neither protected nor rebuilt but was rather neglected and in part disfigured through careless modifications or additions. Resurgence in interest in the project began in the 1950s, when the Weissenhofsiedlung was recognized as an architectural monument in need of protection and restoration, which was ultimately completed in 1987.

The first renewal of postwar modern design was the Liederhalle, designed and built in 1955–56 by Adolf Abel, Rolf Gutbrod, and Blasius Spreng. The Liederhalle was a music center with three large concert halls of various sizes, joined into a common complex through a two-story foyer with a restaurant. A paved courtyard with shallow steps and terraces leads to the squat main entrance on the west front. The exterior of the bastion-like, projecting Mozart Hall is decorated with an overlay of quarzite plates of alternating colors and sizes. The wide wall spaces of the high main building, however, had to be satisfied with a plain segmentation into fields. The rear is pierced with countless rectangular skylights.

The *Neue Staatsgalerie* (New National Gallery of Art) has been considered the most important building in Stuttgart of the last 20 years and as one of the most important new museum buildings constructed in Germany since 1945. It was built between 1979 and 1984 by James Stirling, Michael Wilford, and Associates, London. The first concrete plans for enlargement of the museum arose in 1974, but the present gallery dates from an international competition for the design held in 1977, which set the task of architecturally expanding the state art collection and new construction of a small theater. In total, eleven participants were invited to compete, including seven of the most outstanding from the first competition in 1974 as well as four foreign architectural firms. They were invited to develop proposals with special consideration for urban renewal. In particular, the

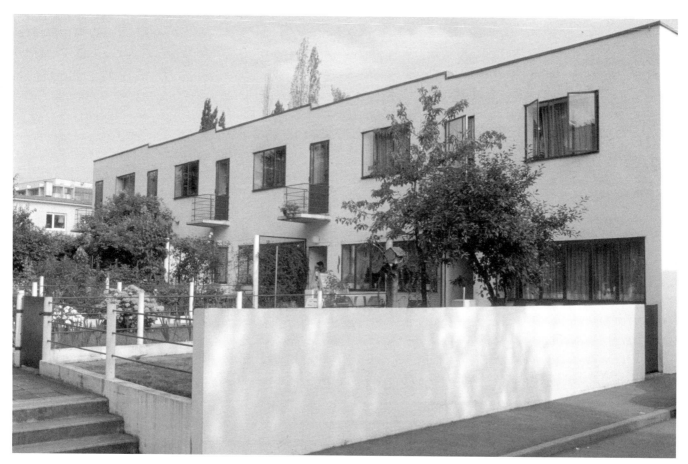

Weissenhof Row Houses, designed by J.J.P. Oud for the Weissenhofsiedlung, Stuttgart (1927)
Photo © Donald Corner and Jenny Young/GreatBuildings.com

architects were challenged to improve green spaces and pedestrian spaces and, in part, ameliorate the scars on the city center infrastructure left from World War II. With the close of the competition in 1977, Stuttgart found itself in the middle of a controversial architectural debate between two different schools of thought and aesthetics: that of Functionalism, which traced its roots in Stuttgart to the Weissenhofsiedlung, and that of Postmodernism, a new import from Great Britain with a marked preference for stylistic pastiche and even whimsy. Immediately adjacent to the preexisting national gallery building, and joined to it by a "bridge" on the gallery level, the New National Gallery is topographically sensitive. Stirling designed a public footpath through the museum complex to integrate the historical buildings of the old National Gallery into the overall conception.

Stirling's epoch-making achievement was to bring together these historicist elements with the modern formal vocabulary of Functionalist architecture such as colored steel construction, visible concrete, or curving forms. Through the contradictions in form and many-layered conception the museum gains in dynamism and seems predestined as a house for the art of the 20th century.

STEPHAN BRAKENSIEK

See also **Corbusier, Le (Jeanneret, Charles-Édouard) (France); Neue Staatsgalerie, Stuttgart; Mies van der Rohe, Ludwig**

(Germany); Oud, J.J.P. (Netherlands); Postmodernism; Weissenhofsiedlung, Deutscher Werkbund, Stuttgart (1927)

Further Reading

Kirsch, Karin, *The Weissenhofsiedlung, experimental housing built for the Deutscher Werkbund, Stuttgart, 1927*. New York: Rizzoli, 1989

Joedicke, Jürgen, *Die Weißenhofsiedlung Stuttgart*. Stuttgart: 1989

Behrendts, W.C., *Der Sieg des neuen Baustils*. Stuttgart: 1927

Bau und Wohnung: die Bauten der Weissenhofsiedlung in Stuttgart, errichtet 1927, hrsg. vom Dt. Werkbund. Stuttgart: Wedekind, 1927 (Reprint Stuttgart 1992)

Innenräume: Räume u. Inneneinrichtungsgegenstände aus d. Werkbundausstellung "Die Wohnung", insbesondere aus den Bauten der städtischen Weißenhofsiedlung in Stuttgart, hrsg. von Werner Gräff. Stuttgart: Wedekind, 1928

Weißenhofsiedlung Stuttgart, red. Bearb. Thomas Schloz., 3. erweiterte Auflage. Stuttgart: IRB, 1991, (IRB-Literaturauslese; 593)

Nägele, Hermann, *Die Restaurierung der Weißenhofsiedlung 1981–87*. Stuttgart: Krämer, 1992

Classen, Helge, *Die Weißenhofsiedlung: Beginn eines neuen Bauens*. Dortmund: Harenberg, 1990

Alfani, Antonio (editor), *Costruire, abitare : gli edifici e gli arredi per la Weissenhofsiedlung di Stoccarda; "Bau und Wohnung" e "Innenräume" (1927–28)*. Roma: Kappa, 1992

Tinelli, Fulvia, *L'involuzione delle tecniche costruttive: dal Weissenhofsiedlung (1927) al Schöne Aussicht (1980)*. Milano: Angeli, 1987

Miller Lane, Barbara, "Architecture and politics in Germany, 1918–1945," 2nd edition, Cambridge, Massachusetts: Harvard University Press, 1985

Rasch, Bodo, Frei Otto, and Berthold Burkhardt (editors), *Fünfzig Jahre Weissenhofsiedlung: eine neue Bauausstellung zum Thema "Wohnen"; eine Dokumentation.* Stuttgart:, 1978

Bartl, Franz, *Stuttgart, Hauptbahnhof: Empfangsgebäude und Bahnsteigüberdachung im Kontext der Architektur- und Konstruktionsentwicklung.* Stuttgart:, 1990

Brunold, Andreas, *Stuttgart: von der Residenz zur modernen Großstadt; Architektur und Städtebau im Wandel der Zeiten.* Tübingen: Silberburg, 1994

Stuttgarter Themen: Architektur in Stuttgart : Antworten auf alte und neue Herausforderungen, Presse- und Informationsamt der Landeshauptstadt Stuttgart (Ed.), Stuttgart 2000

Kähler, Gert (editor), *Bauen in Stuttgart seit 1900*, Braunschweig: Kähler Vieweg Verlag, 1991

Lupfer, Gilbert, *Architektur der fünfziger Jahre in Stuttgart*, Tübingen: Silberburg Verlag, 1997

SUBURBAN PLANNING

The evolution of suburbia as a distinct, and now predominant, terrain of American life and culture is tied to broad shifts throughout American and global culture in the 20th century, particularly in transportation, economics, building technology, ideology of family and home, and leisure. Already by the middle of the 19th century mechanized transport facilitated daily commuting between home and work in major cities. Steam ferries had connected New York to suburban Brooklyn and Staten Island as early as the 1810s, and by mid-century trains extended to New Jersey suburbs such as Llewellyn Park. By the 1870s distinct lines of railroad suburbs extended outward from such cities as New York, Philadelphia, Cincinnati, and Philadelphia. From the opening of the 20th century expanding trolley services filled in a nexus of "streetcar suburbs" surrounding most major cities. Predominantly residential, the typology of rail and streetcar suburbs varied from gated, exclusive tracts of single-family houses on plots of several acres, to "three-decker" and other sorts of multiple-family dwellings, depending on such factors as proximity to the city and the developer's means.

The distinguishing shift in the 20th century was the proliferation of the private automobile, especially from the 1920s onward, and the freedom it afforded for the dispersal of dwellings at distances and densities that previously had been uneconomic. Catering to the growing professional-managerial and other segments of the middle classes, most developers responded with suburban layouts that only repeated low-density 19th-century patterns based on horse and carriage transport, while higher-density multiple-family units such as Sunnyside Gardens (Queens, New York) could take advantage of urban subway connections. But the introduction of faster, limited-access highways and parkways in the 1920s and 1930s, especially in the New York and Los Angeles areas, also forced changes in the scale of suburbia, changes that were only accelerated with the establishment of the interstate highway system in 1956.

Shifts in economic relations were equally crucial. Suburbia primarily evolved at the hands of small-scale speculators, subdivi-ders, and builders who developed tracts ranging from a few houses to several acres at a time, most frequently on a piecemeal basis, quite often according to street plans predetermined by prior subdivision or municipal authorities. With the enormous increase in demand for housing following World War II, as well as the availability of Federal Housing Administration (FHA) mortgages, extensive government infrastructure programs, and standardized subdivision patterns such as those provided by the FHA Land Planning Division, individual large-scale developers now could consolidate in one enterprise the tasks of assembling land parcels, subdividing them into house lots, providing infrastructure and landscaping, providing sites for shopping centers and schools, and in some cases even building all the homes.

Federal government intervention transformed the economics of real estate, with century-long consequences, beginning with establishment of the Home Owners Loan Corporation (HOLC) in 1933 and then the FHA (1934). Endorsing the single family house above all other types, the FHA eventually made it cheaper to own than to rent; and by establishing minimum standards for housing and development, favoring homogeneous tracts of detached, single-family, automobile-dependent dwellings, the FHA contributed substantially to the postwar transformation and standardization of suburbs across the nation. Even during World War II the urgent need to house defense workers had begun to set the pattern for large-scale suburban expansion.

Since the early 18th century origins of modern residential suburbs in the Thames Valley west of London, suburban planning and design have been substantially informed by ideologies of individualism, privacy, and the nuclear family. These basic interests underlie the predisposition of American suburban design toward private lots, single-family houses, distinct front and back yards and, by the mid 20th century, a driveway and garage for one or more cars. While individuality could be reinforced by encouraging economic and environmental homogeneity among large lot owners in 19th-century elite suburbs efforts to maintain individuality in 20th-century middle-class suburbs have produced quite the opposite effect. Uniformity to the point of anonymity, and conformity to the point of oppressive monotony, are exemplified in many subdivisions, especially following World War II, when new production techniques facilitated mass replication of houses of a single type, size, and plan in vast tracts seemingly stamped out in "cookie-cutter" fashion (e.g., in the 1950s in Panorama City, California, or Park Forest, Illinois).

Already in 1931 President Herbert Hoover had proclaimed the private dwelling to be deeply embedded in Americans' consciousness: "I am confident that the sentiment for home ownership is so embedded in the American heart that millions of people who dwell in tenements, apartments, and rented rooms . . . have the aspiration for wider opportunity in ownership of their own homes" (quoted in Jackson 1985, 193–194). This confidence in the private individual as the principal constituent element of American society, and in the private house as the archetypal American dwelling, both of which notions long predate Hoover, have continued to inform shifts and innovations in planning during the last third of the century. Planned Unit Developments (PUDs), gated communities, and similar homogeneous and exclusive subdivision types frequently are marketed explicitly as effective means for articulating the individual residents' status, privilege, and position. Such exclusive enclaves, along with architectural shifts that increasingly have emphasized

withdrawal to indoor spaces, have served to intensify the character of suburbia as a space of consumption, privacy, and the culture of the nuclear family.

Suburban planning also reflects the importance of leisure, evidenced in the visual paradigm to which much of suburbia continues to adhere, a quasi-pastoral setting of lawns, trees, and meandering streets, explicitly differentiated by means of landscaping and zoning from proximate nexuses of commerce, transportation, and labor. Within residential areas, both planning and architecture have accommodated the growing penchant for personal, family, and community leisure activities, commonly through such amenities as community sports fields and recreation centers, backyard barbecues, and household recreation rooms, fitness areas, and entertainment centers.

The progressive theme that informed much of early 20th century planning originated in Ebenezer Howard's *To-morrow: A Peaceful Path to Real Reform* (1898), soon revised as *Garden Cities of To-morrow* (1902). An English manifesto for social reform that took aim at the evils of the "teeming metropolis," Howard's tract was an effort to tame the evils of capitalism by promoting a new approach to community organization that he termed "social individualism." Critical to this process would be a new form of community design, the garden city, which offered an attractive, almost romantic, vision of housing at far lower density than the industrial city, and in far greater visual and ecological harmony with the surrounding countryside, a design that with multiple replications he expected could effect broad-scale social, economic, and political change.

In America as in England, however, the city was not to be economically outmoded or abandoned. Still, in designs for suburban adjuncts to America's growing cities, American designers did look to such figures as Howard and Sir Raymond Unwin, whose *Town Planning in Practice: An Introduction to the Art of Designing Cities and Suburbs* (1909) offered practical examples. What American designers took was a disposition toward medium density, low rise, well landscaped, multiple family dwellings, together with a conviction that such types of design could effect certain social reformist goals. John Nolen based his design for Mariemont (1921), east of Cincinnati, explicitly on English Garden City models, incorporating detached, semidetached, and row houses. His plan combined a formal town center, framed by baroque radiating avenues, with outlying residential areas consisting of curving avenues circumscribing tracts of house plots and parklands. Consistent with the ideals of Howard and Unwin, Mariemont's design incorporated a philanthropic goal of establishing an affordable and healthy working-class community; but unlike the ideal Garden City, Mariemont remained a commuter adjunct to, not a replacement for, the industrial city. Palos Verdes, California, initially developed in the 1920s according to a plan prepared by Frederick Law Olmsted, Jr., was a more ambitious effort at social engineering, incorporating a mix of large and small single-family dwellings along with some multiple family units, grouped into discrete neighborhoods, each with an elementary school and adjacent shopping areas. Olmsted argued that his design, along with the originally isolated location of this development, would make it among the most stable and permanent of communities in an otherwise changing and troublesome era.

The Regional Planning Association of America, founded in 1923, initiated an activist approach to social reform through housing. In 1924–1928 two members of the group, architects Henry Wright and Clarence Stein, working under the auspices of the limited-dividend City Housing Corporation, laid out a section of already grid-platted Queens, New York, within commuting distance of the central city, in an innovative pattern, with low-rise terraces surrounding open interior courtyards. Abandoning the custom of detached dwellings on individual house plots in favor of common interior greenswards this development, called Sunnyside Gardens, was intended to improve both housing and community for working-class people. Wright and Stein's next project afforded comparable innovation for white-collar families with automobiles. Radburn, New Jersey, begun in 1929, was organized as a series of row-house terraces fronting on lawns and walkways, with automobile access diverted to cul-de-sacs at the rear of the terraces. Vehicular traffic thus was separated and screened from pedestrian walkways. Promoted as "A Town for the Motor Age" and "A Town for Children," it remains a well articulated example of a planning type that ultimately succumbed to American predilections for privacy, autonomy, and the trappings of automobile culture. Nevertheless some of the strategies first articulated in Radburn continued to be elaborated in the 1930s New Deal Greenbelt towns (Greenbelt, Maryland, Greendale, Wisconsin, and Greenhills, Ohio), and enjoyed a revival in the 1960s and 1970s in developments such as Columbia, Maryland, and Jonathan, Minnesota.

Apart from the garden city, the other principal paradigm for early 20th century suburbia was the private enclave of single-family dwellings, generally inhabited by members of elite and near-elite social classes. Nineteenth-century exemplars of this type, such as Tuxedo Park, New York (1886), in effect defined themselves as communities of exclusion, often reinforced through gated perimeters. Indeed residence sometimes was limited to those who could pass a social test, such as personal approval by the community's founder, or ability to gain membership in a private association such as the community's country club. While not all subsequent suburbs could even approach the elite tenor of Tuxedo Park, the protection of social homogeneity remained paramount in numerous developments well into the 1920s, notable examples being the Country Club District developed by J.C. Nichols in Kansas City (1922) and the comparable Country Club District in Edina, a suburb of Minneapolis (1924), both of which were explicitly promoted as implements of an exclusive social milieu and lifestyle—amenities that would be conserved through such devices as minimum lot sizes and racial exclusions. Even in subdivisions targeted to a broader economic range of residents, such as Shaker Heights outside of Cleveland (1911 ff.), developers used restrictions against two-family houses, apartments, front porches, and other design and use characteristics to pointed effect in marketing the suburb as a place where "standards" brought status and restrictions safeguarded a lifestyle.

The reformist and privatist-individualist trends in American suburban planning converged, to an extent, in Frank Lloyd Wright's series of designs for a paradigmatic American community that he termed Broadacre City (1913–16). Renewing a long-standing American ideological aversion to the city, Wright's design foresaw wholesale replacement of all cities with uniformly low-density, single-family, automobile-dependent dwellings.

Government too played a role in the shift toward the single-family suburban landscape, first in zoning initiatives concurrent

with municipal reform movements of the 1920s, and then especially in housing programs that were among early efforts to address the Depression. Empowered by a Supreme Court decision enabling a proliferation of zoning codes in the 1920s, local zoning boards intent on refining suburbs' residential character commonly banned or restricted commerce and manufacturing, legislated minimum lot sizes, and otherwise favored single-family dwellings. By establishing both locational and design standards for affordable government-backed loans in the 1930s and 1940s, the HOLC and FHA assured that the bulk of new housing in America would be single-family dwellings located in neighborhoods that were preferentially newer, lower density and, well into the 1950s, racially white.

Small-scale builders and developers continued to produce a considerable portion of post-World War II suburbia, but the demands of the acute postwar housing shortage and the stimulus provided by the Servicemen's Readjustment Act of 1944 (or GI Bill) set the stage for the use of mass-production processes, and production on a larger scale than ever before. The most prominent figure in this transformation was the firm of Levitt and Sons, who prior to 1945 had rapidly mass-produced thousands of homes for the war effort. Their postwar showpiece was the community of Levittown, in the Town of Hempstead on Long Island, where by 1947 they had completed, ready for occupancy, the first of some 17,447 houses. Like many other postwar subdivisions, Levittown was exclusively white; yet there were also a number of African-American subdivisions, mostly in the South, such as Hamilton Park, a suburb of Dallas, and Bunche Park and Richmond Heights, suburbs of Miami.

As developed tracts soon backed up against each other, however, lack of community- and region-wide planning often left little opportunity to alleviate the monotony of the homogeneous domestic environment. Efforts to articulate some sort of community focus often were limited to building shopping centers. As early as the 1920s it was recognized that an elegant, convenient, high-quality retail center could enhance the desirability of a subdivision, as demonstrated by the opening in 1923 of the nation's first automobile-oriented shopping center, Country Club Plaza, as a much-vaunted amenity of J.C. Nichols' subdivision in Kansas City. The need remained, however, to address the lack of civic focus and activity in areas of vast subdivisions. One effort to remedy this was the country's first fully enclosed shopping mall, Southdale Shopping Center (designed by Victor Gruen, 1956) in Edina, Minnesota.

Occasional attempts of a different order in the 1960s and 1970s to restore the full breadth of civic and community life to suburban subdivisions are perhaps epitomized in Reston, Virginia, developed beginning in 1962 by Robert E. Simon. Considerably indebted to examples of contemporary government-funded new town planning in Europe, Simon's private-sector effort envisioned a town with a comparable range of housing opportunities, civic and educational institutions, and possibilities for employment and recreation, all to be kept in harmonious relation with the landscape. Despite major changes of ownership and direction in the 1960s through 1980s, Reston fulfilled much of that vision, becoming a town of seven village clusters plus a town center, and a wide range of recreational facilities, as well as a corporate business center employing over a third of the town's residents, all laid out on a well-landscaped, hierarchized system of major through roads, looping residential streets, and separated pedestrian pathways, serving a mixture of detached houses, townhouses, and apartments.

Reston was part of a shift, beginning in the 1960s, toward suburban planning that aimed to afford a greater sense of identity, community, and security through consistency of design and centralized, long-term management. Some of these efforts were on a deliberately limited scale, as with Planned Unit Developments (PUDs), which in many cases incorporated considerable sensitivity to landscape, community, and design quality, often trading an increase in housing density for more continuous open space between and around the houses. In many of these developments, however, as with larger-scale Master Planned Communities (MPCs), standards of design and rules for land use were appropriated to a central authority, either the developer or a community board empowered to maintain the developer's original restrictions. One of the largest MPCs is the Irvine Ranch, a tract of over 50,000 acres southeast of Los Angeles, originally planned in 1960 by William Pereira as a collection of village clusters centered around a university campus, along with adjacent industrial, commerical, and agricultural tracts. In 1970 Pereira's plan was superseded by the SWA Group, who began by laying out Woodbridge, one of Irvine's earliest villages, in a highly controlled yet picturesque fashion that incorporates a complex combination of mixed housing types and public and private spaces. A recent and controversial example is Celebration, near Orlando, where the Disney Corporation has both imposed rigid design restrictions and retained considerable authority over municipal government and influence in the school system. But perhaps the ascendant form of development at the end of the century is the gated community. Harking back to such smaller-scale prototypes as Llewellyn Park or Tuxedo Park, these enclosed tracts emphasize privacy, security, and in many cases status; but as Blakely and Snyder (1997) have shown they also have the pernicious effect of decoupling residence and community from the civic realm.

However closely planned and managed some communities may be, the predominant mode of suburban development is thoroughly piecemeal, producing the wasteful and chaotic consumption of land known as sprawl. Seeking to reverse this trend on both local and regional bases, the nationwide Congress for the New Urbanism (CNU) has sought since its establishment in 1993 to restructure design, policy, and planning practices in ways that reconcentrate existing communities and incorporate new communities with compact centers, public spaces, coherent plans, and a diverse mix of facilities and activities. Architects working in this vein include the firm of Andres Duany and Elizabeth Plater-Zyberk, and Calthorpe Associates. Parallel efforts, undertaking development in conjunction with explicitly ecological and conservationist objectives, are found in communities such as Prairie Crossing (Grayslake, Illinois), opened in 1994. Here development has been limited to approximately one fourth of a 2500-acre nature preserve, concentrated in ways that safeguard the natural landscape, protect native vegetation and wildlife, conserve energy, and afford long views of open space, while maintaining a sense of place and sustainable community.

JOHN ARCHER

See also **Broadacre City; Duany and Plater-Zyberk (United States); Edge City; Greenbelts and Greenbelt Towns; Gruen,**

Victor David (United States); Levittown, New Jersey and New York

Further Reading

Blakely, Edward J., and Mary Gail Snyder, *Fortress America: Gated Communities in the United States*, Washington, D.C.: The Brookings Institution, and Cambridge, Mass.: Lincoln Institute of Land Policy, 1997.

Fishman, Robert, *Bourgeois Utopias: The Rise and Fall of Suburbia*, New York: Basic Books, 1987.

Garreau, Joel, *Edge City: Life on the New Frontier*, New York: Doubleday, 1991.

Girling, Cynthia L., and Kenneth I. Helphand, *Yard Street Park: The Design of Suburban Open Space*, New York, Chichester, Brisbane, Toronto, and Singapore: John Wiley and Sons, 1994.

Hise, Greg, *Magnetic Los Angeles: Planning the Twentieth-Century Metropolis*, Baltimore and London: Johns Hopkins University Press, 1997.

Jackson, Kenneth T., *Crabgrass Frontier: The Suburbanization of the United States*, New York and Oxford: Oxford University Press, 1985.

Kelly, Barbara M., (editor), *Suburbia Re-Examined*, Westport, Conn.: Greenwood Press, 1989.

Longstreth, Richard, *City Center to Regional Mall: Architecture, the Automobile, and Retailing in Los Angeles, 1920–1950*, Cambridge, Mass., and London: MIT Press, 1997.

Longstreth, Richard, *The Drive-In, the Supermarket, and the Transformation of Commercial Space in Los Angeles, 1914–1941*, Cambridge, Mass., and London: MIT Press, 1999.

McKenzie, Evan, *Privatopia: Homeowner Associations and the Rise of Residential Private Government*, New Haven and London: Yale University Press, 1994.

SUBWAY

The subway is a 19th-century idea realized largely in the 20th century. The industrial revolution was the primary catalyst for the advent of underground transportation; without it the iron horse that pulled the trains, the tunneling technology that bored through the earth, and the iron walls that held those tunnels up would have been impossible. The problem of the subway also had its political and social implications. Mass transit meant reform, for increased mobility freed the working classes from the urban center and gave them greater share of the public realm.

The leader in the industrial revolution, Great Britain came to the forefront of subway design as well. The Metropolitan Railway was opened to the public to much acclaim in 1863. The stations on this first line were architecturally undistinguished; the line's engineers quite naturally borrowed their architectural vocabulary from the established railroads, and so a distinct Underground aesthetic would not be developed until the first years of the 20th century, when consolidation finally allowed a cohesive architectural expression to develop, as ably accomplished by Leslie Green. Green designed more than 50 stations for the Underground; the details of these stations are closely associated with the Arts and Crafts design movement, as extensive tilework unifies the entire station: the exterior, the interior of the booking hall, and the platform. The Underground continued to expand and change throughout the century. After World War I, the lines were routed farther into the suburban hinterlands. Charles Holden designed many of the Under-

ground's stations for this expansion, those on the Northern Line in a stripped classical mode that continued the Underground's signature use of thermal windows. In 1930 Holden traveled throughout Northern Europe, experiencing firsthand Continental modern architecture. His stations for the Piccadilly Line evince his conversion to the modern cause and continued the Underground's excellence in design. Postwar expansions and new lines have not always maintained this architectural excellence, but they have consolidated a uniform corporate identity through the use of supergraphics and typography.

Although the first Continental subway was constructed in Budapest, the Paris Métro is the early European subway best remembered for its architecture. Hector Guimard's stations interpreted plant and animal forms to create an otherworldly art. Guimard himself thought of these designs as being entirely rational, and in fact the Métro was at the time on the cutting edge of French industrial technology, and Guimard's stations are very much industrial products. They were designed to be mass produced, being made of enameled steel and manufactured glass, and yet the form that Guimard adopts is anything but a machine aesthetic and not simple transformations of natural forms. For example, Guimard's lamp standards were designed not after a plant stem but after the sap within the plant stem. Three different station types were designed to give the entire system a coherence and a corporate look. The simplest and most common were the balustrades and signposts, the second topped these balustrades with an iron-and-glass canopy, and the third comprised an entire pavilion into which a ticket booth and newspaper stand were incorporated. Guimard's tenure with the Métro was short-lived, and subsequent designs have been less adventurous, conforming to the engineering requirements of the systems. Opportunities for inventive underground public spaces, such as at the massive interchange at Châtelet, were missed. However, public art and signature graphics emboldened the visual experience of the Métro in the final decades of the century.

The Vienna Stadtbahn, more of a depressed railroad than a true subway for most of its run, is one of the best designed and aesthetically consistent systems in the world; it was Otto Wagner who made it so. Wagner was made the artistic director of the subway system and the Nüssdorf and Kaiserbad Dams in 1894. Few men in Vienna were as well qualified for the task. Wagner had studied civil engineering and understood the interdependent roles that the engineer and the architect must play in order to bring a complex public works project to a successful conclusion. A comprehensive design program prevailed at the Stadtbahn. Wagner and his design team designed the stations, the bridges, the tunnels and cuts, and just about everything except the rolling stock and the locomotives. Wagner built 36 stations from 1894 to 1900, most which survive in some form. All are located in the inner city and along the Wien River. The stations' forms vary according to the site conditions and the mood of the architect, but all share a similar vocabulary and material and are unified by their structural logic, proportion systems, and decorative motifs. Many of the stations are unapologetically classical in their vocabulary, and others are less overtly "architectural." Bridgelike forms are frequent, particularly on the elevated lines. Probably the most famous of the stations along the Stadtbahn is that at the Karlsplatz. The twin entry pavilions are modeled on the Turkish kiosk, a referent equally important to subways under construction in Budapest and New York. This exotic form

fits the Karlsplatz stations perfectly, as the strong curvilinear rooflines of the pavilions respond to the elliptical dome of the Karlskirche across the square. The highly ornamented walls of the pavilions were composed of standardized panels, allowing them, in theory, to be mass produced. Wagner understood the importance of the emerging technical society and embraced it. He was able to reassemble his versatile forms in many ways in order to solve the numerous different sites the Stadtbahn demanded, thus ensuring a corporate look to the enterprise. This is a quality that other systems lacked.

New York's subway also owes its existence and initial appearance to a brilliant engineer. After numerous abortive attempts at subway building on Manhattan, the Interborough Rapid Transit Company finally realized the plans of William Barclay Parsons between 1900 and 1904. Although New York's system was only the second in operation in North America (Boston's subway was inaugurated in 1897), it quickly became the most extensive system in the world. Although the system was largely constructed using excavation techniques perfected in London and Paris, Parson's greatest engineering achievement might be his establishment of a four-track main trunk. Architecturally, the first stations on the line were fairly simple affairs that again combined features of Parisian and London station design. A station's street presence was marked by mass-produced iron-and-glass kiosks, recalling the entry pavilions in Budapest. The stations themselves were largely rectangular in section, as appropriate to their shallow cut-and-cover construction, and distinguished by the forest of steel supports supporting the street above and the terra-cotta and tile murals that identified each stop. The most elaborate station, at City Hall, was designed by Heins and Lafarge and vaulted in Guastavino tile—the effect was intended to induce a spiritual response among the throngs who used the station. As the New York system expanded into Brooklyn and Queens, the architectural qualities of the original line were sacrificed to economy and efficiency. Stations became less uniquely identifiable, and lines in the outer boroughs were as often as not perched on bents several stories above the street, remnants of the el system that was slowly supplanted by the subway across the East River.

While many subway systems purposefully projected a modern, industrial design stance, in Stalin's Moscow political symbolism prevailed over any avant-garde aesthetic. Begun in 1931, construction of the Moscow subway was led by Lazar Kaganovich, the labor boss of the Dnieper Hydroelectric Dam and Nikita Khrushchev, and the labor was supplied by tens of thousands of conscripted unfortunates, thousands of whom died in the works. The initial line was completed in May 1935, but construction continued under accelerated conditions until the Nazi invasion of Russia in the early 1940s. Whereas the engineering of the Moscow subway was quite forward looking, the architectural presentation of the subway stations was by contrast decidedly traditionalist. The classical vocabulary of many of the stations was designed to allude to great moments in Russia's past and was a part of the larger public works effort, the "Columns for the People" campaign. The monumental classical spaces of the subway, such as the rococo foyer of the Komsolskaya station, were intended to demonstrate that the wealth of the nation, once squandered on the nobility and their palaces, was as graciously serving the needs of the proletariat under the Soviet regime. Although Western architects may not have found Moscow's historicist vocabulary worthy of emulation, the Moscow subway did demonstrate that architecturally significant spaces could be achieved five stories underground.

Ironically, the subway most akin to Moscow's in its emphasis on architectural space was built in Washington, D.C. Whereas most postwar subway design aspired to nothing more than functionalism, the Washington, D.C., Metro achieved a meaningful architectural experience; this success is due to the genius of Harry Weese. Weese was trained by both Alvar Aalto and Eliel Saarinen in the grammar of modern architecture, yet he was also the restoration architect of Adler and Sullivan's Auditorium Building in Chicago and Daniel Burnham's Union Station in Washington, D.C. Weese's sensitivity to the classical heritage of the District of Columbia fused with his functionalist sensibilities to produce a dynamic set of station designs that were at once monumental, almost sublime, and yet were produced from a limited set of architectural elements, most notably the deeply coffered concrete vault. Allusions to Washington's classical heritage are made by Weese but are never literal, as in Moscow. With their soaring intersecting groin vaults, the primary interchange stations at Gallery Place and Metro Center are particularly effective and have become memorable spaces in their own right in a city of overscaled interiors.

The formal design of the subway station depended very much on the personal philosophy of the architect. Where that philosophy was in tune with the artistic movements of the day, contemporary architecture resulted. Where the architect was not so moved, nothing in the subway problem prevented a revivalizing aesthetic. The best subway systems hired designers who understood the complex contextual problems of the subway and responded with an architecture that melded the technical requirements of the building type with their own aesthetic vision.

JEFFREY THOMAS TILMAN

See also **Metro Station, Paris; Urban Planning; Wagner, Otto (Austria)**

Further Reading

Bobrick, Benson, *Labyrinths of Iron: A History of the World's Subways*, New York: Newsweek Books, 1981

Borsi, Franco, and Ezio Godoli, *Vienne architecture, 1900*, Paris: Flammarion, 1985; as *Vienna, 1900: Architecture and Design*, translated by Marie-Helene Agueros, New York: Rizzoli, and London: Lund Humphries, 1986

Buddensieg, Tilmann, editor, and John Gabriel, translator, *Berlin 1900–1933: Architecture and Design* (bilingual English-German edition), New York: Cooper-Hewitt Museum, 1987

Edwards, Dennis, and Ron Pigram, *London's Underground Suburbs*, London: Baton Transport, 1986

Fischler, Stan, *Uptown, Downtown: A Trip through Time on New York's Subways*, New York: Hawthorn Books, 1976

Geretsegger, Heinz, Max Peintner, and Walter Pichler, *Otto Wagner, 1841–1918: Unbegrenzte Großstadt, Beginn der modernen Architektur*, Salzburg: Residenz Verlag, 1964; 3rd edition, 1978; as *Otto Wagner, 1841–1918: The Expanding City and the Beginning of Modern Architecture*, translated by Gerald Onn, London: Pall Mall Press, 1964; New York: Praeger, 1970

Graham, F. Lanier, *Hector Guimard*, New York: Museum of Modern Art, 1970

Jackson, Alan A., *London's Metropolitan Railway*, Newton Abbot, Devon, and North Pomfret, Vermont: David and Charles, 1986

Kostina, Olga, "Die Moskauer Metro," in *Tyrannei des Schönen: Architektur der Stalin-Zeit*, edited by Peter Noever, Munich and New York: Prestel, 1994

Menear, Laurence, *London's Underground Stations: A Social and Architectural Study*, Tunbridge Wells, Kent: Midas, 1983

Naylor, Gillian, and Yvonne Brunhammer, *Hector Guimard*, New York: Rizzoli, 1978

SULLIVAN, LOUIS 1856–1924

Architect, United States

Louis Henry Sullivan was the first internationally recognized architect in the United States to pursue the idea of a modern architecture independent of historic styles. He was supremely gifted as a designer of architectural ornament, an important component of almost all his major buildings and central to his thinking about architecture as art. Sullivan was the first American modernist to write extensively on architecture—critically, theoretically, and philosophically. He was the most outstanding creative figure of the Chicago School of the 1880s and 1890s, particularly because of his designs for tall office buildings. His work and thought inspired a number of younger contemporaries throughout his later life, including Frank Lloyd Wright, who was Sullivan's assistant from 1887 to 1893. From 1880 to 1895, Sullivan was continuously associated with Dankmar Adler (1844–1900), whose skills in architectural engineering complemented Sullivan's design abilities to make Adler and Sullivan one of the most extraordinary partnerships in U.S. architectural history.

Louis Sullivan was born in Boston on 3 September 1856, the younger son of Patrick Sullivan, an Irish dancing master, and his wife, Andrienne, a Swiss-born pianist. After graduating from Boston's English High School, Louis studied architecture for one academic year (1872–73) at the Massachusetts Institute of Technology, where his principal teacher was William Robert Ware, who had founded the institute's Department of Architecture in 1865 as the oldest in the United States. Sullivan worked for Frank Furness, at the office of Furness and Hewitt in Philadelphia, from the summer to November 1873. Following his parents to Chicago, Sullivan then worked there in the office of William Le Baron Jenney from December 1873 to June 1874, after which time he went to Paris, where he gained admission to the École des Beaux-Arts in October 1874 as a student in the atelier of Joseph-Auguste-Émile Vaudremer. Sullivan studied at the École only into the spring of 1875, when he took an extended trip to Italy, visiting the Sistine Chapel in Rome and recalling a stay of six weeks in Florence before leaving from Paris to return to the United States in late May 1875. He then resumed work as a draftsman and designer in Chicago, for at least three architectural firms, and independently, between 1875 and about May 1880, by which time he had probably begun his continuous association with Adler, with whom he had worked at least once in 1876. Sullivan became an equal partner in the firm of Adler and Sullivan from 1 May 1883 to July 1895, when Adler briefly left architecture. Afterward, Sullivan practiced in Chicago with a series of assistants (most importantly, George Grant Elmslie, from 1889 to 1909) and then alone until his death there on 14 April 1924, when he was impoverished.

When Sullivan joined Adler, Adler had recently begun independent practice after working with a series of architects in Detroit and Chicago and three years of service in the U.S. Army during the Civil War, partly as a topographical engineer. Adler's skills as a planner, engineer, and acoustic designer and Sullivan's unique abilities as an architect of ornamental, richly colored interiors meant that by 1885 their firm was considered without peer in Chicago in the field of theater design. This led to their being given the commission to design the Chicago Auditorium Building (1886–90), then the largest private architectural project in the city and the structure that did much to launch Chicago's reputation as a major center for early modern architecture. For their client, Ferdinand W. Peck, Adler and Sullivan designed the Auditorium Building as a ten-story block containing a 4,200-seat theater, a 400-room hotel with a set of elaborate public interiors, and rentable stores and offices. The building's massive granite and limestone street fronts, inspired in part by Henry Hobson Richardson's Marshall Field and Co. Wholesale Store (1885–87) in Chicago, combined with the Auditorium's 16-story tower to make the building a prominent landmark on the lakefront at Michigan Avenue and Congress Street. Inside, the Auditorium Theater was meant in part to contrast with the Metropolitan Opera House (1880–83) in New York City, which was planned mainly for its wealthy box holders seated in 122 boxes set in horseshoe-shaped tiers around the theater, which sat a total of 3,045. In the Auditorium, there were only 40 boxes set to the sides of the house, whose vast parquet, balcony, and two upper galleries were meant to accommodate large middle- and working-class audiences for grand opera, orchestral and choral concerts, lectures, and other events. The theater's acoustics, acclaimed by leading singers of the period, depended in large measure on its innovative elliptically arched ceiling, which steps up and out in four segments from the proscenium. The acoustics, mechanical stage equipment, and Sullivan's original program of ornamental plasterwork and stencils, integrated with incandescent electric lighting and ventilation, combined to make the theater one of the world's outstanding rooms for opera.

The Auditorium Theater's opening in December 1889 was a national event that initiated Adler and Sullivan's international reputation. From 1890 to 1895, they designed other theaters inside multistoried business blocks, including the Schiller Theater Building (1890–92, demolished 1961) in Chicago. Sullivan was also the principal designer of the distinctively polychrome Transportation Building at the mostly neoclassical World's Columbian Exposition of 1893. Yet, historically, the firm's most renowned works of the early 1890s were their tall steel-framed office buildings. In addition to the Schiller, Adler and Sullivan's built works of this type were the Wainwright Building (designed 1890, built 1891) in St. Louis, the Union Trust Building (designed 1891–92, built 1892–93) in St. Louis, the Chicago Stock Exchange Building (designed 1892–93, built 1893–94, demolished 1972), and the Guaranty Building (designed 1894–95, built 1895–96) in Buffalo. After Adler left the partnership in July 1895, Sullivan designed the Bayard Building (designed 1897–98, built 1898–99) on Bleecker Street in New York City. Except for the Chicago Stock Exchange, all these tall office buildings had exterior street fronts wherein continuous vertical piers projected forward of windows and horizontal lintels. In his single most famous essay, "The Tall Office Building Artistically Considered," of 1896, Sullivan emphasized the accentuation of verticality in the exterior form of tall office buildings as the appropriate expression of their multistoried height and lofty steel frame. Sullivan's extensive use of terra-cotta ornament on the exteriors

of his tall buildings demonstrated that, unlike some of his European contemporaries and many later modernists, Sullivan did not consider ornament to be an anathema in modern architecture. Rather, he was against the use of overtly historical ornamental and architectural forms. In his essay "Ornament in Architecture," of 1892, Sullivan had emphasized the complementary relationship between structure and ornament in the creation of buildings that embodied what he termed the organic ideal, meaning architecture as living form, analogous to forms in biological nature.

In the aftermath of the dissolution of his partnership with Adler in mid–1895, Sullivan received much professional praise from fellow architects and critics but relatively fewer commissions, especially after 1900, although he continued to write extensively. From his earlier partnership, he retained one major Chicago client, David Mayer, who in 1898 commissioned Sullivan to design the new Schlesinger and Mayer Store, to be a 12-story iron-and-steel-framed department store for retailing on State and Madison Streets at the center of Chicago's shopping district. Built in stages in 1899 and 1903–04, this structure was then acquired by Carson Pirie Scott and Co. and is historically known by that firm's name. The building featured a two-story base of ornamental cast iron (originally envisioned as bronze) framing plate-glass show windows for mercantile display. Above, the upper stories were clad in white terra-cotta (initially designed as white Georgia marble), with each structural bay filled with a Chicago window (a broad, central, fixed pane flanked by an operable sash window on either side). Unlike the subdivided interior floors of tall office buildings, the department store's floors were open lofts in need of maximal daylight. Carson Pirie Scott's upper elevation as the direct expression of its iron-and-steel frame made this building a canonical work of early 20th-century architecture, one often cited in modernist historiography of the Chicago School.

From 1906 to 1919, Sullivan designed a remarkable series of bank buildings in small Midwestern towns that served as centers for surrounding farming regions. At a time when bank buildings in the United States were almost uniformly neoclassical, Sullivan's essays in the type were richly colored, ornamentally elaborate, and highly individual designs. The most architecturally ambitious and historically acclaimed among these buildings was the first of the series, the National Farmers' Bank at Owatonna, Minnesota, designed and built from 1906 to 1908. With the support of the bank's president, Carl K. Bennett, Sullivan, assisted by Elmslie, created a unique structure, nearly cubic in its basic form. Lower walls were faced in cut brownstone as a base below upper walls faced in variably colored paver or tapestry brick, polychrome ornamental terra-cotta, and bands of glazed mosaic. Externally, the bank's form conveyed security of deposits, concentration of wealth, and association with agriculture, all elements of functional character consistent with the building's type and locale. Inside, the bank's main floor is one high spatial volume that receives daylight through a central skylight and the art-glass panels set into the 36-foot-wide arched windows in the south and west upper walls. These sources illuminate the richly colored decorative plasterwork and stenciling that form the borders of the arches set in the opposite north and east walls. These mural arches framed paintings of regional landscapes with dairy cows, the main source of local agricultural wealth and thus of the bank's deposits. Sullivan's later bank

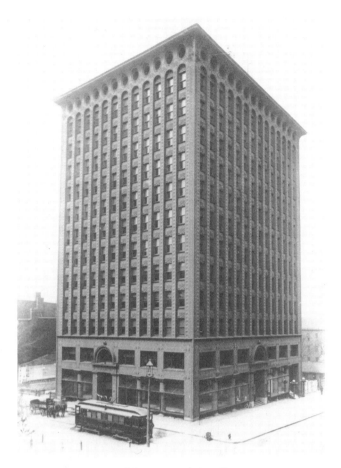

Guaranty Building, Buffalo, New York (1896)
© Buffalo and Erie County Historical Society

buildings explored similar ornamental themes. These surviving (though modified) works include the People's Savings Bank (1909–11) in Cedar Rapids, Iowa; the Purdue State Bank (1913–14) in West Lafayette, Indiana; the Merchants' National Bank (1913–14) in Grinnell, Iowa; the Home Building Association (1914–15) in Newark, Ohio; the People's Savings and Loan Association (1916–18) in Sidney, Ohio; and the Farmers' and Merchants' Union Bank (1919–20) in Columbus, Wisconsin. Sullivan's last multistoried building was the steel-framed dry-goods store (1911–14) for John D. Van Allen and Son in Clinton, Iowa, whose design partly recalls that of Carson Pirie Scott.

As an architectural thinker, Sullivan sought to broaden his influence through his many published writings, which appeared from 1885 until his death. These writings included Sullivan's 52 short essays titled "Kindergarten Chats," first published serially in Cleveland's *Interstate Architect and Builder* from February 1901 to February 1902 and later edited by Sullivan and others in subsequent editions. In these essays, Sullivan emphasized the need for an American architecture as the authentic expression of modern social, economic, cultural, and technical conditions. In this vein, his position is usually understood to be much like that of modernist European architects in the early 20th century. Sullivan's pursuit of these themes made him appear in retrospect to be a "prophet of modern architecture," the subtitle of his first

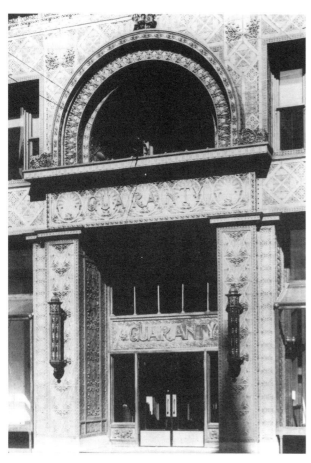

Detail of ornamentation, Guaranty Building
© Buffalo and Erie County Historical Society

Biography

Born in Boston, Massachusetts, 3 September 1856. Attended the Massachusetts Institute of Technology, 1872–73; studied at the École des Beaux-Arts, Paris, 1874–75. Draftsman at the firm of Furness and Hewitt, Philadelphia, 1873; worked for William Le Baron Jenney in Chicago, 1873–74; draftsman in several Chicago offices, including that of Joseph Johnston and John Edelman, 1875–76. Joined the firm of Dankmar Adler & Co., Chicago, about 1880; partner in the firm of Adler and Sullivan, Chicago, 1881–95; Frank Lloyd Wright employed by the firm as draftsman and assistant designer, 1887–93. Went into private practice in Chicago, from 1895. Awarded the Gold Medal, American Institute of Architects, posthumously, 1946. Published several influential works including *Kindergarten Chats* (1901–02) and *The Autobiography of an Idea* (1924). Died in Chicago, Illinois, 14 April 1924.

Selected Works

Auditorium Theater Building, Chicago, 1886–1890
Wainwright Building, St. Louis, Missouri, 1890–1891
Schiller Theater Building (destroyed), Chicago, 1890–1892
Transportation Building (destroyed), World's Columbian Exposition, Chicago, 1891–1893
Union Trust Building, St. Louis, 1891–1893
Stock Exchange Building (destroyed), Chicago, 1892–1894
Guaranty Building, Buffalo, New York, 1894–1896
Bayard Building, New York City, 1897–99
Schlesinger and Mayer Department Store (now Carson Pirie Scott Building), Chicago, 1898–1904
National Farmers' Bank, Owatonna, Minnesota, 1906–1908
People's Savings Bank, Cedar Rapids, Iowa, 1909–1911
Van Allen Dry Goods Store, Clinton, Iowa, 1911–1914
Purdue State Bank, West Lafayette, Indiana, 1913–1914
Merchants' National Bank, Grinnell, Iowa, 1913–1914
Home Building Association, Newark, Ohio, 1914–1915
People's Savings and Loan Association, Sidney, Ohio, 1916–1918
Farmers' and Merchants' Union Bank, Columbus, Wisconsin, 1919–1920
Krause Music Store Facade, Chicago, 1922

Selected Publications

A System of Architectural Ornament According with a Philosophy of Man's Powers, 1924
The Autobiography of an Idea, 1924
"Kindergarten Chats," *Interstate Architect and Builder* (16 February 1901–8 February 1902); as *Kindergarten Chats and Other Writings*, edited by Isabella Athey, 1947
Democracy: A Man-Search, edited by Elaine Hedges, 1961

Further Reading

Andrew, David S., *Louis Sullivan and the Polemics of Modern Architecture: The Present against the Past*, Urbana: University of Illinois Press, 1985
Condit, Carl W., *The Rise of the Skyscraper*, Chicago: University of Chicago Press, 1952
Condit, Carl W, *The Chicago School of Architecture: A History of Commercial and Public Building in the Chicago Area, 1875–1925*, 1964
Frei, Hans, *Louis Henry Sullivan*, Zurich Artemis, 1992
Gregersen, Charles, *Dankmar Adler: His Theaters and Auditoriums*, Athens, Ohio: Swallow Press, Ohio University Press, 1990

biography by Hugh Morrison, originally published in 1935. Yet Sullivan's concern for individual imagination, nature as a prime source of inspiration, botanically inspired ornament, and architectural expression of American ideals of democracy distinguished his work and thought from that of many modernists. In the 1980s, a new cycle of Sullivan scholarship coincided with the rise of Postmodern historicism, and his work was reexamined not only as prophetic of the later modern movement but also for its relation to 19th-century architecture and theory. There was renewed interest in his systems of ornament and color and in his idea of expressing the functional character of building types, a premise taught at the École des Beaux-Arts. Sullivan once cited this school as a chief source of the idea most often associated with him, that "form follows function," an aphorism that Sullivan thought applied to living forms in nature as models for an organic architecture.

JOSEPH M. SIRY

See also **Carson Pirie Scott Store, Chicago; Chicago School; Larkin Building, Buffalo, New York; National Farmers' Bank, Owatonna, Minnesota; Ornament; Wright, Frank Lloyd (United States)**

Jordy, William H., *American Buildings and Their Architects*, volume 3: *Progressive and Academic Ideals at the Turn of the Twentieth Century*, Garden City, New York: Doubleday, 1972; New York. Oxford University Press, 1986

Manieri-Elia, Mario, *Louis Henry Sullivan, 1856–1924*, Milan: Electa, 1995; as *Louis Henry Sullivan*, New York: Princeton Architectural Press, 1996; translated by Antony Shugaar with Carolme Green

Menocal, Narciso, *Architecture as Nature: The Transcendentalist Idea of Louis Sullivan*, Madison: University of Wisconsin Press, 1981

Millett, Larry, *The Curve of the Arch: The Story of Louis Sullivan's Owatonna Bank*, St. Paul: Minnesota Historical Society Press, 1985

Morrison, Hugh, *Louis Sullivan: Prophet of Modern Architecture*, New York: Museum of Modern Art and W.W. Norton, 1935; with introduction and revised list of buildings by Tirmothy J. Samuelson, New York W.W. Norton, 1998

Siry, Joseph M., *Carson Pirie Scott: Louis Sullivan and the Chicago Department Store*, Chicago: University of Chicago Press, 1988

Siry, Joseph M., *The Chicago Auditorium Building: Adler and Sullivan's Architecture and the City*, Chicago: University of Chicago Press, 2002

Sprague, Paul, *The Drawings of Louis Henry Sullivan: A Catalogue of the Frank Lloyd Wright Collection at the Avery Architectural Library*, Princeton, New Jersey: Princeton University Press, 1979

Twombly, Robert, *Louis Sullivan: His Life and Work*, New York: Viking, 1986; Chicago: University of Chicago Press, 1987

Twombly, Robert (editor), *Louis H. Sullivan: The Public Papers*, Chicago: University of Chicago Press, 1988

Twombly, Robert, and Narciso C. Menoral, *Louis Sullivan: The Poetry of Architecture*, New York W.W. Norton, 2000

Van Zanten, David, *Sullivan's City: The Meaning of Ornament for Louis Sullivan*, New York: W.W. Norton, 2000

Weingarden, Lauren S., *Louis H. Sullivan: The Banks*, Cambridge, Massachusetts: MIT Press, 1989

Wit, Wim de (editor), *Louis Sullivan: The Function of Ornament*, New York: W.W. Norton, 1986

SUPERMODERNISM

Critic and historian Hans Ibelings—borrowing from anthropologist Marc Augé—uses the term "supermodernism" (also called "hypermodernism") to describe a style of architecture emerging in the 1990s, characterized by structures that are often airy, minimalist or monolithic, and transparent or translucent and that use an abundance of glass. Although supermodern structures exploit technological innovation, they are generally visually and symbolically simple, with clean lines, a minimalist style, and neutral materials.

Theoretically, Ibelings situates supermodernism in relation to Postmodernism and Deconstructivism and in conjunction with some of the aims of modernism. Ibelings noticed common tendencies in several architectural books published in the mid-1990s: Terence Riley's *Light Construction* (1995), Rodolfo Machado and Rodolphe el-Khoury's *Monolithic Architecture* (1995), Vittorio Savi and Josep Ma Montaner's *Less Is More: Minimalism in Architecture and the Other Arts* (1996), and Daniela Colfranceschi's *Architettura in superfice; Materiali, figure e technologie delle nuove facciate urbane* (1995). The almost simultaneous publication of these texts describing a similar aesthetic led Ibelings to condense formal and theoretical tendencies into a description of a coherent architectural style.

Contributors to this style include contemporary international architectural firms such as Rem Koolhaas's Office of Metropolitan Architecture (OMA), Jean Nouvel, Dominique Perrault, Herzog and De Meuron, and Iñaki Abelos and Juan Herreros. Noteworthy examples of supermodernist architecture include Jean Nouvel's beautifully transparent Cartier Foundation for Contemporary Art and Head Office of Cartier France (1991–94) in Paris as well as his design for the Tour sans Fin (1989), a glass-topped tower to be built in Paris's La Défense. Also significant are Dominque Perrault's new home for the Bibliothèque Nationale (1989–96) in Paris as well as her Hôtel Industriel Berlier (1985–90) in Paris and Koolhaas and OMA's Educatorium (1997), a multipurpose building designed for Utrecht University in the Netherlands.

Supermodernism is a phenomenological architecture, an architecture that appeals to the experience of place rather than to ideas or symbols. Although postmodernist and deconstructivist approaches to architecture often appeal to intellectual and historical relationships among forms, supermodernism suggested a shift toward (perhaps even a return to) the formal qualities of space and the visual and tactile sensations that accompany them. According to Ibelings, the emphasis on space and place rather than on form (or style as an end it itself) contradicts one of the main tenets of postmodern architecture—that a particular building is an often-contradictory composite of symbols or signs that carry cultural and linguistic meanings. Supermodern architecture rejects the desire or need to decode symbols and instead appeals to a range of physical as well as psychological qualities perceived through the experience of the forms. Supermodern buildings reflect neither the history of architecture nor extra-architectural ideas.

The supermodern structure in part appeals to universal concerns (a stronghold of modernist ideology of the earlier part of the century). This emphasis on universality reflects the current interest in globalization, which Ibelings links to homogenization and commodification in art and architecture. Global homogenization has generated a rash of chain stores, internationally recognized products, and expressionless, nondescript architecture in world cities that resemble one another as well as architecture that is no longer built by local architects in local styles.

Linked to globalization is the development of what Augé calls "nonspace." Nonspaces are spaces that "cannot be defined as relational, or historical, or concerned with identity" (Augé, 1995). Rather than social centers where communities gather for collective activity, nonspaces function as common places where groups of people come together yet experience the space separate from others. The current built environment is, according to Augé's somewhat relativist reading, meaningless. However, meaningless space arises as a reaction to three kinds of abundance: an abundance of space, an abundance of signs, and an abundance of individualism. The plethora of nonspaces creates what Augé calls the supermodern condition, an obvious reference to French philosopher Jean-Francois Lyotard's 1979 seminal study *La condition postmoderne: rapport sur le savoir* (The Postmodern Condition: A Report on Knowledge).

Because globalization has increased world travel to a phenomenal extent, the airport perhaps functions as the quintessential nonplace, although supermarkets, hotels, and oversized malls could be added to this list. Ibelings argues that the airport structure has evolved into a universal type he describes as "an exposed

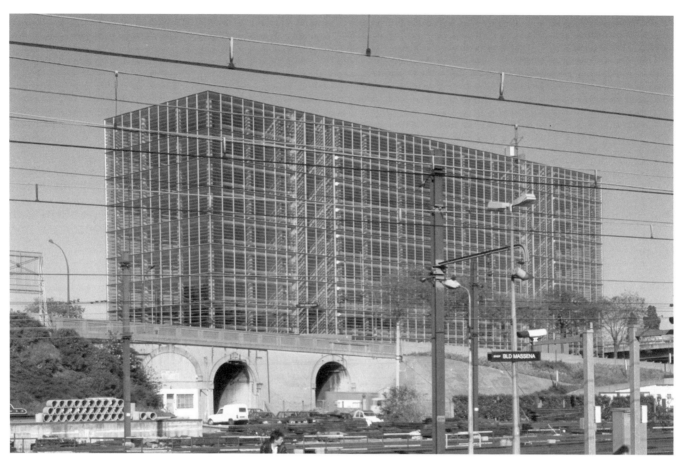

Hotel Industriel Berlier, Paris, designed by Dominique Perrault and Partners (1990)
© Perrault and Partners

steel construction (a space-frame or gigantic trusses), a marked preference for vaulted roofs, a colour palette of grey, white, pale blue and light green and, above all, acres and acres of glass" (1998). Examples of this design include Kansai International Airport Terminal, Osaka (Renzo Piano Building Workshop, 1988–1994); Hong Kong International Airport, Hong Kong, Chek Lap Kok (Foster and Partners, 1992–98); Stansted Airport, Essex, England (Foster and Partners, 1981–91); and Europier, Heathrow Airport, London (Richard Rogers Partnership, 1992–95). Functionally, the contemporary airport encompasses services such as shopping in addition to a means of travel, and further serves as an economic center for the surrounding area, a trend that reflects the transition of the symbolic city center to the periphery.

Supermodernism maintains particular traditions of modernism; namely, an aesthetic of neutrality, minimalism, and abstraction. Yet supermodernist architects seek expressivity; buildings are intended to be as autonomous and obviously separate from their surroundings; as contemporary and new, reflecting the present; as technically innovative; and finally, as a clean slate, an intended break from the past. Nonetheless, contemporary critics and stress the need to not only examine these qualities but to locate them within our contemporary global experience.

LINDA M. STEER

See also **Foster, Norman (England); Herzog, Jacques, and Pierre de Meuron (Switzerland); Hong Kong International Airport, Hong Kong; Kansai International Airport Terminal, Osaka; Koolhaas, Rem (Netherlands); Nouvel, Jean (France); Piano, Renzo (Italy); Postmodernism; Rogers, Richard (England)**

Further Reading

Augé, Marc, *Non-lieux: Introduction à une anthropologie de la surmodernité*, Paris: Seuil, 1992; as *Non-Places: Introduction to an Anthropology of Supermodernity*, translated by John Howe, London and New York: Verso, 1995

Ibelings, Hans, *Supermodernism: Architecture in the Age of Globalization*, Rotterdam: NAi, 1998

Lyotard, Jean-Francois, *La condition postmoderne: rapport sur le savoir*, Paris: Éditions de Minuit, 1979; translated by Geoff Bennington and Brian Massumi as *The Postmodern Condition: A Report on Knowledge*, Minneapolis: University of Minnesota, 1984

Machado, Rodolfo, and Rodolphe el-Khoury (editors), *Monolithic Architecture*, Munich and New York: Prestel, 1995

Riley, Terence, *Light Construction* (exhib. cat.), New York: Museum of Modern Art, 1995

Savi, Vittorio, and Josep M. Montaner, *Less Is More: Minimalisme en arquitectura i d'altres arts; Minimalism in Architecture and the*

Other Arts (exhib. cat.; bilingual Catalan-English edition), Barcelona: Actar, 1996

SUSTAINABILITY AND SUSTAINABLE ARCHITECTURE

Buildings consume one-third of the total energy produced in the United States, produce 40 percent of the carbon dioxide emissions that have been linked to global warming and air pollution, and generate 33 percent of landfill construction waste. These statistics have resulted in a growing trend whereby buildings are designed, constructed, operated, reused, and deconstructed in ways that will enhance human health and protect environmental quality. *Sustainable architecture* is the expression coined for environmentally responsive building practices. It differs from conventional design by considering the environmental impacts of design decisions throughout the entire building life cycle from cradle to cradle instead of cradle to grave. It provides a comprehensive examination of all aspects of architectural design including site selection, energy conservation, passive solar strategies, low-energy systems, building materials, indoor air quality, water conservation, waste minimization, lighting, and use of renewable energies.

The roots of sustainable architecture can be traced to the ancient theoreticians that include Vitruvius, who in *The Ten Books on Architecture* discussed the benefits of designing with the local climate and indigenous materials (Morgan 1960). The skills of preindustrial builders, the mastery of using on-site resources such as proper orientation, thermal mass, shading, ventilation, and local construction materials, were all but abandoned after the invention of artificial lighting and air conditioning. Except for several notable exceptions (i.e., organic movement), architecture of the first half of the 20th century disregarded the environmental context of buildings. The energy crisis brought about by the 1973 Arab oil embargo hastened the return to energy-efficient design. The passive solar architecture movement of the 1970s responded by offering appropriate technical solutions that, for the most part, failed to address broader environmental and architectural concerns. The sustainability movement emerged in the late 1980s as an outgrowth of this period, adding to a heightened environmental awareness determined to achieve more comprehensive and integrated design solutions.

The term *sustainability* has its origins in the 1987 World Commission on Environment and Development report, *Our Common Future*. The concept was central to "a global agenda for change" in current development patterns focusing on both underdeveloped and industrialized countries. The term recognizes the interdependency of economic, social, and environmental factors necessary to sustain life on Earth. The defining quote from this report is: "Sustainable development seeks to meet the needs and aspirations of the present without compromising the ability to meet those of the future" (WCED 1987). Buildings and sites that utilize natural systems to minimize their global, regional, and local environmental impacts on land, energy, water, and materials form the basis of "sustainable" or "green" architecture. Human health, economic affordability, and social equity are also considered attributes of sustainable design.

Sustainable architecture involves both design philosophy and technology. Practitioners in the field have written manifestos, statements of principles, and guidelines to clarify the goals, intentions, and aspirations for sustainable design. One such widely published document is the *Hannover Principles* by William McDonough, named after the World's Fair 2000 city in which the principles were drafted. The statements in this document elucidate the inherent value of nature and our need to seek a more symbiotic relationship with it. Guidelines for sustainable design by contrast tend to focus on applications of design strategies or technologies. The journal *Environmental Building News* of Brattleboro, Vermont, provides one such checklist, which serves as a concise listing of building design and construction practices for any home owner, builder, or designer interested in building sustainability.

Technologies for sustainable architecture form a long, crosscutting list of alternatives that need to be adapted to local environmental conditions. Daylighting design (Guzowski 2000), passive solar heating (Mazria 1979), passive cooling (Givoni 1994), water recycling and reuse, and biological wastewater treatment are primary sustainable design strategies that combine innovations in technology with extensive design knowledge and expertise. Computer tools are still mostly segmented providing design assistance for particular building performance issues such as energy (*Energy-plus, DOE2*, and *Energy-10*) and lighting design (*Lightscape* and *Lumen-micro*). A design tool that links disparate design and analysis components is Lawrence Berkeley National Laboratories' *Building Design Advisor*. The *Green Building Advisor* by the Center for Renewable Energy and Sustainable Technology (CREST), E build, Inc., and Design Harmony, Inc. gives designers qualitative recommendations for sustainable design including bibliographic, video, and electronic resources as well as documented case study buildings.

Selection of building materials is another key focus of sustainable architecture. Construction materials and methods are sought that are low impact throughout the entire material life cycle; that is, the materials should create less environmental damage in their extraction, processing, use, waste, and disposal phases than conventional alternates. Green building materials typically have one or more of the following traits: they are durable, compostable, recyclable, re-usable, and nontoxic to humans. Many of the green building materials not only demonstrate superior environmental performance but also do not degrade indoor air quality when strict adherence to non-toxic content is heeded in installation as well as in the material. Recent history of sick building syndrome calls attention to the health risks of creating sealed buildings with insufficient ventilation and finish materials that cause chemicals to disperse into the indoor environment. In 1996 the American Institute of Architects published their guide to environmental building products called the *Environmental Resource Guide*. This book gave qualitative descriptions of the impacts of common building materials. Alternative building construction materials also play an important role in sustainable design (Elizabeth and Adams 2000). Straw bale (Bainbridge et al. 1994), rammed earth (Easton 1996), cob, recycled tires (Reynolds 1993), and fired ceramics (Khalili 1986) are the most familiar alternatives to conventional construction systems used in sustainable building.

There are a number of exemplary buildings that illustrate the principles of sustainable architecture spanning a wide range of building types, scales, and geographical locations. The examples

presented here highlight the qualities that differentiate sustainable design from conventional practice.

The Center for Regenerative Studies at California State Polytechnic University at Pomona is an example of an integrated design solution demonstrating ecological site planning as well as sustainable building strategies. The project, built on 16 acres across from the main university campus, completed the first phase of construction in 1993 although design ideas originated in the classroom almost 20 years earlier under the tutelage of the late Professor of Landscape Architecture at Cal Poly-Pomona, John Tillman Lyle. Professor Lyle elaborated on the design process and solution in his book, *Regenerative Design for Sustainable Development*. The specific sustainable design strategies applied to the landscape include biological wastewater treatment through pond ecosystems, a solar farm with experimental solar electric technologies, habitat preservation for wildlife, and edible landscapes woven throughout the building site. The buildings were designed by the architectural firm Dougherty and Dougherty as demonstration facilities, with a variety of passive solar heating and cooling strategies. Building materials were selected for their durability, low maintenance, and low embodied energy. Recycled materials were used in the landscapes such as recycled tires for retaining walls and recycled concrete paving for outdoor patio spaces. The Center also enjoys its unique status as a social experiment for participatory student cohousing.

Another example of an integrated building and landscape solution is the passive solar subdivision, Village Homes, in Davis, California, by Mike and Judy Corbett that was started in 1975 (Corbett 1988). This 70-acre site with 220 homes manages storm water drainage using natural landscape features, narrow shaded streets to decrease exterior summer temperatures, a street layout that supports solar access, and edible landscapes throughout. Shared open space is developed between units adding to recreational use as well as a sense of community. Energy consumption for the passive solar homes in this subdivision is less than half that of conventional homes in the surrounding area. Less than 10 per cent of the homes use mechanical cooling, which is a testimonial to passive cooling in a climate that has many days reaching 100 degrees Fahrenheit in summer.

An example of a retail project utilizing the principles of sustainable architecture is the Real Goods Headquarters in Hopland, California. Real Goods, a retailer of renewable energy products, commissioned a building design that reinforced their corporate philosophy toward environmental stewardship. Architects from the Ecological Design Institute of Sausalito, California, designed a straw bale structure finished with "PISÉ" (pneumatically installed stabilized earth). The south-facing semicircular plan optimizes interaction with the sun, with tall clerestory windows on the southeast to capture morning light and shorter clerestories on the southwest to reduce late afternoon solar gain. An exterior trellis protects lower windows from the hot summer sun where visitors can enjoy the evaporative cooling effect from a water fountain in the entrance courtyard. Light shelves on the interior diffuse and reflect light creating a soft glow. Thermal mass is achieved through the concrete floor and interior PISÉ walls. The site has additional sustainable design elements, some built, others planned. There is a solar powered water pump at the entry, flow forms that can be used in water treatment as sculptural water elements, and retention ponds that form part of the landscape ecology. The parking lot utilizes bio-filters to minimize the effects of nonpoint source pollution from automobiles. The restrooms for this complex are touted to passersby on the nearby highway as a "must-see." Waterless urinals, recycled plastic toilet stalls, and reused toilet tank tops as wainscoting are the predominant features. This project and a more general discussion of the design team's sustainable design philosophy are described in *Ecological Design* by Sim Van der Ryn and Stuart Cowan (1996) and *A Place in the Sun* by John Shaeffer (1997).

To illustrate that sustainable design can be achieved in a more extreme climates, the Rocky Mountain Institute in Snowmass, Colorado, offers an excellent example of combining home, office, and indoor farm into an exceptionally energy efficient and aesthetically pleasing environment. The owners, Hunter and Amory Lovins, have created a building that mirrors the resource-efficiency concerns that occupy their professional lives (Hawken, et al. 1999, Lovins 1977). Although the 4000-square-foot building is located in a cold (8700 Fahrenheit heating degree day) climate, it is 99 per cent passively solar heated. The building, built in 1984, uses high-performance window technology, daylighting, energy-efficient electric lighting, high insulation levels, thermal mass, a sunspace, interior water features, and photovoltaics. The building boasts a ten-month payback period in energy savings to recover the initial cost of the energy improvements.

Office buildings, because of their emphasis on lighting and the high monetary value placed on the employees occupying these buildings, are a prime candidate for sustainable design. Worker productivity studies, as well as student performance in sustainable buildings, are beginning to connect design quality and occupant health, as illustrated in the studies by Dr. Judith Heerwagen of Seattle, Washington, and researchers at the Heshong-Mahone Group near Sacramento, California. Two notable office building examples discussed in more detail here are the ING Bank by Alberts and Von Huut and the C.K. Choi Building by Matsuzaki Wright Architects.

The ING Bank (formerly NMB) headquarters building near Amsterdam, the Netherlands is a corporate bank headquarters consisting of 10 vertical towers connected by a serpentine plan linking offices and support spaces. The towers use daylight, stack ventilation, plant materials, water features, and orientation devices to enliven as well as enhance the transition zones between buildings. Office workers are guaranteed natural light either from the exterior windows, with no worker being more than 20 feet from a window, or from the interior borrowed light. Site development includes several gardens placed in part to conceal a parking garage below. The building, built in 1987, is unique in terms of the participatory process used, which involved representatives from all future building occupant groups as well as all members of the design and consultancy teams from the beginning of the process. The 538,000 square foot building is also renowned for using 90 per cent less energy per square meter than the previous bank building, recovering the costs of energy improvements in energy savings after four months and reducing absenteeism by 15 percent (Roodman and Lenssen 1995). The bank is not only energy efficient, but it is also evocative in the variety of spatial experiences and environments it creates.

The C.K. Choi Building at the University of British Columbia utilizes a surprising array of bold and more common sustainable design strategies that are well integrated into the final design

solution. The three-story 30,000-square-foot office building has a long north-south axis to preserve adjacent forest land. Although this could pose a challenge for passive solar heating, the architects skillfully used roof forms to maximize north daylighting while creating a surface for mounting solar electric panels in the future. Reclaimed materials used in the building include salvaged wood trusses from a neighboring building undergoing demolition at the same time and recycled bricks. The architects experimented with a trickle ventilation system at the windows to encourage the infiltration of limited quantities of fresh air and utilized stack ventilation through the daylight atriums to avoid a conventional ducted ventilation system. The immediate landscape utilizes the building's gray water. One of the building's more unusual features for the building type is its use of composting toilets in an office building.

There are many more examples of sustainable office buildings worthy of further examination. These include the Audubon Building in New York City by the Croxton Collaborative, the Building Establishment (BRE) Headquarters in Hertfordshire, England, by Feilden Clegg Architects, the Menara Mesiniaga in Selangor, Malaysia by Kenneth Yeang, the Thoreau Center for Sustainability at the San Francisco Presidio by TLMS Architects, and an environmental studies building at Oberlin College in Ohio by William McDonough.

As seen in these projects, sustainable design goes beyond the energy savings goals of the 1970s by creating buildings that satisfy energy as well as ecological, aesthetic, and functional considerations through the overall design of building envelope, components, systems, and siting. Besides computer analysis of building systems, much of the decision-making and evaluation of sustainable architecture, however, is of a highly qualitative nature. Quantitative assessments that benchmark sustainable buildings for performance is a logical next step in the mainstreaming of sustainable architecture. A few of the current assessment methods are discussed next.

An attempt to combine economic and environmental measures for sustainable building materials has produced a number of computer-based life-cycle assessment tools. BEES, *Building for Environmental and Economic Sustainability*, from the National Institute of Standards and Technology allows comparative analysis of material selections on their environmental merit (e.g., global warming, ozone depletion, embodied energy) as well as their economic cost. Other life-cycle assessment tools, such as the Canadian product ATHENA, allow a detailed environmental accounting of a product throughout its entire manufacturing and use cycles in terms of energy, water, air, and solid waste effects. A concept called the "ecological footprint," developed by Mathis Wackernagel and Bill Rees at the University of British Columbia, considers the far-reaching energy, water, and material resource effects involved in everyday patterns and products of consumption but does so in terms of replacement resources to ameliorate the environmental impact.

Another means for assessing environmental performance of sustainable architecture is through the use of green building rating systems. Rating systems assign building performance categories a value judged against a set of prescribed baseline criteria. Malcolm Wells's 1969 *Wilderness-based Checklist* is one of the earliest rating systems using ecologically based accounting to tally the rewards of designs that improve environmental quality against the penalties of those with the opposite effect. More

recently, the U.S. Green Building Council developed a national rating system called *Leadership in Energy and Environmental Design* (LEED). Regional adaptations to the categories in this system allow jurisdictions, such as cities, to tailor the ratings to their locality. Other examples of rating systems include the Austin, Texas, *Green Builder Program* and *Building Research Establishment Environmental Assessment Method* (BREEAM) in the United Kingdom.

Sustainable architecture developed in response to a cascade of environmental concerns of the late 20th century described by such authors as Rachel Carson, Donella and Dennis Meadows, Aldo Leopold, Buckminister Fuller, David Brower, Amory Lovins, Paul Hawken, and others. A series of international commissions, from the 1987 Bruntland Report to the 1992 Earth Summit's Agenda 21, to the Montreal Protocol and the Kyoto Agreement, have crystallized the global importance of environmental issues that serve as a backdrop for design intervention. These concerns are echoed at the beginning of the 21st century when emerging fields such sustainable architecture, ecological engineering, sustainable agriculture, industrial ecology, and others begin to address the complexities of balancing environmental, economic, and social factors. Design decisions that affect land, energy, water, and material resource consumption, as well as human health and the human spirit, set sustainable design apart from conventional design and will continue to do so for years into the future.

MARGOT KALLY MCDONALD

See also **Energy Efficient Design; Solar Architecture**

Further Reading

Austin's Energy *Green Building Program*, www.ci.austin.tx.us/greenbuilder/

Bainbridge, David, Athena Swentzell Steen, and Bill Steen, *The Straw Bale House*, White River Junction, Vermont: Chelsea Green Publishing, 1994

Banham, Reyer, *The Architecture of the Well-tempered Environment*, 2nd edition, Chicago: University of Chicago Press, 1984

Corbett, Michael, *A Better Place to Live*, Emmaus, Pennsylvania: Rodale Press, 1988

Center for Renewable and Sustainable Technology (CREST), www.crest.org

Easton, David, *The Rammed Earth House*, White River Junction, Vermont: Chelsea Green Publishing, 1996

Elizabeth, Lynne and Cassandra Adams (editors), *Alternative Construction: Contemporary Natural Building Methods*, New York: Wiley, 2000

Environmental Building News, Brattleboro, Vermont, www.BuildingGreen.com

Fathy, Hassan, *Natural Energy and Vernacular Architecture*, Chicago: University of Chicago Press, 1986

Fitch, James Marston with William Bobenhausen, *American Building: The Environmental Forces that Shape It*, New York: Oxford University Press, 1999

Givoni, Baruch, *Passive and Low Energy Cooling of Buildings*, New York: Van Nostrand Reinhold, 1994

Guzowski, Mary, *Daylighting for Sustainable Design*, New York: McGraw-Hill, 2000

Hawken, Paul, Amory Lovins, and Hunter Lovins, *Natural Capitalism*, Boston: Little, Brown, 1999

Holdsworth, Bill and Anthony F. Sealey, *Healthy Buildings*, Essex: Longman Group Ltd, 1992

Hough, Michael, *Cities and Natural Process*, New York: Routledge, 1995

Jones, David Lloyd, *Architecture and the Environment: Bioclimatic Building Design*, New York: Overlook Press, 1998

Khalili, Nader, *Ceramic Houses: How to Build Your Own*, San Francisco: Harper and Row, 1986

Lovins, Amory, *Soft Energy Paths*, San Francisco: Harper and Row, 1977

Lyle, John Tillman, *Regenerative Design for Sustainable Development*, New York: Wiley, 1994

Mazria, Edward, *The Passive Solar Energy Book*, Emmaus, Pennsylvania: Rodale Press, 1979

Melet, Ed, *Sustainable Architecture: Towards a Diverse Built Environment*, Rotterdam: NAI Publishers, 1999

Morgan, Morris Hickey (translator), *Vitruvius: The Ten Books of Architecture*, New York: Dover Publications, 1960

Reynolds, Michael, *Earthship, Vol I., How to Build your Own House*, Taos, New Mexico: Survival Press, 1993

Roodman, David Malin and Nicholas Lenssen, "A Building Revolution: How Ecology and Health Concerns Are Transforming Construction," *World Watch Institute*, paper no. 124, March 1995

Schaeffer, John, *A Place in the Sun: The Evolution of the Real Goods Solar Living Center*, White River Junction, Vermont: Chelsea Green Publishing, 1997

Steele, James, *Sustainable Architecture*, New York: McGraw-Hill, 1997

Todd, Nancy Jack and John Todd, *From Eco-cities to Living Machines*, Berkeley, California: North Atlantic Books, 1994

USGBC, *U.S. Green Building Council*, www.usgbc.org

Vale, Brenda and Robert Vale, *Green Architecture: Design for an Energy Conscious Future*, Boston: Bulfinch Press, 1991

Van der Ryn, Sim and Stuart Cowan, *Ecological Design*, Covelo, California: Island Press, 1996

Venolia, Carol, *Healing Environments*, Berkeley, California: Celestial Arts, 1988

Wackernagel, Mathis and William Rees, *Our Ecological Footprint*, Stony Creek, Connecticut: New Society Publishers, 1996

Wells, Malcolm, *Gentle Architecture*, New York: McGraw-Hill, 1982

Wines, James, *Green Architecture*, New York: Tashen, 2000

World Commission on Environment and Development, *Our Common Future*, New York: Oxford University Press, 1987

Yeang, Ken, *Designing with Nature: The Ecological Basis for Architectural Design*, New York: McGraw-Hill, 1995

Zeiher, Laura C., *The Ecology of Architecture*, New York: Watson-Guptill, 1996

SWEDEN

Swedish architecture at the beginning of the 20th century was characterized by the same search for an appropriate style that was taking place on the European continent at the same time. In addition to a range of stylistic tendencies, architects faced new tasks resulting from social and political changes, housing shortages, rapid urban growth, and the development of new materials and principles of construction. One of the most significant responses to the advent of novel materials and construction techniques came from Ferdinand Boberg, the architect of the 1897 Stockholm Art and Industry Exhibition. Boberg rejected the prevalent adherence to a neo-Renaissance style, instead employing simpler medieval and Romanesque forms and reevaluating the role of ornament (Electricity Works, 1889–92; Rosenbad Bank Building, 1899–1904). Although he did not reject the uses

of ornament, Boberg believed that a building's form should be based on function and that the inherent properties of materials used in its construction should be a primary consideration. These notions would be further developed and find their fullest expression later in the century.

Governed by economic necessity, commercial buildings constructed around the turn of the century employed new, more efficient materials and methods of construction imported from outside Sweden. In 1898, Johan Laurentz constructed the first building for commercial purposes in Stockholm using iron and glass as the major elements for the facade. One year earlier, in 1898, Ernst Stenhammar had used a steel frame to construct a facade devoid of ornament derived from historical references; Stenhammar was also the first Swedish architect to use reinforced concrete in the Myrstedt and Stern Building (1908–10).

Like materials and methods of construction, stylistic tendencies were subject to importation and further contributed to the debate over what was appropriate. One end of the spectrum was represented by Carl Bergsten, whose Industrial Hall at the 1906 Art and Industry Exhibition in Norrköping was clearly influenced by the work of Otto Wagner and other architects active in Vienna at the time, and the other by Georg A. Nilsson, whose stripped-down facades and clear plans anticipated functionalism. Reacting to the former tendency, Carl Westman criticized the Royal Dramatic Theatre in Stockholm, completed in 1908 by

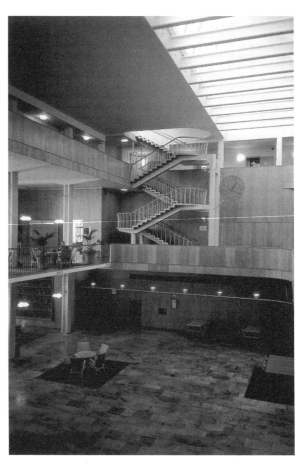

Gothenburg City Hall Extension (1913–37), by Gunnar Asplund
© Kevin Mitchell

Fredrik Lilljekvist, for its adherence to style at the expense of function and the inconsistent use of ornament derived from the Art Nouveau and Jugendstil movements that had developed in continental Europe. Westman's own position was made clear in the Medical Association Building (1904–06) in Stockholm, which is characterized by clear expression of material and simple facade treatment. The work of Westman and those influenced by it, such as Ragnar Östberg (Östermalm Teacher's College, 1906–10; Stockholm Town Hall, 1902–23), Lars Israel Wahlman (Engelbrekt Church, 1905–14), and Sigfrid Ericson (Masthugget Church, 1907–14), has been categorized as part of a movement known as "National Romanticism."

Reactions to National Romanticism included a return to a classical form language, as exemplified in Ivar Tengbom's Enskilda Bank Building (1912–15) and Swedish Match Corporate Headquarters Building (1926–28). During this period, influences from neighboring Denmark were readily apparent and served to inspire the return to classicism, as in Carl Petersen's Faaborg Museum (1912–15). The influence of classicism is apparent in the early work of Gunnar Asplund and Sigurd Lewerentz. Of particular note is the proposed crematorium for Helsingborg designed by Lewerentz and Torsten Stubelius in 1914 and the development of the original proposal for the Woodland Cemetery developed by Lewerentz and Asplund in 1915. While continuing work on the Woodland Cemetery, Asplund completed the Lister County Courthouse (1919–21), a decidedly classical building based on pure geometric forms, and the Stockholm Public Library (1924–28), which can be seen as indicative of the shift from neoclassicism to functionalism.

During the mid-1920s, attention turned to developments occurring on the European continent. One of the major proponents of the ideas developed there was Uno Åhrén, who had traveled to the 1925 Paris Exhibition and reported on the work of Le Corbusier. The 1927 Stuttgart Exhibition and new housing being developed in Germany influenced architects in Sweden at the time, as did the periodical *Kritisk Revy*, published by the Danish architect Poul Henningsen between 1926 and 1928.

Among the earliest functionalist buildings designed by Swedish architects were the industrial structures and housing in a company town known as the Kvarholm Complex in Nacka (1927–34) and the Tiden office building (1929), both designed by the Cooperative movement's architects office headed by Eskil Sundahl. Other significant functionalist buildings included an office building on Drottninggatan in central Stockholm, designed by Wolter Gahn, and the Student's Building (1930) at the Royal College of Technology and the Helsingborg Concert Hall (1932), designed by Sven Markelius.

The 1930s was a time of great change in the social and economic structure of Sweden. High unemployment, housing shortages, and substandard living conditions plagued the country. The response by architects came via the 1930 Stockholm Exhibition and the accompanying manifesto titled *acceptera*, or "accept." The manifesto was written by Gregor Paulsson (director of the Swedish Handicraft Association and general commissioner of the exhibition), Gunnar Asplund, Wolter Gahn, Sven Markelius, Eskil Sundahl, and Uno Åhrén. This document and the exhibition out of which it grew attempted to outline an approach based on "everyday" issues. The main Exhibition Building (1930), designed by Asplund, who was appointed principal architect, clearly reveals his affinity for functionalism. As-

plund would go on to complete other significant buildings in Sweden, including the crematorium and adjoining chapels at the Woodland Cemetery (1935–40), the Bredenberg Department Store (1935), the extension to the Gothenburg Court House (1936), and the National Bacteriological Laboratory (1937).

One of the major themes of the Stockholm Exhibition was housing, and of particular interest were the open-plan terrace houses designed by Uno Åhrén. Problems associated with housing continued to plague Swedish society well into the 20th century, and the Housing Commission was appointed in 1933 to investigate the problems and propose solutions. Out of these investigations came the concept of "collective" housing, and the most significant contributions to this building type were the apartment block on John Ericssongatan by Sven Markelius in 1935 and the Yrkeskvinnornas House (1939) by Albin Stark and Hillevi Svedberg.

Throughout the 1940s, the government worked to establish guidelines for housing. During this time, many architects reacted against the monotony resulting from the rows of parallel blocks of apartments built to solve the housing shortage throughout the 1930s; notable proposals included the first tower block houses in Sweden, known as "star houses" because of their starlike plan configuration, built in Stockholm by Sven Backström and Leif Reinius in 1945. Backström and Reinius were responsible for other inventive proposals, including a large housing area in Gröndal built between 1945 and 1952. The concern for large-scale solutions to housing problems is also manifest in plans for the area of Årsta in Stockholm, initiated in 1942 by Uno Åhrén and continued by Erik and Tore Ahlsén into the 1950s.

The 1940s brought increased international attention to architecture in Sweden as a result of the work of Backström and Reinius and others. Attention was once again focused on Sweden with the publication of *Sweden Builds* in 1950 by G.E. Kidder Smith. In a 1947 article, the English periodical *Architectural Review* labeled the work in Sweden as a part of a movement known as "New Empiricism," which was characterized as a way of building on the basis of experience and a practical knowledge of material traditions. One the most significant contributions came from Nils Tesch, who, just as the previous generation of architects, turned to Denmark for inspiration, particularly the work of Kay Fisker and C.F. Møller. A number of Danish architects had emigrated to Sweden during World War II, and a number of them worked for Tesch, including Erik Asmussen, who would go on to become the main architect for the Anthroposophical movement and complete a series of buildings for this group in Järna between 1968 and 1992.

In 1942, the English architect Ralph Erskine began to work in Sweden. Although clearly influenced by developments in Sweden, Erskine's work is highly expressive and incorporates a wide range of seemingly disparate materials. Of particular significance are the Tourist Hotel in Borgafjäll (1948); a housing, school, and commercial center (1945–55) in Gyttorp; the Luleå Shopping Center (1955); the Byker housing development (1968–82) in Newcastle, England; and a series of buildings done for Stockholm University since 1972.

Many of the large-scale projects initiated in the 1950s would carry over into the 1960s, including the central area of Stockholm and a suburban area of the city known as Vällingby, both based on plans by Sven Markelius. Another large-scale undertaking, the "Million Program," was initiated to construct one mil-

lion dwellings between 1965 and 1974 and exerted great influence on architecture and planning during these years. The center of Stockholm was transformed during the 1960s by the pureglass PUB Department Store (1960) by Erik and Tore Ahlsén, Åhléns Department Store (1964) by Backström and Reinius, and the Culture House, Town Theatre, and Bank of Sweden Building, all designed by Peter Celsing between 1966 and 1976.

Celsing was also responsible for the Härlanda Church, which was awarded as a result of a competition in 1952 and completed in 1958. Just as at Härlanda, Celsing went on to complete a series of simple churches built from dark-fired Helsingborg bricks, including the Church of St. Thomas in Vällingby (1959), Almtuna Church in Uppsala (1959), and Bolinden Church (1960). Although Celsing introduced a building style that explored the role of brick in religious structures, it was Sigurd Lewerentz who demonstrated the full potential of brick construction in religious buildings with St. Mark's Church (1960) and St. Peter's Church (1963–67).

The last building to be constructed by Lewerentz was a small flower kiosk (1969) within the Malmö Eastern Cemetery that he had planned and worked on since 1916. The influence of Lewerentz is apparent in the work of friend and colleague Klas Anshelm, including the Lund Town Hall (1961–66), the Lund Art Gallery (1954–57), the Malmö Art Museum (1976), and the buildings completed for Lund University between 1948 and 1978. Bernt Nyberg, an architect who had worked with both Lewerentz and Anshelm, reveals his indebtedness to both of them in the Lund County Archive (1971), the Höör Chapel (1972), and the "Sparta" student housing complex and Lund University (1964–71).

The oil crisis in 1974 greatly affected Sweden's economy and contributed to the collapse of the Million Program. Large-scale building programs were no longer feasible, and much of the work for architects involved renovations and the upgrading of existing buildings. Economic recovery in the 1980s generated new building commissions resulting from urban-renewal programs and a number of "new towns" planned as an alternative to urban sprawl. Of particular relevance is the area of Skarpnäck on the outskirts of Stockholm.

The search for an appropriate style that characterized turn-of-the-century debates has reappeared in Sweden, accompanied by a multiplicity of approaches and stylistic tendencies. Whereas the Vasa Museum (1990) by Månsson and Dahlbäck was clearly influenced by contemporary architecture based on complex geometries and a divorce of plan and section, architects such as Gunnar Mattsson and Carl Nyrén have adopted a classical form language reminiscent of Postmodern architecture, but with a greater care for material and detailing. The work of contemporary architects Gert Windgårdh, Anders Landström, and Johan Celsing represents efforts to reconcile Postmodernism and the clean lines that characterized Swedish architecture during the 1930s and 1940s.

Although architecture in Sweden during the 20th century has been characterized by intense exchange of ideas with other countries, actual buildings by foreign architects did not appear in the country until the final part of the century, with the notable exception of a series of houses by the Austrian architect Josef Franck in the late 1920s and early 1930s and two apartment complexes by Swiss architects Alfred Roth and Ingrid Wallberg in 1930. Recent buildings by architects from other countries include the Volvo Headquarters (1984) by the American Romaldo Giurgola, the SAS Headquarters (1987) by the Norwegian Niels Torp, and the Malmö Town Library by Henning Larsen from Denmark. In 1990, an international competition for the Museums of Modern Art and Architecture was won by the Spanish architect Rafael Moneo. Completed in 1998, this complex thoughtfully considers the development of architecture in Sweden during the 20th century and offers a significant contribution to the debate about its future directions.

Like other European architects during the latter part of the 20th century, Swedish architects have considered issues of sustainability and ecology. Contributions in this area come from the HSB:S Architects Office at the Understenshöjden Residential Development (1990–95) by Christer Nordström and White architects. With broad-based popular and political support, Sweden has the possibility of developing an economically and ecologically sustainable architecture. However, the question remains whether architects in Sweden can mediate between international influences and the high level of architectural production that has warranted praise from historians and critics of 20th-century architecture.

KEVIN MITCHELL

Further Reading

For an introduction to architecture in Sweden at midcentury, see Kidder Smith. A comprehensive account of Swedish architecture in the 20th century is presented in Caldenby et al. (1998), which also includes brief biographies of significant architects and an extensive bibliography. For in-depth treatments of the work of individual architects, see Coates, Collymore, Dymling, Rudberg, Walton, Wang, and Wrede.

Ahlberg, Hakon, *Swedish Architecture of the Twentieth Century*, London: Benn, 1925

Ahlin, Janne, *Sigurd Lewerentz, arkitekt*, Stockholm: Byggförlaget, 1985; as *Sigurd Lewerentz, Architect, 1885–1975*, Cambridge, Massachusetts: MIT Press, 1987

Andersson, Henrick O. and Fredric Bedoire, *Swedish Architecture: Drawings, 1640–1970; Svensk Arkitektur: Ritningar, 1640–1970* (bilingual English-Swedish edition), Stockholm: Byggförlaget, 1986

Andersson, Henrik O. and Fredric Bedoire, *Stockholm Architecture and Townscape*, Stockholm: Bokförlaget Prisma, 1988

Berglund, Kristina and Hisashi Tanaka (editors), *Swedish Contemporary Architecture; Gendai Sueden kenchiku* (bilingual English-Japanese edition), Tokyo: Process Architecture, 1986

Building Stockholm: Building during the 1980s in Stockholm, Stockholm: Swedish Council for Building Research, 1986

Caldenby, Claes, et al., *Two Churches; Två kyrkor*, Stockholm: Arkitektur Förlag, 1997

Caldenby, Claes, Jöran Lindvall, and Wilfried Wang, *20th-Century Architecture: Sweden*, Munich and New York: Prestel, 1998

Caldenby, Claes and Olof Hultin (editors), *Asplund*, Stockholm: Arkitektur Förlag, 1985; New York: Rizzoli, 1986

Celsing, Peter, *The Facade Is the Meeting between Inside and Outside; Fasaden är mötet mellan ute och inne* (bilingual English-Swedish edition), Helsinki: Museum of Finnish Architecture, 1992

Childs, Marquis William, *Sweden: The Middle Way*, New Haven, Connecticut: Yale University Press, and London: Faber and Faber, 1936; revised and enlarged edition, New Haven, Connecticut: Yale University Press, 1947

Coates, Gary, *Erik Asmussen, Architect*, Stockholm: Byggförlaget, 1997

Collymore, Peter, *The Architecture of Ralph Erskine*, London and New York: Granada, 1982; revised edition, London and New York: Academy Editions, 1994

Constant, Caroline, *The Woodland Cemetery: Toward a Spiritual Landscape: Erik Gunnar Asplund and Sigurd Lewerentz, 1915–1961*, Stockholm: Byggförlaget, 1994

Cruickshank, Dan (editor), *Erik Gunnar Asplund*, London: Architect's Journal, 1988

Dymling, Claes (editor), *Architect Sigurd Lewerentz*, 2 vols., Stockholm: Byggförlaget, 1997

Engfors, Christina, *E.G. Asplund: zrkitekt, vän och kollega*, Stockholm: Arkitektur Förlag, 1990; as *E.G. Asplund: Architect, Friend, and Colleague*, Stockholm: Arkitektur Förlag, 1990

Hald, Arthur, *Swedish Housing*, Stockholm: Swedish Institute, 1949

Holmdahl, Gustav, Sven Ivar Lind, and Kjell Ödeen (editors), *Gunnar Asplund, arkitektur, 1885–1940: ritningar, skisser, och fotografier*, Stockholm: Tidskriften Byggmästaren, 1943; as *Gunnar Asplund, Architect, 1885–1940: Plans, Sketches, and Photographs*, Stockholm: Tidskriften Byggmästaren, 1950; 2nd edition, Stockholm: Byggförlaget, 1981

Hultén, Bertil, *Building Modern Sweden*, London: Penguin, 1951

Hultin, Olof, *Arkitektur i Sverige, 1984–89; Architecture in Sweden, 1984–89* (bilingual English-Swedish edition), Stockholm: Arkitektur Förlag, 1989

Hultin, Olof, *Arkitektur i Sverige, 1990–1994; Architecture in Sweden, 1990–1994* (bilingual English-Swedish edition), Stockholm: Arkitektur Förlag, 1994

Hultin, Olof, *The Complete Guide to Architecture in Stockholm*, Stockholm: Arkitektur Förlag, 1998

Jacobson, Thord Plaenge, and Sven Silow (editors), *Ten Lectures in Swedish Architecture*, Stockholm: s.n., 1949

Johansson, Bengt O.H., *Tallum: Gunnar Asplund's and Sigurd Lewerentz's Woodland Cemetery in Stockholm*, Stockholm: Byggförlaget, 1996

Kidder Smith, G.E., *Sweden Builds: Its Modern Architecture and Land Policy: Background, Development, and Contribution*, New York: Bonnier, and London: Architectural Press, 1950; revised 2nd edition, New York: Reinhold, and London: Architectural Press, 1957

Koopertiva Forbundet, *Swedish Cooperative Wholesale Society's Architect's Office, 1925–1935*, Stockholm: Koopertiva Forbundets Bok Förlag, 1935

Lidberg, Marie Nordin, et al., *Guide to Stockholm Architecture; Arkitekturguide Stockholm* (bilingual English-Swedish edition), Stockholm: Byggförlaget, 1997

Lindvall, Jöran (editor), *The Swedish Art of Building*, Stockholm: Swedish Institute, 1992

Lundahl, Gunilla (editor), *Recent Developments in Swedish Architecture: A Reappraisal*, Stockholm: Swedish Institute, 1983

Rudberg, Eva, *Sven Markelius, Arkitekt*, Stockholm: Arkitektur Förlag, 1989; as *Sven Markelius, Architect*, Stockholm: Arkitektur Förlag, 1989

St. John Wilson, Colin (editor), *Gunnar Asplund, 1885–1940: The Dilemma of Classicism*, London: Architectural Association, 1988

Walton, Ann Thorson, *Ferdinand Boberg, Architect: The Complete Work*, Cambridge, Massachusetts: MIT Press, 1994

Wang, Wilfried, *The Architecture of Peter Celsing*, Stockholm: Arkitektur Förlag, 1996

Wrede, Stuart, *The Architecture of Erik Gunnar Asplund*, Cambridge, Massachusetts: MIT Press, 1980

SWITZERLAND

Like other European countries, Switzerland's architecture was dominated by historicism at the turn of the century. This style emphasized correctness and distinction in design and produced buildings that excelled in formal and aesthetic aspects. The Swiss National Museum (1898) in Zürich by Gustav Gull exemplifies this approach with an irregular, picturesque grouping of building shapes inspired by medieval architecture.

At the beginning of the 20th century, Art Nouveau became the choice for architects intent on expressing a new beginning, a new "spring." In Switzerland, this style emphasized superficial qualities above all else and is found primarily in the decorative treatment of structural parts. Buildings were assembled from heavy elements, in utter contrast to the delicacy of Belgian and Austrian Art Nouveau. These forms were derived from historical styles but transformed into seemingly lighter structures. Through decoration, individual forms merge fluidly into one another. The ornamental treatment emphasizes relationships and influences between parts and focuses on movement expression. This is demonstrated especially in large building complexes that are articulated as pillar architecture, an example of which is the main building of the University of Zürich (1914). Its architect, Karl Moser, was a pivotal figure in early 20th-century architectural development in Switzerland. During the 1920s, he would become a champion of modern architecture, even designing the Church of St. Antonius (1927) in Basel in reinforced-concrete construction.

Modernism in Switzerland presents the efforts of architects to transform an imported style into a nationalized idiom. The machine aestheticism of the International Style seemed to complement Switzerland's propensity to manufacture quality products. Thus, Swiss architects excelled in adapting modernism and did not need to create a distinct version. A close contact with the design cultures surrounding the country has always been a trademark of Swiss architecture. Architects simply experimented with the new constructional means and materials instead of producing creative transformations.

The Swiss national ethos of sobriety manifested itself as a combination of practical reason and moral claims in this style. Rational logic was at the heart of this modernism. Thus, the International Style became a mirror for the Swiss self-view. This view was based on values that were identical to the ideological intentions of modernist architecture. Buildings were solidly constructed in pure, slick cubical forms with flat roofs. In housing settlements, the buildings were differentiated according to typology, and groupings took into consideration the exposure to sunlight. Interiors tended to be open and well lit, thus allowing for grand vistas in rather small spaces. Things inside were placed into the light to allow easy orientation. The buildings used setbacks and had balconies, and the plans are efficiently laid out. The "dwelling for the existence minimum" was a big theme. For modernist architects in Switzerland, dwelling almost defined the profession. The best modernist work in the 1920s and 1930s is found in housing, either in individual structures or in communal settlements. In 1929, the Swiss Werkbund sponsored the Neubühl settlement in Zürich (finished 1932), which continues to be considered a standard.

Apart from having educated one of the masters of the International Style, Le Corbusier, who designed a few exemplary houses in La-Chaux-de-Fonds in an attempt at a regional version of Art Nouveau, Switzerland also boasts a masterpiece of Expressionist architecture, the main alternative to the International Style. Rudolf Steiner's Goetheanum (1928) in Dornach exemplifies this

more intuitive, mystical interpretation of the industrial age. Its amorphous building mass uses a particular formal language, expressing the shell that harbors renewal and whose purpose is to find the way to the spirit. William Lescaze and Sigfried Giedion are two other Swiss names that are synonymous with the International Style.

The political influence of German Fascism during the 1930s created a strong opposition to modernism in Switzerland. The contrasting forces fought over stylistic choices, particularly in the temporary exhibition structures for the national exhibition of 1939 in Zürich. This event became a watershed that pitted sobriety against sentimentality. Ultimately, the authorities compromised by charging modernist Hans Hoffmann with the master plan but distributing individual pavilions to members of both camps. Consequently, regional Romanticism was side by side with a socialist modernism. Famed bridge builder Robert Maillart designed a parabolic reinforced-concrete shed for the Swiss cement industry, and there was also a nostalgic little village containing examples of regional houses. The temporary buildings were constructed in wood and had to represent national contents through associations. Architects were forced to express the spiritual program of the exhibition, which had been set along notions of Swiss community. Architecturally, these political demands produced a mixed bag. Demands of representation and symbolism were made of modernist forms that they were not able to accommodate by their nature. It became clear that soberness was not sufficient as an ideological content. Architecture also had to cater to feelings, not just the intellect. Consequently, architectural images became conventional. Picturesque groupings replaced abstraction, and typological investigations of communal space became important. The previously mentioned Maillart had opened new horizons in modern reinforced-concrete bridge construction. The shape of the supporting arch was used to stabilize the bridge and also became a trademark icon.

However, the slowdown in building activity during World War II allowed the nascent modernist attempts to mature into a competent stylistic expression that provided a solid foundation for future architecture. After the war, the characteristics of building materials and their impact on structure, proportional systems, high quality of execution, and simplicity of form became trademarks of Swiss architecture. Nevertheless, the prewar design elements were reorganized. Rationality was now contrasted with sensuality, feeling, and emotion. Pragmatism was combined with aesthetic design. Human needs and a newly found respect for traditions changed functional design. However, typical Swiss character traits—freedom of thought, high standard of living, justice, and neutrality—are hard to represent and thus have not had a dramatic effect on architecture. Consequently, modernist functionalism continued to be the mainstream of architectural development.

Especially the sculptural vehemence of Le Corbusier's postwar work served as inspiration. Atelier 5's Halen Settlement (1961) in Berne, as well as buildings by Dolf Schneebli, adapted the master's concepts to local patterns of housing. Halen spread collective services over a gently sloped site. Such designs experimented with the sculptural potential of reinforced-concrete construction. Other Swiss architects exploited sloping sites for terraced housing settlements. The Swiss sense for precision and refinement came out in luxuriously detailed adaptations of Mies van der Rohe's steel-and-glass boxes. Some architects excelled in designing for the traditional materials, wood and brick, and exploited them for interesting spatial explorations. Ernst Gisel's Park Theater (1954) in Grenchen is almost a literal copy of Alvar Aalto's Säynätsalo Civic Center.

These propitious beginnings would later fizzle out into empty applications of technology to generate profit. This shoe box architecture was balanced by wildly shaped concrete buildings that were for the most part trivial. There was also a large number of buildings, especially for tourist functions, that used a typical "Heimatstil." Especially large hotels in the mountains were shaped like overfed chalets or other farm and vernacular buildings. Nevertheless, Swiss architects hardly ever indulged in the historicist frivolities that Postmodern architects produced in the United States. Good architecture was still thought to rest on pragmatic principles. Swiss architects chose either to adapt modernist forms to the topography or to expressively interpret the site. An example of the former is the megalomaniac Cité du Lignon (1971) in Geneva. This is a huge apartment building in the form of a bent, one-kilometer-long slab with smooth facades that lacks any human scale.

During the 1960s, urban design in Switzerland was characterized by integrations of new structures into existing environments. Multifunctional buildings expressed the high civilization of the country. Housing settlements of sequential units interspersed with open areas were built. Diversity was felt to be commensurate with the liberal and multicultural Swiss society. Swiss architects also began building in developing countries. Andre Studer's innovative 1954 apartment building in Casablanca is a successful example of the exportation of such Western standards to developing countries. In the Swiss Ticino region, architects such as Luigi Snozzi and Aurelio Galfetti integrated modernist shapes into the rustic landscape and created a strong regionalist typology. There was a rediscovery of primitive architecture, which was praised for its rootedness in topography. The Ticino School advocated an architecture of rational technology, displayed in impeccable details and execution. Their architecture was to focus on its most objective features. This, after all, is what the Swiss generally excel in. The main part of Galfetti's Communal Swimming Pool (1970) in Bellinzona is a footbridge that allows visitors to survey the entire complex. The renovations and remodelings of the castle in Bellinzona have served many an architect to excel in combinations of new and old. Nevertheless, Swiss architects did not advocate taking history only as myth or imagery but also as a source of knowledge and continuity. The Collegiate Church (1966) in Sarnen by Naef, Studer and Studer embedded references to oval baroque plans into its bulging forms. Thus, sculptural shapes on the outside become rich spatial experiences inside.

The younger generation of Ticinese architects, led by Mario Botta, has fashioned for itself an image of craft, even though their buildings are machine built. For these architects, architecture represents through abstraction. It intends to continue the tendencies inherent in the land and in history, thus the title "Tendenzen" of the 1975 exhibition that put this architecture on the map.

The various movements of the 1970s in one way or another provided updated interpretations of modernism. Continuing into the 1980s, Swiss architects produced a good number of qualitatively excellent high-tech buildings. Theo Hotz's Tele-

phone Exchange (1980) in Zürich marks the edge of the city and stands out in its drab environment as a cathedral to technology. Structure and mass of the building enter into a mutual dialogue.

Historic preservation became a significant architectural task as well. An example is the Museum of Contemporary Art (1980) in Basel by K. and W. Steib. The new addition adds a moment of development to the existing context of warehouse buildings.

Emphasis on pure materiality was transmitted from the Ticino School to Herzog and de Meuron and Diener and Diener, two firms that were actively involved in the international reevaluation of Swiss architecture during the late 1980s and early 1990s. However, the globalization of the information age has resulted in an utterly superficial approach to building materials. Herzog and de Meuron's buildings use contrasting materials in an autonomous manner that is no longer structurally determined so that they ultimately lose all meaning. The materials form simple contrasts without ever reaching a synthesis. Together with the abstract forms of their buildings, this produces pure geometry without details. None of the materials is allowed to dominate, and there is no effort to integrate them. Instead, each part is treated as a separate element, and the viewer is charged with their integration. Effects are created only through the materials, not through forms or other conventional features. Thus, imagery is purely material. The buildings then become spiritual expressions; that is, there is no metaphor, no iconography, no personal manner, and no attempt to create a complete, fulfilled form. The buildings present an architecture of entropy in which accepted notions and conventions are not applicable. Through this, the viewer is given a mere projection, just like reality is condensed on thin film in a movie.

However, there is hope yet for Swiss architecture. Successors have taken this aesthetic level of materiality to a more mundane level and attempted to create beautiful buildings with everyday materials, such as wood and brick, and with traditional forms, such as pitched slate roofs. This contemporary architecture rests on the foundations of modernism but also considers the properties of materials and construction as well as the characteristics of the topographical situation. These architects do not see the need to produce original masterworks. It almost seems as if the current generation of Swiss architects has learned the lessons that the modernist architects realized and spread after World War II. The present generation's flag bearer is Peter Zumthor. His architecture is characterized by a virtuoso treatment of materials, first of wood, later also of stone and glass. This is a far cry from the blasé materials of the stars of the 1980s. His Chapel Sogn Benedetg (1989) at Sumvitg imitates stone masonry, but because it uses wood, it reintegrates the building back to the people, making this religious structure look and age as the people's own houses. Wood here gained a layer of symbolism. For Zumthor, architecture is not what is in the materials but what these materials mean. His is an architecture of reduction—to the essential forms and constructions without imposed meanings. It is the building that needs to spark the imagination.

HANS R. MORGENTHALER

Further Reading

The most detailed information on Swiss architecture can be gleaned from the two major architectural periodicals, *Werk, Bauen und Wohnen* and *Archithese.*

Adler, Florian, Hans Girsberger, and Olinde Riege (editors), *Architekturführer Schweiz; Guide d'architecture Suisse; Architectural Guide Switzerland* (trilingual German-French-English edition), Zurich: Artemis, 1978

Altherr, Alfred, *Neue schweizer Architektur; New Swiss Architecture* (bilingual German-English edition), New York: Architectural Book, and London: Tianti, 1965

Bachmann, Jul and Stanislaus von Moos, *New Directions in Swiss Architecture*, New York: Braziller, and London: Studio Vista, 1969

Blaser, Werner, *Architecture 70/80 in Switzerland*, Basel and Boston: Birkhäuser, 1981; 2nd enlarged edition, 1982

Brown-Manrique, Gerardo, *The Ticino Guide*, New York: Princeton Architectural Press, and London: ADT, 1989

Daguerre, Mercedes, *Guida all'architettura del novecento: Svizzera*, Milan: Electa, 1995; as *Birkhäuser Architectural Guide: 20th-Century Switzerland*, Basel and Boston: Birkhäuser, 1997

Giedion, Sigfried (editor), *Moderne schweizer Architektur; Architecture moderne Suisse; Modern Swiss Architecture* (trilingual German-French-English edition), 2 vols., Basel: Werner, 1938

Gubler, Jacques, *Nationalisme et internationalisme dans l'architecture moderne de la Suisse*, Lausanne: Éditions l'Age d'Homme, 1975; 2nd edition, Geneva: Éditions Archigraphie, 1988

Humbel, Carmen, *Junge Schweizer Architekten und Architektinnen; Young Swiss Architects* (bilingual German-English edition), Zurich: Artemis, and Basel and Boston: Birkhäuser, 1995

Kidder Smith, G.E., *Switzerland Builds: Its Native and Modern Architecture*, New York: Bonnier, and London: Architectural Press, 1950

Wronsky, Dieter, *Bauen vor der Stadt: Beispiel, Kanton Basel-Land; Suburban Building: Example, Basel-Country* (bilingual German-English edition), Basel and Boston: Birkhäuser, 1991

Zeller, Christa, *Schweizer Architekturführer; Guide d'architecture Suiss; Guide to Swiss Architecture: 1920–1990* (trilingual German-French-English edition), Stuttgart, Germany: Krämer, and Zurich: Werk-Verlag, 1992

SYDNEY, AUSTRALIA

From the top of the Sydney Harbour Bridge (1932), the city is divided in two by its famous harbor and to the north by the Hawkesbury River, which circles around the back of Sydney and limits the Cumberland Plain, joining the Pacific Ocean at Broken Bay. To the south is Botany Bay, which was proposed as the original site of settlement and later discarded because it lacked a reliable source of fresh water; beyond it, the Illawarra Escarpment shuts the city off to the south, and on the west, the escarpment of the Blue Mountains bars the way to the inland. Sydney is imprisoned by its geography.

The hard Hawkesbury sandstone tabletop on which the city rests has been deeply cut into by water, lifted, and then partly submerged and tilted up at its ocean edge; Port Jackson and Middle Harbour, once separate harbors with their own outlets, are now merged into one extensive harbor that breaks through to the ocean between two lofty heads a little over a mile apart. Sydney occupies a difficult if alluring site, hidden from the oceanside by its narrow entrance.

Following the revolt of the American colonies in 1776, at the suggestion of Joseph Banks, Botany Bay was selected for the site of a new penal settlement to replace what had been lost. The institution was founded in 1788 by 1,487 souls who reached Australia in 11 ships after a prolonged voyage. A little over half

their number were convicts. Captain Phillip, the naval officer in charge of the enterprise, selected a cove 8 kilometers from the entrance on the south shore for the settlement because it possessed the best springwater, and its depth permitted his ships to anchor close to the shore. The developing township was named after British Home Secretary Thomas Townsend, Lord Sydney.

Sydney began as a collection of tents and huts. Organized along military lines, it soon acquired a makeshift, disorderly aspect that provoked successive governors to propose orderly town plans that were resisted by the inhabitants on the principle that the example of civic order in architecture would inspire social discipline and respect.

A small settlement sprang up on the west shore of Sydney Cove known today as The Rocks because it was built against a rocky ridge, one of two that framed the site. The early buildings were primitive: Bricks were laid with clay or mud, the native timber was cranky and iron-hard, and only the she-oak provided fine roof shingles. The Government House, a modest two-story dwelling in a plain Georgian style on the east side of the cove, was occupied by Governor Phillip in June 1789 and was the first building of importance. Walls were whitewashed for additional protection, giving the settlement the air of a Mediterranean village.

During the late 18th and 19th centuries, Australian architecture faithfully mirrored stylistic developments, as it followed the succession of English styles: Georgian, then Regency, followed by Gothic Revival, Victorian, and a diluted version of Arts and Crafts and Art Nouveau. American influence increased after the gold rush, especially in commercial and domestic architecture, causing a split in the sourcing of style influences. The esteem with which such mimicry was greeted depended largely on its fidelity to the original. Architecture was appreciated according to how well it reproduced English models and had an important nostalgic function to re-create a New World version of Old England. Local political and historical factors, the tyranny of distance (which delayed the taking up of new styles), the unavailability of materials, and shortages of skilled craftsmen forced innovation and together distanced Australian architecture from its stylistic models, helping sound a false note of independence. Until recently, the measure of architectural quality has been fidelity of interpretation, not idiosyncratic originality.

Mortimer Lewis (1796–1879), who arrived in Sydney in 1829, was typically schizophrenic in his choice of style, moving fluently between classical and Gothic. An adept at Gothic Revival, this did not prevent him from applying Greek Revival to the courthouse at Darlinghurst, which was his finest essay. He supervised the military-Gothic Government House (1845), de-

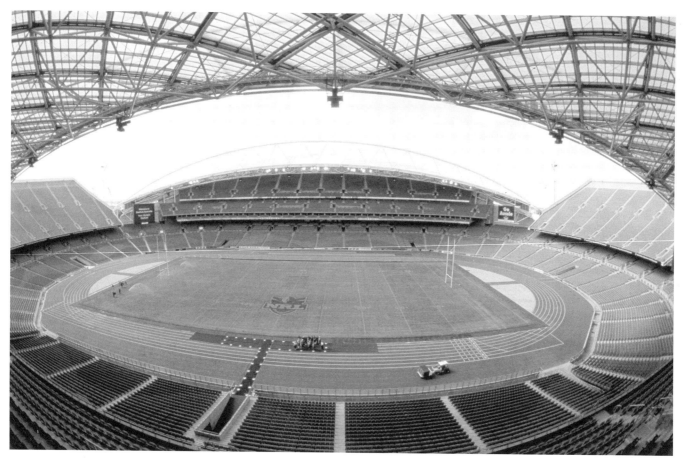

Rugby Field and Stands of Stadium Australia (1998), Homebush Bay, designed for the 2000 Olympic Games
© Australian Picture Library/CORBIS

signed and unsuitably oriented to the northern hemisphere by Edward Blore in England. It supplied a political symbol, an architectural climax, and a harbor focus for the city until the Sydney Opera House (1973) replaced it.

In 1842, wild land speculation led to a collapse of the money market and brought ruin to many people. Following a period of considerable prosperity and optimism, it hit the pastoral economy hard and brought colonial building to a halt. In 1851, the discovery of gold west of Sydney altered the complexion and mood of Australian architecture, bringing with it a new expansionism.

In the decade after 1841, Sydney's population jumped by 14,267 to 44,240. By 1901, half a century later, it would be 481,830. Sydney expanded to the south and west as the wealth of the gold fields flowed back to it. The early Victorian period started innocently enough, incorporating Gothic for ecclesiastical work and schools and classical for public buildings. Saint Andrew's Anglican cathedral by Edmund Blacket was consecrated in 1868, having been finished in stages. A vastly busy William Wardell commenced St. Mary's Cathedral beside Hyde Park in 1865. Commercial buildings set out to catch the eye of customers by what might be called a potpourri style of fanciful frippery. By 1860, terrace houses began to be built in large tracts spreading out from and surrounding the city center.

The Victorian period was notable for the rise of ornament and the blurring of architectural fashions. It was a period of grand public buildings. Sydney's General Post Office (1894) was commenced in 1864 by James Barnet, and Town Hall (1888) by J.H. Wilson set an example for the richer banks and commercial buildings that were to follow. The boom style of the 1880s, Italianate, which touched many residential buildings, had its origin in the English fascination with Romantic traditions and the picturesque. The application of Italianate style to commercial buildings led to the mass production of cast-iron columns and beams, whereas domestic architecture acquired decorative trims, gabled roofs, corner towers, and bull-nosed verandas. The florid phase of High Victorian design, which reached its peak in the 1880s, ended with the 1893 depression, which was sparked by a financial collapse three years earlier in Argentina.

In the 1880s, four stories was the rule for ornate office buildings built with traditional stone and brick exterior walls. The first Otis-type passenger lift was installed in the Farmer's Store (1881). The effect of lifts soon became evident, and by 1892 there were several buildings reaching 10 to 12 stories. Some towers, such as the Lands Department Building (1890) by James Barnet on Bent Street, rose well over 33 meters. Skyscraping got off to a shaky start with Spain and Cosh's Culwalla Chambers (1912), which rose to a height of 52 meters and frightened the city into enacting a height limit of 46 meters, a limit that survived until 1957.

The Australian domestic version of Queen Anne Revival consisting of terra-cotta roofing tiles and exposed deep red bricks was called "Federation." Substantial Federation and Arts and Crafts residences were built in the northern harborside suburbs for the upper-middle class in Mosman and Cremorne, whereas the lower-middle and working classes were housed at Haberfield and Dacey Gardens Estate (Daceyville) west and south of the city.

An outbreak of the bubonic plague caused by poor sanitation led to the reconstruction of port facilities; new standardized wharf structures, such as the Walsh Bay finger wharfs and Woolloomooloo Deep Sea Wharf; and a seawall barrier to prevent rats from coming ashore during the first two decades of the century.

After winning the competition for Australia's capital, Canberra, Walter Burley Griffin (1876–1937), who had previously been Frank Lloyd Wright's office manager in Chicago, settled in Australia. He planned and established the suburb of Castlecrag, where he later built a small cluster of seven houses. His ideas on integrating nature and architecture and his reverence for the native flora produced a unique result.

Wyldefel Gardens (1936), by W.A. Crowl and John Brogon, and Prevost House (1937) at Bellevue Hill, by Sydney Ancher (1904–78), signaled the arrival of modern architecture in Sydney. Wyldefel consisted of 20 terraced garden apartments on either side of a cascading central garden and copied a housing scheme that existed outside Oberammergau, Bavaria. The apartments had flat roofs, round corner glazing, steel windows, and concrete frames. The nautical-style Prevost House was a compact version of Mies van der Rohe's Tugendhat House (1930) at Brno.

The former City Mutual Life Building (1936), an Art Deco design by Emil Sodersten, was the first building in Sydney to be fully air-conditioned. It used a serrated zigzag window treatment and was the most impressive and innovative building at the time. The 1920s and 1930s were eras that saw the building of huge atmospheric cinemas with streamlined interiors in the American style, an example of which is the New Orpheum Theatre (1930) at Cremorne by G.N. Kenworthy.

The weakness that the British showed when challenged by Japanese expansionism in the Pacific during World War II and America's role in avoiding defeat led to a reconsideration of Australia's defense relationship with London and a gradual weakening of ties with the home country. After the war, a mass immigration program from Britain and Europe changed the cultural face of Australia. By 1958, Sydney's population had doubled, from one million in 1926 to two million.

The period since World War II has been one of increasing international influence in Australian architecture, with a shift away from Britain and a much greater awareness of European, Japanese, and American influences. Sydney, situated in the southwest Pacific, was well situated to take advantage of these shifts. Its hedonism and lack of well-considered theory resulted in a superficial borrowing of ideas rather than a deeply considered and well-assimilated style. In the 1950s, a split occurred between the supporters of Frank Lloyd Wright's Romantic organic interpretation, led by what became known afterward as the "Sydney school," a misnomer insofar as it referred to Oak Park, Chicago, not Sydney. Arrayed against the neo-Wrightian camp were the proponents of the European modern cause, with Gropius, Breuer, and Le Corbusier as its exemplars. As a division, it hid a deeper split between those supporting an Australian national identity and those wanting Sydney architecture to be more international. The arrival in 1948 on the Sydney scene of the Viennese-born and Harvard-trained Harry Seidler (1923–) would serve to heighten this division later. The neo-Wrightians in the opposing camp were represented by Peter Muller (Audette House, Castlecrag, 1953; Whale Beach house, 1954, for his family; and the ambitious "Kumale" residence at Palm Beach, 1956), Neville Gruzman (Goodman House, 1956, and Holland

House, 1962, both at Middle Cove), and Bruce Rickard's "Mirrabooka" at Castle Hill (1964). All testify to the extent of Wright's influence at the time.

Seidler's first work was the Rose Seidler House (1950) at Killara, built for his mother. He had designed this house in New York for another client and later relocated it to Killara. Its uncompromising modern character, flat roof, and open planning, as well as its New England modern, Breuer-inspired detailing and contrast of smooth industrial steel windows against rough mass sandstone walls, shocked Sydney residents and provoked wide debate.

Australian architecture since 1945 has largely been about two architects: Harry Seidler (1923–) and Glenn Murcutt (1936–). Both are Sydney architects, and both are committed to modern architectural principles, yet they manage to exemplify the two quite different, if not opposed, architectural currents: a place-based modernism versus a modernist internationalism.

Seidler's career spans 50 years and includes a large number of high-quality houses. In the 1960s, he designed the 183-meter-high Australia Square Tower (1967) with Nervi as his structural consultant and the 65-story MLC Centre (1978). In the 1980s, Seidler became increasingly engaged in office tower projects, resulting in a geometrically disciplined series in Melbourne and Perth as well as Sydney's Grovernor Place (1988) and a radical departure from his customary freestanding approach, the Capita Centre (1990), which, like the Ford Foundation Headquarters (1968) in New York, was based around a garden atrium.

In 1956, Sydney held an international architectural competition for the design of a performing arts center—a long-needed addition to its musical and theater cultural infrastructure. Jørn Utzon, a Dane, won the competition in a field of 230 submissions for a remarkable design that he set about developing from Hellebaek. After three years of intense investigation by his structural consultant, Ove Arup and Partners, for the dramatic shell roofs, Utzon proposed a spherical geometry to suit prefabrication of the elements. In 1966, Utzon withdrew from the project and was replaced by a Sydney consortium led by Peter Hall that completed the project for its opening in October 1973.

Utzon employed Australian assistants; of these, Richard Le Plastrier (1939–) has been the most faithful follower in terms of an anonymous landscape-based, organic domestic idiom. The principal legacy of Utzon was the contribution of his Opera House to the city itself and recognition that as a sculpture it completed and gave the city a climax that oriented it toward the harbor. Utzon's personal influence, which was small, survives through a few of his young Australian assistants, including Richard Le Plastrier. The Sydney Opera House remains unchallenged as Australia's greatest work of architecture and as an international synonym for the city.

Glenn Murcutt's career began with the Marie Short farmhouse (1975) near Kempsey, and although much of his work has been done in Sydney, his best houses are reserved for its fringes or beyond. This has given him an undeserved reputation as a rural designer. In Sydney, his Carpenter house, Point Piper (1982); Stuart Littlemore house, Woollahra (1986); Tom Magney house, Paddington (1990); and Ken Done House, Mosman (1991) testify to his ability to deal with tight city sites and to inject a degree of lyricism and environmental common sense into the urban context.

Compared to Seidler, who ignored local factors in his identification with an international modern tradition inspired by Gropius, Breuer, and Le Corbusier, Murcutt's veranda-inspired spaces and celebration of vernacular verities, such as corrugated iron, glass louvres, and standard ridge ventilators, together with his poetic response to landscape, were widely perceived as distinctively Australian.

Besides giving an enormous stimulus to the Homebush Bay site west of the central business district, the 2000 Olympic Games boosted architectural activity in terms of hotels, rail, airport, and road transport. Barcelona was adopted as a model in terms of the way in which the Olympics could be used to upgrade the city by investing more than $300 million in new pedestrian squares, a Barcelona-derived rail/bus interchange at Central Station (1999), and the Cook and Phillip Park swimming complex (1999), with a 240-meter-long square on its top creating a major new urban plaza and meeting place south of St. Mary's Cathedral. Sculpture walks, new smart lighting, granite paving, and widened footpaths improved the city for pedestrians. Opposed to this is the crass addition of three luxury apartment blocks at Circular Quay East (1999) that obstruct the view of the Opera House and disconnect it from the city.

The 110,000-seat Stadium Australia (1998) is typical of the new Olympic venues: it impresses more by its size, engineering, and straightforward planning than by any imaginative qualities. Only the main Olympic Park railway station (1998) by Hassel Pty Ltd and the Archery 2000 building (1999) by Stutchbury and Pape rise much above the mundane.

Clearly, Sydney is struggling to deal with its size and its uncontrolled expansion to the west and north. The investment in facilities at its center is matched by the poor air quality, road congestion, and underfunding of public transport at its fringes.

PHILIP DREW

Further Reading

There is a lack of reliable general and architectural histories of Sydney. Most sources fall within the category of popular tourist guide. Students researching Sydney's architecture will find Jahn of great benefit, but as an edited work it lacks a coherent voice. Morrison is compact but only concerns itself with contemporary architecture. Clune gives a detailed history of the city center, whereas Fitzgerald supplies a history of the City Council. The Morris book is a readable popular mix of history and biography with an outsider's critical eye for the odd and entertaining. Urban design and planning matters are dealt with by Webber and Winston.

Clune, Frank, *Saga of Sydney: The Birth, Growth, and Maturity of the Mother City of Australia*, Sydney: Halstead Press, 1961; revised edition, Sydney: Angus and Robertson, 1962

Drew, Philip, *Leaves of Iron: Glenn Murcutt: Pioneer of an Australian Architectural Form*, Sydney: Lawbook, 1985; London: Harper Collins, 1993

Fitzgerald, Shirley, *Sydney, 1842–1992*, Sydney: Hale and Iremonger, 1992

Frampton, Kenneth and Philip Drew, *Harry Seidler: Four Decades of Architecture*, London and New York: Thames and Hudson, 1992

Freeland, J.M., *Architecture in Australia: A History*, Melbourne: Cheshire, London: Penguin, and New York: Viking Penguin, 1972

Jahn, Graham, *Sydney Architecture*, Sydney: Watermark Press, 1997

Morris, Jan, *Sydney*, London: Viking, and New York: Random House, 1992

Morrison, Francesca, *Sydney: A Guide to Recent Architecture*, London: Ellipsis, 1997

Rayner, Michael and Philip Graus, *Sydney since the Opera House: An Architectural Walking Guide*, Sydney: Royal Australian Institute of Architects (NSW), 1990

Spearritt, Peter, *Sydney since the Twenties*, Sydney: Hale and Iremonger, 1978; 2nd edition, Sydney: UNSW Press, 1999

Taylor, Jennifer, *Australian Architecture since 1960*, Sydney: Law Book, 1986; 2nd edition, Melbourne: Royal Australian Institute of Architects, 1990

Webber, G. Peter, *The Design of Sydney: Three Decades of Change in the City Centre*, Sydney: Law Book, and Agincourt, Ontario: Carswell, 1988

Winston, Denis, *Sydney's Great Experiment: The Progress of the Cumberland County Plan*, Sydney: Angus and Robertson, 1957

SYDNEY OPERA HOUSE

Designed by Jørn Utzon; completed 1973
Sydney, Australia

The force behind the Sydney Opera House was Eugene Goossens, who was appointed conductor of the Sydney Symphony Orchestra in 1946 and a year later started an "opera house" movement. He was supported by the Labor politician Joseph Cahill (1891–1959), who held the local government portfolio and subsequently became premier of New South Wales in 1952.

The project languished until November 1954, when Cahill sponsored a conference that led to the establishment of a public committee that later agreed to hold an international architectural competition in 1956 for which Jørn Utzon's design was awarded first prize in a field of 230 entries. Utzon's scheme was enthusiastically endorsed by a jury comprising Sir Leslie Martin and Eero Saarinen.

Conceived in the mid-1950s, the Sydney Opera House project brief was formulated as a performing arts center with facilities for opera, concerts, and theater under one roof. The enterprise was fraught with party politics from the outset. It was seen as a project of a Labor Party premier who sought to enlarge access to music and theater for all the citizens of Sydney during a period of acute postwar shortages. Popular opposition arose even within his own party, and Cahill cleverly circumvented these arguments by establishing an Opera House Lottery to pay for the building.

The Opera House supplied Sydney with a much-needed civic climax that recognized the concentrating visual effect of its magnificent harbor and that, in the process, cemented its identity. Today, it is an international architectural icon and is regarded by many people as one of the ten greatest architectural works of the 20th century.

In 1956, when Utzon made his design, there was great interest in shell structures. Vilhelm Lauritzen had built two remarkable shells in Copenhagen before this: the first airport terminal in Kastrup (1939) and the Radio Building's Studio 1 (1945). Utzon's Sydney design resembled these in its adoption of an inner acoustic shell suspended from a heavier outer shell. Felix Candela in Mexico and Eero Saarinen in the United States, in his TWA Terminal (1962), which was designed the same year

with a paired arrangement of balanced flower-petal shells, are other examples.

Both Saarinen and Utzon chose "free" structural forms that lacked circular, rectangular, or parabolic geometries. Although the TWA Terminal kept its free form, Utzon was criticized for his design's lack of geometry, which was essential to standardize the formwork. When, after three years of intense research, Ove Arup and Partners failed to establish a satisfactory mathematical description of the shell shapes after applying parabolic and then elliptical systems, Utzon broke the impasse in mid-1960 by proposing a spherical geometry.

In May 1965, there was a change of government. The incoming minister for public works placed himself in charge of the Opera House project, withheld permission for Utzon to proceed with his scheme to use plywood for the interior acoustic shells and glass wall mullions, and delayed fee payments. In February 1966, Utzon withdrew and was replaced by an Australian team led by Peter Hall, who completed the third stage for the interiors in October 1973. Hall attempted to realize the work as Utzon intended, but a *Review of Programme* submitted in December 1966 recommended that the Major Hall should be a single-purpose hall and that the opera should be transferred to the Minor Hall, thereby eliminating the latter's use as a theater on the grounds that the multipurpose hall would not be functionally satisfactory. The acceptance of this flawed advice resulted in the elimination of grand opera and invalidated the composition of the roofs, whose size had been determined by the volumetric requirements of the interior functions; the demolition of the stage tower and the stage machinery from the Main Hall permanently crippled the Opera House. Its cost rose from $50 million to $102 million, and the building's completion was delayed four years.

The changes to the interiors were attended by a severe aesthetic loss when Peter Hall failed to continue in the same spirit as Utzon. Fortunately, the outside was largely unaffected, and the fame of the Opera House today rests largely on the brilliance of the building's external relationship to its maritime surroundings.

Le Corbusier completed his chapel at Ronchamp in June 1955. It is no accident that the Ronchamp chapel and Utzon's Opera House are formidable sculptural achievements: Le Corbusier reacted to the four horizons and its isolated situation atop a sacred acropolis; Utzon's approach was similar: he visualized a promenade from the city to the Opera House leading to its theaters and heightened its isolation further by pushing it to the end of Bennelong Point to increase the surprise of arrival. Like Le Corbusier, who similarly applied the idea of a "Promenade Architecturale" to Ronchamp, Utzon incorporated a promenade into his architecture to enhance the pedestrian experience and increase the interaction between his building and the site and its surroundings.

Utzon's great concern was to devise the most dramatic route to approach his work by entering it from below and moving upward through its interior spaces to reach the opera and concert and theater halls. The building juts out into the harbor on a platform that he shaped and extended vertically and that contains all the performance services. At its highest, he scooped out a pair of Greek amphitheaters, treating the platform as an artificial hill. With the two stages adjoining the south foyers, the two principal halls, placed lengthwise side by side, have dual foyers

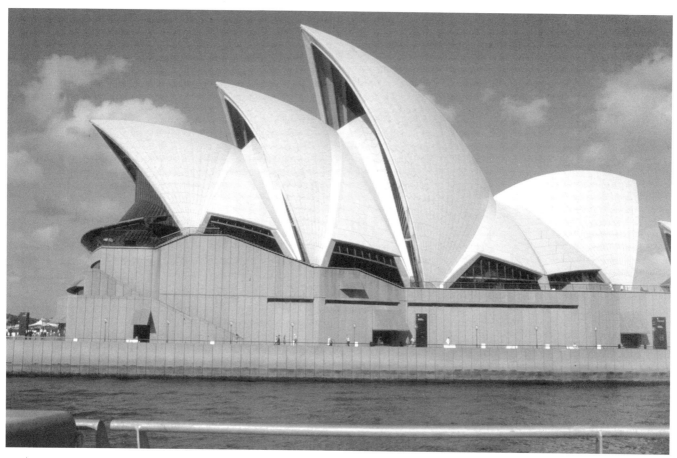

Sydney Opera House (1973)
© GreatBuildings.com

at their north and south ends but are entered along the sides. To reach the halls, patrons climb a monumental external flight of stairs at the front or use an internal staircase to reach the southern foyers and then move around the stage backs and up the platform to access the halls. The north foyers, used at intervals, face the water. The side spaces are pressed between the auditoriums and the V-shaped ribs of the precast-concrete roof vaults.

The glory of the Opera House is its white-tiled roofs surmounting the pink precast-concrete platform. The Main Hall is straddled by three asymmetrical vaults and the Minor Hall by similar smaller vaults, and a separate vault encloses the restaurant on the southwest edge of the platform. Between the two main vault groups, a narrow canyonlike cleavage is formed; below this, a tunnel street gives access to the main under-stage service areas. The open ends of the original shells were intended to be enclosed by gull-wing saddles of suspended glass between hollow plywood tubes, but Utzon's proposal was crudely simplified into stiff glass hoods supported on steel trusses.

The sculptural expressiveness and romantic immersion in the harbor setting went beyond and challenged the prevailing functional ethic of modern architecture in 1957. Its assertion of humanist values rooted in Gunnar Asplund and Alvar Aalto proclaimed a new experiential sensibility that sought to soften the image of a machine aesthetic by an appeal to the simple verities of an anonymous vernacular building. The freshness of the Opera House has not dimmed with time; it seems as ageless as the Australian bush. Utzon was inspired by an anonymous language of technique, the building creating its own style from the perfection of its means in the same way that a yacht achieves beauty through the refinement and ultimate perfection of its shape in meeting the challenge of the sea and wind.

In tying his Opera House so perfectly to its peninsula, Utzon created for Sydney a symbol and identity of such extraordinary power that it is impossible to conceive of the city as complete without it.

PHILIP DREW

Further Reading

Utzon's resistance to scholarly research and documentation and his reticence to cooperate with critical assessment have created severe problems for the serious historian, with the unfortunate consequence that there is a proliferation of errors resulting from an overreliance on secondary source material. There has been far more publication and interpretation than research into establishing reliable facts. The Fromonot account, for instance, is largely a compilation of material copied from *Zodiac* numbers 5, 10, and 14, with additions. Because these issues are rare, their republication in this way is undoubtedly useful. Utzon scholarship remains at an early stage.

The Arup Journal 8, no. 3 (October 1973) (special issue on the Sydney Opera House)

Baume, Michael, *The Sydney Opera House Affair*, Melbourne: Thomas Nelson, 1967

Drew, Philip, *Sydney Opera House: Jørn Utzon*, London: Phaidon Press, 1995

Drew, Philip, *The Masterpiece: Jørn Utzon, a Secret Life*, South Yarra, Victoria: Hardie Grant Books, 1999

Duek-Cohen, Elias, *Utzon and the Sydney Opera House: Statement in the Public Interest*, Sydney: Morgan, 1967

Fromonot, Françoise, *Jørn Utzon et l'Opéra de Sydney*, Paris: Gallimard, 1998; as *Jørn Utzon: The Sydney Opera House*, Corte Madera, California: Gingko, and Milan: Electa, 1998

Messent, David, *Opera House Act One*, Balgowlah, New South Wales, Australia: David Messent Photography, 1997

Nobis, Philip, "Utzon's Interiors for the Sydney Opera House: The Design Development of the Major and Minor Hall, 1958–1966," B.Arch. thesis, University of Technology, Sydney, 1994

"The Sydney Opera House," *Zodiac* 14 (1965)

Sydney Opera House in Its Harbour Setting: Nomination of Sydney Opera House in Its Harbour Setting for Inscription on the World Heritage List, Glebe, New South Wales: Historic Houses Trust of New South Wales, 1996

Yeomans, John, *The Other Taj Mahal*, Harlow: Longmans, 1968

SYMBOLISM

If architecture is as a system of cultural symbols expressing the identity, technology, and condition of a society—or of one group within a particular class or location—at a specific point in time, then the symbolism attributed to individual buildings constitutes one way of interpreting cultural context and the built environment. Form, ornamentation, and the choice of materials are all critical elements articulating symbolic content in architecture.

Symbolism was especially crucial for architecture in the Western world during the 20th century, reflecting the tremendous meaningful changes occurring in everyday life, in spiritual and political values, and in society. Because these changes were both synchronic and diachronic, different styles of architecture were produced and promoted simultaneously by professionally trained architects as well as amateur builders. Sometimes this diversity recorded differences in economics, application, and intention, but in other instances stylistic distinctions reflected profound oppositions in thinking. For example, at the beginning of the century, Beaux-Arts–trained architects produced both Neoclassical and Arts and Crafts–inspired buildings. The structures following in the classical tradition indicated a desire for monumentality, formality, and the continuance of traditional values, societal hierarchies, and building typologies, whereas the Arts and Crafts–inspired buildings used local materials, changes in building form and plan, and motifs selected from medieval vernacular architecture to represent ideals of home, handicraft, and the simplicity of a preindustrialized world in reaction to the political, economic, and social turbulence of the time.

The beginning of the 20th century is also notable for the work of other architects who experimented with form, materials, and ornament to create a new style of architecture expressive of the Zeitgeist. Art Nouveau was one new aesthetic resulting from this exploration exemplified in the organic designs of Victor Horta, Hector Guimard, and Henry van de Velde. These European architects and designers sought inspiration in nature in the same way that their contemporaries, such as Josef Hoffman, Charles Rennie Mackintosh, and Antonio Gaudí, looked to local building traditions for inspiration. Another new aesthetic celebrated the materials and capabilities of industry. The exposed-aluminum rivets in Otto Wagner's Post Office Savings Bank (1904–06) in Vienna and Peter Behrens' steel stanchions in the AEG factory (1908–09) in Berlin are early examples of architects using building components to express innovations in building construction and the wider promise and potential of the machine.

By the 1930s, the machine aesthetic evolved into what came to be called International Style architecture by Henry-Russell Hitchcock and Philip Johnson in the catalogue accompanying the 1932 Museum of Modern Art (New York) exhibition. The machine aesthetic was utopian at its core and aimed at improving the lives of the working classes through the introduction of affordable, utilitarian, machine-produced goods and economic construction. Conventional applied ornamentation, considered a demonstration of the class systems and social ambitions that led to World War I, was rejected as historical and emblematic of an outmoded way of life. In its place, designers substituted factory-sash and ship railings to symbolize their belief in the propensity of new industrialized societies to house populaces in clean, safe, and healthy environments and to address problems scientifically, efficiently, and unemotionally. Consequently, the dramatic change in architecture and aesthetics inherent in the International Style signified a new highly disciplined, standardized, and organized life that, in the extreme, eliminated individual character and emotion and in all phases celebrated the belief that the new architecture appropriately demonstrated the rational thinking and technical capabilities characteristic of the period.

The machine age was also celebrated in the stylized motifs and exotic materials of Art Deco, in the contours and materials of Streamline Moderne, and even in the pared-down simplicity and machine-produced aesthetic of Beaux-Arts–trained architects such as Bertram Goodhue and Paul Cret. The acceptance of the International Style in the United States in the 1930s and after World War II lacked the social purpose and initiative of European modernism and instead became adopted by corporate clients as a symbol of progressive business practices and financial success. This thinking, coupled with the prosperity and pride following World War II, prompted the transformation of regionally expressive, human-scaled American cities to concentrations of curtain-walled skyscrapers placed within recently leveled downtowns in the process of implementing the radical urban-planning ideas of Le Corbusier.

By midcentury, the disruption and destruction of the traditional fabric and the proliferation of high-rises, symbolizing the regularized working and living environments of their inhabitants, failed to produce a vital, rich environment with positive social solutions. In response, architects, including Eero Saarinen, Louis Kahn, and even Le Corbusier (Notre-Dame-du-Haut, Ronchamp, France, 1950–54), introduced dramatic forms in concrete and other materials to create expressive, sculptural, and monumental forms, or architecture as art rather than architecture as social program. This reaction was compounded in 1966 with the publication of Robert Venturi's book, *Complexity and Contradiction*, which condemned the banality and reductivism of

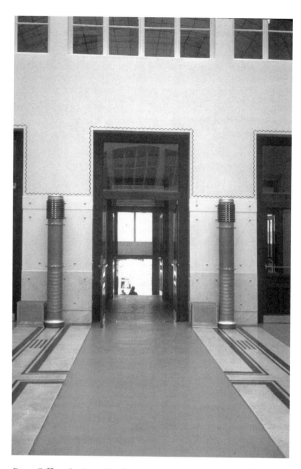

Post Office Savings Bank, Vienna, interior detail of doorway (1906)
© Howard Davis/GreatBuildings.com

to a level of elegance and sublimity in the late 20th-century designs of Tadao Ando, Antoine Predock, and the late Luis Barragán. The most symbolic architecture at the end of the century, however, derives from the fields of philosophy and semiology. Deconstructivism and poststructuralism often use elements from 1920s Constructivism twisted and contorted to signify the end of meaning (absolute knowledge) and the realization of a world pushing technology beyond the limits of human comprehension and control. The fractured, distorted, and dynamic forms suggesting confusion and instability produced by Bernard Tschumi, Peter Eisenman, Coop Himmelb(l)au, and others represent linguistic, archeological, and deconstructive concepts from the philosophy of Jacques Derrida and Michel Foucault. Other architects, however, present a totally different worldview and aesthetic, demonstrated in works associated with Neoclassicism, New Expressionism, and an appreciation of vernacular constructions. Although this wide-ranging inclusiveness might suggest indeterminate architectural chaos, the variety of buildings produced can be understood as symbols of the divergent values and theories of their creators as well as significations of the complexity, multiculturalism, and diversity of contemporary culture.

CAROL A. HRVOL FLORES

See also **AEG Turbine Factory, Berlin; Ando, Tadao (Japan); Art Nouveau (Jugendstil); Arts and Crafts Movement; Barragán, Luis (Mexico); Behrens, Peter (Germany); Chapel of Notre-Dame-du-Haut, Ronchamp, France; Coop Himmelb(l)au (Austria); Cret, Paul Philippe (United States); Deconstructivism; Eisenman, Peter (United States); Foster, Norman (England); Gaudí, Antoni (Spain); Goodhue, Bertram Grosvenor (United States); Hoffmann, Josef (Austria); Hitchcock, Henry-Russell (United States); Horta, Victor (Belgium); International Style; Mackintosh, Charles Rennie (Scotland); Meier, Richard (United States); Post Office Savings Bank, Vienna; Postmodernism; Poststructuralism; Predock, Antoine (United States); Rogers, Richard (England); van de Velde, Henri (Belgium)**

Further Reading

The following readings concentrate on the later half of the 20th-century with writings particularly reinterpreting the modern movement and addressing the theoretical positions and architecture of Postmodernism and poststructuralism. The anthologies by Easthope and McGowan, Fernie, and Nesbitt are of significance because they introduce the ideas and perspectives of several writers on each topic and direct the reader to the larger body of work by each author. In addition, Fernie contains an informative glossary of concepts and bibliographic entries.

Easthope, Anthony and Kate McGowan (editors), *A Critical and Cultural Theory Reader*, Toronto: University of Toronto Press, and Buckingham: Open University Press, 1992
Fernie, Eric (editor), *Art History and Its Methods: A Critical Anthology*, London: Phaidon, 1995
Jameson, Fredric, *Postmodernism; or, The Cultural Logic of Late Capitalism*, Durham, North Carolina: Duke University Press, and London: Verso, 1991
Lagueux, Maurice, "Nelson and Goodman and Architecture," *Assemblage* 35 (April 1998)
Nesbitt, Kate (editor), *Theorizing a New Agenda for Architecture: An Anthology of Architectural Theory, 1965–1995*, New York: Princeton Architectural Press, 1996

modernism and advocated the reintroduction of communicative symbols to produce a richer architecture of multiple meanings, articulations, and intentions. Charles Jencks labeled Venturi's ideas and recommended style as "Postmodern," legitimizing a return to the incorporation of conventional architectural elements, to stylistic references, and to a renewed respect for historical urban context and specific places.

The expansion of architectural ideas and vocabularies in Postmodernism spurred a new pluralism in architecture, reflecting the compound nature and diversification of contemporary conditions and thinking and the perception of architecture as both a cultural product and a cultural symbol. This pluralistic attitude rejects the belief in universal narratives and global solutions and shifts the focus of the designer from the generic to the specific, realized in a conscious attempt to understand the nature of each task and to respond to the needs, problems, and circumstances of the particular client and location.

Some of the forms produced within this environment are outgrowths of modernism, seen in the work of High-Tech architects such as Richard Rogers and Norman Foster, who continue to venerate structural and technological innovation, and in the motifs and early modern aesthetic prominent in the work of Richard Meier. Another outgrowth of modernism is the abstraction and simplicity inherent in the International Style brought

Rose, Margaret, *The Post-modern and the Post-industrial*, Cambridge and New York: Cambridge University Press, 1991

Wigley, Mark, *The Architecture of Deconstruction: Derrida's Haunt*, Cambridge, Massachusetts: MIT Press, 1993

SYNAGOGUE

At the turn of the 20th century, the spirit of integration lay behind much of new synagogue construction in Europe and America. Some examples of the distinctive Moorish-style building continued to be erected, such as the Jerusalem Street Synagogue in Prague (Wilhelm Stiassny and Alois Richter, 1906). Other historic styles such as Romanesque and Gothic (Szeged, Hungary, 1900–03) continued late 19th-century traditions. A few distinctive synagogue designs broke with tradition such as Hector Guimard's striking Art Nouveau Rue Pavée Synagogue in Paris (1911–13), or adapted new traditions, such as the synagogue in Subotica, Yugoslavia (Komor and Jakab, 1901), combining Balkan, Hungarian, and Jewish folk and architectural traditions.

A strong trend toward classicism, however, especially in America, resulted in the notable Congregation Beth El, Detroit (Albert Kahn, 1903), Beth Ahabah, Richmond (Noland and Baskerville, 1904) Mikveh Israel, Philadelphia (William Tachau and Lewis Pilcher, 1909), Temple Society of Concord, Syracuse (Arnold Brunner, 1910), and scores of similar buildings. Brunner's designs for Syracuse and the Henry S. Frank Memorial Synagogue in Philadelphia (1901) were the first synagogues built to directly refer to archaeological finds of ancient synagogues in Palestine.

This form of classical Revivalism, which in most cases resulted in synagogues hardly distinguishable from banks, libraries, and government and university buildings evolved into the more distinctive Byzantine-Revival style, particularly popular after World War I. Here, following the earlier lead of Brunner, patrons and architects justified their designs by likening them to new archaeological finds from Palestine, but they also reinvented the distinctive exoticism that had characterized the Jewish Moorish style begun by Gottfried Semper at Dresden (1838–40) and continued so effectively for more than half a century. Unlike the Moorish style, however, the new Byzantine design emphasized plan and massing over decoration. Free standing buildings were often ingeniously sited in new urban parklike settings, and they often featured open plans that linked main sanctuaries to auxiliary administrative, educational, and social spaces—an innovation already hinted at in Kahn's Classical Beth El of 1903 and that would be more fully developed in the new suburban synagogues and community centers built after World War II. The central dome over the sanctuary space became especially common—it was given many meanings: the cosmos, community, and tradition. A frequent urban variation of this style—especially where synagogues still occupied traditional urban sites, emphasized a single giant facade portal, as at B'nai Jeshurun, New York (Schneider and Herts, 1918) and Temple Emanu-El, New York (Kahn Butler and Stein, 1930). Emanu-El's interior, with its enormous rows of arches, recalls contemporary modern architecture in Italy in its austerity and gigantism.

In Europe, similar simpler architectural forms prevalent in the nascent modern movement were easily adapted for synagogue design. The synagogue of Zilina, Slovakia (Peter Behrens, 1928–30) was, in many ways, a stripped-down version of the Byzantine domed synagogue popular in Hungary and the Balkans. Behrens's design set a half dome on a rectangular block. Within, the dome rises on slender concrete piers from a square set within the rectangular mass. Outside, the ground floor is faced in stone, and the rest of the structure is of reinforced concrete. Despite the use of concrete, the building looks traditional due to its massing and the monumental stairway that leads to the main entrance. Nothing about the building's architecture identifies it as a synagogue. Applied Stars of David set on each exterior corner served this purpose. Like Zelina, the monumental Great Synagogue in Tel Aviv, Israel (c.1930) combined traditional elements such as arched windows and a large central dome with the plain smooth wall surfaces and combined massing of blocklike forms typical in early European modernism. The Yeshurun Synagogue in Jerusalem (Friedmann, Rubin, and Stolzer, 1934–5) eschewed the complex hierarchical arrangement of multiple forms for a simple joining of two main masses—a rectangular block, entered on its long side, with a tall half cylinder housing the sanctuary joined to the rear.

There had been previous experiments with modernism in synagogue design before the war. In Amsterdam, Jewish architect Harry Elte built the Jacob Obrechtplein Synagogue in a Dutch-Cubist style in 1927–28. The building recalls early designs by Frank Lloyd Wright, especially the Unity Temple near Chicago. Perhaps the most radical and most modern synagogue design of the interwar years was that of Plauen, Germany. The synagogue was conceived as a white box elevated on stilts at one end. The arrangement of windows differentiates the discreet functions of the building, much as was done in contemporary industrial buildings.

Also in Amsterdam, the Lekstraat Synagogue (A. Elzas, 1936–37) is a plain stone box with simple square windows that emphasizes only the Ark and Bimah. Elzas won a competition among nine Jewish architects for the commission, which even today ranks as one of the sparest architect designed synagogues. The simplicity of the building's geometry and white concrete walls is offset slightly by the use of stone on the exterior and the introduction of vast amounts of natural light through large windows. Elsewhere, Sir E(van) Owen Williams designed the modern Dollis Hill Synagogue in London with a very open interior with galleries cantilevered from the wall rather than supported by piers of columns. The walls and roof are made of specially designed corrugated concrete that strengthens the structure. Hexagonal and shield-shaped windows recall the Star of David, now an accepted Jewish motif.

American and Canadian Jews had begun an exodus from the urban tenement neighborhoods in the years following World War I leading to new Jewish neighborhoods on city fringes. Large "synagogue-centers" developed to serve the religious and recreational needs of thousands of congregants. These large free-standing monumental buildings in the classical or Byzantine style stood as civic monuments. Immediately after World War II, however, demand for suburban synagogues created a boom of Modern-style community centers, which gave special attention to school facilities.

Modern architecture was preferred as an expression of this new Judaism—for historic, aesthetic, and financial reasons. Prewar trends in synagogue architecture made Jewish communities

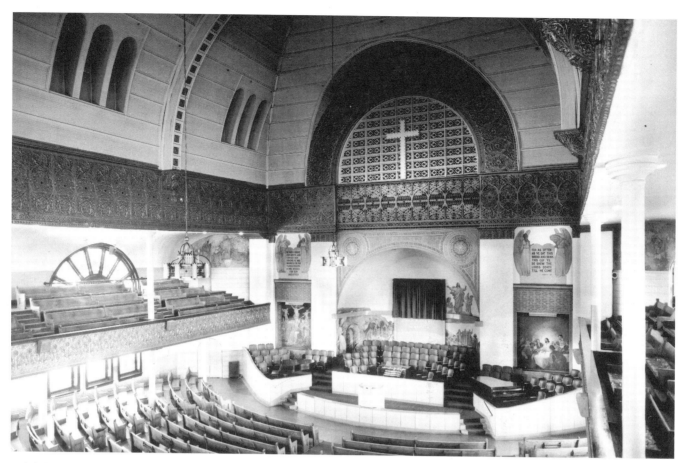

Kehilath Anshe Ma'ariv Synagogue, Cook County, Chicago, IL, designed by Adler and Sullivan
© Historic American Buildings Survey/Library of Congress

receptive to modernism. Byzantine Revival and the Art Deco synagogues were primarily studies in spatial geometry that often emphasized qualities of the building material (most often brick and tile) and limited decoration to flat surface ornament. They emphasized variants on the cube and sphere and utilized natural light as much as possible. They also addressed the modern concerns of adjustable space and incorporation of multiple functions—including social halls, kitchens, gymnasia, swimming pools, libraries, schools, and offices—within a single complex structure.

The full expansion of the sanctuary and multiple-use of spaces was fully developed by Erich Mendelsohn, who developed important concepts for modern synagogue design, including the accentuation of the sanctuary section of a large complex using elevated and curvilinear forms and the creation of adaptable spaces, connectable by sliding partitions to serve diverse functions at different times of the day or year. At B'nai Amoona (St. Louis, 1950) a dramatic parabolic roof rises from the ark wall to the entrance wall, the top of which is glazed, allowing light to pour in over the congregation and onto the bimah and ark. At the Park Synagogue in Cleveland, Mendelsohn designed the sanctuary as a hemispheric dome that rose straight from the ground. B'nai Amoona also included adaptable spaces in a larger plan in which the sanctuary and spillover space were balanced

by a classroom wing across a small open court. Connecting the two sections were a range of offices.

Mendelsohn's designs were quickly understood by Percival Goodman and formed the basis of most suburban synagogue architecture from the late 1940s through the 1980s. Goodman built over 50 synagogues in his lifetime. Although most lack the excitement and drama of Mendelsohn's plans, Goodman incorporated modern sculpture to accentuate certain elements, rather than sculpting space.

Influenced by Mendelsohn and Goodman, and continuing with Frank Lloyd Wright's Beth Shalom Synagogue (Elkins Park, 1959), congregations and architects replaced ties to history through the manipulation of form for symbolic association—often favoring building profiles recalling mountains or tents. Frank Lloyd Wright expressed his intent for the interior of Beth Sholom: "We want to create the kind of building that people, on entering it, will feel as if they were resting in the very hands of God." At Congregation Israel in Glencoe, Illinois (Minoru Yamasaki, 1964), a series of large concrete arches frame the building, but large gaps in the structure fill the sanctuary with filtered light. The interior is spacious, and the use of light, white walls and little ornamentation create a cerebral space. The tall thin gilded ark has been likened to a prayer shawl wrapping the

Torah scrolls, but from the sanctuary entrance it also suggests a single flame—a burning bush or eternal light.

In postwar Europe, of note is the Ruhrallee Synagogue at Essen, Germany (Dieter Knoblauch and Heinz Heise, 1959). Like Mendelsohn's Cleveland synagogue, the primary element in Essen is a hemisphere that rises directly from the ground—there is no visible substructure. The simple unified shape may symbolize the monotheism of Judaism, but it also reflects current trends in architecture—which included a search for pure geometric forms. Inside, the half-dome includes more simple shapes. The ark is a rectangle inscribed within a broad triangle, set into the shell of the hemispheric dome. At the apex of the dome, a Star of David is inscribed, articulated with a series of small round windows that define the shape with light.

The most dramatic postwar European synagogue is in Livorno, Italy (1962), which replaced the famous but totally destroyed Renaissance synagogue. On the outside, the new expressive structure is defined by a series of crooked concrete buttresses, which are connected by concrete walls, appearing to exert intense pressure to keep the building together. This wall allows a large unimpeded interior sanctuary; like the Renaissance predecessor, this synagogue has ranges of seats all around.

In Israel, similar expressive tendencies are found. The synagogue in Beersheba (1961) nestles under a sweeping concrete vault that covers the sanctuary like a turtle shell. The vault is anchored in the ground to either side of the small prayer hall, which is lit by a wall perforated from floor to ceiling by hexagonal openings. Unlike Beersheba, which is so rooted to the earth, the Israel Goldstein Synagogue on the Givat Ram campus of the Hebrew University (Heinz Rau and David Reznik, 1957) appears to float. The windowless synagogue looks something like a giant balloon; its smooth white bulbous form seems to levitate off the ground, at which level it is pierced with wide arched openings that light the entire structure, including the sanctuary, which is encased in the building's upper part. Perhaps the most inventive of modern synagogues is the one at the army officer training school, Mitzpeh Ramon (Zvi Hecker, 1969), set in dreary desert surroundings. The exterior of the small sanctuary is concrete faceted like crystal creating a complex arrangement of colored shapes and patterns.

More recently, the Great Synagogue in Jerusalem (1982) continues the modernist vocabulary of the 1930s, albeit somewhat updated. The main sanctuary is hexagonal, recalling the shape of the Star of David. Unlike most Israeli synagogues, it incorporates some stained glass decoration in five tall, narrow windows over the ark. Common with the Jerusalem synagogue of 1934 and so many other buildings in the city, the Great Synagogue is built of local yellow limestone. For various reasons—tradition, climate, light, and security—Israeli synagogues tend to be built of stone or concrete and look massive, whatever their size. A synagogue at Hadera built in 1935 included a watchtower and courtyard to shelter up to 2,000 people in case of an attack. Although Israeli architects have sensibly not adopted the skin of glass, favored by many synagogue architects in America in the 1960s and 1970s, they have instead experimented with concrete to create sculptural forms.

An exception to abstract expressive and symbolic forms are the many buildings that refer in plan, elevation, detail, or material to the wooden synagogues of Poland, made known in publications since the 1950s. For example, Congregation Sons of Israel in Lakewood, New Jersey (Davis, Brody and Wisniewski, 1963) recalls Polish plan types and building profiles. Louis Kahn mixed pure geometric shapes and volumes at Temple Beth El (Chappaqua, New York, 1972), where the central wood-paneled light shaft recalls the Polish wooden sanctuaries, as does the selective use of wood in Norman Jaffe's Gates of Grove Synagogue (East Hampton, New York, 1989). In the last quarter of the 20th century, stability and even complacency can be found in synagogue architecture throughout the world. Big synagogue projects declined, and resources shifted to the erection of large regional community centers and to Jewish museums and Holocaust memorials. In a reaction to modernism, some communities attempted to recreate the lost intimacy of Old World and inner-city synagogues—often by erecting smaller chapels adjacent to big sanctuaries, and incorporating historical styles or including symbolic elements referring to the lost synagogue culture of the Old World.

Similarly, many new congregations formed, as the traditional segmentation of Judaism was modified with new liturgical variations, including the increased involvement of women in the service—an issue that divided many congregations. The synagogues of new congregations, often small and struggling, were frequently adaptations of existing (nonsynagogue) buildings.

SAMUEL GRUBER

See also **Kahn, Albert (United States); Kahn, Louis (United States); Mendelsohn, Erich (Germany, United States); Yamasaki, Minoru (United States); Wright, Frank Lloyd (United States)**

T

TAFURI, MANFREDO 1935–94

Architectural historian and critic, Italy

Manfredo Tafuri was among the more dominant thinkers of architecture and society in the final third of the 20th century. Tafuri was born in Rome in 1935 to a Jewish mother and Catholic father. His early interests included painting and philosophy. Trained as an architect at the University of Rome, he moved quickly from design to research, becoming involved in issues of planning and urban organization in the early 1960s. In the late 1960s and early 1970s, he wrote a series of penetrating books that became the guides for advanced thinking about architecture in the modern world. In the later 1970s, he shifted his interests to Renaissance architecture, and though his work in that field did not achieve the same following, he became one of its keenest observers.

Although Tafuri studied architecture at the University of Rome, his was not a conventional education. His early years were marked by the formation of oppositional groups. He created seminars and discussion groups and founded a magazine *(Contropiano)* with other disaffected colleagues (notably Alberto Asor Rosa, Mario Tronti, and Massimo Cacciari). At one point Tafuri sought to form a union of architects and architectural students to bring an uncorrupted voice to the discussion of the regulatory plan for Rome. He was an assistant within the architecture department in Rome from 1964 to 1966. From 1966 to 1967, he taught at the University of Palermo. In 1968 he was brought to the University of Venice by Giuseppe Samonà.

The key work of Tafuri's early career was titled *Teorie e storia dell'architettura* (*Theories and History of Architecture*) (1968). There he took a stance against what he called "critica operativa" (operative criticism), the instrumentalization of the past to justify current actions or, more dangerously, the use of the past to validate the potentials of future freedom. In this formulation he leaned heavily on the writings of Martin Heidegger, but he was also very much interested in the writings of Marc Bloch and Lucien Febvre from the French Annales school of history, then little known in Italy.

In 1968 Tafuri took over the leadership of Istituto Universitario di Architettura at the University of Venice. He used it as a forum to bring together specialists from various disciplines in the university to study historical issues and gathered there a brilliant group of architectural historians, including Giorgio Ciucci, Marco de Michelis, Mario Manieri-Elia, and Francesco dal Co. Concerned with practical but fundamental matters of scholarly historical method, he also reached out to other disciplines and quickly developed a series of initiatives. A conference "Socialism: City, Architecture" (1970), for example, examined the nature of urban planning in the 1920s and 1930s in the Soviet Union, and a jointly authored book on the American city titled *La città americana dalla guerra civile al New Deal* (The American City from the Civil War to the New Deal) (1973) took up the nature of development under capitalism. Both were helpful in defining Tafuri's political position in this turbulent period, and he became a significant participant in debates on the role of the Italian Communist Party.

At the same time, Tafuri's work also began to be noticed in the United States. In 1974 he published his first essay in the periodical *Oppositions*, which later published more of his essays as well as those of his Venetian collaborators, most notably Dal Co and Ciucci. He helped to introduce the work of Aldo Rossi in the United States. Tafuri had, naturally, a particular reception in the United States. North American architects were engaged in the critique of modernism and intrigued by the revival of history and theory. Tafuri's first title that was translated into English was *Architecture and Utopia* (1976; Italian edition: *Progetto e utopia: Architettura e sviluppo capitalistico*, 1973), a work that, like *Teorie e storia dell'architettura*, attempted to redefine (and limit) the functions of the architect and historian within contemporary culture. Tafuri brought to American architecture an entirely new language of analysis based on "distance," "alienation," and "masquerade," terms borrowed from European philosophy that presume a tragic view of human history. For Americans accustomed to their own optimistic or descriptive readings of architecture, Tafuri's analyses were startling, and the influence of Tafuri has been traced by Ockman to the work of both Peter Eisenman and John Hejduk. Tafuri's thoughts on the avant-garde and on American architecture were collected in *La sfera e il labirinto: Avanguardie e architettura da Piranesi agli anni '70* (*The Sphere and the Labyrinth: Avant-gardes and Architecture from Piranesi to the 1970s*) (1980; English edition, 1987).

One of the great difficulties in coming to grips with Tafuri's writing is his protean nature. He operated on many fronts simul-

taneously and with equal effect. In the same year as *La città americana*, for example, he published a book on the Via Giulia subtitled *Una utopia urbanistica del '500* (Villa Giulia: An urbanistic utopia of the 1500s) (1973), which followed the fate of a single street through the process of its development starting with Pope Julius II in the early 16th century. From the later 1970s, in fact, Tafuri's interests shifted to a deeper past. *Venezia e il Rinascimento: Religione, scienza, architettura* (Venice and the Renaissance: Religion, Science, Architecture) (1985) and *Ricerca del Rinascimento: Principi, città, architetti* (Renaissance Research: Princes, Cities, Architects) (1992) defined the range of his interests in a total history of the sort that recalls earlier interest in the Annales school.

Efforts to define the stages of Tafuri's career tend to fall into the kinds of Hegelian stylistic categorization that Tafuri himself eschewed. It is true that his later withdrawal from contemporary issues of architecture entailed a retreat from some of the political issues that marked his work in the 1960s. Moreover, his involvement with exhibitions (notably Giulio Romano and Francesco di Giorgio) gives the impression of a return to more traditional forms of biography. Tafuri helped sponsor some of the most conservative scholars of Italian architecture at the University of Venice. All of this has led some to define the later, Renaissance-based period of his scholarly activity as conservative. Yet these decisions were probably strategic and personal rather than principled. Tafuri defined himself as an educator and saw exhibitions, even monographic exhibitions, as a way to raise historical issues to a broader public. Tafuri modeled his own scholarly practice on the architectural team and was anxious to have the best specialists around him.

Tafuri's scholarship concerning the Renaissance remains buoyantly transgressive. Giulio Romano and Francesco di Giorgio, to whom he devoted extensive attention, are figures whose willingness to run against the academic traditions of their own times appealed to him enormously, and he caught their contrary nature very well. He was even able to find the rebelliousness in a drably academic architect such as Antonio da Sangallo the Younger, as is revealed in his posthumously published essay and entries for the corpus of architectural drawings by that architect.

NICHOLAS ADAMS

See also **Eisenman, Peter (United States); Hejduk, John (United States); Rossi, Aldo (Italy)**

Selected Publications

L'architettura moderna in Giappone, Bologna: Cappelli, 1964
La cattedrale di Amiens, Florence: Padua: Marsilio Rome: Laterza Sadea/Sansoni, 1965
Jacopo Sansovino e l'architettura del '500 a Venezia, 1969
La città americana dalla guerra civile al New Deal, 1973; English edition (1979) with Giorgio Ciucci, Francesco dal Co, Mario Manieri-Elia
Via Giulia: una utopia urbanistica del '500 with Luigi Salerno and Luigi Spezzaferro, Rome: Staderini, 1973
Architettura contemporanea, Milan: Electa, 1976; English edition (1979) with Francesco dal Co as Modern Architecture, trans Robert Erich Wolf, NY Abrams 1979
Theories and History of Architecture, New York: Harper and Row, 1976
La sfera e il labirinto: Avanguardie e architettura da Piranesi agli anni '70 Turin: Einaudi, 1980; as *The Sphere and the Labyrinth:*
Avant-gardes and Architecture from Piranesi to the 1970s, translated by Pellegrino d'Acierno and Robert Connolly, Cambridge, Massachusetts: MIT Press, 1987
"Renovatio urbis": Venezia nell'età di Andrea Gritti, 1523–1538, Rome: Officina Edizioni, 1984
Venezia e il Rinascimento: Religione, scienza, architettura, Turin: Einaudi, 1985; as *Venice and the Renaissance: Religion, Science, Architecture*, translated by Jessica Levine, Cambridge, Massachusetts: MIT Press, 1989
Storia dell'architettur italiana 1944–1985, Turin: Einaudi, 1986; as *History of Italian Architecture, 1944–1985*, translated by Jessica Levine, Cambridge, Massachusetts: MIT Press, 1989
Romano, Milan: Electa, 1989, essays and catalog entries
Ricerca del Rinascimento: Principi, città, architetti Turin: Einaudi, 1992
Francesco di Giorgio architetto, edited by Francesco Paolo Fiore and Tafuri, Milan: Electa, 1993, essays and catalog entries
The Architectural Drawings of Antonio da Sangallo the Younger and His Circle, vol. 2 (MIT Press, Cambridge 2000), edited by Nicholas Adams, essay and catalogue entries

Further Reading

Casabella 619/620 (January 1995), titled "Il progetto storico di Manfredo Tafuri/The Historical Project of Manfredo Tafuri," with essays by Vittorio Gregotti, Giorgio Ciucci, Alberto Asor Rosa, Jean-Louis Cohen, Joan Ockman, Francesco Paolo Fiore, and others
Any 25/26 (2000), titled "Being Manfredo Tafuri," with essays by Ignasi de Solà-Morales, Pierluigi Nicolin, Evelina Calvi, Anthony Vidler, K. Michael Hays, Jean-Louis Cohen, Mark Wigley, Kurt W. Forster, Peter Eisenman, and others

TALIESIN WEST
Designed by Frank Lloyd Wright; completed 1937
Scottsdale, Arizona

There were two significant transitional points in Frank Lloyd Wright's long career. One is marked by the abandonment of his first practice in Oak Park and the design of his rural Wisconsin home known as Taliesin (1911–14). The other is marked by his move beyond Wisconsin to the Arizona desert and the construction of Taliesin West (1937). During the early portion of his career, Wright had been engaged with the interior realm of the family and its relationship to the larger society beyond, ideas embodied in his "Prairie house" designs. His move to Taliesin is marked by the study of the relationship of man and mind to landscape. Almost 30 years later, Taliesin West marks the fulfillment of that effort as a giant step forward in Wright's ability to conceive architectural languages as expressions of the human condition.

The "desert compound," as Taliesin West was originally known, consisted of a loosely woven group of enclosures divided roughly into four quadrants by two crossing axes. The orientation of the primary north-south axis in the plan is about 20 feet west of south, facing the afternoon sun. Along with a drafting room, a large room for communal gatherings, and Wright's own study, the compound initially included quarters for the families of the architect and his apprentices, sheltered places for dining and kitchen duties, fireplaces, pools, and gardens. In its original form, these were not so much rooms as places for the designated activi-

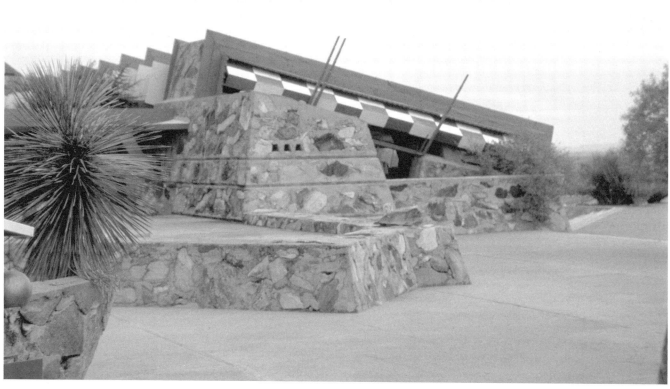

Taliesin West, Scottsdale, Arizona (1937)
© GreatBuildings.com

ties of the Taliesin Fellowship strewn about the desert in an openly ordered pattern.

Taliesin West was built by Wright and the apprentices of his Taliesin Fellowship with minimal help from professional builders. Large stones were gathered from the surrounding landscape and stacked loosely together in battered wooden forms. A lean mixture of concrete and desert sand was poured over the rocks. The resulting recumbent walls are intermingled with level terraces stretching 300 feet across the desert floor, barely protruding above the ground in some cases, in others rising to create cavelike sanctuaries protected from the searing heat of the desert sun. The large drafting and gathering spaces, as well as Wright's private study, were spanned with redwood trusses. These reach across entire sections with skeleton-like repetition, acting as ribs beneath which were hung canvas stretched frames lapped to shed what little rain there was. Similar canvas frames added around the sides and under the eaves could be opened to regulate the presence of sun and wind. The contrast between the heavy raking masonry walls and these floating, light-filled canvas panels formed the architectural backdrop for the activities of the camp.

In its original form, the entire roof structure was disassembled each spring in preparation for the Fellowship's annual move back to Wisconsin. The canvas panels were taken down and stored, leaving only the low stone walls and open redwood frames to suffer the intense heat of the Arizona summer. In later years, as Wright began to stay longer into the summer season, the canvas was replaced by plastic, the open spaces were glazed, and the central parts of the building were eventually air conditioned, making it quite a different place today.

The plan of Taliesin West is organized by the use of two crossing axes that intertwine distant features of the landscape and its history with the pursuit of daily activities in the camp. The pattern of movement along these assumes a quartering of space and experience that was characteristic of Wright's domestic designs going back to his Prairie houses. Here in the desert, the quartered scheme is opened outward in a new way along axes that emerge from the land to direct attention through the man-made forms to the stark beauty of the natural world beyond. His own evaluation is perhaps the most poignant: "The whole opus looked like something we had been excavating, not building"

The entry establishes an axis of movement through the compound, from the public areas of contact with the city and the automobile to private areas of staff and family, cloisters, and walled gardens. The left side of the plan generally contains places of work. The right side of the plan contains places that contact with the stillness of the desert: the apprentice quarters and

Wright's own Usonian dwelling. The pathway between these two spaces is sunk into the ground of the mesa. This pathway, dominated and sheltered by the mountains, brings the viewer into contact with another axis moving downward to the south. The point of crossing of these axes was originally dramatically marked. As the crossing was reached, the earth forced its way through the retaining wall and across a small pool of water directly on axis with the 6,000-foot height of Thompson's Peak in the distance. Here the architectural forms open to the right under a shaded loggia into which one is naturally drawn out of the heat of the Arizona sun. It is from this point that the immensity of the view southward across the desert first becomes apparent. One is drawn by this vista, unavoidably, down a few steps and out again into the full force of the sun to peer upward into the distance.

This experience is reached by a movement downward in plan, from shelter to exposure, from depression in the earth, where you are close to rock and water, to an elevated position in the full glare of the desert sun with almost infinite vista. The upper portions of the plan as originally built were left mostly natural and devoid of buildings and offered controlled views of the wall of mountains to the north. In contrast the lower portions of the plan offer exposure to the distance and to the desert sun. The first axis had led away from civilization into areas of recess, retreat, and privacy. This second movement is more elemental in nature. It leads from physical to ethereal, from solid to open, from earth to sky. Years earlier at Taliesin, the crest of a hill occupied the center of the architectural composition; here in the desert, at Wright's final home, that center was thrown out across the landscape in expression of the timeless quest for the bond that exists between the mind of man and the natural world.

J. MICHAEL DESMOND

See also **Broadacre City; Fallingwater, Bear Run, Pennsylvania; Wright, Frank Lloyd (United States)**

Further Reading

Architectural Forum 68 (January 1938) (special issue on Wright)
Banham, Reyner, "The Wilderness Years of Frank Lloyd Wright," *Journal of the Royal Institute of British Architects* 126 (December 1959)
Egbert, Donald Drew, "The Idea of Organic Expression and American Architecture," in Evolutionary Thought in America, edited by Persons Stow, New Haven, Connecticut: Yale University Press, 1950
Levine, Neil, "Abstraction and Representation in Modern Architecture: The International Style of (and) Frank Lloyd Wright," *AA Files* 11 (Spring 1986)
Levine, Neil, "Frank Lloyd Wright's Own Houses and His Changing Concept of Representation," in *The Nature of Frank Lloyd Wright*, edited by Carol R. Bolton et al., Chicago: University of Chicago Press, 1988
Levine, Neil, *The Architecture of Frank Lloyd Wright* Princeton, New Jersey: Princeton University Press, 1999
Scully, Vincent, *Architecture, the Natural and the Manmade*, New York: St. Martin's Press, 1991
Wright, Frank Lloyd, *An Autobiography*, New York: Duell, Sloan, and Pearce, 1943
Wright, Frank Lloyd, *A Testament*, New York: Horizon Press, 1957

TANGE, KENZO 1913–

Architect, Japan

For the quarter century following World War II, Kenzo Tange was among the world's leading architects; his work defined postwar modernism in Japan. Tange's promising beginning, after graduating from the University of Tokyo in 1938 and then working for Kunio Maekawa for four years, was enhanced by the almost complete disappearance of architectural practice during the latter days of the war. This absence allowed him to return to the University of Tokyo in 1946, and he remained there as a student and member of the faculty until 1974.

In his spectacular debut, winning first place in the Far East Greater Coprosperity Sphere Competition of 1942, Tange engaged the nationalist spirit of the time, gaining recognition through the controversy that emerged. His proposal for a monument to Japan's fallen soldiers, to be built on a long axis beginning at the foot of Mount Fuji, was influenced by Japan's temple precincts. By blending Japanese traditions with European modernism, Tange took a very different position than others of his generation who wholeheartedly embraced an international style.

For many years Tange's work was unabashedly regionalist. Through 1960 Tange defined a new Japan, infused with tradition and optimistically reflecting the utopian hopes of the era. He embraced the symbols Japan's citizens held dear but overlaid them with an enthusiasm for new technologies. This approach is seen in some of his best built works: his first, the Hiroshima Peace Memorial and Museum (1955), was inspired by the *sukiya* character of buildings such as Katsura Imperial Villa; the surface treatments of the facades at both Kagawa Prefectural Offices (1959) and Kurashiki City Hall (1960) drew on Japan's timber traditions, but in concrete used at a monumental scale; and in the later Olympic Stadia (1964, Tokyo), Tange's roofs were structurally remarkable but comfortingly close to the form of Japan's traditional farmhouses. Critics, however, tended to disparage buildings with ties to tradition, favoring more sculptural efforts, such as the Children's Library (1953) at Hiroshima. Tange began to treat traditional nuances as a failing, but today it is those buildings that were initially dismissed by critics that better define his reputation. Yet while Tange's early sculptural works were clumsy, they served as the basis for several extraordinary buildings from the 1960s, including not only the Olympic Stadia but also St. Mary's Cathedral (1964, Tokyo) and the Memorial to Fallen Soldiers (1966).

From the beginning Tange also emphasized the urban and regional scale, using axiality as an ordering device. Throughout the 1950s and 1960s, Tange drew on an emerging political will, reflecting the introduction of democratic ideals through his "mass-human" spaces dedicated to collective activities. Many of his designs for government institutions sandwiched offices between publicly accessible roof terraces (the Kagawa Prefectural Hall had a popular cocktail bar on its rooftop) and an open ground plane slipped through first-floor *pilotis*.

In 1961 Tange founded URTEC, Urbanists and Architects Team, inspired by Gropius's The Architects' Collaborative. His designs from the 1960s tended toward structuralism. Complexes were organized into a three-dimensional system made up of service cores, circulation paths, and bridgelike blocks or figural units dedicated to programmatic needs, with opportunities for

future additions. The most powerful of these is a 1961 plan for Tokyo Bay, developed with students at the University of Tokyo. Participants in this design—among them Fumihiko Maki, Arata Isozaki, Kiyonori Kikutake, and Kisho Kurokawa—went on to shape Japan's most exciting architectural movement, Metabolism. Although none of Tange's urban plans were executed, two notable buildings were completed using similar principles: the Yamanashi Press and Broadcasting Center (1966) and the Shizuoka Press and Broadcasting Center (1970) in Tokyo. The final Metabolist undertaking was Expo '70 in Osaka, the first full-scale demonstration of a Metabolist city. The public received the project more as an entertainment than as a rare opportunity to recognize the value of a comprehensive urban proposal, and the movement collapsed under its failure to be understood.

At roughly the same time, community resistance scrapped Tange's proposal for Yerba Buena (1969) in San Francisco, which was also based on structuralist principles. Suddenly, enormous size was no longer a merit: The architect whose works had deftly represented the conflicts and ideals of Japan's postwar boom found himself out of step. At first Tange found opportunities to work in Europe, but as the West and Japan began to address the ecological fallout of megaprojects, demand for Tange's work shifted to Arab nations and, in the early 1980s, Southeast Asia. At one point 70 to 80 percent of the firm's work came from abroad. His projects from this period often remained unbuilt, and those that were completed took an average of ten years from basic design through execution, making it difficult for Tange to respond to innovations in construction technologies. Furthermore, he was less able to develop a language that reflected the hopes of these unfamiliar cultures, and buildings from this period seem awkwardly fitted to their time and place.

Tange's architecture continued to draw on many earlier themes. He remained concerned with large-scale complexes organized in response to clear principles. In his interiors he often developed a polished monumentality, especially notable in the Akasaka Prince Hotel (1982). His architecture from this period is generally less appreciated, though, as strategies from his earlier work became formulaic. In the final years of his career, however, Tange began again to build symbolically important works in his native country, especially the New Tokyo City Hall (1991) and the United Nations University Building (1992). These buildings, while not as vigorous as works from his youth, retain a monumentality and sense of detail that are clearly related to his earlier masterpieces. Tange also found a way, in the end, to create a large-scale order in the city of Tokyo—not through his revisions to the Tokyo Bay Plan (1986) but in his design of two of Tokyo's tallest buildings. The New Tokyo City Hall and the nearby Tokyo Park Tower can be seen from the megalopolis's farthest suburbs and establish an order in the region that Tange once reserved for Mount Fuji.

DANA BUNTROCK

See also **Isozaki, Arata (Japan); Japan; Kurokawa, Kisho (Japan); Maki, Fumihiko (Japan); Metabolism; Peace Memorial and Museum, Hiroshima; Taniguchi, Yoshio (Japan)**

Biography

Born Imabari, Shikoku, Japan, 1913. Graduated from the University of Tokyo (bachelor's degree, 1938; Ph.D., 1959). Taught at the University of Tokyo, 1946–1974; visiting professor at Massachusetts Institute of Technology, Cambridge, (1959–1960) and Harvard University (1972). Established URTEC in 1961; selected awards include the annual prize of the Japanese Architecture Institute in the years 1954, 1955, 1958, and 1965, including highest honors in 1986. Awarded Royal Gold Medal, the Royal Institute of British Architects (RIBA) in 1965; Gold Medal, American Institute of Architects (AIA), 1966. Received the Pritzker Prize in 1987 and the Praemium Imperiale in 1993. In 1979 Tange was acknowledged as a Person of Merit in Japanese Cultural Achievement and was recognized as a Sacred Treasure (Japan) in 1994.

Selected Works

Children's Library at Hiroshima, 1953
Hiroshima Peace Memorial and Museum, 1955
Tokyo City Hall, 1957
Sogetsu Arts Center, 1958; replaced with a new design by Tange, 1977
Kagawa Prefectural Offices, 1959
Kurashiki City Hall, 1960
WHO headquarters (unbuilt), 1959
Tokyo Bay Plan, 1961; revisited in 1986
Tokyo's Tsukiji district, 1964
St. Mary's Cathedral, Tokyo, 1964
Tokyo Olympic Stadia, 1964
Memorial to Fallen Soldiers, 1966
Yamanashi Press and Broadcasting Center, 1966
Shizuoka Press and Broadcasting Center in Tokyo, 1970
Expo '70 master plan and Festival Plaza, 1970
Akasaka Prince Hotel, 1982
New Tokyo City Hall, 1991
United Nations University, 1992
Shinjuku Park Tower, 1994
Fuji Sankei Communications, 1996

Notable Competition Entries

Far East Greater Coprosperity Sphere Competition (First prize 1942)
Japan–Thai Culture Center (First prize 1943)
Hiroshima Peace Park (First prize 1949)
Tokyo City Hall (First prize 1952)
New Tokyo City Hall (First prize 1986)

Selected Publications

Katsura Tradition and Creation in Japanese Architecture, 1960
A Plan for Tokyo, 1960: Toward a Structural Reorganization, 1961
Ise: Prototype of Japanese Architecture, 1965

Further Reading

A detailed bibliography of Japanese sources is available in Kurita, and a somewhat more limited but easily accessible bibliography of primary and secondary sources in the more recent Bettinotti.

Bettinotti, Massimo (editor), *Kenzo Tange Architecture and Urban Design, 1946–1996*, Milan: Electa, 1996
Boyd, Robin, *Kenzo Tange*, New York: George Braziller, 1962
Kultermann, Udo (editor), *Kenzo Tange Architecture and Urban Design 1946–1969*, Zurich, Switzerland: Verlag Architektur Artemis; New York: Praeger, 1970
Kurita, Isamu (editor), *Gendai Nihon Kenchikuka Zenshu, 10: Tange Kenzo* (Japanese Modern Architects Collection, no. 10: Kenzo Tange), Tokyo: Sanichi [31] Shoubou, 1970

Riani, Paolo, *Kenzo Tange*, London: Hamlyn, 1970
Tange Kenzo: Kenchiku to Toshi (Kenzo Tange: Architecture and the City), Tokyo: Sekai Bunka Sha, 1975
"Sengo Modanizumu Kenchiku no Kiseki: Tange Kenzo to sono Jidai" (The Locus of Postwar Modern Architecture: Kenzo Tange and His Era), a series of interviews of Tange's staff and students, conducted by Dr. Terunobu Fujimori, published in occasional installments since January 1998 in *Shinkenchiku*-
Kenzo Tange Associate: vol. 1, *1946–1979* (originally published as SD vol. 8001); Vol. 2, *–1983* (originally published as SD vol. 8309); vol. 3, *–1987 (originally published as SD vol. 8704); and vol. 4, –1991* (originally published as SD vol. 89105) Tokyo: Kajima Shuppan Kai, 1991

TANIGUCHI, YOSHIO 1937–

Architect, Japan

Yoshio Taniguchi is rare among architects, being steadfastly unwilling to dedicate any effort to promoting his work. He seldom lectures or participates in symposia, he refuses interviews, and he is notoriously difficult to the few journalists and academics who do gain access. However, this taciturn position is justified by his architecture. Although his buildings are certainly photogenic, it is impossible to appreciate their spatial and contextual strengths without physically experiencing them.

Taniguchi's maternal grandfather was one of Japan's earliest architects and later became the head of the Tokyo branch of a major construction company. Taniguchi's father, Yoshiro Taniguchi, was a contemporary of Kunio Maekawa and a respected architect in his own right. Although little known abroad, Yoshiro Taniguchi was entrusted with several commissions on behalf of Japan's royal family, and he also designed notable religious and commemorative structures. Originally inspired by northern European modernism, Taniguchi's father also designed his own house—a laboratory for the father and an inspiration to his son. In some ways Yoshio Taniguchi's work is the fruit of two generations; he shares many objectives with his father, especially an appreciation for serial experience and for compositionally pure organization.

Yoshio Taniguchi holds fond memories of childhood visits to construction sites, but he also feared that his father's reputation stood as too significant a challenge. He initially decided to pursue a related field, taking a degree in mechanical engineering from Keio University in 1960. His father, however, conspired with Kiyoshi Seike to encourage the younger Taniguchi to go to the United States; Taniguchi graduated from Harvard University with a master's degree in architecture in 1964. He was the first Japanese architect to receive licensing following an architectural education exclusively gained abroad, and he took Japan's licensing examinations only following some difficulty.

While at Harvard, Taniguchi met Kenzo Tange, and he joined Tange's office and his Tokyo University research laboratory on his return to Japan in 1965, staying with the firm until 1972. Taniguchi's approach from this period closely resembles his mentor's methods, with an inclination to pursue culturally significant projects, enriching them through collaboration. Taniguchi works frequently with graphic designers, sculptors, and other artists, most notably Gen'ichiro Inokuma and the tea master Hiroshi Teshigahara. Both Taniguchi and his father collaborated with sculptor Isamu Noguchi, and Yoshio Taniguchi is currently on the Noguchi Foundation board. The landscape architect Peter Walker has also worked with Taniguchi, expressing architecture and landscape as a seamlessly integrated art form. Together they have designed the IBM Makuhari Building (1991), the Marugame Museum of Contemporary Art (1991), and the Toyota Municipal Museum of Art (1995).

Taniguchi's first working experiences were as part of a design team (along with Arata Isozaki) working on Tange's plans for the rebuilding of Skopje, Yugoslavia. Two features of this plan, an encircling "City Wall" punctured by prominent "City Gates" at crucial locations, seem to have influenced Taniguchi's work. Embracing protective walls with highlighted entry points recur in his exquisite, carefully proportioned plans. Amplifying this strategy, boxes nested within boxes establish an increasingly removed domain where Taniguchi controls a heightened experience. His architecture is precise, serene, and understated, often informed by contrast. Movement through his earliest buildings juxtaposes centripetal and centrifugal spaces, and in later works, dark alternates with light.

Despite the crisp, modernist appearance of his work, Taniguchi strives for a timeless character and is comfortable embracing Japan's design traditions. Many of his finest works, including the Tsukuba City Theater (1999) and the Tokyo National Museum of Horyuji Treasures (1998), are successors to Katsura Imperial Villa: delicate, complex, and highly refined. His sparing use of exquisitely apt materials demonstrates both artful restraint and subdued elegance. Diaphanous screens, slender columns, and tapered extremities are evident in his frequently published sections and detail drawings and result in an exaggerated thinness. These knifelike planes demarcate expansive, fluid spaces. Buildings extend into their surroundings through the controlled use of *shakkei* (borrowed landscape), and the edge between interior and exterior is often articulated by a stepped configuration said to resemble geese flying in formation, further blurring the distinction between inside and outside.

With the exception of the Tokyo Sea Life Park Aquarium (1989), Taniguchi's work is at its best when it is strictly orthogonal. His architecture is based on movement through an uncompromising three-dimensional spatial matrix, determined not only by an organizing lattice but also by a complex layering of horizontal and vertical planes. Sharply drawn lines link contiguous spaces whereas taut, uninterrupted planes extend from one room to the next. Taniguchi is concerned with the processional character of his buildings and their spaces; as a consequence the quality of light has become increasingly important in his designs. Glowing interiors draw one deeper into these buildings through bounded, cavelike enclosures. He plays with a notable range of light effects, from single beams breaking dim rooms to large, brightly lit volumes. Taniguchi has also experimented with varying degrees of translucency, from the extraordinary clarity resulting from the insubstantial-looking glass cage of the Kasai Rinkai Visitors' Center (1996) to the milky surfaces of the Toyota Museum of Art, achieved with two mullion-free layers of fritted glass.

In 1975 Taniguchi opened his own office, but the intervening years have yielded a relatively small number of published buildings. Most of Taniguchi's buildings are public works, and many of these are art museums, including the Higashiyama Kai'i Gallery for the Nagano Prefectural Shinano Art Museum (1990)

and his competition-winning proposal for the Museum of Modern Art (1997) in New York. Despite the public nature of these commissions, he has been able to develop supportive relationships with his clients. His buildings are often the result of generous budgets and schedules, and a number are repeat projects for the same client. Even among Japanese architects, who enjoy a great deal of support and flexibility during design and construction, Taniguchi's craftsman-like design process and his constant presence on the construction site are considered extreme. As one frequent collaborator has noted, "Every step of the process of design and building is lovingly overseen and often reviewed. No detail remains unconsidered. No idea is unchallenged, often changed even during construction. Basic materials are considered and reconsidered right until their final installation." Taniguchi makes a point of acknowledging the contributions of experienced constructors, and he uses these relationships to exploit the latest material and technological innovations.

The result of his intense focus on each project is a pristine perfection. Taniguchi's dignified and uncompromising architecture has led more than one author to revive the idea of an architectural morality that sets him apart.

DANA BUNTROCK

See also **Japan; Tange, Kenzo (Japan)**

Biography

Born Tokyo, Japan, 1937. Graduated from Keio University, Bachelor's of Mechanical Engineering, 1960, and Harvard University, Master of Architecture, 1963. Taniguchi worked for Kenzo Tange, 1964–72. Established Taniguchi, Takamiya, and Associates in 1975; Taniguchi and Associates was established in 1979. Selected awards include an award from the Architectural Institute of Japan (for the Shiseido Art Museum, 1980), the Japan Academy of Art Prize (for the Ken Domon Museum, 1987), the Togo Murano Memorial Prize (for the Marugame Gen'ichiro Inokuma Museum of Contemporary Art, 1994), and the Public Building Award (for the Tokyo Sea Life Park, 1994). Taniguchi has also won awards from the Building Contractors Society for five of his buildings: Kanazawa Municipal Library (1980), Hotel Appi Grand (1987), Tokyo Sea Life Park (1991), Sakata Kokutai Kinen Gymnasium (1994), and the Marugame Gen'ichiro Inokuma Museum of Contemporary Art (1994).

Selected Works

Shiseido Art Museum, 1978
Ken Domon Photography Museum, Sakata, Japan, 1987
Tokyo Sea Life Park Aquarium, 1989
Higashiyama Kai'i Gallery for the Nagano Prefectural Shinano Art Museum, 1990
IBM Makuhari Building, 1991
Marugame Gen'ichiro Inokuma Museum of Contemporary Art, 1991
Toyota Municipal Museum of Art, Tokyo, 1995
Kasai Rinkai Park Visitors' Center, 1996
Tokyo National Museum of Horyuji Treasures, 1998
Tsukuba City Theater, 1999

Further Reading

Because of Taniguchi's notorious reticence, there is very little available on his work. There are, however, two monographs that offer an up-to-date overview of his work. These are listed first. In addition, two articles attempt to summarize his work, and these are also noted.

Taniguchi, Yoshio, *The Architecture of Yoshio Taniguchi*, Tokyo: Tankosha, 1996, and New York: Harry N. Abrams, 1999
"Yoshio Taniguchi," *Japan Architect* 21 (Spring 1996)
Buntrock, Dana, "Yoshio Taniguchi, Minimalist," *Architecture*, (October)
"The Work of Yoshio Taniguchi," *Casabella* 62 (November 1998)

TAUT, BRUNO 1880–1938
Architect and urban planner, Germany

Bruno Taut was one of the leading architects in the development of a modern architecture in Germany. He worked from a traditional historicist style to a colorful Expressionism before World War I and then helped create a rationalized "New Building" in which he maintained a sense of color and creativity that transcended the austere machine aesthetic and objectivity of his International Style peers. His career can best be divided into four major phases: training and early works, 1903–12; Expressionist experiments, 1912–23; large-scale social housing projects in Berlin, 1924–31; and exile in Russia, Japan, and Turkey, 1932–38.

Taut was born in Königsberg, East Prussia (present-day Kaliningrad, Russia), the son of a merchant and older brother of prominent architect Max Taut. He was educated at the local building college and received further training in the offices of leading contemporary architects Bruno Möhring in Berlin (1903), Theodor Fischer in Stuttgart (1904–08), and the urban designer Theodor Goecke at the Technical University in Berlin (1909). In 1909 Taut opened an office in Berlin with Franz Hoffmann and was joined by his brother Max in 1914, although they maintained separate design practices. The first commissions were for apartment buildings in Berlin in which Taut created abstracted, Secessionist-style compositions within a traditional framework.

In 1912 Taut was appointed advisory architect to the reform-oriented German Garden City Association, which led to commissions for two housing developments: the "Reform" Siedlung (housing estate) in Magdeburg, Germany (1913–14, 1921–23), and the Falkenberg Garden City southeast of Berlin (1913–14). In both developments Taut combined traditional garden city ideals and small, plain pitched-roof houses with brightly colored facades as an inexpensive, expressive way to enliven architecture without traditional historicist ornament.

Beginning in 1912, Taut also received a series of commissions for important experimental exhibition pavilions to advertise new construction materials, including the "Monument to Iron" in Leipzig (1913) and the famous "Glass House" at the Werkbund Exhibition in Cologne (1914). The Glass House, a propaganda building for the German glass industry, contained glass-block floors, a sparkling waterfall, walls lined with brightly colored tiles and prism glass, and a multifaceted, colored-glass dome with reinforced-concrete ribs. The pavilion was dedicated to the

poet Paul Scheerbart, whose fantastical writings praised glass as the material of the future. The important critic and Taut's friend Adolf Behne championed glass in the popular press as the harbinger of a new, modern architecture for the future.

As a committed pacifist, Taut refused to participate in World War I, but in December 1918, within days of the German surrender, he and Walter Gropius formed the short-lived revolutionary Working Council for Art. This was an organization of young artists and architects intent on promoting a visionary new architecture of colorful, magical forms that were free of all the burdens of past traditions, ornament, and materials. Taut publicized his own dreams in several books, including *Alpine Architektur* (1919; *Alpine Architecture*) and *Die Auflösung der Städte* (1920; The Dissolution of Cities), and a series of utopian writings circulated among his friends that were later dubbed the "Crystal Chain Letters." All advocated the dissolution of existing cities in favor of a purified, crystalline architecture of colored glass. Throughout his life Taut used the power of the press to circulate his ideas to a larger audience, writing 21 books and nearly 300 articles over the course of his career.

In 1921 the newly elected socialist government of Magdeburg hired Taut as chief city architect, offering him an opportunity to implement some of his utopian ideas. He oversaw the extension of his own colorful Reform Siedlung, built a large concrete-frame exhibition hall, and initiated a controversial but widely publicized program of colorizing existing urban facades to enliven the drab cityscape of postwar Magdeburg. Rampant inflation and increasing criticism of his avant-garde ideas, however, soon ended his tenure.

The most productive phase of Taut's career began in 1924, when he accepted an offer to oversee the design of large socialized housing developments in Berlin for the communal building association GEHAG in cooperation with the chief city planner of Berlin, Martin Wagner. In seven very productive years, Taut designed more than 10,000 units of affordable housing that proved to be among the most important achievements in public housing of the century. Alongside Wagner, Taut became increasingly committed to rationalized, standardized, and largely prefabricated construction systems, and functional and efficient apartment layouts and furnishings that became models for housing all over the world. Large-scale developments, such as the "Horseshoe" Siedlung in Berlin-Britz (21,374 units, 1925–31) and Onkel Tom's Hütte in Berlin-Zehlendorf (1915 units, 1926–31), were built in a radically modern architecture of mostly flat roofs, unornamented facades (except for Taut's trademark color), and plenty of green space that provided a welcome relief for Berlin's working class. The developments helped alleviate a dire housing shortage and, along with built-in social institutions such as libraries, sports fields, communal laundries, dining facilities, and social clubs, helped promote worker solidarity and the socialist political ideals of Berlin's city government.

The success of these projects earned Taut a prestigious professorship in housing and city planning at the Technical University of Berlin from 1930 to 1932 as well as an honorary membership in the American Institute of Architects. The worldwide economic depression and an increasingly conservative and right-wing press and political machinery, however, once again forced him out of work and office. After 1931 he accepted various offers to work in the young Soviet Union, which had been relatively untouched by the worldwide economic depression and which offered great promise to many important German architects in search of opportunities to implement their dreams of a new architecture for a new socialist society. Taut moved to Russia in 1932 and began plans for a hotel and several institutional buildings as well as a master plan for Moscow. However, political pressure soon forced him on the move again, briefly to Germany, where Adolf Hitler had started to campaign against all modern architects in 1933, and then on to Japan.

Taut stayed in Japan for three years, writing books, designing well-crafted furnishings and household objects, and studying the ancient building traditions of Japan, which he found surprisingly similar to European modern architecture. He was, however, unable to build anything in Japan because of his émigré status. Eager to build, in 1936 Taut once again followed a number of German colleagues and accepted an offer from the Turkish government for a professorship at the Academy of Art in Istanbul and a position in the Ministry of Education. His attempt to combine local Turkish building traditions with European modernism in several university and institutional buildings, and his attempt to use architecture to create a new society for postrevolutionary Turkey, earned him great fame and respect and put Taut back in his element in an adopted homeland. When his life was cut short by failing health in December 1938, he was honored by being the only European buried in the national cemetery.

KAI K. GUTSCHOW

Biography

Born in Königsberg, Germany, 4 May 1880; brother of architect Max Taut. Attended the Baugewerkschule, Königsberg; studied at the Technische Hochschule, Stuttgart under Theodor Fischer 1903–05; studied urban planning under Theodor Goecke at the Technische Hochschule, Charlottenburg, Berlin 1908–09. Married Hedwig Wollgast: 1 child. Worked in the office of Bruno Mehring, Berlin 1900–03; employed in the office of Theodor Fischer, Stuttgart 1904–08. Private practice, Berlin 1908–21; city architect, Magdeburg, Germany 1921–23; partnership with Max Taut and Franz Hoffmann, Berlin 1923–31; advisory architect, GEHAG (Gemeinnützige Heimstätten-, Spar-, und Bau-Aktiengesellschaft) 1924–32; practiced in Moscow 1932–33; practiced in Tokyo 1933–34; worked for Crafts Research Institute, Sendai; practiced in Ankara and Istanbul, Turkey, from 1935; head of architectural office, Turkish Ministry of Education. Professor, Technische Hochschule, Charlottenburg 1930–32; professor of architecture, Academy of Arts, Istanbul. Founding member, Arbeitsrat für Kunst 1918; member, Der Ring 1924. Died in Ankara, 24 December 1938.

Selected Works

Monument to Iron, International Building Trades Exhibition, Leipzig (with Franz Hoffmann), 1913
Garden City Reform, Magdeburg, 1914, 1923
Falkenberg Garden City, Berlin, 1914
Glass House, Werkbund Exhibition, Cologne, 1914
Hufeisensiedlung Housing Estate, Britz, Berlin (stage I with Martin Wagner), 1931

Forest Housing Development, near Onkel Toms Hütte, Zehlendorf,
    Berlin (stage I with Hugo Häring and O.R. Salvisberg), 1931
Bruno Taut House, Ortakoy, Turkey, 1938
Ministry of Culture Exhibition Buildings, International Exposition,
    Izmir, Turkey, 1938
Language and History Faculty Buildings, University of Ankara,
    Turkey, 1938

Selected Publications

Alpine Architektur, 1919; as *Alpine Architecture*, translated by James
    Palmes and Shirley Palmer, 1972
Die Auflösung der Städte, oder die Erde eine gute Wohnung, 1920
Die neue Baukunst in Europa und Amerika, 1929
Nippon mit europäischen Augen gesehen, 1934
Architekturlehre: Grundlagen, Theorie, und Kritik, 1936

Further Reading

Although Taut's papers were destroyed in World War II, the first study
of his socialist-inspired architecture was done by Kurt Junghanns in
communist East Germany. As interest in Expressionism and the "New
Objectivity" of interwar Germany increased over the years, so too did
scholarship on Taut. Bletter, Sharp, and Whyte are good English-
language sources. Speidel's recent catalog for an exhibit in Japan and
Magdeburg provides spectacular color illustrations of Taut's work with
complete reprints of his hard-to-find utopian writings.

Bletter, Rosemarie Haag, "The Interpretation of the Glass Dream:
    Expressionist Architecture and the History of the Crystal
    Metaphor," *Journal of the Society of Architectural Historians* 40/1
    (1981)
Buddensieg, Tilmann (editor), *Berlin, 1900–1933: Architecture and
    Design; Architektur und Design* (bilingual English–German
    edition), New York: Cooper-Hewitt Museum, 1987
Hartmann, Kristiana, "Bruno Taut," in *Baumeister, Architekten,
    Stadtplaner: Biographien zur baulichen Entwicklung Berlins*, edited
    by Wolfgang Ribbe and Wolfgang Schäche, Berlin: Historische
    Kommission zu Berlin, 1987
Jaeger, Roland, "Bau und Buch: 'Ein Wohnhaus' von Bruno Taut,"
    in *Ein Wohnhaus*, edited by Jaeger, Berlin: Gebr. Mann, 1995
Junghanns, Kurt, *Bruno Taut, 1880–1938: Architektur und sozialer
    Gedanke*, Berlin: Henschel, 1970; 3rd edition, Leipzig: Seemann,
    1998
Pehnt, Wolfgang, *Die Architektur des Expressionismus*, Stuttgart,
    Germany: Hatje, 1973; 3rd edition, Ostfildern-Ruit: Hatje,
    1998; as *Expressionist Architecture*, translated by J.A. Underwood
    and Edith Künstner, New York: Praeger, and London: Thames
    and Hudson, 1973
Sharp, Dennis (editor), *Glass Architecture* (by Paul Scheerbart, 1914)
    and Alpine Architecture (by Bruno Taut, 1919), translated by
    James Palmes and Shirley Palmer, New York: Praeger, and
    London: November Books, 1972
Speidel, Manfred (editor), *Bruno Taut: Natur und Fantasie, 1880–
    1938*, Berlin: Ernst, 1995
Taut, Bruno, *Modern Architecture*, London: Studio, and New York:
    Boni, 1929
Thiekötter, Angelika (editor), *Kristallisationen, Splitterungen: Bruno
    Tauts Glashaus*, Basel and Boston: Birkhäuser, 1993
Volkmann, Barbara (editor), *Bruno Taut, 1880–1938*, Berlin:
    Akademie der Künste, 1980
Whyte, Iain Boyd, *Bruno Taut and the Architecture of Activism*,
    Cambridge and New York: Cambridge University Press, 1982
Whyte, Iain Boyd (editor), *The Crystal Chain Letters: Architectural
    Fantasies by Bruno Taut and His Circle*, Cambridge,
    Massachusetts: MIT Press, 1985
Zöller-Stock, Bettina, *Bruno Taut: Die Innenraumentwürfe des
    Berliner Architekten*, Stuttgart, Germany: Deutsch Verlag-Anstalt,
    1993

TÁVORA, FERNANDO 1923–

Architect, Portugal

Fernando Távora can be considered one of the most important
exponents of contemporary Portuguese architecture; he symbolizes the deep cultural renewal that has gradually allowed Portugal
to again play an important role in European architecture. His
poetical language is the fine result of a particular cultural background that has led him to create a new Portuguese architecture
based on a careful dialogue between modernity and tradition.
Most of his works show that he has explored new paths to enhance the traditional values of rural Portuguese architecture:
Each project evokes the past, but his designs follow principles of
modernity, including functional spaces, accurate details, refined
shapes, perfect integration to natural sites, and traditional materials. In other words, Távora's architecture is not "something
different, special, sublime, but work made for man by man."
Thanks to his long teaching experience (university professor,
Faculty of Architecture in Oporto and Coimbra), he has become
one of the main reference points for a new generation of Portuguese architects.

Fully aware of architecture by Le Corbusier and Mies van
der Rohe, Távora sought ways to blend traditional Portuguese
architectural forms with those of the modernists. In 1947 he
wrote an essay titled "O problema da casa portuguesa" (The
Problem of the Portuguese House), in which he explained his
point of view for reinvigorating Portuguese architectural language: "The typical house will provide us with many important
lessons when properly studied, since it is the most functional
and less fanciful; in short it comes closest to the new intentions.
. . . In contemporary architecture, a promising consistency is
looming on the horizon . . . with which Portuguese architecture
should merge, without fear of losing its identity. . . . It does not
fade away like so much smoke; if we do possess this individuality,
nothing will be lost by studying foreign architecture." However,
in the works of this period (1947–52), Távora appears not yet
to be able to adapt these principles to his projects.

Távora's efforts to combine modernity and tradition show
promise in one of his first public projects for Oporto, the Municipal Park of Quinta da Conceição (1960), which included the
simple Tennis Pavilion, his first masterpiece. The park shows
elements of its past: an old monastery, founded in the 15th
century. In the quiet landscape of the old cloister, the chapel
and the pools fit well with the elegant design of new modernist
spaces. Távora himself describes the Tennis Pavilion as the work
of "a young architect torn between reality and dream, the local
and the international, the model and the history." The design
recalls traditional elements of Portuguese rural architecture and
Japanese religious structures. With its balanced proportions and
the use of traditional materials (wooden trusses and white concrete), the small pavilion "contains a certain remote oriental
influence, as does traditional Portuguese architecture from the
sixteenth century onwards."

Távora's experiments continue to blend different elements,
modern and traditional, in the Summer House (1958) in Ofir.

Placed in a Mediterranean pine grove, the house is divided into three functional blocks (living room area, services, and bedroom area) connected by a large covered passage. The whole building evokes local rural architecture with its geometric white surfaces, wooden trusses, red-tiled roof, paved loggias, and colored chimneys.

Throughout his career, Távora has incorporated modern and traditional Portuguese forms to create simple and clean spaces where various cultural references coexist. His literary discussion about architecture carries on and generates other complex works, such as the Gondomar Convent (1971), the Convent of Santa Marinha da Costa Inn (1984), and the Agriculture High School Refoios do Lima (1993). They highlight the evolution of his thinking about traditional and modern architecture in Portugal.

The Gondomar Convent is articulated into various blocks, each fulfilling a different function (dormitories, chapel, meeting rooms, and refectory). Linking buildings with the site, Távora arranged the blocks to follow the natural slope of the landscape. Materials (gray granite, white concrete, and red-tiled roofs) recall local rural architecture and enhance a critical reuse of Portuguese architectural values. The conversion of the 18th-century Convent of Santa Marinha da Costa to a *pousada* (the typical Portuguese inn) allowed Távora to further develop his principles. This project is not a mere restoration of the old walls of the convent but rather a subtle attempt to insert modern structures in an architectural continuity. The conceptual methodology adopted in the restoration of the convent is clearly explained by Távora himself: "The general criterion used was to carry on innovating the already long life of the old building, by preserving its most important areas and creating spaces of quality resulting from the new functional use introduced." The new bedroom section is not a simple addition of forms but rather represents the continuous transformation of the whole building. Popular forms of rural architecture inspired the design of the new parts of the convent: the integration between the old and the new suggests continuity more than rupture. A similar conception was successively adopted for the Refoios do Lima Convent's conversion to the High School for Agriculture (1987). The interior values of the existing structures are unchanged, and the yellow ancient walls are carefully linked with the new buildings.

In summing up Távora's contribution to 20th-century architecture, it is useful to conclude with the words of the critic Manuel Mendes. He asserts that "Távora's architecture is not influenced by any particular architect, by any one particular school or period, it encompasses the whole dimension of memory: his work in its apparent simplicity, is the most original and erudite stylistic research carried out in recent years in Portugal."

STEFANIA ATTI

See also **Corbusier, Le (Jeanneret, Charles-Édouard) (France); Mies van der Rohe, Ludwig (Germany)**

Biography

Távora's thinking about modern and traditional values originated with his upbringing and education. Born in Oporto, Portugal, 25 August 1923, to a rich and well-educated family, he attended the Oporto School of Fine Arts, where he graduated in architecture in 1952.

The discovery of new international architects (Le Corbusier, Gropius, and others) and the principles of the Modern movement caused in Távora a deep change of mind and boosts a new reflection on Portuguese architecture.

Granted a scholarship by the Calouste Gulbenkian Foundation and the Institute for Culture in the United States and Japan. Attended the CIAM summer course at the Faculty of Architecture of Venice. Assistant director at the UIA/Oporto Summer School. Architect for Oporto Town Council, consultant to the Commission for the Urban Renovation of the Ribeira/Barredo project, consultant in the Technical Bureau of the Northern Planning Commission, consultant in the local Technical Bureau of Guimarães Town Council. President of the Ad Hoc Committee of the Faculty of Architecture of Oporto, university professor at the Faculty of Architecture of Oporto and professor at the Department of Architecture of the University of Coimbra. Awarded the First Prize for Architecture by the Calouste Gulbenkian Foundation, the Europa Nostra Award, the 1985 Tourism and Heritage Award, the 1987 National Award for Architecture, and the Golden Medal of the city of Oporto. Doctor Honoris Causa at the University of Coimbra. Member of the Association of Portuguese Architects, the International Union of Architects, the Advisory Committee for Training in the Field of Architecture (European Economic Community). Correspondent of the National Academy of Fine Arts.

His works have been hosted in important exhibitions: Washington (United States), Clermont-Ferrand (France), Brussels (Belgium), Lisbon (Portugal), Milan and Venice (Italy).

Selected Works

Municipal Park of Quinta da Conceiçao, Oporto, 1956–60
Tennis Pavilion of Quinta da Conceiçao, Oporto, 1956–60
Summer House, Ofir, 1957–58
Gondomar Convent, 1961–71
Center and Municipal Building, Aveiro, 1963—67
Covilhã House, Guimarães, 1973–76
Santa Marinha Convent, Guimarães, 1975–84
General Urban Plan of Guimarães, 1980
Renovation of a house in Rua Nova, Guimarães, 1985–87
High School for Agriculture, Refoios do Lima Convent, Ponte de Lima, 1987–93
Urban renovation, Guimarães, 1987–
Police Station, Guimarães, 1988–93
8 de Maio Square, Coimbra, 1993–

Selected Publications

"Regarding the Oporto School," *Casabella* 579 (1991)

Further Reading

Costa, Alexandre Alves, et al., *Fernando Távora*, Lisbon: Blau, 1993
Portas, Nuno, and Manuel Mendes, *Portogallo: Architettura, gli ultimi vent'anni*, Milan: Electa, 1991; as *Portugal: Architecture, 1965–1990*, translated by Anne Guglielmetti, Paris: Éditions du Moniteur, 1992

Italian Architectural Magazines with English Digests:
Angelillo, Antonio, "Agricultural High School in the Convent of Refoios do Lima by Fernanado Tavora" *Casabella*, 595/3 (1992)
Mendes, Manuel, "Recent Portuguese Architecture," *Casabella* 579 (1991)

TAYLOR, ROBERT R. 1868–1942

Architect, United States

Robert R. Taylor, the first professionally trained African American architect, was a designer, teacher, and administrator at Tuskegee Institute (now University) in Alabama.

Taylor was born in Wilmington, North Carolina, to relative privilege for a black southerner. After graduating from the Massachusetts Institute of Technology with a degree in architecture in 1892, he rejected several teaching offers and started an architectural practice in Cleveland, Ohio, which had a black community with long ties to the Wilmington area. Taylor was less immune to the blandishments of Booker T. Washington, who lured him to Tuskegee, which was then a secondary school. Washington had a full understanding of the power of architecture to inspire its inhabitants, instill racial pride, and present the school by photographs in the national press. Washington wanted to showcase black-designed and black-built buildings as well as develop courses in architectural and mechanical drawing. All students in all trades were to draw their projects—stovepipes, wagon wheels, shoes, and carpentry joints—as a precondition to making them. Teachers and ministers as well as those learning

building trades must also be able to draw and then build their own schools, houses, and churches or adapt whatever poor structures they might be assigned in their remote rural destinations. By hiring Taylor, Washington had acquired not only the country's only school-trained black architect but also an able administrator who would soon direct the Boys' Industries Division and manage Tuskegee's building program, serving as its contractor as well as architect.

Taylor's design tracks at Tuskegee remain clear, even with the loss of three major buildings. The Chapel (1898) initially seated 2000 (later 3000) under a hammer-beam roof. Although it burned in 1957, it has lived on as the scene of the hero's epiphany in Ralph Ellison's *Invisible Man*. (Paul Rudolph designed the replacement.) In 1918 a fire took the Slater-Armstrong Memorial Trades Building (1899), and the Huntington Memorial Academic Building (1905) burned recently. Still, enough remains to leave a remarkably attractive campus of gently scaled, white-trimmed brick structures punctuating the green and hilly landscape. Taylor's buildings vary in shape and style, but all have modest detailing that sets off sharp-edged wall surfaces that display Tuskegee's student-made bricks. The trials of getting the school's brickyards started loomed large in Tuskegee's

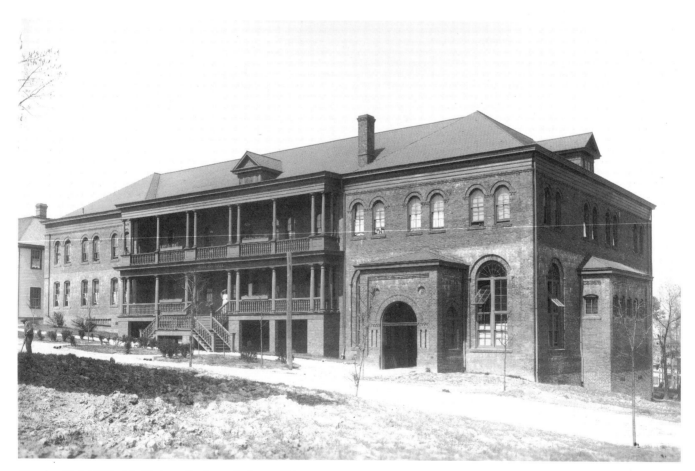

Douglass Hall (1902–04), Tuskegee Institute, Tuskegee, Alabama
Photo by Frances Benjamin Johnson. © Library of Congress

collective memory. Building donors knew that their gifts did triple duty in shelter, student support, and education, as students did most of the construction, learning trades as they earned money.

About two dozen other brick buildings remain that were designed by Taylor and the Architectural Drawing Division. There are many dormitories, a classroom building (now offices), an administration building, Booker T. Washington's house (now a museum), and an unusually elegant Laundry Building (now the George Washington Carver Museum). The exterior of the Girls' Industrial Building still stands, although the interior has been gutted. The Carnegie Library (1902) is fronted by the school's first two-story portico. Critics now interpret southern high classicism as reified white triumphalism based on Jim Crow laws and sanctioned violence. Tuskegee's library portico was built just when a new Alabama constitution denied most black people the vote and just when Booker T. Washington was excoriated throughout the region for taking a meal with Theodore Roosevelt in the White House, thereby seeming to claim social equality. However, even Tuskegee's harshest critics accepted its several classical porticoes and a dome without questioning them for effrontery.

Taylor also designed buildings elsewhere: Carnegie libraries at Livingstone College in Salisbury, North Carolina (1906), and Wiley University in Marshall, Texas (1907); brick school buildings in Cambria, Virginia (1897), and Selma, Alabama (1921); a church in the town of Tuskegee (1907); a Masonic Temple and office building in Birmingham, Alabama (1922); many wooden houses; wooden schools in the countryside; and perhaps a house for C. A. Correa in Mexico City (1908). Taylor did not design all of historic Tuskegee. A white Georgian designed the domed Tompkins Dining Hall (1910), although Taylor did the interiors and supervised construction. Other black architects teaching in the Architectural Drawing Division, such as Walter T. Bailey (trained at the University of Illinois), William S. Pittman (Tuskegee and Drexel Institute), Wallace A. Rayfield (Pratt Institute), Louis H. Persley (Carnegie Institute of Technology), and the office-trained William A. Hazel, also played active design roles. Tuskegee nurtured black architects with teaching jobs and prepared students for architecture schools (Pittman and Charles Brent to Drexel and Vertner W. Tandy to Cornell) or practice (Charles Bowman in Kansas City; Charles T. Russell in Richmond; John A. Lankford in Washington, D.C.; and several others in Puerto Rico and Cuba).

Taylor's life and architecture were, then, closely bound to Tuskegee, which he made into a center of architectural activity for African Americans. Although he left briefly to resume his Cleveland practice, he designed Tuskegee buildings as a part of it. In 1929 the Phelps-Stokes Fund sent him to Liberia to help create the Booker Washington Institute as an "African Tuskegee." The reticent, diplomatic academic administrator observed Liberia's controversial social and economic conditions, proposed a program and staffing, planned the campus, and designed its first buildings. He retired soon after this adventure and spent his remaining years in Wilmington. His son, Robert Rochon Taylor, carried on in some sense, becoming the Chicago Housing Authority administrator for whom the high-rise Robert Taylor Homes were named.

Taylor was too modest or too honest to claim for himself the role of the first black professional, an honor that he might have given his older colleague William A. Hazel (185?–1929). Taylor's architectural reputation was eclipsed during his own lifetime by the stellar Los Angeles career of Paul R. Williams (1894–1980). However, recognition has come recently through the naming of prizes and associations in his honor and by MIT's attention to its first African American graduate.

ELLEN WEISS

Biography

Born in Wilmington, North Carolina, 8 June 1868. Father was a white planter's son who was free before emancipation and had prospered as a coastal trader, merchant, and carpenter/builder. Attended an American Missionary Association school for black children in New England; met Henry and Francis Bacon—the first a future architect, the second a Massachusetts Institute of Technology (MIT) architecture student in 1888; attended MIT, 1888–92; bachelor of science degree in architecture 1892. His thesis was a home for aged Civil War veterans, northern and southern together. Married; son, Robert Rochon Taylor, administrator of the Chicago Housing Administration. In private practice, Cleveland 1892–96; brief private practice, Tuskegee, Alabama. Professor and administrator, Tuskegee Institute (now University), Alabama from 1896; designer and administrator, Booker Washington Institute, Liberia 1929–34. Died in Wilmington, 13 December, 1942.

Selected Works

Grade School, Cambria, Virginia, 1897
Chapel (destroyed), Tuskegee Institute, Alabama, 1898
Slater-Armstrong Memorial Trades Building (destroyed), Tuskegee Institute, 1899
Carnegie Library, Tuskegee Institute, 1902
Huntington Memorial Academic Building (destroyed), Tuskegee Institute, 1905
Carnegie Library, Livingstone College, Salisbury, North Carolina, 1906
Carnegie Library, Wiley University, Marshall, Texas, 1907
Church, Tuskegee, 1907
Grade School, Selma, Alabama, 1921
Masonic Temple, Birmingham, Alabama, 1922

Selected Publications

Further Reading

Dozier, Richard Kevin, "Tuskegee: Booker T. Washington's Contribution to the Education of Black Architects," Ph.D. diss., University of Michigan, 1990
Hudson, Karen E., *Paul R. Williams, Architect: A Legacy of Style*, New York: Rizzoli, 1993
Hutchinson, Louise Daniel, "Building on a Heritage," *American Visions* 4 (1989) (on W.A. Hazel)
Weiss, Ellen, "Robert R. Taylor of Tuskegee: An Early Black American Architect," *Arris: Journal of the Southeast Chapter of the Society of Architectural Historians* 2 (1991)
Weiss, Ellen, *An Annotated Bibliography on African American Architects and Builders*, Philadelphia: Society of Architectural Historians, 1993

TEAM X (NETHERLANDS)

Team X was an architectural group formed in the early 1950s by a number of young European architects. The participants were dissatisfied with the mid-20th-century Modern movement, particularly with the ideals of CIAM (Congrès Internationaux d'Architecture Moderne), with which they had previously been affiliated. Oscar Newman's *CIAM '59 in Otterlo* and Alison Smithson's *The Emergence of Team 10 out of C.I.A.M.* document Team X's official secession from CIAM. Factions that began to appear at the CIAM IX meeting in Aix-en-Provence in 1953 between the old guard and the younger generation anticipated the split. Under that meeting's theme, "Habitat," the younger members contested the simplistic divisions of living, working, leisure, and circulation that had been established in the Athens Charter. Alison Smithson contends in *Team 10 Meetings: 1953–1984* that the first Team X meeting took place during the meeting at Aix-en-Provence. Following the events of CIAM IX, the "youngers" were entrusted with preparing the subject matter for the CIAM X meeting and from then on were known as Team X. Alison and Peter Smithson (England), Aldo van Eyck (Netherlands), Jaap Bakema (Netherlands), Georges Candilis (France), Shadrack Woods (France), John Voelcker (England), and William and Jill Howell (England) were the founding members of Team X. Participants in Team X altered considerably during the group's existence, but in general the group remained small and was defined by its reaction to the inefficiencies of the large CIAM commissions.

Curtis maintains in *Modern Architecture since 1900* that the members of Team X initially advocated the moral convictions of the early Modern movement but were discontented with CIAM's incapacity to respond to growth and change. They felt that culture, climate, and context were not being addressed and opposed the modernist philosophy of "tabula rasa." However, Francis Strauven acknowledges in his article "The Dutch Contribution: Bakema and Van Eyck" that even the method of achieving these mutual goals was not easily agreed on by the members of the group. Bakema and van Eyck, both of whom requested modification of an original draft by the Smithsons of the Doorn Manifesto (January/February 1954), had their suggestions for the document initially ignored. Finally, an appendix to this manifesto, called the "Dutch Supplement," was added.

Few similarities generally existed between Team X members. Individual participants varied in their method of working and in their perception of how a building was produced. Alison Smithson argues in *Team 10 Meetings: 1953–1984* whether even the group's function as a forum for the development of individual architectural concerns was necessary for each architect's work to have advanced.

The most influential manifesto produced by Team X is the *Team 10 Primer*, published in 1962 and edited by Alison Smithson. It consists of a compilation of quotations from its members at the time. John Voelcker and William and Jill Howell were no longer listed as members in *Team 10 Primer*, being replaced by Giancarlo de Carlo (Italy), José Antonio Coderch y de Sentmenat (Spain), C. Pologni (Hungary), Jerzy Soltan (Poland), and S. Wewerka (Germany). Extracts explore issues initiated by the CIAM commissions, such as mass housing and urbanism through the multilevel city, including the Smithson's proposal for the Golden Lane Housing Competition using the concept of "streets in the air." This proposal was strongly influenced by their relationship with Nigel Henderson, a photographer of London's working-class communities, and their involvement in the art collaborative, the Independent Group.

Van Eyck's elaboration of the doorstep metaphor and his criticism of twin phenomena is another important contribution found in *Team 10 Primer*. In the chapter on Van Eyck in *Modern Architecture: A Critical History*, Kenneth Frampton acknowledges how Van Eyck differed from the other participants of Team X in regard to the severity of his critique of the Modern movement. Before his involvement with Team X, Van Eyck had undertaken extensive studies of anthropological concerns through his personal interest in "primitive" cultures.

Formal meetings of Team X members were generally held annually. In 1962 a well-documented Team X meeting occurred at Abbaye Royaumont. Its importance lay in Team X's acknowledged independence from CIAM concerns. Once again the listed participants had changed. Projects presented included the Waterford School in Swaziland by Pancho Guedes (South Africa/Portugal), the Tibro housing project by Ralph Erskine, John Voelcker's Council Offices and proposal for Tilbury House in Maidstone, Peter Smithson's studies of metropolitan London, José Antonio Coderch y de Sentmenat's studies of slums in Barcelona, Christopher Alexander's study of Indian villages, Kurokawa's capsules, Aldo van Eyck's interest in the large-house/little-city image, Jaap Bakema's gallery housing, Giancarlo de Carlo's plans for Milan, Christopher Dean and Brian Richards's studies of Euston Station, Shad Woods's interest in pedestrian avenues, and Georges Candilis's Toulouse-le-Mirail. The records of "Team 10 at Royaumont" differ from those in *Team 10 Primer* in that they chronicle the interactive discourse by participants in the projects presented. The contributions of architects of different nationalities, speaking English to varying degrees, resulted in frustration with this meeting's outcomes.

In 1982 the final Team X family included Alison and Peter Smithson, Aldo van Eyck, Georges Candilis, José Antonio Coderch y de Sentmenat, Giancarlo de Carlo, Jerzy Soltan, Ralph Erskine (Sweden), Manfred Schiedhelm (Germany), Pancho Guedes, and Julian de La Fuente (France). No longer driven to respond to CIAM inadequacies, the group lost effectiveness and was disbanded in 1984.

The contributions made to 20th-century architecture by Team X include the production of important writings such as *Team 10 Primer* and their capacity to reassess the existing canon of the Modern movement. Equally important are the built works and writings of Team X members. In his article "Team 10 after the Sex Pistols," Willem Jan Neutelings acknowledges the impact of Team X on the Dutch architecture that followed, citing a link to Rem Koolhaas's work. Similarly the Smithsons influenced British architecture through Reyner Banham's promotion of them as founders of the Brutalist movement.

See also **Congres Internationaux d'Architecture Moderne (CIAM)**

IGEA TROIANI

Further Reading

Banham, Reyner, *The New Brutalism: Ethic or Aesthetic*, London: The Architectural Press, and New York: Reinhold, 1966

Curtis, William J.R., *Modern Architecture since 1900*, Oxford: Phaidon, and Englewood Cliffs, New Jersey: Prentice-Hall, 1982; 3rd edition, 1996

Frampton, Kenneth, *Modern Architecture: A Critical History*, London: Thames and Hudson, and New York: Oxford University Press, 1980; 3rd edition, London: Thames and Hudson, 1992

Landau, Royston, "The End of the CIAM and the Role of the British," *Rassegna* 14 (1992)

Neutelings, Willem Jan, "Team 10 after the Sex Pistols," *Archis* 8 (1999)

Newman, Oscar (editor), *CIAM '59 in Otterlo*, Stuttgart, Germany: Kramer, and London: Tiranti, 1961; as *New Frontiers in Architecture: CIAM '59 in Otterlo*, New York: Universe Books, 1961

Smithson, Alison (editor), *Team 10 Primer*, London: Studio Vista, and Cambridge, Massachusetts: MIT Press, 1968

Smithson, Alison (editor), *The Emergence of Team 10 out of C.I.A.M.: Documents*, London: Architectural Association, 1982

Smithson, Alison (editor), *Team 10 Meetings: 1953–1984*, Delft: Publikatieburo Bouwkunde, and New York: Rizzoli, 1991

Strauven, Francis, "The Dutch Contribution: Bakema and Van Eyck," *Rassegna* 14 (1992)

"Team 10 in Bonnieux," *Deutsche Bauzeitung* 11/25 (1978)

TECTONICS

The term *tectonics* alludes to the formally expressive capabilities inherent in architectural forms, both as singular components and in relation to the building assembly as a whole. This aspect of architectural form has, therefore, a greater meaning than either the dictionary definition of *tectonic* as merely "pertaining to building or construction in general" or the simple revealing of constructional techniques. Tectonics, in architectural discourse, refers to the poetics of construction in the original Greek sense of poesis as an act of making and revealing.

The term *tectonic* derives from Greek word *tekton*, meaning carpenter or builder, in turn borrowed from the Sanskrit *taksan*, referring to the craft of carpentry and to the use of the ax. Remnants of a similar term can also be found in Vedic, where it again refers to carpentry and to the art of construction in general. This meaning undergoes further evolution as the term passes from being something specific and physical, such as carpentry, to the more generic notion of construction and later to becoming an aspect of poetry.

The history of tectonic form has two major theoretical lines divided roughly between the German lineage of J. J. Winckelmann, Karl Boetticher, Gottfried Semper, and Karl Friedrich Schinkel and the French tradition of Abbé Laugier, Claude Perrault, Jacques-Germain Soufflot, Henri Labrouste, and Eugène-Emmanuel Viollet-le-Duc. Whereas the German architects and writers focused on the post-Enlightenment dilemma of the disjunction between form and spirit as applied to architecture, French thinkers were preoccupied with the expression of statical logic and the rationality of construction procedures insofar as they could be revealed with greater clarity than before using the new materials of iron and concrete informed by the newly developed science of statics.

The first architectural use of the term *tectonics* in German dates from its appearance in Karl Otfried Müller's *Handbuch der Archaologie der Kunst* (1878; Handbook of the Archaeology of Art), wherein he defines *tektonische* as applying to a series of art forms "such as utensils, vases, dwellings and meeting places of men. . . . We call this string of mixed activities tectonic; their

peak is architecture, which mostly through necessity rises high and can be a powerful representation of the deepest feelings." Karl Boetticher, in his *Die Tektonik der Hellenen* (1874; The Tectonic of the Hellenes), elaborated the concept of the tectonic in several ways. At one level he described a process of building made of a series of appropriately interlocking constructional elements. Simultaneously articulated and integrated, this series of joints constituted the body-form, or *Körperbilden*, of the building that enabled construction of the building and made such assemblies symbolic components of an expressive system. At another level Boetticher distinguished between the *Kernform*, or nucleus, and the *Kunstform*, or decorative cladding, the latter having the purpose of representing and symbolizing the status of the work.

The German architect Gottfried Semper was particularly influential in the evolution of tectonics in his work *Die vier Elemente der Baukunst* (1851; The Four Elements of Architecture). Inspired by a Caribbean hut in the Great Exhibition of 1851, Semper evolved the notion of a paradigmatic primitive hut that embodied the four basic tectonic elements of architecture: the earthwork, the hearth, the framework (and roof), and the lightweight enclosing membrane. This model was more anthropological and transcultural than Marc-Antoine Laugier's well-known proposal in his *Essai sur l'architecture* (1755; An Essay in Architecture), which presented a framed pedimented edifice, adopted as an archetype by neoclassical architects. At the same time, Semper divided architectural form into two broader categories: the tectonics of the frame, in which lightweight linear components are in a spatial grid, and the stereotomics of the earthwork, where mass and volume are formed concurrently through the use of heavyweight elements. *Stereotomics* is derived from the Greek terms *stereos*, for solid, and *tomia*, to cut. This distinction between light and heavy is reflected in overall material differences and construction techniques—wood, steel, and other tensile components for the former and brick, stone, reinforced concrete, or their compressive equivalents for the latter. This opposition between iconic construction typologies and their resultant space-forms as a basis for an architectural language is borne out in vernacular building traditions throughout the world. In Semper's *Der Stil in den technischen und tektonischen Künsten, oder praktische Aesthetik* (1879; Style in the Technical and Tectonic Arts, or Practical Aesthetics), he emphasized the joint or the knot, particularly between the stereotomic base of a building and its tectonic frame. Transitions between such elements provided, for Semper, the most extensive opportunities for expression in architecture. With this focus on the joint or knot, he wrote extensively about the nature of the textile arts as the dominant primordial building element that was often preserved over time stylistically in other, more permanent materials, such as stone or wood.

The tectonic in French architectural thought is traceable to Claude Perrault's *Ordonnance des cinq espèces de dolonnes selon la méthode des anciens* (Treatise on the Five Kinds of Columns after the Method of the Ancients, 1783). Perrault proposed a theory of positive versus arbitrary beauty in place of the prevailing academic theory giving the five classical orders precedence over any other aesthetic ideas. He asserted that such academic styles belonged to the realm of arbitrary beauty, whereas symmetry, richness of materials, and precision of execution were the only means of judging a positive or universal form of beauty, qualities

that are tectonic insofar as they are based on material substance and geometric order.

Two Paris masterworks by Henri Labrouste further developed the tectonic with extraordinary grace and clarity: the Bibliothèque Ste.-Geneviève (1850) in Paris and the Bibliothèque Nationale (1875), with the insertion of a prefabricated, fireproof iron framework into an exterior masonry shell, with each element clearly expressed and articulated. The tectonic aspect of this work lay in its attempt to discredit scenographic eclecticism and to establish in its place architecture as an art of construction. Concerned with the economy of structure, he evolved a system of "iron network vaulting" of his own devising—an expressive vocabulary of lightweight iron members and articulated joints that revealed their resistance to gravity in surprising and inventive ways while set within a more traditional heavy outer masonry shell. This syntax was developed further by his pupil Anatole de Baudot in a series of proposals for large-scale, long-span exhibition halls. The last French theorist of the Greco-Gothic ideal was François Auguste Choisy, who, in his *Histoire de l'architecture* (1899; History of Architecture), suggested that great civilizations arrived at their zenith when their essence, subject to geographic and material conditions, became expressed collectively in tectonic form. In part because of the nature of the renowned isometric drawings illustrating this work, Choisy presented the space-form of buildings as inseparable from their mode of construction, thus anticipating the tectonic possibilities of reinforced concrete in the 20th century.

Certain major architects of the 20th century have pursued tectonics as a determinant of architectural form in all or part of their work. The pioneering work of Auguste Perret (1874–1954) was almost exclusively concerned with the expression of the structural frame in opposition to its in-fill. Utilizing the new vocabulary of architectural reinforced concrete, buildings such as the Théâtre des Champs-Elysées (1913) in Paris created a fusion of classical rationalism with the Greco-Gothic ideal. Ludwig Mies van der Rohe (1886–1969) pursued a tectonic form of intense rigor and precision throughout his career, first with brick in a series of houses in Germany and later with steel in such buildings as the Farnsworth House (1950) in Plano, Illinois, and the campus at the Illinois Institute of Technology (1939–57) in Chicago. It is likely that Frank Lloyd Wright (1867–1959) was aware of Semper's writing and developed paradigms in many projects that included Semper's four elements, particularly in the so-called Usonian houses built mainly between 1934 and 1944 and the "textile-block" system of concrete block construction patented in 1923. Louis Kahn (1901–74) gave primacy in his work to understanding the expressive nature of the joint in architecture and emphasized the tectonic element in nearly every project of his career.

In the Kimbell Art Museum (1972) in Fort Worth, Texas, Kahn's manifestation of the Semperian earthwork-and-frame opposition utilized the former as a means of integrating the building into its site and the latter to provide space and reveal light. The work of the Norwegian architect Jørn Utzon has sought to express structure and construction as a major determinant of architectural form in both large- and small-scale projects. These works nearly always seek inspiration from non-European, often vernacular, models and distinguish clearly between the earthwork and roofwork components, the former often accommodating building services within the site and the latter composed of "floating" folded plate or shell-roof structures for the honorific habitable space above the podium. This is clearly manifest in the Sydney Opera House (1973). The tectonic aspect of the work of Carlo Scarpa (1906–78) lies primarily in the extreme emphasis he placed on the constructional joint—its rhetorical amplification and subsequent elaboration—regardless of the building's program or size.

Other architects who have made tectonics an integral part of their work include the Dutch architect H. P. Berlage (1856–1934), who achieved a masterful tectonic synthesis in his Amsterdam Stock Exchange (1903), and the late work of Le Corbusier (1887–1965), where expressive structure began to dominate the character of the work beginning with the Maison Week-End (1935) in St.-Cloud. The Dutch architects Aldo van Eyck and Herman Hertzberger developed the tectonic potential of the reiteration of singular spatial units and highly articulated structural form to create an evolved syntax of architectural form. In England, Foster Associates and the Richard Rogers Partnership have explored the potential of structural efficiency and its expression throughout their respective practices. In Switzerland the work of the Ticino School, as exemplified by Mario Botta and Livio Vacchini, falls easily into this category, as do many late 20th-century Spanish architects, among them Alejandro de la Sota and Bonell and Rius. In Greece the architects Aris Konstantinidis and Dimitris Pikionis worked to successfully unify local regional building and craft traditions with a modern tectonic expression. Finally, the work of Sverre Fehn in Norway as an example of a small practice and that of the Renzo Piano Building Workshop as a large international firm have been producing work that rigorously pursues an architecture rooted in a philosophy of tectonics, work in which the poetics of construction is a primary determinant of form, a determinant that invites adaptation and distortion brought about by exigencies of typological and topographic circumstance.

JOHN CAVA

See also **Berlage, Hendrik Petrus (Netherlands); Fehn, Sverre (Norway); Kahn, Louis (United States); Kimbell Art Museum, Fort Worth, Texas; Mies van der Rohe, Ludwig (Germany); Perret, Auguste (France); Piano, Renzo (Italy); Scarpa, Carlo (Italy); Sydney Opera House; Utzon, Jørn (Denmark)**

Further Reading

Boetticher, Karl, *Die Tektonik der Hellenen*, Berlin: Ernst und Korn, 1874

Choisy, François Auguste, *Histoire de l'architecture*, Paris: Gauthier-Villars, 1899

Laugier, Marc-Antoine, *Essai sur l'architecture*, Paris: N.B. Duchesne, 1755

Müller, Karl Otfried, *Handbuch der Archaologie der Kunst*, Stuttgart: A. Heitz, 1878

Perrault, Claude, *Ordonnance des cinq espèces de dolonnes selon la méthode des anciens*, translated as *Treatise for the Five Kinds of Columns after the Method of the Ancients* by Indra Kagis McEwen, Santa Monica, California: Getty Center for the History of Art and the Humanities, 1993

Semper, Gottfried, *Die vier Elemente der Baukunst*, as translated (*The Four Elements of Architecture*) by Harry Francis Mallgrave and

Wolfgang Herrmann, Cambridge and New York: Cambridge University Press, 1989

Semper, Gottfried, *Der Stil in den technischen und tektonischen Künsten, oder praktische Aesthetik*, Munich: F. Bruckmann, 1879

TENSILE STRUCTURES

The most common tensile structure is a tent, which is a thin, saddle-shaped tension membrane supported by a compression arch or mast. In a tent the fabric carries all or part of the tensile forces. Small tents, made entirely of fabric, are typically supported by masts (columns) or arches. As the span increases, membrane tension forces increase, and the surface area must be subdivided by cables that carry the principal tensile loads with fabric spanning between cables.

If the edge of a tent is flexible (unattached), it is usually shaped into a concave curve to ensure that it remains in tension. Because the edge is a region of high stress, it is usually reinforced with cable that continues to the anchor point. The anchor point may be connected to a guy cable (which transmits tension forces to the foundation), or it may be supported by a mast or compression strut (which transfers compression loads to the ground).

Perhaps the best way to develop an intuitive understanding of appropriate shapes for tents is to experiment with scale models using a stretchy, lightweight double-knit fabric supported by arches, masts, or strings. At the scale of buildings, however, a minimum of stretch is desired; in fact tent fabrics are selected for their resistance to stretch under load (among other qualities). The three-dimensional form represented in the model by the stretched fabric is constructed at full scale by adjusting the shape and location of the individual panels before assembly. This technique is also used in the design and construction of boat sails to ensure the correct aerodynamic shape. In contemporary tent structures, three-dimensional computer models are used to plan the shape of the tent and its individual panels and to calculate internal tensile stresses. For wind stability (as well as longevity), it is essential that tents be designed as double-curvature structures.

Tents are most easily supported by central masts, but this may be functionally undesirable for nonstructural reasons. Catenary cables can be suspended from side masts to support the membrane peaks at several points. Where center supports are used, fabric stress may be reduced by distributing the load over a larger area through the use of a mushroom-shaped mast capital.

Traditionally, tents were considered to be suitable only for temporary structures because of the deterioration of fabrics due to prolonged exposure to sunlight. The development of improved fabrics (notably fiberglass) and coatings that minimize the deterioration due to sunlight (e.g., Dupont Teflon) have increased the useful life of tent fabrics to over 20 years, making them suitable for use on permanent structures.

Tent Case Studies

Riyadh Stadium

Horst Berger, a pioneer in tension structure technology, was the engineer on this graceful project (1986; Riyadh, Saudi Arabia; Fraser, Roberts, and Partners, architects). The structure consists of 24 identical tent modules repeated around a circle to form a ring canopy covering the grandstands. The open center is over the playing field. Like the Munich Olympic Stadium, the masts are positioned behind the seating to maintain the unobstructed view of the playing field from the grandstands, which seat 60,000. The tent covers a total area of 500,000 square feet (46,500 square meters).

The fabric membrane is stretched between ridge cables, valley cables, and catenary edge cables. The ridge cables are connected to the main mast and are radial in plan. The valley cables between the ridge cables are connected to the bottom anchor and stabilize the structure against wind uplift; they are also radial in plan. The outer edge of the ridge cables and the outer edge of the catenary edge cables are held at a fixed point created by the sloping mast and the two triangulated guy cables. The inner end of the membrane is attached to a ring cable that counterbalances the outward thrust of the sloping mast and guys. To make the structure erectable and to provide redundancy and additional stiffness, an additional cable system was added. This consists of adding a suspension cable, a stabilizing cable, and an upper support cable, all aligned with the ridge cable of each module. These, together with the masts, the rear support cables, and the ring cable, form a stable system not requiring the participation of the fabric.

The structure includes a roof-washing system designed to maintain the fabric's 8 percent daylight transmittance and 75 percent solar reflectance. The high solar reflectance, coupled with the natural convection ventilation induced by the openings at the peak, helps maintain spectator comfort. Rain drains outward to the lower anchor points to spill into a perimeter drainage basin. The center ring cable supports speaker and field lighting systems; uplights reflect off the underside of the tent at night to provide general illumination of the grandstands.

Mound Stands, Lord's Cricket Field

When asked to design the new mound stands for the Lord's Cricket Field (1987; London; Michael Hopkins and Partners, architects; Ove Arup and Partners, structural engineers), Hopkins used fabric roofs to create an elegant tent, recalling the temporary structures of the 17th century erected on the green for a Saturday afternoon's cricket match. In collaboration with the engineers, Hopkins devised a steel superstructure above the existing stadium to house two new tiers of seating, a mezzanine level of services, and the elegant roof that characterizes the structure.

Structurally independent of the existing brick terrace, the tent is supported by six 16-inch (406-millimeter)-diameter tubular steel columns that also support a spine of steel girders. Cantilevering from the spine are a series of beams that form the floor of the top level and the ceiling above the viewing boxes. At the back of the building, the beams are connected by plate girders that transfer loads to the vertical steel tension rods placed every 59 feet (18 meters) between the arches of the colonnade.

The top tier of seating is covered by the fabric tent, stressed by a framework of steel struts and catenary cables. Originally intended to be Teflon-coated fiberglass fabric, PVC-coated polyester was finally specified because of fire restrictions. The fabric was cut using computer-generated patterns and ultrasonically welded into seven sections that extend between the six masts.

FULLER MOORE

See also **Hopkins, Michael and Patty (England)**

Further Reading

Berger, Horst, *Light Structures, Structures of Light: The Art and Engineering of Tensile Architecture*, Basel and Boston: Berkhäuser, 1996

Engel, Heino, *Tragsysteme; Structure Systems* (bilingual English-German edition), Stuttgart, Germany: Deutsche Verlags-Anstalt, 1967; as *Structure Systems*, New York: Praeger, 1968

Moore, Fuller, *Understanding Structures*, Boston: WCB/ McGraw-Hill, and London: McGraw-Hill, 1999

Orton, Andrew, *The Way We Build Now: Form, Scale, and Technique*, Wokingham, Berkshire: Van Nostrand Reinhold, 1988

TENSIONED MEMBRANE STRUCTURE

Tensioned structures (from the Latin *tendere*, "to stretch") are ones that resist only tension forces and pull rather than push. A list would include traditional tents, suspension bridges, modern saddle-shaped prestressed membrane and cable roofs, convertible or retractable roofs for temporary covers, air-supported or pneumatic constructions, and combinations of cables and compression struts, referred to as "tensegrity" structures. Some are simply stabilized by their own weight, whereas others resist uplift as well as gravity loadings by being prestressed and having anticlastic surfaces. The majority are either linear or surface structures. A tensioned membrane structure is one in which two dimensions dominate and loads are resisted in a planar manner, such as occurs in tents, membrane, cable-net, and convertible or retractable roofs, and pneumatic constructions.

The origins of tensioned membrane structures arise from three archetypes: tents, suspension bridges, and balloons and airships. Although the tent is the oldest, suspension bridges were more influential. Balloons and airships antedate air-stabilized or pneumatic structures, in which a small pressure differential substitutes for masts or arch supports.

In addition to wire rope and bridge strand for cable or clastic suspended roofs, a number of fabrics are employed, including cotton, canvas, and coated synthetics; of these polyester coated with polyvinyl chloride (PVC) has proven to be the most useful. The experimental introduction of vinyl-coated fiberglass for the shallow cable-reinforced dome of the United States Pavilion at Expo '70 in Osaka, Japan, stimulated the search for longer-lasting fabrics. Teflon-coated fiberglass was used for La Verne College (1973), California, and subsequently for many different building types, the most famous being the Pontiac Silverdome (1975) in Pontiac, Michigan, and the giant King Abdul Aziz International Airport (1980) in Jeddah, Saudi Arabia.

For the most part, nonprestressed or simply suspended cable roofs resemble types of bridges: in a cable-suspended roof, the deck is carried directly on cables in the same manner as in a catenary bridge. The Wuppertal Swimming Pool (1957) and an aircraft hangar at Kempen (1957) both in Germany, are examples. The most famous is the Dulles Airport Terminal (1962) in Washington, D.C. Jørn Utzon adopted similar roofs for the National Assembly Building (1983) in Kuwait City, Kuwait.

Tents and ancient Roman theater *vela* are some of the earliest traditional examples. The Raleigh Arena (1952) in Raleigh, North Carolina, is usually given as a seminal instance of a clastic saddle shape whose prestressed cable roof supplied the prototype for many later structures, such as the Ingalls Hockey Rink (1958) at Yale University in New Haven, Connecticut, and the Sidney Myer Music Bowl (1956) in Melbourne, Australia.

Frei Otto's experimental development of fabric structure marked the 1950s departure from the previous engineering-inspired suspension bridge model and promoted the tent model. Otto was anticipated by a Russian engineer, V. G. Shookhov, who in 1896 designed a series of four steel tents for the Exhibition at Nizhni Novgorod. In his early projects, Otto concentrated his efforts on finding the most efficient minimal surfaces for modest textile pavilions, but when challenged by larger spans in works such as the German Pavilion at Expo '67 in Montreal, he developed a system of flexible prestressed wide-rope cable nets on which he hung the fabric-enclosing membrane. A further step was taken with the 1972 Munich Olympic Stadium, which was significant for its material and technological advances that resulted in the application of computer methods of structural analysis for the first time.

Parallel with this, Otto developed miniature cable tractors that travel on the supporting cables and permit the membrane envelope to be fully stretched or retracted or bunched for automatic storage. After the Bad Hersfeld (Hesse) centrally retracting roof, Otto collaborated on constructing convertible roofs with Roger Taillibert over an open-air theater (1965) at Cannes and a swimming pool at Boulevard Carnot (1967) in Paris.

This construction is possible to do without masts and arches entirely in air-supported membranes, which use a small air-pressure differential to hold up the structure and resist external loads. The two main types are air-inflated structures, consisting of rib and dual-walled structures, and air-supported structures. To these a third, hybrid type that combines features of both can be added.

An English engineer, Frederick William Lanchester, in a suggestion that he made for a field hospital in 1917, was the first to propose that the balloon principle be applied to building. During World War II in the United States, Herbert Stevens proposed that a pneumatic structure be used for aircraft production. The first actual application had to wait until Walter W. Bird, who enclosed radar dishes in the Distant Early Warning Line inside pneumatic bubbles. The success of these "Radomes" led Bird to establish Birdair Structures Incorporated in 1956. Civilian applications followed, including a theater for the Boston Arts Center (1959) and a Portable Exhibition Pavilion for the U.S. Atomic Energy Commission.

With the Brussels World's Fair, pneumatics, which was almost entirely American, crossed the Atlantic with the Pan-American Airways Pavilion (1958). Around this time Frei Otto began making studies of pneumatic forms and cable-reinforced air-supported membranes. The possible range of applications grew to include sports facilities, roofs for stadiums, warehouses, offices, and pavilions at the New York (1963–64) and Osaka (1970) World's Fairs.

PHILIP DREW

See also **Dulles International Airport, Chantilly, Virginia; Expo 1967, Montreal; Expo 1958, Brussels; Jeddah, Saudi Arabia; Otto, Frei (Germany); Utzon, Jørn (Denmark)**

Further Reading

Treatment of this subject tends to be either a technical and mathematical analysis at one extreme, or an enthusiastic but slight analysis on the

other. The following list has been chosen to provide a broad systematic survey of tensile structural development with references to where technical design data can be found.

Blümel, Dieter, *Convertible Roofs; Wandelbare Dächer* (bilingual English–German edition), Stuttgart, Germany: Instituts für Leichte Fläentragwerke, 1972

Boyd, Robin, "Germany," *Architectural Review* 113/846 (August 1967)

Dent, Roger Nicholas, *Principles of Pneumatic Architecture*, London: Architectural Press, 1971; New York: Halsted Press Division, Wiley, 1972

Drew, Philip, *Tensile Architecture*, Boulder, Colorado: Westview Press, and London: Crosby Lockwood Staples, 1979

"The Era of Swoops and Billows," *Progressive Architecture* 61/6 (June 1980)

"Invitation to the Haj," *Progressive Architecture* 63/2 (February 1982)

LSA 86: Lightweight Structures in Architecture: The First International Conference on Lightweight Structures in Architecture, Sydney, August 24–29, 1986: Proceedings, 2 vols., Kensington, New South Wales: Unisearch Limited, University of New South Wales, 1986

"Tensile, Space, Pneumatic," *Zodiac* 21 (1972)

TENT

Traditional tents come in two categories: noble tents, which are affiliated with urban societies belonging to warriors and kings, and nomad tents, which are the property of nomadic and seminomadic pastoralists. Nomad tents are seen in many varieties, including conical skin-covered tents of northern Eurasia and North America, cylindrical felt-covered trellis tents of central Asia, and the black goats' hair tents of the Near and Middle East and North Africa. There are also species of primitive tents, such as the bone tent of northeastern Siberia and the skin and mat tents that survive in North Africa among the Tuareg and others.

Tents arose gradually, often evolving from existing fixed dwellings and huts that had been simplified and lightened under the pressure of nomadism to give the tent cloth a greater structural role in resisting loads imposed by the wind, snow, and rain and to increase the ease of erecting and transporting them.

Tents belonging to urban peoples existed in the ancient world well before Mohammed and are extremely old. Tents are depicted in an Egyptian encampment at the battle of Kadesh in 1285 B.C., and twin semicupola skin tents are illustrated in Assyrian bas-reliefs from 645 B.C. Images of black tents can be seen in the same Assyrian reliefs, and it is very probable that they existed before the 11th century B.C.

Tents come in two basic plan configurations: circular and rectangular. Structurally, the division is elementary as well: frame tents have a limp, unstressed membrane that is hung on a structural supporting frame that carries the imposed loads and is secured by thongs or straps to prevent the membrane from flying off; frameless tents have a load-bearing and load-distributing cover that is supported at points or linear arrangements of compression members, such as struts or arches. Very few traditional nomad tents have wholly, or true, prestressed membranes. The tent cover of the black goats' hair tent is comparatively heavy, and its weight, especially when it is wet, helps stabilize it. However, the cloth is stretched and deformed by rope around its edges to improve its stability under lateral wind loads. Thus, the tent is partly prestressed and partly weight stabilized. Structurally, traditional tents can be divided into unstressed frame tents; stressed tents without frames supported by poles, arches, and horizontal bars or tensile cords or filaments; and any combination of these.

The conical tent fundamentally is a primitive dwelling used by peoples at the hunting stage. It is a circumpolar trait found in the boreal regions of North America and Eurasia. The tent is retained as a summer dwelling by many nomadic and seminomadic herdsmen and even by some sedentary and agricultural tribes. It consists of a conical frame of radially inclined poles in a circle, with their slim upper ends secured at the peak. The pattern of the pole frame and the material used as a cover (but not the basic form) are remarkably uniform. Two, three, or four poles make up the foundation for the secondary poles, which are laid in the V-fork of the crossing. The conical frame tent belongs to the region of northern taiga forest among the Samoyed, Syran, Mansi, Sel'kupi, Ostayak, Vogul, Northern Evenki Tungus, Yeniseians, Khanti, Nganasani, and Lapps in Keti, Upper Yukaghir. Even the Kalmuck of Astrakhan and the Kirghiz use felt-covered conical tents. The tepee of the Great Plains Indians is a late modification of this circumpolar type and displays such essential features of the Eurasian conical frame tent as the central fire, a smoke hole centering on the crossing of the poles, an eastern entrance, and a place of honor opposite the doorway.

The cylindrical felt-covered trellis tent is a further, highly developed frame tent that is found in the vast region surrounding the Volga River and the Anatolian plateau in the west and the Khingan Mountains in the east. The shape and construction of the trellis tent are surprisingly uniform and have remained unchanged over the past four centuries. The two main types are a felt-covered cylindrical walled trellis tent with a conical ribbed roof, found among the Mongol peoples and some Turkic-speaking tribes of northern central Asia, and a convex domical roofed version, found among Turkic-speaking tribes of western and southern Siberia, such as the Kirghiz, Uzbek, and Turkoman.

The black tent type is a frameless tent with a partially stressed membrane with an anticlastic or flat saddlelike surface supported by ridge, arches, or high points and anchored to the ground by long, extended stays. It most resembles the modern prestressed tent and uses the least amount of wood of any type, with the possible exception of Inuit tents. Black tents are distributed in a nearly continuous narrow belt between 25 and 40 degrees north latitude, extending from Mauritania in northwestern Africa to Afghanistan, with the Tibetan group forming an isolated island. This distribution approximates the region of desert vegetation across North Africa and the Middle East and is related to two animals: the goat, from whose hair the tent cloth is woven, and the dromedary, which is used for the tent's transport.

Notable differences exist between the Arabian black tents and tents on the northern fringes of Arabia and North Africa: the cloth tent of the desert Bedouin, the Sba'a and Rwala, has three longitudinal rows of poles supporting a rectangular cloth, with the central row higher than the remainder, giving its characteristic ridge profile. The tents of North Africa differ significantly in having two rather than three rows of poles: a front row and a central row but no back row. The North African black tent

was brought to the region with the Arab expansion in the 11th century B.C. and has a striped awning.

Inuit and Tuareg tents occur in extreme culture-resistance zones and typically are minimal constructions of considerable ingenuity.

Sumptuous tents were introduced into Western Europe in the 12th century A.D. as a result of the Crusades and then spread from France, where their immediate effect was great, and quickly became identified with the tournaments, and warfare that were part of the chivalric tradition in neighboring regions. Tents were symbols for the heavenly city of Jerusalem and the exotic Near East. Tents influenced the design of pavilions and of turret roofs for churches, castles, and palaces (a very fashionable architectural motif) as well as the interior design and decoration of palaces, especially the boudoir. Miniature tents, to symbolize the Old Testament tabernacle, were frequently adopted for reliquaries and monstrances in medieval Christian ritual. Elaborate, fabulously decorated tents were revived in the 15th century, reaching a climax under Francis I and Henry VIII in 1520 at Ardes and later under Emperor Napoleon at the beginning of the 19th century. In the 16th century, the word *pavillon* came to dignify anything likened to a tent—any lightly constructed ornamental building or pleasure house in a garden. Even more widespread was the tent roof that was derived from the conical shape of the parasol-roofed tent or the square pavilion tent with its draped pyramid-shaped canopy.

Tents generally are identified with nomadism, whether a full-blown nomadism; the itinerant nomadism of armies and royal progresses; or that of an individual or groups who are forced by their lifestyle to move often and who, to this end, require a light, portable shelter. The relationship between tents and permanent monumental architecture is a complex two-way one, with exchanges occurring in both directions, reflecting the interdependence between sedentary urban and nomadic pastoral cultures. Because of their symbolic prestige, tent forms have been imitated and preserved in stone buildings and in other durable constructions, resulting in a hybrid class of pseudo-tent buildings, a phenomenon that is very noticeable in France after the Crusades and that spread to Stockholm, Dresden, and Vienna.

PHILIP DREW

Further Reading

Much of the material on tents occurs within ethnographic studies of nomadic life that are not written from an architectural viewpoint but that treat the tent as an expression of culture and weaving technique. The subject of urban tents has received even less attention by comparison, and there are no architectural histories or separate technical accounts of their construction, origin, and development. This selection is biased toward the tents of nomadic peoples and includes some of the more pertinent ethnological reports in addition to popular accounts.

Andrews, P.A., "The Tents of Timur," in *Arts of the Eurasian Steppelands*, edited by Philip Denwood, London: University of London School of Oriental and African Art, 1978

Drew, Philip, *Tensile Architecture*, London: Crosby Lockwood Staples, and Boulder, Colorado: Westview Press, 1979

Ewers, John Canfield, *Murals in the Round: Painted Tipis of the Kiowa and Kiowa-Apache Indians*, Washington, D.C.: Smithsonian Institution Press, 1978

Faegre, Torvald, *Tents: Architecture of the Nomads*, London: John Murray, and Garden City, New York: Anchor Press/Doubleday, 1979

Feilberg, Carl Gunnar, *La Tente noire*, Copenhagen: I Kommission hos Gyldenal, 1944

Laubin, Reginald, and Gladys Laubin, *The Indian Tipi: Its History, Construction, and Use*, Norman: University of Oklahoma Press, and New York: Ballantine, 1957; 2nd edition, Norman: University of Oklahoma Press, 1977

"Tents," *Mimar* 4 (1982)

TERRA-COTTA

Terra-cotta (Italian for "baked earth"), a building material with ancient roots, found its fullest expression in architecture of the first half of the 20th century. Architectural terra-cotta is ceramic or fired clay, most often glazed, used primarily in the 20th century for fireproofing and exterior cladding of buildings. The earliest known use of terra-cotta is in early Mesopotamia, where examples are found from as early as 3200 B.C. Terra-cotta was also used by the ancient Egyptians and the Etruscans as well as the Greeks and the Romans.

Lost with the fall of Rome, the art of terra-cotta was rediscovered in 14th-century Germany and Italy, as exemplified by the work of Luca della Robbia and his family, who introduced polychrome techniques on panels and plaques used as architectural decoration. The techniques for making terra-cotta found their way to England, where unglazed terra-cotta was used as early as the 16th century, mostly as decorative detail on brick and stone buildings. During the 18th century, technological advances resulted in a steady increase in England in the use of terra-cotta, which was noted for its durability and resistance to weathering. Terra-cotta was also admired because of the its ability to mimic the appearance of stone at a fraction of the cost.

By the 19th century, terra-cotta was widely used in England for architectural ornamentation. Its popularity grew because it was available in a range of colors and textures and could be molded with fine detail emulating carved stone. Terra-cotta was also being produced in North America on a limited basis during this period. Factories in New York, Philadelphia, and Chicago produced unglazed terra-cotta for ornamental detail for the facades of buildings, including string courses, capitals, and window surrounds.

Despite its early introduction to the United States, architects and builders tended to be skeptical of the claims for terra-cotta's durability. This began to change after Chicago's Great Fire of 1871. After the devastation of the fire, the emphasis in Chicago and nationwide was to construct buildings that were as fire resistant as possible. Structural terra-cotta provided an extra measure of fireproofing to buildings. At the same time, the last quarter of the 19th century, advances in the terra-cotta manufacture and architectural design that capitalized on the inherent malleability of terra-cotta as a cladding material spurred the growth of the fledgling American industry.

As terra-cotta was receiving acceptance as a building material, dramatic changes were occurring in the technology of building construction. Technological innovations—notably skeleton-frame construction—led to the development of the modern skyscraper. The use of structural metal to form a skeleton on which finish materials could be hung meant that buildings could rise to heights previously unimagined. At the same time, architects were anxious to develop new design motifs to celebrate this new

building type. Architectural terra-cotta proved to be the ideal material. Terra-cotta cost 90 percent less than a piece of ornamental stone and was one-third the weight. In addition, because terra-cotta was molded rather than carved, repeating motifs in a complex design was easily achieved. Variations in surface texture and colors were also possible. One of the earliest structures to use terra-cotta as a cladding material was New York's Flatiron Building (built 1901–03, designed by Daniel Burnham). This 22-story building, the tallest building in the city when it was built, has a stone base, with brick and terra-cotta finishing up the floors above.

Louis Sullivan exploited the plasticity of terra-cotta perhaps better than any other practitioner of his time. The intricate interplay of the design motifs on the facades of Sullivan's commercial buildings and skyscrapers exemplifies terra-cotta's ability to be shaped and molded to fit the architect's design. Because of the material's malleability, architects and designers for the terra-cotta manufacturer often cooperated to produce beautiful systems of wall surfaces and ornament. By the 1910s skyscrapers were soaring to new heights, and terra-cotta was increasingly employed because of its many ornamental and constructional advantages. Both the Woolworth Building in New York, designed by Cass Gilbert and completed in 1913, and Chicago's Wrigley Building of 1924, by Graham, Anderson, Probst, and White, are important examples of buildings fully clad in terra-cotta.

In the early years, the finish color of terra-cotta depended on the color of the clay used. Most terra-cotta manufactured in the United States was gray or buff in color to emulate the stone it was meant to replace. During the early decades of the 20th century, terra-cotta was accepted as a material in its own right, and its success depended less on its ability to imitate other materials. At the same time, architects began to experiment with colored glazes to provide another layer of detail to their designs.

Terra-cotta was adapted as the ideal material for the streamlined Art Deco and Art Moderne styles that became popular after the 1925 Paris Exposition. Improvements in the manufacture of terra-cotta resulted in the introduction of thinner panels that were lighter in weight. Terra-cotta was easily molded into the geometric, stylized, and colorful decorative elements that are found on a variety of small and large buildings from this era. Terra-cotta can be found on myriad commercial structures, small apartment buildings, automobile-related buildings such as garages and showrooms, and movie theaters dating from the early decades of the 20th century.

Terra-cotta was replaced as a structural and as a decorative component by a material that could be produced even less expensively: concrete. Reinforced concrete initially provided the structural fireproofing capabilities of terra-cotta at a reduced price. Eventually, concrete proved to be better suited to the unadorned architecture that became popular at midcentury.

LEAH KONICKI

See also **Art Deco; Chicago School; Flatiron Building, New York City; Ornament; Woolworth Building, New York City**

Further Reading

Slaton, Deborah, and Harry J. Hunderman, "Terra Cotta," in *Twentieth-Century Building Materials: History and Conservation*, edited by Thomas C. Jester, New York: McGraw-Hill, 1995
Tunick, Susan, *Terra Cotta Skyline*, New York: Princeton Architectural Press, 1997
Weaver, Martin E., and F.G. Matero, *Conserving Buildings: Guide to Techniques and Materials*, New York: Wiley, 1993; revised edition, 1997

TERRAGNI, GIUSEPPE 1904–43

Architect, Italy

Giuseppe Terragni was among the most talented and esteemed of the Italian modernist architects working in the period between the world wars. His Casa del Fascio (1936) in Como is generally considered the emblematic modernist building to have been built under the Fascist regime, and his Sant'Elia Nursery School (1937), also in Como, ranks as a tour de force of modern European architecture.

In December 1926 Terragni burst onto the Italian architectural scene with the first of four magazine articles on which he collaborated with six of his contemporaries. These essays, published in the esoteric and unillustrated magazine *La Rassegna Italiana*, later came to be known as the "Rationalist Manifesto." Terragni and his friends of the Gruppo Sette (Group 7) argued in these essays against revivalism in Italian architecture and that rationalism must shape all decisions about form, structure, and function. The avant-garde in Italy were henceforth known as the "rationalists."

Terragni's first major building was the Novocomum Apartment House (1927–29) in Como. A controversial building from the moment of its unveiling, it was hailed as the first rationalist work in Italy. Terragni went on to design a total of 26 built works and numerous unbuilt projects in a 15-year career that was cut short by World War II.

Terragni's undisputed masterpiece—the Casa del Fascio in Como (a local Fascist Party headquarters that the architect named the "Glass House of Fascism")—was begun in 1932 and completed in 1936. The building is a prismatic exercise in modern geometric form and structure, with four different facades that nevertheless together possess compositional coherence and harmony. The building contains a two-story atrium space encased by a system of clerestory windows, one of the first of its kind in Europe and an influence on post–World War II atria. The play of transparency and opacity created by Terragni's use of materials (glass and marble, respectively) results in fascinating visual contradictions. The building was initially condemned by the local Fascist Party chief as being too ordinary for an important state edifice. To appease his critics, Terragni employed an artist and industrial designer, Marcello Nizzoli, to develop a decorative figural design scheme for the building facade. The ensuing panels were never added as envisaged, however.

By 1936 Terragni had built five apartment houses in Milan (in collaboration with Pietro Lingeri) and had gained recognition in the competition for the National Fascist Party Headquarters (1934) in Rome. In 1937–38 he built several significant villas including the Villa Bianca in Seveso and the Sant'Elia Nursery School in Como. Terragni's plan for the nursery school drew on a radical sense of interior transparency, using glass partitions in the design of the flexible free plan derived from Le Corbusier.

In 1938 Terragni and Lingeri designed the Danteum project for Rome. The building was to have been an exercise in the

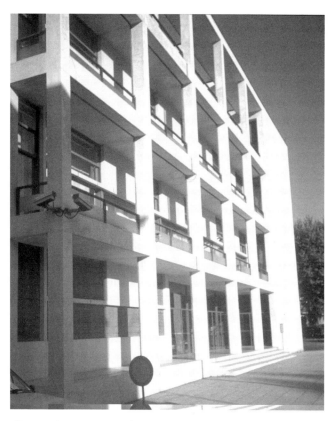

Giuseppe Terragni, Casa del Fascio, Como, Italy (1936)
© Howard Davis/Greatbuildings.com

relation of architecture to literary and political themes, with its composition derived in part from Dante's *Divine Comedy* and its forms referencing the iconography of the resurrected Roman Empire, which Benito Mussolini had declared after the Ethiopian War (1935–41). With its thick marble walls and processional promenade, the Danteum building previsioned much of the massive architecture of the postwar period.

Terragni's last major work—the Casa Giuliani Frigerio Apartment House (1939–40) in Como—was completed by his assistant, Luigi Zuccoli. It was realized when Terragni (now serving in the Italian army) was on his way to the Russian front. At the battle of Stalingrad, he suffered a nervous collapse, and after being returned to Italy in the winter of 1943, he died in Como six days before the coup that deposed Mussolini.

THOMAS SCHUMACHER

See also **Fascist Architecture; Rome, Italy**

Biography

Born in Meda, Italy, 18 April 1904; moved to Como as a child. Attended Liceo Scientifico in Como, graduated 1921; attended Politecnico di Milano, Facoltà di Architettura, 1921–26, degree granted 1926. Founding member, Gruppo 7 1926. Hired Luigi Zuccoli as assistant 1927; formed partnership with Pietro Lingeri, 1933; the pair worked together on competitions, five apart-

ment houses in Milan, and the Danteum Project for Rome. Worked with brother Attilio, an engineer, on buildings in and around Como, 1927–39. Participated in Palazzo Littorio competition, 1934, 1937; won second prize in Palazzo dei Congressi competition, Rome 1939. Founder and editor, *Valori Primordiali* 1937. Inducted into Italian army shortly after the start of World War II, served in the Balkans and the USSR. Died of a brain embolism 19 July 1943. Rumors of suicide have persisted until today, but have not been substantiated.

Selected Works

Novocomum Apartments, Como, 1929
Sala O at the Exhibit of the Fascist Revolution, Rome, 1932
Project for the Competition for the National Fascist Party Headquarters, Rome (with Antonio Carminati, Pietro Lingeri, Enrico Saliva, Luigi Vietti, Marcello Nizzoli, Mario Sironi; unexecuted), 1934
Casa Ghiringhelli, Milan (with Pietro Lingeri), 1935
Casa Toninello, Milan (with Pietro Lingeri), 1935
Tomb of Roberto Sarfatti, Col e'Echele, 1935
Casa del Fascio, Como, 1936
Casa Rustici, Milan (with Pietro Lingeri), 1936
Asilo Sant'Elia, Como, 1937
Danteum, Rome (with Pietro Lingeri; unbuilt), 1938
Casa Giuliani Frigerio, Como (completed by Luigi Zuccoli), 1940

Selected Publications

"Architettura" (with Gruppo 7), *La rassegna italiana* (December 1926)
"Gli stranieri" (with Gruppo 7), *La rassegna italiana* (February 1927)
"Impreparazione, incomprensione, pregiudizi" (with Gruppo 7), *La Rassegna Italiana* (March 1927)
"Una nuova epoca arcaica" (with Gruppo 7), *La Rassegna Italiana* (May 1927)
"Architettura di strato?" and "Lettera sull'architettura," *Ambrosiano* (February 1931)
"La constuzione della Casa del Fascio di Como," *Quadrante* 35 (1936)
"Discorso ai Comaschi," *Ambrosiano* (March 1940)
"Relazione sul Danteum 1938," *Oppositions* 9 (1977)

Further Reading

De Ghirardo, "The Vicenda of the Decoration of the Facade of the Casa del Fascio, Como, 1936–39," *The Art Bulletin* (October 1980)
Eisenman, P., "From Object to Relationship," *Casabella* 344 (January 1970)
Eisenman, P., "From Object to Relationship II," *Perspecta* 13/14 (1971)
Mantero, Enrico, *Giuseppe Terragni e la città del razionalismo italiano*, Bari, Italy: Dedalo, 1969; 2nd edition, 1983
Schumacher, Thomas L., *Il Danteum di Terragni, 1938*, Rome: Officina Edizioni, 1980; 2nd edition, 1983; as *The Danteum: A Study in the Architecture of Literature*, New York: Princeton Architectural Press, 1985; 2nd edition, as *The Danteum: Architecture, Poetics, and Politics under Italian Fascism*, 1993
Schumacher, Thomas L., *Surface and Symbol: Giuseppe Terragni and the Architecture of Italian Rationalism*, New York: Princeton Architectural Press, 1991
Tafuri, M., "Terragni, Subject and Mask," *Oppositions* 11 (1978)
Zevi, Bruno, *Ommagio a Terragni*, Milan: Etas Kompas, 1968
Zevi, Bruno, *Giuseppe Terragni*, Bologna: Zanichelli, 1980; as *Giuseppe Terragni*, London: Triangle, 1989

TERRAZZO

One of the oldest types of flooring, terrazzo was developed by Venetians in the 16th century and was popularized during the late 19th century. Modern terrazzo flooring is composed of 70 percent marble or granite chips (or a combination of both) and 30 percent white, gray, or pigmented Portland cement. After curing, the surface is ground smooth, giving the stone chips a polished surface. Terrazzo flooring is very durable and can be arranged in decorative patterns. During the 1930s terrazzo was very popular for commercial buildings, fitting in well with the Art Deco design then so popular. Public and commercial buildings such as schools, banks, and hospitals and government buildings such as post offices incorporate terrazzo into main corridors and lobby areas. A special type of terrazzo flooring is used in hospital operating rooms.

Terrazzo flooring developed from the first "composition" floors developed by the ancient Greeks. Over time the rubble and charcoal flooring was held together with cement mortar and then developed into flooring of lava cement and charcoal set with marble pieces in imitation of mosaic flooring. This type of flooring was often laid in service areas and on terraces. The name *terrazzo* comes from the Italian word for "terrace."

In Venice, Italy, during the 1500s, a finely finished terrazzo flooring was developed that consisted of the 70–30 marble-to-mortar binder still in use today. After placing the marble chips in the binder matrix, the surface was polished smooth. This type of terrazzo flooring became very popular for use in Italian villas. During the late 19th century, travelers to Italy were impressed by the beauty and function of this flooring. Wealthy travelers, on returning home from Italian excursions, had terrazzo flooring installed in the entrance halls of their homes. The use of terrazzo in public buildings soon became popular as well.

Because of terrazzo's strength, durability, and potential to create decorative patterns reminiscent of mosaic flooring, it became a popular flooring in public and commercial buildings. In particular the use of a pigmented binding matrix made the flooring popular during the Art Deco movement of the 1930s. It is most often used in the same locations that stone flooring would be. Where appearance and durability are needed in high-traffic areas, it is a cost-effective option. Most train stations, movie theaters, fire stations, city and state offices, and schools built during the first third of the 20th century include terrazzo flooring in high-traffic areas.

The original method for installing terrazzo flooring is cast-in-place. It ranges from 1/4 inch (6 mm) to 3 inches (72 mm) thick placed over a mortar bed or secured to the substrate floor using direct bonding. A layer of sand 1/4 inch (6 mm) is used as a cushion when structural movement is anticipated. The sand is covered with a waterproof paper and wire mesh. A 2–1/8-inch (54 mm) concrete slab is poured over the sand. Divider strips are embedded in the concrete with 5/8 inch (16 mm) left exposed. These divider strips help control shrinkage and cracking and allow color changes. They also serve as a guide for installing the topping. Bonded floors, used in areas where structural movement is unlikely (such as corridors, walks, and swimming pool decks), have a total thickness of 1–1/8 inches (29 mm). The base slab is coated with Portland cement to ensure a good bond. The underbase is poured and divider strips are set before the topping is installed.

The terrazzo topping is installed by first coating the underbed with a layer of grout matching the color of the binding matrix. The topping is placed using the divider strips as guides. The topping is sprinkled with marble chips matching the color percentages of the stone in the topping. Heavy rollers compact the topping until most of the water is removed. The surface is then troweled until the divider strips are exposed. The floor must cure for at least six days before grinding and polishing the surface smooth. After curing and first grinding, a light application of grout cement is used to fill voids. The final grinding levels the floor and exposes the 70 percent stone composition. The floor is then cleaned, sealed, and machine buffed to reveal the color and luster of the marble.

Terrazzo floors can also be installed monolithically with the structural slab. Divider strips are placed when the slab is poured and 5/8 inch (16 mm) is left for the terrazzo topping. Curing, grinding, cleaning, sealing, and buffing follow the same procedure as with bonded and sand-cushioned cast-in-place terrazzo.

Although modern terrazzo floors include a mixture of stones capable of taking a high polish, terrazzo originally stuck to marble and granite chips. The advent of linoleum and other durable flooring made the expense of quarrying stone for use in terrazzo, together with the effect of terrazzo's long curing time on tight construction schedules, less desirable to architects and builders. Cheaper alternatives to both budget and schedule caused terrazzo to fall out of popularity during the decades of the mid-20th century. Other disadvantages included the thickness (and thus weight) necessary for terrazzo flooring, and the efforts necessary to prevent cracking as buildings shift and settle.

Developments Expand Terrazzo's Options

Systems for applying thin-set terrazzo and precast terrazzo tiles and products have reawakened an interest in terrazzo flooring. During the last decades of the 20th century, terrazzo flooring in both commercial and residential settings gained popularity.

Thin-set terrazzo reduces the weight of traditional terrazzo by eliminating the underbed. The topping, ranging from 1/4 to 5/8 inch (6 to 16 mm) thick, is bonded directly to the structural slab. The matrix mix, which includes epoxies, polyesters, or latex instead of Portland cement, adds to the adhesion of the topping and shortens the curing time to as little as 24 hours. Divider strips are not necessary, except for color changes and in locations where movement or stress is likely (such as around columns or over beams).

Precast terrazzo tiles also open up options for terrazzo flooring; thus, its renewed popularity. Precast tiles allow easy color changes and patterning and also include additional uses for terrazzo, such as stair treads, risers, bases, and shower receptors. Nonskid finishes are also available. Precast terrazzo products are bonded to surfaces using epoxies and other adhesives as directed by the specific manufacturer.

Special-Use Terrazzo

Conductive terrazzo is commonly used in hospital operating rooms. Acetylene carbon black in the matrix binder as well as the underbed provides a path for electrical conductivity. Static

electricity between people and equipment is absorbed by the acetylene carbon black. This type of terrazzo is also used in some laboratory settings. Acrylic or vinyl emulsions may also be added to the matrix for thin-set terrazzo. These emulsions increase allowable tensile and flexural stresses, allowing the terrazzo topping to be decreased to as little as 1/4 inch (.6 cm). The Portland cement matrix can also be replaced with a plastic matrix, thus expanding use options. Rustic or washed terrazzo provides a pebbly finish rather than a smooth and polished finish. Marble, quartz, onyx, and granite chips are used in a white or colored matrix. After curing, the floor is washed with either water or acid to expose the stone chips, creating the pebble effect.

LISA A. WROBLE

See also **Art Deco**

Further Reading

Detailed information about installation, marble gauges, and mixture ratio is available from contractor and association print sources. Various articles on specific uses of terrazzo are available in trade and association journals.

Gregory, Daniel, "Terrazzo with a Twist," *Sunset* 196/1 (January 1996)

Kerrison, James, "Terrazzo Renewed," *The Canadian Architect* 41 (October 1996)

Watson, Don A., *Construction Materials and Processes*, New York: McGraw-Hill, 1972; 3rd edition, 1986

Williams, Mark, "Failures: Rustic Terrazzo—Case Study," *Progressive Architecture* 67 (February 1986)

TESSENOW, HEINRICH 1876–1950

Architect, Germany

Heinrich Tessenow was born in Rostock in 1876. He was introduced to the art of building by his father, a successful carpenter with whom he worked before studying at the building schools in Neustadt and Leipzig. In 1900 he enrolled at the Technical University in Munich, where he studied architecture under Friedrich von Thiersch. However, he left the university after three semesters and joined the office of the prominent Jugendstil architect Martin Dülfer. Tessenow also worked for Paul Schultze-Naumburg.

Despite the sporadic nature of his own education, Tessenow was an accomplished teacher. After leaving Dülfer's office in 1902, he accepted a position at the Building School in Sternberg. He taught at the Building School in Lüchow and the School of Applied Arts in Trier before accepting a position at the Technical University in Dresden as Dülfer's assistant. From 1913 until 1919, he was a professor at the School of Applied Arts in Vienna. In 1920 he taught at the Academy of Fine Arts in Dresden. In 1926 he was selected by Bruno Paul to lead a master class at the School of Fine and Applied Arts in Berlin. He held a concurrent professorship at the Technical University in the capital.

As an architect Tessenow was fascinated by the problems of mass housing. In 1903 he had developed a housing type with roughcast walls, tiled roofs, and carefully detailed woodwork that was evocative of traditional rural building. Tessenow's aesthetic preferences were suggestive of the Heimatstil (vernacular style) advocated by his former employer, Schultze-Naumburg. How-

ever, Tessenow's residential designs, as exemplified by projects such as his Workers Housing for the Electric Power Station in Trier of 1906, were not merely copies of traditional rural buildings. His workers' houses reflected a pragmatic balance between comfort and affordability. They were carefully designed to encourage efficient lighting and ventilation and typically included sensible built-in furnishings and a garden to provide for a measure of self-sufficiency. For Tessenow the Heimatstil represented a vocabulary of architectural reform. This theme was conveyed in his book *Der Wohnungsbau* (House Building), published in 1909.

In 1910 Tessenow designed his best-known project, the Dalcroze Institute for Rhythmic Dance in the garden city of Hellerau near Dresden. This project, with its severe and attenuated neoclassical forms and simple geometries, represented the translation of the principles of formal abstraction that characterized his houses to a project of substantial scale. The Dalcroze Institute also illustrated the increasing simplicity of Tessenow's projects, a tendency that was also apparent in the houses he designed for Hellerau between 1910 and 1911. These small stucco houses combined his sensitive detailing with creative features, such as the *Patentwand* system for the construction of internally ventilated walls.

In 1916 Tessenow published *Hausbau und Aergleichen* (House Building and Such Things), in which he reiterated his beliefs concerning industry, craft, and the design of modern housing. Although he maintained his dedication to the precedent of vernacular architecture throughout the years of the Weimar Republic, he was an active member of the artistic avant-garde. In 1910 he had joined the Werkbund and in 1921 entered the radical Novembergruppe, whose architectural section was directed by Ludwig Mies van der Rohe. He was also one of the founding members of der Ring. His interest in social progress extended to his own designs, in which he demonstrated an increasing concern for the entire built environment, from furniture through urban planning. In 1925 he designed a school at Klotzsche for the government of the land of Saxony, a regular, symmetrical composition of individual pavilions with pitched tile roofs arranged around expansive courtyards. The plan reflected his theories of urban design, which were also manifested in the residential developments that he composed. The individual building masses at Klotzsche were stark and geometric, with Tessenow's characteristic detailing limited to the door and window surrounds. The same qualities were apparent in his Heinrich-Schütz-Schule in Kassel of 1927. In Kassel, Tessenow dispensed with a pitched roof and designed a loosely symmetrical composition in which the tradition of antique typology was apparent only in the regular disposition of fenestration and the elegant sense of proportion that pervaded the design.

In 1930 Tessenow's design to rebuild Schinkel's Neue Wache in Berlin as a memorial to the fallen of World War I was selected in a competition over submissions by many of Germany's most successful architects, including Peter Behrens, Hans Poelzig, and Mies van der Rohe. His plan was notable for its pervasive simplicity. The interior was a stark, cubic volume lit by a circular oculus placed above a prismatic black stone supporting a bronze wreath in commemoration of the dead. The exquisitely careful detailing of the interior provided a counterpoint to its monumental severity. The drum of the oculus maintained a subtle, elegant compound curve in its profile. A complex molding de-

fined the joint between the metal drum and the stucco ceiling. A similar molding elaborated the joint between the ceiling and the stone veneer of the walls. Tessenow used these abstracted classical details only where they were functionally justified by a change of materials or methods of construction. The interface between the stone walls and the stone pavement was a simple mortar joint. Tessenow's new interior for the Neue Wache represented a distillation of the neoclassical tradition to an essential form that existed in a perfect accord with tectonic and functional requirements.

The nationalistic and racist promotion of the Heimatstil by Paul Schultze-Naumburg and its subsequent association with the ideology of the Nazi government have until recently relegated Tessenow to a position of relative insignificance in the standard histories of 20th-century design. However, during his lifetime Tessenow was an influential author and educator, and his theories were familiar throughout Germany. He was one of the progenitors of the Modern movement. Throughout the first half of the 20th century, his successful solutions to the problem of mass housing in Central Europe served as a point of reference for subsequent experiments in the field, and his transformation of the vocabulary of German neoclassicism as an example of the vitality of traditional forms within the context of modern design.

W. OWEN HARROD

See also **Avant-Garde; Paul, Bruno (Germany); Vernacular Architecture**

Further Reading

De Michelis, Marco, *Heinrich Tessenow, 1876–1950* (exhib. cat.), Milan: Electa, 1991; as *Heinrich Tessenow, 1876–1950*, translated by Ishbel Flett, Frankfurt: Deutsches Architektur-Museum, 1991 (in English)

Grassi, Georgio, "Architecture as Craft," in *On Rigor*, edited by Richard Burdett and Wilfried Wang, Cambridge, Massachusetts: MIT Press, 1989

Hays, Michael, "Tessenow's Architecture as National Allegory: Critique of Capitalism or Protofascism?" in *On Rigor*, edited by Richard Burdett and Wilfried Wang, Cambridge, Massachusetts: MIT Press, 1989

Jessen, Walter, "Introduction to Heinrich Tessenow's *House Building and Such Things*," in *On Rigor*, edited by Richard Burdett and Wilfried Wang, Cambridge, Massachusetts: MIT Press, 1989

Strey, Waltraud, *Die Zeichnungen von Heinrich Tessenow: Der Bestand in der Kunstbibliothek Berlin*, Berlin: Reimer, 1981

Wangerin, Gerda, Gerhard Weiss, and Steen Eiler Rasmussen, *Heinrich Tessenow: Ein Baumeister, 1876–1950. Leben, Lehre, Werk*, Essen, Germany: Bacht, 1976

TESTA, CLORINDO 1923–

Architect and painter, Argentina

If one had to identify Le Corbusier's counterpart in 20th-century Latin America, Clorindo Testa, a major figure in Argentinean architecture in this period, would almost certainly be the choice. He is not referred to here as a "disciple" or "follower," but as a similar personality in terms of his constant innovative and creative capacity, his dialectic and changing relationship to the natural and urban surroundings, his passion for painting and drawing, and his interpretation of society and history in his artistic production. He was the son of an Italian immigrant residing in Argentina, who originated from the town of Ceppaloni. He was born in Naples in 1923 and maintained a persistent emotional relationship with Italy (in 1997 he was declared an honorary citizen of Ceppaloni) despite his full identification with the city of Buenos Aires. He pursued a career in engineering, but his artistic vocation (he started drawing at a very early age) led him to the College of Architecture and Urbanism, where he graduated in 1947. He worked for one year in the Master Plan of the City of Buenos Aires (1948), where he met Ernesto N. Rogers, whose criticism of the "rationalist" project for a collection of residences that was being built definitively distanced him from the rigid designs of the Modern movement. With a scholarship from the College of Architecture and Urbanism, he traveled to Europe, extending his tour for almost three years (1949–52). He did not go to Paris, where Le Corbusier was based, nor did he accept Rogers's offer to work in his Milan studio (BBPR). Painting constituted his principal interest during that period, and he held his first exhibition at the Van Riel Gallery on Florida Street, Buenos Aires (1952).

Associated with the architects Dabinovic, Rossi and Gaido, he obtained various prizes in competitions for public and private works, such as the headquarters of the Argentinean Chamber of Building Contractors (1952), a group of health centers in Misiones (1955), and the Civic Center of Santa Rosa in the province of La Pampa (1956). This ensemble of public buildings, which included the Government House, underwent various successive stages in 1972 (Legislature) and in 1981 (Court and Cultural Center) which illustrate the expressive changes in Testa's language, from the Le Corbusier–inspired Brutalist orthodoxy of exposed concrete and the transparent facades of the canopies to the free and unprejudiced planimetric and volumetric composition of the 1980s decade, foreshadowing the aesthetic values of "supermodernism." From then on, he always worked in teams of professionals from different generations, though his dominant presence could still immediately be identified by the originality of the successive artistic languages used. Two works reached international importance, identified as the expression of Latin American creative freedom even by traditionalist critics such as Nikolaus Pevsner: the Bank of London and South America Head Office (1959–66), in collaboration with the SEPRA studio (an Argentinean version of the SOM) and the National Library, a team project also involving Francisco Bullrich and Alicia Gazzaniga (1962–95). Both buildings are configured by gigantic outer structures of reinforced concrete, a Jurassic exoskeleton according to Berkel and Bos. In the first he created an expanded interior space with hanging trays suggesting an interaction between a Roman cathedral and the dynamism of the Carceri de Piranesi. The library, suspended in air by a base that includes a circulation system, substituted Borges's labyrinth for the image of the Tower of Babel, a metaphor for the integration of universal knowledge.

From the 1960s onward, Testa abandoned Brutalist language and the principle of the autonomy of the "monument," which still continues in the marine shapes of the Central Naval Hospital (1970), in order to work with the multisignifying components of the urban context. Both the Cultural Center of the City of Buenos Aires (with Jacques Bedel and Luis Benedit 1979) and the Design Center in the Recoleta area (1990–93), integrate free forms and a strong chromatism within the preexisting historical

buildings, rescuing the open and unprejudiced discourse of contemporaneity. Simultaneously he was able to introduce in the shopping center's configuration aesthetic attributes similar to those existing in the neighboring Cultural Center. There emerges a constant assimilation of the particular qualities of the surroundings that generate an architectural response, the undulating coastal landscape of the seaside resort La Perla in Mar del Plata (1985–90) or the mimesis with the neighborhood's anonymity in the exterior treatment of the La Paz Sgiar Auditorium (1995–96) in the city of Buenos Aires, whose artistic and spatial values unfold in the interior areas.

In the 1970s he reflected the dark social climate created in Argentina by the military dictatorship and the increment in the contradictions inherent to modern urban life in a series of paintings entitled "The Plague in the City" and "The Plague in Ceppaloni," dramatized by the obsessive use of black and white. In the 1980s chromatism appears in the free forms that identify his artworks and architectural works. It is worth asserting that, despite the spatial and formal control that Testa exerted on his large-scale works—he also carried out urban projects through his participation in the competitions for Puerto Madero (1992), Retiro (1996), and the Acropolis Museum in Athens (1992)—the enigma, the humor, and the unpredictability of his artistic solutions also appear in his designs for smaller residences. This is where architecture, painting, sculpture, and design are unified in the freshness of an achieved poetic synthesis. The Capotesta houses (1983–85) and the Altera art gallery in Pinamar and La Tumbona in Ostende (1985–87) surface as colorful and geometric objets trouvés amid the marine scenery, characterized by the unexpected volumetric "deconstruction" of the original cubic forms. The antithetical dialogue with history reaches its maximum expression with the Ghirardo House in Martínez, Province of Buenos Aires (1992), a Tudor mansion from the 1920s that is penetrated by colorful metallic structures and internally hollowed out with diagonal sliding walls that greatly modify the traditional structure of compartmentalized spaces. Testa thus shows that individual creativity has no end and that the artist's dialogue with his environment implies a persistent rediscovery of the reality that daily surrounds him.

ROBERTO SEGRE

See also **Bank of London and South America, Buenos Aires; Brutalism; Buenos Aires, Argentina; Corbusier, Le (Jeanneret, Charles Édouard) (France); Deconstructivism; Supermodernism**

Biography

His father, an Italian immigrant living in Argentina, decided that Clorindo had to be born in Naples, (10 December 1923). Following the sentimental desire of his family, he never became an Argentine citizen. He returned in 1924 to Buenos Aires where he lived all of his life. After attempting to study naval engineering in La Plata and civil engineering in Buenos Aires, he started to study architecture in 1942 at the University of Buenos Aires, becoming an architect in 1947, and began to work in the Master Plan of Buenos Aires. There he met Ernesto N. Rogers, who had a strong influence on his architectural development. With a fellowship from the School of Architecture, he traveled in Europe between 1949 and 1952, devoting himself to painting more than architecture. As soon as he returned to Buenos Aires, he began his professional career associated with Dabinovic, Rossi and Gaido, and obtained the first prize for the Argentine in Chamber of Building Contractors (1952) and the Civic Center (government building) of Santa Rosa, La Pampa Province. Other buildings for this Center were designed in 1972 and 1981. In partnership with the SEPRA office (Sánchez Elia, Peralta Ramos, Agostini), they won the first prize for the construction of the Bank of London and South America Head Office in Buenos Aires (1959–66). Immediately, associated with Bullrich and Gazzaniga, he obtained the first prize in the competition for the National Library (1962), built between 1971 and 1995. In the early 1970s, he built the Central Naval Hospital (1970–83). In this period, he was mostly devoted to painting activities and obtained several prizes: Punta del Este Bienal, Uruguay (with the Team 5) (1957), Torcuato di Tella International Prize (1961), Second Latin America Kaiser Bienal, Córdoba (1965), Itamaratí Mayor Prize at the XIV São Paulo Bienal (1977), and the Trienal Prize "Architect of America," by FAPA (1987). In the last two decades he designed important buildings: Recoleta Cultural Center of the City of Buenos Aires (1979–80); La Perla beach complex (Mar del Plata, 1985–90), Buenos Aires Design Center (1990–93), and the Soka Gakkai International Auditorium in Buenos Aires (1993–96), nominated in the final selection of the First Mies van der Rohe Latin American Prize (1999). In 1976 he was included in the Buenos Aires Academy of Fine Arts and received a Doctorate Honoris Causa at the University of Buenos Aires (1992), and Honorary Professor at the Faculty of Architecture in Buenos Aires (1996). His paintings were shown in museums and galleries throughout the world, and in 1999 the Museum of Fine Arts in Buenos Aires devoted a complete exhibition to his main design production. In 2000 the Netherlands Institute of Architecture in Rotterdam presented his architectural works in Europe.

Further Reading

Bayón, Damián, and Paolo Gasparini, *The Changing Shape of Latin American Architecture: Conversations with Ten Leading Architects*, Chichester and New York: Wiley, 1979

Bullrich, Francisco, *New Directions in Latin American Architecture*, New York: George Braziller, 1969

Bullrich, Francisco, *Arquitectura Latinoamericana 1930–1970*, Barcelona: G. Gili, 1970

Cuadra, Manuel, and Alfonso Corona Martínez, *Clorindo Testa Architect*, Rotterdam: NAI, 2000

Glusberg, Jorge, *Architectes argentins*, Paris: Institut Français d'Architecture and Centro de Arte y Comunicación, 1980

Glusberg, Jorge, *Clorindo Testa. Pintor y arquitecto*, Buenos Aires: Summa⁺ Libros, 1999

Glusberg, Jorge, and Clorindo Testa, *Hacia una arquitectura topológica*, Buenos Aires: Espacio Editora, 1977

Gutiérrez, Ramón (Coord.), "Clorindo Testa," in *Arquitectura Latinoamericana en el Siglo XX*, Milan-Madrid: Jaca Book, Lunwerg, 1998

Koppmann, Ludovico C., "Clorindo Testa," in *Encyclopedia of Latin American & Caribbean Art*, edited by Jane Turner, London: Macmillan, 2000

Kultermann, Udo, "Clorindo Testa," in *Architekten der dritten Welt. Zwischen Tradition und Neubeginn*, Cologne: Du Mont, 1980

Liernur, Jorge Francisco, "Clorindo Testa: Ilinx," in *America Latina. Architettura, gli ultimi vent'anni*, Milan: Electa Editrice, 1990

Llinás, Julio, *Clorindo Testa*, Buenos Aires: Ediciones Culturales Argentinas, 1962

Segre, Roberto, *América Latina fin de milenio. Raíces y perspectivas de su arquitectura*, Havana: Editorial de Arte y Literatura, 1999

Segre, Roberto, and Rafael López Rangel, *Architettura e territorio nell'America Latina*, Milan: Electa Editrice, 1982

THE ARCHITECTS COLLABORATIVE (TAC) (UNITED STATES)

Formed in December 1945 by Walter Gropius and a number of graduates from the Harvard School of Design, The Architects Collaborative (TAC) was a firm whose output reflected some of the most cherished and derided aspects of postwar architectural design. TAC was a global firm, with offices and projects spanning the globe from Cambridge to Baghdad, and its legacy is predicated primarily on three intertwined elements: the collaborative and democratic principles that guided both the management of the firm and its designs, the prestige associated with Gropius, and the tremendous range (and size) of the firm's work.

In the tradition of the Bauhaus, Gropius and the other architects at TAC worked in collaborative groups headed by "job captains," resisting the postwar trend toward specialization and corporatization. Also in the Bauhaus tradition, the architects of TAC sought to align architecture with the disciplines of art, economics, and sociology. This effort, in theory, enabled architects to treat design as a social process, one responsive to the needs of individual patrons and sites. In the firm's later years, however, many critics argued that TAC simply designed the same solution to any number of different architectural problems, falling into a period of modernist repetition. Although TAC was founded on the notion of challenging the professional tradition of highly individualized firms or ateliers led by a single, famous master architect, in fact it was Gropius's name that was most often associated with the firm. If the anonymity behind the name The Architects Collaborative was supposed to deemphasize Gropius's role in the firm, it might have instead helped to keep TAC's other partners from sharing in both the praise and the criticism leveled at the firm. TAC, at various points, included Jean Fletcher, Norman Fletcher, John Harkness, Sarah Harkness, Robert McMillan, Louis McMillan, Benjamin Thompson, Richard Brooker, Alex Cvijanovic, Herbert Gallagher, William Geddis, Roland Kluver, Peter Morton, and H. Morse Payne, Jr., many of whom had attended the Graduate School of Design at Harvard University during Gropius's tenure there from 1937 to 1953. In 1963 TAC legally incorporated, becoming TAC, Inc.

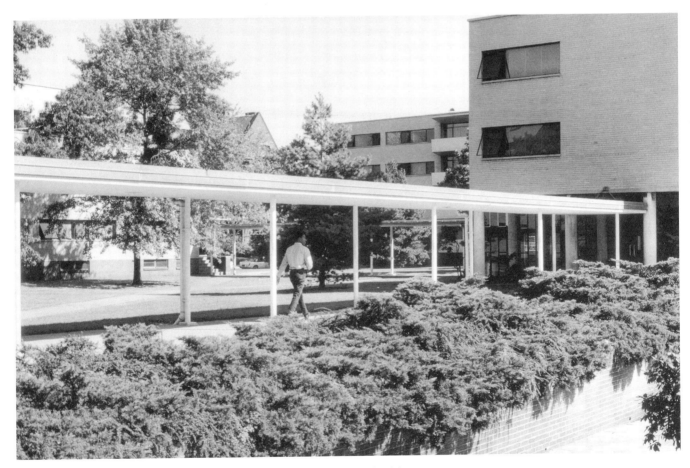

Harvard University Graduate Center, designed by Walter Gropius and TAC (1949)
© G.E. Kidder-Smith, Courtesy of Kidder Smith Collection, Rotch Visual Collections, M.I.T.

Important works from the firm's early years include the Six Moon Hill development (1948) in Lexington, Massachusetts. Eventually home to more than 30 families (and seven of the eight partners in TAC at the time), Six Moon Hill was planned along the standard (soon to become ubiquitous) suburban cul-de-sac road. However, the effort to leave large spaces open for communal use and its equal division of land prices and lot sizes make it an interesting early deviation from the broader trend of postwar suburban development. Perhaps the most famous project from the first 15 years of its history was TAC's design for the Harvard Graduate Center (1949) in Cambridge, Massachusetts. Located on a wedge-shaped lot near the northern edge of the Harvard University campus, the Graduate Center exemplified Gropius's (and, by extension, TAC's) own ambivalent feelings about the relationship between architecture and history. Although the Graduate Center took on the traditional form of the Harvard Yard or academic quad, the appearance of the individual buildings that made up the center seemed to have little to do with their surroundings. Another relevant project from this period was the U.S. Embassy (1956) in Athens, Greece, whose construction signaled the coming widescale adoption of modernism as the symbol of post–World War II American power and prosperity.

By the late 1950s, TAC had largely abandoned small-scale efforts along the lines of Six Moon Hill. Instead the firm became increasingly involved with large corporate commissions. The capitulation of social concerns to the requirements of the marketplace that such a move entailed are strikingly visible in the Pan Am Building (1963) in New York City, designed in collaboration with Emery Roth and Sons and Pietro Belluschi. With a record 2,350,000 square feet of rentable office space, 64 elevators, and 18 escalators, the building's size seemed to obliterate the spaces around it. Responses to the Pan Am Building were largely negative, and today it is for many an example of the worst aspects of an overly programmatic and formal modernist tradition. Critics attacked the building for destroying the historic vistas of Park Avenue and claimed that it destroyed the silhouette of the New York Central Building (Warren and Wetmore, 1929), reducing it to a mere shadow. Gropius seemed baffled by the criticism and responded that he thought that the New York Central Building should be torn down to provide the Pan Am Building with a proper forecourt. The public's refusal to embrace the objective and stylistically neutral design of the Pan Am Building puzzled Gropius, who seemed unable to comprehend the attachment that New Yorkers felt for older urban forms and spaces, an attachment that Gropius considered outdated and archaic.

Significant later commissions undertaken by TAC included the plan for Baghdad University (1958) in Iraq, construction of which was often interrupted because of political instability. The members of TAC had always considered involvement with education one of the defining characteristics of the firm, arguing that sensitive design was an integral element of the learning process. Efforts such as Baghdad University, however, seemed at best a pale effort to incorporate faux regional design elements (in this case Islamic ones) onto a standard steel-framed concrete box. Despite such missteps in 1964 TAC received the Firm Award of the American Institute of Architects (AIA). Eight years later TAC designed the national headquarters of the AIA (Wash-

ington, D.C.). TAC also contributed to the massive Boston development known as Government Center with the design for the JFK Federal Office Building in 1968.

The demise of the firm was precipitated by the death of Gropius in 1969 and the rising influence of Postmodernism in the architectural profession and among the public. Although the reputation of TAC was still quite solid abroad (particularly in the Middle East), in the last two decades of its existence the firm seemed to flounder without the guiding and unifying influence of Gropius. Seemingly unable to adapt or respond to the changing milieu of the architectural world, fewer commissions came to the firm, and for financial reasons the doors finally closed at TAC in 1996.

BENJY FLOWERS

See also **American Institute of Architects; Gropius, Walter (Germany)**

Biography

Established in Cambridge, Massachusetts 1945 by Walter Gropius, Norman Collings Fletcher, Jean Fletcher, John Cheeseman Harkness, Sarah Pillsbury Harkness, Robert Senseman MacMillan, Louis Albert McMillan, and Benjamin Thompson. The Architects Collaborative International was founded in 1960 and dissolved in 1996.

Selected Works

Six Moon Hill, Lexington, Massachusetts, 1948
Harvard University Graduate Center, Cambridge, Massachusetts, 1949
United States Embassy, Athens, 1956
University of Baghdad, 1958
Pan Am Building (consultant architects), New York, 1963
Kennedy Federal Building, Government Center, Boston, 1968
TAC Headquarters, Cambridge, Massachusetts, 1970
American Institute of Architects Headquarters, Washington, D.C., 1973
Bauhaus Archive, Berlin, 1979

Selected Publications

Town Plan for the Development of Self, 1970
A Design Manual for Parking Garages, 1975
Streets: A Program to Develop Awareness of the Street Environment, 1976
Building without Barriers for the Disabled, 1976

Further Reading

Much of the writing about TAC is found in texts largely concerned with Walter Gropius and his career.

"The Architects Collaborative: The Heritage of Walter Gropius," *Process Architecture* 19 (1980)
Giedion, Sigfried, *Walter Gropius: Work and Teamwork,* New York: Reinhold, 1954
Gropius, Walter (editor), *The Architects Collaborative, 1945–1965,* New York: Architectural Book, and London: Tiranti, 1966
Herdeg, Klaus, *The Decorated Diagram: Harvard Architecture and the Failure of the Bauhaus Legacy,* Cambridge, Massachusetts: MIT Press, 1983
McKee, Bradford, "TAC's Demise," *Architecture* 84/12 (1995)

Nerdinger, Winfried, "From Bauhaus to Harvard: Walter Gropius and the Use of History," in *The History of History in American Schools of Architecture, 1865–1975*, edited by Gwendolyn Wright and Janet Parks, New York: The Temple Hoyne Buell Center for the Study of American Architecture and Princeton Architectural Press, 1990

TIMBER FRAME

Timber framing, although largely outmoded by the beginning of the 20th century, not only persevered in its centuries-old, low-technology form but developed as well into high-technology structural systems. Aside from its universal aesthetic appeal, timber construction—eclipsed by steel, concrete, and lightweight wood framing—maintained interest among architects, owners, and builders because of its economy, durability, and ecology.

In the United States, timber framing refers to traditional post-and-beam construction (known as "heavy timber" at the industrial scale). Internationally, however, descriptions of timber-frame buildings often include lightweight wood-stud construction. This discussion considers only the heavier construction—whose columns are usually at least 8 inches by 8 inches, with beams no less than 6 inches by 10 inches—where significant advances were made throughout the past 100 years.

In regions with ready access to timber, vernacular styles of framing with various in-fill materials had become established over the centuries. In Europe and England, timber frames with brick, rubble, or wattle-and-daub walls were ubiquitous. In North America colonial buildings often were clad in wood as well as brick. In tropical Asia and the Pacific islands, wood or other native materials served as sheathing. Japan and China had long traditions of timber temples, palaces, and houses.

Architects of the 20th century working with timber frequently drew on those vernacular references for their own work. At Hvitträsk (1902) near Helsinki, Finland, a housing-studio compound that Eliel Saarinen (1873–1950), Herman Gesellius (1874–1916), and Armas Lindgren (1874–1929) designed for their own use, the architects adapted their country's rustic tradition to create what became known as the National Romantic style.

The English Arts and Crafts movement of the late 19th century continued to influence architects well into the 20th century. Timber was just one of the natural materials used by proponents of the movement. In the United States, California, with its abundance of timber and increasing affluence, generated several timber styles. In the United States, the brothers Charles Sumner Greene (1868–1957) and Henry Mather Greene (1870–1954) ushered in a golden age of timber design with a widely admired series of houses near Los Angeles. Influenced by Japanese and Swiss vernacular timber craft, their Gamble House (1908) in Pasadena may have been the apotheosis of 20th-century timber houses. This sprawling masterpiece revealed the architects' obsessive attention to finishing each exposed structural timber, articulating every handcrafted joint, and specifying the finest wood finishes.

Many architects who worked mostly in other materials used timber to great effect in combination with those materials. The San Francisco Bay Area's most prominent architect, Bernard Maybeck (1882–1957), accented the interior of the First Church of Christ Scientist (1910) in Berkeley, California, with massive decorative timberwork; in his own studio (1924) in Berkeley, the innovative Maybeck used timber framing but added an experimental concrete finish.

In Europe, Austrian architect Adolf Loos (1870–1933) included exposed timber in his Steiner House (1910) in Vienna and, more heavily, in the rustic Khuner Villa (1930) near Payerback, Austria. The modernist Serge Chermayeff (1900–96) designed his house Bentley Wood (1938) in Sussex, England, in timber and brick, an unusual choice for an English country house at that time, which typically would have been all masonry.

Tree heights determined timber spans, and the largest timbers became scarcer as the oldest trees were harvested. Even while steel and concrete increased in popularity, the economy of wood—plentiful and easy to erect—encouraged technological development of timber for increasingly demanding structural purposes. Maybeck had experimented with a timber arch of smaller pieces of wood strapped together. However, not until engineers applied the technology of plywood—an early 20th-century innovation whereby wood veneers were glued together to form a monolithic panel—to heavy timbers did wood become reestablished as a competitive structural component. Relatively small sections of solid timber were laminated together with special glues into one large structural member called a glu-lam (glued-laminated timber).

The economy of laminated timber widened its appeal during the Great Depression of the 1930s. The shortage of steel for buildings during World War II further encouraged the use of timber in structures such as hangars and other utilitarian buildings.

Assembled for beauty as well as structural predictability, glu-lam beams, girders, columns, and trusses began to appear prominently in low-rise, long-span structures, such as buildings for worship, auditoriums, exhibition halls, sports arenas, and recreational buildings. The fact that engineered timber could be pre-bent and custom shaped allowed architects to create dramatic arches, domes, and organic sculptural effects beyond the capabilities of natural timber. Later technologies introduced high-tech connectors to enhance the wood's strength.

In Japan, whose vernacular architecture inspired the Greene brothers and Frank Lloyd Wright, among many others, architects after World War II embraced concrete as their material of choice, yet some evoked natural beauty with occasional spare, timber-frame houses and other small structures. More ambitious was the elegantly spiraling timber-roof structure of the Puppet Theater (1992) in Seiwa, Japan, by Katsuhiro Ishii (b. 1944).

In Finland, a land of ubiquitous timber resources, Heikki Siren (b. 1918) and Kaija Siren (b. 1920) made their mark with the asymmetrical timber trusses at Otaniemi Technical University Chapel (1959, burned 1975) near Helsinki. Other Finnish architects experimented with multistory timber-frame apartment houses during the 1990s. Architects who used the sculptural potential of laminated timber included the Hungarian Imre Makovecz (b. 1935), whose organic buildings included the Farkasret funeral chapel (1977) in Budapest.

Late-century forays with traditional framing into public spaces included Hugh Boyd's 37,000-square-foot Public Market (1998) in Portland, Maine, whose concrete columns carry the largest traditional timber roof in New England. The natural

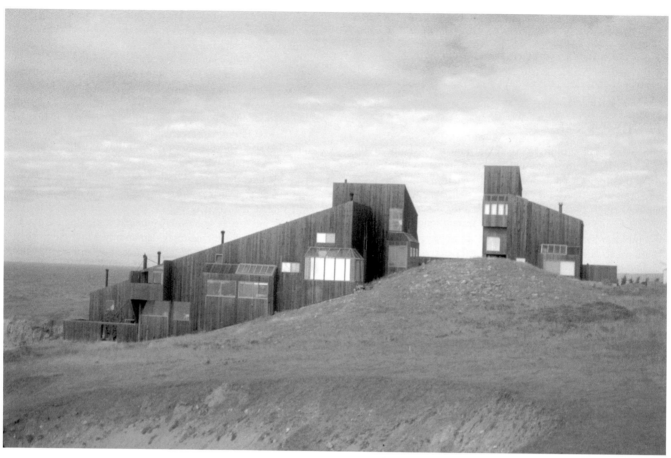

Sea Ranch Condominium, Sea Ranch, California (1964–65), designed by MLTW (Moore, Lyndon, Turnbull and Whitaker)
© GreatBuildings.com

timber beams span up to 40 feet in length. In contrast, the new Globe Theatre (1998) in London re-created the mortise-and-tenon oak timber craft of Shakespearean England, but this time around the wood cladding was treated for fire resistance.

During the 1990s European researchers pioneered the use of timber for new commercial buildings and multistory apartment houses. The British group Timber Research and Development Associates (TRADA) notably included a six-story timber structure (1997) in a testing facility alongside concrete-and-steel structures. Such experiments promised a future for timber framing in building types where fire or structural limitations typically limited its use.

During the last quarter of the century, producers in the United States of off-the-shelf timber components and designs developed a healthy market for "do-it-yourself" timber-frame house kits and even rustic log homes. The affordable option of a timber-frame house enhanced the awareness of this traditional construction type among the general public.

By century's end the conversion of heavy-timber warehouses and other industrial buildings to new uses had become routine in many cities. The resulting lofts with offices, residential spaces,

entertainment venues, and shopping malls popularized a timber-and-masonry aesthetic among urban residents, businesses, and tourists in search of open, flexible spaces with a historic character. These recycled buildings also won favor with proponents of sustainable architecture.

With the focus on sustainable environments and renewable resources, new timber construction qualified as alternative, so-called "green" architecture, as long as the material was harvested from carefully managed forests. While environmental crusades curbed the use of old-growth timber from dwindling ancient forests, ecologically conscious architects and builders turned to timber from managed sources.

By the end of the century, traditional timber was used in combination with efficient new building materials, such as structural insulated panels, and even in composite applications where steel or concrete was integrated with the wood structure.

RANDALL J. VAN VYNCKT

See also **Arts and Crafts Movement; Greene, Henry M. and Charles S. (United States); Loos, Adolf (Austria); Maybeck, Bernard R. (United States); Saarinen, Eliel (Finland);**

Steiner House, Vienna; Sustainability and Sustainable Architecture

TOKYO, JAPAN

In the course of only one century, Tokyo has evolved from a city trying to imitate Western centers to a major metropolis and a center of high-quality architecture. The architectural design work and the theories of contemporary Japanese architects, most of them based in Tokyo, have found interest worldwide. Their projects often reflect the specific architecture and context of Japanese cities, particularly its capital.

Tokyo's urban landscape is characterized by a juxtaposition of high-rise modern business districts and high-density, mixed-function neighborhoods composed mainly of wooden single-family buildings, resembling Asian more than European cities. The nongeometric organization, the multitude of centers, and the cellular addition of neighborhoods have been handed down from Edo, as the city was called before the Meiji Restoration of 1868. The urban layout of the Edo period—its patchwork of extended areas for the warrior class on the *yamanote* highlands and the low-lying *shitamachi* areas, which housed the ordinary people—provided an ideal background for the integration of new functions related to the modernization of the country. The spacious lots and extended green spaces of the daimyo areas permitted the realization of large-scale developments and buildings, such as the government area at Hibiya and the Marunouchi district in the vicinity of the Imperial Palace and Fumihiko Maki's comprehensive design of Hillside Terrace (1969–92).

In contrast to European cities, where buildings often define public places, the liveliest spaces in Tokyo are not given particular architectural form. Infrastructure nodes, such as Shibuya or Ikebukuro on the Yamanote railway ring, are social spaces characterized by a maze of billboards, huge screens, multilevel infrastructure, and a large variety of commercial buildings. Buildings of different scale, height, and age, designed without any concern for aesthetic unity, stand next to one another. The 109 Building (1978) by Minoru Takeyama, with its tall, aluminum-clad tower, exemplifies commercial architecture in Tokyo. A marker in the billboard environment, its facade and layout had to take into account a small wooden restaurant because its owner did not want to sell.

The absence of aesthetic and height control in Tokyo buildings is not a recent development. In 1937, Bruno Taut, in his *Houses and People of Japan*, criticized the chaos of forms and styles, and other westerners have done the same. Recently, this attitude has started to change: Yoshinobu Ashihara and other writers view Tokyo as the urban model for the 21st century, considering the city as the evocation of such recent ideas as chaos theory. Tokyo's architects have made the chaotic urban landscape a central design theme. Maki's Spiral Building (1985), with its collaged and fragmented facade, reflects this, as does Kazuo Shinohara's Centennial Hall (1987) for the Tokyo Institute of Technology.

The reasons for the chaotic appearance of Tokyo are manifold. Tokyo, a wooden city, has been destroyed by fires and earthquakes regularly. In the 20th century alone, the city saw devastation twice in the Great Kanto Earthquake (1923) and

the large-scale bombing in World War II. The city has a tradition of rebuilding, and few old constructions remain. Buildings of the Meiji period (1868–1912) are becoming rare, and major works of postwar modern architecture, including Kenzo Tange's Tokyo City Hall (1957) and Kunio Maekawa's Harumi Apartments (1958), have been demolished. Even Toyo Ito's well-published Nomad Restaurant (1986) disappeared as early as 1990. The permanent threat of another major earthquake, the need to meet recently enacted legal requirements, and high land prices that dwarf construction costs further explain the relative freedom of architecture.

Early Meiji Architecture

When Japan opened its gates to the outside world, it did not have a tradition of monumental public architecture, vistas, and high-rise landmarks comparable with that of major European metropolises. The traditional Japanese prints (*ukiyo-e*) show that natural features in the city's vicinity, such as Mount Fuji, gave a feeling of place. Furthermore, the city did not have a monumental public core: the center was and is occupied by the Imperial Palace and its huge gardens, which are closed to the public.

In the early Meiji period, under the influence of the government, Tokyo became the showcase for the rapid transformation of Japan. The Tsukiji Hotel (1868) and the first Mitsui Bank (1872) by Kisuke Shimizu II illustrate early Meiji attempts to adopt Western (European and American) forms. They were crowned by towers (novelties in Japan) but were not part of the cityscape in the same way as their European counterparts. The buildings were separated from public space through gates and walls, as in traditional daimyo residences. It took years until Japanese architects started to use buildings as public monuments. Even now, vertical markers, such as the Tokyo Tower (1958), do not have the same symbolic value as their Western models. The creation of landmark buildings in Tokyo remains an important topic, taken up particularly by Maki.

Foreign architects, surveyors, or amateurs created many of the early Meiji buildings: an Englishman, Thomas Waters, designed the urban outlay and the brick buildings of the Ginza after a fire in 1872. The Berlin office of Böckmann and Ende projected the Ministry of Justice (1895) and Supreme Court (1896) buildings. A central figure among these foreigners was the English architect Josiah Conder (1852–1920). Author of numerous important buildings, including the Rokumeikan (1883), a government guest house, he was also a professor at the newly founded Tokyo Imperial University, predecessor of the University of Tokyo, where he introduced Western educational concepts.

The first generation of Japanese architects in Tokyo, many of whom had studied with Conder, realized a number of eclectic buildings that include Kingo Tatsuno's Bank of Japan (1896) and his Tokyo Station (1914) as well as the Akasaka Detached Palace (1909) by Tokuma Katayama and the Hyokeikan Museum (1909) in Ueno. By the end of the Meiji period, after two victorious wars, Japan had established itself as a powerful modern state, and Tokyo's architecture was exported to the colonies.

The most recent architectural styles were adopted quickly in Tokyo and other Japanese cities, as the country strove for international recognition. In contrast to colonial situations, tra-

ditional forms were not suppressed. When the need arose in Nara to integrate new large-scale buildings into a traditional setting, a modern Japanese style developed that combined the new scale and function with traditional forms and an overall Japanese look, particularly in the design of the roof and the entrance space. This modern Japanese style quickly spread to Tokyo. The memorial (1930) for the victims of the 1923 earthquake in the form of a pagoda by Chuta Ito and the New Kabuki Theater (1924) by Shinichiro Okada exemplify the combination of new building techniques and materials with traditional forms. Other examples show the adoption of Western style in the facade and the business spaces and the maintenance of traditional spaces for the living areas. The least Western influence occurred in the field of urban planning, as the strong attachment to the land and the scattered character of land ownership hindered redevelopment.

"Modern Style" Architecture in Japan

The start of modern architecture in Japan largely coincided with the presence of Frank Lloyd Wright and the construction of the Imperial Hotel (1923–69, dismantled) in Tokyo, one of the city's best-known buildings because of its size and the name of its architect. The fact that it withstood the Great Kanto Earthquake on the day of its opening further contributed to its fame, even though the "Marubiru" office building (1923), built by the Fuller Company in the Marunouchi district, and other major constructions also withstood the quake. Modern architecture was still rare in Japan at that time, and some of the earliest works, including the Reinanzaka House (1923–24) in Azabu, were produced by Antonin Raymond, a former collaborator with Wright at the Imperial Hotel.

The rapid reconstruction after the 1923 earthquake reinforced the functionalist trends: street widening and replotting took precedence over urban design, and modernist principles were used for public buildings. Examples are Tetsuro Yoshida's Tokyo Central Post Office (1927–31) and several public schools designed by the architectural department of the Tokyo Municipality, including the Yotsuya Fifth Primary School (1934) and the Takanawadai Primary School (1935). Social housing became another field for rationalist design. A nonprofit government foundation, the Dojunkai, was created in 1924 to provide temporary structures for quake relief. It continued to function afterward and provided the city with 2501 ferroconcrete apartment units in 15 new developments between 1926 and 1933. The Aoyama apartments (1926) and some others remain functional today. Many, including the Daikanyama complex (1926), have been demolished for higher-density reconstruction.

Many Japanese architects of the 1910s and 1920s were influenced by German Expressionism and the Viennese Secession. Kikuji Ishimoto's Secessionist-style Asahi Newspaper Offices (1927) at Sukiyabashi was demolished, but Shozo Uchida's Yasuda Hall (1925) at the Imperial University of Tokyo, Hongo, survives as a good example of the North German Expressionist inspiration. The Secessionist Architectural Society (Bunri Ha Kenchiku Kai; 1920–28), founded by six Japanese architects, was a cradle for modernist architecture. Two of its members, Sutemi Horiguchi and Mamoru Yamada, later became major representatives of the International Style. Horiguchi was ac-

knowledged particularly for the Okada Residence (1934), which elegantly integrates traditional Japanese elements and modern Western concepts. Yamada, author of the Expressionist Central Telegraph Office (1925), was the only Japanese architect to have a building—the Electrical Laboratory (1930)—included in the 1932 International Style exhibition of the Museum of Modern Art in New York, marking the entry of Japanese modern architecture on the global scene. Both returned to more traditional forms later, as shown in Horiguchi's Sukiya-style teahouse (1965) in the Minato ward and Yamada's Nippon Budokan (1964), a hall for judo competition with an octagonal pyramidal roof that reinterprets traditional Japanese forms.

Tokyo's architects had intimate contacts with leading modernist designers abroad. Kikuji Ishimoto, a student of Walter Gropius, produced the Shirokiya Department Store (1931) and the Tokyo Airport Office (1932), which reflect his knowledge of works by Erich Mendelsohn and the Bauhaus. Bunzo Yamaguchi worked with Gropius between 1930 and 1932 and, after his Expressionist phase, produced several modernist works in the Tokyo area, such as the Yamada House (1934) in Kita-Kamakura, the Nihon Dental College Hospital (1934), and the Bancho Siedlung (1933), which recalls the Weissenhofsiedlung (1927). Junzo Sakakura and Kunio Maekawa, who studied with Le Corbusier, also realized major works in Tokyo.

In the mid-1930s, the so-called Imperial Crown style (*teikan yoshiki*) became the symbol of Japanese nationalism. The term was developed in the context of the competition for the Imperial Diet Building (1917–19). Although the prize-winning entry was not realized, the term relates to buildings that feature huge Japanese-style roofs, such as Ryoichi Kawamoto's Soldiers' Hall (1934) and Hitoshi (Jin) Watanabe's Imperial Museum (1937) in Ueno and Dai-ichi Seimei Building (1938), used as general headquarters of the American command after World War II.

Architecture in Tokyo after World War II

Tokyo suffered major destruction in the Allied bombings, particularly through fire: 92,778 persons were killed, 129,300 were injured, and 850,000 lost their homes. The reconstruction of the capital symbolized Japan's renewal and revival and was expressed in modernist architecture. Raymond's Reader's Digest Building (1951, demolished 1964) and Sakakura's Prefectural Museum of Modern Art (1951, addition 1966) in Kamakura are major examples. However, the main figures of postwar reconstruction were Tange and Maekawa.

Tange, who had won international recognition with his Hiroshima Peace Center, designed major buildings in Tokyo, including the Tokyo City Hall (1957) and the Tokyo Metropolitan Government Building (1991) in Shinjuku. His Olympic Stadiums (1964), with their suspended roofs, have landmark character and symbolize the major urban transformations of that period.

Maekawa authored several buildings in Tokyo's Ueno Park, including the Metropolitan Festival Hall (1961), a huge cultural center with a powerful protruding roof of exposed concrete; the Tokyo Municipal Museum of Art (1975); and the addition to Le Corbusier's Museum of Western Art (1979). Other architects of roughly the same generation who were influential and revered designers and teachers in Tokyo are Isoya Yoshida, Yoshiro Tani-

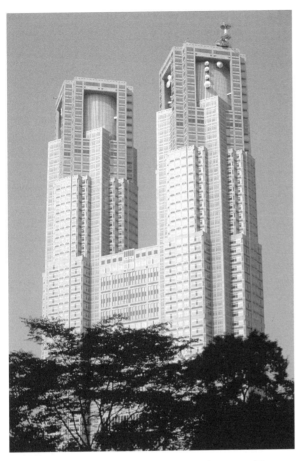

Tokyo City Hall (1957) Shinjuku district, by Kenzo Tange
© Michael S. Yamashita/CORBIS

guchi, Hiroshi Oe, and Togo Murano. Their works drew on a larger range of historical and modern forms and have still to be fully acknowledged in the West.

The economic boom of the 1960s provoked rapid urbanization and overcrowding in Tokyo and other Japanese cities. Confronted with the scarcity of land and carried by their belief in continuing technical and economic development, several visionary projects for Tokyo were developed that suggested extension onto the sea and into the air. Tange's project for a city axis (1960) extending over Tokyo Bay reflected visionary ideas sketched by Kiyonori Kikutake as early as 1958. Several young designers, some of whom had been working on the Tange project, took up these ideas, designing megastructures such as Arata Isozaki's Sky Cities (1961 and 1962), Kisho Kurokawa's Helix City Plan (1961), and Kikutake's Ocean City (1961) and Marine City (1963). These projects were often presented as suggestions for Tokyo, thereby further promoting the capital. Its name was already connected to the emergence of the Metabolist movement at the World Design Conference of 1960.

Several buildings reflecting Metabolist ideas were realized in Tokyo, including the Shizuoka Press and Broadcasting Center (1966–67) by Tange, the Nakagin Capsule Building (1972) by Kurokawa, and later, Kikutake's Edo-Tokyo Museum (1992). No visionary cities were realized, but they prefigured and paral-

leled major transformations of the city at that time: the construction of huge highways and high-speed trains, land reclamation and the extension of the city on artificial islands, and the construction of huge underground passageways and structures, particularly around the stations, are the real megastructures of the city. However, the design of these developments was in the hands mainly of the major construction companies rather than the visionary architects.

The concentration of people and economy in the large centers was reinforced when the traditional height limitation of 31 meters was replaced by a system of floor ratio in the 1961 Building Standards Law. The first skyscraper, the 36-floor Kasumigaseki Building by Yamashita architects and engineers, was completed in 1968. Further skyscrapers rose in the Shinjuku subcenter on the site of a former water purification plant to the west of the station on the Yamanote railway. Based on a development plan from 1960, a skyscraper district came into existence, starting with the Keio Plaza Hotel (1971). Major buildings are the NS-Building (1982) by Nikken Sekkei and the Postmodern Tokyo Metropolitan Government Building (1991) by Tange, which displays two cathedral-like towers and a huge public plaza embraced by wing buildings and the assembly hall.

The most pressing issue for the steadily growing city remained housing. Various policies for decentralization were instigated that led to the creation of new towns, such as the research and university city of Tsukuba outside Tokyo, known for its Center Building (1983) designed by Arata Isozaki. The creation of Tama New Town to the west of Tokyo included the relocation of the Tokyo Metropolitan University, which features several Postmodernist buildings (1991) by Teiichi Takahashi and Daiichi-Kobo.

The negative effects of economic development, including the chaotic landscape of Japanese cities, became obvious in the 1970s, and contemporary architecture responded to this environment in various ways. Toyo Ito's U-shaped House (1976) in Nakano Honcho and Kikoo Mozuna's Mirror Image Hall (1980) mark an introverted attitude, concentrating on the interior space and turning nearly closed facades to the outside. Kazuhiro Ishii's House of 54 Windows (1975) and Takefumi Aida's Toy Bloc Houses of the early 1980s show a more playful response.

High real estate prices and limited sites made it increasingly difficult for people to live in the city. Takamitsu Azuma's Tower House (1967) expresses the difficulties of inner-city private housing: on a basic floor space of 10 square meters, it offers an overall living space of 60 square meters. The lack of buildable land brought about inspiring projects for housing several generations of one family on the same site. Tadao Ando's Kidosaki House (1986) and Riken Yamamoto's Hamlet (1988) demonstrate the possibility of housing three generations in one building complex. Kazuo Shinohara's House under High Voltage Lines (1981) expresses the necessity to use every single site in densely built Tokyo, and Kunihiko Hayakawa's Yoga-A-Flat (1993) addresses the growing diversity of housing needs. Recent small-scale projects, such as Shigeru Ban's Curtain Wall House (1995) and Itsuko Hasegawa's Sumida Culture Factory (1995), illustrate the growing understanding of Tokyo's neighborhoods as a positive life environment.

The land boom of the 1980s paved the ground for expensive and eccentric structures. Shin Takamatsu's machinelike Ima-

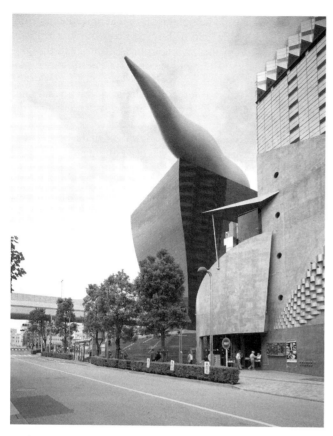

Asahi Beer Hall and Brewery (1989), designed by Philippe Starck
© Angelo Hornak/CORBIS

waterfront of Tokyo Bay: Yokohama started to build Minato Mirai 21 in 1985, and Chiba is developing Makuhari New Town, which features a housing development characterized by strict planning legislation, a rarity in Japan.

Some large-scale interventions have been carried out despite the recession, such as the Tokyo University Komaba Campus redevelopment (1999) by Hiroshi Hara. Further development proposals and futuristic plans are projected for Tokyo, such as sky cities and developments in Tokyo Bay, by Kisho Kurokawa, Shin Takamatsu, and the Shimizu and Takenaka corporations. At the dawn of the 21st century, discussion about relocating the capital city continues.

CAROLA HEIN

See also **Ando, Tadao (Japan); Hasegawa Itsuko (Japan); Kurokawa, Kisho (Japan); Maki, Fumihiko (Japan); Metabolists; Shinohara, Kazuo (Japan); Tange, Kenzo (Japan); Taniguchi, Yoshio (Japan)**

Further Reading

Few books discuss solely the architectural history of Tokyo. Most publications on Japan, however, give a major space to the capital city. Stewart provides the most comprehensive account of modern architecture in Tokyo from the Meiji period to the present. The studies by Fujimori and Inagaki limit themselves to the period from Meiji to 1945. The work by Suzuki, Banham, and Kobayashi is a richly illustrated overview of contemporary architecture in Japan from the postwar period to the 1980s. Bognar discusses the 1980s and 1990s in particular. Yatsuka examines Japanese architectural history in its international context.

Ashihara, Yoshinobu, *The Hidden Order: Tokyo through the Twentieth Century*, Tokyo and New York: Kodansha International, 1989

Berque, Augustin (editor), *La Qualité de la ville: Urbanité française, urbanité nippone*, Tokyo: Maison Franco-Japonaise, 1987

Bognar, Botond, *The Japan Guide*, New York: Princeton Architectural Press, 1995

Bognar, Botond, *Tokyo*, Chichester, West Sussex: Academy Editions, 1997

Cybriwsky, Roman, *Tokyo: The Changing Profile of an Urban Giant*, London: Belhaven, and Boston: G.K. Hall, 1991

Friedman, Mildred (editor), *Tokyo: Form and Spirit*, Minneapolis, Minnesota: Walker Art Center, and New York: Abrams, 1986

Fujimori, Terunobu, *Nihon no kindai kenchiku*, 2 vols., Tokyo: Iwanami Shôten, 1993

Hatsuda, Tôru, et al., *Kindai wafu kenchiku: Dento o koeta sekai*, 2 vols., Tokyo: Kenchiku Chishiki, 1998

Hein, Carola, "Koban in Tokyo: Urban Culture or Trendy Extras?" *Archis*, 8 (1996)

Inagaki, Eizô, *Nihon no kindai kenchiku*, 2 vols., Tokyo: Kajima Shuppankai, 1979

Ishida, Yorifusa, *Tokyo: Urban Growth and Planning, 1868–1988*, Tokyo: Center for Urban Studies, Tokyo Metropolitan University, 1988

"Japan: A Dis-Oriented Modernity," *Casabella*, 608–09 (January–February 1994)

Japan Architect (Summer 1991)

Jinnai, Hidenobu, *Tokyo no kukan jinruigaku*, Tokyo: Chikuma Shobo, 1985; as *Tokyo: A Spatial Anthropology*, translated by Kimiko Nishimura, Berkeley: University of California Press, 1994

Masai, Yasuo, *Atlas Tokyo: Edo/Tokyo through Maps*, Tokyo: Heibonsha, 1986

nishi Motoakasaka Building (1992) and his mainly subterranean Earthtecture (1990), Atsushi Kitagawara's theatrical Rise Cinema Complex (1986), Makoto Sei Watanabe's Aoyama Technical College (1990), Itsuko Hasegawa's futuristic and vernacular design of the Shonandai Cultural Center (1991), and the commercial Collezione (1990) of the Osaka-based architect Tadao Ando became possible during this period. Young emerging architects of the 1990s were given chances to prove themselves in small-scale structures, such as Kazuyo Sejima's Chofu police station (1994). Simultaneously, international architects, including Mario Bellini, Mario Botta, Branson Coates, Peter Eisenman, Norman Foster, Steven Holl, Richard Rogers, and Aldo Rossi, were called on to create landmark buildings, with Philippe Starck's Asahi Beer Hall (1989) being the most visible. The list of Tokyo's grand projects is crowned by Rafael Viñoly's Tokyo International Forum (1996), one of the unique designs in Japan to result from an international competition.

When the economic boom ended, the construction of many large-scale projects was postponed or abandoned. The 1996 Tokyo Frontier World Cities Expo, which was supposed to explore possibilities for the city of the 21st century, was ultimately canceled. In the same waterfront area, the smaller-scale Tokyo Teleport Town, initiated in 1987 as a new subcenter, is taking shape in reduced form. Tange's Fuji Television Building (1997) is one of its most visible markers. The Tokyo waterfront project faces competition from two other major developments on the

Nagao, Shigetake, *The Architect's Guide to Tokyo*, Tokyo: Maruzen, 1996

Popham, Peter, *Tokyo: The City at the End of the World*, Tokyo and New York: Kodansha International, 1985

Reynolds, Jonathon, "Japan's Imperial Diet Building: Debate over Construction of a National Identity," *Art Journal* (Fall 1996)

Ritchie, Donald, *Introducing Tokyo*, Tokyo and New York: Kodansha International, 1987

Seidensticker, Edward, *Low City, High City: Tokyo from Edo to the Earthquake*, London: Allen Lane, and New York: Knopf, 1983

Seidensticker, Edward, *Tokyo Rising: The City since the Great Earthquake*, New York: Knopf, 1990

Speidel, Manfred (editor), *Japanische Architektur: Geschichte und Gegenwart*, Dusseldorf, Germany: Akademie der Architektenkammer Nordrhein-Westfalen, and Stuttgart, Germany: Hatje, 1983

Stewart, David B., *The Making of a Modern Japanese Architecture: 1868 to the Present*, Tokyo and New York: Kodansha International, 1987

Suzuki, Hiroyuki, Reyner Banham, and Katsuhiro Kobayashi, *Contemporary Architecture of Japan, 1958–1984*, London: Architectural Press, and New York: Rizzoli, 1985

Suzuki, Hiroyuki, *Tokyo no "geniusu roki,"* Tokyo: Bungei Shunju, 1990

Tajima, Noriyuki, *Tokyo: A Guide to Recent Architecture*, London: Ellipsis, 1995; New York: Ellipsis Könemann, 1996

Taut, Bruno, *Houses and People of Japan*, Tokyo: Sanseido, 1937

Tokyo: La ville moderne, Tokyo: Museum of Contemporary Art, 1996

Waley, Paul, *Tokyo Now and Then: An Explorer's Guide*, New York: Weatherhill, 1984

Watanabe, Hiroshi, *The Architecture of Tokyo: An Architectural History in 571 Individual Presentations*, Stuttgart, Germany: Edition Axel Menges, 2001

Yatsuka, Hajime, "Internationalism versus Regionalism," in *At the End of the Century*, edited by Richard Koschalek and Elizabeth A.T. Smith, Los Angeles: Museum of Contemporary Art, 1998

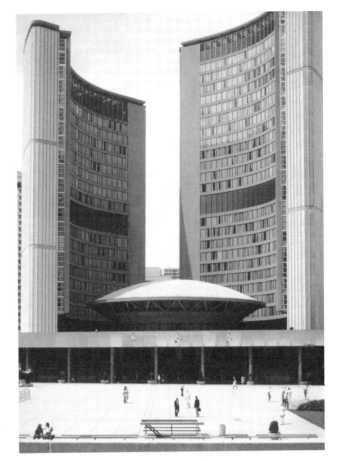

New City Hall, Nathan Phillips Square, Toronto
Photo © Mary Ann Sullivan

TORONTO CITY HALL

Designed by Viljo Revell, completed 1965
Toronto, Ontario

In November 1961 sod was first turned to construct a new city hall, the design of Viljo Revell (1910–64) and the result of the most significant architectural competition in Canadian history. Revell did not live to see his design completed, but its impact continues to shape the evolving character of the city of Toronto to this day. In its evocative fusion of the unfettered reexamination of function and material characteristic of the International Style, with a poised expressionism capable of imparting symbolic presence, New City Hall dramatically broadened the resonant potential of modern architecture to its citizenry. Even more, the design for its accompanying civic square provided Torontonians with a new paradigm for both inhabiting and imagining their unfolding city.

The apparent origin of this fortuitous event lay in a proposal submitted to the city in 1911. John Lyle, a local architect who had trained at the École des Beaux-Arts, envisioned a City Beautiful scheme that included a civic square adjacent to E. J. Lennox's Richardsonian Romanesque city hall (1899). Subsequent proposals for this site followed regularly, but it was not until

1946, with the anticipation of a postwar development boom, that public acquisition of the land was approved by a plebiscite. It was another five years before the city council agreed to build a new city hall, giving the commission to a triumvirate of well-connected and stylistically conservative firms. The subsequent design was met with criticism from members of the city's arts community, who saw in the design a symbol of an "old guard" that had resisted for decades the influence of modernism on painting and sculpture as well as on architecture. Once local papers gave voice to these arguments, public opinion went against the proposal, and it was defeated in a second plebiscite, although yet another vote subsequently reinstated the public's desire for a new building.

Facing possible lawsuits if a fourth architect were hired, Mayor Nathan Philips instead opted for a plan put forward by Eric Arthur, an activist on the faculty of the University of Toronto's School of Architecture. Arthur organized an international competition, with a jury that included Ernesto Rogers, William Holford, and Eero Saarinen. The response saw more than 500 entries, complete with models, from 42 countries. Finnish architect Viljo Revell's winning proposal featured a pair of slender, concave towers, each visibly accommodating one of two tiers of local government. These wings in turn cradled a saucerlike council chamber, all atop a broad, two-story podium.

Revell opened a Toronto office in April 1959 in association with John B. Parkin Partnership. Parkin was a committed modernist who would soon join with Mies van der Rohe in realizing Mies' final, and arguably finest, tower complex, the Toronto-Dominion Centre (1969). Revell and Parkin spent the next two years refining the design and experimenting with details that would accommodate Revell's vision within a North American constructional idiom. The results reveal one of the most thoroughly crafted buildings in Canada from the latter half of the century. The concave surfaces of the single-loaded towers are veiled in an elegantly proportioned stainless-steel curtain wall. The convex sides are clad with windowless precast-concrete panels inlaid with strips of rough-faced Pentelic marble whose fluted surface recalls that of a Doric column. These same marble strips are repeated in the floors of the lobby, embedded in a smooth matrix of black terrazzo. The portly main doors are composed of staggered, laminated strips of oak, with oversize, sculpted door handles of laminated wood.

Approaching the building along the curved front face of the podium, the visitor is enfolded by a double-height colonnade from which the second-floor offices of the mayor and city councillors are clearly visible through floor-to-ceiling glass. Moving inside, the lobby opens up into a clerestory-lit public forum around which an ample circumference of counters allows for contact with municipal services. Graceful curved stairs lead to second-floor offices and committee rooms. At the center of this circular assemblage lies a stepped ceremonial pit, an *umbilicus urbis*, out of which thrusts the massive, flaring column supporting the council chamber, which nonetheless seems to float serenely above the clerestory. Revell intended the chamber to recall a classical theater in which rising tiers of public seating surround concentric rings of council desks. The mayoral dais is framed by a slightly concave, freestanding *scena frons*, itself framed by the gently domed ceiling. Set within the trussed perimeter supporting this dome, a continuous arc of glazing provides a panoramic view of Nathan Philips Square and the downtown core beyond.

The status of Toronto City Hall as the symbolic center of the city is dramatically reinforced by the success of this square. Bordered by an elevated promenade that extends the frontal colonnade, the square's dominant feature transforms seasonally, from fountain pool to a perennially popular ice-skating rink. Henry Moore's *Three-Way Piece No. 2* and a leafy outcropping known as the "Peace Garden" complete the perimeter of a central space occupied by a succession of public concerts, rallies, and demonstrations in addition to art shows and market days. In stark contrast to the common criticism of modernist public space as sterile, Nathan Philips Square is enlivened by a constantly shifting inhabitation both day and night, even during the deepest of Canadian winters. As Dendy and Kilbourn noted in their book *Toronto Observed* (1986), "It is to Viljo Revell and his humanistic concept of ancient and modern city forms, and of urban life itself, that Toronto owes the success of its civic square. Without it the building would have been forever incomplete."

JEFFREY BALMER

See also **City Beautiful Movement; City Hall; Mies van der Rohe, Ludwig (Germany); Revell, Viljo (Finland)**

Further Reading

Bureau of Architecture and Urbanism, *Toronto Modern Architecture, 1945–1965*, Toronto: Coach House Press, 1987

Dendy, William, and William Kilbourn, *Toronto Observed: Its Architecture, Patrons, and History*, Toronto: Oxford University Press, 1986

Fulford, Robert, *Accidental City: The Transformation of Toronto*, Boston: Houghton Mifflin, and Toronto: MacFarlane Walter and Ross, 1996

Kalman, Harold, *A History of Canadian Architecture*, 2 vols., Toronto and New York: Oxford University Press, 1994

McHugh, Patricia, *Toronto Architecture: A City Guide*, Toronto: Mercury Books, 1985; 2nd edition, Toronto: McClelland and Stewart, 1989

TORONTO, ONTARIO

If any one building in Toronto may mark the transition from the 19th century to the next, that building is Old City Hall (1899, E. J. Lennox). Lennox's masterwork marks the culmination in the city of Romanesque Revival, a style influenced by the works of McKim, Mead, and White, and H. H. Richardson, particularly his Allegheny County Courthouse (1884). Other local examples of this genre include the Gooderham House (1892), designed by David Roberts, and the Ontario Legislative Building (1892, known also as "Queen's Park"), by R. A. Waite. These buildings share the robust Richardsonian complement of rusticated stonework, massive rounded arches, steep gabled roofs, and richly ornamented interior woodwork. More generally, Old City Hall marks the culmination of High Victorian Toronto, which, in addition to the Romanesque style, looked toward an eclectic array of Renaissance Revival, Second Empire, Italianate, and Queen Anne. These templates were modified by a web of influences, including a constructional idiom founded on the versatile red and yellow brick produced from local clay pits and the ever-present specter of winter. The most enduring legacy of this period is the near ubiquitous semidetached housing type known as Toronto Bay-n-Gable, variations of which continued to be built throughout the 20th century.

Into the new century, Lennox would continue to match the ambitions of his patrons with the flamboyance of his designs. A case in point is Casa Loma (1911), commissioned by Sir Henry Pellatt, a pioneer in the development of hydroelectric power from Niagara Falls. Here, Lennox forged an elaborate confection composed of French Medieval and early Renaissance that may well have found favor with King Ludwig of Bavaria. Such extravagance was the exception to the rule in Edwardian Toronto, for although the explosive accretion of wealth and population continued along its Victorian trajectory, the opulence of Richardsonian Romanesque gave way to more subtle shades of English domestic architecture. The dominant model for the first two decades of the century was neo-Georgian, all red brick and white trim, although it is in the Cottage style that we recognize two of the city's most significant neighborhood models: Wychwood Park and Riverdale Courts.

Wychwood Park was founded by Marmaduke Matthews, an English-born landscape painter who envisioned an artists' idyll set amid ten acres of ravine land west of Casa Loma. Most of the development dates from after 1907, when the architect Eden Smith, in addition to building his own residence, designed a further half dozen houses in the park. All were executed in the Lutyens-inspired Cottage style, comprising deceptively simple assemblages of sweeping rooflines, stucco walls, and timber de-

tailing. Smith employed this combination throughout other affluent neighborhoods that were then taking shape in the city,
but it is to his credit that he was able to apply the fruit of this
experience to an altogether different challenge. Riverdale Courts
(1914) was the inaugural project of the Toronto Housing Company, a coalition of political and philanthropic organizations
concerned with the lack of affordable housing. Set among a
solidly middle-class area east of the city (and soon to be connected across the Don valley by the Prince Edward Viaduct,
1918), Smith's picturesque Cottage vocabulary provided a palatable image to both residents and neighbors. The original phase
included 208 units, varying in size from one to four bedrooms,
in three-story blocks arranged around quadrangles. These courts
had the double advantage of providing every unit with a
veranda-level entrance while maximizing the amount of land set
aside for lawn and play space. The careful articulation of common and private spaces enabled a balanced sense of community
and provided a role model for many of the successful publicly
assisted in-fill projects built subsequently: the Garden Court
Apartments (1942, Forsey Page and Steele), Sherbourne Lanes
(1976, Diamond and Myers), and the much larger St. Lawrence
Neighborhood (1983, various architects).

The prosperity of Toronto in the early decades of the century
was perhaps most clearly embodied in the head offices of the
banks that grew in importance as both domestic and foreign
investment fueled the development of railways and manufacturing and the exploitation of natural resources. An early example
of this is the Traders' Bank Building (1905), designed by the
New York firm of Carrère and Hastings, which was later known
for the design of the New York Public Library (1911), designed
in association with John M. Lyle. The bank building is composed of a series of layers. A ground level of polished granite
supports a double-height banking hall encased in a Doric colonnade. Above that, eight floors of office space are clad in smooth
stone and punched windows and crowned by a broad cornice.
The Dominion Bank Building (1914), designed by the Toronto
firm of Darling and Pearson, is noteworthy for its pair of banking
halls, the upper hall featuring double-height arcuated piers
suggestive of an Albertian basilica and combined with a richly
coffered timber ceiling. Commissioned by Edmund Walker and
soaring to 34 stories, the Canadian Bank of Commerce Building
(1931) remained the tallest building in the British Empire for
more than 30 years. York and Sawyer, on the heels of its headquarters for the Royal Bank in Montreal (1928), designed a
subtly tapering office shaft clad in piers of buff limestone. The
tower is wrapped by a banking hall, its gilded coffered vault
modeled on the Baths of Caracalla. Across King Street, the construction site of John Lyle's Bank of Nova Scotia (begun 1929,
redesigned by Mathers and Haldenby, 1951) was mothballed,
as the crash of 1929 abruptly halted the upward urge of Canadian banks for a quarter century.

Edmund Walker the banker was also a founding patron of
the Royal Ontario Museum, and for that institution the firm
of Darling and Pearson chose an equally exuberant modern Romanesque style in which to garb its original wing (1914). The
facade features a rich brick and terra-cotta matrix, enlivened by
an articulated profusion of fretwork, corbeling, and friezes, offset
by projecting bays and recessed three-story arched windows.
More typical of public buildings in the first half of the century
was Beaux-Arts classicism, as witnessed by the Toronto Public

Reference Library (1909, with significant additions, 1929), by
A.H. Chapman with Wickson and Gregg, and Union Station
(1927). Although planning for the new station began in 1905,
technical complexities, combined with financial and legal entan-
glements, delayed the opening of the station for a total of 22
years. John Lyle, in collaboration with Ross and McDonald,
architects of Union Station in Ottawa (1912), and Hugh G.
Jones, created one of the most imposing yet urbane public buildings in Canada. As with the Bank of Commerce Building, a
grand vaulted hall is modeled on the Roman imperial baths,
replete with Tennessee marble and Missouri Zumbro. Light
floods this space both through north and south clerestory openings and at the short ends of the hall through four-story arched
windows, their filigree of rippled-glass-and-steel trusswork doing
double duty as glazed corridors bridging office wings flanking
the hall to the east and west.

The most intriguing public building in the city, without re-
servation, is the R. C. Harris water filtration plant (1937),
named for the public works czar responsible for its construction
(he was a kindred spirit of Robert Moses and William Mulhol-
land). Designed by English architect Thomas Pomphrey and
constructed during the leanest years of the Depression, its hydro-
logical panoply of pumps, impellers, Venturi tunnels, and filter
pools is housed in a sumptuous neo-Byzantine fortress. Calling
it "the Palace of Purification," the building is memorialized by
Michael Ondaatje's *In the Skin of a Lion*: "Harris had dreamed
the marble walls, the copper banded roofs. He pulled down
Victoria Park Forest and the essential temple swept up in its
place, built on the slopes towards the lake." The building still
functions with its original equipment, capable of delivering a
billion liters of clean water a day. Its audacity was the exception
to the rule of the middle third of the century, when the city
appeared to have entered a state of suspended animation, its
energies sidetracked by the Depression and the global war.

The arrival of the International Style, that hallmark of postwar economic recovery, was slow to make its mark in Toronto.
A few worthy examples include the Anglo Canada Insurance
Building (1954, James Murray) and the Shell Oil Tower (1955,
George Robb), both since grievously demolished. Peter Dickinson's Benvenuto Place (1955) established a paradigm for modern
apartment dwellings, as the planned community of Don Mills
(begun 1953) did for suburban development. However, it was
not until the onset of the 1960s that a critical mass of influences
and projects decisively marked the second great wave of expansion and experimentation in the city. Benefiting from a massive
buildup in postsecondary education, a new generation of architects sought to advance and adapt modernism in an academic
setting. A supreme example of this synthesis is embodied in
Massey College (1962), a graduate residence of the University
of Toronto. Ron Thom combined the tradition of Collegiate
Gothic (a nearby example, Sproatt and Rolph's elegantly functional Hart House, 1919, was endowed by the same Massey
Foundation that sponsored Thom's design) with modernist influences from the Netherlands into a superbly crafted environment of total design, right down to the silverware, that is reminiscent of Wright's Prairie period. Scarborough College (1965,
John Andrews Architects and Page and Steele), a satellite of
the University of Toronto, challenged existing notions of what
constituted a campus. Arranged along the northern brow of a
forested ravine, the college is essentially a single building extend-

ing along the contours of the valley and interconnected along an internal, temperature-controlled pedestrian spine. The heroic scale of the Brutalist in situ concrete forms, conceived of at the scale of the landscape, is balanced by skillfully modulated spaces of public gathering arranged in succession along the central "street."

At the center of the city, sustained immigration, particularly from southern and Eastern Europe, progressively enriched the realm of public space. The Colonnade (1964, Gerald Robinson) cast in a modernist idiom the often antimodernist concept of mixed use, reflecting in a single complex the more incremental transformations taking shape in neighborhoods such as Yorkville and Kensington Market. The symbolic apotheosis of Toronto's cosmopolitan metamorphosis was the arrival of New City Hall (1965), which saw Finnish architect Viljo Revell's design emerge from a competition field of 520 entries. Unremittingly modern yet sinuously sculptural, the building was matched in impact by its accompanying urban square, which continues to provide a sustained and lively focus to civic events and public gatherings. Equally significant was the Toronto-Dominion Centre (1969, Mies van der Rohe, with John B. Parkin Associates, and Bregman and Hamann), Mies's final, and perhaps finest, corporate tower complex. Set on a gray granite podium, two characteristically prismatic towers offset the supremely elegant banking pavilion, a 150-square-foot clear-span essay in Miesian refinement. Their dramatic effect on the skyline was equaled by an initially more subtle intervention: that of the commercial services buried beneath the podium. Joined with similar underground adjuncts to a cluster of subsequent towers (including Commerce Court, 1972, I. M. Pei, with Page and Steele, and the Royal Bank Plaza, 1976, WZMH Partnership), this concourse grew to encompass most of the subterranean area of the downtown core, including a half dozen subway stations. Along with a similar development in Montreal, it represents a uniquely Canadian response to the nexus of metropolitan life and the forces of nature.

Increasingly identified as the "livable city," Toronto took steps to forestall the blight plaguing American urban centers. Curtailment of the Spadina Expressway saved several historic neighborhoods while simultaneously privileging public over private transportation. Similarly, government-sponsored initiatives favored in-fill and renovation rather than the tabula rasa of "urban renewal" that local transplant Jane Jacobs had castigated in her seminal *Death and Life of Great American Cities*. Situated on artificial landfill, Ontario Place (1971, Craig, Zeidler, and Strong) was a publicly sponsored amusement park inspired by the success of Expo '67 in Montreal. Designed as a showcase for the burgeoning province, Eberhard Zeidler created a broad array of high-tech follies set amid a picturesque landscape of linked islands and lagoons: giant white pods cantilevered on slender pylons several hundred feet above water, a hyperbolic paraboloid "tent" for outdoor concerts (ignobly demolished), and a geodesic sphere containing the first-ever IMAX cinema. It was also instrumental in focusing public attention on the city's shoreline and led to the establishment of Harbourfront (begun 1972)—a 100-acre strip of abandoned piers and warehouses that became Canada's first urban national park. Here, Zeidler's renovation of Queen's Quay Terminal (1983) followed on the heels of the immensely influential Eaton Center (1979, Bregman and Hamann, with the Zeidler Partnership). Connected at both ends to the main subway line running beneath Yonge Street (and to

the subterranean concourse begun by Mies), this urban mall offers a parallel climate-controlled "street," a 900-foot-long glazed vault enclosing five levels of retail from street level down, as many office and parking levels above, and 20 million visitors annually. Like the now ubiquitous profile of the CN Tower (1976, John Andrews, with WZMH Partnership, and E. R. Baldwin), this "street" has served as a lightning rod for critics and boosters alike, joining Revell's City Hall in the pantheon of postcard symbols of the city.

A severe recession in the early 1980s, followed by a lengthy economic downturn through much of the final decade of the 20th century, brought to an end the dynamic experimentation of the postwar period. As elsewhere, although the relative merits of Postmodernism were discussed in academic circles, historicist pastiche began to dominate the sprawl of subdivisions and shopping malls engulfing the exurban hinterland. Notable exceptions buoyed the hopes of conscientious objectors: A. J. Diamond's Central YMCA (1984), a taut assemblage of Platonic volumes with nuanced references to Roman *thermae*, among others, and Mississauga City Hall (1987, Jones and Kirkland Architects), which drew on both vernacular and modernist influences. Financially squeezed local governments lost influence over powerful developers, resulting in projects that ran counter to the spirit of consultation and compromise that had been the cornerstone of the "livable city" formula. The practice of architecture itself increasingly fell to the sway of bottom-line economics of design-build management, eroding the traditional role of the architect. Despite all of this, the city continued to be an enviable place to live, with rich cultural deposits, vibrant neighborhoods, an invigorating waterfront, and an economy poised to meet the challenges of the coming decades. A new generation of architects waits in the wings.

JEFFREY BALMER

See also **Brutalism; Carrère, John Mervin, and Thomas Hastings (United States); Lutyens, Edwin (England); Pei, I.M. (United States); Revell, Viljo (Finland); Toronto City Hall**

Further Reading

Arthur, Eric Ross, *Toronto: No Mean City*, Toronto: University of Toronto Press, 1964; 3rd edition, revised by Stephen A. Otto, 1986

Bureau of Architecture and Urbanism, *Toronto Modern Architecture, 1945–1965*, Toronto: Coach House Press, 1987

Dendy, William, and William Kilbourn, *Toronto Observed: Its Architecture, Patrons, and History*, Toronto: Oxford University Press, 1986

Fulford, Robert, *Accidental City: The Transformation of Toronto*, Boston: Houghton Mifflin, and Toronto: MacFarlane Walter and Ross, 1996

Kalman, Harold, *A History of Canadian Architecture*, 2 vols., Toronto and New York: Oxford University Press, 1994

McHugh, Patricia, *Toronto Architecture: A City Guide*, Toronto: Mercury Books, 1985; 2nd edition, Toronto: McClelland and Stewart, 1989

TORRE, SUSANA 1944–

Architect, theorist, and urban designer, United States

Susana Torre is theorist, educator, practicing architect, urban and interior designer, social activist, and architectural critic.

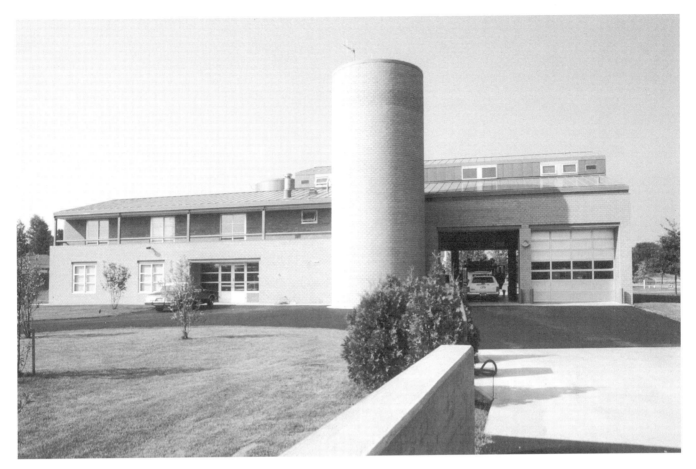

Fire Station Five, Columbus, Indiana (1987)
Photo © Mary Ann Sullivan

Torre has demonstrated her talents in several design competitions and prestigious awards since graduating with an architecture degree from the Universidad de Buenos Aires in 1967. Torre's ability to incorporate allegory and metaphor into complex, plastic forms is nowhere more evident than in her design for the restoration and adaptive reuse of Ellis Island in New York Harbor (1981). She transformed this abandoned relic of immigration into a delightful park of memorable symbols and enjoyable relaxation. Torre's Ellis Island project has been displayed in architectural exhibitions at more than 40 universities and, through numerous publications, educated the general public about architecture's ability to express a culture's narrative histories.

Among her earlier projects, Torre's 1977 design for the offices of Manhattan lawyer Harry Torcyner suggests a pristine orchestration of the relationship between art and architecture. (The space was also designed to house Torcyner's art collection.) Torre subtly used color to amplify the structural grid and employed texture and color to contrast the permanent exterior walls with the flexible interior partitions. Vivid surrealist paintings and primitive objects of art are showcased by sensitively configured architectural spaces.

Two of her commissions—Fire Station Five (1987) at Tipton Lake, Columbus, Indiana, and the Garvey House (1988) in Amagansett, Long Island—embody recognizable yet thoroughly abstracted references to site and context. Fire Station Five's plan is generated by the square. One of the interlocking squares shelters the functional and technical apparatus of the station, whereas another square houses the "human" facilities (sleeping and living areas, kitchen, and offices.) The shape and form of the building echo its suburban and bucolic environment. The exposed steel frame alludes to a barnlike structure meant to house fire trucks. References to silos (the cylindrical stair with a fireman pole and the tower for fire hoses) tie the two functions of the building together formally and physically while making clear reference to Midwest agricultural building traditions. Elegant details and balanced colors augment the architectonic integrity of this admired landmark.

The semicircular two-story Garvey residence gracefully balances vernacular and intellectual traditions. Clad in local cedar, it also pays tribute to the American classicism in architecture through its symmetrical street facade with a central stair tower. The stunning oceanview site ensures direct sunlight all day long.

Torre has integrated her aesthetic concerns with those of education and social reform. In her 1980 studio at Syracuse University's School of Architecture, Torre focused the curriculum on the housing needs of two-income families, asking the students to reexamine the contemporary roles of parents and children. As director of the Architecture Program (1982–85) at

Barnard College, Columbia University, she shaped the educational experiences of many young women. While chairing the Environmental Design Department of the Parsons School of Design (1991–94), she implemented curricula that emphasized social needs of the late 20th century. In collaboration with government agencies and professional offices, she offered a hands-on housing design program for low-income and mentally ill families. The students created plans and models for three sites in Manhattan's Lower East Side and participated in subsequent implementation.

Torre has curated several traveling exhibitions of architecture, including the innovative and acclaimed "Women in American Architecture: A Historic and Contemporary Perspective," displayed at the Brooklyn Museum of Art, New York (1977). The same year Torre organized the traveling exhibition "Childbirth Centers," installed at the New Jersey Institute of Technology, where she was an associate professor (1977–78). A decade later Torre arranged a symposium and traveling exhibition, "Hispanic Traditions in American Architecture and Urbanism," at Columbia University in New York. After touring the United States, this exhibition was shown in Argentina and Spain.

Milka Bliznakov

See also **Contextualism; Columbus, Indiana; Feminist Theory**

Biography

Born in Puan, Argentina, 2 November 1944; attended the Universidad de la Plata, 1961–63; studied at Universidad de Buenos Aires; Edgar Kauffman Foundation Scholar, 1967; earned degree in architecture, 1967; postgraduate studies at Columbia University, New York, 1968–69; Noble Foundation Fellow, 1971–72; J. Clawson Mills Grant, Architectural League of New York 1973. Principal, Architectural Studio, New York, 1978–85; member, editorial board, *Journal of Architectural Education* 1983–85; partner, Wank Adams Slavin Associates, New York, 1985–87; established her firm Susana Torre and Associates, New York, 1988. Cochairperson, assistant professor, and director of design concentration, State University of New York, College of Old Westbury, 1972–76; adjunct professor of architecture at Columbia University, Yale University, Cooper Union for the Advancement of Science and Art, Carnegie Mellon University, and Syracuse University, 1973–80; visiting associate professor, New Jersey Institute of Technology School of Architecture, 1977–78; associate professor of architecture, Columbia Graduate School of Architecture, Planning and Preservation, 1981–89; director, Architecture Program, Barnard College, Columbia University, 1982–85; Sam Gibbons Eminent Scholar in Architecture, FAMU Graduate School of Architecture and Urban Planning, Florida 1990; visiting university professor, University of Sydney, 1990; chairperson, Parsons School of Design, Architecture and Environmental Design Department, New York from 1991. Member, board of directors, Architects, Designers and Planners for Social Responsibility from 1988; vice president of architecture, Architectural League of New York 1989–93; member, board of directors, Architectural League of New York from 1989.

Selected Works

House of Meaning (project), 1972
Law Offices of Harry Torcyner, New York, 1977

Ellis Island Park and Museum, master plan (project), New York, 1981
Clark House, Old Montauk Highway, Petrel Road, Southampton, Long Island, New York, 1981
Schermerhorn Hall, Wallach Fine Arts Center, Columbia University, New York (with WASA Architects and Engineers), 1985
Inner City In-fill Housing, Harlem, New York (project with Parsons School of Design architecture students), 1985
Fordham University Dormitory, Bronx, New York (with WASA Architects and Engineers), 1986
Fire Station Five, Columbus, Indiana (with WASA Architects and Engineers), 1987
Garvey House, Amagansett, Long Island, New York, 1988
Montauk Library, Long Island, New York (with Raymond Beeler), 1991
Housing Prototypes, Lower East Side, New York (project with Parsons School of Design architecture students), 1993
Housing, Avenue D, New York (project with Parsons School of Design architecture students), 1994

Selected Publications

New Urban Settlements, 1970
Women in American Architecture: A Historic and Contemporary Perspective, 1977
"Architecture with People," *Design Quarterly* 109 (1979)
"Inside Out/Outside In," *Process Architecture* 13 (1980)
"Space as a Matrix," *Heresies* 11 (1981)
Susana Torre: Architectural and Urban Design Projects, 1994
"Building on a Divided Ground?" *Oculus* 59/1 (1996)
"The Reward of Experiment," *Harvard Design Magazine* (June 1997)

Further Reading

Most of Susana Torre's work, including drawings, models, and publications by and about her, is preserved in the International Archive of Women in Architecture (IAWA), Special Collections Department, University Library at Virginia Tech in Blacksburg, Virginia.

Castle, Frederick Ted, "Susan Torre and Alan Wexler at Feldman," *Art in America* (April 1985)
Dean, Andrea, "Women in American Architecture: Individual Profiles and a Discussion of Issues," *AIA Journal* (January 1982)
Filler, Martin, "Between Dream and Memory," *House and Garden* 154/1 (1982)
Gustavich, Miriam, "Fire Station No. 5, Columbus, Indiana," *Inland Architect*, 31/5 (1987)
Lorenz, Clare, *Women in Architecture*, London: Trefoil, 1989; New York: Rizzoli, 1990
Morton, David, "Neotypes: Susana Torre," *Progressive Architecture* 58/5 (1977)
Rothschild, Joan, et al. (editors), *Design and Feminism: Re-visioning Spaces, Places, and Everyday Things*, New Brunswick, New Jersey: Rutgers University Press, 1999

TORRE VELASCA (VELASCA TOWER)

Designed by Lodovico, B. di Belgiojoso; completed 1958; Milan, Italy

Completed in 1958, the 26-story Torre Velasca (Velasca Tower) was built by architects Lodovico B. di Belgiojoso (1909–), Enrico Peressutti (1908–76), and Ernesto N. Rogers (1909–69) of the Studio Architetti BBPR in collaboration with structural engineer

Arturo Danusso. Only the second skyscraper to be built in Italy, it followed the Pirelli Tower, designed by Gio Ponti with structural engineer Pier Luigi Nervi, by two years. Milan's two high-rise towers redefined the skyline of the most industrial city in Italy at precisely the moment when modern life began to eclipse the traditional agrarian economy and bleak wartime conditions were giving way to new prosperity. Unlike the Pirelli Tower, located in the vicinity of Milan's Stazione Centrale, and thus somewhat removed from the historic center of the city, the Velasca Tower was situated at the intersection of Corso di Porta Romana and Via Velasca, in the ambit of the unique Gothic Duomo and Giuseppe Mengoni's Galleria Vittorio Emmanuele.

The tower was named after the street, Via Velasca, which in turn had been named for Fernando Velasca, Spanish governor of Milan 1592–1600 and 1610–12. Conceived as a tripartite structure, the building comprises a two-story canopied entrance pavilion at ground level, which houses retail shops; a robust rectangular shaft with central elevator core accommodating commercial office space; and a slightly larger rectangular crown overhanging the central shaft, occupied by private residences and topped by a copper-clad hipped roof. To accommodate the broad base of the structure, war-damaged residential buildings on the site were demolished to expand Via Velasca into the large, open Piazza Velasca that surrounds the tower. In a gesture that echoes Mies van der Rohe's solution for the Seagram Building's (1954–58) plaza in New York, a place of repose was created in the dense urban fabric of Milan. Together, the shaft of the tower and its overhanging crown—which critics have likened to a medieval fortified palace—are visually unified by steel-reinforced concrete ribs that span the height of the building, recalling August Perret's Raynouard Street apartment building in Paris (1932) and his Notre Dame du Raincy (1922). The structure of the Velasca Tower also recalls Pier Luigi Nervi's Palazzetto dello Sport (1957). However, in contrast to the lightness of Nervi's work, the sheer mass of the Velasca Tower asserted a striking monumentality that was mediated by the void of the surrounding piazza.

Designed for the Milan offices of the Società Generale Immobiliare (Real Estate Association), the monumentality of the building suggests longevity and permanence. The reinforced-concrete in-fill panels and vertical ribs evoke the stone architecture of Italy's past at much grander scale, rather than employing the curtain wall introduced in slightly earlier American skyscrapers, including Skidmore, Owings and Merrill's Lever House (New York City, 1951–52) and Mies' Seagram Building. The roof of the overhanging crown is clad with copper and trimmed with ornamental details that recall both the nearby Duomo and medieval fortifications. Even when glass was employed for the tower's fenestration, vast planes of glass that made visible the building's viscera were avoided, and windows were moderately scaled.

Provoking heated debate in local and international architecture circles at a time when skyscrapers were still new to European cities, the distinctive Velasca Tower contradicted the tenets of International Style modern architecture; it appeared anti-modern. The effect of lead architect Ernesto Rogers's rejection of the ethical and aesthetic mandate of modern architecture was no doubt exacerbated by BBPR's decision to present the tower together with the work of Giancarlo de Carlo (Housing in Matera, 1956–57), Ignazio Gardella (Olivetti Cafeteria in Ivrea, 1953–59), and Vico Magistretti (Villa in Arenzano, 1959) at the Otterlo Congrès Internationaux d'Architecture Moderne (CIAM) meeting of 1959. Controversy generated at this meeting concerning the future of Modern architecture ultimately led to the collapse of the organization, and thus the loss of one of the most prominent forums for debate on Modern architecture and urban planning.

Consciously attempting to evoke the ambience of Milan, austere yet sophisticated, urban yet introverted, historic fabric punctuated by gaps and contemporary interventions, BBPR's design for the Velasca Tower sought to make manifest the concept of continuity (*continuità*) that Rogers had adumbrated in his editorial in the December 1953/January 1954 issue of the journal *Casabella*, which he renamed *Casabella-Continuità*. For Rogers continuity referred to historical context in the broad sense, what he termed architecture's "pre-existing environment" (*preesistenze ambientali*). From its founding in 1932, amid heated debate over rationalist architecture and its ties to the Italian Fascist regime, Studio Architetti BBPR took both the classical tradition and the vernacular heritage of the Italian peninsula to be vital sources for modern Italian designers. This position was also pervasive—albeit articulated in different ways—among architects of the postwar period, despite the attempts of the critic and historian Bruno Zevi to promote "organic" architecture. Consideration of context was a necessity for Italian architects operating in war-torn Italy under conditions that forced them to rebuild damaged buildings wherever possible; where older structures

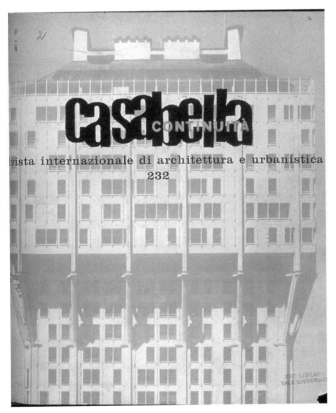

Photograph of Velasca Tower on the cover of *Casabella-Continuitá* (December 1953/January 1954)
Photo courtesy Michelangelo Sabatino

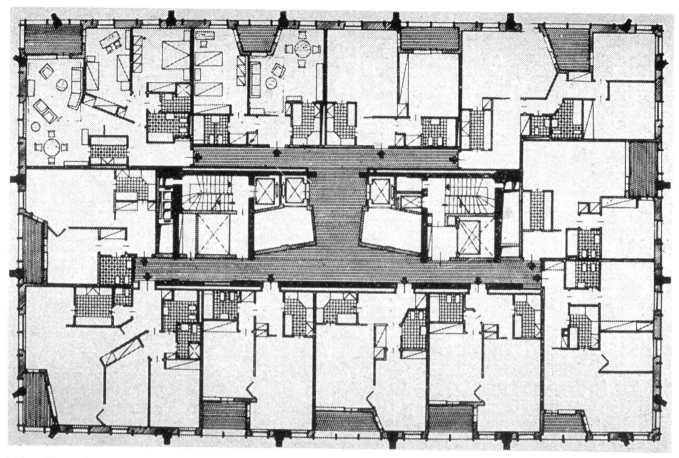

Velasca Tower plan (1958)
Photo courtesy Michelangelo Sabatino

were damaged beyond repair, architects were called on to insert new residential, institutional, or industrial structures into the dense historic urban fabric.

The Velasca Tower was conceived as the remedy for a war-torn site, and no doubt symbolized rebirth in this city that had suffered great losses of its historic building stock during the war. It became a symbol of a revitalized Italy, liberated from the ideological excesses of the Fascist regime and inspired by the hope of rebuilding the country without negating its built heritage.

The Velasca Tower could be compared with late 19th- and early 20th-century tall buildings in New York (e.g., Cass Gilbert's Woolworth Building, 1913), in that it borrowed from historical models such as the medieval fortified castle and tower. The reliance on "traditional" historical types was rejected by modernists in favor of formal innovation. Yet the decision to radically expand the tower's scale and proportions is reminiscent of the striking modernity that one sees, for example, in Adolf Loos's Chicago Tribune Tower Competition entry of 1922.

Departing from the reductive language of international modernism, Studio Architetti BBPR looked to the local context, adapting the built forms of Milan and northern Italy to advanced building technologies to demonstrate that Modern architecture could be representative of the individual as well as the collective,

the local, national, and international. The appropriation of the medieval past was not merely an archaeological exercise. Rogers and his associates sought to reinvent the past in light of the contemporary needs, both spiritual and functional. The fundamental contribution of the Velasca Tower to the history of 20th-century modern architecture lies in its ability to convey the prescient message—against the grain of international modernism—that Modern architecture need not necessarily break with the past but, rather, should aspire to engage in a creative dialogue with it.

MICHELANGELO SABATINO

See also **Lever House, New York; Seagram Building, New York; Woolworth Building, New York**

Further Reading

BBPR La Torre Velasca. Disegni e progetto della Torre Velasca, edited by Leonardo Fiori and Massimo Prizzon, Milan: Editrice Abitare Segesta, 1982

Brunetti, Federico, *BBPR La Torre Velasca a Milano*, Florence: Alinea Editrice, 2000

Kallmann, Gerhard M., "Modern Tower in Old Milan," *Architectural Forum*, 2 (1958)

Rogers, Ernesto N., "Tre problemi di ambientamento," *Casabella-Continuità*, 232 (1959)

TRANSPORTATION PLANNING

Transportation planning in the 20th century grew up with the automobile. Only for the first few years of the century were streetcars able to compete with interest in the automobile. Comprehensive plans that included rail transit, such as those for Llewellyn Park, New Jersey, and Forest Hills Gardens, New York, quickly proved to be the exception. Transportation planning soon became the handmaiden of the automobile, taking it where it wanted to go, often regardless of the consequences.

By the early 1920s, the popularity of the automobile had largely displaced interest in planning for public transportation, which faced declining ridership and loss of profits. Nationwide, voters turned their backs on public transit investments in referenda, sometimes influenced by huge contributions by automobile and parts manufacturers. The automobile quickly became the emblem of the future and national progress. The number of electric streetcars peaked for the century in 1917 at 72,911, and total ridership was greatest in 1923, when 15.7 billion transit trips were taken. The planners' preference was certified at the 1924 National Conference on City Planning when the way of the "horizontal city of the future" was declared—by the automobile.

The sudden tidal wave of automobility swept over cities throughout the 1920s. Suddenly, suburbs began to grow at a much faster rate than cities. As early as 1923, some cities were debating the banning of cars downtown because of congestion. Commuters by automobile quickly outnumbered those by transit. In the early years of the meteoric ascendance of the automobile, transportation planners raced to facilitate its needs. The single answer for congestion was to build more roads, usually in straight radial lines from the center of the city into territories of developable land at the city's edge.

The "good roads" movement gained in popularity. Taking advantage of Progressive Era sentiment against the monopolistic practices of railroads and toll-road operators, the good-roads movement advocated for public ownership and construction of roads. The concept of a continuous national system of highways was instituted in the Federal Aid Highway Act of 1921 with the adoption of a numbered U.S. highway system composed of routes extending across the nation. By the early 1930s, the objective of constructing a system of two-lane roads connecting the centers of population had been largely completed, making it possible to travel across the country on an all-weather highway system.

No one was more aggressive at road building than Robert Moses, who, from 1924, amassed unprecedented power in New York to steamroll thousands of miles of highway building projects. Moses's first parkways were designed for the recreational driver, but by the early 1930s the wide thoroughfares became conduits for commuters. Moses's massive transportation projects, which combined urban expressways, bridges, and tunnels, had an immediate effect of pumping up suburban migration in New York's suburbs, particularly to Westchester and Nassau Counties.

Moses was many things, but he was only figuratively a planner, as he concentrated on building a bureaucratic empire. Many of his massive transportation building projects found their source in the landmark 1929 Regional Plan of New York, a privately funded transportation and development plan for the New York metropolitan region. The plan was a mix of proposals for decentralizing and "decongesting" New York, calling for the expansion of highways and rail links and at the same time recognizing, in Clarence Perry's classic section on neighborhood units, that the automobile was inevitably creating the cellular city.

As Moses drew from the Regional Plan of New York, other large-scale plans attempted to envision and shape the future of automobile transportation. The Regional Plan Association of America (RPAA), composed of the era's most reform-minded planners, including Lewis Mumford, Clarence Stein, and Henry Wright, proposed the idea of the "townless highway," thoroughfares that would "encourage the building of real communities at definite and favorable points off the main road." However, without Moses to take up the idea, the RPAA's plan languished as the Great Depression set in.

With the Federal Aid Highway Act of 1934, Congress authorized funds to state governments for surveys, plans, engineering, and economic analyses for future highway construction projects. By 1940, all states were participating in this program. Transportation planning moved into another realm of influence in 1940 with the opening of the Arroyo Seco Parkway (later the Pasadena Freeway) in Los Angeles (the term "freeway" had been coined initially in 1928 in a *New York Times* article by Edward M. Bassett, a New York planner). Los Angeles' first freeway plan, by Lloyd Aldrich, was not developed until 1939, and by World War II Los Angeles had only 11 miles of freeway. However, Los Angeles soon became the world model of up-to-the-minute modernity in its enthusiastic embrace of transportation planning for the automobile.

The most shining vision of the future of 20th-century transportation, however, was exhibited at the 1939 World's Fair in New York. Rarely has a plan of the future city shown such prescience. The most popular exhibit at the fair was General Motors' Futurama, which attracted long lines of visitors who wanted to visit a future envisioned by America's most successful automobile manufacturer and that resembled nothing so much as the southern California landscape, circa 1955. When Secretary of Defense Charles Wilson asserted that what was good for General Motors "was also good for the country," no voices were heard in dissent. Eventually, more than five million visitors came to the Futurama exhibit to wonder at the expanse of miniature elevated freeways that designer Norman Bel Geddes had created to show the prospects of "modern and efficient city planning—breath-taking architecture—each city block a complete unit in itself [with] broad, one-way thoroughfares—space, sunshine, light and air."

Although the arrival of World War II brought a halt to the rise in automobile ownership and slowed the momentum of transportation planning, significant efforts were made that contributed to the huge surge in highway construction afterward. Congress passed the Federal Aid Highway Act of 1944, financing an interurban system of 32,000 miles that bypassed urban areas. The act immediately created a debate: transportation planners, such as Harold Bartholomew, and power broker Robert Moses wanted to use new roads to attack "urban blight," charting expressways through urban residential areas to entirely redevelop them. However, initially at least, federal aid focused on intercity connections.

The increased interest of the federal government in transportation planning and highway development soon aroused the in-

terest of lobbyists, the most significant of which, the American Road Builders Association, established one of the most effective campaigns in the history of pressure-group politics to advance the cause of federally supported highway building. Members of the group further set out to systematically dismantle municipal streetcar systems in large portions of the country. General Motors, Firestone Tire, Standard Oil of California, and Phillips Petroleum were eventually convicted of antitrust violations for setting up an illegal transportation company, National City Lines Inc., whose purpose was to obtain control of transit companies throughout the Midwest and West and to dismantle streetcars in favor of buses, which were financed by the same manufacturers and suppliers.

In 1953, when the highway lobby sponsored a nationwide essay contest on the need for more highways, the winner was, aptly enough, Robert Moses, who received a $25,000 prize for his essay "How to Plan and Pay for Better Highways." The essay proved to be a preliminary script for more federal funding of highway construction. Although the Eisenhower administration initially had kept highways separate from its 1954 Urban Renewal Act, as had Truman in the original 1949 act, Eisenhower soon became enamored of the prospects for a large-scale highway transportation project.

Eisenhower, whose military success during World War II came on the German autobahns, listened carefully to arguments that a massive federal highway-building project would benefit national defense and stimulate an economic boom. Once again, the debate over "roads fight blight" came to center stage, with many planners insisting that the new highways must penetrate to the center of urban areas to remove slums and improve the connection between outlying suburbs and downtown offices and retail areas.

In June 1956, the Interstate Highway Act was passed with only a single vote in opposition. The $41 billion bill became the largest public works program in the history of the world, setting in place a gigantic imbalance that favored the private automobile over public transit. With an effect befitting its size and cost, the Interstate Highway Act did not by itself create the massive suburbanization that defined the evolution of cities in the second half of century, but it abetted it in an extremely consequential fashion.

By the early 1960s, the automobile was essentially putting other forms of transportation out of business. Between 1950 and 1972, transit patronage declined by 62 percent. Outside of urban areas, it was virtually nonexistent, with only 5 percent of the nation's transit patronage available in rural areas and cities with a population less than 50,000. During the same period, the volume of automobile traffic more than tripled.

It soon became apparent to transportation planners that an undue reliance on the automobile was creating as many problems as it was eliminating. As each new interstate was completed, fresh new problems of displacement, pollution, and congestion arose. Although an entrenched group of planners continued to argue for more highway building, other voices began to be heard in support of the idea of "balanced transportation." In 1962, for example, the San Francisco Bay Area passed a voters' referendum for a 71-mile rail transit system after a prolonged "freeway revolt" had voiced popular dissatisfaction with more and more highway building. The year 1962 also saw the passage of the Federal Aid Highway Act, which mandated local transportation planning.

The Urban Mass Transportation Act of 1964 (UMTA) was the first significant effort of the century to recognize the need to improve and expand public transit. Expenditures increased from approximately $100 million in 1964–65 to approximately $1.3 billion at the end of the 1970s. Under the program, a type of balance was anticipated against the huge federal subsidy for highway building by offering matching funds for capital acquisitions of local transit, and the principal aim was to attain congestion relief by making public transit faster and more comfortable.

The immediate effect of the act was to provide new equipment for public transit buses. However, the act also promoted plans for new rail transit, such as the Bay Area Rapid Transit (BART) in the San Francisco Bay Area. Extensions were funded in New York, Boston, Cleveland, Philadelphia, and Chicago. New rail systems were built in Washington, D.C., Baltimore, Miami, and Atlanta, and planning was begun in Los Angeles and Honolulu.

The ironic consequence of most of these public transit efforts, however, was to spread decentralization of urban downtowns and frequently contribute to the deterioration of central city neighborhoods, often increasing racial segregation. Many of the public transit improvements only facilitated suburban commuting in place of intracity transportation. BART, for example, became a high-speed conduit for financial district office workers from the East Bay suburbs of Contra Costa and Alameda. San Francisco residents were seldom to be found on the bright futuristic cars that sped beneath the city streets. In city after city, the main beneficiaries of the new systems or extensions were suburban commuters, not residents of central cities.

The initial presumption of UMTA was that increased expenditures on capital improvements would relieve traffic congestion. However, by the mid-1970s, planners began to realize the need for a more complex approach. Other influences brought about experiments in vanpooling, dial-a-ride arrangements, and carpool lanes. The principal impetus to these revised approaches was the establishment of the Environmental Protection Agency (EPA). After 1970, pollution in urban areas became a major federal concern, and the EPA sought to develop plans that would diminish traffic in urban areas to reduce pollution, although planners generally continued to ignore the automobile's contribution to urban sprawl. The shift in focus from reducing congestion to reducing pollution brought about certain restrictions on automobiles in central areas, converted downtown streets into pedestrian malls, and reduced downtown speed limits.

Although critics continued to argue that the federal role in transportation planning was only codifying the decentralization of urban areas or providing Band-Aids to the problems of automobile pollution, the notion of balanced transportation continued to be advanced. In 1975, UMTA and the Federal Highway Administration began to require transportation system management plans that had to account for an overall balanced reckoning of transportation needs as a requirement for federal funding. In 1978, requirements were added that focused on the needs of disabled transit riders and residents of densely populated urban areas. During the 1970s, transit planners experimented with a number of varied alternatives to the automobile. In addition to the expansion of bus services and train services, two new modes of transportation came into consideration. The first of these was

personal rapid transit, which attempted to answer the mobility of the automobile with small independent conveyances. Systems were tried in Tampa, in Philadelphia, and at Duke University. The second new mode of transportation was not really new at all: light rail vehicles, as they were newly christened, were really a spiffed-up reinstitution of the old inner-city streetcar systems that had been systematically removed from most urban areas.

Increasingly, the federal role in transportation planning grew more inconsistent during the 1980s. Public transit advocates complained that the government was not doing enough, local jurisdictions complained that it was requiring too much, and congressional representatives increased their opposition to what they termed "big-government intrusion into local affairs." A kind of stalemate ensued throughout the 1980s, with mounting opposition to freeway building by quality-of-life advocates and suburban home owners on the one hand and by public transit advocates faced with reduced federal subsidies for public transit development on the other. Although there were some notable successes of locally funded transit programs, such as in San Diego, California, and a number of other cities that cobbled together funding for new light rail vehicle systems, congestion and sprawl continued to increase as a new phenomenon of "edge cities" grew into the planners' purview with the most far-reaching requirements for automobile commuting yet.

The 1990s saw the influence of numerous state growth-management plans that for the first time addressed the comprehensive relationship of urban growth to balanced transportation principles. States such as Oregon, Florida, Maine, and New Jersey sought to link transportation planning with the wider implications of urban sprawl, loss of open space, and cost of municipal services. Oregon's growth-management plan, the oldest and most far-reaching, called for the establishment of urban growth boundaries to stave off urban sprawl while at the same time increasing the use of public transportation within areas of increased density.

As state growth-management plans began to extend the idea of what balanced transportation meant, federal transportation planning was also influenced. Passage of the Intermodal Surface Transportation Act attempted to put the highway-only approach to transportation planning to rest forever. For the first time, federal transportation planning included significant provisions to balance local land use planning, the environment, historic preservation, and mobility for children, the elderly, and the disabled. Light rail and subway systems, even bicycle and pedestrian travel, were featured as important components of an overall transportation planning approach.

The notion of what transportation planning is or should be has unequivocally grown more complex, increasingly attentive to a wide complex of consequences that flow from the simple act of traveling from one point to another. The pessimist would point to the stranglehold of the automobile on everything from the shape of cities to the air we breathe and conclude that transportation planning has only contributed to the problem. Citing the increased congestion in urban areas, the growing number of gas-guzzling vehicles, and the rampant path of sprawl, the doubter would have ample evidence.

The optimist, however, might point to the incremental progress that is apparent in transportation planning over time, including the increasing interest in what is often called "smart growth" legislation that attempts to address the relationship of transportation planning and land use, and the increased use of public transportation. As the century ended, public transportation ridership was again on the rise, with an equivalent of a million new trips of public transportation ridership, increasing by percentages greater than any other travel modes, including motor vehicle travel. Significantly, these gains were evident in central cities, suburbs, and even rural areas, and the idea of a comprehensive approach to transportation planning shows evidence of spreading with increased levels of influence and acceptance.

RICK ADAMS

Further Reading

Transportation planning is a field that readily tends toward technical methodology, and many of the texts available take a "how to" approach. Nonetheless, several texts attempt to place transportation planning in wider social contexts. Among the best of these are those listed below.

Bottles, Scott L., *Los Angeles and the Automobile: The Making of the Modern City*, Berkeley: University of California Press, 1987

Cervero, Robert, *The Transit Metropolis: A Global Inquiry*, Washington, D.C.: Island Press, 1998

Garreau, Joel, *Edge City: Life on the New Frontier*, New York: Doubleday, 1991

Kay, Jane Holtz, *Asphalt Nation: How the Automobile Took Over America and How We Can Take It Back*, New York: Crown, 1997

Meyer, John R., and Jose A. Gomez-Ibanez, *Autos, Transit, and Cities*, Cambridge, Massachusetts: Harvard University Press, 1981

Mumford, Lewis, *The Highway and the City*, New York: Harcourt Brace, 1963; London: Secker and Warburg, 1964

Newman, Peter, and Jeffrey Kenworthy, *Sustainability and Cities: Overcoming Automobile Dependence*, Washington, D.C.: Island Press, 1998; London: Kogan Page, 1999

Schaeffer, K.H., and Elliott Sclar, *Access for All: Transportation and Urban Growth*, London: Penguin, 1975; New York: Columbia University Press, 1980

TRIBUNE TOWER INTERNATIONAL COMPETITION (1922), CHICAGO

On 10 June 1922—the occasion of the newspaper's diamond (75th) anniversary—the *Chicago Tribune* announced a competition for the building of a new headquarters. Given the title "The Tribune Tower Competition," the competition was conceived of as a vehicle for commemorating the substantial growth and achievements of both the newspaper and the city of Chicago. In statements accompanying the program, site, and submission requirements, the Tribune Building Corporation—the stated "Owner" in the competition documents—hoped for something even grander: an architectural representation of a new time and place befitting the postwar era of limitless and boundless opportunity. Viewing the submissions for the competition, Louis I. Sullivan, the well-known member of the so-called Chicago School of Architecture, registered his own messianic hopes for the future of architecture in an issue of *Architectural Record*. Equating architecture with humanity's redemption, Sullivan gave voice to the highly romanticized, Nietzschean spirit of the time:

The craving for beauty thus set forth by The Tribune is imbued with romance; both that high Romance which is

the essence, the vital impulse, that inheres in all the great works of man in all places and all times, that vibrates in his loftiest thoughts, his heroic deeds, his otherwise inexplicable sacrifices, and which forms the halo of his great compassions, and of the tragedy within the depths of his sorrows. So deeply seated, so persistent, so perennial in the heart of humanity is this ineffable presence, that, suppressed in us, we decay and die. For man is not born to trouble, as the sparks fly upward; he is born to hope and to achieve.

Prominently featured in both trade journals and traditional newspapers, the Tribune Tower Competition engendered extensive debate among national and international architects and advocates of architecture. Perhaps exceeding the Tribune Building Corporation's expectations, notice of the competition provided a touchstone for a vital discussion of contemporary architecture, resulting in debates that considered not only matters of style and taste but social, intellectual, and technological ideals as well. The competition's brief was notable for its conscious attempt to elicit an iconic model for the future both of architecture and of mankind's aspirations for the New World, and all this was to be represented by the skyscraper. In addition, prominent citizens of the city of Chicago—always conscious of their competition with cities on the eastern seaboard—proposed the competition as a challenge to both the city and the world. Appearing with great fanfare in the foremost national and international newspapers, the prominence of the Tribune Building Corporation's flagship newspaper ensured the competition's visibility across the Americas and Europe.

The Tribune Tower Competition brief noted the phenomenal growth of the *Tribune* by chronicling the humble beginnings of the newspaper, growing from a small daily that began with the printing of 400 copies to a circulation of over four million copies per week at the time. Mirroring language used by the *Tribune's* contemporaries—a list that included major corporations and civic-minded cultural and educational institutions—the primary reason for the competition was said to be "the creation of a building that would enhance civic beauty and pride while at the same time augmenting the profile and visibility of the newspaper." As if to downplay the more practical aspects of the competition, the actual building program was outlined in rather mundane if relatively sparse terms: the building was to be "erected on North Michigan Avenue property to house its executive and business departments," with the consideration that the enlarged (and growing) departments in the plant (production) building would also be accommodated. In addition, the building as designed was to provide for the future adaptation and expansion of all departments.

A more significant component of the competition brief was the Tribune Building Corporation's choice of the building site. Underlining the importance of the site—located between numbers 431 and 439 Michigan Avenue just north of the famous downtown Loop—the visibility of the building was stated clearly from the outset: It was to be "situated at the heart of the business and shopping district of Chicago," thus ensuring that the newspaper would be a prominent aspect of the cityscape. By providing an anchor for the development of this particular part of the city, the building was to be thought of as a prominent node in the current and future development of the city and was therefore

seen as simultaneously benefiting both the corporate institution and the general population, a joining of two constituencies in the shared goal of great civic achievement. Accordingly, the site appeared to many civic officials and urban planners to be ideal, if not tinged with an air of inevitability, as the boulevard on which the property fronted (Michigan Avenue) had been substantially improved by the city of Chicago to enable the area's increased visibility relative to other vital areas of the city. Becoming a central component of Chicago's urban fabric, the site was proposed as both the real and the imaginary central node for the financial, social, and political workings of Chicago, a city that many people at the time perceived to be the capital city of the industrialized upper Midwest, the fabled "City of Broad Shoulders." The design and construction of a new office tower to house the region's most important newspaper would seal Chicago's fate as a center of visionary, albeit practical, significance.

In the language of its time, the final aim of the Tribune Tower Competition was stated in vague aesthetic terms. Accordingly, the successful entrant architect was challenged to "erect the most beautiful and distinctive office building in the world." In formulating the mission of the competition, the board of the *Tribune* had sought professional advice, asserting that "this competition has been instituted [with the guidance of] the American Institute of Architects." In recognition of the better-regarded architects of the time and to ensure the highest profile among members of the architectural profession, the competition issued a special invitation to ten architects of national renown, with the rest of the submissions garnered from those responding to a published "general invitation." The winner of the competition was also given the guarantee of being "engaged by the Owner [the Tribune Building Corporation]" for the commission of the winning entry. Although quite specific, the actual submission requirements were relatively minimal: a sketch floor plan at the Michigan Avenue level, showing main entrance lobby, stair and elevator distribution, and the connection of the new building with the plant at one-eighth-inch scale; a typical office floor on a 24-by-36-inch sheet of paper; the Michigan Avenue (west) elevation; the Austin Avenue (south) elevation; a longitudinal section from west to east; and a perspective showing the entire building from the southwest.

The cumulative prize awards for the competition were set at $100,000, an enormous sum of money at the time. The closing of the competition would occur on 1 November 1922, with a one-month grace allowed for drawings arriving from foreign "distant points." By the time of the "absolute closing date" for competition submissions on 1 December 1922 (the date the winners of the competition would be announced), 204 designs had been received by the initial due date, with 49 more designs received "after the competition was closed." In the *Tribune's* publication of the competition entries, 260 submissions were eventually included.

On 23 November 1922, exactly eight days prior to the 1 December closing date, the competition jury, made up of selected architects, city officials, several members of the newspaper's board of directors, and other interested parties (a group collectively referred to as the competition's "advisory committee") met to whittle the large number of entrants to a small group of 12 semifinalists, apparently leaving open the option of considering any late (foreign) entries. With an obvious seriousness of purpose, the same advisory committee announced that

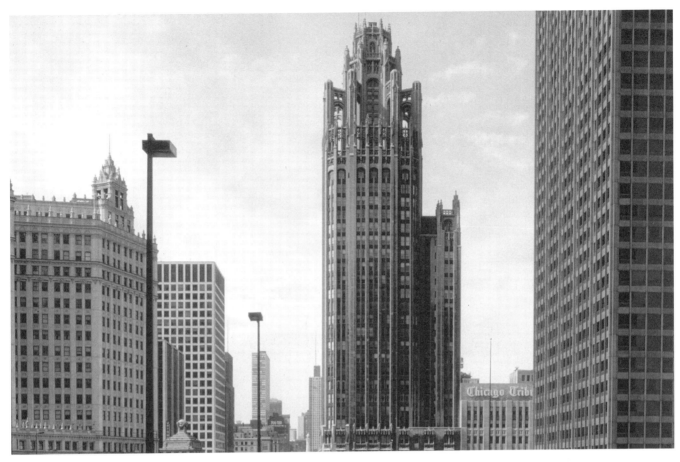

Tribune Tower, Chicago, Illinois, Hood and Howells, 1925
© GreatBuildings.com

it had reached a tentative decision on the final order of prizes on 29 November, when, in what was recorded retrospectively in rather dramatic fashion, "entry number 187 was cleared through customs from Finland" and reassembled for submission. The committee's final decision was finally posted on 3 December 1922. Deemed a unanimous decision, the prize winners were the firms of John Mead Howells and Raymond M. Hood Associates of New York City (first prize, with an award of $50,000); entry number 187 from Finland, the architect Eliel Saarinen (second prize, with an award of $20,000); and the Chicago firm of Holabird and Roche, who were awarded third prize with a cash award of $10,000. The remainder of the prize money was then distributed in $2,000 increments to the ten American architects invited to enter the competition at the outset, invitees that included, among others, firms headed by Bertram Goodhue and James Gamble Rogers; the New York firm Hood and Howells Associates; and two prominent Chicago firms, Holabird and Roche and D. H. Burnham and Company.

At the close of the competition, 23 countries were represented. Announcements of the winners of the competition and further details regarding the entrants and the nature of their work were published in metropolitan newspapers throughout the United States. Newspapers in Europe, including the *Tribune*'s European edition, highlighted the outcome of the compe-

tition; it also received prominent attention in domestic and international architectural trade journals of the time. The publication of the competition results only contributed to the debates surrounding the future of architecture in Europe and the Americas.

Further recognition of the importance of the Tribune Tower Competition continued for some time after the announcement of the competition winners. Multiple requests for the exhibition of the drawings were fielded by the newspaper's offices, including requests from numerous art institutes, associations, and schools; many chapters of the American Institute of Architects; and large universities and educational institutions throughout the United States. In recognition of these requests for a publication or exhibition of the entries, the Tribune Building Corporation agreed to a traveling exhibition featuring drawings by the competition's entrants. The exhibition, accompanied by a publication of record, specifically addressed the competition's educational and cultural potential. In announcing its response to the flurry of requests from across the country, the Tribune Building Corporation issued the following statement on 1 January 1923: "The importance of such an exhibit to furthering the advance of architecture, especially in the study of the skyscraper, cannot well be exaggerated. The designs in some instances have cost the architects competing from 1000 to 10,000 dollars each. With 23

countries represented, the exhibition will show the ideas of the great architects from all parts of the world."

The exhibition consisted of 135 perspective drawings, each drawn on a board measuring 36 by 66 inches in accordance with the original, standard competition requirement. The first exhibit of the competition took place at the University of Illinois, both because of its proximity to the city of Chicago and because it happened to have the largest enrollment of any school of architecture in the country at the time. The program for the exhibition was stated to be primarily educational, with the stated benefit of allowing for the study of the drawings by students and architects. Both the publicity and the expense of the exhibition were borne by the *Tribune*.

The *Tribune*'s accompanying statement about the importance of the original competition and the reason for the traveling exhibit speaks directly to the perception that the Tribune Competition was a signal event—sentiments reflected in Louis Sullivan's observations in *Architectural Record*:

> There never has been such a contest and it is very doubtful that there ever will be another. . . . The greatest architectural contest of history will result not only in achievement of what the Tribune announced as its desire, the most beautiful and distinctive office building in the world, but it will produce many other beautiful buildings. It will give Chicago an architecture gem of the first water and it will add permanently to the resources of the modern architect a mine of new ideas and suggestions. This was the hope of the Tribune and it has been fully realized.

With these words, the Tribune Building Corporation reflected the general optimism of the new century, an optimism that was reflected in the promotion of the "genius" of architecture and its makers. Both Louis Sullivan's and Frank Lloyd Wright's views on architecture, published in popular journal articles and in numerous books, suggest a similar point of view promulgated by advocates of the Chicago style, a school of architecture that viewed architecture as the direct manifestation of the genius of an unfettered and un-self-conscious spirit. The city of Chicago, emblematic of the burgeoning faith in the American Experiment, comprised a time and place in which social, technological, and cultural progress were greeted not only optimistically but also as above reproach. It was in this sense that architecture and urban planning were almost universally—that is, until the spectacular failures of the socially progressive architectural ideals of the post–World War II era—regarded as the material revelation of the destiny and greatness of a new age.

ELIZABETH BURNS GAMARD

See also **Burnham, Daniel H. (United States); Chicago, Illinois; Holabird, William, and Martin Roche (United States); Holabird, William, and John Wellborn Root (United States); Office Building; Skyscraper; Sullivan, Louis (United States); Wright, Frank Lloyd (United States)**

Further Reading

The International Competition for a New Administration Building for the Chicago Tribune, MCMXXII, Chicago: Chicago Tribune, 1923; abridged reprint, as *Chicago Tribune Tower Competition*, New York: Rizzoli, 1980

Pond, Irving K., *The Making of Architecture: An Essay in Constructive Criticism*, Boston: Jones, 1918

Sullivan, Louis, "The Chicago Tribune Competition," *The Architectural Record* 53 (February)

Sullivan, Louis, "Retrospect," in *The Autobiography of an Idea*, by Sullivan, New York: Press of the American Institute of Architects, 1924; reprint, Irvine, California: Reprint Services, 1995

Tigerman, Stanley (editor), *Late Entries to the Chicago Tribune Tower Competition*, New York: Rizzoli, 1980

Zukowsky, John (editor), *Chicago Architecture and Design, 1923–1993*, Munich: Prestel, and Chicago: Art Institute of Chicago, 1993

TRUSS SYSTEMS

Trusses are triangulated frameworks used as spanning or bracing elements in buildings, bridges, transmission towers, and other structures. What distinguishes the truss from other structural forms is precisely its triangulation, from which two benefits accrue: first, the triangular geometry is inherently stable; second, all internal stresses—at least in "ideal" trusses whose bars are pinned together at the vertices of each triangular panel and whose loads are applied only at these pinned joints—are axial, that is, limited to pure tension and pure compression.

Aside from its web of triangular panels, the truss has no intrinsic formal identity. Put another way, it is the specific pattern of internal diagonal, vertical, or horizontal bars (patterns that in many cases bear the names of their 19th-century inventors: Pratt, Howe, Town, Warren, etc.) that makes the structure a truss, not its overall shape. One may design an arch as a truss, a beam or column as a truss, or any number of tower forms—essentially beams cantilevered from the ground plane—as trusses. Advantages of truss construction include the following: (1) large trusses can be assembled from small members pinned together, facilitating production, transportation, and erection; (2) because all internal stresses are axial, with no bending stresses present, the truss is an extremely efficient structural form; (3) because trusses are typically assembled from individual elements bolted, welded, or nailed together, it is relatively easy to customize the overall shape of the truss in relation to external loads and spans, and to adjust the cross-sectional area of each member in relation to anticipated internal stresses.

Trusses have been used for many centuries; Andrea Palladio illustrated truss bridges in his *Four Books of Architecture* as early as 1570. However, it was in the 19th century that industrial expansion—in particular the need for long-span exhibition and market halls, railroad terminals, and bridges—together with the development of engineering theory and improvements in the production of cast and wrought iron, and later steel, provided the motive and means for most of the advances in truss design that were exploited within early 20th-century architecture. For example, the influence of 19th-century iron trusswork in Henri Labrouste's Bibliòteque Nationale Reading Room in Paris (1875) can be seen in the vaulted ceiling above the main concourse in McKim, Mead and White's Pennsylvania Station in New York City (1910); and the tradition of long-span three-hinged arched trusses, epitomized in such 19th-century masterpieces as Contamin and Dutert's Galerie des Machines in Paris (1889), continues in 20th-century structures like Peter Behrens's

AEG Turbine Factory in Berlin (1909) and Tony Garnier's Municipal Slaughterhouse in Lyons, France (1913).

Trusses are seldom found as expressive elements within the canon of mainstream early 20th-century modernism. Like Gothic buttresses, trusses are directly constrained by the geometrical logic of their structural form and, unlike prismatically pure columns and slabs, or expressively cast concrete elements, cannot easily be subsumed within modernism's abstract, formal systems. It is only with Russian Constructivist and derivative projects from the 1920s and 1930s that trusses were first exploited as expressive elements within an explicitly modernist context. Prominent examples include Alexander and Viktor Vesnin's Pravda Building project in Moscow (1923), in which trusses are used as wind-bracing elements within a composition that includes bold text, angled planes, and glazed elevator towers; and Johannes M. Brinkman and L. C. van der Vlugt's Van Nelle Factory in Rotterdam (1930) featuring dynamic horizontal and sloping trussed connecting bridges.

Early 20th-century trusses are also important as infrastructure (bridges) and as industrial (long-span factory roofs), vernacular (ordinary wooden gable roofs), or pragmatic (hidden bracing or support) building elements. Gustav Lindenthal's arched Hell's Gate Bridge in New York City (1916) and Albert Kahn's Glenn Martin Aircraft Plant in Middle River, Maryland (1937), both utilize steel trusses that were the longest spans of their type when constructed. Steel trusswork is commonly employed (and hidden) within the central service "cores" of 20th-century commercial buildings to provide bracing against horizontal wind and earthquake forces. Steel trusses are used to transfer loads over large spans—allowing hotel rooms to be placed on top of lower-floor ballrooms, or office buildings over railroad tracks—without themselves being expressed as part of the architectural form. William LeMessurier's development in the 1960s of a "staggered truss" system is another example of an entirely pragmatic invention utilizing trusses to minimize floor-to-floor dimensions in multistory steel-framed housing or hotel blocks. Pre-engineered, factory-produced triangular wooden trusses made from common lumber connected with toothed metal plates are widely used in 20th-century wood-framed residential roof construction. Open-web steel joists, essentially off-the-shelf trusses first manufactured in the early 1920s, routinely achieved spans of up to 144 feet (44 meters) by the end of the century and are ubiquitous in one-story commercial and industrial buildings. Even precast-concrete trusses, consisting of thin prismatic bars of reinforced concrete joined by steel gusset plates, were proposed for ordinary roof spans in England during World War II, as an expedient response to the short supply of steel.

Where trusses are used deliberately as expressive elements within later 20th-century architecture, it is most often by appropriating and reinterpreting the industrial, off-the-shelf, or pragmatic applications described above. Thus, ordinary steel open-web joists were used in California by architect Raphael Soriano as early as 1938, by Ray and Charles Eames in the influential house they built for themselves in Pacific Palisades, California (1949), and in various industrialized building system designs such as Ezra Ehrenkrantz's School Construction Systems Development (SCSD, 1961). Alvar Aalto's fan-shaped bolted timber trusses supporting the double-skin roof of the Säynätsalo town hall council chamber in Finland (1952) recall, in their detailing, vernacular heavy-timber roof trusses of 19th-century mill build-

ings. Mies van der Rohe's project for a Chicago Convention Hall (1953) visually integrates the diagonal members of its horizontal trusswork within the orthogonal pattern of its exterior curtain wall. Vertical wind-bracing trusses, typically hidden within the framework of tall buildings, are given similar architectural expression on the exterior of Skidmore, Owings and Merrill's Hancock Building in Chicago (1970).

Trusses are commonly featured in so-called High Tech architecture of the late 20th-century. Buildings within this genre reprise to some extent the Constructivists' interest in industrial production, but differ from Constructivist projects in at least two respects: High Tech buildings tend to be less influenced by abstract compositional formulas and often evidence a more theoretically grounded appreciation of structural systems as potential sources of architectural expression. In Renzo Piano and Richard Rogers's Pompidou Center in Paris (1977), virtually the entire architectural concept relies on exposed trusswork. Long-span roof trusses are used as dramatic and expressive elements in innumerable High Tech buildings; examples include Norman Foster's Sainsbury Visual Arts Center near Norwich, England (1978), Michael Hopkins's Research Laboratories for Schlumberger in Cambridge, England (1984), and Nicholas Grimshaw's Waterloo International Rail Terminal (1994) in London, to name but a few.

JONATHAN OCHSHORN

See also **AEG Turbine Factory, Berlin; Pennsylvania Station, New York; Pompidou Center, Paris; Schlumberger Cambridge Research Centre, England; Space Frame; Van Nelle Factory, Rotterdam; Vesnin, Alexander, Leonid, and Viktor (Russia)**

Further Reading

Ambrose, James, *Design of Building Trusses*, New York: Wiley, 1994
Condit, Carl W., *American Building Art: The 20th Century*, New York: Oxford University Press, 1961
Davies, Colin, *High Tech Architecture*, New York: Rizzoli, 1998
Wilkinson, Chris, *Supersheds: The Architecture of Long-Span, Large-Volume Buildings*, Boston: Butterworth, 1996
Yeomans, David T., *The Trussed Roof: Its History and Development*, Aldershot, England: Scolar Press, 1992

TSCHUMI, BERNARD 1944–

Architect, Switzerland and France

Bernard Tschumi's architectural projects are probably best understood in relation to his theoretical writings and ideas, many of which reflect his interest in surrealism and poststructuralism. His sources range from Georges Bataille's writings on philosophy and eroticism to Jacques Derrida's deconstruction as a methodology. A review of a few specific adaptations of these ideas for architecture will help us understand the significantly different way in which Tschumi conceived of the nature and purpose of architecture. Three important theoretical concepts include the pleasures of architecture, strategies of disjunction, and "cross-programming."

The pleasures of architecture, according to Tschumi, are based on the relationships between the physical (body) and the conceptual (mind) rather than the complete absorption of one

mode or experience by the other. Two written works, published to accompany the exhibition of his work at the Museum of Modern Art in New York (*Event-Cities*, 21 April – 5 July 1994), demonstrate this proposition: one text is a collection of his theoretical essays and the other a book of projects (works from his architecture practice). *Event-Cities* establishes the duality of theory and practice that allows for dialectical movement between the physical and the conceptual.

The experience of duality (or "in-between") applies to his architecture as well as his writings. Tschumi relies on the principle of disjunction (a strategy he developed in the 1970s) to reveal the contradictions that exist in architecture between form and function, as well as other oppositions and contradictions. Tschumi argued that habits and conventional assumptions about architecture had to be interrupted or "displaced" in order to make other experiences possible. He employed strategies of shock and defamiliarization to radically shift design paradigms and challenge the viewer.

The theory of disjunction is evident in his critique of the modernist precept that form must follow function. In his explanation of the design for the Parc de la Villette (Paris, 1987–91), for example, Tschumi argued that form and function could ignore or even conflict, and he proceeded to explore this disjunction or rupture by breaking up the space as described in the competition program into volumes placed at the intersections of a superimposed, non–site-specific grid. The volumes were designed as "folies," a play on the double meaning of the French word *folie* (madness or mental imbalance) and *follies*, small pleasure pavilions or ruins popular in 19th-century landscape design.

More important, the shape and form of Tschumi's folies were not determined by specific functions; but rather were ingeniously designed as formal exercises and then modified subsequent to their construction to accommodate specific functions, a process that demonstrated that function could follow form.

Tschumi's later work continued to explore other strategies of disjunction through dis- or cross-programming. The opportunities for new architectural experiences made possible by these concepts ranged from the "unclassifiable" or "unprogrammed" spaces of his later projects such as Kansai Airport (Japan, 1988) and Le Fresnoy National Center for the Contemporary Arts (Tourcoing, France, 1992–98) to those heterogeneous projects that encompass multiple uses or functions, such as the Rouen Concert Hall and Exhibition Center in France and the Columbia University Student Center (Alfred Lerner Hall, New York City, 1994–99). He defined "in-between spaces" as inherently ambiguous; they were not dedicated to a single or specific function. This ambiguity provoked the uncanny, the strange, and the unfamiliar in architecture. Heterogeneous spaces contained several normally unrelated functions simultaneously, such as those he illustrated in *The Manhattan Transcripts* (1981): "the quarterback tangoes on the skating rink; the battalion skates on the tightrope." Heterogeneous spaces are not solely determined by function because life exceeds architecture, according to Tschumi. These spaces invited the multiplicity and diversity of a contemporary fragmented culture.

With the Alfred Lerner Hall at Columbia University, Tschumi attempted to demonstrate these spatial and design principles by containing a series of ramps for circulation between

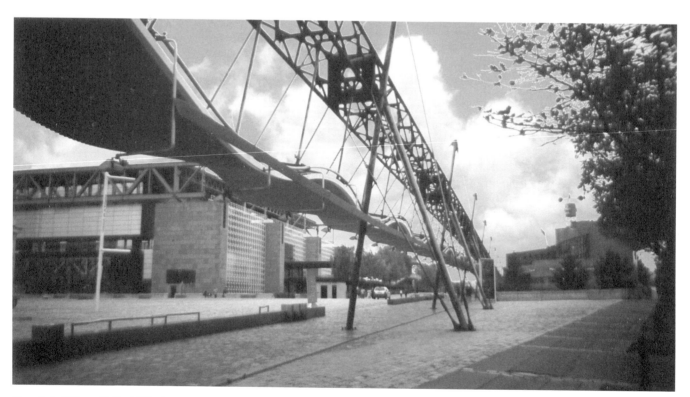

Parc de la Villette, Paris, 1987–91
© Dan Delgado *d2 Arch*

floors, student mailboxes, and several other sitting, standing, and viewing conditions that set up multiple possibilities for social contact.

Shock and disjunction made it possible for subjects to experience and recognize the connections that subjects make between fragments that are artificial and yet habituated in experience and thought. When habits are displaced, new experiences are possible. Tschumi's goal was to redefine the experience of architecture itself.

JEAN LA MARCHE

See also **Deconstructivism; Koolhaas, Rem (Netherlands)**

Biography

Bernard Tschumi was born in Lausanne, Switzerland, 25 January 1944; father was architect Jean Tschumi (1904–62). Graduated with architecture degree from Eidgenössische Technische Hochschule (Federal Institute of Technology) in Zurich, 1969. Taught at Architectural Association in London (1970–79), the Institute for Architecture and Urban Studies in New York (1976), Princeton University (1976, 1980), and the Cooper Union for the Advancement of Science and Art, New York City (1980–83). Dean, Graduate School of Architecture, Planning and Preservation, Columbia University, New York City, 1988–2003. Won international competition for the planning of the Parc de la Villette (Paris, 1983), an award that would propel him into international architectural fame. Appointed chairman, Flushing Meadows Task Force in New York (1987–89); member, Collège International de Philosophie; a chevalier in the Legion d'Honneur; officer, Ordre des Arts et Lettres in France. Received the Grand Prix National d'Architecture of France (1996) and England's Royal Victoria Medal.

Selected Publications

The Manhattan Transcripts: Theoretical Projects, London and New York: Academy Editions/St. Martin's Press, 1981
Architecture and Disjunction, Cambridge, Massachusetts, and London: MIT Press, 1984
La Case vide, London: Architectural Association, 1986
Cinegramme Folie: Le Parc de la Villette New York: Princeton Architectural Press, 1987
Architecture and Disjunction: Collected Essays 1975–1990, Cambridge, Massachusetts: MIT Press, 1994
Event-Cities: Praxis, Cambridge, Massachusetts: MIT Press, 1994

Selected Works

Kansai International Airport, Osaka (competition), 1988
ZKM, Center for Art and Media, Karlsruhe, Germany, 1989
Flushing Meadows Corona Park, Queens, New York, 1989
Parc de la Villette, Paris, France, 1991
Hague Villa, the Netherlands, 1992
School of Architecture, Florida International University, Miami, 1993
Le Fresnoy National Center for the Contemporary Arts, Tourcoing, France, 1998
Columbia University Student Center (Alfred Lerner Hall), New York City, 1999

Further Reading

"Bernard Tschumi 1983–1993," *A + U* (March 1994)
"Bernard Tschumi: Alfred Lerner Hall with Gruzen Samton Architects, New York, New York," *Praxis*, 1 (Fall 1999)
Futagawa, Yukio (editor), *Bernard Tschumi*, G.A. Document Extra, Tokyo: ADA Edita, 1997
Johnson, Philip, and Mark Wigley (editors), *Deconstructivist Architecture*, New York: Museum of Modern Art, 1988
Papadakis, Andreas, Catharine Cooke, and Andrew Benjamin (editors), *Deconstruction: Omnibus Volume*, New York: Rizzoli, 1989
Richardson, Sara S., *Bernard Tschumi: A Bibliography*, Monticello, Illinois: Vance, 1988
Tschumi Le Fresnoy: Architecture In/Between, New York: Monacelli Press, 1999
"Works of Bernard Tschumi", *A + U*, 216 (1988): (1988)

TUGENDHAT HOUSE, BRNO, CZECH REPUBLIC

Designed by Ludwig Mies van der Rohe; completed 1930

Among the most significant private houses of the 20th century, Ludwig Mies van der Rohe's Tugendhat House represents a material unity of steel, stone, and glass. Situated on a slope to provide ample views, the Tugendhat House echoed Mies' use of continuous space first realized in the German Pavilion in Barcelona (1929).

The owners, Grete Weiss Löw-Beer and Fritz Tugendhat, met Mies in Berlin in 1927 before their marriage. They shared a preference for a modern style and an aversion to traditional interiors. After viewing several of Mies' buildings, including the Wolff house in Guben, they commissioned the Berlin architect to design their new house.

In September 1928 Mies went to Brno to view the lot on which the house was to be built, and on the evening of 31 December 1928, the first sketches were discussed. The final design of the house was decided on around July 1929, when work on the foundations was begun. Several changes were made during construction.

The house is built on an incline, with the living area on the southern side with a view of the garden and the Brno cityscape. On the street, or northern side, the house looks unremarkable, presenting a low and closed facade with a wide, covered entry area. The garage and chauffeur's quarters are on the right. On the left are the bedrooms and bathrooms and a terrace with a view of the garden. These private rooms are separated from the entryway by a vestibule that also contains the stairway to the lower floor. The lower floor contains the servants' quarters, kitchen, and pantry on the eastern side, but most of the space is taken up with the living room. That living space, which is not visible from the street, forms the center of the house and functions as dining room, workroom, library, and sitting room. The living area gives access to another terrace on the same level, from which a staircase leads into the garden. The cellars, which can be reached from the kitchen by means of a circular staircase, contains spaces for the furnace, machines to operate the windows, a laundry room, and so on. Originally it also contained a darkroom because Fritz Tugendhat was an amateur filmmaker.

The most remarkable section of the house is the living area, spreading over an area of 223 square meters (about 2400 square feet). Instead of designing a series of closed spaces, Mies chose to build a single continuous space. This freedom in spatial division was made possible by the use of a steel frame, which dispensed with the need for internal supporting walls. Mies had already experimented with this principle in his houses for the Weissenhofsiedlung in Stuttgart of 1927. In Brno his use of steel permitted a different layout for each level, thus providing an exceptional openness of the living space. This openness was reinforced by floor-to-ceiling windows on the southern and western sides. The windows open up the interior space to the outside, much like the German Pavilion.

In the living area, the separate functions are structured and suggested by spatial means and beautiful, pristine materials. A freestanding onyx wall separates the living room from the workroom. A semicircular wooden wall with a Macassar veneer defines the dining area. The arrangement of the furniture also structures the space, marking places for various living functions. Moving it would undermine the "zoning" of the space. In the living space, most of the furniture was metal, including Mies' tube chair from Stuttgart (1927) and his Barcelona armchair (1929). He also designed the sheet-metal "Brno armchair" and the "Brno dining room chair."

The technical facilities of the house were exceptional for the time. Central heating was supplemented in the living area with a forced-hot-air system in the winter that also served as air-conditioning in the summer. In addition the house had built-in humidifiers and air purifiers, a hydraulic system that lowered the living-area windows into the ground, and a light sensor that automatically locked the front door at night.

The house's high cost and the luxurious interior gave rise to criticism. Modernist architects of Brno and Prague objected to the project on the basis of their social convictions. Mies' German origins and the fact that he had succeeded Hannes Meyer at the Bauhaus also played a role in the disapproval from his Czech colleagues. As a consequence Czech architectural circles ignored the house. A different controversy arose in Germany, where *Die Form* asked whether the architectural ideas of Mies determined the lifestyle of the inhabitants to too great a degree. Fritz and Grete Tugendhat denied this in their response, also published in *Die Form*, but admitted that it was not possible to change anything in the interior without disturbing the architect's design.

The inhabitants did not have much time to try out Mies' living concepts. In 1938 the family decided to emigrate to Venezuela as a result of the threatened expansion of the Nazi regime in Germany. The house stood empty for a year before being appropriated by the German occupier. After 1945 the house first became a ballet school and then, in 1950, part of the Brno children's hospital, which used the space for physical therapy. In 1970 the City of Brno took over the house, but renovation on the house did not start until the period 1983–86. The building was freed of additions and adaptations, but the original furniture and equipment were largely lost. In 1995 the restoration of the interior was undertaken, with remakes of the original furnishings. Since 1996 the house has been open to visitors as part of the Brno City Museum.

OTAKAR MÁCEL

See also **German Pavilion, Barcelona (1929); Mies van der Rohe, Ludwig (Germany); Weissenhofsiedlung, Deutscher Werkbund, Stuttgart (1927)**

Further Reading

Drexler, Arthur (editor), *The Mies van der Rohe Archive*, New York and London: Garland, 1986–; see especially part 1, *1910–1937*, vol. 4

Hammer-Tugendhat, Danniela, and Wolf Tegethoff (editors), *Ludwig Mies van der Rohe: Das Haus Tugendhat*, Vienna: Springer, 1998; as *Ludwig Mies van der Rohe: The Tugendhat House*, New York: Springer, 2000

Kudelková, Lenka, and Otakar Mácel, "The Villa Tugendhat in Brno," in *Mies van der Rohe: Architecture and Design in Stuttgart, Barcelona, Brno*, edited by Alexander von Vegesack and Matthias Kries, Milan: Skira Editore, and Weil am Rhein: Vitra Design Museum, 1998

Schulze, Franz, *Mies van der Rohe: A Critical Biography*, Chicago: University of Chicago Press, 1985

Stiller, Adolph (editor), *Das Haus Tugendhat: Ludwig Mies van der Rohe, Brünn, 1930*, Salzburg: Pustet, 1999

TURKEY

As with other areas of cultural production, in Turkey the prevailing theme in both the practice and the discourse of architecture in the 20th century was the tension between a desire to assert a uniquely national character and the quest to become modern by keeping up with international trends in the profession and by responding to the demands of an ever-changing global context. The balance between the two tendencies shifted frequently, remaining a constant source of debate throughout the century. On the basis of overarching similarities in the organization of professional practice and education, the dominant discourses in architecture, the types of buildings commissioned, and the identity of the clients, as well as broader issues concerning national and international politics, economic policies, and ideological orientations, we may divide the time line between the 1890s and the present into four periods. Longer surveys offer further subperiodizations on the basis of the identity of the architects and stylistic preferences. The early Republican years have been divided into First Nationalist (1890s–1927), First International (1927–late 1930s), and Second Nationalist (late 1930s–late 1940s).

1890s to Mid-1920s

The decades preceding the post–World War I collapse and subsequent partition of the Ottoman Empire were defined by turbulent wars followed by waves of mass migration, the encroachment of European imperialism, and formidable economic problems. To remedy these, the Ottoman government implemented various measures designed to modernize the state and its institutions after European models. Similarly, in an effort to raise the standards in professional education, in 1882 the School of Fine Arts (Senayii Nefise), based loosely on the Beaux-Arts model, was founded, followed in 1884 by the School of Engineering (Hendese-i Mülkiye Mektebi), for which faculty were recruited mainly from Germany and Austria. Foreign faculty

from both schools were also commissioned for various projects, many of which were novel building types that housed some new function of the modernizing Ottoman capital. The Ottoman Public Debt Administration (1899), the Imperial College of Medicine (1903), and the Museum of Archaeology (1891–1907) were designed by Alexandre Vallaury of the Fine Arts School, and the Deutsche Bank and the Sirkeci Railroad Terminal (1890) were the work of Professor Jachmund. Among other foreign professionals in Istanbul at the time, Raimondo D'Aronco designed several pavilions at the Yildiz Palace, and Otto Ritter and Helmut Cuno were commissioned to build the Haydarpasa Railroad Terminal (1908). The professional sensibilities of Istanbul's foreign builders differed, depending on their backgrounds. However, when confronted with the challenge of building in a densely packed city with a complex history, a diverse population, and enduring architectural traditions, they typically resorted to incorporating some Ottoman decorative elements into the mainly neoclassical decorative scheme of the interior and exterior surfaces of their buildings while adhering to spatial layouts with the recognizable symmetry and axiality of the Beaux-Arts tradition. Young Ottoman architects trained in the new schools or Europe also experimented with these ideas. Generally known as Ottoman Revivalism, these efforts to incorporate historical references into distinctively modern building programs were comparable to contemporary trends in Europe in terms of discourse and practice. This was evident, for example, in the similarity of the functional layout, volumetric composition, and handling of historical references in Kemalettin Bey's Dördüncü Vakif Hani (1912–26) business complex and Harikzedegan Apartments to their European contemporaries and in Vedad (Tek) Bey's Sirkeci Post Office (1909), which bears a striking resemblance to Otto Wagner's Postal Savings Bank (1904–06) in Vienna.

The conceptual breakdown between the spatial organization and the decorative schemes (in Ottoman Revivalism) also dovetailed conveniently with the tenets of the rising Turkish nationalism, which, albeit artificially, drew a distinction between civilization and culture. The nationalists deemed *civilization* to be a system of objectively formulated universal truths and rules pertaining to practical matters that could be borrowed from the West, but defined *culture* as a subjective system of beliefs and mores that had to be jealously guarded as the core of a distinctively Turko-Islamic identity. Despite its dubious grounding, the analogy was extended into architecture, where new construction technologies and building types were imported as products of Western civilization, whereas the formal repertoire of Ottoman architecture was retained as a vestige of the national culture. Eventually, when the protonationalist Young Turks seized power in 1908, their ambitious initiative to construct administrative and institutional buildings throughout the empire effectively converted Ottoman Revivalism into the official architecture and, more important, replaced its imperial associations with nationalist ones.

After the proclamation of the republic (1923), which marked Turkey's transition to nation-statehood, their credentials as the creators of the nationalist architecture helped Kemal and Vedat Bey and their cohorts secure important commissions for some of the first official buildings of the country's new capital, Ankara.

Kemalettin Bey's Gazi School of Education (1926–30) and Vakif Apartments (1928); Vedat Bey's Parliament Building (1926) and the Ankara Palas Hotel (1924–27); Arif Hikmet's (Koyunoglu) Ministry of Foreign Affairs (1927), Turkish Hearths (1927–30), and Museum of Ethnography (1927–30); and Giulio Mongeri's Agriculture Bank (1926–29) and Labor Bank (1928) stand among the most prominent buildings of the new republic's early years.

Mid-1920s to Late 1940s

Beyond introducing a new political entity, by founding a new republic, Turkey's leaders tried to inaugurate a modern national identity for the country and its people through extensive legal, institutional, and administrative reforms. During this formative period, Turkey's collaboration with longtime ally Germany brought German experts and capital, shaping the principles and direction of the modernization process. Turkey's leaders regarded architecture and urbanism as crucial instruments for rendering their reforms tangible. Thus, building a new capital in Ankara, for which they commissioned a plan from Hermann Jansen (1928–32), was one of their most ambitious undertakings. As the first plan introducing modern planning principles—such as land use zoning and a greenbelt system—on the scale of an entire city, Jansen's plan was regarded as a model for the subsequent development of all Turkish cities.

In architecture, incoming foreign professionals sidelined their Turkish counterparts in obtaining government commissions, as the omission of historicist references in their projects favored them to Turkey's leaders, who by then had moved away from a particularist nationalism with strong Turko-Islamic associations toward a universalist position, seeking to integrate Turkey with Europe. In actuality, the stripped-down Central European Neoclassicism of Theodor Post's Ministry of Health, Ankara (1926–27) or Clemens Holzmeister's ministerial buildings (1929–36) in the new government quarter, to name a few, shared the same Beaux-Arts-inspired compositional principles with nationalist architecture. However, it was more appealing to Turkey's leaders because its restrained unornamented appearance imparted a desirable sense of stately dignity and also because it was less labor intensive and required cheaper materials.

As evidenced by the recruitment of artists, architects, and intellectuals fleeing Nazi persecution alongside those with ties to the German government, the Turkish government was interested more in the expertise and skills of its foreign specialists than in their political associations. Although they rarely found a platform for expressing their political views, émigré architects injected a different strain of modernist sensibilities into Turkey's professional and intellectual discourses both through their involvement in the massive overhaul of higher education and through projects that displayed the trademark traits of German modernism, such as broken masses, interlocking volumes, open plans, and a move away from symmetry and axiality. Bruno Taut's Faculty of Language, History, and Geography (1937) and Trabzon High School (1937–38) and Martin Elsaesser's Sumerbank Headquarters (1937) figure among the prominent examples of the work of German émigrés in Turkey. Moreover,

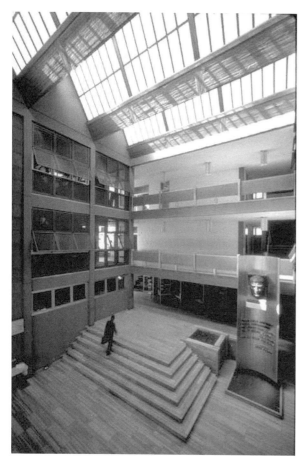

Turkish Historical Society, central court atrium, designed by Turgut Cansever (1966)
© Aga Khan Trust for Culture

Martin Wagner's consultancy for the Istanbul Municipality and Ernst Reuter's tenure in the School of Political Science in Ankara served as a foundation for modern town-planning education in Turkey.

Meanwhile, local architects denounced their exclusion from most major government projects in *Arkitekt*, the first Turkish-language professional journal, which provided information about the latest trends and debates in the profession. *Arkitekt* also promoted the work of Turkish architects, who, as evidenced by Sekip Akalin's Ankara Railroad Terminal (1937), Seyfi Arkan's Palace of Exhibitions (1933), and Harbi Holtan's Istanbul University Observatory (1936), were experimenting with both modernist and neoclassical repertoires. In the late 1930s, Sedad Hakki Eldem, one of the most prolific Turkish architects of the century, spearheaded the Second Nationalist movement, calling for a return to national precedents for inspiration. However, as in the examples of Atatürk's Mausoleum (1942–53, by Emin Onat and Orhan Arda) and the Colleges of Sciences of the Istanbul (1944) and Ankara (1945) universities (by S. H. Eldem and Emin Onat), rather than introducing new spatial ideas, the second wave of nationalists retained their connection to the Beaux-Arts tradition, adhering to the organizational principles of the Central European Neoclassicism of Clemens Holzmeister

and Paul Bonatz. Their references to local traditions took the form of stylized Ottoman decorative elements with a heightened awareness of precedents in civic and domestic architecture in the articulation of masses and plans.

More ubiquitous although less studied in this period are the numerous urban plans and institutional structures (schools, railroad stations, and community centers) that constituted the recurring and recognizable elements of a standardized national landscape. Designed and built by central state agencies, these structures were integral to the nation-building and modernization strategies. Among others, Turkey's first female architects, Leman Tomsu and Munevver Belen, built their careers on these commissions.

Late 1940s to Mid-1980s

In the aftermath of World War II, the onset of the Cold War and the polarization of the international arena into rival blocs brought Turkey closer to the United States politically, economically, and culturally. American experts, capital, and models of modernization replaced those of Germany. The single-party rule ended in 1950, and more liberal economic policies were gradually adopted.

Significant changes also occurred in the architectural profession and education. With more architects graduating and venturing into private practice, the Chamber of Architects was formed in 1950 to protect the interests of the profession and to promote fair practices, especially in government commissions. In 1956, the Middle East Technical University Faculty of Architecture was opened in Ankara, adding American models of professional education to French and German models adopted earlier by the two schools in Istanbul.

During this period, the state continued to be the primary source of projects and jobs, but a growing clientele of private entrepreneurs also began to commission projects, such as factories, hotels, and office buildings. Nevzat Erol's Istanbul City Hall (1953); Skidmore, Owings and Merrill's Istanbul Hilton Hotel (1952, with S. H. Eldem); Bozkurt, Bolak, and Beken's Ulus Business Complex (1954); and Behruz and Altug Cinici's Middle East Technical University campus (starting in 1955) stand out as early examples of the expanding repertoire of architectural practice.

The diversification of projects, the increasing numbers of architects, and changes in education multiplied the stylistic, theoretical, and ethical discourses, especially after the 1960s. The various strains of postwar internationalism with which Turkish architects experimented may be observed in Günay Cilingiroglu's Istanbul Reklam (1969) and Tercuman Press Facilities (1974), Sevki Vanli's M.S.-B. Dormitories (1967–68), Sisa and Tekeli's Lassa Tire Factory (1975–77), and Sargin an Böke's Is Bank Headquarters. Meanwhile, as early as 1962, architects and scholars began to debate questions of contextualism and cultural heritage. Eldem's Zeyrek Social Security Complex (1963–70), Turgut Cansever's Turkish Historical Society (1966), and Cengiz Bektas's Turkish Language Society (1972–78) are examples of projects addressing issues of heritage, context, and regional character. In the 1960s, population increase and waves of internal migration resulted not only in the densification of major metropolitan areas, with speculative apartment buildings emerg-

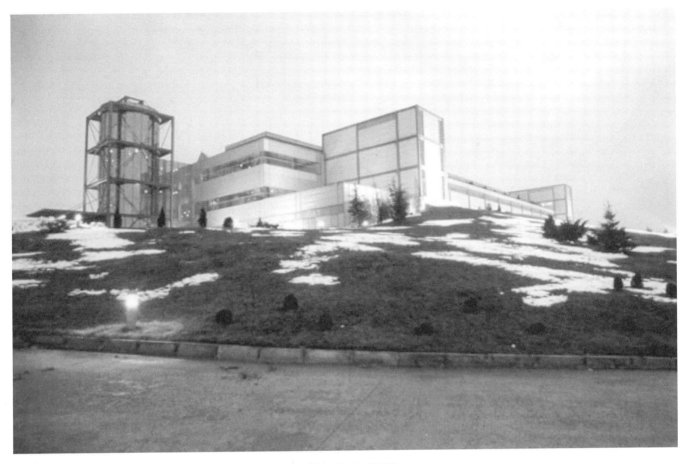

Dogan Media (Printing) Center, designed by Hayati and Murat Tabanlioglu (1997)
© Aga Khan Trust for Culture

ing as the dominant type of urban housing, but also in the growth of squatter settlements around them. Although the academic and professional discourse became highly politicized in response to these problems, little could be implemented to resolve them.

1980s to the Present

Starting in 1980, the introduction of liberal economic measures, designed to integrate Turkey into the globalization process, followed by a military coup that facilitated their implementation, triggered profound changes in society, culture, and politics and widened the gap between the rich and the poor.

The state's role in initiating new projects diminished, but with their newfound autonomy, local governments organized competitions for various projects, such as Davran Eskinat's Ankara Bus Terminal (1995) and Hasan Ozbay and Tamer Basburg's Gaziantep City Hall (1987), among others. Meanwhile, the private sector clearly became the major source of commissions. International partnerships and the influx of foreign capital transformed existing patterns of work and consumption. Like their contemporary counterparts that were mushrooming

around the world, the new building types, which were designed to accommodate emerging uses, were not particularly distinctive by design, yet they stood as a remarkable novelty within the Turkish landscape. Exclusive resort hotels, such as the Sheraton Voyager (1990, by S. Basatemür) and Falez (1990, by Y. and S. Erdemir and S. Akkaya) in Antalya, and holiday villages, such as Pamfilya (by Tuncay Çavdar), burgeoned in coastal regions. Luxury corporate hotels (the Sheraton and Hilton in Ankara and the Swissotel, and Conrad Istanbul), business centers (Dogan Media Center by Aydin Boysan and Hayati and Murat Tabanlioglu and Sabanci Center by Haluk Tümay and Ayhan Böke), and downtown shopping centers (Akmerkez by Han Karabey and Atakule by Ragip Buluç) were built in major cities, which at the same time were challenged by rampant unemployment and massive internal migration. Although squatter settlements encircled many a Turkish metropolis, large housing developments accelerated suburbanization. Such developments include both upscale (MESA Korusitesi and Elvankent) and medium-range (Eryaman and Batikent) ones, gated communities (Mercansaray Evleri and Kemer Country), malls (Galleria Ataköy, 1989, by Hayati Tabanlioglu and Capitol Shopping Center, 1990–93, by Adnan Kazmaoglu and Murat Çilingiroglu), and megastores catering primarily to the upper-middle and upper classes.

In the 1990s, the conversion of Çiragan Palace and Sultan-ahmet Prison into luxury hotels, the gradual gentrification of older urban neighborhoods, and the random formalist replication of traditional motifs in new buildings, as well as a growing interest in miscellaneous traditional artifacts, indicated the increasing commodification of "heritage" in Turkey. As exemplified by the eclectic remix of historical precedents in Kemer Country designed by Elizabeth Plater-Zyberk and Andres Duany, local tradition had become one among many choices available to a select segment of Turkish society with access to the benefits of globalization. Given the relative scarcity of debate about the displacement of meanings in these examples and the rather indiscriminate importation of global trends, such approaches to historical context can hardly be considered critical or regionalist.

Zeynep Kezer

See also **Duany and Plater-Zyberk (United States); Eldem, Sedad Hakki (Turkey); Gürel Family Summer Residence, Çanakkale, Turkey; Istanbul, Turkey; Mosque of the Grand National Assembly, Ankara, Turkey**

Further Reading

Alsaç, Üstün, *Türkiye'deki mimarlik düsüncesinin cumhuriyet dönemindeki evrimi*, Trabzon: Karadeniz Teknik Üniversitesi Mimarlik ve Insaat Fakültesi, 1976

Aslanoglu, Inci, *Erken cumhuriyet dönemi mimarlik*, Ankara: Orta Dogu Teknik Üniversitesi, 1980

Bozdogan, Sibel, *Modernism and Nation Building: Turkish Architectural Culture in the Early Republic*, Seattle: University of Washington Press, 2001

Bozdogan, Sibel, and Resat Kasaba (editors), *Rethinking Modernity and National Identity in Turkey*, Seattle: University of Washington Press, 1997

Holod, Renata, and Ahmet Evin (editors), *Modern Turkish Architecture*, Philadelphia: University of Pennsylvania Press, 1984

Sey, Yildiz (editor), *75 yilda degisen kent ve mimarlik*, Istanbul: Türkiye Ekonomik ve Toplumsal Tarih Vakfi, 1998

Sözen, Metin, *Cumhuriyet dönemi Türk mimarligi, 1923–1983*, Ankara: Türkiye is Bankasi Kültür Yayinlari, 1984

Yavuz, Yildirim, *Mimar Kemalettin ve birinci ulusal mimarlik dönemi*, Ankara: Orta Dogu Teknik Üniversitesi Yayinlari, 1981

TWA AIRPORT TERMINAL

Designed by Eero Saarinen; completed 1962
New York City, New York

Initially known as the Trans World Flight Center, the TWA Airport Terminal rose as one of several stand-alone terminals that made up the original Idlewild Airport (now JFK International) in Queens, a borough of New York City. The TWA Terminal, by Eero Saarinen and Associates, became the culminating work in Saarinen's search for dynamic sculptural expression in reinforced-concrete construction. The architect died during emergency neurosurgery in 1961, the year before the terminal building opened.

The commission from the Trans World Airlines Company was made in 1956, just as Saarinen came to worldwide prominence with the completion of the General Motors Technical Center (1955) in Warren, Michigan—a Mies-inspired scheme

of a corporate-scale campus begun with his father, architect Eliel Saarinen, in the 1940s. The airline company wanted something much bolder from the younger Saarinen for its New York terminal, expecting that its masterpiece would likewise represent the airline's status as the industry leader.

Eero Saarinen had already made clear his self-stated "urge to soar" in architecture, starting with his 1948 competition winner for the Jefferson National Expansion Memorial, colloquially known as the St. Louis Gateway Arch (1964). His quest continued with the thin-shelled triangular concrete roof of the Kresge Auditorium (1955) at the Massachusetts Institute of Technology in Cambridge and at Yale University's Ingalls Hockey Rink (1959) in New Haven, Connecticut. The rink, with its cable-strung roof suspended from a humpbacked central concrete spine, was the forerunner of Saarinen's Dulles International Airport (1962) in Chantilly, Virginia, and of Kenzo Tange's Tokyo Olympic Swim Hall (1964) as much as its formal considerations affected the TWA design.

Saarinen took his cue from its site, positioned at the far corner of the Idlewild property, opposite the airport entry. The building was angled to sweep gently across at sidewalk level to align itself with the curvature of its corner frontage roadway. Inside, behind the encircling arms of the ticket lobby, Saarinen envisioned a shallow rise to a spacious waiting hall from which matched winding staircases would lead passengers to the departure level with its finger ramp out to waiting planes. (A second finger ramp was added by the inheritors of the firm, Kevin Roche and John Dinkeloo.) Passenger movement through the terminal building was to be channeled, gradually but with absolute clarity, by the curved forms of the interior—a circulation process seen by Saarinen as akin in spirit to the science of aerodynamics.

After a year spent working on trial models for the terminal, the chief obstacle for Saarinen and his firm lay in sorting out the best way to put a roof on the building. Along with matters of site and function, structural integrity was the third guiding principle for Saarinen's architectural practice. As a rule he worked closely with the firm's associated engineers. This was particularly the case with Ammann and Whitney, collaborators on the TWA design as well as that for the Dulles Airport. In addition Saarinen was well schooled in the works of Pier Luigi Nervi in Italy and was friends with Minoru Yamasaki, a principal in the firm of Yamasaki, Hellmuth and Leinweber, architects for the St. Louis Air Terminal (1954), with its domed interior spaces.

Saarinen jettisoned earlier TWA roof schemes in favor of a more complex arrangement of four interlocking vaulted segments, set on a perimeter of concrete edge beams. As with Jørn Utzon's counterbalanced roof sails in the Sydney Opera House (the entry that Saarinen supported in that city's commission), a support system had yet to be devised for the terminal roof. The firm and the engineers jointly solved the problem with the introduction of a four-poster arrangement of irregular Y-shaped piers, the front two serving as markers for the terminal entry. Model photographs document how the piers were molded, as if carved from a bar of soap, in keeping with Saarinen's aesthetic vision for the building as a whole, without any loss of structural integrity. A rudimentary version of the various new roof and support elements was recorded as a set of thumbnail sketches preserved as part of the Eero Saarinen Papers at his alma mater, Yale University. Also hearkening back to the Saarinens' Finnish

background, Kevin Roche among others has noted how the shape of the terminal echoes that of an old Norseman's helmet, with its split shell and upturned edge.

Saarinen saw the final composition for the building as somewhat baroque in terms of its fluid, sequential layout, "creating a [comparable] dynamic space . . . but using different play blocks" to create "a total environment" where each part of the design "belonged to the same form-world" (1968). Some architecture critics, notably Vincent Scully, Jr., were initially dismissive of the building but later determined that it had its merits. Art historian Henry-Russell Hitchcock similarly dismissed the building in the *Zodiac* (1962). The flying public had no such reservations.

In a tribute to Saarinen, published by *Architectural Forum* in October 1961, editor Douglas Haskell made fond reference to "Eero's 'big bird' in concrete." Through his final days, even as the terminal roofs were being finished, Saarinen downplayed any zoomorphic interpretations of the building, preferring instead that it be seen and experienced as a visual analogy of flight. Unfortunately, for the terminal building and Saarinen's hopes for it, the nature of air travel has altered dramatically over intervening decades, prompting a host of changes to airport infrastructure. Nearly all the changes have wreaked havoc with the layout of Saarinen's once-expansive interiors. Thirty-three years after Saarinen's last sight of the unfinished building, with both TWA and its flagship terminal reeling in the wake of post-Reagan airline deregulation, architecture critic Herbert Muschamp did find one silver lining for the beleaguered masterwork. In his column of 6 November 1994 for the *New York Times*, "Stay of Execution for a Dazzling Airline Terminal," Muschamp reported that the New York City Council had voted to uphold the air terminal's designation as a municipal landmark.

DAVID NAYLOR

See also **Airport and Aviation Building; Dulles International Airport, Chantilly, Virginia; Gateway Arch, St. Louis, Missouri; Nervi, Pier Luigi (Italy); Saarinen, Eero (Finland); Utzon, Jørn (Denmark)**

Further Reading

A substantial amount of attention was given to the TWA Airport Terminal in two books published in 1962 (the year the building was completed): Allan Temko's monograph and a folio-sized compilation of Saarinen's statements about his work. The latter is heavily illustrated, using mostly photographs made by frequent Saarinen collaborator Ezra Stoller, and was edited by the architect's widow, Aline B. Saarinen and revised for a new edition in 1968. Since the 1960s major coverage has been scarce, aside from a section devoted to the building in the 1984 publication by *A + U* and a three-part 30th anniversary tribute to the TWA Terminal produced by *Progressive Architecture* as a case study for its May 1992 issue.

Brodherson, David, " 'An Airport in Every City': The History of American Airport Design," in *Building for Air Travel: Architecture and Design for Commercial Aviation*, edited by John Zukowsky, Chicago and New York: The Art Institute of Chicago, and Munich: Prestel, 1996

Fisher, Thomas, "Landmarks: TWA Terminal," *Progressive Architecture*, 73 (May 1992)

Leubkeman, Christopher Hart, "Form Swallows Function," *Progressive Architecture*, 73 (May 1992)

Nakamura, Toshio (editor), *Eero Saarinen; Ero Sarinen* (bilingual English–Japanese edition), Tokyo: A + U, 1984

Papademetriou, Peter, "TWA's Influence," *Progressive Architecture*, 73 (May 1992)

Saarinen, Aline B. (editor), *Eero Saarinen on His Work: A Selection of Buildings Dating from 1947 to 1964 with Statements by the Architect*, New Haven, Connecticut: Yale University Press, 1962; revised edition, 1968

Stoller, Ezra, *The TWA Terminal*, New York: Princeton Architectural Press, 1999

Temko, Allan, *Eero Saarinen*, New York: Braziller, and London: Prentice-Hall, 1962

TYPOLOGY

Typology, the study of types or classes of objects, has long served to catalyze debates about both representation and invention. In architecture the types in question may be defined by form (such as central plan churches), by their presumed originary role (such as the "primitive hut"), by program or function (schools and museums), or by a historical sedimentation of characteristics (for example, English terrace housing). "Types" are objects of study, and "typology" is the study of them.

Typology must be exhaustive concerning its chosen class of objects, and thus its limits are as important as its particular content, as when Nikolaus Pevsner opened his *Outline of European Architecture* (1943) by excluding the utilitarian "bicycle shed." Any typology aims to reduce the potentially infinite variety of objects considered. In the most explicitly typological studies of architecture and urban morphology, this gives rise to arrays of diagrams depicting variations in plan, section, and elevation, of which a thorough German tradition is a useful example (Geist, 1983). Related networks of researchers in France, Italy, and the United States continue to work explicitly in a methodological vein known as "typomorphology" (see Vernez Moudon, 1994).

Interest in type among architects and theorists can be understood as the search for a middle ground between the poles of pure invention and blind determinism. Since the beginnings of architectural modernity in the 18th and 19th centuries, advocates of type as a guide or foundation of design have tended to define it by exclusion of these extremes; hence A. C. Quatremère de Quincy's (1755–1849) classic distinction, made in 1829, between the "type" and the "model." The type, for this influential French theoretician, is an ideal schema that is reproduced without copying, whereas the model is to be imitated "as it is." Quatremère's type is above all not a model and cannot be fully incarnated in any single instance; moreover, its various instances might not even resemble one another. Leaving as it does a wide terrain open for formal invention, this notion allies architecture with fine arts such as painting and sculpture, in which such latitude is important. Quatremère's definition has remained a touchstone for many of the succeeding reflections on type.

However, architectural practice, responding to the modern pressure for standardization of all sorts, has made other demands on the idea of type. In particular, the pedagogical approach traced to J. N. L. Durand (1760–1834), who taught architecture to engineering students at the turn of the 19th century, proposes to view the design of a building as a combination of preexisting elements—rooms, colonnades, courtyards, and the like—that could be cataloged, selected, and distributed in a modular, axial

plan arrangement. This so-called rationalist approach finds strong echoes in the literature of professional manuals up to the present day.

At the same time, the structure of architectural commissions has changed under industrialization and the modern state. Where once a single patron, at least symbolically, would have given the order, clients since the 19th century have been increasingly collective—mainly governments and commercial consortia—and have formulated new and complex needs for spaces of production and administration, recorded in the form of detailed written programs. As professional attention has concentrated around considerations of function, they have come to dominate in many contexts over form as a basis for classifying what are now called "building types."

The functional or programmatic type provides a partial answer to Quatremère de Quincy's mysterious contention that works stemming from a common type might not resemble one another. For although the operation of a type must somehow involve a direct shaping of matter to produce a family of similar instances, Quatremère's argument signals a growing distrust of simple resemblance. Such an attitude, surprisingly enough, is not incompatible with Durand's impulse to demote the pictorial (and thereby the aesthetic) from among architecture's first principles. Thus, it is easy enough to find examples of train stations, hospitals, and town halls that belong to the same functional type and yet are dissimilar in plan, elevation, massing, size, or style. If architecture is considered to be determined by criteria that can be written and calculated in programs, then questions of mimesis—literally, what a building looks like—are of secondary importance. On the other hand, the figural characters of the architectural plan and facade remain critical to evaluating designs. In this sense the functional type and its representational or iconic aspects remain intertwined (see Holl, 1980).

Twentieth-century modernism's abstraction is fertile terrain for typological thinking. What unites disparate creations is a negative quality, the exclusion of some aspects in order to leave others visible. Canonically, this is seen in the removal of ornament, which allows the imagination to bracket the building's material specificity and to see it as an actual type instead of merely an instance of one. Such a straightforward reduction is quite close to the basic typological operation of reducing complexity to find the essential traits of a group. Yet what Anthony Vidler (1998) refers to as questions of ontology (essential being), first raised among 18th- and 19th-century theorists, remains heavily implicit in the modernist context as a tension between an "explanation of origins" and a "principle of form."

Hermann Muthesius (1861–1927) argued in the early years of the century that architecture strives toward the typical. As if in direct response to this remark, the facade of Adolph Loos's (1870–1933) Steiner House (1910), with its bare punched windows, eliminates much of the evidence that would allow it to be read in stylistic dialogue with preceding works. This choice to eliminate historically specific ornament—counterbalanced by sensitivity toward materials—is followed through, albeit in otherwise diverse ways, in the work of such later architects as Ludwig Mies van der Rohe (1886–1969) and Louis Kahn (1901–74). All three develop what might be called an essentialist or archetypal dimension, placing particular emphasis on elements that can be argued as present in any work of architecture and can be recognized in all its manifestations: the column, the

wall and its openings, the roof, and the ground plane. Such an attitude, tied to history but opposed to historicism, can be contrasted with the lively interest in prototypes displayed by other modern architects.

Proposing industrial repetition as a substitute for cultural sedimentation, the Modern movement abounds in prototypes intended to launch a kind of typological revolution. These projects are perhaps closer to Quatremère's "model" than to his "type," except insofar as they embrace the idea of variants and adaptation. Le Corbusier's (1887–1965) Dom-ino Houses (1915) seek to define a skeletal substructure on which variation can happen. In fact a great number of Le Corbusier's projects, from the Ville Contemporaine (1922) to the Unité d'Habitation (Marseilles, 1947–52), employ typological reasoning, proposing a typical solution across widely varying circumstances. The strategy is pursued with even greater rigor and persistence by early contemporaries, such as Ludwig Hilbersheimer (1885–1967), who seek to modernize society through architecture of repeated, industrially manufactured housing.

Although these projects rarely continue beyond the level of projects and prototypes, a great deal of post–World War II construction, both in the United States and in Europe, is based on the quasi-industrial repetition of basic types. Issues or considerations of construction and financing have enforced homogeneity in the service of political and financial rather than aesthetic goals. To cite only two well-known cases, the single-family suburban house (see Wright, 1981) and the "typical-plan" office building (see Koolhaas and Mau, 1995) have achieved an ambiguous hegemony, seemingly omnipresent even though widely criticized. This situation in turn has created larger and larger markets such that, even if whole buildings are only rarely mass-produced (see Herbert, 1984), their components certainly are.

Indeed, it is in part this galloping homogeneity and the reliance on top-down or market-driven solutions that elicited a growing critical reaction among architects becoming active in the 1950s and 1960s. The reaction is particularly visible in the group known as Team X, who organized the last of the Congrès Internationaux d'Architecture Moderne (CIAM) in 1956: Aldo Van Eyck (1918–99), Alison and Peter Smithson (1928–93, 1923–), Shadrach Woods (1923–73), Giancarlo de Carlo (1919–), and others. These architects view the imposition of a uniform culture of functional planning and faceless public and banal private housing as a result, among other things, of modernist architecture's abdication of its proper cultural role. They invoke, another kind of typological reasoning whereby, instead of a refined industrial model to be repeated by the thousands, the type could be understood as a collective product issuing from local or regional culture. These architects, practicing what Manfredo Tafuri has referred to as typological criticism, propose an anti-subjective aesthetic, seeing the long collective refinement of cultural artifacts as superior to the work of the individual intellect or the technocratic planner.

However, the debate concerning typology that will be freshest in most English-speaking readers' minds is the one that crystallized around a group of Italian architects who, beginning in the 1960s, promoted a critical reevaluation of traditional architectural and urban form. The group, called La Tendenza (neorationalism), is diverse but has in common an attachment to the idea that correctly conceived buildings and urban spaces would show more affinity with history than with the functional reason-

ing of the moment and might also outlast their current uses to house very different, indeed unforeseeable, ones in the future.

Neorationalism carries the ambiguous charge that already accrues to the different forms of rationalism discernible in architecture: it could be seen as anchored in the rational, that is, what could be explained or considered reasonable. However, it could also be concerned with the exercise of a pure reason, to a point that could in fact be seen as irrational. It is indeed this flip side of the rational that the best-known neorationalist, Aldo Rossi (1931–96), exploited most heavily, especially the ironic, antihumanist projects of the 1970s.

As a representation of the weight of the past on architectural invention, the notion of type has been central through two centuries of debate in architecture. Its lack of precision, while yet purporting to guide practice, has allowed richly differing uses and has kept the notion from becoming the intellectual property of any single group. In architectural and urban history and theory, the study of building types helps to counter the tendency to concentrate on a single building or author. In design practice, type has proven useful both as a workaday professional category and as a point of departure for debates over continuity and innovation. Some sort of typological reasoning is practically indispensable to architecture as an intellectual enterprise.

DAVID VANDERBURGH

See also **Loos, Adolf (Austria); Mies van der Rohe, Ludwig (Germany); Muthesius, Hermann (Germany); Rationalism; Rossi, Aldo (Italy); Steiner House, Vienna; Team X (Netherlands); Unité d'Habitation, Marseilles**

Further Reading

Franck, Karen A., and Linda Schneekloth (editors), *Ordering Space: Type in Architecture and Design*, New York: Van Nostrand Reinhold, 1994

Geist, Johan Friedrich, *Passagen: Ein Bautyp des 19. Jahrunderts*, Munich: Prestel, 1969; as *Arcades: The History of a Building Type*, translated by Jane O. Newman and John H. Smith, Cambridge, Massachusetts: MIT Press, 1983

Herbert, Gilbert, *The Dream of the Factory-Made House: Walter Gropius and Konrad Wachsmann*, Cambridge, Massachusetts: MIT Press, 1984

Holl, Steven, *The Alphabetical City*, New York: Princeton Architectural Press, 1980; second edition, 1987

Koolhaas, Rem, and Bruce Mau, "Typical Plan," in *S, M, L, XL*, edited by Jennifer Sigler, Rotterdam, The Netherlands: 010 Publishers, and New York: Monacelli Press, 1995

Markus, Thomas A., *Buildings and Power: Freedom and Control in the Origin of Modern Building Types*, London: Routledge, 1993

Pevsner, Nikolaus, *A History of Building Types*, Princeton, New Jersey: Princeton University Press, and London: Thames and Hudson, 1976

Rossi, Aldo, *L'architettura dell città*, Padua, Italy: Marsilio, 1966; as *The Architecture of the City*, translated by Diane Ghirardo and Joan Ockman, Cambridge, Massachusetts: MIT Press, 1982

Vernez Moudon, Anne, "Getting to Know the Built Landscape: Typomorphology," in *Ordering Space: Type in Architecture and Design*, edited by Karen A. Franck and Linda Schneekloth, New York: Van Nostrand Reinhold, 1994

Vidler, Anthony, "The Idea of Type: The Transformation of the Academic Ideal, 1750–1830," in *The Oppositions Reader*, edited by Michael Hayes, New York: Princeton Architectural Press, 1998

Wright, Gwendolyn, *Building the Dream: A Social History of Housing in America*, Cambridge, Massachusetts: MIT Press, 1981

U

UNGERS, OSWALD MATHIAS 1926–

Architect, Germany

Born on 12 July 1926 in Kaiseresch (Eifel), Oswald Mathias Ungers helped shape the international architectural scene of the second half of the 20th century. He studied at the Karlsruhe Technical University from 1947 to 1950 under Egon Eiermann, beginning a private practice in Cologne in 1950 and in Berlin in 1964. His work can be divided into three broad categories. His early career saw construction primarily of residences in a Modern style, up to the 1960s. This was followed by a theoretical and conceptual phase, from approximately 1963 to 1980, focusing on major competitions. The last decades of the 20th century provided Ungers with the opportunity for a full elaboration of his architectural ideas and ethos, based on intellectual and spiritual responsibility and the definition of architecture as an autonomous discipline. This commitment, together with his daring use of the cube form, situated him firmly as a leading figure in Postmodernism.

Ungers constructed his early works primarily in the Cologne area, where he opened his first office in 1950. The influence of Eiermann is unmistakable. The elegant lines of his single-family house on Oderweg (1951) in Cologne-Dünnwald or his apartment building on Hültzstrasse (1951) in Cologne-Braunsfeld underline a sleek and sober modernism as regards design and materials. Ungers's residences from a few years later show an influence by the Brutalism movement, inspired by Le Corbusier, including experimentation with new approaches to space as well as material. The multiple-family residence on Brambachstrasse (1955–57) in Cologne-Dellbrück employed his material of choice, rough brick, and represented a departure from the earlier, simple box form typical of modernism. The design of the roof and eaves, situated behind the facade, is a technical feat that he would return to often in later works.

Ungers's move toward new architectural forms and representations is clearest in his apartment building on Belvederstrasse (1958–59) in Cologne-Müngersdorf, where the stacked cubes form the basis of a new exploration of space and volume. Although the house's materials and form reference the neighboring buildings, it stands out as a defiant, new construction. Its expressiveness has caused more than one critic to describe it as part of the German Expressionist movement, a development that plunged Ungers into an analysis of Expressionist architecture. His essay from this period, presented in 1964 in Florence at a symposium on Expressionism, declared his now famous motto "Construction is not utopia, but rather battle." The library "cube house" addition (1989) strengthened the interplay of constructed and free spaces within and between the two buildings, lending the constellation an association of an urban setting and earning it the description of a city in miniature, or a house-city.

The early 1960s provided Ungers with a few larger projects, including the competitions for an art museum (1960) in Düsseldorf and a Roman-Germanic museum (1960) in Cologne. One of his biggest critical failures stems from this period as well, the residential construction of the Märkisches Viertel (1962–67) in Berlin-Wittenau. Initially designed as stacked buildings of 3 to 6 stories, the buildings were actually constructed with 8 to 16 stories, compromising the original statement of the design. This period represented a rupture in Ungers's career, coinciding with an appointment at the Technical University in Berlin, where he taught from 1963 to 1969.

Partly because of a lack of commissions and partly the result of Ungers's desire to reflect on his work, the next years were filled with a "theoretical" construction phase. In 1965 and 1967, he served as a visiting critic at Cornell University. Three projects from these years reflect the new conceptual forms that he had found for his architectural ideals: the design for the Dutch student dormitory (1964) in Enschede, the design for the Berlin museum complex (1965), and the design for the German embassy (1965) in Rome. Using the geometric forms of the circle, square, and triangle, Ungers proceeded to create variations on these basic themes. The result was a harmonious constellation of contrasts and progressions that would influence his work even decades later.

Although Ungers was unable to build most of the projects he designed during this period, usually competition designs, they helped define the possibilities and limits of his architectural thought and practice. Until the late 1970s, he produced numerous plans for major construction projects, including his design for the Berlin-Tegel airport (1966), with its flexible plan for updating the construction according to new airplane models and its emphasis on steel and aluminum. Ungers also entered the

competition for Cologne's Wallraf-Richartz Museum (1975), a design that foresaw the building as an extension of the cathedral area and connected the pedestrian zone with Breslauer Platz. He also began a time of much professional and academic international movement. In 1969 he became chair of the Department of Architecture at Cornell, and he opened an office in New York in 1970 after receiving his license there. In 1973 and 1978, he went to Harvard University as a visiting professor and was also a visiting professor at the University of California, Los Angeles, in 1974–75. In 1976 he opened an office in Frankfurt/Main. He went to the University for Applied Arts in Vienna from 1978 to 1980 and opened another office in Karlsruhe in 1983. He began to work at the university in Düsseldorf in 1986.

The late 1970s heralded a new era of large building projects, including the German Architectural Museum (1979–84) in Frankfurt and the residential complex on Lützowplatz (1979–83) in Berlin, with its bands of vertical window lines topped by triangular gables eliciting the impression of massive, moving arrows punctuating the long wall. Ungers's practice was then inundated with commissions, establishing his signature OMU as an established but dynamic architectural firm. In this new period of construction, Ungers's commitment to the cube form became the basis of almost all his future work. However, despite the reaffirmations of his theoretical plans, Ungers was forced to recognize that the translation of his designs into reality often resulted in compromises that weakened the strength of his structures. In this sense his architectural plans have been in some ways more important than the buildings themselves in elevating him to international status.

The last two decades of the 20th century offered Ungers the opportunity to realize many of his ideas in new forms. In 1990 he exhibited "Kubus," five three-meter-high cubes in a Cologne gallery, demonstrating his mastery of dividing space between concrete forms and emptiness. Numerous publications date from these years as well, including his thoughtful anthology, *Rectangular Houses* (1986). His constructions reflect the near half century of attempts to infuse his designs with uncompromising boldness through imposing geometric forms, such as the Alfred Wegener Institute for Polar Research (1980–84) in Bremerhaven.

Ungers ended the 20th century with a personally satisfying commission: the design of the new Wallraf-Richartz Museum (1996–99) in Cologne. He thereby completed a project for which he had not been selected nearly two decades earlier. Opened in the first month of 2001, the building allowed Ungers to display the many successful techniques he developed during his career, in the city where he had first begun to build. The museum's design alludes to its historic location between the Gürzenichstrasse and the city hall. Here, as in other designs, his building is a massive cube, but it is less imposing than in his other constructions, is less rigorous in its dimensions, and has an almost flowing, elegant quality. Now the newest home to Germany's oldest private art collection, the Wallraf-Richartz Museum is a fitting testimony to Ungers's determination to address the practical challenges of construction and tradition while insisting on architecture's right to self-determination and a building's responsibility to fulfill the individual spiritually and intellectually.

BENITA CAROL BLESSING

See also **Brutalism; Cubism; Expressionism**

Selected Publications

Ungers, Oswald Mathias, *Bauten und Projekte: 1991–1998,* Stuttgart, Germany: Deutsche Verlags-Anstalt, 1998
Ungers, Oswald Mathias, Fritz Neumeyer, and Marco de Michelis, *Oswald Mathias Ungers: Architecture 1951–1990,* 2 vols., Milan: Electa, 1991

Further Reading

Hezel, Dieter (editor), *Architekten: Oswald Mathias Ungers*, Stuttgart, Germany: IRB Verlag, 1990
Jesberg, P., "Zwischen Ratio und Phantasie: Über Oswald Mathias Ungers," *Deutsche Bauzeitschrift*, 40/6 (June)
Kieren, Martin, *Oswald Mathias Ungers* (bilingual English and German text), Zurich: Artemis, 1994

UNITÉ D'HABITATION, MARSEILLES

Designed by Le Corbusier, completed 1952
Marseilles, France

Although it never quite fulfilled its higher social purpose in its short life as public housing, the Unité d'Habitation at Marseilles today is occupied by families who clearly appreciate the building's history and architectural lineage. The first of Le Corbusier's *Unité d'habitation à grandeur conforme* to be realized, the giant, multipurpose complex containing 337 flats was meant to house 1600 people in 23 variants of the typical apartment. The two-story units range in size from small apartments for childless couples to multibedroom small houses for families of eight or more. Based loosely on the horizontal housing blocks on *pilotis* examined in the architect's 1930 book *Cité radieuse* (Radiant City), the Unité d'Habitation at Marseilles, like much of Le Corbusier's domestic architecture, was originally conceived as only part of a larger urban scheme. However, envisioning the need for postwar reconstruction in France, many of his subsequent town plans employed the principles laid out in the *Radiant City* and the Athens Charter of 1943 and contained plans for ultimately unrealized but similar garden cities. After the war, Raoul Dautry, a friend of Le Corbusier's, was appointed the first minister of reconstruction and urbanism and handed Le Corbusier the task of designing new housing in the poverty-stricken port city of Marseilles. Not quite the extensive town-planning project that Le Corbusier was hoping for (French architect and planner Auguste Perret had been drawing up the new urban plan for Le Havre in the meantime), he nonetheless garnered the support of seven subsequent ministers of reconstruction and overcame political instability in the still-Communist Marseilles, countless delays, huge cost overruns, misunderstandings at the site, and harsh criticisms from politicians, doctors, and architects alike. Ultimately, Le Corbusier managed to get an "experimental" tag placed on his plans and thus avoided the constricting zoning ordinances that would have made the building, as it was envisioned, impossible to build.

The self-contained "city" that the architect envisioned for Marseilles relinquished tradition for the convenience of the residents. The garden was on the roof, easily accessible to the nursery school and swimming pool; the "streets" were placed on floors 2, 5, 7, 8, 10, 13, and 16; and shops were placed on parts of the seventh and eighth floors instead of being intertwined with the commercial life of the city outside.

The basic apartment was laid out over two floors with a double-height living room, a kitchen, two bathrooms, two bedrooms for children separated by a movable screen to make for a larger playroom, and a third bedroom for parents. All living rooms faced onto a *bris-soleil*-style balcony that allowed sunlight to enter the apartment in winter and blocked it during the hot summer months. The kitchen is the single, unchanging element throughout the 23 different unit types. The kitchens gave a nod to the materials and beliefs employed by Americans Charles and Ray Eames and George Nelson, utilizing wood and laminated metal for countertops, tables, and cabinets and furthering the relation of the kitchen to the living room by opening the rooms to each other. There were openings from the hallways directly into the refrigerators for the delivery of ice and food, further advancing the ideas of convenience and self-containment.

The building was constructed after the war, a time when building materials were in short supply. Le Corbusier experimented widely with materials in Marseilles and the chapel at Ronchamp, which was being constructed simultaneously. Between these two projects, he fully developed the almost sculptural use of untreated concrete (*béton brut*, literally "raw concrete") as an acceptable building material. The project at Marseilles combined prefabricated-concrete slabs with poured-in-place forms playfully decorated with the patterns of seashells or locally fired tiles. Each apartment is fronted with a wood-framed glass plate inserted behind the concrete facade. The beehive-like structure, as it was once referred to, successfully translates Le Corbusier's original metaphor of the apartment block as bottle rack, in which each apartment was inserted like a bottle into the structure. He even envisioned in future housing units that the apartment units would be constructed off-site and hoisted into place, into the rack. The ground that the "rack" sits on is a table or platform supported by hollow *pilotis* or stilts that provide an area for services beneath the great monolithic structure.

The Unité d'Habitation at Marseilles was Le Corbusier's great experimental site where he applied to the entire structure his Modular measuring scheme. Everywhere, the more rational qualities of Le Corbusier's rambling half-scientific, half-mystical system of measure are employed and illustrated down to the inscribed "modular man" on the side of the building. There is one exception to the Modular rule, and it occurred by mistake; the *bris-soleil* frames on the outside of the building were mismeasured and misproportioned in the construction phase. Le Corbusier decided to have the frames brightly painted in his trademark palette, acknowledging the moment of inspiration that one could find through error.

EUGENIA BELL

See also **Corbusier, Le (Jeanneret, Charles-Édouard) (France)**

Further Reading

Gans, Deborah, *The Le Corbusier Guide*, New York: Princeton Architectural Press, 1987; revised edition, 2000
Jenkins, David, *Unité d'habitation, Marseilles: Le Corbusier*, London: Phaidon, 1993
Le Corbusier, *The Marseilles Block*, translated by Geoffrey Sainsbury, London: Harvill, 1953
Sbriglio, Jaques, *Le Corbusier: L'Unité d'habitation de Marseille*, Marseilles: Editions Parenthèses, 1992

UNITED KINGDOM

When the 20th century opened, the United Kingdom was at the height of its political power and influence and moreover was valued in Europe as a source of ideas in architecture. In terms of modern art, Charles Rennie Mackintosh was seen to be an originator of the Art Nouveau style and became a positive influence on the Secessionist style as it developed in Vienna. During 1898, Adolf Loos wrote many polemical articles in Vienna's *Neue freie Presse* praising English fashion and products. With Hermann Muthesius's publication of *Das englischer Haus* in 1904, Britain seemed to be ahead of continental Europe in providing more flexible models of houses and housing, one of the main strands of modernism in architecture.

However, the development was not confined to matters of taste. In terms of economics, the social structure of Britain had been changing since the onset of the industrial revolution in the later 18th century and had now created the conditions pertaining to a mass culture. Britain had pioneered the development of new industrial products from the time of the Great Exhibition of 1851. The rapid growth of London, following the explosion of the middle class and the concurrent expansion of metropolitan railways, had ensured that Britain was ahead both in achieving

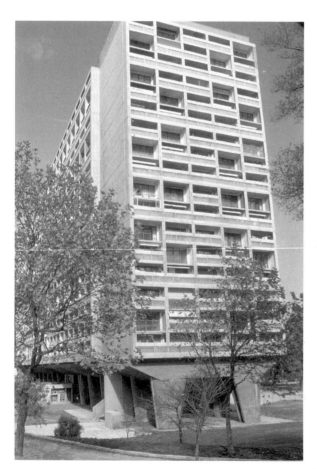

Unité d'Habitation, by Le Corbusier, at Marseilles, France (1946–52)
© Donald Corner and Jenny Young/GreatBuildings.com

urban growth and thereby in being forced to begin dealing with typical 20th-century problems.

The speed with which agricultural land on the outer rim was being consumed by new housing led to anxieties about the loss of food production, and with the publication in 1902 of Ebenezer Howard's *Garden Cities of Tomorrow*, urban growth was for the first time subjected to theory, the theory of limiting it by means of new towns located within a "green belt" of protected countryside. First Letchworth in 1903 and later Welwyn in 1920 confirmed local government acceptance of Howard's thesis as the basis of urban expansion. However, this context also explains why home building in Britain took on a "rural" character because it was conceived as the opposite to city living. No doubt, a love of medieval models and the enormous success of the Arts and Crafts movement promoted by William Morris in the tradition of John Ruskin contributed to this attitude. Vernacular architecture was thought proper for suburban housing and was also adopted by architects working individually for more affluent clients: architects such as C.R. Ashbee, C.F.A. Voysey, Richard Norman Shaw, and Edwin Landseer Lutyens.

However, British culture remained strangely parochial. The French scandal of the new century turned on the Dreyfus case, a question of social identity, but the corresponding British scandal turned on Oscar Wilde, a question of personal identity. Fleeing from social ostracism, Wilde took refuge in France, and France remained the cultural center of Europe. During the years of the Entente Cordiale, French influence became paramount. At a time when even well-to-do people could not afford to build individual town houses, apartment living began to appeal to the middle class, and many apartments serviced by elevators were built in Marylebone and in Battersea, popularly known as "mansion flats." Building apartments rather than one-family houses added more effectively to city fabric, and the popular center around Piccadilly Circus became the focus of Edwardian pretensions. Shaw's style became eclectic, and his Piccadilly Hotel (1905–08) and Regent Street Quadrant are imbued with a heavy classicism. His disciple, Reginald Blomfield, later built two sides of Piccadilly Circus (1913–30) in an elegant French baroque. Mewès and Davis built the Ritz Hotel (1906), of which the grand arcade to Piccadilly is modeled on Percier and Fontaine's rue de Rivoli. It is noteworthy that Lutyens took French models for much of his later rural work, and his imperial work in New Delhi, although highly original, is conceived in a spirit of French grandeur. Between 1901 and 1913, Aston Webb laid out the Rond Point with Queen Victoria's statue, in front of Buckingham Palace, and Admiralty Arch in emulation of the Place de la Concorde and the Arc de Triomphe.

Howard Robertson, architect of the Financial Times Building in London, was the main source of theory in the schools, his *Principles of Composition* being based largely on Guadet. The Beaux-Arts dominated architectural education until the outbreak of World War I, with Robertson at the Architectural Association, Albert Richardson at London University, and Charles Reilly and W.A. Eden at Liverpool University. Where the Arts and Crafts model did not hold, it was the classical model that did. Courtenay Square (1914) in Kennington, by Adshead and Ramsey, is probably the last example of a reduced classicism still executed with conviction. By the 1920s, a neo-Georgian style dominated in architecture, as it did in poetry.

Howard Robertson's influence extended beyond theory, and his participation in the Paris Exposition of 1925 led to a considerable enthusiasm for the Art Deco style, which he promoted during the 1920s. This style is demonstrative and populist without attaining the modernist ideal of renouncing style as much. Many town halls, cinemas, and lidos were built in a lighthearted vein across the country, and the most distinguished probably are those by Oliver Bernard, whose foyers for the Strand Palace Hotel (1929–30) are superb. To this taste was added a liking for decorative brickwork stemming from the influence of W.M. Dudok's Hilversum Town Hall, apparent in the Royal Masonic Hospital (1930–34) by Sir John Burnett Tait and Lorne. The latter firm was typical in veering between a monumental classicism, sometimes with Egyptian overtones, and a reduced moderne, until in 1932 it dipped into a crude streamlined modernism, as exemplified in the Mount Royal Hotel on Oxford Street.

A certain eclecticism was in order. The Hoover Factory in Western Avenue by Wallis Gilbert, in a sort of modernized palatial mode, is the most exuberant instance of the hybrid architecture produced in Britain at this time, but the same architect could come close to an authentic modern idiom in his Daimler Car Hire Garage (1931). Charles Holden could build the Senate House and Library (1932–34) for London University in an inflated if stripped-down classical style and at the same time prefigure the modern in his very controlled work for the Piccadilly Line Underground stations at Arnos Grove and Southgate. Only Joseph Emberton, formerly an assistant to Gordon Tait, achieved genuine modernity with his Yacht Club (1930–32) at Burnham-on-Crouch and two London stores, Simpson's Piccadilly (1934–36) and the HMV Building (1938–39) on Oxford Street.

The Modern style as such did not appear in England until the very end of the 1920s by way of private individuals building villas. A breakthrough was made by the architect Amyas Connell in his famous High and Over (1927–29) at Amersham in Buckinghamshire. It is almost contemporary with Le Corbusier's Les Heures Claires at Poissy and appears to derive its aesthetic from the LaRoche-Jeanneret houses in the rue du Docteur Blanche, which Connell had seen on a visit to Paris in 1926. Here the trefoil plan does not conform to the new rationalism but stems, rather, from Lutyens. The influence of Le Corbusier was furthered by the publication in 1927 of Frederick Etchell's translation of *Vers Une Architecture*. Connell joined with two others to form the Connell, Ward, and Lucas partnership, and throughout the 1930s they produced a number of radical houses in a white-walled modern style, with windows arranged in horizontal runs. Particularly noteworthy is a group of three houses at Saltdean where the flat-roof terrace is approached by an extruded external staircase, as in Le Corbusier's "gratte-ciel" houses at Pessac of 1925. However, they also succeeded in building in the heart of conservative Hampstead a canonic modern house at 66 Frognal.

A wider European horizon was opened up by the arrival of refugees from Hitler's Germany. Walter Gropius, Marcel Breuer, Erick Mendelsohn, and Serge Chermayeff appeared within a short period, and the last two collaborated to build the De La Warr pavilion at Bexhill-on-Sea, Sussex, while Chermayeff also completed a villa (1934) at Rugby, his own house (1935–38) at Bentley Wood near Hallam, and a warehouse for Gilbey's Gin in Camden Town. In several cases, important collaborations

were entered on, with an effect on the future of English practice. Gropius collaborated with E. Maxwell Fry in a house in Chelsea and in several unbuilt university projects as well as the Impington Village College in Cambridgeshire, which became a model for much subsequent English practice. Breuer collaborated with F.R.S. Yorke in a house (1936–37) at Angmering-on-Sea and more famously for an exhibit at the Ideal Home Exhibition of 1936, which projected an ultramodern image of "The Garden City of the Future." Fry succeeded at the same time in invading Hampstead with his own version of modernity, the "Sun House" at 9 Frognal Way, which was well received and prepared the way for a wider acceptance of the Modern style after the war.

There were a few indigenous architects who made their mark in the 1930s and made important contributions to the development of an English modernism: H.S. Goodhart-Rendel (Hays Wharf, 1929–31), George Checkley ("Thurso" house, in Cambridge, 1932), Christopher Nicolson (studio for Augustus John, 1933–34, and the London Gliding Club, Dunstable, 1934–35), Frederick Gibberd (Pullman Curt, Streatham, 1935), Raymond McGrath (house in Chertsey, 1936–37), and David Pleydell-Bouverie (Ramsgate Municipal Airport, 1936–37). It is undeniable, however, that the more original impulses came from abroad: conspicuous were Wells Coates (from Canada), whose Isokon Apartments in Camden, designed for the Pritchards in 1932–34, are still highly desired by young professionals and whose apartments (1934–35) at Brighton are a model of directness and elegance; William Lescaze (from Switzerland), whose buildings (1931–36) for the progressive school at Dartington Hall were architecturally progressive, too; and Erno Goldfinger (from Hungary), who won competitions but whose projects were unbuilt until after the war.

Perhaps most important was the collaboration between the natives Francis Skinner and Lindsey Drake and the Russian émigré Berthold Lubetkin in the partnership called Tecton. Lubetkin not only was energetic but also believed that the functionalist creed to which he subscribed did not deny the architect's right to make art. The Penguin Pool (1932) at the London Zoo is as playful as it is geometric, and the apartment blocks constructed at Highgate—Highpoint I (1933–35) and Highpoint II (1936–38)—are equally virtuoso in their deployment of abstract forms. Published in *The Architectural Review*, these buildings signaled the acceptance of Modern architecture by establishment critics. Its acceptance by the general public had to wait until after World War II.

A young architect who first joined Tecton and later worked on his own account was important in effecting this transition. This was Denys Lasdun. In 1948, still collaborating with Tecton, he began work on an extensive estate of public housing at Hallfield, in Paddington, together with a primary school. The elevations are marked by Lubetkin's preference for breaking the pattern of verticals at alternate floors, but the finesse Lasdun showed here gave him a central role in introducing the Modern style to a wider public.

With the election of a Labour government in 1945, England was motivated by a new spirit of cooperation produced through the war years. This spirit was celebrated in the Festival of Britain (1951), a coordinated group of exhibition buildings on semiderelict land on the south bank of the Thames opposite Charing Cross, highly visible to the public. It was put together with speed and virtuosity under the direction of Hugh Casson. With the installation of a Labour government, municipalities and local authorities were given new powers to clear slums and bomb damage and to expand public investment in building housing, schools, new universities, and even new towns. Architecture in Britain in the 1950s was earnest and populist, taking its cue from the Festival of Britain style. In the eyes of the younger generation, it was condemned as fainthearted.

The Smithsons, Alison and Peter, were the first representatives of the postwar generation. Fiercely critical of the Festival style, they expressed a determination to remake architecture in the name of ordinary people without ceasing to be radical. Their design for housing in the Golden Lane Competition (1952) showed how the access decks for high-rise housing could become "street decks," linking different quarters together with a pedestrian network free from traffic circulation. This was not simply a proposal for housing; rather, it was a fundamental reworking of the city and, in theory, a way of building whole towns. The open-air access deck had been instituted through poor-law housing built by the Peabody Estate in the 1890s, and the system was now adopted by municipalities. The Smithsons provided intellectual leadership for the younger generation, addressing themselves to the architectural establishment as would-be reformers. Their polemic against what they called the "wasteland of the Four Functions" brought an end to the bureaucratic rationalism of CIAM (Congrès Internationaux d'Architecture Moderne) and replaced it with the more self-critical although short-lived meetings of Team X.

Their design for Hunstanton School (1950–54) was broadly Miesian in origin but less monumental, reflecting also the influence of Rudolf Wittkower, who had brought the achievements of Palladio into new focus: if Palladio could create architecture out of farm buildings, surely the modern architect could do it with utilitarian sheds. The light steel structure was used with an extreme economy, and structural walls, pipes, and services were left exposed. The result, in the view of the critic Reyner Banham, was the defining moment of a new approach—the New Brutalism—seeking an absolute honesty by exposing the mechanisms as well as the structure. Although hardly a British invention, Brutalism dominated British architecture for several decades. It was an important influence in the formation of the Archigram Group by Peter Cook in 1962 and led on to the High-Tech style, which by the 1980s had become the dominant style in Britain.

In many respects, the Smithsons' design for the Economist Building (1963–64) represents their considered view of what an honest architecture "without rhetoric" should be. This design broke with commercial grandiosity and showed how a building could be divided into smaller entities that could be more easily absorbed into the city pattern. After the Economist Building, the Smithsons were well placed to become a successful practice. However, this did not happen, and their public housing at Robin Hood Lane was not well received.

The architects were not alone to blame for this. Both Labour and Conservative governments fell into the trap of assessing housing policy in terms of quantity rather than social effectiveness. Many mistakes were made in terms of both social environment and technical construction. In London, the collapse of an apartment block at Ronan Point signaled the end of the belief that reconstruction had been successful. Later, this collapse took on a symbolic significance, roughly equivalent to the tearing

down of the Pruitt Igoe estate in St. Louis. It marked an end to the supposition that progress was inevitable and preordained.

However, this was not just a local phenomenon; it was worldwide in its impact. In the United States, the Vietnam War, in which a powerful industrial nation could not prevail against a determined people, had introduced doubt about the inevitability of technological growth. Europe, too, felt a certain loss of vision after the student events of 1968 and the oil crisis of 1973. Banham was disappointed in the reception of Brutalism by architects and accused them of monumentalism. The influence that led to this tendency was that of Le Corbusier, but it would not have taken hold so quickly had it not been for the advocacy of Leslie Martin. As chief architect of the London County Council (LCC) in 1953, he promoted a rationalized use of the Le Corbusian grid. After the construction of miniature Unité d'Habitation at Roehampton (1951–60), the Le Corbusian style was adopted for much local authority housing in London.

On resigning from the LCC, Leslie Martin founded a new professional school of architecture at Cambridge University. Martin's task was to balance the claims of research and practice and normalize an architecture that could be seen to fit into the traditional campus setting. He took a number of young architects with him who shared his admiration for rational outcomes but who were also able to act with discretion. Among these were Colin St. John Wilson, Patrick Hodgkinson, and Ivor Smith. The influence of Le Corbusier remained primary, but there was also an influence from Alvar Aalto. In Harvey Court (1957–62), a block of student residences for Gonville and Caius College designed with Wilson and Hodgkinson, the structure is in reinforced concrete, but the facing is in brickwork, so that the appearance is softened and adapted to the Cambridge scene. The internal court is also softened by stepping back the accommodation in tiers. Hodgkinson collaborated with Martin in the public housing (1965–73) carried out for Camden Council at the Foundling Estate near Russell Square. Here again, we have a stepped section, with private balconies facing east and west. Quite remarkable is the profiling of the service towers: the tops with their carefully detailed vents have more than a hint of Sant' Elia futurism, and the gable ends reveal a powerful sculptural aspect that comes pretty close to Expressionism.

Another young Cambridge architect heavily influenced by Leslie Martin was Ivor Smith. His fame rests on his role as chief designer to J.L. Womersley, the chief architect to the city of Sheffield, in the construction of housing (1955–65) at Park Hill and Hyde Park, but somewhat problematically it takes on the huge scale of what Banham termed a "megastructure." Another influence in the same direction came from the architect Denys Lasdun, who further adapted the Le Corbusian model by a confident use of the stepped section. His mammoth layout (1962–69) for the University of East Anglia and his residential extensions (1969–70) to Christ's College, Cambridge, both use stepped forms to allow the buildings to melt into the landscape. In another megastructure at Alexandria Road, public housing (1969–79) for the London County Council, the architect Neave Brown created yet another project based on the setback section, but with an explicit ideology not about landscape as such but attempting to recuperate the street as a social space.

The search for a constructional method more suitable for the British climate led to an exploration of brickwork, probably encouraged by Le Corbusier's design for the Maisons Jaoul in Paris. Most visible were the many buildings (1962–75), some using Jaoul-type vaults, constructed by Basil Spence for the University of Sussex. Most influential on other architects was the very precise use of brickwork adopted by the architects Stirling and Gowan, first in their flats (1955–58) at Ham Common and then in their building (1959–63) for the Engineering Faculty at Leicester University, where it was combined with large areas of standard glazing to spectacular effect. After the dissolution of the partnership, Stirling continued this "red-brick" attack on the ancient universities with his History Faculty (1964–67) at Cambridge and the Florey Building (1966–71) at Oxford. Although he built a major extension of the Tate Gallery in London, Stirling was not fully appreciated in Britain during his lifetime. He built in the United States for Rice University, the University of California, and Harvard University, and his Performing Arts Center (1983–88) at Cornell University is a gem of a building. He was appreciated as a master architect in Germany and built there extensively: at Stuttgart (the Neue Staatsgalerie and Music School, 1977–94), at Berlin (the Wissenschaftszentrum, 1979–87), and at Melsungen (the Braun Pharmaceutical Headquarters, 1989–92). He is arguably the most important and distinctive British architect of his generation, and his contribution to world architecture has not yet been fully assessed.

During the 1980s, British architecture was most influential when presented as a continuation of the Brutalist tradition founded by the Smithsons, emphasizing structure and services as principal expression. Important for this outcome were the teaching of Peter Cook and the fantasies of the Archigram Group, which he founded in 1962. Members of this group were employed by Piano and Rogers in making the detailed drawings for the Centre Pompidou (1971–77) in Paris, so there is a direct connection. Rogers's design for Lloyds Headquarters (1978–86) in London was in a similar vein, and specialized industrial buildings in the United States, Wales, and France have confirmed his reputation as a "scientific" architect. More recently, his European Court of Human Rights (1989–94) at Strasbourg and other projects for France show an increasing interest in the use of expressive curves as well as in adapting themselves more cogently to their sites. Designing for buildings in the city center had brought out a need to accommodate to context, and Rogers's commitment to the inner city was confirmed by the publication of his *Reith Lectures* (1995), where he made a strong argument for buildings that will be part of both a sustainable environment and a dense city fabric.

More versatile in his use of industrial components, Norman Foster has become the leading exponent of what is now referred to as the High-Tech style. Originally in partnership with Rogers (and both of their wives) as Team Four, they share a similar approach. He was first recognized for the Willis Faber and Dumas Building (1975) in Ipswich and the Sainsbury Centre for the Visual Arts (1978) at the University of East Anglia. More recently, the elegance of Stansted Airport (1990–91) has made him known to a wider public. The telecommunications tower at Torre di Collserola, near Barcelona, exploits the image of mechanism to great effect, but the Hong Kong and Shanghai Bank (1979–85) in Hong Kong and the Carré d'Art at Nîmes (1984–93) in France, by their very differences, indicate that, for all the emphasis on structure, Foster is sensitive to site conditions and can make appropriate interventions in different contexts. His ability to adjust to existing conditions was proved in the

Sackler Gallery (1985–92) at the Royal Academy and confirmed by his renovations of the German Reichstag and the British Museum, both of which use elegant steel-and-glass structures to modernize classical buildings.

Younger architects who followed the High-Tech line were Farrell and Grimshaw. A partnership at the outset, they split dramatically in 1980, when Terry Farrell adopted a more variable Postmodern approach. His most conspicuous success is Embankment Place, a new commercial construction built above Charing Cross Station and highly visible from the river. Nicholas Grimshaw stayed loyal to the fixed canon of industrial architecture, but his Eurostar Terminal at Waterloo demonstrates great verve in the way it exploits the site conditions to make an expressive space. A near contemporary, Michael Hopkins, made a sophisticated industrial tent (1985) for Schlumberger at Cambridge but has shown great sensitivity with his Mound Stand (1987) at Lords Cricket Ground and the new opera house (1992–94) at Glyndbourne. His new offices for members of Parliament, opposite Big Ben, make the exposed ducting for natural ventilation into a sort of medieval roof, a strange metamorphosis of Louis Kahn's idea that the exposed servicing systems should supply the monumental aspect of a modern building.

It may be possible to deduce from these examples that, in today's United Kingdom, discretion is more important than ideology. Yet the worship of technological know-how pervades British architecture, and a still-younger generation bows to it. Will Alsop, of Alsop and Stormer, has risen to prominence with his Town Hall for Marseilles (Le Grand Bleu), and they have constructed a rail station at North Greenwich, one of the many new stations required to service the Jubilee Line, the only completely new Underground line to be constructed in London since the war, most of which make expressive use of steel and glass. Jan Kaplicky, cofounder with Amanda Levete of the aptly named Future Systems, has so far built little but has received funding from the National Lottery for the construction of a spectacular Eco-Centre at Doncaster. All these architects employ industrial components not as rational expedients but with an eye to their expressive potential. It is possible to speak of a trend that looks to revive the expressive aspects discovered by the Brutalists in the 1950s.

Indeed, with the 20th century now safely completed, the drive to attach architecture firmly to its purely physical determinants seems to have weakened to the point where one can discern a movement to revive the concept of architecture as art, as originally proposed by the Russian Constructivists. This tendency was pronounced in the early work of the Office of Metropolitan Architecture, founded in 1975 by Rem Koolhaas, Madelon Vriesendorp, and Elia Zenghelis, which at its inception practiced from London. From that background, Zaha Hadid has risen to prominence, largely because of the rejection of her winning design for the Cardiff Opera House, which led to a sympathetic reaction in her favor. She now has important commissions on foot in Germany, Italy, and Israel. Her presentations, as distinct from her constructions, are still remarkable insofar as they imitate the weightless qualities of Malevich's paintings. When they are transformed into actual constructions, as with the Fire Station (1993, with Patrik Schumacher) at Vitea in Weil am Rhein, some loss of spirit occurs. Rem Koolhaas, who still maintains an office in London, was the originator of this manner; in con-

struction, however, his projects take on a distinctly surreal aspect, as with his Villa Dall'Ava in Paris (1985–91) and his Convention Hall (1991–97) at the International Business Centre at Lille and still more with his villa at Bordeaux.

Even more equivocal, from the rationalist point of view, are the designs proposed in Britain by the American-Polish architect Daniel Libeskind: an extension to the Victoria and Albert Museum in London and the Imperial War Museum for Manchester. In both cases, the design arises from a distinctly personal impulse: it is conceptual, indeed, but above all it is gestural. These designs are hardly representative of Britain, but the fact that they have been accepted by British cities is highly significant. Now the traditional forms of modernism, supposedly derived from rational procedure and with all the security of an objective judgment, suddenly appear as personal expression, which in principle means subject to whim and open to question. Britain, it appears, has finally joined the rest of the world in accepting the fundamental uncertainty of the postmodern condition.

ROBERT MAXWELL

See also **Archigram; Ashbee, C.R. (England); Breuer, Marcel (United States); Brutalism; Corbusier, Le (Jeanneret, Charles-Édouard) (France); Foster, Norman (England); Grimshaw, Nicholas, and Partners (England); Gropius, Walter (Germany); Hadid, Zaha (Iraq); Loos, Adolf (Austria); Lubetkin and Tecton (England); Lutyens, Edwin (England); Mackintosh, Charles Rennie (Scotland); Postmodernism; Smithson, Peter and Alison (England); Stirling, James (Scotland and England); Voysey, Charles F.A. (England)**

Further Reading

British Architecture, London: Academy Editions, and New York: St. Martin's Press, 1982

Emanuel, Muriel (editor), *Contemporary Architects*, London: Macmillan, and New York: St. Martin's Press, 1980; 3rd edition, New York: St. James Press, 1993

Jones, Edward, and Christopher Woodward, *A Guide to the Architecture of London*, London: Weidenfeld and Nicolson, 1983

Maxwell, Robert, *New British Architecture*, London: Thames and Hudson, 1972

Pevsner, Nikolaus, *Pioneers of the Modern Movement from William Morris to Walter Gropius*, London: Faber, 1936; revised edition, as *Pioneers of Modern Design: From William Morris to Walter Gropius*, London: Penguin, 1975

One Hundred Years of British Architecture, 1851–1951, London: Royal Institute of British Architects, 1951

Sharp, Dennis, *A Visual History of Twentieth Century Architecture*, Greenwich, Connecticut: New York Graphic Society, and London: Heinemann Secker and Warburg, 1972

Thirties: British Art and Design before the War (exhib. cat.), London: Arts Council of Great Britain, 1979

Yorke, Francis Reginald Stevens, *The Modern House in England*, London: Architectural Press, 1937

Zodiac 18 (1968) (special issue on Great Britain)

UNITED NATIONS HEADQUARTERS

New York City, completed 1953

On 26 June 1945, 50 nations founded the United Nations Organization in order to establish international political consultations

for the post–World War II period. In April 1946 the United Nations Secretariat and General Assembly officially replaced the League of Nations based in Geneva. After international diplomatic debates, New York City was chosen to host the United Nations Headquarters. New York's influential city planner Robert Moses proposed to locate the United Nations buildings in a park at Flushing Meadows, Queens, on the site of the 1939 World's Fair, but the businessman John D. Rockefeller offered to buy and donate to the United Nations a site in Manhattan between First Avenue and the East River and East 42nd and 48th Streets. Although this site had accommodated slaughterhouses, and despite the lack of building space for the suborganizations (for example, UNICEF), the Secretariat and General Assembly were placed there. Planning began in 1947, and the buildings were finished in 1953.

A planning commission of ten international architects directed by Wallace K. Harrison had to devise a design that was both significant and functional. Architects and critics regarded the buildings as important models for postwar political representation through architecture. A series of sketches by Le Corbusier, emphatically promoted and refined by the Brazilian modernist and member of the commission Oscar Niemeyer, directed the style debates toward a modern, functionalist design. Only certain American congressmen, who asked for a conservative classical, domed building, and the Russian delegate, who tried to push through Stalinist neoclassicism, opposed the cultural risk of modern architectural representation. Nevertheless, the International Style pattern was legitimized as appropriate for international and modern politics. Already in the 1920s, at the competition for the League of Nations Building in Geneva, the modernist architect Hannes Meyer had promoted a type of transparent architecture without ornament, dedicated only to efficient administration and political representation without any historic monumental references.

European emigrant architects such as Richard Neutra, Walter Gropius, and Mies van der Rohe had prepared the United States to accept modern architecture, and American architectural firms such as Harrison and Abramovitz and Skidmore, Owings and Merrill were professionally prepared to develop large-scale projects such as the United Nations buildings. This European-American coproduction was reflected in the design process. While the basic idea can be traced back to the sketches of Le Corbusier (who felt himself betrayed by his American colleagues), it was Wallace K. Harrison who simplified and elaborated the concept into a professional design for an administration building, thus presenting to the international public a prototype for modern office towers.

The building complex includes a high-rise slab (544 feet high and 72 feet thick) for the Secretariat offices and, on the northern edge of the site, the curving, low horizontal structure of the General Assembly. In 1963 Harrison, Abramovitz and Harris attached a library to its northeastern corner. All architectural elements of the United Nations complex are generously located in open spaces that were expanded to the west by Dag Hammarskjöld Plaza, and part of First Avenue was tunneled in order to reduce traffic noise at the site. Within the dense building context of Manhattan, this urban scheme of high-rise building and openness became prototypical for urban development in New York City and in other cities of the world during the 1950s and 1960s. Lever House, completed one year after the United Nations

buildings; the Seagram Building in Manhattan; and thousands of architectural International Style copies for business uses worldwide produced a new urban order.

The rectangular design of the Secretariat slab with its reflecting curtain wall of green glass in a regular, thin aluminum grid set international design standards for postwar modern architecture. Photographs of it circulated in all international reviews. Representations of the United Nations high-rise building in stamp designs of many countries aesthetically educated postwar planners and citizens worldwide. Only the dynamically rising concrete roof of the Assembly Building breaks with the aesthetic principle of rectangularity. In lieu of applied ornament, the United Nations building complex was equipped with donated works of modern art, among them murals and sculptures by avant-garde artists Fernand Léger and Henry Moore.

Shortly after its completion, the United Nations Secretariat was presented in an exhibition at the Museum of Modern Art as prototypical modern American architecture. In the public debate about the building, the critic Lewis Mumford recognized a specific mixture of Le Corbusian utopianism and American commercialism. Many architects and politicians for different reasons rejected his positive aesthetic evaluation of the transparency and sculptural quality of the slab. Frank Lloyd Wright saw nothing more than a "characterless package" and a gloomy, dismal landmark of International Style in the building, whereas East

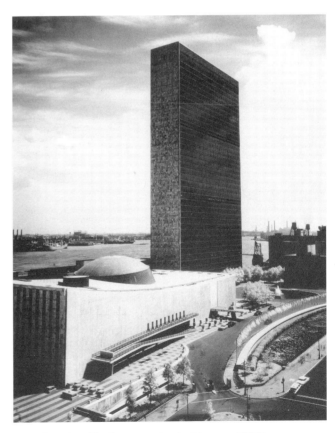

United Nations Headquarters, view looking east (1953)
© Museum of the City of New York and The Port Authority of New York

European politicians refused the modern design for ideological reasons. Stalinist architectural doctrine regarded Western modernism as cultural colonialism of the United States. Other critics were worried about the image of bureaucracy and machinery displayed by the standardized curtain wall and office cells.

When postwar International Style architecture spread to the business districts of New York and other global cities by the end of the 20th century, the aesthetic effect of transparency encoded as political openness and honesty of a peace-oriented world administration became corrupted by commercialization and banality.

The United Nations Secretariat's aesthetics of transparency and regular cubic forms were reinterpreted by late modernism with Kevin Roche and John Dinkeloo's towers, immediately west of the Secretariat, for the hotel and office buildings called 1 and 2 United Nations Plaza (1976, 1983), thus promoting political representation by corporate architecture.

Without the historical background of New York's architectural history and international debates about the political iconography of architecture, the United Nations building complex seems to lack importance, perhaps because of the decreasing political power of this world organization. Nevertheless, the United Nations Secretariat and General Assembly buildings remain landmarks of cultural and political history.

PETER KRIEGER

See also **Aluminum; Corbusier, Le (Jeanneret, Charles-Édouard) (France); Curtain Wall System; Glass; International Style; Lever House, New York City; Meyer, Hannes (Germany); Mies van der Rohe, Ludwig (Germany); Niemeyer, Oscar (Brazil); Roche, Kevin, and John Dinkeloo (United States); Wright, Frank Lloyd (United States)**

Further Reading

Corbusier, Le (Jeanneret, Charles-Édouard), *United Nations Headquarters Report*, New York: United Nations, 1946

Dudley, George, *A Workshop for Peace. Designing the United Nations Headquarters*, New York: Architectural History Foundation, 1994

Hitchcock, Henry-Russell (editor), *Built in USA: Post-war Architecture*, New York: Museum of Modern Art, 1952

Krieger, Peter, "Spiegelnde Curtain Walls als Projektionsflächen für politische Schlagbilder," in *Architektur als politische Kultur. Philosophia Practica*, edited by Hermann Hipp and Ernst Seidl, Berlin: Reimer, 1996

Mumford, Lewis, "U.N. Model and Model U.N.," in *From the Ground Up: Observations on Contemporary Architecture, Housing, Highway Building and Civic Design*, edited by Lewis Mumford, New York: Harcourt Brace, 1956

Ulbricht, Walter, "Das nationale Aufbauwerk und die Aufgaben der deutschen Architektur," in: *Die Aufgaben der Deutschen Bauakademie im Kampf um eine deutsche Architektur. Ansprachen gehalten anläßlich der Eröffnung der Deutschen Bauakademie am 8. Dezember 1951 in Berlin*, edited by Deutsche Bauakademie, Berlin: Henschelverlag, 1952

UNITED STATES

Twentieth-century architecture in the United States exhibits multiple overlapping themes that include historicism, regionalism, and various forms of modernism. Although architects, his-

torians, and critics throughout the 20th century sought continuities, disjuncture appeared more frequently. One attempt at constancy involved reliance on history as the source for design, as in McKim, Mead and White's Pennsylvania Station (1902–10), New York City, and Robert A. M. Stern's Darden Business School (1992–96) at the University of Virginia, Charlottesville. An alternative approach lay with the regionalists or nativists, who sought a unique American expression based on the local vernacular and, often, landscape, such as with Frank Lloyd Wright's early Prairie style houses and Antoine Predock's abstraction of native American forms. The third theme, a quest for a modern architecture, occupied many individuals and includes buildings as diverse as R. M. Schindler's King Road House (Los Angeles, 1921–22), Marcel Breuer's St. John's Abbey (Collegeville, Minnesota, 1953–61), and I. M. Pei's Louvre Pyramid (Paris, 1983–93). All three examples paid homage to abstraction and advanced building materials and techniques. Ideas concerning the American city have ricocheted from grand plazas, as with John Bakewell and Arthur Brown's San Francisco Civic Center and City Hall (1912–16, renovations 1995–99); to setback skyscrapers and elevated roads, pictured by Hugh Ferris's *Metropolis of Tomorrow* (1929); to monolithic towers with little connection to the city, exemplified by John Portman's Renaissance Center (1971–77, Detroit); and finally the ideas of Duany and Plater-Zyberk (Andrés Duany and Elizabeth Plater-Zyberk) for new towns that captured the critical discourse of the 1990s and that make up a movement termed New Urbanism. Instead of singularity, American architecture offers a competition of themes and a bewildering variety of expressions.

American Characteristics

Conditioning American architecture is the unprecedented wealth and standard of living of the country and its emergence as a dominant world power in the 20th century. What would be the nature of American culture and how it would define itself has been a perennial problem as the cult of individuality reigns.

Historicism

The strongest and most continuous theme in American architecture remains an infatuation with history and the employment of imagery from the past. The method of how this past has been quoted—from fidelity to distortion—and the range of appropriation from Colonial to European and Oriental has varied. The semiotician Umberto Eco observed that the American imagination craves the real thing, and to establish that reassurance, Americans fabricate, or reproduce imitations. Architects create buildings in which the quotation is proudly displayed: the English Georgian country houses of David Adler, such as Castle Hill, Ipswich, Massachusetts, (1924–27) or the Roman villa as the basis for the J. Paul Getty Museum (1972–74), Malibu, California, by Langdon, Wilson and Garrett, with Norman Neuerberg as consultant.

The American Renaissance, dominant from, 1890s to the 1930s and led by the firm of McKim, Mead and White and others, posited that American architecture and art could not be invented but, rather, that it should draw upon the classical past

of Europe and America. Out of this approach came the great courts of honor at the various American fairs from Buffalo (1901) to Philadelphia (1926). These courts of honor provided a model of civic architecture and led directly to the City Beautiful Movement and civic centers such as Arthur Brown's in San Francisco and state capitols that lasted well into the Depression, as for example with Cass Gilbert's West Virginia Capitol (Charleston, 1930–32) and John Russell Pope's National Gallery of Art (Washington, D.C., 1936–41).

Opposed to this classicism stood the medieval revival led by Ralph Adams Cram, who argued for the validity of the Gothic and designed over a hundred churches and significant portions of university campuses between 1900 and 1940. Cram succeeded in creating a Boston-based Gothic School that affected thousands of churches across the country, such as Frohman, Robb and Little's (and others) National Cathedral (1906–90) in Washington, D.C.

Colonial Revival, whether Spanish, English, or other nationalities, has proved to be the most lasting historicist approach. The myth of Colonial as the truest, and the earliest, American style had an effect on others that appear to be far removed. The restoration of Colonial Williamsburg (1927–) gave great impetus to Colonial Revival and made the brick Virginia Tidewater Georgian house a national image. In Florida and the Southwest, a Mission and then a Spanish Colonial Revival developed as a localized colonial revival response. Since 1926 towns such as Santa Barbara have continued to rebuild themselves along the lines of a Spanish town, even though that history is mostly fictional.

Recognition of the validity of a historicist approach vacillated in 20th-century America. From 1900 to the 1930s, historicism was the accepted norm, and architectural periodicals showed and promoted historical prototypes. However, beginning in the 1920s, the historical approach came under fire, and by the 1940s the appearance in professional architectural periodicals of buildings in historical dress was rare. From the 1940s through the mid-1970s, serious discussion of historicism as a contemporary approach to design disappeared from the profession, the schools, and writings by most critics and historians. Not all historically based design disappeared, for it thrived with builders and contractors at the suburban house level and also in the hands of many local architects. Allan Greenburg's design for the Brant House (Greenwich, Connecticut, 1979–83), which takes elements of Washington's Mount Vernon, received rave reviews in the professional press, indicating the changed climate. The work of Hartman-Cox Architects (George Hartman and Warren Cox), who began as modernists but turned to preexisting models, received similar praise. Their Georgetown University Law Center Library (Washington, D.C., 1984–89) and their additions to the Chrysler Museum (1982–89) in Norfolk, Virginia, appear as if they have stood since the 1930s.

The recognition of historicism as a valid architectural approach began in the late 1960s with a reevaluation by architects who became known as Postmodernists and by a group of younger historians who began to investigate the hitherto forbidden (i.e., outmoded) Victorian and Beaux-Arts eras. However, the greatest contributing element to the new historicism was the Historic Preservation movement, which gained great support in the 1960s and 1970s because of new federal and local legislation. From 1900 to the 1950s, preservation had a reputation as elit-ist—only concerned with the homes of the wealthy and in recreating historical villages. In the 1960s, however, preservationists questioned urban renewal and the destruction of sections of older cities and whole buildings such as Pennsylvania Station (1961) in New York and the construction of unsympathetic modern structures. A reevaluation of the American built past took place with new recognition of the more recent Victorian, American Renaissance, and Art Deco buildings and even streamlined diners. One effect of the preservation movement has been to direct attention to the validity of historically based design. Within inner cities there developed an acknowledgment of the historic townscape and a contextual approach to design. Kevin Roche, a modernist, continued the original architect Francoise Ier's style for an addition to the Jewish Museum (1989) in New York; in Washington, D.C., for a new building in the Federal Triangle, James I. Freed, of Pei, Cobb, Freed, employed classical orders for the Reagan International Building (1989–98). Older structures were adapted for new purposes, such as The Cannery (San Francisco, 1968) by Joseph Esherick and Quincy Markets (Boston, 1976) by Ben Thompson. These so-called "festival markets" helped influence a semisuccessful attempt to revive main streets across the country.

The New Urbanism movement spearheaded by Duany and Plater-Zyberk at Seaside, Florida, and other places and by the firm Cooper-Robertson (Alexander Cooper and Jaquelin Robertson) and others at Celebration, Florida, draws on nostalgic interpretations of the 19th- and early 20th-century small town. All types of revival houses compete for attention. In a sense these are architectural theme parks—Disneyland as permanent lifestyle. The power of historicism and nostalgia for an earlier time are strong traits in America and have created one of its most enduring legacies.

Regionalism and Nativism

The search for a native American architecture that could be based on the local vernacular or nature has animated many architects. A recognition of localized conditions of environment can be traced far back in American history, but regionalism as a coherent architectural approach owes a debt to the Arts and Crafts philosophy of William Morris and his followers that reached America from the 1870s onward. Simple overall form and complex details became a trademark of both furniture and buildings, which often had wood peg joints and leaded glass windows contrasted with plain woodwork. In England one of the fundamental touchstones was an antimachine, anti-industry attitude and a return of artisans to the production of objects and buildings. Some Americans did adopt a handicraft ethic—especially decorative arts artisans—but overall Americans remained tied to the machine, and the Arts and Crafts aesthetic was widely commercialized in America. Frank Lloyd Wright's 1901 talk, "The Art and Craft of the Machine," noted that the machine could better provide the aesthetic qualities of simplicity and rectilinearity than the hand.

The Arts and Crafts movement in America persisted into the 1920s. Although the overall intention was for a regional response, the movement existed at the national level through the writings of publicists like Gustav Stickley and *The Craftsman* magazine. Stickley and others popularized the concept of the

bungalow, the low-rising story- to-story-and-a-half house that fit easily into the landscape of suburbia and nature. Bungalows appeared from coast to coast and became the archetypal nativist house for the period of 1900 to 1925. In southern California, Irving Gill abstracted the Mission into a simplified concrete type of construction that was remarkable for its absence of details and purity of form. Also in southern California, brothers Charles Sumner and Henry Mather Greene created a very different expression, making the shingle-covered wood bungalow into an exquisite art object of delicately wrought construction. The basis of their design was the local vernacular and the elaboration of wood construction, as in the Gamble house (Pasadena, California, 1906–08). Farther north, in the Bay Area around San Francisco, Bernard Maybeck created his own personalized—and eclectic—regional response, using various foreign and American elements.

The Chicago area, led by Louis Sullivan and Frank Lloyd Wright, created a distinctive regionalism in the Prairie School. Sullivan's early work was large, urban, and commercial, but after 1900 he found such commissions difficult to secure and turned to house and small-town bank designs that fit squarely within the Arts and Crafts regional ethic. His National Farmer's Bank (1907), Owatonna, Minnesota, designed in conjunction with George Grant Elmslie, demonstrated a nativistic and original creation of ornament drawn from nature and geometry. Sullivan represented one side of the Prairie School; his descendants William Gray Purcell and Elmslie followed his lead with essentially boxy forms articulated by openings, structural members, and ornament.

Wright, who had worked for Sullivan, represents the other, better-known side of the Prairie style. Wright openly attempted to recall the landscape through low-rising forms, open spaces, and ornamental details. Except for his earliest buildings and his inexpensive housing solutions, Wright tended to break apart the form, to stretch it out, to articulate the parts into a coherent whole. The Robie House (Chicago, 1906–08) is composed of a series of layers that move upward and outward, pinned to the earth by a large chimney core, and that shelter a continuous living–dining space. Out of Wright's Oak Park Studio came a group of architects such as Walter Burley Griffin, Marion Mahony, and others who elaborated Wright's ideas and helped spread them not only nationwide but internationally.

Wright's career in the United States went into an eclipse between 1914 and 1936; he built little except for works in Tokyo and southern California. This work moves beyond the Arts and Crafts, as Wright attempted to create a native language appropriate to the site. In the Los Angeles area, Wright drew on pre-Columbian Indian forms. Although viewed as a modernist abroad and by many at home, Wright always claimed that his architecture came from American conditions, and he employed the word "organic" as a definition. Fallingwater (Bear Run, Pennsylvania, 1935–37) announced Wright's return to prominence and posited that American modern design should respond to the localized conditions of site. His later Usonian houses and the Guggenheim Museum (New York City, 1943–59) were attempts to forge an American architecture free of either historical or European modern prototypes.

Later followers of Wright in this quest for a nativist American design would include his Taliesin Fellowship, a few of his students, E. Fay Jones, and at some removal, independents like

Bruce Goff. Jones's work has Wrightian forms and details, though with more vertical articulation. His Interdenominational Chapel (1980), Thorncrown, Arkansas, uses wooden uprights and trusses to create a magical space in the middle of a grove. Goff's work has no parallels, for although he admitted to initially being affected by Wright, his designs departed from the essentially geometrical basis of Wright. Goff eccentrically used prows, peaks, towers, carpeted walls, and fringe. His Ford House (Aurora, Illinois, 1947–50) is a round shape with two attached bedroom pods; the form is composed of lower walls of coal embedded with hunks of green glass that carry a Quonset hut frame covered in lapped siding and shingles. The interior, as with most of Goff's work, is unsettling in its unconventionality and exhilarating in its expansiveness.

Another branch of regionalism, more historically based, continued in the 1920s and 1930s with architects such as John Gaw Meem in New Mexico, Robert McGoodwin in Pennsylvania, and Royal Barry Wills in Massachusetts. They designed buildings that eclectically drew on the local vernacular imagery and met modern requirements. The work of these regionalists was accomplished and in many cases distinguished; Wills's work was especially influential because he publicized it through a series of books for homeowners, whereas Meem created an image for an entire region.

Beginning in the 1930s, a new school of abstract regionalism developed in the far west, where architects in southern California (Harwell Hamilton Harris), in the Bay Area (William Wurster), and in Oregon (Pietro Belluschi) drew on the local vernacular of cabins, barns, and ranches and also on the earlier work of Maybeck and the brothers Greene. Harris and Wurster created a "woodsy" California vernacular, using the older ranch house plan, but with open plans and simplified details influenced by the International Style. By the late 1940s, a new West Coast School was openly acknowledged, though it sometimes went under more specific names: the Redwood School, or the Bay Area Group. In the 1950s and 1960s came Joseph Esherick and the firm of Moore, Lyndon, Trumbull and Whitaker. The latter's work at Sea Ranch (1964–74), with Lawrence Halprin, picked up the mid-19th century wooden forms from the nearby Russian settlement at Fort Ross and combined them with landscape sensitivity. Also emerging in the late 1960s and 1970s as part of the counterculture revolution would be a "butcher block," or ad hoc aesthetic of buildings constructed of seemingly random elements for specific sites.

The term "critical regionalism," coined by the critic Kenneth Frampton in 1983, although seeming to indicate a regionalist response, was really a recognition of certain local modernist idioms that had grown up internationally. Placing stress on tectonics and building processes, critical regionalism was really a critique of Postmodernism. Architects sometimes labeled as critical regionalists—Samuel Mockbee and Clark and Menefee—do draw on the local forms, but in a modernist vein. Antoine Predock created in the southwest a compelling abstraction of landscape and indigenous building forms, as in the Fine Arts Center (1985–89), Arizona State University, Tempe. The large geometric forms exude an air of nativist mystery in the harsh sunlight.

Modernism

The quest for a new or modern architecture dominated much of 20th-century American architectural thought. A polemical

warfare existed between factions who attempted to define modern architecture by rigid stylistic criteria. With historical perspective, however, one can see modernism as a broad theme that contains—and continues to have—a number of different thrusts and styles or idioms, which might be labeled decorative, constructive, abstract, and Postmodern. Common to all approaches was a belief that reliance on older historical styles was intellectually bankrupt, given the tremendous social and technological changes that had occurred. A zeitgeist, or a new spirit, had arisen, brought into being by the machine or other technological advances. Architects would be avant-garde, and like painters they should create a new expression. All architectural modernists paid at least lip service to the notion of functionalism, but how it was interpreted differed widely. Few architects belonged exclusively to the decorative, constructive, abstract, or Postmodern approach. Mies van der Rohe argued that his buildings were reflective of their structure with their revealed frame, as with the apartment towers on Lake Shore Drive (Chicago, 1948–51). However, Mies was equally concerned with creating elegant abstract objects irrespective of the revealed frame, as in his Seagram Building (New York City, 1954–58). Similarly, Henry-Russell Hitchcock and Philip Johnson noted the new methods of construction as a basis for *The International Style* (1932), a book they wrote in conjunction with an exhibition at the Museum of Modern Art. However, they argued that the International Style existed irrespective of technology, with its own abstract principles that included the avoidance of applied decoration, volume rather than mass, and regularity rather than symmetry. The International Style is similar to the American Renaissance in the attempt to fix a single national architecture for all purposes. In this concern for a new universal style, some modernists stand out. Mies van der Rohe created forms that could be—and were—built everywhere.

The decorative modernist approach first emerged in the 1920s and 1930s and frequently goes under the name of Art Deco or Art Moderne. Some American architecture was directly influenced by the International Exhibition of Decorative Arts, Paris (1925), and also by the European Secessionist movement. This comes forth most obviously in the ornamental appliqué Eliel Saarinen placed on his Chicago Tribune Tower entry (1922) or in Parkinson and Parkinson's Bullocks-Wilshire Department Store (Los Angeles, 1928). Saarinen's later work remains within the decorative tradition seen especially in his highly colorful Kingswood School (Cranbrook, Michigan, 1929–31). In the later 1930s and 1940s, he evolved a more reticent and simpler modernism, though it was tied to the ornamental texture of materials.

An aspect of the Art Deco was geometrical elements in a setback form with appropriate ornament, which appeared in Bertram Goodhue's Nebraska State Capitol (Lincoln, 1921–31) and then in skyscrapers by Ralph Walker, Raymond Hood, and William Van Alen. The 1916 New York zoning regulations helped in this development because they mandated setbacks in high-rise buildings, and architects across the country imitated the form, irrespective of local zoning regulations. Hugh Ferris, an architectural renderer, showed architects how the setbacks of the tall masses could be molded. Van Alen's Chrysler Building (New York City, 1928–31) combined setbacks with a stainless steel radiating crest. At an urban scale, Raymond Hood, as the leader of a team of architects, planned Rockefeller Center (New York City, 1928–38)—a group of extravagantly decorated setback buildings.

A new decorative approach appeared in the 1950s and 1960s in some works by Philip Johnson, Wallace K. Harrison, Minoru Yamasaki, and Edward Durell Stone. They introduced patterned blocks and screens and also created forms that recalled classicism, as in Stone's United States Embassy (1954) in New Delhi, India. Johnson's Sheldon Museum (1960–63), University of Nebraska, is bounded by decorative, ahistorical pilasters and arches with subtle curves and profiles that are perhaps too graceful.

The Constructivist approach takes as its premise that technology and construction are the major design determinants and should be reflected in the final product. The 19th-century Chicago School, with its emphasis on the revealed frame, was a major influence on American architecture from the 1930s onward. Construction as the form determinant can be seen most prominently in the work of Albert Kahn, a leading factory designer in the first half of the 20th century. He produced large, elegant factories of curtain walls enclosing trusses, columns, and open interior spaces. In California the Case Study housing program of the 1940s and 1950s, led by designers such as Charles Eames and Craig Ellwood, created steel-framed houses out of industrial components. A High-Tech sensibility emerged in which great prominence was given to industrial materials, the structure, and the heating, ventilation, and air conditioning systems. The later work of Ellwood (Art Center College of Design, Pasadena, California, 1977), the early work of Hardy, Holtzman and Pfeiffer (Orchestra Hall, Minneapolis, Minnesota, 1974), and the work of Helmut Jahn (Michigan City, Indiana, Public Library, 1977) all exploited technology both as the basic expression of the building and as ornament.

Far different is the Brutalist approach of Louis Kahn, who saw technology and structure as elements to emphasize, as with the giant laboratory exhausts and reinforced-concrete, prestressed, posttensioned framing elements in the Richards Medical Laboratory (Philadelphia, 1957–61). Kahn acted as a father figure to a group of Philadelphia-based architects such as Romaldo Giurgola. Kahn's work, however, is more than just construction; it is also a concern for light and an employment of abstract references to historical prototypes such as the Italian hill town towers at the Richards Laboratory; the Romanesque barrel vaults at the Kimbell Art Museum, Fort Worth, Texas; or the tapering Egyptian pylons and Renaissance palazzos at the Phillips Exeter Library (Exeter, New Hampshire, 1965–71). As with many creative architects, Kahn escapes any precise classification.

Abstract modernism, the third major direction, is a radical ahistoricism in which all traditional imagery is absent. It first appeared in the work of émigrés such as R. M. Schindler and Richard Neutra. Schindler wanted an architecture that bore no relation to anything of the past and equally avoided contemporary stylisms. His Lovell Beach House (Newport Beach, California, 1924–26) was a series of stacked trays held aloft by a concrete frame and his later houses were exploded boxes of "Space Architecture," as he claimed, perched precariously on hillsides. Schindler fits in no stylistic categories, whereas Richard Neutra was more derivative of the Europe-based International Style. His Lovell Health House (Los Angeles, 1927–29), with its white gunite skin and steel frame, was actually more advanced technologically than its European contemporaries.

Technology was always an important element of abstract modernism, but never a determinant. The arrival in the later 1930s of another group of European émigrés such as Walter Gropius, Marcel Breuer, and Mies van der Rohe helped to make abstract modernism into the dominant American expression. Mies was the more important form-giver, and through his teaching in the College of Architecture at the Illinois Institute of Technology, Chicago—his campus design served as a demonstration—his steel-and-glass expression came to dominate American cities.

American followers of the International Style included George Howe, who with the Swiss émigré William Lescaze designed the PSFS Building (Philadelphia, 1929–32). The PSFS skyscraper, with its cool, high-styled abstraction, became a forerunner of a post–World War II phenomenon—the large, aggressively modern corporate headquarters. Instead of the safety of history as an image to be associated with, corporation presidents now sought the novel and modern. The American firm of Skidmore, Owings and Merrill became the acknowledged leaders of this building type. Under the guidance of designers Gordon Bunshaft and Bruce Graham, Skidmore, Owings and Merrill created crisp and elegant skyscrapers including the Lever House (New York City, 1949–52) and the Sears Tower (Chicago, 1974–76), as well as suburban headquarters such as Connecticut General Life (Bloomfield, Connecticut, 1954–57). The glass office tower assumed political symbolism with the United Nations Headquarters (New York City, 1947–52), designed by Wallace K. Harrison in association with foreign advisers.

Eero Saarinen provided a challenging pluralism of a different style for each commission in contrast to the single-minded steel-and-glass approach. His General Motors Technical Center (Warren, Michigan, 1948–56) suggested a Miesian aesthetic, but he increasingly recognized that form knew no boundaries. In his later works such as the TWA Airport Terminal (1956–62) at New York's John F. Kennedy Airport, or the Dulles Airport Terminal in Chantilly, Virginia (1958–62), Saarinen created tremendously dynamic forms. He also explored a historical contextualism in Morse and Stiles Colleges, Yale University (New Haven, Connecticut, 1958–62), in which the earlier Gothic Revival campus was loosely recalled.

A roughness of concrete and dramatic sculptural form similar to Le Corbusier's late manner at Harvard University's Carpenter Center (Cambridge, Massachusetts, 1960–63) became a popular idiom with a group of architects from the late 1950s through the early 1970s. Paul Rudolph's Yale University Art and Architecture Building (New Haven, Connecticut, 1958–62) echoes both Wright and Le Corbusier in forms. Although Brutalism found a following, more important was the "rebirth of solids" and "a new plasticity," as Marcel Breuer explained it. He exploited the massive concrete frame in a series of large bureaucratic office buildings in the United States and abroad.

From the 1960s onward, minimalist and scaleless exterior forms reflecting the contemporaneous minimal art movement in painting and sculpture became a line of development in abstract modernism. Gordon Bunshaft's Hirshhorn Museum (Smithsonian Institution, Washington, D.C., 1967–74) was essentially a large piece of sculpture—a pure round and monolithic form. Exteriors of buildings appeared to become a single, unified material, such as reflective glass on I. M. Pei and Henry Cobb's John Hancock Buildings (Boston, 1973–77), Kevin Roche's U.N.

Plaza (New York City, 1976–83), or Cesar Pelli's Pacific Design Center (Los Angeles, 1973–75). The reflective glass skin was an American trademark; similarly, long stretches of limestone with few subdivisions, as in Pei's East Wing of the National Gallery (Washington, D.C., 1968–78), also produced this clean, minimal effect.

The "white box" of the 1920s International Style experienced a revival in the 1960s and 1970s via a younger generation. The "New York Five" (Richard Meier, Michael Graves, Peter Eisenman, John Hedjuk, and Charles Gwathmey) were greatly influenced by Le Corbusier's pavilions of the 1920s and by the Anglo-American critic Colin Rowe. All moved on to different work, though Meier retained the most allegiance, showing an ability to inflate the white box into a large and more complicated scale, as with his U.S. Courthouse (Central Islip, New York, 2000).

Postmodernism in the 1970s and 1980s might have been considered a separate theme, but as the term implies, it was (or is) not a total break with modernism, but the opening of a discourse with subjects that modernism had ignored up to that point. Born of a sense of disillusionment and what was termed at the time a "failure" of abstract and technological modernism, Postmodernism frequently exhibited a contextual approach in design and a certain nostalgia for the past that contained analogies with decorative modernism. The term Postmodernism did not receive wide currency until its adoption by proponents such as Robert A. M. Stern and Charles Jencks in the mid-1970s, but its roots go back to the dissatisfaction with modernism seen in the work of Johnson, Stone, and others in the 1950s. Jane Jacobs's *The Death and Life of Great American Cities* (1961) criticized the modernist fascination with isolated buildings. Robert Venturi's *Complexity and Contradiction in Architecture* (1966) and his later (with Denise Scott Brown and Steven Izenour) *Learning from Las Vegas* (1972) were the earliest key texts of the movement. Influenced by the contemporaneous pop art movement, Venturi argued that architects should look to the roadside "strip" and that buildings were primarily "signs" with communicative systems involving nonfunctional elements such as ornament. Symbolism treated with irony became his firm's trademark. Venturi's mother's house (Vanna Venturi House, Philadelphia, Pennsylvania, 1962–64) reflects this approach with raised moldings, an oblique entrance, and a split gable that can be read as a pediment. Venturi and his partners frequently demonstrate a witty streak, as in the play on the 1910s revival of the English Jacobean Revival at Princeton University in their Wu Hall (Princeton, New Jersey, 1980–83). Initially, Charles Moore's architecture of the 1960s had a regionalist orientation, as at Sea Ranch condominiums (Sea Ranch, California, 1964–65); however, Moore also showed a sensibility to history and used ornament in an unorthodox and even distorted manner. A peripatetic teacher at many schools and universities, Moore influenced a tremendous number of younger architects. Stylized references through abstraction and distortion to earlier buildings and forms can be seen as the basis of a group of Postmodernists such as Michael Graves. Graves, who began as a neo-Le Corbusian in his earlier works, retained a modernist search for a distinctive personal language. His Public Services Building (Portland, Oregon, 1980–82), with its unique polychrome pastels and over-scaled and patently false applied classical detail, contains a lurking figurative molding of space and form. Similarly, his Den-

ver Public Library (1995) has a relation to the particularized western mining context but contains its own individuality. Postmodernism's critique of the failure of modernism included its lack of theory that went beyond function and technology. The result was a theory fad that crashed through academia and promoted approaches drawn from other disciplines such as semiotics, anthropology, and gender studies. The most prominent was a form of abstract modernism called deconstructivism, which emerged in the 1980s and drew on French literary theory and philosophy and also on the Russian Constructivism of the 1920s. Deconstructivist architecture existed not as a unified approach but as a group of individuals, including Peter Eisenman, who challenged harmony, unity, and stability by designing buildings or theoretical projects in which forms are rotated, along with the appearance of odd angles, disruptive materials, and a general sense of alienation of the occupant. As shown in his Wexner Center (1985–89), Ohio State University, and the Columbus Convention Center (1989–92)—both in Columbus, Ohio—Eisenman's work is characterized by a progressive distortion and an additive and subtractive design process to create conflict-ridden, unsettling forms.

Avoiding this complex theoretical base, a new wave of abstract modernism far more sculptural and distorted in form emerged in the 1980s and 1990s, as seen in the work of Frank Gehry, Thom Mayne and Morphosis, and Eric Owen Moss—all centered in the Los Angeles area. Gehry's early work, such as his own house (Santa Monica, California, 1977–78, 1992), delighted in collage and the treatment of fragmentary elements in unorthodox ways, including asphalt floors, open stud frames, and chain-link fencing. As Gehry's work developed, it became more sculptural, as with his Advanced Technology Laboratory (1987–92) at the University of Iowa, Iowa City, and the Guggenheim Museum (Bilbao, Spain, 1993–97). The Iowa work is composed of tiled geometrical blocks, whereas in Spain, the 258,000-square-foot museum exudes a strongly organic feel with its long curling surfaces. Partially clad in titanium, the Bilbao structure continues the collage approach with its juncture of various geometries and materials.

Gehry's Guggenheim at Bilbao and other late 20th-century works such as the Korean Presbyterian Church (2000), Queens, New York, by Garofalo, with Lynn and McInturf—with its extruded frame like wings—have been likened to computer-created designs. Certainly, the working drawings and building materials fabrication were done by computer programs. Computers did aid in opening Gehry and Garofalo's vision to new exciting and abstract forms, but computers did not create the fantastic forms that were still products of the designers' imaginations.

At the end of the 20th century, American architecture was as diffuse as Gehry's project for a 40-story-tall new Guggenheim building in New York and Robert A. M. Stern's design for a Public Library in Nashville, Tennessee. Gehry's project is a wild combination of forms, whereas Stern's library recalls Paul Cret's work of the 1930s. They represent an alpha and omega of architecture: two extremely different ideas of what is American. This multiplicity of approaches in American architecture during the 20th century is its ultimate characteristic. The consequence has been many competing themes and approaches with none totally dominant and, indeed, no promise of that occurrence in the near future.

RICHARD GUY WILSON

See also **Art Deco; Art Nouveau (Jugendstil); Arts and Crafts Movement; Breuer, Marcel (United States); Brutalism; Classicism; Cram, Ralph Adams (United States); Cret, Paul Philippe (United States); Deconstructivism; Eisenman, Peter (United States); Ellwood, Craig (United States); Fallingwater, Bear Run, Pennsylvania; Gehry, Frank (United States); Goff, Bruce (United States); Goodhue, Bertram Grosvenor (United States); Greene, Henry M. and Charles S. (United States); Guggenheim Museum, Bilbao, Spain; Guggenheim Museum, New York City; Historicism; International Style; International Style Exhibition, New York (1932); Kahn, Albert (United States); Kahn, Louis (United States); McKim, Mead and White (United States); Moore, Charles (United States); Neutra, Richard (Austria); New York, United States; Pennsylvania Station, New York; Portland Public Services Building, Portland, Oregon; Postmodernism; Prairie School; Predock, Antoine (United States); Robie House, Chicago; Saarinen, Eero (Finland); Schindler, Rudolph M. (Austria, United States); Scott Brown, Denise (United States); Skidmore, Owings and Merrill (United States); Stern, Robert A. M. (United States); TWA Airport Terminal, New York; Vanna Venturi House, Philadelphia; Venturi, Robert (United States); Wanamaker Store, Philadelphia; Wright, Frank Lloyd (United States); Wurster, William (United States)**

Further Reading

Brooks, H. Allen, *The Prairie School; Frank Lloyd Wright and His Midwest Contemporaries*, Toronto: University of Toronto Press, 1972

Condit, Carl, *Chicago, 1930–70: Building, Planning, and Urban Technology*, Chicago: University of Chicago Press, 1974

Ferriss, Hugh, *The Metropolis of Tomorrow*, New York: I. Washburn, 1929

Frampton, Kenneth, *Modern Architecture: A Critical History*, New York: Oxford University Press, 1980

Frampton, Kenneth, and John Cava (editors), *Studies in Tectonic Culture: The Poetics of Construction in Nineteenth and Twentieth Century Architecture*, Cambridge, Massachusetts: MIT Press, 1995

Handlin, David P., *American Architecture*, New York: Thames and Hudson, 1985

Hitchcock, Henry-Russell, *Architecture: Nineteenth and Twentieth Centuries*, third edition, Harmondsworth: Penguin, 1969

Hitchcock, Henry-Russell, and Philip Johnson, *The International Style: Architecture since 1922*, New York: The Museum of Modern Art and W. W. Norton, 1932

Jacobs, Jane, *The Death and Life of Great American Cities*, New York: Random House, 1961

Jencks, Charles A., *The Language of Post-Modern Architecture*, New York: Rizzoli, 1977

Johnson, Philip, and Mark Wigley, *Deconstructivist Architecture*, New York: Museum of Modern Art, 1988

Jordy, William, *American Buildings and Their Architects: Progressive and Academic Ideals at the Turn of the Twentieth Century*, volume 3, Garden City, New York: Doubleday, 1972

Jordy, William, *American Buildings and Their Architects: The Impact of European Modernism in the Mid-Twentieth Century*, volume 4, Garden City, New York: Doubleday, 1972

Kimball, Fiske, *American Architecture*, Indianapolis, Indiana: Bobbs-Merrill, 1928

Mumford, Lewis, *Sticks and Stones: A Study of American Architecture and Civilization*, New York: Boni and Liveright, 1925

Roth, Leland, *American Architecture: A History*, Boulder, Colorado: Westview Press, 2001

Roth, Leland (editor), *America Builds: Source Documents in American Architecture and Planning*, New York: Harper and Row, 1983

Rowe, Colin, and Fred Koetter, *Collage City*, Cambridge, Massachusetts: MIT Press, 1977

Scully, Vincent, *American Architecture and Urbanism*, revised edition, New York: H. Holt, 1988

Stern, Robert A. M. *New Directions in American Architecture*, New York: G. Braziller, 1977

Tallmadge, Thomas E., *The Story of Architecture in America*, revised edition, New York: W.W. Norton, 1936

Upton, Dell, *Architecture in the United States*, New York: Oxford University Press, 1998

Venturi, Robert, *Complexity and Contradiction in Architecture*, New York: Museum of Modern Art, and Garden City, New York: Doubleday, 1966

Venturi, Robert, Denise Scott Brown, and Steven Izenour, *Learning from Las Vegas*, Cambridge, Massachusetts: MIT Press, 1972

Wilson, Richard Guy, *The AIA Gold Medal*, New York: McGraw-Hill, 1984

Wilson, Richard Guy, Dianne Pilgrim, and Dickran Tashijan, *The Machine Age in America, 1918–1941*, New York: Abrams, 1986

Wilson, Richard Guy, and Sidney K. Robinson (editors), *Modern Architecture in America: Visions and Revisions*, Ames: Iowa State University Press, 1991

Wright, Frank Lloyd, *When Democracy Builds*, Chicago: University of Chicago Press, 1945

Wright, Frank Lloyd, *An Organic Architecture: The Architecture of Democracy*, the Sir George Watson lectures of the Sulgrave Manor Board for 1939, London: Lund Humphries, 1970

Zukowsky, John (editor), *Chicago Architecture, 1872–1922: Birth of a Metropolis*, Munich: Prestel-Verlag and Chicago: The Art Institute of Chicago, 1987

Zukowsky, John (editor), *Chicago Architecture and Design, 1923–1993: Reconfiguration of an American Metropolis*, Munich: Prestel-Verlag and Ernest R. Graham Study Center for Architectural Drawings at the Art Institute of Chicago and New York: Neues Publishing, 1993

UNITED STATES AIR FORCE ACADEMY CHAPEL

Designed by Skidmore, Owings and Merrill; completed 1963
Colorado Springs, Colorado

The U.S. Air Force Academy Cadet Chapel, today the most visited man-made structure in Colorado, was once the source of a bitter controversy that extended all the way to the U.S. Congress. Because of this battle, the chapel design, completed by Walter A. Netsch, Jr., of the Chicago office of Skidmore, Owings and Merrill (SOM), was altered and finally completed after five years of planning and four years of construction. SOM was also responsible for the overall design of the campus, which they completed in the International Style. The chapel was to be both literally and figuratively the crowning element of the complex with its pointed profile, symbolizing the surrounding Rocky Mountains or, perhaps more appropriately, a group of upended fighter jets, rising above the other structures of the campus.

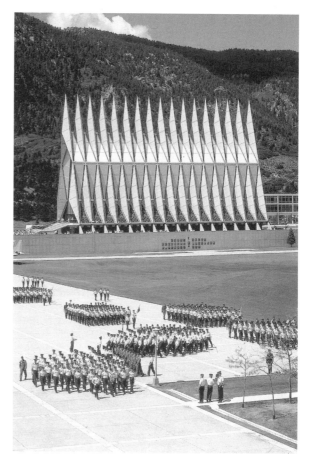

U.S. Air Force Academy Chapel, Colorado Springs
Photo courtesy United States Air Force Academy Headquarters

Netsch's first design for the chapel, a modified A-frame structure with folding concrete plates, was not well received when presented to the public as part of the overall campus design in May 1955. It was labeled an "assembly of wigwams" and a "modernistic cigarette factory." In July 1955, Frank Lloyd Wright led the criticism against the complex when it was presented to Congress, calling the design "half baked" and "resembling a wayside market." Congress held back the necessary funds for the undertaking, but the Air Force fought back, hiring a committee of architectural experts, including Eero Saarinen, Wallace K. Harrison, Welton Becket, and Pietro Belluschi, to help redesign and positively promote the project. Within days, a new scheme, complete with a more traditional chapel design located on a different part of the site, found its way to the Senate floor. Additionally, SOM and the Air Force made it clear that the chapel design was just preliminary and would not be addressed for another four years. The Senate voted to release the monies for the complex, and the Academy was saved, but the future of the chapel's design was uncertain.

Netsch, confident in the quality of his design but distraught over the lack of its acceptance, left for Europe. The trip was not only a much-needed break from the chapel conflict but also a chance to view religious architecture, which he did from Italy to England. Renewed and refreshed, Netsch went back to work

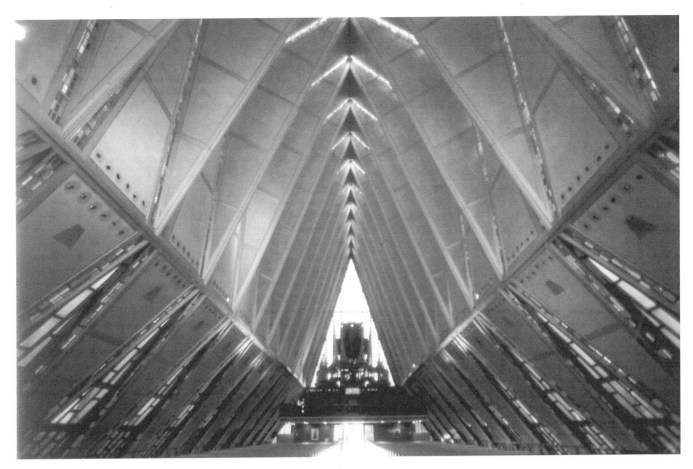

U.S. Air Force Academy Chapel, interior detail of stained glass on ceiling
Photo courtesy United States Air Force Academy Headquarters

on the design of the chapel on his return to the United States. Still, disagreement clouded the process. This time, it was concern over how to provide worship space for three separate faiths: Protestant, Catholic, and Jewish. Should there be three separate chapels, or should there be one chapel that would house all three faiths? Finally, in August of 1957, after a number of design options had been explored, Netsch and SOM presented the chapel's final design to Congress. The building, triangular in profile, was comprised of 19 spires covered with aluminum. The design was modernistic, even industrial, but Congress approved its funding. The Air Force supported Netsch's work by stating that the building would be built as designed, rejuvenating Netsch, who promptly set off with the building's model and plans on a promotional tour across the United States.

Work on the building began under the contractor Robert E. McKee of Santa Fe, New Mexico, on 28 August 1959. The chapel was placed on a podium adjacent to the Academy's Court of Honor. The only change from the final design to the built structure was a reduction in the number of spires from 19 to 17 because of cost constraints. The spires were fashioned from 100 tubular steel-framed tetrahedrons anchored by joints to concrete buttresses. The tetrahedrons, spaced one foot apart to accept interstitial stained glass, were clad in aluminum. Inside,

the chapel was divided into two levels, the upper housing the Protestant chapel and the lower the Catholic, Jewish, and All Faiths chapels. This two-level arrangement might have been impressed on Netsch from his visits to the Sainte-Chapelle in Paris, France, and the monastic church of St. Francis in Assisi, Italy.

The tetrahedrons meet 99 feet above the terrazzo floor of the 900-seat Protestant chapel. Twenty-four thousand pieces of glass, with 35 percent of it chipped to give it a jewellike appearance, fill the spaces between the tetrahedrons. Netsch carefully arranged the layout of the glass by placing the darkest of the 24 shades used at the entrance end of the chapel and progressing to the lighter colors in the front. A special laminated glass fills the triangular spaces at the chapel's northern and southern ends. A 14-foot-tall mosaic reredos completed by the painter-sculptor Lumen Martin Winter, a 46-foot-tall aluminum cross, and a 15-foot marble altar in the shape of a ship fill the liturgical north end.

The major portion of the lower level is reserved for the 500-seat Catholic chapel. The space, accessible from the south on the terrace level, consists of precast-concrete beams and columns filled with blue and amber glass sidewalls. The Baptistery and Blessed Sacrament Chapel are located on either side of the main entrance. The focal point of the space is the sanctuary with

its blue-carpeted, three-step predella; a white marble altar; and Venetian glass reredos. The Catholic chapel takes its name from the marble sculpture of Our Lady of the Skies, one of the two figures in bas-relief on the 18-by-45-foot reredos, the other being the Guardian Angel. Winter was responsible for the reredos, Stations of the Cross, and the six-foot sculptured nickel silver crucifix over the altar.

Adjacent to the Catholic chapel on the north is the 100-seat Jewish chapel. Two separate entrances from the terrace arcade give access to the space. The chapel is circular in form and placed within a square foyer of purple-glass panels alternating with windows of green and blue glass. Cypress stanchions separated by translucent pebble glass separate the foyer from the chapel proper. Ludwig Y. Wolpert of the Jewish Museum in New York City designed the ecclesiastical appointments, including the Holy Ark, menorah, and Eternal Light. To the north of the Jewish chapel is the All Faiths Room, a simple space devoid of ornament and religious symbolism in order to accommodate a variety of faiths. The interior furnishing of each chapel was completed under the guidance of leaders of each faith, including the General Commission on Chaplains in the Armed Services to represent Protestant groups, the National Jewish Welfare Board, and the Roman Catholic Military Ordinariate.

On 22 September 1963, nine years after its original presentation, the Cadet Chapel was dedicated. The dedication did not, however, end the controversy surrounding it. The debate over its new, nontraditional, and modern design was reported again in the architectural and popular press. Indeed, the quest for what is appropriate in religious architecture came from the design of a creator-architect supported by a patron, in this case Walter Netsch designing for the U.S. Air Force. As the Air Force superintendent stated at the building's dedication, "The Cadet Chapel is the architectural and spiritual centerpiece of our academy. As such, it plays a vital role in developing and nurturing the character of our cadets. It is a reminder that we are a nation under God dedicated to the promotion of peace and goodwill among all nations of the world. The young women and men who come to study here do so in order to prepare themselves to protect freedom—freedom which is God's gift to all people."

VICTORIA M. YOUNG

Further Reading

"Air Force Academy Chapel," *Architectural Record*, 132 (December 1962)

Bruegmann, Robert (editor), *Modernism at Mid-Century: The Architecture of the United States Air Force Academy*, Chicago: University of Chicago Press, 1994

Hamilton, C. Mark, "The Air Force Academy Chapel: A Persistent Form in the Face of Controversy," *Architronic*, 4/2 (September 1995)

"Perspectives: Air Academy Chapel Professional Opinion," *Architectural Record*, 122 (December 1957)

Temko, Allan, "The Air Academy Chapel—A Critical Appraisal," *Architectural Forum*, 117 (December 1962) (responses to Temko may be found in the February 1963 issue of *Architectural Forum*)

United States Air Force Academy, *The United States Air Force Academy Cadet Chapel*, Colorado Springs, Colorado: The Academy, 1963

UNITY TEMPLE

Designed by Frank Lloyd Wright; completed 1909
Oak Park, Illinois

Unity Temple is the building for what was originally Unity Church (since 1961 known as the Unitarian-Universalist Church) at 875 Lake Street in the west Chicago suburb of Oak Park, Illinois, designed and built by Frank Lloyd Wright from 1905 to 1909. The structure was Wright's first church and his first building wholly of concrete. Its stark geometry and new material marked it to contemporaries as a work of modern architecture. It is among the most well-known modernist church buildings of the 20th century. Unity Temple is one of Wright's two outstanding nonresidential works of his first mature period before 1910, the other being the Larkin Company Administration Building in Buffalo, New York, designed and built in 1902–06. In his autobiography, Wright wrote of Unity Temple as one of the works that best exemplified his method of design.

Unity Church in Oak Park had previously worshiped in a traditional neo-Gothic wood building with a tall frontal steeple, which was destroyed by fire in a lightning storm in June 1905, just after Wright had returned from his first trip abroad to Japan. Wright had been raised as a Unitarian and was a member of Unity Church during his residence in Oak Park from 1887 to 1909. After the destruction of its older building, Unity Church acquired a more centrally located site and appointed a committee, headed by Rev. Rodney Johonnot, that chose Wright as architect for a new building by September 1905. After much discussion, Unity Church approved Wright's design for Unity Temple in April 1906 for the new site on Oak Park's Lake Street amid the expensive monumental stone buildings of other Protestant churches. In the spring of 1906, construction began on Unity House, the lower rectangular southern part of the building used as a parish hall for social events, and it opened in September 1907. Unity Temple proper, the higher cubic auditorium for worship services on the site's north side, was opened for its first service in October 1908, although work continued into 1909.

Working within a tight site and a minimal budget, Wright planned Unity Temple and Unity House as two semi-independently built volumes with a common central entrance hall between them set back from Lake Street. From this street, paths along either side of Unity Temple lead back and up steps to raised outdoor terraces on the east and west sides of the entrance hall. Above the doors on both sides of the hall is a Unitarian motto of the period, affixed in bronze letters, that reads, "For the Worship of God and the Service of Man," perhaps referring to the distinct functions of Unity Temple and Unity House to either side. Once inside the entrance hall, one proceeds directly south on the same level to enter Unity House. To enter Unity Temple, one moves to the north side of the entrance hall, toward its northeast and northwest corners, into walkways on the same level that extend along the east and west sides of the temple but below its main floor. From these low walkways, or "cloisters" as Wright called them, one rises to the auditorium's main floor via half flights of steps in each of its four corners. From the main floor, other corner steps lead upward to the lower and upper galleries around the auditorium's east, north, and

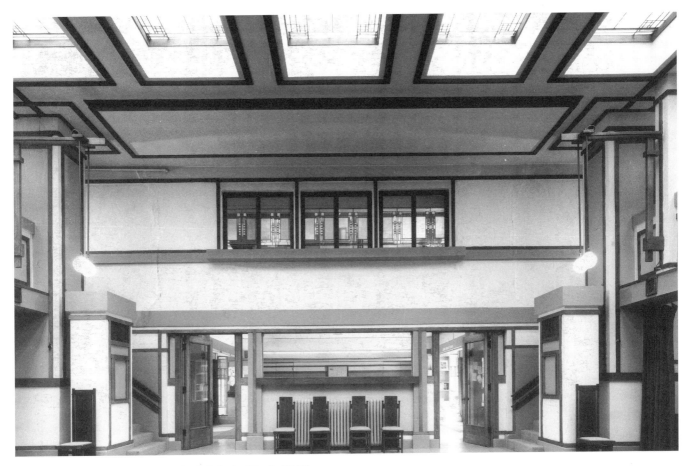

Interior looking north, Unity Temple, Oak Park, Illinois (1909)
© Historic American Buildings Survey/Historic American Engineering Record (Library of Congress)
Photograph by Philip Turner

west sides. These galleries, as well as the pews on the main floor level, address the pulpit in the center of the auditorium's south side, behind which rises the tall organ screen covering the room's central south wall. Worshipers at all levels were to exit the auditorium by filing to either side of the pulpit, where they could greet the minister, and then descend steps back down to the entrance hall.

Unity Temple's auditorium has clerestory windows of mostly clear glass around all four sides and a coffered ceiling of concrete beams filled with panes of colored art glass. The combination of the fully skylit central ceiling and the continuous clerestory windows around all four sides of the space makes Unity Temple's interior consistently bright with daylight. Yet because of the depth of the ceiling coffers and the deep overhang of the roof slabs beyond the clerestory windows, the ambient daylight is even, unlike unmodulated direct sunlight. The overall luminosity of the temple contrasts with the darkness of the low side access "cloisters" so that on entering the temple, one passes through darkness to light. The linear designs for both the clerestory and the skylight glass, like the designs for squared lamps that descend from the central ceiling's four corners, are related to the room's overall square and rectilinear geometry. The whole structure is of concrete, either reinforced with steel rods or encasing steel

beams or trusses. Practically, the choice of concrete created a fireproof church. Symbolically, the monolithic construction conveyed the Unitarian ideal of unity, just as the liberal religious concept of divinity residing in humanity was conveyed in the auditorium's volume (which accommodated 450 worshipers who face one another in a room only 35 feet wide between balcony fronts). Wright used narrow dark-stained oak strips to define the variably tinted planar surfaces of plastered and plain concrete. The colored planes and wood lines create the room's abstract aesthetic with minimal means. In 1984, Unity Temple's original interior colors were restored, as were those of the entrance hall. Outside, Wright used repeated wood formwork for pouring walls, roof slabs, corner stair blocks, and ornamentally cast columns. The original exterior revealed the lines of this wood formwork and the pour layers of the concrete, whose surface featured an aggregate of bird's-eye gravel. In 1973–74, the building's exterior was almost entirely recoated to approximate the original surface, which was retained on the ornamental columns and roof slab soffits.

Although highly original as a design for a church building, Unity Temple might represent Wright's response to a wide range of historic and recent sources. The basic plan of Unity Temple and Unity House joined by the entrance hall recalls that of

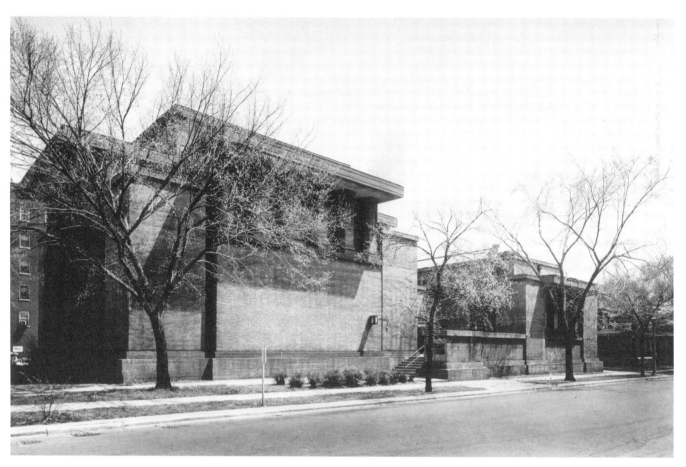

Unity Temple, Oak Park, Illinois (1909)
© James Reber. Photo courtesy The Frank Lloyd Wright Archives

the 17th-century Taiyu-in Mausoleum in Nikko, where Wright stayed briefly in April 1905. Wright's cubic geometry and ornamental columns recall the exterior massing and carved surfaces of Mayan temples known to Wright from at least 1893. A sympathetic response to such non-Western architectures would have been consistent with Unitarian convictions as to the oneness of all human religions and the antiquity of the idea of the unity of divinity. As Wright indicated, Unity Temple's square shape and galleried seating reinterpreted a long tradition of Protestant meetinghouses going back to the 16th century, including nonconformist chapels in Wales and England as well as Puritan colonial meetinghouses in New England. In modernist historiography, Unity Temple's cubic exterior and geometric interior were seen as one forerunner of Dutch De Stijl architecture. Retrospectively, Wright himself emphasized Unity Temple as the work in which he first fully engaged with architectural form as an expression of interior space. In Wright's later oeuvre, the idea of a top-lit sanctuary-like room recurred in such works as his Annie M. Pfeiffer Chapel (1938–41) for Florida Southern College in Lakeland and his Guggenheim Museum (1943–59) in New York City.

JOSEPH M. SIRY

See also **Church; Wright, Frank Lloyd (United States)**

Further Reading

The comprehensive monograph on Unity Temple is by Siry. Wright devoted a section of his autobiography to the building. Other recent sources include discussions of Unity Temple within broader accounts of Wright's work.

Graf, Otto Antonia, *Die Kunst des Quadrats: Zum Werk von Frank Lloyd Wright*, 2 vols., Vienna: Hermann Böhlhaus, 1983 (see especially volume 1)

Laseau, Paul, and James Tice, *Frank Lloyd Wright: Between Principle and Form*, New York: Van Nostrand Reinhold, 1992

Levine, Neil, *The Architecture of Frank Lloyd Wright*, Princeton, New Jersey: Princeton University Press, 1996

McCarter, Robert, *Frank Lloyd Wright*, London: Phaidon, 1997

McCarter, Robert, *Unity Temple: Frank Lloyd Wright*, London: Phaidon, 1997

McCarter, Robert (editor), *Frank Lloyd Wright: A Primer on Architectural Principles*, New York: Princeton Architectural Press, 1991

Nute, Kevin, *Frank Lloyd Wright and Japan: The Role of Traditional Japanese Art and Architecture in the Work of Frank Lloyd Wright*, New York: Van Nostrand Reinhold, and London: Chapman and Hall, 1993

Siry, Joseph M., *Unity Temple: Frank Lloyd Wright and Architecture for Liberal Religion*, New York: Cambridge University Press, 1996

Wright, Frank Lloyd, *An Autobiography*, London and New York: Longman Green, 1932; New York: Duell, Sloan and Pearce, 1943; New York: Horizon Press, 1977

UNIVERSITY LIBRARY, UNIVERSIDAD NACIONAL AUTÓNOMA DE MÉXICO

Designed by Juan O'Gorman, Gustavo Saavedra, and Juan Martínez Velasco; completed 1952
Mexico City, Mexico

The University Library at the Universidad Nacional Autónoma de México (UNAM) in Mexico City was built as both a national book and newspaper repository and the main library of the enormous new University City complex. Since its completion in 1952, the 13-story library, its top ten floors sheathed in figurative stone mosaics, has become the signature building of the University City and one of the iconic images of 21st-century Mexico.

By the 1940s, the 400-year-old University of Mexico's outmoded facilities lay scattered across the capital city. In 1947, the Mexican government acquired 1730 acres of land in the wild, 2000-year-old Pedregal lava field at the city's southern edge—immediately adjacent to the site of Luis Barragán's Jardines del Pedregal, where work was just then beginning. Some 200 million pesos were allocated for the construction of a new,

integrated campus for 25,000 to 30,000 students, and architects Enrique Del Moral, Mario Pani, and Mauricio Campos were commissioned to develop the overall plan and conduct competitions for the individual buildings. In 1950, Carlos Lazo was appointed director general of the project and made responsible for coordinating the efforts of the more than 100 architects, engineers, and artists, and 7000 workmen. Ground was broken for the first buildings that year, and by 20 November 1952, when Mexican President Miguel Alemán officially dedicated the project, the campus was 80 percent complete.

Juan O'Gorman, Gustavo Saavedra, and Juan Martínez Velasco were chosen to design the University Library. O'Gorman led this team and was also the sole designer of the building's mosaics and relief sculpture. During the 1930s, O'Gorman, an accomplished painter, had also been among the most radical exponents in Mexico of European-style functionalist modern architecture—a devoted disciple of Le Corbusier. The stripped-down, reinforced-concrete houses, schools, and factories that he built during those years were underlain by his fervent belief in the universal applicability of Le Corbusier's ideas and by his equally passionate desire to uplift a Mexican nation wracked by years of internecine warfare. By 1936, however, he withdrew from architectural practice, citing what he saw as the sterility and inappropriateness to Mexican culture of the very architec-

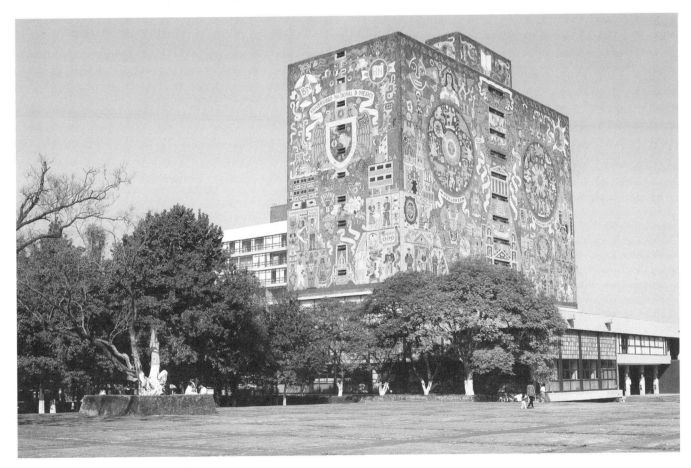

University Library, UNAM, Mexico City
© Royalty-Free/CORBIS

ture that he had advocated and built. When he began designing again in the mid-1940s, it was to assist painter Diego Rivera with the Anahuacalli Museum (1944–66) in Mexico City; built to house Rivera's collection of pre-Columbian art, this was a dense, stone-walled, Mayan Revival–style truncated pyramid with corbeled arches and figurative reliefs. By this time, O'Gorman had discovered the organic architecture of Frank Lloyd Wright—he had stayed at Fallingwater as a guest of the owners and now called Wright the greatest architect of the century—and took this as the inspiration for a Mexican architecture adapted to the peculiarities of site and local culture.

The initial plan for the library submitted by O'Gorman's team called for another truncated pyramid, not unlike Anahuacalli, but larger and cleaner, with translucent onyx windows. This was ultimately rejected for diverging too far from the rectilinear structures that dominated in the central part of the campus. As finally built, the library was composed of two rectangular slabs: a horizontally disposed base surmounted by a tower. Like many of the other buildings on the UNAM campus, the library consists mainly of a reinforced-concrete frame whose interspaces are filled with hollow ceramic tile. The first two stories house reading rooms, offices, and reference and circulation areas. External walls at this level consist of metal-framed glass windows and translucent onyx clerestories. Beyond these are outdoor reading rooms surrounded by heavy stone walls decorated with low-relief sculpture showing Aztec-inspired imagery. Finally, standing directly atop a one-story glass base is the virtually windowless tower containing the book stacks. The ten air-conditioned, fluorescent-lighted stack floors were designed to accommodate 120,000 volumes each, or 1.2 million volumes total.

The building's most striking feature is the 4400 square yards of mosaics completely covering the surface of its tower. Inspired, according to O'Gorman, by the architecture of Antoni Gaudí and the French naifs Fernand Cheval and Raymond Isidore and by Aztec codices and the social realist murals of Rivera and José Clemente Orozco, the library's mosaics depict a history of ideas in Mexico. In this, they are in keeping with the deep and pervasive interest in post–World War II Mexico in defining and giving form to the national character. The north wall is devoted to the Aztecs, the south wall to the Spanish colonial era, and the two narrower end walls to the effects of these two periods on the modern nation. Principal themes represented include religion, humanism, civic life, ceremony, warfare, conquest, education, art, and science. Thirteen different colors of natural stone—brought from all parts of the country and carefully tested for color and durability—were used along with cerulean blue glass. The mosaics were prefabricated in one-meter-square panels, and full-scale drawings were used to guide the placement of the stones and concrete to bind them. Once dried, the panels were lifted and cemented into place on a metal framework fixed to the library walls. O'Gorman touted the mosaics for bringing mural-type imagery outdoors, for blending the building into the landscape (via the colors of the stone), and for their low cost (just over $50,000 for materials and labor).

The library's mosaics, along with the many other mosaics, murals, and sculptures appearing on the campus, were part of a concerted effort to link architecture with the other arts. O'Gorman extolled this "integración plástica," as he called it, as essential to a modern Mexican architecture. Many of Mexico's best-known artists, among them the muralists Rivera and David

Alfaro Siqueiros, supported this integration and worked for it at the University City. Many, however, including several of the artists and architects involved there, were disappointed with the results, seeing the university's artwork as either not integrated enough or as unnecessary, undesirable, and injurious to the architecture. In a scathing critique in the November 1953 issue of *Progressive Architecture*, Sibyl Moholy-Nagy faulted the library for its "continuous mural that leaves not a square inch of the building material free to breathe." Several others at the time, however, both inside and outside Mexico, praised the library as a key element in one of the most ambitious, significant, and successful projects in contemporary world architecture—an architectural coming of age for Mexico in which functional modern forms took on a distinctive localized character. The building continues to serve as UNAM's central library.

KEITH L. EGGENER

See also **Barragán, Luis (Mexico); Corbusier, Le (Jeanneret, Charles-Édouard) (France); Gaudí, Antoni (Spain); Mexico; Mexico City, Mexico; O'Gorman, Juan (Mexico)**

Further Reading

Alvarez Noguera, José Rogelio (editor), *La arquitectura de la Ciudad Universitaria*, Mexico City: Universidad Nacional Autónoma de México, 1994

Arquitectura México, 39 (September 1952) (special issue edited by Mario Pani entitled "Número dedicado a la Ciudad Universitaria")

Burian, Edward R. (editor), *Modernity and the Architecture of Mexico*, Austin: University of Texas Press, 1997

Díaz y de Ovando, Clementina, *La Ciudad Universitaria de México*, 2 vols., Mexico City: Universidad Nacional Autónoma de México, 1980

González Gortazar, Fernando (editor), *La arquitectura méxicana del siglo XX*, Mexico City: Consejo Nacional para la Cultura y las Artes, 1994

Luna Arroyo, Antonio, *Juan O'Gorman: Autobiografiá, antología, juicios críticos y documentación exhaustivo sobre su obra*, Mexico City: Cuadernos Populares de Pintura Méxicana Moderna, 1973

McCoy, Esther, "The New University City of Mexico," *Arts and Architecture* (August 1952)

McCoy, Esther, "Mosaics of Juan O'Gorman," *Arts and Architecture* (February 1964)

Rodríguez Prampolini, Ida, *Juan O'Gorman: Arquitecto y pintor*, Mexico City: Universidad Nacional Autónoma de México, 1982

UNIVERSUM CINEMA, BERLIN

Designed by Eric Mendelsohn; completed 1928 (Schaubühne am Lehninerplatz, reconstruction by Jürgen Sawade, 1978–81)

The Universum Cinema and the WOGA (Wohnhaus-Grundstücks-Verwertungs-Aktien-Gesellschaft) housing complex—Mendelsohn's sole realized urban project—was conceived and built in various phases between 1925 and 1931 on the last undeveloped block along the western section of the Kurfürstendamm in Berlin. The genesis of the project was made difficult by the evolving program and the rivalry with Jürgen Bachmann, another architect hired for his experience in speculative development by the site owner Mosse.

Mendelsohn's first scheme (1925) for a large residential program was quite revolutionary in the context of the bourgeois district, as it integrated the typological advances of the urban (Paul Mebes in Berlin-Stieglitz) and suburban housing reform movement (Taut and Wagner at Berlin Britz). The thin bars of cross-ventilated apartments with common green areas at the back contrasted with the lot-based character of the neighborhood. As construction proceeded at Paulsborner and Albrecht-Achilles streets according to Bachmann's plans (they showed a similar housing layout and interior residential street), Mendelsohn redesigned his scheme.

The motion picture theater and its characteristic semicircular volume on the Kudamm appeared in the second version of 1926. Lined with shops, the "streamlined" interior street or "Basarstrasse" opened on the boulevard; the other end terminated into an ellipse-shaped Revuetheater. In the definitive layout of 1928, Mendelsohn shortened the inner street and framed it with a seven-story 300-room hotel. To the left the circular Kabarett der Komiker was placed behind a restaurant, whereas on the other side, the interior axis of the 1800-seat Universum Cinema was now asymmetrically shifted to accommodate a ring of shops. A long five-story housing bar closed the site along Cicerostrasse (rebuilt in 1980–81). Its multiple entrances servicing two large apartments per floor were marked by slightly projecting curved balconies. Bands of brick-clad walls connected them, thus creating strong horizontal accents terminated by returning semicircular balconies. The half-cylindrical and glazed staircases rhythmically accentuated the garden facade.

Mendelsohn rejected the urban-utopian component of the Expressionist movement as well as advocates of an International Style that espoused purity of aesthetic means over context. He studied in Munich with Theodor Fischer (1862–1938) along with Bruno Taut, Hannes Meyer, J. J. P. Oud, and Ernst May. Under Fischer's tutelage these architects assimilated the lessons of Camillo Sitte, and further kept the street, albeit reinvented, as the primary element of their urban design strategy.

At the WOGA complex, Mendelsohn attempted to interpret the collective memory of the city. His final and genuinely tridimensional arrangement of masses—elevator shafts, stage tower above the screen, vertical hotel—achieved quasi-medieval spatial effects. The bridgelike structure of the hotel brings to mind the Torhaus or gatehouse, a centuries-old sight of the German city and a popular building type that Walter Gropius used at the Bauhaus-Dessau, and Bruno Taut and Otto Salvisberg in their Berlin housing projects. For Mendelsohn it became a recurrent device as seen in his first project for the Deutsche Metallarbeiter-Verbandshaus (1929–30) or in his design for the Alexanderplatz (1931–32). The shape of the Universum also recalled Friedrich Gilly's sketches for a modern theater (1798) inspired by the Théâtre Feydeau in Paris. Mendelsohn's brick-clad volume did not reveal the theater itself as in Gotfried Semper's Opera House in Dresden (1878), but the dramatic foyer was accessed through a recessed entrance between the shops.

The WOGA complex became the point of reference for Martin Wagner's redesign of central Berlin, where the "flow lines" of motorized traffic and the "walking lines" of the pedestrians would smoothly guide the steps of the modern flâneur. This commercial *Grosstadtarchitektur* had to be inexpensive yet striking to capture the buying power of the "distracted" Berliner. From 1924 (*Metropolis*) the facades of the Ufa-Palast and other theaters in Berlin became brilliantly lighted billboards. Mendelsohn made them into architecture (*Reklamearchitektur*, according to Adolf Behne). It was so "cinematic" that its glass walls and rounded corners became the background of *Sunrise*, the first Hollywood film by Murnau in 1927.

Color, form, and light were the ingredients of Mendelsohn's architectural version of Nietzsche's *The Birth of Tragedy*, where "the music of masses in motion was contrasted with the spirit of gravity" (Neumeyer, 1999). The luminous blue of the ceiling dominated the double-height entrance hall, with the futurist glass-enclosed ticket office in the center. The mahogany-red cinema followed Mendelsohn's sketches quite closely: the bright balcony and the ceiling lights made the eyes converge toward the flat screen. For all its modernity, the cinema was still conceived of as a theater, with an orchestra pit and a small fly tower above the screen and its curtain.

The Universum influenced an entire generation of theaters around the world: from Argentina to England (the Odeon cinemas by Harry Weedon) and Tel Aviv, where I. Megidovitch's curved volume of the Kino Esther Cinema at Dizengoff Circle (1938–39) matched Mendelsohn's urban statement. In the United States, two Manhattan interiors prolonged Mendelsohn's experiment in conciseness. Frederick Kiesler's (1890–1965) Film Guild Cinema (1928–30) had a megaphone-shaped auditorium and a curtainless screen in the center of a painted circle; in the New School for Social Research (1929–31) by Joseph Urban (1872–1933), the egg-shaped auditorium displayed a bold set of red and gray colors.

The Ufa Cinema was sold in 1937. Heavily damaged by bombs during the war, it was unsympathetically remodeled several times. Put up for sale in 1975, it was saved by architect Jürgen Sawade, who convinced director Peter Stein and scenographer Karl-Ernst Herrmann to relocate their avant-garde theater, the Schaubühne am Halleschen Ufer. However, the structural problems encountered during construction and Stein's rendition of Gropius's *Totaltheater* eventually imposed a complete reconstruction. In the absence of a fly tower, the entire floor (including the seating) was made up of movable platforms on hydraulic supports. Inaugurated in 1981, the adaptable theater interior bore little relation to the historic facades and volumes. The debate about total reconstruction as legitimate means of urban renewal or historic preservation has been open since, as the controversy about the re-erection of the Berlin Stadtschloss and Schinkel's Bauakademie continues to demonstrate.

JEAN-FRANÇOIS LEJEUNE

See also **Berlin, Germany; Gropius, Walter (Germany); Mendelsohn, Erich (Germany, United States); Oud, J.J.P. (Netherlands); Taut, Bruno (Germany)**

Further Reading

Aulenti, Gae, "Universum theatri," *Casabella*, 46/479 (April 1982)

James, Kathleen, "No Stucco Pastries for Potemkin and Scapa Flow—Metropolitan Architecture in Berlin: the WOGA Complex and the Universum Cinema," in *Eric Mendelsohn Architect 1887–1953*, edited by Regina Stephan, New York: Monacelli Press, 1999

Mendelsohn, Erich, *Der Mendelsohn-Bau am Lehniner Platz: Erich Mendelsohn und Berlin*, Berlin: Hentrich Druck, 1981

Neumeyer, Fritz, "Nietzsche and Modern Architecture," in *Nietzsche and "An Architecture of Our Minds,"* Los Angeles: Getty Research Institute for the History of Art and the Humanities, 1999

Sharp, Dennis, *The Picture Palace and Other Buildings for the Movies*, London: H. Evelyn, 1969

"The Universum Cinema, Berlin: Erich Mendelsohn, Architekt," *Architects' Journal*, 75 supplement (March 8, 1932)

Zevi, Bruno, Manfred Sack, and Vittorio Magnago Lampugnani, "Universum mendelsohniano," *Domus*, 629 (June 1982).

URBAN PLANNING

Cities are mankind's most universal contribution on earth. Throughout human history, it is within cities that mankind has explored all counterpoints of himself in relation to his physical world: man within architecture, man within nature, man as individual and communal being, man and machine, mankind within temple and shelter. From the ancient *urbs* of Rome to the modernity of downtown America, the historical aim of urban planning has been to impose physical order on things that by nature are chaotic. For two millennia, cities have been formed by the seemingly omniscient hand of urban planning or, less fortunately, by the lack thereof. Herein lies the virtually impossible meaning of urban planning.

Defining Urban Planning

Urban planning is both art and social science. It encompasses the contemporary city, the historical site, architecture, the environment, economics, and social interaction. Urban planning constructs the city of today while creating the model of the city that will exist in the next decades. Unlike architecture, urban planning is a public profession dedicated not to individual clients but to the common good, which is a weighty responsibility. Even for an urban planner, it is difficult to define the obligations and limits of the profession. To attempt to define urban planning, this article will limit itself to physical planning, to major Western cities, and to the most influential threads in the history and theory of planning.

Parameters of the subject of physical planning include facilities for housing, transportation, education, health care, and basic urban infrastructure, such as streets, sidewalks, and water supply, down to the most mundane enterprises of sewers and waste disposal. Urban planning, although often unobserved, is operating on the micro- and the macroscale. The city, as we experience its immediate urban form, is composed of street pattern, skyline, vista, and details such as streetscape, signage, and building setbacks. Urban planning must also deal with the larger issues of city form and the distribution of urban land resources through zoning, land use controls, density, and neighborhood considerations. In the urban environment, open space, greenery, and parks are integral to urban planning, and public art enlivens the city; the arts and nature are fundamental to urban design. The context of buildings is an important design element of cities; hence, the relationships of new architecture to existing urban fabric and to historical districts must be respected by the planner. The city must further be considered not in isolation but in its larger regional context. These parameters only begin to define the minimum functional city.

In the greatest of cities, function is only a starting point for urbanism, and urban design reaches higher toward monumentality, achieved through the symbolic meaning of visual configurations and architectural landmarks. We can observe historical examples of planned cities that have exceeded the expectations of function to become symbolic urban spaces in New York, London, Paris, and Rome.

A Brief History of Urban Planning

Modern Western urban planning has its origins in the Roman concept of the *castrum* city, the infinitely logical encampment created in a coherent grid in the Roman provinces, still visible in the antique sections of European towns, such as the City section of London, in the Île de la Cité of Paris, or in Tuscan squares. Thus, the contemporary idea of a city as an entity that can be envisioned, designed, constructed, and administered by a thinking authority, a kind of bureaucratic but benevolent despot (which might be thought of as the theoretical basis of modern city planning), is really quite an ancient concept. After the decline of the Roman Empire, the concept of the ordered city declined as well, as order was more often relegated to the sacred space of the cathedral than to the secular space of the city. In the French town of Chartres, for example, one finds the chaos of the medieval city's streets pushing up against the organized mass of the divinely ordered architectural universe of the cathedral.

The Renaissance, with its rebirth of ancient forms, derived and ultimately monumentalized the Roman ideal of city planning. Michelangelo's plan for the Roman Campidoglio is one of the most complete and perfectly executed plans for a city sector, constructed to front a medieval agglomeration of buildings that themselves had grown up on the edge of the once highly ordered Roman Forum. Although the Campidoglio was intended not as an inhabitable city but as a symbolic urban space, it followed the Roman ideal of the imposition of physical order on chaos. Based on Michelangelo's ingenious geometric patterning and centered on the Roman statue of Marcus Aurelius, this Renaissance masterpiece recalls the order and majesty of ancient Roman planning.

Great baroque urban schemes dwarfed even these Renaissance plans. Bernini's extension of St. Peter's exterior space into Rome via his colonnade set the stage for sweeping baroque urban-planning schemes, with their spatial command and shaping of urban space. Cities extended themselves as medieval city walls were torn down and replaced with dynamic baroque schemes throughout Europe. Whole cities became works of art as urban planning reached its dramatic heights in the 16th and 17th centuries.

The greatest sweep of urban planning, however, was yet to come in the deconstruction and reassemblage of Paris in the 19th century. Paris saw the massive imposition of planning on a chaotic, medieval city with the fervor of Baron von Haussmann's straight, grand *étoile*, or star, of boulevards, with bridges and Napoleonic monuments highlighted. The grand radiating boulevards of Paris created vistas and promenade spaces through the city that we now identify with the French Enlightenment, with clarity and reason in urban design. The influence of French

planning can be felt in the United States in L'Enfant's radiating plan for Washington, D.C.

Urban planning in London is quite a contrast to Paris, for London never experienced an overlaid unifying design but remained instead a kind of crazy quilt city of interconnected sectors, some of which have within them their own individual internal order. In the United States, Boston is the closest analogy to London in form: antique, irrational street patterns contrasting with 19th-century planned sectors. Geometric classicism in urban design had enlightened London from the 18th through the early 19th century in the planning of the west end. London's Bloomsbury, in particular, was developed with order imposed via gridded streets and squares and by the graceful repetition of building forms in the standardized 18th-century row houses.

In opposition to the urbane geometric order of Bloomsbury, however, British urban planning likewise produced plans that were decidedly antiurban and picturesque. The late 19th century in England felt a schism between city and town, urban life and suburban, that developed as a reaction to the tragic consequences of industrialization. Picturesque inventions in urban planning, the schemes for garden cities and suburbs for the amelioration of slums, such as Ebenezer Howard's *Garden Cities of To-morrow* (1902), were alternatives to cities. In the United States, the City Beautiful movement, epitomized by Daniel Burnham's Chicago and San Francisco plans, with their romanticized picturesque curvilinear lines, can be traced to this aesthetic.

Thus, the ideal of the planned city has been seen to move over two millennia from encampment to *étoile*, from geometric griddedness to picturesqueness, and now again will return to the enduring grid, for the most profoundly influential imposition in history of plan on a city is certainly the grid configuration on New York City. The grid of Manhattan, the consummate city, in conjunction with Central Park, created the city plan by which all other cities are judged. The configuration dictates the lives of millions who define their physical space by the plan: "uptown, downtown, east side, west side." The significance of urban planning is demonstrated every day on the streets of New York City, for the concrete canyons of Manhattan, so often romantically sung, are in fact more prosaically the product of New York City's 1811 grid city plan, its 1860s Olmsted park plan, and its 1916 skyscraper zoning laws.

Modern Urban Planning

In the 20th century, there was a tremendous shift in the historical concept of urban planning from art to technics. The practice of urban planning from the mid- to late 20th century had little to do with the artistic grandeur of earlier times and more to do with the technician's approach to the city as a functional entity. Massive urban population growth, the movement from rural to urban areas, two major world wars, the machine economy, the automobile, and the triumph of Marx over monarchy meant that the burden of urban planning became more about the amelioration of living conditions for the masses and less about a carriage ride through the park for those who could afford a carriage.

As urban planning took on the life of the masses, it acquired a new urgency. In the 20th century, theories of urban planning swung in wide and contradictory arcs—with very concrete consequences for cities. From the broad-stroke city plans of Le Corbusier to the curbside observations of Jane Jacobs, the city in the 20th century had seemingly every perceptive perspective and every evil visited on it. There actually exist American cities where one can trace the theoretical swings in urban planning simply by riding a bus across town, seeing the once bright future and the dashed hopes of urban occupants strewn in planned fervor on the landscape. In the East New York section of Brooklyn, where the federally funded Model Cities program collapsed before completion (but not before tearing down all existing buildings), the scarred urban land was left vacant for decades. Urban planning acquired a checkered history in the 20th century. Let us next investigate how this came to be in our times. If good intentions really did make paving, we could put an end to asphalt.

Early 20th-Century Planning

The early 20th century tended toward a utopianism in urban planning that we find bizarre today, exemplified in the metaphorical crystalline city depicted in Fritz Lang's film *Metropolis*. These early utopian planners survived one world war, lived in urban devastation, and were trying to create new cities from the depths of disillusionment with their European past. Certain of the early utopian modernists, such as Walter Gropius and the German Bauhaus designers, had humane aspirations underlying their metaphors, and they tried to bring analysis to tragedy. Empathizing with the proletariat, Gropius sought through planning to bring them the most basic necessities—in his words, "Existenzminimum," or minimum standards for living. He brought to his compassionate stance for the disenfranchised a new scientific standard, attempting for the first time to quantify quality-of-life issues: minimal space requirements, standards of health and hygiene, and light and fresh air in the city.

With their methodological approach, the planners of Germany reconstructed their war-ravaged cities and built some of the largest housing projects for the urban masses ever attempted, the *Siedlungen*, or housing projects, of the 1920s to 1930s. Although perhaps oppressive and mechanistic by today's values, these repetitive plans were humanely intentioned. The modern European ideals of urban planning became international through the meetings of CIAM (Congrès Internationaux d'Architecture Moderne), held in Europe from the 1920s to the 1950s, and were disseminated by J. L. Sert in his prophetically titled *Can Our Cities Survive?* (1942).

The most powerful, although perhaps not the most prudent, voice of CIAM and of 20th-century urbanism in general was, of course, Le Corbusier. Following in the French tradition of Haussmann, through his sweeping unbuilt Parisian plans on paper—the Contemporary City (1922) and the Ville Radieuse (1935)—Le Corbusier reinvented French creative urban design. Although his urban designs were brilliant aesthetic exercises, they were frightening living environments. Le Corbusier's plans are grandiose and potentially destructive of cities that, unlike the German, were not even destroyed by war. Le Corbusier introduced into modern urban planning the fallacy of viewing the city solely as a spatial pattern seen metaphorically and visually from above, forgetting that below, humans seek to live out their sometimes irrational, unpatterned urban lives.

If one were to compare the long-term influence on urban planning of Gropius's Bauhaus functionalism and Le Corbusier's French aestheticism, one might conclude that the derivations of both were harmful to the urban fabric of the 20th century. What differentiates them, however, is intention: the city for the common man or the city for self? While in the history of urban planning we can trace Gropius's methodical study of the angle of the sun as it hit the windows of his *Siedlungen*, we are likewise told the anecdote of Le Corbusier's designing the city of Brasília while sitting in a restaurant, cavalierly scrawling crossed lines on a cocktail napkin. Although there is ample room for ego and self-aggrandizement in architecture, it should have no place in the discipline of urban planning.

Against the European background of the planning debates of CIAM came the work of the most famous American architect of the 20th century, Frank Lloyd Wright, who designed but never built his theoretical Broadacre City in 1938. The "Broadacre" of the title was accurate, for the design allowed each resident one acre of land for subsistence farming, but the word "City" was certainly a misnomer, for Wright's utopia was the very antithesis of the concept of city. It was antiurban in every sense, isolationist in its vision, and totally automobile dependent, so much so that we may credit Broadacre City with spreading the concept of the suburb and inadvertently its concomitant sprawl all over the United States. Wright's vision, born of his agrarian American roots and of the Depression, was not to ameliorate urban problems but to offer an American alternative that would render the city a nasty anachronism of the preautomobile age.

Critiques of Urban Planning

Without question, by the early 20th century, cities in Europe and the United States needed fixing. By necessity, the rise of urban planning as a profession distinct from architecture, economics, and urban sociology was taking root with such major constituents as the New York Regional Planning Association. After utopianism took its last gasp through the planners of the 1939 New York World's Fair, cynicism about cities replaced beliefs in beauty and human aspiration in urban planning. As planning moved away from beauty and toward technology as its goal, it lost its soul. A nadir of urban planning was reached in the mid-20th century with the advent of statistical and technological planning severed from all humanitarian concerns, as Cold War thinking marked city plans destructively with the introduction of military-industrial planning applied to city planning. Cities lost their individual realities as new planners were schooled only in applications of generic models without human content and taught to substitute mindless formulas invented for the design of complex nuclear war machines. Cities, however, are not submarines, and humans are not mathematical models. With the desperation of those who felt inferior to the technologists, urban planners repressed their innate social motivations. Disastrous results, such as the wholesale destruction of neighborhoods as "slum clearance," were often compounded by high-speed freeways cutting through neighborhoods. Worst-case examples left acres of urban land looking bombed.

By the mid-20th century, thoughtful critical voices were emerging as a counterpoint to the grandiose schemes of the utopian 1920s and 1930s and the cynical 1950s and 1960s. Primary among those voices were those of two American planners and their texts of simple messages, Kevin Lynch's *The Image of the City* (1960) and Jane Jacobs's *The Death and Life of Great American Cities* (1961), which together helped turn the tide of city planning toward a closer examination of the existing urban fabric and to the patterns of behavior of its inhabitants. Both had a kind of folksy style that appealed to urban planners, architects, sociologists, and even the general public, so often the enemy of urban planning, and thus both books have continued to be influential for decades.

Lynch was observational and insightful. On the one hand, he explained the nature of cities with a rational model, defining the city as a hierarchy of spaces; on the other hand, he simultaneously presented the irrational side of urban patterns based on humans' uncanny ability to navigate urban space in relation to memory and landmarks. What makes Lynch's approach so novel is that it was based not on a preconceived or imposed model but on actually asking city dwellers how they moved within their physical environment. Jacobs, who wrote literally from the perspective of her own window on her street in lower Manhattan, showed that the social interactions of an active pedestrian street life of a city are the essence of the urban place. She defended the life not only of city people but of city buildings as well, pointing out cogently the significance of retaining old buildings within cities. *The Death and Life of Great American Cities* remains a memorable David-versus-Goliath of wrongheaded urban planning.

Perhaps the quietly successful revolution of Lynch, Jacobs, and others of this bent now needs reexamination, for it is spurring on movements in urban planning that are actually antiurban. Jacobs wanted to preserve old buildings not as historical artifacts or self-consciously arty edifices but as low-rent generators of urban innovation. Instead, we are today boutiqueing our cities out of existence, falsifying the urban fabric. Further, nostalgic but inauthentic new towns spring forth on former desert- and farmland all over the United States, and these false places are controlled by restrictive covenants that are the antithesis of urban life. Beware planners bearing faux cities that, although certainly pretty, by definition cannot ever be real urban environments.

The Future of Urban Planning

The point of urban planning is to encompass the complexity of human experience and to formulate for that experience a physical environment that will be ever self-renewing. Authentic urban places existed in the 20th century, and they give us hope for the life of the city in the 21st century. In London, a supreme example of urbane living is still found in Bloomsbury's squares of parks and row houses and in the 20th-century revival of 17th-century Covent Garden. In Paris, a zenith of 20th-century urban design was achieved by the physical reorganization of the museums, from the Louvre to the Gare d'Orsay along the Seine, relating beauty, urban form, antiquity, and modernism, in the image of I.M. Pei's metaphorical pyramid. In Chicago, the last decade of the 20th century witnessed the expansion of urban beauty, fulfilling again the visions presented to the world in the first decade of the century by Daniel Burnham and Edward H. Ben-

nett in their *Plan of Chicago*. Parkways, boulevards, urban parks, and well-ordered streets display Chicago's vision as a city in a garden. In New York, urban planning has created the scaffolding on which city life thrives. To find urban planning for oneself, experientially, explore the planned places of Manhattan. Walk any day, any season, from Rockefeller Center up Fifth Avenue toward Central Park. Observe the living urban tableau of sleek skyscrapers, hot dog stands, hasty inhabitants, and yellow taxis in counterpoint to the park's oasis of rocks, trees, and sky. Certainly this is as close to the complete human experience of the active and the contemplative, of order amid chaos, of the power of urban planning, as any city experience is ever likely to come.

LESLIE HUMM CORMIER

Further Reading

Jacobs, Jane, *The Death and Life of Great American Cities*, New York: Random House, 1961; London: Jonathan Cape, 1962

Kostof, Spiro, *The City Shaped: Urban Patterns and Meaning through History*, Boston: Little Brown, and London: Thames and Hudson, 1991

Le Corbusier, *Urbanisme*, Paris: Crès, 1924; as *The City of To-morrow and Its Planning*, translated by Frederick Etchells, New York: Payson and Clarke, 1929; reprint, New York: Dover, 1987

Lynch, Kevin, *The Image of the City*, Cambridge, Massachusetts: MIT Press, 1960

Sert, José Luis, *Can Our Cities Survive? An ABC of Urban Problems, Their Analyses, Their Solutions, Based on the Proposals Formulated by the CIAM*, Cambridge, Massachusetts: Harvard University Press, and London: Milford and Oxford University Press, 1942

Wright, Frank Lloyd, *An Autobiography*, book 6, "Broadacre City," Spring Green, Wisconsin: Taliesin, 1943

URBAN RENEWAL

Urban renewal defies simple and brief definition and explanation. Historically, constitutive elements of urban renewal have included planning, zoning, the City Beautiful movement, the modernist ideals of the Congrès Internationaux d'Architecture Moderne (CIAM) and others, the development of public housing, slum clearance, segregation in all of its varieties, the rise of gentrification, the effects of suburbanization on cities, the rise of highways (particularly in the United States), and more recently the construction of festival marketplaces and theories of "new" urbanism. Although renewal has taken on different forms in different locations, it has been mainly a top-down hierarchical process, one that is often criticized by the very communities that it was intended to improve. The central impulse behind urban renewal, and certainly the publicly stated purpose behind all such efforts, is to make a place (a neighborhood or a whole city) better than it was before. It is the method or approach taken to such improvement that lies behind most conflicts over urban renewal.

In the early 20th century, urban renewal was often inspired by an earnest desire to help the poor by improving the conditions in which they labored and lived. A desire to help, however, was also commingled with a variety of widely held beliefs about the relationship between the moral character of a neighborhood's residents and its physical condition. Usually labeled "common sense," these assumptions about the recursive relationship between bad neighborhoods and bad residents (i.e., the poor, recent immigrants, and minorities) were often reinforced by early sociological works attempting to explain the social origins of crime, juvenile delinquency, prostitution, and so on. In the United States, furthermore, the city of the early 20th century was the product of prejudices particular to the late 19th century. With the rise of immigration and urbanization, as Peter Hall notes, "many civic-minded bourgeoisie, faced with increasing ethnic and cultural heterogeneity" and a perceived threat of escalating social disorder, saw as their task "the very preservation of the urban social fabric" (1996).

An American solution to this dilemma—one that had its antecedents in Haussmann's reorganization of Paris under Napoleon III—was the City Beautiful movement, the principles of which are expressed vividly in Daniel Burnham and Edward H. Bennett's Chicago Plan of 1909. Their plan sought to restore a lost (in the eyes of the city's elite) harmonious social order by establishing a dominant neobaroque and Beaux-Arts aesthetic that would dominate not only the design of individual buildings but also the layout of the city as a whole. This City Beautiful design conspicuously embraced hierarchies of race and class, subordinating the pressing need for housing, schools, and sanitation, and instead imagined a future for Chicago in which immigrant machine politics had been expelled and proper Anglo-Saxon order restored. The City Beautiful movement spread both throughout Europe and, under the British raj, to New Delhi, India, with a plan designed by Edwin Lutyens and Herbert Baker.

In his groundbreaking text *The City* (1925), Robert Park stated, "In the great city the poor, the vicious, and the delinquent, crushed in an unhealthful and contagious intimacy, breed in and in, soul and body." Park's assessment, with its treatment of crime and poverty as the result largely of individual pathologies rather than structural inequalities and racism, provided an academic justification for the continued restriction of certain groups to the less-favorable sections of the city. If they ("the poor, the vicious") hoped to move up and out of the slums, they would have to undertake a process of self-improvement, of moral elevation. To eradicate the slums, in such a formulation, required the eradication of the individual traits that produced and sustained slums. Park's analysis, although significantly more nuanced than the mainstream interpretation, still served to justify approaches to urban renewal that treated urban decline as the fault of the disadvantaged, as the result of faulty morals and decaying family structures. It was a view that would remain in circulation (particularly in the United States) for decades.

Following World War II, urban renewal occurred on a global scale as nations began rebuilding after the devastation that the war produced. For some nations, rebuilding in the late 1940s meant repairing not only war damage but also the structural decline that had taken effect during the years of widespread economic depression that preceded the war. In addition, in what was then West Germany, urban renewal also required the development of a new, identifiably democratic building style that would break from the traditions of architecture and urban design established by the Nazi regime (similar efforts on different scales and to different ends were also undertaken in Italy, East Germany, and Japan).

In the United States, the decades following World War II were years when the economic might of the government was

channeled largely into the development of the interstate highway system and efforts to increase the number of Americans who owned their own homes. Both efforts precipitated decades of urban decline. Highways, when they passed into or through a city, invariably did so by smashing through poor and minority neighborhoods. The U.S. Federal Housing Administration (FHA), responsible for insuring the mortgages that allowed middle- and lower-income families to purchase homes, instituted regulations that discriminated against neighborhoods whose residents were poor and/or nonwhite. The FHA rules, prejudiced against heterogeneous neighborhoods and wary of "inharmonious racial or nationality groups" (Jackson, 1985), served to encourage the rapid decline of urban centers by encouraging the flight of capital and the middle class to the suburbs.

In an attempt to counter the decay fostered by such "white flight" and renovate the aging housing stock of cities such as Chicago, New York, and St. Louis, the U.S. government embarked on a campaign to spur urban renewal through the construction of public housing. The limited success and (in some opinions) monumental failure of this effort are encapsulated best by Jane Jacobs's broadside *The Death and Life of Great American Cities* (1961) and writer James Baldwin's assessment that urban renewal constituted in fact "Negro removal." Entire neighborhoods were razed, and massive housing block developments, usually in some derivative form of the International Style, were built (as cheaply as possible) in the poorer neighborhoods of cities across the United States.

By the late 1960s, the United States experienced several waves of urban uprisings. Discontent was centered around racial and economic inequality, conditions that many felt were symptomatic of modernist urban renewal and housing projects. At around the same time, the U.S. government was channeling public funds in ever greater amounts to the war in Vietnam, diverting public money away from the domestic War on Poverty (the broad collection of government programs responsible for many urban-renewal projects) instigated by President Lyndon Johnson. By the late 1970s and early 1980s, the speculative real estate market was taking an increasingly active role in reshaping impoverished neighborhoods. Gentrification, particularly in the United States, has replaced the government as the primary "renovator" of "blighted" neighborhoods. Gentrification is a process that takes advantage of liberal public policy and capital's endless reproductive drive and is, at the dawn of the 21st century, manifested on a global scale, "having emerged widely in the cities of Canada, Australia, New Zealand, and Europe, and more sporadically in Japan, South Africa, and Brazil" (Smith, 1996).

BENJY FLOWERS

Further Reading

Finney, Graham S., "The Architect's Role," *Perspecta*, 29 (1998)

Frieden, Bernard J., and Lynne B. Sagalyn, *Downtown, Inc.: How America Rebuilds Cities*, Cambridge, Massachusetts: MIT Press, 1989

Hall, Peter, *Cities of Tomorrow: An Intellectual History of Urban Planning and Design in the Twentieth Century*, Oxford and New York: Blackwell, 1988; revised edition, 1996

Jackson, Kenneth T., *Crabgrass Frontier: The Suburbanization of the United States*, New York: Oxford University Press, 1985

Jacobs, Jane, *The Death and Life of Great American Cities*, New York: Random House, 1961; London: Jonathan Cape, 1962

Park, Robert, et al., *The City*, Chicago: University of Chicago Press, 1925; reprint, 1984

"Rethinking Regeneration," *World Architecture*, 58 (1997)

Smith, Neil, *The New Urban Frontier: Gentrification and the Revanchist City*, London and New York: Routledge, 1996

Tyrwitt, Jacqueline, José Luis Sert, and Ernesto N. Rogers (editors), *The Heart of the City: Towards the Humanisation of Urban Life*, London: Humphries, and New York: Pellegrini and Cudahy, 1952

UTOPIAN PLANNING

Thomas More's book *Utopia* of 1517 named and inspired a genre of publications concerned with future projections of ideal societies. The term "utopia," in its basic meaning "no place," describes political, economic, and sociocultural structures of a society. One essential part of the utopia concerns the relation between social forms and urban planning. Therefore, the utopia as a literary expression challenged artists, architects, and urban planners to visualize the ambience of ideal communities.

More implicitly "utopia" referred to an increasing interest in designing ideal cities in the 15th and 16th centuries. Based on the Aristotelian idea of architecture and urban planning as practical philosophy or on strict Platonic models of ideal societies in regular geometric city forms, thinkers such as Tommaso Campanella (*Civitas solis*, 1602) and Francis Bacon (*Nova Atlantis*, 1638) developed the philosophical idea of a better society with architectural and urban concepts. Liberated from any reference to existing political pressures, utopias served as imaginative spaces with experimental values for future development. As political imagination allows radical concepts, the utopia as a reflexive and imaginative medium turned out to be very attractive for architects and urban planners all through history.

In the 20th century, utopian thinking and designing constituted one of the most influential sources for cultural development. Economic changes such as the industrialization or political changes caused by two world wars provided, *ex negativo*, utopian planning with a rich material. Already in 1890, when William Morris published his *News from Nowhere*, the consequences of early capitalism challenged alternative models, that is, utopian visions of humane and ecological living conditions in preindustrial town settings. Opposite to that retrospective utopian thinking, artists and architects of the early 20th-century avant-garde, influenced by Nietzschean cultural philosophy and impressed by the first totally industrialized war in 1914, proposed radical visual concepts for the design of a future society, which in postwar times changed from monarchy to democracy (Germany) or communism (Russia).

With few exceptions, such as Camillo Sitte's famous urban manual, future-oriented urban and architectural proposals dominated utopian thinking during the first third of the century. Russian Constructivism (El Lissitzky), Dutch De Stijl (Theo van Doesburg), German Expressionism (Bruno Taut) and Bauhaus (Walter Gropius), or Italian futurism (Antonio Sant'Elia) required the total negation of cultural heritage to present new architectures for a new type of human race.

In perhaps no other architectural ideology does this condition for utopian design emerge more clearly than in the post–World War I writings and drawings of Le Corbusier. His radical pro-

posal for a City of Three Million Inhabitants, situated in a cultural no-man's-land with no traditional references, reveals all the problems of modern utopian planning in the 20th century: a total design of standardized architectural and urban pattern for standardized members of society, thus realizing More's description of total regularity of all cities on the island of Utopia.

The destruction of many European cities during World War II allowed avant-garde architects and planners to transfer utopian wonderlands of architecture into existing spaces. Large-scale projects, such as the urban-renewal programs in the United States, exemplify a kind of utopian planning applied to urban housing. Dense historical networks of urban structures were wiped out in favor of International Style architecture. Out of the cultural critique of totalitarian functionalism (Lewis Mumford, Jane Jacobs, and many others), the retrospective utopia again gained influence. However, the most striking reaction based on insufficient post–World War II planning was the exaggeration of functional and systematic topics of modern planning.

The megastructures in enormous dimensions proposed by architectural groups such as the Metabolists, Archigram, or Superstudio were presented as the ultimate solutions for an overcrowded, polluted, and culturally exhausted planet. More or less seriously elaborated, utopian megastructures at a global scale presented technological instruments as revolutionary sociocultural tools. However, even visions of space colonies (Fritz Haller with the Massachusetts Institute of Technology) could not hide the problems of one-dimensional utopian planning.

Challenged by the lack of complexity of many high-tech utopias, Postmodern ideologies, such as the end of history or the rehabilitation of vulgar commercial culture (Robert Venturi), determined utopian thinking in the 1970s and 1980s. Free exchanges of visual meanings, optical pollution by trademarks, and arbitrary style selections in architecture resulted in a capitalist utopia called Global City.

Revising the history of utopian planning now reveals a basic anthropological pattern: society wants to know and explore the future. Whereas negative utopias or frustrated illusions of modernity request difficult and complex reevalutions of the relations between political and aesthetic ideas, contemporary utopian thinking at the dawn of the 21st century reduces More's model to a mere discussion of surfaces. In this way it seems understandable how the politically encoded forms of Soviet Constructivism could be reduced to the banal and global frame of deconstructivism in the 1990s. Therefore, it might seem reasonable that current architectural and urban-planning theories hardly include political and sociocultural dimensions. Finally, reducing the complex imaginative space of utopia seems to be a consequence of many naive utopian intentions to translate political forms into architectural forms. Utopian planning is more reflection than application. Within this cultural context of the late 20th century, science fiction films and computer and Internet technology gained more importance as utopian media than architectural drawings. Film sets for *Blade Runner* or *The 5th Element* display a negative megapolitan utopia for the masses and thus revitalize utopian reflection.

Computer-aided design is located virtually in the "no place" and, if not reduced to a business superstructure, opens spaces of political imagination and aesthetic critique to a global utopian community.

PETER KRIEGER

See also **Archigram, Bauhaus; Contemporary City for Three Million Inhabitants; Corbusier, Le (Jeanneret, Charles-Édouard) (France); Doesburg, Theo van (Netherlands), Gropius, Walter (Germany); Jacobs, Jane (United States); Sant'Elia, Antonio (Italy); Taut, Bruno (Germany); Venturi, Robert (United States)**

Further Reading

It is recommended to consult any critical edition of More, Thomas, *Utopia* (first ed. 1516), as well as Campanella, Tommaso, *Civitas solis. Idea Reipublicae Philosophicae* (first ed. 1602), and Bacon, Francis, *Nova Atlantis. Fragmentorum alterum* (first ed. 1638). To study the prehistory of 20th-century utopian planning, the reader should consult the writings of Charles Fourier, Morris, William, *News from Nowhere* (first ed. 1890), and Nietzsche, Friedrich, *Vom Nutzen und Nachteil der Historie für das Leben* and *Also sprach Zarathustra*.

Benson, Timothy O. (editor), *Expressionist Utopias: Paradise, Los Angeles Metropolis, Architectural Fantasy*. Los Angeles: County Museum of Art, 1993

Calvino, Italo, *Le città invisibile*, Turin: Einaudi, 1972

Cassirer, Ernst, *An Essay on Man: An Introduction to the Philosophy of Human Culture*, New Haven, Connecticut: Yale University Press, 1944/1979

Horkheimer, Max, and Theodor W. Adorno, *Dialektik der Aufklärung. Philosophische Fragmente*. Amsterdam: Querido, 1947

Hulten, Pontus (editor), *Futurismo & Futurismi*, Milan: 1986

Johnson, Philip, and Mark Wigley, *Deconstructivist Architecture*, New York: Museum of Modern Art, 1988

Klotz, Heinrich (editor), *Vision der Moderne: das Prinzip Konstruktion*. Munich: Prestel, 1986

Koolhaas, Rem, "Singapore. Portait of a Potemkin Metropolis. Songlines . . . or Thirty Years of Tabula Rasa," in Rem Koolhaas, and Bruce Mau, *S, M, L, XL*. Rotterdam: 010 Publishers, 1995

Krieger, Peter, "Totale oder totalitäre Stadt—Fritz Hallers Stadt-Utopien," in *Thesis, Wissenschaftliche Zeitschrift der Bauhaus-Universität Weimar*, 3/4 (1997)

La Biennale di Venezia. 6th International Architecture Exhibition. Sensing the Future. The Architect as Seismograph. Venice and Milan: Electa, 1996

Le Corbusier, *The City of Tomorrow and Its Planning*, New York: Payson and Clarke, 1929

Lissitzky-Küppers, Sophie (editor), *El Lissitzky. Maler, Architekt, Typograph, Fotograf*. Frankfurt/Main, Vienna and Zurich: Büchergilde Gutenberg, 1980

Mannheim, Karl, *Ideology and Utopia*. London: Routledge and Kegan Paul, 1960

Pettena, Gianni (editor), *Radicals. Design and Architecture 1960/75*, Venice: Biennale di Architettura, 1996

Ragon, Michel, *Les Cités de l'avenir*. Barcelona: 1970

Whyte, Ian Bond, and Romana Schneider (editors), *Die gläserne Kette. Briefe von Bruno Taut und Hermann Finsterlin, Hans und Wassili Luckhardt, Wenzel August Hablik und Hans Scharoun, Otto Gröne, Hans Hansen, Paul Goesch und Alfred Brust*. Stuttgart: Hatje, 1996

UTZON, JØRN 1918–

Architect, Denmark

Jørn Utzon occupies a special position in 20th-century architecture that defies simple categorization. As a Dane, he invites com-

parison with German Expressionism, especially Hans Scharoun; his greatest works are in Australia, Kuwait, and Mallorca; and although he gave Gunnar Asplund, Alvar Aalto, and the Dane Kay Fisker as his mentors, his casual spontaneity, his daring, and the absence of a fastidious refinement go against the grain of Danish tradition in much the same way as Asger Jorn's paintings. His architecture is self-consciously sculptural in its appeal, making Utzon more Finnish and European than Danish. Instead of intensely focusing inward in the way that Arne Jacobsen did, Utzon relocated his vision outside Denmark, taking his models from within the modern Scandinavian tradition and from Le Corbusier; this was, at the same time, allied to a new interest in an anonymous vernacular building aesthetic.

His outstanding contribution was the application of an anonymous vernacular expression to repetitive industrial building production disciplined by geometry to create a more varied, flexible, romantic building form that responds to changing human requirements.

Jørn Utzon was born in Copenhagen in 1918 but spent his childhood at Ålborg, where his father, Aage Utzon, was engineering director of the local shipyard. He completed his schooling at the Ålborg Katedralskole in 1936 and was accepted at the Kunstakademiets Arkitektskole in Copenhagen, from which he graduated in 1942. While living in Stockholm, where he stayed for the remainder of the German occupation, he was awarded a minor Royal Academy Gold Medal (1944) for his design for a music academy in Copenhagen. In 1950, Utzon returned to Denmark and started in private practice.

At the Royal Academy, Utzon was exposed to Kay Fisker and to the historian and planner Steen Eiler Rasmussen, whose experiential theory of architecture in his small book *Experiencing Architecture*, published in 1959, Utzon seems subsequently to have adopted.

Utzon traveled extensively in the early years after the war, first a short stint in Alvar Aalto's Munkkiniemi office in 1946, followed by trips to Morocco in 1947 and to the United States and Mexico in 1949. These travel experiences helped solidify his maturing organic approach. From 1945 to 1957, he vigorously participated in many competitions that he combined with extensive travel, absorbing influences from Islamic, Chinese, and Mayan architecture.

He worked alone and with others, including such Danish contemporaries as Tobias Faber and Mogens Irming; however, the most important collaborator was the Norwegian modernist Arne Korsmo. Other influences were Gunnar Asplund (from his time in Sweden) and the organic architecture of Frank Lloyd Wright, Alvar Aalto, and Le Corbusier, whom he met in 1948.

Utzon adopted the additive composition principle of combining standard industrial components that could be augmented by adding extra elements, so that his buildings appear to grow in a manner that crudely mimics the replication of cellular organisms. Utzon was inspired in his architecture by natural phenomena, such as clouds, beech forests, and breaking waves, that he adopted in the early conceptual stage in developing his ideas.

A number of architectural ideas recur in Utzon, the courtyard house being one and the motif of the platform as a technique for relating group forms another. In 1953, with Ib Molegelvang, he won the Skaanske low-cost housing competition for "Scania" house types. His scheme was based on the ancient Chinese courtyard house, and although it was not built, Utzon went on to

design the Kingohusene Housing Estate (1960) near Helsingør and a more elaborate development (1963) at Fredensborg using the courtyard principle. Although these are less known than Sydney's Opera House, they are no less significant, and they demonstrate Utzon's humanitarian commitment to housing innovation. The timber-component house system known as "Espansiva" (1969) took this a step further and attempted to simplify and adapt housing to exploit simple industrial materials and methods. The same concern is apparent in his Utsep Mobler Flexible Furniture (1968) system, which also applied the same additive architecture principle.

Jørn Utzon's world fame rests largely on one work: the Sydney Opera House. Winning the international competition in 1957 thrust him overnight into the international architectural spotlight. Its completion in October 1973 made Sydney instantly recognizable and provided it with an architectural symbol that emphasized the importance of its harbor.

Utzon's Sydney Opera House scheme coincided with Le Corbusier's break with the 1920s cubist aesthetic for the Ronchamp chapel, Notre-Dame-du-Haut, completed in June 1955. Both emphasized the organic quality of their forms inspired by exceptional landscapes: the small plateau and acropolis at Ronchamp and a low-lying sandstone peninsula jutting out into and surrounded on three sides by the harbor in Sydney.

A number of factors help explain the Sydney Opera House's unprecedented originality and use of shell-concrete roofs. The 1930s in Copenhagen witnessed the early development of shell concrete for the Kastrup Airport Terminal (1939) and the Radiohus Building (1946) by Vilhelm Lauritzen. In 1946, Utzon collaborated on a submission in the Crystal Palace International Competition that introduced the identical theme of concert halls with sculptural shell roofs mounted on a common platform.

Although the accusation was justified that progress on the Sydney Opera House was unacceptably slow, it is unlikely that this fact would have provoked the extreme reaction in Europe that it did in Sydney in 1966. The intransigence of Utzon's new political master convinced him that he was no longer trusted, and this caused his withdrawal from the project. At the time this happened, Utzon had overcome the last remaining problems of acoustics and construction in the interiors and was in a position to complete the work in a reasonable time and cost. The client, Davis Hughes, and party politics prevented him from doing so.

The interiors and glass walls enclosing the open ends of the concrete vault roofs, completed by his replacement, Hall Todd and Littlemore, are neither as original nor as daring as Utzon's. The Opera House function was emasculated by relegating opera to the smaller hall, which could no longer function as a drama theater. Acoustic problems have dogged the concert hall and will be expensive, if impossible, to remedy. Despite these shortcomings, the outside is clear proof of Utzon's sculptural genius. It stands as a monument to the human imagination, shared by an entire city, on an extraordinarily sensitive site on the edge of the city where it thrusts into the harbor. Not surprisingly, it has since become the foremost symbol of Sydney around the world.

Of his later works the Bagsvaerd Church (1976) in Copenhagen and the Kuwait National Assembly Building (1983), Kuwait City, Kuwait, provide further evidence of his determination to seek a new anonymous industrial aesthetic using standardized

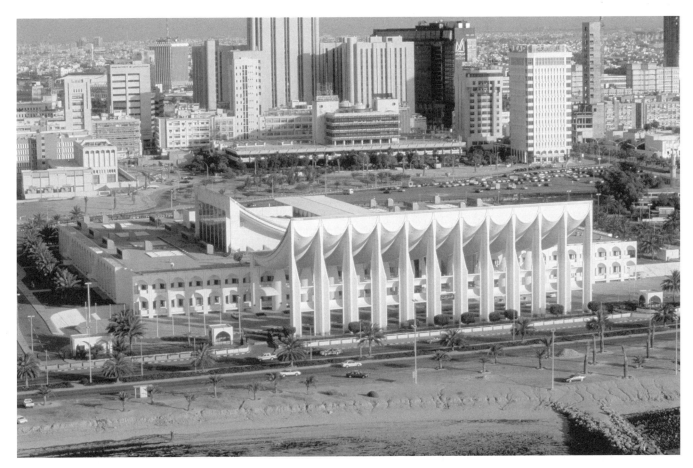

National Assembly Building (1983), Kuwait City, Kuwait
© Yann Arthus-Bertrand/CORBIS

industrial processes that can be varied to match each requirement and that are sensitive to the landscape.

The State Theater complex for Zurich embodied the same lessons of geometry and standardization that Utzon learned in Sydney and that were transferred to Kuwait and, to a lesser extent, to Bagsvaerd Church. At Kuwait, Utzon introduced simply draped concrete sheets similar to Eero Saarinen's Dulles Airport Terminal (1963) but gave them additional sculptural complexity by folding them laterally so that they echo the folds of the Bedouin black tent. The National Assembly Building is an elaborate mix of standard precast-concrete units that Utzon contrasted with his hanging tent roofs looking out across the Persian Gulf and backed by the desert.

The Bagsvaerd Church incorporates a freely unfolding shell of sprayed concrete that is used to support the outer metal roof and that admits a soft, muted, indirect light into the nave. Inspired in part by medieval stave churches, stacked standard precast elements are used for the double-wall frame. Its linear rectangular plan is of great simplicity and elegance. Outside, it looks more like a factory than a church.

One of Utzon's most satisfying small works is "Can Lis" (1973), his cliff house near Santyani on Mallorca. Its expression is firmly rooted in the Mallorcan vernacular but incorporates deep window embrasures that are reminiscent of the south wall of Le Corbusier's Ronchamp chapel to frame the sea vistas. It was conceived as a miniature village of four pavilions jostling one another at various odd angles that add interest to the whole and form mysterious spaces between.

Shy and charming by turns and not unlike the movie actress Greta Garbo, whom he resembles, Utzon adopted the life of a recluse after 1970. Since the 1980s, Utzon has been less active in architecture, his professional involvement being mostly indirect in a series of collaborations with his two architect sons, Jan and Kim Utzon, on unsuccessful large-scale commercial projects to rejuvenate the Copenhagen waterfront, a project for a Danish Museum of Modern Art (1988) in Fredensborg and museums at Bornholm (1988), Skagen, and Samsø Island (1995–), the latter yet to be realized.

PHILIP DREW

Biography

Born in Copenhagen, Denmark, 9 April 1918. Studied under Steen Eiler Rasmussen and Kay Fisker at the Royal Academy of Arts, Copenhagen, 1937–42; degree in architecture 1942; trav-

eled and studied in Europe and North Africa 1947–48 and the United States and Mexico 1949. Assistant architect in the offices of Paul Hedquist and Gunnar Asplund, Stockholm, Sweden 1942–45; assistant architect in the office of Alvar Aalto, Helsinki 1946. In private practice, Copenhagen 1950–52, Sydney 1962–66, United States, Switzerland, and Denmark since 1966; developed a building system, "Espansiva," based on laminated wood sections 1969. Visiting professor, University of Hawaii, Honolulu 1971–75. Honorary fellow, Royal Australian Institute of Architects 1965; honorary fellow, American Institute of Architects 1970. Gold Medal, Royal Institute of British Architects 1978.

Selected Works

Low-Cost Housing (First prize, competition; with Ib Molegelvang), Skaanske, Denmark, 1953
House, Holte, Denmark, 1953
House, near Lake Furesö, Denmark, 1953
Melli Bank, Tehran, 1959
Kingohusene Housing Estate, near Helsingør, Denmark, 1960
Danish Co-operative Building Company Housing Development, Fredensborg, Denmark, 1963
Municipal Theater (First prize, competition), Zurich, 1964
Opera House (First prize, 1957 competition), Sydney, 1966; completed by others, 1973
Utsep Mobler Flexible Furniture (project), 1968
Espansiva Byg A/S Timber, component house system (project), 1969
Jørn Utzon House ("Can Lis"), Porto Petro, Mallorca, 1973
Bagsvaerd Church, Copenhagen, 1976
Kuwait National Assembly Building (First prize, 1973 competition), 1983
Museum of Modern Art (project), Fredensborg, 1988

Selected Publications

Sydney Opera House, 1962
Church at Bagsvaerd, 1981
Tre Generationer, 1988
Jørn Utzon, Houses in Fredensborg, 1991

Further Reading

Utzon's resistance to scholarly research and documentation and his reticence to cooperate with critical assessment has created severe problems for the serious historian, with the unfortunate consequence that there is a proliferation of errors resulting from an overreliance on secondary source material. There has been far more publication and interpretation than research into establishing reliable facts. The Fromonot account, for instance, is largely a compilation of material copied from *Zodiac* numbers 5, 10, and 14, with additions. Because these issues are rare, their republication in this way is undoubtedly useful. Utzon scholarship remains at an early stage.

"Can Lis," *Living Architecture*, 8 (1990)
Drew, Philip, *Third Generation: The Changing Meaning of Architecture*, London: Pall Mall Press, and New York: Praeger, 1972
Drew, Philip, *Sydney Opera House*, London: Phaidon Press, 1995
Drew, Philip, *The Masterpiece: Jørn Utzon, a Secret Life*, South Yarra, Victoria: Hardie Grant Books, 1999
Faber, Tobias, *Jørn Utzon: Houses in Fredensborg*, Berlin: Ernst, 1991
Frampton, Kenneth, "Jørn Utzon: Transcultural Form and the Tectonic Metaphor" in *Studies in Tectonic Culture: The Poetics of Construction in Nineteenth and Twentieth Century Architecture*, Cambridge, Massachusetts: MIT Press, 1995; London: MIT Press, 1996
Fromonot, Françoise, *Jørn Utzon et l'Opéra de Sydney*, Paris: Gallimard, 1998; as *Jørn Utzon: The Sydney Opera House*, Corte Madera, California: Gingko, and Milan: Electa, 1998
Giedion, Sigfried, "Jørn Utzon and the Third Generation" in *Space, Time, and Architecture*, by Giedion, Cambridge, Massachusetts: Harvard University Press, and London: Oxford University Press, 1942; 5th revised and enlarged edition, Cambridge, Massachusetts: Harvard University Press, 1967
"House, Kara Crescent, Bayview," *Content*, 1 (1995)
"Jørn Utzon: A New Personality," *Zodiac*, 5 (1959)
"Jørn Utzons Hus på Mallorca," *Arkitektur DK*, 2 (1996)
"The National Assembly Building, Kuwait," *Living Architecture*, 5 (1986)
"Platforms and Plateaux: Ideas of a Danish Architect," *Zodiac*, 10 (1962)
Sten-Møller, H., "The Light of Heaven, a Church by Jørn Utzon," *Living Architecture*, 1 (1983)
"The Sydney Opera House," *Zodiac*, 14 (1965)
Utzon, Jørn, "Additiv Arkitektur," *Arkitektur*, 1 (1970)

V

VANCOUVER, BRITISH COLUMBIA, CANADA

The city of Vancouver is truly of the 20th century. When the small town of Granville was incorporated as the city of Vancouver in 1886, it had more in common with American cities west of the Rocky Mountains than with the rest of Canada. San Francisco had served as Vancouver's main link to the east before the completion of Canada's transcontinental railway in 1887. Within five years the community of 1000 had grown to nearly 14,000 and the young city became a supply depot and investment center for the Klondike gold rush of 1897–98. From these boomtown beginnings, metropolitan Vancouver is now home to more than 1.8 million people.

During the early 20th century, rapid growth fueled construction of neighborhoods along the street railway and interurban lines. Before 1910 many homes were constructed of a prefabricated, insulated, four-foot modular system, designed and manufactured by the B.C. Mills, Timber, and Trading Company. Known as Vancouver Boxes, these efficient and economical houses were characterized by a single story set on a high foundation, a hip roof with dormer windows, and a broad front veranda. From 1910 until the mid-1920s, the most popular house for middle- and lower-class families was a variant of the California bungalow, typified by front gables, exposed rafter ends, and wall brackets, and often chimneys, porch piers, and foundations of rough brick or stone. These Craftsman homes, a small-scale version of the Queen Anne style, were popular amongst the suburban working classes. At one point South Vancouver was expanding at a rate of 200 families per month, all housed in California bungalows.

In contrast the region's affluent families required large formal estates for entertaining. British expatriates had a fondness for Tudor revivals, English country manors, or Arts and Crafts-style homes. In Point Grey and Shaughnessy Heights, abundantly timbered properties were developed according to the tenets of the City Beautiful movement, creating elegant neighborhoods of parks and scenic drives. In both Victoria (the provincial capital) and Vancouver, one of the most sought-after architects of this era was Samuel Maclure, whose early bungalows were modest versions of the California style—single-storied, wood-framed buildings with cross-axial plans and wood-shingle cladding. Influenced by the art and architecture of Charles F.A. Voysey and Frank Lloyd Wright, Maclure often used Tudor-revival facades to mollify his clients while creating modern designs that maximized the potential of the site and locally available materials.

Thriving business concerns led to the importation of New York and Chicago skyscraper technologies. In 1908 David Spencer and Company built a nine-story department store that was followed by the 13-story Dominion Trust Building in 1910, touted as the most modern and tallest office building in Canada. Originally designed for the Imperial Trust Company by the English-trained architect J.S. Helyer and his son Maurice, the Dominion Trust Building had a brick exterior with yellow terra-cotta features emulating the detailing of classical orders and was capped by a lofty Second Empire–style roof. Others followed, including the W.T. Whiteway's World Building (1912), now known as the Old Sun Tower, whose 17-story corner hexagonal office tower eclipsed the Dominion Trust Building; Parr and Fee's Vancouver Block (1912), with its conspicuous clock atop a central tower; and the Weart Building (1913) by Russell, Babcock and Rice, now known as the Standard Building. The Crédit Foncier Franco-Canadien (1914) by H.L. Stevens and Company offers the most faithful emulation of neoclassical detailing.

In 1914 architect Francis Swales was commissioned to design the Hotel Vancouver to accommodate business travelers and tourists who used the Canadian Pacific Railway. This impressive assembly of cubic forms with intricate Italianate detailing and overhanging roofs dominated the Vancouver skyline until its controversial demolition in 1949. To serve the competing Canadian National Railway, another Hotel Vancouver was built in the Château style by Archibald and Schofield. Although construction had begun in 1929, it was abandoned during the Great Depression, and the hotel was only completed in time for the 1939 Royal Tour. This building's facade was an elegant expression of the restrained modern classicism in vogue at the time. Another example was the new Vancouver City Hall (1936), constructed near recently annexed South Vancouver. The architects, Townley and Matheson, adhered to the modern classical precedents established by other government architecture of the time by stepping down a series of symmetrically arranged cubic forms on opposing sides of a large central tower.

After World War I, Vancouver's thriving port facilities had fostered development of the waterfront and the commercial heart of the city, even during the Depression. The most noteworthy building of this period was J.Y. McCarter and George C. Nairne's Marine Building (1930). Both the 20-story tower and a 10-story wing have richly decorated parapets, executed in pink and green terra-cotta, which contrast with the pale-red brick walls. The striking Art Deco ornamentation incorporates terra-cotta panels illustrating histories of transportation and the Pacific coast.

Economic restraints during World War II limited construction to essential projects. Afterward, however, Vancouver thrived, as veterans returned to the city and foreign demand for Canada's natural resources escalated. The immigration of British-trained architects and the influence of Walter Gropius, Richard Neutra, and Marcel Breuer encouraged the development of modernist building. In 1946 a department of architecture was established at the University of British Columbia under Frederick Lasserre that began to attract international attention. Efforts of early modernists, such as C.B.K. Van Norman, Robert A.D. Berwick, Bertram C. Binning, and Peter Thornton, were quickly overtaken by younger designers like Charles E. Pratt, Ron Thom, and Fred Hollingsworth, who used new lumber products and prefabricated building systems to create a distinctive West Coast style. With an intricate arrangement of flat-roofed terraces stepping down the West Bay hillside, C.E. Pratt demonstrated the West Coast style in a house designed for lumber company executive William S. Brooks (1947). Wood, steel, stone, and large expanses of glass were presented in a manner that highlighted the interrelationship between the building's interior and its natural surroundings.

In commercial building Semmens and Simpson's design for the Vancouver offices of Marwell Construction (1950) won the inaugural round of the national Massey Medal awards in 1952. Components of this scrupulously functional design transcended the normal barriers between exterior and interior. The first Vancouver high-rise constructed since the Depression era was the Burrard Building (1956) by C.K.B. Van Norman and Associates, which used a space-saving curtain wall facade.

The 1963 competition for a new university in the adjacent city of Burnaby relieved the slow pace of local construction. The successful entry by the Vancouver partnership of Arthur Erickson and Geoffrey Massey proved to be the springboard for Arthur Erickson's international career. His scheme for Simon Fraser University revolved around a strong central axis linking all campus buildings and incorporating contemporary approaches to pedagogy. In addition to the campus plan, Erickson and Massey designed the Transportation Centre (1965) and Central Mall (1965), in which massive girders of douglas fir and steel supported a glass canopy. The campus has continued to expand; Erickson also designed a university extension to the West Mall (1994) that remains faithful to the form and materials of the original campus.

The phenomenal growth of Vancouver forced developers to build vertically. High-rise residential buildings, including Rix Reinecke's Ocean Towers (1958), began to dominate the West End skyline following a permissive 1956 zoning amendment. The consequences of the rampant demolition of the 1960s and 1970s were not fully appreciated until much of the city's architectural fabric had been decimated. An emerging heritage conservation movement encouraged reuse and adaptation, one prominent example being the Sylvia Hotel addition, designed by Henriquez Partners. Noted for being the tallest building in the West End until 1958, the Sylvia Court Apartments (1912), designed by W.P. White and converted to a hotel during the 1930s, received heritage designation in 1975. This staid brick, stone, and terra-cotta structure was expanded by Richard Henriquez's tower in 1987.

Economic recession in the 1970s and 1980s proved to be a transitional stage between modernism and regionalism. Just before this construction hiatus, the firm of Rhone and Iredale was awarded the commission for Crown Life Place (1978). Their principal designer, Peter Cardew, created a dramatic V-shaped office tower in the late modern idiom, using green-tinted glass curtain walls. The 1986 Vancouver Centennial and World Exposition spurred development of Granville Island Public Market and transformation of the False Creek industrial area into a livable community. Canada Place (1986) by Zeidler Roberts Partnership hosts public events and welcomes cruise ships. Its multipurpose design incorporates a docking terminal, the Pan-Pacific Hotel, and a row of large display halls, distinctively covered in white sail-shaped fabric.

In the 1990s competing architectural styles dominated, including Paul Merrick's Postmodern Cathedral Place (1991), a controversial complex that replaced McCarter and Nairne's much admired Georgia Medical Dental Building (1929); Moshe Safdie's Vancouver Library Square (1995); and the Chan Centre for the Performing Arts (1997), designed by Bing Thom Architects.

RHODA BELLAMY

See also **Canada; Safdie, Moshe (Canada, Israel)**

Further Reading

Coupland, Douglas, *City of Glass: Douglas Coupland's Vancouver*, Vancouver: Douglas and McIntyre, 2000
Delaney, P. (editor), *Vancouver Representing the Postmodern City*, Vancouver: Arsenal Pulp Press, 1994
Kalman, Harold, Ron Phillips, and Robin Ward, *Exploring Vancouver: The Essential Architectural Guide*, Vancouver: University of British Columbia Press and The Architectural Institute of British Columbia, 1993
Kluckner, Michael, *Vanishing Vancouver*, North Vancouver: Whitecap Books, 1990
Liscombe, Rhodri Windsor (editor), *The New Spirit: Modern Architecture in Vancouver, 1938–1963*, Montreal and Vancouver: Douglas and McIntyre, in association with the Centre Canadien d'Architecture/Canadian Centre for Architecture, 1997
Luxton, Donald, "The Rise and Fall of West Coast Modernism in Greater Vancouver, British Columbia," *APT Bulletin*, 31 (2000)
Macdonald, Bruce, *Vancouver: A Visual History*, Vancouver: Talonbooks, 1992
Roy, Patricia E., *Vancouver: An Illustrated History*, Toronto: James Lorimer, and National Museums of Canada, 1980
Wynn, Graeme, and Timothy Oke (editors), *Vancouver and Its Region*, Vancouver: University of British Columbia Press, 1992

VAN DOESBURG, THEO 1883–1931

Architecture historian, critic, theorist, Netherlands

As founder and polemicist for the Dutch avant-garde group De Stijl, Theo van Doesburg systematically propagated his ideas of

the visual arts, architecture, design, and theory in many forms and forums. Van Doesburg was a critic, poet, novelist, performance artist, teacher, publisher, typographer, and art historian. Instrumental in the development of modern architecture, he was committed to the idea of universal synthesis. Although well known in his lifetime through associations with many international art and architectural groups, he was ultimately unsuccessful in achieving the integration of art and life through the doctrine of Neoplasticism (New Forming). Nonetheless, he was innovative in his ideas that connected art and architecture with cultural and political issues through literature, urbanism, exhibitions, performance, education, and criticism.

Immediately after his service in the Dutch army during World War I, he formed the De Stijl group with the poet Antony Kok, the painters Piet Mondrian and Bart van der Leck, the Hungarian painter and designer Vilmos Huszár, and the architects J.J.P. Oud and Jan Wils. In 1917, he began the journal *De Stijl*, remaining its editor and driving force throughout its irregular publication until 1931. Van Doesburg promoted De Stijl as "The Style," the vehicle to annul the plurality of styles to culminate inevitably in neoplastic synthesis.

Architecturally, van Doesburg enacted this mission by appropriating ideas from painting to several buildings by Oud, Wils, and other Dutch architects. He applied primary colors to window frames and glass panels and developed colored geometric patterns for interiors beginning 1917, simultaneously writing essays and manifestos, launching De Stijl's "Manifesto 1" in 1918. Demanding the reformation of art and culture through collective collaboration, van Doesburg simultaneously emphasized the dystopic condition of the world through his efforts with the Dada artists Kurt Schwitters and Tristan Tzara. As a counterpoint to and groundwork for De Stijl, he wrote essays, sound-poems, and a novel and performed and created art under the Dada pseudonyms I.K. Bonset and Aldo Camini. Hoping to establish a pedagogical base for De Stijl, van Doesburg attempted to infiltrate the Bauhaus in Weimar between 1921 and 1922. When Walter Gropius refused him a teaching position, he formed his own De Stijl architecture course nearby.

Van Doesburg orchestrated De Stijl's international debut at the exhibition *Les Architectes du Groupe "de Styl"* held in the Galerie L'Effort Moderne in Paris in 1923. Here, among several architectural projects by members of the De Stijl group, including Gerrit Rietveld and Ludwig Mies van der Rohe, van Doesburg, in collaboration with Cornelis van Eesteren, developed two theoretical houses in drawings and models influential to the spatial and ideological development of modern architecture. The Maison d'Artiste and the Maison Particuliére were three-dimensional experiments derived from the universalizing forms explored in painting by van Doesburg and Mondrian. Their rectilinear volumes pinwheel about a voided center, emphasizing oblique movement. Their dynamic asymmetries are harmoniously balanced by the primary colors red, blue, and yellow and the noncolors black, white, and gray. Van Doesburg drew several spatially floating axonometrics, or "counter-constructions," from the Maison Particuliére. Unlike the singular fixed vantage point of traditional perspective, these speculative projections allow unlimited points of entry and exit in infinite extension. Van Doesburg photographed the models from below and proposed a sixth elevation for architecture, detached from the specificity of a site. His attempts to define an ungrounded, new con-

ception of space in relation to time were derived from the work of Albert Einstein; van Doesburg owned several books by or about him.

Between 1926 and 1928, van Doesburg transformed two large rooms of an 18th-century building in Strasbourg, France, to the Café Aubette. Designing each as a three-dimensional De Stijl environment, he didactically positioned the rooms in relation to one another. The Small Dance Hall's primary color panels on the walls and ceiling align orthographically with the rectilinear room. Enacting van Doesburg's transition into "Elementarism" and influenced by the oblique "counter-constructions" from the Maison Particuliére, his other room, the Cinema-Dance Hall, features diagonal patterns extending through the room's corners beyond the confines of the space. In the Café Aubette, reconstructed in 1995, the projection of cinema and the oblique gestures of bodies in motion establish the spatial dialogue between art and life. Synthesizing architecture and painting as *Gesamtkunstwerk*, or total work of art, van Doesburg incorporated several different materials into the spaces and designed the menu, furniture, and signs.

Van Doesburg designed and built a house for himself and his wife, Nelly, in Meudon-Val Fleury, outside of Paris, from 1927 to 1930. Intended as a teaching studio and a residence, its main cubic space rests on *pilotis*, suspended over an open terrace. Its narrow site constricted it into a diagonal sectional arrangement. At the same time, van Doesburg planned a series of towers titled "Cité de Circulation." This diagonally oriented collection of 11-story residences, based on previous tower schemes by Le Corbusier, holds four living units per floor, each similar to his Meudon House, pinwheeling around a central open core. A rotated axonometric drawing of the Meudon House demonstrates the interdependence of the two projects—connecting painting to interior to house to city, elevated high above the ground.

MARK STANKARD

See also **Bauhaus; Bauhaus, Dessau; Le Corbusier (Jeanneret, Charles-Édouard) (France); De Stijl, Gropius, Walter (Germany); Mies van der Rohe, Ludwig (Germany); Oud, J.J.P. (Netherlands); Rietveld, Gerrit (Netherlands)**

Biography

Born in Utrecht, Holland, 30 August 1883 as Christiaan Emil Marie Küpper; renamed himself after Dutch stepfather. Began painting and writing art criticism (1908–10); published essays on Leonardo, Michelangelo, and Rembrandt. Served in Dutch army, 1914–16, subsequently settled in Leiden, began collaborating with J.J.P. Oud and Jan Wils. In 1917 formed De Stijl group and publication of the same name (with Piet Mondrian, Vilmos Huszár, Bart van der Leck, and Georges Vantongerloo). Visited Berlin and Weimar (1921), where he met Raoul Hausmann, Mies van der Rohe, Hans Richter, and Le Corbusier; participated in architectural exhibitions, Galerie l'Effort Moderne (1923, Paris) and Ecole Spéciale d'Architecture (Paris, 1924). Collaborated with Jean Arp and Sophie Taueber-Arp for decorations for Café Aubette, Strasbourg, France; returned to Paris (1929), began designing house at Meudon-Val Fleury with Cornelis van Eesteren; published first issue of avant-garde jour-

nal *Art concret* 1929. Died 7 March 1931 of tuberculosis in Davos, Switzerland.

Selected Works

Architektur Projekt (unbuilt), 1923
Counter-Construction Project (drawing), 1923
Café de Unie, Rotterdam, Netherlands, 1925
Café Aubette (interiors), Strasbourg, France, 1928
Architect's House, Meudon-Val Fleury, France, 1930

Selected Publications

Elémentarisme, 1926
De Stijl 1 and *De Stijl 2* (Amsterdam: Athenaeum, 1968). Reprint of the periodical *De Stijl*, edited by Van Doesburg, from 1917 to 1929
On European Architecture: Complete Essays from Het Bouwbedrijf 1924–1931, translated by Charlotte I. Loeb and Arthur L. Loeb, Basel: Birkhäuser Verlag, 1990
Principles of Neo-Plastic Art (1925), translated by Janet Seligman, New York: New York Graphic Society Ltd., 1966

Further Reading

Van Doesburg and De Stijl are synonymous. Many books and articles on De Stijl, listed under that heading, contain further information on Van Doesburg. Doig (1986) and van Straaten (1983, 1988) contain many writings by van Doesburg in Dutch, French, German, and English. The van Doesburg archives, located in Holland and in France, have been thoroughly documented in the publications below.

Baljeu, Joost, *Theo van Doesburg*, New York: Macmillan, 1974
Blotkamp, Carel, "Theo van Doesburg," in *De Stijl: The Formative Years 1917–1922*, edited by Carel Blotkamp, translated by Charlotte I. Loeb and Arthur L. Loeb, Cambridge, Massachusetts: MIT Press, 1986
Doig, Allan, *Theo van Doesburg: Painting into Architecture, Theory into Practice*, Cambridge: Cambridge University Press, 1986
Hedrick, Hannah L., *Theo van Doesburg: Propagandist and Practitioner of the Avante-Garde, 1909–1923*, Ann Arbor, Michigan: UMI Research Press, 1980
Stankard, Mark, "Theo van Doesburg: Architecture at the End of History," *20/1* (Spring 1990)
van Straaten, Evert, *Theo van Doesburg 1883–1931*, The Hague: Staatsuitgeverij, 1983
van Straaten, Evert, *Theo van Doesburg: Painter and Architect*, The Hague: SDU Publishers, 1988

VANNA VENTURI HOUSE, CHESTNUT HILL

Designed by Robert Venturi, completed 1964
Chestnut Hill, Pennsylvania

Robert Venturi's house for his mother in Chestnut Hill, Pennsylvania, marked the formal reintroduction of architectural history into the formulaic modernist practice of architecture. Designed and constructed between 1959 and 1964, the Vanna Venturi house represents the integration of historical precedents, the demonstration of Venturi's architectural theory, and a critique of American domesticity. In a frequently cited description of the house, Venturi explains that it

recognizes complexities and contradictions; it is both complex and simple, open and closed, big and little; some of its elements are good on one level and bad on another; its order accommodates the generic elements of the house in general and the circumstantial elements of a house in particular. (Venturi, 1966)

Concentrating a variety of ideological and formal issues into the approximately 1700-square-foot house, Venturi produced five complete preliminary designs before arriving at the sixth and final scheme.

A house for a family member is a typical early commission for a young architect, and Venturi's achieved notoriety through the carefully composed elevational photograph centered at its entry of Vanna Venturi looking up from her book. As it was exposed to the architectural public, the Vanna Venturi house often was vilified but seldom dismissed. It soon was referenced in the work of other architects, as in the facades of the Phillips Exeter Academy Dining Hall (1972) by Louis Kahn, who was one of Venturi's mentors. By reaching low and broadly to vernacular domestic imagery while rigorously manipulating architectural precedent at a time when architecture had turned its back on history, the Vanna Venturi house profoundly disturbed the status quo of architecture.

Robert Venturi, enacting a genteel form of avante-garde disruption, ushered in Postmodernism with a building and a book to accompany it. *Complexity and Contradiction in Architecture*, written between 1956 and 1964, was Venturi's companion piece for the Vanna Venturi house. In a recent interview, Venturi said, "What I wrote in the book was what I was thinking about while I was drawing the house" (Schwartz, 1992). Venturi published plans for the Vanna Venturi house along with a portfolio of his other work as the last chapter of *Complexity and Contradiction in Architecture*, blurring theory and practice while seamlessly weaving his architecture into the canon of significant historical buildings.

Demonstrating a modern version of the strategy of mannerism—the human desire to impair perfection—Venturi appropriated and critiqued the history of Western architecture while remaining deeply engaged with its modernist tendencies. The Vanna Venturi house quotes freely from the nymphaeum at Andrea Palladio's Villa Barbaro (1554), McKim, Mead and White's Low House (1887), Bruno Taut's Double House (1921), the Casa Girasole by Luigi Moretti (1950), and Venturi's own Beach House project (1959), depicted and discussed in *Complexity and Contradiction in Architecture*. Venturi's Guild House, designed between 1960 and 1963 for the elderly Quaker community in Philadelphia, may be interpreted as a public version of his private house for his mother, an elderly member of the Quaker church. Each building has similar configurations in plan and elevation, and they share similar windows, front arches, taut skins, and a combination of marble and everyday materials.

The uniquely pale green, stuccoed front facade of the Vanna Venturi house presents at first impression a Palladian monumental symmetry. This overall symmetry is shifted and rearranged in asymmetrical elements, such as the slightly off-center actual chimney set within the centered, large-scale chimney block and in the reciprocal distribution of five windows on each half of the house, corresponding to the rooms within. The split pediment challenges the norm of the typical gable-roofed house and vi-

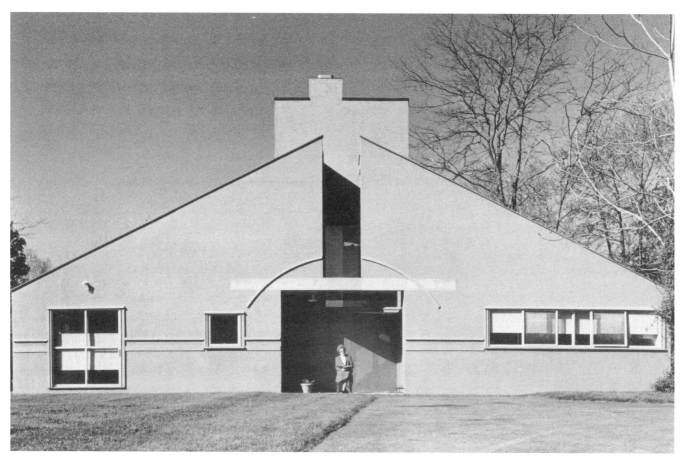

Vanna Venturi House, Chestnut Hill, Pennsylvania, designed by Robert Venturi (1964)
© Rollin La France. Photo courtesy Venturi, Scott Brown and Associates

sually exaggerates the structural capacity of the exposed concrete beam over the entry. Venturi applied a shallow arced dado molding to the facade, split by the central gap and passing over the concrete lintel. The application of thin moldings and the overall simple edges of the house make "the facades look almost like drawings" (Venturi, 1982). Venturi has privileged the perception of the drawn house over the appearance of the house itself. The front facade frequently has been compared to a child's drawing of a generic house, conveying "houseness" in its articulation of the fundamental pragmatic and symbolic elements of house— entry, window, gabled roof, and chimney. Both elementary and complex, the front facade of the Vanna Venturi house displays a tension between its perceived ornament and structure and exhibits Venturi's conception of "superadjacency"—drawing together elements of disparate scales.

The side facades barely exist, leftovers between front and rear. Notched patio spaces at each end minimize their presence. The rear facade combines standard window shapes in a thin-edged floating plane that seems detached from the body of the house. The extended facade wall screens a narrow deck on the upper floor with a "real" arched window behind it, in contrast to the applied arched molding at the front facade.

The plan of the house, which could be contained within a box, is based on an overall symmetry. Similar to the front facade, it diverts into a studied asymmetry. Approaching from the driveway, which is skewed to accommodate a sewer main in the street, the overscaled entry is blocked by the massive chimney. The curved foyer to the right sweeps into the dining area, with its large-scale marble tile floor setting it off from the rest of the house and suggesting a grand vestibule itself. Its high, arched ceiling envelops an independent pipe column. At the focus of the interior, the fireplace and its companion piece—the abruptly narrowing central stair—merge into a codependent entity. The shape of the wall surrounding the overscaled fireplace suggests an enormous version of an elderly woman's shoe, bringing to mind the old woman who lived in a shoe, a figurative domestic association.

The stair to the upper-level bedroom pinches in to accommodate barely one person. The upper level, which Robert Venturi occupied for about three years, contains a tiny utilitarian bathroom and storage spaces tucked under the roof eaves. An even narrower steep stair provides access to clean the high rear window, paint the clerestory, or change the exposed lightbulb. This quotidian finale is pure bathos, extending from elegant refinement to a strategically banal dead end.

From its overall site planning to the ergonomic detail of its stair rail, the Vanna Venturi house simultaneously recalls a typical American residence, gestures to a multitude of historical refer-

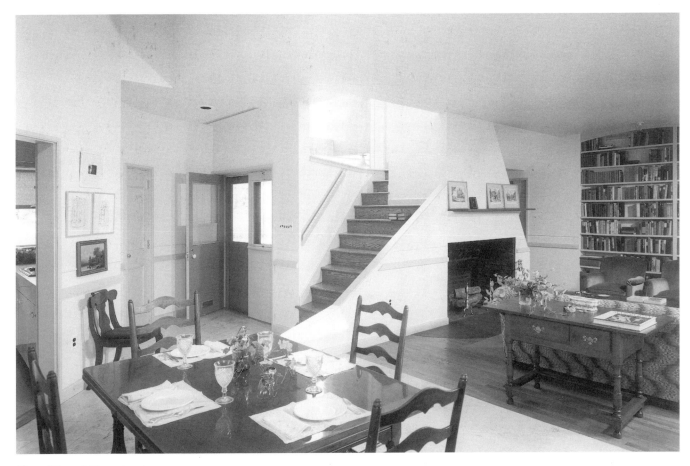

Vanna Venturi House interior
© Rollin La France. Photo courtesy Venturi, Scott Brown and Associates

ences, and deliberately subverts the status of orthodox modern architecture.

MARK STANKARD

Further Reading

Surprisingly, very little was written about the house immediately following its construction. However, it is mentioned and critiqued in a wide range of books and articles on modern and Postmodern architecture and culture by authors ranging from Tom Wolfe to Andrew Benjamin.

Berkeley, Ellen Perry, "Complexities and Contradictions," *Progressive Architecture*, 46/5 (May 1965)
Friedman, Alice T., "It's a Wise Child: The Vanna Venturi House, by Robert Venturi," in *Women and the Making of the Modern House: A Social and Architectural History*, by Friedman, New York: Abrams, 1998
Futagawa, Yukio (editor), *Vanna Venturi House, Chestnut Hill, Philadelphia, Pennsylvania, 1962: Peter Brant House, Greenwich, Connecticut, 1973: Carll Tucker III House, Westchester County, New York, 1975*, Tokyo: A.D.A. Edita, 1976
Schwartz, Frederick, *Mother's House: The Evolution of Vanna Venturi's House in Chestnut Hill*, New York: Rizzoli, 1992
Somol, Robert E., "My Mother the House," *The Princeton Architectural Journal*, 4 (1992)
Venturi, Robert, "House for Mrs. Robert Venturi," *Perspecta*, 9–10 (1965)
Venturi, Robert, *Complexity and Contradiction in Architecture*, New York: Museum of Modern Art, 1966; 2nd edition, New York: Museum of Modern Art, and London: Architectural Press, 1977
Venturi, Robert, "Diversity, Relevance, and Representation in Historicism, or, Plus ça Change . . . Plus a Plea for Pattern All over Architecture, with a Postscript on My Mother's House," *Architectural Record*, 170 (June 1982)
Von Moos, Stanislaus, *Venturi, Rauch, and Scott Brown: Buildings and Projects, 1960–1985*, New York: Rizzoli, 1987

VAN NELLE FACTORY, NETHERLANDS

Designed by J.A. Brinkman and L.C. van der Vlugt
with Mart Stam, Completed 1930
Rotterdam, Netherlands

The Van Nelle factory (1930) in Schiedam, Rotterdam, Netherlands, was designed by the firm of J.A. Brinkman and L.C. van der Vlugt with Mart Stam. Completed between 1926 and 1930, it was admired by fellow modern architects and industrialists alike. The factory complex included industrial buildings for packaging, offices, and warehouse facilities for the Dutch company Van Nelle, renowned for its coffees, teas, and tobaccos. The factory still exists today.

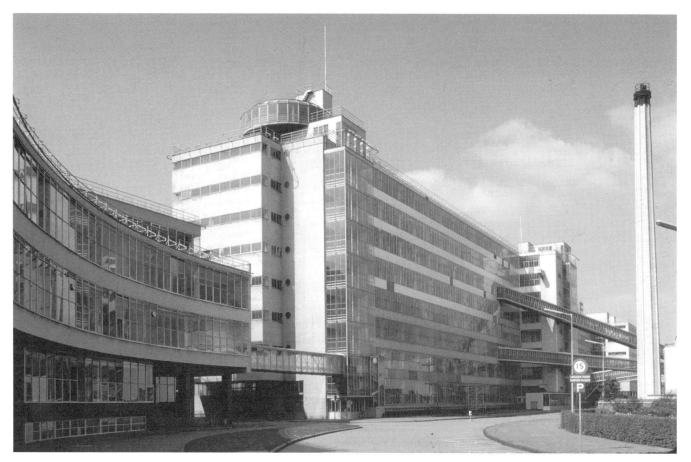

Van Nelle Factory, Rotterdam (1928), by Johannes A. Brinkman and L. C. van der Vlugt
© GreatBuildings.com

Over a ten-year period, the building plans changed and developed because of World War I as well as Van Nelle's need to purchase and unify an appropriate site not being realized until the fall of 1926, the year construction began on the factory buildings. The design for the project was initiated by architect Michiel Brinkman (1873–1925), who died before its completion, so the project was passed on to his young son, J.A. (Jan) Brinkman (1902–49), who, working with a more experienced architect, L.C. (Leendert Cornelis) van der Vlugt (1894–1936), completed the project.

Key in the building's innovative design was the active role of the factory owner, Kees van der Leeuw, who was involved in the design of the complex, the construction methods, and the spatial planning. As a Theosophist, he cared for his employees, which was reflected in his concern to provide them with adequate daylight. This desire paralleled the insight he gained from his 1925 travels to America, where he saw the modern factories of Albert and Moritz Kahn, all noted for their attention to light. His paternalistic view of the happy worker was similar to that of Henry Ford, and he was keen to test the already proven methods of Taylorism in factory organization and employee comfort. His knowledge of Walter Gropius's newly completed Bauhaus building in Dessau and Fagus factory in Germany inspired the transparent design of the Van Nelle factory.

The main entrance with a gatehouse opens onto the complex by means of the sweeping curved facade of the four-story administrative building for the offices and warehouses. A bridge enclosed in glass and steel connects this building to the factory at the second floor, creating the sense of the assembly lines in the flow of the buildings. The ground floor of the office building is set back, with a column supporting the corner curve that sweeps beyond the main rectangular structure. Along the curved facade are the managing director's office, meeting rooms, drafting offices, and sample rooms, and the open rectangular volume has the combined general administrative offices and employee cafeteria. This program and its manifestation demonstrate the architects' interest in Bauhaus principles.

The manufacturing buildings are sited adjacent to the Overschie River for easy transport of goods. The final built scheme, only part of what was originally planned, consists of a main factory block of different heights in one rectangular bar. The boiler house was built separately for safety. An eight-story tobacco factory, a six-story coffee factory, and a three-story tea factory were connected by glazed exterior stair towers. As a vertically organized factory, typical of the early 20th-century type, the production line moved from the upper to the lower floor, with the final product being transferred to the warehouses via exterior conveyor belts in transparent bridges. The roof of the

building is capped with a circular glazed tearoom and viewing platform for visitors and staff.

As an early use of a glass-and-steel curtain wall, the arresting transparent facade is one of the building's genuinely iconic elements. The technical achievements in the design of this glass curtain wall and its construction using machine-made parts led to the further exploration of curtain-wall technologies for many other building types. The vertical mullion elements are steel, sprayed with a zinc coating, and the horizontal spandrels are steel sheets. The effect was of a continuous band of glass and metal in a new industrial aesthetic.

To keep the floors of the factory open for flexible use and to hold the heavy packing machinery, engineer Jan Gerko Wiebenga (1886–1974), who often worked with Van der Vlugt, designed an open system. Using a concrete frame, he placed octagonal concrete mushroom columns on the interior's perimeter within two rows of central columns spaced in 5-by-5.70-meter modules in the tobacco factory and 5.70-by-5.70-meter modules in the other two sections. This design created beamless concrete floor slabs that were cantilevered beyond the perimeter columns and allowed space along the facade for conduits and hallways. The polished concrete floor also contained cables and electric conduits. The last phases of the project included a workers' cafeteria, playing fields, store blocks, and garages. Many years after the Van Nelle factory was constructed, Reyner Banham noted that Mart Stam had played a more significant role in the design of the building than previously considered (footnote in Reyner Banham, *Theory Design in the Machine Age*, Architectural Press, London, 1960).

Van Nelle was seminal as part of the Dutch Nieuwe Bouwen, one of the many groups of European architects who concentrated on the issues of technical progress and modern architecture and who worked to improve the quality of housing and working environments. While providing a decent working environment, the building allowed in plenty of light and air and provided spaces for administrative staff and factory workers, thus being pragmatic in its form to serve the function of the factory. Brinkman and Van der Vlugt went on to design stores for Van Nelle, including housing and commercial buildings.

NINA RAPPAPORT

See also **Factory; Gropius, Walter (Germany); Rotterdam, Netherlands**

Further Reading

De Jonge, Wessel, "A Price and Prize for Van Nelle," *Docomomo Newsletter*, 6 (November 1991)

Derwig, Jan, and Erick Matter, *Functionalism in the Netherlands*, Amsterdam: Architectura en Natura, 1995

Ibelings, Hans, *Niederländische Architektur des 20. Jahrhunderts*, Munich and New York: Prestel, 1995; as *20th-Century Architecture in the Netherlands*, translated by Michael O'Loughlin, Amsterdam: NAi, 1996

"The Van Nelle Factory," *Architectural Record*, 66 (October 1929)

"The Van Nelle Factory," *Architectural Record*, 69 (May 1931)

VAN DE VELDE, HENRI 1863–1957

Architect and interior designer, Belgium

Henri van de Velde was a leading figure of Belgian Art Nouveau. He was born in Antwerp into a family with strong interest in the arts. His father was a pharmacist and a director of the local arts festival. After having contemplated a career as a composer, van de Velde chose to become a painter instead. He studied at the Antwerp Art Academy (1880–83) and at the atelier of Carolys Duran in Paris (1884–85). On his return from Paris in 1886, van de Velde moved to the Belgian countryside, where he started to develop a more holistic approach toward art and environment. In 1887, he discovered pointillism, which allowed him to develop a more analytic approach to painting and form, and from 1890 on, he started to broaden his artistic production to the realm of applied arts, then to interior design, and finally to architecture.

At the same time, van de Velde established himself as a theorist and propagandist. In 1894, he started a series of lectures that promoted the revival of architecture and decorative arts by combining the moral principles of the English Arts and Crafts movement with the acceptance of machine production and social changes. These lectures were published in 1901 under the title *Die Renaissance im Kunstgewerbe* (The Renaissance of Applied Arts). Van de Velde's theoretical position was informed by readings of William Morris, Friedrich Nietzsche, and Leo Tolstoy, in which art and beauty were understood as a significant force for social advancement and cultural renewal.

His first venture into architecture came with his own house, Bloemenwerf (1895–96), in Uccle, near Brussels, where van de Velde, who had no architectural training, collaborated with local craftsmen in a design that is somewhat a combination of a traditional farmhouse and an urban villa. It was van de Velde's first attempt to create a total work of art in which furniture, wallpaper, and even his wife's reform dress are understood as an integral part of architecture.

Van de Velde's reputation spread rapidly in the mid-1890s. The reception was particularly favorable in Germany, and in 1895 the German art dealer Samuel Bing and art critic Julius Meier-Graefe commissioned him to design three room interiors. First exhibited in the Salon Art Nouveau in Paris the same year (and further in 1897 in Dresden), these interiors, characterized by dynamic, curved forms, launched van de Velde's career as a furniture maker and interior designer while also launching a new style: Art Nouveau. Bing and Meier-Graefe played an important part in van de Velde's career, the former becoming van de Velde's dealer in Paris and the latter the first critic to write about his work.

In 1900 Karl Ernst Osthaus invited van de Velde to design the interiors for the Folkwang Museum (1901–04) in Hagen, Germany. Only five years after the completion of their own house, the family moved to Berlin. Contrary to his hopes, Berlin did not offer a breakthrough for other larger projects, and in 1902 he accepted the offer of the duke of Sachsen-Weimar to become the director of the Weimar Kunstgewerblicher Institut. The duke also commissioned van de Velde to design the new school buildings: the Kunstgewerbeschule (school of applied arts, 1904) and the Kunstschule (art school, 1906), which became his first major architectural commissions. During his 12-year tenure at Weimar, van de Velde embraced and inspired the future generation and developed a successful architectural practice. The most notable works from this period include several private villas for Weimar's cultural elite; van de Velde's own second house, called Hohe Pappels (1908); a Tennis Club (1908) in Chemnitz; an interior design of the Nietzsche Archive

(1911); and most notably the theater for the 1914 Werkbund Exhibition in Cologne.

Van de Velde's resignation in 1914 came right after the 1914 Werkbund meeting in Cologne, where he came under a fierce attack by Hermann Muthesius (1861–1927) for representing a reactionary and outdated individualist position and resisting the need for standardized production and typification. Van de Velde recommended Walter Gropius as his successor, thus laying the foundation for the future Bauhaus.

This so-called Werkbund debate is indicative of why many other members of the first generation of the Modern movement, such as Peter Behrens and Frank Lloyd Wright, came to surpass van de Velde in their historical significance as pioneers of 20th-century architecture. However, van de Velde was one of the seminal thinkers around 1890, when 19th-century architectural historicism came into a crisis. Informed by *Einfühlung* (empathy) theory, van de Velde believed that line was the fundamental element of art. According to his motto "a line is a force" (*Kunstgewerbliche Laienpredigten*, 1902), form is an outcome of spontaneous, creative expression based on inner necessity, both structural and emotional. This led to a design strategy based on the combination of constructive and functional logic and dynamic formal expression.

Van de Velde's life after leaving Weimar in 1917 was divided among Switzerland, Holland, and Belgium, where in 1925–47 he held a professorship at the University of Ghent. His mature work includes the Belgian Pavilions for the Paris (1937) and New York (1939) World Exhibitions and the Rijksmuseum Kröller-Müller (1937–54) in Otterlo. After his retirement, van de Velde returned to Switzerland to write his memoirs, *Geschichte meines Lebens* (1962; The Story of My Life), a wonderfully creative testimony of his long and eventful life.

EEVA-LIISA PELKONEN

Biography

Born in Antwerp, 3 April 1863. Attended the Academie voor Schone Kunsten, Antwerp 1880–83; studied painting at the Académie des Beaux-Arts, Antwerp 1882–84 and Paris 1884–85. Painter and interior decorator, Antwerp and Brussels 1885–94. In private practice as an architect and designer, Brussels 1895–98, under the title Société van de Velde 1898–1900; practiced in Berlin 1900–05, Weimar 1906–14, Switzerland 1914–21, Wassenaar, Netherlands 1921–25, and Brussels 1925–47. Lecturer, University of Brussels 1894–95; founder and director, Kunstgewerbeschule (later Bauhaus School), Weimar 1902–14; founder and director, École Nationale Supérieure d'Architecture et des Arts Décoratifs, Brussels 1925–36; professor of architecture, 1925–47, chair of architecture, 1926–35, University of Ghent. Died in Zurich, 25 October 1957.

Selected Works

Bloemenwerf House, Uccle, Belgium, 1896
Interiors, Keller und Reiner Art Gallery, Berlin, 1898
Interiors, Folkwang Museum, Hagen, Germany, 1904
Kunstgewerbeschule, Weimar, 1904
Kunstschule, Weimar, 1906
Hohe Pappels (van de Velde residence), Weimar, 1908
Tennis Club, Chemnitz, Weimar, 1908
Interior, Nietzsche Archive, Weimar, 1911
Theater, Werkbund Exhibition, Cologne, 1914
Belgian Pavilion, World's Fair, Paris, 1937
Belgian Pavilion, World's Fair, New York, 1939
Riksmuseum Kröller-Müller, Otterlo, Belgium, 1954

Selected Publications

Déblaiement d'art, 1894
L'Art futur, 1895
Die Renaissance im Kunstgewerbe, 1901
Der neue Stil, 1906
Vernunftsgemässe Schönheit, 1909
Die drei Sünden wider die Schönheit, 1918
Les Fondements du style moderne, 1933
Geschichte meines Lebens, edited by Hans Curjel, 1962

Further Reading

Delevoy, Robert L., *Henri van de Velde, 1863–1957*, Brussels: Palais des Beaux-Arts, 1963
Delevoy, Robert L., Maurice Culot, and Yvonne Brunhammer, *Pionniers du XXe siècle: Guimard, Horta, van de Velde*, Paris: Tournon, 1971
Hüter, Karl-Heinz, *Henri van de Velde: Sein Werk bis zum Ende seiner Tätigkeit in Deutschland*, Berlin: Akademie-Verlag, 1967
Sembach, Klaus-Jürgen, *Henri van de Velde*, New York: Rizzoli, and London: Thames and Hudson, 1989
Weber, Klaus, *Henri van de Velde: Das buchkünstlerische Werk*, Freiburg im Breisgau: Rombach, 1994

VENICE BIENNALE PAVILIONS

Designed by various architects, 1895–1995
Venice, Italy

The Venice Biennale began in 1895 as an exhibition of international art held every two years in the Castello Gardens at the southeast edge of Venice. Its pavilions, each representing an individual country, perform as autonomous nationalistic objects and as a strategically assembled collection of 20th-century architecture. As an evolving modernist project, new national pavilions accrued between 1895 and 1995, with critical acts of demolition, alteration, addition, refacading, restoration, and re-allocation. The Biennale pavilions, as architectural representations for sovereign nations, can be categorized in terms of Neoclassicism, vernacular nationalism, historicist nationalism, ideological nationalism, and international modernism.

Two fundamental definitions of the word describe these pavilions: "a summerhouse or other decorative building in a garden" and "a temporary stand at an exhibition." Although often dismissed by critics as diminutive pleasure follies or curiosity collections for tourists, they form a permanent extraurban community of 20th-century modernist icons—exterior representational expositions encasing interior mutable exhibitions. Their status oscillates between architectural ambassador and miniature museum for contemporary art.

The original Castello Gardens were constructed on reclaimed marsh between 1808 and 1812 by Giannantonio Selva. In 1895, the Biennale was founded, and its first building, the Palazzo dell'Esposizione (or Central Pavilion) by Enrico Trevisanato,

contained 16 exhibition rooms around a domed space. The artists Marius de Maria and Bartolomeo Bezzi designed its neoclassical facade.

Belgium provided the first national pavilion, or "house of art," in 1907, a contemporary Art Nouveau project by Léon Sneyers. Most of the early pavilions displayed a neoclassical or vernacular character, derived from both museum and villa architecture. The British Pavilion (1909) by Edwin Rickards, built on a prominent hill, quotes Andrea Palladio's 16th-century villas and their modifications as Italianate English country houses. A Venetian architect, Daniele Donghi, designed the Bavarian Pavilion in the same year. Figural ornament was added to its neoclassical facade when it became the German Pavilion in 1912. Géza Maróti's Hungarian Pavilion (1909), a richly ornamented, transplanted vernacular building, was picturesquely sited off the main axis of the Gardens. The neoclassical French Pavilion (1912) by the Venetian architect Fausto Finzi joined Great Britain and Germany at the southeast corner of the Gardens. Ferdinand Boberg designed the Sweden Pavilion in 1912, converted to the Holland Pavilion in 1914. The Central (Italian) Pavilion received a concave Liberty-style facade by Guido Cirilli in 1914. Just before the outbreak of World War I in 1914, the Russian Pavilion, resembling a vernacular Byzantine church, was completed by Aleksej Scusev. In 1924, its facade was accessorized under the new Soviet state with the letters "URSS," a red band, and a hammer and sickle.

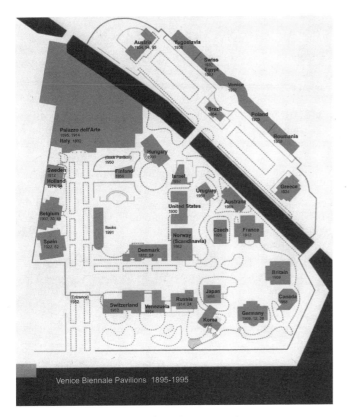

Plan for Venice Biennale Pavilions (1895–1995)
© Mark Stankard

Most pavilions built between World Wars I and II recirculated historicist imagery or conveyed an ideological nationalism. Spain's pavilion (1922) by Javier de Luque featured a Churriguerresque facade displaying its country's 18th-century synthesis of architecture and sculpture. Uniquely, the Czechoslovakian architect Otakar Novotny designed his country's pavilion (1926) as an example of contemporary Czech Cubism. Delano and Aldrich created the United States Pavilion (1930) as a neoclassical colonial version of Thomas Jefferson's neo-Palladian Monticello. Carl Brummer's neoclassical Danish Pavilion (1932) occupied the middle of the Gardens. A Venetian Pavilion for decorative arts (1932) by Brenno Del Giudice was built on the other side of the Canal di Sant'Elena, with flanking pavilions for Poland and Switzerland. Its white, "stile-littorio classicism" followed official state architecture under Mussolini. Identical pavilions for Romania and Yugoslavia were added in 1938, stringing together autonomous nations in a unified structure. Duilio Torres's similar new facade for the Central (Italian) Pavilion (1932) proclaimed itself "Italia" in large block letters. Josef Hoffman's minimalist Austrian Pavilion (1934), north of the Venetian Pavilion, contained an open central arcade and clerestory lighting. The masonry, neo-Byzantine Greek Pavilion (1934) by M. Papandréou was sited axially opposite Austria's pavilion.

Under Hitler, Germany's pavilion was demolished in 1938 and replaced by a monumental "meta-neo-classical" structure by Ernst Haiger. After Germany invaded Austria, Czechoslovakia, Poland, Romania, Hungary, and Yugoslavia, their pavilions were closed. Italy displayed military imagery in the British, French, and United States Pavilions in 1942.

After World War II, the Biennale reopened in 1948. The Venetian architect Virgilio Vallot replaced the facade of the Belgium Pavilion that year. Carlo Scarpa designed several projects for the Biennale, beginning in 1950 with the triangular/trapezoidal Book Pavilion near the Italian Pavilion portico. This pavilion, Scarpa's leaflike Ticket Office (1952), and his Italian Pavilion courtyard (1952) have been destroyed. Significantly, the first post–World War II new pavilion was for Israel (1952), an "international modern" trapezoidal structure by the Tel Aviv architect Zeev Rechter. Bruno Giacometti designed Switzerland's pavilion (1952), a complex assemblage of volumes, sited near the Gardens entry. Egypt occupied the former Swiss Pavilion. The Spanish Pavilion was stripped of its ornament and received a simpler masonry facade by Joaquín Vaquero Palacios in 1952. Carlo Scarpa's innovative Venezuelan Pavilion (1954–56), wedged between those of Switzerland and the Soviet Union, referred to traditional Japanese architecture and the work of Frank Lloyd Wright and Ludwig Mies van der Rohe. In 1954, Gerrit Rietveld designed a new "late De Stijl" Dutch Pavilion, replacing the previous one. Alvar Aalto's wedge-shaped Finnish Pavilion (1956) was similar to Scarpa's Book Pavilion. Painted Finnish blue and white, it was prefabricated and transported to the site. The Le Corbusian Japan Pavilion (1956) by Takamasa Yoshizaka is a concrete box on four massive supports with an Oriental garden on the sloping land below. Denmark's pavilion was extended with a series of brick boxes by Peter Koch in 1958, and Uruguay built a simple new pavilion in the same year. The Italian architects BBPR erected the octagonal Canadian Pavilion (1958) around two existing trees. Several trees were also retained

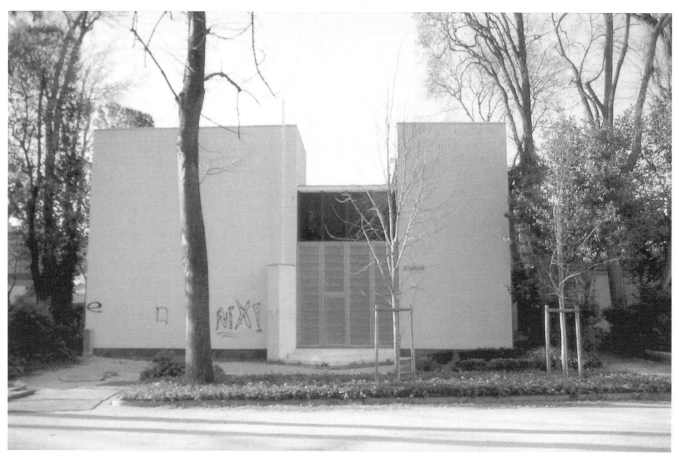

Dutch Pavilion, by Gerrit Rietveld, Venice Biennale (1954)
© Mark Stankard

within the Norway Pavilion (1962) (now for Scandinavia) by Sverre Fehn. The innovative concrete structure remains open to the Gardens and was conceptually derived from the neighboring United States Pavilion. The Brazil Pavilion (1964) by the Venetian Amerigo Marchesin occupies the axial crossing of the pavilions on the island of Sant'Elena.

Louis Kahn proposed designs for a Meeting Hall and a new Italian Pavilion in 1968–69. Little architectural work took place at the Biennale Gardens until the metal-clad, domestic-scaled Australian Pavilion (1988) was built by Philip Cox along the Gardens canal. Slipped within an allée near the Gardens entry, James Stirling and Michael Wilford produced the Book Pavilion, or "bookship," in 1991. In 1995, Josef Hoffman's Austrian Pavilion was significantly altered by the Viennese architects Coop Himmelb(l)au. They infiltrated the historic pavilion with an assemblage of columns, a roof, and a screen. Seok Chul Kim's Korean Pavilion (1995) acknowledges the rising tides by lifting itself up on metal stilts. Its hinged wood screens protect the pavilion during off times—a solution common to both Venice and Korea and a recognition of the ephemeral condition of the Biennale. Many of the pavilions and the Gardens themselves are in poor condition, and as Venice continues to be inundated by the lagoon, this unique collection of 20th-century architecture

requires preservation and the ability to evolve. The Venice Biennale Pavilions serve collectively as a connotative inventory of 20th-century modernism.

MARK STANKARD

Further Reading

Very little has been published in English on the Biennale Pavilions as a whole. Catalogs have been published for each of the Biennale exhibitions; these often contain mentions of the Pavilions, as do reviews in several art periodicals. There are also books on the Austria, Finland, Israel, and Dutch Pavilions and on the works by Scarpa.

Alloway, Lawrence, *The Venice Biennale, 1895–1968,* Greenwich, Connecticut: New York Graphic Society, 1968; London: Faber, 1969
Bazzoni, Romolo, *60 anni della Biennale di Venezia,* Venice: Lombroso, 1962
Irace, Fulvio, "A Venezia, la città per l'arte; A City for Art within the City of Venice," *Abitare,* 270 (December 1988)
Mulazzani, Marco, *I padiglioni della Biennale: Venezia, 1887–1988,* Milan: Electa, 1988; new edition, 1993
Rizzi, Paolo, and Enzo Di Martino, *Storia della Biennale, 1895–1982,* Milan: Electa, 1982
West, Shearer, "National Desires and Regional Realities in the Venice Biennale, 1895–1914," *Art History,* 18/3 (1995)

VENTURI, ROBERT 1925–

Architect, United States

Robert Venturi is the principal partner of Venturi, Scott Brown and Associates with Denise Scott Brown, Steven Izenour, and David Vaughn. He is best known for his architectural ideas outlined in his two influential books, *Complexity and Contradiction in Architecture* (1966) and *Learning from Las Vegas* (1972), written with Scott Brown and Izenour. Both texts critique the often dogmatic and narrow design agenda of modernist architecture and have been viewed as an antidote to the polemics of modernist architects such as Adolf Loos, who famously wrote that "ornament is crime," and Le Corbusier, who authored the classic manifesto *Towards a New Architecture* (1923). Directing 20th-century architects to study the commercial landscape of Main Street and the roadside as well as the classical tradition, Venturi and Scott Brown embrace historicism, decoration, language, and vernacular symbols. *Learning from Las Vegas* in particular argued for the celebration of both "high" and "low" architecture of the past, from the richness of classical Rome to the messiness of the commercial strip. Its emphasis on visual ambiguity, contradiction, dialectic, context, and complexity led to designs that were full of wit and rich in connotations.

Venturi's residential architecture of the 1960s expressed his interest in the vernacular symbols and historical allusions outlined in *Complexity and Contradiction*. The Guild House (1960), a senior citizens apartment complex in Philadelphia, Pennsylvania, referenced the classicism of Andrea Palladio in the design of its facade and pointed to the architecture of commerce with its prominent sign above the entry. The Vanna Venturi House (1962) in Chestnut Hill, Pennsylvania, borrowed from the forms of the American saltbox (shingle style) and emphasized axial symmetry.

The humorous and historical came together in Venturi's creation of Benjamin Franklin's "house" and museum (1973–76) in Independence National Historical Park in Philadelphia. Rather than reconstructing the long-demolished home of Franklin, Venturi and partners designed a vividly colored steel-frame outline of the house, which had been described by Franklin in letters to his wife, and placed the museum in the ground below. The firm has long had an interest in urban design, reflecting its focus on the American landscape. Planning work has included the South Street Rehabilitation Plan (1970) for Philadelphia and the Pennsylvania Avenue Project (1978–79) for Washington, D.C.

Other projects have included industrial design and furniture design as well as exhibitions. "Signs of Life: Symbols in the American City" at the Renwick Gallery in Washington, D.C. (1976) was an exhibit of historical and contemporary signs. The display celebrated the American bicentennial by presenting the rich variety of signage found in the United States. Such work remained consistent with the firm's appreciation of the vernacular and illustrated how Venturi and his partners have refused to limit the application of their ideas to one field.

After 1980 Venturi received a number of large commissions. Such projects, while remaining true to the original theories of the firm, have tended toward the practical, thus helping shed Venturi's reputation for superficial cleverness. Important commissions for universities and museums evidence the office's wider acceptance. Princeton University commissioned three buildings, including Wu Hall (1983), which referenced the style of English manor houses, thus complementing the campus's eclectic mix of buildings. The Sainsbury Wing (1991) of the National Gallery in London alluded to the adjacent classical building yet reconfigured the purist style, referencing Victorian train sheds in the interior. Recent designs continued to reflect the firm's commitment to historical styles and vernacular symbols. The Seattle Art Museum (1991) contained sensitive gallery spaces as well as massive incised lettering along the top of the limestone exterior. The Mielparque Nikko Kirifuri Resort (1997) in Nikko, Japan, reflects the traditional rural architecture of Japan.

The global influence of Venturi and his partner Denise Scott Brown has been widely recognized through extensive writing, teaching, and lecturing. Consistent with an aesthetic of contradiction, Venturi's works deal with both the formal and theoretical intersections of modernism and Postmodernism by engaging with the conditions of contemporary society, construction, and culture.

NICOLAS MAFFEI

See also **Color; Postmodernism; Scott Brown, Denise (United States); Vanna Venturi House, Philadelphia**

Biography

Born in Philadelphia, 25 June 1925. Attended Princeton University, New Jersey 1943–50; bachelor of arts degree 1947; master of fine arts degree 1950; studied at the American Academy, Rome, on a Rome Prize Fellowship 1954–56. Married architect Denise Scott Brown 1967: 1 child. Designer with the firms of Oscar Stonorov, Philadelphia; Eero Saarinen, Bloomfield Hills, Michigan; and Louis I. Khan, Philadelphia 1950–58. Partner with Paul Cope and H. Mather Lippincott, Venturi, Cope and Lippincott, Philadelphia 1958–61; partner with William Short, Venturi and Short, Philadelphia 1961–64; partner with John Rauch from 1964; partner with Rauch and Denise Scott Brown from 1967; Ossabow Island Project, Savannah, Georgia, from 1977; principal, Venturi, Scott Brown and Associates, Philadelphia from 1989. Assistant professor, then associate professor of architecture, University of Pennsylvania, Philadelphia 1957–65; State Department Lecturer in the USSR 1965; architect-in-residence, American Academy, Rome 1966; Charlotte Shepherd Davenport Professor of Architecture, Yale University, New Haven, Connecticut 1966–70; member, Panel of Visitors, School of Architecture and Urban Planning, University of California, Los Angeles 1966–67; visiting critic, Rice University, Houston, Texas 1969; trustee, American Academy, Rome 1969–74; member, board of advisers, department of art and archaeology, Princeton University 1969–72, from 1977; member, board of advisers, School of Architecture and Urban Design, Princeton University from 1977; Walter Gropius Lecturer, Graduate School of Design, Harvard University, Cambridge, Massachusetts 1982. Fellow, American Institute of Architects; fellow, American Academy of Arts and Sciences; fellow, American Academy, Rome; fellow, Accademia Nazionale de San Luca, Rome; honorary fellow, Royal Institute of British Architects; honorary fellow, Royal Incorporation of Architects of Scotland. Gold Medal, American Institute of Architects 1972; Commander, Order of Merit, Italy 1986; Pritzker Prize 1991.

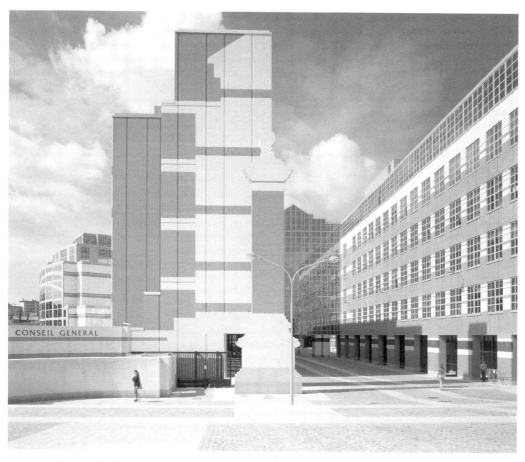

Provincial Capitol Building, Toulouse, France (1999), by Robert Venturi
Photo by Matt Wargo © Venturi, Scott Brown and Associates

Selected Works

Guild House, Philadelphia, 1960
Vanna Venturi House, Chestnut Hill, Pennsylvania, 1962
South Street Rehabilitation Plan for Philadelphia, 1970
Brant House, Greenwich, Connecticut, 1973
Franklin Court, Independence National Historical Park,
    Philadelphia, 1976
Pennsylvania Avenue Project for Washington, 1979
Gordon Wu Hall, Princeton University, New Jersey, 1983
Art Museum, Seattle, 1991
Sainsbury Wing, National Gallery, London, 1991
The Gonda (Goldschmied) Neuroscience and Genetics Research
    Center, Los Angeles, 1997
Mielparque Nikko Kirifuri Resort, Nikko, Japan, 1997
Provincial Capitol Building, Toulouse, France, 1999

Selected Publications

Complexity and Contradiction in Architecture, 1966
Learning from Las Vegas (with Denise Scott Brown and Steven
    Izenour), 1972
A View from the Campidoglio: Selected Essays, 1953–1984 (with
    Denise Scott Brown), edited by Peter Arnell, Ted Bickford, and
    Catherine Bergart, 1984
*Iconography and Electronics upon a Generic Architecture: A View from
    the Drafting Room*, 1996

Further Reading

A + U, 12 (1981) (special issue entitled "Venturi, Rauch, and Scott
    Brown")
Futagawa, Yukio (editor), *Vanna Venturi House, Chestnut Hill,
    Philadelphia, Pennsylvania, 1962: Peter Brant House, Greenwich,
    Connecticut, 1973: Carll Tucker III House, Westchester County,
    New York, 1975*, Tokyo: A.D.A. Edita, 1976
Ghirardo, Diane, *Architecture after Modernism*, New York: Thames
    and Hudson, 1996
Upton, Dell, *Architecture in the United States*, Oxford and New
    York: Oxford University Press, 1998
Von Moos, Stanislaus, *Venturi, Scott Brown and Associates: Buildings
    and Projects, 1986–1998*, New York: Monacelli Press, 1999
Wiseman, Carter, *Shaping a Nation: Twentieth-Century American
    Architecture and Its Makers*, New York: Norton, 1998
The Work of Venturi and Rauch: Architects and Planners (exhib. cat.),
    New York: Whitney Museum of American Art, 1971

VERNACULAR ARCHITECTURE

Although it had been in use among specialists for well over a
century, the term "vernacular architecture" became widely accepted only with its adoption in 1976 by the International

Council on Monuments and Sites (ICOMOS). Other terms persist, such as "traditional," "rural," "regional," "local," "peasant," "folk," and "indigenous" architecture, serving collectively to identify the field of building encompassed by the vernacular. Its original meaning (from the Latin), "the language of the people," is applicable to architecture as an extension of the commonly employed idea of "architecture as language," in which styles of design are analogous to grammar or syntax.

"Arquitectura popular," used in both Spanish- and Portuguese-speaking countries, corresponds to the increasingly prevalent definition of the vernacular as "the architecture *of*, and *by*, the people." With the wider acceptance of the term "vernacular architecture," a distinction is made between buildings that are self-built or community built and used and those that are designed *for* the people, such as fast-food outlets, chain stores, filling stations, and strip malls. Including mobile homes, these latter types, as professionally designed structures for general use, are regarded as popular architecture. As such, they are distinguished from the vernacular, which broadly corresponds to the building traditions depicted in Bernard Rudofsky's exhibition and catalog *Architecture without Architects* (1964) at the Museum of Modern Art, New York. The exhibition emphasized the aesthetic merits of vernacular traditions from nearly 30 countries that had been an inspiration for many architects in the 20th century.

As early as 1910, Frank Lloyd Wright applauded "folk building[s] growing in response to actual needs, fitted into environment by people who knew no better than to fit them to it with native feeling," which were "for us better worth study than all the highly self-conscious academic attempts at the beautiful throughout all Europe" (see Gutheim, 1941). A year later, Le Corbusier was sketching the peasant houses of Serbia and Bulgaria and praising "the *konak*, the Turkish wooden house, ... an architectural masterpiece." He was profoundly drawn to the vernacular buildings of the Greek islands and the Algerian M'Zab, and many architects followed his pursuit of purity and function in the "white" villages of the Mediterranean. Independently, Alvar Aalto in Finland, Michel de Klerk in the Netherlands, and later Luis Barragán in Mexico were among the many architects who drew on regional building for inspiration.

In such cases, the vernacular was a source of stimulation for some and a justification of their design aesthetic for others. Simplicity of form and structure and the moral value of the Mies-inspired truth to materials and economy of means were increasingly established as the modernist architecture par excellence. Following the legacy of Adolf Loos's essay "Ornament and Crime" (1908), vernacular traditions that employed decoration were generally disregarded in favor of reductivism. Vernacular examples offered less to architects who were seeking models of varied spatial experience, but their "fitness for purpose" and, above all, their functionality were seen as paradigms of modern approaches to architectural design.

Undoubtedly, all these qualities could be seen in a wide range of vernacular buildings, from farmhouses to workshops, granaries to cow barns, and lime kilns to windmills that not only helped clarify design objectives in the minds of many architects but also served to reinforce modernist principles. However, although some followed Wright's advice to study "folk building," his somewhat patronizing view of its builders was echoed by many architects and writers who referred to the "spontaneous,"

"unconscious," or "intuitive" building processes. Professional architects studied the vernacular more for their own benefit than for any that might accrue for the survival or protection of the traditions themselves, which in the years following World War II were threatened. The ravages of war, industrialization of building processes, need for mass housing, and universal adoption of Le Corbusian "tower blocks" and "slab blocks" marked the international success of modernism and, in many instances, the imminent demise of many vernacular traditions.

Decline in the vernacular in many Western countries had been evident since the beginning of the 20th century. Largely through voluntary effort, examples of folk and traditional building were salvaged in many countries and displayed in open-air (*Openlucht* or *Freilicht*) museums, the earliest example being the Skansen in Sweden (1897), followed by museums in Maihaugen, Norway; Seurasaari, Finland; Arnhem, Holland; and Lyngby, Denmark. Other policies of protection, such as in situ conservation, relocation, rebuilding, reconstruction, and environmental rehabilitation, were implemented, exemplified in the United States in Old Deerfield; Colonial Williamsburg; the Henry Ford Museum and Greenfield Village in Dearborn, Michigan; Old Sturbridge Village, Massachusetts; Cades Cove, Tennessee; and many other sites.

In Europe, the open-air-museum movement resulted in many thousands of buildings being saved and open to the public in literally hundreds of locations in Scandinavian and Central European countries. Only a few museums opened in Germany and Britain, and none, until the 1980s, opened in Spain, France, or Italy. Although such enterprises did much to conserve specific vernacular buildings, the unfurnished interiors could appear bleak. Many curators solved this problem by depicting a historic period with appropriate artifacts and furniture, or with reenactments of daily life in the form of dioramas. Such methods were instructive, if nostalgic, ensuring the popular success of these museums but associating the vernacular only with past ways of life, having little relevance to the present or the future.

Unfortunately, in most European countries, relatively little continuity of vernacular building was seen in the second half of the 20th century, as the imperative lessened and skills declined in the face of the expansion of the city suburbs and high-rise developments and the industrializing of building components and construction.

Globalization, it might seem, is incompatible with the vernacular, and traditional building of and by the people seems scarce. However, this is not the case. At the middle of the 20th century, the world's population was estimated at 3.5 billion; by the end of the century, the population had almost doubled to six billion. Attempts at urban housing schemes have failed to make a significant impression on the demand for dwellings, as the ever-expanding *bustees*, favelas, *barriadas, bidonvilles, gecekondu*, and other peri-urban squatter settlements in the industrially developing world dramatically demonstrate. Built of scrap materials and frequently illegal, they are the desperate measures taken by migrants to the cities; however, lacking in expression of skills or tradition and meeting no other needs beyond crude and minimal shelter, they are not vernacular.

Of the world's six billion people, a third live in the People's Republic of China, and another billion on the Indian subcontinent. In these countries, housing is mainly vernacular, as it is in Indonesia and Southeast Asia and in much of Africa. The

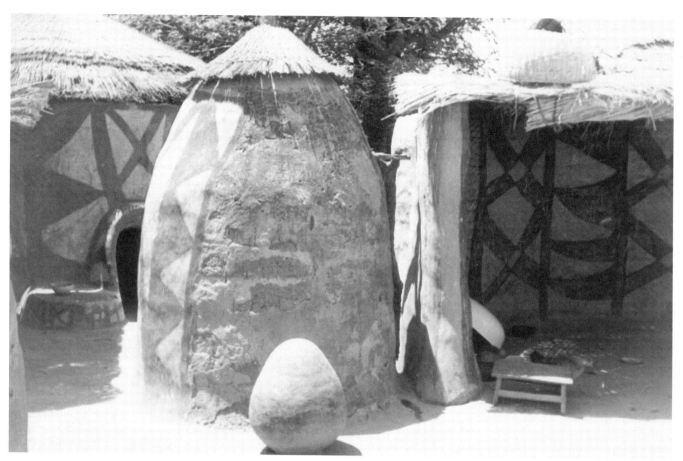

Earth-molded, nontrabeated structures, including granary, shade shelter, and living unit from
Gurunsi culture, northern Ghana
© Paul Oliver

growth in population has been accommodated largely through the absorption of families within existing unmodified structures and through the lateral or vertical extension of others. New building to traditional models has been not only of dwellings but also of innumerable stores, workshops, and religious buildings. It is unknown how many vernacular buildings are extant worldwide, whether old and still in use or of recent date and purpose built. Estimates (that might well be conservative) of around 800 million are cited, representing over 90 percent of the total building stock.

To a great extent, these vernacular traditions have been overlooked by architects and architectural historians. Those histories that acknowledge that architecture is not solely a European and American phenomenon pay attention principally to monumental temples, pagodas, mosques, and palaces, with some reference to colonial or administrative buildings, commercial structures, airports, and stadiums in the International Style of the 20th century. Lack of recognition has served as a disincentive to do original research in vernacular architecture; this was left to the enthusiasm of concerned architects and the personal motivations of devoted amateurs.

Serious recording of vernacular buildings was undertaken in Germany in the late 19th century, in the 1900s by English architects, and more widely in Europe and the United States with the growth of the open-air museums. American research was boosted in the 1930s by the Historic American Buildings Survey (HABS), and subsequently, in France, Portugal, and Romania, intensive national surveys were undertaken, recording the state of the vernacular on a provincial basis. Later, such surveys were conducted in Europe, although often only with institutional support. Methodologically, they followed conventional architectural practices, with plans, elevations, sections, and details being drawn, often with supporting photographic record and sometimes with historical documentation. Frequently, as in France and the United States, a typological approach was taken, although the concept of "type" was for some the identification of function and for others the classification of features, such as plan or roof form.

As early as 1882, British architect W. Simpson published a report on the architecture of the Himalayas, prompting regional officials of the Western colonial powers to occasionally examine the indigenous buildings in their territories. Lacking any agreed program, objectives, or coordination of research, such studies varied greatly in quality and method and were widely dispersed. A concerted study of the vernacular traditions of French Cameroun by architectural students of the École des Beaux-Arts,

published in 1952, marked a significant advance in research in non-Western countries. Preparation of materials, building construction methods, and domestic space use were examined and recorded. Preoccupations with typologies or historic derivation were shown to be largely irrelevant in such contexts, where the respective economies, material resources, and available technologies were important in the determination of their building forms.

In the ensuing years, a number of important studies were made of specific vernacular traditions in parts of Asia, sub-Saharan Africa, the Middle East, North America, and to a lesser extent, Latin America. Often these were local, and researchers had problems developing appropriate methods for comparative studies. Historical resources such as wills, deeds, or parish records used in European research were seldom available, and conventional orthographic techniques were unsuitable for recording cave dwellings, tents, or molded, nontrabeated structures. Comparison of building traditions or the identification of the distribution or diffusion of structural systems or details was hindered by lacunae in research and the lack of comprehensive reference works. Many former studies, although useful in indicating constancy or change in buildings, were superficial visual records. Researchers encountered techniques of, for example, earth construction, which previously had not been subject to scrutiny; craft skills in the working of different kinds of stone, timbers, palms, and fibrous plant materials involved tools and methods of assembly, jointing, and cladding that were largely unclassified or undocumented.

Classification of building forms seemed necessary so that the vast range of vernacular structures could be comprehended. From the domes of the Zulu (southern Africa) to the ring-walled multiple dwellings of the Keijia (southeastern China), they demonstrated both the persistence of systems transmitted over generations and the variety to be found within every tradition. Although the fundamental rectangular prism of trabeated structures and mass-walled stone and adobe and brick structures was widespread, so too were the *rondavels*, or cylindrical units, whose diversity was evident in their compound clusters. Roof forms displayed even greater variety, with gabled, hipped, and half-hipped roofs of diverse pitches evident throughout Europe, from Scotland to Moldavia. Upswept gables that were dispersed throughout insular Southeast Asia, from the Batak of Sumatra to the great saddle roofs of the Toraja of Celebes, were perceived as characteristic of indigenous "styles."

Although the technical problems were not inconsiderable, vernacular studies revealed indigenous methods of climate modification, such as the Egyptian *mashrabiyah*, or balconied window screens, and the "wind scoops," found in hot, arid climates in the Middle East, that transmit cool air to rooms. Hot and humid or monsoon climates require cross ventilation and protection from seasonal precipitation, whereas hurricanes necessitate shallow roof pitches and light construction. In temperate climates, protection is required against heavy rainfall and strong winds, whereas insulation and safeguards against snow loading are necessary in cold conditions. Such means of adaptation led to theories of climatic determinism, with broad principles being defined for settlement forms and building types in certain environments, including desert, savanna, forest, coastal, and insular locations. Exceptions arising from the demands of different economies, whether nomadic or sedentary, pastoral or agricultural, empha-

sized, as Forde had done in the 1930s, the relationship among society, economy, and habitat.

The publication in 1969 of *House Form and Culture* by Amos Rapoport and of the edited collection of case studies *Shelter and Society* marked a new stage in vernacular studies. Although anthropologists such as Lewis H. Morgan and Victor Mindeleff in their researches among Native American tribes in the 1880s had demonstrated the significance of culture in defining building form, their work had been neglected. Now the cultural and anthropological aspects of building were given as much attention as their structural and architectural characteristics. The writings of anthropologists such as Griaule on the Dogon (Mali) and Bourdier on the Kabyle (Algeria), among many others, revealed the importance of kinship, social structures, belief systems, ritual, and symbolism in the vernacular architecture of cultures the world over. Features formerly regarded as styles were now revealed as signifiers of values and expressions of collective identity and were elucidated in, for example, the work of Hugh-Jones (Amazonia), Nabokov and Easton (Native America), and Bourdier and Minh-ha (West Africa).

Anthropologists brought a cultural awareness to the study of vernacular but were seldom familiar with building principles and processes. The need for interdisciplinary dialogue and research inspired in the 1980s the biennial "Built Form and Culture Research" conferences alternating with those of the International Association for the Study of Traditional Environments (IASTE). Both emanated from the United States, but IASTE meetings were also held in Europe and North Africa. Both published proceedings, and books on local vernacular architecture proliferated. Some of these were written by non-Western authors, with the publications of the Aga Khan Award for Architecture (AKAA) providing a forum for Islamic and development studies.

For some years, there had been a growing awareness of the vernacular on the part of architects in the Middle East and Asia. Several endeavored to relate their buildings to local traditions, notably the Egyptian architect Hassan Fathy, whose village of New Gourna in West Luxor used the vault construction skills of Sudanese mud builders. In Turkey, Sedad Hakkí Eldem interpreted traditional models. More widely recognized was the work of the Indian architects Charles Correa and Balkrishna Doshi, whose large-scale projects were modernist in approach but who also designed more modest projects compatible with the local vernacular. Geoffrey Bawa in Sri Lanka, Robi Sularto in Indonesia, and Andre Ravereau in Africa were among the architects who respected regional traditions.

Despite the extent of research, the lack of informed awareness among architects and their clients, whether public or private, of the significance of vernacular traditions has led to disparagement, disregard, and often demolition. By the late 1980s, the need for a comprehensive reference work that could inform both anthropologists and architects and professionals and politicians became increasingly apparent. A ten-year project led eventually to the publication in 1997 of the *Encyclopedia of Vernacular Architecture of the World*, to which researchers from more than 80 countries contributed. Organized on a cultural rather than a national basis, it was unprecedented in bringing together research on the vernacular architecture and its cultural contexts extant on all continents in the 20th century. Principles of building with available resources, the nature of craft skills, environmental conditions and responses, and economies and their bear-

ing on building functions, meaning, symbolism, and motifs are considered in relation to societal systems and building needs. However, attention is drawn to the deficiencies of certain vernacular traditions with regard to services, sanitation, and health.

Much remains to be done, but the question of why such work should be undertaken and acted on must be addressed. Vernacular architecture not only accounted for the vast majority of all buildings up to the 1950s but also met immense housing demands as the world population doubled in the second half of the 20th century. Yet this achievement has never been measured, and neither has the effort in human endeavor or the use of available or renewable resources in building or land. By comparison, officially sanctioned housing, whether government promoted or commercially developed, is minimal in its effect and produced at costs that would be beyond the capacity of most national economies in attempting to meet the demands of the next half century. Although neither acknowledged nor budgeted, vernacular architecture will be essential to meet the housing needs of the projected further doubling of the population. Recognizing this and providing adequate support in services while planning the economic survival of rural communities, developing nations could ensure that appropriate housing can be achieved through vernacular means, as it has been in the past.

PAUL OLIVER

Further Reading

A comprehensive classified bibliography with over 9000 entries is to be found in Oliver 1997; this work covers theories and principles of vernacular architecture and details of publications on regional traditions in all parts of the world. Selected bibliographies are to be found in many of the following works.

Beguin, Jean-Pierre, *L'Habitat au Cameroun: Présentation des principaux types d'habitat*, Paris: Éditions de l'Union Française, 1952

Blier, Suzanne Preston, *The Anatomy of Architecture: Ontology and Metaphor in Batammaliba Architectural Expression*, Cambridge and New York: Cambridge University Press, 1987

Bourdier, Jean-Paul, and Nezar Al-Sayyad (editors), *Dwellings, Settlements, and Tradition: Cross-Cultural Perspectives*, Lanham, Maryland: University Press of America, 1989

Bourdier, Jean-Paul, and Minh-ha Trinh, *Drawn from African Dwellings*, Bloomington: Indiana University Press, 1996

Brunskill, R.W., *Illustrated Handbook of Vernacular Architecture*, London: Faber, 1970; New York: Universe Books, 1971; 4th edition, London: Faber, 2000

Le Corbusier, *Le Voyage d'Orient*, Paris: Éditions Forces Vives, 1966; as *Journey to the East*, edited and translated by Ivan Zaknic, Cambridge, Massachusetts: MIT Press, 1987

Damluji, Salma Samar, *The Valley of Mud Brick Architecture: Shibam, Tarim, and Wadi Hadramut*, Reading, Berkshire: Garnet, 1992

Forde, Cyril Darryl, *Habitat, Economy, and Society*, New York: Harcourt Brace, and London: Methuen, 1934; fifth edition, New York: Dutton, and London: Methuen, 1956

Glassie, Henry H., *Folk Housing in Middle Virginia: A Structural Analysis of Historic Artifacts*, Knoxville: University of Tennessee Press, 1975

Griaule, Marcel, *Dieu d'eau: Entretiens avec Ogotemmêli*, Paris: Éditions du Chêne, 1948; new edition, Paris: Fayard, 1975; as *Conversations with Ogotemmeli: An Introduction to Dogon Religious Ideas*, London: Oxford University Press, 1965; New York: Oxford University Press, 1970

Guidoni, Enrico, *Architettura primitiva*, Milan: Electa, 1975; as *Primitive Architecture*, New York: Abrams, 1978; London: Faber, 1979

Gutheim, Frederick (editor), *Frank Lloyd Wright on Architecture: Selected Writings, 1894–1940*, New York: Duell Sloan and Pearce, 1941

Hugh-Jones, Christine, *From the Milk River: Spatial and Temporal Processes in Northwest Amazonia*, Cambridge and New York: Cambridge University Press, 1979

Mindeleff, Victor, *A Study of Pueblo Architecture in Tusayan and Cibola*, Washington, D.C.: Smithsonian Institution Press, 1891; reprint, 1989

Morgan, Lewis Henry, *Houses and House-Life of the American Aborigines*, Washington, D.C.: Government Printing Office, 1881; reprint, Chicago: University of Chicago Press, 1985

Nabokov, Peter, and Robert Easton, *Native American Architecture*, New York: Oxford University Press, 1989

Oliver, Paul, *Dwellings: The House across the World*, Oxford: Phaidon, and Austin: University of Texas Press, 1987

Oliver, Paul (editor), *Shelter and Society*, London: Barrie and Rockliff the Cresset P., and New York: Praeger, 1969

Oliver, Paul (editor), *The Encyclopedia of Vernacular Architecture of the World*, 3 vols., Cambridge and New York: Cambridge University Press, 1997

Prussin, Labelle (editor), *African Nomadic Architecture: Space, Place, and Gender*, Washington D.C.: Smithsonian Institution Press, 1995

Rapoport, Amos, *House Form and Culture*, Englewood Cliffs, New Jersey: Prentice-Hall, 1969

Rudofsky, Bernard, *Architecture without Architects: A Short Introduction to Non-Pedigreed Architecture*, New York: Museum of Modern Art, and London: Academy Editions, 1964

Turan, Meta (editor), *Vernacular Architecture: Paradigms of Environmental Response*, Aldershot, Berkshire, and Brookfield, Vermont: Avebury, 1990

Upton, Dell, and John Michael Vlach (editors), *Common Places: Readings in American Vernacular Architecture*, Athens: University of Georgia Press, 1986

Waterson, Roxana, *The Living House: An Anthropology of Architecture in South-East Asia*, Singapore, Oxford, and New York: Oxford University Press, 1990

VESNIN, ALEXANDER, LEONID VESNIN, AND VIKTOR VESNIN

Architects, Russia

Among the many architects whose work adhered to the principles of Constructivism, perhaps the most stalwart and productive proponents of the movement were the Vesnin brothers: Leonid (1880–1933), Viktor (1882–1950), and Alexander (1883–1959), all of whom were raised in the town of Iurevets on the Volga River.

Although the brothers went to St. Petersburg at the beginning of the century for their professional education (Leonid graduated from the architectural program at the Academy of Arts in 1909 and Viktor and Alexander from the Institute of Civil Engineering in 1912), their careers were largely connected with Moscow both before and after their graduation. For example, in 1905–07 they worked as assistants to such leading Moscow proponents of the neoclassical revival as Ilarion Ivanov-Schitz and Roman Klein, and in 1909 Leonid worked with the artist V. A. Simonov

in designing a large Arts and Crafts–style house for V. A. Nosen-kov in the Moscow suburbs. Alexander, the most artistically gifted of the three, worked in Vladimir Tatlin's studio between 1912 and 1914 and also revealed a considerable talent as a stage designer.

During the material restrictions of the early postrevolutionary years, the theater stage provided the Vesnins—Alexander in particular—with a means for exploring methods of dynamic construction in space, under the obvious influence of Tatlin. The most remarkable product of this phase was Alexander Vesnin's set design in 1922 for Alexander Tairov's production of *The Man Who Was Thursday* at the Moscow Chamber (Kamernyi) Theater. With its intersecting planes and ramps, the set not only emphasized the dynamic of the actors' motion but also bridged the gap between the theoretical constructions of artists such as El Lissitzky, Kazimir Malevich, and Antoine Pevsner and the practical design of large structures.

The Vesnins' progression from dynamic, avant-garde set constructions to the much larger scale of major architectural projects was soon evident in their 1923 design for the Palace of Labor competition. Although their submission was awarded only third prize, it served as a programmatic statement in the development of a Constructivist aesthetic, combining both monumentality and severe functionalism in the massing of simple geometric shapes in a complex balance. The center of the plan was the oval meeting hall in the form of an amphitheater, 75 by 67 meters in size. The array of radio masts and docking ports for airships around the top was functionally justified despite its futuristic appearance in the context of a war-ravaged country reestablishing a modicum of civilized existence.

In 1925 Alexander and Viktor Vesnin, together with Moisei Ginzburg, founded the Constructivist organization OSA (Organization of Contemporary Architecture). Indeed, the preceding year Alexander had designed the book jacket for Ginzburg's programmatic work *Style and Epoch*. With the quickening tempo of state construction during the late 1920s, all three brothers were actively engaged in projects extending from the Caucasus to the colossal hydroelectric dam across the Dnieper River, the DneproGES, designed by Viktor Vesnin in collaboration with Nikolai Kolli and others. Although each brother maintained a separate, distinct practice, they are best known for the projects they did together.

The brief flourishing of private commerce toward the end of the New Economic Policy (NEP) period is represented in the Vesnins' design of the Mostorg retail department store (1927–29) in central Moscow. Located on an awkward trapezoidal lot in the Krasnaia Presnia working-class district, the store, with its double-glazed facade framed by a ferroconcrete structure, appeared strikingly modern when first constructed in its context of 19th-century brick buildings. It has since suffered by the addition of another story and by a lack of proper maintenance.

Like other major architects of the late 1920s, the Vesnins were much concerned with the creation of institutions for social communication. One of the most modernistic of such designs—and one of the last Constructivist buildings in Moscow—was the club for the Society of Tsarist Political Prisoners, begun in 1931. In addition to meeting rooms and a theater hall, the extensive complex was to contain a museum. In 1934, however, the society was disbanded (an ominous prelude to the Stalinist purges, which would create an altogether new society of political

prisoners), and the larger plans for a museum were eliminated. Even in this truncated and deformed version, the harmony of the pure, undecorated volumetric forms is evident and reflects, if coincidentally, some of the oldest formal traditions in Russian architecture.

The culminating project in the Vesnins' Constructivist oeuvre was an outgrowth of the concept of the workers' club. In order to serve the social needs of the Proletarian district, which contained an automobile factory and workers' settlement in southeast Moscow, the Vesnins designed a large complex of three buildings. The site overlooked the Moscow River and was adjacent to the Simonov Monastery, part of whose walls were razed in the course of constructing the project. Yet the largest part of the ensemble, a theater with a circular hall designed to seat 4000, was never built, nor was the projected sports building. The central element, however—the club building itself—was built between 1931 and 1937. This period was marred by the death of Leonid in 1933 and by the brothers' increasing need to defend their Constructivist designs.

Nonetheless, the Vesnins persevered to a remarkable degree, bending to the system without rejecting the work that stood at the center of the Constructivist movement. In their writings it is clear that Viktor and Alexander Vesnin considered the Proletarian Region Club one of their most significant works, not only for its union of functions—a 1000-seat theater, ballroom, meeting halls, and exhibition space—but also for the way in which form followed function and space flowed effortlessly from one component to another.

The manner in which the design combined an acute aesthetic sensibility with function was particularly important at a time when Constructivism was under attack for its purported inability to recognize the people's aesthetic needs. In the club building, the Vesnins' fluency was reflected on the exterior in such details as the contours of the large rounded bay window over the entrance to the auditorium and a semicircular conservatory extending from the river facade. The club also included a small astronomy observatory, which created an additional visual component for the upper structure. Unfortunately, the interior of the building has been considerably modified since the Vesnins' original design, but the structure itself is still relatively well maintained.

In 1935 the Vesnin brothers attempted a reply to the growing retrospectivist tendency in Stalinist architecture by stating that "the canonization of an old form, however excellent, is a brake on the development of content." At the same time, Viktor and Alexander remained active in the architectural profession, were awarded high state honors, and participated in major competitions, such as the design for the People's Commissariat of Heavy Industry (unrealized). Although structural concepts of the classical revival with which they began their careers appeared in their later designs, they continued to reject the role of monumental painting and sculpture that became so prominent in architecture of the late Stalinist period. To the end they adhered to their belief in the integrity of structure as the determining principle in architectural design.

WILLIAM C. BRUMFIELD

See also **Constructivism; Ginzburg, Moisei (Russia); Monument to the Third International (1920); Russia and the Soviet Union**

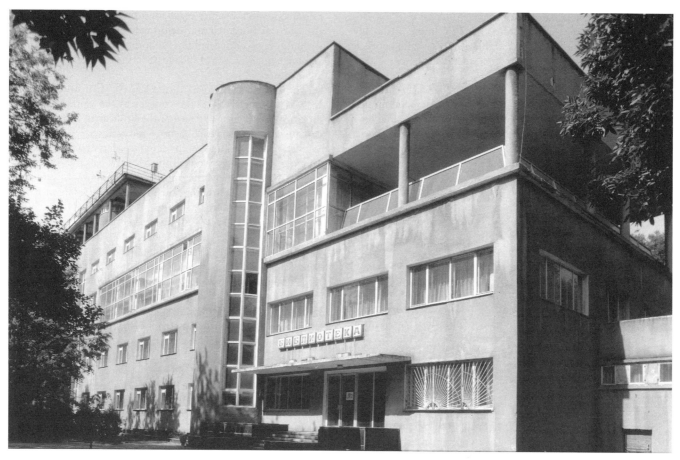

Proletarian Region Club (1937), Moscow, by Alexander, Leonid, and Viktor Vesnin
© William C. Brumfield

Biographies

Alexander Vesnin

Born in Iurevets, Russia, 16 May 1883. Attended the Institute of Civil Engineering, St. Petersburg, 1901–12; studied painting with Yan Tsionglinsky, St. Petersburg, and Konstantin Yuon, Moscow 1909–11; visited Italy and studied Palladio 1913–14. Assistant to Ilarion Ivanov-Schitz, Roman Klein, and O.R. Munts 1909–11; worked in Vladimir Tatlin's studio, The Tower 1912–13. Served in the Russian Army 1916–17. Became involved in stage design 1920; editor, with Moisei Ginzburg, *Sovremennaya arkhitektura* 1926–30; director, architecture studio of the Mussoviet, then the architecture studio of the Commissariat for Heavy Industry and Ministry of Petroleum 1933–35. Professor of painting, VKhUTEMAS, Moscow 1921–24; taught at the Institute of Architecture, Moscow 1930–36. Member, Inkhuk (Russian Institute of Artistic Culture) 1921; founded, with Ginzburg, OSA (Russian Union of Contemporary Architects) 1925; member, All Union Academy of Architecture 1933. Died in Moscow, 7 November 1959.

Leonid Vesnin

Born in Nizhni Novgorod, Russia, 10 December 1880. Studied at the Academy of Fine Arts, St. Petersburg 1901–09. Professor of architectural design, Moscow Higher Technical College. Member, OSA (Russian Union of Contemporary Architects); co-president, Moscow Association of Architects 1922. Received the Order of the Red Banner. Died in Moscow, 8 October 1933.

Viktor Vesnin

Born in Iurevets, Russia, 9 April 1882. Attended the Institute of Civil Engineering, St. Petersburg 1901–1912; visited Italy and studied Palladio 1913–14. Assistant to Ilarion Ivanov-Schitz, Roman Klein, and O.R. Munts 1909–11; director, architecture studio of the Mussoviet, then the architecture studio of the Commissariat for Heavy Industry and Ministry of Petroleum 1933–35. Taught at the Institute of Architecture, Moscow 1930–36. Secretary, Union of Soviet Architects 1937–49; first president, All Union Academy of Architecture 1939–49; member, OSA (Russian Union of Contemporary Architects). Received the Order of Lenin; Gold Medal, Royal Institute of British Architects 1945. Died in Moscow, 17 September 1950.

Alexander, Leonid, and Viktor Vesnin

Collaborated on numerous projects but never established a formal partnership; most active in the period between world wars.

Selected Works

Post Office, Myasnitskaya Street, Moscow, 1911
Sirotkin House, Nizhni Novgorod, 1915

Dynamo Stock Company, Moscow, 1917
Karl Marx Monument (destroyed), Red Square, Moscow, 1919
Palace of Labor (Third prize, competition), Moscow, 1923
Pravda Newspaper Building (unbuilt), Leningrad, 1924
Institute of Mineralogy, Moscow, 1925
Mostorg Department Store, Moscow, 1929
Dnieper Dam and Hydroelectric Station, 1930
Society of Tsarist Political Prisoners Club (incomplete), Moscow, 1934
Film Actors Club, Moscow, 1934
Palace of Culture, Moscow, 1937
Proletarian Region Club, Moscow, 1937

Further Reading

There are many publications in English on the Vesnins' work, most notably Khan-Magomedov's monumental study. A comprehensive Russian selection of their writings from 1922 to 1947 is contained in the Barkhin volume.

Barkhin, M.G., et al. (editors), *Mastera sovetskoi arkhitektury ob arkhitekture* (Masters of Soviet Architecture on Architecture), 2 vols., Moscow: Iskusstvo, 1975

Brumfield, William C., *The Origins of Modernism in Russian Architecture*, Berkeley: University of California Press, 1991

Cooke, Catherine, *Russian Avant-Garde: Theories of Art, Architecture, and the City*, London: Academy Editions, 1995

Ilin, Mikhail, *Vesniny*, Moscow: Izd-vo Akademii Nauk SSSR, 1960

Khan-Magomedov, S.O., *Alexandre Vesnine et le constructivisme russe*, Paris: Sers, 1986; as *Alexander Vesnin and Russian Constructivism*, New York: Rizzoli, and London: Lund Humphries, 1986

Lodder, Christina, *Russian Constructivism*, New Haven, Connecticut: Yale University Press, 1983; third edition, 1987

Riabushin, A.V., and N.I. Smolina, *Landmarks of Soviet Architecture, 1917–1991*, New York: Rizzoli, 1992

Zemtsov, S.M. (editor), *Zodchie Moskvy* (Architects of Moscow), 2 vols., Moscow: Moskovskii Rabochii, 1981–88

VIDHAN BHAVAN (STATE ASSEMBLY BHOPAL)

Designed by Charles Correa, completed 1986
Bhopal, India

The Vidhan Bhavan (1980–86), designed by Charles Correa, sits on a crest that offers magnificent views of the city of Bhopal, the capital of the state of Madhya Pradesh. It houses the state assembly (the lower house with 366 members, the upper house with 75), the offices of the chief minister and other ministers of the cabinet, the speaker, the chief secretary, various committee rooms, and rooms for the supporting staff.

The design is conceived in terms of the circular fortified enclosure within which are housed various buildings that can be accessed from three directions. The formal organization of this complex follows a nine-part layout that the architect attributes to the mandala diagram. Each of the nine parts is distinct, partly because of the function that each section houses and partly because of the iconographic scheme. For example, the Vidhan Sabha (Lower House) is located at the southwest corner within the form of a stupa, representing the stupa at Sanchi, a major architectural monument in the state. The focus of movement is invested in the two axes, whereas the places of congregation—the "Combined Hall," the Vidhan Sabha, the Vidhan Parishad

(Upper House), and the library—are located at the four outer corners. The three main entrances are situated on the two axes, with the legislators' entrance and the VIP entrance for the speaker opposite each other and the public entrance on the southwest axis.

The legislative axis takes one from the legislators' entrance through the foyer and central hall and ends at the legislators' foyer adjacent to the VIP entrance. The Vidhan Sabha and Vidhan Parishad sit on either side at the end. In contrast to this axis, if one follows the more dominant axis of movement, which is supposed to be for public entrance, it seems to have more of a symbolic aspect incorporated into the sequence of movement. It can be compared to the Indian temple, wherein the most sacred element is situated at the very end of the axis—in this case, the cabinet room and the chief minister's office. The architect engages with the images associated with land and water and reverses the traditionally received conceptions along this axis. Here the entrance area is paved in a pattern of waves and has the map of the state on one side, which marks the water body. This entrance plaza leads to the court of the people, which is in the form of a traditional *kund* (water tank). The images associated with the sea are repeatedly employed within the complex, such as the conchlike shapes for the combined hall and the undulating wavelike form for the roofs.

The uniqueness of the project is its use of mythical and historic symbols not only in its organizational scheme but also in its decorative scheme, although the manner in which these symbols are employed in both cases is strictly figurative. The use of folk art in the murals and other artwork in this complex contributes to the revival of traditional art and motifs without an excessive feeling of pastiche. The large murals covering the walls around the *kund* (painted by the finest folk artists of the Bastar region), sculptures such as the green-marbled sculpture of the Goddess of the Narmada River floating above the reflecting pool, and paintings and other artwork found throughout the building are distinct examples of the rich artistic traditions of the state. At the same time, the building is replete with iconic elements, such as the gateway of the Sanchi stupa, which is replicated at the entrance of the Vidhan Sabha.

Although the building has a monumental character, because of the use of a fortified citadel-like enclosure, the architect manages to break down the feeling of a monolithic whole by the use of a series of courtyards, pathways, and halls, thereby creating the feeling of a city within a city. Formally expressed as a unified assembly building, the complex is not so much of the country as it is of the diverse nature of the state of Madhya Pradesh through the use of iconographic elements that are supposed to be emblematic of different aspects of the state.

This project received the Aga Khan Award in 1998 and has been commended by critics for its "heroic scale," "the wide range of spatial experiences that it offers," and its "use of mythical and historical symbols." Although much has been written about the "ritualistic pathway" and the building's being a veritable temple to democracy, the success of these aspects of the building might be overstated. The complex can be seen as one more exploration of what has often been referred to as the "architecture of horizontal planes—of roofs and platforms, open colonnades, verandahs and courtyards," a characteristic seen in a chain of other projects by Correa, such as Bharat Bhavan, the Crafts Museum, and

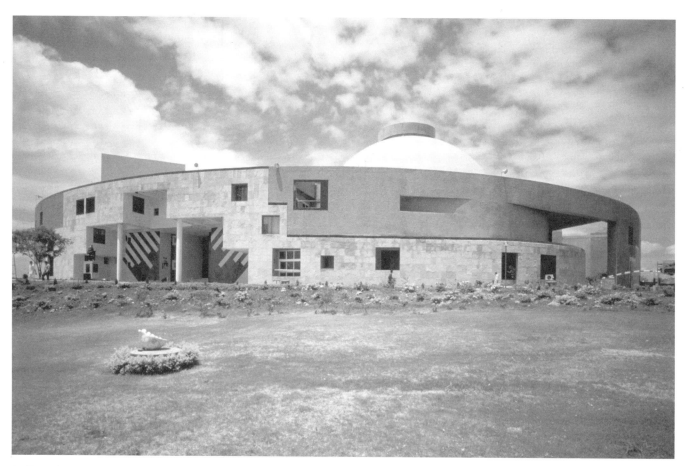

Vidhan Bhavan (State Assembly), Bhopal, India, designed by Charles Mark Correa
© Aga Khan Award for Architecture

especially Jawahar Kala Kendra, which is also organized in a nine-square mandala.

AARATI KANEKAR

See also **Correa, Charles Mark (India); India**

Further Reading

Campbell, Robert, "The Aga Khan Award: Honoring Substance over Style," *Architectural Record*, 186/11 (November 1998)

Charles Correa, Singapore: Concept Media, 1984; revised edition, by Hasan-Uddin Khan, Singapore: Concept Media, and New York: Aperture, 1987

Correa, Charles, and Kenneth Frampton, *Charles Correa*, London: Thames and Hudson, 1996

Davidson, Cynthia (editor), *Legacies for the Future: Contemporary Architecture in Islamic Societies*, London: Thames and Hudson, 1998

Digby-Jones, Penelope, "State of Assembly," *Architecture Review*, 202/1206 (August 1997)

Sorkin, Michael, "The Borders of Islamic Architecture," *Metropolis*, 18/4 (December 1998)

VIENNA SECESSION

The Vienna Secession has attained such an exalted role in the saga of early modern architecture and design that its origins as a society composed mostly of easel painters has been almost forgotten. Like the Munich and Berlin Secessions, which were also formed in the 1890s, the organization—whose official title was the Vereinigung Bildender Künstler Österreichs (Secession) (Association of Austrian Fine Artists [Secession])—was born of a revolt against the artistic establishment, but its objectives were initially as much commercial as ideological. However, it soon emerged at the forefront of the efforts to reform art and architecture, and until the split of the Klimt faction in 1905, it became virtually synonymous with the Vienna Moderne.

The target of the young *revoltés* in Vienna was the Künstlergenossenschaft (Artists' Association), or as it was more commonly known, the Künstlerhaus, a private artists' alliance that, in the absence of a well-developed gallery system, exercised nearly complete control of exhibitions and sales of art. The proximate cause of the rebellion was the reelection of the archconservative Eugen Felix to the presidency of the Künstlerhaus in November 1896. Many of the more radical members, including the painters Josef Engelhart, Carl Moll, and Gustav Klimt and the young architect Joseph Maria Olbrich, already angered by the treatment of impressionists and plein air painters, formed a new, alternate exhibiting society at the beginning of April 1897, and in late May, Klimt and 12 others artists formally resigned from the Künstlerhaus. They were eventually joined by many of the city's

other progressive artists, designers, and architects, including Josef Hoffmann and, in November 1899, Otto Wagner.

From the start, the Secession espoused no single artistic philosophy or style. What united its members instead was a shared rejection of historical realism in painting and revivalism in architecture, and although the Secessionist movement subsequently became closely associated with the Austrian Art Nouveau or Jugendstil (or, as it was often referred to at the time, the Secessionsstil), the association's membership represented a wide array of modernist influences and ideas, from naturalism and impressionism to Art Nouveau and protofunctionalism. The Secession also brought together artists working in a variety of media: painters, sculptors, graphic artists, typographers, and designers, as well as architects. The aims of the group were similarly broad. The formation of the Secession developed, as Klimt expressed in a protest letter to the leadership of the Künstlerhaus,

> out of a recognition of the necessity of bringing artistic life in Vienna into more lively contact with the continuing development of art abroad, and of putting exhibitions on a purely artistic footing, free from any commercial considerations; of thereby awakening in wider circles a purified, modern view of art; and lastly, of inducing a heightened concern for art in official circles. (quoted in Vergo, 1975)

To realize these aspirations, the Secessionists launched their own journal, *Ver Sacrum* (Sacred Spring), in 1898. The title of the journal was drawn from the Roman ritual of consecration of youth in times of national peril, a reflection of the Secessionists' goal of aesthetic and cultural regeneration. Lavishly produced in its early years, *Ver Sacrum* encapsulated the desire of the Secessionists not only to elevate the standards of Austrian artistic production and to embrace the new but also to bring together all the arts. In addition to reproductions of paintings, drawings, graphic design, and architecture, the journal featured music, poetry, and essays by leading Austrian and foreign modernists.

Even more central to this program was the series of exhibitions that the Secessionists organized just before and after the turn of the century. The first of these exhibitions opened in late March 1898. It featured, along with works by the Austrian members of the association, paintings, lithographs, and drawings by Fernand Khnopff, Alphonse Mucha, Auguste Rodin, Giovanni Segantini, James McNeill Whistler, and others. The responsibility for the design and arrangement of the exhibition (held in rented rooms of the Horticultural Society Building on the Parkring) was accorded to Hoffmann and Olbrich, who also outfitted a "*Ver Sacrum* room," the first of a series of spaces combining the newest ideas in the applied arts and interior design. The inaugural exhibition proved to be a huge financial success (despite Klimt and his colleagues' vociferous disavowal of the rampant commercialism of the Künstlerhaus), but it also underscored the need for a permanent exhibition hall. Through various connections with the Vienna city government, the Secessionists succeeded in securing a long-term lease on a parcel of land on the Karlplatz adjacent to the Academy of Fine Arts, and the task of designing the new building was given over to Olbrich.

Olbrich's gallery, which was completed in time for the second exhibition in November 1898, has become the most recognized architectural symbol of the Secession. Emblazoned over its portal are the words of the critic and supporter of the Secession Ludwig

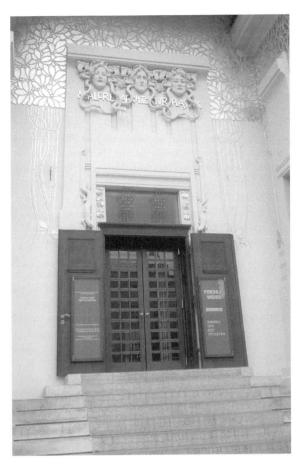

Secession House, detail of door, designed by J.M. Olbrich
© Howard Davis/GreatBuildings.com

Hevesi: "Der Zeit ihre Kunst, der Kunst ihre Freiheit" (To Every Age Its Art, to Art Its Freedom). It was the building's golden dome—an open, gilded ironwork sphere of laurel leaves and berries—however, that drew the immediate attention, as well as the sarcasm, of the Viennese public, who mockingly christened it "the golden cabbage" and "the Mahdi's tomb." However, the revolutionary nature of Olbrich's creation extended beyond its gleaming dome, chaste white walls, and sinuous vegetal graffiti. By relying on a light steel truss and glass roofing system supported by thin columns, Olbrich provided a remarkably open and adaptable space, one that suited perfectly the Secession's ambitious and varied exhibition program.

The second exhibition, like its predecessor, again featured easel art by Viennese and foreign artists. A large area, however, was given over to a group of architectural drawings by Otto Wagner and his students, and an entire room was devoted to a display of applied arts by Olbrich, Hoffmann, Koloman Moser, and others. The emphasis on architecture and the applied arts reflected a conviction within most of the Secession's confraternity of a changing relationship of art and design. Painting and sculpture—previously regarded as a higher form of artistic work—were now displayed on an equal basis with furniture, metal- and glasswork, textiles, and graphic design. Although this trend was evident in avant-garde circles throughout Europe, in

Vienna the striving toward a unification of the arts was even more pronounced, and it accounted for the special character of many of the Secession's subsequent exhibits.

The idea of the *Gesamtkunstwerk*, or total work of art, reached its apotheosis in the 14th exhibition, held from April to June 1902. It featured a single work, a statue of a seated Beethoven by Leipzig artist Max Klinger, which was placed on a carefully framed platform at the far end of the gallery. Surrounding it were murals by Klimt, Roller, and others. Klimt's Beethoven frieze, recently permanently reinstalled in the Secession Building, constituted a visual representation of ideas of the music and ideas of Beethoven's music—perhaps, as some historians have argued, the final, choral movement of Beethoven's Ninth Symphony, which was performed at the exhibit's opening. The installation also included an abstract relief by Hoffmann, one that likewise merged the newest ideas in painting and the decorative arts.

Many of the Secession's early exhibitions also included the works of some of the foremost modernist designers in Europe. The eighth exhibition presented objects by Charles Robert Ashbee, Henri van de Velde, and Charles Rennie Mackintosh and his wife, Margaret Macdonald. Later exhibitions introduced many of the leading young designers in Vienna, among them Joze Plecnik, Robert Örley, and Leopold Bauer.

Before 1901, both the exhibition designs and most of the objects on display evinced the swirling forms of the early, curvilinear Jugendstil. However, by 1901 there was a decided trend toward a new rectilinearity and reductivism in design. This transformation was most evident in the works of Hoffmann and Moser, who together forged what became the emblematic form language of the Secession, a modular, geometricized vocabulary that anticipated the later emergence of functionalism. The era of the geometric Jugendstil in the Secession proved to be short-lived, however. In 1903, Hoffmann and Moser founded their own artists' collective, the Wiener Werkstätte, and they increasingly devoted their time and efforts to its operation. Many of the exhibitions after 1903 also failed to match the quality and inventiveness of the Secession's early years. Among the few significant later exhibitions was the 23rd, which included Wagner's projects for the Steinhof Church and his ill-starred Stadtmuseum.

The decline in standards was in part the result of a growing rift within the Secession that began to manifest itself around 1904. The split was a consequence largely of differing views in the membership over the relative roles of painting and applied arts. Many of the pure painters (*Nur-Maler*) resented the privileged role of Hoffmann and the other *Raumkünstler* (decorative artists), charging that architecture and design were being promoted at the expense of easel art. The Secession had broken into two opposing camps: the Klimt-Gruppe, which included Hoffmann, Moser, Wagner, and most of the other architects and designers, and the pure painters, led by Josef Engelhart. For a time, the two groups continued to coexist, but in 1905 Klimt and most of the other prominent artists, architects, and designers resigned over an argument concerning the Klimt faction's affiliation with a local gallery, leaving the more traditional painters in control. Although the Secession survived as an organization and continued to mount exhibitions, it ceased to be a driving force in Austrian art.

During its heyday, the Vienna Secession provided a vibrant forum for the city's avant-garde to explore the newest currents in art, architecture, and design. For a time, the union succeeded brilliantly in achieving its goals of elevating the standards of Austrian art, establishing contacts abroad, and promoting modernism. However, the Secessionists failed in their bid to win full government support, a situation that would have fateful consequences for Wagner, Klimt, and many of the other progressive members. The position of the Secession in the larger history of modernism is also an ambiguous one. Although Hoffmann, Moser, Olbrich, and the other applied artists were able to foster an extraordinary new design direction, their reliance on traditional craft and deluxe materials ensured that most of the Secession's products would remain inaccessible to a broad spectrum of society. In the end, the growing reliance on industrial production and mass marketing would render their achievements more and more irrelevant. The *Gesamtkunstwerk* ideal of the complete aestheticization of life proved to be unsustainable.

CHRISTOPHER LONG

See also **Art Nouveau (Jugendstil); Ashbee, C. R. (Great Britain); Hoffmann, Josef (Austria); Mackintosh, Charles Rennie (Scotland); Olbrich, Josef Maria (Austria); van de Velde, Henri (Belgium); Wagner, Otto (Austria)**

Further Reading

Ankwicz von Kleehoven 1960, Vergo 1975, and Schorske 1980 provide good brief descriptions of the early years of the Vienna Secession. The most complete account is in Bisanz-Prakken 1999. On the Secession Building itself, see Clark 1967 and Vereinigung Bildender Künstler Wiener Secession, *Die Wiener Secession* 1986, vol. 1. For a discussion of the various exhibition designs see Forsthuber 1991.

Ankwicz von Kleehoven, "Die Anfänge der Wiener Secession," *Alte und moderne Kunst*, 5/6–7 (1960)

Bahr, Hermann, *Secession*, Vienna: L. Rosner, 1900

Bahr, Hermann, *Gegen Klimt*, Vienna: J. Eisenstein, 1903

Bisanz-Prakken, Marian, *Heiliger Frühling. Gustav Klimt und die Anfänge der Wiener Secession, 1895–1905*, Vienna: Albertina/ Christian Brandstätter, 1999

Bubnova, Jaroslava, and Robert Fleck (editors), *Vienna Secession 1898–1998: The Century of Artistic Freedom*, Munich and New York: Prestel, 1998

Clark, Robert Judson, "Olbrich and Vienna," *Kunst in Hessen und am Mittelrhein*, 7 (1967)

Forsthuber, Sabine, *Moderne Raumkunst. Wiener Ausstellungsbauten von 1898 bis 1914*, Vienna: Picus, 1991

Hevesi, Ludwig, *Acht Jahre Secession (März 1897–Juni 1905): Kritik, Polemik, Chronik*, Vienna: Carl Konegen, 1906

Hevesi, Ludwig, *Altkunst—Neukunst—Wien 1894–1908*, Vienna: Carl Konegen, 1909

Nebehay, Christian M. *Ver Sacrum, 1898–1903*, New York: Rizzoli, 1977

Neuwirth, Walter Maria, "Die sieben heroischen Jahre der Wiener Moderne," *Alte und moderne Kunst*, 9/5–6 (1964)

Schorske, Carl E., *Fin-de-siècle Vienna: Politics and Culture*, New York: Knopf, 1980

Shedel, James, *Art and Society: The New Art Movement in Vienna, 1897–1914*, Palo Alto, California: Society for the Promotion of Science, 1981

Varnedoe, Kirk, *Vienna 1900: Art, Architecture, Design* (exhib. cat.), New York: Museum of Modern Art, 1986

Vereinigung Bildender Künstler Wiener Secession, *Die Wiener Secession*, 2 vols., Vienna: Böhlau, 1986

Vergo, Peter, *Art in Vienna, 1898–1918: Klimt, Kokoschka, Schiele, and Their Contemporaries*, London: Phaidon, 1975

Waissenberger, Robert, *Die Wiener Secession*, Vienna: Jugend und Volk, 1971; English edition, *Vienna Secession*, London: Academy, 1977

VIETNAM VETERANS MEMORIAL, WASHINGTON, D.C.

Designed by Maya Lin; completed 1982

From the time of its dedication in 1982, the Vietnam Veterans Memorial in Washington, D.C., has enjoyed a rare combination of both critical and popular acclaim. Perennially one of the most visited sites in the nation's capital, the landscape-and-earthworks construction was the competition-winning design of then-21-year-old Yale University student Maya Ying Lin. On completion the work was also one of the most controversial public landscapes ever executed in the United States. Lin's design was attacked by various conservative cultural and political audiences offended by the memorial's rejection of the officially sponsored neoclassical language of white monuments conventional to the Mall. Despite that vocal minority opinion, the lucid minimal design garnered critical praise as a rare example of the highest quality of public work.

The power of Lin's design resides, at least in part, in its inversion of conventional expectations for memorials on the Mall. In lieu of representing the state-sanctioned official history of U.S. involvement in Vietnam, the Wall (as it came to be known) was conceived and designed as an "open work" intended to be read in multiple ways by diverse audiences. Each participant is capable of reading the Wall's contents relative to the particulars and specifics of his or her own unique experience. Rather than objectifying the state's powerful interest in recording a received history of the war, the Vietnam Veterans Memorial was conceived, financed, and constructed as a memorial by and for the public rather than its government.

Lin's conception encompasses two black, granite-faced retaining walls cut into a mound of earth known as Constitution Gardens. The two sloping wall segments intersect at their highest point, forming an interior angle of 120 degrees, whereas the lower ends are axially aligned with the larger site beyond, effectively grounding the work's geometry in the broader landscape. On the reflective surface of the black stone panels, the names of each of the 58,000 U.S. personnel missing, presumed dead,

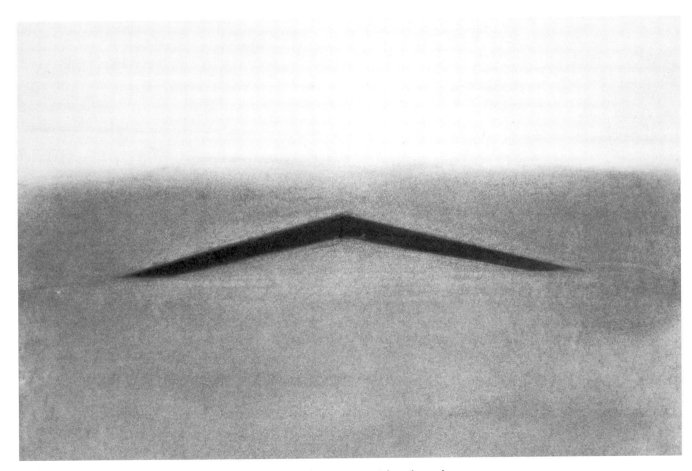

Vietnam Veterans Memorial, architectural drawing (ca. 1980) showing memorial as plan and perspective, with textual description, for competition
© Library of Congress and Maya Lin

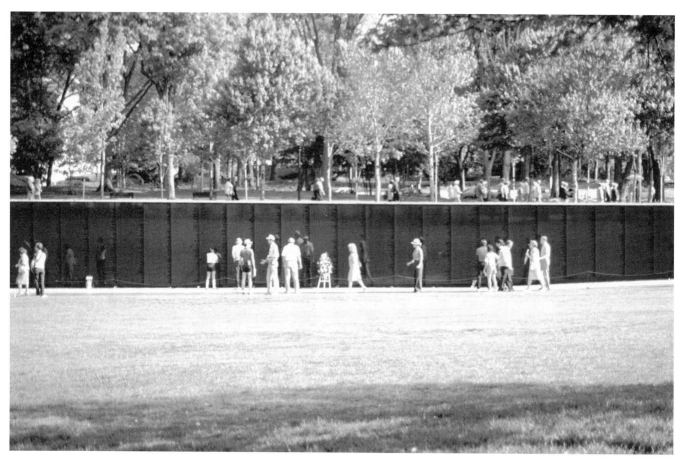

Vietnam Veterans Memorial
Photo © Mary Ann Sullivan

and killed in the Vietnam conflict are inscribed. Organized chronologically, the inscription of those lost suggests the relatedness of those killed at a particular point in time while embedding any particular sought-after name in a sea of adjacent and nearly indistinguishable names. The public and collective experience of searching for a lost friend's or relative's name has sponsored the related material practices of rubbing engraved names to record them on paper and the leaving of memorial objects at the base of the Wall. Although the Wall reinterprets certain well-established American funerary traditions, the closest precedents for the work can be found in cultural developments within minimalist sculpture and land art, both of which found receptive audiences in schools of architecture in the Postmodern era. Lin's design, which earned her a "B" in her class in funerary architecture at Yale, was selected from among more than 1400 entries to an open design competition by a jury of distinguished figures in architecture, landscape, and public art. Lin's conception of an inverted, absent monumentality takes the form of a low wall retaining the earth behind, implicating the surrounding landscape and one's experience of it as the context for the work. By rejecting the contextual clues of the surrounding neoclassical monuments, Lin's design offers an intimate, individually constructed, and ultimately political work of Postmodern landscape sculpture.

Although garnering immediate critical support in the art and design communities, as well as being warmly embraced by untold numbers of veterans, the design was roundly and loudly criticized by culturally conservative constituencies and many political operatives, including several key members of the Republican White House under Ronald Reagan. For many of these conservatives, the Wall was seen as elitist, abstract, and not appropriately representational of what they took to be the legitimately heroic content of the war. At the height of this sentiment, the Wall was infamously referred to as a "black gash of shame" by veteran and Purple Heart recipient Tom Carhart. The memorial's many detractors eventually succeeded in compromising the Wall's simple planar geometry with the addition of a piece of figural sculpture to the site. This sculpture, "The Three Fightingmen" (1984), by Frederick Hart was intended to provide an appropriate literalness that a minority of culturally conservative lay audiences found lacking in the somber power of Lin's "anti-monument." Similar concerns over the Wall's inclusiveness of reading by various constituencies led to the incorporation of a second figural sculpture depicting the sacrifices of women veterans of the Vietnam era. This second sculpture, titled "Vietnam Women's Memorial" (1993), by Glenna Goodacre, although enjoying similar political and financial support for its inclusion

on site, never approached the cultural and critical achievement of Lin's original design while fundamentally compromising its accomplishment. Rather, it is precisely the Wall's clear refusal to engage in an uncritical ahistorical valorization of the Vietnam War that affords multiple viewers the possibility of reading into the work something of their own experience. Understood as an "open text" intended to be read differently depending on the expectations and experience of the viewer, Lin's design offers a subtle and mutable lens through which various political contents might be read. Subsequent public reception of the memorial has been equally kind, and the Wall continues to enjoy broad public support in the United States and internationally as a seminal work of Postmodern landscape. The extraordinary and seemingly unparalleled breakthrough of Lin's design rests precisely on its ability to be read simultaneously by countless individuals implicated in its subject matter toward absolutely diverse political, social, and personal conclusions.

Although the status of the Vietnam Veterans Memorial will continue to change over time, the open interpretive nature of the work ensures its continued relevance well beyond the life expectancy of state-sanctioned monuments whose contents may be rendered redundant by the passage of time. More so than traditional historical representations of official state history, the meaning of the memorial depends on the reading of social and political history by future generations of participants. Whereas

traditional monuments codify for future legibility the consensus view of history concretized by their creators, the Wall constructs a surface of reflection from which changing and multiple viewpoints on historical events might be read.

CHARLES WALDHEIM

See also **Lin, Maya (United States); Memorial**

Further Reading

Beardsley, John, "Personal Sensibilities in Public Places," *Artforum*, 19 (Summer 1981)

Clay, Grady, "The Vietnam Veterans Memorial Competition," *Harvard Magazine*, 87 (1985)

Hass, Kristin Ann, *Carried to the Wall: American Memory and the Vietnam Veterans Memorial*, Berkeley: University of California Press, 1998

Krauss, Rosalind, "Sculpture in the Expanded Field," in *The Anti-Aesthetic: Essays on Postmodern Culture*, edited by Hal Foster, Port Townsend, Washington: Bay Press, 1983

VILLA MAIREA

Designed by Alvar Aalto, completed 1939
Noormarkku, Finland

In 1937, the Finnish industrialist Harry Gullichsen and his wife, Maire, commissioned Alvar Aalto to design a family residence

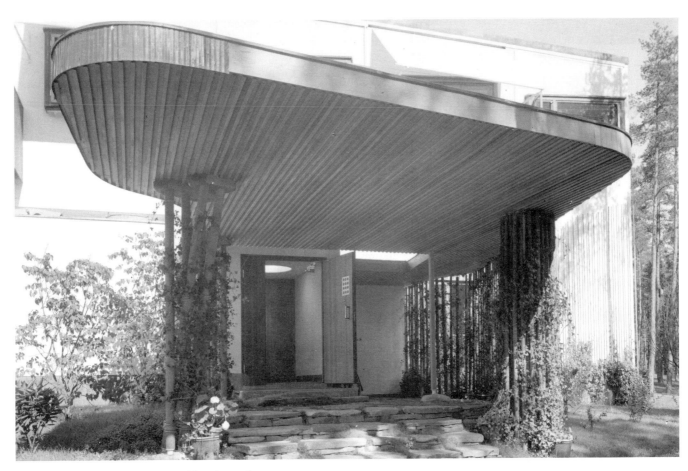

Villa Mairea, main entrance, designed by Alvar Aalto.
Photo © G. Welin/Alvar Aalto Archives

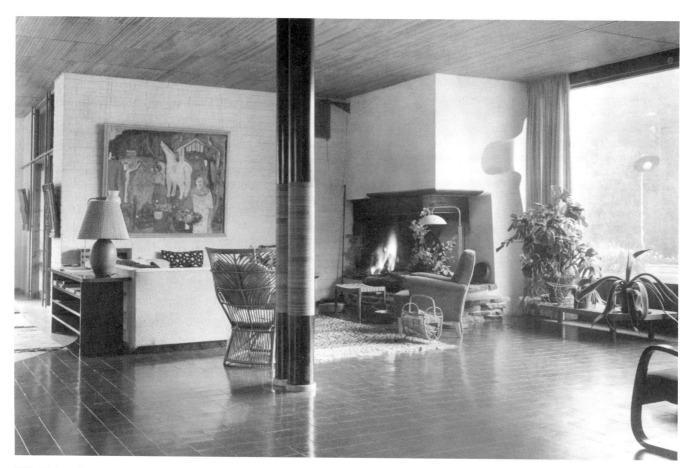

Villa Mairea, living room
Photo © Alvar Aalto Archives

in Noormarkku, Finland, that would be traditionally Finnish yet modern. By this time, Alvar Aalto was well known as a proponent of modern, concrete construction and already famous for his International Style buildings, such as the Tuberculosis Sanitorium in Paimio, Finland. The International Style aesthetic of whiteness and abstraction, with an emphasis on industrial production, was and is fundamentally at odds with the strong traditions of handcraft in Finland. As a result, the Villa Mairea is never quite what it appears to be. Early on, the house was received as a masterpiece but, because of the many apparently contradictory elements, remained problematic as to its meaning and significance.

The first glimpse of its dominant white volume amid pine trees suggests a rigorous modern composition of clear geometries. As one approaches more closely, the free-form entry canopy is the first surprise, contrasting with the "pure" white volume behind. More surprising still, this irregular canopy is screened and supported by lashed bamboolike poles, suggesting primitive, perhaps even Japanese, construction. Here, at the entry, Aalto has announced a dialectic between traditional and modern that is sustained throughout.

Once inside, one's attention is pulled diagonally to the left by the fireplace in the far corner of the living room. Aalto takes the traditional Finnish corner stove, with its extra children's bunk above, and transforms it into something uniquely modern

by converting the stair opening leading to the bunk into a hollowed sculptural profile at the side.

Perhaps the most memorable aspect of the living room is a modern stair of open risers that is elaborately supported and intricately joined to vertical wooden poles. The whole ensemble is adjacent to a large, sliding glass panel leading outside to the rear courtyard. The juxtaposition of stair and glass produces an unexpected result; the view through the stair to the courtyard is reminiscent of looking out through the forest's edge into a landscape beyond. The blurring of the distinction between inside and outside is enhanced by the extensive use of wood in the ceiling and occasional interior columns wrapped in rattan.

At this remove, it is generally accepted that one of Aalto's most significant achievements is this creation of a "forest space." This metaphorical experience of a forest inside his buildings is a reference to the primary experience of his beloved Finland. The living room at the Villa Mairea is the one of the clearest statements of this idea.

Despite the abundant stylistic contradictions, the house is a comfortable, livable home. The interior unfolds as a succession of controlled vistas and carefully formed spaces. Much of this ease results from the L-shaped plan, which is divided into a kitchen–servants' wing and a family–living area. This organization is probably derived from plans of 19th-century aristocratic Scandinavian manor houses, with which Aalto would have been

familiar. Meanwhile, the "L" also forms a courtyard that is reminiscent of much older Finnish peasant farms and faintly of Italian courtyards. Thus, even in the plan, Aalto makes references to other architectures and other places and resolves complex programmatic issues. The combination of conflicting references continues within the courtyard, where there is a traditional sauna combined with a free-form plunge pool. Although the pool is an unfamiliar farm element, the larger reference is to the Finnish landscape with its many lakes. The wooden sauna with its turf roof is a rustic, vernacular structure, and it is connected to the house by a turf-covered breezeway supported by metal pipe columns and a single concrete pier. Countering the sauna, diagonally across the courtyard, is Maire Gullichsen's second-floor study, which is collaged onto the main, white volume of the house. The ambiguous form of the study, sheathed with vertical wood strips, is a combination of crafted material with abstract modern form. Despite the modern elements, the overall effect is to integrate the building with its place. Such an integration is unusual for modern buildings of this period, which usually were treated as objects distinct from their sites.

In all these examples and in the whole of this project, Aalto successfully brought together the opposed worlds of Finnish vernacular and International Style modernism. In so doing, he produced a work that has had a substantial and lasting influence on the history and development of modern architecture. Here, he provided one of the few examples of a "humanized modernism" that recognized the significance and experience of the individual as opposed to focusing on the often dehumanizing effects of industrial technique.

In recent years, the Villa Mairea, with its references to other architectures, times, and traditions, has been a significant touchstone for Postmodernism, whose practitioners see in Aalto's work useful examples of referential and metaphorical design strategies. In particular, various critics have remarked on Aalto's design method as being fundamentally "typological"; that is, designing in plan, elevation, and detail with specific references to historic and basic "types" of architecture. It was Aalto's genius that constantly transformed and mixed those types to produce complex works whose richness, subtlety, and variety set a new standard for architecture.

Despite all the referential games that he played in his buildings, Aalto awakens the viewer to the deep and fundamental connection between humans and the natural world. It is this awareness that remains the moving and transforming core of the Villa Mairea.

LAURENCE KEITH LOFTIN III

Further Reading

There are a number of excellent books available on Alvar Aalto with abundant photographs, commentaries, and bibliographies. The ones listed below contain either excellent commentary on the Villa Mairea in particular or excellent photographic documentation of this remarkable building.

Porphyrios, Demetri, *Sources of Modern Eclecticism: Studies on Alvar Aalto*, London: Academy Editions, and New York: St. Martin's Press, 1982

Reed, Peter, *Alvar Aalto: Between Humanism and Materialism*, New York: Museum of Modern Art, 1998

Trencher, Michael, *The Alvar Aalto Guide*, New York: Princeton Architectural Press, 1996

Weston, Richard, *Alvar Aalto*, London: Phaidon Press, 1995

Weston, Richard, "Between Nature and Culture: Reflections on the Villa Mairea," in *Alvar Aalto: Towards a Human Modernism*, edited by Winfried Nerdinger, Munich, New York, and London: Prestel, 1999

VILLA SAVOYE, POISSY, FRANCE

Designed by Le Corbusier, completed 1930

Le Corbusier (Charles-Édouard Jeanneret) had been living in Paris since 1916, collaborating with Amédée Ozenfant in the production of the review *L'Esprit nouveau*, constructing several private homes, including the La Roche-Jeanneret houses (which would later become the Fondation Le Corbusier), and proposing ambitious projects for mass housing. By 1925, he succeeded in securing official backing for the construction of an experimental housing enclave at Pessac, near Bordeaux—an enterprise that seemed to presage a revolution in the building industry by bringing to construction the benefits of mass production that had made the automobile industry. He now began to receive commissions for luxury villas from families with interests in industry or with American connections. Among these were the designs made for Mongermon, one of the directors of the Voisin car and airplane industries, and in 1926 a villa at Garches for Michael and Sarah Stein.

The process by which Le Corbusier obtained the collaboration of his clients was not an easy one, as his ideas were as much directed to using new materials and developing a new lifestyle as they were to securing satisfied clients. In the case of the commission for the Villa Savoye, which arrived in 1928, the clients rejected his first design but returned to it after he had explored alternatives and presumably after he had succeeded in gaining the confidence not only of Pierre Savoye but of his wife, Emilie, as well. The villa was completed in 1930, at a cost almost double that of the estimate. It was used by the family as a weekend retreat until it was abandoned at the outbreak of war in 1939. However, it was plagued by leaks from the windows, skylights, and flat-roof terraces, and in September 1936 Madame Savoye complained to the architect that "it is raining in my bedroom."

During the war years, the villa was commandeered by the Germans, then by the Americans, and came under threat when the Commune of Poissy planned to absorb the land for the construction of a school. Le Corbusier was forced to make representations in high places, including to his friend André Malraux, minister of cultural affairs, in order to prevent its demolition.

Despite Villa Savoye's rather unsatisfactory history of cost overruns and architectural defects, it was acquired by the government as a national landmark. More than any other of the time, the Villa Savoye embodies the qualities that were to be ascribed to modern architecture produced under functionalism, and as such it has entered into history. In 1938, Henry-Russell Hitchcock and Philip Johnson published their influential book *The International Style* and chose a picture of the Villa Savoye for the dustcover. It embodies the idea of a functional architecture pared down to essentials, and it has, in addition, something exceptional that makes all the difference: a sweet sense of form, and a flair for style. There is a marvelous balance between form and content, each increasing the effect of the other, and so it seems to crystallize the very idea of modernism in architecture.

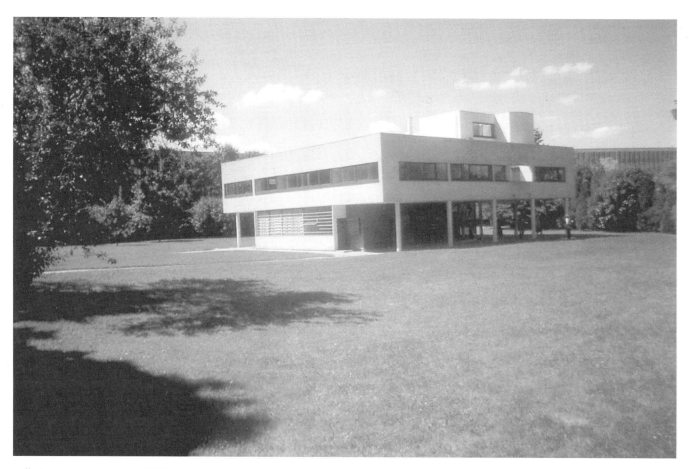

Villa Savoye, Poissy, France (1930)
Photo © Alan Windsor

The villa occupied an extensive field surrounded by a belt of trees. Le Corbusier placed it on the slightly higher ground in the middle of this field, so that it commanded views in all directions, and gave it four similar sides, one for each direction. There is some weight in the critic Colin Rowe's suggestion that it compares with Palladio's Villa Rotunda, just as the villa at Garches can be compared with Palladio's Villa Malcontenta, and there is much about the design that gives it a classical feel, but this aspect has been totally transformed by the idea of the machine aesthetic. To begin with, the frontality of the plan is full of paradox. For a weekend house some 30 kilometers from Paris, the car is obligatory. Instead of directly approaching a front porch, the visitor drives under the house on a gravel surface, sweeps around the back, and stops at the opposite side. The back becomes the front. The ground-floor accommodation is retracted to allow this, and it curves precisely to the sweep of the car.

The entrance door is classically placed on the central axis of the house, but the hall opens out asymmetrically. Directly opposite, instead of the traditional staircase there is a narrow ramp that dives deep into the house before bending back at the half landing. Although the front door, which parts in the center with two sliding leaves, is on the centerline of the house, this axis is also occupied by a row of columns, and on the half landing one crosses this line.

The space of the ramp is fully glazed above, so that it attracts the visitor upward toward the light. Once on the second level, it can be seen that it continues farther upward, on the outside, providing access to the solarium on the roof. The house now appears like an apartment, with all the family accommodations on the raised level, the ground level reserved for the servants' quarters. However, a good slice of this upper level is given to an extensive roof terrace, onto which the living room looks, with large sliding windows facing southwest. There is a Mediterranean feeling about this terrace, with its fixed concrete table ready for the moment of the aperitif. All the family spaces around the house are lit by a continuous band of glazing, the glass omitted where the wall traverses the terrace, so that the appearance on the outside is constant on all sides. The regularity of the outer face is offset by the dynamic thrust of the ramp and the curved roof forms that shelter the solarium from the wind.

In this design, Le Corbusier synthesized elements from his art with elements from his idea of a machine architecture derived from industrial processes. To review the different stages by which he arrives at the final design is to review a tentative process, for it only crystallizes along the way. Yet the finished result is so

imbued with his conviction, so certain in its balance, that it sums up not just an episode but an epoch as well.

ROBERT MAXWELL

See also **Corbusier, Le (Jeanneret, Charles-Édouard) (France); Hitchcock, Henry-Russell (United States); International Style**

Further Reading

Benton, Tim, *The Villas of Le Corbusier, 1920–1930*, New Haven, Connecticut: Yale University Press, 1987

Le Corbusier, Pierre Jeanneret, and Willy Boesiger, *The Complete Architectural Works*, London: Thames and Hudson, 1964

Rowe, Colin, *The Mathematics of the Ideal Villa, and Other Essays*, Cambridge, Massachusetts: MIT Press, 1976

Sbriglio, Jacques, *Le Corbusier: La Villa Savoye; The Villa Savoye* (bilingual English–French edition), Basel: Birkhäuser, 1999

Von Moos, Stanislas, *Le Corbusier: Elemente einer Synthese*, Frauenfeld, Switzerland: Huber, 1968; as *Le Corbusier: Elements of a Synthesis*, Cambridge, Massachusetts: MIT Press, 1979

VILLANUEVA, CARLOS RAÚL 1900–72

Architect, Venezuela

Known as Venezuela's greatest 20th-century architect, Carlos Raúl Villanueva straddled opposing political regimes, cultural milieus, and architectural styles during his long and eclectic career but left no school or followers. His most significant contribution to the country's architecture, a modernist style inflected by Venezuelan vernacular architecture and influenced by the Venezuelan tropical climate, proved too personal to be imitated. Although his residential designs are well known, it is in the public sphere—schools, housing projects, and universities—that Villanueva had the greatest effect. In particular his commitment to implementing his vision of the "synthesis of the arts" in public spaces made his work important to the Venezuelan urban context.

Villanueva began to practice his profession in Caracas in 1929 when he was appointed to the post of architect and director of building in the Ministry of Public Works under the regime of General Juan Vicente Gómez. From this period buildings such as the Plaza de Toros de Maracay (1931–33) and the Museums of Fine Arts and Natural Sciences (1934–35), among others, demonstrate how Villanueva tempered his interest in vanguard European architectural movements with a Neoclassicism designed to appeal to a conservative elite.

The next period of the architect's career is marked by a clearer influence of European modernism, as buildings such as the Gran Colombia School of Caracas (1939; today Francisco Pimentel), lack the ornamentation of earlier projects and instead employ molded reinforced concrete to create curving forms and masses. These buildings also illustrate Villanueva's evolving concern with light and shadow. Demonstrating his early interest in incorporating works of art into buildings, Villanueva integrated a sculpture by Venezuelan modernist sculptor Francisco Narváez into the main wall of the school.

In 1940 Villanueva was named chief architect and consultant of the Banco Obrero (Workers' Bank) of Venezuela, a government institution whose mission was to improve the living conditions of the lower and working classes. One of his first projects was to remodel the neighborhood of El Silencio (1941–43), a barrio in the center of the city known for its high crime and unhygienic, poor housing conditions. With the remodeling of this zone would begin his preoccupation with urban spaces, in particular with the design of large-scale public housing. El Silencio embodied the challenges faced by Villanueva in attempting works on this scale, produced under competing interests and compromised by political circumstances.

In 1944 he commenced work on the University City of Venezuela (Ciudad Universitaria, also known as the Universidad Central de Venezuela [UCV], or Central University of Venezuela), which would not be completed until 1959. At the UCV, Villanueva achieved the apogee of his personal style, a Le Corbusian–derived, Venezuelan-inflected organicism that took as its touchstone the modernist dream of the synthesis of the arts. For Villanueva the creation of this "aesthetic consortium" would enable the city's inhabitants to become truly integrated in aesthetic, spiritual, and functional terms, as he believed that the natural environment of painting and sculpture is "plazas, gardens, public buildings, factories, and airports: all the places where man perceives man as a companion, a partner, a helping hand, a hope, and not as a flower withered by isolation and indifference" (Villanueva, 1957, 11). Although its style has not been duplicated elsewhere, the UCV had a great effect on the course of Venezuelan architecture. In particular, Venezuelan intellectual and political elites came to see modernism as the style most appropriate for embodying Venezuelan identity, and the incorporation of works of art into buildings was an idea taken up by succeeding architects.

Concurrently with his work on the UCV, Villanueva continued his association with the Workers' Bank and the Taller de Arquitectura Banco Obrero (Workers' Bank Architectural Workshop, or TABO). The projects commissioned by the Workers' Bank, beginning in the late 1940s, became larger and more frequent under the regime of Venezuela's last dictator, Marcos Pérez Jiménez (1952–58), ending with some of the largest public housing projects ever built in Latin America by the end of the decade. The most representative of these, Villanueva's housing community "23 de Enero" (23 January 1957), originally named "2 de Diciembre," is usually cited by critics as a turning point in the city's growth. Because of its massive scale, it stood as a concrete symbol of the regime's objective of eradicating the ranchos, or slums, that had sprouted on hillsides, under bridges, and in ravines in Caracas. In projects such as this, Villanueva incorporated elements from different phases of his career, such as the use of polychrome paintings as exterior decoration; window and wall treatments that protected interiors from wind, sun, and rain; and Le Corbusian–derived ideas about rational living spaces.

Villanueva's critics describe his use of modernist styles as superficial and eclectic, and in comparison with the work of other modernist Latin American architects, Villanueva's personal style is less fully realized. However, in context, Villanueva stands out as the first Venezuelan to combine a tropical sensibility with European modernist architecture. For this reason the UCV is regarded as Venezuela's most important architectural monument. This, perhaps, is Villanueva's most important legacy: the incorporation of works of art into architectural projects, particularly in the capital. Large-scale freestanding sculptures and mu-

rals are found all over the city—in private office buildings, plazas, and subway stations and alongside highways—making Caracas a significant public art center on a par with New York City and Paris.

MARGUERITE MAYHALL

See also **Caracas, Venezuela; Ciudad Universitaria Campus and Stadium, Mexico City; Ciudad Universitaria, Caracas**

Biography

Born in London, 30 May 1900, the child of a distinguished Venezuelan family originally from Spain. Educated at École des Beaux-Arts in Paris, graduated 1928; Organized the first Department of Architecture in Venezuela (Ciudad Universitaria) and taught courses as professor in the School of Architecture (1944).

Selected Works

Plaza de Toros de Maracay, Caracas, 1933
Museums of Fine Arts and Natural Sciences, Caracas, 1935
Gran Colombia School of Caracas, 1939
El Silencio barrio project, Caracas, 1943
University City of Venezuela (Ciudad Universitaria), 1959

Selected Publications

La Caracas de ayer y de hoy (The Caracas of Yesterday and Today), Caracas: 1950
"La integración de las artes" (The Integration of the Arts), *Espacio y forma*, no. 3, Caracas: Facultad de Arquitectura de la Universidad Central de Venezuela, 1957
Escritos (Writings), *Espacio y forma*, no. 13, Caracas: Facultad de Arquitectura de la Universidad Central de Venezuela, 1965
Caracas en tres tiempos (Caracas in Three Times), Caracas: Ediciones Cuatricentenario, 1966
Textos escogidos (Selected Writings), Caracas: Universidad Central de Venezuela, Facultad de Arquitectura y Urbanismo, 1980

Further Reading

In addition to his own copious writings, Villanueva gave innumerable public lectures and interviews, many of which have been published in more than one venue. As a result of his significance within the architectural community, and his effect on the Venezuelan landscape, critics and scholars have published frequently on his work as well. Critical analyses of his work, however, are almost nonexistent. In addition, Villanueva's work is not well known outside Latin America, and recent publications in English are therefore scarce. For further bibliography, see the entry on the Ciudad Universitaria.

Galería de Arte Nacional de Venezuela, *Carlos Raúl Villanueva: Un moderno en Sudamérica* (exhib. cat.), Caracas: Galería de Arte Nacional de Venezuela, 2 April–9 July 2000
Moholy-Nagy, Sibyl, *Carlos Raúl Villanueva y la arquitectura de Venezuela* (*Carlos Raúl Villanueva and the Architecture of Venezuela*), Caracas: Editorial Lectura, and New York: Praeger, 1964
Museo de Arte Contemporáneo de Caracas Sofía Imber, *Villanueva el arquitecto* (exhib. cat.), Caracas: Museo de Arte Contemporáneo de Caracas Sofía Imber, 1988
Posani, Juan Pedro, *Arquitecturas de Villanueva* (The Architectural Works of Villanueva), Caracas: Lagoven, 1985

VILLE RADIEUSE (Ca. 1930)
Designed by Le Corbusier

While working on the Tzentrosoyuz (central statistical office) building in 1930, Le Corbusier received an inquiry from the Soviet officials concerning the reorganization of Moscow. His illustrative proposal, entitled "Ville Radieuse" (radiant city), was grounded essentially in individual freedom, exerted no influence in the Soviet Union, and remained a project on paper only. Le Corbusier continued to develop and relentlessly promote Ville Radieuse as a platform on which to present his thoughts about urbanism; it became a theoretical summary of Le Corbusier's most advanced views on town planning and design, eventually evolving into a model of a modern "ideal city" in the best tradition of old-fashioned utopias.

Le Corbusier treated the Moscow inquiry as a case study assessed through a relatively independent theoretical framework: the answers to the questions "were Moscow," but the illustrations (about 20 of them) "were the phenomenon of the organization of life in the city of the machine age, the present age" (Le Corbusier, 1935, p. 90). Essentially, Le Corbusier tried to solve the city as a problem and kept pursuing an absolute formula that would guarantee the highest quality to any urban space. His approach was not wholly new; Ville Radieuse included and refined Le Corbusier's earlier thoughts on urban design, including the Contemporary City for Three Million Inhabitants, the Voisin Plan for Paris, and the ideas expressed in his books *Urbanisme* (The City of To-morrow) and *Precisions*.

This new city was a revised version of his Contemporary City for Three Million Inhabitants, first launched for the Parisian Autumn Salon in 1922. It remained rectangular in form but allowed for lateral growth on both sides of the central communication axis, thus eliminating rigidity, the major shortcoming of the previous model. The business center, in the pattern of sixteen wide-spaced, cruciform skyscrapers, was concentrated at the "top" edge of the plan, tangential to the circular transportation terminal with a heliport on its rooftop. The industrial zone was located at the "bottom" end of the city. Areas of civic and commercial activities flanked the NW–SE communication while serving as a buffer zone to the set-back, residential superblocks. Le Corbusier's preoccupation with a total, wholesome living environment, filled with air, sun, light, and greenery inside and out was presented as an immersion of buildings into the large green areas. Although the "garden city" suburbs and the hierarchic population distribution used in previous models were eliminated, the principles like a multilevel transportation system and a "biological unit," the cell of 14 square meters per occupant, were elaborated on, and a nursery, kindergarten, and primary school were introduced in the "neighborhood unit" of 2,700.

Throughout the 1930s, applying "radiant city" urbanization principles, now formulated as a more universal model of urban planning, Le Corbusier produced a wide variety of unbuilt projects, mostly competition entries for various cities, the majority of which were included in the subsequent book titled *The Radiant City; Elements of a Doctrine of Urbanism to Be Used as the Basis of Our Machine-Age Civilization*.

The book spanned projects from his Voisin Plan for Paris of 1925, which was designed to revitalize the center of the city, to four Latin American cities, among which the site and ambience

of Rio de Janeiro inspired particularly poetic expressions, resulting in the concept of an elevated highway with incorporated housing below; this megastructure was to become a focus of the later plan for Algiers. Although the geometry of Le Corbusier's model seemingly presupposed a flatness of site and indifference to topographic concerns, the scheme was only intended to facilitate the paradigm, whereas some of the most imaginative of Le Corbusier's applications were inspired by the most irregular topographies.

He blamed the migration to cities for some of the gravest urban problems and proposed solving it by redevelopment and revitalization of the rural areas. The resulting concepts for the Radiant Farm and Radiant Village eulogized the modern high-speed connection between the city and country, but his proposed modernization targeted only country living and did not include working conditions.

With the Ville Radieuse, Le Corbusier established some of the 20th century's most memorable and influential urban images and created the concept of urban environment that still underlies much of contemporary design, despite the fact that he was denied urban planning commissions for most of his lifetime. Yet, through the Charter of Athens, a manifesto of the Modern movement, and CIAM gatherings, Le Corbusier promulgated the Ville Radieuse approach to urban planning and design as a recipe for the quality of the living and dwelling environment. His vision presupposed a revolution in dwelling, architecture, and urbanism. That Le Corbusier's romanticized and futuristic urban dreams exerted such influence among generations of architects all over the world was a result of his sophisticated theories that successfully combined a persistent and contagious enthusiasm for the architect's doctrine.

GORDANA KOSTICH-LEFEBVRE

See also **Contemporary City for Three Million Inhabitants; Corbusier, Le (Jeanneret, Charles-Édouard) (France); Voisin Plan for Paris**

Further Reading

Le Corbusier (Jeanneret, Charles-Édouard), *La Ville radieuse, éléments d'une doctrine d'urbanisme pour l'équipement de la civilisation machiniste*, Paris: Éditions de l'Architecture d'Aujourd'hui, 1935; Translated as *The Radiant City; Elements of a Doctrine of Urbanism to Be Used as the Basis of Our Machine-Age Civilization*, New York: Orion Press, 1967

Evenson, Norma, *Le Corbusier: The Machine and the Grand Design*. New York: G. Braziller, 1970

Fishman, Robert, *Urban Utopias in the Twentieth Century: Ebenezer Howard, Frank Lloyd Wright, and Le Corbusier*, Cambridge, Massachusetts: MIT Press, 1977

Frampton, Kenneth, "Le Corbusier and the *ville radieuse* 1928–46," in *Modern Architecture: A Critical History*, London: Themes and Hudson, 1980

VISITOR CENTER

The visitor center is a product of the post–World War II automobile age, welcoming road-weary tourists with promises of comfort, education, and entertainment. Prominently situated at historic areas, national parks, and state borders, the visitor center combines a wide range of functions, such as rest rooms, information kiosks, bookstores, and museum exhibits, that were once housed separately.

The term and concept of "visitor center" were brought into widespread use by the National Park Service during its "Mission 66" building improvement program (1956–66). Under Mission 66 the Park Service promoted 100 newly created visitor centers as the hub of a ten-year, billion-dollar effort to improve tourist and administrative facilities in the national parks. Mission 66 aimed to satisfy an astronomical rise in the number of visitors, growing from 17 million annually in 1940 to 54 million a year by 1954, at park sites that had not been substantially upgraded since the 1930s. Rangers could not handle the massive influx of tourists in the existing structures, small "rustic" buildings often lacking basic conveniences such as air-conditioning or indoor rest rooms.

Under Mission 66, Park Service planners created a prototype design for a new building type—the visitor center—that could be adapted to the unique character and specific requirements of each site. The prototypical visitor center consisted of a compact building equipped with clean rest rooms, public telephones, a large circulation lobby, an information desk, staff offices, and areas for interpretive exhibits. Centers for more popular parks might include an auditorium with regularly scheduled orientation films, a cafeteria, a research room, and a library. A convenient parking area nearby accommodated visitors' automobiles and trailers. These basic elements remain at the core of visitor center planning today.

As the first stop for tourists, the visitor center created a transition zone between the environment outside the park and the natural and cultural features inside. Park planners sited the buildings at strategic points in an effort to funnel tourists through an orientation process, a critical component of the Mission 66 visitor center campaign. Once inside the building, visitors found interpretive exhibits, safety guidelines, educational pamphlets, maps, and a helpful ranger to answer questions. Many of the buildings offered panoramic views of nearby scenic vistas; a well-marked exit might lead to an open patio for an on-site ranger presentation or the first stop on a self-guided tour.

To attract visitors, architects created innovative, high-profile buildings that promised modern facilities in even the most remote locales. Bold dramatic rooflines, wide expanses of glass, overhanging eaves, and prominent entryways raised the visibility, and therefore the appeal, of the buildings to the public. To maintain a contextual continuity, architects incorporated physical or symbolic characteristics of the site in the building design. For example, architect Richard Neutra designed the Visitor Center and Cyclorama Building at Gettysburg National Military Park (1961) as a memorial to Abraham Lincoln and his famous address. The monumental profile of the stark white cylindrical building, displaying such modern design elements as movable sun louvers and a concrete spider-leg, reflects the commemorative character of the 1863 Civil War battlefield and nearby cemetery. Similarly, Romaldo Giurgola of Mitchell/Giurgola Architects conveyed the spirit of innovation in designing a visitor center for the Wright Brothers National Memorial at Kill Devil Hills, North Carolina (1960). The center's sweeping sculptural concrete form rises prominently from the sand dunes and connects the historic past to the present by invoking the character of modern airport terminals of the 1960s.

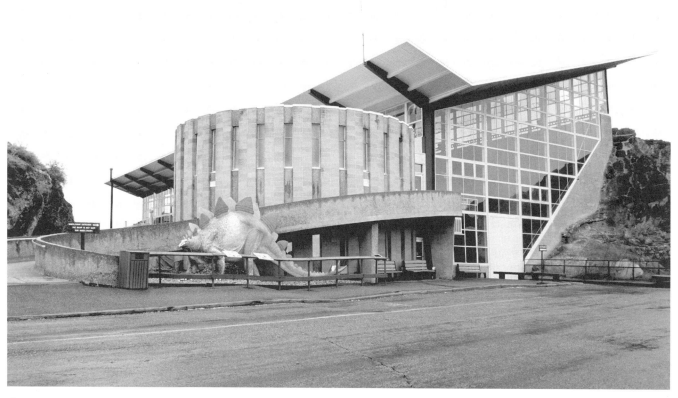

Quarry Visitor Center (1956–58), Dinosaur National Monument, Jensen, Utah
© Christine Madrid French, 2000

The visitor center prototype introduced by the National Park Service in the mid-1950s has been widely adopted by other civic and corporate entities in the decades since. Older structures designed as small-scale museums, information centers, or nature centers were remodeled or replaced by multipurpose facilities; others were simply renamed "visitor centers." In the late 1960s, Pacific Gas and Electric of California established visitor centers at its nuclear power plants as part of a massive pronuclear public relations campaign. British Nuclear Fuels Limited followed quickly with its own center, featuring a life-size model of a nuclear reactor core and a walk-in "Fission Tunnel." Other government agencies, such as the U.S. Bureau of Reclamation and the National Forest Service, followed the Park Service example and created their own system of visitor centers in the 1970s at national recreation areas and national forests.

Once considered gateways to other featured attractions, visitor centers are now marketed as destinations in themselves. It is not unusual to find photographs of visitor centers proudly displayed on postcards or prominently featured in promotional brochures. Indeed, several early examples of the building type are now recognized by leading architects and scholars as American cultural landmarks, worthy of preservation and interpretation.

In the 50 years since its introduction, the visitor center has evolved into an entertainment complex as well as an information service center, combining full-scale museum features, retail outlets, and research facilities. It is a testament to the utility and adaptability of this modern building type that we now consider the visitor center a timeless element of the American roadside landscape.

CHRISTINE MADRID FRENCH

Further Reading

Architectural histories focusing on the development of National Park Service building types are provided by Good (1938) and McClelland (1998). Architect-specific publications provide photographs and descriptions of the Wright Brothers Visitor Center; see Giurgola (1983), and the Gettysburg Cyclorama, see Boesiger (1966). Allaback (2000) focuses on the promotion of the visitor center under the Mission 66 program. Further analyses of the building type are available in magazines and journals dating from 1955 to the present, including Tilson (1993) and Dheere (1999).

Allaback, Sarah, *Mission 66 Visitor Centers: The History of a Building Type*, Washington, D.C.: U.S. Department of the Interior, 2000
Boesiger, W. (editor), *Richard Neutra Buildings and Projects: 1961–66*, New York: Frederick A. Praeger, 1966
Dheere, Jessica Joan, "Portfolio: Four Visitor Centers Subtly Interpret the Landscape, Inviting Park Patrons to Become One with the Wild," *Architectural Record* (October 1999)
Giurgola, Romaldo, and Erhman B. Mitchell, *Mitchell/Giurgola Architects*, New York: Rizzoli, 1983

Good, Albert H., *Park and Recreation Structures*, Washington, D.C.: U.S. Department of the Interior, 1938

McClelland, Linda Flint, *Building the National Parks: Historic Landscape Design and Construction*, Baltimore and London: Johns Hopkins University Press, 1998

Tilson, Donn, "The Shaping of 'Eco-nuclear' Publicity: the Use of Visitors' Centers in Public Relations," *Media Culture and Society* (July 1993)

VOISIN PLAN FOR PARIS (1925)

Designed by Le Corbusier

In the Voisin Plan, Le Corbusier adapted the principles of his Contemporary City for Three Million Inhabitants (1922) to the specific situation of Paris. In 1922 a sketch accompanying the Contemporary City demonstrated an adaptation of the plan to the historic center of Paris. In 1925 the renovation of Paris became the main issue. The plan was exhibited at the Pavilion of Esprit Nouveau at the International Decorative Arts Exhibition of 1925. The pavilion was an architectural manifesto that showcased two projects: a residence type that systematically used standard elements and a study of the principles of standardization in their urban and interurban context. The former was represented by a full-scale model of a unit from the Immeuble Villas block. The latter, the Voisin Plan and the Contemporary City, were featured in an annex of the pavilion. Although a theoretical exercise, the plan was also a concrete proposal aimed at the transformation of Paris and marked the first of Le Corbusier's numerous proposals for Paris, including the Ville Radieuse (Radiant City; ca. 1930) and *Le Destin de Paris* (The Destiny of Paris; 1941). Eugène Hénard's *Études sur les transformations de Paris* (Studies on the Transformations of Paris; 1903–06) was an influential precedent. Somewhat sensational, the radical Voisin Plan was severely denigrated by critics who accused Le Corbusier of wanting to destroy Paris.

The plan addressed the urgent problems facing Paris: overcrowding, traffic congestion, and the lack of office space. Central to the plan was Le Corbusier's conception of the relationship between skyscrapers and traffic routes, based on the principles of high density, open space, and speed. Le Corbusier wrote in *Urbanisme* (*City of Tomorrow*; 1925) that the plan did not provide definitive solutions to the problems of Paris but that its primary aim was to cut through small, uncoordinated efforts at renovation and raise the level of discussion to large-scale reforms that would incorporate contemporary issues. To transform Paris into a modern city, Le Corbusier invoked the tradition of urban planning. Facing the dilemma of medicine or surgery, he referred to the tradition of applying both and chose surgery for the historical center. The projected site was an L-shaped area of 240 hectares located northeast of the Louvre on the Right Bank. Most buildings and streets were to be demolished for the area to be built anew in a rigorous geometric pattern. Only a few isolated, historic buildings were to be preserved: the Louvre, Palais Royal, Place Vendôme, Place de la Concorde, Arc de Triomphe, Opera, and a few churches and town houses.

In the business district on the eastern half of the area facing the Ile de la Cité, 18 cruciform office towers, surrounded by open, green space, were to be built along the axis of the Boulevard Sébastopol. In the western, residential district were to be the setback, or *redent*, blocks, either of the Immeuble-Villas type that form large blocks or covered with immense sheets of glass. Streets were replaced by elevated terraces with shops, cafes, and restaurants for social and commercial functions. Underlying the ideology of creating well-being and happiness through large-scale planning was the political notion that the problems of social disorder could be resolved by the provision of the essential joys of sunlight, greenery, and leisure.

Another essential component of the plan was hygienic and comfortable dwellings. The exhibited full-scale model unit was a standardized modern duplex that, superimposed with other duplexes, formed the apartment block. This seminal building type marked a new approach to architecture. Built in reinforced concrete and Cubist in form, its design centered around spatial proportions and volumes rather than around a two-dimensional facade. Its double-height living area and garden terrace would recur in Le Corbusier's designs. The unit was furnished according to the purist canon of *objets-types* that balanced folk, craft, and machine-made objects.

The name Voisin points to one of the essential aims of the project: the creation of a wide east–west artery parallel to the rue de Rivoli for fast automobile traffic. To finance the Pavilion of Esprit Nouveau, Le Corbusier sent out letters to the biggest names in the automobile industry—Voisin, Michelin, and Citroën—asking them to contribute funds in exchange for publicity. The Voisin car and airplane cartel, which was interested in mass-produced housing, supported the project. Le Corbusier regarded locomotion simultaneously as a modern influence threatening Paris that required reorganization and also as one of the fundamental sources of power for the modern commercial city, as is illustrated by his entrepreneurial aphorism "A city made for speed is a city made for success." Financially, however, as with other aspects of the plan, the construction of the artery was not a viable idea. If enacted, it would have been one of the most costly as well as destructive projects to be carried out in Paris. Financially and politically, the plan was unrealistic.

In the history of urban planning, the Voisin Plan has often been singled out as a symbol of the Modern movement's disregard for the past. However, Le Corbusier's own view was that through the plan the prestigious vestiges of Paris were not only preserved but rescued as well. By opening up the area around the monuments, they were to be protected from the daily urban activities that endangered them. According to this logic, the buildings now became monuments to be conserved and thus were reintegrated into the fabric of the modern city. In this way Le Corbusier's dogmatic project nonetheless underlined the dynamic between renovation and conservation. Moreover, in later plans some of the most radical features of the plan were modified. In 1933 the cruciform skyscraper was replaced with a smaller, Y-shaped type that allowed in more sunlight. In the later plans, these skyscrapers were to be built far from the existing center. Although it was the earlier, cruciform towers that were enthusiastically adopted by planners through the 1960s, other aspects of the plan, such as the Immeuble-Villas unit and the overall call for systematic planning, fundamentally influenced 20th-century architecture.

HAZEL HAHN

See also **Contemporary City for Three Million Inhabitants; Corbusier, Le (Jeanneret, Charles-Édouard) (France); Inter-**

national Exhibition of Decorative Arts, Paris (1925); Ville Radieuse (ca. 1930)

Further Reading

Arrhenius, Thordis, "Restoration in the Machine Age: Themes of Conservation in Le Corbusier's Plan Voisin," *AAfiles*, 38 (1999)

Benton, Tim, *The Villas of Le Corbusier, 1920–1930*, New Haven, Connecticut, and London: Yale University Press, 1987

Curtis, William, *Le Corbusier Ideas and Forms*, London: Phaidon, 1986; New York: Rizzoli, 1986

Frampton, Kenneth, *Le Corbusier*, translated by Frank Straschitz, Paris: Hazan, 1997

Lucan, Jacques (editor), *Le Corbusier, une encyclopédie*, Paris: Centre Georges Pompidou, 1987

Moos, Stanislaus von, *Elements of a Synthesis*, Cambridge, Massachusetts: MIT Press, 1979

Moos, Stanislaus von (editor), *L'Esprit nouveau: Le Corbusier und die Industrie 1920–1925*, Berlin: Ernst und Sohn, 1987

Passanti, Francesco, "The Skyscrapers of the Ville Contemporaine," *Assemblage*, 4 (1987)

Raeburn, Michael, and Victoria Wilson (editors), *Le Corbusier, Architect of the Century* (exhib. cat.), London: Arts Council of Great Britain, 1987

VON MOOS, STANISLAUS 1940–

Architecture historian and critic, Switzerland

In the history of modern architecture, Switzerland is the European country whose role and import have been sorely underplayed and underacknowledged. However, thanks to the assiduous and careful scholarship of Stanislaus von Moos, the Swiss contribution to 20th-century building has been immeasurably enhanced. More than any other Swiss national, Von Moos has maintained a vigorous sponsorship of art and architecture from his native country through a varied program of publishing, curatorial practice, and above all, pedagogy.

Born in Lucerne in 1940, Von Moos studied at the Eidgenössische Technische Hochschule in Zurich and later at the University of Zurich and the Università degli Studi in Florence. From the university he received a Ph.D. with a thesis on military architecture and its impact on 15th- and 16th-century European palaces and villas, later published as *Turm und Bollwerk: Beiträge zu einen politischen Ikonographie der italienischen Renaissancearchitektur* (1974). However, during his studies in Zurich, he had the good fortune to serve as research assistant to Sigfried Giedion, whose *Space, Time, and Architecture* (1941) certainly whetted his appetite for future studies of the modern period in architecture and served as a template for his own major publications.

Von Moos's foray into 20th-century topics began when he was asked to contribute to a series of monographs on notable Swiss men and women, an assignment that would determine the trajectory of his career from that moment forward. Noting the absence in the late 1960s of a comprehensive and critical study of Le Corbusier, Von Moos embarked on such a project, to be published in 1968 as *Le Corbusier; Elemente einer Synthese* (published a decade later in English translation). For the first time since Le Corbusier's death in 1965, and continuing more or less to the present day, Von Moos's chef d'oeuvre was and is the only attempt to understand Le Corbusier's career from a synthetic point of view, encompassing his paintings and graphics, writings, unbuilt projects, and built work. The success of the work is tied to Von Moos's meticulous research and his access (beginning with Giedion) to many of Le Corbusier's compatriots and collaborators.

Le Corbusier: Elements of a Synthesis, the work's English title, is presented as a series of essays on different aspects of Le Corbusier's work, including purism, urbanism, utopian visions, typology, and public commissions. Von Moos writes of Le Corbusier's "visual and poetic approach to reality," a formal reading that allows the author to establish a teleology of Le Corbusier's oeuvre from the Villas Fallet and Schwob (his earliest works in Switzerland), to his purist paintings of the 1920s, to the later works of Chandigarh and La Tourette monastery, foregrounding what Von Moos sees as Le Corbusier's Ruskinian tendency to identify a fundamental order and organization within nature.

As the first book to treat Le Corbusier as a historical subject, *Elements* is responsible for many of the originary ideas about the architect's works; for example, Von Moos indicates the use of continuous typologies for specific building uses, such as the orthogonal box for dwellings, the spiral for museums, and the triangle for assembly halls. In doing so, Von Moos builds on earlier work by Colin Rowe that analyzes Le Corbusier's recycling of themes and motifs in differing projects as a process of "displacement." Thus, the book's strength lies in its central belief in a specific architectural practice's underlying system that found its ultimate epiphany in Le Corbusier's Modulor system of measurement, one that expressed "a common denominator between human proportions and elemental geometry."

Von Moos's interest in architectural polemicists led him to his next major subject: the writings and practice of Robert Venturi. Von Moos had already broached the similarities between Venturi and Le Corbusier in *Elements*, which led him to recognize the attention to typological study that bound these two architects together. While teaching at Harvard University in the early 1970s, Von Moos found in Venturi an introduction to American vernacular architecture; building on the apparent relationship between Le Corbusier's *Towards a New Architecture* (1923) and Venturi's *Complexity and Contradiction in Architecture* (1966)—which share an ahistoricism and privileging of aesthetics over history—he embarked on the first major study of the latter's work (*Venturi, Rauch, and Scott Brown: Buildings and Projects* [1987]).

The book is arranged as an extended essay and catalogue raisonné, with the essay "The Challenge of the Status Quo: 5 Points on the Architecture of VRSB" belying a further debt to Le Corbusier. Von Moos adopts the role of apologist, elucidating one of the first and most extended defenses of Venturi's built work and providing the means away from a narrow vision of Venturi as mere pop theorist and toward one that considers his architecture in a serious manner. As in his treatment of Le Corbusier, thematic and typological motifs (such as the segmented arch, adapted from Louis Kahn) are traced through their use in different contexts as a means of exploring the plastic and fungible quality of architectural themes in Venturi's practice.

Von Moos also fashioned a career as an important curator, having organized important exhibitions devoted to Venturi ("Venturi and Rauch: Architektur im Alltag Amerikas") for the Kunstgewerbemuseum in Zurich (1979) and a major show cele-

brating Le Corbusier's 100th birthday ("L'Esprit nouveau: Le Corbusier und die Industrie, 1920–1925") for the Museum für Gestaltung in Zurich (1987). In the latter exhibition, Von Moos revisited familiar terrain, focusing on Le Corbusier's early theories and their organization around industrial themes. In addition, as curator of the Swiss Pavilion for the 1998 Milan Triennale, he initiated a recuperation of another much maligned figure: the Swiss artist/architect/teacher Max Bill.

Von Moos's work displays an admirable ability to project patriotic pride while avoiding xenophobia. One of his most enduring and selfless projects was as founder and editor in chief of the architectural quarterly *archithese*. From its appearance in 1970 and continuing to the present, this journal has provided a crucial voice for European architectural criticism and theory, with a purview beyond mere Swiss national concerns. As a professor in Europe and abroad, Von Moos has maintained a commitment to pedagogy seemingly at odds with the vast amount of writing and research required of his manifold other projects.

NOAH CHASIN

See also **Corbusier, Le (Jeanneret, Charles-Édouard) (France)**

Biography

Born in Lucerne, 1940. Married; two daughters. Ph.D. from University of Zurich in 1967 (thesis: "Turm und Bollwerk: Beiträge zu einer politischen Ikonographie der italienischen Renaissance-Architektur"). Taught at Harvard University (1971–75); University of Bern, Switzerland (1974–78); Technische Hogeschool, Delft, the Netherlands (1979–83); University of Zurich (1982–present); Princeton University (1997); Graduate Center of the City University of New York (1998). Founding editor of *archithese* (1970–80). Curator of "The Other Twenties: Themes in Art and Advertising" (Harvard University, 1975); "Venturi und Rauch: Architektur im Alltag Amerikas" (Zurich, Berlin, Hannover, Freiburg, Milan, Florence, 1979); "L'Esprit Nouveau: Le Corbusier und die Industrie, 1920–1925 (Zurich, Berlin, Strasbourg, Paris, 1986–87); "Le Corbusier before Le Corbusier" (Baden and New York, 2002–03). Fellowships at Swiss Institute, Rome (1968–70); Institute for Advanced Study, Berlin (1985–86); Getty Center, California (1992–93); CASVA, Washington, D.C. (1996). Schelling Prize for Architectural Theory, Karlsruhe (1998).

Selected Publications

Le Corbusier: Elemente einer Synthese, 1968; as *Le Corbusier: Elements of a Synthesis*, 1979
New Directions in Swiss Architecture, 1969
Turm und Bollwerk: Beiträge zu einer politischen Ikonographie der italienischen Renaissance-Architektur, 1974
Venturi, Rauch, and Scott Brown: Buildings and Projects, 1960–1985, 1987
L'Esprit nouveau: Le Corbusier und die Industrie, 1920–1925 (editor), 1987
"Urbanism and Transcultural Exchanges, 1910–1935," in *Le Corbusier*, edited by H. Allen Brooks, 1987
"Industrieästhetik," *Ars Helvetica*, 11 (1992)
Venturi, Rauch, and Scott Brown: Buildings and Projects, 1986–1998, 1999

Further Reading

Benton, Tim, and Charlotte Benton, "Towards Modernist Classicism," *Werk-archithese*, 65/23–24 (November–December 1978) (special issue)

VOYSEY, CHARLES FRANCIS ANNESLEY 1857–1941
Architect and designer, England

C.F.A. Voysey was, on the one hand, a late product of the English Gothic Revival and, on the other, an original and innovative architect who is regarded today as important for the development of the new architecture of the 20th century. Although he lived long enough to know and to dislike the International Style of the 1920s and 1930s, the publication of Voysey's designs in British, German, Belgian, and Austrian magazines before 1900 was definitely influential on those who formulated the new architecture. Soon after the turn of the century, his work was also noticed, exhibited, and admired in the United States and in Scandinavia. C.R. Mackintosh, whose work Voysey did not like, acknowledged his formative influence. Acknowledged as an enigmatic architect with somewhat ambiguous ties to the English Gothic and Arts and Crafts movements of the 19th century, Voysey nonetheless provided many architects of the first third of the 20th century with a sense of invention and synthesis in his practice of design. Seeking to extract meaning from rural vernacular architecture and from contemporary work by C.R. Ashbee or Arthur H. Mackmurdo, Voysey emphasized simplicity, a principle that mattered to many architects both inside and outside the Modern movement.

He was born at Hessle in Yorkshire, the eldest son of a Church of England clergyman, and his father had a profound influence on him. The Reverend Charles Voysey was a man of resolute faith who was nevertheless eventually expelled from the Anglican Church for heresy: He denied the doctrine of everlasting hell. Reverend Voysey then formed his own Theistic Church based on rational principles. Voysey's religious convictions, firm independence, and unshakable integrity owed much to his father's example. He was taught at home until he was 14 and then attended Dulwich College for two years (1871–73), after which he briefly had a private tutor. As he was a slow learner whose grammar and spelling always remained shaky, his education appears to have been narrow and limited.

At the age of 17, Voysey was articled to John Pollard Seddon and remained in his London office for six years. He then worked briefly (1879) in the office of Saxon Snell, who specialized in hospitals, before spending the next two years with the fashionable country house architect George Devey.

In 1881, at the age of 24, Voysey set up his own practice in Westminster. He was a passionate devotee of the writings of both Pugin and Ruskin, both of whom had been known personally by his father; from them, he developed his conviction that the laws of design and construction should be learned from the study of nature. One of the strongest professional influences on Voysey was that of A.H. Mackmurdo, a protégé of Ruskin's, who introduced Voysey to the design of wallpapers and encouraged him to join the Art Workers' Guild in 1884.

"To be simple is the end, not the beginning of design," Voysey wrote in 1893. He usually drew together the elements of his houses into a single volume, covering this rectangular form with a high-pitched gable or hipped roof of slate. Wall surfaces were plain, characteristically rendered with gray- or white-painted roughcast. Buttresses, incorporated sculpturally into the wall treatment, were needed to support the deep, sweeping roofs. His windows were usually stone mullioned, with metal casements, and arranged in long horizontal groups. Chimney stacks were few and were sculpturally related to the walls and buttresses in material and form.

Voysey's first commission was for The Cottage (1888–89) in Warwickshire, for which he employed roughcast rendering, as his client was a cement manufacturer. From that time on, he preferred this wall treatment; he also almost always used greenish gray slates for roofs, seldom paying attention to local building traditions. His tall, narrow, white and gray house at 14 South Parade (1888–91) in Bedford Park still contrasts sharply with its red-brick, red-tiled neighbors by Norman Shaw, although he was obliged to use the latter materials for his twin town houses, 14 and 16 Hans Road (1891–92).

Similar in style is a superb series of houses in the country: Perrycroft (1893) in Malvern; Lowicks (1894) in Tilford; Annesley Lodge (1895), for his father, in London; Greyfriars (1896),

for the American writer Julian Sturgis, in Surrey; Norney and New Place (both 1897; both in Surrey); and his own house, The Orchard (1899), in Chorleywood. All have cool, spare interiors. The welcoming entrance hall has a fireplace; the staircase rises, usually with a screen of tall, thin, plain, square-sectioned wooden balusters uniting the lower and upper floors. Living rooms usually have inglenook fireplaces, ceramic tiled or paneled with plain marble sheets. In each bedroom, a small ventilator panel of pierced and decorated metal admits fresh air through three narrow slits in the center of the gable outside. Norney and New Place have semicircular, or "bow," windows, a feature that subsequently became very popular in England for small suburban houses. The guttering of the house is characteristically supported at intervals on thin, prominent iron brackets. Doors have long wrought-iron hinge straps terminating in a heart shape and are sometimes pierced with a hole of that shape; another Voysey signature is the sly, almost hidden grotesque caricature of himself or of his client as an unobtrusive profile molding on a staircase or porch bracket. "Simplicity, sincerity, repose, directness and frankness are moral qualities as essential to good architecture as they are to good men," wrote Voysey.

At Broadleys (1898) on Lake Windermere, Voysey's most celebrated masterpiece, he introduced three commanding bow windows to provide maximum enjoyment of the views of the

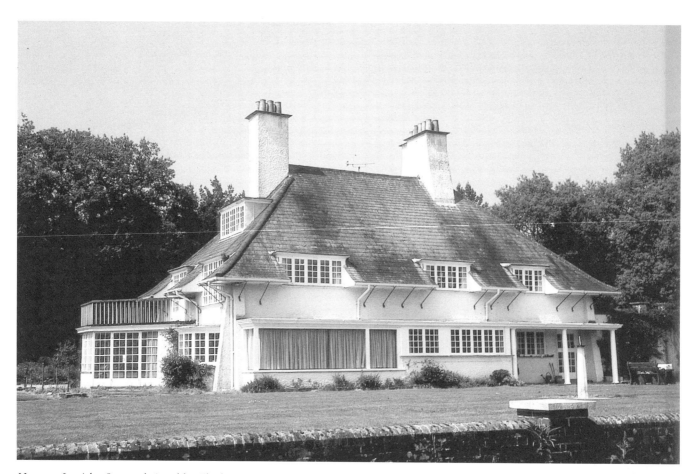

House at Lowicks, Surrey, designed by Charles F.A. Voysey
© Alan Windsor

lake and the mountains beyond; Voysey's houses are always sensitively responsive to their settings.

An exceptional commission was for the Sanderson's Wallpaper Factory (1902) in Chiswick: a three-story rectangular building in which concrete floors resting on steel joists are supported by hollow piers that act also as ventilation shafts. Between these extend large steel-framed windows; there are no walls. The roof is hidden behind a tall parapet of wavy-topped sections between each pier. The whole building is clad in white-glazed bricks, and although quite unlike any of his houses, Voysey's design vocabulary is here perfectly consistent with certain aspects of his style, particularly that of his furniture.

Despite his international fame, Voysey's practice almost ceased after 1914, and for the rest of his long life, apart from a handful of commissions and some extensions to earlier houses, his main income came from designing wallpapers, fabrics, metalwork, and furniture. In 1924, he became master of the Art Workers' Guild. He was awarded the Royal Gold Medal of the Royal Institute of British Architects in 1940.

ALAN WINDSOR

Biography

Born in Hessle, Yorkshire, England, 28 May 1857. Apprenticed to architect J.P. Seddon 1874–79. Married 1885. Chief assistant to J.P. Seddon 1879–80; assistant to architect H. Saxon Snell 1879–80; assistant in the office of George Devey 1880–81. Established a private practice, London 1882; also designed furniture, wallpaper, fabric, tiles, and metalwork. Gold Medal, Royal Institute of British Architects 1940. Died in Winchester, England, 12 February 1941.

Selected Works

The Cottage, Bishop's Intchington, Warwick, 1889
J.W. Forster House, Bedford Park, London, 1891
Grove Town Houses, Kensington, London, 1892
Perrycroft, Malvern, 1893
Lowicks, Tilford, 1894
Annesley Lodge, Hampstead, London, 1895
Sturgis House and Stables (Greyfriars), Surrey, 1896
Norney, Shackleford, Surrey, 1897
New Place, Haslemere, Surrey, 1897
Broadleys and Moorcrag, on Lake Windermere, Lancastershire, 1898
The Orchard, Chorleywood, Hertfordshire, 1899
Sanderson's Wallpaper Factory, Chiswick, 1902

Selected Publications

Reason as a Basis of Art (pamphlet), 1906
Individuality, 1915
The Work of C.F.A. Voysey (exhib. cat.; introduction by Voysey), 1931

Further Reading

Hitchmough makes extensive use of contemporary comment and criticism, and is regarded as the definitive biography. Brandon-Jones's catalog for the Art Gallery, Brighton, illustrates and lists Voysey's work in architecture, furniture, pattern design, and metalwork. Gebhard's book offers a representative selection of Voysey's writings as well as a critical evaluation of his life and work. Davey sets Voysey in the context of his contemporaries.

Brandon-Jones, John (editor), *C.F.A. Voysey: Architect and Designer, 1857–1941*, London: Lund Humphries, 1978
Davey, Peter, *Arts and Crafts Architecture*, London: Architectural Press, 1980; as *Architecture of the Arts and Crafts Movement*, New York: Rizzoli, 1980
Gebhard, David, *Charles F.A. Voysey, Architect*, Los Angeles: Hennesey and Ingalls, 1975
Hitchmough, Wendy, *C.F.A. Voysey*, London: Phaidon, 1995
Simpson, Duncan, *C.F.A. Voysey: An Architect of Individuality*, London: Lund Humphries, 1979; New York: Whitney Library of Design, 1981
Voysey, C.F.A., *Individuality*, London: Chapman and Hall, 1915; reprint, Longmead, Shaftsbury, Dorset: Element Books, 1986

WAGNER, OTTO 1841–1918

Architect, Austria

Otto Wagner's career spanned the transition from 19th-century historical revivalism to the emergence of a new modern architecture. From the mid-1890s to the time of his death at the end of World War I, he occupied a place at the forefront of the modernist assault in Vienna. Yet Wagner's works and ideas were often complex and contradictory, and his position with respect to the modernist program was not infrequently ambiguous. Although he was among the foremost early proponents of a new tectonic rationalism, Wagner never wholly shed traditional notions of style and beauty, and his lifelong ambition, to become the architect to the Habsburg imperial household, stood in glaring opposition to his desire to forge a new building art for the modern metropolis.

Wagner's early years paralleled the development of the Vienna Ringstrasse, and many of his assumptions were shaped by the prevailing ideals and practices of the era. Born in 1841 into a family of wealthy bourgeois bureaucrats, Wagner received his early architectural training at the Vienna Technical University (1857–59) and the Royal Building Academy in Berlin (1860), where he studied with the successors of Karl Friedrich Schinkel. However, it was at the Academy of Fine Arts in Vienna, which Wagner entered in October 1861, where he encountered the two figures who would form his architectural outlook: August Sicardsburg and Eduard van der Nüll. Sicardsburg and van der Nüll, designers of the Vienna Opera House, had long advocated the necessity of finding a "rational expression for modern architecture" (quoted in Graf, 1987). Wagner's later appreciation of utility and his search for a new language of construction arose from their teachings, and it was to van der Nüll that he attributed his refined facility for drawing.

After completing his education at the Academy in 1863, Wagner embarked on his architectural career. Early on, however, he found few commissions for public projects, and he worked instead on a series of apartment houses, a number of which he financed himself as speculative ventures. Many of these buildings were executed in a "free Renaissance" style, and this new astringent and innovative classicism became the young Wagner's hallmark. By the late 1880s, Wagner was considered the preeminent builder of tenement houses in Vienna, but his attempts to secure more prestigious works remained mostly fruitless. Among the notable exceptions were his Orthodox Synagogue (1871–76) in Budapest and the Österreichische Länderbank (1882–84) in Vienna. The former was executed in a neo-Moorish idiom and the latter in Wagner's more characteristic Renaissance style, but in both buildings the outer historicist skin concealed what were—in material, constructional, and spatial terms—already remarkably modern buildings. Wagner, however, continued to experiment with more conventional ideas of monumentality and form, as his neobaroque *Artibus* project of 1880 powerfully demonstrates, and it was not until the early 1890s that he fully emerged in the guise of an architectural reformer.

Wagner's transformation followed in the wake of his successful entry into the Vienna city-planning competition held in 1893. Drawing on his own growing sense of the primacy of functionality, Wagner's proposal emphasized the creation of an extensive urban rail network as well as the regulation of the Danube Canal and the Wien River. Wagner's straightforward response to the problems of traffic and urban expansion drew widespread praise, and as a consequence, he was named chief architect of the municipal railway system in 1894. The work, which continued until 1901, not only required Wagner to design more than 30 stations but also involved the siting and design of a series of bridges, tunnels, and viaducts. Wagner's first stations, executed in brick and stucco with pronounced classical detailing, reflected traditional ideas of building "art." However, as construction progressed, he began to explore a more stripped and utilitarian idiom. After 1897, Wagner also investigated the possibilities of the new Jugendstil language, which he combined with elements of Renaissance and baroque classicism. In some instances, such as the twin stations on the Karlsplatz that he produced in collaboration with his younger protégé, Josef Maria Olbrich, Wagner's solutions pointed toward a new mode of building—a light iron skeleton framing thin slabs of marble—that anticipated the constructions of the 1920s and beyond. Yet other features of Wagner's designs reveal his continuing allegiance to the past: the private railway pavilion he designed for the imperial family at the Schönbrunn Palace—despite its ebullient iron *porte-cochère*—was still firmly rooted in the "style architecture" of the Ringstrasse era, and many of his other stations

included features—swags, statuary, wreaths, and rustication—intended to disguise or aestheticize their structural details.

In 1894, shortly after beginning work on the city railway project, Wagner was appointed professor of architecture at the Academy of Fine Arts. Although the chair, previously occupied by the noted Ringstrasse architect Carl von Hasenauer, was reserved for a "convinced representative of classical Renaissance," Wagner in his inaugural address called for a new, "realist" approach to the problem of modern building:

> Our living conditions and methods of construction must be fully and completely expressed if architecture is not to be reduced to caricature. The realism of our time must pervade the developing work of art. It will not harm it, nor will any decline of art ensue as a consequence of it; rather it will breathe a new and pulsating life into forms, and in time conquer new fields that today are still devoid of art—for example that of engineering. (quoted in Mallgrave, 1993)

He sounded these same themes again in his book, *Modern Architecture*, which appeared the following year. Conceived as both textbook and manifesto, the work assailed the inability of 19th-century "style architecture" to meet the needs of modern urban life. Wagner called instead for a visual language suited to the new age, one that could fulfill the requirements of the expanding metropolis. Wagner's insistence on pragmatism, like his chosen motto for the *Stadtbahn* project (borrowed from Gottfried Semper), *artis sola domina necessitas* (Necessity is the only master of art), however, merely concealed his own lofty "artistic" ideals: he maintained that the mission of the architect was to find a means of reconciling the realistic and utilitarian with the forms of artistic expression and that it was only through this mediation that mere building could be elevated to *Baukunst* (building art).

Wagner sought to communicate these ideas not only through his works but also in his teachings. Between 1894 and 1912, he devoted a significant portion of his time and energy to his "Special class"—the so-called *Wagnerschule*, or Wagner School—at the Academy; and his students, who included Josef Hoffmann, Joze Plecnik, Jan Kotera, Pavel Janák, Rudolf Perco, Karl Ehn, and Hubert and Franz Gessner, among others, subsequently assumed a central position in the avant-garde in Central Europe. Despite Wagner's stated conviction that truthful and logical construction should constitute the basis for architecture's renewal, however, many of his students were more taken with his language of form, which emphasized the importance of masking or wrapping the internal structure in an outer aesthetic veil. This idea, adapted by Wagner from Semper's theory of *Bekleidung*, or "dressing," emphasized the use of poetic forms or symbols to

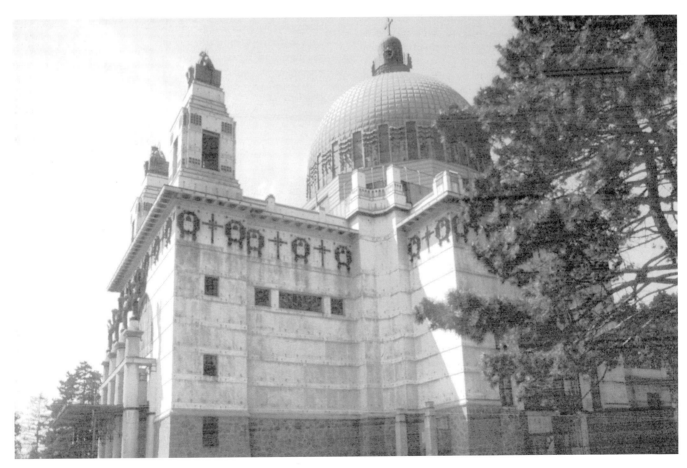

Church of St. Leopold am Steinhof (1907)
Photo © Mary Ann Sullivan

represent themes that could not be expressed through structure alone. Such an approach stood in direct opposition to later concepts of modernism, which advocated clarity and rationality, yet it had a profound and lasting impact on a whole range of younger Central European architects and designers, who reshaped it to articulate a wide array of social, cultural, and economic messages.

In Wagner's own work, this tactic of *Bekleidung* assumed various guises. In 1898–99, in a pair of adjacent buildings on the Linke Wienzeile, it appeared in the form of a florid Jugendstil idiom, the ornament often reduced to two-dimensional graphics or low-relief appliqué. By the early years of the 20th century, however, Wagner had abandoned this language in favor of a stripped, utilitarian classicism, which he combined with geometric forms. His Postal Savings Bank (1904–06, 1910–12), for example, still observed the conventions of a rusticated base and elaborate cornice, but he added to it elements of the new rectilinear Jugendstil. Consistent with his belief in the necessity of adopting new forms of construction, Wagner employed reinforced concrete for the floors of this large office block and made extensive use of aluminum, which he exploited both for its structural qualities and for its aesthetic values. Yet the most dramatic feature of its exterior, the aluminum-headed pins that appear to affix the thin stone panels to the walls while reinforcing the impression of tectonic play, were as much symbolic as structural. Although the pins (which were actually iron but clad in lead with polished aluminum caps so that they would not discolor the marble) served a purpose—to support the underlying mortar—they were also intended to express solidity and stability and thus to reinforce the idea of the building's "dress."

If the Postal Savings Bank betokened a new *Nutzstil*, or utilitarian style, Wagner's unrealized designs for the Franz Josef-Stadtmuseum (city museum) suggested how past and new forms might be fused to fashion a modern monumentality. Wagner labored on the project for more than a decade, from 1900 to 1912, producing a number of variant designs. However, despite his efforts to forge a "modern way of building" that retained the monumental grandeur associated with 19th-century architecture, his building failed to find official or public acceptance—a telling reminder of how strongly Wagner's aesthetic, even in its most traditional form, ran counter to the contemporary taste.

Around 1905, Wagner produced two further examples of the stone-panel-and-aluminum-pin idiom he had announced in the Postal Savings Bank: the Church of St. Leopold am Steinhof (1905–07) and the Kaiserbad Control House (1904–05) on the Danube Canal. However, in his subsequent designs he returned to a highly simplified, functional language. This last phase of his work is perhaps best exemplified by the residential apartment building (1909–10) at Neustiftgasse 40, which, with its clear, blocklike form and regular fenestration, pointed firmly in the direction of a developing modularity.

This gesture toward a new practical aesthetic similarly informed the design of the housing blocks depicted in Wagner's Project for the Future Twenty-second District of Vienna, published in his work *Die Grosstadt* (1911; The Metropolis). The 23-page pamphlet laid out Wagner's mature ideas on city planning, describing in precise terms both an architectural and an economic solution to the problem of the expanding city. He argued that future growth could be financed through municipal control of public utilities and by permitting the city authorities to buy and sell properties. To enable the city to grow, he called for new urban districts of 100,000 to 150,000 inhabitants, with both dwellings and places of work in close proximity to allow residents to work and reside in the same area. Each district would have a formal "air center" for its public and cultural institutions surrounded by uniform apartment buildings. The basic street system would follow a grid, and radial arteries and circular belts of roads and rail would provide connections with the center and other districts. Monumentality would not be achieved by the individual residential blocks but would arise out of their regularity and repetition.

Die Grosstadt was by turns both practical and utopian, but in its advocacy of rational approaches to the problem of the modern city, it was consistent with Wagner's fundamental belief that purpose should be a primary determinant of form. Wagner's vision of modernism, however, although emphasizing the principle of functionality, was considerably more complex and variegated. Despite his emphasis on the constructional and practical aspects of building, he sought at the same time to perpetuate the monumental and representational values of the old architecture as a means to maintain a link with the past. In addition, he remained committed to the ideals of architectural quality and art that, by the end of his life, were rapidly losing currency. Nonetheless, Wagner stands as one of the great early modernist form givers, and his influence reached far into the 20th century.

CHRISTOPHER LONG

Biography

Born in Penzing, Austria, 13 July 1841. Studied at the Technische Hochschule, Vienna 1857–59; attended the Bauakademie, Berlin 1860–61; studied with Eduard van der Nüll and August Sicard von Siccardsburg at the Akademie der Bildenden Künste, Vienna 1861–63. Worked in the studio of Ludwig Förster, Vienna; employed as a master builder for Theophilus Hanser, Vienna 1867. In private practice, Vienna from 1869; assistant to Josef Maria Olbrich 1894. Professor, Akademie der Bildenden Künste, Vienna from 1894; started the Wagnerschule. Founding member, Vienna Secession 1897. Died in Vienna, 11 April 1918.

Selected Works

Synagogue, Budapest, 1876
Länderbank, Vienna, 1884
Stadtbahn System (Karlsplatz Station with Josef Maria Olbrich), Vienna, 1899
Apartment Houses, 38–40 Linke Wienzeile, Vienna, 1899
Quayside Installations, Danube Canal, Vienna, 1905
Postal Savings Bank Office (two stages), Vienna, 1906, 1912
Church of St. Leopold am Steinhof, Vienna, 1907
Kaiserbund Dam, Vienna, 1908
Apartment House, 40 Neustiftgasse, Vienna, 1910

Selected Publications

Einige Skizzen: Projekte und ausgeführte Bauwerke, 4 vols., 1895–1914; as *Sketches, Projects, and Executed Buildings*, 1987
Moderne Architektur, 1896; as *Modern Architecture*, translated by Harry Francis Mallgrave, 1988
Wagnerschule: Projekte, Studien und Skizzen aus der Spezialschule für Architektur des Oberbaurats Otto Wagner, 1902–1907, 1910
Die Grosstadt, 1911

Die Qualität des Baukünstlers, 1912
Die Baukunst unserer Zeit, 4th edition, 1914

Further Reading

Asenbaum, Paul, *Otto Wagner: Möbel und Innenräume*, Salzburg: Residenz, 1984

Bernabei, Giancarlo, *Otto Wagner*, Bologna, Italy: Zanichelli, 1983

Doumato, Lamia, *Otto Wagner, 1841–1918*, Monticello, Illinois: Vance Bibliographies, 1983

Geretsegger, Heinz, Max Peintner, and Walter Pichler, *Otto Wagner, 1841–1918: Unbegrenzte Groszstadt, Beginn der modernen Architektur*, Salzburg: Residenz, 1964; 3rd edition, 1978; as *Otto Wagner, 1841–1918: The Expanding City, the Beginning of Modern Architecture*, London: Pall Mall Press, 1964; New York: Praeger, 1970

Graf, Otto Antonia, *Die vergessene Wagnerschule*, Vienna: Jugend und Volk, 1969

Graf, Otto Antonia, *Masterdrawings of Otto Wagner* (exhib. cat.), New York: Drawing Center, and Vienna: Otto Wagner-Archiv, 1987

Graf, Otto Antonia, *Otto Wagner*, 7 vols., Vienna: Böhlau, 1985–2000

Haiko, Peter and Renata Kassal-Mikula (editors), *Otto Wagner und das Kaiser Franz Josef-Stadtmuseum: Das Scheitern der Moderne in Wien* (exhib. cat.), Vienna: Eigenverlag der Museen der Stadt Wien, 1988

Hollein, Hans, *Otto Wagner*, Tokyo: ADA, 1978

Horvat-Pintaric, V., *Vienna, 1900: The Architecture of Otto Wagner*, New York: Dorset Press, and London: Studio Editions, 1989

Lux, Joseph August, *Otto Wagner*, Munich: Delphin, 1914

Mallgrave, Harry Francis (editor), *Otto Wagner: Reflections on the Raiment of Modernity*, Santa Monica, California: Getty Center for the History of Art and the Humanities, 1993

Müller, Ines, *Die Otto Wagner-Synagoge in Budapest*, Vienna: Löcker, 1992

Otto Wagner, Vienna 1841–1918: Designs for Architecture (exhib. cat.), Oxford: Museum of Modern Art, 1985

Peichl, Gustav, *Die Kunst des Otto Wagner*, Vienna: Akademie der Bildenden Künste, 1984

Pozzetto, Marco, *La Scuola di Wagner, 1894–1912*, Trieste, Italy: Comune di Trieste, 1979

Tietze, Hans, *Otto Wagner*, Vienna: Rikola Verlag, 1922

Varnedoe, Kirk, *Vienna 1900: Art, Architecture, and Design* (exhib. cat.), New York: Museum of Modern Art, 1986

WANAMAKER STORE

Designed by Daniel H. Burnham, completed 1911
Philadelphia, Pennsylvania

The point-and-click mentality of on-line shopping and the average neighborhood mall of the late 20th century are worlds away from what was designed to be an elegant, social, and even educational experience in the first department stores. This spirit was manifest in Philadelphia's Wanamaker's Store. Its patron, John Wanamaker, was a clever businessman who helped to revolutionize retailing in the United States and, while making himself rich, gained the respect and loyalty of generations of Philadelphians who saw his building as more than a department store: Wanamaker's was a monument to the entrepreneurial spirit, deserved success, and benevolence of John Wanamaker.

In 1861 Wanamaker opened a men's apparel shop in Philadelphia with an idea that he could improve the current American

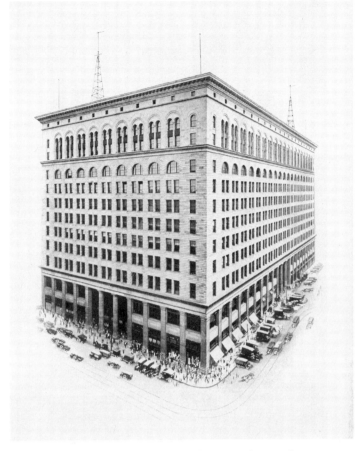

John Wanamaker Building, aerial view of the store showing the Running Track and Game Courts of the Meadowbrook Athletic "Field", Philadelphia, PA
Photo courtesy Friends of the Wanamaker Organ, Bryn Mawr, Pennsylvania

system based on haggling and narrow specialization; by 1876 the business was successful enough to fill an abandoned railroad depot, offering over two acres of floor area and a variety of goods, proving the effectiveness of Wanamaker's introduction of such French retailing principles as accommodating browsing, exchanges and returns, and clearly marking all goods with the same price for all. By the turn of the 20th century, Wanamaker had determined to build a new, even larger establishment. After acquiring a lot on Market Street in downtown Philadelphia adjacent to the Second Empire City Hall, he looked for an architect who could house and give proper expression to his flourishing business on this prestigious site. With dozens of large-scale buildings, high-rises, and planning projects to his credit, Chicago architect Daniel Hudson Burnham was certainly capable of an adequate solution for as big a building as Wanamaker proposed. Burnham's experience and success with this new building type, as with such clients as Marshall Field, the Gimbel Brothers, Edward Filene, and Selfridge of London, made him the acknowledged leader of department store architecture. In addition to his technical and aesthetic talents, Wanamaker must have admired an architect who shared his vision: Wanamaker observed of

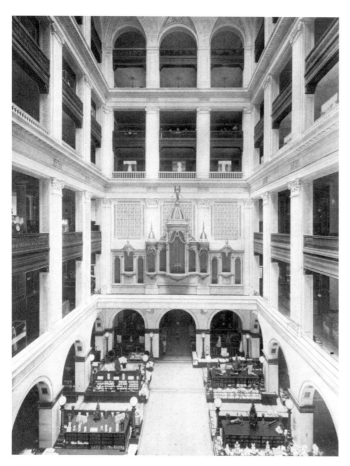

John Wanamaker Building, interior Grand Court
Photo courtesy Friends of the Wanamaker Organ, Bryn Mawr,
Pennsylvania

Burnham, "I think he never had from his boyhood a small idea in his head" (Appel, 1930).

Ground was broken in February 1902. Constructed across eight years, the new building was phased such that the older store emptied a section at a time into it without ever halting business; parts of the new store opened successively in 1905, 1908, and 1910. Its grand opening was held in 1911, Wanamaker's jubilee year in business. The dedication was celebrated in the highest style of any commercial building to date, its trappings indicative of the public character of this privately financed building and 30,000 people in attendance. Of special note was speaker William H. Taft; because U.S. presidents usually bestowed the decorum of their office only on occasions meant to improve or enhance the public welfare, the Wanamaker Store was interpreted on par with such progressive, civic-minded, and publicly oriented projects as the opening of railroads or the celebration of a historical event. Taft glorified the store as "one of the most important instrumentalities in modern life for the promotion of comfort among people" by bringing under one roof at low and fixed prices all of life's necessities (Appel, 1930). Wanamaker, too, lauded the societal importance of his store and compared it with great building projects of the past: unlike the Colosseum—an architectural masterpiece but an otherwise "empty shell"—he compared his store with the Cooper Union, the Carnegie Institute, and Girard College, each a gift of education from a businessman. At Wanamaker's, space was set aside for workers to complete high school degrees. More generally, customers with a world of goods at their fingertips could learn the geography and produce of different countries along with economic lessons; they also had access to free concerts and Wanamaker's own art collection, drawn from the Paris salons, which adorned the store.

The building's form was expressive of its cultured mission. Like many of his earlier office blocks and department stores (especially Marshall Field's, 1902, in Chicago), Burnham conceived the Wanamaker Store after the model of a Renaissance *palazzo* in plan and elevation. Hewn of Maine granite, the tripartite facades feature a three-story base with large squared openings glazed with broad plate-glass display windows. Above, seven nearly identical floors, articulated with paired windows between piers and topped with arched windows, express the building's repetitive steel structure in a pattern reminiscent of H.H. Richardson's Marshall Field Wholesale Store (1885). A classical cornice two stories tall caps the building. With another three additional stories below street level, the hulking mass commanded a full city block, its footprint measuring roughly 500 by 250 feet. Hailed as the most monumental commercial structure in the world, the $10 million store housed two million square feet of retailing space from which one could buy literally anything, including automobiles and airplanes.

A model of corporate efficiency, the store was the first in America to employ a pneumatic tube system, telephone service, and a ventilation fan system and to provide a restaurant and U.S. parcel post delivery. The display areas were spacious and well illuminated (power was furnished by Wanamaker's own power plant on Ludlow Street), arranged logically around a courtyard to provide ease of navigation through the huge store. Although the functionality of the floor area was of prime concern to Burnham and Wanamaker, both saw the building as more than a place to buy and sell. The building's focus is a centralized Grand Court rising 150 feet to its ceiling and surrounded by arcaded galleries opening from the first seven floors, whose ceiling heights range from 15 to 25 feet. Giant Ionic and Corinthian columns, a marble floor, and classical ornaments in plaster and Keene cement articulate the space in which Wanamaker deposited two souvenirs from the 1903 St. Louis World's Fair: a large bronze eagle sculpture that became a landmark in itself (Philadelphians have met under its beak for generations) and a great pipe organ, advertised as the second largest in the world, on which daily concerts were performed. The balcony at its base accommodated 100 musicians. In an attempt to make the retail experience elegant and uplifting, as well as to educate the public in music, concerts were also provided in the 1,500-seat Egyptian Room, which was adorned with columns based on those at Karnak, on sphinxes, and on other Egyptian motifs. A smaller auditorium also fitted with an organ, the mahogany-paneled Greek Room, seated 600 among sturdy Doric pilasters and columns. In keeping with the Gilded Age's interest in period rooms, the store also featured a Byzantine Hall, Empire Room, and Moorish Room for special goods, further conjoining cultural lessons with retail merchandising, the overall goal of Wanamaker's.

JHENNIFER A. AMUNDSON

Further Reading

Hendrickson offers a fine account of the social and business history of the department store in America. Brief architectural considerations of the Wanamaker Building are included in Tatum and in Hines. The most complete description of the building appears in the *Golden Book of the Wanamaker Stores*, a 500-page work that combines a history of Philadelphia and of the evolution of retail commerce in the United States with Wanamaker's philosophies on life and business.

Appel, Joseph H., *The Business Biography of John Wanamaker*, New York: Macmillan, 1930

Appel, Joseph Herbert, and Leigh Mitchell Hodges (compilers), *Golden Book of the Wanamaker Stores, Jubilee Year, 1861–1911*, Philadelphia, Pennsylvania: John Wanamaker, 1911

Conwell, Russell H., *The Romantic Rise of a Great American*, New York and London: Harper, 1924

Hendrickson, Robert, *The Grand Emporiums*, New York: Stein and Day, 1979

Hines, Thomas S., *Burnham of Chicago, Architect and Planner*, New York: Oxford University Press, 1974

Tatum, George, *Penn's Great Town*, Philadelphia: University of Pennsylvania Press, 1961

WAREHOUSE

Warehouses, buildings that provide storage for commercial gain, have had two primary functional mandates—the provision of storage space on floors with a high load capacity and the facilitation of the movement of goods and freight with materials-handling equipment—since the mid-19th century, when the building type and term became common. Nevertheless, warehouses underwent fundamental changes in form as well as in architectural presence during the 20th century.

General-purpose, cold-storage, bonded, and household-goods warehouses, as well as industry-specific facilities, were in use by the turn of the 20th century. At that time the typical warehouse was a loft structure of five stories in which goods were moved with platform elevators. The interior framing of these structures consisted of wood, cast-iron, and wrought-iron members combined to support heavy floor loads. Masonry warehouses were often divided by interior firewalls into a series of discrete spaces, and such divisions were sometimes expressed on their exteriors through piers and fenestration patterns. These warehouses had enough windows to light the interior without the introduction of the fire hazard of lanterns and to allow for conversion of the building to other uses; as electric lighting became more commonly used in warehouses, the number of window openings was reduced. Exterior, raised loading platforms sheltered by sheet-metal awnings and series of wide doorways articulated the street levels of warehouses.

A functional yet expressive tone of architectural styling for warehouses was set during the 19th century. The sturdy brick forms and detailing of the *Rundbogenstil*, with piers, arcades, corbeled brick cornices, and arched window openings, were often selected to express both a warehouse's stability and strength and its important role in commerce. In a series of articles that appeared in the *Architectural Record*, the critic Russell Sturgis drew attention to early 20th-century warehouse design that offered a similar clear expression of structure and monumentality and was not cluttered with any applied ornament. Many ware-houses built during the first half of the 20th century exhibited architectural presence and expressed this aesthetic sensibility as utilitarian purpose tempered references to current styles.

During the first decades of the 20th century, warehouses reflected both the continued success of capitalism and advances in building arts as the warehouses became even larger and stronger and incorporated new materials-handling methods. The use of expensive steel beams was often limited to the framing of wide bays on the ground floor for the accommodation of rail and motor vehicles. Reinforced concrete, however, was widely adopted because it was strong and fire resistant. The United States Army Supply Base (1918) in Brooklyn, New York, designed by architect Cass Gilbert, consisted of a pair of reinforced-concrete loft buildings that flanked a covered rail siding commanded by a traveling crane. The facility was widely admired because of its materials-handling system as well as for the way in which Gilbert carefully modeled the stark concrete facades to convey great scale and strength. Another American project, the Starrett-Lehigh Building (1930–31) in New York City, designed by Cory and Cory with Yasuo Matsui, associate architect, demonstrated the ultimate development of the multi-story warehouse both in the vertical movement of goods and in the architectural expression of function. This structure covered an entire block and rose to a height of 19 stories. Its steel-framed central service and circulation core, which served as a "vertical street" to bring trucks to each warehouse floor, was articulated by soaring pilasters. More dominant in the design, however, were the flanking lofts. Their walls were slightly cantilevered beyond the exterior columns to permit horizontal bands of windows and rounded corners. With its interpretation of European architectural modernism of the day, the Starrett-Lehigh Building earned notice in the Museum of Modern Art's "Modern Architecture: International Exhibition" of 1932.

A new preference for the horizontal movement of goods, the relocation of warehousing operations to sites outside of urban cores, and a heightened desire to minimize warehousing costs led to dramatic changes for warehouses during the middle third of the century. Experimentation with platform trucks during the 1930s demonstrated the advantages of one-story facilities; after World War II, forklift trucks and pallets that "unitized" goods storage and shipment became the modern tools of warehousing. The warehouse design problem changed to become a matter of limiting initial costs and choosing the best size and shape of a one-story structure that would have masonry bearing walls and a lightweight flat roof. Ceiling heights of 20 feet or more and smooth floors were provided to accommodate forklift trucks and pallets. An office area with a public entry and fenestration was positioned to screen the rest of the building from the street or to occupy a corner of the building. Freight doors, truck docks, and railroad sidings became the only features of the other sides of these windowless warehouses. Brick and other siding materials enclosed bland, unstyled warehouses intended to blend in with nearby commercial and industrial structures.

During the late 20th century, warehousing operations and buildings continued to evolve in response to a just-in-time manufacturing philosophy and the development of distribution networks that used a smaller number of larger warehouses. Even more emphatically, the warehouse building became perceived as merely a means to protect the storage medium and materials-handling systems that were the important components of the

operation. To serve Europe, Nike, Inc., developed a pair of side-by-side distribution centers (1994–95) near Meerhout, Belgium, that are representative of the quite large facilities developed during the 1990s. The structures enclose one million square feet and cover 23 acres as they accommodate high-bay storage that rises to a height of nearly 100 feet.

Yet even as most new warehouses became little-noticed background buildings in industrial developments and port areas, older urban warehouses were rehabilitated for new uses. Since the 1970s warehouses with style and versatile loft floors in Copenhagen, London, New York, and many other cities have provided space for people to live and work in lively mixed-use neighborhoods and waterfront areas.

BETSY HUNTER BRADLEY

Further Reading

Architectural historians and critics have seldom turned their attention to the warehouse. Some books on industrial architecture, such as Bradley, address both the functional and aesthetic aspects of warehouses. Works by engineers on facilities design (Harmon; Heragu) are useful to trace changes in warehousing practice and operation. Architectural periodicals remain the best source for warehouse design trends. American warehouses in historic districts and redevelopment areas have often been documented in local preservation agency reports, such as the New York City Landmarks Preservation Commission's SoHo and TriBeCa Historic District Designation Reports.

Bradley, Betsy Hunter, *The Works: The Industrial Architecture of the United States*, New York: Oxford University Press, 1999
Buildings for Industry, New York: Dodge, 1957
Harmon, Roy L., *Reinventing the Warehouse: World Class Distribution Logistics*, New York: Free Press and Macmillan International, and Toronto, Ontario: Macmillan Canada, 1993
Heragu, Sunderesh, *Facilities Design*, Boston: PWS, 1997
Shockley, Jay, *Starrett-Lehigh Building, 601–625 West 26th Street, Borough of Manhattan: Built 1930–31: Russell G. and Walter M. Cory, Architects: Yasuo Matsui, Associate Architect: Purdy & Henderson, Consulting Engineers*, New York: New York City Landmarks Preservation Commission, 1986
SoHo—Cast Iron Historic District Designation Report, New York: New York City Landmarks Preservation Commission, 1973
Sturgis, Russell, "The Warehouse and Factory: Architecture," *Architectural Record*, 15 (January–February 1904)
Sturgis, Russell, "Some Recent Warehouses," *Architectural Record*, 23 (May 1908)
TriBeCa South Historic District: Designation Report, New York: New York City Landmarks Preservation Commission, 1992

WASHINGTON, D.C.

A discussion of Washington, D.C., architecture must begin with the city plan developed by Pierre Charles L'Enfant in 1791, for it established a strong context of geometry, scale, and hierarchy. L'Enfant's plan overlaid an orthogonal grid of streets with diagonal avenues. The narrower, orthogonal streets serve as utilitarian means of access, whereas the wide, tree-lined avenues connect open-space nodes. The heights of buildings along all Washington thoroughfares are limited by law so that no building can be taller than the Capitol.

L'Enfant's plan established a monumental federal precinct surrounded by smaller-scaled mercantile and residential precincts. The Capitol was placed on the highest hill within a Congress Garden, linked by Pennsylvania Avenue to the White House, set in the President's Park. On the axis west from the Capitol to the Potomac River was the Grand Avenue, now the Mall, a vast open space lined with federal buildings. This area developed haphazardly until the Senate Park Commission Plan of 1901 established a clear master plan. Since 1972 the Pennsylvania Avenue Development Corporation has redesigned this avenue and controlled development along its north side.

The context for architecture in the federal precinct was established early by the Capitol and the White House: neoclassical, light-colored stone, figural, symmetrical, and monumental. All the early buildings of the 20th century, the memorials and museums, were designed in this idiom. In the last half of the century, architects struggled with these contextual restrictions and found ways to vary the materials and alter the stylistic formula.

The context for architecture in the mercantile precinct changed the most during the 20th century from low-scale mixed use to high-density commercial. It is highly varied, with examples from all eras of the city's history. Metro, Washington's rapid transit and subway system, was opened in 1976 with handsome stations dominated by concrete barrel vaults consistently designed by Harry Weese and Associates of Chicago.

The first part of the 20th century, from 1900 to 1940, was a very active period of design and construction, primarily within the federal precinct. A great number of high-quality buildings were built as the federal government acted on the recommendations of the Senate Park Commission. The first act was to remove the train station from the Mall and to construct a new one west of the Capitol. The Beaux-Arts–inspired Union Station and Columbia Plaza were completed in 1908 as designed by the noted Chicago architect Daniel Burnham.

This was followed by development of the Mall, capitol square, and the federal triangle. The Lincoln Memorial (1922) by Henry Bacon, on axis with the Capitol, features the marble statue of Abraham Lincoln by Daniel Chester French. The Jefferson Memorial (1943) by John Russell Pope, on axis with the White House, features the enormous statue of Thomas Jefferson by Rudolph Evans. New buildings added to capitol square included the Supreme Court Building (1935) between twin buildings for the House and the Senate built in 1908. New buildings along the north side of the Mall were the National Museum of Natural History (1911) and the National Gallery of Art (1941). The federal triangle was developed as an ensemble of large neoclassical buildings featuring the National Archives (1935) by John Russell Pope. Defining the north side of the Mall west of the White House were Constitution Hall (1939), the Organization of American States (1910), the Federal Reserve Building (1937), the National Academy of Sciences (1924), and the American Pharmaceutical Association (1933). This series of white pavilions set within a verdant landscape and designed by very notable architects is probably the most handsome series of buildings along one avenue in Washington.

The most glorious building commenced during this era is the Washington National Cathedral (1907–90) by Henry Vaughn and George Bodley, the last Gothic cathedral structure to be built in the world.

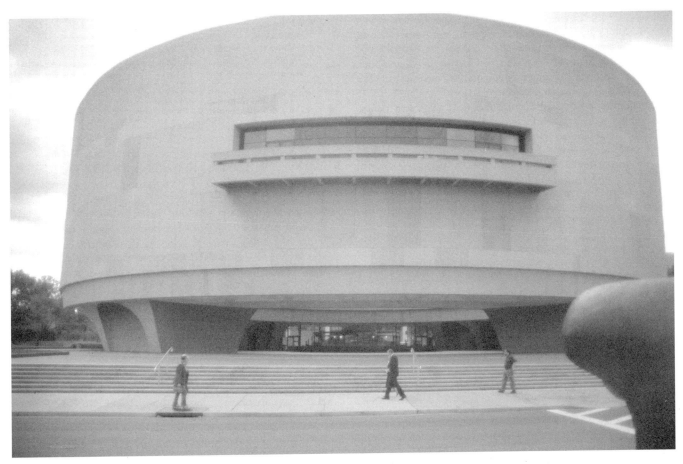

Hirshhorn Museum (1974), designed by Gordon Bunshaft (Skidmore, Owings, and Merrill)
© Ernest and Kathleen Meredith/GreatBuildings.com

From 1945 to 1960, the country and city were recovering from the aftermath of World War II. Much good architecture was destroyed during the urban-renewal era of the 1950s for the sake of highways or real estate development. The historic preservation movement abated this destruction, but it still did occur many times, with only historic pieces of blocks and buildings saved and incorporated into new development. The replacement buildings usually were not noteworthy. Modern architecture was introduced to Washington during this period in the work of architects Joseph Abel, Charles Goodman, and Chloethiel Woodard Smith.

From 1960 to 2000, both the quality and the quantity of architecture in Washington increased substantially. Two early buildings from this period worth noting are the exquisite Pre-Columbian Museum (1963) at Dumbarton Oaks by Philip Johnson and the boldly curvilinear Watergate (1965) by Luigi Moretti.

During this era, the firms of Hartman-Cox and Keyes Condon Florance (KCF) developed an approach to developer architecture that was sympathetic to the Washington urban context while also exploring inventive design expressions. George Hartman and Warren Cox began their practice designing very modern buildings, such as the Euram Building (1971) on Dupont Circle and the National Permanent Building (1976) at 18th Street and Pennsylvania Avenue. They progressed to a number of contextual commercial projects that incorporated historic buildings, such as Sumner School (1986) and 1001 Pennsylvania Avenue, NW (1986). Their two best projects are One Franklin Square (1990) and Market Square (1990). The former, on Franklin Square, strongly defines the north side of this space and adds two pyramid-topped towers. The latter, on Pennsylvania Avenue across from the National Archives, is suitably neoclassical and incorporates the Navy Memorial.

KCF began as Keyes Lethbridge Condon, designing the modern curvilinear housing of Columbia Plaza (1967). The firm then became Keyes Condon Florance, designing urbanistically appropriate buildings with strong street walls, such as Lafayette Square (1991). Many of their projects have been at street intersections that they exploit. A good example is at 2401 Pennsylvania Avenue, NW (1980), with its curved windows and balconies. The firm then changed partners to become Florance Eichbaum Esocoff King and designed the Art Deco office building at 1100 New York Avenue, incorporating the Greyhound bus station as an entry. Three other firms that have been developing a Washington style of abstract contextualism are Shalom Baranes Associates, David M. Schwarz, and Weinstein Associates.

The most influential out-of-town firm has been I.M. Pei and Partners, now Pei, Cobb, Freed and Partners. Their work began with urban-renewal projects in the southwest part of the city: Town Center Plaza (1962) and L'Enfant Plaza (1968). This was

followed by the East Building of the National Gallery of Art (1978), a tour de force of monumental abstract forms encompassing an exhilarating atrium. The United States Holocaust Memorial Museum (1993), designed by James Ingo Freed, maintains a balance between monumentality and contextual resolution with a highly energized central space. Their latest project is the enormous Ronald Reagan Building (1998), which completes the federal triangle. Here, Freed's exterior is more influenced by the monumental neoclassical context, whereas the engaging interior public space is very modern in expression.

The international firm of Skidmore, Owings and Merrill (SOM) has had a strong influence on Washington architecture because it maintained a local office for many years under the direction of partner David Childs. During this period it produced some of the refined modern office buildings for which it is known. These include the Inter-American Development Bank at 1300 New York Avenue, NW (1983), with its spectacular atrium, and 1201 Pennsylvania Avenue, NW (1984), with its triangular atrium. The best-known and most controversial building by SOM is the circular concrete Hirshhorn Museum (1974) on the Mall, designed by partner Gordon Bunshaft.

Washington has also been the locus for numerous buildings by well-known architects from around the world. Although these buildings have usually challenged their context, they add an element of surprise attraction that enlivens the cityscape. The earliest of these projects is the Brutalist concrete Department of Housing and Urban Development (1968) by Marcel Breuer. Later projects include the boxlike, white-marble Kennedy Center for the Performing Arts (1971) by Edward Durell Stone; the stark steel Martin Luther King, Jr., Memorial Library (1972) by Mies van der Rohe; and the marble-and-glass cubes of the National Air and Space Museum (1976) by Hellmuth, Obata and Kassabaum.

Because Washington is the national capital, it has embassies that add another aspect of architectural interest, as they try to reflect the spirit of their country. The earliest of these is the British Embassy (1931) by Sir Edwin Lutyens, a quirky interpretation of an English country house. The Canadian Chancery (1989) by Arthur Erickson is in the most prominent location on Pennsylvania Avenue between the Capitol and the White House. It is a gray-marble building of varied forms with an open courtyard facing John Marshall Park. The recent Embassy of Finland (1994) by Heikkinen and Komonen has attracted much attention for its deference to the natural setting, utilizing transparent screens.

Washington is a city with architecture that abides by its civic role. The strong context was established at its founding by the L'Enfant plan and continues to be followed. The building masses form clearly defined streets and open spaces, and the materials and colors are contextually appropriate. There is a civility to the architecture that gives this city more design integrity than any other American city.

MICHAEL J. BEDNAR

Further Reading

Highsmith, Carol M., and Ted Landphair, *Pennsylvania Avenue: America's Main Street*, Washington, D.C.: American Institute of Architects Press, 1988

Kousoulas, Claudia D., and George W. Kousoulas, *Contemporary Architecture in Washington, D.C.*, Washington, D.C.: Preservation Press, and New York: Wiley, 1995

Longstreth, Richard (editor), *The Mall in Washington, 1791–1991*, Washington, D.C.: National Gallery of Art, 1991

Scott, Pamela, and Antoinette J. Lee, *Buildings of the District of Columbia*, New York: Oxford University Press, 1993; Oxford: Oxford University Press, 1994

Weeks, Christopher, *AIA Guide to the Architecture of Washington, D.C.*, 3rd edition, Baltimore, Maryland: Johns Hopkins University Press, 1994

WISSA WASSEF, RAMSES 1911–74

Architect, Egypt (Africa)

Ramses Wissa Wassef was born into a prominent and cultured Francophile Coptic (Egyptian Christian) family in Cairo. His father was an influential member of the nationalist Wafd Party and one of the founders of the École des Beaux-Arts in Cairo, which opened, in the teeth of opposition from the office of the British consul-general in Egypt, in 1908. Wissa Wassef completed his education in France and studied architecture at the École des Beaux-Arts in Paris, where he received his diploma in 1935. His diploma project, "The Potter's House in Old Cairo," already revealed his interest in and knowledge of the traditional crafts of his homeland.

On returning to Egypt in 1936, Wissa Wassef was appointed professor of the art and history of architecture in the Department of Architecture of the School of Fine Arts, Cairo. The Department of Architecture at the School of Fine Arts, in Zamalek on Gezira Island between the two arms of the Nile near Cairo, was the first modern school of architecture to be founded in Egypt. Presently incorporated in the University of Helwan (Zamalek Campus), the school continues the arts-and-crafts tradition pioneered by Hassam Fathy and Wissa Wassef.

Wissa Wassef had followed Hassan Fathy as head of the Department of Architecture at the School of Fine Arts, and both men shared a passion for the traditional vernacular architecture of their native land. Field study visits into the rural areas of the Nile delta and of Lower and Upper Egypt were annual events for students of the School of Architecture under their direction; and for both men, the traditional architecture of Nubia, the southernmost region of Egypt above and around the Aswan Dam, became and remained a perennial source of inspiration. Wissa Wassef was primarily a teacher, fired by the desire to communicate his love and profound knowledge of architecture and of arts and crafts generally not only to his architecture students but also to children. He stated, "I had this vague conviction that every human being was born an artist, but that his gifts could be brought out only if artistic creation were encouraged by the practising of a craft from early childhood" (see de Stefano, n.d.).

In 1941 Wissa Wassef was commissioned by a social welfare organization to design a small primary school in the Coptic quarter of Old Cairo. This provided him with the opportunity to test his conviction, and he persuaded the management committee to let him teach weaving to the children after school. He chose weaving, a craft about which he knew very little, as the first craft to teach young children because he believed that the simple techniques could be easily learned and that the craft process would enable children to develop and express their innate creativity through producing colorful visual images. His pupils,

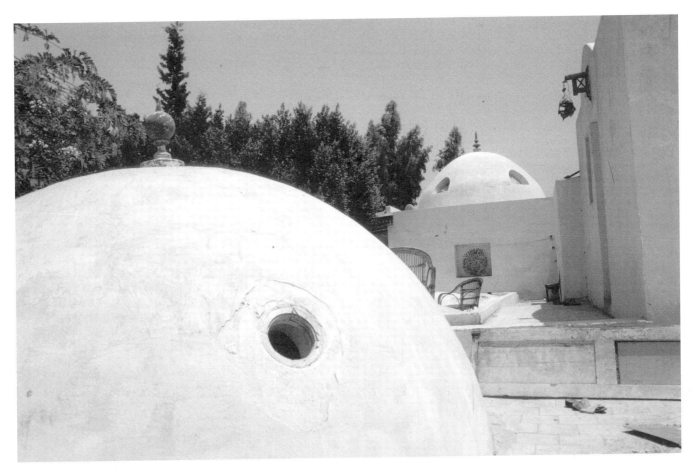

El-Dar Restaurant, view from the roof showing its mud-brick dome
© Aga Khan Trust for Culture

children from the humblest homes, were producing work that gave them both great satisfaction and a potential source of income, and so within a few years he resolved to build his own school and craft training center where he could realize his vision of a cooperative of artist-craftsmen, living and working in the local community. His wife, Sophie Habib Gorgy, was a sculptor and shared his enthusiasm and his vision. In 1951, they purchased a small plot of land on the outskirts of the village of Harraniya, a few miles south of Giza on the west bank of the Nile, and began to build the school that was eventually to bear his name, the Ramses Wissa Wassef Arts Centre. He devoted the greater part of the rest of his life, especially after his retirement from the School of Fine Arts in 1969, to its completion.

Although primarily a teacher, Wissa Wassef was a sensitive and accomplished architect, and his built works are many and varied. Apart from the Arts Centre at Harraniya, his best-known works are the Mahmoud Mokhtar Sculpture Museum (1962–64) in Cairo, the Church of al-Mar'ashali in Zamalek, Cairo, and the Virgin Mary Church in Cairo. He designed and built several houses for private clients, including the Ina Magar Country Home (1969), Adam Hennen Residence (1968), the Mohi Houssin Residence (1970), and his own house in Agouza. In 1968, Wissa Wassef incorporated traditional Nubian structures

in the design of El-Dar Restaurant in Giza, Egypt, that he built of mud brick with vault and dome technology.

In 1961, he was awarded a National Prize for the Arts for the stained-glass windows he designed and made for the National Festival Hall in Cairo and in 1964 a National Prize for the Arts for the design of the Mahmoud Mokhtar Sculpture Museum.

ANTHONY D.C. HYLAND

See also **Cairo, Egypt; Ramses Wissa Wassef Arts Centre, Giza, Egypt**

Biography

Born in Cairo, 9 November 1911; father was a lawyer and politician. Studied architecture, École des Beaux-Arts, Paris 1929–35; bachelor's degree 1935. Married Sophie Habib Gorgy, 1948: 2 children. Bought land in Harraniya, near Giza, and built the Harraniya Arts Centre later the Ramses Wissa Wassef Arts Centre 1951–70. Professor of the art and the history of architecture, College of Fine Arts, Cairo 1936–69. The Ramses Wissa Wassef Arts Centre received the Aga Khan Award for Architecture in 1983. Died in Cairo 1974.

Selected Works

Primary School, Church of St. Barbara, Old Cairo (Misr El-Adima), 1941

Harraniya Weaving (Craft) Village (with Hassan Fathy), Giza, Egypt, 1957

Mahmoud Mokhtar Sculpture Museum, Cairo, Egypt, 1964

Adam Hennen Residence, Giza, Egypt, 1968

El-Dar Restaurant, Giza, Egypt, 1968

Mohi Houssin Residence, Giza, Egypt, 1970

Harraniya Art Center (Ramses Wissa Wassef Arts Centre), Harraniya, Egypt, 1970

Coptic Cathedral, Zamalek

Coptic Cathedral, Heliopolis

Ramses Wissa Wassef House, Agouza

Further Reading

De Stefano, E.A., *Threads of Life: A Journey in Creativity: Ramses Wissa Wassef Arts Centre*, Giza, Egypt: Ramses Wissa Wassef Arts Centre, n.d.

Kultermann, Udo, "Contemporary Arab Architecture: The Architects of Egypt," *Mimar*, 4 (1982)

WEISSENHOFSIEDLUNG, DEUTSCHER WERKBUND (STUTTGART, 1927)

Exhibition by various architects, 1927
Stuttgart, Germany

The Weissenhofsiedlung was one of the most significant architectural exhibitions of the 20th century. It brought together for the first time the work of some of the most influential and progressive European designers from the early decades of the century. The exposition, held in Stuttgart, Germany, in 1927, focused on "Die Wohnung" (the Dwelling). Initiated by the Deutscher Werkbund and financed by the city of Stuttgart, it presented current ideas in modern residential design. The central feature of the event was a development of 21 domestic buildings located on the Weissenhof hillside overlooking the city. Over a half million people visited the Siedlung during the summer of 1927.

The full-scale model housing development was only one part of the exhibition. Domestic products and furniture were displayed together in the exhibit "The Interior Design of the House," located at Gewerbeplatz in Stuttgart. The exhibit featured the Spiegelglashalle, a plate-glass hall designed by Lilly Reich and Ludwig Mies van der Rohe that consisted of wall planes of various glass materials—a predecessor to Mies's German Pavilion designed two years later for the Barcelona Exposition. The "International Exhibition of Modern Architecture: Designs and Models," held in the center of Stuttgart, contained plans, drawings, models, and photographs of foreign buildings that reflected the new architectural ideas promoted in the designs of the Siedlung. A third group of exhibits, located at a site adjacent to the Weissenhof estate, demonstrated the attributes of recently developed building materials and new methods of construction, including industrial prefabrication.

The initial underlying social goal of the exhibition was to present modern solutions to the urgent need for low- and middle-income housing. Event organizers sought to demonstrate ways to reduce housing costs and improve living conditions through the use of recently introduced building materials and construction methods. Many of the 17 architects involved in the Siedlung, however, ignored the basic economic objective of the show and created designs more appropriate for affluent families. Many of the individual housing units even contained maid's quarters.

Participating designers came from Austria, Holland, Switzerland, Belgium, and Germany. Organizers hired Mies van der Rohe as artistic director, and Richard Döcker served as technical director. Other architects who contributed designs for the development included Peter Behrens, Le Corbusier and his partner Pierre Jeanneret, Josef Frank, Walter Gropius, Ludwig Hilberseimer, J.J.P. Oud, Hans Poelzig, Adolf Rading, Hans Scharoun, Adolf Schneck, Mart Stam, Bruno Taut, and Max Taut. A house designed by the Belgian architect Victor Bourgeois located adjacent to the development was also incorporated into the exhibition.

Most of the buildings in the Siedlung were situated on streets that curved along the Weissenhof hillside. The designs featured flat, unadorned facades; flat roofs; ribbon windows; and pipe railing. Although the basic, formal characteristics of the buildings suggested a great sense of unity among the designers, the unique nature of each of their architectural ideologies was apparent in the details. Individual designers focused on different aspects of modern housing. Mies van der Rohe designed a four-story block of terrace apartments that served as the centerpiece of the exhibition. Inside, he showed how universal spaces could be adapted to meet individual needs. Le Corbusier illustrated his own ideas for the modern dwelling in two houses of reinforced concrete that he designed with Pierre Jeanneret. The architect realized the concept of his Citrohan House in the first residence, whereas the second house featured the five points of architecture discussed in his 1923 treatise *Towards a New Architecture*. Some designers, such as Gropius, Stam, and Max Taut, explored newly available building materials and ideas regarding prefabrication. Others, such as Scharoun, Poelzig, and Schneck, were more interested in producing functional layouts that could better meet the needs of the modern family. Although the facades of the Weissenhof buildings appear neutral in black-and-white photographs, in reality many of the walls were originally painted in shades of yellow, blue, and other colors. Bruno Taut, Max Taut, and Le Corbusier all incorporated intense colors in their designs. Bruno Taut, for example, specified different saturated hues for the individual walls of his small, single-family residence, leading one critic to describe the vivid colors as coming right out of a paint box.

The architecture of the Weissenhofsiedlung was strongly rejected by the National Socialists in Germany, who labeled it the "product of 'cultural Bolshevists.'" The event was better received in European and American design journals. The success of the Siedlung led to a succession of similar housing exhibitions in Germany and elsewhere across Central Europe, including events in Prague, Brno, and Vienna. Progressive European architects used these exhibitions to present and debate their modern design ideologies. Their desire to further develop such dialogue led to the formation of CIAM (Congrès Internationaux d'Architecture Moderne) in 1929, which provided a platform for designers to discuss developing ideas in modern architecture. The formal unity of the designs included in the Siedlung contributed to the concept of an International Style in modern architecture that was heavily promoted five years later by Henry Russell Hitch-

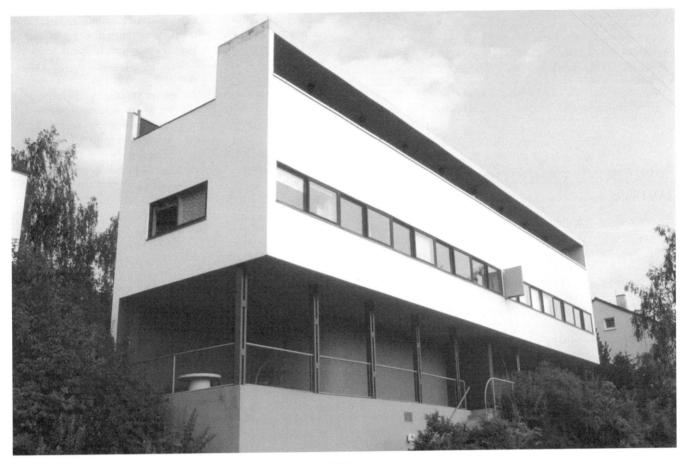

House for Weissenhofsiedlung, designed by Le Corbusier, Stuttgart (1927)
Photo © Donald Corner and Jenny Young/GreatBuildings.com

cock and Philip Johnson in the "Modern Architecture—International Exposition" show held at the Museum of Modern Art in 1932. The exhibit and subsequent book featured several buildings from the Weissenhofsiedlung.

The site of the Weissenhof development was sold to the German state in 1938 for use by the military. Bombs destroyed houses located in the center of the estate in 1944. New houses replaced these and several other residences that were torn down after World War II. At the end of the century, only 11 of the original buildings remained standing. The Siedlung underwent an extensive restoration in the mid-1980s that was completed in time for a 60th anniversary celebration of the exhibition. Today the development continues to attract visitors interested in experiencing full-scale examples of progressive modern housing designs from the mid-1920s.

LISA D. SCHRENK

See also **Corbusier, Le (Jeanneret, Charles-Édouard) (France); Deutscher Werkbund; Gropius, Walter (Germany); Mies van der Rohe, Ludwig (Germany); Oud, J.J.P. (the Netherlands); Poelzig, Hans (Germany); Taut, Bruno (Germany)**

Further Reading

Badovici, Jean, *L'Architecture vivante en Allemagne: La Cité jardin du Weissenhof à Stuttgart*, Paris: Morancé, 1928

Classen, Helge, *Die Weissenhofsiedlung: Beginn eines neuen Bauens*, Dortmund, Germany: Harenberg, 1990

DIA Serie I: *Die Weissenhofsiedlung: Architektur und Architekten*, Stuttgart: Landesbildstelle Württemberg, 1990

DIA Serie II: *Die Weissenhofsiedlung: Innenräume: Impulse für unser Jahrhundert* (text by Karin Kirsch), Stuttgart: Landesbildstelle Württemberg, 1990

Gleinig, Wolf Rainer, *Der Weissenhof im Dritten Reich*, Weinsberg: Kunow, 1983

Joedicke, Jürgen, *Die Weissenhofsiedlung*, Stuttgart: Kramer, 1968; 3rd edition, as *Die Weissenhofsiedlung; The Weissenhof Colony; La Cité de Weissenhof, Stuttgart* (trilingual English-German-French edition), 1984

Joedicke, Jürgen, *Weissenhofsiedlung Stuttgart*, Stuttgart: Karl Krämer, 1968; 2nd edition, 1989

Kirsch, Karin, *Die Weissenhofsiedlung: Werkbund Ausstellung "Die Wohnung," Stuttgart 1927*, Stuttgart: Deutsche Verlags-Anstalt, 1987; as *The Weissenhofsiedlung: Experimental Housing Built for the Deutscher Werkbund, Stuttgart, 1927*, New York: Rizzoli, 1989

Kirsch, Karin, *Kleiner Führer durch die Weissenhofsiedlung: Ein Denkmal der modernen Architektur*, Stuttgart: Deutsche Verlags-Anstalt, 1991

Menrad, Anreas, "Die Weissenhof-Siedlung-farbig: Quellen, Befunde und die Revision eines Klischees," *Deutsche Kunst und Denkmalpflege*, 34/1 (1986)

Nägele, Hermann, *Die Restaurierung der Weissenhofsiedlung, 1981–1987*, Stuttgart: Kramer, 1992

Pommer, Richard and Christian F. Otto, *Weissenhof 1927 and the Modern Movement in Architecture*, Chicago: University of Chicago Press, 1991

Rasch, Heinz, and Bodo Rasch, *Wie bauen? Bau und Einrichtung der Werkbundsiedlung am Weissenhof in Stuttgart 1927*, Stuttgart: Wedekind, 1927

Roth, Alfred, *Zwei Wohnhäuser von Le Corbusier und Pierre Jeanneret*, Stuttgart: Wedekind, 1927; reprint, Stuttgart: Kramer, 1977

WERKBUND EXHIBITION, COLOGNE (1914)

The Werkbund Exhibition held in Cologne, Germany, on the eve of World War I was the first major manifesto of the Deutscher Werkbund (DWB; German Work Association), an organization founded in 1907 by artists, architects, and industrialists to address the problem of form and design in the industrial age. The exhibit sought to show the world the Werkbund's successful attempt to ally the creative potential of art with the modern power of industry to create more aesthetically pleasing and higher-quality products and thereby raise German exports in an increasingly competitive world market. Architecturally, the exhibit gained nearly instant fame through a number of very innovative exhibit pavilions built by some of Germany's most distinguished architects as well as the theoretical "Werkbund Debate," which greatly influenced the future of modern German design and architecture after the war.

Much like a world's fair, the exhibition was a microcosm of prewar German culture, products, and know-how designed by more than 1000 Werkbund members. The vast exhibits contained "everything from couch cushions to city building," as a contemporary slogan proclaimed. The primary exhibits featured architecture and applied arts, but there were also displays on sport, women's fashion, religious art, colonial wares, worker housing, factories, cabaret, cinema, transportation, theater, garden design, funerary sculpture, and much more. A large amusement park was integrated into the exhibit to provide entertainment and eating establishments for the more than one million visitors who came. The city built advanced mass transit systems to ensure easy access to the fairgrounds from all over the world.

Although the city of Cologne previously had very few connections to the Werkbund, by agreeing to pay for the exhibit, and with its strategic location in the center of one of Germany's most industrialized regions and close to the French border, Cologne proved to be an ideal host for this exhibit of the pride of German industry. Intent on success, the organizers commissioned the famed architect and designer Peter Behrens to create the overall exhibit organization and hired only the biggest-name architects to design the various pavilions. The main festival hall by Behrens, the primary exhibit building by Theodor Fischer, several buildings by Hermann Muthesius, the Austrian Pavilion by Josef Hoffmann, as well as most of the other buildings at the fair were all designed in a spare form of German Neoclassicism, a formal vocabulary based on established traditions and conventions that regained popularity after the exuberant, individualist Art Nouveau style at the turn of the century. Other buildings were more purely classical or Renaissance in style, and a mock vernacular town was built in a stylized version of local brick architectural traditions to introduce visitors to regional culture.

There were, however, three major exceptions to these conservative designs. One of the first buildings that visitors saw on entering the fairgrounds that received much attention in the press was the small "Glass House" designed by Bruno Taut to display products of the German glass industry. It was intended as a poetic essay in glass block, colored glass, tile, mirrors, light, and water that were to show off the completely new aesthetic that could be achieved by a more intense use of glass in the building industry. A theater with an innovative, flexible stage configuration, designed by the Belgian designer Henri van de Velde, was equally popular. It featured bold geometric volumes, softened through some flowing curves in plan and in the main facade, as well as some sculptural reliefs by Hermann Obrist that recalled the Art Nouveau style of a few years earlier. Finally, toward the rear of the exhibit, Walter Gropius designed a model Werkbund factory and office building with a symmetrical brick facade inspired by American technology and the designs of Frank Lloyd Wright but flanked by two daring concrete spiral stairs cantilevered inside glass cylinders. The rear elevation of the same building featured a glass curtain wall that looked out over a large courtyard and exhibit hall crammed full of modern machines and engineering, including some Pullman car interiors by Gropius.

The contrast between the rather conventional, classicized designs and the more individualized, artistically daring buildings formed the backdrop to a very heated debate that erupted almost without warning at the exhibit. During his opening speech, Muthesius, the vice president of the Werkbund, outlined a series of ten programmatic points to direct the future of the Werkbund's efforts. He called for more standardized, typical, and conventionalized forms in architecture and industrial design to counter the rampant individualism and arbitrary forms that he perceived in the modern, industrialized consumer culture around him. On the basis of interpretations of the knotty word *Typisierung* (meaning "type" or "standardize") used by Muthesius, many historians have given him credit for anticipating the standardization and machine aesthetic that were to become hallmarks of avant-garde design and International Style modern architecture after World War I in Germany. Stanford Anderson, however, has more perceptively argued that Muthesius intended to reinforce the conservative statement made by the classicism of his own buildings and that he surely spoke for many of the reform-minded architects present.

Others at the exhibit, however, disagreed completely with Muthesius and were outraged that he voiced these ideas as Werkbund policy. The next day, speaking for a group of younger architects, including Gropius and Taut, van de Velde proposed ten "countertheses" that insisted that the road to success for the Werkbund lay not in fostering standards, norms, or conventions but rather in the creative, individual artistic talents of designers in search of innovative forms and production techniques. Those historians who have seen Muthesius's remarks as an early call for standardization have criticized van de Velde's countertheses as a retreat to earlier, Romantic sensibilities about artistic genius espoused by Art Nouveau rather than as the more general recantation of stultifying norms that Anderson credits him with.

The intense debate between the Muthesius and van de Velde camps concerning the future of Werkbund policy raged on until the exhibition suddenly closed its doors on 1 August 1914, just as the German kaiser declared war on Russia and on nearby

France and, with it, the beginning of World War I. Although discussion halted in the fervor of war, the legacy of the debate continued for decades. Blaming German industry for much of the devastation of the Great War and with the revolutionary zeal to replace everything that was old, established, and conservative after the war, the younger architects took over the Werkbund in 1919 and insisted on van de Velde's theses that individual artistic design was the key to modern design. Paradoxically, however, through the writings of critics such as Adolf Behne and Adolf Loos, the Werkbund, alongside the Bauhaus and modern architects and designers all over Germany, began to connect the search for new artistic forms with an increasingly rational, standardized, and industrially mass-produced aesthetic. The uniform International Style architecture that became the norm for most of the Western world just before and after World War II thus combined aspects of both the artistic and the standardized sides of the famous Werkbund debate initiated at the Cologne exhibit.

KAI K. GUTSCHOW

See also **Art Nouveau; Bauhaus; Bauhaus, Dessau; Hoffmann, Josef (Austria); International Style; Loos, Adolf (Austria); Muthesius, Hermann (Germany); Taut, Bruno (Germany); van de Velde, Henri (Belgium); Wright, Frank Lloyd (United States)**

Further Reading

The catalog *Der westdeutsche Impuls*, edited by Herzogenrath, is the most complete overall description and analysis of the 1914 exhibit, whereas his other work listed offers a reprint of the exhibit catalog. Conrads's book includes English translations of Muthesius's and van de Velde's theses. Campbell offers the most complete account of the Werkbund in English, though Schwartz's work offers a more intensive interpretation of the consumer and commodity culture inspired by the Werkbund. Anderson's article, part of a large body of work on the role of "convention" in modern architecture, revises the traditional interpretations of the Muthesius–van de Velde debate.

Anderson, Stanford, "Deutscher Werkbund—The 1914 Debate: Hermann Muthesius versus Henry van de Velde," in *Companion to Contemporary Architectural Thought*, edited by Ben Farmer and Hentie J. Louw, London and New York: Routledge, 1993

Banham, Reyner, "Germany: Industry and Werkbund," in *Theory and Design in the First Machine Age*, by Banham, London: Architectural Press, and New York: Praeger, 1960

Behrendt, Walter Curt, "Die Deutsche Werkbund Ausstellung in Köln," *Kunst und Künstler*, 12/12 (September 1914)

Burckhardt, Lucius (editor), *The Werkbund: History and Ideology, 1907–1933*, translated by Pearl Sanders, Woodbury, New York: Barron's, 1980; as *The Werkbund: Studies in the History and Ideology of the Deutscher Werkbund, 1907–1933*, translated by Pearl Sanders, London: The Design Council, 1980

Campbell, Joan, *The German Werkbund: The Politics of Reform in the Applied Arts*, Princeton, New Jersey: Princeton University Press, 1978

Conrads, Ulrich (compiler), *Programme und Manifeste zur Architektur des 20. Jahrhunderts*, Berlin: Ullstein, 1964; as *Programs and Manifestoes on 20th-Century Architecture*, translated by Michael Bullock, Cambridge, Massachusetts: MIT Press, 1970

Deutsche Form im Kriegsjahr: Die Ausstellung Köln 1914, Munich: Bruckmann, 1915

Fischer, Wend (editor), *Zwischen Kunst und Industrie: Der Deutsche Werkbund* (exhib. cat.), Munich: Die Neue Sammlung, Staatliches Museum für Angewandte Kunst, 1975

Herzogenrath, Wulf (editor), *Frühe Kölner Kunstausstellungen: Sonderbund 1912, Werkbund 1914, Pressa USSR 1928*, Cologne: Wienand, 1981

Herzogenrath, Wulf, Dirk Teuber, and Angelika Thiekötter (editors), *Der Westdeutsche Impuls, 1900–1914: Kunst und Umweltgestaltung im Industriegebiet: Die Deutsche Werkbund-Ausstellung, Köln, 1914*, Cologne: Kölnischer Kunstverein, 1984

Junghanns, Kurt, *Der Deutsche Werkbund: Sein erstes Jahrzehnt*, Berlin: Henschelverlag Kunst und Gesellschaft, 1982

Schwartz, Frederic, *The Werkbund: Design Theory and Mass Culture before the First World War*, New Haven, Connecticut: Yale University Press, 1996

WILLIAMS, AMANCIO (1913–89)

Architect, Argentina

Amancio Williams is considered one of the most significant architects in Argentina's history. His work is characterized by recurring modernist themes: the use of technology to generate lyrical forms, concern for hygienic and functional issues, and minimal application of ornament. The thematic schemes of Le Corbusier and the classicist tendency and attention to detail of Mies van der Rohe also influenced his projects. Williams's work addressed the concept of type or paradigmatic space. Over time these concepts were explored, refined, and often expressed through the building section. Aspects of modern life can be seen in his development typologies, such as the "Housing in Space" project, the large cultural complex, the office tower, the airport, the hospital, and the exhibit space. Williams's projects are identified and qualified through the integration of type, structure, architecture, and site.

From 1948 to 1951, Williams served as construction supervisor for Le Corbusier's Currutchet House project in La Plata, Argentina. Williams produced most of the construction documents for this house and supervised the project's structural and concrete work.

In his Housing in Space project (1943), Williams explored the relationship between site and climate. Williams's new approach toward creating a settlement is revealed in the manner in which the units are stepped to maximize light and ventilation, and a gentle curving roof offers broader views for all residents.

The House over the Brook (1945) in Mar del Plata synthesized many significant ideas for Williams. Designed for his father, a musician, it remains one of his few built projects. Williams described this house, which embodies his classicist attitudes, as "a form in space that cannot deny nature . . . concrete—its material—is exposed, and textured by mechanical and chemical procedures: form, structure and quality are thus here the same thing" (Frampton, p. 10). Two pillars support the bridgelike structure, and the curvature of the building responds to the landscape. The manner in which the house spans the brook is related to Maillart's bridge (1933) over the Schwanbach River. It exemplifies Williams's belief in the confluence of engineering and architecture. The interior displays his concern for detail and his poetic sensibility toward the use of materials.

Structural typology also plays a crucial role in Williams's proposal for the Airport of Buenos Aires (1945). The solution is logical in its simplicity. Located 8 kilometers from the city,

the airport was proposed to sit on massive slabs resembling airplane wings and was supported by enormous pillars embedded into the shallow river. The proposal connected the airport with the city via a platform, beneath which hung all airport circulation and services.

The Suspended Office Building project (1946) was designed in collaboration with Janello, Janello and Butler. This suspended skyscraper, designed for a site in Buenos Aires, is the most paradigmatic among all Williams's projects. Four concrete columns support two beams from which hang a steel framework for 28 floors divided into three sectors. The first slab was suspended 18 meters above the entrance, thereby generating a covered open space for a densely populated area of the city. The interior had flexible partitions, a structural type that was developed decades later by Sir Norman Foster in the Hong Kong and Shanghai Bank Buildings.

In Williams's Hall for Visual Spectacle and Sound in Space (1953), the development of the typology is determined not by the location but rather by objective scientific study. Research that investigated the propagation of sound in space was used to shape the auditorium and optimize acoustics for all listeners. Rotating a vertical axis generated the shell; thus, it created a mushroomlike amphitheater capable of providing a variety of visual spectacles.

Since the late 1940s, Williams produced a series of projects that studied the relationships between program–function, site–structure, and climate–city. Several of these, executed from 1951 to 1966, employed concrete building shells of minimum thickness. Others in the early 1960s rearticulated his strategies for the use of high roof structures. In both cases the structures consisted of thin building shells or roofs that were supported by large columns.

The shells in several projects acted as umbrellas that either grouped together or isolated spaces. They were carefully calculated to incorporate alternative functions to easily accommodate production processes and responded to differing contexts and programs. Among these proposals are the Hospitals in Corrientes, the proposals for Mbucuruyá and Curuzu-Cuatia (1948–53), the Gas Station (1955) in Avellaneda, the Industrial School (1960) in Olavarría, the House (1960) in Punta del Este, and the Bunge and Born Exhibition Stand (1966).

The series of projects employing high roof structures is part of Williams's research and innovative attitude toward design. In these cases individual shells are replaced with continuous large roof structures supported by few columns. Horizontal panels or glass membranes hang from the roof to offer protection from the climate and provide continuity with the existing context. The basic structural components generate ample space that can accommodate diverse programs and activities. Examples of this approach are the factory building proposal (1962) for Iggam, a small furniture shop (1962) in Buenos Aires, and a monument (1964) for the city of Berlin.

Many of Williams's later major projects were also unrealized. Among these is an urban proposal for a linear city of 300 kilometers in length by 6 kilometers in width. It is modeled after Le Corbusier's approach to urban design, with the buildings supported by *pilotis*, thereby reclaiming the ground space to promote greater contact with nature. An additional unrealized project is Williams's design for a 200-meter-high cross standing over the river (1988). It was to be situated on a large platform outside the port of Buenos Aires.

In 1981 the critic Kenneth Frampton wrote that Williams "was an enigmatic figure . . . a brilliant designer whose influence has been totally disproportionate to the extent of his own rather limited output" (Frampton, 1981). A renewed interest in architectural typology and Latin American architecture led to Williams's work being exhibited at Harvard University in 1987. The exhibit contributed to a greater understanding and deeper appreciation of Williams's contribution to modern architecture.

JOSE BERNARDI

See also **Argentina; Buenos Aires, Argentina; Corbusier, Le (Jeanneret, Charles-Édouard) (France); Foster, Norman (England); Maillart, Robert (Switzerland)**

Biography

Born in Buenos Aires, 19 February 1913, son of the composer Alberto Williams. Studied engineering and aviation before graduating as an architect from the University of Buenos Aires (1941); opened his architectural practice in Buenos Aires in 1942. His work was mostly experimental, and very few of his projects were ever built. Williams was one of the Argentinean members of CIAM (Congrès Internationaux d'Architecture Moderne). Died in Buenos Aires, 14 October 1989.

Selected Works

Housing in Space (project), 1943
House over the Brook, Mar del Plata, Argentina, 1945
Airport of Buenos Aires (project), 1945
Suspended Office Building (project), 1946
Hall for Visual Spectacle and Sound in Space (project), 1953

Further Reading

Frampton, Kenneth, *Casabella*, 468 (1981)
Glusberg, Jorge, *Breve historia de la arquitectura argentina*, Vol. 2. Buenos Aires: Editorial Claridad, 1991
Irace, Fulvio, "Amancio Williams," Abitare, 342 (1995)
Pronsato, Graciela, and Roberto Capelli, *7 + 1 Lamparas de la arquitectura argentina* (7 + 1 Lamps of Argentinean Architecture), La Plata: Ediciones Capro, 1993
Silvetti, Jorge (editor), *Amancio Williams*, New York and Cambridge, Massachusetts: Rizzoli and Harvard University Graduate School of Design, 1987

WILLIAMS, E. OWEN 1890–1969

Architectural engineer, England

Considered to be one of the individuals responsible for the establishment of modern architecture, Sir (Evan) Owen Williams is best known as the civil engineer who introduced structural methods pioneered in Europe, notably by the Swiss engineer Robert Maillart, into Great Britain. Williams was one of a number of architects who were skeptical about the imitators and vulgarizers of the new modern architecture who lacked integrity. As early as 1932, he denounced "Facadism" as forgery.

Born in Tottenham, London, Williams studied at the University of London before working for Electric Tramways between 1905 and 1911. He served as chief aircraft designer for Wells Aviation until World War I, setting up an independent engineering practice in 1919. From about 1930 on, Williams dispensed with the collaboration of a consulting architect and produced his own designs, building up a successful practice specializing in industrial and commercial buildings using reinforced-concrete frame construction.

In 1924 Williams was appointed consulting engineer for the British Empire Exhibition, Wembley, in association with architect Sir John Simpson, with whom he collaborated on the design of Wembley Stadium (1925). Williams's reinforced-concrete design for the Dorchester Hotel (1930) in London was thought far too advanced, and Curtis Green was employed to devise a suitably restrained and elegant facade.

In the 1930s Williams designed a number of bridges in reinforced concrete, working mostly with the architect Maxwell Ayrton, but it was his design for the Boots Factory (1932) in Beeston, Nottingham, that was to be one of the most remarkable buildings of the Modern movement in Britain. New constructional techniques were employed on a more complete, vast, and uncompromising scale than in any other European building. Williams, an engineer with a sophisticated tectonic sensibility, showed how ideally fitted "mushroom" construction was for industrial buildings. The use of reinforced-concrete columns from which the concrete floor slabs spring outward in all directions created wider spans and allowed movement of goods around unobstructed voids. The floors are entirely supported by a row of these columns down each wing of the building, and the external walls, relieved of their load-bearing responsibilities, are glass clad from floor to ceiling. The central space was a sort of nave interrupted by cross galleries and top lit by a thin-glass, brick-and-concrete membrane roof. The effect was assertive and tough yet ennobling, a quality that understandably endeared it to the so-called New Brutalists of the 1950s.

The laboratory of a cement factory (1932) at Thurrock in Essex is a simple rectangular building. Reinforced-concrete benches, suitably clad, run round the walls with a shelf above, and the walls are opaque to this level, with glass above with slender concrete mullions. Powerful electric lamps were employed to provide an equivalent to daylight. The warehouse for Lilley and Skinner (1933) again used "mushroom" columns and slab construction. Long horizontal bands run between the windows, which wrap around the corners of the building. The Empire Swimming Pool (1934) at Wembley, the largest hall to be built in England to date, covered a space of 341 feet by 236.5 feet. The pool was constructed with a reinforced-concrete frame and used a grid system; the use of standardized units contributed to the speed of its eight-month construction. The Pioneer Health Centre (1935) in Peckham, London, was privately developed and financed and became famous as a pioneer social and health enterprise. Its founders believed that physical disorders were the result of environmental factors. The flexible space created in this rectangular three-story structure of reinforced concrete provided opportunities for various physical, social, and cultural activities. Members could meet and discuss their problems with trained staff who could give diagnoses and advice. The ultimate aim was not to cure conventional diseases but, rather, through preventive action, to sustain the health of the community. Various parts of the building were grouped around a central swimming pool, covered by a steeply pitched glass roof. The gymnasium was on the left, the theater on the right, and between them the children's covered playground with sliding glazing designed to make it an open-air space. On the first floor were spacious lounges with their shallow, bowed bays, cafeteria, and kitchen. The second floor housed medical rooms, a library, a study, and rest rooms. Unfortunately, because of a lack of support, the center closed in March 1950.

Williams was consulting engineer for Ellis and Clarke, who designed the Daily Express Buildings in Fleet Street, London (1932), Manchester (1939), and Glasgow. His other work included Dollis Hill Synagogue (1938) in London and a proposal (1935) for a new Wateroo Bridge. Postwar work includes all bridges on the M1 motorway and the maintenance headquarters at Heathrow Airport in London.

HILARY GRAINGER

See also **Airport and Aviation Building; Brutalism; Reinforced Concrete**

Further Reading

Cottam, D., F. Newby, S. Rosenberg, and G. Stamp, *Sir Owen Williams*, London: Architectural Association, 1986.
Gold, M., "Sir Owen Williams, K.B.E.," *Zodiac* (1968)
Rosenberg, S., W. Chalk, and S. Mullin, "Sir Owen Williams," *Architectural Design* (July 1969)
The Architecural Review (May 1935)

WILLIAMS, PAUL REVERE 1894–1980
Architect, United States

A native of Los Angeles, Paul Revere Williams designed some of the most distinctive residences and public structures known throughout the United States during a long and distinguished career. His achievements paralleled the growth of Los Angeles, where his eclectic practice varied from designing homes for the city's elite, including famous figures of the entertainment industry, to important institutional and commercial landmarks. These accomplishments reflect his mastery for adapting a multitude of revival and modern styles to the culture of southern California's Mediterranean climate. His success is also notable considering that Williams was the first African American architect licensed in California (1921) and the first to be accepted as a member of the American Institute of Architects (AIA) (1923). His recognition as a master designer, member of numerous civic and government bodies, and mentor to generations of minority architects led to his induction as the first African American Fellow of the AIA (1957).

On graduation from the University of Southern California, Williams worked for another noted Los Angeles architect, John C. Austin (1920–22), expanding his knowledge while working on major civic structures, including the 5000-seat Shrine Auditorium (1922) and numerous public schools. His association with Austin led to a collaboration on many future projects and a lifelong friendship. Recognizing his diverse skills as a city planner, Williams was appointed to Los Angeles's first planning com-

mission (1920), beginning service on what would amount to more than a dozen public bodies during his 60-year career at the local, state, and federal levels. By 1923 Williams opened his own practice, Paul R. Williams and Associates, Architects, in the fashionable Stock Exchange Building at the core of a booming Los Angeles. His first projects were for politician and developer Senator Frank J. Flint for his new development of Flintridge in the hills overlooking Pasadena.

Williams adapted to the cultural racial biases of his times, including restrictions against his living in most of the communities where he designed homes. Nonetheless, he designed many cultural institutions and businesses for the booming African American community at or below cost to improve opportunity and activities in his community of south-central Los Angeles. These included many neighborhood YMCAs (1925–27) and churches, including the Second Baptist Church (1924). His client roster included Hollywood royalty and elite of the booming region. So great were his talents in diminishing the boundaries to success that he would create sketches for Anglo clients upside down, sitting opposite so as not to come into close contact with them. This so impressed many skeptics that he rarely lost a commission because of the color of his skin.

Prejudices aside, Williams was able to design comfortable surroundings that evoked a sense of grandeur while maintaining a human scale. Past experience with master architects taught Williams a deep respect for the varied revival-style structures that were in vogue throughout his practice. This, in turn, influenced the fashion-conscious of Hollywood to seek out his design sensibilities.

Following World War II, Williams embraced modernism like most of his contemporaries, but with a style and grace that evoked the balanced classical compositions of the prewar period. This can best be seen in his addition to the Beverly Hills Hotel (1947–51), the Los Angeles County Courthouse and Hall of Administration (1955), and the Frank Sinatra residence (1956). The postwar years also saw expansion with allied offices in Bogotá, Colombia, and Washington, D.C. The number of commissions for public and commercial structures following World War II eclipsed his prewar residential commissions, with his offices swelling to more than 60 draftsmen. It was during this period that one of his greatest landmarks was designed in association with Pereira and Luckman and Welton Becket Associates: the Los Angeles International Airport Theme Building (1961–65).

After a prosperous career, Williams spent his final years lecturing around the world about dedication to one's desires and the obstacles that must be overcome to achieve them. He continued his practice until the mid-1970s, taking on projects that

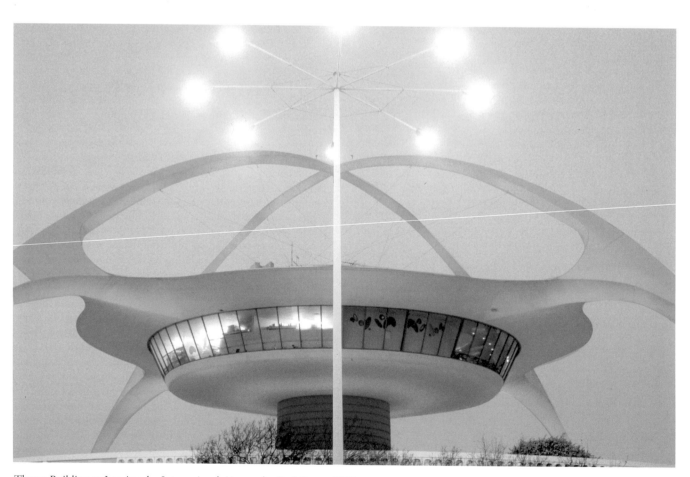

Theme Building at Los Angeles International Airport, by Paul Revere Williams
© Joseph Sohm; Chromo Sohm Inc./CORBIS

more closely resembled those from his practice during the first two decades of his career. Williams understood more keenly than most design professionals that many outside influences affected how and what is built. His dedication to improving design went well beyond the drafting room tables.

JEFFREY B. SAMUDIO

Biography

Born Los Angeles, 18 February 1894, son of poor recent immigrants from the southern United States, orphaned at an early age. Attended Los Angeles Polytechnic High School; attended the Los Angeles School of Art and the Beaux-Arts School of Design Atelier 1912–16; winner of the Beaux-Arts Medal and First Prize for a Neighborhood Center in Pasadena, California. Attended the University of Southern California School of Engineering, specializing in structural design and engineering 1916–19. Married Della Mae Givens 27 June 1917. Member of the first Los Angeles Planning Commission 1920–28; certified as an architect, state of California 1921. Established firm of Paul R. Williams, Architect 1922; became member of the Southern California Chapter of the American Institute of Architects 1923; appointed to the National Monuments Committee by President Calvin Coolidge 1929; appointed to the first Los Angeles Housing Commission 1933–41. Won first AIA award for design of the Music Corporation of America corporate offices (1937), Beverly Hills, in 1939; received honorary doctorate of science degree, Lincoln University, Missouri. Enlisted as a navy architect during World War II 1942–45. First major public buildings 1940–41, Long Beach Naval Station; followed after the war with major additions to the Los Angeles General Hospital 1947; also that year he was appointed to the board, serving as vice president, then director of Broadway Federal Savings and Loan, the oldest federal savings and loan headed by African Americans west of the Mississippi. Appointed by governor, and later chief justice of the Supreme Court, Earl Warren, to the California Housing Commission 1949–55. Received honorary doctor of architecture degree, Howard University (presented by President Truman); appointed to the National Commission on Housing by President Eisenhower 1953. Retired from practice following his commission to design a sorority house at his alma mater, USC 1973. Died in Los Angeles, 23 January 1980.

Selected Publications

Small Homes of Tomorrow, 1945
New Homes for Today, 1946

Further Reading

Hudson, Karen E., *Paul R. Williams, Architect: A Legacy of Style*, Rizzoli, 1993
Hudson, Karen E., *The Will and the Way*, New York: Rizzoli, 1994

WILLIAMS, TOD (1943–) AND BILLIE TSIEN (1949–)

Architects, United States

The architecture of Tod Williams and Billie Tsien has been characterized as one that is preoccupied with the craft of making.

Working together in practice in New York, these two architects have developed particular interests in the inherent qualities of materials that they have combined with investigations of the details of the physical and philosophical nature of construction. They have explored these interests through a range of projects that originated in designs for exhibitions and performance and that have subsequently developed to embrace more conventional architectural commissions that have included houses, educational facilities, and civic buildings.

After studying architecture at Princeton University and working for Richard Meier for six years, Tod Williams opened his own office in 1974. Billie Tsien's first degree was in fine arts, and she went on to study architecture at the University of California, Los Angeles, before joining Williams. Together they have developed a practice that has been significantly influenced by their backgrounds in architecture and fine art. However, theirs is also a practice that reflects a collaborative effort that grows out of their relationship as a married couple, and they have frequently spoken of their interest in "bringing together the issues of life and architecture."

In their early work, Williams and Tsien experimented with materials in the designs for installations at the Museum of the Chinese in the Americas in New York and elsewhere. They used unconventional materials and also reconsidered how familiar materials could be used in unfamiliar ways. For an exhibition of Noguchi's Akari lanterns, they used obsidian with lit fiberglass screens, and a project that was developed with the Elisa Monte Dance Company in New York advanced the ideas of large screens to create a dynamic backdrop for the staging of dance productions.

These investigations informed their subsequent architectural work. The design for new galleries at the Phoenix Art Museum explored the use of glass and metal and of different aggregates in the making of the concrete for the building. The systems of construction were also developed to define paths of movement that organize the new galleries and link them into an existing building. This consideration of the path as an organizing element in architecture and also as a place of meeting and social interaction has become increasingly influential in their work. In the planning of the Neurosciences Institute in La Jolla, California, a theoretical and clinical research campus for the study of the brain, Williams and Tsien designed places of informal meeting that are integrated with spaces for work by creating a series of paths that become meandering walks through the building. These paths also integrate the institute into a surrounding natural landscape framed by the Santa Rosa Mountains.

In the development and design of the Cranbrook Estate in Michigan, the architect Eliel Saarinen, together with his client George Booth, established a strong relationship among landscape, art, and architecture. It was a relationship that was also reflected in the organization of a curriculum that sought to connect the mental and the physical through the integration of academic and athletic activities there. Increases in enrollment at Cranbrook prompted the need for new and improved facilities, and Williams and Tsien were commissioned to prepare a plan for new buildings there to provide gymnasiums, exercise rooms, and a swimming pool. Their design developed ideas of movement and path embodied in their earlier designs for academic buildings in California, at Princeton, and at the University of Virginia. The coeducational natatorium at Cranbrook has been

planned to connect to existing buildings, and large occuli and doors enable the building to be opened up during spring and summer. These devices successfully connect the building to the landscapes of the Cranbrook Estate. The first building in this phased development, which was completed in 1999, is one of the most successful new educational buildings in the United States.

Commissions to design houses for sites in New York City, Long Island, and Phoenix have enabled Williams and Tsien to explore these issues of materiality, path, and the integration of building with site at another scale. These explorations are particularly successful in the houses in Phoenix and Long Island, which were completed in 1997 and 1999, respectively.

In 1998 Williams and Tsien received a commission to design the Museum of Folk Art in New York. This project develops these ideas within the confines of a restricted site on Fifty-third Street. Of necessity the scheme organizes the galleries as a series of spaces that are linked vertically. An elevator is itself designed as a gallery. Internally, a series of shafts are also cut through the building to link spaces and define the paths that connect them with natural light. The facade on the 40-foot-wide street frontage, proposed as a folded plane of white bronze panels, is mainly solid. Not only does the fold give the museum a greater presence on the street, but the material was selected to reflect the dynamism of changing light throughout the day. This new museum opened in 2001.

In its preoccupation with materials and the details of fabrication, the work of Williams and Tsien recalls that of Charles and Ray Eames. By working closely together, they have been able to develop interests in the craft of making architecture and shaping space to a level that articulates an important alternative to corporate practice and the overwhelmingly generic buildings that frequently result from industrial production.

BRIAN CARTER

Selected Publications

Works, 2G Monographs, 1999

Further Reading

Carter, Brian, and Annette LeCuyer (editors), *Tod Williams Billie Tsien*, Ann Arbor: Michigan Architecture Papers, 1998
M.S., "Walden Revisited," *The Architectural Review* (September 1999)

WILSON, (SIR) COLIN ST. JOHN 1922–

Architect, England

Colin Wilson, with his firm of Colin St. John Wilson and Partners, founded in 1971, is responsible for the largest and most expensive (£511 million) architectural commission in Britain—the British Library—which on its completion in 1998 had been some 36 years in the making. Wilson faced hostility and ridicule during the design and construction, but his courage and confidence finally brought vindication—today the British Library enjoys immense popularity and prestige. While this monumental building constitutes Wilson's chief constructed architectural legacy, as an educator and persuasive author, Wilson has had an effect on architecture that transcends his numerically modest built output. He has been a very important voice for those who care about integrity more than fashion and who believe that architecture should serve human needs over time, be embellished by use, served in and provide a frame in which human actions are made manifest.

Educated at Cambridge University and University College, London, after wartime naval service, Wilson served in the Housing Division of the London County Council (LCC) between 1950 and 1955, when public housing was the most important task on the architectural agenda in a Britain still recovering from wartime damages. After a year with the developer John De Vere Hunt, Wilson moved to Cambridge at the invitation of Leslie Martin, principal architect at the LCC before his appointment in 1956 as professor at the School of Architecture, to teach and to associate with him on architectural projects.

Initially, Wilson had been captivated by Le Corbusier, especially his sculptural post war Brutalist work. Thus, Wilson's extension to the Architecture School at Cambridge has the textured roughness of Le Corbusier's Unité d'Habitation (Marseilles, 1946–52) and the Maisons Jaoul (Paris, 1952–56). Ultimately, however, Alvar Aalto would be much more influential. Wilson often quotes the Finnish master's observation about modern architecture of the heroic period, made when Aalto received the RIBA Medal in 1957: "Like all revolutions it starts with enthusiasm and stops with some sort of Dictatorship" (*Architectural Reflections*, p. 84). Thus, Wilson began to seek an alternative tradition for modern architecture, which he found in the work of other Scandinavians like Sigurd Lewerentz and Gunnar Asplund, as well as German organicists like Hugo Häring and Hans Scharoun. Aalto's immediate effect can be recognized in Harvey Court at Gonville and Caius College, Cambridge, in the dominant materials of brick (rather than the prevailing *béton brut*), natural wood, and copper; in the arrangement of a raised courtyard (as at the Town Hall, Säynatsalo, 1950–52) with a pyramidal skylight admitting light to below; and in the way the stairs are expressed (both devices also recalling Aalto's Baker House at the Massachusetts Institute of Technology, 1946–49). Although at Harvey Court the image of La Tourette also lingered, increasingly it was Aalto and the German Expressionists who excited Wilson's admiration. Thus, the fan shape of the William Stone Building at Peterhouse College (1960–64) brings to mind one of Aalto's favorite motifs.

In his designs and his writings, Wilson vigorously combats the leading tendency of the 1980s and 1990s to view architecture as autonomous and as a discipline, a mode of abstract thinking, that exists outside the practice of making buildings and creating space. Wilson has also set himself against "inauthenticity," which he has found both in the modernism of the International Style and in Postmodernism. Probity is a revered quality, and Wilson seeks an ethical dimension that is hardly new; its sources can be found in A. W. N. Pugin and John Ruskin no less than H. P. Berlage or Aalto—all intellectual forebears.

Nourished on a diet of astute English critics of widely varied opinions, including Ruskin, Geoffrey Scott, and Adrian Stokes, Wilson is passionate about architecture without being narrow-minded or doctrinaire. He is also a bibliophile, and it is appropriate that he should have become a specialist in redefining the program of the contemporary library. Thus, with Martin he designed three libraries for Oxford University (1959–64), with Long he worked on the National Libraries Feasibility Study as

well as the libraries for the Bishops' School and for Queen Mary College, and he acted as consultant for the Harold Washington Library in Chicago by Hammond Beeby Babka.

At the same time, Wilson is also profoundly involved in the visual arts as painter, draftsman, and sculptor; as museum trustee; and as collector. He has been the intimate friend, and often mentor, of many artists: Peter Blake, Eduardo Paolozzi, R. J. Kitaj, Howard Hodgkin, Richard Hamilton, and William Turnbull, among others; his extensive collection of their work has been promised to the Pallant House Gallery in Chichester, for which he designed an extension.

In 1994 Wilson suggested that Long and their associate Rolfe Kentish establish a new partnership to supplement the existing firm, and he subsequently has involved himself with projects by Long and Kentish. Although many laurels have come his way since the opening of the British Library—for example, a knighthood and an exhibition at the British Pavilion of the Venice Biennale (1996), as well as numerous invitations to teach and lecture—Wilson is still deeply engaged in shaping architectural practice to embody his deeply felt principles.

HELEN SEARING

See also **Aalto, Alvar (Finland); Asplund, Erik Gunnar (Sweden); Banham, Reyner (United States); British Library, London; Congrès Internationaux d'Architecture Moderne (CIAM, 1927–); Corbusier, Le (Jeanneret, Charles-Édouard) (France); Häring, Hugo (Germany); International Style; Loos, Adolf (Austria); Scharoun, Hans (Germany); Unité d'Habitation, Marseilles**

Biography

Born Cheltenham, England, 14 March 1922. Corpus Christi College, Cambridge 1940–42; master's degree 1942. Bartlett School of Architecture, University of London 1946–49; diploma of architecture 1949. Royal Naval Volunteer Reserve 1942–46. Housing Division, Architects' Department, London County Council 1950–55; development office of John De Vere Hunt 1955–56. Private partnership with Leslie Martin 1956–70. Senior partner, Colin St. John Wilson and Partners, London, since 1971. Partner, Long and Kentish, since 1994. Instructor, School of Architecture, Cambridge University 1956–59; professor and head of School of Architecture, Cambridge 1975–1989. Visiting critic Yale University School of Architecture 1960, 1964, 1983, 1985, 2000; William Henry Bishop Visiting Professor jointly with M. J. Long 2002; Bemis Visiting Professor of Architecture, MIT 1970–72. Trustee Tate Gallery 1973–80; National Gallery, London 1977–80.

Selected Works

Own Practice
Wilson apartment conversion, Primrose Hill, London, 1952
City Center Project for Team X Meeting (with Peter Carter), 1956
Extension, School of Architecture, Cambridge University (with Alex Hardy), 1959
Pair of houses (one the Wilson house), Grantchester Road, Cambridge, 1964
Cornford House, Madingley, Cambridge (with M. J. Long), 1967
Civic and Social Center, St. John's Gardens, Liverpool (with M. J. Long), 1970

With Sir Leslie Martin
Housing, St. Pancras, London, 1957
Harvey Court Residential Building, Gonville and Caius College, Cambridge, 1962
William Stone Residential Building, Peterhouse College, Cambridge, 1962
Three Libraries, Oxford University, 1964
Library, British Museum, Bloomsbury, London, 1964
Colin St. John Wilson and Partners
New Extension, British Museum, London (1st project, 1970; 2nd project, constructed, 1973–79), 1979
Bishop Wilson Memorial Library, Bishops' School, Springfield, Essex, 1984
New Wing, Johnson House, Barton Road, Cambridge, 1986
Queen Mary College Library, University of London, 1989
Home for the Deaf, Annaly House, Wandsworth, London, 1995
Extension to Pallant House Gallery, Chichester, 1999

Selected Publications

The Design and Construction of the British Library, London: The British Library, 1998
The Other Tradition of Modern Architecture, London: Academy Editions, 1995
Architectural Reflections: Studies in the Philosophy and Practice of Architecture, Oxford: Butterworth, 1992

Further Reading

Banham, Reyner, *The New Brutalism*, London: Architectural Press, 1966
Frampton, Kenneth, R. B. Kitaj, and Martin Richardson, *Colin St. John Wilson*, London: Royal Institute of British Architects, 1997
Maxwell, Robert, *New British Architecture*, New York: Praeger, 1973
Searing, Helen "The Other Tradition," *Constructs*, New Haven: Yale University School of Architecture, 2000.

WOOD

The dramatic technological, environmental, political, and economic changes that occurred during the 20th century irrevocably changed the way in which wood is used in all types of building. Three major themes can be discerned: improved technology and accelerating scientific research have resulted in novel uses for wood as well as in structural and decorative substitutes for wood; improved transportation, rising demand, and freer trade have created large, new worldwide markets for all types of timber and wood fiber; and, despite constantly shifting styles, steady change in construction technology has reduced wood's relevance to architecture.

The immense investment of energy, time, and wealth in scientific research by governments, businesses, and universities throughout the 20th century bore fruit in practically every field of endeavor, and wood, despite its seemingly elemental nature, was not neglected. The fundamental innovations of the 20th century were to devise new ways to break wood down into its boards, strips, strands, fibers, and even molecules and to concoct new and better ways to reattach these components. Another breakthrough, although of questionable environmental merit, was the gradual development of improved techniques for planting, growing, and harvesting trees. These innovations had the net result of increasing both the usefulness and the value of wood in society. They also permitted, for the first time, many physical weaknesses of wood to be significantly ameliorated.

Except for scarce "old growth" timber, which can be up to 10 feet in diameter and over 100 feet in length, trees produce lumber that is not very long, very straight, or very stable. Premodern carpentry accommodated the slender, flexible, environmentally sensitive nature of wood by devising intricate, labor-intensive methods of combining small pieces of wood to create architectural surfaces and structural frames. Carpenters in the 20th century, by contrast, were able to use many new wood products that are, in theory, infinitely wide, flat, long, stiff, uniform, and stable. The most famous example of this is plywood, actually a trade name for a Douglas fir product that was first exhibited at the Lewis and Clark Centennial Exposition of 1905. Plywood is best known because, by the middle of the 20th century, it was being used for everything from furniture designed by Frank Lloyd Wright to P.T. boats, but it is just one of many different types of composite wood panels made up of layers of wood veneer glued together. Because the layers of veneer are laid at cross angles to one another, plywood warps, shrinks, and cracks very little. Although it is sold today primarily in panels four feet wide by eight feet long, it can theoretically be manufactured to any dimension and in virtually any thickness. Many types of veneer panel were being manufactured in limited quantities during the 19th century, but the growing usefulness of composite wood panels in the 20th century depended primarily on the increasing strength, durability, and water resistance of the adhesives.

Composite panels could also be made from straw, wood, sugarcane, or practically any other kind of vegetable fiber. Such products as Masonite, Homasote, Celotex, Insulite, and Presdwood were developed and produced throughout the 20th century and offered builders some of the same advantages as plywood, namely, perfect uniformity of size and strength, extreme economy, and tremendous structural efficiency. Because these products had limited insulating quality—and also because they were cheap, easy to produce, and manufactured from agricultural or lumber waste products—they were in extremely high demand during World War II. As the Masonite Man boasted in a wartime advertisement:

> Many a U.S. fighting man, from the north pole to the tropics, lives and works in a Quonset Hut, lined entirely with Masonite Presdwood. The entire lining for a Hut is shipped easily in one compact crate . . . painted and ready to install. These Masonite Presdwood walls resist both the frigid blasts of the Arctic and the heat, humidity and insects of the equator.

Another product that achieved popularity and importance in the 20th century was the "glue-lam" timber. The first recorded use of glued laminated arches was in Basel, Switzerland, in 1893. In 1901 the first patent was awarded to Otto Hetzer of Weimar, Germany. Thereafter, glued laminated arches were known in Europe as the Hetzer construction method. In the United States, the first glued laminated timbers were manufactured by Max C. Hanisch, Sr., a German immigrant and the founder of the Unit Structures Corporation of Peshtigo, Wisconsin, in 1934. The principle of the glue-laminated beam was probably first employed by Bronze Age fletchers who manufactured bows of extreme flexibility and power by gluing thin strips of animal horn together. In the case of the glue-lam timber, however, scientists in the 20th century developed efficient ways to laminate small, dry boards together to create, in theory, infinitely long, deep timbers of uniform cross section and stable composition. Glue-lam timbers could also be bent into any shape, increasing the variety of architectural effects that could be achieved.

In the past several decades, numerous variations on these two themes have been developed in an effort to reduce costs, preserve timber, increase efficiency, and raise profits. Oriented strand board, Para-lam timbers, pre-primed plywood siding, and truss-joists, to list just four among hundreds of brand-new products, utilize super-strong new waterproof adhesives and small, thin, dry boards or even mill scraps. The advantage of all this innovation has been constantly increasing speed of construction, vastly increased efficiency in the use of diminishing timber resources, ever lighter-weight structures, and lower building costs. The drawback to all these new products is greater fire hazard, slimmer margins of engineering safety, shorter life spans, and a reliance on an increasing number of synthetic glues and preservative chemicals.

Throughout the 20th century, but particularly after World War II, many nations and regions began to export formerly untapped timber resources, and many developing nations established strong new wood-manufacturing industries. Increased trade in the 20th century had two major effects: the largest Western economies were benefited from the increased availability of foreign wood species, were formerly tiny, insular economies were being affected by international trends in construction, timber harvesting, and manufacturing.

The international timber trade is at least as old as recorded history. In biblical times the ceiling of Solomon's temple was reputedly framed of cedar beams imported from Lebanon. During the Middle Ages, most of the highest-quality oak boards used in England for doors and furniture were brought by ship from the Baltic. One result of growing trade in the 20th century, however, was the availability of larger and comparatively less expensive quantities of foreign timber than ever before. The species might be exotic, such as teak from Myanmar or mahogany from Brazil, valued by shipbuilders, cabinetmakers, and other specialty secondary industries, or they might simply be inexpensive softwood for framing, such as the huge quantities of fir, spruce, hemlock, and pine pouring onto the world market from Canada, Russia, and other Baltic countries. Naturally, this increased trade was largely a result of rising demand. Annual world demand for all types of wood is expected to rise in 2010 to approximately 2.7 billion cubic meters, according to the United Nations. This is approximately 15 percent higher than the world's production capacity in 1997.

Increased international trade also increased pressure in many markets to standardize or to adopt new techniques. In Japan, for example, where carpentry is a ferociously defended traditional craft, pressures were mounting to incorporate Western-style framing because of its low cost and its efficient earthquake resistance. This was contrary both to popular opinion in Japan, where traditionally framed structures are believed to flex and bend with earth tremors, and to carpenters' preferred methods of work. Nevertheless, the effectiveness of Western-style framing was demonstrated during the Kobe earthquake of 1995. Following the terrible devastation, engineers in Japan noted that modern American-style plywood boxes had proven quite durable, whereas many traditionally framed postwar buildings had performed poorly. American-style platform framing, however, relies

on standardized kiln-dried lumber and plywood, which American lumber companies are eager to begin exporting to Japan in larger quantities. Japanese carpenters and lumber companies, on the other hand, would much prefer to import select American logs and process the lumber themselves, thereby preserving jobs and, they believe, increasing quality. The serious consideration in Japan of the adoption of Western-style framing, Western lumber dimensions, and offshore labor exemplifies the power of international trends to change even the most entrenched traditional local uses of wood in construction. Such shifts have occurred throughout the world.

Probably the most interesting—and misleading—force that influenced wood's use in the 20th century was the fluctuating popularity of many different fads, trends, styles, and practitioners of architecture. These influences are difficult to disentangle from simultaneous technological, economic, and political changes and indeed were usually precipitated by the more powerful shifts of the world at large.

One of the most notable shifts of the early 20th century was a worldwide move away from romantic, historicizing styles of building to the International Style. In the United States, this meant that Richardsonian Romanesque, Neoclassical, Craftsman, Edwardian, Art Nouveau, and a host of other styles of building were slowly overcome by the machinery of the building itself. This shift was not merely stylistic. As Henry-Russell Hitchcock noted as early as 1928, "Indeed a client, while he may ask for a Tudor or a Georgian or even a Maya design, is unlikely to permit any serious sacrifice of *le comfort moderne* to the exigencies of a past style" (Hitchcock, 1928).

In retrospect, it was inevitable that as the building became filled with more and more lighting, heating, cooling, communication, and transportation equipment, not to mention a strong new steel skeleton, it would divide into at least three parts: guts, bones, and skin. The inconsistency of having fresh, young, vigorous guts and bones sealed in a leathery old skin from a previous millennium slowly became more objectionable until advocates of the International Style proposed a solution: the entire building ought to be a new, up-to-date machine for living.

Naturally, this shift had a powerful influence on how wood was used in architecture. Where the Greene brothers, Charles Rennie Mackintosh, and Victor Horta glorified the skill of the craftsman, the physical beauty of architectural materials, and the expense and complexity of fabricating architecture, the International Style celebrated the economy, simplicity, and directness of mass-produced materials and components. Metals, glass, concrete, plastics, and rubber became the preferred palette of leading architects from the 1930s on. Wood was acceptable if it was served up in flat, straight, square, uniform, repetitive chunks—in other words, if it imitated the stripped-down, mass-produced aesthetic of the other parts of the machine. Frank Lloyd Wright expressed the disgust that many modern architects felt toward traditional wooden embellishments very clearly when he wrote:

Wood, therefore, has more human outrage done upon it than man has ever done, even upon himself. . . . In his search for novelty, wood in his hands has been joined and glued, braced and screwed, boxed and nailed, turned and tortured, scroll sawed, beaded, fluted, suitably furbelowed and flounced at the carpenter's party—enough to please even him. By the aid of "modern" machines the carpenter-artist got it into Eastlake composites of trim and furniture, into Usonian jigger porches and corner-towers eventuating into candle snuffer domes or what would you have?; got it all over Queen Anne houses outside and inside—the triumph of his industrial ingenuity—until carpentry and millwork became synonymous with butchery and botchwork. (Wright, 1928)

According to Wright, the machine itself was not to blame—it could easily produce the smooth, rectangular, geometrically pure pieces that he and many other modernists desired and put to use in Wright's Prairie-style houses and many other buildings. Naturally, therefore, the scientific and technological advances in the use of wood during the early 20th century appealed to modern architects, and they made excellent use of new materials and techniques.

What is not obvious, perhaps even to the architects and critics of the Modern movement themselves, is that some of the best-known and most contentious commentators of the 20th century were merely running a few steps ahead of the pack, ten moist fingers to the wind. Far more influential—and ultimately irresistible in its power—was the tide of economics and technology that swept everything architectural in its wake. Rising labor costs, decreasing quality of timber resources, sudden enormous wartime demands, the growth and monopolization of wood industries, and, most important, the growing dominance of mechanical systems have been far more influential than any style or architect despite what some might say about Alvar Aalto's plywood chairs or Tadao Ando's rustic wall treatments. According to Kenneth Frampton, two-thirds of the total budget of any large building built in the 1990s is expended on mechanical and electrical provisions of one kind or another, from air-conditioning to piped information.

This observation has many implications. First, combined with the fact that most large buildings today are framed in steel, it means that high-status architecture utilizes very little wood and consequently has practically no influence on the lumber industry. Custom-furnishings manufacturers provide the entire (small) package of fittings, furnishings, trim, and moldings. Wherever possible in their design, they will substitute a cheaper synthetic material, such as plastic laminate or metal. Where wood is absolutely required, it will usually be a thin veneer over a particleboard backing. Second, because most "vernacular" structures—everything from tract homes to taco stands—are designed with absolute economy and relatively short life expectancies, lumber manufacturers are in cutthroat competition to produce the cheapest possible structural components—and these vernacular wood-framed buildings, designed by builders and engineers, make up nearly 86 percent of all American structures and a growing percentage of new structures worldwide. The innovations of the lumber industry, consequently, will rarely reflect the stylistic or philosophical attitudes of architects, and because architects have little reason to be interested in the lumber industry anyway, only contractors, engineers, and environmentalists will be left to argue over how scarce timber resources ought to be used, protected, or augmented. In short, wood has moved out of the purview of the most influential architects.

The main difficulty in an analysis of any topic as broad as the 20th-century use of wood is to distinguish causes from effects. Scientists and engineers in the 20th century created marvelous

new uses for wood and surprising new ways to reconfigure wood. Large new supplies of timber came onto the world market from all corners of the world; and, most noticeably to those of us who are architects and historians of architecture, there were extremely novel and exciting new applications for wood devised in the 20th century. No one who has visited one of Alvar Aalto's buildings can fail to be impressed by his sensitive handling of a material as mundane as birch plywood, and no one who has stood in a modern church sanctuary vaulted by glue-lam beams can fail to be impressed by their warmth, clarity, and dramatic effect. However, wood is rarely a major component in high-status architecture. Wood's flexibility, warmth, beauty, and dynamic vitality are used by leading architects only as special effects. Instead of being revered as the essential, expensive, natural material that it once was, it has become another cheap mass-produced commodity sold by the truckload to weekend do-it-yourselfers and tract home builders. Scientific technology, which facilitated so many exciting changes in wood's use throughout the 20th century, eventually brought forth other materials and systems. Those new systems, namely, electrical, plumbing, insulating, heating, communication, and transportation, have assumed prominence in construction projects of all types, and they, far more than any structural or decorative material, will continue to be primary architectural influences throughout the 21st century.

A. GORDON MACKAY

See also **Aalto, Alvar (Finland); Ando, Tadao (Japan); Craftsman Style; Greene, Henry M. and Charles S. (United States); Hitchcock, Henry-Russell (United States); Horta, Victor (Belgium); Mackintosh, Charles Rennie (Scotland); Wright, Frank Lloyd (United States)**

Further Reading

Elliott, Cecil D., *Technics and Architecture: The Development of Materials and Systems for Buildings*, Cambridge, Massachusetts: MIT Press, 1992

Haygreen, John G., *Forest Products and Wood Science: An Introduction*, Ames: Iowa State University Press, 1982; 3rd edition, 1996

Hitchcock, Henry-Russell, Jr., "Modern Architecture: I. The Traditionalists and the New Tradition," *Architectural Record* (April 1928)

Jester, Thomas C., editor, *Twentieth-Century Building Materials: History and Conservation*, New York: McGraw-Hill, 1995

Schniewind, Arno P., *Concise Encyclopedia of Wood and Wood-Based Materials*, Cambridge, Massachusetts: MIT Press, and Oxford: Pergamon, 1989

Wilson, Forrest, "Wood: Holding Its Place through Decades of Change," *Architecture: The AIA Journal*, 87/2 (February 1988)

Wright, Frank Lloyd, "In the Cause of Architecture: IV. The Meaning of Materials—Wood," *Architectural Record* (May 1928)

WOOLWORTH BUILDING, NEW YORK CITY

Designed by Cass Gilbert; completed 1913

The Woolworth Building in New York was designed by the architect Cass Gilbert during 1910–13. Frank Woolworth, the founder of the popular F.W. Woolworth Company, undertook the project in 1910, after having expanded his business from a single store in Lancaster, Pennsylvania, established in 1879 to a chain of 318 stores. That year, he selected a site at Broadway and Park Place, across from the Brooklyn Bridge and Fronting City Hall Park. For the purposes of financing his skyscraper, Woolworth formed a limited partnership, the Broadway-Park Place Company, with Irving National Exchange Bank.

Woolworth chose Gilbert as the project's architect after Gilbert designed the Broadway Chambers (1896–1900) and the West Street buildings (1905–07), achieving renown for his skyscrapers. Gilbert's West Street Building, his first "skyscraper Gothic" design, featured rational verticals inspired by Louis Sullivan's Bayard Building and a pinnacled, picturesque crown.

Woolworth selected the Victoria Tower at the Houses of Parliament in London, a perpendicular Gothic tower, as the model for his skyscraper. Gilbert's objective, however, was to create a "civic" or "commercial" identity for the headquarters of the F.W. Woolworth Company. This he based on his study of the secular Gothic *hotels des villes*, cloth halls, and belfries of medieval Flanders. Woolworth also envisioned his project as a "giant signboard." In November 1911, he merged his chain with those of competitors to create the F.W. Woolworth Company,

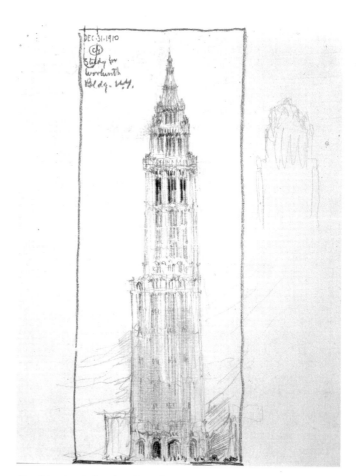

Graphite sketch for elevation of Woolworth Building, by Cass Gilbert
© Library of Congress

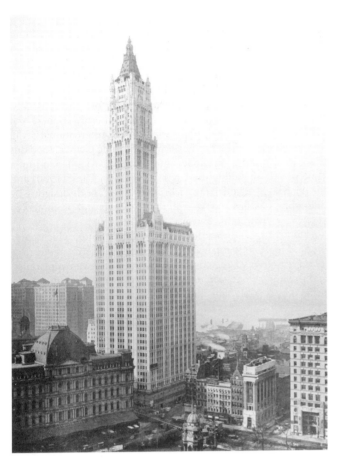

Woolworth Building, New York (1913)
© Museum of the City of New York. Gift of Collection LeRoy Barton

with a new total of 597 stores; his new retailing empire stretched from England across the Atlantic to the American shores of the Pacific.

The Woolworth Building's final design, which Gilbert completed in January 1911, had Gothic verticals showing a heightened energy and rhythm. An ingenious system of portal arch wind bracing, designed by the project's structural engineer, Gunvald Aus, made possible the exterior's soaring, attenuated, and diaphanous qualities. Flamboyant Gothic canopies, the gables of the crown, the tower's recessing stages, and the culminating tourelles—all of which were modeled in ivory-colored terracotta—enhanced the design's picturesqueness in the city. Gilbert used accenting blues, greens, and yellows to suggest depth and shadows in the elevations and to relate the tower to the surroundings of clouds and sky.

Woolworth, who chose to build in an already overbuilt market for office space, devised strategies for advertising the Woolworth Building to prospective tenants. He and his press agent, Hugh McAtemney, exploited the skyscraper's design and construction as the "world's highest" in an aggressive program of publicity. They had President Woodrow Wilson push a telegraphic button in Washington, D.C., on 24 April 1913, staging the skyscraper's opening as a great lighting spectacle. In January 1915 Woolworth installed a permanent lighting scheme that he hailed as a "standing advertisement." Woolworth also developed the tower as a sensational pinnacle observatory, which drew up to 1000 visitors a day and became an important landmark in the tourist's itinerary of the city.

The Woolworth Building's lobby-arcade, designed as an entrance to both the F.W. Woolworth Company and Irving National Bank, was one of the most opulent and colorful in the city. A cross between a Romanesque cathedral nave and the early Christian mausoleum of Galla Placidia, it featured C. Paul Jennewein's murals "Labor" and "Commerce." The interior's semipublic spaces, among them Irving National Bank's "Elizabethan" banking hall, the "medieval German" Rathskeller, and Woolworth's own Napoleonic "Empire style" executive offices on the 24th story, enriched the experience of office work with environments of fantasy that evoked the treasures of Europe. Offices for tenants were unusually light filled, and some had ceilings 20 feet high. Tenant conveniences included 18 stores in the lobby-arcade, direct access to two adjacent subway lines, and 26 high-speed electric elevators outfitted with Ellithorpe air cushions. Woolworth and McAtemney touted the skyscraper as "the highest, safest, and most perfectly appointed office structure in the world" (*Real Estate Record*, p. 587).

The Woolworth Building was christened the "Cathedral of Commerce" by the Reverend S. Parkes Cadman in 1916, and during the vibrant economy of the 1920s, it was viewed at home and abroad as a symbol of America's optimism, progress, and material success. After the Depression, however, it became a lightning rod for modernist historians, who chided its Gothic ornament as out of step with the times. It was named a national historical landmark in 1983 and subsequently underwent two restorations, the first by the Ehrenkrantz Group in 1978–80 and the second by Beyer Blinder Belle, Architects and Planners, in 1998–99.

GAIL FENSKE

See also **Gilbert, Cass (United States); New York, New York, United States; Skyscraper**

Further Reading

Koeper (1969) examines the Woolworth Building in relation to the evolution of the Gothic style in skyscrapers, and Jones (1982) argues that Gilbert's design for the building showed his indebtedness to the architectural cultures of both the Midwest and the East. Fenske (1988) analyzes Woolworth and Gilbert's project in the context of the skyscraper as a building type, the urbanization of New York, and the objectives of the City Beautiful movement.

Fenske, Gail, "The 'Skyscraper Problem' and the City Beautiful: The Woolworth Building," Ph.D. dissertation, MIT, 1988
Irish, Sharon, *Cass Gilbert, Architect: Modern Traditionalist*, New York: Monacelli Press, 1999
Jones, Robert Allen, "Cass Gilbert's Career in New York," Ph.D. disserataion, Case Western Reserve University, 1976; New York: Arno Press, 1982
Koeper, Howard Frederick, "The Gothic Skyscraper: A History of the Woolworth Building and Its Antecedents," Ph.D. dissertation, Harvard University, 1969

Landau, Sarah, and Condit, Carl, *Rise of the New York Skyscraper, 1865–1913*, New Haven and London: Yale University Press, 1996

Real Estate Record and Builders' Guide, 89 (March 23, 1912)

WORLD TRADE CENTER, NEW YORK CITY

Designed by Minoru Yamasaki; completed 1976, destroyed 11 September 2001

The design and building of the World Trade Center complex (1966–76) comprised a unique architectural vision, the application of innovative technology, and public interest. Conceived of as a public project in 1960 by the Port Authority Commissions of New York and New Jersey, the World Trade Center was intended to unite private and public interests in trade and commerce in one major building complex. Among the goals were bringing together government agencies and international trade businesses, rehabilitating the appearance of the lower Manhattan financial district, and attracting new businesses to the blighted downtown neighborhood by adding more modern office space. The building site, encompassing 16 acres located on the far west side of Manhattan along the Hudson River, was chosen as a prominent place for an important architectural statement. The convergence of major transportation routes from northern Manhattan, Brooklyn, and New Jersey was also a consideration for conceiving a central trade center. The selection of Minoru Yamasaki, a Michigan-based architect with no experience in designing skyscrapers, over other major figures in International Style design offered a distinctive vision of modern architecture to the landscape of lower Manhattan. The Port Authority's mandate for more than ten million square feet of space required the additional assistance of Emery Roth, a noted builder of many large-scale commercial and residential projects in New York City.

Minoru Yamasaki, born in 1912 in Seattle, presented an architectural style that showed a preference for subtly ornamented modern structures set within open plaza spaces. After several experimental models, Yamasaki presented a design for a World Trade Complex that included a pair of giant towers, surrounded by three smaller buildings: a hotel, the first in lower Manhattan since 1836; a large above-ground plaza; and a subterranean shopping and transportation concourse. A below-ground parking garage was the site of a terrorist attack in 1993, foreshadowing the devastating destruction of the two towers by terrorist attacks on 11 September 2001.

The plaza and underground spaces reflected Yamasaki's concern for the functional needs of people in an urban setting and were intended to serve as a contemplative open space for public respite from the noise and congestion of the narrow, crowded streets of lower Manhattan. The placement of the twin towers at angles to one another offset the importance of the plaza and drew attention to the buildings themselves. Encased in new Alcoa aluminum and rising more than 110 stories to 1368 feet, to become the tallest buildings in New York City since the Empire State Building, the towers were intended to be seen from a distance as gleaming monoliths, symbolic of the power of New York commerce.

Closer views of the twin-tower complex, particularly from street level, show that the steel-encased piers commenced on the open ground floor area as expansive, glass-filled spaces that narrowed into Gothic arches and rose to the top of the structure. The subtle Gothic design imposed on the exterior and visible in lower interior lobby areas related to Yamasaki's personal aesthetic interest in architectural elements, most notably the arch, borrowed from notable buildings of the past—in this case from Venetian architecture. In his incorporation of historic details, Yamasaki transformed the meaning and interpretation of the modern glass skyscraper, popularized in the International Style. As a result the appearance of the World Trade Center stood out from other notable skyscrapers built in lower Manhattan in the same period, including the Chase Manhattan Bank (1960) and the Marine Midland Bank (1967) buildings, both designed by Skidmore, Owings and Merrill, the architects and promoters of glass skyscraper architecture in New York City.

The construction of the World Trade Center, which commenced in 1966, contained many feats of modern engineering. The excavation of the site alone required innovative planning and the implementation of new technologies. The prime waterfront property, actually landfill extending about 600 feet from the original shoreline, required that the foundations for the two towers be dug to a very deep level to reach the bedrock of Manhattan Island. The depth of the digging, to 75 feet, or about six stories below the bottom of the adjacent Hudson River, also caused the underground train service to be temporarily elevated,

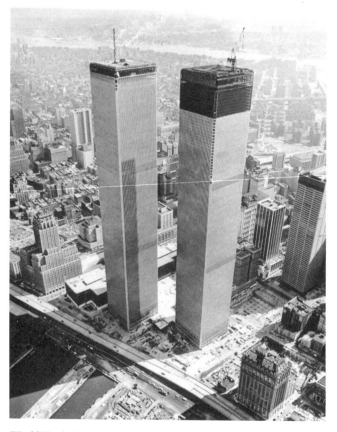

World Trade Center towers under construction, 27 March 1972
Photograph by T. Sheehan © Museum of the City of New York and The Port Authority of New York

but it was not disrupted at any point during construction. A slurry wall system, previously used for the construction of subway tunnels, was implemented to anchor the concrete foundations to heavy steel plates that were bolted into the bedrock. The dirt dug for the foundations led to the creation of a new neighborhood along the riverbank that became another notable new neighborhood: Battery Park City.

The construction of the twin towers also required engineering ingenuity. The structural engineering firm Skilling, Helle, Christiansen, Robertson coordinated the buildings to be built from the inside out, starting at the elevator cores. Through tests conducted on models of the towers in wind tunnels, a shock-absorbing damping system was devised to minimize the swaying of the tall buildings in high-wind conditions.

The elevator system was sectionalized into three separate banks. Express elevators were designed to reach sky lobbies constructed at various intervals, where passengers would then board another set of local elevators to reach the intervening floors. The result was greater efficiency in terms of both the movement of people and the opening up of more valuable floor space for office rental. The exterior walls were constructed with prefabricated panels combining two horizontal windows and three vertical windows, producing a uniform pattern of fifty-eight 22-inch-wide windows spread across each facade and separated by spandrels and columns. Prefabrication was also introduced in the floor framing. The exterior walls were also designed to be load bearing. With the assistance of Skilling, Helle, Christiansen, Robertson, a bracing system of vierendrel trusses, consisting of horizontal and vertical members, was incorporated into the exterior wall design, applying a nontraditional kind of stabilizing system that appeared to be lighter and did not diminish usable interior space.

With more than 30 million visitors reported to have made the vertical journey to the observation deck on the 107th floor of the second tower, the World Trade Center more than fulfilled Yamasaki's expressed confidence that the monoliths would be experienced as some of the most significant and loved New York City buildings. The numbers of visitors and tourists alike who continue to be drawn to the site in downtown New York City, which is still undergoing repair and reconstruction as of 2003, indicates the symbolic and iconic resonance the World Trade Center buildings maintained for a quarter of a century.

EVIE T. JOSELOW

See also **Empire State Building, New York City; International Style; New York (NY), United States; Skidmore, Owings and Merrill (United States); Skyscraper; Yamasaki, Minoru (United States)**

Further Reading

Darton, Eric, *Divided We Stand: A Biography of New York's World Trade Center*, New York: Basic Books, 1999

Gillespie, Angus Kress, *Twin Towers: The Life of New York City's World Trade Center*, New Brunswick, New Jersey: Rutgers University Press, 1999

White, Anthony G., and Minoru Yamasaki, *Minoru Yamasaki: A Selected Bibliography*, Monticello, Illinois: Vance Bibliographies, 1990

Yamasaki, Minoru, *A Life in Architecture*, New York: Weatherhill, 1979

WRIGHT, FRANK LLOYD 1867–1959

Architect and designer, United States

Frank Lloyd Wright remains America's most original, influential, and significant architect. His works are more popular today, more than a century after he began his practice in 1893 and more than 40 years after his death, than they were at any time during his lifetime. During his 72-year career, Wright designed more than 600 built works and 600 unbuilt projects, employing an astonishing range of forms and methods, yet he always described his life's work as being one singular effort, emphasizing the fundamental and unchanging ordering principles that consistently determined his work from beginning to end.

The first of these fundamental ordering principles, and by far the most important, was the primacy of the space of inhabitation, which he called "the space within." Wright's concepts for architectural space evolved first in his designs for interior spaces and were only later projected or expressed in the exterior forms. For Wright, the spatial composition must be determined by the experience of the inhabitants and not by some preconceived formal order. The second principle was that space is given its essential character through its construction. Wright believed that the way a space is experienced is directly related to the way it is constructed and that the architect must work with "the nature of materials." The third principle was that architecture takes place in nature, where interior and exterior space are woven together to make an integral whole. The relationship between architecture and the landscape was of fundamental importance to Wright, and he believed that the design of a building should start with the ground from which it was to grow. Wright designed buildings not simply as freestanding forms but as contributing elements in the larger order of both the landscape and the city.

Wright was raised in a household where the rigorously structured study of natural forms, the Unitarian faith, the ideas of American Transcendental philosophy, and the Froebel kindergarten training methods were all powerfully present. These complementary systems of thought had in common the belief that the material and spiritual worlds could not be separated but were in fact one and the same. Emerson had written that "all form is an effect of character," and Wright came to believe that every physical form had spiritual and moral meaning. Wright's development as an architect involved the evolution of this moral imperative through the search for a more principled relation to historical form, for a monumentality appropriate to the young American nation, and for a systematic yet personal process of architectural design.

Wright's education as an architect took place in Chicago from 1888 until 1893, when he apprenticed for his mentor, Louis Sullivan. In his public lectures at this time, Sullivan was calling attention to the absence of an appropriate American architecture but also warning against efforts to speed its arrival by transplanting European historical styles onto the American continent. Rejecting imported Beaux-Arts classicism, Sullivan held that any truly organic American architecture would develop only on a regional basis, with variations dependent on local climate, landscape, building methods, and materials. Wright, who would later fulfill this prophecy of Sullivan's, assisted Sullivan in his search for alternatives to what they believed to be the exhausted European classical tradition, analyzing the patterns

from Islamic, Oriental, and Celtic sources presented by Owen Jones in *The Grammar of Ornament*.

In 1893, the year Wright started his own practice, he saw the efforts of Sullivan's Chicago School style overwhelmed by the classical architecture dictated for the World's Columbian Exposition of 1893 in Chicago. This academic classicism, as defined by the Beaux-Arts School in Paris, was canonically uniform, explicitly noncontextual, and intended to be the same around the world—the first true "International Style." For Wright, it was this universal applicability, as something that had nothing to do with the particular character of a place, that would always be unacceptable and that led him to later oppose International Style modernism as forcefully as he now opposed Beaux-Arts classicism.

Yet, even as Wright attacked the Beaux-Arts as a superficial style, he was directly engaging its source, integrating the formal order underlying the architecture of classical antiquity into his work of the Prairie period (1895–1915). In the first comprehensive national publication of his work in 1908, "In the Cause of Architecture," written when he was 40 years old, Wright challenged the academic classicists' exclusive control over historical form. He argued that his designs, with their symmetry, axial planning, and hierarchical ordering from earth to sky, but without any classical forms, demonstrated a more principled manner of relating and remaining true to the architectural forms inherited from history. Although Wright characterized the appearance of his buildings as radical in comparison with the prevalent classicism, he noted that his designs were the result of reverential yet rigorous analyses of the great architecture of the past.

While this battle raged in the professional publications, Wright was in fact well on his way to winning the war by establishing a truly American architecture, one based on his perfection of a particularly American building type, the single-family suburban house. By 1910, when his designs were first extensively published in Europe, Wright had completed more than 150 built works, the vast majority of them houses. The prairie house was first defined in Wright's two prototypes published in *Ladies' Home Journal* in 1901 and built out in the Ward Willits House (1902), the Thomas Hardy House (1905), the Robert Evans House (1908), and the Avery Coonley House (1908). The Frederick Robie House (1909) was Wright's greatest urban residential design, engaging its compressed site to create a dynamic sequence of interlocking spaces, culminating in the famous living room and dining room, joined by their common ceiling, which passes through the open center of the fireplace. The Darwin Martin House (1904), five structures comprising a series of interpenetrating cruciform spaces woven into the landscape, was Wright's greatest suburban residential design, its plan an astonishingly resolved masterpiece of formal composition and the inhabitation of its exquisitely articulated interior spaces a comforting yet profoundly meaningful experience.

In Wright's prairie house, the solid fireplace mass anchored the center while the space opened out in all directions at eye level, the outriding walls and overhanging eaves acting to layer the house into the earth, giving the suburban site a geometric order so that the house and the landscape were inextricably bound to each other. Wright's prairie houses combined the formal order of symmetrical planning with the dynamism of interpenetrating spaces to produce the open, multifunctioning interiors, integrated with surrounding nature, that have since become the most popular characteristic of modern domestic architecture. Wright's prairie houses crystallized a uniquely American interpretation of the dwelling place, allowing the inhabitant to experience both comfort and inspiration, shelter and outlook, freedom and order.

In addition to the reinvention of the American house, Wright's Prairie period also produced new forms for public architecture. At the time Wright left Sullivan's office, an appropriate monumental form for American public architecture had not yet emerged. The legacy of the steel-framed office tower, which Wright had received from Sullivan and the Chicago School, had proved totally incapable of giving monumental form to the architecture of the public realm. As a manifestation of the economic determinism of scale and massing, the universal planning grid, and the production of uniform interior spaces to be "styled" later by tenants, the Chicago frame skyscraper was a projection of private commercial interests at a scale heretofore given only to public buildings yet without any of the essential qualities necessary for monumentality.

Wright understood monumentality to originate in the fundamental uniqueness of each place, regardless of its scale within the city. This understanding was reflected in Wright's work only a year after leaving Sullivan's office with his project for the Monolithic Concrete Bank (1894), a diminutive single-room edifice that nevertheless had the powerful presence of an Egyptian temple. In his repeatedly revised designs for the All Souls Church, later renamed the Abraham Lincoln Center (1897–1905), Wright transformed the spatial uniformity of Sullivan's skyscrapers into a monumental form that precisely articulated on the exterior the diverse functional spaces of the interior.

Wright achieved his fully developed vision of an appropriate monumentality for public buildings with his design and construction of the Larkin Building (1904) and Unity Temple (1906). The plans of these two buildings were simple rectangles, with mezzanines surrounding and overlooking a central multistory space, lit by high clerestory windows and continuous skylights and allowing no views out at eye level. On the exterior these buildings were closed and solid and possessed a severity of form unlike anything else of their time, seeming to relate more to the stark rectilinearity of ancient monuments.

For Wright the monumentality appropriate to American public spaces would inevitably take the form of an introverted compound, seen from the outside as a grouping of powerful independent masses bound together by mutual purpose. Entry occurred between these masses, leading to a low, dark, horizontal, rotating movement sequence that compressed and then released the occupant into the tall, light, hidden, vertical central space. The singularity of the central space, and the manner in which it fused form, structure, material, and experience, were profoundly monumental. The entire spatial and ornamental program for Wright's public buildings, from plans and massing to furniture and carpet patterns, was given order through developments of the square and cube, which Wright considered to be the most perfect of geometries. Wright intended that his public buildings be experienced as sacred spaces, whatever their function, their introspective interiors flooded from above with transcendent light to create a morally edifying effect for those inhabiting the public place.

Wright went through a personal and professional crisis in 1909, closing his Oak Park office, abandoning his family, and

taking up residence in Italy. There, he and a select group of draftsmen prepared drawings for publication by the Wasmuth Company, a German publishing house that was to issue a set of drawings of Wright's work in 1910 and a book of photographs of Wright's built works in 1911 that together were to exercise considerable influence in Europe. That year, Wright returned to the United States and began construction on his home and studio, called Taliesin (1911), outside Spring Green, Wisconsin. Like his favorite of the prairie houses, the Coonley House, Taliesin was organized around an exterior garden courtyard, framing but not completely enclosing the brow of the hill on which it was built. This courtyard house type was developed by Wright in response to commissions, such as those for the unbuilt Henry Ford (1909) and Harold McCormick (1907) Houses and the Aline Barnsdall "Hollyhock" House (1917–20), built around the brow of Olive Hill in Los Angeles, which called for far larger compositions than what could be organized within the pyramidal massing of the prototypical prairie house.

During this same period, from 1909 to 1920, Wright designed a series of public buildings that focused on interior garden courtyards. In contrast to his courtyard houses, which were inevitably asymmetrical and informal in plan, these public courtyard buildings were rigorously symmetrical, illustrating Wright's use of symmetry to distinguish between the public and the private realms. The Midway Gardens (1913), an indoor and outdoor garden for music and dining, is perhaps Wright's most completely resolved total work of art, for here he designed not only the architecture but also the band shell, interiors, furniture, dishes, sculpture, decorations, and landscaping. The Imperial Hotel (1914–22), a commission that required Wright to live in Japan during its construction, was a composition of monumental grandeur, unlike anything else in Wright's opus. This massive building was designed by Wright to float on a field of structural piers sunk into the unstable soil, an innovative seismic precaution almost immediately tested when the Imperial Hotel survived the devastating 1923 Tokyo earthquake.

Wright engaged new materials with almost every design, yet reinforced concrete proved to be the most consistently challenging to him. Despite his early success with reinforced concrete in Unity Temple, Wright remained critical of concrete's lack of inherent order and its ability to be formed into any shape at the whim of the designer; unlike all other construction materials, concrete did not exhibit a "nature" that would determine its appropriate use. In 1906, the same year that construction began on Unity Temple, Wright designed what he later called "the first block house," developing the concrete-block system of construction that he would realize 17 years later. The Alice Millard House (1923), the John Storer House (1923), the Charles Ennis House (1923), and the Samuel Freeman House (1923), all built in Los Angeles, were constructed using concrete blocks cast in custom-designed forms. In these houses, Wright succeeded in finding a means of expression suitable to reinforced concrete, the modular order imparted to the concrete blocks giving character to this previously formless material.

In 1932, during the Great Depression in the United States, Wright was already 65 years old, having written his autobiography while building only two houses since 1923. It is thus understandable that both the American public and the architectural establishment assumed that Wright had retired from active practice. However, Wright was already laying the foundations for

the most remarkable resurgence in architectural history, and he would go on to construct almost twice as many designs in the next 27 years as he had built in the preceding 40. Pivotal in this resurgence were the publication of Wright's *Autobiography*, which brought new clients, and Wright's opening of the Taliesin Fellowship, an apprenticeship school and office housed in the new Drafting Room (1932) addition to Hillside School (1902) at Taliesin, which provided both the architectural and the farming workforce. The astonishing works that Wright designed in 1934–37 effectively reestablished his dominance of the American architectural profession. With their publication in the January 1938 issue of *Architectural Forum* and *Time* magazine, Wright was again hailed as the greatest living architect.

The Edgar Kaufmann House (1937), called Fallingwater, together with his own winter home and studio, Taliesin West (1938), exemplified Wright's belief that architecture is born of its place and thus can never be the product of an "International Style," as European modernism was represented in 1932 at the Museum of Modern Art. Fallingwater, built above a mountain stream in southwestern Pennsylvania, is Wright's greatest "natural" house, a place where man can truly be at home in nature. Taliesin West, built in the desert outside Scottsdale, Arizona, celebrated both the ephemerality of life, with its canvas roofs that had to be replaced seasonally, and the permanence of place, with its boulders cast into the concrete walls, still showing the carvings of the original Native American inhabitants of this landscape.

The Johnson Wax Building (1939) is Wright's great "cathedral of work," with its innovative thin-shell concrete columns standing in small brass shoes that delicately touch the floor of the central top-lit workroom, clad in streamlined brick and lit by tube glass laid up like bricks in clerestories and skylights. Like his own Drafting Room at Taliesin, employees work here in a room that feels as if it is in the forest, among the column trees, in the light filtering down through the skylight leaves. Although dedicated to work and not worship, the central room of the Johnson Wax Building illustrates the way in which Wright celebrated everyday rituals and functions by housing them in sacred spaces. It is without question one of the greatest spaces in architectural history.

Broadacre City (1934) was Wright's visionary proposal for a pattern of land development that sought to establish an ordered pattern of cultivation and inhabitation for the enormous scale of the Jeffersonian grid while providing every household a place in nature. A complete plan for the future expansion of America's communities, it had public, commercial, and religious structures woven into its underlying fabric of single-family houses, giving the suburb an appropriate and precise spatial and social order. The Herbert Jacobs House (1937) was the first of Wright's "Usonian" houses, small and affordable homes for the rapidly growing American middle class that were to be placed on one-acre sites to form the basic pattern of Broadacre City. In the last 20 years of his life, Wright designed hundreds of these Usonian houses for various climates and construction types, each one a masterpiece of spatial generosity within remarkably small total floor areas. Broadacre City was Wright's counterproposal to the traditional city, to the isolation of agrarian life, and to the sprawling spread of the developer's speculative suburb.

The last ten years of Wright's life were incredibly productive, with hundreds of designs emerging from Taliesin for virtually

every conceivable building type. Among the best of this last period was the Solomon Guggenheim Museum (1943–59), built facing Central Park in New York City. A glorious expression of the plastic formal possibilities of reinforced concrete, the Guggenheim Museum also explored dynamic spatial and experiential territory, suspending the art and its spectators in a continuously spiraling volume that opens toward the sky. The Beth Sholom Synagogue (1954), with its seating within a folded concrete base anchored to the earth and its roof a translucent tent scaled to the heavens, is a powerful summary of man's condition as both permanent dweller and perpetual wanderer. Finally, the Marin County Civic Center (1957–66), a series of horizontal planes bridging between the low hills, although unfinished at his death, is perhaps Wright's most brilliant site design.

Despite the extraordinary public commissions of his last years, it could be argued that Wright's greatest accomplishment remained his designs for hundreds of modest, inexpensive, yet spatially rich and experientially powerful Usonian houses. In a surprisingly humble definition, Wright had early on stated his belief that architecture was the background or framework for the daily life that takes place within it. Wright's system of design was measured, scaled, and calibrated precisely by the human body and its experience, and although the geometric rigor of Wright's planning is well known, the esteem in which he held the concepts of use and comfort is not widely understood. The intellectual and formal order of Wright's designs was balanced by the physical and spiritual engagement of the inhabitant: For Wright, architecture was understood to be the shared discipline of principled place making. It could be argued that Wright's achievement was virtually unmatched in the 20th century, which produced a rich assortment of new architectural forms but few systematic conceptions that link spatial form and order to human occupation and experience.

ROBERT MCCARTER

Biography

Born in Richland Center, Wisconsin, 8 June 1867. Attended the School of Engineering, University of Wisconsin, Madison 1885–87. Married 1) Catherine Lee Tobin 1889 (separated 1909; divorced): 6 children; lived with Mrs. Mamah Bortwich Cheney 1909–1914 (died in Taliesin fire); married 2) Miriam Noel 1915 (separated 1924; died 1927); married 3) Olgivanna Lazovich 1925: 1 child; sons Lloyd and John became architects, son David joined a firm manufacturing concrete blocks like those used by Wright. Junior draftsman for Allen D. Conover, Madison 1885–87; junior draftsman for Lyman Silsbee, Chicago 1887; assistant architect, 1888–89, head of planning and design department, 1889–93, Adler and Sullivan, Chicago. Partnership with Cecil Corwin, Chicago 1893–96; private practice in Oak Park, Illinois 1896–97 and Chicago 1897–1909; traveled in Europe and stayed in Fiesole, Italy 1909–11. Built first Taliesin house and studio and resumed practice, Spring Green, Wisconsin 1911; reopened Chicago office 1912; Taliesin partially destroyed by fire and rebuilt as Taliesin II 1914; established an office in Tokyo in conjunction with work on the Imperial Hotel 1915–20; compiled the Spaulding Collection of Japanese Prints while in Japan; worked on the first concrete "texture block" houses, California 1921–24; Taliesin II partially destroyed by

fire and rebuilt as Taliesin III 1925; worked in La Jolla, California 1928; established his southwestern headquarters, Ocatillo, in Chandler, Arizona 1928–29; founded the Wright Foundation Fellowship at Taliesin 1932 with annual winter transfers of fellowship activities from Wisconsin to Chandler, Arizona 1933–38 and Scottsdale, Arizona after 1938; worked on major theoretical studies for Broadacre City from 1933; built Taliesin West, near Scottsdale, Arizona 1938; continued to practice in Wisconsin and Arizona until 1959; his students formed Taliesin Associated Architects to complete works after his death. Honorary member, Académie Royale des Beaux-Arts, Brussels 1927; honorary member, Akademie Royal der Künste, Berlin 1929; honorary member, National Academy of Brazil 1932; honorary member, Royal Institute of British Architects 1941; honorary member, National Academy of Architects, Uruguay 1942; honorary member, National Academy of Architects, Mexico 1943; honorary member, National Academy of Finland 1946; member, National Institute of Arts and Letters 1949; honorary member, Royal Academy of Fine Arts, Stockholm 1953. Royal Gold Medal, Royal Institute of British Architects 1941; Gold Medal, American Institute of Architects 1949. Died in Phoenix, Arizona, 9 April 1959.

Selected Works

Frank Lloyd Wright House and Studio, Oak Park, Illinois, 1889–1911
Charnley House, Astor Street, Chicago (with Louis Sullivan), 1891
Monolithic Concrete Bank, Chicago, 1894
Hillside Home School Buildings, near Spring Green, Wisconsin, 1902
Willits House, Highland Park, Illinois, 1902
Martin House, Buffalo, 1904
Larkin Company Administration Building (destroyed), Buffalo, 1904
All Souls Church (now Abraham Lincoln Center), Chicago, 1905
Hardy House, Racine, Wisconsin, 1905
Unity Temple, Oak Park, Illinois, 1906
McCormick House (unbuilt), 1907
Evans House, Chicago, 1908
Coonley House and Annexes, Riverside, Illinois, 1908–12
Robie House, South Woodlawn, Chicago, 1909
Ford House (unbuilt), 1909
Taliesin, near Spring Green, Wisconsin, 1911; remodeled 1914, 1925
Midway Gardens (destroyed), Chicago, 1913
Barnsdall House and Annexes, Los Angeles, 1917–20
Imperial Hotel, Tokyo, 1922
Millard House (La Miniatura), Pasadena, 1923
Storer House, Los Angeles, 1923
Ennis House, Los Angeles, 1923
Freeman House, Los Angeles, 1923
Taliesin Fellowship Complex, near Spring Green, Wisconsin, 1932
Broadacre City model and exhibition plans, 1934
Jacobs House I, Madison, 1937
Kaufmann House (Fallingwater), Bear Run, Pennsylvania, 1937
Taliesin West, near Scottsdale, Arizona, 1938
S.C. Johnson and Son Company Administration Building and Annexes, Racine, Wisconsin, 1939
S.C. Johnson Research Tower, Racine, Wisconsin, 1944
Beth Sholom Synagogue, Elkins Park, Pennsylvania, 1954
Solomon R. Guggenheim Museum, New York, 1959
Marin County Civic Center, San Raphael, California, 1966

Selected Publications

The Japanese Print: An Interpretation, 1912
Experimenting with Human Lives, 1923

The Life Work of the American Architect Frank Lloyd Wright, 1925
Modern Architecture, 1931
Two Lectures on Architecture, 1931
An Autobiography, 1932
The Disappearing City, 1932; revised edition as *When Democracy Builds*, 1945; as *The Living City*, 1958
Architecture and Modern Life (with Baker Brownell), 1937
An Organic Architecture: The Architecture of Democracy, 1939
Frank Lloyd Wright on Architecture: Selected Writings 1894–1940, edited by Frederick Gutheim, 1941
Genius and the Mobocracy, 1949
The Future of Architecture, 1953
The Natural House, 1954
An American Architecture, edited by Edgar Kaufmann, 1955
The Story of the Tower, 1956
A Testament, 1957
Drawings for a Living Architecture, 1959
The Solomon R. Guggenheim Museum, 1960
Frank Lloyd Wright: Writings and Buildings, edited by Edgar Kaufmann, Jr., and Ben Raeburn, 1960
The Drawings of Frank Lloyd Wright, edited by Arthur Drexler, 1962
Buildings, Plans and Designs, 1963
Frank Lloyd Wright: His Life, His Work, His Words, edited by Olgivanna Lloyd Wright, 1966
Architectural Essays from the Chicago School, 1967
Frank Lloyd Wright: The Early Work, 1968
In the Cause of Architecture: Essays by Frank Lloyd Wright for the Architectural Review 1908–1952, edited by Frederick Gutheim, 1975
Letters to Apprentices: Frank Lloyd Wright, edited by Bruce Brooks Pfeiffer, 1982
Letters to Architects: Frank Lloyd Wright, edited by Bruce Brooks Pfeiffer, 1984
The Guggenheim Correspondence, edited by Bruce Brooks Pfeiffer, 1986
Frank Lloyd Wright: Letters to Clients, edited by Bruce Brooks Pfeiffer, 1986
Studies and Executed Buildings by Frank Lloyd Wright, edited by Vincent Scully, 1986
Modern Architecture: Being the Kahn Lectures for 1930, 1990

Further Reading

Three comprehensive monographs exist on Wright. The earliest, Hitchcock, although not including the work of Wright's last two decades, is the only monograph written with Wright's direct involvement and approval. Levine 1996 and McCarter 1997 vary dramatically in approach, with the former placing Wright in the larger context of art-historical interpretations, whereas the latter documents the experience of inhabiting the spaces of Wright's built works. Both of these monographs benefit from access to Wright's archival material after its organization and selected publication by Bruce Brooks Pfeiffer, documented in Futagawa 1984–88 (12 vols.). Wright's own writings, including his *An Autobiography*, are collected in Wright 1992–95 (5 vols.). A comprehensive catalog of all Wright's built work is contained in Storrer. Several essay collections offer appropriately varied views of Wright, including Riley 1994, McCarter 1991, and Bolon, Nelson, and Seidel 1988. Finally, a number of excellent single-building or building-type studies exist, such as Sergeant 1976, which, due to their narrow focus, allow a sufficiently extended analysis to capture the richness of Wright's individual designs.

Bolon, Carol, Robert Nelson, and Linda Seidel (editors), *The Nature of Frank Lloyd Wright*, Chicago: University of Chicago Press, 1988
Futagawa, Yukio (editor), *Frank Lloyd Wright Monograph*, text by Bruce Brooks Pfeiffer, 12 vols., Tokyo: A.D.A. Edita, 1984–88
Hitchcock, Henry-Russell, *In the Nature of Materials, 1887–1941: The Buildings of Frank Lloyd Wright*, New York: Duell, Sloan and Pearce, 1942; with new foreword and bibliography, New York: Da Capo Press, 1973
Levine, Neil, *The Architecture of Frank Lloyd Wright*, Princeton, New Jersey: Princeton University Press, 1996
McCarter, Robert, *Frank Lloyd Wright*, London: Phaidon Press, 1997
McCarter, Robert (editor), *Frank Lloyd Wright: A Primer on Architectural Principles*, New York: Princeton Architectural Press, 1991
Riley, Terrance (editor), *Frank Lloyd Wright, Architect*, New York: Museum of Modern Art, 1994
Sergeant, John, *Frank Lloyd Wright's Usonian Houses*, New York: Whitney Library of Design, 1976
Storrer, William Allin, *The Frank Lloyd Wright Companion*, Chicago: University of Chicago Press, 1993
Wright, Frank Lloyd, *Frank Lloyd Wright Collected Writings*, edited by Bruce Brooks Pfeiffer, 5 vols., New York: Rizzoli, 1992–95

WU LIANGYONG 1922–

Architect, China

Wu Liangyong was born in 1922 in Nanjing. He received his Bachelor of Architecture degree from the National Central University in Chongqing in 1944 and completed his Master of Architecture and Urban Design degree under Eliel Saarinen at Cranbrook Academy in Cranbrook, Michigan, in 1949. On his return to China in 1950, he joined the faculty of the Department of Architecture at Tsinghua University, a major school in China for technical and engineering studies.

Wu has been recognized as a leading architectural designer and urban planner in China, especially since the 1970s. He played a major role in the replanning and design of Tiananmen Square, located in the center of Beijing. Surrounding the square are the National Congress Hall and the National Museum of History. In 1976 Wu worked with a team of five senior architects to win the competition for the design of the National Library of China. In the projects he has designed, he strives to combine traditional spirit in architecture with modern construction to create a new form of Chinese contemporary architecture.

Wu's most well-known project in urban and architectural preservation is the New Courtyard House Complex (1987) at Juer Hutong, located in northeastern Beijing. Facing the challenges of rapid economic growth, the single-story courtyard houses, which were the major housing form for the old city of Beijing, had been in danger of disappearing entirely from the city to make room for high-rise apartments. Wu and his design and research group selected a typical neighborhood in the eastern district of Beijing as an experimental project. It bears the main features of a multicourtyard system of housing with multiple—usually three—stories in the structures to accommodate more residents. The salvation of this traditional housing form turned out to be a success. The Juer Hutong project won the World Habitat Award from the United Nations in 1993 and the Gold Medal in Architecture from the Architects' Regional Council in 1992.

Wu worked as a designer and planner for several cities in China: Beijing, Handan, Beidaihe, Baoding, and Tangshan in the north; Beihai, Guilin, and Liuzhou in the south; Jiuquan in

the west; and Suzhou and Wuxi in the east. Zhangjiagang is a newly planned city, and Wu worked there in 1993. He focused on Beijing for research in city design and planning; he is on the committee for capital planning as a consultant for the municipal government, helping in the strategic planning of the city. He also participates in policy making and research on historic preservation for the city.

As an educator in architecture, Wu led the School of Architecture at Tsinghua University as the dean from 1977 to 1983. He was invited by the eminent architectural scholar Liang Sicheng to participate in the founding of the school in 1946. Wu has since then been one of the school's most influential professors. He has formed two research centers at Tsinghua: the Institute of Architecture and Urban Studies and the Center for Human Settlements. He serves as the director of both; many design and research projects were completed by the centers under his directorship. The Institute of Confucianism in Qufu, Confucius's hometown, is one of the most recent projects that they have completed.

Wu's teaching covers studio instruction and lectures on theory and history of cities. His *A Brief History of Ancient Chinese City Planning* (1986) is the first English-language book on the topic ever published by a scholar of mainland China. Wu used this book as a main reference when he taught at Gesamthochschule in Kassel, Germany. His teaching extended to the seminar courses in Beijing for mayors. Wu was awarded the Jean Tschumi Prize by the UIA (Union Internationate des Architect) in 1996 for his renowned contributions in architectural education.

A Theory of Integral Architecture (2001) advanced Wu's ideas in China for dealing with design issues in a global perspective. His book *A General Theory of Architecture* (1990, Beijing; 1992, Taipei) discusses human settlements, world urbanism, China's responses to the challenges of environmental changes, and architectural regionalism, among many other topics. Wu proposes that architectural studies in China should employ "holistic thinking" and "cross-disciplinary research." In that sense architectural and urban studies in China should be combined closely in a system but should remain general: architecture and its humanistic presence of time and space, architecture and its geographical presence of time and space, architecture as the presence of culture and tradition, technical essence in architecture, and finally, architecture as a cultural expression for its aesthetic forms. Wu uses diagrammatic charts to illustrate his theory, and he concludes that the general theory is a new subject that he calls a "science of human settlement." He further distinguishes his theory as a "new regionalism."

China opened the door to the world after the Cultural Revolution that took place between 1966 and 1976, and it resumed its international connections to the architectural world in the mid-1970s. Wu has performed a major role in representing China's architectural professionals in world organizations and conferences. In addition to his busy schedule as visiting professor and research fellow in the United States and Europe, he served as a vice president of UIA (1987–90) and the president of the World Society of Ekistics. He is an honorary fellow of the American Institute of Architects and an honorary fellow of the Royal Institute of British Architects, among other professional memberships. Most recently, in the summer of 1999, he co-chaired

the Beijing conference of UIA and drafted the UIA Beijing Charter.

YUNSHENG HUANG

Biography

Born in Nanjing, Jiangsu Province, China, 7 May 1922. Attended National Central University, Chongqing (bachelor's degree 1944), and Cranbrook Academy, Cranbrook, Michigan (master's degree 1949). Married Yao Tongzhen, a landscape architect. Taught part-time at Lawrence Institute of Technology, Detroit, Michigan, 1949–50; then lifelong professor at the School of Architecture, Tsinghua University, Beijing 1951–; visiting scholar, Cambridge University 1995; visiting professor, University of Hong Kong 1983; visiting professor, University of California, Berkeley, 1988; and other universities. Has exhibited artwork in China, Australia, the United States, and Germany.

Selected Works

Automobile Body Design Building, GM Technical Research Center, Detroit, Michigan, 1950
New East Wing of the Beijing Hotel, 1973
"Beijing 2000" Urban Design Plan, Shichahai District, Beijing, 1979
New Courtyard House Complex at Juer Hutong, Beijing, 1987
Extension of the National Museum of History, Beijing, 1994

Selected Publications

A Brief History of Ancient Chinese City Planning, 1986
A General Theory of Architecture, 1990 (in Chinese)
Reflection at the Turn of the Century: The Future of Architecture, 1999 (in Chinese)
Rehabilitating the Old City of Beijing: A Project in the Ju'er Hutong Neighbourhood, 1999

Further Reading

Most articles about Wu Liangyong are in Chinese journals.
American Institute of Architects Memo, 9 (January 1990) (special issue)
Liang, Ssu-ch'eng, *A Pictorial History of Chinese Architecture*, Cambridge, Massachusetts: MIT Press, 1984

WURSTER, WILLIAM 1895–1973

Architect, United States

William Wurster was a chief exponent of the "Bay Region School" of architecture in the United States. His development as an architect coincided with the years of the Great Depression (1929–35) and his maturation with the years 1935–42, preceding World War II. Wurster's architecture, like that of his contemporaries Pietro Belluschi, Harwell Hamilton Harris, and O'Neil Ford, exemplified a form of rooted and indigenous modernism that flourished in the United States before the internationalist orientation of the 1950s. Wurster and his contemporaries believed that architecture, whether designed for the Northwest, the Pacific coast, or the Southwest, should visibly express the identity of a region.

Between 1913 and 1918, Wurster visited works by well-known Bay Region architects, among them Bernard Maybeck,

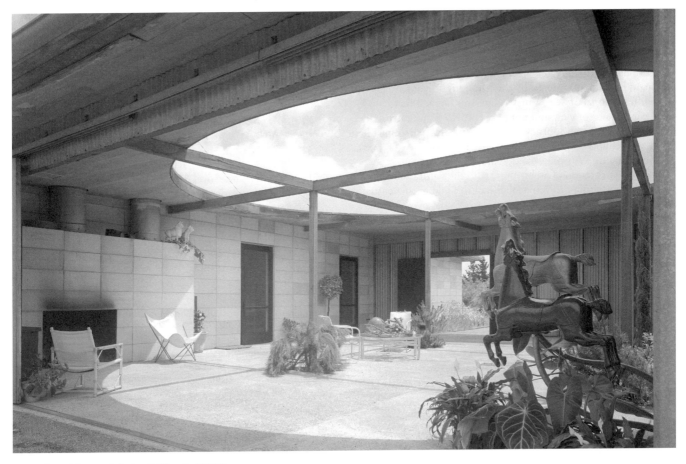

Saxon Pope House, Orinda, California (1940)
Ezra Stoller © Esto

Ernest Coxhead, and Willis Polk. Wurster especially appreciated Maybeck's Christian Science Church, which synthesized Beaux-Arts ornamental exuberance with experimental building techniques and the Arts and Crafts ideals of simplicity, authenticity, and naturalism. Wurster traveled to Paris in 1922 and from there departed on sketching tours throughout Europe during 1922–23. Italy and Spain were key destinations: Their vernacular traditions and rural landscapes held significance for California. After his return William Adams Delano assisted Wurster with the financing of his own office in Berkeley in 1924 and with introductions to some of Wurster's most important early clients.

Wurster launched his career with the Gregory Farmhouse (1927–28) near Santa Cruz. Designed for Mrs. Warren (Sadie) Gregory, whom Wurster met through a friend of Delano's, the Farmhouse was widely published and functioned as a clear visual statement of Wurster's architectural principles. First, both Wurster and his client envisioned an architectural character of crafted simplicity and calculated understatement. Wurster, who was committed to the "cleanliness" of wood carpentry and inspired by the vernacular structures in California's gold-mining towns and early Monterey, conceived and detailed a composition that was both ranchlike and modern yet conscientiously devoid of any particular style. Finally, Wurster devised numerous strategies for integrating the house with its country setting. Each individual room, for instance, opened onto a *corredor*, or terrace, some of which served as "outdoor rooms," and the house's L-shaped plan framed a central courtyard, recalling at once European manor houses, Italian villas, and the Spanish-influenced adobe houses of old Monterey.

During the years following the Gregory commission, Wurster continued to refine his modern regionalist approach. In the early 1930s he designed 13 houses for Pasatiempo, a country club and residential community near Monterey Bay, among them the MacKenzie-Field House (1931). Wurster's Pasatiempo houses, which he viewed as antidotes to an overmechanized urban life, showed that he continued to develop his vernacular-inspired architectural vocabulary, simple yet refined techniques of wood construction, integration of indoor and outdoor spaces, and sensitivity to the natural surroundings. The Voss House (1931) in the countryside of Big Sur, with a profile embedded in the landscape, kitchen "cave," and direct confrontation of the ocean vista, epitomized Wurster's search for a modern architecture that embodied the California yearning for the simple yet "good" life in the open.

By the mid-1930s Wurster's practice was well established. As his regionalist sensibility matured, his houses also became more consistently modernist and abstract. Wurster's Clark House

(1937) in Aptos, which had cubic volumes and flush planar surfaces, and his Saxton Pope House (1940) in Orinda, with powerful geometries and construction in concrete block and corrugated steel, exemplified his new, starker approach. These houses suggested a greater affinity with the European avant-garde, at the time promoted by the Museum of Modern Art as the "International Style." Wurster, however, argued that "modern" was a point of view and not a style. In 1937 Wurster made his second European journey, with the objective of seeing the modern architecture of Scandinavia and, in particular, the work of Alvar Aalto. Wurster valued Aalto's "humanist" approach; that is, his integration of architecture with the natural surroundings and his attention to vernacular resources and to the sensuality of craftsmanship in wood. After Wurster discovered Aalto's own house on the outskirts of Helsinki, the two architects visited Aalto's Savoy Restaurant, Sunila Pulp Mill, and Paimio Sanatorium; they discussed their shared philosophical viewpoints and established a friendship that lasted throughout their lives.

During the 1930s, Wurster became increasingly involved with the problem of low-cost housing. His designs for individual minimum dwellings, such as his "Unit Steel House" (1937) for the Soule Steel Company, along with housing communities such as Valencia Gardens (1939) in San Francisco, a 246-unit project, demonstrated his command of a range of housing scales. In 1939 Wurster met Catherine Bauer, whose *Modern Housing* (1934) had become the seminal work on the subject. They married in 1940, and Bauer's emphasis on the virtues of large-scale projects and rationalized construction techniques, along with her study of garden communities such as Radburn, influenced Wurster's approach to designing communities for war workers in the early 1940s. Among these were his Carquinez Heights (1941) in Vallejo. In this project and others, such as Chabot Terrace (1942) in Vallejo and Parker Homes (1943) in Sacramento, Wurster aspired to integrate current thinking on standardized housing with his own long-standing commitment to the client and to the environmental specifics of landscape, climate, and views.

GAIL FENSKE

See also **Aalto, Alvar (Finland); Maybeck, Bernard R. (United States)**

Biography

Born in Stockton, California, 20 October 1895. Studied at the University of California, Berkeley 1912–13; worked in a surveyor's office 1913–14; studied naval architecture and marine engineering at the University of California 1914–16; went to sea as an engineer 1916–18; finished studies at the University of California 1919–20; bachelor's degree in architecture 1920; traveled in Europe 1922–23. Married Catherine Bauer 1940 (died 1964): 1 child. Assistant in the office of E. B. Brown, Stockton 1910; worked for the firm of John Reid, Jr., San Francisco 1920; employed by the Filtration Division, City of Sacramento, California, under architect Charles Dean 1921–22; worked for the firm of Delano and Aldrich, New York 1923–24; returned to California to design a filtration plant for East Bay Water Company 1924–25. In private practice, San Francisco 1926–43; partner, with Theodore Bernardi and Donn Emmons, Wurster, Bernardi, and Emmons, San Francisco from 1945. Fellow, Harvard Graduate School of Design 1943–44; dean, School of Architecture and Planning, Massachusetts Institute of Technology, Cambridge 1944–50; dean, College of Architecture, 1950–59, dean, College of Environmental Design, 1959–63, dean emeritus, 1963–73, University of California, Berkeley. Chairman, Architects Advisory Committee, United States National Housing Agency 1942; chairman, 1949–50, California State, Member, 1959–67, National Capitol Park and Planning Commission; member, Architectural Advisory Panel, Office for Foreign Buildings, United States State Department 1958–63. Fellow, American Institute of Architects; fellow, American Academy of Arts and Sciences; fellow, Royal Academy of Fine Arts, Copenhagen; member, Akademie der Künste, Berlin; honorary corresponding member, Royal Institute of British Architects; affiliate, American Institute of Planners. Gold Medal, American Institute of Architects 1969. Died in Berkeley, 19 September 1973.

Selected Works

Gregory Farmhouse, Santa Cruz, California, 1928
MacKenzie-Field House, Monterey Bay, California, 1931
Voss House, Big Sur, California, 1931
Clark House, Aptos, California, 1937
"Unit Steel House" (project), Soule Steel Company, 1937
Housing Development, Valencia Gardens, San Francisco, 1939
Saxton Pope House, Orinda, California, 1940
Carquinez Heights, Vallejo, California, 1941
Chabot Terrace, Vallejo, 1942
Parker Homes, Sacramento, 1943

Selected Publications

"From Log Cabin to Modern House," *New York Times Magazine* (20 January 1946)
"When Is a Small House Large," *House and Garden* (August 1947)
"Architectural Education," *AIA Journal* (January 1948)
"Architecture Broadens Its Base," *AIA Journal* (July 1948)
"The Outdoors in Residential Design," *Architectural Forum* (September 1949)
"Row House Vernacular and High Style Monument," *Architectural Report* (August 1958)
"College Planning," *Architectural Record* (September 1959)

Further Reading

Michelson provides a definitive account of Wurster's career and includes a house-by-house bibliography, a list of Wurster's writings, and a chronology. Treib's exhibition catalog expands Michelson's account with eight essays that situate Wurster's career within the broader social and intellectual milieu of the United States. Hille provides complete visual documentation of Wurster's key residential works.

Fenske, Gail, "Lewis Mumford, Henry-Russell Hitchcock, and the Bay Region Style," in *The Education of the Architect: Historiography, Urbanism, and the Growth of Architectural Knowledge. Essays Presented to Stanford Anderson*, edited by Martha D. Pollak, Cambridge, Massachusetts: MIT Press, 1997
Gregory, Daniel P., "An Indigenous Thing: The Story of William Wurster and the Gregory Farmhouse," *Places*, 7 (Fall 1990)
Hille, R. Thomas, *Inside the Large Small House: The Residential Design Legacy of William W. Wurster*, New York: Princeton Architectural Press, 1994
Michelson, Alan Richard, "Towards a Regional Synthesis: The Suburban and Country Residences of William Wilson Wurster, 1922–1964," Ph.D. dissertation, Stanford University, 1993

Peters, Richard C., "The Integrity Is Implicit, the Sincerity Intense: William Wilson Wurster, Gold Medalist, 1969," *AIA Journal*, 51 (May 1969)

Riess, Suzanne B., interviewer, *William Wilson Wurster, 1895–1973 (d. Sept. 19, 1973): College of Environmental Design, University of* *California, Campus Planning, and Architectural Practice*, Berkeley: University of California Press, 1964

Treib, Marc (editor), *An Everyday Modernism: The Houses of William Wurster* (exhib. cat.), San Francisco: San Francisco Museum of Modern Art, and Berkeley: University of California Press, 1995

Y

YAAMA MOSQUE, TAHOUA, NIGER
Designed by Falké Barmou, completed 1982

The Yaama Mosque is a mud-brick building, but it is one that is strikingly different from the Dyula-type mosques found in Mali. This is an example of a building built in a local style but whose growth over time shows a desire for monumentality in size, form, and the complexity of its decoration. It also emphasizes that there can be monuments within a vernacular style of architecture.

A mud-brick and tamped-earth building, the mosque was designed by mason and farmer Falké Barmou in a semidesert region of Niger. Twenty years in the making, this Friday mosque was completed in 1982. The client and the construction team was the community of Yaama.

The mosque is squarish in plan. The initial building was a hypostyle hall, a field of closely spaced heavy columns whose visual weight lends the building's interior a somber air. The building was initially roofed with a simple post-and-lintel system. In 1975 Barmou took advantage of the need to fix a leaking roof to replace the ceiling with a livelier vaulted system. Barmou had traveled to Dakar and to Mecca and thus was exposed to, and incorporated into his work, many building techniques.

Frequently referred to simply as "Hausa," Labelle Prussin feels that a more accurate term is "Fulani-Hausa." Her term acknowledges the dual influences of the nomadic Fulani, a Fulbe-speaking people who migrated into the region, which today lies in northern Nigeria and Niger. The Hausa were the sedentary people native to the area.

Barmou used one of the most significant features of Hausa architecture: arches, vaults, and domes made of bundled and bent reeds covered with a mud-and-straw mortar. On top of these groin vaults, sticks are laid in a basket-weave pattern. When he replaced the roof, Barmou also removed a central column that created a central space over which he added a dome. This imposition of a central dome into the hypostyle hall shows the interconnectedness of mosque architecture with multidomed Byzantine Christian churches, such as St. Mark's in Venice.

This vaulted-and-domed construction system demonstrates the continuity into a permanent kind of architecture of tech-niques derived from less-exalted kinds of architecture, such as tents and straw huts. With temporary structures a material (fabric, hides, or straw) is laid over a framework. Prussin writes, "The Fulani-Hausa dome can be construed as a visual synthesis of several contradictory aspirations into a unified image: mobility, identity with Islam, and sedentarization" (Prussin, 1986).

The largest element in the project is the hypostyle prayer hall. As is customary with mosques, a mihrab, or prayer niche, occupies the middle of the qibla wall (qibla denotes the direction toward Mecca). As there is a central row of columns, in the Yaama Mosque the mihrab is slightly off center so that it lies at the end of a visual axis. A low perimeter wall creates an enclosed compound that can be used as an overflow area for prayers.

Some mosques (e.g. Djenné and Niono) are rectangular in plan, and the entry is in the center of one of the long sides. This allows rows of worshipers to extend laterally as far as possible. Other mosques are square in plan, something that Prussin argues relates to the Islamic magic square. The magic square is an arrangement of numbers in a graphic pattern found in a variety of Islamic arts. A typical example is a three-by-three nine-house square. Both the overall plan of Yaama and the square-based dome are similar in form to the Islamic magic square.

The roof is made of bundles of sticks that are visible on the interior although skim coated with mud on the exterior. This kind of architecture, built of local materials and using local craftsmen, was sustainable before the term *sustainability* achieved its current popularity. This building was literally built by the community.

There are four corner towers, all different in form. The towers are divided into vertical zones with setbacks. An initial simplicity has been augmented over time by an increasing desire to add detail and monumentality, particularly considering the towers. Over time, there has been an increasing concern for aesthetics and decoration.

None of the four towers, however, functions as a minaret. A minaret, the tower from which worshipers are called to prayer, is not an essential part of a mosque. Minarets are frequently significant vertical elements in the design of Ottoman and Middle Eastern mosques.

The selection of the Yaama Mosque for an Aga Khan Award in 1986 provoked a controversy within the Islamic architectural

community. One of six winners, it was controversial, but not because of any perceived failings of this particular mosque. By excluding projects such as airports and skyscrapers, dissenting members of the judging panel felt that the overall message sent by the Aga Khan Awards was overtly nostalgic and traditional. Islamic architecture did not, they argued, have to be anti-Western, antimodern, and antitechnology.

The Yaama Mosque reconciles local tradition and a modern Islam with a grace and ease that were lacking in the Aga Khan Award debacle. At once restrained and massive, delicate and decorative, this project shows the creative energy that still exists within traditional African building techniques.

MARK HINCHMAN

Further Reading

Campbell, Robert, "The Aga Khan Awards for 1987 Raise Issues of Tradition," *Architecture* (January 1987)

Holod, Renata, and Hasan-Uddin Khan (editors), *The Contemporary Mosque: Architects, Clients, and Designs since the 1950s*, New York: Rizzoli, 1997; as *The Mosque and the Modern World: Architects, Patrons, and Designs since the 1950s*, London: Thames and Hudson, 1997

"Permeating Excellence: Third Cycle of the Aga Khan Award for Architecture," *Arts and the Islamic World*, 4 (Autumn/Winter 1986)

Prussin, Labelle, *Hatumere: Islamic Design in West Africa*, Berkeley: University of California Press, 1986

"Yaama Mosque, Niger," *Architectural Review*, 180 (November 1986)

"Yaama Mosque, Niger," *The Architectural Record*, 175 (January 1987)

YAMASAKI, MINORU 1912–86

Architect, United States

Driven by the sincere belief that architecture should make daily life more beautiful and emotionally fulfilling, Japanese-American architect Minoru Yamasaki developed a highly ornamental architecture that drew on his world travels for inspiration. Although other architects (notably Edward Durell Stone and Philip Johnson) also explored the combination of modernist forms and materials with historicist motifs and elements, Yamasaki's ornamental eclecticism (drawing from a variety of sources, from mosques to Gothic cathedrals) set him apart from his contemporaries. Although the sheer size of Yamasaki's best-known work, the World Trade Center Towers (1976) in New York overwhelmed its neo-Gothic ornament, the majority of his architecture reflected an interest in human scale and lightness of materials.

This approach pervades the McGregor Memorial Conference Center (1958) at Wayne State University in Detroit, which Yamasaki adorned with triangular arches and inverted pyramidal canopies over a glass atrium, all surrounded by a series of fountains and platforms. Although derived from his genuine desire to harmonize architecture with humanity, this preoccupation with ornament and surface effects has led many critics to deride his work as self-indulgent, formalist, and overly decorative. Regardless of these criticisms, Yamasaki enjoyed considerable suc-cess with a public weary of the anonymity of glass-and-steel modernism constructed in the second half of the 20th century.

The 33 orange brick blocks of Yamasaki's Pruitt Igoe Houses (1952–55) in St. Louis seem an unlikely beginning for an architect committed to an architecture of serenity and delight (Yamasaki even excluded the project from his autobiography). The award-winning design for low-income public housing was praised for its modernist features (including window-lined galleries intended to serve as outdoor socializing areas, reminiscent of Le Corbusier) and cost-efficient design. However, in reality, the housing project was a spectacular failure, plagued by crime, low occupancy, vandalism, and ill-functioning services. The buildings' demolition in 1972 received worldwide coverage and was seen as representing the ultimate failure of the social engineering and functionalist rhetoric of modernism.

Even with the initially positive reception of the Pruitt Igoe housing project, Yamasaki would depart radically from such doctrinaire modernism for the rest of his career. Contemporary to the design of Pruitt Igoe, Yamasaki, Hellmuth, and Leinweber received the commission for a new airport for the city of St. Louis. Intended to serve the demands of air travel while functioning as a monumental entrance to the city, the soaring concrete groin vaults of Lambert Airport (1956) recalled the grandeur of American railroad depots in the early 20th century, such as New York's Grand Central Station. The sweeping and elegant concrete vaults of the Terminal Building established Yamasaki's international reputation and introduced a new idiom for airport design (further refined and developed in the works of Eero Saarinen).

Following the success of Lambert Airport, Yamasaki increasingly incorporated overt Gothic-, Islamic-, and Japanese-inspired ornament into his architecture. The elaborately patterned aluminum screen walls at the Reynolds Metals Regional Sales Office (1959) in Southfield, Michigan, demonstrate his interest in exotic patterns, whereas the concrete ogee arches and canopies of the Dhahran Air Terminal (1961) in Dhahran, Saudi Arabia, attempted to harmonize with the surroundings. Among his most elaborate works was the enormously popular Federal Science Pavilion (1962) at the Seattle World's Fair, which consisted of a series of lacy canopies with parabolic arches, rendered in a kind of space-age neo-Gothic style.

Yamasaki's particular blend of ornament and modernist structure ensured him a prominent place in the architecture of the United States and throughout the world. His architecture was chosen to represent the United States with the U.S. Pavilion (1959) at the World Agricultural Fair in New Delhi. Additionally, Yamasaki was invited to design the Founders Hall (1983) in Shinji Shumeikai, Shiga prefecture, Japan. Overall, Yamasaki was one of a few architects who dared to question the modernist mantra "Less is more." Through his inventive combination of historicist motifs and elements, Yamasaki created an architecture that addressed far more than its overt functions, striving to make modern architecture enjoyable to a broad spectrum of the public.

MATTHEW S. ROBINSON

See also **Johnson, Philip (United States); Ornament; Pruitt Igoe Housing, St. Louis, Missouri; Skyscraper; Stone, Edward Durell (United States); World Trade Center, New York City**

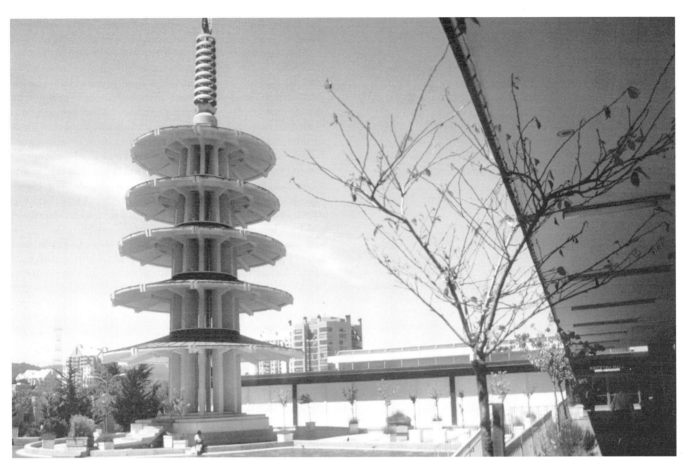

Japan Center, San Francisco (1968)
Photo © Mary Ann Sullivan

Biography

Born in Seattle, Washington, 1 December 1912. Studied at the University of Washington, Seattle 1930–34; bachelor's degree in architecture 1934; attended New York University 1934–35. Worked as a designer for Githens and Keally, New York 1935–37; designer for Shreve, Lamb and Harmon, New York 1937–43; designer for the firm of Harrison and Fouilhoux, New York 1943–44; designer for Raymond Loewy Associates, New York 1944–45; chief architectural designer, Smith, Hinchman and Grylls, Detroit, Michigan 1945–49. Principal, Minoru Yamasaki and Associates, Troy, Michigan from 1949; partnership with Joseph Leinweber, Yamasaki, Leinweber and Associates, Detroit 1949–55; partnership with Leinweber and George Hellmuth, Leinweber, Yamasaki and Hellmuth, St. Louis, Missouri 1949–55. Instructor at New York University 1935–36 and Columbia University, New York 1943–45. Fellow, American Institute of Architects 1960; fellow, American Academy of Arts and Sciences 1960. Died in Detroit, 6 February 1986.

Selected Works

Pruitt Igoe Housing Project (destroyed), St. Louis, Missouri, 1955
Terminal Building, Lambert Airport, St. Louis, Missouri, 1956

McGregor Memorial Community Conference Center, Wayne State University, Detroit, Michigan, 1958
Reynolds Metals Regional Sales Office, Southfield, Michigan, 1959
U.S. Pavilion, World Agricultural Fair, New Delhi, 1959
Dhahran Air Terminal, Dhahran, Saudi Arabia, 1961
Federal Science Pavilion, World's Fair, Seattle, Washington, 1962
Japan Center, San Francisco, Calfornia, 1968
World Trade Center, New York City (with Emery Roth and Sons; destroyed), 1976
Rainier Square Bank Tower (architectural design and detailing only), Seattle, Washington, 1977
Saudi Arabian Monetary Agency Headquarters, Riyadh, 1982
Founders Hall, Shinji Shumeikai, Shiga prefecture, Japan, 1983

Selected Publications

Minoru Yamasaki: The Architect and His Use of Sculpture as an Integral Part of Design (exhib. cat.), 1967
A Life in Architecture, 1979

Further Reading

Unfortunately, there is a relative dearth of information concerning the life and architecture of Minoru Yamasaki. The primary source for information about Yamasaki is his autobiography, *A Life in Architecture* (1979), which offers insight into his practice and philosophy of architec-

ture. Articles by Veronese, Huxtable, and a host of others position Yamasaki in the context of the late 1950s and early 1960s. Yamasaki enjoyed a degree of prominence in the American press, appearing on the cover of *Time* magazine in 1963; the accompanying article, "The Road to Xanadu," balances a sympathetic appraisal of his architecture with more critical statements by his fellow architects. Other than some ongoing commentary surrounding the World Trade Center Towers, Yamasaki is infrequently discussed by critics and historians.

Huxtable, Ada Louise, "Minoru Yamasaki's Recent Buildings," *Art in America*, 50 (Winter 1962)

"The Road to Xanadu," *Time* (18 January 1963)

Veronese, Giulia, "Minoru Yamasaki, Edward Durell Stone," *Zodiac*, 8 (1961)

YUGOSLAVIA

Although Yugoslavia existed as an official state through much of the 20th century, its architecture has been commonly presented through separate, regional surveys rather than general overviews. On the basis of the major political events of the century, three phases can be considered distinctive in terms of architectural analysis: the period before the creation of Yugoslavia in 1918, the interwar period of the kingdom of Yugoslavia, and the period after World War II, when the country was officially the Socialist Federal Republic of Yugoslavia.

Constituted on territory shared through the centuries by two quite different empires, the Habsburg and the Ottoman, Yugoslavia had unequal potential for the development of modernity in its eastern and western regions. However, the modern age was brought to the whole country from the same source: the Central European metropolis. Being in Austro-Hungarian territory at the turn of the century, buildings in Slovenia, Croatia, and Bosnia-Herzegovina were designed either by foreign builders or by domestic architects educated at leading schools of the empire. On the other hand, Serbia and Montenegro, emancipated from the Ottoman government in the mid-19th century, passed through an intense transformation, catching up with the trends of contemporary Europe. The first Serbian architects to bring modern architectural features to the kingdom of Serbia (independent from 1878) were educated in Vienna, similar to their fellows from the western regions.

The turning point in Slovenian architecture was the earthquake of 1895, after which the cultural capital of Slovenia, Ljubljana, was rebuilt following the plans of Camillo Sitte and Max Fabiani. Besides shaping the modern urban structure of Ljubljana, Max Fabiani (1865–1962) brought the Viennese Secession to Slovenia, designing many public and residential buildings, such as Hribar House (1905), Bamberg Palace (1906–07), and the girls' school Mladika (1906–07).

The first decades of 20th-century architecture in Croatia are associated with the name of Viktor Kovacic (1874–1924), a student of Otto Wagner, who initiated an enthusiastic struggle against "dogmatic historicism." Joining a group of young artists and writers, the founders of the Zagreb magazine *Zivot* (Life), Kovacic published a manifesto titled "Modern Architecture" in its first issue of 1900. Whereas his projects such as Frank House (1910) and the Church of St. Blaz (1913) vary the recognizable idiom of the Wagnerschule, other chief examples of the Croatian Secession, such as Ignjat Fischer's Sanatorium (1908) and Rudolf Lubinsky's University Library (1913), both in Zagreb, pres

ent a closer interpretation of the Viennese "geometric" forerunner.

After the Austrian occupation of Bosnia-Herzegovina of 1878, the favored style for new public buildings, chosen to present the distinctiveness of the mixed population, was the pseudo-Moorish. Richly decorated edifices in Sarajevo, such as Wittek and Ivekovic's City Hall (1892–96, almost destroyed in the civil war, 1992–95) or the Evangelistic Church (1899), designed by the leading architect of the time, Karlo Parzik (1857–1942), exemplify the popular within-the-empire trend of compiling "exotic," pseudo-Moorish and neo-Byzantine elements with the forms of Western Medieval Revival. With exceptions such as Jan Kotera's Slavija Bank (1910–11) in Sarajevo, whose pure geometric forms anticipated his "revolutionary" Urbánek's Mozarteum Building in Prague, characteristic Secessionist buildings in Bosnia-Herzegovina were a mixture of eclectic features and new decorative motifs, as on the Post Office in Sarajevo (1907–13, severely damaged in the civil war, 1992–95), designed by Josip Vancas (1859–1932).

Before the establishment of an architectural program at Belgrade Technical Faculty in 1897, the first generation of Serbian architects earned their degrees from universities in Vienna, Munich, Berlin, Karlsruhe, and Zurich, bringing back both the academic traditions as well as the new, turn-of-the-century tendencies. The Secession appeared in Serbia in two different manners, one of which came as a synthesis of the eclectic method and modern architectural elements (e.g., large continuous glass screens, characteristic railings, and floral decoration) that can be seen on Svetozar Jovanovic's Officers Union (1908) in Belgrade. The other Secessionist manner, represented in the work of Branko Tanazevic (1876–1945), such as the Telephone Exchange (1907–08) and the Ministry of Education (1912–13), both in Belgrade, was closely related to the turn-of-the-century National Romanticism of the Central European countries that introduced modern, stylized folk motifs as the new forms of expression. This mode of Serbian Secession was a further step in the creation of a "true" national idiom, already announced in the academic neo-Byzantine designs of the earlier generation of Theophil von Hansen's pupils.

After the formation of the Kingdom of Serbs, Croats, and Slovenes in 1918 (in 1929 renamed the Kingdom of Yugoslavia), building was intensive in the strongest economic centers, Ljubljana and Zagreb, and especially brisk in Belgrade, the capital of the entire country. The significant event was the foundation of architectural schools at the Technical Faculty of Ljubljana, led by Joze Plecnik (1872–1957) and Ivan Vurnik (1884–1971); at the Technical Faculty of Zagreb, guided by Viktor Kovacic and Edo Schön (1877–1949); and at the Academy of Fine Arts, also in Zagreb, conceived by the radically modern Drago Ibler (1894–1964). At the same time, the architectural faculty at the Technical University of Belgrade was strengthened by a generation of professors who faithfully continued academic traditions. The architectural character of the three national capitals of the Kingdom of Serbs, Croats, and Slovenes (Belgrade, Zagreb, and Ljubljana) reflected their different cultural climates and political aspirations. Whereas Belgrade's desire to grow into the capital of a major nation was promoted by the forms of "late academicism" and the architectural face of Ljubljana was changed with enthusiasm to demonstrate Slo-

vene national character, Zagreb became the only strong center of the architectural avant-garde of that time.

Different methods of dealing with historical vocabulary dominated the architectural production of Yugoslavia during the interwar period. In addition to Belgrade, where academic historicism determined the architectural scene during the 1920s and resulted in noteworthy projects, such as those by Nikola Nestorovic (1868–1957), including the University Library (1919–26, with Dragutin Djordjevic) and the Technical Faculty (1925–31, with Branko Tanazevic), the eclectic method was also employed by architects from the other regions. The Mortgage Bank (1923) in Zagreb, designed by one of the most remarkable Croatian modernists, Hugo Ehrlich (1879–1936), who became well known as Adolf Loos's collaborator on the Villa Karma, on Lake Geneva, confirms that the strict line between the eclecticist and the modernist cannot be drawn. For the academic tradition, the writings of Belgrade architect Milutin Borisavljevic (Miloutine Borissavliévitch, 1889–1970) were the only theoretical statements from interwar Yugoslavia to receive a world reputation.

The Wagnerschule associates, Joze Plecnik and Viktor Kovacic, originated recognizable modes of modern expression without denying historical references. Plecnik's achievements in Ljubljana, Zale Cemetery (1939–40) and the National University Library (1936–40), as well as Kovacic's works in Zagreb, among them his masterpiece, the Stock Exchange (1922–27), can be considered distinguished examples of European modernism in general.

A specific modern idiom of treating the past through the transformation of folk motifs—a National Romantic variant of the Art Deco—arose in Yugoslav regions, as among the majority of "small" European nations, from an attempt to create a unique national style. A colorful facade of the Trade Union Bank (1922) in Ljubljana, decorated with painted motifs reminiscent of peasant fabrics, informs Ivan Vurnik's vivid approach of generating a Slovene national style. In Serbia, an established agenda of shaping a national style found its passionate devotee in Momir Korunovic (1883–1969). His most famous buildings, Post Office No. 2 (1927–28) and the Postal Ministry (1927–30), demonstrate his method of mixing motifs from folk art with elements from Serbian medieval architecture.

Zagreb was the only Yugoslav center to accept the avant-garde ideas of European functionalism. Most of the leading Croatian architects of the time were either educated in the avant-garde European schools or worked with some of the most famous European architects: Loos, Behrens, Poelzig, and Le Corbusier. Peter Behrens's involvement with the reconstruction of the Elsafluid Building in 1927 had a special impact on Zagreb's architectural scene. Two architectural groups, Zemlja and Radna Grupa Zagreb (RGZ), became leading generators of the new climate, working both on new, radical designs and on architectural publications and exhibitions. The members of RGZ took an active role in CIAM (Congrès Internationaux d'Architecture Moderne) of 1933 in Athens, opposing, with their own proposals, the charter advanced by Le Corbusier.

One of the rare examples of Belgrade functionalism is the Union Bank (1929–30), the masterpiece of Croatian architect Hugo Ehrlich. In contrast to the "monumental modernism" of the 1930s, which was gladly received by Serbian architects, functionalism found only a few followers: Djordje Tabakovic (1897–1971) in Novi Sad; Nikola Dobrovic (1897–1967), who

built mainly outside Serbia; and Milan Zlokovic (1898–1965), whose University Children's Clinic (1933–40) in Belgrade is the main avant-garde accomplishment. Works of Dragisa Brasovan (1887–1965), among them the Government Building (1930–39) of the Danube Region in Novi Sad and the Air Force Headquarters (1935, damaged in the NATO bombing of 1999) in Zemun, offer key examples of the monumental Modern idiom, created through a refined juxtaposition of Expressionism and "purified" Neoclassicism. The Albania Palace (1938–40) in Belgrade, designed by a team of architects from Zagreb and Belgrade, and especially the Yugoslavian Pavilion at the Paris International Exhibition of 1937, by Croatian architect Josip Seissel (1904–87), are outstanding examples of this "monumental manner."

After World War II, the political system in Yugoslavia was radically changed. First associated with the politics of the Eastern bloc, "Tito's socialism" shifted its course, breaking with Stalinist politics. Because of the immense loans taken from the West from the 1950s until the late 1970s, the potential for a high standard of architectural productions was better than in other Eastern European countries. Being socialistic in content and capitalistic in form, Yugoslavian architecture of the post–World War II period dealt with a series of "socialistic" programs, such as collective housing, community centers, houses of culture, and partisan memorials (best represented through the work of Bogdan Bogdanovic), trying to keep abreast with current architectural trends in Western Europe. The urban planning associated with the controlled economy found its best expression in radical plans for new city districts, among which the one for New Belgrade was the most ambitious.

One of the rare examples of designs from the late 1940s, when Soviet models were still recommended, is the Federal Executive Government Building (1947–61) in Belgrade, begun according to a project by a group of architects from Zagreb, although its "Eastern" monumental features modified into the International Style during the construction as a result of the political shift. During the 1950s and early 1960s, the International Style dominated architectural production. Le Corbusier's vocabulary occurred in works of his assistants, Juraj Neidhardt from Sarajevo and the Slovene Edvard Ravnikar, but emerged more obviously in Milorad Macura's Military Printing House (1953) in Belgrade and Drago Galic's Apartment Block (1953–56) in Zagreb. The "constructional aesthetic" of Pier Luigi Nervi found its reinterpretations in Vladimir Turina's Dinamo Stadium (1954) in Zagreb as well as in Milorad Pantovic's new Belgrade Fair (1956–57). A new, more individualistic and expressive trend of the international architecture appeared at the very end of the 1950s with Vjenceslav Richter's Pavilion for Expo '58 in Brussels, Nikola Dobrovic's Secretariat of National Defense (1957–63, severely damaged in the NATO bombing of 1999), and Ivan Antic's Museum of Contemporary Art (1960–65, with Ivanka Raspopovic), the latter two in Belgrade. The most striking architectural events in Yugoslavia of the time were the last meeting of CIAM, held in Dubrovnik in 1956, and Kenzo Tange's engagement with the reconstruction of the Macedonian capital, Skopje, after the earthquake of 1963.

Yugoslav architects accepted the diversity of the late 1960s and 1970s following the manners of Brutalism, late modern Expressionism, structuralism, regionalism, High-Tech, and so on. Different Brutalist expressions can be summarized through

a couple of remarkable examples, such as those in Skopje after the earthquake, including Alfred Roth's Elementary School (1967), Janko Konstantinov's Telecommunication Center (1971–74), and Marko Music's University Complex (1974), as well as through others, in smaller Yugoslavian cities, including Svetlana Radevic's Hotel Podgorica (1965–67) in the Montenegrin capital of Podgorica, Milan Sosteric's Bakery (1971) in Makarska, Mladen Vodicka's City Library (1976) in Karlovac, and the Military High School (1975) in Ljubljana, designed by the group Studio 7. Application of the High-Tech vocabulary found its best interpretations in Stojan Maksimovic's Center Sava (1977–79) in Belgrade, Milan Mihelic's Telephone Exchange (1978) in Ljubljana, Boris Magas's Stadium Poljud (1979) in Split, and Stanko Kristl's City Hospital (1979) in Izola. Designs of Bosnian architect Zlatko Ugljen include the National Theater (1978, with Jahiel Finci) in Zenica, Hotel Ruza (1978) in Mostar, and the White Mosque (1980) in Visoko, for which he received the Aga Khan Award of 1983 and which represents one the most respected works of the time.

Various Postmodern modes of the late 1970s and 1980s were welcome among architects of different generations. The leading designs of the new wave, related to the trends introduced by Aldo Rossi, Richard Meier, James Stirling, and the Berlin IBA, are associated with the names of Milos Bonca, the group Kras, Penezic and Rogina, Branko Siladjin, and Petar Vulovic. As a consequence of the civil war and the breakup of the country in the last decade of the 20th century, a possible summary of Yugoslavian architecture of the 1990s includes more examples of destruction than of construction.

TANJA DAMLJANOVIC

Further Reading

With the exception of the post–World War II period, general surveys of the architecture of Yugoslavia hardly exist. Architectural monographs dealing with the most influential figures from specific former-Yugoslav regions serve as the best point of departure.

Kultermann, Udo, *Zeitgenössische Architektur in Osteuropa*, Cologne: DuMont Buchverlag, 1985

Mambriani, Alberto, *L'architettura moderna nei Paesi Balcanici*, Bologna: Cappelli Editore, 1969

Manevic, Zoran, et al., *Arhitektura XX vijeka* (Architecture of the 20th Century), Belgrade: Prosveta, 1986

Music, Marjan, "The Architecture of the Twentieth Century," in *Art Treasures of Yugoslavia*, edited by Oto Bihalji-Merin, New York: Abrams, 1969

Straus, Ivan, *Arhitektura Jugoslavije, 1945–1990* [Architecture in Yugoslavia, 1945–1990], Sarajevo: Svjetlost, 1991

Z

ZEVI, BRUNO 1918–2000

Architectural historian, Italy

Bruno Zevi's formation as Italy's foremost architectural historian in the immediate postwar period is closely linked with his early political activity. Born into a distinguished Jewish family, Zevi studied at the Faculty of Architecture in Rome before the introduction of the Fascist racial laws induced him to move to London. Zevi then left Europe for the United States, studying at Columbia University in New York and Harvard University's Graduate School of Design, then under the directorship of Walter Gropius, earning a bachelor's degree in 1942.

A significant amount of Zevi's time abroad was spent in antiFascist activities, such as radio transmissions and the publication in Boston of the Carlo Rosselli–inspired *Quaderni italiani* (Italian Notebooks). The network of contacts he developed on such occasions brought him in touch with some influential Italian intellectuals, notably the art historians Carlo Ludovico Ragghianti and Lionello Venturi; hence the openness of Zevi's cultural background and some of the peculiarities of his later intellectual engagement.

After returning to Rome in 1944, Zevi became critically engaged in a cultural battle for a renewal of Italian architecture. *Towards an Organic Architecture*, his first book, was published in 1945. The title echoed Le Corbusier's *Vers Une Architecture*, but the additional adjective, "organic," hinted at the need to enrich the functionalist theories on which the many branches of European architectural research in the 1920s and 1930s had been based. The book was essentially a comparison of two worlds: Europe and the United States. In both, Zevi argued, recent developments in modern architecture had paved the way for a "humanisation" of the new language, a general tendency best illustrated by the domestic buildings of Frank Lloyd Wright and the work of Alvar Aalto and other Scandinavian architects. Italy was implicitly invited to follow the same route, and in 1945 Zevi founded the Association for Organic Architecture (APAO). For a time the association's local branches were a focal point for some of the architects who hoped to play a leading role in the country's reconstruction.

Three years later his *How to Look at Architecture* was the result of a more ambitious approach that reflected Zevi's familiarity with Benedetto Croce's writing on aesthetics and his growing interest in the Vienna School of art history. Despite the long discussions about the peculiarities of architecture compared with other forms of artistic expression, the book was mainly a reflection on the purpose and methodology of architectural history. Zevi showed how the tools of modern architectural criticism (in particular a notion of "space" partly inspired by an analysis of Wright's buildings) could serve as the basis for a new approach to the whole history of Western architecture. In his view, the gap that existed between modern architectural design and academic architectural history needed to be bridged to forge a link between the study of classical and medieval buildings and the daily battle for a better built world.

In line with this principle, in 1948 Zevi began to teach architectural history at the universities in Venice (1948–63) and Rome (1948–51, 1963–79) and became more actively involved in the daily debates in the Italian architectural press. His ponderous *History of Modern Architecture*, originally published in 1950 as a completely rewritten version of his 1945 book, still stands as his most important work as a historian. It was the first comprehensive historical narrative about the origins and the development of the Modern movement to be published in Italy and one of the most original and sympathetic European studies on the subject to appear in the postwar period. Substantially revised in 1975 and 1996, the book was crucial in deciding the fortunes of architectural history as a discipline in the Italian academic world, a secondary effect well documented by the biographies of scholars such as Leonardo Benevolo and Manfredo Tafuri.

The core themes of *History* are still central to most of Zevi's subsequent studies, such as the ones on De Stijl architecture (1953) and Erich Mendelsohn (1970). Other essays from the 1950s and 1960s further extended the chronological boundaries of his research, focusing on a group of Renaissance architects, including Ferrara's "planner" Biagio Rossetti (1960) and Michelangelo Buonarroti. However, Zevi's prescriptive, operational approach to history increasingly began to show its limitations. His original sensitivity toward the visual analysis of buildings became constricted within an oversimplified, barely evolving conceptual framework based on a handful of binary opposites: classicism versus anticlassicism, symmetry versus asymmetry, spatial (and political) freedom versus dictatorship. It is therefore not surprising that Zevi's most acclaimed and challenging book after *History* was not a historical one but rather an essay about

the methodology of architectural design: the brilliant *The Modern Language of Architecture*, published in 1973.

After Zevi's involvement with the Partito d'Azione (Party of Action) between 1944 and 1947, he still occasionally became involved in politics and was elected to Parliament as a member of the Radical Party in 1987. In the late 1990s, renewed interest in his work gave him the opportunity to become editor of a second series of architectural studies (Turin: Testo e Immagine, 1996–), following the one he had edited for Dedalo Editions (73 titles between 1978 and 1985). He also worked on a few historical overviews, the last of which was published in 1998 with the title *Counterhistory and History of Architecture*.

FILIPPO DE PIERI

See also **Fascist Architecture; Tafuri, Manfredo (Italy); Wright, Frank Lloyd (United States)**

Biography

Born in Rome, 22 January 1918. Studied at Faculty of Architecture, Rome, 1936–39; Architectural Association's School of Architecture, London, 1939; Columbia University, New York City, 1939–40; Harvard University, Cambridge, Massachusetts, 1940–42. Married Tullia Calabi, 1940. Moved to London, 1943–44; worked for the Office of Chief Engineer of the European Headquarters of the U.S. Army (February–July 1944). Returned to Rome, July 1944. Worked for the United States Information Service (USIS), 1945–46; founded the Associazione per l'architettura organica (APAO), 1945–50. Co-editor of the review *Metron*, 1945–55. Professional partnership with the architects Luigi Piccinato, Enrico Tedeschi, Cino Calcaprina, Silvio Radiconcini, 1946. Taught at the Faculty of Architecture in Venice, 1948–63. General Secretary of the Istituto Nazionale di Urbanistica (INU), 1951–69. Editor of the review *L'architettura-cronache e storia* (1955–2000); architectural critic of the magazine *L'Espresso* (1955–2000). Professional partnership with Errico Ascione and Vittorio Gigliotti, 1961. Taught architectural history at the Faculty of Architecture in Rome, 1963–79 (resignation). Honorary Fellow of the American Institute of Architects (1968); president of the Comité International des Critiques d'Architecture (CICA), 1978–. Editor of the series Universale di Architettura, Bari: Dedalo Libri (1978–85). Elected to the Chamber of Deputies in the ranks of the Radical Party, 1987. Degree *honoris causa*, Technion, Haifa, Israel, 1990. Honorary Fellow of the Royal Architectural Institute of Canada, 1990. Died in Rome, 9 January 2000.

Selected Publications

Verso un'architettura organica. Saggio sullo sviluppo del pensiero architettonico negli ultimi cinquant'anni, Turin: Einaudi, 1945; published as *Towards an Organic Architecture*, London: Faber and Faber, 1950

Frank Lloyd Wright, Milan: Il Balcone, 1947; expanded edition, 1955

Saper vedere l'architettura. Saggio sull'interpretazione spaziale dell'architettura, Turin: Einaudi, 1948; republished as *Architecture as Space. How to Look at Architecture*, translated by Milton Gendel, New York: Horizon Press, 1957; 3rd edition, New York: Da Capo Press, 1993

Erik Gunnar Asplund, Milan: Il Balcone, 1948

Architettura e storiografia. Le matrici antiche del linguaggio moderno, Milan: Politecnica Tamburini, 1950; expanded edition, Turin: Einaudi, 1974; reprinted in *Leggere, scrivere, parlare architettura*, Venice: Marsilio, 1997

"Frank Lloyd Wright and the Conquest of Space," *Magazine of Art* (May 1950)

Storia dell'architettura moderna, Turin: Einaudi, 1950; 5th edition, revised and expanded, Turin: Einaudi, 1975; 10th edition, revised and expanded, 2 vols., Turin: Einaudi, 1996

Poetica dell'architettura neoplastica. Il linguaggio della scomposizione quadridimensionale, Milan: Tamburini, 1953; revised and expanded edition, Turin: Einaudi, 1974; reprinted in *Leggere, scrivere, parlare architettura*, Venice: Marsilio, 1997

Richard Neutra, Milan: Il Balcone, 1954

"Architettura," in *Enciclopedia universale dell'arte*, volume I, 1958; revised and expanded edition, *Architectura in nuce*, Venice and Rome: Istituto per la Collaborazione Culturale, 1960

Biagio Rossetti, architetto ferrarese. Il primo urbanista moderno europeo, Turin: Einaudi, 1960; reissued as *Saper vedere l'urbanistica. Ferrara di Biagio Rossetti, la prima città moderna europea*, Turin: Einaudi, 1971 and 1997

Michelangiolo architetto (exhib. cat.), with contributions by Giulio Carlo Argan, Franco Barbieri, Lionello Puppi, Paolo Portoghesi, and Bruno Zevi, Turin: Einaudi, 1964

"History as a Method of Teaching Architecture," in *The History, Theory and Criticism of Architecture*, edited by Marcus Whiffen, papers from the 1964 AIA-ACSA Teacher Seminar (Cranbrook), Cambridge, Massachusetts: MIT Press, 1965

Erich Mendelsohn, opera completa. Architettura e immagini architettoniche, Milan: Etas Kompass, 1970; Turin: Testo e Immagine, 1997

Cronache di architettura, 24 vols., Bari: Laterza, 1970–75, 1978–81

Il linguaggio moderno dell'architettura. Guida al codice anticlassico, Turin: Einaudi, 1973; reprinted in *Leggere, scrivere, parlare architettura*, Venice: Marsilio, 1997; republished as *The Modern Language of Architecture*, Seattle: University of Washington Press, 1978; New York, Van Nostrand Reinhold, 1981

Zevi su Zevi, Milan: Magma, 1977; Venice: Marsilio, 1993

Frank Lloyd Wright, Bologna: Zanichelli, 1979

Giuseppe Terragni, Bologna: Zanichelli, 1980

Linguaggi dell'architettura contemporanea, Milan: Etas Libri, 1993

Storia e controstoria dell'architettura in Italia, 3 vols., Rome: Newton Compton, 1997

Controstoria e storia dell'architettura, 3 vols., Rome: Newton Compton, 1998

Further Reading

"Architectural Criticism after Zevi," *Zodiac*, (1999), essays by Carlo Olmo, Jean-Louis Cohen, Ignasi de Solà-Morales, Stanislaus von Moos, and others

Fullaondo, Juan Daniel, and Muñoz, Maria Teresa, *Zevi*, Madrid: Kain, 1992

Oppenheimer Dean, Andrea, *Bruno Zevi on Modern Architecture*, New York: Rizzoli, 1983

Pigafetta, Giorgio, *Architettura moderna e ragione storica: La storiografia italiana sull'architettura moderna, 1928–1976*, Milan: Guerini, 1993

Tafuri, Manfredo, *Theories and History of Architecture*, New York: Harper and Row, 1979 (originally published as *Teorie e storia dell'architettura*, Bari: Laterza, 1968)

Tournikiotis, Panayotis, *The Historiography of Modern Architecture*, Cambridge, Massachusetts, and London: MIT Press, 1999

ZONNESTRAAL SANATORIUM 1926–31

Hilversum, Netherlands

Thought to be a symbol of the solidarity of the Dutch working-class movement at the turn of the century, the Zonnestraal Sana-

torium in Hilversum is considered one of the most complex and influential buildings of its time. Deemed one of the major works by its designer, Johannes (Jan) Duiker (1890–1935), the Sanatorium has long been associated with the Modern architectural movement in the Netherlands.

An independent and innovative architect, Duiker studied at Delft University of Technology with Bernhard Bijvoet (1889–1979), with whom he later became partners. Together they worked in the office of their former professor, Henri Evers, architect of the Rotterdam City Hall. Much of Duiker's early influence can be attributed to Evers, Hendrik Petrus Berlage and the Amsterdam School, and the American architect Frank Lloyd Wright. Duiker garnered later influence from the developing International Style and the Nieuwe Bouwen movement while employing new building materials and methods in the integration of architecture and science. It is believed that Duiker was also somewhat influenced by the De Stijl movement; however, he was more a proponent of the "nonaesthetic" Modern architecture and not the movement's "decorative facade architecture," feeling that it only concealed inferior floor plans. As a result, he became the movement's principal antagonist, further illustrated by his lack of exposure in their periodical, choosing rather to subscribe to the philosophies of the functionalist De 8, later known as the De 8 and Opbouw group.

Choosing functionality over aesthetic appearances, Duiker produced his own functionalist idiom, which became stronger and more expressive as his design philosophy developed. His quest for an ideal structural form created a dichotomy between simplistic and complex avant-garde architecture that was influential enough to have inspired Ludwig Mies van der Rohe's Tuberculosis Sanatorium (1929–33) at Paimio, Finland. Duiker's unfortunate early death at the age of 45 meant that his design repertoire was not as extensive as that of his peers. This and the demolition of much of what he did design are perhaps the reasons for his apparent international obscurity. As a result, his remaining architecture has suffered from indifference and neglect.

After winning the competition for elderly housing in Alkmaar (1917), the socially conscious Duiker and Bijvoet desired to improve the quality of lower-income health facility construction. Through associations with Berlage, Duiker and Bijvoet were retained by the Koperen Stelen Fonds (KSF) foundation—a group of diamond workers organized in 1905 whose motto was "renewed vitality"—to design a convalescent facility for their tuberculosis-infected colleagues. Through fund-raising efforts by the foundation and by Delft professor Henri ter Meulen, in 1919 the KSF purchased the Pampahoeve, a country estate west of Hilversum. Designs were temporarily postponed, however, after the diamond industry collapse in 1920.

Duiker, collaborating with structural engineer Jan Gerko Wiebenga, utilized the newest structural technology, creating a cantilever system that produced a buoyant and rhythmically tectonic architecture. Resting on concrete blocks, the skeletal structure of the buildings consists of a three-meter (ten-foot) grid with structural columns every nine meters. Concrete was generously used in the floor slabs and the prefabricated paneled walls that were installed between steel I sections at each floor. Although still in its infancy, reinforced concrete and the prefabricated-concrete building systems played a monumental

role in the development of the Sanatorium as well as the rest of Duiker's architecture.

The Zonnestraal Sanatorium consists of three large buildings: the main building, the Henri ter Meulen Pavilion, and the Dresselhuys Pavilion, along with various smaller outbuildings. The main building was begun in 1928 and was used to house the general facilities of the complex. The functions were grouped together by their practical relationships, dividing the boiler house/bathroom, the kitchen, the medical facility, and the infirmary into four distinct linear sections. The cruciform-shaped upper floor spans three of the four lower buildings, creating a unified mass.

Flanking the main building are two independent pavilions. Also functionally distinct, each consists of a square central form connecting two long wings that flare out at different angles to provide maximum sunlight to the southern-exposed patient rooms and terraces. The Henri ter Meulen Pavilion was constructed in 1928, along with the skeleton of the Dresselhuys Pavilion, completed in 1931. Nowhere in the complex is Duiker's coalescence of structure, form, and space so evident as in the pavilions. Structurally identical to the main building, the rhythmic grid system provides the convalescent living spaces.

Between the years of 1919 and 1932, many outbuildings were constructed as part of the complex. Dormitory huts were built in 1929 for patients who were at the end of their convalescence, allowing them to transition out of the hospital setting. For economic and occupational therapy reasons, the convalescents themselves constructed a number of these buildings. Following the trends of the Amsterdam School, the first eight small utilitarian buildings, constructed in 1919–20, were timber-floored load-bearing brick structures. When construction resumed in 1924, Duiker's conversion to concrete was evident.

Most other buildings went unrealized. The most unusual was the Adamas diamond-polishing works (1928), designed to prepare the healed convalescents for their return to society. Construction, however, went no further than the reinforced-concrete skeleton. Its notable feature was the unusual roof, consisting of alternating asymmetrical sawtooth projections.

Unfortunately, the Sanatorium's insufficiently prepared steel framing and structural members proved unsuitable for the Dutch climate. After World War II, the complex was expanded, but without any regard to Duiker's original design concept. Along with an apparent lack of interest in his architecture, by the 1970s the complex was in serious decline. Recently restored, however, it is now listed as a national monument. The Zonnestraal Sanatorium was the culmination of Duiker and Bijvoet's utopian yet avant-garde design philosophy. By using the latest structural technology, both the architects and the buildings were significantly innovative for their time.

ELISABETH BAKKER-JOHNSON

See also **Amsterdam School; Berlage, Hendrik Petrus; Concrete; De Stijl; Duiker, Johannes; Modernism; Wright, Frank Lloyd**

Further Reading

A fairly comprehensive, albeit brief, history of Duiker and his architectural accomplishments can be found in Molema (1989). More detailed information on the Sanatorium is provided by De Beek, et al. (1996)

and Milelli (1978). Ibelings (1995) and Overy (1991) offer insight into the stylistic developments of the period.

De Beek, Aimée, Sabine Berndsen, and Camiel Berns, *Zeer aangenaam Verblijf: Het Dienstbodenhuis van J. Duiker op Sanatorium Zonnestraal* (A Space of Their Own: The Servants' House by J. Duiker at Zonnestraal Sanatorium), Rotterdam: Uitgeverij 010, 1996

Ibelings, Hans, *20th Century Architecture in the Netherlands*, Rotterdam: Netherlands Architecture Institute, 1995

Milelli, Gabriele, *Zonnestraal, il sanatorio di Hilversum* (Zonnestraal, the Hilversum Sanatorium), Bari: Dedalo Libri, 1978

Molema, Jan, Jan Duiker: Obras y proyectos (Jan Duiker: Works and Projects), Rotterdam: Uitgeverij 010, 1989

Molema, Jan, and Peter Bak, *Jan Gerko Wiebenga: Apostel van het Nieuwe Bouwen* (Jan Gerko Wiebenga: An Apostle of the New Buildings Movement), Rotterdam: Uitgeverij 010, 1987

Overy, Paul, *De Stijl*, New York: Thames and Hudson, 1991

ZUMTHOR, PETER 1943–

Architect, Switzerland

Switzerland today represents one of the most important centers of modern architectural thought and practice, and Peter Zumthor has been among the major architects representing the country since the 1980s. Zumthor presents in his work not only beautiful form and masterly construction but the sensitive control of material and space achieved only by gaining intimate knowledge of all these factors.

Trained as a cabinetmaker, Zumthor studied design instead of architecture at Basel's school of arts and crafts. He has concentrated on adapting the rural form and materials of his headquarters, the Swiss canton of Graubuden, and he has built a small but captivating oeuvre almost exclusively in his adopted home since his arrival there in 1967. Zumthor has said that he "creates spaces with soul" that become part of the everyday and stand in opposition to the "general artificiality of the world" (*Peter Zumthor, Works*, 1998). He argues his case to great effect in all of his projects, including the Sogn Benedegt Chapel, a shingled, leaf-shaped church perched high in the misty Surselva Mountains. A weathered, earthy, and private place, the form is derived from the lemniscate, an algebraic figure-8-shaped curve that when proportionately shortened also determines the section. A delicate band of windows ringing the top of the building ensures steady natural light. The chapel is an artful combination of rationality and poetry existing in an almost dreamlike setting.

The architect's atelier in Haldenstein draws on the contrast between softly finished local wood and brushed steel details to highlight the beauty in each. The humble building, though sited in the middle of town, lends no notion to its purpose. The modern addition to a traditional farmhouse in Versam, Switzerland, is an example of Zumthor's seamless straddling of old and new, tradition and modernization, and his dedication to rooting buildings to the landscape. The architect was able to match almost perfectly the wood of the original building and made a modern addition for a family without interrupting the spirit of the old house.

The much publicized and much photographed thermal baths in Vals revisit the importance and sheer pleasure of bathing known in ancient Roman baths. The entire structure looks almost prehistoric, as if it emerged from the ground, and is constructed entirely of whole slabs of locally quarried, gray gneiss laid one on top of another, to a great monolithic effect. The beauty of the spa is awe-inspiring, as is its perfection in plan and construction. The sensuality of the color, the water, the sounds echoed in the chamber of the bath seem all but mathematically engineered by the architect—a stunning feat matched by few, if any, other of his projects.

If the spa at Vals is all subterranean mystery, then Zumthor's first non-Swiss site, the Kunsthaus in Bregenz, Austria, is all light and transparency. Nestled beside a lake, the glass box of a modern art museum goes from white to blue to glowing yellow during the course of day to night. The light skin of the building allows but a peek into the frame and at the silhouettes of the staircases between galleries. The glass panels of the museum's skin are not perforated and hang on a system of metal brackets held in place by large, modified clamps. Lighting is controlled by the amount of natural light entering the building at any given time through the massive glass skin of the structure. The interior floors and walls of the gallery levels are concrete and uniquely climate controlled by the circulation of water to the gallery floors and walls from an underground stream.

Zumthor's plan for the Swiss Pavilion at the Hannover Expo 2000 was meant to echo a lumberyard in its use of piles of timber in parallel walls and the notion that the lumber will be sold after the close of the exposition. The multidimensional use of the space speaks to all the senses: lines of poetry are projected on the walls, and small troupes of dancers and musicians perform in the space, making it a living, beating organism.

The architect has succeeded by trying the "obvious but difficult solutions" first. Those solutions make architecture the medium it is: construction, materials, earth and sky, structure. He handles each with respect to create structures true to their surroundings, reflective of their culture, and representative of an architect craftsman who blends invention and sensitivity, intuition and intelligence.

EUGENIA BELL

Biography

Peter Zumthor was born in 1943 near Basel, Switzerland. The son of a furniture manufacturer, he was trained as a cabinetmaker. He enrolled at the Pratt Institute in New York as a visiting student in architecture and design in 1966, and opened his own architecture practice in Haldenstein, Graubunden, in 1979. He has taught at the Academy of Architecture in Mendrisio, Switzerland, the University of Zurich, and the Southern California Institute of Architecture.

Selected Publications

Three Concepts: Thermal Bath Vals, Art Museum Bregenz, "Topography of Terror," Berlin: Architekturgale Luzern, and Basel: Birkhauser, 1997

Peter Zumthor, Works: Buildings and Projects, 1979–1997, Basel: Birkhauser, 1998

Thinking Architecture, Basel: Birkhauser, 1998

Therme Vals, Vals, Graubunden, Switzerland, 1990–96

Swiss Pavilion for the Hannover Exposition, Germany, 2000

Further Reading

Zumthor, Peter, Plinio Bachmann, et al., *Soundbodybook*, Basel: Birkhauser, 2000

Notes on Contributors

Adams Annmarie. School of Architecture, McGill University, Montreal, Quebec. Articles contributed to *Encyclopedia of 20th-Century Architecture*: Hospital.

Adams, Nicholas. Department of Art, Vassar College, New York. Articles contributed to *Encyclopedia of 20th-Century Architecture*: Elevator; Erskine, Ralph (England); Grand Central Station, New York; Museum of Modern Art, New York; Stockholm Public Library; Stockholm, Sweden; Tafuri, manfredo (Italy).

Adams, Rick. Columbia University, New York. Articles contributed to *Encyclopedia of 20th-Century Architecture*: Campus Planning; Regional Planning; Roadway Systems; Transportation Planning.

Addington, Michelle D. Faculty of Architecture, Harvard University. Articles contributed to *Encyclopedia of 20th-Century Architecture*: Heating, Ventilation, and Air Conditioning (HVAC).

Al-Hathloul, Saleh. Independent scholar, Riyadh, Saudi Arabia. Articles contributed to *Encyclopedia of 20th-Century Architecture*: Riyadh, Saudi Arabia; Saudi Arabia.

Amundson, Jennifer A. Department of Architecture, Judson College. Articles contributed to *Encyclopedia of 20th-Century Architecture*: Burnham, Daniel H. (United States); Classicism; Demolition; Glass Skyscraper (1920–21); Hilberseimer, Ludwig (United States and Germany); Wanamaker Store, Philadelphia.

Archer, John. Department of Cultural Studies, University of Minnesota, Minneapolis. Articles contributed to *Encyclopedia of 20th-Century Architecture*: Suburban Planning.

Ashraf, Kazi. Department of Architecture, University of Hawaii at Manoa. Articles contributed to *Encyclopedia of 20th-Century Architecture*: Dhaka, Bangladesh; Islam, Muzharul (Bangladesh).

Atti, Stefania. Independent scholar, Ferrara, Italy. Articles contributed to *Encyclopedia of 20th-Century Architecture*: Lisbon, Portugal; Távora, Fernando (Portugal).

Bakker-Johnson, Elizabeth. Independent scholar, New York. Articles contributed to *Encyclopedia of 20th-Century Architecture*: Dudok, Willem Marinus (Netherlands); Eigen Haard Housing Estate, Amsterdam; Hilversum Town Hall, Netherlands; Open-Air School, Amsterdam; Zonnestraal Sanatorium, Hilversum.

Balmer, Jeffrey. Department of Architecture, Iowa State University, Ames. Articles contributed to *Encyclopedia of 20th-Century Architecture*: Toronto City Hall; Toronto (Ontario), Canada.

Bassnett, Sarah C. Binghamton University, New York. Articles contributed to *Encyclopedia of 20th-Century Architecture*: Eames, Charles and Ray (United States); Institutes/Associations.

Bednar, Michael. School of Architecture, University of Virginia, Charlottesville. Articles contributed to *Encyclopedia of 20th-Century Architecture*: National Gallery of Art, East Building, Washington, DC; Plaza; Washington (DC) United States.

Bell, Eugenia. Bell & Weiland Publishers, New York. Articles contributed to *Encyclopedia of 20th-Century Architecture*: Calatrava, Santiago (Spain); Chapel of Notre-Dame-du-Haut, Ronchamp, France; Diener and Diener (Switzerland); Fagus Werk, Alfeld Germany; Unite d'Habitation, Marseilles Cité Radieuse; Zumthor, Peter (Switzerland).

Bellamy, Rhoda. Nova Arcadia Heritage, Ontario, Canada. Articles contributed to *Encyclopedia of 20th-Century Architecture*: Aga Khan Award (1977–); Arquitectonica (United States); Canada; Revell, Viljo (Finland); Vancouver (BC), Canada.

Bernardi, Jose. School of Design, Arizona State University, Tempe. Articles contributed to *Encyclopedia of 20th-Century Architecture*: Alvarez, Mario Roberto (Argentina); Argentina; Buenos Aires, Argentina; Chile; Dieste, Eladio (Uruguay); Kalach, Alberto (Mexico); Manteola, Sánchez Gómez, Santos, Solsona, Viñoly (Argentina); Soleri, Paolo (United States); Williams, Amancio (Argentina).

Bhatt, Vikram. School of Architecture, McGill University, Montreal. Articles contributed to *Encyclopedia of 20th-Century Architecture*: Ahmedabad, India; Doshi, Balkrishna (India).

Black, Brian. Pennsylvania State University, Altoona. Articles contributed to *Encyclopedia of 20th-Century Architecture*: Agricultural Buildings; Automobile; Restaurant; Stadium.

Blessing, Benita Carol. Articles contributed to *Encyclopedia of 20th-Century Architecture*: Cologne, Germany; Ungers, Oswald Mathias (Germany).

Bliznakov, Milka T. College of Architecture and Urban Studies, Virginia Polytechnic Institute and State University. Articles contributed to *Encyclopedia of 20th-Century Architecture*: Ginzburg, Moisei (Russia); Torre, Susana (United States).

Bosley, Edward. School of Architecture, University of Southern California. Articles contributed to *Encyclopedia of 20th-Century Architecture*: Greene, Henry M. and Charles S. (United States).

Boyle, Bernard. School of Architecture and Humanities, Arizona State University, Tempe. Articles contributed to *Encyclopedia of 20th-Century Architecture*: Brutalism.

Bozdogan, Sibel. Massachusetts Institute of Technology. Articles contributed to *Encyclopedia of 20th-Century Architecture*: Eldem, Sedad Hakki (Turkey).

Bradley, Betsy. Case Western Reserve University, Cleveland, Ohio. Articles contributed to *Encyclopedia of 20th-Century Architecture*: Warehouse/Storage Facility.

Brakensiek, Stephan. Independent scholar, Dortmund, Germany. Articles contributed to *Encyclopedia of 20th-Century Architecture*: Poelzig, Hans (Germany); Stuttgart, Germany.

Bretler, Marc Itamar. Independent scholar, Lausanne, Switzerland. Articles contributed to *Encyclopedia of 20th-Century Architecture*: Mallet-Stevens, Robert (France).

Brumfield, William C. German and Slavic Department, Tulane University, New Orleans, Louisiana. Articles contributed to *Encyclopedia of 20th-Century Architecture*: Constructivism; Golosov, Ilya (Russia); Moscow, Russia; Russia/Soviet Union; Shekhtel, Fedor (Russia); St. Petersburg, Russia; Vesnin, Alexander, Leonid, and Viktor (Russia).

Buelinckx, Hendrika. College of Architecture, Texas Technical University. Articles contributed to *Encyclopedia of 20th-Century Architecture*: Belgium; Brussels, Belgium.

Bunk, Brian. Independent scholar, Northampton, Massachusetts. Articles contributed to *Encyclopedia of 20th-Century Architecture*: Puig i Cadafalch, Josep (Catalan); Studio Per (Spain).

Buntrock, Dana. Department of Architecture, University of California, Berkeley. Articles contributed to *Encyclopedia of 20th-Century Architecture*: Church on the Water, Hokkaido, Japan; Hasegawa Itsuko (Japan); Ito, Toyo (Japan); Metabolists; Metropolitan Festival Hall, Tokyo; Peace Memorial and Museum, Hiroshima; Sejima, Kazuyo (Japan); Tange, Kenzo (Japan); Taniguchi, Yoshio (Japan).

Burns, Carol. Taylor MacDougall Burns Architects, Boston, Massachusetts. Articles contributed to *Encyclopedia of 20th-Century Architecture*: Mobile Home.

Busbea, Larry. Independent scholar, New York. Articles contributed to *Encyclopedia of 20th-Century Architecture*: Grande Arche de La Défense, Paris; Structuralism.

Campbell, Douglas G. Department of Fine Arts, George Fox University, Oregon. Articles contributed to *Encyclopedia of 20th-Century Architecture*: Portland Public Services Building, Portland, Oregon; Saarinen, Eliel (Finland).

Carr, Angela. Department of Art History, Carleton University, Ottawa, Ontario. Articles contributed to *Encyclopedia of 20th-Century Architecture*: Church; Department Store.

Carranza, Luis E. School of Architecture, Rogers William University, Rhode Island. Articles contributed to *Encyclopedia of 20th-Century Architecture*: Norten, Enrique (Mexico); O'Gorman, Juan (Mexico).

Carso, Kerry Dean. Boston University. Articles contributed to *Encyclopedia of 20th-Century Architecture*: Boston (MA), United States.

Carter, Brian. School of Architecture, University of Michigan. Articles contributed to *Encyclopedia of 20th-Century Architecture*: Arup, Ove (England); Boots Factory, Nottingham, England; Patkau, Patricia and John (Canada); Roche, Kevin, and John Dinkeloo (United States); Williams, Tod, and Billie Tsien (United States).

Castriota, Leonardo. School of Architecture, Federal University of Minas Gerais. Articles contributed to *Encyclopedia of 20th-Century Architecture*: Levi, Rino (Brazil); Poststructuralism.

Castro, Ricardo. School of Architecture, McGill University, Montreal. Articles contributed to *Encyclopedia of 20th-Century Architecture*: Lewerentz, Sigurd (Sweden); Plecnik, Joze (Yugoslavia); Salmona, Rogelio (Colombia).

Cava, John M. Department of Architecture, University of Oregon. Articles contributed to *Encyclopedia of 20th-Century Architecture*: Hodgetts and Fung; Tectonics.

Chalana, Manish. College of Architecture and Planning, Univeristy of Colorado. Articles contributed to *Encyclopedia of 20th-Century Architecture*: Greenbelts and Greenbelt Towns; New Delhi, India.

Chapman, Michael. Department of Architecture, University of Newcastle, New South Wales, Australia. Articles contributed to *Encyclopedia of 20th-Century Architecture*: Abraham, Raimund (Austria and United States); Bank of London and South America, Buenos Aires; Brasília, Brazil; Palace of the Soviets Competition (1931); Shanghai World Financial Center, Shanghai.

Chappell, Sally A. Kitt. Independent scholar, Chicago, Illinois. Articles contributed to *Encyclopedia of 20th-Century Architecture*: Graham, Anderson, Probst, and White (United States).

Chasin, Noah. Independent scholar, New York. Articles contributed to *Encyclopedia of 20th-Century Architecture*: Eyck, Aldo Van (The Netherlands); Hertzberger, Herman (Netherlands); Malagueira Quarter, Évora, Portugal; Von Moos, Stanislaus (Switzerland).

Chattopadhyay, Swati. History of Art and Architecture, University of California, Santa Barbara. Articles contributed to *Encyclopedia of 20th-Century Architecture*: Correa, Charles Mark (India); India; Plan of New Delhi.

Cheng, Renee. College of Architecture and Landscape Architecture, University of Minnesota. Articles contributed to *Encyclopedia of 20th-Century Architecture*: Gehry, Frank (United States); Guggenheim Museum, Bilbao; Petronas Towers, Kuala Lumpur; Reichstag, Berlin.

Cody, Jeffrey. Department of Architecture, Chinese University of Hong Kong. Articles contributed to *Encyclopedia of 20th-Century Architecture*: HONGKONG AND SHANGHAI BANK, SHANGHAI; LU YANZHI (CHINA).

Collins, Christiane Crasemann. Independent scholar, West Falmouth, Massachusetts. Articles contributed to *Encyclopedia of 20th-Century Architecture*: HEGEMANN, WERNER (GERMANY).

Constant, Caroline. Taubman College of Architecture + Urban Design, University of Michigan. Articles contributed to *Encyclopedia of 20th-Century Architecture*: GRAY, EILEEN (IRELAND AND FRANCE).

Cormier, Leslie Humm. Faculty, Department of Visual and Media Arts, Emerson College, Boston, Massachusetts. Articles contributed to *Encyclopedia of 20th-Century Architecture*: BREUER, MARCEL (UNITED STATES); GROPIUS, WALTER (GERMANY); INTERNATIONAL STYLE; LINCOLN CENTER, NEW YORK; MUSEUM; NEW YORK (NY), UNITED STATES; SEAGRAM BUILDING, NEW YORK; SERT, JOSEP LLUÍS (UNITED STATES); URBAN PLANNING.

Craig, Robert M. College of Architecture, Georgia Institute of Technology. Articles contributed to *Encyclopedia of 20th-Century Architecture*: ART DECO; MAYBECK, BERNARD R. (UNITED STATES); MORGAN, JULIA (UNITED STATES); PORTMAN, JOHN C. (UNITED STATES); STICKLEY, GUSTAV (UNITED STATES).

Crosnier Leconte, Marie-Laure. Independent scholar, Levallois, France. Articles contributed to *Encyclopedia of 20th-Century Architecture*: GUADET, JULIEN (FRANCE).

Dagenhart, Richard. College of Architecture, Georgia Institute of Technology. Articles contributed to *Encyclopedia of 20th-Century Architecture*: DE KLERK, MICHEL (NETHERLANDS); KOOLHAAS, REM (NETHERLANDS).

Dalvesco, Rebecca. School of Design, Arizona State University. Articles contributed to *Encyclopedia of 20th-Century Architecture*: ARCOSANTI, ARIZONA; FULLER, RICHARD BUCKMINSTER (UNITED STATES); GLACIER MUSEUM, FJAERLAND FJORD, NORWAY; NORWAY; SAFDIE, MOSHE (CANADA, ISRAEL).

Damljanovic, Tanja. Independent scholar, Belgrade, Serbia, and Montenegro. Articles contributed to *Encyclopedia of 20th-Century Architecture*: YUGOSLAVIA.

Daniel, Ronn. School of Art and Art History, James Madison University, Harrisonburg, Virginia. Articles contributed to *Encyclopedia of 20th-Century Architecture*: BANHAM, REYNER (UNITED STATES); PARKING GARAGE; SHRINE OF THE BOOK, JERUSALEM.

Dargavel, Richard. Manchester Metropolitan University, Manchester, England. Articles contributed to *Encyclopedia of 20th-Century Architecture*: FEHN, SVERRE (NORWAY).

Davidson, Lisa. Historian, National Park Service Washington, D.C. Articles contributed to *Encyclopedia of 20th-Century Architecture*: APARTMENT BUILDING; HOTEL; RESORT HOTEL.

Davis, Timothy. National Park Service Washington, D.C. Articles contributed to *Encyclopedia of 20th-Century Architecture*: PARKWAYS.

De Pieri, Filippo. Department of Architecture, Politecnico di Torino, Italy. Articles contributed to *Encyclopedia of 20th-Century Architecture*: ZEVI, BRUNO (ITALY).

Desmond, John Michael. Department of Architecture, Louisiana State University. Articles contributed to *Encyclopedia of 20th-Century Architecture*: JOHNSON WAX BUILDING, RACINE, WISCONSIN; TALIESIN WEST, NEAR PHOENIX, ARIZONA.

Diniz Moreira, Fernando. Department of Fine Arts, University of Pennsylvania. Articles contributed to *Encyclopedia of 20th-Century Architecture*: FEDERAL CAPITAL COMPLEX, BRASÍLIA.

Draper, Joan E. College of Architecture and Planning, University of Colorado, Boulder. Articles contributed to *Encyclopedia of 20th-Century Architecture*: CHICAGO (ILLINOIS), UNITED STATES.

Dreller, Sarah M. Independent scholar, San Francisco. Articles contributed to *Encyclopedia of 20th-Century Architecture*: ARCHITECTURAL PHOTOGRAPHY.

Drew, Philip. Author, New South Wales, Australia. Articles contributed to *Encyclopedia of 20th-Century Architecture*: AIRPORT AND AVIATION BUILDING; NORBERG-SCHULZ, CHRISTIAN (NORWAY); OTTO, FREI (GERMANY); SIREN, HEIKKI AND KAIJA (FINLAND); SYDNEY, AUSTRALIA; SYDNEY OPERA HOUSE; TENSIONED MEMBRANE STRUCTURE; TENT; UTZON, JØRN (DENMARK).

Dunham-Jones, Ellen. School of Architecture, Massachusetts Institute of Technology. Articles contributed to *Encyclopedia of 20th-Century Architecture*: EDGE CITY; SEASIDE, FLORIDA.

Eaton, Leonard K. Author. Articles contributed to *Encyclopedia of 20th-Century Architecture*: BIRKERTS, GUNNAR (UNITED STATES); PRAIRIE SCHOOL; PURCELL, WILLIAM GRAY, AND GEORGE GRANT ELMSLIE (UNITED STATES).

Eckert, Kathryn B. Author. Articles contributed to *Encyclopedia of 20th-Century Architecture*: CRANBROOK, MICHIGAN.

Edwards, Clive. School of Art and Design, Loughborough University, Leicestershire, England. Articles contributed to *Encyclopedia of 20th-Century Architecture*: ALUMINUM.

Eggener, Keith L. Department of Art History and Archaeology, University of Missouri, Columbia. Articles contributed to *Encyclopedia of 20th-Century Architecture*: BARRAGÁN, LUIS (MEXICO); UNIVERSITY LIBRARY, UNAM, MEXICO CITY.

Elleh, Nnamdi. Department of Art History, Northwestern University, Evanston, Illinois. Articles contributed to *Encyclopedia of 20th-Century Architecture*: ABUJA, FEDERAL CAPITAL COMPLEX OF NIGERIA; HASSAN II MOSQUE, CASABLANCA; OUR LADY OF PEACE BASILICA, YAMOUSSOUKRO, IVORY COAST.

Esperdy, Gabrielle. School of Architecture, New Jersey Institute of Technology. Articles contributed to *Encyclopedia of 20th-Century Architecture*: ALUMINAIRE HOUSE, LONG ISLAND, NEW YORK; COLUMBUS INDIANA), UNITED STATES; LAPIDUS, MORRIS (UNITED STATES); LUBETKIN AND TECTON (ENGLAND).

Farmer, Graham. School of Architecture Planning and Landscape, University of Newcastle upon Tyne, England. Articles contributed to *Encyclopedia of 20th-Century Architecture*: SOLAR ARCHITECTURE (PASSIVE).

Farnham, Katherine Larson. John Milner Associates. Articles contributed to *Encyclopedia of 20th-Century Architecture*: PENNSYLVANIA STATION, NEW YORK CITY; ROW HOUSE.

Fausch, Deborah. Department of Art History, University of Illinois at Chicago. Articles contributed to *Encyclopedia of 20th-Century Architecture*: SCOTT BROWN, DENISE (UNITED STATES).

Fedders, Kristin. Office of Fine Arts, Earlham College, Richmond, Indiana. Articles contributed to *Encyclopedia of 20th-Century Architecture*: ARCHIGRAM; RANCH HOUSE.

Fenske, Gail. Independent scholar, Winchester, Massachusetts. Articles contributed to *Encyclopedia of 20th-Century Architecture*: GILBERT, CASS (UNITED STATES); WOOLWORTH BUILDING, NEW YORK CITY; WURSTER, WILLIAM (UNITED STATES).

Feuerstein, Marcia F. College of Architecture and Urban Studies, Virginia Polytechnic and State University, Blacksburg. Articles contributed to *Encyclopedia of 20th-Century Architecture*: BAUHAUS, DESSAU.

Fisher, Roger C. School of Architecture, University of Pretoria, South Africa. Articles contributed to *Encyclopedia of 20th-Century Architecture*: AFRICA: SOUTHERN AND CENTRAL AFRICA.

Fleming, Steven. School of Architecture and Built Environment, The University of Newcastle, Australia. Articles contributed to *Encyclopedia of 20th-Century Architecture*: SALK INSTITUTE, LA JOLLA, CALIFORNIA.

Flores, Carol A. College of Architecture and Planning, Ball State University, Muncie, Indiana. Articles contributed to *Encyclopedia of 20th-Century Architecture*: GETTY CENTER, LOS ANGELES; ORNAMENT; SYMBOLISM.

Flowers, Benjamin. University of Minnesota. Articles contributed to *Encyclopedia of 20th-Century Architecture*: CORPORATE OFFICE PARK/ESTATE/CAMPUS; THE ARCHITECTS COLLABORATIVE (TAC) (UNITED STATES); URBAN RENEWAL.

Foggle Plotkin, Andrea. Author Newton, Massachusetts. Articles contributed to *Encyclopedia of 20th-Century Architecture*: HOLABIRD, WILLIAM, AND JOHN WELLBORN ROOT (UNITED STATES); L'INNOVATION DEPARTMENT STORE, BRUSSELS; MONUMENT TO THE THIRD INTERNATIONAL (1920).

Frank, Suzanne. New York Institute of Technology. Articles contributed to *Encyclopedia of 20th-Century Architecture*: INSTITUTE FOR ARCHITECTURE AND URBAN STUDIES.

French, Christine Madrid. Author, Charlottesville, Virginia. Articles contributed to *Encyclopedia of 20th-Century Architecture*: VISITOR CENTER.

Froehlich, Dietmar E. College of Architecture, University of Houston. Articles contributed to *Encyclopedia of 20th-Century Architecture*: COOP HIMMELB(L)AU (AUSTRIA); CZECH, HERMANN (AUSTRIA).

Gale, Dennis. Joseph C. Cornwall Center for Metropolitan Studies, Rutgers-The State University of New Jersey, Newark. Articles contributed to *Encyclopedia of 20th-Century Architecture*: CITY BEAUTIFUL MOVEMENT.

Gamard, Elizabeth Burns. School of Architecture, Tulane University, New Orleans, Louisiana. Articles contributed to *Encyclopedia of 20th-Century Architecture*: BAUHAUS; DEUTSCHER WERKBUND; HÄRING, HUGO (GERMANY); HOLOCAUST MEMORIAL MUSEUM, WASHINGTON, DC; KAHN, ALBERT (UNITED STATES); POST OFFICE SAVINGS BANK, VIENNA; RICOLA FACTORY, LAUFEN, SWITZERLAND; SCHAROUN, HANS (GERMANY); TRIBUNE TOWER INTERNATIONAL COMPETITION, CHICAGO (1922).

Garner, John. School of Architecture, University of Illinois-Urbana, Champaign. Articles contributed to *Encyclopedia of 20th-Century Architecture*: FACTORY/INDUSTRIAL TOWN PLANNING; GRAIN ELEVATOR.

Gelernter, Mark. College of Architecture and Planning, University of Colorado at Denver. Articles contributed to *Encyclopedia of 20th-Century Architecture*: REGIONALISM.

Gilderbloom, John. Urban Studies Institute, University of Louisville, Kentucky. Articles contributed to *Encyclopedia of 20th-Century Architecture*: CUBA.

Glassman, Paul. New York School of Interior Design. Articles contributed to *Encyclopedia of 20th-Century Architecture*: AT&T BUILDING, NEW YORK; GLASS HOUSE, NEW CANAAN, CONNECTICUT; GUGGENHEIM MUSEUM, NEW YORK; HOWE, GEORGE, AND WILLIAM LESCAZE (UNITED STATES).

Gold, Martin. School of Architecture, University of Florida, Gainesville, Florida. Articles contributed to *Encyclopedia of 20th-Century Architecture*: ACOUSTICS; LIGHTING.

Gomez, Javier Alvarez-Tostado. Department of Architecture, Louisiana State University. Articles contributed to *Encyclopedia of 20th-Century Architecture*: EXPO 1992 SEVILLE CUADRA.

Gournay, Isabelle. School of Architecture, Planning, and Preservation, University of Maryland. Articles contributed to *Encyclopedia of 20th-Century Architecture*: COHEN, JEAN-LOUIS (FRANCE); MONTREAL (QUEBEC), CANADA.

Grainger, Hilary J. School of Art and Design, Staffordshire University, England. Articles contributed to *Encyclopedia of 20th-Century Architecture*: BAKER, HERBERT (ENGLAND); DARMSTADT, GERMANY; FOSTER, NORMAN (ENGLAND); GARDEN CITY MOVEMENT; GRIMSHAW NICHOLAS AND PARTNERS (ENGLAND); HOLABIRD, WILLIAM, AND MARTIN ROCHE (UNITED STATES); LE HAVRE, FRANCE; LUTYENS, EDWIN (ENGLAND); McKIM, MEAD AND WHITE (UNITED STATES); NOTRE DAME, LE RAINCY; PERRET, AUGUSTE (FRANCE); WILLIAMS, E. OWEN (ENGLAND).

Grash, Valerie. Department of Fine Arts, University of Pittsburgh at Johnstown. Articles contributed to *Encyclopedia of 20th-Century Architecture*: CHICAGO SCHOOL; KOHN PEDERSON FOX (UNITED STATES); SKIDMORE, OWINGS AND MERRILL (UNITED STATES); SKYSCRAPER.

Gruber, Samuel. Jewish Heritage Research Center, Syracuse, New York. Articles contributed to *Encyclopedia of 20th-Century Architecture*: SYNAGOGUE.

Gruskin, Nancy. Cambridge, Massachusetts. Articles contributed to *Encyclopedia of 20th-Century Architecture*: RAYMOND ELEANOR (UNITED STATES).

Gutschow, Kai K. School of Architecture, Carnegie Mellon University, Pittsburgh, Pennsylvania. Articles contributed to *Encyclopedia of 20th-Century Architecture*: FRANKFURT, GERMANY; GERMANY; TAUT, BRUNO (GERMANY); WERKBUND EXHIBITION, COLOGNE (1914).

Gyure, Dale Allen. College of Architecture and Design, Lawrence Technological University, Southfield, Michigan. Articles contributed to *Encyclopedia of 20th-Century Architecture*: EMPIRE STATE BUILDING, NEW YORK; GAS STATION.

Hadaya, Hagit. Independent scholar, Ottawa, Canada. Articles contributed to *Encyclopedia of 20th-Century Architecture*: ISRAEL; MOSQUE; PONTI, GIO (ITALY).

Hahn, Hazel. College of Arts and Sciences, Seattle University, Washington. Articles contributed to *Encyclopedia of 20th-Century Architecture*: CITÉ INDUSTRIELLE, UNE (1901–04); CONTEMPORARY CITY FOR THREE MILLION INHABITANTS; DOM-INO HOUSES (1914–15); HELSINKI, FINLAND; VOISIN PLAN FOR PARIS.

Hale, Jonathan. Institute of Architecture, University of Nottingham, England. Articles contributed to *Encyclopedia of 20th-Century Architecture*: HOPKINS, MICHAEL AND PATTY (ENGLAND); PERRAULT, DOMINIQUE (FRANCE); SMITHSON, PETER AND ALISON (ENGLAND).

Hammann, Ralph. School of Architecture, University of Arizona, Tucson. Articles contributed to *Encyclopedia of 20th-Century Architecture*: MENIL COLLECTION, HOUSTON, TEXAS; OFFICE BUILDING; PLATE GLASS; PREFABRICATION.

Handa, Rumiko. Department of Architecture, University of Nebraska. Articles contributed to *Encyclopedia of 20th-Century Architecture*: ANDO, TADAO (JAPAN); GATEWAY ARCH, ST. LOUIS, MISSOURI; JAPAN; KOSAKU BUNKA RENMEI (JAPANESE WERKBUND); OLYMPIC STADIUM; TOKYO (1964).

Harding, Anneliese. Author, Wellesley, Massachusetts. Articles contributed to *Encyclopedia of 20th-Century Architecture*: GROPIUS HOUSE, LINCOLN, MASSACHUSETTS.

Harrod, W. Owen. Architect, Austin, Texas. Articles contributed to *Encyclopedia of 20th-Century Architecture*: PAUL, BRUNO (GERMANY); TESSENOW, HEINRICH (GERMANY).

Hart, Linda. Southern California Institute of Architecture, Los Angeles. Articles contributed to *Encyclopedia of 20th-Century Architecture*: ARCHITECTURAL DRAWING; COMPETITIONS; PRITZKER ARCHITECTURE PRIZE.

Hartoonian, Gevork. Faculty of Architecture, University of Canberra, Australia. Articles contributed to *Encyclopedia of 20th-Century Architecture*: MODERNISM.

Hashem, Zouheir A. School of Architecture, University of Nevada, Las Vegas. Articles contributed to *Encyclopedia of 20th-Century Architecture*: JEDDAH, SAUDI ARABIA; PLASTICS; SPACE FRAME; STRUCTURAL SYSTEMS.

Heathcott, Joseph. Department of History, Washington University, St. Louis, Missouri. Articles contributed to *Encyclopedia of 20th-Century Architecture*: PRUITT IGOE HOUSING, ST. LOUIS, MISSOURI.

Hein, Carola. Program in Growth and Structure of Cities, Bryn Mawr College, Bryn Mawr, Pennsylvania. Articles contributed to *Encyclopedia of 20th-Century Architecture*: KANSAI INTERNATIONAL AIRPORT TERMINAL, OSAKA; KYOTO, JAPAN; MAKI, FUMIHIKO (JAPAN); TOKYO, JAPAN.

Hendrix, John. School of Art, Architecture, and Historic Preservation, Roger Williams University, Bristol, Rhode Island. Articles contributed to *Encyclopedia of 20th-Century Architecture*: AULENTI, GAE (ITALY); BENEVOLO, LEONARDO (ITALY); GREGOTTI, VITTORIO (ITALY); NERVI, PIER LUIGI (ITALY); PORTOGHESI, PAOLO (ITALY).

Heynen, Hilde. Katholieke Universiteit Leuven, Belgium. Articles contributed to *Encyclopedia of 20th-Century Architecture*: AVANT-GARDE; MAY, ERNST (GERMANY); POSTMODERNISM.

Hietkamp, Lenore. Department of Art History, University of Washington. Articles contributed to *Encyclopedia of 20th-Century Architecture*: PARK HOTEL, SHANGHAI.

Hinchman, Mark. Department of Architecture, University of Nebraska. Articles contributed to *Encyclopedia of 20th-Century Architecture*: ALLIANCE FRANCO-SÉNÉGALAISE, KAOLACK, SENEGAL; GREAT MOSQUE OF NIONO, MALI; YAAMA MOSQUE, TAHOUA, NIGER.

Ho, Puay-peng. Department of Architecture, Chinese University of Hong Kong, China. Articles contributed to *Encyclopedia of 20th-Century Architecture*: BANK OF CHINA TOWER, HONG KONG; CHINA.

Hoekstra, Rixt. Institute for Art and Architectural History, Rijksuniversiteit Groningen, Netherlands. Articles contributed to *Encyclopedia of 20th-Century Architecture*: HISTORIOGRAPHY.

Huang, Yunsheng. School of Architecture, University of Virginia, Charlottesville. Articles contributed to *Encyclopedia of 20th-Century Architecture*: WU LIANGYONG (CHINA).

Hyland, Anthony D.C. Department of Architecture, National University of Science and Technology, Zimbabwe. Articles contributed to *Encyclopedia of 20th-Century Architecture*: AFRICA: NORTHERN AFRICA; EARTHEN BUILDING; FATHY, HASSAN (AFRICA); PEVSNER, NIKOLAUS (ENGLAND); RAMSES WISSA WASSEF ARTS CENTRE, GIZA, EGYPT; WASSEF WISSA (AFRICA).

Jackson, Neil. School of Civil Engineering, University of Leeds, England. Articles contributed to *Encyclopedia of 20th-Century Architecture*: ELLWOOD, CRAIG (UNITED STATES); FREY, ALBERT (UNITED STATES).

Jenner, Ross. School of Architecture, University of Auckland, New Zealand. Articles contributed to *Encyclopedia of 20th-Century Architecture*: SANT'ELIA, ANTONIO (ITALY); SCARPA, CARLO (ITALY).

Johansson, Britt-Inger. Department of Art History, University of Uppsala Sweden. Articles contributed to *Encyclopedia of 20th-Century Architecture*: CONCERT HALL, HÄLSINGBORG, SWEDEN; GRUNDTVIG CHURCH, COPENHAGEN.

Johnson, Donald Leslie. University of South Australia. Articles contributed to *Encyclopedia of 20th-Century Architecture*: BROADACRE CITY (1934–35); RATIONALISM; SEIDLER, HARRY (AUSTRALIA).

Joselow, Evie T. Chief of Research, Commission for Art Recovery, New York. Articles contributed to *Encyclopedia of 20th-Century Architecture*: JEWISH MUSEUM, BERLIN; WORLD TRADE CENTER, NEW YORK.

Kalner, Scott. Independent scholar, Philadelphia, Pennsylvania. Articles contributed to *Encyclopedia of 20th-Century Architecture*: ADAPTIVE RE-USE; GLASGOW SCHOOL OF ART, GLASGOW.

Kanekar, Aarati. Department of Architecture and Interior Design, University of Cincinnati. Articles contributed to *Encyclopedia of 20th-Century Architecture*: ENTREPRENEURSHIP DEVELOPMENT INSTITUTE, AHMEDABAD; HIGH MUSEUM OF ART, ATLANTA, GEORGIA; INDIAN INSTITUTE OF MANAGEMENT, AHMEDABAD; NATIONAL ASSEMBLY BUILDING, SHER-E-BANGLA NAGAR, DHAKA; VIDHAN BHAVAN (STATE ASSEMBLY), BHOPAL.

Kariouk, Paul. School of Architecture, Carleton University, Ontario, Canada. Articles contributed to *Encyclopedia of 20th-Century Architecture*: FERRISS, HUGH (UNITED STATES).

Kezer, Zeynep. School of Architecture, University of British Columbia, Canada. Articles contributed to *Encyclopedia of 20th-Century Architecture*: MOSQUE OF THE GRAND NATIONAL ASSEMBLY, ANKARA, TURKEY; TURKEY.

Khan, Hasan-Uddin. Department of Architecture, Massachusetts Institute of Technology. Articles contributed to *Encyclopedia of 20th-Century Architecture*: ARDALAN, NADER (IRAN); BAWA, GEOFFREY (SRI LANKA); CHADIRJI, RIFAT (IRAQ); GÜREL FAMILY SUMMER RESIDENCE, ÇANAKKALE, TURKEY; IRAN; REWAL, RAJ (INDIA); SOUTHEAST ASIA.

Koeck, Monika. University of Cambridge, England. Articles contributed to *Encyclopedia of 20th-Century Architecture*: BÖHM, GOTTFRIED (GERMANY).

Koeck, Richard. Independent scholar, Norman, Oklahoma. Articles contributed to *Encyclopedia of 20th-Century Architecture*: PIANO, RENZO (ITALY).

Konicki, Leah. Independent scholar, Covington, Kentucky. Articles contributed to *Encyclopedia of 20th-Century Architecture*: TERRA-COTTA.

Kostich-Lefebvre, Gordana. Fine Arts Division, University of Pennsylvania. Articles contributed to *Encyclopedia of 20th-Century Architecture*: MEMPHIS (GROUP) (ITALY); VILLE RADIEUSE (C. 1930).

Kremers, Jack. Department of Architecture, Judson College, Elgin, Illinois. Articles contributed to *Encyclopedia of 20th-Century Architecture*: BOSTON CITY HALL; SEARS TOWER, CHICAGO.

Krieger, Peter. Instituto de Investigaciones Estéticas, U.N.A.M., Mexico City. Articles contributed to *Encyclopedia of 20th-Century Architecture*: CIUDAD UNIVERSITARIA CAMPUS AND STADIUM, MEXICO CITY; CONTEXTUALISM; UNITED NATIONS HEADQUARTERS, NEW YORK; UTOPIAN PLANNING.

Krinsky, Carol Herselle. Department of Fine Arts, New York University. Articles contributed to *Encyclopedia of 20th-Century Architecture*: BUNSHAFT, GORDON (UNITED STATES); CHRYSLER BUILDING, NEW YORK; HAJ TERMINAL, JEDDAH AIRPORT; LEVER HOUSE, NEW YORK; ROCKEFELLER CENTER, NEW YORK.

Krutulis, Rima. Independent scholar, Chicago, Illinois. Articles contributed to *Encyclopedia of 20th-Century Architecture*: EGYPTIAN REVIVAL.

Kruty, Paul. Department of Architecture, University of Illinois at Urbana-Champaign. Articles contributed to *Encyclopedia of 20th-Century Architecture*: HORTA, VICTOR (BELGIUM); PLAN OF CANBERRA.

Kuhlmann, Dörte. Department of Architecture, Vienna University of Technology, Austria. Articles contributed to *Encyclopedia of 20th-Century Architecture*: AALTO, ALVAR (FINLAND); GOFF, BRUCE (UNITED STATES); HOLLEIN, HANS (AUSTRIA); PIETILÄ, REIMA AND RAILI (FINLAND).

Kvan, Thomas. Faculty of Architecture, University of Hong Kong, China. Articles contributed to *Encyclopedia of 20th-Century Architecture*: COMPUTERS AND ARCHITECTURE; HONG KONG, CHINA; HONG KONG INTERNATIONAL AIRPORT, HONG KONG.

La Marche, Jean. Department of Architecture, University at Buffalo, New York. Articles contributed to *Encyclopedia of 20th-Century Architecture*: HOUSE; LIBESKIND, DANIEL (UNITED STATES); TSCHUMI, BERNARD (FRANCE).

Langdon, Philip. Author, New Haven, Connecticut. Articles contributed to *Encyclopedia of 20th-Century Architecture*: ROADSIDE ARCHITECTURE.

Langmead, Donald. School of Architecture, University of South Australia. Articles contributed to *Encyclopedia of 20th-Century Architecture*: OUD, J.J.P. (NETHERLANDS).

Lara, Fernando. Federal University of Minas Gerais, Brazil. Articles contributed to *Encyclopedia of 20th-Century Architecture*: BRAZIL; BURLE MARX, ROBERTO (BRAZIL); PAMPULHA BUILDINGS, BELO HORIZONTE, BRAZIL; RIO DE JANEIRO, BRAZIL.

Larrañaga, Enrique. Architect, Miami Beach, Florida. Articles contributed to *Encyclopedia of 20th-Century Architecture*: CARACAS, VENEZUELA.

Lawrence, Attila. School of Architecture, University of Nevada. Articles contributed to *Encyclopedia of 20th-Century Architecture*: HELSINKI RAILWAY STATION, FINLAND; METRO STATION, PARIS.

Leach, Neil. Department of Architecture and Civil Engineering, University of Bath, England. Articles contributed to *Encyclopedia of 20th-Century Architecture*: DECONSTRUCTIVISM.

LeCuyer, Annette. Department of Architecture, The State University of New York at Buffalo. Articles contributed to *Encyclopedia of 20th-Century Architecture*: MIRALLES, ENRIC, AND CARME PINÓS (SPAIN); POMPIDOU CENTER, PARIS; SCHLUMBERGER CAMBRIDGE RESEARCH CENTRE, ENGLAND.

Lefaivre, Liane. Department of Architecture, Technical University of Delft, the Netherlands. Articles contributed to *Encyclopedia of 20th-Century Architecture*: BÒ BARDI, LINA (BRAZIL).

Lejeune, Jean-François. School of Architecture, University of Miami, Florida. Articles contributed to *Encyclopedia of 20th-Century Architecture*: CELEBRATION, FLORIDA; UNIVERSUM CINEMA, BERLIN.

Lewittes, Deborah. Architectural historian, New York. Articles contributed to *Encyclopedia of 20th-Century Architecture*: CHANNEL 4 HEADQUARTERS, LONDON; CONNELL, AMYAS, COLIN LUCAS, AND BASIL WARD (ENGLAND); HIGHPOINT 1 APARTMENT BLOCK, LONDON.

Lindman, Timo. Architect, New York. Articles contributed to *Encyclopedia of 20th-Century Architecture*: HEIKKINEN AND KOMONEN (FINLAND); PALLASMAA, JUHANI (FINLAND).

Lizon, Peter. College of Architecture and Design, The University of Tennessee Knoxville. Articles contributed to *Encyclopedia of 20th-Century Architecture*: CZECH REPUBLIC/CZECHOSLOVAKIA; LOVELL HEALTH HOUSE, LOS ANGELES; PRAGUE, CZECH REPUBLIC.

Loeffler, Jane. University of Maryland. Articles contributed to *Encyclopedia of 20th-Century Architecture*: EMBASSY.

Loftin, Laurence Keith. College of Architecture and Planning, University of Colorado, Denver. Articles contributed to *Encyclopedia of 20th-Century Architecture*: EINSTEIN TOWER, POTSDAM, GERMANY; VILLA MAIREA, NOORMARKKU, FINLAND.

Lombard, Joanna. School of Architecture, University of Miami, Florida. Articles contributed to *Encyclopedia of 20th-Century Architecture*: DUANY AND PLATER-ZYBERK (UNITED STATES).

Long, Christopher. School of Architecture, University of Texas at Austin. Articles contributed to *Encyclopedia of 20th-Century Architecture*: AUSTRIA; FRANK, JOSEF (AUSTRIA); NEUTRA, RICHARD (AUSTRIA); OLBRICH, JOSEF MARIA (AUSTRIA); STEINER HOUSE, VIENNA; VIENNA SECESSION; WAGNER, OTTO (AUSTRIA).

Lorance, Loretta. Graduate School and University Center, City University of New York. Articles contributed to *Encyclopedia of 20th-Century Architecture*: HADID, ZAHA (IRAQ); SMITH, CHLOETHIEL WOODARD (UNITED STATES).

Lord, Jill Marie. Independent scholar, New York. Articles contributed to *Encyclopedia of 20th-Century Architecture*: GWATHMEY, CHARLES, AND ROBERT SIEGEL (UNITED STATES); HAMLIN, TALBOT (UNITED STATES).

Mácel, Otakar. Department of Architecture, Delft University of Technology, Netherlands. Articles contributed to *Encyclopedia of 20th-Century Architecture*: CUBISM; KARL MARX HOF, VIENNA; MELNIKOV, KONSTANTIN (RUSSIA); TUGENDHAT HOUSE, BRNO, CZECH REPUBLIC.

Maciuika, John V. Architectural History Department, University of Virginia, Charlottesville. Articles contributed to *Encyclopedia of 20th-Century Architecture*: MUTHESIUS, HERMANN (GERMANY).

MacKay, A. Gordon. Foxcroft School, Middleburg, Virginia. Articles contributed to *Encyclopedia of 20th-Century Architecture*: ENGINEERED LUMBER; WOOD.

Madanipour, Ali. Global Urban Research Unit, University of Newcastle upon Tyne, England. Articles contributed to *Encyclopedia of 20th-Century Architecture*: NEW TOWNS MOVEMENT.

Maffei, Nicolas. Norwich School of Art and Design, England. Articles contributed to *Encyclopedia of 20th-Century Architecture*: VENTURI, ROBERT (UNITED STATES).

Maxwell, Robert. Maxwell Scott Architects, London, England. Articles contributed to *Encyclopedia of 20th-Century Architecture*: ABSTRACTION; ROGERS, RICHARD (ENGLAND); ROWE, COLIN (UNITED STATES); STIRLING, JAMES (SCOTLAND AND ENGLAND); UNITED KINGDOM; VILLA SAVOYE, POISSY, FRANCE.

Mayhall, Marguerite K. Department of Fine Arts, Kean University, New Jersey. Articles contributed to *Encyclopedia of 20th-Century Architecture*: CIUDAD UNIVERSITARIA, CARACAS; VILLANUEVA, CARLOS RAUL (VENEZUELA).

Mayo, James. School of Architecture and Urban Design, University of Kansas. Articles contributed to *Encyclopedia of 20th-Century Architecture*: COUNTRY CLUB.

McCarter, Robert. Department of Architecture, University of Florida. Articles contributed to *Encyclopedia of 20th-Century Architecture*: FALLINGWATER, BEAR RUN, PENNSYLVANIA; KAHN, LOUIS (UNITED STATES); SARASOTA SCHOOL; WRIGHT, FRANK LLOYD (UNITED STATES).

McDonald, Margot. Department of Architecture California Polytechnic State University, San Luis Obispo. Articles contributed to *Encyclopedia of 20th-Century Architecture*: CLIMATE; SUSTAINABILITY/SUSTAINABLE ARCHITECTURE.

Meister, Michael. Department of History of Art, University of Pennsylvania. Articles contributed to *Encyclopedia of 20th-Century Architecture*: SANTOS, ADÈLE NAUDÉ (SOUTH AFRICA).

Meneguello, Cristina. Department of History, State University of Campinas, Brazil. Articles contributed to *Encyclopedia of 20th-Century Architecture*: SÃO PAULO, BRAZIL.

Merlino, Kathryn Rogers. Department of Architecture, University of Washington. Articles contributed to *Encyclopedia of 20th-Century Architecture*: HOLL, STEVEN (UNITED STATES).

Meyers, Andrew. Department of History, Ethical Culture Fieldston School, New York. Articles contributed to *Encyclopedia of 20th-Century Architecture*: NEW YORK WORLD'S FAIR (1939).

Mical, Thomas. Department of Architecture, University of Oklahoma, Norman. Articles contributed to *Encyclopedia of 20th-Century Architecture*: HEJDUK, JOHN (UNITED STATES); JAHN, HELMUT (UNITED STATES); MORPHOSIS (UNITED STATES); ROSSI, ALDO (ITALY).

Miller, Char. Department of Public and International Affairs, George Mason University, Virginia. Articles contributed to *Encyclopedia of 20th-Century Architecture*: COLQUHOUN, ALAN (ENGLAND); LINCOLN MEMORIAL, WASHINGTON, DC; POPE, JOHN RUSSELL (UNITED STATES).

Miller, Christopher. Department of Architecture, Judson College Elgin, Illinois. Articles contributed to *Encyclopedia of 20th-Century Architecture*: CLASSICISM.

Miller, Naomi. Department of Art History, Boston University. Articles contributed to *Encyclopedia of 20th-Century Architecture*: DE CARLO, GIANCARLO (ITALY).

Miller, William C. School of Architecture, University of Utah. Articles contributed to *Encyclopedia of 20th-Century Architecture*: ASPLUND, ERIK GUNNAR (SWEDEN); BLOMSTEDT, AULIS (FINLAND); FINLAND; PAIMIO SANATORIUM, NEAR TURKU, FINLAND.

Millette, Daniel. Department of Architecture, University of British Columbia, Canada. Articles contributed to *Encyclopedia of 20th-Century Architecture*: CHOISY, AUGUSTE (FRANCE).

Mitchell, Kevin. School of Architecture and Design, The American University of Sharjah, United Arab Emirates. Articles contributed to *Encyclopedia of 20th-Century Architecture*: DENMARK; MARKELIUS, SVEN (SWEDEN); MINISTRY OF FOREIGN AFFAIRS, RIYADH, SAUDI ARABIA; RASMUSSEN, STEEN EILER (DENMARK); SWEDEN.

Monson, Christopher. Department of Architecture, Mississippi State University. Articles contributed to *Encyclopedia of 20th-Century Architecture*: COLOR.

Moore, Fuller. Miami University. Articles contributed to *Encyclopedia of 20th-Century Architecture*: TENSILE STRUCTURES.

Moore, Steven. School of Architecture, University of Texas at Austin. Articles contributed to *Encyclopedia of 20th-Century Architecture*: ENERGY-EFFICIENT DESIGN; ENVIRONMENTAL ISSUES.

Moravánszky, Ákos. Institute for the History and Theory of Architecture, Zürich, Switzerland. Articles contributed to *Encyclopedia of 20th-Century Architecture*: BUDAPEST, HUNGARY; HUNGARY; MEDGYASZAY, ISTVÁN (HUNGARY); MOLNAR, FARKAS (HUNGARY).

Moravánszky-Gyöngy, Katalin. Independent scholar, Zürich, Switzerland. Articles contributed to *Encyclopedia of 20th-Century Architecture*: BUDAPEST, HUNGARY; HUNGARY; MEDGYASZAY, ISTVÁN (HUNGARY); MOLNAR, FARKAS (HUNGARY).

Morgan, Keith N. Department of Art History, Boston University. Articles contributed to *Encyclopedia of 20th-Century Architecture*: PLATT, CHARLES ADAMS (UNITED STATES).

Morgenthaler, Hans. Department of Architecture, University of Colorado, Denver. Articles contributed to *Encyclopedia of 20th-Century Architecture*: BOTTA, MARIO (SWITZERLAND); EXPRESSIONISM; MENDELSOHN, ERICH (GERMANY AND UNITED STATES); SWITZERLAND.

Morton, Patricia. Department of the History of Art, University of California, Riverside. Articles contributed to *Encyclopedia of 20th-Century Architecture*: FEMINIST THEORY; PRIMITIVISM.

Moy, Catherine. Venturi, Scott Brown, and Associates, Philadelphia, Pennsylvania. Articles contributed to *Encyclopedia of 20th-Century Architecture*: KUROKAWA, KISHO (JAPAN); LIN, MAYA (UNITED STATES).

Mumford, Eric. School of Architecture, Washington University, St. Louis, Missouri. Articles contributed to *Encyclopedia of 20th-Century Architecture*: ATHENS CHARTER (1943); CONGRÈS INTERNATIONAUX D'ARCHITECTURE MODERNE (CIAM, 1927–); FRAMPTON, KENNETH (UNITED STATES).

Naylor, David. Department of Architecture, The University of Queensland, Australia. Articles contributed to *Encyclopedia of 20th-Century Architecture*: DULLES INTERNATIONAL AIRPORT, CHANTILLY, VIRGINIA; TWA AIRPORT TERMINAL, NEW YORK.

Nesbitt, Kate. Author, Charlottesville, Virginia. Articles contributed to *Encyclopedia of 20th-Century Architecture*: GULLICHSEN, KRISTIAN (FINLAND); JACOBSEN, ARNE (DENMARK); LARSEN, HENNING (DENMARK).

Neumann, Dietrich. Department of History of Art and Architecture, Brown University, Providence, Rhode Island. Articles contributed to *Encyclopedia of 20th-Century Architecture*: CATALAN (GUASTAVINO) VAULTS.

Notaro, Anna. School of American and Canadian Studies, University of Nottingham, England. Articles contributed to *Encyclopedia of 20th-Century Architecture*: ROME, ITALY.

Oberholzer, Mark. Department of Architecture, Rice University Houston, Texas. Articles contributed to *Encyclopedia of 20th-Century Architecture*: MAILLART, ROBERT (SWITZERLAND).

Ochshorn, Jonathan. Department of Architecture, Cornell University, Ithaca, New York. Articles contributed to *Encyclopedia of 20th-Century Architecture*: BRICK; CURTAIN WALL SYSTEM; STEEL; STONE; TRUSS SYSTEMS.

Olivarez, Jennifer Komar. Minneapolis Institute of Arts, Minnesota. Articles contributed to *Encyclopedia of 20th-Century Architecture*: FISKER, KAY (DENMARK); PERKINS AND WILL (UNITED STATES).

Oliver, Paul. School of Architecture, Centre for International Vernacular Studies, England. Articles contributed to *Encyclopedia of 20th-Century Architecture*: VERNACULAR ARCHITECTURE.

Olsen, Patrice. Department of History, Illinois State University. Articles contributed to *Encyclopedia of 20th-Century Architecture*: CANDELA, FELIX (MEXICO); GONZÁLEZ DE LÉON, TEODORO AND ABRAHAM ZABLUDOVSKY (MEXICO); LEGORRETA, RICARDO (MEXICO); MEXICO CITY, MEXICO; MORAL, ENRIQUE DEL, (MEXICO).

Ostwald, Michael. School of Architecture and Built Envrionment, The University of Newcastle, Callaghan, Australia. Articles contributed to *Encyclopedia of 20th-Century Architecture*: AMUSEMENT PARK; BOFILL, RICARDO (SPAIN); CULTURAL CENTRE JEAN MARIE TJIBARO-NOUMIA, NEW CALEDONIA; MEIER, RICHARD (UNITED STATES); PARLIAMENT BUILDING, CHANDIGARH; SHINOHARA, KAZUO (JAPAN).

Ott, Randall. Department of Architecture, University of Colorado at Boulder. Articles contributed to *Encyclopedia of 20th-Century Architec-*

ture: BERLIN, GERMANY; GERMAN PAVILION, BARCELONA (1929); MEYER, HANNES (GERMANY).

Papademetriou, Peter C. School of Architecture, New Jersey Institute of Technology. Articles contributed to *Encyclopedia of 20th-Century Architecture*: AMBASZ, EMILIO (ARGENTINA AND UNITED STATES); SAARINEN, EERO (FINLAND).

Pelkonen, Eeva-Liisa. School of Architecture, Yale University New Haven, Connecticut. Articles contributed to *Encyclopedia of 20th-Century Architecture*: KADA, KLAUS (AUSTRIA); VELDE, HENRI VAN DE (BELGIUM).

Perrotta, Marc. Independent scholar, Columbus, Ohio. Articles contributed to *Encyclopedia of 20th-Century Architecture*: BUS TERMINAL.

Phipps, Linda. Independent scholar, Oakland, California. Articles contributed to *Encyclopedia of 20th-Century Architecture*: COSTA, LÚCIO (BRAZIL); HARRISON, WALLACE K., AND MAX ABRAMOVITZ (UNITED STATES); NIEMEYER, OSCAR (BRAZIL); NITZSCHKE, OSCAR (FRANCE).

Picard, Michèle. Canadian Center for Architecture, Montreal. Articles contributed to *Encyclopedia of 20th-Century Architecture*: EXPO '67, MONTREAL; HABITAT '67, MONTREAL.

Pizzi, Marcela. Faculty of Architecture and Town Planning, University of Chile. Articles contributed to *Encyclopedia of 20th-Century Architecture*: SANTIAGO, CHILE.

Popescu, Carmen. Independent scholar, Paris, France. Articles contributed to *Encyclopedia of 20th-Century Architecture*: BUCHAREST, ROMANIA; ROMANIA.

Prakash, Vikramaditya. Department of Architecture, University of Washington. Articles contributed to *Encyclopedia of 20th-Century Architecture*: CHANDIGARH, INDIA.

Prigmore, Kathryn. Einhorn Yaffee Prescott Architecture and Engineering P.C., Washington, D.C. Articles contributed to *Encyclopedia of 20th-Century Architecture*: ESCALATOR.

Pursell, Timothy. University of Alaska, Fairbanks. Articles contributed to *Encyclopedia of 20th-Century Architecture*: BERLAGE, HENDRIK PETRUS (NETHERLANDS); DÜSSELDORF, GERMANY; PALAIS STOCLET, BRUSSELS.

Quinan, Jack. Department of Art History, The State University of New York at Buffalo. Articles contributed to *Encyclopedia of 20th-Century Architecture*: LARKIN BUILDING, BUFFALO, NEW YORK.

Randolph, Dennis. Calhoun County Community Development, Battle Creek, Michigan. Articles contributed to *Encyclopedia of 20th-Century Architecture*: STEEL FRAME CONSTRUCTION.

Rappaport, Nina. Independent scholar, New York. Articles contributed to *Encyclopedia of 20th-Century Architecture*: BENNETON FACTORY, ITALY; FACTORY; FIAT WORKS, TURIN; OLIVETTI FACTORY, BUENOS AIRES; RENAULT DISTRIBUTION CENTER, SWINDON, ENGLAND; VAN NELLE FACTORY, ROTTERDAM.

Riedinger, Edward A. Ohio State University, Columbus. Articles contributed to *Encyclopedia of 20th-Century Architecture*: LISBON WORLD EXPOSITION (1998); DE MOURA, EDUARDO SOUTO (PORTUGAL).

Robinson, Matthew S. Pennsylvania State University, University Park. Articles contributed to *Encyclopedia of 20th-Century Architecture*: EXPO 1958, BRUSSELS; FALLOUT SHELTER; GRUEN, VICTOR DAVID

(United States); Stone, Edward Durell (United States); Yamasaki, Minoru (United States).

Rodríguez-Camilloni, Humberto. College of Architecture and Urban Studies, Virginia Polytechnic Institute and State University, Blacksburg. Articles contributed to *Encyclopedia of 20th-Century Architecture*: Scully, Vincent (United States).

Rohan, Tim. Department of Art, University of Massachusetts, Amherst. Articles contributed to *Encyclopedia of 20th-Century Architecture*: Rudolph, Paul (United States).

Rujivacharakul, Vimalin. Department of Architecture, University of California, Berkeley. Articles contributed to *Encyclopedia of 20th-Century Architecture*: Baiyoke Tower, Bangkok; Bangkok, Thailand.

Rylance, Keli. Department of Art and Design, University of Wisconsin-Stout. Articles contributed to *Encyclopedia of 20th-Century Architecture*: Barcelona, Spain; Spain.

Sabatino, Michelangelo. School of Architecture, Yale University, New Haven, Connecticut. Articles contributed to *Encyclopedia of 20th-Century Architecture*: Torre Velasca, Milan.

Salny, Stephen. Architectural and design historian, Baltimore, Maryland. Articles contributed to *Encyclopedia of 20th-Century Architecture*: Adler, David (United States).

Samson, M. David. Department of Humanities and Arts, Worcester Polytechnic Institute, Massachusetts. Articles contributed to *Encyclopedia of 20th-Century Architecture*: Hitchcock, Henry-Russell (United States); International Style Exhibition, New York (1932); Johnson, Philip (United States).

Samudio, Jeffrey B. Design Aid Architects, Hollywood, California. Articles contributed to *Encyclopedia of 20th-Century Architecture*: Williams, Paul (United States).

Sanchez, Alfonso. Independent scholar, Mexico. Articles contributed to *Encyclopedia of 20th-Century Architecture*: Mexico.

Sarkis, Hashim. Department of Urban Planning and Design, Harvard University, Cambridge, Massachusetts. Articles contributed to *Encyclopedia of 20th-Century Architecture*: Beirut, Lebanon; Lynch, Kevin (United States).

Sauls, Allison. Department of Art, Missouri Western State College. Articles contributed to *Encyclopedia of 20th-Century Architecture*: Museum of Modern Art, Frankfurt; Pilgrimage Church at Neviges.

Schrenk, Lisa. Department of Art History, University of California, Davis. Articles contributed to *Encyclopedia of 20th-Century Architecture*: Century of Progress Exposition, Chicago (1933); Concrete Shell Structure; National Farmers' Bank, Owatonna, Minnesota; Weissenhofsiedlung, Deutscher Werkbund (Stuttgart, 1927).

Schulze, Franz. Department of Art, Lake Forest College, Lake Forest, Illinois. Articles contributed to *Encyclopedia of 20th-Century Architecture*: Farnsworth House, Plano, Illinois; Mies van der Rohe, Ludwig (Germany).

Schumacher, Thomas. School of Architecture, Planning, and Preservation, University of Maryland. Articles contributed to *Encyclopedia of 20th-Century Architecture*: Moretti, Luigi (Italy); Terragni, Giuseppe (Italy).

Schwarzer, Mitchell. California College of Arts and Crafts, San Francisco. Articles contributed to *Encyclopedia of 20th-Century Architecture*: Gill, Irving (United States); Loos, Adolf (Austria).

Searing, Helen. Smith College, Northampton, Massachusetts. Articles contributed to *Encyclopedia of 20th-Century Architecture*: Abteiberg Municipal Museum, Mönchengladbach, Germany; Amsterdam, The Netherlands; Amsterdam School; Art Nouveau (Jugendstil); British Library, London; Duiker Johannes (Netherlands); Glasgow School; Goody, Joan (United States); International Exhibition of Decorative Arts, Paris (1925); Lasdun, Denys (England); London, England; Netherlands; Neue Staatsgalerie, Stuttgart; Polshek, James Stewart (United States); Rotterdam, Netherlands; Sainsbury Wing, National Gallery, London; Stern, Robert A.M. (United States); Wilson, Colin St. John (England).

Segre, Roberto. Faculty of Architecture and Urbanism, Federal University of Rio de Janeiro, Brazil. Articles contributed to *Encyclopedia of 20th-Century Architecture*: Church of St. Francis of Assisi, Brazil; Favela; Romañach, Mario (Cuba); National Art Schools, Havana, Cuba; Testa, Clorindo (Argentina).

Sekler, Eduard F. Professor Emeritus, Harvard University, Cambridge, Massachusetts. Articles contributed to *Encyclopedia of 20th-Century Architecture*: Hoffmann, Josef (Austria).

Shanken, Andrew M. Department of Art, Oberlin College, Ohio. Articles contributed to *Encyclopedia of 20th-Century Architecture*: Giedion, Sigfried (Switzerland); Glass; Memorial.

Sieira, Maria. Independent scholar, New York. Articles contributed to *Encyclopedia of 20th-Century Architecture*: Nouvel, Jean (France); Representation.

Simon, Madlen. College of Architecture, Planning and Design, Kansas State University. Articles contributed to *Encyclopedia of 20th-Century Architecture*: Education of Architects Schools.

Siry, Joseph. Department of Art and Art History, Wesleyan University, Connecticut. Articles contributed to *Encyclopedia of 20th-Century Architecture*: Carson Pirie Scott Store, Chicago; Plan of Chicago, Illinois; Sullivan, Louis (United States); Unity Temple, Oak Park, Illinois.

Smith, Cynthia Duquette. Department of Communication and Culture, Indiana University, Bloomington. Articles contributed to *Encyclopedia of 20th-Century Architecture*: Ashbee, C.R. (England); Bungalow; Craftsman Style; Levittown, New Jersey and New York.

Sobti, Manu. College of Architecture, Georgia Institute of Technology. Articles contributed to *Encyclopedia of 20th-Century Architecture*: Maidan.

Sokol, David M. Department of Art History, University of Illinois, Chicago. Articles contributed to *Encyclopedia of 20th-Century Architecture*: Jacobs, Jane (United States).

Speck, Lawrence W. School of Architecture, University of Texas at Austin. Articles contributed to *Encyclopedia of 20th-Century Architecture*: Herzog, Jacques, and Pierre de Meuron (Switzerland); Houston, (TX), United States; Kimbell Art Museum, Fort Worth, Texas; Moore, Charles (United States).

Sprague, Paul. Author, Rockledge, Florida. Articles contributed to *Encyclopedia of 20th-Century Architecture*: ROBIE HOUSE, CHICAGO.

Stankard, Mark. Department of Architecture, Iowa State University. Articles contributed to *Encyclopedia of 20th-Century Architecture*: DE STIJL; DOESBURG, THEO VAN (NETHERLANDS); VANNA VENTURI HOUSE, PHILADELPHIA; VENICE BIENNALE PAVILIONS, ITALY.

Steer, Linda. Department of Art History, Binghamton University, New York. Articles contributed to *Encyclopedia of 20th-Century Architecture*: SUPERMODERNISM

Steinhardt, Nancy. Department of Asian and Middle Eastern Studies, University of Pennsylvania. Articles contributed to *Encyclopedia of 20th-Century Architecture*: LIANG SICHENG (CHINA).

Suzuki, Hiroyuki. Faculty of Engineering, University of Tokyo, Japan. Articles contributed to *Encyclopedia of 20th-Century Architecture*: ISOZAKI, ARATA (JAPAN).

Swanson, Randy. College of Architecture, University of North Carolina, Charlotte. Articles contributed to *Encyclopedia of 20th-Century Architecture*: CENTER FOR INTEGRATED SYSTEMS, STANFORD UNIVERSITY; EXHIBITION BUILDING; RESEARCH CENTER.

Thompson, Jennifer. Princeton Architectural Press, New York. Articles contributed to *Encyclopedia of 20th-Century Architecture*: CARRÈRE, JOHN MERVIN, AND THOMAS HASTINGS (UNITED STATES).

Thompson, W. P. Department of Architecture, University of Manitoba, Canada. Articles contributed to *Encyclopedia of 20th-Century Architecture*: COLLINS, PETER (CANADA).

Thorne, Martha. Department of Architecture, The Art Institute of Chicago. Articles contributed to *Encyclopedia of 20th-Century architecture*: JIRICNA, EVA (ENGLAND); MONEO, RAFAEL (SPAIN); NAVARRO BALDWEG, JUAN (SPAIN); SIZA VIEIRA, ÁLVARO J.M. (PORTUGAL); SOTA, ALEJANDRO DE LA (SPAIN).

Tilman, Jeffrey Thomas. School of Architecture and Interior Design, University of Cincinnati. Articles contributed to *Encyclopedia of 20th-Century Architecture*: CITY HALL; EXPOSITION UNIVERSELLE, PARIS (1900); HISTORICISM; LAS VEGAS, NEVADA, UNITED STATES; PANAMA PACIFIC EXPOSITION, SAN FRANCISCO (1915); SUBWAY.

Tomlan, Michael A. Department of City and Regional Planning, Cornell University. Articles contributed to *Encyclopedia of 20th-Century Architecture*: HISTORIC PRESERVATION.

Toure, Diala. University of California, Berkeley. Articles contributed to *Encyclopedia of 20th-Century Architecture*: BUREAUX D'ETUDES HENRI CHOMETTE (FRANCE AND WEST AFRICA).

Tournikiotis, Panayotis. School of Architecture, National Technical University of Athens, Greece. Articles contributed to *Encyclopedia of 20th-Century Architecture*: GREECE; NEORATIONALISM.

Townsend, Gavin Edward. Department of Art, University of Tennessee at Chattanooga. Articles contributed to *Encyclopedia of 20th-Century Architecture*: SHAW, HOWARD VAN DOREN (UNITED STATES).

Triff, Kristin. Department of Fine Arts, Trinity College, Connecticut. Articles contributed to *Encyclopedia of 20th-Century Architecture*: CASA MILÀ, BARCELONA; MIAMI, (FL) UNITED STATES.

Troiani, Igea. School of Architecture, Queensland University of Technology, Australia. Articles contributed to *Encyclopedia of 20th-Century*

Architecture: CODERCH Y DE SENTMENAT, ANTONIO, JOSÉ (SPAIN); TEAM X (NETHERLANDS).

Trowles, Peter. Glasgow School of Art, Scotland. Articles contributed to *Encyclopedia of 20th-Century Architecture*: MACKINTOSH, CHARLES RENNIE (SCOTLAND).

Trubiano, Franca. Department of Fine Arts, University of Pennsylvania. Articles contributed to *Encyclopedia of 20th-Century Architecture*: EXHIBITION HALL, TURIN; FASCIST ARCHITECTURE; LIBERA, ADALBERTO (ITALY).

Turan, Belgin. Department of Architecture, Middle East Technical University, Ankara, Turkey. Articles contributed to *Encyclopedia of 20th-Century Architecture*: ISTANBUL, TURKEY; SOCIAL SECURITY COMPLEX, ISTANBUL.

Turnbull, Jeffrey John. Faculty of Architecture, Building and Planning, University of Melbourne, Australia. Articles contributed to *Encyclopedia of 20th-Century Architecture*: AUSTRALIA; CANBERRA, AUSTRALIA; GRIFFIN, WALTER BURLEY, AND MARION MAHONY GRIFFIN (UNITED STATES); MELBOURNE, AUSTRALIA.

Udovicki-Selb, Danilo François. School of Architecture, University of Texas at Austin. Articles contributed to *Encyclopedia of 20th-Century Architecture*: AEG TURBINE FACTORY, BERLIN; FUTURISM; PERRIAND, CHARLOTTE (FRANCE).

Valentine, Maggie. School of Architecture, University of Texas, San Antonio. Articles contributed to *Encyclopedia of 20th-Century Architecture*: LOS ANGELES (CA), UNITED STATES; MOVIE THEATER.

Van Slyck, Abigail A. Department of Architectural Studies, Connecticut College. Articles contributed to *Encyclopedia of 20th-Century Architecture*: LIBRARY; PHOENIX PUBLIC LIBRARY, ARIZONA; SCHOOL.

Van Vliet, Willem. College of Architecture and Planning, University of Colorado, Boulder. Articles contributed to *Encyclopedia of 20th-Century Architecture*: ORDINANCES: ZONING; PUBLIC HOUSING.

Van Vynckt, Randall J. Author, Chicago. Articles contributed to *Encyclopedia of 20th-Century Architecture*: TIMBER FRAME.

Vanderburgh, David J. T. Unité Architecture, Universite Catholique de Louvain, Louvain-la-Neuve, Belgium. Articles contributed to *Encyclopedia of 20th-Century Architecture*: PRISON; TYPOLOGY.

Vinegar, Aron. Department of Art History and Communication Studies, McGill University, Montreal, Canada. Articles contributed to *Encyclopedia of 20th-Century Architecture*: GARNIER, TONY (FRANCE).

Volait, Mercedes. Université François-Rabelais, Tours, France. Articles contributed to *Encyclopedia of 20th-Century Architecture*: CAIRO, EGYPT; GABR, A. LABIB (AFRICA).

Waldheim, Charles. School of Architecture, University of Illinois at Chicago. Articles contributed to *Encyclopedia of 20th-Century Architecture*: ILLINOIS INSTITUTE OF TECHNOLOGY, CHICAGO; O'HARE AIRPORT, CHICAGO; VIETNAM VETERANS MEMORIAL, WASHINGTON, DC.

Walker, Paul. Faculty of Architecture, Building and Planning, University of Melbourne, Australia. Articles contributed to *Encyclopedia of 20th-Century Architecture*: NEW ZEALAND.

Walters, David. College of Architecture, University of North Carolina, Charlotte. Articles contributed to *Encyclopedia of 20th-Century*

Architecture: Città Nuova (1914); Glasgow, Scotland; New Urbanism; Ordinances: Design; Pelli, Cesar (Argentina and United States).

Webb, Bruce. College of Architecture, University of Houston. Articles contributed to *Encyclopedia of 20th-Century Architecture*: Best Products Showroom, Houston; Disney Theme Parks; Motel.

Weiss, Ellen. School of Architecture, Tulane University New Orleans, Louisiana. Articles contributed to *Encyclopedia of 20th-Century Architecture*: Taylor, Robert R. (United States).

Weisser, Amy. Dia Center for the Arts, New York. Articles contributed to *Encyclopedia of 20th-Century Architecture*: Barnes, Edward Larrabee (United States).

Wheeler Borum, Katherine. School of Architecture and Planning, Massachusetts Institute of Technology. Articles contributed to *Encyclopedia of 20th-Century Architecture*: Berlin Philharmonic Concert Hall; Rietveld, Gerrit (Netherlands); Schröder-Schräder House, Utrecht, Netherlands.

White, Jerry. University of California. Articles contributed to *Encyclopedia of 20th-Century Architecture*: Concrete; Eyre, Wilson (United States); Masonry Bearing Wall; Power Plant; Precast Concrete; Reinforced Concrete; Shopping Center.

Whiting, Sarah. Faculty of Architecture, Harvard University. Articles contributed to *Encyclopedia of 20th-Century Architecture*: Eisenman, Peter (United States); Goldberg, Bertrand (United States).

Wiederspahn, Peter H. Department of Architecture, Northeastern University, Boston. Articles contributed to *Encyclopedia of 20th-Century Architecture*: Chareau, Pierre (France); Maison de Verre, Paris.

Williams, Celeste. College of Architecture, University of Houston, Texas. Articles contributed to *Encyclopedia of 20th-Century Architecture*: Himmelb(l)au, Coop (Austria); Czech, Hermann (Austria).

Wilson, Christopher. Faculty of Art, Design and Architecture, Bilkent University, Ankara, Turkey. Articles contributed to *Encyclopedia of 20th-Century Architecture*: Berlin Wall, Berlin; Casa Malaparte, Capri; Philadelphia (PA), United States; Railroad Station; Royal Institute of British Architects.

Wilson, Richard Guy. School of Architecture, University of Virginia, Charlottesville. Articles contributed to *Encyclopedia of 20th-Century Ar-

chitecture: Schindler, Rudolph M. (Austria and United States); United States.

Windsor, Alan. Author, London, England. Articles contributed to *Encyclopedia of 20th-Century Architecture*: Behrens, Peter (Germany); Le Corbusier (Jeanneret, Charles-Édouard) (France); Paris, France; Voysey, Charles F.A. (England).

Wiseman, Carter. Author, Westport, Connecticut. Articles contributed to *Encyclopedia of 20th-Century Architecture*: Cram, Ralph Adams (United States); Cret, Paul Philippe (United States); Goodhue, Bertram Grosvenor (United States); Hood, Raymond (United States); Pei, I.M. (United States).

Wojtowicz, Robert. Department of Art, Old Dominion University, Norfolk, Virginia. Articles contributed to *Encyclopedia of 20th-Century Architecture*: Mumford, Lewis (United States).

Wroble, Lisa A. Author, Plymouth, Michigan. Articles contributed to *Encyclopedia of 20th-Century Architecture*: American Institute of Architects; Gaudí, Antoni (Spain); Terrazzo.

Young, Victoria. Department of Art History, University of St. Thomas, St. Paul, Minnesota. Articles contributed to *Encyclopedia of 20th-Century Architecture*: Predock, Antoine (United States); U.S. Air Force Chapel, Colorado Springs.

Young, William H. Department of American Studies, Lynchburg College, Lynchburg, Virginia. Articles contributed to *Encyclopedia of 20th-Century Architecture*: American Foursquare.

Zabel, Craig. Department of Art History, Pennsylvania State University, University Park. Articles contributed to *Encyclopedia of 20th-Century Architecture*: Flatiron Building, New York.

Zapatka, Christian. Architect and author, Washington, DC. Articles contributed to *Encyclopedia of 20th-Century Architecture*: Agrest, Diana, and Mario Gandelsonas (United States); Graves, Michael (United States).

Zipf, Catherine W. Independent scholar, San Francisco, California. Articles contributed to *Encyclopedia of 20th-Century Architecture*: Arts and Crafts Movement; Feng Shui; Huxtable, Ada Louise (United States); Imperial Hotel, Tokyo.

Zygas, K. Paul. School of Architecture, Arizona State University, Tempe. Articles contributed to *Encyclopedia of 20th-Century Architecture*: Leonidov, Ivan Ilich (Russia).

INDEX

Note: Main encyclopedia entries are indicated by **bold** type. Figures are indicated by *italicized* type. Plates are indicated by the letters *i* (Volume 1), *ii* (Volume 2), and *iii* (Volume 3). Plates can be found in the middle of each volume.

Aalto, Alvar, **1–4**; acoustical ray tracing diagrams, 11; churches by, 256; comparison with Blomstedt, 148; Finnish Pavilion (1956), 1398; industrial town planning, 435; influence in Denmark, 354, 355; influence in United Kingdom, 1362; Jyväskylä Workers' Club, 1, 460, *461*; Massachusetts Institute of Technology, Baker dormitory, 2, 159, 207; Paimio Sanatorium, 517, **967–69**, 1469; relation with environmental issues, 410; relation with William Wurster, 1459; renovations to his works, 574; Sunila Pulp Mill, *2ii*; town halls by, 265; Turun Sanomat Newspaper Building, 461; use of wood, 1449; Villa Mairea, 2, 438, 937, **1414–16**; work in Finland, 462; work in Helsinki, 601, 602

Abbott, Berenice, 60

Abby Aldrich Rockefeller Sculpture Garden, 893, 897

Abdelhalim, Abdelhalim I., Cultural Park for Children in Cairo, *202*, 203

Abdul Raouf Hasan Khalil Museum, *710*

Abraham, Raimund, **4–5**

Abramovitz, Max. *See* Harrison and Abramovitz

abstract art, 5–6

abstraction, **5–7**; in domestic architecture, 656; importance to modernism, 860; Kazuyo Sejima's works, 1194; Richard Neutra's work, 918

Abstract Modernism in United States, 1368

Abteiberg Municipal Museum, **7–9**, *8*, 635, 1049

Abuja, Federal Capital Territory of Nigeria, **9–10**; design model, *10*

Academic Bookshop in Helsinki, 602

Academic Bookstore in Stockholm, 574

acoustics, **10–12**; Aalto's ceilings, 1, 2; Berlin Philharmonic Concert Hall, 143

adaptive re-use, **12–14**; awards for, 25; Boston, 160; of convents, by Fernando Tàvora, 1308; Cummins Engine Company building, 282; Ellis Island, 1336; factory to recreation center, 150–51; Fiat Works (Turin), 1012; Gasometers in Vienna, 307–8; by Giancarlo De Carlo, 345; Glass Palace, 1103; Grand Rapids Art Museum, 42; Paris, 979; projects in Chile, 248; railroad station buildings, 1078; Rovaniemi Art Museum, 972; Tate Gallery of Modern Art, 607; timber buildings, 1327; warehouses, 1433

Addis-Ababa, 191

additive architecture principle, 1385

adhesives, 406, 407; mortar, 819

Adler, Dankmar. *See* Adler and Sullivan

Adler, David, **14–16**

Adler and Sullivan, 1275; Auditorium Building, Chicago, 11, 655, 1275; Kaehilath Anshe Ma'ariv Synagogue, *1297*

adobe, 383, 385

Advanced Factory Units, 558–59

AEG Turbine Factory, **17–18**, *18*, 269, 1243

aeronautical forms: Air Force Academy Chapel, Colorado Springs, 256; Ciudad Universitaria auditorium, Caracas, 268; Kansai International Airport Terminal, 727–29; Lyon-Satolas Station for Lyon Airport, 1078; TWA terminal in New York City, 1150

Africa. *See* Northern Africa; Southern and Central Africa; West Africa

African American architects, 1309, 1310, 1442

African architects, 19, 193

Afrocentricity, 25

Aftimos, Yousif, 129

Aga Khan Award, **25–26**; impact on Northern Africa, 21. *See also* Pritzker Architecture Prize

Agrest, Diana, 454, 678. *See also* Agrest and Gandelsonas

Agrest and Gandelsonas, **26–29**, *1i*

agricultural buildings, **29–30**; as models for country clubs, 319; in Wright's Broadacre City, 177. *See also* grain elevators

Ahmedabad, India, **30–32**; Balkrishna Doshi's projects, 367; Entrepreneurship Development Institute, **407–8**; Indian Institute of Management, **676–77**

AIA (American Institute of Architects). *See* American Institute of Architects (AIA)

air circulation. *See* heating, ventilation, and air conditioning (HVAC)

airfield design, 33

air-inflated structures, 1265

airports and aviation buildings, **32–35**, 1462; as nonplaces, 1278; use of concrete shells, 296

Alamar, 331

Alamillo Bridge, 203

Alcoa Building, 40, 590, 935, 1212

Alexandra Road complex, 788

al-Faisaliah Center, *1170*

Algeria, 19, 20

Al-Ghadir Mosque, *688*

Algiers, Le Corbusier's plan for, 21

al-Kindi Plaza in Riyadh, 1169

Allgemeine Elektricitäts Gesesells (AEG). *See* AEG Turbine Factory

Alliance Française, 938

Alliance Franco-Sénéfalaise, **35–36**; exterior, *36*, *1i*

All India Handloom Board Pavilion, 314–15

Alls Souls Church (Abraham Lincoln Center), 1453

All-Star Sports and Music Resorts, 67–68

Alpine Architecture (Taut), 426

Al-Sharq Waterfront in Kuwait City, *63*

Altamira Building, 215

Altera Art Gallery, 1323

Alter Palmero Plaza towers, 816

Alton West, 788

Altounian, Mardiros, 129

Aluar Housing Project, 816

Aluminaire House, **36–38**, *38–39*, 474; exterior, *37*

aluminum, **38–40**; facade details, 1045; Otto Wagner's use of aluminum pins, 1429; space frames, 1233; use in Berlin Philharmonic Concert Hall, 142; use in Getty Museum, 498; use

aluminum (continued)
  in U.S. Air Force Academy Chapel, 1382. *See also* Aluminaire
    House
Aluminum City Terrace townhouse, *169*
Alvarado Palace, 164
Álvarez, Augusto H., 844
Alvarez, Mario Roberto, **40–41**, 66
Alvorada Palace, 449
al-Wakil, Abd al-Wahid, 883
Ambasz, Emilio, **41–43**
American Academy in Rome, *825*
American Foursquare, **43–45**. *See also* bungalows; ranch houses; row
    houses
American Hotel, 47
American influence: Cairo, 201–2, 203; Caracas, 215–16; Chile,
    247; Denmark, 354; on European architecture, 274; Germany,
    496; Japan, 670; London, 789; Montreal, 866; New Zealand,
    932; Shanghai, 241; on Swedish architecture, 1257; Turkey, 1351
American Institute of Architects (AIA), 389, 679; **45–46;** Climate
    Control Project, 271; "Guidelines for Architectural Design
    Competitions," 284; national headquarters, *46;* reaction to
    prefabrication, 39
American modernism: Aluminaire House, 38; Sullivan's prescription
    for, 1453
American Pharmaceutical Association Building, 1038
American Radiator Building, 647; exterior, *648*
American Shingle style, *1186*
American Spirit of Architecture (Hamlin), 585
American University of Cairo, Desert Research Center, 444
American Vitruvius: An Architects' Handbook of Civic Art
    (Hegemann), 597
Amstel Bridge, 135
Amsterdam, Netherlands, **46–49;** Eigen Haard Housing Estate,
    392–93; Open-Air School, **953–55**
Amsterdam School, **49–50**, 346, 912–13. *See also* De Stijl
Amsterdam Stock Exchange, 135, 171
amusement parks, **50–52**
"analogous architecture," 1133
Anderson, William Pierce. *See* Graham, Anderson, Probst, and
    White
Ando, Tadao, **52–55**, 740; Chapel of the Sea, 259; Church of the
    Light, 293; Church on the Water, **258–59;** Theater on the
    Water, 259; use of concrete, 293; work in Tokyo, 1331
Andreu, Paul, 251, 540
Anglo-Palestine Bank in Jerusalem, 836
Anthony House, 823
Anthroposophical movement, 1284
anti-architecture groups, 57–58
Antonakakis, Dimitris and Suzana, 550
apartment building complexes: Alison and Peter Smithson's
    innovations, 1361; Byker Wall, 412; futurist, *261;* Les Espaces
    D'Abraxas, 152–53; St. Petersburg (Leningrad), 1236, 1237,
    1238; Vancouver, 1390
Apartment Building Petrusgasse, 339
apartment buildings, **55–57**, 473; in Brussels, 179; high-rise, 55
Apartment House in Moscow, *507*
Apartments, Mercatorplein, *913*
Aquapolis, 839
arcades, Las Vegas Fremont Street, 751

archaeological projects: Northern Africa, 21; Society for Commercial
    Archaeology, 1118
Archbishopric Museum, 451
arches: AEG Turbine Factory, 17,18; by Antoni Gaudí, 487, 488;
    AT&T Building, 85; Egyptian architecture, 390; Gateway Arch
    (St. Louis), **486–87;** Gateway to the West, 1149; Grande Arche
    de la Défense, **540–42;** Helsinki Railway Station, 604, 605; India
    Gate, 920; Shekhtel's multistoried, 1202; steel truss system, 1264.
    See also memorials
Archigram, **57–58**, 306, 789, 1361, 1362; comparison with
    Metabolists, 839
Architect, The: Reconstructing Her Practice (Hughes), 454
Architectural Design magazine, 469
architectural drawing, **58–59**; Auguste Choisy's technique, 252;
    futurist examples, *261;* Hugh Ferriss's technique, 457; by Mario
    Gandelsonas, 28; by Morphosis, 877; by Paul Rudolph, 1142; by
    Raimund Abraham, 4; and representation, 1097; Steven Holl's
    diagrams, 634. *See also* computer-aided design
architectural photography, **59–61**, 1097
architectural technology, 389. *See also* technology
architectural theories: Adolf Loos, 790–91; Agrest and Gandelsonas,
    28; Bernard Tschumi, 1346–47; Colin St. John Wilson, 1445–46;
    "de-architecture," 145; Hermann Czech, 338; Herzog and de
    Meuron, 1108; Jørn Utzon's additive principle, 1385; Josep Puig i
    Cadafalch, 1072; Julien Gaudet, 568; Mario Blomstedt, 148–49;
    Peter Collins' history of, 275; Raimund Abraham, 4–5; Sigfried
    Giedion, 97–98; Talbot Faulkner Hamlin, 585; Venturi and Scott
    Brown's, 1183–84; Vittorio Gregotti's influence on, 554–55; Wu
    Liangyong's "new regionalism," 1457
architecture: as an "affair of the elite," 635; as communal art form,
    1072; as dramatic backdrop for life, 1208; as language, 1043,
    1048, 1049; as a natural organism, 1044; "of silence," 602–3; as
    "society of rooms," 723–24; as vehicle for social change, 933
Architecture: Nineteenth and Twentieth Centuries (Hitchcock), 625
Architecture and Feminism, 454
Architecture and Nature movement, 1043
Architecture of the Well Tempered Environment (Banham), 107
Architecture without Architects exhibition, 1402
arcology, 61
Arcosanti, Arizona, **61–62**, 1224, 1225; Crafts III Building, *62*
arctic climate construction, 209, 412
Ardalan, Nader, **62–65**, 689–90
ARDEV (The Architects of Devetsil), 1053
Argentina, **66–67**
Argentina Televisor Color, 815
Argentinian architecture, 1322
Arhus University, 465; Main Building, *354*
Arizona State University, Nelson Fine Arts Center, 1057
Ark, The (London), 412
Arneberg, Arnstein, 939
Arnoff Center for Design and Art, *279, 2i*
ARO Building, *183*
Arquitectonica, **67–69**, 684, 851–52
Arroyo Silo Parkway, 1119
Art Center College of Design in Pasadena, 399
Art Deco, **69–72**, 866; Ali Labib Gabr's use, 481; Argentina, 65;
    Brazil, 165; Buenos Aires, 186; Cairo, 201–2, 202; Chile, 247;
    Chrysler Building, 253; city halls, 264; and Egyptian revival
    styles, 391; Empire State Building lobby, 404; Hong Kong, 641;
    India, 30, 671; Indonesia, 1228; Josef Hoffman's relation with,

629; Los Angeles, 795; Mexico, 843; Miami, Florida, 850, 851; Netherlands, 913; New York City, 927; New Zealand, 932; Northern Africa, 20; ornament, 958; Park Hotel, 982; relation with Art Nouveau, 74; Rio de Janeiro, 1112; Santiago, Chile, 1160; skyscrapers in Boston, 158; United Kingdom, 1360; United States, 1368; use of terracotta, 1318; use of terrazzo, 1320

Arthur Norman House, 89

"artistic will," 17

art moderne. *See* Art Deco

art museums. *See* museums

Art Nouveau (Jugendstil), **72–75**; Argentina, 65; aspect of Einstein Tower, 394; Austria, 91–92; Belgium, 131, 1396; Berlage's opposition to, 136; Bruno Paul's role, 988; Brussels, 178, 970; Cairo, 201; Catalan adaptation, 223; Chile, 247; curvilinear *vs.* rectilinear, 912; Czechoslovakia, 341; Germany, 495; Hungary, 662; influence of primitivism on, 1062; Istanbul, 697; London, 787; Melbourne, 829; Netherlands, 912; New York City, 926; ornament, 958; Palais Stoclet as example, 970; Paris, 840, 977; poster, *73*; Prague, 1053; relation with Expressionism, 425; relation with Glasgow School, 510; relation with Vienna Secession, 1410; Romania, 1129; Russia and Soviet Union, 1145; Switzerland, 1286; in Van Nelle Factory, 1396; Victor Horta's contribution to, 650, 782; Vienna, 970

Arts and Crafts Movement, **75–78**, 1258–59; Australia, 89; Budapest, 185; and environmental issues, 409; Glasgow School relation with, 510; Herbert Baker's domestic work, 102; Hungary, 663; influence on London subway, 1273; influence on Pompidou Center, 1035; London, 787; Melbourne, 829; need for liberation from, 6; Peter Behrens's analysis of, 343; relation with Art Noveau, 72, 73; relation with Prairie School, 1054; relation with primitivism, 1062; relation with regionalism, 1091; Southern and Central Africa, 22; United States, 1366–67; use of timber framing, 1326. *See also* bungalows; Craftsman Style

Arup, Ove, **78–80**

Asahi Beer Hall and Brewery, *1329*

Ashbee, C.R., **80–81**, 343. *See also* Arts and Crafts Movement

Asiad Village, 673–74

Asian architecture, 672

Asian Games Building, 1106

Asilomar Conference Center, 875; Phoebe Apperson Hearst Administration Building, *1091*

Asmussen, Erik, 1284

Aso Hill (Abuja), 9

Asplund, Erik Gunnar, **81–84**, 1257; Gothenburg City Hall Extension, *1283*; influence in Sweden, 1284; Stockholm Public Library, 82, 269, **1255–56**, *7iii*

Association for Organic Architecture, 1467

associations. *See* institutes and associations

Astrodome, 659, 1240

ATC (Argentina Televisora Color) Building, *187*

ATC (Argentina Televisor Color), 815

Atheneum (Meier), 827

Athens Charter, **86–87**, 297

Atlanta, Georgia, works by John C. Portman Jr., 1040

Atlanta, Georgia High Museum of Art, **608–10**

Atlanta, Georgia Merchandise Mart, 1040

Atlántida Church, 362

Atlantis Condominiums, 67

Atlantis in Miami, 684

atmospheric theaters, 890

Atomium (Molecule Building), *420*

atriums. *See also* courtyards in architecture; plazas: Aalto's Academic Bookstore, 574; Academic Bookshop, 602; Ardalan's use of, 64; Asplund's use of, 83; glass, 518; glass-canopied, 84; High Museum of Art, 609; in hotels, 1040–41; Hyatt Regency Hotels, 655; Lever House, 759; multistory, 474; National Gallery of Art, East Building, 906; Old Post Office Building in Washington, D.C., 12; Turkish Historical Society, *1351*; vertical, 571

AT&T Building, **84–86**, 621, 716, 1217; exterior, *85*

Auditorium Annex, Chicago, *633*

Auditorium Building, 655, 1275; acoustics, 11

auditoriums. *See also* concert halls; theaters: Ciudad Universitaria, Caracas, 268

Auev Workers' Club, *527*

Aukrust Museum, 451

Aulenti, Gae, **87–89**; designs for exhibitions, 87; Gare d'Orsay, 12

Austral Group, 65–66

Australia, **89–91**; Art Deco, 70–71; Australian National University, 212–13

Australian architects, 90; work abroad, 90–91

Australian architecture, 1289

Austria, **91–94**

Austrian architecture, 719

Austrian Pavilion for International Exhibition of Decorative Arts in Paris, 629

autobahns, 985

automobiles, **94–97**; effect on house design, 657; effect on storefront window design, 1205; glass used in, 516; impact on regional planning, 1087; impact on restaurants, 1101–2; pavilions at New York World's Fair (1939), 931; place in Voisan Plan for Paris (1925), 1422–23; separation from pedestrians, 304–5; and suburban planning, 1270. *See also* Futurism; gas stations; parking garages; roadway systems; visitor centers

avante-garde, **97–99**; Adolf Loos, 792; Austria, 93; Berlin, 137, 138; Brussels houses and housing development, 178; Church of St. Francis of Assisi, 257–58; Einstein Tower, 393; Hannes Meyer, 848; Heinrich Tessenow, 1321; impact of Bank of London and South America on, 110; Otto Wagner's influence on Central Europe, 1428; Philip Johnson, 715, 716; Robert Mallet-Stevens's role, 814; Rome, 478; Soviet Union, 830

Avenida Bolivar, *216*

Avenue de los Presidentes, El Vedado, *1028*

Avery Fisher Hall, acoustics, 11

Avery Index to Architectural Periodicals, 585

awards, 25–26. *See also* Aga Khan Award; competitions; institutes and associations; Pritzker Architecture Prize; Reynolds Company, 30

azulejos, 973

Babson Stable and Service Building, *1074*

Bacardi and Company buildings, 213

Backer, Lars, 940

Bacon, Henry, Lincoln Memorial, **779–81**

Badovici, Jean, 544

Badran, Rasem, *1114*

Baer, Steve, 410

Bagdad, Iraq, 231

Bagdad Conference Palace, 1209

Bagdad University, 1325

Bagsvaerd Church, 1386

Baiyoke Tower, **101–2**

Bakas, Sergio. *See* Arquitectonica

Baker, Herbert, 22, **102–4**, 1020; relationship with Edwin Lutyens, 801–2; work in New Delhi, 919

Baker School, 23

Balboa Park Tower in San Diego, 532

Bal-Tic-Tac ballroom, 478

Banco de México Building, 845

Bang, Ove, 940

Bangkok, Thailand, **104–7**

Bangladesh College of Arts and Crafts, 360

Bangladesh Polytechnic Institutes, 692

Banham, Peter Reyner, **107–8**, 365, 427, 1223

Bank Austria Client Service Center in Vienna, 340

Bankinter Building, 865

Bank of America Tower, 993, *6ii*

Bank of Buenos Aires Headquarters, 815

Bank of China Tower, **108–10**, 455–56, 992, *1215*

Bank of London and South America, Buenos Aires, **110–11**, 187, 1322

Bank of Mexcio Building in Veracruz, 844

Bank of Montreal, *867*

Bank of the Southwest Tower, 706

banks: banking halls, 415; first in China, 249; by Louis Sullivan, 1276; Philadelphia, 1009; by Purcell and Elmslie, 1074; Toronto, 1334

Banque de Luxembourg's headquarters, 68

Banque du Liban et d'Outre Mer, *129*

Barbican Estate, 788

Barbizon Apartment Hotel, *70*

Barcelona, Spain, **111–14**. *See also* International Exhibition (Barcelona 1929)

Barcelona Anti-Tubercular Dispensary, 1196

Barcelona Chairs, 854

Barcelona School, 113, 1234, 1267

Bardi's Bowl (chair), 151

Barkhin, Grigory, Izvestiia Building, *1147*

Barmou, Falké, Yaama Mosque, **1461–62**

Barnes, Edward Larrabee, **114–16**

Barnes House, 987

barns, 29; as billboards, 30

Baroque style: Brazil, 165, 166; in Christian Norberg-Schulz's works, 936; churches, 254; Memphis Group's innovations, 835

Barr, Alfred H., Jr., 685

Barragán, Luis, **116–18**, 845; Casa Cristo, *117*; Cuadra San Cristóbal, **327–29**, *2i*; relation with environmental issues, 410; use of color, 279

Basel, Switzerland, 361

Bash House, 577

Basil Street Workers Housing, 938

Bass House, 1144

Bastei restaurant, 277

Bauer, Catherine, 1459

Bauhaus, **118–21**, 388, 495; chair, *119*; color theory, 278–79; factories, 433; Henri van de Velde's role, 1396; influence in Israel, 695; influence in Spain, 1234; influence on the Architects Collaborative, 1324; relation with Cubism, 333; relation with International Style, 681, 682, 683; relation with primitivism, 1063; ties with constructivists, 303. *See also* Bauhaus Dessau

Bauhaus Dessau, **121–23**; Hannes Meyer's directorate, 849; Ludwig Mies van der Rohe's relation with, 854; move of Bauhaus to, 120; night view from North, *122*. *See also* Bauhaus

Bavinger House, 523, 1063

Bawa, Geoffrey, **123–25**

Bay Region School (San Francisco, California), 1457

bay windows, 709

beach hotels, by Geoffrey Bawa, 124

beach houses by Paul Rudolph, 1142

beam-and-mast system, 1096

beauty in architecture, 648, 705

Beaux-Arts classicism: ateliers, 388; campus planning, 206, 207; Caracas, 215; department stores, 356; Frank Lloyd Wright's rejection, 1453; impact of New York World's Fair (1939), 929; London, 787; Montreal, 866; New York City, 926–27; Rome, 1131

Beelman, Claude, *793*

Behne, Adolf, 1174

Behnisch, Gunter: Hysolar Research Institute, *1099*; Olympic Games Tent in Munich, *1239, 1240*

Behrens, Peter, **125–28**; AEG Turbine Factory, **17–18**, 269, 1243; curtain-wall system, 433; exhibition buildings, 1439; impact on Düsseldorf, 377; project at International Exhibition of Decorative Arts (Paris 1925), 680; relation with Deutscher Werkbund, 357; Synagogue of Zilina, 1296; time at Darmstadt artists' colony, 343, 344; work in Czechoslovakia, 342; work in Frankfurt, 473

Behrens House, *126*

Beijing, China, 250

Beirut, Lebanon, **128–30**

Beit Nassif, 709

Belém Cultural Centre, 783

Belfort Theater, 944

Belgiojoso, Lodovico B. di, 1337

Belgium, **130–32**; Art Nouveau (Jugendstil), 1396; Social Democratic Workers' Party headquarters, 73

Belo Horizonte, Brazil: Church of St. Francis of Assisi, **257–58**; Pampulha Buildings, **973–74**

Benedictine Monastery in Las Condes Santiago de Chile, 248

Benetton Factory, **134–35**

Benevolo, Leonardo, **132–34**, 623, 624

Ben Franklin Parkway, *1008*, 1009

Benjamin, Walter, 98

Benjamin Franklin's "house" and museum, 1400

Benjamin Henry Latrobe (Hamlin), 585

Bennett, Edward H., 1018; Plan of Chicago, 1379, 1380

Bentley Wood, 1326

Bergpolder, 1136

Berlage, Hendrik Petrus, **135–37**, 912; Amsterdam Stock Exchange, 171; Apartments, Mercatorplein, *913*; Bourse, 47; influence on European architecture, 372; Plan for Amsterdam South, 47; relation with Amsterdam School, 49; tectonics, 1313

Berlin, Germany, **137–42**. *See also* Berlin wall; AEG Turbine Factory, **17–18**, 269, 1243; housing projects by Bruno Taut, 1306; Reichstag, **1092–95**; Universum Cinema, **1375–76**; Werner Hegemann's writings on, 597

Berlin architects, 138

Berlin National Gallery, 854

Berlin Philharmonie, **142–44**, 1176; acoustics, 11, 143; exterior, *143*

Berlin Wall, 140–41, **144–45**

Berman House, 1192

Bernhard, Karl, 17

Best Products Showroom, **145–46**; exterior, *146*

Beth Shalom Synagogue (Wright), 1297, 1455

Beverly Hills Hotel, 1443

Bianchi House, 161

Biedermeier Revival, 1248

Big Duck, The, *1117*, 1118

Bijlmermeer, 48

Bijvoet, Bernard, 373

Bill, Max, 1424

Binet, René, 424

Bingham House, 822

Bioclimatic Chart, 271

Birkerts, Gunnar, **146–48**

black brick, 647

black colleges, 388

Blacker House, 552

Black Mountain College plan, 207

Blair House, 14

Bloemenwerf, 130, 1396

Blomstedt, Aulis, **148–50**, 462, 463–64

Bò Bardi, Lina, **150–52**, 167

Boccaro, Charles, *20*

Boccioni, Umberto, 394

Bodley, George, 1433

Bofill, Ricardo, **152–54**, 621, 1049, 1258

Bogardus, James, 1060

Bohigas Guardiola, Oriol, 113, 114

Böhm, Dominikus, *277*, 278

Böhm, Gottfried, **154–55**; church design, 256; Pilgrimage Church at Neviges, **1015–16**

Boley Building, 516

Bolt, Beranek and Newman, 11

bond patterning, 819

Bonet, Pep, 1266

Boots Pure Drugs Factory, **155–56**, 1442

Boston, Massachusetts, **158–60**; high-tech corridor on Route 128, 386; urban development, 1377

Boston City Hall, **156–58**, 159, 265; competition, 285–86; *exterior*, 157

Boston Government Services Center, 1144

Boston Public Library, 158, *771*

Boston Symphony Hall, 11

Botta, Mario, **160–63**, 1287

Bourne End, 298

Bourne-White, Margaret, 60

Bourse, 47

Bouwma, S.J., 913

bow windows, 1425, 1426

Boyd, Robin, 90, 830

Brandstron, Howard, 775

Brasília, **163–65**; impact on Rio de Janerio, 1112; Niemeyer's role, 934; Rino Levi's proposal for, 761. *See also* Federal Capital Complex, Brasília

Braun Headquarters, 1254

Brazil, 40, **165–68**; Church of St. Francis of Assisi, **257–58**

Brazilian architects, 165

Brazilian architecture, 318, 569, 973

Brazilian influence: on African architecture, 24; on Israel architects, 695–96

Brazilian Pavilion at New York World's Fair (1939), 931, 934

Breuer, Marcel, **167–70**, *1137*; Bauhaus chair, 119; Black Mountain College plan, 207; relation with International Style, 682; Whitney Museum of American Art, *1260*

brick, **170–73**; Aalto's use of, 2; apparently collapsing, 145; Behren's use of, 127; Berlage's use of, 135; black, 647; curtain walls, 337; Dutch varieties, 912; glass bricks, 229; Holland brick, 14; Michel de Klerk's use of, 392; reinforced, 362; at Tuskegee Institute, 1310; use in Expressionism, 426; use in United Kingdom, 1362; white, 647

bridges: Amstel, 135; by E. Owen Williams, 1442; glass, 237; Paolo Soleri's drawings, 1225; by Robert Maillart, 808; by Santiago Calatrava, 203–4; Seville, 422; truss systems, 1264

Brief History of Ancient Chinese City Planning, A (Wu Liangyong), 1457

Briley, Jenifer. *See* Arquitectonica

Brinkman, Johannes Andreas, 1136; Van Nelle Factory, Rotterdam, **1394–96**

Brion-Vega Tomb and Cemetery, 1172; Chapel, *1172*; entrance and meditation pavilion, *1173*

British architects, 155–56, 180; Archigram, 57

British architecture, 1220

British influence: Cairo, 201; New Zealand, 932

British Library, **173–75**, 1445; exterior, *174*

British Museum, Great Court, *467, 468, 6i*

British Pavilion at Expo '92, 559

Broadacre City, **175–78**, 1378–79, 1454–55; map of regional layout, *177*; model, *176*

Broadgate, 789

Bronx River Parkway, 985

Bronx Zoo, African Habitat, 935

Brooklyn Institute of Arts and Sciences, 824

Brown Decades, The (Mumford), 891

Bruder, Will, Phoenix Public Library, **1010–12**

Brunei, 1230

Brussels, Belgium, **178–80**; L'Innovation Department Store, **781–82**

Brussels Exposition (1958), 416, **419–20**

Brutalism, **180–82**; Alan Colquhoun's relation with, 280; Argentina, 66; Australia, 90; Boston City Hall design, 157; Brasília Federal Capital Complex, 449; Canberra, 213; Israel, 697; London, 788; of Marcel Breuer, 169; Netherlands, 914; New Zealand, 932; Oswald Mathias Ungers's work, 1357; Paul Rudolph's relation with, 1142; Peter and Alison Smithson's works, 1220; of Peter Reyner Banham, 107; relation with primitivism, 1063; Southern and Central Africa, 24; that used brick, 172; United Kingdom, 1361; United States, 1368; use of concrete, 293; Yugoslavia, 1465–66

Bryant Park, 1027

Bryggman, Erik, 461, 462

Bucharest, Romania, **182–84**

Buck House, 1177

Budapest, Hungary, **184–86**

Buenos Aires, Argentina, **186–88**; Agrest and Gandelsonas apartment buildings, 28; Olivetti Factory, **951–52**

Buenos Aires Airport proposal, 1440–41

building demolition. *See* demolition

building envelopes, thin-skin, 1150

building materials: sustainability and sustainable architecture: at Chicago World's Fair (1933), 230; and climate, 272; computer quantification of, 288; Dutch, 50; effect on house design, 657; and energy-efficient design, 405; Finnish, 601; "green," 1280; Hans Poelzig's symbolic use of, 1031; Hassan II Mosque minaret, 592, 593; James Stewart Polshek's use of metal, 1033; Kazuyo Sejima's innovative use, 1194; light-emitting surfaces, 775; Middle Eastern, 709; Renzo Piano's experiments, 1012; responses to light, 522; semiprecious stones, 972; symbolism, 1288; used by Frank Lloyd Wright, 669; used by Itsuko Hasegawa, 590; used by Tadao Ando, 52–53; used in Expressionism, 426; used in prefabrication, 1060. *See also* locally available materials use

buildings, companionability among, 169, 174, 541, 906, 968, 1176. *See also* sites, compatibility with buildings

Buildings of England series (Pevsner), 1006

built-in furniture, 1181

bungalows, 96, **188–89**; Australian, 89; California, 188; Los Angeles, 794; Midwestern, 188; origins of, 920. *See also* American Foursquare; ranch houses; row houses

Bunshaft, Gordon, **189–91**; Hirshhorn Museum, 190, 1213, 1369, *1434*, 1435; Lever House, 190, 518, 596, **759–60**, 928, 1212, 1216–17; National Commercial Bank Headquarters, 710; work in United States, 1369

Bureaux d'Etudes Henri Chomette, **191–93**

Bürger, Peter, 97, 98

Burle Marx, Roberto, **193–94**

Burnham, Daniel Hudson, **194–98**, 534, 1008, 1228; Flatiron Building, **466–67**, 1318; Monadnock Building, 171, 391, 819; Plan of Chicago, 1018, 1379, 1380; Wanamaker Store, **1430–32**; World's Columbian Exposition (Chicago 1893), 262

bus terminals, **198–99**; Art Deco, 71; platform design, 198; relationship with rail stations, 198, 199

Byker Wall, 412, *413*, 1048

Byzantine Museum in Thessaloniki, *549*

Byzantine Revival style in synagogues, 1296

cable nets, 960

cable-suspended systems, 1264

Caesar's Palace, 750

Cafe Aubette, 349

Cafe Museum in Vienna, 791

Cairo, Egypt, 19, 20, 21, **201–2**

Calatrava, Santiago, **202–4**, 1235; bridges for Expo 1992, 422; church design, 255; Gare Do Oriente, 783, *784, 785*; Lyon-Satolas Station for Lyon Airport, 1078

Caldwell, Alfred, 668

California, Craftsman style, 322

California chic homes, 399

"California style" architects, 490

Calthorpe, Peter, 922

Cambridge, England: city center, 412; Schlumberger Cambridge Research Center, **1178–79**

Campo Volantin Footbridge, *204*

camps for children, 114

"camp" style, 1143

campus planning, **205–8**; Australia, 212–13; Belgium, 132; Boston, Massachusetts, 159; by Cass Gilbert, 502; International Style, 1381; by Joan Edelman Goody, 533; by Ralph Adams Cram, 323; by Wallace K. Harrison, 589

Canada, **208–11**

Canada chancery in Berlin, 401

Canada Place, 1390

Canadian architects, 208

Canadian architecture, 987, 988

Canadian Clay and Glass Gallery, 987

Canberra, Australia, **211–13**; Plan, **1016–18**

Candela, Félix, **213–15**; church design, 255; first shell building, 267; use of concrete shells, 296

"Can Lis," 1386

Cansever, Turgut, *1351*

Cape Dutch Revival, 22

Cape Town, South Africa, 102

capital cities: Abuja, **9–10**; Basília, **163–65**; Canberra, **1016–18**; Caracas, **215–17**; Chandigarh, India, **235–36**; New Delhi, **919–20**, **1019–21**; Sher-e-Banglanagar complex, **902–4**; in Southern and Central Africa, 25

Capitalism's impact on architecture: along with architectural photography, 60; antagonism with high culture, 17; in China, 982; Garden City Movement, 1271; Manfedo Tafuri's writings on, 1299; Plan of Chicago, 1019; roadside architecture, 1116; skyscrapers, 1004; Thailand, 106; Turkey, 1353; utopian plan of Global City, 1384

Capitol Park, 1218

Capitol Theatre in Melbourne, 557

Capotesta houses, 1323

Capri, 221

Caracas, Venezuela, **215–17**; Ciudad Universitaria, **267–69**

Cardiff Bay Opera House, 581

carioca school, 1112

Carlo Felice Theater in Genoa, 1134

Carlyle Hotel, *851*

Carnegie Hall Tower, 993–94

Carnegie Libraries, 771

Carpenter Center for the Visual Arts, 159, *310*

Carrère and Hastings, **217–19**, 975

Carson Pirie Scott Store, **219–21**, 1276; exterior, *220*

Carter House, *556*

Cartier Museum, 942; exterior, *943*

Casa Agustí, 112

Casa Albert Lleó i Morera, *112*

Casa Antoni Amatller, 1071, 1072; detail, *1071*

Casa Astrea, 874

Casa Batllo, *488*

Casablanca, 20, 21; Hassan II Mosque, **592–94**

Casa Cristo, *117*

Casa de les Punxes, 1072

Casa del Fascio, 1318, *1319*

Casa Girasole, Rome, 874, *874*

Casa Malaparte, **221–23**, 768, *4i* interior, *222*

Casa Martí, 1071

Casa Milà, **223–25**; exterior, *223, 224, 5i*

Casa Regás and Belvedere Giorgina, 1267

Casa Rotunda, 162

Casa Terrades, 1072

Casa Ugalde, 273

Casa Vittoria, Isla de Pantelleria, 1267

Case Study Houses, 381, 795, 1244

CASFPI tower, 816

Casio del Fascio, 443

Castel Beranger, *959*

Castilla-León Congress Center, 908

cast iron. *See also* cast steel: spheroidal graphite, 1096

Castle Hill, 14

castles, adaptive reuse, 13

"castle" style of Edwin Lutyens, 801

cast steel, 1035

Catalan architects, 273, 857, 1195

Catalan architecture, 111, 1071

Catalan craft revival, 224

Catalan (Guastavino) vaults, 111, 224, **225–26**

Catalan modernisme, 111

"Cathedral of Commerce, The," 1450

Cathedral of St. John the Divine, 255

CBS Building. *See* Columbia Broadcasting System Headquarters

Cedars-Sinai Comprehensive Cancer Clinic, 878

Celebration, Florida, **226–27**, 1272

cement, 290; white, 911. *See also* concrete

Cement Hall at Swiss National Exhibition (1939), 809

cemeteries, 858; by Sigurd Lewerentz, 764, 765. *See also* Brion-Vega
    Tomb and Cemetery

Cemetery of San Cataldo, 1134

Centraal Beheer Insurance offices, 605–6, 946

Central European architecture, 730

Central Institute of Educational Technology, *1107*

Central Post Office of Paris, 568

Central Station of Stuttgart, 1268

Central University Campus in Caracas, 215

Centro Escolar Benito Juarez, 947

Centrust Tower, 852

Century of Progress Exposition (Chicago 1933), **229–31**, *230*, 242

CEPAL (Comisión Económica Para America Latina), 247–48

Ceramica Artistica Solimene, 1225

Chadirji, Rifat, **231–34**

chairs: Barcelona Chairs, 854; Bardi's Bowl, 151; Bauhaus, *119*;
    Marcel Breuer cantilevered, 168; Superleggera, 1038

Chame-Chame House, 151

Chandigarh, India, **235–36**

Changing Ideals in Modern Architecture, 1750–1950 (Collins), 622

Channel 4 Headquarters, London, **236–37**; windows, *236*

"Chaos and Machine" (Shinohara), 1204

Chapel of Capuchinas Sacramentarias, 327

Chapel of Notre-Dame-du-Haut, **237–39**, 256; exterior, *238*

Chapel of St. Ignatius in Seattle, Washington, 634

Chapel of the Sea, 259

Chareau, Pierre, **239–40**; Maison De Verre, **810–11**

Charles Lang Freer House, 431

Charter of the New Urbanism, 922

Chassagne stone, 68

Chassé Theatre in Breda, 606

Château d'Eau, 424

Château style, 210

Chatterjee, Sris Chandra, 672

Checkhov Museum, 1202

Chemosphere House, 795

Chen, Zhi, **240–41**

Chermayeff, Serge, 1326

Cheung Kong Centre, 642

Chiado National Gallery, 784

Chiat/Day in Venice, 490

Chicago, Illinois, **241–44**; Carson Pirie Scott Store, **219–21**;
    Century of Progress Exposition (1933), **229–31**; Daniel Hudson
    Burnham's work in, 195; Plan of 1909, 196–97, 242, 263, **1018–
    19**; Postmodernism, 246; Sears Tower, **1188–89**; urban
    development, 1378. *See also* Chicago School

Chicago Board of Trade, 630

Chicago Convention Hall, 1346

Chicago Daily News Building, 242, 630

Chicago Exposition (1933–34), 416

Chicago School, **244–46**, 632; influence in Chile, 247; skyscrapers,
    1215

"Chicago Style" skyscrapers, 1199

Chicago Tribune Competition. *See* Tribune Tower International
    Competition (Chicago 1922)

Chicago window, 244, 632

Chick House, 822

Children's Home in Amsterdam, 428

Chile, **246–49**

Chilean architecture, 248

Chile House, 426

China, **249–51**

Chinese architects, 250, 269, 992. *See also* feng shui

Chinese architecture, 241, 642–43, 765, 1198, 1456

"Chippendale" skyscraper, 84, *85*

Chocolate Factory in Blois, 943

Choisy, Auguste, **251–52**

Choy, Jose Antonio, 331

Chrysler Building, **252–54**, 927, 1216; competition with Empire
    State Building, 403

churches, **253–57**; Art Deco, 70; Brasília, 934; China, 249;
    Cologne, Germany, 277–78; Cuba, 330; Denmark, 355; by
    Eladio Dieste, 362; Finland, 463; by Gottfried Böhm, 154; in
    Muurame (Alvar Aalto), 1; by Prairie School architects, 1054;
    Southern and Central Africa, 24; Sweden, 1285; by Tadeo Ando,
    53–54

Church in Rárósmulyad, 826

Church of Saint-Joseph in Le Havre, 755

Church of St. Francis of Assisi, **257–58**, 974

Church of St. Leopold am Steinhof, *1428*

Church of the Holy Spirit in Ottakring, 1029

Church of the Light, 53–54, 293

Church of the Sagrada Familia, 489

Church of the Virgen de la Medalla Milagroso, 214

Church on the Water, **258–59**

CIAM (Congrès Internationaux de l'Architecture Moderne). *See*
    Congrès Internationaux de l'Architecture Moderne (CIAM)

Çinici, Behruz and Can, Mosque of the Grand National Assembly,
    884–86

circulation. *See* paths of movement

Cirici, Cristian, 1266

Cité de Circulation, 1391

Cité de Refuge, 517

Cité Industrielle, Une, **259–60**

Citicorp Center, 684

Cities and the Wealth of Nations (Jacobs), 703

Citrohan House, 366

Città Nuova, **260–62**

City, The (Park), 1380

City Beautiful Movement, **262–64**; application to shopping centers,
    1205; Ben Franklin Parkway, 1009; and campus planning, 206;

City Beautiful Movement (continued)
Cass Gilbert's involvement in, 502; influence on Seaside, Florida, 1190; relation with urban renewal, 1380; United States, 1366; use in colonial capitals, 919; Vancouver, 1389. *See also* memorials

city centers; Ahmedabad, India, 30; Athens Charter position on, 86; Beirut, 130; Cambridge, England, 412; Glasgow, 514; Hilberseimer's approach to, 613; Ho Chi Minh City, 1230. *See also* redevelopment projects

"City for 10 Million People," 839

City for Three Million Inhabitants. *See* Contemporary City for Three Million Inhabitants

city halls, **264–66**; Denmark, 354; plaza design near, 1027–28. *See also* Boston City Hall; Toronto City Hall

City in History, The (Mumford), 891

city planning. *See* urban planning

City Planning: Housing (Hegemann), 598

Ciudad Universitaria, Caracas, **267–69**

Ciudad Universitaria Campus and Stadium, Mexico City, **266–67**

Civic Center, Bucharest, 184

Civic Opera Building, 535

Civil Government Offices in Tarragona, 1226

Civil Rights Memorial in Montgomery, 776, 777

cladding, 170; AT&T Building, 84, 85; brick, 171, 172; brick and steel, 172; copper, 607; on Getty Museum, 498; plastic, 1022; porcelain-enameled steel panels, 1117; purpose of thin skin, 594; relation to curtain-wall system, 335; Shanghai World Financial Center, 1198; steel, 1246; stone, 1259; stone veneer *vs.* brick, 172; terra cotta, 135; theories of, 629; titanium, 571

Clark House, *15*, 1459

Clark/Maple Gasoline Service Station, 525

Clason, Isak Gustaf, 1256

Classicism, **269–70**; Asplund's motifs, 81–82; Auguste Choisy's writings, 252; Australia, 89; Bucharest, 184; Cairo, 202; churches, 254; of Daniel Hudson Burham, 197; effect of Sant'Elia's drawings on, 262; Finland, 460; Gio Ponti's use of, 1036; Joseph Maria Odbrich's move towards, 950; in Kenzo Tange's works, 989; Nordic, 601; Norway, 939; Robert Stern's affinity for, 1248; Southern and Central Africa, 22; synagogues, 1296; in Tony Garnier's work, 483, 484; at Tuskegee Institute, 1310; in works of Cass Gilbert, 502

classroom acoustics, 11

claustra walls, 35

Cleveland, Ohio, Plan, 263

Cleveland Terminal Group buildings, 534

client-centered architects, 590; James Stewart Polshek, 1033; Richard Neutra, 918

climate, **270–73**; and construction in United Kingdom, 1362; global changes in, 272; housing experiments by Coderch, 273; relation with site, 1440, 1441; and use of Mediterranean architecture in Finland, 462. *See also* arctic climate construction; desert climate construction; wind pressure design

climate control, 46; Bauhaus, Dessau, 121; Benetton Factory, 135; British library, London, 174–75; with canvas, 1301; indigenous methods of, 1404; relation with curtain walls, 336; at Rocky Mountain Institute, 1281; shopping centers, 1205; stadiums, 1240; street with, 1335; telescope temperature control, 1213; U.S. Embassy in New Delhi, 1262; using patios, 813. *See also* energy-efficient design; heating, ventilation, and air conditioning (HVAC); solar architecture

Clotet, Lluis, 1266

clubhouse designs, 320; by McKim, Mead and White, 824; by Stepanovich Melnikov, 831

"cluster" blocks, 753

CNIT, Palais des Expositions, 979

CNU (Congress for the New Urbanism), 369

Cobb, Henry Ives, 206

Coca-Cola Bottling Plant in Los Angeles, 795

Cocoon, 1142

Cocoon House, 1166

Coderch y de Sentmenat, José Antonio, 112, 113, **273–74**

Cogan Residence, 578

Cohen, Jean-Louis, **274–75**

Colisee buildings in Nimes, *738*

Collage City (Rowe and Koetter), 306

Collins, Peter, **275–76**, 622

Cologne, Germany, **276–78**

Colonial Revival, 1085; United States, 1366

colored concrete, 361

color photography, 60

colors, **278–80**; adding to concrete, 291, 292; Baiyoke Towers, 101; Bruno Taut's urban design with, 1306; Frank Gehry's use of, 491; Hassan II Mosque, 593; Josep Lluis Sert's use of, 1196; Luis Barragán's use of, 116, 845; Portland Public Services Building, 1040; Susana Torre's use of, 1336; Theo van Doesburg's use of, 1391; use at Fagus Werk, 436; use at gas stations, 485; use at Panama-Pacific International Exposition in San Francisco, 975; use at Schröoder-Schräder House, 1182; use by Gwathmey and Siegel, 577, 578; use by Ralph Erskine, 412; used at Weissenhofsiedlung (Stuttgart 1927), 1437; used by Glasgow School, 510; use for structural balance, 1038; use in Woolworth Building, 1450; use of discordant, 222

Colquhoun, Alan, **280–81**

Columbia Broadcasting System Headquarters, 1150, 1216

Columbia University: Alfred Lerner Hall, 1347–48; Low Library, 927; plan, 206

Columbus, Indiana, **281–84**; Gateway Study, *282*

columns: by Antoni Gaudí, 487, 488, 489; Cranbrook Academy, 972; Great Mosque of Niono, 546; High Museum of Art, 609; of ivory, 964; Johnson Wax Administrative Building, 313, *714*, 715; at Lincoln Memorial, 780; memorial, 833–34; "mushroom," 1442; Sainsbury Wing, National Gallery, London, 1155; tall buildings as, 620; tilted, 40

comfort, human. *See also* climate control: Eileen Gray's emphasis, 544

commercial buildings, definition, 12

Commercial Center of Fountivegge, 1134–35

commercialism. *See* Capitalism's impact on architecture

Commerzbank Tower, 474, 1224

Commissariat of Agriculture in Moscow, *302*

Commons shopping center, Columbus, Indiana, *565*

communication via architecture, 57

Communist impact on architecture: Bucharest, 183–84; Budapest, 185; China, 250; Cuba, 330–31; East Germany, 496; Hungary, 663–64; Prague, 1053; use of demolition, 352

community and architecture, 1186; communities of builders, 1461; exclusionary communities, 1270, 1271; shopping centers as community centers, 565. *See also* paths of movement

community centers. *See* cultural centers

community/individual relationship through architecture, 142, 362, 605

company towns, 434–35

competitions, **284–87**. *See also* awards

Complexity and Contradiction in Architecture (Venturi), 1047, 1294–95, 1369, 1400

computer-aided design, 59, 287–88; climate data software, 271, 272; Frank Gehry's use of, 491, 492; for Guggenheim Museum (Bilbao), 571; lighting, 775; Morphosis's use of, 878; Peter D. Eisenman's use of, 395, 396; sustainable architecture tools, 1280; of tensile structures, 1314; for utopian planning, 1384

computers and architecture, **287–89**

Concert Hall, Hälsingborg, Sweden, **289–90**

concert halls: acoustics, 10–11, 11; seating, 142

concrete, **290–94**; colored, 361; corrugated, 1296; Edward Stone's screen walls, 1262; ferro-cement, 418–19; first use of precast, 1061; high-strength, 1005–6; influence on factory design, 433; István Medgyaszay's work with, 826; Knitlock system, 557; Louis Kahn's use of, 1156; magnesite, 746; mixed with coquina stone, 217; mixed with marble aggregate, 529; Ove Arup experiments with, 78; Paul Rudolf's use of, 1142, 1144; Pier Luigi Nervi's construction techniques, 910; for private house, 150; in PVC pipes, 36; Soleri's experiments with, 61; and stone walls, 1260; trusses, 1346; use at Fiat Works (Turin), 459; use in Brutalism, 180; use in grain elevators, 538. *See also* reinforced concrete

concrete-shell structure, **294–96**; Philips Pavilion, 292–93; Shrine of the Dome, 1207

Condition Postmoderne, La (Lyotard), 1049

Condominium Apartments in Acapulco, 1192

Coney Island, 52; Destruction of Dreamland, *51*

Congregation Beth El in Detroit, 1296

Congrès Internationaux de l'Architecture Moderne (CIAM), **296–98**, 587; Athens meeting, 549; British branch, 298; Frankfurt congress, 473; Hungarian group, 663, 863; influence in Spain, 1234; influence on urban planning, 1378; Japanese branch, 736; Norwegian branch, 450, 940; Pruitt-Igoe Public Housing Project impact on, *1067*. *See also* Athens Charter; Frank, Josef

Congress for the New Urbanism (CNU), 369, 922, 1272

Conklin House, 431

Connell, Ward and Lucas, **298–99**

construction management, **299–301**; computer use for, 288–89

Construction Management at Risk system, 300

construction techniques: Arts and Crafts Movement, **75–78**; "bundled tubes," 1188; of E. Owen Williams, 1442; Empire State Building, 404; innovations in Mexico, 843; innovative concrete, 952; of Paolo Soleri, 1225; precast construction, **1056–57**; at Pruitt-Igoe Public Housing Project, 1066; of Ramses Wissa Wassef, 1436; School of Construction Technicians, 947; skeletal, 37; of Skidmore Owings and Merrill, 1211, 1212; St. Petersburg (Leningrad), 1236; thin-skin building envelopes, 1150; using wood, 1448; welded buildings, 40; wooden stud frame, 1177; World Trade Center, 1452. *See also* construction management; masonry bearing walls; prefabrication; steel-frame construction; structural systems

Constructivism, **301–4**; Berlin, 140; demise, 969; in Ilya Golosov's work, 526, 527; impact on Czechoslovakia, 341; influence on James Stirling, 917; of Ivan Ilich Leonidov, 758; Moisei Ginzburg's contribution to, 506; Monument to the Third International in, 869; Moscow, 879; Netherlands, 913; relation with Bauhaus, 119; relation with Futurism, 478; relation with modernism, 861–62; Russia, 1146, 1147; St. Petersburg

(Leningrad), 1236–37; United States, 1368; use of trusses for expression, 1346; of Vesnin brothers, 1405–6

contemporary art. *See* modern art and architecture

Contemporary Arts Center in Cincinnati, 581

Contemporary City for Three Million Inhabitants, **304–5**, 366, 1383–84; relation with Ville Radieuse, 1419

Contemporary Museum of Art in Los Angeles, 693

Contextualism, **305–6**; Aalto's exemplary work of, 3; of Alvaro Siza, 1210; of Antoine Predock, 1057; by Arne Emile Jacobsen, 705; of Dominique Perrault, 999, 1001; of Enric Miralles and Carme Pinós, 857; exceptions to, in Romania, 1129; and house design, 657–58; Johannes Duiker's exception, 955; Malaysia, 994; of Moshe Safdie, 1153; Paul Rudolph's six determinants of form, 1142; relation with historicism, 621; of Richard Rogers, 1127; Social Security Complex, Istanbul, 1222

contour planning, 434

convenience stores, 486

convention-facilities, 654

Conway, Patricia, 453, 732

Conway Building, 241

Cook, Peter, **306–7**, 1361, 1362. *See also* Archigram

Coonley House, 1122

Coop Himmelblau, **307–9**; Falkenstrasse Roof Construction Project in Vienna, 93; Groninger Museum, *3i*; "Open House," 657; relation with Deconstructivism, 350, *351*

Copan Building, *1165*

Copenhagen, Plan, 1082

Copenhagen, Denmark, 353; Grundtvig Church, 567

Copenhagen Town Hall, 264

Copley Square: buildings, *159*, 160; redesign, 1027

copper roof shingles, 228

coquina stone, 217

coral reef building materials, 709

Le Corbusier, (Jeanneret, Charles-Edouard), **309–13**; Ahamedabad buildings, 30, 31; appreciation of Eileen Gray's work, 545; appreciation of vernacular buildings, 1402; buildings at Weissenhofsiedlung (Stuttgart 1927), 1437, *1438*; Carpenter Center for the Visual Arts, 159, *310*; Chapel at Ronchamp, 1292; Chapel of Notre-Dame-du-Haut, **237–39**, 256; Contemporary City for Three Million Inhabitants, **304–5**, 366, 1383–84; Dom-ino Houses, 292, 304, 310, **365–67**, 656; "Five Points of a New Architecture," 311; impact in Chile, 247, 248; influence in Brazil, 318; influence in Buenos Aires, 186; influence in Hungary, 663; influence in Israel, 696; influence of Choisy on, 252; Maisons Jaoul at Neuilly-sur-Seine, 172; opinion of Fiat Works (Turin), 459; opinion of Highpoint I, 611–12; Palace of the Soviets Competition entry, 969, *970*; Paris architects who inspired, 977; Paris buildings, 978; Parliament Building, *6ii*; pavilion at International Exhibition of Decorative Arts (Paris 1925), 680; Philips Pavilion, 419; photography, 59, 1097; praise of Algerian pisé buildings, 385; redesign of Chandigarh plan, 235; relation with Brutalism, 180–81; relation with Cubism, 333; relation with environmental issues, 410; relation with International Style, 681, 682; relation with primitivism, 1063; role in CIAM, 297, 298; tectonics in works of, 1313; typological reasoning, 1355; Unite d'Habitation, 56, 312, **1358–59**; urban planning designs, 1378; use of color, 279; use of concrete, 292; use of concrete shells, 296; use of glass, 517; views on urbanism, 1419; Villa Savoye, 31, **1416–18**; Ville Radieuse, **1419–20**;

Le Corbusier, (Jeanneret, Charles-Edouard) (continued)
    Voisin Plan for Paris, 311, **1422–23**; work in Brazil, 165;
    writings about airport architecture, 33. *See also* Athens Charter
Córdoba, 66
cornice on Flatiron Building, 466
Cornich Mosque, 710
Corning Museum of Glass, *147*, 148
corporate logos, 485; by Erich Mendelsohn, 836
corporate plazas, 1028
corporate visitor centers, 1421
corprorate office park, estate, and campus, **313–14**; in edge cities,
    386
Correa, Charles, **314–17**; Ghandi Smarak Sangrahalaya, 31, 315;
    relation with environmental issues, 411; use of traditional building
    methods, 1404; Vidhan Bhavan (State Assembly), **1408–9**, *7iii*;
    work in India, 673, 674
Cosanti, 1225
Costa, Lúcio, 165, 166, **317–19**, 931, 1112; Brasília plan, 163;
    Ministry of Education Building in Rio de Janeiro, *318*; work on
    Brasília, 447
Cottage style in Toronto, 1333
country clubs, **319–21**
Court of the Universe, 975
courtyards in architecture: Alliance Franco-Sénéfalaise, 35; bungalow
    court, 188; Entrepreneurship Development Institute in India,
    407–8; Frank Lloyd Wright's public buildings, 1454; Jørn
    Utzon's use of, 1385; Ministry of Foreign Affairs, Riyadh, 856;
    traditional Chinese architecture, 249
Cowles House, 114
Crabtree, William, 787
Craftsman Style, **321–22**; of Gustav Stickley, **1250–52**
Cram, Ralph Adams, **322–24**, 1366; Boston works, 158; campus
    planning, 206; Cathedral of St. John the Divine, 323; Rice
    University, 658
Cranbrook, Michigan, **324–25**
Cranbrook Academy, 972; renovation, 1445
Crawford House, 878
Creanga, Horia, 183
Cret, Paul Philippe, **325–27**, 1009; campus planning, 206; influence
    on Chinese architects, 765
critical regionalism, 152, 1367; Cultural Centre Jean Marie Tjibaou,
    335; effect on use of concrete, 293; Kenneth Frampton's theory
    of, 470; relation with environmental issues, 410; relation with
    Historicism, 621
Croly, Herbet, 1026
Crow Island School, 997, 1180, *1180*; exterior, *1180*
Crown Hall, Illinois Institute of Technology, 667, *668*
Crystal Cathedral, 256
Crystal Chain, 426
Crystal Palace, 417
crystals, use in Expressionism, 426
Cuadra San Cristóbal, **327–29**; exterior, *328*
Cuba, **329–32**; use of Catalan vaults, 225
Cuban architecture, 1127
Cuban Pavilion at Expo '67, 422
Cubism, **332–34**, 384, 1097; impact on architectural drawing, 58–
    59; impact on Czechoslovakia, 341; influence in Prague, 1053;
    influence in Riyadh, 1113; influence on Amsterdam School, 913;
    influence on Gropius House, 560; influence on Michael Graves,
    542; relation with International Style, 683

Cueto House, 1127
CUJAE, 331
Cultural Center, Le Havre, *933*
cultural centers: Alliance Franco-Sénéfalaise, **35–36**; mosques, 884
Cultural Centre Jean Marie Tjibaou-Noumia, **334–35**, *3ii*; interior,
    335
Cultural Congress Center Concert Hall, 11
Cultural Park for Children in Cairo, *202*, 203
culture: architectural, 358; *vs.* capitalism, 17
Cummins Engine Company, 281–82
Cunha Lima House, 569
Cuno House, 127
curtain wall system, **335–37**; adaptation, in Brussels, 179;
    aluminum, 39, 40; Bank of China Tower, 109; concrete, Bank of
    London and South America, Buenos Aires, 110; effect on interior
    climate control, 594; "floating," 436; glass, 121, 337, 515, 516,
    517, 519, 994; as image-making device, 943, 944; Institut du
    Monde Arabe, 980; by Peter Behrens, 433; tinted Thermopane
    glass, 590
Curtis, Louis S., 516
curved rooms, 8
curvilinear Art Nouveau (Judendstil), 72, 74, 912
Cushicle, 57
Cuypers, Eduard, 49
cyburbia, 386
cylindrical forms, 427; brick fireplace, 521; grain elevators, 538;
    staircase with wall of glass, 527
Czech, Hermann, **337–40**
Czech Republic and Czechoslovakia, **340–42**

Dacca. *See* Dhaka, Bangladesh
Dalcroze Institute for Rhythmic Dance, 1321
Dallas Museum of Art, 115
Dangler, Henry C., 14
Danish architects, 355
Danish architecture, 704
Danteum project for Rome, 1318–19
Dar-al-Islam, 445
Darmstadt, Germany, **343–44**
Darvich, Djhanguir, 690
Darwin Martin House, 1453
De 8, 47–48
Death and Life of Great American Cities, The (Jacobs), 616, 703,
    1047
De Bazel, Karel P.C., 372
de Beauvoir, Simone, 453
De Bijenkorf, *1137*
De Carlo, Giancarlo, **344–46**
Deconstructivism, **350–52**, 1295; architectural drawings of, 59;
    Daniel Libeskind's work, 768; Denmark, 355; exhibit at Modern
    Museum of Art, New York, 717; and house design, 657;
    Hungary, 664; ornament, 959; relation with Contextualism, 306;
    relation with Cubism, 333; United States, 1369–70; use of brick,
    172; Zaha M. Hadid's contribution to, 581
decorated shed, 29, 751, 1183
Defense Corps Building in Jyväskylä, 1
de Klerk, Michel, **346–48**; Eigen Haard Housing Estate, **392–93**,
    8i; Expressionist work, 427
De-La-War Pavilion, 836
Delft School, 914, 1137

De Lijnbaan, 1137

de Meuron, Pierre. *See* Herzog and De Meuron

"Democracity," 930

democracy, representation in buildings: Brasília Federal Capital Complex, 448; at Canberra, 1017; embassies, 401; Reichstag, 1092

demolition, **352–53**; Berlin, 141; Istanbul, 699; Pruitt-Igoe Public Housing Project, *1067*. *See also* adaptive reuse

Denmark, **353–56**

Denver Art Museum, *1037*

Denver Park Mayfair East Apartments, 819

Denver Public Library, 543

department stores, **356–57**; Art Deco, 70; Cairo, 201; Carson Pirie Scott Store, **219–21**; Chicago, 632; Czechoslovakia, 341, 342; designs by Eva Jircna, 713; escalators, 414; European, 782; Germany, 377, 494, 497; by Graham, Anderson, Probst and White, 535; parking garages, 983; Philadelphia, 1008. *See also* plate glass

Depression Moderne, 929

Derrida, Jacques, 350, 351, 395

desert climate construction, 1168; by Erich Mendelsohn, 836; Haj Terminal, Jeddah Airport, 584; Riyadh, 855, 856

Desert Research Centre, 445

design: Adolf Loos Raumplan, 792; alterations on-site, 124; asymmetrical, 683; Barnes's theory, 115; Birkerts's process, 147–48; Bruno Zevi's writings, 1468; buffalo-shaped house, 524; Charles Voysey's work, 1424–26; charrett process, 1189; by Chloethiel Woodard Smith, 1218; Ciudad Universitaria, Caracas auditorium, 268; community involvement, 412; controversy over Church of St. Francis of Assisi, 257–58; in cultural context, 27–28; effect of plastic on, 1022; Entrepreneurship Development Institute in India, 407–8; evolution of public housing, 1070; fan-plan motif of Alvar Aalto, 2, 1445; of Frank Lloyd Wright, 1054; Frank Lloyd Wright's rectilinearity, 1121; gender and sex in, 453–54; of Gordon Bunshaft, 190; Gropius' Bauhaus, Dessau, 121; Heikkinen and Komonen's technique, 599; Henning Larsen's whimsical, 747; Herzog and de Meuron's approach, 1109; as image not text, 42; impact of lighting of, 774; as interdisciplinary discourse, 41; of Itsuko Hasegawa, 591; John Hejduk's technique, 599–600; Kazuo Shonhara's emphasis on chaos, 1203–4; Kazuyo Sejima's residential, 1194; Kenzo Tange's structural, 1302; mosques, 546; Ove Arup's totally integrated, 79–80; of Raj Rewal, 1106; of Rem Koolhaas, 734–35; Scandinavian modern, 471; Shanghai World Financial Center, 1198; Steven Holl's conceptual, 634; theory of Hermann Muthesius, 898; timeliness of, 53; as way to better living, 381. *See also* computer-aided design; construction techniques; energy-efficient design; ordinances

Despotopoulos, Ionnais, 548

Dessau Bauhaus. *See* Bauhaus Dessau

De Stijl, **348–50**, 912–13; Berlage's relation with, 136; impact in Rotterdam, 1136; impact on architectural drawing, 59; influence in Schröder-Schräder House, 1182; J.J.P. Oud's role, 962–63; Johannes Duiker's relation with, 374; Norway, 940; ornament, 958; Theo van Doesburg's role, 1391; Thomas Gerrit Rietveld's importance, 1109; use of color, 278. *See also* Amsterdam School

Detroit Public Library, 503

Deutsche Bank, *473*

Deutscher Werkbund, **357–59**, 495; influence of Hermann Muthesius on, 898. *See also* Nihon Kosaku Bunka Renmei (Japanese Werkbund); Weissenhofsiedlung (Stuttgart 1927)

Deutscher Werkbund Exhibition (Cologne 1914), 415

Deutscher Werkbund Exhibition (Stuttgart 1927), 359

Dhaka, Bangladesh, **359–61**; National Assembly Building, **902–4**

Dharmala Sakti Office, *1228*, 1230

4D house (Fuller), 39, 475

Diagoon Houses, 606

Diamond Series Houses, 600

Diba, Kamran, 689

Diener and Diener, **361–62**

Dieste, Eladio, 225, **362–63**

diners, 1116

Dinkeloo, John, 1123, 1124

Diplomatic Quarter in Riyadh, 1115, 1170

Dipoli Student and Conference Center, 1014

Director's House at Dessau Colony, 564

"disappearing" column memorial, 833

Disney Corporation Headquarters, 621

Disney theme parks, **363–65**, 862

display designs: by Eva Jircna, 713; Williams and Tsien's museum exhibits, 1444

disposable architecture, 57, 230

Djenne conservation project, *384*

Dogan Media (Printing) Center, *1352*

Dome House, 1225

Domènech i Montanar, Luis, 111, *112*

Dome of Discovery, 39–40; alloy girders, *39*

domes: aluminum, 39–40; Brasília Federal Capital Complex, 448; Church in Rárósmulyad, 826; copper-cladded, 604; floating concrete, 908; geodesic dome structure, 476; glass, 251, 515; Hagia Sophia, 254; Hassan II Mosque minaret, 592, 593; King Saud Mosque, 710, 883; Millennial Dome at Greenwich, 1127, 1164; mud-brick, *1436*; on Olbrich's Vienna Secession exhibition hall, 950, *951*; of reeds, mud, and straw, 1461; Reichstag, 1094; in ring-beam moat, 213; Shrine of the Book, 1206, *1207*; stadium, 1240; structures for, 1263, 1264; synagogues, 1296

Dom-ino Houses, 292, 304, 310, **365–67**, 656

Domino's Pizza World Headquarters, 147

Dominus Winery, 607–8

Donnelley and Sons, 1199

Donnènech I Montaner, Lluis, 225; Palau de la Música, *226*

Doshi, Balkrishna V., **367–69**, 674, 675, 1404; Ahmedabad buildings, 31

double-glazed glass, 517

Douglas House, 827

Dover Sun House, 1086

Drake University Science and Pharmacy buildings, 1099

drawn glass, 516

Dreyfus, Henry, 930

drive-in restaurants and theaters, 95, 1116–17

Duany and Plater-Zyberk, **369–71**, 956, 1353, 1366; Seaside, Florida, 369, 922, *923*, **1189–92**

duck, 751, 1183

ducts, 595; Salk Institute, 1156

Dudok, Willem Marinus, 334, **371–73**, 913; Hilversum Town Hall, 265, **614–15**; Town Hall for Hilversum, 265

Duhart, Emilio, 247–48

Duiker, Johannes, **373–75**, 1469; Open Air School, **953–55**

Dujarric, Patric, Alliance Franco-Sénéfalaise, **35–36**, *1i*

Dulles International Airport, Chantilly, Virginia, 375–77, 644

Düsseldorf, Germany, **377–79**

Dutch architects, 915, 1227
Dutch architecture, 48, 135, 912; in southern Africa, 22
Dutch Expressionism, 426, 427
Dutch Functionalism, 913, 914, 1396
Dutch Pavilion, *1399*
Dutch structuralism, 429
Dymaxion Airocean World Map, 476
Dymaxion House, 475, 476, 1244

Eames, Charles and Ray, **381–83**, 1346; Case Study Houses, 1244; documentary on Dulles International Airport, 376; relationship with Eero Saarinen, 1149
Eames House, 381, *382*, 1346
earthen building, **383–86**, 1168; by Hassan Fathy, 444; mud-dried bricks, 546; Vietnam Veterans Memorial, 1412; Yaama Mosque, 1461
Earth House, 1225
Earthworks, 776
East Berlin architecture, 140–41
Eastern Columbia Building, *793*
East Germany, 496
Eastland Mall in Detroit, 566
Eaton, Norman, 24
Eaton Center, 1335
École des Beaux-Arts, 388, 568
Ecological Design Institute of Sausalito, 1281
"Eco"-logic types, 410–11
ecology, 405
ecotourism, 52
edge cities, **386–87**, 1342; Northpark, 1041
educational institutions, **387–90**
Edwardian architecture, 786, 787
egalitarian architecture, 49
Egyptian architects, 19, 21, 444, 445
Egyptian Revival style, **390–92**
Ehime Prefectural Museum of General Science, 738
Ehn, Karl, Karl Marxhof, **729–31**
Ehrencrantz, Ezra, 1178, 1180, 1346
Ehrenhof, 378
Eigen Haard Housing Estate, **392–93**, 427; exterior, *393, 8i*
Einstein Tower, **393–94**; as Expressionist work, 426
Eisenman, Peter, **394–96**; Arnoff Center for Design and Art, *279, 2i*; designs, 306; House VI, 657; importance in United States, 1370; Institute for Architecture and Urban Studies, **677–78**; relation with Deconstructivism, 350; use of color, 280; Wexner Center for the Visual Arts, 172, 777
Ekelund, Hilding, 461
El-Dar Restaurant, *1436*
Eldem, Sedad Hakkí, **396–98**, 699, 1351; Social Security Complex, **1222–23**; use of traiditional building methods, 1404
electric light, 774
"electropolis," 138
elevation, 58
elevators, **398–99**; effect on Sears Tower, 1188; exposed, 237; parking garage, 984; platform, 1432; use for air circulation, 595; in World Trade Center, 1452
el-Khoury, Pierre, Banque du Liban et d'Outre Mer, *129*
Elkins, Frances, 15–16
Ellwood, Craig, **399–400**
Ellwood houses, 399, *400*

Elmslie, George Grant, **1073–75**
El Pedregal, 117, 847
El-Wakil, Abdel Wahid, King Saud Mosque, 710
Embarcadero Center, 1041
embassies, **400–403**
Emergency Services College in Kuopio, 599
Emery House, 557
Emory University, R. Howard Dobbs Center, *1041*, 1042
emotional architecture, 327, 329, 821, 976
Empire State Building, **403–4**, 927, 1216; competition with Chrysler Building, 253; exterior, *404*
Empire State Plaza, *589*
Empire style, 23
Empire Swimming Pool, 1442
Endell House, 1175
energy-efficient design, 336, 404–6; Canada, 209; and climate, 271; impact of wind farms on landscape, 1052; by Joan Edelman Goody, 533; by Michael and Patty Hopkins, 649; with plastic, 1022; precast concrete, 1061. *See also* solar architecture
engineered lumber, **406–7**. *See also* wood
engineers, architects' relations with, 45–46
Enoch Pratt Free Library, 772
Enso-Gutzeit Headquarters, 3, 574
Entelechy I and II, 1042
Entertainments Tower, 57
entrance, AT&T Building, 84–85
entrances, Frank Lloyd Wright buildings, 714
Entrepreneurship Development Institute, **407–8**; exterior, *408*
environmental design: by Balkrishna Doshi, 367; Barragán's mix of, 117; combined with cultural sensitivity, 123; David Victor Gruen's interest in, 565; by Michael and Patty Hopkins, 650; by Paolo Soleri, 1225; rainwater collection, 239; Ramses Wissa Wassef Arts Centre, **1079–80**; suburban developments, 1272; by Vincent Scully Jr., 1186
environmental issues, **408–11**; conservation, 21; Kenneth Frampton's writings, 470; power plants, 1052; skyscrapers, 1216; Social Security Complex, Istanbul, 1222; sustainability assessment methods, 1282. *See also* energy-efficient design; sustainability and sustainable architecture
environmental technology. *See* climate control
EPCOT, 364
ergonomic design, 767, 768
Erickson, Arthur, 1390
Ernst Ludwig Haus, 950
Erskine, Ralph, **411–14**, 1048, 1258, 1284
Ervi, Aarne, 462
escalators, **414–15**; external, 237
Ethiopia, 191
Ethiopian embassy, 403
EUR'42, 443, 1132
Euro Disney, 365
European architecture: Arts and Crafts Movement, 77; department store design, 356; Garden City Movement in, 482–83; in Southern and Central Africa, 22–23
European Court of Human Rights, 1127
European influence: on American architects, 1140, 1299; Bangkok architecture, 104; Buenos Aires, 186; Cairo, 201–2, 203; in Iran, 688; in Melbourne, 829; in Mexico, 843; Montreal, 867; New York City, 928; Turkey, 1350; United Kingdom, 1260, 1359; United States, 1369; Vancouver, 1390

European Parliament in Brussels, 179

E.1027 villa, 544

evolving architecture, 338, 339

E-Walk redevelopment project, 68

exclusionary zoning, 957

exhibition building, **415–16**; Art Nouveau, 73; Czech contributions to, 342; Fascist architecture and, 443; Gae Aulenti's designs, 87; by Hodgetts and Fung, 626; by Josef Hoffman, 629; Joseph Maria Olbrich's Vienna Secession, 950, *951*; Panama-Pacific International Exposition, San Francisco, 975, 976. *See also* pavilions

Exhibition Hall, Turin, Italy, **416–19**; interior, *418*

Exhibit of the Fascist Revolution (1932), 443

exoskeletons, 1242

Experience Music Project in Seattle, 491

Expiatory Temple of the Holy Family, 489

Expo 1967, Montreal, 210, 416, **420–22**, 1232. *See also* Habitat 1967, Montreal

Expo 1992, Seville, 416, **422–23**

Expo 1958 (Brussels), 416, **419–20**

Expo in Barcelona, 1234

exposed elevators, 398–99

Exposition des Arts et Techniques (1937), 978

Exposition Universelle, Paris (1900), 415, **423–25**

Expressionism, **425–28**; in Alvar Aalto's works, 3; Australia, 90, 91; Bauhaus, 119; Berlin, 137, 138; Canada, 210; in church design, 255; in Einstein Tower, 394; Erich Mendelsohn's relation with, 835; Finland, 462–63; Germany, 495, 496–97; Grundtvig Church, Copenhagen, 567; in Hans Poelzig's work, 1031; impact on architectural drawing, 59; influence of primitivism on, 1062; Kyoto, Japan, 740; Melbourne, 829, 830; Norway, 940; Oswald Mathias Ungers's analysis, 1357; in Paul Rudolph's works, 1142; relation of skyscrapers to, 6–7; relation with functionalism, 1175; roots in Cologne, Germany, 276; Switzerland, 1286–87; using brick, 171

Expressionist House of Culture, 2, *3*

Extremadura Government Offices at Mérida, 908

exurbs, 386

Eyecatcher, 1023

Eykelenboom, Walter, 422

Eyre, Wilson, **430–31**

Fabiani, Max, 1464

fabrics used for tensioned membrane structures, 1315; Canada Place, 1390

facades: of Alvar Aalto, 3; by Antoni Gaudí, 488–89; Art Deco, 69; cast-iron, 1060; Ciudad Universitaria Campus and Stadium, Mexico City, 267; Cubism and, 333; divorced from function, 50; of Erich Mendelsohn, 836; glass, 109; Great Mosque of Niono, 546, *547*; indeterminate, 145; integrating old and new, 83; Larkin Building, 746; L'Innovation Department Store, 782; Mario Botta's buildings, 162; Museum of Folk Art in New York, 1445; Museum of Modern Art, New York, 896, *897*; by Oscar Nitzchke, 935; Paris, 977; Prudential Building, 40; of Rifat Chadirji, 231; tenements in Glasgow, 514; Vanna Venturi House, 1392, *1393*

factories, **433–34**; adaptive reuse, 13; AEG Turbine Factory, Berlin, **17–18**; Behrens', 127; Boots Factory, **155–56**; brick-walled, 171; Gothic style, 1199; planning, **434–35**. *See also* industrial buildings

Fagus Werk, **435–36**, *1ii*

Fair Store, *998*

Fakhoury, Pierre, Our Lady of Peace Basilica, **964–65**

Falk Apartment Building, 1177

Falkenstrasse Roof Construction Project in Vienna, 93

Fallingwater, **436–38**, 1454; exterior, *436*; interior, *436*

fallout shelters, **438–40**

fan/heating systems, 594

farm buildings. *See* agricultural buildings

Farmer, Graham, 410

Farnsworth House, **440–42**, 656, 854–55, 1244; comparison with Glass House, 716; exterior, *441, 442*

Farrell, Terry, 789, 1363

Fascist architecture, **442–44**, 1131; Adalberto Libera's relation with, 767; Antonio Sant'Elia and, 1158; Casa del Fascio, 1318; influence in Switzerland, 1287; Italian pavilion at Century of Progress Exposition (Chicago 1933), 229; of Luigi Moretti, 874; relation with Expressionism, 427; stone, 1259

Fathy, Hassan, 21, **444–46**; Beit Nassif, 709; influence on Africa, 24; relation with environmental issues, 411; use of traditional building methods, 1404; work with adobe, 385

Fauvism, 384

favelas, **446–47**; Rio de Janerio example, *446*; São Paulo, Brazil, 1165

Federal Capital Complex, Brasília, 167, **447–50**; exterior, *448, 449*; Lúcio Costa's role, 318–19, 447

Federal Granary Building, 808

Federal Reserve Bank in Minneapolis, 147

Federal Science Pavilion at Seattle World's Fair, 1462

Federation style in Australia, 1290

Fehn, Sverre, **450–52**; Glacier Museum, 451, **508–9**; Norway Pavilion (1962), 1399; Norwegian Pavilion, 420; Villa Busk, *939*

Felix Nussbaum Haus, *769*

Fellowship House, 517

feminist theory, **452–55**; house design, 658; and shopping centers, 1205

feng shui, **455–56**; of Bank of China Tower, 109

Fergus Factory, 563

Ferriss, Hugh, 71, **456–58**, 955

ferro-cement, 418–19, 911; Renzo Piano's use at Menil Collection, 837

Festival of Britain, 788

Fiat Works (Turin), **458–59**, 1012; exterior, *458*

fiberboard, 406

fiber-optic light, 775

fiber-reinforced plastic, 1022, 1023

Field Museum of Natural History, 534

film sets, 625; amusement park similarities, 50; Robert Mallet-Stevens work, 814

Financial Times Printing Plant in London, 434, 559

Finland, **459–64**; Aalto's relationship with, 3; Villa Mairea, 2, 438, 973, **1414–16**

Finlandia Concert Hall, 602

Finnish architects, 462, 463

Finnish architecture, 148, 574, 600, 972

Finnish Embassy, in New Delhi, 1014

Finnish Embassy in Washington, D.C., 599

Finnish National Theatre annex, 1208

Finnish Parliament House, 460

Finnish Pavilion (Aalto, 1956), 1398

Finnish Pavilion at Paris Expo (1990), 424, 459, 1151

Finnish Pavilion Brussels World Fair, 1014
Finnish Pavilion New York World's Fair (1939), 931
Finnish Science Center, 598
fins, glass, 519
Finsbury Health Centre, 799, *800*
Fire Station Five, 1336; exterior, *1336*
First Christian Church, *1151, 1152*
First Christian Church, Columbus, Indiana, 281
First Church of Christ, Scientist, Berkeley, 322, *822*, 823, 1326
First National Bank of Chicago, 997–98
First Source Center, *707*
First Unitarian Church, Rochester, New York, 724
First Unitarian Meeting House in Madison, 256
Fischer, Theodor, 357, 586–87; exhibition buildings, 1439
Fishdance Restaurant, 490
Fisker, Kay, 353, **464–65**; project at International Exhibition of Decorative Arts (Paris 1925), 680
Fitch, James Marston, 271
Flamingo Hotel, 749
Flatiron Building, **466–67**, 1318; exterior, *466*
Flemish architects, 132
Fletcher, A.L., 234
float glass, 52
Floating Mosque, The, 592
flooring, barns, 29
floor plans, 58
Florida Southern College plan, 207
fluorescent lighting, 774
Folger Shakespeare Library, *326, 327*
Fontainbleau Hotel, 1101
Football Stadium in Mendoza, 815, *816*
Foote House, 875
Forbidden City, 766
Ford, Henry, 176–77, 722
Ford House, 523, 524, 1367
Ford Plant Offices, Highland Park, *721*, 722
form: accidental, 1003; in James Stirling's work, 1253, 1354
form and function, contradictions between, 1347
form as expression: of function, 218; Guggenheim Museum (Bilbao), 7
form follows function, 220, 909; Alan Colquhoun's focus on, 281; British Library, London, 175; Constructivism, 301; disadvantage of, 746; in factory building, 433; Frank Lloyd Wright's belief in, 1083; Louis Sullivan's belief about, 1277; served *vs.* servant spaces, 724
forms: Alvar Aldo's fan-motif, 2, 1445; Art Nouveau (Jugendstil), 72; balloon-frame, 29; cantilever, 168; connection with technique, 252; crystal, 17; cylindrical, 162, 723; cylindrical void, 734; describing digitally, 288; dodecagon, 53; equality with space, 82; Expressionist, 426; harmony among, 506; indeterminacy of, 43; James Stewart Polshek's use of square, 1032–3022; late 20th-century skyscraper, 109; nonorthoganal, 525; paraboloid, in churches, 255; polyhedral-based structures, 1243; pyramidal, 164; schism with content, 146; shell, 213; spiral, 869; used by Arata Isozaki, 693, 694; used by Wallace K. Harrison, 589; Wright's spiral, 572. *See also* form follows function; nautical forms
Forms and Functions of Twentieth Century Architecture (Hamlin), 585
Fort-Brescia, Bernado. *See* Arquitectonica
Foster, Norman, 405, **467–69**, 474, 640, 649–50, 789; Al-Faisaliah Center, *1170*; construction techniques, 1178; Hong Kong and

Shanghai Bank Corporate Headquarters, *946*; Reichstag, **1092–95**; Renault Distribution Centre, 469, **1096–97**; Sainsbury Centre, 1243; solar architecture, 1224; Stansted airport, *33, 34*; works of, 1362–1633
Foster and Partners: British Museum, *6i*; Chek Lap Kok airport terminal, 34; Hong Kong International Airport, **643–45**
Foundation Beyler Museum, 1013
Foundation Miro, *1196*
Fountainbleau Hotel, 743; gardens, *744*
Fox, Sheldon, 732
Fragrant Hill Hotel, 250, 992
Frampton, Kenneth, **469–71**, 623; critique of postmodernism, 1050; relation with environmental issues, 410; study of streets, 678; on Sverre Fehn's work, 509
France, New Urbanism in, 924
Frank, Josef, **471–72**; "accidentism," 339
Frankfurt, Germany, **472–74**
Frankfurt Museum, 610
Frank Sinatra residence, 1443
Franz Josef-Stadtmuseum, 1429
Fraser University, 1390
Freed, James Ingo, 621; Holocaust Memorial Museum (Washington, D.C.), 632, **637–39**
Freedom Lane Housing in Amsterdam, *347*
French architects, 182; in Algeria, 19
French architecture: Jean-Louis Cohen's writings, 274; Peter Collins's writings, 275
French influence: Southeast Asia, 1227–28; United Kingdom, 1360; United States, 14, 568
Fresh School for the Health Child, 374
Frey, Albert, **474–75**; Aluminaire House, **36–38**, 38–39
Frey House 1, 474
Frey House 2, 475
Friedrichstrasse department store, 943
Fry, Maxwell, 1180
Fukuoka Prefectural International Hall, 43
Fuller, Richard Buckminster, **475–78**; 4D house, 39, 475; Dymaxion House, 475, 476, 1244; Dymaxion Principle, 405, 410; Triton City, 1153; U.S. Pavilion at Expo 1967, *421, 422*
Fuller Building. *See* Flatiron Building
Fuller House, 1058
Functionalisim, relation with abstraction, 6
Functionalism, 1103; Aalto's conversion to, 1; Amsterdam, 48; Asplund's, 82–83; Berlin, 137; Blomstedt's, 149; Czechoslovakia, 342; Denmark, 353; Farkas Molnár's role, 863; Finland, 460–62, 967; Gunnar Asplund's manifesto, 1257; Helsinki, 601; "integrated," 529; Johannes Duiker, 373, 1469; Juan O'Gorman, **946–47**; Kay Fisker, 464–65; London, 787; Mexico, 844; Mexico City, 847; Netherlands, 913, 914, 1396; Norway, 940; pioneering work of, 289; relation with Expressionism, 427; Richard Rogers, 1126; Romania, 1130; in Rotterdam, 1136; Russia, 1147; Sven Markelius's work, 818; Switzerland, 1287; Tokyo, 1329; in Viljo Gabriel Revell's work, 1104; of Villa Savoye, 1416; Walter Gropius's contribution to, 562; Yugoslavia, 1465. *See also* form follows function
Fung, Hsin-Ming, **625–27**
furniture, 28; built-in, 188–89; by Charlotte Perriand, 1002; by Eileen Gray, 544; Stickley, 1250
Futurama exhibit, 1340

Futurism, **478–79**, 1158; and expositions, 416; impact on architectural drawing, 58–59; impact on Berlin architecture, 137; Italian, 260; of Ville Radieuse, 1420

Gabr, A. Labib, **481–82**
Gage Building, 632
Galacia City of Culture, 396
Galeria Jardin, 40–41
Gallaratese, 1134
Gamble House, 77, 552, 553, 794, 1062; drawing for, *553*; use of timber framing, 1326
Gandelsonas, Mario. *See* Agrest and Gandelsonas
Garage Ponthieu, 1001
garages, 96
Garatti, Vittorio, 901
garden apartments, 55
garden city developments: Belgium, 131; Brussels, 178; Canada, 209; Northern Africa, 19
Garden City Movement, **482–83**, 1271; Bruno Taut's work, 1305; Hong Kong, 641; impact on Chandigarh, 234; impact on Disney theme parks, 364; importance to United Kingdom, 1360; influence on New Towns Movement, 921; Marktown, 1200; Montreal, 866; New Delhi, 1020; relation with industrial town planning, 434; Santiago, Chile, 1160. *See also* greenbelts and greenbelt towns
garden suburbs, Australia, 89
Gare Do Oreinte, 783, *784, 785*
Gare d'Orsay, 12, 424, 979
Garnier, Tony, **483–85**; project at International Exhibition of Decorative Arts (Paris 1925), 680; Une Cité Industrielle, **259–60**
Garvey House, 1336
Gasometers in Vienna, 307–8
gas stations, 96, **485–86**, 1116. *See also* automobiles
GATCPAC (Grup d'Artistes i Tècnics Catalans pe Progrés de l'Arquitectra Contemporània), 112
Gateway Arch (St. Louis), **486–87**, 1245
Gateway Center in Minneapolis, 1059
Gateway to the West, 1149
Gatti Wool Factory, 1095
Gatwick airport terminal, 32–33, 34
Gaudet, Julien, **568–69**, 1091
Gaudí, Antoni, 111, **487–90**; Casa Milà, **223–25**, 489, *5i*; Sagrada Familia, *1234*
Gaussa vault, 362
Geddes, Bel, 71, 986; Futurama exhibit, 1340
Gehry, Frank, **490–92**; campus plan, 207; Der Neue Zolhof, *378, 379*; Festival Disney concourse, 365; influence in Los Angeles, 795; National Netherlands Building, 1053; relation with Deconstructivism, 350; relation with environmental issues, 411; University of Iowa, Advanced Technology Laboratory, 1370; use of color, 280; work in Czechoslovakia, 342. *See also* Guggenheim Museum (Bilbao)
Gehry House, 490, *491*, 571
General Archives of Columbia, 1157
General Motors Technical Center, 1100, 1150
Genoa harbor revitalization, 1012
gentrification, 1381
geodesic domes, *421, 422, 476*; Fuller's conception, 476, 1263 (*See also* space frames)

geometric aspects of architecture: Austrian architecture, 92; Baiyoke Towers, 101; Behrens's use of, 126; Berlage's use of, 135; Bernard Tschumi's work, 1347; Botta's use of, 162; cube-based house, 577–78; Eisenman's use of, 395; Frank Lloyd Wright's work, 1454; Hans Poelzig's use of forms in design, 1031; Henri van de Velde's design strategy, 1396; Irving John Gill's work, 504; Islamic architecture, 63, 994; Kazuo Shonhara's work, 1203–4; Kisho Kurokawa's work, 738; Kyoto Symphony Hall, 740; Michel de Klerk's, 392; multiples of a square, 67; of Muzharul Islam, 692; National Gallery of Art, East Building, 906; Netherlands, 912; Oswald Mathias Ungers's work, 1357, 1358; Philip Johnson's work, 716; in rationalism, 1083, 1084; Stepahnovich Melnikov, 831; by Susana Torre, 1336; Thailand, 105; used by Heikkinen and Komonen, 599; Vittorio Gregotti's view on, 554; works by Corbusier, Le (Jeanneret, Charles-Edouard), 1423; Zaha M. Hadid's forms, 581
Georgeakopoulos, Periklis, 549
George Washington Memorial Parkway, *1119*
Gerhardt, Paul, Marmon Hupmobile Auto showroom, *391*
German architects, 1030
German Architectural Museum in Frankfurt, 1358
German architecture, 377; East *vs.* West Berlin, 140–41; influence of Hermann Muthesius, 898; in Southern and Central Africa, 22–23
German Architecture Museum, 497
German Arts and Crafts Society. *See* Deutscher Werkbund
German Embassy, St. Petersburg, 127
German Pavilion, Expo 1967 Montreal, 960
German Pavilion (Barcelona 1929), **492–94**, 682, 854; exterior, *493*; use of glass, 517
German Romanticism, Hugo Häring's work, 586
Germany, **494–98**; environmentalism, 409; industrial town planning, 434–35
Gerz, Jochen, 833–34
Gesamtkunstwerk (total work of art), 1411
GESOLEI exposition, 378
Getty Center, **498–500**, 827, 894; exterior, *499*; interior, *500*
Getty Villa in Malibu, 894
Ghandi Smarak Sangrahalaya, 31
Ghirardo House, 1323
Giedion, Sigfried, 97–98, **500–502**; on Aldo Van Eyck's work, 428; on Brasília, 449; on International Style, 427; "new regionalism," 940
Gifu Kitagata Apartments, 1194
Gilbert, Cass, 206, **502–4**, 1215, 1255; campus planning, 206; Woolworth Building, 502, 1215, **1449–51**
Gill, Irving John, **504–6**; work in Los Angeles, 794
Ginzberg, Moisei, **506–8**, 1147; Palace of the Soviets Competition entry, 969; relation with Constructivism, 301, 302–3; work with Vesnin brothers, 1406
Girault, Charles, 424
Giurgola, Romaldo, 212
Glacier Museum, 451, **508–9**, 940
Glasgow, Scotland, **513–15**
Glasgow School, **509–11**
Glasgow School of Art (Scotland), **511–13**, 805; exterior, *513*
Glaspalast, 276
glass, **515–19**; bricks, 229; bridge, 237; Corning Museum of Glass, *147*, 148; curtain walls, 121, 337, 515, 516, 517, 519, 994; fins, 519; floors, 1046; heat absorbing, 760; Helmet Jahn's use of, 708;

glass (continued)
  importance to American architecture, 1369; Klaus Kada's
    experiments with, 719–20; laminates, 519; in plastic, 1023; Toyo
    Ito's use of, 700; undulating, 522; use in Expressionism, 426; use
    in Penn Station, 515; Walter Gropius' use of, 563; wired, 516; in
    Zuev Workers' Club, 527. See also plate glass
glass block, 810
Glass Chain (chain letters), 1175
glass curtain walls, Van Nelle Factory, 1395
Glass House (Bardi), 150
Glass House (Johnson), 517, **519–21**, 656, 1244, *1ii*; comparison
    with Farnsworth House, 716; interior, *520*
Glass House (Taut), 1305–6, 1439
Glass Palace, 462, 1103
Glass Pavilion, 426, 515
Glass Skyscraper, **521–22**
Glenn Martin Aircraft Plant, 1242
Global City, 1384
glue-laminated timber, 406. See also laminated timber; wood
GM (General Motors) Technical Center, 314
Goetheanum, 427, 1286–87
Goetz Gallery, 607
Goff, Bruce, 409, **522–24**, 795, 1367
Goldberg, Bertrand, 243, **524–26**
golf course design, 320
Golosov, Ilya, **526–28**, 1147
Golosov, Panteleimon, 527
Gómez, Javier Sánchez, 815
Gondomar Convent, 1308
Gön Leather Product Factory, *698, 699*
González de Léon, Teodoro, **528–30**, 845
Goodhue, Bertram Grosvenor, 323, **530–32**
"good roads" movement, 1340
Goodwin, Philip L., 896
Goody, Joan, **532–34**
Gotardi, Roberto, 901
Göteborg Law Courts Annex, 83
Gothenburg City Hall Extension, *1283*
Gothic Deco, 70
Gothic Revival, 620, 1062
Gothic Style: arches in World Trade Center, 1451; Auguste Choisy's
    writings, 252; Boston, 158; Chicago, 242, 243; churches, 254,
    255; college campuses, 206–7; factories, 1199; last cathedral in,
    1433; "Mediterranean Gothic," 489; Ralph Adams Cram, **322–
    24**; skyscrapers, 1215, 1450; United States, 1366; use of glass,
    515
government-sponsored projects: Abuja, Federal Capital Territory of
    Nigeria, **9–10**; apartment buildings, 56; Art Deco, 69; Canada,
    208; effect on urban blight in United States, 1380; historic
    preservation, 617; India, 673; Mexico, 529; mosques, 883; New
    Deal works in Chicago, 242; New Zealand, 932; Northern Africa,
    21; Romania, 1130; Spain, 1234; Tapiola, 1104; U. S.
    government buildings, 12; in U.S., during the Depression, 985;
    Vietnam Veterans Memorial's difference from, 1412. See also
    Chandigarh, India; Fascist architecture; regional planning
Graham, Anderson, Probst, and White, 241, **534–37**
grain elevators, **537–38**; importance to Canada, 209
Grand Central Terminal, **538–40**; perspective drawing, *539*
Grande Arche de la Défense, **540–42**, *541, 5ii*
Grand Ecran, Le, 980

Grand Rapids (Michigan) Art Museum, 42
Grand Union Walk Housing, *559*
Grange-Blanche Hospital, 484
Granja Sanitaria, 947
Granville Island Public Market, 1390
Graves, Michael, 364, 365, **542–44**; Denver Public Library, 1369–
    70; Humana Building, *620*; Portland Public Services Building,
    542, **1039–40**, 1369; relation with historicism, 621; relation with
    Postmodernism, 1048
Gray, Eileen, **544–46**
Graz architects, 719
Graz School, 93
Great Mosque of Djenne, Mali, 385
Great Mosque of Niono, **546–48**; facade, *547*
Great Synagogue in Jerusalem, 1298
Greece, **548–51**
Greek Revival Architecture in America (Hamlin), 585
Green, Leslie, 1273
"green" architecture. See sustainability and sustainable architecture
greenbelts and greenbelt towns, **551–52**; Canberra, 212; Cologne,
    Germany, 277; New Deal towns, 1271; relation with Garden City
    Movement, 482; relation with regional planning, 1087–88
Greene, Charles Sumner, 552, 554. See also Greene and Greene
Greene, Henry Mather, 552, 554. See also Greene and Greene
Greene, Herb, 524
Greene and Greene, 322, **552–53**, 1092, 1367; Arts and Crafts
    designs, 77; use of timber framing, 1326
Greene King Beer Warehouse, 649, 650
Gregory Farmhouse, 1458
Gregotti, Vittorio, **554–55**
Greyhound Bus Terminal in Louisville, Kentucky, *198*
Griffin, Marion (Lucy) Mahony, **555–58**, 829
Griffin, Walter Burley, **555–58**, 829, 1290; Plan of Canberra, 212,
    1016–18
Grimshaw, Nicholas, and Partners, 405, 434, **558–60**, 1363
Groep 32, 914
Groniger Museum East Pavilion, 307, *3ii*
Groote Schuur, 102
Gropius, Walter, **562–65**; Bauhaus Dessau, **121–23**; Black
    Mountain College plan, 207; exhibition buildings, 1439; Fagus
    Werk, **435–36**, *1ii*; impact in Boston, 158–59; Impington Village
    College, 1180; influence on Deutscher Werkbund, 358; Palace of
    the Soviets Competition entry, 969; relation with Expressionism,
    138; role in The Architects Collaborative, 1324; urban planning
    goals, 1378; work with Bruno Taut, 1306; work with Peter
    Behrens, 126–27. See also Bauhaus
Gropius House, **560–62**, 564; exterior, *561*
Grosses Schauspielhaus, 1031
Groundswell (1993), 777
"group form," 811
Group R (Barcelona), 112–13
Gruen, Victor, 1205
Gruen, Victor David, **565–66**
Grundtvig Church, Copenhagen, 567, *2ii*
Grup d'Artistes i Tècnics Catalans pe Progrés de l'Arquitectra
    Contemporània (GATCPAC), 112
Gruppo 7, 767
Guadalajara, Mexico, 116
Guaranty Building, *1276, 1277*
Guastavino, Rafael, 225

Guastavino tile, 1274
Guedes, Joaquim, **569–70**
Guggenheim Museum (Bilbao), 7, 306, 490, **570–72**; effect on Deconstructivism, 351; exterior, *570*; skycourt, *571, 7i*
Guggenheim Museum (New York), **572–74**, 746, 928, 1455; exterior, *573*
Guggenheim Museum (Vienna and Salzburg), 636
Guild House in Philadelphia, 172, 1392, 1400
Guimard, Hector: Castel Beranger, *959*; Metro Stations in Paris, **840–41**
Gullichsen, Kristian, **574–75**
Gürel Family Summer Residence, **575–76**; exterior, *576*
Gustavo Gili Publishing House, 113
Gut Garkau, *588*
Guy, Simon, 410
Gwathmey, Charles, 573, **576–78**
Gwathmey Residence and Studio, 577, 578

Haas House, 636; interior, *636*
Habermas, Jürgen, 1049–50
Habitat 1967, Montreal, 210, 422, **579–81**, 867–68, 1153; exterior, *580*; interior, 581
Hadassah Hospital in Jerusalem, 836
Hadid, Zaha M., **581–83**, 641, 1363; relation with Deconstructivism, 350, 351
Hague, The, 266
Haj Terminal, Jeddah Airport, **583–85**, 710, 1171, 1213
Hakata Bay Oriental Hotel and Resort, 994
Hall, Peter, 1292
Hall for Visual Spectacle and Sound in Space, 1441
Hallidie Building, 516
Hamburger Vorhalle, 126
Hamlin, Talbot Faulkner, **585–86**
Hammerstrasse Apartment Complex, 361
Hammond Compound, 1086
HAMS Code (Gorden Cullen), 956
Hancock Tower, 518
Hannover Principles (McDonough), 1280
Harbour Square, 1218
Hardboard, 406
Häring, Hugo, **586–88**; relationship with Hans Scharoun, 1175
Harris, Harwell Hamilton, 517
Harrison and Abramovitz, **588–90**, 1125; acoustical design, 11; Alcoa Building, 40, 935; Avery Fisher Hall, 11; Lincoln Center, **778–79**; United States Embassy in Cuba, 330
Hartman-Cox, 1434
Harvard University: Center for Study of World Religions, 1197; Fogg Art Museum Lecture Hall, 11; Graduate Center, *1324*, 1325; Josep Lluis Sert's works, 1197. *See also* Carpenter Center for the Visual Arts
Hasegawa, Itsuko, **590–92**, 1331
Hassan II Mosque, **592–94**
Hass House, 93
Hastings, Thomas. *See* Carrère and Hastings
Hatton House and Guest House, 474
Havana, Cuba, National Art Schools, **901–2**
Havana architecture, 329
Hawley, Christine, 307
Haystack Mountain School of Crafts, 114–15
Healey Guest House, 1142

Hearthstone, the, 875
heating, ventilation, and air conditioning (HVAC), **594–96**; air circulation, 594; costs in construction, 1448; and design of Kansai International Airport Terminal, 727; and glass, 518; Haj Terminal, Jeddah Airport, 584; health risks of sealed buildings, 1280; Hong Kong International Airport, 645; hotels, 655; innovation at Maison De Verre, 810; Jeddah homes, 709; Lever House, 760; Olivetti Factory, 952; Phoenix Central Library, 1010; plate glass and, 1025; Pompidou Center, 979; Reichstag reconstruction, 1094; Rietveld's "core" house idea, 1109; stadiums, 1314; using courtyards for, 407; Wright's Larkin Building, 746. *See also* energy-efficient design; lighting
Hecker, Zvi, 696
Hedrich-Blessing, 60
Hegemann, Werner, **596–98**
Heikkinen, Mikku, 355, **598–99**
Hejduk, John, **599–600**
Heliopolis, 201
Helix City Plan for Tokyo, 737, 839
Helsingborg Concert Hall, 817
Helsinki, Finland, **600–603**
Helsinki Finnish Worker's Institute, 149
Helsinki Railway Station, 460, 601, **603–5**, 1077, 1151; exterior, *604*
Helsinki Technical University Otaniemi Chapel, 601
Henneberry Press Building, 1199
Hennebique, François, 459; work with concrete, 290, 292
Hennebique frame, 365
heritage preservation. *See* historic preservation
Herman Miller Distribution Centre, 558
Herman Miller Furniture Company, 382, 383
Heron, Ron, 57
Hershey Sports Arena, 295
Hertzberger, Herman, **605–6**, 946
Hervanta Congregational, Leisure and Shopping Center, in New Delhi, 1014
Herzog, Jacques. *See* Herzog and De Meuron
Herzog, Thomas, 405
Herzog and de Meuron, **606–8**; Ricola Storage Building, **1108–9**
Heurtley House, *1055*
High and Over, 298
High Museum of Art, **608–10**; exterior, *610*; interior, *609*
Highpoint 1 Apartment Block, 78, **610–12**, 799; exterior, *611*
highrise. *See* apartment buildings; skyscrapers
High-Tech style, 558, 1295; Belgium, 132; Canada, 211; Hungary, 664; influence of Craig Ellwood on, 399; influence of Olivetti Factory on; *Insitut du Monde Arabe*, 943; Kyoto, Japan, 740; London, 788, 789; Michael and Patty Hopkins, 649; Norman Foster's work, 467; origins, 1361; ornament, 959; pavilions at Expo 1992, Seville, 423; Pompidou Center, 1035; and power plants, 1051; Ralph Erskine, 413; Renault Distribution Centre, 1096; Richard Rogers, 237, 1126; Schlumbeger Cambridge Research Center, 1178; Southeast Asia, 1230; United Kingdom, 1362–63; United States, 1368; use of aluminum, 40; use of trusses, 1346; Yugoslavia, 1466. *See also* machine aesthetic
highway building, 94, 96
Hilberseimer, Ludwig, **612–13**
Hill House, 76–77, 805, *806, 5i*
Hillside Terrace Complex in Tokyo, 811
Hilversum Community Bath, *372*

Hilversum Sanatorium Zonnestraal, 374, **1468–70**

Hilversum Town Hall, 265, **614–15**, 913

Hiroshima Peace Memorial and Museum, **989–90**, 1302

Hirshhorn Museum and Sculpture Garden, 190, 1213, 1369, *1434*, 1435

Hispanic American architecture exhibit, 1337

historical context of architecture: in Aldo Rossi's work, 1135; Benevolo's exploration of, 133; Brussels, 179; city halls, 264; importance in United States, 1365; Manfredo Tafuri's writings, 1299; meaning from, 161; mosques, 883, 885; Sullivan's search for independence from, 1275

historical revivalism, Austria, 91–92

Historicism, **619–22**; Edward Durell Stone use of, 1261; of Edwin Lutyens, 802; Istanbul, 698; Joseph Maria Olbrich's relation with, 950. *See also* typology

historicist design, 619

historic preservation, **616–19**; awards for, 26; Belgium, 132; Boston, 160; British Library, London, 173; Canada, 211; Chicago, 243; Fascist architecture, 443; Germany, 497; Glasgow, 514; by Joan Edelman Goody, 533; Mexico, 845; Northern Africa, 21; Palace of Fine Arts, 976; Paris, 980; by Philip Johnson, 716; as reaction to globalism, 1092; roadside architecture, 1118; Savannah, Georgia, 1027; St. Petersburg, 1238; United States, 1366; Vincent Scully's advocacy, 1186. *See also* adaptive reuse; demolition; redevelopment projects

historiography, **622–24**

History of Modern Architecture (Zevi), 1467

Hitchcock, Henry-Russell, 619, **624–25**; influence on Collin Rowe, 1140; International Style Exhibition, **685–87**

Hitler, Adolf, 139

Ho Chi Minh City, 1230

Hodgetts and Fung, **625–27**

Hoffmann, Josef (Franz Maria), 92, **627–30**; exhibition buildings, 1439; Palais Stoclet, 130–31, 656, **970–72**; project at International Exhibition of Decorative Arts (Paris 1925), 680; relation with Deutscher Werkbund, 357; role in Vienna Secession, 1410, 1411

Höger, Fritz, 426

Holabird, William, and Martin Roche, **632–33**; Marquette Building, 241; Stevens Hotel, 654

Holabird, William, and Root, John Wellborn, **630–32**; Chicago Daily News Building, 242

Holberseimer, Ludwig, 668

Holden, Charles, 787

Holl, Steven, 325, **633–35**

Holland House, 135

Hollein, Hans, 93, **635–37**; Abteiberg Municipal Museum, **7–9**, 635, 1049; Haas House, 90; Museum of Modern Art, Frankfurt, **894–96**; Retti Candle Shop, 90

Hollyhock, 1176

Holocaust Memorial Museum, 621, **637–39**; Hall of Witness, *638*; rear facade, *639*

Holocaust Museum in Berlin, 7

Holy Prophet Mosque of Medina, *1169*

homosexual style, 1143–44

Hong Kong: Bank of China Tower, **108–10**; Chek Lap Kok airport terminal, 34

Hong Kong, China, **639–43**; Bank of China Tower, **108–10**, 455–56, 922, *1215*

Hong Kong and Shanghai Bank Corporation Headquarters, 469, 640, **645–47**, *946*; exterior, *646*

Hong Kong Bank, 455

Hong Kong Club, 641, *643*, 1192, *4iii*

Hong Kong International Airport, *640*, 642, **643–45**

Hong Kong Peak Club, 581

Hood, Raymond, 90, **647–49**, 687, *3iii*; Rockefeller Center, 927, 1028, **1124–26**

Hopewell Baptist Church in Oklahoma, 523

Hopkins, Michael and Patty, **649–50**, 1363; Schlumberger Cambridge Research Centre, **1178–79**

Horta, Victor, **650–52**, 840; and Art Nouveau, 73; L'Innovation Department Store, **781–82**; Tassel House, 130

hospitals, **652–54**; by Bertrand Goldberg, 526; Greece, 548–49; by Rino Levi, 761; sanatoriums, 954; use of terrazzo, 1320

Hotel Camino Real, 756

Hôtel Du Mobilier National, 1001

Hotel Flamingo, *750*

Hotel Industriel Berlier, 999, *1279*

Hotel Kempinski, 708

Hotel Metropole, 879

Hotel Nacional, 329

hotels, **654–55**; Canadian railway, 210; escalators, 415; near Disney theme parks, 364, 543; Northern Africa, 21

Hotel Santiago in Cuba, 331

Hotel Sylvia, 1390

Hotel Vancouver, 1389

House and Garden in Valle Del Bravo, 726

House and Garden magazine, 430

House at Kuwahara, 591

House at Lowicks, Surrey, *1425*

House for Stephan Riabushinskii, *1201, 1202*

House in Aspen, Colorado, *1090*

House LE, 293, 938

House of Culture in Helsinki, 2, *3*

House of Glass (Chareau), 239, 240

House of Michaelerplatz, *791, 792*

House of Rain, 908

"House of the Future" by Peter and Alison Smithson, 1220

"House of Tomorrow" (Keck), 1224

House-on-Hill (Celia Tobin Clark House), *15*

House on the Mesa, 686

House Over the Brook, 1440

houses, **655–58**; Art Nouveau (Jugendstil), 72; Bauhaus, 119; Belgium, 130, 131; Brussels, 179; Bucharest, 182; existing vernacular, 1402–3; by Frank Lloyd Wright, 1453; as group of "found objects," 28; "house as a city," 1162; India, 671, 672; Levittown, *763*; Muthesius' suburban *Landhaus*, 898; by Purcell and Elmslie, 1074; steel in, 1244–45; use of plate glass, 1025; zones within, 430. *See also* mobile homes

Houses N and R i Valle de Bravo, 937, 938

House Stekhoven, 1162

House under High Voltage Lines, 1331

House VI (Eisenman), 657

housing: Athens Charter position on, 86; created from industrial properties, 13; exhibits at International Style Exhibition, 686–87; low-density, 202, 203; uses of prefabrication, 1060

Housing Complex in Novazzano, 162

housing developments: by Adèle Naudé Santos, 1162–63; Hong Kong, 641; of Josef Frank, 471; by Kay Fisker, 464; London, 788; low-rise, 355; Moscow, 830; Vienna, 729

housing estates: Amsterdam, 48; Arquitectonica's, 67; Australia, 90; Barragán's, 116, 117; Bauhaus, 120, 121; Behrens's, 126–27; Levittown, 95; low-scaled density, 138; Southwark, London, 56

housing for displaced persons, 1337; India, 31; Tokyo, 1329

housing for workers, 816, 1136; by Ali Labib Gabr, 481; Berlin, 138; Cuba, 1127; by Heinrich Tessenow, 1321; India, 673–74; by J.J.P. Oud, 963; by John Irving Gill, 505; Malagueira Housing Quarter, **813–14**; Marktown, 1200; Mexico, 872, 938; Mexico City, 846; Russia, 1146; Sunila, 2; Sunnyside Gardens, 1271; by Viljo Gabriel Revell, 1104; by William Wurster, 1459

Housing in Space, 1440

housing projects: Amsterdam, 47; Barcelona, 112, 113; by Bruno Taut, 1306; Budapest, 185; Caracas, 216; by Carlos Raúl Villanueva, 1418; by Corbusier, Le (Jeanneret, Charles-Edouard), 1422; Cuba, 331; East and West Berlin, 140; Eric Mendelsohn, 1375; by Heinrich Tessenow, 1321; multifunction, 847; new town of Tapiola, 149; by Rogelio Salmona, 1157; Stockholm, 1258; Sweden, 1284; Switzerland, 1286; Turkey, 1352

Houston, Texas, **658–60**; Best Products Showroom, **145–46**; Menil Collection, **837–38**

Houston Astrodome, 1240

Howard, Ebenezer, 482; New Towns Movement, **920–21**

Howard Johnson's motel, 887; restaurants, 1102

Howe, George, and William Lescaze, **660–62**; PSFS Building, 13

Howe and Lescaze, 1008; design for Museum of Modern Art, New York, 896; Philadelphia Savings Fund Society (PSFS) Building, 1216; PSFS Building, 661

Hubertus House, 429

Hughes, Francesa, 454

Humana Building, 542, 543, 620

humanistic approach to architecture, 997; of Alvar Aalto, 1416; of Josep Lluis Sert, 1195; Moshe Safdie, 1153; of William Wurster, 1459

humanitarian considerations. See social responsibility of architecture

Hungary, **662–64**; industrial town planning, 434–35

Husser House, 1120–21

Huxtable, Ada Louise, 658, **664–65**

HVAC (heating, ventilation, and air conditioning). See heating, ventilation, and air conditioning (HVAC)

Hvitträsk, 1151

Hyatt Hotel in Atlanta, 518, 1040–41

Hydraulic Museum of the Segura River Mills, 908

hypermodernism. See supermodernism

Hysolar Research Institute, 1099

Ibelings, Hans, 1278–79

IBM headquarters in Buenos Aires, 41

IBM tower, 115

IDS Center in Minneapolis, 716

Igualada Cemetery, 858

Illinois grain elevator and office, 537

Illinois Institute of Technology, 207, **667–69**; Chemistry Laboratory, 1098; Crown Hall, 854; master plan, 854; student center, 708

Image of the City, The (Lynch), 802, 1379

Imperial Crown style in Tokyo, 1330

Imperial Hotel, 1329, 1454

Imperial Hotel (Tokyo), **669–71**; exterior, 670

Imperial Palace in Addis-Ababa, 191

impermanence in architecture, 700

Impington Village College, 1180

inclusionary zoning ordinances, 958

Independence Mall, 1009

Independent Group in London, 106

India, **671–76**; Vidhan Bhavan (State Assembly), **1408–9**

India Gate, 920

Indian architects, 31, 671

Indian architecture, 317, 367, 671, 1106; Western influences, 30

Indian Institute of Management, **676–77**, 724; exterior, 676

Indira Gandhi Institute for Development, 672, 674

indirect light, 775

Indonesian architecture, 1228, 1229

industrial buildings: by Albert Kahn, 721–22; definition, 12; by Graham, Anderson, Probst and White, 536; in Hungary, 664; by Kristian Gullichsen, 574; by Nicholas Grimshaw, 558; plastic, 1023; by Ricardo Legorreta, 756. See also factories; mill buildings

industrial product designs, 43

industrial town planning, **434–35**

ING Bank Headquarters, 1281

Inland Revenue Headquarters in Nottingham, 649

Inland Steel Building, 242–43, 1212

Inn River bridge, 809

Inside Architecture (Vittorio), 554, 555

Institut du Monde Arabe, 943, 980

Institute for Architecture and Urban Studies, 27, **677–78**

Institute for Lightweight Structures, 961

Institute of Confucianism, 1457

Institute of Indology, 367

institutes and associations, **678–80**

Insurgentes Theater, 938

interior design: Aluminaire House, 37; churches, 254; by Eva Jiricna, 713; floating floor slabs, 110; Glasgow School, 510; by Griffin and Griffin, 557; Henri van de Velde, 1396; Jewish Museum, Berlin, 712; Le Corbusier's functionalist approach, 1002; office space, 946; by Patricia Conway, 732–33; space designated by furniture, 1349; Unité d'Habitation, 1359; use of woven metal textiles, 1000; Williams and Tsien's museum exhibits, 1444; Yale University, Art and Architecture Building, 1143. See also climate control; furniture; lobbies

International Exhibition (Barcelona 1929), 111; German Pavilion, 415, **492–94**

International Exhibition of Decorative Arts (Paris 1925), 65, **680–81**

International Institute of Appropriate Technology, 445

International Movement for Rational Architecture (MIAR), 443

International Situationism, 98

International Style, **681–85**; apartment buildings, 56; Argentina, 66; Austria, 92; Bangkok, 105; Banham's writings about, 107; Belgium, 131–32; Bruno Paul's projects, 988; Brutalism's rejection of, 180; Budapest, 185; Cairo, 202–3; Canada, 210; Caracas, 215; Chile, 247; China, 249, 251; churches, 256; college campuses, 207; department stores, 356–57; Frank Lloyd Wright's rejection, 1453; gas stations, 95; Germany, 496; Henry-Russell Hitchcock Jr. contribution to, 624; Hong Kong, 641; houses, 1025; Hungary, 664; impact on architectural photography, 60; impact on use of wood, 1448; India, 30; Istanbul, 699; Kisho Kurokawa's reaction against, 737–38; Las Vegas, 749; Lubetkin and Tecton's works, 799; Mexico, 844; Mexico City, 847, 848; Moscow, 881; Netherlands, 913; New York City, 927–28; Northern Africa, 20; ornament, 958; Philadelphia, 1008; relation

International Style (continued)
   with Expressionism, 427; Rotterdam, 1136; Santiago, Chile, 1161; São Paulo, Brazil, 1165; Saudi Arabia, 710; of Studio Per, 1266; Switzerland, 1286; Toronto, 1334; Toronto City Hall, 1332; Torre Velasca break from, 1338; and U.N. Headquarters design, 1364; use of stone, 1259; Yugoslavia, 1465. *See also* regionalism
International Style Exhibition (New York 1932), **685–87**
Inter-University Center for Astronomy and Astrophysics, *315, 316, 317–18*
Inventure Place, Inventors Hall of Fame, *1033*
Iran, **687–91**
Iranian architects, 688
iron: ironwork at Glasgow School of Art (Scotland), 511; prefabrication with, 1060; symbolism, 868; use in Paris Metro Station, 841; Victor Horta's use of, 782. *See also* cast iron; steel
Irwin, Robert, 499
Irwin Union Bank and Trust, Columbus, Indiana, 281–82
Islam, Muzharul, *360*, 361, **691–92**
Islamic architects, 26
Islamic architecture, 63, 687; geometric aspects, 994; symbolism, 1005. *See also* maidans; mosques
Isozaki, Arata, **692–94**, 839, *893*, 1049, 1084
Israel, **694–97**
Israeli architects, 695
Israeli Museum, 1206
Istanbul, Turkey, **697–99**; Sedad Hakkí Eldem's projects, 397; Social Security Complex, **1222–23**
Italian architects, 87, 1036, 1318, 1355–56
Italian architecture, 133; and Fascism, 443
Italian Rationalism Movement, 1084
Italy, Benetton Factory, **134–35**
Ito, Toyo, **699–701**; Kazuyo Sejima's relation with, 1195
Ivory Coast, Africa, Our Lady of Peace Basilica, **964–65**
Izenour, Stephen, 750, 1118
Izvestiia Building, *1147*

Jacobs, Jane, **703–4**, 1047; *Death and Life of Great American Cities, The*, 616, 703, 1047
Jacobsen, Arne Emil, 354, **704–6**
Jahangirnagar University, 692; student dormitories, *691*
Jahn, Helmut, **706–9**
Jami Masjid, *1020*
Jansen, Hermann, 1350
Jansen House, 1177
Japan, Church on the Water, **258–59**
Japan Center, San Francisco, *1463*
Japanese architects, 590, 736, 737, 740, 1194, 1328; Tadao Ando, **52–55**
Japanese architecture, 736, 738; influence on Abuja in Nigeria, 10; Kenzo Tange's views of, 990; use of aluminum, 40
Japanese influence: on American architects, 1032, 1054, 1062; in American architecture, 524; on Charlotte Perriand, 1003; Denmark, 354
Jardines del Pedregal, 117
Jazz Moderne, Australia, 90
Jeanneret, Charles-Edouard. *See* Corbusier, Le (Jeanneret, Charles-Edouard)
Jecquier, Emilio, 247

Jeddah, Saudi Arabia, **709–11**; Haj Terminal, Jeddah Airport, **583–85**, 710, 1171, 1213
Jefferson Memorial, 1038
Jencks, Charles, 1047
Jensen-Klimt, Peder Vilhelm, Grundtvig Church, 567, *2ii*
Jerusalem, Israel: Ashbee's work, 81; Erich Mendelsohn's work, 836; Moshe Safdie's work, 1153; Shrine of the Book, **1206–8**
Jewish Museum, Berlin, **711–12**, 768; exterior, *711, 4ii*; interior, *712*
Jiricna, Eva, **712–13**
Johannesburg, 24, 102
John F. Kennedy Airport, TWA Terminal, 375
John F. Kennedy Library, exterior, *991*, 991–92
John Hancock Center, 242, 246, *683*, 684, 1212; windows, 992
Johns Hopkins University, 205, 206
Johnson, Philip, **715–18**; Abby Aldrich Rockefeller Sculpture Garden, 893; admiration for Farnsworth House; AT&T Building, **84–86**, 621, 716, 1217; "camp" style, 1143; church design, 256; Glass House, **519–21**, 1244, *1ii*; International Style Exhibition, **685–87**; memorial for commuters, 833; Museum of Modern Art renovation, 896, 897; New York State Theater, 778; postmodern origins, 1188; relation with International Style, 683–84; relation with J.J.P. Oud, 963; relation with postmodernism, 1049; use of glass, 517; work in Houston, Texas, 659
Johnson and Burgee, AT&T Building, 1217
Johnson Wax Administration Building, 313, **713–15**, 746, 1095, 1454
joinery: aesthetics of, 1312, 1313; beam-and-mast system, 1096; Craftsman, 321; Griffin house, 557; space frame, 1232; truss, 1246; used in Glacier Museum, 509; wood, 406
Jourdaine, Franz, Samaritaine Department Store, *978*
Joypurhat Housing, 692
Juer Hutong project, 1457
Jugendstil. *See* Art Nouveau (Jugendstil)
Jujol i Gilbert, Josep Ma, 111
Jurkovic, Dusan, 341
JVC Center in Guadalajara, 308
Jyväskylä Workers' Club, 1, 460, *461*

Kada, Klaus, **719–20**
Kaehilath Anshe Ma'ariv Synagogue, *1297*
Kafka's Castle, 152
Kahn, Albert, **720–22**, 931, *1iii*; Altamira Building, 215; Congregation Beth El in Detroit, 1296; Glenn Martin Aircraft Plant, 1242
Kahn, Julius, 720
Kahn, Louis I., **722–26**; air circulation designs, 595; Capital Complex project in Dhaka, 359, 361; classicism style of, 269; Indian Institute of Management, **676–77**; influence in Africa, 24; influence in Denmark, 354; influence on Balkrishna Doshi, 367; Kimbell Art Museum, **731–32**; "Monumentality," 486; National Assembly Building, Dhaka, **902–4**; question about brick, 170; relation with rationalism, 1084; relation with Robert Venturi, 1392; Salk Institute, 293, 653, 724, 1099, **1156–57**; tectonics in works of, 1313; Temple Beth El, 1298; University of Pennsylvania, Richards Medical Research Building, 172, 723–24, 1099; use of brick, 172; work in Philadelphia, 1009; works in United States, 1368
Kalach, Alberto, **726–27**
Kalinin Prospekt (New Arbat buildings), *881*

Kallmann, Gerhard, 156
Kandinsky, Wassily, 119, 302, 303
Kansai International Airport Terminal, 34, **727–29**, 1012; exterior, *728*
Karfik, Vladimir, 341
Kärjensivu Rowhouse, 1104
Karl Marxhof, **729–31**; exterior, *730*
Karmi, Dov, 695
Kasai Rinkai Visitors' Center, 1304
Kaufhaus Tietz Building, 276
Kaufmann House, *918*, 919
Kemaleddin, 698
Kemper Arena in Kansas City, 706
Kentlands, Maryland, *370*
Keyes Condon Florance (KCF), 1434
Kharkov, constructivism in, 303
Kiasma Museum, *634*
Kiesler and Bartos, Shrine of the Book, **1206–8**
Kikutake, Kiyonori, 838, 839
Kimbell Art Museum, 724, **731–32**, 1313; interior, *731*; lighting, 774
King Abdul Aziz Historic Center, *1114*
King Saud Mosque, 710, *883*
King's Road House, 794, 1176, *1177*
Klauder, Charles Zeller, 206–7
Klee, Paul, 119
Kleines Café/Little Cafe, 338, *339*
Klimt, Gustav, 629, 1409, 1410, 1411
Klint, P.V. Jensen, 353
Knesset in Jerusalem, *696*
Knights of Columbus Headquarters, *1123*
Knitlock concrete tile system, 557, 829
knowledge-based design processes, 288
Knowles, Edward, 156
Knutsen, Knut, 940
Kocher, Lawrence, 36
Kohn, A. Eugene, 732
Kohn Pederson Fox, **732–34**; Proctor and Gamble Headquarters, *314*; Shanghai World Financial Center, **1197–98**
Kolonihavehus, 999
Komonen, Markku, 355, **598–99**
Konstantinidis, Aris, 550
Koolhaas, Rem, **734–36**, 914
Koppers Building, 535
Korean architecture, 1229
Korean War Veterans Memorial, 834
Korsmo, Arne, 940
Kosaku Bunka Renmei (Japanese Werkbund), **736–37**
Kotera, Jan, 341
Kovicic, Viktor, 1465
Kramer, Piet, 427
Kreis, Wilhelm, 377, 378
Krier, Leon, 270, 922, 923, 924; neo-Rationalism of, 909
Kroeller-Mueller project, 853
Krokos, Kyriakos, 550; Byzantine Museum, *549*
Kromhout, Willem, 47
Kuala Lumpur, Malaysia, Petronas Towers, **1004–6**, 1230
"Kubus," 1358
Kulczewsky, Luciano, 247
Kunsthaus, 1470

Kurokawa, Kisho, **737–39**, 838, 839
Kursaal Cultural Center, 865
Kuwait City, waterside development, *63*, 64
Kyoto, Japan, **739–41**
Kyoto Station Building, 740

laboratories. *See* research centers
La Città Nuova, 1158, *1159, 1160*
LACMA Pavilion for Japanese Art, *523*
Lafayette Park in Detroit, 855
Laguna West, 922
Lake Shore Drive Apartments, *245, 246*, 854
Lakeside Press Building, 1199
Laloux, Victor, 424
Lambert Airport in St. Louis, 1462
laminated timber, 1326, 1447; in architecture, 936; integration of houses with, 1166; Panama-Pacific International Exposition in San Fancisco, 975; relation with European schools, 1179. *See also* glue-laminated timber; wood landscape
landscape design: Abuja, Federal Capital Complex of Nigeria, 9–10; by Alberto Kalach, 726, 727; Brazil, 194; country clubs, 320; feng shui, 455; gardens of Charles A. Platt, 1026; by Maya Lin, 776; "rooms," 124. *See also* Contextualism; nature integrated with buildings
Land Title Building, 1008
land use regulations. *See* zoning ordinances
La Nouvelle Maison, 131
Lapidus, Morris, **743–45**, 851, 1101
Lapsipalatsi Building. *See* Glass Palace
Laredo Transit Center, 199
large-scale projects: Arquitectonica, 67; Denmark, 353. *See also* multifunction complexes
Larkin Building, 715, **745–46**, 1453; exterior, *745*
Larsen, Henning, **746–48**; Ministry of Foreign Affairs, Riyadh, **855–57**, 1171
Lasdun, Denys, **752–54**, 1361, 1362
Las Vegas, **748–52**; Fremont Street Experience Light and Sound Show, 1233
Laszlo, Hudec, Park Hotel, **980–82**
La Tendenza, 1355–56
Latin America: influence of CIAM on, 297; modernism, 40; need for different architectural solutions, 362
Latin American architecture, 248, 1441
Latinoamericana Tower, 844
Latvian National Library, 148
L'Aubette in Strasbourg, 6
League of Nations Building in Geneva, 285
Learning from Las Vegas, 750, 1118, 1183
Lebanese architects, 129, 130
Lechner, Ödön, 662
Le Corbusier: Elements of a Synthesis (Von Moos), 1423
LED lamps, 775
Legorreta, Ricardo, **755–57**, *4ii*
Le Havre, France, **754–55**
Leicester University, Engineering Building, *181*
Lenin Institute, 757
Lenin Memorial, *833*
Lenningrad, Constructivism in, 303
Leonidov, Ivan Ilich, **757–59**
Leon Roos House, 822

Le Parc tower in Buenos Aires, 41

Les Arcades Du Lac, 152, *153*

lesbian views and architecture, 454

Lescaze, William, **660–62**

Les Espaces D'Abraxas, 152–53

Letchworth, 434, 482

Lethaby, W.R., 75

Lever House, 190, 518, 596, **759–60**, 928, 1212, 1216–17; exterior, *759*

Levi, Rino, **760–62**

Le Viaduc, 152

Levittown, 96, **762–64**, 1272; aerial view, *95*

Lewerentz, Sigurd, 354, **764–65**

Liang Sicheng, **765–66**

Libera, Adalberto, 478, **766–68**; Casa Malaparte, **221–23**, *4i*

Libeskind, Daniel, **768–70**; Holocaust Museum in Berlin, 7; Jewish Museum, Berlin, **711–12**, *4ii*, 768; relation with Deconstructivism, 350

libraries, **770–73**; Aalto's compared with Larsen's, 748; Ciudad Universitaria, Mexico City, 267; by Colin St. John Wilson, 1446. *See also* Phoenix Central Library

Libya, 20

Liebknecht-Luxemburg Memorial, 853

Liederhall in Stuttgart, 1268

light as building material: Birkert's use of, 147–48; Cartier Museum, 942–43; Fumihiko Maki's use of, 812; Getty Museum, 499; Hans Poelzig's "light architecture," 1031; Peter Zumthor's use of, 1470; Renzo Piano's use, 1013; Toyo Ito's work, 700

lighting, **773–76**; Boston City Hall, 158; British Library, London, 174; Church of St. Francis of Assisi, 257; in department stores, 220; in factories, 156, 1395; in Frank Lloyd Wright's works, 1373; at Glasgow School of Art, 511; Hilversum Town Hall, 615; Hong Kong, 642; by internal light court, 745; Kimbell Art Museum, 732; light as raw material, 35; L'Innovation Department Store, 782; Louis Kahn's relating with structure, 724; in museums, 917; neon, 229; Phoenix Central Library, 1010–11; Sainsbury Wing, National Gallery, London, 1155; by Steven Holl, 634; use by Yoshio Taniguchi, 1304; Westin Times Square Hotel, 68

Lighting Center, 937

lightweight frames: aluminum, 37; by Frei Otto, 960

lightweight structures, Ove Arup's use of, 79

Lilla Bommen, 412

Lille Grand Palais, *735*

limestone blocks of coral, 709

Lin, Maya, **776–78**; Vietnam Veterans Memorial, **1412–14**

Lincoln Center, **778–79**; plaza, *779*

Lincoln Memorial, **779–81**; exterior, *780*

linguistics and architecture, 92

L'Innovation Department Store, **781–82**

Liperi Rehabilitation Centre for War Consumptives, 1104

Lippo Centre, 642

Lisbon, Portugal, **782–84**

Lisbon Ismaili Center, 1106

Lisbon World Exhibition (1998), 783

Lisbon World Exposition (1998), **784–86**

Lissitzky, El, 303, 1146; relation with constructivism, 301; relation with De Stijl, 349

live-work units, 1163

living memorials, 832, 833

Ljubljana, Jože Plecnik's work in, 1030

Lloyd's of London, 595, 1126; exterior, *1126*

load-bearing walls, 819

lobbies: AT&T Building, 85–86; Berlin Philharmonic Concert Hall, 142; Channel 4 Headquarters, London, 237; Chrysler Building, 253; Empire State Building, 404; Grand Central Terminal, 539–40; by Helmut Jahn, 706; hotel atrium, 655; Lyons Opera House, 943. *See also* atriums; waiting areas

locally available materials use: Alliance Franco-Sénéfalaise, 36; by Alvaro Siza, 1210; awards for, 26; Bank of London and South America, Buenos Aires, 110; by Fernando Tàvora, 1308; Petronas Towers in Malaysia, 1006; Ramses Wissa Wassef Arts Centre, 1079; Spain, 1234

Loews Philadelphia Hotel. *See* PSFS Building

Loewy House, 474

London, England, **786–90**; Sainsbury Wing, National Gallery, **1154–56**; subway, 1273; Survey of London, 81; urban development, 1377; urban redevelopment, 1379

London: The Unique City (Rasmussen), 1082

London Zoo: Gorilla House and Penguin Pool, 78, 799; Penguin Pool, 611

Loos, Adolf, **790–93**; impact on vernacular traditions, 1402; impact on Viennese modernism, 92; influence on Czechoslovakia, 341, 342; modernism of, 861; *Raumplan*, 339; Steiner House, 790, **1247–48**; use of timber framing, 1326; view of ornament, 656

Lord's Cricket Field, 649, 650, 1314, 1363

Los Angeles, California, **793–96**; Art Deco, 70; Banham's ideal of, *108*; freeways, 985, 1119; transportation planning, 1340

Los Angeles: The Architecture of Four Ecologies (Banham), 107

Los Angeles Country Courthouse and Hall of Administration, 1443

Los Angeles International Airport, Theme Building, *1443*, 1443–44, *8iii*

Los Angeles Museum of Art, Shin'enKan Museum, 524

Los Angeles Museum of Contemporary Art, 490

Los Angeles Public Library, 532

Louvre pyramid, 391, 518, 894, 992

Lovell beach house, 796, 1176, 1368

Lovell Health House, 795, **796–97**, 918, *5ii*; drawing, *797*

low-cost housing: Adèle Naudé Santos's model for, 1162; by Balkrishna Doshi, 367; Charles Correa's, 316; Le Corbusiersier's plan, 311; exhibits at Expo 1967, 422; India, 367, 674; by Irving John Gill, 504; Malagueira Housing Quarter, **813–14**; Mexico, 844; Mexico City, 528; by Michel De Klerk, 346; Paris, 1012; by Tony Garnier, 484; using pisé, 385; by William Wurster, *1459*. *See also* public housing; urban planning

Lowell Mills, 13

low-tech architecture, 24

Loyola Law School campus, 490–91

Lubetkin, Berthold, 78

Lubetkin and Tecton, **799–801**; Highpoint 1 Apartment Block, 78, **610–12**

Lucas, Colin. *See* Connell, Ward, and Lucas

Lucile Halsell Conservatory, main courtyard, *42*

Luckenwalde Hat Factory, 138

Lume Media Center, 599

Luna Park, Coney Island, 52

Lunuganga, 124; garden at, *124*

Lutyens, Edwin, **801–2**; classicism in works of, 269; Cottage style, 1333; Empire style buildings, 23; relationship with Herbert Baker,

102; relation with regionalism, 1091; use of earthen materials, 384; work in London, 787; work in New Delhi, 919, 1019
Luxor Casino and Hotel in Las Vegas, 391
Lu Xun Memorial Museum, 241
Lu Yanzhi, **797–99**
Lyle, John M., 210, 1334
Lynch, Kevin, **802–4**, 1379
Lyons, France: Garnier's public buildings, 260; Tony Garnier's work, 484
Lyon-Satolas Station for Lyon Airport, 1078
Lyons Opera House, 943
Lyotard, Jean-François, 1049

MacDonald, Frances, 509; Art nouveau poster, *73*
MacDonald, Margaret, 509
machine aesthetic, 1294; AEG Turbine Factory, 18; Art Deco, 69; Arts and Crafts Movement resistance to, 75; Banham's writings about, 107; cities, 1419; furniture by Charlotte Perriand, 1002; in Kazuo Shonhara's work, 1203–4; Moisei Ginzberg's design, 506; roadside attractions, 1116; role of steel, 1242; Villa Savoye, 1417; in Walter Gropius's work, 562. *See also* Futurism
Mackintosh, Charles Rennie, 509, **805–7**, 1091; Glasgow School of Art (Scotland), **511–13**; Hill House, 76–77, *5i*
Mackintosh Room at Glasgow School of Art, *512*
Madison Square Presbyterian Church in New York City, 824
Madonna Inn, 888
Maeght Museum, 1196–97
Maekawa, Kuno, Metropolitan Festival Hall, **842**
magnesite, 746
Mahmoud Mokhtar Sculpture Museum, 1436
Mahony, Marion, 1120
maidans, **807–8**. *See also* piazza theme; plazas
Maillart, Robert, **808–10**, 1095; use of concrete, 292
Maison Cubist project, 332
Maison d'Artiste, 348, 349, 1391
Maison de la Culture in Le Havre, 755
Maison de la Publicité, 935
Maison de Verre, 239, 240, **810–11**
Maison du Peuple, 73, 651
Maison Particuliére, 348, 349, 1391
Maisons Jaoul at Neuilly-sur-Seine, 172, 978
Majolikahaus, *74*
Maki, Fumihiko, **811–13**, 838, 839
Makovecz, Imre, 185, 664
Malagueira Quarter, Evora, Portugal, **813–14**
Malaysian architecture, 1228
Malevich, Kazimir, 1146
Mali: Great Mosque of Djenne, 385; Great Mosque of Niono, 546
Mallet-Stevens, Robert, **814–15**; project at International Exhibition of Decorative Arts (Paris 1925), 680
Managua Cathedral, *756, 4ii*
"Manhattan Modern," 927
Manteola, Flora, 815
Manteola, Sánchez Gómez, Santos, Solsona, Viñoly, **815–17**
manufacturing facilities. *See* industrial buildings
Maravillas Gymnasium, 1226
marble: undulating, 1045, white, 971. *See also* terrazzo
Marina City in Chicago, 243, *525*
Marin County Civic Center, 1455
Marinette, Fillipo Tomaso, 260
Marinetti, Filippo Tomaso, 478

Markelius, Sven, **817–18**; Hälsingborg, Sweden Concert Hall, **289–90**; Vällingby, 1284
Market Square in Lake Forest, 1200, 1205
Marktown, 1200
Marmon Hupmobile Auto showroom, *391*
Marquette Building in Chicago, 241
Marrakesh Regional Military Hospital, *20*
Marriot Marquis, 1041
MARS (Modern Architectural Research) Group, 298, 299, 787, 799
Mary Cooper Jewett Arts Center, 1142
Máscara de la Medusa, 600
Masonic Temples, 391
Masonite, 406
masonry: Bruno Taut's opinion, 522; curtain wall system, 336
masonry bearing walls, **819–20**; containing concrete, 1260; limits of, 1246. *See also* stone
Massachusetts Institute of Technology: Baker Dormitory, 2, 159, 207; Kresge Auditorium, *295*, 296; Kresge Chapel, 256
Massey, Geoffrey, 1390
masted tension structures, 1243
master plans, 206
materialism *vs.* high culture, 17, 53
Mathewson House, 823
Mätyniemi, 1015
May, Cliff, 795
May, Ernst, 472–73, **820–21**, 1179–80
Maybeck, Bernard R., **821–24**, 1091; Church of Christ, Scientist, Berkeley, 322, 822, 823, 1326; experiments with concrete, 290; use of timber framing, 1326
Mayer, Albert, 234, 235; Fagus Werk, **435–36**
Mayne, Thom, 877, 878
Mazloum, Djahanguir, *688*
McClurg Building, 632
McCormick Place Convention Center, 706
McDonough, William, 1280
McGraw-Hill Building, 648
McKim, Mead and White, **824–25**; acoustical design, 11; approach to American architecture, 1365; Bank of Montreal, *867*; Boston Public Library, 158; Boston Symphony Hall, 11; campus plans, 206; Court of the Universe, *415*, 975; General Post Office in New York, 927; Hotel Nacional, 329; Pennsylvania Station, New York City, 269, 270; use of glass, 515
McKinnell, Michael, 156
McMath Solar Telescope at Kitt Peak, 1213
McNair, James Herbert, 509
Mead, William Rutherford. *See* McKim, Mead and White
mechanical innovations, introduction into architecture, 261
Mechanization Takes Command (Giedion), 501
Medgyaszay, István, 663, **825–26**
medieval architecture aesthetic, 75, 76
Mediterranean style: in Israel, 695; in Los Angeles, 794; in Miami, Florida, 850
megastructures, 261, 1362; and utopian planning, 1384
Meier, Richard, 573, **827–29**; Getty Center, **498–500**, 827, 894; The Hague, 266; High Museum of Art, **608–10**
Melbourne, Australia, **829–30**
Melbourne School, 90, 830
Melnikhov House, The (Pallasmaa), 972
Melnikov, Konstantin, **830–32**, 879, 970; project at International Exhibition of Decorative Arts (Paris 1925), 680

Melrose Community Center (Bronx, New York), *27, 1i*

Memorial da América Latina, 1165

Mémorial de la Déportation, 979

memorials, **832–34**; Art Deco Anzac Memorial, 71; "disappearing" column, 833; by Edwin Lutyens, 802; Gateway Arch (St. Louis), **486–87**; by Herbert Baker, 102, 103; Jefferson Memorial, 1038; by Lu Yanzhi, 797, 798; by Maya Lin, 776; by Otto Wagner, 832; by Paul Philippe Cret, 326; by Ricardo Bofill, 152; Sun Yat-sen Memorial Hall, 797, 798; Victims of Japanese Massacre, 251; at visitor centers, 1420, *1421*; World Trade Center, 769

Memory Foundations, 769. *See also* monuments

Memphis Group, Italy, **834–35**

Mendelsohn, Erich, 516, **835–37**, 1297; Einstein Tower, **393–94**; Expressionist work, 426; Luckenwalde Hat Factory, 138; Palace of the Soviets Competition entry, 969; photographs, 59; Universum Cinema, **1375–76**; views of Rotterdam, 1135; work in Israel, 695

Menil Collection, 659, **837–38**

Mercadal, Fernando García, 1233

Mesaggio, 1158, 1159

Messeturm, 708

Metabolists, 693, 699, 737, **838–40**, 1303; Fumihiko, Maki, **811–13**; influence in Tokyo, 1330; In Japan, 739–40

metal curtain wall panels, 337

Metron, 66

Metropolis of Tomorrow, The (Ferriss), 456

Metropolitan Chapel, 163–64

Metropolitan Festival Hall, Tokyo, **842**

Metropolitan Government Building in Tokyo, 1330

Metropolitan Life Building, 775

Metropolitan Museum of Art, New York extension, 1123

Metro Station, Paris, 423–24, **840–41**, 1273; entrance, *841*

Mexican architects, 116, 213

Mexican architecture, 327, 528, 872, 937

Mexican School of Architecture, 843

Mexico, **842–46**

Mexico City, 843, **846–48**; architects, 116; Ciudad Universitaria Campus and Stadium, **266–67**

Mexico House II, 878

Meyer, Hannes, **848–50**

Meyerson Symphony Center, 992

MGM Grand Hotel, 750

Miami, Florida, **850–52**

Miami architects, 852

Miami Beach, Florida, 70; Art Deco District, 1184; urban renewal, 744

MIAR (International Movement for Rational Architecture), 443

Middle School in Morbio Inferiore, 162

Midway Gardens, 1454

Mies van der Rohe, Ludwig, **852–55**; approach to architecture, 1368; buildings at Weissenhofsiedlung (Stuttgart 1927), 1437; Chicago Convention Hall, 1346; church design, 256; furniture, 521; German Pavilion (Barcelona 1929), 415, **492–94**; Glass Chain crystal, 138; Glass Skyscraper, **521–22**; Illinois Institute of Technology, 207, **667–69**; Illinois Institute of Technology, Chemistry Laboratory, 1098; impact on Chicago, 242–43, 244, 245–46; International Style, 682–83; Lake Shore Drive Apartments, *245*, 246; move to Bauhaus, 120; Neue Nationalgalerie, *138*; Paimio Sanatorium, 1469; plazas, 1028; relation with De Stijl, 348; Seagram Building, **1187–88**; skyscrapers, 1216; Spiegelglashalle, 1437; tectonics in works of,

1313; Toronto-Dominion Centre, 1335; Tugendhat House, **1348–49**, *5iii*; use of brick, 171; use of color, 279; use of glass, 516; Westmount Square, 867; work in Czechoslovakia, 342. *See also* Farnsworth House; Seagram Building

Miho Museum, 992

Milan, Italy Torre Velasca, **1337–39**

mill buildings, adaptive re-use, 13

Millennial Dome at Greenwich, 1127, 1264

Mills College: El Campanil, 875; library, 875

Milwaukee Art Museum *3i*; expansion project, 204; Santiago Quadracci pavilion, *205*

minimalist architecture: Brussels, 179; Germany, 496; Helsinki, 602; relation with ornament, 959

Minimalist style, Flemish architects, 132

Ministry of Education Building in Rio de Janeiro, 194

Ministry of Foreign Affairs, Riyadh, *747, 748*, **855–57**, 1171; courtyard, *856*

Ministry of Heavy Industry, 758

Ministry of Social Welfare and Employment in The Hague, 606

Minneapolis, Minnesota, twin cities regional planning council, 1088

Minnesota State Capitol, 502

Minta, Lassiné, Great Mosque of Niono, 546

Mirage, 751

Miralles, Enric, **857–59**

Miró Museum, 1196–97

Miró studio, 112

Mission Revival, 1062

Mission style architecture, 228; country clubs, 320

Mito Art Tower, The, 693

mobile architecture, 426

mobile homes, **859–60**

Moda en Casa, 938

model city, 226

Model Factory for Werkbund Exhibition (Cologne 1914), 563

models: Antoni Gaudí's use of, 489; Bauhaus, 120; Broadacre City, *176*; by Morphosis, 877

Modern Architecture: A Critical History (Frampton), 623

Modern Architecture (Tafuri), 623

modern art and architecture, 5–6; Cubism, **332–34**

Modern Art Museum of Fort Worth, *54*

"Modern Classicism," 929

Modern Housing (Bauer), 1459

modernism, **860–63**. *See also* Futurism; and abstraction, 6–7; Ada Louise Huxtable's writings, 665; apartment buildings, 56; Australia, 90; Austria, 93; Bangkok, 104, 105; Brazil, 194, 1111; Brazilian, 165–68; Bucharest, 183; Buenos Aires, 186–87; Cairo, 201; Chile, 247; concept of space and order, 1166; effect on country clubs, 321; Finland, 461; Finnish, 148; inner contradiction seen by Norberg-Schulz, 936; Iran, 688; Latin America, 40; Manhattan, 928; metaphor of health, 967, 1224; Norway, 940; Ralph Adams Crams's view of, 324; relation with avante-garde, 97; relation with roadside attractions, 1116; relation with supermodernism, 1279; relation with typology, 1355; of Seagram Building, 1187; Switzerland, 1286; Thailand, 102; view of brick, 170–71

modernisme architects, 1071; Barcelona, 111

modernismo, 223, 225

modernist nationalism: China, 249–50; United States, 600

modernity, difference from moderism, 861

Modern Movement: airport buildings, 32–33; Argentina, 65–66; Banham's writings about, 107; Bruno Paul's role, 988; Bruno Zevi's writings, 1467; Canada, 210; Caracas, 215–16; Cuba, 329; Heinrich Tessenow's relation with, 1322; and historic preservation, 618; historiography, 622–23; impact of Nikolaus Pevsner on, 1006; impact on architectural drawing, 58–59; importance of CIAM to, 296; influence of Auguste Choisy, 251; Juhani Uolevi Pallasmaa's writings, 972; ornament, 959; relation to avant-garde, 97; relation with Arts and Crafts Movement, 77; relation with historicism, 620; relation with rationalism, 1084; Southern and Central Africa, 24; United Kingdom, 1360, 1361; in United States, 36. *See also* Functionalism

modern regionalism, 192, 1128

modern vernacular: of Alvar Aalto, 1416; of Fernando Tàvora, 1307, 1308; Kyoto, Japan, 739; Saudi Arabia, 1169

modular systems: Blomstedt's use of, 149; Habitat '67, Montreal, 579; Kisho Kurokawa's interest in, 737; library, 772, 1010; Molnár's sliding walls, 863, 864; office, 605–6; precast construction, 1057; at Renault Distribution Centre, 1096; research centers, 1099

Moduli 225, 972

Moerdyk, Gerhard, 23–24

Moholy-Nagy, Sibyl, 1375

Mohrmann House, 1175

Molchow House, 1151

Molnar, Farkas, **863–64**

Monadnock Building, 171, 391, 819

Mondrian, Piet, 348

Moneo Vallés, José Rafael, 325, **864–66**, 1078, 1258; Museums of Modern Art and Architecture in Sweden, 1285

monolithic earth construction, 383

Monte Carlo seaside project (Archigram), 58

Montreal, Canada, **866–68**. *See also* Expo 1967, Montreal

monumental architecture: Exposition des Arts et Techniques (1937), 978; Grande Arche de la Défense, **540–42**; Henning Larsen's work, 748; Hungary, 662; Indonesia, 1229; of Kenzo Tange, 1302, 1303; Louis Kahn's view of, 723; Melbourne, 830; Mexico City, 847, 848; Moscow, 879; Philippines, 1229; relationship with tents, 1317; Romania, 1131; Sigfried Giedion's writings, 501; use of stone, 1258; Willem Marinus Dudok's view, 615; Wright's understanding of, 1453–54

monuments: Berlin Wall designation as, 145; at Brasilia, 164; by Raimund Abraham, 5; vernacular style, 1461; Washington Monument, 543. *See also* memorials

Monument to the Resistance, 1134

Monument to the Third International, **868–70**

Moore, Charles, 365, 621, **870–72**, 1369; relation with postmodernism, 1048

Moorish style: at Panama-Pacific International Exposition in San Francisco, 975; in Sarajevo, 1464; synagogues, 1296

Moral, Enrique del, **872–73**

Moravian architecture, 341

Moretti, Luigi, **873–75**; Stock Exchange Tower, 867

Morgan, Julia, 388, **875–77**, 1092

Morgan Library, 824

Morocco, urban development, 20

Morphosis, **877–79**, 1084; relation with Deconstructivism, 350

Morris, William, 75, 76, 77

mortar, 819

Moscow, Russia, **879–82**; constructivism in, 301–3; Moisei Ginzburg's model for, 507; Monument to the Third International, **868–70**; style moderne, 1145; subway, 1274; subway escalators, 414–15

Moscow Art Theater, 1201

Moscow Insurance Society on Old Square, 1202

Moscow State University, 880–881, *880*

Moser House, *628*

Moses, Robert, 94, 985, 1087, 1340

Mosque, Rome, *1044*

Mosque of the Grand National Assembly, **884–86**; facade, *885*; main entrance, *886*

mosques, **882–84**; in Dhaka, 360; Southern and Central Africa, 24

Moss, Eric Owen, 1051

Mostorg Department Store, 1406

motels, 95, **887–88**; as roadside attractions, 1117

Motherwell Studio, 240

Mound Stand at Lord's Cricket Ground, 649, 650, 1314, 1363

movie theaters, **888–90**; Coop Himmelblau design, 307; influence of Universum Cinema on, 1376; marquee, *889*

moving walkways, 414

Mt. Hope, New Jersey Elementary School, 1181

MTV Studios, 878

Müller, Karl-Heinrich, 379

multifunction complexes: Baiyoke Towers, 101; Beirut apartment buildings, 129; bus terminals, 199; Canada Place, 1390; disjunctive, 1347; Glass Palace, 1103; by John C. Portman Jr., 1041; parking garages in, 984; Rockefeller Center, 1124; stadiums as, 1239–49; Switzerland, 1287; Unité d'Habitation, 1358

Multiple-Prime Contracting system, 300

multiplex theaters, 890

Mumford, Lewis, 501, 518, 551, 686, **890–92**; regional planning, 1087

municipal codes. *See* ordinances

Municipal Stadium in Lyon, 484

Municipal Stadium of Florence, 910

Municipal Theater General San Martin, 40

Murphy, C.F., 948

Musée des Travaux Publics, 1001

Musée d'Orsay, 87, *88*, 979

Museum for the Decorative Arts in Frankfurt, 827–28

Museum Insel Hombroich, 379

Museum of Antiquities, Cairo, 201

Museum of Contemporary Art, Barcelona, *828*

Museum of Contemporary Art, Los Angeles, *893*

Museum of Contemporary Art in Helsinki, 634

Museum of Finnish Architecture, 464

Museum of Folk Art in New York, 1445

Museum of Modern Art, Copenhagen, 355

Museum of Modern Art, Frankfurt, 636, **894–96**; exterior, *895*

Museum of Modern Art, New York, 893, **896–98**; Ambasz' influence, 41–42; "Deconstructivist Architecture" exhibition, 350, 351; 1959 exhibition, impact on Art Nouveau, 75; guest house, 520; International Style Exhibition, **685–87**; Philip Johnson's work at, 715–16, *716*

Museum of Modern Art, San Francisco, *161*

Museum of São Paulo, 150–51; exterior, *151*

museums, **892–94**; adaptive re-use of buildings for, 12, 13; Aulenti's exhibition space designs, 87–88; design, 7; by Edward Larrabee

museums (continued)
    Barnes, 115; by Frank Gehry, 490; lighting in, 917; in New York City, 928; open-air, 1402; Paris, 979; Philadelphia, 1009
Museums of Modern Art and Architecture in Sweden, 1285
music and architecture, 149, 373; Hans Hollein, 7; Mies' metaphor, 516; Paolo Portoghesi's work, 1044; Steven Holl, 634; Willem Marinus Dudok, 614
Muthesius, Hermann, **898–99**, 1355; exhibition buildings, 1439; relation with Deutscher Werkbund, 357, 358
Muuratsalo Summer House, 2–3

Nagakin Capsule Tower, 737, 738
Nairobi, Kenya, 24
Najdi style, 1113
Nakagin Capsule Building, 839
Narkomfin Building, 302–3
National Archives in Washington, D.C., *1039*
National Archives of Canada, 211
National Art Schools, Havana, **901–2**; School of Visual Arts, *902*
National Assembly Building, Dhaka, **902–4**; exterior, *903*
National Assembly Building Kuwait City, *1386*
National Building Museum, 12
National Center for Atmospheric Research (NCAR), 991
National Commercial Bank Headquarters, 710
National Commercial Bank in Jeddah, *190*
Nationale-Nederlanden Building, 490, 571
National Exhibition of 1939 in Zürich, 1287
National Farmers' Bank, **904–6**, 1276; interior, *905*
National Gallery of Art, 1038; East Building, 894, **906–7**, 992; East Building interior, *907*
National Gallery of Canada, 1153
National Grand Theater of China, 251
National Library and Archives in Dhaka, 692
National Library of Argentina, 1322
National Library of China, 1456
National Library of France, 999, *1000*
National Mall in Washington, D.C., 781
National Museum of Anthropology, Mexico, 844
National Museum of Modern Art in Kyoto, 811
National Museum of Roman Art, 865
National Netherlands Building, 1053
National Park Service, U.S., 985, 1420
National Pensions Institute in Helsinki, 2
National Queen Sirikit Convention Center, 106
National Romanticism, 81; Budapest, 185; city halls, 264; Finland, 459; Hungary, 662, 663; Norway, 939; Sweden, 1284; use of timber framing, 1326; Yugoslavia, 1465
National Romantic movement, Finland, 600, 601
National School Theater in Mexico City, 938
national style: Budapest, 185; Cairo, 202; Canadian, 210; Cuba, 329; Thailand, 105; United States, 1453
National Theater in Prague, 1053
National Trust for Historic Preservation, 618
National University in Mexico, National Library, 947
nature: in Ando's architecture, 53; as architect, 6; balancing the forces of, 455; bringing into the city, 305; inspiration from, 72, 73–74
nature integrated with buildings, 42–43, 194, 258, 1458; Adèle Naudé Santos' work, 1162; Alberto Kalach's use of patios, 726; Alvar Aalto, 2; Antoine Predock's work, 1058; Atocha Station in

Madrid, 1078; Bruce Alonzo Goff's work, 523; Chloethiel Woodard Smith's works, 1218; churches, 256; Ciudad Universitaria Stadium, Mexico City, 267; Cuba, 331; Frank Lloyd Wright's works, 1452; Getty Museum, 499; Glacier Museum, 509; Gürel Family Summer Residence, 575–76; House-on-Hill, 15; Itsuko Hasegawa's work, 591; Kazuyo Sejima's work, 1194; Menil Collection, 838; Nicholas Grimshaw's work, 559–60; Our Lady of Peace Basilica, *965*; Palais Stoclet, 971; Reima and Raili Pietilä's work, 1014–15; in Sverre Fehn's work, 450; tree in facade, 66; use at Schröder-Schräder House, 1182; use of glass to simulate, 1081; Yoshio Taniguchi's works, 1304. *See also* Contextualism
Naumann, Friedrich, 357
nautical forms, 239; The Ark in London, 412; church design with, 256; Coca-Cola Bottling Plant in Los Angeles, 795; in Expressionist work, 427; House of Maria Melero, 329; Kölnsiche Zeitung, 277; Lisbon World Expo, 783, 785–86; by Reima Pietilä, 602; Seamen's Church Institute in New York, 1032
Navarro Baldeweg, Juan, **907–8**
Navrongo Cathedral in Ghana, 385
Nazi effects on architecture, 443–44; Berlin, 139–40; book burning, 598; Cologne, Germany, 277–78; Germany, 496; Nazi use of stripped classicism, 269
Nebraska State Capitol, 531
necoclassical style, City Beautiful movement, 262
Negro House, 726
neighborhood conservation, 616–17
neo-avant-garde, 98
neobaroque style: Hungary, 663; London, 787; New Delhi, 672
neoclassical revival style, Moscow, 879
Neoclassicism: in Auguste Perret's work, 1001; Bangkok, 104; Barcelona architects, 112, 113; Boston, 158; Brazil, 165; Canada, 208; Chicago, 242; China, 249; Denmark, 353; effect of UER'42, 443; Hong Kong Shanghai Bank, 646; Hungary, 664; of John Russell Pope, 1038; in Kay Fisker's work, 464; Le Harve, France, 754; Northern Africa, 20; Norway, 939; Philadelphia, 1009; in Plan of Chicago, 1019; Russia, 1145; Turkey, 1350; use of stone, 1258; in Washington, D.C., 1433
neo-Colonial style: Argentina, 65; Brazil, 165; Mexico, 843; Mexico City, 846; Rio de Janeiro, 1112
neo-Gothic style, Canada, 209
neon signs, 96
Neoplasticism (New Forming), 1391
neorationalism, **909**, 1048, 1355–56
neorealism, 1132
neo-Russian style, 879, 1202
neovernacular, London, 789
"neovernacular design," 924
Nervi, Pier Luigi, **910–11**; church design, 256; Exhibition Hall, Turin, Italy, **416–19**; Gatti Wool Factory, 1095; George Washington Bridge Bus Terminal, 199; influence on Harry Seidler, 1192; Olympic Stadium in Rome, 1132; pavilions by, 416; Stock Exchange Tower, 867; structural innovations, 1037; use of concrete, 293; work in Paris, 979; work in Yugoslavia, 1465
Netherlands, **912–15**
Netherlands Exhibition Hall (1969), *963*
Netherlands Pavilion at Expo 1967, 422
Netherlands Pavilion for Venice Biennale, 1109–10
Netsch, Walter, 243, 1381

Neue Nationalgalerie, detail, *138*

Neue Staatsgalerie, **916–17**; compared with Museum Abteiberg, 9; exterior, *916*

Neue Vahr Apartment building, 3

Neue Wache, 1321–22

Neue Zolhof, Der, *378, 379*

Neumann, Alfred, 696

Neurosciences Institute in La Jolla, 1444

Neutra, Richard, **917–19**; influence in Cuba, 330; influence on suburban housing, 1081; Lovell Health House, 796, *5ii*; relation with environmental issues, 410; relation with International Style, 682; work in Los Angeles, 795

Neviges Pilgrimage Church, **1015–16**

New Austrian Cultural Institute in Manhattan, 5

New Brutalism. *See* Brutalism

New Caledonia Cultural Centre Jean Marie Tjibaou, **334–35**

New City, The: Principles of Planning (Hilberseimer), 612

New Courtyard House Complex, 1456–57

New Delhi, India, **919–20**; Raj Rewal's work in, 1106

New Delhi Embassy, 401, *402*

New England Merchants National Bank in Boston, 115

New Farm in Surrey, 298

New Gourna, 445

New National Gallery of Art in Stuttgart, 1268–69

New Objectivity, 137, 989; "constructed organicist" version, 1175; Hannes Meyer's work, 848. *See also* Functionalism

New Petersburg Apartment Building, *1238*

"new regionalism," 940

New School for Social Research, 928

New Theatre in Oslo, 939

new town developments: Ankara, 1350; Ardalan's, 63; Chandigarh, India, **235–36**; Coldspring, Maryland, 1153; downside of, 1379; Fascist, 443; Finland, 462; Heliopolis, 201; Iran, 689; near Glasgow, Scotland, 514; Northern Africa, 21; Stockholm, 1258; Sweden, 1285; Tapiola, 149; Tokyo, 1330–31; Tyrone, New Mexico, 531; in the USSR, 820; Vällingby, 818. *See also* Arcosanti, Arizona; utopian planning

New Towns Movement, **919–20**

New Urbanism, **921–25**, 1049: Colin Rowe's influence, 1140; effect of ordinances on, 956; and historic preservation, 618; Jane Jacobs's influence, 703; relation with Disney theme parks, 365; relation with Historicism, 621; Romania, 1131; roots in Contextualism, 306; Seaside, Florida example, 1189; second generation example, 226; United States, 1366. *See also* greenbelts and greenbelt towns

New York City, **925–29**; Ada Louise Huxtable's writings, 665; AT&T Building, **84–86**, 621, 716, 1217; Carrère and Hastings' works in, 218; Empire State Building, 253, **403–4**, 927, 1216; Flatiron Building, **466–67**; Guggenheim Museum (New York), **572–74**, 746, 928, 1455; Master Plan, 677; Regional Plan of 1923, 1087; Rem Koolhaas writings, 734; Rockefeller Center, 927, 1028, **1124–26**; Seagram Building, **1187–88**; skyline, *926*; skyscrapers, 1215; subway, 1274; TWA Airport Terminal, **1353–54**; United Nations Headquarters, 765, 818, 928, **1963–65**; urban development, 1378; Woolworth Building, 502, 1215, **1449–51**; World Trade Center, 769, 1217, **1451–52**

New York Daily News Building, 647

New Yorker magazine "Sky Line," 891

New York Exposition of 1939, 416

"New York Five," 394, 542, 578, 827, 1369

New York Museum of Natural History, Rose Center for Earth and Space, 1033

New York New York (hotel), 751

New York Public Library, 217–18; exterior, *218*

New York State Theater, 778

New York World's Fair (1939), **929–31**

New Zealand, **932–33**

New Zealand architects, 932

Niagara City Performing Arts Center, 591

Niagara Falls Power Generating Station, 208

nickelodeons, 889

Niedecken, George, 1120

Niemeyer, Oscar, **933–34**; Capela de Pampulha, 166–67; Church of St. Francis of Assisi, **257–58**; collaboration with Lúcio Costa, 318; Copan Building, *1165*; impact on Brazil, 166; Memorial da América Latina, 1165; National Congress Complex, *8iii*; Pampulha Buildings, **973–74**; relation with Brasília, 163, 164; work in Rio de Janeiro, 1112

Nieuwe Bouwen. *See* Dutch Functionalism

Nieuwe Kunst. *See* Art Nouveau (Jugendstil)

Nigeria, Abuja, Federal Capital Territory, **9–10**

night lighting, 775

Nihon Kosaku Bunka Renmei (Japanese Werkbund), 736–37

Nishizawa, Ryue, 1195

Nitzschke, Oscar, **934–36**

Noguchi, Isamu, 990

"nonspace," 1278

Norberg-Schulz, Christian, **936–37**

Nordic architecture, 81, 508, 936

Nordic Classicism, 149

Nordic Romanticism, Hungary, 663

Nordiska Museum, 1256

Norten, Enrique, 293, **937–38**

North Christian Church, Columbus, Indiana, 281

Northern Africa, **19–21**

Northern moderne, 1236

North Korean architecture, 1229

North Pole Mobile Ice Cream Store, 525

Norton, Enrique, use of concrete, 293

Norway, **938–41**

Norwegian influence in Australia, 936

Norwegian Pavilion (Sverre Fehn), 420, 450, 940

Notre Dame, Le Raincy, **941–44**, 1001; exterior, *942*

Nottingham, England, Boots Pure Drugs Factory, **155–56**

Nottingham University, 649, 650

Nouvel, Jean, **942–44**, 980

Novecento architecture in Hungary, 663

Novia Icària (Olympic Village, 1992), 114

Novocomum Apartment House in Como, 1318

Nuestra Señora de Guadalupe shrine, 844

Nyrop, Martin, 353

Oakland Cathedral, 204

Oakland Museum, 1123

observatories: Einstein Tower, **393–94**, 426; McMath Solar Telescope at Kitt Peak, 1213. *See also* shell designs

Ocean Terminal, 641

office buildings, **945–46**; skyscrapers; with basilica-based plan, 155; Chicago, 241; corporate office park, estate, and campus, **313–14**; Louis Sullivan's, 1276; New York City building code, 253;

office buildings (continued)
    plastic, 1023; by Ralph Erskine, 412; sustainable design, 1281–82.
    See also Johnson Wax Administration Building
O'Gorman, Juan, 844, **946–48**; University Library, UNAM, Mexico
    City, 267, **1373–75**
O'Hare International Airport, **948–50**; United Airlines Terminal,
    707, *949*
Ohgimi Beach House, 1162
Ohio State University, Wagner Center for the Visual Arts, *395*
Olbrich, Josef Maria, 91–92, 343, 344, 377, **950–51**; relation with
    Deutscher Werkbund, 357; relation with Vienna Secession, 1409,
    1410, 1411; Secession Building door detail, *1410, 6iii*
Old Post Office Building in Washington, D.C., 12
Old Stone Town, Zanzibar, Tanzania, *23*
Olgyay, Victor and Alada, 405
Olivetti Factory, **951–52**
Olmsted, Frederick Law, 985
Olsen Line Passenger Terminal in London, 468
Olympic Games in Sydney, 1291
Olympic Games Tent in Munich, *1239, 1240*
Olympic Stadium, Australia, *1289*
Olympic Stadium, Caracas, 267–68
Olympic Stadium, Munich (1971), 960, *961*
Olympic Stadium, Rome, 1132
Olympic Stadium, Tokyo, **952–53**
Olympic Velodrome and Swimming Pool, Berlin, 999, *3iii*
Olympic Village housing, Rome, 874–75
Ontario Place amusement park, 1335
Onyx Center, 944
Open Air School, Amsterdam, **953–55**; front entry, *954*
Open City in Chile, 248
open-plan schools, 1180–81
Opéra de la Bastille, *979*
Oporto, Tennis Pavilion by Fernando Tàvora, 1307
Orangery at Prague Castle, 713
ordinances, **955–57**; affecting Getty Museum, 498; affecting
    Highpoint I Apartments, 610; alliterative to, 227; design, **955–
    57**; in Glasgow, Scotland, 513; Hong Kong, 642; lack of, in
    Tokyo, 1328; for roadside architecture, 1118; Seaside, Florida,
    1189; suburban developments, 1272; Washington, D.C., 1433.
    See also zoning ordinances
organic functionalists, 587
organicism: in Australia, 90, 91; of Bruno Zevi, 1467; of Carlos
    Raúl Villanueva, 1418; and environmental issues, 409; of Frank
    Lloyd Wright, 669; Gunnar Birkerts's, 146; of Hugo Häring,
    567, 586; in Hungary, 664; of Jørn Utzon, 1385; of Juan
    O'Gorman, 946–47; Wright's transmission to Europe, 244
oriented strand board (OSB), 406, 407
ornament, **958–60**; Adolf Loos's aphorism about, 1400; Adolf
    Loos's rejection of, 1248; Alliance Franco-Sénéfalaise, 35; of
    Antoni Gaudí, 487, 488; Art Deco, 71; Art Nouveau (Jugendstil),
    72; Berlage's views on, 135; Casa Milà, 224; Chrysler Building,
    253; Classicism, 269; Edward Durell Stone's use of, 1261;
    Egyptian architecture, 390; feminine and masculine, 454; Hassan
    II Mosque, 592; by Holabird and Root, 630; Hong Kong and
    Shanghai Bank, 646–47; Indian, 673; Josep Puig i Cadafalch's use
    of, 1072; Louis Sullivan's views about, 1276; by Minoru
    Yamasaki, 1462; in mosques, 882; neo-Russian style, 1202;
    Portland Public Services Building, 1040; Stockholm Public
    Library, 1255; terracotta, 1318; in theaters, 890; used by Hans

Poelzig, 1031; used by Purcell and Elmslie, 1074, 1075; use in
    Art Deco, 1368; Viennese, 1172; Wanamaker Department Store,
    1431; when structure not expressive, 1428–29
Ort, Carlos, Opéra de la Bastille, *979*
orthographic projections, 58
OSA (Organization of Contemporary Architecture), 1406
OSB (oriented strand board), 406, 407
Osborn House, 114
Östberg, Ragnar, 1256
Otaka, Masato, 839, 842
Otaniemi Chapel, 259
Otis, Elisha Graves, 398
Otis Elevator Company, 414
Ottawa Civic Hospital, *653*
Otto, Frei, **960–62**; fabric structure experiments, 1315; West
    German Pavilion, 422
Ottoman architecture, 697, 1222, 1350
Oud, J.J.P., 334, **962–64**, 1136; relation with De Stijl, 348, 349;
    Weissenhof Row Houses, *1269*
Our Lady of Peace Basilica, Yamoussoukro, **964–65**
Ove Arup, 1096, 1178, 1291, 1314; energy-efficient design, 405;
    Menil Collection, 659; relation with environmental issues, 410
Oxford Ice Rink, 559
oya (lava stone), 669

Pailais de la Découverte, 935
Paimio Sanatorium, 517, **967–69**, 1469; elevation, *968*
Palace Hotel in Helsinki, 1104
Palace of Culture in Moscow, 758
Palace of Electricity, 424
Palace of Fine Arts, 821, *975, 976*
Palace of the Soviets Competition, **969–70**
palaces, Bangkok, 105
Palacio Güell, 488–89
Palacios y Ramilo, Antonio, 1233
Palais des Beaux-Arts, 652
Palais Stoclet, 656, **970–72**; exterior, *971*
Palau de la Música, 226
Palau Sant Jordi Sports Palace, *693, 694*
Palazetto Dello Sport, Rome, *910*
palazzo: Casa Girasole as, 874; impact on department stores, 356;
    influence on department stores, 1431; influence on embassies,
    402; model for libraries, 772; relation of Flatiron Building to,
    468; Santiago, Chile, 1160
Palazzo a Vela, 1012
Palazzo Hotel and Restaurant Complex, Il, 1135
Palladio, Andrea, 521
Pallasmaa, Juhani, 463, **972–73**
Palmer and Turner, 645
Palmer House Hotel, 632–33
Palmolive Building, 630
Palm Springs City Hall, 475
Palumbo, Lord Peter, 441–42
Pampulha Buildings, **973–74**; Church of St. Francis of Assisi, **257–
58**
Panama Pacific Exposition (San Francisco 1915), 415, **974–77**;
    Bertram Grosvenor Goodhue's buildings, 531; Court of the
    Universe, *415*
Pan Am Building, 684, 928, 1325
Pan American Union Building, 326

Pan-American Village, 331
Pani, Mario, 847, 872
Pantheon of Liberty and Democracy, 164
paper architecture, 635
parade grounds, 444; Baghdad, 808
Paradise Garden concept, 886
paradise garden theme, 63
Para-lam timber, 406
Parc de la Vilette, 350, *1347*
Parc Güell, 489
Paris, France, **977–80**; Voisin Plan for Paris; buildings by Le
   Corbusier, 978; Le Corbusier's plan for, 305; Metro Stations,
   840–41; urban planning, 1377; Voisin Plan for Paris, **1422–23**
Paris Exposition (1900), 415, **423–25**, 977
Paris Exposition (1937), 416
Park, Robert, 1380
Parker, Barry, 1164
Park Hotel, **980–82**; exterior, *981*
parking garages, 94, **982–84**; beneath plazas, 1027; Miami example,
   983; for row houses, 1139. *See also* warehouse and storage
   facilities
parkways, **984–86**, 1119; Benjamin Franklin, 263; New Delhi,
   1020–21; system of "green fingers," 227
Parliamentary Complex in Kotte, 124
Parliament Building, Chandigarh, **986–88**, *7ii*
Parliament Complex, Dhaka, 359, 361
Parliament House, Canberra, 212
Parliament House, Helsinki, 601, *602*
Parliament Library in New Delhi, 1106
participatory design, 1048
particleboard, 406, 407
Pasadena City Hall, 620
Pasadena Freeway, 985
Pasatiempo houses, 1458
Patel, Bimal, Entrepreneurship Development Institute, **407–8**
paths of movement: Bawa's work, 124; Channel 4 Headquarters,
   London, 237; Charles Correa's shifting axis, 315; effects of
   escalators, 414, 415; Holocaust Memorial Museum, Washington,
   D.C., 637; Pennsylvania Station, 995; in Peter and Alison
   Smithson's works, 1220, 1351; Reichstag, 1094; at Seaside,
   Florida, 1191; Taliesin West, 1301; Toyo Ito's work, 700; Yoshio
   Taniguchi's buildings, 1304. *See also* parkways
patio as transitional space, 844, 845
Patkau, Patricia and John, 211, **987–88**
Patscenter, 1099
Paul, Bruno, 357, **988–89**
Pavilion de la Musique, 935
Pavilion de l'Espirit Nouveau, 681
Pavilion of Cosmic Rays, 267
Pavilion of Portugal, 783, 786
Pavilion of Tourism, 680
pavilion-plan hospitals, 652
pavilions: All India Handloom Board, 314–15; Barcelona (1929),
   492–94; Chicago World's Fair (1933), **229–31**; concrete, 292–
   93; Disney theme parks, 364; by José Antonio Coderch y de
   Sentmenat, 273; Ludwig Mies van der Rohe's clear-span, 854;
   New York World's Fair (1939), *930*, 931; by Peter Behrens, 126,
   127; set into landscape, 124; Shrine of the Book, 1206; by
   Stepahnovich Melnikov, 831; styles at Panama-Pacific
   International Exposition in San Francisco, 976; by Sverre Fehn,

450–51; Taut's Glaspalast, 276; Venice Biennale (1895–1995),
   1397–99; World's Fair, Expo 1967, 210. *See also* exhibition
   building; tents
Peabody Studio, 1085
Peace Chapel for Juniata College, 776
Peace Memorial and Museum, Hiroshima, **989–90**
Peachtree Center, 1041
Peak Club, 641
Peak Tram Station Tower, *644*
Pearl Harbor fallout shelter, *439*
Pederson, William, 732
Pedestrian movement. *See* paths of movement
Pedrera, La, 489
Pei, I.M., 981, **990–93**; Bank of China Tower, **108–10**, 455–56,
   922, *1215*; Central Station project in Montreal, 867; Centrust
   Tower, 852; Fragrant Hill Hotel, 250, 992; Hancock Tower, 518;
   Hong Kong Bank, 455; influence in Washington, D.C., 1434–35;
   Louvre pyramid, 391, 518, 894; National Gallery of Art, East
   Building, 894; National Gallery of Art, East Building
   (Washington, D.C.), 894; relation with International Style, 684;
   use of concrete shells, 296
Pelli, Cesar, 642, 775, **993–95**, *5ii*; Petronas Towers, 994, **1004–6**
Pennsylvania Convention Center in Philadelphia, 13
Pennsylvania Station, 269, 270, 515, 927, **995–97**; interior, *996*
Pennsylvania style architecture, 430
Pension Building in Washington, D.C., 12
Penzoil Place Building, *659*, 716
people of color, women in architecture, 453
people of color in architecture schools, 388
Peressutti, Enrico, 1337
Periera, William, 207
Perkins, Lawrence Bradford, 997, 998
Perkins and Will, 949, **997–99**, 1170; Mt. Hope, New Jersey
   Elementary School, 1181
Perls House, 853
Perrault, Dominique, **999–1000**, *3iii*
Perret, Auguste, 620, 754, 977, **1001–2**; Notre Dame, Le Raincy,
   941–42; project at International Exhibition of Decorative Arts
   (Paris 1925), 680; tectonics in works of, 1313; use of concrete,
   292
Perriand, Charlotte, **1002–4**
Persico, Edoardo, 459
perspective drawings, 58
Peterlee New Town, 800
Peters House, 557
Petit Palais, 424
Petronas Towers, 994, **1004–6**; exterior, *1005*
Peugeot Tower in Buenos Aires, 1105
Pevsner, Nikolaus, 501, **1006–7**, 1354; views on historicism, 619,
   620; writings relating to historiography, 623
phenomenological approach to architecture, 936; Structuralism's
   rejection of, 1264; supermodernism, 1278
Philadelphia, Pennsylvania, **1007–9**; architects, 431; Benjamin
   Franklin Parkway, 263; Wanamaker Store, **1430–32**
Philadelphia City Hall, 1006
Philadelphia Crosstown Community Plan, 1184
Philadelphia Savings Fund Society (PSFS) Building, 1008, 1216
Philippines architecture, 1228, 1229
Philips pavilion, 419
Phillips Exeter Academy, *323*, 1392

Phoenix Art Museum, 1444

Phoenix Central Library, **1010–12**; exterior, *1011*; interior, *1010*

Piano, Renzo, **1012–14**; Cultural Centre Jean Marie Tjibaou, **334–35**, *3ii*; energy-efficient design, 405; Kansai International Airport Terminal, 34, **727–29**; Menil Collection, 659, **837–38**; Pompidou Center, **1034–36**; relation with environmental issues, 410; solar architecture, 1224; use of color, 279

Piazza d'Italia, 1048

piazza theme: Aalto's, 2. *See also* maidans

pictorial projections, 58–59

pictorial zoning ordinances, 956

Pietilä, Reima and Raili, 462–63, 602, **1014–15**

Pikionis, Dimitris, 549

pile footings, 230

Pilgrimage Church at Neviges, **1015–16**; exterior, *1016*; interior, *1015*

Pink House, 67

Pinós, Carme, **857–59**

Pinseau, Michel, Hassan II Mosque, **592–94**

Pinto e Sotto Major Bank, 1210

Pioneer Health Centre, 1442

Pirelli Skyscraper, 1037

pisé, 383

Pittsburgh University, 207

Plan Architects, Baiyoke Tower, **101–2**

planetariums. *See* observatories

Plan for Berlin, Speer's, 140

Plan for Chicago, Illinois, 196–97

Plan for Copenhagen, 1082

Plan for Magnitogorsk, 758

Plan for St. Petersburg (Leningrad), 1237

Plan for Venice Biennale Pavilions, *1398*

Plan for Washington, D.C. 1902, 195–96

Plan of Canberra, 212, **1016–18**

Plan of Chicago, **1018–19**, 1379, 1380

Plan of New Delhi, **1019–21**

Plan of Riyadh, 1113

Plan of Washington, D.C., 1433

plantations, American, 29

plants. *See* factories

plaster finishes over brick, 171–72

plastic, **1021–23**; roofs of, 1096; space frames, 1233; spray, 1142

Plastic Integration movement, 844

plate glass, 516, **1023–25**; hall (Spiegelglashalle), 1437

Plater-Zyberk, Elizabeth. *See* Duany and Plater-Zyberk

platform canopies, 199

Platform I and II, 1194

Platt, Charles A., **1025–27**

Plattenhaus Typ 1018, 989

playgrounds, 597

Plaza and PPG Skyscraper, *1024*

plazas, **1027–29**; around Boston City Hall, 158; in Cuba, 330; Peace Memorial and Museum, Hiroshima, 989; Salk Institute, 1156; Seagram Building, 1187. *See also* atriums

Plecnik, Jože, **1029–30**

plexiglas, 1144

Plischke, Ernst, 932

Plug-In City, 57, 154

Plymouth Building in Chicago, *1199*

plywood, 406, 1326, 1447; in Frank Gehry's work, 490. *See also* wood

pneumatic structures, 1315

Poelzig, Hans, 396, **1030–32**; work in Frankfurt, 473

Poggioli, Renato, 97, 98

Pohja Insurance Building, 460

Point West Place, 1048

Polish wood synagogues, 1298

politics, architecture disassociated from, 181

Polk, William, 516

Polshek, James Stewart, **1032–34**

Pompéia Factory, 150

Pompidou Center, 279, 979, 1012, **1034–36**, 1126; competition, 286; exterior, *1035*; link with Archigram, 1362; use of steel, 1243; use of trusses, 1346

Ponti, Gio, **1036–38**

Poole House, 14

pop-art-affiliated architects, 107; Denise Scott Brown, 1184; John C. Portman Jr., 1042; Peter and Alison Smithson, 1220; Robert Arthur Morgan Stern, 1248

Pope, John Russell, **1038–39**

porches, 44

Porro, Ricado, 901

portable structures: amusement park, 50. *See also* lightweight frames

Portcullis House, 649, 650

Porte de Concorde, 424

Portland, Oregon, regional planning, 1088

Portland Building, 621

Portland Public Service Building, 542, **1039–40**, 1048, 1369; exterior, *1045*

Portman, John C., Jr., 399, **1040–43**

Porto, Portugal, Eduardo Souto de Moura's work, 1231

Portoghesi, Paolo, **1043–45**, 1048, 1132

Portuguese architecture, 1231, 1307

Posokhin, Mikhail, 881

post and beam system, 1263

Postindustrial metropolitan development, 386

Postmodernism, 862, **1047–50**, 1156, *1295*; Ada Louise Huxtable's writings, 665; Alan Colquhoun's relation with, 280; Amsterdam, 48; Argentina, 66; Austria, 93; Bangkok, 106; Boston, 160; Brazil, 167–68; Canada, 209; Canberra, 213; Charles Willard Moore's work, 870; Chicago, 243, 246; college campus design, 207; corporate headquarters buildings, 314; and Disney theme parks, 363; founders, 870; Hans Hollein's work, 635; and historic preservation, 618; Hong Kong, 642; and house design, 656–57; Hungary, 664; influence of Stockholm Public Library on, 1256; influence of Villa Mairea on, 1416; influence on utopian planning, 1384; Iran, 690; Japan, 692; John C. Portman Jr. works, 1041–42; Juhani Uolevi Pallasmaa's view of, 972; Kenneth Frampton's critique, 470; Kohn Pederson Fox's work, 733; London, 788–89; Melbourne, 830; Memphis Group influence on, 835; Miami, Florida, 851–52; Montreal, 868; of Museum of Modern Art, Frankfurt, 895; Norway, 940–40; ornament, 35, 959; Paolo Portoghesi's role, 1043; Philip Johnson's work, **715–18**, 1188; Portland Public Service Building, 1039; relation with abstraction, 6–7; relation with classicism, 270; relation with Contextualism, 306; relation with historicism, 621; relation with primitivism, 1063; relation with representation, 1097; relation with Structuralism, 1266; Ricardo Bofill, **152–54**; Robert Stern, 1248; Rome, 1132; Santiago, Chile, 1162; São Paulo, Brazil,

1165; SITE group, 145; skyscrapers, 1217; Spain, 1235; tenements in Glasgow, 514; United Kingdom, 1363; United States, 1369; use of brick, 172; use of color, 279–80; use of stone, 1259–60; Vancouver, 1390; Venturi and Scott Brown, 1156; Vietnam Veterans Memorial, 1413; West Berlin, 141; Yugoslavia, 1466

Postmodernism (Portoghesi), 1044

Post Office and Telecommunications Building in Leon, Spain, 1227

Post Office and Telecommunications Building in Rome, *767, 768*

Post Office Savings Bank, Vienna, 515, **1045–47**, *1295*; exterior, *1046*; use of aluminum in, 38

poststructuralism, 1295; Bernard Tschumi's interest in, 1346

Poststructuralist architecture, 959, 1265, 1266

postwar reconstruction: Athens Charter and, 87; Berlin, 140, 141; Cologne, Germany, 277, 278; Dom-ino Houses, 366; Finland, 149; Germany, 496; industrial town planning, 435; Italy, 1339; Lebanon, 130; Rotterdam, 1137; Tokyo, 1330; Vienna, 92

Potsdamer Platz, 1013

Poulsson, Magnus, 939

Power, Ethel, 1085

Power in Buildings: An Artist's View of Contemporary Architecture (Ferriss), 457

power plants, 261, **1051–52**; by Graham, Anderson, Probst and White, 536; Niagra Falls Power Generating Station, 208

Prague, Czech Republic, 341, **1052–54**; Cubism's roots in, 332, 333; Jože Plecnik's work in, 1029

prairie houses, 1453

Prairie School, 556, **1054–56**; adherents, 1054; National Farmers' Bank influence on, 905; Purcell and Elmslie's relation with, 1073, 1074; relation with Craftsman Style, 322

Pratt House, 552

Pravda Building, 527

precast construction, **1056–57**; ferro-cement, 418–19; Phoenix Central Library, 1010; prestressed concrete, 292–93; Sydney Opera House, 1293; terazzo tiles, 1320. *See also* concrete-shell structure

Predock, Antoine, 621, **1057–59**; Stanford University, Center for Integrated Systems, **227–29**

prefabrication, **1059–61**; agricultural buildings, 29; Aluminaire House, 37; aluminum, 38, 40; of Bertrand Goldberg, 524; building materials used for, 230; bungalow, 189; Canada, 209; Cuba, 331; Dom-ino Houses, 365; for factories, 434; fallout shelter, 439; and fortification of buildings, 22; houses, 657; housing exhibits at Expo 1967, 422; mass-produced houses, 44; Module 335 system, 574; Oscar Nitzchke's interest in, 935; Palais Stoclet, 971; for Pompidou Center, 1035; protest against, 664; public dissatisfaction with, 185; Russia, 1148; at Schlumbeger Cambridge Research Center, 1178; in schools, 1180; Vancouver Boxes, 1389; World Trade Center, 1452. *See also* postwar reconstruction; precast construction; space frames

preservation. *See* historic preservation

President's House for Illustrious Guests, 1157

prestressing process, 1056

Pretoria Railway Station, *103*

Pretoria Regionalism, 24

Pretoria Union Buildings, 102

Primitivism, **1061–63**

Prince Narissaranuwattiwongs, 104, *105*

Princeton University, 206; Ralph Adams Cram's work at, 323; Whig Hall, 577

Princeton University, Department of Music extension, 908

Principia College, 822, 823

prisons, **1063–65**

Pritzker Architecture Prize, **1065**. *See also* Aga Khan Award

privacy in buildings, 113, 709; modules for, 810; Saudi culture, 1169; and suburban planning, 1270; wooden screens for balconies, 856

private buildings: adaptive re-use, 13; definition, 12

Probst, Ernest. *See* Graham, Anderson, Probst, and White

Proctor and Gamble Headquarters, *314, 733*

professional associations, 679

Project for a Villa (Tschumi), 657

project planning, 300

project scheduling, 300; software, 2

Proletarian Region Club, 1406

promedades, 1292

Prouvé, Jean, 39, 451, 979

Provincial Capitol Building, Toulouse, *1401*

Prudential Building, 40, 243, 684

Pruitt Igoe Public Housing, 352, 656, **1065–69**, 1462; exterior, *1067*

PSFS Building, 661; adaptive re-use, 13; exterior, *661*

public buildings: Alvar Aalto's, 3; Belgium, 131; Brussels, 178–79, 179; Bucharest, 183, 184; Canberra, 213; definition, 12; by Gottfried Böhm, 154–55; Itsuko Hasegawa's view of, 591

public housing, 56, **1069–71**; Behrens' writings about, 127; Berlin, 138–39; by Chloethiel Woodard Smith, 1218; failure of American, 1381; Germany, 495–96; Gifu Kitagata Apartments, 1194; Venezuela, 1418. *See also* low-cost housing; Pruitt Igoe Public Housing; urban renewal

public parks, 152

public transportation, 1341

Puig i Cadafalch, Josep, **1071–73**, *8ii*

punched metal, 591

Purcell and Elmslie, **1073–1075**

Quarry Visitor Center, *1421*

Quebec Museum of Civilization, 1153

Queens, New York, 1271

Quonset hut, 29, 1447; use for building shell, 240

Rabat, 20, 21

Rachel Raymond House, 1085

racial exclusionism in suburban development, 1271, 1272

Radio House, 1031

Radna Grupa Zabreb (RGZ), 1465

Ragdale House, 1200

railroad stations, **1077–79**; adaptive re-use of, 12–13; bus terminal relationship with, 198, 199; futurist example, *261*; by Herzog and De Meuron, 607; influence of Grand Central Terminal, 538; Santiago, Cuba, 331. *See also* airports and aviation buildings

railway hotels in Canada, 210

Raja Mahmadabad Library Project, 557

ramps: at Fiat Works (Turin), 459; High Museum of Art, 609, 610; at Neue Staatsgalerie, 916–17; parking garage, 983; of plastic, 1022

Ramses Wissa Wassef Arts Centre, 385, **1079–80**, *8ii*

ranch houses, 96, **1080–81**; bungalows; row houses. *See also* American Foursquare

Rasmussen, Steen Eiler, **1081–83**

Rationalism, **1083–85**; approach to design, 1354–55; Argentina, 65; Barcelona architects, 112, 113; Belgium, 131; Berlage's, 135; Bucharest, 184; Budapest, 185; Chile, 247; Cuba, 1127; Czechoslovakia, 341; effect of Universal Expostion 1942, 443; Finland, 462; Frank Lloyd Wright's works, 1083; Gio Ponti's contribution, 1036; of Giuseppe Tarragni, 1318; Greece, 548; Hannes Meyer's work, 848; Hans Poelzig's influence, 1031; Italian, 767; Itsuko Hasegawa's relation with, 591; Mario Roberto Alvarez's, 40–41; and modernism, 148; Santiago, Chile, 1160; Soviet Union, 301, 302. *See also* Functionalism

Rautatalo Office Building, 3

Raymond, Eleanor, **1085–86**

Reading Railroad station in Philadelphia, 12–13

rebars, 819

reconstruction projects, James Stewart Polshek's work with landmarks, 1032

rectilinear Art Nouveau (Jugendstil), 72, 74, 912; Glasgow School, 510

recycled architecture, 187, 522, 912

Red Blue Chair, 349, *1110*

redevelopment projects: Chicago, 242–43; Columbus, Indiana, 282–83; Düsseldorf, 378, 379; by Eduardo Souto de Moura, 1231; E-Walk, 68; Harbor Point, Boston, 533; Kyoto, Japan, 740; Le Havre, 1001; Miami Beach, Florida Art Deco District, 1184; Paris, 980; in Rio de Janeiro, 1112; Riyadh, 1115; Sverdlovsk, 1147. *See also* historic preservation; postwar reconstruction; urban renewal

Red House, 76

Reed, Charles A., 539

Reed House, 15–*16*

reeds as building material, 1461

Reeth, Bob van, 132

Regent Theater in New York City, 889

regionalism, **1089–92**; abstract, 1367; Art Deco, 71; Australia, 91; Barcelona, 113; Bardi's, 151; Brazil, 167; Canada, 209; in city halls, 264; critical, 1367; effect of ranch houses on, 1081; in hotels, 888; Hungary, 664; Mexico, 845; Phoenix Central Library, 1011; in resort hotels, 1100–1101; United States, 430; of William Wurster, 1458. *See also* International Style; vernacular architecture

regional modernism, 861; Iran, 690; of Kenzo Tange, 1302; Rifat Chadirji's search for, 231; Sarasota School, **1166–67**; Spain, 1235

regional planning, **1086–89**. *See also* transportation planning

Reichstag, **1092–95**; exterior, *1093*; interior, *1094*

reinforced concrete, **1095–96**; Auguste Perret's use of, 1001; first church in Vienna, 1029; first house in England with, 298; first use in Paris, 977; Frank Lloyd Wright's use of, 1454; Johannes Duiker's use of, 1469; Pier Luigi Nervi's experiments, 1037; popularity in Russia, 1146; Robert Maillart's use of, 808; safety against earthquakes, 819; steel-reinforced, 291–92; use at Notre Dame, Le Raincy, 941; use by E. Owen Williams, 1442; use by Irving John Gill, 504; use by Johannes Duiker, 374; use for Dom-ino Houses, 365; use in Switzerland, 1287; use in TWA Airport Terminal in New York, 1353

Reliance Building, 195, *1246*

Reliance Controls Factory, 468, 1126

Renaissance Center, 1041

Renault Distribution Centre, 469, **1096–97**

Renault Factory in Durango, 756

renovation projects: Bank Austria Client Service Center in Vienna, 340; libraries, 773; by Lina Bò Bardi, 151; Metropolitan Museum

of Art, New York extension, 1123; Reichstag, 1093–95; Ronacher Theater in Vienna, 307; by Williams and Tsien, 1445

Renzo Piano Building Workshop, 1012–13

representation, **1097–98**; importance in design process, 1109

research centers, **1098–1100**; use of terrazzo, 1321; by Wu Liangyong, 1457. *See also* Cambridge, England, Schlumberger Cambridge Research Center; Stanford University, Center for Integrated Systems

resort hotels, **1100–1101**; Miami, Florida, 850, 851; Morris Lapidus' work, 743; Southeast Asia, 1230; Turkey, 1352. *See also* Las Vegas

resorts, 21; Disney theme parks; Arquitectonica, 67–68; Czechoslovakia, 341; Seaside, Florida, **1189–92**. *See also* amusement parks

restaurants, **1101–3**; by Hermann Czech, 338; impact of automobiles on, 95; by Morphosis, 878; as roadside attractions, 1116

Revell, Viljo, 461, 462, **1103–5**; Glass Palace, 462; Toronto City Hall, **1332–33**

Revival architecture: Egyptian, 390; relation with historicism, 621; use of glass, 516

Rewal, Raj, 673–74, **1106–8**

Riabushinskii buildings, 1202

RIBA Headquarters Building, 1141

Rice University, 658, 659

Richardson Romanesque style city halls, 264

Ricola Storage Building, **1108–9**

Riech, Lilly, 1437

Rietveld, Thomas Gerrit, **1109–11**; Dutch Pavilion, *1399*; Red Blue Chair, 349, *1110*; relation with De Stijl, 348, 349; Schröder-Schräder House, 6, 348, 349, 1109, **1181–82**

Ring, 587–88

Rio de Janeiro, Brazil, 194, **1111–13**; favelas, **446–47**

Riphahn, Wilhelm, 277

Riverside Plaza, Chicago, 631

Riyadh, Saudi Arabia, **1113–15**; Stadium, 1314

roadside architecture, **1115–18**; Art Deco, 69. *See also* gas stations; visitor centers

roadway systems, 94, 96, **1118–20**. *See also* parkways

Roberts, Zeidler, 1399

Robertson, Howard, 1360

Robie House, 77, 322, 656, **1120–23**, 1367; exterior, *1121*; interior, *1122*

"robot architecture," 1230

Roche, Kevin, 1123, 1124, 1366

Roche, Martin. *See* Holabird, William, and Martin Roche

Roche and Dinkeloo, **1123–24**; work in Columbus, Indiana, 281–82, 283; work on Dulles International Airport, 375

Rockefeller Center, 927, 1028, **1124–26**; plaza, *1125*

Rockefeller Chapel at University of Chicago, 531

Rock 'n' Roll Hall of Fame, 992

Rodchenko, Alexander, 301

Rogers, Ernesto N., 1337

Rogers, Richard, 468, **1136–37**, 1362; Channel 4 Headquarters, London, **236–37**; High-Tech style, 1051; Pompidou Center, **1034–36**; use of color, 279. *See also* Pompidou Center

Romañach, Mario, **1127–28**

Romania, **1128–31**

Romanian architects, 182, 184

Romantic modernists, 860–61

Romantic Nationalism: Finland, 603; Southern and Central Africa, 24

Rome, Italy, **1131–33**

Römerstadt, 820

Romney, Hervin A.R. *See* Arquitectonica

Ronacher Theater, 307

roofs: advances at Chicago World's Fair (1933), 230; by Amancio Williams, 1441; automobile test track on, 459; Baiyoke Tower, 102; Berlin Philharmonic Concert Hall, 142; Boots Factory, 156; broken pediment of AT&T Building, 84; cable-suspended, 1315; cantilevered overarching, 740; Chinese-style, 249, 250; city parks on, 591; contrasts and unity among, 134; copper-sheathed, 228; copper-trimmed, 604; covered sidewalk and plaza, Caracas, 268; curving sheet-metal, 1247; Dulles International Airport, 375, *376*; of Félix Candela, 213, 214; General Archives of Columbia, 1157; George Washington Bridge Bus Terminal, 199; glass, 740, 995, 1013; Gropius House, 561; Hong Kong International Airport, 644; Hungarian-style, 664; inverted, 973; Kansai International Airport Terminal, 727; by Kenzo Tange, 1302; Le Corbusier's exposed structure, 969; made of sticks, 1461; Menil Collection, 837; Museum of Modern Art, Frankfurt, 895; Olympic Stadium, Tokyo, 953; by Otto Frei, 960; Pilgrimage Churche at Neviges, 1015; pitched, 123–24; plastic, 1022, 1096; reflective, 584; shell designs, 1385; split pediment, 1392, *1393*; steel, 1245; suspended rubberized, 1166; Teflon, 649; tensile, 1178; trusses as expressive elements of, 1346; Turin Exhibition Hall by Pier Luigi Nervi, 419; use of steel for, 1242; water cascade over, 42

Rookery Building, 195

Root, John Wellborn. *See* Holabird, William, and Root, John Wellborn

Rosa-Jochmann-School, 339–40

Rose Seidler House, 90

Rossi, Aldo, **1133–35**; critique of modernism, 1047; neo-Rationalism of, 909, 1356; work at Celebration, Florida, 227

Rotterdam, Netherlands, **1135–38**; J.J.P. Oud's work in, 963; Van Nelle Factory, Rotterdam, **1394–96**

Rotunda, La, 521

Rotundi, Michael, 877, 878, 879

Rovaniemi Airport Terminal, 599

Rovaniemi Art Museum, 972

Rowe, Colin, **1140–41**; writings about cities, 306

row houses, **1138–40**; Art Deco, 71; in Brussels, 179; International Style, 95; Kärjensivu Rowhouse, 1104; suburban, 1271. *See also* American Foursquare

Royal College of Physicians, 753

Royal Danish Embassy in London, 704

Royal Institute of British Architects (RIBA), 679, **1141–42**

Royal National Theater in London, *753*

Royal Theatre of Copenhagen, 451

Rudnev, Lev, 881

Rudofsky, Bernard, 1402

Rudolph, Paul, 256, **1142–45**, 1166, 1230; Tuskegee Institute plan, 207; Yale University, Art and Architecture Building, 291

Rue de Meaux Apartments, 1012

Russia and Soviet Union, **1145–48**

Russian architects, 1200

Russian architectural drawing, 59

Russian Monumental style in China, 250

Russian Suprematism, 6

Ruusuvuori, Aarno, 462

Ryerson Townhouse, 14

Saarinen, Aline, 377

Saarinen, Eero, **1149–50**; Bell Telephone Corporate Headquarters, 518; church design, 256; Columbia Broadcasting System Headquarters, 1216; Dulles International Airport, **375–77**, 644; Gateway Arch (St. Louis), **486–87**, 1245; Kresge Auditorium, *295*, 296; TWA Airport Terminal, **1353–54**, *5iii*; use of concrete shells, 296; Vivian Beaumont Theater, 778; work in United States, 1369; work with Charles Eames, 381

Saarinen, Eliel, 460, 601, **1150–53**; Crow Island School, 243, *1180*; Drake University Science and Pharmacy buildings, 1099; Finnish Pavilion at Paris Expo (1990), 424; First Christian Church, Columbus, Indiana, 281; General Motors Technical Center, 1100; GM Technical Center, 314; Helsinki Railway Station, 460, 601, **603–5**, 1077, 1151; Irwin Union Bank and Trust, Columbus, Indiana, 281–82; North Christian Church, Columbus, Indiana, 281; work at Cranbrook, Michigan, 324, 325; work in Columbus, Indiana, 282

Saarinen, Lily Swann, 486

Saavedra, Gustavo, University Library, UNAM, Mexico City, **1373–75**

Sabine, Wallace Clement, 11

Sack House, 823

Sadao, Shoji, *421*

Safdie, Moshe, 696, 697, **1153–54**, 1390; Habitat 1967, Montreal, 210, 422, **579–81**

safety: in bus terminals, 199; against earthquakes, 819; Hong Kong International Airport, 645; inside buildings, 594; lighting for, 774; at Pruitt-Igoe Public Housing Project, 1066; retrofitting historic properties, 618; usefulness of plastic, 1023; Wright's earthquake designs, 669. *See also* fallout shelters; terrorism

Sagrada Familia, *1234*

Sahat al-Kindi Plaza, *3ii*

Saigon South, 1213

Sainsbury Centre, 468–69, 1243

Sainsbury Supermarket Development in Camden Town, 559

Sainsbury Wing, National Gallery, London, **1154–56**, *1155*

Saishunkan Seiyaku Women's Dormitory, 1194

Salginatobel Bridge, 809

Salish community school at Agassiz, 987

Salk Institute, 293, 653, 724, 1099, **1156–57**, *1iii*

Salmona, Rogelio, **1157–58**

Salto, Uruguay, 363

Samaritaine Department Store, *978*

Sami Center in Karasjok, 941

Sami Museum and Northern Lapland Visitors Center, 972

Sanatorium Purkersdorf, 628

Sanderson's Wallpaper Factory in Chiswick, 1426

sandstone: piers, 437; Raj Rewal's use of, 1106; as veneer, 228

San Francisco, California: Museum of Modern Art, *161*; Plan, 263. *See also* Panama Pacific Exposition (San Francisco 1915)

Sangath, 367, *368*, 674

San Martin Cultural Center, 40

San Nicola Sports Stadium, 1012

San Simeon, 875, 876

Santacilia, Carlos Obregón, 843

Santa EfigQafenia Viaduct, *166*

Sant'Elia, Antonio, **1158–60**; Città Nuova drawings, 260. *See also* Futurism

Sant'Elia Nursery School, 1318
Santiago, Chile, **1160–62**; downtown, *1161*
Santiago, Cuba train station, 331
Santiago Hotel in Cuba, 330
Santos, Adèle Naudé, **1162–64**
Santos, Josefina, 815
São Paulo, Brazil, **1164–66**; Bardi's works, 150–51
São Paulo School, 167
Sarasota School, **1166–67**
SAS Hotel in Denmark, 354
Saudia Arabian architecture, 709, 1113
Saudi Arabia, **1167–71**
Saudi Arabian architects, 1114–15, 1169
Savannah, Georgia, heritage preservation, 1027
Saxton Pope House, 1459
Sayin, Nevzat, *698*, *699*
Säynätsalo Town Hall, 2
Scandinavian architects, 81, 508, 1445
Scandinavian architecture, 936
Scandinavian modern design, 471
Scarborough College, 1334–35
Scarpa, Alfra and Tobia, Benetton Factory, Italy, **134–35**
Scarpa, Carlo, **1171–74**
Scharoun, Hans, 138, 140, 588, **1174–76**. *See also* Berlin
    Philharmonie
Scheerbart, Paul, 515
Scheu House, 790
Schindler, Rudolph M., 794, **1176–78**, 1368
Schindler-Chase House, 1176
Schlumberger Cambridge Research Centre, 649, 650, 1099, **1178–79**
Scholl House, 471
Schönbühl Apartments, 3
School of Oporto, 1231
schools, **1179–81**; Greece, 548; Hong Kong, 642; by Ralph Adams
    Cram, 323; use of plate glass for, 1025; Walter Gropius's designs
    for, 564–65. *See also* campus planning; educational institutions
schools of architecture: North Africa, 19–20, 21; Southern and
    Central Africa, 25
Schreiner House, 451
Schröder-Schräder House, 6, 348, 349, 1109, **1181–82**
Schultze-Naumburg, Paul, 357
Schumacher, Fritz, 277
Scientific Data Systems in El Segundo, 399
Scott, Foresman, and Company Headquarters, 997
Scott Brown, Denise, 453, 621, 750, 1118, 1155, **1182–85**, *1iii*
Scottish domestic architecture, 76–77
Scully, Vincent, **1185–87**; opinion of Adolf Loos's work, 1248
sculptural approach to architecture, 154, 239
sculpture and architecture, 427
Seagram Building, 518, 854, 928, **1187–88**; compared with AT&T
    Building, 84; exterior view, *1187*
Seamen's Church Institute in New York, 1032
Sea Palace Paradise Garden, 63
Sea Ranch Condominium I project, 870, *1327*, 1367
Sears Tower, 242, 684, **1188–89**, 1212–13, 1217; exterior, *1189*
Seaside, Florida, 369, 922, **1189–92**; houses, *1190*; urban code for,
    923
"Seaside Code" ordinances, 956
Seattle Exposition (1962), 416

Secession Building, 950, *951*; door detail, *1410*
Secessionism: Cairo, 201; Germany, 495; relation with Glasgow
    School, 510; Robert Mallet-Stevens relation with, 814
Secondary School at Hunstanton, 180
Second Bangkok International Airport, 708
Second Nationalist movement in Turkey, 1351
Second Sex, The (de Beauvoir), 453
Sedes Sapientiae Building, *761*
Seidler, Harry, 90, 641, *643*, **1192–94**, 1290–91, *4iii*
Seinäjoki Civil Guard Building, 1
Sejima, Kazuyo, **1194–95**
Semper, Gottfried, 357, 1312
Sendai Mediatheque proposal by Ito, 700
Senegal Alliance Franco-Sénéfalaise, *36*
Serbian Secession, 1464
Sert, Josep Lluís, 112, 297, **1195–97**
served *vs.* servant spaces, 724, 1247
Seventeenth Church of Christ, Scientist, 243
Seville, Spain, 203; Expo '92, 416, **422–23**
Sex of Architecture, The (Agrest), 454
Shalev-Gerz, Esther, 833
Shanghai, China: Park Hotel, **980–82**; Zhi Chen projects, 240
Shanghai Grand Theater, 251
Shanghai World Financial Center, 733, **1197–98**
shapes. *See* forms; geometric aspects of architecture
Sharon, Eldan, 696
Shaw, Howard Van Doren, 14, 242, **1199–1200**, 1205
Shchusev, Aleksei, Commissariat of Agriculture in Moscow, *302*
shear walls in skyscrapers, 1263
Shedd Aquarium, 534
Shekhtel, Fedor, 1145, **1200–1203**
shell designs, 1264, 1292; roofs, 1385. *See also* concrete-shell
    structure
Shingle Style, The (Scully), 1185
Shingle-style houses, remodeling by Robert Stern, 1248
Shinohara, Kazuo, 590, **1203–4**, 1331
Shin Takamatsu, 740
shipping container houses, 524–25
Shonandai Culture Center, 590
shop-house mosques, 884
shopping centers, 1118, **1204–6**; Commercial Center of
    Fountivegge, 1134–35; De Lijnbaan, 1137; designed by Eladio
    Dieste, 363; first in United States, 1200; impact of automobile,
    96; suburban developments, 1272; Turkey, 1352; by Victor David
    Gruen, 565. *See also* department stores
shopping malls, 96, 1205; escalators, 414
Shopping Towns USA: The Planning of Shopping Centers (Gruen),
    566
showroom design, 87; Bernard R. Maybeck, 823; Best Products,
    145–46; Memphis Group, 835; shopping center windows, 1205
Shreve, Lamb and Harmon, Empire State Building, **403–4**, 927
Shrine of the Book, **1206–8**; exterior, *1207*
Shun Tak Centre and Macau Ferry Terminal, 641
Shustar New Town, 689; street, *689*
sick-building syndrome, 411
Sief Palace, 1014
Siegel, Robert, 573, **576–78**
signage, development of, 96; by Jean Nouvel, 944; Las Vegas, 751;
    by Oscar Nitzchke, 935; Robert Venturi's writing, 1400
Silicon Valley, California, 314, 386

Silk Mill, 80

silt as building material, 61

Silver Hut, 700, 1194

Simpson, Vernon, 391

simulation. *See* virtual reality

Singapore architecture, 1228–29

Singer Sewing Machine Company Headquarters, 1236, *1237*

Sin Mao Tower, *1212*

Sirén, Heikki and Kaija, 462, **1208–9**; Otaniemi Chapel, 259

Siren, J.S., Helsinki Parliament House, 601, *602*

SITE, 145; Best Products Showroom, **145–46**; use of brick, 172

site location: country clubs, 320; ecological site planning, 1281; of Heikki and Kaija Sirén's works, 1208; Holocaust Memorial Museum, Washington, D.C., 637; importance to Alberto Kalach, 726; importance to resort hotels, 1100; Kimbell Art Museum, 732; Mies' German Pavilion, 492; Petronas Towers in Malaysia, 1006; visitor centers, 1420; Wright's Fallingwater, 437. *See also* Contextualism; nature integrated with buildings

sites, compatibility with buildings, 161; Adler's concern for, 14; Asplund's concern for, 81. *See also* Contextualism

Six Moon Hill development, 1325

Sixth Street House, 878

Siza, Alvaro, 783, **1210–11**

Skandia Cinema, 82

Skansen Restaurant in Oslo, 940

Skidmore Owings and Merrill, 789, **1211–14**; Alcoa Building, 40, 590, 935, 1212; Chicago School influence on, 246; church design, 256; Columbus, Indiana City Hall, 283; Haj Terminal, Jeddah Airport, **583–85**, 710, 1171, 1213; Jin Mao Towers, *2iii*; Hirshhorn Museum and Sculpture Garden, 190, 1213, 1369, *1434*, 1435; influence in Washington, D.C., 1435; Inland Steel Building, 242–43, 1212; Istanbul Hilton Hotel, 1351; John Hancock Center, 242, 246, *683*, 684, 992, 1212; Lever House, 596, **759–560**, 1212, 1216–17; plan for Canberra, 213; Sears Tower, 242, **1188–89**, 1212–13, 1217; U.S. Air Force Academy Chapel, 1213, **1381–83**; work at Lincoln Center, 778; work in United States, 1369

skybridges, 1006

skycourts, 67, *571*

Sky House, 839

skyscrapers, **1214–18**; aluminum in, 38; Alvar Aalto's views on, 3; Art Deco, 70; Bangkok, 101–2, 106; Bank of China Tower, **108–10**; Barnes's, 115; Belgium, 131; Boston, 158; brick, 1157; Buenos Aires, 41, 66, 188; by Cass Gilbert, 502–3; Cesar Pelli's writings, 993; China, 251; Chrysler Building, **252–54**; city halls, 264; Empire State Building, **403–4**; first European, 1136; Flatiron Building, **466–67**; Frankfurt, 472, 473; Frank Lloyd Wright's view of, 175, 176; Germany's first, 377; glass, 518; by Harry Seidler, 1192; by Helmut Jahn, 706; Holabird and Roche, 632; Holabird and Root, 630; hotels, 653, 980; by Kohn Pedersen Fox, 732; London, 788; by Ludwig Mies van der Rohe, 853; Melbourne, 830; Mexico City, 848; Montreal, 866; Moscow, 880, 1147; opposition of cruciform tower to, 304; Paris, 979; by Philip Johnson, 716; postmodern, 84; by Rino Levi, 761; Rotterdam, 1136; Santiago, Chile, 1160; São Paulo, Brazil, 1165; Saudi Arabia, 1168; shear walls, 1263; suspended, 1441; tallest in world, 1198; with terracota cladding, 1318; Tokyo, 1330; Toronto, 210; use of steel, 1242; Vancouver, 1389. *See also* Chicago School; elevators; office buildings

skywalks, 740

slate, 508

slaughterhouses, 484

slip-slab construction, 1057

Slovak architecture, 341

Slovenian architects, 1029

Slovenian architecture, 1464

slums. *See* favelas; tenement houses; urban renewal

Smith, Chloethiel Woodard, **1218–20**

Smith House, 827

Smithson, Peter and Alison, 180, **1220–22**, 1311, 1361

Socialist realism, 185, 969

social responsibility of architecture, 98, 244, 1033; awards, 26; Berlage's, 135–36; conflict with Structuralism, 1265–66; Group R in Barcelona, 113

Social Security Complex in Istanbul, 397, **1222–23**; exterior, *1223*

social stratification: in Brasília plan, 164; brick and, 172; of City Beautiful Movement, 1380; in Plan of New Delhi, 1019, 1021

software. *See* computer-aided design

Sogn Benedegt Chapel, 1470

Solana Village Center, 756

solar architecture, 272, **1223–24**; Eleanor Raymond's use of, 1086; by Paolo Solari, 61; protection against sunlight, 24; Village Homes in Davis, California, 1281. *See also* energy-efficient design; sustainability and sustainable architecture

Soleri, Paolo, **1224–26**; Arcosanti, Arizona, **61–62**, 1225; Cosanti, 1225; experiments with concrete, 291

Solomon R. Guggenheim Museum. *See* Guggenheim Museum

Solsona, Justo, 815

Solvay House, 651

SOMISA Building, 40

Sonsbeck Pavilion in Arnhem, 1110

Sony Center in Berlin, 708

Sony Corporation. *See* AT&T Building

Sörenson, Erik Christian, 355

SOS Children's Village International, *192*

Sota, Alejandro de la, **1226–27**

Sottsass, Ettore, Jr., 834

South African architecture, 102

South American architecture, 1219

South Bronx Community Center, 28

Southdale Mall in Minnesota, 1205

Southeast Asia, **1127–1231**; Paul Rudolf's work, 1144

Southern and Central Africa, **22–25**; Neoclassicism using local materials, 102

South in Architecture, The (Mumford), 891

South Korean architecture, 1229

Southside Settlement Community Center, *626*

Souto de Moura, Eduardo, 783, **1231–32**

Soviet architecture, 526; Jean-Louis Cohen's writings, 274. *See also* Constructivism

Soviet Central Union of Consumer Cooperatives Headquarters, 312

Soviet influence, on Berlin, 140

Soviet realism, Romania, 1130

Soviet Union. *See* Russia and Soviet Union

space: African sense of, 25; Bawa's visual effects using, 124; Bruno Zevi's writings, 1467; Coop Himmelblau's, 93; designing for escalators, 415; effect on social interaction, 152; equality with form, 82; experiments with breaking up, 87; fluid, 700; fragmentation, 600; Frank Gehry's unusual use of, 490; Frank

space: African sense of (continued)
Lloyd Wright's concepts for, 1452; importance of emptiness, 258; interlocking spaces of different heights, 366; Jean Nouvel's illusory, 943, 944; Josep Lluis Sert's use of, 1196; Morphosis view of, 878; "nonspace," 1278; playful use of horizontal and vertical planes, 105; relationship with motion, 1003; served *vs.* servant, 724, 1247; simulation, 50, 52; Theo van Doesburg's conception of, 1391; unencumbered by structural elements, 150

Space, Time, and Architecture (Giedion), 501

space frames, **1232–33**; aluminum domes, 39–40; in Kahn's Yale Art Gallery, 595; Kisho Kurokawa's modular metal, 737

Spa design, 1470

Spain, **1233–36**

Spangan, 1136

Spanish architects, 864, 1226

Spanish architecture, 1266; Coderch's contribution to, 273

Spanish colonial revival style, 329

Spanish influence, in Southeast Asia, 1228

Spanish Pavilion (1937), 1196

spatial experience: Ando's, 53; Berlin Philharmonic Concert Hall, 142; Church on the Water, 258; created by Bernard Tschumi, 1347; Cuadra San Cristóbal surrealist, 328–29; in Enrique Norten's work, 938; experiments with brick, 171; Fallingwater, 437; Getty Museum, 499; in Henning Larsen's work, 748; importance in supermodernism, 1278; Metropolitan Festival Hall in Tokyo, 842; of Mies' German Pavilion, 494; of Universum Cinema, **1375–76**

Spear, Laurinda. *See* Arquitectonica

Spear House, 67, 851

Speer, Alfred, 140, 443–44

Spiegelglashalle, 1437

Spiral Building, 811

spiritual nature in architecture, 54, 358

St. Augustine, Florida, 217

St. Batholomew's Episcopal Church in New York City, 531

St. John's Presbyterian Church in Berkeley, *876*

St. Joseph's Church at Le Harve, *1001*

St. Louis, Missouri Gateway Arch, **486–87**

St. Maria Königin, *277*, 278

St. Mary's Cathedral in San Francisco, 256

St. Mary's Cathedral (Tokyo), *4iii*

St. Pancras Chambers, 173–74

St. Petersburg (Leningrad), Russia, 1145, **1236–39**, *1237*

St. Petri's Church, 765

St. Thomas Episcopal Church in New York City, 323, 531

stadiums, **1239–41**; airport likenesses, 32; Russia, 1148; tensile structures, 1314. *See also* concrete-shell structure

Stafford, Jim, 877

stained glass, 965, 1015, 1436

staircases: Ando's embedded meaning, 53; at Bentota Beach Hotel, 124; Casa Malaparte, 221–22; enclosed by glass, 515; freestanding, *16*; by Hannes Meyer, 849; Joseph Store in London, 713; Pilgrimage Church at Neviges, **1015–16**

Stam, Mart, Van Nelle Factory, Rotterdam, **1394–96**

standardization: advantages for architecture, 972; Dutch architecture, 912; of housing in Finland, 602; motels, 888; in Romania, 1130; in Russia, 1147–48; in suburban developments, 1270. *See also* typology

Standing Conference of Public Enterprises (SCOPE) office building, 1106

Stanford University, 206; Center for Integrated Systems, **227–29**

Stansted Airport Terminal, 469, 644, 645; exterior, *33*

Starck, Philippe, *1329*

State Bank in Fribourg, 162

State Circus, *1130*

state growth management plans, 1342

State Parliament in Düsseldorf, 378

state-sponsored projects. *See* government-sponsored projects; urban renewal

State Theater complex in Zurich, 1386

State University of New York, Albany, 1262

State University of New York at Stony Brook, Health Sciences Center, 526

Stauffacher Bridge, 808

steam heating, 594

steel, **1241–45**; Australian structural experiments, 90; cast steel, 1035; concrete reinforcement, 290, 291–92; trusses, 1346. *See also* cast steel

steel cables, 953, 1243, 1264; nets, 960

steel-frame construction, **1245–47**; in Chicago, 244, 245; Eames House, 381; Farnsworth House, 441; Lovell Health House, 796; of Ludwig Mies van der Rohe, 667

Steiglitz, Alfred, 59

Steiner, Rudolf, 427; Goetheanum, **1286–87**

Steiner House, 790, **1247–48**, 1326

Stem, Allen, 539

Stenhammar, Ernst, 1283

stereotomics of the earthwork, 1312

Stern, Robert Arthur Morgan, 365, 410, 621, **1248–50**; relation with postmodernism, 1048

Stevens Hotel, 654

Stickley, Gustav, 77, **1250–52**; United States, 1366–67

Stickley furniture, 1250

Sticks and Stones (Mumford), 891

Stick style, 45

Stirling, James, 789, 1049, **1252–54**, 1362; Leicester University, Engineering Building, *181*; Neue Staatsgalerie, 9, **916–17**; New National Gallery of Art in Stuttgart, 1268–69

Stock Exchange Tower, 867

Stockholm, Sweden, **1256–58**

Stockholm City Hall, 264, *265*, 1256–57

Stockholm Public Library, 82, 269, **1255–56**, *7iii*

Stockholm University at Frescati, 412

Stockmann Department Store, 460; addition, 574

Stoclet House, 628–29

stone, **1258–61**; Chassagne stone, 68; concrete as alternative to, 292; Diener and Diener's use of, 361; Ethiopian, 403; Juan O'Gorman's use of rocks, 947; oya (lava stone), 669; tepetate, 726; used in Mies German Pavilion, 493; used in Washington, D.C., 1433; veneer panels, 337

Stone, Edward Durell, 896, **1261–63**; American Pavilion, 419; New Delhi Embassy, 401, *402*

Stone Cloud House, 293

Stonehill House, 14

storefront mosques, 884

storefront theaters, 889

Stradelhofen Station in Zurich, 203

Streamline Moderne, 69, 929, 1294; bus terminals, 199; in Los Angeles, 795. *See also* aeronautical forms

Stretto House, 634. *See also* aeronautical forms

strip architecture, 96, 145, 146, 1102

stripped Classicism, 269; of Paul Philippe Cret, 326, 327

Struckus House, 795

Structuralism, **1264–66**; Dutch School, 605; in Henning Larsen's work, 747; Hungary, 664; Netherlands, 914; of Vesnin brothers, 1406

structural systems, **1263–64**; airport terminals, 32; analogies applied to, 620; of Antoni Gaudí, 489; of Arne Emil Jacobsen, 704; Bank of China Tower, 109; Bardi's Taba Guaianases Building, 150; Bauhaus, Dessau, 121–22; Benetton Factory, 134; Casa Milà, 223, 224; cast iron, 1060; ceiling at Phoenix Public Library, 1010, 1011; Eladio Dieste's innovations, 362; exoskeletal, 1178, 1242; Frei Otto's lightweight, 960; Hong Kong and Shanghai Bank, 646, 647; innovations in Melbourne, 829, 839; innovative use of masonry skins, 994; interlocking rooms on multiple levels, 92; Kazuyo Sejima's innovations, 1195; load-bearing brick, 171, 172; as masculine, 454; megastructures, 61–62; as ornament, 958–59; Pier Luigi Nervi's writings about, 911; poetics of, 1312; in research centers, 1098; at Schlumbeger Cambridge Research Center, 1178; steel, 1243; straw bale, 1281; towers, 68; Toyo Ito, 700; use of plastic, 1023; Van Nelle Factory, 1396; of Wallace K. Harrison, 590; without columns or load-bearing walls, 952, 953; in Woolworth Building, 1450; Zonnestraal Sanatorium, 1469. *See also* joinery; roofs

stucco, 337

Studio Architetti BBPR, 1337, 1338

studio design education, 389

Studio Per, **1266–68**

Stuttgart, Germany, **1268–70**

style moderne, 1145

suburban developments, 658; Bangkok, 106; Chicago, 242; Denis Scott Brown's interest in, 1183–84; department stores, 357; Finland, 460, 462; impact of automobile on, 96; relation with roadway systems, 1120; relation with urban renewal, 1380–81; Riyadh, 1113; row houses, 1139; São Paulo, Brazil, 1164; Six Moon Hill, 1325; Stockholm, 1258. *See also* edge cities; Levittown; ranch houses

suburban houses, by Michel De Klerk, 346

suburban planning, **1270–73**; shopping center, 1204. *See also* transportation planning

subways, **1273–75**; and suburban planning, 1270

Sullivan, Louis, **1275–78**; belief in regionalism, 1453; Carson Pirie Scott Store, **219–21**, 1276; Guaranty Building, *1277*; importance to American architecture, 1367; influence on Chicago School, 244; National Farmers' Bank, **904–6**, 1276; relation with Prairie School, 1054; relation with rationalism, 1083; Wainwright Building, 171

Sumida Culture Factory, 1331

Summer House in Ofir, 1307–8

Summerlin, 751

Sunnyside Gardens, 1271

Sun Yat-sen Mausoleum, 797, 798

Sun Yat-sen Memorial Hall, 797, 798

"superadjacency," 1393

superblocks, *612*, 729, 762

Superleggera chair, 1038

supermodernism, 999, **1278–80**; Clorindo Testa's relation with, 1322

Supreme Court Building in Jerusalem, 697

Suspended Office Building, 1441

sustainability and sustainable architecture, **1280–83**; awards for, 25; and climate, 272; and energy-efficient design, 405; HVAC systems and, 596; Norway, 941; plastic and, 1022; in Reichstag reconstruction, 1094; Renzo Piano's work, 1013; Southern and Central Africa, 25; United Kingdom, 1362; use of timber for, 1327. *See also* solar architecture

Suvikumpu Housing Project, 1014

Sverdlovsk, Constructivism in, 303

Swales, Francis, 1389

Sweden, **1283–86**; functionalism in, 82; Hälsingborg Concert Hall, **289–90**; Sigurd Lewerentz's work, 764

Swedish architecture, 1283

swimming pools: by Alvaro Siza, 1210; by E. Owen Williams, 1442; by Julia Morgan, 875, 876

Swiss architects, 160

Swiss architecture, 1288, 1423, 1470

Swiss Pavilion at Cité Universitaire, 312

Swiss Pavilion at Hannover Expo (2000), 1470

Switzerland, **1286–88**

Sydney, Australia, **1288–92**

Sydney Opera House, 90, **1292–94**; competition, 285; exterior, *1293*; Ove Arup's design work, 79

Sydney School, 90, 1290

symbiosis in architecture, 737, 738

"symbolic romanticism" movement, 526

symbolism, **1294–96**; Asian architecture, 123–24; bamboo, 109; building materials, 1031, 1288; in Carlo Scarpa's work, 1173; Chinese, 251; church, 254, 256; concrete in Wright's Unity Temple, 1373; of the elevator, 398; Ellis Island, 1336; and Expressionism, 425; Finnish, 1208; Frank Gehry's whimsical, 490, 571; Glacier Museum, 509; Glasgow School, 510; glass, 515; of government buildings, 158; Grande Arche de la Défense, **540–42**; Holocaust Memorial Museum, Washington, D.C., 637, 638; huts or "cases," 334; Islamic, 63, 1461; Islamic architecture, 1005; Kenzo Tange's work, 953, 1302; male/female, 454; marine imagery, 69; mathematical, 53; Ministry of Foreign Affairs, Riyadh, 856; Monument to the Third International, 868, 869; mosques, 885; "over vast space," 1183; prairie, 524; pre-Islamic, 547; Seagram Building, 1187; Sears Tower, 1188; Shrine of the Book, 1206, 1208; skyscrapers, 982; steel, 1241; synagogues, 1297–98; tents, 1317; TWA Airport Terminal in New York, 1353–54; of United Nations Headquarters, 1364–65; Velasca Tower, 1339; Vidhan Bhavan (State Assembly), **1408–9**; World Trade Tower, 1451, 1452; of Zonnestraal Sanatorium, 1468. *See also* nautical forms; ornament

synagogues, **1296–98**

synergy, 475

Taba Guaianases Building, 150

TAC (The Architects Collaborative). *See* The Architects Collaborative (T.A.C.)

Tafuri, Manfredo, 97, 99, 623, 678, **1299–1300**

Taliesin, 1454

Taliesin West, **1300–1302**; exterior, *1301*

Taller de Arquitectura, 621

Tally's Electric Theatre in Los Angeles, 888

Tampere Main Library, 1014

Tange, Kenzo, 1114, **1302–4**; Abuja, Federal Capital Territory of Nigeria, 9–10; "City for 10 Million People," 839; first European building, 980; Olympic Stadium, Tokyo, **952–53**; Peace

Tange, Kenzo (continued)
    Memorial and Museum, Hiroshima, **989–90**; Tokyo City Hall,
    266, *1328*; urban planning in Southeast Asia, 1230; work in
    Tokyo, 1330; work in Yugoslavia, 1465
Taniguchi, Yoshio, 893, 897, **1304–5**
Tapiola, 149, 462, 1104
Tassel House, 73, 130, 651, 1062; exterior, *651*
Tatar houses, 506
Tate Gallery of Modern Art, 607; Core Gallery for the Turner
    Collection, *1253*; interior, *607*
Tatlin, Vladimir, Monument to the Third International, **868–70**
Taut, Bruno, **1305–7**; Alpine Architecture, 426; Expressionist
    works, 426; Glaspalast, 276; Glass House, 1305–6, 1439; Glass
    Pavilion, 426; Istanbul residence, 699; observations of Japanese
    architecture, 736; relationship with Hans Scharoun, 1174–75; use
    of glass, 515; use of Ottoman walling technique, 397; work in
    Turkey, 1350; writings about Japan, 1328
Tavanasa Bridge, 809
Tàvora, Fernando, **1307–9**
Taylor, Robert R., **1309–10**
Teague, Harry, *1090*
teahouse design, 738
Team 10, 737, 1167. *See also* Team X
Team Disney Building, 694
Team X, 344, 605, 914, **1310–12**
Team X Primer, 1220, 1311
Teatro del Mondo, 1134
TÉBE Building, 826
Technical University at Otaniemi, Chapel, 1208
Technion, 696
technoburb, 386
technology: architectural, 389; Berlin's embrace of, 137–38; Centre
    for Alternative Technology, 1224; and cultural values, 17; effect
    on country clubs, 321; effect on house design, 657, 658; glass
    production, 516; Gropius's philosophy, 121; in Hodgetts and
    Fung projects, 626; impact on agricultural landscape, 29–30;
    impact on truth in architecture, 1098; importance of welding,
    1243; inseparability from architecture, 301; Maya Lin's use of,
    776; and modernism, 861; for sustainable architecture, 1280;
    transfer, 558, 1005; urban impact of military technology, 276;
    Wanamaker's pioneering use, 1431
Tecton. *See* Lubetkin and Tecton
Tectonics, **1312–14**
Teflon, 584, 649, 1099, 1178; alternative, 1314
Tehran Center for Celebration of Music, 63
Tehran Center for Management Studies, 63
Tejeda House, 872
Tek, Vedat, 698
TELEVISA Services Building, 938
Tempe à Pailla, 544, *545*
temperature. *See* climate
Temple Beth El (Louis Kahn), 1298
temples in Bangkok, 105–6
Templeton Factory in Glasgow, 13
tenement houses, 55; Berlin, 137; Glasgow, 513–14. *See also* favelas
Tennessee Valley Authority (TVA), 1088
tensegrity structures, 1315
tensile structures, **1314–15**. *See also* tents
tensioned membrane structures, 1243, **1315–16**
Tent City, 533

tents, **1316–17**; tent structures, 1264, 1314. *See also* tensile
    structures
tepetate (stone), 726
terminal buildings in airports, 32–33, 34
terracotta, **1317–18**; bricks, 648; cladding, 135; use of, in
    Woolworth Building, 1450
Terragni, Giuseppe, 767, 1084, **1318–19**
terrazzo, 1262, **1320–21**
Territorial Executive Committee Building, *1146*
terrorism: airport design, 34, 728; embassy design, 401, 402. *See also*
    fallout shelters
Tessenow, Heinrich, **1321–22**
Testa, Clorindo, 66; Bank of London and South America, Buenos
    Aires, **110–11**, 187, 1322
Texas Houses (John Hejduk), 600
tezontle sand, 529
Thai architects, 102, 104, 1230
Thai architecture, 1227, 1229
The Architects Collaborative (TAC), **1324–26**; American Institute
    of Architects Headquarters, *46*
Theater Français, 568
Theater on the Water, 259
theaters, 753; drive-in, 95–96; Egyptian revival style, 391; by István
    Medgyaszay, 826; by Mario Roberto Alvarez, 40
theater set design: Alexander Vesnin, 1406; Fedor Shekhtel, 1201;
    Gae Aulenti, 87–88
Théâtre des Champs-Elysées, 1001
theme parks, 50; by Hodgetts and Fung, 626; Las Vegas, 751
Theory and Design in the First Machine Age (Banham), 107
Thermal Baths in Vals, 1470
Thirtieth Street Station in Philadelphia, 534
Thompson Center, 707
Thorsen House, 552
Three Arms Zone (Abuja), 10
Three-Slab House, 378
throwaway architecture, 57
Thyssen Tower, 378
Tiananmen Square, 1456
Ticino school, 161
Tietz Department Store, 377
tiles: Catalan vault, 225; terrazzo, 1320; use at University Library,
    UNAM, Mexico City, 1375; use by Antoni Gaudí, 489; use in
    grain elevators, 538
tiles (azulejos), 973
Tilyou, George, 52
timber framing, **1326–28**. *See also* engineered lumber
Time-Life Building, 1125
tinted glass, 518, 1025
Tishler House, 1177
titanium, 571
Tobacco Monopoly Offices and Warehouse Complex, 231, *232, 233*
Tokyo, Japan, **1328–32**; Metropolitan Festival Hall, **842**
Tokyo architects, 740, 1203
Tokyo Bay Plan, 1303
Tokyo City Hall, 266, *1328*
Tokyo Dome, 1264
Tokyo Forum Project, 1126
Tomek House, 1121
TOPO (1991), 776
topographical architecture, 857

Toronto, Ontario, **1333–35**

Toronto City Hall, 1105, **1332–33**; exterior, *1332*

Torre, Susana, **1335–37**

Torre Velasca, **1337–39**; exterior, *1338*; plan, *1339*

toughened glass, 518

tourism. *See* hotels; resorts

Tournikiotis, Panayotis, 623, 624

tower forms, 427; clock tower, Hilversum Town Hall, *615*; double-helix, 693; Great Mosque of Niono, 547; Helsinki Railway Station, 604; Holocaust Memorial Museum, Washington, D.C., 637; Mills College El Campanil, 875; Notre Dame, Le Raincy, 942; Rockefeller Center, 648; Saudi Arabia, 1168; in Soviet Union, 869

Tower of Jewels, 975

Tower of Winds, 700

towers. *See* skyscrapers

Townscape movement, 924

Toyota Museum of Art, 1304

Traditional architecture. *See* Classicism; Vernacular architecture

Traditional Design Build, 300

Train Shed in Chiasso, 808

transportation planning, **1340–42**; Athens Charter position on, 86–87; Chicago, 1018; escalators in, 414–15; Hong Kong, 641; multiuse terminals, 540; and new urbanism, 922; and precast construction, 1057; saving historic roads, 617; streets, 677–78; underground project in Caracas, 217; in Voisin Plan for Paris (1925), 1422–23. *See also* automobiles; parkways; suburban planning

Transvaal Group, 24

Travail (Zola), 483

travertine, 498

Trenton Jewish Community Center Bath House, 723

Tribune Review Publishing Company Building, 724

Tribune Tower, *1344*, *3iii*

Tribune Tower International Competition (Chicago 1922), 245, 285, 1215–16, **1342–45**

trigrams, 455

Tripoli, 20

Triton City, 1153

tropical climate construction, 104, 106, 334–35; Bank of China Tower, 109; Miami, Florida, 851; skyscrapers, 761

Tropical Deco, 70, 850

Trucco, Giacomo Mattê, Fiat Works (Turin), **458–59**

truss systems, 1246, 1263–64, **1345–46**; at Taliesin West, 1301; World Trade Center, 1452

truth in architecture, 75, 392

Tschumi, Bernard, **1346–48**; Project for a Villa, 657; relation with Deconstructivism, 350

Tsien, Billie, 325, **1444–45**

Tugendhat House, 492, 854, **1348–49**, *5iii*; use of glass, 517

Tugwell, Rexford, 551

Turbine Hall at Moabit, 127

Turin, Italy: Exhibition Hall by Peir Luigi Nervi, **416–19**; Fiat Works, **458–59**

Turin Expositions, 416

Turkey, **1349–53**; Bruno Taut's work in, 1306

Turkish architecture, 396–98; houses, 575

Turkish Historical Society, *1351*

"Turkish house" idea of Eldem, 396, 397

Turkish houses, 699, 1222

Turrell, James, 775

Turtle Bay Exploration Center bridge, 203–4

Turtle Creek House, 1058

Tuskegee Institute, Douglass Hall, *1309*

Tuskegee Institute plan, 207

Tusquets, Oscar, 1266

TWA Airport Terminal, New York, **1353–54**, *5iii*

Twaiq Palace, 1169

Twitchell, Ralph, 1166

typology, **1354–56**; Amancio Williams's development of, 1440; relation with neorationalism, 909

Tzelepis, Panos, 549

Tzonis, Alexander, 550

Uehara House, 1203

UFA Cinema Center in Dresden, 307

UFA Palast, *351*

Ugljen, Zlatko, 1466

Ukiyo-e Museum, 1203

Une cité moderne, 814

UNESCO: Headquarters in Paris, 169, 978–79; teahouse, 1003

UNESCO world heritage list, 122–23

Ungers, Oswald Mathias, **1357–58**

Union Bank in Basel, 162

Union Building, 646

Union Industrial Argentina, 816

Union Internationale des Architectes (UIA), 679; guidelines for architecture competitions, 284

Union of South Africa, 23

Union Station in Chicago, 534

Union Station in St. Louis, 12

Union Station in Washington, D.C., *196*

Unishelter, 524–25

Unitarian Church of All Souls, 556

Unitary urbanism, 98

Unité d'Habitation, 56, 312, **1358–59**; kitchens, 1003

Unité d'Habitation, exterior, *1359*

United Kingdom, **1359–63**; New Urbanism, 924

United Nations Headquarters, 765, 818, 928, *1364*, **1963–65**

United States, **1365–71**; Arts and Crafts Movement, 77; city halls, 264, 265; department store design, 356; Foreign Buildings Operations (FBO), 401; state capitol buildings, 824; state capitol cities, 263

United States Air Force Academy Chapel. *See* U.S. Air Force Academy Chapel

United States architects, 172

United State Schools for Fine and Applied Arts, 988–98

United States Customs House in New York, 502

United States Embassy in Athens, 1325

United States Embassy in Cuba, 330

United States Embassy in Lima, 68

United States Embassy in New Delhi, 1261–62

United States National Park Service, 617–18

United States Post Office in D.C., 534

United States Supreme Court Building, *503*

Unity Temple, 746, **1371–73**, 1453; exterior, *1372*; interior, *1371*

Universal Exposition of 1942, 443

Universidad Nacional Autónoma del México (UNAM) master plan, 872

Université de Montréal, 210

universities. *See* campus planning
University City, Mexico City, 844
University City of Venezuela, 1418
University Library, UNAM, Mexico City, **1373–75**; exterior, *1374*
University of Bath, 1220
University of British Columbia, C.K. Choi Building, 1281–82
University of California at Berkeley, 206; Hearst Hall, 822; Hearst Memorial Gym and Pool, 875; Men's Faculty Club, 822
University of California at Irvine plan, 207
University of California at Santa Cruz, 207; Kresge College, 870, *871*
University of Chicago plan, 206
University of Cincinnati, Arnoff Center for Design and Art, *279*
University of Ghent, Library Building, 131
University of Hong Kong, Kadoorie Biological Sciences Building, 642
University of Illinois, Chicago Circle campus, 207, 243
University of Imam Sadegh, 63
University of Iowa, Advanced Technology Laboratory, 1370
University of London in Bloomsbury extensions, 754
University of Michigan, Law School, 147
University of Nebraska: Sheldon Memorial Art Gallery, *717*; Wick Alumni Center, *577*
University of Pennsylvania: Addams Hall and Fine Arts Building, 938; Richards Medical Research Building, 172, 723–24, 1099; Wynn Commons, *1iii*
University of Texas at Austin, 206
University of Virginia, Darden Graduate School of Business, *1249*
University of Wyoming, American Heritage Center and Art Museum, *1058*
Universum Cinema, **1375–76**
Unwin, Raymond, 1164
urban development, 61; Bagdad, 232; Buenos Aires, 187–88; Lisbon, 783; role of stadiums, 1241; Saudi Arabia, 1168; Spain, 1235. *See also* cities; suburban developments
urban heat islands, 272
urban planning, 956, **1376–80**; Abuja, Federal Capital Territory of Nigeria, 9–10; by Adalberto Libera, 768; Ada Louise Huxtable's writings, 665; by Adèle Naudé Santos, 1162; Aldo Rossi's writings, 1133; in the Arctic, 412; Beirut, 129, 130; Benevolo's writings about, 133; Berlage's idea, 135–36; Broadacre City, **175–78**; Canberra, **1016–18**; Caracas, 217; Chandigarh, 234, 235; Chicago, **1018–19**; China, 1456; CIAM approach to, 86; Contemporary City for Three Million Inhabitants, **304–5**; by Coop Himmelblau, 307; critiques of, 1379; by Daniel Hudson Burnham, 195–96; by Denise Scott Brown, 1184; Dessau, 121; Disney's superiority, 364; by Duany and Plater-Zyberk, 369; by Ernst May, 820; by Heinrich Tessenow, 1321; Hodgetts and Fung proposals, 625; Hugh Ferriss's contribution, 456–57; Islamic principles, 1170; by Joaquim Guedes, 569; Josep Lluis Sert's writings, 1195; Kevin Lynch's writings, 802–3; Kuala Lumpur, 1227; Lewis Mumford's writings, 891; Ludwig Karl Hilberseimer's writings, 612; by Mario Romañach, 1128; by Morphosis, 878; neoclassical, 754; New Delhi, **1019–21**; Otto Wagner's writings, 1429; parkways, 985; plan for Brasilia, 163; by Robert Venturi, 1400; Saigon South, 1213; Sigfried Giedion's writing, 501; Steen Eiler Rasmussen's writings, 1082; by Sven Markelius, 818; Tony Garnier's impact, 483; Une Cité Industrielle, **259–60**; use at Getty Museum, 498; Vision Plan for Des Moines, Iowa, 28; Voisin Plan for Paris (1925), 1422;

Werner Hegemann's involvement, 596, 597; Yugoslavia, 1465. *See also* cities; City Beautiful Movement; Contextualism; Garden City Movement; industrial town planning; regional planning
Urban Prospect, The (Mumford), 891
urban renewal, **1380–81**; apartment building, 56; Barcelona School typology for, 113; Boston, 159–60; Cairo, 203; by Chloethiel Woodard Smith, 1218; failure of, 1068; Glasgow, 514; by I.M. Pei, 1434–35; Jane Jacobs's writings, 703; Montreal, 867; by Morris Lapidus, 744; of plazas, 1027; Riyadh, 1171; Rotterdam, 1137–38; of row houses, 1139; Spain, 1235; St. Louis, 1066; Sweden, 1285; as utopian planning, 1384; Victor Gruen's interest in, 565; Vincent Scully Jr., writings, 1186; West Berlin, 1134. *See also* adaptive re-use; demolition; favelas; historic preservation; ordinances
urban sprawl, 386; antidote, 1082
"urban villages," 924
Urbino, Italy, 344, 345
Uruguay, 225, 363
U.S. Air Force Academy Chapel, 1213, **1381–83**; exterior, *1381*; interior, *1382*
U.S. Army Supply Base in Brooklyn, 503
U.S. Military Academy at West Point, 323, 530
U.S. National Park Service, 985, 1420
U.S. Pavilion at Expo '67, *421*, 422
U.S. Steel Headquarters, 590
Usonian houses, 1081, 1367, 1455
utopian planning, **1383–84**; Abraham's technology-driven, 4; Arcosanti, 61; Brasília, **163–65**; Benevolo's writings about, 133; Contemporary City for Three Million Inhabitants, **304–5**; by Hans Scharoun, 1174; by Ivan Ilich Leonidov, 758; Lewis Mumford's writings, 891; of Ludwig Mies van der Rohe, 1187; Molnar's KOLVÁROS project, 863; Stepahnovich Melnikov, 831; Une Cité Industrielle, 260, 262; Zonnestraal Sanatorium, 1468–69. *See also* Garnier, Tony; new town developments
Utopia Pavilion, 783, 786
Utzon, Jørn, 1291, **1384–87**; influence on Sverre Fehn, 450; Sydney Opera House, 79, 90, 285, 296, 1291, **1292–94**; tectonics in works of, 1313; work in Denmark, 354

Vällingby, 818, 1284
Valsamakis, Nikos, 550
Van Alen, William. *See* Chrysler Building
Vancouver, Canada, **1389–90**
van der Vlugt, L.C., 1136; Van Nelle Factory, Rotterdam, **1394–96**
van de Velde, Henri, 73, **1396–97**; Bloemenwerf, 130; exhibition buildings, 1439; influence in Belgium, 131; La Nouvelle Maison, 131; reaction to Deutscher Werkbund, 358; University of Ghent, Library Building, 131
van Doesburg, Theo, **1390–92**, *8i*; abstract art and architecture, 6; Cafe Aubette, 349; J.J.P. Oud's relation with, 962; L'Aubette dance hall, 6; relation with Bauhaus, 119; role in De Stijl, 348
van Eesteren, Cornelis, 48, 348
Van Eetvelde House, 651
van Eyck, Aldo, **428–30**, 1311; impact on Amsterdam, 48; writings about cities, 306
Vanna Venturi House, 279, 1369, **1392–94**, 1400; exterior, *1393*; interior, *1394*
Van Nelle Factory, Rotterdam, 1136, **1394–96**; exterior, *1395*
Van Roosmalen House, 132
Vaughn, Henry, 1433

vaults: AT&T Building, 84–85; of Félix Candela, 213; Gaussa, 362; Gothic rib, 254, 255; Lambert Airport in St. Louis, 1462; self-supporting, 363; steel truss system, 1264; undulating barrel, 644; Washington D.C. subway, 1274. *See also* steel-frame construction

Velasca Tower. *See* Torre Velasca

Velasco, Juan Martínez, University Library, UNAM, Mexico City, **1373–75**

Venetian (hotel), 751

Venezuelan architecture, 1418

Venice Biennale Pavilions, **1397–99**

Venice II, 878

Ventana Vista Elementary School, 1058

ventilation. *See* heating, ventilation, and air conditioning (HVAC)

Venturi, Rauch, and Scott Brown: Buildings and Projects (Von Moos), 1423

Venturi, Robert, 1118, **1400–1401**; *Complexity and Contradiction in Architecture*, 1047, 1294–95, 1369, 1400; Guild House in Philadelphia, 172, 1392; Las Vegas book, 750; "less is bore," 959; partnership with Denise Scott Brown, *1183*; relation with environmental issues, 409–10; relation with historicism, 621; relation with International Style, 684; relation with Paul Rudolf, 1144; Sainsbury Wing, National Gallery, London, 1155; use of color, 279; Vanna Venturi House, 279, 1369, **1392–94**, 1400; work in Philadelphia, 1009; writings about cities, 306

vernacular architecture, **1401–5**; American, 1367; awards, 26; Barcelona, 111; Bawa's, 124–25; Cairo, 202; Canada, 208; desert, 64; India, 672; linked to new decorative program, 35; Maori, 932; Mexico, 755, 1375; Miami, Florida, 851; pavilions at Expo 1992, Seville, 422; postmodern interest in, 1048; Ramses Wissa Wassef's passion for, 1435; Robert Venturi's appreciation of, 1400; rural Catalan houses, 1072; Scandinavian, 81; Switzerland, 1287; Thailand, 106; timber framing, 1326; United States, 45; use by Heinrich Tessenow, 1321; use of stone, 1260–61; use of wood, 1448–49. *See also* modern vernacular; regionalism

vernacular modernism: by Rogelio Salmona, 1157; in Studio Per's works, 1267

Vesnin, Alexander, 1405, 1406, 1407. *See also* Vesnin, Alexander, Leonid, and Viktor

Vesnin, Alexander, Leonid, and Viktor, 970, 1147, **1405–8**; relation with constructivism, 302, 303

Vesnin, Leonid, 1405, 1406, 1407. *See also* Vesnin, Alexander, Leonid, and Viktor

Vesnin, Viktor, 1405, 1406, 1407. *See also* Vesnin, Alexander, Leonid, and Viktor

Via Galilei, 767

Viceroy's House, 920

Viceroy's Palace in New Delhi, 1021

Victorian Gothic, Canada, 209

video game environments, 52, 625

Vidhan Bhavan (State Assembly), **1408–9**; exterior, *1409, 7iii*

Vieira, Alvaro Siza, Malagueira Housing Quarter, **813–14**

Vienna, Austria: Hans Hollein's work in, 635; Karl Marxhof, **729–31**; Post Office Savings Bank, 515, **1045–47**; Stadtbahn (subway), 1273–74; Steiner House, 790, **1247–48**

Vienna residential and office development, *338*; by Josef Hoffmann, 629

Vienna Secession, 1029, **1409–12**, *6iii*; influence in Tokyo, 1330; Josef Hoffman's relation with, 628; members, 1045; Olbrich's exhibition hall, 950, *951*; in Slovenia, 1464

Viennese architects, 627

Viennese Moderne, 91

Vietnam Veterans' Memorial, 776, 777, 834, **1412–14**; drawing, *1412*; visitors at, *1413*

Viipuri Library, 2, 772; lecture hall, *2*

Viipuri Railroad Station, 1151

Viking Ship Museum, 355

Villa Amore, 28

Villa Beer, 471

Villa Busk, 451, *939*

Villa Capra, 521

Village Matteotti, 345

Villa in the Forest, 1194

Villa Mairea, 2, 438, 973, **1414–16**; living room, *1415*; main entrance, *1414*

Villa Noailles, 814

Villanueva, Carlos Raúl, 215, 216, **1418–19**; Ciudad Universitaria, Caracas, **267–69**

Villa Savoye, **1416–18**; exterior, *1417*; influence on other buildings, 31

Villa Schwob, 310, 366

Ville Radieuse, 304, **1419–20**

Vimanmek Palace, 104, *105*

Viñoly, Rafael, 815

Violich, Francis, 215–16

Viollet-le-Duc, E.E., 72, 74, 1083; influence on churches, 254–55

Virginia Polytechnic Institute, Carol M. Newman Library Addition, *1183*

virtual reality, 52, 862

Viscaya, 850

visitor centers, **1420–22**. *See also* roadside architecture

Vitra Firestation, *582*

Vittorio Emanuele II monument, 1131

Vivian Beaumont Theater, 778

Voisin Plan for Paris, 311, **1422–23**

Voldparken estate, 464–65

von Haussmann, Baron, 1377

Von Moos, Stanislaus, **1423–24**

von Spreckelsen, Johann Otto, Grande Arche de la Défense, **540–42**, *5ii*

Voss House, 1458

Voysey, Charles F.A., 384, 1091, **1424–26**

333 Wacker Drive, *733*

Wacoal Media Center, 811, *812*

Wagner, Otto, **1427–30**; impact on Austria, 91; influence in Vienna, 1029; Majolikahaus, *74*; memorials by, 832; Post Office Savings Bank, 38, 515, **1045–47**; role in Vienna Secession, 1410, 1411; use of glass, 515; Vienna Stadtbahn (subway), 1273–74

Wagner Center for the Visual Arts, *395*

Wagner School, 1428

Wainwright Building, 171

waiting areas: bus terminal, 199; Union Station in Chicago, 534. *See also* lobbies

Walden–7, 152

Waldorf Schools, 427

Walker Art Center, 115

Walking City, 57

Wall Houses, 600

Wallot, Paul, 1092

Wallraf-Richartz Museum, 278, 1358

walls: Ando's primary, 52; buildings as, 463; clapboard siding for interior, 562; claustra walls, 35; Cuadra San Cristóbal, 328; curvilinear, 224, 225, 394, 577; curvilinear glass, 237; glass, 521, 720; importance to amusement parks, 52; of Kristian Gullichsen, 574; made of glass, 517; made of recycled materials, 523; made of sugar cane waste, 331; masonry-bearing, **819–20**; Mies' use in German Pavilion, 493; movable interior house, 355, 1182; movable interior office, 135; Ottoman, 397; plate glass, 1025; stone, 1259; stone and concrete, 1260; Taliesin West, 1301; tilted, 572; timber rib, 334–35; undulating, 8; using as screens, 1037; by Yoshio Taniguchi, 1304. *See also* curtain wall system

Walt Disney World in Florida, 363

Walter Dodge House, 504, *505*

Wanamaker Store, **1430–32**; exterior, *1430*; interior, *1431*

Ward, Basil. *See* Connell, Ward, and Lucas

warehouse and storage facilities, **1432–33**

Warren, Whitney, 539

Washington, D.C., **1433–35**; adaptive-reuse in, 12; Chloethiel Woodard Smith works, 1218; Embassy Row buildings, 402; Frank Lloyd Wright's views about, 1038; John Russell Pope's work, 1039; McMillan Plan, 781; parkway system, 985; Plan, 263; plan, 195; subway, 1274; Vietnam Veterans Memorial, **1412–14**

Washington National Cathedral, 1433

Wassef, Ramses Wissa, **1435–37**

watercolor renderings, 59

waterfront revitalization, 617

Watergate Complex in Washington, D.C., 873, 875

Waterloo Station: Continental Train Platform, *1078*; International Terminal addition, 559

wattle and daub construction, 383

Wayfarer's Chapel in Los Angeles, 794

Wayne State University McGregor Memorial Conference Center, 1462

Webb, Mike, 57

Webb, Philip, 76

Weese, Harry, 243, 281

Weimar Bauhaus, 118

Weisman, Leslie Kanes, 454

Weissenhof Row Houses, *1269*

Weissenhofsiedlung (Stuttgart 1927), 471, 597, 681–82, 1175, 1268, **1437–39**; House by Le Corbusier, *1348*; J.J.P. Oud's Weissenhof Row Houses, *1269*

welding, importance of, 1243

Welwyn Garden City Company, 482

Werdermühle, 1031

Werkbund Exhibition (Cologne 1914), 127, **1439–40**; Gropius' Model Factory, 563

Werner, Eduard, 435

Wertheim Department Store, 494

West Africa: Bureaux d'Etudes Henri Chomette, **191–93**; French cultural centers, 35; Yaama Mosque, **1461–62**. *See also* Great Mosque of Niono; Northern Africa; Southern and Central Africa

West Berlin architecture, 140–41

Westenstrasse 1/DG Bank Headquarters Building, 733

Western influence: China, 249–50; in China, 251; on Indian architecture, 30; Istanbul, 697; Kyoto, Japan, 739; Moscow, 881

West German Pavilion (Frei Otto), 422

Westin Peachtree Plaza Hotel, 1041

Westin Times Hotel at Times Square, *68*

Westmount Square, 867

Wetmore, William, 539

Wexner Center for the Visual Arts, 172, 777

White, Howard Judson. *See* Graham, Anderson, Probst, and White

White, Stanford. *See* McKim, Mead and White

white brick, 647

white cement, 911

white marble, 971

White Mosque, 1466

White U, 700, 1194

Whitney Museum of American Art, 169, *1260*; extension, 543

Wichita House, 476

Wiebenga, Jan Gerko, 373

Wiedenhofer-Hof, 471

Wieizmann House, 836

Wilford, Michael, Neue Staatsgalerie, **916–17**

Wilgus, William J., 539

Wilhelmine style, 22

Wilhelm Marx House, 377

Will, Philip, 997, 998–99

Williams, Amancio, **1440–41**

Williams, E. Owen, **1441–42**; Boots Pure Drugs Factory, **155–56**, 1442

Williams, Paul Revere, **1442–44**, *8iii*

Williams, Tod and Billie Tsien, 325, **1444–45**

Willis Faber Dumas Building, *336*, 468

Wilson, Colin St. John, 173, **1445–46**

Wilson, George Leopold: Hong Kong and Shanghai Bank Corporation Headquarters, 469, 640, **645–47**, 946

Wilson House, 1177

Winarsky-Hof, 471

Winckelmann, Johann Joachim, *623*

windows: American Foursquare house, 44; bay, 709; bow, 1425, 1426; Chicago, 220, 244, 632; by Erich Mendelsohn, 836; IDESTA system, 764; John Hancock Building, 992; with metal mesh screens, 236; periscope, 148; relation with curtain walls, 336; that must stay closed, 596; types of glass in, 516; use of asymmetrical, 511; vertical bands of, 436

wind pressure design, 734, 1212, 1246, 1247, 1263; computer-aided, 1314; portal arch, 1450; trusses in, 1346; typhoons, 109; World Trade Center, 1452

Winslow House, 16

Winton Guest House, 571

wire-mesh reinforcement, 1095

Wiseman House, 1249

Wissa Wassef, Ramses, Ramses Wissa Wassef Arts Centre, **1079–80**

Wolfe House, 1177

women architects, 87; associations for, 679; Denise Scott Brown, **1182–85**; Eleanor Raymond, 1085; Eva Jiricna, **712–13**; in Finland, 460; Glasgow School, 510; Goody, Joan, **532–34**; Itsuko Hasegawa, **590–92**; Joan Edelman Goody, 532; Kazuyo Seijima, 1194; Lina Bò Bardi, **150–52**; Susana Torres's exhibition of, 1337

women in architecture, 453

women in architecture schools, 388

Women's Table, The, 776, 777

Woo, Kyu Sung, 293

wood, **1446–49**; Dusan Jurkovic's use of, 341; Heikki and Kaija Sirén's use of, 1209; Maybeck's redwood houses, 822; Sverre

Fehn's use of, 450; synagogues, 1298; teakwoods, 709; truss system, 1301; use at Byker Wall, 413; use in Cultural Centre Jean-Marie Tjibaou, 334. *See also* engineered lumber

Woodbury County Courthouse in Sioux City, 1074

wooden screens (mashrabiyah), 1168

Woodland Cemetery in Stockholm, 764

Woodland Chapel in Stockholm, *82*, 1257; interior, *83*

Woodland Crematorium, 83

Woolworth Building, 502, 1215, **1449–51**; drawing, *1449*; exterior, *1450*

Work, Robert, 14

workers' clubs, 526–28, 1406

Workers' Neighborhood of Lyanóu, 1127

Working Council for Art, 1306

World Bank Building in New Delhi, 1106

World Exhibition (Brussels 1958), 131

World's Columbian Exposition (Chicago 1893), 195, 205, 262, 824

World Trade Center, 1217, **1451–52**, 1462; exterior, *1451*; memorial, 769

Wright, Frank Lloyd, **1452–56**; Beth Shalom Synagogue, 1297, 1455; Broadacre City, **175–78**, 1378–79; designs for Chicago World's Fair, 230; Fallingwater, **436–38**, 1454; First Unitarian Meeting House in Madison, 256; Florida Southern College plan, 207; on "folk buildings," 1402; Guggenheim Museum, **572–74**, 746, 928, 1455; Heurtley House, *1055*; House on the Mesa, 686; impact in Chicago, 242; Imperial Hotel, **669–771**, 1329; influence on Sedad Hakkí Eldem, 396; Johnson Wax Administrative Building, 313, **713–15**; Johnson Wax Building, 1095; Larkin Building, 715, **745–46**; load-bearing brick structures, 171; Nakoma Country Club plan, 321; opinion of U.N. Headquarters, 1364; opinion of U.S. Air Force Academy Chapel, 1381; Prairie School work, 1054; precast system, 1060; relation with Arts and Crafts Movement, 77; relation with environmental issues, 409; relation with regionalism, 1091; Robie House, 77, 322, 656, **1120–23**, 1367; skyscrapers, 1217; Taliesin West, **1300–1302**; tectonics in works of, 1313; Unity Temple, Oak Park, Illinois, 746, **1371–73**; Usonian houses, 1081, 1367, 1455; views about Washington, D.C., 1038; views about way wood was used, 1448; work in Los Angeles, 794

Wrigley Building, 534–35; exterior, *535*

Wu Liangyong, **1456–57**

Wurster, William, **1457–60**

Wyldefel Gardens, 1290

Wyntoon, 822, 876

Yaama Mosque, **1461–62**

Yale University: Art and Architecture Building, 291, 1142, *1143*, 1144; Art Gallery, 595; campus additions, 207; Center for British Art, *724; Women's Table, The*, 776

Yamasaki, Minoru, 1113, **1462–64**; Pruitt Igoe Housing, **1065–69**, 1462; World Trade Center, 769, 1217, **1451–52**, 1462

Yanbu Industrial City, 1170

yellow brick, 567

Yerba Buena Gardens, *1163*; Zeum and Rooftop Complex, 1163

Yeshivat Porat Joseph Rabbinical College, 1153

Yugoslavia, **1464–66**

Zabludovsky, Abraham, **528–30**, 845

Zacherl House, 1029

Zanuso, Marco, Olivetti Factory, **951–52**

Zenetos, Takis, 550

Zeppelin Field, 444

Zevi, Bruno, 623, 874, 1338, **1467–68**

Zimbabwe, 385

Zlin Architecture construction system, 341

Zola, Emile, 483

"Zoning Envelopes: First through Fourth Stages," 955

zoning ordinances, **957–58**; affecting Seagram Building, 1187; Amsterdam, 47; apartment building, 56; Caracas, 217; by Duany and Plater-Zyberk, 369; effect on Lever House, 759; effect on New Urbanism in the United States, 924; Europe, 133; Hong Kong, 641; Hugh Ferriss' four stages, *456*; Israel, 695; lack of, in Houston, Texas, 658; New York City, 115, 253, 403. *See also* ordinances

Zonnestraal Sanatorium, **1468–70**

Zumthor, Peter, 1288, **1470**

Zurich Tower, *993*

FOR REFERENCE

Do Not Take From This Room

DATE DUE

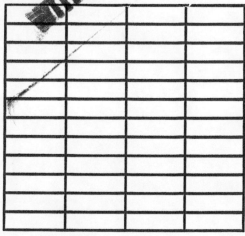

LIBRARY
SOUTHWESTERN OREGON
COMMUNITY COLLEGE

1988 Newmark Avenue

Coos Bay, OR 97420

COOS COOPERATIVE

3 2881 00736148 3   ICO